Infectious Diseases of the Fetus and Newborn Infant

Infectious Diseases of the Fetus and Newborn Infant

SEVENTH EDITION

JACK S. REMINGTON, MD
Professor Emeritus, Department of Medicine,
Division of Infectious Diseases and Geographical Medicine,
Stanford University School of Medicine, Stanford,
California,
Marcus Krupp Research Chair Emeritus,
Research Institute, Palo Alto Medical Foundation,
Palo Alto, California

JEROME O. KLEIN, MD
Professor of Pediatrics, Boston University School of
Medicine, Maxwell Finland Laboratory for Infectious
Diseases, Boston Medical Center, Boston, Massachusetts

CHRISTOPHER B. WILSON, MD
Director, Discovery
Global Health Program
Bill & Melinda Gates Foundation, Seattle, Washington

VICTOR NIZET, MD
Professor of Pediatrics and Pharmacy, University of
California, San Diego School of Medicine, Skaggs School
of Pharmacy and Pharmaceutical Sciences, Rady
Children's Hospital, San Diego, La Jolla, California

YVONNE A. MALDONADO, MD
Professor of Pediatrics and Health Research and Policy,
Chief, Division of Pediatric Infectious Diseases, Stanford
University School of Medicine, Berger-Raynolds Packard
Distinguished Fellow, Lucile Salter Children's Hospital
at Stanford, Palo Alto, California

ELSEVIER
SAUNDERS

ELSEVIER
SAUNDERS

1600 John F. Kennedy Blvd.
Ste 1800
Philadelphia, PA 19103-2899

ISBN: 978-1-4160-6400-8

INFECTIOUS DISEASES OF THE FETUS AND NEWBORN INFANT, 7E

Copyright © 2011, 2006, 2001, 1995, 1990, 1983, 1976, **by Saunders, an imprint of Elsevier Inc.**

Notice

Knowledge and best practice in this field are constantly changing. As new research and experience broaden our knowledge, changes in practice, treatment and drug therapy may become necessary or appropriate. Readers are advised to check the most current information provided (i) on procedures featured or (ii) by the manufacturer of each product to be administered, to verify the recommended dose or formula, the method and duration of administration, and contraindications. It is the responsibility of the practitioner, relying on his or her own experience and knowledge of the patient, to make diagnoses, to determine dosages and the best treatment for each individual patient, and to take all appropriate safety precautions. To the fullest extent of the law, neither the Publisher nor the Editors assume any liability for any injury and/or damage to persons or property arising out of or related to any use of the material contained in this book.

The Publisher

Library of Congress Cataloging-in-Publication Data
Infectious diseases of the fetus and newborn infant / [edited by] Jack S. Remington ... [et al.]. – 7th ed.
 p. ; cm.
 Includes bibliographical references and index.
 ISBN 978-1-4160-6400-8
 1. Communicable diseases in newborn infants. 2. Communicable diseases in pregnancy–Complications.
3. Fetus–Diseases. 4. Neonatal infections. I. Remington, Jack S., 1931-
 [DNLM: 1. Communicable Diseases. 2. Fetal Diseases. 3. Infant, Newborn, Diseases. 4. Infant,
Newborn. WC 100 I42 2011]
 RJ275.I54 2011
 618.92′01–dc22

2010014728

Acquisitions Editor: Judith A. Fletcher
Developmental Editor: Rachel Miller
Project Manager: Jagannathan Varadarajan
Design Direction: Steven Stave
Publishing Services Manager: Hemamalini Rajendrababu

Printed in the United States of America

Last digit is the print number: 9 8 7 6 5 4 3 2 1

To Those Most Dear to Us
Francoise
J.S.R.

Linda, Andrea, Bennett, Adam, Zachary, Alex, Evan, and Dana
J.O.K.

Sherryl, Alyssa and Bryan, Amelia and Floyd, and Helen
C.B.W.

To my parents, Pierre and Maria; Christine, Oliver and Alex
V.N.

Lauren, Stephen, Lindsey, Alfonso and Aida, Ann, and Ramiro
Y.A.M.

And to the mentors, colleagues, fellows, and students who have enriched our academic and personal lives,
and to the physicians and the women and infants with infectious diseases for whom they care

Silence

The gentle silence of the dandelion seed
floating on
a wisp of warm air

of the violet
opening
to the morning sun

of the motion of
the butterfly's wings
as it sucks the nectar
of a cherry blossom

The silence is broken
by the cries
of all of the infants destroyed
and the anguish of their mothers
whose tears cannot reverse
what the organism has wrought

The quiet silence of the womb
harboring an unborn child
awaiting its first breath
of deserved normality

Not the sad silence
of deafness
or
of retardation
or
of blindness
Nor of the sad silence
of the grave

How can we silence the sad silence?
                    Jack (2005)

LIST OF CONTRIBUTORS

Stuart P. Adler, MD
Professor
Department of Pediatrics
Virginia Commonwealth University
Medical College of Virginia Campus
Richmond, Virginia

Charles A. Alford, Jr., MD†
Professor Emeritus
Department of Pediatrics
University of Alabama School of Medicine
Birmingham, Alabama

Ann M. Arvin, MD
Professor
Department of Pediatrics and
Microbiology and Immunology
Stanford University
Stanford, California

Elizabeth D. Barnett, MD
Associate Professor of Pediatrics
Boston University School of Medicine
Section of Pediatric Infectious Diseases
Boston Medical Center
Boston, Massachusetts

Catherine M. Bendel, MD
Associate Professor
Department of Pediatrics
University of Minnesota
Minneapolis, Minnesota

Daniel K. Benjamin, Jr., MD, PhD, MPH
Professor of Pediatrics
Duke University
Durham, North Carolina

Robert Bortolussi, MD, FRCPC
Professor
Department of Pediatrics and
Microbiology & Immunology
Dalhousie University;
Medical Staff
Department of Pediatrics
IWK Health Centre
Halifax, Nova Scotia, Canada

John S. Bradley, MD
Professor of Clinical Pediatrics
Department of Pediatrics
Division of Infectious Diseases
University of California;
Director
Department of Infectious Diseases
Rady Children's Hospital
San Diego, California

William Britt, MD
Charles A. Alford Endowed Chair in Pediatric
Infectious Diseases
Professor
Department of Pediatrics, Microbiology, and
Neurobiology
University of Alabama School of Medicine
Birmingham, Alabama

James D. Cherry, MD, MSc
Distinguished Professor of Pediatrics
Department of Pediatrics
David Geffen School of Medicine at UCLA;
Attending Physician
Department of Pediatrics
Division of Infectious Diseases
Mattel Children's Hospital at UCLA
Los Angeles, California

Thomas G. Cleary, MD
Professor
Center for Infectious Diseases
Division of Epidemiology
University of Texas School of Public Health
Houston, Texas

Susan E. Coffin, MD, MPH
Associate Professor of Pediatrics
Division of Infectious Diseases
University of Pennsylvania School
of Medicine;
Hospital Epidemiologist and Medical
Director, Infection Prevention & Control
Children's Hospital of Philadelphia
Philadelphia, Pennsylvania

Louis Z. Cooper, MD
Professor Emeritus of Pediatrics
Department of Pediatrics
College of Physicians and Surgeons
of Columbia University
New York, New York

James E. Crowe, Jr., MD
Ingram Professor of Research
Department of Pediatrics
Microbiology and Immunology
Vanderbilt University School of Medicine;
Director
Vanderbilt Vaccine Center
Vanderbilt University School of Medicine
Nashville, Tennessee

Andrea T. Cruz, MD, MPH
Assistant Professor of Pediatrics
Baylor College of Medicine;
Attending Physician
Department of Pediatrics
Texas Children's Hospital
Houston, Texas

Carl T. D'Angio, MD
Associate Professor
Pediatrics and Medical Humanities
University of Rochester
School of Medicine and Dentistry;
Attending Neonatologist
Golisano Children's Hospital
University of Rochester Medical Center
Rochester, New York

Gary L. Darmstadt, MD, MS
Director, Family Health
Global Health Program
Bill and Melinda Gates Foundation
Seattle, Washington

Toni Darville, MD
Professor of Pediatrics and Immunology
Department of Pediatric Infectious Diseases
University of Pittsburgh Medical Center;
Chief, Infectious Diseases
Department of Pediatrics
Children's Hospital of Pittsburgh
Pittsburgh, Pennsylvania

George Desmonts, MD†
Chief (Retired)
Laboratoire de Sérologie Néonatale et de
Recherche sur la Toxoplasmose
Institut de Puériculture
Paris, France

Simon Dobson, MD, MBBS, MRCP [UK], FRCPC
Department of Pediatrics
Division of Infectious
& Immunological Diseases
University of British Columbia;
Attending Physician
British Columbia Children's Hospital
Vancouver, BC, Canada

Morven S. Edwards, MD
Professor of Pediatrics
Baylor College of Medicine;
Attending Physician
Texas Children's Hospital
Houston, Texas

†Deceased

Joanne E. Embree, MD, FRCP(C)
Professor and Head
Department of Medical Microbiology
University of Manitoba;
Section Head
Pediatric Infectious Diseases
Department of Pediatrics and Child Health
Children's Hospital
Winnipeg, Manitoba, Canada

Amy J. Gagnon, MD
Instructor/Fellow, Maternal-Fetal Medicine
Department of Obstetrics and Gynecology
University of Colorado Denver School of
Medicine
Aurora, Colorado

Michael A. Gerber, MD
Professor of Pediatrics
University of Cincinnati College of Medicine;
Attending, Division of Infectious Diseases
Cincinnati Children's Hospital Medical
Center
Cincinnati, Ohio

Anne A. Gershon, MD
Professor
Department of Pediatrics
Columbia University College of Physicians
and Surgeons;
Attending Physician
Department of Pediatrics
Morgan Stanley Children's Hospital of NY
Presbyterian Hospital
New York, New York

Ronald S. Gibbs, MD
Professor and E. Stewart Taylor Chair
Associate Dean, Continuing Medical
Education
Department of Obstetrics and Gynecology
University of Colorado Denver School of
Medicine
Denver, Colorado

Kathleen M. Gutierrez, MD
Assistant Professor
Department of Pediatrics
Division of Pediatric Infectious Disease
Stanford University
Stanford, California

R. Doug Hardy, MD
Department of Pediatric Infectious Diseases
Medical City Children's Hospital;
Department of Infectious Diseases
Medical City Dallas Hospital;
Department of Adult and Pediatric
Infectious Diseases
ID Specialists, P.A.
Dallas, Texas

Wikrom Karnsakul, MD
Assistant Professor
Department of Pediatrics
Division of Pediatric Gastroenterology and
Nutrition
Johns Hopkins University School of Medicine
Baltimore, Maryland

Jerome O. Klein, MD
Professor of Pediatrics
Boston University School of Medicine
Maxwell Finland Laboratory for Infectious
Diseases
Boston Medical Center
Boston, Massachusetts

William C. Koch, MD, FAAP, FIDSA
Associate Professor of Pediatrics
Division of Infectious Diseases
Virginia Commonwealth University School of
Medicine;
Attending Physician
Virginia Commonwealth University
Children's Medical Center
Richmond, Virginia

Tobias R. Kollmann, MD, PhD
Department of Pediatrics
Division of Infectious
& Immunological Diseases
University of British Columbia;
Attending Physician
British Columbia Children's Hospital
Vancouver, BC, Canada

Paul Krogstad, MD, MS
Professor of Pediatrics and Molecular and
Medical Pharmacology
Department of Pediatrics
David Geffen School of Medicine
at UCLA;
Attending Physician
Department of Pediatrics
Division of Infectious Diseases
Mattel Children's Hospital at UCLA
Los Angeles, California

David B. Lewis, MD
Professor of Pediatrics
Chief, Division of Immunology and Allergy
Department of Pediatrics
Stanford University School of Medicine
Stanford, California;
Attending Physician at Lucile Salter Packard
Children's Hospital
Palo Alto, California

Sarah S. Long, MD
Professor of Pediatrics
Drexel University College of Medicine;
Chief, Section of Infectious Diseases
St. Christopher's Hospital for Children
Philadelphia, Pennsylvania

Timothy L. Mailman, MD, FRCPC
Associate Professor of Pediatrics
Department of Pediatrics
Dalhousie University;
Chief, Department of Pathology and
Laboratory Medicine
Department of Pathology and
Laboratory Medicine
IWK Health Centre
Halifax, Nova Scotia, Canada

Yvonne A. Maldonado, MD
Professor of Pediatrics and Health Research
and Policy
Chief, Division of Pediatric Infectious
Diseases
Stanford University School of Medicine
Berger-Raynolds Packard Distinguished
Fellow
Lucile Salter Children's Hospital at Stanford
Palo Alto, California

Rima McLeod, MD
Professor, The University of Chicago
Departments of Surgery (Ophthalmology &
Visual Science) and Pediatrics (Infectious
Diseases)
Committee on Molecular Medicine, Genetics
Immunology, Institute of Genomics and
Systems Biology and The College
Medical Director, Toxoplasmosis Center
University of Chicago Medical Center
Chicago, Illinois

Julia A. McMillan, MD
Professor, Vice Chair for Education
Associate Dean for Graduate Medical
Education
Department of Pediatrics
Johns Hopkins University School
of Medicine;
Department of Pediatrics
Johns Hopkins Children's Center
Baltimore, Maryland

James P. Nataro, MD, PhD, MBA
Benjamin Armistead Shepherd Professor
Chair, Department of Pediatrics
University of Virginia
Charlottesville, Virginia

Victor Nizet, MD
Professor of Pediatrics and Pharmacy
University of California
San Diego School of Medicine
Skaggs School of Pharmacy and
Pharmaceutical Sciences
Rady Children's Hospital
San Diego, La Jolla, California

Pearay L. Ogra, MD
Emeritus Professor
School of Medicine and Biomedical Sciences
State University of New York
University at Buffalo
Buffalo, New York;
Former John Sealy Distinguished Chair
Professor and Chair Pediatrics
University of Texas Medical Branch at
Galveston
Galveston, Texas

Miguel L. O'Ryan
Full Professor and Director
Microbiology and Mycology Program
Institute of Biomedical Sciences
Faculty of Medicine
University of Chile
Santiago, Chile

Gary D. Overturf, MD
Professor of Pediatrics and Pathology
Department of Pediatrics
University of New Mexico;
Emeritus Chief of Pediatric
Infectious Diseases
Department of Pediatrics
Childrens Hospital of New Mexico;
Medical Director, Infectious Diseases
Department of Infectious Diseases
and Microbiology
TriCore Reference Laboratories
Albuquerque, New Mexico

Stanley A. Plotkin, MD
Emeritus Professor
Department of Pediatrics
University of Pennsylvania;
Former Chief
Department of Infectious Diseases
Children's Hospital
Philadelphia, Pennsylvania

Octavio Ramilo, MD
Henry G. Cramblett Chair in Pediatric
Infectious Diseases
Professor
Department of Pediatrics
The Ohio State University
College of Medicine;
Chief
Department of Infectious Diseases
Nationwide Children's Hospital
Columbus, Ohio

Susan E. Reef, MD
Medical Epidemiologist
Centers for Disease Control and Prevention
Atlanta, Georgia

Jack S. Remington, MD
Professor Emeritus, Department of Medicine
Division of Infectious Diseases and
Geographical Medicine
Stanford University School of Medicine
Stanford, California;
Marcus Krupp Research Chair
Emeritus
Research Institute, Palo Alto Medical
Foundation
Palo Alto, California

Kathleen B. Schwarz, BA, MAT, MD
Professor of Pediatrics
Johns Hopkins University School of Medicine;
Director
Johns Hopkins Pediatric Liver Center
Baltimore, Maryland

Eugene D. Shapiro, MD
Professor
Departments of Pediatrics, Epidemiology and
Investigative Medicine
Yale University School of Medicine;
Attending Physician
Children's Hospital at Yale-New Haven
New Haven, Connecticut

Avinash K. Shetty, MD
Associate Professor
Department of Pediatrics
Wake Forest University Health Sciences;
Attending Physician
Department of Pediatric Infectious Diseases
Brenner Children's Hospital
Winston-Salem, North Carolina

Jeffrey R. Starke, MD
Professor of Pediatrics
Baylor College of Medicine;
Infection Control Officer
Texas Children's Hospital
Houston, Texas

Barbara J. Stoll, MD
Jr. Professor and Chair
Department of Pediatrics
Emory University School of Medicine;
SVP and Chief Academic Officer
Department of Administration
Children's Healthcare of Atlanta
Atlanta, Georgia

Kelly C. Wade, MD, PhD, MSCE
Assistant Professor of Clinical Pediatrics
Department of Pediatrics
University of Pennsylvania;
Neonatologist
Department of Pediatrics
Children's Hospital of Philadelphia
Philadelphia, Pennsylvania

Geoffrey A. Weinberg, MD
Professor of Pediatrics
University of Rochester School of Medicine &
Dentistry;
Director, Pediatric HIV Program
Golisano Children's Hospital & Strong
Memorial Hospital
Rochester, New York

Richard J. Whitley, MD
Professor
Department of Pediatrics
University of Alabama at Birmingham
Birmingham, Alabama

Christopher B. Wilson, MD
Director, Discovery
Global Health Program
Bill & Melinda Gates Foundation
Seattle, Washington

Anita K. M. Zaidi, MBBS, SM
Professor
Department of Pediatrics and Child Health
Aga Khan University
Karachi, Pakistan

Theoklis E. Zaoutis, MD, MSCE
Associate Professor
Pediatrics and Epidemiology
University of Pennsylvania
School of Medicine;
Associate Chief
Division of Infectious Diseases
The Children's Hospital of Philadelphia
Philadelphia, Pennsylvania

PREFACE

Major advances in biology and medicine made during the past several decades have contributed greatly to our understanding of infections that affect the fetus and newborn. As the medical, social, and economic impact of these infections becomes more fully appreciated, the time is again appropriate for an intensive summation of existing information on this subject. Our goal for the seventh edition of this text is to provide a complete, critical, and contemporary review of this information. We have directed the book to all students of medicine interested in the care and well-being of children, and hope to include among our readers medical students, practicing physicians, microbiologists, and health care workers. We believe the text to be of particular importance for infectious disease specialists; obstetricians and physicians who are responsible for the pregnant woman and her developing fetus; pediatricians and family physicians who care for newborn infants; and primary care physicians, neurologists, audiologists, ophthalmologists, psychologists, and other specialists who are responsible for children who suffer the sequelae of infections acquired in utero or during the first month of life.

The scope of this book encompasses infections of the fetus and newborn, including infections acquired in utero, during the delivery process, and in early infancy. When appropriate, sequelae of these infections that affect older children and adults are included as well. Infection in the adult is described when pertinent to recognition of infection in the pregnant woman and her developing fetus and newborn infant. The first chapter provides an introductory overview of the subsequent chapters, general information, and a report on new developments and new challenges in this area. Each subsequent chapter covers a distinct topic in depth, and when appropriate touches on issues that overlap with the theme of other chapters or refers the reader to those chapters for relevant information. Chapters in Sections II, III, and IV cover specific types of infection, and each includes a review of the history, microbiology, epidemiology, pathogenesis and pathology, clinical signs and symptoms, diagnosis, prognosis, treatment, and prevention of the infection. Chapters in Sections I and V address issues of a more general nature. The length of the chapters varies considerably. In some instances, this variation is related to the available fund of knowledge on the subject; in others (e.g., the chapters on host defense, toxoplasmosis, neonatal diarrhea, varicella, measles, and mumps), the length of the chapter is related to the fact that recent comprehensive reviews of these subjects are not otherwise available.

For J.S.R. and J.O.K., it has been an extraordinary experience and privilege over the past 40 years to be participants in reporting the advances in understanding and management of the infectious diseases of the fetus and newborn infant. Consider the virtual elimination in the developed world of some infectious diseases (e.g., rubella, early-onset group B streptococcal diseases); the recognition of new diseases (e.g., *Borrelia*, HIV); the increased survival and vulnerability to infection of the very low birth weight infant; the introduction of new antimicrobial agents, in particular antiviral and antifungal drugs; and increased emphasis on immunization of women in the childbearing years to prevent transmission of disease to the fetus and neonate. Of particular importance now and in the future is the recognition of the universality of infectious diseases. Of particular concern is the continued high mortality rates of infectious diseases for infants in the first weeks of life. Increased efforts are important to extrapolate advances in care of the pregnant woman and her newborn infant from developed countries to regions with limited resources.

The first, second, third, fourth, fifth, and sixth editions of this text were published in 1976, 1983, 1990, 1995, 2001, and 2006. As of this writing, in summer 2010, it is most interesting to observe the changes that have occurred in the interval since publication of the last edition. New authors provide fresh perspectives. Major revisions of most chapters suggest the importance of new information about infections of the fetus and newborn infant.

Each of the authors of the different chapters is a recognized authority in the field and has made significant contributions to our understanding of infections in the fetus and newborn infant. Most of these authors are individuals whose major investigative efforts on this subject have taken place during the past 25 years. Almost all were supported, in part or totally, during their training period and subsequently, by funds obtained from the National Institutes of Health or from private agencies such as March of Dimes and Bill & Melinda Gates Foundation. The major advances of this period would not have been possible without these funding mechanisms and the freedom given to the investigators to pursue programs of their own choosing. The advances present in this text are also a testimony to the trustees of agencies and the legislators and other federal officials who provided research funds from the 1960s to the present day.

Two of us (J.S.R. and J.O.K.) were Fellows at the Thorndike Memorial Laboratory (Harvard Medical Unit, Boston City Hospital) in the early 1960s under the supervision of Maxwell Finland. Although subsequently we worked in separate areas of investigation on the two coasts, one of us as an internist and the other as a pediatrician, we maintained close contact, and, because of a mutual interest in infections of the fetus and newborn infant and their long-term effects, we joined our efforts to develop this text. Christopher B. Wilson joined us in editing the sixth and now seventh editions. Chris trained in immunology and infectious diseases in Palo Alto with J.S.R., and since J.S.R. and J.O.K. consider themselves as sons of Maxwell Finland, Chris is representative of the many grandsons and granddaughters of Dr. Finland. Joining us for this edition are two new editors, Yvonne A. Maldonado and Victor Nizet. Bonnie is an expert in pediatric HIV infection and is the Chief of the Division of Pediatric Infectious Diseases at Stanford University School of Medicine. Victor is an expert in the molecular pathogenesis of gram-positive bacterial infections and Chief of the Division of Pharmacology and Drug Discovery in the Departments of Pediatrics and the Skaggs School of Pharmacy and Pharmaceutical Sciences at the University of California, San Diego.

We are indebted to our teachers and associates, and especially to individuals such as Dr. Maxwell Finland, who guided our training and helped to promote our development as physician-scientists through the early stages of our careers. We also wish to express our appreciation to Sarah Myers, and Judith Fletcher, Rachel Miller and Jagannathan Varadarajan of Elsevier, for guiding this project to a successful conclusion, and to Ms. Nancy Greguras for her editorial assistance.

Jack S. Remington
Jerome O. Klein
Christopher B. Wilson
Victor Nizet
Yvonne A. Maldonado

CONTENTS

SECTION I GENERAL INFORMATION 1

1 CURRENT CONCEPTS OF INFECTIONS OF THE FETUS
AND NEWBORN INFANT 2
Yvonne A. Maldonado ◌ Victor Nizet
◌ Jerome O. Klein ◌ Jack S. Remington
◌ Christopher B. Wilson

2 NEONATAL INFECTIONS: A GLOBAL PERSPECTIVE 24
Gary L. Darmstadt ◌ Anita K. M. Zaidi ◌ Barbara J. Stoll

3 OBSTETRIC FACTORS ASSOCIATED WITH INFECTIONS OF THE
FETUS AND NEWBORN INFANT 51
Amy J. Gagnon ◌ Ronald S. Gibbs

4 DEVELOPMENTAL IMMUNOLOGY AND ROLE OF HOST
DEFENSES IN FETAL AND NEONATAL SUSCEPTIBILITY
TO INFECTION 80
David B. Lewis ◌ Christopher B. Wilson

5 HUMAN MILK 191
Christopher B. Wilson ◌ Pearay L. Ogra

SECTION II BACTERIAL INFECTIONS 221

6 BACTERIAL SEPSIS AND MENINGITIS 222
Victor Nizet ◌ Jerome O. Klein

7 BACTERIAL INFECTIONS OF THE RESPIRATORY TRACT 276
Elizabeth D. Barnett ◌ Jerome O. Klein

8 BACTERIAL INFECTIONS OF THE BONES AND JOINTS 296
Gary D. Overturf

9 BACTERIAL INFECTIONS OF THE URINARY TRACT 310
Sarah S. Long ◌ Jerome O. Klein

10 FOCAL BACTERIAL INFECTIONS 322
Gary D. Overturf

11 MICROORGANISMS RESPONSIBLE FOR NEONATAL
DIARRHEA 359
Miguel L. O'Ryan ◌ James P. Nataro
◌ Thomas G. Cleary

12 GROUP B STREPTOCOCCAL INFECTIONS 419
Morven S. Edwards ◌ Victor Nizet

13 LISTERIOSIS 470
Robert Bortolussi ◌ Timothy L. Mailman

14 STAPHYLOCOCCAL INFECTIONS 489
Victor Nizet ◌ John S. Bradley

15 GONOCOCCAL INFECTIONS 516
Joanne E. Embree

16 SYPHILIS 524
Tobias R. Kollmann ◌ Simon Dobson

17 BORRELIA INFECTIONS: LYME DISEASE AND RELAPSING
FEVER 564
Eugene D. Shapiro ◌ Michael A. Gerber

18 TUBERCULOSIS 577
Jeffrey R. Starke ◌ Andrea T. Cruz

19 CHLAMYDIA INFECTIONS 600
Toni Darville

20 MYCOPLASMAL INFECTIONS 607
R. Doug Hardy ◌ Octavio Ramilo

SECTION III VIRAL INFECTIONS 621

21 HUMAN IMMUNODEFICIENCY VIRUS/ACQUIRED
IMMUNODEFICIENCY SYNDROME IN THE INFANT 622
Avinash K. Shetty ◌ Yvonne A. Maldonado

22 CHICKENPOX, MEASLES, AND MUMPS 661
Anne A. Gershon

23 CYTOMEGALOVIRUS 706
William Britt

24 ENTEROVIRUS AND PARECHOVIRUS INFECTIONS 756
James D. Cherry ◌ Paul Krogstad

25 HEPATITIS 800
Wikrom Karnsakul ◌ Kathleen B. Schwarz

26 HERPES SIMPLEX VIRUS INFECTIONS 813
Kathleen M. Gutierrez ◌ Richard J. Whitley
◌ Ann M. Arvin

27 HUMAN PARVOVIRUS 834
Stuart P. Adler ◌ William C. Koch

28 RUBELLA 861
Stanley A. Plotkin ◌ Susan E. Reef
◌ Louis Z. Cooper ◌ Charles A. Alford, Jr.

29 SMALLPOX AND VACCINIA 899
Julia A. McMillan

30 LESS COMMON VIRAL INFECTIONS 905
Yvonne A. Maldonado

SECTION IV PROTOZOAN, HELMINTH, AND FUNGAL
INFECTIONS 917

31 TOXOPLASMOSIS 918
Jack S. Remington ◌ Rima McLeod
◌ Christopher B. Wilson ◌ George Desmonts

32 LESS COMMON PROTOZOAN AND HELMINTH
INFECTIONS 1042
Yvonne A. Maldonado

33 CANDIDIASIS 1055
Catherine M. Bendel

34 PNEUMOCYSTIS AND OTHER LESS COMMON FUNGAL
INFECTIONS 1078
Yvonne A. Maldonado

SECTION V DIAGNOSIS AND MANAGEMENT 1125

35   HEALTHCARE–ASSOCIATED INFECTIONS IN THE
      NURSERY 1126
      Susan E. Coffin ☉ **Theoklis E. Zaoutis**

36   LABORATORY AIDS FOR DIAGNOSIS OF NEONATAL
      SEPSIS 1144
      Geoffrey A. Weinberg ☉ **Carl T. D'Angio**

37   CLINICAL PHARMACOLOGY OF ANTI-INFECTIVE DRUGS 1160
      Kelly C. Wade ☉ **Daniel K. Benjamin, Jr.**

38   PREVENTION OF FETAL AND EARLY LIFE INFECTIONS
      THROUGH MATERNAL–NEONATAL IMMUNIZATION 1212
      James E. Crowe, Jr.

INDEX 1231

GENERAL INFORMATION

SECTION OUTLINE

1 Current Concepts of Infections of the Fetus and Newborn Infant 2

2 Neonatal Infections: A Global Perspective 24

3 Obstetric Factors Associated with Infections in the Fetus and Newborn Infant 51

4 Developmental Immunology and Role of Host Defenses in Fetal and Neonatal Susceptibility to Infection 80

5 Human Milk 191

CURRENT CONCEPTS OF INFECTIONS OF THE FETUS AND NEWBORN INFANT

Yvonne A. Maldonado ❂ Victor Nizet ❂ Jerome O. Klein
❂ Jack S. Remington ❂ Christopher B. Wilson

CHAPTER OUTLINE

Overview 2
Infections of the Fetus 3
    Pathogenesis 3
    Efficiency of Transmission of Microorganisms from Mother
        to Fetus 10
    Diagnosis of Infection in the Pregnant Woman 10
    Diagnosis of Infection in the Newborn Infant 13
    Prevention and Management of Infection in the Pregnant
        Woman 13

Infections Acquired by the Newborn Infant during Birth 15
    Pathogenesis 15
    Microbiology 16
    Diagnosis 16
    Management 17
    Prevention 18
Infections of the Newborn Infant in the First Month of Life 19
    Pathogenesis and Microbiology 19

OVERVIEW

Current concepts of pathogenesis, microbiology, diagnosis, and management of infections of the fetus and newborn infant are briefly reviewed in this chapter. This first section of the book contains chapters providing a global perspective on fetal and neonatal infections and chapters addressing obstetric factors, immunity, host defenses, and the role of human breast milk in fetal and neonatal infections. Chapters containing detailed information about specific bacterial, viral, protozoan, helminthic, and fungal infections follow in subsequent sections. The final section contains chapters addressing nosocomial infections, the diagnosis and therapy of infections in the fetus and neonate, and prevention of fetal and neonatal infections through immunization of the mother or neonate.

Changes continue to occur in the epidemiology, diagnosis, prevention, and management of infectious diseases of the fetus and newborn infant since publication of the last edition of this book. Some of these changes are noted in Table 1–1 and are discussed in this and the relevant chapters.

Substantial progress has been made toward reducing the burden of infectious diseases the fetus and newborn infant. The incidence of early-onset group B streptococcal disease has been reduced by aggressive use of intrapartum chemoprophylaxis and, in particular, by the culture-based chemoprophylaxis strategy now recommended for universal use in the United States. Vertical transmission of human immunodeficiency virus (HIV) has been reduced by identification of the infected mother and subsequent treatment, including the use of brief regimens that are practical in countries with high prevalence but limited resources. There has been a commitment of resources by government agencies and philanthropies, such as the Bill and Melinda Gates Foundation, the Clinton Foundation, Save the Children among others, to combat global infectious diseases in mothers and children. Use of polymerase chain reaction (PCR) techniques in etiologic diagnosis has expanded, permitting more rapid and specific identification of microbial pathogens. Finally, in the United States, national legislation on postpartum length of hospital stay has been enacted to prevent insurers from restricting insurance coverage for hospitalization to less than 48 hours after vaginal deliveries or 96 hours after cesarean deliveries.

Setbacks in initiatives to reduce the global burden of infectious disease in the fetus and newborn infant include the continuing increase in the prevalence of HIV infection in many developing countries, particularly among women, and the lack of finances to provide effective treatment for these women and their newborn infants. In the United States, setbacks include the increase in antimicrobial resistance among nosocomial pathogens and in the incidence of invasive fungal infections among infants of extremely low birth weight.

Use of the Internet has grown further, allowing access to information hitherto unavailable to physicians or parents. Physicians may obtain current information about diseases and management and various guidelines for diagnosis and treatment. Interested parents who have access to the Internet can explore various Internet sites that present a vast array of information and misinformation. As an example of the latter, a case of neonatal tetanus was associated with the use of cosmetic facial clay (Indian Healing Clay) as a dressing on an umbilical cord stump. The product had been publicized as a healing salve by midwives on an Internet site on "cordcare." [1] Because much of the information on the Internet is from commercial sources and parties with varying interests and expertise, physicians should assist interested parents and patients in finding Internet sites of value. Internet sites pertinent to infectious diseases of the fetus and newborn infant are listed in Table 1–2.

DOI: 10.1016/B978-1-4160-6400-8.00001-8

TABLE 1-1 Changes in Epidemiology and Management of Infectious Diseases of the Fetus and Newborn Infant

Epidemiology	Increased viability of very low birth weight infants at risk for invasive infectious diseases
	Increased number of multiple births (often of very low birth weight) because of successful techniques for management of infertility
	Global perspective of vertically transmitted infectious diseases
	Early discharge from the nursery mandated by insurance programs reversed by legislation to ensure adequate observation for infants at risk for sepsis
Diagnosis	Polymerase chain reaction assay for diagnosis of infection in mother, fetus, and neonate
	Decreased use of fetal blood sampling and chorionic villus sampling for diagnosis of infectious diseases
Prevention	Intrapartum antibiotic prophylaxis widely implemented to prevent early-onset group B streptococcal infection
	Antiretroviral therapy in pregnancy to prevent transmission of HIV to fetus
Treatment	Antiretroviral therapy in mother to treat HIV infection in fetus
	Antitoxoplasmosis therapy in mother to treat infection in fetus
	Spread within nurseries of multiple antibiotic-resistant bacterial pathogens
	Increased use of vancomycin for β-lactam–resistant gram-positive infections
	Increased use of acyclovir for infants with suspected herpes simplex infection

HIV, human immunodeficiency virus.

TABLE 1-2 Useful Internet Sites for Physicians Interested in Infectious Diseases of the Fetus and Newborn Infant

Agency for Healthcare Research and Quality	http://www.ahrq.gov
American Academy of Pediatrics	http://www.aap.org
American College of Obstetricians and Gynecologists	http://www.acog.org
Centers for Disease Control and Prevention	http://www.cdc.gov
Food and Drug Administration	http://www.fda.gov
Immunization Action Coalition	http://www.immunize.org
Information on AIDS Trials	http://www.aidsinfo.nih.gov
Morbidity and Mortality Weekly Report	http://www.cdc.gov/mmwr
National Center for Health Statistics	http://www.cdc.gov/nchs
General Academic Information	http://www.googlescholar.com

Vital statistics relevant to infectious disease risk in neonates in the United States for 2005 are listed in Table 1-3 [2]. The disparities in birth weight, prenatal care, and neonatal mortality among different racial and ethnic groups are important to note.

The number of infectious diseases in fetuses and newborn infants must be extrapolated from selected studies (see chapters on diseases). Approximately 1% of newborn infants excrete cytomegalovirus (CMV), greater than 4% of infants are born to mothers infected with *Chlamydia trachomatis*, and bacterial sepsis develops in 1 to 4 infants per 1000 live births. Since the institution of intrapartum chemoprophylaxis in the United States, the number of infants with early-onset group B streptococcal disease has declined, with reduction in incidence from approximately 1.5 cases to 0.34 case per 1000 live births, and the incidence is expected to decline further with the universal adoption of the culture-based strategy [3,4]. In the United States, the use of maternal highly active antiretroviral treatment and peripartum chemoprophylaxis has led to a reduction in the rate of mother-to-child transmission of HIV from approximately 25% of infants born to mothers who received no treatment to 2%; less complex but practical regimens of intrapartum prophylaxis have helped to reduce the rate of HIV transmission in the developing world [5–7]. Among sexually transmitted diseases, the rate of congenital syphilis had declined substantially in the United States to 13.4 per 100,000 live births in 2000 [8]; however, after 14 years of decline, the rate of congenital syphilis increased in 2006 and 2007 from 9.3 to 10.5 cases per 100,000 live births, in parallel to the increase in the syphilis rates among the general population [9]. Immunization has virtually eliminated congenital rubella syndrome in newborn infants of mothers who were themselves born in the United States, but cases continue to occur in infants of foreign-born mothers; 24 of 26 infants with congenital rubella born between 1997 and 1999 were born to foreign-born mothers, and 21 of these were born to Hispanic mothers [10]. Efforts led by the Pan American Health Organization to eliminate congenital rubella syndrome in the Americas by 2010 may be successful [11].

Consequences of perinatal infections vary depending on whether the infection occurs in utero or during the intrapartum or postpartum periods. Infection acquired in utero can result in resorption of the embryo, abortion, stillbirth, malformation, intrauterine growth restriction, prematurity, or the untoward sequelae of chronic postnatal infection. Infection acquired during the intrapartum or early postpartum period may result in severe systemic disease that leads to death or persistent postnatal infection. In utero infection and intrapartum infections may lead to late-onset disease. The infection may not be apparent at birth, but may manifest with signs of disease weeks, months, or years later, as exemplified by chorioretinitis of *Toxoplasma gondii* infection, hearing loss of rubella, and immunologic defects that result from HIV infection. The immediate and the long-term effects of these infections constitute a major problem throughout the world.

INFECTIONS OF THE FETUS
PATHOGENESIS

Pregnant women not only are exposed to infections prevalent in the community, but also are likely to reside with young children or to associate with groups of young children, which represents a significant additional factor in exposure to infectious agents. Most infections in pregnant women affect the upper respiratory and gastrointestinal

TABLE 1–3 Vital Statistics Relevant to Newborn Health in the United States in 2005*

		Racial/Ethnic Origin of Mother		
	All Races	**Non-Hispanic White**	**Non-Hispanic Black**	**Hispanic**
Mother				
<20 yr old	10.2	7.3	17	14.1
≥40 yr old	2.7	3	2.2	2
Unmarried	36.9	25.3	69.9	48
Diabetes during pregnancy	3.9	3.7	3.5	3.8
Cesarean section delivery	30.3	30.4	32.6	29
Infant				
Birth weight				
VLBW†	1.49	1.21	3.27	1.20
LBW†	8.2	7.3	14	6.9
Gestational age				
Very preterm‡	2.03	1.64	4.17	1.79
Preterm‡	12.6	11.7	18.4	12.1

*All values are in percent births.
†VLBW, very low birth weight (<1500 g); LBW, low birth weight (<2500 g).
‡Very preterm <32 weeks' gestation; preterm <37 weeks' gestation.
Modified from Martin JA, Kung HC, Mathews TJ, et al. Annual Summary of Vital Statistics—2006. Pediatrics 121:788-801, 2008.

tracts, and either resolve spontaneously without therapy or are readily treated with antimicrobial agents. Such infections usually remain localized and have no effect on the developing fetus. The infecting organism may invade the bloodstream, however, and subsequently infect the placenta and fetus.

Successful pregnancy is a unique example of immunologic tolerance—the mother must be tolerant of her allogeneic fetus (and vice versa). The basis for maternal-fetal tolerance is not completely understood, but is known to reflect local modifications of host defenses at the maternal-fetal interface and more global changes in immunologic competence in the mother. Specific factors acting locally in the placenta include indoleamine 2,3-dioxygenase, which suppresses cell–mediated immunity by catabolizing the essential amino acid tryptophan, and regulatory proteins that prevent complement activation [12,13]. As pregnancy progresses, a general shift from T helper type 1 (T_H1) cell–mediated immunity to T helper type 2 (T_H2) responses also occurs in the mother, although this description probably constitutes an overly simplistic view of more complex immunoregulatory changes [14,15]. Nonetheless, because T_H1 cell-mediated immunity is important in host defense against intracellular pathogens, the T_H2 bias established during normal gestation may compromise successful immunity against organisms such as *T. gondii*. In addition, it has been proposed that a strong curative T_H1 response against an organism may overcome the protective T_H2 cytokines at the maternal-fetal interface, resulting in fetal loss.

Transplacental spread and invasion of the bloodstream after maternal infection is the usual route by which the fetus becomes infected. Uncommonly, the fetus may be infected by extension of infection in adjacent tissues and organs, including the peritoneum and the genitalia, during parturition, or as a result of invasive methods for the

diagnosis and therapy of fetal disorders, such as the use of monitors, sampling of fetal blood, and intrauterine transfusion.

Microorganisms of concern are listed in Table 1–4 and include those identified in the acronym *TORCH*: *T. gondii*, rubella virus, CMV, and herpes simplex virus (HSV) (as a point of historical interest, the *O* in TORCH originally stood for "other infections/pathogens," reflecting an early appreciation of this possibility). A new acronym is needed to include other, well-described causes of in utero infection: syphilis, enteroviruses, varicella-zoster virus (VZV), HIV, Lyme disease (*Borrelia burgdorferi*), and parvovirus. In certain geographic areas, *Plasmodium* and *Trypanosoma cruzi* are responsible for in utero infections. *ToRCHES CLAP* (see Table 1–4) is an inclusive acronym. Case reports indicate other organisms that are unusual causes of infections transmitted by a pregnant woman to her fetus, including *Brucella melitensis* [16], *Coxiella burnetii* (Q fever) [17], *Babesia microti* (babesiosis) [18], human T-cell

TABLE 1–4 Suggested Acronym for Microorganisms Responsible for Infection of the Fetus: ToRCHES CLAP

To	*Toxoplasma gondii*
R	Rubella virus
C	Cytomegalovirus
H	Herpes simplex virus
E	Enteroviruses
S	Syphilis (*Treponema pallidum*)
C	Chickenpox (varicella-zoster virus)
L	Lyme disease (*Borrelia burgdorferi*)
A	AIDS (HIV)
P	Parvovirus B19

AIDS, acquired immunodeficiency syndrome; HIV, human immunodeficiency virus.

lymphotropic virus types I and II (although the main route of transmission of these viruses is through breast-feeding) [19,20], hepatitis G and TT viruses [21,22], human herpesvirus 6 [23,24], and dengue [25].

Before rupture of fetal membranes, organisms in the genital tract may invade the amniotic fluid and produce infection of the fetus. These organisms can invade the fetus through microscopic defects in the membranes, particularly in devitalized areas overlying the cervical os. It also is possible that microorganisms gain access to the fetus from descending infection through the fallopian tubes in women with salpingitis or peritonitis, or from direct extension of an infection in the uterus, such as myometrial abscess or cellulitis. Available evidence does not suggest, however, that transtubal or transmyometrial passage of microbial agents is a significant route of fetal infection.

Invasive techniques that have been developed for in utero diagnosis and therapy are potential sources of infection for the fetus. Abscesses have been observed in infants who had scalp punctures for fetal blood sampling or electrocardiographic electrodes attached to their scalps. Osteomyelitis of the skull and streptococcal sepsis have followed local infection at the site of a fetal monitoring electrode [26]; HSV infections at the fetal scalp electrode site also have been reported. Intrauterine transfusion for severe erythroblastosis diagnosed in utero also has resulted in infection of the fetus. In one case, CMV infection reportedly resulted from intrauterine transfusion [27]; in another instance, contamination of donor blood with a gram-negative coccobacillus, *Acinetobacter calcoaceticus*, led to an acute placentitis and subsequent fetal bacteremia [28].

Fetal infection in the absence of rupture of internal membranes usually occurs transplacentally after invasion of the maternal bloodstream. Microorganisms in the blood may be carried within white blood cells or attached to erythrocytes, or they may be present independent of cellular elements.

Microbial Invasion of the Maternal Bloodstream

The potential consequences of invasion of the mother's bloodstream by microorganisms or their products (Fig. 1–1) include (1) placental infection without infection of the fetus, (2) fetal infection without infection of the placenta, (3) absence of fetal and placental infection, and (4) infection of placenta and fetus.

Placental Infection without Infection of the Fetus

After reaching the intervillous spaces on the maternal side of the placenta, organisms can remain localized in the placenta without affecting the fetus. Evidence that placentitis can occur independently of fetal involvement has been

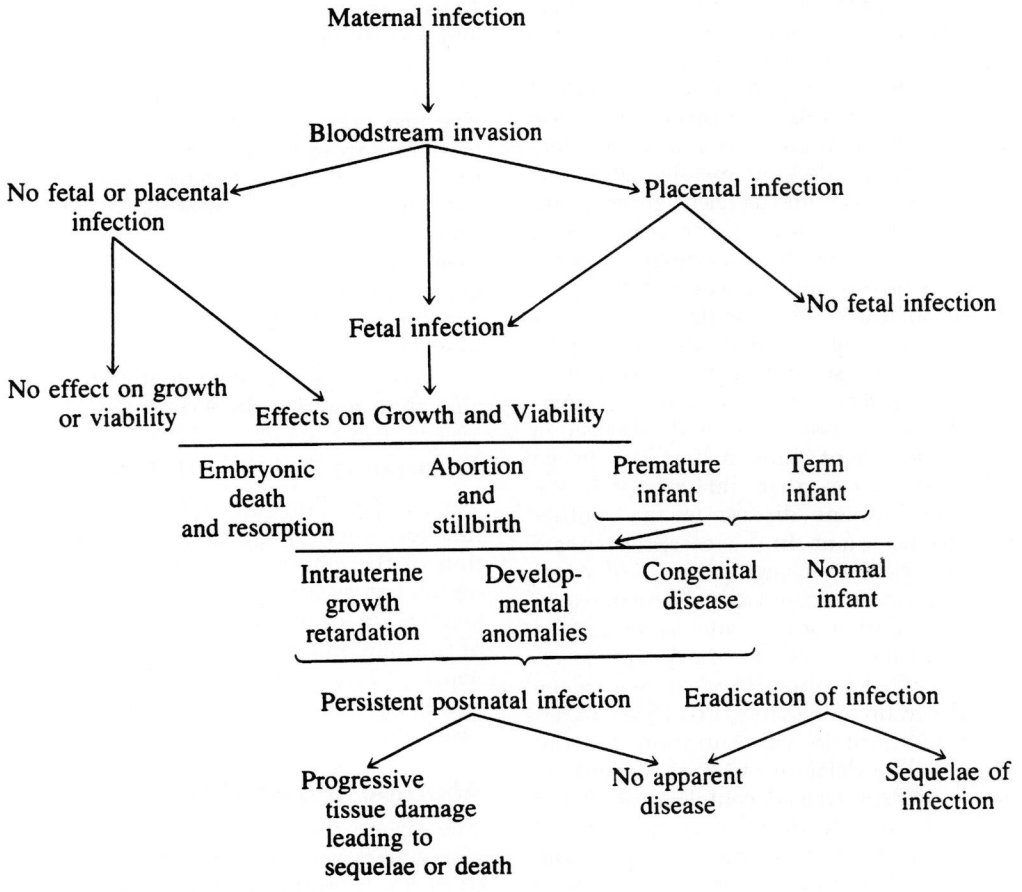

FIGURE 1–1 Pathogenesis of hematogenous transplacental infections.

shown after maternal tuberculosis, syphilis, malaria, coccidioidomycosis, CMV, rubella virus, and mumps vaccine virus infection. The reasons for the lack of spread to the fetus after placental infection are unknown. Defenses of the fetus that may operate after placental infection include the villous trophoblast, placental macrophages, and locally produced immune factors such as antibodies and cytokines.

Fetal Infection without Infection of the Placenta

Microorganisms may traverse the chorionic villi directly through pinocytosis, placental leaks, or diapedesis of infected maternal leukocytes and erythrocytes. Careful histologic studies usually reveal areas of placentitis sufficient to serve as a source of fetal infection, however.

Absence of Fetal and Placental Infection

Invasion of the bloodstream by microorganisms is common in pregnant women, yet in most cases neither fetal nor placental infection results. Bacteremia may accompany abscesses or cellulitis, bacterial pneumonia, pyelonephritis, appendicitis, endocarditis, or other pyogenic infections; nevertheless, placental or fetal infection as a consequence of such bacteremias is rare. In most cases, the fetus is likely protected through efficient clearance of microbes by the maternal reticuloendothelial system and circulating leukocytes.

Many bacterial diseases of the pregnant woman, including typhoid fever, pneumonia, sepsis caused by gram-negative bacteria, and urinary tract infections, may affect the developing fetus without direct microbial invasion of the placenta or fetal tissues. Similarly, protozoal infection in the mother, such as malaria, and systemic viral infections, including varicella, variola, and measles, also may affect the fetus indirectly. Fever, anoxia, circulating toxins, or metabolic derangements in the mother concomitant with these infections can affect the pregnancy, possibly resulting in abortion, stillbirth, and premature delivery.

The effects of microbial toxins on the developing fetus are uncertain. The fetus may be adversely affected by toxic shock in the mother secondary to *Staphylococcus aureus* or *Streptococcus pyogenes* infection. Botulism in pregnant women has not been associated with disease in infants [29,30]. A unique case of Guillain-Barré syndrome in mother and child shows that infection-induced, antibody-mediated autoimmune disease in the mother may be transmitted to her infant. In this case, the disease was diagnosed in the mother during week 29 of pregnancy. A healthy infant was delivered vaginally at 38 weeks of gestation, while the mother was quadriplegic and on respiratory support. On day 12 of life, the infant developed flaccid paralysis of all limbs with absence of deep tendon reflexes, and cerebrospinal fluid (CSF) examination revealed increased protein concentration without white blood cells [31]. The delay in onset of paralysis in the infant seemed to reflect transplacentally transferred blocking antibodies specifically directed at epitopes of the mature, but not the fetal, neuromuscular junction. The infant improved after administration of intravenous immunoglobulin [32].

The association of maternal urinary tract infection with premature delivery and low birth weight is a well-studied example of a maternal infection that adversely affects growth and development of the fetus, despite no evidence of fetal or placental infection. Asymptomatic bacteriuria in pregnancy has been linked to increased numbers of infants with low birth weight [33,34]. In one early study, when the bacteriuria was eliminated by appropriate antibiotic therapy, the incidence of pyelonephritis was lower in the women who received treatment, yet the rate of premature and low birth weight infants was the same among the women in the treatment group as among women without bacteriuria [35]. A meta-analysis concluded that antibiotic treatment is effective in reducing the risk of pyelonephritis in pregnancy and the risk for preterm delivery, although the evidence supporting this latter conclusion is not as strong [36]. The basis for the premature delivery and low birth weight of infants of mothers with bacteriuria remains obscure [37].

Infection of Placenta and Fetus

Microorganisms may be disseminated from the infected placenta to the fetal bloodstream through infected emboli of necrotic chorionic tissues, or through direct extension of placental infection to the fetal membranes with secondary amniotic fluid infection and aspiration by the fetus.

Infection of the Embryo and Fetus

Hematogenous transplacental spread may result in death and resorption of the embryo, abortion and stillbirth of the fetus, and live birth of a premature or term infant who may or may not be healthy. The effects of fetal infection may appear in a live-born infant as low birth weight (resulting from intrauterine growth restriction), developmental anomalies, congenital disease, or none of these. Infection acquired in utero may persist after birth and cause significant abnormalities in growth and development that may be apparent soon after birth or may not be recognized for months or years. The variability of the effects of fetal infection is emphasized by reports of biovular twin pregnancies that produced one severely damaged infant and one infant with minimal or no detectable abnormalities [38–43].

Embryonic Death and Resorption

Various organisms may infect the pregnant woman in the first few weeks of gestation and cause death and resorption of the embryo. Because loss of the embryo usually occurs before the woman realizes she is pregnant or seeks medical attention, it is difficult to estimate the incidence of this outcome for any single infectious agent. The incidence of early pregnancy loss after implantation from all causes has been estimated to be 31%. The proportion of cases of loss because of infection is unknown [44].

Abortion and Stillbirth

The earliest recognizable effects of fetal infection are seen after 6 to 8 weeks of pregnancy and include abortion and stillbirth. Intrauterine death may result from overwhelming fetal infection, or the microorganisms may interfere with organogenesis to such an extent that the development of functions necessary for continued viability is interrupted. The precise mechanisms responsible for early spontaneous termination of pregnancy are unknown; in many cases, it is difficult to ascertain whether fetal death caused or resulted from the expulsion of the fetus.

Numerous modifying factors probably determine the ultimate consequence of intrauterine infection, including virulence or tissue tropism of the microorganisms, stage of pregnancy, associated placental damage, and severity of the maternal illness. Primary infection is likely to have a more important effect on the fetus than recurrent infection [45]. Recurrent maternal CMV infection is less severe than primary infection and is significantly less likely to result in congenital CMV infection of the fetus. Available studies do not distinguish between the direct effect of the microorganisms on the developing fetus and the possibility of an indirect effect attributable to illness or poor health of the mother.

Prematurity

Prematurity is defined as the birth of a viable infant before week 37 of gestation. Premature birth may result from almost any agent capable of establishing fetal infection during the last trimester of pregnancy. Many microorganisms commonly responsible for prematurity are also implicated as significant causes of stillbirth and abortion (Table 1–5).

Previous studies have shown that women in premature labor with bacteria-positive amniotic fluid cultures have elevated levels of multiple proinflammatory cytokines in their amniotic fluid [46–51]. In many patients with elevated levels of interleukin-6 (IL-6), results of amniotic fluid culture were negative. Premature births are invariably observed, however, in women in premature labor having positive amniotic fluid culture and elevated amniotic fluid levels of IL-6.

To clarify further the role of elevated levels of IL-6 in amniotic fluid, Hitti and colleagues [47] amplified bacterial 16S recombinant RNA (rRNA) encoding DNA by PCR to detect infection in amniotic fluid in women in premature labor whose membranes were intact. In patients who were culture-negative by amniotic fluid testing, PCR assay detected bacterial infection in significantly more patients with elevated IL-6 levels. These data suggest that 33% of women in premature labor with culture-negative amniotic fluid but with elevated IL-6 levels may have infected amniotic fluid. The investigators concluded that the association between infected amniotic

TABLE 1–5 Effects of Transplacental Fetal Infection on the Fetus and Newborn Infant

| Organism | Disease | | | | |
	Prematurity	Intrauterine Growth Restriction/Low Birth Weight	Developmental Anomalies	Congenital Disease	Persistent Postnatal Infection
Viruses	CMV	CMV	CMV	CMV	CMV
	HSV	Rubella	Rubella	Rubella	Rubella
	Rubeola	VZV*	VZV	VZV	VZV
	Smallpox	HIV*	Coxsackievirus B*	HSV	HSV
	HBV		HIV*	Mumps*	HBV
	HIV*			Rubeola	HIV
				Vaccinia	
				Smallpox	
				Coxsackievirus B	
				Poliovirus	
				HBV	
				HIV	
				LCV	
				Parvovirus	
Bacteria	*Treponema pallidum*			*T. pallidum*	*T. pallidum*
	Mycobacterium tuberculosis			*M. tuberculosis*	*M. tuberculosis*
	Listeria monocytogenes			*L. monocytogenes*	
	Campylobacter fetus			*C. fetus*	
	Salmonella typhi			*S. typhi*	
				Borrelia burgdorferi	
Protozoa	*Toxoplasma gondii*	*T. gondii*		*T. gondii*	*T. gondii*
	Plasmodium*	*Plasmodium*		*Plasmodium*	*Plasmodium*
	Trypanosoma cruzi	*T. cruzi*		*T. cruzi*	

Association of effect with infection has been suggested and is under consideration.
CMV, cytomegalovirus; HBV, hepatitis B virus; HIV, human immunodeficiency virus; HSV, herpes simplex virus; LCV, lymphocytic choriomeningitis virus; VZV, varicella-zoster virus.

fluid and premature labor may be underestimated on the basis of amniotic fluid cultures. They suggested that the broad-spectrum bacterial 16S rDNA PCR assay may be useful for detecting infection of amniotic fluid. Even in cases in which cultures and PCR assay have failed to detect infection, elevated levels of amniotic fluid IL-6 are clearly associated with an increased risk of preterm delivery [52]. Although this finding likely reflects infection undetected by either technique, it is possible that factors other than infection contribute to preterm labor and elevated amniotic fluid IL-6 levels.

Intrauterine Growth Restriction and Low Birth Weight

Infection of the fetus may result in birth of an infant who is small for gestational age. Although many maternal infections are associated with low birth weight infants and infants who are small for gestational age, causal evidence is sufficient only for congenital rubella, VZV infection, toxoplasmosis, and CMV infection.

The organs of infants dying with congenital rubella syndrome or congenital CMV infection contain reduced numbers of morphologically normal cells [53,54]. By contrast, in infants who are small for gestational age with growth deficit from noninfectious causes, such as maternal toxemia or placental abnormalities, the parenchymal cells are normal in number, but have a reduced amount of cytoplasm, presumably because of fetal malnutrition [55,56].

Developmental Anomalies and Teratogenesis

CMV, rubella virus, and VZV cause developmental anomalies in the human fetus. Coxsackieviruses B3 and B4 have been associated with congenital heart disease. Although the pathogenetic mechanisms responsible for fetal abnormalities produced by most infectious agents remain obscure, histologic studies of abortuses and congenitally infected infants have suggested that some viruses render these effects through mediating cell death, alterations in cell growth, or chromosomal damage. Lesions resulting indirectly from the microorganisms through inflammatory activation must be distinguished from defects that arise from a direct effect of the organisms on cell and tissue growth in the developing embryo or fetus. Inflammation and tissue destruction, rather than teratogenic activity, seem to be responsible for the widespread structural abnormalities characteristic of congenital syphilis, transplacental HSV and VZV infection, and toxoplasmosis. Infants with congenital toxoplasmosis may have microcephaly, hydrocephalus, or microphthalmia, but these manifestations usually result from an intense necrotizing process involving numerous organisms and are more appropriately defined as lesions of congenital infection, rather than as effects of teratogenic activity of the organism.

Some mycoplasmas [57] and viruses [58,59] produce chromosomal damage in circulating human lymphocytes or in human cells in tissue culture. The relationship of these genetic aberrations to the production of congenital abnormalities in the fetus is unknown.

Congenital Disease

Clinical evidence of intrauterine infections, resulting from tissue damage or secondary physiologic changes caused by the invading organisms, may be present at birth or may manifest soon thereafter or years later. The clinical manifestations of infection acquired in utero or at delivery in the newborn infant are summarized in Table 1–6. Signs of widely disseminated infection may be evident during the neonatal period in infants with congenital rubella; toxoplasmosis; syphilis; or congenital CMV, HSV, or enterovirus infection. These signs include jaundice, hepatosplenomegaly, and pneumonia, each of which reflects lesions caused by microbial invasion and proliferation, rather than by defects in organogenesis. Although these signs of congenital infection are not detected until the neonatal period, the pathologic processes responsible for their occurrence have been progressing for weeks or months before delivery. In some infants, the constellation of signs is sufficient to suggest the likely congenital infection (Table 1–7). In other infants, the signs are transient and self-limited and resolve as neonatal defense mechanisms control the spread of the microbial agent and tissue destruction. If damage is severe and widespread at the time of delivery, the infant is likely to die.

It is frequently difficult to determine whether the infection in the newborn infant was acquired in utero, intrapartum, or postpartum. If the onset of clinical signs after birth occurs within the minimal incubation period for the disease (e.g., 3 days for enteroviruses, 10 days for VZV and rubella viruses), it is likely that the infection was acquired before delivery. The interval between malaria exposure in the mother and congenital malaria in the infant can be prolonged; one case of congenital malaria resulting from *Plasmodium malariae* occurred in an infant born in the United States 25 years after the mother had emigrated from China [60]. Children with perinatal HIV infection can be diagnosed by 6 months of age using a DNA (or RNA) PCR method, which has largely replaced other approaches for viral detection [61]. A variable fraction (less than half) of children with perinatal HIV contract the infection in utero, depending on the setting and maternal treatment [62]. Virus-negative infants who later become virus-positive may have been infected in the intrapartum or early postpartum period.

Healthy Infants

Most newborn infants infected in utero by rubella virus, *T. gondii*, CMV, HIV, or *Treponema pallidum* have no signs of congenital disease. Fetal infection by a limited inoculum of organisms or with a strain of low virulence or pathologic potential may underlie this low incidence of clinical disease in infected infants. Alternatively, gestational age may be the most important factor in determining the ultimate consequences of prenatal infection. When congenital rubella and toxoplasmosis are acquired during the last trimester of pregnancy, the incidence of clinical disease in the infected infants is lower than when microbial invasion occurs during the first or second trimester. Congenital syphilis results from exposure during the second or third, but not the first, trimester.

TABLE 1–6 Clinical Manifestations of Neonatal Infection Acquired In Utero or at Delivery

Rubella Virus	Cytomegalovirus	*Toxoplasma gondii*	Herpes Simplex Virus	*Treponema pallidum*	Enteroviruses
Hepatosplenomegaly	Hepatosplenomegaly	Hepatosplenomegaly	Hepatosplenomegaly	Hepatosplenomegaly	Hepatosplenomegaly
Jaundice	Jaundice	Jaundice	Jaundice	Jaundice	Jaundice
Pneumonitis	Pneumonitis	Pneumonitis	Pneumonitis	Pneumonitis	Pneumonitis
Petechiae or purpura	Petechiae or purpura	Petechiae or purpura	Petechiae or purpura	Petechiae or purpura	Petechiae or purpura
Meningoencephalitis	Meningoencephalitis	Meningoencephalitis	Meningoencephalitis	Meningoencephalitis	Meningoencephalitis
Hydrocephalus	Hydrocephalus	Hydrocephalus*	Hydrocephalus	Adenopathy	Adenopathy
Adenopathy	Microcephaly*	Microcephaly	Microcephaly	Maculopapular exanthems*	Maculopapular exanthems
Hearing deficits	Intracranial calcifications*	Maculopapular exanthems	Maculopapular exanthems	Bone lesions*	Paralysis*
Myocarditis	Hearing deficits	Intracranial calcifications*	Vesicles*	Glaucoma	Myocarditis*
Congenital defects*	Chorioretinitis or retinopathy	Myocarditis	Myocarditis	Chorioretinitis or retinopathy	Conjunctivitis or keratoconjunctivitis
Bone lesions*	Optic atrophy	Bone lesions	Chorioretinitis or retinopathy	Uveitis	
Glaucoma*		Chorioretinitis or retinopathy*	Cataracts		
Chorioretinitis or retinopathy*		Cataracts	Conjunctivitis or keratoconjunctivitis*		
Cataracts*		Optic atrophy			
Microphthalmia		Microphthalmia			
		Uveitis			

Has special diagnostic significance for this infection.

TABLE 1–7 Syndromes in the Neonate Caused by Congenital Infections

Microorganism	Signs
Toxoplasma gondii	Hydrocephalus, diffuse intracranial calcification, chorioretinitis
Rubella virus	Cardiac defects, sensorineural hearing loss, cataracts, microcephaly, "blueberry muffin" skin lesions, hepatomegaly, interstitial pneumonitis, myocarditis, disturbances in bone growth, intrauterine growth restriction
CMV	Microcephaly, periventricular calcifications, jaundice, petechiae or purpura, hepatosplenomegaly, intrauterine growth restriction
HSV	Skin vesicles or scarring, eye scarring, microcephaly or hydranencephaly, vesicular skin rash, keratoconjunctivitis, meningoencephalitis, sepsis with hepatic failure
Treponema pallidum	Bullous, macular, or eczematous skin lesions involving palms and soles; rhinorrhea; dactylitis and other signs of osteochondritis and periostitis; hepatosplenomegaly; lymphadenopathy
VZV	Limb hypoplasia, cicatricial skin lesions, ocular abnormalities, cortical atrophy
Parvovirus B19	Nonimmune hydrops fetalis
HIV	Severe thrush, failure to thrive, recurrent bacterial infections, calcification of basal ganglia

CMV, cytomegalovirus; HIV, human immunodeficiency virus; HSV, herpes simplex virus; VZV, varicella-zoster virus.

Absence of clinically apparent disease in the newborn may be misleading. Careful observation of infected but healthy-appearing children over months or years often reveals defects that were not apparent at birth. The failure to recognize such defects early in life may be due to the inability to test young infants for the sensory and developmental functions involved. Hearing defects identified years after birth may be the only manifestation of congenital rubella. Significant sensorineural deafness and other central nervous system deficiencies have affected children with congenital CMV infection who were considered to

be normal during the neonatal period. In utero infection with *Toxoplasma*, rubella, and CMV may have manifestations that are difficult to recognize, including failure to thrive, visual defects, and minimal to severe brain dysfunction (including motor, learning, language, and behavioral disorders). Infants infected with HIV are usually asymptomatic at birth and for the first few months of life. The median age of onset for signs of congenital HIV infection is approximately 3 years, but many children remain asymptomatic for more than 5 years. Signs of perinatal infection related to HIV include failure to thrive, persistent diarrhea, recurrent suppurative infections, and diseases associated with opportunistic infections that occur weeks to months or years after birth. Of particular concern is a report by Wilson and colleagues [63] showing stigmata of congenital *T. gondii* infection, including chorioretinitis and blindness, in almost all of 24 children at follow-up evaluations; the children had serologic evidence of infection, but were without apparent signs of disease at birth and did not receive treatment or received inadequate treatment.

Because abnormalities may become obvious only as the child develops and fails to reach appropriate physiologic or developmental milestones, it is crucial to perform careful and thorough follow-up examinations to infants born to women with known or suspected infections during pregnancy.

Persistent Postnatal Infection

Microbial agents may continue to survive and replicate in tissues for months or years after in utero infection. Rubella virus and CMV have been isolated from various body fluid and tissue compartments over long periods from healthy-appearing children and children with abnormalities at birth. Progressive tissue destruction has been shown in some congenital infections, including rubella; toxoplasmosis; syphilis; tuberculosis; malaria; and CMV, HSV, and HIV infection. Recurrent skin and eye infections can occur as a result of HSV infection acquired in utero or at the time of delivery. A progressive encephalitis occurred in children with congenital rubella infection; stable clinical manifestations of congenital infection over many years was followed by deterioration of motor and mental functions at ages 11 to 14 years [64,65]. Rubella virus was subsequently isolated from the brain biopsy specimen of a 12-year-old child. Finally, fetal parvovirus B19 infection can persist for months after birth with persistent anemia because of suppressed hematopoiesis [66].

The mechanisms responsible for maintaining or terminating chronic fetal and postnatal infections are only partially understood. Humoral immune responses, as determined by measurement of either fetal IgM antibodies or specific IgG antibodies that develop in the neonatal period, seem to be intact in almost all infants (see Chapter 4). The importance of cell-mediated immunity, cytokines, complement, and other host defense mechanisms remains to be defined; at present, there is insufficient evidence to support a causal relationship between deficiencies in any one of these factors and persistent postnatal infection. All of the diseases associated with persistent postnatal infection—with the exception of rubella, but including syphilis; tuberculosis; malaria; toxoplasmosis; hepatitis; and CMV, HSV, VZV, and HIV infections—can also produce prolonged and, in certain instances, lifelong infection when acquired later in life.

EFFICIENCY OF TRANSMISSION OF MICROORGANISMS FROM MOTHER TO FETUS

The efficiency of transmission from the infected, immunocompetent mother to the fetus varies among microbial agents and can vary with the trimester of pregnancy.

In utero transmission of rubella virus and *T. gondii* occurs mainly during primary infection, whereas in utero transmission of CMV, HIV, and *T. pallidum* can occur in consecutive pregnancies. The risk of congenital rubella infection in fetuses of mothers with symptomatic rubella was high in the first trimester (90% before 11 weeks of gestation), declined to a nadir of 25% at 23 to 26 weeks, and then increased to 67% after 31 weeks. Infection in the first 11 weeks of gestation was uniformly teratogenic, whereas no birth defects occurred in infants infected after 16 weeks of gestation [67]. By contrast, the frequency of stillbirth and clinical and subclinical congenital *T. gondii* infection among offspring of women who acquired the infection during pregnancy was lowest in the first trimester (14%), increased in the second trimester (29%), and was highest in the third trimester (59%) [68].

Congenital CMV infection results from primary and recurrent infections. On the basis of studies in Birmingham, Alabama, and other centers, Whitley and Stagno and their colleagues [69,70] estimate that 1% to 4% of women have primary infection during pregnancy, 40% of these women transmit the infection to their fetuses, and 5% to 15% of the infants have signs of CMV disease. Congenital infection as a result of recurrent CMV infection occurs in 0.5% to 1% of live births, but less than 1% of the infected infants have clinically apparent congenital disease.

The transmission rate of HIV infection from an untreated mother to the fetus is estimated to be about 25%, but the data are insufficient to identify efficiency of transmission by trimester. Risk of transmission does not seem to be greater in mothers who acquire primary infection during pregnancy than in mothers who were infected before they became pregnant [71].

DIAGNOSIS OF INFECTION IN THE PREGNANT WOMAN

Clinical Diagnosis

Symptomatic or Clinical Infection

In many instances, infection in the pregnant woman and congenital infection in the newborn infant can be suspected on the basis of clinical signs or symptoms. Careful examination can be sufficient to suggest a specific diagnosis, particularly when typical clinical findings are accompanied by a well-documented history of exposure (see Tables 1–6 and 1–7).

Asymptomatic or Subclinical Infection

Many infectious diseases with serious consequences for the fetus are difficult or impossible to diagnose in the mother solely on clinical grounds. Asymptomatic or subclinical infections may be caused by rubella virus, CMV, *T. gondii*, *T. pallidum*, HSV, and HIV. Most women infected with these organisms during pregnancy have no apparent signs of disease; only 50% of women infected with rubella virus have a rash, and although occasional cases of CMV mononucleosis are recognized, these constitute a very small proportion of women who acquire primary CMV infection during pregnancy. Similarly, the number of women with clinical manifestations of toxoplasmosis is less than 10%, and few women have systemic illness associated with primary HSV infection. The genital lesions associated with HSV infection and syphilis often are not recognized.

Recurrent and Chronic Infection

Some microorganisms can infect a susceptible person more than once, and when such reinfections occur in a pregnant woman, the organism can affect the fetus. These reinfections generally are associated with waning host immunity, but low levels of circulating antibodies may be detectable. Such specific antibodies would be expected to provide some protection against hematogenous spread and transplacental infection. Fetal disease has followed reexposure of immune mothers, however, to vaccinia [72], variola [73], and rubella [74] viruses.

In addition, an agent capable of persisting in the mother as a chronic asymptomatic infection could infect the fetus long after the initial infection. Such delayed infection is common for congenital CMV and HIV infections, which have been observed in infants from consecutive pregnancies in the same mother. Reports of infection of the fetus as a result of chronic maternal infection have been cited in cases of malaria [75], syphilis [76], hepatitis [77], herpes zoster [43] and herpes simplex [78], and *T. gondii* infection [79]. In the case of *T. gondii*, congenital transmission from a chronically infected woman occurs almost solely when the woman is immunocompromised during pregnancy.

Preconceptional Infection

The occurrence of acute infection immediately before conception may result in infection of the fetus, and the association may go unrecognized. Congenital rubella has occurred in the fetus in cases in which the mother was infected 3 weeks to 3 months before conception. A prolonged viremia or persistence of virus in the maternal tissues may be responsible for infection of the embryo or fetus. The same has occurred rarely in cases of maternal infection with *T. gondii* [80].

Isolation and Identification of Infectious Agents
General Approach

Diagnostic tests for microorganisms or infectious diseases are part of routine obstetric care; special care is warranted for selected patients with known or suspected exposure to the infectious agent or clinical signs of infection. Table 1–8 lists diagnostic tests and interventions that may be required in the event of a diagnosis. The specific interventions for each disease are discussed in subsequent chapters.

The most direct mode of diagnosis is isolation of the microbial agent from tissues and body fluids such as blood, CSF, or urine. Isolation of the agent must be considered in context with its epidemiology and natural history in the host. Isolation of an enterovirus from stool during the summer months may represent colonization, rather than significant infection, with risk of hematogenous spread to

TABLE 1–8   Management of Infections in the Pregnant Woman

Microorganism	Diagnostic Test	First Visit	Third Trimester	At Delivery	Intervention*
Routine Care					
Mycobacterium tuberculosis	Tuberculin skin test	+			Therapy
Gonorrhea	Culture or antigen	+	+		Therapy
Hepatitis B	Serology	+			HBIG and hepatitis B vaccine to the infant within 12 hours of birth†
Chlamydia	Antigen	+	+		Therapy
Syphilis	Serology	+	+	+	Therapy
Rubella	Serology	+			Postpartum vaccine
Group B streptococcus	Culture		+		Intrapartum prophylaxis
Herpes simplex	Examination	+	+	+	Cesarean section‡
	Culture				Therapy
Special Care if Exposed or with Clinical Signs					
HIV	Serology	+			Therapy
Parvovirus	Ultrasound				Intrauterine transfusion
	Serology				
Toxoplasmosis	Serology				Therapy
	PCR assay (amniotic fluid)				
VZV	Serology				Therapy
	Cytology				

*See appropriate chapters.
†Hepatitis B immunoglobulin only in neonates born to women with high-risk factors, and hepatitis B vaccine for neonate.
‡When signs or symptoms of active genital HSV are present at the onset of labor.
HIV, human immunodeficiency virus; PCR, polymerase chain reaction; VZV, varicella-zoster virus.
Modified from table prepared by Riley L, Fetter S, Geller D, Boston City Hospital and Boston University School of Medicine.

the fetus. Isolation of an enterovirus from an atypical body fluid or identification of a significant increase in antibody titer would be necessary to define an acute infectious process.

Tests for the presence of hepatitis B virus (HBV) surface antigen (HBsAg) should be performed in all pregnant women. The Centers for Disease Control and Prevention (CDC) has estimated that 16,500 births occur each year in the United States to women who are positive for HBsAg. Infants born to HBsAg-positive mothers may have a 90% chance of acquiring perinatal HBV infection. If maternal infection is identified soon after birth, use of hepatitis B immunoglobulin combined with hepatitis B vaccine is an effective mode of prevention of infection. For these reasons, the Advisory Committee on Immunization Practices of the U.S. Public Health Service [81] and the American Academy of Pediatrics [82] recommend universal screening of all pregnant women for HBsAg.

Because the amniotic fluid contains viruses or bacteria shed from the placenta, skin, urine, or tracheal fluid of the infected fetus, this fluid, which can be obtained during gestation with less risk than fetal blood sampling, may also be used to detect the infecting organism by culture, antigen detection test, or PCR assay. Amniocentesis and analysis of desquamated fetal cells in the amniotic fluid have been used for the early diagnosis of genetic disorders for some time. The seminal publication by Daffos and colleagues in 1983 [83], in which fetal blood sampling for prenatal diagnosis was first described, provided a method for diagnosing various infections in the fetus that previously could be diagnosed only after birth. Their methods were widely adopted and have contributed significantly to our understanding of the immune response of the fetus to various pathogens, including rubella virus, VZV, CMV, and T. gondii [84–87], and to a more objective approach to treating infection in the fetus before birth.

Fetal blood sampling and amniocentesis are performed under ultrasound guidance. The method is not free of risk; amniocentesis alone carries a risk of fetal injury or death of 1% [50,88], and fetal blood sampling carries a risk of approximately 1.4% [89]. Amniotic fluid may be examined for the presence of the infecting organism or its antigens, DNA, or RNA. Fetal blood can be examined for the same factors and antibodies formed by the fetus against the pathogen (e.g., IgA or IgM antibodies that do not normally cross the placental barrier). Fetal blood sampling is usually performed during or after week 18 of gestation. A fetus diagnosed with infection with a specific pathogen or who is at high risk for infection (e.g., the fetus of a nonimmune woman who acquired infection with T. gondii or rubella virus during pregnancy) may be followed by ultrasound examination to detect abnormalities such as dilation of the cerebral ventricles.

Isolation, Culture, and Polymerase Chain Reaction Assay

Isolation of CMV and rubella virus [90] and demonstration of HBsAg [91] from amniotic fluid obtained by amniocentesis have been reported. As PCR techniques have proved to be sensitive and specific for diagnosing many infections in the pregnant woman, fetus, and newborn, in many instances isolating the infectious agent to make a definitive diagnosis is no longer necessary with use of PCR techniques. PCR methods decrease the time to diagnosis and increase the sensitivity for diagnosis of many infectious agents, as exemplified by the prenatal diagnosis of infections caused by parvovirus [92,93], CMV [94–96], T. gondii [97,98], and rubella virus [99,100].

As with all diagnostic testing, caution is required in interpreting the results of prenatal PCR testing, however, because the sensitivity of PCR results on amniotic fluid is uncertain. One third of cases of congenital toxoplasmosis yield a negative result on amniotic fluid PCR assay [98,100], and infants with congenital rubella may have negative amniotic fluid PCR assay results, but positive fetal blood tests. Also, false-positive rates of 5% for viral DNA detection in fluids obtained for genetic testing have been observed when congenital fetal infection was not suspected or documented. Combined diagnostic approaches in which PCR is used in concert with fetal serology and other diagnostic modalities (e.g., serial fetal ultrasonography) to test amniotic fluid and fetal blood may offer the greatest sensitivity and predictive power in cases in which congenital infection is suspected and this information is important in management decisions [98,101].

Cytologic and Histologic Diagnosis

Review of cytologic preparations and tissue sections may provide a presumptive diagnosis of certain infections. Cervicovaginal smears or cell scrapings from the base of vesicles are valuable in diagnosing VZV and HSV infections. Typical changes include multinucleated giant cells and intranuclear inclusions. These morphologic approaches have largely been replaced, however, by more specific testing methods, such as direct immunofluorescence techniques or immunoperoxidase staining to detect VZV, HSV, and CMV infection. The diagnosis of acute toxoplasmosis can be made from characteristic histologic changes in lymph nodes or by demonstration of the tachyzoite in biopsy or autopsy specimens of infected tissues.

Detailed descriptions of the changes associated with infections of the placenta are presented in a monograph by Fox [102]. Examination of the placental parenchyma, the membranes, and the cord may provide valuable information for diagnosis of the infection and identification of the mode of transmission to the fetus (in utero or ascending infection).

Serologic Diagnosis

The serologic diagnosis of infection in the pregnant woman most often requires demonstration of elevated antibody titer against the suspected agent. Ideally, the physician should have available information about the patient's serologic status at the onset of pregnancy to identify women who are unprotected against T. pallidum, T. gondii, and rubella virus or who are infected with HBV or HIV. Many obstetricians have adopted this valuable practice.

Difficulties in interpreting serologic test results seldom arise when patients are seen shortly after exposure or at the onset of symptoms. In certain infections (e.g., rubella, toxoplasmosis), a relatively rapid increase in antibody levels may preclude the demonstration, however, of a significant increase in titer in patients who are tested more than 7 days after the onset of the suspected illness. In these circumstances, a diagnosis may be obtained through the measurement of antibodies that increase more slowly over several weeks. Demonstration of IgA and IgE antibodies (in addition to the more conventional use of tests for IgG and IgM antibodies) is useful in the early diagnosis of infection in the pregnant woman, fetus, and newborn, and this should serve as an impetus to commercial firms to make these methods more widely available for health care providers. The same pertains to IgG avidity tests, which have proved accurate in ruling out recently acquired infection with *T. gondii* [103], CMV [104,105], and rubella virus [106,107]. At present, these tests require special techniques and are not performed routinely by most laboratories, so local or state health departments should be consulted for further information regarding their availability.

Use of Skin Tests

Routine skin tests for diagnosis of tuberculosis should be considered a part of prenatal care. Tuberculin skin tests can be administered to the mother without risk to the fetus.

Universal Screening

Prenatal care in the United States includes routine screening for serologic evidence of syphilis and rubella infection; culture or antigen evidence of *Chlamydia trachomatis*, group B streptococcus, or HBV infection; screening for urinary tract infection; and skin testing for tuberculosis. Evidence that treatment of the HIV-infected mother significantly reduces virus transmission to the fetus has led to recommendations by the U.S. Public Health Service and others for universal HIV screening for all pregnant women in the United States. Current CDC guidelines support voluntary HIV testing under conditions that simplify consent procedures, while preserving a woman's right to refuse testing [5,108,109].

Pregnant women with known HIV infection should be monitored and given appropriate treatment to enhance mother and fetal well-being and to prevent maternal-to-fetal transmission. Pregnant women should be examined carefully for the presence of HIV-related infections, including gonorrhea, syphilis, and *C. trachomatis*. Baseline antibody titers should be obtained for opportunistic infections, such as *T. gondii*, which are observed commonly in HIV-infected women and which may be transmitted to their fetuses. More detailed information on management of the HIV-infected pregnant woman and her infant is given in Chapter 21.

DIAGNOSIS OF INFECTION IN THE NEWBORN INFANT

Infants with congenital infection as a result of rubella virus, CMV, HSV, *T. gondii*, or *T. pallidum* may present similarly with one or more of the following abnormalities: purpura, jaundice, hepatosplenomegaly, pneumonitis, and meningoencephalitis. Some findings have specific diagnostic significance (see Tables 1–5 and 1–6).

In certain congenital infections, the organism may be isolated from tissues and body fluids. Infants may excrete CMV and rubella virus in the urine for weeks to months after birth. *T. pallidum* may be found in the CSF, in nasal secretions, and in syphilitic skin lesions. In infants with congenital HIV infection, approximately 30% to 50% are culture-positive or PCR assay–positive at birth, but nearly 100% are positive by 4 to 6 months of life.

Serologic tests are available through state or commercial laboratories for the TORCH group of microorganisms (*T. gondii*, rubella virus, CMV, and HSV) and for certain other congenitally acquired infections. To distinguish passively transferred maternal IgG antibody from antibody produced by the neonate in response to infection in utero, it is necessary to obtain two blood specimens from the infant. Because the half-life of IgG is approximately 3 weeks, the first sample is obtained soon after birth, and the second sample should be obtained at least two half-lives, or approximately 6 weeks, after the first specimen.

IgA, IgE, and IgM antibodies do not cross the placenta. Antigen-specific IgA, IgE, and IgM antibodies in the infant's blood provide evidence of current infection, but few commercial laboratories employ reliable assays for these antibodies for the purpose of identifying congenital infections (as described in a Public Health Advisory from the U.S. Food and Drug Administration outlining the limitations of *Toxoplasma* IgM commercial test kits).

Although most congenital infections occur as a single entity, many HIV-infected mothers are coinfected with other infectious agents that may be transmitted to the newborn. A neonate born to a mother with HIV infection should be considered at risk for other sexually transmitted infections, such as syphilis, gonorrhea, and *C. trachomatis* infection. Coinfection also has been documented for CMV [110,111].

PREVENTION AND MANAGEMENT OF INFECTION IN THE PREGNANT WOMAN

Prevention of Infection

The pregnant woman should avoid contact with individuals with communicable diseases, particularly if the pregnant woman is known to be seronegative (e.g., for CMV) or has no prior history of the disease (e.g., with VZV). In some cases, specific measures can be taken. The pregnant woman should avoid intercourse with her sexual partner if he has a vesicular lesion on the penis that may be associated with HSV, or if he is known or suspected to be infected with HIV.

Pregnant women should avoid eating raw or undercooked lamb, pork, and beef because of risk of *T. gondii* contamination. They also should avoid contact with cat feces or objects or materials contaminated with cat feces because these are highly infectious if they harbor oocysts of *T. gondii* (see Chapter 31). Pregnant women should not eat unpasteurized dairy products (including all soft cheeses), prepared meats (hot dogs, deli meat, and paté), and undercooked poultry because these foods often contain *Listeria monocytogenes* (see Chapter 13).

Immunization

Routine immunization schedules for infants and children with currently available live vaccines, including measles, poliomyelitis, mumps, and rubella, should confer protection against these infections throughout the childbearing years.

Public health authorities and obstetricians generally agree that immunization during pregnancy poses only theoretical risks to the developing fetus. Nevertheless, pregnant women should receive a vaccine only when the vaccine is unlikely to cause harm, the risk for disease exposure is high, and the infection would pose a significant risk to the mother (e.g., influenza) or fetus (e.g., tetanus) [112]. The following are important considerations regarding immunization of the pregnant woman:

- The only vaccines routinely recommended for administration during pregnancy in the United States, when indicated for either primary or booster immunization, are vaccines for tetanus, diphtheria, and influenza [113]. These and other inactivated vaccines, including typhoid fever vaccine, are not considered hazardous to the pregnant woman or her fetus and often provide major benefit when indicated. An example is the use of tetanus toxoid vaccines in areas of the world where unsterile delivery and cord care practices may cause infection and high risk of fatality in the newborn. In the United States, pregnant women are at increased risk for influenza-like illness requiring hospitalization compared with nonpregnant women of similar age. For this reason, routine immunization of pregnant women at the onset of the influenza season is recommended by the Advisory Committee on Infectious Diseases of the CDC [113]. In women at increased risk for certain serious bacterial infections, such as invasive pneumococcal or meningococcal disease (e.g., women with sickle cell disease or HIV infection), immunization should precede pregnancy where possible. If immunization has not occurred before pregnancy, and the risk is significant (e.g., with a meningococcal outbreak in the community), women should be vaccinated.
- Pregnancy is a contraindication to administration of all live vaccines except when susceptibility and exposure are highly probable, and the disease to be prevented constitutes a greater threat to the woman and her fetus than a possible adverse effect of the vaccine. Yellow fever vaccine is indicated for pregnant women who are at substantial risk for imminent exposure to infection (e.g., with international travel). A report of IgM antibodies to yellow fever in the infant of a woman immunized during pregnancy suggests that transplacental transmission of the yellow fever vaccine virus does occur, although the incidence of congenital infection is unknown [114].
- Varicella vaccine should not be administered to pregnant women because the possible effects on fetal development are unknown. When women of childbearing age, including postpubertal girls, are immunized, pregnancy should be avoided for at least 2 months after immunization.
- Because several weeks can elapse before pregnancy is evident, vaccines indicated for any woman of childbearing age should be administered with caution and selectivity. Evidence that prolonged virus shedding occurs after immunization with live virus vaccine suggests that, where possible, pregnancy should be avoided for 2 to 3 months after administration of any live immunizing agent.
- The risk to the mother or fetus from immunization of members of the immediate family or other intimate contacts is uncertain. The use of attenuated measles, rubella, mumps, and varicella vaccines rarely results in transmission of these viruses to susceptible subjects in the immediate environment, but household spread of attenuated polioviruses through contact with recently vaccinated, susceptible individuals in the family is common. From March 1995 through March 2003, 509 pregnant women whose pregnancy outcomes were documented were inadvertently given varicella vaccine (VARIVAX Pregnancy Registry). No offspring had congenital varicella, and the rate of congenital anomalies was no greater than that in the general population. The presence of a pregnant woman in the household is not a contraindication to varicella immunization of a child in that household, and women who are susceptible to varicella should be vaccinated postpartum.

Use of Immunoglobulin

Human immune serum globulin administered after exposure to rubella, varicella, measles, or hepatitis A virus may modify clinical signs and symptoms of disease, but has not proved to be consistently effective in preventing disease, and presumably viremia, in susceptible individuals. Human immune serum globulin is of undetermined value in protecting the fetus of a susceptible woman against infection with these viruses. Use after maternal exposure to rubella virus should be limited to women to whom therapeutic abortion is unacceptable, in the event of documented infection during pregnancy.

Antimicrobial Therapy

Almost without exception, antimicrobial agents administered systemically to the mother pass to the fetus. Clinical management of pregnant women with acute infections amenable to therapy should be the same as management of nonpregnant patients, but should include particular attention to the possible effects of the antimicrobial drug on the fetus. Pregnant women with recently acquired acute toxoplasmosis, Lyme disease, and syphilis should undergo treatment as outlined in the specific chapters devoted to those topics. Women who are colonized with *C. trachomatis* or group B streptococci may receive treatment under selected circumstances (discussed in the next section).

A landmark study by Connor and colleagues [115] showed reduction of mother-to-infant transmission of HIV from 25.5% to 8.3% using zidovudine in women who had peripheral CD4$^+$ T lymphocyte counts greater than 200 cells/μL and were mildly symptomatic. The currently recommended treatment regimen in the United States is oral zidovudine administered to pregnant women beginning at 14 to 34 weeks of gestation and continuing throughout pregnancy, intravenous zidovudine during labor and delivery, and oral zidovudine to the newborn for the first 6 weeks of life (see Chapter 21). This complex and costly regimen is not feasible for resource-limited countries, but studies in Uganda using a single dose of nevirapine administered to the mother during labor and a single dose to the neonate before discharge provided a model for simpler and effective prophylactic therapy [116]. More recent recommendations from the World Health Organization include the use of simple, short course combination prophylactic therapeutic regimens which are effective and prevent development of antiretroviral resistance among infants with breakthrough infections [117].

INFECTIONS ACQUIRED BY THE NEWBORN INFANT DURING BIRTH
PATHOGENESIS

The developing fetus is protected from the microbial flora of the maternal genital tract. Initial colonization of the newborn and of the placenta usually occurs after rupture of maternal membranes. If delivery is delayed after membranes rupture, the vaginal microflora can ascend and in some cases produce inflammation of fetal membranes, umbilical cord, and placenta. Fetal infection also can result from aspiration of infected amniotic fluid. Some viruses are present in the genital secretions (HSV, CMV, HBV, or HIV) or blood (HBV, hepatitis C virus, or HIV). If delivery occurs shortly after rupture of the membranes, the infant can be colonized during passage through the birth canal. Various microorganisms may be present in the maternal birth canal, as summarized in Table 1–8, including gram-positive cocci (staphylococci and streptococci); gram-negative cocci (*Neisseria meningitidis* [rarely] and *Neisseria gonorrhoeae*); gram-negative enteric bacilli (*Escherichia coli, Proteus* species, *Klebsiella* species, *Pseudomonas* species, *Salmonella,* and *Shigella*); anaerobic bacteria; viruses (CMV, HSV, rubella virus, and HIV); fungi (predominantly *Candida albicans*); *C. trachomatis*; mycoplasmas; and protozoa (*Trichomonas vaginalis* and *T. gondii*). As indicated in Table 1–8, some of these organisms are significantly associated with disease in the newborn infant, whereas others affect the neonate rarely, if at all.

The newborn is initially colonized on the skin; mucosal surfaces including the nasopharynx, oropharynx, conjunctivae, umbilical cord, and external genitalia; and the gastrointestinal tract (from swallowing of infected amniotic fluid or vaginal secretions). In most infants, the organisms proliferate at these sites without causing illness. A few infants become infected by direct extension from the sites of colonization (e.g., otitis media from nasopharyngeal colonization). Alternatively, invasion of the bloodstream can ensue, with subsequent dissemination of infection. The umbilical cord was a particularly common portal of entry for systemic infection before local disinfection methods became routine because the devitalized tissues are an excellent medium for bacterial growth, and because the thrombosed umbilical vessels provide direct access to the bloodstream. Microorganisms also can infect abrasions or skin wounds. At present, the most frequent routes for bloodstream invasion are the lung from aspirated infected amniotic fluid or vaginal contents and the gastrointestinal tract from transmigration of microbial flora across the gut wall.

Infants who develop bacterial sepsis often have specific risk factors not evident in infants who do not develop significant infections. Among these factors are preterm delivery at a gestational age less than 37 weeks, low birth weight, prolonged rupture of maternal membranes, maternal intra-amniotic infection, traumatic delivery, and fetal anoxia. Relative immaturity of the immune system is considered to be one factor increasing risk of infection during the neonatal period. The role of host defenses in neonatal infection is discussed in detail in Chapter 4.

Preterm birth is the most significant risk factor for acquisition of infections in infants immediately before or during delivery or in the nursery. Because of the increasing number of infants with extremely low birth weight and very low birth weight, infection remains a cause of morbidity and mortality. Expansion of treatments for infertility has continued to increase the number of pregnancies with multiple births, and a gestational age of less than 28 weeks is common following these treatments. A summary of 6215 very low birth weight neonates (birth weight 401 to 1500 g) from the National Institute of Child Health and Human Development Neonatal Research Network reported that 21% had one or more episodes of blood culture–positive, late-onset sepsis [119]. Infection rate was inversely correlated with birth weight and gestational age, and infected infants had a significantly prolonged mean hospital stay (79 days) compared with uninfected infants (60 days). Also, infants with late-onset sepsis were significantly more likely to die than uninfected infants (18% versus 7%), especially if they were infected with gram-negative organisms (36%) or fungi (32%) [119].

The value of certain defense mechanisms remains controversial. Vernix caseosa contains antimicrobial proteins (see Chapter 4), and retention of vernix probably provides a protective barrier to the skin. Breast milk influences the composition of the fecal flora by suppression of *E. coli* and other gram-negative enteric bacilli and encouragement of *Lactobacillus* growth. In addition, breast milk contains secretory IgA, lysozymes, white blood cells, and lactoferrin (an iron-binding protein that significantly inhibits the growth of *E. coli* and other microorganisms); however, the role of these constituents in mitigating colonization and systemic infection in the neonate acquired at or shortly after birth is uncertain (see Chapter 5).

The virulence of the invading microorganism is also a factor in the pathogenesis of neonatal sepsis. Certain phage types of *S. aureus* (types 80 and 81) were responsible for most cases of disease in the staphylococcal pandemic of the 1950s. Phage group 2 *S. aureus* strains have been responsible for staphylococcal scalded skin syndrome sometimes seen in neonates (toxic epidermal necrolysis). Other evidence suggests that the K1 capsular antigens of *E. coli* and type III strains of group B streptococcus possess virulence properties that enhance their propensity for invasion of the blood-brain barrier during bacteremia compared with non-K1 and non–type III strains.

MICROBIOLOGY

The agents responsible for early-onset (before 7 days) neonatal sepsis are found in the maternal birth canal [120,121]. Most of these organisms are considered to be saprophytic, but occasionally can be responsible for maternal infection and its sequelae, including endometritis and puerperal fever. The microbial flora of the adult female genital tract and their association with neonatal infection and disease are reviewed in Table 1–9.

Before the introduction of the sulfonamides and penicillin in the 1940s, gram-positive cocci, particularly group A streptococci, were responsible for most cases of neonatal sepsis. After the introduction of antimicrobial agents, gram-negative enterics, in particular *E. coli*, were the predominant causes of serious bacterial infections of the newborn. An increase in serious neonatal infection caused by group B streptococci was noted in the early 1970s, and group B streptococci and *E. coli* continue to be the most frequent causative agents for early-onset neonatal sepsis and late-onset sepsis in term infants. By contrast, late-onset (after 7 days) sepsis in preterm neonates remaining in the neonatal intensive care unit for weeks or months is typically caused by commensal organisms (e.g., coagulase-negative staphylococci and *Enterococcus*) and organisms acquired from the mother and from the nursery environment.

The bacteria responsible for neonatal sepsis are discussed in Chapter 6. Mycoplasmas, anaerobic bacteria, and viruses (including HSV, HBV, CMV, and HIV) that colonize the maternal genital tract also are acquired during birth.

DIAGNOSIS

Review of the maternal record provides important clues for diagnosis of infection in the neonate. Signs of illness during pregnancy; exposure to sexual partners with transmissible infections; and results of cultures (e.g., for *C. trachomatis*, *N. gonorrhoeae*, or group B streptococci), serologic tests (e.g., for HIV infection, rubella, HBV, hepatitis C virus, or syphilis), and tuberculin skin tests or chest radiographs should be identified in the pregnancy record. The delivery chart should be checked for peripartum events that indicate risk of sepsis in the neonate, including premature rupture of membranes; prolonged duration (>18 hours) of rupture of membranes; evidence of fetal distress and fever; or other signs of maternal infection such as bloody diarrhea, respiratory or gastrointestinal signs (i.e., enterovirus), indications of large concentrations of pathogens in the genitalia (as reflected in bacteriuria caused by group B streptococci), and evidence of invasive bacterial infections in prior pregnancies.

TABLE 1–9   Association of Neonatal Disease with Microorganisms Present in the Maternal Birth Canal

Organism	Significant	Uncommon	Rare
Bacteria	Group A streptococci	*Staphylococcus aureus*	*Lactobacillus*
	Group B streptococci	α-hemolytic streptococci	*Staphylococcus epidermidis*
	Enterococcus	*Proteus* species	*Gardnerella vaginalis*
	Escherichia coli	*Klebsiella* species	*Corynebacterium*
	Neisseria gonorrhoeae	*Pseudomonas* species	*Bacillus subtilis*
	Listeria monocytogenes	*Salmonella* species	
		Shigella species	
		Alkaligenes faecalis	
		Neisseria meningitidis	
		Haemophilus influenzae	
		Haemophilus parainfluenzae	
		Vibrio fetus	
Anaerobic bacteria		*Bacteroides*	*Peptostreptococcus*
		Clostridium species	*Veillonella*
Chlamydia	Chlamydia trachomatis		*Bifidobacterium*
			Eubacterium
Mycoplasma			*Mycobacterium tuberculosis*
			Mycoplasma hominis
			Ureaplasma urealyticum
Viruses	CMV	HIV	Rubella virus
	HSV		HPV
	HBV		LCV
Fungi	*Candida albicans*	*Coccidioides immitis*	*Candida glabrata*
	Chlamydia trachomatis	*Mycoplasma hominis*	*Saccharomyces*
		Ureaplasma urealyticum	
Protozoa		*Toxoplasma gondii*	
		Trichomonas vaginalis	

CMV, cytomegalovirus; HBV, hepatitis B virus; HIV, human immunodeficiency virus; HPV, human papillomavirus; HSV, herpes simplex virus; LCV, lymphocytic choriomeningitis virus.

The clinical diagnosis of systemic infection in the newborn can be difficult because the initial signs of infection may be subtle and nonspecific. Not only are the signs of infectious and noninfectious processes similar, but also the signs of in utero infection are indistinguishable from signs of infections acquired during the birth process or during the first few days of life. Respiratory distress, lethargy, irritability, poor feeding, jaundice, emesis, and diarrhea are associated with various infectious and non-infectious causes.

Some clinical manifestations of neonatal sepsis, such as hepatomegaly, jaundice, pneumonitis, purpura, and meningitis, are common to many infections acquired in utero or during delivery. Certain signs are related to specific infections (see Tables 1–6 and 1–7). Many signs of congenital infection are not evident at birth. HBV infection should be considered in an infant with onset of jaundice and hepatosplenomegaly between 1 and 6 months of age; CMV infection acquired at or soon after delivery is associated with an afebrile protracted pneumonitis; enterovirus infection should be considered in an infant with CSF pleocytosis in the first months of life. Most infants with congenital HIV infection do not have signs of disease during the first months of life. Uncommonly, signs may be present at birth. Srugo and colleagues [122] described an infant with signs of meningoencephalitis at 6 hours of life; HIV was subsequently isolated from CSF.

Most early-onset bacterial infections are nonfocal except in the circumstance of respiratory distress at or shortly after birth, in which the chest radiograph reveals pneumonia. Focal infections are frequent with late-onset neonatal sepsis and include otitis media, pneumonia, soft tissue infections, urinary tract infections, septic arthritis, osteomyelitis, and peritonitis. Bacterial meningitis is of particular concern because of the substantial mortality rate and the significant morbidity in survivors. Few infants have overt meningeal signs, and a high index of suspicion and examination of the CSF are required for early diagnosis.

Available routine laboratory methods provide limited assistance in the diagnosis of systemic infections in the newborn infant. In bacterial sepsis, measurement of the total white blood cell count can be variable and supports a diagnosis of bacterial sepsis only if it is high ($>30,000$ cells/mm^3) or very low (<5000 cells/mm^3). Immunoglobulin is produced by the fetus and newborn infant in response to infection, and increased levels of IgM have been measured in the serum of newborns with infections (i.e., syphilis, rubella, cytomegalic inclusion disease, toxoplasmosis, and malaria) acquired transplacentally. Increased levels of IgM also result from postnatally acquired bacterial infections. Not all infected infants have increased levels of serum IgM, however, and some infants who do have elevated concentrations of total IgM are apparently uninfected. Identification of increased levels of total IgM in the newborn suggests an infectious process acquired before or shortly after birth, but this finding is not specific and is of limited assistance in diagnosis and management.

Because inflammation of the placenta and umbilical cord may accompany peripartum sepsis, pathologic examination of sections of these tissues may assist in the diagnosis of infection in the newborn. Histologic evidence of inflammation also is noted in the absence of evidence of neonatal sepsis, however. In the immediate postnatal period, gastric aspirate, pharyngeal mucus, or fluid from the external ear canal has been used to delineate exposure to potential pathogens, but is not useful in the diagnosis of neonatal sepsis.

Isolation of microorganisms from a usually sterile site, such as blood, CSF, or skin vesicle fluid, or from a suppurative lesion or a sterilely obtained sample of urine remains the only valid method of diagnosing systemic infection. Aspiration of any focus of infection in a critically ill infant (e.g., needle aspiration of middle ear fluid in an infant with otitis media or from the joint or metaphysis of an infant with osteoarthritis) should be performed to determine the etiologic agent. In infants with very low birth weight, commensal microorganisms, such as coagulase-negative staphylococci, *Enterococcus*, or *Candida*, isolated from a usually sterile body site should be considered pathogens until proven otherwise. Culture of infectious agents from the nose, throat, skin, umbilicus, or stool indicates colonization; these agents may include the pathogens that are responsible for the disease, but in themselves do not establish the presence of active systemic infection.

PCR assay is useful to detect the nucleic acid of various important pathogens including viruses and *Pneumocystis jiroveci*. When appropriate, serologic studies should be performed to ascertain the presence of in utero or postnatal infection. Serologic tests for HIV, rubella, parvovirus B19, *T. gondii*, and *T. pallidum* are available through local or state laboratories. For some of these infections (e.g., rubella), the serologic assay measures IgG. To distinguish passively transferred maternal antibody from antibody derived from infection in the neonate, it is necessary to obtain two blood specimens from the infant. Because the half-life of IgG is estimated to be 23 days, the first sample is obtained soon after birth, and the second sample should be obtained at least two half-lives, or approximately 6 weeks, after the first specimen. Measurement of IgM antibody provides evidence of current infection in the neonate, but none of these assays has proven reliability at present.

MANAGEMENT

Successful management of neonatal bacterial sepsis depends on a high index of suspicion based on maternal history and infant signs, prompt initiation of appropriate antimicrobial therapy while diagnostic tests are performed, and meticulous supportive measures. If the physician suspects bacterial infection in a newborn, culture specimens should be obtained, and treatment with appropriate antimicrobial agents should be initiated immediately. Generally, initial therapy must provide coverage against gram-positive cocci, particularly group B and other streptococci, and gram-negative enteric bacilli. Ampicillin is the preferred agent with effectiveness against gram-positive cocci and *L. monocytogenes*. The choice of therapy for gram-negative infections depends on the current pattern of antimicrobial susceptibility in the local community. Most experts prefer ampicillin and gentamicin therapy for early-onset presumptive sepsis, with the addition of cefotaxime for presumptive bacterial meningitis [123]. Intrapartum antimicrobial therapy can yield drug concentrations in the blood of the newborn infant sufficient to suppress growth of group B streptococci and possibly other susceptible organisms in blood obtained for culture. The requirement for more than one blood specimen for the microbiologic diagnosis of early-onset sepsis places a substantial burden on the clinician.

An algorithm has been devised to guide empirical management of neonates born to mothers who received intrapartum antimicrobial prophylaxis for prevention of early-onset group B streptococcal infection [124]. These infants may be divided into three management groups:

1. Neonates who have signs of sepsis or neonates whose mothers are colonized with group B streptococci and have chorioamnionitis should receive a full diagnostic evaluation with institution of presumptive treatment.
2. Term neonates who appear healthy and whose mothers received penicillin, ampicillin, or cefazolin 4 or more hours before delivery do not require further evaluation or treatment.
3. Healthy-appearing term neonates whose mothers received prophylaxis less than 4 hours before delivery and neonates born at less than 35 weeks of gestation whose mothers received prophylaxis of any duration before delivery should be observed for 48 hours or longer and should receive a limited evaluation, including white blood cell count and differential and blood culture [124].

Infants in the first two categories are readily identified, but assignment of infants to the third category is often problematic because of the vague end points. Recommendations for prevention and treatment of early-onset group B streptococcal infection are discussed in Chapter 12.

The choice of antibacterial drugs should be reviewed when results of cultures and susceptibility tests become available. The clinician should take care to select drugs that have been studied for appropriate dose, interval of dosing, and safety in neonates, especially very low birth weight infants, and that have the narrowest antimicrobial spectrum that would be effective (see Chapter 37). The duration of therapy depends on the initial response to the appropriate antibiotics—typically 10 days in most infants with sepsis, pneumonia, or minimal or absent focal infection; a minimum of 14 days for uncomplicated meningitis caused by group B streptococci or *L. monocytogenes*; and 21 days for gram-negative enteric bacilli [124]. The clinical pharmacology of antibiotics administered to the newborn infant is unique and cannot be extrapolated from adult data on absorption, excretion, and toxicity. The safety of new antimicrobial agents is a particular concern because toxic effects may not be detected until several years later (see Chapter 37).

Development of antimicrobial drug resistance in microbial pathogens is a constant concern. Group B streptococci remain uniformly susceptible to penicillins and cephalosporins, but many isolates now are resistant to erythromycin and clindamycin [125]. Administration of one or two doses of a penicillin or cephalosporin as part of a peripartum prophylactic regimen for prevention of group B streptococcal infection in the neonate should not significantly affect the genital flora, but monitoring should be continued to detect alterations in flora and antibiotic susceptibility. Because the nursery is a small, closed community, development of resistance is a greater concern with nosocomial infections than with infections acquired in utero or at delivery.

Despite the use of appropriate antimicrobial agents and optimal supportive therapy, mortality from neonatal sepsis remains substantial. To improve survival and decrease the severity of sequelae in survivors, investigators have turned their attention to studies of adjunctive modes of treatment that supplement the demonstrated deficits in the host defenses of the infected neonate. These therapies include use of standard hyperimmune immunoglobulins, leukocyte growth factors, and pathogen-specific monoclonal antibody preparations.

Antiviral therapies are available for newborns infected with HSV (acyclovir), VZV (acyclovir), and HIV. Acyclovir and zidovudine for HIV are well tolerated in pregnant women. Because early use of acyclovir for herpes simplex infections in neonates has been associated with improved outcome, physicians may choose to begin therapy for presumptive HSV disease and reevaluate when information on clinical course and results of cultures and PCR assay become available.

A phase II trial examining safety, pharmacodynamics, and efficacy of ganciclovir treatment for symptomatic congenital CMV infection established the safe dose in infants and showed an antiviral effect with suppression of viruria [126,127]. Neutropenia (63%), thrombocytopenia, and altered hepatic enzymes were noted in most of the infants, with nearly half of the infants requiring dosage adjustments because of severe neutropenia. A phase III randomized, controlled trial of intravenous ganciclovir for 6 weeks in 100 CMV-infected infants with central nervous system involvement at birth maintained hearing or showed hearing improvement in 84% of infants who received ganciclovir compared with 41% of control infants (see Chapter 23).

PREVENTION
Immunoprophylaxis

Passive immunoprophylaxis with specific hyperimmune immunoglobulin or monoclonal antibody preparations is indicated for the prevention of hepatitis B, varicella and respiratory syncytial virus infection in infants at risk for these infections. Details are provided in Chapter 38.

Universal immunization of infants with hepatitis B vaccine has been recommended by the American Academy of Pediatrics since 1992 [128]. Prior strategies of selective vaccination in high-risk populations and serologic screening of all pregnant women for HBsAg had little impact on control of HBV infections or their sequelae, and public health authorities believe that infant immunization offers the most feasible approach to universal protection and eventual eradication of the disease. Infants born to HBsAg-positive women should be immunized at birth and receive hepatitis B immunoglobulin at or shortly after birth. This prevention strategy may be improved if a birth dose of hepatitis B vaccine is universally recommended, providing additional coverage for infants whose maternal records are incorrect or unavailable before hospital discharge.

Chemoprophylaxis

After administration to the mother, antimicrobial agents capable of crossing biologic membranes can achieve pharmacologic concentrations in the fetus comparable with concentrations in well-vascularized maternal tissues. Prevention of group B streptococcal infection in the newborn by administration of ampicillin to the mother was shown by Boyer and colleagues [129] and other investigators in 1983 (see Chapter 12). A prevention strategy initially recommended by the American Academy of Pediatrics in 1992[130] was revised in 1997, and current recommendations from the CDC are endorsed by the American Academy of Pediatrics, the American College of Obstetricians and Gynecologists, and the American Academy of Family Physicians. These organizations recommend universal culture screening of all pregnant women at 35 to 37 weeks of gestation and administration of intravenous penicillin during labor [3].

Fetal drug concentrations can exceed 30% of the maternal blood concentrations [131], and concentrations bactericidal against group B streptococci can be achieved in amniotic fluid 3 hours after a maternal dose (see Chapters 12 and 37). Parenteral antimicrobial therapy administered to the mother in labor essentially treats the fetus earlier in the course of the intrapartum infection. If the fetus has been infected, the regimen is treatment, not prophylaxis, and for some infected fetuses the treatment administered in utero is insufficient to prevent early-onset group B streptococcal disease [132]. Although the prophylactic regimen has decreased the incidence of early-onset group B streptococcal disease (by >80% in a Pittsburgh survey [133], the regimen has had no impact on the incidence of late-onset disease [3].

Other modes of chemoprophylaxis administered to the neonate include ophthalmic drops or ointments for prevention of gonococcal ophthalmia and zidovudine to infants born to HIV-infected mothers. Administration of antibacterial agents to infants with minimal or ambiguous clinical signs is considered therapy for presumed sepsis and should not be considered prophylaxis.

INFECTIONS OF THE NEWBORN INFANT IN THE FIRST MONTH OF LIFE

When fever or other signs of systemic infection occur in the first weeks or months of life, various sources of infection should be considered: (1) congenital infections with onset in utero; (2) infections acquired during the birth process from the maternal genital tract; (3) infections acquired in the nursery; (4) infections acquired in the household after discharge from the nursery; and (5) infection that suggests an anatomic defect, underlying immunologic disease, or metabolic abnormality.

PATHOGENESIS AND MICROBIOLOGY
Congenital Infections

Signs of congenital infection may not appear for weeks, months, or years after birth. Diagnosis and management are discussed in the disease chapters.

Infections Acquired during Delivery

Although maternal intrapartum prophylaxis has reduced the incidence of early-onset group B streptococcal disease, it has not altered the incidence of late-onset disease [3,133], with signs occurring from 6 to 89 days of life, up to 6 months of age in infants with very low birth weight. The pathogenesis of late-onset group B streptococcal disease remains obscure, but it is likely that even when vertical transmission from the mother at birth is prevented, exposure to either the mother (in whom colonization resumes after delivery) or other colonized family members and caregivers can serve as a source for colonization through direct contact. It is unknown why sepsis develops without warning in an infant who has no risk factors for sepsis and was well for days to weeks; this concern also is relevant in infants who acquire late-onset disease as a result of *E. coli* and *L. monocytogenes*.

Nursery-Acquired Infections

After arrival in the nursery, the newborn may become infected by various pathways involving either human carriers or contaminated materials and equipment. Human sources in the hospital include personnel, mothers, and other infants. The methods of transmission may include the following:

- Respiratory droplet spread from adults or other newborn infants. Outbreaks of respiratory virus infections, including influenza, respiratory syncytial, and parainfluenza viruses, in prolonged-stay nurseries are frequent [132]. Methods for identification and control are provided in Chapter 35.
- Carriage of the microorganism on the hands of hospital personnel. A study has suggested that the hands may be not only a means of transmission, but also a significant reservoir of bacteria [134].
- Suppurative lesions. Although spread of staphylococcal and streptococcal infections to infants or mothers may be associated with asymptomatic carriers, the most serious outbreaks have been caused by a member of the medical or nursing staff with a significant lesion.
- Human milk. CMV, HIV, HSV, human T-cell lymphotropic virus type I [135], human T-cell lymphotropic virus type II [136], and HBsAg have been identified in mother's milk and may be transmitted to the neonate by this route. CMV-infected milk from banks can be dangerous for infants lacking passively transferred maternal antibody.

Breast milk transmission of HIV is of concern because of the importance of breast-feeding in providing nutrition and immunologic protection in the first year of life. Breast milk has been documented as the likely source of HIV infection in neonates whose mothers were transfused with HIV-infected blood after delivery or in whom disease developed postpartum through sexual contact [137]. These acute infections must be differentiated from the usual event, in which the mother is infected throughout pregnancy. Infection during the acute period occurs before development of antibody and may be a time when breast milk has a high titer of transmissible virus.

Because of the importance of breast-feeding for infant nutrition in developing countries, the World Health

Organization initially recommended that women in developing countries be encouraged to breast-feed despite HIV status [138]. By contrast, in the United States and Western Europe, HIV-infected mothers were discouraged from breast-feeding because other forms of nutrition were available [139]. In July 1998, the United Nations revised its position and issued recommendations to discourage HIV-infected women from breast-feeding, recognizing that many infants were infected by the breast milk of HIV-infected mothers. The recommendation also noted that in some regions and cultures, women are stigmatized for not breast-feeding, and alternatives such as formula are unaffordable or unsafe. The number of antenatal women in developing countries that lack resources for prevention in pregnancy has reached alarming proportions: 70% of women at a prenatal clinic in Zimbabwe and 30% of women in urban areas in six African countries were infected. The United Nations survey indicated that by 2000, breast-feeding would be responsible for more than one third (>200,000) of children newly infected with HIV unless some attempts were made to limit this route of transmission [140]. Current efforts to prevent breast-feeding transmission include improved dissemination of prophylactic regimens for pregnant women and their newborns [117]. However, availability of such regimens appears to be limited to ~45% of HIV infected pregnant women in low and middle income countries [118].

Infection of breast milk by bacterial pathogens such as *S. aureus*, group B streptococci, *L. monocytogenes* [141], and *Salmonella* species can result in neonatal disease. Bacteria that are components of skin flora, including *Staphylococcus epidermidis* and α-hemolytic streptococci, are frequently cultured from freshly expressed human milk and are unlikely to be associated with disease in the breast-fed infant. If these bacteria are allowed to multiply in banked breast milk, infection of the neonate is theoretically possible, but no substantive data have supported this possibility.

Other possible sources of infection in the nursery include the following:

- Blood used for replacement or exchange transfusion in neonates should be screened for safety using validated, efficacious methods, including tests for hepatitis B antigen, hepatitis C, HIV antibody, CMV antibody, and *Plasmodium* species in malaria-endemic areas.
- Equipment has been implicated in common-source nursery outbreaks, usually including contaminated solutions used in nebulization equipment, room humidifiers, and bathing solutions. Several gram-negative bacteria, including *Pseudomonas aeruginosa*, *Serratia marcescens*, and *Flavobacterium*, have been termed "water bugs" because of their ability to multiply in aqueous environments at room temperature. In recent years, few solution-related or equipment-related outbreaks caused by these organisms have been reported because of the scrupulous infection control practices enforced in most intensive care nurseries.
- Catheterization of the umbilical vein and artery has been associated with sepsis, umbilical cellulitis, and abscess formation, but careful hygienic practices with insertion of these devices make these complications rare. Intravenous alimentation using central venous catheters has been lifesaving for some infants, but also is associated with increased risk for catheter-related bacteremia or fungemia.
- Parenteral feeding with lipid emulsions has been associated with neonatal sepsis caused by coagulase-negative staphylococci and *Candida* species. Strains of staphylococci isolated from infected ventricular shunts or intravascular catheters produce a slime or glycocalyx that promotes adherence and growth of colonies on the surfaces and in the walls of catheters manufactured with synthetic polymers. The slime layer also protects the bacteria against antibiotics and phagocytosis. The introduction of lipid emulsion through the venous catheter provides nutrients for growth of the bacteria and fungi [142].

Hand hygiene remains the most important element in controlling the spread of infectious diseases in the nursery (see Chapter 35). Hand hygiene measures should be implemented before and after every patient contact. Surveys of hospital employees indicate that rigorous adherence to hand hygiene, although the most simple of infection control techniques, is still lacking in most institutions. A study by Brown and colleagues [143] in a Denver neonatal intensive care unit indicated that compliance with appropriate hand-washing techniques was low for medical and nursing personnel. Compliance was monitored using a direct observation technique; of 252 observed encounters of nurses, physicians, and respiratory therapists with infants, 25% of the personnel broke contact with the infant by touching self (69%) or touching another infant (4%), and 25% did not wash before patient contact.

Waterless, alcohol-based hand hygiene products are routinely used in nurseries, with surveys indicating their rapid acceptance by nursery personnel including physicians. Their ease of application and time saved through reduction in the need for hand washing should increase adherence with hand hygiene recommendations.

Early patient discharge at 24 or 48 hours was common several years ago as hospitals and third-party payers have attempted to reduce costs of health care. A cohort study of more than 300,000 births in Washington documented that newborns discharged home early (before 30 hours after birth) were at increased risk for rehospitalization during the first month of life; the leading causes were jaundice, dehydration, and sepsis, with onset within 7 days after discharge. Among 1253 infants who were rehospitalized within the first month of life, sepsis was the cause in 55 infants (4.4%) who were discharged early, in contrast to 42 infants (3.4%) who were discharged late [144]. These and other reports, combined with corrective legislation in many states, have led to recommendations that newborns remain hospitalized at least 48 hours after vaginal birth and 72 hours after cesarean section delivery.

Community-Acquired Infections

The newborn infant is susceptible to many of the infectious agents that colonize other members of the household and caregivers. The physician should consider illnesses in these contacts before discharging an infant from the hospital. If signs of an infectious disease develop after 15 to 30 days of life in an infant who was healthy at discharge and had no significant risk factors during gestation or delivery, the infection was probably acquired from a household or community contact. Suppurative lesions related to *S. aureus* in a household member can expose an infant to a virulent strain that causes disseminated infection. A careful history of illness in family members can suggest the source of the infant's disease (e.g., respiratory viruses, skin infections, a prolonged illness with coughing).

An infant also can be a source of infection for household contacts. An infant with congenital rubella syndrome can shed virus for many months and is a significant source of infection for susceptible close contacts. The same is true for an infant with vesicular lesions of herpes simplex or a syphilitic infant with rhinitis or skin rash.

Infections That Indicate Underlying Abnormalities

Infection may serve as a first clue indicating an underlying anatomic, metabolic, or immune system abnormality. Infants with galactosemia, iron overload, chronic granulomatous disease, and leukocyte adhesion defects are susceptible to certain invasive gram-negative infections. Genitourinary infection in the first months of life can suggest an anatomic or a physiologic defect of the urinary tract. Similarly, otitis media in the first month of life may be an indication of a midline defect of the palate or a eustachian tube dysfunction. Meningitis caused by non-neonatal pathogens (e.g., coagulase-negative staphylococci) can be a clue to the presence of a dermoid sinus tract to the intradural space. In infants with underlying humoral immune defects, systemic infections may not develop until passively acquired maternal antibody has dissipated. Because the half-life of IgG is about 3 weeks, such infections are likely to occur after 3 months of age.

REFERENCES

[1] U.S. Food and Drug Administration, Med. Bull. (8) Summer, (1998).

[2] E. Arias, et al., Annual summary of vital statistics—2002, Pediatrics 112 (2003) 1215–1230.

[3] S. Schrag, et al., Prevention of perinatal group B streptococcal disease. Revised guidelines from CDC, MMWR Recomm. Rep. 51 (2002) 1–22.

[4] C.R. Phares, et al., Epidemiology of invasive group B streptococcal disease in the United States, 1999–2005, JAMA 299 (2008) 2056–2065.

[5] HIV testing and prophylaxis to prevent mother-to-child transmission in the United States, Pediatrics 122 (2008) 1127–1134.

[6] J.L. Sullivan, Prevention of mother-to-child transmission of HIV—what next? J. Acquir. Immune Defic. Syndr. 34 (Suppl. 1) (2003) S67–S72.

[7] WHO Expert Consultation on New and Emerging Evidence on the Use of Antiretroviral Drugs for the Prevention of Mother-to-Child Transmission of HIV, Geneva, November 17–19, (2008). Available at http://www.who.int/hiv/topics/mtct/mtct_conclusions_consult.pdf Accessed January 20, 2009.

[8] Congenital syphilis—United States, 2000, MMWR Morb. Mortal. Wkly Rep. 50 (2001) 573–577.

[9] Sexually Transmitted Disease Surveillance, 2007 Syphilis, 2008. Available at http://cdc.gov/std/stats07/syphilis.htm. Accessed January 20, 2009.

[10] Control and prevention of rubella: evaluation and management of suspected outbreaks, rubella in pregnant women, and surveillance for congenital rubella syndrome, MMWR Recomm. Rep. 50 (2001) 1–23.

[11] Progress toward elimination of rubella and congenital rubella syndrome—the Americas, 2003–2008, MMWR Morb. Mortal. Wkly Rep. 57 (2008) 1176–1179.

[12] A.L. Mellor, et al., Indoleamine 2, 3-dioxygenase, immunosuppression and pregnancy, J. Reprod. Immunol. 57 (2002) 143–150.

[13] C. Xu, et al., A critical role for murine complement regulator crry in feto-maternal tolerance, Science 287 (2000) 498–501.

[14] G. Gaunt, K. Ramin, Immunological tolerance of the human fetus, Am. J. Perinatol. 18 (2001) 299–312.

[15] G. Chaouat, et al., A brief review of recent data on some cytokine expressions at the materno-foetal interface which might challenge the classical TH1/TH2 dichotomy, J. Reprod. Immunol. 53 (2002) 241–256.

[16] S. Chheda, S.M. Lopez, E.P. Sanderson, Congenital brucellosis in a premature infant, Pediatr. Infect. Dis. J. 16 (1997) 81–83.

[17] A. Stein, D. Raoult, Q fever during pregnancy: a public health problem in southern France, Clin. Infect. Dis. 27 (1998) 592–596.

[18] D.L. New, et al., Vertically transmitted babesiosis, J. Pediatr. 131 (1997) 163–164.

[19] T. Fujino, Y. Nagata, HTLV-I transmission from mother to child, J. Reprod. Immunol. 47 (2000) 197–206.

[20] R.B. Van Dyke, et al., Mother-to-child transmission of human T-lymphotropic virus type II, J. Pediatr. 127 (1995) 924–928.

[21] M. Schroter, et al., Detection of TT virus DNA and GB virus type C/hepatitis G virus RNA in serum and breast milk: determination of mother-to-child transmission, J. Clin. Microbiol. 38 (2000) 745–747.

[22] H.H. Feucht, et al., Vertical transmission of hepatitis G, Lancet 347 (1996) 615–616.

[23] O. Adams, et al., Congenital infections with human herpesvirus 6, J. Infect. Dis. 178 (1998) 544–546.

[24] M. Lanari, et al., Congenital infection with human herpesvirus 6 variant B associated with neonatal seizures and poor neurological outcome, J. Med. Virol. 70 (2003) 628–632.

[25] J.K. Chye, et al., Vertical transmission of dengue, Clin. Infect. Dis. 25 (1997) 1374–1377.

[26] G.D. Overturf, G. Balfour, Osteomyelitis and sepsis: severe complications of fetal monitoring, Pediatrics 55 (1975) 244–247.

[27] P.A. King-Lewis, S.D. Gardner, Congenital cytomegalic inclusion disease following intrauterine transfusion, BMJ 2 (1969) 603–605.

[28] J.M. Scott, A. Henderson, Acute villous inflammation in the placenta following intrauterine transfusion, J. Clin. Pathol. 25 (1972) 872–875.

[29] E.H. St Clair, J.H. DiLiberti, M.L. O'Brien, Observations of an infant born to a mother with botulism. Letter to the editor, J. Pediatr. 87 (1975) 658.

[30] L. Robin, D. Herman, R. Redett, Botulism in pregnant women, N. Engl. J. Med. 335 (1996) 823–824.

[31] G.J. Luijckx, et al., Guillain-Barré syndrome in mother and newborn child, Lancet 349 (1997) 27.

[32] B. Buchwald, et al., Neonatal Guillain-Barré syndrome: blocking antibodies transmitted from mother to child, Neurology 53 (1999) 1246–1253.

[33] R.L. Naeye, Causes of the excessive rates of perinatal mortality and prematurity in pregnancies complicated by maternal urinary-tract infections, N. Engl. J. Med. 300 (1979) 819–823.

[34] W.E. Savage, S.N. Hajj, E.H. Kass, Demographic and prognostic characteristics of bacteriuria in pregnancy, Medicine (Baltimore) 46 (1967) 385–407.

[35] C.W. Norden, E.H. Kass, Bacteriuria of pregnancy—a critical appraisal, Annu. Rev. Med. 19 (1968) 431–470.

[36] F. Smaill, Antibiotics for asymptomatic bacteriuria in pregnancy, Cochrane Database Syst. Rev. CD000490, (2001).

[37] L.K. Millar, S.M. Cox, Urinary tract infections complicating pregnancy, Infect. Dis. Clin. North Am. 11 (1997) 13–26.

[38] W.T. Shearer, Cytomegalovirus infection in a newborn dizygous twin, J. Pediatr. 81 (1972) 1161–1165.

[39] J.H. Stokes, H. Beerman, Modern Clinical Syphilology, Diagnosis, Treatment, Case Study, WB Saunders, Philadelphia, 1968.

[40] C.G. Ray, R.J. Wedgwood, Neonatal listeriosis: six case reports and a review of the literature, Pediatrics 34 (1964) 378–392.

[41] J.P. Marsden, C.R.M. Greenfield, Inherited smallpox, Arch. Dis. Child. 9 (1934) 309.

[42] R.M. Forrester, V.T. Lees, G.H. Watson, Rubella syndrome: escape of a twin, BMJ 5500 (1966) 1403.

[43] G.V. Feldman, Herpes zoster neonatorum, Arch. Dis. Child. 27 (1952) 126–127.

[44] A.J. Wilcox, et al., Incidence of early loss of pregnancy, N. Engl. J. Med. 319 (1988) 189–194.

[45] B.J. Brabin, Epidemiology of infection in pregnancy, Rev. Infect. Dis. 7 (1985) 579–603.

[46] S.L. Hillier, et al., The relationship of amniotic fluid cytokines and preterm delivery, amniotic fluid infection, histologic chorioamnionitis, and chorioamnion infection, Obstet. Gynecol. 81 (1993) 941–948.

[47] J. Hitti, et al., Broad-spectrum bacterial rDNA polymerase chain reaction assay for detecting amniotic fluid infection among women in premature labor, Clin. Infect. Dis. 24 (1997) 1228–1232.

[48] R. Romero, et al., The diagnostic and prognostic value of amniotic fluid white blood cell count, glucose, interleukin-6, and Gram stain in patients with preterm labor and intact membranes, Am. J. Obstet. Gynecol. 169 (1993) 805–816.

[49] R. Romero, et al., A comparative study of the diagnostic performance of amniotic fluid glucose, white blood cell count, interleukin-6, and Gram stain in the detection of microbial invasion in patients with preterm premature rupture of membranes, Am. J. Obstet. Gynecol. 169 (1993) 839–851.

[50] E.C. Roper, et al., Genetic amniocentesis: gestation-specific pregnancy outcome and comparison of outcome following early and traditional amniocentesis, Prenat. Diagn. 19 (1999) 803–807.

[51] B. Jacobsson, et al., Microbial invasion and cytokine response in amniotic fluid in a Swedish population of women in preterm labor, Acta Obstet. Gynecol. Scand. 82 (2003) 120–128.

[52] A.Y. El-Bastawissi, et al., Amniotic fluid interleukin-6 and preterm delivery: a review, Obstet. Gynecol. 95 (2000) 1056–1064.

[53] R.L. Naeye, W. Blanc, Pathogenesis of congenital rubella, JAMA 194 (1965) 1277–1283.

[54] R.L. Naeye, Cytomegalic inclusion disease: the fetal disorder, Am. J. Clin. Pathol. 47 (1967) 738–744.

[55] R.L. Naeye, J.A. Kelly, Judgment of fetal age. 3. The pathologist's evaluation, Pediatr. Clin. North Am. 13 (1966) 849–862.

[56] R.L. Naeye, Infants of prolonged gestation: a necropsy study, Arch. Pathol. 84 (1967) 37–41.

[57] A.C. Allison, G.R. Paton, Chromosomal abnormalities in human diploid cells infected with mycoplasma and their possible relevance to the aetiology of Down's syndrome (mongolism), Lancet 2 (1966) 1229–1230.

[58] W.W. Nichols, The role of viruses in the etiology of chromosomal abnormalities, Am. J. Hum. Genet. 18 (1966) 81–92.

[59] J. Nusbacher, K. Hirschhorn, L.Z. Cooper, Chromosomal abnormalities in congenital rubella, N. Engl. J. Med. 276 (1967) 1409–1413.

[60] Congenital malaria in children of refugees—Washington, Massachusetts, Kentucky, MMWR Morb. Mortal. Wkly. Rep. 30 (1981) 53–55.

[61] S. Nesheim, et al., Quantitative RNA testing for diagnosis of HIV-infected infants, J. Acquir. Immune Defic. Syndr. 32 (2003) 192–195.

[62] R. Balasubramanian, S.W. Lagakos, Estimation of the timing of perinatal transmission of HIV, Biometrics 57 (2001) 1048–1058.

[63] C.B. Wilson, et al., Development of adverse sequelae in children with subclinical congenital Toxoplasma infection, Pediatrics 66 (1980) 767–774.

[64] J.J. Townsend, et al., Progressive rubella panencephalitis: late onset after congenital rubella, N. Engl. J. Med. 292 (1975) 990–993.

[65] M.L. Weil, et al., Chronic progressive panencephalitis due to rubella virus simulating subacute sclerosing panencephalitis, N. Engl. J. Med. 292 (1975) 994–998.

[66] G.G. Donders, et al., Survival after intrauterine parvovirus B19 infection with persistence in early infancy: a two-year follow-up, Pediatr. Infect. Dis. J. 13 (1994) 234–236.

[67] E. Miller, J.E. Cradock-Watson, T.M. Pollock, Consequences of confirmed maternal rubella at successive stages of pregnancy, Lancet 2 (1982) 781–784.

[68] G. Desmonts, J. Couvreur, Congenital toxoplasmosis: a prospective study of the offspring of 542 women who acquired toxoplasmosis during pregnancy, in: O. Thalhammer, K. Baumgarten, A. Pollack (Eds.), Pathophysiology of Congenital Disease, Georg Thieme, Stuttgart, 1979, pp. 51–60.

[69] K.B. Fowler, et al., The outcome of congenital cytomegalovirus infection in relation to maternal antibody status, N. Engl. J. Med. 326 (1992) 663–667.

[70] S. Stagno, R.J. Whitley, Herpesvirus infections of pregnancy. Part I. Cytomegalovirus and Epstein-Barr virus infections, N. Engl. J. Med. 313 (1985) 1270–1274.

[71] A. Roongpisuthipong, et al., HIV seroconversion during pregnancy and risk for mother-to-infant transmission, J. Acquir. Immune Defic. Syndr. 26 (2001) 348–351.

[72] D.M. Green, S.M. Reid, K. Rhaney, Generalised vaccinia in the human foetus, Lancet 1 (1966) 1296–1298.

[73] R. Sharma, D.K. Jagdev, Congenital smallpox, Scand. J. Infect. Dis. 3 (1971) 245–247.

[74] T. Eilard, O. Strannegard, Rubella reinfection in pregnancy followed by transmission to the fetus, J. Infect. Dis. 129 (1974) 594–596.

[75] B. Harvey, J.S. Remington, A.J. Sulzer, IgM malaria antibodies in a case of congenital malaria in the United States, Lancet 1 (1969) 333–335.

[76] N.A. Nelson, V.R. Struve, Prevention of congenital syphilis by treatment of syphilis in pregnancy, JAMA 161 (1956) 869–872.

[77] A.J. Zuckerman, P.E. Taylor, Persistence of the serum hepatitis (SH-Australia) antigen for many years, Nature 223 (1969) 81–82.

[78] A.J. Nahmias, C.A. Alford, S.B. Korones, Infection of the newborn with herpesvirus hominis, Adv. Pediatr. 17 (1970) 185–226.

[79] G. Desmonts, J. Couvreur, P. Thulliez, Congenital toxoplasmosis: 5 cases of mother-to-child transmission of pre-pregnancy infection, Presse Med. 19 (1990) 1445–1449.

[80] N. Vogel, et al., Congenital toxoplasmosis transmitted from an immunologically competent mother infected before conception, Clin. Infect. Dis. 23 (1996) 1055–1060.

[81] Hepatitis B virus: a comprehensive strategy for eliminating transmission in the United States through universal childhood vaccination. Recommendations of the Immunization Practices Advisory Committee (ACIP), MMWR Recomm. Rep. 40 (1991) 1–25.

[82] L.K. Pickering (Ed.), Red Book: Report of the Committee on Infectious Diseases, American Academy of Pediatrics, Elk Grove Village, Ill, 2003.

[83] F. Daffos, M. Capella-Pavlovsky, F. Forestier, Fetal blood sampling via the umbilical cord using a needle guided by ultrasound: report of 66 cases, Prenat. Diagn. 3 (1983) 271–277.

[84] F. Daffos, et al., Prenatal diagnosis of congenital rubella, Lancet 2 (1984) 1–3.

[85] F. Daffos, et al., Prenatal management of 746 pregnancies at risk for congenital toxoplasmosis, N. Engl. J. Med. 318 (1988) 271–275.

[86] P. Hohlfeld, et al., Cytomegalovirus fetal infection: prenatal diagnosis, Obstet. Gynecol. 78 (1991) 615–618.

[87] L. Grangeot-Keros, et al., Prenatal and postnatal production of IgM and IgA antibodies to rubella virus studied by antibody capture immunoassay, J. Infect. Dis. 158 (1988) 138–143.

[88] F.W. Hanson, et al., Ultrasonography-guided early amniocentesis in singleton pregnancies, Am. J. Obstet. Gynecol. 162 (1990) 1376–1381.

[89] A. Ghidini, et al., Complications of fetal blood sampling, Am. J. Obstet. Gynecol. 168 (1993) 1339–1344.

[90] R. Skvorc-Ranko, et al., Intrauterine diagnosis of cytomegalovirus and rubella infections by amniocentesis, Can. Med. Assoc. J. 145 (1991) 649–654.

[91] G. Papaevangelou, et al., Hepatitis B antigen and antibody in maternal blood, cord blood, and amniotic fluid, Arch. Dis. Child 49 (1974) 936–939.

[92] T.J. Torok, et al., Prenatal diagnosis of intrauterine infection with parvovirus B19 by the polymerase chain reaction technique, Clin. Infect. Dis. 14 (1992) 149–155.

[93] P. Wattre, et al., A clinical and epidemiological study of human parvovirus B19 infection in fetal hydrops using PCR Southern blot hybridization and chemiluminescence detection, J. Med. Virol. 54 (1998) 140–144.

[94] T. Lazzarotto, et al., Prenatal indicators of congenital cytomegalovirus infection, J. Pediatr. 137 (2000) 90–95.

[95] T. Lazzarotto, et al., Congenital cytomegalovirus infection in twin pregnancies: viral load in the amniotic fluid and pregnancy outcome, Pediatrics 112 (2003) 153–157.

[96] M.G. Revello, et al., Improved prenatal diagnosis of congenital human cytomegalovirus infection by a modified nested polymerase chain reaction, J. Med. Virol. 56 (1998) 99–103.

[97] P. Hohlfeld, et al., Prenatal diagnosis of congenital toxoplasmosis with a polymerase-chain-reaction test on amniotic fluid, N. Engl. J. Med. 331 (1994) 695–699.

[98] S. Romand, et al., Prenatal diagnosis using polymerase chain reaction on amniotic fluid for congenital toxoplasmosis, Obstet. Gynecol. 97 (2001) 296–300.

[99] T.J. Bosma, et al., Use of PCR for prenatal and postnatal diagnosis of congenital rubella, J. Clin. Microbiol. 33 (1995) 2881–2887.

[100] F. Gay-Andrieu, et al., Fetal toxoplasmosis and negative amniocentesis: necessity of an ultrasound follow-up, Prenat. Diagn. 23 (2003) 558–560.

[101] G. Enders, et al., Prenatal diagnosis of congenital cytomegalovirus infection in 189 pregnancies with known outcome, Prenat. Diagn. 21 (2001) 362–377.

[102] H. Fox, Pathology of the Placenta, WB Saunders, Philadelphia, 1978.

[103] O. Liesenfeld, et al., Effect of testing for IgG avidity in the diagnosis of Toxoplasma gondii infection in pregnant women: experience in a U.S. reference laboratory, J. Infect. Dis. 183 (2001) 1248–1253.

[104] G. Nigro, M.M. Anceschi, E.V. Cosmi, Clinical manifestations and abnormal laboratory findings in pregnant women with primary cytomegalovirus infection, Br. J. Obstet. Gynaecol. 110 (2003) 572–577.

[105] M.G. Revello, G. Gerna, Diagnosis and management of human cytomegalovirus infection in the mother, fetus, and newborn infant, Clin. Microbiol. Rev. 15 (2002) 680–715.

[106] J.W. Tang, et al., Prenatal diagnosis of congenital rubella infection in the second trimester of pregnancy, Prenat. Diagn. 23 (2003) 509–512.

[107] J. Gutierrez, et al., Reliability of low-avidity IgG and of IgA in the diagnosis of primary infection by rubella virus with adaptation of a commercial test, J. Clin. Lab. Anal. 13 (1999) 1–4.

[108] Revised recommendations for HIV screening of pregnant women, MMWR Recomm. Rep. 50 (2001) 63–85.

[109] ACOG Committee Opinion No. 418, Prenatal and perinatal human immunodeficiency virus testing: expanded recommendations, Obstet. Gynecol. 112 (2008) 739–742.

[110] M.M. Mussi-Pinhata, et al., Congenital and perinatal cytomegalovirus infection in infants born to mothers infected with human immunodeficiency virus, J. Pediatr. 132 (1998) 285–290.

[111] D.L. Thomas, et al., Perinatal transmission of hepatitis C virus from human immunodeficiency virus type 1-infected mothers. Women and Infants Transmission Study, J. Infect. Dis. 177 (1998) 1480–1488.

[112] Immunization during pregnancy, ACOG Technical Bulletin, vol. 64, American College of Obstetrics and Gynecology, Washington, DC, 1982.

[113] Centers for Disease Control and Prevention, Prevention and control of influenza. Recommendations of the Advisory Committee on Immunization Practices, MMWR Recomm. Rep. 50 (2001) 1–44.

[114] T.F. Tsai, et al., Congenital yellow fever virus infection after immunization in pregnancy (see comments), J. Infect. Dis. 168 (1993) 1520–1523.

[115] E.M. Connor, et al., Reduction of maternal-infant transmission of human immunodeficiency virus type 1 with zidovudine treatment. Pediatric AIDS Clinical Trials Group Protocol 076 Study Group, N. Engl. J. Med. 331 (1994) 1173–1180.

[116] J.B. Jackson, et al., Intrapartum and neonatal single-dose nevirapine compared with zidovudine for prevention of mother-to-child transmission of HIV-1 in Kampala, Uganda: HIVNET 012 randomised trial, Lancet 354 (2003) 795–802.

[117] WHO Rapid advice: use of antiretroviral drugs for treating pregnant women and preventing HIV infection in infants. Available at http://www.who.int/hiv/pub/mtct/rapid_advice_mtct.pdf. Accessed June 10, 2010.

[118] http://www.who.int/hiv/topics/mtct/en/index.html. Accessed June 10, 2010.

[119] B.J. Stoll, et al., Late-onset sepsis in very low birth weight neonates: the experience of the NICHD neonatal research network, Pediatrics 110 (2002) 285–291.

[120] T. Roseberry, Microorganisms Indigenous to Man, McGraw-Hill, New York, 1962.

[121] S.L. Gorbach, et al., Anaerobic microflora of the cervix in healthy women, Am. J. Obstet. Gynecol. 117 (1973) 1053–1055.

[122] I. Srugo, et al., Meningoencephalitis in a neonate congenitally infected with human immunodeficiency virus type 1, J. Pediatr. 120 (1992) 93–95.

[123] M.S. Edwards, C.J. Baker, Bacterial infections in the neonate, in: S.S. Long, L.K. Pickering, C.G. Prober (Eds.), Principles and Practice of Pediatric Infectious Diseases, Churchill Livingstone, Philadelphia, 2002.

[124] M. Fernandez, M.E. Hickman, C.J. Baker, Antimicrobial susceptibilities of group B streptococci isolated between 1992 and 1996 from patients with bacteremia or meningitis, Antimicrob. Agents Chemother. 42 (1998) 1517–1519.

[125] D.J. Biedenbach, J.M. Stephen, R.N. Jones, Antimicrobial susceptibility profile among β-haemolytic *Streptococcus* spp. Collected in SENTRY antimicrobial surveillance program—North America, 2001, Diagn. Microbiol. Infect. Dis. 46 (2003) 291–294.

[126] R.J. Whitley, et al., Ganciclovir treatment of symptomatic congenital cytomegalovirus infection: results of a phase II study. National Institute of Allergy and Infectious Diseases Collaborative Antiviral Study Group, J. Infect. Dis. 175 (1997) 1080–1086.

[127] D.W. Kimberlin, et al., Effect of ganciclovir therapy on hearing in symptomatic congenital cytomegalovirus disease involving the central nervous system: a randomized, controlled trial, J. Pediatr. 98 (2003) 16–25.

[128] American Academy of Pediatrics Committee on Infectious Diseases, Universal hepatitis B immunization, Pediatrics 89 (1992) 795–800.

[129] K.M. Boyer, et al., Selective intrapartum chemoprophylaxis of neonatal group B streptococcal early-onset disease. I. Epidemiologic rationale, J. Infect. Dis. 148 (1983) 795–801.

[130] American Academy of Pediatrics Committee on Infectious Diseases and Committee on Fetus and Newborn, Guidelines for prevention of group B streptococcal (GBS) infection by chemoprophylaxis, Pediatrics 90 (1992) 775–778.

[131] M.A. MacAulay, M. Abou-Sabe, D. Charles, Placental transfer of ampicillin, Am. J. Obstet. Gynecol. 96 (1966) 943–950.

[132] S.E. Moisiuk, et al., Outbreak of parainfluenza virus type 3 in an intermediate care neonatal nursery, Pediatr. Infect. Dis. J. 17 (1998) 49–53.

[133] B.S. Brozanski, et al., Effect of a screening-based prevention policy on prevalence of early-onset group B streptococcal sepsis, Obstet. Gynecol. 95 (2000) 496–501.

[134] M.A. Knittle, D.V. Eitzman, H. Baer, Role of hand contamination of personnel in the epidemiology of gram-negative nosocomial infections, J. Pediatr. 86 (1975) 433–437.

[135] M. Nagamine, et al., DNA amplification of human T lymphotropic virus type I (HTLV-I) proviral DNA in breast milk of HTLV-I carriers. Letter to the editor, J. Infect. Dis. 164 (1991) 1024–1025.

[136] W. Heneine, et al., Detection of HTLV-II in breastmilk of HTLV-II infected mothers. Letter to the editor, Lancet 340 (1992) 1157–1158.

[137] D.T. Dunn, et al., Risk of human immunodeficiency virus type 1 transmission through breastfeeding (see comments), Lancet 340 (1992) 585–588.

[138] World Health Organization, Breast feeding/breast milk and human immunodeficiency virus (HIV), Wkly. Epidemiol. Rec. 33 (1987) 245.

[139] American Academy of Pediatrics Work Group on Breastfeeding, Breastfeeding and the use of human milk, Pediatrics 100 (1997) 1035–1039.

[140] L.K. Altman, AIDS brings a shift on breast-feeding, in: The New York Times, 1998, pp 1 and 6.

[141] M. Svabic-Vlahovic, et al., Transmission of *Listeria monocytogenes* from mother's milk to her baby and to puppies. Letter to the editor, Lancet 2 (1988) 1201.

[142] J.O. Klein, From harmless commensal to invasive pathogen—coagulase-negative staphylococci, N. Engl. J. Med. 323 (1990) 339–340.

[143] J. Brown, et al., High rate of hand contamination and low rate of hand washing before infant contact in a neonatal intensive care unit, Pediatr. Infect. Dis. J. 15 (1996) 908–910.

[144] L.L. Liu, et al., The safety of newborn early discharge: the Washington State experience, JAMA 278 (1997) 293–298.

NEONATAL INFECTIONS: A GLOBAL PERSPECTIVE

Gary L. Darmstadt ✪ Anita K. M. Zaidi ✪ Barbara J. Stoll

CHAPTER OUTLINE

Global Burden of Neonatal Infections   24
    Infection as a Cause of Neonatal Death   24
    Incidence of Neonatal Sepsis, Bacteremia, and Meningitis and
        Associated Mortality   25
    Bacterial Pathogens Associated with Infections in Different
        Geographic Regions   26
    Incidence of Group B Streptococcal Colonization and Infection   27
    Antimicrobial Resistance in Neonatal Pathogens   28
    Nosocomial Infections   28
    Hospital Infection Control   28
Neonatal Infections   29
    Acute Respiratory Infections   29
    Diarrhea   30
    Omphalitis   30
    Tetanus   31
    Ophthalmia Neonatorum   32
    Human Immunodeficiency Virus Infection   33

    Tuberculosis   35
    Malaria   37
Indirect Causes of Neonatal Death Related to Infection   39
Strategies to Prevent and Treat Infection in Neonates   39
    Maternal Immunization to Prevent Neonatal Disease   40
    Neonatal Immunization   41
    Antenatal Care and Prevention of Neonatal Infection   41
    Intrapartum and Delivery Care and Prevention of Neonatal
        Infection   42
    Postnatal Care and Prevention of Neonatal Infection   42
    Breast-Feeding   42
    Management of Neonatal Infection   43
    Identification of Neonates with Infection   43
    Antibiotic Treatment of Neonates with Infection   43
    Integrated Management of Neonatal Illness   44
    Maternal Education and Socioeconomic Status   45
Conclusion   45

One of the greatest challenges in global public health is to eliminate the gaps between high-income and low-income countries in health care resources, access to preventive and curative services, and health status outcomes. Although child and infant mortality burden has declined substantially in recent decades [1,2], neonatal mortality, especially deaths in the first week of life, has changed relatively little [3]. Worldwide, an estimated 3.8 million neonatal deaths occur annually, accounting for 41% of deaths in children younger than age 5 years [4]. Of these deaths, 99% occur in low-income and middle-income countries [3], in the context of poverty, high-risk newborn care practices, poor care seeking and access to quality care, and poorly functioning health systems. Causes of neonatal mortality, especially in low-income countries, are difficult to ascertain, partly because many of these deaths occur at home, unattended by medical personnel, in settings without vital registration systems, and partly because critically ill neonates often present with nondiagnostic signs and symptoms of disease.

Serious infections, intrapartum-related neonatal deaths (i.e., "birth asphyxia") [5], and complications of prematurity are the major direct causes of neonatal death worldwide [3]. Malnutrition and low birth weight (LBW) underlie most of these deaths [6]. Globally, serious neonatal infections cause an estimated 36% of neonatal deaths [3]. In settings with very high mortality (neonatal mortality rate >45 per 1000 live births), neonatal infections are estimated to cause 40% to 50% of all neonatal deaths [3,7]. Neonatal mortality related to infection could

be substantially reduced by simple, known preventive interventions before and during pregnancy, labor, and delivery, and by preventive and curative interventions in the immediate postnatal period and in the early days of life [8–12]. This chapter reviews the global burden of infectious diseases in the newborn, direct and indirect causes of neonatal mortality attributed to infection, specific infections of relevance in low-income and middle-income countries, and strategies to reduce the incidence of neonatal infection and morbidity and mortality in infants who do become infected.

GLOBAL BURDEN OF NEONATAL INFECTIONS

INFECTION AS A CAUSE OF NEONATAL DEATH

Most infectious-related neonatal deaths are due to bacterial sepsis and meningitis, respiratory infection, neonatal tetanus, diarrhea, and omphalitis. Neonatal deaths caused by infection may occur early in the neonatal period, in the first 7 days of life, and are usually attributable to infection acquired during the peripartum process. Late neonatal deaths, occurring from 8 to 28 days of life, are most commonly due to acquisition of pathogens from the environment in which the vulnerable newborn is placed.

In low-income and middle-income countries, because most births and neonatal deaths occur at home and are not attended by medical personnel, deaths are underreported, and information on cause of death is often incomplete. Very few published studies worldwide present detailed surveillance data on numbers of births and neonatal deaths and on probable causes of death. Although hospital-based studies are important for accurately determining causes of morbidity and mortality, they may not reflect what is happening in the community, and because of selection bias, they may not be representative of the population. One review summarized 32 community-based studies that were published during 1990-2007 [13]. Infection-specific mortality was found to range from 2.7 per 1000 live births in South Africa to 38.6 per 1000 live births in Somalia. Overall, 8% to 80% (median 36.5%, interquartile range 26% to 49%) of all neonatal deaths in developing countries were found to be attributable to infections [13]. Significant data gaps exist, however, especially from countries with low resources. There is a need for carefully conducted population-based studies that assess the number and causes of neonatal deaths in low-income and middle-income countries.

In the absence of better data, global estimates for causes of neonatal deaths have been derived through statistical modeling, extrapolating from evidence available from several countries at different levels of development and neonatal mortality rates [14]. According to these estimates, infections are the largest cause of neonatal mortality, accounting for 36% of all neonatal deaths; sepsis, pneumonia, and meningitis together account for 26% of neonatal deaths, whereas tetanus and diarrhea account for 7% and 3% [3]. This translates to 1.4 million neonatal deaths from infections, most of which can be averted with appropriate prevention and management [8,15].

INCIDENCE OF NEONATAL SEPSIS, BACTEREMIA, AND MENINGITIS AND ASSOCIATED MORTALITY

Hospital and community-based studies from low-income and middle-income countries were reviewed to determine the incidence of neonatal sepsis, bacteremia, and meningitis; the case-fatality rates (CFRs) associated with these infections; and the spectrum of bacterial pathogens in different regions of the world. Cases reported occurred among infants born in hospitals or homes, and infants referred from home or other health facilities. Investigators reviewed 77 studies from low-income and middle-income countries [16–91] published during 1980-2009 to evaluate neonatal sepsis and meningitis in different

geographic regions. Of these studies, 62 were primarily reports of neonatal sepsis, and 18 presented data on bacterial meningitis. Most studies did not distinguish among maternally acquired, community-acquired, and nosocomial infections. Table 2–1 summarizes data by region.

In all regions, clinically suspected sepsis was responsible for a substantial burden of disease, with high CFRs reported in most studies. Overall, incidence of clinical neonatal sepsis ranged from 2 to 29.8 per 1000 live births. A carefully conducted population-based surveillance study from Mirzapur, a rural part of Bangladesh, attempted to capture all births and all cases of sepsis in a well-defined population through active, household-level surveillance [41]. The incidence of clinically suspected neonatal infection was approximately 50 per 1000 live births [41]. Reported CFRs for neonatal sepsis in the above-mentioned reviewed studies [16–91] ranged from 1% to 69%. Only six studies reported CFRs less than 10%, whereas most of the studies reported sepsis-associated CFRs greater than 30%.

Information on incidence rates of neonatal bacteremia (sepsis confirmed by isolation of bacteria from the blood) from developing countries is extremely limited. Berkley and associates [30] reported a bacteremia rate of 5.5 per 1000 live births in rural Kenya, which is most likely an underestimate because only infants presenting to their referral hospital from the surrounding catchment area were included, and no active case-finding through community surveillance was conducted. In Mirzapur, Bangladesh, active population-based, household-level newborn illness surveillance detected an incidence rate of bacteremia of 3 per 1000 person-neonatal periods [41], a rate that is comparable with incidence of early-onset neonatal sepsis reported in the United States and incidence of neonatal sepsis reported in Israel [51,92,93].

Fewer studies on neonatal meningitis were available to evaluate incidence and CFRs by region. The incidence of neonatal meningitis ranged from 0.33 to 7.3 per 1000 live births (average 1 per 1000 live births), with CFRs ranging from 13% to 59%.

Using these hospital and community-based rates and estimates from the United Nations of approximately 122,266,000 births per year in the low-income and middle-income countries of the world [94], we estimate that 245,000 to 3,668,000 cases of neonatal sepsis and 40,000 to 900,000 cases of neonatal meningitis occur in developing countries each year. The range is large because of the imprecision of available data.

TABLE 2–1 Incidence and Case-Fatality Rate (CFR) for Sepsis and Meningitis from Hospital and Community-Based Studies in Low-Income and Middle-Income Countries

Region	Incidence of Sepsis (Cases per 1000 Live Births)	CFR (%)	Incidence of Meningitis (Cases per 1000 Live Births)	CFR (%)
India/Pakistan/Southeast Asia/Pacific	2.4-29.8	2-69	0.63-7.3	45
Sub-Saharan Africa	6-22.9	27-56	0.7-1.9	18-59
Middle East/North Africa	1.8-12	13-45	0.33-1.5	16-32
Americas/Caribbean	2-9	1-31	0.4-2.8	13-35

Data updated from Stoll BJ. The global impact of neonatal infection. Clin Perinatol 24:1, 1997.

BACTERIAL PATHOGENS ASSOCIATED WITH INFECTIONS IN DIFFERENT GEOGRAPHIC REGIONS

Historical reviews from developed countries have shown that the predominant organisms responsible for neonatal infections change over time [95,96]. Prospective microbiologic surveillance is important to guide empirical therapy and to identify potential targets for vaccine development, to identify new agents of importance for neonates, to recognize epidemics, and to monitor changes over time. The organisms associated with neonatal infection are different in different geographic areas, reinforcing the need for local microbiologic surveillance. In areas where blood cultures in sick neonates cannot be performed, knowledge of the bacterial flora of the maternal genital tract may serve as a surrogate marker for organisms causing early-onset neonatal sepsis, meningitis, and pneumonia. Most studies on the causes of neonatal sepsis and meningitis are hospital reviews that include data on infants born in hospitals and infants transferred from home or other facilities.

A more recent review highlighted the scarcity of data on pathogens associated with neonatal sepsis and meningitis in low-income and middle-income countries [97]. This review found 63 studies published during 1980-2007 that reported etiologic data from low-income and middle-income countries [97]. The review also included findings from the Young Infant Clinical Signs Studies and community-based data from Karachi. Only 12 of these studies focused on community-acquired infections. In most of the remaining studies, it was difficult to determine whether infections were of maternal origin or were hospital-acquired or community-acquired. Because of insufficient information provided, assumptions of community-acquired infections were made if this was implied by the study setting. The possible inclusion of some nosocomial infections cannot be ruled out. Also, the infants' ages at the time of infection were not always specified. The studies varied in the detail with which culture methods were presented.

Table 2–2 gives further details about the distribution of organisms by geographic region. The review found 19 studies that reported etiologic data for the entire neonatal period. In the aggregated data of these studies, the ratio of gram-negative to gram-positive organisms was 1.6:1, and *Staphylococcus aureus*, *Escherichia coli*, and *Klebsiella* species collectively caused almost half of all infections. This pattern was consistent across all regions except Africa, where gram-positive organisms were predominant owing to higher frequency of *S. aureus*, *Streptococcus pneumoniae*, and *Streptococcus pyogenes*.

The etiology of early-onset neonatal sepsis in low-income and middle-income countries was presented in 44 facility-based studies. One fourth of all episodes of

TABLE 2–2   Etiology of Community-Acquired Neonatal Sepsis in Low-Income and Middle-Income Countries by Region

Organism Isolated	Africa		East Asia and Pacific		Middle East and Central Asia		South Asia		All Regions	
	No.	%	No.	%	No.	%	No.	%	No.	%
Total	1058	100	915	100	256	100	365	100	2594	100
Staphylococcus aureus	112	10.6	146	16.0	51	19.9	36	9.9	345	13.3
Streptococcus pyogenes	71	6.7	8	0.9	2	0.8	3	0.8	84	3.2
Group B streptococci	161	15.2	2	0.2	20	7.8	26	7.1	209	8.1
Group D streptococci or *Enterococcus*	4	0.4	—	—	13	5.1	22	6.0	39	1.5
Group G streptococci	1	0.1	1	0.1	—	—	—	—	2	0.1
Streptococcus pneumoniae	129	12.2	4	0.4	7	2.7	7	1.9	147	5.7
Other *Streptococcus* species or unspecified	3	0.3	40	4.4	1	0.4	43	11.8	87	3.4
Other gram-positive organisms	72	6.8	—	—	—	—	2	0.6	74	2.9
All gram-positive organisms	553	52.3	201	22.0	94	36.7	139	38.1	987	38.1
Klebsiella species	82	7.8	134	14.6	49	19.1	85	23.3	350	13.5
Escherichia coli	94	8.9	237	26.0	68	26.6	44	12.1	443	17.1
Pseudomonas species	7	0.7	134	14.6	8	3.1	37	10.1	186	7.2
Enterobacter species	3	0.3	52	5.7	8	3.1	15	4.1	78	3.0
Serratia species	—	—	39	4.3	2	0.8	—	—	41	1.6
Proteus species	5	0.5	—	—	7	2.7	1	0.3	13	0.5
Salmonella species	118	11.2	4	0.4	—	—	2	0.6	124	4.8
Citrobacter species	—	—	—	—	—	—	4	1.1	4	0.2
Haemophilus influenzae	12	1.1	1	0.1	2	0.8	1	0.3	16	0.6
Neisseria meningitidis	11	1.0	—	—	3	1.2	—	—	14	0.5
Acinetobacter species	—	—	94	10.3	2	0.8	13	3.6	109	4.2
Other gram-negative organisms	132	12.5	19	2.1	1	0.4	20	5.5	172	6.6
All gram-negative organisms	464	43.9	714	78.0	150	58.6	222	60.8	1550	59.8
Other organisms	41	3.9	—	—	12	4.7	4	1.1	57	2.2

Adapted from Zaidi AK, et al. Pediatr Infect Dis J 28(1 Suppl):S10-S18, 2009.

early-onset neonatal sepsis were caused by *Klebsiella* species, 15% were caused by *E. coli*, 18% were caused by *S. aureus*, 7% were caused by group B streptococci (GBS), and 12% were caused collectively by *Acinetobacter* species and *Pseudomonas* species The overall ratio of gram-negative organisms to gram-positive organisms was 2:1. In African countries, the ratio of gram-positive organisms to gram-negative organisms was equal, however, with a larger proportion of infections caused by *S. aureus* and GBS. *Pseudomonas* species and *Acinetobacter* species were found to be more common in East Asia, Pacific, and South Asian countries. *S. aureus* was uncommon in East Asia and Latin America compared with other regions.

The review also found 11 studies that reported etiologic data on community-acquired infections occurring between 7 and 59 days of life. Almost half of the isolates in this age group were from the large World Health Organization (WHO)–sponsored multicenter Young Infant Study conducted in the early 1990s in four developing countries: Ethiopia, The Gambia, Papua New Guinea, and the Philippines [71,98-104]. The ratio of gram-negative to gram-positive organisms in this group was 0.8:1, with higher proportions of *Salmonella* species, *Haemophilus influenzae*, *S. pneumoniae*, and *S. pyogenes* compared with the first week of life [97].

Although data are limited, studies involving home-delivered infants or infants from maternity hospitals and rural referral hospitals found gram-negative organisms to be more than three times as common as gram-positive organisms (ratio of 3:1 among home births, 3.5:1 among rural referral hospitals) [97]. Three gram-negative bacteria (*E. coli*, *Klebsiella* species, and *Pseudomonas* species) accounted for 43% to 64% of all infections, and gram-positive *S. aureus* accounted for 8% to 21% of all infections. Among infants born at home, gram-negative organisms were responsible for 77% of all neonatal infections. In Mirzapur, Bangladesh, among home-born newborns identified through population-based household surveillance, half of all culture-proven episodes of suspected sepsis were due to gram-negative organisms, including *Klebsiella* species, *Pseudomonas* species, *Acinetobacter* species, and *Enterobacter* species. Among gram-positive cultures, *S. aureus* was the most common isolate, responsible for one third of all positive cultures [41].

INCIDENCE OF GROUP B STREPTOCOCCAL COLONIZATION AND INFECTION

The spectrum of organisms presented in this review differs from what is known from developed countries. Although GBS remains the most important bacterial pathogen associated with early-onset neonatal sepsis and meningitis in many developed countries (especially among term infants) [105], studies from developing countries present a different picture. The most striking finding in the review was the significantly lower rates of GBS sepsis in South Asia, Central Asia, East Asia, Middle East, and the Pacific, in contrast to the relatively high rate reported from Africa (Table 2–2).

It is unclear why neonates in many low-income and middle-income countries are rarely infected with GBS.

The most important risk factor for invasive GBS disease in the neonate is exposure to the organism via the mother's genital tract. Other known risk factors include young maternal age, preterm birth, prolonged rupture of the membranes, maternal chorioamnionitis, exposure to a high inoculum of a virulent GBS strain, and a low maternal serum concentration of antibody to the capsular polysaccharide of the colonizing GBS strain [106]. In the United States, differences in GBS colonization rates have been identified among women of different ethnic groups that seem to correlate with infection in newborns.

In an attempt to understand the low rates of invasive GBS disease reported among neonates in many low-income and middle-income countries, Stoll and Schuchat [107] reviewed 34 studies published during 1980-1998 that evaluated GBS colonization rates in women. These studies reported culture results from 7730 women, with an overall colonization rate of 12.7%. Studies that used culture methods that were judged to be appropriate found significantly higher colonization rates than the studies that used inadequate methods (675 of 3801 women [17.8%] versus 308 of 3929 women [7.8%]). When analyses were restricted to studies with adequate methods, the prevalence of colonization by region was Middle East/North Africa, 22%; Asia/Pacific, 19%; sub-Saharan Africa, 19%; India/Pakistan, 12%; and Americas, 14%.

The distribution of GBS serotypes varied among studies. GBS serotype III, the most frequently identified invasive serotype in the West, was identified in all studies reviewed and was the most frequently identified serotype in one half of the studies. GBS serotype V, which has been recognized only more recently as a cause of invasive disease in developed countries [108], was identified in studies from Peru [109] and The Gambia [110]. Monitoring serotype distribution is important because candidate GBS vaccines are considered for areas with high rates of disease.

With estimated GBS colonization rates among women in low-income and middle-income countries of about 18%, higher rates of invasive neonatal disease than have been reported would be expected. Low rates of invasive GBS disease in some low-income and middle-income countries may be due to lower virulence of strains, genetic differences in susceptibility to disease, as-yet unidentified beneficial cultural practices, or high concentrations of transplacentally acquired protective antibody in serum (i.e., a mother may be colonized, but have protective concentrations of type-specific GBS antibody).

In low-income and middle-income countries, where most deliveries occur at home, infants with early-onset sepsis often get sick and die at home or are taken to local health care facilities, where a diagnosis of possible sepsis may be missed, or where blood cultures cannot be performed. In these settings, there may be underdiagnosis of infection by early-onset pathogens, including GBS. In the WHO Young Infants Study [98], 1673 infants were evaluated in the first month of life; only 2 had cultures positive for GBS. The absence of GBS in this study cannot be explained by the evaluation of insufficient numbers of sick neonates (360 of the 1673 infants were <1 week of age).

Increasing evidence suggests that heavy colonization with GBS increases the risk of delivering a preterm infant with LBW [111]. Population differences in the prevalence of heavy GBS colonization have been reported in the United States, where African Americans have a significantly higher risk of heavy colonization. If heavy colonization is more prevalent among women in low-income and middle-income countries and results in an increase in numbers of preterm infants with LBW, GBS-related morbidity may appear as illness and death related to prematurity. By contrast, heavy colonization could increase maternal type-specific GBS antibody concentrations, resulting in lower risk of neonatal disease. Further studies in low-income and middle-income countries are needed to explore these important issues.

ANTIMICROBIAL RESISTANCE IN NEONATAL PATHOGENS

Increasing rates of resistance to antimicrobial agents among common pathogens involved in neonatal infections are being observed in low-income and middle-income countries [112]. Very limited published information is available, however, on antimicrobial resistance patterns among neonatal pathogens from community settings where a large proportion of births take place at home. A review identified only 10 studies during 1990-2007, including 2 unpublished, that contributed resistance data from community settings in low-income and middle-income countries, primarily regarding *Klebsiella* species, *E. coli*, and *S. aureus* [112]. Compared with data from hospital settings, resistance rates were lower in community-acquired infections. Greater than 70% of isolates of *E. coli* were resistant to ampicillin, and 13% were resistant to gentamicin. All *Klebsiella* species were resistant to ampicillin, and 60% were resistant to gentamicin [112]. Resistance to third-generation cephalosporins was uncommon, and methicillin-resistant *S. aureus* occurred rarely [112]. Additional data on antimicrobial resistance patterns of neonatal pathogens encountered in home-delivered infants are needed to develop evidence-based guidelines for management.

By contrast, a wealth of data from hospitals from low-income and middle-income countries show alarming antimicrobial resistance rates among neonatal pathogens in hospital nurseries. A large review showed that more than 70% of neonatal isolates from hospitals of low-income and middle-income countries were resistant to ampicillin and gentamicin—the recommended regimen for the management of neonatal sepsis [113,114]. Resistance was also documented against expensive second-line and third-line agents; 46% of *E. coli* and 51% of *Klebsiella* species were found to be resistant to the third-generation cephalosporin, cefotaxime [114]. Equally disturbing was the high prevalence of methicillin-resistant *S. aureus* isolates, especially in South Asia, where it constituted 56% of all isolates [114]. Also, pan-resistant *Acinetobacter* species infections are widely reported [115,116]. In these settings with constrained resources, many of these multidrug-resistant pathogens are untreatable.

NOSOCOMIAL INFECTIONS

Hospitals in low-income and middle-income countries are ill-equipped to provide hygienic care to vulnerable newborn infants. A review of the rates of neonatal infections among hospital-born infants in low-income and middle-income countries found the rates to be 3 to 20 times higher than observed in industrialized countries [114]. A high proportion of infections in the early neonatal period were due to *Klebsiella* species, *Pseudomonas* species, and *S. aureus*, rather than organisms typically associated with the maternal birth canal, suggesting acquisition from the hospital environmental, rather than the mother [114]. Overall, gram-negative rods were found to be predominant, constituting 60% of all positive cultures from newborns. *Klebsiella* species were found to be the major pathogens, present in 23% of cases, followed by *S. aureus* (16.3%) and *E. coli* (12.2%) [114].

High nosocomial infection rates observed among hospital-born infants in low-income and middle-income countries are attributable to lack of aseptic delivery and hand hygiene; lack of essential supplies such as running water, soap, and gloves; equipment shortages; lack of sterilization facilities; lack of knowledge and training regarding adequate sterilization; overcrowded and understaffed health facilities, and inappropriate and prolonged use of antibiotics [114].

HOSPITAL INFECTION CONTROL

Lack of attention to infection control increases the newborn's risk of acquiring a nosocomial pathogen from the hospital environment [114]. Urgent attention to improving infection control practices in hospitals that care for mothers and newborns is required if survival gains from promoting institutional delivery are to be fully realized. Several cost-effective strategies to reduce infection transmission in hospitals of low-income and middle-income countries have been discussed in a review of hospital-acquired neonatal infections [114].

Hand hygiene remains the most important infection control practice. In many low-income and middle-income countries, hospital delivery wards and nurseries lack sinks and running water, however. For such settings, alcohol-based hand rubs are an attractive option. Several studies have shown the efficacy of use of hand rubs by hospital staff in reducing rates of colonization and infection among neonates [117,118]. Although commercially available alcohol-based hand gels are expensive, costs may be offset by significant reduction in nosocomial infections. Also, low-cost solutions can be prepared by hospital pharmacies by combining 20 mL of glycerine, sorbitol, glycol, or propylene with 980 mL of greater than 70% isopropanol [114]. Addition of 0.5% chlorhexidine prolongs the bactericidal effect, but increases expense [114].

Aseptic technique during intrapartum care for the mother and sterile cord cutting are other important areas of intervention. Reducing the number of vaginal examinations reduces the risk of chorioamnionitis. A systematic review of the use of vaginal chlorhexidine treatment included two large, nonrandomized, nonblinded hospital-based trials from Malawi and Egypt that reported neonatal outcomes [119–121]. Both trials found that the use of 0.25% chlorhexidine wipes during vaginal examinations and application of another wipe for the neonate soon after birth significantly reduced early neonatal deaths (in Egypt, 2.8% versus 4.2% in intervention versus control groups, $P = .01$) and neonatal mortality caused by infections (in Malawi, odds ratio 0.5, 95% confidence interval [CI] 0.29-0.88; in Egypt, 0.22% versus 0.84% in intervention versus control groups, $P = .004$) [122,123]. A hospital-based trial from South Africa found no impact, however, of maternal vaginal and newborn skin cleansing with chlorhexidine on rates of neonatal sepsis or the vertical acquisition of potentially pathogenic bacteria among neonates [124].

Topical application of emollients that serve to augment the barrier for invasion of pathogenic microbes through immature skin of premature infants has also shown promise. Daily applications of sunflower seed oil in very premature infants hospitalized in Bangladesh and Egypt have been shown to reduce nosocomial infections and mortality [125–127].

Appropriate measures are also needed to address infection transmission that may occur through reuse of critical items that come into contact with sterile body sites, mucous membranes, or broken skin. Improper sterilization and defective reprocessing of these items has been associated with higher rates of *Pseudomonas* infections in a study from Indonesia [128]. A study from Mexico identified several faults in the reprocessing chain, such as inadequate monitoring of sterilization standards and use of inappropriate sterilization agents [129].

Fluid reservoirs such as those used in suctioning and respiratory care can also be a source of infection in critical care areas. Targeted respiratory tract care with focused education campaigns has been found to be effective in reducing infection rates in developing countries [130]. In the face of outbreaks, point sources of contamination, such as intravenous fluids and medications, must be investigated and eliminated. Systematic reviews have found no evidence of the benefit of routine gowning by health personnel or infant attendants in hospital nurseries [131].

Several studies have also examined the impact of "bundled" or packaged interventions in controlling hospital-acquired infections among children in developing countries. These packages include several infection control interventions such as use of alcohol-based hand rubs, bedside checklists to monitor adequate infection control practices, appropriate antibiotic use policies, simple algorithms for effective treatment of neonatal sepsis, decreasing the degree of crowding in wards, increase in the number of infection control nurses, and establishing guidelines for appropriate handling of intravenous catheters and solutions. Although the results from these studies have varied in the degree of success, they all have reported decreases in nosocomial infections through implementation of such interventions [132].

NEONATAL INFECTIONS
ACUTE RESPIRATORY INFECTIONS

Onset of pneumonia in neonates may be early (acquired during birth from organisms that colonize or infect the maternal genital tract) or late (acquired later from organisms in the hospital, home, or community). Although only a few studies of the bacteriology of neonatal pneumonia have been performed, the findings suggest that organisms causing disease are similar to organisms that cause neonatal sepsis [133,134]. The role of viruses in neonatal pneumonia, especially in low-income and middle-income countries, is unclear. More recent studies from developed countries suggest that viruses, including respiratory syncytial virus, parainfluenza viruses, adenoviruses, and influenza viruses, contribute to respiratory morbidity and mortality, especially during epidemic periods [135,136]. Maternal influenza vaccination during pregnancy in Bangladesh reduced febrile respiratory illnesses in their young infants by one third compared with infants of mothers not receiving influenza vaccine, suggesting an important role for influenza viruses in neonatal acute respiratory infections (ARIs) [137].

Because of similarities in presentation, pneumonia in neonates is very difficult to differentiate from neonatal sepsis or meningitis, and all three diseases are often grouped under one category and treated similarly. Assessing the true burden of neonatal respiratory infections is very difficult. In a review of the magnitude of mortality from ARI in low-income and middle-income countries, Garenne and coworkers [138] estimated that 21% of all ARI deaths in children younger than 5 years occur in the neonatal period (1254 of 6041 ARI deaths in 12 countries). In a carefully conducted community-based study in rural India published in 1993, Bang and associates [139] determined that 66% of ARI deaths in the first year of life occurred in the neonatal period.

It is difficult to determine the incidence of neonatal ARIs in low-income and middle-income countries because many sick neonates are never referred for medical care. In a large community-based study of ARIs in Bangladeshi children, the highest incidence of ARIs was in children younger than 5 months of age [137]. In the study by Bang and associates [139], there were 64 cases of pneumonia among 3100 children (incidence of 21 per 1000), but this finding underestimates the true incidence because it was known that many neonates were never brought for care. A community-based study conducted by English and colleagues [47] in Kenya found the incidence of pneumonia to be 81 per 1000 for children younger than 2 months. The risk of pneumonia and of ARI-related death increases in infants who have LBW or are malnourished and in infants who are not breast-fed [140,141]. In a study of infants with LBW in India [142] in which infants were visited weekly and mothers queried about disease, there were 61 episodes of moderate to severe ARI among 211 infants with LBW and 125 episodes among 448 infants with normal birth weight. Although 33% of episodes of ARI occurred in infants with LBW, 79% of the deaths occurred in this weight group.

Management of pneumonia in neonates follows the same principles as management of neonatal sepsis because the presentation is difficult to distinguish clinically from sepsis. A respiratory rate greater than 60/min in an infant younger than 2 months has been proposed as a sensitive sign of serious illness and possible pneumonia by WHO, but concerns about low specificity secondary to conditions such as transient tachypnea of the newborn and upper respiratory infections remain to be addressed [143].

DIARRHEA

Although diarrheal diseases are important killers of infants younger than 1 year, most deaths resulting from diarrhea during infancy occur in infants 6 to 12 months old [144,145]. Worldwide, only 3% of deaths in the neonatal period are attributed to diarrhea [3]. The high prevalence of breast-feeding in the first month of life in low-income and middle-income countries most likely protects breast-fed newborns from diarrhea [146,147].

Huilan and associates [148] studied the agents associated with diarrhea in children from birth to 35 months of age from five hospitals in China, India, Mexico, Myanmar, and Pakistan. The investigators studied 3640 cases of diarrhea, 28% of which occurred in infants younger than 6 months. Data on the detection of rotavirus, enterotoxigenic *E. coli*, and *Campylobacter* species were provided by age. Of these agents, 5% of isolates (17 of 323) were from neonates. Some studies report high diarrhea rates in the neonatal period, however. Black and colleagues [149] performed community studies of diarrheal epidemiology and etiology in a periurban community in Peru. The incidence of diarrhea was 9.8 episodes per child in the first year of life and did not differ significantly by month of age (0.64 to 1 episode per child-month). Mahmud and colleagues [150] prospectively followed a cohort of 1476 Pakistani newborns from four different communities. Of infants evaluated in the first month of life, 18% (180 of 1028) had diarrhea.

Although most infants in low-income and middle-income countries are born at home, infants born in hospitals are at risk for nosocomial diarrheal infections. Aye and coworkers [151] studied diarrheal morbidity in neonates born at the largest maternity hospital in Rangoon, Myanmar. Diarrhea was a significant problem, with rates of 7 cases per 1000 live births for infants born vaginally and 50 per 1000 for infants delivered by cesarean section. The difference in diarrhea rates was attributed to the following: Infants born by cesarean section remained hospitalized longer, were handled more by staff members and less by their own mothers, and were less likely to be exclusively breast-fed.

Rotavirus is one of the most important causes of diarrhea among infants and children worldwide, occurring most commonly in infants 3 months to 2 years. In low-income and middle-income countries, most rotavirus infections occur early in infancy [152,153]. There are few reports of rotavirus diarrhea in newborns [154]. In most cases, neonatal infection seems to be asymptomatic, and neonatal infection may protect against severe diarrhea in subsequent infections [155–157]. Neonates are generally infected with unusual rotavirus strains that may be less virulent and may serve as natural immunogens [158]. Exposure to the asymptomatic rotavirus I321 strain in particular has been shown to confer protection against symptomatic diarrheal episodes caused by rotavirus among neonates [159].

Infection among neonates may be more common, however, than was previously thought. Cicirello and associates [158] screened 169 newborns at six hospitals in Delhi, India, and found a rotavirus prevalence of 26%. Prevalence increased directly with length of hospital stay.

More recently, Ramani and colleagues [160] found the prevalence of rotavirus among neonates with gastrointestinal symptoms to be 55% in a tertiary hospital in south India. The high prevalence of neonatal infections in India (and perhaps in other countries with low resources) could lead to priming of the immune system and have implications for vaccine efficacy. Several community-based studies reviewed earlier presented data on diarrhea as a cause of neonatal death [161–170]. In these studies, diarrhea was responsible for 1% to 12% of all neonatal deaths. In 9 of the 10 studies, 70 of 2673 neonatal deaths (3%) were attributed to diarrhea. Although diarrhea is more common in infants after 6 months of age, it is a problem in terms of morbidity and mortality for neonates in low-income and middle-income countries.

OMPHALITIS

In low-income and middle-income countries, aseptic delivery techniques and hygienic cord care have markedly decreased the occurrence of omphalitis, or umbilical infection. Prompt diagnosis and antimicrobial therapy have decreased morbidity and mortality in cases of omphalitis. Omphalitis continues to be an important problem, however, where clean delivery and hygienic cord care practices remain a challenge, particularly among the world's 60 million home births, which account for nearly half of all births, and for many facility-based births in settings with low resources [171,172]. The necrotic tissue of the umbilical cord is an excellent medium for bacterial growth. The umbilical stump is rapidly colonized by bacteria from the maternal genital tract and from the environment. This colonized necrotic tissue, in close proximity to umbilical vessels, provides microbial pathogens with direct access to the bloodstream. Invasion of pathogens via the umbilicus may occur with or without the presence of signs of omphalitis, such as redness, pus discharge, swelling, or foul odor [173,174].

Omphalitis is associated with increased risk of mortality [175]. Omphalitis may remain a localized infection or may spread to the abdominal wall, the peritoneum, the umbilical or portal vessels, or the liver. Infants who present with abdominal wall cellulitis or necrotizing fasciitis have a high incidence of associated bacteremia (often polymicrobial) and a high mortality rate [172,176,177].

Limited data are available on risk factors and incidence of umbilical infections from low-income and middle-income countries, especially from community settings [169,171,178–183]. Overall, incidence of omphalitis in hospital-based studies has ranged from 2 to 77 per 1000 hospital-born infants, with CFR ranging from 0% to 15%. Mullany and colleagues [174] defined clinical algorithms for identification of umbilical infections and reported a 15% incidence of mild omphalitis, defined as the presence of moderate redness (<2 cm extension of redness onto the abdominal skin at the base of the cord stump), and a 1% incidence of severe omphalitis, defined as severe redness with pus, among 15,123 newborn infants identified in rural Nepal through community-based household surveillance [173,178].

A key risk factor for development of omphalitis in the community included topical applications of potentially unclean substances (e.g., mustard oil). Hand washing with the soap in the clean delivery kit by the birth attendant before assisting with the delivery, consistent hand washing by the mother, and the practice of skin-to-skin care reduced the risk of omphalitis. In Pemba, Tanzania, 9550 cord assessments in 1653 infants identified an omphalitis rate of 1%, based on a definition of moderate to severe redness with pus discharge, to 12%, based on the presence of pus and foul odor [171].

Microbiologic data on causes of omphalitis are particularly lacking. Güvenç and associates [182] identified 88 newborns with omphalitis at a university hospital in eastern Turkey over a 2-year period. Gram-positive organisms were isolated from 68% of umbilical cultures, gram-negative organisms were isolated from 60%, and multiple organisms were cultured in 28% of patients. Airede [179] studied 33 Nigerian neonates with omphalitis. Aerobic bacteria were isolated from 70%, and anaerobic bacteria were isolated from 30%. Of the aerobic isolates, 60% were gram-positive organisms, and polymicrobial isolates were common. Faridi and colleagues [181] in India identified gram-negative organisms more frequently than gram-positive organisms (57% versus 43%), but *S. aureus* was the most frequent isolate (28%). In a study from Papua New Guinea, umbilical cultures were performed in 116 young infants with signs suggestive of omphalitis. The most frequently isolated organisms were group A β-hemolytic streptococci (44%), *S. aureus* (39%), *Klebsiella* species (17%), *E. coli* (17%), and *Proteus mirabilis* (16%) [102]. In infants with omphalitis and bacteremia, *S. aureus*, group A β-hemolytic streptococci, and *Klebsiella pneumoniae* were isolated from both sites. In Thailand, postdischarge follow-up cultures from 180 newborns yielded a positive culture in all cases, most commonly for *Klebsiella* species (60%), *E. coli* (37%), *Enterobacter* species (32%), and *S. aureus* [184]. In Oman, cultures from 207 newborns with signs of omphalitis yielded a positive culture in 191 cases; 57% were positive for *S. aureus*, 14% were positive for *E. coli*, and 10% were positive for *Klebsiella* species [185]. Community-based data on etiology of omphalitis in low-income and middle-income countries are lacking.

The method of caring for the umbilical cord after birth affects bacterial colonization, time to cord separation, and risk for infection and mortality [186–188]. Hygienic delivery and postnatal care practices, including hand washing and clean cord care, are important interventions to reduce risk of omphalitis and death [10,188]. Clean birth kits, which package together items such as a sterile blade, sterile cord tie, and soap, are promoted in many settings, especially for home births, although evidence for impact of birth kits on reducing rates of omphalitis and neonatal mortality is limited [189–194]. WHO currently recommends the practice of clean cord care, although it is acknowledged that antiseptics might benefit infants in settings where harmful substances are traditionally applied [195].

There is little evidence for optimal cord care practices to prevent cord infections and mortality in the community, although it is generally agreed that application of antimicrobial agents to the umbilical cord reduces bacterial colonization [188]. The effect of such agents on reducing infection is less clear [120,121,186,188]. During a study of pregnancy in a rural area of Papua New Guinea, Garner and colleagues [196] detected a high prevalence of neonatal fever and umbilical infection, which were associated with the subsequent development of neonatal sepsis. They designed an intervention program for umbilical cord care that included maternal health education and umbilical care packs containing acriflavine spirit and new razor blades. Neonatal sepsis was significantly less frequent in the intervention group.

More recently, Mullany and associates [173] showed a 75% reduction (95% CI 47% to 88%) in severe umbilical cord infections and a 24% reduction (95% CI −4% to 55%) in all-cause neonatal mortality in a large (*N* = 15,123) community-based trial of 4% chlorhexidine cord cleansing, applied once daily for 8 of the first 10 days of life, compared with dry cord care. In infants enrolled within the first 24 hours of life, mortality was significantly reduced by 34% (95% CI 5% to 54%) in the chlorhexidine cord cleansing group. In a third study arm, soap and water did not reduce infection or mortality risk compared with dry cord care. Chlorhexidine treatment delayed cord separation by about 1 day; however, this was not associated with increased risk of omphalitis [197]. Data are awaited from additional studies of the impact of chlorhexidine cord cleansing on neonatal mortality from Pakistan, Bangladesh, Zambia, and Tanzania.

TETANUS

Neonatal tetanus, caused by *Clostridium tetani*, is an underreported "silent" illness. Because it attacks newborns in the poorest countries of the world in the first few days of life, often while they are still confined to home, because it has a high and rapid CFR (85% untreated) [198], and because the newborns have poor access to medical care, the disease may go unrecognized [199–201]. The surveillance case definition of neonatal tetanus is straightforward—the ability of a newborn to suck at birth and for the first few days of life, followed by inability to suck starting between 3 and 10 days of age, spasms, stiffness, convulsions, and death [14].

Neonatal tetanus is a completely preventable disease. It can be prevented by immunizing the mother before or during pregnancy or by ensuring a clean delivery, clean cutting of the umbilical cord, and proper care of the cord in the days after birth [10]. Clean delivery practices have additional benefits, including prevention of other maternal and neonatal infections in addition to tetanus. Tetanus threatens mothers and infants, and tetanus-related mortality is a complication of induced abortion and childbirth in unimmunized women [202]. Immunization of women with at least three doses of tetanus toxoid vaccine provides complete prevention against maternal and neonatal tetanus.

The Maternal and Neonatal Tetanus Elimination Initiative of United Nations Children's Fund (UNICEF), WHO, United Nations Population Fund, and other partners, established in 1999, has led to the vaccination of more than 90 million women of childbearing age against tetanus, either through vaccination campaigns or during routine antenatal care visits. During 2000-2009,

14 countries and 15 states in India eliminated tetanus. In 2008, 81 million doses of tetanus vaccine were administered to mothers through routine antenatal care. An estimated 74% of women of childbearing age in developing countries are now adequately protected from tetanus, associated with marked and rapid declines in global deaths attributed to tetanus, from an estimated 787,000 in 1988 to 215,000 in 1999 and 128,000 in 2004 [203]. Progress continues, although the elimination of maternal and neonatal tetanus remains a global goal.

OPHTHALMIA NEONATORUM

Ophthalmia neonatorum, defined as purulent conjunctivitis in the first 28 days of life, remains a common problem in many low-income and middle-income countries. The risk of infection in the neonate is directly related to the prevalence of maternal infection and the frequency of ocular prophylaxis. Infants born in areas of the world with high rates of sexually transmitted diseases (STDs) are at greatest risk.

Data on incidence and bacteriologic spectrum from specific countries are limited. Although a wide array of agents are cultured from infants with ophthalmia neonatorum [204–206], *Neisseria gonorrhoeae* (the gonococcus) and *Chlamydia trachomatis* are the most important etiologic agents from a global perspective [205,207–212] and share similar mechanisms of pathogenesis. Infection is acquired from an infected mother during passage through the birth canal or through an ascending route. Infection caused by one agent cannot be distinguished from infection caused by another agent by clinical examination; both produce a purulent conjunctivitis. Gonococcal ophthalmia may appear earlier, however, and is typically more severe than chlamydial conjunctivitis. Untreated gonococcal conjunctivitis may lead to corneal scarring and blindness, whereas the risk of severe ocular damage is low with chlamydial infection. Without ocular prophylaxis, ophthalmia neonatorum develops in 30% to 42% of infants born to mothers with untreated *N. gonorrhoeae* infection [208,210,211] and in approximately 30% of infants exposed to *Chlamydia* [210].

A 5-year study from Iran showed *S. aureus* to be the major organism responsible for ophthalmia neonatorum [213]. Similar predominance of *S. aureus* has been reported from Argentina and Hong Kong [214,215]. The reasons for these differences in etiology are not well understood, and data from countries with the lowest resources are unavailable.

Strategies to prevent or ameliorate ocular morbidity related to ophthalmia neonatorum include (1) primary prevention of STDs, (2) antenatal screening for and treatment of STDs (particularly gonorrhea and *Chlamydia* infection), (3) eye prophylaxis at birth, and (4) early diagnosis and treatment of ophthalmia neonatorum [211]. For developing countries, eye prophylaxis soon after birth is the most cost-effective and feasible strategy in settings where STD rates are high. Eye prophylaxis is used primarily to prevent gonococcal ophthalmia. Primary prevention of STDs in low-income and middle-income countries is limited, although promotion of condom use has been successful in reducing STDs in some countries [216,217]. Screening women at prenatal and STD clinics and treating based on a syndromic approach (i.e., treat for possible infections in all women with vaginal discharge without laboratory confirmation) is cost-effective, but may lead to overtreatment of uninfected women and missed cases.

Eye prophylaxis consists of cleaning the eyelids and instilling an antimicrobial agent into the eyes as soon after birth as possible. The agent should be placed directly into the conjunctival sac (using clean hands), and the eyes should not be flushed after instillation. Infants born vaginally and by cesarean section should receive prophylaxis. Although no agent is 100% effective at preventing disease, the use of 1% silver nitrate solution (introduced by Credé in 1881) [218] dramatically reduced the incidence of ophthalmia neonatorum. This inexpensive agent is still widely used in many parts of the world. The major problems with silver nitrate are that it may cause chemical conjunctivitis in 50% of infants, and it has limited antimicrobial activity against *Chlamydia* [211,219,220]. In low-income and middle-income countries where heat and improper storage may be a problem, evaporation and concentration are particular concerns. Although 1% tetracycline and 0.5% erythromycin ointments are commonly used and are as effective as silver nitrate for the prevention of gonococcal conjunctivitis, these agents are more expensive and unavailable in many parts of the world. Silver nitrate seems to be a better prophylactic agent in areas where penicillinase-producing *N. gonorrhoeae* is a problem [221].

The ideal prophylactic agent for settings with low resources would have a broad antimicrobial spectrum and be available and affordable. Povidone-iodine is an inexpensive, nontoxic topical agent that is potentially widely available. More recent studies suggest that it may be useful in preventing ophthalmia neonatorum. A prospective masked, controlled trial of ocular prophylaxis using 2.5% povidone-iodine solution, 1% silver nitrate solution, or 0.5% erythromycin ointment was conducted in Kenya [222]. Of 3117 neonates randomly assigned, 13.1% in the povidone-iodine group versus 15.2% in the erythromycin group and 17.5% in the silver nitrate group developed infectious conjunctivitis ($P < .01$). The high rates of infection in this study despite ocular prophylaxis are striking. Although there was no significant difference among agents in prevention of gonococcal ophthalmia ($\leq 1\%$ for each agent), povidone-iodine was most effective in preventing chlamydial conjunctivitis. A 2003 study by the same group compared prophylaxis with 1 drop and with 2 drops of the povidone-iodine solution instilled in both eyes at birth in 719 Kenyan neonates. No cases of *N. gonorrhoeae* infection were identified. Double application did not change the rates of infection with *C. trachomatis* (4.2% and 3.9%) [223].

Although the antimicrobial spectrum of povidone-iodine is wider than that of the other topical agents [224], and antibacterial resistance has not been shown [156], published data on the efficacy of povidone-iodine against penicillinase-producing *N. gonorrhoeae* are not yet available. A solution of 2.5% povidone-iodine might also be useful as an antimicrobial agent for cord care—of relevance in the prevention of omphalitis (see earlier).

Another trial in Iran compared the efficacy of topical povidone-iodine with erythromycin as prophylactic agents for ophthalmia neonatorum compared with no prophylaxis [225]. Among 330 infants studied, ophthalmia neonatorum developed in 9% of neonates receiving povidone-iodine versus 18% of neonates receiving erythromycin and 22% of neonates receiving no prophylaxis. Further studies are needed to establish the safety and efficacy of povidone-iodine in low-income and middle-income countries.

The frequency of practice of ocular prophylaxis in low-income and middle-income countries is unknown. In consideration of the high rates of STDs among pregnant women in many countries with low resources, eye prophylaxis is an important blindness prevention strategy. For infants born at home, a single dose of antimicrobial agent for ocular prophylaxis could be added to birth kits and potentially distributed to trained birth attendants during antenatal care, although more information about the feasibility and acceptability of this approach is needed. The strategy of ocular prophylaxis is more cost-effective than early diagnosis and appropriate treatment. In areas of the world in which access to medical care is limited, and effective drugs are scarce or unavailable, it may be the only viable strategy.

No prevention strategy is 100% effective. Even with prophylaxis, 5% to 10% of infants develop ophthalmia. All infants with ophthalmia must be given appropriate treatment, even if they received prophylaxis at birth. A single dose of either ceftriaxone (25 to 50 mg/kg intravenously or intramuscularly, not to exceed 125 mg) or cefotaxime (100 mg/kg intravenously or intramuscularly) is effective therapy for gonococcal ophthalmia caused by penicillinase-producing *N. gonorrhoeae* and non-penicillinase-producing *N. gonorrhoeae* strains [221]. Gentamicin and kanamycin also have been shown to be effective therapeutic agents and may be more readily available in some settings. Rarely, gonococcal infection acquired at birth may become disseminated, resulting in arthritis, septicemia, and meningitis. Neonates with disseminated gonococcal disease require systemic therapy with ceftriaxone or cefotaxime (25 to 50 mg/kg once daily) or cefotaxime (25 mg/kg intramuscularly or intravenously twice daily) for 7 days (for arthritis or sepsis) or 10 to 14 days (for meningitis). If a lumbar puncture cannot be performed (and meningitis cannot be ruled out) in an infant with evidence of dissemination, the longer period of therapy should be chosen [221]. Infants with chlamydial conjunctivitis should receive a 2-week course of oral erythromycin (50 mg/kg per day in four divided doses). After the immediate neonatal period, oral sulfonamides may be used [221].

HUMAN IMMUNODEFICIENCY VIRUS INFECTION

The Joint United Nations Programme on HIV/AIDS (UNAIDS) and WHO estimate that in 2007 approximately 33 million people worldwide were infected with human immunodeficiency virus (HIV), and new infections were occurring at a rate of approximately 2.7 million per year [226]. Most HIV infections occur in low-income and middle-income countries; more than 90% of infected individuals live in sub-Saharan Africa, Asia, Latin America, or the Caribbean. Women are particularly vulnerable to HIV infection; worldwide, approximately 50% of cases occur in women. The proportion of women infected with HIV has increased in many regions; women represent approximately 60% of HIV infections in sub-Saharan Africa. An estimated 370,000 children were infected with HIV in 2007, mostly by mother-to-infant transmission in utero, at the time of delivery, or through breast-feeding [226].

Because HIV increases deaths among young adults, the acquired immunodeficiency syndrome (AIDS) epidemic has resulted in a generation of AIDS orphans. In 2007, it was estimated that 15 million children younger than 15 years of age have been orphaned by AIDS, most in sub-Saharan Africa [226–228]. It is well known that maternal mortality increases neonatal and infant deaths, independent of HIV infection. Global estimates for 2007, including the number of people living with HIV/AIDS, the number newly infected, and total AIDS deaths, are presented in Table 2–3.

Transmission—Reducing the Disparity between Low-Income and High-Income Countries

Risk factors for mother-to-infant transmission of HIV include maternal health and severity of disease, obstetric factors, maternal coinfection with other STDs, prematurity or LBW, and infant feeding practices (Table 2–4). In most developed countries, evidence-based interventions including use of antiretroviral drugs, elective cesarean section before the onset of labor and before rupture of membranes, and avoidance of breast-feeding have reduced vertical transmission of HIV to 1% to 2%, with virtual elimination of transmission in some settings [229–232]. Without interventions, it is estimated that 20% to 45% of infants may become infected [233]. Rates of transmission remain high in settings with low resources, where there has been limited progress in increasing services for the prevention of mother-to-infant transmission of HIV [234]. In 2001, United Nations member states committed to the goal of reducing the

TABLE 2–3 Statistics on the World Epidemic of Human Immunodeficiency Virus and Acquired Immunodeficiency Syndrome (HIV/AIDS): 2007

	Estimate	Range
All people living with HIV/AIDS	33 million	30.3-36.1 million
Adults living with HIV/AIDS	30.8 million	28.2-34 million
Women living with HIV/AIDS	15.5 million	14.2-16.9 million
Children living with HIV/AIDS	2 million	1.9-2.3 million
All people newly infected with HIV	2.7 million	2.2-3.2 million
Children newly infected with HIV	0.37 million	0.33-0.41 million
All AIDS deaths	2 million	1.8-2.3 million
Child AIDS deaths	0.27 million	0.25-0.29 million

Adapted from Report on the AIDS Epidemic. Geneva, WHO, UNAIDS, 2008.

TABLE 2–4 Risk Factors Associated with Mother-to-Infant Transmission of Human Immunodeficiency Virus (HIV)

Risk Factor	Possible Mechanism of Mother-to-Infant Transmission of Infection
Maternal Health	
Advanced HIV disease	High viral load and low CD4 T cells
Primary HIV infection	High viral load; lack of immune response
No maternal antiretroviral treatment	High viral load
Obstetric Factors	
Vaginal delivery	Exposure to HIV-infected genital secretions
Episiotomies and vaginal tears	Exposure to HIV-infected blood
Instrumental deliveries	Exposure of breached infant skin to secretions containing HIV
Chorionic villus biopsy or amniocentesis	Increased risk of placental microtransfusion
Fetal electrode monitoring	Breach in infant skin and exposure to infected secretions
Prolonged rupture of fetal membranes	Prolonged exposure to HIV-infected secretions
Chorioamnionitis	Ascending infection
Low birth weight	Impaired fetal or placental membranes
Prematurity	Impaired fetal or placental membranes
Maternal Coinfection	
Malaria (placental malaria)	Increased viral load, disruption in placental architecture
HSV-2	Increased plasma viral load, increased shedding of HIV in genital secretions, genital ulcers
Other STDs	Genital ulcerations and exposure to HIV-infected blood or genital secretions
Infant Feeding	
Breast-feeding	Mastitis, cell-free and cell-associated virus
Mixed feeding	Contaminated formula or water used in preparing formula may cause gastroenteritis leading to microtrauma to infant's bowel, which provides entry to HIV virus
Miscellaneous Factors	
Infant-mother HLA concordance	HLA molecules on the surface of HIV-infected maternal cells are recognized as "self" by cytotoxic T lymphocytes or NK cells of the infant and are less likely to be destroyed
Maternal HLA homozygosity	Increased viral load
Presence of CCR5 Δ32 mutation in T cells of exposed infants	Decreased susceptibility to HIV infection

HLA, human leukocyte antigen; HSV-2, herpes simplex virus type 2; NK, natural killer; STDs, sexually transmitted diseases.
Adapted from Paintsil E, Andiman A. Update on successes and challenges regarding mother-to-child transmission of HIV. Curr Opin Pediatr 21:94-101, 2009.

proportion of infants infected with HIV by 50% by 2010 [235]; although progress has been made, this goal has not been achieved.

Breast-Feeding and Human Immunodeficiency Virus

Although breast-feeding by HIV-positive mothers is discouraged in Europe and North America, where safe and affordable alternatives to breast milk are available, the issue of breast-feeding and HIV is much more complicated in developing countries, where breast-feeding has proven benefits and where artificial feeding has known risks. Benefits of breast-feeding include decreased risk of diarrhea and other infectious diseases, improved nutritional status, and decreased infant mortality [236,237]. Research conducted over 20 years has increased understanding of mother-to-infant transmission of HIV through breast milk [238–240]. Risk factors for transmission of HIV via breast milk include maternal factors (e.g., recent infection or advanced maternal disease, low CD4 counts, viral load in breast milk and plasma, mastitis or breast abscess, and duration of breast-feeding); infant factors (e.g., prematurity,

oral thrush, and being fed breast milk and non–breast milk alternatives resulting in "mixed" infant feeding); and viral factors (viral load, clade C) [238]. Three interventions have been shown to reduce late mother-to-infant transmission via breast-feeding: complete avoidance of breast-feeding, exclusive breast-feeding rather than mixed feeding, and antiretroviral prophylaxis for the lactating mother and for the infant who is breast-feeding [238–241].

In 2009 WHO updated their recommendations on HIV and infant feeding to help decision makers in different countries develop their own policies regarding feeding practices in the context of HIV infection [241]. The statement addresses several issues: the human rights perspective, prevention of HIV infection in women, the health of mothers and children, and elements for establishing a policy on HIV status and infant feeding. The document recommends that the choice of feeding option should depend on the mother's individual circumstances. All HIV-infected mothers should be counseled about the risks and benefits of feeding options and supported in their choice. Exclusive breast-feeding is recommended for the first 6 months of life, introducing appropriate complementary foods thereafter, and continue breastfeeding for the first 12 months of life. Breastfeeding should then only stop once a nutritionally adequate and safe diet without breast milk can be provided. In addition, antiretroviral therapy to prevent perinatal HIV transmission should be provided to the pregnant woman as early as the 14th week of gestation and then to her infant throughout the breastfeeding period. The document also emphasizes that information and education on mother-to-infant transmission of HIV should be directed to the general public and to affected communities and families. A major challenge will be to implement these policies in developing countries where the bulk of perinatal HIV infections occur and where resources to follow these guidelines are limited.

Prevention of Human Immunodeficiency Virus Infection in Low-Income and Middle-Income Countries

Primary prevention of HIV infection among women of childbearing age is the most successful but most difficult way to prevent the infection of infants. Improving the social status of women, educating men and women, ensuring access to information about HIV infection and its prevention, promoting safer sex through condom use, social marketing of condoms, and treating other STDs that increase the risk of HIV transmission are potential strategies that have been successful in reducing HIV infection. A goal for health services in low-income and middle-income countries is to provide interventions to reduce sexual transmission of HIV, with special focus on reducing infections during pregnancy and among women who are breast-feeding, and to prevent unintended pregnancies among women infected with HIV.

Prevention of Human Immunodeficiency Virus Transmission from an Infected Mother to Her Infant

Antiretroviral Strategies

The era of antiretroviral therapy to reduce vertical transmission of HIV began in 1994 with publication of the Pediatric AIDS Clinical Trials Groups (ACTG) Protocol 076 [242]. This trial, performed in the United States and France, showed that zidovudine administered orally to HIV-infected pregnant women with no prior treatment with antiretroviral drugs during pregnancy, beginning at 14 to 34 weeks of gestation and continuing throughout pregnancy, and then intravenously during labor to the mother, and orally to the newborn for the first 6 weeks of life, reduced perinatal transmission by 67.5%, from 25.5% (95% CI 18.4% to 32.5%) to 8.3% (95% CI 3.9% to 12.8%). The regimen was recommended as standard care in the United States and quickly became common practice. Studies have shown that various antiretroviral regimens among pregnant women can reduce mother-to-infant transmission of HIV. These studies have shown that it is feasible to provide antiretroviral therapy and prophylaxis to women in low-income and middle-income countries and substantially reduce mother-to-infant transmission throughout the world [234,243–245].

Antiretroviral therapy requires the identification of HIV-infected women early enough in pregnancy to allow them access to therapy. A system for voluntary, confidential HIV counseling and testing must be in place. In 2007, only 18% of pregnant women in low-income and middle-income countries where data were available had been tested for HIV, however, and only 33% of pregnant women infected with HIV were treated with antiretroviral drugs including therapy to prevent vertical transmission of HIV [234].

Cesarean Section

Meta-analyses of North American and European studies performed in the late 1990s found that elective cesarean section reduced the risk of mother-to-infant transmission of HIV by more than 50% [246,247]. For mothers on highly active antiretroviral therapy and with low viral loads, the benefits of delivery by cesarean section for reducing perinatal transmission of HIV are uncertain, especially in settings with low resources where risks of operative complications are high [248].

Integrated Health Care Programs

Successful programs to reduce mother-to-infant transmission of HIV require integration with health care services for women and children. These programs provide early access to adequate antenatal care, voluntary and confidential counseling and HIV testing for women and their partners, antiretroviral drugs during pregnancy and delivery for HIV-positive women, improved care during labor and delivery, counseling for HIV-positive women regarding choices for infant feeding, and support for HIV-positive women with ongoing health care and antiretrovirals for life and follow-up for their infants (Table 2–5).

Human Immunodeficiency Virus and Child Survival

Although there have been tremendous gains in child survival over the past 3 decades, with reductions worldwide in deaths resulting from diarrhea, pneumonia, and vaccine-preventable diseases [1,249], the AIDS epidemic threatens to undermine this dramatic trend in some countries in sub-Saharan Africa [250]. In sub-Saharan Africa, AIDS has become a leading cause of death among infants and children, although globally it causes only 3% of deaths in children younger than 5 years of age [1,249]. There is a complex link between increasing mortality of children younger than 5 years old and high rates of HIV prevalence in adults, related to mother-to-infant transmission of HIV and the compromised ability of parents who are ill themselves to care for young children [251].

With success of programs to prevent mother-to-infant transmission of HIV, increasing numbers of infants who are exposed to HIV but uninfected are being born [252]. A challenge for health care systems is to ensure that these infants have access to health care and remain healthy. Programs for HIV/AIDS prevention and treatment have been developed largely as vertical programs that now need to be linked to broader efforts to improve maternal, neonatal, and child health care in low-income and middle-income countries.

TUBERCULOSIS

Tuberculosis affects 13.9 million people worldwide and remains a major global public health threat, causing the deaths of 0.5 million women annually [203]. After

TABLE 2–5   Essential Services for High-Quality Maternal Care

Routine Quality Antenatal and Postpartum Care for All Women Regardless of HIV Status

Health education; information on prevention and care for HIV and sexually transmitted infections including safer sex practices; and pregnancy including antenatal care, birth planning and delivery assistance, malaria prevention, optimal infant feeding, family planning counseling and related services

Provider-initiated HIV testing and counseling, including HIV testing and counseling for women of unknown status at labor and delivery or postpartum

Couple and partner HIV testing and counseling including support for disclosure

Promotion and provision of male and female condoms

HIV-related gender-based violence screening

Obstetric care, including history taking and physical examination

Maternal nutritional support

Counseling on infant feeding

Psychosocial support

Birth planning and birth preparedness (including pregnancy and postpartum danger signs), including skilled birth attendants

Tetanus vaccination

Iron and folic acid supplementation

Syphilis screening and management of sexually transmitted diseases

Risk reduction interventions for injecting drug users

Additional Services for Women Living with HIV

Additional counseling and support to encourage partner testing, adoption of risk reduction and disclosure

Clinical evaluation, including clinical staging of HIV disease

Immunologic assessment (CD4 cell count) where available

ART when indicated

Counseling and support on infant feeding based on knowledge of HIV status

Antiretroviral prophylaxis for prevention of mother-to-infant transmission of HIV provided during antepartum, intrapartum, and postpartum periods

Co-trimoxazole prophylaxis where indicated

Additional counseling and provision of services as appropriate to prevent unintended pregnancies

Supportive care, including adherence support

Additional counseling and provision of services as appropriate to prevent unintended pregnancies

Tuberculosis screening and treatment when indicated; preventive therapy (isoniazid prophylaxis) when appropriate

Advice and support on other prevention interventions such as safe drinking water

Supportive care including adherence support and palliative care and symptom management

Additional Services for All Women Regardless of HIV Status in Specific Settings

Malaria prevention and treatment

Counseling, psychosocial support, and referral for women who are at risk of or have experienced violence

Counseling and referral for women with a history of harmful alcohol or drug use

Deworming

Consider retesting late in pregnancy where feasible in generalized epidemics

Essential Postnatal Care for HIV-Exposed Infants and Young Children

Completion of antiretroviral prophylaxis regimen as necessary

Routine newborn and infant care including routine immunization and growth monitoring

Co-trimoxazole prophylaxis

Early HIV diagnostic testing and diagnosis of HIV-related conditions

Continued infant feeding counseling and support, especially after HIV testing and at 6 mo

Nutritional support throughout the first year of life including support for optimal infant feeding practices and provision of nutritional supplements and replacement foods if indicated

ART for children living with HIV, when indicated

Treatment monitoring for all children receiving ART

Isoniazid prophylaxis when indicated

Counseling on adherence support for caregivers

Malaria prevention and treatment where indicated

Diagnosis and management of common childhood infections and conditions and integrated management of childhood illness

Diagnosis and management of tuberculosis and other opportunistic infections

Continued

TABLE 2-5   Essential Services for High-Quality Maternal Care—cont'd

Antiretroviral Regimens Recommended by World Health Organization (WHO) for Treating Pregnant Women and Preventing HIV Infection in Infants: Promoting More Efficacious Antiretroviral Regimens
WHO recommends ART for all pregnant women who are eligible for treatment. Initiation of ART in pregnant women addresses not only their health needs, but also significantly reduces HIV transmission to their infants. In addition, by securing the health of women, it also improves child well-being and survival
For pregnant women with HIV who do not yet require ART, antiretroviral prophylactic regimens are recommended for prevention of mother-to-infant transmission. Two regimens are recommended by WHO: Option A: MOTHER: Antepartum zidovudine (AZT, from as early as 14 weeks gestation); single dose nevirapine (NVP) at onset of labor; AZT and lamivudine (3TC) during labor and delivery and for 7 days postpartum. If mother received >4 weeks of AZT antepartum, can omit single dose NVP, AZT and 3TC. INFANT: Breastfeeding infants should receive daily NVP from birth until 1 week after all exposure to breastmilk has ended; Non-breastfeeding infants should receive AZT or NVP for 6 weeks. Option B: MOTHER: Triple antiretroviral drug therapy from 14 weeks gestation until 1 week after all exposure to breastmilk has ended. INFANT: Breastfeeding infants should receive daily NVP for 6 weeks and non-breastfeeding infants should receive AZT or NVP for 6 weeks.

ART, antiretroviral therapy; HIV, human immunodeficiency virus.
WHO. Rapid Advice: Use of antiretroviral drugs for treating pregnant women and preventing HIV infection in infants. http://www.who.int/hiv/pub/mtct/rapid_advice_mtct.pdf. Last accessed June 20, 2010.

HIV/AIDS, tuberculosis is the second leading cause of death from infectious causes of women of childbearing age (15 to 44 years old), with an estimated 228,000 deaths occurring annually in this population [253]. Most worldwide disability-adjusted life years (99.4%) and deaths (99.6%) resulting from tuberculosis occur in low-income and middle-income countries [203,253]. Tuberculosis during pregnancy may have adverse consequences for the mother and infant, including increased risk of miscarriage, prematurity, LBW, and neonatal death [254–257]. Adverse perinatal outcomes are increased in mothers who have late diagnosis or incomplete or irregular therapy [254]. Ideally, diagnosis and treatment of tuberculosis in women should occur before pregnancy.

The lung remains the most common site of infection; however, the prevalence of extrapulmonary tuberculosis is increasing. Although congenital tuberculosis is rare, the fetus may become infected by hematogenous spread in a woman with placentitis, by swallowing or aspirating infected amniotic fluid, or by direct contact with an infected cervix at delivery [257]. The most common route of infection of the neonate is through airborne transmission of *Mycobacterium tuberculosis* from an infected, untreated mother to her infant. Infected newborns are at particularly high risk of developing severe disease, including fulminant septic shock with disseminated intravascular coagulation and respiratory failure [257,258].

The resurgence of tuberculosis and the increased risk of tuberculosis among individuals who are infected with HIV are well known. In areas where HIV is endemic, tuberculosis rates are increasing [259,260]. Pregnant women who are coinfected with HIV may be at increased risk for placental or genital tuberculosis, resulting in an increased risk of transmission to the fetus [261]. Additionally, neonates born with tuberculosis/HIV coinfection have been shown to be at higher risk of severe, rapidly progressive HIV disease [262]. In areas of the world where tuberculosis and HIV are endemic, the key to preventing neonatal tuberculosis is early identification of maternal tuberculosis and HIV serostatus, based primarily on maternal history and relevant investigations of the mother and newborn [263].

MALARIA

From a global perspective, malaria is one of the most important infectious diseases. Half of the world's population live in areas with malaria risk. The disease is mainly confined to poorer tropical areas of Africa, Asia, and Latin America. An estimated 85% of all malaria deaths in 2006 occurred in children younger than 5 years old, amounting to 760,000 deaths in children younger than 5 years [264]. Countries in sub-Saharan Africa account for more than 90% of malaria cases and 88% of malaria cases among children younger than 5 years [264]. Each year, approximately 24 million African women become pregnant in malaria-endemic areas and are at risk for malaria during pregnancy [265]. Four species of the malaria parasite infect humans: *Plasmodium falciparum, Plasmodium vivax, Plasmodium ovale,* and *Plasmodium malariae. P. falciparum* is responsible for the most severe form of disease and is the predominant parasite in tropical Africa, Southeast Asia, the Amazon area, and the Pacific. Groups at greatest risk for severe disease and death are young nonimmune children, pregnant women (especially primigravidas), and nonimmune adults [266].

Malaria in Pregnancy

Preexisting levels of immunity determine susceptibility to infection and severity of disease [265–269]. In areas of high endemicity or high stable transmission, where there are high levels of protective immunity, the effects of malaria on the mother and fetus are less severe than in areas where malaria transmission is low or unstable (i.e., sporadic, periodic). It is unclear why pregnant women (even with preexisting immunity) are at increased risk for malaria. The most severe maternal complications (cerebral malaria, pulmonary edema, renal failure) occur in women previously living in nonendemic areas who have little or no immunity and are most frequent with infections caused by *P. falciparum.* Severe malaria may result in pregnancy-related maternal death.

Malaria parasitemia is more common, and the parasite burden tends to be higher in pregnant than in nonpregnant women [267,268]. This increase in prevalence and density of parasitemia is highest in primiparous women and decreases with increasing parity [268]. The greater severity in primiparous women from endemic areas seems to be attributable in part to a pregnancy-restricted *P. falciparum* variable surface protein present on parasitized erythrocytes; because primiparous women have not been previously exposed to this antigen, they lack immunity to it, allowing this protein to bind to placental chondroitin sulfate and parasitized erythrocytes to become sequestered in the placenta [270]. The parasite burden is highest in the second trimester and decreases with increasing gestation [269,271,272]. The most important effects of malaria on pregnant women are severe anemia [267] and placental infection [265–269,273,274]. The prevalence of anemia can be 78%, and anemia is more common and more severe in primigravidas [273].

Perinatal Outcome

Perinatal outcome is directly related to placental malaria. Malaria is associated with an increase in spontaneous abortions, stillbirths, preterm delivery, and intrauterine growth restriction, particularly in areas where malaria is acquired by nonimmune women [269,275,276]. Reported rates of fetal loss range from 9% to 50% [268]. The uteroplacental vascular space is thought to be a relatively protected site for parasite sequestration and replication [274,277]. Placental malaria is characterized by the presence of parasites and leukocytes in the intervillous space, pigment within macrophages, proliferation of cytotrophoblasts, and thickening of the trophoblastic basement membrane [273]. Placental infection may alter the function of the placenta, reducing oxygen and nutrient transport and resulting in intrauterine growth restriction, and may allow the passage of infected red blood cells to the fetus, resulting in congenital infection. In primigravidas living in endemic areas, placental malaria occurs in 16% to 63% of women, whereas in multigravidas, the prevalence is much lower at 12% to 33% [267,268].

The most profound effect of placental malaria is the reduction of birth weight [269,278,279]. *P. falciparum* and *P. vivax* infection during pregnancy are associated with a reduction in birth weight [280]. Steketee and associates [278] estimated that in highly endemic settings, placental malaria may account for approximately 13% of cases of LBW secondary to intrauterine growth restriction. In Africa, malaria is thought to be an important contributor to LBW in the almost 3.5 million infants with LBW born annually [281]. Malaria is one of the few preventable causes of LBW. Because LBW is a major determinant of neonatal and infant mortality in developing countries, malaria may indirectly increase mortality by increasing LBW [282].

Congenital Malaria

Transplacental infection of the fetus also may occur. It is relatively rare in populations with prior immunity (0.1% to 1.5%) [267], but more common in nonimmune mothers. It is thought that the low rate of fetal infection concomitant with a high incidence of placental infection is due in part to protection from transplacental maternal antibodies [283,284].

The clinical characteristics of neonates with congenital malaria (i.e., malaria parasitemia on peripheral blood smear) include fever, respiratory distress, pallor, anemia, hepatomegaly, jaundice, and diarrhea. There is a high mortality rate with congenital infection [285]. The global burden of disease related to congenital malaria is unknown.

Prevention and Treatment of Malaria in Pregnancy

Pregnant women living in malaria-endemic areas need access to services that can provide prompt, safe, and effective treatment for malaria. Among at-risk pregnant populations in areas with stable or high transmission, WHO recommends that malaria control strategies include antenatal care, at least two doses of intermittent preventive treatment with sulfadoxine-pyrimethamine during the second and third trimesters, early and consistent use of insecticide-treated bednets during pregnancy through the postpartum period, effective case management of malaria, and screening and treatment of anemia frequently resulting from malaria infection [286,287]. In areas with low transmission, case management is emphasized [287].

Prophylaxis and Treatment Using Antimalarial Drugs

Chloroquine, the safest, cheapest, and most widely available antimalarial drug, has been the agent of choice for the prevention and treatment of malaria in pregnancy [288]. In all areas where *P. falciparum* is prevalent, the parasite is at least partially resistant to chloroquine, however, and resistance to sulfadoxine-pyrimethamine, the first-line drug for intermittent preventive treatment in pregnancy, is increasing [289,290]. There are a limited number of safe and effective antimalarials available for use in pregnancy. For a drug to be considered safe, it must be safe for the mother, safe for the fetus, and ideally safe for the breast-feeding infant [288,291]. New drug development has been impeded by the fact that pregnant women have been excluded for ethical reasons from drug development programs because of the justified fear of risks to the fetus [292,293].

A 2002 systematic review of prevention versus therapy in pregnant women examined studies on the effectiveness of prompt therapy for malaria infection, prophylaxis with antimalarial drugs to prevent infection, and reduced exposure to mosquito-borne infection by using insecticide-treated bednets [294]. Chemoprophylaxis is associated with reduced maternal disease, including anemia and placental infection. One study found that the incidence of placental malaria is reduced by prophylaxis, even when chloroquine is used in areas with chloroquine-resistant malaria [295]. In addition, a large systematic review showed prophylaxis to have a positive effect on birth weight, risk of preterm delivery, and neonatal mortality (relative risk [RR] 0.73, 95% CI 0.53 to 0.99) [296].

A major problem with chemoprophylaxis and prompt therapy for known or suspected infection is that it is often difficult to deliver services to pregnant women, especially women who live in areas remote from health centers. Intermittent preventive treatment involves two or three doses of a safe and effective antimalarial given to women in malaria-endemic areas with the presumption that they are at high risk of malaria infection. Studies from Africa have shown that intermittent preventive treatment can reduce the incidence of malaria and its adverse consequences [297,298]. These interventions are particularly important and cost-effective in pregnancy and have been estimated to reduce all-cause neonatal mortality by 32% [10,299,300]. In 2000, WHO recommended intermittent preventive treatment with sulfadoxine-pyrimethamine in malaria-endemic areas where *P. falciparum* is resistant to chloroquine and sensitive to sulfadoxine-pyrimethamine

[301]. This drug is effective in a single dose, is not bitter, and is relatively well tolerated. In areas where malaria transmission is lower and *P. vivax* and *P. falciparum* are a problem, finding an appropriate drug regimen is more difficult [302]. In these areas and where *P. falciparum* is resistant to sulfadoxine-pyrimethamine, further research on the safety and efficacy of alternative antimalarial drugs for prevention and treatment of malaria in pregnancy, including artemisinin-based combination therapies, is urgently needed [293].

Prevention Using Insecticide-Treated Bednets

Although the benefits of antimalarial chemoprophylaxis have been established, poor compliance and increasing drug resistance have led to trials of alternative prevention strategies [303]. The use of insecticide-treated bednets has been successful in reducing childhood morbidity and mortality in malaria-endemic areas [304–306]. A systematic review of use of insecticide-treated bednets during pregnancy in Africa associated their use with a reduced risk of placental malaria in all pregnancies (RR 0.79, 95% CI 0.63 to 0.98), reduced risk of LBW (RR 0.77, 95% CI 0.61 to 0.98), and reduced risk of fetal loss in the first to fourth pregnancy (RR 0.67, 95% CI 0.47 to 0.97) [307]. The use of social marketing and incentive initiatives such as voucher and discounted net programs have increased bednet coverage and use [308,309]. An additional benefit of bednet use is protection of the neonate, who almost always sleeps with the mother in these settings [308]. A pooled analysis of studies of insecticide-treated bednet use in early childhood found a reduction in all-cause child mortality associated with the use of insecticide-treated bednets (RR 0.82, 95% CI 0.76-0.89) [15]. Although there is clear evidence of the impact of insecticide-treated bednets in Africa, further data are needed from trials of insecticide-treated bednets in Latin America and Asia and areas of high *P. vivax* transmission [307].

Malaria Control Strategies and Challenges

Comprehensive malaria prevention and treatment strategies implementing the interventions recommended by WHO can have dramatic effects on child health outcomes. A program that achieved high coverage of multiple malaria control measures in Equatorial Guinea was associated with reduced prevalence of malaria infection (odds ratio 0.31, 95% CI 0.2 to 0.46) and led to an overall reduction in mortality in children younger than 5 years from 152 per 1000 to 55 per 1000 births (hazard ratio 0.34, 95% CI 0.23-0.49) [310].

Studies have shown an association between malaria and HIV in pregnancy with an increase in the risk of maternal malaria and of placental malaria in HIV-positive mothers, although the influence of malaria on the clinical course of HIV infection remains unclear [311–313]. There is some suggestion that coinfection with malaria and HIV infection in pregnancy may be linked with increased mother-to-infant transmission of HIV, perinatal and early infant mortality, and morbidity after the neonatal period [314,315]. Intermittent preventive treatment with sulfadoxine-pyrimethamine is less effective in preventing malaria in HIV-infected

women than in women without HIV infection, underscoring the need for research to expand the arsenal of safe and effective antimalarials and to understand interactions between antimalarial and antiretroviral drugs [314]. Effective, practical, and well-tolerated strategies are needed to prevent and treat malaria in HIV-infected women.

INDIRECT CAUSES OF NEONATAL DEATH RELATED TO INFECTION

In addition to direct infectious causes of neonatal deaths, a vast array of indirect causes contribute to infectious deaths in developing countries. These contributory factors have socioeconomic and medical roots. Sociocultural factors include poverty; illiteracy; low social status of women; lack of political power (for women and children) and lack of will in individuals who have power; gender discrimination (for mother and neonate); harmful traditional or cultural practices; poor hygiene; lack of clean water and sanitation; the cultural belief that a sick newborn is doomed to die, and that the family is powerless to alter fate; the family's inability to recognize danger signs in the newborn; inadequate access to high-quality medical care (because it is unavailable or unaffordable, or because of lack of transport for emergency care) or the lack of supplies or appropriate drugs; and maternal death [316–319]. Medical factors that may also contribute to an infectious neonatal death include poor maternal health; untreated maternal infections (including STDs, urinary tract infection, and chorioamnionitis); failure to immunize the mother fully against tetanus; unhygienic and inappropriate management of labor and delivery; unsanitary cutting and care of the umbilical cord; failure to promote early and exclusive breast-feeding; and prematurity or LBW or both [316,317,320–322]. To promote change, families must be empowered and mobilized to identify illness and to seek care. Health care workers (of all levels) must know what to do and must have the resources to support needed therapy. Better maternal care—preventive and curative—is preventive medicine for the newborn.

Coordinated activities are needed to bring about change that is sustainable by countries on their own over the long-term. A multidisciplinary approach—bringing together people with different interests, from different backgrounds, different agencies, different government ministries—is needed to seek solutions to problems and to implement change at the local level. Finally, global acknowledgment is needed that this is the right thing to do (i.e., a moral imperative), and with this acknowledgment the long-term commitment of substantial funding to help provide needed services to countries with low resources and high maternal and neonatal mortality. A major remaining challenge is to link science and medicine with social solutions through a global commitment to long-term, long-lasting change so that improvements in maternal and newborn health can be achieved and sustained.

STRATEGIES TO PREVENT AND TREAT INFECTION IN NEONATES

Strategies to prevent or reduce neonatal infections and to reduce morbidity and mortality in newborns in whom infection develops involve putting into practice what is known and creating innovative ways to make these interventions feasible in a developing country context. Use of simple, cost-effective technologies that are potentially available and feasible for use in the community and at first-level health facilities could have a major impact in reducing morbidity and mortality related to neonatal infection. Public health, medical, and social interventions all have a role to play in reducing the global burden of neonatal infection. Several potential interventions are reviewed here (Table 2–6).

MATERNAL IMMUNIZATION TO PREVENT NEONATAL DISEASE

There is growing interest in the possibility of using maternal immunization to protect neonates and very young infants from infection through passively acquired transplacental antibodies or breast milk antibodies, or both (for additional information, see Chapter 38) [323,324].

TABLE 2–6 Interventions to Reduce Neonatal Infections or to Reduce Infection-Associated Mortality in Low-Income and Middle-Income Countries

Periconceptional Care

Folic acid supplementation to prevent neural tube defects (and associated risk of infectious morbidity and mortality)

Antenatal Care

Tetanus immunization

Maternal influenza immunization

Primary prevention of sexually transmitted disease, including HIV infection, through maternal education and safer sex using condoms

Diagnosis and treatment of sexually transmitted diseases (e.g., syphilis), urinary tract infection (including detection and treatment of asymptomatic bacteriuria), malaria, and tuberculosis

Intermittent presumptive treatment for malaria

Sleeping under insecticide-treated bednet

Balanced protein-energy supplements in populations with insecure food sources

Intrapartum and Delivery Care

Skilled maternal and immediate newborn care

Antibiotics for preterm premature rupture of membranes

Corticosteroids for preterm labor (to prevent respiratory distress syndrome and hyaline membrane disease)

Optimal management of complications including fever, premature rupture of membranes, and puerperal sepsis

Clean delivery

Clean cutting of umbilical cord and clean cord care

Immediate breast-feeding

Postnatal Care

Immediate, exclusive breast-feeding

Hand washing

Thermal care to prevent and manage hypothermia

Skin-to-skin care

Emollient therapy (e.g., sunflower seed oil for very preterm infants)

Case management for pneumonia

Data from Darmstadt et al [10,12], and Bhutta et al [15].

Immunization of pregnant women with tetanus toxoid has dramatically reduced cases of neonatal tetanus and is the classic example of maternal immunization and subsequent passive immunization to protect the newborn and the mother. Because most IgG antibody is transported across the placenta in the last 4 to 6 weeks of pregnancy, maternal immunization to prevent neonatal disease through transplacental antibodies is most promising for term rather than preterm newborns because the former would have adequate antibody levels at birth. Boosting breast milk antibodies by immunizing the mother is a potential strategy for reducing infection in term and preterm infants.

Routine influenza vaccination is recommended for women who are or will be pregnant during the influenza season [325]. Despite the fact that no study to date has shown an increased risk of either maternal complications or adverse fetal outcomes associated with inactivated influenza vaccination [326], compliance remains poor. A study in Bangladesh[327] revealed a greater burden of influenza in infants than had been predicted and showed that maternal influenza vaccination provided significant protection to infants and their mothers. Vaccinating mothers against influenza reduced laboratory-proven influenza in their infants by 68% from birth to 6 months of age and reduced episodes of maternal influenza-like illnesses by 35%. To achieve protection, influenza vaccines would need to be administered during each pregnancy. This vaccination would require strengthening of current antenatal immunization programs, which have limited reach, and education on the benefits of the vaccine to overcome the general reluctance to intervene in healthy pregnant women.

Other vaccines currently being developed or field tested to reduce or prevent neonatal infection by maternal immunization include vaccines against GBS, *S. pneumoniae*, and *H. influenzae* [328–337]. Because most neonatal GBS disease—especially the most severe—occurs in the first hours of life, maternal immunization to provide passive protection to the neonate is a potentially important strategy. A problem with GBS vaccines has been poor immunogenicity, resulting in more recent interest in the potential of conjugate vaccines [338]. GBS polysaccharide-tetanus toxoid conjugates are safe in adults and elicit antibody levels above what is likely to be passively protective for neonates [331,332]. Multivalent vaccines, which could provide protection against multiple GBS serotypes, are particularly promising [330].

Pneumococcal polysaccharide vaccines have been administered safely to pregnant women [334,336]. A study from Bangladesh reported that pneumococcal vaccination during pregnancy increased type-specific IgG serum antibody in mothers and their infants [335]. Cord blood levels of antibody were about half those of the mothers, with IgG1 subclass antibodies preferentially transferred to the infants. The estimated antibody half-life in the infants was 35 days. Immunization increased breast milk antibody as well. In a study of the 23-valent pneumococcal vaccine given to women before pregnancy, neither mothers nor infants had significantly elevated pneumococcus-specific antibody at delivery [335]. The study in Bangladesh of the impact of maternal influenza vaccination on risk of maternal and infant respiratory illness used vaccination of mothers with 23-valent polysaccharide vaccine for the control group [327]. If passive immunization does not interfere with active immunization of young infants, vaccination of pregnant women could potentially be used to prevent pneumococcal disease in early infancy; however, this requires further research.

Additional studies of the safety, efficacy, and effectiveness of immunizing pregnant women with specific vaccines are needed. Studies must address issues of safety to the mother, fetus, and young infant. Vaccines are not routinely tested for safety in pregnant women, so most safety data come from animal studies or postlicensure pregnancy registries and adverse event reporting systems. Based on accumulated evidence, vaccines against diphtheria, tetanus, and influenza have been recommended for use in pregnancy. Studies must assess protection against specific diseases (e.g., sepsis, pneumonia, meningitis) and protection against all causes of neonatal and infant mortality. Local epidemiology must also be considered because HIV and malaria can reduce the amount of antibody transferred to the fetus, decreasing the benefits of maternal immunization programs in highly endemic areas. The subsequent response of the infant to active immunization also must be evaluated, to ensure that passive immunization does not interfere with the infant's ability to mount an immune response. In low-income and middle-income countries, studies must be done in settings in which it is possible to maintain surveillance throughout infancy.

NEONATAL IMMUNIZATION

Protection of young infants against vaccine-preventable diseases requires vaccines that are immunogenic in early life (for additional information, see Chapter 38) [339]. Bacillus Calmette-Guérin (BCG), hepatitis B, and oral poliovirus vaccine are currently given to neonates within the first days of life in many low-income and middle-income countries. The BCG vaccine, developed early in the 20th century, is a live attenuated strain of *Mycobacterium bovis*. WHO promotes the use of BCG in newborns to prevent tuberculosis, and this vaccine is widely used in developing countries in which tuberculosis is a common and potentially lethal disease. Although approximately 3 billion doses have been given, the efficacy of this vaccine is still debated. Vaccine efficacy in many prospective trials and case-control studies of vaccine use at all ages ranges from possibly harmful to 90% protective [340].

One meta-analysis of BCG studies in newborns and infants concluded that the vaccine was effective and reduced infection in children by more than 50% [341]. It was estimated that the 100 million BCG vaccinations given to infants in 2002 prevented nearly 30,000 cases of tuberculous meningitis (5th to 95th centiles, 24,063 to 36,192) in children during their first 5 years of life, or 1 case for every 3435 vaccinations (2771 to 4177), and 11,486 cases of miliary tuberculosis (7304 to 16,280), or 1 case for every 9314 vaccinations (6172 to 13,729) [342]. At a cost of US$2 to 3 per dose, BCG vaccination costs US$206 (US$150 to 272) per year of healthy life gained, considered highly cost-effective. BCG reduced the risk of pulmonary tuberculosis, tuberculosis meningitis, disseminated tuberculosis, and

death from tuberculosis. Factors that may explain the variability of responses to BCG vaccination in different studies and populations include use of a wide variety of vaccine preparations, regional differences in environmental flora that may alter vaccine response, and population differences [323]. The safety of BCG in immunocompromised patients (e.g., patients with HIV infection) is of significant concern, and WHO has now made HIV infection in infants a full contraindication to BCG vaccination [343].

Hepatitis B vaccination of newborns has proved that neonatal immunization can prevent neonatal infections and their sequelae [344]. Studies from developed and developing countries have shown that hepatitis B vaccine administered in the immediate newborn period can significantly reduce the rate of neonatal infection and the development of a chronic hepatitis B surface antigen (HBsAg) carrier state [345]. The efficacy of vaccine alone (without hepatitis B immunoglobulin) has allowed developing countries that cannot screen pregnant women and do not have hepatitis B immunoglobulin to make a major impact in reducing the infection of newborns. WHO recommends that all countries include hepatitis B vaccine in their routine childhood immunization programs [346].

With the global problem of increasing antibiotic resistance, maternal and neonatal immunization have become even more important strategies to pursue. In low-income and middle-income countries, issues of vaccine cost, availability, and efficacy in the field are particularly pressing and are major barriers to the use of vaccines that are known to be safe and effective. Global Alliance for Vaccines and Immunisation (GAVI), established in 1999 with funding from the Bill and Melinda Gates Foundation, is working to address these issues. Since 2000, more than 200 million children have been immunized with vaccines funded by GAVI, and more than 3.4 million premature deaths have been averted [347].

ANTENATAL CARE AND PREVENTION OF NEONATAL INFECTION

The care and general well-being of the mother are inextricably linked to the health of her newborn. Antenatal care can play an important role in the prevention or reduction of neonatal infections [348]. Preventive and curative interventions directed toward the mother can have beneficial effects on the fetus and newborn. Tetanus immunization of the pregnant woman is an essential component of any developing country's antenatal care program and, as discussed earlier, prevents neonatal tetanus [349,350]. The diagnosis and treatment of STDs—especially syphilis, gonorrhea, and chlamydial infection—can have a significant impact on neonatal morbidity and mortality [351,352]. In areas of the world in which syphilis is endemic, congenital syphilis may be an important cause of neonatal morbidity and mortality [353]. Antenatal treatment of gonorrhea and chlamydial infection can prevent neonatal infection with these agents—ophthalmia neonatorum (for gonorrhea and chlamydial infection), disseminated gonorrhea, and neonatal respiratory disease (for chlamydial infection) [351,352]. STDs and maternal urinary tract infection increase the mother's risk of puerperal sepsis, with its associated increased risk of neonatal sepsis. In malaria-endemic areas, treatment of maternal malaria can have an impact on newborn health, particularly through a reduction in the incidence of LBW [354].

Antenatal care also is an important setting for maternal education regarding danger signs during pregnancy, labor, and delivery—especially maternal fever, prolonged or premature rupture of the membranes, and prolonged labor—and danger signs to watch for in the newborn. It is the time and place for the mother to plan where and by whom she will be delivered and for the health care worker to stress the importance of a clean delivery, preferably with a skilled birth attendant.

INTRAPARTUM AND DELIVERY CARE AND PREVENTION OF NEONATAL INFECTION

It is universally recognized that poor aseptic techniques during labor and delivery, including performing procedures with unclean hands and unclean instruments and unhygienic cutting of the umbilical cord, are major risk factors for maternal and neonatal infections [348]. It is essential to promote safe and hygienic practices at every level of the health care system where women deliver (home, first-level health clinic, district or referral hospital). Proper management of labor and delivery can have a significant impact on the prevention of neonatal infection. It is important to emphasize the need for clean hands; clean perineum; clean delivery surface; clean instruments; clean cord care; avoidance of harmful traditional practices; prevention of unnecessary vaginal examinations; prevention of prolonged labor; and optimal management of pregnancy complications including prolonged rupture of the membranes, maternal fever, and chorioamnionitis or puerperal sepsis [355].

POSTNATAL CARE AND PREVENTION OF NEONATAL INFECTION

The birth attendant is responsible for observation of the newborn at and after birth and deciding that the newborn is healthy and ready to be "discharged" to the care of the mother. It is important to link postpartum care of the mother with surveillance and care of the newborn. Postnatal visits should be used for health education and negotiation of improved household practices and to detect and treat the sick newborn and to evaluate the mother. Birth attendants need to be trained to identify problems in the newborn, to treat simple problems (e.g., skin infections), and to refer newborns with conditions that are potentially life-threatening (e.g., suspected sepsis). Birth attendants should provide all new mothers with breast-feeding support and give advice regarding personal hygiene and cleanliness and other prevention strategies, such as clean cord care, thermal care, and immunization. Improvement in domestic hygiene should be encouraged, including sanitary disposal of wastes, use of clean water, and hand washing, so that the newborn enters a clean home and is less likely to encounter pathogenic organisms. Community interventions need to be designed and modified to meet the needs of mothers and newborns in different settings in different countries with varying policies on the role of frontline workers in the recognition and management of infections.

Despite its importance, postnatal care is one of the most neglected aspects of maternal and newborn care in low-income and middle-income countries. Although numerous simple, low-cost preventive interventions are available that can avert a substantial proportion of deaths attributed to infections—including immediate and exclusive breast-feeding, thermal care, hand washing, clean cord care, and skin-to-skin care [8,10,12,15]—few data are available on coverage with postnatal care (i.e., a postnatal visit with a health care provider within 2 days of delivery). In 12 African countries, more recent Demographic Health Survey data indicated that less than 10% of newborns, on average, received an early postnatal care visit [356].

The importance of early postnatal care was highlighted in a study in Sylhet, Bangladesh, where, overall, a 34% reduction (95% CI 7% to 53%) in neonatal mortality was achieved through implementation of maternal and neonatal interventions aimed primarily at prevention and treatment of infections delivered by community health workers through antenatal and postnatal home visits [357]. Further analysis revealed, however, that a 64% reduction (95% CI 45% to 77%) in mortality was seen among the newborns who had an early postnatal home visit within the first 2 days of life, whereas no impact on mortality was found among the newborns who were visited only after the first 2 days [358]. Another study found that promotion of healthy, preventive household newborn care practices (e.g., birth preparedness, clean delivery, breast-feeding, clean cord and skin care, thermal care) through home visitation and community meetings by trained community health workers in a very high mortality setting in Uttar Pradesh, India, resulted in a 54% reduction (95% CI 40% to 65%) in all-cause neonatal mortality [359]. Serious infections seemed to be the most important cause of death that was averted.

BREAST-FEEDING

The promotion of early and exclusive breast-feeding is one of the most important interventions for the maintenance of newborn health and the promotion of optimal growth and development [355]. Breast-feeding is especially important in developing countries, where safe alternatives to breast milk are often unavailable or too expensive. Poor hygiene and a lack of clean water and clean feeding utensils make artificial formula a significant vehicle for the transmission of infection. Breast milk has many unique anti-infective factors, including secretory IgA antibodies, lysozyme, and lactoferrin (for additional information, see Chapter 5). In addition, breast milk is rich in receptor analogues for certain epithelial structures that microorganisms need for attachment to host tissues, an initial step in infection [360]. Many studies have shown that breast-feeding reduces the risk of infectious diseases, including neonatal sepsis, diarrhea, and possibly respiratory tract infection [361–366], and that breast-feeding protects against infection-related neonatal and infant mortality [8,10,367–370].

The HIV epidemic has raised questions about the safety of breast-feeding in areas in which there is a high prevalence of HIV infection among lactating women [371–381]. HIV can be transmitted through breast-feeding. A major question for any setting is whether the benefits of breast-feeding outweigh the risk of postnatal transmission of HIV through breast milk [373]. For many areas of the world, where infectious diseases, especially diarrheal diseases, are a primary cause of infant death, breast-feeding, even when the mother is HIV-infected, remains the safest mode of infant feeding. As noted earlier, all HIV-infected mothers should be counseled, however, about the risks and benefits of feeding options and supported in their choice.

MANAGEMENT OF NEONATAL INFECTION

If the mother develops a puerperal infection, the newborn requires special attention and should be treated for presumed sepsis [348]. Prolonged rupture of the membranes, maternal fever during labor, and chorioamnionitis are particular risk factors for early-onset neonatal sepsis and pneumonia [382–384]. Ideally, high-risk infants who are born at home should be referred to the nearest health care facility for observation and antibiotic therapy. In practice, this referral may be either impossible or unacceptable to the family, as evidenced by high rates of noncompliance with referral in many settings [27,357,359], and ways to deliver care to the mother and the newborn in the home must be developed and evaluated.

IDENTIFICATION OF NEONATES WITH INFECTION

If untreated, infections in newborns can rapidly become severe and life-threatening. Early identification and appropriate treatment of newborns with infection are crucial to survival. In low-income and middle-income countries, where access to care may be limited, diagnosis and treatment are particularly difficult. Maternal and neonatal factors that increase risk of infection in the newborn must be recognized. These factors include maternal infections during pregnancy (STDs, urinary tract infection, others); premature or prolonged rupture of membranes; prolonged labor; fever during labor; unhygienic obstetric practices or cord care; poor hand-washing practices; prematurity or LBW; artificial feeding; and generally unhygienic living conditions [316,317,320].

In areas without sophisticated technology and the diagnostic help of laboratory tests and radiographic studies, treatment decisions must be made on the basis of the history and findings on physical examination. The WHO Young Infants Study was designed to identify clinical predictors of serious neonatal infections; this study enrolled more than 3000 sick infants younger than 2 months of age who presented to health facilities in Ethiopia, The Gambia, Papua New Guinea, and the Philippines [385]. In multivariable analysis, 14 signs were independent predictors of severe disease: reduced feeding ability, absence of spontaneous movement, temperature greater than 38° C, drowsiness or unconsciousness, a history of a feeding problem or change in activity, state of agitation, the presence of lower chest indrawing (retractions), respiratory rate greater than 60/min, grunting, cyanosis, a history of convulsions, a bulging fontanelle, and slow digital capillary refill. The presence of any one of these signs had a sensitivity for severe disease (sepsis, meningitis, hypoxemia, or radiologically proven pneumonia) of 87% and a specificity of 54%; reducing the list to nine signs reduced sensitivity only slightly (83%), but significantly improved specificity (62%) [385].

More recently, 8899 young infants who presented to health facilities in six countries (India, Bangladesh, Pakistan, Ghana, South Africa, Bolivia) with a complaint of illness were enrolled in a second Young Infant Clinical Signs Study. Seven signs were found to be associated with severe illness requiring referral level care in the first week of life: history of difficulty feeding, history of convulsions, movement only when stimulated, respiratory rate of 60 breaths/min or more, severe chest indrawing, and temperature of 37.5° C or greater or less than 35.5° C. These signs had a sensitivity and specificity of 85% and 75% in infants less than 1 week old. Studies in Bangladesh have sought to validate the ability of community health workers to use the clinical signs recommended by the WHO Young Infant Studies during routine household surveillance to identify neonates needing referral level care.

In Sylhet, 288 newborns were assessed independently for the presence of clinical signs suggestive of very severe disease by community health workers and by study physicians. Compared with the physician's gold standard assessment, community health workers correctly classified very severe disease in newborns with a sensitivity of 91%, specificity of 95%, and kappa value of 0.85 (P < .001) [386]. In Mirzapur, Bangladesh, classification of very severe disease by community health workers showed a sensitivity of 73%, a specificity of 98%, a positive predictive value of 57%, and a negative predictive value of 99% [387]. In addition to clinical signs, community health workers gathered historical information on neonatal illness. A history of a feeding problem, as reported by the mother to a physician, was significantly associated with the presence of a severe feeding problem (particularly a lack of ability to suck) as assessed by community health workers. Because assessing breast-feeding is complex, time-consuming, and difficult for male physicians owing to cultural sensitivity, a reported history may substitute for an observed feeding problem in the algorithm, substantially simplifying the assessment. Trained and supervised community health workers seem to be able to use a diagnostic algorithm to identify severely ill newborns with high validity.

ANTIBIOTIC TREATMENT OF NEONATES WITH INFECTION

The drugs most frequently used at present to treat suspected severe neonatal infections are a combination of penicillin or ampicillin and an aminoglycoside (usually gentamicin) [388]. WHO continues to recommend that young infants (from birth to 2 months of age) with signs of severe infection should be referred for inpatient care and treated with intravenous broad-spectrum antibiotics—a combination of a benzyl penicillin and an aminoglycoside such as gentamicin for 10 to 14 days.

If 90% of neonates with infections received timely and appropriate antibiotic therapy, it is estimated that 30% to 70% of global neonatal deaths attributed to infections could be averted [10]. Most infants with suspected serious infections in developing countries do not currently receive adequate treatment, however; inpatient care is not feasible for most families either because treatment is available only in tertiary care facilities that are inaccessible or because hospitalization is unaffordable or unacceptable to families [27,357]. In many settings, placement and management of an intravenous line is impossible, and parenteral antibiotic therapy must be delivered by intramuscular injections. In this context, extended-interval gentamicin regimens have been recommended as the preferred mode of aminoglycoside dosing [389–391], and evidence is accumulating that procaine penicillin may be a feasible alternative to multiple daily dosing regimens with ampicillin [392].

Eliminating the need for multiple daily contacts with the patient to deliver antibiotics makes it more feasible for frontline workers in settings with low resources potentially to treat neonates with suspected infections, either at peripheral health facilities or possibly even in the home [392]. Further efforts are under way to identify even simpler antibiotic treatment regimens that require fewer injections over the course of treatment. Antibiotics available for treatment of serious neonatal infections in developing countries have been reviewed more recently [393,394].

Ideally, antibiotic therapy should be tailored to the specific microbiologic needs of a particular patient or, if patient-level data are unavailable, for the geographic region based on local surveillance data, especially if blood cultures are not performed and cannot be used to guide therapy, as is the case in most low-income and middle-income countries. In reality, surveillance data also are generally unavailable, however. In addition, issues related to drug supply, availability, quality, and cost must be addressed. The problem of antibiotic resistance is now recognized to be a global problem, and the emergence of antibiotic-resistant pathogens is particularly alarming in hospitals in countries with low resources. The widespread availability of antibiotics in many low-income and middle-income countries, even directly to families outside contact with the formal health system, and indiscriminate and inappropriate antibiotic use in the health and agriculture sectors contribute to this problem.

Appropriate treatment of neonatal infections is one of the most important child survival interventions [10]. In areas where it is impossible to deliver parenteral antibiotic therapy in a health facility, community-based case management is emerging as a viable alternative to facility-based care [10–12,27,357,386,387,395–399]. More recent data suggest that well-trained and supervised primary health care workers, including community health workers conducting routine household surveillance, are capable of identifying and treating sick newborns [386,387,400]. In a pooled analysis of five controlled trials of community-based management of neonatal pneumonia (four using co-trimoxazole, one using ampicillin or penicillin), all-cause neonatal mortality was reduced by 27% (95% CI 18% to 35%), and pneumonia-specific mortality was reduced by 42% (95% CI 22% to 57%) [401]. A 62% reduction in neonatal mortality was also shown in a non-randomized controlled study in rural Maharashtra, India, in which village health workers conducted home visits and identified and treated neonates with suspected serious infections with a combination of oral co-trimoxazole and injectable gentamicin. CFR declined from 16.6% before the intervention to 2.8% after the intervention ($P < .05$).

Similarly, in a cluster randomized controlled trial in rural Sylhet, Bangladesh, community health workers identified sick newborns and referred them to a health facility for treatment. If the family refused referral, the community health workers provided treatment in the home with injectable procaine penicillin and gentamicin, resulting in a 34% reduction (95% CI 7% to 53%) in neonatal mortality compared with the control arm where the usual services of the Government of Bangladesh and various private providers were available. In Sylhet, although only 32% of referrals of sick newborns to the hospital by community health workers were complied with, another 42% accepted injectable antibiotic treatment at home, indicating that with the addition of home-based treatment, approximately three fourths of sick neonates received curative antibiotic treatment from qualified providers or community health workers. CFR for treatment of neonates with suspected serious infections was 14.2% at health facilities and 4.4% in the hands of the community health workers. After controlling for differences in background characteristics and illness signs among treatment groups, newborns treated by community health workers had a hazard ratio of 0.22 (95% CI 0.07 to 0.71) for death during the neonatal period and newborns treated by qualified providers had a hazard ratio of 0.61 (95% CI 0.37 to 0.99) compared with newborns who received no treatment or were treated by untrained providers [392].

INTEGRATED MANAGEMENT OF NEONATAL ILLNESS

An integrated approach to the sick child, including the young infant, has been developed by WHO and UNICEF [402]. This strategy promotes prompt recognition of disease, appropriate therapy using standardized case management, referral of serious cases, and prevention through improved nutrition (breast-feeding of the neonate), and immunization. This approach stresses diagnosis using simple clinical signs, defined through the Young Infant Clinical Signs Studies, that can be taught to health care workers at all levels. The health care worker assesses the infant by questioning the mother and examining the infant; classifies the illness as serious or not; and determines if the infant needs urgent treatment and referral, specific treatment and advice, or only simple advice and home management. The importance of breast-feeding is stressed, and follow-up instructions are given. All young infants are checked for specific danger signs that equate with need for emergency care and urgent referral. Because the signs of serious bacterial infection in the newborn are not easily recognized, every young infant with danger signs is given treatment for a possible bacterial infection.

MATERNAL EDUCATION AND SOCIOECONOMIC STATUS

Maternal education, literacy, and overall socioeconomic status are powerful influences on the health of the mother and the newborn [403–406]. Education of girls must be promoted and expanded so that women of reproductive age know enough to seek preventive services, understand the implications of danger signs during labor and delivery and in their newborns, and recognize that they must obtain referral care for obstetric or newborn complications. Improvements in education and socioeconomic status are linked. They may affect child health by allowing the mother a greater voice in the family with greater decision-making power, making her better informed about domestic hygiene, disease prevention, or disease recognition, or enhancing her ability to seek medical attention outside the home and to comply with medical advice.

CONCLUSION

Neonatal infections cause a massive burden of mortality and morbidity, most of which occur in low-income and middle-income countries in settings characterized by high-risk household practices, poor care seeking and access to quality care, and weak health systems. Surveillance for infections is lacking, but limited data indicate that antibiotic resistance is increasing. Many preventive and curative interventions are available, however, which if implemented effectively at large scale could avert most neonatal deaths around the world secondary to serious infections. Development of new and adapted tools and technologies holds promise for expanding the availability and impact of interventions to prevent deaths secondary to infections. Implementation challenges continue to limit coverage with interventions, however. Renewed commitment is needed to deliver evidence-based interventions at the community level and at health facilities, integrated with maternal and child health programs.

ACKNOWLEDGMENTS

The authors are grateful to Dr. Rachel Haws for her excellent assistance with article references and editing of the chapter.

REFERENCES

[1] R.E. Black, S.S. Morris, J. Bryce, Where and why are 10 million children dying every year? Lancet 361 (2003) 2226–2234.

[2] J. Bryce, et al., Reducing child mortality: can public health deliver? Lancet 362 (2003) 159–164.

[3] J.E. Lawn, S. Cousens, J. Zupan, 4 million neonatal deaths. When? Where? Why? Lancet 365 (2005) 891–900.

[4] K.J. Kerber, et al., Continuum of care for maternal, newborn, and child health: from slogan to service delivery, Lancet 370 (2007) 1358–1369.

[5] J.E. Lawn, et al., Two million intrapartum-related stillbirths and neonatal deaths. Where, why, and what can be done, Int. J. Gynaecol. Obstet. 28 (2009) 28.

[6] Z.A. Bhutta, et al., What works? Interventions for maternal and child under-nutrition and survival, Lancet 371 (2008) 417–440.

[7] A.H. Baqui, et al., Rates, timing and causes of neonatal deaths in rural India: implications for neonatal health programmes, Bull. World Health Organ. 84 (2006) 706–713.

[8] T. Adam, et al., Cost effectiveness analysis of strategies for maternal and neonatal health in developing countries, BMJ 331 (2005) 1107.

[9] Z.A. Bhutta, et al., Management of newborn infections in primary care settings. A review of the evidence and implications for policy, Pediatr. Infect. Dis. J. 28 (Suppl. 5) (2009) S22–S30.

[10] G.L. Darmstadt, et al., Evidence-based, cost-effective interventions. How many newborn babies can we save, Lancet 365 (2005) 977–988.

[11] G.L. Darmstadt, R.E. Black, M. Santosham, Research priorities and postpartum care strategies for the prevention and optimal management of neonatal infections in less developed countries, Pediatr. Infect. Dis. J. 19 (2000) 739–750.

[12] G.L. Darmstadt, et al., Saving newborn lives in Asia and Africa: cost and impact of phased scale-up of interventions within the continuum of care, Health Policy Plan. 23 (2008) 101–117.

[13] D. Thaver, A.K. Zaidi, Burden of neonatal infections in developing countries: a review of evidence from community-based studies, Pediatr. Infect. Dis. J. 28 (Suppl. 1) (2009) S3–S9.

[14] J.E. Lawn, K. Wilczynska-Ketende, S.N. Cousens, Estimating the causes of 4 million neonatal deaths in the year 2000, Int. J. Epidemiol. 35 (2006) 706–718.

[15] Z.A. Bhutta, et al., Alma-Ata: Rebirth and Revision 6 Interventions to address maternal, newborn, and child survival. What difference can integrated primary health care strategies make, Lancet 372 (2008) 972–989.

[16] E.A. Adejuyigbe, et al., Septicaemia in high risk neonates at a teaching hospital in Ile-Ife, Nigeria, East Afr. Med. J. 78 (2001) 540–543.

[17] M. Adhikari, Y.M. Coovadia, D. Singh, A 4-year study of neonatal meningitis: clinical and microbiological findings, J. Trop. Pediatr. 41 (1995) 81–85.

[18] C.G. Aiken, The causes of perinatal mortality in Bulawayo, Zimbabwe, Cent. Afr. J. Med. 38 (1992) 263–281.

[19] A.I. Airede, Neonatal septicaemia in an African city of high altitude, J. Trop. Pediatr. 38 (1992) 189–191.

[20] A.I. Airede, Neonatal bacterial meningitis in the middle belt of Nigeria, Dev. Med. Child Neurol. 35 (1993) 424–430.

[21] E.J. Al-Zwaini, Neonatal septicaemia in the neonatal care unit, Al-Anbar governorate, Iraq, East. Mediterr. Health J. 8 (2002) 509–514.

[22] Z. Ali, Neonatal meningitis: a 3-year retrospective study at the Mount Hope Women's Hospital, Trinidad, West Indies, J. Trop. Pediatr. 41 (1995) 109–111.

[23] Z. Ali, Neonatal bacterial septicaemia at the Mount Hope Women's Hospital, Trinidad, Ann. Trop. Paediatr. 24 (2004) 41–44.

[24] M. Anyebuno, M. Newman, Common causes of neonatal bacteraemia in Accra, Ghana, East Afr. Med. J. 72 (1995) 805–808.

[25] B. Aurangzeb, A. Hameed, Neonatal sepsis in hospital-born babies: bacterial isolates and antibiotic susceptibility patterns, J. Coll. Physicians Surg. Pak. 13 (2003) 629–632.

[26] A.T. Bang, et al., Burden of morbidities and the unmet need for health care in rural neonates—a prospective observational study in Gadchiroli, India, Indian Pediatr. 38 (2001) 952–965.

[27] A.T. Bang, et al., Effect of home-based neonatal care and management of sepsis on neonatal mortality: field trial in rural India, Lancet 354 (1999) 1955–1961.

[28] A.T. Bang, et al., Is home-based diagnosis and treatment of neonatal sepsis feasible and effective? Seven years of intervention in the Gadchiroli field trial (1996 to 2003), J. Perinatol. 25 (Suppl. 1) (2005) S62–S71.

[29] Y. Bell, et al., Neonatal sepsis in Jamaican neonates, Ann. Trop. Paediatr. 25 (2005) 293–296.

[30] J.A. Berkley, et al., Bacteremia among children admitted to a rural hospital in Kenya, N. Engl. J. Med. 352 (2005) 39–47.

[31] Z.A. Bhutta, et al., Neonatal sepsis in Pakistan: presentation and pathogens, Acta. Paediatr. Scand. 80 (1991) 596–601.

[32] Z.A. Bhutta, K. Yusuf, Neonatal sepsis in Karachi: factors determining outcome and mortality, J. Trop. Pediatr. 43 (1997) 65–70.

[33] N.Y. Boo, C.Y. Chor, Six year trend of neonatal septicaemia in a large Malaysian maternity hospital, J. Paediatr. Child Health 30 (1994) 23–27.

[34] G. Campagne, et al., Epidemiology of bacterial meningitis in Niamey, Niger, 1981–96, Bull. World Health Organ. 77 (1999) 499–508.

[35] B. Chacko, I. Sohi, Early onset neonatal sepsis, Indian J. Pediatr. 72 (2005) 23–26.

[36] T. Chotpitayasunondh, Bacterial meningitis in children: etiology and clinical features, an 11-year review of 618 cases, Southeast Asian J. Trop. Med. Public Health 25 (1994) 107–115.

[37] K. Chugh, et al., Bacteriological profile of neonatal septicemia, Indian J. Pediatr. 55 (1988) 961–965.

[38] Y.M. Coovadia, et al., Hospital-acquired neonatal bacterial meningitis: the impacts of cefotaxime usage on mortality and of amikacin usage on incidence, Ann. Trop. Paediatr. 9 (1989) 233–239.

[39] A.S. Daoud, et al., The changing face of neonatal septicaemia, Ann. Trop. Paediatr. 15 (1995) 93–96.

[40] A.S. Daoud, et al., Neonatal meningitis in northern Jordan, J. Trop. Pediatr. 42 (1996) 267–270.

[41] G.L. Darmstadt, et al., Population-based incidence and etiology of community-acquired neonatal bacteremia in Mirzapur, Bangladesh: an observational study, J. Infect. Dis. 200 (2009) 906–915.

[42] P.K. Das, et al., Clinical and bacteriological profile of neonatal infections in metropolitan city based medical college nursery, J. Indian Med. Assoc. 97 (1999) 3–5.

[43] P.K. Das, et al., Early neonatal morbidity and mortality in a city based medical college nursery, Indian J. Public Health 42 (1998) 9–14.

[44] A. Dawodu, K. al Umran, K. Twum-Danso, A case control study of neonatal sepsis: experience from Saudi Arabia, J. Trop. Pediatr. 43 (1997) 84–88.

[45] A.H. Dawodu, C.E. Effiong, Neonatal morbidity and mortality among Nigerian infants in a special-care baby unit, East Afr. Med. J. 60 (1983) 39–45.

[46] A.Y. Elzouki, T. Vesikari, First international conference on infections in children in Arab countries, Pediatr. Infect. Dis. 4 (1985) 527–531.

[47] M. English, et al., Signs of illness in Kenyan infants aged less than 60 days, Bull. World Health Organ. 82 (2004) 323–329.

[48] S.J. Etuk, et al., Perinatal outcome in pregnancies booked for antenatal care but delivered outside health facilities in Calabar, Nigeria, Acta Trop. 75 (2000) 29–33.

[49] A. Gebremariam, Neonatal meningitis in Addis Ababa: a 10-year review, Ann. Trop. Paediatr. 18 (1998) 279–283.

[50] B. Ghiorghis, Neonatal sepsis in Addis Ababa, Ethiopia: a review of 151 bacteremic neonates, Ethiop. Med. J. 35 (1997) 169–176.

[51] D. Greenberg, et al., A prospective study of neonatal sepsis and meningitis in southern Israel, Pediatr. Infect Dis. J. 16 (1997) 768–773.

[52] P. Gupta, et al., Clinical profile of *Klebsiella* septicemia in neonates, Indian J. Pediatr. 60 (1993) 565–572.

[53] I.E. Haffejee, et al., Neonatal group B streptococcal infections in Indian (Asian) babies in South Africa, J. Infect. 22 (1991) 225–231.

[54] K.N. Haque, A.H. Chagia, M.M. Shaheed, Half a decade of neonatal sepsis, Riyadh, Saudi Arabia, J. Trop. Pediatr 36 (1990) 20–23.

[55] I. Kago, et al., Neonatal septicemia and meningitis caused by gram-negative bacilli in Yaonde: clinical, bacteriological and prognostic aspects, Bull. Soc. Pathol. Exot. 84 (5 Pt 5) (1991) 573–581.

[56] G. Karthikeyan, K. Premkumar, Neonatal sepsis: *Staphylococcus aureus* as the predominant pathogen, Indian J. Pediatr. 68 (2001) 715–717.

[57] K.A. Karunasekera, D.R. Jayawardena, N.P. Chandra, The use of commercially prepared 10% dextrose reduces the incidence of neonatal septicaemia, Ceylon Med. J. 42 (1997) 207–208.

[58] S.L. Kaushik, et al., Neonatal sepsis in hospital born babies, J. Commun. Dis. 30 (1998) 147–152.

[59] S.P. Khatua, et al., Neonatal septicemia, Indian J. Pediatr. 53 (1986) 509–514.

[60] A. Koutouby, J. Habibullah, Neonatal sepsis in Dubai, United Arab Emirates, J. Trop. Pediatr. 41 (1995) 177–180.

[61] A. Kuruvilla, Neonatal septicaemia in Kuwait, J. Kuwait Med. Assoc. 14 (1980) 225–231.

[62] K.A. Kuruvilla, et al., Bacterial profile of sepsis in a neonatal unit in south India, Indian Pediatr. 35 (1998) 851–858.

[63] E. Leibovitz, et al., Sepsis at a neonatal intensive care unit: a four-year retrospective study (1989–1992), Isr. J. Med. Sci. 33 (1997) 734–738.

[64] N.L. Lim, et al., Bacteraemic infections in a neonatal intensive care unit—a nine-month survey, Med. J. Malaysia 50 (1995) 59–63.

[65] A.C. Longe, J.A. Omene, A.A. Okolo, Neonatal meningitis in Nigerian infants, Acta Paediatr. Scand. 73 (1984) 477–481.

[66] E. Mansour, et al., Morbidity and mortality of low-birth-weight infants in Egypt, East. Mediterr. Health J. 11 (2005) 723–731.

[67] N. Modi, C. Kirubakaran, Reasons for admission, causes of death and costs of admission to a tertiary referral neonatal unit in India, J. Trop. Pediatr. 41 (1995) 99–102.

[68] A.O. Mokuolu, N. Jiya, O.O. Adesiyun, Neonatal septicaemia in Ilorin: bacterial pathogens and antibiotic sensitivity pattern, Afr. J. Med. Sci. 31 (2002) 127–130.

[69] G.P. Mondal, et al., Neonatal septicaemia among inborn and outborn babies in a referral hospital, Indian J. Pediatr. 58 (1991) 529–533.

[70] M.T. Moreno, et al., Neonatal sepsis and meningitis in a developing Latin American country, Pediatr. Infect. Dis. J. 13 (1994) 516–520.

[71] L. Muhe, et al., Etiology of pneumonia, sepsis and meningitis in infants younger than three months of age in Ethiopia, Pediatr. Infect. Dis. J. 18 (Suppl. 10) (1999) S56–S61.

[72] U.K. Namdeo, et al., Bacteriological profile of neonatal septicemia, Indian Pediatr. 24 (1987) 53–56.

[73] K.J. Nathoo, P.R. Mason, T.H. Chimbira, Neonatal septicaemia in Harare Hospital: aetiology and risk factors. The Puerperal Sepsis Study Group, Cent. Afr. J. Med. 36 (1990) 150–156.

[74] K.J. Nathoo, et al., Neonatal meningitis in Harare, Zimbabwe: a 2-year review, Ann. Trop. Paediatr. 11 (1991) 11–15.

[75] E. Nel, Neonatal meningitis: mortality, cerebrospinal fluid, and microbiological findings, J. Trop. Pediatr. 46 (2000) 237–239.

[76] A. Ohlsson, T. Bailey, F. Takieddine, Changing etiology and outcome of neonatal septicaemia in Riyadh, Saudi Arabia, Acta Paediatr. Scand. 75 (1986) 540–544.

[77] A. Ohlsson, F. Serenius, Neonatal septicaemia in Riyadh, Saudi Arabia, Acta Paediatr. Scand. 70 (1981) 825–829.

[78] A.A. Okolo, J.A. Omene, Changing pattern of neonatal septicaemia in an African city, Ann. Trop. Paediatr. 5 (1985) 123–126.

[79] J.A. Owa, O. Olusanya, Neonatal bacteraemia in Wesley Guild Hospital, Ilesha, Nigeria, Ann. Trop. Paediatr. 8 (1988) 80–84.

[80] W. Prasertsom, et al., Early versus late onset neonatal septicemia at Children's Hospital, J. Med. Assoc. Thai. 73 (1990) 106–110.

[81] A. Rajab, J. De Louvois, Survey of infection in babies at the Khoula Hospital, Oman, Ann. Trop. Paediatr. 10 (1990) 39–43.

[82] P.Y. Robillard, et al., Neonatal bacterial septicemia in a tropical area: four-year experience in Guadeloupe (French West Indies), Acta Paediatr. 82 (1993) 687–689.

[83] P.Y. Robillard, et al., Evaluation of neonatal sepsis screening in a tropical area, part I: major risk factors for bacterial carriage at birth in Guadeloupe, West Indian Med. J. 49 (2000) 312–315.

[84] C.J. Rodriguez, et al., Neonatal sepsis: epidemiologic indicators and relation to birth weight and length of hospitalization time, An. Esp. Pediatr. 48 (1998) 401–408.

[85] S. Saxena, et al., Bacterial infections among home delivered neonates: clinical picture and bacteriological profile, Indian Pediatr. 17 (1980) 17–24.

[86] P.P. Sharma, et al., Bacteriological profile of neonatal septicemia, Indian Pediatr. 24 (1987) 1011–1017.

[87] N. Sinha, A. Deb, A.K. Mukherjee, Septicemia in neonates and early infancy, Indian J. Pediatr. 53 (1986) 249–256.

[88] N. Tafari, A. Ljungh-Wadstrom, Consequences of amniotic fluid infections: early neonatal septicaemia, Ciba Foundation Symposium, Amsterdam, 1979, pp. 55–67.

[89] S.S. Tallur, et al., Clinico-bacteriological study of neonatal septicemia in Hubli, Indian J. Pediatr. 67 (2000) 169–174.

[90] N.A. Wong, L.P. Hunt, N. Marlow, Risk factors for developing neonatal septicaemia at a Malaysian hospital, J. Trop. Pediatr. 43 (1997) 54–58.

[91] D. Yardi, S. Gaikwad, L. Deodhar, Incidence, mortality and bacteriological profile of septicemia in pediatric patients, Indian J. Pediatr. 51 (1984) 173–176.

[92] T.B. Hyde, et al., Trends in incidence and antimicrobial resistance of early-onset sepsis: population-based surveillance in San Francisco and Atlanta, Pediatrics 110 (2002) 690–695.

[93] A. Schuchat, et al., Risk factors and opportunities for prevention of early-onset neonatal sepsis: a multicenter case-control study, Pediatrics 105 (1 Pt 1) (2000) 21–26.

[94] The State of the World's Children 2009, UNICEF, New York, 2009.

[95] R. Bennett, et al., Changes in the incidence and spectrum of neonatal septicemia during a fifteen-year period, Acta Paediatr. Scand. 74 (1985) 687–690.

[96] I.M. Gladstone, et al., A ten-year review of neonatal sepsis and comparison with the previous fifty-year experience, Pediatr. Infect. Dis. J. 9 (1990) 819–825.

[97] A.K. Zaidi, et al., Pathogens associated with sepsis in newborns and young infants in developing countries, Pediatr. Infect. Dis. J. 28 (1 Suppl. 1) (2009) S10–S18.

[98] WHO Young Infants Study Group, The bacterial etiology of serious infections in young infants in developing countries—results of a multicenter study, Pediatr. Infect. Dis. J. (Suppl. 18) (1999) S17–S22.

[99] WHO Young Infants Study Group, Clinical prediction of serious bacterial infections in young infants in developing countries, Pediatr. Infect. Dis. J. (Suppl. 18) (1999) S23–S31.

[100] WHO Young Infants Study Group, Conclusions from the WHO multicenter study of serious infections in young infants, Pediatr. Infect. Dis. J. (Suppl. 18) (1999) S32–S34.

[101] S.R. Gatchalian, et al., Bacterial and viral etiology of serious infections in very young Filipino infants, Pediatr. Infect. Dis. J. (Suppl. 18) (1999) S50–S55.

[102] D. Lehmann, et al., The bacterial and viral etiology of severe infection in children aged less than three months in the highlands of Papua New Guinea, Pediatr. Infect. Dis. J. (Suppl. 18) (1999) S42–S49.

[103] D. Lehmann, et al., High rates of *Chlamydia trachomatis* infections in young Papua New Guinean infants, Pediatr. Infect. Dis. J. (Suppl. 18) (1999) S62–S69.

[104] E.K. Mulholland, et al., Etiology of serious infections in young Gambian infants, Pediatr. Infect. Dis. J. (Suppl 18) S35–S41.

[105] M.R. Moore, S.J. Schrag, A. Schuchat, Effects of intrapartum antimicrobial prophylaxis for prevention of group-B-streptococcal disease on the incidence and ecology of early-onset neonatal sepsis, Lancet 3 (2003) 201–213.

[106] Centers for Disease Control and Prevention, Prevention of perinatal group B streptococcal disease. Revised Guidelines from CDC, MMWR. Morb. Mortal. Wkly. Rep. 51 (2002) 1–22.

[107] B.J. Stoll, A. Schuchat, Maternal carriage of group B streptococci in developing countries, Pediatr. Infect. Dis. J. 17 (1998) 499–503.

[108] H.M. Blumberg, et al., Invasive group B streptococcal disease: the emergence of serotype V, J. Infect. Dis. 173 (1996) 365–373.

[109] T.S. Collins, et al., Group B streptococcal colonization in a developing country: its association with sexually transmitted disease and socioeconomic factors, Am. J. Trop. Med. 59 (1998) 633–636.

[110] R.O. Suara, et al., Carriage of group B streptococci in pregnant Gambian mothers and their infants, J. Infect. Dis. 70 (1994) 1316–1319.

[111] J.A. Regan, et al., Colonization with group B streptococci in pregnancy and adverse outcome. VIP Study Group, Am. J. Obstet. Gynecol. 174 (1996) 1354–1360.

[112] D. Thaver, S.A. Ali, A.K. Zaidi, Antimicrobial resistance among neonatal pathogens in developing countries, Pediatr. Infect. Dis. J. 28 (Suppl. 1) (2009) S19–S21.

[113] Management of the child with a serious infection or severe malnutrition, Guidelines for care at the first-referral level in developing countries, World Health Organization, Geneva, 2000.

[114] A.K. Zaidi, et al., Hospital-acquired neonatal infections in developing countries, Lancet 365 (2005) 1175–1188.

[115] P.C. Chan, et al., Control of an outbreak of pandrug-resistant *Acinetobacter baumannii* colonization and infection in a neonatal intensive care unit, Infect. Control Hosp. Epidemiol. 28 (2007) 423–429.

[116] W. Zingg, K.M. Posfay-Barbe, D. Pittet, Healthcare-associated infections in neonates, Curr. Opin. Infect. Dis. 21 (2008) 228–234.

[117] S.M. Brown, et al., Use of an alcohol-based hand rub and quality improvement interventions to improve hand hygiene in a Russian neonatal intensive care unit, Infect. Control Hosp. Epidemiol. 24 (2003) 172–179.

[118] P.C. Ng, et al., Combined use of alcohol hand rub and gloves reduces the incidence of late onset infection in very low birthweight infants, Arch. Dis. Child. Fetal. Neonatal. Ed. 89 (2004) F336–F440.

[119] R.L. Goldenberg, et al., Use of vaginally administered chlorhexidine during labor to improve pregnancy outcomes, Obstet. Gynecol. 107 (2006) 1139–1146.

[120] E.M. McClure, et al., The use of chlorhexidine to reduce maternal and neonatal mortality and morbidity in low-resource settings, Int. J. Gynaecol. Obstet. 97 (2007) 89–94.

[121] L.C. Mullany, G.L. Darmstadt, J.M. Tielsch, Safety and impact of chlorhexidine antisepsis interventions for improving neonatal health in developing countries, Pediatr. Infect. Dis. J. 25 (2006) 665–675.

[122] T.E. Taha, et al., Effect of cleansing the birth canal with antiseptic solution on maternal and newborn morbidity and mortality in Malawi: clinical trial, BMJ 315 (1997) 216–219.

[123] A.F. Bakr, T. Karkour, Effect of predelivery vaginal antisepsis on maternal and neonatal morbidity and mortality in Egypt, J. Womens Health (Larchmt) 14 (2005) 496–501.

[124] C.L. Cutland, et al., Chlorhexidine maternal-vaginal and neonate body wipes in sepsis and vertical transmission of pathogenic bacteria in South Africa: a randomised, controlled trial, Lancet 19 (2009) 19.

[125] G.L. Darmstadt, et al., Topically applied sunflower seed oil prevents invasive bacterial infections in preterm infants in Egypt: a randomized, controlled clinical trial, Pediatr. Infect. Dis. J. 23 (2004) 719–725.

[126] G.L. Darmstadt, et al., Effect of topical treatment with skin barrier-enhancing emollients on nosocomial infections in preterm infants in Bangladesh: a randomised controlled trial, Lancet 365 (2005) 1039–1045.

[127] G.L. Darmstadt, et al., Effect of skin barrier therapy on neonatal mortality rates in preterm infants in Bangladesh: a randomized, controlled, clinical trial, Pediatrics 121 (2008) 522–529.

[128] E. Rhinehart, D.A. Goldmann, E.J. O'Rourke, Adaptation of the Centers for Disease Control guidelines for the prevention of nosocomial infection in a pediatric intensive care unit in Jakarta, Indonesia, Am. J. Med. 91 (1991) 213S–220S.

[129] M. Zaidi, M. Angulo, J. Sifuentes-Osornio, Disinfection and sterilization practices in Mexico, J. Hosp. Infect. 31 (1995) 25–32.

[130] D.E. Berg, et al., Control of nosocomial infections in an intensive care unit in Guatemala City, Clin. Infect. Dis. 21 (1995) 588–593.

[131] J. Webster, M.A. Pritchard, Gowning by attendants and visitors in newborn nurseries for prevention of neonatal morbidity and mortality, Cochrane Database Syst. Rev. (3) (2003) CD003670.

[132] G.L. Darmstadt, et al., Infection control practices reduce nosocomial infections and mortality in preterm infants in Bangladesh, J. Perinatol. 25 (2005) 331–335.

[133] S. Misra, et al., Clinical and bacteriological profile of neonatal pneumonia, Indian J. Med. Res. 93 (1991) 366–370.

[134] A.K. Patwari, et al., Aetiology of pneumonia in hospitalized children, J. Trop. Pediatr. 42 (1996) 15–19.

[135] A.S. Monto, Lehmann, Acute respiratory infections (ARI) in children: prospects for prevention, Vaccine 16 (1998) 1582–1588.

[136] D. Ploin, et al., Influenza burden in children newborn to eleven months of age in a pediatric emergency department during the peak of an influenza epidemic, Pediatr. Infect. Dis. J. 22 (2003) S218–S222.

[137] K. Zaman, et al., Acute respiratory infections in children: a community-based longitudinal study in rural Bangladesh, J. Trop. Pediatr. 43 (1997) 133–137.

[138] M. Garenne, C. Ronsmans, H. Campbell, The magnitude of mortality from acute respiratory infections in children under 5 years in developing countries, World Health Stat. Q. 45 (1992) 180–191.

[139] A.T. Bang, et al., Pneumonia in neonates: can it be managed in the community? Arch. Dis. Child. 68 (1993) 550–556.

[140] C.G. Victora, et al., Potential interventions for the prevention of childhood pneumonia in developing countries: improving nutrition, Am. J. Clin. Nutr. 70 (1999) 309–320.

[141] S. Arifeen, et al., Exclusive breastfeeding reduces acute respiratory infection and diarrhea deaths among infants in Dhaka slums, Pediatrics 108 (2001) e67.

[142] N. Datta, et al., Application of case management to the control of acute respiratory infections in low-birth-weight infants: a feasibility study, Bull. World Health Organ. 65 (1987) 77–82.

[143] Young Infants Clinical Signs Study Group, Clinical signs that predict severe illness in children under age 2 months: a multicentre study, Lancet 371 (2008) 135–142.

[144] C. Bern, et al., The magnitude of the global problem of diarrhoeal disease: a ten-year update, Bull. World Health Organ. 70 (1992) 705–714.

[145] J.D. Snyder, M.H. Merson, The magnitude of the global problem of acute diarrhoeal disease: a review of active surveillance data, Bull. World Health Organ. 60 (1982) 605–613.

[146] J. Golding, P.M. Emmett, I.S. Rogers, Gastroenteritis, diarrhoea and breast feeding, Early Hum. Dev. 49 (Suppl. l) (1997) S83–S103.

[147] S.R. Huttly, S.S. Morris, V. Pisani, Prevention of diarrhoea in young children in developing countries, Bull. World Health Organ. 75 (1997) 163–174.

[148] S. Huilan, et al., Etiology of acute diarrhoea among children in developing countries: a multicentre study in five countries, Bull. World Health Organ. 89 (1991) s49–s55.

[149] R.E. Black, et al., Incidence and etiology of infantile diarrhea and major routes of transmission in Huascar, Peru, Am. J. Epidemiol. 129 (1989) 785–799.

[150] A. Mahmud, et al., Early child health in Lahore, Pakistan, VII. diarrhoea, Acta Paediatr. Suppl. 390 (1993) 79–85.

[151] D.T. Aye, et al., Neonatal diarrhea at a maternity hospital in Rangoon, Am. J. Public Health 81 (1991) 480–481.

[152] F. Espinoza, et al., Rotavirus infections in young Nicaraguan children, Pediatr. Infect. Dis. J. 16 (1997) 564–571.

[153] U.D. Parashar, et al., Rotavirus, Emerg. Infect. Dis. 4 (1998) 1–10.

[154] I.E. Haffejee, The epidemiology of rotavirus infections: a global perspective, J. Pediatr. Gastroenterol. Nutr. 20 (1995) 275–286.

[155] M.K. Bhan, et al., Protection conferred by neonatal rotavirus infection against subsequent diarrhea, J. Infect. Dis. 168 (1993) 282–287.

[156] R.F. Bishop, et al., Clinical immunity after neonatal rotavirus infection: a prospective longitudinal study in young children, N. Engl. J. Med. 309 (1983) 72–76.

[157] T.K. Fischer, et al., Protective immunity after natural rotavirus infection: a community cohort study of newborn children in Guinea-Bissau, west Africa, J. Infect. Dis. 186 (2002) 593–597.

[158] H.G. Cicirello, et al., High prevalence of rotavirus infection among neonates born at hospitals in Delhi, India: predisposition of newborns for infection with unusual rotavirus, Pediatr. Infect. Dis. J. 13 (1994) 720–724.

[159] R.R. Vethanayagam, et al., Possible role of neonatal infection with the asymptomatic reassortant rotavirus (RV) strain I321 in the decrease in hospital admissions for RV diarrhea, Bangalore, India, 1988–1999, J. Infect. Dis. 189 (2004) 2282–2289.

[160] S. Ramani, et al., Rotavirus infection in the neonatal nurseries of a tertiary care hospital in India, Pediatr. Infect. Dis. J. 27 (2008) 719–723.

[161] S. Bhatia, Patterns and causes of neonatal and postneonatal mortality in rural Bangladesh, Stud. Fam. Plann. 20 (1989) 136–146.

[162] A. De Francisco, et al., The pattern of infant and childhood mortality in Upper River Division, The Gambia, Ann. Trop. Paediatr. 13 (1993) 345–352.

[163] S.K. Garg, et al., Neonatal mortality in Meerut district, Indian J. Med. Sci. 47 (1993) 222–225.

[164] M.S. Islam, et al., Infant mortality in rural Bangladesh: an analysis of causes during neonatal and postneonatal periods, J. Trop. Pediatr. 28 (1982) 294–298.

[165] B.S. Kandeh, Causes of infant and early childhood deaths in Sierra Leone, Soc. Sci. Med. 23 (1986) 297–303.

[166] S.R. Khan, et al., Early child health in Lahore, Pakistan, X: mortality, Acta Paediatr. 390 (Suppl) (1993) 109–177.

[167] R.H. Knobel, W.S. Yang, M.S. Ho, Urban-rural and regional differences in infant mortality in Taiwan, Soc. Sci. Med. 39 (1994) 815–822.

[168] V. Kumar, N. Datta, S.S. Saini, Infant mortality in a rural community development block in Haryana, Indian J. Pediatr. 49 (1982) 795–802.

[169] P.K. Singhal, et al., Neonatal morbidity and mortality in ICDS urban slums, Indian Pediatr. 27 (1990) 485–488.

[170] C. Sivagnanasundram, N. Sivarajah, A. Wijayaratnam, Infant deaths in a health unit area of Northern Sri Lanka, J. Trop. Med. Hyg. 88 (1985) 401–406.

[171] L.C. Mullany, et al., Incidence and risk factors for newborn umbilical cord infections on Pemba Island, Zanzibar, Tanzania, Pediatr. Infect. Dis. J. 28 (2009) 503–509.

[172] A.H. Cushing, Omphalitis: a review, Pediatr. Infect. Dis. 4 (1985) 282–285.

[173] L.C. Mullany, et al., Topical applications of chlorhexidine to the umbilical cord for prevention of omphalitis and neonatal mortality in southern Nepal: a community-based, cluster-randomised trial, Lancet 367 (2006) 910–918.

[174] L.C. Mullany, et al., Development of clinical sign based algorithms for community based assessment of omphalitis, Arch. Dis. Child Fetal. Neonatal. Ed. 91 (2006) F99–F104.

[175] L.C. Mullany, et al., Risk of mortality subsequent to umbilical cord infection among newborns of southern Nepal: cord infection and mortality, Pediatr. Infect. Dis. J. 28 (2009) 17–20.

[176] R.S. Sawin, et al., Early recognition of neonatal abdominal wall necrotizing fasciitis, Am. J. Surg. 167 (1994) 481–484.

[177] M. Samuel, et al., Necrotizing fasciitis: a serious complication of omphalitis in neonates, J. Pediatr. Surg. 29 (1994) 1414–1416.

[178] L.C. Mullany, et al., Risk factors for umbilical cord infection among newborns of southern Nepal, Am. J. Epidemiol. 165 (2007) 203–211.

[179] A.I. Airede, Pathogens in neonatal omphalitis, J. Trop. Pediatr. 38 (1992) 129–131.

[180] N. Bhardwaj, S.B. Hasan, High perinatal and neonatal mortality in rural India, J. R. Soc. Health. vol 113, (1993) 60–63.

[181] M.M. Faridi, A. Rattan, S.H. Ahmad, Omphalitis neonatorum, J. Indian Med. Assoc. 91 (1993) 283–285.

[182] H. Güvenç, et al., Neonatal omphalitis is still common in eastern Turkey, Scand. J. Infect. Dis. 23 (1991) 613–616.

[183] H. Güvenç, et al., Omphalitis in term and preterm appropriate for gestational age and small for gestational age infants, J. Trop. Pediatr. 43 (1997) 368–372.

[184] S. Chamnanvanakij, et al., A randomized study of 3 umbilical cord care regimens at home in Thai neonates: comparison of time to umbilical cord separation, parental satisfaction and bacterial colonization, J. Med. Assoc. Thai. 88 (2005) 967–972.

[185] K.P. Sawardekar, Changing spectrum of neonatal omphalitis, Pediatr. Infect. Dis. J. 23 (2004) 22–26.

[186] J. Rush, I. Chalmers, M. Enkin, Care of the new mother and baby, in: I. Chalmers, M. Enkin, M.J. Keirse (Eds.), Effective Care in Pregnancy and Childbirth, Oxford University Press, New York, 1989, pp. 1333–1346.

[187] J.E. Baley, A.A. Fanaroff, Neonatal infections, I: infection related to nursery care practices, in: J.C. Sinclair, M.B. Bracken (Eds.), Effective Care of the Newborn Infant, Oxford University Press, New York, 1992, pp. 454–476.

[188] L.C. Mullany, G.L. Darmstadt, J.M. Tielsch, Role of antimicrobial applications to the umbilical cord in neonates to prevent bacterial colonization and infection: a review of the evidence, Pediatr. Infect. Dis. J. 22 (2003) 996–1002.

[189] Z.P. Balsara, et al., Impact of clean delivery kit use on clean delivery practices in Beni Suef Governorate, Egypt J. Perinatol. 29 (2009) 673–679.

[190] G.L. Darmstadt, et al., Impact of clean delivery kit use on newborn umbilical cord and maternal puerperal infections in Egypt. J. Health Popul. Nutr. 27 (2009) 746–754.

[191] A.H. Jokhio, H.R. Winter, K.K. Cheng, An intervention involving traditional birth attendants and perinatal and maternal mortality in Pakistan, N. Engl. J. Med. 352 (2005) 2091–2099.

[192] F. Mosha, et al., Evaluation of the effectiveness of a clean delivery kit intervention in preventing cord infection and puerperal sepsis among neonates and their mothers in rural Mwanza Region, Tanzania, Tanzan. Health Res. Bull. 7 (2005) 185–188.

[193] V. Tsu, Nepal Clean Home Delivery Kit: Evaluation of the Health Impact, PATH, Seattle, WA, 2000.

[194] S. Winani, et al., Use of a clean delivery kit and factors associated with cord infection and puerperal sepsis in Mwanza, Tanzania, J. Midwifery Womens Health 52 (2007) 37–43.

[195] WHO, Care of the Umbilical Cord, World Health Organization, Geneva, 1998.

[196] P. Garner, et al., Avoiding neonatal death: an intervention study of umbilical cord care, J. Trop. Pediatr. 40 (1994) 24–28.

[197] L.C. Mullany, et al., Impact of umbilical cord cleansing with 4.0% chlorhexidine on time to cord separation among newborns in southern Nepal: a cluster-randomized, community-based trial, Pediatrics 118 (2006) 1864–1871.

[198] G. Stroh, et al., Measurement of mortality from neonatal tetanus in Burma, Bull. World Health Organ. 65 (1987) 309–316.

[199] W.U.W. Bank, State of the World's Vaccines and Immunization, World Health Organization, Geneva, 2002.

[200] UNICEF, The Progress of Nations 2000, UNICEF, New York, 2000.

[201] WHO, Maternal and Neonatal Tetanus Elimination by 2005: Strategies for Achieving and Maintaining Elimination, World Health Organization, Geneva, 2000.

[202] R. Rochat, H.H. Akhter, Tetanus and pregnancy-related mortality in Bangladesh, Lancet 354 (1999) 565.

[203] WHO, The Global Burden of Disease: 2004 Update, World Health Organization, Geneva, 2008.

[204] H. Nsanze, et al., Ophthalmia neonatorum in the United Arab Emirates, Ann. Trop. Paediatr. 16 (1996) 27–32.

[205] K.K. Pandey, et al., Clinico-bacteriological study of neonatal conjunctivitis, Indian J. Pediatr. 57 (1990) 527–531.

[206] M. Verma, J. Chhatwal, P.V. Varughese, Neonatal conjunctivitis: a profile, Indian Pediatr. 31 (1994) 1357–1361.

[207] L. Fransen, et al., Ophthalmia neonatorum in Nairobi, Kenya: the roles of *Neisseria gonorrhoeae* and *Chlamydia trachomatis*, J. Infect. Dis. 153 (1986) 862–869.

[208] F. Galega, D. Heymann, B. Nasah, Gonococcal ophthalmia neonatorum: the case for prophylaxis in tropical Africa, Bull. World Health Organ. 62 (1984) 95–98.

[209] M. Laga, A. Meheus, P. Piot, Epidemiology and control of gonococcal ophthalmia neonatorum, Bull. World Health Organ. 67 (1989) 471–477.

[210] M. Laga, et al., Epidemiology of ophthalmia neonatorum in Kenya, Lancet 2 (1986) 1145–1148.

[211] M. Laga, et al., Prophylaxis of gonococcal and chlamydial ophthalmia neonatorum: a comparison of silver nitrate and tetracycline, N. Engl. J. Med. 318 (1988) 653–657.

[212] A. Sergiwa, et al., Ophthalmia neonatorum in Bangkok: the significance of *Chlamydia trachomatis*, Ann. Trop. Paediatr. 13 (1993) 233–236.

[213] E. Amini, M. Ghasemi, K. Daneshjou, A five-year study in Iran of ophthalmia neonatorum: prevalence and etiology, Med. Sci. Monit. 14 (2008) CR90–CR96.

[214] K. Chang, V. Cheng, N. Kwong, Neonatal haemorrhagic conjunctivitis: a specific sign of chlamydial infection, Hong Kong Med. J. 12 (2006) 27–32.

[215] S. Di Bartolomeo, et al., [Neonatal conjunctivitis in a hospital at Gran Buenos Aires: last 5 years up-date], Rev. Argent. Microbiol. 37 (2005) 139–141.

[216] R. Hanenberg, et al., Impact of Thailand's HIV-control programme as indicated by the decline of sexually transmitted diseases, Lancet 344 (1994) 243–246.

[217] K. Nelson, et al., Changes in sexual behavior and decline in HIV infection among young men in Thailand, N. Engl. J. Med. 335 (1996) 297–303.

[218] K.S.F. Credé, Die Verhütung der Augenentzündung der Neugeborenen, Arch. Gynekol. 17 (1881) 50–53.

[219] M.R. Hammerschlag, et al., Efficacy of neonatal ocular prophylaxis for the prevention of chlamydial and gonococcal conjunctivitis, N. Engl. J. Med. 320 (1989) 768–772.

[220] D. Zanoni, S. Isenberg, L. Apt, A comparison of silver nitrate with erythromycin for prophylaxis against ophthalmia neonatorum, Clin. Pediatr. 31 (1992) 295–298.

[221] 2000 Red Book: Report of the Committee on Infectious Diseases, twenty fifth ed., American Academy of Pediatrics, Chicago, 2000.

[222] S.J. Isenberg, L. Apt, M. Wood, A controlled trial of povidone-iodine as prophylaxis against ophthalmia neonatorum, N. Engl. J. Med. 332 (1995) 562–566.

[223] S. Isenberg, et al., A double application approach to ophthalmia neonatorum prophylaxis, Br. J. Ophthalmol. 87 (2003) 1449–1452.

[224] W. Benevento, et al., The sensitivity of *Neisseria gonorrhoeae*, *Chlamydia trachomatis*, and herpes simplex type II to disinfection with povidone-iodine, Am. J. Ophthalmol. 109 (1990) 329–333.

[225] Z. Ali, et al., Prophylaxis of ophthalmia neonatorum comparison of Betadine, erythromycin and no prophylaxis, J. Trop. Pediatr. 53 (2007) 388–392.

[226] WHO/UNAIDS, Report on the AIDS Epidemic, World Health Organization & UNAIDS, Geneva, 2008.

[227] UNICEF, The State of the World's Children, UNICEF, New York, 2009.

[228] UNICEF, Africa's Orphaned Generations, UNICEF, New York, 2003.

[229] Mother-to-child transmission of HIV infection in the era of highly active antiretroviral therapy, Clin. Infect. Dis. 40 (2005) 458–465.

[230] B.L. Anderson, S. Cu-Uvin, Pregnancy and optimal care of HIV-infected patients, Clin. Infect. Dis. 48 (2009) 449–455.

[231] L.M. Mofenson, Advances in the prevention of vertical transmission of human immunodeficiency virus, Semin. Pediatr. Infect. Dis. 14 (2003) 295–308.

[232] L. Navér, et al., Children born to HIV-1-infected women in Sweden in 1982–2003: trends in epidemiology and vertical transmission, J. Acquir. Immune. Defic. Syndr. 42 (2006) 484–489.

[233] K.M. De Cock, et al., Prevention of mother-to-child HIV transmission in resource-poor countries: translating research into policy and practice, JAMA 283 (2000) 1175–1182.

[234] WHO/UNICEF, The Interaction Task Team (IATT) on Prevention of HIV Infection in Pregnant Women, Mothers and Their Children. Guidance on Global Scale-up of the Prevention of Mother-to-Child Transmission of HIV: Towards Universal Access for Women, Infants and Young Children and Eliminating HIV and AIDS among Children, World Health Organization, Geneva, 2007.

[235] United Nations General Assembly, Final declaration of commitment on HIV/AIDS (A/s-26/L.2), United Nations, New York, 2001.

[236] Effect of breastfeeding on infant and child mortality due to infectious diseases in less developed countries: a pooled analysis. WHO Collaborative Study Team on the Role of Breastfeeding on the Prevention of Infant Mortality, Lancet 355 (2000) 451–455.

[237] G. Jones, et al., How many child deaths can we prevent this year? Lancet 362 (2003) 65–71.

[238] H. Coovadia, Current issues in prevention of mother-to-child transmission of HIV-1, Curr. Opin. HIV AIDS 4 (2009) 319–324.

[239] T. Horvath, et al., Interventions for preventing late postnatal mother-to-child transmission of HIV, Cochrane Database Syst. Rev. 21 (2009) CD006734.

[240] L. Kuhn, C. Reitz, E.J. Abrams, Breastfeeding and AIDS in the developing world, Curr. Opin. Pediatr. 21 (2009) 83–93.

[241] WHO. Rapid Advice: Infant Feeding in the Context of HIV http://www.who.int/hiv/pub/paediatric/advice/en/index.html. Last accessed June 20, 2010.

[242] E.M. Connor, et al., Reduction of maternal-infant transmission of human immunodeficiency virus type 1 with zidovudine treatment. Pediatric AIDS Clinical Trials Group Protocol 076 Study Group, N. Engl. J. Med. 331 (1994) 1173–1180.

[243] E. Paintsil, W.A. Andiman, Update on successes and challenges regarding mother-to-child transmission of HIV, Curr. Opin. Pediatr. 21 (2009) 94–101.

[244] A. Spensley, et al., Preventing mother-to-child transmission of HIV in resource-limited settings: the Elizabeth Glaser Pediatric AIDS Foundation experience, Am. J. Public Health 99 (2009) 631–637.

[245] WHO, HIV/AIDS Programme. Antiretroviral Drugs for Treating Pregnant Women and Preventing HIV Infection in Infants: Towards Universal Access, World Health Organization, Geneva, 2010.

[246] The mode of delivery and the risk of vertical transmission of human immunodeficiency virus type 1—a meta-analysis of 15 prospective cohort studies. The International Perinatal HIV Group, N. Engl. J. Med. 340 (1999) 977–987.

[247] J.S. Read, M.K. Newell, Efficacy and safety of cesarean delivery for prevention of mother-to-child transmission of HIV-1, Cochrane Database Syst. Rev. 19 (2005) CD005479.

[248] J.S. Read, Cesarean section delivery to prevent vertical transmission of human immunodeficiency virus type 1: associated risks and other considerations, Ann. N. Y. Acad. Sci. 918 (2000) 115–121.

[249] J. Bryce, et al., WHO estimates of the causes of death in children, Lancet 365 (2005) 1147–1152.

[250] E. Menu, et al., Mother-to-child transmission of HIV: developing integration of healthcare programmes with clinical, social and basic research

studies. Report of the International Workshop held at Chobe Marina Lodge, Kasane, Botswana, 21–25 January 2003, Acta Paediatr. 92 (2003) 1343–1348.

[251] J.V. Bennett, M.F. Rogers, Child survival and perinatal infections with human immunodeficiency virus, Am. J. Dis. Child. 145 (1991) 1242–1247.

[252] S. Filteau, The HIV-exposed, uninfected African child, Trop. Med. Int. Health 14 (2009) 276–287.

[253] WHO, Women and Health: Today's Evidence, Tomorrow's Agenda, World Health Organization, Geneva, 2009.

[254] R. Figueroa-Damián, J.L. Arredondo-García, Neonatal outcome of children born to women with tuberculosis, Arch. Med. Res. 32 (2001) 66–69.

[255] N. Jana, et al., Perinatal outcome in pregnancies complicated by pulmonary tuberculosis, Int. J. Gynecol. Obstet. 44 (1994) 119–124.

[256] K.C. Smith, Congenital tuberculosis: a rare manifestation of a common infection, Curr. Opin. Infect. Dis. 15 (2002) 269–274.

[257] J.R. Starke, Tuberculosis: an old disease but a new threat to the mother, fetus, and neonate, Clin. Perinatol. 24 (1997) 107–127.

[258] M.A. Mazade, et al., Congenital tuberculosis presenting as sepsis syndrome: case report and review of the literature, Pediatr. Infect. Dis. J. 20 (2001) 439–442.

[259] S.D. Lawn, G. Churchyard, Epidemiology of HIV-associated tuberculosis, Curr. Opin. HIV AIDS 4 (2009) 325–333.

[260] S.S. Abdool Karim, et al., HIV infection and tuberculosis in South Africa: an urgent need to escalate the public health response, Lancet 374 (2009) 921–933.

[261] M. Adhikari, T. Pillay, D. Pillay, Tuberculosis in the newborn: an emerging disease, Pediatr. Infect. Dis. J. 16 (1997) 1108–1112.

[262] T. Pillay, et al., Severe, rapidly progressive human immunodeficiency virus type 1 disease in newborns with coinfections, Pediatr. Infect. Dis. J. 20 (2001) 404–410.

[263] M. Adhikari, Tuberculosis and tuberculosis/HIV co-infection in pregnancy, Semin. Fetal. Neonatal. Med. 14 (2009) 234–240.

[264] WHO, WHO Global Malaria Programme. World Malaria Report 2008, World Health Organization, Geneva, 2008.

[265] R.W. Steketee, et al., The problem of malaria and malaria control in pregnancy in sub-Saharan Africa, Am. J. Trop. Med. Hyg. 55 (1996) 2–7.

[266] C.E. Shulman, E.K. Dorman, Importance and prevention of malaria in pregnancy, Trans. R. Soc. Trop. Med. Hyg. 97 (2003) 30–35.

[267] B.J. Brabin, An analysis of malaria in pregnancy in Africa, Bull. World Health Organ. 61 (1983) 1005–1016.

[268] I.A. McGregor, Epidemiology, malaria, and pregnancy, Am. J. Trop. Med. Hyg. 33 (1984) 517–525.

[269] F. Nosten, et al., Malaria during pregnancy in an area of unstable endemicity, Trans. R. Soc. Trop. Med. Hyg. 85 (1991) 424–429.

[270] P.E. Duffy, Plasmodium in the placenta: parasites, parity, protection, prevention and possibly preeclampsia, Parasitology 134 (Pt 13) (2007) 1877–1881.

[271] H.M. Gilles, et al., Malaria, anaemia and pregnancy, Ann. Trop. Parasitol. 63 (1969) 245–263.

[272] O.A. Egwunyenga, J.A. Ajayi, D.D. Duhlinska-Popova, Malaria in pregnancy in Nigerians: seasonality and relationship to splenomegaly and anaemia, Indian J. Malariol. 34 (1997) 17–24.

[273] A. Matteelli, et al., The placenta and malaria, Ann. Trop. Med. Parasitol. 91 (1997) 803–810.

[274] I.A. McGregor, M.E. Wilson, W.Z. Billewicz, Malaria infection of the placenta in The Gambia, West Africa: its incidence and relationship to stillbirth, birthweight and placental weight, Trans. R. Soc. Trop. Med. Hyg. 77 (1983) 232–244.

[275] B.J. Okoko, G. Enwere, M.O. Ota, The epidemiology and consequences of maternal malaria: a review of immunological basis, Acta Trop. 87 (2003) 193–205.

[276] B.J. Okoko, et al., Influence of placental malaria infection on fetal outcome in the Gambia: twenty years after Ian Mcgregor, J. Health Popul. Nutr. 20 (2002) 4–11.

[277] R.M. Galbraith, et al., The human maternal-foetal relationship in malaria, II: histological, ultrastructural and immunopathological studies of the placenta, Trans. R. Soc. Trop. Med. Hyg. 74 (1980) 61–72.

[278] R.W. Steketee, et al., The effect of malaria and malaria prevention in pregnancy on offspring birthweight, prematurity, and intrauterine growth retardation in rural Malawi, Am. J. Trop. Med. Hyg. 55 (1996) 33–41.

[279] P. Bouvier, et al., Seasonality, malaria, and impact of prophylaxis in a West African village, II: effect on birthweight, Am. J. Trop. Med. Hyg. 56 (1997) 384–389.

[280] F. Nosten, et al., Effects of Plasmodium vivax malaria in pregnancy, Lancet 354 (1999) 546–549.

[281] M.S. Kramer, Determinants of low birth weight: methodological assessment and metaanalysis, Bull. World Health Organ. 65 (1987) 663–737.

[282] C. Luxemburger, et al., Effects of malaria during pregnancy on infant mortality in an area of low malaria transmission, Am. J. Epidemiol. 154 (2001) 459–465.

[283] C. Chizzolini, et al., Isotypic analysis, antigen specificity, and inhibitory function of maternally transmitted Plasmodium falciparum-specific antibodies in Gabonese newborns, Am. J. Trop. Med. Hyg. 45 (1991) 57–64.

[284] P. Nguyen-Dinh, et al., Rapid spontaneous postpartum clearance of Plasmodium falciparum parasitemia in African women, Lancet 2 (1988) 751–752.

[285] S.E. Ibhanesebhor, Clinical characteristics of neonatal malaria, J. Trop. Pediatr. 41 (1995) 330–333.

[286] B.J. Brabin, et al., Monitoring and evaluation of malaria in pregnancy—developing a rational basis for control, Malar. J. 7 (7 Suppl. 1) (2008) S6.

[287] WHO/AFRO, A Strategic Framework for Malaria Prevention and Control during Pregnancy in the African Region, World Health Organization Regional Office for Africa, Brazzaville, 2004.

[288] M.S. Wolfe, J.F. Cordero, Safety of chloroquine in chemosuppression of malaria during pregnancy, BMJ 290 (1985) 1466–1467.

[289] UNICEF, The Progress of the Nations 1997, UNICEF, New York, 1997.

[290] F.O. ter Kuile, A.M. van Eijk, S.J. Filler, Effect of sulfadoxine-pyrimethamine resistance on the efficacy of intermittent preventive therapy for malaria control during pregnancy: a systematic review, JAMA 297 (2007) 2603–2616.

[291] R.D. Newman, et al., Safety, efficacy and determinants of effectiveness of antimalarial drugs during pregnancy: implications for prevention programmes in Plasmodium falciparum-endemic sub-Saharan Africa, Trop. Med. Int. Health 8 (2003) 488–506.

[292] F. Nosten, et al., Editorial: Maternal malaria: time for action, Trop. Med. Int. Health 8 (2003) 485–487.

[293] F. Nosten, et al., Antimalarial drugs in pregnancy: a review, Curr. Drug Saf. 1 (2006) 1–15.

[294] P. Garner, A.M. Gulmezoglu, Prevention versus treatment for malaria in pregnant women, Cochrane Database Syst. Rev. 2 (2000) CD000169.

[295] M. Cot, et al., Effect of chloroquine chemoprophylaxis during pregnancy on birth weight: results of a randomized trial, Am. J. Trop. Med. Hyg. 46 (1992) 21–27.

[296] P. Garner, A.M. Gulmezoglu, Drugs for preventing malaria in pregnant women, Cochrane Database Syst. Rev. 18 (2006) CD000169.

[297] C.E. Shulman, et al., Intermittent sulphadoxine-pyrimethamine to prevent severe anaemia secondary to malaria in pregnancy: a randomised placebo-controlled trial, Lancet 353 (1999) 632–636.

[298] L.J. Schultz, et al., Evaluation of maternal practices, efficacy, and cost-effectiveness of alternative antimalarial regimens for use in pregnancy: chloroquine and sulfadoxine-pyrimethamine, Am. J. Trop. Med. Hyg. 55 (Suppl. 1) (1996) 87–94.

[299] R.W. Steketee, et al., The burden of malaria in pregnancy in malaria-endemic areas, Am. J. Trop. Med. Hyg. 64 (Suppl. 1–2) (2001) 28–35.

[300] C.A. Goodman, P.G. Coleman, A.J. Mills, The cost-effectiveness of antenatal malaria prevention in sub-Saharan Africa, Am. J. Trop. Med. Hyg. 64 (Suppl. 1–2) (2001) 45–56.

[301] WHO Expert Committee on Malaria, WHO Technical Report Series Number 892, World Health Organization, Geneva, 2000.

[302] R.W. Steketee, Malaria prevention in pregnancy: when will the prevention programme respond to the science, J. Health Popul. Nutr. 20 (2002) 1–3.

[303] D.L. Heymann, et al., Antenatal chloroquine chemoprophylaxis in Malawi: chloroquine resistance, compliance, protective efficacy and cost, Trans. R. Soc. Trop. Med. Hyg. 84 (1990) 496–498.

[304] P.L. Alonso, et al., The effect of insecticide-treated bed nets on mortality of Gambian children, Lancet 337 (1991) 1499–1502.

[305] C.G. Nevill, et al., Insecticide-treated bednets reduce mortality and severe morbidity from malaria among children on the Kenyan coast, Trop. Med. Int. Health 1 (1996) 139–146.

[306] F.N. Binka, et al., Impact of permethrin impregnated bednets on child mortality in Kassena-Nankana district, Ghana: a randomized controlled trial, Trop. Med. Int. Health 1 (1996) 147–154.

[307] C. Gamble, J.P. Ekwaru, F.O. ter Kuile, Insecticide-treated nets for preventing malaria in pregnancy, Cochrane Database Syst. Rev. 19 (2006) CD003755.

[308] T. Marchant, et al., Socially marketed insecticide-treated nets improve malaria and anaemia in pregnancy in southern Tanzania, Trop. Med. Int. Health 7 (2002) 149–158.

[309] K. Hanson, et al., Household ownership and use of insecticide treated nets among target groups after implementation of a national voucher programme in the United Republic of Tanzania: plausibility study using three annual cross sectional household surveys, BMJ 339 (2009) b2434.

[310] I. Kleinschmidt, et al., Marked increase in child survival after four years of intensive malaria control, Am. J. Trop. Med. Hyg. 80 (2009) 882–888.

[311] H. Brahmbhatt, et al., The effects of placental malaria on mother-to-child HIV transmission in Rakai, Uganda, AIDS 17 (2003) 2539–2541.

[312] J. Ladner, et al., Malaria, HIV and pregnancy, AIDS 17 (2003) 275–276.

[313] A.M. van Eijk, et al., HIV increases the risk of malaria in women of all gravidities in Kisumu, Kenya, AIDS 17 (2003) 595–603.

[314] V. Briand, C. Badaut, M. Cot, Placental malaria, maternal HIV infection and infant morbidity, Ann. Trop. Paediatr. 29 (2009) 71–83.

[315] C. Ticconi, et al., Effect of maternal HIV and malaria infection on pregnancy and perinatal outcome in Zimbabwe, J. Acquir. Immune. Defic. Syndr. 34 (2003) 289–294.

[316] J.R. Bale, B.J. Stoll, A.O. Lucas (Eds.), Improving Birth Outcomes: Meeting the Challenge in the Developing World, Institute of Medicine, The National Academy Press, Washington, DC, 2003.

[317] The State of the World's Newborns, A Report from Saving Newborn Lives, Save the Children, Washington, DC, 2001.

[318] The World's Women 1995, Trends and Statistics. Social Statistics and Indicators, United Nations, New York, 1995.

[319] K. Tomasevski, Women and Human Rights, Zed Books, Atlantic Highlands, NJ, 1993.

[320] Mother-baby package, Implementing safe motherhood in countries, World Health Organization, Division of Family Health, Maternal Health and Safe Motherhood Programme, Geneva, 1994.

[321] Maternal and Perinatal Infections, A Practical Guide: Report of a WHO Consultation, WHO/MCH/91.10. World Health Organization, Geneva, 1991.

[322] Maternal Care for the Reduction of Perinatal and Neonatal Mortality, World Health Organization, Geneva, 1986.

[323] G.W. Fischer, M.G. Ottolini, J.J. Mond, Prospects for vaccines during pregnancy and in the newborn period, Clin. Perinatol. 24 (1997) 231–249.

[324] M. Vicari, B. Dodet, J. Englund, Protection of newborns through maternal immunization, Vaccine 21 (2003) 3351.

[325] H5N1 avian influenza: first steps towards development of a human vaccine, Wkly. Epidemiol. Rec. 80 (2005) 277–278.

[326] P.D. Tamma, et al., Safety of influenza vaccination during pregnancy, Am. J. Obstet. Gynecol. 20 (2009) 20.

[327] K. Zaman, et al., Effectiveness of maternal influenza immunization in mothers and infants, N. Engl. J. Med. 359 (2008) 1555–1564.

[328] C.J. Baker, et al., Immunization of pregnant women with a polysaccharide vaccine of group B streptococcus, N. Engl. J. Med. 319 (1988) 1180–1185.

[329] C.J. Baker, M.S. Edwards, Group B streptococcal conjugate vaccines, Arch. Dis. Child. 88 (2003) 375–378.

[330] C.J. Baker, et al., Safety and immunogenicity of a bivalent group B streptococcal conjugate vaccine for serotypes II and III, J. Infect. Dis. 188 (2003) 66–73.

[331] C.J. Baker, M.A. Rench, P. McInnes, Immunization of pregnant women with group B streptococcal type III capsular polysaccharide-tetanus toxoid conjugate vaccine, Vaccine 21 (2003) 3468–3472.

[332] F.Y. Lin, et al., Level of maternal antibody required to protect neonates against early-onset disease caused by group B streptococcus type Ia: a multicenter, seroepidemiology study, J. Infect. Dis. 184 (2001) 1022–1028.

[333] K. Mulholland, et al., Maternal immunization with *Haemophilus influenzae* type b polysaccharide-tetanus protein conjugate vaccine in The Gambia, JAMA 275 (1996) 1182–1188.

[334] T.J. O'Dempsey, et al., Immunization with a pneumococcal capsular polysaccharide vaccine during pregnancy, Vaccine 14 (1996) 963–970.

[335] M. Santosham, et al., Safety and antibody persistence following *Haemophilus influenzae* type b conjugate or pneumococcal polysaccharide vaccines given before pregnancy in women of childbearing age and their infants, Pediatr. Infect. Dis. J. 20 (2001) 931–940.

[336] N.S. Shahid, et al., Serum, breast milk, and infant antibody after maternal immunisation with pneumococcal vaccine, Lancet 346 (1995) 1252–1257.

[337] J.A. Englund, et al., *Haemophilus influenzae* type b-specific antibody in infants after maternal immunization, Pediatr. Infect. Dis. J. 16 (1997) 1122–1130.

[338] F. Michon, et al., Group B streptococcal type II and III conjugate vaccines: physicochemical properties that influence immunogenicity, Clin. Vaccine Immunol. 13 (2006) 936–943.

[339] A. Marchant, M. Newport, Prevention of infectious diseases by neonatal and early infantile immunization: prospects for the new millennium, Curr. Opin. Infect. Dis. 13 (2000) 241–246.

[340] P.G. Smith, Case-control studies of the efficacy of BCG against tuberculosis. International Union Against Tuberculosis, in: XXVIth IUAT World Conference on Tuberculosis and Respiratory Diseases, 1987, Professional Postgraduate Services International, Singapore, 1987, pp. 73–79.

[341] G.A. Colditz, et al., The efficacy of bacillus Calmette-Guerin vaccination of newborns and infants in the prevention of tuberculosis: meta-analyses of the published literature, Pediatrics 96 (1995) 29–35.

[342] B.B. Trunz, P. Fine, C. Dye, Effect of BCG vaccination on childhood tuberculous meningitis and miliary tuberculosis worldwide: a meta-analysis and assessment of cost-effectiveness, Lancet 367 (2006) 1173–1180.

[343] A.C. Hesseling, et al., Consensus statement on the revised World Health Organization recommendations for BCG vaccination in HIV-infected infants, Int. J. Tuberc. Lung. Dis. 12 (2008) 1376–1379.

[344] G. Delage, S. Remy-Prince, S. Montplaisir, Combined active-passive immunization against the hepatitis B virus: five-year follow-up of children born to hepatitis B surface antigen-positive mothers, Pediatr. Infect. Dis. J. 12 (1993) 126–130.

[345] F.E. Andre, A.J. Zuckerman, Review: protective efficacy of hepatitis B vaccines in neonates, J. Med. Virol. 44 (1994) 144–151.

[346] WHO, World Health Organization Expanded Programme on Immunization: global advisory group, Wkly. Epidemiol. Rec. 3 (1992) 11–16.

[347] WHO, State of the World's Vaccines and Immunization, third ed., World Health Organization, Geneva, 2009.

[348] WHO, The Prevention and Management of Puerperal Infections, World Health Organization, Geneva, 1992.

[349] WHO, The Global Elimination of Neonatal Tetanus: Progress to Date, Bull. WHO 72 (1994) 155–164.

[350] WHO/UNICEF, Maternal care for the reduction of perinatal and neonatal mortality. A Joint WHO/UNICEF Statement, World Health Organization, Geneva, 1986.

[351] A.C. Gerbase, J.T. Rowley, T.E. Mertens, Global epidemiology of sexually transmitted diseases, Lancet 351 (Suppl. 3) (1998) 2–4.

[352] P. Moodley, A.W. Sturm, Sexually transmitted infections, adverse pregnancy outcome and neonatal infection, Semin. Neonatol. 5 (2000) 255–269.

[353] D.G. Walker, G.J. Walker, Forgotten but not gone: the continuing scourge of congenital syphilis, Lancet Infect. Dis. 2 (2002) 432–436.

[354] B. Kuate Defo, Epidemiology and control of infant and early childhood malaria: a competing risks analysis, Int. J. Epidemiol. 24 (1995) 204–217.

[355] B.J. Stoll, The global impact of neonatal infection, Clin. Perinatol. 24 (1997) 1–21.

[356] Partnership for Maternal, Newborn and Child Health, Opportunities for Africa's Newborns: Practical Data, Policy and Programmatic Support for Newborn Care in Africa, Partnership for Maternal, Newborn and Child Health, Cape Town, South Africa, 2006.

[357] A.H. Baqui, et al., Effect of community-based newborn-care intervention package implemented through two service-delivery strategies in Sylhet district, Bangladesh: a cluster-randomised controlled trial, Lancet 371 (2008) 1936–1944.

[358] A.H. Baqui, et al., Effect of timing of first postnatal care home visit on neonatal mortality in Bangladesh: a observational cohort study, BMJ 339 (339) (2009) b2826.

[359] V. Kumar, et al., Effect of community-based behaviour change management on neonatal mortality in Shivgarh, Uttar Pradesh, India: a cluster-randomised controlled trial, Lancet 372 (2008) 1151–1162.

[360] L.A. Hanson, et al., Breast feeding: overview and breast milk immunology, Acta Paediatr. Jpn. 36 (1994) 557–561.

[361] R.N. Ashraf, et al., Breast feeding and protection against neonatal sepsis in a high risk population, Arch. Dis. Child. 66 (1991) 488–490.

[362] K.H. Brown, et al., Infant-feeding practices and their relationship with diarrheal and other diseases in Huascar (Lima), Peru, Pediatrics 83 (1989) 31–40.

[363] I. De Zoysa, M. Rea, J. Martines, Why promote breastfeeding in diarrhoeal disease control programmes? Health Policy Plan. 6 (1991) 371–379.

[364] R.G. Feachem, M.A. Koblinsky, Interventions for the control of diarrhoeal diseases among young children: promotion of breast-feeding, Bull. World Health Organ. 62 (1984) 271–291.

[365] W.P. Glezen, Epidemiological perspective of breastfeeding and acute respiratory illnesses in infants, Adv. Exp. Med. Biol. 310 (1991) 235–240.

[366] I. Narayanan, et al., Randomised controlled trial of effect of raw and holder pasteurised human milk and of formula supplements on incidence of neonatal infection, Lancet 2 (1984) 1111–1113.

[367] J.P. Habicht, J. DaVanzo, W.P. Butz, Does breastfeeding really save lives, or are apparent benefits due to biases? Am. J. Epidemiol. 123 (1986) 279–290.

[368] S.P. Srivastava, V.K. Sharma, S.P. Jha, Mortality patterns in breast versus artificially fed term babies in early infancy: a longitudinal study, Indian Pediatr. 31 (1994) 1393–1396.

[369] C.G. Victora, et al., Infant feeding and deaths due to diarrhea: a case-control study, Am. J. Epidemiol. 129 (1989) 1032–1041.

[370] C.G. Victora, et al., Evidence for protection by breast-feeding against infant deaths from infectious diseases in Brazil, Lancet 2 (1987) 319–322.

[371] J. Bertolli, et al., Estimating the timing of mother-to-child transmission of human immunodeficiency virus in a breast-feeding population in Kinshasa, Zaire, J. Infect. Dis. 174 (1996) 722–726.

[372] R. Bobat, et al., Breastfeeding by HIV-1-infected women and outcome in their infants: a cohort study from Durban, South Africa, AIDS 11 (1997) 1627–1633.

[373] H. Brahmbhatt, R.H. Gray, Child mortality associated with reasons for non-breastfeeding and weaning: is breastfeeding best for HIV-positive mothers? AIDS 17 (2003) 879–885.

[374] D.T. Dunn, et al., Risk of human immunodeficiency virus type 1 transmission through breastfeeding, Lancet 340 (1992) 585–588.

[375] E.R. Ekpini, et al., Late postnatal mother-to-child transmission of HIV-1 in Abidjan, Cote d'Ivoire, Lancet 349 (1997) 1054–1059.

[376] M.G. Fowler, M.L. Newell, Breast-feeding and HIV-1 transmission in resource-limited settings, J. Acquir. Immune Defic. Syndr. 30 (2002) 230–239.

[377] A.P. Kourtis, et al., Breast milk and HIV-1: vector of transmission or vehicle of protection? Lancet Infect. Dis. 3 (2003) 786–793.

[378] J. Kreiss, Breastfeeding and vertical transmission of HIV-1, Acta Paediatr. (Suppl. 421) (1997) 113–117.

[379] B.H. Tess, et al., Breastfeeding, genetic, obstetric and other risk factors associated with mother-to-child transmission of HIV-1 in Sao Paulo State, Brazil. Sao Paulo Collaborative Study for Vertical Transmission of HIV-1, AIDS 12 (1998) 513–520.

[380] P. Van de Perre, Postnatal transmission of human immunodeficiency virus type 1: the breast-feeding dilemma, Am. J. Obstet. Gynecol. 173 (1995) 483–487.

[381] WHO/UNAIDS, HIV and Infant Feeding: A Policy Statement Developed Collaboratively by UNAIDS, WHO, and UNICEF, WHO/UNAIDS, Geneva, 1998.

[382] M. Raghavan, et al., Perinatal risk factors in neonatal infections, Indian J. Pediatr. 59 (1992) 335–340.

[383] A.I. Airede, Prolonged rupture of membranes and neonatal outcome in a developing country, Ann. Trop. Paediatr. 12 (1992) 283–288.

[384] A.A. Asindi, J.A. Omene, Prolonged rupture of membrane and neonatal morbidity, East Afr. Med. J. 57 (1980) 707–711.

[385] M.W. Weber, et al., Predictors of neonatal sepsis in developing countries, Pediatr. Infect. Dis. J. 22 (2003) 711–717.

[386] A.H. Baqui, et al., Community-based validation of assessment of newborn illnesses by trained community health workers in Sylhet district of Bangladesh, Trop. Med. Int. Health 5 (2009) 5.

[387] G.L. Darmstadt, et al., Validation of community health workers' assessment of neonatal illness in rural Bangladesh, Bull. World Health Organ. 87 (2009) 12–19.

[388] J.O. Klein, Bacterial sepsis and meningitis, in: J.S. Remington, J.O. Klein (Eds.), Infectious Diseases of the Fetus and Newborn Infant, fifth ed., WB Saunders, Philadelphia, 2000, pp. 943–998.

[389] G.L. Darmstadt, et al., Determination of extended-interval gentamicin dosing for neonatal patients in developing countries, Pediatr. Infect. Dis. J. 26 (2007) 501–507.

[390] G.L. Darmstadt, et al., Extended-interval dosing of gentamicin for treatment of neonatal sepsis in developed and developing countries, J. Health Popul. Nutr. 26 (2008) 163–182.

[391] M. Hossain, et al., Simplified gentamicin dosing for treatment of sepsis in Bangladeshi neonates, J. Health Popul. Nutr. 27 (2009) 640–645.

[392] A.H. Baqui, et al., Effectiveness of home-based management of newborn infections by community health workers in rural Bangladesh, Pediatr. Infect. Dis. J. 28 (2009) 304–310.

[393] G.L. Darmstadt, M. Batra, A.K. Zaidi, Oral antibiotics in the management of serious neonatal bacterial infections in developing country communities, Pediatr. Infect. Dis. J. 28 (Suppl. 1) (2009) S31–S36.

[394] G.L. Darmstadt, M. Batra, A.K. Zaidi, Parenteral antibiotics for the treatment of serious neonatal bacterial infections in developing country settings, Pediatr. Infect Dis. J. 28 (Suppl. 1) (2009) S37–S42.

[395] A.H. Baqui, et al., A population-based study of hospital admission incidence rate and bacterial aetiology of acute lower respiratory infections in children aged less than five years in Bangladesh, J. Health Popul. Nutr. 25 (2007) 179–188.

[396] Z.A. Bhutta, et al., Community-based interventions for improving perinatal and neonatal health outcomes in developing countries: a review of the evidence, Pediatrics 115 (Suppl. 2) (2005) 519–617.

[397] R.A. Haws, et al., Impact of packaged interventions on neonatal health: a review of the evidence, Health Policy Plan. 22 (2007) 193–215.

[398] A.T. Bang, et al., Neonatal and infant mortality in the ten years (1993 to 2003) of the Gadchiroli field trial: effect of home-based neonatal care, J. Perinatol. 25 (1 Suppl. 1) (2005) S92–S107.

[399] P.J. Winch, et al., Intervention models for the management of children with signs of pneumonia or malaria by community health workers, Health Policy Plan. 20 (2005) 199–212.

[400] G.L. Darmstadt, et al., Household surveillance of severe neonatal illness by community health workers in Mirzapur, Bangladesh: coverage and compliance with referral, Health Policy Plan. 25 (2010) 112–124.

[401] S. Sazawal, R.E. Black, Effect of pneumonia case management on mortality in neonates, infants, and preschool children: a meta-analysis of community-based trials, Lancet Infect. Dis. 3 (2003) 547–556.

[402] WHO, Integrated management of the sick child, Bull. World Health Organ. 73 (1995) 735–740.

[403] The World Bank, World Development Report 1993: Investing in Health, Oxford University Press, New York, 1993.

[404] G.T. Bicego, J.T. Boerma, Maternal education and child survival: a comparative study of survey data from 17 countries, Soc. Sci. Med. 36 (1993) 1207–1227.

[405] J.K. van Ginneken, J. Lob-Levyt, S. Gove, Potential interventions for preventing pneumonia among young children in developing countries: promoting maternal education, Trop. Med. Int. Health 1 (1996) 283–294.

[406] C.G. Victora, et al., Maternal education in relation to early and late child health outcomes: findings from a Brazilian cohort study, Soc. Sci. Med. 34 (1992) 899–905.

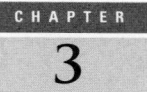

CHAPTER 3

OBSTETRIC FACTORS ASSOCIATED WITH INFECTIONS OF THE FETUS AND NEWBORN INFANT

Amy J. Gagnon ◎ Ronald S. Gibbs

CHAPTER OUTLINE

Intra-amniotic Infection   52
  Pathogenesis   52
  Microbiology   53
  Diagnosis   54
  Chronic Intra-amniotic Infection   55
  Management   55
  Short-Term Outcomes   57
  Long-Term Outcome   58
  Conclusion   59
Infection as a Cause of Preterm Birth   59
  Histologic Chorioamnionitis and Prematurity   60
  Clinical Infection and Prematurity   60
  Association of Lower Genital Tract Organisms or Infections with Prematurity   61
  Amniotic Fluid Cultures in Preterm Labor   61
  Biochemical Links of Prematurity and Infection   62
  Antibiotic Trials   62

Premature Rupture of Membranes   64
  Definition   64
  Incidence   65
  Etiology   65
  Diagnosis   65
  Natural History   66
  Complications   66
  Approach to Diagnosis of Infection   67
  Treatment of Preterm Premature Rupture of Membranes before Fetal Viability   68
  Treatment of Preterm Premature Rupture of Membranes in Early Third Trimester   69
  Recurrence of Preterm Premature Rupture of Membranes   72
  Prevention of Preterm Premature Rupture of Membranes   73
  Special Situations   73
  Treatment of Term Premature Rupture of Membranes   73

Early-onset neonatal infections often originate in utero. Risk factors for neonatal sepsis include prematurity, premature rupture of the membranes (PROM), and maternal fever during labor (which may be caused by clinical intra-amniotic infection [IAI]). This chapter focuses on these major obstetric conditions. In addition to these three "classic" topics, we discuss information indicating that intrauterine exposure to bacteria is linked to major neonatal sequelae, including cerebral palsy, bronchopulmonary dysplasia, and respiratory distress syndrome (RDS).

INTRA-AMNIOTIC INFECTION

Clinically evident intrauterine infection during the latter half of pregnancy develops in 1% to 10% of pregnant women and leads to increased maternal morbidity and perinatal morbidity and mortality. Generally, the diagnosis is clinically based on the presence of fever and other signs and symptoms, such as maternal or fetal tachycardia, uterine tenderness, foul odor of the amniotic fluid, and maternal leukocytosis. Although not invariably present, rupture of membranes or labor typically occurs in cases of clinically evident IAI. Older retrospective studies report rates of IAI of 1% to 2% [1]. Subsequent prospective studies report rates of 4% to 10% [2–5]. Numerous terms have been applied to this infection, including chorioamnionitis, amnionitis, intrapartum infection, amniotic fluid infection, and IAI. We use IAI to distinguish this clinical syndrome from bacterial colonization of amniotic fluid (also referred to as microbial invasion of the amniotic cavity) and from histologic inflammation of the placenta (i.e., histologic chorioamnionitis). When citing authors who use alternative expressions, however, we defer to their terminology.

IAI can refer to a histologic, subclinical, or clinical diagnosis. Histologic IAI is defined by infiltration of the fetal membranes by polymorphonuclear leukocytes and occurs much more often than clinically apparent infection. This diagnosis can be made in 20% of term deliveries and more than 50% of preterm deliveries [6]. Pettker and colleagues [7] evaluated the ability of microbiologic and pathologic examination of the placenta to diagnose IAI accurately and found that microbiologic studies of the placenta show poor accuracy to diagnose IAI (as defined by positive amniotic fluid cultures). They concluded that the presence of histologic chorioamnionitis is a sensitive, but not specific, test to diagnose intra-amniotic inflammation.

PATHOGENESIS

Before labor and membrane rupture, amniotic fluid is nearly always sterile. The physical and chemical barriers formed by intact amniotic membranes and cervical mucus are usually effective in preventing entry of bacteria. With the onset of labor or with membrane rupture, bacteria from the lower genital tract typically enter the amniotic cavity. With increasing interval after rupture of membranes, the numbers of bacteria can increase. This ascending route is the most common pathway for development of IAI [1]. In 1988, Romero and coworkers [1a] described four stages of ascending IAI (Fig. 3–1). Shifts in vaginal or cervical flora and the presence of pathologic bacteria in the cervix represent stage I. Bacterial vaginosis may also be classified as stage I. In stage II, bacteria ascend from the vagina or cervix into the decidua, the specialized endometrium of pregnancy. The inflammatory response here allows organisms to invade the amnion and chorion leading to chorioamnionitis. In state III, bacteria invade chorionic vessels (choriovasculitis) and migrate through the amnion into the amniotic cavity to cause IAI. When in the amniotic cavity, bacteria may gain access to the fetus through several potential mechanisms, culminating in stage IV; fetal bacteremia, sepsis, and pneumonia may result [8].

Occasional instances of documented IAI in the absence of rupture of membranes or labor support a presumed

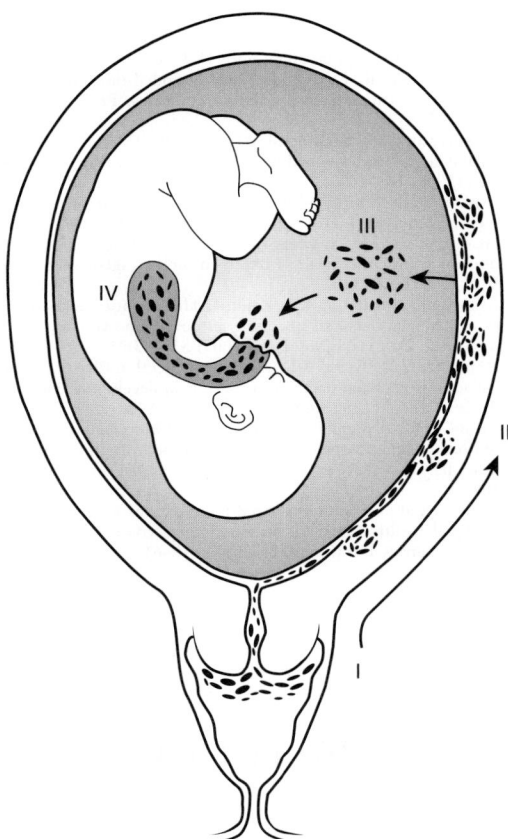

FIGURE 3–1 Stages of ascending infection. (*Adapted from Romero R, Mazor M. Infection and preterm labor: pathways for intrauterine infections. Clin Obstet Gynecol 31:558, 1988.*)

hematogenous or transplacental route of infection. IAI without labor and without rupture of membranes may be caused by *Listeria monocytogenes* [9–13]. Maternal sepsis caused by this aerobic gram-positive rod often manifests as a flulike illness and may result in fetal demise. In an outbreak caused by "Mexican-style" cheese contaminated with *Listeria*, several maternal deaths occurred [14]. Other virulent organisms, such as group A streptococci, may lead to a similar blood-borne infection [15].

IAI may develop as a consequence of obstetric procedures such as cervical cerclage, diagnostic amniocentesis, cordocentesis (percutaneous umbilical cord blood sampling), or intrauterine transfusion. The absolute risk is small with all these procedures. With cervical cerclage, data regarding infectious complications are sparse; reported rates range from 1% to 18%, with increasing rate with advanced dilation [16–18]. After diagnostic amniocentesis, rates of IAI range from 0% to 1% [19,20]. With intrauterine transfusion, infection is reported to develop in approximately 10%. Chorioamnionitis is a rare complication of chorionic villus sampling. Although IAI is very rare after percutaneous umbilical blood sampling, and the fetal loss rate accompanying this procedure is only 1% to 2%, infection is responsible for a high percentage of losses and may lead to life-threatening maternal complications [21].

Two large studies of risk factors for IAI identified characteristics of labor as the major risk factors by logistic regression analysis. These features included low parity, increased number of vaginal examinations in labor, increased duration of labor, increased duration of membrane rupture, and internal fetal monitoring [1,4]. Other data from a randomized trial of active management of labor showed that chorioamnionitis occurs less frequently when labor management features early diagnosis of abnormalities and early intervention [5]. Although internal fetal monitoring is associated with IAI, it should be employed if it enables practitioners to diagnose and treat abnormalities more efficiently.

Risk factors for IAI have been stratified for term versus preterm pregnancies [22]. For patients at term with IAI, the study investigators observed, by logistic regression analysis, that the independent risk factors were membrane rupture for longer than 12 hours (odds ratio [OR] 5.81), internal fetal monitoring (OR 2.01), and more than four vaginal examinations in labor (OR 3.07). For preterm pregnancies, these three risk factors were identified again as being independently associated with IAI, but with differing ORs. Specifically, in the preterm pregnancies, membrane rupture for longer than 12 hours was associated with an OR of 2.49; internal fetal monitoring, OR of 1.42; and more than four examinations in labor, OR of 1.59. One interpretation of these data regarding risk factors among preterm pregnancies is that there was some other risk factor not detected in this survey. Additionally, meconium staining of the amniotic fluid has been associated with an increased risk of chorioamnionitis (4.3% versus 2.1%) [23]. Prior spontaneous and elective abortion (at <20 weeks) in the immediately preceding pregnancy also has been associated with development of IAI in the subsequent pregnancy (OR 4.3 and OR 4.0) [24].

In 1996, a multivariable analysis showed the importance of chorioamnionitis in neonatal sepsis [25]. The OR for neonatal sepsis accompanying clinical chorioamnionitis was 25, whereas for preterm delivery, membrane rupture for longer than 12 hours, endometritis, and colonization with group B streptococcus (GBS), an ORs all were less than 5.

Although Naeye had reported an association between recent coitus and development of chorioamnionitis defined by histologic study [26], further analysis of the same population refuted this association [27]. Other studies have not shown any relationship between coitus and PROM, premature birth, or perinatal death [28].

MICROBIOLOGY

The cause of IAI is often polymicrobial, involving aerobic and anaerobic organisms. Sperling and colleagues [72] reported a microbiologic controlled study of amniotic fluid cultures from patients with IAI versus patients without IAI. Patients with IAI were more likely to have 10^2 colony-forming units (CFU)/mL of any isolate, any number of high virulence isolates, and more than 10^2 CFU/mL of a high-virulence isolate (e.g., GBS, *Escherichia coli*, and enterococci). The isolation of low-virulence organisms, such as lactobacilli, diphtheroids, and *Staphylococcus epidermidis*, was similar in the IAI and control groups [29]. Table 3–1 shows the most common amniotic fluid isolates found in more than 400 cases of IAI.

Although GBS and *E. coli* were isolated with only modest frequency (15% and 8%), they are strongly associated with either maternal or neonatal bacteremia. When GBS

TABLE 3–1   Microbes Isolated in Amniotic Fluid from Cases of Intra-amniotic Infection*

Microbe	Representative % Isolated
Genital Mycoplasmas	
Ureaplasma urealyticum	47-50
Mycoplasma hominis	31-35
Anaerobes	
Prevotella bivia	11-29
Peptostreptococcus	7-33
Fusobacterium species	6-7
Aerobes	
Group B streptococci	12-19
Enterococci	5-11
Escherichia coli	8-12, 55
Other aerobic gram-negative rods	5-10
Gardnerella vaginalis	24

*Data from references [13, 27, 28, 33], and [40]. See text.

was found in the amniotic fluid of women with IAI, maternal or neonatal bacteremia was detected in 25% of the cases. When *E. coli* was found, maternal or neonatal bacteremia was detected in 33%. These rates of bacteremia are significantly higher ($P < .05$) than the 10% rate for all organisms and the 1% rate for anaerobes (see Chapter 2). Although *Gardnerella vaginalis* was isolated with high frequency, its pathogenic role is unclear. In a case-control study, *G. vaginalis* was isolated with similar frequencies in IAI and control cases (24 of 86 [28%] versus 18 of 86 [21%]), and there was no detectable maternal antibody response to this organism.

Neisseria gonorrhoeae rarely has been reported to cause amnionitis [30,31]. Data related to the role of *Chlamydia trachomatis* in infections of amniotic fluid are conflicting. Martin and coworkers prospectively studied perinatal mortality in women whose pregnancies were complicated by antepartum maternal *Chlamydia* infections [32]. Two of the six fetal deaths in the *Chlamydia*-positive group were associated with chorioamnionitis compared with one of eight in the control group. Wager and colleagues showed that the rate of occurrence of intrapartum fever was higher in patients with *C. trachomatis* infection (9%) than in patients without *C. trachomatis* isolated from the cervix (1%) [33]. These data must be interpreted with caution because of the limited number of patients and because the control group may not have been sufficiently similar to the infected group. *C. trachomatis* has not been isolated from amniotic cells or placental membranes of patients with IAI [34,35].

In a controlled study of IAI, 35% of amniotic fluid samples from 52 patients with IAI yielded *Mycoplasma hominis*, whereas only 8% of amniotic fluid samples from the 52 matched controls had *M. hominis* ($P < .001$). *Ureaplasma urealyticum* was isolated from the amniotic fluid from 50% of the infected and uninfected patients. *M. hominis* is present more commonly in the amniotic fluid of infected patients, but usually in association with other bacteria of known virulence. In a subsequent study, *M. hominis* was found in the blood of 2% of women with IAI and with *M. hominis* in the amniotic fluid. The rate of serologic response was significantly greater than that in asymptomatic control women or infected women without IAI in the amniotic fluid ($P < .001$). These results suggest that the pathogenic potential of *M. hominis* is high.

Goldenberg and colleagues found that 23% of neonates who were born between 23 and 32 weeks of gestation had positive umbilical blood cultures for genital mycoplasmas (*U. urealyticum* and *M. hominis*) [36]. Patients with spontaneous preterm delivery had a significantly higher rate of blood cultures positive for *U. urealyticum* or *M. hominis* or both than patients with indicated preterm delivery (34.7% versus 3.2%; $P < .0001$) The earlier the gestational age at delivery, the more likely the culture was positive. In addition, newborns with a positive blood culture had a higher frequency of a neonatal systemic inflammatory response syndrome, higher serum concentrations of interleukin (IL)-6, and more frequent histologic evidence of placental inflammation than neonates with negative cultures.

The aforementioned studies support the idea that genital mycoplasmas can cause fetal and neonatal morbidity. Considering this notion, a crucial question is why genital mycoplasmas gain access to the amniotic cavity in some, but not most, pregnant women.

Pregnant women seem particularly susceptible to infection with *L. monocytogenes*, an organism that has caused regular outbreaks of infection often associated with contaminated cheeses and other dairy products. The infection is especially dangerous in immunocompromised hosts (fetuses, neonates, and immunocompromised children or adults). Several outbreaks of *L. monocytogenes*–associated febrile gastroenteritis have been reported among healthy adults, but only at doses of 10^5 CFU or greater [37–40]. A study using rhesus monkeys as a surrogate for pregnant women indicated that oral exposure to 10^7 CFU of *L. monocytogenes* resulted in about 50% stillbirths [41]. In 2002, an outbreak of listeriosis in the United States that was responsible for three stillbirths was linked to eating sliceable turkey deli meat [42].

Evidence has shown that maternal bacterial vaginosis is causally linked to IAI [43]. The evidence may be categorized as follows: (1) The microorganisms in bacterial vaginosis and in IAI are similar (anaerobes and mycoplasmas plus *G. vaginalis*), (2) bacterial vaginosis is associated with the isolation of organisms in the chorioamnion, and (3) bacterial vaginosis is associated with development of clinical chorioamnionitis in selected populations [44–46]. It has been shown that treatment of bacterial vaginosis in high-risk populations prenatally decreases the risk of chorioamnionitis and other pregnancy outcomes [47]. In the large trial of Maternal-Fetal Medicine Units Network of the National Institutes of Child Health and Development (NICHD), screening and treatment did not lead to benefit, however, either in the overall patient population or in the secondary analysis of women with prior preterm birth [48]. Subsequently, an American College of Obstetricians and Gynecologists Practice Bulletin on assessment of risk factors for preterm birth advocated that screening and treatment of high-risk or low-risk women would not be expected to reduce the overall rate of preterm birth [49]. In certain populations of high-risk women, such as women with prior preterm birth and bacterial vaginosis early in pregnancy, many experts still recommend treatment of bacterial vaginosis diagnosed early in pregnancy [50].

The role of viruses in causing IAI is unclear. Yankowitz and associates evaluated fluid from 77 mid-trimester genetic amniocenteses by polymerase chain reaction (PCR) assay for the presence of adenovirus, enterovirus, respiratory syncytial virus, Epstein-Barr virus, parvovirus, cytomegalovirus, and herpes simplex virus. Six samples were positive (three adenovirus, one parvovirus, one cytomegalovirus, and one enterovirus), and two resulted in pregnancy loss, one at 21 weeks (adenovirus) and one at 26 weeks (cytomegalovirus) [51]. More recently, primary or reactivated adeno-associated virus-2 infection (maternal IgM seropositivity) early in pregnancy was associated with spontaneous preterm delivery [52].

DIAGNOSIS

Diagnosis of IAI requires a high index of suspicion because the clinical signs and symptoms may be subtle. Usual laboratory indicators of infection, such as positive stains for organisms or leukocytes and positive culture results, are found more frequently than clinically evident infection. Microorganisms are easily grown in culture from amniotic fluid or chorioamniotic membranes using standard techniques.

Antepartum Criteria

The clinical criteria used to make the diagnosis of clinical IAI varies among centers, but often includes maternal fever, maternal tachycardia, fetal tachycardia, uterine tenderness, and foul-smelling amniotic fluid [2]. Maternal leukocytosis (peripheral white blood cell count >15,000/mm^3) supports the diagnosis of clinical IAI. The presence of a left shift (i.e., an increase in the proportion of neutrophils, especially immature forms) is particularly suggestive of clinical IAI. One caveat is that the recent administration of corticosteroids may cause a mild leukocytosis [53]. The increase is caused by demarginated mature neutrophils, however, and the presence of immature forms still suggests infection.

Other causes of fever in the parturient patient include epidural analgesia, concurrent infection of the urinary tract or other organ systems, dehydration, illicit drug use, and other rare conditions. The differential diagnosis of fetal tachycardia includes prematurity, medications, arrhythmias, and hypoxia. Possible causes of maternal tachycardia include drugs, hypotension, dehydration, anxiety, intrinsic cardiac conditions, hypothyroidism, and pulmonary embolism. Foul-smelling amniotic fluid and uterine tenderness, although more specific signs, occur in only a few cases. Bacteremia occurs in less than 10% of cases.

Direct examination of the amniotic fluid may provide important diagnostic information. Samples can be collected transvaginally by aspiration of an intrauterine pressure catheter, by needle aspiration of the forewaters, or by amniocentesis. Outside of research protocols, transabdominal amniocentesis is the most common technique.

Of the rapid diagnostic tests that evaluate IAI, amniotic fluid glucose is the most specific for predicting a positive amniotic fluid culture [54]. Kiltz and colleagues found that an amniotic fluid glucose of less than or equal to 5 mg/dL had a positive predictive value of 90%, whereas a glucose of greater than 20 mg/dL had a negative predictive value of 98% [55]. With intermediate values (i.e., 14 to 15 mg/dL), the likelihood of a positive amniotic culture is 30% to 50%. Hussey and associates prospectively evaluated Gram stain and showed that it is 80% sensitive and 91% specific when a positive result is considered in the presence of white blood cells or bacteria [56]. These investigators concluded that the combination of Gram stain with amniotic fluid glucose level is superior to any individual test.

Amniotic fluid IL-6 is even more sensitive and specific than amniotic fluid glucose and Gram stain [57,58]. IL-6 is an immunostimulatory cytokine and a key mediator of fetal host response to infection. At the present time, this test is not typically available outside of research protocols.

PCR, a molecular biologic technique that amplifies the signal of small amounts of DNA, is likely to change the future of diagnosis of IAI. Several studies have evaluated amniotic fluid samples using PCR techniques. PCR assay has a higher sensitivity than culture for detection of microorganisms in the amniotic fluid, particularly in patients whose amniotic fluid is culture-negative but other markers indicate evidence of an inflammatory response [59–63].

The term amniotic fluid "sludge" has been proposed to describe "free floating hyperechogenic material within the amniotic fluid in close proximity to the uterine cervix." [64] When aspirated, this "sludge" often resembles pus and may show aggregation of epithelial and white blood cells and bacteria on Gram stain. In one retrospective case-control study, patients with "sludge" had a significantly higher rate of spontaneous preterm delivery; a higher frequency of clinical chorioamnionitis, histologic chorioamnionitis, and funisitis; a higher frequency of preterm PROM; and a shorter median ultrasound-to-delivery interval [65]. The presence of amniotic fluid "sludge" was an independent explanatory variable for the occurrence of spontaneous preterm delivery, preterm PROM, microbial invasion of the amniotic cavity, and histologic chorioamnionitis. In addition, the combination of a cervical length less than 25 mm and "sludge" conferred an OR of 14.8 for spontaneous preterm delivery at less than 28 weeks and an OR of 9.9 for spontaneous preterm delivery at less than 32 weeks.

Rates of IAI are probably underestimated with preterm PROM because severe oligohydramnios may preclude successful sampling. The rate of positive amniotic fluid cultures for microorganisms is higher with preterm PROM (32.4%) than with preterm labor with intact membranes (12.8%) [63]. Additionally, women in labor on hospital admission generally do not have their amniotic fluid sampled, but have been shown to have higher rates of microbial invasion of the amniotic cavity (39%) than women not in labor (25%). When women do enter labor, the risk of microbial invasion of the amniotic cavity is even higher at 75% [66].

Neonatal Criteria

Most cases of early-onset neonatal sepsis originate in utero. Immediately after delivery, the diagnosis of septicemia is difficult because the neonate's response to infection is impaired, and the reaction is often nonspecific. The earliest signs are often subtle and include changes in color, tone, activity, and feeding patterns; poor temperature control; or simply a general feeling that the neonate is "not doing well." Other possible early signs are abdominal distention, apnea, and jaundice, but they may not appear until later stages, or they may even be seen in healthy premature newborns. Late signs include grunting, dyspnea, cyanosis, arrhythmias, hepatosplenomegaly, petechiae, seizures, bulging fontanelles, and irritability. Focal signs of meningitis or pneumonia may also develop [29].

Laboratory Criteria in the Placenta and Newborn or Stillborn Infant

Examination of the cord, placenta, or membranes for a leukocytic infiltrate has been suggested as another technique to identify infants at risk for infection. Placental inflammation or funisitis or both are found far in excess of proven cases of sepsis, however, and the technique is cumbersome [7]. In a stillborn with suspected IAI, a blood sample should be obtained to attempt to isolate the infecting microbe. This technique should also be applied in cases of stillbirth with unknown cause.

CHRONIC INTRA-AMNIOTIC INFECTION

Some evidence suggests that IAI may exist as a chronic condition. Several studies have performed microbiologic studies of mid-trimester genetic amniocentesis fluid. Risk of adverse pregnancy outcome is increased when patients are asymptomatic, but have positive results on such studies at mid-trimester amniocentesis compared with patients with culture-negative fluid [59]. Similarly, amniotic fluid IL-6 concentrations were found to be significantly higher in patients experiencing a loss after mid-trimester amniocentesis than in patients delivering at term [67,68].

Emerging evidence also suggests that chronic inflammation may be present in maternal serum. Goldenberg and colleagues showed elevated granulocyte colony-stimulating factor at 24 weeks and 28 weeks in women subsequently delivering prematurely [69].

Building on the idea that infection could be present before conception, Andrews and associates [70] performed a prospective, randomized trial to evaluate whether inter-conceptional antibiotics (azithromycin and metronidazole) decreased the rate of preterm birth. In their population of women with a recent early spontaneous birth, administration of these antibiotics did not significantly reduce the rate of subsequent preterm birth. In a subsequent subgroup analysis, this group found that neither baseline endometrial microbial colonization nor plasma cell endometritis was a risk factor for adverse pregnancy outcome. Colonization with specific microbes interacted with the antibiotics to increase adverse outcomes [71]. Interconceptional antibiotics are not recommended at this time in an attempt to reduce subsequent preterm delivery.

MANAGEMENT

Traditionally, the effectiveness of management of IAI has been viewed in terms of short-term maternal and neonatal outcomes, including maternal sepsis, neonatal sepsis, pneumonia, meningitis, and perinatal death. This section discusses the management principles of these short-term outcomes.

In the past, there was debate regarding timing of antibiotic administration, but it has now become standard to begin treatment during labor, as soon as possible after the maternal diagnosis of IAI is made. Three studies, including a randomized clinical trial, have shown benefits from intrapartum antibiotic therapy compared with immediate postpartum treatment (Table 3–2) [72–74]. In a large, nonrandomized allocation of intrapartum versus immediate postpartum treatment, the former treatment was associated with a significant decrease in neonatal bacteremia (2.8% versus 19.6%; $P < .001$) and a reduction in neonatal death from sepsis (0.9% versus 4.3%; $P = .07$) [72]. Another large study showed an overall reduction in neonatal sepsis ($P = .06$), especially bacteremia caused by GBS (0% versus 4.7%; $P = .004$), with use of intrapartum treatment [73].

In a randomized clinical trial, Gibbs and associates showed that intrapartum treatment provided maternal benefits (decreased hospital stay, lower mean temperature postpartum) and neonatal benefits (decrease in sepsis [0% versus 21%; $P = .03$] and decreased hospital stay). In this study, neonates received one set of blood cultures and a chest x-ray film. Cerebrospinal fluid specimens were obtained only from infants with referable signs or symptoms. All infants received identical regimens consisting of intravenous ampicillin and gentamicin begun within 1 to 2 hours of birth and continued for at least 72 hours. If bacteremia or neonatal pneumonia was diagnosed, antibiotics were continued for 10 days [74]. Initiation of intrapartum antibiotics leads to a decrease in neonatal death from sepsis and an improved maternal outcome. These benefits seem to outweigh any theoretical arguments (e.g., obscuring positive neonatal cultures) against intrapartum treatment in cases of IAI.

Pharmacokinetic studies [75] done during early pregnancy show that ampicillin concentrations in maternal and fetal sera are comparable 60 to 90 minutes after administration (Fig. 3–2). Penicillin G levels in fetal serum are one third the maternal levels 120 minutes after administration [76]. In addition, ampicillin has some activity against *E. coli*. Ampicillin is preferable to penicillin G for treatment of IAI. When used in combination with an

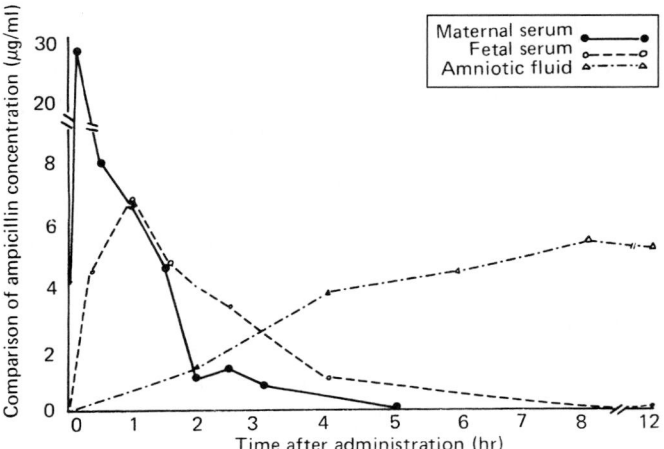

FIGURE 3–2 Ampicillin levels achieved with systemic administration to the mother. *(From Bray RE, Boe RW, Johnson WL. Transfer of ampicillin into fetus and amniotic fluid from maternal plasma in late pregnancy. Am J Obstet Gynecol 96:938, 1966.)*

aminoglycoside, ampicillin should be administered first because it has a broader antimicrobial spectrum.

In late pregnancy, gentamicin also crosses the placenta rapidly, but peak fetal levels may be low, especially if maternal levels are subtherapeutic [77]. Traditionally, an initial gentamicin dose of at least 1.5 to 2 mg/kg followed by 1 to 1.5 mg/kg every 8 hours is used because of the potential for unfavorable gentamicin kinetics. Locksmith and colleagues [78] evaluated maternal and fetal serum drug levels between women who received the standard gentamicin dosing versus once-daily dosing (5 mg/kg every 24 hours). The authors found that the once-daily dosing regimen resulted in fetal serum peak levels that were closer to optimal neonatal values. No adverse effects of once-daily dosing were seen. Achieving the same gentamicin levels in the fetus as are targeted in the newborn infant seems worthy of future investigation.

Clindamycin achieves peak concentrations in maternal blood within minutes after injection and in fetal blood shortly thereafter. In pharmacokinetic studies later in pregnancy, peak clindamycin concentrations were approximately one half of maternal peaks, but the former were still within therapeutic ranges [77].

TABLE 3–2 Comparative Studies of Intrapartum versus Postpartum Maternal Antibiotic Therapy in Treatment of Intra-amniotic Infection

Author, Year	Design/Setting	No. Patients	Maternal Intrapartum Antibiotic Regimen	Benefits of Intrapartum Treatment
Sperling et al [28], 1987	Retrospective/public teaching hospital in San Antonio, TX	257	Penicillin G plus gentamicin IV	NNS reduced from 19.6% in postpartum treatment group to 2.8% in intrapartum treatment group ($P = .001$)
Gilstrap et al, 1988	Retrospective/public teaching hospital in Dallas, TX	273	Varied*	NNS reduced from 5.7% in postpartum treatment group to 1.5% in intrapartum treatment group ($P = .06$); group B streptococcal bacteria reduced from 5.7% to 0% ($P = .004$)
Gibbs et al, 1988	Randomized clinical trial/same as Sperling (1987)	45	Ampicillin plus gentamicin IV	NNS reduced from 21% to 0%; maternal morbidity also decreased ($P = .05$)

Antibiotic regimens noted as 47% received ampicillin or penicillin in combination with gentamicin and clindamycin; 22%, ampicillin or penicillin with gentamicin; 20%, cefoxitin; and 11%, other antibiotics.

IV, intravenously; NNS, neonatal sepsis confirmed by blood culture.

As an alternative, a newer penicillin or cephalosporin with excellent activity against aerobic gram-negative bacteria might be used. There is little published experience with these other antibiotics in IAI, however. In cases of clinical chorioamnionitis, one study showed that clindamycin, mezlocillin, ampicillin, cefoxitin, and gentamicin all penetrated into cord blood and placental membranes, with achievement of therapeutic concentrations in cord blood [79].

The traditional antibiotic choice in cases of IAI includes a combination of a broad-spectrum penicillin with an aminoglycoside, plus clindamycin in some cases (e.g., cesarean delivery or apparent sepsis). Because of expense and complexity, there has been interest in treatment of IAI with a single agent. In view of the typical causative microbes, there are several reasonable choices for single-drug treatment, such as extended-spectrum penicillin (piperacillin, tazobactam) or extended-spectrum cephalosporins (cefotetan). More recent studies have addressed the issue of duration of antibiotic therapy postpartum in cases of IAI. One randomized trial compared single-dose versus multidose postpartum treatment of mothers and reported that single-dose treatment was accompanied by a shorter time to discharge (33 hours versus 57 hours; $P = .001$) [80]. The single-dose group had a nearly threefold increase in failure of therapy, but this did not achieve statistical significance (11% versus 3.7%; $P = .27$). Although not statistically significant, this threefold increase in "failed therapy" elicits concern regarding single-dose postpartum therapy for IAI.

In a study of antibiotic therapy after cesarean delivery for chorioamnionitis, Turnquest and associates [29] randomly assigned patients to receive no scheduled postoperative antibiotics or clindamycin and gentamicin until they were afebrile (for a minimum of at least 24 hours.) All patients received ampicillin in labor, and clindamycin and gentamicin, one dose each preoperatively. No patients in either group developed an abscess or were readmitted for endometritis. Although there was no significant difference in endometritis (14.8% in patients with no routine antibiotic versus 21.8% in patients who received clindamycin and gentamicin), there was a 2.5-fold increase in wound infection rate in patients who did not receive scheduled postpartum antibiotics (5% versus 1.8%).

A subsequent study randomly assigned postpartum patients with chorioamnionitis to receive ampicillin (2 g every 6 hours) and gentamicin (1.5 mg/kg every 8 hours) until afebrile and asymptomatic for 24 hours (control group) or to receive only the next scheduled dose of each antibiotic [81]. In this study, 40% of patients delivered by cesarean section. All patients received ampicillin and gentamicin intrapartum; patients who underwent cesarean delivery also received clindamycin (900 mg) at cord clamping. Patients in the control group had clindamycin continued every 8 hours until antibiotics were discontinued, whereas patients in the study group received only the one dose of clindamycin. The primary outcome was failure of treatment, defined as one temperature elevation after the first postpartum antibiotics dose of 39° C or more than two temperatures of 38.4° C, at least 4 hours apart. These two regimens had similar rates of failure. Based on the information related here, it seems that when antibiotic treatment is initiated early, a short course of therapy in the puerperium is sufficient therapy in most patients.

SHORT-TERM OUTCOMES

With regard to timing of delivery, short-term outcome does not depend on duration of chorioamnionitis [2,82–85]. Cesarean delivery usually is reserved for standard obstetric indications, not for IAI itself. No critical interval from diagnosis of amnionitis to delivery could be identified. Specifically, neither prenatal mortality nor maternal complications correlated with more prolonged intervals from diagnosis of chorioamnionitis to delivery, yet all patients delivered within 4 to 12 hours. Nearly all of these cases described pregnancy at or near term, however. Rates of cesarean section are two to three times higher among patients with IAI than in the general population, owing to patient selection (most cases occur in women with dystocia already diagnosed) and a poor response to oxytocin [86,87].

We use a combination of an intravenous penicillin and intravenous gentamicin as soon as the diagnosis of IAI is made [2,88]. Several studies have reported good results with similar regimens [82]. When a cesarean section is necessary, clindamycin should be added postpartum to these antibiotics to cover anaerobic microbes that are associated with post–cesarean section infection and because of high failure rate (20%) with penicillin and gentamicin therapy after cesarean section [1]. Other initial regimens with cefoxitin alone or ampicillin plus a newer cephalosporin may be equally effective, but no comparative trials have been performed.

Since 1979, retrospective studies have shown a vastly improved perinatal outcome compared with perinatal outcomes reported in older studies. Gibbs and colleagues reported a retrospective study of 171 patients with IAI in whom therapy (with penicillin G and kanamycin) usually was begun at the time of diagnosis [1]. The mean gestational age of the neonate was 37.7 weeks. There were no maternal deaths, and bacteremia was found in only 2.3% of mothers. Among women with IAI, the rate of cesarean delivery was increased approximately threefold to 35%, mainly because of dystocia. The outcome was good in all mothers. There was only one episode of septic shock, with no pelvic abscesses or maternal deaths. Similar results were reported from Los Angeles County Hospital [89].

Gibbs and colleagues found that when IAI is present, perinatal mortality rate (140 per 1000 births) was approximately seven times the overall perinatal mortality rate for infants weighing more that 499 g (which was 18.2 per 1000 births) [1]. None of the perinatal deaths was clearly attributable to infection, however; of live-born infants weighing more than 1000 g, none died of infection. In the study by Koh and coworkers, the perinatal mortality rate was lower (28.1 per 1000 births), which probably reflected the higher mean gestational age (39.3 weeks) [89]. There were no intrapartum fetal deaths and only four neonatal deaths. No deaths were due to infection. Neither perinatal nor maternal complications correlated with more prolonged diagnosis-to-delivery intervals. Because patients who underwent cesarean section had more complicated courses, it was concluded that cesarean section should be reserved for patients with standard obstetric indications.

Yoder and colleagues later reported a prospective, case-control study of 67 neonates with microbiologically confirmed IAI at term [88]. There was only one perinatal death, which was unrelated to infection. Cerebrospinal fluid culture results were negative for all 49 infants tested, and there was no clinical evidence of meningitis. Findings on chest radiographs were interpreted as possible pneumonia in 20% of patients and as unequivocal pneumonia in only 4%. Neonatal bacteremia was documented in 8%. There was no significant difference in the frequency of low Apgar scores between the IAI and control groups.

Two other retrospective studies have been confirmatory. Looff and Hager reported the outcomes of 104 pregnancies with clinical chorioamnionitis [82]. The mean gestational age was 36 weeks. The perinatal mortality rate was 123 per 1000 births. Nearly all of the excess mortality was attributed to prematurity, rather than to sepsis. These authors also reported an increase in the cesarean delivery rate. Hauth and coworkers reviewed data for 103 pregnancies with clinical chorioamnionitis at term [83]. The mean interval from diagnosis of amnionitis to delivery was 3.1 hours, which confirmed the absence of a critical interval for delivery. In this study, the overall perinatal mortality rate was 9.7 per 1000 births, and the cesarean delivery rate was 42%.

Neonates born prematurely have a higher frequency of complications if their mothers have IAI. Garite and Freeman noted that the perinatal death rate was significantly higher in 47 preterm neonates with IAI than in 204 neonates with similar birth weights, but without IAI [90]. The group with IAI also had a significantly higher percentage (13% versus 3%; $P < .05$) with RDS and total infection. A larger but similar comparative study of 92 patients with chorioamnionitis and 606 controls of similar gestational age also showed significant increases in mortality, RDS, intraventricular hemorrhage (IVH), and clinically diagnosed sepsis in the group with chorioamnionitis (Table 3–3) [91]. When Sperling and associates stratified outcomes in cases of IAI by birth weight, cases with low birth weight were associated with more frequent maternal bacteremia (13.5% versus 4.9%; $P = .06$), early-onset neonatal sepsis (16.2% versus 4.1%; $P = .005$), and neonatal death from sepsis (10.8% versus 0; $P < .001$) [92].

In a retrospective, case-control study, Ferguson and coworkers reported neonatal outcome after chorioamnionitis [93]. Of newborns, 70% weighed less than 2500 g. In 116 matched pairs, the authors found more deaths (20% versus 11%), more sepsis (7% versus 2%), and more asphyxia (27% versus 16%) in the group with chorioamnionitis. None of these differences, achieved statistical significance.

Chorioamnionitis has been previously considered a maternal infection. Increasing evidence indicates, however, that the fetus is primarily involved in the inflammatory response leading to premature delivery. Fetal inflammatory response syndrome, well described by Yoon and colleagues, characterizes preterm PROM and spontaneous preterm labor, with a systemic proinflammatory cytokine response resulting in earlier delivery and with an increased risk of complications [94]. Additionally, these investigators showed an association between the fetal inflammatory cascade and fetal white matter damage [95]. It is unclear, however, whether cytokines mediate this damage or directly cause the damage, or whether infection itself is responsible for the damage. Cytokines also can be stimulated by many noninfectious insults, such as hypoxia, reperfusion injury, and toxins [96].

IAI has a significant adverse effect on the mother and neonate. Outcome largely depends on the involved microbes (with E. coli and GBS more likely to result in maternal or neonatal bacteremia), birth weight (with low birth weight infants faring more poorly), and timing of antibiotic therapy (with intrapartum administration improving outcome.)

LONG-TERM OUTCOME

Hardt and colleagues studied long-term outcomes in preterm infants (weighing <2000 g) born after a pregnancy with chorioamnionitis and found a significantly lower mental development index (Bayley score) for the infants than seen in preterm control infants (104 ± 18 versus 112 ± 14; $P = .017$) [97]. Morales reported 1-year follow-up of preterm infants born after pregnancy with chorioamnionitis and of control infants. Differences in mental and physical development were not observed, but adjustments were made for IVH and RDS, both of which were more frequent in the amnionitis group [91].

Intriguing new information strongly suggests that intrauterine exposure to bacteria is associated with long-term serious neonatal complications, including cerebral palsy or its histologic precursor, periventricular leukomalacia (PVL), and major pulmonary problems of bronchopulmonary dysplasia and RDS. The unifying hypothesis states that intrauterine exposure of the fetus to infection leads to abnormal fetal production of proinflammatory cytokines; this leads to fetal cellular damage in the brain, lung, and, potentially, other organs. This fetal inflammatory response syndrome has been likened to systemic inflammatory response syndrome in adults. The evidence linking infection to cerebral palsy may be summarized as follows:

1. Intrauterine exposure to maternal or placental infection is associated with an increased risk of cerebral palsy in preterm and term infants [98–101].

TABLE 3–3 Perinatal Outcome in Preterm Amnionitis (Intra-amniotic Infection)

Measure (%)	Amnionitis*		Control*	
	Garite [88] (n = 47)	Morales [89] (n = 92)	Garite [88] (n = 204)	Morales [89] (n = 606)
Perinatal death	13	25	3[†]	6[†]
Respiratory distress syndrome	34	62	16[†]	35[†]
Total infections	17	28	7[†]	11[†]
Intraventricular hemorrhage	NR	56	NR[†]	22[†]

*At centers reporting these results, there were active referral services. In these series of consecutive patients with preterm premature rupture of membranes, patients with amnionitis are compared with patients without amnionitis.
[†]Rates are significantly lower than for amnionitis group in corresponding study.
NR, not reported.

2. Clinical chorioamnionitis in infants with very low birth weight is significantly associated with an increase in PVL ($P = .001$) [102].
3. The levels of inflammatory cytokines are increased in the amniotic fluid of infants with white matter lesions (PVL), and there is overexpression of these cytokines in neonatal brain with PVL [103].
4. Experimental intrauterine infection in animal models leads to brain white matter lesions [104,105].
5. Marked inflammation of the fetal side of the placenta is associated with adverse neurologic outcomes. Coexisting evidence of infection and thrombosis, particularly on the fetal side of the placenta, is associated with a heightened risk of cerebral palsy or neurologic impairment in term and preterm infants. Additionally, histologic funisitis is associated with an increased risk of subsequent cerebral palsy (OR 5.5, 95% confidence interval [CI] 1.2 to 24.5) [102,106–108]. This risk underscores the importance of sending placentas to pathology for gross and microscopic examination in the setting of IAI.

The association between IAI and cerebral palsy differs for term and preterm infants. A review article outlined the controversies in this area, including the associations among microbiologic, clinical, and histologic chorioamnionitis [109]. Additionally, emerging evidence points to genetic predispositions to inflammation and thrombosis. Cytokine polymorphisms also may be linked to cerebral palsy [96].

In addition to cellular and tissue damage in the fetal brain, an overexuberant cytokine response induced by bacteria may damage other fetal tissues, such as the lung, contributing to RDS and bronchopulmonary dysplasia [110]. In support of this hypothesis, a case-control study of infants with and without RDS was conducted. Infants with RDS were significantly more likely to have elevated levels of amniotic fluid tumor necrosis factor (TNF)-α, a positive culture of the amniotic fluid, and severe histologic chorioamnionitis ($P < .05$ for each association). Elevated amniotic fluid IL-6 levels were also twice as common in the group with RDS, but this association did not achieve statistical significance. Preterm fetuses with elevated cord blood IL-6 concentrations (>11 pg/mL) were more likely to develop RDS (64% versus 24%; $P < .005$) than preterm fetuses without elevated cord IL-6 levels. Rates of occurrence of bronchopulmonary dysplasia also were increased (11% versus 5%), but the observed difference was not statistically significant [111]. Curley and associates found elevated matrix metalloproteinase (MMP)-9 concentration in bronchoalveolar lavage fluid in preterm neonates with pregnancies complicated by chorioamnionitis compared with age-matched uninfected controls. These investigators hypothesized that increased MMP levels in the lung cause destruction of the extracellular matrix, breaking down type IV collagen in the basement membrane and leading to the failure of alveolarization and to the fibrosis components of chronic lung disease [112].

More recently, genetic predisposition toward exuberant host response to tissue injury has been described. Proinflammatory cytokine polymorphisms such as TNF-α 308 relate to bacterial endotoxin and an increased risk of preterm delivery [113–115].

IAI has significant adverse effects on the mother and neonate, but vigorous antibiotic therapy and reasonable prompt

TABLE 3–4   Proposed Prevention Strategies for Clinical Intra-amniotic Infection

Prompt management of dystocia
Induction of labor with premature rupture of membranes at term
Antibiotic prophylaxis with preterm premature rupture of membranes
Antibiotic prophylaxis with preterm labor, but with intact membranes
Antibiotic prophylaxis for group B streptococcal infection
Prenatal treatment of bacterial vaginosis
Chlorhexidine vaginal irrigations in labor
Infection control measures

delivery result in an excellent short-term prognosis, especially for the mother and term neonate. With the combination of prematurity and amnionitis, serious sequelae are more likely for the neonate. Newer information suggests that intrauterine infection is linked to major neonatal long-term complications. A complex interplay of cytokine genotypes may contribute to long-term complications as well.

CONCLUSION

The unanswered question remains: Why does IAI develop in some patients and not in others? Investigations of maternal and fetal genotypes for proinflammatory markers, among others, and study of mucosal immunity and host response may help to answer this important question and clarify when neonatal damage occurs. Satisfactory therapeutic approaches cannot be developed until we understand the answers to these questions.

Prevention

As categorized in Table 3–4, numerous approaches have been proposed for the prevention of IAI. Among these, prompt management of dystocia has been shown to decrease chorioamnionitis and to shorten labor and reduce cesarean section rate [5]. Similarly, induction in women with PROM at term most likely results in fewer maternal infections than may occur with expectant management [115]. Antibiotic prophylaxis for patients with preterm PROM decreases chorioamnionitis and other complications [116,117]. Treatment for bacterial vaginosis in high-risk women decreases the incidence of preterm birth. Antibiotic prophylaxis for patients in preterm labor (but with intact membranes) does not seem to decrease frequency of chorioamnionitis [118]. Intrapartum prophylaxis for the prevention of neonatal sepsis with GBS is now a national standard in patients with GBS colonization or in patients with specific high risks. It is presumed that this approach also decreases chorioamnionitis, but there are no definitive data to support this. Prenatal treatment of bacterial vaginosis in low-risk women, chlorhexidine vaginal washes in labor, and specific infection control measures have not been shown to be effective [22,119–122].

INFECTION AS A CAUSE OF PRETERM BIRTH

Preterm birth is a leading perinatal problem in the United States, and rates continue to increase. In 2005, the rate of preterm birth before 37 completed weeks of gestation

TABLE 3–5 Evidence for Relationship between Preterm Births and Subclinical Genitourinary Tract Infection

The incidence of histologic chorioamnionitis is increased after preterm birth

The incidence of clinical infection is increased after preterm birth in the mother and neonate

Some lower genital tract microbes or infections are associated with increased risk of preterm birth

Biochemical mechanisms link prematurity and infection

Infection and inflammation cause cytokine release and prostaglandin production

Bacteria and bacterial products induce preterm delivery in animal models

Amniotic fluid tests for bacteria are positive in some patients in premature labor

Some antibiotic trials have shown a decrease in numbers of preterm births

increased to 12.7%, an increase of 20% since 1990 and 9% since 2000 [123]. Preterm infants account for 70% of all perinatal deaths and half of long-term neurologic morbidity.

In most cases, the underlying cause of premature labor is not evident. Evidence from many sources points to a relationship between preterm birth and genitourinary tract infections (Table 3–5) [124,125]. In addition to the genitourinary tract, infection leading to preterm birth may arise in a more remote site, such as the lung or periodontal tissues [126–129]. Newer information has suggested that subclinical infection is responsible not only for preterm birth, but also for many serious neonatal sequelae, including PVL, cerebral palsy, RDS, bronchopulmonary dysplasia, and necrotizing enterocolitis [96,98–110].

HISTOLOGIC CHORIOAMNIONITIS AND PREMATURITY

Over the past 3 decades, one of the most consistent observations is that placentas in premature births are more likely to show evidence of inflammation (i.e., histologic chorioamnionitis) (Fig. 3–3). In a series of 3500 consecutive placentas, Driscoll found infiltrates of polymorphonuclear cells in 11% [130]. Clinically evident infection developed in only a few of the women in the study, but the likelihood of neonatal sepsis and death was increased [131].

An association has been established between histologic chorioamnionitis and chorioamnion infection (defined as a positive culture) [131]. ORs of 2.8 to 14 have been reported, this relationship being stronger among preterm deliveries than among term deliveries. Overall, the organisms found in the chorioamnion are similar to organisms found in the amniotic fluid in cases of clinical IAI. This array of organisms supports an ascending route for chorioamnion infection in most cases.

Although it is uncertain how histologic chorioamnionitis and membrane infection cause preterm delivery or preterm PROM, studies suggest that they lead to weakening of the membranes (as evidenced by lower bursting tension, less work to rupture, and less elasticity [132] in vitro) and to production of prostaglandins by the amnion [133,134].

The rate of histologic chorioamnionitis increases with decreasing gestational age at delivery. In one study, when birth weight was greater than 3000 g, the percentage of placentas showing histologic chorioamnionitis was less

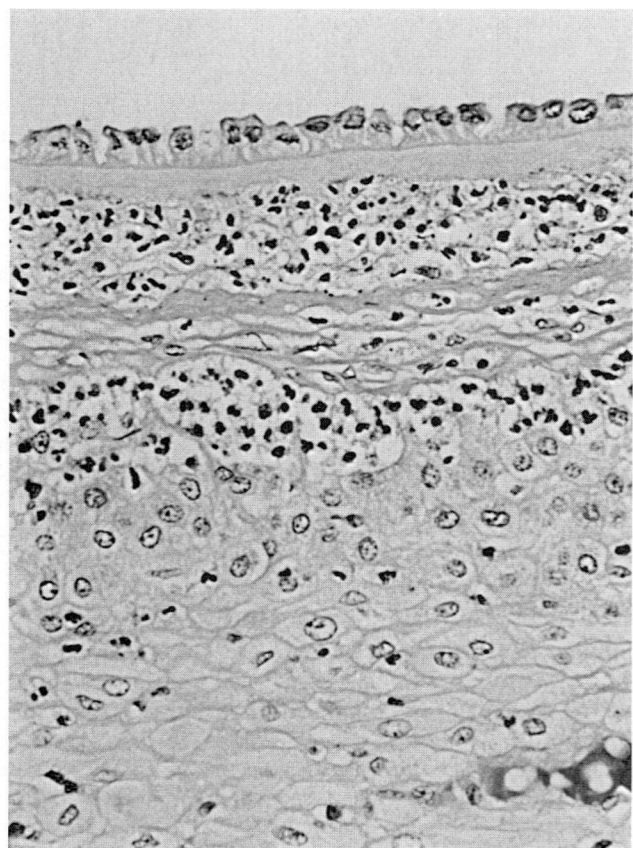

FIGURE 3–3 Infiltrates of polymorphonuclear cells are seen in fetal membranes. Inflammation of placenta and membranes has been consistently observed more often after preterm births than after term births.

than 20%; when birth weight was less than 1500 g, the percentage was 60% to 70% [135].

CLINICAL INFECTION AND PREMATURITY

Premature infants and women who previously gave birth to premature infants are more likely to develop clinically evident infection [136]. In a large study of more than 9500 deliveries, confirmatory evidence showed that chorioamnionitis, endometritis, and neonatal infection all were significantly increased in preterm pregnancies, even after correcting for the presence of PROM [137]. These observations suggest that subclinical infection led to the labor and that infection became clinically evident after delivery. Some investigators argue that there is no causal relationship, but that infection develops more frequently in premature infants because they are compromised hosts, or because they have more invasive monitoring in the nursery.

Strong evidence supports the relationship between preterm birth and genitourinary tract infections. Untreated bacteriuria in pregnancy leads to acute pyelonephritis in 20% to 40% of patients; pyelonephritis has a significantly increased risk of fetal morbidity and mortality. Untreated acute pyelonephritis is associated with a 30% risk of preterm labor and delivery. A meta-analysis [138] showed that women with asymptomatic bacteriuria had a 60% higher rate of low birth weight (95% CI 1.4 to 1.0) and a 90% higher rate of preterm delivery (95% CI 1.3 to 1.9).

Mounting evidence indicates that periodontal disease is associated with preterm birth. A meta-analysis [139] stated that a "likely association" existed between periodontitis and preterm birth or low birth weight, with approximately a twofold increased risk for preterm birth in patients with periodontal disease. As Stamilio and colleagues pointed out [140], the validity of the meta-analytic results is limited by the quality of studies that comprise the analysis. In addition, association does not always correspond to causation. Finally, we can never conclude that an association leads to proof of efficacy for an intervention. Based on all of the available information, the authors do not recommend dental interventions as preventive therapy for preterm birth.

ASSOCIATION OF LOWER GENITAL TRACT ORGANISMS OR INFECTIONS WITH PREMATURITY

Premature birth has been associated with isolation of several organisms from the maternal lower genital tract and with subclinical infections, as listed in Table 3–6. A large collaborative study including more than 4500 patients showed that lower genital tract colonization with *U. urealyticum* is not associated with preterm birth; this organism is one of the most commonly isolated in the amniotic fluid of women in preterm labor. Similarly, cervical infection with *C. trachomatis* is not associated with preterm birth [141].

Other lower genital tract or urinary infections, including infections caused by *N. gonorrhoeae* and *Trichomonas vaginalis* and bacteriuria, are associated with preterm birth, however. Several studies found increased OR for preterm birth among women with *T. vaginalis* infection [125]. In the large Vaginal Infections and Prematurity Study, lower genital tract carriage of *T. vaginalis* at mid-pregnancy was significantly associated with preterm low birth weight. Preterm low birth weight occurred in 7.1% of women with *T. vaginalis*

compared with 4.5% of women without *T. vaginalis* (OR 1.6, 95% CI 1.3-1.9) [142]. Bacterial vaginosis, characterized by high concentrations of anaerobes, *G. vaginalis*, and genital mycoplasmas, with a corresponding decrease in the normal vaginal lactobacilli, confers an approximately twofold to threefold increase in spontaneous premature birth. It is unclear whether bacterial vaginosis causes preterm delivery by leading to subclinical infection, or whether bacterial vaginosis acts locally in the lower genital tract infections because it is associated with increased concentrations of elastase, mucinase, and sialidase (hydrolytic enzymes associated with increased risks of adverse pregnancy outcomes) [143–148].

Macones and colleagues presented evidence that an interaction between genetic susceptibility and environmental factors (i.e., bacterial vaginosis) increased the risk of spontaneous preterm birth. Specifically, they showed that maternal carriers of TNF-2 were at significantly increased risk of spontaneous preterm birth (OR 2.7, 95% CI 1.7-4.5). The association between TNF-2 and preterm birth was modified by the presence of bacterial vaginosis; mothers with a "susceptible" genotype and bacterial vaginosis had an increased OR of preterm birth compared with mothers who did not (OR 6.1, 95% CI 1.9-21.0) [149].

Maternal genital tract colonization with GBS may lead to neonatal sepsis, especially when birth occurs prematurely, or when the membranes have been ruptured for prolonged intervals. In addition, Regan and coworkers [150] found an association between colonization of the cervix with these organisms and premature birth. These investigators noted delivery at less than 32 weeks in 1.8% of the total population, but in 5.4% of women colonized with GBS (*P* < .005). PROM also occurred significantly more often in the colonized group (15.3% versus 8.1%; *P* < .005). Of six studies evaluating the association between GBS genital colonization and preterm labor or delivery, five found no association [125].

In contrast with the conflicting data regarding genital colonization with GBS, GBS bacteriuria has been consistently associated with preterm delivery, and treatment of this bacteriuria resulted in a marked reduction in prematurity (37.5% in the placebo group versus 5.4% in the treatment group) [151–153]. In a randomized treatment trial of erythromycin versus placebo in women colonized with GBS, erythromycin use was not shown to be effective in prolonging gestation or increasing birth weight [154].

Current recommendations for prevention of perinatal infection with GBS from the U.S. Centers for Disease Control and Prevention (CDC) are for intrapartum treatment only, with the exception of GBS bacteriuria, which should be treated antepartum. The 2002 CDC guidelines recommend adoption of universal screening. The universal screening approach involves screening women at 35 to 37 weeks of gestation with proper collection and culture techniques, followed by intrapartum treatment for all women with positive cultures [155].

TABLE 3–6 Association of Lower Genitourinary Tract Infections with Preterm Birth

Infection	Odds Ratio for Preterm Birth (95% Confidence Interval)
Ureaplasma urealyticum	1.0 (0.8-1.2)[a]
Chlamydia trachomatis	0.7 (0.36-1.37)[b,c]
Neisseria gonorrhoeae	531 (1.57-17.9)[d]
Trichomonas vaginalis	1.3 (1.1-1.4)[e]
Bacterial vaginosis	1.3 (1.1-1.4)[f]
Bacteriuria	1.64 (1.35-1.78)[g]

[a]Data from Carey JC, et al. Antepartum cultures for Ureaplasma urealyticum are not useful in predicting pregnancy outcome. Am J Obstet Gynecol 164:728, 1991.
[b]Data from Sweet RL, et al. Chlamydia trachomatis infection and pregnancy outcome. Am J Obstet Gynecol 156:824, 1987.
[c]Data from Harrison HR, et al. Cervical Chlamydia trachomatis and mycoplasmal infections in pregnancy. JAMA 250:1721, 1983.
[d]Data from Elliott B, et al. Maternal gonococcal infection as a preventable risk factor for low birth weight. J Infect Dis 161:531, 1990.
[e]Data from Cotch MF, et al. Trichomonas vaginalis associated with low birth weight and preterm delivery. Sex Transm Dis 24:353, 1997.
[f]Data from Leitich H, et al. Bacterial vaginosis as a risk factor for preterm delivery: a meta-analysis. Am J Obstet Gynecol 189:139, 2003.
[g]Data from Romero R, et al. Meta-analysis of the relationship between asymptomatic bacteriuria and preterm delivery/low birth weight. Obstet Gynecol 73:567, 1989.

AMNIOTIC FLUID CULTURES IN PRETERM LABOR

Among patients with signs and symptoms of preterm labor, the probability of finding a positive result on tests for bacteria depends on several factors: the specimen tested, the population under investigation, and the technique used for microbial detection. When standard culture techniques have been used for the amniotic fluid of patients clinically defined as being in preterm labor, the likelihood of positive cultures ranges from 0% to 25%. Yet with culture of the amniotic fluid of patients in preterm labor who deliver a preterm infant within 72 hours of the amniocentesis, the likelihood of a positive result has been 22%. With use of more sensitive assays such as PCR, the probability of finding bacteria in the amniotic fluid of patients in preterm labor has been 30% to 55% [60–62,125,156]. Because bacteria are likely to be present in the amniotic membranes before appearing in the amniotic fluid, the rate of positive cultures of the membranes for patients in preterm labor has been 32% to 61%. Histologic evidence of chorioamnion infection is extremely common, being found in approximately 80% of placentas after birth of infants weighing 1000 g or less.

BIOCHEMICAL LINKS OF PREMATURITY AND INFECTION

The widely accepted working hypothesis is that bacteria ascending into the uterine cavity are able to stimulate cytokine activity directly. IL-1, IL-6, and TNF-α, the proinflammatory cytokines, have been shown to be produced by the fetal membranes, decidua, and myometrium. Patients with elevated levels of these cytokines in the amniotic fluid have shorter amniocentesis-to-delivery intervals than patients without elevated cytokine levels. Levels also are elevated when preterm labor is associated with IAI [156]. Similarly, Gomez and associates [157] showed that elevated fetal plasma levels of IL-6 in patients with preterm PROM, but not in labor, had a higher rate of delivery within 48 hours compared with patients who delivered more than 48 hours after cordocentesis. These important findings suggest that a fetal inflammatory cytokine response triggers spontaneous preterm delivery.

Immunomodulatory cytokines, such as IL-1 receptor antagonist (IL-1ra), IL-10, and transforming growth factor (TGF)-β, play a regulatory role in the cytokine response, allowing for a downregulation of this response [158]. IL-1ra has been shown in humans to increase in response to IAI [159]. Murtha and coworkers showed that maternal carriage of at least one copy of the IL-1ra allele 2 is associated with increased risk of preterm birth [159]. Similarly, Mulherin and colleagues reported that common genetic variants in proinflammatory cytokine genes could influence the risk for spontaneous preterm birth. They found that selected TNF-α haplotypes were associated with spontaneous preterm birth in African American and white subjects [160]. IL-10 inhibits IL-1β–induced preterm labor in a rhesus model [161].

Animal models have been used to evaluate cytokine-mediated initiation of preterm birth. Romero and colleagues showed that systemic administration of IL-1 induced preterm birth in a murine model [162]. Similarly, Kaga and coworkers gave low-dose lipopolysaccharide intraperitoneally to preterm mice, causing preterm delivery [163]. Again using a murine model, other investigators showed preterm birth after intrauterine inoculation of *E. coli*.

Other investigators have used inoculation of live bacteria to study the infection-cytokine-preterm birth pathway. In rabbits, we found that intrauterine inoculation of *E. coli*,

Fusobacterium species, or GBS led to rapid induction of labor at 70% gestation with an accompanying increase in histologic infiltrate and elaboration of TNF-α into the amniotic fluid. More recently, using our rabbit model, we showed that intrauterine inoculation of the anaerobe *Prevotella bivia* at 70% gestation led to establishment of a "chronic" infection in 64% of animals, with preterm birth occurring in 33% [164]. Also, using a rhesus monkey model, Gravett and colleagues inoculated GBS at 78% gestation and found resulting increases in amniotic fluid cytokines and prostaglandins followed by a progressive cervical dilation [165].

ANTIBIOTIC TRIALS

Antibiotic treatment trials may be categorized into three general types as follows: (1) antibiotics given during prenatal care to patients at increased risk of preterm delivery; (2) antibiotics given adjunctively with tocolytics to women in preterm labor; and (3) antibiotics given to women with preterm PROM, but not yet in labor. In the prototype of the first category of antibiotic trial, Kass and colleagues [166] and McCormack and associates [167] noted a reduction in the percentage of low birth weight infants delivered of women who received oral erythromycin for 6 weeks in the third trimester compared with infants delivered of women who were given a placebo. These results were not confirmed in a National Institutes of Health–sponsored, multi-institutional study. More than 1100 women with genital *U. urealyticum* were randomly assigned to receive placebo or erythromycin beginning at 26 to 28 weeks of gestation and continuing until 35 weeks. No improvement was detected in any outcome measure, including no difference in birth weight, low birth weight, or prematurity rate (Table 3–7). Treatment of *U. urealyticum* in pregnancy to prevent prematurity remains experimental.

Two retrospective, nonrandomized studies have reported reductions in PROM, low birth weight, and preterm labor through antenatal treatment of *C. trachomatis* infection [168, 169]. In the first study, patients successfully treated for *C. trachomatis* had significantly lower rates of PROM and premature labor than patients who failed to have *C. trachomatis* eradicated. In the second study, adverse outcome was assessed among three large groups: *C. trachomatis*–positive

TABLE 3–7 Randomized Trial of Erythromycin for Treatment of Vaginal *Ureaplasma urealyticum* Infection in Pregnancy

Outcome	Treatment Group		P Value
	Erythromycin (*n* = 605)	Placebo (*n* = 576)	
Birth weight (g, mean ± SD)	3302 ± 557	3326 ± 558	NS
Birth weight <2500 g (%)	7	6	NS
Gestational age at delivery ≥36 wk (%)	8.6	8.2	NS
Premature rupture of membranes at ≥36 wk (%)	2.5	2.5	NS
Stillbirth (%)	0.5	0.5	NS
Neonatal death (%)	0.2	0	NS

NS, not significant; SD, standard deviation.

but untreated (*n* = 1110), *C. trachomatis*–positive and treated (*n* = 1327), and *C. trachomatis*–negative (*n* = 9111). The *C. trachomatis*–positive but untreated group had PROM and low birth weight significantly more often and had higher perinatal mortality than the other two groups. The only randomized treatment trial for *C. trachomatis* in pregnancy led to conflicting results, however [170]. In this latter study, the rate of pregnancies resulting in low birth weight infants was reduced in three of the five centers, but not significantly reduced in the remaining two. A more recent study by the NICHD Maternal-Fetal Medicine Units Network found that treatment of *C. trachomatis* in the mid-trimester was not associated with a decreased frequency of preterm birth [141]. At the present time, it is standard of care to treat women with *C. trachomatis* infection, not as much to prevent preterm labor, but to prevent spread of the sexually transmitted disease.

Treatment with metronidazole should be offered to women who have symptomatic *T. vaginalis* infection in pregnancy to relieve maternal symptoms and prevent spread of a sexually transmitted disease [171]. Metronidazole is safe for use in the first trimester of pregnancy [172]. When pregnant women with asymptomatic *T. vaginalis* infection at 24 to 29 weeks of gestation were randomly assigned to receive treatment with either metronidazole or placebo, rates of delivery at less than 37 weeks and at less than 37 weeks because of preterm labor were increased in the group given metronidazole (relative risk 1.8 [95% CI 1.2 to 2.7] for delivery at <37 weeks and relative risk 3.0 [95% CI 1.5 to 5.9] for delivery at <37 weeks because of preterm labor) [173].

Because of the consistent association of bacterial vaginosis with preterm birth, several treatment trials have been carried out in pregnant women. A meta-analysis reported no significant reduction in preterm delivery when women with bacterial vaginosis were given antibiotic therapy as part of prenatal care. Similarly, there is no significant reduction in preterm labor with treatment for bacterial vaginosis in women at low risk for preterm birth. In the subset of women with previous preterm birth and treatment for at least 7 days with an oral regimen, there was a significant reduction in preterm delivery (OR 0.42, 95% CI 0.27 to 0.67). Following the meta-analysis, the PREMET study [174], a randomized controlled trial, concluded that oral metronidazole does not reduce early preterm birth in high-risk women (selected by history and a positive vaginal fetal fibronectin test). Whether vaginal treatment of bacterial vaginosis is effective in preventing preterm birth is unclear. In the meta-analysis, no benefit was obtained by vaginal treatment [175]. Subsequent trials supported the idea, however, that a course of clindamycin cream early in pregnancy leads to a decreased incidence of preterm birth [176,177].

Among women in preterm labor with intact membranes, there have been several studies and meta-analyses studying the effect of various antibiotic regimens. The ORACLE II study showed no delay in delivery or no improvement in a composite outcome that included neonatal death, chronic lung disease, or cerebral anomaly [178]. In the Cochrane meta-analysis, 7428 women in 11 trials were assessed. As shown in Table 3–8, the use of antibiotics did not decrease preterm birth delivery within

TABLE 3–8 Risk of Selected Adverse Outcomes with Use of Antibiotics in Preterm Labor with Intact Membranes

Outcome	RR* (95% Confidence Interval)
Preterm birth	0.99 (0.92-1.05)
Delivery within 48 hr	1.04 (0.89-1.23)
Perinatal mortality	1.22 (0.88-1.70)
Neonatal death	1.52 (0.99-2.34)

*Relative risk (RR) <1.0 favors antibiotics, and RR >1.0 favors controls. RR is statistically significant if the 95% confidence interval excludes 1.0.
From King J, Flenady V. Prophylactic antibiotics for inhibiting preterm labour with intact membranes. Cochrane Database Syst Rev (1), 2003.

48 hours or perinatal mortality. The relative risk for neonatal death in the antibiotic treatment group was 1.52 (95% CI 0.99 to 2.34). There was a significant reduction in postpartum intrauterine infection with use of antibiotics, but this reduction was not seen as sufficient justification for widespread use of antibiotics in preterm labor.

In a subanalysis, the reviewers looked at trials employing antibiotics that were active against anaerobes (i.e., metronidazole or clindamycin). There were significant benefits in delivery within 7 days and in neonatal intensive care unit admissions. These benefits were not accompanied, however, by significant reductions in major end points such as preterm birth, perinatal mortality, or neonatal sepsis.

There have been several large trials among patients with preterm PROM. In 2003, the Cochrane Library updated its meta-analysis of these trials. In 13 trials comprising 6000 patients, antibiotics in this clinical setting had consistent benefits. Among women given antibiotics, delivery within 48 hours, delivery within 7 days, or development of chorioamnionitis was less likely. Their neonates were less likely to have infection or sepsis (Table 3–9).

Lack of consistent findings in these antibiotic trials raises the question of why antibiotics have been effective in so few clinical situations. One likely explanation is that a true effective antibiotic may be "diluted out" by inclusion in the trials of patients in whom premature labor is not due to infection, such as patients in preterm labor at 34 to 37 weeks. Another likely explanation is that when clinical signs and symptoms of preterm labor begin, the complex biochemical reactions have progressed too far to be stopped by antibiotic therapy alone.

Widespread use of antibiotics for the purpose of prolonging a premature pregnancy raises concerns

TABLE 3–9 Risk of Selected Adverse Outcomes with Use of Antibiotics for Preterm Premature Rupture of Membranes

Outcome	RR* (95% Confidence Interval)
Delivery within 48 hr	0.71 (0.58-0.87)
Delivery within 7 days	0.8 (0.71-0.9)
Chorioamnionitis	0.57 (0.37-0.86)
Neonatal infection	0.68 (0.53-0.87)
Abnormalities on cerebral ultrasound examination	0.82 (0.68-0.98)

*Relative risk (RR) <1.0 favors antibiotics, and RR >1.0 favors controls. RR is statistically significant if the 95% confidence interval excludes 1.0.
Data from ***.

TABLE 3–10 Consensus on Use of Antibiotics to Prevent Preterm Birth

Opinion	Comment
During Prenatal Care	
Treat *Neisseria gonorrhoeae* and *Chlamydia trachomatis* infection	Screening and treatment of these two sexually transmitted organisms should follow standard recommendations to prevent spread to sexual partner(s) and the newborn. Published nonrandomized trials show improved pregnancy outcome with treatment.
Treat bacteriuria, including group B streptococcal bacteriuria	Screening and treatment for bacteriuria is a standard practice to prevent pyelonephritis. A meta-analysis concluded that bacteriuria is directly associated with preterm birth.
Screen for and treat bacterial vaginosis in patients at high risk for preterm birth. In these high-risk women, treat with an oral metronidazole for ≥1 wk	A meta-analysis has shown benefit with this treatment in women with high-risk pregnancies.
Treat symptomatic *Trichomonas vaginalis* infection to relieve maternal symptoms, but do not screen for or treat asymptomatic trichomoniasis	This opinion is based on randomized trials in asymptomatic infected women.
Do not treat *Ureaplasma urealyticum* genital colonization	One double-blind treatment trial that corrected for confounding infections showed no benefit.
Do not treat group B streptococcal genital colonization	One double-blind treatment trial showed no benefit.
With Preterm Labor and Intact Membranes	
Give group B streptococcal prophylaxis to prevent neonatal sepsis	As recommended by Centers for Disease Control and Prevention and American College of Obstetricians and Gynecologists.
Do not give antibiotics routinely to prolong pregnancy	A meta-analysis concluded that antibiotics gave no neonatal benefit.
With Preterm Premature Rupture of Membranes	
Give group B streptococcal prophylaxis to prevent neonatal sepsis	As recommended by Centers for Disease Control and Prevention and American College of Obstetricians and Gynecologists.
Give additional antibiotics in pregnancies at 24 to 32 wk	Meta-analyses concluded that there was substantial benefit to the neonate.

regarding selection of resistant organisms and masking of infection. To date, evidence of selection pressure has been limited mainly to infants with very low birth weight [179]. Masking infection is now of great concern, especially in view of evidence that intrauterine exposure to bacteria is associated with long-term adverse neonatal outcomes including cerebral palsy and PVL [99,110].

For reasons other than prevention of preterm birth, detection and treatment of *N. gonorrhoeae*, *C. trachomatis*, and bacteriuria are appropriate. Table 3–10 summarizes our recommendations for use of antibiotics to prevent preterm birth. Future research is urgently needed, however, to identify markers in women who are in preterm labor as a result of infection, in whom intervention with antibiotics or other novel therapies is most likely to be beneficial. In addition, detection of women genetically predisposed to infection-induced preterm birth is important. Some investigators have identified associations between polymorphisms in the cytokine gene complexes including TNF-α and preterm PROM or spontaneous preterm birth [113–115,180].

PREMATURE RUPTURE OF MEMBRANES

PROM is a common but poorly understood problem. Because there is little understanding of its etiology, management has been largely empirical, and obstetricians have been sharply divided over what constitutes the best approach to care [181–184]. The problem is complex. Gestational age and demographic factors influence the outcome with PROM. Therapeutic modalities added within the past 2 decades include corticosteroids, tocolytics, and more potent antibiotics, but their place in therapy is controversial. Of major importance is the marked improvement in survival of infants with low birth weight. This chapter emphasizes developments since 1970. The literature has been reviewed periodically.

DEFINITION

Lack of standard, clear terminology has hindered understanding of PROM. Most authors define PROM as rupture at any time before the onset of contractions, but "premature" also carries the connotation of preterm pregnancy. To avoid confusion, we reserve "preterm" to refer to rupture occurring at a gestational age less than 37 weeks. Others using the expression "prolonged rupture of the membranes" have used the same acronym, PROM.

The latent period is defined as the time from membrane rupture to onset of contractions. It is to be distinguished from the latent phase, which designates the phase of labor that precedes the active phase. "Conservative" or "expectant" management refers to the period of watchful waiting when IAI has been clinically excluded in the setting of PROM.

In addition to IAI, terms used to describe maternal or perinatal infections during labor include fever in labor, intrapartum fever, chorioamnionitis, amnionitis, and intrauterine infection. In most reports, clinical criteria used for these diagnoses include fever, uterine irritability or tenderness, leukocytosis, and purulent cervical discharge. After delivery, maternal uterine infection is referred to an endometritis, endomyometritis or metritis. These clinical diagnoses usually are based on fever and uterine tenderness. In a few studies, presumed maternal infections were confirmed by blood and genital tract cultures.

For neonates, the most common term used to report infection is neonatal sepsis. Some authors use a positive blood or cerebrospinal fluid culture result, whereas others use clinical signs of sepsis without bacteriologic confirmation.

INCIDENCE

In several reports, the incidence of PROM has ranged from 3% to 7% of total deliveries [185,186], whereas PROM related to preterm birth has occurred in approximately 1% of all pregnancies [10–12]. In some referral centers, preterm PROM accounted for 30% of all preterm births. Despite some progress in prolonging the latent period after preterm PROM and possible prevention of recurrence (e.g., by use of progesterone or by treating bacterial vaginosis), preterm PROM remains a leading contributor to the overall problem of premature birth.

ETIOLOGY

Several clinical variables have been associated with PROM [187,188], including cervical incompetence, cervical operations and lacerations, multiple pregnancies, polyhydramnios, antepartum hemorrhage, and heavy smoking. In most instances, none of these clinical variables are present, however. No association has been found between the frequency of PROM and maternal age, parity, maternal weight, fetal weight and position, maternal trauma, or type of maternal work [181,189]. The NICHD Maternal-Fetal Medicine Units Network found that the combination of short cervical length, previous preterm birth caused by preterm PROM, and positive fetal fibronectin screening results was highly associated with preterm delivery caused by preterm PROM in the current gestation [190].

Physical properties of membranes that rupture prematurely also have been investigated. Studies of the collagen content of amnion in patients with PROM have led to conflicting results, perhaps because of important differences in methodology. Patients with Ehlers-Danlos syndrome, a hereditary defect in collagen synthesis, are at increased risk of preterm PROM. Other reports have shown that membranes from women with PROM are thinner than membranes from women without PROM [189]. Using in vitro techniques to measure rupturing pressure, investigators have found that the membranes from patients with PROM withstand either the same or higher pressure before bursting than do membranes from women without PROM [191,192]. Such observations have suggested a local defect at the site of rupture, rather than a diffuse weakening, in membranes that rupture before labor. These studies of physical properties should be interpreted with caution because of differences in measuring techniques, possible deterioration of membrane preparations, and need for proper controls.

In addition to being a possible cause of premature labor, subclinical infection may be a cause of PROM (see previous section). Acute inflammation of the placental membranes is twice as common when membranes rupture within 4 hours

before labor than when they rupture after the onset of labor, which suggests that this "infection" may be the cause of PROM [193]. Supporting this hypothesis, increases in amniotic fluid MMP-1, MMP-8, and MMP-9 and decreases in MMP-1 and MMP-2 inhibitors have been shown in women experiencing preterm PROM [194,195].

Several reports have suggested a relationship among coitus, histologic inflammation, and PROM. In additional analyses, two successive singleton pregnancies in each of 5230 women (10,460 pregnancies) were considered [196]. Preterm PROM occurred in only 2% of 773 pregnancies when there was no recent coitus and histologic chorioamnionitis, but it occurred in 23% of 96 pregnancies when both of these features were present. A causal role of coitus or infection was not established, however, because there may have been other factors that were not considered. Evaluation of successive pregnancies would not have eliminated these confounding variables. In the South African black population, the rates of histologic chorioamnionitis and PROM were increased when coitus had occurred within the last 7 days. Use of a condom during coitus resulted in less placental inflammation. In addition, PROM occurred more often ($P > .01$) when there had been male orgasm during coitus [197]. Because organisms may attach to sperm, it has been hypothesized that sperm carry organisms into the endocervix or uterus.

Further evidence is provided by bacteriologic studies. Patients with PROM before term or with prolonged membrane rupture are more likely to have anaerobes in endocervical cultures than women without PROM at term [198,199]. These observations may be interpreted as showing that subclinical anaerobic "infection" leads to PROM. The increased presence of anaerobes in cervical cultures may reflect hormonal or other influences at different stages of gestation, however.

Investigations of risk factors for preterm PROM are likely to provide insight into the etiology of this condition. In the largest case-control study, Harger and colleagues reported 341 cases and 253 controls [200]. Only three independent variables were associated with preterm PROM in a logistic regression analysis: previous preterm delivery (OR 2.5, 95% CI 1.4 to 2.5), uterine bleeding in pregnancy, and cigarette smoking. OR accompanying bleeding increased with bleeding in late pregnancy and with the number of trimesters in which bleeding occurred (OR for first-trimester bleeding 2.4, 95% CI 1.9 to 23; OR for bleeding in more than one trimester 7.4, 95% CI 2.2 to 26). For cigarette smoking, OR was higher for women who continued smoking (OR 2.1, 95% CI 1.4 to 3.1) than for women who stopped (OR 1.6, 95% CI 0.8 to 3.3). Because previous preterm pregnancy is a historical feature and little can be done to prevent bleeding in pregnancy, this study provides an additional reason to encourage all patients, especially women of reproductive age, to stop smoking. Finally, in most cases, the specific etiology of preterm PROM is unknown.

DIAGNOSIS

In most cases, PROM is readily diagnosed by history, physical findings, and simple laboratory tests such as determination of pH (Nitrazine [phenaphthazine] test

[Bristol-Myers Squibb, Princeton, NJ]) or detection of ferning. Although these tests are accurate in approximately 90% of cases, they yield false-positive and false-negative results, especially in women with small amounts of amniotic fluid in the vagina. If the patient is not going to be delivered immediately, a digital examination should be deferred because examination may introduce bacteria into the uterus and shorten the latent phase.

Other biochemical and histochemical tests and intra-amniotic injection of various dyes have been suggested, but they have not gained wide acceptance. Indigo carmine blue (1 mL diluted in 9 mL of sterile normal saline solution) can be injected into the amniotic fluid, and a sponge can be placed into the vagina and inspected 30 minutes later for dye. Methylene blue should not be used because of reported methemoglobinemia in the fetus. This test is invasive, and the accuracy of diagnosis is unknown.

An immunoassay for placenta α_1-microglobulin (abundant in amniotic fluid, but barely detectable in normal cervicovaginal secretions) has been approved for detecting PROM. Initial reports have found high diagnostic accuracy [29,201].

Ultrasound examination also has been used as a diagnostic technique because oligohydramnios supports a diagnosis of PROM. Oligohydramnios has many additional causes, however. Ultrasound examination should be considered in the context of the entire clinical picture.

NATURAL HISTORY

The onset of regular uterine contractions occurs within 24 hours after membrane rupture in 80% to 90% of term patients [2]. The latent period exceeds 24 hours in 19% of patients at term and exceeds 48 hours in 12.5% [200,202]. Only 3.6% of term patients do not begin to labor within 7 days [200].

Before term, latent periods are longer among patients with PROM. Confirming earlier studies, more recent investigations have shown latent periods of 24 hours in 57% to 83% [202,203], of 72 hours in 15% to 26% [204–206], and of 7 days in 19% to 41% of patients [202,204]. There is an inverse relationship between gestational age and of patients with latent periods of 3 days [205]. There is also an inverse relationship between advancing gestation and a decreased risk of chorioamnionitis. One third of women with pregnancies between 25 and 32 weeks of gestation had latent periods of 3 days, whereas for pregnancies between 33 and 34 weeks and between 35 and 37 weeks, the values were 16% and 4.5%. In 53 cases of PROM at 16 to 25 weeks (mean 22.6 weeks), the median length of time from PROM to delivery was 6 days (range 1 to 87 days, mean 17 days) [207]. In a population-based study of 267 cases of PROM before 34 weeks, 76% of women were already in labor at the time of admission, and an additional 5% had an indicated delivery. Only 19% were candidates for expectant management, and of these women, 60% went into labor within 48 hours [208]. The natural history of PROM reveals that labor usually develops within a few days.

In a few cases of PROM, the membranes can "reseal," especially with rupture of membranes after amniocentesis. With expectant management, 2.8% to 13% may anticipate the cessation of leakage of amniotic fluid [209,210].

COMPLICATIONS

Analysis of complications described in more recent studies is complex because of differences in study design. Table 3–11 summarizes complications observed in studies with more than 100 infants. Direct comparisons of data from one study to another require extreme caution. The wide-ranging differences are attributable to major differences in populations at risk, gestational age, definitions, and management.

The most common complication among cases with PROM before 37 weeks is RDS, which is found in 10% to 40% in neonates. (A few studies have reported RDS in 60% to 80% of newborns.) Neonatal sepsis was documented in less than 10%, whereas amnionitis (based on clinical criteria only) occurred in 4% to 60% [211]. Endometritis developed in 3% to 29% of patients in most reports, but it is unclear whether patients with amnionitis are included in the endometritis category. In selected groups, such as women who undergo cesarean section after PROM, endometritis can occur in 70% of patients. Abruptio placentae after PROM is reported in 4% to 6% of cases, severalfold higher than the rate of 0.5% to 1% in the general population [212].

When latent periods in preterm pregnancies are prolonged, pulmonary hypoplasia is an additional neonatal complication. Although the rate of pulmonary hypoplasia seems to depend on the gestational age of PROM and the remaining amount of amniotic fluid surrounding the fetus, reported rates vary [213–215]. Vergani and colleagues reported that if severe oligohydramnios is present, there is nearly a 100% probability of lethal pulmonary hypoplasia when PROM occurs before 23 weeks [215]. Other investigators reported that the incidence of pulmonary hypoplasia is approximately 60% when rupture occurs before 19 weeks, however [216]. Nimrod and associates showed a 27% incidence of pulmonary hypoplasia in cases in which PROM occurred before 26 weeks and with long intervals (e.g., >5 weeks) between

TABLE 3–11 Complications in Newborns after Premature Rupture of Membranes*

Complication	Rate (%)
Perinatal mortality, overall	0–43
Term	0–2.5
All preterm	2–43
1000-1500 g	29
1501-2500 g	7
RDS, all preterm	10–42
1000-1500 g	42
1501-2500 g	7
Infection	
Amnionitis	4–33
Maternal (overall)	3–29
Endometritis	3–29
Neonatal sepsis	0–7
Neonatal overall (including clinically diagnosed sepsis)	3–281

*Studies with >100 infants.
RDS, respiratory distress syndrome.

rupture and delivery [214]. Other studies showed a lower incidence of pulmonary hypoplasia [213]. Pulmonary hypoplasia is rare if PROM occurs after 26 weeks of gestation [215]. Pulmonary hypoplasia is poorly predicted antenatally by ultrasound examination [213]. Ultrasound estimates of interval fetal lung growth include lung length, chest circumference, chest circumference–abdominal circumference ratio, or chest circumference–femur length ratio.

In addition to the risk of pulmonary hypoplasia, an additional 20% of neonates had fetal skeletal deformities as a result of compression. Nonskeletal restriction deformities of prolonged intrauterine crowding similar to features of Potter syndrome include abnormal facies with low-set ears and epicanthal folds. Limbs may be malpositioned and flattened [217].

Low Apgar scores (<7 at 5 minutes of life) are noted in 15% to 64% of live-born infants [186,187,218–219]. This complication is most common among infants with very low birth weight. Other complications of PROM, especially in preterm pregnancies, include malpresentation, cord prolapse, and congenital anomalies. In view of the long list of potential hazards, it is not surprising that premature infants surviving after PROM often are subject to prolonged hospitalization.

Perinatal mortality depends mainly on gestational age. The wide variation in results for preterm infants reflects different groupings of gestational ages. It is uncertain whether infants with PROM have higher mortality than infants of the same gestational age without PROM.

Causes of perinatal death may be determined by examining data from four large series (Table 3–12) [185,188,220]. Two of these studies included stillbirths; two studies excluded them. Overall, RDS was the leading cause of death. Deaths were presumed to be due to hypoxia when there was an antepartum or intrapartum death of a very small infant. In frequency and severity, RDS was a greater threat than infection to the preterm fetus.

Maternal mortality as a complication of PROM is rare. Studies have documented only one maternal death (related to chorioamnionitis, severe toxemia, and cardiorespiratory arrest) in more than 3000 women with PROM [221]. Case reports of maternal death from sepsis complicating PROM appear sporadically [222].

TABLE 3–12   Primary Causes of Death among Preterm Infants Born with Premature Rupture of Membranes

Cause	% of Perinatal Deaths*
RDS	29-70
Infection	3-19
Congenital anomaly	9-27
Asphyxia-anoxia	5-46[†]
Others[‡]	9-27

Overall perinatal mortality was 13% to 24%.
[†]*Includes stillbirths with birth weight 500 to 1000 g.*
[‡]*Includes atelectasis, erythroblastosis fetalis, intracranial hemorrhage, and necrotizing enterocolitis.*
RDS, respiratory distress syndrome.
Data from references [277, 305, 306], and Romero R, Kadar N, Hobbins JC. Infection and labor. Am J Obstet Gynecol 157:815, 1987.

APPROACH TO DIAGNOSIS OF INFECTION

Because of the frequency and potential severity of maternal and fetal infections after PROM, various tests have been studied as predictors of infection. One review critically appraised eight tests and found no test to be ideal [223]. A rectovaginal culture for GBS should be taken, unless the GBS status is already known. In addition, all patients with preterm PROM should receive a thorough physical examination focusing on possible evidence of chorioamnionitis. Digital examination should be avoided in patients with PROM, unless delivery is imminent. In a comparison of outcomes, women with digital examination after PROM had a significantly shorter latent period (2.5 ± 4 days versus 11.3 ± 13.4 days; $P < .001$), more maternal infections (44% versus 33%; $P = .09$), and more positive amniotic fluid cultures (11 of 25 [44%] versus 10 of 63 [16%]; $P < .05$) [224].

Abnormal physical examination findings that could support a diagnosis of chorioamnionitis include maternal or fetal tachycardia; uterine tenderness; and detection of a purulent, foul-smelling discharge. Temperature is often a late sign of chorioamnionitis, especially in preterm PROM.

Several authors have evaluated the use of amniocentesis and microscopic examination of amniotic fluid. Analyses for possible IAI include performing a Gram stain; glucose concentration; and cultures for anaerobes, aerobes, and genital mycoplasmas. A low amniotic fluid glucose can predict a positive amniotic fluid culture. When the glucose is greater than 20 mg/dL, the likelihood of a positive culture is less than 5%; when glucose is less than 5 mg/dL, the likelihood of a positive culture approaches 90% [55,225]. In addition, an elevated IL-6 in amniotic fluid may be the most sensitive predictor of intrauterine infection. Measurement of IL-6 in amniotic fluid is not a widely available test at this time, however.

Clinical infection is more common in women with positive smears or cultures, but 20% to 30% of these women or their newborns had no clinical evidence of infection [226–229]. In addition, amniocentesis may potentially be accompanied by trauma, bleeding, initiation of labor, or introduction of infection, although Yeast and colleagues reported no increase in onset of labor and no trauma in their retrospective series [230]. Table 3–13 summarizes the diagnostic and prognostic value of several tests of amniotic fluid.

Because the value of amniocentesis in patients with preterm PROM has not been determined precisely, most practitioners do not employ this test routinely for several reasons. Most patients with PROM and positive amniotic fluid culture results are in labor within 48 hours, and culture results are often delayed and available after the fact. Because some patients have positive culture results with no clinical evidence of infection, there is concern regarding unnecessary delivery of preterm infants. Finally, it has not been shown that clinical decisions based on data from amniocentesis lead to an improved perinatal outcome. Feinstein and colleagues evaluated 73 patients with preterm PROM who underwent amniocentesis [231]. When the Gram stain or culture result was positive, delivery was accomplished. Results were compared with 73 matched controls from a historical group. Compared with controls, patients managed by amniocentesis had less clinically diagnosed amnionitis (7% versus 20%, $P < .05$) and

TABLE 3-13 Diagnostic Values of Amniotic Fluid Testing in Detection of Positive Amniotic Fluid Culture in Patients with Preterm Labor and Intact Membranes

Diagnostic Index	Sensitivity	Specificity	Positive Predictive Value	Negative Predictive Value
Gram stain	7/11 (63.64%)	108/109 (99.08%)	7/8 (87.50%)	108/112 (96.43%)
IL-6 (≥11.30 ng/mL)	11/11 (100%)	90/109 (82.57%)	11/30 (36.67%)	90/90 (100%)
WBC count (≥50 cells/mm³)	7/11 (63.64%)	103/109 (94.50%)	7/13 (53.85%)	103/107 (96.26%)
Glucose (≤14 mg/dL)	9/11 (81.82%)	80/109 (81.65%)	9/29 (31.03%)	89/91 (97.80%)
Gram stain plus WBC count (≥50 cells/mm³)	10/11 (90.91%)	102/109 (93.58%)	10/17 (58.82%)	102/103 (99.03%)
Gram stain plus glucose (≤14 mg/dL)	10/11 (90.91%)	88/109 (80.73%)	10/31 (32.26%)	88/89 (98.88%)
Gram stain plus IL-6 (≥11.30 ng/mL)	11/11 (100%)	89/109 (81.65%)	11/31 (35.48%)	89/89 (100%)
Gram stain plus glucose (≤14 mg/dL) plus WBC count (≥50 cells/mm³)	10/11 (90.91%)	85/109 (77.98%)	10/34 (29.41%)	85/86 (98.84%)
Gram stain plus WBC count (≥50 cells/mm³) plus IL-6 (≥11.30 ng/mL)	11/11 (100%)	87/109 (79.82%)	11/33 (33.33%)	87/87 (100%)
Gram stain plus glucose (≤14 mg/dL) plus IL-6 (≥11.30 ng/mL)	11/11 (100%)	78/109 (71.56%)	11/42 (26.19%)	78/78 (100%)
Gram stain plus WBC count (≥50 cells/mm³) plus IL-6 (≥11.30 ng/mL) plus glucose (≤14 mg/dL)	11/11 (100%)	76/109 (69.72%)	11/44 (25.00%)	76/76 (100%)

IL-6, interleukin-6; WBC, white blood cell.
Data from Romero R, et al. The diagnostic and prognostic value of amniotic fluid white blood cell count, glucose, interleukin-6, and Gram stain in patients with preterm labor and intact membranes. Am J Obstet Gynecol 169:805, 1993.

fewer low Apgar scores for their infants at 5 minutes (3% versus 12%, $P < .05$). There were no significant differences, however, in rates of overall infection (22% versus 30%), "possible neonatal sepsis" (12% versus 14%), or perinatal deaths (1% versus 3%).

Although there were apparent advantages to management by amniocentesis, controlled studies have serious limitations, and no significant decreases in overall infection or perinatal mortality were found. In a small comparative study of expectant management versus the use of amniocentesis, Cotton and associates reported a significantly shorter neonatal hospital stay in the amniocentesis group ($P < .01$), but more than 25% of patients were excluded because no amniotic fluid pocket was seen [232]. Also, there were no significant differences in rates of maternal infection, neonatal sepsis, or neonatal death. Ohlsson and Wang found Gram stain and culture of amniotic fluid to have a modest positive predictive value for clinical chorioamnionitis [226]. Clear evidence for the widespread use of amniocentesis in PROM is unavailable. In view of information regarding the association of cerebral palsy and infection, these issues should be reinvestigated in a controlled fashion.

Noninvasive procedures such as measuring the level of maternal serum C-reactive protein, measuring the level of IL-6 in vaginal secretions, and assessment of amniotic fluid volume have also been suggested as predictors of infection. Several groups have evaluated C-reactive protein as such a predictor [233–237]. An elevated level of C-reactive protein in serum from patients with PROM has a modest positive predictive value for histologic amnionitis (40% to 96%), but its predictive value for clinically evident infection is poor (10% to 45%). The value of a normal level of C-reactive protein for predicting absence of clinical chorioamnionitis is better (80% to 97%). In view of the low predictive value of a positive test, a decision to attempt delivery based solely on an elevated C-reactive protein level does not seem wise.

Kayem and colleagues [238] evaluated the diagnostic value of an IL-6 bedside test of vaginal secretions for neonatal infection in cases of preterm PROM. They showed that the sensitivity of this new test of IL-6 for the prediction of neonatal infection was 79% (95% CI 65 to 92), and its specificity was 56% (95% CI 42 to 70). Similar to evaluation of IL-6 in amniotic fluid, this immunochromatographic test is not widely available.

Women who have PROM with oligohydramnios seem to be at increased risk for clinically evident infection, but the positive predictive value is modest (33% to 47%). In 1985, Gonik and coworkers noted that "amnionitis" developed in 8 (47%) of 17 patients with no pocket of amniotic fluid larger than 1 × 1 cm on ultrasound examination, whereas amnionitis developed in 3 (14%) of 22 patients with adequate pockets (i.e., >1 × 1 cm) ($P < .05$) [239]. To improve the predictability of these tests, Vintzileos and colleagues used a biophysical profile that included amniotic fluid volume, fetal movement and tone, fetal respirations, and a nonstress test [240]. Positive predictive value of the biophysical profile has been variable (31% to 60% for clinical chorioamnionitis and 31% to 47% for neonatal sepsis) [226].

TREATMENT OF PRETERM PREMATURE RUPTURE OF MEMBRANES BEFORE FETAL VIABILITY

Because fetal viability is nil throughout nearly all of the second trimester, the traditionally recommended approach to PROM in this period of gestation has been to induce labor. Retrospective reports have provided pertinent data on expectant management for PROM before fetal viability, however [208,241–244]. As expected, the latent period is relatively long (mean 12 to 19 days, median 6 to 7 days). Although maternal clinically evident infections were common (amnionitis in 35% to 59% and endometritis in 13%

to 17%) in these reports, none of these infections were serious; however, maternal death from sepsis has been reported [243,244]. There was an appreciable neonatal survival rate of 13% to 50%, depending on gestational age at membrane rupture and duration of the latent period. In cases with PROM at less than 23 weeks, the perinatal survival rate was 13% to 47%; with PROM at 24 to 26 weeks, it was 50% [243,244]. The incidence of stillbirth is greater (15%) with mid-trimester preterm PROM than with later preterm PROM (1%). The incidence of lethal pulmonary hypoplasia is 50% to 60% when membrane rupture occurs before 19 weeks [213].

With appropriate counseling, expectant management may be offered even in the second trimester for selected cases of PROM (Table 3–14). As neonatal survival in the previable periods continues to improve, the numbers of infants with moderate to severe disabilities remains substantial [245]. These concerns should be clearly communicated to the mother before delivery. As discussed subsequently, a plan for GBS surveillance and treatment also would be indicated.

TABLE 3–14 Summary of Management Plans for Premature Rupture of Membranes

Management	Evidence
In Second Trimester (<26-28 wk)	
Induction	
Expectant management	Retrospective works show high maternal infection rate but 13-50% neonatal survival
In Early Third Trimester (26-34 wk)	
Tocolytics to delay delivery	Randomized trials show no important benefits
Corticosteroids to accelerate lung maturity 32 wk	CDC consensus statement recommends use between 24 and 32 wk
Antibiotics for prophylaxis of neonatal group B streptococcal infection	Efficiency established in randomized trial
Antibiotics to prolong latent period	Risk-benefit ratio unresolved; limit to randomized trials; optimal duration of antibiotics unresolved
Expectant management	Approach followed most commonly; if premature rupture of membranes occurs >32 wk, randomized trials show no neonatal benefit to expectant management
At or Near Term (>35 wk)	
Early induction, within 12-24 hr	
Late induction, after approximately 24 hr	
Expectant management until labor or infection develops	Evidence supports early induction and expectant management
Prostaglandin E_1 and E_2 preparations to ripen cervix and induce labor	Randomized trials and historical data support safety and efficacy

CDC, Centers for Disease Control and Prevention.

Investigational Treatment Measures

Highly experimental protocols are investigating the possibility of extrinsic materials to promote resealing of the amniotic membranes. This idea stems from the use of a blood patch for treatment of spinal headache [246]. An aggressive interventional protocol for early mid-trimester PROM using a gelatin sponge for cervical plugging in patients with spontaneous or iatrogenic preterm PROM at less than 22 weeks with significant oligohydramnios (maximum vertical pocket <1.5 cm) evaluated transabdominal or transcervical placement of the gelatin sponge. This measure was in addition to broad-spectrum antibiotic therapy and cervical cerclage. Eight of 15 women undergoing the procedure reached a late enough stage in gestation to allow fetal viability, and 3 (30%) infants survived to hospital discharge. Three of the surviving infants had talipes equinovarus, and two had bilateral hip dysplasia and torticollis.

Quintero [247] introduced an "amniopatch" consisting of autologous or heterologous platelets and cryoprecipitate through a 22-gauge needle intra-amniotically into seven patients with preterm PROM 16 to 24 weeks after fetoscopy or genetic amniocentesis and reported a fetal survival rate of 42.8% (three of seven). Of the remaining patients, two had unexplained fetal death, one miscarried, and a fourth had underlying bladder outlet obstruction that prevented resealing of membranes. With spontaneous rupture of membranes, zero of 12 patients have had resealing of their membranes [246]. Quintero speculated that with spontaneous rupture of membranes, rupture sites are larger, are located over the internal cervical os, are less amenable to patching, and are more susceptible to ascending infection and weakening of the lower portion of the membranes by proinflammatory agents.

To address the larger defect with spontaneous preterm PROM, Quintero and colleagues investigated the use of an "amnio graft," achieved by laser-welding the amniotic membranes using Gore-Tex materials and a collagen-based graft material (Biosis) and combined use with a fibrin glue, with variable success in animal models and selected patients [246–248]. Use of a fibrin sealant was associated with a 53.8% survival rate when the sealant was placed transcervically. In their study, mean gestational age at rupture of membranes was 19 weeks 4 days; at treatment, 20 weeks 5 days; and at delivery, 27 weeks 4 days, with a mean latency of 48 days from initial rupture to delivery. Additional research in this area is necessary to establish the safety and efficacy of this modality.

TREATMENT OF PRETERM PREMATURE RUPTURE OF MEMBRANES IN EARLY THIRD TRIMESTER

Management is most controversial at the gestational age interval of 24 to 34 weeks. New information has become available, however, and sophisticated meta-analyses have been performed. Controversial components of therapy, including corticosteroids, tocolytics, and antibiotics are reviewed here. Specific situations, such as herpes simplex virus and human immunodeficiency virus (HIV) infection and cerclage coexisting with PROM, are reviewed later.

Some studies reported significant (or nearly significant) decreases in the occurrence of RDS, but others found no significant decrease when corticosteroids were used in patients with PROM [249–258]. There are major difficulties in interpreting these studies. In some of the more rigorously designed studies of corticosteroid use, the numbers of patients with PROM were small. The real differences may have been missed (a beta error). In most studies, there were at least small decreases in the incidence of RDS in the corticosteroid group. A wide range of gestational ages was studied. The minimum number of weeks of gestation for entry into a study was 25 to 32, and the maximum was 32 to 37. Because an equal effect of corticosteroids on the rate of RDS is unlikely at all gestational age intervals, real differences may have been missed in some intervals because data for these intervals were combined with data for other gestational ages. Finally, experiments measuring the surfactant-inducing potency of corticosteroids suggest differences in the efficacy of various corticosteroid preparations and various dosages.

Several studies, including three meta-analyses, have attempted to resolve the confusion [259–261]. The authors reached differing conclusions. Ohlsson concluded that in preterm PROM, corticosteroid treatment "cannot presently be recommended to prevent RDS . . . outside a randomized controlled trial [259]. The reasons underlying this conclusion are that the evidence that it decreases RDS is weak and its use increases incidence of endometritis and may increase neonatal infections." Crowley concluded that corticosteroids were effective in preventing RDS after preterm PROM (OR 0.44, 95% CI 0.32 to 0.60) and that they were not associated with a significant increase in perinatal infection (OR 0.84, 95% CI 0.57 to 1.23) or neonatal infection (OR 1.61, 95% CI 0.9 to 3.0) [260]. Lovett and colleagues, in a prospective, double-blind trial of treatment for preterm PROM, used corticosteroids in all patients. They also found significant decreases in mortality, sepsis, and RDS rates and increased birth weight when corticosteroids and antibiotics were given compared with use of corticosteroids alone. Lewis and coworkers investigated use of ampicillin-sulbactam in preterm PROM and randomly assigned patients to receive weekly corticosteroids versus placebo between 24 and 34 weeks. They found a decrease in RDS (44% versus 18%; $P = .03$ or 0.29, 95% CI 0.10% to 0.82%) in the corticosteroid treatment group with no increase in maternal or neonatal infection complications [261].

Leitich and associates concluded that corticosteroids seem to diminish the beneficial effects of antibiotics in the treatment of preterm PROM. This conclusion was based on the results of their meta-analysis of five randomized trials of antibiotics and preterm PROM without corticosteroids. They found nonsignificant differences in mortality, sepsis, RDS, IVH, and necrotizing enterocolitis when antibiotics and corticosteroids were used. By contrast, when antibiotics without corticosteroids were used, they found a significant decrease in chorioamnionitis (OR 0.37, $P = .0001$), postpartum endometritis (OR 0.47, $P = .03$), neonatal sepsis (OR 0.27, $P = .002$), and IVH (OR 0.48, $P = .02$) [262].

The National Institutes of Health Consensus Development Panel in 1995 recommended that corticosteroids be given in the absence of IAI to women with preterm PROM at less than 30 to 32 weeks of gestation because the benefits of corticosteroids may outweigh the risk at this gestational age, particularly of IVH. Because the number of patients

receiving corticosteroids with PROM at more than 32 weeks of gestation was small, the consensus panel chose to restrict its recommendation to less than 32 weeks of gestation. Recommended dosing includes betamethasone, 12 mg intramuscularly every 24 hours for two doses, or dexamethasone, 6 mg every 12 hours for four doses. The consensus panel reconvened in 2000 and reconfirmed their original recommendations. Repeat dosing of steroids was not recommended outside of randomized trials. A 2006 Cochrane Update on antenatal corticosteroids recommended a single course of corticosteroids for women at 24 to 34 weeks of gestation in whom there is reason to anticipate early delivery, including women with ruptured membranes. Weighing the hypothetical risk of increased infection when corticosteroids are used in preterm PROM, we use 32 weeks as the upper gestational age limit for use.

Lee and associates also evaluated use of weekly steroids in a randomized double-blind trial in women at 24 to 32 weeks of gestation with preterm PROM compared with a single course of steroids. Although investigators found no differences in the overall composite neonatal morbidity between the groups (34.2% versus 41.8%), they did find an increased rate of chorioamnionitis in the weekly course group (49.4% versus 31.7%; $P = .04$). In the group with gestational age at delivery of 24 to 27 weeks, there was a significant reduction in RDS from 100% in the single course group to 26.5% ($P = .001$) in the weekly course group [263]. Guinn and colleagues found no decrease in neonatal morbidity with serial weekly courses of betamethasone compared with single course therapy [236]. In the secondary analysis of this multicenter, randomized trial of weekly courses of antenatal corticosteroids versus single course therapy, this same group reported that multiple courses were associated with an increase in the rate of chorioamnionitis [263]. Based on the available information, antenatal steroid therapy in preterm PROM should be limited to a single course.

Antibiotics

Patients with preterm PROM are candidates for prophylaxis against GBS [264–266]. In addition, one innovative report noted use of combination antibiotics in an asymptomatic patient with preterm PROM because of bacterial colonization of the amniotic fluid, which was detected by amniocentesis. A second amniocentesis 48 hours after therapy revealed a sterile culture [267].

Some studies of preterm pregnancies have found an increased rate of amnionitis to be associated with an increasing length of latent period [186,220,268], whereas others [219] have not. In patients with preterm PROM, digital vaginal examination should be avoided until labor develops, although transvaginal or transperineal ultrasound can be used safely to assess cervical length without increasing the risk of infection [269]. Some studies noted that prolonged rupture of membranes decreased the incidence of RDS [188,221], others noted no significant effect [185,204,219,220,250,270,271]. These discrepancies may be explained by differences in experimental design (e.g., grouping of various gestational ages and using different sample sizes) or in definitions of clinical complications.

Antibiotics in several classes have been found to prolong pregnancy and reduce maternal and neonatal morbidity in the setting of preterm PROM [272]. Two large multicenter clinical trials with different approaches had adequate power to evaluate the utility of antibiotics in the setting of preterm PROM. Mercer and Arheart [116] evaluated the use of antibiotics in PROM with a meta-analysis. They evaluated such outcomes as length of latency, chorioamnionitis, postpartum infection, neonatal survival, neonatal sepsis, RDS, IVH, and necrotizing enterocolitis. Several classes of antibiotics were used, including penicillins and cephalosporins, although few studies used either tocolytics or corticosteroids. Benefits of antibiotics in this analysis included a significant reduction in chorioamnionitis, IVH, and confirmed neonatal sepsis. There was a significant decrease in the number of women delivering within 1 week of membrane rupture (OR 0.56, CI 0.41 to 0.76), but no significant differences were seen in necrotizing enterocolitis, RDS, or mortality. The evidence currently supports use of antibiotics in preterm PROM to prolong latency and to decrease maternal and neonatal infectious complications, but further studies to select the preferred agent have yet to be performed.

The NICHD Maternal-Fetal Medicine Units Network conducted a large, multicenter trial of antibiotics after PROM, but did not use tocolytics or corticosteroids. Patients with preterm PROM between 24 and 32 weeks were included. Patients were randomly assigned to receive aggressive intravenous antibiotic therapy consisting of ampicillin (2 g intravenously every 6 hours) and erythromycin (250 mg intravenously every 6 hours) for the first 48 hours, followed by 5 days of oral therapy of amoxicillin (250 mg every 8 hours) and enteric-coated erythromycin (333 mg orally every 8 hours) or placebo. Antibiotic treatment resulted in prolongation of pregnancy. Twice (50%) as many patients in the antibiotic treatment group remained pregnant after 7 days, and 21-day composite neonatal morbidity was reduced in the antibiotic treatment group from 53% to 44% ($P < .05$). In addition, individual neonatal comorbid conditions occurred less often in the antibiotic treatment group, including RDS (40.5% versus 48.7%), stage 3/4 necrotizing enterocolitis (2.3% versus 5.8%), patent ductus arteriosus (11.7% versus 20.2%), and bronchopulmonary dysplasia (13% versus 20.5%) ($P < .05$ for each). Occurrence rates for specific infections including neonatal GBS-associated sepsis (0% versus 1.5%), overall neonatal sepsis (8.4% versus 15.6%), and pneumonia (2.9% versus 7%) all were significantly less ($P < .05$) in the antibiotic treatment group.

The second large trial was the multicenter, multiarm ORACLE trial of oral antibiotics in women with preterm PROM at less than 37 weeks. More than 4000 patients were randomly assigned to receive oral erythromycin, amoxicillin/clavulanic acid, erythromycin and amoxicillin/clavulanic acid, or placebo for up to 10 days. All of the antibiotic regimens prolonged pregnancy compared with placebo. Amoxicillin/clavulanic acid increased the risk for neonatal necrotizing enterocolitis (1.9% versus 0.5%; $P = .001$), however, and this regimen is now advised against. The investigators showed a significant decrease in perinatal morbidity, RDS, and necrotizing enterocolitis with use of ampicillin and erythromycin [117].

Egarter and associates found in a meta-analysis of seven published studies a 68% reduction of neonatal sepsis and a 50% decreased risk of IVH in infants born to mothers receiving antibiotics after preterm PROM. They did not find any significant differences, however, in either RDS or neonatal mortality [273].

The Cochrane Library has reviewed antibiotic use in preterm PROM in more than 6000 women in 19 trials. This meta-analysis also found that antibiotic use in preterm PROM was associated with an increased latent period at 48 hours and 7 days and reduction in major neonatal comorbid conditions or indicators such as neonatal infection, surfactant use, oxygen therapy, and abnormalities on head ultrasound examination before hospital discharge. There was an increased risk of necrotizing enterocolitis in the two trials involving 2492 infants in which co-amoxiclav was administered to the mother (relative risk 4.6, 95% CI 1.98 to 10.72). Another trial in the meta-analysis compared erythromycin with co-amoxiclav; the investigators found fewer deliveries at 48 hours in the co-amoxiclav group, but no difference at 7 days. The trial also found a decrease in necrotizing enterocolitis when erythromycin rather than co-amoxiclav was used (relative risk 0.46, 95% CI 0.23 to 0.94) [274]. The investigators in this trial recommended that co-amoxiclav should be avoided in the setting of preterm PROM.

Owing to concerns of emergence of resistant organisms, another question involves duration of antibiotic therapy in preterm PROM. Two small trials have evaluated this question. Segel and associates compared 3 days and 7 days of ampicillin in patients at 24 to 33 weeks with preterm PROM. In 48 patients, there was no difference in 7-day latency and no difference in rates of chorioamnionitis, postpartum endometritis, and neonatal morbidity and mortality [275]. Lewis and colleagues studied 3 days versus 7 days of ampicillin/sulbactam (3 g intravenously every 8 hours) and similarly found no difference in outcomes between groups [276]. Both of these studies are small, so this important question remains unanswered. We use 7 days of antibiotics, usually ampicillin and erythromycin, following the dosing from the NICHD trial.

Tocolytics and Development of Respiratory Distress Syndrome

Older studies suggested a decrease in the rate of RDS with use of β-adrenergic drugs, but in the National Collaborative Study, use of tocolytics in patients with ruptured membranes increased the likelihood of RDS by about 350% [277]. In addition, two small randomized controlled trials assessed use of tocolytics in the presence of PROM [278,279]. Both trials found no significant increase in time to delivery or in birth weight and no decrease in RDS or neonatal hospital stay. These studies did not use antibiotics or corticosteroids, however. Tocolytics have been shown to prolong pregnancy by about 48 hours in patients with intact membranes, but their efficacy with preterm PROM is unclear. In a patient with preterm PROM and contractions, IAI should be ruled out before consideration of tocolytics. Tocolytics could be considered in the early third trimester to maximize the impact of antenatal corticosteroids (48-hour delay) on neonatal morbidity and mortality. Continuing tocolysis beyond the 48-hour window is contraindicated because of an increase in chorioamnionitis and endometritis [280]. Interested readers are referred to a review of this subject [281].

Determination of Fetal Lung Maturity

Some clinicians determine the status of fetal pulmonary maturity and proceed with delivery if the lungs are mature. Amniotic fluid may be collected by amniocentesis or from the posterior vagina. Either the presence of phosphatidylglycerol or a lecithin/sphingomyelin ratio higher than 2 in amniotic fluid has been reported to be a good predictor of pulmonary maturity. In a series of patients with PROM before 36 weeks, Brame and MacKenna determined whether phosphatidylglycerol was present in the vaginal pool and delivered patients when there was presence of phosphatidylglycerol, spontaneous labor, or evidence of sepsis [282]. Of 214 patients, 47 had phosphatidylglycerol present initially and were delivered. Of the remaining 167, 36 (21%) were subsequently found to have phosphatidylglycerol and were induced or delivered by cesarean section. Evidence of maternal infection developed in 8 (5%) and spontaneous labor developed in 123 (74%) of the 167 patients. Phosphatidylglycerol in amniotic fluid from the vagina reliably predicted fetal lung maturity; however, its absence did not mean that RDS would develop. Of 131 patients who did not show phosphatidylglycerol in the vaginal pool in any sample, 82 (62%) were delivered of infants who had no RDS. Lewis and colleagues also showed the presence of a mature Amniostat-FLM (Hana Biologies, Irvine, CA) in a vaginal pool sample from 18% of 201 patients, and none developed RDS.

Intentional Preterm Induction in Mid–Third Trimester

Even with PROM, delivery of a premature infant simply because the lungs show biochemical maturity may be questioned in view of other potential hazards of prematurity and the potential difficulties of the induction. Two articles have examined this controversial issue. With respect to the new information regarding the association among preterm PROM, chorioamnionitis, and subsequent development of cerebral palsy, the use of intentional mid–third trimester induction is receiving increased attention.

Mercer and colleagues compared expectant management and immediate induction in 93 pregnancies complicated by PROM between 32 and 36 weeks and 6 days, when mature fetal lung profiles were documented. They found significant prolongation of latent period and of maternal hospitalization, increased neonatal length of stay, and increased antimicrobial use in the expectant management group despite no increase in documented neonatal sepsis. These investigators concluded that in women with preterm PROM at 32 through 36 weeks with a mature fetal lung profile, immediate induction of labor reduces the duration of hospitalization in the mother and neonate [218,283].

Cox and Leveno similarly studied pregnancies complicated by preterm PROM at 30 to 34 weeks of gestation. Consenting patients were randomly assigned to one of two groups: expectant management versus immediate induction. Corticosteroids, tocolytics, and antibiotics were not used in either group. Fetal lung profiles were not determined. The investigators found a significant

difference in birth weight or frequency of IVH, necrotizing enterocolitis, neonatal sepsis, RDS, or perinatal death. They concluded that there were no clinically significant neonatal advantages to expectant management of ruptured membranes and decreased antepartum hospitalization in women managed with immediate induction [284].

A more recent review evaluated 430 women with preterm PROM and evaluated maternal and neonatal outcomes. They found that expectant management of women at 34 weeks and beyond is of limited benefit [285]. Based on all available data, we routinely proceed with induction of labor at 34 weeks in patients with preterm PROM and no other indication for earlier delivery.

Fetal Surveillance

Because of concerns regarding cord compression and cord prolapse and the development of intrauterine and fetal infection, daily fetal monitoring in the setting of preterm PROM has been studied. Vintzileos and colleagues showed that infection developed when the nonstress test became nonreactive 78% of the time compared with only 14% when the nonstress test remained reactive [286]. Biophysical profile score of 6 or less also predicted perinatal infection [287]. As a result, we recommend daily monitoring with nonstress tests. If the nonstress test is nonreactive, further work-up with biophysical profile should be performed. Because there are currently no large studies evaluating outpatient management of preterm PROM, we recommend hospitalization until delivery.

Conclusion

Despite availability of more recent data and sophisticated meta-analyses, we believe the evidence supports the use of expectant management in the absence of IAI and in the absence of documented fetal lung maturity in the third trimester until 34 completed weeks. If expectant management is chosen, corticosteroids to enhance fetal organ maturation should be given until 32 weeks. In addition, broad-spectrum antibiotics consisting of ampicillin and erythromycin should be administered for 7 days. Bacterial vaginosis, if present, should also be treated. Tocolytics generally should be avoided. Daily fetal surveillance is also recommended. Appropriate prophylaxis for GBS in this high-risk group is strongly encouraged during labor. From a cost-effectiveness standpoint, Grable and others looked at preterm PROM between 32 and 36 weeks. Using their decision analysis based on 1996 cost data, they weighed the costs of maternal hospitalization, latency, infection, and minor and major neonatal morbidity versus that of immediate induction. These investigators found that it is most effective to delay delivery by 1 week between 32 and 34 weeks and to induce at presentation at or after 35 weeks [288,289].

RECURRENCE OF PRETERM PREMATURE RUPTURE OF MEMBRANES

Recurrence of preterm PROM in a subsequent pregnancy after an index pregnancy complicated by preterm PROM has been estimated to be 13.5% to 44%. In Lee and colleagues' population-based case-control study, OR for recurrent preterm PROM was 20.6 and for recurrent preterm birth was 3.6. The estimated gestational age of index preterm PROM is poorly predictive, however, of subsequent timing of recurrent events. The other two studies had higher recurrence of risks, but probably included transferred patients, so that the study populations constituted a more select group [196,290–292].

PREVENTION OF PRETERM PREMATURE RUPTURE OF MEMBRANES

Because preterm PROM often is accompanied by maternal and neonatal adverse events, prevention of preterm PROM is desirable. Prediction of preterm PROM was evaluated in a large prospective trial, the Preterm Prediction Study [292], sponsored by the NICHD Maternal-Fetal Medicine Units Network. Prior preterm birth and preterm birth secondary to preterm PROM were associated with subsequent preterm birth. In nulliparas, preterm PROM is associated with medical complications, work in pregnancy, symptomatic contractions, bacterial vaginosis, and low body mass index. In nulliparas and multiparas, a cervix found to be shorter than 25 mm by endovaginal ultrasound examination was associated with preterm PROM. A positive fetal fibronectin also was predictive of preterm PROM in nulliparas (16.7%) and multiparas (25%). Multiparas with a prior history of preterm birth, a short cervix, and a positive fetal fibronectin had a 31-fold higher risk of PROM and delivery before 35 weeks compared with women without these risk factors (25% versus 0.8%; $P = .001$) [190]. Progesterone therapy seems to be effective in reducing the risk of recurrent preterm birth secondary to PROM or preterm labor [293–295].

SPECIAL SITUATIONS

Cerclage and Preterm Premature Rupture of Membranes

Classic obstetric dogma has suggested immediate removal of the cervical cerclage stitch when preterm PROM occurs. Risks associated with the retained stitch include maternal infection from bacterial proliferation emanating from the foreign body and cervical lacerations consequent to progression of labor despite the retained stitch. Small retrospective studies have shown conflicting results. At present, there are not enough data in the literature to recommend removal or retention of the suture. If there is no evidence of IAI or preterm labor in very premature gestations, one could consider leaving the stitch in during corticosteroid administration while there is uterine quiescence [296–300].

Preterm Premature Rupture of Membranes and Herpes Simplex Virus

In a retrospective review from 1986-1996 of 29 patients with preterm PROM and a history of recurrent genital herpes, there were no cases of neonatal herpes. The 95% CI suggests, however, that the risk of vertical transmission could be 10%. The mean estimated gestational age at membrane rupture was 27.7 weeks. Mean estimated gestational age at development of maternal herpetic lesion was 28.7 weeks. With continued expectant management, mean estimated gestational age at delivery was 30.6 weeks in the study group. Of the 29 patients, 13 (45%) were delivered by cesarean section. Additionally, although delivery was performed

for obstetric indication only, 8 of 13 patients undergoing cesarean section had active lesions as the only or a secondary indication for cesarean section. In this study, risk of neonatal death from complications of prematurity was 10%. Risk of major neonatal morbidity was 41%. The risks of major morbidity and mortality would have been considerably higher had there been iatrogenic delivery at the time of development of the herpetic lesion.

It seems prudent when there is a history of recurrent herpes simplex virus infection to continue expectant management in a significantly preterm gestation. In the setting of primary herpes (or nonprimary first episode), with the higher viral loads that entails, early delivery may prevent vertical transmission, but this has not been specifically studied. Only eight of the patients in this study received acyclovir treatment. Use of acyclovir for symptomatic outbreaks would theoretically reduce the risk of transmission and decrease the number of cesarean sections performed for presence of active lesions at the time of delivery [301]. Additionally, Scott and associates showed a decreased cesarean section rate in term patients with a history of recurrent herpes simplex virus infection [302].

Human Immunodeficiency Virus and Preterm Premature Rupture of Membranes

There are no specific data regarding the subset of patients with preterm PROM who are seropositive for HIV. With highly active antiretroviral therapy (HAART) and a low viral load, expectant management of preterm PROM after clinical exclusion of IAI might be considered because the complications of prematurity with gestational age of less than 32 weeks, and certainly less than 28 weeks, are significant. With continued HAART, the risk of vertical transmission should remain low. The physician should discuss and document potential risks and benefits with the mother regarding the possibility of vertical transmission or neonatal morbidity and mortality. Intravenous infusion of zidovudine should be initiated at admission because latency can be unpredictable short in many patients with preterm PROM [303]. After a period of observation and no evidence of spontaneous preterm labor, intravenous zidovudine may be discontinued and oral HAART continued.

TREATMENT OF TERM PREMATURE RUPTURE OF MEMBRANES

Approximately 8% of pregnant women at term experience PROM, although contractions begin spontaneously within 24 hours of membrane rupture in 80% to 90% of patients [211]. After more than 24 hours elapses following membrane rupture at term, the incidence of neonatal infection is approximately 1%, but this risk increases to 3% to 5% when clinical chorioamnionitis is diagnosed [304]. For many years, the practice in most institutions had been to induce labor in term patients within approximately 12 hours of PROM, primarily because of concerns about development of chorioamnionitis and neonatal infectious complications. More recently, three studies have shown that in most patients, expectant management can be safely applied. The designs of these three reports were different.

Kappy and associates reported a retrospective review in a private population [202]. Duff and colleagues performed a randomized study of indigent patients with unfavorable cervix characteristics (<2 cm dilated, <80% effaced) and with no complications of pregnancy (e.g., toxemia, diabetes, previous cesarean section, malpresentation, meconium-stained fluid) [305]. In the patients assigned to the induction group, initiation of induction generally was 12 hours after rupture of membranes. The excess cesarean deliveries in the induction group were for failed induction. In the induction group, there was a higher probability of IAI. In the study by Conway and colleagues, all patients were observed until the morning after admission [306]. Induction of labor was then undertaken if the patient was not in labor.

Wagner and coworkers provided another variant by comparing early induction (at 6 hours after preterm PROM) with late induction (at 24 hours after PROM) [307]. In their population at a Kaiser Permanente hospital, the results favored early induction by shortening maternal hospital stay and decreasing neonatal sepsis evaluations. More recent work also has evaluated use of oral and vaginal prostaglandin preparations (prostaglandins E_1 and E_2) to ripen the cervix or induce labor after PROM at term. These preparations seem to be effective in shortening labor without increasing maternal or neonatal infection [308–310].

Hannah and colleagues evaluated four management schemes in women with PROM at term: (1) immediate induction with oxytocin, (2) immediate induction with vaginal prostaglandin E_2, (3) expectant management for up to 4 days followed by oxytocin induction, and (4) expectant management followed by prostaglandin E_2 induction. Although no differences in cesarean section rates or frequency of neonatal sepsis were found, an increase in chorioamnionitis was noted in the expectant management groups, and all deaths not caused by congenital anomalies occurred in the expectant management group. Patient satisfaction was higher in the immediate induction group. A secondary analysis showed five variables as independent predictors of neonatal sepsis: clinical chorioamnionitis (OR 5.89), presence of GBS (OR 3.08), seven to eight vaginal examinations (OR 2.37), duration of ruptured membranes 24 to 48 hours (OR 1.97), greater than 48 hours from membrane rupture to active labor (OR 2.25), and maternal antibiotics before delivery (OR 1.63) [311].

A more recent study investigated how the interval of membrane rupture and delivery affects the risk of neonatal sepsis and whether duration of labor (defined as the interval between onset of regular contractions and delivery) influences the risk [312]. The investigators showed that the risk of neonatal sepsis increased independently and nearly linearly with duration of membrane rupture up to 36 hours, with an OR of 1.29 for each 6-hour increase in membrane rupture duration. The risk also increased with increasing birth weight, increasing gestational age, primiparity, and male infant gender. Duration of labor was not an independent risk factor for neonatal sepsis.

We endorse immediate induction with oxytocin in women with PROM at term if the condition of the cervix is favorable and the patient is willing. If the condition of the cervix is unfavorable, induction with appropriate doses of prostaglandins may be used before use of oxytocin. Intrapartum antibiotic prophylaxis against GBS should be used according to the 2002 CDC guidelines [264], which emphasize universal screening of all gravidas at 35 to 37 weeks. All seropositive women should receive intravenous antibiotics in labor.

Changes in the 2002 recommendations over the previous guidelines also include antibiotic guidelines for patients with high-risk and low-risk penicillin allergy and checking sensitivities owing to emerging antibiotic resistance, particularly resistance of erythromycin and clindamycin to GBS.

REFERENCES

[1] R.S. Gibbs, M.S. Castillo, P.J. Rodgers, Management of acute chorioamnionitis, Am. J. Obstet. Gynecol. 136 (1980) 709–713.
[1a] R. Romero, M. Mazor, Infection and preterm labor: pathways for intrauterine infections, Clin Obstet Gynecol 31 (1988) 558.
[2] R.S. Gibbs, P. Duff, Progress in pathogenesis and management of clinical intraamniotic infection, Am. J. Obstet. Gynecol. 164 (1991) 1317–1326.
[3] E.R. Newton, T.J. Prihoda, R.S. Gibbs, Logistic regression analysis of risk factors for intra-amniotic infection, Obstet. Gynecol. 73 (1989) 571–575.
[4] D.E. Soper, C.G. Mayhall, H.P. Dalton, Risk factors for intraamniotic infection: a prospective epidemiologic study, Am. J. Obstet. Gynecol. 161 (1989) 562–566 discussion 6–8.
[5] J.A. Lopez-Zeno, A.M. Peaceman, J.A. Adashek, M.L. Socol, A controlled trial of a program for the active management of labor, N. Engl. J. Med. 326 (1992) 450–454.
[6] K.H. van Hoeven, A. Anyaegbunam, H. Hochster, et al., Clinical significance of increasing histologic severity of acute inflammation in the fetal membranes and umbilical cord, Pediatr. Pathol. Lab. Med. 16 (1996) 731–744.
[7] C.M. Pettker, I.A. Buhimschi, L.K. Magloire, A.K. Sfakianaki, B.D. Hamar, C.S. Buhimschi, Value of placental microbial evaluation in diagnosing intra-amniotic infection, Obstet. Gynecol. 109 (2007) 739–749.
[8] R. Romero, J. Espinoza, T. Chaiworapongsa, K. Kalache, Infection and prematurity and the role of preventive strategies, Semin. Neonatol. 7 (2002) 259–274.
[9] H.L. Halliday, T. Hirata, Perinatal listeriosis–a review of twelve patients, Am. J. Obstet. Gynecol. 133 (1979) 405–410.
[10] P.G. Shackleford, Listeria revisited, Am. J. Dis. Child. 131 (1977) 391.
[11] A.D. Fleming, D.W. Ehrlich, N.A. Miller, G.R. Monif, Successful treatment of maternal septicemia due to Listeria monocytogenes at 26 weeks' gestation, Obstet. Gynecol. 66 (1985) 52S–53S.
[12] E.S. Petrilli, G. D'Ablaing, W.J. Ledger, Listeria monocytogenes chorioamnionitis: diagnosis by transabdominal amniocentesis, Obstet. Gynecol. 55 (1980) 5S–8S.
[13] M. Boucher, M.L. Yonekura, Perinatal listeriosis (early-onset): correlation of antenatal manifestations and neonatal outcome, Obstet. Gynecol. 68 (1986) 593–597.
[14] Listeriosis outbreak associated with Mexican-style cheese–California, MMWR Morb. Mortal. Wkly Rep. 34 (1985) 357–359.
[15] G.R. Monif, Antenatal group A streptococcal infection, Am. J. Obstet. Gynecol. 123 (1975) 213.
[16] D. Charles, W.R. Edwards, Infectious complications of cervical cerclage, Am. J. Obstet. Gynecol. 141 (1981) 1065–1071.
[17] J.H. Harger, Comparison of success and morbidity in cervical cerclage procedures, Obstet. Gynecol. 56 (1980) 543–548.
[18] A.G. Mitra, V.L. Katz, W.A. Bowes Jr., S. Carmichael, Emergency cerclages: a review of 40 consecutive procedures, Am. J. Perinatol. 9 (1992) 142–145.
[19] R.G. Burnett, W.R. Anderson, The hazards of amniocentesis, J. Iowa Med. Soc. 58 (1968) 133.
[20] K.A. Eddleman, F.D. Malone, L. Sullivan, et al., Pregnancy loss rates after midtrimester amniocentesis, Obstet. Gynecol. 108 (2006) 1067–1072.
[21] I. Wilkins, G. Mezrow, L. Lynch, E.J. Bottone, R.L. Berkowitz, Amnionitis and life-threatening respiratory distress after percutaneous umbilical blood sampling, Am. J. Obstet. Gynecol. 160 (1989) 427–428.
[22] D.E. Soper, C.G. Mayhall, J.W. Froggatt, Characterization and control of intraamniotic infection in an urban teaching hospital, Am. J. Obstet. Gynecol. 175 (1996) 304–309 discussion 9–10.
[23] S.H. Tran, A.B. Caughey, T.J. Musci, Meconium-stained amniotic fluid is associated with puerperal infections, Am. J. Obstet. Gynecol. 189 (2003) 746–750.
[24] M.A. Krohn, M. Germain, K. Muhlemann, D. Hickok, Prior pregnancy outcome and the risk of intraamniotic infection in the following pregnancy, Am. J. Obstet. Gynecol. 178 (1998) 381–385.
[25] M.K. Yancey, P. Duff, P. Kubilis, P. Clark, B.H. Frentzen, Risk factors for neonatal sepsis, Obstet. Gynecol. 87 (1996) 188–194.
[26] R.L. Naeye, Coitus and associated amniotic-fluid infections, N. Engl. J. Med. 301 (1979) 1198–1200.
[27] M.A. Klebanoff, R.P. Nugent, G.G. Rhoads, Coitus during pregnancy: is it safe? Lancet 2 (1984) 914–917.
[28] J.L. Mills, S. Harlap, E.E. Harley, Should coitus late in pregnancy be discouraged, Lancet 2 (1981) 136–138.
[29] R.L. Sweet, R.S. Gibbs, Infectious diseases of the female genital tract, fifth ed., Lippincott Williams & Wilkins, Philadelphia, 2009.
[30] C.W. Nickerson, Gonorrhea amnionitis, Obstet. Gynecol. 42 (1973) 815–817.
[31] H.H. Handsfield, W.A. Hodson, K.K. Holmes, Neonatal gonococcal infection. I. Orogastric contamination with Neisseria gonorrhoea, JAMA 225 (1973) 697–701.
[32] D.H. Martin, L. Koutsky, D.A. Eschenbach, et al., Prematurity and perinatal mortality in pregnancies complicated by maternal Chlamydia trachomatis infections, JAMA 247 (1982) 1585–1588.

[33] G.P. Wager, D.H. Martin, L. Koutsky, et al., Puerperal infectious morbidity: relationship to route of delivery and to antepartum Chlamydia trachomatis infection, Am. J. Obstet. Gynecol. 138 (1980) 1028–1033.

[34] G.A. Pankuch, P.C. Appelbaum, R.P. Lorenz, J.J. Botti, J. Schachter, R.L. Naeye, Placental microbiology and histology and the pathogenesis of chorioamnionitis, Obstet. Gynecol. 64 (1984) 802–806.

[35] Y. Dong, P.J. St Clair, I. Ramzy, K.S. Kagan-Hallet, R.S. Gibbs, A microbiologic and clinical study of placental inflammation at term, Obstet. Gynecol. 70 (1987) 175–182.

[36] R.L. Goldenberg, W.W. Andrews, A.R. Goepfert, et al., The Alabama Preterm Birth Study: umbilical cord blood Ureaplasma urealyticum and Mycoplasma hominis cultures in very preterm newborn infants, Am. J. Obstet. Gynecol. 198 (43) (2008) e1–e5.

[37] P. Aureli, G.C. Fiorucci, D. Caroli, et al., An outbreak of febrile gastroenteritis associated with corn contaminated by Listeria monocytogenes, N. Engl. J. Med. 342 (2000) 1236–1241.

[38] C.B. Dalton, C.C. Austin, J. Sobel, et al., An outbreak of gastroenteritis and fever due to Listeria monocytogenes in milk, N. Engl. J. Med. 336 (1997) 100–105.

[39] D.M. Frye, R. Zweig, J. Sturgeon, et al., An outbreak of febrile gastroenteritis associated with delicatessen meat contaminated with Listeria monocytogenes, Clin. Infect. Dis. 35 (2002) 943–949.

[40] M.K. Miettinen, A. Siitonen, P. Heiskanen, H. Haajanen, K.J. Bjorkroth, H.J. Korkeala, Molecular epidemiology of an outbreak of febrile gastroenteritis caused by Listeria monocytogenes in cold-smoked rainbow trout, J. Clin. Microbiol. 37 (1999) 2358–2360.

[41] M.A. Smith, K. Takeuchi, G. Anderson, et al., Dose-response model for Listeria monocytogenes-induced stillbirths in nonhuman primates, Infect. Immun. 76 (2008) 726–731.

[42] Outbreak of listeriosis–northeastern United States, 2002, MMWR Morb. Mortal. Wkly Rep. 51 (2002) 950–951.

[43] R.S. Gibbs, Chorioamnionitis and bacterial vaginosis, Am. J. Obstet. Gynecol. 169 (1993) 460–462.

[44] H.M. Silver, R.S. Sperling, P.J. St Clair, R.S. Gibbs, Evidence relating bacterial vaginosis to intraamniotic infection, Am. J. Obstet. Gynecol. 161 (1989) 808–812.

[45] M.G. Gravett, H.P. Nelson, T. DeRouen, C. Critchlow, D.A. Eschenbach, K.K. Holmes, Independent associations of bacterial vaginosis and Chlamydia trachomatis infection with adverse pregnancy outcome, JAMA 256 (1986) 1899–1903.

[46] E.R. Newton, J. Piper, W. Peairs, Bacterial vaginosis and intraamniotic infection, Am. J. Obstet. Gynecol. 176 (1997) 672–677.

[47] H. McDonald, P. Brocklehurst, J. Parsons, R. Vigneswaran, Antibiotics for treating bacterial vaginosis in pregnancy, Cochrane Database Syst. Rev. (2003) CD000262.

[48] J.C. Carey, M.A. Klebanoff, J.C. Hauth, et al., Metronidazole to prevent preterm delivery in pregnant women with asymptomatic bacterial vaginosis. National Institute of Child Health and Human Development Network of Maternal-Fetal Medicine Units, N. Engl. J. Med. 342 (2000) 534–540.

[49] ACOG Practice Bulletin, Assessment of risk factors for preterm birth. Clinical management guidelines for obstetrician-gynecologists. Number 31, October 2001. (Replaces Technical Bulletin number 206, June 1995; Committee Opinion number 172, May 1996; Committee Opinion number 187, September 1997; Committee Opinion number 198, February 1998; and Committee Opinion number 251, January 2001), Obstet. Gynecol. 98 (2001) 709–716.

[50] J.D. Iams, R. Romero, J.F. Culhane, R.L. Goldenberg, Primary, secondary, and tertiary interventions to reduce the morbidity and mortality of preterm birth, Lancet 371 (2008) 164–175.

[51] J. Yankowitz, C.P. Weiner, J. Henderson, S. Grant, J.A. Towbin, Outcome of low risk pregnancies with evidence of intraamniotic viral infection detected by PCR on amniotic fluid obtained at second trimester genetic amniocentesis. J. Soc. Gynecol. Invest. (1996) 3: 132A.

[52] F. Arechavaleta-Velasco, L. Gomez, Y. Ma, et al., Adverse reproductive outcomes in urban women with adeno-associated virus-2 infections in early pregnancy, Hum. Reprod. 23 (2008) 29–36.

[53] R.K. Edwards, Chorioamnionitis and labor, Obstet. Gynecol. Clin. North Am. 32 (2005) 287–296, x.

[54] P.C. Greig, J.M. Ernest, L. Teot, Low amniotic fluid glucose levels are a specific but not a sensitive marker for subclinical intrauterine infections in patients in preterm labor with intact membranes, Am. J. Obstet. Gynecol. 171 (1994) 365–370; discussion 70–1.

[55] R.J. Kiltz, M.S. Burke, R.P. Porreco, Amniotic fluid glucose concentration as a marker for intra-amniotic infection, Obstet. Gynecol. 78 (1991) 619–622.

[56] M.J. Hussey, E.S. Levy, X. Pombar, P. Meyer, H.T. Strassner, Evaluating rapid diagnostic tests of intra-amniotic infection: Gram stain, amniotic fluid glucose level, and amniotic fluid to serum glucose level ratio, Am. J. Obstet. Gynecol. 179 (1998) 650–656.

[57] A.Y. El-Bastawissi, M.A. Williams, D.E. Riley, J. Hitti, J.N. Krieger, Amniotic fluid interleukin-6 and preterm delivery: a review, Obstet. Gynecol. 95 (2000) 1056–1064.

[58] R. Figueroa, D. Garry, A. Elimian, K. Patel, P.B. Sehgal, N. Tejani, Evaluation of amniotic fluid cytokines in preterm labor and intact membranes, J. Matern. Fetal Neonatal. Med. 18 (2005) 241–247.

[59] W.W. Andrews, J.C. Hauth, R.L. Goldenberg, R. Gomez, R. Romero, G.H. Cassell, Amniotic fluid interleukin-6: correlation with upper genital tract microbial colonization and gestational age in women delivered after spontaneous labor versus indicated delivery, Am. J. Obstet. Gynecol. 173 (1995) 606–612.

[60] J. Hitti, D.E. Riley, M.A. Krohn, et al., Broad-spectrum bacterial rDNA polymerase chain reaction assay for detecting amniotic fluid infection among women in premature labor, Jackson Hole, WY, Clin. Infect. Dis. 24 (1997) 1228–1232.

[61] E. Oyarzun, M. Yamamoto, S. Kato, R. Gomez, L. Lizama, A. Moenne, Specific detection of 16 micro-organisms in amniotic fluid by polymerase chain reaction and its correlation with preterm delivery occurrence, Am. J. Obstet. Gynecol. 179 (1998) 1115–1119.

[62] G.R. Markenson, R.K. Martin, M. Tillotson-Criss, K.S. Foley, R.S. Stewart Jr., M. Yancey, The use of the polymerase chain reaction to detect bacteria in amniotic fluid in pregnancies complicated by preterm labor, Am. J. Obstet. Gynecol. 177 (1997) 1471–1477.

[63] L.F. Goncalves, T. Chaiworapongsa, R. Romero, Intrauterine infection and prematurity, Ment. Retard. Dev. Disabil. Res. Rev. 8 (2002) 3–13.

[64] R. Romero, J.P. Kusanovic, J. Espinoza, et al., What is amniotic fluid 'sludge'? Ultrasound Obstet. Gynecol. 30 (2007) 793–798.

[65] J.P. Kusanovic, J. Espinoza, R. Romero, et al., Clinical significance of the presence of amniotic fluid 'sludge' in asymptomatic patients at high risk for spontaneous preterm delivery, Ultrasound Obstet. Gynecol. 30 (2007) 706–714.

[66] R. Romero, R. Quintero, E. Oyarzun, et al., Intraamniotic infection and the onset of labor in preterm premature rupture of the membranes, Am. J. Obstet. Gynecol. 159 (1988) 661–666.

[67] R. Romero, H. Munoz, R. Gomez, et al., Two-thirds of spontaneous abortion/fetal deaths after genetic amniocentesis are the results of pre-existing subclinical inflammatory process of the amniotic cavity, Am. J. Obstet. Gynecol. 172 (1995) 261.

[68] K.D. Wenstrom, W.W. Andrews, T. Tamura, M.B. DuBard, K.E. Johnston, G.P. Hemstreet, Elevated amniotic fluid interleukin-6 levels at genetic amniocentesis predict subsequent pregnancy loss, Am. J. Obstet. Gynecol. 175 (1996) 830–833.

[69] R.L. Goldenberg, W.W. Andrews, B.M. Mercer, et al., The preterm prediction study: granulocyte colony-stimulating factor and spontaneous preterm birth. National Institute of Child Health and Human Development Maternal-Fetal Medicine Units Network, Am. J. Obstet. Gynecol. 182 (2000) 625–630.

[70] W.W. Andrews, R.L. Goldenberg, J.C. Hauth, S.P. Cliver, R. Copper, M. Conner, Interconceptional antibiotics to prevent spontaneous preterm birth: a randomized clinical trial, Am. J. Obstet. Gynecol. 194 (2006) 617–623.

[71] A.T. Tita, S.P. Cliver, A.R. Goepfert, et al., Clinical trial of interconceptional antibiotics to prevent preterm birth: subgroup analyses and possible adverse antibiotic-microbial interaction, Am. J. Obstet. Gynecol. 197 (367) (2007) e1–e6.

[72] R.S. Sperling, R.S. Ramamurthy, R.S. Gibbs, A comparison of intrapartum versus immediate postpartum treatment of intra-amniotic infection, Obstet. Gynecol. 70 (1987) 861–865.

[73] L.C. Gilstrap 3rd, K.J. Leveno, S.M. Cox, J.S. Burris, M. Mashburn, C.R. Rosenfeld, Intrapartum treatment of acute chorioamnionitis: impact on neonatal sepsis, Am. J. Obstet. Gynecol. 159 (1988) 579–583.

[74] R.S. Gibbs, M.J. Dinsmoor, E.R. Newton, R.S. Ramamurthy, A randomized trial of intrapartum versus immediate postpartum treatment of women with intra-amniotic infection, Obstet. Gynecol. 72 (1988) 823–828.

[75] R.E. Bray, R.W. Boe, W.L. Johnson, Transfer of ampicillin into fetus and amniotic fluid from maternal plasma in late pregnancy, Am. J. Obstet. Gynecol. 96 (1966) 938–942.

[76] D. Charles, Dynamics of antibiotic transfer from mother to fetus, Semin. Perinatol. 1 (1977) 89–100.

[77] A.J. Weinstein, R.S. Gibbs, M. Gallagher, Placental transfer of clindamycin and gentamicin in term pregnancy, Am. J. Obstet. Gynecol. 124 (1976) 688–691.

[78] G.J. Locksmith, A. Chin, T. Vu, K.E. Shattuck, G.D. Hankins, High compared with standard gentamicin dosing for chorioamnionitis: a comparison of maternal and fetal serum drug levels, Obstet. Gynecol. 105 (2005) 473–479.

[79] L.C. Gilstrap 3rd, R.E. Bawdon, J. Burris, Antibiotic concentration in maternal blood, cord blood, and placental membranes in chorioamnionitis, Obstet. Gynecol. 72 (1988) 124–125.

[80] S.J. Chapman, J. Owen, Randomized trial of single-dose versus multiple-dose cefotetan for the postpartum treatment of intrapartum chorioamnionitis, Am. J. Obstet. Gynecol. 177 (1997) 831–834.

[81] R.K. Edwards, P. Duff, Single additional dose postpartum therapy for women with chorioamnionitis, Obstet. Gynecol. 102 (2003) 957–961.

[82] J.D. Looff, W.D. Hager, Management of chorioamnionitis, Surg. Gynecol. Obstet. 158 (1984) 161–166.

[83] J.C. Hauth, L.C. Gilstrap 3rd, G.D. Hankins, K.D. Connor, Term maternal and neonatal complications of acute chorioamnionitis, Obstet. Gynecol. 66 (1985) 59–62.

[84] A. Locatelli, P. Vergani, A. Ghidini, et al., Duration of labor and risk of cerebral white-matter damage in very preterm infants who are delivered with intrauterine infection, Am. J. Obstet. Gynecol. 193 (2005) 928–932.

[85] D.J. Rouse, M. Landon, K.J. Leveno, et al., The Maternal-Fetal Medicine Units cesarean registry: chorioamnionitis at term and its duration-relationship to outcomes, Am. J. Obstet. Gynecol. 191 (2004) 211–216.

[86] P. Duff, R. Sanders, R.S. Gibbs, The course of labor in term patients with chorioamnionitis, Am. J. Obstet. Gynecol. 147 (1983) 391–395.

[87] R.K. Silver, R.S. Gibbs, M. Castillo, Effect of amniotic fluid bacteria on the course of labor in nulliparous women at term, Obstet. Gynecol. 68 (1986) 587–592.

[88] P.R. Yoder, R.S. Gibbs, J.D. Blanco, Y.S. Castaneda, P.J. St Clair, A prospective, controlled study of maternal and perinatal outcome after intra-amniotic infection at term, Am. J. Obstet. Gynecol. 145 (1983) 695–701.

[89] K.S. Koh, F.H. Chan, A.H. Monfared, W.J. Ledger, R.H. Paul, The changing perinatal and maternal outcome in chorioamnionitis, Obstet. Gynecol. 53 (1979) 730–734.

[90] T.J. Garite, R.K. Freeman, Chorioamnionitis in the preterm gestation, Obstet. Gynecol. 59 (1982) 539–545.

[91] W.J. Morales, The effect of chorioamnionitis on the developmental outcome of preterm infants at one year, Obstet. Gynecol. 70 (1987) 183–186.

[92] R.S. Sperling, E. Newton, R.S. Gibbs, Intraamniotic infection in low-birth-weight infants, J. Infect. Dis. 157 (1988) 113–117.

[93] M.G. Ferguson, P.G. Rhodes, J.C. Morrison, C.M. Puckett, Clinical amniotic fluid infection and its effect on the neonate, Am. J. Obstet. Gynecol. 151 (1985) 1058–1061.

[94] B.H. Yoon, R. Romero, J.S. Park, et al., The relationship among inflammatory lesions of the umbilical cord (funisitis), umbilical cord plasma interleukin 6 concentration, amniotic fluid infection, and neonatal sepsis, Am. J. Obstet. Gynecol. 183 (2000) 1124–1129.

[95] B.H. Yoon, J.K. Jun, R. Romero, et al., Amniotic fluid inflammatory cytokines (interleukin-6, interleukin-1beta, and tumor necrosis factor-alpha), neonatal brain white matter lesions, and cerebral palsy, Am. J. Obstet. Gynecol. 177 (1997) 19–26.

[96] C.S. Gibson, A.H. MacLennan, P.N. Goldwater, G.A. Dekker, Antenatal causes of cerebral palsy: associations between inherited thrombophilias, viral and bacterial infection, and inherited susceptibility to infection, Obstet. Gynecol. Surv. 58 (2003) 209–220.

[97] N.S. Hardt, M. Kostenbauder, M. Ogburn, M. Behnke, M. Resnick, A. Cruz, Influence of chorioamnionitis on long-term prognosis in low birth weight infants, Obstet. Gynecol. 65 (1985) 5–10.

[98] D.J. Murphy, S. Sellers, I.Z. MacKenzie, P.L. Yudkin, A.M. Johnson, Case-control study of antenatal and intrapartum risk factors for cerebral palsy in very preterm singleton babies, Lancet 346 (1995) 1449–1454.

[99] J.K. Grether, K.B. Nelson, Maternal infection and cerebral palsy in infants of normal birth weight, JAMA 278 (1997) 207–211.

[100] Y.W. Wu, J.M. Colford Jr., Chorioamnionitis as a risk factor for cerebral palsy: A meta-analysis, JAMA 284 (2000) 1417–1424.

[101] Y.W. Wu, G.J. Escobar, J.K. Grether, L.A. Croen, J.D. Greene, T. B. Newman, Chorioamnionitis and cerebral palsy in term and near-term infants, JAMA 290 (2003) 2677–2684.

[102] J.M. Alexander, L.C. Gilstrap, S.M. Cox, D.M. McIntire, K.J. Leveno, Clinical chorioamnionitis and the prognosis for very low birth weight infants, Obstet. Gynecol. 91 (1998) 725–729.

[103] B.H. Yoon, R. Romero, C.J. Kim, et al., High expression of tumor necrosis factor-alpha and interleukin-6 in periventricular leukomalacia, Am. J. Obstet. Gynecol. 177 (1997) 406–411.

[104] B.H. Yoon, C.J. Kim, R. Romero, et al., Experimentally induced intrauterine infection causes fetal brain white matter lesions in rabbits, Am. J. Obstet. Gynecol. 177 (1997) 797–802.

[105] L.A. Patrick, L.M. Gaudet, A.E. Farley, J.P. Rossiter, L.L. Tomalty, G. N. Smith, Development of a guinea pig model of chorioamnionitis and fetal brain injury, Am. J. Obstet. Gynecol. 191 (2004) 1205–1211.

[106] R.W. Redline, M.A. O'Riordan, Placental lesions associated with cerebral palsy and neurologic impairment following term birth, Arch. Pathol. Lab. Med. 124 (2000) 1785–1791.

[107] R.W. Redline, D. Wilson-Costello, E. Borawski, A.A. Fanaroff, M. Hack, Placental lesions associated with neurologic impairment and cerebral palsy in very low-birth-weight infants, Arch. Pathol. Lab. Med. 122 (1998) 1091–1098.

[108] J. Lau, F. Magee, Z. Qiu, J. Hoube, P. Von Dadelszen, S.K. Lee, Chorioamnionitis with a fetal inflammatory response is associated with higher neonatal mortality, morbidity, and resource use than chorioamnionitis displaying a maternal inflammatory response only, Am. J. Obstet. Gynecol. 193 (2005) 708–713.

[109] R.E. Willoughby Jr., K.B. Nelson, Chorioamnionitis and brain injury, Clin. Perinatol. 29 (2002) 603–621.

[110] J. Hitti, M.A. Krohn, D.L. Patton, et al., Amniotic fluid tumor necrosis factor-alpha and the risk of respiratory distress syndrome among preterm infants, Am. J. Obstet. Gynecol. 177 (1997) 50–56.

[111] R. Gomez, R. Romero, F. Ghezzi, B.H. Yoon, M. Mazor, S.M. Berry, The fetal inflammatory response syndrome, Am. J. Obstet. Gynecol. 179 (1998) 194–202.

[112] A.E. Curley, D.G. Sweet, C.M. Thornton, et al., Chorioamnionitis and increased neonatal lung lavage fluid matrix metalloproteinase-9 levels: implications for antenatal origins of chronic lung disease, Am. J. Obstet. Gynecol. 188 (2003) 871–875.

[113] A.K. Roberts, F. Monzon-Bordonaba, P.G. Van Deerlin, et al., Association of polymorphism within the promoter of the tumor necrosis factor alpha gene with increased risk of preterm premature rupture of the fetal membranes, Am. J. Obstet. Gynecol. 180 (1999) 1297–1302.

[114] M.R. Genc, S. Gerber, M. Nesin, S.S. Witkin, Polymorphism in the interleukin-1 gene complex and spontaneous preterm delivery, Am. J. Obstet. Gynecol. 187 (2002) 157–163.

[115] P.E. Ferrand, S. Parry, M. Sammel, et al., A polymorphism in the matrix metalloproteinase-9 promoter is associated with increased risk of preterm premature rupture of membranes in African Americans, Mol. Hum. Reprod. 8 (2002) 494–501.

[116] B.M. Mercer, K.L. Arheart, Antimicrobial therapy in expectant management of preterm premature rupture of the membranes, Lancet 346 (1995) 1271–1279.

[117] B.M. Mercer, M. Miodovnik, G.R. Thurnau, et al., Antibiotic therapy for reduction of infant morbidity after preterm premature rupture of the membranes. A randomized controlled trial. National Institute of Child Health and Human Development Maternal-Fetal Medicine Units Network, JAMA 278 (1997) 989–995.

[118] C. Egarter, H. Leitich, P. Husslein, A. Kaider, M. Schemper, Adjunctive antibiotic treatment in preterm labor and neonatal morbidity: a meta-analysis, Obstet. Gynecol. 88 (1996) 303–309.

[119] D.A. Eschenbach, P. Duff, J.A. McGregor, et al., 2% Clindamycin vaginal cream treatment of bacterial vaginosis in pregnancy (abstract), in: Annual Meeting of the infectious Diseases Society for Obstetrics and Gynecology, 1993.

[120] D.J. Rouse, J.C. Hauth, W.W. Andrews, B.B. Mills, J.E. Maher, Chlorhexidine vaginal irrigation for the prevention of peripartal infection: a placebo-controlled randomized clinical trial, Am. J. Obstet. Gynecol. 176 (1997) 617–622.

[121] K.M. Sweeten, N.L. Eriksen, J.D. Blanco, Chlorhexidine versus sterile water vaginal wash during labor to prevent peripartum infection, Am. J. Obstet. Gynecol. 176 (1997) 426–430.

[122] D.J. Rouse, S. Cliver, T.L. Lincoln, W.W. Andrews, J.C. Hauth, Clinical trial of chlorhexidine vaginal irrigation to prevent peripartal infection in nulliparous women, Am. J. Obstet. Gynecol. 189 (2003) 166–170.

[123] J.A. Martin, B.E. Hamilton, P.D. Sutton, et al., Births: final data for 2005, Natl. Vital. Stat. Rep. 56 (2007) 1–103.

[124] H. Minkoff, Prematurity: infection as an etiologic factor, Obstet. Gynecol. 62 (1983) 137–144.

[125] R.S. Gibbs, R. Romero, S.L. Hillier, D.A. Eschenbach, R.L. Sweet, A review of premature birth and subclinical infection, Am. J. Obstet. Gynecol. 166 (1992) 1515–1528.

[126] R.S. Gibbs, The relationship between infections and adverse pregnancy outcomes: an overview, Ann. Periodontol. 6 (2001) 153–163.

[127] K. Jarjoura, P.C. Devine, A. Perez-Delboy, M. Herrera-Abreu, M. D'Alton, P.N. Papapanou, Markers of periodontal infection and preterm birth, Am. J. Obstet. Gynecol. 192 (2005) 513–519.

[128] K.A. Boggess, P.N. Madianos, J.S. Preisser, K.J. Moise Jr., S. Offenbacher, Chronic maternal and fetal Porphyromonas gingivalis exposure during pregnancy in rabbits, Am. J. Obstet. Gynecol. 192 (2005) 554–557.

[129] R. Lopez, Periodontal disease and adverse pregnancy outcomes, Evid. Based Dent. 9 (2008) 48.

[130] S.G. Driscoll, The placenta and membranes, in: D. Charles, M. Finlands (Eds.), Obstetrical and Perinatal Infections, Lea & Febiger1973p. 532.

[131] P. Russell, Inflammatory lesions of the human placenta: I. Clinical significance of acute chorioamnionitis, Am. J. Diagn. Gynecol. Obstet. 1 (1979) 127.

[132] J.N. Schoonmaker, D.W. Lawellin, B. Lunt, J.A. McGregor, Bacteria and inflammatory cells reduce chorioamniotic membrane integrity and tensile strength, Obstet. Gynecol. 74 (1989) 590–596.

[133] A. Bernal, D.J. Hansell, T.Y. Khont, et al., Prostaglandin E production by the fetal membranes in unexplained preterm labour and preterm labor associated with chorioamnionitis, Br. J. Obstet. Gynaecol. 96 (1989) 1133.

[134] R.F. Lamont, F. Anthony, L. Myatt, L. Booth, P.M. Furr, D. Taylor-Robinson, Production of prostaglandin E2 by human amnion in vitro in response to addition of media conditioned by microorganisms associated with chorioamnionitis and preterm labor, Am. J. Obstet. Gynecol. 162 (1990) 819–825.

[135] S.L. Hillier, J. Martius, M. Krohn, N. Kiviat, K.K. Holmes, D.A. Eschenbach, A case-control study of chorioamnionic infection and histologic chorioamnionitis in prematurity, N. Engl. J. Med. 319 (1988) 972–978.

[136] N.H. Daikoku, D.F. Kaltreider, T.R. Johnson Jr., J.W. Johnson, M.A. Simmons, Premature rupture of membranes and preterm labor: neonatal infection and perinatal mortality risks, Obstet. Gynecol. 58 (1981) 417–425.

[137] K. Seo, J.A. McGregor, J.I. French, Preterm birth is associated with increased risk of maternal and neonatal infection, Obstet. Gynecol. 79 (1992) 75–80.

[138] R. Romero, M. Mazor, Infection and preterm labor, Clin. Obstet. Gynecol. 31 (1988) 553–584.

[139] J.N. Vergnes, M. Sixou, Preterm low birth weight and maternal periodontal status: a meta-analysis, Am. J. Obstet. Gynecol. 196 (135) (2007) e1–e7.

[140] D.M. Stamilio, J.J. Chang, G.A. Macones, Periodontal disease and preterm birth: do the data have enough teeth to recommend screening and preventive treatment? Am. J. Obstet. Gynecol. 196 (2007) 93–94.

[141] W.W. Andrews, M.A. Klebanoff, E.A. Thom, et al., Midpregnancy genitourinary tract infection with Chlamydia trachomatis: association with subsequent preterm delivery in women with bacterial vaginosis and Trichomonas vaginalis, Am. J. Obstet. Gynecol. 194 (2006) 493–500.

[142] S.L. Hillier, R.P. Nugent, D.A. Eschenbach, et al., Association between bacterial vaginosis and preterm delivery of a low-birth-weight infant. The Vaginal Infections and Prematurity Study Group, N. Engl. J. Med. 333 (1995) 1737–1742.

[143] A.M. Briselden, B.J. Moncla, C.E. Stevens, S.L. Hillier, Sialidases (neuraminidases) in bacterial vaginosis and bacterial vaginosis-associated microflora, J. Clin. Microbiol. 30 (1992) 663–666.

[144] J.A. McGregor, J.I. French, W. Jones, et al., Bacterial vaginosis is associated with prematurity and vaginal fluid mucinase and sialidase: results of a controlled trial of topical clindamycin cream, Am. J. Obstet. Gynecol. 170 (1994) 1048–1059 discussion 59–60.

[145] J.N. Schoonmaker, B.D. Lunt, D.W. Lawellin, J.I. French, S.L. Hillier, J. A. McGregor, A new proline aminopeptidase assay for diagnosis of bacterial vaginosis, Am. J. Obstet. Gynecol. 165 (1991) 737–742.

[146] S. Cauci, J. Hitti, C. Noonan, et al., Vaginal hydrolytic enzymes, immunoglobulin A against Gardnerella vaginalis toxin, and risk of early preterm birth among women in preterm labor with bacterial vaginosis or intermediate flora, Am. J. Obstet. Gynecol. 187 (2002) 877–881.

[147] S. Cauci, P. Thorsen, D.E. Schendel, A. Bremmelgaard, F. Quadrifoglio, S. Guaschino, Determination of immunoglobulin A against Gardnerella vaginalis hemolysin, sialidase, and prolidase activities in vaginal fluid: implications for adverse pregnancy outcomes, J. Clin. Microbiol. 41 (2003) 435–438.

[148] S. Cauci, J. McGregor, P. Thorsen, J. Grove, S. Guaschino, Combination of vaginal pH with vaginal sialidase and prolidase activities for prediction of low birth weight and preterm birth, Am. J. Obstet. Gynecol. 192 (2005) 489–496.

[149] G.A. Macones, S. Parry, M. Elkousy, B. Clothier, S.H. Ural, J.F. Strauss 3rd, A polymorphism in the promoter region of TNF and bacterial vaginosis: preliminary evidence of gene-environment interaction in the etiology of spontaneous preterm birth, Am. J. Obstet. Gynecol. 190 (2004) 1504–1508 discussion 3A.

[150] J.A. Regan, S. Chao, L.S. James, Premature rupture of membranes, preterm delivery, and group B streptococcal colonization of mothers, Am. J. Obstet. Gynecol. 141 (1981) 184–186.

[151] M. Moller, A.C. Thomsen, K. Borch, et al., Rupture of fetal membranes and premature delivery associated with group B streptococci in urine of pregnant women, Lancet 2 (1989) 69.

[152] C.P. White, E.G. Wilkins, C. Roberts, D.C. Davidson, Premature delivery and group B streptococcal bacteriuria, Lancet 2 (1984) 586.

[153] A.C. Thomsen, L. Morup, K.B. Hansen, Antibiotic elimination of group-B streptococci in urine in prevention of preterm labour, Lancet 1 (1987) 591–593.

[154] M.A. Klebanoff, J.A. Regan, A.V. Rao, et al., Outcome of the Vaginal Infections and Prematurity Study: results of a clinical trial of erythromycin among pregnant women colonized with group B streptococci, Am. J. Obstet. Gynecol. 172 (1995) 1540–1545.

[155] Prevention of perinatal group B streptococcal disease: a public health perspective. Centers for Disease Control and Prevention, MMWR Recomm. Rep. 45 (1996) 1–24.

[156] R. Romero, M. Sirtori, E. Oyarzun, et al., Infection and labor. V. Prevalence, microbiology, and clinical significance of intraamniotic infection in women with preterm labor and intact membranes, Am. J. Obstet. Gynecol. 161 (1989) 817–824.

[157] R. Gomez, F. Ghezzi, R. Romero, H. Munoz, J.E. Tolosa, I. Rojas, Premature labor and intra-amniotic infection. Clinical aspects and role of the cytokines in diagnosis and pathophysiology, Clin. Perinatol. 22 (1995) 281–342.

[158] P.L. Fidel Jr., R. Romero, M. Ramirez, et al., Interleukin-1 receptor antagonist (IL-1ra) production by human amnion, chorion, and decidua, Am. J. Reprod. Immunol. 32 (1994) 1–7.

[159] A.P. Murtha, A. Nieves, E.R. Hauser, et al., Association of maternal IL-1 receptor antagonist intron 2 gene polymorphism and preterm birth, Am. J. Obstet. Gynecol. 195 (2006) 1249–1253.

[160] S.A. Engel, H.C. Erichsen, D.A. Savitz, J. Thorp, S.J. Chanock, A.F. Olshan, Risk of spontaneous preterm birth is associated with common proinflammatory cytokine polymorphisms, Epidemiology 16 (2005) 469–477.

[161] M.G. Gravett, Interleukin-10 (IL-10) inhibits interleukin-Iβ (IL-1β) induced preterm labor in Rhesus monkeys (abstract), in: Annual Meeting of the Infectious Diseases Society for Obstetrics and Gynecology, 1998.

[162] R. Romero, M. Mazor, B. Tartakovsky, Systemic administration of interleukin-1 induces preterm parturition in mice, Am. J. Obstet. Gynecol. 165 (1991) 969–971.

[163] N. Kaga, Y. Katsuki, M. Obata, Y. Shibutani, Repeated administration of low-dose lipopolysaccharide induces preterm delivery in mice: a model for human preterm parturition and for assessment of the therapeutic ability of drugs against preterm delivery, Am. J. Obstet. Gynecol. 174 (1996) 754–759.

[164] R.S. Gibbs, R.S. McDuffie Jr., M. Kunze, et al., Experimental intrauterine infection with Prevotella bivia in New Zealand White rabbits, Am. J. Obstet. Gynecol. 190 (2004) 1082–1086.

[165] M.G. Gravett, S.S. Witkin, G.J. Haluska, J.L. Edwards, M.J. Cook, M. J. Novy, An experimental model for intraamniotic infection and preterm labor in rhesus monkeys, Am. J. Obstet. Gynecol. 171 (1994) 1660–1667.

[166] E.H. Kass, W.M. McCormack, J.S. Lin, B. Rosner, A. Munoz, Genital mycoplasmas as a cause of excess premature delivery, Trans. Assoc. Am. Physicians 94 (1981) 261–266.

[167] W.M. McCormack, B. Rosner, Y.H. Lee, A. Munoz, D. Charles, E.H. Kass, Effect on birth weight of erythromycin treatment of pregnant women, Obstet. Gynecol. 69 (1987) 202–207.

[168] I. Cohen, J.C. Veille, B.M. Calkins, Improved pregnancy outcome following successful treatment of chlamydial infection, JAMA 263 (1990) 3160–3163.

[169] G.M. Ryan Jr., T.N. Abdella, S.G. McNeeley, V.S. Baselski, D.E. Drummond, Chlamydia trachomatis infection in pregnancy and effect of treatment on outcome, Am. J. Obstet. Gynecol. 162 (1990) 34–39.

[170] D.H. Martin, D.A. Eschenbach, M.F. Cotch, et al., Double-Blind Placebo-Controlled Treatment Trial of Chlamydia trachomatis Endocervical Infections in Pregnant Women, Infect. Dis. Obstet. Gynecol. 5 (1997) 10–17.

[171] Sexually transmitted diseases treatment guidelines 2002. Centers for Disease Control and Prevention, MMWR Recomm. Rep. 51 (2002) 1–78.

[172] P. Burtin, A. Taddio, O. Ariburnu, T.R. Einarson, G. Koren, Safety of metronidazole in pregnancy: a meta-analysis, Am. J. Obstet. Gynecol. 172 (1995) 525–529.

[173] M.A. Klebanoff, J.C. Carey, J.C. Hauth, et al., Failure of metronidazole to prevent preterm delivery among pregnant women with asymptomatic Trichomonas vaginalis infection, N. Engl. J. Med. 345 (2001) 487–493.

[174] A. Shennan, S. Crawshaw, A. Briley, et al., A randomised controlled trial of metronidazole for the prevention of preterm birth in women positive for cervicovaginal fetal fibronectin: the PREMET Study, BJOG 113 (2006) 65–74.

[175] H. Leitich, M. Brunbauer, B. Bodner-Adler, A. Kaider, C. Egarter, P. Husslein, Antibiotic treatment of bacterial vaginosis in pregnancy: a meta-analysis, Am. J. Obstet. Gynecol. 188 (2003) 752–758.

[176] R.F. Lamont, S.L. Duncan, D. Mandal, P. Bassett, Intravaginal clindamycin to reduce preterm birth in women with abnormal genital tract flora, Obstet. Gynecol. 101 (2003) 516–522.

[177] R.F. Lamont, S.R. Sawant, Infection in the prediction and antibiotics in the prevention of spontaneous preterm labour and preterm birth, Minerva Ginecol. 57 (2005) 423–433.

[178] S.L. Kenyon, D.J. Taylor, W. Tarnow-Mordi, Broad-spectrum antibiotics for spontaneous preterm labour: the ORACLE II randomised trial. ORACLE Collaborative Group, Lancet 357 (2001) 989–994.

[179] B.J. Stoll, N. Hansen, A.A. Fanaroff, et al., Changes in pathogens causing early-onset sepsis in very-low-birth-weight infants, N. Engl. J. Med. 347 (2002) 240–247.

[180] D.S. Dizon-Townson, H. Major, M. Varner, K. Ward, A promoter mutation that increases transcription of the tumor necrosis factor-alpha gene is not associated with preterm delivery, Am. J. Obstet. Gynecol. 177 (1997) 810–813.

[181] G.C. Gunn, D.R. Mishell Jr., D.G. Morton, Premature rupture of the fetal membranes. A review, Am. J. Obstet. Gynecol. 106 (1970) 469–483.

[182] R.S. Gibbs, J.D. Blanco, Premature rupture of the membranes, Obstet. Gynecol. 60 (1982) 671–679.

[183] T.J. Garite, Premature rupture of the membranes: the enigma of the obstetrician, Am. J. Obstet. Gynecol. 151 (1985) 1001–1005.

[184] ACOG practice bulletin, Premature rupture of membranes. Clinical management guidelines for obstetrician-gynecologists. Number 1, June 1998. American College of Obstetricians and Gynecologists, Int. J. Gynaecol. Obstet. 63 (1998) 75–84.

[185] H.S. Bada, L.C. Alojipan, B.F. Andrews, Premature rupture of membranes and its effect on the newborn, Pediatr. Clin. North Am. 24 (1977) 491–500.

[186] J.A. Fayez, A.A. Hasan, H.S. Jonas, G.L. Miller, Management of premature rupture of the membranes, Obstet. Gynecol. 52 (1978) 17–21.

[187] G. Evaldson, A. Lagrelius, J. Winiarski, Premature rupture of the membranes, Acta Obstet. Gynecol. Scand. 59 (1980) 385–393.

[188] T.R. Eggers, L.W. Doyle, R.J. Pepperell, Premature rupture of the membranes, Med. J. Aust. 1 (1979) 209–213.

[189] R. Artal, R.J. Sokol, M. Neuman, A.H. Burstein, J. Stojkov, The mechanical properties of prematurely and non–prematurely ruptured membranes. Methods and preliminary results, Am. J. Obstet. Gynecol. 125 (1976) 655–659.

[190] B.M. Mercer, R.L. Goldenberg, P.J. Meis, et al., The Preterm Prediction Study: prediction of preterm premature rupture of membranes through clinical findings and ancillary testing. The National Institute of Child Health and Human Development Maternal-Fetal Medicine Units Network, Am. J. Obstet. Gynecol. 183 (2000) 738–745.

[191] E. Parry-Jones, S. Priya, A study of the elasticity and tension of fetal membranes and of the relation of the area of the gestational sac to the area of the uterine cavity, Br. J. Obstet. Gynaecol. 83 (1976) 205–212.

[192] N.S. Al-Zaid, M.N. Bou-Resli, G. Goldspink, Bursting pressure and collagen content of fetal membranes and their relation to premature rupture of the membranes, Br. J. Obstet. Gynaecol. 87 (1980) 227–229.

[193] R.L. Naeye, E.C. Peters, Causes and consequences of premature rupture of fetal membranes, Lancet 1 (1980) 192–194.

[194] F. Vadillo-Ortega, A. Hernandez, G. Gonzalez-Avila, L. Bermejo, K. Iwata, J.F. Strauss 3rd, Increased matrix metalloproteinase activity and reduced tissue inhibitor of metalloproteinases-1 levels in amniotic fluids from pregnancies complicated by premature rupture of membranes, Am. J. Obstet. Gynecol. 174 (1996) 1371–1376.

[195] E. Maymon, R. Romero, P. Pacora, et al., Human neutrophil collagenase (matrix metalloproteinase 8) in parturition, premature rupture of the membranes, and intrauterine infection, Am. J. Obstet. Gynecol. 183 (2000) 94–99.

[196] R.L. Naeye, Factors that predispose to premature rupture of the fetal membranes, Obstet. Gynecol. 60 (1982) 93–98.

[197] R.L. Naeye, S. Ross, Coitus and chorioamnionitis: a prospective study, Early Hum. Dev. 6 (1982) 91–97.

[198] G. Creatsas, M. Pavlatos, D. Lolis, D. Aravantinos, D. Kaskarelis, Bacterial contamination of the cervix and premature rupture of membranes, Am. J. Obstet. Gynecol. 139 (1981) 522–525.

[199] V.E. Del Bene, E. Moore, M. Rogers, A.K. Kreutner, Bacterial flora of patients with prematurely ruptured membranes, South. Med. J. 70 (1977) 948–950 54.

[200] J.H. Harger, A.W. Hsing, R.E. Tuomala, et al., Risk factors for preterm premature rupture of fetal membranes: a multicenter case-control study, Am. J. Obstet. Gynecol. 163 (1990) 130–137.

[201] S.E. Lee, J.S. Park, E.R. Norwitz, K.W. Kim, H.S. Park, J.K. Jun, Measurement of placental alpha-microglobulin-1 in cervicovaginal discharge to diagnose rupture of membranes, Obstet. Gynecol. 109 (2007) 634–640.

[202] K.A. Kappy, C.L. Cetrulo, R.A. Knuppel, et al., Premature rupture of the membranes at term. A comparison of induced and spontaneous labors, J. Reprod. Med. 27 (1982) 29–33.

[203] K.A. Kappy, C.L. Cetrulo, R.A. Knuppel, et al., Premature rupture of the membranes: a conservative approach, Am. J. Obstet. Gynecol. 134 (1979) 655–661.

[204] K.K. Christensen, P. Christensen, I. Ingemarsson, et al., A study of complications in preterm deliveries after prolonged premature rupture of the membranes, Obstet. Gynecol. 48 (1976) 670–677.

[205] D.J. Nochimson, R.H. Petrie, B.L. Shah, et al., Comparisons of conservation and dynamic management of premature rupture of membranes/premature labor syndrome: new approaches to the delivery of infants whih may minimize the need for intensive care, Clin. Perinatol. 7 (1979) 17.

[206] J.W. Johnson, N.H. Daikoku, J.R. Niebyl, T.R. Johnson Jr., V.A. Khouzami, F.R. Witter, Premature rupture of the membranes and prolonged latency, Obstet. Gynecol. 57 (1981) 547–556.

[207] J.M. Miller Jr., J.E. Brazy, S.A. Gall, M.C. Crenshaw Jr., F.R. Jelovsek, Premature rupture of the membranes: maternal and neonatal infectious morbidity related to betamethasone and antibiotic therapy, J. Reprod. Med. 25 (1980) 173–177.

[208] J. Taylor, T.J. Garite, Premature rupture of membranes before fetal viability, Obstet. Gynecol. 64 (1984) 615–620.

[209] S.M. Cox, M.L. Williams, K.J. Leveno, The natural history of preterm ruptured membranes: what to expect of expectant management, Obstet. Gynecol. 71 (1988) 558–562.

[210] J.W. Johnson, R.S. Egerman, J. Moorhead, Cases with ruptured membranes that "reseal" Am. J. Obstet. Gynecol. 163 (1990) 1024–1030; discussion 30–2.

[211] B.M. Mercer, Management of premature rupture of membranes before 26 weeks' gestation, Obstet. Gynecol. Clin. North Am. 19 (1992) 339–351.

[212] R. Gonen, M.E. Hannah, J.E. Milligan, Does prolonged preterm premature rupture of the membranes predispose to abruptio placentae? Obstet. Gynecol. 74 (1989) 347–350.

[213] A. Rotschild, E.W. Ling, M.L. Puterman, D. Farquharson, Neonatal outcome after prolonged preterm rupture of the membranes, Am. J. Obstet. Gynecol. 162 (1990) 46–52.

[214] C. Nimrod, F. Varela-Gittings, G. Machin, D. Campbell, R. Wesenberg, The effect of very prolonged membrane rupture on fetal development, Am. J. Obstet. Gynecol. 148 (1984) 540–543.

[215] P. Vergani, A. Ghidini, A. Locatelli, et al., Risk factors for pulmonary hypoplasia in second-trimester premature rupture of membranes, Am. J. Obstet. Gynecol. 170 (1994) 1359–1364.

[216] B.M. Mercer, Premature rupture of membranes, ACOG Practice Bulletin (1998).

[217] M.R. Lauria, B. Gonik, R. Romero, Pulmonary hypoplasia: pathogenesis, diagnosis, and antenatal prediction, Obstet. Gynecol. 86 (1995) 466–475.

[218] B.M. Mercer, Preterm premature rupture of membranes, Obstet. Gynecol. 101 (2003) 178–193.

[219] R.P. Perkins, The neonatal significance of selected perinatal events among infants of low birth weight. II. The influence of ruptured membranes, Am. J. Obstet. Gynecol. 142 (1982) 7–16.

[220] J. Schreiber, T. Benedetti, Conservative management of preterm premature rupture of the fetal membranes in a low socioeconomic population, Am. J. Obstet. Gynecol. 136 (1980) 92–96.

[221] R.L. Berkowitz, R.D. Kantor, G.J. Beck, J.B. Warshaw, The relationship between premature rupture of the membranes and the respiratory distress syndrome. An update and plan of management, Am. J. Obstet. Gynecol. 131 (1978) 503–508.

[222] N.H. Daikoku, D.F. Kaltreider, V.A. Khouzami, M. Spence, J.W. Johnson, Premature rupture of membranes and spontaneous preterm labor: maternal endometritis risks, Obstet. Gynecol. 59 (1982) 13–20.

[223] J.F. Jewett, Committee on maternal welfare: prolonged rupture of the membranes, N. Engl. J. Med. 292 (1975) 752.

[224] D.F. Lewis, C.A. Major, C.V. Towers, T. Asrat, J.A. Harding, T.J. Garite, Effects of digital vaginal examinations on latency period in preterm premature rupture of membranes, Obstet. Gynecol. 80 (1992) 630–634.

[225] R. Romero, B.H. Yoon, M. Mazor, et al., The diagnostic and prognostic value of amniotic fluid white blood cell count, glucose, interleukin-6, and gram stain in patients with preterm labor and intact membranes, Am. J. Obstet. Gynecol. 169 (1993) 805–816.

[226] A. Ohlsson, E. Wang, An analysis of antenatal tests to detect infection in preterm premature rupture of the membranes, Am. J. Obstet. Gynecol. 162 (1990) 809–818.

[227] T.J. Garite, R.K. Freeman, E.M. Linzey, P. Braly, The use of amniocentesis in patients with premature rupture of membranes, Obstet. Gynecol. 54 (1979) 226–230.

[228] F.J. Zlatnik, D.P. Cruikshank, C.R. Petzold, R.P. Galask, Amniocentesis in the identification of inapparent infection in preterm patients with premature rupture of the membranes, J. Reprod. Med. 29 (1984) 656–660.

[229] A.M. Vintzileos, W.A. Campbell, D.J. Nochimson, P.J. Weinbaum, D.T. Escoto, M.H. Mirochnick, Qualitative amniotic fluid volume versus amniocentesis in predicting infection in preterm premature rupture of the membranes, Obstet. Gynecol. 67 (1986) 579–583.

[230] J.D. Yeast, T.J. Garite, W. Dorchester, The risks of amniocentesis in the management of premature rupture of membranes, Am. J. Obstet. Gynecol. 149 (1984) 505–508.

[231] S.J. Feinstein, A.M. Vintzileos, J.G. Lodeiro, W.A. Campbell, P.J. Weinbaum, D.J. Nochimson, Amniocentesis with premature rupture of membranes, Obstet. Gynecol. 68 (1986) 147–152.

[232] D.B. Cotton, B. Gonik, S.F. Bottoms, Conservative versus aggressive management of preterm rupture of membranes. A randomized trial of amniocentesis, Am. J. Perinatol. 1 (1984) 322–324.

[233] M.I. Evans, S.N. Hajj, L.D. Devoe, N.S. Angerman, A.H. Moawad, C-reactive protein as a predictor of infectious morbidity with premature rupture of membranes, Am. J. Obstet. Gynecol. 138 (1980) 648–652.

[234] H.F. Farb, M. Arnesen, P. Geistler, G.E. Knox, C-reactive protein with premature rupture of membranes and premature labor, Obstet. Gynecol. 62 (1983) 49–51.

[235] P. Hawrylyshyn, P. Bernstein, J.E. Milligan, S. Soldin, A. Pollard, F.R. Papsin, Premature rupture of membranes: the role of C-reactive protein in the prediction of chorioamnionitis, Am. J. Obstet. Gynecol. 147 (1983) 240–246.

[236] D.A. Guinn, M.W. Atkinson, L. Sullivan, et al., Single vs weekly courses of antenatal corticosteroids for women at risk of preterm delivery: A randomized controlled trial, JAMA 286 (2001) 1581–1587.

[237] Y. Romem, R. Artal, C-reactive protein as a predictor for chorioamnionitis in cases of premature rupture of the membranes, Am. J. Obstet. Gynecol. 150 (1984) 546–550.

[238] G. Kayem, F. Goffinet, F. Batteux, P.H. Jarreau, B. Weill, D. Cabrol, Detection of interleukin-6 in vaginal secretions of women with preterm premature rupture of membranes and its association with neonatal infection: a rapid immunochromatographic test, Am. J. Obstet. Gynecol. 192 (2005) 140–145.

[239] B. Gonik, S.F. Bottoms, D.B. Cotton, Amniotic fluid volume as a risk factor in preterm premature rupture of the membranes, Obstet. Gynecol. 65 (1985) 456–459.

[240] A.M. Vintzileos, W.A. Campbell, D.J. Nochimson, M.E. Connolly, M.M. Fuenfer, G.J. Hoehn, The fetal biophysical profile in patients with premature rupture of the membranes–an early predictor of fetal infection, Am. J. Obstet. Gynecol. 152 (1985) 510–516.

[241] S.N. Beydoun, S.Y. Yasin, Premature rupture of the membranes before 28 weeks: conservative management, Am. J. Obstet. Gynecol. 155 (1986) 471–479.

[242] C.A. Major, J.L. Kitzmiller, Perinatal survival with expectant management of midtrimester rupture of membranes, Am. J. Obstet. Gynecol. 163 (1990) 838–844.

[243] M. Moretti, B.M. Sibai, Maternal and perinatal outcome of expectant management of premature rupture of membranes in the midtrimester, Am. J. Obstet. Gynecol. 159 (1988) 390–396.

[244] M.J. Dinsmoor, R. Bachman, E.I. Haney, M. Goldstein, W. Mackendrick, Outcomes after expectant management of extremely preterm premature rupture of the membranes, Am. J. Obstet. Gynecol. 190 (2004) 183–187.

[245] Pediatrics AAo, Perinatal care at the threshold of viability, Pediatrics 96 (1995) 974.

[246] R.A. Quintero, Treatment of previable premature ruptured membranes, Clin. Perinatol. 30 (2003) 573–589.

[247] R.A. Quintero, W.J. Morales, M. Allen, P.W. Bornick, J. Arroyo, G. LeParc, Treatment of iatrogenic previable premature rupture of membranes with intra-amniotic injection of platelets and cryoprecipitate (amniopatch): preliminary experience, Am. J. Obstet. Gynecol. 181 (1999) 744–749.

[248] A.C. Sciscione, J.S. Manley, M. Pollock, et al., Intracervical fibrin sealants: a potential treatment for early preterm premature rupture of the membranes, Am. J. Obstet. Gynecol. 184 (2001) 368–373.

[249] H.W. Taeusch Jr., F. Frigoletto, J. Kitzmiller, et al., Risk of respiratory distress syndrome after prenatal dexamethasone treatment, Pediatrics 63 (1979) 64–72.

[250] A.N. Papageorgiou, M.F. Desgranges, M. Masson, E. Colle, R. Shatz, M.M. Gelfand, The antenatal use of betamethasone in the prevention of respiratory distress syndrome: a controlled double-blind study, Pediatrics 63 (1979) 73–79.

[251] Effect of antenatal dexamethasone administration on the prevention of respiratory distress syndrome, Am. J. Obstet. Gynecol. 141 (1981) 276–287.

[252] T.J. Garite, R.K. Freeman, E.M. Linzey, P.S. Braly, W.L. Dorchester, Prospective randomized study of corticosteroids in the management of premature rupture of the membranes and the premature gestation, Am. J. Obstet. Gynecol. 141 (1981) 508–515.

[253] J.M. Barrett, F.H. Boehm, Comparison of aggressive and conservative management of premature rupture of fetal membranes, Am. J. Obstet. Gynecol. 144 (1982) 12–16.

[254] P.L. Schmidt, M.E. Sims, H.T. Strassner, R.H. Paul, E. Mueller, D. McCart, Effect of antepartum glucocorticoid administration upon neonatal respiratory distress syndrome and perinatal infection, Am. J. Obstet. Gynecol. 148 (1984) 178–186.

[255] J.D. Iams, M.L. Talbert, H. Barrows, L. Sachs, Management of preterm prematurely ruptured membranes: a prospective randomized comparison of observation versus use of steroids and timed delivery, Am. J. Obstet. Gynecol. 151 (1985) 32–38.

[256] G.F. Simpson, G.M. Harbert Jr., Use of beta-methasone in management of preterm gestation with premature rupture of membranes, Obstet. Gynecol. 66 (1985) 168–175.

[257] L.H. Nelson, P.J. Meis, C.G. Hatjis, J.M. Ernest, R. Dillard, H.M. Schey, Premature rupture of membranes: a prospective, randomized evaluation of steroids, latent phase, and expectant management, Obstet. Gynecol. 66 (1985) 55–58.

[258] W.J. Morales, N.D. Diebel, A.J. Lazar, D. Zadrozny, The effect of antenatal dexamethasone administration on the prevention of respiratory distress

syndrome in preterm gestations with premature rupture of membranes, Am. J. Obstet. Gynecol. 154 (1986) 591–595.

[259] A. Ohlsson, Treatments of preterm premature rupture of the membranes: a meta-analysis, Am. J. Obstet. Gynecol. 160 (1989) 890–906.

[260] P.A. Crowley, Antenatal corticosteroid therapy: a meta-analysis of the randomized trials, 1972 to 1994, Am. J. Obstet. Gynecol. 173 (1995) 322–335.

[261] D.F. Lewis, K. Brody, M.S. Edwards, R.M. Brouillette, S. Burlison, S.N. London, Preterm premature ruptured membranes: a randomized trial of steroids after treatment with antibiotics, Obstet. Gynecol. 88 (1996) 801–805.

[262] H. Leitich, C. Egarter, K. Reisenberger, A. Kaider, P. Berghammer, Concomitant use of glucocorticoids: a comparison of two metaanalyses on antibiotic treatment in preterm premature rupture of membranes, Am. J. Obstet. Gynecol. 178 (1998) 899–908.

[263] M.J. Lee, J. Davies, D. Guinn, et al., Single versus weekly courses of antenatal corticosteroids in preterm premature rupture of membranes, Obstet. Gynecol. 103 (2004) 274–281.

[264] Services USDoHaH, Prevention of Perinatal group B streptococcal disease: revised guidelines from CDC, MMWR Morb. Mortal. Wkly Rep. 51 (RR11) (2002) 1.

[265] H. Minkoff, P. Mead, An obstetric approach to the prevention of early-onset group B beta-hemolytic streptococcal sepsis, Am. J. Obstet. Gynecol. 154 (1986) 973–977.

[266] K.M. Boyer, S.P. Gotoff, Prevention of early-onset neonatal group B streptococcal disease with selective intrapartum chemoprophylaxis, N. Engl. J. Med. 314 (1986) 1665–1669.

[267] R. Romero, A.L. Scioscia, S.C. Edberg, J.C. Hobbins, Use of parenteral antibiotic therapy to eradicate bacterial colonization of amniotic fluid in premature rupture of membranes, Obstet. Gynecol. 67 (1986) 15S–17S.

[268] D.W. Thibeault, G.C. Emmanouilides, Prolonged rupture of fetal membranes and decreased frequency of respiratory distress syndrome and patent ductus arteriosus in preterm infants, Am. J. Obstet. Gynecol. 129 (1977) 43–46.

[269] M.F. Schutte, P.E. Treffers, G.J. Kloosterman, S. Soepatmi, Management of premature rupture of membranes: the risk of vaginal examination to the infant, Am. J. Obstet. Gynecol. 146 (1983) 395–400.

[270] M.F. Block, O.R. Kling, W.M. Crosby, Antenatal glucocorticoid therapy for the prevention of respiratory distress syndrome in the premature infant, Obstet. Gynecol. 50 (1977) 186–190.

[271] M.D. Jones Jr., L.I. Burd, W.A. Bowes Jr., F.C. Battaglia, L.O. Lubchenco, Failure of association of premature rupture of membranes with respiratory-distress syndrome, N. Engl. J. Med. 292 (1975) 1253–1257.

[272] S. Kenyon, M. Boulvain, J. Neilson, Antibiotics for preterm rupture of the membranes: a systematic review, Obstet. Gynecol. 104 (2004) 1051–1057.

[273] C. Egarter, H. Leitich, H. Karas, et al., Antibiotic treatment in preterm premature rupture of membranes and neonatal morbidity: a metaanalysis, Am. J. Obstet. Gynecol. 174 (1996) 589–597.

[274] S. Kenyon, M. Boulvain, J. Neilson, Antibiotics for preterm rupture of membranes, Cochrane Database Syst. Rev. (2003) CD001058.

[275] S.Y. Segel, A.M. Miles, B. Clothier, S. Parry, G.A. Macones, Duration of antibiotic therapy after preterm premature rupture of fetal membranes, Am. J. Obstet. Gynecol. 189 (2003) 799–802.

[276] D.F. Lewis, C.D. Adair, A.G. Robichaux, et al., Antibiotic therapy in preterm premature rupture of membranes: Are seven days necessary? A preliminary, randomized clinical trial, Am. J. Obstet. Gynecol. 188 (2003) 1413–1416; discussion 6–7.

[277] L.B. Curet, A.V. Rao, R.D. Zachman, et al., Association between ruptured membranes, tocolytic therapy, and respiratory distress syndrome, Am. J. Obstet. Gynecol. 148 (1984) 263–268.

[278] T.J. Garite, K.A. Keegan, R.K. Freeman, M.P. Nageotte, A randomized trial of ritodrine tocolysis versus expectant management in patients with premature rupture of the membranes at 25 to 30 weeks of gestation, Am. J. Obstet. Gynecol. 157 (1987) 388–393.

[279] C.P. Weiner, K. Renk, M. Klugman, The therapeutic efficacy and cost-effectiveness of aggressive tocolysis for premature labor associated with premature rupture of the membranes, Am. J. Obstet. Gynecol. 159 (1988) 216–222.

[280] G. Decavalas, D. Mastrogiannis, V. Papadopoulos, V. Tzingounis, Short-term verus long-term prophylactic tocolysis in patients with preterm premature rupture of the membranes, Eur. J. Obstet. Gynecol. Reprod. Biol. 59 (1995) 143–147.

[281] T. Fontenot, D.F. Lewis, Tocolytic therapy with preterm premature rupture of membranes, Clin. Perinatol. 28 (2001) 787–796, vi.

[282] R.G. Brame, J. MacKenna, Vaginal pool phospholipids in the management of premature rupture of membranes, Am. J. Obstet. Gynecol. 145 (1983) 992–1000.

[283] B.M. Mercer, L.G. Crocker, N.M. Boe, B.M. Sibai, Induction versus expectant management in premature rupture of the membranes with mature amniotic fluid at 32 to 36 weeks: a randomized trial, Am. J. Obstet. Gynecol. 169 (1993) 775–782.

[284] S.M. Cox, K.J. Leveno, Intentional delivery versus expectant management with preterm ruptured membranes at 30–34 weeks' gestation, Obstet. Gynecol. 86 (1995) 875–879.

[285] J.M. Lieman, C.G. Brumfield, W. Carlo, P.S. Ramsey, Preterm premature rupture of membranes: is there an optimal gestational age for delivery? Obstet. Gynecol. 105 (2005) 12–17.

[286] A.M. Vintzileos, W.A. Campbell, D.J. Nochimson, P.J. Weinbaum, The use of the nonstress test in patients with premature rupture of the membranes, Am. J. Obstet. Gynecol. 155 (1986) 149–153.

[287] M.L. Hanley, A.M. Vintzileos, Biophysical testing in premature rupture of the membranes, Semin. Perinatol. 20 (1996) 418–425.

[288] I.A. Grable, Cost-effectiveness of induction after preterm premature rupture of the membranes, Am. J. Obstet. Gynecol. 187 (2002) 1153–1158.

[289] R.W. Naef 3rd, J.R. Allbert, E.L. Ross, B.M. Weber, R.W. Martin, J.C. Morrison, Premature rupture of membranes at 34 to 37 weeks' gestation: aggressive versus conservative management, Am. J. Obstet. Gynecol. 178 (1998) 126–130.

[290] T. Lee, M.W. Carpenter, W.W. Heber, H.M. Silver, Preterm premature rupture of membranes: risks of recurrent complications in the next pregnancy among a population-based sample of gravid women, Am. J. Obstet. Gynecol. 188 (2003) 209–213.

[291] T. Asrat, D.F. Lewis, T.J. Garite, et al., Rate of recurrence of preterm premature rupture of membranes in consecutive pregnancies, Am. J. Obstet. Gynecol. 165 (1991) 1111–1115.

[292] B.M. Mercer, R.L. Goldenberg, A.H. Moawad, et al., The preterm prediction study: effect of gestational age and cause of preterm birth on subsequent obstetric outcome. National Institute of Child Health and Human Development Maternal-Fetal Medicine Units Network, Am. J. Obstet. Gynecol. 181 (1999) 1216–1221.

[293] E.B. da Fonseca, R.E. Bittar, M.H. Carvalho, M. Zugaib, Prophylactic administration of progesterone by vaginal suppository to reduce the incidence of spontaneous preterm birth in women at increased risk: a randomized placebo-controlled double-blind study, Am. J. Obstet. Gynecol. 188 (2003) 419–424.

[294] P.J. Meis, M. Klebanoff, E. Thom, et al., Prevention of recurrent preterm delivery by 17 alpha-hydroxyprogesterone caproate, N. Engl. J. Med. 348 (2003) 2379–2385.

[295] J.R. Petrini, W.M. Callaghan, M. Klebanoff, et al., Estimated effect of 17 alpha-hydroxyprogesterone caproate on preterm birth in the United States, Obstet. Gynecol. 105 (2005) 267–272.

[296] I. Blickstein, Z. Katz, M. Lancet, B.M. Molgilner, The outcome of pregnancies complicated by preterm rupture of the membranes with and without cerclage, Int. J. Gynaecol. Obstet. 28 (1989) 237–242.

[297] J.D. Yeast, T.R. Garite, The role of cervical cerclage in the management of preterm premature rupture of the membranes, Am. J. Obstet. Gynecol. 158 (1988) 106–110.

[298] J. Ludmir, T. Bader, L. Chen, C. Lindenbaum, G. Wong, Poor perinatal outcome associated with retained cerclage in patients with premature rupture of membranes, Obstet. Gynecol. 84 (1994) 823–826.

[299] T.M. Jenkins, V. Berghella, P.A. Shlossman, et al., Timing of cerclage removal after preterm premature rupture of membranes: maternal and neonatal outcomes, Am. J. Obstet. Gynecol. 183 (2000) 847–852.

[300] T.F. McElrath, E.R. Norwitz, E.S. Lieberman, L.J. Heffner, Perinatal outcome after preterm premature rupture of membranes with in situ cervical cerclage, Am. J. Obstet. Gynecol. 187 (2002) 1147–1152.

[301] C.A. Major, C.V. Towers, D.F. Lewis, T.J. Garite, Expectant management of preterm premature rupture of membranes complicated by active recurrent genital herpes, Am. J. Obstet. Gynecol. 188 (2003) 1551–1554; discussion 4–5.

[302] L.L. Scott, P.J. Sanchez, G.L. Jackson, F. Zeray, G.D. Wendel Jr., Acyclovir suppression to prevent cesarean delivery after first-episode genital herpes, Obstet. Gynecol. 87 (1996) 69–73.

[303] D.H. Watts, Management of human immunodeficiency virus infection in pregnancy, N. Engl. J. Med. 346 (2002) 1879–1891.

[304] J.S. Gerdes, Clinicopathologic approach to the diagnosis of neonatal sepsis, Clin. Perinatol. 18 (1991) 361–381.

[305] P. Duff, R.W. Huff, R.S. Gibbs, Management of premature rupture of membranes and unfavorable cervix in term pregnancy, Obstet. Gynecol. 63 (1984) 697–702.

[306] D.I. Conway, W.J. Prendiville, A. Morris, D.C. Speller, G.M. Stirrat, Management of spontaneous rupture of the membranes in the absence of labor in primigravid women at term, Am. J. Obstet. Gynecol. 150 (1984) 947–951.

[307] M.V. Wagner, V.P. Chin, C.J. Peters, B. Drexler, L.A. Newman, A comparison of early and delayed induction of labor with spontaneous rupture of membranes at term, Obstet. Gynecol. 74 (1989) 93–97.

[308] S.F. Meikle, M.E. Bissell, W.L. Freedman, R.S. Gibbs, A retrospective review of the efficacy and safety of prostaglandin E2 with premature rupture of the membranes at term, Obstet. Gynecol. 80 (1992) 76–79.

[309] T.A. Mahmood, M.J. Dick, N.C. Smith, A.A. Templeton, Role of prostaglandin in the management of prelabour rupture of the membranes at term, Br. J. Obstet. Gynaecol. 99 (1992) 112–117.

[310] D.A. Ray, T.J. Garite, Prostaglandin E2 for induction of labor in patients with premature rupture of membranes at term, Am. J. Obstet. Gynecol. 166 (1992) 836–843.

[311] P.G. Seaward, M.E. Hannah, T.L. Myhr, et al., International multicenter term PROM study: evaluation of predictors of neonatal infection in infants born to patients with premature rupture of membranes at term. Premature Rupture of the Membranes, Am. J. Obstet. Gynecol. 179 (1998) 635–639.

[312] A. Herbst, K. Kallen, Time between membrane rupture and delivery and septicemia in term neonates, Obstet. Gynecol. 110 (2007) 612–618.

CHAPTER

4

DEVELOPMENTAL IMMUNOLOGY AND ROLE OF HOST DEFENSES IN FETAL AND NEONATAL SUSCEPTIBILITY TO INFECTION

David B. Lewis ⊛ Christopher B. Wilson

CHAPTER OUTLINE

Epithelial Barriers 83
  Antimicrobial Peptides 83
  Skin 83
  Gastrointestinal Tract 83
  Respiratory Tract 84
  Summary 85
Complement and Other Humoral Mediators of Innate Immunity 85
  Collectins and Pentraxins 85
  Complement 86
  Summary 87
Phagocytes 88
  Hematopoiesis 88
  Phagocyte Production by the Bone Marrow 88
Neutrophils 89
  Production 89
  Migration to Sites of Infection or Injury 90
  Migration of Neonatal Neutrophils 91
  Phagocytosis 92
  Killing 92
  Neutrophil Clearance and Resolution of Neutrophilic
    Inflammation 93
  Effects of Immunomodulators 93
  Summary 93
Eosinophils 93
Mononuclear Phagocytes 93
  Production and Differentiation of Monocytes and Resident Tissue
    Macrophages 93
  Migration to Sites of Infection and Delayed Hypersensitivity
    Responses 94
  Antimicrobial Properties of Monocytes and Macrophages 94
  Antimicrobial Activity and Activation of Neonatal Monocytes and
    Macrophages 95
  Mononuclear Phagocytes Produce Cytokines and Other Mediators
    That Regulate Inflammation and Immunity 95
  Cytokine Production Induced by Engagement of Toll-like
    Receptors and Other Innate Immune Pattern Recognition
    Receptors 96
  Cytokine Production, Toll-like Receptors, and Regulation of Innate
    Immunity and Inflammation by Neonatal Monocytes and
    Macrophages 98
  Summary 100
Dendritic Cells—the Link between Innate and Adaptive
  Immunity 101
  Properties and Functions of Conventional Dendritic Cells 101
  Fetal Conventional Dendritic Cells 102
  Properties and Functions of Adult and Neonatal Plasmacytoid
    Dendritic Cells 103
  Summary 103

Natural Killer Cells 103
  Overview and Development 103
  Natural Killer Cell Receptors 104
  Natural Killer Cell Cytotoxicity 105
  Natural Killer Cell Cytokine Responsiveness and Dependence 105
  Natural Killer Cell Cytokine and Chemokine Production 106
  Natural Killer Cells of the Maternal Decidua and Their Regulation
    by Human Leukocyte Antigen G 106
  Natural Killer Cell Numbers and Surface Phenotype in the Fetus and
    Neonate 106
  Fetal and Neonatal Natural Killer Cell–Mediated Cytotoxicity and
    Cytokine Production 107
  Summary 107
T Cells and Antigen Presentation 107
  Overview 107
  Antigen Presentation by Classic Major Histocompatibility
    Complex Molecules 108
  Nonclassic Antigen Presentation Molecules 110
  Prothymocytes and Early Thymocyte Differentiation 111
  Intrathymic Generation of T-Cell Receptor Diversity 113
  T-Cell Receptor Excision Circles 115
  Thymocyte Selection and Late Maturation 116
  Naïve T Cells 117
  Ontogeny of Naïve T-Cell Surface Phenotype 118
  Homeostatic Proliferation 120
  Naïve T-Cell Activation, Anergy, and Costimulation 121
  Differentiation of Activated Naïve T Cells into Effector
    and Memory Cells 124
  Production of Cytokines, Chemokines, and Tumor Necrosis
    Factor–Ligand Proteins by Neonatal T Cells 127
  T–Cell Mediated Cytotoxicity 131
  Effector T-Cell Migration 132
  Termination of T-Cell Effector Response 132
  Unique Phenotype and Function of Fetal T-Cell Compartment 133
  Regulatory T Cells 134
  Natural Killer T Cells 135
  γδ T Cells 136
  Antigen-Specific T-Cell Function in the Fetus and Neonate 138
  T-Cell Response to Congenital Infection 139
  T-Cell Response to Postnatal Infections and Vaccination
    in Early Infancy 140
  Summary 141
B Cells and Immunoglobulin 141
  Overview 141
  Early B-Cell Development and Immunoglobulin Repertoire
    Formation 142
  B-Cell Maturation, Preimmune Selection, and Activation 144
  B-Cell Activation and Immune Selection 145

Memory B Cells   147
B Cells as Antigen-Presenting Cells   147
Switching of Immunoglobulin Isotype and Class and Antibody
   Production   148
Marginal Zone and IgM⁺IgD⁺CD27⁺ B Cells   150
B-1 Cells and Natural IgM   151
T Cell–Dependent and T Cell–Independent Responses
   by B Cells   151
Specific Antibody Response by the Fetus to Maternal Immunization
   and Congenital Infection   153

Postnatal Specific Antibody Responses   154
Maternally Derived IgG Antibody   156
Immunoglobulin Synthesis by the Fetus and Neonate   157
Summary   158
Host Defense against Specific Classes of Neonatal
Pathogens   159
   Extracellular Microbial Pathogens: Group B Streptococci   159
   Viruses: Herpes Simplex Virus   162
   Nonviral Intracellular Pathogens: *Toxoplasma gondii*   169

The human fetus and neonate are unduly susceptible to infection with a wide variety of microbes, many of which are not pathogenic in more mature individuals. This susceptibility results from limitations of innate and adaptive (antigen-specific) immunity and their interactions. This chapter focuses on the ontogeny of the immune system in the fetus, neonate, and young infant and the relationship between limitations in immune function and susceptibility to specific types of infection.

The immune system includes innate protective mechanisms against pathogens provided by the skin, respiratory and gastrointestinal epithelia, and other mucosa; humoral factors such as cytokines (Tables 4–1 and 4–2) and complement components (Fig. 4–1); and innate and adaptive immune mechanisms mediated by hematopoietic cells, including mononuclear phagocytes, granulocytes, dendritic cells (DCs), and lymphocytes. Certain nonhematopoietic cells, such as follicular DCs and thymic epithelial cells, also play important roles in adaptive immunity.

Innate immunity, in contrast to adaptive immunity to be discussed later, does not require prior exposure to be immediately effective and is equally efficient on primary and subsequent encounter with a microbe, but does not provide long-lasting protection against reinfection. Innate defenses consist of fixed epithelial barriers and resident tissue macrophages, which act immediately or within the first minutes to hours of encounter with a microbe. These "frontline" defenses are sufficient for protection from most microbes in the environment, which do not produce disease in healthy individuals. If the microbial insult is too great, or the organism is able to evade these initial

TABLE 4–1 Major Human Cytokines and Tumor Necrosis Factor (TNF) Family Ligands: Structure, Cognate Receptors, and Receptor-Mediated Signal Transduction Pathways

Cytokine Family	Members	Structure	Cognate Receptor Family	Proximal Signal Transduction Pathways
IL-1	IL-1α, IL-1β, IL-18 (IL-1γ), IL-1 receptor antagonist	β-trefoil, monomers; processed and secreted	IL-1 receptor	IRAK, JNK
Hematopoietin	IL-2 through IL-7, IL-9 through IL-13, IL-15, IL-17, IL-19, IL-29, CSFs, oncostatin-M, IFNs (α, β, γ, and others); class II subfamily consists of IL-10, IL-19, IL-20, IL-22, IL-24, IL-26, IFNs	Four α-helical; monomers except for IL-5 and IFNs (homodimers) and IL-12, IL-23, and IL-27 (heterodimers); secreted	Hematopoietin receptors	JAK tyrosine kinases/STAT, Src and Syk tyrosine kinases
TNF ligand	TNF-α, lymphotoxin-α, lymphotoxin-β, CD27L, CD30L, CD40L, OX40L, TRAIL, others	β-jellyroll, homotrimers; type II membrane proteins and secreted	TNF receptor family	TRAFs and proteins mediating apoptosis
TGF-β	TGF-β1, TGF-β2, TGF-β3, bone morphogenetic proteins	Cysteine knot; processed and secreted	TGF-β receptors type 1 and type 2 heterodimers (intrinsic serine threonine kinases)	Smad proteins
Chemokines		Three-stranded β-sheet; all but fractalkine are secreted	Seven membrane-spanning domains	G protein–mediated
CXC ligand subfamily	CXCL1-14, CXCL16		CXCR1 through CXCR6	
CC ligand subfamily	CCL1-5, CCL7, CCL8, CCL11, CCL13 through CCL28		CCR1 through CCR10	
C ligand subfamily	XCL1 (lymphotactin), XCL2 (SCM-1β)		XCR1	
CX3C ligand subfamily	CX3CL (fractalkine)		CX3CR1	

CSF, colony-stimulating factors; IFN, interferon; IL, interleukin; IRAK, IL-1 receptor–associated serine/threonine kinase; JNK, c-Jun N-terminal kinase; STAT, signal transducer and activator of transcription; TGF, transforming growth factor; TRAFs, TNF-α receptor–associated factors; TRAIL, TNF-related apoptosis–inducing ligand.

TABLE 4–2   Immunoregulatory Effects of Select Cytokines, Chemokines, and Tumor Necrosis Factor (TNF) Ligand Family Proteins

Cytokine	Principal Cell Source	Major Biologic Effects
IL-1α, IL-1β	Many cell types; Mϕ are a major source	Fever, inflammatory response, cofactor in T- and B-cell growth
IL-2	T cells	T-cell > B-cell growth, increased cytotoxicity by T and NK cells, increased cytokine production and sensitivity to apoptosis by T cells, growth and survival of regulatory T cells
IL-3	T cells	Growth of early hematopoietic precursors (also known as multi-CSF)
IL-4	T cells, mast cells, basophils, eosinophils	Required for IgE synthesis; enhances B-cell growth and MHC class II expression; promotes T-cell growth and T_H2 differentiation, mast cell growth factor; enhances endothelial VCAM-1 expression
IL-5	T cells, NK cells, mast cells, basophils, eosinophils	Eosinophil growth, differentiation, and survival
IL-6	Mϕ, fibroblasts, T cells	Hepatic acute-phase protein synthesis, fever, T- and B-cell growth and differentiation
IL-7	Stromal cells of bone marrow and thymus	Essential thymocyte growth factor
IL-8 (CXCL8)	Mϕ, endothelial cells, fibroblasts, epithelial cells, T cells	Chemotaxis and activation of neutrophils
IL-9	T cells, mast cells	T-cell and mast cell growth factor
IL-10	Mϕ, T, cells, B cells, NK cells, keratinocytes, eosinophils	Inhibits cytokine production by T cells and mononuclear cell inflammatory function; promotes B-cell growth and isotype switching, NK-cell cytotoxicity
IL-11	Marrow stromal cells, fibroblasts	Hematopoietic precursor growth, acute-phase reactants by hepatocytes
TNF-α	Mϕ, T cells, and NK cells	Fever and inflammatory response effects similar to IL-1, shock, hemorrhagic necrosis of tumors, and increased VCAM-1 expression on endothelium; induces catabolic state
CD40 ligand (CD154)	T cells, lower amounts by B cells and DCs	B-cell growth factor; promotes isotype switching, promotes IL-12 production by dendritic cells, activates Mϕ
Fas ligand	Activated T cells, NK cells retina, testicular epithelium	Induces apoptosis of cells expressing Fas, including effector B and T cells
Flt-3 ligand	Bone marrow stromal cells	Potent DC growth factor; promotes growth of myeloid and lymphoid progenitor cells in conjunction with other cytokines
G-CSF	Mϕ, fibroblasts, epithelial cells	Growth of granulocyte precursors
GM-CSF	Mϕ, endothelial cells, T cells	Growth of granulocyte-Mϕ precursors and dendritic cells, enhances granulocyte-Mϕ function and B-cell antibody production
CCL3 (MIP-1α)	Mϕ, T cells	Mϕ chemoattractant; T-cell activator
CCL5 (RANTES)	Mϕ, T cells, fibroblasts, epithelial cells	Mϕ and memory T-cell chemoattractant; enhances T-cell activation; blocks HIV coreceptor
TGF-β	Mϕ, T cells, fibroblasts, epithelial cells, others	Inhibits Mϕ activation; inhibits T_H1 T-cell responses

CSF, colony-stimulating factor; DC, dendritic cell; G-CSF, granulocyte colony-stimulating factor; GM-CSF, granulocyte-macrophage colony-stimulating factor; HIV, human immunodeficiency virus; IL, interleukin; Mϕ, mononuclear phagocytes; MHC, major histocompatibility complex; NK, natural killer; TGF, transforming growth factor; VCAM-1, vascular cell adhesion molecule-1.

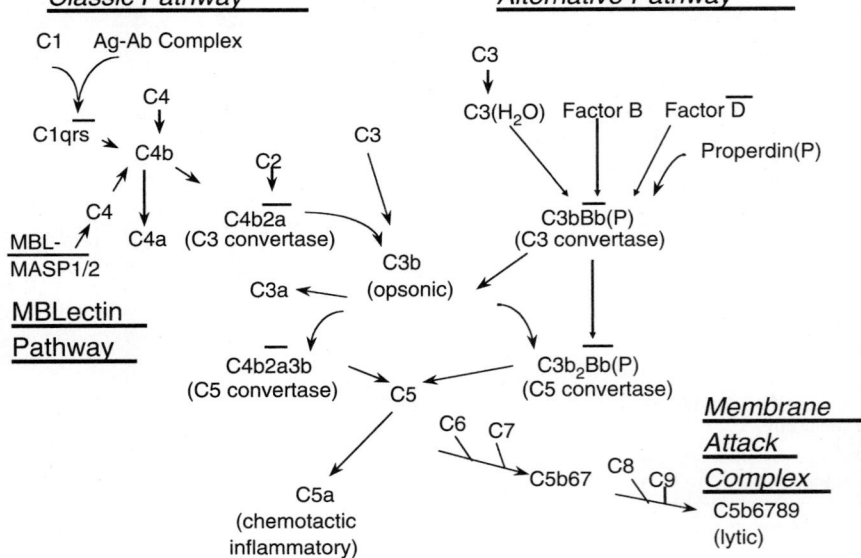

FIGURE 4–1 Complement activation. Classic and mannan-binding lectin (MBL) pathways of activation intersect with the alternative pathway at C3. MBL pathway of activation is identical to the classic pathway starting with the cleavage of C4. When C3 is activated, this is followed by activation of the terminal components, which generate the membrane attack complex (C5b6789). Enzymatically active proteases, which serve to cleave and activate subsequent components, are shown with an *overbar*.

defenses, these cells release mediators that incite an inflammatory response, through which soluble and cellular defenses are recruited and help to limit or eradicate the infection over the next hours to days and to initiate the antigen-specific immune response that follows.

EPITHELIAL BARRIERS

Epithelia form a crucial physical and chemical barrier against infection. Tight junctions between epithelial cells prevent direct entry of microbes into deeper tissues, and physical injury that disrupts epithelial integrity can greatly increase the risk for infection. In addition to providing a physical barrier, mechanical and chemical factors and colonization by commensal microbes contribute to the protective functions of the skin and of the mucosal epithelia of the gastrointestinal and respiratory tract.

ANTIMICROBIAL PEPTIDES

A general feature of epithelial defenses is the production of one or more antimicrobial peptides, which include the α-defensins, β-defensins and the cathelicidin LL-37. Defensins and cathelicidin have direct antimicrobial activity against gram-positive and gram-negative bacteria and some fungi, viruses, and protozoa [1–4]. Some of these antimicrobial peptides also exhibit proinflammatory and immunomodulatory activities.

There are six known human α-defensins: human neutrophil proteins (HNP) 1 through 4 and human defensins (HD) 5 and 6. HNP1 through HNP4 are expressed in leukocytes (white blood cells). HD5 and HD6 are produced and secreted by Paneth cells, located at the base of crypts in the small intestine. HD5 has antimicrobial activity against gram-positive and gram-negative bacteria and *Candida albicans*. There are at least six human β-defensins (hBD), but only four (hBD-1 through hBD-4) have been well characterized. hBD-1 is constitutively expressed by skin keratinocytes, whereas exposure to bacteria or proinflammatory cytokines, including tumor necrosis factor (TNF)-α and interleukin (IL)-1 (see Tables 4–1 and 4–2), induces expression of hBD-2 and hBD-3 in keratinocytes and hBD-4 in lung epithelial cells. hBD-1 and hBD-2 are active against gram-negative bacteria and streptococci, but are less active against *Staphylococcus aureus*, whereas hBD-3 is broadly active against gram-positive and gram-negative bacteria and *Candida* species. The cathelicidin LL-37 is expressed in leukocytes, and its expression is induced by microbes and proinflammatory cytokines in epithelial cells of the skin, gut, and respiratory tract; LL-37 is active against gram-positive and gram-negative bacteria, but less active against *S. aureus* than hBD-3 [5].

SKIN

The barrier function of the skin is mediated primarily by its outermost layer, the stratum corneum, which consists of keratinocytes and the lipid-rich matrix that surrounds them [6]. These lipids, particularly ceramides, inhibit microbial growth, as does the low pH environment they help to create. The lipid content and acidic pH of the skin

are established postnatally reaching maturity by 2 to 4 weeks in term neonates, but at a later age in premature neonates. Epithelial integrity and the antimicrobial barrier this provides are easily disrupted at this age. The skin of neonates is also coated by a water, protein, and lipid-rich material, the vernix caseosa. The skin is rapidly colonized by environmental bacteria after birth, creating a normal flora of commensal bacteria that help to prevent colonization by pathogens. This flora normally consists of coagulase-negative staphylococci, micrococci, and other species [7]. Contemporary genomics-based analyses of the flora of adult skin indicate that these and related gram-positive species represent only approximately 25% of the normal flora, with corynebacteria and other Actinobacteria predominating [8], but such approaches have not been applied to study the ontogeny of neonatal skin colonization.

Antimicrobial peptides are expressed by neonatal keratinocytes and present in the vernix caseosa. As in adults, the stratum corneum of skin from normal term neonates contains hBD-1 [9]. Neonatal skin also contains hBD-2 and LL-37 [9,10], which are absent or present only in very low amounts in the skin of normal adults. The mechanisms underlying the apparent constitutive production of hBD-2 and LL-37 by neonatal keratinocytes are unknown, but their presence may help to provide an immediate barrier against bacterial invasion during the initial exposure of the neonate to environmental microbes. The expression of LL-37 by the stratum corneum does not seem to be further upregulated in neonates with erythema toxicum, but this antimicrobial peptide is expressed by neutrophils, eosinophils, and DCs that are found in the dermis in this condition, which is thought to be triggered by colonizing bacteria. Vernix caseosa may augment skin defenses. Although the presence of LL-37 in vernix caseosa is controversial, being detected by one group, but not by another, both groups showed it to contain HNP1 through HNP3 and additional antibacterial proteins, including lysozyme [11,12].

GASTROINTESTINAL TRACT

The proximal gastrointestinal epithelium of the mouth and esophagus consists of a squamous epithelium, whereas the stomach, small intestine, and colon have a columnar epithelium with microvilli, which, along with intestinal peristalsis, help to maintain the longitudinal movement of fluid. The acidic pH of the stomach acts as a chemical barrier in adults. Gastric acidification is not yet fully developed in neonates, but digestion of milk lipids by gastric lipases may compensate in part by generating free fatty acids [13]. The gastrointestinal tract is coated with a mucin-rich glycocalyx, which forms a viscous coating that helps to protect the epithelium and to which commensal intestinal bacteria bind [14]. The composition of the intestinal glycocalyx in neonates differs from adults and may contribute to differences in commensal flora.

The application of high-throughput, comprehensive, culture-independent molecular approaches to assess microbial diversity has shown that the commensal intestinal flora of humans is a highly diverse ecologic system consisting of approximately 10^{14} microorganisms, representing the most abundant and diverse microbial community in the human body and exceeding the numbers and genetic content of human cells in an individual [8]. In adults, colonic and stool flora are dominated by gram-negative anaerobic bacteria (*Bacteroides*) and two phyla of gram-positive bacteria (Actinobacteria, Firmicutes), and aerobic gram-negative bacteria (e.g., *Escherichia coli*) are present in much lower abundance. The composition of stool flora in the first year of life is highly dynamic. Based on a longitudinal study of 14 term infants from whom serial samples were collected from birth to 1 year of age, the flora of individual infants differs substantially from one infant to another in the first months of life, initially most closely resembling the maternal fecal, vaginal, or breast milk flora [15]. This interindividual variability typically diminishes over time and by 1 year of age converges on a pattern similar to that found in adults. By contrast to older findings, which were based on culture-based methods, the flora of breast-fed infants was not dominated by bifidobacteria, which were rare in the first months after birth and thereafter represent only a small fraction of the total flora.

Although these findings are limited to a few healthy infants, they suggest that earlier views regarding normal stool and colonic flora and perhaps flora in other portions of the intestinal tract require revision. Future studies applying such approaches to compare systematically the flora of breast-fed infants versus formula-fed infants, infants delivered by different routes, infants born prematurely, and infants residing in the hospital versus the home should help us to understand better how such factors affect the intestinal flora and, perhaps, risk for necrotizing enterocolitis and other inflammatory, infectious, or allergic diseases in neonates and infants.

The dynamic interaction between host and microbe in the gut has an important impact on nutrition, intestinal homeostasis, and development of innate and adaptive immunity [14]. Such immunity restricts these microbes to the gut and primes the immune system to respond properly to dangerous microbes, while dampening the response to the normal flora, harmless environmental antigens, and self-antigens to prevent self-injury. Certain intestinal epithelial cells play special roles in intestinal immunity: Goblet cells produce mucus, Paneth cells (located at the base of small intestinal crypts) secrete antimicrobial factors, and M cells deliver by transcytosis a sample of the distal small intestinal microbiota to antigen-presenting DCs located beneath the epithelium; some DCs (the nature and function of which are discussed later) also directly sample the intestinal lumen of the distal small intestine.

The intestinal epithelium can directly recognize and respond to microbes using a limited set of invariant cell surface, endosomal, and cytosolic innate immune pattern recognition receptors, including toll-like receptors (TLRs) and others described later (see "Cytokine Production Induced by Engagement of Toll-like Receptors and Other Innate Immune Pattern Recognition Receptors"). How commensals prime innate and adaptive immunity in the gut without inducing deleterious inflammation, and how potentially dangerous pathogens are discriminated from harmless commensals are areas of active investigation. This discrimination is made in part by the location of commensals versus pathogens. Intestinal epithelial cells normally express little or no TLRs on their luminal surface—where they are in contact with commensals. Conversely, pathogens that invade through or between epithelial cells can be recognized by endosomal TLRs, cytosolic innate immune recognition receptors, and TLRs located on the basolateral surface of epithelial cells. Certain commensal bacteria inhibit signaling and inflammatory mediator production downstream of these receptors [14,16] or induce anti-inflammatory cytokine production [17], actively suppressing gut inflammation.

Adaptation of the intestinal epithelium to avoid unwarranted inflammatory responses to the normal flora is developmentally regulated or environmentally regulated, or both. Human 20- to 24-week fetal small intestinal organ cultures produced much more of the proinflammatory cytokine IL-8 (see Tables 4–1 and 4–2) when exposed to bacterial lipopolysaccharide (LPS) or IL-1 than similar cultures from infants or adults [18]. Studies in neonatal mice suggest that a general dampening of inflammatory signaling in intestinal epithelium occurs in response to postnatal colonization with commensal bacteria [19], but developmental differences may also be a factor. If so, and if this is also true in humans, such differences may contribute to aberrant intestinal inflammation in preterm neonates with necrotizing enterocolitis [20].

Intestinal epithelial cells produce and secrete defensins and other antimicrobial factors. Epithelial cells of the esophagus, stomach, and colon constitutively produce hBD-1 and the cathelicidin LL-37 and produce hBD-2, hBD-3, and hBD-4 in response to infection and inflammatory stimuli [21]. Intrinsic host defense of the small intestine is provided by Paneth cells, which constitutively produce HD5 and lysozyme [3]. The abundance of HD5 in the neonatal small intestine correlates with the abundance of Paneth cells—present but much less abundant in the fetus at mid-gestation than at term, which is much less abundant than in adults. These data suggest that intrinsic small intestinal defenses may be compromised in human neonates, particularly when preterm. A study in mice suggests another possibility, however. The intestinal epithelium of neonatal mice expresses abundant amounts of cathelicidin, which is lost by 14 days of postnatal age, by which time Paneth cells expressing murine defensins reach adult numbers [22]. It is unknown whether a similar "switch" in intestinal antimicrobial defenses occurs in humans.

RESPIRATORY TRACT

The respiratory tract is second only to the gut in epithelial surface area. The upper airways and larger airways of the lung are lined by pseudostratified ciliated epithelial cells, with smaller numbers of mucin-producing goblet cells, whereas the alveoli are lined by nonciliated type I pneumocytes and by smaller numbers of surfactant-producing type II pneumocytes. Airway surface liquid and mucociliary clearance mechanisms provide an important first line of defense. Airway surface liquid contains numerous antimicrobial factors, including lysozyme, secretory leukoprotease inhibitor, defensins and cathelicidin

LL-37, and surfactant apoproteins A and D (SP-A, SP-D) [23]. Collectively, these factors likely account for the lack of microbes in the lower respiratory tract of normal individuals.

Lung parenchymal cells express a diverse set of TLRs and other innate immune receptors. Lower airway epithelial cells express and respond to ligands for TLR2, TLR4, and TLR5 [23–25]. The subcellular localization of these TLRs; the expression and localization of other TLRs; and the relative contribution of TLR-mediated microbial recognition by airway epithelial cells, other lung parenchymal cells, and lung macrophages are incompletely understood and areas of active investigation. Although, to our knowledge, there are no data carefully comparing TLR expression and function in the airways of the human fetus and neonate versus human adults, data from neonatal sheep (and rodents) indicate development differences. TLR2 and TLR4 are expressed in the lungs of fetal sheep in the latter part of gestation—messenger RNA (mRNA) abundance increases from 20% of adult values at the beginning of the third trimester to 50% at term [26]. TLR4 mRNA was present in the airway epithelium and parenchyma, whereas TLR2 expression was found primarily in inflammatory cells after intra-amniotic administration of LPS, which resulted in increased expression of TLR2 and TLR4. TLR3 expression was approximately 50% of adult values and unchanged in response to LPS. Similar developmental differences have been observed in mice [27].

Airway epithelial cells express hBD-1 constitutively and hBD-2, hBD-3, and LL-37 in response to microbial stimuli and inflammatory cytokines, including IL-1 [23]. Lung explants from term, but not preterm, fetuses expressed hBD-2 and smaller amounts of hBD-1, although the amounts even at term seemed to be less than at older ages, but did not contain hBD-3 mRNA [28]. By contrast, LL-37 mRNA was present and seemed not to vary at these ages. Consistent with these findings, tracheal aspirates from mechanically ventilated term, but not preterm, neonates contained hBD-2, whereas lower amounts of LL-37 were found in similar amounts in aspirates from preterm neonates. Another study found no difference in the abundance of hBD-1, hBD-2, and LL-37 in aspirates from ventilated neonates ranging in age from 22 to 40 weeks.

SP-A and SP-D are produced by type II pneumocytes and by Clara cells, which are progenitors of ciliated epithelial cells located at the bronchoalveolar junction. SP-A and SP-D are members of the collectin family. Collectins bind to carbohydrates, including mannose, glucose, and fucose, found on the surface of gram-positive and gram-negative bacteria, yeasts, and some viruses, including respiratory syncytial virus (RSV) [23,29]. When bound, collectins can result in aggregation of microbes, which may inhibit their growth or facilitate their mechanical removal, or can opsonize microbes (i.e., facilitate their ingestion by phagocytic cells). Mice lacking SP-A have impaired lung clearance of group B streptococci (GBS), *Haemophilus influenzae*, *Pseudomonas aeruginosa*, and RSV [30,31]. Mice lacking SP-D also exhibit impaired clearance of RSV [31] and *P. aeruginosa* [30], and although they clear GBS normally, lung inflammation in response to this infection is more intense (reviewed by Grubor and colleagues [23] and Haagsman and colleagues [29]). SP-A and SP-D are detectable in human fetal lungs by 20 weeks of gestation [32], and amounts apparently increase with increasing fetal maturity and in response to antenatal steroid administration [33,34].

SUMMARY

The skin of neonates, particularly preterm neonates, is more readily disrupted and lacks the protection provided by an acidic pH until approximately 1 month of postnatal age. Counterbalancing these factors is the constitutive production in neonates of a broader array of antimicrobial peptides by the skin epithelium and the presence of such peptides in the vernix caseosa. The lack of an acidic pH in the stomach may facilitate the establishment of the protective commensal flora, which at birth varies substantially from infant to infant, converging by 1 year of age to resemble adult flora. The lack of gastric acidity and diminished numbers of antimicrobial peptide–producing Paneth cells in the small intestine of preterm and, to a lesser degree, term neonates may increase their risk for enterocolitis and invasion by pathogens; these deficits may be counterbalanced by more robust production of antimicrobial peptides by other intestinal epithelial cells, but as yet this has been shown only in animal models. Innate defenses of the respiratory epithelium—TLRs, antimicrobial peptides, and SP-A and SP-D—are maturing in the last trimester. Consequently, these defenses may be compromised in preterm infants. Reduced numbers of resident alveolar macrophages may impair lung innate defenses further in preterm infants (see "Mononuclear Phagocytes").

COMPLEMENT AND OTHER HUMORAL MEDIATORS OF INNATE IMMUNITY
COLLECTINS AND PENTRAXINS

C-reactive protein (CRP) and mannose-binding lectin (MBL) are soluble proteins that can bind to structures found on the surface of microbes and infected or damaged host cells and facilitate their clearance by phagocytes. Both are produced by the liver. Their concentrations in the blood increase in response to infection and tissue injury as part of the acute-phase response, allowing them to contribute to early host defense to infection and the clearance of damaged cells.

CRP is a member of the pentraxin family of proteins [35], which binds to phosphocholine and other lipids and carbohydrates on the surface of certain gram-positive bacteria, particularly *Streptococcus pneumoniae*, fungi, and apoptotic host cells. It does not cross the placenta. Term and preterm neonates can produce CRP as well as adults [36]. Values of CRP in cord blood from term infants are low, increasing to concentrations found in adult blood in the first days of life, paralleling a postnatal increase in serum IL-6 and microbial colonization [37].

MBL (similar to SP-A and SP-D described earlier) is a member of the collectin family and binds to carbohydrates, including mannose, glucose, and fucose, on the surface of bacteria, yeasts, and some viruses [38]. When bound, MBL activates complement and enhances phagocytosis by neutrophils and macrophages. Engagement of MBL is impeded by capsular polysaccharides of most virulent bacterial pathogens. The gene encoding MBL is highly polymorphic, and as a result concentrations of MBL in healthy adults vary widely (undetectable to approximately 10 μg/mL), with approximately 40% of Europeans having low MBL and approximately 5% having little or no MBL in the blood [39,40]. MBL-deficient individuals beyond the neonatal period who are otherwise immunocompetent have a slightly higher rate of respiratory tract infections between 6 and 17 months of age, but are not otherwise predisposed to infection.

MBL abundance in neonates is affected by three interacting variables: MBL genotype, gestational age, and postnatal age. In neonates with wild-type MBL genotype, MBL concentrations are 50% to 75% of those in adults and reach adult values by 7 to 10 days of age in term neonates and 20 weeks of age in preterm neonates [41,42]. Concentrations are more than fivefold lower and these increases are less evident in neonates with variant MBL genotypes. Preterm neonates with low concentrations of MBL found in those with variant genotypes seem to be at greater risk for sepsis or pneumonia [40,42,43]. Although the rigor of the criteria by which sepsis was defined and the seriousness of the causative agent varied in these studies, it seems that neonates with values less than 0.4 μg/mL are at greater risk compared with neonates of similar gestational age or birth weight [43].

COMPLEMENT

The complement system is composed of serum proteins that can be activated sequentially through one of three pathways—the classic, MBL, and alternative pathways—each of which leads to the generation of activated C3, C3 and C5 convertases, and the membrane attack complex (see Fig. 4–1) [44].

Classic and Mannan-Binding Lectin Pathways

Activation of the classic pathway is initiated when antibodies capable of engaging C1q to their Fc portion (IgM, IgG1, IgG2, and IgG3 in humans) form a complex with microbial (or other) antigens. The formation of complexes alters the conformation of IgM and juxtaposes two IgG molecules, which creates an appropriate binding site for C1q. This is followed by the sequential binding of C1r and C1s to C1q. C1s can cleave C4 followed by C2, and the larger fragments of these bind covalently to the surface of the microbe or particle, forming the classic pathway C3 convertase (C2aC4b). C3 convertase cleaves C3, liberating C3b, which binds to the microbe or particle, and C3a, which is released into the fluid phase.

This pathway can also be activated before the development of antibody by CRP. When CRP binds to the surface of a microbe, its conformation is altered such that it can bind C1q and activate the classic pathway [45]. Similarly, when MBL engages the surface of a microbe, its confirmation is altered, creating a binding site for MASP1

and MASP2, which are the functional equivalents of C1r and C1s. MASP2 cleaves C4 and C2 leading to the formation of the C3 convertase.

Alternative Pathway

The alternative pathway is activated constitutively by the continuous low-level hydrolysis of C3 in solution, creating a binding site for factor B. This complex is cleaved by factor D, generating C3b and Bb. If C3b and Bb bind to a microorganism, they form a more efficient system, which binds and activates additional C3 molecules, depositing C3b on the microbe and liberating C3a into the fluid phase. This interaction is facilitated by factor P (properdin) and inhibited by alternative pathway factors H and I. The classic pathway, by creating particle-bound C3b, also can activate the alternative pathway, amplifying complement activation. This amplification step may be particularly important in the presence of small amounts of antibody. Bacteria vary in their capacity to activate the alternative pathway, which is determined by their ability to bind C3b and to protect the complex of C3b and Bb from the inhibitory effects of factors H and I. Sialic acid, a component of many bacterial polysaccharide capsules, including those of GBS and *E. coli* K1, favors factor H binding. Many bacterial pathogens are protected from the alternative pathway by their capsules. Antibody is needed for efficient opsonization of such organisms.

Terminal Components, Membrane Attack Complex, and Biologic Consequences of Complement Activation

Binding of C3b on the microbial surface facilitates microbial killing or removal, through the interaction of C3b with CR1 receptors on phagocytes. C3b also is cleaved to C3bi, which binds to the CR3 receptor (Mac-1, Cd11b-CD18) and CR4 receptor (CD11c-CD18). C3bi receptors are β_2 integrins, which are present on neutrophils, macrophages, and certain other cell types and play a role in leukocyte adhesion. Along with IgG antibody, which binds to Fcγ receptors on phagocytes, C3b and C3bi promote phagocytosis and killing of bacteria and fungi.

Bound C3b and C4b and C2a or bound C3b and Bb form C5 convertases, which cleave C5. The smaller fragment, C5a, is released into solution. The larger fragment, C5b, triggers the recruitment of the terminal components, C6 to C9, which together form the membrane attack complex. This complex is assembled in lipid-containing cell membranes, which include the outer membrane of gram-negative bacteria and the plasma membrane of infected host cells. When assembled in the membrane, this complex can lyse the cell. This lysis seems to be a central defense mechanism against meningococci and systemic gonococcal infection. Certain gram-negative organisms have mechanisms to impede complement-mediated lysis, and gram-positive bacteria are intrinsically resistant to complement-mediated lysis because they do not have an outer membrane. As a result, in contrast to the important role of complement-mediated opsonization, complement-mediated lysis may play a limited role in defense against common neonatal bacterial pathogens.

The soluble fragments of C5, C5a, and, to a more limited degree, C3a and C4a cause vasodilation and increase vascular permeability. C5a also is a potent chemotactic factor for phagocytes. In addition to these roles for complement in innate immunity, complement facilitates B-cell responses to T cell–dependent antigens, as discussed in the section on B cells and immunoglobulin.

Complement in the Fetus and Neonate

Complement components are synthesized by hepatocytes and, for some components, by macrophages. Little, if any, maternal complement is transferred to the fetus. Fetal synthesis of complement components can be detected in tissues at 6 to 14 weeks of gestation, depending on the specific complement component and tissue examined [46].

Table 4–3 summarizes published reports on classic pathway complement activity (CH_{50}) and alternative pathway complement activity (AP_{50}) and individual complement components in neonates. Substantial interindividual variability is seen, and in many term neonates, values of individual complement components or of CH_{50} or AP_{50} are within the adult range. Alternative pathway activity and components are more consistently decreased than classic pathway activity and components. The most marked deficiency is in the terminal complement component C9, which

correlates with poor killing of gram-negative bacteria by serum from neonates. The C9 deficiency in neonatal serum seems to be a more important factor in the inefficient killing of E. coli K1 than the deficiency in antigen-specific IgG antibodies [47]. Preterm infants show a greater and more consistent decrease in classic and alternative pathway complement activity and components [48]. Mature infants who are small for gestational age have values similar to those for healthy term infants [49]. The concentration of most complement proteins increases postnatally and reaches adult values by 6 to 18 months of age [50].

Opsonization is the process whereby soluble factors present in serum or other body fluids bind to the surface of microbes (or other particles) and enhance their phagocytosis and killing. Some organisms are effective activators of the alternative pathway, whereas others require antibody to activate complement. Depending on the organism, opsonic activity reflects antibody, MBL, CRP, classic or alternative complement pathway activity, or combinations of these, and the efficiency with which neonatal sera opsonize organisms is quite variable. Although opsonization of S. aureus was normal in neonatal sera in all studies [51–53], opsonization of GBS [52,54], S. pneumoniae [53], E. coli [52,55], and other gram-negative rods [52,55] was decreased against some strains and in some studies, but not in others.

Neonatal sera generally are less able to opsonize organisms in the absence of antibody. This difference is compatible with deficits in the function of the alternative and MBL pathways [56–58] and with the moderate reduction in alternative pathway components. This difference is not due to a reduced ability of neonatal sera to initiate complement activation through the alternative pathway [59]. Neonatal sera also are less able to opsonize some strains of GBS in a classic pathway–dependent but antibody-independent manner [54,60]. The deficit in antibody-independent opsonization is accentuated in sera from premature neonates and may be impaired further by the depletion of complement components in septic neonates.

Sera from term neonates generate less chemotactic activity than adult sera. This diminished activity reflects a defect in complement activation, rather than lack of antibody [61–63]. These observations notwithstanding, preterm and term neonates do generate substantial amounts of activated complement products in response to infection in vivo [64].

TABLE 4–3 Summary of Published Complement Levels in Neonates

Complement Component	Mean % of Adult Levels	
	Term Neonate	Preterm Neonate
CH_{50}	56-90 (5)*	45-71 (4)
AP_{50}	49-65 (4)	40-55 (3)
CIq	61-90 (4)	27-58 (3)
C4	60-100 (5)	42-91 (4)
C2	76-100 (3)	67-96 (2)
C3	60-100 (5)	39-78 (4)
C5	73-75 (2)	67 (1)
C6	47-56 (2)	36 (1)
C7	67-92 (2)	72 (1)
C8	20-36 (2)	29 (1)
C9	<20-52 (3)	<20-41 (2)
B	35-64 (4)	36-50 (4)
P	33-71 (6)	16-65 (3)
H	61 (1)	—
C3bi	55 (1)	—

*Number of studies.

References

Johnston RB, Stroud RM. Complement and host defense against infection. J Pediatr 90:169-179, 1977.

Notarangelo LD, et al. Activity of classical and alternative pathways of complement in preterm and small for gestational age infants. Pediatr Res 18:281-285, 1984.

Davis CA, Vallota EH, Forristal J. Serum complement levels in infancy: age related changes. Pediatr Res 13:1043-1046, 1979.

Lassiter HA, et al. Complement factor 9 deficiency in serum of human neonates. J Infect Dis 166:53-57, 1992.

Wolach B, et al. The development of the complement system after 28 weeks' gestation. Acta Paediatr 86:523-527, 1997.

Zilow G, et al. Quantitation of complement component C9 deficiency in term and preterm neonates. Clin Exp Immunol 97:52-59, 1994.

SUMMARY

Compared with adults, neonates have moderately diminished alternative complement pathway activity, slightly diminished classic complement pathway activity, and decreased abundance of some terminal complement components. Neonates with much reduced concentrations of MBL resulting from genetic variation and prematurity seem to be at greater risk for sepsis or pneumonia. Consistent with these findings, neonatal sera are less effective than adult sera in opsonization when concentrations of specific antibody are limiting and in the generation of complement-derived chemotactic activity; these differences are greater in preterm than in term neonates. These deficiencies, in concert with phagocyte deficits described subsequently, may contribute to delayed inflammatory responses and impaired bacterial clearance in neonates.

PHAGOCYTES
HEMATOPOIESIS

Phagocytes and all leukocytes of the immune system are derived from self-renewing, pluripotent hematopoietic stem cells (HSCs), which have the capacity for indefinite self-renewal (Fig. 4–2). Most circulating HSCs in cord blood and adult bone marrow are identified by their $CD34^+CD45^+CD133^+CD143^+$ surface phenotype combined with a lack of expression of CD38 and markers found on specific lineages of mature leukocytes (e.g., they lack CD3, a T-cell marker, and are CD34 positive and lineage marker negative [$CD34^+Lin^-$]) [65,66]. HSCs are generated during ontogeny from embryonic para-aortic tissue, fetal liver, and bone marrow [67]. The yolk sac, which is extraembryonic, is a major site of production of primitive erythrocytes and some primitive mononuclear phagocytes starting at about the third week of embryonic development. HSCs that give rise to erythrocyte and all nonerythroid hematopoietic cell lineages appear in the fetal liver after 4 weeks of gestation and in the bone marrow by 11 weeks of gestation

[67]. Liver-mediated hematopoiesis ceases by 20 weeks of gestation [67], with the bone marrow becoming the sole site of hematopoiesis thereafter. All major lineages of hematopoietic cells that are part of the immune system are present in the human by the beginning of the second trimester.

HSCs can subsequently differentiate into common lymphoid progenitors or common myeloid-erythroid progenitors (see Fig. 4–2). Common lymphoid progenitors give rise to T, B, and natural killer (NK) lymphocytes (discussed in later sections). Common myeloid-erythroid progenitors give rise to the megakaryocyte, erythroid, and myeloid lineages. Myeloid and lymphoid cells represent the two largely distinct but functionally interrelated immune cell lineages, with one cell type—DCs—seeming to provide a developmental and functional bridge between these lineages (see "Dendritic Cells—the Link between Innate and Adaptive Immunity").

PHAGOCYTE PRODUCTION BY THE BONE MARROW

Phagocytes are derived from a common precursor myeloid stem cell, which often is referred to as the colony-forming unit–granulocyte-monocyte (CFU-GM) (see Fig. 4–2).

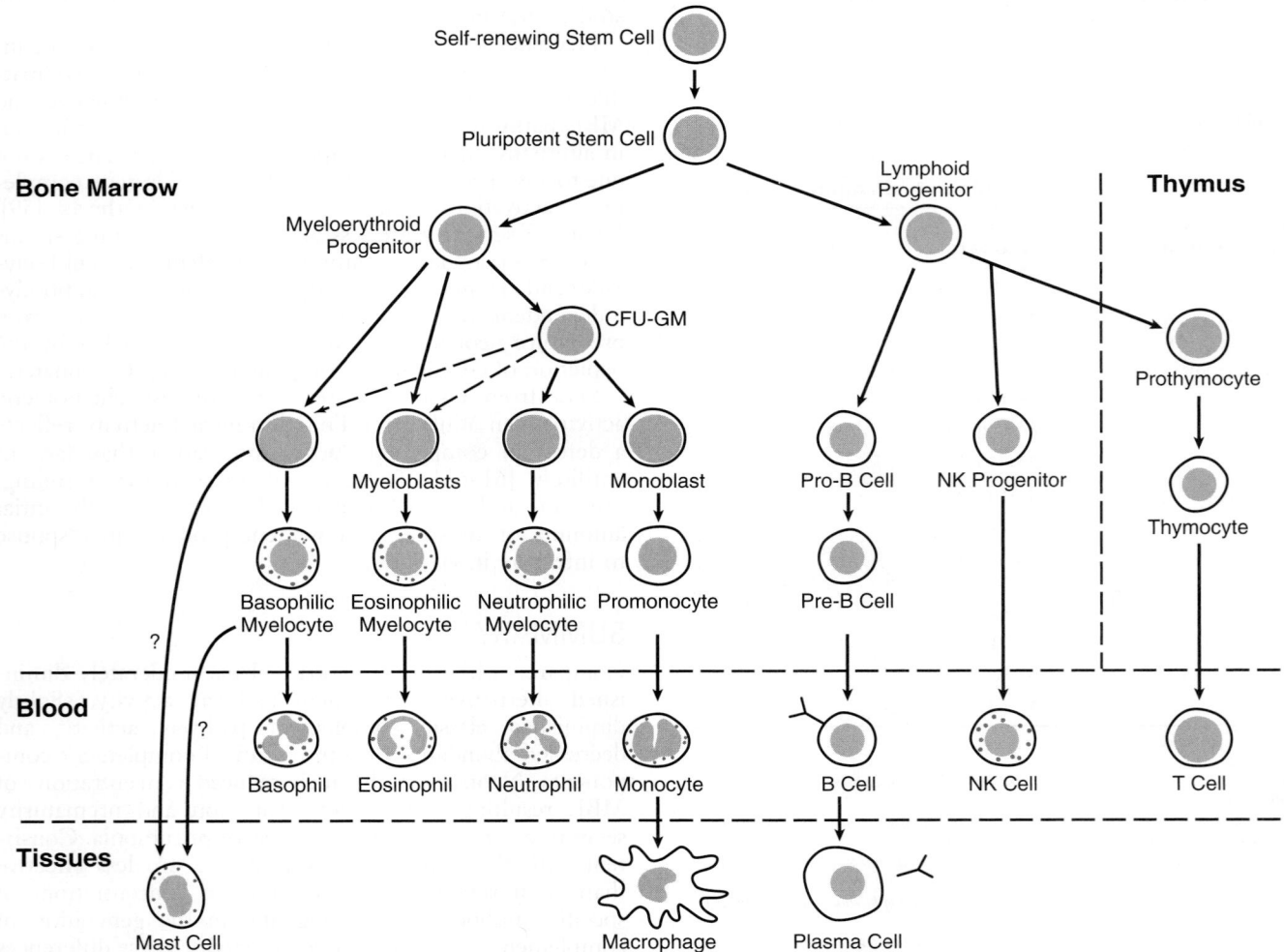

FIGURE 4–2 Myeloid and lymphoid differentiation and tissue compartments in which they occur. CFU-GM, colony-forming unit–granulocyte-macrophage.

The formation of myeloid stem cells from pluripotent HSCs and further differentiation of the myeloid precursor into mature granulocytes and monocytes are governed by bone marrow stromal cells and soluble colony-stimulating factors (CSFs) and other cytokines (see Table 4–2) [68,69]. Factors that act primarily on early HSCs include stem cell factor (also known as steel factor or c-Kit ligand) and Flt-3 ligand. The response to these factors is enhanced by granulocyte colony-stimulating factor (G-CSF) and thrombopoietin, hematopoietic growth factors originally identified by their ability to enhance the production of neutrophils (G-CSF) and platelets (thrombopoietin). IL-3 and IL-11 augment the effects of these factors on CFU-GM. Other factors act later and are more specific for given myeloid lineages. granulocyte-macrophage colony-stimulating factor (GM-CSF) acts to increase the production of neutrophils, eosinophils, and monocytes; G-CSF acts to increase neutrophil production; macrophage colony-stimulating factor (M-CSF) acts to increase monocyte production; and IL-5 enhances eosinophil production.

The precise role of these mediators in normal steady-state hematopoiesis is becoming clearer, primarily as a result of studies in mice with targeted disruptions of the relevant genes. Genetic defects in the production of biologically active stem cell factor or its receptor c-Kit lead to mast cell deficiency and severe anemia, with less severe defects in granulocytopoiesis and in formation of megakaryocytes [70]. Deficiency for Flt-3 ligand and c-Kit has a more severe phenotype than for either alone, indicating partial redundancy in their function. Deficient production of M-CSF is associated with some diminution in macrophage numbers and a marked deficiency in maturation of osteoclasts (presumably from monocyte precursors), which results in a form of osteopetrosis [71]. Mice and humans with mutations in the G-CSF receptor are neutropenic (although they do not completely lack neutrophils) and have fewer multilineage hematopoietic progenitor cells [68]. By contrast, GM-CSF receptor deficiency does not cause neutropenia, but instead causes pulmonary alveolar proteinosis in humans and mice [72]. IL-5 deficiency results in an inability to increase the numbers of eosinophils in response to parasites or allergens. Hematopoietic growth factors apparently play complex and, in some cases, partially overlapping roles in normal steady-state production of myeloid cells.

In response to an infectious or inflammatory stimulus, the production of G-CSF and GM-CSF and certain other of these growth factors is increased, resulting in increased production and release of granulocytes and monocytes. Similarly, when given exogenously, these factors enhance production and function of the indicated cell lineages [69].

NEUTROPHILS
PRODUCTION

Polymorphonuclear leukocytes or granulocytes, including neutrophils, eosinophils, and basophils, are derived from CFU-GM. Neutrophils are the principal cells of interest in relation to defense against pyogenic pathogens. The first identifiable committed neutrophil precursor is the myeloblast, which sequentially matures into myelocytes, metamyelocytes, bands, and mature neutrophils. Myelocytes and more mature neutrophilic granulocytes cannot replicate and constitute the postmitotic neutrophil storage pool [73]. The postmitotic neutrophil storage pool is an important reserve because these cells can be rapidly released into the circulation in response to inflammation. Mature neutrophils enter the circulation, where they remain for approximately 8 to 10 hours and are distributed equally and dynamically between circulating cells and cells adherent to the vascular endothelium. After leaving the circulation, neutrophils do not recirculate and die after approximately 24 hours. Release of neutrophils from the marrow may be enhanced in part by cytokines, including IL-1, IL-17 and TNF-α, in response to infection or inflammation [74,75].

Neutrophil precursors are detected at the end of the first trimester, appearing later than macrophage precursors [76]. Mature neutrophils are first detected by 14 to 16 weeks of gestation, but at mid-gestation the numbers of postmitotic neutrophils in the fetal liver and bone marrow remain markedly lower than in term newborns and adults [77]. By term, the numbers of circulating neutrophil precursors are 10-fold to 20-fold higher in the fetus and neonate than in the adult, and neonatal bone marrow also contains an abundance of neutrophil precursors [78,79]. The rate of proliferation of neutrophil precursors in the human neonate seems to be near maximal [78,80], however, suggesting that the capacity to increase numbers in response to infection may be limited.

At birth, neutrophil counts are lower in preterm than in term neonates and in neonates born by cesarean section without labor. Within hours of birth, the numbers of circulating neutrophils increase sharply [81–83]. The number of neutrophils normally peaks shortly thereafter, whereas the fraction of neutrophils that are immature (bands and less mature forms) remains constant at about 15%. Peak counts occur at approximately 8 hours in neonates greater than 28 weeks' gestation and at approximately 24 hours in neonates less than 28 weeks' gestation, then decline to a stable level by approximately 72 hours in neonates without complications. Thereafter, the lower limit of normal for term and preterm neonates is approximately 2500/μL and 1000/μL; the upper limit of normal is approximately 7000/μL for term and preterm neonates under most conditions, but may be higher (approximately 13,000/μL) for neonates living at higher altitudes, as observed in neonates living at approximately 1500 m elevation in Utah [83].

Values may be influenced by numerous additional factors. Most important is the response to sepsis. Septic infants may have normal or increased neutrophil counts. Sepsis and other perinatal complications, including maternal hypertension, periventricular hemorrhage, and severe asphyxia, can cause neutropenia, however, and severe or fatal sepsis often is associated with persistent neutropenia, particularly in preterm neonates [78,84,85]. Neutropenia may be associated with increased margination of circulating neutrophils, which occurs early in response to infection [73]. Neutropenia that is sustained often reflects depletion of the neonate's limited postmitotic neutrophil storage pool. Septic neutropenic neonates in whom the neutrophil storage pool is depleted are more likely to die than neonates with normal neutrophil storage pools [85]. Leukemoid reactions also are observed at a frequency of approximately 1% in term neonates in the absence of an identifiable cause. Such reactions apparently reflect increased neutrophil production [86].

Circulating G-CSF levels in healthy infants are highest in the first hours after birth, and levels in premature neonates are generally higher than levels in term neonates [87–89]. Levels decline rapidly in the neonatal period and more slowly thereafter. One study reported a direct correlation between circulating levels of G-CSF and the blood absolute neutrophil count, although this finding has not been confirmed in other studies [87,88]. Plasma G-CSF levels tend to be elevated in neonates with infection [89], although some studies have found considerable overlap with the levels of neonates without infection [90]. Although the cause of neutropenia in these neonates was not described, these observations raise the possibility that deficient G-CSF production might be a contributory factor to neutropenia in some neonates. Mononuclear cells and monocytes from mid-gestation fetuses and premature neonates generally produce less G-CSF and GM-CSF after stimulation in vitro than comparable adult cell types, whereas cells from term neonates produce amounts that are similar to or modestly less than amounts produced by cells of adults [91–95].

MIGRATION TO SITES OF INFECTION OR INJURY

After release from the bone marrow into the blood, neutrophils circulate until they are called on to enter infected or injured tissues. Neutrophils adhere selectively to endothelium in such tissues, but not in normal tissues. The adhesion and subsequent migration of neutrophils through blood vessels into tissues and to the site of infection results from a multistep process, which is governed by the pattern of expression on their surface of adhesion molecules and receptors for chemotactic factors and by the local patterns and gradients of adhesion molecule and chemotactic factors in the tissues.

The adhesion molecules involved in neutrophil migration from the blood into tissues include selectins, integrins, and the molecules to which they adhere (Table 4–4) [96]. The selectins are named by the cell types in which they are primarily expressed: L-selectin by leukocytes, E-selectin by endothelial cells, and P-selectin by platelets and endothelial cells. L-selectin is constitutively expressed on leukocytes and seems to bind to tissue-specific or inflammation-specific, carbohydrate-containing ligands on endothelial cells. E-selectin and P-selectin are expressed on activated, not resting, endothelial cells or platelets. E-selectin and P-selectin bind to sialylated glycoproteins on the surface of leukocytes, including P-selectin

TABLE 4–4 Selected Pairs of Surface Molecules Involved in T Cell–Antigen-Presenting Cell (APC) Interactions

T Cell Surface Molecule	T Cell Distribution	Corresponding Ligands on APCs	APC Distribution
CD2	Most T cells; higher on memory cells, lower on adult naïve and neonatal T cells	LFA-3 (CD58), CD59	Leukocytes
CD4	Subset of αβ T cells with predominantly helper activity	MHC class II β chain	Dendritic cells, Mφ, B cells, others (see text)
CD5	All T cells	CD72	B cells, Mφ
CD8	Subset of αβ T cells with predominantly cytotoxic activity	MHC glass I heavy chain	Ubiquitous
LFA-1 (CD11a/CD18)	All T cells; higher on memory cells, lower on adult naïve and neonatal T cells	ICAM-1 (CD54)	Leukocytes (ICAM-3 > ICAM-1, ICAM-2) and endothelium (ICAM-1, ICAM-2); most ICAM-1 expression requires activation
		ICAM-2 (CD102)	
		ICAM-3 (CD50)	
CD28	Most CD4$^+$ T cells, subset of CD8$^+$ T cells	CD80 (B7-1)	Dendritic cells, Mφ, activated B cells
		CD86 (B7-2)	
ICOS	Effector and memory T cells; not on resting naïve cells	B7RP-1 (B7h)	B cells, Mφ, dendritic cells, endothelial cells
VLA-4 (CD49d/CD29)	All T cells; higher on memory cells, lower on adult naïve and neonatal T cells	VCAM-1 (CD106)	Activated or inflamed endothelium (increased by TNF, IL-1, IL-4)
ICAM-1 (CD54)	All T cells; higher on memory cells, lower on adult virgin and neonatal T cells	LFA-1 (CD11a/CD18)	Leukocytes
CTLA-4 (CD152)	Activated T cells	CD80	Dendritic cells, Mφ, activated B cells, activated T cells
		CD86	
CD40 ligand (CD154)	Activated CD4$^+$ T cells; lower on neonatal CD4$^+$ T cells	CD40	Dendritic cells, Mφ, B cells, thymic epithelial cells
PD-1	Activated CD4$^+$ and CD8$^+$ T cells	PD-L1, PD-L2	Dendritic cells, Mφ, B cells, regulatory T cells

CTLA-4, cytotoxic T-lymphocyte antigen-4; ICAM, intercellular adhesion molecule; ICOS, inducible costimulator; IL, interleukin; LFA, leukocyte function antigen; Mφ, mononuclear phagocytes; MHC, major histocompatibility complex; PD, programmed death [molecule]; VCAM, vascular cell adhesion molecule; VLA-4, very late antigen-4.

glycoprotein ligand-1. L-selectin binds to glycoproteins and glycolipids, which are expressed on vascular endothelial cells in specific tissues. The integrins are a large family of heterodimeric proteins composed of an α and a β chain. β_2 integrins LFA-1 (CD11a through CD18) and Mac-1 (CD11b through CD18) play a crucial role in neutrophil function because neutrophils do not express other integrins in substantial amounts. β_2 integrins are constitutively expressed on neutrophils, but their abundance and avidity for their endothelial ligands are increased after activation of neutrophils in response to chemotactic factors. Their endothelial ligands include intercellular adhesion molecule (ICAM)-1 and ICAM-2. Both are constitutively expressed on endothelium, but ICAM-1 expression is increased markedly by exposure to inflammatory mediators, including IL-1, TNF-α, and LPS.

Chemotactic factors may be derived directly from bacterial components, such as n-formylated-Met-Leu-Phe (fMLP) peptide; from activated complement, including C5a; and from host cell lipids, including leukotriene B$_4$ (LTB$_4$) [97]. In addition, a large family of chemotactic cytokines (chemokines) are synthesized by macrophages and many other cell types (see Tables 4–1 and 4–2). Chemokines constitute a cytokine superfamily with more than 50 members known at present, most of which are secreted and of relatively low molecular weight [98]. Chemokines attract various leukocyte populations, which bear the appropriate G protein–linked chemokine receptors. They can be divided into four families according to their pattern of amino-terminal cysteine residues: CC, CXC, C, and CX3C (X represents a noncysteine amino acid between the cysteines).

A nomenclature for the chemokines and their receptors has been adopted, in which the family is first denoted (e.g., CC), followed by L for ligand (the chemokine itself) and a number or followed by R (for receptor) and a number. Functionally, chemokines also can be defined by their principal function—in homeostatic or inflammatory cell migration—and by the subsets of cells on which they act. Neutrophils are attracted by the subset of CXC chemokines that contain a glutamine-leucine-arginine motif, including the prototypic neutrophil chemokine CXLC8, also known as IL-8.

These adhesion molecules and chemotactic factors act in a coordinated fashion to allow neutrophil recruitment. In response to injury or inflammatory cytokines, E-selectin and P-selectin are expressed on the endothelium of capillaries or postcapillary venules. Neutrophils in the blood adhere to these selectins in a low-avidity fashion, allowing them to roll along the vessel walls. This step is transient and reversible, unless a second, high-avidity interaction is triggered. At the time of the low-avidity binding, if neutrophils also encounter chemotactic factors released from the tissues or from the endothelium itself, they rapidly upregulate the avidity and abundance of LFA-1 and Mac-1 on the neutrophil cell surface. This process results in high-avidity binding of neutrophils to endothelial cells, which, in the presence of a gradient of chemotactic factors from the tissue to the blood vessel, induces neutrophils to migrate across the endothelium and into the tissues. Neutrophils must undergo considerable deformation to allow diapedesis through the endothelium. Migration through the tissues also is likely to be facilitated by the reversible adhesion and deadhesion between ligands on the neutrophil surface, including the integrins, and components of the extracellular matrix, such as fibronectin and collagen.

The profound importance of integrin-mediated and selectin-mediated leukocyte adhesion is illustrated by the genetic leukocyte adhesion deficiency syndromes [99]. Deficiency of the common β_2 integrin chain results in inability of leukocytes to exit the bloodstream and reach sites of infection and injury in the tissues. Affected patients are profoundly susceptible to infections with pathogenic and nonpathogenic bacteria and may present in early infancy with delayed separation of the umbilical cord, omphalitis, and severe bacterial infection without pus formation. A related syndrome—leukocyte adhesion deficiency syndrome type II—is due to a defect in synthesis of the carbohydrate selectin ligands.

MIGRATION OF NEONATAL NEUTROPHILS

The ability of neonatal neutrophils to migrate from the blood into sites of infection and inflammation is reduced or delayed, and the transition from a neutrophilic to mononuclear cell inflammatory response is delayed [76]. This diminished delivery of neutrophils may result in part from defects in adhesion and chemotaxis.

Adhesion of neonatal neutrophils under resting conditions is normal or at most modestly impaired, whereas adhesion of activated cells is deficient [100,101]. Adhesion and rolling of neonatal neutrophils to activated endothelium under conditions of flow similar to those found in capillaries or postcapillary venules is variable, but on average approximately 50% of that observed with adult neutrophils [102,103]. This decreased adhesion seems to reflect, at least in part, decreased abundance and shedding of L-selectin and decreased binding of neonatal neutrophils to P-selectin [102,103]. Resting neonatal and adult neutrophils have similar amounts of Mac-1 and LFA-1 on their plasma membrane, but neonatal neutrophils have a reduced ability to upregulate expression of these integrins after exposure to chemotactic agents [102–104]. Reduced integrin upregulation is associated with a parallel decrease in adhesion to activated endothelium or ICAM-1 [105]. Two studies have concluded, however, that expression of Mac-1 and LFA-1 is not reduced on neonatal neutrophils, and that diminished expression observed in other studies may be an artifact of the methods used to purify neutrophils [106,107]. Nonetheless, the preponderance of data suggests that a deficit in adhesion underlies in part the diminished ability of neonatal neutrophils to migrate through endothelium into tissues, and these defects are greater in preterm neonates [102,105].

In nearly all studies in which neutrophil migration has been examined in vitro, chemotaxis of neonatal neutrophils was less than that of adult neutrophils. Some studies have found that chemotaxis remains less than that of adult cells until 1 to 2 years of age, whereas others have suggested more rapid maturation [61,108]. The response of neonatal neutrophils to various chemotactic factors, such as fMLP, LTB$_4$, and neutrophil-specific chemokines including IL-8, is reduced [109–111]. Chemotactic factor binding and dose response patterns of neonatal neutrophils seem to be similar to adult neutrophils, whereas downstream processes, including expression of Rac2, increases in free intracellular calcium concentration ($[Ca^{2+}]_i$) and inositol phospholipid generation, and change in cell membrane potential, are impaired [112–114]. An additional factor may be the reduced deformability of neonatal neutrophils, which may limit their ability to enter the tissues after binding to the vascular endothelium [101,115]. Decreased generation of chemotactic factors in neonatal serum [61,116] may compound the intrinsic chemotactic deficits of neonatal neutrophils. The generation of other chemotactic agents, such as LTB_4, by neonatal neutrophils seems to be normal, however [117]. It has also been hypothesized that the relatively greater production by neonatal phagocytes and DCs of the cytokine IL-6 (see later), which impedes neutrophil migration into tissues, may dampen neutrophil recruitment [118], but this notion has not been tested.

PHAGOCYTOSIS

Having reached the site of infection, neutrophils must bind, phagocytose, and kill the pathogen [119]. Opsonization greatly facilitates this process. Neutrophils express on their surface receptors for multiple opsonins, including receptors for the Fc portion of the IgG molecule (Fcγ receptors)—FcγRI (CD64), FcγRII (CD32), and FcγRIII (CD16) [120]. Neutrophils also express receptors for activated complement components C3b and C3bi [121], which are bound by CR1, CR3 (CD11b-CD18) and CR4 (CD11c-CD18). Opsonized bacteria bind and cross-link Fcγ and C3b-C3bi receptors. This cross-linkage transmits a signal for ingestion and for the activation of the cell's microbicidal mechanisms.

Under optimal in vitro conditions, neutrophils from healthy neonates bind and ingest gram-positive and gram-negative bacteria as well as or only slightly less efficiently than adult neutrophils [115,122,123]. The concentrations of opsonins are reduced in serum from neonates, in particular preterm neonates, however, and when concentrations of opsonins are limited [51], neutrophils from neonates ingest bacteria less efficiently than neutrophils from adults. Consistent with this finding, phagocytosis of bacteria by neutrophils from preterm, but not term, neonates is reduced compared with adult neutrophils when assayed in whole blood [124–126]. Why neonatal neutrophils have impaired phagocytosis when concentrations of opsonins are limiting is incompletely understood. Basal expression of receptors for opsonized bacteria is not greatly different. Neutrophils from neonates, particularly preterm neonates, express greater amounts of the high-affinity FcγRI, lesser amounts of FcγRIII, and similar or slightly reduced amounts of FcγRII at birth compared with adults; values in preterm neonates approach values of term neonates by 1 month of age [127]. Expression of complement receptors on neutrophils from term neonates and adults is similar, but reduced expression of CR3 on neutrophils from preterm neonates has been reported in some studies [107,127]. Neutrophils from preterm neonates also are less able to upregulate CR3 in response to LPS and chemotactic factors [128–130]. Lower expression of proteins involved in the engulfment process, including Rac2 as noted earlier, may also contribute to impaired phagocytosis when concentrations of opsonins are limited.

KILLING

After ingestion, neutrophils kill ingested microbes through oxygen-dependent and oxygen-independent mechanisms. Oxygen-dependent microbicidal mechanisms are of central importance, as illustrated by the severe compromise in defenses against a wide range of pyogenic pathogens (with the exception of catalase-negative bacteria) observed in children with a genetic defect in this system [131]. Children with this disorder have a defect in one of several proteins that constitute the phagocyte oxidase, which is activated during receptor-mediated phagocytosis. The assembly of the oxidase in the plasma membrane results in the generation and delivery of reactive oxygen metabolites, including superoxide anion, hydrogen peroxide, and hydroxyl radicals. These oxygen radicals along with the granule protein myeloperoxidase are discharged into the phagocytic vacuole, where they collaborate in killing ingested microbes. In addition to this oxygen-dependent pathway, neutrophils contain other granule proteins with potent microbicidal activity, including the defensins HNP1 through HNP4, the cathelicidin LL-37, elastase, cathepsin G, and bactericidal permeability-increasing protein, a protein that binds selectively to and helps to kill gram-negative bacteria [1,132–134].

Oxygen-dependent and oxygen-independent microbicidal mechanisms of neonatal and adult neutrophils do not differ greatly [115,123]. Generation of superoxide anion and hydrogen peroxide by neutrophils from term neonates is generally similar to or greater than that by adult cells in response to soluble stimuli [135,136]. Although a modest reduction in the generation of reactive oxygen metabolites by neutrophils from preterm compared with term neonates was seen in response to some strains of coagulase-negative staphylococci, this was not observed with other strains or with a strain of GBS and is of uncertain significance [137]. By contrast, LPS primes adult neutrophils for increased production of reactive oxygen metabolites, but priming is much reduced with neonatal neutrophils, which could limit their efficacy in response to infection in vivo [130,138]. Studies of oxygen-independent microbicidal mechanisms of neonatal neutrophils are less complete. Compared with adult neutrophils, neonatal neutrophils contain and release reduced amounts of bactericidal permeability-increasing protein (approximately two-fold to threefold) and lactoferrin (approximately twofold), but contain or release comparable amounts of myeloperoxidase, defensins, and lysozyme [115,123,139,140].

Consistent with these findings, killing of ingested gram-positive and gram-negative bacteria and *Candida* organisms by neutrophils from neonates and adults is generally similar [115,123]. Variable and usually mildly decreased bactericidal activity has been noted, however, against *P. aeruginosa* [141], *S. aureus* [142], and certain strains of GBS [143–145]. Deficits in killing of engulfed microbes by neonatal neutrophils are more apparent at high ratios of bacteria to neutrophils [146], as is killing by neutrophils from sick or stressed neonates (i.e., neonates born prematurely or who have sepsis, respiratory impairment, hyperbilirubinemia, premature rupture of membranes, or hypoglycemia) [147,148]. Whether killing by neonatal than adult neutrophils is more severely compromised by comparable illnesses is uncertain, however.

NEUTROPHIL CLEARANCE AND RESOLUTION OF NEUTROPHILIC INFLAMMATION

Neutrophils undergo apoptosis 1 to 2 days after egress from the bone marrow and are efficiently cleared by tissue macrophages without producing inflammation or injury. In the context of infection or sterile inflammation, their survival is prolonged by colony-stimulating factors and other inflammatory mediators, allowing them to aid in microbial clearance, while augmenting or perpetuating tissue injury. Studies from several groups have shown that spontaneous and anti-Fas–induced apoptosis of isolated neonatal neutrophils is reduced when these cells are cultured in vitro [76,149–151], although this was not observed in one study in which neutrophil survival in whole blood for a shorter time was assessed [152]. The greater survival of neonatal than adult neutrophils was associated with reduced expression of the apoptosis-inducing Fas receptor and proapoptotic members of the Bcl-2 family, but whether these differences account for the greater survival is uncertain [149]. The increased survival of neonatal neutrophils has led some authorities to speculate that this may help to compensate for the neonate's limited neutrophil storage pool in protection against infection, but also contributes to persistent untoward inflammation and tissue injury [76].

EFFECTS OF IMMUNOMODULATORS

After systemic treatment with G-CSF and GM-CSF, the number of neutrophils increases in neonates, as does expression of CR3 on these cells [80]. The increased numbers likely reflect increased production and survival [149,151]. GM-CSF and interferon (IFN)-γ enhance the chemotactic response of neonatal neutrophils [80,153], although at high concentrations GM-CSF inhibits chemotaxis, while augmenting oxygen radical production [154]. The methylxanthine pentoxifylline exhibits a biphasic enhancement of chemotaxis by neonatal neutrophils [115]. Of potential concern, indomethacin, which is used clinically to facilitate ductal closure in premature neonates, impairs chemotaxis of cells from term and preterm neonates [155].

SUMMARY

The most critical deficiency in phagocyte defenses in the term and particularly preterm neonate is the limited ability to accelerate neutrophil production in response to infection. This age-specific limitation seems to result in large part from a limited neutrophil storage pool and perhaps a more limited ability to increase neutrophil production in response to infection. Impaired migration of neutrophils into tissues is likely also to be a factor, whereas phagocytosis and killing do not seem to be greatly impaired. Persistent inflammation and tissue injury may result from impaired clearance of infection and protracted neutrophilic inflammation after the infection is cleared.

EOSINOPHILS

In adults and older children, eosinophils represent a small percentage of the circulating granulocytes. In the healthy fetus and neonate, eosinophils commonly represent a larger percentage (10% to 20%) of total granulocytes than in adults [156,157]. Numbers of eosinophils increase postnatally, peaking at 3 to 4 weeks of postnatal life. A relative increase in the abundance of eosinophils in inflammatory exudates of various causes is also seen in neonates, paralleling their greater numbers in the circulation [103]. Eosinophil-rich inflammatory exudates do not suggest the presence of allergic disease or helminth infection as strongly as they do in older individuals. The degree of eosinophilia is greater yet in preterm neonates and in neonates with Rh disease, total parenteral nutrition, and transfusions [158]. This physiologic neonatal eosinophilia is not associated with increased amounts of circulating IgE [159]. The basis for the eosinophilic tendency of the neonate is unknown. By contrast to the diminished migration of neonatal neutrophils, neonatal eosinophils exhibit greater spontaneous and chemotactic factor–induced migration than adult eosinophils [157]. Their greater numbers and ability to migrate may contribute to the relatively greater abundance of eosinophils in neonatal inflammatory infiltrates, including those seen in physiologic conditions such as erythema toxicum (see "Epithelial Barriers").

MONONUCLEAR PHAGOCYTES
PRODUCTION AND DIFFERENTIATION OF MONOCYTES AND RESIDENT TISSUE MACROPHAGES

Together, monocytes and tissue macrophages are referred to as mononuclear phagocytes. Blood monocytes are derived from bone marrow precursors (monoblasts and promonocytes). Under steady-state conditions, monocytes are released from the bone marrow within 24 hours and circulate in the blood for 1 to 3 days before moving to the tissues [160], where they differentiate into tissue macrophages or conventional DCs (cDCs). All monocytes express CD14, which serves as a coreceptor for recognition of LPS by TLR4/MD-2. CD14 is commonly used as a lineage marker for these cells because they are the only cell type that expresses it in high amounts. Monocytes also express the human leukocyte antigen (HLA) HLA-DR and can present antigens to CD4 T cells, although the amounts expressed and efficiency of antigen presentation are less than by DCs. Monocytes are heterogeneous. A small subset (approximately 10% in adults) of monocytes expresses CD16 (FcγRIII). This monocyte subset expresses more of the surface major histocompatibility complex (MHC) class II molecule HLA-DR (MHC molecules and their functions are discussed subsequently in "Antigen Presentation by Classic Major Histocompatibility Complex Molecules"), produces greater amounts of proinflammatory cytokines, and more readily differentiates into DCs after entry into tissues than the CD16-negative subset [161].

Macrophages are resident in tissues throughout the body, where they have multiple functions, including the clearance of dead host cells, phagocytosis and killing of microbes, secretion of inflammatory mediators, and presentation of antigen to T cells. The functions of macrophages are readily modulated by cytokines, and macrophages can fuse to form multinucleated giant cells. The estimated life span of macrophages in the tissues is 4 to 12 weeks, and they are capable of limited replication in situ [162,163].

Macrophages are detectable by 4 weeks of fetal life in the yolk sac and are found shortly thereafter in the liver and then in the bone marrow [164]. The capacity of the fetus and the neonate to produce monocytes is at least as great as that of adults [165]. The numbers of monocytes per volume of blood in neonates are equal to or greater than the numbers in adults [166]. Neonatal blood monocytes express approximately 50% as much HLA-DR as adult monocytes, and a larger fraction of neonatal monocytes lack detectable HLA-DR [161]. A similar fraction of neonatal, infant, and adult monocytes are CD16$^+$, so the diminished expression of HLA-DR cannot be attributed to the absence of this subset.

The numbers of tissue macrophages in human neonates are less well characterized. Limited data in humans, which are consistent with data in various animal species, suggest that the lung contains few macrophages until shortly before term [167]. Postnatally, the numbers of lung macrophages increase to adult levels by 24 to 48 hours in healthy monkeys [168]. A similar increase occurs in humans, although the data are less complete and by necessity derived from individuals with clinical problems necessitating tracheobronchial lavage [169]. The blood of premature neonates contains increased numbers of pitted erythrocytes or erythrocytes containing Howell-Jolly bodies [170], suggesting that the ability of splenic and liver macrophages to clear these effete cells, and perhaps microbial cells, may be reduced in the fetus and premature infant.

MIGRATION TO SITES OF INFECTION AND DELAYED HYPERSENSITIVITY RESPONSES

Similar to neutrophils, mononuclear phagocytes express the adhesion molecules L-selectin and β_2 integrins. These cells also express substantial amounts of the $\alpha_4\beta_1$ integrin (VLA-4), allowing them, in contrast to neutrophils, to adhere efficiently to endothelium expressing vascular cell adhesion molecule (VCAM)-1, the ligand for VLA-4 [171]. Interaction of VLA-4 with VCAM-1 allows monocytes to enter tissues in states in which there is little or no neutrophilic inflammation. As in neutrophils, monocyte chemotaxis, integrin avidity, and strength of vascular adhesion are regulated by chemotactic factors, including fMLP, C5a, LTB$_4$, and chemokines. Chemokines that are chemotactic for neutrophils are not generally chemotactic for monocytes, and vice versa. Monocytes respond to a range of CC chemokines, such as CCL2 (MCP-1) [98].

The acute inflammatory response is characterized by an initial infiltration of neutrophils that is followed within 6 to 12 hours by the influx of mononuclear phagocytes [160]. The orchestration of this sequential influx of leukocytes seems to be governed by the temporal order in which specific inflammatory cytokines, chemokines, and endothelial adhesins are expressed, with some data suggesting an important role for IL-6 in this transition [172]. Some inflammatory responses, including delayed-type hypersensitivity (DTH) reactions induced by the injection of antigens (e.g., purified protein derivative [PPD]) to which the individual is immune (i.e., has developed an antigen-specific T-cell response), are characterized by the influx of mononuclear phagocytes and lymphocytes with very minimal or no initial neutrophilic phase [173].

The influx of monocytes into sites of inflammation, including DTH responses, is delayed and attenuated in neonates compared with adults [174–176]. This is true even when antigen-specific T-cell responses are evident in vitro, suggesting that decreased migration of monocytes and lymphocytes into the tissues is responsible for the poor response in neonates. Whether this delay results from impaired chemotaxis of neonatal monocytes or impaired generation of chemotactic factors or both is unresolved [61,62,108,177].

ANTIMICROBIAL PROPERTIES OF MONOCYTES AND MACROPHAGES

Although neutrophils ingest and kill pyogenic bacteria more efficiently, resident macrophages are the initial line of phagocyte defense against microbial invasion in the tissues. When the microbial insult is modest, these cells are sufficient. If not, they produce cytokines and other inflammatory mediators to direct the recruitment of circulating neutrophils and monocytes from the blood. Monocytes and macrophages express receptors that bind to microbes, including FcγRI, FcγRII, and FcγRIII that bind IgG-coated microbes[120]; FcαR that binds IgA-coated microbes[178]; and CR1 and CR3 receptors that bind microbes coated with C3b and C3bi [179]. Microbes bound through these receptors are efficiently engulfed by macrophages and when ingested can be killed by microbicidal mechanisms, including many of the mechanisms also employed by neutrophils and discussed in the preceding section. Mononuclear phagocytes generate reactive oxygen metabolites, but in lesser amounts than neutrophils. Circulating monocytes, but not tissue macrophages, contain myeloperoxidase, which facilitates the microbicidal activity of hydrogen peroxide. The expression of microbicidal granule proteins differs in mononuclear phagocytes and neutrophils; for example, human mononuclear phagocytes express β-defensins, but not α-defensins [180].

The microbicidal activity of resident tissue macrophages is relatively modest. This limited activity may be important in allowing macrophages to remove dead or damaged host cells and small numbers of microbes without excessively damaging host tissues. In response to infection, macrophage microbicidal and proinflammatory functions are enhanced in a process referred to as macrophage activation [123,181]. Macrophage activation results from the integration of signals from TLRs and other innate immune pattern recognition receptors (discussed later) and receptors for activated complement components, immune complexes, cytokines, and ligands produced by other immune cells, including IFN-γ, CD40 ligand, TNF-α and GM-CSF [181,182].

The increased antimicrobial activity of activated macrophages results in part from increased expression of FcγRI, enhanced phagocytic activity, and increased production of reactive oxygen metabolites. Other antimicrobial mechanisms induced by activation of these cells include the catabolism of tryptophan by indoleamine 2,3-dioxygenase, scavenging of iron, and production of nitric oxide and its metabolites by inducible nitric oxide synthase. The last is a major mechanism by which activated murine macrophages inhibit or kill various intracellular pathogens. The role of nitric oxide in the antimicrobial activity of human macrophages is controversial, however. Activated mononuclear phagocytes also secrete numerous noncytokine products that are potentially important in host defense mechanisms. These include complement components, fibronectin, and lysozyme.

Activation of macrophages plays a crucial role in defense against infection with intracellular bacterial and protozoan pathogens that replicate within phagocytic vacuoles. Support for this notion comes from studies in humans and mice with genetic deficiencies that impair the activation of macrophages by IFN-γ. Humans with genetic defects involving IL-12, which induces IFN-γ production by NK and T cells; the IL-12 receptor; the IFN-γ receptor; or the transcription factor STAT-1, which is activated via the IFN-γ receptor, experience excessive infections with mycobacteria and *Salmonella* [39]. Deficiency of TNF-α or its receptors in mice and treatment of humans with antagonists of TNF-α also impair antimycobacterial defenses [183,184]. Patients with the X-linked hyper-IgM syndrome, which is due to a defect in CD40 ligand, are predisposed to disease caused by *Pneumocystis jiroveci* and *Cryptosporidium parvum*, in addition to the problems they experience from defects in antibody production (see section on T-cell help for antibody production) [185]. These findings are consistent with the notion that IFN-γ–mediated, TNF-α–mediated, and CD40 ligand–mediated macrophage activation is important in host defense against these pathogens, and that these molecules activate macrophages, at least in part, in a nonredundant manner.

By contrast to this canonical pathway of macrophage activation, macrophages exposed to cytokines produced by T helper type 2 (T_H2) cells, which are induced by infection with parasitic helminths, are activated in an alternative manner [181]. These alternatively activated macrophages dampen acute inflammation, impede the generation of reactive nitrogen products, attenuate proinflammatory T-cell responses, and foster fibrosis through the production of arginase and other mediators. Although best characterized in mice, this alternative pathway is likely to be relevant in humans as well.

ANTIMICROBIAL ACTIVITY AND ACTIVATION OF NEONATAL MONOCYTES AND MACROPHAGES

Monocytes from human neonates and adults ingest and kill *S. aureus*, *E. coli*, and GBS with similar efficiency [143,177,186–188]. Consistent with these findings, the production of microbicidal oxygen metabolites by neonatal and adult monocytes is similar [187,189–192]. Neonatal and adult monocytes, monocyte-derived macrophages, and fetal macrophages are comparable in their ability to prevent herpes simplex virus (HSV) from replicating within them [193,194]. Although neonatal monocytes may be slightly less capable of killing HSV-infected cells than adult monocytes in the absence of antibody, they are equivalent in the presence of antibody [195,196].

The ability of neonatal and adult monocyte-derived macrophages (monocytes cultured in vitro) to phagocytose GBS, other bacteria, and *Candida* through receptors for mannose and fucose, IgG, and complement components is similar. Despite comparable phagocytosis, neonatal monocyte-derived macrophages kill *Candida* and GBS less efficiently. GM-CSF, but not IFN-γ, activates neonatal monocyte-derived macrophages to produce superoxide anion and to kill these organisms, whereas both of these cytokines activate adult macrophages [197–199]. The lack of response to IFN-γ by neonatal macrophages was associated with normal binding to its receptor, but decreased activation of STAT-1 [197]. Macrophages obtained from aspirated bronchial fluid of neonates were found to be less effective at killing the yeast form of *C. albicans* than bronchoalveolar macrophages from adults [200]. To our knowledge, this result has not been reproduced, and the decreased effectiveness could reflect differences in the source of cells. Nonetheless, similar studies with alveolar macrophages from newborn and particularly premature newborn monkeys, rabbits, and rats also have shown reduced phagocytic or microbicidal activity [201–206]. In contrast to these reports of decreased antimicrobial activity and failure of macrophage activation by IFN-γ, blood monocytes and IFN-γ–treated monocyte-derived and placental macrophages from neonates kill and restrict the growth of *Toxoplasma gondii* as effectively as cells from adults [207,208].

MONONUCLEAR PHAGOCYTES PRODUCE CYTOKINES AND OTHER MEDIATORS THAT REGULATE INFLAMMATION AND IMMUNITY

Monocytes and macrophages produce cytokines, chemokines, colony-stimulating factors, and other mediators in response to ligand binding by TLRs and other pattern recognition receptors expressed by these cells (described in the next section), by cytokines produced by other cell types, by activated complement components and other mediators, and by engagement of CD40 on their surface by CD40 ligand expressed on activated helper T cells [181,182]. These include the cytokines IL-1, TNF-α, IL-6, and α and β IFNs (type I IFNs), which induce the production of prostaglandin E_2, which induces fever [209,210], accounting for the antipyretic effect of drugs that inhibit prostaglandin synthesis. Fever may have a beneficial role in host resistance to infection by inhibiting the growth of certain microorganisms and by enhancing host immune responses [211]. TNF-α, IL-1, IL-6, and type I IFNs also act on the liver to induce the acute-phase response, which is associated with decreased albumin synthesis and increased synthesis of certain complement components, fibrinogen, CRP, and MBL. G-CSF, GM-CSF, and M-CSF enhance the production of their respective target cell populations, increasing the numbers of phagocytes available.

At sites of infection or injury, TNF-α and IL-1 increase endothelial cell expression of adhesion molecules, including E-selectin, P-selectin, ICAM-1, and VCAM-1; increase endothelial cell procoagulant activity; and enhance neutrophil adhesiveness by upregulating β_2 integrin expression [96]. IL-6 may help to terminate neutrophil recruitment into tissues and to facilitate a switch from an inflammatory infiltrate rich in neutrophils to one dominated by monocytes and lymphocytes [172]. IL-8 and other related CXC chemokines that share with IL-8 an N-terminal glu-leu-arg motif enhance the avidity of neutrophil β_2 integrins for ICAM-1 and attract neutrophils into the inflammatory-infectious focus; CC chemokines play a similar role in attracting mononuclear phagocytes and lymphocytes. These and additional factors contribute to edema, redness, and leukocyte infiltration, which characterize inflammation.

In addition to secreting cytokines that regulate the acute inflammatory response and play a crucial role in host defense to extracellular bacterial and fungal pathogens, monocytes and macrophages (and DCs—see later) produce cytokines that mediate and regulate defense against intracellular viral, bacterial, and protozoan pathogens. Type I IFNs directly inhibit viral replication in host cells [212,213], as do IFN-γ and TNF-α [214]. IL-12, IL-23, and IL-27 are members of a family of heterodimeric cytokines that help to regulate T-cell and NK-cell differentiation and function [215]. IL-12 is composed of IL-12/23 p40 and p35, IL-23 is composed of IL-12/23 p40 and p19, and IL-27 is composed of EBI-3 and p28 [215,216]. IL-12, in concert with IL-15 and IL-18 [217,218], enhances NK-cell lytic function and production of IFN-γ and facilitates the development of CD4 T helper type 1 (T_H1) and CD8 effector T cells, which are discussed more fully in "Differentiation of Activated Naïve T Cells into Effector and Memory Cells," and which play a crucial role in control of infection with intracellular bacterial, protozoal, and viral pathogens. IFN-γ activates macrophages, allowing them to control infection with intracellular pathogens, and enhances their capacity to produce IL-12 and TNF-α, which amplify IFN-γ production by NK cells and cause T cells to differentiate into IFN-γ–producing T_H1 cells [219,220]. IL-27 also facilitates IFN-γ production, while inducing the expression of IL-10, which dampens inflammatory and T_H1 responses to limit tissue injury. By contrast, IL-23 favors IL-17–producing T_H17 T-cell responses, in which IL-17 promotes neutrophil production, acute inflammation, and defense of extracellular pathogens.

The production of cytokines by mononuclear phagocytes normally is restricted temporally and anatomically to cells in contact with microbial products, antigen-stimulated T cells, or other agonists. When produced in excess, these cytokines are injurious [221,222]. When excess production of proinflammatory cytokines occurs systemically, septic shock and disseminated intravascular coagulation may ensue, underscoring the importance of closely regulated and anatomically restricted production of proinflammatory mediators.

Tight control of inflammation normally is achieved by a combination of positive and negative feedback regulation. TNF-α, IL-1, and microbial products that induce their production also cause macrophages to produce cytokines that attenuate inflammation and dampen immunity, including IL-10 [223] and IL-1 receptor antagonist [224]. Inflammation is also attenuated by the production of anti-inflammatory lipid mediators, including lipoxins and arrestins [225].

CYTOKINE PRODUCTION INDUCED BY ENGAGEMENT OF TOLL-LIKE RECEPTORS AND OTHER INNATE IMMUNE PATTERN RECOGNITION RECEPTORS

Monocytes, macrophages, DCs, and other cells of the innate immune system discriminate between microbes and self [226], or things that are "dangerous" and "not dangerous," [227] through invariant innate immune pattern recognition receptors. These receptors recognize microbial structures (commonly referred to as pathogen-associated molecular patterns) or molecular danger signals produced by infected or injured host cells. Recognition is followed by signals that activate the innate immune response.

Toll-like Receptors

TLRs are a family of structurally related proteins and are the most extensively characterized set of innate immune pattern recognition receptors. Ten different TLRs have been defined in humans [228–230]. Their distinct ligand specificities, subcellular localization, and patterns of expression by specific cell types are shown in Table 4–5 [231–234].

TLR4 forms a functional LPS receptor with MD-2, a soluble protein required for surface expression of the TLR4/MD-2 receptor complex [230,235]. This complex also recognizes the fusion protein of RSV. CD14, which is expressed abundantly on the surface of monocytes and exists in a soluble form in the plasma, facilitates recognition by the TLR4/MD-2 complex and is essential for recognition of smooth LPS present on pathogenic gram-negative bacteria [236]. TLR4-deficient and MD-2–deficient mice are hyporesponsive to LPS [237,238] and susceptible to infection with *Salmonella typhimurium* and *E. coli* [239–242]. TLR2, which forms a heterodimer with TLR1 or TLR6, recognizes bacterial lipopeptides, lipoteichoic acid, and peptidoglycan, and this recognition is facilitated by CD14. TLR2 has a central role in the recognition of gram-positive bacteria and contributes to recognition of fungi, including *Candida* species [229,243,244]. TLR5 recognizes bacterial flagellin [245]. Consistent with their role in recognition of microbial cell surface structures, these TLRs are displayed on the cell surface.

By contrast, TLR3, TLR7, TLR8, and TLR9 recognize nucleic acids: TLR3 binds double-stranded RNA, TLR7 and TLR8 bind single-stranded RNA, and TLR9

TABLE 4–5   Human Toll-like Receptors (TLRs)

TLR	Microbial Ligands	Site of Interaction with Ligand	Signal Transduction/Effector Molecules	Expression by Antigen-Presenting Cells
TLR-1	See TLR-2	Cell surface	MyD88-dependent induction of cytokines	Monocytes and B cells > cDCs
TLR-2	Bacterial peptidoglycan, lipoteichoic acid and lipopeptides; mycobacterial lipoarabinomannan, recognition of some ligands is mediated by TLR2/TLR-1 or TLR2/TLR-6 heterodimers	Cell surface	MyD88-dependent induction of cytokines	Monocytes and cDCs > B cells
TLR-3	Double-stranded RNA	Endosome	TRIF-dependent induction of type I IFNs and cytokines	cDCs
TLR-4	LPS, RSV	Cell surface	MyD88-dependent and TRIF-dependent induction of cytokines; TRIF-dependent induction of type I IFNs	Monocytes > cDCs
TLR-5	Flagellin	Cell surface	MyD88-induced cytokines	Monocytes > cDCs
TLR-6	See TLR-2	Cell surface	MyD88-dependent induction of cytokines	Monocytes and cDCs, B cells > pDCs
TLR-7	Single-stranded RNA, imidazoquinoline drugs	Endosome	MyD88-dependent induction of type I IFNs and cytokines	pDCs and B cells >> cDCs > monocytes
TLR-8	Single-stranded RNA, imidazoquinoline drugs	Endosome	MyD88-dependent induction of type I IFNs and cytokines	Monocytes and cDCs
TLR-9	Unmethylated CpG DNA	Endosome	MyD88-dependent induction of cytokines and type I IFNs	pDCs and B cells
TLR-10	Unknown	Unknown	Unknown	B cells > cDCs and pDCs

cDCs, conventional dendritic cells; IFN, interferon; LPS, lipopolysaccharide; pDCs, plasmacytoid dendritic cells; RSV, respiratory syncytial virus.

binds nonmethylated CpG-containing DNA. These TLRs apparently function primarily in antiviral recognition and defense [231,246,247]. TLR9 also contributes to defense against bacteria and protozoans [248,249]. These TLRs preferentially recognize features of nucleic acids that are more common in microbes than mammals, but their specificity may be based on location as much as nucleic sequence: TLR3, TLR7, TLR8, and TLR9 detect nucleic acids in a location where they should not be found—acidified late endolysosomes. Individuals or mice lacking TLR3, TLR9, or a protein (UNC93B) required for proper localization of these TLRs to endosomes are unduly susceptible to infection with cytomegalovirus (CMV) and HSV [250,251].

A conserved cytoplasmic TIR (Toll/interleukin-receptor) domain links TLRs to downstream signaling pathways by interacting with adapter proteins, including MyD88 and TRIF [252–254]. MyD88 is involved in signaling downstream of all TLRs with the exception of TLR3. TLR signaling via MyD88 leads to the activation and translocation of the transcription factor nuclear factor κB (NFκB) to the nucleus and to the induction or activation by ERK/p38/JNK mitogen-activated protein kinases of other transcription factors, resulting in the production of the proinflammatory cytokines TNF, IL-1, and IL-6.

In addition to these transcription factors, activation of IRF3 or IRF7 or both is required for the induction of type I IFNs, which are key mediators of antiviral innate immunity. Activation of IRF3 and the production of type I IFNs downstream of TLR4 depend on TRIF. TRIF is also essential for the activation of IRF3 and for the production of type I IFNs and other cytokines via TLR3. Conversely,

TLR7, TLR8, and TLR9 use the adapter MyD88 to activate IRF7 and to induce the production of type I IFNs and other cytokines [255–258]. Consistent with their role in detection of bacterial, but not viral, structures, TLR2 and TLR5 do not induce type I IFNs.

Similar to the production of type I IFNs, the production of IL-12 and IL-27 (but not of the structurally related cytokine IL-23) is dependent on IRF3 and IRF7. Consequently, signals via TLR3, TLR4, and TLR7/8, but not via TLR2 and TLR5, can induce the production of these two cytokines; by contrast, each of these TLRs except TLR3, which signals exclusively via TRIF, can induce the production of IL-23. IL-23 promotes the production of IL-17 and IL-22, which contribute to host defenses to extracellular bacterial and fungal pathogens, whereas IL-12 and IL-27 stimulate IFN-γ production by NK cells and facilitate defense against viruses and other intracellular pathogens. Through the concerted regulation of IL-12, IL-27, and type I IFNs, IRF3 and IRF7 link TLR recognition to host defenses against intracellular pathogens. Production of the anti-inflammatory and immunomodulatory cytokine IL-10 depends on STAT3 activation in addition to NFκB and mitogen-activated protein kinase activation [259].

Other Innate Immune Pattern Recognition Receptors

Nucleotide binding domain–containing and leucine-rich repeat–containing receptors (NLRs) are a family of 23 proteins (in humans) [260,261]. These include NOD1, NOD2, and NALP3, which recognize components of bacterial peptidoglycan. NALP3 is also involved in responses to components of gram-positive bacteria, including bacterial RNA and DNA [262]; products of injured host cells such as uric acid; and noninfectious foreign substances, including asbestos and the widely used adjuvant alum [263,264]. IPAF is involved in responses to *Salmonella*. NOD1 and NOD2 can activate mitogen-activated protein kinase and NFκB pathways and proinflammatory cytokines in synergy with TLRs [215]. By contrast, NALP3 and IPAF activate a macromolecular complex known as the inflammasome, leading to the activation of caspase 1, which is required for secretion of the proinflammatory cytokines IL-1β and IL-18.

C-type lectin receptors are a family of proteins, which include DC-SIGN, a receptor on DCs that is involved in their interaction with human immunodeficiency virus (HIV), and the macrophage mannose receptor, Dectin-1, and Dectin-2, which are expressed by DCs and macrophages. Dectin-1 and Dectin-2 act together with TLR2 ligands present on fungi to induce the production of cytokines, including TNF-α, IL-6, and IL-10. The yeast form induces IL-12 and IL-23, whereas the hyphal form induces only IL-23 [265]. The mechanistic basis for these differences is presumed to involve differential signaling via Dectin-1 and Dectin-2 in combination with TLR2, but this remains to be shown.

There are three members of the retinoic acid inducible gene (RIG)-I–like receptor (RLR) family—RIG-I, MDA-5, and LGP2 [247,266,267]. RLRs are present in the cytoplasm of nearly all mammalian cells, where they provide rapid, cell-intrinsic, antiviral surveillance. RIG-I is important for host resistance to a wide variety of RNA viruses, including influenza, parainfluenza, and hepatitis C virus, whereas MDA-5 is important for resistance to picornaviruses. RIG-I and MDA-5 interact with a common signaling adapter (MAVS or IPS-1), which, similar to TRIF in the TLR3/4 pathway, induces the phosphorylation of IRF3 to stimulate production of type I IFNs.

Decoding the Nature of the Threat through Combinatorial Receptor Engagement

The differing molecular components of specific microbes result in the engagement of different combinations of innate immune recognition receptors. The innate immune system uses combinatorial receptor recognition patterns to decode the nature of the microbe and tailors the ensuing early innate response and the subsequent antigen-specific response to combat that specific type of infection. Extracellular bacteria engage TLR2, TLR4, or TLR5 on the cell surface and activate NLRs, providing a molecular signature of this type of pathogen. This leads to the production of proinflammatory cytokines and IL-23 to recruit neutrophils and support the development of a T_H17 type T-cell response (see "Differentiation of Activated Naïve T Cells into Effector and Memory Cells").

Fungal products engage TLR2 and Dectins, leading to a similar response [254,265,268]. Conversely, virus recognition via TLR3, TLR7, TLR8, TLR9, and RLRs stimulates the production of type I IFNs and IFN-induced chemokines (e.g., CXCL10), which induce and recruit CD8 and T_H1 cells. Nonviral intracellular bacterial pathogens also induce type I IFNs, which collaborate

with signals from cell surface TLRs and NLRs to induce the production of IL-12 and IL-27, resulting in T_H1 type responses. The importance of these innate sensing mechanisms is underscored by strategies that pathogenic microbes have evolved to evade them and the mediators they induce (for examples, see Yoneyama and Fujita [267] and Haga and Bowie [269]).

CYTOKINE PRODUCTION, TOLL-LIKE RECEPTORS, AND REGULATION OF INNATE IMMUNITY AND INFLAMMATION BY NEONATAL MONOCYTES AND MACROPHAGES

Much of the older literature suggested that neonatal blood mononuclear cells (BMCs), consisting of monocytes, DCs, B lymphocytes, T lymphocytes, and NK lymphocytes, and monocytes were less efficient in general in the production of cytokines in response to LPS, other (often impure) TLR ligands, or whole bacteria. More recently, because of simplicity and a desire to minimize manipulations that might activate or alter the functions of these cells, many studies have been done with whole blood to which TLR ligands are added directly ex vivo. For the most part, findings from these studies are consistent with the studies done using BMCs cultured in medium containing serum or plasma. The studies shown for whole blood and BMCs in Table 4–6 report cytokines assayed in culture supernatants of whole blood or BMCs that have been stimulated with TLR agonists. Responses to TLR2 and TLR4 agonists are grouped for simplicity and because in many of the studies done years ago the LPS used was contaminated with TLR2 agonists. Because of the more than 10-fold greater abundance of monocytes compared with DCs in blood and BMCs, and the limited production by lymphocytes of cytokines in response to TLR agonists, monocytes are likely to be the predominant source for most of these cytokines. This is not true, however, for stimuli that act via TLRs (e.g., TLR3 and TLR9) or cytokines (e.g., type I IFNs) that monocytes do not produce or produce poorly.

The preponderance of the currently available data does not support the notion of a general inability of neonatal monocytes and DCs to produce cytokines, but rather suggests a difference in the nature of their response. There is a clear, substantial, and with rare exception consistent deficit in the production of cytokines involved in protection against intracellular pathogens, including type I IFNs, IL-12, and IFN-γ in response to TLR agonists (see Table 4–6). Similarly, type I IFN production in response to HSV [270] and parainfluenza virus is reduced [271,272]. This reduced production likely reflects impaired IL-12 and type I IFN production by neonatal DCs, however, and impaired IL-12–induced and type I IFN–induced IFN-γ production by NK cells. The production by neonatal BMCs of IL-18, a cytokine that acts in concert with IL-12 and type I IFNs to induce IFN-γ production by NK cells, is also modestly reduced (approximately 65% of adult cells) [273]. In one study, IL-12 production by adult and neonatal BMCs was similar when they were stimulated with whole gram-positive

TABLE 4–6 Toll-like Receptor (TLR)–Induced Cytokine Production by Neonatal versus Adult Cells*

	Whole Blood			Blood Mononuclear			Monocytes		cDCs/moDCs			pDCs	
	TLR2/4	TLR3	TLR8	TLR2/4	TLR3	TLR8	TLR2/4	TLR8	TLR2/4	TLR3*	TLR8	TLR7	TLR9
Proinflammatory, T_H17, Extracellular Pathogens													
TNF-α	≤[†]	~	~	≤	≤	~	≤	~	≤	≤	~	<	<
IL-1	~		>	~		~	~		≤				
IL-6	>	>	>	≤	~	>	≤	~	~	≤	~	~	
IL-23	≤	>		≤		>	≤		≤	~	>		
IL-8	≤					~	>			≤	~		
Type I, T_H1, Intracellular Pathogens													
IL-12	<<	<<	<<	<<		<<			<<	<<	<<		
IFN-α/β	<<	≤	<<		≤	<<			<<	≤		<<	<<
IFN-γ	<<	<<	<<	<<	<<	<<							
CXCL9/10	<<								<<				
Anti-inflammatory, Immunoregulatory													
IL-10	>		>	≤		≤	≤		~	~	~		

cDCs, conventional dendritic cells; moDCs, monocyte-derived dendritic cells; pDCs, plasmacytoid dendritic cells; TLR, Toll-like receptor.
*Results are for moDCs, flow cytometric detection of IL-1 in cDCs present in whole blood, or are inferred to be from cDCs because only they among blood cells express TLR3 in substantial amounts and respond to stimulation with poly I:C.
†Production by cells from term neonates compared with adult cells.

References

Whole Blood
Cohen L, Haziot A, Shen DR, et al. CD14-independent responses to LPS require a serum factor that is absent from neonates. J Immunol 155:5337-5342, 1995.
Seghaye MC, et al. The production of pro- and anti-inflammatory cytokines in neonates assessed by stimulated whole cord blood culture and by plasma levels at birth. Biol Neonate 73:220-227, 1998.
Yachie A, et al. Defective production of interleukin-6 in very small premature infants in response to bacterial pathogens. Infect Immun 60:749-753, 1992.
Dembinski J, et al. Cell-associated interleukin-8 in cord blood of term and preterm infants. Clin Diagn Lab Immunol 9:320-323, 2002.
Levy O, et al. Selective impairment of TLR-mediated innate immunity in human newborns. J Immunol 173:4627-4634, 2004.
Drohan L, et al. Selective developmental defects of cord blood antigen-presenting cell subsets. Hum Immunol 65:1356-1369, 2004.
De Wit D, et al. Impaired responses to Toll-like receptor 4 and Toll-like receptor 3 ligands in human cord blood. J Autoimmun 21:277-281, 2003.
Keski-Nisula L, et al. Stimulated cytokine production correlates in umbilical arterial and venous blood at delivery. Eur Cytokine Netw 15:347-352, 2004.
Forster-Waldl E, et al. Monocyte toll-like receptor 4 expression and LPS-induced cytokine production increase during gestational aging. Pediatr Res 58:121-124, 2005.
Sadeghi K, et al. Immaturity of infection control in preterm and term newborns is associated with impaired toll-like receptor signaling. J Infect Dis 195:296-302, 2007.
Aksoy E, et al. Interferon regulatory factor 3-dependent responses to lipopolysaccharide are selectively blunted in cord blood cells. Blood 109:2887-2893, 2007.
Levy O. et al. The adenosine system selectively inhibits TLR-mediated TNF-alpha production in the newborn. J Immunol 177:1956-1966, 2006.
Levy O, et al. Unique efficacy of Toll-like receptor 8 agonists in activating human neonatal antigen-presenting cells. Blood 108:1284-1290, 2006.
Angelone DF, et al. Innate immunity of the human newborn is polarized toward a high ratio of IL-6/TNF-alpha production in vitro and in vivo. Pediatr Res 60:205-209, 2006.
Kollmann TR, et al. Neonatal innate TLR-mediated responses are distinct from those of adults. J Immunol 183:7150-7160, 2009.

Blood Mononuclear Cells
Liechty KW, et al. Production of interleukin-6 by fetal and maternal cells in vivo during intra-amniotic infection and in vitro after stimulation with interleukin-1. Pediatr Res 29:1-4, 1991.
Prescott SL, et al. Clinical effects of probiotics are associated with increased interferon-gamma responses in very young children with atopic dermatitis. Clin Exp Allergy 35:1557-1664, 2005.
Taniguchi T, et al. Fetal mononuclear cells show a comparable capacity with maternal mononuclear cells to produce IL-8 in response to lipopolysaccharide in chorioamnionitis. J Reprod Immunol 23:1-12, 1993.
Lee SM, et al. Decreased interleukin-12 (IL12) from activated cord versus adult peripheral blood mononuclear cells and upregulation of interferon-gamma, natural killer, and lymphokine-activated killer activity by IL-12 in cord blood mononuclear cells. Blood 88:945-954, 1996.
Levy O, et al. The adenosine system selectively inhibits TLR-mediated TNF-alpha production in the newborn. J Immunol 177:1956-1966, 2006.
Levy O, et al. Unique efficacy of Toll-like receptor 8 agonists in activating human neonatal antigen-presenting cells. Blood 108:1284-1290, 2006.
Yerkovich ST, et al. Postnatal development of monocyte cytokine responses to bacterial lipopolysaccharide. Pediatr Res 62:547-552, 2007.
Kollmann TR, et al. Neonatal innate TLR-mediated responses are distinct from those of adults. J Immunol 183:7150-7160, 2009.

Monocytes
Burchett SK, et al. Regulation of tumor necrosis factor/cachectin and IL-1 secretion in human mononuclear phagocytes. J Immunol 140:3473-3481, 1988.
Schibler KR, et al. Defective production of interleukin-6 by monocytes: a possible mechanism underlying several host defense deficiencies of neonates. Pediatr Res 31:18-21, 1992.
Rowen JL, Smith CW, Edwards MS. Group B streptococci elicit leukotriene B4 and interleukin-8 from human monocytes: neonates exhibit a diminished response. J Infect Dis 172:420-426, 1995.
Hebra A, et al. Intracellular cytokine production by fetal and adult monocytes. J Pediatr Surg 36:1321-1326, 2001.
Schultz C, et al. Enhanced interleukin-6 and interleukin-8 synthesis in term and preterm infants. Pediatr Res 51:317-322, 2002.
Aksoy E, et al. Interferon regulatory factor 3-dependent responses to lipopolysaccharide are selectively blunted in cord blood cells. Blood 109:2887-2893, 2007.
Levy O, et al. Selective impairment of TLR-mediated innate immunity in human newborns. J Immunol 173:4627-4634, 2004.
Levy O, et al. Unique efficacy of Toll-like receptor 8 agonists in activating human neonatal antigen-presenting cells. Blood 108:1284-1290, 2006.
Angelone DF, et al. Innate immunity of the human newborn is polarized toward a high ratio of IL-6/TNF-alpha production in vitro and in vivo. Pediatr Res 60:205-209, 2006.
Yerkovich ST, et al. Postnatal development of monocyte cytokine responses to bacterial lipopolysaccharide. Pediatr Res 62:547-552, 2007.
Kollmann TR, et al. Neonatal innate TLR-mediated responses are distinct from those of adults. J Immunol 183:7150-7160, 2009.

cDCs/moDCs
Goriely S, et al. A defect in nucleosome remodeling prevents IL-12(p35) gene transcription in neonatal dendritic cells. J Exp Med 199:1011-1016, 2004.
Langrish CL, et al. Neonatal dendritic cells are intrinsically biased against Th-1 immune responses. Clin Exp Immunol 128:118-123, 2002.
Upham JW, et al. Development of interleukin-12-producing capacity throughout childhood. Infect Immun 70:6583-6588, 2002.
Drohan L, et al. Selective developmental defects of cord blood antigen-presenting cell subsets. Hum Immunol 65:1356-1369, 2004.
ven den Eijnden S, et al. Preferential production of the IL-12(p40)/IL-23(p19) heterodimer by dendritic cells from human newborns. Eur J Immunol 36:21-16, 2006.
Aksoy E, et al. Interferon regulatory factor 3-dependent responses to lipopolysaccharide are selectively blunted in cord blood cells. Blood 109:2887-2893, 2007.
Krumbiegel D, Zepp F, Meyer CU. Combined Toll-like receptor agonists synergistically increase production of inflammatory cytokines in human neonatal dendritic cells. Hum Immunol 68:813-822, 2007.
Kollmann TR, et al. Neonatal innate TLR-mediated responses are distinct from those of adults. J Immunol 183:7150-7160, 2009.

pDCs
De Wit D, et al. Blood plasmacytoid dendritic cell responses to CpG oligodeoxynucleotides are impaired in human newborns. Blood 103:1030-1032, 2004.
Gold MC, et al. Human neonatal dendritic cells are competent in MHC class I antigen processing and presentation. PLoS ONE 2:e957, 2007.
Danis B, et al. Interferon regulatory factor 7-mediated responses are defective in cord blood plasmacytoid dendritic cells. Eur J Immunol 38:507-517, 2008.
Kollmann TR, et al. Neonatal innate TLR-mediated responses are distinct from those of adults. J Immunol 183:7150-7160, 2009.

or gram-negative bacteria [274], suggesting that activation of neonatal cells with particles that contain multiple TLR and NLR ligands may be sufficient to overcome this deficit.

With the exception of TNF-α, production by neonatal cells of cytokines central to host defense against extracellular bacterial and fungal pathogens, acute inflammation, and T$_H$17-type responses seems not to be greatly decreased and in some cases is more robust. IL-1 production by cells from term neonates and adults is similar or at most marginally reduced, whereas neonatal cells generally produce more IL-6, IL-8, and IL-23. In more limited studies with cells from preterm neonates, production of IL-8 in response to LPS was also greater than production by adult cells [275], whereas production of TNF-α and IL-6 was reduced [271,276–278]. A similar deficit in TNF-α production is evident in response to stimulation with TLR2, TLR3, and TLR5 agonists [279,280], particularly when whole blood is used or BMCs or monocytes are cultured in high (≥50%) concentrations of neonatal serum. By contrast, TNF-α production in response to TLR8 agonists or whole gram-positive or gram-negative bacteria is similar [274]. Although some early studies suggested that the production of the immunoregulatory and anti-inflammatory cytokine IL-10 by neonatal cells was reduced [281,282], most studies have found greater production of IL-10 by whole blood and equal or greater production by BMCs [271,274,280,283,284].

The basis for lower production of certain cytokines by neonatal monocytes and macrophages in response to microbial products that signal through TLRs is incompletely understood. Cell surface expression of TLR2 and TLR4 by adult and neonatal monocytes is similar [161,279,284–288], and expression of CD14, which facilitates responses to LPS and TLR2 agonists, is similar or at most slightly reduced on neonatal monocytes [161,279,285,287,289–291]. To our knowledge, there are no published data on the expression of other TLR proteins by neonatal monocytes. By reverse transcriptase polymerase chain reaction analysis, neonatal and adult monocytes contain similar amounts of TLR1 through TLR9, MD-2, CD14, MyD88, TIRAP, and IRAK4 mRNA [279]; however, monocytes are known not to express TLR3 or TLR9, clouding the interpretation of some of these findings.

One group reported that neonatal monocytes have reduced amounts of MyD88 protein [287], but found no difference between adult and neonatal monocytes in LPS-induced activation of ERK1/2 and p38 kinases and phosphorylation and degradation of IκB, events that are downstream of MyD88 [287]. Decreased expression of MyD88 is insufficient to explain the diminished induction of HLA-DR and CD40 on neonatal monocytes in response to LPS [161] or of CD40 and CD80 on neonatal monocyte-derived dendritic cells (moDCs) in response to LPS and poly I:C [271] because these TLR ligands induce costimulatory molecules by TRIF-dependent and type I IFN–dependent, but MyD88-independent pathways [228,231,292,293]. Others reported diminished activation of p38 kinase in monocytes and production of TNF in response to the TLR4 ligand LPS, but not in response to TLR8 ligands [279,285,294]; these studies were done

using whole blood or cells cultured in high concentrations of autologous plasma, in contrast to the study reporting no difference in p38 activation.

Levy and colleagues [37,279] concluded that differences between neonatal and adult plasma in addition to cell intrinsic differences contribute to decreased production of TNF-α and greater or equal production of IL-6 in response to LPS and TLR2 agonists by neonatal versus adult monocytes. Compared with blood from healthy adults, neonatal cord blood contains lower amounts of soluble CD14 and similar or modestly reduced amounts of soluble LPS-binding protein; concentrations of CD14 and LPS-binding protein increase to adult levels in the first week of life and increase further in response to infection, as they do in adults [295].

The reduced amounts of these two proteins may account for the earlier observation that neonatal cord blood contains lower amounts of a soluble protein, which facilitates the response of monocytes to LPS [289]. The addition of soluble CD14 to neonatal plasma did not restore TNF-α production by neonatal monocytes, however. Rather, the authors proposed that elevated concentrations of adenosine in cord blood plasma, in concert with increased intracellular concentrations of cyclic adenosine monophosphate (cAMP) induced in neonatal monocytes by adenosine, inhibit TNF and enhance IL-6 and IL-10 production by these cells [37]. Adenosine is induced by hypoxia, suggesting that the elevated adenosine concentrations may be a transient phenomenon alleviated shortly after birth. Perhaps consistent with this possibility, the robust production of IL-6, IL-8, and IL-10 in response to stimulation with LPS and IFN-γ by neonatal BMCs was found to be transient and replaced by decreased production at 1 month of age [284]. These findings have not yet been replicated and were obtained with cryopreserved cells, and the potential contribution of adenosine to these differences is unknown. The relative similarity of findings regarding cytokine production using whole blood and BMCs cultured in heterologous serum and the absence of differences in TNF-α production in response to TLR8 agonists under any conditions suggest that cell intrinsic factors are substantially responsible for the differences between adult and neonatal cells.

SUMMARY

Monocytes and macrophages are detected in early fetal life and are present in blood and tissues by late gestation in amount similar to adults. An exception is lung alveolar macrophages, which are few in number before birth, increase rapidly after birth in term neonates, but may be delayed in preterm neonates. Recruitment of monocytes to sites of infection and inflammation is slower than in adults. Ingestion and killing of pathogens by neonatal monocytes is as competent as in adults, but neonatal macrophages may be less efficient and be activated less efficiently by IFN-γ. Although expression by neonatal and adult monocytes of TLRs and other innate immune receptors seems not to differ greatly, their responses to stimulation via these receptors differ. In response to most, but not all, microbial stimuli, neonatal BMCs produce (1) substantially lower amounts of IL-12 and type I IFNs, which are cytokines produced primarily by DCs and important for defense against intracellular pathogens; (2) moderately less TNF-α; (3) similar or greater amounts of other proinflammatory cytokines and IL-23, which are cytokines produced primarily by monocytes and important in defense against extracellular bacterial and fungal pathogens; and (4) similar or greater amounts of the anti-inflammatory and immunoregulatory cytokine IL-10.

DENDRITIC CELLS—THE LINK BETWEEN INNATE AND ADAPTIVE IMMUNITY

In addition to resident macrophages, all tissues contain resident DCs. DCs are also found in the blood, where they represent approximately 0.5% to 1% of BMCs in adults. DCs derive their name from the characteristic cytoplasmic protrusions or dendrites found on mature DCs. DCs do not express cell surface molecules used to identify other white blood cell lineages, but they do express class II MHC molecules (e.g., HLA-DR), and mature DCs express much greater amounts of class II MHC than any other cell type [161,296–298]. (MHC and HLA molecules are discussed in "Antigen Presentation by Classic Major Histocompatibility Complex Molecules"). DCs are lineage marker–negative (Lin$^-$), HLA-DR$^+$ mononuclear cells and can be identified and purified on this basis.

DCs are heterogeneous. The major subtypes in humans are cDCs, often referred to as myeloid DCs, which are CD11c$^+$CD123$^-$, and plasmacytoid DCs (pDCs), which are CD11c$^-$CD123$^+$. Both of these DC subsets are derived from bone marrow progenitors that give rise to other lymphoid and myeloid cell lineages [299], although the precise lineage relationships remain controversial [300]. Production and survival of cDCs is enhanced by GM-CSF, and cells similar, although not identical, to cDCs can be generated by culturing monocytes in GM-CSF plus IL-4 to produce moDCs. By contrast, pDCs express IL-3 receptors (CD123 is IL-3Rα), and IL-3 enhances their survival in vitro. Langerhans cells are a unique type of DC found only in the epidermis, where they can be differentiated from dermal cDCs by their expression of Langerin and S100 antigens and by intracellular Birbeck granules [300,301].

Langerhans cells and dermal cDCs are found in fetal skin by 16 weeks of gestation [302], and immature cDCs are found in the interstitium of solid organs by this age. Cells with the features of immature pDCs are found in fetal lymph nodes by 19 to 21 weeks of gestation [303]. DCs constitute a similar fraction (0.5% to 1%) of BMCs in neonates, children, and adults, but pDCs predominate in cord blood, constituting about 75% of the total, whereas cDCs constitute about 75% of the total in adults [161,304–307]. The absolute number of cDCs remains constant from the neonatal period into adulthood, whereas the fraction and absolute number of pDCs decline with increasing postnatal age, reaching numbers similar to adults at 5 years of age or older [306]. The biologic significance of the predominance of pDCs in the neonatal circulation is uncertain.

PROPERTIES AND FUNCTIONS OF CONVENTIONAL DENDRITIC CELLS

cDCs play a unique and essential role in the initiation and modulation of the adaptive immune response. cDCs in the blood and uninflamed tissues are immature, in that they express low to moderate amounts of MHC class I and class II molecules on their surface. In the steady-state conditions that prevail in uninfected individuals, there is a constant low-level turnover of cDCs. New cDCs enter from the blood, and others migrate via lymphatics to secondary lymphoid tissues where they play a central role in maintaining a state of tolerance to self-antigens by presenting them to T cells in the absence of costimulatory signals required for T-cell activation [308]. In response to infection, the influx of immature cDCs and monocytes, which can give rise to immature cDCs, from the blood is induced by inflammatory chemokines produced by resident tissue macrophages and cDCs. In these tissues, immature cDCs take up microbes and microbial antigens and at the same time are induced to express on their surface the CCR7 chemokine receptor and to lose expression of receptors for chemokines present in the tissues. This change in chemokine receptor expression enhances cDC migration via lymphatics to T cell–rich areas of the draining lymph nodes, which constitutively express chemokines that bind to CCR7 (CCL19, CCL21).

Concomitant with their migration to the draining lymph nodes, DCs mature. As they do, uptake of microbes and antigens ceases, and antigenic peptides derived from previously internalized microbes and antigens are displayed on their cell surface in the groove of MHC class I and class II molecules. These peptide–MHC complexes are present on the surface of mature DCs in great abundance, as are the costimulatory molecules, CD40, CD80 (B7-1), and CD86 (B7-2), which together allow these cells to present antigens to T cells in a highly effective manner (see "Antigen Presentation") [309]. DCs not only play a crucial role in T-cell activation, but they also influence the quality of the T-cell response that ensues through the production of cytokines [231,310,311]. IL-12, IL-27, and type I IFNs instruct naïve CD4 T cells to produce IFN-γ and to differentiate into T_H1 cells, which help to protect against viruses and other intracellular pathogens, whereas IL-6, TGF-β, and IL-23 induce naïve T cells to become T_H17 cells, which help to protect against extracellular bacteria and fungi, and T_H2 cells develop in the absence of these cytokines and the presence of thymic stromal lymphopoietin (TSLP) produced by epithelial cells [312]. The function and localization of cDCs are highly plastic and rapidly modulated in response to infection and inflammation, which allows them to induce and instruct the nature of the T-cell response.

DC migration and maturation can be triggered by various stimuli, including pathogen-derived products that are recognized directly by innate immune receptors; by cytokines, including IL-1, TNF-α, and type I IFNs (see Tables 4–1 and 4–2); and by engagement of CD40 on the DC surface by CD40 ligand (CD154) on the surface of activated CD4 T cells (see Table 4–4). cDCs express multiple TLRs [231,232,261,266], but do not express

TLR9 (see Table 4–5) and consequently are not activated by unmethylated CpG DNA, a potent inducer of IFN-α production by pDCs. In contrast to pDCs (and monocytes), cDCs express TLR3 (see Table 4–5), however, which, along with RIG-I, allows them to produce type I IFNs and other cytokines in response to double-stranded RNAs, including poly I:C (polyinosinic:polycytidylic acid).

FETAL CONVENTIONAL DENDRITIC CELLS

Expression of MHC class II (HLA-DR), CD40, CD80, and CD86 on neonatal and on adult blood cDCs is similar [161,271,304]. Consistent with these findings, cord blood DCs can stimulate allogeneic cord blood T cells in vitro [305,313,314]. Whether neonatal cDCs are proficient in processing and presenting foreign antigens to T cells, however, or are as effective as adult cells in doing so is unclear from these studies. When blood was stimulated with LPS or poly I:C, neonatal cDCs matured less completely, upregulating HLA-DR and CD86 to a similar degree, but CD40 and CD80 less than adult cDCs [271]. Decreased maturation of neonatal blood cDCs was also observed in response to pertussis toxin [315]. By contrast to blood cDCs, neonatal moDCs (commonly used as a more readily available, but possibly imperfect surrogate for neonatal cDCs) have decreased allostimulatory activity; have lower expression of HLA-DR, CD40, and CD80; and upregulate CD86 expression less in response to LPS or a TLR7/8 agonist than adult moDCs [219,316–319]. Impaired upregulation of CD86 was not observed when neonatal moDCs were stimulated with these two agonists in combination or with poly I:C, suggesting that these limitations in neonatal moDC function may be overcome in certain contexts [319].

The available data regarding cytokine production by neonatal cDCs, or by moDCs used as surrogate for cDCs, are consistent with the trends observed in studies comparing neonatal whole blood and BMCs: Neonatal cDCs and moDCs produce much lower amounts of type I/T_H1–inducing cytokines, moderately less of the proinflammatory cytokine TNF-α, and comparable or greater amounts of other proinflammatory and T_H17-inducing cytokines and the anti-inflammatory and immunoregulatory cytokine IL-10 (Fig. 4–3). Data regarding cytokine production by cDCs are sparse and have been obtained by flow cytometric detection of intracellular cytokines after stimulation of whole blood or BMCs with TLR agonists. In these studies, neonatal cDCs were approximately 50% as efficient as adult cDCs at producing TNF-α in response LPS. Less difference was seen in TNF-α production in response to TLR8 agonists, and IL-1α and IL-6 production were similar in response to both (see Table 4–6) [161,320].

Because poly I:C activates cells of the blood primarily via TLR3, and cDCs are the only cells in blood that express substantial amounts of TLR3, one can infer that the modestly diminished production of type I IFNs and markedly diminished production of IL-12 by poly I:C–stimulated whole blood and BMCs reflects production by cDCs [271,320]. Likewise, the production of IFN-γ by poly I:C–stimulated neonatal whole blood and BMCs likely reflects diminished IL-12 and type I IFN production by cDCs, which results in diminished production of IFN-γ by neonatal NK cells (see "Natural Killer Cells").

These inferences and other data indicating a selective reduction in type I/T_H1 T cell–inducing cytokine by neonatal cells are supported by data from studies done with moDCs. With the exception of one study [321], neonatal moDCs have been shown consistently to produce much less IL-12 in response to LPS, poly I:C, and TLR8 ligands or engagement of CD40 than adult moDCs [318,319,322]. This is paralleled by reduced production of type I IFNs and of the IFN-dependent chemokines CXCL9, CXCL10, and CXCL11 [323]. Neonatal cDCs [320] and moDCs [318,323] produce comparable amounts of the p40 component common to IL-12 and IL-23, but much reduced amounts of the p35 component specific for IL-12. Diminished p35 production seems to result from a defect in IRF3 binding to and remodeling of the IL-12 promoter, whereas more proximal aspects of signaling resulting in IRF3 translocation from the cytoplasm to the nucleus seem to be intact [288,323].

Because IRF3 is also required for the production of type I IFNs in response to LPS or poly I:C, this IRF3 defect is also likely to be an important factor in the diminished production of type I IFNs. The basis for this IRF3 defect is incompletely understood. Stimulation with whole gram-positive or gram-negative bacteria induces substantial and equal IL-12 production by adult and neonatal BMCs, however [274]. Although neonatal moDCs stimulated with live *Mycobacterium bovis* bacillus Calmette-Guérin (BCG) [324]

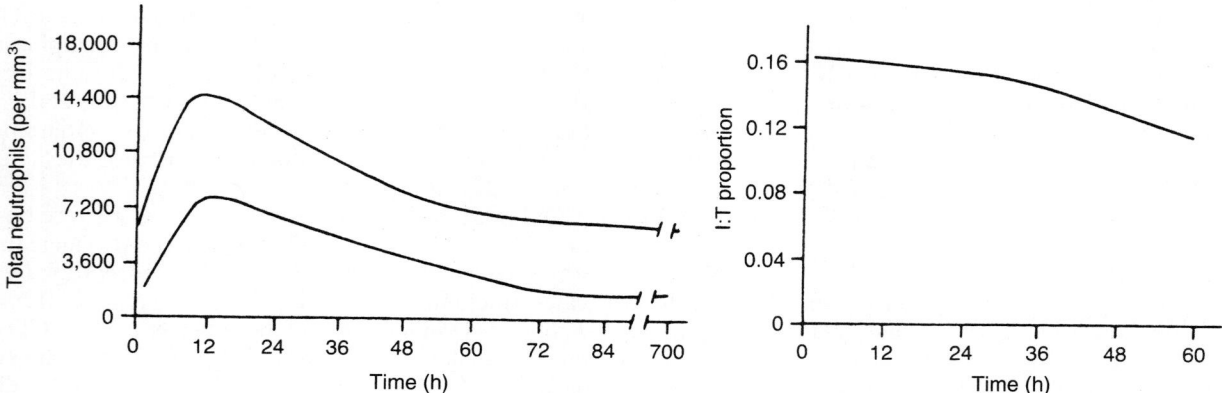

FIGURE 4–3 Change in total number of neutrophils (*left*) and in ratio of immature to total neutrophils (I:T) (*right*) in the neonate. (*Data from Manroe BL, et al. The neonatal blood count in health and disease, I: reference values for neutrophilic cells. J Pediatr 95:89-98, 1979.*)

or with a TLR8 agonist plus LPS or poly I:C secreted much less IL-12 than adult moDCs, when moDCs were stimulated with these combinations of TLR ligands in cultures also containing autologous naïve CD4 T cells, comparable, IL-12–dependent IFN-γ production was observed [319]. Together, these observations suggest that defective production of IFN-γ–inducing cytokines, including IL-12, by neonatal DCs can be overcome by combined signaling from TLRs, NLRs, and direct physical interactions between T cells and DCs. This suggestion has not been tested directly, however.

PROPERTIES AND FUNCTIONS OF ADULT AND NEONATAL PLASMACYTOID DENDRITIC CELLS

Immature pDCs are found in the blood, secondary lymphoid organs, and particularly inflamed lymph nodes [296,301]. The predominant function of pDCs is not antigen presentation to T cells, but rather the production of cytokines that help to protect against viral infection directly and through the induction of type I/T$_H$1 T-cell responses. Consistent with this function, pDCs do not seem to employ NLRs, C-type lectin receptors, or RLRs to recognize and respond to microbes. Rather, recognition and response are triggered through the two TLRs they express in abundance, TLR7 and TLR9 (see Table 4–5), allowing them to respond to single-stranded RNA from RNA viruses such as influenza and unmethylated CpG DNA from bacteria and viruses such as HSV [325–327].

Early studies showed diminished numbers of neonatal versus adult white blood cells producing IFN-α in response to HSV [270]. That this deficiency was attributable to diminished production by pDCs was shown more recently [304,328]. Reduced type I IFN production by neonatal pDCs was also observed in response to CMV. Neonatal pDCs also produce less type I IFNs in response to unmethylated CpG oligonucleotides and to synthetic TLR7 ligands [328]. This defect in type I IFN production seems to result in part from impaired activation and translocation of IRF7 to the nucleus [328]. Consistent with these findings, production of the NF-κB–dependent cytokine TNF-α is more modestly reduced, and production of IL-6 is comparable to adult pDCs [328].

Although pDCs in the blood and uninflamed tissues have a very limited capacity for antigen uptake and presentation, stimulation of these cells via TLR7 or TLR9 results in their upregulation of CCR7 and migration to T cell–rich areas of lymph nodes, upregulation of HLA-DR and costimulatory molecules, and increased capacity to present antigen to T cells. Neonatal blood pDCs express lower amounts of HLA-DR, CD40, CD80, CD86, and CCR7 after stimulation with TLR7 or TLR9 agonists than adults pDCs [304,328,329].

SUMMARY

DCs are detectable by 16 weeks of gestation. At birth, the concentration of cDCs is similar and the concentration of pDCs greater than in adult blood. Although adult and neonatal blood cDCs and moDCs express on their surface the MHC class II molecule HLA-DR and costimulatory molecules in similar abundance, expression by neonatal DCs

increases less in response to stimulation via TLRs. TLR-stimulated neonatal cDCs and moDCs generally produce substantially less IL-12 and type I IFNs, cytokines that contribute to early innate defenses and subsequent T cell–mediated defenses against intracellular pathogens, although they produce proinflammatory cytokines and IL-23, which are important in defense against extracellular bacterial and fungal pathogens, much more efficiently. Neonatal pDCs are also selectively deficient in the production of type I IFNs and IFN-dependent chemokines. These differences may limit the ability of neonatal DCs to activate naïve pathogen-specific T cells and in particular to induce IFN-γ–producing T$_H$1 T-cell responses, rather than T$_H$17 or T$_H$2 T-cell responses. Neonatal DCs may be able, however, to produce IL-12 and support IFN-γ production by neonatal T cells in response to combinatorial activation of innate immune receptors and in contact with T cells.

NATURAL KILLER CELLS
OVERVIEW AND DEVELOPMENT

NK cells are large granular lymphocytes with cytotoxic function, which, in contrast to T and B lymphocytes, are part of the innate rather than adaptive immune system. In clinical practice, NK cells are usually defined as cells that express CD56, a molecule of uncertain function, but not CD3 (i.e., CD56$^+$CD3$^-$) [330]. Virtually all circulating NK cells from adults also express the NK cell–specific NKp30 and NKp46 receptors [331,332]. They also express CD2 and CD161, and approximately 50% express CD57 [333,334], but these molecules are found on other cell types as well.

The fetal liver produces NK cells by 6 weeks of gestation, but the bone marrow is the major site for NK-cell production from late gestation onward. NK cells are derived from CD34$^+$ bone marrow cells that lack surface molecules specific for other cell lineages (i.e., CD34$^+$Lin$^-$ cells), but expressing CD7 or CD38 [335,336]. These CD34$^+$CD7$^+$Lin$^-$ cells can also differentiate into NK cells and DCs, depending on the culture conditions employed, suggesting the existence of a common T/NK/lymphoid DC progenitor [337,338]. The precise point at which there is an irreversible commitment to NK-cell lineage development is unclear. In vitro studies suggest an NK lineage cell developmental sequence in which CD161 is acquired early in NK development [339]. At the next developmental stage, NKp30, NKp46, 2B4, and NKG2D are expressed on the cell surface [340,341], followed by members of the killer cell inhibitor receptor (KIR) family, CD94-NKG2A, CD2, and CD56; the function of these molecules is discussed in the sections that follow.

NK cells are functionally defined by their natural ability to lyse virally infected or tumor target cells in a non–HLA-restricted manner that does not require prior sensitization [342]. NK cells preferentially recognize and kill cells with reduced or absent expression of self-HLA class I molecules, a property referred to as natural cytotoxicity. This is in contrast to cytotoxic CD8 T cells, which are triggered to lyse targets after the recognition of foreign antigenic peptides bound to self-HLA class I molecules or self-peptides bound to foreign HLA class I molecules. NK cells also have the ability to kill target cells that are coated with IgG antibodies, a process known as antibody-dependent cellular cytotoxicity (ADCC). ADCC requires the recognition of IgG bound to the target cell by the NK cell FcγRIIIB receptor (CD16) [343].

Mature NK cells can be subdivided into CD56^{hi}CD16^{lo} and CD56^{lo}CD16^{hi} populations [344,345]. CD56^{hi}CD16^{lo} cells usually are only a minority of mature NK cells in the circulation, but express CCR7 and L-selectin and predominate in lymph node tissue. CD56^{hi}CD16^{lo} cells have limited cytotoxic capacity, but produce cytokines and chemokines efficiently, whereas the inverse is true for CD56^{lo}CD16^{hi} NK cells [346]. These features suggest that the CD56^{hi}CD16^{lo} subset could regulate lymph node T cells and DCs through cytokine secretion. Developmental studies suggest that CD56^{hi}CD16^{lo} NK cells are less mature than CD56^{lo}CD16^{hi} NK cells, but the precise precursor product relationship of these subsets under various conditions in vivo has not been firmly established.

NK cells are particularly important in the early containment of viral infections, especially with pathogens that may initially avoid control by adaptive immune mechanisms. Infection of host cells by the herpesvirus group, including HSV, CMV, and varicella-zoster virus (VZV), and some adenoviruses leads to decreased surface expression of HLA class I molecules, which is discussed in more detail in "Host Defense against Specific Classes of Neonatal Pathogens." Viral protein–mediated decreases in expression of HLA class I may limit the ability of CD8 T cells to lyse virally infected cells and to clonally expand from naïve precursors. These virus-mediated effects may be particularly important during early infection, when CD8 T cells with appropriate antigen specificity are present at a low frequency. By contrast, decreased HLA class I expression facilitates recognition and lysis by NK cells. The importance of NK cells in the initial control of human herpesvirus infections is suggested by the observation that individuals with selective deficiency of NK cell numbers or function are prone to severe infection with HSV, CMV, and VZV [347].

NATURAL KILLER CELL RECEPTORS

NK-cell cytotoxicity is regulated by a complex array of inhibitory and activating receptor-ligand interactions with target cells (Fig. 4–4). NK-cell activation is inhibited by recognition of HLA class I molecules expressed on nontransformed, uninfected cells; this recognition is presumed to provide a net inhibitory signal that predominates over activating signals. Infection of the host target cell can reduce the amount of HLA class I on the cell surface, reducing inhibitory signaling, and upregulate other molecules that promote NK-cell activation, such as MHC class I–related chains A and B (MICA and MICB).

There are two major families of NK-cell receptors that recognize HLA class I molecules in humans: KIR and CD94-containing C-type lectin families [348,349]. KIRs with a long cytoplasmic domain transmit signals that inhibit NK-cell activation; most, although not all, NK cells express one or more inhibitory KIRs on their surface. Most NK cells, including all NK cells not expressing any inhibitory KIRs, also express inhibitory CD94-NKG2A receptors [350]. KIRs bind to polymorphic HLA-B, HLA-C, or HLA-A molecules [349], whereas CD94-NKG2A binds to HLA-E, which is monomorphic (HLA molecules are discussed in "Antigen Presentation by Classic and Nonclassic Major Histocompatibility Complex Molecules"). Because HLA-E reaches the cell surface only when its peptide-binding groove is occupied by hydrophobic peptides derived from the leader

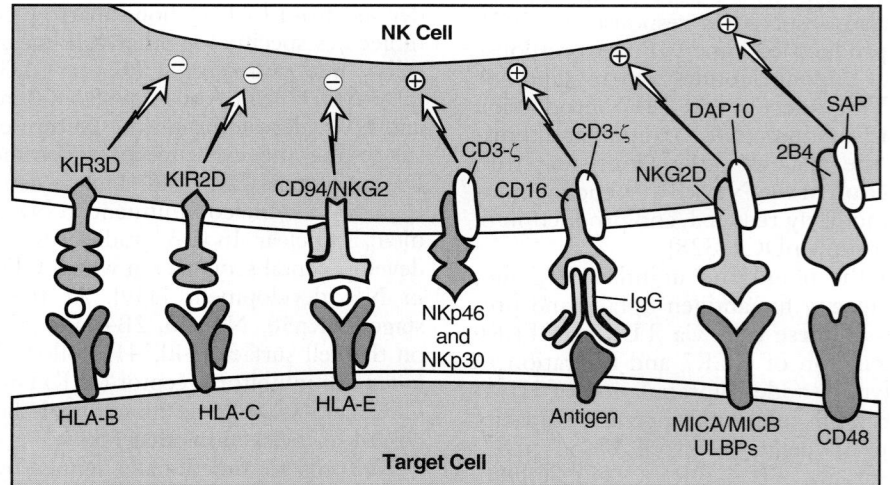

FIGURE 4–4 Positive and negative regulation of natural killer (NK) -cell cytotoxicity by receptor/ligand interactions. NK-cell cytotoxicity is inhibited by engagement of killer inhibitory receptors (KIR) by major histocompatibility complex (MHC) class I molecules, such as HLA-B and HLA-C. In addition, NK cells are inhibited when CD94/NKG2 complex, a member of the C-type lectin family, on the NK cell is engaged by HLA-E. HLA-E binds hydrophobic leader peptides derived from HLA-A, HLA-B, and HLA-C molecules and requires these for its surface expression. HLA-E surface expression on a potential target cell indicates the overall production of conventional MHC class I molecules. These inhibitory influences on NK-cell cytotoxicity are overcome if viral infection of the target cell results in decreased MHC class I and HLA-E levels. NK-cell cytotoxicity is positively regulated by the engagement of NKG2D, which interacts with MICA, MICB, and ULBPs; 2B4, which interacts with CD48; and natural cytotoxicity receptors, such as NKp30 and NKp46, for which the ligands on the target cell are unknown. CD16 is an Fc receptor for IgG and mediates antibody-dependent cellular cytotoxicity against cells coated with antibody (e.g., against viral proteins found on the cell surface). Positive receptors mediate their intracellular signals via associated CD3-ζ, FcER1, DAP10, or DAP12 proteins. MICA and MICB, MHC class I -related chains A and B; ULBPs, UL16-binding proteins (UL16 is a cytomegalovirus protein).

sequences of HLA-A, HLA-B, and HLA-C molecules [351], the amount of HLA-E on the cell surface reflects the overall levels of HLA-A, HLA-B, and HLA-C molecules on that cell [352].

In addition to CD94-NKG2A, a third group of inhibitory receptors that broadly recognize HLA class I molecules are the leukocyte immunoglobulin-like receptors B1 and B2 (LILRB1 and LILRB2). LILRB1 and LILRB2, also referred to as LIR1/CD85J and LIR2/CD85d, bind to HLA-A, HLA-B, and HLA-C molecules and the nonconventional class I molecules HLA-E, HLA-F, and HLA-G. HLA-G is the only HLA class I molecule constitutively expressed on the surface of fetal trophoblast. The interaction of LILRB1 and LILRB2 with HLA-G is thought to protect the placenta from injury by maternal NK cells [353].

Countering the effects of these inhibitory receptors are multiple types of activating receptors. NKG2D is found on NK cells and on certain T-cell populations. NKG2D recognizes MICA and MICB and UL16-binding proteins (ULBPs). MICA and MICB are nonclassic HLA class I molecules that are expressed on stressed or infected cells [354]. ULPBs are a group of HLA class I–like molecules expressed on many cell types that were first identified and named based on their ability to bind to the human CMV UL16 viral protein. In CMV infection, the secretion of UL16 probably limits NK cell–mediated and T cell–mediated activation by binding to ULBPs on the surface of the infected cell. Little is known of how ULBP expression is regulated during infection in vivo.

NK cells also express NKp30, NKp44, and NKp46. NKp44 and NKp46 can trigger NK cell cytotoxicity through their recognition of influenza virus hemagglutinin and Sendai (parainfluenza family) virus hemagglutinin-neuraminidase [355]. The importance of such NK cell recognition in influenza infection in vivo is unknown, however, and may be limited by the ability of NK cells to reach the respiratory epithelial cell, the major cell type that is productively infected. These receptors also recognize ligands on tumor cells and cells infected with herpesviruses, but the nature of the ligands is unknown.

The proteins 2B4 (CD244) and NTBA are members of the signaling lymphocyte activation molecule (SLAM) protein family and are expressed on most NK cells [356]. 2B4 binds to CD48, whereas the ligand for NTBA remains unclear. 2B4 and NTBA engagement triggers NK-cell activation through SLAM-associated protein (SAP), an intracellular adapter protein. X-linked lymphoproliferative syndrome is due to genetic deficiency of SAP and results in severe, often life-threatening infection from primary Epstein-Barr virus (EBV) infection, with a high associated risk for the development of lymphoma or chronic hypogammaglobulinemia [356]. SAP deficiency allows alternative molecules, the SH2-domain–containing phosphatases (SHPs), to bind the cytoplasmic tails of 2B4 and NTBA. This results in inhibition of NK-cell function, rather than merely the loss of activating function, a mechanism that may contribute to the severity and sequelae of EBV infection in these patients.

Finally, NK cells may express KIRs with short cytoplasmic tails, which, in contrast to their counterparts with long cytoplasmic tails, activate NK cells [357]. In contrast

to CD94-NKG2A, CD94-NKG2C is an activating receptor complex [358]. These activating KIRs and CD94-NKG2C and their respective inhibitory forms have identical or very similar ligand specificities. How NK cells integrate the effects on natural cytotoxicity of these multiple inhibitory and activating receptors, particularly receptors that recognize the same or similar ligands, is unclear.

NATURAL KILLER CELL CYTOTOXICITY

Target cell killing by NK cells can be divided into a binding phase and an effector phase. Numerous receptor-ligand pairs may help to mediate the initial binding, including the interaction between β_2 integrins and ICAM-1 and between CD2 and CD58 [359]. Some of these interactions may also play a role in triggering NK-cell activation, but the receptors described in the previous section seem to be the primary regulators of activation.

After binding and activation, NK cells release perforin and granzymes from preformed cytotoxic granules into a synapse formed between the NK cell and its target, leading to death by apoptosis of the target cell. NK cell–mediated cytotoxicity also may be mediated by Fas-ligand [360] or TNF-related apoptosis–inducing ligand (TRAIL) [361] expressed on the activated NK-cell surface. Fas–Fas-ligand interactions apparently are not essential for human NK-cell control of viral infections because individuals with dominant-negative mutations in Fas or Fas-ligand develop autoimmunity, but do not experience an increased severity of virus infections [362]. In contrast to natural cytotoxicity, in which perforin/granzyme–dependent mechanisms seem to be predominant, ADCC seems to use perforin/granzyme–dependent and Fas-ligand–dependent cytotoxic mechanisms [363].

NATURAL KILLER CELL CYTOKINE RESPONSIVENESS AND DEPENDENCE

NK-cell proliferation and cytotoxicity are enhanced in vitro by cytokines produced by T cells (IL-2, IFN-γ), antigen-presenting cells (APCs) (IL-1, IL-12, IL-18, and type I IFNs), and nonhematopoietic cells (IL-15, stem cell factor, Flt3 ligand, IFN-β). IL-15, which seems crucial for the development of NK cells, also promotes the survival of mature NK cells and, similar to IL-12, increases the expression of perforin and granzymes [364,365]. NK-cell cytotoxicity in vivo is modestly decreased in mice genetically deficient in IFN-γ [366], IL-12 [367], or IL-18 [368] and markedly depressed in mice with combined IL-12 and IL-18 deficiency. These findings suggest that IL-12 and IL-18 largely act in a nonredundant fashion to help maintain NK-cell cytotoxicity in vivo, and this maintenance is mediated, at least in part, by the induction of IFN-γ by these cytokines. IL-23 and IL-27 are more recently described members of the IL-12 cytokine family [216]. Although their effects on NK-cell function in vivo are incompletely understood, a report suggests that a subset of NK cells found in mucosa-associated lymphoid tissue (MALT) responds to IL-23 by producing cytokines, including IL-22, that help to protect the gut from bacterial pathogens [345].

NATURAL KILLER CELL CYTOKINE AND CHEMOKINE PRODUCTION

NK cells are also important producers of IFN-γ and TNF-α in the early phase of the immune response to viruses, and IFN-γ may promote the development of CD4 T cells into T$_H$1 effector cells (see "Differentiation of Activated Naïve T Cells into Effector and Memory Cells"). NK cell–mediated IFN-γ production may be induced by the ligation of surface β$_1$ integrins on the NK cell surface [369] and by the cytokines IL-1, IL-12, and IL-18 [370], which are produced by DCs and mononuclear phagocytes. The combination of IL-12 and IL-15 also potently induces NK cells to produce the CC chemokine MIP-1α (CCL-3) [371], which may help to attract other types of mononuclear cells to sites of infection, where NK cell–mediated lysis occurs [372].

NK cells from HIV-infected individuals also are able to produce various CC chemokines, including MIP-1α, MIP-1β (CCL-4), and RANTES (CCL-5), in response to treatment with IL-2 alone; these chemokines may help prevent HIV infection of T cells and mononuclear phagocytes by acting as antagonists of the HIV coreceptor CCR5 [373]. NK cells also can be triggered to produce a similar array of cytokines during ADCC in vitro, but the role of such ADCC-derived cytokines in regulating immune responses in vivo is poorly defined. Some cytokine-dependent mechanisms by which NK cells, T cells, and APCs may influence each other's function, such as in response to infection with viruses and other intracellular pathogens, are summarized in Figure 4–5.

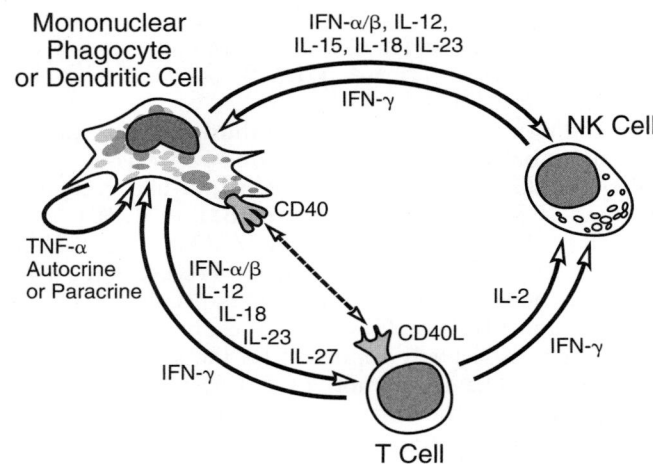

FIGURE 4–5 **Cytokines link innate and antigen-specific immune mechanisms against intracellular pathogens.** Activation of T cells by antigen-presenting cells, such as dendritic cells and mononuclear phagocytes, results in the expression of CD40 ligand and the secretion of cytokines, such as interleukin (IL)-2 and interferon (IFN)-γ. Mononuclear phagocytes are activated by IFN-γ and the engagement of CD40 with increased microbicidal activity. Mononuclear phagocytes produce tumor necrosis factor (TNF)-α, which enhances their microbicidal activity in a paracrine or autocrine manner. Mononuclear phagocytes also secrete the cytokines IFN-α/β, IL-12, IL-15, IL-18, IL-23, and IL-27. These cytokines promote T$_H$1 effector cell differentiation, and most also promote activation of natural killer (NK) cells. IL-15 (*not shown*) also is particularly important for the generation of effector and memory CD8 T cells. NK-cell activation is augmented further by IL-2 and possibly by IL-21, which are produced by CD4 T cells. Activated NK-cells secrete IFN-γ, which enhances mononuclear phagocyte activation and T$_H$1 effector cell differentiation further.

NATURAL KILLER CELLS OF THE MATERNAL DECIDUA AND THEIR REGULATION BY HUMAN LEUKOCYTE ANTIGEN G

The maternal decidua contains a prominent population of NK cells, which may help contribute to the maintenance of pregnancy. NK cells belonging to the CD56^{hi}CD16^{lo} subset, which have a high capacity for cytokine production, but low capacity for cytotoxicity, predominate. Murine studies suggest that maternal NK cell–derived cytokines, such as IFN-γ, may help to remodel the spiral arteries of the placenta. Although the NK cell populations of the decidua have a low capacity for cytotoxicity, their presence in a tissue lacking expression of HLA-A, HLA-B, and HLA-C molecules could potentially contribute to placental damage and fetal rejection. As noted previously, the expression by human fetal trophoblast of HLA-G is thought to protect this tissue from attack by maternal NK cells through binding to the inhibitory receptors LILRB1 and LILRB2 [353].

NATURAL KILLER CELL NUMBERS AND SURFACE PHENOTYPE IN THE FETUS AND NEONATE

NK cells become increasingly abundant during the second trimester [333,374], and at term their numbers in the neonatal circulation (approximately 15% of total

lymphocytes) are typically the same as or greater than in adults [333]. The fraction of CD56^{hi}CD16$^{-/lo}$ (approximately 10%) and CD56^{lo}CD16$^+$ NK cells (approximately 90%) is also similar [375,376]. Earlier studies of cell surface molecule expression on neonatal NK cells varied in their conclusions regarding the expression of molecules involved with adhesion, activation, inhibition, and cytotoxic mediators by neonatal NK cells. More recent studies using newer, more reliable methods suggest that neonatal NK cells have decreased expression of ICAM-1, but similar expression of other adhesion molecules; similar or greater expression of the inhibitory CD94-NKG2A complex, but reduced expression of the inhibitory LILRB1 (LIR1) receptor; similar or greater expression of the activating NKp30 and NKp46 receptors; similar or slightly reduced expression of the activating NKG2D receptor; and similar reduced surface expression of CD57 [375,376]. The abundance of the cytotoxic molecules perforin and granzyme B and FasL and TRAIL is as great or greater in neonatal NK cells as in adult NK cells [376]. These findings suggest that neonatal NK cells differ phenotypically from, and are not simply immature versions of, adult NK cells. Congenital viral or *T. gondii* infection during the second trimester can increase the number of circulating NK cells [374], which have phenotypic features of activated cells [377].

FETAL AND NEONATAL NATURAL KILLER CELL–MEDIATED CYTOTOXICITY AND CYTOKINE PRODUCTION

The cytotoxic function of NK cells increases progressively during fetal life to reach values approximately 50% (range 15% to 60% in various studies) of the values in adult cells at term, as determined in assays using tumor cell targets and either unpurified or NK cell–enriched preparations [333,376,378,379]. Reduced cytotoxic activity by neonatal NK cells has been observed in studies using cord blood from vaginal or cesarean section deliveries or peripheral blood obtained 2 to 4 days after birth [380]. Full function is not achieved until at least 9 to 12 months of age.

Decreased cytotoxic activity by neonatal NK cells compared with adult cells also is consistently observed with HSV-infected and CMV-infected target cells [381,382]. By contrast, neonatal and adult NK cells have equivalent cytotoxic activity against HIV-1–infected cells [383]. These results suggest that ligands on the target cell or the target cell's intrinsic sensitivity to induction of apoptosis may influence fetal and neonatal NK-cell function. The mechanisms of these pathogen-related differences are unclear, but may contribute to the severity of neonatal HSV infection. Paralleling the reduction in natural cytotoxic activity of neonatal cells, ADCC of neonatal mononuclear cells is approximately 50% of that of adult mononuclear cells, including against HSV-infected targets.

The reduced cytotoxic activity of neonatal NK cells seems not to reflect decreased expression of cytotoxic molecules, but instead may result from diminished adhesion to target cells, perhaps as a result of decreased expression of ICAM-1 or diminished recycling of cells to kill multiple targets [376,379,384]. The mechanisms responsible for diminished neonatal NK-cell cytotoxicity have not been conclusively defined, however. Cytokines including IL-2, IL-12, IL-15, IFN-α, IFN-β, and IFN-γ can augment the cytotoxic activity of neonatal NK cells, as they do for adult NK cells [378,385–387], and neonatal NK cells are as cytotoxic as adult NK cells when both have been treated with IL-15 [376]. Consistent with the ability of IL-2 and IFN-γ to augment their cytolytic activity, neonatal NK cells express on their surface receptors for IL-2/IL-15 and IFN-γ in numbers that are equal to or greater than those of adult NK cells [388]. Treatment of neonatal NK cells with ionomycin and phorbol myristate acetate (PMA) also enhances natural cytotoxicity to levels present in adult NK cells [389]. This increase is blocked by inhibitors of granule exocytosis, indicating that decreased release of granules containing perforin and granzyme may contribute to reduced neonatal NK-cell cytotoxicity. Finally, decreased neonatal NK-cell cytotoxicity is not determined at the level of the precursor cells of the NK-cell lineage: Donor-derived NK cells appear early after cord blood transplantation, with good cytotoxicity effected through the perforin/granzyme and Fas–Fas-ligand cytotoxic pathways [390].

Neonatal NK cells produce IFN-γ as effectively as adult NK cells in response to exogenous IL-2, IL-12, and IL-18; HSV [391]; and polyclonal stimulation with ionomycin and PMA [375,376,391,392], but fewer neonatal NK cells express TNF-α than adult NK cells after ionomycin and PMA stimulation [392]. Neonatal NK cells produce chemokines that suppress the growth of HIV strains that use CCR5 as a coreceptor to infect CD4 T cells, but not strains that use CXCR4 as a receptor [373].

SUMMARY

NK cells appear early during gestation and are present in normal numbers by mid-gestation to late gestation. Certain phenotypic features of NK cells differ, however, from features of adult NK cells. Neonatal NK cells seem to be as capable as adult cells of producing IFN-γ and chemokines that inhibit the ability of CCR5-trophic HIV strains to infect CD4 T cells, but may produce less TNF-α and chemokines that inhibit infection by CXCR4-trophic strains of HIV. Compared with adult NK cells, neonatal NK cells have decreased cytotoxicity to many types of target cells, including HSV-infected and CMV-infected cells, but not HIV-infected cells. Neonatal NK-cell cytotoxicity can be augmented by incubation with cytokines such as IL-15 in vitro, suggesting a potential immunotherapeutic strategy.

T CELLS AND ANTIGEN PRESENTATION
OVERVIEW

T cells are so named because most of these cells originate in the thymus. Along with B cells, which in mammals develop in the bone marrow, T cells compose the adaptive or antigen-specific immune system. T cells play a central role in antigen-specific immunity because they directly mediate and regulate cellular immune responses and play a crucial role in facilitating antigen-specific humoral immune responses by B cells. Most T cells recognize antigen in the form of peptides bound to MHC molecules on APCs. Antigen-specific T-cell receptors (TCRs) are heterodimeric molecules composed of either α and β chains ($\alpha\beta$-TCRs) (Fig. 4–6) or γ and δ chains ($\gamma\delta$-TCRs), with the amino-terminal portion of each of these chains variable and involved in antigen recognition. This variability is generated, in large part, as a result of TCR gene rearrangement of variable (V), diversity (D), and joining (J) segments. The TCR on the cell surface is invariably associated with the nonpolymorphic complex of CD3 proteins, which include CD3-γ, CD3-δ, CD3-ϵ, and CD3-ζ (see Fig. 4–6). The cytoplasmic domains of proteins of the CD3 complex include 10 immunoreceptor tyrosine-based activation motifs (ITAMs), which serve as docking sites for the lck and ZAP-70 (CD3-ζ–associated protein of 70 kDa) intracellular tyrosine kinases that transduce proximal activation signals to the interior of the cell after the TCR has been engaged by antigen.

Most T cells that bear $\alpha\beta$-TCR (or $\alpha\beta$ T cells) also express on their surface the CD4 or CD8 coreceptors in a mutually exclusive manner and are commonly referred to as CD4 or CD8 T cells. Nearly all CD8 T cells recognize protein antigens in the form of peptide fragments that are 7 to 9 amino acids in length bound to MHC class I molecules of the classic type (HLA-A, HLA-B, and HLA-C in humans). CD4 T cells recognize antigen

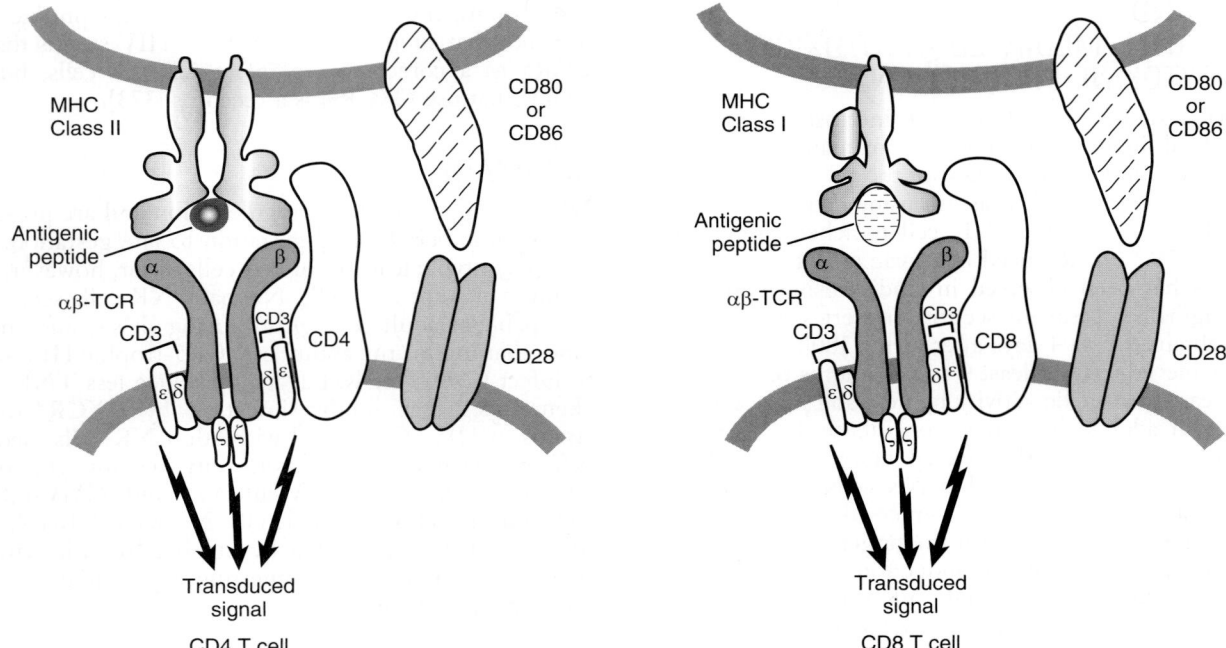

FIGURE 4–6 T-cell recognition of antigen and activation. αβ T-cell receptor (αβ-TCR) recognizes antigen presented by the antigen-presenting cell (APC) in the form of antigenic peptides bound to major histocompatibility complex (MHC) molecules on the APC surface. Most CD4⁺ T cells recognize peptides bound to MHC class II, whereas most CD8⁺ T cells recognize peptides bound to MHC class I. This MHC restriction is the result of a thymic selection process and is due in part to an intrinsic affinity of the CD4 and CD8 molecules for the MHC class II and class I molecules. When antigen is recognized, the CD3 protein complex, which is invariably associated with αβ-TCR, acts as docking site for tyrosine kinases that transmit activating intracellular signals. Interaction of the T-cell CD28 molecule with either CD80 (B7-1) or CD86 (B7-2) provides an important costimulatory signal to the T cell leading to complete activation, rather than partial activation or functional inactivation (anergy).

presented by MHC class II molecules (HLA-DR, HLA-DP, and HLA-DQ in humans); most of these antigens are in the form of peptide fragments typically 12 to 22 amino acids in length. MHC class II presentation of certain zwitterionic bacterial polysaccharides, such as those derived from *Bacteroides fragilis*, can also occur [17].

APCs, which include DCs, mononuclear phagocytes, and B cells, constitutively express MHC class I and class II molecules, which allows them to present antigenic peptides to CD8 and CD4 T cells. DCs are particularly important for presentation to T cells that are antigenically naïve and that have not been previously activated by foreign antigen. γδ T cells, which mainly recognize stress-induced molecules rather than peptide–MHC complexes, have distinct immune functions from αβ T cells and are discussed later in a separate section.

ANTIGEN PRESENTATION BY CLASSIC MAJOR HISTOCOMPATIBILITY COMPLEX MOLECULES

Major Histocompatibility Complex Class Ia

MHC class Ia proteins are heterodimers of a heavy chain that is polymorphic and a monomorphic light chain, β_2-microglobulin. Antigenic peptides 8 to 10 amino acids in length bind to a cleft formed by two domains of the heavy chain (Fig. 4–7; see also Fig. 4–6). There are three different types of MHC class Ia molecules—HLA-A,

HLA-B, and HLA-C; all three types are highly polymorphic, and 548, 936, and 300 different molecularly defined alleles have been described for HLA-A, HLA-B, and HLA-C [393]. The greatest degree of polymorphism is found in the region encoding the antigenic cleft, which results in there being considerable differences among individuals in their ability to present antigenic peptides to T cells. The CD8 molecule has an affinity for a non-variable domain of the heavy chain that is not involved in binding peptide and that contributes to T-cell activation.

Most peptides bound to MHC class Ia molecules are derived from proteins synthesized de novo within host cells (see Fig. 4–7), with the bulk derived from recently translated proteins, rather than as a result of turnover of stable proteins. This helps minimize any delay in detecting pathogen-derived peptides that may result from recent infection [394]. In uninfected cells, these peptides are derived from host proteins; that is, they are self-peptides. Recently synthesized host proteins that are targeted for degradation (e.g., because of misfolding or defective post-translational modification) are a major source of self-peptides that bind to MHC class Ia. After intracellular infection, such as with a virus, peptides derived from viral proteins endogenously synthesized within the cell bind to and are presented by MHC class Ia. Antigenic peptides are derived predominantly by enzymatic cleavage of proteins in the cytoplasm by the proteasome. A specific peptide transporter or pump, the

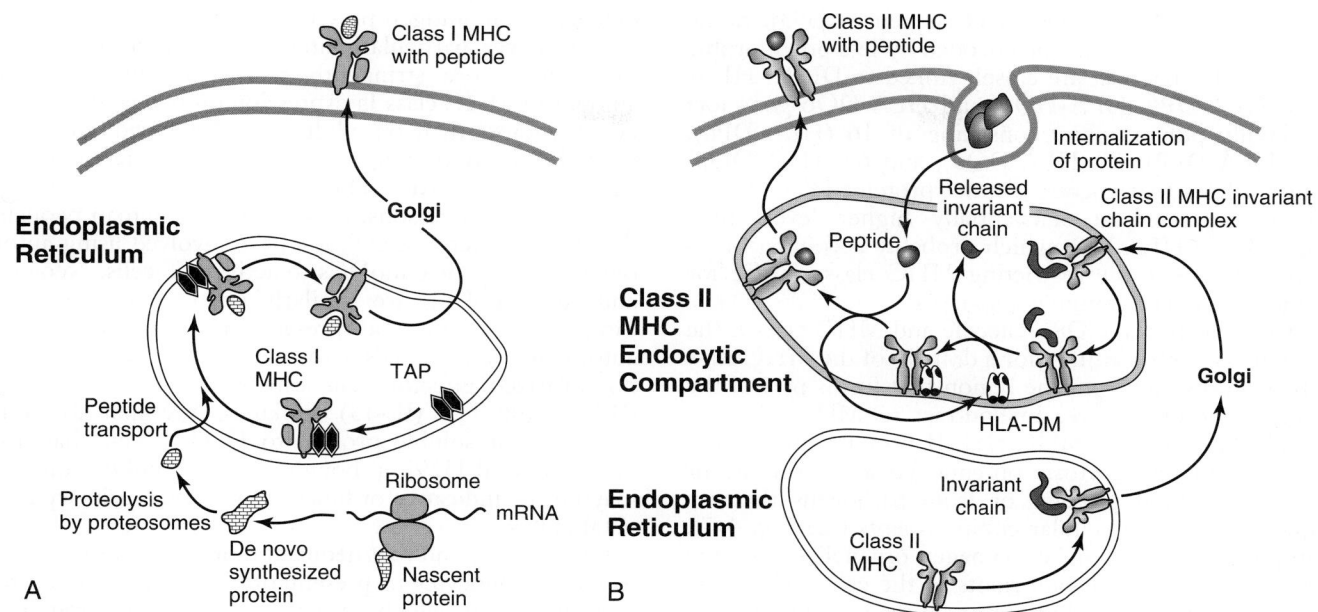

FIGURE 4–7 Intracellular pathways of antigen presentation. A, Foreign peptides that bind to major histocompatibility complex (MHC) class I are predominantly derived from cytoplasmic proteins synthesized de novo within the cell. Viral proteins entering cells after fusion of an enveloped virus with the cell membrane may also enter this pathway. Dendritic cells are particularly efficient at taking up proteins for the MHC class I pathway by micropinocytosis or macropinocytosis. These cells can also transfer proteins taken up as part of necrotic or apoptotic debris into the MHC class I pathway, a process known as cross-presentation. Cytoplasmic proteins are degraded by proteasomes into peptides, which enter into the endoplasmic reticulum via the transporter associated with antigen processing (TAP) system. Peptide binding by de novo synthesized MHC class I occurs within the endoplasmic reticulum. **B,** Foreign peptides that bind to MHC class II are mainly derived from internalization proteins found in the extracellular space or that are components of cell membrane. The invariant chain binds to recently synthesized MHC class II and prevents peptide binding until a specialized cellular compartment for MHC class II peptide loading is reached. In this compartment, the invariant chain is proteolytically cleaved and released, and peptides derived from internalized proteins may now bind to MHC class II. The HLA-DM molecule facilitates the loading of peptide within this compartment. In dendritic cells, proteins that enter into the MHC class II antigen presentation pathway can be transferred to the MHC class I pathway by cross-presentation.

transporter associated with antigen processing (TAP), shuttles peptides formed in the cytoplasm to the endoplasmic reticulum, where peptides are able to bind to recently synthesized MHC class Ia molecules. Peptide binding stabilizes the association of the heavy chain with β_2-microglobulin in this compartment and allows the complex to transit to the cell surface.

MHC class Ia molecules and the cell components required for peptide generation, transport, and MHC class Ia binding are virtually ubiquitous in the cells of vertebrates. The advantage to the host is that cytotoxic CD8 T cells can recognize and lyse cells infected with intracellular pathogens in most tissues. The abundance of MHC class I molecules is increased by exposure to type I IFNs and IFN-γ, which also can induce the expression of modest amounts of MHC class Ia molecules on cell types that normally lack expression, including neuronal cells.

DCs are unique in their ability to present antigenic peptides on MHC class Ia molecules by an additional pathway, known as cross-presentation, in which extracellular proteins that are taken up as large particles (phagocytosis), as small particles (macropinocytosis), or in soluble form (micropinocytosis) are transferred from endocytic vesicles to the cytoplasm. When these proteins are in the cytoplasm, they undergo proteasome-mediated degradation and loading onto MHC class Ia molecules through TAP. Cross-presentation is essential for the

induction of primary CD8 T-cell responses directed toward antigens of pathogens that do not directly infect APCs (e.g., most viruses) and cannot be directly loaded into the MHC class Ia pathway. Cross-presentation is enhanced by exposure of DCs to type I IFNs [395]. UNC-93B1, a protein that is important for TLR signaling and antiviral host defense (see section on TLRs earlier and antiviral host defenses later), has also been implicated as playing a role in cross-presentation by murine APCs [396], but it is unclear if this applies to human APC cross-presentation. Cross-presentation may also be facilitated by the nicotinamide adenine dinucleotide phosphate (NADPH) oxidase complex [397], which helps limit acidification that can destroy protein-derived epitopes.

Major Histocompatibility Complex Class II

In MHC class II molecules, an α and a β chain contribute to the formation of the antigenic peptide-binding groove (see Fig. 4–7). The three major types of human MHC class II molecules—HLA-DR, HLA-DP, and HLA-DQ—are highly polymorphic, particularly in the region encoding the peptide-binding cleft. In humans and primates, HLA-DR allelic diversity is mediated solely by the HLA-DR β chain because the HLA-DR α chain is monomorphic. HLA-DRβ protein is encoded mainly at the DRB1 locus, for which there are 556 known alleles that encode distinct amino acid sequences [393]. Some HLA-DRβ proteins may be encoded by less polymorphic loci, such DRB3, that are closely linked to DRB1. HLA-DPα, HLA-DPβ, HLA-DQα, and HLA-DQβ gene loci are highly polymorphic, consisting of 16 (HLA-DPα), 115 (HLA-DPβ), 25 (HLA-DQα), and 69 (HLA-DQβ) known alleles that encode distinct proteins [393]. HLA-DR is expressed at substantially higher levels than HLA-DP or HLA-DQ, which probably accounts for its predominance as the restricting MHC class II type for many CD4 T-cell immune responses.

Analogous to the CD8 molecule and MHC class I, the CD4 molecule has affinity for a domain of the MHC class II β chain distinct from the region that forms part of the peptide-binding groove. In contrast to MHC class Ia, peptides that bind to MHC class II proteins are derived mostly from phagocytosis or endocytosis of soluble or membrane-bound proteins or from pathogens that are sequestered in intracellular compartments (see Fig. 4–7). Autophagy, which removes damaged organelles from the cytoplasm and provides nutrients to the cell during starvation, also may be an important source of peptides.

In the absence of foreign proteins, most peptides bound to MHC class II molecules are self-peptides derived from proteins found on the cell surface or secreted by the cell. Newly synthesized MHC class II molecules associate in the endoplasmic reticulum with a protein called the invariant chain, which impedes their binding of endogenous peptides in this compartment. The loading of exogenously derived peptides and the removal of invariant chain from MHC class II are facilitated by HLA-DM (see Fig. 4–7), a nonpolymorphic heterodimeric protein, and likely occur in a late phagolysosomal compartment. Most MHC class II peptides are 14 to 18 amino acids in length, although they can be substantially longer.

The distribution of MHC class II in uninflamed tissues is much more restricted than MHC class Ia, with constitutive MHC class II mainly limited to APCs, such as DCs, mononuclear phagocytes, and B cells. Limiting MHC class II expression in most situations to these cell types makes teleologic sense because the major function of these professional APCs is to process foreign antigen for recognition by CD4 T cells. Many other cell types can be induced to express MHC class II and, in some cases, present antigen to CD4 T cells, as a consequence of tissue inflammation or exposure to cytokines, particularly IFN-γ, but also TNF-α or GM-CSF (see Tables 4–1 and 4–2).

Major Histocompatibility Complex Molecule Expression and Antigen Presentation in the Fetus and Neonate

The expression of MHC class I and class II molecules by fetal tissues is evident by 12 weeks of gestation, and all of the major APCs, including mononuclear phagocytes, B cells, and DCs [398], are present by this time. Fetal tissues are vigorously rejected after transplantation into non–MHC-matched hosts, indicating that surface MHC expression is sufficient to initiate an allogeneic response, probably by host cytotoxic CD8 T cells. This vigorous allogeneic response does not exclude more subtle deficiencies in antigen presentation in the fetus and neonate, however, particularly under more physiologic conditions that more stringently test APC function. The amount of MHC class Ia expression on neonatal lymphocytes is lower than on adult cells [399], and this could limit the ability of lymphocytes infected by pathogens to be lysed by cytotoxic CD8 T cells.

For technical reasons, most studies of human neonatal dendritic antigen presentation have involved using autologous or allogeneic moDCs to activate T cells. Neonatal and adult moDCs are similarly efficient in processing exogenous protein and present antigenic peptides to autologous naïve T cells with similar efficiency to become nonpolarized effector cells capable of producing T_H1 (IFN-γ) and T_H2 (IL-13) cytokines. A similar ability to cross-present soluble protein to CD8 T cells has also been reported [329], although neonatal moDC function may not be indicative of function of human primary neonatal cDCs.

One study found that neonatal monocytes were inferior to adult monocytes in presentation of either whole protein antigen, in which antigen processing was required, or exogenous peptide to HLA-DR–expressing T-cell hybridomas [400]. This inferiority was not accounted for by decreased expression of either MHC class II or costimulatory molecules, such as CD80 or CD86, by neonatal monocytes, and because this applied to whole protein and exogenously added peptides, a defect only in antigen processing is unlikely. The precise mechanisms are unclear, but could involve neonatal monocyte limitations in adhesion to or immunologic synapse formation with T cells [400] (discussed in "Memory T-Cell Activation"). A substantial fraction of MHC class II molecules on neonatal, but not adult, B cells are "empty"—that is, they lack peptides in the binding groove [401]. Neonatal B cells may be functionally limited as APCs.

NONCLASSIC ANTIGEN PRESENTATION MOLECULES

HLA-E

HLA-E is a nonclassic and essentially monomorphic class Ib MHC molecule similar to conventional MHC class Ia in its dependency on the proteasome for the generation of peptides and its obligate association with β2-microglobulin. In contrast to conventional MHC class Ia molecules, HLA-E preferentially binds hydrophobic peptides, including peptides derived from the amino-terminal leader sequences of most alleles of HLA-A, HLA-B, and HLA-C [402]. Low levels of HLA-E surface expression can be detected on most cell types, consistent with the nearly ubiquitous distribution of HLA-A, HLA-B, and HLA-C and the TAP system. An important role for HLA-E is to interact with the CD94-containing receptors on NK lymphocytes and to regulate their function (see earlier section on NK-cell inhibitory receptors). HLA-E is also expressed by fetal-derived extravillous trophoblasts of the human placenta. Because trophoblast cells lack expression of most conventional MHC class Ia molecules, the surface expression of HLA-E may limit the lysis of these cells by maternal or fetal NK cells [403].

HLA-G

HLA-G, which, similar to HLA-E, is expressed at high levels by human cytotrophoblasts within the maternal uterine wall, has limited polymorphism, but otherwise is quite similar to MHC class Ia in its association with β_2-microglobulin and structure. HLA-G occurs as either an integral membrane protein or a secreted isoform [404]. Similar to HLA-E, HLA-G is capable of engaging regulatory receptors on NK cells and may serve to limit NK cell–mediated cytotoxicity against trophoblasts (see "Natural Killer Cells of the Maternal Decidua and Their Regulation by Human Leukocyte Antigen G"). In this context, the hydrophobic leader sequence of HLA-G may provide a peptide that is particularly effective for HLA-E–mediated regulation of NK cell cytotoxicity [403]. Soluble HLA-G is present at relatively high levels in the serum of pregnant women [404] and in lower amounts in cord blood and in the peripheral blood of nonparous women and men. The in vivo function of soluble HLA-G is unclear, but it may inhibit immune responses. Consistent with this proposed function, soluble HLA-G (and class Ia molecules) can induce Fas (CD95)-dependent apoptosis of activated CD8 T cells, by engaging CD8 and increasing surface expression of Fas-ligand (CD95L) [405,406].

Major Histocompatibility Complex Class I–Related Chains A and B

MICA and MICB have limited but clear homology with conventional MHC class I molecules. In contrast to conventional MHC class I, they lack a binding site for CD8, are not associated with β_2-microglobulin, and do not seem to be involved with the presentation of peptide antigens. Instead, these molecules are expressed on stressed intestinal epithelial cells, such as cells experiencing heat shock, and on other cell types in response to infection with viruses, such as cells of the herpesvirus group. The expression of MICA and MICB transcripts in the unstressed cell is under negative control by cellular microRNAs, which themselves are downregulated by stress [407]. MICA and MICB are ligands for NKG2D found on most NK cells, some CD8 T cells, and certain populations of $\gamma\delta$ T cells (e.g., cells expressing Vγ9Vδ2 TCRs) [408]. NKG2D can either directly activate or act in concert with TCR-mediated signals to activate the cells that express it [409].

CD1

The human CD1 locus includes five nonpolymorphic genes—CD1a through CD1e. CD1 molecules associate with β_2-microglobulin, but have limited structural homology with either MHC class I or MHC class II proteins. In humans, they are expressed mainly on APCs, including DCs. CD1a, CD1b, and CD1c are involved in the presentation of diverse types of lipids unique to microorganisms, such as mycolic acids, glucose monomycolate, sulfolipid, phosphatidyl mannosides, and mannosylated lipoarabinomannan or mycobacteria, to clonally diverse T cells [410]. CD1d, in contrast, presents lipid antigens to natural killer T (NKT) cells, a specialized T-cell population with a highly restricted $\alpha\beta$-TCR repertoire (discussed in more detail subsequently) [411]. The microbial lipids presented by CD1d include diverse microbial sources, such as *Borrelia burgdorferi*, *Sphingomonas* species, and *Leishmania donovani*. CD1e, which is expressed only intracellularly, facilitates antigen processing of the mycobacterial lipid hexamannosylated phosphatidyl-*myo*-inositol, so that it can be displayed on the APC cell surface in association with CD1b [410].

Antigen processing and loading of CD1 molecules involves endocytic pathways, at least some of which intersect with pathways involved in peptide loading of MHC class II molecules [410]. The CD1 molecules also are capable of presenting self-lipids, such as phosphatidylinositol and G_{M1} ganglioside. This recognition of self-lipids, which typically involves lower affinity interactions with CD1 than that of microbial-derived ligands, may be involved in the positive selection of CD1-restricted T cells in the thymus, analogous to the process by which peptide–MHC complexes with relatively low affinity for the TCR play such a role (see later section on thymocyte development). Little is known of the adequacy of antigen presentation by CD1 molecules in the human fetus or neonate.

PROTHYMOCYTES AND EARLY THYMOCYTE DIFFERENTIATION

Thymic Ontogeny

With the exception of a subset of the T cells found in the gut and perhaps the liver, most $\alpha\beta$ T cells develop from immature progenitor cells within the unique microenvironment of the thymus. The thymus does not have a population of self-replenishing stem cells and requires a continual input of thymocyte progenitor cells (prothymocytes) to maintain thymocytopoiesis. The entry of prothymocytes from the circulation into the thymus seems to occur cyclically rather than continuously, resulting in waves of thymocyte development.

The thymic rudiment (lacking hematopoietic cells) arises from the endoderm of the third pharyngeal pouch [412] at weeks 4 to 5 of gestation. An interstitial deletion of a 1.5- to 3-Mb region of the human chromosome 22q11.2 region is the most frequent genetic cause of DiGeorge syndrome and velocardiofacial syndrome and results in hypoplasia of tissues deriving from the third pharyngeal pouches, including the thymus [413]. A murine model suggests that haploinsufficiency for two genes located within the human 22q11.2 deleted segment—Tbx1 and Crkl—are responsible for this hypoplasia [414].

The prothymocyte is an early derivative of, but not identical to, a fully totipotent HSC. The human prothymocyte of the fetal bone marrow has a CD7$^+$CD34^{hi}CD45RA^{hi}Lin$^-$ (lacking markers for the mature T-cell, B-cell, NK-cell, erythroid cell, and myeloid cell lineages) surface phenotype [415]. This cell population is replaced in the postnatal bone marrow by a CD7$^-$CD10$^+$CD24$^-$CD34Lin$^-$ cell population as the likely major prothymocyte population [416]. Human fetal prothymocytes not only have T-cell differentiation potential, but also retain the capacity to differentiate along B-cell, NK-cell, and myeloid cell, but not erythroid cell lineages [415]. Whether postnatal human prothymo-cytes retain a capacity for myeloid and erythroid lineage differentiation is controversial [416,417].

The first waves of human fetal CD7+ prothymocytes probably enter into the thymic rudiment when it lacks a vasculature at about 8 weeks of gestation [415], with later ones entering through postcapillary venules at the cortical medullary junction. These prothymocytes derive from the bone marrow, and the human fetal liver does not seem to play a role in producing prothymocytes [415]. Newly entering prothymocytes rapidly encounter perivascular thymic epithelial cells [415] that express the Delta-like ligands. These ligands engage Notch 1 on the prothymocyte cell to promote its T-cell lineage commitment rapidly, as evidenced by the expression of T cell–specific genes and the suppression of B-cell development. The rapid induction of the expression of these T cell–specific genes may be facilitated by their having an open chromatin structure starting at the HSC stage [418]; this chromatin configuration likely continues through the prothymocyte stage.

Intrathymic cellular progeny of the entering prothymo-cyte gives rise to the three major subsets of thymocytes characteristic of the second-trimester and third-trimester fetal and postnatal human thymus (Fig. 4–8). These subsets are named according to their pattern of surface expression of CD4 and CD8 and are characterized further by their surface expression of αβ-TCR complexes. Thymocytes can be classified as double-negative (CD4−CD8−), which express little or no CD4 or CD8 (hence, double-negative) or αβ-TCR–CD3 (and sometimes referred to as triple-negative) and are direct products of the entering prothymocyte; double-positive (CD4hiCD8hi), which express medium levels of αβ-TCR–CD3 and are derived from the most mature double-negative cells; and single-positive (CD4hiCD8− and CD4−CD8hi), which express high levels of αβ-TCR–CD3 and are derived from double-positive cells. In humans, there is also an intermediate stage between double-negative and double-positive thymocytes that is characterized by a CD4loCD8−CD3− (immature single-positive) surface phenotype [419].

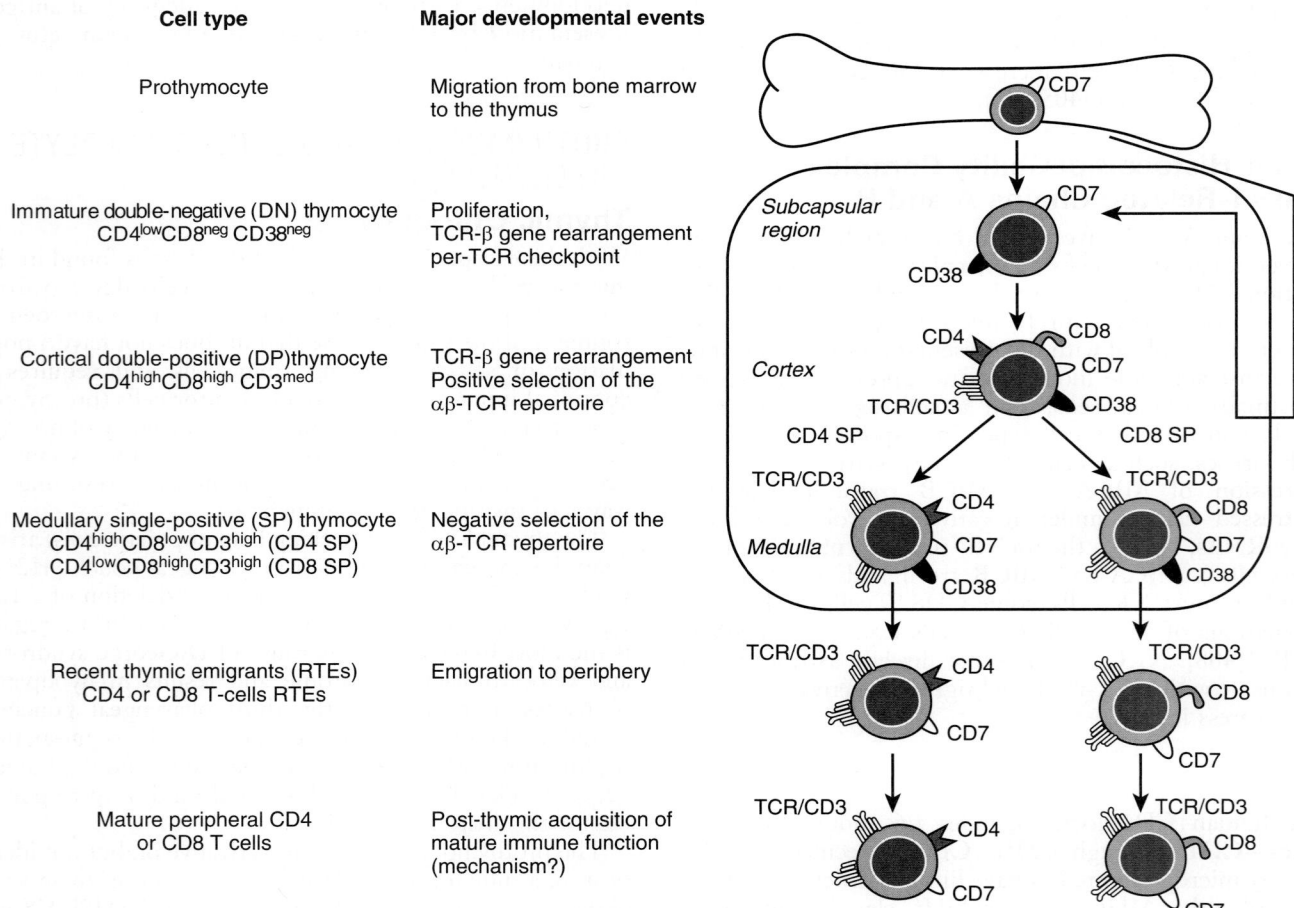

Cell type	Major developmental events
Prothymocyte	Migration from bone marrow to the thymus
Immature double-negative (DN) thymocyte CD4lowCD8neg CD38neg	Proliferation, TCR-β gene rearrangement per-TCR checkpoint
Cortical double-positive (DP)thymocyte CD4highCD8high CD3med	TCR-β gene rearrangement Positive selection of the αβ-TCR repertoire
Medullary single-positive (SP) thymocyte CD4highCD8lowCD3high (CD4 SP) CD4lowCD8highCD3high (CD8 SP)	Negative selection of the αβ-TCR repertoire
Recent thymic emigrants (RTEs) CD4 or CD8 T-cells RTEs	Emigration to periphery
Mature peripheral CD4 or CD8 T cells	Post-thymic acquisition of mature immune function (mechanism?)

FIGURE 4–8 Putative stages of human αβ T-cell receptor–positive (TCR+) thymocyte development. Prothymocytes from the bone marrow or fetal liver, which express CD7, enter the thymus via vessels at the junction between the thymic cortex and medulla. They differentiate to progressively more mature αβ-TCR+ thymocytes, defined by their pattern of expression of αβ-TCR/CD3 complex, CD4, CD8, and CD38. TCR-α and TCR-β chain genes are rearranged in the outer cortex. Positive selection occurs mainly in the central thymic cortex by interaction with thymic epithelial cells, and negative selection occurs mainly in the medulla by interaction with thymic dendritic cells. Following these selection processes, medullary thymocytes emigrate into the circulation and colonize the peripheral lymphoid organs as CD4+ and CD8+ T cells with high levels of αβ-TCR/CD3 complex. These recent thymic emigrants (RTEs) also contain signal joint T-cell receptor excision circles (sjTRECs), which are a circular product of TCR gene rearrangement. Most RTEs probably lack CD38 surface expression. In contrast, in neonates, most peripheral T cells retain surface expression of CD38 and have high amounts of sjTRECs compared with adult peripheral T cells.

A fetal triple-negative (CD3$^-$CD4$^-$CD8$^-$) thymocyte population that is also CD1a$^-$CD7$^+$CD34^{hi}CD45RA^{hi} likely includes prothymocytes that have recently immigrated into the thymus [415]. In the postnatal thymus, this most recent thymic immigrant population is replaced by a triple-negative population that is CD1a$^-$CD7$^-$CD10$^+$ CD34^{hi}CD45RA^{hi}. Triple-negative thymocytes undergo progressive differentiation that involves alterations in expression of CD34, CD38, and CD1a in which the progeny of recent thymic immigrants progressively differentiate into CD1a$^+$CD34$^-$CD38$^-$, CD1a$^+$CD34$^-$CD38$^+$, and CD1a$^+$CD34$^+$CD38$^+$ thymocytes to become CD4^{lo}CD8$^-$CD3$^-$ (immature single-positive) cells [417]. During this differentiation, thymocytes move outward in the cortex toward the subcapsular region, a process that is accompanied by proliferation driven by the binding of Wnt, IL-7, and Flt3-ligand to their specific receptors on the thymocyte cell surface [420]. When thymocytes reach the outer cortex, they reverse course and move from the outer to the inner cortex as double-positive thymocytes [421]. Finally, double-positive cells become single-positive thymocytes in the medulla, which exit the thymus as mature but naïve (i.e., they have not yet encountered and are naïve to the antigen they are capable of recognizing) T cells probably through blood vessels located in the medulla (see Fig. 4–8).

Thymocytes expressing proteins that are characteristic of T-lineage cells, including CD4, CD8, and αβ-TCR–CD3 complex, are found shortly after the initial colonization at 8.5 weeks of gestation [422]. By 12 weeks of gestation, the pattern of expression of numerous other proteins expressed by thymocytes, such as CD2, CD5, CD38, and the CD45 isoforms, matches the pattern in the postnatal thymus. Concurrently, a clear architectural separation between the thymic cortex and medulla is evident [423], with Hassall corpuscles observable in the thymic medulla shortly thereafter [424]. By 14 weeks of gestation, the three major human thymocyte subsets (double-negative [CD4$^-$CD8$^-$], double-positive [CD4$^+$CD8$^+$], and mature single-positive [CD4$^+$CD8$^-$ and CD4$^-$CD8$^+$]) characteristic of the postnatal thymus are found (see Fig. 4–8). Fetal thymocyte expression of the chemokine receptors CXCR4 and CCR5, which also are major coreceptors for entry of HIV-1, has been found by 18 to 23 weeks of gestation [425] and is likely to be present earlier.

Thymic cellularity increases dramatically during the second and third trimesters. Transient thymic involution, mainly the loss of cortical double-positive (CD4^{hi}CD8^{hi}) thymocytes, which is evident within 1 day after birth, probably begins at the end of the third trimester [426]. This involution may be a consequence of the elevation in circulating levels of glucocorticoids that occurs during the third trimester before delivery. Thymic recovery is evident by 1 month after delivery and is paralleled by a sharp decline in glucocorticoid levels within hours after birth [426]. This transient involution is followed by a resumption of increased thymic cellularity, with peak cellularity and thymus size probably attained at about 1 year of age [427]. When complete thymectomy is performed during the first year of life, subsequent circulating numbers of CD4 and CD8 T cells are decreased, indicating the importance of postnatal thymocyte production for the maintenance of the peripheral T-cell compartment [428].

There is gradual replacement of thymic cellularity of the cortex and medulla by fat after early childhood, with single-positive thymocytes within the medulla being relatively spared compared with cortical double-positive thymocytes [429]. Nevertheless, the thymus remains active in T-cell production through the fourth decade of life [430–433] and is capable of increasing its output of antigenically naïve T cells in response to severe T-cell lymphopenia (e.g., after intense cytoablative chemotherapy or treatment with highly active combination antiretroviral therapy for HIV infection) [434]. The mechanisms by which increased thymocytopoiesis is triggered by severe lymphopenia are unclear, but may include increased production of IL-7, which is plausible as IL-7 administration increases output of recent thymic emigrants (RTEs) in healthy adults [435].

INTRATHYMIC GENERATION OF T-CELL RECEPTOR DIVERSITY
Overview

T (and B) lymphocytes undergo a unique developmental event—the generation of a highly diverse repertoire of antigen receptors through DNA recombination, a process referred to as V(D)J recombination. This diversity is generated through the random rearrangement and juxtaposition into a single exon of variable (V), diversity (D), and joining (J) segments to form in each cell a unique TCR α and TCR β gene sequence (Fig. 4–9). The process of V(D)J recombination is restricted to immature T-lineage and B-lineage cells, the only cell types that express the two recombination-activating genes, *RAG1* and *RAG2*. Recombination of the TCR genes is restricted further to cells of the T-lymphocyte rather than B-lymphocyte lineage by mechanisms (e.g., histone acetylation) that allow RAG access to the TCR genes only in T-cell progenitors. The RAG proteins are critically involved in the initiation of the recombination process—they recognize and cleave conserved sequences flanking each V, D, and J segment.

Other proteins, including a high-molecular-weight, DNA-dependent protein kinase and its associated Ku70 and Ku80 proteins, DNA ligase IV and its associated XRCC4 protein, Artemis, and Cernunnos-XLF, perform nonhomologous DNA end-joining (NHEJ) repair of the cleaved V(D)J segments [436]. In contrast to RAG proteins, these other proteins involved in NHEJ DNA repair are expressed in most cells and are involved in repair of double-stranded DNA breaks induced by cell damage, such as radiation. Genetic deficiency of any of the proteins involved in the rearrangement process results in a form of severe combined immunodeficiency (SCID) because T-cell and B-cell development depends on the surface expression of rearranged TCR (T cell) and immunoglobulin (B cell) genes [437].

The complementarity-determining regions (CDRs) of the TCR and immunoglobulin molecules are those that are involved in forming the three-dimensional structure that binds with antigen. The V segments encode the CDR1 and CDR2 regions for both TCR chains. The CDR3 region, where the distal portion of the V segment joins the (D)J segment, is a particularly important

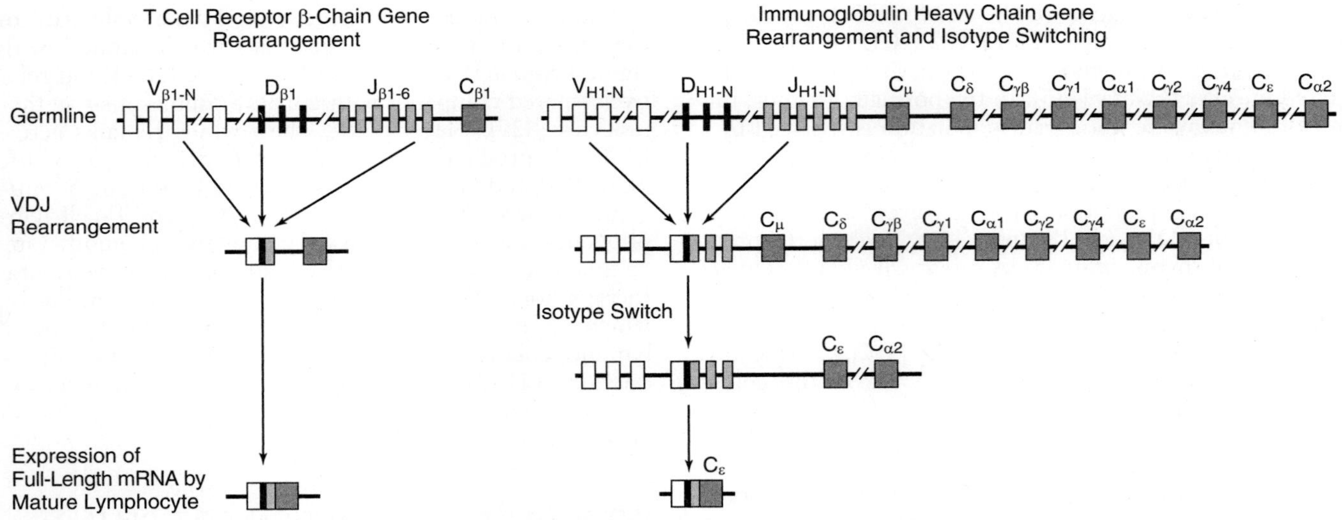

FIGURE 4–9 **T-cell receptor (TCR) and immunoglobulin genes are formed by rearrangement in immature lymphocytes.** TCR-β chain gene and the immunoglobulin heavy chain genes are shown as examples. A similar process is involved with rearrangement of the TCR-α, TCR-γ, and TCR-δ chain genes and with immunoglobulin light chain genes. Rearrangement involves the joining of dispersed segments of V (variable), D (diversity), and J (joining) gene segments with the deletion of intervening DNA. This process allows expression of a full-length mRNA transcript that can be translated into a functional protein, provided that there are no premature translational stop codons. Immunoglobulin heavy chain genes undergo an additional rearrangement called isotype switching, in which the C (constant) region segment is changed without alteration of the antigen combining site formed by the V, D, and J segments. The isotype switch from IgM to IgE is shown.

source of αβ-TCR diversity for peptide-MHC recognition and is the center of the antigen-binding site for peptide–MHC complexes. CDR3 (also known as junctional) diversity is achieved by multiple mechanisms. These mechanisms include the following:

1. The addition of one or two nucleotides that are palindromic to the end of the cut gene segment (termed P-nucleotides); these nucleotides are added as part of the process of asymmetric repairing of "hairpin" ends (the two strands of DNA are joined at the ends) that are generated by RAG endonuclease activity

2. The activity of terminal deoxytransferase (TdT; also referred to as deoxynucleotidyltransferase terminal), which randomly adds nucleotides (called N-nucleotides) to the ends of segments undergoing rearrangement; TdT addition is a particularly important mechanism for diversity generation because every three additional nucleotides encodes a potential codon, potentially increasing repertoire diversity by a factor of 20

3. Exonuclease activity that results in a variable loss of nucleotide residues, as part of the DNA repair process

Together, the mechanisms for generating diversity can theoretically result in 10^{15} types of αβ-TCR. In reality, the final repertoire of naïve T cells in the adult human circulation is on average a total of 10^6 different TCR β chains, each pairing on average with at least 25 different TCR α chains [438]. This results in a maximum of about 10^8 different combinations of TCR α and TCR β chains for the naïve T-cell αβ-TCR repertoire. Because in young adults the body has approximately 2×10^{11} CD4 T cells

and 1×10^{11} CD8 T cells [439,440], of which about 50% belong to the naïve subset, the average clonal size (all clones express an identical αβ-TCR) for a naïve T cell is approximately 500 to 1000 [438,441].

RAG expression is present by the double-negative thymocyte stage, with the TCR-γ chain and TCR-δ chain genes typically undergoing rearrangement first [442]. The TCR β gene becomes accessible to RAG proteins before the TCR α gene, and it is the first to undergo rearrangement (a small fraction of double-negative cells may undergo productive rearrangements of the TCR γ and TCR δ genes; this is discussed in more detail in the section on γδ T cells). The TCR β chain D segment first rearranges to a downstream J segment, with the deletion of intervening DNA. This is followed by rearrangement of a V segment to the DJ segment, resulting in a contiguous (VDJ) β chain gene segment, which is joined to the constant (C) region segment by mRNA splicing. If a VDJ segment lacks premature translation stop codons, the TCR β chain protein may be expressed on the thymocyte surface in association with a pre-TCR α chain protein (pre-Tα) and the CD3 complex proteins [443]. This pre-Tα complex signals intracellularly and instructs the thymocyte to increase its surface expression of CD4 and CD8, to start rearrangement of the TCR α chain gene, and to stop rearrangement of the other TCR β chain allele [444]. This inhibition of TCR β chain gene rearrangement results in allelic exclusion, so that greater than 99% of αβ T cells express only a single type of TCR β chain gene [445]. Pre-Tα complex signaling also results in multiple rounds of cell division of the thymocyte [446], which improves the chances that some of the progeny would have a productive TCR-β and TCR-α gene rearrangement.

Rearrangement of the TCR α chain gene occurs at the double-positive stage and involves the joining of V segments directly to J segments, without intervening D segments. If successful, this leads to the expression of a TCR αβ heterodimer on the cell surface in association with CD3 proteins to form the TCR-CD3 complex. Allelic exclusion is ineffective for the TCR α chain gene, and it is estimated that one third of peripheral human αβ T cells may express two types of TCR α chains [447]. RAG protein expression normally ceases in cortical thymocytes, limiting TCR gene rearrangement to thymic development.

Fetal and Neonatal T-Cell Receptor Repertoire

The generation of the αβ-TCR repertoire by the process of V(D)J recombination of TCR β and TCR α genes probably occurs within a few days after colonization of the thymus by prothymocytes. The usage of D and J segments in rearrangement of the TCR β chain gene in the thymus at approximately 8 weeks of gestation is less diverse than at 11 to 13 weeks of gestation or subsequently [448–450]. This restriction is not explained by an effect of positive or negative selection in the thymus because it applies to D-to-J rearrangements, which are not expressed on the immature thymocyte cell surface [448–451]. The CDR3 region of the TCR β chain transcripts is reduced in length and sequence diversity in the human fetal thymus between 8 and 15 weeks of gestation. This is probably due to decreased amounts of the TdT enzyme, which performs N-nucleotide addition during V(D)J recombination [448–452]. TdT is detectable by 13 weeks of gestation, and fetal TdT activity and CDR3 length increase during the second trimester [448–450].

Exonuclease activity ("nucleotide nibbling"), in which there is variable trimming of the length of V(D)J segments before their joining by Artemis and, possibly, a long isoform of TdT, remains relatively constant from the second trimester onward [452]. Vα and Vβ segment usage in the thymus and peripheral lymphoid organs is diverse [449–451,453]. The αβ-TCR repertoire of cord blood T cells that is expressed on the cell surface is characterized by a diversity of TCR β usage and CDR3 length that is similar to that of antigenically naïve T cells in adults and infants, indicating that the functional preimmune repertoire is fully formed by birth [454–457].

Because the CDR3 region of the TCR chains is a major determinant of antigen specificity [458], decreased CDR3 diversity, in conjunction with restricted usage of V(D)J segments, theoretically could limit recognition of foreign antigens by the fetal αβ-TCR repertoire, particularly during the first trimester. The effects of any potential "holes" in the αβ-TCR repertoire of the human fetus from limitations in CDR3 are likely to be subtle, however, particularly after the second trimester, when V segment usage is diverse. This is suggested by the fact that the T-cell response to immunization and viral challenge generally is normal in mice that are completely deficient in TdT as a result of selective gene targeting [459].

Analysis of the TCR repertoire suggests that there is greater oligoclonal expansion of αβ T cells during the third trimester, particularly after 28 weeks of gestation, than in adults, and that these oligoclonal expansions involve a variety of different Vβ segment families [460]. Whether this oligoclonal expansion is antigen-driven, such as by a response to maternally derived immunoglobulins (e.g., immunoglobulin idiotypes) [461], or, more likely, is a form of homeostatic proliferation is unknown.

T-CELL RECEPTOR EXCISION CIRCLES

The V(D)J recombination process that joins the TCR gene segments also generates double-stranded circular DNA by-products of the intervening sequences, known as T-cell receptor excision circles (TRECs). TRECs seem to be stable throughout the life of a T-lineage lymphocyte. Because they lack a DNA origin of replication, TRECs are diluted at the population level by cell proliferation [462]. The level of DβJβ TRECs, which are formed during Dβ to Jβ rearrangement of the TCR-β gene locus during the double-negative stage of thymocyte development, is at the highest concentration in this cell population [463].

The marked thymocyte proliferation after surface expression of a TCR-β/pre-Tα complex is indicated by the observation that double-positive thymocytes lacking αβ-TCR/CD3 surface complexes (and have not yet achieved a productive TCR-α gene rearrangement) have only 4% of the concentration of DβJβ TRECs per cell as do double-negative cells [463]; this suggests that about four to five mitoses occur between these two stages of thymocyte development. At the double-positive αβ-TCR/CD3⁻ stage of thymocyte development, most TCR-α gene loci first undergo a rearrangement that deletes much of the TCR-δ gene locus, which is located between clusters of Vα and Jα segments. This rearrangement forms a signal joint (sj) between the δRec segment and the downstream ψJα segment and a sjTREC that contains the deleted Dδ, Jδ, and Cδ segments (Fig. 4–10); this irreversibly commits the TCR-α/δ gene locus undergoing this rearrangement to the αβ-TCR differentiation pathway [464]. This rearrangement is followed by a second V(D)J recombination event, discussed in the previous section, in which Vα is joined to Jα to form a recombined Vα-Jα-Cα gene segment and a coding joint (cj)TREC.

sjTRECs, which are the result of sj forming between a δRec segment and a downstream ψJα segment in the TCR-α gene (see Fig. 4–10), have been the predominant type of TREC assayed in human studies. In most αβ T cells, both TCR-α/δ gene loci have undergone δRec/ψJα joining, with the maximal theoretical level of sjTREC content per T-lineage cell being 2. The highest levels of sjTRECs that have been measured are 1.5 copies/cell for CD4⁺CD8⁺αβ-TCR/CD3⁻ human fetal thymocytes [465,466]. As fetal thymocytes progress to the CD4⁺CD8⁺CD3^mid and the mature single-positive (CD4⁺CD8⁻CD3^hi or CD4⁻CD8⁺ CD3^hi) stages, the sjTREC content declines to 0.7 copies/ cell and 0.6 copies/cell [465,466]. This indicates that the maturation of double-positive into single-positive thymocytes, which occurs by the process of positive selection described subsequently, is accompanied by approximately one cell division.

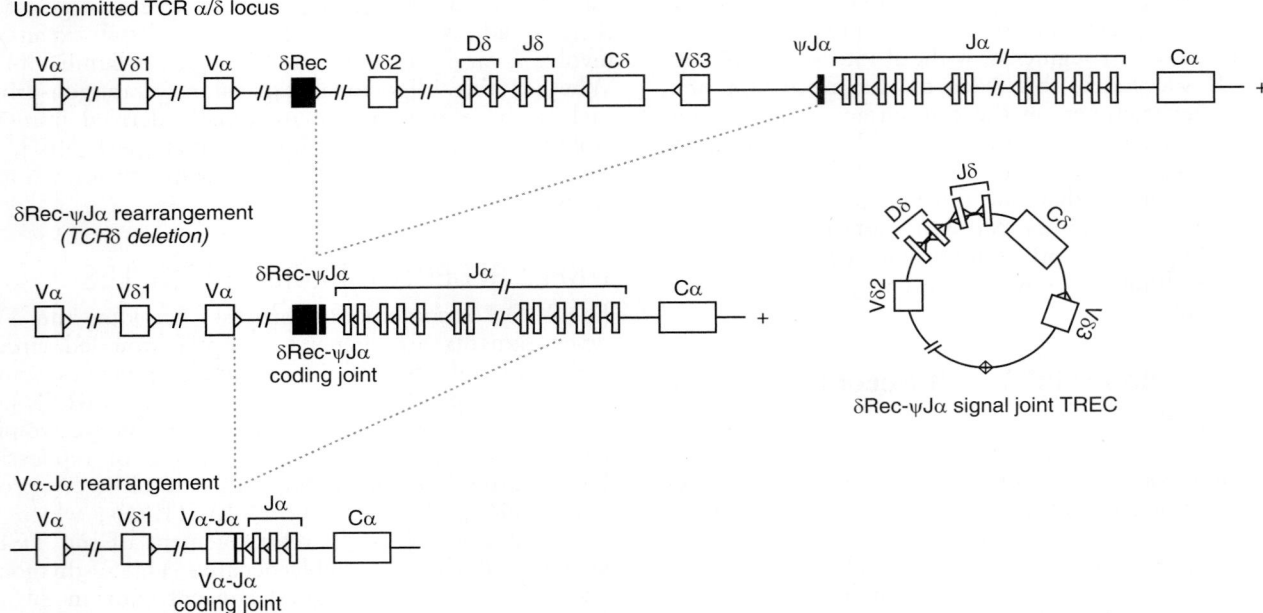

FIGURE 4–10 Sequential rearrangements in the T-cell receptor (TCR)-α/δ locus generate signal joint T-cell receptor excision circles (sjTRECs) and Vα-Jδ rearrangements. Rearrangement of δRec to Jα segment results in a commitment to αβ-TCR lineage because this deletes the C and J segments that are necessary to encode a productive TCR-δ chain. δRec-ψJα rearrangement also generates sjTREC, which is commonly used for monitoring peripheral T-cell populations for their recent thymic origin. δRec-ψJα rearrangement is followed by TCR-α (Vα-Jδ) rearrangements, which, if productive, result in expression of αβ-TCR on the thymocyte cell surface. Most thymocytes that express αβ-TCRs have molecular evidence of nonproductive rearrangements of portions of TCR-δ gene locus (*not shown*).

The sjTREC content of neonatal CD4 T cells is significantly higher than adult antigenically naïve CD4 T cells, indicating that a greater fraction of the adult naïve CD4 T-cell subset has undergone cell division, most likely in the form of homeostatic proliferation, than in the neonate. Such homeostatic proliferation, in which the naïve CD4 T cells retain their characteristic surface phenotype (i.e., CD45RA^hi L-selectin^hi), seems to occur as PTK7+ CD4 RTEs mature into PTK7− naïve CD4 T cells because the sjTREC content of PTK7+ CD4 RTEs is significantly higher than that of PTK7− naïve CD4 T cells [433]. The ratio of sjTRECs and DβJβ TRECs (generated during Dβ to Jβ gene segment rearrangement) in peripheral naïve T cells has also been used to infer the relative amount of intrathymic proliferation occurring between the double-negative and double-positive stages of thymic development, with higher values indicating greater amounts of proliferation [463]. In certain states, such as HIV infection, this ratio is reduced in peripheral T cells, indicating that the infection has a deleterious impact on the intrathymic production of T cells [463].

THYMOCYTE SELECTION AND LATE MATURATION
Positive and Negative Selection

Thymocytes that have successfully rearranged and express αβ-TCRs have a CD4^hi CD8^hi surface phenotype (see Fig. 4–8) and undergo a selective process that tests the appropriateness of their TCR specificity, known as positive selection [444]. Positive selection requires that the αβ-TCR recognize self-peptides bound to MHC molecules displayed on epithelial cells of the thymic cortex. If the TCR has sufficient, but not too high, affinity for self-peptide–MHC complexes, the thymocyte receives a signal allowing its survival. If this signal is absent or weak, the thymocyte dies by apoptosis as a result of activation of caspases, a family of intracellular cysteine proteases. Too strong a signal in the thymic cortex also may not result in effective positive selection.

Studies indicate that the default pathway of maturation of a positively selected double-positive thymocyte is to become to a mature CD4− CD8^hi single-positive cell. If the double-positive thymocyte receives a relatively strong signal via the αβ-TCR/CD3 complex, however, this increases the expression of the GATA-3 transcription factor, which induces the ThPOK transcription factor. ThPOK acts to help upregulate its own expression and prevent the loss of CD4 expression by binding to and inhibiting silencer elements in both of these genes [467]. This action directs the double-positive thymocyte to become a CD4^hi CD8− single-positive cell and ultimately a naïve CD4 T cell. Positive selection also extinguishes *RAG* gene expression, terminating further TCR-α rearrangement. Effective positive selection by MHC class I and MHC class II molecules requires that cortical thymic epithelial cells express the proteolytic enzyme cathepsin L [468] and a novel β5t catalytic subunit of the proteasome [469]. This requirement most likely reflects the importance of generating a specialized set of peptides for positive selection, although the identities of these peptides remain to be defined.

Positively selected CD4^hi CD8− and CD4− CD8^hi thymocytes enter the medulla, where they undergo a second selection process called negative selection, in which they are eliminated by apoptosis if their TCR has too high an affinity for self-peptide–MHC complexes expressed on medullary DCs [470]. Negative selection helps eliminate $\alpha\beta$ T cells with TCRs that could pose a risk of autoimmune reactions and is an important influence on the final TCR repertoire. Thymic epithelial cells found in the medulla express a diverse array of tissue-specific self-antigens (e.g., insulin, myelin basic protein) that help in this elimination. Individual thymic medullary epithelial cells express only some of these self-antigen proteins, and this expression is acquired in an apparently stochastic manner.

The protein encoded by the autoimmune regulator (AIRE) gene plays a key role in enhancing the expression of these tissue-specific proteins by thymic epithelial cells. AIRE may act as a transcriptional coactivator that interacts with components of the RNA polymerase to overcome the inhibitory influence of unmethylated histones in the region of the transcriptional start site [471]. The importance of AIRE is indicated by the high frequency of autoimmune endocrine disease in patients with AIRE gene defects, particularly hypoadrenalism, hypoparathyroidism, and type 1 diabetes mellitus. AIRE may play a similar role in inducing peripheral T-cell tolerance by increasing the expression of tissue-specific antigens by lymph node stromal cells. As a net result of the failure to rearrange productively the TCR α or TCR β chain gene, the lack of positive selection, or the occurrence of negative selection, only about 2% to 3% of the progeny of hematopoietic lymphoid precursors that enter the thymus emerge as mature single-positive thymocytes.

Because the region forming the peptide-binding groove of MHC molecules is highly polymorphic in humans (see section on basic aspects of antigen presentation), a result of positive selection is that T cells have a strong preference for recognizing a particular foreign peptide bound to self-MHC, rather than to the MHC of an unrelated person. The fact that TCR has intrinsic affinity for MHC molecules [472] accounts for the ability of an APC bearing foreign MHC molecules to activate a substantial proportion (several percent) of T cells—the allogeneic response. In the allogeneic response, T cells are activated by novel antigen specificities that are thought to result from the combination of a foreign MHC with multiple self-peptides [473]. Because these self-peptide–foreign MHC specificities are not expressed in the thymus, T cells capable of recognizing them have not been eliminated by the negative selection process in the medulla.

Thymocyte Growth and Differentiation Factors

The factors within the thymic microenvironment that are essential for thymocyte development include key cytokines produced by thymic epithelial cells, such as IL-7. Individuals lacking a functional IL-7 receptor, owing to a genetic deficiency of either the IL-7 receptor α chain or the common γ chain (γc) cytokine receptor (CD132) with which the α chain associates, have abortive thymocyte development and lack mature $\alpha\beta$ T cells [437]. A similar phenotype is observed with genetic deficiency

of JAK-3 tyrosine kinase, which is associated with the cytoplasmic domain of the γc cytokine receptor and delivers activation signals to the interior of the cell [474]. Human fetal B-cell development is spared in these human genetic immunodeficiencies, although a lack of γc-dependent cytokine receptors, such as that for IL-21, results in these B cells having intrinsic functional defects.

Thymocyte Postselection Maturation

CD4^{hi}CD8$^-$ and CD4$^-$CD8^{hi} thymocytes are the most mature $\alpha\beta$ T-lineage cell population in the thymus and predominate in the thymic medulla. Many of the functional differences between peripheral CD4 and CD8 T cells apparently are established during the later stages of thymic maturation, presumably as a result of differentiation induced by positive selection: Mature CD4^{hi}CD8$^-$ thymocytes are similar to peripheral CD4 T cells, in that they are enriched in cells that can secrete certain cytokines, such as IL-2, and provide help for B cells in producing immunoglobulin [475,476]. CD4$^-$CD8^{hi} thymocytes are similar to peripheral CD8 T cells, in that they have a relatively limited ability to produce IL-2, but when primed by antigen are effective in mediating cytotoxic activity [475]. In preparation for thymic emigration, the last stages of single-positive thymocyte maturation include increased levels of the Kruppel-like factor 2 (KLF-2) transcription factor, which seems to increase the thymocyte expression of the sphingosine 1-phosphate receptor [477]. Thymocytes are then directed to emigrate into the blood or lymph or both; blood and lymph have high concentrations of sphingosine 1-phosphate compared with the medulla.

NAÏVE T CELLS
CD4 and CD8 Recent Thymic Emigrants

Mature CD4^{hi}CD8$^-$ and CD4$^-$CD8^{hi} single-positive thymocytes enter into the circulation as RTEs, joining the antigenically naïve CD4 and CD8 $\alpha\beta$ T-cell compartments (see Fig. 4–8). In humans, RTEs of the CD4 T-cell lineage are identified by their expression of protein tyrosine kinase 7 (PTK7), a member of the receptor tyrosine kinase family [433]. The function of PTK7 in immune function is unclear (Lewis DB, unpublished observations, 2009), and this protein has no known ligands and seems to be a catalytically inactive kinase because it lacks a functional adenosine triphosphate (ATP) binding cassette in its cytoplasmic domain [478]. Approximately 5% of circulating naïve CD4 T cells from healthy young adults are PTK7$^+$, and these cells are highly enriched in their sjTREC content compared with PTK7$^-$ naïve CD4 T cells, but otherwise have a similar surface phenotype [433]. As expected for an RTE cell population, PTK7$^+$ naïve CD4 T cells have a highly diverse $\alpha\beta$-TCR repertoire similar to that of the overall naïve CD4 T-cell population and rapidly decline in the circulation after complete thymectomy (performed for the treatment of myasthenia gravis) [433]. As described subsequently, PTK7$^+$ naïve CD4 T cells (hereafter referred to as PTK7$^+$ CD4 RTEs) from healthy adults have reduced activation-dependent function compared with PTK7$^-$ naïve CD4 T cells.

Virtually all CD4 T cells and most CD8 T cells of the neonate express high levels of surface protein and mRNA transcripts for PTK7, which is a marker for CD4 RTEs in older children and adults [433] (Lewis DB, unpublished observations, 2009). Although this high level of PTK7 expression by neonatal naïve CD4 T cells may be explained in part by their being highly enriched in RTEs, it is likely that PTK7 expression is regulated differently in neonatal CD4 T cells compared with adult naïve CD4 T cells based on two observations: First, there is a higher level of expression of PTK7 per neonatal naïve CD4 T cell compared with adult PTK7 CD4 RTEs [433]. Second, there are few, if any, PTK7$^-$ cells among circulating neonatal naïve CD4 T cells even though studies of older children undergoing complete thymectomy suggest that most PTK7$^+$ CD4 RTEs are converted to PTK7$^-$ naïve CD4 T cells over a 3-month period [433], and at least some neonatal T cells are likely to have emigrated from the thymus more than 6 months previously.

The expression of CD103 ($\alpha_E\beta_7$ integrin) seems to be a marker for CD8, but not CD4 T-lineage RTEs [466]. As for PTK7$^+$ CD4 RTEs, the thymic dependence of this circulating CD8 RTE population has been shown by the impact of complete thymectomy [466], and these cells are relatively enriched in sjTRECs compared with CD103$^-$ naïve CD4 T cells. It is unclear whether CD103$^+$ naïve CD8 T cells in the adult circulation differ in function from that of the CD103$^-$ naïve CD8 T-cell subset.

Naïve T-Cell Entry into Lymphoid Tissue, Recirculation, and Survival

Human naïve CD4 T cells have a CD45RA^{hi}CD45RO^{lo}-CD27^{hi}L-selectin^{hi}α$_4$β$_1$–CD11a^{dim} surface phenotype [479]. Naïve T cells, including RTEs, preferentially home to the secondary lymphoid tissue, which includes the lymph nodes, spleen, Peyer patches, and MALT, and then recirculate along with the rest of the antigenically naïve CD4 and CD8 T-cell compartments. Egress of RTEs from the thymus and of naïve T cells and B cells from secondary lymphoid tissue requires that these cell types express sphingosine 1-phosphate receptors. Sphingosine 1-phosphate, the receptor ligand, is at higher concentrations in the blood and lymph than in the thymus and secondary lymphoid tissue, which directs these cells to exit the tissues and enter into these fluids [480]. Bronchus-associated lymphoid tissue, a type of MALT, typically appears only after birth and is another potential site for naïve T-cell homing and recirculation [481].

Development of secondary lymph node tissues depends on signaling by lymphotoxin (LT) α and β members of the TNF cytokine gene family (see Table 4–1). Peripheral lymphoid organogenesis involves lymphoid tissue inducer cells, which are CD45$^+$CD4$^+$CD3$^-$ and express surface LTαβ$_2$ trimers engaging the LTβ receptor on stromal cells. Stromal cells are induced to become stromal organizers by increasing their expression of adhesion molecules (VCAM-1, ICAM-1, and MAdCAM-1) and of chemokines (CXCL13, CCL19, and CCL21), which attracts naïve B cells and T cells and more lymphoid tissue inducer cells, ultimately resulting in fully formed peripheral lymph nodes [482].

As described for DCs, migration of fully mature naïve T cells and RTEs, both of which express high levels of the CCR7 chemokine receptor and L-selectin [433], into the peripheral lymphoid organs is determined in part by the local patterns and gradients of chemokine receptor ligands in tissues (see Tables 4–1 and 4–2) and ligands for adhesion molecules. L-selectin, which is constitutively expressed on many types of leukocytes, including naïve and certain subsets of memory T cells, binds to multivalent carbohydrate ligands displayed on specific protein or lipid backbones on the cell surface. T-cell surface expression of L-selectin allows their binding to the peripheral lymph node addressin, which is expressed on the surface of the specialized high endothelium of the postcapillary venules in the peripheral lymph nodes, Peyer patches, and tonsils [483]. Tethered to the surface of the high endothelium of the postcapillary venules is the chemokine CCL21, which binds to CCR7 on the surface of RTEs and naïve T cells. CCL21 and another CCR7 ligand, CCL19, are produced by stromal cells and perhaps some APCs in the lymph node. The engagement of CCR7 on naïve T cells by CCL21 triggers signals leading to an increase in the affinity of LFA-1, allowing the naïve T cells to bind avidly to the LFA-1 ligands ICAM-1 and ICAM-2 on the vascular endothelium. This stops T-cell rolling, allowing the T cell to undergo diapedesis across the endothelium and to enter the T-cell zones of the lymph node. CCL19 is produced there by DCs, resulting in the juxtaposition of naïve T cells and DCs [483].

Based on elegant studies in mice, the survival of naïve T cells in the periphery has been shown to be dependent on two major exogenous factors. The first is continuous interaction with self-peptide–MHC complexes, which seems to be particularly important for the survival of the antigenically naïve T-cell populations [484]. Whether this survival signal is analogous to positive selection in the thymus in its requirements for a diverse self-peptide repertoire is unclear. The second major factor seems to be signals provided by IL-7 binding to IL-7 receptors on naïve CD4 and CD8 T cells [484]. It is unclear if human naïve T cells have similar requirements for their survival in the periphery, and, if so, whether RTEs and more mature naïve T cells differ in their dependence on these αβ-TCR/CD3 and cytokine receptor signals.

ONTOGENY OF NAÏVE T-CELL SURFACE PHENOTYPE

Circulating T cells are detectable by 12.5 weeks of gestation, showing the emigration of mature T-lineage cells from the thymus [485]. By 14 weeks of gestation, CD4 and CD8 T cells are found in the fetal liver and spleen, and CD4 T cells are detectable in lymph nodes [486]. The percentage of T cells in the fetal or premature circulation gradually increases during the second and third trimesters of pregnancy through approximately 6 months of age [486], followed by a gradual decline to adult levels during childhood [487]. The ratio of CD4 to CD8 T cells in the circulation is relatively high during fetal life (about 3.5) and gradually declines with age [487]. The levels of expression of the αβ-TCR, CD3, CD4, CD5, CD8, and

CD28 proteins on fetal and neonatal αβ T cells are similar to those in adult T cells (Lewis DB, unpublished data, 2008) [488].

CD31

CD31, also known as platelet endothelial cell adhesion molecule-1 (PECAM-1), is expressed in large amounts on most adult peripheral CD4 T cells that have a naïve (CD45RA^{hi}) surface phenotype, but is absent or decreased on most memory CD4 T cells. A small fraction of CD45RA^{hi} CD4 T cells that are CD31^{lo} appears and gradually increases with aging, especially after adulthood, and these cells have very low sjTREC content and an oligoclonal rather than polyclonal αβ-TCR repertoire compared with either PTK7^{+} CD4 RTEs (which are uniformly CD31^{hi}) or PTK7^{-} CD31^{hi} naïve CD4 T cells [489,490]. It has been argued that these CD31^{lo} naïve CD4 T cells are the result of homeostatic proliferation of CD31^{hi} naïve CD4 T cells, rather than reversion of memory/effector cells to a CD45RA surface phenotype because these cells lack a capacity to express cytokines characteristic of memory/effector cells, such as IFN-γ. The origin of the cells constituting this CD31^{lo} subset might be clarified by more extensive phenotyping, including gene expression profiling.

Most neonatal CD45RA^{hi} T cells are CD31^{hi}, but approximately 10% to 20% have been reported to be CD31^{lo} [491]. It is unclear if the neonatal CD31^{lo} subset of naïve CD4 T cells has low levels of sjTRECs similar to that found in adult CD31^{lo} naïve CD4 T-cell subset, which would suggest that these cells have undergone extensive proliferation compared with most neonatal CD4 T cells. Alternatively, a finding of high sjTREC content in CD31^{lo} naïve CD4 T cells of the neonate would suggest that this population may be an immature population that gives rise to CD31^{hi} naïve CD4 T cells. Because neonatal CD4 T cells are uniformly PTK7^{hi}, and PTK7 expression by adult CD4 RTEs is lost in an in vitro model of homeostatic proliferation using a cytokine cocktail [433], the latter possibility seems to be more likely.

CD38

CD38 is an ectoenzyme that generates cyclic adenosine diphosphate (ADP)–ribose, a metabolite that induces intracellular calcium mobilization. It is expressed on most thymocytes, some activated peripheral blood T cells and B cells, plasma cells, and DCs. In contrast adult naïve T cells, virtually all peripheral fetal and neonatal T cells express very high levels of the CD38 molecule [492,493], suggesting that peripheral T cells in the fetus and neonate may represent a thymocyte-like immature transitional population. There is no substantial difference in CD38 expression by adult circulating PTK7^{+} CD4 RTEs and PTK7^{-} naïve CD4 T cells [433], indicating that this persistence of high levels of CD38 expression is unique to the naïve T-cell compartment of the fetus and neonate. In contrast with circulating fetal and neonatal T cells, a significant fraction of T cells in the fetal spleen between 14 and 20 weeks of gestation lack CD38 expression [494], which suggests that CD38 may be downregulated on entry into secondary lymphoid tissue.

As discussed subsequently, a significant fraction of splenic CD4 T cells in the fetus seem to belong to the regulatory T-cell subset, and it is plausible that this subset may have only relatively low levels of CD38 expression, based on analysis of adult regulatory T cells (Tregs) [495]. Neonatal CD4 T cells lose expression of CD38 after in vitro culture with IL-7 for 10 days [496], which implies that this cytokine promotes further maturation independently of engagement of the αβ-TCR–CD3 complex. The precursor-product relationship between CD38^{+} and CD38^{-} peripheral naïve T cells in humans is unclear.

The role of CD38 in the function of human T cells and other cell types also is unknown. In mice, CD38 is required for chemokine-mediated migration of mature DCs into secondary lymphoid tissue, and as a consequence, CD38 deficiency impairs humoral immunity to T-cell–dependent antigens. Mice, in contrast with humans, have relatively low levels of thymocyte expression of CD38, and CD38 deficiency in these animals does not have a clear impact on thymocyte development or intrinsic T-cell function.

CD45 Isoforms

Circulating T cells in the term and preterm (22 to 30 weeks of gestation) neonate and in the second-trimester and third-trimester fetus predominantly express a CD45RA^{hi}CD45RO^{lo} surface phenotype [493,497,498], which also is found on antigenically naïve T cells of adults. About 30% of circulating T cells of the term neonate are CD45RA^{lo}CD45RO^{lo} [499], a surface phenotype that is rare or absent in circulating adult T cells. Because these CD45RA^{lo}CD45RO^{lo} T cells are functionally similar to neonatal CD45RA^{hi}CD45RO^{lo} T cells and become CD45RA^{mid}CD45RO^{lo} T cells when incubated in vitro with fibroblasts [499], they seem to be immature thymocyte-like cells, rather than naïve cells that have been activated in vivo to express the CD45RO isoform.

Most studies have found that the healthy neonate and the fetus in late gestation lack circulating CD45RO^{hi} T cells, consistent with their limited exposure to foreign antigens. A lack of surface expression of other memory/effector markers, such as β$_1$ integrins (e.g., VLA-4) and, in the case of CD8 T cells, KIRs [500] and CD11b [501,502], also is consistent with an antigenically naïve population predominating in the healthy neonate.

A postnatal precursor-product relationship between CD45RA^{hi}CD45RO^{lo} and CD45RA^{lo}CD45RO^{hi} T cells is suggested by the fact that the proportion of αβ T cells with a memory/effector phenotype and the capacity of circulating T cells to produce cytokines, such as IFN-γ, gradually increase, whereas the proportion of antigenically naïve T cells decreases, with increasing postnatal age [487,503]. These increases in the ability to produce cytokines and expression of the CD45RO^{hi} phenotype presumably are due to cumulative antigenic exposure and T-cell activation, leading to the generation of memory T cells from antigenically naïve T cells.

In premature or term neonates who are stressed, a portion of circulating T-lineage cells are CD3^{lo} and coexpress CD1, CD4, and CD8 [492], a phenotype characteristic of immature thymocytes of the cortex

[504]. It is likely that stress results in the premature release of cortical thymocytes into the circulation, but the immunologic consequences of this release are unclear.

A few, although still a substantial proportion, T cells in the second-trimester fetal spleen are CD45RA^{lo}CD45RO^{hi}, a T-cell population that is absent from the spleen of young infants [498]. These fetal CD45RO^{hi} T cells have a diverse αβ-TCR repertoire and express high levels of CD25 (IL-2 receptor α chain) and proliferate with IL-2 [499]. In contrast to adult CD45RO^{hi} T cells, these fetal spleen CD45RO^{hi} T cells express low surface levels of CD2 and LFA-1 and proliferate poorly after activation with either anti-CD2 or anti-CD3 monoclonal antibody (mAb), suggesting that they are not fully functional [498]. As discussed in "Regulatory T Cells of the Fetus and Neonate," many features of this cell population are consistent with their being Tregs, which have been shown to be prominent in the spleen and lymph nodes of the fetus [505,506]. The extent to which these fetal spleen CD45RO^{hi} T cells contribute to the postnatal (Treg or non-Treg) peripheral T-cell compartment is unknown.

HOMEOSTATIC PROLIFERATION
Spontaneous Naïve Peripheral T-Cell Proliferation

Naïve T cells may undergo proliferation by processes that are distinct from the processes of full activation by cognate antigen and appropriate costimulation, and such proliferative processes may make a significant contribution to expansion of the peripheral T-cell pool during development. Based on flow cytometric analysis of expression of the Ki67 antigen, a significantly higher fraction of naïve (CD45RO^{lo}) CD4 and CD8 T cells in the third-trimester fetus and the term neonate are spontaneously in cell cycle than the fraction of adult naïve T cells [441]. The highest levels are observed at 26 weeks of gestation, and these gradually decline with gestational age. Even at term, the frequencies reported for naïve CD4 and CD8 T cells—approximately 1.4% and 3.2%—are sevenfold those of adult naïve T cells and are substantially higher than the frequencies observed for adult CD45RO^{hi} T cells [441]. These results are supported by other in vitro assays of mitosis, such as the incorporation of tritiated (^{3}H)-thymidine or the loss of fluorescence after labeling cell membranes with carboxyfluorescein succinimidyl ester (CFSE) [507] (Lewis DB, unpublished results, 2008).

A substantial proportion of CD4 and CD8 T cells of the neonate express the killer cell lectin-like receptor G1 (KLRG1) [508], an inhibitory receptor that is also expressed by NK cells and that interacts with cadherins. These KLRG1$^+$ neonatal T cells have naïve surface phenotype, a normal proliferative response to anti-CD3 and CD28 mAb, and a diverse αβ-TCR repertoire, but a reduced sjTREC content compared with their KLRG1$^-$ counterparts [508]. Based on these findings, it is plausible that the KLRG1$^+$ subset of naïve T cells of the neonate may be enriched for cells that have undergone homeostatic proliferation.

Although the mechanism underlying this proliferation of human fetal and neonatal naïve T cells is unclear, it differs from the mechanism in rodent models of homeostatic proliferation, including in the neonatal mouse [509], in that the proliferation occurs in the absence of peripheral lymphopenia. As discussed next, one potential explanation for this increased spontaneous proliferation is an increased sensitivity of fetal and neonatal T cells to cytokines, such as IL-7, which is also a feature of circulating PTK7$^+$ CD4 RTEs of adults [433]. Future studies are needed to determine if spontaneously proliferating naïve T cells in fetus and neonate (and proliferating PTK7$^+$ CD4 RTEs in adults) have a diverse TCR repertoire (as would be predicted by a model of generalized increased sensitivity to cytokines), and whether they can be distinguished from noncycling cells by other markers, such as those that are induced during naïve T-cell proliferation in the setting of peripheral lymphopenia, and by reduced sjTREC content.

Antigen-Independent Naïve T-Cell Proliferation in Response to IL-7 and IL-15

Murine studies show that the homeostatic proliferation in the lymphopenic host and survival of naïve CD4 and CD8 T cells depends on IL-7 [434]. Human neonatal naïve CD4 T cells are capable of higher levels of polyclonal cell proliferation than adult naïve CD4 T cells in response to IL-7 [441,510-512]; it is plausible that IL-7–dependent proliferation could account for the high rate of spontaneous CD4 T-cell proliferation in the human fetus and neonate and contribute to the normal and rapid expansion of the peripheral CD4 T-cell compartment at this age. The increased IL-7 proliferative response is associated with increased expression of the CD127 (IL-7 receptor α chain component) by neonatal naïve CD4 T cells compared with adult naïve CD4 T cells [510,512,513], although surface expression of the other component of the IL-7 receptor, the γc cytokine receptor, was decreased on neonatal naïve CD4 T cells compared with adult naïve T cells in one study [512]. This increased expression of the IL-7 receptor α chain by neonatal naïve CD4 T cells is not observed for PTK7$^+$ CD4 RTEs in adults [433], indicating that the increased responsiveness of RTEs to IL-7 may be mediated by a different mechanism (see next).

Murine studies also indicate that positive selection results in a dramatic upregulation of the IL-7 receptor α chain and the γc cytokine receptor on CD3^{hi} (mature) CD4–single-positive and CD8–single-positive thymocytes [513]. In vitro thymic organ culture experiments suggest that IL-7 plays a key role in the postselection expansion of the single-positive thymocyte population by a mechanism that does not involve αβ-TCR engagement [513]. Human CD4–single-positive thymocytes have also been shown to have an increased proliferative response to IL-7 [514], suggesting that this increased IL-7 sensitivity also applies to late thymocyte maturation in humans. These observations, taken with the finding that human PTK7$^+$ CD4 RTEs also have an increased proliferative response to IL-7 compared with PTK7$^-$ naïve CD4 T cells even though there are no differences in surface expression of either component of the IL-7 receptor [433] (Lewis DB, unpublished observations, 2009), suggest that the mechanism for this increased

IL-7 sensitivity by neonatal CD4 T cells is (1) likely to be downstream of cytokine receptor binding and (2) shared with mature CD4+CD8− thymocytes and PTK7+ CD4 RTEs.

Whether IL-7 not only contributes to extrathymic expansion of naïve CD4 T cells, but also influences their maturation is unclear. IL-7 treatment of neonatal naïve CD4 T cells for relatively long periods (7 or 14 days) does not decrease expression of CD45RA or L-selectin and does not increase the expression of CD45RO [496,510,515,516]. The extent to which IL-7 treatment, alone, of neonatal naïve CD4 T cells results in acquisition of a phenotype with selective features of naïve and memory/effector cells remains contentious: Results are conflicting regarding whether IL-7 treatment increases surface expression of CD11a, a memory/effector cell marker; the activation-dependent proteins CD25 and CD40 ligand; or the capacity of neonatal CD4 T cells to produce T_H1 and T_H2 cytokines [496,510]. IL-7 in combination with a cocktail of other cytokines (IL-6, IL-10, IL-15, and TNF-α) has been shown to result in the loss of PTK7 surface expression by adult PTK7+ CD4 RTEs, but it is unknown if PTK7 downregulation is accompanied by an increased capacity for T_H1 effector function by adult RTEs and if this downregulation occurs with such treatment of neonatal T cells.

Naïve CD4 and CD8 T-cell survival in adults requires interactions between the $\alpha\beta$-TCR and self-peptide/MHC molecules on immature DCs and engagement of the T-cell IL-7 receptor by IL-7 on fibroblastic reticular cells found in the T-cell zone of secondary lymphoid organs; IL-15 may also play a role in CD8 T-cell survival [484]. Human neonatal naïve CD8 T cells are more responsive to treatment with a combination of IL-7 and IL-15 than is the analogous adult cell population, as indicated by loss of CFSE staining with culture after in vitro labeling [441]. Whether this enhanced effect is related to increased levels of IL-15 receptors on neonatal T cells is unknown. Also unclear are the effects of treatment with this combination of cytokines on neonatal naïve CD8 T-cell phenotype and function.

NAÏVE T-CELL ACTIVATION, ANERGY, AND COSTIMULATION

If naïve T cells encounter DCs presenting cognate peptide–MHC complexes, they stop migrating and remain in the lymph node. If they do not encounter such DCs, they migrate through the lymph node to the efferent lymph and return to the bloodstream. Naïve T cells continually circulate between the blood and secondary lymphoid tissues, allowing them the opportunity to sample APCs continuously for their cognate antigen. Because they regulate this homeostatic recirculation of naïve T cells, CCL19 and CCL21 are referred to as homeostatic chemokines.

When naïve CD4 T cells first encounter foreign peptide–MHC complexes during a primary immune response, they extinguish expression of LKLF, a transcription factor that maintains naïve T cells in a resting state [517], allowing them to become activated. The TCR-CD3 complex is linked to an intricate and highly interconnected complex of kinases, phosphatases, and adapter molecules that together transduce signals in response to engagement of the TCR and, in $\alpha\beta$ T cells, the appropriate CD4 or CD8 coreceptor by cognate peptide–MHC complexes (Fig. 4–11; see also Fig. 4–6) [518]. Lipid rafts play a crucial role in facilitating the assembly of signaling complexes at specific regions of the plasma membrane at high local concentrations; these complexes

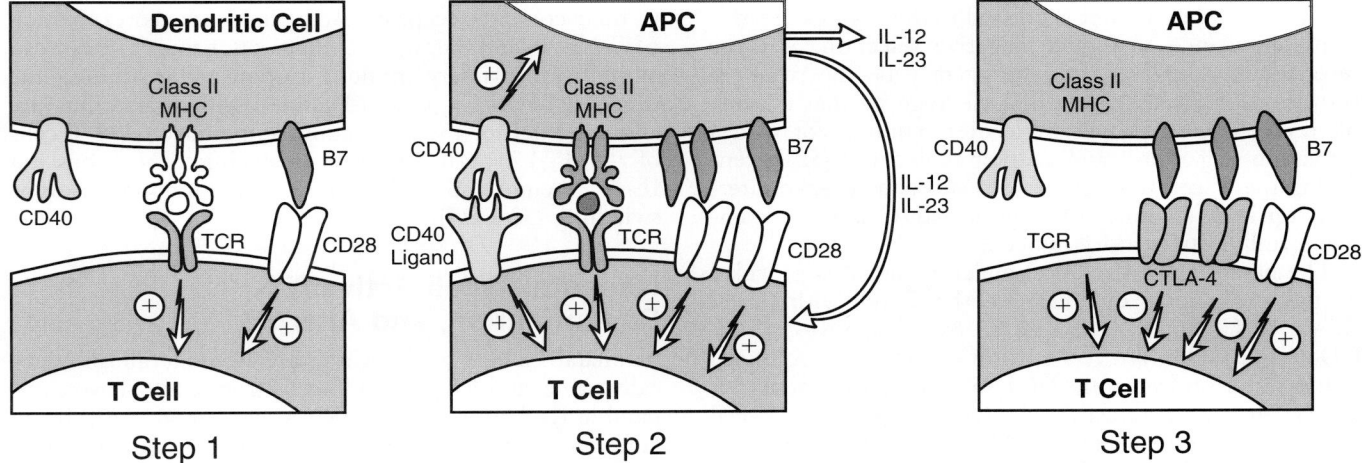

FIGURE 4–11 **T cell–antigen-presenting cell (APC) interactions early during the immune response to peptide antigens.** Major histocompatibility complex (MHC) class II–restricted response by CD4+ T cells is shown as an example. Dendritic cells are probably the most important APC for antigenically naïve T cells and constitutively express CD80 or CD86 (B7 molecules), CD40, and MHC class II molecules on their cell surface. Engagement of $\alpha\beta$ T-cell receptor ($\alpha\beta$-TCR) on the CD4+ T cell by antigenic peptides bound to MHC molecules on the dendritic cell, in conjunction with costimulation by B7 (CD80/86) interactions with CD28 interactions, leads to T-cell activation (*Step 1*). The activated T cell expresses CD40 ligand (CD154) on its surface, which engages CD40 on the dendritic cell; this increases B7 expression on the dendritic cell, enhancing T-cell costimulation (*Step 2*). CD40 engagement also activates the dendritic cell to produce cytokines, such as interleukin (IL)-12. IL-12 promotes the proliferation and differentiation of T cells into T_H1-type effector cells that produce high levels of interferon (IFN)-γ and low or undetectable amounts of IL-4. CTLA-4 (CD152) is expressed on T cells during later stages of T-cell activation. Engagement of CTLA-4 by B7 molecules on the APC delivers negative signals that help terminate T-cell activation (*Step 3*).

contained in lipid microdomains recruit adapters and signal-transducing proteins [519]. Proximal activation events include the activation of the Lck and ZAP-70 tyrosine kinases and phospholipase C followed by elevation of inositol triphosphate, which leads to the release of calcium into the cytoplasm from the endoplasmic reticulum. This increase in $[Ca^{2+}]_i$ is sensed by the STIM1 protein of the endoplasmic reticulum, which interacts with and opens calcium-release activated calcium channels of the cell membrane, resulting in a 10-fold increase in $[Ca^{2+}]_i$ and full T-cell activation [520].

An increased calcium concentration activates calcineurin, allowing the translocation of nuclear factor of activated T cells (NFAT) transcription factors from the cytosol to the nucleus. Concurrent activation of the extracellular signal-regulated kinase/mitogen-activated protein kinase (ERK/MAPK) pathway enhances activation of other transcription factors, including activator protein-1/activating transcription factor. T-cell activation also activates the NFκB transcription factor by a pathway that involves protein kinase C-θ and the CARMA1/Bcl10/Malt1 trimolecular complex [518]. Collectively, these transcription factors induce the transcription of genes encoding key proteins for activation, such as cytokines (e.g., IL-2); cell cycle regulators; and, in cytotoxic T cells, proteins involved in killing other cells, such as perforins.

Full naïve T-cell activation that leads to cytokine production and cell proliferation requires that signaling through the trimolecular αβ-TCR–peptide–MHC complex exceed a specific threshold and costimulatory signaling pathways. Low-affinity interactions that do not trigger full T-cell activation, particularly in the absence of costimulation, may lead to a state of long-term unresponsiveness to subsequent stimulation, which is referred to as anergy. Anergy may help maintain tolerance by mature T cells to certain self-antigens—in particular, self-antigens that are not expressed in the thymus in sufficient abundance to induce negative selection. A more recent study suggests that anergy may be the result of activation of caspase 3 and the cleavage by that enzyme of intracellular signaling molecules required for T-cell activation (e.g., Vav1 and adapter molecules) [521], rendering the T cell unresponsive to subsequent encounters with optimal amounts of peptide–MHC antigen complexes and costimulatory molecules.

The best-characterized costimulatory signal is provided by the engagement of CD28 on the T cell with CD80 (B7-1) or CD86 (B7-2) on APCs (see Table 4–4) [522]. CD80 and CD86 are related proteins that are expressed at low levels on immature DCs, mononuclear phagocytes, and B cells and increased levels after LPS exposure, B-cell receptor cross-linking, and CD40 signaling (see Fig. 4–11). APCs primed by these factors and, in particular, mature DCs express high levels of CD80 and CD86. CD80 and CD86 bind to CD28, which is constitutively expressed on T cells, reducing the strength or duration of TCR signaling needed for full activation [522]. Another B7 family member, inducible costimulator (ICOS)–ligand and its receptor on T cells, ICOS, which is homologous to CD28, are important for driving the differentiation of activated T cells into specialized effector lineages, such as

T_H17 cells and T follicular helper cells (T_{FH}), which are discussed in more detail subsequently. Other members of the family such as PD-1 ("programmed death-1") and PD-2 when engaged on the T cell by PD-ligands act to dampen the T-cell response by inducing T-cell apoptosis [522].

Activated T cells are induced to express high-affinity IL-2 receptor complexes composed of the IL-2R α and β chains and γc. Engagement of the IL-2 receptor complex by IL-2, acting as an autocrine and a paracrine growth factor, triggers T cells to undergo multiple rounds of proliferation, expanding the numbers of antigen-specific T cells, and to differentiate into effector T cells (Fig. 4–12). IL-2–mediated proliferation leads to an expansion in the numbers of the responding T-cell population, which is a key feature of antigen-specific immunity. In the absence of prior exposure, the frequency of T lymphocytes capable of recognizing and responding to that antigen is small, generally less than 1:100,000, but in response to infection can increase to greater than 1:20 for CD8 T cells and greater than 1:1000 for CD4 T cells in less than 1 week [523].

Activated T cells, especially those of the CD4 T-cell subset, also express on their surface CD40 ligand (CD154 or TNFSF5), a member of the TNF ligand family (see Tables 4–1 and 4–4) that engages the CD40 molecule on B cells, DCs, and mononuclear phagocytes [524,525]. As mentioned previously, CD40 engagement induces the expression of CD80 and CD86 on these APCs and induces DCs to produce IL-12 family heterodimeric cytokines, such as IL-12p70 (see Fig. 4–11). Interactions between CD40 and CD40 ligand seem to play an important role in vivo in the expansion of CD4 T cells during a primary immune response, but may be less crucial for expansion of CD8 T cells. Several other members of the TNF ligand family can be expressed on activated T cells and may stimulate APC function by binding to their cognate receptors. Activation-induced expression of TNF ligand family members on naïve T cells can amplify the primary immune responses by priming the function of APCs. CD40-ligand/CD40 interactions are also essential for the generation of memory CD4 T cells of the T_H1 type (capable of producing IFN-γ, but not IL-4), memory B cells, and immunoglobulin isotype switching [524,525].

Neonatal T-Cell Activation, Costimulation, and Anergy

Neonatal CD4 T cells, which are virtually all antigenically naïve, and naïve CD4 T cells from adults have comparable IL-2 protein and mRNA expression and rates of IL-2 gene transcription if strong (and potentially nonphysiologic) activators of T cells are used, such as calcium ionophores or mitogenic lectins combined with phorbol esters [526–528]. Neonatal T cells also produce IL-2 and proliferate as well as adult T cells in response to anti-CD3 mAb if optimal CD28 costimulation is provided [529], indicating that CD28-mediated signaling is intact. Decreased IL-2 production by neonatal T cells has been observed using more physiologic activation conditions, however. Compared with adult naïve CD4

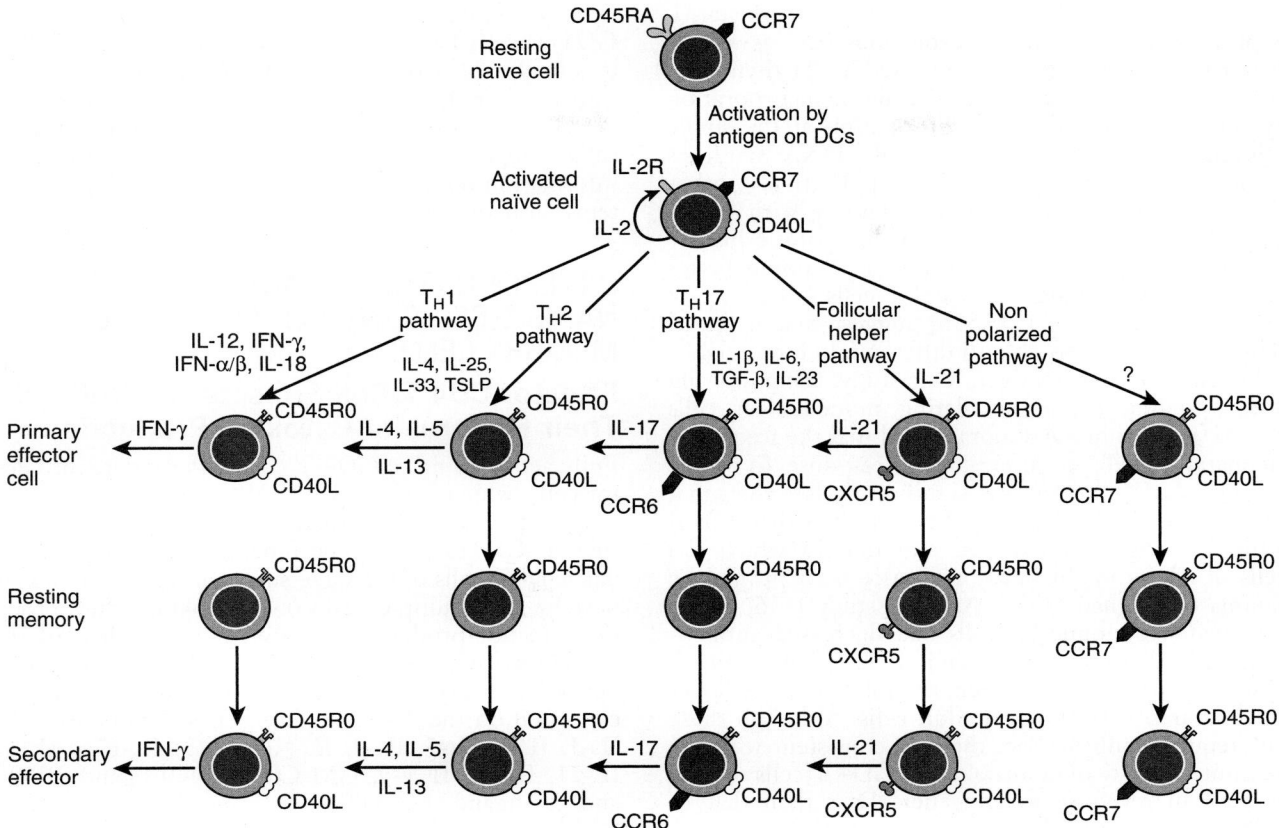

FIGURE 4–12 Differentiation of antigenically naïve CD4$^+$ T cells into T$_H$1, T$_H$2, unpolarized, and T follicular helper effector and memory T cells. Antigenically naïve CD4$^+$ T cells express high levels of the CD45RA isoform of the CD45 surface protein tyrosine phosphatase. They are activated by antigen presented by APC to express CD40-ligand and IL-2 and to undergo clonal expansion and differentiation, which is accompanied by expression of the CD45RO isoform and loss of the CD45RA isoform. Most effector cells die by apoptosis, but a small fraction of these cells persist as memory cells that express high levels of CD45RO. Exposure of expanding effector cells to IL-12, interferon (IFN)-γ, and type I interferon favors their differentiation into T$_H$1 effector cells that secrete IFN-γ, whereas exposure to IL-4 and dendritic cells that have been exposed to thymic stromal lymphopoietin (TSLP), IL-25, and IL-31 favors their differentiation into T$_H$2 effector cells that secrete IL-4, IL-5, and IL-13. Many memory cells are nonpolarized and do not express either T$_H$1 or T$_H$2 cytokines. They may be enriched for cells that continue to express the CCR7 chemokine receptor, which favors their recirculation between the blood and the lymph nodes and spleen. T follicular helper cells, which express high levels of CXCR5, move into B-cell follicle areas where they express CD40 ligand and provide help for B-cell responses. The signals that promote the accumulation of memory T follicular helper cells and their capacity to produce cytokines are poorly understood. Memory cells rechallenged with antigen undergo rapid clonal expansion into secondary effector cells that mediate the same functions as the initial memory population. Most secondary effector cells eventually die by apoptosis.

T cells, neonatal naïve CD4 T cells produced less IL-2 mRNA and expressed fewer high-affinity IL-2 receptors in response to stimulation with anti-CD2 mAb [530–532].

These differences were abrogated when phorbol ester, which bypasses proximal signaling pathways and directly activates the Ras signaling pathway, was included [530], suggesting that the capacity to express IL-2 and high-affinity receptors is not absolutely limited for neonatal cells, but signals leading to their induction may not be transmitted efficiently. Similarly, the production of IL-2 by neonatal naïve CD4 T cells was reduced compared with production by adult CD45RA^{hi} CD4 T cells after allogeneic stimulation with adult moDCs, a system that closely mimics physiologic T-cell activation by foreign peptide/self-MHC complexes [533]. Together, these observations argue that neonatal cells may be intrinsically limited in their ability to be physiologically activated for IL-2 production.

The ability of activated T cells to divide efficiently in response to IL-2 depends on the expression of the high-affinity IL-2 receptor, which consists of CD25 (IL-2 receptor α chain), β chain (shared with the IL-15 receptor), and the γc cytokine receptor (shared with the specific receptors for IL-4, IL-7, IL-9, IL-15, and IL-21). In contrast with IL-2 production, neonatal T cells seem to express similar or higher amounts of CD25 after stimulation with anti-CD3 mAb [526]. This finding is consistent with the signal transduction pathways leading to the induction of CD25 being distinct from the pathways involved in IL-2 production, and with neonatal T cells having a relatively selective limitation in signals required for cytokine production, rather than a generalized limitation acting at an early step of the activation cascade. Basal expression of the γc cytokine receptor by neonatal T cells is lower than that by either adult CD45RA^{hi} or CD45RO^{hi} T cells [534]. The importance of this finding is unclear because activated neonatal T cells proliferate in response to exogenous IL-2 as well as or better than adult T cells, as indicated by ^{3}H-thymidine incorporation [526]. Radioactive thymidine incorporation assays do not provide mitotic information at the single cell level, however, and examine only DNA synthesis and not actual cell proliferation. The application of other techniques, such as cell membrane staining with CFSE [507], which allows an assessment of the mitotic history of individual cells, should be helpful in defining better the replicative potential of neonatal T cells.

Two in vitro studies [535,536] suggest that neonatal T cells may also be less able to differentiate into effector cells in response to neoantigen. One study, using limiting dilution techniques and circulating mononuclear cells from CMV-nonimmune donors, found that the frequency of neonatal T cells proliferating in response to whole inactivated CMV antigen was significantly less than that of adult T cells [535]. A pitfall of this study is that it used a complex antigen preparation and one to which the T cells of adults might have previously been primed by infections other than CMV. Another study [536] found that neonatal mononuclear cells had decreased antigen-specific T-cell proliferation and IL-2 production in response to a protein neoantigen, keyhole limpet hemocyanin, compared with those in adult cells. Although these results require confirmation, they are consistent with the more limited ability of neonatal naïve CD4 T cells to produce IL-2 in response to allogeneic DCs than that of adult naïve cells [533].

Superantigens activate T cells by binding to a portion of the TCR β chain outside of the peptide antigen recognition site, but otherwise mimic activation by peptide–MHC complexes in most respects. Neonatal T cells differ from adult naïve CD45RA^{hi} T cells in their tendency to become anergic rather than competent for increased cytokine secretion after priming with bacterial superantigen bound to MHC class II–transfected murine fibroblasts [537]. This anergic tendency is developmentally regulated because CD4^{hi}CD8$^-$ thymocytes, the immediate precursors of antigenically naïve CD4 T cells, also are prone to anergy when treated under these conditions [538]. Consistent with this anergic tendency, newborns with toxic shock syndrome–like exanthematous disease, in which the Vβ2-bearing T-cell population is markedly expanded in vivo by the superantigen TSST-1, have a greater fraction of anergic Vβ2-bearing T cells than is found in adults with TSST-1–mediated toxic shock syndrome [539].

Some studies also have found that neonatal, but not adult, CD4 T cells primed by alloantigen, in the form of EBV-transformed human B cells, become nonresponsive to restimulation by alloantigen or by a combination of anti-CD3 and anti-CD28 mAbs [385,540]. Preliminary studies implicate a lack of Ras signaling as the basis for this reduced responsiveness [540]. These results, taken with results using bacterial superantigen, suggest that neonatal and, presumably, fetal T cells have a greater tendency to become anergic, particularly under conditions in which production of inflammatory mediators or costimulation (e.g., by CD40, CD80, or CD86 on the APC) may be limited.

ICOS expression by circulating neonatal and adult CD4 T cells has been reported to be similar [541], but it is unclear if neonatal CD4 T cells are as responsive to signals after ICOS-ligand engagement as adult CD4 T cells (i.e., for the differentiation into $T_{H}17$ and T_{FH} cells, which are discussed next). There is also limited information on the expression of PD and PD-ligand proteins on neonatal T cells.

DIFFERENTIATION OF ACTIVATED NAÏVE T CELLS INTO EFFECTOR AND MEMORY CELLS

Effector CD4 T-Cell Subsets Are Defined by Their Patterns of Cytokine Production

Fully activated naïve CD4 T cells differentiate into effector cells, which have a CD45RA^{lo}CD45RO^{hi} surface phenotype and increased expression of adhesion molecules, such as CD11a [542]. The functions of effector T cells, particularly cells of the CD4 subset, are mediated in large part by the multiple additional cytokines they produce that are not produced by naïve T cells. Most of these cytokines are secreted, although some (e.g., some members of the TNF ligand family) may be predominantly expressed on the T-cell surface. These cytokines include IL-3, IL-4, IL-5, IL-9, IL-10, IL-13, IL-17A, IL-17F, IL-21, IL-22, IFN-γ, GM-CSF, CD40 ligand, TNF-α, and Fas-ligand [543,544].

Table 4–2 summarizes the major immunomodulatory effects of T cell–derived cytokines and of cytokines produced by other cell types that act on T cells. IFN-γ is the signature cytokine produced by $T_{H}1$ effector cells, which also produce substantial amounts of IL-2, lymphotoxin-α, and TNF-α, but little or no IL-4, IL-5, IL-13, IL-17, or IL-21. By contrast, IL-4 is the signature cytokine of $T_{H}2$ cells, which also produce IL-5, IL-9, and IL-13, but little or no IFN-γ, IL-2, IL-17, or IL-21. Human $T_{H}17$ cells secrete IL-17A and IL-17F, two members of the IL-17 family. A minor subset of human $T_{H}17$ cells expresses IL-22 and IFN-γ; in contrast to murine $T_{H}17$ cells, most human $T_{H}17$ cells express TNF-α, but not IL-6 [545]. T_{FH} are particularly efficient producers of IL-21, a cytokine that may also be involved in their generation from naïve CD4 T cells [546]. Cells producing effector cytokines of $T_{H}1$ and $T_{H}2$ types are commonly referred to as $T_{H}0$ cells, which often are seen after vaccination with protein antigens or after viral infections, such as influenza virus or CMV [547]. The generation of $T_{H}0$ cells in vitro seems to be favored by the presence of large amounts of IL-2 in the absence of cytokines that polarize differentiation toward particular effector cell subsets. Most circulating adult memory CD4 T cells seem to be nonpolarized (i.e., not belonging to the $T_{H}1$, $T_{H}2$, $T_{H}17$, or T_{FH} subsets) based on their capacity for cytokine expression and their expression of chemokine receptors [548]. These nonpolarized memory cells can likely give rise to more polarized cell subsets with appropriate instructional signals, which are described subsequently.

In addition to their differing cytokine profiles, the four effector subsets differ in their repertoire of chemokine receptors, and this has an important influence on their localization and function in vivo. Human T_H1 cells preferentially express CCR5 and CXCR3. In contrast, most T_H2 cells express CCR4, but only a few T_H1 cells do [548]. The expression of CCR5 by most T_H1 cells and monocytes allows these two cell types to be concurrently recruited to sites of inflammation [549], which may enhance the activation of mononuclear phagocytes by T_H1-derived IFN-γ. The ligands for CCR4, CCL17, and CCL22 are commonly expressed by leukocytes at sites of allergic disease, which attracts T_H2 cells that contribute to allergic pathogenesis. Most human T_H17 cells express CCR6 [545], which helps target these cells to tissues, such as inflamed gastrointestinal epithelium that produce high levels of CCL20, the sole ligand for CCR6 [550]. T_{FH} cells are defined by their expression of CXCR5, whose sole ligand is CXCL13, a chemokine produced by stromal cells of the B-cell follicle. This CXCR5/CXCL13 interaction helps retain T_{FH} in the B-cell follicles where they can provide help for antibody production [551].

Regulation of CD4 Effector T-Cell Subset Differentiation

The cytokine milieu encountered by activated naïve CD4 T cells and the key master transcriptional regulatory factors this milieu induces play a dominant role in directing T_H subset differentiation [312]. T_H1 effector development is favored by the exposure to high levels of IL-12p70 and IL-18 produced by APCs and to IFN-γ produced by NK cells and other T cells (see Fig. 4–6) and the induction of the T-bet transcription factor. In humans, but less so in mice, type I IFNs also promote T_H1 differentiation, although they cannot replace IL-12 in this process [552]. The importance of these cytokines in the development of robust T_H1 responses is shown by the limited T_H1 responses observed in patients with defects of IL-12 or IL-12 receptor signaling [553,554]. T_H2 development is favored when CD4 T cells initially are activated in the presence of IL-4, TSLP, IL-25, and IL-33 (an IL-1 family member), which are derived from epithelial sources [555], particularly in the absence of IL-12, IL-18, type I IFNs, or IFN-γ (see Fig. 4–12). The usual source of IL-4 in this context is uncertain. GATA-binding protein–3 is a master regulator of T_H2 T-cell development [312]. T_H17 cell development is favored by exposure to IL-1β, IL-6, and TGF-β and IL-21, IL-23, and TNF-α [556], and requires RORγt and RORα as master transcriptional regulators. $T_{FH}1$ cell development in mice, and likely in humans, depends on IL-21 binding to IL-21 receptors on activated naïve CD4 T cells and on ICOS/ICOS-ligand interactions between CD4 T cells and B cells [546]. The transcriptional regulation of T_{FH} differentiation is less well characterized than for the other T_H effector subsets, but c-Maf may play a role in promoting T_{FH} and T_H17 development, at least in mice, by increasing IL-21 production [557].

CD4 T-Cell Help for Antibody Production

CD4 T cells play a crucial role in the regulation of B-cell proliferation, immunoglobulin class switching, affinity maturation, and memory B-cell generation in response to proteins or protein conjugates. The enhancement of B-cell responses is commonly referred to as T-cell help. This process is critically dependent on the recognition through the αβ-TCR of cognate peptide–MHC complexes on B cells, and on multiple contact-dependent interactions (see Fig. 4–11) between members of the TNF ligand–TNF receptor families (see Table 4–1) and the CD28-B7 families (see Table 4–4). Recently activated CD4 T cells that express CXCR5 migrate to B-cell follicles and provide key help for antibody production as T_{FH} cells that secrete IL-21 and express surface CD40 ligand (see Fig. 4–12) [551]. CXCR5 is the receptor for CXCL13 (BCA-1), a chemokine produced by stromal cells of the B-cell follicle. The function of these T_{FH} cells in providing B-cell help is discussed in more detail in the section on naïve B-cell activation, clonal expansion, immune selection, and T-cell help.

The importance of cognate T-cell help is illustrated by the phenotype of patients with X-linked hyper-IgM syndrome, who have genetic defects in the expression of CD40 ligand [525]. In affected individuals, the marked paucity of immunoglobulin isotypes other than IgM and inability to generate memory B-cell responses indicate that these responses critically depend on the engagement of CD40 on B cells by CD40 ligand (CD154) on T cells. Engagement of CD40 on B cells in conjunction with other signals provided by cytokines, such as IL-4 and IL-21, markedly enhances immunoglobulin production and class switching and B-cell survival [558].

Activated and memory CD4 T cells also express ICOS, a receptor for ICOS-ligand, which is constitutively expressed on B cells and various other cell types. ICOS costimulates the T-cell response and promotes the development of T_H2 and T_{FH} responses. ICOS-ligand engagement on the B cell by ICOS also is important for enhancing the production of IgG. The identification of ICOS deficiency as a cause of common variable immunodeficiency, in which there is profound hypogammaglobulinemia and poor antibody responses to vaccination [559], shows the importance of ICOS–ICOS-ligand interactions in humans. Other interactions, such as between LFA-1 and CD54 (ICAM-1), may enhance T cell–dependent B-cell responses [560], an idea supported by the finding that humans with CD18 deficiency, which is a component of the LFA-1 integrin, have depressed antibody responses after immunization [561].

Soluble cytokines produced by activated T cells influence the amount and type of immunoglobulin produced by B cells. Experiments in mice in which the IL-2, IL-4, IL-5, or IFN-γ gene or, in some cases, their specific receptors and associated STAT signaling molecules have been disrupted by gene targeting suggest that these cytokines are important for the proper regulation of B-cell immunoglobulin isotype expression. Inactivation of the IL-4 gene, components of the high-affinity IL-4 receptor, or the STAT-6 protein involved in IL-4 receptor signal transduction results in a greater than 90% decrease in IgE production, whereas the production of other antibody isotypes is largely unperturbed [562]. IL-21 secretion by T cells may be important for immunoglobulin production by B cells not only because of direct effects on B-cell antibody secretion, but also because of IL-21 promoting $T_{FH}1$ development in an autocrine or paracrine manner [546].

Overview of Memory T Cells

Although greater than 90% of antigen-specific effector T cells generated during a robust primary immune response die, a fraction of effector cells persist as memory T cells. Memory T cells account for the enhanced secondary T-cell response to subsequent challenge—this reflects the substantially greater frequency of antigen-specific memory T cells (approximately 1:100 to 1:10,000) compared with antigen-specific T cells in a naïve host (approximately 1:100,000 for most antigens) and the enhanced functions of memory T cells compared with naïve T cells [563]. Memory T cells retain many of the functions of the effector T cells that characterized the immune response from which the memory T cells arose. These functions include a reduced threshold for activation and the ability to produce more rapidly the effector cytokines that characterized the effector T-cell subset from which they arose (i.e., T_H1, T_H2, T_H17, or T_{FH} cells). Turnover of human memory T cells occurs slowly, but more rapidly than turnover of naïve T cells [563]. Memory T cells apparently persist (in humans most likely for decades) in the absence of further contact with foreign antigenic peptide–MHC complexes [484].

Murine experiments indicate that memory CD4 T cells are derived from a small subset of effector T cells that survive and persist [564]. An origin from effector cells is consistent with the estimation that human memory T cells arise from naïve T-cell precursors after an average of 14 cell divisions as assessed based on telomere length [565], which shortens with lymphocyte cell division [566]. One model proposes that effector and memory T-cell lineages may be generated from the two progeny of a single cell division of an activated naïve CD4 or CD8 T cell because the two daughter cells have unequal partitioning of the proteins involved in cell signaling, cell differentiation, and the asymmetric cell division process itself [567]. Humans genetically deficient in CD40 ligand have reduced CD4 T-cell recall responses to previously administered protein vaccines [568,569], indicating that CD40–CD40 ligand–mediated signals are most likely essential for memory CD4 T-cell generation or maintenance or both.

Similar to effector cells, most human memory CD4 T cells can be distinguished from naïve cells by their surface expression of the CD45RO rather than the CD45RA isoform of CD45 (see Fig. 4–12) [563]. In addition, memory and effector T cells typically express higher levels of adhesion molecules, such as the $\alpha_4\beta_1$ and CD11a/CD18 integrins, than levels observed on naïve T cells (see Table 4–4) [542,570]. About 40% of circulating adult CD4 T cells have this CD45RA^{lo}CD45RO^{hi} ($\alpha_4\beta_1^{hi}$) memory/effector surface phenotype, and a fraction of these cells are L-selectin^{hi}, most of which belong to the central memory cell subset [571] (discussed subsequently). In persistent viral infection, a subset of memory CD4 T cells expresses PD-1, and this expression is associated with impaired T-cell function in cases of HIV-1 infection.

Activation and propagation of CD45RA^{hi}CD45RO^{lo} CD4 T cells in vitro results in their acquisition of memory/effector cell–like features, including a lower threshold for activation; a CD45RA^{lo}CD45RO^{hi} phenotype in most cases; an enhanced ability to produce effector cytokines (e.g., IFN-γ, IL-4, IL-17, or IL-21); and an increased ability to provide help for B-cell antibody production. These findings support the notion that CD45RA^{hi} T cells are precursors of CD45RO^{hi} T cells and that this differentiation occurs after T-cell activation; in addition, these findings are consistent with the observation that the CD45RA^{lo}CD45RO^{hi} cell subset consists mainly of memory T cells that respond to recall antigens [563].

Memory CD8 T cells are similar to T cells of the CD4 subset in expressing a CD45RA^{lo}CD45RO^{hi} surface phenotype and in possessing an enhanced capacity to produce multiple cytokines compared with that in their naïve precursors and molecules involved in cell-mediated cytotoxicity, such as perforins and granzymes [572]. In addition, in contrast to memory CD4 T cells, a substantial subset of these CD45RO^{hi} CD8 T cells expresses CD11b, CD57, KIRs, and NK-G2D [573,574]. As discussed in the earlier section on NK cells, KIRs bind self–HLA-A, self–HLA-B, or self–HLA-C alleles and deliver an inhibitory signal into the cell and are expressed at high levels on most or all human NK cells. KIR expression by T cells may regulate effector function, such as cytotoxicity, by increasing the threshold for activation by antigenic peptide–MHC complexes, but human KIR$^+$ CD8 T cells seem to have equivalent function as CD8 T cells of the KIR$^-$ subset [575]. NKG2D expression may serve as a means to enhance CD8 T-cell effector function [574].

Human effector CD8 T cells also can be distinguished from circulating naïve CD8 T cells by surface phenotype. Most human CD8 effector cells have a CD45RA^{hi} CD27$^-$CD28$^-$ surface phenotype and a high capacity to mediate cytotoxicity directly (high levels of intracellular perforin and granzyme staining) and to produce T_H1-type effector cytokines, including TNF-α and IFN-γ [542,572]. By contrast, naïve CD8 T cells have a CD45RA^{hi} CD27$^+$CD28$^+$ surface phenotype and a limited ability to mediate cytotoxicity and to secrete these cytokines.

Compared with naïve T cells, memory T cells generally have a lower activation threshold, are less dependent on these costimulatory signals, and can commit to proliferate after engagement of $\alpha\beta$-TCR more quickly than naïve T cells [576]. This increased responsiveness of memory T cells compared with naïve T cells reflects a reprogramming of gene expression by epigenetic changes, such as DNA methylation, histone modifications, and chromatin remodeling and alterations in transcription factors [577].

The tissue localization of memory T cells is determined by differential expression of adhesion molecules and chemokine receptors. Distinct central (lymphoid homing) and effector (nonlymphoid tissue homing) memory T-cell populations in humans have been identified [571]. Central memory T cells express CCR7 receptor and high levels of L-selectin, whereas, in contrast, most effector memory T cells lack CCR7 and express low levels of L-selectin. Most effector memory T cells express adhesion molecules other than L-selectin that help target them to specific tissues. In humans, the generation of T_H1 and T_H17 CCR7^{lo} (effector memory) CD4 T cells is impaired in genetic deficiency of the IL-12Rβ1 chain [553,578], a component for signaling via the IL-12 receptor (required for T_H1 development) and the IL-23 receptor (which enhances T_H17 immunity). Central memory CD4 T cells typically show reduced antigen-specific expression of certain cytokines, such as IFN-γ, compared with the effector memory subset, whereas IL-2 production is similar or higher by the central memory subset compared with effector memory CD4 T cells [579,580].

The central memory pool may be a larger fraction of the memory pool for CD4 than for CD8 T cells. Human central memory CD4 T cells also have a lower turnover [581] and are more responsive to maintenance signals provided by cytokines, such as IL-2 and IL-7, compared with effector memory CD4 T cells [582]. Although the precursor-product relationship between central and effector memory T cells is controversial [542], there is strong evidence that central memory CD4 T cells are the precursors of effector memory cells, at least in primates. In chronic simian immunodeficiency virus infection, a progressive decline in central memory CD4 T cells ultimately results in effector memory CD4 T-cell insufficiency and increased viral-induced disease [583].

Turnover of memory CD4 and CD8 T cells seems to be much more frequent than turnover of their naïve counterparts, suggesting that the process is a dynamic one [563]. In contrast to naïve T cells, the maintenance of memory T cells seems not to require continued contact with self-peptide–MHC complexes, but does require IL-7 and IL-15 [484]. Most memory CD4 T cells require both cytokines for survival, whereas most memory CD8 T cells require IL-15, but not IL-7 for survival [484]. IL-7 also may be required to promote the transition of effector CD8 T cells to memory cells, although signaling via specific IL-7 receptors is insufficient for this conversion [584].

Memory T-Cell Activation

When memory T cells reencounter antigenic peptide–MHC complexes ("recall antigen") as part of the secondary response, they are activated and undergo expansion and differentiation into a secondary effector population (see Fig. 4–12). The secondary immune response to recall antigen is typically more rapid and robust than the primary response to an antigen that has never been encountered previously. This difference is due to the greater frequency of antigen-specific memory T cells than of naïve T cells with TCRs that recognize the same antigenic peptides and to the enhanced function of these memory T cells and their secondary effector progeny. This increased responsiveness of memory T cells is the result of reprogramming of gene expression by epigenetic changes such as DNA methylation, histone modifications, chromatin remodeling of genes involved in effector functions such as IFN-γ genetic locus [585], and alterations in transcription factors [586,587]. In addition, there are alterations of the proximal signaling cascade that may reduce the activation threshold for memory T cells compared with naïve T cells [588]. The quality of the effector immune response may also be enhanced. Individual secondary effectors generated from memory CD8 T cells may express perforin and effector cytokines, whereas primary effectors generated from naïve CD8 T cells may express either perforin or cytokines, but not both [589].

Postnatal Ontogeny of Memory CD4 T-Cell Subsets

The memory CD4 T-cell subset in infants and young children has a significantly higher ratio of central memory to effector memory CD4 T cells than that observed in adults [579]. The frequency of effector memory CD4 T cells that can produce IFN-γ and the amount of IFN-γ produced per cell in response to bacterial superantigen are similar in the blood of infants and young children and adults, however [579]. This finding indicates that effector memory cells generated during infancy are functionally similar to those of adults. It is likely that the greater proportion of central memory cells also applies to memory CD4 T-cell responses that occur in the first few months of life, but this remains to be shown. The mechanism responsible for the greater fraction of central memory cells in infants and children is unclear. One possibility is that the decreased proportion of effector memory CD4 T cells may reflect reduced activity of IL-12–dependent T_H1 pathway because effector memory CD4 T cells are markedly reduced in IL-12Rβ1 deficiency, which ablates IL-12p70 [553].

PRODUCTION OF CYTOKINES, CHEMOKINES, AND TUMOR NECROSIS FACTOR–LIGAND PROTEINS BY NEONATAL T CELLS

CD4 T-Cell Cytokine Production

In contrast to IL-2, the production of most other cytokines or their cognate mRNAs by unfractionated neonatal T cells or the CD4 T-cell subset seems to be reduced after short-term stimulation, including with anti-CD3 mAb, mitogen, or pharmacologic agents (e.g., the combination of calcium ionophore and phorbol ester) compared with that in adult T cells. For most cytokines (IL-3, IL-4, IL-5, IL-6, IL-10, IL-13, IFN-γ, and GM-CSF), this is a marked reduction [91,92,528,590,591]; for a few, such as TNF-α [592], the reduction is modest. As with neonatal T cells, naïve T cells from adults have a reduced capacity to produce most of these cytokines compared with adult memory/effector T cells [593–596], although adult naïve T cells may produce substantial amounts of IL-13 [597]. The low capacity of neonatal T cells to produce IFN-γ and IL-4 is due to an almost complete absence of IFN-γ and IL-4 mRNA-expressing cells [528], which is paralleled by a lack of cells expressing detectable levels of these cytokines after polyclonal activation and analysis by flow cytometry after intracellular staining [392,598,599]. Together, these results suggest that much of the apparent deficiency in cytokine production by neonatal T cells is accounted for by the fact that almost all neonatal T cells are naïve and lack antigenic experience.

Highly purified naïve CD4 T cells from neonates also have a reduced capacity to produce IFN-γ in vitro compared with adult naïve CD4 T cells after more prolonged stimulation with the same pool of moDCs from multiple unrelated blood donors [533]. This finding strongly suggests that the capacity of neonatal naïve CD4 T cells to produce IFN-γ is intrinsically more limited, even when a potent, physiologic APC population is used for antigen presentation.

In contrast to short-term stimulation, IL-10 production by anti-CD3 mAb and IL-2–stimulated neonatal CD4 T cells may be substantially higher than by adult naïve CD4 T cells after more prolonged incubation [600]. Whether these IL-10–producing neonatal CD4 T cells are derived from non-Treg versus natural Treg cell populations is uncertain, but, regardless, increased production of IL-10 by T cells in vivo would be expected to inhibit APC and effector T-cell function [601].

CD8 T-Cell Cytokine and Chemokine Production

Cytokine production by neonatal CD8 T cells has not been as well characterized as for the CD4 T-cell subset. The lack of a memory (CD45RO^{hi}) CD8 T-cell subset in the neonate seems to account for reduced production of the chemokine CCL-5 (RANTES) by neonatal T cells compared with adult cells [602]. A striking result, which needs to be confirmed, is that neonatal naïve CD8 T cells produce substantially more IL-13, which is characteristic of T$_H$2 immune responses, than that produced by analogous adult cells after stimulation with anti-CD3 and anti-CD28 mAbs and exogenous IL-2 [603]. It would be of interest to determine if this unusual cytokine profile also applies to antigen-specific immune responses mediated by neonatal CD8 T cells, such as to viral pathogens.

Postnatal Ontogeny of Cytokine Production

Neonatal T cells have been intensively studied for their cytokine secretion phenotype, but relatively little is known regarding the postnatal ontogeny of T-cell cytokine production during the first year of life. A study using phytohemagglutinin as a stimulus found that the capacity of peripheral blood lymphocytes obtained from newborns was similar to umbilical vein cord blood in having a low capacity to produce IFN-γ, IL-4, and IL-10 [604]. The capacity of peripheral blood lymphocytes to produce all three of these cytokines gradually increased during the first year of life [604], consistent with the acquisition of increased cytokine production as a result of the progressive acquisition of memory T cells resulting from exposure to foreign antigens.

CD40 Ligand

Durandy and colleagues [605] reported that a substantial proportion of circulating fetal T cells between 19 and 31 weeks of gestation expressed CD40 ligand in vitro in response to polyclonal activation. Whether fetal T cells that can express CD40 ligand have a distinct surface phenotype from T cells lacking this capacity is unclear. By contrast, T cells from fetuses of later gestational age and from neonates have a much more limited capacity to produce CD40 ligand after activation with calcium ionophore and phorbol ester [605–608].

Expression of CD40 ligand by activated neonatal CD4 T cells remains reduced for at least 10 days postnatally, but is almost equal to adult cells by 3 to 4 weeks after birth [605] (Lewis DB, unpublished data, 2000). In most of these studies, activated neonatal CD4 T cells of cord blood expressed markedly lower amounts of CD40 ligand surface protein and mRNA than either adult CD45RA^{hi} or CD45RO^{hi} CD4 T cells [605–608]. Decreased CD40 ligand expression may not be due to the lack of a memory/effector population in the neonatal T-cell compartment, but may represent a true developmental limitation in cytokine production.

Decreased CD40 ligand production by neonatal T cells also has been documented in the mouse [609], suggesting that it may be a feature of RTEs. Consistent with this idea, human CD4^{hi}CD8$^-$ thymocytes, the immediate precursors of RTEs, also have a low capacity to express CD40 ligand [608,610]. Adult PTK7$^+$ CD4 RTEs have similar levels of CD40 ligand expression as PTK7$^-$ naïve CD4 T cells [433], however, indicating that the capacity for activation-induced CD40-ligand expression is upregulated before thymic emigration or shortly thereafter, at least in adults. As with most T cell–derived cytokines characteristic of effector cells [91], when neonatal T cells are strongly activated in vitro into an effector-like T-cell population, they acquire a markedly increased capacity to produce CD40 ligand on restimulation, showing that this reduction is not a fixed phenotypic feature [605,608].

In view of the importance of CD40 ligand in multiple aspects of the immune response [524,525], limitations in CD40 ligand production could contribute to decreased antigen-specific immunity mediated by T$_H$1 effector cells and B cells in the neonate. The initial studies showing a relative deficiency of CD40 ligand expression by neonatal T cells used calcium ionophore and phorbol ester for stimulation, a combination that maximizes the production of CD40 ligand, but that may not accurately mimic physiologic T-cell activation. Reduced CD40 ligand surface expression by purified neonatal naïve CD4 T cells compared with that observed in adult naïve CD4 T cells also has been observed after stimulation with various stimuli that engage the αβ-TCR–CD3 complex either alone or in combination with anti-CD28 mAb [611], suggesting that this reduction is likely to be applicable to physiologic T-cell activation. Similar results have been independently obtained for anti-CD3 and anti-CD28 mAb stimulation using unfractionated neonatal and adult T cells [612]. Others have found equivalent levels of CD40 ligand expression by neonatal and adult T cells using anti-CD3 mAb stimulation [613,614], however, suggesting that the particular in vitro conditions used (e.g., the particular anti-CD3 mAb and cell culture conditions) may influence the outcome of the assay.

The ability of neonatal and adult T cells to produce CD40 ligand in response to allogeneic stimulation, a condition that should closely mimic T-cell activation through the recognition of foreign peptide–MHC complexes, has also been studied. Neonatal CD4 T cells stimulated allogeneically can express some CD40 ligand and induce IL-12 production by DCs after 3 days of culture, but the ability of adult T cells to do so was not evaluated for comparison [615]. Another study found that CD40 ligand expression by neonatal T cells was similar to that by adult T cells after 5 days of allogeneic stimulation with irradiated adult moDCs [616]. By contrast, another study [533] found that CD40 ligand expression by purified neonatal naïve CD4 T cells was substantially less than in adult naïve CD4 T cells after 24 to 48 hours of stimulation. This reduced CD40 ligand production was accompanied by reduced IL-12p70 production (by moDCs) and IL-2 and IFN-γ production (by naïve CD4 T cells). Together, these findings suggest that CD40 ligand surface expression initially may be more limited for neonatal naïve CD4 T cells, but that with continued priming, at least in vitro, this can be overcome with variable results [533,615,616]. The differentiation of neonatal naïve CD4 T cells into T$_H$1 effector cells by CD40 ligand–dependent and IL-12–dependent processes may be limited during the early stages of T-cell differentiation.

Other Tumor Necrosis Factor Family Ligands

Fas-ligand, another member of the TNF ligand family, plays a key role in inducing apoptotic cell death on target cells that express Fas on the surface. Human Fas or Fas-ligand deficiency is associated with antibody-mediated autoimmunity and lymphoid hyperplasia, rather than defects in viral clearance [617]. Neonatal T cells have decreased Fas-ligand expression after anti-CD3 and anti-CD28 mAb stimulation compared with adult cells [612]. Neonatal and adult CD4 T cells express similar surface levels of Fas [541]. Iwama and colleagues [618] reported that circulating levels of Fas-ligand are elevated in newborns, but the cellular source of this protein and its functional significance are unclear. The role of Fas–Fas-ligand interactions in regulating apoptosis of neonatal T cells is discussed in the section on neonatal T-cell apoptosis.

Mechanisms for Decreased Cytokine, Chemokine, and Tumor Necrosis Factor– Ligand Production by Neonatal T Cells

For many cytokine and TNF-ligand genes, a key event leading to de novo gene transcription is an activation-induced increase in the concentration of $[Ca^{2+}]_i$, which is required for NFAT nuclear location and transcriptional activity [619]. Certain studies comparing adult and neonatal unfractionated or CD4 T cells have suggested that neonatal T cells have substantial limitations in proximal signal transduction events that are required for the cytokine and TNF-ligand expression. These limitations include a generalized decrease in the overall level of activation-induced tyrosine phosphorylation of intracellular proteins compared with that in unfractionated adult T cells [620]; decreased activation-induced phosphorylation of CD3-ε; decreased phosphorylation and enzyme activity of the Lck and ZAP-70 tyrosine kinases and the ERK2, JNK, and p38 kinases [612]; reduced basal expression of protein kinase C β1, ε, θ, and ζ [621]; and reduced basal and activation-induced levels of phospholipase C isoenzymes [622].

It is unclear if the above-described reported deficiencies in proximal signal transduction events apply specifically to neonatal naïve T cells, but not to adult naïve T cells, because these studies used unfractionated adult T cells.

In one study in which such a direct comparison was made, purified neonatal naïve CD4 T cells had a substantially reduced increase in $[Ca^{2+}]_i$ after anti-CD3 mAb cross-linkage compared with that observed in identically treated adult naïve cells [611]. Although the mechanism for this reduced calcium response remains to be defined, it is plausible that this reduction may account in part for reduced neonatal T-cell expression of genes positively regulated by NFAT, such as secreted cytokines and, as discussed later on, CD40 ligand.

Another study [623] found that the combination of activation by anti-CD3 and anti-CD26 mAb was markedly less effective for inducing proximal signaling events, such as phosphorylation of lck, and proliferation for neonatal T cells compared with adult naïve T cells. This poor activation by anti-CD26 mAb was associated with CD26 being located outside lipid raft microdomains in neonatal T cells, whereas in activated adult naïve T cells CD26 was a lipid raft component. Although the importance of CD26 in physiologic T-cell activation is uncertain, these observations are of interest because they suggest that further analysis of the composition of the lipid raft microdomains of neonatal versus adult naïve T cells may provide addition insights into limitations of neonatal T-cell activation.

Reduced IL-4 and IFN-γ mRNA expression by polyclonally activated neonatal CD4 and CD8 T cells compared with that observed in adult T cells is due primarily to reduced transcription of these cytokine genes. These differences in cytokine mRNA expression do not seem to reflect solely differences in proximal signal transduction because they have been observed not only after activation through the αβ-TCR–CD3 complex [91], but also after activation with ionomycin and PMA [528], which bypass proximal signal transduction events. IFN-γ and IL-4 are expressed mainly by memory/effector T-cell populations, rather than by the naïve T-cell populations [594]; the reduced expression of these cytokines by neonatal T cells can be accounted for by the lack of memory/effector cells in the circulating neonatal T-cell population. For many genes, including the IFN-γ gene, DNA methylation of the locus represses transcription by decreasing the ability of transcriptional activator proteins to bind to regulatory elements, such as promoters and enhancers [624]. Reduced expression of IFN-γ by neonatal T cells may also result in part from greater methylation of DNA in the IFN-γ gene locus in neonatal and adult naïve T cells than in adult memory T cells [625,626]. With a detailed understanding of epigenetic alterations of the IFN-γ gene locus during T-cell development and by naïve versus memory T cells [585], a comparison of naïve T cells from neonates and adults for these epigenetic modifications may provide new insights as to mechanisms for decreased IFN-γ expression by neonatal T cells.

In addition to decreased cytokine gene transcription, decreased cytokine mRNA stability may play a role in reduced cytokine production by neonatal T cells. Decreased IL-3 production by neonatal T cells seems to be due mainly to reduced IL-3 mRNA stability, rather than to decreased gene transcription [627]. The mechanism for this reduced mRNA stability is unclear.

Decreased mRNA stability also has been observed for other cytokines after stimulation of cord BMCs [282], but whether this also holds for purified neonatal T cells has not been addressed.

Cytokine Production by Neonatal T Cells after Short-Term In Vitro Differentiation

The generation of effector T cells from naïve precursors in response to antigen in vivo can be mimicked by in vitro stimulation, such as by engagement of the αβ-TCR–CD3 complex in conjunction with accessory cells (non–T cells contained in peripheral BMCs) and exogenous cytokines. Neonatal T cells, if polyclonally activated under conditions that favor repeated cell division (strong activation stimuli in common with the provision of exogenous IL-2), resemble antigenically naïve adult T cells in efficiently acquiring the characteristics of effector cells. These characteristics include a $CD45RA^{lo}CD45RO^{hi}$ surface phenotype, an enhanced ability to be activated by anti-CD2 or anti-CD3 mAb, and an increased capacity to produce cytokines (e.g., IL-4, IFN-γ) [91,628–630].

Although neonatal CD4 T cells can be effectively primed for expression of effector cytokines by strong mitogenic stimuli and provision of cytokines, such as IL-2, as already noted, their capacity to differentiate into T_H1 effector cells under more physiologic conditions may be more limited. Neonatal naïve CD4 T cells stimulated with allogeneic DCs were found to have decreased frequency of $IFN-γ^+$ cells, based on intracellular cytokine staining, compared with that observed in adult naïve CD4 T cells in response to short-term (i.e., 24 to 48 hours' duration) stimulation by allogeneic DCs [533].

This decreased expression of IFN-γ by neonatal CD4 T cells activated under these more physiologic conditions of DC-mediated allogeneic stimulation probably is due to several factors. First, neonatal CD4 T cells are less effective than adult naïve cells at inducing the cocultured DCs to produce IL-12p70 [533], a key cytokine for promoting T_H1 differentiation and IFN-γ production [554]. This reduced IL-12 production is attributable, at least in part, to reduced expression of CD40 ligand by neonatal CD4 T cells in response to allogeneic stimulation using DCs [533] because engagement of CD40 on DCs by CD40 ligand is an important mechanism for inducing IL-12 production [631]. Second, CD40 ligand is also important in the acquisition of antigen-specific CD4 T cells, including cells with T_H1 immune function [568,569]. Third, neonatal CD4 T cells may have decreased expression of certain transcription factors, such as the NFATc2 protein [632,633], although this finding is controversial [634]; such a reduction could limit the induction of IFN-γ gene transcription and IL-2 and CD40 ligand expression in response to T-cell activation [635]. Fourth, the greater methylation of DNA of the IFN-γ genetic locus in neonatal T cells than in adult naïve T cells may also contribute to a reduced and delayed acquisition of IFN-γ production after activation in vitro [626]. Together, these mechanisms intrinsic to the T cell and immaturity of cDC function (see earlier) may account for the delayed acquisition of IFN-γ production by antigen-specific CD4 T cells

after infection in the neonatal period (see later section on antigen-specific T-cell function in the fetus and neonate).

In contrast to impaired T_H1 generation by neonatal CD4 T cells, it has been argued that there is skewing toward T_H2 development in the human fetus and neonate similar to what has been observed in neonatal mice [636]. There is also considerable interest in using the production of T_H2 cytokines by cord BMCs or T cells as a predictor of the later development of atopic disease [637]. Purified naïve ($CD45RA^{hi}$) neonatal T cells proliferate substantially more in response to IL-4 than do analogous adult cells [638], suggesting a way by which neonatal T cells might be more prone to become T_H2 effectors. Studies by Delespesse and associates [491] also suggest that neonatal and adult $CD45RA^{hi}$ CD4 T cells may differ in their tendency to become T_H2-like effector cells under certain conditions in vitro; when these cells were primed using a combination of anti-CD3 mAb, a fibroblast cell line expressing low amounts of the CD80 costimulatory molecule, and exogenous IL-12, production of IL-4 by neonatal CD4 T cells was enhanced compared with adult cells. These investigators found that the neonatal effector T cells generated had a substantially lower capacity to produce IFN-γ than adult cells, and these differences persisted even when endogenous IL-4 was blocked with an anti–IL-4 receptor antibody [639].

Such skewing is not evident for increased production of IL-4 by neonatal CD4 T cells compared with adult naïve CD4 T cells after stimulation with allogeneic DCs [533]. Also, many studies equate IL-13 with IL-4 as an indicator of a T_H2 response. There is substantial evidence, however, that IL-13 and IL-4 are not invariably coexpressed, suggesting that they may have distinct roles in immune function rather than being equivalent indicators of a T_H2 response. IL-13, in contrast to IL-4, is produced by adult $CD454RA^{hi}$ and $CD45RO^{hi}$ CD4 T cells [597] and is expressed at high levels by neonatal CD8 T cells [603].

Cytokine Production after Long-Term In Vitro Generation of Effector CD4 T Cells

Activated neonatal CD4 T cells can be differentiated in vitro into either T_H1-like or T_H2-like effector cells by incubation for several days to weeks with IL-12 and anti-IL-4 antibody or with IL-4 and anti-IL-12 antibody [491,640–643]. Consistent with this ability to differentiate into T_H1 cells, activated neonatal and adult naïve CD4 T cells upregulate expression of the IL-12Rβ1 and IL-12Rβ2 chains similarly [640,644]. In many cases, IL-2 is added after the initial activation phase to promote survival and expansion of the effector cells. Treatment of neonatal T cells with IL-4 and anti–IL-12 upregulates GATA-3 [645], the master transcription factor promoting T_H2 effector generation [312]. Treatment of neonatal CD4 T cells with the combination of IL-12 is effective at inducing T-bet, the master transcriptional regulator promoting T_H1 effector generation [642]. Mature single-positive ($CD4^{hi}CD8^-$ or $CD4^-CD8^{hi}$) fetal thymocytes obtained by 16 weeks of gestation can be also differentiated into either T_H1 or T_H2 effector cells by such cytokine treatment [646], indicating that the capacity to acquire a polarized cytokine profile is established early in fetal life. This tendency of neonatal CD4 T cells to develop a T_H2-like or T_H0-like cytokine profile may not apply to more physiologic conditions of stimuli, however, because no IL-4 production by neonatal naïve CD4 T cells was detected in response to allogeneic DC stimulation [533].

IL-17–producing T cells, indicative of T_H17 generation, can be generated from neonatal cord blood CD4 T cells, but not from adult naïve CD4 T cells [647]. These IL-17–producing cells generated in vitro are similar to cells in the adult circulation in their expression of RORγt, a key transcription factor required for T_H17 generation in vivo, and their high levels of expression of the CCR6 chemokine receptor [647]. The capacity for neonatal CD4 T cells to become T_H17 cells is limited to a small CD161$^+$ subset that is absent from the circulating adult naïve CD4 T-cell compartment. Despite its expression of CD161 (also known as NK1.1 in mice), which is expressed on NK and NKT cells, this CD161$^+$ T-cell population is distinct from NKT cells by its diverse αβ-TCR repertoire and in being MHC class II–restricted rather than CD1d-restricted in its activation [647]. One possibility to explain these age-related differences is that the CD161$^+$ population may preferentially home after birth to sites known to be rich for the generation of T_H17 cells, such as gastrointestinal mucosa, and not subsequently recirculate. The capacity of neonatal CD4 T cells to differentiate in vitro into T_{FH} cells has not yet been defined.

T CELL–MEDIATED CYTOTOXICITY

T cell–mediated cytotoxicity involves two major pathways of killing of cellular targets either through the secretion of the perforin and granzyme cytotoxins or through the engagement of Fas by Fas-ligand (Fig. 4–13). The growing use of cord blood for hematopoietic cell transplantation and the finding that its use is associated with reduced graft-versus-host disease compared with that seen with adult bone marrow have led to great interest in the capacity of neonatal T cells to mediate cytotoxicity and to potentiate graft rejection.

Early studies mostly used unfractionated mononuclear cells as a source of killer cells in various non–antigen-specific assays, such as lectin-mediated cytotoxicity or redirected cytotoxicity using anti-CD3 mAb. Reduced cytotoxicity was observed with lectin-activated cord blood lymphocytes, particularly if purified T cells were used [648,649]. T cells also can be sensitized in vitro for cytotoxicity using allogeneic stimulator cells followed by testing for cytotoxic activity against allogeneic target cells. Using this approach, most studies have found that neonatal T cells are moderately less effective than adult T cells as cytotoxic effector cells [650–653]. As with the acquisition of T_H1 effector function by neonatal CD4 T cells, more substantial defects in T cell–mediated cytotoxicity by neonatal T cells after allogeneic priming is observed when no exogenous cytokines, such as IL-2 [654,655], are added, suggesting that this decreased cytolytic activity might be physiologically significant in vivo.

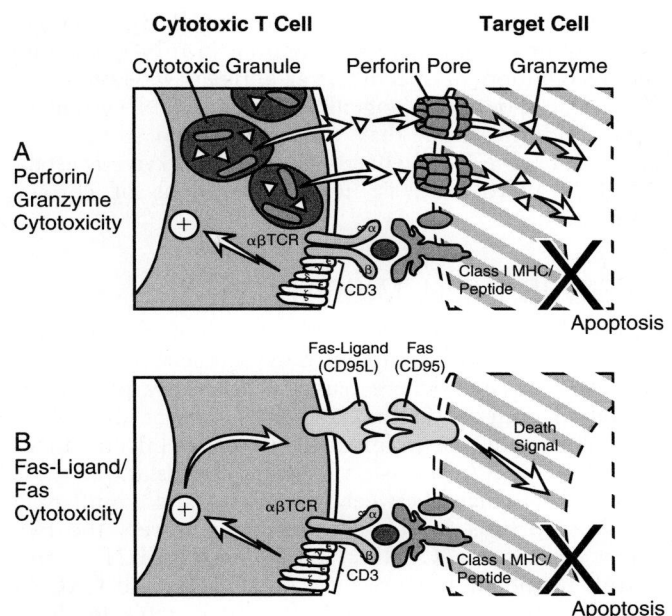

FIGURE 4–13 Two major mechanisms of antigen-specific major histocompatibility complex (MHC) class I–restricted T cell–mediated cytotoxicity. Engagement of αβ T-cell receptor (αβ-TCR) of CD8$^+$ T cells by antigenic peptides bound to MHC class I molecules on the target cell leads to T-cell activation and target cell death. **A,** Cytotoxicity may occur by extracellular release of the contents of cytotoxic granules from the T cell, including perforins, granzymes, and other cytotoxins, such as granulysin. Perforins introduce pores by which granzymes can enter into the target cell leading to the triggering of apoptosis and cell death. **B,** Activation of T cells results in their surface expression of Fas ligand which engages Fas on the target cell, resulting in the delivery of death signal culminating in apoptosis. Other related molecules, such as TRAIL (TNF-related apoptosis-inducing ligand), may also play a role in cytotoxicity.

The mechanism for reduced neonatal T cell–mediated cytotoxicity is poorly understood. Two studies have found that only a low percentage of neonatal CD8 T cells constitutively express perforin, whereas approximately 30% of adult CD8 T cells contain this protein [656,657]. By contrast, another study found that approximately 30% of neonatal T cells expressed perforin, a frequency that was similar to the frequency for adult T cells [658].

Effector and memory CD8 T cells kill more efficiently than antigenically naïve T cells after stimulation with lectin or anti-CD3 mAb [659] or after allogeneic sensitization [570,660]. The apparent deficiency of neonatal cytotoxic T lymphocyte (CTL) activity after in vitro activation or priming may partially reflect the absence among neonatal CD8 T cells of effector and memory cells [542].

Until more recently, the capacity of fetal T cells to mediate cytotoxicity has not received as much scrutiny, despite its relevance to the development of fetal therapy using HSCs. CD8 T cells bearing αβ-TCRs can be cloned as polyclonal lines from human fetal liver by 16 weeks of gestation [661,662]. These CD8 T-cell lines have proliferative activity in response to allogeneic stimulation, but their reactivity toward HLA antigens and their cytolytic activity are unknown. More compelling are studies documenting robust fetal effector CD8 T-cell responses, including clonal expansion and perforin expression, in response to congenital CMV infection [663], although these responses may include limitations in IFN-γ secretion and recognition of specific viral antigens [664,665] (see "T-Cell Response to Congenital Infection"). Nevertheless, these findings show that the capacity to generate a functional CD8 T-cell effector population in vivo is established in utero, at least under conditions of chronic stimulation.

EFFECTOR T-CELL MIGRATION

As already noted, the differential expression of chemokine receptors by T cells is important in their selective trafficking either to sites where naïve T cells may potentially encounter antigen for the first time, such as the spleen and lymph nodes, or to inflamed tissues for effector functions [98]. CCR7 expression by naïve T cells allows these cells to recirculate between the blood and uninflamed lymphoid organs, which constitutively express the two major ligands for CCR7: CCL19 and CCL21. Naïve T cells in the adult express CCR1, CCR7, and CXCR4 on their surface and have low to undetectable levels of CCR5. The role served by CCR1 and CXCR4 expression on naïve T cells is unclear, and CCR1 may be nonfunctional in this cell type [666]. Neonatal naïve T cells have a phenotype similar to those of adult naïve cells except that they lack CCR1 surface expression. Also, in contrast to adult naïve T cells, they do not increase CXCR3 expression, and they do not decrease CCR7 expression, after activation by means of anti-CD3 and anti-CD28 mAbs [488,667]. The CCR7 expressed on neonatal T cells is functional and mediates chemotaxis of these cells in response to CCL19 and CCL21 [668]. These results suggest that activated neonatal T cells may be limited in their capacity to traffic to nonlymphoid tissue sites of inflammation and, instead, may continue to recirculate between the blood and peripheral lymphoid organs.

CCR5 recognizes numerous chemokines that are produced at high levels by leukocytes at sites of inflammation, including CCL2 (MIP-1α), CCL4 (MIP-1β), and CCL5 (RANTES), and is an important chemokine receptor for the entry of T cells into inflamed or infected tissues. Neonatal T cells can increase their surface expression of CCR5 by treatment with either mitogen or IL-2 [669]. The observation that CCR5 is expressed by fetal mesenteric lymph node T cells during the second trimester of pregnancy [424] suggests that this CCR5 can be upregulated in vivo by a mechanism that does not involve antigenic stimulation. CCR5 expression on CD4 T cells gradually increases after birth, in parallel with the appearance of memory cells, suggesting that this process occurs in vivo as part of memory cell generation [670].

Neonatal naïve CD4 T cells also have the capacity after long-term in vitro differentiation to acquire expression of chemokines characteristic of T_H1 or T_H2 effectors after exposure to polarized cytokine milieu (IL-12 and anti–IL-4 for T_H1 and IL-4 and anti–IL-12 for T_H2). The T_H1 effectors generated in vitro tend to express CXCR3, CCR5, and CX3CR1, whereas T_H2 effectors tend to express CCR4 and, to a lesser extent, CCR3 [671–673]. Studies of freshly isolated memory CD4 T cells suggest that expression of CXCR3 and CCR4 may be more accurate predictors of cells with T_H1 and T_H2 cytokine profiles [548,674]. In many cases, a combination of chemokine receptors—for example, CXCR3 and CCR5 for the T_H1 cytokine producers—may be the most predictive of highly polarized patterns of cytokine production by memory T cells [548].

TERMINATION OF T-CELL EFFECTOR RESPONSE

To prevent excessive immune responses, mechanisms for terminating the T-cell response operate on multiple levels. CD45 is a protein tyrosine phosphatase that promotes T-cell activation by counteracting the phosphorylation of tyrosine residues that inhibit the function of tyrosine kinases involved in T-cell activation, such as Lck. Because dimerization of CD45 impedes its phosphatase activity, it is possible that the preferential expression of the low-molecular-weight CD45RO isoform on effector CD4 T cells may facilitate CD45 dimerization and attenuate the immune response [675]. T-cell activation is also limited by the engagement of cytotoxic T lymphocyte antigen-4 (CTLA-4) (i.e., CD152) on the T cell by CD80 and CD86 on the APC. CTLA-4 is expressed mainly on the T-cell surface during the later stages of activation. How CTLA-4 acts to terminate T-cell activation is controversial and includes its competition with CD28 for costimulatory B7 family members and potential ligand-independent mechanisms [676]. The engagement of the B7 family member PD-1 on activated T cells by its B7 family ligands PDL1 (B7-H1) and PDL2, expressed on APCs (see Table 4–4) and in certain tissues, also dampens the effector T-cell response, particularly within parenchymal tissues [522,676]. As discussed next, most effector T cells generated during a robust immune response to infection are eliminated by apoptosis, which is important in preventing autoimmune pathology.

Regulation of T-Cell Expansion by Apoptosis

The elimination of effector T cells by apoptosis is important for lymphocyte homeostasis; a failure of this process results in autoimmunity and severe immunopathology, such as hemophagocytosis [677]. Activated T cells express surface Fas molecules [678] and downregulate expression of the intracellular Bcl-2 and Bcl-xL proteins that protect against apoptosis [679]. Effector T cells may also have increased expression of other Bcl-2 family members that antagonize Bcl-2 and Bcl-xL, such as Bad and Bim, or that directly promote apoptosis downstream, such as Bax and Bcl-xS [677]. The balance between the activity of prosurvival and proapoptotic Bcl-2 family members determines whether the integrity of mitochondria is maintained to prevent the release proteins that trigger apoptosis, such as cytochrome c. This net apoptotic tendency is countered by signals through the IL-2 receptor complex, which maintains or increases expression of Bcl-XL, making effector T cells highly dependent on IL-2 (or other cytokines that signal through the γc cytokine receptor) for their survival [677].

Apoptosis can be studied using effector T cells that are generated in vitro from naïve precursors either by acutely withdrawing exogenous cytokines, such as IL-2, used in effector generation, or by reactivating the effector cells (e.g., using anti-CD3 mAb). This Bcl-2-regulated pathway of apoptosis can also be induced by cytotoxic drugs, such as glucocorticoids. In addition, activated T cells upregulate their expression of Fas and other receptors, such as the p55 (type I) and p75 (type II) TNF-α receptors (TNFRs), which contain cytoplasmic death domains. The ligation of Fas by Fas-ligand on another cell results in the activation of a death receptor–regulated pathway of apoptosis, and a similar process occurs with the engagement of other surface TNFRs [677,680].

An early event in the death receptor–regulated pathway is the activation of caspase-8, a member of a group of proteases that are primarily involved in the regulation of apoptosis and that is associated with the cytoplasmic domains of death receptors. The Bcl-2-regulated and death receptor–regulated pathways of apoptosis have a final common pathway in which downstream effector caspases (caspase-3, caspase-6, and caspase-7) proteolytically cleave a group of proteins that irrevocably commit the cell to undergo apoptosis. These include activation of caspase-activated DNase, which is involved in the internucleosomal cleavage of genomic DNA into 200- to 300-bp fragments that are characteristic of apoptosis [677].

Circulating mononuclear cells from cord blood, including naïve CD4 T cells, are more prone than cells from the adult circulation to undergo spontaneous apoptosis in vitro [511,515,681,682]. The mechanism is most likely mediated by the Bcl-2-regulated pathway of apoptosis and probably does not involve Fas engagement because Fas levels are low to undetectable on freshly isolated neonatal lymphocytes, including CD4 and CD8 T cells [682–685]; high levels of Fas expression are limited mainly to memory/effector cells, which are largely absent in the neonatal circulation [684]. The increased tendency of neonatal naïve CD4 and unfractionated T cells to undergo apoptosis may be related to their expression of a lower ratio of Bcl-2 (antiapoptotic) to Bax (proapoptotic) protein compared with that in adult T cells [511,686]. Neonatal naïve T cells have a more marked decrease than adult T cells in expression of Bcl-2 and Bcl-XL (also antiapoptotic) after 7 days in culture without exogenous cytokines [515]. Treatment of neonatal naïve CD4 T cells with IL-7 can block spontaneous apoptosis [496,515,516], and this effect is accompanied by increased expression of Bcl-2 and Bcl-XL [496,515]. The tendency for neonatal T cells to undergo apoptosis spontaneously in mononuclear cell culture can also be blocked by incubation with insulin-like growth factor-I (IGF-I) [682], but the mechanism involved is unclear. The circulating levels of soluble Fas, soluble TNF, and soluble p55 TNFR increase in the first several days after birth [687], and it has been proposed that the apoptotic tendency of neonatal lymphocytes may be downregulated in the immediate postnatal period by these factors.

Although neonatal T cells have an increased tendency to undergo spontaneous apoptosis, their activation in vitro (priming) may render them less prone than adult cells to undergo apoptosis by Fas-ligand or TNF-α engagement, probably because they express less Fas, p55 TNFR, TNFR-associated death domain (TRADD) (which associates in the cytoplasm with pro–caspase 8),

and effector caspases such as caspase-3 that are involved in this process [686,688]. By contrast, restimulation of primed neonatal T cells using anti-CD3 mAb induces greater apoptosis than occurs with use of similarly treated adult T cells; this anti-CD3 mAb–induced pathway in neonatal cells seems to be Fas-independent [688].

These results suggest a mechanism by which the clonal expansion of neonatal T cells might be limited after activation through the αβ-TCR–CD3 complex and the means to counteract this apoptotic tendency, such as administration of IL-2, other exogenous γc cytokine receptor–using cytokines, or IGF-I or IL-6 (which is induced by IGF-I in cultures of neonatal mononuclear cell culture) [689]. It is unclear, however, whether adult naïve T cells primed under the same conditions as for neonatal T cells retain the tendency of unfractionated adult T cells for greater Fas-mediated and p55 TNFR–mediated apoptosis and reduced anti-CD3 mAb–mediated apoptosis. A tendency for greater apoptosis after anti-CD3 activation mAb stimulation of neonatal CD4 T cells does not seem to be due to their consisting mainly of RTEs because no significant differences have been found between the frequency of apoptotic cells after CD3 and CD28 mAb stimulation of adult PTK7+ CD4 RTEs and PTK7− naïve CD4 T cells (Lewis DB, unpublished observations, 2008).

Neonatal circulating mononuclear cells, probably including T cells, also are more prone than adult mononuclear cells to undergo apoptosis after engagement of MHC class I achieved by mAb treatment [681], apparently by a mechanism independent of Fas–Fas-ligand interactions. The physiologic importance of the spontaneous and MHC class I–induced apoptotic pathways for fetal lymphocytes is unclear. It is plausible that an increased tendency of fetal T lymphocytes to undergo apoptosis after engagement of MHC class I might be a mechanism to maintain tolerance against noninherited maternal alloantigens.

An important caveat of most of the above-described studies of T-cell apoptosis is that they have mainly used cord blood from term deliveries as a T-cell source. It is unclear if this proapoptotic tendency of neonatal naïve T cells applies to the fetus or early postnatal period and, if so, if it is influenced by prematurity and circulating levels of glucocorticoids. In most studies, there also has not been a direct comparison of neonatal T cells, which are predominantly antigenically naïve, with antigenically naïve adult T cells. Non-Treg populations have not been assessed separately from neonatal Tregs, which seem to be intrinsically resistant to apoptosis (see later).

UNIQUE PHENOTYPE AND FUNCTION OF FETAL T-CELL COMPARTMENT

As discussed in the sections on CD45 isoforms and regulatory T cells of the fetus and neonate, a substantial proportion of splenic T cells of the second-trimester fetus, but not the young infant, are CD45RA^{lo}CD45RO^{hi} [498]. Most likely, these fetal T cells, which have a diverse αβ-TCR repertoire, are mainly Tregs because they have phenotypic features (e.g., high levels of surface CD25) and functional features (e.g., high proliferative responses to IL-2, but limited activation by anti-CD3 mAb) [498] that are suggestive of this T-cell subset [505,506].

It is unclear if the CD45RA^{hi}CD45RO^{lo} subset of the second-trimester fetus has substantial differences from circulating or splenic T cells of the neonate in terms of function after mAb stimulation.

Mucosal T cells are present in the fetal intestine by 15 to 16 weeks of gestation, and these cells have the capacity to secrete substantial amounts of IFN-γ after treatment with anti-CD3 mAb in combination with exogenous IFN-α [690]. IFN-α helps direct differentiation of naïve CD4 T cells, including cells of the neonate, toward a T$_H$1 effector cytokine profile dominated by production of IFN-γ, and not IL-4, IL-5, or IL-13 [640], although it does not replace a requirement for IL-12p70 in this context. A similar mechanism may occur in these fetal explant cultures. Although it is unclear what T-cell type is the major source of IFN-γ in this tissue, these observations suggest the possibility that a similar T$_H$1 skewing of T-cell responses might occur in cases of fetal viral infection involving the intestine in which type I IFN (IFN-α/β) is induced.

Fetal Extrathymic T-Cell Differentiation

The human fetal liver contains rearranged VDJ transcripts of the TCR β chain by 7.5 weeks of gestation, and pre-Tα transcripts can be found at 6 weeks of gestation [661,662]. This raises the possibility that extrathymic differentiation of αβ-TCR–bearing T cells could occur in the fetal liver before such differentiation in the thymus. In the adult liver, CD4^{hi}CD8$^-$ and CD4$^-$CD8$^-$ T cells with characteristics distinct from those of NKT cells (which also may have, in part, an extrathymic origin) have been described in conjunction with detection of transcripts for pre-Tα and *RAG* genes. It is possible that some liver T cells may be generated in situ even in adults.

Extrathymic differentiation of αβ T cells may occur in the fetal intestine because the lamina propria of the fetal intestine contains CD3$^-$CD7$^+$ lymphocytes expressing pre-Tα transcripts by 12 to 14 weeks of gestation, and these cells have the capacity to differentiate into αβ T cells [691]. Although it is unclear if these CD3$^-$CD7$^+$ precursor cells have a thymic or other origin, the Vβ repertoire of αβ T-lineage cells in the fetal intestine differs substantially from that of contemporaneous fetal αβ T-lineage cells found in the circulation, suggesting their independent origin [691]. Extrathymic intestinal T-cell development has been shown to occur in mice in specialized structures of the small intestine (cryptopatches), but no analogous structures containing immature lymphocytes have been observed in humans [692]. In humans, the lamina propria and epithelium of the jejunum are potential sites of extrathymic T-cell development in adults, in that immature lymphocytes with markers indicative of T-lineage commitment (CD2$^+$CD7$^+$ CD3$^-$) are found at these sites. These cells colocalize with transcripts for pre-Tα and *RAG-1* gene [693], consistent with this tissue being a site of T-cell differentiation.

REGULATORY T CELLS
Overview

Regulatory T cells (Tregs) are αβ T cells that are crucial for inhibiting immune responses to autoantigens, transplantation antigens, and antigens derived from normal endogenous bacterial flora of the gut and may be important in maintenance of maternal-fetal tolerance [694–697]. Tregs are highly enriched within the small fraction of circulating human CD4 T cells that are CD25^{hi}, express the Foxp3 transcription factor, and lack expression of CD127 (IL-7 receptor α chain) [698]. CD25 is the IL-2 receptor α chain, which, in conjunction with the IL-2 receptor β chain and the γc cytokine receptor, constitutes the high-affinity IL-2 receptor. CD25^{hi} CD4 Tregs depend on IL-2 and high-affinity IL-2 receptors for their generation and maintenance[699] and signaling via the STAT5b pathway [700].

In addition to CD25^{hi} CD4 Tregs, other cell types with regulatory activity include certain subsets of CD8 or CD4$^-$CD8$^-$ T cells and of B cells. CD25^{hi} CD4 Tregs can be generated in the thymus (referred to as natural Tregs) or from peripheral CD4 T cells (referred to as adaptive Tregs). Human natural Tregs may be generated from CD4$^+$CD8$^-$ medullary thymocytes by a process of "secondary positive selection," in which these cells interact with thymic DCs displaying high levels of self-antigen and costimulatory molecules. These DCs are proposed to display high levels of costimulatory molecules as a result of their exposure to TSLP, an IL-7-like cytokine, produced by thymic epithelial cells of Hassall corpuscle [701].

Natural Tregs predominate in the healthy fetus and neonate, require the Foxp3 transcription factor for their intrathymic development, and have a circulating surface phenotype similar to that of most non-Treg naïve CD4 T cells (i.e., CD45RA^{hi}CD45RO^{lo}Fas$^-$) [702]. Genetic deficiency of Foxp3 (IPEX (immunodysregulation polyendocrinopathy enteropathy X-linked) syndrome) results in an absence of circulating Tregs and early postnatal or congenital onset of a severe T cell–mediated autoimmune disease (enteritis, type 1 diabetes mellitus, and other autoimmune endocrinopathies) [703].

After in vitro activation with CD3 and CD28 mAbs, these naïve CD25^{hi} CD4 Tregs have decreased expression of CD45RA and increased expression of CD45RO, Fas, and glucocorticoid-induced TNF receptor (GITR) [702]. CD25^{hi} CD4 Tregs with this activated phenotype predominate in adults. Although adaptive CD25^{hi} CD4 Tregs have generally been thought to be derived from naïve Tregs or conventional naïve CD4 T cells, or both, more recent studies suggest that in adults most circulating Tregs may have originate from memory CD4 T cells [704].

Treg-mediated suppression requires activation through the αβ-TCR (e.g., antigenic peptide–MHC), but thereafter, Treg–mediated suppression is not antigen-specific. Mechanisms of inhibition may include the production of cytokines, such as IL-10, TGF-β, or IL-35 (a novel heterodimeric cytokine consisting of the IL-12/IL-23p40 and EBI-3); expression of surface molecules, such as CTLA-4; and competition for cytokines (e.g., IL-2) on which effector T-cell responses are dependent [705]. Tregs may also "regulate" effector T-cell responses by killing other T cells or APCs or both [698].

Fetal and Neonatal Regulatory T Cells

CD25^{hi} CD4 Tregs, as assessed by their lack of CD127 expression and enrichment for Foxp3 mRNA or protein expression [533,702,706], constitute about 5% to 10% of circulating CD4 T cells in neonates [707–709], including premature neonates [541]. Most likely, these circulating Tregs are predominantly produced intrathymically based on their naïve phenotype (i.e., CD45RA^{hi}CD45RO^{lo}Fas$^-$) [702], whereas most circulating adult Tregs have a phenotype indicating prior activation suggesting that they are induced rather than natural Tregs [710]. These neonatal CD25^{hi} CD4 Tregs are resistant to Fas-ligand–mediated apoptosis, as would be expected because of their limited Fas expression [702].

CD4$^+$CD8$^+$ intrathymic precursors of CD25^{hi} CD4 Tregs are identifiable in the fetal thymus by 13 to 17 weeks of gestation and display an antigenically naïve surface phenotype (CD45RA^{hi}CD45RO^{lo}CD69$^-$Fas$^-$ GITR$^-$) [505]. After leaving the thymus, these Foxp3$^+$ CD25^{hi} CD4 Tregs enter into the fetal lymph nodes and spleen, where they acquire a phenotype indicative of activation (CD45RA^{lo} CD45RO^{hi}CD69$^+$Fas$^+$GITR$^+$ intracytoplasmic CTLA-4$^+$). Despite their strikingly different surface phenotypes, the mature intrathymic CD25^{hi} CD4 Treg precursors and the Tregs found in peripheral lymphoid tissue have a similar ability to suppress the activation of autologous CD25$^-$ CD4 T cells in vitro [505]. A large fraction of these CD25$^-$ CD4 and CD8 T cells in fetal lymphoid tissue express CD69 and secrete IFN-γ in the absence of CD25^{hi} CD4 Tregs, indicating that they are previously activated effector cells [506].

Taken together, the above-described results suggest that natural Tregs in the human fetus acquire the capacity for suppression in the thymus before their emigration to the periphery. After entering into the peripheral lymphoid tissues, they apparently encounter potentially autoreactive CD25$^-$ CD4 T cells and gain Treg activity. This implies that peripheral non-Treg T cells in the fetus have an $\alpha\beta$-TCR repertoire that is highly enriched for autoreactive specificities, an idea supported by studies of the murine neonatal peripheral T-cell compartment [711].

In normal human pregnancy, maternal cells are routinely detectable in the fetal lymph nodes, where they seem to be responsible for the induction of fetal Tregs that are specific for maternal alloantigens [697]. Tregs with this maternal alloantigen specificity seem to persist until at least early adulthood and are likely to have an impact on the regulation of postnatal immune responses [697]. In contrast to the fetus, Foxp3$^+$ CD25^{hi} CD4 Tregs are rare in mesenteric lymph node tissue of healthy adults [506]. This suggests that there is a dramatic postnatal decline in Tregs of the peripheral lymphoid organs, which might reflect a reduced requirement postnatally for Treg-mediated peripheral tolerance of the naïve T cells. These findings, which suggest a high level of CD25^{hi} CD4 Treg activity in the fetus, may also account for the presence at birth of autoimmune disease, such as type 1 diabetes, in some cases of genetic deficiency of Foxp3, a disorder in which natural Treg development is ablated [703].

Most studies [541,708,709], but not all [712,713], have found that cord blood CD25^{hi} CD4 Tregs have a similar ability as adult peripheral Tregs to inhibit CD25$^-$ T-cell activation. One study also found that reduced Treg activity in the cord blood may be a risk factor for children subsequently to develop allergic disease [714].

NATURAL KILLER T CELLS
Overview

A small population of circulating human T cells expresses $\alpha\beta$-TCR and CD161 (NKR-P1A), the human orthologue of the mouse NK1.1 protein. These features and others, such as CD56 and CD57 surface expression and a developmental dependence on the cytokine IL-15, also are characteristic of NK cells, as described earlier. For this reason, these T cells frequently are referred to as NKT cells. Similar to murine T cells expressing NK1.1, human NKT cells have a restricted repertoire of $\alpha\beta$-TCR (TCR α chains containing the Vα24Jα18 segments in association with TCR-β chains containing Vβ11 segments) [715,716] and mainly recognize antigens presented by the nonclassic MHC molecule, CD1d, rather than by MHC class I or class II molecules. CD1d-restricted antigens that can be recognized by NKT cells include certain lipid molecules, such as α-galactosylceramide (an artificial but potent stimulator of these cells derived from the sea sponge), and less well-characterized antigens derived from several species of bacteria (e.g., *Sphingomonas*) [411].

Murine studies indicate that NKT cells may be derived from CD4^{hi}CD8^{hi} double-positive thymocytes by the interaction of their $\alpha\beta$-TCR with CD1d [715,716]. NKT-cell development in humans and mice also depends on signaling via the SLAM family, which uses SAP for intracellular signaling. NKT cells are absent in X-linked lymphoproliferative syndrome, which is due to a genetic deficiency of SAP [717].

NKT cells have the ability to secrete high levels of IL-4 and IFN-γ and to express Fas-ligand and TRAIL on their cell surface on primary stimulation, a capacity not observed with most antigenically naïve $\alpha\beta$ T cells [411]. This rapid ability to secrete cytokines such as IFN-γ is due to these cells constitutively expressing IFN-γ mRNA with cell activation resulting in the rapid translation of cytokine mRNA into protein that is secreted [585]. Activated NKT cells, including NKT cells of humans, may also be major sources of IL-17 and IL-21 and have certain T$_H$17-like features such as constitutive expression of RORγt and functional IL-23 receptors [718,719]. NKT cells can potentially be an early source of cytokines that are characteristically secreted by T$_H$1, T$_H$2, T$_H$17, or T$_{FH}$ cells. Some NKT cells also secrete IL-10 after activation [720], which may partly mediate their regulatory activity on other effector cell populations. NKT cells are also enriched for preformed cytoplasmic stores of perforin and granzymes [720] that allows them to carry out cell-mediated cytotoxicity rapidly, in contrast to naïve CD8 T cells, which initially lack such cytotoxic capacity and acquire it only after their differentiation into effector cells.

In adults, NKT cells that express the Vα24$^+$ $\alpha\beta$-TCR can be divided into CD4$^+$(CD8$^-$) and CD4$^-$CD8$^-$ cell subsets. The CD4$^+$Vα24$^+$ subset has higher levels of L-selectin (CD62L) and lower surface expression of CD11a and secretion of IFN-γ and cytotoxins (perforin and granzyme A) than the CD4$^-$CD8$^-$Vα24$^+$ subset [720,721]. This suggests that the CD4$^+$Vα24 NKT cells may preferentially recirculate in secondary lymphoid tissue and act as regulatory cells, whereas CD4$^-$CD8$^-$Vα24

NKT cells may mainly serve as effector cells at sites of extralymphoid tissue inflammation.

Although the physiologic role of NKT cells in host defense remains poorly understood, they may provide an important source of early cytokines that influence the later phases of innate immunity and the nature of the subsequent adaptive immune response [411]. The ability of NKT cells to produce large amounts of cytokines in response to IL-12 alone or other cytokines raises the possibility that antigen recognition by the invariant αβ-TCR may not play a role in this early innate response, but rather be required only for the intrathymic development of these NKT cells. NKT cells have also been implicated as negative regulators of certain T cell–mediated immunopathologic responses [715,716], such as in certain autoimmune diseases, graft-versus-host disease after hematopoietic cell transplantation, and asthma [722].

Natural Killer T Cells of the Neonate

Only small numbers of NKT cells (<1% of circulating T cells) are present in the neonatal circulation, but these subsequently increase with aging [723]. This finding suggests that NKT cells may undergo postnatal expansion (e.g., in relation to exposure to a ubiquitous antigen presented by CD1d molecules), or that their production by the thymus or at extrathymic sites occurs mainly postnatally. Neonatal NKT cells are similar to adult NKT cells in having a memory/effector–like cell surface phenotype, including expression of CD25, the CD45RO isoform, and a low level of expression of L-selectin [724,725]. In the case of murine NKT cells, many of these activation phenotypic features are found on NKT cells during intrathymic development, indicating that these are a result of differentiation rather than prior antigenic stimulation in the periphery before birth [715,716].

The neonatal NKT-cell population can be activated and expanded in vitro using a combination of anti-CD3 and anti-CD28 mAbs and cytokines [726] or by incubation with autologous DCs pulsed with α-galactosylceramide [727]. Although neonatal NKT cells have a surface phenotype similar to that of adult NKT cells, they produce only limited amounts of IL-4 or IFN-γ on primary stimulation, indicating functional immaturity [724]. This decreased capacity may be due to mechanisms similar to those for the reduced IFN-γ mRNA production by neonatal CD4 T cells, such as decreased levels of the NFATc2 transcription factor or increased methylation of the IFN-γ genetic locus (see earlier). A limitation in the rapid translation of preformed IFN-γ mRNA is also possible, although this has not been evaluated for neonatal NKT cells.

After in vitro expansion, neonatal NKT cells produce higher levels of IL-4 and lower amounts of IFN-γ than produced by similarly treated adult NKT cells [726]. The combination of reduced effector function and a memory/effector–like cell surface phenotype by neonatal (and likely fetal) NKT cells has led to the proposal [724] that these cells may have encountered self-antigens in extralymphoid tissue and as a result have become tolerized rather than effector cells. Such a process of extralymphoid tolerization for neonatal T cells in the mouse has been described [728], but it is unclear if this occurs for human fetal T cells or

NKT cells. An alternative possibility is that activated fetal NKT cells may serve as negative regulators of autoreactive CD4 and CD8 T cells. This memory/effector–like surface phenotype may also be a general characteristic of the generation of NKT cells within the thymus [715,716].

The cytokine profile of neonatal NKT cells shows greater plasticity than that of adult NKT cells. Expansion of the neonatal NKT-cell population and priming using either cDCs or pDCs in conjunction with phytohemagglutinin, IL-2, and IL-7 result in an IL-4–predominant or an IFN-γ–predominant cytokine expression profile. By contrast, similarly treated adult NKT cells retain their ability to produce both cytokines [726], suggesting that these cells have lost the ability to adopt a polarized T_H1 or T_H2 phenotype after birth.

The capacity of neonatal and infant NKT cells to mediate cytotoxicity directly has not been reported. Neonatal CD56$^+$ T cells constitutively express less perforin than adult cells [657]. Because the CD56$^+$ T-cell population is highly enriched in CD1d-restricted NKT cells, NKT-cell cytotoxicity probably is limited at birth and gradually increases with age. Culturing of neonatal NKT cells in vitro for several weeks results in acquisition of potent cytotoxic activity [727,729], indicating that developmental limitations can be overcome after expansion and differentiation.

γδ T CELLS
Phenotype and Function

γδ T cells, which express a TCR heterodimer consisting of a γ and a δ chain in association with the CD3 complex proteins, are rarer than αβ T cells in most tissues, including the blood where they constitute approximately 1% to 10% of circulating T cells in adults. A major exception is the intestinal epithelium, where they predominate. Although some γδ-TCRs can recognize conventional peptide antigens presented by MHC, most directly recognize three-dimensional nonprotein or protein structures. The antigen-combining site of the γδ-TCR shares some structural features with that of immunoglobulin molecules [730], which is consistent with preferential recognition of three-dimensional structures by both of these receptors.

Human γδ T cells expressing the Vγ9Vδ2 (using an older but still commonly employed nomenclature for Vγ segments) can proliferate and secrete cytokines, cytotoxins (perforins, granzymes, granulysin), and growth factors after recognition of phosphoantigens (i.e., nonpeptidic pyrophosphomonoester compounds). These phosphoantigens can be derived from mycobacteria and other bacterial species or from cellular isopentenyl phosphates that are involved in cholesterol biosynthesis from mevalonate [731]. The cellular levels of isopentenyl phosphates can be increased by metabolic stress from intracellular infection, after treatment with certain drugs (e.g., aminobisphosphonates), or after oncogenic transformation [731]. The precise mechanism by which the Vγ9Vδ2 TCR recognizes exogenous or endogenous phosphoantigens is unclear, but does not involve MHC class I or class II or CD1 recognition and may instead require ATP synthase, a mitochondrial enzyme that can translocate to the cell surface [732]. Many Vγ9Vδ2 T cells express NKG2D, which recognizes the MHC class I–like molecule MICA [733], and enhances antigen-dependent effector function [408]. Such enhancement in vivo may be a consequence of the induction of MICA on APCs by mycobacteria and other pathogens [408].

This in vitro activation of γδ T cells probably is relevant in vivo because increased numbers are found in the skin lesions of patients with leprosy and in the blood of patients with malaria and acute and chronic herpesvirus infections. Resident γδ T cells of the murine skin produce keratinocyte growth factors and IGF-I that help maintain epithelial integrity during stress [734]. The observation that MICA or MICB is expressed in the skin of patients with acute graft-versus-host disease is consistent with a similar role for human γδ T cells [735].

γδ T cells also may have important immunosurveillance function for malignancy because murine cutaneous γδ T cells can kill skin carcinoma cells by a mechanism that involves engagement of NKG2D by Rae-1 and H60 [736], which have homology with human MICA. Many human epithelial cell tumors express NKG2D ligands and can be lysed by human γδ T cells in vitro [737], which indicates that γδ T cells have a potential role in tumor immunotherapy. Murine studies also suggest that distinct subpopulations of γδ T cells appearing at sites of infection either decrease inflammatory responses to pathogens, such as *Listeria*, by killing activated macrophages by Fas-ligand–mediated cytotoxicity or contribute to macrophage activation [738].

Most activated γδ T cells express high levels of perforin, serine esterases, Fas-ligand, and granulysin and are capable of cytotoxicity against tumor cells and other cell targets, such as infected cells [739]. γδ T cells also can secrete various cytokines in vitro, including TNF-α, IFN-γ, IL-4, and IL-17 [731,740], and chemokines that may help recruit inflammatory cells to the tissues. Cytokine production can be potently activated by products from live bacteria, such as isobutylamine [741], and by type I IFN or by agents that potently induce it, such as oligonucleotides containing unmethylated CpG motifs [742]. Human Vγ2Vδ2 γδ T cells after adoptive transfer into SCID mice can mediate rapid and potent antibacterial activity against gram-positive and gram-negative bacteria, with protection associated with the production of IFN-γ [741].

Only about 2% to 5% of T-lineage cells of the thymus and peripheral blood express γδ-TCR in most individuals [743]. In contrast to in most αβ T cells, whose development requires an intact thymus, a significant proportion of γδ T cells can develop by a thymic-independent pathway, and normal numbers of γδ T cells are found in cases of complete thymic aplasia [743] and in the human fetus before the first waves of thymically derived T cells [744]. This may be explained, at least in part, by the differentiation of γδ T cells directly from primitive lymphohematopoietic precursor cells found in the small intestine, as has been shown in the mouse [745].

Ontogeny of γδ T-Cell Receptor Gene Rearrangements

The human TCR γ and δ chain genes undergo a programmed rearrangement of dispersed segments analogous to that of the TCR β and TCR α chain genes. Most circulating adult human γδ T cells lack evidence of TCR-β chain gene rearrangement [746], indicating that commitment to this lineage mainly is the result of a double-negative thymocyte expressing a productive TCR-γ and TCR-δ chain gene rearrangement. This expression results in strong cell signaling that suppresses TCR β chain rearrangement [747]. Alternatively, if the TCR β chain gene is productively rearranged (not the TCR-γ and TCR-δ genes), signals from the pre-TCR complex and Notch signaling favor progression to the CD4+CD8+ stage where positive selection can occur [748]. Most γδ T cells lack surface expression of either CD4 or CD8α/CD8β heterodimers, consistent with their not undergoing a process of positive selection that is obligatory for αβ T cells. Whether human γδ T cells undergo negative selection is unclear.

Rearranged TCR δ genes are first expressed extrathymically in the liver and primitive gut between 6 and 9 weeks of gestation [749,750]. Rearrangement of the human TCR γ and TCR δ genes in the fetal thymus begins shortly after its colonization with lymphoid cells, with TCR δ protein detectable by 9.5 weeks of gestation [751]. γδ T cells constitute about 10% of the circulating T-cell compartment at 16 weeks, a percentage that gradually declines to less than 3% by term [497,752].

Although there is potential for the formation of a highly diverse γδ-TCR repertoire, peripheral γδ T cells use only a few V segments, which vary with age and with tissue location. These can be divided into two major groups, Vγ9Vδ2 cells and Vδ1 cells, in which a Vδ1-bearing TCR δ chain predominantly pairs with a TCR γ chain using a Vγ segment other than Vγ9. Most γδ-TCR+ thymocytes in the first trimester express Vδ2 segments. This is followed by γδ-TCR+ thymocytes that express Vδ1, which predominate at least through infancy in the thymus. Most circulating fetal and neonatal γδ T cells also are Vδ1-bearing, with only about 10% bearing Vδ2 [723], and these Vδ1 cells constitute the predominant γδ T-cell population of the small intestinal epithelium after birth. In contrast to the early gestation fetal thymus and the fetal and neonatal circulation, Vδ2 T cells predominate in the fetal liver and spleen early during the second trimester [590,753] and appear before αβ TCR+ thymocytes [751,754], suggesting that they are produced extrathymically by the fetal liver.

As indicated by TCR spectratyping, the TCR δ chains using either Vδ1 or Vδ2 segments usually are oligoclonal at birth [755,756]. Because this oligoclonality also is characteristic of the adult γδ T-cell repertoire, this is not due to postnatal clonal expansion, but reflects an intrinsic feature of this cell lineage. By age 6 months, γδ T cells bearing Vγ9 Vδ2 segments become predominant and remain so during adulthood [757], probably because of their preferential expansion in response to ubiquitous antigens, such as endogenous bacterial flora.

Ontogeny of γδ T-Cell Function

Antigenically naïve and experienced subsets of γδ T cells can be distinguished using markers commonly applied to αβ T cells; naïve γδ T cells can be identified by their CD45RA^{hi}CD45RO^{lo}CD27^{hi}CD1a^{lo} surface phenotype [758]. By these criteria, circulating γδ T cells of the neonate are predominantly antigenically naïve [758].

Although neonatal γδ T cells proliferate in vitro in response to mycobacterial lipid antigens [759], they express lower levels of serine esterases than adult γδ T cells, suggesting they are less effective cytotoxic cells [760]. γδ T-cell clones derived from cord blood also have a markedly reduced capacity to mediate cytotoxicity against tumor cell extracts [752]. Because these neonatal clones also have lower CD45RO surface expression than observed in the adult clones, their reduced activity may reflect their antigenic naïveté. In contrast to freshly isolated neonatal αβ T cells, activation and propagation of these fetal and neonatal γδ T cells in culture (e.g., with exogenous IL-2) do not enhance their function. The function of fetal liver γδ T cells is unclear, although one report suggests that they have cytotoxic reactivity against maternal MHC class I [754] and may prevent engraftment of maternal T cells.

ANTIGEN-SPECIFIC T-CELL FUNCTION IN THE FETUS AND NEONATE
Delayed Cutaneous Hypersensitivity, Graft Rejection, and Graft-versus-Host Disease

Skin test reactivity to cell-free antigens assesses a form of DTH reaction that requires the function of antigen-specific CD4 T cells. Skin test reactivity to common antigens such as *Candida*, streptokinase-streptodornase, and tetanus toxoid usually is not detectable in neonates [761–763]. Absence of such reactivity reflects a lack of antigen-specific sensitization because in vitro T-cell reactivity to these antigens also is absent. When leukocytes, and presumably antigen-specific CD4 T cells, from sensitized adults are adoptively transferred to neonates, children, or adults, only neonates fail to respond to antigen-specific skin tests [764]. This finding indicates that the neonate may be deficient in other components of the immune system required for DTH reaction, such as APCs and production of inflammatory chemokines or cytokines. Such deficiencies may account, at least in part, for diminished skin reactivity in the neonate after specific sensitization or after intradermal injection with T-cell mitogens [175,765]. Diminished skin reactivity to intradermally administered antigens persists postnatally up to 1 year of age [765].

Neonates, including premature neonates, are capable of rejecting foreign tissues, such as skin grafts, although rejection may be delayed compared with adults [766]. Experiments using human–SCID mouse chimeras also suggest that second-trimester human fetal T cells are capable of becoming cytotoxic effector T cells in response to foreign antigens and in rejecting solid tissue allografts [767]. Clinical transplantation of fetal blood from one unaffected fraternal twin to another did not result in marrow engraftment, despite a sharing of similar MHC haplotypes; instead, there was a postnatal recipient cytotoxic T-cell response against donor leukocytes [768]. A T-cell response to alloantigens can also be detected in newborns after in utero irradiated red blood cell transfusions from unrelated donors [769,770]. Fetal T cells seem similar to neonatal T cells in being able to mediate allogeneic responses in vivo, including graft rejection.

Another indication that neonatal T cells can mediate allogeneic responses is the fact that blood transfusions rarely induce graft-versus-host disease in the neonate. Rare cases of persistence of donor lymphocytes and of graft-versus-host disease have developed after intrauterine transfusion in the last trimester and in transfused premature neonates, however [771–774]. Because the infusion of fresh leukocytes induces partial tolerance to skin grafts [766], tolerance for transfused lymphocytes might occur by a similar mechanism, predisposing the fetus or neonate to graft-versus-host disease. Together, these observations suggest a partial immaturity in T-cell and inflammatory mechanisms required for DTH reaction and for graft rejection.

T-Cell Reactivity to Environmental Antigens

Specific antigen reactivity theoretically can develop in the fetus by exposure to antigens transferred from the mother, by transfer of antigen-specific cellular maternal lymphocytes, or by infection of the fetus itself. Several studies suggest that fetal T cells have become primed to environmental or dietary protein allergens as a result of maternal exposure and transfer to the fetus [775–778]. A criticism of these studies is that the antigen-specific proliferation is low compared with the basal proliferation of cord BMCs. In addition, many of these studies used antigen extracts rather than defined recombinant proteins or peptides, and these may have nonspecific stimulatory effects.

Prenatal sensitization has been assessed by antigen-induced incorporation of ^{3}H-thymidine and cytokine and cytokine mRNA production by cord BMCs [778–781]. In some studies, the production of IL-10 in these cultures is high relative to that of the classic T_H2 cytokines (IL-4, IL-5, IL-9, and IL-13). IFN-γ production was 100-fold higher than IL-4 production, a ratio that is nonetheless still reduced compared with adult cells. This cytokine profile has been interpreted as a T_H2-biased response or a regulatory T-cell (IL-10–dominant) response. Its frequent occurrence suggests that T_H2 priming per se may be a normal outcome of fetal exposure to such antigens [778,779]. Consistent with this idea, a follow-up study found no significant relationship between T_H2 priming of fetal T cells to environmental antigens and the risk of developing atopic disease by 6 years of age [782].

Prenatal priming of T cells by environmental allergens can be shown by 20 weeks of gestation, based on their proliferative responses to seasonal allergens [783]. These responses are weak, however, and the cytokine profile was not reported. In one study, protein allergen–specific T-cell proliferation detected at birth was more common when allergen exposure occurred in the first or second trimester rather than in the third trimester [777]. This finding could reflect decreased maternal-fetal transport of antigen during late pregnancy or an intrinsic capacity of early and late gestation fetal T cells to be primed.

Fetal T-Cell Sensitization to Maternally Administered Vaccines and Maternally Derived Antigens

In contrast to protein allergens, there is only one report in which antigen-specific fetal T-cell priming to influenza vaccination has been detected using a flow cytometric assay after staining of T cells with fluorochrome-labeled influenza hemagglutinin peptide/HLA-DR (MHC class II) tetramers influenza [784]. This study, which needs to be confirmed, contrasts with one in which maternal vaccination during the last trimester of pregnancy with tetanus toxoid or inactivated influenza virus A or B did not result in detectable neonatal T-cell responses using lymphocyte blastogenesis assays [785].

The use of corroborating assays that are reliable for the detection of very low frequencies of T cells, such as enzyme-linked immunospot (ELISPOT) assays, might allow a better definition of the extent of fetal T-cell sensitization by maternal vaccination. In any case, the neonatal CD4 T-cell responses induced by maternal immunization are of a much lower frequency that postnatal vaccination responses in children [786], and their durability is unknown. Together, these findings suggest that fetal sensitization to foreign proteins may be relatively inefficient, particularly when exposure is temporally limited. Whether this reflects relatively inefficient maternal-fetal transfer of protein antigens or intrinsic limitations of the fetus for antigen presentation and T-cell priming, or both, is unclear. Even if it is assumed that the capacity for fetal T cells to be primed by foreign antigens is similar to that of antigenically naïve adult T cells, the immune response to maternally derived foreign vaccine proteins by fetal T cells would be expected to be poor compared with the maternal response because antigen probably enters into the fetal circulation with little, if any, accompanying activation of the innate response required for efficient T-cell activation.

Growing evidence suggests that fetal T-cell sensitization can occur in cases of antigen exposure owing to chronic infection of the mother with parasites or viruses. Parasite (schistosomal, filarial, and plasmodial) antigen-specific cytokine production by peripheral blood lymphocytes, probably of T-cell origin, was detectable at birth in infants without congenital infection who were born to infected mothers [787,788]. This apparent T-cell immunity persisted for at least 1 year after birth in the absence of postnatal infection with parasites and was associated with downregulation of *Mycobacterium bovis* BCG-specific IFN-γ production after neonatal administration of BCG vaccine [787]. These results suggest that fetal exposure to parasitic antigens without infection can downregulate subsequent postnatal T$_H$1 responses to unrelated antigens. HIV peptide–specific IL-2 production by cord blood CD4 T cells also has been reported in uninfected infants born to HIV-infected mothers, suggesting that fetal T-cell sensitization can occur in cases of chronic viral infection of the mother without congenital infection [789].

Maternal Transfer of T-Cell Immunity to the Fetus

The older literature contains many reports of cord blood lymphocyte proliferation or cytokine production in response to antigens that the fetus is presumed not to have encountered. These antigen responses (e.g., for PPD, *Mycobacterium leprae*, measles, or rubella) have been attributed to passive transfer of T-cell immunity from the mother. The responses usually are weak and may

represent laboratory artifacts, rather than true sensitization, because complex antigen mixtures were used that likely may activate T cells in a non-MHC–restricted manner. Although maternal-to-fetal transfer of leukocytes, particularly T cells, occurs, their number in the fetus is very low (usually <0.1%) [790], unless the neonate or infant has a severe defect of T cells that normally prevents maternal T-cell engraftment, such as SCID [791]. Detectable antigen-specific cellular immunity by conventional assays is unlikely for immunocompetent neonates. Reports of T-cell responses in healthy neonates as a result of transfer of maternal immunity should remain suspect, unless the T-cell population is identified and its antigen specificity and MHC restriction are shown.

T-CELL RESPONSE TO CONGENITAL INFECTION
CD4 T Cells

Pathogen-specific T-cell proliferative responses and cytokine responses (IL-2 and IFN-γ) in infants and children with congenital infection (e.g., with *Treponema pallidum*, CMV, VZV, or *T. gondii*) are markedly decreased compared with such responses in infants and children with postnatal infection or are absent entirely [792–797]. These assays mainly detected CD4 T-cell responses because antigen preparations (e.g., whole cell lysates of virally infected cells) and APC populations (e.g., peripheral blood monocytes and B cells as the predominant APCs with few cDCs) were used that favor activation of MHC class II–restricted rather than MHC class I–restricted responses. These reduced CD4 T-cell responses are particularly true with first-trimester or second-trimester infections. With severe infections in the first trimester, a direct deleterious effect on T-cell development is possible. T cells from infants and children with congenital toxoplasmosis retain the ability, however, to respond to alloantigen, mitogen, and, in one case, tetanus toxoid [797].

The adaptive immune responses to *Plasmodium falciparum* antigens have been evaluated using cord blood from neonates in an area with a high rate of fetal exposure to maternally derived malaria antigens. Malaria antigen–induced CD4 T-cell cytokine production (IFN-γ, IL-4, and IL-13) was detectable in these neonates [788,798], but not in samples from neonates in North America [788]. The limited ability of the fetus to mount CD4 T-cell responses to pathogen-derived antigens is not absolute, and dual T$_H$1-type and T$_H$2-type immune responses can develop after some congenital infections or fetal exposure to pathogenic antigens from the mother.

The reduced CD4 T-cell responses seen in many types of congenital infection may be the result of antigen-specific unresponsiveness (e.g., anergy, deletion, or ignorance—the failure of the CD4 T cell to be initially activated by antigen). As discussed earlier, it is unlikely that a decreased TCR repertoire limits these immune responses, particularly after the second trimester onward. Decreased responses do not occur to all pathogens; in one study, 10-year-old children congenitally infected with mumps had DTH reactions to mumps antigen, indicating persistence of mumps-specific memory/effector T cells [799].

CD8 T Cells

CD8 T-cell responses to congenital infections seem to be relatively robust, which is in marked contrast to responses of CD4 T cells. In congenital CMV infection, high frequencies of CMV-specific CD8 T cells were detectable by staining with CMV peptide–MHC class I tetramers, and these cells showed perforin expression, cytolytic activity, and oligoclonal $\alpha\beta$-TCR expansion IFN-γ, similar to cells of chronically infected adults [663]. More recent studies found that although the CMV-infected fetus and the transmitter mother had similar levels of activated, effector/memory, and memory CMV-specific CD8 T cells, there was impaired secretion by fetal CD8 T cells of IFN-γ in response to CMV antigen or CD3 and CD28 mAb stimulation [664,665], and this impairment was associated with decreased viral clearance. Similarly, in HIV-1 infection, an expansion of HIV-specific cytotoxic T cells was detected at birth, indicating that fetal T cells were activated by viral antigens [800]. In another case of in utero HIV infection, HIV-specific T cell–mediated cytotoxicity was detected at age 4 months and persisted for several years despite a high HIV viral load [801].

Congenital infection with *Trypanosoma cruzi* also results in a marked expansion of CD8 T cells over CD4 T cells, with evidence of oligoclonality of the TCR repertoire, indicating that this is antigen-driven [802]. These CD8 T cells are enriched in markers for activation (HLA-DR^{hi}), memory (CD45RO^{hi}), and end-stage effector (CD28$^-$) cells and for cytotoxicity (perforin$^+$) and have markedly greater capacity to produce IFN-γ and TNF-α than is seen in CD8 T cells from uninfected newborns; compared with CD8 T cells, CD4 T cells in these congenitally infected newborns seem to have undergone much less clonal expansion and acquisition of effector function [802]. Congenital infection with viruses or *T. gondii* during the second and third trimesters may result in the appearance of CD45RO^{hi} memory T cells and an inverse ratio of CD4 to CD8 T cells [803–805], findings that also suggest that fetal CD8$^+$ T cells are activated and expanded in response to serious infection. These alterations in CD45RO expression by T cells in congenital infection may persist at least through early infancy [806,807].

T-CELL RESPONSE TO POSTNATAL INFECTIONS AND VACCINATION IN EARLY INFANCY

CD4 T Cells

Postnatal infection with HSV results in antigen-specific proliferation and cytokine (IL-2 and IFN-γ) production by CD4 T cells. These responses are substantially delayed, however, compared with responses in adults with primary HSV infection [808,809]. It is unclear at what postnatal age the kinetics of this response becomes similar to that in adults. Studies of CMV-specific CD4 T-cell immunity (expression of IL-2, IFN-γ, and CD40 ligand) in older infants and young children with primary infection found substantially reduced responses compared with adults with infection of similar duration [579]. This reduced CD4 T-cell response was associated with persistent shedding of the virus into secretions [579]. It is likely

that reduced CMV-specific CD4 T-cell responses also apply to the neonate and young infant with perinatal or postnatally acquired infection, who also persistently shed the virus for several years after acquisition. As in congenital CMV infection [663–665], older infants and young children with primary CMV infection had robust CMV-specific CD8 T-cell responses similar to those in adults [579,810,811].

Infants 6 to 12 months old also show reduced IL-2 production in response to tetanus toxoid than observed in older children and adults [812]. This finding suggests that antigen-specific memory CD4 T-cell generation or function is decreased during early infancy. It is unclear whether this reflects limitations in antigen processing, T-cell activation and costimulation, or proliferation and differentiation.

In contrast to postnatally acquired herpesvirus infections or inactivated vaccine antigens, BCG vaccination at birth versus 2 months or 4 months of age was equally effective in inducing CD4 T-cell proliferative and IFN-γ responses to PPD, extracellular *Mycobacterium tuberculosis* antigens, and *M. tuberculosis* intracellular extract [813, 814]. The responses were robust not only at 2 months after immunization, but also at 1 year of age, and no skewing toward T_H2 cytokine production was noted, even by PPD-specific CD4 T-cell clones [813,814]. Early postnatal administration of BCG vaccine does not result in decreased vaccine-specific T_H1 responses, tolerance, or T_H2 skewing. How these responses compare with responses in older children and adult vaccinees is unknown. Early BCG vaccination also may influence antigen-specific responses to unrelated vaccine antigens. BCG given at birth increased T_H1-specific and T_H2-specific responses and antibody titers to hepatitis B surface antigen (HBsAg) given simultaneously [814]. BCG given at birth did not enhance the T_H1 response to tetanus toxoid given at 2 months of age, but did increase the T_H2 response (IL-13 production). It is likely that BCG vaccination may accelerate DC maturation, so that these cells can augment either T_H1 or T_H2 responses.

The T cell–specific response to oral poliovirus vaccine (OPV), another live vaccine, suggests a decreased T_H1 response. Infants given OPV at birth and at 1, 2, and 3 months of age show lower OPV-specific CD4 T-cell proliferation and IFN-γ production and have fewer IFN-γ–positive cells compared with adults who were immunized as children but not recently reimmunized [815]. By contrast, their antibody titers were higher than titers in adults, suggesting that CD4 T-cell help for B cells is not impaired. It is plausible that OPV may be less effective at inducing a T_H1 response than BCG in neonates and young infants because of its limited replication, site of inoculation, or ability to stimulate APCs in a manner conducive to T_H1 immunity, relative to BCG, which induces persistent infection in the recipient.

Although neonates and young infants have been suggested to have skewing of CD4 T-cell responses toward a T_H2 cytokine profile, this may be an oversimplification. The tetanus toxoid–specific response after vaccination indicates that T_H1 (IFN-γ) and T_H2 (IL-5 and IL-13) memory responses occur, particularly after the third vaccine dose at 6 months of age [547]. The tetanus toxoid–specific T_H1

response may transiently decrease by 12 months of age; T_H2 responses are not affected [547,816].

CD8 T cells

CD8 T-cell responses to CMV infection acquired in utero [663] or during infancy and early childhood [579,800,810] are robust, and it is likely that this also applies for infection acquired perinatally or during early infancy. Cytotoxic responses to HIV in perinatally infected infants suggest that CD8 T cells capable of mediating cytotoxicity have undergone clonal expansion in vivo by 4 months of age [817]. The cytotoxicity may be reduced and delayed in appearance compared with adults, however [818]. There is also decreased HIV-specific CD8 T-cell production of IFN-γ by young infants after perinatal HIV infection [819] and an inability to generate HIV-specific cytotoxic T cells after highly active antiretroviral therapy [820]. When evaluated beyond infancy, cytolytic activity directed to HIV envelope proteins was commonly detected, but cytolytic activity directed against gag or pol proteins was rarely detected [800], suggesting that the antigenic repertoire of cytotoxic CD8 T cells was less diverse than in adults.

HIV-1 infection may inhibit antigen-specific immunity by depleting circulating DCs, impairing antigen presentation, decreasing thymic T-cell output, and promoting T-cell apoptosis. In addition, maintenance of HIV-specific CD8 T cells with effector function depends on HIV-specific CD4 T cells and may be selectively and severely impaired by the virus. Regardless of the precise mechanism, the suppressive effects of HIV-1 on cytotoxic responses may be relatively specific for HIV-1 because HIV-infected infants who lack HIV-specific cytotoxic T cells may maintain cytolytic T cells against EBV and CMV [819,820]. Some of the inhibitory effects of HIV-1 infection also may occur in HIV-exposed but uninfected infants born to HIV-infected mothers [821,822].

In one older study, RSV-specific cytotoxicity was more pronounced and frequent in infants 6 to 24 months of age than in younger infants [823]. These results, which need to be repeated using more current assays, suggest that the CD8 T-cell response to RSV gradually increases with postnatal age. Murine studies indicate that RSV infection suppresses CD8 T cell–mediated effector activity (IFN-γ production and cytolytic activity) and that only transient memory CD8 T-cell responses occur after infection. Longitudinal studies of CD8 T-cell immunity to RSV in children and adults after primary and secondary infection would be of interest to determine if this immunoevasive mechanism applies to humans.

SUMMARY

T-cell function in the fetus and neonate is impaired compared with adults. Diminished functions include T-cell participation in cutaneous DTH reaction and, as also discussed in the next section, T-cell help for B-cell differentiation. Selectively decreased cytokine production by fetal and neonatal T cells, such as decreased IFN-γ secretion and expression of CD40 ligand, may contribute to these deficits. In the case of IFN-γ, the predominance in the fetus and neonate of RTEs may contribute to this

immaturity in cytokine secretion. The repertoire of $\alpha\beta$-TCR probably is adequate except in early gestation. After fetal or neonatal infection, the acquisition of CD4 T-cell antigen-specific responses typically is delayed. In vitro studies suggest that deficiencies of DC function and activation and differentiation of antigenically naïve CD4 T cells into memory/effector T cells may be contributory. In contrast with diminished CD4 T-cell function, CD8 T cell–mediated cytotoxicity and cytokine production in response to strong chronic stimuli, such as congenital CMV infection or allogeneic cells, seem to be intact in the fetus and neonate. The mother does not transfer T cell–specific immunity to the fetus. T-cell sensitization to environmental allergens may occur during fetal life and with maternal vaccination, but such sensitization must be confirmed in future studies.

B CELLS AND IMMUNOGLOBULIN
OVERVIEW

Mature B cells are lymphocytes that are identifiable by their surface expression of immunoglobulin. Immunoglobulin, which is synonymous with antibody, is a heterotetrameric protein consisting of two identical heavy chains and two identical light chains linked by disulfide bonds (Fig. 4–14). As with the TCR, the amino-terminal

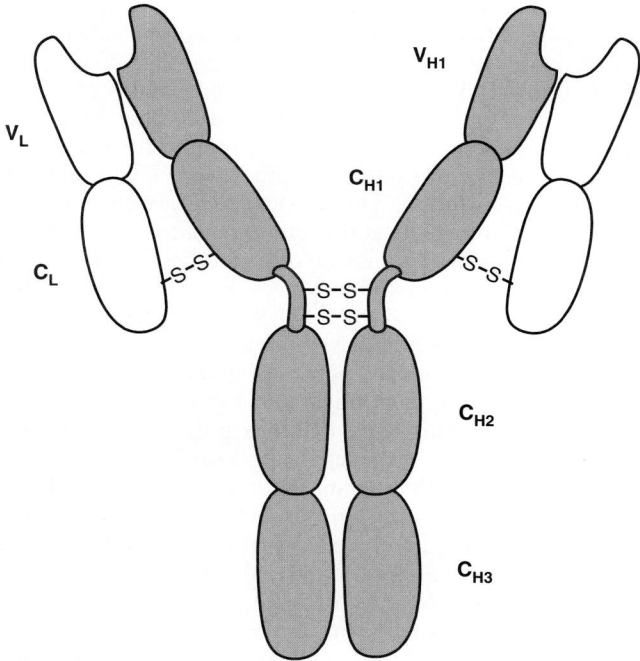

FIGURE 4–14 Structure of immunoglobulin molecule. An immunoglobulin molecule consists of two heavy chains (*dark shading*) and two light chains (*unshaded*) linked together by disulfide bonds. The antigen-combining site is formed by amino-terminal region of the heavy and light chains contained in the V_H and V_L domains of the heavy and light chains. For IgG, IgD, and IgA, the constant region C_H3 domain of the heavy chain encodes isotype or subclass specificity, which determines the ability of the immunoglobulin to fix complement, bind to Fc receptors, and be actively transported from the mother to the fetus during gestation. IgM and IgE (*not shown*) are structurally similar except that they contain an additional C_H4 domain conferring these properties, and they lack a hinge region.

portion of the antibody chains is highly variable as a consequence of the assembly of V, D, and J gene segments (heavy chain) or V and J segments (light chain) to a monomorphic constant (C) region. These amino-terminal regions of a pair of heavy and light chains form the antigen-binding fragment (Fab) portion of immunoglobulin, which contains the antigen-binding site (see Fig. 4–14).

As with the TCR, the variable region of each chain can be subdivided into three hypervariable CDR1, CDR2, and CDR3 regions and four intervening, less variable framework regions. The three-dimensional folding of the antibody molecules results in the approximation of the three CDR regions into a contiguous antigen recognition site, with CDR3 located at the center and the CDR1 and CDR2 regions forming the outer border of the site [824,825]. Antibody molecules are distinct from the αβ-TCR, however, in that they typically recognize antigens found on intact proteins or other molecules, such as complex carbohydrates. The B-cell recognition of antigen is typically highly sensitive to its three-dimensional structure.

The constant regions of the heavy and light chains consist of three constant heavy (CH) domains and one constant light (CL) domain (see Fig. 4–14). The heavy chains also have a hinge region at which the two halves are joined by disulfide bonds. The heavy chain C region is the Fc portion of immunoglobulin and contains sites that determine complement fixation, placental transport, and binding to leukocyte Fc receptors. The portion of the heavy chain C region encoded by the last exon of heavy chain gene defines antibody isotype or isotype subclass, of which there are nine in humans: IgM, IgD, IgG1, IgG2, IgG3, IgG4, IgA1, IgA2, and IgE. Light chains comprise two types, κ and λ, each containing a distinct type of C region. In isotype switching, the C region at the carboxy terminus of the immunoglobulin heavy chain gene is replaced with another isotype-specific segment, but the antigen-combining site at the amino terminus is preserved.

In addition to their secretion of antibodies, mature B cells express MHC class II and may participate in antigen processing and presentation to CD4 T cells. They may also serve as a source of effector cytokines (e.g., IFN-γ) and as suppressors of immune responses (regulatory B cells).

In cases in which the antigen has multiple and identical surface determinants (e.g., complex polysaccharides, certain viral proteins with repetitive motifs) and multiple surface immunoglobulins are cross-linked, antigen binding alone may be sufficient to induce B-cell activation without cognate (direct cell-cell interaction) help from T cells. In this case, other signals derived from non–T cells, such as cytokines, or from microorganisms, such as bacterial lipoproteins or bacteria-derived DNA containing unmethylated CpG motifs, may enhance antibody responses [826].

EARLY B-CELL DEVELOPMENT AND IMMUNOGLOBULIN REPERTOIRE FORMATION
Pro–B Cell and Pre–B Cell Maturation

The pro-B cell is the most immature cell type that is known to have differentiated along the B lineage. Human pro-B cells of the adult bone marrow have a CD10^{hi}CD19$^-$CD34^{hi} surface phenotype. They also express intracellular Pax5, RAG, TdT, and CD79 proteins and undergo D-to-J and then V-to-DJ immunoglobulin heavy chain gene rearrangements [827]. D-to-J heavy chain gene rearrangements also may occur in immature lymphocytes that are not committed to the B lineage, but V-to-DJ rearrangement may be a characteristic feature of committed B-lineage cells. In cases in which the immunoglobulin heavy chain is productively rearranged, it is expressed cytoplasmically and on the B-lineage cell surface as part of the pre–B-cell receptor (BCR) complex, which consists of a surrogate light chain (a VpreB and a λ5/14.1 segment) in association with Ig-α (CD79a) and Ig-β (CD79b) heterodimers. Expression of the pre-BCR complex defines the pre–B-cell stage, and pre-B cells have a CD10^{hi}CD19^{hi} surface phenotype. CD34 expression decreases during the pro–B cell to pre–B cell transition [827].

The heavy chain gene usually rearranges first, initially with a joining of a D segment to a J segment [828]. D-to-J heavy chain gene rearrangement and protein expression are followed by the joining of a V segment to the D-to-J segment. Productive V(D)J rearrangement results in the expression of full-length heavy chain protein in the cytoplasm. In humans, the first easily recognized pre-B cells are those that contain cytoplasmic IgM heavy chains, but no light chains or surface immunoglobulin. The expression of the pre-BCR by the pre-B cell blocks rearrangement of the other heavy chain gene allele (allelic exclusion) and results in proliferation of the pre-B cell for four to five divisions, with concurrent downregulation of RAG and TdT activity [829].

The human pro–B cell to pre–B cell transition depends on the ability to form a functional pre-BCR complex. This transition is blocked by mutations in the Cμ segment of the heavy chain gene, Ig-α, Ig-β, the cytoplasmic Btk tyrosine kinase, or the SLP-65 (also known as B-cell linker) cytoplasmic adapter protein, all of which compromise pre-BCR signal transduction. No known ligand for the human pre-BCR has been defined, and much of its extracellular domain of heavy chain is dispensable for its function. This suggests that the pre-BCR may have ligand-independent basal signaling function [830]. Such ligand-independent function is supported by a structural study that found that the human pre-BCR receptor can dimerize in the absence of any ligand and probably cannot recognize antigens because of steric blockade of the heavy chain binding site by the surrogate light chain [831]. After a burst of cell proliferation, the pre-B cell exits from cycling, upregulates RAG and TdT activity, and promotes immunoglobulin light chain rearrangement.

After the expression of the pre-BCR, a similar process of gene rearrangement subsequently occurs to assemble light chain genes from V and J segments. Allelic exclusion also usually acts at the light chain level, so that only a single type of light chain is produced. κ light chain gene rearrangement usually occurs first, and if κ chain gene rearrangement is productive, this apparently permits λ chain gene rearrangement to proceed [832]. Approximately 60% of human immunoglobulin molecules use κ light chains, and the remainder use λ light chains [833]. If rearrangement and expression of a complete κ or λ light chain subsequently occur, a functional immunoglobulin molecule is assembled and expressed as surface immunoglobulin. The end result of allelic exclusion is that a B cell usually synthesizes only a single immunoglobulin protein. Compared with the heavy chain, allelic exclusion of immunoglobulin light chains is "leaky" such that 0.2% to 0.5% of circulating B cells express a κ and a λ light chain in their surface IgM [834].

Pre-B cells are first detected in the human fetal liver and omentum by 8 weeks of gestation and in the fetal bone marrow by 13 weeks of gestation [835]. Between 18 and 22 weeks of gestation, pro-B cells or pre-B cells also can be detected in the liver, lung, and kidney [836]. These findings raise the possibility that B-cell lymphopoiesis may occur in these organs in situ at this stage of fetal development. By mid-gestation, the bone marrow is the predominant site of pre–B cell development [837]. B-cell lymphopoiesis occurs solely in the bone marrow after 30 weeks of gestation and for the remainder of life [836]. The neonatal circulation contains higher levels of $CD34^+CD38^-$ progenitor cells that are capable of differentiating into B cells than are found in the bone marrow compartment of children or adults [838]. Cord blood has circulating $IgM^-CD34^+CD19^+Pax-5^+$ B-cell progenitors cells that span the early B cell, pro–B cell, and pre–B cell stages of development; CD10 expression by these circulating B-cell progenitor cells is variable [839].

V(D)J Recombination of the Immunoglobulin Gene Loci

Analogous to the β chain of the TCR, the heavy immunoglobulin chain is encoded by V, D, J, and C regions. Approximately 164 V and 37 D gene segments are dispersed over 1100 kb of DNA upstream of the JC region, with nine different J segments located near the C region. Antibody gene rearrangement is required to bring the V, D, and J regions together to form a single exon that is juxtaposed to the C region so that the gene can be expressed (see Fig. 4–9). The same recombinase enzyme complex required for TCR gene rearrangement, including the RAG-1 and RAG-2 proteins, mediates this process. The assembly of the κ and λ light chain genes from multiple potential segments is similar except that D segments are not used.

As in the TCR chains, the CDR1 and CDR2 regions of the antigen-combining site are encoded entirely by the V segments, and the CDR3 is encoded at the junction of the V, D, and J segments. Antibody diversity, similar to TCR diversity, is generated by the juxtaposition of various combinations of V, D, and J segments and by imprecision in the joining process itself owing to exonucleolytic activity, random nucleotide addition by the TdT enzyme, and resolution of hairpin ends as P nucleotides. In the case of the heavy chain gene, D-to-D joining can also occur, and D segments also can rearrange by inversion or deletion. Together, these mechanisms permit a theoretical immunoglobulin repertoire of more than 10^{12} specificities to be generated from less than 10^3 somatic gene segments. For reasons that are unclear, however, immunoglobulin heavy chain V segment usage by immature pre-B cells and antigenically naïve B cells seems to be dominated by

relatively few segments [840,841]. Actual immunoglobulin diversity is less than would be predicted if segment usage were completely random. As in the case of the TCR genes, the CDR3 region seems to be the most important source of diversity. Further diversification is possible later in B-cell differentiation by processes known as receptor editing and somatic mutation, which are described later.

V(D)J Segment Usage of the Fetus and Neonate

The primary or preimmune immunoglobulin repertoire, which consists of all antibodies that can be expressed before encounter with antigen, is determined by the number of different B-cell clones with distinct antigen specificity and is limited during the initial stages of B-cell development in the fetus compared with that in the adult. In the early gestation to mid-gestation human fetus, the set of V segments used to generate the heavy chain gene is smaller than in the adult [842,843]. The V segments are scattered throughout the heavy chain gene locus [844]. Differences in the usage of particular heavy chain D and J segments between the first and second trimesters and term also have been identified [845]. These developmental differences are intrinsic, rather than the result of environmental influences, because they occur in immature B-cell precursors lacking a pre-BCR complex.

By the third trimester, the V and D segment heavy chain gene repertoire of peripheral B cells seems to be similar to that of the adult, although there may be overrepresentation of certain segments [846,847] and underuse of certain JH segments [847]. Certain heavy chain V segments expressed in adult B cells are not found in neonatal B cells [848,849], but it is unlikely that this severely limits the neonatal humoral immune response. Other V segments, such as V_{H3}, are present at a greater frequency in the preimmune immunoglobulin repertoire [849,850]. This increased representation may confer on antibody molecules the ability to bind protein A of *S. aureus*, providing some intrinsic protection during the perinatal period.

CDR3 Length and Terminal Deoxytransferase

The length of the CDR3 region of the immunoglobulin heavy chain, which is formed at the junction of the V segment with the D and J segments, is shorter in the mid-gestation fetus than at birth [851] or in adulthood [852]. This is due, in part, to decreased TdT, which is responsible for N-nucleotide additions. This decreased TdT expression is an intrinsic property of neonatal $CD34^+$ precursor cells not yet committed to the B lineage because in vitro differentiation of B-lineage cells from neonatal $CD34^+$ cells results in lower amounts of TdT than are present in similar cells from adults [853].

Of heavy chain CDR3 regions in fetal B cells, 25% lack N additions, and in the remaining regions, the size of the N-nucleotide additions is smaller than for neonatal or adult CDR3 regions. The CDR3 region is the most hypervariable portion of immunoglobulins, and a short CDR3 region significantly reduces the diversity of the fetal immunoglobulin repertoire [848]. The CDR3 region of the heavy chain gene remains relatively short at the beginning of the third trimester and gradually increases in length until birth [846,854,855]. Because the CDR3 region is at the center of the antigen-binding pocket of the antibody [856], reduced CDR3 diversity could limit the efficiency of the antibody response. The importance of shortened CDR3 regions by themselves in limiting antibody responses is doubtful, however, because gene knockout mice lacking TdT produce normal antibody responses after immunization or infection [459]. Although a combination of lack of TdT and limitations in V and D usage could limit the ability of the fetal B cells to recognize a full spectrum of foreign antigens, particularly before mid-gestation, such a "hole in the repertoire" has not been documented.

In mice, premature expression of TdT during fetal development achieved by transgenesis was detrimental in adulthood by preventing the appearance of certain natural (preimmune) antibody specificities (e.g., reactive with phosphorylcholine), which increased the susceptibility of the animals to bacterial infection [857]. The combination of decreased TdT activity and the preferential usage of DH7-27, which is the shortest of the DH segments, results in particularly short CDR3 regions in the human fetus and neonate [847]. It has been proposed that these limitations in CDR3 length combined with preferential usage of VH6-1 may be important in generating natural IgM antibody specificities, such as for single-stranded DNA, that may be protective in the fetus and neonate (e.g., by helping eliminate fetal apoptotic cells) [847].

B-CELL MATURATION, PREIMMUNE SELECTION, AND ACTIVATION

Receptor Editing, Clonal Deletion, and Clonal Anergy

Immature B cells of the bone marrow that have successfully generated a productive heavy and light chain express these as IgM on the cell surface. A large proportion of these surface immunoglobulins are autoreactive (i.e., they bind with relatively high affinity to molecules on other cell types within the bone marrow microenvironment and peripheral lymphoid organs) [858]. Such self-reactivity and BCR signaling at this stage of development maintains RAG activity with the result that the B cell frequently undergoes a secondary V-to-J light chain rearrangement [859]. This involves V segments located 5' and J segments that are located 3' to the current VJ rearrangement. If this eliminates surface immunoglobulin autoreactivity, the lack of BCR-mediated cell signaling turns off RAG activity, and the B cell enters into the circulation as a new emigrant (transitional) B cell to complete its maturation. If not, additional light chain rearrangement can occur.

Analysis of patients with genetic immunodeficiencies of signaling pathways involved in TLR recognition unexpectedly found an accumulation of autoreactive B cells, indicating that IRAK-4–dependent and MyD88-dependent signaling is involved in the receptor editing process [860]. Replacement of V heavy chain gene segments with previously unrearranged upstream V segments is also possible [861], but this is a rare form of editing for human B cells. Most immature autoreactive B cells can be converted to nonautoreactivity by receptor editing, allowing most B cells with productive immunoglobulin heavy chain rearrangements to contribute to the final repertoire.

The persistently autoreactive B cells are probably eliminated by a process of clonal deletion, which involves apoptosis induced by strong BCR signaling [858], or anergy, in which the B cells are functionally inactivated. A more recent study [862] has identified a distinct naïve B-cell subset of IgD$^+$IgM$^-$CD27$^-$ cells that has the BCR antigen specificity (predominantly autoreactive) and intracellular signaling characteristics (reduced capacity to increase intracellular calcium and increase tyrosine phosphorylation) indicative of anergic B cells. In healthy adults, these IgD$^+$IgM$^-$ anergic B cells constitute about 3% of all circulating B cells.

In contrast to IgM$^+$ adult B cells in the peripheral lymphoid organs, most of which also express surface IgD, first-trimester fetal B cells express IgM without IgD [863]. Such IgM$^+$IgD$^-$ B cells constitute a transitory stage between pre-B cells and mature IgM$^+$IgD$^+$ B cells. Murine studies have shown that exposure of transitional IgM$^+$IgD$^-$ B cells to antigens, including antigens found in the adult bone marrow, results in clonal anergy rather than activation [864]. The susceptibility of transitional IgM$^+$IgD$^-$ cells to clonal anergy maintains B-cell tolerance to soluble self-antigens present at high concentrations. Antigen exposure in utero may induce B-cell tolerance, rather than an antibody response, and may account for the observation that early congenital infection sometimes results in pathogen-specific defects in immunoglobulin production. In some cases, such as congenital mumps, these defects may occur despite apparently normal T-cell responses [799], suggesting a direct inhibitory effect on B-cell function.

An analysis of productive and nonproductive λ light chain gene repertoire of the human fetal spleen at 18 weeks of gestation found evidence of receptor editing, indicating that B cells encounter self-antigens that mediate negative selection in early ontogeny [865,866]. Similar findings apply to the κ light chain repertoire of cord blood B cells [866]. Together, these findings suggest that the preimmune fetal immunoglobulin repertoire is significantly shaped by self-antigens.

New Emigrant (Transitional) versus Fully Mature Naïve B Cells

The initial expression of surface immunoglobulin by B-lineage cells is in the form of IgM and IgD isotypes. This is the result of alternative mRNA splicing of the exons of the heavy chain gene. In adults, these IgM^{hi}IgD^{hi} transitional B cells can be identified in the bone marrow and circulation by their high levels of expression of CD24, CD38, CD5, and CD10 and low levels of Bcl-2 and the ABCB1 transporter [867–870]. These cells also are enriched for Ki67 staining, indicating they have recently undergone proliferation. CD5, CD10, CD24, CD38, and Ki67 staining decline, and ABCB1 is upregulated as new emigrant B cells mature into naïve B cells

[867]. Analogous to T-lineage cells, these circulating transitional B cells can be considered as recent bone marrow emigrants (new emigrants) that undergo a post–bone marrow phase of peripheral maturation into fully mature naïve B cells. Murine studies indicate that transitional B cells mainly undergo further maturation into naïve B cells in the spleen. Although the sites of this maturation process in humans is unknown, it seems to be B-cell activating factor of the tumor necrosis factor family (BAFF)–dependent [871].

The maturation of new emigrant B cells into fully mature, antigenically naïve B cells includes negative selection of B cells with autoreactive BCRs that have entered into the periphery and that have somehow escaped central tolerance mechanism in the bone marrow. Although the mechanisms involved in this secondary checkpoint for B-cell tolerance remain poorly understood, it may involve, at least in part, the death of autoreactive B cells because of their greater dependence on BAFF for survival than nonautoreactive B cells [860]. This peripheral tolerance checkpoint also seems to require CD4 T cell–derived signals, as the proportion of B cells that have autoreactive BCRs is significantly increased in antigenically naïve B cells of patients with genetic defects affecting CD40 ligand or MHC class II [872]. It is plausible that the increased frequency of autoreactive naïve B cells in patients with MHC class II deficiency may reflect decreased numbers of MHC class II–restricted $CD25^+$ CD4 Tregs in these individuals [860].

New emigrant B cells may also be subject to the influence of positive selection, which in mice can influence whether a B cell differentiates into particular B-cell subsets, such as follicular B cells versus marginal zone B cells, which are discussed subsequently. Positive selection requires an intact BCR complex and presumably involves some interaction of the antigen-combining site of the BCR with self-molecules or tonic signaling by the BCR complex [830], or both. In contrast with positive selection of thymocytes, which involves mainly cortical epithelial cells that present self-peptides, the nature and cellular sources of the ligands involved remain obscure. Evidence for positive selection of B cells in the human in fetal life comes from comparisons of the immunoglobulin repertoire of pre-B cells and transitional B cells versus the immunoglobulin repertoire of mature naïve B cells [873].

Follicular B-Cell Maturation

New emigrant B cells that escape negative selection and have undergone positive selection are directed by poorly understood pathways to become fully mature naïve $IgM^{hi}IgD^{hi}CD27^{lo/-}ABCB1^+$ follicular B cells [867,874]. Follicular B cells include most of the B cells that are involved in adaptive immune responses to T-dependent antigens, such as proteins and protein-carbohydrate conjugates, and are the predominant naïve B-cell subset of cells in the circulation or secondary lymphoid tissue. Marginal zone and B-1 B cells, which have distinct roles from follicular B cells in immunity, are discussed separately.

Similar to naïve T cells, the naïve B-cell subset has a very slow rate of turnover in vivo [867,875] and expression of CXCR4, CXCR5, and CCR7, which promotes

their recirculation between the follicles of the peripheral lymphoid organs, including the spleen, lymph nodes, and Peyer patches, and the blood and lymph [876]. The CXCR5 chemokine receptor recognizes CXCL13, which is produced within the follicles and promotes entry into and retention by the follicle [877]. Other B-cell functions that concurrently mature include a decreased tendency to undergo apoptosis after BCR engagement, an increased responsiveness to T-cell help (e.g., CD40 ligand and soluble cytokines, such as IL-21), increased expression of CD86, and maturation of intracellular signaling in response to BCR engagement. In addition to secondary lymphoid tissue, follicular B cells may also home to the perisinusoidal areas of bone marrow, which are also enriched in DCs that may provide important signals for B-cell survival. Perisinusoidal bone marrow B cells are poised to respond rapidly to blood-borne antigens, such as those derived from *Salmonella*, and produce antigen-specific IgM in a T-independent manner [878].

Fetal and Neonatal B-Cell Frequency and Surface Phenotype

B cells expressing surface IgM are present by 10 weeks of gestation [835]. The frequency of B cells in tissues rapidly increases, so that by 22 weeks of gestation, the proportion of B cells in the spleen, blood, and bone marrow is similar to that in the adult [863]. The concentration of B cells in the circulation is higher during the second and third trimesters than at birth and declines further by adulthood [879].

Circulating neonatal B cells are highly enriched in the new emigrant cell subset [867] based on their $IgM^+IgD^+CD24^+CD38^+ABCB1^-$ surface phenotype and high levels of CD5, CD10, and Ki67. Approximately 70% to 75% of cord blood B cells are new emigrants, and 25% to 30% are fully naïve B cells [867,880]. $CD27^+$ B cells, which include most memory B cells in adults, are low to undetectable in cord blood, consistent with the antigenic naïvete of the healthy newborn. Together, these findings account for earlier reports of higher levels of IgM, CD5, CD10, and CD38 surface expression and lower levels of CD11a, CD21, CD44, CD54 (ICAM-1), and L-selectin [881–886] in cord blood B cells than in the adult circulation Most fetal spleen B cells express CD5 and CD10 [827,887], indicating that new emigrant B cells predominate in the spleen. As for RTEs, the predominance of new emigrant B cells in the fetus and neonate is consistent with the likely high level of production of B cells at this age.

Unfractionated neonatal B cells and $CD27^-/IgM^+$ adult B cells of the circulation have similar levels of surface IgD, CD19, CD22, CD23, CD40, CD44, CD80, CD81, CD86, CCR6, and CXCR5 [881,884–886,888–891], but neonatal B cells may have modestly lower levels of CCR7 [881]. The frequency of new emigrant B cells in the circulation gradually declines with age.

B-CELL ACTIVATION AND IMMUNE SELECTION

As with T cells, B cells receive additional regulatory signals from the engagement of surface molecules other than the BCR that act as either costimulatory or inhibitory molecules. Of the costimulatory molecules, a complex consisting of CD19, CD21, and CD81 is best defined [892,893]. CD21, also known as complement receptor 2, binds the CD3d fragment of the C3 complement component. CD19 transmits intracellular activation signals after complement binding to CD21. Effective signaling after engagement of the BCR requires that key proximal signaling molecules are appropriately compartmentalized by means of lipid rafts, which are specialized cholesterol and glycosphingolipid microdomains of the plasma cell membrane [894]. In this context, CD81 may be particularly important for partitioning CD19/CD21/BCR complexes into lipid rafts so that antigen engagement is effective for B-cell activation [895].

The encounter of naïve B cells with antigen recognized by the surface immunoglobulin triggers their activation and proliferation under appropriate conditions. In contrast to αβ T cells, which recognize antigen in the form of processed fragments bound to the antigen-presenting grooves of MHC molecules, most B-cell surface immunoglobulins recognize antigen in a nondenatured form so that antigen recognition is highly sensitive to any alterations in the three-dimensional shape, such as post-translational modifications. Naïve B cells may encounter such nondenatured antigens presented by cDCs shortly after the B cell enters the lymph node or spleen via high endothelial venules before it enters the follicle [896]. Alternatively, naïve B cells entering the follicle may have soluble antigens shuttled to them by other B cells [897] or presented by follicular DCs, resident nonhematopoietic cells of the follicle. The relative importance of these different mechanisms for antigen presentation to naïve B cells likely varies depending on the nature of the antigen and the sites at which it is acquired by APCs.

B cells are activated to proliferate and differentiate into antibody-secreting cells after surface immunoglobulin binds antigen. The surface immunoglobulin molecule is invariably associated with the nonpolymorphic membrane proteins, Ig-α (CD79a) and Ig-β (CD79b), which, in conjunction with surface immunoglobulin, constitute the BCR. Ig-α and Ig-β, which are structural and functional homologs of the CD3 complex proteins, are expressed as disulfide-linked heterodimers, and contain ITAM motifs in their cytoplasmic tails. ITAMs act as docking sites for signaling molecules, such as the Lyn and Syk tyrosine kinases, that ultimately signal to alter gene transcription and initiate an activation program.

As with naïve T cells, activation of naïve B cells by BCR engagement has a high signal threshold compared with that of memory cells, a feature that may prevent inappropriate activation by low-affinity self-antigens. This is followed by activation of the phospholipase C/protein kinase C, Ras, and NFκB/Rel pathways that ultimately alter gene transcription. The CD19 molecule also has a cytoplasmic domain that serves as a docking site for several tyrosine kinases that provide costimulation when the CD19/CD21 complex is engaged by complement fragments, such as C3d. Engagement of CD40 on the B cell by CD40-ligand on the CD4 T cell also contributes to activation by inducing NF-κB/Rel transcription factor pathway. In the case of protein antigens, BCR engagement is followed by antigen internalization and entry into

the MHC class II antigen presentation pathway. Activation also increases B-cell expression of CCR7, which promotes B-cell movement toward the outer border of the T-cell zone [898], and of OX40 ligand (TNFSF4) and CD30 ligand (TNFSF8) [899], which can provide T-cell costimulation.

Negative Regulation of B-Cell Signaling

As for T cells, the activation of B cells is tightly regulated, and several surface molecules provide inhibitory signals that ensure that full activation requires overcoming a high signaling threshold, limiting the risk of activation by low-affinity autoantigens. These include CD22 and CD72, both of which contain intracellular ITIM motifs that when phosphorylated recruit tyrosine phosphatases (e.g., SHP-1 and SHP-2) and inositol phosphatases (e.g., SHIP-1) that limit B-cell activation signals via the BCR and costimulatory molecules (e.g., CD21) [900]. In addition, B cells express FcRγIIb, an ITIM-containing Fc receptor that mediates negative signaling when antibody simultaneously engages this receptor via its Fc moiety and binds to antigen on the BCR surface [120]. Surface expression of FcγRIIb is reduced on neonatal B cells [885,901], possibly rendering them less subject to the inhibitory effect of antigen-antibody complexes.

CD4 T-Cell Help for Naïve B-Cell Activation

For B cells to be activated effectively and to produce antibody against protein and protein-carbohydrate conjugate antigens requires help from CD4 T cells in most cases. This help is in the form of soluble cytokines, such as IL-21 [868], and of cell surface–associated signals, such as CD40 ligand, which is transiently expressed on the surface of activated CD4 T cells [524,525]. In T cell–dependent activation, antigenically naïve CD4 T cells probably are first activated by DCs independently of B cells [902]. CD4 T cells that are activated by DCs bearing antigenic peptide–MHC class II complexes and CD80-CD86 costimulatory molecules express CD40 ligand, OX40, ICOS, and CXCR5 [903]. These activated CD4 T cells may leave the lymphoid organ to become effector or memory T cells or become CD4 T cells specialized to provide help to B cells.

CD4 T cells destined to leave the lymphoid organ and to enter sites of tissue inflammation and participate in inflammatory responses (e.g., T$_H$1 cytokine secretion) are P-selectin^{hi}, CXCR3$^+$, and CXCR5$^-$. By contrast, CD4 T cells that are retained in the lymph node and that eventually enter the follicle as T$_{FH}$ cells are P-selectin$^-$ and CXCR3$^-$, but express CXCR5. This CXCR5 expression promotes movement of these CD4 T cells to the outer border of the T-cell zone, to contact antigen-activated B cells at the edge of the follicular zone [877]. Here, CD4 T-cell activation is reinforced by recognition of antigenic peptides displayed on MHC class II molecules of the B cell, and the interaction of CD40 ligand and OX40 on the T cell with CD40 and OX40 ligand on the B cell enhances B-cell activation. OX40 engagement of the CD4 T cell also promotes its differentiation into a T$_{FH}$ cell by increasing or helping retain the expression of CXCR5. These CXCR5^{hi} CD4 T cells enter into the follicle, where they provide help to B cells as T$_{FH}$

cells by expressing CD40 ligand, secreting IL-21 and other cytokines, and providing ICOS-dependent B-cell costimulation [551].

As discussed earlier, surface levels of CD40 ligand by circulating neonatal CD4 T cells is reduced compared with that by naïve adult CD4 T cells. Although this reduction could limit B-cell help for antibody responses, it is unclear if such reductions apply to T_{FH} cells of the neonate and infant in vivo.

B-Cell Selection in Germinal Centers of the Follicle

During the initial immune response, most antigenically naïve follicular B cells are derived from clones expressing antibody variable regions with relatively low affinity for antigen. As in the case of the TCR, activation through the BCR is not an all-or-none phenomenon. High-affinity binding to IgM of the BCR may allow B-cell proliferation to occur in the absence of any T-cell help, whereas lower affinity binding may result in proliferation only in the presence of additional T cell–derived signals. Antigen-specific B cells proliferate strongly within the B-cell follicle, leading to the formation of germinal centers. The more avidly the B cell binds antigen, the stronger is the stimulus to proliferate. The major source of antigen for triggering the extensive B-cell proliferation of the germinal center may be provided by antigen complexed with antibody bound to Fc receptors on follicular DCs, although this point is controversial [904]. The follicular DC is a nonhematopoietic cell type that seems to have the unusual capacity to bind antigen-antibody complexes for long periods on their cell surface. As already noted, follicular B cells may also receive antigen from other B cells that enter into the follicle or by their interactions with DCs on entry into the lymph node from the circulation [904]. True germinal centers in the spleen and lymph nodes are absent during fetal life, but appear during the first months after postnatal antigenic stimulation [905].

Somatic Hypermutation

Immunoglobulin variants are generated among germinal center B cells by the process of somatic hypermutation, in which immunoglobulin genes accumulate apparently random point mutations within productively rearranged V, D, and J segments. These variants undergo a selection process favoring B cells that bear surface immunoglobulin with high affinity for antigen. Such high-affinity immunoglobulin provides high levels of BCR signaling, favoring germinal center B-cell survival, rather than a default pathway of apoptosis. Somatic hypermutation requires an activation-induced cytidine deaminase (AID), which apparently is expressed only by germinal center B cells. AID deaminates deoxycytidine residues in single-stranded DNA to deoxyuridines, which are processed by DNA replication, base excision, or mismatch repair to restore normal base pairing between the two DNA strands, resulting in somatic hypermutation [525]. The effects of the mutator are focused on the variable region of immunoglobulin and its immediate flanking sequences. The peak of somatic mutation is approximately 10 to 12 days after immunization with a protein antigen [906]. Somatic mutation is an important means for increasing antibody affinity, but it may also result in the acquisition of autoimmunity. Human B cells with newly acquired autoreactivity as a result of somatic mutation are not subject to receptor editing or other tolerance mechanisms [907].

Most neonatal and fetal immunoglobulin heavy chain gene variable regions seem not to have undergone somatic mutation [849,851], consistent with the predominance of antigenically naïve new emigrant B cells in the fetus and neonate. By contrast, somatic mutations are detectable in some neonatal B cells expressing IgG or IgA transcripts [855], and the mutational frequency per length of DNA is similar to that of adult B cells. In contrast to follicular B cells, in which somatic hypermutation seems to occur only in germinal centers, a subset of marginal zone IgM+IgD+CD27+ B cells shows somatic hypermutation in the fetus before the appearance of germinal centers. In this context, extrafollicular somatic hypermutation seems to serve as a means to broaden the preimmune immunoglobulin repertoire of this B-cell subset.

MEMORY B CELLS

Germinal center B cells that receive appropriate survival signals leave the germinal center to persist as memory B cells. Most follicular memory B cells are CD27hi and have undergone isotype switching so that they are IgM−IgD− [908]. They also lack the ABCB1 naïve B-cell marker [867]. The turnover of memory B cells is approximately fivefold higher than naïve B cells based on their high levels of labeling in vivo and expression of the Ki67 antigen [867,875]. A fraction of memory B cells are CD27−ABCB1− cells, most of which express BCRs that have undergone isotype switching to IgG1 or IgG3, but not to IgG2 or IgA [867]. Human memory B cells are also heterogeneous in their expression of CD19, CD21, CD24, CD25, CD38, and FcRH4 (an inhibitory receptor), and these markers can be used to define additional memory B-cell subsets [909].

The engagement of CD40 on germinal center B cells by CD40 ligand on T cells is absolutely required for memory B-cell generation. Efficient memory B-cell generation requires the binding by CD21 on B cells of C3 complement components, such as C3d [892]. When a memory B cell is generated, further somatic mutation of its immunoglobulin genes apparently does not occur. Memory B cells enter the recirculating lymphocyte pool, where they preferentially colonize the skin and mucosa, sites that are likely to have direct contact with antigen, and the marginal zone of the spleen, where they are poised to respond to bloodborne antigens. When memory B cells are generated, they seem to persist indefinitely even in the absence of any subsequent exposure to the inciting antigen [910]. Memory B cells are typically not detectable in the circulation of the healthy fetus or neonate, consistent with limited B-cell exposure to foreign antigens in utero.

B CELLS AS ANTIGEN-PRESENTING CELLS

B cells express all of the proteins of the MHC class II antigen presentation pathway and can serve as APCs to CD4 T cells. Memory B cells are probably more effective than antigenically naïve B cells in simulating CD4 T cells because they constitutively express higher surface levels of CD80 or CD86 molecules that provide T-cell costimulation. Interactions between ICOS on the T cell and ICOS-ligand on the B cell may also be essential for inducing naïve CD4 T cells to differentiate into T_{FH} cells [551]. Surface immunoglobulin–protein complexes internalized from the cell surface are probably the preferential source of protein for antigenic peptides presented to T cells by B cells. The internalized proteins are degraded to peptides, which can be presented back on the B-cell surface bound to MHC class II molecules. Because the surface immunoglobulin–antigen interaction is of high affinity, B-cell antigen presentation theoretically permits CD4 T cells to be activated at relatively low concentrations of antigen. The observation that CD4 T-cell T_H1 immunity is intact in patients with X-linked agammaglobulinemia is consistent, however, with the notion that DCs, rather than B cells, play the central role in MHC class II antigen presentation [911].

Circulating neonatal B cells have lower levels of MHC class II than observed for adult splenic B cells [912], but proliferate at least as well as adult splenic B cells after MHC class II engagement [912]. Circulating third-trimester fetal and adult B cells were reported to express similar amounts of MHC class II [913]. There is limited information, however, regarding the capacity of fetal and neonatal B cells to serve as APCs for CD4 T cells.

SWITCHING OF IMMUNOGLOBULIN ISOTYPE AND CLASS AND ANTIBODY PRODUCTION
Isotype Switching

Human B cells produce five isotypes of antibody: IgM, IgD, IgG, IgA, and IgE. The IgG and IgA isotypes can be divided into the IgA1 and IgA2 and the IgG1, IgG2, IgG3, and IgG4 subclasses. During their process of differentiation into plasma cells, B cells are able to change from IgM to other antibody isotypes without changing antigen specificity (see Fig. 4–9). With the exception of IgD expression, this switching usually involves isotype recombination, the genetic replacement of the IgM-specific portion of the constant region (Cμ) of the heavy chain with a new isotype-specific gene segment. As in V(D)J recombination, the intervening DNA is excised as a large circle. Isotype recombination is mediated by switch regions that are positioned immediately upstream of each of the isotype-specific C regions, with the exception of IgD. Successive multiple isotype switching by a single B cell also can occur (e.g., IgM to IgA to IgG to IgE).

Genetic studies of hyper-IgM syndrome, in which there is a generalized block in isotype switching from IgM to other isotypes, have revealed that the process requires interactions between CD40 ligand on the T cell and CD40 on the B cell, the AID gene product (which also is required for somatic hypermutation), and the uracil N-glycolyase (UNG) enzyme [525]. There are also CD40-independent signals for such switching, such as provided by TLR9 found in the B-cell endosomal compartment binding to unmethylated CpG DNA (e.g., derived from bacteria) [914]. The molecular biology of switch recombination is complex, but similar to V(D)J recombination, involves double-stranded DNA breaks, in this case induced by the sequential action of AID, UNG, and an apurinic/apyrimidinic endonuclease [915], rather than the RAG proteins. These breaks are repaired by the NHEJ proteins involved in V(D)J recombination and additional proteins [916]. Secreted cytokines derived from T cells or other cell types play an important role in promoting or inhibiting switching to a specific isotype. IL-4 or IL-13 is absolutely required for isotype switching to IgE, a process that can be inhibited by the presence of IFN-γ [917]. In some instances, hormones also may play a role in isotype switching. Vasoactive intestinal peptide in conjunction with CD40 engagement can induce human B cells to produce high levels of IgA1 and IgA2 [918].

During a primary immune response, isotype switching by B cells seems to occur shortly after these cells enter into the follicle [919]. These B cells may have received the requisite T cell–derived signals (i.e., cytokines and CD40 ligand) during their interaction with T cells at the border between the follicle and T-cell zones. Switch recombination after primary immunization is evident in peripheral lymphoid tissue 4 days after immunization with protein antigen and peaks at 10 to 18 days [920]. Switch recombination also is triggered during memory B-cell responses, is detectable within 24 hours of secondary immunization, and peaks at 3 to 4 days [921].

Generation of Plasma Cells and the Molecular Basis for Immunoglobulin Secretion

Some activated B cells become plasmablasts and migrate to extrafollicular regions of the lymph node or spleen, where they become short-lived plasma cells that mainly produce IgM. Differentiation of these plasma cells does not require, and may be inhibited by, the CD40 ligand–CD40 interaction. In the absence of CD40 engagement, germinal center B cells that have survived the selection process probably differentiate to memory B-cell populations. Lanzavecchia and colleagues [910] suggested that memory B cells have a low threshold to become relatively long-lived plasma cells in an antigen-dependent manner, and that this antigen-independent conversion and antigen-independent division within the memory B-cell pool accounts for the typically lifelong maintenance of serologic (antibody) memory in humans after natural infection. In this case, the level of memory B cells attained after infection or vaccination would be the main determinant of antibody levels. Human memory B cells can differentiate into plasma cells in response to antigen-independent mechanisms, such as exposure to oligonucleotides containing unmethylated CpG DNA or activated T cells [922]. Such polyclonal activation of memory B cells has been proposed to maintain levels of specific antibody for a lifetime after memory B-cell responses have been generated [910].

Plasma cell generation from B cells involves the down-regulation of the Bcl6 protein and the upregulation of the B lymphocyte–induced maturation protein-1 (BLIMP1) and X box binding protein 1 (XBP1) transcription factors [923]. XBP1 drives B cell differentiation into a fully mature plasma cell that is capable of extremely high levels of antibody production [924]. The membrane-bound form of immunoglobulin is slightly longer than the secreted form and contains a carboxy-terminal region that anchors the molecule in the cell membrane. Plasma cell differentiation results in a switch to a secretory form of immunoglobulin that lacks this membrane-anchoring segment and the loss of surface immunoglobulin expression as a result of a change in splicing of the heavy chain mRNA. Plasma cells, rather than mature B cells, account for most of the secreted antibody during primary and secondary immune responses.

B cell differentiation into plasma cells is also likely accompanied by increases in CXCR4 expression, which helps target these cells to niches in the bone marrow containing stromal cells that secrete the CXCR4 ligand SDF-1 [925]. Plasma cells are concentrated in peripheral lymphoid tissue, liver, and bone marrow and in lymphoid tissue of the gastrointestinal and respiratory tracts.

Isotype Switching and Immunoglobulin Production by Fetal and Neonatal B Cells

Early in vitro studies of neonatal immunoglobulin production used pokeweed mitogen, a polyclonal activator of T cells and B cells. In this system, immunoglobulin production was low compared with immunoglobulin production in adults, and mixing experiments suggested that neonatal T cells acted as suppressors of immunoglobulin production by either adult or neonatal B cells. Further fractionation of the T-cell populations in this assay suggested that in the absence of memory/effector T cells, antigenically naïve (CD45RA^{hi}CD45RO^{lo}) CD4$^+$ T cells of either the neonate or the adult acted as suppressors of antibody production [628]. The relevance of the suppression to neonatal B-cell responses in vivo is unclear, however. Priming of neonatal or adult antigenically naïve CD4 T cells in vitro resulted in their acquisition of a CD45RA^{lo}CD45RO^{hi} phenotype and, concurrently, an ability to enhance rather than suppress pokeweed mitogen–induced immunoglobulin production [628]. This increased capacity for B-cell help probably reflects the fact that priming of naïve T cells enhances expression of CD40 ligand and cytokines needed for T cell–dependent help for B-cell responses.

When B cells are activated by exogenous cytokines (e.g., IL-4, IL-10, or cytokine-containing supernatants from activated T cells) and a cellular source of CD40 ligand (e.g., CD40 ligand expressing fibroblasts) or EBV infection, neonatal B-cell production of IgM, IgG1, IgG2, IgG3, IgG4, and IgE is similar to that in adult antigenically naïve B cells [608,926–928]. This is not unexpected because neonatal B cells are highly enriched in new emigrant B cells [867,869,870,880], and this B-cell subset in adults and fully mature naïve B cells are similarly efficient in undergoing isotype switching and secreting switched antibody [880]; neonatal B cells treated under these conditions also have robust signaling based on tyrosine phosphorylation of STAT6 by IL-4 and of STAT3 by IL-21 and secrete high levels of IgE [929]. Isotype switching is associated with cell division, and neonatal and adult B cells show a similar acquisition of

switching starting after the third cell division [930]. Pre-B cells have the capacity for isotype switching even during fetal ontogeny. Isotype switching and IgE and IgG4 production by fetal B and pre-B cells at 12 weeks of gestation can be induced in vitro [931]. IgA1 and IgA2 are produced in similar amounts by antigenically naïve fetal and adult B cells on stimulation with anti-CD40 antibody and vasoactive intestinal peptide hormone. Fetal pre-B cells also can synthesize IgA under these conditions [917]. When human fetal or neonatal B cells develop in, or are adoptively transferred into, SCID mice, they are capable of isotype switching and immunoglobulin production if appropriate T cell–derived signals are present [767,932,933].

Other studies suggest that isotype switching and antibody production by fetal and neonatal B cells is limited compared with these processes in antigenically naïve (IgM$^+$IgD$^+$) adult B cells. Durandy and colleagues [605] found that IgM, IgG, and IgE production by fetal B cells at mid-gestation was substantially lower than that of neonatal or adult B cells, suggesting an intrinsic hyporesponsiveness to CD40 or cytokine receptor engagement or both. Neonatal B cells produce substantially less IgA than adult naïve B cells in the presence of adult T cells stimulated by anti-CD3 mAb (as a source of CD40 ligand) and exogenous cytokines, such as IL-10 [934]. These limitations of fetal and neonatal isotype switching and antibody production probably reflect intrinsic limitations of B-cell function, particularly when T-cell help may be limited. Such limited production is not due to decreased activation or proliferation because neonatal B cells proliferate normally in response to engagement of CD40 or surface IgM or both [886].

Neonatal T cells activated for a few hours provide less help for neonatal B-cell immunoglobulin production and isotype switching than do similarly treated adult T cells [608]. Because this help probably is through CD40 ligand, reduced expression of CD40 ligand (or similar activation-induced molecules) by naïve neonatal T cells in the first few hours after activation may limit fetal and neonatal B-cell immune responses. Whether decreased neonatal DC function also contributes to diminished B-cell responses has not been determined.

Between 8 and 11 weeks of gestation, transcripts for IgA and IgG can be detected in the liver [935], and synthesis of IgM and IgG has been detected by 12 weeks of gestation in fetal organ cultures [936]. By 16 weeks of gestation, fetal bone marrow B cells expressing surface immunoglobulin of all heavy chain isotypes are detectable [937]. Immunoglobulin-secreting plasma cells are detectable by week 15 of gestation, and plasma cells secreting IgG and IgA are detectable by 20 and 30 weeks of gestation [938]. The stimulus for isotype switching during fetal development is unclear because in the adult, isotype switching typically occurs in response to B-cell activation by foreign protein antigens. These findings in bone marrow contrast with a flow cytometric study, in which nonspecific binding was carefully excluded, and neonatal B cells expressing surface IgG or IgA were below the limit of detectability (i.e., <1% of circulating B cells) [939].

Generally, neonatal B cells can differentiate into IgM-secreting plasma cells as efficiently as adult cells.

T cell–dependent immunoglobulin production by neonatal B cells is more readily inhibited, however, by agents that increase intracellular cAMP, such as prostaglandin E_2 [940].

MARGINAL ZONE AND $IgM^+IgD^+CD27^+$ B CELLS

The human spleen has distinct anatomic sites that may play specialized roles in the production of antibody against blood-derived particulate antigens and purified repetitive carbohydrate antigens. Important examples of such carbohydrate antigens are the capsular polysaccharides of pathogenic bacteria, such as *S. pneumoniae*, *Neisseria meningitidis*, and *H. influenzae*. Antigens and leukocytes enter the spleen through vascular sinusoids located in the red pulp that are in proximity to the marginal zone area. The white pulp area contains periarteriolar sheaths of lymphocytes, mainly T cells, and periarteriolar follicles, which are mainly B cells. These are surrounded by a microanatomic site known as the marginal zone that contains loose clusters of B cells, DCs, macrophages, and some CD4 T cells and that are in direct contact with the blood.

B cells of the human marginal zone of the adult spleen are predominantly $IgM^+IgD^+CD27^+$ and have BCRs encoded by somatically mutated immunoglobulin genes. B cells with this phenotype are of interest because they seem to mediate most of the IgM antibody response to unconjugated polysaccharides [941], which are T-independent type II antigens. In contrast to the murine marginal zone B cells, which do not seem to recirculate when they arise in the spleen from new emigrant B cells, the human adult circulation and tonsils have substantial numbers of B cells of a similar phenotype of those in the marginal zone. Somatic hypermutation is thought to be limited to B cells undergoing activation in germinal centers; however, $IgM^+IgD^+CD27^+$ B cells retain their somatic hypermutated immunoglobulin receptors in genetic disorders that prevent germinal center formation, such as deficiency of CD40, CD40 ligand, ICOS, and SH2D1A (SAP) [525,942], arguing for the existence of a germinal center–independent pathway.

Marginal zone B cells have unique phenotypic and functional properties that may be important in their production of IgM in response to blood-borne particulate antigens, such as bacteria, in addition to their having direct access to the blood and to circulating DCs that may bear these antigens [943]. Compared with naïve follicular B cells, marginal zone B cells express higher levels of CD21, which may facilitate the binding of C3d-coated blood-borne antigens, such as encapsulated bacteria [944]. Marginal zone B cells are also more readily activated by non-BCR signals, such as LPS, and more rapidly become effector cells than naïve follicular B cells after activation. This enhanced reactivity may be important in their being able to respond to purified polysaccharide antigens in the absence of T-cell signals [945]. Marginal zone B cells also seem "poised" to differentiate rapidly into IgM^+ plasmablasts [943] because of their constitutive expression of BLIMP-1, which promotes plasma cell differentiation [946].

The hyposplenic or asplenic state invariably compromises the human antibody response to purified polysaccharides, such as capsular polysaccharide components of the 23-valent pneumococcal vaccine. Splenic marginal zone B cells may be required for the generation of antibody responses to purified polysaccharide antigens, accounting for the loss of these responses with splenectomy. This loss could also be due to the removal of other cell types, however, or a specialized splenic microenvironment required for the purified polysaccharide antigens. This immune response does not absolutely require T-cell help (see section on development of B-cell capacity to respond to T cell–dependent and T cell–independent antigens). Immunization with T-independent antigens before human splenectomy maintains the capacity of the immune system to respond to these antigens subsequently [947]. This finding suggests that the activation of splenic B cells recognizing polysaccharide antigens may result in their migration and persistence in other lymphoid organs. The pathways by which capsular polysaccharide antigens reach the marginal zone are unknown, and the role that human marginal zone DCs or macrophages play in activating marginal zone B cells to produce antibody to purified polysaccharides is poorly understood. How human splenic marginal zone B cells involved in the response to purified polysaccharide antigens differentiate from naïve precursors also is unclear.

Marginal Zone B Cells of the Fetus and Neonate

$IgM^+IgD^+CD27^+$ B cells are detectable at birth in relatively low numbers and gradually increase to adult levels by approximately 2 to 3 years of age. $IgM^+IgD^+CD27^+$ B cells have a diverse immunoglobulin repertoire similar to that of conventional naïve B cells, rather than a more skewed repertoire typical for memory B cells that have undergone isotype switching. Together, these observations argue that $IgM^+IgD^+CD27^+$ B cells are distinct from conventional follicular B cells in that somatic hypermutation occurs outside of germinal centers and generates a mutated immunoglobulin sequence as part of a preimmune mechanism. Consistent with this idea, $IgM^+IgD^+CD27^+$ B cells with somatically mutated immunoglobulin genes are detectable in the circulation, liver, mesenteric lymph nodes, spleen, and bone marrow by 14 weeks of gestation [948], even though germinal centers and presumably antigen exposure are absent until after birth.

Somatic hypermutation of this fetal B-cell population may occur in the mesenteric lymph nodes and liver because these tissues express the AID enzyme required for this process, whereas fetal spleen tissue does not. The somatic hypermutation does not seem to require T-cell help because it occurs normally in human $IgM^+IgD^+CD27^+$ B cells developing from human HSCs in RAG-2/common γ chain knockout mice, which lack T cells [948]. Although the marginal zone of the spleen does not achieve its mature configuration until about 2 years of age, $IgM^+IgD^+CD27^+$ B cells have been identified in the marginal zone at 8 months of age [949]. If the $IgM^+IgD^+CD27^+$ marginal zone B-cell population is required for the responses to unconjugated polysaccharides, the inability of infants younger than 2 years of age to respond to such vaccines is not accounted for by an absence of this splenic B-cell subset. Rather, the deficiency is likely to be due at least in part to a qualitative defect in this IgM+IgD+CD27+ B-cell subset or in the APCs involved in its activation, such as the macrophages and DCs of the marginal zone. One such factor may be the reduced expression on B cells from preterm and, to a lesser degree, term neonates of receptors for BAFF and APRIL (a proliferation-inducing ligand) [950]. These cytokines are produced by APCs, are similar in structure to CD40 ligand, and are essential for T-independent responses to polysaccharide antigens. It is unclear, however, whether this observation also applies to the marginal zone B-cell subset of neonates.

B-1 CELLS AND NATURAL IgM

In mice, a B-cell subset that has been termed B-1 has a distinct tissue distribution restricted largely to the peritoneal and pleural cavities and special functional features, such as a tendency for polyreactive antibody specificities, particularly of the IgM isotype, compared with the bulk of B cells, which are termed B-2. The murine B-1 subset can be divided further into B-1a cells, in which CD5 is expressed on the cell surface, and B-1b cells, in which CD5 expression is limited to the RNA level. The B-2 lineage includes most peripheral B cells of the secondary lymphoid organs and most marginal zone B cells of the spleen. The identification of a distinct precursor B-lineage cell population for murine B-1 cells in the fetal murine bone marrow [951] has confirmed that B-1 and B-2 are distinct cell lineages, but an analogous human B-1 committed precursor cell population has not yet been identified.

Murine naïve B-1 cells and marginal zone B cells are important contributors to the early and rapid production of IgM in response to blood-borne particulate antigens and to other T-independent antigens [952]. B-1 cells are commonly reactive with self-antigens, such as DNA, and foreign antigens, such as viral proteins or bacteria-derived products such as phosphorylcholine. In mice, B1a cells seem to be essential for the production of natural antibodies that provide protection against encapsulated bacteria, whereas B1b cells are essential for producing anticapsular antibodies in response to immunization [953].

A distinct feature of human fetal and neonatal B cells is the high frequency of CD5 expression compared with unfractionated circulating adult B cells. More than 40% of B cells in the fetal spleen, omentum, and circulation at mid-gestation are CD5+ [954–956]; CD5+ B cells also are present in the neonatal circulation [487] and gradually decline with postnatal age [954]. Fetal and newborn CD5+ B cells express IgM antibodies that are polyreactive, including reactivity with self-antigens, such as DNA [954,955,957], and this has been interpreted as the fetal and neonatal B-cell compartment being enriched for B-1 cells. More recent studies indicate, however, that the high level of CD5 expression by human fetal and cord blood B cells and the polyreactivity of their IgM are fully accounted for by a high frequency of new emigrant B cells in early ontogeny [869,870,958]. It is unclear whether the frequency, distribution, and function of B-1 cells differ in the human fetus and neonate compared with the adult; this requires the development of new markers that can distinguish human B-1 cells from B-2 cells.

In mice, B-1 cells constitute the major source of the low amounts of circulating "natural" IgM present at birth produced in the absence of antigenic stimulation, and animals lacking the ability to secrete natural IgM have an increased susceptibility to acute peritonitis from endogenous bacteria [959]. Although natural IgM antibodies are of low affinity, they can activate complement, which may allow antigenically naïve B cells to become activated as a result of receiving costimulation via CD21. In addition to a role in host defense, natural IgM may also play a role in removing apoptotic cells [847].

As discussed subsequently ("Immunoglobulin Synthesis by the Fetus and Neonate"), total circulating IgM is very low in the fetus and healthy newborn. Nevertheless, antigen microarrays have revealed that most cord blood sera have IgM that reacts with multiple self-antigens, such as single-stranded DNA, whereas such reactivity is lacking in maternal IgM [960]. Some autoreactivity was observed with cord blood IgA, although to a much lesser degree than for IgM. The importance of natural IgM in human host defense in the fetus and neonate and its B-cell source is unclear.

T CELL–DEPENDENT AND T CELL–INDEPENDENT RESPONSES BY B CELLS
Overview
The chronology of the response to various antigens differs, depending on the need for cognate T-cell help (Table 4–7). Largely on the basis of findings in murine studies, antigens

TABLE 4–7 Hierarchy of Antibody Responsiveness

Species	Type of Antigen	Examples of Antigen	Age at Onset of Antibody Response
Mouse	T cell–dependent	TNP-KLH	Birth
	T cell–independent type I	TNP–*Brucella abortus*	Birth
	T cell–independent type II	TNP-Ficoll	Delayed (2-3 wk of age)
Human	T cell–dependent	Tetanus toxoid, HBsAg, *Haemophilus influenzae* conjugate vaccine, bacteriophage φX174	Birth
	T cell–independent type I	TNP–*B. abortus*	Birth
	T cell–independent type II	Bacterial capsular polysaccharides (*H. influenzae* type b, *Neisseria meningitidis*, *Streptococcus pneumoniae*, GBS)	Delayed (6-24 mo of age)

GBS, group B streptococci; HBsAg, hepatitis B surface antigen; KLH, keyhole limpet hemocyanin; TNP, trinitrophenol.
Adapted from Stiehm ER, Fudenberg HH. Serum levels of immune globulins in health and disease: a survey. Pediatrics 37:715, 1966.

can be divided into antigens dependent on a functional thymus and cognate help (direct cell-cell interactions) provided by mature αβ T cells (T-dependent antigens) and antigens partially or completely independent of T-cell help (T-independent antigens). T-independent antigens can be divided further into T-independent type I and T-independent type II, in accordance with their dependence on cytokines produced by T cells (or other cells).

Most proteins are T-dependent antigens requiring cognate T-cell–B-cell interaction for production of antibodies (other than small amounts of IgM). The antibody response to T-dependent antigens is characterized by the generation of memory B cells with somatically mutated, high-affinity immunoglobulin and the potential for isotype switching.

T-independent type I antigens are antigens that bind to B cells and directly activate them in vitro to produce antibody without T cells or exogenous cytokines. In the human, one such T-independent type I antigen is fixed *Brucella abortus*. T-independent type II antigens are mostly polysaccharides with multiple identical subunits and certain proteins that contain multiple determinants of identical or similar antigenic specificity. Responses to these antigens are enhanced in vitro and in vivo by cytokines, including IL-6, IL-12, IFN-γ, and GM-CSF [961-964]. NK cells, T cells, NKT cells, macrophages, and DCs may provide these cytokines. T-independent type II responses also are enhanced by bacterially derived TLR ligands, including LPS, lipoproteins, and unmethylated CpG DNA [963,965–967].

The response to T-independent type II antigens is characterized by the lack of B-cell memory and is restricted largely to the IgM and IgG_2 isotypes [883]. The IgM response to T-independent type II antigens seems to be mediated mainly by $IgM^+IgD^+CD27^+$ B cells, which have a high degree of somatic hypermutation of their immunoglobulin genes that seems to be generated before their encountering antigen. Immunization with T-independent type II antigens may result in the appearance of additional somatic hypermutations of the antibody produced by $IgM^+IgD^+CD27^+$ B cells [968], although whether this represents the expansion of previously mutated clones that were undetectable before immunization versus additional somatic hypermutations is unclear. Such additional antigen-induced somatic hypermutation is a controversial mechanism because most studies have found that $IgM^+IgD^+CD27^+$ B cells of the spleen and circulation have undetectable levels of the AID enzyme, which is absolutely required for somatic hypermutation.

Response to T Cell–Dependent Antigens

The capacity of the neonate to respond to T-dependent antigens is well established at birth (see Table 4–7) and is only modestly reduced compared with the response in the adult. Several mechanisms, alone or in combination, may be responsible for this modest reduction, including decreased DC interactions or function with CD4 T cells or B cells, limitations in CD4 T-cell activation and expansion into a T helper/effector cell population, impaired cognate interactions between CD4 T cells and B cells,

or an intrinsic B-cell defect. Another possibility is that T-dependent antigens preferentially upregulate CD22, which raises the threshold for B-cell activation, on neonatal compared with adult B cells [884]. Because neonatal B cells are highly enriched for the new emigrant subset, it is plausible that this subset may be less effective at responding to T-dependent antigens than fully mature naïve B cells, which predominate in the non–memory B-cell compartment of adults.

Most studies of the neonatal immune response to T-dependent antigens have not evaluated antibody affinity, a reflection of somatic mutation, or isotype expression. Such responses, particularly isotype switching, might be limited early in the immune response because of decreased CD40 ligand expression by CD4 T cells [608,611,969]. Studies are needed to determine if reductions in CD40 ligand expression by antigen-specific T cells also occur in response to neonatal vaccination and, if so, whether such reduced expression correlates with reduced memory B-cell development, decreased isotype switching, and somatic hypermutation. An additional factor that may contribute to the modest reduction in T-dependent antibody production is the reduced expression on B cells (nearly all of which are naïve $IgM^+IgD^+CD27^+$ follicular B cells) from preterm and, to a lesser degree, term neonates of receptors for BAFF and APRIL, which help promote T-dependent differentiation into plasma cells and plasma cell survival [950].

Response to T Cell–Independent Antigens

Antibody production by human neonatal B cells to a T-independent type I antigen in vitro (*B. abortus*) is only modestly reduced (see Table 4–7) [970]. This reduction may reflect a decreased ability of antigen-activated B cells to proliferate, rather than a decreased precursor frequency of antigen-specific clones [970].

In humans and mice, the response to T-independent type II antigens is the last to appear chronologically (see Table 4–7). This helps to account for the neonate's susceptibility to infection with encapsulated bacteria, such as GBS, and the poor response to polysaccharide antigens from other capsulated bacterial pathogens until approximately 2 to 3 years of age. The poor response in neonates is associated with their relatively low levels of circulating $IgM^+IgD^+CD27^+$ B cells, which are characteristically found in the marginal zone of the spleen and other extrafollicular sites, such as the tonsils. More recent studies have documented these cells in the marginal zone region of the spleen and blood in substantial numbers during the first 2 years of life, however, arguing that the poor response to T-independent type II antigens is not simply a quantitative defect of this B-cell subset. Rather, the decreased responses to T-independent type II antigens during early childhood probably reflect an intrinsic immaturity of $IgM^+IgD^+CD27^+$ B cells, perhaps including decreased expression of BAFF and APRIL receptors [950] or decreased function of other cell types that support their differentiation and function.

Decreased expression of CD21 on neonatal B cells has been proposed as a possible mechanism for limitations in T-independent type II response in the neonate

[971,972]. CD19 is expressed in association with CD21, the type 2 complement receptor, and serves to transduce B cell–activating signals when CD21 is engaged by C3 complement components [892], inducing polysaccharide-reactive B cells to proliferate in vivo. Genetic disruption experiments in mice support the idea that the type 2 complement receptor, which includes CD21 and CD35 in mice, is important for T-independent type II antibody responses to pathogens, such as *S. pneumoniae* [944]. In vitro studies of human splenic tissue suggest that T-independent type II antigens activate complement and bind C3 and then localize to the marginal zone splenic B cells expressing complement receptors [883]. Whether IgM+IgD+CD27+ B cells of the neonate and young infant have reduced CD21 expression compared with B cells of older children and adults is unclear, however.

Human neonatal B cells show a marked decrease in CD22 expression after engagement of IgM, a stimulus used to mimic a T-independent type II antigen [884]. Because CD22 is a negative regulator of B-cell activation, however, this finding does not explain the diminished response, unless it results in hyperresponsive neonatal B cells prone to apoptosis.

Dextran-conjugated anti-immunoglobulin mAbs have been used to mimic the events in T-independent type II antibody responses in vitro [963]. Human neonatal B cells respond to this stimulus as well as adult B cells, suggesting that the lack of the neonatal T-independent type II response is not due to an intrinsic limitation in their activation via surface immunoglobulin cross-linking [973]. B cells that respond to dextran-conjugated anti-immunoglobulin mAbs may be enriched for B cell types, such as new emigrant B cells and fully mature naïve B cells, that are functionally distinct, however, from IgM+IgD+CD27+ B cells that respond to polysaccharides or other T-independent type II antigens.

The response of human cord blood and adult peripheral blood B cells to CpG oligonucleotides is similar in terms of cell proliferation, the production of chemokines (CCL3 [MIP-1α] and CCL4 [MIP-1β]), and upregulation of CD86 and MHC class II expression [881]. This indicates that neonatal B-cell expression of TLR9 is similar to that of the adult, and the TLR9 signaling pathway, which involves MyD88, is intact. These findings are consistent with a more recent study [968] showing that new emigrant B cells of the adult and neonate express high levels of TLR9 and are capable of secreting IgM and IgG after stimulation with CpG oligonucleotides in the absence of added exogenous cytokines, including detectable levels of antipneumococcal polysaccharide IgM antibody. This stimulus also increases new emigrant B-cell expression of AID and BLIMP-1, consistent with the acquisition of the ability to secrete isotype-switched IgG plasma cells and the acquisition of a plasmablast surface phenotype by a substantial cell fraction [968].

Some of these CpG oligonucleotide–stimulated new emigrant B cells of the neonate acquire a CD27+IgM+ surface phenotype reminiscent of the IgM+IgD+CD27+ B-cell subset of the marginal zone of the spleen and circulation [968] (see "Marginal Zone B Cells of the Spleen and IgM+IgD+CD27+ B Cells" earlier). These observations raise the possibility that new emigrant B cells in the neonate and young infant may give rise to the IgM+IgD+CD27+ B-cell subset implicated in the IgM response to T-independent type II antigens and that this maturation may be enhanced by exposure to bacterial-derived products, such as CpG-containing DNA, in an antigen-independent manner.

A striking feature of the IgM+IgD+CD27+ B-cell subset is its high degree of preimmune somatic hypermutation of the immunoglobulin genes; an analysis of the immunoglobulin repertoire of IgM+IgD+CD27+ B cells generated from adult or cord blood new emigrant B cells would be of interest in future studies. This hypothesized postnatal pathway for IgM+IgD+CD27+ B-cell maturation is distinct from a pathway that is operative in the fetus in which these somatically hypermutated preimmune IgM+ B cells are generated in a sterile environment [948]. Finally, the TLR9 pathway also is capable of inducing naïve adult B cells to produce IL-12p70, a key cytokine for promoting T_H1 differentiation as discussed earlier, but it is unknown whether neonatal B cells are also capable of IL-12p70 production under these conditions.

SPECIFIC ANTIBODY RESPONSE BY THE FETUS TO MATERNAL IMMUNIZATION AND CONGENITAL INFECTION

Response to Fetal Immunization in Animal Models

Early studies by Silverstein and colleagues [974] of the antibody response of fetal sheep and rhesus monkeys to immunization with foreign proteins were conceptually important in establishing two major features of the ontogeny of B-cell immune competence for T cell–dependent antigens in larger mammals. First, immune competence for T cell–dependent antigens is established early during fetal ontogeny: Primary immunization of fetal rhesus monkeys between 103 and 127 days of gestation (out of a total of 160 days) with sheep red blood cells, a T cell–dependent antigen, results in the formation of sheep red blood cell–reactive B cells in the spleen; reimmunization 3 weeks later results in a rapid antibody response using IgG. In fetal sheep, the antibody response to bacteriophage φX174 occurs 40 days after conception [975], and isotype switching is evident during the fetal response.

Together, these findings suggest that the B-cell responses to protein antigens, including isotype switching and probably memory cell generation, are functional during fetal life. Second, these responses occur in a predictable, stepwise fashion for particular antigens. In fetal sheep, the antibody responses to keyhole limpet hemocyanin and lymphocytic choriomeningitis virus are first detectable at about 80 and 120 days after conception [975]. These differences in the responsiveness to particular antigens are not explained by limitations in the repertoires of surface immunoglobulin or αβ-TCRs.

No correlation exists between the physical or chemical characteristics of particular antigens and their immunogenicity during ontogeny. Bacteriophage φX174 and bacteriophage T4 are particulate antigens that should interact in a similar manner. In fetal sheep, however, bacteriophage T4 becomes immunogenic 60 days after φX174 does so. Baboon fetuses immunized with HBsAg vaccine have a robust IgG antibody response, and this response is boosted by postnatal immunization [976].

Response to Maternal Immunization

In studies by one group of investigators, antibody responses by the human fetus may occur after maternal immunization with tetanus toxoid during the third trimester but not earlier, as shown by the presence of IgM tetanus antibodies at birth [977,978]. Whether tetanus-specific IgG responses at birth were reduced, as suggested by reports of reduced CD4 T-cell responses to tetanus vaccine in young infants [812], is unclear. Infants with tetanus-specific antibodies at birth had enhanced secondary antibody responses after tetanus immunization, indicating that fetal antigen exposure was a priming event, rather than a tolerizing one [977]. Englund and associates [785] were unable to show neonatal tetanus toxoid–specific IgM antibody or T-cell proliferation after maternal tetanus toxoid vaccination in the third trimester. Similarly, no fetal response to maternal immunization with inactivated trivalent influenza vaccine was noted [785]. Another study found, however, that maternal immunization with a split influenza vaccine during the second and third trimesters of pregnancy resulted in detectable IgM-specific responses to influenza proteins in cord blood [784]. If adequate fetal antibody responses to maternal vaccination with polysaccharide-protein conjugate vaccines occurred, such vaccines could be used during pregnancy to ensure that protective antibody levels were present at birth.

Response to Intrauterine Infection

Specific antibody may be present at birth to agents of intrauterine infection, including rubella virus, CMV, HSV, VZV, and *T. gondii*, and often can be used to diagnose congenital infection. Not all fetuses have an antibody response to intrauterine infection, however; specific IgM antibody was undetectable in 34% of infants with congenital rubella [979], 19% to 33% of infants with congenital *T. gondii* infection [980,981], and 11% of infants with congenital CMV infection [982]. When congenital infection is severe during the first or second trimester, antibody production may be delayed until late childhood [799]. This delay may reflect a lack of T-cell help because antigen-specific T-cell responses often are reduced in parallel with B-cell responses.

Congenital *T. gondii* infection may lead to detectable IgE and IgA anti–*T. gondii* antibodies at birth or during early infancy [983]. Similarly, filaria-specific or schistosome-specific IgE is present in the sera of most newborns after maternal filiariasis or schistosomiasis [984]. T cell–dependent isotype switching and immunoglobulin production occur during fetal life, at least for certain pathogens. With some infectious agents, such as *T. gondii*, IgA or IgE antibodies may be more sensitive than IgM antibodies for diagnosis of congenital infection. The titers of IgA and IgE anti–*T. gondii* antibodies may be lower at

20 to 30 weeks of gestation than after birth [985–987], however, indicating that their production is delayed in the context of congenital infection.

POSTNATAL SPECIFIC ANTIBODY RESPONSES

Specific Antibody Responses by the Neonate and Young Infant to Protein Antigens

Immunization of neonates usually elicits or at least primes for a protective response to protein antigens, including tetanus and diphtheria toxoids [988], OPV [989], *Salmonella* flagellar antigen [990,991], bacteriophage φX174 [992], and HBsAg (with hepatitis B vaccine) [993]. The response to some vaccines may be less vigorous in the neonate, however, than in older children or adults. A diminished primary response to recombinant hepatitis B vaccine has been noted in term neonates lacking maternally derived HBsAg antibody compared with the response in unimmunized children and adults [993,994]. The ultimate anti-HBsAg titers achieved in neonates after secondary and tertiary immunizations are similar to titers in older children, indicating that neonatal immunization does not result in tolerance [993]. If initial immunization is delayed until 1 month of age, the antibody response to primary hepatitis B vaccination is increased and nearly equivalent to that in older children, suggesting that the developmental limitations responsible for reduced antibody responses are transient [993,995]. Similarly, 2-week-old infants immunized with a single dose of diphtheria or tetanus toxoid showed delayed production of specific antibody compared with older infants, but by 2 months of age, their response was similar to the response of 6-month-old infants [996]. The switch from IgM to IgG also may be delayed after neonatal vaccination for some (e.g., *Salmonella* H vaccine) [991], but not all (e.g., bacteriophage φX174) [992], antigens. Immunization of infants born to HIV-infected mothers with recombinant HIV-1 gp120 vaccine in MF59 adjuvant, beginning at birth, also resulted in high antibody titers, indicating that early postnatal vaccination is not tolerigenic [997].

In contrast to other vaccines, in newborns given whole-cell pertussis vaccination, not only may they show a poor initial antibody response, but also their subsequent antibody response to certain antigenic components, such as pertussis toxin, may be less than in infants initially immunized at 1 month of age or older [998–1000], suggesting low-level tolerance. Whole-cell pertussis vaccine immunization of premature infants (born at 28 to 36 weeks of gestation) at 2 months of age elicited responses similar to those in 2-month-old term infants [989], indicating that this putative tolerigenic period wanes rapidly and is relatively independent of gestational age. This low-level tolerance was restricted to the pertussis component of the whole-cell pertussis vaccine because an inhibitory effect has not been observed after administration of diphtheria or tetanus toxoid [988] or hepatitis B vaccine given within 48 hours of birth [993].

A more recent study [1001] also found that neonatal immunization with acellular pertussis vaccine combined with diphtheria and tetanus toxoids resulted in lower subsequent pertussis-specific antibody responses than when vaccination was delayed. In contrast, and for unclear reasons, no such inhibition of pertussis-specific antibody responses was observed when the acellular pertussis vaccine was administered alone shortly after birth [1002,1003]. Administration of OPV at birth enhanced rather than inhibited the response to subsequent immunization, also indicating that immunization through the mucosal route does not produce tolerance [1004].

The antibody response to measles vaccine given at 6 months of age is significantly less than when the vaccine is given at 9 or 12 months of age, even when the inhibitory effect of maternal antibody is controlled for [1005]. This decreased response is not due to a lack of measles-specific T cells because measles antigen–specific T-cell proliferation and IL-12 and IFN-γ proliferation were similar in the three age groups [1005–1007]. Although the basis for this reduced response is unknown, early vaccination in infants 6 months of age does not impair the antibody and T-cell response after a second dose of vaccine at 12 months [1008]. Thus, there is no evidence for a tolerigenic effect from early measles vaccination.

Specific Antibody Responses by the Term Neonate to Polysaccharide and Polysaccharide-Protein Conjugates

In contrast to the response to protein antigens, the newborn's response to polysaccharide antigens is absent or severely blunted, as shown by an inability to mount an antibody response to unconjugated H. influenzae type b (Hib) polysaccharide vaccine or to group B streptococcal capsular antigens after infection. The response to some polysaccharide antigens can be shown by 6 months of age, but the response to vaccination with Hib, most pneumococcal serotype polysaccharides, and N. meningitidis type C is poor until 18 to 24 months of age [1009]. The delayed postnatal appearance of marginal zone B cells in the spleen has been proposed to account for this delayed response (see "Development of B-Cell Capacity to Respond to T-Cell–Dependent and T-Cell–Independent Antigens"), although this suggestion is controversial, as noted in the preceding sections.

Covalent conjugation of Hib capsular polysaccharide to a protein carrier renders it immunogenic in infants 2 months of age and primes for an enhanced antibody response to unconjugated vaccine given at 12 months of age. Because the response to the unconjugated vaccine usually is poor at this age, the conjugate vaccine acts by inducing Hib polysaccharide–specific B-cell memory [1010]. Similarly, the administration of a single dose of Hib polysaccharide–tetanus toxoid conjugate to term neonates at a few days of age may enhance the antibody response to unconjugated Hib polysaccharide vaccine at 4 months [1011]. This enhanced response is weak, however, and does not occur when the neonate is primed with tetanus toxoid followed by immunization with conjugate vaccine at 2 months of age [1012]. Although administration of a single dose of Hib polysaccharide–meningococcal outer membrane protein complex conjugate at 2 months of age is highly immunogenic, administration to term neonates induces persistent unresponsiveness to subsequent

immunizations throughout the first year of life [1013,1014]; the basis for this unresponsiveness is unknown.

Coupling of the Hib polysaccharide to a protein carrier converts a T-independent type II antigen to a T-dependent antigen [1015]. This change is accompanied by an enhanced magnitude and higher avidity antibody response on subsequent boosting, presumably resulting from T-dependent memory B-cell generation and somatic hypermutation. The early interactions between T cells and B cells in response to such carbohydrate-protein conjugate vaccines are summarized in Figure 4–15. Conjugation of Hib polysaccharide to tetanus or diphtheria toxoid does not change the repertoire of the antibodies produced from that of the free polysaccharide [1010,1016]. Vaccination with protein–capsular polysaccharide conjugate vaccines containing polysaccharides of S. pneumoniae (types 4, 6B, 9V, 14, 18C, 19F, and 23F in the Danish nomenclature) [1017] and N. meningitidis (types A and C) [1018] is immunogenic in infants 2 months of age and primes them for subsequent memory responses.

Antibody Responses by the Premature Infant to Immunization

Preterm neonates of 24 weeks of gestation or greater produce antibody to protein antigens such as diphtheria toxoid, diphtheria-pertussis-tetanus vaccine, and oral and inactivated poliovirus vaccines as well as term neonates when the vaccines are administered at 2, 4, and 6 months of age [989,1019–1022]. The antibody response in

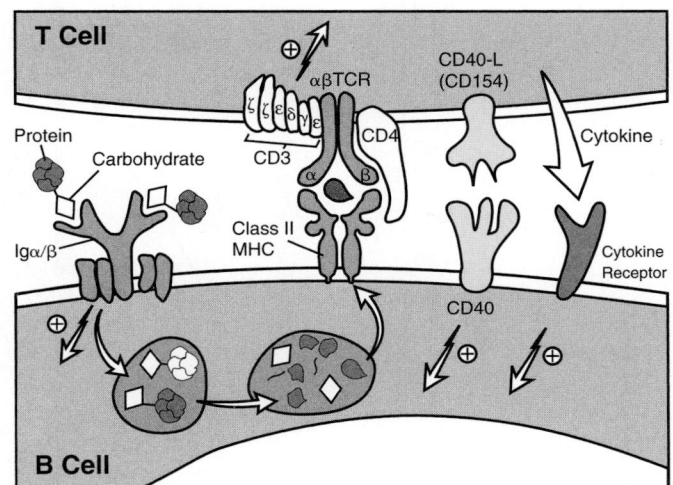

FIGURE 4–15 Interactions between B cells and T cells in response to vaccines consisting of purified carbohydrate (e.g., bacterial capsular polysaccharide) covalently linked to protein carrier. The carbohydrate moiety of the conjugate is bound by surface immunoglobulin on B cells, resulting in internalization of the conjugate. Peptides derived from the protein moiety of the conjugate are presented by major histocompatibility complex (MHC) class II on the B cell resulting in the activation of the T cell and expression of CD40 ligand. Engagement of CD40 on the B cell by CD40 ligand, in conjunction with cytokines secreted by the T cell, results in carbohydrate-specific B-cell proliferation, immunoglobulin isotype switching, secretion of antibody, and memory B-cell generation.

premature infants to multiple doses of hepatitis B vaccine, initially administered at birth, is reduced compared with term infants [1023,1024]. These titers are substantially increased if immunization of the premature infant is delayed until 5 weeks of age, indicating the importance of postnatal age over a particular body weight [1025]. The benefits of such a delay for long-term hepatitis B–specific antibody levels persist for at least the first 3 years of life [1026].

The antibody levels after three doses of Hib polysaccharide–tetanus conjugate vaccine are significantly less in premature infants than in term infants when vaccination is begun at 2 months of age [1027,1028]. This reduced antibody response occurs particularly in premature infants with chronic lung disease [1029], in whom it may result in part from glucocorticoid treatment.

MATERNALLY DERIVED IgG ANTIBODY

The transfer of IgG to the fetus depends on the recognition of maternal IgG through its Fc domain. IgG is internalized by the syncytiotrophoblast, possibly by pinocytosis, and binds to FcRn (also known as the Brambell receptor, FcRB) in the early endosome [1030]. FcRn is a unique β_2-microglobulin–associated nonpolymorphic member of the MHC class I family, which lacks a functional peptide-binding groove and instead uses a different region of the

molecule to bind the Fc domain of IgG [1031]. IgG bound to FcRn undergoes transcytosis across the syncytiotrophoblast and is released into the fetal circulation. In addition to the syncytiotrophoblast, FcRn is widely expressed by nonplacental tissues, where it binds to pinocytosed IgG and recycles it to the circulation [1030]. This recycling system accounts for the very long half-life of IgG.

Maternal IgG and FcRn expression can be detected in placental syncytiotrophoblasts during the first trimester [1032], but transport does not occur until about 17 weeks of gestation. The maternally derived placental cytotrophoblast, which is found between the syncytiotrophoblast and the fetal endothelium during the first trimester, may act as a barrier to IgG transport. This cytotrophoblast layer becomes discontinuous as the villous surface area expands during the second trimester [1032].

IgG is detectable in the fetus by 17 weeks of gestation, after which circulating concentrations increase steadily, reaching half of the term concentration by about 30 weeks and equaling that of the mother by about 38 weeks [1033,1034]. In some instances, fetal IgG concentrations may exceed IgG concentrations of the mother [1035,1036].

The fetus synthesizes little IgG—the concentration in utero is almost solely maternally derived (Fig. 4–16) [1037]. Accordingly, the degree of prematurity is reflected in proportionately lower neonatal IgG concentrations. The IgG_2 concentration in cord blood relative to the

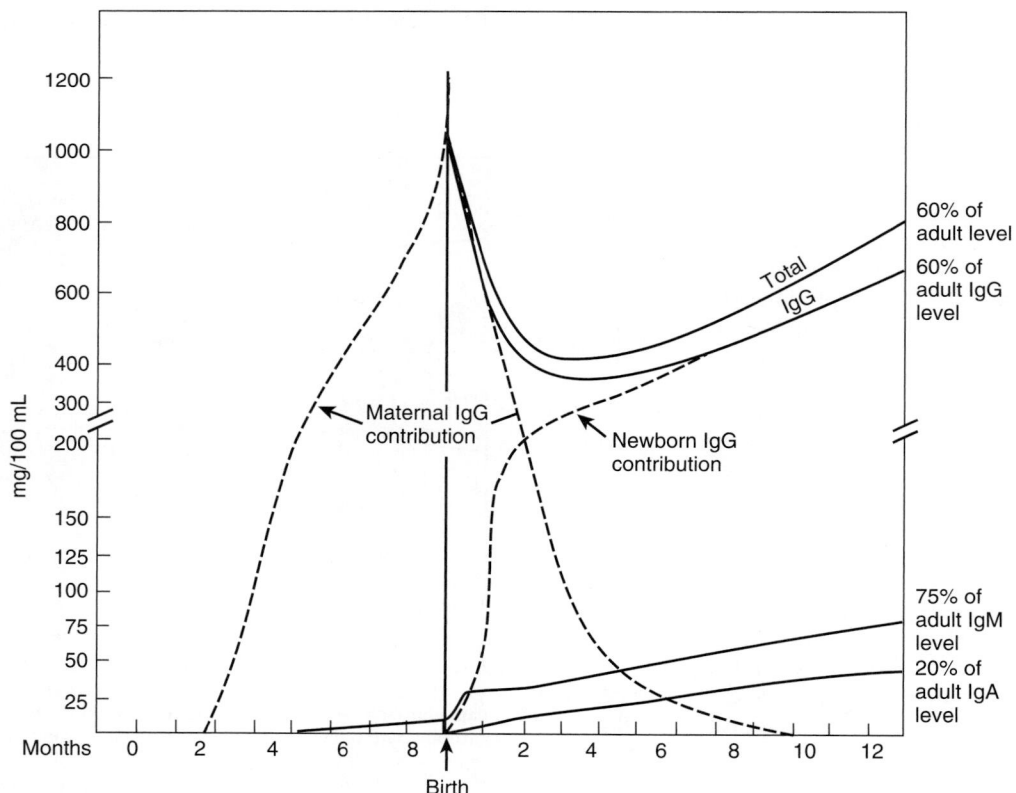

FIGURE 4–16 **Immunoglobulin (IgG, IgM, and IgA) levels in the fetus and in the infant in the first year of life.** IgG of the fetus and newborn infant is solely of maternal origin. Maternal IgG disappears by age 9 months, by which time endogenous synthesis of IgG by the infant is well established. IgM and IgA of the neonate are entirely endogenously synthesized because maternal IgM and IgA do not cross the placenta. *(Data from Saxon A, Stiehm ER. The B-lymphocyte system. In Stiehm ER [ed]. Immunologic Disorders in Infants and Children, 3rd ed. Philadelphia, WB Saunders, 1989, pp 40-67.)*

concentration in maternal blood is low at birth, particularly in preterm infants, whereas the overall fetal-to-maternal ratio is usually near 1.0 for the other IgG subclasses [1038–1040]. The low IgG_2 concentration seems to reflect a relatively low affinity of FcRn for IgG_2. IgM, IgA, IgD, and IgE do not cross the placenta. Evidence for transamniotic transfer of IgG to the fetus also is lacking [1036].

Placental Transfer of Specific Antibodies

The fetus receives IgG antibodies against antigens to which the mother has been exposed by infection or vaccination. In mothers immunized with Hib capsular polysaccharide antigen at 34 to 36 weeks of gestation, concentrations of anticapsular antibody are high, resulting in protective antibody levels in infants for approximately the first 4 months of life. In the absence of recent immunization or natural exposure, the maternal antibody IgG antibody titer may be too low to protect the neonate. Protection of the infant may be absent even if the mother is protected because she has memory B cells and can mount a rapid recall antibody response on infectious challenge. In addition, if maternal antibodies are primarily IgM, such as antibodies to *E. coli* and *Salmonella* [990,991], the fetus would not be protected because IgM does not traverse the placenta. Finally, premature infants may not receive sufficient amounts of IgG for protection because the bulk of maternal IgG is transferred to the fetus after 34 weeks of gestation [1041], accounting for the greater susceptibility of premature neonates compared with term neonates to certain infections, such as with VZV [1042].

Inhibition of Neonatal Antibody Responses by Maternal Antibodies

Maternal antibody also may inhibit the production by the fetus or newborn of antibodies of the same specificity. This inhibition varies with the maternal antibody titer and with the type and amount of antigen. Maternal antibody markedly inhibits the response to measles and rubella vaccine, but not mumps vaccine [1043]; this is the reason for delaying measles-mumps-rubella (MMR) vaccine until at least 12 months of age in the developed world. Inhibition of the response to these live-attenuated viral vaccines may result in part from the binding of maternal antibody to immunogenic epitopes, inhibiting antigen binding to surface immunoglobulin on the antigen-specific B cells of the infant (i.e., masking), and from reduced replication of vaccine virus.

Maternal antibodies also may inhibit the response of the neonate and young infant to certain nonreplicating vaccines, such as whole-cell pertussis vaccine [1000], diphtheria toxoid [1044], *Salmonella* flagellar antigen [991], and inactivated poliovirus vaccine [1045], but not others, such as Hib conjugate vaccine [1046]. Maternal antibody may mask the immunogenic epitope, and formation of maternal IgG antibody–antigen complexes may inhibit activation of B cells via surface immunoglobulin by simultaneous engagement of the inhibitory FcγRII receptor by the IgG component of the complex [120]. Alternatively, maternal antibody may lead to the rapid clearance of vaccine antigen and decreased immunogenicity. Maternal antibodies may enhance, rather than inhibit, the T-cell response to postnatal vaccination, as in the case of tetanus toxoid [1047]. Finally, for certain antibodies, such as anti-HbsAg, neither maternal antibodies nor hepatitis B immune globulin administration has a substantial inhibitory effect on the newborn's immune response to hepatitis B vaccination.

IMMUNOGLOBULIN SYNTHESIS BY THE FETUS AND NEONATE
IgG

IgG is the predominant immunoglobulin isotype at all ages (Table 4–8) [1048]. In adults, IgG1 is the predominant subclass, accounting for approximately 70% of total IgG; IgG2, IgG3, and IgG4 account for approximately 20%, 7%, and 3% of the total [1049]. Passively derived maternal IgG is the source of virtually all of the IgG subclasses detected in the fetus and neonate. Because the IgG

TABLE 4–8 Levels of Immunoglobulins in Sera of Normal Subjects by Age*

Age	IgG mg/dL	IgG % Adult Level	IgM mg/dL	IgM % Adult Level	IgA mg/dL	IgA % Adult Level	Total Immunoglobulins mg/dL	Total Immunoglobulins % Adult Level
Newborn	1031 ± 200[†]	89 ± 17	11 ± 5	11 ± 5	2 ± 3	1 ± 2	1044 ± 201	67 ± 13
1-3 mo	430 ± 119	37 ± 10	30 ± 11	30 ± 11	21 ± 13	11 ± 7	418 ± 127	31 ± 9
4-6 mo	427 ± 186	37 ± 16	43 ± 17	43 ± 17	28 ± 18	14 ± 9	498 ± 204	32 ± 13
7-12 mo	661 ± 219	58 ± 19	54 ± 23	55 ± 23	37 ± 18	19 ± 9	752 ± 242	48 ± 15
13-24 mo	762 ± 209	66 ± 18	58 ± 23	59 ± 23	50 ± 24	25 ± 12	870 ± 258	56 ± 16
25-36 mo	892 ± 183	77 ± 16	61 ± 19	62 ± 19	71 ± 37	36 ± 19	1024 ± 205	65 ± 14
3-5 yr	929 ± 228	80 ± 20	56 ± 18	57 ± 18	93 ± 27	47 ± 14	1078 ± 245	69 ± 17
6-8 yr	923 ± 256	80 ± 22	65 ± 25	66 ± 25	124 ± 45	62 ± 23	1112 ± 293	71 ± 20
9-11 yr	1124 ± 235	92 ± 20	79 ± 33	80 ± 33	131 ± 60	66 ± 30	1334 ± 254	85 ± 17
12-16 yr	946 ± 124	82 ± 11	59 ± 20	60 ± 20	148 ± 63	74 ± 32	1153 ± 169	74 ± 12
Adult	1158 ± 305	100 ± 26	99 ± 27	100 ± 27	200 ± 61	100 ± 31	1457 ± 353	100 ± 24

*The values were derived from measurements made for 296 normal children and 30 adults. Levels were determined by the radial diffusion technique, using specific rabbit antisera to human immunoglobulins.
[†]1 SD.
Adapted from Stiehm ER, Fudenberg HH. Serum levels of immune globulins in health and disease: a survey. Pediatrics 37:715, 1966.

plasma half-life is about 21 days, these maternally derived levels decline rapidly after birth. IgG synthesized by the neonate and IgG derived from the mother are approximately equal at 2 months of age, and by 10 to 12 months of age, the IgG is nearly all derived from synthesis by the infant. As a consequence of the decline in passively derived IgG and increased synthesis of IgG, values reach a nadir of approximately 400 mg/dL in term infants at 3 to 4 months of age and increase thereafter (see Table 4–8 and Fig. 4–16). The premature infant has lower IgG concentrations at birth, which reach a nadir at 3 months of age; mean IgG values of 82 mg/dL and 104 mg/dL are observed in infants born at 25 to 28 weeks of gestation and 29 to 32 weeks of gestation.

By 1 year, the total IgG concentration is approximately 60% of that in adults. IgG3 and IgG1 subclasses reach adult concentrations by 8 years, whereas IgG2 and IgG4 reach adult concentrations by 10 and 12 years of age [1050]. As discussed earlier, maternal IgG may inhibit certain postnatal antibody responses by binding to FcγRII receptors and by rapidly clearing or masking potential antigens. The slow onset of IgG synthesis in the neonate is predominantly an intrinsic limitation of the neonate, however, rather than of maternal antibody; a similar pattern of IgG development was observed in a neonate born to a mother with untreated agammaglobulinemia [1051].

The slow increase in IgG2 concentrations parallels the poor antibody response to bacterial polysaccharide antigens, which are predominantly IgG2 [1052]. The postpartum order in which adult levels of isotype expression are achieved closely parallels the chromosomal order of the heavy chain gene segments that encode these isotypes. Postnatal regulation of isotype switching is mediated partly at the heavy chain gene locus. Although passive maternal antibody plays an important role in protection, it limits the value of immunoglobulin and antibody levels in the diagnosis of immunodeficiency or infection in the young infant.

IgM

IgM is the only isotype besides IgG that binds and activates complement. IgM has a half-life in the blood of 5 days. The concentration of IgM in the blood increases from a mean of 6 mg/dL in infants born at less than 28 weeks of gestation to 11 mg/dL in infants born at term [1053,1054], which is approximately 8% of the maternal IgM level. This IgM, which is likely to be preimmune (i.e., not the result of a B-cell response to foreign antigens), is enriched for polyreactive antibodies. Murine studies suggest that such natural IgM plays an important role in innate defense against infection, allowing time for the initiation of antigen-specific B-cell response; it also enhances antigen-specific B-cell responses through its ability to fix complement and costimulate B-cell activation through CD21 [892]. Some human neonatal IgM is monomeric and nonfunctional, however, as opposed to its usual pentameric functional form [1055,1056].

Postnatal IgM concentrations increase rapidly for the first month and then more gradually thereafter, presumably in response to antigenic stimulation (see Fig. 4–16 and Table 4–8). By 1 year of age, values are approximately

60% of those in adults. The postnatal increase is similar in premature and in term infants [1055]. Elevated (>20 mg/dL) IgM concentrations in cord blood suggest possible intrauterine infections [1057], but many infants with congenital infections have normal cord blood IgM levels [982].

IgA

IgA does not cross the placenta, and its concentration in cord blood usually is 0.1 to 5 mg/dL, approximately 0.5% of the levels in maternal sera [1054]. Concentrations are similar in term and in premature neonates [1053], and IgA1 and IgA2 are present. IgA has a half-life in the blood of 6 days.

At birth, the frequency of IgA1-bearing and IgA2-bearing B cells is equivalent. Subsequently, a preferential expansion of the IgA1-bearing cell population occurs [1058]. Concentrations in serum increase to 20% of those in adults by 1 year of age and increase progressively through adolescence (see Table 4–8). Increased cord blood IgA concentrations are observed in some infants with congenital infection [1057] and is common in infants infected with HIV by vertical transmission. Secretory IgA is present in substantial amounts in the saliva by 10 days after birth [1059].

IgD

IgD is detectable by sensitive techniques in serum from cord blood in term and premature infants [1053,1060]. Mean serum levels at birth are approximately 0.05 mg/dL [1054] and increase during the first year of life [1061]. IgD is also detectable in the saliva of newborn infants [1059]. Circulating or salivary IgD have no clear functional role because mice in which IgD expression has been eliminated by gene targeting seem to be normal. Surface IgD can replace surface IgM in B-cell function in the mouse.

IgE

Although IgE synthesis by the fetus is detectable at 11 weeks, concentrations of IgE in cord blood are typically low, with a mean of approximately 0.5% of that of maternal levels [1054]. This IgE is of fetal origin, and concentrations are higher in infants born at 40 to 42 weeks of gestation than in infants born at 37 to 39 weeks [1054]. The rate of postnatal increase varies and is greater in infants predisposed to allergic disease or greater environmental exposure to allergens [1062,1063]. The concentration of IgE at birth seems to have limited predictive value for later development of atopic disease for most individuals [1063,1064].

SUMMARY

The neonate is partially protected from infection by passive maternal IgG antibody, predominantly transferred during the latter third of pregnancy. Fetal IgG concentrations are equal to or higher than maternal concentrations at term. The inability of the neonate to produce antibodies in response to polysaccharides, particularly bacterial capsular polysaccharides, limits resistance to bacterial pathogens to which the mother has little or no IgG antibody. The basis for this defect is unclear, but it may reflect an intrinsic limitation of B-cell function or a deficiency in the anatomic microenvironment required for B cells to become activated and differentiate into plasma cells. By contrast, the neonatal IgM response to most protein antigens is intact and only slightly limited for IgG responses to certain vaccines.

A clear difference between neonates and older infants has been observed in the magnitude of the antibody response to most protein neoantigens, but this difference rapidly resolves after birth. The predominance of transitional B cells in the fetus and neonate may account in part for limitations in function. A limited antibody response of premature infants to immunization with protein antigens occurs during the first month of life, but not subsequently. Chronologic (i.e., postnatal) age is a more important determinant of antibody responses to T-dependent antigens than gestational age. Isotype expression by B cells after immunization with T-dependent antigens is limited by altered T-cell function, such as reduced CD40 ligand production, and intrinsic limitations of B-cell maturation and function. These limitations are exaggerated in the fetus.

HOST DEFENSE AGAINST SPECIFIC CLASSES OF NEONATAL PATHOGENS
EXTRACELLULAR MICROBIAL PATHOGENS: GROUP B STREPTOCOCCI
Overview of Host Defense Mechanisms

Infection of the neonate with GBS in most cases results from aspiration of infected amniotic or vaginal fluid, followed by adherence to and subsequent invasion through the respiratory mucosa. Initial colonization is influenced by the organism's ability to adhere to mucosal epithelial cells. Physical disruption of the mucosal epithelium may not be required for tissue invasion because GBS can enter into the cytoplasm of cultured respiratory epithelial cells by an actin microfilament–dependent process [202]. Specific secretory IgA antibody and fibronectin may decrease bacterial adherence to the mucosa. As noted in "Antimicrobial Peptides," epithelial cells in the skin, tongue, and airways express β-defensins and the cathelicidin LL-27, which are active against GBS [1–4].

When GBS cross the mucosal epithelium and enter the tissues, phagocytes and opsonins become the critical elements of defense. Antibody and complement opsonize the bacteria for phagocytosis and killing by neutrophils and macrophages, but similar to all gram-positive bacteria, these organisms are resistant to lysis by complement. GBS and strains of *E. coli* that cause serious neonatal infections possess type-specific polysaccharide capsules, which impede or block antibody-independent activation of the alternative and MBL complement pathways [54,60,1065]. Consistent with this notion, there is an inverse correlation between the degree of encapsulation and the deposition of C3b on type III GBS through the alternative pathway [1066], although some studies have not found an effect of capsule on complement deposition [1067].

Efficient complement activation leading to deposition of C3b and C3bi on the bacterial surface depends on type-specific anticapsular IgG antibody [1068]. Consistent with these findings, susceptibility to infection with type III GBS is essentially limited to infants lacking type-specific antibody (see Chapter 12). Complement also plays an important role. In animal models, complement components C3 and C4 are required for protection before the development of type-specific antibodies, suggesting that antibody-independent activation of the C4 complement component by the MBL pathway may be involved, whereas C3, but not C4, is required when type-specific antibodies are produced [1069]. IgG-coated and, in the lung, surfactant apoprotein A–coated bacteria are ingested by phagocytes, and ingestion is augmented by C3b and C3bi.

Small numbers of GBS may be cleared by resident lung macrophages [202]. If the bacteria are not cleared, neutrophils and monocytes are recruited to the site of infection by chemotactic factors, including fMLP, C5a, LTB$_4$, and chemokines (e.g., CXCL8) [1070]. Many strains of GBS contain an enzyme, C5a-ase, which degrades human C5a [1071]. In addition to recruitment of neutrophils from the circulation, release of the mature neutrophil storage pool and upregulation of neutrophil production by the bone marrow may be required to provide sufficient numbers of neutrophils to contain the infection. As described in previous sections, entry of neutrophils and monocytes into tissues depends on the upregulation of adhesion molecules on the vascular endothelium by inflammatory mediators and cytokines and chemotactic factor–induced increases in the abundance and avidity of integrins on neutrophils and monocytes. Chemotactic factors also prime neutrophils and macrophages to ingest and kill GBS more efficiently. When ingested, GBS are exposed to a variety of potentially microbicidal products, including reactive oxygen metabolites, acidic pH, elastase, cathepsin G, and cationic proteins, as discussed previously. IL-12 facilitates IFN-γ production, and both cytokines enhance the resistance of neonatal rats to GBS infection [1072,1073]. The mechanism by which IFN-γ enhances resistance is unknown, and it is unknown whether IFN-γ contributes to protection in humans.

In cases in which GBS overwhelm neonatal defenses, septic shock may result, and this is the most frequent cause of death resulting from systemic infection owing to GBS in neonates. Septic shock results from systemic overproduction of inflammatory mediators, including TNF-α, IL-1, and IL-6, by phagocytes and other host cells. Encapsulated and unencapsulated type III GBS induce production of these cytokines by human monocytes in vitro [1074]. Lipoproteins released by GBS induce inflammatory mediator production after binding to TLR2 plus TLR6; other components of GBS induce these mediators through an as-yet undefined TLR or TLR-related receptor [1075]. GBS also likely activate NLRs, although this has not been directly shown. Neutralization of TNF-α enhances survival in animal models, even when begun 12 hours after inoculation with these organisms [1076]. Similarly, administration of IL-10, which inhibits production of TNF-α and other proinflammatory cytokines, enhances survival in animals [1077]. These findings suggest that excessive proinflammatory cytokine production is deleterious in the context of

GBS infection, but this has not been shown in human neonates. Treatment of sepsis in adults with a soluble TNF-α antagonist led to increased mortality in adults [1078].

Neonatal Defenses

With rare exceptions [1079], neonatal GBS infection occurs only in infants who do not receive protective amounts of GBS type-specific antibodies from their mothers [1068,1080]. Although the concentrations of GBS type-specific IgG antibodies in cord sera are usually slightly less than in maternal sera at term, term neonates born to mothers with protective concentrations of IgG antibodies generally are protected. In infants born before 34 weeks of gestation, the amounts of GBS type-specific antibodies often are markedly less than in the mother [1081]; preterm neonates may not be protected even though their mothers' serum contains protective amounts of IgG antibodies.

Production of type-specific antibodies by infected neonates is unlikely to contribute to protection. Infected neonates commonly do not make detectable type-specific antibodies during the first month after infection; a few transiently synthesize IgM, but not IgG antibodies [1082]. By 3 months of postnatal age, sera from uninfected infants and from infants who had previous type III GBS infection usually contain type-specific IgM antibodies [1083,1084]. It is unclear, however, that these antibodies require the exposure of normal infants to type III GBS; they could develop naturally or result from a cross-reactive immune response to another source of antigens to which the infant is exposed postnatally.

In the absence of type-specific antibodies, subtle but cumulative deficits in numerous other host defense mechanisms probably contribute to the neonate's susceptibility to GBS. Type III GBS efficiently adhere to mucosal epithelial cells of neonates, particularly ill neonates [1085,1086]. Production of β-defensin and LL-37 antimicrobial peptides that are active against GBS by the skin of neonates is robust [9,10]. Production of these peptides by respiratory epithelial cells seems to be less, however, than that of adult cells at term and to be more clearly reduced in preterm neonates [28]. At birth, neonates also lack secretory IgA. Reduced amounts of surfactant apoprotein A in the lungs of preterm neonates, a paucity of alveolar macrophages in the lungs of term and particularly preterm neonates before birth, and diminished phagocytosis and killing of bacteria by these cells may also enable GBS to invade via the respiratory tract. Limitations in the generation of chemotactic factors or deficits in the chemotactic responses of neonatal neutrophils, or both, may result in delayed recruitment of neutrophils to sites of infection. When they reach sites of infection, neonatal neutrophils may kill bacteria less efficiently because of limited amounts of opsonins, because the local bacterial density has reached high levels, or because the microbicidal activity of neutrophils is decreased in certain neonates. To compound the problem, rapidly progressive infection can deplete the limited marrow neutrophil reserve.

Although the lack of type-specific antibodies and a multitude of subtle deficits in neonatal defenses together likely contribute to the neonate's predisposition to GBS disease, why does disease develop in less than 10% of infants who lack type-specific antibodies and are born to colonized mothers? At present, the answer to this question is incomplete. Among neonates who lack type-specific antibodies, the risk for development of GBS disease seems to be greater in neonates born to mothers with high-density genital tract colonization or GBS amnionitis and may vary with the virulence of the strain. It also is likely that variations in host defense competence between individuals contribute, such as differences in antibody-independent complement activation, and that these deficits are greater in more premature neonates [1087].

Immunologic Interventions for Neonatal Group B Streptococcal Sepsis

As summarized in the preceding section, the principal host defense deficits that predispose the neonate to infections with GBS and other extracellular microbial pathogens seem to be a deficiency of opsonins, particularly protective antibodies, and a limited capacity to increase neutrophil production and mobilize neutrophils to sites of infection. Attempts have been made to address both of these deficits through immunologic interventions. There is at present no conclusive evidence, however, that any form of immunologic intervention for prevention or adjunctive therapy of bacterial or fungal infections in the neonate improves outcome.

Prevention

Selective intrapartum chemoprophylaxis with penicillin or ampicillin has reduced the rate of early-onset disease owing to GBS by approximately 80%, but had no impact on the incidence of late-onset disease [1088]. This observation supports the importance of developing a vaccine that could be used to immunize women before conception or in the early part of the third trimester. Studies have shown that 80% to 93% of adults immunized with type Ia, Ib, II, III, and V capsular polysaccharide–protein conjugate vaccines respond with approximately fourfold titer increases, with geometric mean titers ranging from 2.7 μg/mL for type III to 18.3 μg/mL for type Ia [1089]. Vaccines that induce protective antibodies against shared protein antigens also show promise [1090]. Although this approach may not supplant the need to provide intrapartum chemoprophylaxis for very preterm neonates—born at less than 34 weeks of gestation before receiving passive maternal antibodies in amounts sufficient to provide protection—it is estimated that such an approach would prevent more than half of all neonatal GBS disease [1088].

Numerous studies have evaluated the efficacy of intravenous immunoglobulin (IVIG) for the prevention of nosocomial or late-onset pyogenic infections in premature neonates. A 1997 meta-analysis of 12 randomized controlled trials, which included 4933 infants, showed a slight but statistically significant reduction in the incidence of sepsis ($P < .02$) [1091]. A more recent meta-analysis by the Cochrane collaboration in 2001, which included 19 randomized controlled trials with a total of 4986 infants, found a 3% reduction in sepsis ($P = .02$) [1092]. The stringency with which sepsis was defined in these studies varied. Perhaps more important, IVIG prophylaxis had no effect on mortality rates.

A multicenter randomized controlled trial in premature neonates at increased risk because of total IgG concentrations less than 400 mg/dL found no significant reduction in sepsis or other tangible benefit of IVIG prophylaxis. Similarly, a trial of prophylactic administration of a polyclonal IVIG preparation derived from donors with high titers of antibody to surface adhesins of *S. aureus* and *Staphylococcus epidermidis* showed no impact on the incidence of sepsis attributable to these organisms, *Candida*, or other agents and no effect on mortality [1093]. The authors of these reports and others [1094] concluded that IVIG is not indicated for prophylaxis in preterm neonates and neonates with low birth weight because there is no effect on long-term outcome and little or no effect on short-term outcomes.

Recombinant G-CSF and GM-CSF augment granulocyte production and function in neonatal animals and provide some protection against challenge with pyogenic bacteria, including GBS, in neonatal animal models. These findings prompted clinical trials to determine if administration of recombinant G-CSF or GM-CSF to human neonates would result in increased levels of circulating neutrophils and protect at-risk neonates from sepsis. Four randomized trials of prophylaxis with recombinant GM-CSF and one comparative observational study of prophylaxis with recombinant G-CSF were conducted [80,1095–1097]. These studies showed that G-CSF and GM-CSF increase circulating neutrophil counts and seem to be well tolerated.

The most recent and largest randomized trial of 280 neonates and a meta-analysis of the results from the four GM-CSF trials showed no reduction in the rate of sepsis or mortality [1096]. The small, nonrandomized observational study found that prophylactic administration of G-CSF to neutropenic infants with low birth weight born to mothers with preeclampsia led to a reduction in proven bacterial infections in these patients [1098]. No randomized controlled trials with G-CSF have been conducted, however, so its utility as a prophylactic agent is essentially untested. The evidence does not support the prophylactic use of G-CSF or GM-CSF in neonates.

Adjunctive Therapy of Pyogenic Infections

Passive Antibody

Over the past 2 decades, various studies have been performed to determine whether IVIG would improve the outcome in neonates with suspected or proven sepsis. These studies have differed in design and have been performed in countries with differing rates of neonatal sepsis, management approaches, and preparations of IVIG. The Cochrane collaboration performed a meta-analysis of 13 randomized controlled trials from seven countries involving neonates with suspected or proven invasive bacterial or fungal infections [1092]. In the six trials ($N = 318$ subjects) that included neonates with clinically suspected infection, IVIG had a marginal effect on mortality rate (relative risk 0.63, 95% confidence interval 0.41% to 1.00%, $P = .05$). In the seven trials ($N = 262$ subjects) that evaluated outcome only in neonates subsequently proven to have invasive infections, mortality also was marginally reduced by IVIG (relative risk 0.51, 95%

confidence interval 0.31% to 0.98%, $P = .04$). The authors concluded that the marginal statistical significance and the variability in study design and quality do not allow firm conclusions to be made at the present time. To address this uncertainty, an international neonatal immunotherapy study with a target enrollment of approximately 5000 has been proposed [1094]. Nonetheless, there is currently insufficient evidence to support the routine use of IVIG in the management of neonatal sepsis.

Neutrophil Transfusions

Neutrophil transfusions enhance survival rate in certain animal models of neonatal sepsis, but the clinical efficacy of neutrophil transfusion in human neonates with sepsis is uncertain. Three of five controlled studies showed statistically significant improvement in the survival rate for neonates receiving granulocyte transfusions compared with infants not receiving this therapy [1095]. Nonetheless, small sample sizes and differences in entry criteria for treatment and control groups, in methods of neutrophil preparation, in numbers of neutrophils per transfusion, in numbers of transfusions, and in bacterial pathogens causing disease preclude a meaningful meta-analysis of these studies. Although neutrophil storage pool depletion has been used as a selection criterion for neonates for whom transfusion may be beneficial, the difficulty in ascertainment of neutrophil storage pool size in clinical practice and the failure of this parameter to predict outcome in some studies make this measure an imperfect criterion in clinical practice. The utility of neutrophil transfusions is compromised further by the difficulty in obtaining these cells in a timely fashion and the potential complications of transfusions, including the risk of infection. For these reasons, neutrophil transfusions cannot be recommended as routine therapy for neonates with suspected or proven sepsis.

Colony-Stimulating Factors

Administration of G-CSF to human neonates 26 to 40 weeks of gestational age with presumed early-onset sepsis was shown to increase significantly the numbers of circulating neutrophils, bone marrow neutrophil storage pool size, and neutrophil expression of CR3 receptors (CD11b through CD18) without adverse effects [1099–1101]. The 2003 Cochrane meta-analysis of all causes of mortality in 257 infants with suspected sepsis from seven randomized clinical trials showed, however, that survival was not improved by adjunctive treatment with G-CSF or GM-CSF; G-CSF was used in most of these studies [1172]. A subset analysis from three of these studies that included 97 infants with neutropenia (absolute neutrophil count <1700/mm^3) showed an apparent reduction in mortality (relative risk 0.34, 95% confidence interval 0.12% to 0.92%). In an earlier meta-analysis of five studies involving 73 neonates who received G-CSF and 82 controls by Bernstein and colleagues [1102], the mortality rate was significantly reduced ($P < .05$), but if data from two nonrandomized trials were excluded, there was no significant difference (observed risk 0.43, 95% confidence interval 0.14% to 1.23%, $P = .13$). No significant adverse effects of G-CSF adjunct therapy were noted in these studies; also, one long-term follow-up study found no adverse effects. As with the meta-analyses of adjunct therapy of neonatal sepsis with IVIG, data regarding the use of G-CSF for adjunctive therapy of neonatal sepsis indicate that it is safe and might be useful in some situations. Nonetheless, evidence is currently insufficient to support the routine use of G-CSF or GM-CSF as adjunctive therapy in septic neonates.

Summary

Substantial advances have occurred in the understanding of factors that compromise the neonate's defenses against bacterial infections. As a result of this information, numerous clinical trials have evaluated the use of IVIG, G-CSF, or GM-CSF for the prophylaxis or adjunctive treatment of neonatal infections. The results from these studies have been disappointing or inconclusive. To date, there is no established role for these or any other immunologic therapy in the prevention or treatment of bacterial or fungal infections in human neonates. The existing data are sufficient to conclude that the prophylactic use of IVIG is not cost-effective and that such use of GM-CSF is not beneficial. Conversely, randomized clinical trials to test the potential benefit of IVIG in septic neonates or G-CSF in septic, neutropenic neonates, or combinations of these agents as adjunctive therapies for neonatal sepsis may be indicated.

VIRUSES: HERPES SIMPLEX VIRUS
Overview of Host Defense Mechanisms

Effective viral host defense mechanisms of vertebrates typically depend on a combination of innate and adaptive immune mechanisms that are highly interlinked. Because viruses replicate intracellularly and potentially infect a wide range of cell types, generic antiviral mechanisms, such as those involving type I IFNs, are crucial for early control of infection. Innate and adaptive cellular mechanisms that control or block infection within cells, such as by NK cells and CD8 T cells, prevent spread of virus from cell to cell and are crucial for effective host defense. Antibody and complement also may modify viral expression, especially by preventing spread of virus into the central nervous system, but in most tissues the cellular immune response is crucial for control of viral replication and the elimination of virally infected cells. This section focuses on host defenses operative against HSV-1 and HSV-2, both of which cause strikingly more severe primary disease in neonates than in immunocompetent adults [1103].

HSV-1 and HSV-2 mostly are collectively referred to here as HSV because these two viruses are very closely related and, in most instances, have very similar pathogenic properties. HSV infection is severe in term infants infected at the time of parturition and in the uncommon cases when it is acquired in utero. Characteristically, HSV infection in neonates spreads rapidly to produce either disseminated or central nervous system disease. Enteroviral infections also are severe and may be fatal when acquired in the perinatal period and, similar to HSV infections, have a propensity to produce

disseminated or central nervous system disease. Another similarity between HSV and enteroviral infections is that infection acquired after the neonatal period (after age 4 weeks) is typically effectively controlled, suggesting that common developmental limitations in antiviral immunity are responsible. Deficiencies in the function of neonatal NK cells and DCs probably are important contributors to poor early control of infection by the innate immune response. Neonates also may develop crucial antigen-specific T-cell responses to the virus too slowly to prevent the virus from producing irreparable tissue injury or death.

Innate Immunity

The antiviral immune response generally can be divided into two phases. The first is an early, nonspecific phase (typically the first 5 to 7 days in HSV infection) involving innate immune mechanisms. This is followed by a later, antigen-specific phase involving adaptive immunity mediated by T cells and B cells and their products [1104]. The early phase is critical because infection either may be successfully contained or may disseminate throughout the host.

Interferons, Cytokines, and Their Induction by Toll-like Receptors

HSV triggers high levels of type I IFN secretion by pDCs in a TLR9-dependent fashion [325] as the HSV double-stranded DNA genome is unmethylated at CpG dinucleotide residues. The secretion of high levels of IFN-α by pDCs results in a systemic antiviral state by binding to type I IFN receptors, which are almost ubiquitously expressed. This antiviral state enhances local adaptive immune responses, such as those mediated by B cells and T cells, as a result of a direct effect on these cells in secondary lymphoid tissue [1105]. The type I IFN receptor mediates its effects by the binding of a heterotrimeric complex of STAT-1, STAT-2, and IRF-9 to IFN-stimulated response elements (ISREs) of genomic DNA, influencing gene transcription [250]. STAT-1 also can homodimerize and bind to γ-IFN–activating sequences, which induce a distinct set of genes from the genes using ISREs. Because these STAT-1 homodimers (but not other STATs) and γ-IFN–activating sequence–regulated genes are activated when IFN-γ binds to its specific receptor, type I IFN may potentially induce genes that are characteristic of IFN-γ responses, but not vice versa. For antiviral host defense in humans, including to HSV, only the ISRE genes seem to be critical, however [1106,1107]. IL-28 and IL-29 (also known as IFNs λ), which are also induced by HSV infection and TLR9 engagement, also provide ISRE gene–dependent antiviral immunity after binding to a unique receptor distinct from the receptor for type I IFN [1108].

HSV induces the production of type I IFN and other cytokines after engagement of TLR3, which is expressed in cDCs, but not pDCs; fibroblasts; epithelial cells; and resident cells of the central nervous system, including microglia, astrocytes, and oligodendrocytes. Because TLR3 preferentially recognizes double-stranded RNA or surrogates, such as poly I:C, but not DNA, its recognition of HSV may be the result of a symmetric transcription process that generates abundant amounts of viral double-stranded RNA [1109]. Genetic deficiency of either TLR3, owing to a dominant-negative–acting heterozygous mutation [1110], or UNC-93B [1111] results in a selective vulnerability of humans to primary HSV-1 encephalitis and not other infections. UNC-93B is a highly conserved 12-membrane spanning protein that is found in the endoplasmic reticulum and that is required for signaling for TLR3, TLR7, and TLR9. The importance of TLR3 in limiting the development of HSV encephalitis may be due to its higher levels of expression in the central nervous system than other TLRs that can recognize HSV.

Some HSV strains induce cytokine production by mononuclear cells and DCs in a TLR2-dependent manner [1112]. The TLR2 ligands expressed by HSV are unclear, but glycoproteins are plausible candidates because other herpesvirus glycoproteins, such as those of CMV, are recognized by TLR2 [1113]. The importance of TLR2 in human HSV infection also is suggested by the observation that certain genetic TLR2 polymorphisms are associated with increased shedding of HSV-2 and the frequency of genital lesions caused by this virus [1114]. A murine model of lethal HSV1 encephalitis infection found that brain inflammation and mortality were reduced in TLR2-deficient compared with wild-type neonatal mice [1112]. This protective effect of TLR2 deficiency was associated with markedly reduced levels of serum IL-6 and of brain tissue CCL2 compared with levels found in wild-type animals. There was a strong trend toward there being higher levels of HSV1 in brain tissue in TLR2-deficient animals early after infectious challenge, although this did not achieve statistical significance. Together, these results suggest that the TLR2-dependent induction of cytokines and chemokines by HSV can result in deleterious levels of proinflammatory cytokines and chemokines. A single study [1115] has also reported that cord BMCs produce substantially higher levels of IL-6 and IL-8 than adult peripheral BMCs in response to HSV infection in vitro, although whether this increased response is dependent on TLR2 has not been evaluated.

Circulating and Cerebrospinal Fluid Levels of Cytokines and Chemokines in Human Herpes Simplex Virus Infection

Substantial amounts of type I IFNs are found in the tissues of HSV-infected humans, such as the cerebrospinal fluid of adults, children, and neonates with HSV encephalitis [1116–1118]. Although HSV efficiently induces type I IFN production, the virus is relatively resistant to its antiviral effects. This relative resistance may account for the limited effectiveness of type I IFNs in treating recurrences of established HSV infections, such as of the eye. The resistance may be due in part to the ability of the HSV ICP34.5 protein to interfere with the production of and cellular responsiveness to type I IFNs [1119]. HSV infection of certain human cell types also may inhibit type I IFN–mediated activation of the JAK/STAT pathway by inducing increased suppressor of cytokine signaling-3 [1120].

IFN-γ, which also has antiviral activity on numerous cell types, could also play a role in early innate immune control of HSV infection by its secretion from NK cells, NKT cells, and $\gamma\delta$ T cells before the appearance of HSV-specific CD4 and CD8 T cells. There is little information on the circulating levels of IFN-γ in primary HSV infection or HSV reactivation in humans. Neither form of HSV infection seems to be more severe in individuals who have IFN-γ receptor genetic defects [554] or STAT1 mutations that selectively compromise IFN-γ–dependent STAT1 homodimer-directed transcription [1106]. An increased severity of HSV or other herpesvirus infections has also not been observed in genetic deficiency of the IL-12Rβ1 subunit, which impairs IL-12p70–dependent generation of T_H1 cells and IL-23–dependent T_H17 immunity [553,554,578].

Circulating IL-6 and soluble TNFR1 levels are markedly elevated in human neonates with systemic HSV infection, as is the circulating viral load, which can reach extremely high levels (i.e., a mean of 10^6 viral genomes/mL of blood) [1121,1122]. The highest levels of these proteins and viral load are observed in cases that have a fatal outcome [1121,1122], but evidence for a direct involvement of soluble TNFR1, IL-6, or other cytokines that are elevated in the circulation in the morbidity or mortality of disseminated HSV in neonates [1103] is lacking. Although "overexuberant" cytokine and chemokine production, possibly by a TLR-dependent mechanism, could contribute to the sepsis-like syndrome, it is equally or more plausible that the sepsis-like syndrome of disseminated HSV is simply a reflection of an overwhelming viral infection, as indicated by the extremely high viral load [1121,1122], evidence of extensive coagulative necrosis of liver [1103], and detectable circulating levels of cytochrome c (also suggestive of extensive cell death) [1122]. The sensitivity of the liver to coagulative necrosis is not unique to the neonate and is part of the pathogenesis of cases of HSV hepatitis after primary infection in pregnant women and apparently immunocompetent adults. This suggests the importance of the prevention of HSV dissemination to the liver by innate or adaptive immune responses. A more complete assessment of circulating levels of cytokines and chemokines in neonatal HSV, particularly disseminated and central nervous system disease, might be helpful in understanding of disease pathogenesis and identifying particular cytokines that might be useful in adjunctive therapy (see later).

The induction of chemokines is an important early step in attracting leukocytes to mediate antiviral immune mechanisms and initiate antigen uptake and processing for the generation of the adaptive immune response. Elevated cerebrospinal fluid levels of the CC chemokines CCL2, CCL3, and CCL5 (RANTES) and of CXCL8 also have been documented in cases of adult human HSV encephalitis [1123], suggesting their role in central nervous system inflammation, but similar information for neonatal infection is limited.

Mononuclear Phagocytes

Macrophages are likely to play an important role in the early and local containment of HSV infection by their secretion of cytokines and chemokines. HSV can directly infect mononuclear phagocytes in vitro, but the resultant infection usually is nonpermissive and does not result in viral replication. Such nonreplicative infection may result in apoptosis [1124], which could limit antiviral immune mechanisms, such as cytokine production. The in vitro production of other cytokines by cells of the innate immune system that enhance NK-cell and T_H1 T-cell responses may be decreased in neonates. IL-12 and IL-15 production by mononuclear cells (presumably mainly by monocytes) from term neonates after stimulation with LPS was approximately 25% of that by adult cells [1125,1126]. Whether such cytokines are produced in amounts sufficient to limit NK-cell or T-cell immunity in neonates with HSV infection is unknown.

Dendritic Cells

The in vivo role of human DCs in the control of HSV is poorly understood. HSV can efficiently replicate in immature, but not mature, moDCs, and infection decreases expression of cytokines, such as IL-12 and type I IFN [1127], and markers indicative of DC maturity, such as CD83 [1128]. These decreases are associated with a limited capacity of these cells to activate T cells in vitro [1127]. Similar limitations in type I IFN production and the capacity to activate T cells may apply to murine DCs that are exposed to HSV [1129]. Together, these findings suggest that DCs are not effectively activated by HSV infection and may be direct cellular targets of HSV-mediated immunosuppression. It is unclear, however, how frequently DCs are infected in vivo with HSV in humans. In addition, as a potential countermeasure against viral immunosuppression, human DCs can take up HSV-infected DCs that are undergoing apoptosis and effectively cross-present HSV antigens to CD8 T cells [1130,1131]. Based on murine studies, it is plausible that apoptotic HSV-infected Langerhans cells of the skin may be taken up by cDCs, which cross-present antigens to CD8 T cells in the draining lymph nodes [1132].

Little is known concerning the innate immune response during primary HSV infection in neonates, including that mediated by DCs. An older study [270] found that type I IFN production by peripheral BMCs and the frequency of IFN-α–producing cells (assayed by the ELISPOT technique) in response to fixed HSV were diminished compared with adults, particularly for prematurely born infants. The major cell type that produces type I IFN in this assay are pDCs, and, consistent with these results, a more recent study found diminished production of type I IFNs by neonatal pDCs in response to HSV-1, CMV, and TLR7 and TLR9 ligands [328]. The mechanisms for reduced cytokine production by neonatal pDCs may include decreased nuclear translocation of IRF7, most likely because of block in TLR-induced IRF7 phosphorylation.

Given the association of mutations of TLR3 in humans with an increased susceptibility to primary HSV encephalitis [1110], the function of TLR3 signaling in the neonate is of particular interest. TLR3 mRNA expression is upregulated by the differentiation of adult peripheral blood monocytes into moDCs, whereas cord blood monocytes have minimal increases in TLR3 after in vitro differentiation into DCs [1133]. Reduced TLR3

expression or TLR3-mediated signaling may also apply to cDCs of the neonate because circulating adult cDCs have substantially greater increases in CD40 and CD80 expression compared with cord blood cDCs in response to treatment with the TLR3 ligand poly I:C [271]. Whole-blood levels of IFN-α are also substantially lower in cord blood compared with adult peripheral blood after poly I:C treatment [271], and cDCs are likely to be the major source of IFN-α in this assay. Because poly I:C treatment of either monocytes or moDCs results in significantly greater increases in TLR3 mRNA expression by adult cells compared with neonatal cells [1133], these developmental differences in TLR3-mediated responses may be accentuated further after TLR3 ligand exposure in vivo. The mechanisms underlying reduced TLR3 gene expression by neonatal monocytes and cDCs and their relationship to the levels of TLR3 protein are unclear; whether such decreases apply to nonhematopoietic cells, such as those of the central nervous system, also is unclear.

Studies of signaling by other TLRs, such as TLR4 of neonatal mDCs and TLR9 of neonatal pDCs, suggest that neonatal DCs may have limitations in IRF3-regulated and IRF7-regulated transcription. In the case of IRF3, the ability of IRF3 that translocates to the nucleus to bind to DNA and to associate with transcriptional coactivators may be impaired; for IRF7, TLR-induced nuclear translocation may be reduced [328]. Because IRF3 is crucial for the production of IFN-β by TLR3 signaling, and IRF7 is key for IFN-α production by pDC TLR9 signaling [1134], these developmental limitations in IRF-dependent transcription could impair antiviral protection mediated by type I IFNs in neonatal HSV infection.

Natural Killer Cells

NK cells provide a particularly important restraint on viral replication and dissemination before the appearance of adaptive immunity, as shown by the severity of primary infections with herpesviruses, including HSV and VZV, in patients with a selective lack of NK cells [1135]. Although the initial disease is severe, NK cell–deficient patients are able to clear virus eventually, presumably by T cell–mediated immunity (Lewis DB, Wilson CB, unpublished data). The importance of human NK cells in the control of HSV is also suggested by the markedly impaired NK-cell function of patients with Wiskott-Aldrich syndrome, who are highly prone to develop severe primary HSV infection [1135]. NK cell–derived cytokines, such as IFN-γ and TNF-α, have direct antiviral effects on HSV replication, and IFN-γ also increases MHC expression (class I and class II), which facilitates antigen presentation to CD4 and CD8 T cells. The presence of NK cell–derived IFN-γ during the early phases of naïve T-cell activation also may increase expression of the T-bet transcription factor and may favor T-cell differentiation into T_H1 cells. NK cells may accomplish this bias toward T_H1 differentiation of naïve CD4 T cells by localizing to antigenically stimulated lymph nodes in a CXCR3-dependent manner [1136]. IL-15, which has a key role in NK-cell development, is also a potent activator of NK cells for enhanced cytotoxicity against most herpes-viruses, including HSV [1137]. Exposure of human peripheral BMCs to HSV also upregulates NK-cell cyto-toxicity by an IL-15–dependent mechanism [1138].

As discussed earlier, fetal and neonatal NK cells have reduced cytotoxic activity compared with NK cells of adults, including against HSV-infected [1139] or CMV-infected target cells [382]. The addition of activating cytokines to neonatal NK cells, such as IFN-α or IFN-γ, does not reliably increase cytolytic activity against HSV-infected targets, whereas adult NK cells have consistent and substantially increased cytotoxicity [1139]. Paralleling the reduction in natural cytotoxic activity of neonatal cells, ADCC of neonatal mononuclear cells is approximately 50% of that of adult mononuclear cells, including against HSV-infected targets [1104]. Decreased ADCC mediated by purified neonatal NK cells seems to be caused in part by an adhesion defect in the presence of antibody [378]. Cytokine production by NK cells is another potentially important mechanism of host defense against HSV. Neonatal NK cells produce IFN-γ as effectively as adult NK cells in response to exogenous IL-2 and HSV [1140] or to polyclonal stimulation with iono-mycin and PMA [599]. The adequacy of neonatal NK-cell production of these and other cytokines in response to physiologic stimulation (e.g., with HSV-infected cell targets in the absence of exogenous cytokines) is unknown.

Regardless of the precise mechanism, reduced NK-cell cytolytic activity may be an important contributor to the pathogenesis of neonatal HSV infection as indicated in a neonatal murine model in which adoptively transferred human mononuclear cells from adults, but not neonates, provided protection after adoptive transfer [1104]. This model has also implicated deficits in IFN-γ production by neonatal mononuclear cells in limiting protection because the addition of IFN-γ restores the protection. The role of IFN-γ in controlling HSV infections in humans is unclear, however, because severe primary or recurrent HSV infection has not been reported as a major complication of patients with genetic deficiency of IFN-γ receptors or acquired autoantibodies against IFN-γ. No studies have directly compared NK-cell function against HSV targets in neonates versus adults with primary HSV infection, including after treatment with various immunostimulatory cytokines.

γδ T Cells

γδ T cells, particularly cells bearing Vγ9Vδ2 TCRs, obtained from HSV-seropositive donors can lyse HSV-infected cells in a non-MHC–restricted manner. Vγ9Vδ2 γδ T cells are also a major portion of the T cells that infiltrate sites of human genital HSV infection [1141]. As is generally true for the Vγ9Vδ2 cell subset, these T cells are not HSV-specific, but recognize intracellular-derived metabolites that are produced in increased amounts as a result of cellular stress (see previous chapter section on γδ T cells). γδ T-cell clones derived from these intralesional T cells are capable of secreting IFN-γ, TNF-α, IL-8, CCL3, and CCL5 [1141], suggesting that they may exert antiviral activity and maintain inflammation at these sites of infection. The importance of γδ T cells in limiting

HSV infection in humans, including neonates, is unclear, however, because immunodeficient states that selectively involve this cell lineage have not been identified.

Adaptive Immunity

Adaptive immune responses mediated by HSV antigen–specific T cells and B cells are first detected 5 to 7 days after the onset of primary HSV infection in adult humans, with the peak response achieved at approximately 2 to 3 weeks after infection [808,809,1142]. Antigen-specific immunity does not eradicate infection (i.e., achieve sterile immunity), but rather terminates active viral replication and the acute infection. T cells play the crucial role in resolution of active HSV infection and the maintenance of viral latency. The general importance of T cells in the control of human HSV and other herpesvirus infections is indicated by the increased susceptibility of individuals with quantitative or qualitative T-cell defects to these infections. The relative importance of CD4 and CD8 T cells in HSV infections in humans, including at particular sites, is uncertain, however. B cells do not seem to be able to provide protection in the absence of T cells.

Viral Inhibition of Antigen Presentation and Effect on T-Cell Immune Response

In view of the importance of MHC class I antigen presentation in antiviral control, it is not surprising that many herpesviruses, including HSV and CMV, have accumulated multiple gene products to inhibit MHC class I antigen presentation. Inhibition of the MHC class I pathway limits not only CD8 T cell–mediated cytotoxicity, but also the generation of CTL from naïve CD8 T cells, although the presence of HSV-specific CD8 T cells at sites of infection shows that this inhibition is ultimately overcome. HSV encodes a viral host shutoff protein that is an RNA endonuclease and is required for viral pathogenicity. This viral protein preferentially destroys cellular mRNA and decreases host cell protein synthesis, including MHC class I molecules. This downregulation of MHC class I limits CD8 T cell–mediated cytotoxicity of HSV-infected target cells, such as fibroblasts and keratinocytes [1143]. HSV also produces an immediate early ICP47 protein that binds to the TAP transporter and prevents the loading of peptides onto MHC class I molecules and the transport of MHC class I molecules to the cell surface [1144].

The importance of selective inhibition of MHC class I antigen presentation in the pathogenicity of HSV has not yet been formally tested in vivo, but NK cells and HSV antigen–specific CD4 T cells are detected earlier than antigen-specific CD8 T cells in lesions of adult humans with recurrent HSV-2 disease [1145]. IFN-γ produced by infiltrating NK and CD4 T cells may help override the inhibitory effects of ICP47 on MHC class I expression, allowing the subsequent eradication of virus by CD8 T cells, which increase in lesions around the time of viral clearance. When HSV-specific CD8 T cells arrive at local sites of infection, they may persist, providing relative resistance to reinfection. HSV infection also results in marked reductions in the expression of invariant chains, which is required for MHC class II maturation during antigen processing and its ultimate expression on the cell surface. The RNA endonuclease activity of the viral host shutoff protein may also decrease MHC class II expression directly. Together, these mechanisms may account for the observation that HSV infection in mice results in central nervous system lesions in which MHC class II expression remains intracellular, reducing the chance of detection by CD4 T cells [1146].

In addition to its well-known inhibition of MHC class I antigen presentation, HSV infection of neonatal monocytes [1147], moDCs [1148], or B cells [1149] can block the ability of these cells to activate CD4 T cells. As discussed previously, the extent to which HSV directly infects DCs and other APCs in vivo is unclear.

CD4 T Cells

CD4 T cells may help control HSV infection by directly lysing HSV-infected cells that express viral peptides on MHC class II molecules [1145,1150,1151] and by inhibiting viral replication through the production of IFN-γ, TNF-α, and CD40 ligand. The IFN-γ–mediated increase in expression of the molecules involved in MHC class I antigen presentation also may help override the inhibition of MHC class I antigen presentation by HSV. Consistent with this idea, CD4 T cells and mononuclear phagocytes, and not CD8 T cells, are prominent initially in HSV-infected skin; later, CD8 T cells predominate [1145], most likely because CD4 T-cell IFN-γ production has restored surface expression of HSV peptides presented by MHC class I. CD40 ligand expression by CD4 T cells also is probably essential for HSV-specific antibody production by B cells and antibody isotype switching and for the ability of CD4 T cells to become long-term memory T cells [568], including those of the T_H1 subset [1152]. In rare patients with CD40 deficiency, production of IFN-γ by pDCs is decreased in response to HSV infection in vitro [1153], which strongly supports the idea that CD40 engagement by CD40 ligand contributes to human antiviral immunity. CD4 T cells also likely promote the generation and survival of anti-HSV effector CD8 T cells, as suggested by a large body of murine studies [1154]. They may even serve as APCs to HSV-specific CD8 T cells by bearing viral peptide/MHC complexes acquired from conventional APCs [1155].

CD4 T cells in HSV-seropositive adults have been identified in the circulation at a low frequency [1156] and from sites of recurrent infection in the skin, cervix, cornea, and retina. These CD4 T cells seem to be broad in their target recognition, with peptide epitopes derived from envelope glycoproteins, tegument (the layer between the envelope and capsid), and capsid [1157]. The HSV-specific circulating CD4 T-cell response has a predominant T_H1 cytokine profile [1158], consistent with the ability of the virus to induce type I IFN and IL-12p70 at sites of infection (discussed earlier), and this cytokine profile likely applies to HSV-specific CD4 T cells of the tissues. CD4 T cells with cytotoxic activity have been readily isolated from HSV seropositive adults by in vitro expansion from the circulation of HSV-infected individuals but their actual circulating frequency is unknown. Cytotoxicity is directed against various viral

proteins, including glycoproteins of the lipid envelope, such as gB, gC, and gD [1151,1159,1160], and these viral glycoproteins may enter into the MHC class II antigen–processing endocytic pathway after first fusing with the host cell membrane. The kinetics of appearance of CD4 T cells in the tissues after primary HSV infection in adults is unknown.

In two studies in which T-cell responses in neonates and adults with primary HSV infection were compared [808,809], HSV-specific proliferation of peripheral BMCs and production of IFN-γ and TNF-α were markedly diminished and delayed in the neonates compared with these measures in the adults. The neonates did not achieve adult levels of these responses for 3 to 6 weeks after clinical presentation, whereas the adults developed robust responses within 1 week. In both studies, HSV antigen–specific responses by peripheral BMCs used viral antigen preparations that are processed mainly by the MHC class II pathway, rather than the class I pathway, mainly assaying CD4 T-cell function.

Other reports indicate that antigen-specific CD4 T-cell responses commonly are slow to develop in neonates infected perinatally or in utero with CMV [793,794]. Delayed CD4 T-cell responses to primary CMV infection also have been observed for older infants and young children compared with such responses in adults [579], suggesting that limitations in developing CD4 T-cell responses to at least some herpesviruses may continue beyond the neonatal period. Because, as discussed earlier, CD4 T cells provide multiple effector functions that may be crucial for the resolution of HSV infection—including direct antiviral cytokine production and help for CD8 T cells and B cells—this marked lag in development of HSV-specific CD4 T-cell responses in neonates could be an important contributor to the tendency of neonatal HSV infection to disseminate and to cause prolonged disease.

The basis for the delayed development of HSV antigen–specific CD4 T cells in neonates is unknown, but could reflect limitations intrinsic to these cells or limitations in APC function or both. Because immature DCs are primed for efficient antigen presentation by engagement of their CD40 molecule by CD40 ligand expressed by activated T cells, or by exposure to microbes or inflammatory cytokines induced by microbes, lack of prior exposure to microbes, which occurs in a cumulative manner after birth, might contribute to the increased susceptibility of the neonate to infection with HSV. A study showing reduced basal DC function in adult mice lacking functional TLR4 supports the idea that postnatal exposure to microbial products may contribute to the maturation of DC function [1161].

Intrinsic limitations in CD4 T-cell function might also contribute to the reduced and delayed HSV-specific CD4 T-cell immune response, such as decreased CD40 ligand by activated naïve CD4 T cells [533]. Other mechanisms intrinsic to the neonatal CD4 T cell, such as a decreased capacity to elevate $[Ca^{2+}]_I$ [611] and greater methylation of the IFN-γ gene [626], might also contribute. The tendency of activated neonatal CD4 T cells to become anergic, rather than develop into effector cells after exposure to bacterial superantigens [538], might also apply to HSV and contribute to the impaired antigen-specific response. The neonatal murine model of HSV suggests that Tregs may contribute to the attenuated primary CD4 (and CD8) T-cell response [1162]. Whether Tregs play a similar inhibitory role in human primary HSV infection, including in neonates, is unclear, but Tregs can suppress recall responses by CD4 T cells to HSV antigens in vitro in adults [1163].

Neonates also have been reported to have a lower frequency of precursor T cells capable of responding to HSV and CMV [1164]. This finding is unlikely to be due to a limitation in the diversity of the αβ-TCR repertoire [454,456,457] and is more likely to be an artifact of in vitro culture conditions that may favor the survival of adult rather than neonatal T cells.

CD8 T Cells

The efficient clearance of most viral infections depends on CD8 T cell–mediated cytotoxicity, in which infected target cells are induced to undergo apoptosis by the secretion of perforin and granzymes or the engagement of Fas by Fas-ligand (see Fig. 4–13). Direct evidence for the importance of CD8 T cells in the control of herpesvirus infections in humans comes from studies showing that the adoptive transfer of donor-derived CD8 T cells against CMV or EBV provides protection of hematopoietic cell transplant recipients from primary infection with these viruses. Murine studies indicate that CD8 T cells are key in resolving established lytic infections of the skin and nerves and in preventing spread of HSV from reactivation of sensory neurons. These roles also likely apply to the human CD8 T-cell response because HSV-specific CD8 T cells with features of effector memory cells are highly concentrated around sensory ganglia, such as those of the trigeminal nerve [1165]. Latent HSV infection is associated with a persistent and compartmentalized response that is likely directly involved in maintaining latency. These CD8 T cells may rely principally on nonlytic mechanisms for preventing HSV reactivation, including the production of IFN-γ; HSV may also express antiapoptotic proteins that also protect the neuron from CD8 T-cell perforin/granzyme B-mediated cell death [1166].

In HSV-seropositive adults with chronic infection, HSV-specific CD8 T cells are found mainly at sites of local recurrence of virus, such as the skin adjacent to the genital tract and the cervix [1167] and the cornea [1168]. At sites of healed genital lesions, CD8 T cells seem to persist, and studies suggest that HSV reactivation is frequent, but asymptomatic [1169] owing to active control by these local T-cell populations [1167]. By contrast, HSV-specific CD8 T cells are not detectable in the circulation with use of intracellular cytokine staining after stimulation with whole HSV [1156], but can be expanded in vitro from the blood of HSV-immune donors. An analysis of CD8 T cells using ELISPOT assays and overlying peptide pools have revealed a much broader CD8 T-cell response in individuals with genital HSV-2 infection, which includes all virion components [1170]. As for CD4 T cells, the CD8 T-cell immune response to primary HSV infection in adults is not well characterized.

To the best of our knowledge, there are no published studies of antigen-specific cytotoxic T-cell responses in the fetus, neonate, or young infant in response to HSV. This lack reflects, in part, the technical difficulties of performing classic cytotoxicity assays, which require HLA-matched or autologous virally infected target cells. This limitation might be overcome by newer approaches, such as detection of viral antigen–specific CD8 T cells identified using HSV peptide–class I HLA tetramers, particularly at local sites of HSV replication, such as cutaneous lesions [1171]. The kinetics of accumulation and tissue distribution of HSV-specific CD8 T cells in primary HSV infection is unknown. In a murine model of primary neonatal HSV using a replication-defective virus, which limits any adverse effects on T-cell priming from overwhelming infection, CD8 T cells with full effector activity, such as IFN-γ secretion, were slow to develop compared with HSV-infected adult mice [1162].

As discussed in detail in the section on T-cell response to congenital infection, studies of congenital CMV infection using CMV peptide–HLA-A2 tetramers found a robust response in the fetus, neonate, and young infant in terms of frequency of CD8 T cells and their function [663]. Although this finding suggests that strong stimulation, particularly if persistent, may induce virus-specific CD8 T-cell responses in the fetus, it does not exclude a potential lag in the appearance of CD8 T cells in the fetus or perinatally infected infant compared with adults with primary CMV. More recent studies suggest that CMV-specific CD8 T cells of the fetus may not be as diverse in terms of recognition of viral antigens and may have reduced IFN-γ secretion compared with the cells of pregnant women [665].

Evidence from perinatal HIV-1 infection also suggests such a lag in the appearance of CD8 T cell–mediated cytotoxicity and cytokine production, recognizing a diverse repertoire of viral antigens compared with adults with primary HIV-1 infection [818,820,1172]. The potential for a general lag in CD8 T-cell immunity also is suggested by older studies, which found that naïve CD8 T cells of the fetus and neonate generate less CTL activity than analogous adult cells after activation and culture in vitro. As indicated by the data on HSV-specific CD4 T-cell responses, a lag of days to weeks in the development of HSV-specific CD8 T-cell immunity after primary infection would likely be a major contributor to the morbidity of this infection in neonates.

Chemotactic and Homing Receptor Expression by Viral Antigen–Specific T Cells

In established HSV infection, most recurrences of viral replication occur in keratinocytes found at epithelial sites, such as the skin and genitourinary mucosa. During these recurrences, virus-specific CD4 T cells and NK cells may infiltrate the sites by 48 hours after the appearance of lesions. Infiltration by these cells is followed several days later by the appearance of virus-specific CD8 T cells, which is associated with viral clearance [1145]. Many of the HSV-specific CD8 T cells at these sites express CLA [1173], an adhesion molecule that is involved in homing of T cells to skin and other tissues that contain keratinocytes, and it is likely that HSV-specific T cells that enter other sites of viral replication, such as the central nervous system during HSV encephalitis, use a distinct combination of homing and chemotactic receptors (e.g., CCR2 and CCR5) to achieve selective trafficking [1174]. Other chemokine and homing receptor combinations are likely to be involved in trafficking of HSV-specific T cells to the liver and gastrointestinal tract in cases of disseminated disease.

Human neonatal naïve T cells differ from cells of adults in that they do not increase CXCR3 expression and decrease CCR7 expression after activation by anti-CD3 and anti-CD28 monoclonal antibodies [488,667]. CXCR3 facilitates T-cell trafficking to inflamed tissues that have been exposed to IFN-γ, whereas CCR7 mediates entry into lymphoid tissues in response to the CCL19 and CCL21 chemokines. These findings suggest that activated neonatal T cells may be limited in their capacity to traffic to nonlymphoid sites of inflammation, such as sites of HSV infection.

B-Cell Immunity and Antibody-Dependent Cellular Cytotoxicity

Although preexisting antibody (e.g., that induced by vaccination) can prevent certain viral infections, antibody probably plays a limited role in the control of viral infections that are established. This limitation probably also applies to human herpesvirus infections because patients with X-linked agammaglobulinemia, who lack mature B cells and antibody production, generally are not more susceptible to these pathogens. Nonetheless, antibody may serve an auxiliary role in HSV host defense, particularly when cellular components of the response are deficient, such as in the human neonate. Antibody also may be important for prevention of dissemination of viral infections to the central nervous system, as has been well documented in agammaglobulinemic or hypogammaglobulinemic patients, who can develop paralytic poliomyelitis or severe chronic encephalitis with echoviruses or coxsackieviruses [1175].

Human HSV infection results in the induction of antibodies against a diverse set of HSV proteins, including surface glycoproteins involved in cell attachment and entry [1176]. The production of most HSV-specific antibodies by B cells is T cell–dependent. If antibody is passively acquired, as in the case of maternal-to-fetal transfer, humoral immunity may exist independently of T-cell immunity. Under relatively physiologic conditions, IgG and alternative pathway complement components can coat the surfaces of some viruses, including HSV, effectively neutralizing their infectivity, possibly by preventing their attachment or fusion with cell membranes. Antibodies also can react with viral proteins found on the surface of infected cells, and IgG and complement components can lyse in vitro human cells infected with many different viruses, including HSV. The importance of complement in viral host defense in humans is uncertain, however, because serious viral infection is not a feature seen in patients with severe inherited complement deficiency [1177].

A potentially more effective system for the elimination of virus-infected cells by specific antibody is by ADCC, with NK cells probably being the most efficient ADCC effector cells [1178]; the specificity of cytotoxicity is probably due to the specific recognition by antibody of viral antigens present on the infected cell surface. In vitro,

ADCC requires relatively low concentrations of antibody and occurs rapidly (within hours), making it less likely that the virus would have had sufficient time to produce infectious particles. ADCC mediated by all types of effector cells is upregulated by cytokines, such as IFN-γ, type I IFNs, IL-12, and IL-15 [1179–1181]. In vitro ADCC activity correlates in some cases with protection against serious viral infections in humans and in animal models, but it is uncertain to what extent this protection is due to ADCC occurring in vivo.

Neonates have a modestly reduced antibody response, particularly for IgG, compared with older infants to most protein neoantigens, whereas IgM responses are similar. These decreased responses and isotype switching may be due, at least in part, to decreased expression of CD40 ligand by neonatal naïve CD4 T cells during their initial interaction with APCs [533]. Although these limitations in antibody response to T cell–dependent antigens may resolve by early infancy, they probably apply to HSV-specific antibodies made in response to neonatal HSV infection. Assuming that HSV-specific antibody that is neutralizing or involved in ADCC contributes to the control of primary HSV infection in humans, it is possible that limitations in isotype switching from IgM to IgG or a slower rate of somatic hypermutation of IgG responses could contribute to the severity of neonatal infection.

The neonate also is partially protected from infection by passive maternal IgG antibody, transferred predominantly during the third trimester of pregnancy. Fetal IgG concentrations are equal to or higher than maternal concentrations after 34 weeks of gestation, reflecting active transport mechanisms. In newborns with gestational age less than 38 weeks, a greater fraction of this maternally derived HSV-specific IgG may enter into the central nervous system [1182], reflecting a generally less effective blood-brain barrier. The risk of transmission of HSV from mother to infant in cases of primary or initial maternal infection is much higher (approximately 35%) than in cases of recurrent maternal infection. This difference may reflect in part lesser amounts of virus in the maternal genital tract in recurrent infection, but also may be due to protection by passively acquired HSV type-specific antibody, particularly to glycoprotein G [1183].

Kohl and colleagues [1184] also have shown that HSV-infected infants with greater concentrations of ADCC antibody had less severe disease compared with other infants with HSV infection. In otherwise healthy adults and older children with primary HSV infection, who by definition lack antibody to HSV, severe disease does not develop, as it does in neonates with primary infection. This finding indicates that the deficits intrinsic to the neonate are the important factors predisposing to severe infection. Nevertheless, passively acquired antibody may play a role in decreasing transmission or ameliorating disease severity.

Adjunctive Therapy and Vaccination for Herpesvirus Infections

The foregoing studies raise the possibility that neonates could be passively protected by administration of antibody to HSV, particularly antibody that would facilitate ADCC. In vitro studies also suggest that polyclonal antibodies or mAbs could potentially be protective by directly blocking HSV transmission from neurons to epithelial cells [1185]. Passive antibody can provide substantial protection from a low-inoculum HSV challenge in the absence of type I IFN signaling and T cells and B cells, by IL-12–dependent and IFN-γ–dependent mechanisms [1186], at least in mice. Human mAbs, murine mAbs that have been humanized, or specific hyperimmunoglobulin could potentially be employed for this purpose. The phage display technique has been used to select human mAbs with an ability to neutralize either HSV-1 or HSV-2 effectively at a relatively low concentration in vitro [1187], but it remains to be seen if these or related antibodies would be efficacious in limiting the extent of primary HSV infection in humans.

The unique capacity of IFN-γ to endow human neonatal BMCs with the ability to protect neonatal mice from infection suggests that exogenous IFN-γ also may be a potentially useful means to enhance the human neonate's resistance to HSV. In the experimental models described by Kohl [1104], passive immunotherapy must be given before or at the time of infection, however. Such therapy, if administered after infection is established, may be less effective, at least in controlling virally induced tissue damage. In addition, unanticipated fatal toxicity from early studies administering IL-12 to adult cancer patients [1188] indicates caution in the use of exogenous cytokine therapy in the seriously ill neonate; this is particularly true for IFN-γ because IL-12–induced IFN-γ has been implicated as the cause of such IL-12 toxicity [1189]. There is as yet no direct evidence that the initial innate immune response of the neonate to HSV infection is deficient in terms of cytokine production (e.g., for IL-12, TNF-α, and IFN-γ) derived from cells other than T cells.

Additional concerns about the use of exogenous cytokines comes from one study [1115] that reported cord BMCs produce substantially higher levels of IL-6 and IL-8 than adult peripheral BMCs in response to HSV infection in vitro. Based on this observation and results from a murine HSV model in which inflammation and mortality were reduced in TLR2-deficient neonatal mice [1112], it is argued that HSV induces overexuberant levels of proinflammatory cytokines in a TLR2-dependent manner, contributing to the sepsis-like syndrome of disseminated neonatal HSV infection. Consistent with this idea, circulating IL-6 and soluble TNFR1 levels are highly elevated in neonates with disseminated HSV infection, but the importance of IL-6 in neonatal HSV infection morbidity and mortality is unclear. More complete evaluation of the circulating levels of cytokines and chemokines in neonatal HSV might help to address the importance of impaired production versus overproduction of these immune regulators in pathogenesis.

Facilitating the more rapid development of antigen-specific CD4 and CD8 T cells with appropriate effector function might be a more physiologic approach, allowing these cells and the cytokines they produce to localize properly to the sites of infection. Further elucidation of the cellular and molecular mechanisms that underlie the lag in the development of antigen-specific immunity in the neonate in response to HSV may help in devising therapies to overcome these limitations in host defenses.

Vaccination

Preventing the acquisition of genital HSV infection by women of childbearing age would markedly reduce neonatal HSV infection. HSV-2 vaccines employing recombinant glycoproteins, such as glycoprotein D2 in combination with alum and monophosphoryl lipid adjuvants, were effective in preventing acquisition of infection in women, but not men, who were initially HSV-2–seronegative [1190]. The reason for these sex differences is unclear, but HSV-seropositive women have been shown to have higher levels of HSV glycoprotein D–specific CD4 T cells than men [1160]. Although these vaccines have induced high levels of IgG antibodies against the glycoprotein immunogens, these antibodies may not efficiently mediate ADCC [1191]. If ADCC is important in preventing maternal-to-neonatal HSV transmission, these vaccines are unlikely to be beneficial in reducing neonatal HSV disease when used in the context of women who are already HSV-2–seropositive. With the growing recognition of the importance of HSV-specific CD8 T cells in maintaining latency and limiting shedding and spread from sites of reactivation, numerous strategies are also being pursued to increase the CD8 T-cell response to other HSV proteins [1192].

NONVIRAL INTRACELLULAR PATHOGENS: *TOXOPLASMA GONDII*
Host Defense Mechanisms

In addition to viruses, certain nonviral intracellular pathogens can replicate within cells and cause severe fetal or neonatal infection. These pathogens include *Salmonella* species, *Listeria monocytogenes*, and *M. tuberculosis*, which are facultative intracellular pathogens, and *T. gondii* and *Chlamydia trachomatis*, which are obligate intracellular pathogens. In contrast to pyogenic bacteria, for which phagocytosis usually results in death, phagocytosis of these pathogens is a means of entry into an intracellular haven. Each of these pathogens readily infects tissue macrophages of the reticuloendothelial system. In addition, *T. gondii* can infect virtually any nucleated mammalian cell type, and this nonspecificity has important consequences for the pathogenesis of toxoplasmosis. The following discussion of host defense mechanisms focuses primarily on *T. gondii*. Relevant information from studies of *L. monocytogenes* is included.

During acute toxoplasmosis in humans, replication of tachyzoites occurs intracellularly. A 30-kDa tachyzoite surface protein, P30, seems to be involved in the initial attachment of *T. gondii* to host cells [1193]. Antibodies frequently are made against this protein after infection and constitute a basis for serodiagnosis [1193,1194]. Intracellular *T. gondii* organisms are found principally in specialized parasitophorous vacuoles [1195]. These vacuoles, from which lysosomal components and host plasma membrane proteins are excluded, allow the free exchange of nutrients with the host cell cytoplasm, facilitating parasite replication [1196]. Cellular invasion by tachyzoites occurs without generating a respiratory burst in human macrophages [1197] or activating microbicidal nitric oxide production in murine macrophages [1198].

In response to adverse intracellular conditions that slow its replication [1199], the tachyzoite is induced to convert into a less metabolically active form, the bradyzoite. Bradyzoites can persist in many tissues for years or decades in the form of cysts. As discussed later, limiting chronic *T. gondii* infection to this quiescent state depends on antigen-specific cellular immunity; acquired T-cell immunodeficiency can allow bradyzoites to reconvert to tachyzoites that resume invasive infection.

Murine studies suggest that the control of acute infection by *T. gondii* and other nonviral intracellular pathogens is critically dependent on IFN-γ and T_H1 T cells, which activate macrophages to control the infection [1200,1201]. In the early stages of infection, *T. gondii* tachyzoites or products they secrete induce DCs or mononuclear phagocytes to produce cytokines, including IL-1, IL-12, IL-15, IL-18, and TNF. These cytokines induce NK cells to produce IFN-γ. NK cell–derived IFN-γ increases toxoplasmacidal activity of mononuclear phagocytes, helping to limit the initial extent of infection. IFN-γ produced by NK cells, in conjunction with IL-12 and IL-18 produced by mononuclear phagocytes and DCs, also favors the differentiation of antigen-specific $CD4^+$ T cells into T_H1 effector T cells that secrete large amounts of IFN-γ. T_H1 effector T cells produce IFN-γ that contains the parasite during the late phase of acute infection and helps limit the spread of infection in tissues should *T. gondii* bradyzoites later reactivate into tachyzoites. T cells and the IFN-γ they produce and IL-12, IL-15, and IL-23 produced by non–T cells that sustain T_H1 responses all seem to be essential for the lifelong control of reactivation, as shown from studies in chronically infected mice. In addition, IL-27 plays a crucial role in preventing the induction of T_H17 responses and the severe neuroinflammation they induce.

T. gondii actively inhibits these protective responses in several ways. *T. gondii* inhibits signaling pathways involved in the induction of IL-12 and TNF-α [1202]. This inhibition may account for the observation that infection of human mononuclear phagocytes and DCs with *T. gondii* induces very little IL-12, whereas the production of IL-12 can be markedly upregulated by engagement of CD40 on these cells by CD40 ligand on activated T cells [1202–1204]. Inhibition of IL-12 and TNF-α production by *T. gondii* may allow it to evade initial activation of protective immunity or may be an important mechanism by which the organism avoids inducing an excessive and potentially lethal inflammatory response [1202,1205]. Consistent with the latter possibility, *T. gondii* counters the induction of proinflammatory cytokines in mice by inducing the production of IL-27 and IL-10, which dampen the production of IL-17, IL-12, TNF-α, and IFN-γ and prevent lethal inflammatory responses to *T. gondii* [1201,1206].

The crucial role of macrophages in resistance to intracellular nonviral pathogens was first shown in animal studies of *L. monocytogenes* in which depletion of macrophages increased susceptibility [1207]. In the first days of infection, the rate at which monocytes are recruited to the site of infection and the microbicidal activity of these cells correlate with the control of *T. gondii* in animals [1208]. Infection of human monocytes by *T. gondii*

tachyzoites also results in the induction of CD80 and increased expression of CD86 [1203]. The increased expression of these costimulatory molecules may enhance proliferation and IFN-γ production by T cells early in *T. gondii* infection and may assist in the differentiation of T_H1 effector cells from naïve T cells [1203].

Generally, the microbicidal activity of human monocytes against *T. gondii* is greater than that of macrophages [1209,1210]. In vitro studies with mononuclear phagocytes or microglial cells, which are mononuclear phagocytes of the central nervous system, show that oxidative and nonoxidative mechanisms are involved in limiting intracellular *T. gondii* replication. Cytokines are critical regulators of mononuclear phagocyte activity. IFN-γ produced by activated T cells and NK cells activates macrophage toxoplasmacidal activity in concert with CD40 ligand and TNF-α [1200,1211]. Activated macrophages kill and limit the intracellular replication of *T. gondii* by oxygen-dependent and oxygen-independent mechanisms. The latter include the induction of the enzyme indoleamine 2,3-dioxygenase, which leads to tryptophan degradation and deprives replicating *T. gondii* of this essential nutrient [1212,1213]. The relative importance of these mechanisms in humans is unclear.

The critical importance of $CD4^+$ T lymphocytes in protection against *T. gondii* is shown by the increased prevalence and severity of infection in patients with acquired immunodeficiency syndrome (AIDS). Similarly, mice with genetic T-cell immunodeficiencies are unable to control this infection. The importance of $CD4^+$ and $CD8^+$ T cells in mice depends on the phase of infection. In acute infection, $CD8^+$ T cells seem to be more protective than $CD4^+$ T cells [1214]. Both populations are necessary to limit the extent of central nervous system infection in the brain [1215], and $CD4^+$ T cells are required for the development of long-term protective immunity [1216].

Although antibodies seem to play little or no role in defense against *L. monocytogenes* [1217], antibodies probably make some contribution to defense against *T. gondii*. Nonetheless, T cell–deficient mice are much more susceptible than antibody-deficient animals and are not protected by antibody. The fact that *T. gondii* encephalitis in adult patients with AIDS typically develops by recrudescence of latent infection despite the presence of preexisting anti–*T. gondii* antibodies [1218] underscores the importance of T cells rather than B cells in the control of chronic infection with this pathogen.

Fetal and Neonatal Defenses

Information regarding the innate immune response of the human fetus and neonate to *T. gondii* is limited. Neonatal monocytes can ingest and kill *T. gondii* [207,208]. Monocyte-derived and placental macrophages from human neonates are activated by IFN-γ to kill or restrict the growth of *T. gondii* as effectively as cells from adults [207,1219]. Nonetheless, it is likely that other limitations in innate immunity contribute to the increased susceptibility of the human fetus to *T. gondii* infection. Studies in neonatal rodents, which are highly susceptible to infection with *L. monocytogenes*, are consistent with this possibility. Administration of recombinant IFN-γ to neonatal mice or rats before or at the time of infection protects them from acute infection and allows the development of protective immunity [1220,1221]. By contrast, administration of TNF-α protects adult, but not neonatal, rats, whereas coadministration of suboptimal doses of IFN-γ and TNF-α protects neonates. In these studies, acquisition of resistance to infection correlated with acquisition of adult competence for TNF-α production [1220]. The ontogeny of the immune responses in neonatal rodents and humans is substantially different, however, and the relevance of these findings for the human fetus and neonate is unclear.

Because T cell–mediated immunity plays a paramount and lifelong role in the control of *T. gondii* infection after acquisition of infection, differences in T-cell responses by the fetus and neonate (described in detail in chapter section on "T-Cell Development and Function in the Fetus and Neonate") are likely to be an important factor in their greater susceptibility compared with adults. In humans, *T. gondii*, similar to congenital viral pathogens such as CMV, is much more likely to produce severe fetal injury when the mother acquires primary infection early in pregnancy. The most severely damaged infants are likely to have acquired infection during the first trimester, when their numbers of T cells and their αβ-TCR repertoire for antigen recognition are limited compared with the fetus in the latter half of gestation. Nonetheless, αβ-TCR repertoire limitations are unlikely to be an important predisposing factor in most cases of congenital toxoplasmosis because severe sequelae do occur in fetuses infected during mid-gestation to late gestation, and sequelae ultimately develop in most infants infected at any time during gestation. Similarly, *L. monocytogenes* infection occurring in infants in the latter part of gestation usually is severe. This line of evidence suggests that mechanisms acting to contain *T. gondii* and *L. monocytogenes* infection are still immature in late gestation and at term relative to the mechanisms of older individuals.

These immature mechanisms are likely to include T-cell extrinsic differences, including diminished production of IL-12, type I IFNs and other T_H1 promoting cytokines by fetal and neonatal APCs, and T-cell intrinsic differences, which are described in detail in the section "T-Cell Development and Function in the Fetus and Neonate." These differences may include the greater tendency for neonatal T cells to acquire or sustain IL-10 and IL-4 production, relative to IFN-γ production, and lesser initial expression of CD40 ligand. Together, these differences may impede their ability to activate macrophages. In the case of IFN-γ, the predominance in the fetus and neonate of RTEs may contribute to this immaturity in cytokine secretion.

As noted subsequently, the acquisition of antigen-specific CD4 T-cell responses in utero in response to infection with *T. gondii* and other causes of congenital infection is often delayed. In vitro studies suggest that deficiencies of DC function and activation and differentiation of naïve $CD4^+$ T cells into memory/effector T cells may be contributory. Particularly in the mid-gestation fetus, Tregs are abundant and fully functional relative to other T cells and may help to delay the development of

antigen-specific T-cell responses. The relatively less efficient induction of CXCR3, which is a hallmark of T_H1 cells and aids in their recruitment into infected tissues, and tendency to retain expression of CCR7, which facilitates continued trafficking to lymph nodes, may impair the delivery of neonatal CD4 effector T cells to sites of *T. gondii* infection. The severe brain injury observed in congenital *T. gondii* infection may result from unchecked parasite growth owing to impaired T_H1 immunity, impaired regulation of neuroinflammation, or both. In this regard, it would be interesting to know whether the congenitally infected fetus and neonate have impaired IL-27 production and excessive T_H17 responses, which have been associated with excessive neuroinflammation in mice [1206], but there are at present no data addressing this possibility.

T. gondii–specific memory $CD4^+$ T-cell responses may be delayed in their appearance in congenital toxoplasmosis and may not be detectable until weeks or months after birth. McLeod and colleagues [797] found that lymphocyte proliferation in response to *T. gondii* antigens, which primarily detects responses by $CD4^+$ T cells, was below the limit of detection in 11 of 25 congenitally infected infants younger than 1 year of age. The most severely affected infants were more likely to have undetectable or low antigen-specific T-cell responses. When memory T cells were first detected by lymphocyte proliferation assays in congenitally infected children, their capacity to produce IL-2 and IFN-γ often was less than that of memory T cells from adults with postnatal *T. gondii* infection [797].

Results consistent with these were reported by another group [1222]. Fatoohi and colleagues [1223] found that anti–*T. gondii* T-cell responses (determined using a different and less standardized assay) were lower in eight congenitally infected infants younger than 1 year of age than in individuals with acquired *T. gondii* infection and congenitally infected children studied when they were older than 1 year of age. Nonetheless, anti–*T. gondii* T-cell responses were detectable in most of the congenitally infected infants younger than 1 year of age by this assay. Ciardelli and coworkers [1224] also found that greater than 90% of congenitally infected infants less than 90 days of age had detectable T-cell proliferation and IFN-γ production in response to *T. gondii* antigen. The basis for the differences between these studies is unknown. Nonetheless, these data suggest that antigen-specific $CD4^+$ T-cell responses may develop more slowly or be diminished in some infants with congenital *T. gondii* infection.

A similar impairment or lag, or both, in the development of antigen-specific $CD4^+$ T-cell responses has been observed in infants with congenital infection caused by *T. pallidum*, CMV, VZV, or rubella virus [793–797,1225,1226] and, as discussed earlier, in neonates infected postnatally with HSV [809,811]. Similarly, Tu and colleagues [579] found that antigen-specific CD4+ T-cell responses may be low in infants and young children with postnatally acquired CMV infection until active viral replication ceases, whereas antigen-specific $CD8^+$ T-cell responses are detectable much earlier. The basis for the initially poor $CD4^+$ T-cell response in these infections is unknown. Regardless of the precise mechanisms, these findings suggest that infection of the immunologically immature fetus may lead in some cases to complete or partial antigen-specific unresponsiveness that may persist for some time after birth.

At least some neonates and young infants with congenital *T. gondii* infection show increased expansion of the Vγ2Vδ2-bearing γδ T-cell population, most of which express a CD45RA^lo^CD45RO^hi^ surface phenotype, indicating prior activation in vivo [808]. An analysis of a few patients found that αβ T cells in congenitally infected neonates show a poor proliferative response to stimulation by peripheral BMCs infected with viable or irradiated *T. gondii* organisms [808]. Other functions, such as the secretion of cytokines by these cells, were not assessed, and rigorous age-matched controls were not employed. These results suggest, however, that αβ T cells in infants with congenital toxoplasmosis may be anergic.

Although the foregoing results suggest that multiple aspects of cell-mediated immunity against *T. gondii* organisms are compromised in the human fetus and neonate, particularly in early gestation, antigen-specific antibody responses to *T. gondii* are commonly detectable (see Chapter 31 for more details). Antibodies to the P30 *T. gondii* antigen are frequently detectable in the fetus and neonate after congenital infection and are useful for serodiagnosis. Anti-P30 IgA antibodies are found in most neonates after congenital infection, whereas anti-P30 IgM antibodies are found in a few [1194,1228]. *T. gondii*–specific IgE antibodies may also be demonstrable within the first 2 months of life in congenitally infected infants [1229]. Anti-P30 IgA and IgE antibodies are not unique to the fetus and neonate, but also are common in older individuals with acquired toxoplasmosis. Together, these results suggest that isotype switching of antibodies from IgM to the IgA and IgE isotypes can occur in utero, particularly in the face of continuing antigenic stimulation. Because IL-4 produced by CD4^+^ T cells is likely to be required for the production of protein antigen-specific IgE antibodies, these results suggest that the CD4^+^ T-cell response to *T. gondii* organisms in the fetus may include the production of IL-4.

Implications for Immunologic Intervention

The findings in human neonates, in concert with the results of studies in rodents, suggest that correction of the deficits in NK-cell function, cytokine production, and T-cell responses could facilitate treatment of infections with intracellular pathogens, such as *T. gondii*. Several limitations are apparent, however. Treatment of neonatal rats with IFN-γ after infection with *L. monocytogenes* is established is ineffective, whereas concomitant therapy or pretreatment is effective [1230]. In the case of congenital infection with *T. gondii*, therapy would need to be initiated and maintained in utero, when maternal infection is often asymptomatic, and there is no obvious way by which this could be safely targeted to the fetus. Data in mouse models suggest that increased production of IFN-γ during maternal infection may contribute to fetal loss as a result of maternal rejection of the fetus as a foreign allograft [1231]. After birth, it may be possible

to provide exogenous IFN-γ (or perhaps TNF-α, IL-12, or IL-15), but the same caveats noted for treatment in cases of viral infection would apply. There are at present no safe and effective vaccines against *T. gondii*, and none is likely to be available in the near future [1232].

REFERENCES

[1] K. De Smet, R. Contreras, Human antimicrobial peptides: defensins, cathelicidins and histatins, Biotechnol. Lett. 27 (2005) 1337–1347.

[2] M.H. Braff, et al., Cutaneous defense mechanisms by antimicrobial peptides, J. Invest. Dermatol. 125 (2005) 9–13.

[3] N.H. Salzman, M.A. Underwood, C.L. Bevins, Paneth cells, defensins, and the commensal microbiota: a hypothesis on intimate interplay at the intestinal mucosa, Semin. Immunol. 19 (2007) 70–83.

[4] M.E. Selsted, A.J. Ouellette, Mammalian defensins in the antimicrobial immune response, Nat. Immunol. 6 (2005) 551–557.

[5] K.O. Kisich, et al., The constitutive capacity of human keratinocytes to kill *Staphylococcus aureus* is dependent on beta-defensin 3, J. Invest. Dermatol. 127 (2007) 2368–2380.

[6] A.A. Larson, J.G. Dinulos, Cutaneous bacterial infections in the newborn, Curr. Opin. Pediatr. 17 (2005) 481–485.

[7] D.L. Carr, W.E. Kloos, Temporal study of the staphylococci and micrococci of normal infant skin, Appl. Environ. Microbiol. 34 (1977) 673–680.

[8] L. Dethlefsen, M. McFall-Ngai, D.A. Relman, An ecological and evolutionary perspective on human-microbe mutualism and disease, Nature 449 (2007) 811–818.

[9] G. Marchini, et al., The newborn infant is protected by an innate antimicrobial barrier: antimicrobial peptides are present in the skin and vernix caseosa, Br. J. Dermatol. 147 (2002) 1127–1134.

[10] R.A. Dorschner, et al., Neonatal skin in mice and humans expresses increased levels of antimicrobial peptides: innate immunity during development of the adaptive response, Pediatr. Res. 53 (2003) 566–572.

[11] H. Yoshio, et al., Antimicrobial polypeptides of human vernix caseosa and amniotic fluid: implications for newborn innate defense, Pediatr. Res. 53 (2003) 211–216.

[12] H.T. Akinbi, et al., Host defense proteins in vernix caseosa and amniotic fluid, Am. J. Obstet. Gynecol. 191 (2004) 2090–2096.

[13] D.S. Newburg, Innate immunity and human milk, J. Nutr. 135 (2005) 1308–1312.

[14] D. Artis, Epithelial-cell recognition of commensal bacteria and maintenance of immune homeostasis in the gut, Nat. Rev. Immunol. 8 (2008) 411–420.

[15] C. Palmer, et al., Development of the human infant intestinal microbiota, PLoS Biol. 5 (2007) e177.

[16] M.T. Tien, et al., Anti-inflammatory effect of *Lactobacillus casei* on *Shigella*-infected human intestinal epithelial cells, J. Immunol. 176 (2006) 1228–1237.

[17] S.K. Mazmanian, D.L. Kasper, The love-hate relationship between bacterial polysaccharides and the host immune system, Nat. Rev. Immunol. 6 (2006) 849–858.

[18] N.N. Nanthakumar, et al., Inflammation in the developing human intestine: a possible pathophysiologic contribution to necrotizing enterocolitis, Proc. Natl. Acad. Sci. U S A 97 (2000) 6043–6048.

[19] M. Lotz, et al., Postnatal acquisition of endotoxin tolerance in intestinal epithelial cells, J. Exp. Med. 203 (2006) 973–984.

[20] S.C. Gribar, et al., No longer an innocent bystander: epithelial toll-like receptor signaling in the development of mucosal inflammation, Mol. Med. 14 (2008) 645–659.

[21] J. Wehkamp, J. Schauber, E.F. Stange, Defensins and cathelicidins in gastrointestinal infections, Curr. Opin. Gastroenterol. 23 (2007) 32–38.

[22] S. Menard, et al., Developmental switch of intestinal antimicrobial peptide expression, J. Exp. Med. 205 (2008) 183–193.

[23] B. Grubor, D.K. Meyerholz, M.R. Ackermann, Collectins and cationic antimicrobial peptides of the respiratory epithelia, Vet. Pathol. 43 (2006) 595–612.

[24] A. Muir, et al., Toll-like receptors in normal and cystic fibrosis airway epithelial cells, Am. J. Respir. Cell Mol. Biol. 30 (2004) 777–783.

[25] A.K. Mayer, et al., Differential recognition of TLR-dependent microbial ligands in human bronchial epithelial cells, J. Immunol. 178 (2007) 3134–3142.

[26] N.H. Hillman, et al., Toll-like receptors and agonist responses in the developing fetal sheep lung, Pediatr. Res. 63 (2008) 388–393.

[27] K. Harju, V. Glumoff, M. Hallman, Ontogeny of Toll-like receptors Tlr2 and Tlr4 in mice, Pediatr. Res. 49 (2001) 81–83.

[28] T.D. Starner, et al., Expression and activity of beta-defensins and LL-37 in the developing human lung, J. Immunol. 174 (2005) 1608–1615.

[29] H.P. Haagsman, et al., Surfactant collectins and innate immunity, Neonatology 93 (2008) 288–294.

[30] E. Giannoni, et al., Surfactant proteins A and D enhance pulmonary clearance of *Pseudomonas aeruginosa*, Am. J. Respir. Cell Mol. Biol. 34 (2006) 704–710.

[31] A.M. LeVine, et al., Surfactant protein-d enhances phagocytosis and pulmonary clearance of respiratory syncytial virus, Am. J. Respir. Cell Mol. Biol. 31 (2004) 193–199.

[32] M.T. Stahlman, et al., Immunolocalization of surfactant protein-D (SP-D) in human fetal, newborn, and adult tissues, J. Histochem. Cytochem. 50 (2002) 651–660.

[33] A. Stray-Pedersen, et al., Post-neonatal drop in alveolar SP-A expression: biological significance for increased vulnerability to SIDS? Pediatr. Pulmonol. 43 (2008) 160–168.

[34] A. Hilgendorff, et al., Host defence lectins in preterm neonates, Acta Paediatr. 94 (2005) 794–799.

[35] A. Mantovani, et al., Pentraxins in innate immunity: from C-reactive protein to the long pentraxin PTX3, J. Clin. Immunol. 28 (2008) 1–13.

[36] E. Ainbender, et al., Serum C-reactive protein and problems of newborn infants, J. Pediatr. 101 (1982) 438–440.

[37] D.F. Angelone, et al., Innate immunity of the human newborn is polarized toward a high ratio of IL-6/TNF-alpha production in vitro and in vivo, Pediatr. Res. 60 (2006) 205–209.

[38] D.P. Eisen, R.M. Minchinton, Impact of mannose-binding lectin on susceptibility to infectious diseases, Clin. Infect. Dis. 37 (2003) 1496–1505.

[39] J.L. Casanova, L. Abel, The human model: a genetic dissection of immunity to infection in natural conditions, Nat. Rev. Immunol. 4 (2004) 55–66.

[40] F.N. Frakking, et al., Low mannose-binding lectin (MBL) levels in neonates with pneumonia and sepsis, Clin. Exp. Immunol. 150 (2007) 255–262.

[41] Y.L. Lau, et al., Mannose-binding protein in preterm infants: developmental profile and clinical significance, Clin. Exp. Immunol. 102 (1995) 649–654.

[42] A.B. Dzwonek, et al., The role of mannose-binding lectin in susceptibility to infection in preterm neonates, Pediatr. Res. 63 (2008) 680–685.

[43] F. de Benedetti, et al., Low serum levels of mannose binding lectin are a risk factor for neonatal sepsis, Pediatr. Res. 61 (2007) 325–328.

[44] J.D. Lambris, D. Ricklin, B.V. Geisbrecht, Complement evasion by human pathogens, Nat. Rev. Microbiol. 6 (2008) 132–142.

[45] A.A. Manfredi, et al., Pentraxins, humoral innate immunity and tissue injury, Curr. Opin. Immunol. 20 (2008) 538–544.

[46] P.F. Kohler, Maturation of the human complement system, I: onset time and sites of fetal C1q, C4, C3, and C5 synthesis, J. Clin. Invest. 52 (1973) 671–677.

[47] H.A. Lassiter, et al., Complement factor 9 deficiency in serum of human neonates, J. Infect. Dis. 166 (1992) 53–57.

[48] R.B. Johnston Jr., et al., Complement in the newborn infant, Pediatrics 64 (1979) 781–786.

[49] L.D. Notarangelo, et al., Activity of classical and alternative pathways of complement in preterm and small for gestational age infants, Pediatr. Res. 18 (1984) 281–285.

[50] C.A. Davis, E.H. Vallota, J. Forristal, Serum complement levels in infancy: age related changes, Pediatr. Res. 13 (1979) 1043–1046.

[51] M.E. Miller, Phagocyte function in the neonate: selected aspects, Pediatrics 64 (1979) 709–712.

[52] J.H. Dossett, R.C. Williams Jr., P.G. Quie, Studies on interaction of bacteria, serum factors and polymorphonuclear leukocytes in mothers and newborns, Pediatrics 44 (1969) 49–57.

[53] S.P. Geelen, et al., Deficiencies in opsonic defense to pneumococci in the human newborn despite adequate levels of complement and specific IgG antibodies, Pediatr. Res. 27 (1990) 514–518.

[54] M.S. Edwards, et al., Deficient classical complement pathway activity in newborn sera, Pediatr. Res. 17 (1983) 685–688.

[55] J.A. Winkelstein, L.E. Kurlandsky, A.J. Swift, Defective activation of the third component of complement in the sera of newborn infants, Pediatr. Res. 13 (1979) 1093–1096.

[56] E.L. Mills, B. Bjorksten, P.G. Quie, Deficient alternative complement pathway activity in newborn sera, Pediatr. Res. 13 (1979) 1341–1344.

[57] Y. Kobayashi, T. Usui, Opsonic activity of cord serum—an evaluation based on determination of oxygen consumption by leukocytes, Pediatr. Res. 16 (1982) 243–246.

[58] L. Marodi, et al., Opsonic activity of cord blood sera against various species of microorganism, Pediatr. Res. 19 (1985) 433–436.

[59] D. Adamkin, et al., Activity of the alternative pathway of complement in the newborn infant, J. Pediatr. 93 (1978) 604–608.

[60] M.E. Eads, et al., Antibody-independent activation of C1 by type Ia group B streptococci, J. Infect. Dis. 146 (1982) 665–672.

[61] S.G. Pahwa, et al., Cellular and humoral components of monocyte and neutrophil chemotaxis in cord blood, Pediatr. Res. 11 (1977) 677–680.

[62] R. Raghunathan, et al., Phagocyte chemotaxis in the perinatal period, J. Clin. Immunol. 2 (1982) 242–245.

[63] D.C. Anderson, et al., Impaired chemotaxigenesis by type III group B streptococci in neonatal sera: relationship to diminished concentration of specific anticapsular antibody and abnormalities of serum complement, Pediatr. Res. 17 (1983) 496–502.

[64] E.P. Zilow, et al., Alternative pathway activation of the complement system in preterm infants with early onset infection, Pediatr. Res. 41 (1997) 334–339.

[65] M.Z. Ratajczak, Phenotypic and functional characterization of hematopoietic stem cells, Curr. Opin. Hematol. 15 (2008) 293–300.

[66] V.J. Jokubaitis, et al., Angiotensin-converting enzyme (CD143) marks hematopoietic stem cells in human embryonic, fetal, and adult hematopoietic tissues, Blood 111 (2008) 4055–4063.

[67] M. Tavian, B. Peault, The changing cellular environments of hematopoiesis in human development in utero, Exp. Hematol. 33 (2005) 1062–1069.

[68] D. Metcalf, Cellular hematopoiesis in the twentieth century, Semin. Hematol. 36 (1999) 5–12.

[69] M. Wadhwa, R. Thorpe, Haematopoietic growth factors and their therapeutic use, Thromb. Haemost. 99 (2008) 863–873.

[70] K.M. Zsebo, et al., Stem cell factor is encoded at the Sl locus of the mouse and is the ligand for the c-kit tyrosine kinase receptor, Cell 63 (1990) 213–224.

[71] W. Wiktor-Jedrzejczak, et al., Total absence of colony-stimulating factor 1 in the macrophage-deficient osteopetrotic op/op mouse, Proc. Natl. Acad. Sci. U S A 87 (1990) 4828–4832.

[72] T. Suzuki, et al., Familial pulmonary alveolar proteinosis caused by mutations in CSF2RA, J. Exp. Med. 205 (2008) 2703–2710.

[73] R.I. Walker, R. Willemze, Neutrophil kinetics and the regulation of granulopoiesis, Rev. Infect. Dis. 2 (1980) 282–292.

[74] W.L. Furman, W.M. Crist, Biology and clinical applications of hemopoietins in pediatric practice, Pediatrics 90 (1992) 716–728.

[75] S. von Vietinghoff, K. Ley, Homeostatic regulation of blood neutrophil counts, J. Immunol. 181 (2008) 5183–5188.

[76] J.M. Koenig, M.C. Yoder, Neonatal neutrophils: the good, the bad, and the ugly, Clin. Perinatol. 31 (2004) 39–51.

[77] J. Laver, et al., High levels of granulocyte and granulocyte-macrophage colony-stimulating factors in cord blood of normal full-term neonates, J. Pediatr. 116 (1990) 627–632.

[78] R.D. Christensen, Hematopoiesis in the fetus and neonate, Pediatr. Res. 26 (1989) 531–535.

[79] R.K. Ohls, et al., Neutrophil pool sizes and granulocyte colony-stimulating factor production in human mid-trimester fetuses, Pediatr. Res. 37 (1995) 806–811.

[80] M.C. Banerjea, C.P. Speer, The current role of colony-stimulating factors in prevention and treatment of neonatal sepsis, Semin. Neonatol. 7 (2002) 335–349.

[81] A. Mouzinho, et al., Revised reference ranges for circulating neutrophils in very-low-birth-weight neonates, Pediatrics 94 (1994) 76–82.

[82] B.L. Manroe, et al., The neonatal blood count in health and disease, I: reference values for neutrophilic cells, J. Pediatr. 95 (1979) 89–98.

[83] N. Schmutz, et al., Expected ranges for blood neutrophil concentrations of neonates: the Manroe and Mouzinho charts revisited, J. Perinatol. 28 (2008) 275–281.

[84] W.D. Engle, et al., Circulating neutrophils in septic preterm neonates: comparison of two reference ranges, Pediatrics 99 (1997) E10.

[85] R.D. Christensen, D.A. Calhoun, L.M. Rimsza, A practical approach to evaluating and treating neutropenia in the neonatal intensive care unit, Clin. Perinatol. 27 (2000) 577–601.

[86] D.A. Calhoun, J.F. Kirk, R.D. Christensen, Incidence, significance, and kinetic mechanism responsible for leukemoid reactions in patients in the neonatal intensive care unit: a prospective evaluation, J. Pediatr. 129 (1996) 403–409.

[87] A. Ishiguro, et al., Reference intervals for serum granulocyte colony-stimulating factor levels in children, J. Pediatr. 128 (1996) 208–212.

[88] J.A. Wilimas, et al., A longitudinal study of granulocyte colony-stimulating factor levels and neutrophil counts in newborn infants, J. Pediatr. Hematol. Oncol. 17 (1995) 176–179.

[89] P. Gessler, et al., Serum concentrations of granulocyte colony-stimulating factor in healthy term and preterm neonates and in those with various diseases including bacterial infections, Blood 82 (1993) 3177–3182.

[90] C. Kennon, et al., Granulocyte colony-stimulating factor as a marker for bacterial infection in neonates, J. Pediatr. 128 (1996) 765–769.

[91] S. Ehlers, K.A. Smith, Differentiation of T cell lymphokine gene expression: the in vitro acquisition of T cell memory, J. Exp. Med. 173 (1991) 25–36.

[92] B.K. English, et al., Decreased granulocyte-macrophage colony-stimulating factor production by human neonatal blood mononuclear cells and T cells, Pediatr. Res. 31 (1992) 211–216.

[93] K.R. Schibler, et al., Production of granulocyte colony-stimulating factor in vitro by monocytes from preterm and term neonates, Blood 82 (1993) 2478–2484.

[94] M.S. Cairo, et al., Decreased stimulated GM-CSF production and GM-CSF gene expression but normal numbers of GM-CSF receptors in human term newborns compared with adults, Pediatr. Res. 30 (1991) 362–367.

[95] J.S. Buzby, et al., Increased granulocyte-macrophage colony-stimulating factor mRNA instability in cord versus adult mononuclear cells is translation-dependent and associated with increased levels of A + U-rich element binding factor, Blood 88 (1996) 2889–2897.

[96] K. Ley, et al., Getting to the site of inflammation: the leukocyte adhesion cascade updated, Nat. Rev. Immunol. 7 (2007) 678–689.

[97] L. Harvath, Neutrophil chemotactic factors, EXS 59 (1991) 35–52.

[98] I.F. Charo, R.M. Ransohoff, The many roles of chemokines and chemokine receptors in inflammation, N. Engl. J. Med. 354 (2006) 610–621.

[99] M. Bunting, et al., Leukocyte adhesion deficiency syndromes: adhesion and tethering defects involving beta 2 integrins and selectin ligands, Curr. Opin. Hematol. 9 (2002) 30–35.

[100] D.C. Anderson, B.J. Hughes, C.W. Smith, Abnormal mobility of neonatal polymorphonuclear leukocytes: relationship to impaired redistribution of surface adhesion sites by chemotactic factor or colchicine, J. Clin. Invest. 68 (1981) 863–874.

[101] D.C. Anderson, et al., Impaired motility of neonatal PMN leukocytes: relationship to abnormalities of cell orientation and assembly of microtubules in chemotactic gradients, J Leuk Biol 36 (1984) 1–15.

[102] D.C. Anderson, et al., Diminished lectin-, epidermal growth factor-, complement binding domain-cell adhesion molecule-1 on neonatal neutrophils underlies their impaired CD18-independent adhesion to endothelial cells in vitro, J. Immunol. 146 (1991) 3372–3379.

[103] J.B. Smith, et al., Expression and regulation of L-selectin on eosinophils from human adults and neonates, Pediatr. Res. 32 (1992) 465–471.

[104] L.T. McEvoy, H. Zakem-Cloud, M.F. Tosi, Total cell content of CR3 (CD11b/CD18) and LFA-1 (CD11a/CD18) in neonatal neutrophils: relationship to gestational age, Blood 87 (1996) 3929–3933.

[105] D.C. Anderson, et al., Impaired transendothelial migration by neonatal neutrophils: abnormalities of Mac-1 CD11b/CD18-dependent adherence reactions, Blood 76 (1990) 2613–2621.

[106] N. Rebuck, A. Gibson, A. Finn, Neutrophil adhesion molecules in term and premature infants: normal or enhanced leucocyte integrins but defective L-selectin expression and shedding, Clin. Exp. Immunol. 101 (1995) 183–189.

[107] M. Adinolfi, et al., Ontogeny of human complement receptors CR1 and CR3: expression of these molecules on monocytes and neutrophils from maternal, newborn and fetal samples, Eur. J. Immunol. 18 (1988) 565–569.

[108] R.B. Klein, et al., Decreased mononuclear and polymorphonuclear chemotaxis in human newborns, infants, and young children, Pediatrics 60 (1977) 467–472.

[109] C. Dos Santos, D. Davidson, Neutrophil chemotaxis to leukotriene B4 in vitro is decreased for the human neonate, Pediatr. Res. 33 (1993) 242–246.

[110] N.D. Tan, D. Davidson, Comparative differences and combined effects of interleukin-8, leukotriene B4, and platelet-activating factor on neutrophil chemotaxis of the newborn, Pediatr. Res. 38 (1995) 11–16.

[111] S.E. Fox, et al., The effects and comparative differences of neutrophil specific chemokines on neutrophil chemotaxis of the neonate, Cytokine 29 (2005) 135–140.

[112] F. Sacchi, H.R. Hill, Defective membrane potential changes in neutrophils from human neonates, J. Exp. Med. 160 (1984) 1247–1252.

[113] P. Santoro, et al., Impaired d-myo-inositol 1,4,5-triphosphate generation from cord blood polymorphonuclear leukocytes, Pediatr. Res. 38 (1995) 564–567.

[114] V.M. Meade, et al., Rac2 concentrations in umbilical cord neutrophils, Biol. Neonate 90 (2006) 156–159.

[115] H.R. Hill, Biochemical, structural, and functional abnormalities of polymorphonuclear leukocytes in the neonate, Pediatr. Res. 22 (1987) 375–382.

[116] A. Boner, B.J. Zeligs, J.A. Bellanti, Chemotactic responses of various differentiational stages of neutrophils from human cord and adult blood, Infect. Immun. 35 (1982) 921–928.

[117] Y. Kikawa, Y. Shigematsu, M. Sudo, Leukotriene B4 biosynthesis in polymorphonuclear leukocytes from blood of umbilical cord, infants, children, and adults, Pediatr. Res. 20 (1986) 402–406.

[118] O. Levy, et al., The adenosine system selectively inhibits TLR-mediated TNF-alpha production in the human newborn, J. Immunol. 177 (2006) 1956–1966.

[119] D.M. Underhill, A. Ozinsky, Phagocytosis of microbes: complexity in action, Annu. Rev. Immunol. 20 (2002) 825–852.

[120] F. Nimmerjahn, J.V. Ravetch, Fc-receptors as regulators of immunity, Adv. Immunol. 96 (2007) 179–204.

[121] T. Takai, et al., Augmented humoral and anaphylactic responses in Fc gamma RII-deficient mice, Nature 379 (1996) 346–349.

[122] S. Bektas, B. Goetze, C.P. Speer, Decreased adherence, chemotaxis and phagocytic activities of neutrophils from preterm neonates, Acta Paediatr. Scand. 79 (1990) 1031–1038.

[123] R.B. Johnston Jr., Function and cell biology of neutrophils and mononuclear phagocytes in the newborn infant, Vaccine 16 (1998) 1363–1368.

[124] T. Fujiwara, et al., Plasma effects on phagocytic activity and hydrogen peroxide production by polymorphonuclear leukocytes in neonates, Clin. Immunol. Immunopathol. 85 (1997) 67–72.

[125] A.E. Falconer, R. Carr, S.W. Edwards, Impaired neutrophil phagocytosis in preterm neonates: lack of correlation with expression of immunoglobulin or complement receptors, Biol. Neonate 68 (1995) 264–269.

[126] A.E. Falconer, R. Carr, S.W. Edwards, Neutrophils from preterm neonates and adults show similar cell surface receptor expression: analysis using a whole blood assay, Biol. Neonate 67 (1995) 26–33.

[127] G. Fjaertoft, et al., CD64 (Fcgamma receptor I) cell surface expression on maturing neutrophils from preterm and term newborn infants, Acta Paediatr. 94 (2005) 295–302.

[128] P. Henneke, et al., Impaired CD14-dependent and independent response of polymorphonuclear leukocytes in preterm infants, J Perinat. Med. 31 (2003) 176–183.

[129] D.H. Jones, et al., Subcellular distribution and mobilization of MAC-1 CD11b/CD18 in neonatal neutrophils, Blood 75 (1990) 488–498.

[130] G. Qing, K. Rajaraman, R. Bortolussi, Diminished priming of neonatal polymorphonuclear leukocytes by lipopolysaccharide is associated with reduced CD14 expression, Infect. Immun. 63 (1995) 248–252.

[131] B.H. Segal, et al., Genetic, biochemical, and clinical features of chronic granulomatous disease, Medicine (Baltimore) 79 (2000) 170–200.

[132] C.G. Vinuesa, et al., Recirculating and germinal center B cells differentiate into cells responsive to polysaccharide antigens, Eur. J. Immunol. 33 (2003) 297–305.

[133] O. Levy, Antibiotic proteins of polymorphonuclear leukocytes, Eur. J. Haematol. 56 (1996) 263–277.

[134] D. Yang, O. Chertov, J.J. Oppenheim, Participation of mammalian defensins and cathelicidins in anti-microbial immunity: receptors and activities of human defensins and cathelicidin (LL-37), J. Leukoc. Biol. 69 (2001) 691–697.

[135] T. Strunk, et al., Differential maturation of the innate immune response in human fetuses, Pediatr. Res. 56 (2004) 219–226.

[136] U.H. Chudgar, G.W. Thurman, D.R. Ambruso, Oxidase activity in cord blood neutrophils: a balance between increased membrane associated cytochrome b558 and deficient cytosolic components, Pediatr. Blood Cancer 45 (2005) 311–317.

[137] M. Bjorkqvist, et al., Defective neutrophil oxidative burst in preterm newborns on exposure to coagulase-negative staphylococci, Pediatr. Res. 55 (2004) 966–971.

[138] W. Al-Hertani, et al., Human newborn polymorphonuclear neutrophils exhibit decreased levels of MyD88 and attenuated p38 phosphorylation in response to lipopolysaccharide, Clin. Invest. Med. 30 (2007) E44–E53.

[139] I. Nupponen, et al., Extracellular release of bactericidal/permeability-increasing protein in newborn infants, Pediatr. Res. 51 (2002) 670–674.

[140] O. Levy, et al., Impaired innate immunity in the newborn: newborn neutrophils are deficient in bactericidal/permeability-increasing protein, Pediatrics 104 (1999) 1327–1333.

[141] P. Cocchi, L. Marianelli, Phagocytosis and intracellular killing of *Pseudomonas aeruginosa* in premature infants, Helv. Paediatr. Acta 22 (1967) 110–118.

[142] R. Coen, O. Grush, E. Kauder, Studies of bactericidal activity and metabolism of the leukocyte in full-term neonates, J. Pediatr. 75 (1969) 400–406.

[143] I.D. Becker, et al., Bactericidal capacity of newborn phagocytes against group B beta-hemolytic streptococci, Infect. Immun. 34 (1981) 535–539.

[144] J. Stroobant, et al., Diminished bactericidal capacity for group B streptococcus in neutrophils from "stressed" and healthy neonates, Pediatr. Res. 18 (1984) 634–637.

[145] A.O. Shigeoka, et al., Defective oxidative metabolic responses of neutrophils from stressed neonates, J. Pediatr. 98 (1981) 392–398.

[146] E.L. Mills, et al., The chemiluminescence response and bactericidal activity of polymorphonuclear neutrophils from newborns and their mothers, Pediatrics 63 (1979) 429–434.

[147] W.C. Wright Jr., et al., Decreased bactericidal activity of leukocytes of stressed newborn infants, Pediatrics 56 (1975) 579–584.

[148] A.O. Shigeoka, J.I. Santos, H.R. Hill, Functional analysis of neutrophil granulocytes from healthy, infected, and stressed neonates, J. Pediatr. 95 (1979) 454–460.

[149] N. Hanna, et al., Effects of ibuprofen and hypoxia on neutrophil apoptosis in neonates, Biol. Neonate 86 (2004) 235–239.

[150] E.J. Molloy, et al., Labor promotes neonatal neutrophil survival and lipopolysaccharide responsiveness, Pediatr. Res. 56 (2004) 99–103.

[151] E.J. Molloy, et al., Granulocyte colony-stimulating factor and granulocyte-macrophage colony-stimulating factor have differential effects on neonatal and adult neutrophil survival and function, Pediatr. Res. 57 (2005) 806–812.

[152] C.A. Liu, et al., Higher spontaneous and TNFalpha-induced apoptosis of neonatal blood granulocytes, Pediatr. Res. 58 (2005) 132–137.

[153] H.R. Hill, N.H. Augustine, H.S. Jaffe, Human recombinant interferon gamma enhances neonatal polymorphonuclear leukocyte activation and movement, and increases free intracellular calcium, J. Exp. Med. 173 (1991) 767–770.

[154] M.S. Cairo, et al., Recombinant human granulocyte-macrophage colony-stimulating factor primes neonatal granulocytes for enhanced oxidative metabolism and chemotaxis, Pediatr. Res. 26 (1989) 395–399.

[155] S. Kamran, et al., In vitro effect of indomethacin on polymorphonuclear leukocyte function in preterm infants, Pediatr. Res. 33 (1993) 32–35.

[156] F. Forestier, et al., Hematological values of 163 normal fetuses between 18 and 30 weeks of gestation, Pediatr. Res. 20 (1986) 342–346.

[157] A. Moshfegh, et al., Neonatal eosinophils possess efficient Eotaxin/IL-5- and N-formyl-methionyl-leucyl-phenylalanine-induced transmigration in vitro, Pediatr. Res. 58 (2005) 138–142.

[158] A.M. Bhat, J.W. Scanlon, The pattern of eosinophilia in premature infants: a prospective study in premature infants using the absolute eosinophil count, J. Pediatr. 98 (1981) 612.

[159] A.D. Rothberg, et al., Eosinophilia in premature neonates: phase 2 of a biphasic granulopoietic response, S. Afr. Med. J. 64 (1983) 539–541.

[160] R. van Furth, J.A. Raeburn, T.L. van Zwet, Characteristics of human mononuclear phagocytes, Blood 54 (1979) 485–500.

[161] L. Drohan, et al., Selective developmental defects of cord blood antigen-presenting cell subsets, Hum. Immunol. 65 (2004) 1356–1369.

[162] W.G. Hocking, D.W. Golde, The pulmonary-alveolar macrophage (first of two parts), N. Engl. J. Med. 301 (1979) 580–587.

[163] W.G. Hocking, D.W. Golde, The pulmonary-alveolar macrophage (second of two parts), N. Engl. J. Med. 301 (1979) 639–645.

[164] E. Kelemen, M. Jaanossa, Macrophages are the first differentiated blood cells formed in human embryonic liver, Exp. Hematol. 8 (1980) 996–1000.

[165] Y. Ueno, et al., Characterization of hemopoietic stem cells CFUc in cord blood, Exp. Hematol. 9 (1981) 716–722.

[166] A.G. Weinberg, et al., Neonatal blood cell count in health and disease, II: values for lymphocytes, monocytes, and eosinophils, J. Pediatr. 106 (1985) 462–466.

[167] E. Alenghat, J.R. Esterly, Alveolar macrophages in perinatal infants, Pediatrics 74 (1984) 221–223.

[168] R.F. Jacobs, et al., Age-dependent effects of aminobutyryl muramyl dipeptide on alveolar macrophage function in infant and adult Macaca monkeys, Am. Rev. Respir. Dis. 128 (1983) 862–867.

[169] M.J. Blahnik, et al., Lipopolysaccharide-induced tumor necrosis factor-alpha and IL-10 production by lung macrophages from preterm and term neonates, Pediatr. Res. 50 (2001) 726–731.

[170] R. Freedman, et al., Development of splenic reticuloendothelial function in neonates, J. Pediatr. 96 (1980) 466–468.

[171] E.C. Butcher, Leukocyte-endothelial cell recognition: three or more steps to specificity and diversity, Cell 67 (1991) 1033–1036.

[172] S.A. Jones, Directing transition from innate to acquired immunity: defining a role for IL-6, J. Immunol. 175 (2005) 3463–3468.

[173] A.D. Luster, The role of chemokines in linking innate and adaptive immunity, Curr. Opin. Immunol. 14 (2002) 129–135.

[174] J.D. Bullock, et al., Inflammatory response in the neonate re-examined, Pediatrics 44 (1969) 58–61.

[175] J.W. Uhr, J. Dancis, C.G. Neumann, Delayed-type hypersensitivity in premature neonatal humans, Nature 187 (1960) 1130–1131.

[176] S. Smith, R.F. Jacobs, C.B. Wilson, The immunobiology of childhood tuberculosis: a window on the ontogeny of cellular immunity, J. Pediatr. 131 (1997) 16–26.

[177] W.L. Weston, et al., Monocyte-macrophage function in the newborn, Am. J. Dis. Child. 131 (1977) 1241–1242.

[178] R.C. Monteiro, J.G. Van De Winkel, IgA Fc receptors, Annu. Rev. Immunol. 21 (2003) 177–204.

[179] H. Sengelov, Complement receptors in neutrophils, Crit. Rev. Immunol. 15 (1995) 107–131.

[180] L.A. Duits, et al., Expression of beta-defensin 1 and 2 mRNA by human monocytes, macrophages and dendritic cells, Immunology 106 (2002) 517–525.

[181] S. Gordon, Alternative activation of macrophages, Nat. Rev. Immunol. 3 (2003) 23–35.

[182] A. Aderem, Role of Toll-like receptors in inflammatory response in macrophages, Crit. Care Med. 29 (2001) S16–S18.

[183] T.H. Ottenhoff, et al., Genetics, cytokines and human infectious disease: lessons from weakly pathogenic mycobacteria and salmonellae, Nat. Genet. 32 (2002) 97–105.

[184] J. van Ingen, et al., Mycobacterial disease in patients with rheumatic disease, Nat. Clin. Pract. Rheumatol. 4 (2008) 649–656.

[185] T.H. Watts, M.A. DeBenedette, T cell co-stimulatory molecules other than CD28, Curr. Opin. Immunol. 11 (1999) 286–293.

[186] R.R. Dretschmer, et al., Chemotactic and bactericidal capacities of human newborn monocytes, J. Immunol. 117 (1976) 1303–1307.

[187] C.S. Hawes, A.S. Kemp, W.R. Jones, In vitro parameters of cell-mediated immunity in the human neonate, Clin. Immunol. Immunopathol. 17 (1980) 530–536.

[188] J.P. Orlowski, L. Sieger, B.F. Anthony, Bactericidal capacity of monocytes of newborn infants, J. Pediatr. 89 (1976) 797–801.

[189] C.P. Speer, et al., Oxidative metabolism in cord blood monocytes and monocyte-derived macrophages, Infect. Immun. 50 (1985) 919–921.

[190] C.P. Speer, et al., Phagocytic activities in neonatal monocytes, Eur. J. Pediatr. 145 (1986) 418–421.

[191] C.P. Speer, et al., Phagocytosis-associated functions in neonatal monocyte-derived macrophages, Pediatr. Res. 24 (1988) 213–216.

[192] M.E. Conly, D.P. Speert, Human neonatal monocyte-derived macrophages and neutrophils exhibit normal nonopsonic and opsonic receptor-mediated phagocytosis and superoxide anion production, Biol. Neonate 60 (1991) 361–366.

[193] S. Plaeger-Marshall, et al., Replication of herpes simplex virus in blood monocytes and placental macrophages from human neonates, Pediatr. Res. 26 (1989) 135–139.

[194] L. Mintz, et al., Age-dependent resistance of human alveolar macrophages to herpes simplex virus, Infect. Immun. 28 (1980) 417–420.

[195] S. Kohl, Herpes simplex virus immunology: problems, progress, and promises, J. Infect. Dis. 152 (1985) 435–440.

[196] H. Milgrom, S.L. Shore, Assessment of monocyte function in the normal newborn infant by antibody-dependent cellular cytotoxicity, J. Pediatr. 91 (1977) 612–614.

[197] L. Marodi, Deficient interferon-gamma receptor-mediated signaling in neonatal macrophages, Acta Paediatr. 91 (Suppl.) (2002) 117–119.

[198] L. Marodi, R. Kaposzta, E. Nemes, Survival of group B streptococcus type III in mononuclear phagocytes: differential regulation of bacterial killing in cord macrophages by human recombinant gamma interferon and granulocyte-macrophage colony-stimulating factor, Infect. Immun. 68 (2000) 2167–2170.

[199] L. Marodi, et al., Candidacidal mechanisms in the human neonate. Impaired IFN-gamma activation of macrophages in newborn infants, J. Immunol. 153 (1994) 5643–5649.

[200] J.B. D'Ambola, et al., Human and rabbit newborn lung macrophages have reduced anti-*Candida* activity, Pediatr. Res. 24 (1988) 285–290.

[201] T. Ganz, et al., Newborn rabbit alveolar macrophages are deficient in two microbicidal cationic peptides, MCP-1 and MCP-2, Am. Rev. Respir. Dis. 132 (1985) 901–904.

[202] T.R. Martin, et al., The effect of type-specific polysaccharide capsule on the clearance of group B streptococci from the lungs of infant and adult rats, J. Infect. Dis. 165 (1992) 306–314.

[203] J.A. Bellanti, L.S. Nerurkar, B.J. Zeligs, Host defenses in the fetus and neonate: studies of the alveolar macrophage during maturation, Pediatrics 64 (1979) 726–739.

[204] J.D. Coonrod, M.C. Jarrells, R.B. Bridges, Impaired pulmonary clearance of pneumococci in neonatal rats, Pediatr. Res. 22 (1987) 736–742.

[205] M.P. Sherman, et al., Role of pulmonary phagocytes in host defense against group B streptococci in preterm versus term rabbit lung, J. Infect. Dis. 166 (1992) 818–826.

[206] G. Kurland, et al., The ontogeny of pulmonary defenses: alveolar macrophage function in neonatal and juvenile rhesus monkeys, Pediatr. Res. 23 (1988) 293–297.

[207] C.B. Wilson, J.E. Haas, Cellular defenses against *Toxoplasma gondii* in newborns, J. Clin. Invest. 73 (1984) 1606–1616.

[208] J.D. Berman, W.D. Johnson Jr., Monocyte function in human neonates, Infect. Immun. 19 (1978) 898–902.

[209] M.P. Glauser, Pathophysiologic basis of sepsis: considerations for future strategies of intervention, Crit. Care Med. 28 (2000) S4–S8.

[210] C. Gabay, I. Kushner, Acute-phase proteins and other systemic responses to inflammation, N. Engl. J. Med. 340 (1999) 448–454.

[211] C.A. Dinarello, J.G. Cannon, S.M. Wolff, New concepts on the pathogenesis of fever, Rev. Infect. Dis. 10 (1988) 168–189.

[212] M.G. Katze, Y. He, M. Gale Jr., Viruses and interferon: a fight for supremacy, Nat. Rev. Immunol. 2 (2002) 675–687.

[213] T. Taniguchi, A. Takaoka, The interferon-alpha/beta system in antiviral responses: a multimodal machinery of gene regulation by the IRF family of transcription factors, Curr. Opin. Immunol. 14 (2002) 111–116.

[214] U. Boehm, et al., Cellular responses to interferon-gamma, Annu. Rev. Immunol. 15 (1997) 749–795.

[215] S. Goriely, M. Goldman, The interleukin-12 family: new players in transplantation immunity? Am. J. Transplant. 7 (2007) 278–284.

[216] R.A. Kastelein, C.A. Hunter, D.J. Cua, Discovery and biology of IL-23 and IL-27: related but functionally distinct regulators of inflammation, Annu. Rev. Immunol. 25 (2007) 221–242.

[217] K. Palucka, J. Banchereau, How dendritic cells and microbes interact to elicit or subvert protective immune responses, Curr. Opin. Immunol. 14 (2002) 420–431.

[218] L. Eckmann, M.F. Kagnoff, Cytokines in host defense against *Salmonella*, Microbes Infect. 3 (2001) 1191–1200.

[219] M. Moser, K.M. Murphy, Dendritic cell regulation of TH1-TH2 development, Nat. Immunol. 1 (2000) 199–205.

[220] K.M. Murphy, S.L. Reiner, The lineage decisions of helper T cells, Nat. Rev. Immunol. 2 (2002) 933–944.

[221] T. Calandra, P.Y. Bochud, D. Heumann, Cytokines in septic shock, Curr. Clin. Top. Infect. Dis. 22 (2002) 1–23.

[222] A.S. Cross, S.M. Opal, A new paradigm for the treatment of sepsis: is it time to consider combination therapy? Ann. Intern. Med. 138 (2003) 502–505.

[223] K.W. Moore, et al., Interleukin-10 and the interleukin-10 receptor, Annu. Rev. Immunol. 19 (2001) 683–765.

[224] C.A. Dinarello, Blocking IL-1 in systemic inflammation, J. Exp. Med. 201 (2005) 1355–1359.

[225] C.N. Serhan, N. Chiang, T.E. Van Dyke, Resolving inflammation: dual anti-inflammatory and pro-resolution lipid mediators, Nat. Rev. Immunol. 8 (2008) 349–361.

[226] R. Medzhitov, P. Preston-Hurlburt, C.A. Janeway Jr., A human homologue of the *Drosophila* Toll protein signals activation of adaptive immunity, Nature 388 (1997) 394–397.

[227] P. Matzinger, Tolerance, danger, and the extended family, Annu. Rev. Immunol. 12 (1994) 991–1045.

[228] S. Akira, K. Takeda, Functions of toll-like receptors: lessons from KO mice, C. R. Biol. 327 (2004) 581–589.

[229] N.J. Gay, M. Gangloff, Structure and function of Toll receptors and their ligands, Annu. Rev. Biochem. 76 (2007) 141–165.

[230] M.S. Jin, J.O. Lee, Structures of the toll-like receptor family and its ligand complexes, Immunity 29 (2008) 182–191.

[231] A. Iwasaki, R. Medzhitov, Toll-like receptor control of the adaptive immune responses, Nat. Immunol. 5 (2004) 987–995.

[232] M. Rehli, Of mice and men: species variations of Toll-like receptor expression, Trends Immunol. 23 (2002) 375–378.

[233] M. Gilliet, W. Cao, Y.J. Liu, Plasmacytoid dendritic cells: sensing nucleic acids in viral infection and autoimmune diseases, Nat. Rev. Immunol. 8 (2008) 594–606.

[234] N. Kadowaki, et al., Subsets of human dendritic cell precursors express different toll-like receptors and respond to different microbial antigens, J. Exp. Med. 194 (2001) 863–869.

[235] Y. Nagai, et al., Essential role of MD-2 in LPS responsiveness and TLR4 distribution, Nat. Immunol. 3 (2002) 667–672.

[236] Z. Jiang, et al., CD14 is required for MyD88-independent LPS signaling, Nat. Immunol. 6 (2005) 565–570.

[237] A. Poltorak, et al., Defective LPS signaling in C3H/HeJ and C57BL/10ScCr mice: mutations in Tlr4 gene, Science 282 (1998) 2085–2088.

[238] S.T. Qureshi, et al., Endotoxin-tolerant mice have mutations in Toll-like receptor 4 (Tlr4), J. Exp. Med. 189 (1999) 615–625.

[239] A.D. O'Brien, et al., Genetic control of susceptibility to *Salmonella typhimurium* in mice: role of the LPS gene, J. Immunol. 124 (1980) 20–24.

[240] A.D. O'Brien, et al., Additional evidence that the Lps gene locus regulates natural resistance to *S. typhimurium* in mice, J. Immunol. 134 (1985) 2820–2823.

[241] A.S. Cross, et al., Pretreatment with recombinant murine tumor necrosis factor alpha/cachectin and murine interleukin 1 alpha protects mice from lethal bacterial infection, J. Exp. Med. 169 (1989) 2021–2027.

[242] O. Takeuchi, et al., Differential roles of TLR2 and TLR4 in recognition of gram-negative and gram-positive bacterial cell wall components, Immunity 11 (1999) 443–451.

[243] S. Akira, Mammalian Toll-like receptors, Curr. Opin. Immunol. 15 (2003) 5–11.

[244] K. Takeda, T. Kaisho, S. Akira, Toll-like receptors, Annu. Rev. Immunol. 21 (2003) 335–376.

[245] F. Hayashi, et al., The innate immune response to bacterial flagellin is mediated by Toll-like receptor 5, Nature 410 (2001) 1099–1103.

[246] D.M. Klinman, Use of CpG oligodeoxynucleotides as immunoprotective agents, Expert Opin. Biol. Ther. 4 (2004) 937–946.

[247] A. Pichlmair, C. Reis e Sousa, Innate recognition of viruses, Immunity 27 (2007) 370–383.

[248] U. Bhan, et al., TLR9 is required for protective innate immunity in Gram-negative bacterial pneumonia: role of dendritic cells, J. Immunol. 179 (2007) 3937–3946.

[249] P. Parroche, et al., Malaria hemozoin is immunologically inert but radically enhances innate responses by presenting malaria DNA to Toll-like receptor 9, Proc. Natl. Acad. Sci. U S A 104 (2007) 1919–1924.

[250] V. Sancho-Shimizu, et al., Genetic susceptibility to herpes simplex virus 1 encephalitis in mice and humans, Curr. Opin. Allergy Clin. Immunol. 7 (2007) 495–505.

[251] B. Beutler, E.M. Moresco, The forward genetic dissection of afferent innate immunity, Curr. Top. Microbiol. Immunol. 321 (2008) 3–26.

[252] L.A. O'Neill, A.G. Bowie, The family of five: TIR-domain-containing adaptors in Toll-like receptor signalling, Nat. Rev. Immunol. 7 (2007) 353–364.

[253] L.A. O'Neill, Fine tuning' TLR signaling, Nat. Immunol. 9 (2008) 459–461.

[254] S. Goriely, M.F. Neurath, M. Goldman, How microorganisms tip the balance between interleukin-12 family members, Nat. Rev. Immunol. 8 (2008) 81–86.

[255] T. Kawai, et al., Interferon-alpha induction through Toll-like receptors involves a direct interaction of IRF7 with MyD88 and TRAF6, Nat. Immunol. 5 (2004) 1061–1068.

[256] M. Jurk, et al., Human TLR7 or TLR8 independently confer responsiveness to the antiviral compound R-848, Nat. Immunol. 3 (2002) 499.

[257] F. Heil, et al., Species-specific recognition of single-stranded RNA via toll-like receptor 7 and 8, Science 303 (2004) 1526–1529.

[258] K. Honda, et al., Role of a transductional-transcriptional processor complex involving MyD88 and IRF-7 in Toll-like receptor signaling, Proc. Natl. Acad. Sci. U S A 101 (2004) 15416–15421.

[259] Y. Huang, et al., IRAK1 serves as a novel regulator essential for lipopolysaccharide-induced interleukin-10 gene expression, J. Biol. Chem. 279 (2004) 51697–51703.

[260] T.D. Kanneganti, M. Lamkanfi, G. Nunez, Intracellular NOD-like receptors in host defense and disease, Immunity 27 (2007) 549–559.

[261] L.A. O'Neill, Innate immunity: squelching anti-viral signalling with NLRX1, Curr. Biol. 18 (2008) R302–R304.

[262] D.A. Muruve, et al., The inflammasome recognizes cytosolic microbial and host DNA and triggers an innate immune response, Nature 452 (2008) 103–107.

[263] S.C. Eisenbarth, et al., Crucial role for the Nalp3 inflammasome in the immunostimulatory properties of aluminium adjuvants, Nature 453 (2008) 1122–1126.

[264] V. Hornung, et al., Silica crystals and aluminum salts activate the NALP3 inflammasome through phagosomal destabilization, Nat. Immunol. 9 (2008) 847–856.

[265] E.V. Acosta-Rodriguez, et al., Surface phenotype and antigenic specificity of human interleukin 17-producing T helper memory cells, Nat. Immunol. 8 (2007) 639–646.

[266] T. Saito, M. Gale Jr., Differential recognition of double-stranded RNA by RIG-I-like receptors in antiviral immunity, J. Exp. Med. 205 (2008) 1523–1527.

[267] M. Yoneyama, T. Fujita, Structural mechanism of RNA recognition by the RIG-I-like receptors, Immunity 29 (2008) 178–181.

[268] S. LeibundGut-Landmann, et al., Syk- and CARD9-dependent coupling of innate immunity to the induction of T helper cells that produce interleukin 17, Nat. Immunol. 8 (2007) 630–638.

[269] I.R. Haga, A.G. Bowie, Evasion of innate immunity by vaccinia virus, Parasitology 130 (Suppl.) (2005) S11–S25.

[270] B. Cederblad, T. Riesenfeld, G.V. Alm, Deficient herpes simplex virus-induced interferon-alpha production by blood leukocytes of preterm and term newborn infants, Pediatr. Res. 27 (1990) 7–10.

[271] D. De Wit, et al., Impaired responses to toll-like receptor 4 and toll-like receptor 3 ligands in human cord blood, J. Autoimmun. 21 (2003) 277–281.

[272] P. Neustock, et al., Failure to detect type 1 interferon production in human umbilical cord vein endothelial cells after viral exposure, J. Interferon Cytokine Res. 15 (1995) 129–135.

[273] T.R. La Pine, et al., Defective production of IL-18 and IL-12 by cord blood mononuclear cells influences the T helper-1 interferon gamma response to group B streptococci, Pediatr. Res. 54 (2003) 276–281.

[274] H. Karlsson, C. Hessle, A. Rudin, Innate immune responses of human neonatal cells to bacteria from the normal gastrointestinal flora, Infect. Immun. 70 (2002) 6688–6696.

[275] C. Schultz, et al., Enhanced interleukin-6 and interleukin-8 synthesis in term and preterm infants, Pediatr. Res. 51 (2002) 317–322.

[276] T. Taniguchi, et al., Fetal mononuclear cells show a comparable capacity with maternal mononuclear cells to produce IL-8 in response to lipopolysaccharide in chorioamnionitis, J. Reprod. Immunol. 23 (1993) 1–12.

[277] K.R. Schibler, et al., Defective production of interleukin-6 by monocytes: a possible mechanism underlying several host defense deficiencies of neonates, Pediatr. Res. 31 (1992) 18–21.

[278] S.K. Burchett, et al., Regulation of tumor necrosis factor/cachectin and IL-1 secretion in human mononuclear phagocytes, J. Immunol. 140 (1988) 3473–3481.

[279] O. Levy, et al., Selective impairment of TLR-mediated innate immunity in human newborns: neonatal blood plasma reduces monocyte TNF-alpha induction by bacterial lipopeptides, lipopolysaccharide, and imiquimod, but preserves the response to R-848, J. Immunol. 173 (2004) 4627–4634.

[280] T.R. Kollmann, et al., Deficient MHC class I cross-presentation of soluble antigen by murine neonatal dendritic cells, Blood 103 (2004) 4240–4242.

[281] M. Chang, et al., Transforming growth factor-beta 1, macrophage inflammatory protein-1 alpha, and interleukin-8 gene expression is lower in stimulated human neonatal compared with adult mononuclear cells, Blood 84 (1994) 118–124.

[282] S. Chheda, et al., Decreased interleukin-10 production by neonatal monocytes and T cells: relationship to decreased production and expression of tumor necrosis factor-alpha and its receptors, Pediatr. Res. 40 (1996) 475–483.

[283] M.C. Seghaye, et al., The production of pro- and anti-inflammatory cytokines in neonates assessed by stimulated whole cord blood culture and by plasma levels at birth, Biol. Neonate 73 (1998) 220–227.

[284] S.T. Yerkovich, et al., Postnatal development of monocyte cytokine responses to bacterial lipopolysaccharide, Pediatr. Res. 62 (2007) 547–552.

[285] K. Sadeghi, et al., Immaturity of infection control in preterm and term newborns is associated with impaired toll-like receptor signaling, J. Infect. Dis. 195 (2007) 296–302.

[286] E. Forster-Waldl, et al., Monocyte toll-like receptor 4 expression and LPS-induced cytokine production increase during gestational aging, Pediatr. Res. 58 (2005) 121–124.

[287] S.R. Yan, et al., Role of MyD88 in diminished tumor necrosis factor alpha production by newborn mononuclear cells in response to lipopolysaccharide, Infect. Immun. 72 (2004) 1223–1229.

[288] S. Goriely, et al., A defect in nucleosome remodeling prevents IL-12(p35) gene transcription in neonatal dendritic cells, J. Exp. Med. 199 (2004) 1011–1016.

[289] L. Cohen, et al., CD14-independent responses to LPS require a serum factor that is absent from neonates, J. Immunol. 155 (1995) 5337–5342.

[290] E. Liu, et al., Changes of CD14 and CD1a expression in response to IL-4 and granulocyte-macrophage colony-stimulating factor are different in cord blood and adult blood monocytes, Pediatr. Res. 50 (2001) 184–189.

[291] B. Kampalath, R.P. Cleveland, L. Kass, Reduced CD4 and HLA-DR expression in neonatal monocytes, Clin. Immunol. Immunopathol. 87 (1998) 93–100.

[292] K. Hoebe, B. Beutler, LPS, dsRNA and the interferon bridge to adaptive immune responses: Trif, Tram, and other TIR adaptor proteins, J. Endotoxin Res. 10 (2004) 130–136.

[293] K. Hoebe, et al., Upregulation of costimulatory molecules induced by lipopolysaccharide and double-stranded RNA occurs by Trif-dependent and Trif-independent pathways, Nat. Immunol. 4 (2003) 1223–1229.

[294] O. Levy, et al., Unique efficacy of Toll-like receptor 8 agonists in activating human neonatal antigen-presenting cells, Blood 108 (2006) 1284–1290.

[295] R. Berner, et al., Elevated levels of lipopolysaccharide-binding protein and soluble CD14 in plasma in neonatal early-onset sepsis, Clin. Diagn. Lab. Immunol. 9 (2002) 440–445.

[296] M. Colonna, Alerting dendritic cells to pathogens: the importance of Toll-like receptor signaling of stromal cells, Proc. Natl. Acad. Sci. U S A 101 (2004) 16083–16084.

[297] K.P. MacDonald, et al., Characterization of human blood dendritic cell subsets, Blood 100 (2002) 4512–4520.

[298] K. Lore, et al., Toll-like receptor ligands modulate dendritic cells to augment cytomegalovirus- and HIV-1-specific T cell responses, J. Immunol. 171 (2003) 4320–4328.

[299] F. Ishikawa, et al., The developmental program of human dendritic cells is operated independently of conventional myeloid and lymphoid pathways, Blood 110 (2007) 3591–3660.

[300] J. Bancherau, et al., Immunobiology of dendritic cells, Annu. Rev. Immunol. 18 (2000) 767–811.

[301] M. Cella, et al., Plasmacytoid monocytes migrate to inflamed lymph nodes and produce large amounts of type I interferon, Nat. Med. 5 (1999) 919–923.

[302] M. Drijkoningen, et al., Epidermal Langerhans' cells and dermal dendritic cells in human fetal and neonatal skin: an immunohistochemical study, Pediatr. Dermatol. 4 (1987) 11–17.

[303] J. Olweus, et al., Dendritic cell ontogeny: a human dendritic cell lineage of, Proc. Natl. Acad. Sci. U S A 94 (1997) 12551–12556.

[304] D. De Wit, et al., Blood plasmacytoid dendritic cell responses to CpG oligodeoxynucleotides are impaired in human newborns, Blood 103 (2004) 1030–1032.

[305] F.E. Borras, et al., Identification of both myeloid CD11c+ and lymphoid CD11c– dendritic cell subsets in cord blood, Br. J. Haematol. 113 (2001) 925–931.

[306] N. Teig, et al., Age-related changes in human blood dendritic cell subpopulations, Scand. J. Immunol. 55 (2002) 453–457.

[307] M.M. Hagendorens, et al., Differences in circulating dendritic cell subtypes in cord blood and peripheral blood of healthy and allergic children, Clin. Exp. Allergy 33 (2003) 633–639.

[308] R.M. Steinman, D. Hawiger, M.C. Nussenzweig, Tolerogenic dendritic cells, Annu. Rev. Immunol. 21 (2003) 685–711.

[309] A. Lanzavecchia, F. Sallusto, Regulation of T cell immunity by dendritic cells, Cell 106 (2001) 263–266.

[310] C. Pasare, R. Medzhitov, Toll pathway-dependent blockade of CD4+CD25+ T cell-mediated suppression by dendritic cells, Science 299 (2003) 1033–1036.

[311] C. Pasare, R. Medzhitov, Toll-dependent control mechanisms of CD4 T cell activation, Immunity 21 (2004) 733–741.

[312] J. Zhu, W.E. Paul, CD4 T cells: fates, functions, and faults, Blood 112 (2008) 1557–1569.

[313] R.V. Sorg, G. Kogler, P. Wernet, Functional competence of dendritic cells in human umbilical cord blood, Bone Marrow Transplant. 22 (Suppl. 1) (1998) S52–S54.

[314] R.V. Sorg, G. Kogler, P. Wernet, Identification of cord blood dendritic cells as an immature CD11c– population, Blood 93 (1999) 2302–2307.

[315] S. Tonon, et al., *Bordetella pertussis* toxin induces the release of inflammatory cytokines and dendritic cell activation in whole blood: impaired responses in human newborns, Eur. J. Immunol. 32 (2002) 3118–3125.

[316] Z. Zheng, et al., Generation of dendritic cells from adherent cells of cord blood with granulocyte-macrophage colony-stimulating factor, interleukin-4, and tumor necrosis factor-alpha, J. Hematother. Stem Cell Res. 9 (2000) 453–464.

[317] E. Liu, et al., Decreased yield, phenotypic expression and function of immature monocyte-derived dendritic cells in cord blood, Br. J. Haematol. 113 (2001) 240–246.

[318] S. Goriely, et al., Deficient IL-12(p35) gene expression by dendritic cells derived from neonatal monocytes, J. Immunol. 166 (2001) 2141–2146.

[319] D. Krumbiegel, F. Zepp, C.U. Meyer, Combined Toll-like receptor agonists synergistically increase production of inflammatory cytokines in human neonatal dendritic cells, Hum. Immunol. 68 (2007) 813–822.

[320] C.B. Wilson, T.R. Kollmann, Induction of antigen-specific immunity in human neonates and infants, Nestle Nutr. Workshop Ser. Pediatr. Program 61 (2008) 183–195.

[321] J.W. Upham, et al., Development of interleukin-12-producing capacity throughout childhood, Infect. Immun. 70 (2002) 6583–6588.

[322] C.L. Langrish, et al., Neonatal dendritic cells are intrinsically biased against Th-1 immune responses, Clin. Exp. Immunol. 128 (2002) 118–123.

[323] E. Aksoy, et al., Interferon regulatory factor 3-dependent responses to lipopolysaccharide are selectively blunted in cord blood cells, Blood 109 (2007) 2887–2893.

[324] E. Liu, H.K. Law, Y.L. Lau, BCG promotes cord blood monocyte-derived dendritic cell maturation with nuclear Rel-B up-regulation and cytosolic I kappa B alpha and beta degradation, Pediatr. Res. 54 (2003) 105–112.

[325] J. Lund, et al., Toll-like receptor 9-mediated recognition of herpes simplex virus-2 by plasmacytoid dendritic cells, J. Exp. Med. 198 (2003) 513–520.

[326] A. Krug, et al., Herpes simplex virus type 1 activates murine natural interferon-producing cells through toll-like receptor 9, Blood 103 (2004) 1433–1437.

[327] J.M. Lund, et al., Recognition of single-stranded RNA viruses by Toll-like receptor 7, Proc. Natl. Acad. Sci. U S A 101 (2004) 5598–5603.

[328] B. Danis, et al., Interferon regulatory factor 7-mediated responses are defective in cord blood plasmacytoid dendritic cells, Eur. J. Immunol. 38 (2008) 507–517.

[329] M.C. Gold, et al., Human neonatal dendritic cells are competent in MHC class I antigen processing and presentation, PLoS ONE 2 (2007) e957.

[330] L.L. Lanier, Natural killer cell receptor signaling, Curr. Opin. Immunol. 15 (2003) 308–314.

[331] R. Biassoni, et al., Human natural killer cell receptors: insights into their molecular function and structure, J. Cell. Mol. Med. 7 (2003) 376–387.

[332] J.H. Phillips, et al., Ontogeny of human natural killer NK cells: fetal NK cells mediate cytolytic function and express cytoplasmic CD3 epsilon,delta proteins, J. Exp. Med. 175 (1992) 1055–1066.

[333] T. Nakazawa, K. Agematsu, A. Yabuhara, Later development of Fas ligand-mediated cytotoxicity as compared with granule-mediated cytotoxicity during the maturation of natural killer cells, Immunology 92 (1997) 180–187.

[334] M.A. Cooper, T.A. Fehniger, M.A. Caligiuri, The biology of human natural killer-cell subsets, Trends Immunol. 22 (2001) 633–640.

[335] B. Blom, P.C. Res, H. Spits, T cell precursors in man and mice, Crit. Rev. Immunol. 18 (1998) 371–388.

[336] F. Colucci, M.A. Caligiuri, J.P. Di Santo, What does it take to make a natural killer? Nat. Rev. Immunol. 3 (2003) 413–425.

[337] A. Poggi, et al., Expression of human NKRP1A by CD34+ immature thymocytes: NKRP1A-mediated regulation of proliferation and cytolytic activity, Eur. J. Immunol. 26 (1996) 1266–1272.

[338] T. Hori, et al., Human fetal liver-derived CD7+CD2lowCD3–CD56– clones that express CD3 gamma, delta, and epsilon and proliferate in response to interleukin-2 (IL-2), IL-3, IL-4, or IL-7: implications for the relationship between T and natural killer cells, Blood 80 (1992) 1270–1278.

[339] C. Vitale, et al., Analysis of the activating receptors and cytolytic function of human natural killer cells undergoing in vivo differentiation after allogeneic bone marrow transplantation, Eur. J. Immunol. 34 (2004) 455–460.

[340] S. Sivori, et al., Early expression of triggering receptors and regulatory role of 2B4 in human natural killer cell precursors undergoing in vitro differentiation, Proc. Natl. Acad. Sci. U S A 99 (2002) 4526–4531.

[341] M.C. Mingari, et al., Interleukin-15-induced maturation of human natural killer cells from early thymic precursors: selective expression of CD94/NKG2-A as the only HLA class I-specific inhibitory receptor, Eur. J. Immunol. 27 (1997) 1374–1380.

[342] L. Ruggeri, et al., Effectiveness of donor natural killer cell alloreactivity in mismatched hematopoietic transplants, Science 295 (2002) 2097–2100.

[343] C.A. Biron, K.S. Byron, J.L. Sullivan, Severe herpesvirus infections in an adolescent without natural killer cells, N. Engl. J. Med. 320 (1989) 1731–1735.

[344] R. Jacobs, et al., CD56bright cells differ in their KIR repertoire and cytotoxic features from CD56dim NK cells, Eur. J. Immunol. 31 (2001) 3121–3127.

[345] M. Cella, et al., A human natural killer cell subset provides an innate source of IL-22 for mucosal immunity, Nature 457 (2009) 722–725.

[346] M.J. Loza, B. Perussia, The IL-12 signature: NK cell terminal CD56+high stage and effector functions, J. Immunol. 172 (2004) 88–96.

[347] J.S. Orange, et al., Viral evasion of natural killer cells, Nat. Immunol. 3 (2002) 1006–1012.

[348] K. Natarajan, et al., Structure and function of natural killer cell receptors: multiple molecular solutions to self, nonself discrimination, Annu. Rev. Immunol. 20 (2002) 853–885.

[349] P. Parham, Taking license with natural killer cell maturation and repertoire development, Immunol. Rev. 214 (2006) 155–160.

[350] L.L. Lanier, NK cell receptors, Annu. Rev. Immunol. 16 (1998) 359–393.

[351] C.A. O'Callaghan, Natural killer cell surveillance of intracellular antigen processing pathways mediated by recognition of HLA-E and Qa-1b by CD94/NKG2 receptors, Microbes Infect. 2 (2000) 371–380.

[352] B.A. Croy, et al., Update on pathways regulating the activation of uterine natural killer cells, their interactions with decidual spiral arteries and homing of their precursors to the uterus, J. Reprod. Immunol. 59 (2003) 175–191.

[353] E. Morel, T. Bellon, HLA class I molecules regulate IFN-gamma production induced in NK cells by target cells, viral products, or immature dendritic cells through the inhibitory receptor ILT2/CD85j, J. Immunol. 181 (2008) 2368–2381.

[354] P. Engel, M.J. Eck, C. Terhorst, The SAP and SLAM families in immune responses and X-linked lymphoproliferative disease, Nat. Rev. Immunol. 3 (2003) 813–821.

[355] J. Wu, et al., Intracellular retention of the MHC class I-related chain B ligand of NKG2D by the human cytomegalovirus UL16 glycoprotein, J. Immunol. 170 (2003) 4196–4200.

[356] M.R. Snyder, C.M. Weyand, J.J. Goronzy, The double life of NK receptors: stimulation or co-stimulation? Trends Immunol. 25 (2004) 25–32.

[357] L.L. Lanier, On guard—activating NK cell receptors, Nat. Immunol. 2 (2001) 23–27.

[358] M. Carretero, et al., Mitogen-activated protein kinase activity is involved in effector functions triggered by the CD94/NKG2-C NK receptor specific for HLA-E, Eur. J. Immunol. 30 (2000) 2842–2848.

[359] T.I. Arnon, et al., The mechanisms controlling the recognition of tumor- and virus-infected cells by NKp46, Blood 103 (2004) 664–672.

[360] Y. Oshimi, et al., Involvement of Fas ligand and Fas-mediated pathway in the cytotoxicity of human natural killer cells, J. Immunol. 157 (1996) 2909–2915.

[361] L. Zamai, et al., Natural killer (NK) cell-mediated cytotoxicity: differential use of TRAIL and Fas ligand my immature and mature primary human NK cells, J. Exp. Med. 188 (1998) 2375–2380.

[362] P.D. Arkwright, et al., Cytomegalovirus infection in infants with autoimmune lymphoproliferative syndrome (ALPS), Clin. Exp. Immunol. 121 (2000) 353–357.

[363] C.M. Eischen, et al., Fc receptor-induced expression of Fas ligand on activated NK cells facilitates cell-mediated cytotoxicity and subsequent autocrine NK cell apoptosis, J. Immunol. 156 (1996) 2693–2699.

[364] J.P. Lodolce, et al., IL-15 receptor maintains lymphoid homeostasis by supporting lymphocyte homing and proliferation, Immunity 9 (1998) 669–676.

[365] O. Salvucci, et al., Differential regulation of interleukin-12- and interleukin-15-induced natural killer cell activation by interleukin-4, Eur. J. Immunol. 26 (1996) 2736–2741.

[366] D.K. Dalton, et al., Multiple defects of immune cell function in mice with disrupted interferon-gamma genes, Science 259 (1993) 1739–1742.

[367] J. Magram, et al., IL-12-deficient mice are defective but not devoid of type 1 cytokine responses, Ann. N Y Acad. Sci. 795 (1996) 60–70.

[368] K. Takeda, et al., Defective NK cell activity and Th1 response in IL-18-deficient mice, Immunity 8 (1998) 383–390.

[369] F. Mainiero, et al., Integrin-mediated ras-extracellular regulated kinase (ERK) signaling regulates interferon gamma production in human natural killer cells, J. Exp. Med. 188 (1998) 1267–1275.

[370] C.A. Hunter, R. Chizzonite, J.S. Remington, IL-1 beta is required for IL-12 to induce production of IFN-gamma by NK cells: a role for IL-1 beta in the T cell-independent mechanism of resistance against intracellular pathogens, J. Immunol. 155 (1995) 4347–4354.

[371] E.M. Bluman, et al., Human natural killer cells produce abundant macrophage inflammatory protein-1 alpha in response to monocyte-derived cytokines, J. Clin. Invest. 97 (1996) 2722–2727.

[372] C.H. Tay, E. Szomolanyi-Tsuda, R.M. Welsh, Control of infections by NK cells, Curr. Top. Microbiol. Immunol. 230 (1998) 193–220.

[373] H.B. Bernstein, et al., Neonatal natural killer cells produce chemokines and suppress HIV replication in vitro, AIDS Res. Hum. Retroviruses 20 (2004) 1189–1195.

[374] K.F. Bradstock, C. Luxford, P.G. Grimsley, Functional and phenotypic assessment of neonatal human leucocytes expressing natural killer cell-associated antigens, Immunol. Cell. Biol. 71 (1993) 535–542.

[375] Y. Sundstrom, et al., The expression of human natural killer cell receptors in early life, Scand. J. Immunol. 66 (2007) 335–344.

[376] J.H. Dalle, et al., Characterization of cord blood natural killer cells: implications for transplantation and neonatal infections, Pediatr. Res. 57 (2005) 649–655.

[377] E. Braakman, et al., Expression of CD45 isoforms by fresh and activated human gamma delta T lymphocytes and natural killer cells, Int. Immunol. 3 (1991) 691–697.

[378] S. Kohl, M. Sigouroudinia, E.G. Engleman, Adhesion defects of antibody-mediated target cell binding of neonatal natural killer cells, Pediatr. Res. 46 (1999) 755–759.

[379] G.D. Georgeson, et al., Natural killer cell cytotoxicity is deficient in newborns with sepsis and recurrent infections, Eur. J. Pediatr. 160 (2001) 478–482.

[380] J.D. Merrill, M. Sigaroudinia, S. Kohl, Characterization of natural killer and antibody-dependent cellular cytotoxicity of preterm infants against human immunodeficiency virus-infected cells, Pediatr. Res. 40 (1996) 498–503.

[381] B.J. Webb, et al., The lack of NK cytotoxicity associated with fresh HUCB may be due to the presence of soluble HLA in the serum, Cell. Immunol. 159 (1994) 246–261.

[382] C.J. Harrison, J.L. Waner, Natural killer cell activity in infants and children excreting cytomegalovirus, J. Infect. Dis. 151 (1985) 301–307.

[383] M. Jenkins, J. Mills, S. Kohl, Natural killer cytotoxicity and antibody-dependent cellular cytotoxicity of human immunodeficiency virus-infected cells by leukocytes from human neonates and adults, Pediatr. Res. 33 (1993) 469–474.

[384] T. McDonald, et al., Natural killer cell activity in very low birth weight infants, Pediatr. Res. 31 (1992) 376–380.

[385] J. Gaddy, G. Risdon, H.E. Broxmeyer, Cord blood natural killer cells are functionally and phenotypically immature but readily respond to interleukin-2 and interleukin-12, J. Interferon Cytokine Res. 15 (1995) 527–536.

[386] Q.H. Nguyen, et al., Interleukin (IL)-15 enhances antibody-dependent cellular cytotoxicity and natural killer activity in neonatal cells, Cell. Immunol. 185 (1998) 83–92.

[387] P. Han, et al., Phenotypic analysis of functional T-lymphocyte subtypes and natural killer cells in human cord blood: relevance to umbilical cord blood transplantation, Br. J. Haematol. 89 (1995) 733–740.

[388] S.J. Lin, et al., Effect of interleukin-15 and Flt3-ligand on natural killer cell expansion and activation: umbilical cord vs. adult peripheral blood mononuclear cells, Pediatr. Allergy Immunol. 11 (2000) 168–174.

[389] R. Condiotti, A. Nagler, Effect of interleukin-12 on antitumor activity of human umbilical cord blood and bone marrow cytotoxic cells, Exp. Hematol. 26 (1998) 571–579.

[390] Z. Brahmi, et al., NK cells recover early and mediate cytotoxicity via perforin/granzyme and Fas/FasL pathways in umbilical cord blood recipients, Hum. Immunol. 62 (2001) 782–790.

[391] A. Nomura, et al., Functional analysis of cord blood natural killer cells and T cells: a distinctive interleukin-18 response, Exp. Hematol. 29 (2001) 1169–1176.

[392] S. Schatt, W. Holzgreve, S. Hahn, Stimulated cord blood lymphocytes have a low percentage of Th1 and Th2 cytokine secreting T cells although their activation is similar to adult controls, Immunol. Lett. 77 (2001) 1–2.

[393] IMGT/HLA, database (http://www.ebi.ac.uk/imgt/hla/), accessed 12-09.

[394] J.W. Yewdell, Plumbing the sources of endogenous MHC class I peptide ligands, Curr. Opin. Immunol. 19 (2007) 79–86.

[395] A. Le Bon, D.F. Tough, I. Type, interferon as a stimulus for cross-priming, Cytokine Growth Factor Rev. 19 (2008) 33–40.

[396] K. Tabeta, et al., The Unc93b1 mutation 3d disrupts exogenous antigen presentation and signaling via Toll-like receptors 3, 7 and 9, Nat. Immunol. 7 (2006) 156–164.

[397] A.R. Mantegazza, et al., NADPH oxidase controls phagosomal pH and antigen cross-presentation in human dendritic cells, Blood 112 (2008) 4712–4722.

[398] S. Fossum, The life history of dendritic leukocytes (DL), Curr. Top. Pathol. 79 (1989) 101–124.

[399] C.A. Keever, et al., Characterization of the alloreactivity and anti-leukemia reactivity of cord blood mononuclear cells, Bone Marrow Transplant. 15 (1995) 407–419.

[400] D.H. Canaday, et al., Class II MHC antigen presentation defect in neonatal monocytes is not correlated with decreased MHC-II expression, Cell. Immunol. 243 (2006) 96–106.

[401] F. Garban, et al., Detection of empty HLA class II molecules on cord blood B cells, Blood 87 (1996) 3970–3976.

[402] J.D. Miller, et al., Analysis of HLA-E peptide-binding specificity and contact residues in bound peptide required for recognition by CD94/NKG2, J. Immunol. 171 (2003) 1369–1375.

[403] A. Ishitani, N. Sageshima, K. Hatake, The involvement of HLA-E and -F in pregnancy, J. Reprod. Immunol. 69 (2006) 101–113.

[404] J.S. Hunt, Stranger in a strange land, Immunol. Rev. 213 (2006) 36–47.

[405] S. Fournel, et al., Cutting edge: soluble HLA-G1 triggers CD95/CD95 ligand-mediated apoptosis in activated CD8+ cells by interacting with CD8, J. Immunol. 164 (2000) 6100–6104.

[406] P. Contini, et al., Soluble HLA-A,-B,-C and -G molecules induce apoptosis in T and NK CD8+ cells and inhibit cytotoxic T cell activity through CD8 ligation, Eur. J. Immunol. 33 (2003) 125–134.

[407] N. Stern-Ginossar, et al., Human microRNAs regulate stress-induced immune responses mediated by the receptor NKG2D, Nat. Immunol. 9 (2008) 1065–1073.

[408] H. Das, et al., MICA engagement by human Vgamma2Vdelta2 T cells enhances their antigen-dependent effector function, Immunity 15 (2001) 83–93.

[409] S. Gonzalez, V. Groh, T. Spies, Immunobiology of human NKG2D and its ligands, Curr. Top. Microbiol. Immunol. 298 (2006) 121–138.

[410] D.C. Barral, M.B. Brenner, CD1 antigen presentation: how it works, Nat. Rev. Immunol. 7 (2007) 929–941.

[411] E. Tupin, Y. Kinjo, M. Kronenberg, The unique role of natural killer T cells in the response to microorganisms, Nat. Rev. Microbiol. 5 (2007) 405–417.

[412] J. Gordon, et al., Functional evidence for a single endodermal origin for the thymic epithelium, Nat. Immunol. 5 (2004) 546–553.

[413] G. Hollander, et al., Cellular and molecular events during early thymus development, Immunol. Rev. 209 (2006) 28–46.

[414] D.L. Guris, et al., Dose-dependent interaction of Tbx1 and Crkl and locally aberrant RA signaling in a model of del22q11 syndrome, Dev. Cell 10 (2006) 81–92.

[415] R. Haddad, et al., Dynamics of thymus-colonizing cells during human development, Immunity 24 (2006) 217–230.

[416] E.M. Six, et al., A human postnatal lymphoid progenitor capable of circulating and seeding the thymus, J. Exp. Med. 204 (2007) 3085–3093.

[417] F. Weerkamp, et al., Human thymus contains multipotent progenitors with T/B lymphoid, myeloid, and erythroid lineage potential, Blood 107 (2006) 3131–3137.

[418] J. Maes, et al., Lymphoid-affiliated genes are associated with active histone modifications in human hematopoietic stem cells, Blood 112 (2008) 2722–2729.

[419] D.L. Kraft, I.L. Weissman, E.K. Waller, Differentiation of CD3–4–8– human fetal thymocytes in vivo: characterization of a CD3–4+8– intermediate, J. Exp. Med. 178 (1993) 265–277.

[420] F.J. Staal, T.C. Luis, M.M. Tiemessen, WNT signalling in the immune system: WNT is spreading its wings, Nat. Rev. Immunol. 8 (2008) 581–593.

[421] A. Misslitz, G. Bernhardt, R. Forster, Trafficking on serpentines: molecular insight on how maturating T cells find their winding paths in the thymus, Immunol. Rev. 209 (2006) 115–128.

[422] E. Horst, et al., The ontogeny of human lymphocyte recirculation: high endothelial cell antigen (HECA-452) and CD44 homing receptor expression in the development of the immune system, Eur. J. Immunol. 20 (1990) 1483–1489.

[423] N.E. Gilhus, R. Matre, O. Tonder, Hassall's corpuscles in the thymus of fetuses, infants and children: immunological and histochemical aspects, Thymus 7 (1985) 123–135.

[424] S.G. Kitchen, J.A. Zack, Distribution of the human immunodeficiency virus coreceptors CXCR4 and CCR5 in fetal lymphoid organs: implications for pathogenesis in utero, AIDS Res. Hum. Retroviruses 15 (1999) 143–148.

[425] P. Vandenberghe, et al., In situ expression of B7/BB1 on antigen-presenting cells and activated B cells: an immunohistochemical study, Int. Immunol. 5 (1993) 317–321.

[426] S.B. Ramos, et al., Phenotypic and functional evaluation of natural killer cells in thymectomized children, Clin. Immunol. Immunopathol. 81 (1996) 277–281.

[427] F. Weerkamp, et al., Age-related changes in the cellular composition of the thymus in children, J. Allergy Clin. Immunol. 115 (2005) 834–840.

[428] C.D. Baroni, et al., The human thymus in ageing: histologic involution paralleled by increased mitogen response and by enrichment of OKT3+ lymphocytes, Immunology 50 (1983) 519–528.

[429] J.F. Poulin, et al., Direct evidence for thymic function in adult humans, J. Exp. Med. 190 (1999) 479–486.

[430] C.L. Mackall, et al., Age, thymopoiesis, and CD4+ T-lymphocyte regeneration after intensive chemotherapy, N. Engl. J. Med. 332 (1995) 143–149.

[431] F.T. Hakim, et al., Age-dependent incidence, time course, and consequences of thymic renewal in adults, J. Clin. Invest. 115 (2005) 930–939.
[432] N. Vrisekoop, et al., Sparse production but preferential incorporation of recently produced naive T cells in the human peripheral pool, Proc. Natl. Acad. Sci. U S A 105 (2008) 6115–6120.
[433] C.J. Haines, et al., Human CD4+ T cell recent thymic emigrants are identified by protein tyrosine kinase 7 and have reduced immune function, J. Exp. Med. 206 (2009) 275–285.
[434] M. Guimond, T.J. Fry, C.L. Mackall, Cytokine signals in T-cell homeostasis, J. Immunother. 28 (2005) 289–294.
[435] C. Sportes, et al., Administration of rhIL-7 in humans increases in vivo TCR repertoire diversity by preferential expansion of naive T cell subsets, J. Exp. Med. 205 (2008) 1701–1714.
[436] M.R. Lieber, et al., Flexibility in the order of action and in the enzymology of the nuclease, polymerases, and ligase of vertebrate non-homologous DNA end joining: relevance to cancer, aging, and the immune system, Cell Res. 18 (2008) 125–133.
[437] R.H. Buckley, Molecular defects in human severe combined immunodeficiency and approaches to immune reconstitution, Annu. Rev. Immunol. 22 (2004) 625–655.
[438] T.P. Arstila, et al., A direct estimate of the human alphabeta T cell receptor diversity, Science 286 (1999) 958–961.
[439] J. Westermann, R. Pabst, Distribution of lymphocyte subsets and natural killer cells in the human body, Clin. Invest. 70 (1992) 539–544.
[440] A.T. Haase, Population biology of HIV-1 infection: viral and CD4+ T cell demographics and dynamics in lymphatic tissues, Annu. Rev. Immunol. 17 (1999) 625–656.
[441] S.O. Schonland, et al., Homeostatic control of T-cell generation in neonates, Blood 102 (2003) 1428–1434.
[442] W.A. Dik, et al., New insights on human T cell development by quantitative T cell receptor gene rearrangement studies and gene expression profiling, J. Exp. Med. 201 (2005) 1715–1723.
[443] S. Yamasaki, T. Saito, Molecular basis for pre-TCR-mediated autonomous signaling, Trends Immunol. 28 (2007) 39–43.
[444] H. von Boehmer, Selection of the T-cell repertoire: receptor-controlled checkpoints in T-cell development, Adv. Immunol. 84 (2004) 201–238.
[445] E. Padovan, et al., Normal T lymphocytes can express two different T cell receptor beta chains: implications for the mechanism of allelic exclusion, J. Exp. Med. 181 (1995) 1587–1591.
[446] A.R. Ramiro, et al., Regulation of pre-T cell receptor (pT alpha-TCR beta) gene expression during human thymic development, J. Exp. Med. 184 (1996) 519–530.
[447] E. Padovan, et al., Expression of two T cell receptor alpha chains: dual receptor T cells, Science 262 (1993) 422–424.
[448] J.F. George Jr., H.W. Schroeder Jr., Developmental regulation of D beta reading frame and junctional diversity in T cell receptor-beta transcripts from human thymus, J. Immunol. 148 (1992) 1230–1239.
[449] F.M. Raaphorst, et al., Non-random employment of V beta 6 and J beta gene elements and conserved amino acid usage profiles in CDR3 regions of human fetal and adult TCR beta chain rearrangements, Int. Immunol. 6 (1994) 1–9.
[450] F.M. Raaphorst, et al., Usage of TCRAV and TCRBV gene families in human fetal and adult TCR rearrangements, Immunogenetics 39 (1994) 343–350.
[451] A. Bonati, et al., T-cell receptor beta–chain gene rearrangement and expression during human thymic ontogenesis, Blood 79 (1992) 1472–1483.
[452] T.H. Thai, J.F. Kearney, Distinct and opposite activities of human terminal deoxynucleotidyltransferase splice variants, J. Immunol. 173 (2004) 4009–4019.
[453] B.A. Vandekerckhove, et al., Thymic selection of the human T cell receptor V beta repertoire in SCID-hu mice, J. Exp. Med. 176 (1992) 1619–1624.
[454] L. Garderet, et al., The umbilical cord blood alphabeta T-cell repertoire: characteristics of a polyclonal and naïve but completely formed repertoire, Blood 91 (1998) 340–346.
[455] M.A. Hall, J.L. Reid, J.S. Lanchbury, The distribution of human TCR junctional region lengths shifts with age in both CD4 and CD8 T cells, Int. Immunol. 10 (1998) 1407–1419.
[456] Z.C. Kou, et al., T-cell receptor Vbeta repertoire CDR3 length diversity differs within CD45RA and CD45RO T-cell subsets in healthy and human immunodeficiency virus-infected children, Clin. Diagn. Lab. Immunol. 7 (2000) 953–959.
[457] R. van den Beemd, et al., Flow cytometric analysis of the Vbeta repertoire in healthy controls, Cytometry 40 (2000) 336–345.
[458] M.M. Davis, The evolutionary and structural 'logic' of antigen receptor diversity, Semin. Immunol. 16 (2004) 239–243.
[459] S. Gilfillan, et al., Efficient immune responses in mice lacking N-region diversity, Eur. J. Immunol. 25 (1995) 3115–3122.
[460] R.L. Schelonka, et al., T cell receptor repertoire diversity and clonal expansion in human neonates, Pediatr. Res. 43 (1998) 396–402.
[461] J. Grunewald, C.H. Janson, H. Wigzell, Biased expression of individual T cell receptor V gene segments in CD4+ and CD8+ human peripheral blood T lymphocytes, Eur. J. Immunol. 21 (1991) 819–822.
[462] M.L. Dion, R.P. Sekaly, R. Cheynier, Estimating thymic function through quantification of T-cell receptor excision circles, Methods Mol. Biol. 380 (2007) 197–213.
[463] M.L. Dion, et al., HIV infection rapidly induces and maintains a substantial suppression of thymocyte proliferation, Immunity 21 (2004) 757–768.
[464] M.D. Hazenberg, et al., T cell receptor excision circles as markers for recent thymic emigrants: basic aspects, technical approach, and guidelines for interpretation, J. Mol. Med. 79 (2001) 631–640.
[465] Y. Okamoto, et al., Effects of exogenous interleukin-7 on human thymus function, Blood 99 (2002) 2851–2858.
[466] R.D. McFarland, et al., Identification of a human recent thymic emigrant phenotype, Proc. Natl. Acad. Sci. U S A 97 (2000) 4215–4220.
[467] J.J. Bell, A. Bhandoola, Putting ThPOK in place, Nat. Immunol. 9 (2008) 1095–1097.
[468] K. Honey, et al., Cathepsin L regulates CD4+ T cell selection independently of its effect on invariant chain: a role in the generation of positively selecting peptide ligands, J. Exp. Med. 195 (2002) 1349–1358.
[469] S. Murata, Y. Takahama, K. Tanaka, Thymoproteasome: probable role in generating positively selecting peptides, Curr. Opin. Immunol. 20 (2008) 192–196.
[470] K.A. Hogquist, T.A. Baldwin, S.C. Jameson, Central tolerance: learning self-control in the thymus, Nat. Rev. Immunol. 5 (2005) 772–782.
[471] P. Peterson, T. Org, A. Rebane, Transcriptional regulation by AIRE: molecular mechanisms of central tolerance, Nat. Rev. Immunol. 8 (2008) 948–957.
[472] J. Zerrahn, W. Held, D.H. Raulet, The MHC reactivity of the T cell repertoire prior to positive and negative selection, Cell 88 (1997) 627–636.
[473] D. Housset, B. Malissen, What do TCR-pMHC crystal structures teach us about MHC restriction and alloreactivity? Trends Immunol. 24 (2003) 429–437.
[474] M. Pesu, et al., Jak3, severe combined immunodeficiency, and a new class of immunosuppressive drugs, Immunol. Rev. 203 (2005) 127–142.
[475] R. Ceredig, A.L. Glasebrook, H.R. MacDonald, Phenotypic and functional properties of murine thymocytes, I: precursors of cytolytic T lymphocytes and interleukin 2-producing cells are all contained within a subpopulation of "mature" thymocytes as analyzed by monoclonal antibodies and flow microfluorometry, J. Exp. Med. 155 (1982) 358–379.
[476] R. Ceredig, et al., Precursors of T cell growth factor producing cells in the thymus: ontogeny, frequency, and quantitative recovery in a subpopulation of phenotypically mature thymocytes defined by monoclonal antibody GK-1.5, J. Exp. Med. 158 (1983) 1654–1671.
[477] M.A. Weinreich, K.A. Hogquist, Thymic emigration: when and how T cells leave home, J. Immunol. 181 (2008) 2265–2270.
[478] P. Blume-Jensen, T. Hunter, Oncogenic kinase signalling, Nature 411 (2001) 355–365.
[479] S.C. De Rosa, L.A. Herzenberg, M. Roederer, 11-color, 13-parameter flow cytometry: identification of human naive T cells by phenotype, function, and T-cell receptor diversity, Nat. Med. 7 (2001) 245–248.
[480] S.R. Schwab, J.G. Cyster, Finding a way out: lymphocyte egress from lymphoid organs, Nat. Immunol. 8 (2007) 1295–1301.
[481] B. Xu, et al., Lymphocyte homing to bronchus-associated lymphoid tissue (BALT) is mediated by L-selectin/PNAd, alpha4beta1 integrin/VCAM-1, and LFA-1 adhesion pathways, J. Exp. Med. 197 (2003) 1255–1267.
[482] M.F. Vondenhoff, G. Kraal, R.E. Mebius, Lymphoid organogenesis in brief, Eur. J. Immunol. 37 (Suppl. 1) (2007) S46–S52.
[483] R. Forster, A.C. Davalos-Misslitz, A. Rot, CCR7 and its ligands: balancing immunity and tolerance, Nat. Rev. Immunol. 8 (2008) 362–371.
[484] C.D. Surh, J. Sprent, Homeostasis of naive and memory T cells, Immunity 29 (2008) 848–862.
[485] G.S. Pahal, et al., Normal development of human fetal hematopoiesis between eight and seventeen weeks' gestation, Am. J. Obstet. Gynecol. 183 (2000) 1029–1034.
[486] U. Settmacher, et al., Characterization of human lymphocytes separated from fetal liver and spleen at different stages of ontogeny, Immunobiology 182 (1991) 256–265.
[487] I. Hannet, et al., Developmental and maturational changes in human blood lymphocyte subpopulations, Immunol. Today 13 (1992) 218.
[488] K. Sato, et al., Chemokine receptor expressions and responsiveness of cord blood T cells, J. Immunol. 166 (2001) 1659–1666.
[489] S. Kimmig, et al., Two subsets of naïve T helper cells with distinct T cell receptor excision circle content in human adult peripheral blood, J. Exp. Med. 195 (2002) 789–794.
[490] S. Kohler, et al., Post-thymic in vivo proliferation of naive CD4+ T cells constrains the TCR repertoire in healthy human adults, Eur. J. Immunol. 35 (2005) 1987–1994.
[491] G. Delespesse, et al., Maturation of human neonatal CD4+ and CD8+ T lymphocytes into Th1/Th2 effectors, Vaccine 16 (1998) 1415–1419.
[492] M. Wilson, et al., Ontogeny of human T and B lymphocytes during stressed and normal gestation: phenotypic analysis of umbilical cord lymphocytes from term and preterm infants, Clin. Immunol. Immunopathol. 37 (1985) 1–12.
[493] A. Tsegaye, et al., Immunophenotyping of blood lymphocytes at birth, during childhood, and during adulthood in HIV-1-uninfected Ethiopians, Clin. Immunol. 109 (2003) 338–346.
[494] G.E. Asma, R.L. Van den Bergh, J.M. Vossen, Use of monoclonal antibodies in a study of the development of T lymphocytes in the human fetus, Clin. Exp. Immunol. 53 (1983) 429–436.
[495] N.I. Rallon, et al., Level, phenotype and activation status of CD4+FoxP3+ regulatory T cells in patients chronically infected with human immunodeficiency virus and/or hepatitis C virus, Clin. Exp. Immunol. 155 (2009) 35–43.

[496] J. Hassan, D.J. Reen, IL-7 promotes the survival and maturation but not differentiation of human post-thymic CD4+ T cells, Eur. J. Immunol. 28 (1998) 3057–3065.

[497] M. Peakman, et al., Analysis of lymphocyte phenotypes in cord blood from early gestation fetuses, Clin. Exp. Immunol. 90 (1992) 345–350.

[498] J.A. Byrne, A.K. Stankovic, M.D. Cooper, A novel subpopulation of primed T cells in the human fetus, J. Immunol. 152 (1994) 3098–3106.

[499] M. Bofill, et al., Immature CD45RA(low) RO(low) T cells in the human cord blood, I: antecedents of CD45RA+ unprimed T cells, J. Immunol. 152 (1994) 5613–5623.

[500] A. D'Andrea, L.L. Lanier, Killer cell inhibitory receptor expression by T cells, Curr. Top. Microbiol. Immunol. 230 (1998) 25–39.

[501] M. Azuma, et al., Requirements for CD28-dependent T cell-mediated cytotoxicity, J. Immunol. 150 (1993) 2091–2101.

[502] M. Azuma, J.H. Phillips, L.L. Lanier, CD28– lymphocytes: antigenic and functional properties, J. Immunol. 150 (1993) 1147–1159.

[503] L. Frenkel, Y.J. Bryson, Ontogeny of phytohemagglutinin-induced gamma interferon by leukocytes of healthy infants and children: evidence for decreased production in infants younger than 2 months of age, J. Pediatr. 111 (1987) 97–100.

[504] H. Spits, Development of alphabeta T cells in the human thymus, Nat. Rev. Immunol. 2 (2002) 760–772.

[505] T. Cupedo, et al., Development and activation of regulatory T cells in the human fetus, Eur. J. Immunol. 35 (2005) 383–390.

[506] J. Michaelsson, et al., Regulation of T cell responses in the developing human fetus, J. Immunol. 176 (2006) 5741–5748.

[507] A.B. Lyons, Analysing cell division in vivo and in vitro using flow cytometric measurement of CFSE dye dilution, J. Immunol. Methods 243 (2000) 147–154.

[508] I. Marcolino, et al., Frequent expression of the natural killer cell receptor KLRG1 in human cord blood T cells: correlation with replicative history, Eur. J. Immunol. 34 (2004) 2672–2680.

[509] B. Min, et al., Neonates support lymphopenia-induced proliferation, Immunity 18 (2003) 131–140.

[510] T. Fukui, et al., IL-7 induces proliferation, variable cytokine-producing ability and IL-2 responsiveness in naïve CD4+ T-cells from human cord blood, Immunol. Lett. 59 (1997) 21–28.

[511] J. Hassan, D.J. Reen, Human recent thymic emigrants—identification, expansion, and survival characteristics, J. Immunol. 167 (2001) 1970–1976.

[512] V. Dardalhon, et al., IL-7 differentially regulates cell cycle progression and HIV-1-based vector infection in neonatal and adult CD4+ T cells, Proc. Natl. Acad. Sci. U S A 98 (2001) 9277–9282.

[513] K.J. Hare, E.J. Jenkinson, G. Anderson, An essential role for the IL-7 receptor during intrathymic expansion of the positively selected neonatal T cell repertoire, J. Immunol. 165 (2000) 2410–2414.

[514] H. Okazaki, et al., IL-7 promotes thymocyte proliferation and maintains immunocompetent thymocytes bearing alpha beta or gamma delta T-cell receptors in vitro: synergism with IL-2, J. Immunol. 143 (1989) 2917–2922.

[515] M.V. Soares, et al., IL-7-dependent extrathymic expansion of CD45RA+ T cells enables preservation of a naïve repertoire, J. Immunol. 161 (1998) 5909–5917.

[516] L.M. Webb, B.M. Foxwell, M. Feldmann, Putative role for interleukin-7 in the maintenance of the recirculating naïve CD4+ T-cell pool, Immunology 98 (1999) 400–405.

[517] A.F. Buckley, C.T. Kuo, J.M. Leiden, Transcription factor LKLF is sufficient to program T cell quiescence via a c-Myc-dependent pathway, Nat. Immunol. 2 (2001) 698–704.

[518] J.E. Smith-Garvin, G.A. Koretzky, M.S. Jordan, T cell activation, Annu. Rev. Immunol. 27 (2009) 591–619.

[519] M.L. Dustin, Visualization of cell-cell interaction contacts—synapses and kinapses, Adv. Exp. Med. Biol. 640 (2008) 164–182.

[520] S. Feske, Calcium signalling in lymphocyte activation and disease, Nat. Rev. Immunol. 7 (2007) 690–702.

[521] I. Puga, A. Rao, F. Macian, Targeted cleavage of signaling proteins by caspase 3 inhibits T cell receptor signaling in anergic T cells, Immunity 29 (2008) 193–204.

[522] M.E. Keir, et al., PD-1 and its ligands in tolerance and immunity, Annu. Rev. Immunol. 26 (2008) 677–704.

[523] B. Spellberg, J.E. Edwards Jr., Type 1/type 2 immunity in infectious diseases, Clin. Infect. Dis. 32 (2001) 76–102.

[524] S.A. Quezada, et al., CD40/CD154 interactions at the interface of tolerance and immunity, Annu. Rev. Immunol. 22 (2004) 307–328.

[525] L.D. Notarangelo, et al., Defects of class-switch recombination, J. Allergy Clin. Immunol. 117 (2006) 855–864.

[526] C.B. Wilson, et al., Decreased production of interferon-gamma by human neonatal cells: intrinsic and regulatory deficiencies, J. Clin. Invest. 77 (1986) 860–867.

[527] D.B. Lewis, A. Larsen, C.B. Wilson, Reduced interferon-gamma mRNA levels in human neonates: evidence for an intrinsic T cell deficiency independent of other genes involved in T cell activation, J. Exp. Med. 163 (1986) 1018–1023.

[528] D.B. Lewis, et al., Cellular and molecular mechanisms for reduced interleukin 4 and interferon-gamma production by neonatal T cells, J. Clin. Invest. 87 (1991) 194–202.

[529] M. Cayabyab, J.H. Phillips, L.L. Lanier, CD40 preferentially costimulates activation of CD4+ T lymphocytes, J. Immunol. 152 (1994) 1523–1531.

[530] J. Hassan, et al., Signalling via CD28 of human naïve neonatal T lymphocytes, Clin. Exp. Immunol. 102 (1995) 192–198.

[531] J. Hassan, E. Rainsford, D.J. Reen, Linkage of protein kinase C-beta activation and intracellular interleukin-2 accumulation in human naïve CD4 T cells, Immunology 92 (1997) 465–471.

[532] J. Hassan, D.J. Reen, Cord blood CD4+CD45RA+ T cells achieve a lower magnitude of activation when compared with their adult counterparts, Immunology 90 (1997) 397–401.

[533] L. Chen, A.C. Cohen, D.B. Lewis, Impaired allogeneic activation and T-helper 1 differentiation of human cord blood naive CD4 T cells, Biol. Blood Marrow Transplant. 12 (2006) 160–171.

[534] S. Saito, et al., Expression of the interleukin-2 receptor gamma chain on cord blood mononuclear cells, Blood 87 (1996) 3344–3350.

[535] B.A. Chilmonczyk, et al., Characterization of the human newborn response to herpesvirus antigen, J. Immunol. 134 (1985) 4184–4188.

[536] J. Hassan, D.J. Reen, Reduced primary antigen-specific T-cell precursor frequencies in neonates is associated with deficient interleukin-2 production, Immunology 87 (1996) 604–608.

[537] N. Takahashi, et al., Evidence for immunologic immaturity of cord blood T cells: cord blood T cells are susceptible to tolerance induction to in vitro stimulation with a superantigen, J. Immunol. 155 (1995) 5213–5219.

[538] K. Imanishi, et al., Post-thymic maturation of migrating human thymic single-positive T cells: thymic CD1a-CD4+ T cells are more susceptible to anergy induction by toxic shock syndrome toxin-1 than cord blood CD4+ T cells, J. Immunol. 160 (1998) 112–119.

[539] N. Takahashi, et al., Immunopathophysiological aspects of an emerging neonatal infectious disease induced by a bacterial superantigen, J. Clin. Invest. 106 (2000) 1409–1415.

[540] P. Porcu, J. Gaddy, H.E. Broxmeyer, Alloantigen-induced unresponsiveness in cord blood T lymphocytes is associated with defective activation of Ras, Proc. Natl. Acad. Sci. U S A 95 (1998) 4538–4543.

[541] Y. Takahata, et al., CD25+CD4+ T cells in human cord blood: an immunoregulatory subset with naive phenotype and specific expression of forkhead box p3 (Foxp3) gene, Exp. Hematol. 32 (2004) 622–629.

[542] V. Appay, et al., Phenotype and function of human T lymphocyte subsets: consensus and issues, Cytometry A 73 (2008) 975–983.

[543] L.H. Glimcher, Lineage commitment in lymphocytes: controlling the immune response, J. Clin. Invest. 108 (2001) s25–s30.

[544] R.M. Locksley, The roaring twenties, Immunity 28 (2008) 437–439.

[545] H. Liu, C. Rohowsky-Kochan, Regulation of IL-17 in human CCR6+ effector memory T cells, J. Immunol. 180 (2008) 7948–7957.

[546] J.S. Silver, C.A. Hunter, With a little help from their friends: interleukin-21, T cells, and B cells, Immunity 29 (2008) 7–9.

[547] J. Rowe, et al., Heterogeneity in diphtheria-tetanus-acellular pertussis vaccine-specific cellular immunity during infancy: relationship to variations in the kinetics of postnatal maturation of systemic Th1 function, J. Infect. Dis. 184 (2001) 80–88.

[548] C.H. Kim, et al., Rules of chemokine receptor association with T cell polarization in vivo, J. Clin. Invest. 108 (2001) 1331–1339.

[549] A. Viola, B. Molon, R.L. Contento, Chemokines: coded messages for T-cell missions, Front. Biosci. 13 (2008) 6341–6353.

[550] I.R. Williams, CCR6 and CCL20: partners in intestinal immunity and lymphorganogenesis, Ann. N Y Acad. Sci. 1072 (2006) 52–61.

[551] C. King, S.G. Tangye, C.R. Mackay, T follicular helper (TFH) cells in normal and dysregulated immune responses, Annu. Rev. Immunol. 26 (2008) 741–766.

[552] H.J. Ramos, et al., IFN-alpha is not sufficient to drive Th1 development due to lack of stable T-bet expression, J. Immunol. 179 (2007) 3792–3803.

[553] A.M. Cleary, et al., Impaired accumulation and function of memory CD4 T cells in human IL-12 receptor beta 1 deficiency, J. Immunol. 170 (2003) 597–603.

[554] O. Filipe-Santos, et al., Inborn errors of IL-12/23- and IFN-gamma-mediated immunity: molecular, cellular, and clinical features, Semin. Immunol. 18 (2006) 347–361.

[555] S.A. Saenz, B.C. Taylor, D. Artis, Welcome to the neighborhood: epithelial cell-derived cytokines license innate and adaptive immune responses at mucosal sites, Immunol. Rev. 226 (2008) 172–190.

[556] T. Korn, et al., IL-17 and Th17 cells, Annu. Rev. Immunol. 27 (2009) 485–517.

[557] A.T. Bauquet, et al., The costimulatory molecule ICOS regulates the expression of c-Maf and IL-21 in the development of follicular T helper cells and T(H)-17 cells, Nat. Immunol. 10 (2009) 167–175.

[558] R. Ettinger, S. Kuchen, P.E. Lipsky, The role of IL-21 in regulating B-cell function in health and disease, Immunol. Rev. 223 (2008) 60–86.

[559] A.A. Schaffer, et al., Deconstructing common variable immunodeficiency by genetic analysis, Curr. Opin. Genet. Dev. 17 (2007) 201–212.

[560] H.D. Ochs, et al., The role of adhesion molecules in the regulation of antibody responses, Semin. Hematol. 30 (1993) 72–79.

[561] K. Takeda, et al., Essential role of Stat6 in IL-4 signalling, Nature 380 (1996) 627–630.

[562] R.S. Geha, H.H. Jabara, S.R. Brodeur, The regulation of immunoglobulin E class-switch recombination, Nat. Rev. Immunol. 3 (2003) 721–732.

[563] P.C. Beverley, Kinetics and clonality of immunological memory in humans, Semin. Immunol. 16 (2004) 315–321.

[564] L.E. Harrington, et al., Memory CD4 T cells emerge from effector T-cell progenitors, Nature 452 (2008) 356–360.

[565] N.P. Weng, et al., Human naïve and memory T lymphocytes differ in telomeric length and replicative potential, Proc. Natl. Acad. Sci. U S A 92 (1995) 11091–11094.

[566] N. Rufer, et al., Telomere length dynamics in human lymphocyte subpopulations measured by flow cytometry, Nat. Biotechnol. 16 (1998) 743–747.

[567] J.T. Chang, et al., Asymmetric T lymphocyte division in the initiation of adaptive immune responses, Science 315 (2007) 1687–1691.

[568] R. Ameratunga, et al., Defective antigen-induced lymphocyte proliferation in the X-linked hyper-IgM syndrome, J. Pediatr. 131 (1997) 147–150.

[569] J. Levy, et al., Clinical spectrum of X-linked hyper-IgM syndrome, J. Pediatr. 131 (1997) 47–54.

[570] D. Hamann, et al., Phenotypic and functional separation of memory and effector human CD8+ T cells, J. Exp. Med. 186 (1997) 1407–1418.

[571] A. Lanzavecchia, F. Sallusto, Understanding the generation and function of memory T cell subsets, Curr. Opin. Immunol. 17 (2005) 326–332.

[572] V. Appay, S.L. Rowland-Jones, Lessons from the study of T-cell differentiation in persistent human virus infection, Semin. Immunol. 16 (2004) 205–212.

[573] C.W. McMahon, D.H. Raulet, Expression and function of NK cell receptors in CD8+ T cells, Curr. Opin. Immunol. 13 (2001) 465–470.

[574] K. Ogasawara, L.L. Lanier, NKG2D in NK and T cell-mediated immunity, J. Clin. Immunol. 25 (2005) 534–540.

[575] L.T. van der Veken, et al., Functional analysis of killer Ig-like receptor-expressing cytomegalovirus-specific CD8+ T cells, J. Immunol. 182 (2009) 92–101.

[576] A. Lanzavecchia, F. Sallusto, Progressive differentiation and selection of the fittest in the immune response, Nat. Rev. Immunol. 2 (2002) 982–987.

[577] V. Kalia, et al., Differentiation of memory B and T cells, Curr. Opin. Immunol. 18 (2006) 255–264.

[578] L. de Beaucoudrey, et al., Mutations in STAT3 and IL12RB1 impair the development of human IL-17-producing T cells, J. Exp. Med. 205 (2008) 1543–1550.

[579] W. Tu, et al., Persistent and selective deficiency of CD4+ T cell immunity to cytomegalovirus in immunocompetent young children, J. Immunol. 172 (2004) 3260–3267.

[580] M. Stubbe, et al., Characterization of a subset of antigen-specific human central memory CD4+ T lymphocytes producing effector cytokines, Eur. J. Immunol. 38 (2008) 273–282.

[581] D.C. Macallan, et al., Rapid turnover of effector-memory CD4(+) T cells in healthy humans, J. Exp. Med. 200 (2004) 255–260.

[582] C. Riou, et al., Convergence of TCR and cytokine signaling leads to FOXO3a phosphorylation and drives the survival of CD4+ central memory T cells, J. Exp. Med. 204 (2007) 79–91.

[583] A. Okoye, et al., Progressive CD4+ central memory T cell decline results in CD4+ effector memory insufficiency and overt disease in chronic SIV infection, J. Exp. Med. 204 (2007) 2171–2185.

[584] T.W. Hand, M. Morre, S.M. Kaech, Expression of IL-7 receptor alpha is necessary but not sufficient for the formation of memory CD8 T cells during viral infection, Proc. Natl. Acad. Sci. U S A 104 (2007) 11730–11735.

[585] J.R. Schoenborn, C.B. Wilson, Regulation of interferon-gamma during innate and adaptive immune responses, Adv. Immunol. 96 (2007) 41–101.

[586] L.S. Berenson, N. Ota, K.M. Murphy, Issues in T-helper 1 development—resolved and unresolved, Immunol. Rev. 202 (2004) 157–174.

[587] L.H. Glimcher, et al., Recent developments in the transcriptional regulation of cytolytic effector cells, Nat. Rev. Immunol. 4 (2004) 900–911.

[588] M.R. Chandok, et al., A biochemical signature for rapid recall of memory CD4 T cells, J. Immunol. 179 (2007) 3689–3698.

[589] H. Veiga-Fernandes, et al., Response of naive and memory CD8+ T cells to antigen stimulation in vivo, Nat. Immunol. 1 (2000) 47–53.

[590] G.T. Erbach, et al., Phenotypic characteristics of lymphoid populations of middle gestation human fetal liver, spleen and thymus, J. Reprod. Immunol. 25 (1993) 81–88.

[591] C. Schultz, et al., Reduced IL-10 production and -receptor expression in neonatal T lymphocytes, Acta Paediatr. 96 (2007) 1122–1125.

[592] B.K. English, et al., Production of lymphotoxin and tumor necrosis factor by human neonatal mononuclear cells, Pediatr. Res. 24 (1988) 717–722.

[593] G. Dolganov, et al., Coexpression of the interleukin-13 and interleukin-4 genes correlates with their physical linkage in the cytokine gene cluster on human chromosome 5q23-31, Blood 87 (1996) 3316–3326.

[594] D.B. Lewis, et al., Restricted production of interleukin 4 by activated human T cells, Proc. Natl. Acad. Sci. U S A 85 (1988) 9743–9747.

[595] M. Salmon, G.D. Kitas, P.A. Bacon, Production of lymphokine mRNA by CD45R+ and CD45R− helper T cells from human peripheral blood and by human CD4+ T cell clones, J. Immunol. 143 (1989) 907–912.

[596] F.M. Kloosterboer, et al., Similar potential to become activated and proliferate but differential kinetics and profiles of cytokine production of umbilical cord blood T cells and adult blood naive and memory T cells, Hum. Immunol. 67 (2006) 874–883.

[597] T. Jung, et al., Interleukin-13 is produced by activated human CD45RA+ and CD45RO+ T cells: modulation by interleukin-4 and interleukin-12, Eur. J. Immunol. 26 (1996) 571–577.

[598] M. Krampera, et al., Progressive polarization towards a T helper/cytotoxic type-1 cytokine pattern during age-dependent maturation of the immune response inversely correlates with CD30 cell expression and serum concentration, Clin. Exp. Immunol. 117 (1999) 291–297.

[599] M. Krampera, et al., Intracellular cytokine profile of cord blood T- and NK-cells and monocytes, Haematologica 85 (2000) 675–679.

[600] E. Rainsford, D.J. Reen, Interleukin 10, produced in abundance by human newborn T cells, may be the regulator of increased tolerance associated with cord blood stem cell transplantation, Br. J. Haematol. 116 (2002) 702–709.

[601] D.M. Mosser, X. Zhang, Interleukin-10: new perspectives on an old cytokine, Immunol. Rev. 226 (2008) 205–218.

[602] D. Hariharan, et al., C-C chemokine profile of cord blood mononuclear cells: RANTES production, Blood 95 (2000) 715–718.

[603] L.M. Ribeiro-do-Couto, et al., High IL-13 production by human neonatal T cells: neonate immune system regulator? Eur. J. Immunol. 31 (2001) 3394–3402.

[604] A. Vigano, et al., Differential development of type 1 and type 2 cytokines and beta-chemokines in the ontogeny of healthy newborns, Biol. Neonate 75 (1999) 1–8.

[605] A. Durandy, et al., Undetectable CD40 ligand expression on T cells and low B cell responses to CD40 binding agonists in human newborns, J. Immunol. 154 (1995) 1560–1568.

[606] D. Brugnoni, et al., Ineffective expression of CD40 ligand on cord blood T cells may contribute to poor immunoglobulin production in the newborn, Eur. J. Immunol. 24 (1994) 1919–1924.

[607] R. Fuleihan, D. Ahern, R.S. Geha, Decreased expression of the ligand for CD40 in newborn lymphocytes, Eur. J. Immunol. 24 (1994) 1925–1928.

[608] S. Nonoyama, et al., Diminished expression of CD40 ligand by activated neonatal T cells, J. Clin. Invest. 95 (1995) 66–75.

[609] V. Flamand, et al., CD40 ligation prevents neonatal induction of transplantation tolerance, J. Immunol. 160 (1998) 4666–4669.

[610] R. Fuleihan, D. Ahern, R.S. Geha, CD40 ligand expression is developmentally regulated in human thymocytes, Clin. Immunol. Immunopathol. 76 (1995) 52–58.

[611] P. Jullien, et al., Decreased CD154 expression by neonatal CD4+ T cells is due to limitations in both proximal and distal events of T cell activation, Int. Immunol. 15 (2003) 1461–1472.

[612] K. Sato, H. Nagayama, T.A. Takahashi, Aberrant CD3- and CD28-mediated signaling events in cord blood, J. Immunol. 162 (1999) 4464–4471.

[613] J.B. Splawski, et al., CD40 ligand is expressed and functional on activated neonatal T cells, J. Immunol. 156 (1996) 119–127.

[614] D.J. Reen, Activation and functional capacity of human neonatal CD4 T-cells, Vaccine 16 (1998) 1401–1408.

[615] Y. Ohshima, G. Delespesse, T cell-derived IL-4 and dendritic cell-derived IL-12 regulate the lymphokine-producing phenotype of alloantigen-primed naïve human CD4 T cells, J. Immunol. 158 (1997) 629–636.

[616] N.C. Matthews, et al., Sustained expression of CD154 (CD40L) and proinflammatory cytokine production by alloantigen-stimulated umbilical cord blood T cells, J. Immunol. 164 (2000) 6206–6212.

[617] J.B. Oliveira, S. Gupta, Disorders of apoptosis: mechanisms for autoimmunity in primary immunodeficiency diseases, J. Clin. Immunol. 28 (Suppl. 1) (2008) S20–S28.

[618] H. Iwama, et al., Serum concentrations of soluble Fas antigen and soluble Fas ligand in mother and newborn, Arch. Gynecol. Obstet. 263 (2000) 108–110.

[619] M. Oh-hora, A. Rao, Calcium signaling in lymphocytes, Curr. Opin. Immunol. 20 (2008) 250–258.

[620] H. Ansart-Pirenne, et al., Defective IL2 gene expression in newborn is accompanied with impaired tyrosine-phosphorylation in T cells, Pediatr. Res. 45 (1999) 409–413.

[621] C.S. Hii, et al., Selective deficiency in protein kinase C isoenzyme expression and inadequacy in mitogen-activated protein kinase activation in cord blood T cells, Biochem. J. 370 (2003) 497–503.

[622] S. Miscia, et al., Inefficient phospholipase C activation and reduced Lck expression characterize the signaling defect of umbilical cord T lymphocytes, J. Immunol. 163 (1999) 2416–2424.

[623] S. Kobayashi, et al., Association of CD26 with CD45RA outside lipid rafts attenuates cord blood T-cell activation, Blood 103 (2004) 1002–1010.

[624] D.R. Fitzpatrick, C.B. Wilson, Methylation and demethylation in the regulation of genes, cells, and responses in the immune system, Clin. Immunol. 109 (2003) 37–45.

[625] A.J. Melvin, et al., Hypomethylation of the interferon-gamma gene correlates with its expression by primary T-lineage cells, Eur. J. Immunol. 25 (1995) 426–430.

[626] G.P. White, et al., Differential patterns of methylation of the IFN-gamma promoter at CpG and non-CpG sites underlie differences in IFN-gamma gene expression between human neonatal and adult CD45RO− T cells, J. Immunol. 168 (2002) 2820–2827.

[627] Y. Suen, et al., Dysregulation of lymphokine production in the neonate and its impact on neonatal cell mediated immunity, Vaccine 16 (1998) 1369–1377.

[628] L.T. Clement, Isoforms of the CD45 common leukocyte antigen family: markers for human T-cell differentiation, J. Clin. Immunol. 12 (1992) 1–10.

[629] A. Hayward, M. Cosyns, Proliferative and cytokine responses by human newborn T cells stimulated with staphylococcal enterotoxin B, Pediatr. Res. 35 (1994) 293–298.

[630] H. Pirenne, et al., Comparison of T cell functional changes during childhood with the ontogeny of CDw29 and CD45RA expression on CD4+ T cells, Pediatr. Res. 32 (1992) 81–86.

[631] M. Cella, et al., Ligation of CD40 on dendritic cells triggers production of high levels of interleukin-12 and enhances T cell stimulatory capacity: T-T help via APC activation, J. Exp. Med. 184 (1996) 747–752.

[632] S. Kadereit, et al., Reduced NFAT1 protein expression in human umbilical cord blood T lymphocytes, Blood 94 (1999) 3101–3107.

[633] A. Kiani, et al., Regulation of interferon-gamma gene expression by nuclear factor of activated T cells, Blood 98 (2001) 1480–1488.

[634] R.M. O'Neill, D.J. Reen, Equivalent functional nuclear factor of activated T cell 1 mRNA and protein expression in cord blood and adult T cells, Transplantation 76 (2003) 1526–1528.

[635] F. Macian, C. Lopez-Rodriguez, A. Rao, Partners in transcription: NFAT and AP-1, Oncogene 20 (2001) 2476–2489.

[636] B. Adkins, Heterogeneity in the CD4 T cell compartment and the variability of neonatal immune responsiveness, Curr. Immunol. Rev. 3 (2007) 151–159.

[637] J. Lange, et al., High interleukin-13 production by phytohaemagglutinin- and Der p 1-stimulated cord blood mononuclear cells is associated with the subsequent development of atopic dermatitis at the age of 3 years, Clin. Exp. Allergy 33 (2003) 1537–1543.

[638] E. Early, D. Reen, Antigen-independent responsiveness to interleukin-4 demonstrates differential regulation of newborn human T cells, Eur. J. Immunol. 26 (1996) 2885–2889.

[639] D.M. Bullens, et al., Naïve human T cells can be a source of IL-4 during primary immune responses, Clin. Exp. Immunol. 118 (1999) 384–391.

[640] L. Rogge, et al., Selective expression of an interleukin-12 receptor component by human T helper 1 cells, J. Exp. Med. 185 (1997) 825–831.

[641] T. Sornasse, et al., Differentiation and stability of T helper 1 and 2 cells derived from naïve human neonatal CD4+ T cells, analyzed at the single-cell level, J. Exp. Med. 184 (1996) 473–483.

[642] E. Ylikoski, et al., IL-12 up-regulates T-bet independently of IFN-gamma in human CD4+ T cells, Eur. J. Immunol. 35 (2005) 3297–3306.

[643] C.E. Demeure, et al., In vitro maturation of human neonatal CD4 T lymphocytes, II: cytokines present at priming modulate the development of lymphokine production, J. Immunol. 152 (1994) 4775–4782.

[644] M. Bofill, et al., Differential expression of the cytokine receptors for human interleukin (IL)-12 and IL-18 on lymphocytes of both CD45RA and CD45RO phenotype from tonsils, cord and adult peripheral blood, Clin. Exp. Immunol. 138 (2004) 460–465.

[645] C. Macaubas, P.G. Holt, Regulation of cytokine production in T-cell responses to inhalant allergen:GATA-3 expression distinguishes between Th1- and Th2-polarized immunity, Int. Arch. Allergy Immunol. 124 (2001) 176–179.

[646] E. Yamaguchi, J. de Vries, H. Yssel, Differentiation of human single-positive fetal thymocytes in vitro into IL-4- and/or IFN-gamma- producing CD4+ and CD8+ T cells, Int. Immunol. 11 (1999) 593–603.

[647] L. Cosmi, et al., Human interleukin 17-producing cells originate from a CD161+CD4+ T cell precursor, J. Exp. Med. 205 (2008) 1903–1916.

[648] U. Andersson, et al., Humoral and cellular immunity in humans studied at the cell level from birth to two years of age, Immunol. Rev. 57 (1981) 1–38.

[649] R.G. Lubens, et al., Lectin-dependent T-lymphocyte and natural killer cytotoxic deficiencies in human newborns, Cell. Immunol. 74 (1982) 40–53.

[650] L.S. Rayfield, L. Brent, C.H. Rodeck, Development of cell-mediated lympholysis in human foetal blood lymphocytes, Clin. Exp. Immunol. 42 (1980) 561–570.

[651] C. Granberg, T. Hirvonen, Cell-mediated lympholysis by fetal and neonatal lymphocytes in sheep and man, Cell. Immunol. 51 (1980) 13–22.

[652] G. Risdon, J. Gaddy, H.E. Broxmeyer, Allogeneic responses of human umbilical cord blood, Blood Cells 20 (1994) 566–570.

[653] D.T. Harris, In vitro and in vivo assessment of the graft-versus-leukemia activity of cord blood, Bone Marrow Transplant. 15 (1995) 17–23.

[654] C. Barbey, et al., Characterisation of the cytotoxic alloresponse of cord blood, Bone Marrow Transplant. 22 (1998) S26–S30.

[655] A. Slavcev, et al., Alloresponses of cord blood cells in primary mixed lymphocyte cultures, Hum. Immunol. 63 (2002) 155–163.

[656] C. Berthou, et al., Cord blood T lymphocytes lack constitutive perforin expression in contrast to adult peripheral blood T lymphocytes, Blood 85 (1995) 1540–1546.

[657] K. Kogawa, et al., Perforin expression in cytotoxic lymphocytes from patients with hemophagocytic lymphohistiocytosis and their family members, Blood 99 (2002) 61–66.

[658] D. Rukavina, et al., Age-related decline of perforin expression in human cytotoxic T lymphocytes and natural killer cells, Blood 92 (1998) 2410–2420.

[659] R. de-Jong, et al., Human CD8+ T lymphocytes can be divided into CD45RA+ and CD45RO+ cells with different requirements for activation and differentiation, J. Immunol. 146 (1991) 2088–2094.

[660] A.N. Akbar, et al., Human CD4+CD45RO+ and CD4+CD45RA+ T cells synergize in response to alloantigens, Eur. J. Immunol. 21 (1991) 2517–2522.

[661] M.C. Renda, et al., Evidence of alloreactive T lymphocytes in fetal liver: implications for fetal hematopoietic stem cell transplantation, Bone Marrow Transplant. 25 (2000) 135–141.

[662] M.C. Renda, et al., In utero fetal liver hematopoietic stem cell transplantation: is there a role for alloreactive T lymphocytes, Blood 96 (2000) 1608–1609.

[663] A. Marchant, et al., Mature CD8(+) T lymphocyte response to viral infection during fetal life, J. Clin. Invest. 111 (2003) 1747–1755.

[664] M.A. Elbou Ould, et al., Cellular immune response of fetuses to cytomegalovirus, Pediatr. Res. 55 (2004) 280–286.

[665] B. Pedron, et al., Comparison of CD8+ T cell responses to cytomegalovirus between human fetuses and their transmitter mothers, J. Infect. Dis. 196 (2007) 1033–1043.

[666] K. Sato, et al., An abortive ligand-induced activation of CCR1-mediated downstream signaling event and a deficiency of CCR5 expression are associated with the hyporesponsiveness of human naïve CD4+ T cells to CCL3 and CCL5, J. Immunol. 168 (2002) 6263–6272.

[667] R.D. Berkowitz, et al., CXCR4 and CCR5 expression delineates targets for HIV-1 disruption of T cell differentiation, J. Immunol. 161 (1998) 3702–3710.

[668] K. Christopherson, Z. Brahmi, R. Hromas, Regulation of naïve fetal T-cell migration by the chemokines Exodus-2 and Exodus-3, Immunol. Lett. 69 (1999) 269–273.

[669] H. Mo, et al., Expression patterns of the HIV type 1 coreceptors CCR5 and cells and monocytes from cord and adult blood, AIDS Res. Hum. Retroviruses 14 (1998) 607–617.

[670] P. Auewarakul, et al., Age-dependent expression of the HIV-1 coreceptor CCR5 on CD4+ lymphocytes in children, J. Acquir. Immune Defic. Syndr. 24 (2000) 285–287.

[671] A. Langenkamp, et al., Kinetics of dendritic cell activation: impact on priming of TH1, TH2 and nonpolarized T cells, Nat. Immunol. 1 (2000) 311–316.

[672] R. Bonecchi, et al., Differential expression of chemokine receptors and chemotactic responsiveness of type 1 T helper cells (Th1s) and Th2s, J. Exp. Med. 187 (1998) 129–134.

[673] P. Fraticelli, et al., Fractalkine (CX3CL1) as an amplification circuit of polarized Th1 responses, J. Clin. Invest. 107 (2001) 1173–1181.

[674] J. Chipeta, et al., Neonatal (cord blood) T cells can competently raise type 1 and 2 immune responses upon polyclonal activation, Cell. Immunol. 205 (2000) 110–119.

[675] M.L. Hermiston, Z. Xu, A. Weiss, CD45: a critical regulator of signaling thresholds in immune cells, Annu. Rev. Immunol. 21 (2003) 107–137.

[676] B.T. Fife, J.A. Bluestone, Control of peripheral T-cell tolerance and autoimmunity via the CTLA-4 and PD-1 pathways, Immunol. Rev. 224 (2008) 166–182.

[677] A. Strasser, The role of BH3-only proteins in the immune system, Nat. Rev. Immunol. 5 (2005) 189–200.

[678] A.N. Akbar, et al., The significance of low bcl-2 expression by CD45RO T cells in normal individuals and patients with acute viral infections: the role of apoptosis in T cell memory, J. Exp. Med. 178 (1993) 427–438.

[679] B.H. Nelson, D.M. Willerford, Biology of the interleukin-2 receptor, Adv. Immunol. 70 (1998) 1–81.

[680] M.D. Tibbetts, L. Zheng, M.J. Lenardo, The death effector domain protein family: regulators of cellular homeostasis, Nat. Immunol. 4 (2003) 404–409.

[681] A. El Ghalbzouri, et al., An in vitro model of allogeneic stimulation of cord blood: induction of Fas independent apoptosis, Hum. Immunol. 60 (1999) 598–607.

[682] W. Tu, P.T. Cheung, Y.L. Lau, Insulin-like growth factor 1 promotes cord blood T cell maturation and inhibits its spontaneous and phytohemagglutinin-induced apoptosis through different mechanisms, J. Immunol. 165 (2000) 1331–1336.

[683] B. Drenou, et al., Characterisation of the roles of CD95 and CD95 ligand in cord blood, Bone Marrow Transplant. 22 (1998) S44–S47.

[684] M. Potestio, et al., Age-related changes in the expression of CD95 (APO1/FAS) on blood lymphocytes, Exp. Gerontol. 34 (1999) 659–673.

[685] T.B. Kuntz, et al., Fas and Fas ligand expression in maternal blood and in umbilical cord blood in preeclampsia, Pediatr. Res. 50 (2001) 743–749.

[686] S. Aggarwal, et al., TNF-alpha-induced apoptosis in neonatal lymphocytes: TNFRp55 expression and downstream pathways of apoptosis, Genes Immun. 1 (2000) 271–279.

[687] A. Malamitsi-Puchner, et al., Evidence for a suppression of apoptosis in early postnatal life, Acta Obstet. Gynecol. Scand. 80 (2001) 994–997.

[688] S. Aggarwal, et al., Programmed cell death (apoptosis) in cord blood lymphocytes, J. Clin. Immunol. 17 (1997) 63–73.

[689] H.K. Law, et al., Insulin-like growth factor I promotes cord blood T cell maturation through monocytes and inhibits their apoptosis in part through interleukin-6, BMC Immunol 9 (2008) 74.

[690] G. Monteleone, et al., Interferon-alpha drives T cell-mediated immunopathology in the intestine, Eur. J. Immunol. 31 (2001) 2247–2255.

[691] D. Howie, et al., Extrathymic T cell differentiation in the human intestine early in life, J. Immunol. 161 (1998) 5862–5872.

[692] M. Moghaddami, A. Cummins, G. Mayrhofer, Lymphocyte-filled villi: comparison with other lymphoid aggregations in the mucosa of the human small intestine, Gastroenterology 115 (1998) 1414–1425.

[693] A. Bas, S.G. Hammarstrom, M.L. Hammarstrom, Extrathymic TCR gene rearrangement in human small intestine: identification of new splice forms of recombination activating gene-1 mRNA with selective tissue expression, J. Immunol. 171 (2003) 3359–3371.

[694] V.R. Aluvihare, M. Kallikourdis, A.G. Betz, Regulatory T cells mediate maternal tolerance to the fetus, Nat. Immunol. 5 (2004) 266–271.

[695] D.A. Somerset, et al., Normal human pregnancy is associated with an elevation in the immune suppressive CD25+ CD4+ regulatory T-cell subset, Immunology 112 (2004) 38–43.

[696] T. Tilburgs, et al., Evidence for a selective migration of fetus-specific CD4+CD25bright regulatory T cells from the peripheral blood to the decidua in human pregnancy, J. Immunol. 180 (2008) 5737–5745.

[697] J.E. Mold, et al., Maternal alloantigens promote the development of tolerogenic fetal regulatory T cells in utero, Science 322 (2008) 1562–1565.

[698] M.G. Roncarolo, M. Battaglia, Regulatory T-cell immunotherapy for tolerance to self antigens and alloantigens in humans, Nat. Rev. Immunol. 7 (2007) 585–598.

[699] S. Sakaguchi, et al., Regulatory T cells and immune tolerance, Cell 133 (2008) 775–787.

[700] A.C. Cohen, et al., Cutting edge: decreased accumulation and regulatory function of CD4+ CD25(high) T cells in human STAT5b deficiency, J. Immunol. 177 (2006) 2770–2774.

[701] Y.J. Liu, A unified theory of central tolerance in the thymus, Trends Immunol. 27 (2006) 215–221.

[702] B. Fritzsching, et al., Naive regulatory T cells: a novel subpopulation defined by resistance toward CD95L-mediated cell death, Blood 108 (2006) 3371–3378.

[703] H.D. Ochs, E. Gambineri, T.R. Torgerson, IPEX, FOXP3 and regulatory T-cells: a model for autoimmunity, Immunol. Res. 38 (2007) 112–121.

[704] M. Vukmanovic-Stejic, et al., Human CD4+ CD25hi Foxp3+ regulatory T cells are derived by rapid turnover of memory populations in vivo, J. Clin. Invest. 116 (2006) 2423–2433.

[705] P. Pandiyan, et al., CD4+CD25+Foxp3+ regulatory T cells induce cytokine deprivation-mediated apoptosis of effector CD4+ T cells, Nat. Immunol. 8 (2007) 1353–1362.

[706] T. Fuchizawa, et al., Developmental changes of FOXP3-expressing CD4+CD25+ regulatory T cells and their impairment in patients with FOXP3 gene mutations, Clin. Immunol. 125 (2007) 237–246.

[707] W.R. Godfrey, et al., Cord blood CD4(+)CD25(+)-derived T regulatory cell lines express FoxP3 protein and manifest potent suppressor function, Blood 105 (2005) 750–758.

[708] K. Wing, et al., CD4+CD25+FOXP3+ regulatory T cells from human thymus and cord blood suppress antigen-specific T cell responses, Immunology 115 (2005) 516–525.

[709] N. Seddiki, et al., Persistence of naive CD45RA+ regulatory T cells in adult life, Blood 107 (2006) 2830–2838.

[710] A.N. Akbar, et al., The dynamic co-evolution of memory and regulatory CD4+ T cells in the periphery, Nat. Rev. Immunol. 7 (2007) 231–237.

[711] H. Smith, et al., Neonatal thymectomy results in a repertoire enriched in T cells deleted in adult thymus, Science 245 (1989) 749–752.

[712] W. Fujimaki, et al., Comparative study of regulatory T cell function of human CD25CD4 T cells from thymocytes, cord blood, and adult peripheral blood, Clin. Dev. Immunol. (2008) Article ID 305859.

[713] B. Schaub, et al., Impairment of T-regulatory cells in cord blood of atopic mothers, J. Allergy Clin. Immunol. 121 (2008) 1491–1499.

[714] M. Smith, et al., Children with egg allergy have evidence of reduced neonatal CD4(+)CD25(+)CD127(lo/−) regulatory T cell function, J. Allergy Clin. Immunol. 121 (2008) 1460–1466.

[715] A. Bendelac, P.B. Savage, L. Teyton, The biology of NKT cells, Annu. Rev. Immunol. 25 (2007) 297–336.

[716] D.I. Godfrey, S.P. Berzins, Control points in NKT-cell development, Nat. Rev. Immunol. 7 (2007) 505–518.

[717] P.L. Schwartzberg, et al., SLAM receptors and SAP influence lymphocyte interactions, development and function, Nat. Rev. Immunol. 9 (2009) 39–46.

[718] A.V. Rachitskaya, et al., Cutting edge: NKT cells constitutively express IL-23 receptor and RORgammat and rapidly produce IL-17 upon receptor ligation in an IL-6-independent fashion, J. Immunol. 180 (2008) 5167–5171.

[719] J.M. Coquet, et al., IL-21 is produced by NKT cells and modulates NKT cell activation and cytokine production, J. Immunol. 178 (2007) 2827–2834.

[720] J.K. Sandberg, N. Bhardwaj, D.F. Nixon, Dominant effector memory characteristics, capacity for dynamic adaptive expansion, and sex bias in the innate Valpha24 NKT cell compartment, Eur. J. Immunol. 33 (2003) 588–596.

[721] J.K. Sandberg, et al., Selective loss of innate CD4(+) V alpha 24 natural killer T cells in human immunodeficiency virus infection, J. Virol. 76 (2002) 7528–7534.

[722] O. Akbari, J.L. Faul, D.T. Umetsu, Invariant natural killer T cells in obstructive pulmonary diseases, N. Engl. J. Med. 357 (2007) 193–194, author reply 194–195.

[723] N. Musha, et al., Expansion of CD56+ NK T and gamma delta T cells from cord blood of human neonates, Clin. Exp. Immunol. 113 (1998) 220–228.

[724] A. D'Andrea, et al., Neonatal invariant Valpha24+ NKT lymphocytes are activated memory cells, Eur. J. Immunol. 30 (2000) 1544–1550.

[725] H.J. van Der Vliet, et al., Human natural killer T cells acquire a memory-activated phenotype before birth, Blood 95 (2000) 2440–2442.

[726] N. Kadowaki, et al., Distinct cytokine profiles of neonatal natural killer T cells after expansion with subsets of dendritic cells, J. Exp. Med. 193 (2001) 1221–1226.

[727] M. Hagihara, et al., Killing activity of human umbilical cord blood-derived TCRValpha24(+) NKT cells against normal and malignant hematological cells in vitro: a comparative study with NK cells or OKT3 activated T lymphocytes or with adult peripheral blood NKT cells, Cancer Immunol. Immunother. 51 (2002) 1–8.

[728] J. Alferink, et al., Control of neonatal tolerance to tissue antigens by peripheral T cell trafficking, Science 282 (1998) 1338–1341.

[729] Y. Ueda, et al., The effects of alphaGalCer-induced TCRValpha24 Vbeta11(+) natural killer T cells on NK cell cytotoxicity in umbilical cord blood, Cancer Immunol. Immunother. 52 (2003) 625–631.

[730] H. Li, et al., Structure of the Vdelta domain of a human gammadelta T-cell antigen receptor, Nature 391 (1998) 502–506.

[731] S. Beetz, et al., Innate immune functions of human gammadelta T cells, Immunobiology 213 (2008) 173–182.

[732] M. Bonneville, E. Scotet, Human Vgamma9Vdelta2 T cells: promising new leads for immunotherapy of infections and tumors, Curr. Opin. Immunol. 18 (2006) 539–546.

[733] V. Groh, et al., Recognition of stress-induced MHC molecules by intestinal epithelial gammadelta T cells, Science 279 (1998) 1737–1740.

[734] J. Jameson, W.L. Havran, Skin gammadelta T-cell functions in homeostasis and wound healing, Immunol. Rev. 215 (2007) 114–122.

[735] M. Gannage, et al., Induction of NKG2D ligands by gamma radiation and tumor necrosis factor-alpha may participate in the tissue damage during acute graft-versus-host disease, Transplantation 85 (2008) 911–915.

[736] M. Girardi, et al., Regulation of cutaneous malignancy by gammadelta T cells, Science 294 (2001) 605–609.

[737] P. Wrobel, et al., Lysis of a broad range of epithelial tumour cells by human gamma delta T cells: involvement of NKG2D ligands and T-cell receptor- versus NKG2D-dependent recognition, Scand. J. Immunol. 66 (2007) 320–328.

[738] D. Tramonti, et al., Evidence for the opposing roles of different gamma delta T cell subsets in macrophage homeostasis, Eur. J. Immunol. 36 (2006) 1729–1738.

[739] F. Dieli, et al., Biology of gammadelta T cells in tuberculosis and malaria, Curr. Mol. Med. 1 (2001) 437–446.

[740] C.L. Roark, et al., Gammadelta T cells: an important source of IL-17, Curr. Opin. Immunol. 20 (2008) 353–357.

[741] L. Wang, et al., Antibacterial effect of human V gamma 2V delta 2 T cells in vivo, J. Clin. Invest. 108 (2001) 1349–1357.

[742] S. Rothenfusser, et al., Distinct CpG oligonucleotide sequences activate human gamma delta T cells via interferon-alpha/-beta, Eur. J. Immunol. 31 (2001) 3525–3534.

[743] J. Borst, et al., Tissue distribution and repertoire selection of human gamma delta T cells: comparison with the murine system, Curr. Top. Microbiol. Immunol. 173 (1991) 41–46.

[744] L.D. McVay, S.R. Carding, Extrathymic origin of human gamma delta T cells during fetal development, J. Immunol. 157 (1996) 2873–2882.

[745] H. Saito, et al., Generation of intestinal T cells from progenitors residing in gut cryptopatches, Science 280 (1998) 275–278.

[746] M.L. Joachims, et al., Human alpha beta and gamma delta thymocyte development: TCR gene rearrangements, intracellular TCR beta expression, and gamma delta developmental potential—differences between men and mice, J. Immunol. 176 (2006) 1543–1552.

[747] T. Kreslavsky, et al., T cell receptor-instructed alphabeta versus gammadelta lineage commitment revealed by single-cell analysis, J. Exp. Med. 205 (2008) 1173–1186.

[748] A.I. Garbe, H. von Boehmer, TCR and Notch synergize in alphabeta versus gammadelta lineage choice, Trends Immunol. 28 (2007) 124–131.

[749] L.D. McVay, et al., The generation of human gammadelta T cell repertoires during fetal development, J. Immunol. 160 (1998) 5851–5860.

[750] L.D. McVay, S.R. Carding, Generation of human gammadelta T-cell repertoires, Crit. Rev. Immunol. 19 (1999) 431–460.

[751] B.F. Haynes, C.S. Heinly, Early human T cell development: analysis of the human thymus at the time of initial entry of hematopoietic stem cells into the fetal thymic microenvironment, J. Exp. Med. 181 (1995) 1445–1458.

[752] J.F. Bukowski, C.T. Morita, M.B. Brenner, Recognition and destruction of virus-infected cells by human gamma delta CTL, J. Immunol. 153 (1994) 5133–5140.

[753] K.W. Wucherpfennig, et al., Human fetal liver gamma/delta T cells predominantly use unusual rearrangements of the T cell receptor delta and gamma loci expressed on both CD4+CD8− and CD4−CD8− gamma/delta T cells, J. Exp. Med. 177 (1993) 425–432.

[754] Y. Miyagawa, et al., Fetal liver T cell receptor gamma/delta+ T cells as cytotoxic T lymphocytes specific for maternal alloantigens, J. Exp. Med. 176 (1992) 1–7.

[755] K. Beldjord, et al., Peripheral selection of V delta 1+ cells with restricted T cell receptor delta gene junctional repertoire in the peripheral blood of healthy donors, J. Exp. Med. 178 (1993) 121–127.

[756] J. Shen, et al., Oligoclonality of Vdelta1 and Vdelta2 cells in human peripheral blood mononuclear cells: TCR selection is not altered by stimulation with gram-negative bacteria, J. Immunol. 160 (1998) 3048–3055.

[757] C.M. Parker, et al., Evidence for extrathymic changes in the T cell receptor gamma/delta repertoire, J. Exp. Med. 171 (1990) 1597–1612.

[758] S.C. De Rosa, et al., Ontogeny of gamma delta T cells in humans, J. Immunol. 172 (2004) 1637–1645.

[759] I. Tsuyuguchi, et al., Increase of T-cell receptor gamma/delta-bearing T cells in cord blood of newborn babies obtained by in vitro stimulation with mycobacterial cord factor, Infect. Immun. 59 (1991) 3053–3059.

[760] M.D. Smith, et al., T gamma delta-cell subsets in cord and adult blood, Scand. J. Immunol. 32 (1990) 491–495.

[761] R.W. Steele, et al., Screening for cell-mediated immunity in children, Am. J. Dis. Child. 130 (1976) 1218–1221.

[762] A.I. Munoz, D. Limbert, Skin reactivity to *Candida* and streptokinase-streptodornase antigens in normal pediatric subjects: influence of age and acute illness, J. Pediatr. 91 (1977) 565–568.

[763] M.L. Franz, J.A. Carella, S.P. Galant, Cutaneous delayed hypersensitivity in a healthy pediatric population: diagnostic value of diphtheria-tetanus toxoids, J. Pediatr. 88 (1976) 975–977.

[764] W. Warwick, R.A. Good, R.T. Smith, Failure of passive transfer of delayed hypersensitivity in the newborn human infant, J. Lab. Clin. Med. 56 (1960) 139–147.

[765] R.J. Bonforte, et al., Phytohemagglutinin skin test: a possible in vivo measure of cell-mediated immunity, J. Pediatr. 81 (1972) 775–780.

[766] R. Fowler Jr., W.K. Schubert, C.D. West, Acquired partial tolerance to homologous skin grafts in the human infant at birth, Ann. N Y Acad. Sci. 87 (1960) 403–428.

[767] M. Rouleau, et al., Antigen-specific cytotoxic T cells mediate human fetal pancreas allograft rejection in SCID-hu mice, J. Immunol. 157 (1996) 5710–5720.

[768] F. Orlandi, et al., Evidence of induced non-tolerance in HLA-identical twins with hemoglobinopathy after in utero fetal transplantation, Bone Marrow Transplant. 18 (1996) 637–639.

[769] H.E. Vietor, et al., Alterations in cord blood leukocyte subsets of patients with severe hemolytic disease after intrauterine transfusion therapy, J. Pediatr. 130 (1997) 718–724.

[770] H.E. Vietor, et al., Intrauterine transfusions affect fetal T-cell immunity, Blood 90 (1997) 2492–2501.

[771] J.L. Naiman, et al., Possible graft-versus-host reaction after intrauterine transfusion for Rh erythroblastosis fetalis, N. Engl. J. Med. 281 (1969) 697–701.

[772] R. Parkman, et al., Graft-versus-host disease after intrauterine and exchange transfusions for hemolytic disease of the newborn, N. Engl. J. Med. 290 (1974) 359–363.

[773] R.S. Berger, S.L. Dixon, Fulminant transfusion-associated graft-versus-host disease in a premature infant, J. Am. Acad. Dermatol. 20 (1989) 945–950.

[774] O. Flidel, et al., Graft versus host disease in extremely low birth weight neonate, Pediatrics 89 (1992) 689–690.

[775] Z. Szepfalusi, et al., Prenatal allergen contact with milk proteins, Clin. Exp. Allergy 27 (1997) 28–35.

[776] S. Prescott, et al., Developing patterns of T cell memory to environmental allergens during the first two years of life, Int. Arch. Allergy Immunol. 113 (1997) 75–79.

[777] K. Van-Duren-Schmidt, et al., Prenatal contact with inhalant allergens, Pediatr. Res. 41 (1997) 128–131.

[778] S. Prescott, et al., Transplacental priming of the human immune system to environmental allergens: universal skewing of initial T cell responses toward the Th2 cytokine profile, J. Immunol. 160 (1998) 4730–4737.

[779] S.L. Prescott, et al., Reciprocal age-related patterns of allergen-specific T-cell immunity in normal vs. atopic infants, Clin. Exp. Allergy 28 (1998) 39–44.

[780] R.L. Miller, et al., Prenatal exposure, maternal sensitization, and sensitization in utero to indoor allergens in an inner-city cohort, Am. J. Respir. Crit. Care Med. 164 (2001) 995–1001.

[781] G. Devereux, A.M. Hall, R.N. Barker, Measurement of T-helper cytokines secreted by cord blood in response to allergens, J. Immunol. Methods 234 (2001) 13–22.

[782] S.L. Prescott, et al., The value of perinatal immune responses in predicting allergic disease at 6 years of age, Allergy 58 (2003) 1187–1194.

[783] Z. Szepfalusi, et al., Transplacental priming of the human immune system with environmental allergens can occur early in gestation, J. Allergy Clin. Immunol. 106 (2000) 530–536.

[784] D. Rastogi, et al., Antigen-specific immune responses to influenza vaccine in utero, J. Clin. Invest. 117 (2007) 1637–1646.

[785] J.A. Englund, et al., Maternal immunization with influenza or tetanus toxoid vaccine for passive antibody protection in young infants, J. Infect. Dis. 168 (1993) 647–656.

[786] A.M. Zeman, et al., Humoral and cellular immune responses in children given annual immunization with trivalent inactivated influenza vaccine, Pediatr. Infect. Dis. J. 26 (2007) 107–115.

[787] I. Malhotra, et al., Helminth- and bacillus Calmette-Guérin-induced immunity in children sensitized in utero to filariasis and schistosomiasis, J. Immunol. 162 (1999) 6843–6848.

[788] C.L. King, et al., Acquired immune responses to *Plasmodium falciparum* merozoite surface protein-1 in the human fetus, J. Immunol. 168 (2002) 356–364.

[789] L. Kuhn, et al., T-helper cell responses to HIV envelope peptides in cord blood: against intrapartum and breast-feeding transmission, AIDS 15 (2001) 1–9.

[790] Y. Lo, et al., Two-way traffic between mother and fetus: biologic and clinical implications, Blood 88 (1996) 4390–4395.

[791] S.M. Muller, et al., Transplacentally acquired maternal T lymphocytes in severe combined immunodeficiency: a study of 121 patients, Blood 98 (2001) 1847–1851.

[792] P.S. Friedmann, Cell-mediated immunological reactivity in neonates and infants with congenital syphilis, Clin. Exp. Immunol. 30 (1977) 271–276.

[793] S.E. Starr, et al., Impaired cellular immunity to cytomegalovirus in congenitally infected children and their mothers, J. Infect. Dis. 140 (1979) 500–505.

[794] R.F. Pass, et al., Specific cell-mediated immunity and the natural history of congenital infection with cytomegalovirus, J. Infect. Dis. 148 (1983) 953–961.

[795] E. Buimovici-Klein, L.Z. Cooper, Cell-mediated immune response in rubella infections, Rev. Infect. Dis. 7 (1985) S123–S128.

[796] S.G. Paryani, A.M. Arvin, Intrauterine infection with varicella-zoster virus after maternal varicella, N. Engl. J. Med. 314 (1986) 1542–1546.

[797] R. McLeod, et al., Phenotypes and functions of lymphocytes in congenital toxoplasmosis, J. Lab. Clin. Med. 116 (1990) 623–635.

[798] S. Metenou, et al., Fetal immune responses to *Plasmodium falciparum* antigens in a malaria-endemic region of Cameroon, J. Immunol. 178 (2007) 2770–2777.

[799] J.M. Aase, et al., Mumps-virus infection in pregnant women and the immunologic response of their offspring, N. Engl. J. Med. 286 (1972) 1379–1382.

[800] K. Luzuriaga, et al., HIV-1-specific cytotoxic T lymphocyte responses in the first year of life, J. Immunol. 154 (1995) 433–443.

[801] C. Brander, et al., Persistent HIV-1-specific CTL clonal expansion despite high viral burden post utero HIV-1 infection, J. Immunol. 162 (1999) 4796–4800.

[802] E. Hermann, et al., Human fetuses are able to mount an adultlike CD8 T-cell response, Blood 100 (2002) 2153–2158.

[803] P. Hohlfeld, et al., *Toxoplasma gondii* infection during pregnancy: T lymphocyte subpopulations in mothers and fetuses, Pediatr. Infect. Dis. J. 9 (1990) 878–881.

[804] B. Thilaganathan, et al., Fetal immunological and haematological changes in intrauterine infection, Br. J. Obstet. Gynaecol. 101 (1994) 418–421.

[805] T. Bruning, A. Daiminger, G. Enders, Diagnostic value of CD45RO expression on circulating T lymphocytes of fetuses and newborn infants with pre-, peri- or early post-natal infections, Clin. Exp. Immunol. 107 (1997) 306–311.

[806] C. Michie, et al., Streptococcal toxic shock-like syndrome: evidence of superantigen activity and its effects on T lymphocyte subsets in vivo, Clin. Exp. Immunol. 98 (1994) 140–144.

[807] T. Hara, et al., Human V delta 2+ gamma delta T-cell tolerance to foreign antigens of *Toxoplasma gondii*, Proc. Natl. Acad. Sci. U S A 93 (1996) 5136–5140.

[808] W.M. Sullender, et al., Humoral and cell-mediated immunity in neonates with herpes simplex virus infection, J. Infect. Dis. 155 (1987) 28–37.

[809] S.K. Burchett, et al., Diminished interferon-gamma and lymphocyte proliferation in neonatal and postpartum primary herpes simplex virus infection, J. Infect. Dis. 165 (1992) 813–818.

[810] S.F. Chen, et al., Antiviral CD8 T cells in the control of primary human cytomegalovirus infection in early childhood, J. Infect. Dis. 189 (2004) 1619–1627.

[811] L. Gibson, et al., Human cytomegalovirus proteins pp65 and immediate early protein 1 are common targets for CD8(+) T cell responses in children with congenital or postnatal human cytomegalovirus infection, J. Immunol. 172 (2004) 2256–2264.

[812] M. Clerici, et al., Analysis of T helper and antigen-presenting cell functions in cord blood and peripheral blood leukocytes from healthy children of different ages, J. Clin. Invest. 91 (1993) 2829–2836.

[813] A. Marchant, et al., Newborns develop a Th1-type immune response to *Mycobacterium bovis* bacillus Calmette-Guérin vaccination, J. Immunol. 163 (1999) 2249–2255.

[814] M.O. Ota, et al., Influence of *Mycobacterium bovis* bacillus Calmette-Guérin on antibody and cytokine responses to human neonatal vaccination, J. Immunol. 168 (2002) 919–925.

[815] J. Vekemans, et al., T cell responses to vaccines in infants: defective IFN-gamma production after oral polio vaccination, Clin. Exp. Immunol. 127 (2002) 495–498.

[816] J. Rowe, et al., Antigen-specific responses to diphtheria-tetanus-acellular pertussis vaccine in human infants are initially Th2 polarized, Infect. Immun. 68 (2000) 3873–3877.

[817] Y. Riviere, F. Buseyne, Cytotoxic T lymphocytes generation capacity in early life with particular reference to HIV, Vaccine 16 (1998) 1420–1422.

[818] C.A. Pikora, et al., Early HIV-1 envelope-specific cytotoxic T lymphocyte responses in vertically infected infants, J. Exp. Med. 185 (1997) 1153–1161.

[819] Z.A. Scott, et al., Infrequent detection of HIV-1-specific, but not cytomegalovirus-specific, CD8(+) T cell responses in young HIV-1-infected infants, J. Immunol. 167 (2001) 7134–7140.

[820] K. Luzuriaga, et al., Early therapy of vertical human immunodeficiency virus type 1 (HIV-1) infection: control of viral replication and absence of persistent HIV-1-specific immune responses, J. Virol. 74 (2000) 6984–6991.

[821] S.D. Nielsen, et al., Impaired progenitor cell function in HIV-negative infants of HIV-positive mothers results in decreased thymic output and low CD4 counts, Blood 98 (2001) 398–404.

[822] C. Chougnet, et al., Influence of human immunodeficiency virus–infected maternal environment on development of infant interleukin-12 production, J. Infect. Dis. 181 (2000) 1590–1597.

[823] Y. Chiba, et al., Development of cell-mediated cytotoxic immunity to respiratory syncytial virus in human infants following naturally acquired infection, J. Med. Virol. 28 (1989) 133–139.

[824] J.L. Xu, M.M. Davis, Diversity in the CDR3 region of V(H) is sufficient for most antibody specificities, Immunity 13 (2000) 37–45.

[825] H.W. Schroeder Jr., Similarity and divergence in the development and expression of the mouse and human antibody repertoires, Dev. Comp. Immunol. 30 (2006) 119–135.

[826] J.J. Mond, J.F. Kokai-Kun, The multifunctional role of antibodies in the protective response to bacterial T cell-independent antigens, Curr. Top. Microbiol. Immunol. 319 (2008) 17–40.

[827] T.W. LeBien, et al., Multiparameter flow cytometric analysis of human fetal bone marrow B cells, Leukemia 4 (1990) 354–358.

[828] H. Kubagawa, et al., Light-chain gene expression before heavy-chain gene rearrangement in pre-B cells transformed by Epstein-Barr virus, Proc. Natl. Acad. Sci. U S A 86 (1989) 2356–2360.

[829] I.L. Martensson, R.A. Keenan, S. Licence, The pre-B-cell receptor, Curr. Opin. Immunol. 19 (2007) 137–142.

[830] J.G. Monroe, ITAM-mediated tonic signalling through pre-BCR and BCR complexes, Nat. Rev. Immunol. 6 (2006) 283–294.

[831] A.J. Bankovich, et al., Structural insight into pre-B cell receptor function, Science 316 (2007) 291–294.

[832] A. Brauninger, et al., Regulation of immunoglobulin light chain gene rearrangements during early B cell development in the human, Eur. J. Immunol. 31 (2001) 3631–3637.

[833] B.B. Blomberg, et al., Regulation of human lambda light chain gene expression, Ann. N Y Acad. Sci. 764 (1995) 84–98.

[834] C. Giachino, E. Padovan, A. Lanzavecchia, Kappa+lambda+ dual receptor B cells are present in the human peripheral repertoire, J. Exp. Med. 181 (1995) 1245–1250.

[835] N. Solvason, et al., The fetal omentum in mice and humans: a site enriched for precursors of CD5 B cells early in development, Ann. N Y Acad. Sci. 65 (1992) 10–20.

[836] C. Nunez, et al., B cells are generated throughout life in humans, J. Immunol. 156 (1996) 866–872.

[837] N. Nishimoto, et al., Normal pre-B cells express a receptor complex of mu heavy chains and surrogate light-chain proteins, Proc. Natl. Acad. Sci. U S A 88 (1991) 6284–6288.

[838] J. Arakawa-Hoyt, et al., The number and generative capacity of human B lymphocyte progenitors, measured in vitro and in vivo, is higher in umbilical cord blood than in adult or pediatric bone marrow, Bone Marrow Transplant. 24 (1999) 1167–1176.

[839] E. Sanz, et al., Human cord blood CD34+Pax-5+ B-cell progenitors: single-cell analyses of their gene expression profiles, Blood 101 (2003) 3424–3430.

[840] A.K. Stewart, et al., High-frequency representation of a single VH gene in the expressed human B-cell repertoire, J. Exp. Med. 177 (1993) 1227.

[841] P. Kraj, et al., The human heavy chain Ig V region gene repertoire is biased at all stages of B cell ontogeny, including early pre-B cells, J. Immunol. 158 (1997) 5824–5832.

[842] H.J. Schroeder, J.L. Hillson, R.M. Perlmutter, Early restriction of the human antibody repertoire, Science 238 (1987) 791–793.

[843] A.M. Cuisinier, et al., Preferential expression of VH5 and VH6 immunoglobulin genes in early human B-cell ontogeny, Scand. J. Immunol. 30 (1989) 493–497.

[844] M.E. Schutte, et al., Deletion mapping of Ig VH gene segments expressed in human CD5 B cell lines: JH proximity is not the sole determinant of the restricted fetal VH gene repertoire, J. Immunol. 149 (1992) 3953–3960.

[845] H.W. Schroeder Jr., G.C. Ippolito, S. Shiokawa, Regulation of the antibody repertoire through control of HCDR3 diversity, Vaccine 16 (1998) 1383–1390.

[846] M. Zemlin, et al., Regulation and chance in the ontogeny of B and T cell antigen receptor repertoires, Immunol. Res. 26 (2002) 265–278.

[847] E. Meffre, J.E. Salmon, Autoantibody selection and production in early human life, J. Clin. Invest. 117 (2007) 598–601.

[848] I. Sanz, Multiple mechanisms participate in the generation of diversity of human H chain CDR3 regions, J. Immunol. 147 (1991) 1720–1729.

[849] F. Mortari, et al., The human cord blood antibody repertoire: frequent usage of the VH7 gene family, Eur. J. Immunol. 22 (1992) 241–245.

[850] G.J. Silverman, M. Sasano, M. Wormsley, Age-associated changes in binding of human B lymphocytes to a VH3-restricted unconventional bacterial antigen, J. Immunol. 151 (1993) 5840–5855.

[851] F.M. Raaphorst, et al., Restricted utilization of germ-line VH3 genes and short diverse third complementarity-determining regions CDR3 in human fetal B lymphocyte immunoglobulin heavy chain rearrangements, Eur. J. Immunol. 22 (1992) 247–251.

[852] F.M. Raaphorst, et al., Human Ig heavy chain CDR3 regions in adult bone marrow pre-B cells display an adult phenotype of diversity: evidence for structural selection of DH amino acid sequences, Int. Immunol. 9 (1997) 1503–1515.

[853] Y. Hirose, et al., B-cell precursors differentiated from cord blood CD34+ cells are more immature than those derived from granulocyte colony-stimulating factor-mobilized peripheral blood CD34+ cells, Immunology 104 (2001) 410–417.

[854] A.M. Cuisinier, et al., Rapid expansion of human immunoglobulin repertoire VH, V kappa, V lambda expressed in early fetal bone marrow, New Biol. 2 (1990) 689–699.

[855] F. Mortari, J.Y. Wang, H.J. Schroeder, Human cord blood antibody repertoire: mixed population of VH gene segments and CDR3 distribution in the expressed C alpha and C gamma repertoires, J. Immunol. 150 (1993) 1348–1357.

[856] E.A. Padlan, Anatomy of the antibody molecule, Mol. Immunol. 31 (1994) 169–217.

[857] C.L. Benedict, J.F. Kearney, Increased junctional diversity in fetal B cells results in a loss of protective anti-phosphorylcholine antibodies in adult mice, Immunity 10 (1999) 607–617.

[858] H. Wardemann, M.C. Nussenzweig, B-cell self-tolerance in humans, Adv. Immunol. 95 (2007) 83–110.

[859] M. Jankovic, et al., RAGs and regulation of autoantibodies, Annu. Rev. Immunol. 22 (2004) 485–501.

[860] I. Isnardi, et al., IRAK-4- and MyD88-dependent pathways are essential for the removal of developing autoreactive B cells in humans, Immunity 29 (2008) 746–757.

[861] Z. Zhang, VH replacement in mice and humans, Trends Immunol. 28 (2007) 132–137.

[862] J.A. Duty, et al., Functional anergy in a subpopulation of naive B cells from healthy humans that express autoreactive immunoglobulin receptors, J. Exp. Med. 206 (2009) 139–151.

[863] S. Gupta, et al., Ontogeny of lymphocyte subpopulations in human fetal liver, Proc. Natl. Acad. Sci. U S A 73 (1976) 919–922.

[864] E.S. Metcalf, N.R. Klinman, In vitro tolerance induction of neonatal murine B cells, J. Exp. Med. 143 (1976) 1327–1340.

[865] J. Lee, N.L. Monson, P.E. Lipsky, The V lambda J lambda repertoire in human fetal spleen: evidence for positive selection and extensive receptor editing, J. Immunol. 165 (2000) 6322–6333.

[866] H.J. Girschick, P.E. Lipsky, The kappa gene repertoire of human neonatal B cells, Mol. Immunol. 38 (2002) 1113–1127.

[867] S. Wirths, A. Lanzavecchia, ABCB1 transporter discriminates human resting naive B cells from cycling transitional and memory B cells, Eur. J. Immunol. 35 (2005) 3433–3441.

[868] R. Ettinger, et al., IL-21 induces differentiation of human naive and memory B cells into antibody-secreting plasma cells, J. Immunol. 175 (2005) 7867–7879.

[869] A.K. Cuss, et al., Expansion of functionally immature transitional B cells is associated with human-immunodeficient states characterized by impaired humoral immunity, J. Immunol. 176 (2006) 1506–1516.

[870] A. Marie-Cardine, et al., Transitional B cells in humans: characterization and insight from B lymphocyte reconstitution after hematopoietic stem cell transplantation, Clin. Immunol. 127 (2008) 14–25.

[871] J.E. Stadanlick, M.P. Cancro, BAFF and the plasticity of peripheral B cell tolerance, Curr. Opin. Immunol. 20 (2008) 158–161.

[872] M. Herve, et al., CD40 ligand and MHC class II expression are essential for human peripheral B cell tolerance, J. Exp. Med. 204 (2007) 1583–1593.

[873] H.P. Brezinschek, R.I. Brezinschek, P.E. Lipsky, Analysis of the heavy chain repertoire of human peripheral B cells using single-cell polymerase chain reaction, J. Immunol. 155 (1995) 190–202.

[874] U. Klein, K. Rajewsky, R. Kuppers, Human immunoglobulin (Ig)M+IgD+ peripheral blood B cells expressing the CD27 cell surface antigen carry somatically mutated variable region genes: CD27 as a general marker for somatically mutated (memory) B cells, J. Exp. Med. 188 (1998) 1679–1689.

[875] D.C. Macallan, et al., B-cell kinetics in humans: rapid turnover of peripheral blood memory cells, Blood 105 (2005) 3633–3640.

[876] C.D. Allen, J.G. Cyster, Follicular dendritic cell networks of primary follicles and germinal centers: phenotype and function, Semin. Immunol. 20 (2008) 14–25.

[877] C.D. Allen, T. Okada, J.G. Cyster, Germinal-center organization and cellular dynamics, Immunity 27 (2007) 190–202.

[878] A. Cariappa, et al., Perisinusoidal B cells in the bone marrow participate in T-independent responses to blood-borne microbes, Immunity 23 (2005) 397–407.

[879] C. Schultz, et al., Maturational changes of lymphocyte surface antigens in human blood: comparison between fetuses, neonates and adults, Biol. Neonate 78 (2000) 77–82.

[880] D.T. Avery, et al., IL-21-induced isotype switching to IgG and IgA by human naive B cells is differentially regulated by IL-4, J. Immunol. 181 (2008) 1767–1779.

[881] L. Tasker, S. Marshall-Clarke, Functional responses of human neonatal B lymphocytes to antigen receptor cross-linking and CpG DNA, Clin. Exp. Immunol. 134 (2003) 409–419.

[882] C. Parra, E. Rold’an, J.A. Brieva, Deficient expression of adhesion molecules by human CD5− B lymphocytes both after bone marrow transplantation and during normal ontogeny, Blood 88 (1996) 1733–1740.

[883] G.T. Rijkers, et al., Infant B cell responses to polysaccharide determinants, Vaccine 16 (1998) 1396–1400.

[884] D. Viemann, et al., Differential expression of the B cell-restricted molecule CD22 B lymphocytes depending upon antigen stimulation, Eur. J. Immunol. 30 (2000) 550–559.

[885] P.J. Macardle, et al., The antigen receptor complex on cord B lymphocytes, Immunology 90 (1997) 376–382.

[886] A. Gagro, et al., CD5-positive and CD5-negative human B cells converge to an indistinguishable population on signalling through B-cell receptors and CD40, Immunology 101 (2000) 201–209.

[887] J. Punnonen, et al., Induction of isotype switching and Ig production by CD5+ and CD10+ human fetal B cells, J. Immunol. 148 (1992) 3398–3404.

[888] S.R. Elliott, et al., Expression of the costimulator molecules, CD80, CD86, CD28, and CD152, on lymphocytes from neonates and young children, Hum. Immunol. 60 (1999) 1039–1048.

[889] S.R. Elliott, et al., Expression of the costimulator molecules, CD40 and CD154, on lymphocytes from neonates and young children, Hum. Immunol. 61 (2000) 378–388.

[890] C.A. Thornton, J.A. Holloway, J.O. Warner, Expression of CD21 and CD23 during human fetal development, Pediatr. Res. 52 (2002) 245–250.

[891] R. Krzysiek, et al., Regulation of CCR6 chemokine receptor expression and responsiveness to macrophage inflammatory protein-3alpha/CCL20 in human B cells, Blood 96 (2000) 2338–2345.

[892] R.C. Rickert, Regulation of B lymphocyte activation by complement C3 and the B cell coreceptor complex, Curr. Opin. Immunol. 17 (2005) 237–243.

[893] R. Roozendaal, M.C. Carroll, Complement receptors CD21 and CD35 in humoral immunity, Immunol. Rev. 219 (2007) 157–166.

[894] N. Gupta, A.L. DeFranco, Lipid rafts and B cell signaling, Semin. Cell. Dev. Biol. 18 (2007) 616–626.

[895] A. Cherukuri, et al., The tetraspanin CD81 is necessary for partitioning of coligated CD19/CD21-B cell antigen receptor complexes into signaling-active lipid rafts, J. Immunol. 172 (2004) 370–380.

[896] H. Qi, et al., Extrafollicular activation of lymph node B cells by antigen-bearing dendritic cells, Science 312 (2006) 1672–1676.

[897] K.A. Pape, et al., The humoral immune response is initiated in lymph nodes by B cells that acquire soluble antigen directly in the follicles, Immunity 26 (2007) 491–502.

[898] T. Okada, J.G. Cyster, B cell migration and interactions in the early phase of antibody responses, Curr. Opin. Immunol. 18 (2006) 278–285.

[899] P.J. Lane, et al., CD4+CD3− cells regulate the organization of lymphoid tissue and T-cell memory for antibody responses, Int. J. Hematol. 83 (2006) 12–16.

[900] L. Nitschke, The role of CD22 and other inhibitory co-receptors in B-cell activation, Curr. Opin. Immunol. 17 (2005) 290–297.

[901] C.F. Jessup, et al., The Fc receptor for IgG (Fc gamma RII; CD32) on human neonatal B lymphocytes, Hum. Immunol. 62 (2001) 679–685.

[902] M.D. Cahalan, I. Parker, Choreography of cell motility and interaction dynamics imaged by two-photon microscopy in lymphoid organs, Annu. Rev. Immunol. 26 (2008) 585–626.

[903] A. Langenkamp, et al., Kinetics and expression patterns of chemokine receptors in human CD4+ T lymphocytes primed by myeloid or plasmacytoid dendritic cells, Eur. J. Immunol. 33 (2003) 474–482.

[904] F.D. Batista, N.E. Harwood, The who, how and where of antigen presentation to B cells, Nat. Rev. Immunol. 9 (2009) 15–27.

[905] B. Zheng, G. Kelsoe, S. Han, Somatic diversification of antibody responses, J. Clin. Immunol. 16 (1996) 1–11.

[906] J. Jacob, et al., Intraclonal generation of antibody mutants in germinal centres, Nature 354 (1991) 389–392.

[907] T. Tiller, et al., Autoreactivity in human IgG+ memory B cells, Immunity 26 (2007) 205–213.

[908] T. Okada, et al., Chemokine requirements for B cell entry to lymph nodes and Peyer's patches, J. Exp. Med. 196 (2002) 65–75.

[909] I. Sanz, et al., Phenotypic and functional heterogeneity of human memory B cells, Semin. Immunol. 20 (2008) 67–82.

[910] A. Lanzavecchia, et al., Understanding and making use of human memory B cells, Immunol. Rev. 211 (2006) 303–309.

[911] A. Amedei, et al., Preferential Th1 profile of T helper cell responses in X-linked (Bruton's) agammaglobulinemia, Eur. J. Immunol. 31 (2001) 1927–1934.

[912] F. Garban, et al., Signal transduction via human leucocyte antigen class II molecules distinguishes between cord blood, normal, and malignant adult B lymphocytes, Exp. Hematol. 26 (1998) 874–884.

[913] C.A. Jones, J.A. Holloway, J.O. Warner, Phenotype of fetal monocytes and B lymphocytes during the third trimester of pregnancy, J. Reprod. Immunol. 56 (2002) 45–60.

[914] A. Jegerlehner, et al., TLR9 signaling in B cells determines class switch recombination to IgG2a, J. Immunol. 178 (2007) 2415–2420.

[915] J. Stavnezer, J.E. Guikema, C.E. Schrader, Mechanism and regulation of class switch recombination, Annu. Rev. Immunol. 26 (2008) 261–292.

[916] L. Du, et al., Involvement of Artemis in nonhomologous end-joining during immunoglobulin class switch recombination, J. Exp. Med. 205 (2008) 3031–3040.

[917] H. Kimata, M. Fujimoto, Induction of IgA1 and IgA2 production in immature human fetal B cells and pre-B cells by vasoactive intestinal peptide, Blood 85 (1995) 2098–2104.

[918] A. Cerutti, The regulation of IgA class switching, Nat. Rev. Immunol. 8 (2008) 421–434.

[919] K.A. Pape, et al., Visualization of the genesis and fate of isotype-switched B cells during a primary immune response, J. Exp. Med. 197 (2003) 1677–1687.

[920] H.D. Ochs, J. Winkelstein, Disorders of the B-cell system, in: E.R. Stiehm (Ed.), Immunologic Disorders in Infants and Children, WB Saunders, Philadelphia, 1996, pp. 296–338.

[921] H.D. Ochs, D. Hollenbaugh, A. Aruffo, The role of CD40L (gp39)/CD40 in T/B cell interaction and primary immunodeficiency, Semin. Immunol. 6 (1994) 337–341.

[922] M. Maruyama, K.P. Lam, K. Rajewsky, Memory B-cell persistence is independent of persisting immunizing antigen, Nature 407 (2000) 636–642.

[923] S.A. Diehl, et al., STAT3-mediated up-regulation of BLIMP1 is coordinated with BCL6 down-regulation to control human plasma cell differentiation, J. Immunol. 180 (2008) 4805–4815.

[924] A.L. Shaffer, et al., XBP1, downstream of Blimp-1, expands the secretory apparatus and other organelles, and increases protein synthesis in plasma cell differentiation, Immunity 21 (2004) 81–93.

[925] K. Moser, et al., Stromal niches, plasma cell differentiation and survival, Curr. Opin. Immunol. 18 (2006) 265–270.

[926] J. Banchereau, et al., Molecular control of B lymphocyte growth and differentiation, Stem Cells (Dayt) 12 (1994) 278–288.

[927] D.C. Servet, et al., Delayed IgG2 humoral response in infants is not due to intrinsic T or B cell defects, Int. Immunol. 8 (1996) 1495–1502.

[928] K.O. Gudmundsson, et al., Immunoglobulin-secreting cells in cord blood: effects of Epstein-Barr virus and interleukin-4, Scand. J. Immunol. 50 (1999) 21–24.

[929] D.T. Avery, et al., STAT3 is required for IL-21-induced secretion of IgE from human naive B cells, Blood 112 (2008) 1784–1793.

[930] S.G. Tangye, et al., Isotype switching by human B cells is division-associated and regulated by cytokines, J. Immunol. 169 (2002) 4298–4306.

[931] J. Punnonen, B.G. Cocks, J.E. de Vries, IL-4 induces germ-line IgE heavy chain gene transcription in human fetal pre-B cells: evidence for differential expression of functional IL-4 and IL-13 receptors during B cell ontogeny, J. Immunol. 155 (1995) 4248–4254.

[932] Y. Ueno, et al., T-cell-dependent production of IgG by human cord blood B cells in reconstituted SCID mice, Scand. J. Immunol. 35 (1992) 415–419.

[933] B.A. Vandekerckhove, et al., Human Ig production and isotype switching in severe combined immunodeficient-human mice, J. Immunol. 151 (1993) 128–137.

[934] J. Splawski, K. Yamamoto, P. Lipsky, Deficient interleukin-10 production by neonatal T cells does not expalin their ineffectiveness at promoting neonatal B cell differentiation, Eur. J. Immunol. 28 (1998) 4248–4256.

[935] B. Baskin, K.B. Islam, C.I. Smith, Characterization of the CDR3 region of rearranged alpha heavy chain genes in human fetal liver, Clin. Exp. Immunol. 112 (1998) 44–47.

[936] D. Gitlin, A. Biasucci, Development of gamma G, gamma A, gamma M, beta IC-beta IA, Ca 1 esterase inhibitor, ceruloplasmin, transferrin, hemopexin, haptoglobin, fibrinogen, plasminogen, alpha 1-antitrypsin, orosomucoid, beta-lipoprotein, alpha 2-macroglobulin, and prealbumin in the human conceptus, J. Clin. Invest. 48 (1969) 1433–1446.

[937] H.M. Dosch, et al., Concerted generation of Ig isotype diversity in human fetal bone marrow, J. Immunol. 143 (1989) 2464–2469.

[938] W.E. Gathings, H. Kubagawa, M.D. Cooper, A distinctive pattern of B cell immaturity in perinatal humans, Immunol. Rev. 57 (1981) 107–126.

[939] J.F. Wedgwood, et al., Umbilical cord blood lacks circulating B lymphocytes expressing surface IgG or IgA, Clin. Immunol. Immunopathol. 84 (1997) 276–282.

[940] J.B. Splawski, P.E. Lipsky, Prostaglandin E2 inhibits T cell-dependent Ig secretion by neonatal but not adult lymphocytes, J. Immunol. 152 (1994) 5259–5267.

[941] S. Kruetzmann, et al., Human immunoglobulin M memory B cells controlling *Streptococcus pneumoniae* infections are generated in the spleen, J. Exp. Med. 197 (2003) 939–945.

[942] D.M. Tarlinton, F. Batista, K.G. Smith, The B-cell response to protein antigens in immunity and transplantation, Transplantation 85 (2008) 1698–1704.

[943] M. Balazs, et al., Blood dendritic cells interact with splenic marginal zone B cells to initiate T-independent immune responses, Immunity 17 (2002) 341–352.

[944] K.M. Haas, et al., Complement receptors CD21/35 link innate and protective immunity during Streptococcus pneumoniae infection by regulating IgG3 antibody responses, Immunity 17 (2002) 713–723.

[945] A. Zandvoort, W. Timens, The dual function of the splenic marginal zone: essential for initiation of anti-TI-2 responses but also vital in the general first-line defense against blood-borne antigens, Clin. Exp. Immunol. 130 (2002) 4–11.

[946] G. Martins, K. Calame, Regulation and functions of Blimp-1 in T and B lymphocytes, Annu. Rev. Immunol. 26 (2008) 133–169.

[947] P.L. Amlot, A.E. Hayes, Impaired human antibody response to the thymus-independent antigen, DNP-Ficoll, after splenectomy: implications for postsplenectomy infections, Lancet 1 (1985) 1008–1011.

[948] F.A. Scheeren, et al., T cell-independent development and induction of somatic hypermutation in human IgM+ IgD+ CD27+ B cells, J. Exp. Med. 205 (2008) 2033–2042.

[949] S. Weller, et al., Somatic diversification in the absence of antigen-driven responses is the hallmark of the IgM+ IgD+ CD27+ B cell repertoire in infants, J. Exp. Med. 205 (2008) 1331–1342.

[950] K. Kaur, et al., Decreased expression of tumor necrosis factor family receptors involved in humoral immune responses in preterm neonates, Blood 110 (2007) 2948–2954.

[951] R. Montecino-Rodriguez, H. Leathers, K. Dorshkind, Identification of a B-1 B cell-specified progenitor, Nat. Immunol. 7 (2006) 293–301.

[952] F. Martin, J.F. Kearney, B1 cells: similarities and differences with other B cell subsets, Curr. Opin. Immunol. 13 (2001) 195–201.

[953] K.M. Haas, et al., B-1a and B-1b cells exhibit distinct developmental requirements and have unique functional roles in innate and adaptive immunity to *S. pneumoniae*, Immunity 23 (2005) 7–18.

[954] N.M. Bhat, et al., The ontogeny and functional characteristics of human B-1 CD5+ B cells, Int. Immunol. 4 (1992) 243–252.

[955] T.J. Kipps, B.A. Robbins, D.A. Carson, Uniform high frequency expression of autoantibody-associated crossreactive idiotypes in the primary B cell follicles of human fetal spleen, J. Exp. Med. 171 (1990) 189–196.

[956] J.H. Antin, et al., Leu-1+ (CD5+) B cells: a major lymphoid subpopulation in human fetal spleen: phenotypic and functional studies, J. Immunol. 136 (1986) 505–510.

[957] Z.J. Chen, et al., Polyreactive antigen-binding B cells are the predominant cell type in the newborn B cell repertoire, Eur. J. Immunol. 28 (1998) 989–994.

[958] G.P. Sims, et al., Identification and characterization of circulating human transitional B cells, Blood 105 (2005) 4390–4398.

[959] M. Boes, et al., A critical role of natural immunoglobulin M in immediate defense against systemic bacterial infection, J. Exp. Med. 188 (1998) 2381–2386.

[960] Y. Merbl, et al., Newborn humans manifest autoantibodies to defined self molecules detected by antigen microarray informatics, J. Clin. Invest. 117 (2007) 712–718.

[961] D.M. Ambrosino, N.R. Delaney, R.C. Shamberger, Human polysaccharide-specific B cells are responsive to pokeweed mitogen and IL-6, J. Immunol. 144 (1990) 1221–1226.

[962] C.C. Peeters, et al., Interferon-gamma and interleukin-6 augment the human in vitro antibody response to the Haemophilus influenzae type b polysaccharide, J. Infect. Dis. 165 (1992) S161–S162.

[963] C.M. Snapper, J.J. Mond, A model for induction of T cell-independent humoral immunity in response to polysaccharide antigens, J. Immunol. 157 (1996) 2229–2233.

[964] R.M. Buchanan, B.P. Arulanandam, D.W. Metzger, IL-12 enhances antibody responses to T-independent polysaccharide vaccines in the absence of T and NK cells, J. Immunol. 161 (1998) 5525–5533.

[965] C.M. Snapper, et al., Bacterial lipoproteins may substitute for cytokines in the humoral immune response to T cell-independent type II antigens, J. Immunol. 155 (1995) 5582–5589.

[966] R.L. Chelvarajan, et al., CpG oligodeoxynucleotides overcome the unresponsiveness of neonatal B cells to stimulation with the thymus-independent stimuli anti-IgM and TNP-Ficoll, Eur. J. Immunol. 29 (1999) 2808–2818.

[967] J. Huggins, et al., CpG DNA activation and plasma-cell differentiation of CD27− naive human B cells, Blood 109 (2007) 1611–1619.

[968] F. Capolunghi, et al., CpG drives human transitional B cells to terminal differentiation and production of natural antibodies, J. Immunol. 180 (2008) 800–808.

[969] A. Durandy, et al., Undetectable CD40 ligand expression on T cells and low B cell, J. Immunol. 154 (1995) 1560–1568.

[970] B. Golding, A.V. Muchmore, R.M. Blaese, Newborn and Wiskott-Aldrich patient B cells can be activated by TNP-Brucella abortus: evidence that TNP-Brucella abortus behaves as a T-independent type 1 antigen in humans, J. Immunol. 133 (1984) 2966–2971.

[971] A.W. Griffioen, et al., Role of CR2 in the human adult and neonatal in vitro antibody response to type 4 pneumococcal polysaccharide, Cell. Immunol. 143 (1992) 11–22.

[972] W. Timens, T. Rozeboom, S. Poppema, Fetal and neonatal development of human spleen: an immunohistological study, Immunology 60 (1987) 603–609.

[973] S.M. Halista, et al., Characterization of early activation events in cord blood B cells after stimulation with T cell-independent activators, Pediatr. Res. 43 (1998) 496–503.

[974] A.M. Silverstein, R.A. Prendergast, C.J. Parshall Jr., Cellular kinetics of the antibody response by the fetal rhesus monkey, J. Immunol. 104 (1970) 269–271.

[975] A. Silverstein, Ontogeny of the immune response: a perspective, in: M.D. Cooper, D.H. Dayton (Eds.), Development of Host Defenses, Raven Press, New York, 1977, pp. 1–10.

[976] A.M. Watts, et al., Fetal immunization of baboons induces a fetal-specific antibody response, Nat. Med. 5 (1999) 427–430.

[977] T.J. Gill, et al., Transplacental immunization of the human fetus to tetanus by immunization of the mother, J. Clin. Invest. 72 (1983) 987–996.

[978] Y. Vanderbeeken, et al., In utero immunization of the fetus to tetanus by maternal vaccination during pregnancy, Am. J. Reprod. Immunol. Microbiol. 8 (1985) 39–42.

[979] G. Enders, Serologic test combinations for safe detection of rubella infections, Rev. Infect. Dis. 7 (1985) S113–S122.

[980] Y. Naot, G. Desmonts, J.S. Remington, IgM enzyme-linked immunosorbent assay test for the diagnosis of congenital Toxoplasma infection, J. Pediatr. 98 (1981) 32–36.

[981] B.F. Chumpitazi, et al., Diagnosis of congenital toxoplasmosis by immunoblotting and relationship with other methods, J. Clin. Microbiol. 33 (1995) 1479–1485.

[982] P.D. Griffiths, et al., Congenital cytomegalovirus infection: diagnostic and prognostic significance of the detection of specific immunoglobulin M antibodies in cord serum, Pediatrics 69 (1982) 544–549.

[983] J.M. Pinon, et al., Detection of specific immunoglobulin E in patients with toxoplasmosis, J. Clin. Microbiol. 28 (1990) 1739–1743.

[984] C.L. King, et al., B cell sensitization to helminthic infection develops in utero in humans, J. Immunol. 160 (1998) 3578–3584.

[985] G. Desmonts, et al., Prenatal diagnosis of congenital toxoplasmosis, Lancet 1 (1985) 500–504.

[986] P. Stepick-Biek, et al., IgA antibodies for diagnosis of acute congenital and acquired toxoplasmosis, J. Infect. Dis. 162 (1990) 270–273.

[987] A. Decoster, et al., Anti-P30 IgA antibodies as prenatal markers of congenital toxoplasma infection, Clin. Exp. Immunol. 87 (1992) 310–315.

[988] J. Dengrove, et al., IgG and IgG subclass specific antibody responses to diphtheria and tetanus toxoids in newborns and infants given DTP immunization, Pediatr. Res. 20 (1986) 735–739.

[989] P. Smolen, et al., Antibody response to oral polio vaccine in premature infants, J. Pediatr. 103 (1983) 917–919.

[990] C. Fink, et al., The formation of macroglobulin antibodies, II: studies on neonatal infants and older children, J. Clin. Invest. 41 (1962) 1422–1428.

[991] R. Smith, D.V. Eitzman, The development of the immune response, Pediatrics 33 (1964) 163–183.

[992] J. Uhr, et al., The antibody response to bacteriophage in newborn premature infants, J. Clin. Invest. 41 (1962) 1509–1513.

[993] D.J. West, Clinical experience with hepatitis B vaccines, Am. J. Infect. Control 17 (1989) 172–180.

[994] S.S. Lee, et al., A reduced dose approach to hepatitis B vaccination for low-risk newborns and preschool children, Vaccine 13 (1995) 373–376.

[995] D.P. Greenberg, Pediatric experience with recombinant hepatitis B vaccines and relevant safety and immunogenicity studies, Pediatr. Infect. Dis. J. 12 (1993) 438–445.

[996] J. Dancis, J.J. Osborn, H.W. Kunz, Studies of the immunology of the newborn infant, IV: antibody formation in the premature infant, Pediatrics 12 (1953) 151–157.

[997] E.J. McFarland, et al., Human immunodeficiency virus type 1 (HIV-1) gp120-specific antibodies in neonates receiving an HIV-1 recombinant gp120 vaccine, J. Infect. Dis. 184 (2001) 1331–1335.

[998] J. Peterson, Immunization in the young infant: response to combined vaccines: I-IV, Am. J. Dis. Child. 81 (1951) 484–491.

[999] R. Provenzano, L.H. Wetterow, C.L. Sullivan, Immunization and antibody response in the newborn infant, I: pertussis inoculation within twenty-four hours of birth, N. Engl. J. Med. 273 (1965) 959–965.

[1000] L.J. Baraff, et al., Immunologic response to early and routine DTP immunization in infants, Pediatrics 73 (1984) 37–42.

[1001] N.B. Halasa, et al., Poor immune responses to a birth dose of diphtheria, tetanus, and acellular pertussis vaccine, J. Pediatr. 153 (2008) 327–332.

[1002] C. Belloni, et al., Immunogenicity of a three-component acellular pertussis vaccine administered at birth, Pediatrics 111 (2003) 1042–1045.

[1003] M. Knuf, et al., Neonatal vaccination with an acellular pertussis vaccine accelerates the acquisition of pertussis antibodies in infants, J. Pediatr. 152 (2008) 655–660.

[1004] B.D. Schoub, et al., Monovalent neonatal polio immunization—a strategy for the developing world, J. Infect. Dis. 157 (1988) 836–839.

[1005] H.A. Gans, et al., Deficiency of the humoral immune response to measles vaccine in infants immunized at age 6 months, JAMA 280 (1998) 527–532.

[1006] H.A. Gans, et al., IL-12, IFN-gamma, and T cell proliferation to measles in immunized infants, J. Immunol. 162 (1999) 5569–5575.

[1007] H. Gans, et al., Immune responses to measles and mumps vaccination of infants at 6, 9, and 12 months, J. Infect. Dis. 184 (2001) 817–826.

[1008] H.A. Gans, et al., Humoral and cell-mediated immune responses to an early 2-dose measles vaccination regimen in the United States, J. Infect. Dis. 190 (2004) 83–90.

[1009] D.H. Smith, et al., Responses of children immunized with the capsular polysaccharide of Hemophilus influenzae, type b, Pediatrics 52 (1973) 637–644.

[1010] D.M. Granoff, et al., Induction of immunologic memory in infants primed with Haemophilus influenzae type b conjugate vaccines, J. Infect. Dis. 168 (1993) 663–671.

[1011] J. Eskola, H. Kayhty, Early immunization with conjugate vaccines, Vaccine 16 (1998) 1433–1438.

[1012] J.M. Lieberman, et al., Effect of neonatal immunization with diphtheria and tetanus toxoids on antibody responses to Haemophilus influenzae type b conjugate vaccines, J. Pediatr. 126 (1995) 198–205.

[1013] H.L. Keyserling, C. Wickliffe, ICAAC Abstracts, American Society of Microbiology, (1990), Atlanta, GA.

[1014] J.I. Ward, et al., ICAAC Abstracts, American Society for Microbiology, (1992), New Orleans, LA.

[1015] Y. Schlesinger, D.M. Granoff, Avidity and bactericidal activity of antibody elicited by different Haemophilus influenzae type b conjugate vaccines. The Vaccine Study Group, JAMA 267 (1992) 1489–1494.

[1016] E.E. Adderson, et al., Restricted Ig H chain V gene usage in the human antibody response to Haemophilus influenzae type b capsular polysaccharide, J. Immunol. 147 (1991) 1667–1674.

[1017] K.K. Hsu, S.I. Pelton, Heptavalent pneumococcal conjugate vaccine: current and future impact, Expert Rev. Vaccines 2 (2003) 619–631.

[1018] L.O. Conterno, et al., Conjugate vaccines for preventing meningococcal C meningitis and septicaemia, Cochrane Database Syst. Rev. (3) (2006) CD001834.

[1019] J.C. Bernbaum, et al., Response of preterm infants to diphtheria-tetanus-pertussis immunizations, J. Pediatr. 107 (1985) 184–188.

[1020] B.A. Koblin, et al., Response of preterm infants to diphtheria-tetanus-pertussis vaccine, Pediatr. Infect. Dis. J. 7 (1988) 704–711.

[1021] S.C. Adenyi-Jones, et al., Systemic and local immune responses to enhanced-potency inactivated poliovirus vaccine in premature and term infants, J. Pediatr. 120 (1992) 686–689.

[1022] H. Shinefield, et al., Efficacy, immunogenicity and safety of heptavalent pneumococcal conjugate vaccine in low birth weight and preterm infants, Pediatr. Infect. Dis. J. 21 (2002) 182–186.

[1023] Y.L. Lau, et al., Response of preterm infants to hepatitis B vaccine, J. Pediatr. 121 (1992) 962–965.

[1024] M.S. Freitas da Motta, et al., Immunogenicity of hepatitis B vaccine in preterm and full term infants vaccinated within the first week of life, Vaccine 20 (2002) 1557–1562.

[1025] S.C. Kim, et al., Immunogenicity of hepatitis B vaccine in preterm infants, Pediatrics 99 (1997) 534–536.

[1026] N. Linder, et al., Hepatitis B vaccination: long-term follow-up of the immune response of preterm infants and comparison of two vaccination protocols, Infection 30 (2002) 136–139.

[1027] D.P. Greenberg, et al., Immunogenicity of Haemophilus influenzae type b tetanus toxoid conjugate vaccine in young infants. The Kaiser-UCLA Vaccine Study Group, J. Infect. Dis. 170 (1994) 76–81.

[1028] P.T. Heath, et al., Hib vaccination in infants born prematurely, Arch. Dis. Child. 88 (2003) 206–210.

[1029] L.K. Washburn, et al., Response to Haemophilus influenzae type b conjugate vaccine in chronically ill premature infants, J. Pediatr. 123 (1993) 791–794.

[1030] D.C. Roopenian, S. Akilesh, FcRn: the neonatal Fc receptor comes of age, Nat. Rev. Immunol. 7 (2007) 715–725.

[1031] M. Firan, et al., The MHC class I-related receptor, FcRn, plays an essential role in the maternofetal transfer of gamma-globulin in humans, Int. Immunol. 13 (2001) 993–1002.

[1032] N.E. Simister, Human placental Fc receptors and the trapping of immune complexes, Vaccine 16 (1998) 1451–1455.

[1033] P.F. Kohler, R.S. Farr, Elevation of cord over maternal IgG immunoglobulin: evidence for an active placental IgG transport, Nature 210 (1966) 1070–1071.

[1034] J.P. Gusdon Jr., Fetal and maternal immunoglobulin levels during pregnancy, Am. J. Obstet. Gynecol. 103 (1969) 895–900.

[1035] R.W. Pitcher-Wilmott, P. Hindocha, C.B. Wood, The placental transfer of IgG subclasses in human pregnancy, Clin. Exp. Immunol. 41 (1980) 303–308.

[1036] M. Landor, Maternal-fetal transfer of immunoglobulins, Ann. Allergy Asthma Immunol. 74 (1995) 279–283.

[1037] L. Martensson, H.H. Fudenberg, Gm genes and gamma G-globulin synthesis in the human fetus, J. Immunol. 94 (1965) 514–520.

[1038] F.C. Hay, M.G. Hull, G. Torrigiani, The transfer of human IgG subclasses from mother to foetus, Clin. Exp. Immunol. 9 (1971) 355–358.

[1039] V.A. Oxelius, N.W. Svenningsen, IgG subclass concentrations in preterm neonates, Acta Paediatr. Scand. 73 (1984) 626–630.

[1040] A. Malek, R. Sager, H. Schneider, Maternal-fetal transport of immunoglobulin G and its subclasses during the third trimester of human pregnancy, Am. J. Reprod. Immunol. 32 (1994) 8–14.

[1041] A. Morell, et al., IgG subclasses and antibodies to group B streptococci, pneumococci, and tetanus toxoid in preterm neonates after intravenous infusion of immunoglobulin to the mothers, Pediatr. Res. 20 (1986) 933–936.

[1042] N. Linder, et al., Placental transfer and decay of varicella-zoster virus antibodies in preterm infants, J. Pediatr. 137 (2000) 85–89.

[1043] H. Sato, et al., Transfer of measles, mumps, and rubella antibodies from mother to infant: its effect on measles, mumps, and rubella immunization, Am. J. Dis. Child. 133 (1979) 1240–1243.

[1044] B. Vahlquist, Response of infants to diphtheria immunization, Lancet 1 (1949) 16–18.

[1045] F. Perkins, R. Yetts, W. Gaisford, Response of infants to a third dose of poliomyelitis vaccine given 10 to 12 months after primary immunization, BMJ 1 (1959) 680–682.

[1046] C. Panpitpat, et al., Elevated levels of maternal anti-tetanus toxin antibodies do not suppress the immune response to a Haemophilus influenzae type b polyribosylphosphate-tetanus toxoid conjugate vaccine, Bull. World Health Organ. 78 (2000) 364–371.

[1047] J. Rowe, et al., Enhancement of vaccine-specific cellular immunity in infants by passively acquired maternal antibody, Vaccine 22 (2004) 3986–3992.

[1048] E.R. Stiehm, H.H. Fudenberg, Serum levels of immune globulins in health and disease: a survey, Pediatrics 37 (1966) 715–727.

[1049] S.I. Lee, D.C. Heiner, D. Wara, Development of serum IgG subclass levels in children, Monogr. Allergy 19 (1986) 108–121.

[1050] H.D. Ochs, R.J. Wedgwood, IgG subclass deficiencies, Annu. Rev. Med. 38 (1987) 325–340.

[1051] R.H. Kobayashi, C.J. Hyman, E.R. Stiehm, Immunologic maturation in an infant born to a mother with agammaglobulinemia, Am. J. Dis. Child. 134 (1980) 942–944.

[1052] D.M. Granoff, et al., Antibody responses to Haemophilus influenzae type b polysaccharide vaccine in relation to Km 1 and G2m 23 immunoglobulin allotypes, J. Infect. Dis. 154 (1986) 257–264.

[1053] L.L. Cederqvist, L.C. Ewool, S.D. Litwin, The effect of fetal age, birth weight, and sex on cord blood immunoglobulin values, Am. J. Obstet. Gynecol. 131 (1978) 520–525.

[1054] O.M. Avrech, et al., Efficacy of the placental barrier for immunoglobulins: correlations between maternal, paternal and fetal immunoglobulin levels, Int. Arch. Allergy Immunol. 103 (1994) 160–165.

[1055] M. Allansmith, et al., The development of immunoglobulin levels in man, J. Pediatr. 72 (1968) 276–290.

[1056] J.E. Perchalski, L.W. Clem, P.J. Small, 7S gamma-M immunoglobulins in normal human cord serum, Am. J. Med. Sci. 256 (1968) 107–111.

[1057] C.J. Alford, S. Stagno, D.W. Reynolds, Diagnosis of chronic perinatal infections, Am. J. Dis. Child. 129 (1975) 455–463.

[1058] M.E. Conley, et al., Differentiation of human B cells expressing the IgA subclasses as demonstrated by monoclonal hybridoma antibodies, J. Immunol. 125 (1980) 2311–2316.

[1059] B.M. Seidel, et al., Determination of secretory IgA and albumin in saliva of newborn infants, Biol. Neonate 78 (2000) 186–190.

[1060] S.H. Josephs, R.H. Buckley, Serum IgD concentrations in normal infants, children, and adults and in patients with elevated IgE, J. Pediatr. 96 (1980) 417–420.

[1061] A. Haraldsson, et al., Serum immunoglobulin D in infants and children, Scand. J. Immunol. 51 (2000) 415–418.

[1062] M. Bazaral, H.A. Orgel, R.N. Hamburger, IgE levels in normal infants and mothers and an inheritance hypothesis, J. Immunol. 107 (1971) 794–801.

[1063] G. Edenharter, et al., Cord blood-IgE as risk factor and predictor for atopic diseases, Clin. Exp. Allergy 28 (1998) 671–678.

[1064] W.T. Chang, et al., Predictability of early onset atopic dermatitis by cord blood IgE and parental history, Acta Paediatr. Taiwan 46 (2005) 272–277.

[1065] G. Pluschke, M. Achtman, Degree of antibody-independent activation of the classical complement pathway by K1 Escherichia coli differs with O antigen type and correlates with virulence of meningitis in newborns, Infect. Immun. 43 (1984) 684–692.

[1066] M.B. Marques, et al., Prevention of C3 deposition by capsular polysaccharide is a virulence mechanism of type III group B streptococci, Infect. Immun. 60 (1992) 3986–3993.

[1067] J.R. Campbell, C.J. Baker, M.S. Edwards, Deposition and degradation of C3 on type III group B streptococci, Infect. Immun. 59 (1991) 1978–1983.

[1068] C.J. Baker, M.S. Edwards, Group B streptococcal conjugate vaccines, Arch. Dis. Child. 88 (2003) 375–378.

[1069] M.R. Wessels, et al., Studies of group B streptococcal infection in mice deficient in complement component C3 or C4 demonstrate an essential role for complement in both innate and acquired immunity, Proc. Natl. Acad. Sci. U S A 92 (1995) 11490–11494.

[1070] A. Matsukawa III., et al., Chemokines and other mediators, 8. Chemokines and their receptors in cell-mediated immune responses in the lung, Microsc. Res. Tech. 53 (2001) 298–306.

[1071] J.F. Bohnsack, et al., A role for C5 and C5a-ase in the acute neutrophil response to group B streptococcal infections, J. Infect. Dis. 175 (1997) 847–855.

[1072] V. Cusumano, et al., Neonatal hypersusceptibility to endotoxin correlates with increased tumor necrosis factor production in mice, J. Infect. Dis. 176 (1997) 168–176.

[1073] G. Mancuso, et al., Role of interleukin 12 in experimental neonatal sepsis caused by group B streptococci, Infect. Immun. 65 (1997) 3731–3735.

[1074] P.A. Williams, et al., Production of tumor necrosis factor by human cells in vitro and in vivo, induced by group B streptococci, J. Pediatr. 123 (1993) 292–300.

[1075] J. Wennekamp, P. Henneke, Induction and termination of inflammatory signaling in group B streptococcal sepsis, Immunol. Rev. 225 (2008) 114–127.

[1076] L.B. Givner, L. Gray, T.M. O'Shea, Antibodies to tumor necrosis factor-alpha: use as adjunctive therapy in established group B streptococcal disease in newborn rats, Pediatr. Res. 38 (1995) 551–554.

[1077] V. Cusumano, et al., Interleukin-10 protects neonatal mice from lethal group B streptococcal infection, Infect. Immun. 64 (1996) 2850–2852.

[1078] C.J. Fisher Jr., et al., Treatment of septic shock with the tumor necrosis factor receptor:Fc fusion protein. The Soluble TNF Receptor Sepsis Study Group, N. Engl. J. Med. 334 (1996) 1697–1702.

[1079] V.G. Hemming, et al., Assessment of group B streptococcal opsonins in human and rabbit serum by neutrophil chemiluminescence, J. Clin. Invest. 58 (1976) 1379–1387.

[1080] F.Y. Lin, et al., Level of maternal antibody required to protect neonates against early-onset disease caused by group B streptococcus type Ia: a multicenter, seroepidemiology study, J. Infect. Dis. 184 (2001) 1022–1028.

[1081] K.K. Christensen, et al., Correlation between serum antibody-levels against group B streptococci and gestational age in newborns, Eur. J. Pediatr. 142 (1984) 86–88.

[1082] C.J. Baker, M.S. Edwards, D.L. Kasper, Role of antibody to native type III polysaccharide of group B streptococcus in infant infection, Pediatrics 68 (1981) 544–549.

[1083] M.S. Edwards, et al., Patterns of immune response among survivors of group B streptococcal meningitis, J. Infect. Dis. 161 (1990) 65–70.

[1084] K.M. Boyer, M.E. Klegerman, S.P. Gotoff, Development of IgM antibody to group B streptococcus type III in human infants, J. Infect. Dis. 165 (1992) 1049–1055.

[1085] T.J. Nealon, S.J. Mattingly, Role of cellular lipoteichoic acids in mediating adherence of serotype III strains of group B streptococci to human embryonic, fetal, and adult epithelial cells, Infect. Immun. 43 (1984) 523–530.

[1086] R.A. Broughton, C.J. Baker, Role of adherence in the pathogenesis of neonatal group B streptococcal infection, Infect. Immun. 39 (1983) 837–843.

[1087] J. Kallman, et al., Impaired phagocytosis and opsonisation towards group B streptococci in preterm neonates, Arch. Dis. Child. Fetal Neonatal Ed. 78 (1998) F46–F50.

[1088] H.T. Jordan, et al., Revisiting the need for vaccine prevention of late-onset neonatal group B streptococcal disease: a multistate, population-based analysis, Pediatr. Infect. Dis. J. 27 (2008) 1057–1064.

[1089] C.M. Healy, C.J. Baker, Prospects for prevention of childhood infections by maternal immunization, Curr. Opin. Infect. Dis. 19 (2006) 271–276.

[1090] D. Maione, et al., Identification of a universal group B streptococcus vaccine by multiple genome screen, Science 309 (2005) 148–150.

[1091] H.B. Jenson, B.H. Pollock, Meta-analyses of the effectiveness of intravenous immune globulin for prevention and treatment of neonatal sepsis, Pediatrics 99 (1997) E2.

[1092] A. Ohlsson, J.B. Lacy, Intravenous immunoglobulin for preventing infection in preterm and/or low-birth-weight infants, Cochrane Database Syst. Rev. (2001) CD000361.

[1093] M. DeJonge, et al., Clinical trial of safety and efficacy of INH-A21 for the prevention of nosocomial staphylococcal bloodstream infection in premature infants, J. Pediatr. 151 (2007) 260–265 265 e261.

[1094] INIS Study, International Neonatal Immunotherapy Study, Non-specific intravenous immunoglobulin therapy for suspected or proven neonatal sepsis: an international, placebo controlled, multicentre randomised trial, BMC Pregnancy Childbirth 8 (2008) 52.

[1095] M. Suri, et al., Immunotherapy in the prophylaxis and treatment of neonatal sepsis, Curr. Opin. Pediatr. 15 (2003) 155–160.

[1096] R. Carr, N. Modi, C. Dore, G-CSF and GM-CSF for treating or preventing neonatal infections, Cochrane Database Syst. Rev. (2003) CD003066.

[1097] R. Carr, et al., Granulocyte-macrophage colony stimulating factor administered as prophylaxis for reduction of sepsis in extremely preterm, small for gestational age neonates (the PROGRAMS trial): a single-blind, multicentre, randomised controlled trial, Lancet 373 (2009) 226–233.

[1098] P. Kocherlakota, E.F. La Gamma, Preliminary report: rhG-CSF may reduce the incidence of neonatal sepsis in prolonged preeclampsia–associated neutropenia, Pediatrics 102 (1998) 1107–1111.

[1099] J. Rosenthal, et al., A two-year follow-up of neonates with presumed sepsis treated with recombinant human granulocyte colony-stimulating factor during the first week of life, J. Pediatr. 128 (1996) 135–137.

[1100] E.R. Gillan, et al., A randomized, placebo-controlled trial of recombinant human granulocytes colony stimulating factor administration in newborn infants with presumed sepsis: significant induction of peripheral and bone marrow neutrophilia, Blood 84 (1994) 1427–1433.

[1101] V. Drossou-Agakidou, et al., Administration of recombinant human granulocyte-colony stimulating factor to septic neonates induces neutrophilia and enhances the neutrophil respiratory burst and beta2 integrin expression. Results of a randomized controlled trial, Eur. J. Pediatr. 157 (1998) 583–588.

[1102] H.M. Bernstein, et al., Administration of recombinant granulocyte colony-stimulating factor to neonates with septicemia: a meta-analysis, J. Pediatr. 138 (2001) 917–920.

[1103] D.W. Kimberlin, Herpes simplex virus infections of the newborn, Semin. Perinatol. 31 (2007) 19–25.

[1104] S. Kohl, The neonatal human's immune response to herpes simplex virus infection: a critical review, Pediatr. Infect. Dis. J. 8 (1989) 67–74.

[1105] M.G. Tovey, C. Lallemand, G. Thyphronitis, Adjuvant activity of type I interferons, Biol. Chem. 389 (2008) 541–545.

[1106] S. Dupuis, et al., Impairment of mycobacterial but not viral immunity by a germline human STAT1 mutation, Science 293 (2001) 300–303.

[1107] S. Dupuis, et al., Impaired response to interferon-alpha/beta and lethal viral disease in human STAT1 deficiency, Nat. Genet. 33 (2003) 388–391.

[1108] G. Uze, D. Monneron, IL-28 and IL-29: newcomers to the interferon family, Biochimie 89 (2007) 729–734.

[1109] M. Kozak, B. Roizman, RNA synthesis in cells infected with herpes simplex virus, IX: evidence for accumulation of abundant symmetric transcripts in nuclei, J. Virol. 15 (1975) 36–40.

[1110] S.Y. Zhang, et al., TLR3 deficiency in patients with herpes simplex encephalitis, Science 317 (2007) 1522–1527.

[1111] A. Casrouge, et al., Herpes simplex virus encephalitis in human UNC-93B deficiency, Science 314 (2006) 308–312.

[1112] E.A. Kurt-Jones, et al., Herpes simplex virus 1 interaction with Toll-like receptor 2 contributes to lethal encephalitis, Proc. Natl. Acad. Sci. U S A 101 (2004) 1315–1320.

[1113] K.W. Boehme, M. Guerrero, T. Compton, Human cytomegalovirus envelope glycoproteins B and H are necessary for TLR2 activation in permissive cells, J. Immunol. 177 (2006) 7094–7102.

[1114] P.Y. Bochud, et al., Polymorphisms in TLR2 are associated with increased viral shedding and lesional rate in patients with genital herpes simplex virus type 2 infection, J. Infect. Dis. 196 (2007) 505–509.

[1115] E.A. Kurt-Jones, J. Belko, C. Yu, et al., The role of toll-like receptors in herpes simplex infection in neonates, J. Infect. Dis. 191 (2005) 746–748.

[1116] P. Lebon, G. Ponsot, J. Aicardi, Early intrathecal synthesis of interferon in herpes encephalitis, Biomedicine 31 (1979) 267–271.

[1117] E. Dussaix, et al., Intrathecal synthesis of different alpha-interferons in patients with various neurological diseases, Acta Neurol. Scand. 71 (1985) 504–509.

[1118] P. Lebon, et al., Interferon gamma in acute and subacute encephalitis, BMJ (Clin. Res. Ed.) 296 (1988) 9–11.

[1119] R.J. Duerst, L.A. Morrison, Herpes simplex virus 2 virion host shutoff protein interferes with type I interferon production and responsiveness, Virology 322 (2004) 158–167.

[1120] S. Yokota, et al., Induction of suppressor of cytokine signaling-3 by herpes simplex virus type 1 contributes to inhibition of the interferon signaling pathway, J. Virol. 78 (2004) 6282–6286.

[1121] H. Kimura, Y. Ito, M. Futamura, et al., Quantitation of viral load in neonatal herpes simplex virus infection and comparison between type 1 and type 2, J. Med. Virol. 67 (2002) 349–353.

[1122] J. Kawada, et al., Evaluation of systemic inflammatory responses in neonates with herpes simplex virus infection, J. Infect. Dis. 190 (2004) 494–498.

[1123] A. Rosler, et al., Time course of chemokines in the cerebrospinal fluid and serum during herpes simplex type 1 encephalitis, J. Neurol. Sci. 157 (1998) 82–89.

[1124] M. Fleck, et al., Herpes simplex virus type 2 infection induced apoptosis in peritoneal macrophages independent of Fas and tumor necrosis factor-receptor signaling, Viral Immunol. 12 (1999) 263–275.

[1125] S. Lee, et al., Decreased interleukin-12 (IL-12) from activated cord blood versus adult peripheral blood mononuclear cells and upregulation of interferon-gamma, natural killer, and lymphokine-activated killer activity by IL-12 in cord blood mononuclear cells, Blood 88 (1996) 645–654.

[1126] J.X. Qian, et al., Decreased interleukin-15 from activated cord versus adult peripheral blood mononuclear cells and the effect of interleukin-15 in upregulating antitumor immune activity and cytokine production in cord blood, Blood 90 (1997) 3106–3117.

[1127] G. Pollara, et al., Herpes simplex virus infection of dendritic cells: balance among activation, inhibition, and immunity, J. Infect. Dis. 187 (2003) 165–178.

[1128] M. Kummer, et al., Herpes simplex virus type 1 induces CD83 degradation in mature dendritic cells with immediate-early kinetics via the cellular proteasome, J. Virol. 81 (2007) 6326–6338.

[1129] P. Bjorck, Dendritic cells exposed to herpes simplex virus in vivo do not produce IFN-alpha after rechallenge with virus in vitro and exhibit decreased T cell alloreactivity, J. Immunol. 172 (2004) 5396–5404.

[1130] L. Bosnjak, et al., Herpes simplex virus infection of human dendritic cells induces apoptosis and allows cross-presentation via uninfected dendritic cells, J. Immunol. 174 (2005) 2220–2227.

[1131] N. Novak, W.M. Peng, Dancing with the enemy: the interplay of herpes simplex virus with dendritic cells, Clin. Exp. Immunol. 142 (2005) 405–410.

[1132] R.S. Allan, et al., Epidermal viral immunity induced by CD8alpha+ dendritic cells but not by Langerhans cells, Science 301 (2003) 1925–1928.

[1133] A. Porras, et al., Developmental and epigenetic regulation of the human TLR3 gene, Mol. Immunol. 46 (2008) 27–36.

[1134] T. Kawai, S. Akira, Antiviral signaling through pattern recognition receptors, J. Biochem. 141 (2007) 137–145.

[1135] J.S. Orange, Human natural killer cell deficiencies, Curr. Opin. Allergy Clin. Immunol. 6 (2006) 399–409.

[1136] A. Martin-Fontecha, et al., Induced recruitment of NK cells to lymph nodes provides IFN-gamma for T(H)1 priming, Nat. Immunol. 5 (2004) 1260–1265.

[1137] J. Gosselin, et al., Interleukin-15 as an activator of natural killer cell-mediated antiviral response, Blood 94 (1999) 4210–4219.

[1138] L.M. Fawaz, E. Sharif-Askari, J. Menezes, Up-regulation of NK cytotoxic activity via IL-15 induction by different viruses: a comparative study, J. Immunol. 163 (1999) 4473–4480.

[1139] P.J. Leibson, et al., Impaired neonatal natural killer-cell activity to herpes simplex virus: decreased inhibition of viral replication and altered response to lymphokines, J. Clin. Immunol. 6 (1986) 216–224.

[1140] A.R. Hayward, M. Herberger, D. Saunders, Herpes simplex virus–stimulated interferon-γ production by newborn mononuclear cells, Pediatr. Res. 20 (1986) 398–401.

[1141] G.M. Verjans, et al., Isopentenyl pyrophosphate-reactive Vgamma9Vdelta 2 T helper 1-like cells are the major gammadelta T cell subset recovered from lesions of patients with genital herpes, J. Infect. Dis. 190 (2004) 489–493.

[1142] W.E. Lafferty, L.A. Brewer, L. Corey, Alteration of lymphocyte transformation response to herpes simplex virus infection by acyclovir therapy, Antimicrob. Agents Chemother. 26 (1984) 887–891.

[1143] D.M. Koelle, et al., Herpes simplex virus infection of human fibroblasts and keratinocytes inhibits recognition by cloned CD8+ cytotoxic T lymphocytes, J. Clin. Invest. 91 (1993) 961–968.

[1144] D. Bauer, R. Tampe, Herpes viral proteins blocking the transporter associated with antigen processing TAP—from genes to function and structure, Curr. Top. Microbiol. Immunol. 269 (2002) 87–99.

[1145] D.M. Koelle, et al., Clearance of HSV-2 from recurrent genital lesions correlates with infiltration of HSV-specific cytotoxic T lymphocytes, J. Clin. Invest. 101 (1998) 1500–1508.

[1146] G.A. Lewandowski, D. Lo, F.E. Bloom, Interference with major histocompatibility complex class II-restricted antigen presentation in the brain by herpes simplex virus type 1: a possible mechanism of evasion of the immune response, Proc. Natl. Acad. Sci. U S A 90 (1993) 2005–2009.

[1147] A.R. Hayward, G.S. Read, M. Cosyns, Herpes simplex virus interferes with monocyte accessory cell function, J. Immunol. 150 (1993) 190–196.

[1148] M. Salio, et al., Inhibition of dendritic cell maturation by herpes simplex virus, Eur. J. Immunol. 29 (1999) 3245–3253.

[1149] S. Barcy, L. Corey, Herpes simplex inhibits the capacity of lymphoblastoid B cell lines to stimulate CD4+ T cells, J. Immunol. 166 (2001) 6242–6249.

[1150] D.M. Koelle, et al., Direct recovery of herpes simplex virus (HSV)-specific T lymphocyte clones from recurrent genital HSV-2 lesions, J. Infect. Dis. 169 (1994) 956–961.

[1151] A.A. Chentoufi, et al., Asymptomatic human CD4+ cytotoxic T-cell epitopes identified from herpes simplex virus glycoprotein B, J. Virol. 82 (2008) 11792–11802.

[1152] A. Jain, et al., Defects of T-cell effector function and post-thymic maturation in X-linked hyper-IgM syndrome, J. Clin. Invest. 103 (1999) 1151–1158.

[1153] S. Fontana, et al., Functional defects of dendritic cells in patients with CD40 deficiency, Blood 102 (2003) 4099–4106.

[1154] M.A. Williams, et al., Developing and maintaining protective CD8+ memory T cells, Immunol. Rev. 211 (2006) 146–153.

[1155] E. Adamopoulou, et al., Human CD4+ T cells displaying viral epitopes elicit a functional virus-specific memory CD8+ T cell response, J. Immunol. 178 (2007) 5465–5472.

[1156] H. Asanuma, et al., Frequencies of memory T cells specific for varicella-zoster virus, herpes simplex virus, and cytomegalovirus by intracellular detection of cytokine expression, J. Infect. Dis. 181 (2000) 859–866.

[1157] D.M. Koelle, L. Corey, Recent progress in herpes simplex virus immunobiology and vaccine research, Clin. Microbiol. Rev. 16 (2003) 96–113.

[1158] M.A. Carmack, et al., T cell recognition and cytokine production elicited by common and type-specific glycoproteins of herpes simplex virus type 1 and type 2, J. Infect. Dis. 174 (1996) 899–906.

[1159] M. Kim, et al., Immunodominant epitopes in herpes simplex virus type 2 glycoprotein D are recognized by CD4 lymphocytes from both HSV-1 and HSV-2 seropositive subjects, J. Immunol. 181 (2008) 6604–6615.

[1160] X. Zhang, et al., Gender-dependent HLA-DR-restricted epitopes identified from herpes simplex virus type 1 glycoprotein D, Clin. Vaccine Immunol. 15 (2008) 1436–1449.

[1161] K. Dabbagh, et al., Toll-like receptor 4 is required for optimal development of Th2 immune responses: role of dendritic cells, J. Immunol. 168 (2002) 4524–4530.

[1162] M.A. Fernandez, et al., Neonatal CD8+ T cells are slow to develop into lytic effectors after HSV infection in vivo, Eur. J. Immunol. 38 (2008) 102–113.

[1163] G.A. Diaz, D.M. Koelle, Human CD4+ CD25 high cells suppress proliferative memory lymphocyte responses to herpes simplex virus type 2, J. Virol. 80 (2006) 8271–8273.

[1164] A.R. Hayward, et al., Specific immunity after congenital or neonatal infection with cytomegalovirus or herpes simplex virus, J. Immunol. 133 (1984) 2469–2473.

[1165] G.M. Verjans, et al., Selective retention of herpes simplex virus-specific T cells in latently infected human trigeminal ganglia, Proc. Natl. Acad. Sci. U S A 104 (2007) 3496–3501.

[1166] S. Divito, T.L. Cherpes, R.L. Hendricks, A triple entente: virus, neurons, and CD8+ T cells maintain HSV-1 latency, Immunol. Res. 36 (2006) 119–126.

[1167] D.M. Koelle, L. Corey, Herpes simplex: insights on pathogenesis and possible vaccines, Annu. Rev. Med. 59 (2008) 381–395.

[1168] J. Maertzdorf, et al., Restricted T cell receptor beta-chain variable region protein use by cornea-derived CD4+ and CD8+ herpes simplex virus-specific T cells in patients with herpetic stromal keratitis, J. Infect. Dis. 187 (2003) 550–558.

[1169] K.E. Mark, et al., Rapidly cleared episodes of herpes simplex virus reactivation in immunocompetent adults, J. Infect. Dis. 198 (2008) 1141–1149.

[1170] N. Hosken, et al., Diversity of the CD8+ T-cell response to herpes simplex virus type 2 proteins among persons with genital herpes, J. Virol. 80 (2006) 5509–5515.

[1171] J. Zhu, et al., Virus-specific CD8+ T cells accumulate near sensory nerve endings in genital skin during subclinical HSV-2 reactivation, J. Exp. Med. 204 (2007) 595–603.

[1172] A.Y. Park, P. Scott, IL-12: keeping cell-mediated immunity alive, Scand. J. Immunol. 53 (2001) 529–532.

[1173] D.M. Koelle, et al., Expression of cutaneous lymphocyte-associated antigen by CD8(+) T cells specific for a skin-tropic virus, J. Clin. Invest. 110 (2002) 537–548.

[1174] A. Nansen, et al., CCR2+ and CCR5+CD8+ T cells increase during viral infection and migrate to sites of infection, Eur. J. Immunol. 30 (2000) 1797–1806.

[1175] P.P. Sanna, D.R. Burton, Role of antibodies in controlling viral disease: lessons from experiments of nature and gene knockouts, J. Virol. 74 (2000) 9813–9817.

[1176] D.F. Westra, et al., Natural infection with herpes simplex virus type 1 (HSV-1) induces humoral and T cell responses to the HSV-1 glycoprotein H:L complex, J. Gen. Virol. 81 (2000) 2011–2015.

[1177] J.E. Figueroa, P. Densen, Infectious diseases associated with complement deficiencies, Clin. Microbiol. Rev. 4 (1991) 359–395.

[1178] S. Kohl, et al., Human monocyte-macrophage–mediated antibody-dependent cytotoxicity to herpes simplex virus–infected cells, J. Immunol. 118 (1977) 729–735.

[1179] K.C. Petroni, L. Shen, P.M. Guyre, Modulation of human polymorphonuclear leukocyte IgG Fc receptors and Fc receptor-mediated functions by IFN-γ and glucocorticoids, J. Immunol. 140 (1988) 3467–3472.

[1180] S.J. Lin, et al., Effect of interleukin (IL)-12 and IL-15 on activated natural killer (ANK) and antibody-dependent cellular cytotoxicity (ADCC) in HIV infection, J. Clin. Immunol. 18 (1998) 335–345.

[1181] V. Poaty-Mavoungou, et al., Enhancement of natural killer cell activation and antibody-dependent cellular cytotoxicity by interferon-alpha and interleukin-12 in vaginal mucosae Sivmac251-infected Macaca fascicularis, Viral Immunol. 15 (2002) 197–212.

[1182] T. Osuga, et al., Transfer of specific IgG and IgG subclasses to herpes simplex virus across the blood-brain barrier and placenta in preterm and term newborns, Acta Paediatr. 81 (1992) 792–796.

[1183] R.L. Ashley, et al., Herpes simplex virus-2 (HSV-2) type-specific antibody correlates of protection in infants exposed to HSV-2 at birth, J. Clin. Invest. 90 (1992) 511–514.

[1184] S. Kohl, et al., Neonatal antibody-dependent cellular cytotoxic antibody levels are associated with the clinical presentation of neonatal herpes simplex virus infection, J. Infect. Dis. 160 (1989) 770–776.

[1185] Z. Mikloska, P.P. Sanna, A. Cunningham, Neutralizing antibodies inhibit axonal spread of herpes simplex virus type 1 to epidermal cells in vitro, J. Virol. 73 (1999) 5934–5944.

[1186] S. Vollstedt, et al., Interleukin-12- and gamma interferon-dependent innate immunity are essential and sufficient for long-term survival of passively immunized mice infected with herpes simplex virus type 1, J. Virol. 75 9596–9600.

[1187] R. Burioni, et al., Recombinant human Fab to glycoprotein D neutralizes infectivity and prevents cell-to-cell transmission of herpes simplex viruses 1 and 2 in vitro, Proc. Natl. Acad. Sci. U S A 91 (1994) 355–359.

[1188] J. Cohen, IL-12 deaths: explanation and a puzzle, Science 270 (1995) 908.

[1189] J.P. Leonard, et al., Effects of single-dose interleukin-12 exposure on interleukin-12-associated toxicity and interferon-gamma production, Blood 90 (1997) 2541–2548.

[1190] L.R. Stanberry, et al., Glycoprotein-D-adjuvant vaccine to prevent genital herpes, N. Engl. J. Med. 347 (2002) 1652–1661.

[1191] S. Kohl, et al., Limited antibody-dependent cellular cytotoxicity antibody response induced by a herpes simplex virus type 2 subunit vaccine, J. Infect. Dis. 181 (2000) 335–339.

[1192] D.M. Koelle, Vaccines for herpes simplex virus infections, Curr. Opin. Investig. Drugs 7 (2006) 136–141.

[1193] J.R. Mineo, et al., Antibodies to Toxoplasma gondii major surface protein SAG-1, P30 inhibit infection of host cells and are produced in murine intestine after peroral infection, J. Immunol. 150 (1993) 3951–3964.

[1194] A. Decoster, Detection of IgA anti-P30 SAG1 antibodies in acquired and congenital toxoplasmosis, Curr. Top. Microbiol. Immunol. 219 (1996) 199–207.

[1195] L.D. Sibley, Toxoplasma gondii: perfecting an intracellular life style, Traffic 4 (2003) 581–586.

[1196] J.C. Schwab, C.J. Beckers, K.A. Joiner, The parasitophorous vacuole membrane surrounding intracellular Toxoplasma gondii functions as a molecular sieve, Proc. Natl. Acad. Sci. U S A 91 (1994) 509–513.

[1197] C.B. Wilson, V. Tsai, J.S. Remington, Failure to trigger the oxidative metabolic burst by normal macrophages: possible mechanism for survival of intracellular pathogens, J. Exp. Med. 151 (1980) 328–346.

[1198] L.B. Adams, et al., Microbiostatic effect of murine-activated macrophages for Toxoplasma gondii: role for synthesis of inorganic nitrogen oxides from l-arginine, J. Immunol. 144 (1990) 2725–2729.

[1199] W. Bohne, J. Heesemann, U. Gross, Reduced replication of Toxoplasma gondii is necessary for induction of bradyzoite-specific antigens: a possible role for nitric oxide in triggering stage conversion, Infect. Immun. 62 (1994) 1761–1767.

[1200] A. Sher, et al., Induction and regulation of IL-12-dependent host resistance to Toxoplasma gondii, Immunol. Res. 27 (2003) 521–528.

[1201] P.J. Gaddi, G.S. Yap, Cytokine regulation of immunopathology in toxoplasmosis, Immunol. Cell. Biol. 85 (2007) 155–159.

[1202] E.Y. Denkers, L. Kim, B.A. Butcher, In the belly of the beast: subversion of macrophage proinflammatory signalling cascades during Toxoplasma gondii infection, Cell. Microbiol. 5 (2003) 75–83.

[1203] C.S. Subauste, CD154 and type-1 cytokine response: from hyper IgM syndrome to human immunodeficiency virus infection, J. Infect. Dis. 185 (2002) S83–S89.

[1204] P. Scott, C.A. Hunter, Dendritic cells and immunity to leishmaniasis and toxoplasmosis, Curr. Opin. Immunol. 14 (2002) 466–470.

[1205] D. Sacks, A. Sher, Evasion of innate immunity by parasitic protozoa, Nat. Immunol. 3 (2002) 1041–1047.

[1206] J.S. Stumhofer, et al., Interleukin 27 negatively regulates the development of interleukin 17-producing T helper cells during chronic inflammation of the central nervous system, Nat. Immunol. 7 (2006) 937–945.

[1207] E.R. Unanue, Macrophages, NK cells and neutrophils in the cytokine loop of Listeria, resistance, Res. Immunol. 147 (1996) 499–505.

[1208] R. McLeod, et al., Immune response of mice to ingested Toxoplasma gondii: a model of toxoplasma infection acquired by ingestion, J. Infect. Dis. 149 (1984) 234–244.

[1209] H.W. Murray, et al., Human mononuclear phagocyte antiprotozoal mechanisms: oxygen-dependent vs oxygen-independent activity against intracellular Toxoplasma gondii, J. Immunol. 134 (1985) 1982–1988.

[1210] C.B. Wilson, J.S. Remington, Activity of human blood leukocytes against Toxoplasma gondii, J. Infect. Dis. 140 (1979) 890–895.

[1211] L.D. Sibley, et al., Tumor necrosis factor-alpha triggers antitoxoplasmal activity of IFN-gamma primed macrophages, J. Immunol. 147 (1991) 2340–2345.

[1212] S.M. Thomas, et al., IFN-gamma-mediated antimicrobial response: indoleamine 2,3-dioxygenase-deficient mutant host cells no longer inhibit intracellular Chlamydia spp. or Toxoplasma growth, J. Immunol. 150 (1993) 5529–5534.

[1213] W. Dai, et al., Human indoleamine 2,3-dioxygenase inhibits Toxoplasma gondii growth in fibroblast cells, J. Interferon Res. 14 (1994) 313–317.

[1214] Y. Suzuki, et al., Interferon-gamma: the major mediator of resistance against *Toxoplasma gondii*, Science 240 (1988) 516–518.

[1215] C.R. Brown, R. McLeod, Class I MHC genes and CD8+ T cells determine cyst number in *Toxoplasma gondii* infection, J. Immunol. 145 (1990) 3438–3441.

[1216] F.G. Araujo, Depletion of L3T4+CD4+ T lymphocytes prevents development of resistance to *Toxoplasma gondii* in mice, Infect. Immun. 59 (1991) 1614–1619.

[1217] B.T. Edelson, E.R. Unanue, Immunity to *Listeria* infection, Curr. Opin. Immunol. 12 (2000) 425–431.

[1218] B.J. Luft, et al., Toxoplasmic encephalitis in patients with acquired immune deficiency syndrome, JAMA 252 (1984) 913–917.

[1219] C.B. Wilson, Congenital nonbacterial infections: diagnosis, treatment and prevention, Perinatol Neonatol 9 (1985) 9.

[1220] R. Bortolussi, K. Rajaraman, B. Serushago, Role of tumor necrosis factor-alpha and interferon-gamma in newborn host defense against *Listeria monocytogenes* infection, Pediatr. Res. 32 (1992) 460–464.

[1221] Y. Chen, A. Nakane, T. Minagawa, Recombinant murine gamma interferon induces enhanced resistance to *Listeria monocytogenes* infection in neonatal mice, Infect. Immun. 57 (1989) 2345–2349.

[1222] S. Guglietta, et al., Age-dependent impairment of functional helper T cell responses to immunodominant epitopes of *Toxoplasma gondii* antigens in congenitally infected individuals, Microbes Infect. 9 (2007) 127–133.

[1223] A.F. Fatoohi, et al., Cellular immunity to *Toxoplasma gondii* in congenitally infected newborns and immunocompetent infected hosts, Eur. J. Clin. Microbiol. Infect. Dis. 22 (2003) 181–184.

[1224] L. Ciardelli, et al., Early and accurate diagnosis of congenital toxoplasmosis, Pediatr. Infect. Dis. J. 27 (2008) 125–129.

[1225] N. Hayashi, et al., Flow cytometric analysis of cytomegalovirus-specific cell-mediated immunity in the congenital infection, J. Med. Virol. 71 (2003) 251–258.

[1226] R. Cauda, et al., Congenital cytomegalovirus: immunological alterations, J. Med. Virol. 23 (1987) 41–49.

[1227] J. Li, G. Huston, S.L. Swain, IL-7 promotes the transition of CD4 effectors to persistent memory cells, J. Exp. Med. 198 (2003) 1807–1815.

[1228] J. Huskinson, P. Thulliez, J.S. Remington, *Toxoplasma* antigens recognized by human immunoglobulin A antibodies, J. Clin. Microbiol. 28 (1990) 2632–2636.

[1229] S.Y. Wong, et al., Role of specific immunoglobulin E in diagnosis of acute *Toxoplasma* infection and toxoplasmosis, J. Clin. Microbiol. 31 (1993) 2952–2959.

[1230] R. Bortolussi, et al., Neonatal *Listeria monocytogenes* infection is refractory to interferon, Pediatr. Res. 29 (1991) 400–402.

[1231] L. Krishnan, et al., T helper 1 response against *Leishmania major* in pregnant C57BL/6 mice increases implantation failure and fetal resorptions: correlation with increased IFN-gamma and TNF and reduced IL-10 production by placental cells, J. Immunol. 156 (1996) 653–662.

[1232] J.L. Garcia, Vaccination concepts against *Toxoplasma gondii*, Expert Rev. Vaccines 8 (2009) 215–225.

HUMAN MILK*

Christopher B. Wilson ⊛ Pearay L. Ogra

CHAPTER OUTLINE

Physiology of Lactation   192
  Developmental Anatomy of the Mammary Gland   192
  Endocrine Control of Mammary Gland Function   192
  Secretory Products of Lactation: Nutritional Components
    of Human Colostrum and Milk   194
Resistance to Infection   198
  Component Mechanisms of Defense: Origin and Distribution   198
  Soluble Products   198

  Cellular Elements   201
  Other Defense Factors   203
  Milk and Altered Pregnancy   207
Benefits and Risks of Human Milk   207
  Benefits   207
  Potential Risks   210
Current Trends in Breast-Feeding   213
Summary and Conclusions   213

Mother's milk delivered naturally through breast-feeding has been the sole source of infant nutrition in mammalian species for millions of years. Since human beings learned to domesticate cattle about 10,000 years ago, nonhuman mammalian milk also has been used to supplement or replace maternal milk in human infants. The development and widespread use of commercially prepared infant formula products have been phenomena of the 20th century and notably of the past 6 decades. Such products provide an alternative to breast-feeding that is useful in certain situations. Nonetheless, compelling evidence shows that breast-feeding is an ideal source of infant nutrition, whose use is associated with lower rates of postneonatal infant mortality in the United States and in other parts of the world [1–3]. Human milk helps to protect infants against a wide variety of infections; helps to reduce the risk for allergic and autoimmune diseases, the risk of obesity and its complications, and the risk for certain types of neoplasms later in life; and has been associated with slightly better performances on tests of cognitive development in some studies [3]. For these reasons, the American Academy of Pediatrics (AAP) and the World Health Organization (WHO) recommend that in the absence of specific contraindications (see "Benefits and Risks of Human Milk"), healthy term infants should be exclusively breast-fed or fed expressed breast milk beginning within the first hour after birth through 6 months of age [1,3].

---

* This chapter is rededicated to Lars A. Hansen, MD, PhD, the discoverer of sIgA in human milk, the father of modern "mother's milk feeding practices," and a remarkable human being.

Over the past few decades, the immune responses at intestinal and respiratory mucosal surfaces to local infections have been intensely studied. These investigations have led to the development of concepts of immunity on mucosal surfaces of gastrointestinal, respiratory, and genitourinary tracts and identification of mucosa-associated lymphoid tissue and local mechanisms of defense that are distinct from the internal (systemic) immune system. This chapter reviews existing information on major aspects of the physiologic, nutritional, immunologic, and anti-infective components of the products of lactation. Evidence on the contribution of human milk to the development of immunologic integrity in the infant and its influence on the outcome of infections and other host-antigen interactions is also discussed.

PHYSIOLOGY OF LACTATION
DEVELOPMENTAL ANATOMY OF THE MAMMARY GLAND

The rudimentary mammary tissue undergoes several developmental changes during morphogenesis and lactogenesis: In the 4-mm human embryo, the breast tissue appears as a tiny mammary band on the chest wall [4,5]; by the 7-mm embryonic stage, the mammary band develops into the mammary line, along which eventually develops the true mammary anlage; by the 12-mm stage, a primitive epithelial nodule develops; by the 30-mm stage, the primitive mammary bud appears. These initial phases of development occur in both genders (Table 5–1). Further development in the male apparently is limited, however, by androgenic or other male-associated substances [6,7]. Castration in male rat embryos early in gestation leads to female breast development, whereas ovariectomy in female rat embryos does not alter the course of development of the mammary anlage. Toward the end of pregnancy, initial phases of fetal mammary differentiation seem to occur under the influence of placental and transplacentally acquired maternal hormones, with transient development of the excretory and lactiferous ductular systems. Such growth, differentiation, and secretory activities are transient and regress soon after birth [7,8].

At thelarche, and later on at menarche, true mammary growth and development begin in association with rapidly increasing levels of estrogens, progesterone, growth hormone, insulin, adrenocorticosteroids, and prolactin [8,9]. Estrogens seem to be important for the growth and development of the ductular system, and progestins apparently are important for lobuloalveolar development (see Table 5–1). Final differentiation of the breast associated with growth and proliferation of the acinar lobes and alveoli continues to be influenced by the levels of estrogen and progesterone. Other peptide hormones, such as prolactin, insulin, and placental chorionic somatomammotropin, appear to be far more important for the subsequent induction and maintenance of lactation (see Table 5–1).

Prolactin secretion from the pituitary gland seems to be under neural control, and the increasing innervation of the breast observed throughout pregnancy apparently is regulated by estrogens [9]. Intense neural input in virgin and parturient, but not in currently pregnant, mammals has been shown to result in lactation. Lactation in goats can be induced by milking maneuvers. Adoptive breast-feeding also is well documented in primitive human societies. Sudden and permanent cessation of suckling can result in the termination of milk secretion and involution of the breast to the prepregnant state as the concentrations of prolactin decline. Estrogen and progesterone also may amplify the direct effects of prolactin or may induce additional receptors for this peptide hormone on appropriate target tissues in the breast.

ENDOCRINE CONTROL OF MAMMARY GLAND FUNCTION

Breast tissue is responsive to hormones, even as a rudimentary structure, as illustrated by the secretion of "witch's milk" by male and female newborns in response to exposure to maternal secretion of placental lactogen, estrogens, and progesterone [5]. The secretion of this early milk ceases after exposure to maternal hormones has waned. Sexual differentiation, marked by puberty, is the next major stage in mammary development. As pointed out earlier, androgens inhibit the development of mammary tissue in males, whereas the development of mammary tissue in females depends on estrogen, progesterone, and pituitary hormones [10]. The postpubertal mammary gland undergoes cyclical changes in response to the release of hormones that occurs during the menstrual cycle. The last stage of development occurs during menopause, when the decline in estrogen secretion results in some atrophy of mammary tissue.

During the menstrual cycle, the mammary gland responds to the sequential release of estrogen and progesterone with a hyperplasia of the ductal system that

TABLE 5–1 Possible Endocrine Factors in Growth of Human Female Mammary Glands

Clinical State	Growth Characteristics	Maturational Hormones
Prenatal	Rudimentary	None
Infancy	Rudimentary	None
Puberty	Growth and budding of milk ducts	Growth hormone, prolactin-estrogen, corticosteroids, prolactin (high doses)
Pregnancy	Growth of acinar lobules and alveoli	Estrogen, progesterone, prolactin, growth hormone, corticosteroids
Parturition	Alveolar growth	Prolactin, corticosteroids
Lactational growth of tissue	None	None
Secretory products	Casein, α-lactalbumin	Prolactin, insulin, corticosteroids

continues through the secretory phase and declines with the onset of menstruation. The concentration of prolactin modestly increases during the follicular stage of the menstrual cycle, but remains constant during the secretory phase [11]. Prolactin secretion seems to be held in readiness for the induction and maintenance of lactation.

Initiation and Maintenance of Lactation

Pregnancy is marked by profound hormonal changes reflecting major secretory contributions from the placenta, the hypothalamus, and the pituitary gland, with contributions from many other endocrine glands (e.g., pancreas, thyroid, and parathyroid). Increased estrogen and progesterone levels during pregnancy stimulate secretion of prolactin from the pituitary, whereas placental lactogen seems to inhibit the release of a prolactin-inhibiting factor from the hypothalamus. Prolactin, lactogen, estrogen, and progesterone all aid in preparing the mammary gland for lactation. Initially in gestation, an increased growth of ductule and alveolobular tissue occurs in response to estrogen and progesterone. In the beginning of the second trimester, secretory material begins to appear in the luminal cells. By the middle of the second trimester, mammary development has proceeded sufficiently to permit lactation to occur should parturition take place.

When the infant is delivered, a major regulatory factor, the placenta, is lost, and new regulatory factors including the maternal-infant interaction and neuroendocrine regulation are gained for control of lactation. Loss of placental hormone secretion results in an endocrine hypothalamic stimulation of prolactin release from the anterior pituitary gland and neural stimulation of oxytocin from the posterior pituitary. The stimulation of the nipple by suckling activates a neural pathway that results in release of prolactin and oxytocin. Prolactin is responsible for stimulating milk production, whereas oxytocin stimulates milk ejection (the combination is known as the let-down reflex). Oxytocin also stimulates uterine contractions, which the mother may feel while she is breast-feeding; this response helps to restore the uterus to prepregnancy tone. Milk production and ejection depend on the complex interaction of stimulation by the infant's suckling, neural reflex of the hypothalamus to such stimulation, release of hormones from the anterior and posterior pituitary, and response of the mammary gland to these hormones to complete the cycle.

Milk Secretion

Milk is produced as the result of synthetic mechanisms within the mammary gland and the transport of components from blood. Milk-specific proteins are synthesized in the mammary secretory cells, packaged in secretory vesicles, and exocytosed into the alveolar lumen. Lactose is secreted into the milk in a similar manner, whereas many monovalent ions, such as sodium, potassium, and chloride, depend on active transport systems based on sodium-potassium adenosine triphosphatases (Na^+,K^+-ATPases). In some situations, the mammary epithelium, which may behave as a "mammary barrier" between interstitial fluid derived from blood and the milk because of the lack of space between these cells, may "leak," permitting direct diffusion of components into the milk.

This barrier results in the formation of different pools or compartments of milk components within the mammary gland and is responsible for maintaining gradients of these components from the blood to the milk.

Lipid droplets can be observed within the secretory cells of the mammary gland and are surrounded by a milk fat globule membrane. These fat droplets seem to fuse with the apical membrane of the secretory cells and to be exocytosed or "pinched off" into the milk [10]. Some whole cells also are found in milk, including leukocytes, macrophages, lymphocytes, and broken or shed mammary epithelial cells. The mechanisms by which these cells enter the milk are complex and include, among others, specific cellular receptor-mediated homing of antigen-specific lymphocytes.

As the structure of the mammary gland is compartmentalized, so is the structure of milk. The gross composition of milk consists of cytoplasm encased by cellular membranes in milk fat globule membranes (fat compartments composed of fat droplets), a soluble compartment containing water-soluble constituents, a casein-micelle compartment containing acid-precipitable proteins with calcium and lactose, and a cellular compartment. The relative amounts of these components change during the course of lactation, generally with less fat and more protein in early lactation than in late lactation. The infant consumes a dynamic complex solution that has physical properties permitting unique separation of different functional constituents from one another, presumably in forms that best support growth and development.

Lactation Performance

Successful lactation performance depends on continued effective contributions from the neural, endocrine, and maternal-infant interactions that were initiated at the time of delivery. The part of this complex behavior most liable to inhibition is the mother-child interaction. Early and frequent attachment of the infant to the breast is mandatory to stimulate the neural pathways essential to maintaining prolactin and oxytocin release.

A healthy newborn infant placed between the mother's breasts locates a nipple and begins to suck spontaneously within the first hour of birth [12]. This rapid attachment to the mother may reflect olfactory stimuli from the breast received by the infant at birth [13]. Frequent feedings are necessary for the mother to maintain an appropriate level of milk production for the infant's proper growth and development. Programs to support lactation performance must emphasize proper maternal-infant bonding, relaxation of the mother, support for the mother, technical assistance to initiate breast-feeding properly and to cope with problems, and reduction of environmental hindrances. Such hindrances may include lack of rooming-in in the hospital, use of supplemental formula feeds, and lack of convenient day care for working mothers.

Lactation ceases when suckling stops; any behavior that reduces the amount of suckling by the infant initiates weaning or the end of lactation. Introduction of water in bottles or of one or two bottles of formula a day may begin the weaning process regardless of the time after parturition, but can be most damaging to the process when the mother-infant dyad is first establishing lactation.

SECRETORY PRODUCTS OF LACTATION: NUTRITIONAL COMPONENTS OF HUMAN COLOSTRUM AND MILK

Colostrum and milk contain a rich diversity of nutrients, including electrolytes, vitamins, minerals, and trace metals; nitrogenous products; enzymes; and immunologically specific cellular and soluble products. The distribution and relative content of various nutritional substances found in human milk are presented in Table 5–2. The chemical composition often exhibits considerable variation among lactating women and in the same woman at different times of lactation [14], and between samples obtained from mothers of infants with low birth weight and from mothers of full-term infants [15,16]. Mature milk contains the following average amounts of major chemical constituents per deciliter: total solids, 11.3 g; fat, 3 g; protein, 0.9 g; whey protein nitrogen, 760 mg; casein nitrogen, 410 mg; α-lactalbumin, 150 mg; serum albumin, 50 mg; lactose, 7.2 g; lactoferrin, 150 mg; and lysozyme, 50 mg.

Human milk contains relatively low amounts of vitamins D and E (see Table 5–2) and little or no β-lactoglobulin (the major whey protein in bovine milk). The fat globule membrane seems to have a high content of oleic acid, linoleic acid, phosphatidylpeptides, and inositol [17]. In addition, a binding ligand that promotes absorption of zinc has been identified in human milk [18,19]. Temporal studies have indicated that concentrations of many chemical components, especially nitrogen, calcium, and sodium, decrease significantly as the duration of lactation increases [20,21]. Several components have been found to change in concentration as a function of water content, however, because their total daily output seems to be remarkably constant, at least during the first 8 weeks of lactation [22,23].

Milk production progresses through three distinct phases, characterized by the secretion of colostrum, transitional (early) milk, and mature milk. Colostrum comprises lactational products detected just before and for the first 3 to 4 days of lactation. It consists of yellowish, thick fluid, with a mean energy value of greater than 66 kcal/dL and contains high concentrations of immunoglobulin, protein, fat, fat-soluble vitamins, and ash. Transitional milk usually is produced between days 5 and 14 of lactation, and mature milk is produced thereafter. The concentrations of many nutritional components decline as milk production progresses to synthesis of mature milk. The content of fat-soluble vitamins and proteins decreases as the water content of milk increases. Conversely, levels of lactose, fat, and water-soluble vitamins and total caloric content have been shown to increase as lactation matures [24,25].

As the result of several manufacturing errors, the nutrient composition of infant formulas has been legislated [26], resulting in the paradoxical situation that human milk may not always meet the recommended standards for some nutrients, whereas infant formulas may exceed the recommendation. Human milk nutrient composition varies with time of lactation (colostrum versus early milk versus mature milk) and, to some extent, maternal nutritional status. The appropriate amounts of each nutrient must be considered within these constraints.

TABLE 5–2   Distribution of Secretory Products in Human Colostrum and Milk*

Water	86%-87.5%
Total Solids	11.5 g
Nutritional Components	
Lactose	6.9-7.2 g
Fat	3-4.4 g
Protein	0.9-1.03 g
α-lactalbumin	150-170 mg
β-lactoglobulin	Trace
Serum albumin	50 mg
Electrolytes, Minerals, Trace Metals	
Sodium	15-17.5 mg
Potassium	51-55 mg
Calcium	32-43 mg
Phosphorus	14-15 mg
Chloride	38-40 mg
Magnesium	3 mg
Iron	0.03 mg
Zinc	0.17 mg
Copper	15-105 μg
Iodine	4.5 μg
Manganese	1.5-2.4 μg
Fluoride	5-25 μg
Selenium	1.8-3.2 μg
Boron	8-10 μg
	Total 0.15-2 g
Nitrogen Products	
Whey protein nitrogen	75-78 mg
Casein protein nitrogen	38-41 mg
Nonprotein nitrogen	25% of total nitrogen
Urea	0.027 g
Creatinine	0.021 g
Glucosamine	0.112 g
Vitamins	
C	4.5-5.5 mg
Thiamine (B1)	12-15 μg
Niacin	183.7 μg
B6	11-14 μg
B12	<0.05 μg
Biotin	0.6-0.9 μg
Folic acid	4.1-5.2 μg
Choline	8-9 mg
Inositol	40-46 mg
Pantothenic acid	200-240 μg
A (retinol)	54-56 μg
D	<0.42 IU
E	0.56 μg
K	1.5 μg

*Estimates based on amount per deciliter.

Minerals

The mineral content of human milk is low relative to that of infant formulas and very low compared with cow's milk, from which most formulas are prepared; although human milk is sufficient to support growth and development, it also represents a fairly low solute load to the developing kidney. The levels of major minerals tend to decline during lactation, with the exception of magnesium, but with considerable variability among women tested [27]. Sodium, potassium, chloride, calcium, zinc, and phosphorus all seem to be more bioavailable in human milk than in infant formulas, reflecting their lower concentrations in human milk. Iron is readily bioavailable to the infant from human milk, but may have to be supplemented later in lactation [28,29]. Preterm infants fed human milk may need supplements of calcium and sodium [30].

Vitamins

Human milk contains sufficient vitamins to maintain infant growth and development, with the caveat that water-soluble vitamins are particularly dependent on maternal intake of these nutrients [31]. Preterm infants may require supplements of vitamins D, E, and K when fed human milk [32,33]. The low content of vitamin D in human milk has been related to the development of rickets in a few breast-fed infants, as discussed later [34]. The AAP currently recommends that all breast-fed infants receive 200 IU of oral vitamin D drops daily beginning in the first 2 months of life and continuing until adequate amounts of vitamin D are provided through daily consumption by the infant of fortified formula or milk [3].

Carbohydrates and Energy

Lactose is the primary sugar found in human milk and usually is the carbohydrate chosen for the preparation of commercial formulas. Lactose supplies approximately half the energy (of a total 67 kcal/dL) taken in by the infant from human milk. Lactose (a disaccharide of glucose and galactose) also may be important to the neonate as a carrier of galactose, which may be more readily incorporated into gangliosides in the central nervous system than galactose derived from glucose in the neonate [35]. Also, glycogen may be synthesized more efficiently from galactose than from glucose in the neonate because of the relatively low activity of glucokinase in early development [36]. Human milk also contains other sugars, including glucose and galactose and more than 100 different oligosaccharides [37]. These oligosaccharides may have protective functions for the infant, especially with respect to their ability to bind to gastrointestinal pathogens [38].

Lipids

Fats provide almost half of the calories in human milk, primarily in the form of triacylgycerols (triglycerides) [33]. These lipids are supplied in the form of fat globules enclosed in plasma membranes derived from the mammary epithelial cells [39]. The essential fatty acid linoleic acid supplies about 10% of the calories derived from the lipid fraction. Triacylglycerols serve as precursors for prostaglandins, steroids, and phospholipids and as carriers for fat-soluble vitamins. The lipid profiles of human milk differ dramatically from the lipid profiles of commercial formulas, and despite considerable adaptation of such formulas, human milk lipids are absorbed more efficiently by the infant.

Cholesterol, an important lipid constituent of human milk (12 mg/dL), usually is found in only trace amounts in commercial formulas. It has been suggested that cholesterol may be an essential nutrient for the neonate [40]. A lack of cholesterol in early development may result in turning on of cholesterol-synthetic mechanisms that are difficult to turn off later in life, influencing induction of hypercholesterolemia [41]. Some studies suggest that breast-feeding of the neonate is associated with lowered adult serum cholesterol levels and reduced deaths from ischemic heart disease [42].

Interest has increased in the role that long-chain polyunsaturated fatty acids may play in human milk, especially docosahexaenoic acid and arachidonic acid. These long-chain polyunsaturated fatty acids are not found in unsupplemented infant formulas, but are present in human milk. They are structural components of brain and retinal membranes and may be important for cognitive and visual development. In addition, they may have a role in preventing atopy [43]. Numerous studies have found that infants fed formula without docosahexaenoic acid or arachidonic acid have reduced red blood cell amounts of these fatty acids [44–46]; however, findings in visual and cognitive functional studies in term infants have been inconsistent [47,48]. These studies have been complicated by the finding of slower growth in some preterm infants fed formulas supplemented with long-chain polyunsaturated fatty acids [45,46]. The inconsistent findings in infants fed supplemented formula may reflect the difficulty in determining the optimal amounts of docosahexaenoic acid and arachidonic acid and their precursors linoleic and linolenic acids in such supplemented formulas. These lipids seem to be best delivered from human milk.

Protein and Nonprotein Nitrogen

The exact protein content of mature human milk is variable, but is around 1 g/dL, in contrast to infant formulas, which usually contain 1.5 g/dL; the milk from mothers who deliver preterm infants may have slightly more protein [49]. The nutritionally available protein may be less than 1 g/dL—possibly 0.8 g/dL—as a result of the proportion of proteins that is used for non-nutritional purposes. In addition, human milk contains a considerably greater percentage of nonprotein nitrogen (25% of the total nitrogen) compared with formulas (5% of the total nitrogen) [50].

Human milk protein is primarily whey predominant (acid-soluble protein), whereas formulas prepared from bovine milk classically reflect the 18% whey–82% casein protein composition in that species. The whey-to-casein protein ratio in humans may change during lactation, with the whey component ranging from 90% (early milk) to 60% (mature milk) to 50% (late milk) [51]. Formulas for preterm infants have been reconstituted from bovine milk to provide 60% whey and 40% casein proteins; all major formulas for term infants in the United States are now bovine whey-protein–predominant preparations, in an attempt to make them closer to human milk in composition. These differences in protein quality are reflected by differences in the plasma and urine amino acid responses of infants fed human milk or formulas that are casein-protein–predominant or whey-protein–predominant [52–54]. Generally, term infants do not respond with the dramatic differences seen in preterm infants when fed formulas with different protein quality [55–58].

The nonprotein nitrogen component of human milk contains various compounds that may be important to the development of the neonate: polyamines, nucleotides, creatinine, urea, free amino acids, carnitine, and taurine [59]. The significance of the presence of these components is not always clear, but when they are not fed, as in the case of infant formulas that contain little taurine [52] or of soy formulas that contain little carnitine [60], apparent deficiencies that may influence the development of the infant occur. Taurine is important for bile salt conjugation and for support of appropriate development of the brain and retina [40], whereas carnitine seems to be important for appropriate fatty acid metabolism [61].

Nucleotides, in particular, seem to bridge the gap between the nutritional and the immunologic roles of human milk components. Human milk contains most of these compounds in the form of polymeric nucleotides or nucleic acids [62,63], whereas formulas contain nucleotides (when they are supplemented) only in the monomeric forms (Table 5–3). Nucleotides seem to enhance intestinal development, promote iron absorption, and modify lipid metabolism in their nutritional role [64]. These compounds perform an immunologic function by promoting killer cell cytotoxicity and interleukin (IL)-2 production by stimulated mononuclear cells from infants either breast-fed or fed nucleotide-supplemented formulas [65].

Nucleotide supplementation also has been reported to reduce the number of episodes of infant diarrhea in a group of infants of lower socioeconomic status in Chile, in a manner analogous to that for protection afforded by human milk [66]. In 1998, it was reported that nucleotide-supplemented formulas promoted the immune response of infants to *Haemophilus influenzae* type b polysaccharide immunization at 7 months of age, and a similar response was observed for diphtheria immunization [67]. Infants fed human milk for more than 6 months showed a similar response and exhibited an enhanced titer response to oral polio vaccine; this latter response was not observed in the group fed nucleotide-supplemented formula [67]. Nucleotides are emerging as nutritional and immunologic components of human milk.

Nutritional Proteins

As noted, the nutritional proteins in human milk are classified as either whey (acid-soluble) or casein (acid-precipitable). Within these two classes of proteins, several specific proteins are responsible for supporting the nutritional needs of the infant.

Human casein is composed primarily of β-casein and κ-casein, although the actual distribution of these two proteins is unclear [68]. By contrast, bovine milk contains α_{s1}-casein and α_{s2}-casein (neither of which is found in human milk), in addition to β-casein and κ-casein [69]. These two human milk casein proteins seem to account for approximately 30% of the protein found in human milk, in contrast to the earlier calculation of 40% (the amount commonly used to prepare reconstituted, so-called humanized formulas from bovine milk, which normally contains 82% casein proteins).

The whey-protein fraction contains all of the proposed functional proteins in human milk (immunoglobulins, lysozyme, lactoferrin, enzymes, cytokines, peptide hormones), in addition to the major nutritional protein, α-lactalbumin. Whey proteins compose approximately 70% of human milk proteins, in contrast to 18% in bovine milk. Although α-lactalbumin is the major whey protein in human milk, β-lactoglobulin is the major whey protein in bovine milk (and is not found in human milk) [50]. A consistent fraction of human milk whey protein is composed of serum albumin. Its source is unclear; some evidence indicates that it may be synthesized in the mammary gland [70]. Most of the serum albumin probably is synthesized outside the mammary gland, however.

Milk proteins are characterized by their site of synthesis and are species specific. Proteins such as α-lactalbumin and β-lactoglobulin are species and organ specific, whereas proteins such as serum albumin are species specific, but not organ specific [71]. The net result of these differences in proteins used for nutrition by the neonate is that different amounts of amino acids are ingested by the neonate, depending on the source of milk; even reconstitution of the whey and casein classes of proteins from one species in a ratio similar to that of another species does not result in an identical amino acid intake. These differences are reflected in plasma amino acid profiles of infants fed commercial milks versus human milk, regardless of the ratios of reconstitution [54].

Bioactive Proteins and Peptides

Although a major proportion of human milk protein is composed of the nutritional proteins just described, many of the remaining proteins subserve a variety of functions, other than or in addition to the nutritional support of the neonate. These proteins include carrier proteins, enzymes, hormones, growth factors, immunoglobulins, and cytokines (the latter two are discussed later in "Resistance to Infection"). Whether these proteins are still functional after they have been ingested by the neonate has not always been established, but it is clear that human

TABLE 5-3 Nucleotides in Human Milk and Supplemented Formula

	Human Milk*	Human Milk†	Formula*
Nucleic acid (%)	48	42	4
Nucleotides (%)	36	52	81
Nucleosides (%)	8	7	15
Total (μmol/L)	402	163	141

*See reference 63.
†See reference 62.

milk supplies a mixture that is potentially far more complex than just nutritional substrate.

Carrier Proteins

Many nutrients are supplied to the neonate bound to proteins found in human milk. This binding may play an important role in making these nutrients bioavailable. Lactoferrin is an iron-binding protein (a property that also may play a role in its bacteriostatic action) that is apparently absorbed intact by the infant [72]. Lactoferrin may be important in the improved absorption of iron by the infant from human milk compared with iron from cow's milk preparations, which contain little lactoferrin [28]. Lactoferrin also may bind other minerals, including zinc and manganese, although the preferred mineral form seems to be the ferric ion.

Numerous other proteins seem to be important as carriers of vitamins and hormones. Folate-binding, vitamin B_{12}–binding, and vitamin D–binding proteins all have been identified in human milk. These proteins apparently have some resistance to proteolysis, especially when they are saturated with the appropriate vitamin ligand [73]. Serum albumin acts as a carrier of numerous ligands, whereas α-lactalbumin acts as a carrier for calcium. Finally, proteins that bind thyroid hormone and corticosteroids have been reported to be present in human milk [74,75], although serum albumin may partially fulfill this function.

Enzymes

The activity of more than 30 enzymes has been detected in human milk [76]. Most of these enzymes seem to originate from the blood, with a few originating from secretory epithelial cells of the mammary gland. Little is known about the role of these enzymes, other than lysozyme and the lipases, in human milk. The enzymes found in human milk range from ATPases to antioxidant enzymes, such as catalase, to phosphatases and glycolytic enzymes. Although these enzymes have important roles in normal body metabolism, it is unclear how many of them either function in the milk itself or survive ingestion by the neonate to function in the neonate.

Lysozyme seems to have a part in the antibacterial function of human milk, whereas the lipases have a more nutrient-related role in modulating fat metabolism for the neonate. Two lipases have been identified in human milk: a lipoprotein lipase and a bile salt–stimulated lipase [77]. Lipoprotein lipase seem to be involved in determining the pattern of lipids found in human milk by regulating uptake into milk at the level of the mammary gland. Human milk bile salt–stimulated lipase is an acid-stable protein that compensates for the low activity of lipases secreted into the digestive tract during early development [78]. These two enzymes regulate the amount and the pattern of lipid that appears in milk and the extremely efficient absorption of lipid by the infant. Human milk lipid is absorbed much more readily than lipid from commercial milk formulas despite the many adaptations that have been made to improve absorption, illustrating the effective mechanisms supported by the lipases.

Hormones and Growth Factors

Peptide, steroid hormones, and growth factors have been identified in trace amounts in human milk, although as with most enzymes, it is unclear to what degree they function in the neonate who has ingested the milk. As discussed previously, binding proteins for corticosteroids and thyroxine have been identified in milk and, by extrapolation from observations of other milk components, may play a role in making these bioactive compounds more readily available to the infant.

Among the hormones identified in human milk are insulin, oxytocin, calcitonin, and prolactin. Most of these hormones apparently are absorbed by the infant, but their role in in vivo function is unclear [79]. Breast-fed infants seem to have a different endocrine response from that of formula-fed infants, presumably reflecting the intake of hormones from human milk [80]. The advantages or disadvantages to the infant of these responses are unknown.

Human milk also contains a rich mixture of growth factors, including epidermal growth factor, nerve growth factor, and transforming growth factor-β [81]. In addition, various gastrointestinal peptides have been identified in human milk. Presumably, the supply of these various factors to the infant through milk compensates for their possible deficiency in the infant during early development.

The composition of human milk provides a complex and complete nutritional substrate to the neonate. Human milk supplies not only individual nutrients, but also enzymes involved in metabolism, carriers to improve absorption, and hormones that may regulate metabolic rates. Commercial formulas have not yet been developed to the point that they can provide an analogous complete nutritional system.

Special Considerations for the Premature Neonate

Many of the benefits of human milk evident in term neonates are also evident in preterm neonates with very low birth weight (<1500 g) fed unfortified human milk; the incidence of necrotizing enterocolitis also seems to be reduced [82–84]. Nonetheless, the content of calcium, phosphorus, protein, sodium, vitamins, and energy in unfortified human milk may be inadequate to meet the needs of the very low birth weight preterm neonate, and if used as an exclusive source of nutrients, unfortified human milk may be associated with impaired growth and nutrient deficiencies. Meta-analysis of studies comparing these premature infants fed unfortified or fortified human milk found that fortified milk was associated with greater increases in weight, length, and head circumference and better nitrogen balance and bone mineral content without an increase in feeding intolerance or complications [83,85].

The feeding of fortified human milk does not seem to be associated with a substantially increased rate of feeding intolerance or with a reduction in the beneficial effects of human milk on rates of infections or necrotizing enterocolitis [84]. The quality of the data regarding the utility of fortified human milk is still limited, however, and additional research is needed to define better means by which to provide the benefits of human milk to these preterm infants, while meeting their specific nutritional requirements.

RESISTANCE TO INFECTION
COMPONENT MECHANISMS OF DEFENSE: ORIGIN AND DISTRIBUTION

Fresh human milk contains a wealth of components that provide specific and nonspecific defenses against infectious agents and environmental macromolecules (Table 5–4). These component factors include cells such as T and B lymphocytes, polymorphonuclear neutrophils (i.e., polymorphonuclear leukocytes), and macrophages; soluble products, especially immunoglobulins; secretory immunoglobulin A (sIgA); immunomodulatory cytokines and cytokine receptors; components of the complement system; several carrier proteins; enzymes; and numerous endocrine hormones or hormone-like substances. Additional soluble factors that are active against streptococci, staphylococci, and tumor viruses also have been identified [24,86]. Epidermal growth factor promotes growth of mucosal epithelium and maturation of intestinal brush border.

The developmental characteristics of sIgA have been studied more extensively than those of other components [87–89]. On the basis of available information, most IgA-producing cells observed in milk have their origin in the precursor immunocompetent cells in the gut-associated lymphoid tissue (GALT) and bronchus-associated lymphoid tissue (BALT). Exposure of IgA precursor B lymphocytes in GALT or BALT to microbial and dietary antigens in the mucosal lumen is an important prerequisite for their initial activation and proliferation. Such antigen-sensitized cells eventually are transported through the systemic circulation to other mucosal surfaces, including the mammary glands, and, as plasma cells, initiate the synthesis of immunoglobulin against specific antigens previously experienced in the mucosa of the respiratory or alimentary tract [87]. It has been proposed that T cells observed in the milk also may be derived from GALT and BALT in a manner similar to that of IgA-producing cells. Little or no information is available regarding the site

of origin of other cellular or soluble immunologic components normally present in human milk. Specific antibody and cellular immune reactivity against many respiratory and enteric bacterial and viral pathogens and ingested food proteins also is present in human breast milk (Table 5–5).

SOLUBLE PRODUCTS
IgA

As observed in other peripheral mucosal sites, the major class of immunoglobulin in human colostrum and milk is 11S sIgA. Other isotypes—7S IgA, IgG, IgM, IgD, and IgE—also are present. The 11S IgA exists as a dimer of two 7S IgA molecules linked together by a polypeptide chain, the J-chain, and is associated with a nonimmunoglobulin protein referred to as the secretory component. The sIgA protein constitutes about 75% of the total nitrogen content of human milk. The IgA dimers produced by plasma cells at the basal surface of the mammary epithelium are bound by the polymeric immunoglobulin receptor on the basolateral surface of mammary epithelial cells, which transports them through these cells, where they are released into the alveolar spaces as an 11S IgA dimer associated with a portion of the polymeric immunoglobulin receptor referred to as the secretory component [90].

Sequential quantitation of class-specific immunoglobulin in human colostrum and milk has shown that the highest levels of sIgA and IgM are present during the first few days of lactation (Fig. 5–1). Levels of IgA are 4 to 5 times greater than levels of IgM, 20 to 30 times greater than levels of IgG, and 5 to 6 times greater than levels of serum IgA [89]. As lactation progresses, IgA declines to levels of 20 to 27 mg per gram of protein, and IgM levels decline to 3.5 to 4.1 mg/g protein. IgG levels do not show any significant change during early and late lactation and usually are maintained in the range of 1.4 to 4.9 mg/g protein (see Fig. 5–1). Although a dramatic and rapid decline in milk IgA and IgM occurs during the first week of life, this

TABLE 5–4 Immunologically and Pharmacologically Active Components and Hormones Observed in Human Colostrum and Milk

Soluble	Cellular	Hormones and Hormone-like Substances
Immunoglobulin sIgA (11S), 7S IgA, IgG, IgM, IgE, IgD, secretory component	T lymphocytes	Epidermal growth factors
Cytokines (see Table 5–8)	B lymphocytes	Prostaglandins
Histocompatibility antigens	Neutrophils	Neurotensin
Complement	Macrophages	Relaxin
Chemotactic factors	Epithelial cells	Somatostatin
Properdin		Bombesin
α-fetoprotein		Gonadotropins
Folate uptake enhancer		Ovarian steroids
Carrier proteins		Thyroid-releasing hormone
Lactoferrin		Thyroid-stimulating hormone
Transferrin		Thyroxine and triiodothyronine
B_{12}-binding protein		Adrenocorticotropin
Lysozyme		Corticosteroids
Lipoprotein lipase		Corticoid-binding protein
Leukocyte enzymes		Insulin

TABLE 5–5 Specific Antibody or Cell-Mediated Immunologic Reactivity in Human Colostrum and Milk

Bacteria	Viruses	Other
Escherichia coli	Rotavirus	*Candida albicans*
Salmonella	Rubella virus	*Giardia* species
Shigella species	Poliovirus types 1, 2, 3	*Entamoeba histolytica*
Vibrio cholerae	Echoviruses	Food proteins
Bacteroides fragilis	Coxsackieviruses A and B	
Streptococcus pneumoniae	Respiratory syncytial virus*	
Bordetella pertussis	Cytomegalovirus*	
Clostridium tetani and *Clostridium difficile*	Influenza A virus	
Corynebacterium diphtheriae	Herpes simplex virus type 1	
Streptococcus mutans	Arboviruses	
Haemophilus influenzae type B	Semliki Forest virus	
Mycobacterium tuberculosis *	Ross River virus	
	Japanese B virus	
	Dengue virus	
	Human immunodeficiency virus	
	Hepatitis A and B viruses	

Evidence of reactivity for antibody and cellular immunity.

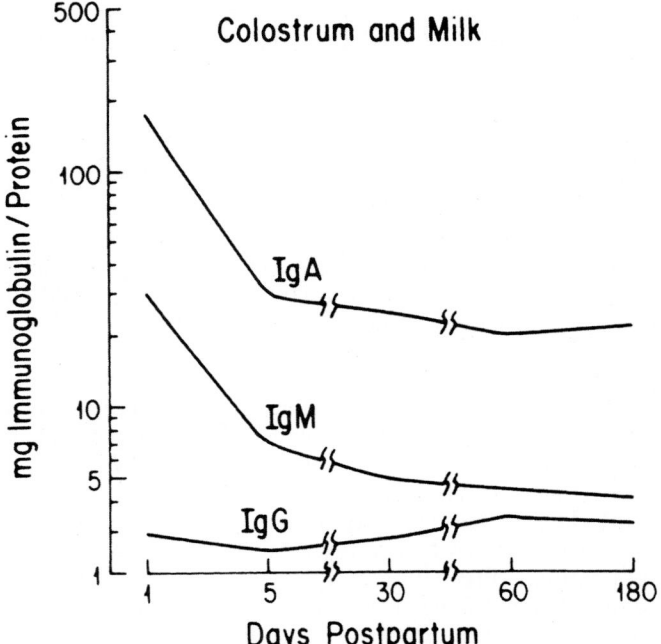

FIGURE 5–1 Comparison of mean levels of IgG, IgA, and IgM in colostrum and milk at different intervals after onset of lactation in mothers who were breast-feeding. *(Data from Ogra SS, Ogra PL. Immunologic aspects of human colostrum and milk, II: characteristics of lymphocyte reactivity and distribution of E-rosette forming cells at different times after the onset of lactation. J Pediatr 92:550-555, 1978.)*

decrease is more than balanced by an increase in the volume of milk produced as the process of lactation becomes established (Table 5–6; see Fig. 5–1).

IgA antibodies found in milk possess specificity for infectious agents endemic to or pathogenic for the intestinal and respiratory tracts (see Table 5–4). These antibodies may be present in the milk in the absence of specific circulating IgA. In a study in which pregnant women were given oral feedings of *Escherichia coli* O83, development of IgA antibody in human milk was evident in the absence of detectable serum antibody-specific responses [91]. In another study, investigators observed similar responses in animal models using intrabronchial immunization with *Streptococcus pneumoniae*. These and other studies [92–95] have strongly supported the concept of a bronchomammary, and enteromammary, axis of immunologic reactivity in the breast.

Despite the elegance of studies that have defined the mechanisms of IgA cell trafficking from GALT and BALT to the mammary glands, the actual number of B cells or IgA plasma cells in the mammary glands is sparse. Colostrum and milk may contain large amounts of IgA (11 g in colostrum and 1 to 3 g per day in later milk), as shown in Table 5–6. The reasons underlying the apparent disparity between the content of immunoglobulin-producing cells and concentrations of immunoglobulin are unknown. The disparity may be related to the unique hormonal environment of the mammary glands. The hormones that have been consistently observed in human milk are listed in Table 5–4.

The effects of pregnancy-related and lactation-related hormones on regulation of immunologic reactivity present in the resting and lactating breast have been examined [96]. In a study of immunoglobulin production in the nonlactating human breast, several interesting findings were noted [97]. Few mononuclear cells were present in the nonlactating breast of nulliparous and of parous women, although IgA-containing cells predominated. Synthesis of IgA seemed to be slightly increased in the parous women. IgA was found in the mammary tissues during the proliferative stage of the menstrual cycle in the nulliparous women and during the luteal phase in the parous women. The number of IgA-producing cells in the nonlactating breast was observed to increase with

TABLE 5–6 Level of Immunoglobulins in Colostrum and Milk and Estimates of Delivery of Lactational Immunoglobulins to the Breast-Feeding Neonate*

Day Postpartum	Percentage of Total Proteins Represented by Immunoglobulin			Output of Immunoglobulin (mg/24 hr)		
	IgG	IgM	IgA	IgG	IgM	IgA
1	7	3	80	80	120	11,000
3	10	45	45	50	40	2000
7	1–2	4	20	25	10	1000
7–28	1–2	2	10–15	10	10	1000
<50	1–2	0.5–1	10–15	10	10	1000

Estimates based on the available data for total immunoglobulin and daily protein synthesis (see references 8, 87, and 88).

parity. These findings suggest that the immunologic makeup of the nonlactating and the lactating breast may be significantly influenced by the hormonal milieu.

In another study of virgin mice given exogenously administered hormones [98], an extended exposure to estrogen, progesterone, and prolactin was necessary for maximal increments in IgA-producing plasma cells in the breast. Similarly, castrated males exposed to these hormones became moderately receptive to mammary gland homing of cells specific for IgA synthesis. As would be expected, testosterone eliminated female breast receptivity to these cells. These studies suggest the existence of a hormonally determined homing mechanism in the mammary gland for class-specific, immunoglobulin-producing cells.

More recent studies have proposed another possible influence of lactational hormones on immunocompetent cells. In limited observations, combinations of prolactin with estrogen and progesterone (in concentrations observed normally at the beginning of parturition) seemed to have an amplifying effect on the synthesis and secretion of IgA from peripheral blood lymphocytes [99]. This observation raises the possibility that the high levels of sIgA observed in colostrum and milk may be partly the result of selective, hormonally mediated proliferation of antigen-sensitized IgA cells in the peripheral blood. The immunoglobulin could acquire a secretory component during its passage through the mammary epithelium and eventually appear in the colostrum or milk as mature sIgA. Although the appearance of sIgA antibody in milk characteristically follows antigenic exposure in GALT or BALT, the precise nature of the IgA content in milk seems to be determined by various other factors operating in the mucosal lymphoid tissue. These factors include the dendritic cell and regulatory T-cell network in GALT and possibly in BALT [100,101], the nature of antigens (soluble proteins versus particulate microbial agents) [102], and the route of primary versus secondary antigenic exposure [103].

It has been estimated that the breast-fed infant may consistently receive about 1 g of IgA each day, and approximately 1% of this amount of IgM and IgG [104,105]. The estimates of lactational immunoglobulin delivered to the breast-fed infant at different periods of lactation are presented in Table 5–6. Most ingested IgA is eliminated in the feces, although 10% may be absorbed from the intestine into the circulation within the first 18

to 24 hours after birth [106]. Feces of breast-fed infants contain functional antibodies present in the ingested milk [107]. Other studies support the finding of prolonged survival of milk IgA in the gastrointestinal tract. Infants fed human milk have shown the presence of all immunoglobulin classes in the feces. Fecal IgA content was three to four times greater than that of IgM after human milk feeding. Comparative studies on survival of human milk IgA and bovine IgG in the neonatal intestinal tract have suggested that the fecal content of IgA may be 14 to 20 times greater after human milk feeding than that of bovine IgG after feeding of bovine immunoglobulin [108].

Endogenous production of sIgA by the infant's mucosal immune system increases progressively in the postnatal period [109]. Nonetheless, breast-fed infants have substantially greater concentrations of fecal sIgA than formula-fed infants. Prentice and colleagues [110] found approximately 10-fold and approximately 4-fold higher concentrations of sIgA in the stools of breast-fed infants compared with formula-fed infants at 6 and 12 weeks of postnatal age, even though only approximately 15% to 20% of ingested sIgA appeared in the feces.

Direct information about the role of milk IgA in antimicrobial defense is available in several studies. sIgA interferes with bacterial adherence to cell surfaces [111]. Colostrum and milk can inhibit the activity of *E. coli* and *Vibrio cholerae* enterotoxins in experimental settings [112]. The antitoxic activity of human milk seems to correlate well with its IgA content, but not with its IgM and IgG content. Precoating of *V. cholerae* with specific sIgA protects infant mice from disease [113]. Similar results have been obtained by using specific purified milk sIgA in preventing *E. coli*–induced and *Shigella dysenteriae*–induced disease in rabbits [114]. Less definite, but suggestive, is a study conducted with human milk feeding relative to the intestinal replication of orally administered live poliovirus vaccine [115]. This study found that breast-feeding may reduce the degree of seroconversion for poliovirus antibody in the vaccinated infants. Because antipolio IgA is present in human milk and colostrum, the investigators concluded that specific IgA may bind poliovirus and influence viral replication in the intestinal mucosa. Extensive experience with oral polio immunization worldwide has not found a convincing association, however, between breast-feeding and live vaccine failures. Other studies have shown that the magnitude of poliovirus replication in the intestine is determined by the presence and level of preexisting sIgA antibody. With high levels of intestinal IgA antibody, little or no replication of vaccine virus was observed in the gut. With lower levels, varying degrees of viral replication could be shown [116].

Epidemiologic studies strongly support the notion that breast-feeding protects the infant against infectious diseases (see "Benefits and Risks of Human Milk"). It is impossible in these studies, however, to dissect the relative contribution of sIgA from the contributions of other soluble or cellular components present in colostrum and milk.

IgG and IgM

Normal neonates exhibit characteristic paucity or lack of serum IgA and sIgA during the first 7 to 10 days after birth. At that time, the presence of IgM and IgG in milk may be important to compensate for immunologic functions not present in the mucosal sites. IgG and IgM participate in complement fixation and specific bactericidal activity, functions not associated with IgA. Studies done after oral feeding of immune serum globulin (mostly IgG) suggested that IgG may survive in the gastrointestinal tract of infants with low birth weight [117]. Other immunoglobulin isotypes in milk also may be able to serve as effective substitutes for IgA in the neonates of IgA-deficient mothers in prevention of infection with enteric or respiratory pathogens.

IgE and IgD

Investigations have failed to show local synthesis of IgE in the breast [118–120]. Although IgE may be detected in 40% of colostrum and milk samples, the concentrations are extremely low, and many samples of colostrum and milk contain no IgE activity when paired samples of serum contain high IgE levels. IgD has been detected in most colostrum and milk samples. It has been suggested that nursing women with high serum IgD levels are more likely to have high IgD concentrations in their milk. The possibility of some local production of IgE and IgD cannot be ruled out [120].

CELLULAR ELEMENTS

Human colostrum and milk contain lymphocytes, monocytes-macrophages, neutrophils, and epithelial cells [121]. Early colostrum contains the highest concentration of cells, approximately 1×10^6 to 3×10^6 cells/mL. By the end of the first week of lactation, cell concentration is of the order of 10^5 cells/mL. Total cell numbers delivered to the newborn throughout lactation may remain constant, however, when adjustments are made for the increase in volume of milk produced [89]. The two major cell populations in human milk—macrophages and neutrophils—are difficult to distinguish by common staining methods because of numerous intracytoplasmic inclusions. More accurate estimates made by flow cytometry analysis suggest that the relative percentages of neutrophils, macrophages, and lymphocytes in early milk samples are approximately 80%, 15%, and 4% [122,123]. The remaining cells are present in smaller amounts, especially in the absence of active suckling, engorgement, or local breast infection.

Macrophages

Histochemically, the milk macrophage differs from the blood monocyte in showing decreased peroxidase staining, with increased lysosomes and significant amounts of immunoglobulin, especially IgA, in the cytoplasm [124–126]. The intracellular immunoglobulin in macrophages represents 10% of milk IgA [127]. Kinetic studies on the release of IgA by human milk macrophages suggest that immunoglobulin release by macrophages, in contrast to immunoglobulin release by other phagocytic cells, is a time-dependent phenomenon and is not significantly influenced by the use of secretagogues or stimulants, such as phorbol myristate acetate [127]. Active phagocytosis is associated, however, with significant increase in release of IgA [128].

The precise functions of macrophages in colostrum or milk have not been fully explored. These cells have been suggested as potential transport vehicles for IgA [126,129]. Milk macrophages possess phagocytic activity against *Staphylococcus aureus*, *E. coli*, and *Candida albicans*, with possible cytocidal activity against the first two organisms [130]. Milk macrophages participate in antibody-dependent, cell-mediated cytotoxicity for herpes simplex virus type 1–infected cells [131]. Infection of milk macrophages by respiratory syncytial virus results in the production of the proinflammatory cytokines IL-1β, IL-6, and tumor necrosis factor (TNF)-α [132]. These cells also are involved in various other biosynthetic and excretory activities, including production of lactoferrin, lysozyme [133], components of complement [134], properdin factor B, epithelial growth factors, and T lymphocyte–suppressive factors [87]. Milk macrophages also have been suggested to be important in regulation of T-cell function [135,136].

Lymphocytes

Milk contains a few lymphocytes; 80% are T cells, and 4% to 6% are B cells [123]. The small number of B cells reflects the sessile nature of these cells, which enter the lamina propria of the mammary gland to transform into plasma cells. Although several investigators have been unable to show in vitro antibody synthesis by milk lymphocytes, studies performed with colostral B cells transformed by Epstein-Barr virus showed production of IgG and J-chain–containing IgM and IgA [137]. A small population of CD16+ natural killer (NK) cells also can be identified in most milk samples, but cannot be accurately quantitated [123]. In functional studies, colostral cells exhibit NK cytotoxicity, however, which is enhanced by interferon (IFN) and IL-2. Colostral cells also elicit antibody-dependent and lectin-dependent cellular cytotoxic responses. The NK and the antibody-dependent and lectin-dependent responses in colostral cells have been observed to be significantly lower than those of autologous peripheral blood cells. Reduced cellular cytotoxicity of colostral cells also has been observed against virus-infected targets and certain bacteria. With several specific virus-infected targets, colostrum and milk cells conspicuously lack cellular cytotoxicity compared with autologous peripheral blood cells. There is also an apparent exclusion of cytolytic T cells in the milk that are specific for certain human leukocyte antigens (HLA) [138,139].

TABLE 5-7 Lymphocyte Subpopulations in Human Milk and Autologous Blood*

Lymphocyte Subpopulation	Human Milk	Blood
CD3+[†]	83 ± 11	75 ± 7
CD3+ CD4+[†]	36 ± 13	44 ± 6
CD3+ CD8+[†]	43 ± 12	27 ± 4
CD4+/CD8+[‡]	0.88 ± 0.35	1.70 ± 0.45
CD19+[†]	6 ± 4	14 ± 5

*Expressed as mean ± standard deviation (SD).
[†]Expressed as percentage of total lymphocytes.
[‡]Ratio of CD3+/CD4+ to CD3+/CD8+ lymphocytes.
Adapted from Wirt DP, et al. Activated-memory T lymphocytes in human milk. Cytometry 13:282-290, 1992.

Most T lymphocytes in colostrum and milk are mature CD3+ cells. CD4+ (helper) and CD8+ (cytotoxic) populations are present in human milk, with a proportion of CD8+ T cells higher than that found in human blood (Table 5-7). The CD4+/CD8+ ratio in milk is significantly lower than the ratio observed in peripheral blood and is not due to an increase of CD8+ cells in the peripheral blood of women during the postpartum period. Colostral and milk T lymphocytes manifest in vitro proliferative responses on stimulation with numerous mitogens and antigens. Several studies have shown a selectivity in lymphocyte stimulation responses in colostral and milk lymphocytes to various antigens compared with peripheral blood lymphocyte responses [140,141]. Antigens such as rubella virus stimulate T lymphocytes in secretory sites and milk and in systemic sites [140]. By contrast, E. coli K1 antigen, whose exposure is limited to mucosal sites, produces stimulation of lymphoproliferative responses only in milk lymphocytes. These findings support the concept of select T-cell populations in the mammary gland.

In addition to antigen selectivity, a general hyporesponsiveness to mitogenic stimulation of milk lymphocytes relative to peripheral blood lymphocytes has been observed [136,140]. The decreased reactivity of milk lymphocytes to phytohemagglutinin may be partly the result of a relative deficiency of certain populations of T cells in milk. Macrophage–T cell interactions also have been postulated to be responsible for this relative hyporesponsiveness [140], although it is unknown whether the effects are the result of decreased helper or increased regulatory function. Studies have shown that milk lymphocytes exhibit reduced responses to allogeneic cells, but display good ability to stimulate alloreactivity [138]. Generally, the T-cell proliferative responses to phytohemagglutinin and tetanus toxoid in breast-fed infants seem to be significantly higher than the responses in bottle-fed infants, possibly secondary to the presence of maternally derived cell growth factors and other lymphokines in human milk [136,142].

Virtually all CD4+ and CD8+ T cells in milk bear the CD45 isoform CD45RO that is associated with immunologic memory [123,143]. In addition, the proportion of T cells that display other phenotypic markers of activation, including CD25 (IL-2R) and HLA-DR, is much greater

than that in blood [123,144]. Consistent with their memory phenotype, T cells in human milk produce IFN-γ [143]. A significantly greater number of CD4+ T cells in colostrum express the CD40 ligand (CD40L), which helps these cells provide help for B-cell antibody production and macrophage activation (see Chapter 4 for more details) compared with autologous or heterologous blood T cells [145]. The function of these memory T cells in the recipient human infant is currently unknown, however. Mucous membrane sites in the alimentary or respiratory tract, or both, of the recipient infant would seem to be potential entry sites for human milk leukocytes. Very few memory T cells are detected in blood in infancy [146]. It is possible that maternal memory T cells in milk may help compensate for the developmental delay in their production in the infant.

The proportion of T lymphocytes bearing the γδ T-cell receptor (γδ-TCR) is approximately two times greater in colostrum than in blood [147,148]. Human γδ-TCR+ cells populate organized lymphoid tissues and represent half of the intraepithelial lymphocytes in the gut [149]. The intestinal epithelia may have a selective affinity for γδ-TCR+ cells and provide a favorable environment for maternal T cells in milk to be transferred to the breast-fed infant. Evidence from experimental animal studies indicates that milk lymphocytes enter tissues of the neonate [150–153], but this has not been shown in humans.

In humans, possible transfer of maternal T-cell reactivity to tuberculin protein from the mother to the neonate through the process of breast-feeding has been suggested [106,154,155]. The implications of these observations are that maternal cellular products or soluble mediators of cellular reactivity may be transferred passively to the neonate through breast-feeding. The occurrence of such phenomena in humans has not been studied carefully, and there is no direct evidence that milk T cells, either αβ-TCR+ or γδ-TCR+, play a role in the transfer of adoptive immunoprotection to the recipient infant. Similarly, there is at present no evidence to suggest that there is any immunologic risk to the human neonate of maternal T cells ingested through breast-feeding.

Neutrophils

Milk contains numerous neutrophils. Although the absolute counts in actively nursing mothers exhibit considerable variability among different samples, highest numbers are generally observed during the first 3 to 4 days of lactation. The numbers of neutrophils decrease significantly after 3 to 4 weeks of lactation, and only rare neutrophils are observed in samples collected after 60 to 80 days postpartum. Leukocytes in human milk seem to be metabolically activated. Although the neutrophils are phagocytic and produce toxic oxygen radicals, they do not respond well to chemoattractants by increasing their adherence, polarity, or directed migration in in vitro systems [156]. This diminished response was found to be due to prior activation in that the neutrophils in milk displayed a phenotypic pattern that is typical of activated neutrophils. The expression of CD11b, the α chain subunit of Mac-1, was increased, and the expression of L-selectin was decreased [122].

Epithelial Cells

On the basis of their anatomic distribution, epithelial cells in the human mammary gland can be classified into two main types: myoepithelial and luminal. Epithelial cells of both types seem to be more heterogeneous, however, on histologic and physicochemical testing [138,157,158]. They include secretory cells, which contain abundant rough endoplasmic reticulum, lipid droplets, and Golgi apparatus. The secretory cells apparently produce casein micelle. The squamous epithelial cells usually are seen in the regions of the cutaneous junction of the nipples, especially near the galactophores. The ductal or luminal cells, which exist in clusters, have many short microvilli, tight junctions, and remnants of desmosomes [157,158].

In human milk, relatively few epithelial cells are observed in the early phases of lactation. Most epithelial cells appear after 2 to 3 weeks and are seen in appreciable numbers, even 180 to 200 days after the onset of lactation. With the possible exception of the synthesis of secretory component and casein and possibly other products, with which secretory epithelial cells have been associated in the stroma of the mammary gland, the role of epithelial cells in the milk remains to be defined.

Possible Functions of Cellular Elements

The information reviewed so far provides strong evidence for the existence of numerous dynamic cellular reactions in the mammary gland, colostrum, and milk. The specific functional role, collectively or individually, for the epithelial cells, monocytes, neutrophils, or lymphocytes in the mammary gland or the milk remains to be defined. In view of the high degree of selectivity and the differences in the quantitative and functional distribution of cellular elements, it is suggested that the mammary gland, similar to mucosal surfaces, may function partitioned from the cellular elements in peripheral blood, in a manner similar to that for other peripheral sites (e.g., the genital tract) of the mucosal immune system. It is unknown, however, whether the characteristic proportions of macrophages, T lymphocytes, other cytotoxic cells, or epithelial cells are designed for any specific functions localized to the mammary gland in the lactating mother or to epithelium or lumen of the intestinal or respiratory mucosa of the breast-feeding infant, or both.

The observations on the transfer of delayed hypersensitivity reactions in human neonates and of graft-versus-host reactivity in the rat raise the possibility that milk cells may function as important vehicles in transfer of maternal immunity to neonates. The potential beneficial and harmful roles of such cell-mediated transfer through the mucosal routes need to be investigated further. The paucity of NK and other cytotoxic cells in the colostrum may have a role for the breast-feeding neonate, especially in influencing the antigen processing and uptake of replicating microorganisms and their immune response at systemic or mucosal levels or both. Although further elucidation of the functions of these cellular elements in the mammary glands and the suckling neonate is needed, it is likely that their presence in the milk represents a highly selective phenomenon and not a mere contamination with peripheral blood cells.

OTHER DEFENSE FACTORS
Direct-Acting Antimicrobial Agents
General Features

The defense agents in human milk, although biochemically diverse, share the following features: (1) They usually are common to mucosal sites. (2) They are adapted to resist digestion in the gastrointestinal tract of the recipient infant. (3) They protect by noninflammatory mechanisms. (4) They act synergistically with each other or with factors produced by the infant. (5) Most components of the immune system in human milk are produced throughout lactation and during gradual weaning. (6) There is often an inverse relationship between the production of these factors in the mammary gland and their production by the infant during the same time frames of lactation and postnatal development. As lactation proceeds, the concentration of many factors in human milk declines. Concomitantly, the mucosal production of these factors increases in the developing infant. Whether the inverse relationship between these processes is due to feedback mechanisms, or the processes are independent, is unclear.

Carbohydrate Components

Human milk contains several oligosaccharides and glyco-conjugates, including monosialogangliosides that are receptor analogues for heat-labile toxins produced by *V. cholerae* and *E. coli* [159]; fucose-containing oligosaccharides that inhibit the hemagglutinin activity of the classic strain of *V. cholerae* [160]; fucosylated oligosaccharides that protect against heat-stable enterotoxin of *E. coli* [161]; mannose-containing, high-molecular-weight glycoproteins that block the binding of the El Tor strain of *V. cholerae* [159]; and glycoproteins and glycolipids that interfere with the binding of colonization factor (CFA/II) fimbriae on enterotoxigenic *E. coli* [162]. The inhibition of toxin binding is associated with acidic glycolipids containing sialic acid (gangliosides). Although the quantities of total gangliosides in human milk and in bovine milk are similar, the relative frequencies of each type of ganglioside in milk from these two species are distinct.

More than 50 types of monosialylated oligosaccharides have been identified in human milk, and new types are still being recognized [163]. Monosialoganglioside 3 constitutes about 74% of total gangliosides in human milk, but the percentage is much lower in bovine milk [164,165]. Also, the level of the enterotoxin receptor ganglioside G_{M1} is 10 times greater in human milk than in bovine milk [165]. This difference may be clinically important because G_{M1} inhibits enterotoxins of *E. coli* and *V. cholerae* [166]. Also, intact human milk fat globules and the mucin from the membranes of these structures inhibit the binding of S-fimbriated *E. coli* to human buccal epithelial cells [167].

Oligosaccharides in human milk also interfere with the attachment of *H. influenzae* and *S. pneumoniae* [168]. In this regard, *N*-acetylglucosamine (GlcNAc) (1-3) Gal-disaccharide subunits block the attachment of *S. pneumoniae* to respiratory epithelium. Human milk can interfere with the binding of human immunodeficiency virus (HIV) envelope antigen gp120 to CD4 molecules on T cells [169]. Some evidence from animal models suggests that the oligosaccharides and glycoconjugates in human milk protect in vivo [170–172], but relevant clinical data are scarce [173] and transmission of HIV through breast-feeding is a well-established means for mother-to-infant transmission of HIV (see "Benefits and Risks of Human Milk").

In addition to the direct antimicrobial effects of the carbohydrates in human milk, nitrogen-containing oligosaccharides, glycoproteins, and glycopeptides are growth promoters for *Lactobacillus bifidus* var. *pennsylvanicus* [174,175,176]. The ability of human milk to promote the growth of *L. bifidus* may reside in the oligosaccharide moiety [177] and peptides [178] of caseins. It seems that these factors are responsible to a great extent, however, for the predominance of *Lactobacillus* species in the bacterial flora of the large intestine of the breast-fed infant. These bacteria produce large amounts of acetic acid, which aids in suppressing the multiplication of enteropathogens. It also has been reported that *Lactobacillus* species strain GG aids in the recovery from acute rotavirus infections [179] and may enhance the formation of circulating cells that produce specific antibodies of the IgG, IgA, and IgM isotypes and serum levels of those antibodies [180].

Generation of Antiviral, Antiparasitic Lipids from Substrata in Human Milk

Human milk supplies defense agents from fat as it is partially digested in the recipient's alimentary tract. Fatty acids and monoglycerides produced from milk fats by bile salt–stimulated lipase or lipoprotein lipase in human milk [78], lingual/gastric lipase from the neonate from birth, or pancreatic lipase after a few weeks of age are able to disrupt enveloped viruses [181,182]. These antiviral lipids may aid in preventing coronavirus infections of the intestinal tract [183] and may defend against intestinal parasites such as *Giardia lamblia* and *Entamoeba histolytica* [184,185].

Proteins

The principal proteins in human milk that have direct antimicrobial properties include the following.

α-Lactalbumin

α-Lactalbumin is a major component of the milk proteins and may possess some important functions of immunologic defense. This protein appears as large complexes of several α-lactalbumin molecules, which can induce apoptosis in transformed embryonic and lymphoid cell lines.

Lactoferrin

Lactoferrin, the dominant whey protein in human milk, is a single-chain glycoprotein with two globular lobes, both of which display a site that binds ferric iron [186]. More than 90% of the lactoferrin in human milk is in the form of apolactoferrin (i.e., it does not contain ferric iron) [187], which competes with siderophilic bacteria and fungi for ferric iron [188–192] and disrupts the proliferation of these microbial pathogens. The epithelial growth-promoting activities of lactoferrin in human milk also

may aid in the defense of the recipient infant [193]. The mean concentration of lactoferrin in human colostrum is 5 to 6 mg/mL [194]. As the volume of milk production increases, the concentration decreases to about 1 mg/mL at 2 to 3 months of lactation [194,195].

Because of its resistance to proteolysis [196–198], the excretion of lactoferrin in stool is higher in infants fed human milk than in infants fed cow's milk [72,199–201]. The mean intake of milk lactoferrin per day in healthy breast-fed, full-term infants is about 260 mg/kg at 1 month of lactation and 125 mg/kg by 4 months [199]. The quantity of lactoferrin excreted in the stools of low-birth-weight infants fed human milk is approximately 185 times that excreted in stools of infants fed a cow's milk formula [202]. That estimate may be too high, however, because of the presence of immunoreactive fragments of lactoferrin in the stools of infants fed human milk [203]. Consistent with this suggestion, Prentice and colleagues [110] found that only approximately 1% of lactoferrin ingested in breast milk was excreted intact in stool by 6 weeks of postnatal age.

In addition, a significant increment in the urinary excretion of intact and fragmented lactoferrin occurs as a result of human milk feedings [110,203,204]. Stable isotope studies suggest that the increments in urinary lactoferrin and its fragments are principally from ingested human milk lactoferrin [205].

Lysozyme

Relatively high concentrations of lysozyme single-chain protein are present in human milk [194,195,206]. This 15-kDa agent lyses susceptible bacteria by hydrolyzing β-1,4 linkages between *N*-acetylmuramic acid and 2-acetylamino-2-deoxy-D-glucose residues in cell walls [207]. Lysozyme is relatively resistant to digestion by trypsin or denaturation owing to acid. The mean concentration of lysozyme is about 70 μg/mL in colostrum [194], about 20 μg/mL at 1 month of lactation, and 250 μg/mL by 6 months [195]. The approximate mean daily intake of milk lysozyme in healthy, full-term, completely breast-fed infants is 3 to 4 mg/kg at 1 month of lactation and 6 mg/kg by 4 months [199].

Few studies have been conducted to examine the fate of human milk lysozyme ingested by the infant. The amount of lysozyme excreted in the stools of low-birth-weight infants fed human milk is approximately eight times that of the amount excreted in the stools of infants fed a cow's milk formula [202], but the urinary excretion of this protein does not increase as a result of human milk feedings.

Fibronectin

Fibronectin, a high-molecular-weight protein that facilitates the uptake of many types of particulates by mononuclear phagocytic cells, is present in human milk (mean concentration in colostrum is 13.4 mg/L) [208]. The in vivo effects and fate of this broad-spectrum opsonin in human milk are unknown.

Complement Components

The components of the classic and alternative pathways of complement are present in human milk, but the concentrations of these components except C3 are exceptionally low [209,210].

Anti-inflammatory Agents

Although a direct anti-inflammatory effect of human milk has not been shown in vivo, numerous clinical observations suggest that breast-feeding protects the recipient infant from injury to the intestinal or respiratory mucosa [211,212]. This protection may be partly due to the more rapid elimination or neutralization of microbial pathogens in the lumen of the gastrointestinal tract by specific or broad-spectrum defense agents from human milk, but other features of human milk suggest that this is not the sole explanation. Proinflammatory mediators are poorly represented in human milk [213]. By contrast, human milk contains a host of anti-inflammatory agents [214], including a heterogeneous group of growth factors with cytoprotective and trophic activity for the mucosal epithelium, antioxidants, antiproteases, cytokines and cytokine receptors and antagonists, and other bioactive agents that inhibit inflammatory mediators or block the selected activation of leukocytes. Similar to the antimicrobial factors, some of these factors are well adapted to operate in the hostile environment of the recipient's alimentary tract.

Growth factors in human milk include epidermal growth factor [215,216], transforming growth factor-α and transforming growth factor-β [217,218], lactoferrin [193], and polyamines [219,220]. These and a host of hormones [221], including insulin-like growth factor, vascular endothelial growth factor, growth hormone–releasing factor, hepatocyte growth factor, prolactin, leptin, and cortisol [222], may affect the growth and maturation of epithelial barriers, limit the penetration of pathogenic microorganisms and free antigens, and prevent allergic sensitization. Corticosterone, a glucocorticoid that is present in high concentrations in rat milk, speeds gut closure in the neonatal rat [223]. Although macromolecular absorption does not seem to be as marked in the human neonate [224–226], the function of the mucosal barrier system in early infancy is important to host defense, and this system may be affected by factors in human milk. In this regard, the maturation of the intestinal tract as measured by mucosal mass, DNA, and protein content of the small intestinal tract seems to be influenced by milk, particularly early milk secretions [227].

Antioxidant activity in colostrum has been shown to be associated with an ascorbate compound and uric acid [228]. In addition, two other antioxidants present in human milk, α-tocopherol [229,230] and β-carotene [230], are absorbed into the circulation by the recipient gastrointestinal mucosa. Serum vitamin E concentrations increase in breast-fed infants from a mean of 0.3 mg/mL at birth to approximately 0.9 mg/mL on day 4 of life [229].

Very high concentrations of the pleiotropic anti-inflammatory and immunoregulatory cytokine IL-10, which attenuates dendritic cell, macrophage, T-cell, and NK-cell function, have been shown in samples of human milk collected during the first 80 hours of lactation [231]. IL-10 is present not only in the aqueous phase of the milk, but also in the lipid layer. Its bioactive properties were confirmed by the finding that human milk samples inhibited blood lymphocyte proliferation and that this property was greatly reduced by treatment with anti–IL-10 antibody. Mice with a targeted disruption in the IL-10 gene, when raised under conventional housing conditions, spontaneously develop a generalized enterocolitis that becomes apparent at the age of 4 to 8 weeks (time of weaning) [232]. These observations suggest that IL-10 in rat milk, and perhaps in human milk, may play a crucial role in the homeostasis of the immature intestinal barrier by regulating aberrant immune responses to foreign antigens.

Soluble cytokine receptors and cytokine receptor antagonists also are potent anti-inflammatory agents. Human colostrum and mature milk have been shown to contain biologically active levels of IL-1 receptor antagonist (IL-1Ra) and soluble TNF-α receptors I and II (sTNF-αRI and sTNF-αRII) [233]. The in vivo relevance of these observations also has been shown in a chemically induced colitis model of rats. Animals with colitis fed human milk had significantly lower neutrophilic inflammation than animals fed either chow or infant formula [234]. Similar "protective" effects were seen in rats with colitis fed an infant formula supplemented with IL-1Ra [234], suggesting that this anti-inflammatory agent present in milk may contribute to the broad protection against different injuries provided by human milk feeding.

The presence in human milk of platelet-activating factor acetylhydrolase (PAF-AH), the enzyme that catalyzes the degradation and inactivation of PAF, is intriguing [235]. Elevated serum concentrations of PAF have been found in rat and human neonates with necrotizing enterocolitis, whereas the concentrations of PAF-AH were found to be significantly lower than in control (unaffected) neonates [236,237]. Serum concentrations of PAF-AH at birth are less than concentrations in adults and gradually increase [237]. The enzyme is actively transferred from the mucosal to the serosal fluid in intestine of neonatal rats, particularly in the earliest postnatal period [238]. Other anti-inflammatory factors present in human milk include an IgE-binding factor, related antigenically to FcεRII (the lower affinity receptor for IgE), that suppresses the in vitro synthesis of human IgE [239] and the glycophosphoinositol-containing molecule protectin (CD59) that inhibits insertion of the complement membrane attack complex to cell targets [240]. The in vivo fate and effects of these anti-inflammatory factors in human milk are still poorly understood.

Modulators of the Immune System

Several seemingly unrelated types of observations suggest that breast-feeding modulates the development of the immune system of the recipient infant.

- Prospective and retrospective epidemiologic studies have shown that breast-fed infants are at less risk for development of certain chronic immunologically mediated disorders later in childhood, including allergic diseases [241], Crohn disease [242], ulcerative colitis [243], insulin-dependent diabetes mellitus [244], and some lymphomas [245].
- Humoral and cellular immune responses to specific antigens (i.e., vaccines) given during the first year of life seem to develop differently in breast-fed and in formula-fed infants. Several studies have reported increased serum antibody titers to *H. influenzae* type b

polysaccharide [246], oral poliovirus [247], tetanus [248], and diphtheria toxoid [249] immunizations in breast-fed infants. In regard to cell-mediated immunity, breast-fed infants given bacille Calmette-Guérin vaccine at birth or later show a significantly higher lymphocyte transformation response to purified protein derivative than infants who were never breast-fed [249]. Maternal renal allografts survive better in individuals who were breast-fed than in individuals who were not [250–252]. In this respect, the in vitro allogeneic responses between the blood lymphocytes of mothers (stimulating cells) and their infants (responding cells), as measured by an analysis of the frequencies of cytotoxic T lymphocyte (CTL) precursors directed against HLA alloantigens (CTL allorepertoire), are low in breast-fed infants [253].

- Increased levels of certain immune factors in breast-fed infants, which could not be explained simply by passive transfer of those substances, also suggest immunomodulatory activity of human milk. Breast-fed infants produce higher blood levels of IFN in response to respiratory syncytial virus infection [254]. It also was found that the increments in blood levels of fibronectin that were achieved by breast-feeding could not be due to the amounts of that protein in human milk [208]. In addition, it was found that human milk feeding led to a more rapid development in the appearance of sIgA in external secretions [202,204,110,248,255], some of which, such as urine, are far removed anatomically from the route of ingestion [204,110].
- Breast milk inhibits the response of human adult and fetal intestinal epithelial cells, dendritic cells, and monocytes to ligand-induced activation by toll-like receptor 2 and TLR3, but augments activation via TLR4 and TLR5 [256]. Inhibition of activation via TLR2 seemed to be mediated by a soluble form of this receptor [257], whereas augmentation of TLR4 signaling was associated with an as yet uncharacterized protein. These immunomodulatory activities were not present in infant formula. These results suggest that breast milk can modulate the gut innate immune recognition of and response to microbes, which may affect the nature of the gut microbial flora (e.g., microbiome) and risk for disease in early and later life [258,259].

These and other observations suggest that the ability of human milk to modulate the development of the infant's own mucosal and systemic immune systems may be associated with immunoregulatory factors present in colostrum and in more mature milk. Several different types of immunomodulatory agents can be identified in human milk [214]. Among the numerous substances with proven or potential ability to modulate the infant immune response are prolactin [260], α-tocopherol [229], lactoferrin [261], nucleotides [67], anti-idiotypic sIgA [262], and cytokines [263]. It is evident that many of these factors in milk have other primary biologic functions, as in the case of hormones or growth factors, and that their potential as immunoregulatory agents overlaps with their antimicrobial or anti-inflammatory properties [214].

Cytokines in Human Milk

In the 1990s, several cytokines, chemokines, and growth factors that mediate the effector phases of natural and specific immunity were discovered in human milk, and many more have been identified subsequently (Table 5–8). Human milk displays numerous biologic activities characteristic of cytokines, including the stimulation of growth, differentiation of immunoglobulin production by B cells [125,264,265], enhancement of thymocyte proliferation [266], inhibition of IL-2 production by T cells [267], and suppression of IgE production [239]. IL-1β [268] and TNF-α [269] were the first two cytokines quantified in human milk. In colostrum, TNF-α is present mainly in fractions of molecular weight of 80 to 195 kDa, probably bound to its soluble receptors [233]. Milk TNF-α is secreted by milk macrophages [269,270] and by the mammary epithelium [271].

IL-6 was first shown in human milk by a specific bioassay [272]. In this study, anti–IL-6–neutralizing antibodies inhibited IgA production by colostrum mononuclear cells, suggesting that IL-6 may be involved in the production of IgA in the mammary gland. The presence of IL-6 in milk also has been shown by immunoassays [269,271,273,274]. Similarly, IL-6 is localized in high-molecular-weight fractions of human milk [273]. The association of IL-6 with its own receptor has not been studied in milk, although the expression of IL-6 receptor by the mammary epithelium [271] and in secreted form in the milk [233] may explain the high molecular weight of this cytokine in human milk. The expression of IL-6 messenger ribonucleic acid (mRNA) and protein in milk cells and in the mammary gland epithelium suggests that milk mononuclear cells and the mammary gland are likely major sources of this cytokine [270,271,275].

The presence of IFN-γ in human milk also has been reported [148,271,274], although some investigators have found significant levels of IFN-γ only in milk samples obtained from mothers whose infants had been delivered

TABLE 5–8 Cytokines, Chemokines, and Colony-Stimulating Factors in Human Milk

Cytokines	Chemokines	Colony-Stimulating Factors
IL-1β	CXCL1	G-CSF
IL-2	CXCL8 (IL-8)	GM-CSF
IL-4	CXCL9	M-CSF
IL-6	CXCL10	Erythropoietin
IL-7	CCL2	
IL-8	CCL5	Interferons
IL-10	CCL11	
IL-13		
IL-15	TGF-β	
IFN-γ		
TNF-α		

G-CSF, granulocyte colony-stimulating factor; GM-CSF, granulocyte-macrophage colony-stimulating factor; IL, interleukin; M-CSF, monocyte colony-stimulating factor; TGF-β, transforming growth factor-β; TNF-α, tumor necrosis factor-α.
Adapted from references 277 and 278 and other sources.

by cesarean section. The significance of this observation is unclear at present. IFN-γ bioactivity and its association with specific subsets of milk T cells also remains to be determined [148]. (The presence and possible function of IL-10 in human milk are discussed in "Anti-inflammatory Agents.")

Chemokines are a novel class of small cytokines with discrete target cell selectivity that are able to recruit and activate different populations of leukocytes (see Chapter 4). Chemokines are grouped into families, which are defined by the spacing between cysteine residues (see Chapter 4). CXC chemokines, in which cysteine pairs are separated by one amino acid, and CC chemokines, in which paired cysteines are adjacent to each other, are found in human milk. Certain CXC chemokines that contain an ELR motif, including CXCL8 (also known as IL-8) and CXCL1 (GRO-α), predominantly attract neutrophils, whereas basophils, eosinophils, dendritic cells, monocytes, and specific subsets of T and B lymphocytes are attracted by specific CC chemokines and non-ELR CXC chemokines. The presence of many CXC and CC chemokines has been described in human milk (see Table 5–8) [275–278].

Colony-stimulating factors—highly specific protein factors that regulate cell proliferation and differentiation in the process of hematopoiesis—are also present in human milk [148,279–282]. The concentrations of monocyte colony-stimulating factor in particular seem to be 10-fold to 100-fold higher in human milk than in serum, and monocyte colony-stimulating factor evidently is produced by epithelial cells of the ducts and alveoli of the mammary gland under the regulatory activity of female sex hormones [281].

Although it is tempting to speculate that cytokines present in milk may be able to interact with mucosal tissues in the respiratory and alimentary tracts of the recipient infant, the functional expression of specific receptors for cytokines on epithelial or lymphoid cells in the airway and gastrointestinal mucosa has not been fully explored [214]. A receptor-independent mechanism of cytokine uptake by the gastrointestinal mucosa during the neonatal period has not been shown to date.

Whether and to what extent cytokines in breast milk contribute to the beneficial effects of human milk in the gut and elsewhere is largely unknown. Indirect evidence suggests that IL-7, which is a growth factor for T-cell progenitors (and for memory T cells), in breast milk may support thymic growth. Thymus size was found to be larger in breast-fed than in formula-fed 4-month-old infants in Denmark [283], and thymus size and IL-7 content of breast milk were directly correlated with each other in exclusively breast-fed infants in the Gambia [284]. In the latter study, reduced breast milk content of IL-7 was observed in the "hungry season" in association with reduced thymus size and thymic production of T cells; however, whether IL-7 in breast milk was absorbed intact and causally related to greater thymus size or was merely a surrogate for other factors cannot be determined from this study.

MILK AND ALTERED PREGNANCY

Several investigators have examined the effects of prematurity, early weaning, galactorrhea, and maternal malnutrition on the process of lactation. The immunologic aspects of these studies have focused largely on evaluation of the total content of sIgA and specific antibody activity. As described previously, the mammary secretions of the nonlactating breast contain sIgA, although the amount seems to be much lower than in the lactating breast [285]. Mammary secretions of patients with galactorrhea seem to contain sIgA in concentrations similar to those of normal postpartum colostrum [286]. Although malnutrition has been associated with reduced secretory antibody response in other external secretions, maternal malnutrition does not seem to affect the total sIgA concentration or antimicrobial-specific antibody activity in the milk [287]. By contrast, as noted in the preceding paragraph, poor maternal nutrition in the "hungry season" in the Gambia was associated with decreased thymus size [284].

The nutritional and immunologic composition of milk from mothers of premature infants seems to be significantly different from that of milk from mothers of infants born at term [16,49,195,288]. Comparative studies conducted during the first 12 weeks of lactation suggest that the mean concentrations of lactoferrin and lysozyme are higher in preterm than in term milk. sIgA is the predominant immunoglobulin in preterm and in term milk, although the sIgA concentration seems to be significantly higher in preterm milk collected during the first 8 to 12 weeks of lactation. sIgA antibody activity against certain organisms (*E. coli* somatic antigen) in the preterm milk was observed to be less than, or at best similar to, that found in term milk. In addition, the number of lymphocytes and macrophages in milk seems to be lower at 2 weeks, but significantly higher at 12 weeks in milk from mothers with preterm (born at 34 to 38 weeks of gestational age) infants than in milk from mothers with full-term infants [288]. The authors of these investigations have proposed that some of the observed changes may reflect the lower volume of milk produced by mothers delivered of preterm infants. The possibility remains that changes in the immunologic profile of preterm milk may be a consequence of inadequate stimulation by the preterm infant, alterations in the maternal hormonal milieu, or other factors underlying premature delivery itself.

BENEFITS AND RISKS OF HUMAN MILK
BENEFITS
Gastrointestinal Homeostasis and Prevention of Diarrhea

Development of mucosal integrity in the gut seems to depend on maturation of the mucosal tissue itself and the establishment of a normal gut flora. The former represents an anatomic and enzymatic blockage to invasion of microorganisms and antigens, and the latter represents an inhibition of colonization by pathogenic bacteria. Although permeability of the neonatal gut to immunoglobulin is short-lived, damaged neonatal gut is permeable to a host of other proteins and macromolecules for several weeks or longer. Large milk protein peptides and bovine serum albumin have been shown to enter the circulation and to induce a circulating antibody response. The inflamed or ischemic gut is even more porous to antigens and pathogens. Various proven and presumed mechanisms for the role of sIgA and the normal flora have been proposed to compensate for these temporary inadequacies.

Breast-feeding has been strongly implicated in supporting gastrointestinal homeostasis in the neonate and in establishing normal gut flora. Observations have shown a reduced rate of diarrheal disease in breast-fed infants, even in the face of contamination of the fed milk with *E. coli* and *Shigella* species [289]. A preventive and therapeutic role for breast-feeding also has been suggested in nursery outbreaks of diarrheal disease caused by enteropathogenic strains of *E. coli* [290] and rotavirus [291]. Breast-feeding plays an inhibitory role in the appearance of *E. coli* O83 agglutinins found in the feces of colonized infants. In addition, the diverse serotypes of aerobic, gram-negative bacilli present in the oropharynx and the gastrointestinal tract of the neonate may serve as a source of antigen to boost the presensitized mammary glands, leading to a further modulation of specific bacterial growth in the mucosa [292]. The precise role of antibody that blocks adherence of these pathogens to the gut and the effects of other factors, such as lactoperoxidase, lactoferrin, lysozyme, and the commensal flora, in those situations are uncertain.

Extensive epidemiologic evidence supports the "prophylactic value" of breast-feeding, particularly exclusive breast-feeding. in the first 6 months of life with the addition of complementary feeding thereafter, in the prevention or amelioration of diarrheal disease in infants and young children in developed and developing nations and is summarized in several reviews [1,3,86,87,293]. Ample experimental animal data on the value of specific colostral antibody in preventing diarrheal illness are available from studies of colostral deprivation. These include colibacteriosis associated with *E. coli* K88 in swine; rotaviral gastroenteritis in cattle, swine, and sheep; and diarrheal illness associated with transmissible gastroenteritis of swine [294]. In humans, cholera is rare in infancy, especially in endemic areas where the prevalence of breast-feeding is high. The experience with an outbreak of cholera in the Persian Gulf lends support to the possibility that the absence of breast-feeding is an important variable in increasing the risk of cholera in infancy.

A few reports have claimed that nursery outbreaks of diarrhea associated with enteropathogenic strains of *E. coli* can be interrupted by use of breast milk. Conflicting data exist regarding prevention of human rotaviral infection and disease. Evaluation of nursery outbreaks of rotaviral disease has suggested that the incidence of infection and of illness was lower in breast-fed infants, but the incidence of symptoms in formula-fed infants also was very low. Studies done in Japan have noted a fivefold decrease in incidence of rotaviral infection among breast-fed infants younger than 6 months. Most rotavirus infections in neonates are asymptomatic, regardless of breast-feeding or bottle-feeding [295–297]. On the basis of careful clinical observations, Bishop and coworkers[298] in Australia first questioned the positive effects of breast-feeding in rotavirus infection.

More recent case-control studies of enteric viral infections in breast-fed infants have suggested that breast-feeding may protect infants from hospitalization rather than from infection itself [299,300]. Longitudinal follow-up of a large cohort of infants during a community outbreak of rotavirus has shown that attack rates of rotavirus infection were similar in breast-fed and in bottle-fed infants. The frequency of clinical disease with diarrhea seemed to be significantly lower in breast-fed infants, however. The protection observed in these patients was more a reflection of altered microbial flora from breast-feeding than of specific immunologic protection against rotavirus. Breast milk contains sIgA directed against rotavirus, with the greatest concentrations in colostrum and lower amounts in mature milk; neutralization of rotavirus by breast milk correlates imperfectly with antibody concentrations measured by enzyme immunoassay, suggesting that other factors present in milk contribute to rotavirus neutralization [301]. It seems that breast-feeding provides significant protection against diarrheal disease, although the mechanisms of such protection remain to be more fully defined [299,300].

Necrotizing Enterocolitis

Necrotizing enterocolitis is a complex illness of the stressed premature infant, often associated with hypoxia, gut mucosal ischemia, and necrolysis and death [302,303]. Clinical manifestations have occasionally been associated with bacteremia and invasion by gram-negative bacilli, particularly *Klebsiella pneumoniae*, into the intestinal submucosa. Clinical manifestations include abdominal distention, gastric retention, and bloody diarrhea. Classic radiographic findings include air in the bowel wall (pneumatosis intestinalis), air in the portal system, and free infradiaphragmatic air (signifying perforation). Treatment involves decompression, systemic antibiotics, and, often, surgery [304–306].

Numerous studies have suggested a beneficial role of breast milk in preventing or modifying the development of necrotizing enterocolitis in high-risk human infants. Some pediatric centers have claimed virtual absence of necrotizing enterocolitis in breast-fed infants; however, many instances of the failure of milk feeding to prevent human necrotizing enterocolitis also have been reported [307]. Outbreaks of necrotizing enterocolitis related to *Klebsiella* and *Salmonella* species secondary to banked human milk feedings have been documented [124,308,309]. In an asphyxiated neonatal rat model of necrotizing enterocolitis, the entire syndrome could be prevented with feeding of maternal milk. The crucial factor in the milk seemed to be the cells, probably the macrophages [124]. It also is possible that antibody and nonspecific factors play a role, as does establishment of a gut flora. Prophylactic oral administration of immunoglobulin has been found to have a profound influence on the outcome of necrotizing enterocolitis in well-controlled studies [309]. Penetration of the gut by pathogens and antigens is increased with ischemic damage, and noncellular elements of milk may aid in blockage of this transit [310].

Necrotizing enterocolitis is a complex disease entity whose pathogenesis and cause remain to be defined.

Although breast-feeding may be protective, many other factors are related to the mechanism of mucosal injury and the pathogenesis of this syndrome.

Neonatal Sepsis

The incidence of bacteremia among premature infants fed breast milk has been suggested to be significantly lower than that among premature infants receiving formula feedings or no feeding [311–313]. A decrease in the incidence of neonatal sepsis, including sepsis associated with gram-negative bacilli and *E. coli* serotype K1, also has been linked to breast-feeding [314–316]; antibody and compartmentalized cellular reactivity to this serotype have been shown in human colostrum. Other studies have failed, however, to show clear evidence of protection against systemic infection in breast-fed infants [317–319]. A review of the evidence for protection of very low birth weight neonates from late-onset sepsis through the use of human milk suggested that the quality of the current evidence was insufficient to show a beneficial effect [320], although other authors have reached different conclusions [84,321].

Prevention of Atopy and Asthma

One of the most challenging developments in human milk research has been the demonstration in breast-fed infants of a reduced incidence of diseases with autoregulated or dysregulated immunity, long after the termination of breast-feeding [241–245]. Since the first report in 1936 [322], numerous published studies have addressed the effect of infant feeding on the development of atopic disease and asthma. Beneficial results of breast-feeding as prophylaxis against atopy have been observed in most of the studies; however, in others, beneficial effects were reported only in infants with a genetically determined risk for atopic disease. Finally, no beneficial effect at all or even an increased risk has been suggested in some breast-fed infants.

Kramer [323], in an extensive meta-analysis of 50 studies published before 1986 that focused on infant feeding and atopic disease, attempted to shed some light on the controversy. Of the 13 studies on asthma included in this analysis, 7 claimed a protective effect of breast-feeding, whereas 6 claimed no protection. Several serious methodologic drawbacks have been noted in this analysis, however. In many of the studies analyzed, early infant feeding history was obtained months or years after the feeding period, ascertainment of the infant feeding history was obtained by interviewers who were aware of the disease outcome, or insufficient duration and exclusivity of breast-feeding were documented; all were confounding variables that considered inappropriate "exposure standards." Nonblind ascertainment of disease outcome was found to be the most common violation of the "outcome standards."

Kramer's analysis also found that failure to control for confounding variables was a common violation in "statistical analysis standards" identified in several studies. The effect of infant feeding on subsequent asthma may be confounded by other variables that are associated with infant feeding and with unique investigational conditions. Factors that seem to have the greatest potential for confounding effects include family history of atopic disease,

socioeconomic status, and parental cigarette smoking. Only 1 of 13 studies on asthma included in the meta-analysis adequately controlled for these confounding factors. Three of the studies that did not show a protective effect of breast-feeding on asthma had inadequate statistical power. The effect of infant feeding on the severity of outcome and on the age at onset of the disease was virtually ignored in most of the studies [323].

Although this extensive meta-analysis may suggest some uncertainty about the prophylactic benefit of breast-feeding, other studies strongly support a positive effect of breast-feeding on the development of atopic disease and asthma. The first study [241] consisted of prospective, long-term evaluation from infancy until age 17 years; the prevalence of atopy was significantly higher in infants with short-duration (<1 month) or no breast-feeding, which increased to a demonstrable difference by age 17 years, than in infants with intermediate-duration (1 to 6 months) or prolonged (>6 months) breast-feeding. The differences in the prevalence of atopy persisted when the groups were divided according to positive or negative atopic heredity. The atopy manifestations in the different infant feeding groups did not remain constant with age. In particular, respiratory allergy, including asthma, increased greatly in prevalence up to age 17 years, with a prevalence of 64% in the group with short-duration or no breast-feeding [241].

In the second study, a prospective, longitudinal study of the prevalence and risk factors for acute and chronic respiratory illness in childhood, the investigators examined the relationship of infant feeding to recurrent wheezing at age 6 years and the association with lower respiratory tract illnesses with wheezing early in life [324]. Children who were never breast-fed had significantly higher rates of recurrent wheezing at 6 years of age. Increasing duration of breast-feeding beyond 1 month was not associated with significantly lower rates of recurrent wheezing. The effect of breast-feeding was apparent for children with and without wheezing lower respiratory tract illnesses in the first 6 months of life. In contrast with the findings of the first study, however, the effect of breast-feeding was significant only among nonatopic children [324].

The exact mechanisms by which breast-feeding seems to confer long-lasting protection against allergic sensitization are poorly understood. It is likely, however, that multiple synergistic mechanisms may be responsible for this effect, including (1) maturation of the recipient gastrointestinal and airway mucosa, promoted by growth factors present in human milk [216–218]; (2) inhibition of antigen absorption by milk sIgA [325]; (3) reduced incidence of mucosal infections and consequent sensitization to bystander antigens [326]; (4) changes in the microbial flora of the intestine of breast-fed infants [302]; and (5) direct immunomodulatory activity of human milk components on the recipient infant [214].

Numerous earlier and more recent studies have greatly contributed to the understanding of macromolecular transport across the immature gut and its consequences in terms of the generation of circulating antibody or immune complexes, the processes that are blocked predominantly by sIgA, the glycocalyx, and the intestinal enzymes. These mucosal immunologic events have been the basis for the concept of immune exclusion. Immune exclusion is not absolute, however, because uptake of some antigens across the gut may be enhanced rather than blocked by interaction with antibody at the mucosal surface. Beginning with the observations of IgA-deficient patients, it has become clear that the absence of the IgA barrier in the gut is associated with an increased incidence of circulating antibodies directed against many food antigens and an increased occurrence of atopic-allergic diseases [325]. Some studies have noted complement activation in serum after feeding of bovine milk to children with cow's milk allergy. The neonate is similar in some respects to the IgA-deficient patient [327], and increased transintestinal uptake of food antigen with consequent circulating antibody formation in the premature infant has been reported [328]. Other studies have suggested that early breast-feeding, even of short duration, is associated with a decreased serum antibody response to cow's milk proteins [226]. Prolonged breast-feeding not only may partially exclude foreign antigens through immune exclusion, but may also, because the mother's milk is the infant's sole food, prevent their ingestion [329]. Intact bovine milk proteins and other food antigens and antibodies have been observed, however, in samples of colostrum and milk [8].

Other Benefits

Epidemiologic evidence suggests that bacterial and viral respiratory infections are less frequent and less severe among breast-fed infants in various cultures and socioeconomic settings [330,331]. Antibodies and immunologic reactivity directed against herpes simplex virus, respiratory syncytial virus, and other infectious agents [92,102,164,331,332] and that protect against enterovirus infections [333] have been quantitated in colostrum and milk. Adoptive experiments in suckling ferrets have shown that protection of the young against respiratory syncytial virus can be transferred in colostrum containing specific antibody. The neonatal ferret gut is quite permeable, however, to macromolecules and permits passage of large quantities of virus-specific IgG. In the absence of either documented antibody or cellular transfer in the human neonate across the mucosa, any mechanisms of protection against respiratory syncytial virus and other respiratory pathogens remain obscure.

Data are lacking in humans regarding passive protection on other mucosal surfaces, such as the eye, ear, or genitourinary tract. Some epidemiologic evidence suggests that recurrence of otitis media with effusion is strongly associated with early bottle-feeding and that breast-feeding may confer protection against otitis media with effusion for the first 3 years of life [334]. Foster feeding–acquired antibody to herpes simplex virus has been found to result in significant protection against reinfection challenge in experimental animal studies [332].

Numerous other benefits have been associated with breast-feeding, including natural contraception during active nursing [335] and protection against sudden infant death syndrome [336], diabetes [337], obesity [338], and

high cholesterol level and ischemic heart disease later in life [42]. Of particular more recent interest has been the association of breast-feeding with improved intellectual performance in older children. Several studies have shown enhanced cognitive outcome in breast-fed children, although controversy exists regarding the mechanisms by which such improved performance may occur [339–341]. Health benefits for the mother also may be associated with breast-feeding: A reduced incidence of breast cancer has been noted in women who have lactated [342].

POTENTIAL RISKS
Noninfectious Risks

Human milk is the optimal form of nutrition for healthy term infants in almost all situations. The failure to initiate lactation properly during early breast-feeding may present a risk of dehydration to the infant because insufficient fluids may be ingested. Inappropriate introduction of bottles and pacifiers also may interfere with proper induction of lactation. Later in lactation, introduction of bottles may induce premature weaning as the result of a reduction in the milk supply.

Some circumstances have been identified in which breast-feeding is contraindicated and others have been identified in which continued breast-feeding should be conducted with caution to protect the infant [3]. Infants with inherited metabolic diseases may require alternative forms of nutrition: neonates with classic galactosemia owing to deficiency of galactose-1-phosphate uridyltransferase should receive lactose-free milk (lactose is a glucose-galactose disaccharide); infants with phenylketonuria may receive some human milk to support their requirement for phenylalanine, but often may be better managed by use of specially prepared commercial milks. Mothers who have received radionuclides for diagnostic or therapeutic purposes should use alternative forms of nutrition for the days to weeks required for these compounds to be eliminated, as should mothers receiving certain chemotherapeutic and immunosuppressive agents and actively using drugs of abuse, including amphetamines, cocaine, heroin, and phencyclidine [343]. Low-level maternal exposure to environmental chemicals and tobacco smoking should be avoided as much as possible, but are not a contraindication to breast-feeding.

Antimicrobial agents taken by mothers only rarely represent a contraindication to breast-feeding. As first principles, antimicrobials that may be safely given to infants may be safely given to their lactating mothers, and blood concentrations that may be achieved through breast milk ingestion are lower than therapeutic doses used in infants [344]. Breast-feeding by mothers receiving chloramphenicol is contraindicated because its use may be associated with fatal complications in newborn infants. The effects of metronidazole are uncertain, but to minimize exposure to this drug, which is mutagenic in bacteria, mothers receiving single-dose therapy should discontinue breast-feeding for 12 to 24 hours [343]. Excretion of antibiotics in human milk is also discussed in Chapter 37. For up-to-date information regarding drugs and lactation, the reader should consult http://www.toxnet.nlm.nih.gov/cgi-bin/sis/htmlgen?LACT.

Several instances of specific nutrient deficiencies in breast-fed infants have been described, specifically related to lack of vitamin K, vitamin D, vitamin B$_{12}$, folic acid, vitamin C, and carnitine. In each of these instances, several case reports have appeared warning against deficiencies that have resulted in clinical consequences to the neonate. Hemorrhagic disease reported in a few breast-fed infants was successfully treated with vitamin K [345]. These infants did not receive vitamin K at birth. Mothers who practice unusual dietary habits, such as strict vegetarianism, may have reduced levels of vitamin B$_{12}$ and folic acid in their milk, and deficiencies in breast-fed infants of such mothers have been reported [346,347]. Cases of rickets in breast-fed infants have been reported, particularly during winter among infants not exposed to the sun [34,348]. Deficiency of carnitine, a nutrient responsible for modulating fat absorption, also has been reported to result in clinical symptoms in breast-fed infants in mothers ingesting unusual diets [61,349]. These concerns can best be addressed in almost all cases by counseling mothers regarding nutritional practices and by the provision of supplemental vitamins and other micronutrients when appropriate; this is the case in the developed world and even more so in the developing world where the untoward consequences of not breast-feeding are particularly great [293].

Management of hyperbilirubinemia associated with breast-feeding has been an area of some controversy. Present recommendations are for continued breast-feeding with efforts to increase the volume of milk ingested, with the provision that with severe hyperbilirubinemia a brief interruption of breast-feeding might be appropriate [3].

Infectious Risks

Human milk may contain infectious agents that are secreted into the milk; enter milk during lactation; or are acquired when milk is improperly collected, stored, and later fed to the infant. Formal training and evaluation of breast-feeding practices by trained caregivers is the best way to reduce these risks; routine culture or heat treatment of a mother's milk even when it is stored and later used to feed her infant is not cost-effective [3].

Stored milk is now commonly used to feed infants when their mothers are unable to breast-feed directly because of work or travel constraints or when the infant is premature or otherwise unable to breast-feed effectively. Inadvertent feeding of stored milk from other than the birth mother has occurred in nurseries. If this occurs, the AAP recommends that this be handled in the same manner as if accidental exposure to blood or other body fluids has occurred [344] (see Chapter 35 for additional information).

In the United States, the Human Milk Banking Association of North America (http://www.hmbana.org/) collects human donor milk for the purpose of administration to infants whose mothers' milk is unavailable or inadequate. Members of this association follow guidelines formulated in consultation with the U.S. Food and Drug Administration (FDA) and Centers for Disease Control and Prevention. These guidelines help to ensure that donors are screened for transmissible infections and that the milk is carefully collected, processed, and stored. Using these practices, donor milk is collected and pooled and subjected to Holder pasteurization (62.5° C) for 30 minutes, which reliably kills bacteria and inactivates HIV and cytomegalovirus (CMV) and eliminates or substantially reduces the amounts of other viruses. The pooled milk is tested to ensure that it meets standards and is frozen for later distribution and use.

Bacterial Infections

Transmission of bacterial pathogens, including *S. aureus*, group B streptococci, mycobacteria, and other species, may occur through breast-feeding (Table 5–9). Mastitis and breast abscesses may be associated with substantial concentrations of bacteria in the mother's milk. Generally, feeding an infant from a breast affected by an abscess is not recommended [344]. Infant feeding on the affected breast may be resumed, however, 24 to 48 hours after drainage and the initiation of appropriate antibiotic therapy. Mastitis usually resolves with appropriate antimicrobial therapy and with continued lactation, even if feeding from the affected breast is temporarily interrupted.

TABLE 5–9 Infectious Agents Transmitted through Breast-Feeding

Organism	Transmission	Disease	Intervention
Cytomegalovirus	+	VLBW infants	Consider risk/benefit
Hepatitis B virus	+	+	HBIG/hepatitis B vaccine
Hepatitis C virus	HIV+ mothers only	?	See text
Herpes simplex virus	+	+	See text
HIV	+	+	U.S.: Do not breastfeed*
HTLV-1	+	±	U.S.: Do not breastfeed*
HTLV-2	+	±	U.S.: Do not breastfeed*
Rubella virus	+	0	None
West Nile virus	±	±	None
Group B streptococci	+	±	See text
Staphylococcus aureus	+	±	See text
Mycobacterium tuberculosis	+	−	See text

*In many other parts of the world, the benefits of breast-feeding often outweigh the risks of alternative methods of infant feeding. See text for discussion of risk versus benefit in other parts of the world.
HBIG, hepatitis B immunoglobulin; HIV, human immunodeficiency virus; HTLV, human T-lymphotropic virus; VLBW, very low birth weight.

In both of these conditions, feeding from the unaffected breast need not be interrupted.

Mothers with active tuberculosis should refrain from breast-feeding for at least 2 weeks or longer after institution of appropriate treatment if they are considered contagious. This recommendation also applies to the uncommon situation where mastitis or breast abscess is caused by *Mycobacterium tuberculosis* [344].

Viral Infections

Viruses that have been detected in human milk include CMV, hepatitis B (HBV) and hepatitis C (HCV) viruses, herpes simplex virus, HIV-1, human T-lymphotropic virus 1 (HTLV-1) and HTLV-2, rubella virus, and West Nile virus (see Table 5–9) [344]. It is unknown whether varicella virus is secreted into human milk. Although some of these viruses do present a risk to the infant, for most, but not all, the benefits of breast-feeding to the infant are greater than the risk.

Cytomegalovirus Infection

CMV infection is a common perinatal infection. The virus is shed in the milk in about 25% of infected mothers. Although breast-feeding from infected mothers may result in seroconversion in 70% of breast-feeding neonates, the infection often is not associated with clinical symptoms of disease. Infants with very low birth weight (<1500 g) may exhibit evidence of clinical disease, however, with thrombocytopenia, neutropenia, or hepatosplenomegaly seen in 50% of very low birth weight infants infected through breast-feeding. The decision to breast-feed a premature infant by an infected mother should be based on weighing the potential benefits of human milk versus the risk of CMV transmission [344].

Hepatitis B Virus Infection

Hepatitis B surface antigen has been detected in milk of HBV-infected mothers. Nevertheless, breast-feeding does not increase the risk of HBV infection among these infants. Infants born to HBV-positive mothers should receive hepatitis B immunoglobulin and the recommended series of hepatitis B vaccine without any delay in the institution of breast-feeding [344].

Hepatitis C Virus Infection

The RNA of HCV and antibody to HCV have been detected in the milk from infected mothers. Transmission via breast-feeding has not been documented in anti-HCV–positive, anti-HIV–negative mothers, but is a theoretical possibility about which these mothers should be informed before deciding whether they will breast-feed. According to current guidelines, HCV infection does not contraindicate breast-feeding [344].

Herpes Simplex Virus Type 1

Herpes simplex virus transmission directly from maternal breast lesions to infants has been shown. Women with lesions on one breast may feed from the other unaffected breast, making sure that lesions on the other breast or on other parts of the body are covered and using careful hand hygiene [344].

Human Immunodeficiency Virus Type 1

Numerous studies have shown HIV in milk [350–354]. The findings include isolation of HIV from milk supernatants collected from symptom-free women and from cellular fractions of maternal milk, recovery of HIV virions in the histiocytes and cell-free extracts of milk by electron microscopy, and detection of viral DNA by polymerase chain reaction in greater than 70% of samples from HIV-seropositive lactating women.

Transmission of HIV through breast-feeding may account for one third to one half of all HIV infections globally, with risk of transmission being approximately 15% when breast-feeding continues beyond the first year of life [355,356]. The risk of postnatal HIV transmission seems to be constant throughout the first 18 months of life; risk is cumulative as duration of breast-feeding increases [357]. Risk of transmission via breast milk is greater when maternal HIV infection is acquired during lactation; when viral load is greater or maternal disease is more advanced; when infants are breast-fed and formula-fed; when the mother has bleeding or cracked nipples, mastitis, or a breast abscess; and when the infant has thrush or certain other coinfections (see Chapter 21 for more details).

Current recommendations from the AAP [344] and other authorities [358] state that in populations such as that of the United States, in which the risk of death from infectious diseases and malnutrition is low and in which safe and effective alternative sources of feeding are readily available, HIV-infected women should be counseled not to breast-feed their infants and not to donate milk. One report found that highly active antiretroviral therapy administered during pregnancy or postpartum suppresses HIV RNA, but not DNA in breast milk [359]. At present, the AAP recommends that infants of HIV-infected mothers in the United States receiving highly active antiretroviral therapy should not be breast-fed.

Despite the potential risk of HIV infection in infants of HIV-infected breast-feeding mothers, consideration of cessation of breast-feeding must be balanced against the other beneficial effects described in this chapter. In areas of the world where infectious diseases and malnutrition are important causes of death early in life, the beneficial effects of breast-feeding often outweigh the potential risk of HIV transmission through breast-feeding. Studies in such settings have shown that HIV-free survival at 7 months of age is similar in exposed infants that were breast-fed or formula-fed from birth [360–362]. Studies in Africa show that mothers who exclusively breast-feed in the first 6 months of life have reduced risk of HIV transmission compared with mothers who supplement breast-feeding with other foods and milk sources [360,361,363]. In areas of the world where the burden of infectious diseases and malnutrition is high and where alternatives to breast milk that provide adequate nutrition are unacceptable, affordable, feasible, and safe, exclusive breast-feeding is recommended by the WHO and other authorities for women whose HIV status is unknown and for women known to be HIV-infected [293,344,358,364]. The WHO policy also stresses the need for continued support for breast-feeding by mothers who are HIV-negative, improved access to HIV counseling and testing, and government efforts to ensure uninterrupted access to nutritionally adequate human milk substitutes [344].

Human T-Lymphotropic Viruses 1 and 2

HTLV-1 is endemic in Japan, the Caribbean, and parts of South America. This infection can be transmitted from mother to infant, and transmission occurs primarily through breast-feeding. HTLV-2 infection has been identified in some Native Americans and Native Alaskans and in some injection drug abusers in the United States and Europe. Mother-to-infant transmission of HTLV-2 has been shown, although the frequency with which this occurs and the route of transmission are uncertain. Women in the United States who are known to be seropositive for HTLV-1 or HTLV-2 should not breast-feed. Routine screening for HTLV-1 and HTLV-2 is not recommended [344].

Rubella

Rubella virus has been recovered from milk after natural and vaccine-associated infection. It has not been associated with significant disease in infants, although transient seroconversion has been frequently shown. No contraindication to breast-feeding exists in women recently immunized with currently licensed rubella vaccines.

West Nile Virus Infection

The RNA of West Nile virus has been detected in human milk, and seroconversion in breast-feeding infants also has been observed. Although West Nile virus can be transmitted in milk, the extent of transmission in humans remains to be determined. Most infants and children infected with the virus to date have been asymptomatic or have had minimal disease [344]. Because the risk is uncertain, the AAP recommends that women in endemic areas may continue to breast-feed.

CURRENT TRENDS IN BREAST-FEEDING

International and national organizations have endorsed breast-feeding as the optimal means of feeding for healthy term infants [344]. The percentage of mothers initiating breast-feeding in developing countries generally is 80% or greater and often 90% or greater. The health and economic consequences for bottle-fed infants in these countries are severe, however. In the United States, at one point in the early 1970s, the rate of breast-feeding initiation was 25%. The rate of initiation since that time has increased but fluctuated over time. In a survey (IFPS II) conducted by the FDA in 2005-2007, 83% of respondents initiated breast-feeding [365].

In contrast to this favorable trend, the recommendation for exclusive breast-feeding for the first 6 months of life in the United States and internationally is uncommonly followed. In the United States, supplemental feeding was often initiated in the hospital in the immediate postpartum period, and by 3 months of age more than 61% of infants had received formula [365]. Similarly, although

breast-feeding initiation approaches 100% in developing nations in Africa, Asia, and the Caribbean, the rates of exclusive breast-feeding for the first 6 months of life are approximately 50% and approximately 30% for infants less than 2 months and 2 to 5 months of age [1].

Within the United States, various demographic patterns seem to be associated with breast-feeding behavior. Older mothers, mothers with a college education, and mothers with higher incomes all are more likely to breast-feed. African American and Hispanic mothers, mothers of lower socioeconomic status who are participants in the Women, Infants, and Children (WIC) program of the U.S. Department of Health and Human Services, and mothers who live in the southern regions of the United States are much less likely to breast-feed. The low rate of breast-feeding for mothers enrolled in WIC is of particular concern because that agency has a specific policy to encourage breast-feeding. Many states now depend on formula manufacturer rebates to fund part of their WIC programs, however, creating a conflict of interest. The disturbing part of the demographic pattern of breast-feeding in the United States is that the infants of lower socioeconomic status mothers, who would accrue the greatest health and economic benefits from breast-feeding, are those least likely to be breast-fed.

Although demographic studies indicate who is breast-feeding, they do not explain the behavioral differences among groups of mothers. One of the more complete models designed to explain breast-feeding behavior includes components that address maternal attitudes and family, societal, cultural, and environmental variables [366]. Individual studies have shown that the maternal decision-making process is closely related to the social support and influence that come from the family members surrounding the mother [367]. The husband in particular seems to have a strong positive influence, whereas the mother's mother may have a negative influence on the breast-feeding decision. Social support seems to be different among ethnic groups, as are maternal attitudes; such differences may provide one explanation for differences in breast-feeding behavior among ethnic groups [368,369]. Higher rates of exclusive breast-feeding have been observed for infants born in U.S. hospitals who follow the practices recommended by the WHO/United Nations Children's Fund Baby-friendly Hospital Initiative, which emphasizes 10 steps that promote successful breast-feeding [370].

SUMMARY AND CONCLUSIONS

Human milk contains a wide variety of soluble and cellular components with a diverse spectrum of biologic functions. The major milk components identified to date exhibit antimicrobial, anti-inflammatory, proinflammatory, and immunoregulatory functions; cytotoxicity for tumor cells; ability to repair tissue damage; receptor analogue functions; and other metabolic effects. The biologic activities of different milk components are summarized in Table 5–10.

Polymorphonuclear leukocytes, macrophages, lymphocytes, and epithelial cells are observed in human milk, but their functions in milk are unknown. It is possible that their primary task is the antimicrobial defense of the

TABLE 5–10 Possible Role of Soluble and Cellular Factors Identified in Human Milk

Factor	Antimicrobial	Anti-inflammatory	Proinflammatory	Immunoregulatory	Other
Immunoglobulin (sIgA)	+++	++	—	++	++
Other immunoglobulins	+++	+	++	+	—
T-lymphocyte products	+++	++	++	—	—
PMNs, macrophages	++	—	+	++	—
Lactoferrin	+++	+++	—	—	—
α-Lactalbumin	—	++	—	—	—
Carbohydrates					
Oligosaccharides	++	++	—	—	++
Glycoconjugates	++	++	—	—	++
Glycolipids	—	—	—	—	—
Lipid and fat globules	++	—	—	—	—
Nucleotides	+	—	—	++	++
Defensins	+	—	—	+	—
Lysozymes	±	—	—	—	—
Cytokines, chemokines					
TGF-β	—	++	++	++	—
IL-10	—	++	++	++	—
IL-1β	—	++	++	++	—
TNF-α	—	—	—	++	—
IL-6	—	—	—	++	—
IL-7	—	—	—	(prothymus)	—
Others	—	—	—	++	—
Prostaglandins	—	++	—	—	—
Leptin*	—	—	—	++	++
Antiproteases	—	++	—	—	—
Other growth factors	—	++	—	++	—
sTLR-2, sCD14	—	+++	—	++	—

*IL-1α, TNF-β, and IL-6 are associated with increased levels of leptin.
+ to +++ = minimal to moderate effect; — = no known effect; ±= equivocal.

IL, interleukin; PMNs, polymorphonuclear neutrophils; sIgA, secretory IgA; TGF, transforming growth factor; TLR, toll-like receptor; TNF, tumor necrosis factor.

mammary gland itself. These cells may help to promote tolerance to their mothers' HLA allotype, which may have implications regarding immune responsiveness and allograft rejection [371].

The bulk of the antimicrobial effects of human milk are associated with milk immunoglobulin, especially the sIgA isotype, which makes up to 80% of all immunoglobulins in the human body. Milk antibodies seem to provide protection against many intestinal pathogens, such as *Campylobacter*, *Shigella*, *E. coli*, *V. cholerae*, *Giardia*, and rotavirus, and against respiratory pathogens such as respiratory syncytial virus. Milk antibodies also effectively neutralize toxins and various human viruses. The role of small amounts of IgG and IgM in milk is uncertain. Milk IgA antibodies generally induce antimicrobial protection in the absence of any inflammation. Lactoferrin, lysozyme, α-lactalbumin, and other milk proteins and carbohydrates and lipids also contribute to the antimicrobial and immunomodulatory properties of human milk. Milk also contains numerous cytokines, chemokines, growth factors, soluble TLRs, and CD14, which modulate inflammatory and immunologic responses in the gut.

The passive transfer of the diversity of maternal biologic experiences to the neonate through the process of breast-feeding represents an essential component of the survival mechanism in the mammalian neonate. For millions of years, maternal products of lactation delivered through the process of breast-feeding have been the sole source of nutrition and immunity during the neonatal period and early infancy for all mammals, including the human infant. During the past 150 to 300 years, human societies have undergone remarkable changes, which have had a major impact on the basic mechanisms of maternal-neonatal interaction, breast-feeding, and the environment. Such changes include introduction of sanitation and nonhuman milk and formula feeds for neonatal nutrition, use of antimicrobial agents, introduction of processed foods, and exposure to newer environmental macromolecules and dietary antigens. The introduction of such human-made changes in the neonatal environment has had a profound impact on human homeostatic mechanisms, while allowing new insights into the role of breast-feeding in the developing human neonate.

Comparative analysis of natural (traditional) forms of breast-feeding and artificial feeding modalities has shown that natural breast-feeding is associated with significant reduction in infant mortality and morbidity; protection against acute infectious diseases; and possible protection against allergic disorders and autoimmune disease, acute and chronic inflammatory disorders, obesity, diabetes mellitus and other metabolic disorders, allograft rejection, and development of many malignant conditions in childhood or later in life. This information has been reviewed by Hanson in an elegant monograph [372] and by others [86]. Despite the overwhelmingly protective role attributed to natural breast-feeding and the evolutionary advantages related to the development of lactation, several infectious agents have acquired, during the course of evolution, the ability to evade immunologic factors in milk and to use milk as the vehicle for maternal-to-infant transmission. The potential for the acquisition of infections, including HIV, HTLV, CMV, and possibly other pathogens, highlights potential hazards of breast-feeding in some clinical situations. It is reasonable to conclude that the development of lactation, the hallmark of mammalian evolution, is designed to enhance the survival of the neonate of the species and that breast-feeding may have a remarkable spectrum of immediate and long-term protective functions.

REFERENCES

[1] R.E. Black, et al., Maternal and child undernutrition: global and regional exposures and health consequences, Lancet 371 (2008) 243–260.
[2] A. Chen, W.J. Rogan, Breastfeeding and the risk of postneonatal death in the United States, Pediatrics 113 (2004) e435–e439.
[3] L.M. Gartner, et al., Breastfeeding and the use of human milk, Pediatrics 115 (2005) 496–506.
[4] K. Kratochwil, Experimental analysis of the prenatal development of the mammary gland, in: N. Kretchmer, E. Rossi, F. Sereni (Eds.), Milk and Lactation, Modern Problems in Paediatrics, vol. 15, S. Karger, Basel, 1975, pp. 1–15.
[5] H. Vorherr, The Breast: Morphology, Physiology and Lactation, Academic Press, New York, 1974.
[6] A.S. Goldman, B. Shapiro, F. Neumann, Role of testosterone and its metabolites in the differentiation of the mammary gland in rats, Endocrinology 99 (1976) 1490–1495.
[7] D.L. Kleinberg, W. Niemann, E. Flamm, Primate mammary development: effects of hypophysectomy, prolactin inhibition, and growth hormone administration, J. Clin. Invest. 75 (1985) 1943–1950.
[8] S.S. Ogra, P.L. Ogra, Components of immunologic reactivity in human colostrum and milk, in: P.L. Ogra, D. Dayton (Eds.), Immunology of Breast Milk, Raven Press, New York, 1979, pp. 185–195.
[9] J.L. Pasteels, Control of mammary growth and lactation by the anterior pituitary: an attempt to correlate classic experiments on animals with recent clinical findings, in: N. Kretchmer, E. Rossi, F. Sereni (Eds.), Milk and Lactation, Modern Problems in Paediatrics, vol. 15, S. Karger, Basel, 1975, pp. 80–95.
[10] T.B. Mepham, Physiology of Lactation. Milton Keynes, Open University Press, England, 1987.
[11] A.G. Frantz, Prolactin, N. Engl. J. Med. 298 (1978) 201–207.
[12] A.M. Widström, et al., Gastric suction in healthy newborn infants, Acta Paediatr. Scand. 76 (1987) 566–572.
[13] H. Varendi, R.H. Porter, J. Winberg, Does the newborn baby find the nipple by smell? Lancet 344 (1994) 989–990.
[14] B. Lönnerdal, E. Forsum, L. Hambraeus, The protein content of human milk, I: a transversal study of Swedish normal mothers, Nutr. Rep. Int. 13 (1976) 125–134.
[15] R.J. Schanler, W. Oh, Composition of breast milk obtained from mothers of premature infants as compared to breast milk obtained from donors, J. Pediatr. 96 (1980) 679–681.
[16] L. Sann, F. Bienvenu, C. Lahet, Comparison of the composition of breast milk from mothers of term and preterm infants, Acta Paediatr. Scand. 70 (1981) 115–116.
[17] L. Mata, Breast-feeding: main promoter of infant health, Am. J. Clin. Nutr. 31 (1978) 2058–2065.
[18] L.S. Hurley, B. Lonnerdal, A.G. Stanislowski, Zinc citrate, human milk and acrodermatitis enteropathica, Lancet 1 (1979) 677–678.
[19] C.D. Eckert, M.V. Sloan, J.R. Duncan, Zinc binding: a difference between human and bovine milk, Science 195 (1977) 789–790.
[20] S.J. Fomon, Infant Nutrition, second ed., WB Saunders, Philadelphia, 1974.
[21] C.W. Woodruff, The science of infant nutrition and the art of infant feeding, JAMA 240 (1978) 657–661.
[22] R. Moran, et al., Epidermal growth factor concentrations and daily production in breast milk during seven weeks post delivery in mothers of premature infants, Pediatr. Res. 16 (1982) 171A.
[23] R. Moran, et al., The concentration and daily output of trace elements, vitamins and carnitine in breast milk from mothers of premature infants for seven postnatal weeks, Pediatr. Res. 16 (1982) 172A.
[24] P.L. Ogra, H.L. Greene, Human milk and breast-feeding: an update on the state of the art, Pediatr. Res. 16 (1982) 266–271.
[25] H.L. Greene, M.E. Courtney, Breast-feeding and infant nutrition, in: P.L. Ogra (Ed.), Neonatal Infections: Nutritional and Immunologic Interactions, Grune & Stratton, Orlando, FL, 1984, pp. 265–284.
[26] Code of Federal Regulations, Title 21, Pat 107, 100. U.S. Government Printing Office, Washington, DC, 1992, p. 84.
[27] R.R. Anderson, Variations in major minerals of human milk during the first 5 months of lactation, Nutr. Res. 12 (1992) 701–711.
[28] U.M. Saarinen, M.A. Siimes, P.R. Dallman, Iron absorption in infants: high bioavailability of breast milk iron as indicated by extrinsic tag method of iron absorption and by the concentration of serum ferritin, J. Pediatr. 91 (1977) 36–39.
[29] J.A. McMillan, et al., Iron absorption from human milk, simulated human milk, and proprietary formulas, Pediatrics 60 (1977) 896–900.
[30] S. Fomon, E. Ziegler, H. Vasquez, Human milk and the small premature infant, Am. J. Dis. Child. 131 (1977) 463–467.
[31] C. Gopalan, B. Belavady, Nutrition and lactation, Fed. Proc. 20 (1961) 177–184.
[32] M.K. Gorten, E.R. Cross, Iron metabolism in premature infants, II: prevention of iron deficiency, J. Pediatr. 64 (1964) 509–520.
[33] American Academy of Pediatrics Committee on Nutrition. Nutritional needs of low-birth-weight infants, Pediatrics 60 (1977) 519–530.
[34] P. O'Connor, Vitamin D-deficiency rickets in two breast-fed infants who were not receiving vitamin D supplementation, Clin. Pediatr. 16 (1977) 361–363.
[35] H.W. Moser, M.L. Karnovsky, Studies on the biosynthesis of glycolipids and other lipids of the brain, J. Biol. Chem. 234 (1959) 1990–1997.
[36] R.M. Kliegman, E.L. Miettinen, S. Morton, Potential role of galactokinase in neonatal carbohydrate assimilation, Science 220 (1983) 302–304.
[37] D.S. Newburg, S.H. Neubauer, Carbohydrate in milks: analysis, quantities and significance, in: J.G. Jensen (Ed.), Handbook of Milk Composition, Academic Press, San Diego, 1995, pp. 273–349.
[38] D.S. Newburg, Do the binding properties of oligosaccharides in milk protect human infants from gastrointestinal bacteria? J. Nutr. 127 (1997) 980S–984S.
[39] R.G. Jensen, A.M. Ferris, C.J. Lammi-Keefe, Lipids in human milk and infant formulas, Annu. Rev. Nutr. 12 (1992) 417–441.
[40] D.K. Rassin, N.C. Räihä, G.E. Gaull, Protein and taurine nutrition in infants, in: E. Lebenthal (Ed.), Textbook of Gastroenterology and Nutrition in Infancy, Raven Press, New York, 1989, pp. 391–401.
[41] R. Reiser, Z. Sidelman, Control of serum cholesterol homeostasis by cholesterol in the milk of the suckling rat, J. Nutr. 102 (1972) 1009–1016.
[42] C.H. Fall, et al., Relation of infant feeding to adult serum cholesterol concentration and death from ischaemic heart disease, BMJ 304 (1992) 801–805.
[43] E. Galli, et al., Analysis of polyunsaturated fatty acids in newborn sera: a screening tool for atopic disease, Br. J. Dermatol. 130 (1994) 752–756.
[44] S.M. Innis, N. Auestad, J.S. Siegman, Blood lipid docosahexaenoic acid in term gestation infants fed formulas with high docosahexaenoic acid, low eicosapentaenoic acid fish oil, Lipids 31 (1996) 617–625.
[45] S.E. Carlson, et al., Visual acuity and fatty acid status of term infants fed human milk and formulas with and without docosahexaenoate and arachidonate from egg yolk lecithin, Pediatr. Res. 39 (1996) 882–888.
[46] S.E. Carlson, S.H. Werkman, E.A. Tolley, Effect of long-chain n-3 fatty acid supplementation on visual acuity and growth of preterm infants with and without bronchopulmonary dysplasia, Am. J. Clin. Nutr. 63 (1996) 687–689.
[47] N. Auestad, et al., Visual acuity, erythrocyte fatty acid composition and growth in term infants fed formulas with long chain polyunsaturated fatty acids for one year, Pediatr. Res. 41 (1997) 1–10.
[48] E.E. Birch, et al., Visual acuity and the essentiality of docosahexaenoic acid and arachidonic acid in the diet of term infants, Pediatr. Res. 44 (1998) 201–209.
[49] S.J. Gross, J. Geller, R.M. Tomarelli, Composition of breast milk from mothers of preterm infants, Pediatrics 68 (1981) 490–493.
[50] L. Hambraeus, Proprietary milk versus human breast milk in infant feeding: a critical appraisal from the nutritional point of view, Pediatr. Clin. North Am. 24 (1977) 17–36.
[51] C. Kunz, B. Lönnerdal, Re-evaluation of the whey protein/casein ratio of human milk, Acta Paediatr. 81 (1992) 107–112.
[52] A.L. Järvenpää, et al., Milk protein quantity and quality in the term infant, II: effects on acidic and neutral amino acids, Pediatrics 70 (1982) 221–230.
[53] L.M. Janas, M.F. Picciano, T.F. Hatch, Indices of protein metabolism in term infants fed human milk, whey-predominant formula, or cow's milk formula, Pediatrics 75 (1985) 775–784.
[54] T.A. Picone, et al., Growth, serum biochemistries, and amino acids of term infants fed formulas with amino acid and protein concentrations similar to human milk, J. Pediatr. Gastroenterol. Nutr. 9 (1989) 351–360.
[55] D.K. Rassin, et al., Milk protein quantity and quality in low-birth-weight infants, II: effects on selected essential and nonessential amino acids in plasma and urine, Pediatrics 59 (1977) 407–422.

[56] D.K. Rassin, et al., Milk protein quantity and quality in low-birth-weight infants, IV: effects on tyrosine and phenylalanine in plasma and urine, J. Pediatr. 90 (1977) 356–360.

[57] G.E. Gaull, et al., Milk protein quantity and quality in low-birth-weight infants, III: effects on sulfur-containing amino acids in plasma and urine, J. Pediatr. 90 (1977) 348–355.

[58] N.C. Räihä, et al., Milk protein quantity and quality in low-birth-weight infants, I: metabolic responses and effects on growth, Pediatrics 57 (1976) 659–674.

[59] G.E. Gaull, et al., Human milk as food, Adv. Perinatal. Med. 2 (1982) 47–120.

[60] M. Novak, et al., Acetyl-carnitine and free carnitine in body fluids before and after birth, Pediatr. Res. 13 (1979) 10–15.

[61] E. Schmidt-Sommerfeld, et al., Carnitine and development of newborn adipose tissue, Pediatr. Res. 12 (1978) 660–664.

[62] L. Thorell, L.B. Sjoberg, O. Hernell, Nucleotides in human milk: sources and metabolism by the newborn infant, Pediatr. Res. 40 (1996) 845–852.

[63] J.L. Leach, et al., Total potentially available nucleotides of human milk by stage of lactation, Am. J. Clin. Nutr. 61 (1995) 1224–1230.

[64] R. Uauy, Dietary nucleotides and requirements in early life, in: E. Lebenthal (Ed.), Textbook of Gastroenterology and Nutrition in Infancy, Raven Press, New York, 1989, pp. 265–280.

[65] J.D. Carver, et al., Dietary nucleotide effects upon immune function in infants, Pediatrics 88 (1991) 359–363.

[66] O. Brunser, et al., Effect of dietary nucleotide supplementation on diarrhoeal disease in infants, Acta Paediatr. 83 (1994) 188–191.

[67] L. Pickering, et al., Modulation of the immune system by human milk and infant formula containing nucleotides, Pediatrics 101 (1998) 242–249.

[68] B. Lönnerdal, E. Forsum, Casein content of human milk, Am. J. Clin. Nutr. 41 (1985) 113–120.

[69] C. Kunz, B. Lönnerdal, Casein micelles and casein subunits in human milk, in: S.A. Atkinson, B. Lönnerdal (Eds.), Protein and Non-Protein Nitrogen in Human Milk, CRC Press, Boca Raton, FL, 1989, pp. 9–27.

[70] B.O. Phillippy, R.D. McCarthy, Multi-origins of milk serum albumin in the lactating goat, Biochim. Biophys. Acta 584 (1979) 298–303.

[71] R. Jenness, Biosynthesis and composition of milk, J. Invest. Dermatol. 63 (1974) 109–118.

[72] G. Spik, et al., Characterization and properties of the human and bovine lactoferrins extracted from the faeces of newborn infants, Acta Paediatr. Scand. 71 (1982) 979–985.

[73] N.M. Trugo, M.J. Newport, Vitamin B12 absorption in the neonatal piglet, II: resistance of the vitamin B12-binding protein in cow's milk to proteolysis in vivo, Br. J. Nutr. 54 (1985) 257–267.

[74] L.V. Oberkotter, et al., Tyroxine-binding proteins in human breast milk similar to serum thyroxine-binding globulin, J. Clin. Endocrinol. Metab. 57 (1983) 1133–1139.

[75] D.W. Payne, L.H. Peng, W.H. Pearlman, Corticosteroid-binding proteins in human colostrum and milk and rat milk, J. Biol. Chem. 251 (1976) 5272–5279.

[76] B. Blanc, Biochemical aspects of human milk—comparison with bovine milk, World Rev. Nutr. Diet. 36 (1981) 1–89.

[77] T. Olivecrona, O. Hernell, Human milk lipases and their possible role in fat digestion, Padiatr. Pädol. 11 (1976) 600–604.

[78] M. Hamosh, Lingual and breast milk lipases, Adv. Pediatr. 29 (1982) 33–67.

[79] O. Koldovsky, W. Thomburg, Peptide hormones and hormone-like substances in milk, in: S.A. Atkinson, B. Lönnerdal (Eds.), Protein and Non-Protein Nitrogen in Human Milk, CRC Press, Boca Raton, FL, 1989, pp. 53–65.

[80] A. Lucas, et al., Breast vs bottle: endocrine responses are different with formula feeding, Lancet 1 (1980) 1267–1269.

[81] O. Koldovsky, Strbák V Hormones and growth factors in human milk, in: J.G. Jensen (Ed.), Handbook of Milk Composition, Academic Press, San Diego, 1995, pp. 428–436.

[82] C.A. Boyd, M.A. Quigley, P. Brocklehurst, Donor breast milk versus infant formula for preterm infants: systematic review and meta-analysis, Arch. Dis. Child Fetal Neonatal Ed. 92 (2007) F169–F175.

[83] M.A. Quigley, et al., Formula milk versus donor breast milk for feeding preterm or low birth weight infants, Cochrane Database Syst. Rev. (4) (2007) CD002971.

[84] R.J. Schanler, The use of human milk for premature infants, Pediatr. Clin. North Am. 48 (2001) 207–219.

[85] C.A. Kuschel, J.E. Harding, Multicomponent fortified human milk for promoting growth in preterm infants, Cochrane Database Syst. Rev. (1) (2004) CD000343.

[86] M.H. Labbok, D. Clark, A.S. Goldman, Breastfeeding: maintaining an irreplaceable immunological resource, Nat. Rev. Immunol. 4 (2004) 565–572.

[87] G.A. Losonsky, P.L. Ogra, Mucosal immune system, in: P.L. Ogra (Ed.), Neonatal Infections: Nutritional and Immunologic Interactions, Grune & Stratton, Orlando, FL, 1984, pp. 51–65.

[88] P.L. Ogra, G.A. Losonsky, Defense factors in products of lactation, in: P.L. Ogra (Ed.), Neonatal Infections: Nutritional and Immunologic Interactions, Grune & Stratton, Orlando, FL, 1984, pp. 67–68.

[89] S.S. Ogra, P.L. Ogra, Immunologic aspects of human colostrum and milk, I: distribution characteristics and concentrations of immunoglobulins at different times after the onset of lactation, J. Pediatr. 92 (1978) 546–549.

[90] F.E. Johansen, R. Braathen, P. Brandtzaeg, J. The, chain is essential for polymeric Ig receptor-mediated epithelial transport of IgA, J. Immunol. 167 (2001) 5185–5192.

[91] R.M. Goldblum, et al., Antibody forming cells in human colostrum after oral immunization, Nature 257 (1975) 797–799.

[92] J.M. Fishaut, et al., The broncho-mammary axis in the immune response to respiratory syncytial virus, J. Pediatr. 99 (1981) 186–191.

[93] F. Orskov, Sorenson KB. Escherichia coli serogroups in breast-fed and bottle-fed infants, Acta Pathol. Microbiol. Scand. [B] 83 (1975) 25–30.

[94] J. van Genderen, Diphtheria-antitoxin in Kolostrum und Muttermilch bei Menschen, Z. Immunitatsforsch. Allerg. Klin. Immunol. 83 (1934) 54–59.

[95] P.C. Montgomery, et al., The secretory antibody response: anti-DNP antibodies induced by dinitrophenylated type III pneumococcus, Immunol. Commun. 3 (1974) 143–156.

[96] M. Lamm, et al., Mode of induction of an IgA response in the breast and other secretory sites by oral antigen, in: P.L. Ogra, D. Dayton (Eds.), Immunology of Breast Milk, Raven Press, New York, 1979, pp. 105–114.

[97] J. Drife, et al., Immunoglobulin synthesis in the "resting" breast, BMJ 2 (1976) 503–506.

[98] P. Weisz-Carrington, et al., Hormonal induction of the secretory immune system in the mammary gland, Proc. Natl. Acad Sci. U. S. A. 75 (1978) 2928–2932.

[99] J.C. Cumella, P.L. Ogra, Pregnancy associated hormonal milieu and bronchomammary cell traffic, in: M. Hamosh, A.S. Goldman (Eds.), Human Lactation 2, Plenum Publishing, New York, 1986, pp. 507–524.

[100] D. Artis, Epithelial-cell recognition of commensal bacteria and maintenance of immune homeostasis in the gut, Nat. Rev. Immunol. 8 (2008) 411–420.

[101] J.L. Coombes, F. Powrie, Dendritic cells in intestinal immune regulation, Nat. Rev. Immunol. 8 (2008) 435–446.

[102] B.A. Peri, et al., Antibody content of rabbit milk and serum following inhalation or ingestion of respiratory syncytial virus and bovine serum albumin, Clin. Exp. Immunol. 48 (1982) 91–101.

[103] G.A. Losonsky, et al., Effect of immunization against rubella on lactation products, I: development and characterization of specific immunologic reactivity in breast milk, J. Infect. Dis. 145 (1982) 654–660.

[104] D.B. McClelland, J. McGrath, R.R. Samson, Antimicrobial factors in human milk: studies of concentration and transfer to the infant during the early stages of lactation, Acta Paediatr. Scand. Suppl. 271 (1978) 1–20.

[105] J. Pitt, The milk mononuclear phagocyte, Pediatrics 64 (1979) 745–749.

[106] S.S. Ogra, D. Weintraub, P.L. Ogra, Immunologic aspects of human colostrum and milk, III: fate and absorption of cellular and soluble components in the gastrointestinal tract of the newborn, J. Immunol. 119 (1977) 245–248.

[107] J.F. Kenny, M.I. Boesman, R.H. Michaels, Bacterial and viral coproantibodies in breast-fed infants, Pediatrics 39 (1967) 201–213.

[108] B. Haneberg, Immunoglobulins in feces from infants fed human or bovine milk, Scand. J. Immunol. 3 (1974) 191–197.

[109] C. Weemaes, et al., Development of immunoglobulin A in infancy and childhood, Scand. J. Immunol. 58 (2003) 642–648.

[110] A. Prentice, et al., The nutritional role of breast-milk IgA and lactoferrin, Acta Paediatr. Scand. 76 (1987) 592–598.

[111] D.B. McClelland, et al., Bacterial agglutination studies with secretory IgA prepared from human gastrointestinal secretions and colostrum, Gut 13 (1972) 450–458.

[112] O.A. Stoliar, et al., Secretory IgA against enterotoxins in breast milk, Lancet 1 (1976) 1258–1261.

[113] E.J. Steele, W. Chicumpa, D. Rowley, Isolation and biological properties of three classes of rabbit antibody in Vibrio cholerae, J. Infect. Dis. 130 (1974) 93–103.

[114] J.R. Cantey, Prevention of bacterial infections of mucosal surfaces by immune secretory IgA, Adv. Exp. Med. Biol. 107 (1978) 461–470.

[115] S.A. Plotkin, et al., Oral poliovirus vaccination in newborn African infants: the inhibitory effect of breast-feeding, Am. J. Dis. Child. 111 (1966) 27–30.

[116] P.L. Ogra, D.T. Karzon, The role of immunoglobulins in the mechanism of mucosal immunity to virus infection, Pediatr. Clin. North Am. 17 (1970) 385–390.

[117] P. Blum, et al., Survival of oral human immune serum globulin in the gastrointestinal tract of low birth weight infants, Pediatr. Res. 15 (1981) 1256–1260.

[118] S.L. Bahna, M.A. Keller, D.C. Heiner, IgE and IgD in human colostrum and plasma, Pediatr. Res. 16 (1982) 604–607.

[119] M.A. Keller, et al., Local production of IgG4 in human colostrum, J. Immunol. 130 (1983) 1654–1657.

[120] M.A. Keller, et al., IgD in human colostrum, Pediatr. Res. 19 (1985) 122–126.

[121] C.W. Smith, A.S. Goldman, The cells of human colostrum, I: in vitro studies of morphology and functions, Pediatr. Res. 2 (1968) 103–109.

[122] S.E. Keeney, et al., Activated neutrophils and neutrophil activators in human milk: increased expression of CD116 and decreased expression of L-selectin, J. Leukoc. Biol. 54 (1993) 97–104.

[123] D.P. Wirt, et al., Activated-memory T lymphocytes in human milk, Cytometry 13 (1992) 282–290.

[124] J. Pitt, B. Barlow, W.C. Heird, Protection against experimental necrotizing enterocolitis by maternal milk, I: role of milk leucocytes, Pediatr. Res. 11 (1977) 906–909.

[125] B.K. Pittard III., Differentiation of cord blood lymphocytes into IgA-producing cells in response to breast milk stimulatory factor, Clin. Immunol. Immunopathol. 13 (1979) 430–434.

[126] W.B. Pittard III., S.H. Polmar, A.A. Fanaroff, The breast milk macrophage: potential vehicle for immunoglobulin transport, J. Reticuloendothel. Soc. 22 (1977) 597–603.

[127] J. Clemente, et al., Intracellular immunoglobulins in human milk macrophages: ultrastructural localization and factors affecting the kinetics of immunoglobulin release, Int. Arch. Allergy Appl. Immunol. 80 (1986) 291–299.

[128] E.A. Weaver, et al., Enhanced immunoglobulin A release from human colostral cells during phagocytosis, Infect. Immun. 34 (1981) 498–502.

[129] W.B. Pittard, K. Bill, Immunoregulation by breast milk cells, Cell Immunol. 42 (1979) 437–441.

[130] J.E. Robinson, B.A. Harvey, J.F. Sothill, Phagocytosis and killing of bacteria and yeast by human milk after opsonization in aqueous phase of milk, BMJ 1 (1978) 1443–1445.

[131] S. Kohl, et al., Human colostral antibody dependent cellular cytotoxicity against herpes simplex virus infected cells mediated by colostral cells, J. Clin. Lab. Immunol. 1 (1978) 221–224.

[132] S. Sone, et al., Enhanced cytokine production by milk macrophages following infection with respiratory syncytial virus, J. Leukoc. Biol. 61 (1997) 630–636.

[133] C.H. Kirkpatrick, et al., Inhibition of growth of *Candida albicans* by iron-unsaturated lactoferrin: relation to host defense mechanisms in chronic mucocutaneous candidiasis, J. Infect. Dis. 124 (1971) 539–544.

[134] G.J. Murillo, A.S. Goldman, The cells of human colostrum, II: synthesis of IgA and B-1C, Pediatr. Res. 4 (1970) 71–75.

[135] E. Diaz-Uanen, R.C. Williams Jr., T and B lymphocytes in human colostrum, Clin. Immunol. Immunopathol. 3 (1974) 248–255.

[136] J.R. Oksenberg, E. Persity, C. Brautbar, Cellular immunity in human milk, Am. J. Reprod. Immunol. Microbiol. 8 (1985) 125–129.

[137] L.A. Hanson, et al., Protective factors in milk and development of the immune system, J. Pediatr. 75 (1985) 172–175.

[138] P.L. Ogra, S.S. Ogra, Cellular aspects of immunologic reactivity in human milk, in: L.A. Hanson (Ed.), Biology of Human Milk. Nestlé Nutrition Workshop Series, vol. 15, Raven Press, New York, 1988, pp. 171–184.

[139] M.P. Nair, et al., Comparison of the cellular cytotoxic activities of colostral lymphocytes and maternal peripheral blood lymphocytes, J. Reprod. Immunol. 7 (1985) 199–213.

[140] S.S. Ogra, P.L. Ogra, Immunologic aspects of human colostrum and milk, II: characteristics of lymphocyte reactivity and distribution of E-rosette forming cells at different times after the onset of lactation, J. Pediatr. 92 (1978) 550–555.

[141] M.J. Parmely, A.E. Beer, R.E. Billingham, In vitro studies on the T-lymphocyte population of human milk, J. Exp. Med. 144 (1976) 358–370.

[142] H. Shinmoto, et al., IgA specific helper factor in human colostrum Clin, Exp. Immunol. 66 (1986) 223–230.

[143] A. Bertotto, et al., Human breast milk T lymphocytes display the phenotype and functional characteristics of memory T cells, Eur. J. Immunol. 20 (1990) 1877–1880.

[144] C.E. Gibson, et al., Phenotype and activation of milk-derived and peripheral blood lymphocytes from normal and coeliac subjects, Immunol. Cell. Biol. 69 (1991) 387–391.

[145] A. Bertotto, et al., CD40 ligand expression on the surface of colostral T cells, Arch. Dis. Child. 74 (1996) F135–F136.

[146] A.R. Hayward, J. Lee, P.C. Beverley, Ontogeny of expression of UCHL1 antigen on TcR-1+ (CD4/8) and TcR+ T cells, Eur. J. Immunol. 19 (1989) 771–773.

[147] A. Bertotto, et al., Lymphocytes bearing the T cell receptor γδ in human breast milk, Arch. Dis. Child. 65 (1990) 1274–1275.

[148] B.A. Eglinton, D.M. Roberton, A.G. Cummins, Phenotype of T cells, their soluble receptor levels, and cytokine profile of human breast milk, Immunol. Cell. Biol. 72 (1994) 306–313.

[149] L.K. Trejdosiewicz, Intestinal intraepithelial lymphocytes and lympho-epithelial interactions in the human gastrointestinal mucosa, Immunol. Lett. 32 (1992) 13–19.

[150] J.R. Head, A.E. Beer, R.E. Billingham, Significance of the cellular component of the maternal immunologic endowment in milk, Transplant. Proc. 9 (1977) 1465–1471.

[151] L. Jain, et al., In vivo distribution of human milk leucocytes after ingestion by newborn baboons, Arch. Dis. Child. 64 (1989) 930–933.

[152] K.L. Schnorr, L.D. Pearson, Intestinal absorption of maternal leukocytes by newborn lambs, J. Reprod. Immunol. 6 (1984) 329–337.

[153] I.J. Weiler, W. Hickler, R. Spenger, Demonstration that milk cells invade the neonatal mouse, Am. J. Reprod. Immunol. 4 (1983) 95–98.

[154] J.A. Mohr, R. Leu, W. Mabry, Colostral leukocytes, J. Surg. Oncol. 2 (1970) 163–167.

[155] J.J. Schlesinger, H.D. Covelli, Evidence for transmission of lymphocyte response to tuberculin by breast-feeding, Lancet 2 (1977) 529–532.

[156] L.W. Thorpe, et al., Decreased response of human milk leukocytes to chemoattractant peptides, Pediatr. Res. 20 (1986) 373–377.

[157] R. Dulbecco, et al., Epithelial cell types and their evolution in the rat mammary gland determined by immunological markers, Proc. Natl. Acad. Sci. U. S. A. 80 (1983) 1033–1037.

[158] R. Allen, et al., Developmental regulation of cytokeratins in cells of the rat mammary gland studies with monoclonal antibodies, Proc. Natl. Acad. Sci. U. S. A. 81 (1984) 1203–1207.

[159] J. Holmgren, A.M. Svennerholm, C. Ahren, Nonimmunoglobulin fraction of human milk inhibits bacterial adhesion (hemagglutination) and enterotoxin binding of *Escherichia coli* and *Vibrio cholerae*, Infect. Immun. 33 (1981) 136–141.

[160] J. Holmgren, A.M. Svennerholm, M. Lindblad, Receptor-like glyco-compounds in human milk that inhibit classical and El Tor *Vibrio cholerae* cell adherence (hemagglutination), Infect. Immun. 39 (1983) 147–154.

[161] D.S. Newburg, et al., Fucosylated oligosaccharides of human milk protect suckling mice from heat-stable enterotoxin of *Escherichia coli*, J. Infect. Dis. 162 (1990) 1075–1080.

[162] J. Holmgren, et al., Inhibition of bacterial adhesion and toxin binding by glycoconjugate and oligosaccharide receptor analogues in human milk, in: A.S. Goldman, S.A. Atkinson, L.N. Hanson (Eds.), Human Lactation 3: The Effects of Human Milk on the Recipient Infant, Plenum Press, New York, 1987, pp. 251–259.

[163] G. Grönberg, et al., Structural analysis of five new monosialylated oligosaccharides from human milk, Arch. Biochem. Biophys. 296 (1992) 597–610.

[164] A. Laegreid, A.B. Kolsto Otnaess, K. Bryn, Purification of human milk gangliosides by silica gel chromatography and analysis of trifluoroacetate derivatives by gas chromatography, J. Chromatogr. 377 (1986) 59–67.

[165] A. Laegreid, A.B. Kolsto Otnaess, J. Fuglesang, Human and bovine milk: comparison of ganglioside composition and enterotoxin-inhibitory activity, Pediatr. Res. 20 (1986) 416–421.

[166] A. Laegreid, A.B. Kolsto Otnaess, Trace amounts of ganglioside GM1 in human milk inhibit enterotoxins from *Vibrio cholerae* and *Escherichia coli*, Life Sci. 40 (1987) 55–62.

[167] H. Schroten, et al., Inhibition of adhesion of S-fimbriated *Escherichia coli* to buccal epithelial cells by human milk fat globule membrane components: a novel aspect of the protective function of mucins in the nonimmunoglobulin fraction, Infect. Immun. 60 (1992) 2893–2899.

[168] B. Andersson, et al., Inhibition of attachment of *Streptococcus pneumoniae* and *Haemophilus influenzae* by human milk and receptor oligosaccharides, J. Infect. Dis. 153 (1986) 232–237.

[169] D.S. Newburg, et al., A human milk factor inhibits binding of human immunodeficiency virus to the CD4 receptor, Pediatr. Res. 31 (1992) 22–28.

[170] A.B. Otnaess, A.M. Svennerholm, Non-immunoglobulin fraction in human milk protects rabbit against enterotoxin-induced intestinal fluid secretion, Infect. Immun. 35 (1982) 738–740.

[171] S. Ashkenazi, D.S. Newburg, T.G. Cleary, The effect of human milk on the adherence of enterohemorrhagic *E. coli* to rabbit intestinal cells, in: J. Mesteky, C. Blair, P.L. Ogra (Eds.), Immunology of Milk and the Neonate, Plenum Press, New York, 1991, pp. 173–177.

[172] T.G. Cleary, J.P. Chambers, L.K. Pickering, Protection of suckling mice from the heat-stable enterotoxin of *Escherichia coli* by human milk, J. Infect. Dis. 148 (1983) 1114–1119.

[173] R.L. Glass, et al., Protection against cholera in breast-fed children by antibodies in breast milk, N. Engl. J. Med. 308 (1983) 1389–1392.

[174] P. György, et al., Undialyzable growth factors for *Lactobacillus bifidus* var. *pennsylvanicus*: protective effect of sialic acid bound to glycoproteins and oligosaccharides against bacterial degradation, Eur. J. Biochem. 43 (1974) 29–33.

[175] A. Bezkorovainy, D. Grohlich, J.H. Nichols, Isolation of a glycopeptide fraction with *Lactobacillus bifidus* subspecies *pennsylvanicus* growth-promoting activity from whole human milk casein, Am. J. Clin. Nutr. 32 (1979) 1428–1432.

[176] J.H. Nichols, A. Bezkorovainy, R. Paque, Isolation and characterization of several glycoproteins from human colostrum whey, Biochim. Biophys. Acta 412 (1975) 99–108.

[177] A. Bezkorovainy, N. Topouzian, *Bifidobacterium bifidus* var. *pennsylvanicus* growth promoting activity of human milk casein and its derivates, Int. J. Biochem. 13 (1981) 585–590.

[178] C. Liepke, et al., Human milk provides peptides highly stimulating the growth of bifidobacteria, Eur. J. Biochem. 269 (2002) 712–718.

[179] E. Isolauri, et al., A human *Lactobacillus* strain (*Lactobacillus* GG) promotes recovery from acute diarrhea in children, Pediatrics 88 (1991) 90–97.

[180] M. Kaila, et al., Enhancement of the circulating antibody secreting cell response in human diarrhea by a human *Lactobacillus* strain, Pediatr. Res. 32 (1992) 141–144.

[181] H. Thormar, et al., Inactivation of enveloped viruses and killing of cells by fatty acids and monoglycerides, Antimicrob. Agents Chemother. 31 (1987) 27–31.

[182] J.K. Welsh, et al., Effect of antiviral lipids, heat, and freezing on the activity of viruses in human milk, J. Infect. Dis. 140 (1979) 322–328.

[183] S. Resta, et al., Isolation and propagation of a human enteric coronavirus, Science 229 (1985) 978–981.

[184] F.D. Gillin, D.S. Reiner, M.J. Gault, Cholate-dependent killing of *Giardia lamblia* by human milk, Infect. Immun. 47 (1985) 619–622.

[185] F.D. Gillin, D.S. Reiner, C.S. Wang, Human milk kills parasitic protozoa, Science 221 (1983) 1290–1292.

[186] B.F. Anderson, et al., Structure of human lactoferrin at 3.1-resolution, Proc. Natl. Acad. Sci. U. S. A. 84 (1987) 1769–1773.

[187] G.B. Fransson, B. Lonnerdal, Iron in human milk, J. Pediatr. 96 (1980) 380–384.

[188] R.R. Arnold, M.F. Cole, J.R. McGhee, A bactericidal effect for human milk lactoferrin, Science 197 (1977) 263–265.

[189] J.J. Bullen, H.J. Rogers, L. Leigh, Iron-binding proteins in milk and resistance of *Escherichia coli* infection in infants, BMJ 1 (1972) 69–75.

[190] G. Spik, et al., Bacteriostasis of a milk-sensitive strain of *Escherichia coli* by immunoglobulins and iron-binding proteins in association, Immunology 35 (1978) 663–671.

[191] S. Stephens, et al., Differences in inhibition of the growth of commensal and enteropathogenic strains of *Escherichia coli* by lactoferrin and secretory immunoglobulin A isolated from human milk, Immunology 41 (1980) 597–603.

[192] J. Stuart, S. Norrel, J.P. Harrington, Kinetic effect of human lactoferrin on the growth of *Escherichia coli*, Int. J. Biochem. 16 (1984) 1043–1047.

[193] B.L. Nichols, et al., Human lactoferrin stimulates thymidine incorporation into DNA of rat crypt cells, Pediatr. Res. 21 (1987) 563–567.

[194] R.M. Goldblum, et al., Human milk banking, II: relative stability of immunologic factors in stored colostrum, Acta Paediatr. Scand. 71 (1981) 143–144.

[195] A.S. Goldman, et al., Immunologic factors in human milk during the first year of lactation, J. Pediatr. 100 (1982) 563–567.

[196] R.D. Brines, J.H. Brock, The effect of trypsin and chymotrypsin on the in vitro antimicrobial and iron-binding properties of lactoferrin in human milk and bovine colostrum, Biochim. Biophys. Acta 759 (1983) 229–235.

[197] R.R. Samson, C. Mirtle, D.B. McClelland, The effect of digestive enzymes on the binding and bacteriostatic properties of lactoferrin and vitamin B12 binder in human milk, Acta Paediatr. Scand. 69 (1980) 517–523.

[198] G. Spik, J. Montreuil, Études comparatives de la structure de la tranferrine de la lactotransferrine humaines: finger-printing des hydrolytes protéasiques des deux glycoproteides, C. R. Seances. Soc. Biol. Paris. 160 (1996) 94–98.

[199] N.F. Butte, et al., Daily ingestion of immunologic components in human milk during the first four months of life, Acta Paediatr. Scand. 73 (1984) 296–301.

[200] L.A. Davidson, B. Lonnerdal, Lactoferrin and secretory IgA in the feces of exclusively breast-fed infants, Am. J. Clin. Nutr. 41 (1985) 852A.

[201] L.A. Davidson, B. Lonnerdal, The persistence of human milk proteins in the breast-fed infant, Acta Paediatr. Scand. 76 (1987) 733–740.

[202] R.J. Schanler, et al., Enhanced fecal excretion of selected immune factors in very low birth weight infants fed fortified human milk, Pediatr. Res. 20 (1986) 711–715.

[203] A.S. Goldman, et al., Molecular forms of lactoferrin in stool and urine from infants fed human milk, Pediatr. Res. 27 (1990) 252–255.

[204] R.M. Goldblum, et al., Human milk feeding enhances the urinary excretion of immunologic factors in birth weight infants, Pediatr. Res. 25 (1989) 184–188.

[205] T.W. Hutchens, et al., Origin of intact lactoferrin and its DNA-binding fragments found in the urine of human milk-fed preterm infants: evaluation of stable isotopic enrichment, Pediatr. Res. 29 (1991) 243–250.

[206] A.S. Goldman, et al., Immunologic components in human milk during weaning, Acta Paediatr. Scand. 72 (1983) 133–134.

[207] D.M. Chipman, N. Sharon, Mechanism of lysozyme action, Science 165 (1969) 454–465.

[208] H.E. Friss, et al., Plasma fibronectin concentrations in breast-fed and formula fed neonates, Arch. Dis. Child. 63 (1988) 528–532.

[209] M. Ballow, et al., Developmental aspects of complement components in the newborn, Clin. Exp. Immunol. 18 (1974) 257–266.

[210] S. Nakajima, A.S. Baba, N. Tamura, Complement system in human colostrum, Int. Arch. Allergy Appl. Immunol. 54 (1977) 428–433.

[211] A.S. Cunningham, D.B. Jelliffe, E.F. Jelliffe, Breast-feeding and health in the 1980s: a global epidemiologic review, J. Pediatr. 118 (1991) 659–666.

[212] R.I. Glass, B.J. Stoll, The protective effect of human milk against diarrhea, Acta Paediatr. Scand. 351 (1989) 131–136.

[213] A.S. Goldman, et al., Anti-inflammatory properties of human milk, Acta Paediatr. Scand. 75 (1986) 689–695.

[214] R.P. Garofalo, A.S. Goldman, Expression of functional immunomodulatory and anti-inflammatory factors in human milk, Clin. Perinatol. 26 (1999) 361–377.

[215] G. Carpenter, Epidermal growth factor is a major growth-promoting agent in human milk, Science 210 (1980) 198–199.

[216] M. Klagsbrun, Human milk stimulates DNA synthesis and cellular proliferation in cultured fibroblasts, Proc. Natl. Acad. Sci. U. S. A. 75 (1978) 5057–5061.

[217] M. Okada, et al., Transforming growth factor (TGF)-α in human milk, Life. Sci. 48 (1991) 1151–1156.

[218] S. Saito, et al., Transforming growth factor-beta (TGF-β) in human milk, Clin. Exp. Immunol. 94 (1993) 220–224.

[219] J. Sanguansermsri, P. György, F. Zilliken, Polyamines in human and cow's milk, Am. J. Clin. Nutr. 27 (1974) 859–865.

[220] N. Romain, et al., Polyamine concentration in rat milk and food, human milk, and infant formulas, Pediatr. Res. 32 (1992) 58–63.

[221] O. Koldovsky, et al., Hormones in milk: their presence and possible physiological significance, in: A.S. Goldman, S.A. Atkinson, L.N. Hanson (Eds.), Human Lactation 3: The Effects of Human Milk on the Recipient Infant, Plenum Press, New York, 1987, pp. 183–193.

[222] J.K. Kulski, P.E. Hartmann, Milk insulin, GH and TSH: relationship to changes in milk lactose, glucose and protein during lactogenesis in women, Endocrinol. Exp. 17 (1983) 317–326.

[223] S. Teichberg, et al., Development of the neonatal rat small intestinal barrier to nonspecific macromolecular absorption, II: role of dietary corticosterone, Pediatr. Res. 32 (1992) 50–57.

[224] L.T. Weaver, W.A. Walker, Uptake of macromolecules in the neonate, in: E. Lebenthal (Ed.), Textbook of Gastroenterology and Nutrition in Infancy, Raven Press, New York, 1989, pp. 731–748.

[225] I. Axelsson, et al., Macromolecular absorption in preterm and term infants, Acta Paediatr. Scand. 78 (1989) 532–537.

[226] E.J. Eastham, et al., Antigenicity of infant formulas: role of immature intestine on protein permeability, J. Pediatr. 93 (1978) 561–564.

[227] E.M. Widdowson, V.E. Colombo, C.A. Artavanis, Changes in the organs of pigs in response to feeding for the first 24 h after birth, II: the digestive tract, Biol. Neonate. 28 (1976) 272–281.

[228] E.S. Buescher, S.M. McIlheran, Colostral antioxidants: separation and characterization of two activities in human colostrum, J. Pediatr. Gastroenterol. Nutr. 14 (1992) 47–56.

[229] J.E. Chappell, T. Francis, M.T. Clandinin, Vitamin A and E content of human milk at early stages of lactation, Early Hum. Dev. 11 (1985) 157–167.

[230] E.M. Ostrea Jr., et al., Influence of breast-feeding on the restoration of the low serum concentration of vitamin E and β-carotene in the newborn infant, Am. J. Obstet. Gynecol. 154 (1986) 1014–1017.

[231] R. Garofalo, et al., Interleukin-10 in human milk, Pediatr. Res. 37 (1995) 444–449.

[232] R. Kühn, et al., Interleukin-10-deficient mice develop chronic enterocolitis, Cell 25 (1993) 263–274.

[233] E.S. Buescher, I. Malinowska, Soluble receptors and cytokine antagonists in human milk, Pediatr. Res. 40 (1996) 839–844.

[234] C. Grazioso, et al., Anti-inflammatory effects of human milk on chemically induced colitis in rats, Pediatr. Res. 42 (1997) 639–643.

[235] M. Furukawa, H. Narahara, J.M. Johnston, The presence of platelet-activating factor acetylhydrolase activity in milk, J. Lipid. Res. 34 (1993) 1603–1609.

[236] M.S. Caplan, A. Kelly, W. Hsueh, Endotoxin and hypoxia-induced intestinal necrosis in rats: the role of platelet activating factor, Pediatr. Res. 31 (1992) 428–434.

[237] M.M. Caplan, et al., Serum PAF acetylhydrolase increases during neonatal maturation, Prostaglandins 39 (1990) 705–714.

[238] M. Furukawa, R.A. Frenkel, J.M. Johnston, Absorption of platelet-activating factor acetylhydrolase by rat intestine, Am. J. Physiol. 266 (1994) G935–G939.

[239] M. Sarfati, et al., Presence of IgE suppressor factors in human colostrum, Eur. J. Immunol. 16 (1986) 1005–1008.

[240] L. Bjørge, et al., Identification of the complementary regulatory protein CD59 in human colostrum and milk, Am. J. Reprod. Immunol. 35 (1996) 43–50.

[241] U.M. Saarinen, M. Kajosaari, Breast-feeding as prophylaxis against atopic disease: prospective follow-up study until 17 years old, Lancet 346 (1995) 1065–1069.

[242] S. Koletzko, et al., Role of infant feeding practices in development of Crohn's disease in childhood, BMJ 298 (1989) 1617–1618.

[243] S. Koletzko, et al., Infant feeding practices and ulcerative colitis in childhood, BMJ 302 (1991) 1580–1581.

[244] E.J. Mayer, et al., Reduced risk of IDDM among breast-fed children, Diabetes 37 (1988) 1625–1632.

[245] M.K. Davis, D.A. Savitz, B. Grauford, Infant feeding in childhood cancer, Lancet 2 (1988) 365–368.

[246] H.F. Pabst, D.W. Spady, Effect of breast-feeding on antibody response to conjugate vaccines, Lancet 336 (1990) 269–270.

[247] M. Hahn-Zoric, et al., Antibody responses to parenteral and oral vaccines are impaired by conventional and low protein formula as compared to breast-feeding, Acta Paediatr. Scand. 79 (1990) 1137–1142.

[248] S. Stephens, et al., In-vivo immune responses of breast- and bottle-fed infants to tetanus toxoid antigen and to normal gut flora, Acta Paediatr. Scand. 73 (1984) 426–432.

[249] H.F. Pabst, et al., Effect of breast-feeding on immune response to BCG vaccination, Lancet 1 (1989) 295–297.

[250] D.A. Campbell Jr., Maternal donor-related transplants: influence of breast-feeding on reactivity to the allograft, Transplant. Proc. 15 (1983) 906–909.

[251] D.A. Campbell Jr., et al., Breast-feeding and maternal-donor renal allografts, Transplantation 37 (1984) 340–344.

[252] W.E. Kois, et al., Influence of breast-feeding on subsequent reactivity to a related renal allograft, J. Surg. Res. 37 (1984) 89–93.

[253] L. Zhang, et al., Influence of breast-feeding on the cytotoxic T cell allorepertoire in man, Transplantation 52 (1991) 914–916.

[254] Y. Chiba, et al., Effect of breast-feeding on responses of systemic interferon and virus-specific lymphocyte transformation in infants with respiratory syncytial virus infection, J. Med. Virol. 21 (1987) 7–14.

[255] S. Stephens, Development of secretory immunity in breast-fed and bottle fed infants, Arch. Dis. Child. 61 (1986) 263–269.

[256] E. LeBouder, et al., Modulation of neonatal microbial recognition: TLR-mediated innate immune responses are specifically and differentially modulated by human milk, J. Immunol. 176 (2006) 3742–3752.

[257] E. LeBouder, et al., Soluble forms of Toll-like receptor (TLR)2 capable of modulating TLR2 signaling are present in human plasma and breast milk, J. Immunol. 171 (2003) 6680–6689.

[258] R.E. Ley, D.A. Peterson, J.I. Gordon, Ecological and evolutionary forces shaping microbial diversity in the human intestine, Cell 124 (2006) 837–848.

[259] L. Wen, et al., Innate immunity and intestinal microbiota in the development of Type 1 diabetes, Nature 455 (2008) 1109–1113.

[260] R.R. Gala, Prolactin and growth hormone in the regulation of the immune system, Proc. Soc. Exp. Biol. Med. 198 (1991) 513–527.

[261] J.H. Nuijens, P.H. van Berkel, F.L. Schanbacher, Structure and biological action of lactoferrin, J. Mammary Gland. Biol. Neoplasia 1 (1996) 285–295.

[262] M. Hahn-Zoric, et al., Anti-idiotypic antibodies to polio virus in commercial immunoglobulin preparations, human serum, and milk, Pediatr. Res. 33 (1993) 475–480.

[263] R.P. Garofalo, A.S. Goldman, Cytokines, chemokines, and colony-stimulating factors in human milk: the 1997 update, Biol. Neonate. 74 (1998) 134–142.

[264] P. Juto, Human milk stimulates B cell function, Arch. Dis. Child. 60 (1985) 610–613.

[265] M.H. Julius, M. Janusz, J. Lisowski, A colostral protein that induces the growth and differentiation of resting B lymphocytes, J. Immunol. 140 (1988) 1366–1371.

[266] O. Soder, Isolation of interleukin-1 from human milk, Int. Arch. Allergy. Appl. Immunol. 83 (1987) 19–23.

[267] J.W. Hooton, et al., Human colostrum contains an activity that inhibits the production of IL-2, Clin. Exp. Immunol. 86 (1991) 520–524.

[268] C. Munoz, et al., Interleukin-1 beta in human colostrum, Res. Immunol. 141 (1990) 501–513.

[269] H.E. Rudloff, et al., Tumor necrosis factor-α in human milk, Pediatr. Res. 31 (1992) 29–33.

[270] U. Skansen-Saphir, A. Linfors, U. Andersson, Cytokine production in mononuclear cells of human milk studied at the single-cell level, Pediatr. Res. 34 (1993) 213–216.

[271] F. Basolo, et al., Normal breast epithelial cells produce interleukins-6 and 8 together with tumor-necrosis factor: defective IL-6 expression in mammary carcinoma, Int. J. Cancer. 55 (1993) 926–930.

[272] S. Saito, et al., Detection of IL-6 in human milk and its involvement in IgA production, J. Reprod. Immunol. 20 (1991) 267–276.

[273] H.E. Rudloff, et al., Interleukin-6 in human milk, J. Reprod. Immunol. 23 (1993) 13–20.

[274] V. Bocci, et al., Presence of interferon-α and interleukin-6 in colostrum of normal women, Lymphokine. Cytokine. Res. 12 (1993) 21–24.

[275] M.D. Srivastava, et al., Cytokines in human milk, Res. Commun. Mol. Pathol. Pharmacol. 93 (1996) 263–287.

[276] M.F. Bottcher, M.C. Jenmalm, B. Bjorksten, Cytokine, chemokine and secretory IgA levels in human milk in relation to atopic disease and IgA production in infants, Pediatr. Allergy Immunol. 14 (2003) 35–41.

[277] M.W. Groer, M.M. Shelton, Exercise is associated with elevated proinflammatory cytokines in human milk, J. Obstet. Gynecol. Neonatal Nurs. 38 (2009) 35–41.

[278] Y. Takahata, et al., Detection of interferon-gamma-inducible chemokines in human milk, Acta Paediatr. 92 (2003) 659–665.

[279] S.K. Sinha, A.A. Yunis, Isolation of colony stimulating factor from milk, Biochem. Biophys. Res. Commun. 114 (1983) 797–803.

[280] W.S. Gilmore, Human milk contains granulocyte-colony stimulating factor (G-CSF), Eur. J. Clin. Nutr. 48 (1994) 222–224.

[281] T. Hara, et al., Identification of macrophage colony-stimulating factor in human milk and mammary epithelial cells, Pediatr. Res. 37 (1995) 437–443.

[282] A. Gasparoni, et al., Granulocyte-macrophage colony stimulating factor in human milk, Eur. J. Pediatr. 156 (1996) 69.

[283] H. Hasselbalch, et al., Decreased thymus size in formula-fed infants compared with breastfed infants, Acta Paediatr. 85 (1996) 1029–1032.

[284] P.T. Ngom, et al., Improved thymic function in exclusively breastfed infants is associated with higher interleukin 7 concentrations in their mothers' breast milk, Am. J. Clin. Nutr. 80 (2004) 722–728.

[285] P.L. Yap, et al., Milk protein concentrations in the mammary secretions of non-lactating women, J. Reprod. Immunol. 3 (1981) 49–58.

[286] P.L. Yap, E.A. Pryde, D.B. McClelland, Milk protein concentrations in galactorrhoeic mammary secretions, J. Reprod. Immunol. 1 (1980) 347–357.

[287] B.S. Carlsson, et al., Escherichia coli-O antibody content in milk from healthy Swedish mothers from a very low socioeconomic group of a developing country, Acta Paediatr. Scand. 65 (1976) 417–423.

[288] A.S. Goldman, et al., Effects of prematurity on the immunologic system in human milk, J. Pediatr. 101 (1982) 901–905.

[289] L.J. Mata, R.G. Wyatt, The uniqueness of human milk: host resistance to infection, Am. J. Clin. Nutr. 24 (1971) 976–986.

[290] S. Svirsky-Gross, Pathogenic strains of coli (O;111) among prematures and the cause of human milk in controlling the outbreak of diarrhea, Ann. Pediatr. (Paris) 190 (1958) 109–115.

[291] R.H. Yolken, et al., Secretory antibody directed against rotavirus in human milk—measurement by means of an ELISA, J. Pediatr. 93 (1978) 916–921.

[292] R. Lodinova, V. Jouya, Antibody production by the mammary gland in mothers after oral colonization of their infants with a nonpathogenic strain E. coli 083, Acta Paediatr. Scand. 66 (1977) 705–708.

[293] Z.A. Bhutta, et al., What works? Interventions for maternal and child undernutrition and survival, Lancet 371 (2008) 417–440.

[294] W. Sandine, et al., Lactic acid bacteria in food and health: a review with special references to enteropathogenic Escherichia coli as well as certain enteric diseases and their treatment with antibiotics and lactobacilli, J. Milk Food Technol. 35 (1972) 691–702.

[295] R.F. Bishop, et al., The aetiology of diarrhea in newborn infants, Ciba. Found. Symp. 42 (1976) 223–236.

[296] D.J. Cameron, et al., Noncultivable viruses and neonatal diarrhea: fifteen-month survey in a newborn special care nursery, J. Clin. Microbiol. 8 (1978) 93–98.

[297] A.M. Murphy, M.B. Albrey, E.B. Crewe, Rotavirus infections of neonates, Lancet 2 (1977) 1149–1150.

[298] R.F. Bishop, et al., Diarrhea and rotavirus infection associated with differing regimens for postnatal care of newborn babies, J. Clin. Microbiol. 9 (1979) 525–529.

[299] L.C. Duffy, et al., The effects of infant feeding on rotavirus-induced gastroenteritis: a prospective study, Am. J. Public. Health 76 (1986) 259–263.

[300] L.C. Duffy, et al., Modulation of rotavirus enteritis during breast-feeding, Am. J. Dis. Child. 140 (1986) 1164–1168.

[301] M.T. Asensi, C. Martinez-Costa, J. Buesa, Anti-rotavirus antibodies in human milk: quantification and neutralizing activity, J. Pediatr. Gastroenterol. Nutr. 42 (2006) 560–567.

[302] I.D. Frantz III, et al., Necrotizing enterocolitis, J. Pediatr. 86 (1975) 259–263.

[303] M.J. Bell, R.D. Feigen, J.L. Ternberg, Changes in the incidence of necrotizing enterocolitis associated with variation of the gastrointestinal microflora in neonates, Am. J. Surg. 138 (1979) 629–631.

[304] L.S. Book, et al., Clustering of necrotizing enterocolitis: interruption by infection-control measures, N. Engl. J. Med. 297 (1977) 984–986.

[305] G.L. Bunton, et al., Necrotizing enterocolitis, Arch. Dis. Child. 52 (1977) 772–777.

[306] R.M. Kliegman, W.B. Pittard, A.A. Fanaroff, Necrotizing enterocolitis in neonates fed human milk, J. Pediatr. 95 (1979) 450–453.

[307] G. Stout, et al., Necrotizing enterocolitis during the first week of life: a multicentered case-control and cohort comparison study, J. Perinatol. 28 (2008) 556–560.

[308] R.R. Moriartey, et al., Necrotizing enterocolitis and human milk, J. Pediatr. 94 (1979) 295–296.

[309] M.M. Eibl, et al., Prophylaxis of necrotizing enterocolitis by oral IgA-IgG: review of a clinical study in low birth weight infants and discussion of pathogenic role of infection, J. Clin. Immunol. 10 (1990) 72S–77S.

[310] J. Pitt, Necrotizing enterocolitis: a model for infection-immunity interaction, in: P.L. Ogra (Ed.), Neonatal Infections: Nutritional and Immunologic Interactions, Grune & Stratton, Orlando, FL, 1984, pp. 173–184.

[311] R.J. Weinberg, Effect of breast-feeding on morbidity in rotavirus gastroenteritis, Pediatrics 74 (1984) 250–253.

[312] Research Subcommittee of the South-East England Faculty. The influence of breast-feeding on the incidence of infectious illness during the first year of life, Practitioner 209 (1972) 356–362.

[313] M.E. Fallot, J.L. Boyd, F.A. Oski, Breast-feeding reduces incidence of hospital admissions for infection in infants, Pediatrics 65 (1980) 1121–1124.

[314] M.A. Hylander, D.M. Strobino, R. Dhanireddy, Human milk feedings and infection among very low birth weight infants, Pediatrics 102 (1998) E38.

[315] M.P. Glode, et al., Neonatal meningitis due to Escherichia coli K1, J. Infect. Dis. 136 (Suppl.) (1977) S93–S97.

[316] J. Ellestad-Sayed, et al., Breast-feeding protects against infection in Indian infants, Can. Med. Assoc. J. 120 (1979) 295–298.

[317] M.S. Elger, A.R. Rausen, J. Silverio, Breast vs. bottle feeding, Clin. Pediatr. 23 (1984) 492–495.

[318] J.P. Habicht, J. DaVanzo, W.P. Butz, Does breast-feeding really save lives, or are apparent benefits due to biases? Am. J. Epidemiol. 123 (1986) 279–290.

[319] H. Bauchner, J.M. Leventhal, E.D. Shapiro, Studies of breast-feeding and infections: how good is the evidence? JAMA 256 (1986) 887–892.

[320] A. de Silva, P.W. Jones, S.A. Spencer, Does human milk reduce infection rates in preterm infants? A systematic review, Arch. Dis. Child Fetal Neonatal Ed. 89 (2004) F509–F513.

[321] L. Furman, Yes, human milk does reduce infection rates in very low birth-weight infants, Arch. Dis. Child Fetal Neonatal Ed. 91 (1) (2006) F78.

[322] C.G. Grulee, H.N. Sanford, The influence of breast and artificial feeding on infantile eczema, J. Pediatr. 9 (1936) 223–225.

[323] M.S. Kramer, Does breast-feeding help protect against atopic disease? Biology, methodology, and a golden jubilee of controversy, J. Pediatr. 112 (1988) 181–190.

[324] A.L. Wright, et al., Relationship of infant feeding to recurrent wheezing at age 6 years, Arch. Pediatr. Adolesc. Med. 149 (1995) 758–763.

[325] L.A. Hanson, et al., Secretory IgA antibodies against cow's milk proteins in human milk and their possible effect in mixed feeding, Int. Arch. Allergy Appl. Immunol. 54 (1977) 457–462.

[326] I.S. Uhnoo, et al., Effect of rotavirus infection and malnutrition on uptake of dietary antigen in the intestine, Pediatr. Res. 27 (1990) 153–160.

[327] P. Brandtzaeg, The secretory immune system of lactating human mammary glands compared with other exocrine organs, Ann. N. Y. Acad. Sci. 409 (1983) 353–382.

[328] C.H. Rieger, R.M. Rothberg, Development of the capacity to produce specific antibody to an ingested food antigen in the premature infant, J. Pediatr. 87 (1975) 515–518.

[329] L. Businco, et al., Prevention of atopic disease in "at risk newborns" by prolonged breast-feeding, Ann. Allergy 51 (1983) 296–299.

[330] M. Downham, et al., Breast-feeding protects against respiratory syncytial virus infections, BMJ 2 (1976) 274–276.

[331] R. Scott, et al., Human antibody dependent cell-mediated cytotoxicity against target cells infected with respiratory syncytial virus, Clin. Exp. Immunol. 28 (1977) 19–26.

[332] S. Kohl, L.S. Loo, The relative role of transplacental and milk immune transfer in protection against lethal neonatal herpes simplex virus infection in mice, J. Infect. Dis. 149 (1984) 38–42.

[333] K. Sadeharju, et al., Maternal antibodies in breast milk protect the child from enterovirus infections, Pediatrics 119 (2007) 941–946.

[334] U.M. Saarinen, Prolonged breast-feeding as prophylaxis for recurrent otitis media, Acta Paediatr. Scand. 71 (1982) 567–571.

[335] R.V. Short, Breast-feeding, Sci. Am. 250 (1984) 35–41.

[336] M. Gunther, The neonate's immunity gap, breast-feeding and cot death, Lancet 1 (1975) 441–442.

[337] D.J. Pettitt, et al., Breast-feeding and incidence of non-insulin-dependent diabetes mellitus in Pima Indians, Lancet 350 (1997) 166–168.

[338] M.S. Kramer, Do breast-feeding and delayed introduction of solid foods protect against subsequent obesity? J. Pediatr. 98 (1981) 883–887.

[339] B. Rodgers, Feeding in infancy and later ability and attainment: a longitudinal study, Dev. Med. Child. Neurol. 20 (1978) 421–426.

[340] W.J. Rogan, B.C. Gladen, Breast-feeding and cognitive development, Early Hum. Dev. 31 (1993) 181–193.

[341] L.J. Horwood, D.M. Fergusson, Breast-feeding and later cognitive and academic outcomes, Pediatrics 101 (1998) 99.

[342] K. Katsouyani, et al., A case-control study of lactation and cancer of breast, Br. J. Cancer 73 (1996) 814–818.

[343] Transfer of drugs and other chemicals into human milk, Pediatrics 108 (2001) 776–789.

[344] Human Milk, L.K. Pickering (Ed.), Red Book: Report of the Committee on Infectious Diseases, American Academy of Pediatrics, Elk Grove Village, IL, 2009.

[345] M.E. O'Connor, et al., Vitamin K deficiency and breast-feeding, Am. J. Dis. Child. 137 (1983) 601–602.

[346] E. Zmora, R. Gorodescher, J. Bar-Ziv, Multiple nutritional deficiencies in infants from a strict vegetarian commune, Am. J. Dis. Child. 133 (1979) 141–144.

[347] S.B. Nau, G.B. Stickler, J.C. Hawort, Serum 25-hydroxyvitamin D in infantile rickets, Pediatrics 57 (1976) 221–225.

[348] M.C. Higinbotham, L. Sweetman, W.L. Nyhan, A syndrome of methylmalonic aciduria, homocystinuria, megaloblastic anemia and neurologic abnormalities in a vitamin B12-deficient breast-fed infant of a strict vegetarian, N. Engl. J. Med. 299 (1978) 317–323.

[349] C. Kanaka, B. Schütz, K.A. Zuppinger, Risks of alternative nutrition in infancy: a case report of severe iodine and carnitine deficiency, Eur. J. Pediatr. 151 (1992) 786–788.

[350] L. Thiry, et al., Isolation of AIDS virus from cell-free breast milk of three healthy virus carriers. Letter to the editor, Lancet 2 (1985) 891–892.

[351] M.W. Vogt, et al., Isolation of HTLV-III/LAV from cervical secretions of women at risk of AIDS. Letter to the editor, Lancet 1 (1986) 525–527.

[352] M. Bucens, J. Armstrong, M. Stuckey, Virologic and electron microscopic evidence for postnatal HIV transmission via breast milk (abstract), Fourth International Conference on AIDS, Stockholm, 1988.

[353] M. Pezzella, et al., The presence of HIV-1 genome in human colostrum from asymptomatic seropositive mothers, vol. 6, International Conference on AIDS, 1990, p. 165.

[354] A. Ruff, et al., Detection of HIV-1 by PCR in breast milk, vol. 7, International Conference on AIDS, 1991, p. 300.

[355] M.G. Fowler, et al., Reducing the risk of mother-to-child human immunodeficiency virus transmission: past successes, current progress and challenges, and future directions, Am. J. Obstet. Gynecol. 197 (Suppl. 3) (2007) S3–S9.

[356] A.P. Kourtis, et al., Prevention of human immunodeficiency virus-1 transmission to the infant through breastfeeding: new developments, Am. J. Obstet. Gynecol. 197 (Suppl. 3) (2007) S113–S122.

[357] A. Coutsoudis, et al., Late postnatal transmission of HIV-1 in breast-fed children: an individual patient data meta-analysis, J. Infect. Dis. 189 (2004) 2154–2166.

[358] W.T. Shearer, Breastfeeding and HIV infection, Pediatrics 121 (2008) 1046–1047.

[359] R.L. Shapiro, et al., Highly active antiretroviral therapy started during pregnancy or postpartum suppresses HIV-1 RNA, but not DNA, in breast milk, J. Infect. Dis. 192 (2005) 713–719.

[360] H.M. Coovadia, R.M. Bland, Preserving breastfeeding practice through the HIV pandemic, Trop. Med. Int. Health 12 (2007) 1116–1133.

[361] H.M. Coovadia, et al., Mother-to-child transmission of HIV-1 infection during exclusive breastfeeding in the first 6 months of life: an intervention cohort study, Lancet 369 (2007) 1107–1116.

[362] I. Thior, et al., Breastfeeding plus infant zidovudine prophylaxis for 6 months vs formula feeding plus infant zidovudine for 1 month to reduce mother-to-child HIV transmission in Botswana: a randomized trial: the Mashi Study, JAMA 296 (2006) 794–805.

[363] P.J. Iliff, et al., Early exclusive breastfeeding reduces the risk of postnatal HIV-1 transmission and increases HIV-free survival, AIDS 19 (2005) 699–708.

[364] C.M. Wilfert, M.G. Fowler, Balancing maternal and infant benefits and the consequences of breast-feeding in the developing world during the era of HIV infection, J. Infect. Dis. 195 (2007) 165–167.

[365] L.M. Grummer-Strawn, K.S. Scanlon, S.B. Fein, Infant feeding and feeding transitions during the first year of life, Pediatrics 122 (Suppl. 2) (2008) S36–S42.

[366] A. Bentovim, Shame and other anxieties associated with breast-feeding: a systems theory and psychodynamic approach, Ciba Found. Symp. 45 (1976) 159–178.

[367] T. Baranowski, et al., Social support, social influence, ethnicity and the breast-feeding decision, Soc. Sci. Med. 17 (1983) 1599–1611.

[368] T. Baranowski, et al., Attitudes toward breast-feeding, J. Dev. Behav. Pediatr. 7 (1986) 367–372.

[369] T. Baranowski, et al., Expectancies of infant-feeding methods among mothers in three ethnic groups, Psychol. Health 5 (1990) 59–75.

[370] A. Merewood, et al., Breastfeeding rates in US Baby-Friendly hospitals: results of a national survey, Pediatrics 116 (2005) 628–634.

[371] A. Deroche, et al., Regulation of parental alloreactivity by reciprocal F1 hybrids: the role of lactation, J. Reprod. Immunol. 23 (1993) 235–245.

[372] L.A. Hanson, Immunobiology of Human Milk: How Breastfeeding Protects Babies, Pharmasoft Publishing, Amarillo, TX, 2004.

BACTERIAL INFECTIONS

SECTION OUTLINE

6 Bacterial Sepsis and Meningitis   222

7 Bacterial Infections of the Respiratory Tract   276

8 Bacterial Infections of the Bones and Joints   296

9 Bacterial Infections of the Urinary Tract   310

10 Focal Bacterial Infections   322

11 Microorganisms Responsible for Neonatal Diarrhea   359

12 Group B Streptococcal Infections   419

13 Listeriosis   470

14 Staphylococcal Infections   489

15 Gonococcal Infections   516

16 Syphilis   524

17 *Borrelia* Infections: Lyme Disease and Relapsing Fever   564

18 Tuberculosis   577

19 *Chlamydia* Infections   600

20 Mycoplasmal Infections   607

BACTERIAL SEPSIS AND MENINGITIS

Victor Nizet ⊛ Jerome O. Klein

CHAPTER OUTLINE

Bacteriology 223
  Group B Streptococci 225
  Group A Streptococci 226
  Streptococcus pneumoniae 228
  Other Streptococci 228
  Enterococcus Species 229
  Staphylococcus aureus and Coagulase-Negative
    Staphylococci 229
  Listeria monocytogenes 230
  Escherichia coli 230
  Klebsiella species 230
  Enterobacter species 231
  Citrobacter species 231
  Serratia marcescens 232
  Pseudomonas aeruginosa 232
  Salmonella species 232
  Neisseria meningitidis 232
  Haemophilus influenzae 233
  Anaerobic Bacteria 233
  Neonatal Tetanus 234
  Mixed Infections 234
  Uncommon Bacterial Pathogens 234
Epidemiology 235
  Incidence of Sepsis and Meningitis 235
  Characteristics of Infants Who Develop Sepsis 235
  Nursery Outbreaks or Epidemics 238
Pathogenesis 239
  Host Factors Predisposing to Neonatal Bacterial Sepsis 240
  Infection in Twins 241
  Umbilical Cord as a Focus of Infection 241
  Administration of Drugs to the Mother before Delivery 242
  Administration of Drugs Other than Antibiotics to the Neonate 243
Pathology 243
Clinical Manifestations 243
  Fever and Hypothermia 246
  Respiratory Distress 247
  Jaundice 247

Organomegaly 247
  Gastrointestinal Signs 248
  Skin Lesions 248
  Neurologic Signs 248
Diagnosis 248
  Maternal History 248
  Microbiologic Techniques 248
  Laboratory Aids 255
Management 255
  Choice of Antimicrobial Agents 255
  Current Practice 256
  Continuation of Therapy When Results of Cultures
    Are Available 256
  Management of an Infant Whose Mother Received Intrapartum
    Antimicrobial Agents 257
  Treatment of an Infant Whose Bacterial Culture Results
    Are Negative 258
  Management of an Infant with Catheter-Associated Infection 258
  Treatment of Neonatal Meningitis 258
  Management of an Infant with a Brain Abscess 258
  Treatment of an Infant with Meningitis Whose Bacterial Culture
    Results Are Negative 259
  Treatment of Anaerobic Infections 259
  Adjunctive Therapies for Treatment of Neonatal Sepsis 259
Prognosis 260
Prevention 261
  Obstetric Factors 261
  Chemoprophylaxis 261
  Maternal Factors 261
  Immunoprophylaxis 261
  Decontamination of Fomites 263
  Epidemiologic Surveillance 263
Sepsis in the Newborn Recently Discharged from the Hospital 263
  Congenital Infection 263
  Late-Onset Infection 263
  Infections in the Household 263
  Fever in the First Month of Life 264

Bacterial sepsis in the neonate is a clinical syndrome characterized by systemic signs of infection and accompanied by bacteremia in the first month of life. Meningitis in the neonate is usually a sequela of bacteremia and is discussed in this chapter because meningitis and sepsis typically share a common cause and pathogenesis. Infections of the bones, joints, and soft tissues and of the respiratory, genitourinary, and gastrointestinal tracts can be accompanied by bacteremia, but the cause, clinical features, diagnosis, and management of these infections are sufficiently different to warrant separate discussions. Bloodstream and central

nervous system (CNS) infections caused by group B streptococci (GBS), *Staphylococcus aureus* and coagulase-negative staphylococci (CoNS), *Neisseria gonorrhoeae*, *Listeria monocytogenes*, *Salmonella* species, Treponema pallidum, and Borrelia borderforrii, and *Mycobacterium tuberculosis* are described in detail in individual chapters. Chapter 2 describes the features of neonatal sepsis and meningitis in developing regions of the world.

The two patterns of disease—early onset and late onset—have been associated with systemic bacterial infections during the first month of life (Table 6–1). Early-onset disease

TABLE 6–1 Characteristics of Early-Onset and Late-Onset Neonatal Sepsis

Characteristic	Early-Onset*	Late-Onset[†]
Time of onset (days)	0-6	7-90
Complications of pregnancy or delivery	+	±
Source of organism	Mother's genital tract	Mother's genital tract; postnatal environment
Usual clinical presentation	Fulminant	Slowly progressive or fulminant
	Multisystem	Focal
	Pneumonia frequent	Meningitis frequent
Mortality rate (%)	3-50[‡]	2-40[‡]

*Many studies define early-onset sepsis as sepsis that occurs in the first 72 hours of life; others define it as sepsis that occurs in the first 5 or 6 days of life.
[†]Very small premature infants may have late-onset sepsis beyond 90 days of life.
[‡]Higher mortality rates in earlier studies.

typically manifests as a fulminant, systemic illness during the first 24 hours of life (median age of onset approximately 6 hours), with most other cases manifesting on the second day of life. Infants with early-onset disease may have a history of one or more obstetric complications, including premature or prolonged rupture of maternal membranes, preterm onset of labor, chorioamnionitis, and peripartum maternal fever, and many of the infants are premature or of low birth weight. Bacteria responsible for early-onset disease are acquired hours or days before delivery from the birth canal during delivery after overt or occult rupture of membranes. The mortality rate varies from 3% to 50% in some series, especially with gram-negative pathogens.

Late-onset disease has been variably defined for epidemiologic purposes as occurring after 72 hours to 6 days (e.g., group B streptococcus) of life. Very late onset infection secondary to group B streptococcus (disease in infants >3 months old) is discussed in Chapter 12. Term infants with late-onset infections can have a history of obstetric complications, but these are less characteristic than in early-onset sepsis or meningitis. Bacteria responsible for late-onset sepsis and meningitis include organisms acquired from the maternal genital tract and organisms acquired after birth from human contacts or infrequently from contaminated hospital equipment or materials when prolonged intensive care is needed for a neonate. The mortality rate usually is lower than for early-onset sepsis but can range from 2% to 40%, with the latter figure typically for infants of very low birth weight with gram-negative sepsis.

Because different microorganisms are responsible for disease by age at onset, the choice of antimicrobial agents also differs. Some organisms, such as *Escherichia coli*, groups A and B streptococci, and *L. monocytogenes*, can be responsible for early-onset and late-onset infections, whereas others, such as *S. aureus*, CoNS, and *Pseudomonas aeruginosa*, rarely cause early-onset disease and typically are associated with late-onset disease. The survival of very low birth weight infants with prolonged stays in the neonatal intensive care unit (NICU) has been accompanied by

increased risk for nosocomial or hospital-associated infections and for very late onset disease (see Chapter 35) [1].

BACTERIOLOGY

The changing pattern of organisms responsible for neonatal sepsis is reflected in a series of reports by pediatricians at the Yale–New Haven Hospital covering the period 1928-2003 (Table 6–2) [2–8]. Before development of the sulfonamides, gram-positive cocci including *S. aureus* and β-hemolytic streptococci caused most cases of neonatal sepsis. With the introduction of antimicrobial agents, gram-negative enteric bacilli, particularly *E. coli*, became the predominant cause of serious infection in the newborn. Reports for the periods 1966-1978 and 1979-1988 document the increase in importance of GBS and *E. coli* as agents of neonatal sepsis. In a more recent analysis from 1989-2003, CoNS species, predominantly *Staphylococcus epidermidis*, emerged as the most commonly identified agent of neonatal sepsis, with GBS, *E. coli*, *Enterococcus faecalis*, *S. aureus*, and *Klebsiella* species also occurring with substantial frequency. Later reports also document the problem of sepsis in very premature and low birth weight infants who have survived with the aid of sophisticated life-support equipment and advances in neonatal intensive care—CoNS are particularly threatening in these infants. Emerging data from the same center indicate that although intrapartum antibiotic prophylaxis protocols have reduced the overall incidence of early-onset sepsis, they may be influencing a higher proportion of septicemia attributable to ampicillin-resistant *E. coli* [9].

The etiologic pattern of microbial infection observed at Yale Medical Center also has been reported in studies of neonatal sepsis carried out at other centers during the same intervals (Table 6–3). Studies indicate that GBS and gram-negative enteric bacilli, predominantly *E. coli*, were the most frequent pathogens for sepsis, but other organisms were prominent in some centers. *S. aureus* was an important cause of sepsis in the mid-1980s in Finland [10] and East Africa [11] and a more recently significant pathogen in Connecticut [7] and southern Israel [12]. *S. epidermidis* was responsible for 53% of cases in Liverpool [13], and CoNS account for 35% to 48% of all late-onset sepsis in very low birth weight infants across the United States [14,15] and in Israel [16]. *Klebsiella* and *Enterobacter* species were the most common bacterial pathogens in Tel Aviv [17]. Sepsis and focal infections in neonates in developing countries are discussed further in Chapter 2.

A survey of five university hospitals in Finland [10] provides data about the association of the etiologic agent and mortality based on age at onset of sepsis (Table 6–4) and birth weight (Table 6–5). Infants with sepsis onset during the first 24 hours of life and weighing less than 1500 g at birth had the highest mortality rate.

The mortality rates for neonatal sepsis over time are documented in the Yale Medical Center reports. In the preantibiotic era, neonatal sepsis usually was fatal. Even with the introduction of penicillins and aminoglycosides in the reports from 1944-1965, death resulted from sepsis in most infants. Concurrent with the introduction of NICUs and technologic support for cardiorespiratory

TABLE 6–2   Bacteria Causing Neonatal Sepsis at Yale–New Haven Hospital, 1928-2003

Organism	No. Cases						
	1928-1932*	1933-1943[†]	1944-1957[†]	1958-1965[‡]	1966-1978[§]	1979-1988[¶]	1989-2003[¶]
β-hemolytic streptococci	15	18	11	8	86	83	155
Group A	—	16	5	0	0	0	0
Group B	—	2	4	1	76	64	86
Group D (*Enterococcus*)	—	0	1	7	9	19	65
Viridans streptococci	—	—	—	—	—	11	10
Staphylococcus aureus	11	4	8	2	12	14	70
Staphylococcus epidermidis	—	—	—	—	—	36	248
Streptococcus pneumoniae	2	5	3	2	2	2	0
Haemophilus species	—	—	—	1	9	9	5
Escherichia coli	10	11	23	33	76	46	106
Pseudomonas aeruginosa	1	0	13	11	5	6	33
Klebsiella and *Enterobacter* species	0	0	0	8	28	25	97
Others	0	6	4	9	21	38	54
Total number of cases	*39*	*44*	*62*	*73*	*239*	*270*	*784*
Mortality rate for years	87%	90%	67%	45%	26%	16%	3%

*Data from Dunham.[2]
[†]Data from Nyhan and Fousek.[3]
[‡]Data from Gluck et al.[4]
[§]Data from Freedman et al.[5]
[¶]Data from Gladstone et al.[6]
[¶]Data from Bizzarro et al.[8]

and metabolic functions beginning in the early 1970s, the mortality rate was reduced to 16%. By 1989-2003, mortality from neonatal sepsis in this academic medical center was rare, occurring in only 3% of cases. A decline in the incidence of early-onset sepsis, commonly associated with more virulent pathogens, coupled with an increase in late-onset and "late-late" onset sepsis from CoNS and other commensal species (which together now account for nearly half of all cases), has contributed to the improved survival figures, along with continued advances in care and monitoring of critically ill infants.

The Yale data also provide information about the microorganisms responsible for early-onset and late-onset bacterial sepsis (Table 6–6). GBS were responsible for most early-onset disease. CoNS, *S. aureus*, *E. coli*, *Enterococcus* species, and *Klebsiella* species were the major pathogens of late-onset disease; a wide variety of gram-positive cocci and gram-negative bacilli are documented as causes of bacterial sepsis in infants after age 30 days.

The incidence of neonatal sepsis showed a strong inverse correlation to birth weight in the latest Yale cohort: birth weight greater than 2000 g, 0.2%; 1500 to 1999 g, 2.5%; 1000 to 1499 g, 9.4%; 750 to 999 g, 14.8%; and less than 750 g, 34.8%. Survival of very low birth weight infants (<1500 g) has been accompanied by an increased risk for invasive, nosocomial, or health care–associated bacterial infection as a cause of morbidity and mortality. The danger of sepsis is documented in a multicenter trial that enrolled 2416 very low birth weight infants in a study of the efficacy of intravenous

immunoglobulin in preventing nosocomial infections [18]. Of the very low birth weight infants, 16% developed septicemia at a median age of 17 days, with an overall mortality rate of 21% and hospital stay that averaged 98 days; infants without sepsis had an overall mortality rate of 9% and 58-day average length of stay. Stoll and colleagues [19] reported patterns of pathogens causing early-onset sepsis in very low birth weight infants (400 to 1500 g) in the centers participating in the National Institute of Child Health and Human Development (NICHD) Neonatal Research Network. Compared with earlier cohorts, a marked reduction in group B streptococcal infections (from 5.9 to 1.7 per 1000 live births) and an increase in *E. coli* infections (3.2 to 6.8 per 1000 live births) were noted, although the overall incidence of neonatal sepsis in this population did not change.

Organisms responsible for bacterial meningitis in newborns are listed in Table 6–7, which summarizes data collected from 1932-1997 at neonatal centers in the United States [20–23], The Netherlands [24], Great Britain [25,26], and Israel [12]. Gram-negative enteric bacilli and GBS currently are responsible for most cases. Organisms that cause acute bacterial meningitis in older children and adults—*Streptococcus pneumoniae*, *Neisseria meningitidis*, and type b and nontypable *Haemophilus influenzae*—are relatively infrequent causes of meningitis in the neonate [27]. A nationwide survey of causative agents of neonatal meningitis in Sweden in 1976-1983 indicated a shift from bacterial to viral or unidentified microorganisms, with lower attributable mortality rates [28].

TABLE 6-3   Surveys of Neonatal Bacteremia

Country or Region	Site	Year of Publication	Reference
United States	New Haven	1933	2
		1958	3
		1966	4
		1981	5
		1990	6
		2001	7
		2005	8
	New York	1949	735
	Minneapolis	1956	736
	Nashville	1961	737
	Baltimore	1965	738
	Los Angeles	1981	264
	Indianapolis	1982	77
	Philadelphia	1985	169
	Kansas City	1987	96
	Multicenter	1998	18
	Eastern Virginia	2000	14
	Multicenter	2002	15
Canada	Montreal	1985	78
Europe	Finland	1985	10
		1989	258
	Liverpool	1985	13
	Göttingen	1985	286
	Göteborg	1990	257
	London	1981	287
		1991	25
	Mallorca	1993	265
	Denmark	1991	259
	Norway	1998	739
Middle East	Tel Aviv	1983	17
	Beer-Sheva	1997	12
	Israel	2002	16
Africa	Nigeria	1984	11
	Ethiopia	1997	740
	South Africa	1998	741
Asia	Hyderabad	1985	742
Australia	South Brisbane	1997	743

GROUP B STREPTOCOCCI

Group B β-hemolytic streptococci were implicated in human disease shortly after the precipitin-grouping technique was described [29]. For the past 3 decades, GBS have been the most common organisms causing invasive disease in neonates throughout the United States and western Europe (see Chapter 12).

Streptococcus agalactiae, the species designation of GBS, has a characteristic colonial morphology on suitable solid media. The organism produces a mucoid colony with a narrow zone of β-hemolysis on sheep blood agar media. GBS can be differentiated immunochemically on the basis of their type-specific polysaccharides. Ten capsular types—Ia, Ib, II, III, IV, V, IV, VI, VII, and VIII—have been characterized, and most invasive human isolates can be classified as one of these types, with serotypes Ia, III, and V the most prevalent in many more recent epidemiologic surveys.

GBS have been isolated from various sites and body fluids, including throat, skin, wounds, exudates, stool, urine, cervix, vagina, blood, joint, pleural or peritoneal fluids, and cerebrospinal fluid (CSF). The organisms frequently are found in the lower gastrointestinal and genital tracts of women and men and in the lower gastrointestinal and upper respiratory tracts of newborns. Patterns of early-onset, late-onset, and very late onset disease have been associated with GBS (see Table 6–1). Early-onset disease manifests as a multisystem illness with rapid onset typically during the first 1 or 2 days of life and is frequently characterized by severe respiratory distress. The pathogenesis is presumed to be similar to that of other forms of early-onset sepsis of neonates. The mortality rate is currently estimated at 8%, but was 50% in the 1970s [30].

Clinical manifestations of late-onset neonatal sepsis are more insidious than the manifestations of early-onset disease, and meningitis is frequently a part of the clinical picture. Some infants with meningitis have a fulminant onset, however, with rapid progression to centrally mediated apnea. Many infants with late-onset sepsis are products of a normal pregnancy and delivery and have no problems in the nursery. It is uncertain whether group B streptococcal infection was acquired at the time of birth and carried until disease developed, was acquired after delivery from the mother or other household contacts, or

TABLE 6-4   Bacteremia in Finnish Neonates Related to Times of Onset of Signs and Mortality

Organism	Mortality for Onset of Signs at					
	<24 hr		24 hr–7 day		8-20 day	
	No. Died/Total	%	No. Died/Total	%	No. Died/Total	%
Group B streptococci	28/93	30	0/26	0	1/11	0
Escherichia coli	8/26	31	14/45	31	3/10	30
Staphylococcus aureus	3/14	21	7/64	11	1/12	8
Other	15/47	32	9/55	16	4/7	57
Total	*54/180*	*30*	*30/190*	*16*	*9/40*	*23*

Data from Vesikari R, et al. Neonatal septicemia. Arch Dis Child 60:542-546, 1985.

TABLE 6-5   Bacteremia in Finnish Neonates Related to Birth Weight and Mortality

	Mortality for Onset of Signs at					
	<1500 g		1500-2500 g		>2500 g	
Organism	No. Died/Total	%	No. Died/Total	%	No. Died/Total	%
Group B streptococci	11/15	73	10/36	20	8/79	10
Escherichia coli	11/15	73	8/19	42	6/47	13
Staphylococcus aureus	4/9	44	4/26	15	3/55	5
Other	12/18	67	7/21	33	9/70	13
Total	*38/57*	*67*	*29/102*	*28*	*26/251*	*10*

Data from Vesikari R, et al. Neonatal septicemia. Arch Dis Child 60:542-546, 1985.

TABLE 6-6   Microbiology of Neonatal Sepsis at Yale–New Haven Hospital, 1989-2003

	No. Isolates				
	Age When Cultured (days)				
Microorganism	0-4	5-30	>30	Transported Infants	Total
Staphylococcus aureus	8	18	20	24	70
Coagulase-negative staphylococci	6	119	42	81	248
Group B streptococci	53	12	7	14	86
Enterococcus species	5	21	23	33	82
Viridans streptococci	0	3	3	4	10
Stomatococcus species	0	0	0	1	1
Bacillus species	1	0	1	0	2
Listeria monocytogenes	1	0	0	0	1
Escherichia coli	25	27	12	41	106
Klebsiella pneumoniae	0	20	9	18	47
Klebsiella oxytoca	0	7	8	4	19
Enterobacter aerogenes	0	1	3	4	8
Enterobacter agglomerans	0	3	1	0	4
Enterobacter cloacae	0	7	5	7	19
Serratia marcescens	0	6	10	7	23
Pseudomonas aeruginosa	2	14	4	13	33
Acinetobacter species	1	0	2	1	4
Proteus mirabilis	0	1	1	1	3
Citrobacter freundii	1	0	0	1	2
Haemophilus influenzae	5	0	0	0	5
Bacteroides species	0	0	1	2	3
Yersinia enterocolitica	0	1	0	2	3
Other gram-negative rods	0	3	0	1	4
Candida and other fungi/yeast	3	41	16	18	78
Total	*112*	*304*	*169*	*277*	*862*

Data from Bizzaro MJ, et al. Seventy-five years of neonatal sepsis at Yale: 1928-2003. Pediatrics 116:595, 2005.

was acquired from other infants or personnel in the nursery. In late-onset infection, most strains belong to serotype III. The mortality rate, estimated at 3%, is lower than the mortality for early-onset disease. With increasing survival of extremely low birth weight (<1000 g) infants, very late onset disease (>89 days) has been described [16].

In addition to sepsis and meningitis, other manifestations of neonatal disease caused by GBS include pneumonia, empyema, facial cellulitis, ethmoiditis, orbital cellulitis, conjunctivitis, necrotizing fasciitis, osteomyelitis, suppurative arthritis, and impetigo. Bacteremia without

systemic or focal signs of sepsis can occur. Group B streptococcal infection in pregnant women can result in peripartum infections, including septic abortion, chorioamnionitis, peripartum bacteremia, septic pelvic thrombophlebitis, meningitis, and toxic shock syndrome [31].

GROUP A STREPTOCOCCI

Streptococcal puerperal sepsis has been recognized as a cause of morbidity and mortality among parturient women since the 16th century [32–36]. Neonatal group A

TABLE 6-7 Bacteria Associated with Neonatal Meningitis in Selected Studies

Organism	Boston, 1932-1957, 77 Cases[20]	Los Angeles, 1963-1968, 125 Cases[21]	Houston, 1967-1972, 51 Cases[22]	Multihospital Survey,* 1971-1973, 131 Cases[7,44]	The Netherlands, 1976-1982, 280 Cases[24]	Great Britain, 1985-1987, 329 Cases[25]	Dallas, 1969-1989, 257 Cases[45]	Israel, 1986-1994, 32 Cases[31†]	Great Britain, 1996-1997, 144 Cases[45]
β-hemolytic streptococci (group not stated)	9	12	—	—	—	—	—	—	—
β-hemolytic streptococci									
Group A	—	—	1	2	—	—	—	—	—
Group B	—	—	18	41	68	113	134	6	69
Group D	—	—	—	2	4	9	—	2	1
Staphylococcus epidermidis or coagulase-negative staphylococci	—	5	—	3	—	—	—	—	2
Staphylococcus aureus	12	1	3	1	7	4	—	—	—
Streptococcus pneumoniae	7	4	3	2	6	21	18	—	8
Listeria monocytogenes	—	6	5	7	12	21	—	—	7
Escherichia coli	25	44	16‡	50	132	2	42	4	26
Pseudomonas aeruginosa	4	1	2	2	4	3	—	1	—
Klebsiella and Enterobacter species	3	13	‡	3	19	8	10	4	—
Proteus species	2	5	‡	4	5	8	3	2	1
Haemophilus species	—	2	2	3	2	12	—	—	—
Neisseria meningitidis	1	—	—	1	3	14	—	—	6
Salmonella species	2	4	1	3	3	2	4	—	1
Miscellaneous	12	28	—	7	15	32	46	—	23

*Survey of 16 newborn nurseries participating in neonatal meningitis study of intrathecal gentamicin under the direction of Dr. George McCracken, Jr.
†Authors report an additional nine cases of gram-positive and six cases of gram-negative meningitis with organisms not otherwise specified.
‡Authors report 16 cases related to enteric bacteria, including E. coli, Proteus species, and Klebsiella-Enterobacter group.

streptococcal infection now is reported infrequently [37–43], but it can occur rarely in epidemic form in nurseries [37,44–47]. The reemergence of virulent group A streptococcal infections during the last 3 decades, including invasive disease and toxic shock syndrome, has been reflected in more case reports of severe disease in pregnant women and newborns.

Group A streptococcal disease in the mother can affect the fetus or newborn in two clinical patterns. Maternal streptococcal bacteremia during pregnancy can lead to in utero infection resulting in fetal loss or stillbirth; alternatively, acquisition of group A streptococci from the maternal genital tract can cause early-onset neonatal sepsis similar to early-onset group B streptococcal disease. In the first form of disease, previously healthy pregnant women with influenza-like signs and symptoms have been reported. This presentation rapidly progressed to disseminated intravascular coagulopathy and shock, with high mortality and risk to the fetus or newborn [48–50].

The features of 38 cases of neonatal invasive group A streptococcal infection from the literature were catalogued in 2004 [51]. Overall mortality rate in neonatal invasive group A streptococcal infection was significantly high (31%). Most of these infants presented with early-onset infection (62%), with many occurring in the first 48 hours of life. A specific focus of group A streptococcal infection was documented in three quarters of cases—42% of neonates had pneumonia, sometimes complicated by empyema, and 17% had a toxic shock syndrome–like presentation. Among the cases of early-onset group A streptococcal infection, puerperal sepsis or toxic shock-like syndrome in the mother during the peripartum period was an associated factor in 62% of cases. In late-onset cases of neonatal group A streptococcal infection reviewed in this series, soft tissue infections, meningitis, and pneumonia were among the reported clinical manifestations. A review by Greenberg and colleagues [52] in 1999 on 15 cases of group A streptococcal neonatal infection yielded similar statistics on clinical presentations and mortality.

In addition to sepsis, meningitis, and toxin-mediated disease in the neonate, focal infections, including cellulitis, omphalitis, Ludwig angina [53], pneumonia, and osteomyelitis, have been reported. Because all group A streptococci are susceptible to β-lactam antibiotics, the current strategy for prevention or treatment of infections caused by GBS also could apply to infections caused by group A streptococci.

STREPTOCOCCUS PNEUMONIAE

Although pneumococcal infections in the neonate are unusual occurrences, they are associated with substantial morbidity and mortality [54–61]. Bortolussi and colleagues [54] reported five infants with pneumococcal sepsis who had respiratory distress and clinical signs of infection on the first day of life. Three infants died, two within 12 hours of onset. S. pneumoniae was isolated from the vaginas of three of the mothers. Radiographic features were consistent with hyaline membrane disease or pneumonia or both. The clinical features were strikingly similar to features of early-onset group B streptococcal infection, including the association of prolonged interval after rupture of membranes, early-onset respiratory distress, abnormal chest radiographs, hypotension, leukopenia, and rapid deterioration. Fatal pneumococcal bacteremia in a mother 4 weeks postpartum and the same disease and outcome in her healthy term infant, who died at 6 weeks of age, suggested an absence of protective antibody in the mother and the infant [55].

Hoffman and colleagues from the United States Multicenter Pneumococcal Surveillance Group [59] identified 20 cases of neonatal S. pneumoniae sepsis or meningitis in a review of 4428 episodes of pneumococcal infection at eight children's hospitals from 1993-2001. Ninety percent of the infants were born at term, with a mean age at the onset of infection of 18.1 days. Only two of the mothers had clinically apparent infections at the time of delivery. Eight neonates had meningitis, and 12 had bacteremia; 4 of the bacteremic neonates also had pneumonia. The most common infecting pneumococcal serotypes were 19 (32%), 9 (18%), and 18 (11%). Penicillin and ceftriaxone nonsusceptibility were observed in 21.4% and 3.6% of isolates. Three deaths (15%) occurred, all within 36 hours of presentation. A case report of peripartum transmission of penicillin-resistant S. pneumoniae underlines concern that the increasing use of peripartum ampicillin to prevent group B streptococcal disease in neonates may result in an increase in neonatal infections caused by β-lactam–resistant organisms [60].

OTHER STREPTOCOCCI

Human isolates of group C and G streptococci form large β-hemolytic colonies that closely resemble those of group A streptococcus and share many virulence genes, including genes encoding surface M proteins and the cytotoxin streptolysin S. Group C streptococci have been associated with puerperal sepsis, but neonatal sepsis or meningitis related to these organisms is rare [62–65]. Likewise, group G streptococci are an infrequent cause of neonatal sepsis and pneumonia [66–70]. Maternal intrapartum transmission was the likely source for most cases [68], and concurrent endometritis and bacteremia in the mother and sepsis in the neonate have been reported [69]. Dyson and Read [68] found very high rates of colonization in neonates born at New York Hospital in a 1-year survey of discharge cultures in 1979; the monthly incidence of cultures of group G streptococci from the nose and umbilicus ranged from 41% to 70%. During this period, group B streptococcal colonization was only 1% to 11% [68].

Viridans streptococci are a heterogeneous group of α-hemolytic and nonhemolytic streptococci that are constituents of the normal flora of the respiratory and gastrointestinal tracts of infants, children, and adults. There are several classification schemata for these streptococci, and they may bear different designations in the literature. Streptococcus bovis is capable of causing neonatal sepsis and meningitis that is clinically similar to sepsis caused by GBS [71–73]. Rare cases of neonatal sepsis caused by Streptococcus mitis have been reported [74,75].

Viridans streptococci accounted for 23% of isolates from cultures of blood and CSF obtained from neonates at the Jefferson Davis Hospital, Houston; only GBS were more common (28%) as a cause of neonatal sepsis [76]. In this series, most infants had early-onset infection with clinical features similar to sepsis caused by other pathogens, but 22.6% had no signs of infection. One infant had meningitis. The case-fatality rate was 8.8%. Sepsis related to viridans streptococci also has been reported from Finland [10], Liverpool [13], Indianapolis [77], and Montreal [78]. Among ventilated neonates in a NICU in Ankara, Turkey, the most prominent bacteria in bronchioalveolar lavage cultures were multidrug-resistant viridans streptococci (66%), and these were also one of the most common bloodstream isolates (29%) in the same population [79]. It is clear from these studies that isolation of viridans streptococci from the blood culture of a neonate suspected to have sepsis cannot be considered a contaminant, as is the case in many other patient populations.

ENTEROCOCCUS SPECIES

Members of the genus *Enterococcus* (*E. faecalis* and *Enterococcus faecium*) were formerly classified as group D streptococci; but in the mid-1980s, genomic DNA sequence analysis revealed that taxonomic distinction was appropriate, and a unique genus was established [80]. Enterococci are differentiated from nonenterococci by their ability to grow in 6.5% sodium chloride broth and to withstand heating at 60° C for 30 minutes.

Most cases of enterococcal sepsis in the neonate are caused by *E. faecalis*, with a smaller number caused by *E. faecium* [71,72,81–84]. In 4 years beginning in 1974, 30 neonates with enterococcal sepsis occurred among 30,059 deliveries at Parkland Memorial Hospital in Dallas [81]. During this period, enterococci were second only to GBS (99 cases) and were more common than *E. coli* (27 cases) as a cause of neonatal sepsis. The clinical presentation in most cases was similar to early-onset sepsis of any cause [83]. Among infants with respiratory distress as a prominent sign of infection, chest radiographs were similar to radiographs showing the hyaline membrane–appearing pattern of group B streptococcal infection. Enterococcal bacteremia during 10 years beginning in January 1977 was reported in 56 neonates from Jefferson Davis Hospital in Houston, Texas [85]. Early-onset disease was a mild illness with respiratory distress or diarrhea; late-onset infection often was severe with apnea, bradycardia, shock, and increased requirement for oxygen and mechanical ventilation; many cases were nosocomial [85]. A large series of 100 cases of enterococcal bacteremia in neonates over a 20-year period at New York Hospital–Cornell Medical Center was evaluated by McNeeley and colleagues [82]. The presence of a central venous catheter (77%) and a diagnosis of necrotizing enterocolitis (33%) were common characteristics.

Enterococcus species generally are resistant to cephalosporins and are only moderately susceptible to penicillin G and ampicillin; they require the synergistic activity of penicillin at high dosage and an aminoglycoside for maximal bactericidal action. Nonenterococcal strains are susceptible to penicillin G, ampicillin, and most cephalosporins. Vancomycin-resistant *Enterococcus* has been reported from NICUs, causing illnesses clinically indistinguishable from vancomycin-sensitive strains [82]; these resistant strains raise concerns about the efficacy of antimicrobial agents currently approved for use in neonates [86]. Use of high doses of ampicillin is one option, but other drugs, including the newer streptogramin combination of quinupristin and dalfopristin and the oxazolidinone, linezolid, may be suggested by the susceptibility pattern (see Chapter 37).

STAPHYLOCOCCUS AUREUS AND COAGULASE-NEGATIVE STAPHYLOCOCCI

S. aureus and CoNS, especially *S. epidermidis*, colonize skin and mucosa. Isolation of *S. aureus* from tissue, blood, or other body fluid usually is clearly associated with disease. Most episodes of sepsis caused by *S. aureus* are hospital acquired, and mortality can be high (23% among 216 Swedish neonates with *S. aureus* bacteremia during the years 1967-1984), with low birth weight as the most important risk factor [87]. More recently, reports of pneumonia and other severe nosocomial infection in neonates caused by community-acquired methicillin-resistant *S. aureus* strains, including the epidemic USA300 clone, have been documented [88,89]. Molecular epidemiologic techniques have established direct transmission of community-acquired methicillin-resistant *S. aureus* between postpartum women [90] and among NICU patients [91].

CoNS include more than 30 different species. *S. epidermidis* is the dominant species of CoNS responsible for neonatal sepsis, but other species, including *Staphylococcus capitis*, *Staphylococcus hemolyticus* and *Staphylococcus hominis*, have been identified as causes of sepsis in newborns [92]. A well-documented increased incidence of CoNS sepsis [8,14–16,18] has accompanied the increased survival of very low birth weight and extremely low birth weight infants with developmentally immature immune systems and prolonged stay in NICUs. CoNS infections have been associated with the introduction of invasive procedures for maintenance and monitoring of the infants, in particular, long-term vascular access devices. Levels of serum complement and transplacental anti-CoNS IgG are inversely correlated with gestational age, and this relative deficiency in preterm infants contributes to their suboptimal opsonization and impaired bacterial killing of CoNS [93]. Because CoNS are present on the skin, isolation of these organisms from a single culture of blood can represent skin contamination, but also can indicate bloodstream invasion. Collection of two cultures of blood at separate sites can assist in differentiating skin or blood culture bottle contamination from bloodstream invasion in an infant with suspected late-onset sepsis [94], and adoption of a standard practice of two blood cultures can reduce the number of neonates diagnosed with CoNS and exposed to intravenous antibiotic therapy [95]. The significance of a positive blood culture yielding CoNS is discussed below in "Microbiologic Techniques."

Many episodes of sepsis caused by CoNS are associated with the use of vascular catheters. *S. epidermidis* and other CoNS species can adhere to and grow on surfaces of synthetic polymers used in the manufacture of catheters. Strains obtained from infected ventricular shunts or intravenous catheters produce a mucoid substance (i.e., slime or glycocalyx) that stimulates adherence of microcolonies to various surfaces in the environment and on epithelial surfaces, ultimately leading to establishment of a biofilm [96,97]. In addition to this adhesin function, the slime may protect staphylococci against antibiotics and host defense mechanisms such as macrophage phagocytosis [98]. Parenteral nutrition with a lipid emulsion administered through a venous catheter with organisms adherent to the polymer provides nutrients for growth of the bacteria, leading to invasion of the bloodstream when the organisms reach an inoculum of sufficient size [99]. Disease in newborn infants caused by *S. aureus* and CoNS is discussed in detail in Chapter 14.

LISTERIA MONOCYTOGENES

The potential of *L. monocytogenes* to contaminate food products and the resultant danger to immunocompromised patients and pregnant women was reconfirmed in a 2002 outbreak involving 46 patients in eight states. This outbreak resulted in seven deaths of adults and miscarriages or stillbirths in three pregnant women [100]. *Listeria* can be found in unprocessed animal products, including milk, meat, poultry, cheese, ice cream, and processed meats, and on fresh fruits and vegetables. The organism possesses several virulence factors that allow it to infect the fetal placental unit, survive and replicate within human cells, and achieve cell-to-cell spread [101]. Although most people exposed to *L. monocytogenes* do not develop illness, pregnant women can suffer fetal loss, and neonates can develop early-onset or late-onset sepsis and meningitis. Neonatal disease resulting from *Listeria* is discussed in detail in Chapter 13.

ESCHERICHIA COLI

E. coli is second only to GBS as the most common cause of early-onset and late-onset neonatal sepsis and meningitis [9,102–104]. Coliform organisms are prevalent in the maternal birth canal, and most infants are colonized in the lower gastrointestinal or respiratory tracts during or just before delivery. The antigenic structure of *E. coli* is complex; members of this species account for more than 145 different somatic (O) antigens, approximately 50 flagellar (H) antigens, and 80 different capsular (K) antigens. Although there is a wide genetic diversity of human commensal isolates of *E. coli*, strains causing neonatal pathology are derived from a limited number of clones [105]. One of these, the O18:K1:H7 clone, is distributed globally, whereas others such as O83:K1 and O45:K1 are restricted to a smaller subset of countries [106]. The presence of a 134-kDa plasmid encoding iron aquisition systems and other putative virulence genes is characteristic of several of these clones, and loss of the plasmid reduces the virulence more than 100-fold in a neonatal rat model of *E. coli* meningitis [107].

The K1 capsular antigen present in certain strains of *E. coli* is uniquely associated with neonatal meningitis [108–110]. K1 antigen is polysialic acid that is immunochemically identical to the capsular antigen of group B *N. meningitidis*. McCracken and coworkers [109] found K1 strains in the blood or CSF of 65 of 77 neonates with meningitis related to *E. coli*. These strains also were cultured from the blood of some infants (14 of 36) and adults (43 of 301) with sepsis, but without meningitis. The K1 capsular antigen was present in 88% of 132 strains from neonates with *E. coli* meningitis reported from The Netherlands [24]. Infants with meningitis caused by K1 strains had significantly higher mortality and morbidity rates than infants with meningitis caused by non-K1 *E. coli* strains [110]. The severity of disease was directly related to the presence, amount, and persistence of K1 antigen in CSF. Strains of *E. coli* with K1 antigen were isolated from cultures of stool of 7% to 38% (varying with time and location of the study) of healthy newborns and from approximately 50% of nurses and mothers of the infants [110,111]. The K1 strains have been present in the birth canal of mothers and subsequently in cultures from their newborns, indicating that these newborn infants acquired the organisms vertically from their mothers [111,112]. High rates of carriage of K1 strains by nursery personnel indicate, however, that postnatal acquisition of the K1 strains in the nursery also may occur [110,111].

The pathogenesis of *E. coli* K1 infection is hypothesized to begin with bacterial penetration of the gastrointestinal epithelium to enter the circulation, and efficient transcytosis of gastrointestinal epithelial cell monolayers by the pathogen has been shown in tissue culture [113]. Next the organisms can establish high-grade bacteremia in the immunosusceptible neonate through the complement resistance properties of its *O*-lipopolysaccharide and K1 capsule–mediated impairment of opsonophagocytic killing [114]. Finally, the pathogen possesses a series of surface protein determinants (e.g., OmpA, IbeA-C, CNF1) that mediate binding to and invade brain endothelial cells, as shown in human tissue culture experiments and the neonatal rat model of meningitis [115].

KLEBSIELLA SPECIES

Klebsiella is a genus of Enterobacteriaceae that has emerged as a significant nosocomial pathogen in neonates [116,117]. The four recognized species include *Klebsiella pneumoniae*, *Klebsiella oxytoca*, *Klebsiella terrigena*, and *Klebsiella planticola*. *K. pneumoniae*, the most common human pathogen, and *K. oxytoca* cause neonatal infections of the bloodstream, urinary tract, CNS, lung, skin, and soft tissues [118–120]. Previously thought to be a nonpathogenic organism inhabiting soil and water, *K. planticola* has been implicated as a cause of neonatal sepsis [121,122].

In a 4-year retrospective study from Israel [123], *Klebsiella* species caused 31% of late-onset neonatal sepsis. *Klebsiella* was also the most common single agent in a review of sepsis in Jamaican neonates [124]. Greenberg and colleagues [12] performed an 8-year prospective study of neonatal sepsis and meningitis at Soroka University Medical Center during 1986-1994; 49 (20%) of 250 cases were caused by *K. pneumoniae*, with a mortality rate of 29%. Risk factors for infection included prematurity, very low birth weight, prolonged rupture of membranes (>24 hours), and cesarean section or instrument delivery. *Klebsiella* species seem to be common causes of liver abscess complicating bacteremia in neonates [125].

The reservoirs for transmission of *Klebsiella* infections include the hands of health care workers and the gastrointestinal tracts of hospitalized infants. Multidrug resistance, in the form of extended-spectrum β-lactamase production, of *Klebsiella* strains causing neonatal infections and nursery outbreaks has become a substantial problem in some nurseries and is associated with increased morbidity and mortality [126–128]. Enhanced infection control measures and changes in use of routine broad-spectrum antibiotics can reduce the frequency of these serious infections.

ENTEROBACTER SPECIES

Among the *Enterobacter aerogenes* (i.e., *Aerobacter aerogenes*) species, *Enterobacter cloacae*, *Enterobacter sakazakii*, and *Enterobacter hormaechei* have caused sepsis and a severe form of necrotizing meningitis in neonates [129–134]. In 2008, the taxonomy of *E. sakazakii* was revised, resulting in identification of five species belonging to a new genus, *Cronobacter* [135]. For purposes of this chapter, the discussion of earlier articles retains the designation of *E. sakazakii*.

Enterobacter septicemia was the most common nosocomial infection in neonates at the Ondokuz Mayis University Hospital in Samsun, Turkey, from 1988-1992 [136]. Willis and Robinson [130] reviewed 17 cases of neonatal meningitis caused by *E. sakazakii*; cerebral abscess or cyst formation developed in 77% of the infants, and 50% of the infants died. Bonadio and colleagues [131] reviewed 30 cases of *E. cloacae* bacteremia in children, including 10 infants younger than 2 months. The high frequency of multidrug resistance among isolates from patients in the NICUs was attributed to routine extended-spectrum cephalosporin usage [137]. An outbreak of *E. sakazakii* in a French NICU in 1994 involved 17 cases including 7 neonates with necrotizing enterocolitis, 1 case of sepsis, and 1 case of meningitis; 8 infants were colonized, but asymptomatic; there were 3 deaths. Four separable pulse types of *E. sakazakii* were identified, but the deaths were attributable to only one [138]. In a review of *Enterobacter* sepsis in 28 neonates from Taiwan, thrombocytopenia (66%) and increased band-form neutrophils (41%) were common laboratory features, with a reported clinical outcome of 11% mortality, 14% meningitis, and 7% brain abscess [139].

In addition to the gastrointestinal tracts of hospitalized infants and hands of health care personnel, sources and modes of transmission of *Enterobacter* infections in the neonate include contaminated infant formula [140–143], contaminated total parenteral nutrition fluid [144,145], bladder catheterization devices [144], and contaminated saline [146]. Effective infection control measures require reinforcement of procedures including proper hand hygiene, aseptic technique, isolation protocols, and disinfection of environmental surfaces.

CITROBACTER SPECIES

Organisms of the genus *Citrobacter* are gram-negative bacilli that are occasional inhabitants of the gastrointestinal tract and are responsible for disease in neonates and debilitated or immunocompromised patients. The genus has undergone frequent changes in nomenclature, making it difficult to relate the types identified in reports of newborn disease over the years. In 1990, *Citrobacter koseri* replaced *Citrobacter diversus* [147]. For the purposes of this chapter, *C. koseri* replaces *C. diversus*, even though the original article may refer to the latter name.

Citrobacter species are responsible for sporadic and epidemic clusters of neonatal sepsis and meningitis, and *C. koseri* is uniquely associated with brain abscesses [147–155]. Neonatal disease can occur as early-onset or late-onset presentations. Brain abscesses caused by *C. koseri* have been reported in a pair of twins [156]. Doran [147] reviewed outbreaks of *C. koseri* in NICUs resulting in sepsis and meningitis, septic arthritis, and skin and soft tissue infections. Other focal infections in neonates caused by *Citrobacter* species include bone, pulmonary, and urinary tract infections [147].

During the period 1960-1980, 74 cases of meningitis caused by *Citrobacter* species were reported to the Centers for Disease Control and Prevention (CDC) of the U.S. Public Health Service [148]. In 1999, Doran [147] reviewed an additional 56 cases of neonatal meningitis caused by *Citrobacter* species. Combining results from the two studies, brain abscess developed in 73 (76%) of 96 patients for whom information was available. The pathogenesis of brain abscess caused by *C. koseri* is uncertain; cerebral vasculitis with infarction and bacterial invasion of necrotic tissues is one possible explanation [153]. Studies in the neonatal rat model suggest that the ability of *C. koseri* to survive phagolysosome fusion and persist intracellularly within macrophages could contribute to the establishment of chronic CNS infection and brain abscess [157]. Such persistence of *C. koseri* in the CNS is well illustrated by a case report of recovery of the organism from CSF during a surgical procedure 4 years after treatment of neonatal meningitis [152]. The mortality rate for meningitis resulting from *Citrobacter* species was about 30%; most of the infants who survived had some degree of mental retardation. A review of 110 survivors of meningitis caused by *Citrobacter* revealed only 20 infants who were believed to have structurally intact brains and age-appropriate development [147].

Citrobacter species usually are resistant to ampicillin and variably susceptible to aminoglycosides. Historically, most infants were treated with a combination of penicillin or cephalosporin plus an aminoglycoside. Surgical drainage has been used in some cases with variable success. Choosing antimicrobial agents with the most advantageous susceptibility pattern and selected surgical drainage seems to be the most promising approach to therapy, but no one regimen has been found to be more successful than another. Plasmid profiles, biotypes, serotypes, and chromosomal restriction endonuclease digests are useful as epidemiologic markers for the study of isolates of *C. koseri*. Morris and colleagues [154] used these markers to investigate an outbreak of six cases of neonatal meningitis caused by *C. koseri* in three Baltimore hospitals from 1983-1985. Identification of a specific outer membrane protein associated with strains isolated from CSF but uncommon elsewhere can provide a marker for virulent strains of *C. koseri* according to some investigators [155].

SERRATIA MARCESCENS

Similar to other members of Enterobacteriaceae, *Serratia marcescens* increasingly is associated with hospital-acquired infections in infants in the NICU [158–160]. Late-onset sepsis has occurred in infants infected from health care equipment [160–163], the hands of heath care workers [164], milk bottles [159], aqueous solutions such as theophylline [159], hand hygiene washes [160], and lipid parenteral feeds [162]. The gastrointestinal tracts of hospitalized infants provide a reservoir for transmission and infection [161]. Investigation of an outbreak of multi-drug-resistant *S. marcescens* in the NICU identified exposure to inhalational therapy as an independent risk factor for acquisition [165].

In a review by Campbell and colleagues [166] of neonatal bacteremia and meningitis caused by *S. marcescens*, 11 (29%) of 38 infants had meningitis as a complication of bacteremia. Mean gestational age was 28 weeks, and mean birth weight was 1099 g. All patients required mechanical ventilation, 90% had central venous catheters in situ, 90% had received prior antibiotics, 50% had a prior intraventricular hemorrhage, 40% had a hemodynamically significant patent ductus arteriosus treated medically or surgically, and 20% had necrotizing enterocolitis with perforation. All patients were treated for a minimum of 21 days with combination antimicrobial therapy that included a third-generation cephalosporin or a ureido-penicillin and an aminoglycoside, typically gentamicin. Three of 10 patients died. Four of the seven survivors developed severe hydrocephalus requiring ventriculoperitoneal shunt placement and had poor neurologic outcome. Poor neurologic outcome also was documented in a report of *S. marcescens* brain abscess resulting in multicystic encephalomalacia and severe developmental retardation [167].

PSEUDOMONAS AERUGINOSA

P. aeruginosa usually is a cause of late-onset disease in infants who are presumably infected from their endogenous flora or from equipment, aqueous solutions, or occasionally the hands of health care workers. An outbreak of *P. aeruginosa* sepsis in a French NICU was associated with contamination of a milk bank pasteurizer [168]. Stevens and colleagues [169] reported nine infants with *Pseudomonas* sepsis, four of whom presented in the first 72 hours of life. In three of these infants, the initial signs were of respiratory distress, and chest radiographs were consistent with hyaline membrane disease. Noma (i.e., gangrenous lesions of the nose, lips, and mouth) in a neonate has been associated with bacteremia caused by *P. aeruginosa* [170].

A retrospective review of sepsis in infants admitted over the 10-year period 1988-1997 to the NICU at Children's Hospital of the King's Daughters in Norfolk, Virginia, identified 825 cases of late-onset sepsis [14]. Infants with *Pseudomonas* sepsis had the highest frequency of clinically fulminant onset (56%), and 20 of the 36 (56%) infants with *Pseudomonas* sepsis died within 48 hours of collection of blood culture.

P. aeruginosa conjunctivitis in the neonate is a danger because it is rapidly destructive to the tissues of the eye and because it may lead to sepsis and meningitis. Shah and Gallagher [171] reviewed the course of 18 infants at Yale–New Haven Hospital NICU who had *P. aeruginosa* isolated from cultures of the conjunctiva during 10 years beginning in 1986. Five infants developed bacteremia, including three with meningitis, and two infants died. A cluster of four fatal cases of *P. aeruginosa* pneumonia and bacteremia among neonates in 2004 was traced by genotypic fingerprinting to their shared exposure to a health care worker experiencing intermittent otitis externa [172].

SALMONELLA SPECIES

Non-Typhi *Salmonella* infection is an uncommon cause of sepsis and meningitis in neonates, but a significant proportion of cases of *Salmonella* meningitis occur in young infants. The CDC observed that approximately one third of 290 *Salmonella* isolates from CSF reported during 1968-1979 were from patients younger than 3 months, and more than half were from infants younger than 1 year [173]. A 21-year review of gram-negative enteric meningitis in Dallas beginning in 1969 identified *Salmonella* as the cause in 4 of 72 cases [23]. Investigators from Turkey reported seven cases of neonatal meningitis caused by *Salmonella* during the years 1995-2001 [174]. Two of the five survivors developed communicating hydrocephalus, and one had a subdural empyema. In a case of neonatal meningitis caused by *Salmonella enterica* serotype Agona, the pathogen was isolated simultaneously from the newborn's CSF, parental fecal samples, and the mother's breast milk [175].

Reed and Klugman [176] reviewed 10 cases of neonatal typhoid that occurred in a rural African hospital. Six of the infants had early-onset sepsis with acquisition of the organism from the maternal genital tract, and four had late-onset infection with acquisition from a carrier or an environmental source. Two neonates developed meningitis, and three died.

NEISSERIA MENINGITIDIS

Although *N. meningitidis* is a leading cause of bacterial sepsis and meningitis among children and adolescents, it rarely is associated with invasive infection in neonates [12, 26, 177]. *N. meningitidis* may colonize the female genital tract [178–180] and has been associated with pelvic inflammatory disease [181]. The infant can be infected at delivery by organisms present in the maternal genital tract, or intrauterine infection can result during maternal meningococcemia [182]. Meningococcal sepsis is rare in neonates, but more than 50 cases (including 13 from the preantibiotic era) have been described [183–185]. Early-onset and late-onset forms [178, 179, 185] of meningococcal sepsis in neonates have been reported. Purpura similar to meningococcemia in older children has been observed in a 15-day-old infant [186] and a 25-day-old infant [187].

Shepard and colleagues [185] from the CDC reported 22 neonates with invasive meningococcal disease from a 10-year active, population-based surveillance of 10 states with diverse populations and more than 31 million persons. The average annual incidence was 9 cases per 100,000 people (versus 973.8 per 100,000 for GBS). Sixteen patients had meningitis, and 6 of these also had meningococcemia. Six patients had early-onset disease. The overall mortality rate was 14%. Ten isolates were serogroup B, four were serogroup C, three were serogroup Y, one was nongroupable, and four were unavailable. A case of meningococcal meningitis in a 2-week-old infant was successfully treated with no evidence of neurologic sequelae [188].

HAEMOPHILUS INFLUENZAE

Because of the introduction of *H. influenzae* type b conjugate vaccines in 1988, there has been a substantial decrease in the incidence in *H. influenzae* type b disease in infants and children in the United States and many other countries [189–191]. Given the estimated proportion of individuals who are completely immunized, the decrease in *H. influenzae* type b invasive disease has exceeded expectations. The reduction in *H. influenzae* carriage associated with vaccination and the consequent decreased transmission from immunized children to unimmunized infants and children likely explains this effect [192–194].

Despite increased reporting of invasive infections caused by nontypable *H. influenzae* in adults and older children [195–197], such infections in neonates remain uncommon [198–201]. Five clinical syndromes have been associated with neonatal disease caused by *H. influenzae*: (1) sepsis or respiratory distress syndrome, (2) pneumonia, (3) meningitis, (4) soft tissue or joint infection, and (5) otitis media or mastoiditis. The overall mortality rate was 5.5% for 45 cases reviewed by Friesen and Cho [202]; the mortality rate was 90% for 20 infants with a gestation lasting less than 30 weeks. Clinical and epidemiologic characteristics were similar to neonatal disease caused by GBS, including early-onset (≤24 hours of birth) and late-onset presentations, signs simulating respiratory distress syndrome, and a high mortality rate. Autopsy of infants with bacteremia related to nontypable *H. influenzae* and signs of respiratory distress syndrome revealed hyaline membranes with gram-negative coccobacilli within the membranes, similar to findings of hyaline membranes secondary to GBS [203].

Examination of placentas from mothers of infants with sepsis caused by nontypable *H. influenzae* revealed acute chorioamnionitis and acute villitis in some [199]. *H. influenzae* also has been responsible for maternal disease, including bacteremia, chorioamnionitis [204], acute or chronic salpingitis, and tubo-ovarian abscess [200]. A cluster of eight cases of early-onset infections over 53 months caused by β-lactamase–negative, nontypable *H. influenzae* was reported from an NICU in Israel [205]. In this series, a presentation resembling pneumonia rather than classic respiratory distress syndrome characterized the infants' respiratory problems. Neonatal sepsis caused by *Haemophilus parainfluenzae* [206–208] and *Haemophilus aphrophilus* [209] has been reported.

ANAEROBIC BACTERIA

Improvements in techniques for isolation and identification of the various genera and species of anaerobic bacteria have provided a better understanding of the anaerobic flora of humans and their role in disease [210]. With the exception of *Clostridium tetani* and *Clostridium botulinum*, all of the anaerobic bacteria belong to the normal flora of humans. Anaerobes are present on the skin, in the mouth, in the intestines, and in the genital tract. They account for the greatest proportion of the bacteria of the stool. All are present in the intestines and have been isolated from the external genitalia or vagina of pregnant and nonpregnant women [211–213]. Newborns are colonized with these organisms during or just before delivery. A review of the literature on neonatal bacteremia caused by anaerobic bacteria by Brook [214] in 1990 included 179 cases, with a mortality rate of 26%. *Bacteroides* and *Clostridium* species were the most common isolates. Predisposing factors for infection included premature rupture of membranes, preterm delivery, and necrotizing enterocolitis.

Anaerobic bacteria have been isolated from the blood of newborns with sepsis [212,215,216], from various organs at autopsy [217], from an infant with an adrenal abscess [218], from an infant with an infected cephalhematoma [219], and from infants with necrotizing fasciitis of the scalp associated with placement of a scalp electrode [220]. Feder [221] reviewed meningitis caused by *Bacteroides fragilis*; seven of nine reported cases occurred in neonates.

The incidence of neonatal sepsis caused by anaerobic bacteria is uncertain, but more recent data available from surveys suggest the incidence is low (<5%) [12,14,214]. Noel and colleagues [215] identified 29 episodes of anaerobic bacteremia in neonates in the intensive care unit at New York Hospital during 18 years. Chow and coworkers [217] analyzed 59 cases of neonatal sepsis associated with anaerobic pathogens and classified them into four groups: (1) transient bacteremia after premature rupture of membranes and maternal amnionitis, (2) sepsis after postoperative complications, (3) fulminant septicemia (in the case of clostridial infections), and (4) intrauterine death associated with septic abortion. The mortality rate associated with neonatal anaerobic sepsis reported in the literature ranges from 4% to 38% [217,222,223].

Serious infections of the bloodstream or CNS of neonates caused by *Bacillus cereus* have been reported [224,225] and in certain cases have proven intractable and refractory to antibiotic therapy [226,227]. One outbreak of *B. cereus* infections in an NICU was traced to contamination of balloons used in mechanical ventilation [228]. *B. fragilis* has been identified as a cause of pneumonia, sepsis, or meningitis in the immediate newborn period [229–231].

Infections caused by *Clostridium* species can be localized, as in the case of omphalitis [232], cellulitis, and necrotizing fasciitis [233], or can manifest as sepsis or meningitis [234]. Disease in neonates has been related to *Clostridium perfringens, Clostridium septicum, Clostridium sordellii, Clostridium butyricum, Clostridium tertium,* and *Clostridium paraputrificum* [235]. The presenting signs usually are similar to signs of other forms of bacterial sepsis. Chaney [234] reported a case of bacteremia caused by *C. perfringens* in a mother and neonate in which the neonate had classic features of adult clostridial sepsis, including active hemolysis, hyperbilirubinemia, and hemoglobinuria. Motz and colleagues [236] reviewed five cases of clostridial meningitis resulting from *C. butyricum* and *C. perfringens*. Clostridial sepsis has a high mortality rate [234].

NEONATAL TETANUS

Neonatal tetanus is caused by the gram-positive anaerobic spore-forming bacillus *C. tetani*. The organism is present in soil and can be present in human and animal feces. Infection usually occurs after contamination of the umbilical stump. Maternal and neonatal tetanus are important causes of mortality in developing countries, resulting in an estimated 180,000 deaths annually [237]. In the United States, tetanus in the newborn is exceedingly rare [238]. Since 1984, only three cases of neonatal tetanus have been reported [238–240]. The most recent case, reported from Montana in 1998, was an infant born to an unimmunized mother; the parents used a *C. tetani*–contaminated clay powder to accelerate drying of the umbilical cord. The use of this product had been promoted on an Internet site on "cord care" for use by midwives [241].

In many developing countries, the incidence and mortality of neonatal tetanus remain startlingly high [242–245]. Mustafa and colleagues [246] conducted a retrospective neonatal tetanus survey among rural and displaced communities in the East Nile Province in the Sudan and observed an incidence of neonatal tetanus of 7.1 cases per 1000 live births, more than double that reported from the stable rural community (3.2 per 1000). In both communities, coverage with two doses of tetanus toxoid was about 58%. Mortality attributable to neonatal tetanus in Djakarta in 1982 was 6.9 deaths per 1000 live births, and in the island provinces of Indonesia, it was 10.7 deaths per 1000 live births [247]. Among 62 cases of neonatal tetanus in Ethiopia, 90% were born at home, and 70% lacked antenatal care [245]. Three quarters of infants in this series died in the hospital, and risk factors for fatal outcome included an incubation period of less than 1 week, onset of symptoms less than 48 hours, tachycardia, and fever [245]. The mortality rate for neonates with tetanus in Lima, Peru, was 45% and was not improved with use of intrathecal tetanus antitoxin [248]. A meta-analysis of intrathecal therapy in tetanus suggested benefit in adults, but not in neonates [249].

Application of contaminated materials to the umbilical cord is associated with deep-rooted customs and rituals in developing countries. A case-control study to identify risk factors for neonatal tetanus in rural Pakistan identified application of ghee (i.e., clarified butter from the milk of water buffaloes or cows) to the umbilical wound as the most important risk factor [250]. Although commercial ghee is available in Pakistan, the ghee used in rural areas is made at home from unpasteurized milk. Oudesluys-Murphy [251] observed that application of some materials, including ghee and a stone wrapped in wet cloth, increased the risk of neonatal tetanus among Yoruba women, but that other practices of cord care decreased the incidence, including searing of the cord with heat in China during the Ming dynasty and use of a candle flame to scar the cord in Guatemala. Neonatal tetanus is a preventable disease; use of hygienic techniques at delivery and a program of tetanus toxoid immunization of children and young adults, particularly of pregnant women, are effective in eliminating this lethal disease [251–254].

MIXED INFECTIONS

Multiple organisms frequently are present in brain, liver, or lung abscesses; aspirates in the lung after pneumonia; or pleural empyema. Such mixed infections infrequently are found in cultures of the blood or CSF, however. When several species are found, the significance of each is uncertain because it is possible that one or more of the organisms in a mixed culture is a contaminant.

Bacteremia with more than one organism occurs in patients with immunodeficiency, major congenital abnormalities, or contamination of a body fluid with multiple organisms, as is present in peritonitis typically as a sequela of severe necrotizing enterocolitis in a very low birth weight infant. Neonatal meningitis caused by *S. pneumoniae* and *Acinetobacter calcoaceticus* [255] and sepsis caused by *P. aeruginosa* and *Yersinia enterocolitica* [256] have been reported. Although included in a series of cases of neonatal sepsis by some investigators, mixed cultures are not identified by most. Mixed infections were reported by Tessin and coworkers [257] in 5% of 231 Swedish neonates, by Vesikari and associates [258] in 4% of 377 Finnish infants, and by Bruun and Paerregaard [259] in 7% of 81 Danish neonates. Faix and Kovarik [260] reviewed the records of 385 specimens of blood or CSF submitted to the microbiology laboratories at the University of Michigan Medical Center for the period of September 1971 to June 1986. More than one organism was present in 38 specimens from 385 infants in the NICU; 15 (3.9%) infants had multiple pathogens associated with clinical signs of sepsis or meningitis. The mortality rate was high (60%).

Factors predisposing to mixed infection included prolonged rupture of membranes (>24 hours); total parenteral nutrition; necrotizing enterocolitis; presence of an intravascular catheter or ventriculostomy; and entities associated with multiple pathogens, including peritonitis, pseudomembranous colitis, and hepatic necrosis. Chow and colleagues [217] reported polymicrobial bacteremia in eight newborns with anaerobic coisolates or aerobic and anaerobic organisms in combination. Jarvis and associates [261] reported an outbreak of polymicrobial bacteremia caused by *K. pneumoniae* and *E. cloacae* associated with use of a contaminated lipid emulsion.

Mixed infections also can include bacteria and viruses or bacteria and fungi, typically *Candida*, in the situation of intravascular central catheter or peritoneal infections associated with bowel perforation. Sferra and Pacini [262] reported mixed viral-bacterial meningitis in five patients, including neonates with CSF isolates of enterovirus and GBS in a 10-day-old infant and enterovirus and *Salmonella* in a 12-day-old infant.

UNCOMMON BACTERIAL PATHOGENS

Numerous additional bacterial pathogens have been identified as rare or uncommon causes of neonatal sepsis and meningitis. These are listed in Table 6–8 with their references and were reviewed by Giacoia [263].

TABLE 6-8 Unusual Pathogens Responsible for Neonatal Sepsis and Meningitis

Organism	Reference
Achromobacter species	745-747
Acinetobacter species	748-752
Bacillus anthracis	753
Bacillus cereus	225, 226, 228, 754
Borrelia (relapsing fever)	755, 756
Brucella species	757, 758
Burkholderia cepacia	759-761
Burkholderia pseudomallei	762
Campylobacter species	718, 763
Capnocytophaga species	764-766
Corynebacterium species	767, 768
Edwardsiella tarda	769-771
Escherichia hermanii	772, 773
Chryseobacterium (Flavobacterium) species	774, 775
Gardnerella vaginalis	776, 777
Helicobacter cinaedi	778
Lactobacillus species	779, 780
Leptospira species	781, 782
Leuconostoc species	783, 784
Morganella morganii	785-787
Mycoplasma hominis	788
Ochrobactrum anthropi	789
Pantoea agglomerans	790
Pasteurella species	715, 791, 792
Plesiomonas species	793-795
Proteus mirabilis	796-798
Pseudomonas pseudomallei	799
Psychrobacter immobilis	800
Ralstonia pickettii	801
Rothia dentocariosa	802
Shigella sonnei	803-805
Staphylococcus capitis	806
Stomatococcus mucilaginosus	807
Vibrio cholerae	808, 809
Yersinia enterocolitica	810, 811
Yersinia pestis	812

EPIDEMIOLOGY
INCIDENCE OF SEPSIS AND MENINGITIS

The reported incidence of neonatal sepsis varies from less than 1 to 8.1 cases per 1000 live births [12,116,123, 257,264–269]. A 2-year study of 64,858 infants from the Atlanta metropolitan area beginning in January 1982 (Table 6–9) reported an incidence of early-onset group B streptococcal disease of 1.09 per 1000 live births and an incidence of 0.57 per 1000 live births for late-onset disease [267]. The increased usage of intrapartum antibiotic prophylaxis for women with group B streptococcal colonization with or without other risk factors associated with neonatal group B streptococcal disease has been associated with a 70% reduction in the incidence of early-onset group B streptococcal sepsis to 0.44 per 1000 live births in 1999, a rate comparable to that of late-onset sepsis (see Chapter 12) [7].

The incidence of meningitis usually is a fraction of the number of neonates with early-onset sepsis. During the 8-year period 1986-1994 at the Soroka University Medical Center in southern Israel, Greenberg and colleagues [12] found incidences of neonatal bacterial sepsis of 3.2 cases per 1000 live births and of meningitis of 0.5 case per 1000 live births. Certain pathogens that cause bloodstream invasion, such as GBS, *E. coli*, and *L. monocytogenes*, are more likely to be accompanied by meningeal invasion than others (e.g., *S. aureus*). Meningitis is more frequent during the first month of life than in any subsequent period (see Table 6–6).

CHARACTERISTICS OF INFANTS WHO DEVELOP SEPSIS

Host susceptibility, socioeconomic factors, obstetric and nursery practices, and the health and nutrition of mothers are important in the pathogenesis of neonatal sepsis and meningitis. Infants who develop sepsis, particularly early-onset disease, usually have a history of one or more risk factors associated with the pregnancy and delivery that significantly increase the risk for neonatal infection. These factors include preterm delivery or low birth weight, premature rupture of membranes (i.e., rupture before the onset of labor), prolonged time of rupture of membranes, maternal peripartum infection, septic or traumatic delivery, and fetal hypoxia.

TABLE 6-9 Incidence and Mortality of Group B Streptococcal Disease by Birth Weight, Atlanta 1982-1983

Birth Weight	Total Births	Early Onset		Late Onset	
		Cases/(Deaths)	Cases/1000	Cases/(Deaths)	Cases/1000
<1500 g	835	5 (1)	5.99	0	0
1500-2499 g	4380	11 (2)	2.51	6 (0)	1.37
>2500 g	59,303	53 (5)	0.89	23 (0)	0.39

Data from Schuchat A, et al. Population-based risk factors for neonatal group B streptococcal disease: results of a cohort study in metropolitan Atlanta. J Infect Dis 162:672, 1990.

Birth Weight

The factor associated most significantly with enhanced risk for bacterial sepsis and meningitis in neonates is low birth weight (see Tables 6–5 and 6–9) [12,18,270–272]. Infection is the most common cause of death in infants with very low birth weight [271,272]. With the exception of infection caused by GBS, it is unusual for a term infant to develop early-onset sepsis after an uneventful pregnancy and delivery. In a study in England and Wales, neonates weighing less than 2000 g at birth acquired meningitis six times more frequently than infants weighing more than 2000 g [26]. The lower the infant's birth weight, the higher is the incidence of sepsis (see Table 6–5). An Israeli study of 5555 very low birth weight infants documented the increased risk of late-onset sepsis with decreasing birth weight; late-onset sepsis occurred in 16.8% of neonates with a birth weight of 1250 to 1500 g, 30.6% of neonates weighing 1000 to 1249 g, 46.4% of neonates weighing 750 to 999 g, and 53% of neonates weighing less than 750 g at birth [16]. In a study of infants in Atlanta (see Table 6–9), the importance of birth weight was identified as a predisposing factor for development of early-onset and late-onset sepsis. If very low birth weight infants survived the first days of life, rates of sepsis decreased, but remained elevated [267]; 16% of 2416 infants with birth weights of 501 to 1500 g who were enrolled in a study sponsored by NICHD developed sepsis at a median of 17 days of age [18].

Risk Factors of Infant and Mother

The relative importance of other factors associated with systemic infection in the newborn is more difficult to define. In their prospective study of 229 infants with sepsis and meningitis, Greenberg and coworkers [12] found that certain conditions were common: 130 (57%) were premature (<37 weeks' gestation), 64 (28%) were delivered by cesarean section or instrumental delivery, 43 (19%) had an Apgar score of less than 7 at 5 minutes, and 27 (2%) had a prolonged (>24 hours) interval after rupture of maternal membranes. Investigators in Pakistan [273] found that maternal urinary tract infection, maternal fever, vaginal discharge, and vaginal examinations during labor were maternal factors significantly associated with neonatal early-onset sepsis, whereas low Apgar scores at birth and the need for endotracheal intubation were significant neonatal risk factors.

Attack rates for early-onset group B streptococcal sepsis in a study from Chicago [274] were affected by birth weight, duration of rupture of membranes, and occurrence of maternal peripartum fever. Infants with one or more of these perinatal risk factors had an attack rate of 8 per 1000 live births and a mortality rate of 33% compared with infants without such risk factors, who had an attack rate of 0.6 per 1000 live births and a mortality rate of 6% (Table 6–10).

Maternal fever during labor or after delivery suggests a concurrent infectious event in the mother and infant, but noninfectious events may be responsible for maternal fever. Use of epidural analgesia for pain relief during labor is associated with increases in maternal temperature.

TABLE 6–10 Relationship of Attack Rates and Fatalities of Neonatal Group B Streptococcal Early-Onset Disease to Perinatal Characteristics

Characteristic	Attack Rate per 1000 Live Births	Mortality Rate (%)
Birth weight (g)		
<1000	26	90
1001-1500	8	25
1501-2000	9	29
2001-2500	4	33
>2500	1	3
Rupture of membranes (hr)		
<18	1	20
19-24	6	27
25-48	9	18
>48	11	33
Peak intrapartum temperature (° C)		
<37.5	2	29
>37.5	7	17
Perinatal risk factors		
Present	7.6	33
Absent	0.6	6
Total no. infants = 32.384	2	26

Data from Boyer KM, et al. Selective intrapartum chemoprophylaxis of neonatal group B streptococcal early-onset disease, I: epidemiologic rationale. J Infect Dis 148:795-801, 1983.

Intrapartum fever of more than 38° C (>100.4° F) occurred an average of 6 hours after initiation of epidural anesthesia in 14.5% of women receiving an epidural anesthetic compared with 1% of women not receiving an epidural agent; the rate of fever increased from 7% in women with labors of less than 6 hours to 36% in women with labors lasting longer than 18 hours. There was no difference in the incidence of neonatal sepsis in the infants born to 1045 women who received epidural analgesia (0.3%) compared with infants born to women who did not have epidural analgesia (0.2%) [275]. Fetal core temperature may be elevated during maternal temperature elevation, and increased temperature may be present transiently in the neonate after delivery.

Ethnicity

The Collaborative Perinatal Research Study provides historical information on 38,500 pregnancies [276]; selected data for white and black women are presented in Table 6–11. Black women had a higher rate of premature rupture of membranes lasting more than 24 hours (21.4%) compared with white women (10.8%), black women had a higher rate of puerperal infection (4.1%) compared with white women (3.6%), and more black infants weighed less than 2500 g at birth (13.4%) compared with white infants (7.1%). More recent published data concur with the data observed 30 years ago. The National Center for Health Statistics reported continued

TABLE 6–11   Selected Characteristics of Women, Their Pregnancies, and Newborns (NINDS 1972)*

Characteristic	Percent with Characteristics	
	White Women	Black Women
Premature rupture of membranes: time from rupture to onset of labor (hr)		
<8	70.9	56.7
8-23	18.3	21.9
24-48	5.4	11.7
≥49	5.4	9.7
Puerperal infection	3.6	4.1
Type of delivery		
Vaginal vertex	91.7	92.4
Vaginal breech	3.3	2.6
Cesarean section	4.9	5
Birth weight <2500 g	7.1	13.4
Neutrophilic infiltration of		
Amnion	9	7.9
Chorion	13.1	15.6
Umbilical vein	14.6	7.5

*Approximately 18,700 white women and 19,800 black women were evaluated.
Data from Niswander KR, Gordon M. The women and their pregnancies. The Collaborative Perinatal Study of the National Institute of Neurological Diseases and Stroke. U.S. Department of Health, Education and Welfare Publication No. (NIH) 73-379. Washington, DC, U.S. Government Printing Office, 1972.*

TABLE 6–12   Incidence of Fetal and Neonatal Infections by Sex

Infection	No. Infants		Ratio of Male to Female
	Male	Female	
Intrauterine infections			
Syphilis	118	134	0.89
Tuberculosis	15	14	1.07
Toxoplasmosis	118	103	1.14
Listeriosis	26	37	0.70
Perinatal sepsis			
Gram-negative organisms	82	34	2.41
Gram-positive organisms	58	31	1.87
Perinatal meningitis			
Gram-negative organisms	126	44	2.87
Gram-positive organisms	45	39	1.15

Data based on a review of the literature and study of Johns Hopkins Hospital case records, 1930-1963. From Washburn TC, Medearis DN Jr, Childs B. Sex differences in susceptibility to infections. Pediatrics 35:57, 1965.

disparities between blacks and whites in maternal and infant health indicators [277]. In 1996, significant differences were found between blacks and the general population in terms of neonatal mortality (9.6 deaths versus 4.8 deaths per 1000 live births), low birth weight (13% versus 7.4%), and severe complications of pregnancy (23 complications versus 14 complications per 100 deliveries). A review of the literature from 1966-1994 reported significantly increased rates of severe histologic chorioamnionitis, maternal fever during labor, prolonged rupture of membranes, and early neonatal mortality from sepsis in blacks compared with whites [278].

In a study of group B streptococcal disease in infants from the Atlanta metropolitan area [267], black infants had a higher incidence than nonblack infants of early-onset disease; the risk of late-onset disease was 35 times greater in black than in white infants. After controlling for other significant risk factors, such as low birth weight and maternal age younger than 20 years, 30% of early-onset disease and 92% of late-onset disease could be attributed to black race. The increased incidence of group B streptococcal disease in blacks of all ages was observed in a survey by the CDC in selected counties in California, Georgia, and Tennessee and the entire state of Oklahoma. The rate of disease of 13.5 cases per 100,000 blacks was significantly higher than the 4.5 cases per 100,000 whites. In neonates with early-onset infection, 2.7 cases per 1000 live births occurred in blacks, and 1.3 cases per 1000 live births occurred in whites [279]. Maternal factors such as socioeconomic status, nutrition, recently acquired sexually transmitted diseases, or racial

differences in maternally acquired protective antibodies may result in the increased risk of group B streptococcal disease among blacks.

Gender

Historical data have suggested that there is a predominance of male neonates affected by sepsis and meningitis, but not by in utero infections (Table 6–12) [280,281]. This difference may partially reflect the fact that female infants had lower rates of respiratory distress syndrome (i.e., hyaline membrane disease) than male infants. Torday and colleagues [282] studied fetal pulmonary maturity by determining lecithin-to-sphingomyelin ratios and concentrations of saturated phosphatidylcholine and cortisol in amniotic fluid of fetuses of 28 to 40 weeks' gestation. Female infants had higher indices of pulmonary maturity than male infants. These data provide a biochemical basis for the increased risk of respiratory distress syndrome in male infants and the possible role of these factors of pulmonary maturation in the development of pulmonary infection. Later studies failed to confirm a significant increased risk for bacterial sepsis and meningitis among male infants [12,283–285].

Geographic Factors

The cause of neonatal sepsis varies from hospital to hospital and from one community to another. These differences probably reflect characteristics of the population served, including unique cultural features and sexual practices, local obstetric and nursery practices, and patterns of antimicrobial agent usage. The bacteriology of neonatal sepsis and meningitis in western Europe* and Jamaica [288] is generally similar to that in the United States.

*References 10, 13, 25, 257–259, 265, 286, 287.

In tropical areas, a different pattern can be observed [289–291]. In Riyadh, Saudi Arabia, from 1980-1984, *E. coli*, *Klebsiella* species, and *Serratia* species were the dominant causes of neonatal sepsis; GBS was an infrequent cause [291]. Later data from this geographic location revealed *E. coli* and CoNS were the most common pathogens, however, causing early-onset and late-onset sepsis [292].

Every year, 4 million neonatal deaths occur. About one third of the deaths are due to sepsis [293,294]. The highest numbers of neonatal deaths are in South Central Asian countries and sub-Saharan Africa. The global perspective of neonatal sepsis is discussed in Chapter 2. The most common isolates responsible for neonatal sepsis vary by country, but include a wide spectrum of gram-negative and gram-positive species, the most common of which are *E. coli*, *S. aureus*, *Pseudomonas*, and *Klebsiella* [295]. Multidrug-resistant strains are an increasing threat to intervention programs [296,297].

GBS is the most frequent cause of early-onset and late-onset sepsis in the United States, but the rates and risk factors for maternal and neonatal GBS colonization and disease vary in different communities [298–300]. Amin and colleagues [298] in the United Arab Emirates evaluated 563 pregnant women from similar socioeconomic and ethnic backgrounds and reported a GBS colonization rate of 10.1%. In Athens, Greece, maternal and neonatal colonization rates were 6.6% and 2.4% with a vertical transmission rate of 22.5% [299]. Middle-class women followed in the private practice setting were more frequently colonized with GBS than women followed in a public hospital. No association was found between colonization with GBS and maternal age, nationality, marital status, previous obstetric history, cesarean section, infant birth weight, or preterm birth.

Stoll and Schuchat [300] reviewed data on female genital colonization with GBS from 34 reports in the literature and emphasized the importance of appropriate specimen collection and inoculation into selective (antibiotic-containing) broth media in the ascertainment of accurate colonization rates. Analysis of data from studies employing adequate methods revealed regional GBS colonization rates of 12% in India and Pakistan, 19% in Asian and Pacific countries, 19% in sub-Saharan Africa, 22% in the Middle East and North Africa, and 14% in the Americas. A comparison of studies that did and did not use selective broth media revealed significantly higher GBS colonization rates in the populations where selective broth media was employed to assess colonization. Other reasons for varying rates of GBS colonization and disease may include socioeconomic factors or differences in sexual practices, hygiene, or nutrition.

Socioeconomic Factors

The lifestyle pattern of mothers, including cultural practices, housing, nutrition, and level of income, seems to be important in determining infants at risk for infection. The most significant factors enhancing risk for neonatal sepsis are low birth weight and prematurity, and the incidence of these is inversely related to socioeconomic status. Various criteria for determining socioeconomic status have been used, but no completely satisfactory and reproducible standard is available. Maternal education, resources, and access to health care can affect the risk of neonatal sepsis. A CDC report [301] evaluating the awareness of perinatal group B streptococcal infection among women of childbearing age in the United States revealed that women with a high school education or less; women with a household income of less than $25,000; and women reporting black, Asian/Pacific Islander, or other ethnicity had lower awareness of perinatal GBS infections than other women.

Procedures

Most infants with very low birth weight have one or more procedures that place them at risk for infection. Any disruption of the protective capability of the intact skin or mucosa can be associated with infection. In a multicenter study of NICU patients, increased risk of bacteremia was associated with parenteral nutrition, mechanical ventilation, peripherally inserted central catheters, peripheral venous catheters, and umbilical artery catheters [302].

NURSERY OUTBREAKS OR EPIDEMICS

The nursery is a small community of highly susceptible infants where patients have contact with many adults, including parents, physicians, nurses, respiratory therapists, and diagnostic imaging technicians (see Chapter 35). Siblings may enter the nursery or mothers' hospital suites and represent an additional source of infection. In these circumstances, outbreaks or epidemics of respiratory and gastrointestinal illness, most of which is caused by nonbacterial agents, can occur. Spread of microorganisms to the infant occurs by droplets from the respiratory tracts of parents, nursery personnel, or other infants. Organisms can be transferred from infant to infant by the hands of health care workers. Individuals with open or draining lesions are especially hazardous agents of transmission.

Staphylococcal infection and disease are a concern in many nurseries in the United States (see Chapters 14 and 35). Epidemics or outbreaks associated with contamination of nursery equipment and solutions caused by *Proteus* species, *Klebsiella* species, *S. marcescens*, *Pseudomonas* species, and *Flavobacterium* also have been reported. An unusual and unexplained outbreak of early-onset group B streptococcal sepsis with an attack rate of 14 per 1000 live births occurred in Kansas City during January through August of 1990 [303].

Molecular techniques to distinguish among bacterial strains are an important epidemiologic tool in the investigation of nursery outbreaks. Previously, methods to determine strain relatedness relied on antibiotic susceptibility patterns, biochemical profiles, and plasmid or phage analysis [154,304]. More recent techniques permit the discrimination of strains based on bacterial chromosomal polymorphisms. Pulse-field gel electrophoresis, ribotyping, multilocus sequence typing, and polymerase chain reaction–based methods are widely used tools to assign strain identity or relatedness [305–307].

Antimicrobial agents play a major role in the ecology of the microbial flora in the nursery. Extensive and prolonged use of these drugs eliminates susceptible strains and allows for proliferation of resistant subpopulations of neonatal flora. There is selective pressure toward colonization by microorganisms that are resistant to the antimicrobial agents used in the nurseries and, because of cross-resistance patterns, to similar drugs within an antimicrobial class.

A historical example of the selective pressure of a systemic antimicrobial agent is provided by Gezon and coworkers [45] in their use of benzathine penicillin G to control an outbreak of group A streptococcal disease. All infants entering the nursery during a 3-week period were treated with a single intramuscular dose of penicillin. Before institution of this policy, most strains of *S. aureus* in the nursery were susceptible to penicillin G. One week after initiation of the prophylactic regimen and for the next 2 years, almost all strains of *S. aureus* isolated from newborns in this nursery were resistant to penicillin G.

During a 4-month period in 1997, van der Zwet and colleagues [308] investigated a nosocomial nursery outbreak of gentamicin-resistant *K. pneumoniae* in which 13 neonates became colonized and 3 became infected. Molecular typing of strains revealed clonal similarity of isolates from eight neonates. The nursery outbreak was terminated by the substitution of amikacin for gentamicin in neonates when treatment with an aminoglycoside was believed to be warranted. Development of resistance in gram-negative enteric bacilli also has been documented in an Israeli study after widespread use of aminoglycosides [309].

Extensive or routine use of third-generation cephalosporins in the nursery, especially for all neonates with suspected sepsis, can lead to more rapid emergence of drug-resistant gram-negative enteric bacilli than occurs with the standard regimen of ampicillin and an aminoglycoside. Investigators in Brazil [126] performed a prospective investigation of extended-spectrum β-lactamase–producing *K. pneumoniae* colonization and infection during the 2-year period 1997-1999 in the NICU. A significant independent risk factor for colonization was receipt of a cephalosporin and an aminoglycoside. Previous colonization was an independent risk factor for infection. In India, Jain and coworkers [137] concluded that indiscriminate use of third-generation cephalosporins was responsible for the selection of extended-spectrum β-lactamase–producing, multiresistant strains in their NICU, where extended-spectrum β-lactamase production was detected in 86.6% of *Klebsiella* species, 73.4% of *Enterobacter* species, and 63.6% of *E. coli* strains. Nosocomial infections in the nursery and their epidemiology and management are discussed further in Chapter 35.

PATHOGENESIS

The developing fetus is relatively protected from the microbial flora of the mother. Procedures disturbing the integrity of the uterine contents, such as amniocentesis [310], cervical cerclage [311,312], transcervical chorionic villus sampling [313], or percutaneous umbilical blood sampling [310,314], can permit entry of skin or vaginal organisms into the amniotic sac, however, causing amnionitis and secondary fetal infection.

Initial colonization of the neonate usually occurs after rupture of the maternal membranes [280,315]. In most cases, the infant is colonized with the microflora of the birth canal during delivery. If delivery is delayed, vaginal bacteria may ascend the birth canal and, in some cases, produce inflammation of the fetal membranes, umbilical cord, and placenta [316]. Fetal infection can result from aspiration of infected amniotic fluid [317], leading to stillbirth, premature delivery, or neonatal sepsis [310,316, 318,319]. The organisms most commonly isolated from infected amniotic fluid are GBS, *E. coli* and other enteric bacilli, anaerobic bacteria, and genital mycoplasmas [310,318].

Studies have reported that amniotic fluid inhibits the growth of *E. coli* and other bacteria because of the presence of lysozyme, transferrin, immunoglobulins (IgA and IgG, but not IgM), zinc and phosphate, and lipid-rich substances [319–325]. The addition of meconium to amniotic fluid in vitro has resulted in increased growth of *E. coli* and GBS in some studies [326,327]. In other in vitro studies of the bacteriostatic activity of amniotic fluid, the growth of GBS was not inhibited [328–330]. Bacterial inhibition by amniotic fluid is discussed further in Chapter 3.

Infection of the mother at the time of birth, particularly genital infection, can play a significant role in the development of infection in the neonate. Transplacental hematogenous infection during or shortly before delivery (including the period of separation of the placenta) is possible, although it is more likely that the infant is infected just before or during passage through the birth canal. Among reports of concurrent bacteremia in the mother and neonate are cases caused by *H. influenzae* type b [331], *H. parainfluenzae* [208], *S. pneumoniae* [58,332], group A streptococcus [42], *N. meningitidis* [182], *Citrobacter* species [333], and *Morganella morgagnii* [334]; concurrent cases of meningitis have been reported as caused by *S. pneumoniae* [335], *N. meningitidis* [182], and GBS [336]. Many neonates are bacteremic at the time of delivery, which indicates that invasive infection occurred antepartum [337]. Infants with signs of sepsis during the first 24 hours of life also have the highest mortality rate [10]. These data suggest the importance of initiating chemoprophylaxis for women with group B streptococcal colonization or other risk factors for invasive disease in the neonate at the time of onset of labor (see Chapter 12) [338].

Microorganisms acquired by the newborn just before or during birth colonize the skin and mucosal surfaces, including the conjunctivae, nasopharynx, oropharynx, gastrointestinal tract, umbilical cord, and, in the female infant, the external genitalia. Normal skin flora of the newborn includes CoNS, diphtheroids, and *E. coli* [339]. In most cases, the microorganisms proliferate at the initial site of attachment without resulting in illness. Occasionally, contiguous areas may be infected by direct extension (e.g., sinusitis and otitis can occasionally occur from upper respiratory tract colonization).

Bacteria can be inoculated into the skin and soft tissue by obstetric forceps, and organisms may infect these tissues if abrasions or congenital defects are present. Scalp abscesses can occur in infants who have electrodes placed during labor for monitoring of heart rate [85,340,341]. The incidence of this type of infection in the hands of experienced clinicians is generally quite low (0.1% to 5.2%), however [342]. A 10-year survey of neonatal enterococcal bacteremia detected 6 of 44 infants with scalp abscesses as the probable source of their bacteremia [85]. The investigators were unable to deduce from the data available whether these abscesses were associated with fetal scalp monitoring, intravenous infusion, or other procedures that resulted in loss of the skin barrier.

Transient bacteremia can accompany procedures that traumatize mucosal membranes such as endotracheal suctioning [343]. Invasion of the bloodstream also can follow multiplication of organisms in the upper respiratory tract or other foci. Although the source of bacteremia frequently is inapparent, careful inspection can reveal a focus, such as an infected circumcision site or infection of the umbilical stump, in some neonates. Metastatic foci of infection can follow bacteremia and can involve the lungs, kidney, spleen, bones, or CNS.

Most cases of neonatal meningitis result from bacteremia. Fetal meningitis followed by stillbirth [344] or hydrocephalus, presumably because of maternal bacteremia and transplacentally acquired infection, has been described, but is exceedingly rare. Although CSF leaks caused by spiral fetal scalp electrodes do occur, no cases of meningitis have been traced to this source [345,346]. After delivery, the meninges can be invaded directly from an infected skin lesion, with spread through the soft tissues and skull sutures and along thrombosed bridging veins [315], but in most circumstances, bacteria gain access to the brain through the bloodstream to the choroid plexus during the course of sepsis [344]. Infants with developmental defects, such as a midline dermal sinus or myelomeningocele, are particularly susceptible to invasion of underlying nervous tissue [23].

Brain abscesses can result from hematogenous spread of microorganisms (i.e., septic emboli) and proliferation in tissue that is devitalized because of anoxia or vasculitis with hemorrhage or infarction. Certain organisms are more likely than others to invade nervous tissue and cause local or widespread necrosis [23]. Most cases of meningitis related to *C. koseri* (formerly *C. diversus*) and *E. sakazakii* are associated with formation of cysts and abscesses. Other gram-negative bacilli with potential to cause brain abscesses include *Proteus, Citrobacter, Pseudomonas, S. marcescens*, and occasionally GBS [155,166,347–349]. Volpe [350] commented that bacteria associated with brain abscesses are those that cause meningitis with severe vasculitis.

HOST FACTORS PREDISPOSING TO NEONATAL BACTERIAL SEPSIS

Infants with one or more predisposing factors (e.g., low birth weight, premature rupture of membranes, septic or traumatic delivery, fetal hypoxia, maternal peripartum infection) are at increased risk for sepsis. Microbial factors such as inoculum size [351] and virulence properties of the organism [310] undoubtedly are significant. Immature function of phagocytes and decreased inflammatory and immune effector responses are characteristic of very small

infants and can contribute to the unique susceptibility of the fetus and newborn (see Chapter 4).

Metabolic factors are likely to be important in increasing risk for sepsis and severity of the disease. Fetal hypoxia and acidosis can impede certain host defense mechanisms or allow localization of organisms in necrotic tissues. Infants with hyperbilirubinemia can have impairment of various immune functions, including neutrophil bactericidal activity, antibody response, lymphocyte proliferation, and complement functions (see Chapter 4). Indirect hyperbilirubinemia that commonly occurs with breast-feeding jaundice rarely is associated with neonatal sepsis [352]. Late-onset jaundice and direct hyperbilirubinemia can be the result of an infectious process. In one study from Turkey, more than one third of infants with late-onset direct hyperbilirubinemia had culture-proven sepsis, with gram-negative enteric bacteria including *E. coli* the most common etiologic agent [353]. Evidence of diffuse hepatocellular damage and bile stasis has been described in such infected and jaundiced infants [354,355].

Hypothermia in newborns, generally defined as a rectal temperature equal to or less than 35° C (≤95° F), is associated with a significant increase in the incidence of sepsis, meningitis, pneumonia, and other serious bacterial infections [356–359]. In developing countries, hypothermia is a leading cause of death during the winter. Hypothermia frequently is accompanied by abnormal leukocyte counts, acidosis, and uremia, each of which can interfere with resistance to infection. The exact cause of increased morbidity in infants presenting with hypothermia is poorly understood, however. In many infants, it is unclear whether hypothermia predisposes to or results from bacterial infection. In a large outbreak of *S. marcescens* neonatal infections affecting 159 cases in Gaza City, Palestine, hypothermia was the most common presenting symptom, recorded in 38% of cases [360].

Infants with galactosemia have increased susceptibility to sepsis caused by gram-negative enteric bacilli, in particular *E. coli* [361–363]. Among eight infants identified with galactosemia by routine newborn screening in Massachusetts, four had systemic infection caused by *E. coli* [362]. Three of these four infants died of sepsis and meningitis; the fourth infant, who had a urinary tract infection, survived. A survey of state programs in which newborns are screened for galactosemia revealed that among 32 infants detected, 10 had systemic infection, and 9 died of bacteremia. *E. coli* was the infecting organism in nine of the infants. Galactosemic neonates seem to have an unusual predisposition to severe infection with *E. coli*, and bacterial sepsis is a significant cause of death among these infants. Depressed neutrophil function resulting from elevated serum galactose levels is postulated to be a possible cause of their predisposition to sepsis [364,365]. The gold standard for diagnosis of classic galactosemia is measurement of galactose-1-phosphate uridyltransferase activity in erythrocytes, and the sole therapy is galactose restriction in the diet [366]. Shurin [364] observed that infants became ill when serum galactose levels were high when glucose levels were likely to be low, and that susceptibility to infection diminished when dietary control was initiated.

Other inherited metabolic diseases have not been associated with a higher incidence of neonatal bacterial infection. A poorly documented increase in the relative frequency of sepsis has been observed in infants with hereditary fructose intolerance [367]. Infants with methylmalonic acidemia and other inborn errors of branched-chain amino acid metabolism manifest neutropenia as a result of bone marrow suppression by accumulated metabolites; however, no increased incidence of infection has been described in this group of infants [368,369].

Iron may have an important role in the susceptibility of neonates to infection, but this is controversial. Iron added to serum in vitro enhances the growth of many organisms, including *E. coli*, *Klebsiella* species, *Pseudomonas* species, *Salmonella* species, *L. monocytogenes*, and *S. aureus*. The siderophore Iron is a proven virulence factor for the bacteremic phase of *E. coli* K1 sepsis and meningitis in the neonatal rat infection model [370]. The iron-binding proteins lactoferrin and transferrin are present in serum, saliva, and breast milk. The newborn has low levels of these proteins, however [371]. The iron-sequestering capacity of oral bovine lactoferrin supplementation may be one contributing factor to its reported efficacy in prophylaxis of bacterial sepsis in very low birth weight infants [372].

Barry and Reeve [373] showed an increased incidence of sepsis in Polynesian infants who were treated with intramuscular iron as prophylaxis for iron deficiency anemia. The regimen was shown to be effective in preventing anemia of infancy, but an extraordinary increase in bacterial sepsis occurred. The incidence of sepsis in newborns receiving iron was 17 cases per 1000 live births, whereas the incidence of sepsis in infants who did not receive iron was 3 cases per 1000 live births; during a comparable period, the rate of sepsis for European infants was 0.6 case per 1000 live births. Special features of sepsis in the infants who received iron soon after birth were late onset, paucity of adverse perinatal factors, and predominance of *E. coli* as the cause of sepsis. During the period studied, *E. coli* was responsible for 26 of 27 cases of sepsis in iron-treated Polynesian infants and for none of three cases of sepsis in the infants who did not receive iron. Results of this study were similar to the experience reported by Farmer [374] for New Zealand infants given intramuscular iron. The incidence of meningitis caused by *E. coli* increased fivefold in infants who received iron and decreased when the use of iron was terminated. Conventional iron-supplemented human milk fortifiers seem to be safe and do not contribute to a higher rate of sepsis in preterm infants [375].

INFECTION IN TWINS

Studies have suggested a higher risk for contracting ascending intrauterine infection in the first than the second born of twins [376,377]. Comparing delivery methods, no difference was observed in the incidence of neonatal sepsis in twins delivered in the vertex/vertex position compared with cases requiring uterine manipulation (vertex/breech extraction) [378]. Vaginal delivery of twin A followed by cesarean delivery of twin B may be associated with a higher rate of endometritis and neonatal

sepsis, however, compared with cases in which both twins are delivered by cesarean section [379].

Pass and colleagues [380] showed that low birth weight twins were at higher risk for group B streptococcal infection than low birth weight singletons; infection developed in 3 of 56 twin births, or 53.5 cases per 1000 live births, compared with infections in 7 of 603 singleton births, or 11.6 cases per 1000 live births. Edwards and associates [381] studied group B streptococcal infection in 12 index cases of multiple gestations. Early-onset disease occurred in both twins in one pair and in one twin in five other pairs; late-onset infection occurred in both twins in two pairs and in one twin in four other pairs. Cases of late-onset group B streptococcal disease in twin pairs occurred closely in time to one another: 19 and 20 days of age in one set and 28 and 32 days of age in the other set. In another case report of late-onset group B streptococcal infection in identical twins, twin A had fulminant fatal meningitis, whereas twin B recovered completely. GBS isolates proved to be genetically identical; clinical variables associated with the adverse outcome in twin A were longer duration of fever before antibiotics and the development of neutropenia [382].

In twins, the presence of virulent organisms in the environment, especially the maternal genital tract; the absence of specific maternal antibodies; and their similar genetic heritage probably contribute to the risk for invasive infection. It seems logical that twins, particularly if monochorionic, should have high rates of simultaneous early-onset infection, but it is particularly intriguing that some cases of late-onset disease occur in twins almost simultaneously. Late onset sepsis in a twin warrants close observation and consideration of cultures and presumptive therapy in the asymptomatic twin [383, 384a].

Infections in twins, including disease related to *Treponema pallidum*, echoviruses 18 and 19, and *Toxoplasma gondii*, are discussed in Chapters 16, 24, and 31. Neonatal infections in twins have been caused by group A streptococci (case report of streptococcal sepsis in a mother and infant twins) [384], *Salmonella* species [385], *Salmonella E. coli* [384a], *C. koseri* (brain abscesses in twins) [156], malaria [386,387], coccidioidomycosis [388], cytomegalovirus infection [389–391], and rubella [392].

UMBILICAL CORD AS A FOCUS OF INFECTION

Historically, the umbilical cord was a particularly common portal of entry for systemic infection in newborns, and infection by this route can still occur. The devitalized tissue is an excellent medium for bacterial growth, the recently thrombosed umbilical vessels provide access to the bloodstream, the umbilical vein is a direct route to the liver, and the umbilical artery and urachus are pathways to the pelvis [393]. Epidemics of erysipelas, staphylococcal disease, tetanus, and gas gangrene of the umbilicus were common in the 19th century. The introduction of simple hygienic measures in cord care resulted in a marked reduction of omphalitis [394]. In 1930, Cruickshank [395] wrote, "in Prague, before antiseptic and aseptic dressing of the cord was introduced, sepsis neonatorum was as common as puerperal sepsis ... after the introduction of cord dressing in the hospital the number of newborn children developing fever sank from 45% to 11.3%." [396]

Closure of the umbilical vessels and the subsequent aseptic necrosis of the cord begins soon after the infant takes the first breath. The umbilical arteries contract; the blood flow is interrupted; and the cord tissues, deprived of a blood supply, undergo aseptic necrosis. The umbilical stump acquires a rich flora of microorganisms. Within hours, the umbilical stump is colonized with large numbers of gram-positive cocci, particularly *Staphylococcus* species, and shortly thereafter with fecal organisms [396,397]. These bacteria can invade the open umbilical wound, causing a localized infection with purulent discharge and, as a result of delayed obliteration of the umbilical vessels, bleeding from the umbilical stump. From this site, infection can proceed into the umbilical vessels, along the fascial planes of the abdominal wall, or into the peritoneum (Fig. 6–1) [396,398,399].

Although umbilical discharge or an "oozing" cord is the most common manifestation of omphalitis, periumbilical cellulitis and fasciitis are the conditions most often associated with hospitalization [398]. Infants presenting with fasciitis have a high incidence of bacteremia, intravascular coagulopathy, shock, and death [398]. Edema of the umbilicus and peau d'orange appearance of the surrounding abdominal skin, signaling obstruction of the underlying lymphatics, can be an early warning sign, whereas the pathognomonic purplish blue discoloration implies advanced necrotizing fasciitis [393]. Septic embolization arising from the infected umbilical vessels is

uncommon, but can produce metastatic spread to various organs, including the lungs, pancreas, kidneys, and skin [394]. Such emboli can arise from the umbilical arteries and from the umbilical vein, because final closure of the ductus venosus and separation of the portal circulation from the inferior vena cava and the systemic circulation are generally delayed until day 15 to 30 of life [400].

Although omphalitis is now a rare infection in developing countries, it is a significant cause of mortality in developing countries. Topical application of chlorhexidine to the umbilical chord was shown to decrease the incidence of omphalitis in neonates in southern Nepal [400a]. Complications of omphalitis include various infections, such as septic umbilical arteritis [394,401], suppurative thrombophlebitis of the umbilical or portal veins or the ductus venosus [401–403], peritonitis [399,401,402,404], intestinal gangrene [399], pyourachus (infection of the urachal remnant) [405], liver abscess, endocarditis, pyelophlebitis [399,406], and subacute necrotizing funisitis [407]. Some of these infections can occur in the absence of signs of omphalitis [394,401].

ADMINISTRATION OF DRUGS TO THE MOTHER BEFORE DELIVERY

Almost all antimicrobial agents cross the placenta. Antimicrobial drugs administered to the mother at term can alter the initial microflora of the neonate and can complicate the diagnosis of infection in the neonate. Chapter 37 reviews the clinical pharmacology of antimicrobial agents administered to the mother.

Studies have shown that corticosteroid administration to mothers in preterm labor to enhance pulmonary maturation in the fetus resulted in a significant decrease in the incidence and severity of neonatal respiratory distress syndrome, but an increase in maternal infection, particularly endometritis, compared with placebo [408]; however, the impacts of this practice on the risk of neonatal infection differed among early studies [408,409]. Roberts and Dalziel [410] more recently performed a large meta-analysis of 21 randomized controlled studies from the Cochrane Pregnancy and Childbirth Group Trials register, comprising 3885 pregnant women and 4269 infants, and concluded that antenatal corticosteroid administration (betamethasone, dexamethasone, or hydrocortisone) given to women expected to deliver singleton or multiple pregnancies, whether labor was spontaneous, induced by membrane rupture, or electively induced, was associated with multiple favorable outcomes, including reduced neonatal death (relative risk 0.69), intensive care admissions (relative risk 0.80) and systemic infections in the first 48 hours of life (relative risk 0.56).

Substance abuse during pregnancy can affect immune function in the neonate. Significant abnormalities in T-cell function and an apparent increased incidence of infections have been found during the first year of life among infants born to alcohol-addicted [411–413] and heroin-addicted [414,415] mothers. The adverse effects of cocaine and opiates on placental function, fetal growth and development, and prematurity also may predispose to a greater likelihood of neonatal infection [415,416]. Drug abuse is a multifactorial problem; it is virtually impossible to separate the consequences of direct pharmacologic effects on the fetus from the consequences secondary to

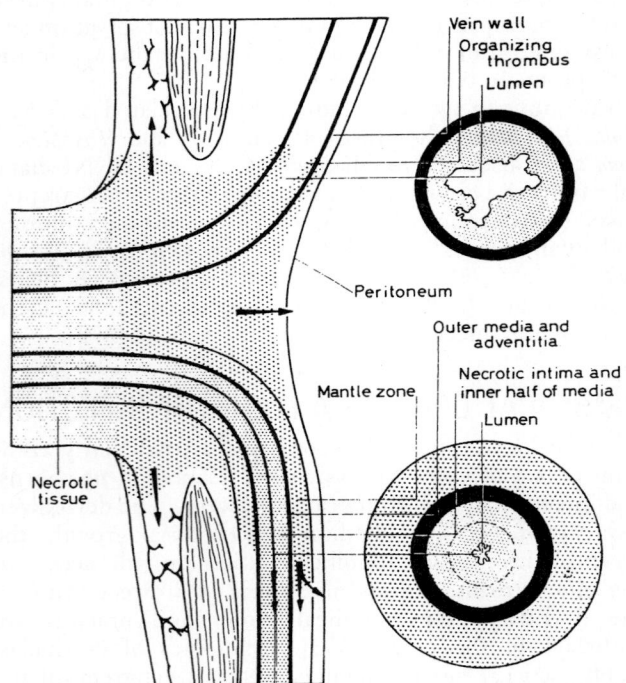

FIGURE 6–1 After birth, the necrotic tissue of the umbilical stump separates. This provokes some inflammation, which is limited by a fibroblastic reaction extending to the inner margin of the *coarsely stippled area*. The inner half of the media and the intima of the umbilical arteries become necrotic, but this does not stimulate an inflammatory reaction. *Arrows* indicate routes by which infection may spread beyond the granulation tissue barriers. Organisms invading the thrombus in the vein may disseminate by emboli. (*From Morison JE. Foetal and Neonatal Pathology, 3rd ed. Washington, DC, Butterworth, 1970.*)

inadequate nutrition, lack of prenatal care, and infectious medical complications encountered in addicted pregnant women [415,416].

ADMINISTRATION OF DRUGS OTHER THAN ANTIBIOTICS TO THE NEONATE

Administration of indomethacin to neonates for the closure of a patent ductus arteriosus has been associated with a higher incidence of sepsis and necrotizing enterocolitis in the indomethacin-treated groups compared with infants treated with surgery or other medications [417–419]. The mechanism by which indomethacin predisposes low birth weight infants to sepsis is unknown [420]. A meta-analysis of studies comparing ibuprofen with indomethacin for patent ductus arteriosus closure did not identify differences in the incidence of sepsis, mortality, or duration of hospitalization [421].

O'Shea and colleagues [420] described the outcomes of very low birth weight (500 to 1250 g) infants given dexamethasone at 15 to 25 days of age for the prevention of chronic lung disease. Among 61 infants treated with tapering doses of dexamethasone for 42 days, there was no increase in the incidence of sepsis or the number of sepsis evaluations in the treatment group compared with a control population. Further trials of dexamethasone administration for prophylaxis of chronic lung disease in very low birth weight infants confirmed a lack of increased risk for sepsis [422].

A strong association between intravenous lipid administration to newborns and bacteremia caused by CoNS has been established [99,423]. The role of lipid as a nutritional source for the bacteria, mechanical blockage of the catheter by deposition of lipid in the lumen, and the effect of lipid emulsions on the function of neutrophils and macrophages each might contribute to the observed increased risk for bacteremia. Avila-Figueroa and colleagues [423] identified exposure to intravenous lipids at anytime during hospitalization as the most important risk factor (odds ratio 9.4) for development of CoNS bacteremia in very low birth weight infants, calculating that 85% of these bacteremias were attributable to lipid therapy. A randomized trial found that changing intravenous tubing for lipid infusion in neonates every 24 hours instead of every 72 hours may reduce bloodstream infections and mortality by approximately 50% [424].

More recently, a surprisingly strong association between ranitidine therapy in neonates admitted to one NICU and the risk of late-onset bacterial sepsis was reported [425]. The mechanism for such an association is unclear, but warrants further analysis.

PATHOLOGY

Infants with severe and rapidly fatal sepsis generally have minimal or no histologic indication of an infectious process [315,426]. Findings typical of bacteremia, such as multiple disseminated abscesses of similar size, purulent vasculitis, and intravascular identification of bacteria, are evident in a few infants [426]. Shock accompanying sepsis sometimes causes findings such as periventricular leukomalacia and intraventricular hemorrhage, scattered areas of nonzonal hepatic necrosis, renal medullary hemorrhage, renal

cortical or acute tubular necrosis, and adrenal hemorrhage and necrosis. Evidence of disseminated intravascular coagulopathy, manifested by strands of interlacing fibrin in the vessels or by a well-demarcated subarachnoid fibrinous hematoma, also can be present [344,426]. The pathology of infections of the respiratory, genitourinary, and gastrointestinal tracts and focal suppurative diseases is discussed in subsequent chapters.

The pathology of neonatal meningitis [344,427,428] and brain abscess [429,430] is similar to that in older children and adults. The major features are ventriculitis (including inflammation of the choroid plexus), vasculitis, cerebral edema, infarction, cortical neuronal necrosis, and periventricular leukomalacia; chronic pathologic features include hydrocephalus, multicystic encephalomalacia and porencephaly, and cerebral cortical and white matter atrophy [431]. Significant collections of purulent material can be present in the sulci and subarachnoid space, particularly around the basal cisterns, of infants with meningitis. Because the fontanelles are open, exudative material can collect around the base of the brain without a significant increase in intracranial pressure. Hydrocephalus may result from closure of the aqueduct or the foramina of the fourth ventricle by purulent exudate or by means of inflammatory impairment of CSF resorption through the arachnoid channels [344,432]. Ventriculitis has been described in 20% to 90% of cases [23,344,432] and often is the reason for persistence of bacteria in CSF when obstruction ensues and for a slow clinical recovery [433]. Acute inflammatory cells infiltrate the ependymal and subependymal tissues, causing destruction of the epithelial lining of the ventricles. Hemorrhage, venous thrombosis, and subdural effusions often are present.

Brain abscesses and cysts in the neonate are distinguished by the large size of the lesions and poor capsule formation. They occur most frequently in association with meningitis caused by *C. koseri*, *E. sakazakii*, *S. marcescens*, and *Proteus mirabilis* and usually are located in the cerebrum, involving several lobes [155,166,347,429]. These organisms characteristically give rise to a hemorrhagic meningoencephalitis caused by intense bacterial infiltration of cerebral vessels and surrounding tissues. The resulting vascular occlusion is followed by infarction and widespread necrosis of cerebral tissue with liquefaction and formation of multiple loculated abscesses and cysts [347,350].

CLINICAL MANIFESTATIONS

Signs of fetal distress can be the earliest indication of infection in neonates with sepsis, beginning at or soon after delivery. Fetal tachycardia in the second stage of labor was evaluated as a sign of infection by Schiano and colleagues [434]. Pneumonia or sepsis occurred in 3 of 8 infants with marked fetal tachycardia (>180 beats/min), in 7 of 32 infants with mild tachycardia (160 to 179 beats/min), and in 1 of 167 infants with lower heart rates. Maternal risk factors such as premature rupture of membranes, foul-smelling amniotic fluid, and evidence of acute placental inflammation are associated with increased risk of neonatal sepsis and should prompt detailed evaluation of the newborn [435,436].

A low Apgar score, suggesting distress at or before delivery, also has been correlated with sepsis and associated adverse outcomes in the newborn period [435,437]. Infants delivered vaginally had a 56-fold higher risk of sepsis when the Apgar score was less than 7 at 5 minutes compared with infants with higher Apgar scores [438]. Among infants born after rupture of the amniotic membranes for 24 hours or more, St. Geme and colleagues [316] found a significant increase in the risk for perinatal bacterial infection in infants with an Apgar score of less than 6 at 5 minutes, but found no association with fetal tachycardia (>160 beats/min).

The Apgar score is well characterized in term infants, but less so in premature infants, who have higher attack rates for sepsis. Because low Apgar scores (<3 at 1 minute, <6 at 5 minutes) were significantly associated with low birth weight and shorter gestation, the use of the score is less valuable as an indicator of sepsis in premature than in term infants [439].

The earliest signs of sepsis often are subtle and nonspecific. Poor feeding, diminished activity, or "not looking well" can be the only early evidence that infection is present. More prominent findings are respiratory distress; apnea; lethargy; fever or hypothermia; jaundice; vomiting; diarrhea; and skin manifestations, including petechiae, abscesses, and sclerema [440]. The nonspecific and subtle nature of the signs of sepsis in newborns is even more problematic in identifying sepsis in infants with very low birth weight. In a study by Fanaroff and colleagues [18], the clinical signs of late-onset sepsis in 325 infants weighing 501 to 1500 g at birth included increasing apnea and bradycardia episodes (55%), increasing oxygen requirement (48%), feeding intolerance, abdominal distention or guaiac-positive stools (46%), lethargy and hypotonia (37%), and temperature instability (10%). Unexplained metabolic acidosis (11%) and hypoglycemia (10%) were the most common laboratory indicators of the metabolic derangement accompanying sepsis.

Bonadio and coworkers [441] attempted to determine the most reliable clinical signs of sepsis in more than 200 febrile infants from birth to 8 weeks old. They found that changes in affect, peripheral perfusion, and respiratory status best identified infants with serious bacterial infection. Alterations in feeding pattern, level of alertness, level of activity, and muscle tone also were present; however, these signs were less sensitive indicators. More recently, Kudawla and associates [442] developed a scoring system for late-onset neonatal sepsis in infants weighing 1000 to 2500 g. Clinical parameters included lethargy, tachycardia, grunting, abdominal distention, increased prefeed residual gastric aspirates, fever, and chest retractions. These data needed to be combined with laboratory parameters such as elevated C-reactive protein or absolute neutrophil or band count to achieve high sensitivity and specificity.

Focal infection involving any organ can occur in infants with sepsis, but most often (excluding pneumonia or meningitis), this occurs in neonates with late-onset rather than early-onset disease. Evaluation of infants with suspected bacteremia must include a careful search for primary or secondary foci, such as meningitis, pneumonia, urinary tract infection, septic arthritis, osteomyelitis, peritonitis, or soft tissue infection.

Serious bacterial infections are uncommon in neonates without any clinical evidence of illness [441], even among infants with maternal risk factors for infection [443].

Occasionally, bacteremia occurs without clinical signs [444–446]. Albers and associates [444] described case histories of three infants without signs of illness for whom blood cultures were performed as part of a nursery study involving 131 infants. Blood was obtained from peripheral veins at different times during the first 10 days of life. The same pathogen was isolated repeatedly (i.e., three, three, and two times) from the blood of the three infants even though they remained well. The infants subsequently were treated with appropriate antimicrobial agents. Bacteremia caused by GBS can occur with minimal or no systemic or focal signs [446–448], and it may be sustained over several days [449]. Most healthy-appearing infants with group B streptococcal bacteremia were born at term and had early-onset (<7 days old) infection. Similarly, among 44 neonates with enterococcal bacteremia, 3 of 18 with early-onset infection but none with late-onset infection appeared well [85]. The true incidence of bacteremia without clinical signs is uncertain because few cultures of blood are performed for infants who show no signs of sepsis.

Table 6–13 lists the common clinical signs of neonatal bacterial sepsis. Clinical signs of neonatal bacterial meningitis are presented in Table 6–14. Noninfectious conditions with clinical manifestations similar to those of sepsis are listed in Table 6–15.

TABLE 6–13 Clinical Signs of Bacterial Sepsis

Clinical Sign	Percent of Infants with Sign
Hyperthermia	51
Hypothermia	15
Respiratory distress	33
Apnea	22
Cyanosis	24
Jaundice	35
Hepatomegaly	33
Lethargy	25
Irritability	16
Anorexia	28
Vomiting	25
Abdominal distention	17
Diarrhea	11

Data from references 3, 4, 737, and 738.

TABLE 6–14 Clinical Signs of Bacterial Meningitis

Clinical Sign	Percent of Infants with Sign
Hypothermia or fever	62
Lethargy or irritability	52
Anorexia or vomiting	48
Respiratory distress	41
Bulging or full fontanelle	35
Seizures	31
Jaundice	28
Nuchal rigidity	16
Diarrhea	14

Data from references 20, 26, 430, and 450.

TABLE 6–15   Differential Diagnosis: Clinical Signs Associated with Neonatal Sepsis and Some Noninfectious Conditions

Respiratory Distress (Apnea, Cyanosis, Costal and Sternal Retraction, Rales, Grunting, Diminished Breath Sounds, Tachypnea)

Transient tachypnea of the newborn

Respiratory distress syndrome

Atelectasis

Aspiration pneumonia, including meconium aspiration

Pneumothorax

Pneumomediastinum

CNS disease: hypoxia, hemorrhage

Congenital abnormalities, including tracheoesophageal fistula, choanal atresia, diaphragmatic hernia, hypoplastic lungs

Congenital heart disease

Cardiac arrhythmia

Hypothermia (neonatal cold injury)

Hypoglycemia

Neonatal drug withdrawal syndrome

Medication error with inhaled epinephrine

Temperature Abnormality (Hyperthermia or Hypothermia)

Altered environmental temperature

Disturbance of CNS thermoregulatory mechanism, including anoxia, hemorrhage, kernicterus

Hyperthyroidism or hypothyroidism

Neonatal drug withdrawal syndrome

Dehydration

Congenital adrenal hyperplasia

Vaccine reaction (Hepatitis B Vaccine)

Jaundice

Breast milk jaundice

Blood group incompatibility

Red blood cell hemolysis, including blood group incompatibility, G6PD deficiency

Resorption of blood from closed space hemorrhage

Gastrointestinal obstruction, including pyloric stenosis

Extrahepatic or intrahepatic biliary tract obstruction

Inborn errors of metabolism, including galactosemia, glycogen storage disease type IV, tyrosinemia, disorders of lipid metabolism, peroxisomal disorders, defective bile acid synthesis (trihydroxycoprostanic acidemia)

Hereditary diseases, including cystic fibrosis, α_1-antitrypsin deficiency, bile excretory defects (Dubin-Johnson syndrome, Rotor syndrome, Byler disease, Aagenaes syndrome)

Hypothyroidism

Prolonged parenteral hyperalimentation

Hepatomegaly

Red blood cell hemolysis, including blood group incompatibility, G6PD deficiency

Infant of a diabetic mother

Inborn errors of metabolism, including galactosemia, glycogen storage disease, organic acidemias, urea cycle disorders, hereditary fructose intolerance, peroxisomal disorders

Biliary atresia

Congestive heart failure

Benign liver tumors, including hemangioma, hamartoma

Malignant liver tumors, including hepatoblastoma, metastatic neuroblastoma, congenital leukemia

Gastrointestinal Abnormalities (Anorexia, Regurgitation, Vomiting, Diarrhea, Abdominal Distention)

Gastrointestinal allergy

Overfeeding, aerophagia

Intestinal obstruction (intraluminal or extrinsic)

Necrotizing enterocolitis

Hypokalemia

Hypercalcemia or hypocalcemia

TABLE 6–15   Differential Diagnosis: Clinical Signs Associated with Neonatal Sepsis and Some Noninfectious Conditions—cont'd

Hypoglycemia
Inborn errors of metabolism, including galactosemia, urea cycle disorders, organic acidemias
Ileus secondary to pneumonia
Congenital adrenal hyperplasia
Gastric perforation
Neonatal drug withdrawal syndrome

Lethargy

CNS disease, including hemorrhage, hypoxia, or subdural effusion
Congenital heart disease
Neonatal drug withdrawal syndrome
Hypoglycemia
Hypercalcemia
Familial dysautonomia

Seizure Activity (Tremors, Hyperactivity, Muscular Twitching)

Hypoxia
Intracranial hemorrhage or kernicterus
Congenital CNS malformations
Neonatal drug withdrawal syndrome
Hypoglycemia
Hypocalcemia
Hyponatremia, hypernatremia
Hypomagnesemia
Inborn errors of metabolism, including urea cycle disorders, organic acidemias, galactosemia, glycogen storage disease, peroxisomal disorders
Pyridoxine deficiency

Petechiae, Purpura, and Vesiculopustular Lesions

Birth trauma
Blood group incompatibility
Neonatal isoimmune thrombocytopenia
Maternal idiopathic thrombocytopenic purpura
Maternal lupus erythematosus
Drugs administered to mother
Giant hemangioma (Kasabach-Merritt syndrome)
Thrombocytopenia with absent radii syndrome
Disseminated intravascular coagulopathy
Coagulation factor deficiencies
Congenital leukemia
Child abuse
Cutaneous histiocytosis

CNS, central nervous system; G6PD, glucose-6-phosphate dehydrogenase.

FEVER AND HYPOTHERMIA

The temperature of an infant with sepsis may be elevated, depressed, or normal [447–453]. In a multicenter survey of nearly 250 infants with early-onset group B streptococcal bacteremia, approximately 85% had a normal temperature (36° C to 37.2° C [96.8° F to 99° F]) at the time of their admission to the NICU [447]. Comparing temperatures by gestational age, it was observed that term infants were more likely to have fever than preterm infants (12% versus 1%), whereas preterm infants more frequently had hypothermia (13% versus 3%). Phagocytes of an infant born after an uncomplicated labor can produce adult concentrations of interleukin-1, a potent pyrogen. The phagocytes of infants born after cesarean section have a markedly suppressed ability to produce this pyrogen [454]. In the studies reviewed in Table 6–13, approximately half of the infants had fever. Hypothermia, which was mentioned in one study, occurred in 15% of the infants.

Fever is variably defined for newborns. A temperature of 38° C (100.4° F) measured rectally generally is accepted as the lower limit of the definition of fever. Although some clinical studies indicate that axillary [455], skin-mattress [456], and infrared tympanic membrane thermometry [457] are accurate and less dangerous than rectal measurements for obtaining core temperature, the reliability of these methods, particularly in febrile infants, has been questioned [458–460]. A study established that statistically significant differences are present between the rectal and axillary temperatures obtained in newborns during the first 4 days of life even with the same electronic temperature device [461]. The current method of choice for determining the presence of fever in neonates is a rectal temperature taken at a depth of 2 to 3 cm past the anal margin. In infants with suspected sepsis without fever, it has been shown that a difference between core (rectal) and skin (sole of the foot) temperature of more than 3.5° C can be a more useful indicator of infection than measurement of core temperature alone [453].

There is no study of temperatures in neonates that is prospective, assesses all infants (febrile and afebrile), includes rectal and axillary temperatures, includes preterm and term infants, and requires positive cultures of blood or other body fluids to define invasive bacterial infection. Voora and colleagues [462] observed 100 term infants in Chicago with an axillary or rectal temperature of equal to or greater than 37.8° C ($\geq$100.1° F) during the first 4 days of life, and Osborn and Bolus [463] conducted a retrospective review of 2656 term infants in Los Angeles. Both groups of investigators reported that temperature elevation in healthy term infants was uncommon. Approximately 1% of neonates born at term had at least one episode of fever, measured as equal to or greater than 37.8° C ($\geq$100.1° F) per axilla [462]. Temperature elevation infrequently was associated with systemic infection when a single evaluation occurred. None of 64 infants in these two studies who had a single episode of fever developed clinical evidence of systemic infection (cultures of blood or other body fluids were not obtained). By contrast, temperature elevation that was sustained for more than 1 hour frequently was associated with infection. Of seven infants with sustained fever in the study by Osborn and Bolus [463], five had proven bacterial or viral infections. Of 65 infants reported by Voora and colleagues [462], 10 had documented systemic bacterial disease. Temperature elevation without other signs of infection was infrequent. Only one infant (with cytomegalovirus infection) of the five Los Angeles infants had fever without other signs. Only 2 infants (with bacteremia caused by E. coli or GBS) of the 10 Chicago infants with fever and proven bacterial disease had no other signs of infection.

In addition to infection, fever may be caused by an elevation in ambient temperature, dehydration, retained blood or extensive hematoma, and damage to the temperature-regulating mechanisms of the CNS. Less common noninfectious causes of fever are hyperthyroidism, cystic fibrosis, familial dysautonomia, and ectodermal dysplasia. When thermoregulatory devices that monitor and modify infant temperature are introduced, the use of fever or hypothermia as a diagnostic sign of sepsis sometimes is impeded.

RESPIRATORY DISTRESS

Signs of respiratory distress, including tachypnea, grunting, flaring of the alae nasi, intercostal retractions, rales, and decreased breath sounds, are common and important findings in the infant suspected to have sepsis. Respiratory distress syndrome and aspiration pneumonia must be considered in the differential diagnosis. Apnea is one of the most specific signs of sepsis, but usually occurs in the setting of a fulminant onset or after other nonspecific signs have been present for hours or days. Clinical signs of cardiovascular dysfunction, including tachycardia, arrhythmia, and poor peripheral perfusion, that occur in the absence of congenital heart disease are sensitive and specific signs of sepsis.

JAUNDICE

Jaundice is present in approximately one third of infants with sepsis and is a common finding in infants with urinary tract infection [353,464–468]. It can develop suddenly or subacutely and occasionally is the only sign of sepsis. Jaundice usually decreases after institution of appropriate antimicrobial therapy. It occurs in septic infants regardless of the type of bacterial pathogen.

ORGANOMEGALY

The liver edge is palpable in premature infants and can extend to 2 cm below the costal margin in healthy term infants. Ashkenazi and colleagues [469] evaluated liver size in healthy term infants examined within 24 hours of birth and again at 72 to 96 hours. Measurements ranged from 1.6 to 4 cm below the costal margin, and there was no significant difference between early and late examinations. Reiff and Osborn [470] suggested that determination of liver span by palpation and percussion is a more reliable technique than identifying the liver projection below the costal margin. Hepatomegaly is a common sign of in utero infections and of some noninfectious conditions, such as cardiac failure and metabolic diseases, including galactosemia and glycogen storage disease. Tender hepatomegaly can be a sign of bacterial liver abscess in neonates, a potential complication of misplaced central umbilical catheters [125]. Splenomegaly is less common than hepatomegaly and infrequently is mentioned in reports of bacterial sepsis of the newborn [471].

Lymph nodes infrequently are palpable in newborns unless they are infected with viruses, spirochetes, or protozoa. Bamji and coworkers [472] examined 214 healthy neonates in New York and identified palpable nodes at one or more sites in one third of the infants. Embree and Muriithi [473] examined 66 healthy term Kenyan neonates during the first 24 hours of life and found palpable axillary nodes (27.7%), but no palpable inguinal nodes. Adenopathy is a sign of congenital infection caused by rubella virus, T. gondii, T. pallidum, and enteroviruses. Adenitis can occur in drainage areas involved with bacterial soft tissue infection. Although adenopathy is not an important sign of systemic bacterial infection in neonates, cellulitis-adenitis syndrome, a rare clinical manifestation of late-onset group B streptococcal infection in infants, is a condition in which local inflammation can be the only initial sign of sepsis that can include concurrent meningitis [474–476].

GASTROINTESTINAL SIGNS

Gastrointestinal disturbances, including poor feeding, regurgitation or vomiting, large gastric residuals in infants fed by tube, diarrhea, and abdominal distention, are common and significant early signs of sepsis. The first indications of illness can be a change in feeding pattern or lethargy during feedings.

SKIN LESIONS

Various skin lesions can accompany bacteremia, including cellulitis, abscess, petechiae, purpuric lesions, sclerema, erythema multiforme, and ecthyma. These lesions are described in Chapter 10.

NEUROLOGIC SIGNS

The onset of meningitis in the neonate is accompanied by identical signs of illness as observed in infants with sepsis. Meningitis can be heralded by increasing irritability, alteration in consciousness, poor tone, tremors, lip smacking, or twitching of facial muscles or an extremity. Seizures were present in 31% of the infants reviewed in Table 6–14, but Volpe [350] identified seizures, in many cases subtle, in 75% of infants with bacterial meningitis. Approximately half of the seizures were focal, and at their onset, they usually were subtle. Focal signs, including hemiparesis; horizontal deviation of the eyes; and cranial nerve deficits involving the seventh, third, and sixth cranial nerves, in that order of frequency, can be identified [350]. Because cranial sutures in the neonate are open and allow for expansion of the intracranial contents and for increasing head size, a full or bulging fontanelle can be absent [448,477]. The presence of a bulging fontanelle is not related to gestational age. Among 72 newborns with gram-negative enteric bacillary meningitis, a bulging fontanelle was seen in 18% of term infants and 17% of preterm infants [23]. Nuchal rigidity, an important sign in older children and adults, is uncommon in neonates [23].

In addition to the physical findings observed in infants with meningitis, several investigators have reported the occurrence of fluid and electrolyte abnormalities associated with inappropriate antidiuretic hormone secretion, including hyponatremia, decreased urine output, and increased weight gain [432,438]. Occasionally, the onset of meningitis has been followed by a transient or persistent diabetes insipidus [477].

Early clinical signs of brain abscess in the newborn are subtle and frequently unnoticed by the physician or parent. Presenting signs include signs of increased intracranial pressure (e.g., emesis, bulging fontanelle, enlarging head size, separated sutures), focal cerebral signs (e.g., hemiparesis, focal seizures), and acute signs of meningitis. Of six infants with brain abscesses described by Hoffman and colleagues [429], two were febrile, two had seizures, and five had increased head size. Other focal infections in the nervous system include pneumococcal endophthalmitis in a neonate with meningitis [478], pseudomonal endophthalmitis in a

premature neonate with late-onset sepsis [479], and epidural abscess caused by *S. aureus* in 3-week-old [480], 4-week-old [481], and 7-week-old infants [482].

DIAGNOSIS

The diagnosis of systemic infection in the newborn is difficult to establish on the basis of clinical findings alone. A history of one or more risk factors for neonatal sepsis associated with the pregnancy and delivery often is associated with early-onset infection, but there can be no clues before the onset of subtle signs in a term infant who develops late-onset sepsis. The extensive list of conditions that must be considered in the differential diagnosis for the various signs that are associated with sepsis or meningitis and noninfectious conditions is presented in Table 6–15. Laboratory tests to assist in the diagnosis of sepsis are discussed in Chapter 36.

MATERNAL HISTORY

Many infants, particularly infants born prematurely, who develop systemic infection just before or shortly after delivery are born to women who have one or more risk features for early-onset sepsis in their infants. These features include preterm labor, premature rupture of the membranes at any time during gestation, prolonged rupture of membranes, chorioamnionitis, prolonged labor, intrauterine scalp electrodes, and traumatic delivery. The following features are identified by the American College of Obstetrics and Gynecology (ACOG) as the basis for identification of women who should receive intrapartum antibiotic prophylaxis to prevent early-onset group B streptococcal disease:[483,484]

1. Antenatal colonization with GBS
2. Unknown group B streptococcal colonization status and
    a. Preterm labor (<37 weeks' gestation)
    b. Fever during labor (defined by temperature of ≥38° C [≥100.4° F])
    c. Rupture of membranes for 18 or more hours
3. Urine culture that grows GBS during the current pregnancy
4. Prior delivery of a neonate with invasive group B streptococcal infection

MICROBIOLOGIC TECHNIQUES

Isolation of microorganisms from a usually sterile site, such as the blood, CSF, urine, other body fluids (e.g., peritoneal, pleural, joint, middle ear), or tissues (e.g., bone marrow, liver, spleen) remains the most valid method of diagnosing bacterial sepsis. Infectious agents cultured from the nose, throat, external auditory canal, skin, umbilicus, or stool indicate colonization and can include organisms that cause sepsis, but isolation of a microorganism from these sites does not establish invasive systemic infection. The limited sensitivity, specificity, and predictive value of body surface cultures in the NICU was documented using a database of 24,584 cultures from 3371 infants by Evans and colleagues [485]. These investigators strongly discouraged the use of cultures from these sites in diagnosing neonatal sepsis because of their poor correlation with the pathogen in the blood and their expense.

Culture of Blood

Isolation of a pathogenic microorganism from the blood or other body fluid is the only method to establish definitively the diagnosis of neonatal bacteremia/sepsis.

Methods

Technology has evolved from manually read, broth-based methods to continuously monitored, automated blood culture systems that use enriched media for processing of blood culture specimens. Automated and semiautomated systems for continuous blood culture monitoring are standard in laboratories in the United States [486–488]. Before the widespread use of automated blood-culturing systems, direct plating was the most often employed method of isolating bacteria. Positive cultures were recognized by growth of colonies on agar and provided a rapid means to obtaining quantitative blood culture results from pediatric patients. St. Geme and colleagues [489] used this technique to investigate the distinction of sepsis from contamination in cultures of blood growing CoNS.

Time to Detection of a Positive Blood Culture

Bacterial growth is evident in most cultures of blood from neonates within 48 hours [490–492]. With use of conventional culture techniques and subculture at 4 and 14 hours, only 4 of 105 cultures that had positive results (one GBS and three S. aureus) required more than 48 hours of incubation [491]. By use of a radiometric technique (BACTEC 460), 40 of 41 cultures that grew GBS and 15 of 16 cultures with E. coli were identified within 24 hours [492]. Controlled experiments suggest that delayed entry of the collected blood culture bottle into the automated blood culture machine can significantly prolong the time to positivity for common newborn pathogens [493].

Optimal Number of Cultures

The optimal number of cultures to obtain for the diagnosis of bacteremia in the newborn is uncertain. A single blood culture from an infant with sepsis can be negative, but most studies suggest a sensitivity of 90% or slightly more. Sprunt [494] suggested the use of two blood cultures "not primarily to increase the yield of organisms …" but to "minimize the insecurity and debates over the meaning of the findings." In a study by Struthers and colleagues [95], it was estimated that in 5% of neonates a second blood culture failed to substantiate the presence of CoNS leading to an 8% reduction in antibiotic use. In the high-risk neonate, there is no doubt the need to initiate therapy promptly can make this practice difficult.

Optimal Volume of Blood

The optimal volume of blood needed to detect bacteremia in neonates has not been determined. Neal and colleagues [495] evaluated the volume of neonatal blood submitted for culture by physicians who were unaware of the study and found that the mean blood volume per patient was 1.05 mL. Dietzman and coworkers [496] suggested that 0.2 mL of blood was sufficient to detect bacteremia caused by E. coli. The relationship between colony counts of E. coli from blood cultures from infants with sepsis and meningitis and mortality was evaluated. Meningitis occurred only in neonates with more than 1000 colonies of E. coli per milliliter of blood. These data of Dietzman and coworkers [496] are supported by experimental results indicating that common pediatric pathogens can be reliably recovered from 0.5 mL of blood even when cultured at blood-to-broth ratios of 1:100 [497,498]. Several more recent studies have found, however, that in the circumstance of low inoculum bacteremia (<10 colony-forming units/mL of blood), the collection of only 0.5 mL of blood proved inadequate for the reliable detection of common pathogens [499–502]. If one blood culture is to be collected before antimicrobial therapy is initiated, a volume of 1 mL or more seems to ensure the greatest sensitivity.

Cultures of Blood from Umbilical Vessels and Intravascular Catheters

Umbilical vessel and intravascular catheters are essential in the care of neonates in the NICU and are preferred blood culture sampling sites [503–505]. Results of cultures of blood obtained from indwelling umbilical or central venous catheters can present ambiguities in interpretation (e.g., contamination versus catheter colonization versus systemic infection). Obtaining blood cultures from a peripheral vessel and catheters in an ill-appearing neonate is useful in the interpretation of results. A prospective study of semiquantitative catheter tip cultures in a Brazilian NICU found that a cutoff point of approximately 100 colony-forming units was predictive of clinically significant catheter-related infections, of which CoNS accounted for 75% of cases [506].

Distinguishing Clinically Important Bacteremia from Blood Culture Contamination

The increased use of intravascular catheters in neonates has resulted in an increase in the incidence of bacteremia, particularly bacteremia caused by CoNS, and uncertainty regarding the significance of some results. Investigators have considered criteria based on clinical signs and microbiologic factors.

Yale investigators [6] used the following criteria to define the role of commensal organisms in neonatal sepsis: one major clinical sign, such as apnea, bradycardia, or core temperature greater than 38° C or less than 36.5° C documented at the time the blood culture was obtained, plus another blood culture positive for the same organism obtained within 24 hours of the first or an intravascular access device in place before major clinical signs occurred. Some microbiologic features can be useful in differentiating sepsis from contamination, as follows:

1. *Time to growth in conventional media*: The longer the time needed to detect growth (>2 to 3 days), the more likely that skin or intravascular line contamination was present.

2. *Number of cultures positive*: If peripheral and intra-vascular catheter specimens are positive, the presence of the organism in the blood is likely; if the catheter specimen alone is positive, intravascular line colonization may have occurred; if multiple cultures from an indwelling vascular catheter are positive, or if a single culture is positive and the patient has had a clinical deterioration, a bloodstream infection must be presumed.

3. *Organism type*: Organisms that are part of skin flora (e.g., diphtheroids, nonhemolytic streptococci, CoNS) suggest contamination in certain cases as described previously, whereas known bacterial pathogens must be considered to be associated with sepsis. Contamination is more likely when multiple species grow in one blood culture bottle, different species grow in two bottles, or only one of several cultures before or during antimicrobial therapy is positive.

4. *Clinical signs*: If the infant is well without use of antibiotics, growth of a commensal organism from a blood culture is more likely to be a contaminant.

In an attempt to resolve the question of sepsis versus contamination, investigators have used multiple-site blood cultures [507], comparisons of results of cultures of blood and cultures of skin at the venipuncture site [508], and quantitative blood cultures [491]. These techniques are of investigational interest, but the results do not suggest that any one is of sufficient value to be adopted for clinical practice. Healy and colleagues [509] suggest that isolation of CoNS of the same species or antimicrobial susceptibility from more than one blood culture or from one blood culture obtained from an indwelling catheter or a peripheral vessel and a normally sterile body site represents true infection if the patient is a premature infant with signs of clinical sepsis. At present, management of a sick premature infant, especially a very low birth weight infant, with a positive blood culture for CoNS requires that the organism be considered a pathogen and managed with appropriate antimicrobial agents. If the infant is well, the microbiologic results given earlier should be considered in the decision to continue or discontinue use of an antimicrobial agent. Another culture of blood should be obtained when the initial culture result is ambiguous.

Buffy-Coat Examination

The rapid diagnosis of bacteremia by identification of microorganisms in the buffy leukocyte layer of centrifuged blood is a method used for many years and has been evaluated for use in newborn infants [510–516]. By using Gram and methylene blue stains of the buffy-coat preparation, immediate and accurate information was obtained for 37 (77%) of 48 bacteremic, clinically septic infants in the four studies [511–513,515]. Positive results were found for gram-positive and gram-negative organisms. In contrast to findings reported for adult populations [517], there were no false-positive results among almost 200 infants with negative blood cultures. Failure to identify organisms was attributed to extreme neutropenia in several patients.

The large inoculum of microorganisms in the blood of neonates with sepsis most probably explains the excellent sensitivity of leukocyte smears. Smears can be positive with 50 colonies per milliliter of *S. aureus* in the peripheral blood; approximately 50% of neonates with *E. coli* bacteremia have higher concentrations [496]. *Candida* and *S. epidermidis* septicemia in young infants also have been diagnosed by this method [518–521]. Rodwell and associates reported that bacteria were identified in peripheral blood smears in 17 of 19 infants with septicemia; however, they [522] were able to identify bacteria in direct blood smears, however, for only 4 of 24 bacteremic neonates. It is likely that the disparity in these results reflects differences in patient populations or distribution of etiologic agents or both. Buffy-coat examination of blood smears has been infrequently used in laboratories since the introduction of automated systems for continuous blood culture monitoring.

Culture of Urine

Infants with sepsis can have a urinary tract origin or a concomitant urinary tract infection. The yield from culture of urine is low in early-onset sepsis and most often reflects metastatic spread to the bladder from the bacteremia, but in late-onset infection, the yield is substantially higher. Visser and Hall [523] found positive cultures of urine in only 1.6% of infants with early-onset sepsis compared with 7.4% of infants with late-onset sepsis. DiGeronimo [524] performed a chart review of 146 clinically septic infants who had cultures of blood and urine. Of 11 infants with positive blood cultures, only one infant with GBS bacteremia had a positive urine culture. These data suggest that cultures of urine yield very limited information about the source of infection in infants with signs of sepsis before age 7 days. In contrast, urine should be collected for culture from infants with suspected late-onset sepsis before initiation of antimicrobial therapy. The presence of elevated leukocyte counts ($\geq$10 per high-power field) in urine of infants less than 90 days of age is an accurate predictor of urinary tract infections complicated by bacteremia [525].

Because of the difficulty in collecting satisfactory clean-voided specimens of urine from newborns, bladder catheterization or suprapubic needle aspiration of bladder urine frequently is performed. These methods are simple and safe, and suprapubic bladder aspiration avoids the ambiguities inherent in urine obtained by other methods [526–528]. If a suprapubic aspirate cannot be performed for technical or medical reasons, catheterization is a satisfactory method of obtaining urine, although ambiguous results can occur because of contamination from the urethra, especially in very low birth weight neonates. Application of a clinical pain scoring system employing a blinded observer and video recording found suprapubic aspiration to produce more discomfort than transurethral catheterization in female and circumcised male infants younger than 2 months of age [529].

Cultures of Tracheal Aspirates and Pharynx

Because of the association of pneumonia and bacteremia, investigators have sought to determine the risk of sepsis on the basis of colonization of the upper respiratory tract.

Lau and Hey [530] found that among ventilated infants who became septic, the same organism usually was present in cultures of tracheal aspirate and blood. Growth of a bacterial pathogen from a tracheal aspirate culture does not predict which infants will develop sepsis, however. Similarly, cultures of the pharynx or trachea do not predict the causative organism in the blood of a neonate with clinical sepsis [531]. A review of the literature by Srinivasan and Vidyasagar [532] suggests endotracheal aspirates are of poor sensitivity (approximately 50%), modest specificity (approximately 80%), and poor positive predictive value. Unless the patient has a change in respiratory status documented clinically and radiographically, routine use of cultures from the pharynx or trachea provide low diagnostic yield and seem unjustified given their expense.

Diagnostic Needle Aspiration and Tissue Biopsy

Direct aspiration of tissues or body fluids through a needle or catheter is used for the diagnosis of a wide variety of infectious and noninfectious diseases [533]. Aspiration of an infectious focus in lung, pleural space, middle ear, pericardium, bones, joints, abscess, and other sites provides immediate and specific information to guide therapy. Biopsy of the liver or bone marrow can assist in diagnosing occult infections, but this rarely is necessary.

Autopsy Microbiology

Two factors must be considered in interpreting bacterial cultures obtained at autopsy: the frequent isolation of organisms usually considered to be nonpathogenic and the difficulty of isolating fastidious organisms such as anaerobic bacteria. To minimize these problems, it is important that specimens be collected with proper aseptic technique and as early as possible after death.

It is a common belief that organisms in the intestinal and respiratory tracts gain access to tissues after death, but it also is possible that bacteremia occurs shortly before death and is not a postmortem phenomenon. Eisenfeld and colleagues [534] identified the same organisms in specimens obtained before and within 2 hours after death. Confusion in the interpretation of results of bacteriologic cultures often is obviated by the review of slides prepared directly from tissues and fluids. If antimicrobial treatment was administered before death, organisms can be observed on a smear even though they are not viable. Pathogens would be expected to be present in significant numbers and accompanied by inflammatory cells, whereas contaminants or organisms that invade tissues after death, if they are seen, would be present in small numbers with no evidence of an inflammatory process [535,536].

Rapid Techniques for Detection of Bacterial Antigens in Body Fluid Specimens

In the 1970s, the limulus lysate assay for detection of endotoxin produced by gram-negative bacteria based on a gelation reaction between lysates of *Limulus* (horseshoe crab) amebocytes and bacterial endotoxin was investigated for diagnosis of neonatal meningitis with equivocal results [537–541]. Counterimmunoelectrophoresis also was used successfully for detecting the capsular polysaccharide antigens of various pathogenic bacteria, including *S. pneumoniae*, *N. meningitidis*, *H. influenzae*, and GBS (see Chapter 12) in CSF, serum, and urine. Less complex and more rapid detection methods have replaced these two assays.

Latex agglutination detection now is preferred because of its speed, simplicity, and greater sensitivity for selected organisms. Kits designed to detect cell wall or capsular or cell wall antigen released into body fluids are commercially available. Latex agglutination assays have been shown to be of potential benefit in early detection of bacterial antigens in CSF of patients with acute meningitis, which may be of increased importance in the era of intrapartum antibiotic prophylaxis and its potential interference with culture yield. Among the prevalent bacterial pathogens in neonatal infections, only GBS is routinely analyzed by latex agglutination. *N. meningitidis* group B shares a common capsular antigen, however, with the neonatal meningitis pathogen *E. coli* serotype K1, which should allow cross-identification of the latter using a meningococcal latex reagent [542]. The sensitivity of latex agglutination methods for identifying infants with group B streptococcal meningitis ranges from 73% to 100% for CSF and 75% to 84% for urine [543]. Possible cross-reactions have occurred when concentrated urine was tested. GBS cell wall antigen can occasionally cross-react with antigens from *S. pneumoniae*, CoNS, enterococci, and gram-negative enteric bacteria, including *P. mirabilis* and *E. cloacae*.

False-positive results in urine for a positive latex agglutination test for GBS often were caused by contamination of bag specimens of urine with the streptococci from rectal or vaginal colonization [544]. The poor specificity of GBS antigen detection methods used with urine led to the U.S. Food and Drug Administration (FDA) recommendation in 1996 that these methods not be employed except for testing of CSF and serum.

Lumbar Puncture and Examination of Cerebrospinal Fluid

Because meningitis can accompany sepsis with no clinical signs to differentiate between bacteremia alone and bacteremia with meningitis, a lumbar puncture should be considered for examination of CSF in any neonate before initiation of therapy. Of infants with sepsis, 15% have accompanying meningitis. The overall incidence of bacterial meningitis is less than 1 case per 1000 infants, but the incidence for low birth weight (<2500 g) infants or premature infants is severalfold higher than the incidence for term infants. Data from NICHD Neonatal Research Network surveyed 9641 very low birth weight infants who survived 3 days or more: 30% had one or more lumbar punctures, and 5% of infants who had lumbar puncture had late-onset meningitis [545]. For the diagnosis of some noninfectious CNS diseases in neonates (e.g., intracranial hemorrhage), cranial ultrasonography and, occasionally, computed tomography (CT) or magnetic resonance imaging (MRI) are the techniques of choice. Among infants with hypoxic-ischemic encephalopathy, lumbar puncture should be considered only for infants in whom meningitis is a possible diagnosis.

Some investigators suggest that too many healthy term infants have a diagnostic evaluation for sepsis, including lumbar puncture, based solely on maternal risk features and that lumbar puncture rarely provides clinically useful information. Other investigators have questioned the role of lumbar puncture on admission in the premature infant with respiratory distress and found that the yield of the procedure is very low [546–548]. Of more than 1700 infants with respiratory distress syndrome evaluated for meningitis, bacterial pathogens were identified in CSF of only 4. Three of the four infants with meningitis were bacteremic with the same pathogen [548].

A large, retrospective study assessed the value of lumbar puncture in the evaluation of suspected sepsis during the first week of life and found that bacteria were isolated from 9 of 728 CSF specimens, but only one infant was believed to have bacterial meningitis [549]. Fielkow and colleagues [550] found no cases of meningitis among 284 healthy-appearing infants who had lumbar puncture performed because of maternal risk factors, whereas 2.5% of 799 neonates with clinical signs of sepsis had meningitis regardless of maternal risk factors. The value of lumbar puncture has been established for infants with clinical signs of sepsis, but lumbar puncture performed because of maternal risk features in a healthy-appearing neonate is less likely to be useful.

The considerations are quite different for very low birth weight neonates (400 to- 1500 g), as documented in a study by Stoll and colleagues [545] performed through NICHD Neonatal Research Network. One third (45 of 134) of these high-risk neonates with meningitis has negative blood cultures. Lower gestational age and prior sepsis were important risk factors for development of meningitis, which carried a significant risk of mortality compared with uninfected infants (23% versus 2%). These results indicate the critical importance of lumbar puncture and suggest that meningitis may be significantly underdiagnosed in very low birth weight infants [545].

Method of Lumbar Puncture

Lumbar puncture is more difficult to perform in neonates than in older children or adults; traumatic lumbar punctures resulting in blood in CSF are more frequent, and care must be taken in the infant who is in respiratory distress. Gleason and colleagues [551] suggested that the procedure be performed with the infant in the upright position or, if performed in the flexed position, be modified with neck extension. Pinheiro and associates [552] evaluated the role of locally administered lidocaine before lumbar puncture and found that the local anesthesia decreased the degree of struggling of the infant. Other investigators concluded, however, that local anesthesia failed to influence physiologic changes in the neonate undergoing lumbar puncture [553]. Fiser and colleagues [554] suggested that the administration of oxygen before lumbar puncture prevents most hypoxemia resulting from this procedure in infants.

The physician can choose to withhold or delay lumbar puncture in some infants who would be placed at risk for cardiac or respiratory compromise by the procedure. Weisman and colleagues [555] observed that transient hypoxemia occurred during lumbar puncture performed in the lateral position (i.e., left side with hips flexed to place knees to chest), but occurred less frequently when the infant was in a sitting position or modified lateral position (i.e., left side with hips flexed to 90 degrees). Reasons for withholding lumbar puncture in older children, such as signs of increased intracranial pressure, signs of a bleeding disorder, and infection in the area that the needle would traverse to obtain CSF, are less likely to be concerns in the neonate.

Ventricular puncture should be considered in an infant with meningitis who does not respond clinically or microbiologically to antimicrobial therapy because of ventriculitis, especially with obstruction between the ventricles and lumbar CSF. Ventriculitis is diagnosed on the basis of elevated white blood cell count (>100 cells/mm³) or identification of bacteria by culture, Gram stain, or antigen detection. Ventricular puncture is a potentially hazardous procedure and should be performed only by a physician who is an expert in the technique.

If a Lumbar Puncture Is Not Performed

Is it sufficient to culture only blood and urine for the diagnosis of neonatal bacterial meningitis? Visser and Hall [556] showed that the blood culture was sterile when CSF yielded a pathogen in 6 (15%) of 39 infants with bacterial meningitis. Franco and colleagues [557] reported that in 26 neonates with bacterial meningitis, only 13 had a positive blood culture. In surveys from two large databases—NICUs managed by the Pediatrix Medical Group [558] and NICHD Neonatal Research Network [545]—results were similar: One third of infants at 34 or more weeks estimated gestation with meningitis and one third of very low birth weight neonates with meningitis had negative blood cultures. A significant number of infants with meningitis do not have this diagnosis established unless lumbar puncture is performed.

Ideally, lumbar puncture should be performed before the initiation of antimicrobial therapy, but there are alternative strategies for infants who may not tolerate the procedure. If the physician believes that lumbar puncture would endanger the infant with presumed sepsis and meningitis, therapy should be initiated after blood (and urine for late-onset illness) is obtained for culture. After the infant is stabilized, lumbar puncture should be performed. Even several days after the start of antibiotic therapy, CSF pleocytosis and abnormal CSF chemistry assays usually should identify the presence or absence of an inflammatory reaction, although CSF culture may be sterile.

Examination of Cerebrospinal Fluid

The cell content and chemistry of CSF of healthy newborn infants differ from those of older infants, children, and adults (Table 6–16). The values vary widely during the first weeks of life, and the normal range must be considered in evaluation of CSF in infants suspected to have meningitis [559–568]. The cell content in CSF of a neonate is higher than in older infants. Polymorphonuclear leukocytes often are present in CSF of normal newborns,

TABLE 6–16 Hematologic and Chemical Characteristics of Cerebrospinal Fluid in Healthy Term Newborns: Results of Selected Studies

Study (Year)	No. Patients	Age (Days)	White Blood Cells (mm³)*	Neutrophils (mm³)*	Glucose (mg/dL)*	Protein (mg/dL)*
Naidoo[559] (1968)	135	1	12 (0-42)	7 (0-26)	48 (38-64)	73 (40-148)
	20	7	3 (0-9)	2 (0-5)	55 (48-62)	47 (27-65)
Sarff[560] (1976)	87	Most <7	8.2 ± 7.1, median 5 (0-32)	61	52 (34-119)	90 (20-170)
Bonadio[561] (1992)	35	0-4 wk	11 ± 10.4, median 8.5	0.4 ± 1.4, median 0.15	46 ± 10.3	84 ± 45.1
	40	4-8 wk	7.1 ± 9.2, median 4.5	0.2 ± 0.4, median 0	46 ± 10	59 ± 25.3
Ahmed[562] (1996)	108	0-30	7.3 ± 13.9, median 4	0.8 ± 6.2, median 0	51.2 ± 12.9	64.2 ± 24.2

(*Expressed as mean with range (number in parentheses) or ± standard deviation unless otherwise specified.)
Data from Ahmed A, et al. Cerebrospinal fluid values in the term neonate. Pediatr Infect Dis J 15:298, 1996.

TABLE 6–17 Hematologic and Chemical Characteristics of Cerebrospinal Fluid in Healthy Very Low Birth Weight Newborns

Birth Weight (g)	Age (Days)	No. Samples	Red Blood Cells (mm³)*	White Blood Cells (mm³)*	Neutrophils (%)*	Glucose (mg/dL)*	Protein (mg/dL)*
<1000	0-7	6	335 (0-1780)	3 (1-8)	11 (0-50)	70 (41-89)	162 (115-222)
	8-28	17	1465 (0-19,050)	4 (0-14)	8 (0-66)	68 (33-217)	159 (95-370)
	29-84	15	808 (0-6850)	4 (0-11)	2 (0-36)	49 (29-90)	137 (76-260)
1000-1500	0-7	8	407 (0-2450)	4 (1-10)	4 (0-28)	74 (50-96)	136 (85-176)
	8-28	14	1101 (0-9750)	7 (0-44)	10 (0-60)	59 (39-109)	137 (54-227)
	29-84	11	661 (0-3800)	8 (0-23)	11 (0-48)	47 (31-76)	122 (45-187)

*Expressed as mean with range (number in parentheses) or +/- standard deviation unless otherwise specified.
Data from Rodriguez AF, Kaplan SL, Mason EO. Cerebrospinal fluid values in the very low birth weight infant. J Pediatr 116:971, 1990.

whereas more than a single polymorphonuclear neutrophil in CSF of older infants or children should be considered abnormal. Similarly, protein concentration is higher in preterm than in term infants and highest in very low birth weight infants (Table 6–17) [568].

In term infants, total protein concentration decreases with age, reaching values of healthy older infants (<40 mg/dL) before the third month of life. In low birth weight infants or preterm infants, CSF leukocyte and protein concentrations decline with postnatal age, but may not decline to normal values for older infants for several months after birth [569]. CSF glucose levels are lower in neonates than in older infants and can be related to lower concentrations of glucose observed in blood. Healthy term infants may have blood glucose levels of 30 mg/dL, and preterm infants may have levels of 20 mg/dL [568]. The physiologic basis for the higher concentration of protein and the increased numbers of white blood cells in CSF of healthy, uninfected preterm and term infants is unknown. Explanations that have been offered include possible mechanical irritation of the meninges during delivery and increased permeability of the blood-brain barrier.

In nearly all of the studies of CSF in newborns, "normal" or "healthy" refers to the absence of clinical manifestations at the time of examination of CSF. Only the study by Ahmed and colleagues [562] included in the definition of normal the absence of viral infection, defined by lack of evidence of cytopathic effect in five cell lines and negative polymerase chain reaction for enteroviruses. None of the studies included information about the health of the infant after the newborn period. It now is recognized that infants with congenital infections, such as rubella, cytomegalovirus infection, toxoplasmosis, acquired immunodeficiency syndrome (AIDS), and syphilis, can have no signs of illness during the newborn period. Observations of these infants over the course of months or years can reveal abnormalities that are inapparent at birth. Until more data are available, it seems prudent to observe carefully infants with white blood cells greater than 20 per mm³ or protein level greater than 100 mg/dL in CSF and, if clinical signs indicate, to obtain paired serum samples for serologic assays and viral cultures from body fluids or tissues for congenital CNS infections (i.e., *T. gondii*, rubella virus, cytomegalovirus, herpes simplex virus, human immunodeficiency virus [HIV], and *T. pallidum*).

In newborns with bacterial meningitis, there can be thousands of white blood cells in CSF, and polymorphonuclear leukocytes predominate early in the course of the disease [20,560]. The number of white blood cells in CSF can vary greatly in infants with gram-negative and gram-positive meningitis. The median number of cells per cubic millimeter in CSF of 98 infants with gram-negative meningitis was more than 2000 (range 6 to 40,000), whereas the median number of cells per cubic millimeter in 21 infants with group B streptococcal meningitis was less than 100 (range 8 to >10,000) [560]. The concentration of glucose in CSF usually is less than two thirds of the concentration in blood. The concentration of protein can be low (<30 mg/dL) or very high (>1000 mg/dL). CSF parameters observed in the healthy term neonate can overlap with those observed in the infant with meningitis.

A Gram stain smear of CSF should be examined for bacteria, and appropriate media should be inoculated with the CSF specimen. Sarff and colleagues [560] detected organisms in Gram stain smears of CSF in 83% of infants with group B streptococcal meningitis and in 78% of infants with gram-negative meningitis. After initiation of appropriate antimicrobial therapy, gram-positive bacteria usually clear from CSF within 36 hours, whereas in some patients with meningitis caused by gram-negative enteric bacilli, cultures can remain positive for many days [567].

Microorganisms can be isolated from CSF that has normal white blood cell and chemistry test values. Visser and Hall [556] reported normal CSF parameters (cell count <25; protein level <200 mg/dL) in 6 (15%) of 39 infants with culture-proven meningitis. Subsequent examination of CSF identified an increase in the number of cells and in the protein level. Presumably, the initial lumbar puncture was performed early in the course of meningitis before an inflammatory response occurred. Other investigators reported isolation of enterovirus [570] and S. pneumoniae [571] from the CSF of neonates in the absence of pleocytosis.

Identification of bacteremia without meningitis defined by the absence of pleocytosis or isolation of a pathogen from culture of CSF can be followed by meningeal inflammation on subsequent examinations. Sarman and colleagues [572] identified six infants with gram-negative bacteremia and initial normal CSF who developed evidence of meningeal inflammation 18 to 59 hours after the first examination. Although the investigators suggest that a diagnosis of gram-negative bacteremia in the neonate warrants repeat lumbar puncture to identify the optimal duration of therapy, this recommendation could be broadened to include all infants with bacteremia and initial negative studies of CSF. Dissemination of the organisms from the blood to the meninges can occur after the first lumbar puncture before sterilization of the blood by appropriate antimicrobial therapy occurs. This dissemination is especially likely to occur in neonates with intense bacteremia where sterilization by β-lactam agents (i.e., third-generation cephalosporins) depends on the inoculum.

Smith and colleagues [573] performed a large cohort study of CSF parameters in preterm neonates with meningitis. Analysis of first lumbar puncture of 4632 neonates less than 34 weeks' gestation found significant differences in culture-proven meningitis cases versus controls in CSF leukocyte count (110 cells/mm³ versus 6 cells/mm³), total protein (217 mg/dL versus 130 mg/dL), and glucose (43 mg/dL versus 49 mg/dL). The sensitivity for predicting meningitis was only 71%, however, for CSF leukocyte count greater than 25 cells/mm³, 61% for CSF protein greater than 170 mg/dL, and 32% for CSF glucose less than 24 mg/dL. The positive predictive value for each of these parameters was low (4% to 10%), emphasizing the critical need for CSF culture to establish the diagnosis of meningitis. In terms of excluding meningitis, a normal CSF protein was the most useful parameter because 96% of premature neonates with meningitis had CSF protein greater than 90 mg/dL [573].

Investigators have sought a sensitive and specific CSF metabolic determinant of bacterial meningitis with little success. Among products that have been evaluated and found to be inadequate to distinguish bacterial meningitis from other neurologic disease (including cerebroventricular hemorrhage and asphyxia) are γ-aminobutyric acid [574], lactate dehydrogenase [575], and creatine kinase brain isoenzyme [576]. Cyclic-3',5'-adenosine monophosphate was elevated in CSF of neonates with bacterial meningitis compared with CSF of infants who had nonbacterial meningitis or a control group [577]. Elevated CSF concentrations of C-reactive protein have been reported for infants older than 4 weeks with bacterial meningitis [578]; however, the test was found to be of no value in neonates [579,580]. Current investigations of the proinflammatory cytokines interleukin-6 and interleukin-8 indicate that there is a cytokine response in CSF after birth asphyxia and that these assays are not useful in detecting infants with meningitis [581,582].

Traumatic Lumbar Puncture

A traumatic lumbar puncture can result in blood in CSF and can complicate the interpretation of the results for CSF white blood cell count and chemistries. Schwersenski and colleagues [549] found that 13.8% of 712 CSF specimens obtained during the first week of life were bloody and that an additional 14.5% were considered inadequate for testing.

If the total number of white blood cells compared with the number of red blood cells exceeds the value for whole blood, the presence of CSF pleocytosis is suggested. Some investigators have found that the observed white blood cell counts in bloody CSF were lower than would be predicted based on the ratio of white blood cells to red blood cells in peripheral blood; the white blood cells lyse more rapidly than red blood cells, or the number of white blood cells is decreased for other reasons [583–586]. Several formulas have been used in an attempt to interpret cytologic findings in CSF contaminated by blood [587–589]. None of the corrections applied to bloody CSF can be used with confidence, however, for excluding meningitis in the neonate [590–592]. In a cohort study of lumbar punctures performed at 150 neonatal units from 1997-2004, 39.5% (2519 of 6374) were traumatic, and 50 of these infants were found to have meningitis by culture. The authors found that adjustment of the leukocyte count to account for blood contamination resulted in loss of sensitivity and only marginal gain in specificity, and would not aid in the diagnosis of bacterial (or fungal) meningitis [593].

Protein in CSF usually is elevated after a traumatic lumbar puncture because of the presence of red blood cells. It has been estimated in older children and adults that an increase of 1 mg/dL in CSF protein occurs for every 1000 red blood cells/μL. The concentration of glucose does not seem to be altered by blood from a traumatic lumbar puncture; a low CSF glucose concentration should be considered an important finding even when associated with a traumatic lumbar puncture.

Because a "bloody tap" is difficult to interpret, it may be valuable to repeat the lumbar puncture 24 to 48 hours later. If the results of the second lumbar puncture reveal a normal white blood cell count, bacterial meningitis can be excluded. Even if performed without trauma or apparent bleeding, CSF occasionally can be ambiguous because white blood cells can be elicited by the irritant effect of blood in CSF.

Brain Abscess

Brain abscess is a rare entity in the neonate, usually complicating meningitis caused by certain gram-negative bacilli. CSF in an infant with a brain abscess can show a pleocytosis of a few hundred cells with a mononuclear predominance and an elevated protein level. Bacteria may not be seen by Gram stain of CSF if meningitis is not present. Sudden clinical deterioration and the appearance of many cells (>1000/mm^3), with most polymorphonuclear cells, suggest rupture of the abscess into CSF.

LABORATORY AIDS

Historically, aids in the diagnosis of systemic and focal infection in the neonate include peripheral white blood cell and differential counts, platelet counts, acute-phase reactants, blood chemistries, histopathology of the placenta and umbilical cord, smears of gastric or tracheal aspirates, and diagnostic imaging studies. New assays for diagnosis of early-onset sepsis, including serum concentrations of neutrophil CD 11b [594], granulocyte colony-stimulating factor [595], interleukin receptor antagonist [596], interleukin-6 [597–599], procalcitonin [600–602], serum amyloid A [603], and prohepcidin [604], show promise for increased sensitivity and specificity compared with other laboratory assessments, such as white blood cell count, absolute neutrophil count, and acute-phase reactants. Proinflammatory cytokines, including interleukin-1, interleukin-6, and tumor necrosis factor-α, have been identified in serum and CSF in infants after perinatal asphyxia, raising doubts about the specificity of some of these markers [581,582,605,606]. Mehr and Doyle [607] reviewed the more recent literature on cytokines as aids in the diagnosis of neonatal bacterial sepsis. These assays and procedures are discussed in detail in Chapter 36.

Attention has focused more recently on the use of real-time polymerase chain reaction technologies, often based on the 16S ribosomal RNA sequence of leading pathogens, as a tool for the accelerated culture-independent diagnosis of neonatal sepsis. Compared with the gold standard of blood culture, the evaluation of sensitivity and specificity of PCR technologies and their consequent clinical utility has ranged from equivocal [608,609] to highly promising [610,611]. Continued rapid advances in nucleic acid–based diagnostics are certain to be explored in this important clinical arena.

MANAGEMENT

If the maternal history or infant clinical signs suggest the possibility of neonatal sepsis, blood and CSF (all infants) and cultures of urine and other clinically evident focal sites should be collected (all infants with suspected late-onset infection). If respiratory abnormalities are apparent or respiratory status has changed, a radiograph of the chest should be performed. Because the clinical manifestations of sepsis can be subtle, the progression of the disease can be rapid, and the mortality rate remains high compared with mortality for older infants with serious bacterial infection, presumptive treatment should be initiated promptly. Many infants who have a clinical course typical of bacterial sepsis are treated empirically because of the imperfect sensitivity of a single blood culture in the diagnosis of sepsis.

CHOICE OF ANTIMICROBIAL AGENTS
Initial Therapy for Presumed Sepsis

The choice of antimicrobial agents for the treatment of suspected sepsis is based on knowledge of the prevalent organisms responsible for neonatal sepsis by age of onset and hospital setting and on their patterns of antimicrobial susceptibility. Initial therapy for the infant who develops clinical signs of sepsis during the first few days of life (early-onset disease) must include agents active against gram-positive cocci, particularly GBS, other streptococci, and *L. monocytogenes*, and gram-negative enteric bacilli. Treatment of the infant who becomes septic while in the nursery after age 6 days (late-onset disease) must include therapy for hospital-acquired organisms, such as *S. aureus*, gram-negative enteric bacilli, CoNS (in very low birth weight infants), and occasionally *P. aeruginosa*, and for maternally acquired etiologic agents.

GBS continue to exhibit significant in vitro susceptibility to penicillins and cephalosporins. Of 3813 case isolates in active population-based surveillance by the CDC from 1996-2003, all were sensitive to penicillin, ampicillin, cefazolin, and vancomycin [612]. New reports in the United States and Japan have identified GBS strains with reduced β-lactam susceptibility, however, and first-step mutations in the PBPx2 protein reminiscent of the emergence of β-lactam resistance in pneumococci decades ago [613,614]. In the CDC surveillance, GBS resistance to clindamycin (15%) and erythromycin (30%) also was noted to be increasing [612].

In vitro studies [615–617] and experimental animal models of bacteremia [618,619] indicate that the bactericidal activity of ampicillin and penicillin against GBS and *L. monocytogenes* is enhanced by the addition of gentamicin (synergy). Some physicians prefer to continue the combination of ampicillin and gentamicin for 48 to 72 hours, but when GBS is identified as the etiologic agent, the drug of choice for therapy is penicillin administered intravenously for the remainder of the treatment regimen. There are no clinical data to indicate that continuing an aminoglycoside in combination with a penicillin after 72 hours results in more rapid recovery or improved outcome for infected neonates (see Chapter 12).

Most strains of *S. aureus* that cause disease in neonates produce β-lactamase and are resistant to penicillin G and ampicillin. Many of these organisms are susceptible to penicillinase-resistant penicillins, such as nafcillin, and to first-generation cephalosporins. Methicillin-resistant staphylococci that are resistant to other penicillinase-resistant penicillins and cephalosporins have been encountered in many nurseries in the United States. Antimicrobial susceptibility patterns must be monitored by surveillance of staphylococcal strains causing infection and disease in each NICU. Bacterial resistance must be considered whenever staphylococcal disease is suspected or confirmed in a patient, and empirical vancomycin therapy should be initiated until the susceptibility pattern of the organism is known. Virtually all staphylococcal strains isolated from neonates have been susceptible to vancomycin. Synergistic activity is provided by the combination of an aminoglycoside (see Chapter 14). Vancomycin-resistant and glycopeptide-resistant *S. aureus* has been reported from Japan and the United States, but none of these strains has been isolated from neonates.

CoNS can cause systemic infection in very low birth weight infants and in neonates with or without devices such as an intravascular catheter or a ventriculoperitoneal shunt. Vancomycin is the drug of choice for treatment of serious CoNS infections. If daily cultures from an indwelling device continue to grow CoNS, removal of the foreign material probably is necessary to cure the infection.

Enterococcus species are only moderately susceptible to penicillin and highly resistant to cephalosporins. Optimal antimicrobial therapy for neonatal infections caused by *Enterococcus* includes ampicillin or vancomycin in addition to an aminoglycoside, typically gentamicin or tobramycin.

L. monocytogenes is susceptible to penicillin and ampicillin and resistant to cephalosporins. Ampicillin is the preferred agent for treating *L. monocytogenes*, although an aminoglycoside can be continued in combination with ampicillin if the patient has meningitis. Specific management of *L. monocytogenes* infection is discussed in Chapter 13.

The choice of antibiotic therapy for infections caused by gram-negative bacilli depends on the pattern of susceptibility for these isolates in the nursery that cares for the neonate. These patterns vary by hospital or community and by time within the same institution or community. Although isolates from neonates should be monitored to determine the emergence of new strains with unique antimicrobial susceptibility patterns, the general pattern of antibiotic susceptibility in the hospital is a good guide to initial therapy for neonates. Aminoglycosides, including gentamicin, tobramycin, netilmicin, and amikacin, are highly active in vitro against virtually all isolates of *E. coli*, *P. aeruginosa*, *Enterobacter* species, *Klebsiella* species, and *Proteus* species.

Role of Third-Generation Cephalosporins and Carbapenems

The third-generation cephalosporins, cefotaxime, ceftriaxone, and ceftazidime, possess attractive features for therapy for bacterial sepsis and meningitis in newborns, including excellent in vitro activity against GBS and *E. coli* and other gram-negative enteric bacilli. Ceftazidime is highly active in vitro against *P. aeruginosa*. None of the cephalosporins is active against *L. monocytogenes* or *Enterococcus*, and activity against *S. aureus* is variable. The third-generation cephalosporins provide concentrations of drug at most sites of infection that greatly exceed the minimum inhibitory concentrations of susceptible pathogens, and there is no dose-related toxicity. Clinical and microbiologic results of studies of sepsis and meningitis in neonates suggest that the third-generation cephalosporins are comparable to the traditional regimens of penicillin and an aminoglycoside (see Chapter 37) [620–623]. Because ceftriaxone can displace bilirubin from serum albumin, it is not recommended for use in neonates unless it is the only agent effective against the bacterial pathogen. Meropenem is a broad-spectrum carbapenem antibiotic with extended-spectrum antimicrobial activity including *P. aeruginosa* and excellent CSF penetration that appears safe and efficacious in the neonate for treatment of most nosocomial gram-negative pathogens [624].

The rapid development of resistance of gram-negative enteric bacilli when cefotaxime is used extensively for presumptive therapy for neonatal sepsis suggests that extensive use of third-generation or fourth-generation cephalosporins can lead to rapid emergence of drug-resistant bacteria in nurseries [625]. Also of concern, studies have identified a principal risk factor for development of invasive infection with *Candida* and other fungi in preterm neonates to be extended therapy with third-generation cephalosporins [626,627]. Empirical use of cefotaxime in neonates should be restricted to infants with evidence of meningitis or with gram-negative sepsis. Continued cefotaxime therapy should be limited to infants with gram-negative meningitis caused by susceptible organisms or infants with ampicillin-resistant enteric infections [628].

CURRENT PRACTICE

The combination of ampicillin and an aminoglycoside, usually gentamicin or tobramycin, is suitable for initial treatment of presumed early-onset neonatal sepsis [629]. If there is a concern for endemic or epidemic staphylococcal infection, typically occurring beyond 6 days of age, the initial treatment of late-onset neonatal sepsis should include vancomycin.

The increasing use of antibiotics, particularly in NICUs, can result in alterations in antimicrobial susceptibility patterns of bacteria and can necessitate changes in initial empirical therapy. This alteration of the microbial flora in nurseries where the use of broad-spectrum antimicrobial agents is routine supports recommendations from the CDC for the judicious use of antibiotics. The hospital laboratory must regularly monitor isolates of pathogenic bacteria to assist the physician in choosing the most appropriate therapy. The clinical pharmacology and dosage schedules of the various antimicrobial agents considered for neonatal sepsis are provided in Chapter 37.

CONTINUATION OF THERAPY WHEN RESULTS OF CULTURES ARE AVAILABLE

The choice of antimicrobial therapy should be reevaluated when results of cultures and susceptibility tests become available. The duration of therapy depends on the initial response to the appropriate antibiotics, but should be 10 days, with sepsis documented by positive culture of blood and minimal or absent focal infection. The usual duration of therapy for infants with meningitis caused by GBS gram-negative enteric bacilli is 21 days. In complicated cases of neonatal meningitis, the proper duration of therapy may be prolonged and is best determined in consultation with an infectious diseases specialist.

The third-generation cephalosporins, cefotaxime, ceftriaxone, and ceftazidime, have important theoretical advantages for treatment of sepsis or meningitis compared with therapeutic regimens that include an aminoglycoside. In contrast to the aminoglycosides, third-generation cephalosporins are not associated with ototoxicity and nephrotoxicity. Little toxicity from aminoglycosides occurs when use is brief, however, or, when continued for the duration of therapy, if serum trough levels are maintained at less than 2 µg/mL. Because cephalosporins have no dose-related toxicity, measurements of serum concentrations, which are required with the use of aminoglycosides beyond 72 hours or in infants with renal insufficiency, are unnecessary. Routine use of cephalosporins for presumptive sepsis therapy in neonates often leads to problems with drug-resistant enteric organisms, however. Extensive use of third-generation cephalosporins in the nursery could result in the emergence of resistance caused by de-repression of chromosomally mediated β-lactamases [630].

Cefotaxime is preferred to other third-generation cephalosporins for use in neonates because it has been used more extensively [621–623] and because it does not affect the binding of bilirubin [630,631]. Ceftazidime or meropenem in combination with an aminoglycoside should be used in therapy for *P. aeruginosa* meningitis because of excellent in vitro activity and good penetration into CSF. Use of ceftriaxone in the neonate should be determined on a case-by-case basis because of its ability to displace bilirubin from serum albumin and result in biliary sludging.

MANAGEMENT OF AN INFANT WHOSE MOTHER RECEIVED INTRAPARTUM ANTIMICROBIAL AGENTS

Antimicrobial agents commonly are administered to women in labor who have risk factors associated with sepsis in the fetus, including premature delivery, prolonged rupture of membranes, fever, or other signs of chorioamnionitis or group B streptococcal colonization. Antimicrobial agents cross the placenta and achieve concentrations in fetal tissues that are parallel to concentrations achieved in other well-vascularized organs. Placental transport of antibiotics is discussed in more detail in Chapter 37.

Protocols for prevention of infection with GBS in the newborn by administration of a penicillin to the mother were published in 1992 by ACOG [632] and the American Academy of Pediatrics (AAP) [633]. These guidelines were revised in 1996 by the CDC [634]; in 1997 by the AAP [635]; and in 2002 by the CDC [636], AAP, and ACOG [484]. More recent data suggest that nearly 50%

of women receive intrapartum chemoprophylaxis because of the presence of one or more risk factors for neonatal sepsis or because of a positive antenatal screening culture for GBS [637].

When ampicillin or penicillin is administered to the mother, drug concentrations in the fetus are more than 30% of the concentrations in the blood of the mother [638]. Concentrations of penicillin, ampicillin, and cefazolin that are bactericidal for GBS are achieved in the amniotic fluid approximately 3 hours after completion of a maternal intravenous dose. Parenteral antibiotic therapy administered to a mother with signs of chorioamnionitis in labor essentially is treating the fetus early in the course of the intrapartum infection [639,640]. For some infected fetuses, the treatment administered in utero is insufficient, however, to prevent signs of early-onset group B streptococcal disease. Although maternal intrapartum prophylaxis has been associated with a 75% decrease in the incidence of early-onset group B streptococcal disease since 1993 [641,642], the regimen has had no impact on the incidence of late-onset disease [643].

The various algorithms prepared to guide empirical management of the neonate born to a mother with risk factors for group B streptococcal disease who received intrapartum antimicrobial prophylaxis for prevention of early-onset group B streptococcal disease focus on three clinical scenarios [641–644]:

1. Infants who have signs of sepsis should receive a full diagnostic evaluation and should be treated, typically with ampicillin and gentamicin, until laboratory studies are available.
2. Infants born at 35 or more weeks' gestation who appear healthy and whose mothers received intrapartum prophylaxis with penicillin, ampicillin, or cefazolin for 4 or more hours before delivery do not have to be evaluated or treated, but should be observed in the hospital for 48 hours.
3. Infants who are less than 35 weeks' gestation who appear healthy and whose mothers received penicillin, ampicillin, or cefazolin for less than 4 hours before delivery should receive a limited evaluation, including a blood culture and a complete blood cell count with a differential count, and be observed for 48 hours in the hospital. The same management probably is necessary for infants of any gestation whose mothers received vancomycin for prophylaxis because nothing is known about the amniotic fluid penetration of this drug or its efficacy in preventing early-onset group B streptococcal disease.

The first two clinical scenarios are readily identified, but the third category often leads to controversy regarding optimal management. Recommendations for prevention and treatment of early-onset group B streptococcal infection are discussed in detail in Chapter 12.

Management of the infant born to a mother who received an antimicrobial agent within hours of delivery must include consideration of the effect of the drug on cultures obtained from the infant after birth. Intrapartum therapy provides some treatment of the infant in utero, and variable concentrations of drug are present in the infant's body fluids. If the infant is infected and the bacterial pathogen is susceptible to the drug administered to the mother, cultures of the infant can be sterile despite a clinical course suggesting sepsis.

TREATMENT OF AN INFANT WHOSE BACTERIAL CULTURE RESULTS ARE NEGATIVE

Whether or not the mother received antibiotics before delivery, the physician must decide on the subsequent course of therapy for the infant who was treated for presumed sepsis and whose bacterial culture results are negative. If the neonate seems to be well and there is reason to believe that infection was unlikely, treatment can be discontinued at 48 hours. If the clinical condition of the infant remains uncertain and suspicion of an infectious process remains, therapy should be continued as outlined for documented bacterial sepsis unless another diagnosis becomes apparent. Significant bacterial infection can occur without bacteremia. Squire and colleagues [645] found that results of premortem blood cultures were negative in 7 (18%) of 39 infants with unequivocal infection at autopsy. Some infants with significant systemic bacterial infection may not be identified by the usual single blood culture technique. The physician must consider this limitation when determining length of empirical therapy. If treatment for infection is deemed necessary, parenteral administration for 10 days is recommended.

MANAGEMENT OF AN INFANT WITH CATHETER-ASSOCIATED INFECTION

Investigators in Connecticut found that multiple catheters, low birth weight, low gestational age at birth, and low Apgar scores were significant risk factors for late-onset sepsis [504]. Benjamin and colleagues [505] reported a retrospective study at Duke University from 1995-1999 of all neonates who had central venous access. The goal of the Duke study was to evaluate the relationship between central venous catheter removal and outcome in bacteremic neonates. Infants bacteremic with *S. aureus* or a gram-negative rod who had their catheter retained beyond 24 hours had a 10-fold higher rate of infection-related complications than infants in whom the central catheter was removed promptly. Compared with neonates who had three or fewer positive intravascular catheter blood cultures for CoNS, neonates who had four consecutive positive blood cultures were at significantly increased risk for end-organ damage and death. In neonates with infection associated with a central venous catheter, prompt removal of the device is advised, unless there is rapid clinical improvement and sterilization of blood cultures after initiation of therapy.

TREATMENT OF NEONATAL MENINGITIS

Because the pathogens responsible for neonatal meningitis are largely the same as the pathogens that cause neonatal sepsis, initial therapy and subsequent therapy are similar. Meningitis caused by gram-negative enteric bacilli can pose special management problems. Eradication of the pathogen often is delayed, and serious complications can occur [23,119,348,632]. The persistence of gram-negative bacilli in CSF despite bactericidal levels

of the antimicrobial agent led to the evaluation of lumbar intrathecal [646] and intraventricular [647] gentamicin. Mortality and morbidity were not significantly different in infants who received parenteral drug alone or parenteral plus intrathecal therapy [646]. The study of intraventricular gentamicin was stopped early because of the high mortality in the parenteral plus intraventricular therapy group [647].

Feigin and colleagues [629] reviewed the management of meningitis in children, including neonates. Ampicillin and penicillin G, initially with an aminoglycoside, are appropriate antimicrobial agents for treating infection caused by GBS. Cefotaxime has excellent in vitro and in vivo bactericidal activity against many microorganisms responsible for neonatal meningitis [621]. Treatment of enteric gram-negative bacillary meningitis should include cefotaxime and an aminoglycoside until results of susceptibility testing are known.

If meningitis develops in a low birth weight infant who has been in the nursery for a prolonged period or in a neonate who has received previous courses of antimicrobial therapy for presumed sepsis, alternative empirical antibiotic regimens should be considered. Enterococci and antibiotic-resistant gram-negative enteric bacilli are potential pathogens in these settings. A combination of vancomycin, an aminoglycoside, and cefotaxime may be appropriate. Ceftazidime or meropenem in addition to an aminoglycoside should be considered for *P. aeruginosa* meningitis.

Other antibiotics may be necessary to treat highly resistant organisms. Meropenem [648], ciprofloxacin [649–651], or trimethoprim-sulfamethoxazole [652,653] can be the only antimicrobial agents active in vitro against bacteria that are highly resistant to broad-spectrum β-lactam antibiotics or aminoglycosides. Some of these drugs require careful monitoring because of toxicity to the newborn (see Chapter 37), and ciprofloxacin has not been approved for use in the United States in infants. Definitive treatment of meningitis caused by gram-negative enteric bacilli should be determined by in vitro susceptibility tests; consultation with an infectious diseases specialist can be helpful.

Use of dexamethasone as adjunctive treatment in childhood bacterial meningitis has been recommended based on reduction of neurologic sequelae in infants and children, in particular hearing loss and especially in cases of *H. influenzae* type b meningitis. Only one randomized controlled study exists for neonates; in 52 full-term neonates, mortality (22% dexamethasone versus 28% controls) and morbidity at 24 months (30% versus 39%) were not significantly different between groups [654]. If cultures of blood and CSF for bacterial pathogens by usual laboratory techniques are negative in the neonate with meningitis, the differential diagnosis of aseptic meningitis must be reviewed, particularly in view of diagnosing treatable infections (Table 6–18).

MANAGEMENT OF AN INFANT WITH A BRAIN ABSCESS

If purulent foci or abscesses are present, they should be drained. Some brain abscesses resolve with medical therapy alone, however [348,655]. Brain abscesses can be

TABLE 6–18 Infectious and Noninfectious Causes of Aseptic Meningitis* in Neonates

Cause	Disease
Infectious Agent	
Bacteria	Partially treated meningitis
	Parameningeal focus (brain or epidural abscess)
	Tuberculosis
Viruses	Herpes simplex meningoencephalitis
	Cytomegalovirus
	Enteroviruses
	Rubella
	Acquired immunodeficiency syndrome
	Lymphocytic choriomeningitis
	Varicella
Spirochetes	Syphilis
	Lyme disease
Parasites	Toxoplasmosis
	Chagas disease
Mycoplasma	Mycoplasma hominis infection
	Ureaplasma urealyticum infection
Fungi	Candidiasis
	Coccidioidomycosis
	Cryptococcosis
Noninfectious Causes	
Trauma	Subarachnoid hemorrhage
	Traumatic lumbar puncture
Malignancy	Teratoma
	Medulloblastoma
	Choroid plexus papilloma and carcinoma

*Aseptic meningitis is defined as meningitis in the absence of evidence of a bacterial pathogen detectable in cerebrospinal fluid by usual laboratory techniques.

polymicrobial or result from organisms that uncommonly cause meningitis, such as *Citrobacter* [148,150], *Enterobacter* [130], *Proteus* [348], and *Salmonella* species [651]. Aspiration of the abscess provides identification of the pathogens to guide rational antimicrobial therapy.

TREATMENT OF AN INFANT WITH MENINGITIS WHOSE BACTERIAL CULTURE RESULTS ARE NEGATIVE

In the absence of a detectable bacterial pathogen, an aggressive diagnostic approach is necessary for the infant with meningitis, defined by CSF pleocytosis and variable changes in the concentration of CSF protein and glucose. The most frequent cause of aseptic or nontuberculous bacterial meningitis in the neonate is prior antimicrobial therapy resulting in negative blood and CSF cultures. Congenital infections need to be excluded. Treatable diseases, such as partially treated bacterial disease and meningoencephalitis caused by herpes simplex virus, syphilis, cytomegalovirus, toxoplasmosis, Lyme disease in regions where *Borrelia* is prevalent, tuberculosis, and malignancy, need to be considered in the differential diagnosis. The history of illness and contacts in the mother and family members and epidemiologic features, such as animal exposures and recent travel, should be explored. Reexamination of the infant for focal signs of disease, including special techniques such as ophthalmologic examination, and appropriate diagnostic imaging studies of the long bones, skull, and brain can provide further information in determining the source of infection. Treatment of possible bacterial or nonbacterial causes of aseptic meningitis may be necessary before the results of culture, polymerase chain reaction, or serology tests are available to indicate the diagnosis.

TREATMENT OF ANAEROBIC INFECTIONS

The importance of anaerobic bacteria as a cause of serious neonatal infection is uncertain. *Clostridium*, *Peptococcus*, and *Peptostreptococcus* are highly sensitive to penicillin G, but *B. fragilis* usually is resistant. If anaerobic organisms are known or suspected to be responsible for infection (as in peritonitis), initiating therapy with a clinically appropriate agent, such as clindamycin, metronidazole, meropenem, ticarcillin, or piperacillin/tazobactam, is warranted.

ADJUNCTIVE THERAPIES FOR TREATMENT OF NEONATAL SEPSIS

Despite appropriate antimicrobial and optimal supportive therapy, mortality rates resulting from neonatal sepsis remain high, especially for infants with very low birth weight. With the hope of improving survival and decreasing the severity of sequelae in survivors, investigators have considered adjunctive modes of treatment, including granulocyte transfusion, exchange transfusion, and the use of standard intravenous immunoglobulin (IVIG) or pathogen-specific polyclonal or monoclonal antibody reagents for deficits in neonatal host defenses. These therapies are discussed in further detail in Chapter 4. Pentoxifylline has been documented to reduce plasma tumor necrosis factor-α concentrations in premature infants with sepsis and to improve survival, but the number of infants treated (five of five survived) and number of controls (one of four survived) were too small to provide more than a suggestion of efficacy [656]. In neutropenic infants with sepsis, the administration of granulocyte colony-stimulating factor and human granulocyte-macrophage colony-stimulating factor has had variable effects on outcome [657–660]. Although the results of selected studies indicate that some of these techniques improved survival, the potential adverse effects (e.g., graft-versus-host reaction, pulmonary leukocyte sequestration) are sufficiently concerning to warrant further study in experimental protocols.

IVIG preparations have been assessed for adjunctive therapy for neonatal sepsis based on the hypothesis that infected infants lack circulating antibodies against bacterial pathogens and that IVIG can provide some antibody for protection. Ohlsson and Lacy [661] performed a meta-analysis of 553 neonates with suspected infection who had been enrolled in randomized clinical trials in seven countries through 2003 to evaluate the effect of

IVIG on subsequent outcomes. The results revealed a borderline significant reduction in mortality (relative risk 0.63, 95% confidence interval 0.40 to 1.00). In the studies in which analysis was restricted to neonates with subsequently proven systemic bacterial infection, a statistically significant reduction of mortality was identified (relative risk 0.55, 95% confidence interval 0.31 to 0.98). Based on these preliminary encouraging data from diverse studies, an ongoing, placebo-controlled multicenter trial in low birth weight or ventilated neonates (INIS [International Neonatal Immunotherapy Study]) is comparing the adjunctive use of 10 mg/kg of IVIG versus placebo at the time of suspected infection and 48 hours later; mortality and major disability at 2 years are the major outcome variables [662].

PROGNOSIS

Before the advent of antibiotics, almost all infants with neonatal sepsis died [5]. Dunham [2] reported that physicians used various treatments, including "erysipelas serum" and transfusions, without altering the course of the disease. The introduction of sulfonamides and penicillin and later introduction of broad-spectrum antibiotics such as chloramphenicol and streptomycin decreased the mortality rate to about 60% [3,5]. During this period, some infants undoubtedly died because of treatment with high dosages of chloramphenicol, which can cause cardiovascular collapse (i.e., gray baby syndrome).

The introduction of the aminoglycosides, first with kanamycin in the early 1960s and gentamicin late in that decade, vastly improved therapy for bacteremia caused by gram-negative organisms, the leading cause of sepsis at that time [6]. These therapies, together with an improved understanding of neonatal physiology and advances in life-support systems, combined to result in a steady decrease in neonatal mortality in the United States [6] and in Europe [257,258,286,663] during the period 1960-1985. Mortality rates for sepsis, including infants of all weights and gestational ages, decreased from 40% to 50% in the 1960s [4,6,286,663] to 10% to 20% in the 1970s and 1980s [6,10,258,447,663]. Population-based surveillance of selected counties in the United States conducted by the CDC from 1993-1998 reported 2196 cases of neonatal sepsis caused by GBS, of which 92 (4%) were fatal [643].

The postnatal age at which infection occurs, previously thought to be of prognostic significance, has become less important within the past 2 decades. Fulminant sepsis, with signs of illness present at birth or during the first day of life, has a high mortality rate, ranging from 14% to 20% [6,12,258,288] to 70% [664]. When infections occurring during the first 24 hours of life, most of which are caused by GBS, are excluded from the analysis, however, the percentage of deaths resulting from early-onset sepsis does not differ significantly from late-onset infection.* Mortality from sepsis is higher for preterm than for term infants in virtually all published studies,† but is

approximately the same for all major bacterial pathogens (see Tables 6–4 and 6–5) [10,257].

In more recent surveys, the mortality rate for neonatal meningitis has declined from 25% [10,24,665,666] to 10% to 15% [12,23,26,667,668]. This decrease represents a significant improvement from prior years, when studies reported a case-fatality rate of more than 30% [21,431,648,649,669]. Mortality is greater among preterm than term infants [12,23,26,670].

Significant sequelae develop in 17% to 60% of infants who survive neonatal meningitis caused by gram-negative enteric bacilli or GBS [23,665–668]. These sequelae include mental and motor disabilities, convulsive disorders, hydrocephalus, hearing loss, and abnormal speech patterns. The most extensive experience with the long-term observation of infants who had group B streptococcal meningitis as neonates was reported by Edwards and colleagues [670]. During the period 1974-1979, 61 patients were treated, and 21% died. Of the 38 survivors who were available for evaluation at 3 years of age or older, 29% had severe neurologic sequelae, 21% had minor deficits, and 50% were functioning normally. Presenting factors that were associated with death or severe disability included comatose or semicomatose state, decreased perfusion, total peripheral white blood cell count less than 5000/mm³, absolute neutrophil count less than 1000/mm³, and CSF protein level greater than 300 mg/dL.

Another study evaluating 35 newborns who survived GBS meningitis over 3 to 18 years showed more favorable outcomes with 60% of survivors considered normal at the time of follow-up compared with sibling controls, 15% with mild to moderate neurologic residua, and 25% with major sequelae [669]. Franco and coworkers [668] reported the results of frequent and extensive neurologic, developmental, and psychometric assessments on a cohort of 10 survivors of group B streptococcal meningitis followed for 1 to 14 years. The investigators found that one child had severe CNS damage; five children, including one with hydrocephalus, had mild academic or behavioral problems; and four children were normal.

The neurodevelopmental outcomes described for infants with gram-negative bacillary meningitis are similar to the outcomes reported for group B streptococcal meningitis. Unhanand and colleagues [23] reported findings from their 21-year experience with gram-negative meningitis at two hospitals in Dallas, Texas. Of 72 patients less than 28 days old at the onset of symptoms, there were 60 survivors, 43 of whom were followed and evaluated for at least 6 months. Neurologic sequelae, occurring alone or in combination, were described in 56% and included hydrocephalus (approximately 30%), seizure disorder (approximately 30%), developmental delay (approximately 30%), cerebral palsy (25%), and hearing loss (15%). At follow-up, 44% of the survivors were developmentally normal at follow-up. Among infants with gram-negative bacillary meningitis, thrombocytopenia, CSF white blood cell count greater than 2000/mm³, CSF protein greater than 200 mg/dL, CSF glucose-to-blood glucose ratio of less than 0.5, prolonged (>48 hours) positive CSF cultures, and elevated endotoxin and interleukin-1 concentrations in CSF were indicators of a poor outcome

---

*References [6, 10, 85, 257, 258, 286, 447].

†References [7, 10, 12, 18, 257, 258, 446, 447].

[23,433,541,671]. Investigators in England and Wales [668] found that independent predictors of adverse outcome 12 hours after admission were the presence of seizures, coma, ventilatory support, and leukopenia.

CT reveals a high incidence of CNS residua among newborns with meningitis. McCracken and colleagues [672] reported that of CT scans performed in 44 infants with gram-negative bacillary meningitis, only 30% of the scans were considered normal. Hydrocephalus was found in 20% of cases; areas of infarct, cerebritis, diffuse encephalomalacia, or cortical atrophy were found in 30%; brain abscess was found in about 20%; and subdural effusions were found in 7%. Two or more abnormalities were detected in about one third of infants.

The prognosis of brain abscess in the neonate is guarded because about half of these children die, and sequelae such as hydrocephalus are common among survivors. Of 17 children who had brain abscess during the neonatal period and were followed for at least 2 years, only 4 had normal intellect and were free of seizures [348]. In neonates with brain abscess, the poor outcome probably is caused by destruction of brain parenchyma as a result of hemorrhagic infarcts and necrosis.

PREVENTION
OBSTETRIC FACTORS

Improvement in the health of pregnant women with increased use of prenatal care facilities has led to lower rates of prematurity. Increased use of antenatal steroids in pregnant women with preterm labor and of surfactant in their infants has resulted in significantly fewer cases of respiratory distress syndrome. More appropriate management of prolonged interval after rupture of maternal membranes, maternal peripartum infections, and fetal distress has improved infant outcomes. Because these factors are associated with sepsis in the newborn, improved care of the mother should decrease the incidence of neonatal infection. The development of neonatal intensive care expertise and units with appropriate equipment has resulted in the survival of very low birth weight infants. Increasingly, obstetric problems are anticipated, and mothers are transferred to medical centers with NICUs before delivery.

CHEMOPROPHYLAXIS

The use of antibiotics to prevent infection can be valuable when they are directed against specific microorganisms for a limited time. In the neonate, the use of silver nitrate eye drops or intramuscular ceftriaxone to prevent gonococcal ophthalmia, vaccination with bacillus Calmette-Guérin or prophylactic use of isoniazid to reduce morbidity from tuberculosis in infants who must return to endemic areas, and use of hexachlorophene baths to prevent staphylococcal disease have been recognized as effective modes of chemoprophylaxis. The value of using antimicrobial agents against unknown pathogens in infants believed to be at high risk of infection or undergoing invasive procedures is uncertain. Studies of penicillin administered to the mother during labor for prevention of neonatal disease caused by GBS are reviewed earlier and in Chapter 12.

Prophylaxis using low-dose vancomycin as a strategy to prevent late-onset sepsis in high-risk neonates has been the subject of several more clinical investigations [673–676]. A meta-analysis incorporating these studies found that low-dose prophylactic vancomycin reduced the incidence of total neonatal nosocomial sepsis and specifically CoNS sepsis in preterm infants, but that mortality and length of NICU stay did not differ between the treatment and placebo groups [677]. A potential confounding factor in these studies is that low-dose vancomycin in the intravenous infusion may itself have prevented recovery of pathogens from blood cultures drawn from the central lines. Because clear clinical benefits have not been shown, the rationale for routine prophylaxis with intravenous vancomycin cannot presently outweigh the theoretical concern of selection for antibiotic-resistant pathogens (e.g., vancomycin-resistant enterococci).

An intriguing alternative approach was studied in a randomized prospective trial by Garland and colleagues [678]—the use of a vancomycin-heparin lock solution in peripherally inserted central catheters in neonates with very low birth weight and other critically ill neonates. The study found the antibiotic lock solution to be associated with a marked reduction in the incidence of catheter-associated bloodstream infections (5% versus 30% in controls), providing proof-of-principle for wider investigation of this method that reduces systemic antibiotic exposure [678].

MATERNAL FACTORS

The antiviral and antibacterial activity of human milk has been recognized for many years [679–682] and is discussed extensively in Chapter 5. Evidence that breast-feeding defends against neonatal sepsis and gram-negative meningitis was first reported more than 30 years ago from Sweden [683]. Studies done in Pakistan have shown that even partial breast-feeding seems to be protective among neonates in a resource-limited nation with a high neonatal mortality rate from clinical sepsis [684]. In a study from Georgetown University, very low birth weight infants fed human milk had a significant reduction in sepsis or meningitis compared with very low birth weight infants exclusively fed formula (odds ratio 0.47, 95% confidence interval 0.23 to 0.95) [685].

Breast-fed infants have a lower incidence of gastroenteritis, respiratory illness, and otitis media than formula-fed infants. A protective effect of breast-feeding against infections of the urinary tract also has been suggested [686]. Breast-feeding is also associated with general immunostimulatory effects as evidenced by larger thymus size [687] and improved antibody responses to immunization [688,689]. Lactoferrin is the major whey protein in human milk and has immunomodulatory activities A study of bovine lactoferrin supplementation in very low birth weight neonates identified efficacy in decreasing the incidence of late-onset sepsis. The decrease occurred for gram-positive bacteremia and fungemia [372].

IMMUNOPROPHYLAXIS

The immaturity of the neonatal immune system is characterized by decreased levels of antibody against common pathogens; decreased complement activity, especially alternative pathway components; diminished polymorpho-nuclear leukocyte production, mobilization, and function; diminished T-lymphocyte cytokine production to many antigens; and reduced levels of lactoferrin and transferrin [686]. Recognition of these factors has resulted in attempts at therapeutic intervention aimed specifically at each component of the deficient immune response [690].

Infants are protected from infection by passively trans-ferred maternal IgG. To enhance the infant's ability to ward off severe infections, immunization of pregnant women and women in their childbearing years has been selectively adopted [688,691–693]. Programs in countries with limited resources to immunize pregnant women with tetanus toxoid have markedly decreased the incidence of neonatal tetanus. Investigational programs for immuniza-tion of pregnant women with polysaccharide pneumo-coccal, *H. influenzae* type b, and group B streptococcal vaccines aim to provide infants with protection in the first months of life. Studies of safety and immunogenicity of polysaccharide conjugate vaccines for GBS show promise of a reduction in incidence of late-onset and early-onset disease in newborns [693]. Use of vaccines in pregnant women is discussed in Chapter 38.

Several clinical trials have explored the use of IVIG to correct the antibody deficiency of neonates, particularly very preterm newborns, and reduce the incidence of sep-sis. In 1994, the NICHD Neonatal Research Network reported a randomized clinical trial of 2416 subjects to determine the effects of prophylactic IVIG on the risk of sepsis in premature neonates [694]. No reduction in mortality, morbidity, or incidence of nosocomial infec-tions was achieved by IVIG administration. The use of hyperimmune IVIG preparations and human monoclonal antibodies to prevent specific infections (e.g., CoNS, *S. aureus*) in high-risk neonates is also an area of active exploration; however, although these products seem to be safe and well tolerated, no reduction in staphylococcal infection was documented in two more recent large, ran-domized multicenter studies [695,696]. A systematic meta-analysis of 19 published studies through 2003 including approximately 5000 infants calculated that IVIG prophylaxis provided a 3% to 4% reduction in nos-ocomial infections, but did not reduce mortality or other important clinical outcomes (e.g., necrotizing enterocoli-tis, length of hospital stay) [697]. The costs of IVIG and the value assigned to these clinical outcomes are expected to dictate use; basic scientists and clinicians need to explore new avenues for prophylaxis against bacterial infection in this special patient population [697].

An older study by Sidiropoulos and coworkers [698] explored the potential benefit of low-dose (12 g in 12 hours) or high-dose (24 g daily for 5 days) IVIG given to pregnant women at risk for preterm delivery because of chorioamnionitis. Cord blood IgG levels were doubled in infants older than 32 weeks' gestational age whose mothers received the higher dosage schedule, but were unaffected in infants born earlier, suggesting little or no placental transfer of IVIG before the 32nd week of gesta-tion. Among the infants delivered after 32 weeks, 6 (37%) of 16 born to untreated mothers developed clinical, labo-ratory, or radiologic evidence of infection and required antimicrobial therapy, whereas none of 7 infants born to treated mothers became infected. Although this study suggests that intrauterine fetal prophylaxis can be benefi-cial in selected cases, widespread use of IVIG for all women having premature onset of labor is not feasible because of uncertain timing before delivery, widespread shortages of IVIG, and cost.

The decreased number of circulating polymorphonu-clear leukocytes and reduced myeloid reserves in the bone marrow of newborns have been ascribed to impaired production of cytokines, interleukin-3, granulocyte colony-stimulating factor, granulocyte-macrophage col-ony-stimulating factor, tumor necrosis factor-α, and interferon-γ [699,700]. Considerable experience with in vitro myeloid cell cultures and animal models [701,702] suggested that cytokine or growth factor therapy to stim-ulate myelopoiesis could be an effective aid in preventing sepsis among newborns with hereditary or acquired con-genital neutropenia. Individual studies of prophylactic granulocyte-macrophage colony-stimulating factor in neonates were inconsistent in showing that absolute neu-trophil counts are increased or that the incidence of sepsis is reduced [659,660,703]. A single-blind, multicenter randomly controlled trial of granulocyte-macrophage colony-stimulating factor in 280 infants at 31 weeks' ges-tation or less showed that although neutrophil counts increased more rapidly in the treatment group in the first 11 days after study initiation, there were no differences in the incidence of sepsis or improved survival associated with these changes [704]. Although therapy of severe con-genital neutropenia with granulocyte colony-stimulating factor reverses neutropenia, demonstrable functional defi-ciency of the neutrophils persists, and this probably explains why these neonates remain at significantly ele-vated risk of infection [705].

The amino acid glutamine has been recognized as important for gut and immune function in critically ill adults, and more recent attention has focused on its potential benefit to neonates, especially because it is not included in standard intravenous amino acid solutions. A large, multicenter double-blind clinical trial of glutamine supplementation was found not to decrease the incidence of sepsis or the mortality in extremely low birth weight infants [706], and this failure to provide a statistically significant benefit was borne out in a meta-analysis of seven rando-mized trials including more than 2300 infants [707].

A few studies have examined the effect of probiotic administration of *Lactobacillus* or *Bifidobacterium* species, generally intended as prophylaxis against necrotizing enterocolitis in neonates, on the secondary outcome of systemic bacterial infection, yielding conflicting results [708–710]. A meta-analysis of nine randomized trials comprising 1425 infants suggested that enteral supple-mentation of probiotic bacteria reduced the risk of severe necrotizing enterocolitis, but there was no evidence of a comparable beneficial effect on the incidence of nosoco-mial sepsis [711].

The iron-binding glycoprotein lactoferrin is a compo-nent of the innate immune system produced at mucosal sites and activated in response to infection or inflamma-tion. By restricting microbial iron access and through the direct cell wall lytic activity of its component peptides, lactoferrin exhibits broad-spectrum antimicrobial activity

[712]. Bovine lactoferrin, sharing 77% homology with the human protein, has been granted "generally recognized as safe" (GRAS) status by the FDA. A randomized study of bovine lactoferrin supplementation in very low birth weight neonates showed a reduced rate of a first episode of late-onset sepsis in the treatment group (risk ratio 0.34, 95% confidence interval 0.17 to 0.70) [372]. This simple, promising intervention warrants further exploration as a tool to reduce the incidence of nosocomial infection in this extremely high-risk population.

DECONTAMINATION OF FOMITES

Because contamination of equipment poses a significant infectious challenge for the newborn, disinfection of all materials that are involved in the care of the newborn is an important responsibility of nursery personnel. The basic mechanisms of large pieces of equipment must be cleaned appropriately or replaced because they have been implicated in nursery epidemics. The use of disposable equipment and materials packaged in individual units, such as containers of sterile water for a nebulization apparatus, are important advances in the prevention of infection. The frequency of catheter-associated CoNS sepsis has led to attempts to prevent bacterial colonization of intravascular catheters through use of attachment-resistant polymeric materials, antibiotic impregnation, and immunotherapy directed against adherence factors [713]. These procedures are reviewed in Chapter 35.

EPIDEMIOLOGIC SURVEILLANCE
Endemic Infection

Nursery-acquired infections can become apparent days to several months after discharge of the infant. A surveillance system that provides information about infections within the nursery and involves follow-up of infants after discharge should be established. Various techniques can be used for surveillance and are reviewed in Chapter 35.

Epidemic Infection

The medical and nursing staff must be aware of the possibility of outbreaks or epidemics in the nursery. Prevention of disease is based on the level of awareness of personnel. Infection in previously well infants who lack high-risk factors associated with sepsis must be viewed with suspicion. Several cases of infection occurring within a brief period caused by the same or an unusual pathogen and occurring in close physical proximity should raise concern about the possibility of a nursery outbreak. Techniques for management of infection outbreaks in nurseries are discussed in Chapter 35.

SEPSIS IN THE NEWBORN RECENTLY DISCHARGED FROM THE HOSPITAL

When fever or other signs of systemic infection occur in the first weeks after the newborn is discharged from the nursery, appropriate management requires consideration of the possible sources of infection. Infection acquired at birth or from a household contact is the most likely cause. Congenital infection can be present with signs of disease that are detected after discharge. Late-onset infection from microorganisms acquired in the nursery can occur weeks or occasionally months after birth. Infection can occur after discharge because of underlying anatomic, physiologic, or metabolic abnormalities.

Newborns are susceptible to infectious agents that colonize or cause disease in other household members. If an infant whose gestation and delivery were uneventful is discharged from the nursery and develops signs of an infectious disease in the first weeks of life, the infection was probably acquired from someone in the infant's environment. Respiratory and gastrointestinal infections are common and can be accompanied by focal disease such as otitis media. A careful history of illnesses in household members can suggest the source of the infant's infection.

CONGENITAL INFECTION

Signs of congenital infection can appear or be identified after discharge from the nursery. Hearing impairment caused by congenital rubella or cytomegalovirus infection can be noticed by a parent at home. Hydrocephalus with gradually increasing head circumference caused by congenital toxoplasmosis is apparent only after serial physical examinations. Chorioretinitis, jaundice, or pneumonia can occur as late manifestations of congenital infection. A lumbar puncture may be performed in the course of a sepsis evaluation. CSF pleocytosis and increased protein concentration can be caused by congenital infection and warrant appropriate follow-up diagnostic studies.

LATE-ONSET INFECTION

Late-onset infection can manifest after the first week to months after birth as sepsis and meningitis or other focal infections. GBS (see Chapter 12) is the most frequent cause of late-onset sepsis in the neonate, followed by *E. coli*. Organisms acquired in the nursery also can cause late-onset disease. Skin and soft tissue lesions or other focal infections, including osteomyelitis and pneumonia from *S. aureus*, can occur weeks after birth. The pathogenesis of late-onset sepsis is obscure in many cases. The reason why an organism becomes invasive and causes sepsis or meningitis after colonizing the mucous membranes; skin; or upper respiratory, genitourinary, or gastrointestinal tracts remains obscure. Nosocomially acquired or health care–associated organisms are discussed in further detail in Chapter 35.

INFECTIONS IN THE HOUSEHOLD

Infection can be associated with an underlying anatomic defect, physiologic abnormality, or metabolic disease. An infant who fails to thrive or presents with fever can have a urinary tract infection as the first indication of an anatomic abnormality. Infants with lacrimal duct stenosis or choanal atresia can develop focal infection. Sepsis caused by gram-negative enteric bacilli occurs frequently in infants with galactosemia (see "Pathogenesis").

The infected infant can be an important source of infection to family members. In one study in New York [714], 12.6% of household contacts developed suppurative lesions during the 10-month period after introduction into the home of an infant with a staphylococcal lesion. The incidence of suppurative infections in household contacts of infants without lesions was less than 2%. Damato and coworkers [713] showed colonization of neonates with enteric organisms possessing R factor–mediated resistance to kanamycin and persistence of these strains for more than 12 months after birth. During the period of observation, one third of the household contacts of the infants became colonized with the same strain.

Infections in infants have been associated with bites or licks from household pets. *Pasteurella multocida* is part of the oral flora of dogs, cats, and rodents. A review of 25 cases of *P. multocida* infection in the neonatal period found animal exposure to cats or dogs or both in 52% of cases, most of which did not involve bites or trauma; the balance were believed to represent vertical transmission from an infected mother [715]. In one case report, a 5-week-old infant with *P. multocida* meningitis frequently was licked by the family dog, and the organism was identified in cultures of the dog's mouth, but not of the parents' throats [716]. *P. multocida* sepsis and meningitis was reported in 2-month-old twin infants after household exposure to a slaughtered sheep [717]. A neonatal case of *Campylobacter jejuni* sepsis was proven genetically to result from transmission from the family dog [718]. The epidemiologic link between cats and dogs and infection in young infants suggests that parents should limit contact between pets and infants.

FEVER IN THE FIRST MONTH OF LIFE

Reviews of fever in the first weeks of life indicate that elevation of temperature (>38.8° C [>101.8° F]) [719–724] is relatively uncommon. When fever occurs in the young infant, the incidence of severe disease, including bacterial sepsis, meningitis, and pneumonia, is sufficiently high to warrant careful evaluation and conservative management [719,725]. Approximately 12% of all febrile (>38° C [>100.4° F]) neonates presenting to emergency departments are found to have a serious bacterial infection [726,727]. Important pathogens in neonatal age groups include *GBS* and *E. coli*, and occult bacteremia and urinary tract infections are the most common foci of disease [726,727].

A careful history of the pregnancy, delivery, nursery experience, interval since discharge from the nursery, and infections in the household should be obtained. Physical examination should establish the presence or absence of signs associated with congenital infection and late-onset diseases. Culture of blood and urine should be done if no other focus is apparent, and culture of CSF and a chest radiograph should be considered if the infant is believed to have systemic infection. Risk stratification algorithms have been evaluated to incorporate ancillary clinical testing in hopes of supplementing the often incomplete picture that emerges from history and physical examination [725].

The "Rochester criteria" for analysis of febrile infants, originally proposed by Dagan and colleagues [722], used criteria such as normal peripheral leukocyte count (5000 to 15,000/mm^3), normal absolute band neutrophil count (<1500/mm^3) and absence of pyuria to identify low-risk patients. When Ferrera and coworkers [721] retrospectively applied these criteria to the subset of patients in their first 4 weeks of life, 6% of the neonates fulfilling low-risk criteria had serious bacterial infections. Similarly, when groups of febrile newborns were retrospectively stratified as low risk by the "Philadelphia criteria" [728] or "Boston criteria" [729] developed for older infants, it became apparent that 3.5% to 4.6% of the neonates with a serious bacterial infection would have been missed [726,727].

Consequently, because of the inability to predict serious bacterial infections accurately in this age group, a complete sepsis evaluation should be performed and includes a culture of blood, urine, and CSF; a complete blood cell and differential count; examination of CSF for cells, glucose, and protein; and a urinalysis. Although a peripheral blood cell count is routinely ordered, it is not sufficiently discriminatory to preclude the mandatory collection of blood for culture [730,731]. In contrast to older infants [732], the presence of signs consistent with a viral upper respiratory tract infection in the neonate does not obviate the need for a full diagnostic evaluation. Neonates infected with respiratory syncytial virus had equivalent rates of serious bacterial infection as neonates testing negative for the virus [733]. More recent data suggest, however, that febrile infants less than 60 days of age positive for influenza virus infection may have lower rates of bacteremia and urinary tract infection than similar infants without influenza infection [734]. Because of the high rates of serious bacterial infections, guidelines prepared by Baraff and colleagues [719] for the management of infants and children with fever without source state that all febrile infants younger than 28 days should be hospitalized for parenteral antibiotic therapy, regardless of the results of laboratory studies.

ACKNOWLEDGMENTS

Drs. S. Michael Marcy, Carol Baker, and Debra L Palazzi contributed to this chapter in earlier editions. The authors are indebted to these scholars for their roles in the preparation of this chapter.

REFERENCES

[1] R.P. Gaynes, et al., Nosocomial infections among neonates in high-risk nurseries in the United States, Pediatrics 93 (1996) 357.
[2] E.C. Dunham, Septicemia in the newborn, Am. J. Dis. Child. 45 (1933) 229.
[3] W.L. Nyhan, M.D. Fousek, Septicemia of the newborn, Pediatrics 22 (1958) 268.
[4] L. Gluck, H.F. Wood, M.D. Fousek, Septicemia of the newborn, Pediatr. Clin. North. Am. 13 (1966) 1131.
[5] R.M. Freedman, et al., A half century of neonatal sepsis at Yale, Am. J. Dis. Child. 35 (1981) 140.
[6] I.M. Gladstone, et al., A ten-year review of neonatal sepsis and comparison with the previous fifty-year experience, Pediatr. Infect. Dis. J. 9 (1990) 819.
[7] R.S. Baltimore, et al., Early-onset neonatal sepsis in the era of group B streptococcal prevention, Pediatrics 108 (2001) 1094.
[8] M.J. Bizzarro, et al., Seventy-five years of neonatal sepsis at Yale: 1928–2003, Pediatrics 116 (2005) 595–602.
[9] M.J. Bizzarro, et al., Changing patterns in neonatal *Escherichia coli* sepsis and ampicillin resistance in the era of intrapartum antibiotic prophylaxis, Pediatrics 121 (2008) 689–696.

[10] R. Vesikari, et al., Neonatal septicemia, Arch. Dis. Child. 60 (1985) 542.

[11] I. Winfred, The incidence of neonatal infections in the nursery unit at the Ahmadu Bello University Teaching Hospital, Zaria, Nigeria, East Afr. Med. J. 61 (1984) 197.

[12] D. Greenberg, et al., A prospective study of neonatal sepsis and meningitis in Southern Israel, Pediatr. Infect. Dis. J. 16 (1997) 768.

[13] O.J. Hensey, C.A. Hart, R.W.I. Cooke, Serious infection in a neonatal intensive care unit: a two-year survey, J. Hyg. (Camb) 95 (1985) 289.

[14] M.G. Karlowicz, E.S. Buescher, A.E. Surka, Fulminant late-onset sepsis in a neonatal intensive care unit, 1988–1997, and the impact of avoiding empiric vancomycin therapy, Pediatrics 106 (2000) 1387.

[15] B.J. Stoll, et al., Late-onset sepsis in very low birth weight neonates: the experience of the NICHD neonatal research network, Pediatrics 110 (2002) 285.

[16] I.R. Makhoul, et al., Epidemiology, clinical, and microbiological characteristics of late-onset sepsis among very low birth weight infants in Israel: a national survey, Pediatrics 109 (2002) 34.

[17] J. Karpuch, M. Goldberg, D. Kohelet, Neonatal bacteremia: a 4-year prospective study, Isr. J. Med. Sci. 19 (1983) 963.

[18] A.A. Fanaroff, et al., Incidence, presenting features, risk factors and significance of late onset septicemia in very low birth weight infants, Pediatr. Infect. Dis. 17 (1998) 593.

[19] B.J. Stoll, et al., Changes in pathogens causing early-onset sepsis in very-low-birth-weight infants, N. Engl. J. Med. 347 (2002) 240–247.

[20] M. Ziai, R.J. Haggerty, Neonatal meningitis, N. Engl. J. Med. 259 (1958) 314.

[21] A.W. Mathies Jr., P.F. Wehrle, Management of Bacterial Meningitis, WB Saunders, Philadelphia, 1974.

[22] M.D. Yow, et al., Initial antibiotic management of bacterial meningitis, Medicine (Baltimore) 52 (1973) 305.

[23] M. Unhanand, et al., Gram-negative enteric bacillary meningitis: a twenty-one-year experience, J. Pediatr. 122 (1993) 15.

[24] C.J.J. Mulder, L. van Alphen, H.C. Zanen, Neonatal meningitis caused by *Escherichia coli* in the Netherlands, J. Infect. Dis. 150 (1984) 935.

[25] J. de Louvois, et al., Infantile meningitis in England and Wales: a two year study, Arch. Dis. Child. 66 (1991) 603.

[26] D.E. Holt, et al., Neonatal meningitis in England and Wales: 10 years on, BMJ 84 (2001) F85.

[27] M.T. Moreno, et al., Neonatal sepsis and meningitis in a developing Latin American country, Pediatr. Infect. Dis. J. 13 (1994) 516.

[28] R. Bennhagen, N.W. Svenningsen, A.N. Bekassy, Changing pattern of neonatal meningitis in Sweden: a comparative study 1976 vs. 1983, Scand. J. Infect. Dis. 19 (1987) 587.

[29] R.C. Lancefield, Serologic differentiation of human and other groups of hemolytic streptococci, J. Exp. Med. 57 (1933) 571.

[30] C.J. Baker, et al., Suppurative meningitis due to streptococci of Lancefield group B: a study of 33 infants, J. Pediatr. 82 (1973) 724.

[31] P.M. Schlievert, J.E. Gocke, J.R. Deringer, Group B streptococcal toxic shock-like syndrome: report of a case and purification of an associated pyrogenic toxin, Clin. Infect. Dis. 17 (1993) 26.

[32] D. Charles, B. Larsen, Streptococcal puerperal sepsis and obstetric infections: a historical perspective, Rev. Infect. Dis. 8 (1986) 411.

[33] I. Loudon, Puerperal fever, the streptococcus, and the sulphonamides, 1911–1945, BMJ 295 (1987) 485.

[34] B.P. Watson, An outbreak of puerperal sepsis in New York City, Am. J. Obstet. Gynecol. 16 (1928) 159.

[35] J.F. Jewett, et al., Childbed fever: a continuing entity, JAMA 206 (1968) 344.

[36] W.R. McCabe, A.A. Abrams, An outbreak of streptococcal puerperal sepsis, N. Engl. J. Med. 272 (1965) 615.

[37] J.R. Campbell, et al., An outbreak of M serotype 1 group A streptococcus in neonatal intensive care unit, J. Pediatr. 129 (1996) 396.

[38] V.K. Wong, H.T. Wright Jr., Group A β-hemolytic streptococci as a cause of bacteremia in children, Am. J. Dis. Child. 142 (1988) 831.

[39] D.J. Murphy Jr., Group A streptococcal meningitis, Pediatrics 71 (1983) 1.

[40] M.H. Rathore, L.L. Barton, E.L. Kaplan, Suppurative group A β-hemolytic streptococcal infections in children, Pediatrics 89 (1992) 743.

[41] M. Wilschanski, et al., Neonatal septicemia caused by group A beta-hemolytic streptococcus, Pediatr. Infect. Dis. J. 8 (1989) 536.

[42] N.R. Panaro, L.I. Lutwick, E.K. Chapnick, Intrapartum transmission of group A streptococcus, Clin. Infect. Dis. 17 (1993) 79.

[43] L.M. Mahieu, et al., Congenital streptococcal toxic shock syndrome with absence of antibodies against streptococcal pyrogenic exotoxins, J. Pediatr. 127 (1995) 987.

[44] C.C. Geil, W.K. Castle, E.A. Mortimer, Group A streptococcal infections in newborn nurseries, Pediatrics 46 (1970) 849.

[45] H.M. Gezon, M.J. Schaberg, J.O. Klein, Concurrent epidemics of *Staphylococcus aureus* and group A streptococcus disease in a newborn nursery-control with penicillin G and hexachlorophene bathing, Pediatrics 51 (1973) 383.

[46] G. Peter, J. Hazard, Neonatal group A streptococcal disease, J. Pediatr. 87 (1975) 454.

[47] J.D. Nelson, H.C. Dillon Jr., J.B. Howard, A prolonged nursery epidemic associated with a newly recognized type of group A streptococcus, J. Pediatr. 89 (1976) 792.

[48] U. Acharya, C.A.R. Lamont, K. Cooper, Group A beta-hemolytic streptococcus causing disseminated intravascular coagulation and maternal death, Lancet 1 (1988) 595.

[49] J. Kavi, R. Wise, Group A beta-hemolytic streptococcus causing disseminated intravascular coagulation and maternal death, Lancet 1 (1988) 993.

[50] G.R. Swingler, et al., Disseminated intravascular coagulation associated with group A streptococcal infection in pregnancy, Lancet 1 (1988) 1456.

[51] I. Miyairi, et al., Neonatal invasive group A streptococcal disease: case report and review of the literature, Pediatr. Infect. Dis. J. 23 (2004) 161–165.

[52] D. Greenberg, et al., Neonatal sepsis caused by *Streptococcus pyogenes*—resurgence of an old etiology? Pediatr. Infect. Dis. J. 18 (1999) 479.

[53] P. Patamasucon, J.D. Siegel, G.H. McCracken Jr., Streptococcal submandibular cellulitis in young infants, Pediatrics 67 (1981) 378.

[54] R. Bortolussi, T.R. Thompson, P. Ferrieri, Early-onset pneumococcal sepsis in newborn infants, Pediatrics 60 (1977) 352.

[55] P.J. Shaw, D.L. Robinson, J.G. Watson, Pneumococcal infection in a mother and infant, Lancet 2 (1984) 47.

[56] H. Westh, L. Skibsted, B. Korner, *Streptococcus pneumoniae* infections of the female genital tract and in the newborn child, Rev. Infect. Dis. 12 (1990) 416.

[57] E.N. Robinson Jr., Pneumococcal endometritis and neonatal sepsis, Rev. Infect. Dis. 12 (1990) 799.

[58] B.R. Hughes, J.L. Mercer, L.B. Gosbel, Neonatal pneumococcal sepsis in association with fatal maternal pneumococcal sepsis, Aust. N. Z. J. Obstet. Gynaecol. 41 (2001) 457.

[59] J.A. Hoffman, et al., Streptococcus pneumoniae infections in the neonate, Pediatrics 112 (2003) 1095.

[60] L.C. McDonald, K. Bryant, J. Snyder, Peripartum transmission of penicillin-resistant *Streptococcus pneumoniae*, J. Clin. Microbiol. 41 (2003) 2258–2260.

[61] R.A. Primhak, M.S. Tanner, R.C. Spencer, Pneumococcal infection in the newborn, Arch. Dis. Child. 69 (1993) 317–318.

[62] P. Stewardson-Krieger, S.P. Gotoff, Neonatal meningitis due to group C beta hemolytic streptococcus, J. Pediatr. 90 (1977) 103.

[63] R.J. Quinn, et al., Meningitis caused by *Streptococcus dysgalactiae* in a preterm infant, Am. J. Clin. Pathol. 70 (1978) 948–950.

[64] J.A. Hervas, et al., Neonatal sepsis and meningitis due to *Streptococcus equisimilis*, Pediatr. Infect. Dis. J. 4 (1985) 694.

[65] M. Arditi, et al., Group C β-hemolytic streptococcal infections in children: nine pediatric cases and review, Rev. Infect. Dis. 11 (1989) 34.

[66] C.J. Baker, Unusual occurrence of neonatal septicemia due to group G streptococcus, Pediatrics 53 (1974) 568.

[67] P.C. Appelbaum, et al., Neonatal sepsis due to group G streptococci, Acta Paediatr. Scand. 69 (1980) 599.

[68] A.E. Dyson, S.E. Read, Group G streptococcal colonization and sepsis in neonates, J. Pediatr. 99 (1981) 944.

[69] H. Carstensen, C. Pers, O. Pryds, Group G streptococcal neonatal septicemia: two case reports and a brief review of the literature, Scand. J. Infect. Dis. 20 (1988) 407.

[70] R. Auckenthaler, P.E. Hermans, J.A. Washington II., Group G streptococcal bacteremia: clinical study and review of the literature, Rev. Infect. Dis. 5 (1983) 196.

[71] C.R. Fikar, J. Levy, *Streptococcus bovis* meningitis in a neonate, Am. J. Dis. Child. 133 (1979) 1149.

[72] D.L. Headings, et al., Fulminant neonatal septicemia caused by *Streptococcus bovis*, J. Pediatr. 92 (1978) 282.

[73] P.J. Gavin, et al., Neonatal sepsis caused by *Streptococcus bovis* variant (biotype II/2): report of a case and review, J. Clin. Microbiol. 41 (2003) 3433–3435.

[74] G.E. Bignardi, D. Isaacs, Neonatal meningitis due to *Streptococcus mitis*, Rev. Infect. Dis. 11 (1989) 86.

[75] H.H. Hellwege, et al., Neonatal meningitis caused by *Streptococcus mitis*, Lancet 1 (1984) 743.

[76] R.A. Broughton, R. Krafka, C.J. Baker, Non-group D alpha-hemolytic streptococci: new neonatal pathogens, J. Pediatr. 99 (1981) 450.

[77] S.P. Kumar, M. Delivoria-Papadopoulos, Infections in newborn infants in a special care unit, Ann. Clin. Lab. Sci. 15 (1985) 351.

[78] L. Spigelblatt, et al., Changing pattern of neonatal streptococcal septicemia, Pediatr. Infect. Dis. J. 4 (1985) 56.

[79] A. Gunlemez, et al., Multi-resistant viridans streptococcal pneumonia and sepsis in the ventilated newborn, Ann. Trop. Paediatr. 24 (2004) 253–258.

[80] W. Ludwig, et al., The phylogenetic position of *Streptococcus* and *Enterococcus*, J. Gen. Microbiol. 131 (1985) 543–551.

[81] J.D. Siegel, G.H. McCracken Jr., Group D streptococcal infections, J. Pediatr. 93 (1978) 542.

[82] D.F. McNeeley, F. Saint-Louis, G.J. Noel, Neonatal enterococcal bacteremia: an increasingly frequent event with potentially untreatable pathogens, Pediatr. Infect. Dis. J. 15 (1996) 800.

[83] J.B. Alexander, G.P. Giacoia, Early onset nonenterococcal group D streptococcal infection in the newborn infant, J. Pediatr. 93 (1978) 489.

[84] K. Bavikatte, et al., Group D streptococcal septicemia in the neonate, Am. J. Dis. Child. 133 (1979) 493.

[85] S.R.M. Dobson, C.J. Baker, Enterococcal sepsis in neonates: features by age at onset and occurrence of focal infection, Pediatrics 85 (1990) 165.

[86] D.F. McNeeley, et al., An investigation of vancomycin-resistant *Enterococcus faecium* within the pediatric service of a large urban medical center, Pediatr. Infect. Dis. J. 17 (1998) 184.

[87] F. Espersen, et al., *Staphylococcus aureus* bacteremia in children below the age of one year, Acta Paediatr. Scand. 78 (1989) 56.

[88] C. Eckhardt, et al., Transmission of methicillin-resistant *Staphylococcus aureus* in the neonatal intensive care unit from a patient with community-acquired disease, Infect. Control Hosp. Epidemiol. 24 (2003) 460–461.

[89] S. Yee-Guardino, et al., Recognition and treatment of neonatal community-associated MRSA pneumonia and bacteremia, Pediatr. Pulmonol. 43 (2008) 203–205.

[90] L. Saiman, et al., Hospital transmission of community-acquired methicillin-resistant *Staphylococcus aureus* among postpartum women, Clin. Infect. Dis. 37 (2003) 1313–1319.

[91] M.D. David, et al., Community-associated methicillin-resistant *Staphylococcus aureus*: nosocomial transmission in a neonatal unit, J. Hosp. Infect. 64 (2006) 244–250.

[92] S.M. Wang, et al., *Staphylococcus capitis* bacteremia of very low birth weight premature infants at neonatal intensive care units: clinical significance and antimicrobial susceptibility, J. Microbiol. Immunol. Infect. 32 (1999) 26–32.

[93] T. Strunk, et al., Neonatal immune responses to coagulase-negative staphylococci, Curr. Opin. Infect. Dis. 20 (2007) 370–375.

[94] S. Baumgart, et al., Sepsis with coagulase-negative staphylococci in critically ill newborns, Am. J. Dis. Child. 137 (1983) 461.

[95] S. Struthers, et al., A comparison of two versus one blood culture in the diagnosis and treatment of coagulase-negative staphylococcus in the neonatal intensive care unit, J. Perinatol. 22 (2002) 547–549.

[96] R.T. Hall, et al., Characteristics of coagulase negative staphylococci from infants with bacteremia, Pediatr. Infect. Dis. J. 6 (1987) 377.

[97] M. Otto, Virulence factors of the coagulase-negative staphylococci, Front. Biosci. 9 (2004) 841–863.

[98] A.L. Shiau, C.L. Wu, The inhibitory effect of *Staphylococcus epidermidis* slime on the phagocytosis of murine peritoneal macrophages is interferon-independent, Microbiol. Immunol. 42 (1998) 33–40.

[99] J. Freeman, et al., Association of intravenous lipid emulsion and coagulase-negative staphylococcal bacteremia in neonatal intensive care units, N. Engl. J. Med. 323 (1990) 301.

[100] Centers for Disease Control and Prevention, Public health dispatch: outbreak of listeriosis—Northeastern United States 2002, MMWR Morb. Mortal. Wkly. Rep. 51 (2002) 950.

[101] K.M. Posfay-Barbe, E.R. Wald, Listeriosis, Semin. Fetal. Neonatal. Med. 14 (2009) 228–233.

[102] S.J. Schrag, et al., Risk factors for invasive, early-onset *Escherichia coli* infections in the era of widespread intrapartum antibiotic use, Pediatrics 118 (2006) 570–576.

[103] J. Raymond, et al., Evidence for transmission of *Escherichia coli* from mother to child in late-onset neonatal infection, Pediatr. Infect. Dis. J. 27 (2008) 186–188.

[104] S.M. Soto, et al., Comparative study of virulence traits of *Escherichia coli* clinical isolates causing early and late neonatal sepsis, J. Clin. Microbiol. 46 (2008) 1123–1125.

[105] E. Bingen, et al., Phylogenetic analysis of *Escherichia coli* strains causing neonatal meningitis suggests horizontal gene transfer from a predominant pool of highly virulent B2 group strains, J. Infect. Dis. 177 (1998) 642.

[106] S. Bonacorsi, E. Bingen, Molecular epidemiology of *Escherichia coli* causing neonatal meningitis, Int. J. Med. Microbiol. 295 (2005) 373–381.

[107] C. Peigne, et al., The plasmid of *Escherichia coli* strain S88 (O45:K1:H7) that causes neonatal meningitis is closely related to avian pathogenic *E. coli* plasmids and is associated with high-level bacteremia in a neonatal rat meningitis model, Infect. Immun. 77 (2009) 2272–2284.

[108] J.B. Robbins, et al., *Escherichia coli* K1 capsular polysaccharide associated with neonatal meningitis, N. Engl. J. Med. 290 (1974) 1216.

[109] G.H. McCracken Jr., et al., Relation between *Escherichia coli* K1 capsular polysaccharide antigen and clinical outcome in neonatal meningitis, Lancet 2 (1974) 246.

[110] G.H. McCracken Jr., L.D. Sarff, Current status and therapy of neonatal *E. coli* meningitis, Hosp. Pract. 9 (1974) 57.

[111] L.D. Sarff, et al., Epidemiology of *Escherichia coli* K1 in healthy and diseased newborns, Lancet 1 (1975) 1099.

[112] G. Peter, J.S. Nelson, Factors affecting neonatal *E. coli* K1 rectal colonization, J. Pediatr. 93 (1978) 866.

[113] J.L. Burns, et al., Transcytosis of gastrointestinal epithelial cells by *Escherichia coli* K1, Pediatr. Res. 49 (2001) 30–37.

[114] Y. Xie, K.J. Kim, K.S. Kim, Current concepts on *Escherichia coli* K1 translocation of the blood-brain barrier, FEMS Immunol. Med. Microbiol. 42 (2004) 271–279.

[115] S.H. Huang, M.F. Stins, K.S. Kim, Bacterial penetration across the blood-brain barrier during the development of neonatal meningitis, Microbes. Infect. 2 (2000) 1237–1244.

[116] J.A. Hervás, et al., Increase of *Enterobacter* in neonatal sepsis: a twenty-two-year study, Pediatr. Infect. Dis. J. 20 (2001) 1134.

[117] A. Gupta, Hospital-acquired infections in the neonatal intensive care unit—*Klebsiella pneumoniae*, Semin. Perinatol. 26 (2002) 340.

[118] S.K. Sood, D. Mulvihill, R.S. Daum, Intrarenal abscess caused by *Klebsiella pneumoniae* in a neonate: modern management and diagnosis, Am. J. Perinatol. 6 (1989) 367.

[119] S. Basu, et al., An unusual case of neonatal brain abscess following *Klebsiella pneumoniae* septicemia, Infection 29 (2001) 283.

[120] H. Ozkan, et al., Perianal necrotizing fasciitis in a neonate, Indian J. Pediatr. 64 (1997) 116.

[121] R. Podschun, H. Acktun, J. Okpara, Isolation of *Klebsiella planticola* from newborns in a neonatal ward, J. Clin. Microbiol. 36 (1998) 2331.

[122] G.L. Westbrook, et al., Incidence and identification of *Klebsiella planticola* in clinical isolates with emphasis on newborns, J. Clin. Microbiol. 38 (2000) 1495.

[123] E. Leibovitz, et al., Sepsis at a neonatal intensive care unit: a four-year retrospective study (1989–1992), Isr. J. Med. Sci. 33 (1997) 734.

[124] Y. Bell, et al., Neonatal sepsis in Jamaican neonates, Ann. Trop. Paediatr. 25 (2005) 293–296.

[125] E. Simeunovic, et al., Liver abscess in neonates, Pediatr. Surg. Int. 25 (2009) 153–156.

[126] C.L. Pessoa-Silva, et al., Extended-spectrum beta-lactamase-producing *Klebsiella pneumoniae* in a neonatal intensive care unit: risk factors for infection and colonization, J. Hosp. Infect. 53 (2003) 198.

[127] E. Roilides, et al., Septicemia due to multiresistant *Klebsiella pneumoniae* in a neonatal unit: a case-control study, Am. J. Perinatol. 17 (2000) 35.

[128] P.W. Stone, et al., Attributable costs and length of stay of an extended-spectrum beta-lactamase-producing *Klebsiella pneumoniae* outbreak in a neonatal intensive care unit, Infect. Control Hosp. Epidemiol. 24 (2003) 601.

[129] M.B. Kleiman, et al., Meningoencephalitis and compartmentalization of the cerebral ventricles caused by *Enterobacter sakazakii*, J. Clin. Microbiol. 14 (1981) 352.

[130] J. Willis, J.E. Robinson, *Enterobacter sakazakii* meningitis in neonates, Pediatr. Infect. Dis. J. 7 (1988) 196.

[131] W.A. Bonadio, D. Margolis, M. Tovar, *Enterobacter cloacae* bacteremia in children: a review of 30 cases in 12 years, Clin. Pediatr. 30 (1991) 310.

[132] S. Harbarth, et al., Outbreak of *Enterobacter cloacae* related to understaffing, overcrowding, and poor hygiene practices, Infect. Control Hosp. Epidemiol. 20 (1999) 598.

[133] P.J. Wenger, et al., An outbreak of *Enterobacter hormaechei* infection and colonization in an intensive care nursery, Clin. Infect. Dis. 24 (1997) 1243.

[134] C.L. da Silva, et al., *Enterobacter hormaechei* bloodstream infection at three neonatal intensive care units in Brazil, Pediatr. Infect. Dis. J. 21 (2002) 175.

[135] C. Iversen, et al., *Cronobacter* gen. nov., a new genus to accommodate the biogroups of *Enterobacter sakazakii*, and proposal of *Cronobacter sakazakii* gen. nov., comb. nov., *Cronobacter malonaticus* sp. nov., *Cronobacter turicensis* sp. nov., *Cronobacter muytjensii* sp. nov., *Cronobacter dublinensis* sp. nov., *Cronobacter genomospecies* 1, and of three subspecies, *Cronobacter dublinensis* subsp. *dublinensis* subsp. nov., *Cronobacter dublinensis* subsp. *lausannensis* subsp. nov. and *Cronobacter dublinensis* subsp. *lactaridi* subsp. nov, Int. J. Syst. Evol. Microbiol. 58 (2008) 1442–1447.

[136] N. Gurses, *Enterobacter* septicemia in neonates, Pediatr. Infect. Dis. J. 14 (1995) 638.

[137] A. Jain, et al., Prevalence of extended-spectrum beta-lactamase-producing gram-negative bacteria in septicaemic neonates in a tertiary care hospital, J. Med. Microbiol. 52 (2003) 421.

[138] S. Townsend, E. Hurrell, S. Forsythe, Virulence studies of *Enterobacter sakazakii* isolates associated with a neonatal intensive care unit outbreak, BMC Microbiol. 8 (2008) 64.

[139] H.N. Chen, et al., Late-onset *Enterobacter cloacae* sepsis in very-low-birth-weight neonates: experience in a medical center, Pediatr Neonatol 50 (2009) 3–7.

[140] H.L. Muytjens, L.A.A. Kollee, *Enterobacter sakazakii* meningitis in neonates: causative role of formula? Pediatr. Infect. Dis. J. 9 (1990) 372.

[141] F.R. Noriega, et al., Nosocomial bacteremia caused by *Enterobacter sakazakii* and *Leuconostoc mesenteroides* resulting from extrinsic contamination of infant formula, Pediatr. Infect. Dis. J. 9 (1990) 447.

[142] D. Drudy, et al., *Enterobacter sakazakii*: an emerging pathogen in powdered infant formula, Clin. Infect. Dis. 42 (2006) 996–1002.

[143] *Cronobacter* species isolation in two infants—New Mexico, 2008, MMWR Morb. Mortal. Wkly. Rep. 58 (2009) 1179–1183.

[144] T.F. Fok, et al., Risk factors for *Enterobacter* septicemia in a neonatal unit: case-control study, Clin. Infect. Dis. 27 (1998) 1204.

[145] A.T. Tresoldi, et al., Enterobacter cloacae sepsis outbreak in a newborn unit caused by contaminated total parenteral nutrition solution, Am. J. Infect. Control. 28 (2000) 258.

[146] H.S. Cheng, et al., Outbreak investigation of nosocomial *Enterobacter cloacae* bacteraemia in a neonatal intensive care unit, Scand. J. Infect. Dis. 32 (2000) 293.

[147] T.I. Doran, The role of *Citrobacter* in clinical disease of children: review, Clin. Infect. Dis. 28 (1999) 384.

[148] D.R. Graham, J.D. Band, *Citrobacter diversus* brain abscess and meningitis in neonates, JAMA 245 (1981) 1923.

[149] D.R. Graham, et al., Epidemic nosocomial meningitis due to *Citrobacter diversus* in neonates, J. Infect. Dis. 144 (1981) 203.

[150] A.M. Kaplan, et al., Cerebral abscesses complicating neonatal *Citrobacter freundii* meningitis, West. J. Med. 127 (1977) 418.

[151] F.Y.C. Lin, et al., Outbreak of neonatal *Citrobacter diversus* meningitis in a suburban hospital, Pediatr. Infect. Dis. J. 6 (1987) 50.

[152] S.C. Eppes, et al., Recurring ventriculitis due to *Citrobacter diversus*: clinical and bacteriologic analysis, Clin. Infect. Dis. 17 (1993) 437.

[153] S.D. Foreman, et al., Neonatal *Citrobacter* meningitis; pathogenesis of cerebral abscess formation, Ann. Neurol. 16 (1984) 655.

[154] J.G. Morris, et al., Molecular epidemiology of neonatal meningitis due to *Citrobacter diversus*: a study of isolates from hospitals in Maryland, J. Infect. Dis. 154 (1986) 409.

[155] M.W. Kline, E.O. Mason Jr., S.L. Kaplan, Characterization of *Citrobacter diversus* strains causing neonatal meningitis, J. Infect. Dis. 157 (1988) 101.

[156] O. Etuwewe, et al., Brain abscesses due to *Citrobacter koseri* in a pair of twins, Pediatr. Infect. Dis. J. 28 (2009) 1035.

[157] S.M. Townsend, et al., *Citrobacter koseri* brain abscess in the neonatal rat: survival and replication within human and rat macrophages, Infect. Immun. 71 (2003) 5871–5880.

[158] O. Assadian, et al., Nosocomial outbreak of *Serratia marcescens* in a neonatal intensive care unit, Infect. Control Hosp. Epidemiol. 23 (2002) 457.

[159] F. Fleisch, et al., Three consecutive outbreaks of *Serratia marcescens* in a neonatal intensive care unit, Clin. Infect. Dis. 34 (2002) 767.

[160] T.N. Jang, et al., Use of pulsed-field gel electrophoresis to investigate an outbreak of *Serratia marcescens* infection in a neonatal intensive care unit, J. Hosp. Infect. 48 (2001) 13.

[161] M.T. Newport, et al., Endemic *Serratia marcescens* infection in a neonatal intensive care nursery associated with gastrointestinal colonization, Pediatr. Infect. Dis. 4 (1985) 160.

[162] P. Berthelot, et al., Investigation of a nosocomial outbreak due to *Serratia marcescens* in a maternity hospital, Infect. Control Hosp. Epidemiol. 20 (1999) 233.

[163] M.M. Cullen, et al., *Serratia marcescens* outbreak in a neonatal intensive care unit prompting review of decontamination of laryngoscopes, J. Hosp. Infect. 59 (2005) 68–70.

[164] M. Zaidi, et al., Epidemic of *Serratia marcescens* bacteremia and meningitis in a neonatal unit in Mexico City, Infect. Control Hosp. Epidemiol. 10 (1989) 14.

[165] L.L. Maragakis, et al., Outbreak of multidrug-resistant *Serratia marcescens* infection in a neonatal intensive care unit, Infect. Control Hosp. Epidemiol. 29 (2008) 418–423.

[166] J.R. Campbell, T. Diacovo, C.J. Baker, *Serratia marcescens* meningitis in neonates, Pediatr. Infect. Dis. J. 11 (1992) 881.

[167] M. Ries, et al., Brain abscesses in neonates—report of three cases, Eur. J. Pediatr. 152 (1993) 745.

[168] C. Gras-Le Guen, et al., Contamination of a milk bank pasteuriser causing a *Pseudomonas aeruginosa* outbreak in a neonatal intensive care unit, Arch. Dis. Child. Fetal Neonatal Ed. 88 (2003) F434–F435.

[169] D.C. Stevens, M.B. Kleiman, R.L. Schreiner, Early-onset *Pseudomonas* sepsis of the neonate, Perinatol. Neonatol. 6 (1982) 75.

[170] S.P. Ghosal, P.C. SenGupta, A.K. Mukherjee, Noma neonatorum: its aetiopathogenesis, Lancet 2 (1978) 289.

[171] S.S. Shah, P.G. Gallagher, Complications of conjunctivitis caused by *Pseudomonas aeruginosa* in a newborn intensive care unit, Pediatr. Infect. Dis. J. 17 (1999) 97.

[172] A. Zawacki, et al., An outbreak of *Pseudomonas aeruginosa* pneumonia and bloodstream infection associated with intermittent otitis externa in a healthcare worker, Infect. Control Hosp. Epidemiol. 25 (2004) 1083–1089.

[173] Centers for Disease Control, Reported isolates of *Salmonella* from CSF in the United States, 1968–1979, J. Infect. Dis. 143 (1981) 504.

[174] M. Totan, et al., Meningitis due to *Salmonella* in preterm neonates, Turk. J. Pediatr. 44 (2002) 45.

[175] F.J. Cooke, et al., Report of neonatal meningitis due to *Salmonella enterica* serotype *Agona* and review of breast milk-associated neonatal *Salmonella* infections, J. Clin. Microbiol. 47 (2009) 3045–3049.

[176] R.P. Reed, K.P. Klugman, Neonatal typhoid fever, Pediatr. Infect. Dis. J. 13 (1994) 774.

[177] A. Schuchat, et al., Bacterial meningitis in the United States in 1995, N. Engl. J. Med. 337 (1997) 970.

[178] W.A. Sunderland, et al., Meningococcemia in a newborn infant whose mother had meningococcal vaginitis, J. Pediatr. 81 (1972) 856.

[179] R.N. Jones, J. Stepack, A. Eades, Fatal neonatal meningococcal meningitis: association with maternal cervical-vaginal colonization, JAMA 236 (1976) 2652.

[180] S.M. Fiorito, et al., An unusual transmission of *Neisseria meningitidis*: neonatal conjunctivitis acquired at delivery from the mother's endocervical infection, Sex. Transm. Dis. 28 (2001) 29.

[181] D.J. Cher, et al., A case of pelvic inflammatory disease associated with *Neisseria meningitidis* bacteremia, Clin. Infect. Dis. 17 (1993) 134.

[182] Z.A. Bhutta, I.A. Khan, Z. Agha, Fatal intrauterine meningococcal infection, Pediatr. Infect. Dis. J. 10 (1991) 868.

[183] K. Chugh, C.K. Bhalla, K.K. Joshi, Meningococcal abscess and meningitis in a neonate, Pediatr. Infect. Dis. J. 7 (1988) 136.

[184] C.A. Arango, M.H. Rathore, Neonatal meningococcal meningitis: case reports and review of literature, Pediatr. Infect. Dis. J. 15 (1996) 1134.

[185] C.W. Shepard, N.E. Rosenstein, M. Fischer, Active Bacterial Core Surveillance Team. Neonatal meningococcal disease in the United States, 1990 to 1999, Pediatr. Infect. Dis. J. 22 (2003) 418.

[186] F.P. Manginello, et al., Neonatal meningococcal meningitis and meningococcemia, Am. J. Dis. Child. 133 (1979) 651.

[187] H.W. Clegg, et al., Fulminant neonatal meningococcemia, Am. J. Dis. Child. 134 (1980) 354.

[188] M.C. Falcao, et al., Neonatal sepsis and meningitis caused by *Neisseria meningitidis*: a case report, Rev. Inst. Med. Trop. Sao. Paulo. 49 (2007) 191–194.

[189] W.G. Adams, et al., Decline of childhood *Haemophilus influenzae* type b (Hib) disease in the Hib vaccine era, JAMA 269 (1993) 221.

[190] H. Peltola, T. Kilpi, M. Anttila, Rapid disappearance of *Haemophilus influenzae* type b meningitis after routine childhood immunization with conjugate vaccines, Lancet 340 (1992) 592.

[191] K.M. Bisgard, et al., *Haemophilus influenzae* invasive disease in the United States, 1994–1995: near disappearance of a vaccine-preventable childhood disease, Emerg. Infect. Dis. 4 (1998) 229.

[192] A.K. Takala, et al., Reduction of oropharyngeal carriage of *Haemophilus influenzae* type b (Hib) in children immunized with Hib conjugate vaccine, J. Infect. Dis. 164 (1991) 982.

[193] T.V. Murphy, et al., Decreased *Haemophilus* colonization in children vaccinated with *Haemophilus influenzae* type b conjugate vaccine, J. Pediatr. 122 (1993) 517.

[194] J.C. Mohle-Boetani, et al., Carriage of *Haemophilus influenzae* type b in children after widespread vaccination with *Haemophilus influenzae* type b vaccines, Pediatr. Infect. Dis. J. 12 (1993) 589.

[195] G. Urwin, et al., Invasive disease due to *Haemophilus influenzae* serotype f: clinical and epidemiologic characteristics in the *H. influenzae* serotype b vaccine era, Clin. Infect. Dis. 22 (1996) 1069.

[196] P.T. Heath, et al., Non-type b *Haemophilus influenzae* disease: clinical and epidemiologic characteristics in the *Haemophilus influenzae* type b vaccine era, Pediatr. Infect. Dis. J. 20 (2001) 300.

[197] D.G. Perdue, L.R. Bulkow, G.B. Gellin, Invasive *Haemophilus influenzae* disease in Alaskan residents aged 10 years and older before and after infant vaccination programs, JAMA 283 (2000) 3089.

[198] L.L. Barton, R.D. Cruz, C. Walentik, Neonatal *Haemophilus influenzae* type C sepsis, Am. J. Dis. Child. 136 (1982) 463.

[199] P. Campognone, D.B. Singer, Neonatal sepsis due to nontypeable *Haemophilus influenzae*, Am. J. Dis. Child. 140 (1986) 117.

[200] R.J. Wallace Jr., et al., Nontypable *Haemophilus influenzae* (biotype 4) as a neonatal, maternal and genital pathogen, Rev. Infect. Dis. 5 (1983) 123.

[201] T.J. Falia, et al., Population-based study of non-typeable *Haemophilus influenzae* invasive disease in children and neonates, Lancet 341 (1993) 851.

[202] C.A. Friesen, C.T. Cho, Characteristic features of neonatal sepsis due to *Haemophilus influenzae*, Rev. Infect. Dis. 8 (1986) 777.

[203] L.D. Lilien, et al., Early-onset *Haemophilus* sepsis in newborn infants: clinical, roentgenographic, and pathologic features, Pediatrics 62 (1978) 299.

[204] K. Silverberg, F.H. Boehm, *Haemophilus influenzae* amnionitis with intact membranes: a case report, Am. J. Perinatol. 7 (1990) 270.

[205] S. Hershckowitz, et al., A cluster of early neonatal sepsis and pneumonia caused by nontypable *Haemophilus influenzae*, Pediatr. Infect. Dis. J. 23 (2004) 1061–1062.

[206] J.S. Bradley, *Haemophilus parainfluenzae* sepsis in a very low birth weight premature infant: a case report and review of the literature, J. Perinatol. 19 (1999) 315.

[207] R.N. Holt, et al., Three cases of *Hemophilus parainfluenzae* meningitis, Clin. Pediatr. (Phila) 13 (1974) 666.

[208] S.H. Zinner, et al., Puerperal bacteremia and neonatal sepsis due to *Hemophilus parainfluenzae*: report of a case with antibody titers, Pediatrics 49 (1972) 612.

[209] A. Miano, et al., Neonatal *Haemophilus aphrophilus* meningitis, Helv. Paediatr. Acta 31 (1977) 499.

[210] S.L. Gorbach, J.G. Bartlett, Anaerobic infections, N. Engl. J. Med. 290 (1974) 1177.

[211] S.L. Gorbach, et al., Anaerobic microflora of the cervix in healthy women, Am. J. Obstet. Gynecol. 117 (1973) 1053.

[212] A.W. Chow, L.B. Guze, Bacteroidaceae bacteremia: clinical experience with 112 patients, Medicine (Baltimore) 53 (1974) 93.

[213] S.M. Finegold, Anaerobic infections, Surg. Clin. North. Am. 60 (1980) 49.

[214] I. Brook, Bacteremia due to anaerobic bacteria in newborns, J. Perinatol. 10 (1990) 351.

[215] G.J. Noel, D.A. Laufer, P.J. Edelson, Anaerobic bacteremia in a neonatal intensive care unit: an eighteen year experience, Pediatr. Infect. Dis. J. 7 (1988) 858.

[216] S. Mitra, D. Panigrahi, A. Narang, Anaerobes in neonatal septicaemia: a cause for concern, J. Trop. Pediatr. 43 (1997) 153.

[217] A.W. Chow, et al., The significance of anaerobes in neonatal bacteremia: analysis of 23 cases and review of the literature, Pediatrics 54 (1974) 736.

[218] S. Ohta, et al., Neonatal adrenal abscess due to *Bacteroides*, J. Pediatr. 93 (1978) 1063.

[219] Y.H. Lee, R.B. Berg, Cephalhematoma infected with *Bacteroides*, Am. J. Dis. Child. 121 (1971) 72.

[220] S.F. Siddiqi, P.M. Taylor, Necrotizing fasciitis of the scalp: a complication of fetal monitoring, Am. J. Dis. Child. 136 (1982) 226.

[221] H.M. Feder Jr., *Bacteroides fragilis* meningitis, Rev. Infect. Dis. 9 (1987) 783.

[222] J.R. Harrod, D.A. Stevens, Anaerobic infections in the newborn infant, J. Pediatr. 85 (1974) 399.

[223] L.M. Dunkle, T.J. Brotherton, R.D. Feigin, Anaerobic infections in children: a prospective survey, Pediatrics 57 (1976) 311.

[224] H.M. Feder Jr., et al., *Bacillus* species isolates from cerebrospinal fluid in patients without shunts, Pediatrics 82 (1988) 909–913.

[225] N.J. Hilliard, R.L. Schelonka, K.B. Waites, *Bacillus cereus* bacteremia in a preterm neonate, J. Clin. Microbiol. 41 (2003) 3441–3444.

[226] A.B. John, et al., Intractable *Bacillus cereus* bacteremia in a preterm neonate, J. Trop. Pediatr. 53 (2007) 131–132.

[227] R. Tuladhar, et al., Refractory *Bacillus cereus* infection in a neonate, Int. J. Clin. Pract. 54 (2000) 345–347.

[228] W.C. Van Der Zwet, et al., Outbreak of *Bacillus cereus* infections in a neonatal intensive care unit traced to balloons used in manual ventilation, J. Clin. Microbiol. 38 (2000) 4131–4136.

[229] M.D. Yohannan, et al., Congenital pneumonia and early neonatal septicemia due to *Bacteroides fragilis*, Eur. J. Clin. Microbiol. Infect. Dis. 11 (1992) 472–473.

[230] G.L. Keffer, G.R. Monif, Perinatal septicemia due to the Bacteroidaceae, Obstet. Gynecol. 71 (1988) 463–465.

[231] H.M. Feder Jr., *Bacteroides fragilis* meningitis, Rev. Infect. Dis. 9 (1987) 783–786.

[232] A.I. Airede, Pathogens in neonatal omphalitis, J. Trop. Pediatr. 38 (1992) 129.

[233] A. Kosloske, et al., Cellulitis and necrotizing fasciitis of the abdominal wall in pediatric patients, J. Pediatr. Surg. 16 (1981) 246.

[234] N.E. Chaney, *Clostridium* infection in mother and infant, Am. J. Dis. Child. 134 (1980) 1175.

[235] R.P. Spark, D.A. Wike, Nontetanus clostridial neonatal fatality after home delivery, Ariz. Med. 40 (1983) 697.

[236] R.A. Motz, A.G. James, B. Dove, *Clostridium perfringens* meningitis in a newborn infant, Pediatr. Infect. Dis. J. 15 (1996) 708.

[237] M.H. Roper, J.H. Vandelaer, F.L. Gasse, Maternal and neonatal tetanus, Lancet 370 (2007) 1947–1959.

[238] F.B. Pascual, et al., Tetanus surveillance—United States, 1998–2000, MMWR. Surveill. Summ. 52 (2003) 1.

[239] A.S. Craig, et al., Neonatal tetanus in the United States: a sentinel event in the foreign-born, Pediatr. Infect. Dis. J. 16 (1997) 955.

[240] S. Kumar, L.M. Malecki, A case of neonatal tetanus, South. Med. J. 84 (1991) 396.

[241] Centers for Disease Control, Neonatal tetanus—Montana, 1998, MMWR. Morb. Mortal. Wkly. Rep. 47 (1998) 928.

[242] J. Vandelaer, et al., Tetanus in developing countries: an update on the Maternal and Neonatal Tetanus Elimination Initiative, Vaccine 21 (2003) 3442.

[243] A. Quddus, et al., Neonatal tetanus: mortality rate and risk factors in Loralai District, Pakistan Int. J. Epidemiol. 31 (2002) 648.

[244] C.D. Idema, et al., Neonatal tetanus elimination in Mpumalanga Province, South Africa, Trop. Med. Int. Health 7 (2002) 622.

[245] S. Amsalu, S. Lulseged, Tetanus in a children's hospital in Addis Ababa: review of 113 cases, Ethiop. Med. J. 43 (2005) 233–240.

[246] B.E. Mustafa, et al., Neonatal tetanus in rural and displaced communities in the East Nile Province, J. Trop. Pediatr. 42 (1996) 110.

[247] R.B. Arnold, T.I. Soewarso, A. Karyadi, Mortality from neonatal tetanus in Indonesia: results of two surveys, Bull. World Health Organ. 64 (1986) 259.

[248] J.I.H. Herrero, R.R. Beltran, A.M.M. Sanchanz, Failure of intrathecal tetanus antitoxin in the treatment of tetanus neonatorum, J. Infect. Dis. 164 (1991) 619.

[249] E. Abrutyn, J.A. Berlin, Intrathecal therapy in tetanus, JAMA 266 (1991) 2262.

[250] H.P. Traverso, et al., Ghee application to the umbilical cord: a risk factor for neonatal tetanus, Lancet 1 (1989) 486.

[251] A.M. Oudesluys-Murphy, Umbilical cord care and neonatal tetanus, Lancet 1 (1989) 843.

[252] Centers for Disease Control and Prevention. Progress toward the global elimination of neonatal tetanus, 1989–1993, JAMA 273 (1995) 196.

[253] R.E. Black, D.H. Huber, G.T. Curlin, Reduction of neonatal tetanus by mass immunization of nonpregnant women: duration of protection provided by one or two doses of aluminum-adsorbed tetanus toxoid, Bull. World Health Organ. 58 (1980) 927.

[254] F. Schofield, Selective primary health care: strategies for control of disease in the developing world. XXII. Tetanus: a preventable problem, Rev. Infect. Dis. 8 (1986) 144.

[255] D.S. Gromisch, et al., Simultaneous mixed bacterial meningitis in an infant, Am. J. Dis. Child. 119 (1970) 284.

[256] L. Pacifico, et al., Early-onset *Pseudomonas aeruginosa* sepsis and *Yersinia enterocolitica* neonatal infection: a unique combination in a preterm infant, Eur. J. Pediatr. 146 (1987) 192.

[257] I. Tessin, B. Trollfors, K. Thiringer, Incidence and etiology of neonatal septicaemia and meningitis in western Sweden 1975–1986, Acta Paediatr. Scand. 79 (1990) 1023.

[258] T. Vesikari, et al., Neonatal septicaemia in Finland 1981–85, Acta Paediatr. Scand. 78 (1989) 44.

[259] B. Bruun, A. Paerregaard, Septicemia in a Danish neonatal intensive care unit, 1984 to 1988, Pediatr. Infect. Dis. J. 10 (1991) 159.

[260] R.G. Faix, S.M. Kovarik, Polymicrobial sepsis among intensive care nursery infants, J. Perinatol. 9 (1989) 131.

[261] W.R. Jarvis, et al., Polymicrobial bacteremia associated with lipid emulsion in a neonatal intensive care unit, Pediatr. Infect. Dis. J. 2 (1983) 203.

[262] T.J. Sferra, D.L. Pacini, Simultaneous recovery of bacterial and viral pathogens from CSF, Pediatr. Infect. Dis. J. 7 (1988) 552.

[263] G.P. Giacoia, Uncommon pathogens in newborn infants, J. Perinatol. 14 (1994) 134.

[264] J.E. Hodgman, Sepsis in the neonate, Perinatol Neonatol 5 (1981) 45.

[265] J.A. Hervás, et al., Neonatal sepsis and meningitis in Mallorca, Spain, 1977–1991, Clin. Infect. Dis. 16 (1993) 719.

[266] Public Health Laboratory Service Report. Neonatal meningitis: a review of routine national data 1975–83, BMJ 290 (1985) 778.

[267] A. Schuchat, et al., Population-based risk factors for neonatal group B streptococcal disease: results of a cohort study in metropolitan Atlanta, J. Infect. Dis. 162 (1990) 672.

[268] L. Cordero, M. Sananes, L.W. Ayers, Bloodstream infections in a neonatal intensive-care unit: 12 years' experience with an antibiotic control program, Infect. Control Hosp. Epidemiol. 20 (1999) 242.

[269] E. Persson, et al., Septicaemia and meningitis in neonates and during early infancy in the Goteborg area of Sweden, Acta Paediatr. 91 (2002) 1087.

[270] C. Simon, et al., Neonatal sepsis in an intensive care unit and results of treatment, Infection 19 (1991) 146.

[271] B.J. Stoll, N. Hansen, Infections in VLBW infants: studies from the NICHD Neonatal Research Network, Semin. Perinatol. 27 (2003) 293.

[272] L. Barton, J.E. Hodgman, Z. Pavlova, Causes of death in the extremely low birth weight infant, Pediatrics 103 (1999) 446.

[273] Z.A. Bhutta, K. Yusuf, Early-onset neonatal sepsis in Pakistan: a case control study of risk factors in a birth cohort, Am. J. Perinatol. 14 (1997) 577.

[274] K.M. Boyer, et al., Selective intrapartum chemoprophylaxis of neonatal group B streptococcal early-onset disease, I: epidemiologic rationale, J. Infect. Dis. 148 (1983) 795.

[275] E. Lieberman, et al., Epidural analgesia, intrapartum fever, and neonatal sepsis evaluation, Pediatrics 99 (1997) 415.

[276] K.R. Niswander, M. Gordon, The women and their pregnancies, The Collaborative Perinatal Study of the National Institute of Neurological Diseases and Stroke. U.S. Department of Health, Education and Welfare Publication No. (NIH) 73-379. U.S. Government Printing Office, Washington, DC, 1972.

[277] National Center for Health Statistics. Healthy People 2000. Maternal and Infant Health Progress Review, (1999) Live broadcast from Washington, DC, May 5, 1999.

[278] K. Fiscella, Race, perinatal outcome, and amniotic infection, Obstet. Gynecol. Surv. 51 (1996) 60.

[279] Centers for Disease Control and Prevention. Group B streptococcal disease in the United States, 1990: report from a multistate active surveillance system, In CDC Surveillance Summaries, November 20, 1992. MMWR. Morb. Mortal. Wkly. Rep. 41 (1992) 25.

[280] K. Benirschke, S. Driscoll, The Pathology of the Human Placenta, Springer-Verlag, New York, 1967.

[281] T.C. Washburn, D.N. Medearis Jr., B. Childs, Sex differences in susceptibility to infections, Pediatrics 35 (1965) 57.

[282] J.S. Torday, et al., Sex differences in fetal lung maturation, Am. Rev. Respir. Dis. 123 (1981) 205.

[283] A. Sinha, D. Yokoe, R. Platt, Epidemiology of neonatal infections: experience during and after hospitalization, Pediatr. Infect. Dis. J. 22 (2003) 244.

[284] A. Schuchat, et al., Risk factors and opportunities for prevention of early-onset neonatal sepsis: a multicenter case-control study, Pediatrics 105 (2000) 21.

[285] A.H. Sohn, et al., Prevalence of nosocomial infections in neonatal intensive care unit patients: results from the first national point-prevalence study, J. Pediatr. 139 (2001) 821.

[286] C. Speer, et al., Neonatal septicemia and meningitis in Gottingen, West Germany, Pediatr. Infect. Dis. J. 4 (1985) 36.

[287] O. Battisi, R. Mitchison, P.A. Davies, Changing blood culture isolates in a referral neonatal intensive care unit, Arch. Dis. Child. 56 (1981) 775.

[288] D.E. MacFarlane, Neonatal group B streptococcal septicaemia in a developing country, Acta Paediatr. Scand. 76 (1987) 470.

[289] A.K. Ako-Nai, et al., The bacteriology of neonatal septicaemiae in Ile-Ife, Nigeria, J. Trop. Pediatr. 45 (1999) 146.

[290] K.A. Kuruvilla, et al., Bacterial profile of sepsis in a neonatal unit in South India, Indian Pediatr. 35 (1998) 851.

[291] A. Ohlsson, T. Bailey, F. Takieddine, Changing etiology and outcome of neonatal septicemia in Riyadh, Saudi Arabia, Acta Paediatr. Scand. 75 (1986) 540.

[292] R.A. Kilani, M. Basamad, Pattern of proven bacterial sepsis in a neonatal intensive care unit in Riyadh-Saudi Arabia: a 2-year analysis, J. Med. Liban. 48 (2000) 77.

[293] R. Knippenberg, et al., Systematic scaling up of neonatal care in countries, Lancet 365 (2005) 1087–1098.

[294] J.E. Lawn, S. Cousens, J. Zupan, 4 million neonatal deaths. When? Where? Why? Lancet 365 (2005) 891–900.

[295] S. Vergnano, et al., Neonatal sepsis: an international perspective, Arch. Dis. Child. Fetal Neonatal Ed. 90 (2005) F220–F224.

[296] S. Rahman, et al., Multidrug resistant neonatal sepsis in Peshawar, Pakistan, Arch. Dis. Child. Fetal Neonatal Ed. 87 (2002) F52–F54.

[297] B. Blomberg, et al., High rate of fatal cases of pediatric septicemia caused by gram-negative bacteria with extended-spectrum beta-lactamases in Dar es Salaam, Tanzania, J. Clin. Microbiol. 43 (2005) 745–749.

[298] A. Amin, Y.M. Abdulrazzaq, S. Uduman, Group B streptococcal serotype distribution of isolates from colonized pregnant women at the time of delivery in United Arab Emirates, J. Infect. 45 (2002) 42.

[299] M. Tsolia, et al., Group B streptococcus colonization of Greek pregnant women and neonates: prevalence, risk factors and serotypes, Clin. Microbiol. Infect. 9 (2003) 832.

[300] B.J. Stoll, A. Schuchat, Maternal carriage of group B streptococci in developing countries, Pediatr. Infect. Dis. J. 17 (1998) 499.

[301] K. Cogwill, et al., Report from the CDC. Awareness of perinatal group B streptococcal infection among women of childbearing age in the United States, 1999 and 2002, J. Womens Health 12 (2003) 527.

[302] C.M. Beck-Sague, et al., Blood stream infections in neonatal intensive care unit patients: results of a multicenter study, Pediatr. Infect. Dis. J. 13 (1994) 1110.

[303] W.G. Adams, et al., Outbreak of early onset group B streptococcal sepsis, Pediatr. Infect. Dis. J. 12 (1993) 565.

[304] T. Cheasty, et al., The use of serodiagnosis in the retrospective investigation of a nursery outbreak associated with *Escherichia coli* O157:H7, J. Clin. Pathol. 51 (1998) 498.

[305] C. Hoyen, et al., Use of real time pulsed field gel electrophoresis to guide interventions during a nursery outbreak of *Serratia marcescens* infection, Pediatr. Infect. Dis. J. 18 (1999) 357.

[306] D.M. Olive, P. Bean, Principles and applications of methods for DNA-based typing of microbial organisms, J. Clin. Microbiol. 37 (1999) 1661.

[307] A. Dent, P. Toltzis, Descriptive and molecular epidemiology of gram-negative bacilli infections in the neonatal intensive care unit, Curr. Opin. Infect. Dis. 16 (2003) 279.

[308] W.C. van der Zwet, et al., Nosocomial outbreak of gentamicin-resistant *Klebsiella pneumoniae* in a neonatal intensive care unit controlled by a change in antibiotic policy, J. Hosp. Infect. 42 (1999) 295.

[309] R. Raz, et al., The elimination of gentamicin-resistant gram-negative bacteria in newborn intensive care unit, Infection 15 (1987) 32.

[310] R.S. Gibbs, P. Duff, Progress in pathogenesis and management of clinical intraamniotic infection, Am. J. Obstet. Gynecol. 164 (1991) 1317.

[311] D. Charles, W.R. Edwards, Infectious complications of cervical cerclage, Am. J. Obstet. Gynecol. 141 (1981) 1065.

[312] J.M. Aarts, J.T. Brons, H.W. Bruinse, Emergency cerclage: a review, Obstet. Gynecol. Surv. 50 (1995) 459.

[313] M. Fejgin, et al., Fulminant sepsis due to group B beta-hemolytic streptococci following transcervical chorionic villi sampling, Clin. Infect. Dis. 17 (1993) 142.

[314] I. Wilkins, et al., Amnionitis and life-threatening respiratory distress after percutaneous umbilical blood sampling, Am. J. Obstet. Gynecol. 160 (1989) 427.

[315] J.E. Morison, Foetal and Neonatal Pathology, third ed., Butterworth, Washington, DC, 1970.

[316] J.W. St Geme Jr., et al., Perinatal bacterial infection after prolonged rupture of amniotic membranes: an analysis of risk and management, J. Pediatr. 104 (1984) 608.

[317] W.A. Blanc, Pathways of fetal and early neonatal infection: viral placentitis, bacterial and fungal chorioamnionitis, J. Pediatr. 59 (1961) 473.

[318] S.L. Hillier, et al., Microbiologic causes and neonatal outcomes associated with chorioamnion infection, Am. J. Obstet. Gynecol. 165 (1991) 955.

[319] P.R. Yoder, et al., A prospective, controlled study of maternal and perinatal outcome after intra-amniotic infection at term, Am. J. Obstet. Gynecol. 145 (1983) 695.

[320] B. Larsen, I.S. Snyder, R.P. Galask, Bacterial growth inhibition by amniotic fluid, I: in vitro evidence for bacterial growth-inhibiting activity, Am. J. Obstet. Gynecol. 119 (1974) 492.

[321] J.L. Kitzmiller, S. Highby, W.E. Lucas, Retarded growth of E. coli in amniotic fluid, Obstet. Gynecol. 41 (1973) 38.

[322] P. Axemo, et al., Amniotic fluid antibacterial activity and nutritional parameters in term Mozambican and Swedish pregnant women, Gynecol. Obstet. Invest. 42 (1996) 24.

[323] T.M. Scane, D.F. Hawkins, Antibacterial activity in human amniotic fluid: relationship to zinc and phosphate, Br. J. Obstet. Gynaecol. 91 (1984) 342.

[324] M.A. Nazir, et al., Antibacterial activity of amniotic fluid in the early third trimester: its association with preterm labor and delivery, Am. J. Perinatol. 4 (1987) 59.

[325] S.M. Baker, N.N. Balo, F.T. Abdel Aziz, Is vernix a protective material to the newborn? A biochemical approach, Indian J. Pediatr. 62 (1995) 237.

[326] A.L. Florman, D. Teubner, Enhancement of bacterial growth in amniotic fluid by meconium, J. Pediatr. 74 (1969) 111.

[327] I.A. Hoskins, et al., Effects of alterations of zinc-to-phosphate ratios and meconium content on group B streptococcus growth in human amniotic fluid in vitro, Am. J. Obstet. Gynecol. 157 (1988) 770.

[328] C. Altieri, et al., In vitro survival of *Listeria monocytogenes* in human amniotic fluid, Zentralbl. Hyg. Umweltmed. 202 (1999) 377.

[329] G. Evaldson, C.E. Nord, Amniotic fluid activity against *Bacteroides fragilis* and group B streptococci, Med. Microbiol. Immunol. 170 (1981) 11.

[330] A.I. Eidelman, et al., The effect of meconium staining of amniotic fluid on the growth of *Escherichia coli* and group B streptococcus, J. Perinatol. 22 (2002) 467.

[331] G. Marston, E.R. Wald, *Hemophilus influenzae* type b sepsis in infant and mother, Pediatrics 58 (1976) 863.

[332] M.M. Tarpay, D.V. Turbeville, H.F. Krous, Fatal *Streptococcus pneumoniae* type III sepsis in mother and infant, Am. J. Obstet. Gynecol. 136 (1980) 257.

[333] J.M. Mastrobattista, V.M. Parisi, Vertical transmission of a *Citrobacter* infection, Am. J. Perinatol. 14 (1997) 465.

[334] T. Boussemart, et al., *Morganella morganii* and early-onset neonatal infection, Arch. Pediatr. 11 (2004) 37.

[335] B. Tempest, Pneumococcal meningitis in mother and neonate, Pediatrics 53 (1974) 759.

[336] J. Grossman, R.L. Tompkins, Group B beta-hemolytic streptococcal meningitis in mother and infant, N. Engl. J. Med. 290 (1974) 387.

[337] S.P. Pyati, et al., Penicillin in infants weighing two kilograms or less with early-onset group B streptococcal disease, N. Engl. J. Med. 308 (1983) 1383.

[338] M.C. Maberry, L.C. Gilstrap, Intrapartum antibiotic therapy for suspected intraamniotic infection: impact on the fetus and neonate, Clin. Obstet. Gynecol. 34 (1991) 345.

[339] L.M. Sacks, J.C. McKitrick, R.R. MacGregor, Surface cultures and isolation procedures in infants born under unsterile conditions, Am. J. Dis. Child. 137 (1983) 351.

[340] I. Brook, E.H. Frazier, Microbiology of scalp abscess in newborn, Pediatr. Infect. Dis. J. 11 (1992) 766.

[341] R.M. Freedman, R. Baltimore, Fatal *Streptococcus viridans* septicemia and meningitis: a relationship to fetal scalp electrode monitoring, J. Perinatol. 10 (1990) 272.

[342] L. Cordero, C.W. Anderson, F.P. Zuspan, Scalp abscess: a benign and infrequent complication of fetal monitoring, Am. J. Obstet. Gynecol. 146 (1983) 126.

[343] W. Storm, Transient bacteremia following endotracheal suctioning in ventilated newborns, Pediatrics 65 (1980) 487.

[344] D.B. Singer, Infections of Fetuses and Neonates, Blackwell Scientific Publications, Boston, 1991.

[345] Y. Sorokin, et al., Cerebrospinal fluid leak in the neonate—complication of fetal scalp electrode monitoring: case report and review of the literature, Isr. J. Med. Sci. 26 (1990) 633.

[346] P. Nieburg, S.J. Gross, Cerebrospinal fluid leak in a neonate with fetal scalp electrode monitoring, Am. J. Obstet. Gynecol. 147 (1983) 839.

[347] R.C. Nagle, et al., Brain abscess aspiration in nursery with ultrasound guidance, J. Neurosurg. 65 (1986) 557.

[348] D. Renier, et al., Brain abscesses in neonates: a study of 30 cases, J. Neurosurg. 69 (1988) 877.

[349] T. Jadavji, R.P. Humphreys, C.G. Prober, Brain abscesses in infants and children, Pediatr. Infect. Dis. 4 (1985) 394.

[350] J.J. Volpe, Neurology of the Newborn, second ed., WB Saunders, Philadelphia, 1987.

[351] H.C. Dillon, S. Khare, B.M. Gray, Group B streptococcal carriage and disease: a 6-year prospective study, J. Pediatr. 110 (1987) 31.

[352] M.J. Maisels, E. Kring, Risk of sepsis in newborns with severe hyperbilirubinemia, Pediatrics 90 (1992) 741.

[353] F. Tiker, et al., Early onset conjugated hyperbilirubinemia in newborn infants, Indian J. Pediatr. 73 (2006) 409–412.

[354] B.A. Haber, A.M. Lake, Cholestatic jaundice in the newborn, Clin. Perinatol. 17 (1990) 483.

[355] J.C. Rooney, D.J. Hills, D.M. Danks, Jaundice associated with bacterial infection in the newborn, Am. J. Dis. Child. 122 (1971) 39.

[356] R. Dagan, R. Gorodischer, Infections in hypothermic infants younger than 3 months old, Am. J. Dis. Child. 138 (1984) 483.

[357] R.B. Johanson, et al., Effect of post-delivery care on neonatal body temperature, Acta Paediatr. 81 (1992) 859.

[358] M. Michael, D.J. Barrett, P. Mehta, Infants with meningitis without CSF pleocytosis, Am. J. Dis. Child. 140 (1986) 851.

[359] A.S. El-Radhy, et al., Sepsis and hypothermia in the newborn infant: value of gastric aspirate examination, J. Pediatr. 104 (1983) 300.

[360] A.M. Al Jarousha, et al., An outbreak of *Serratia marcescens* septicaemia in neonatal intensive care unit in Gaza City, Palestine, J. Hosp. Infect. 70 (2008) 119–126.

[361] P.H. Barr, Association of *Escherichia coli* sepsis and galactosemia in neonates, J. Am. Board. Fam. Pract. 5 (1992) 89.

[362] H.L. Levy, et al., Sepsis due to *Escherichia coli* in neonates with galactosemia, N. Engl. J. Med. 297 (1977) 823.

[363] S. Kelly, Septicemia in galactosemia, JAMA 216 (1971) 330.

[364] S.B. Shurin, *Escherichia coli* septicemia in neonates with galactosemia, Letter to the editor N. Engl. J. Med. 297 (1977) 1403.

[365] R.H. Kobayashi, B.V. Kettelhut, A. Kobayashi, Galactose inhibition of neonatal neutrophil function, Pediatr. Infect. Dis. J. 2 (1983) 442.

[366] A.M. Bosch, Classical galactosaemia revisited, J. Inherit. Metab. Dis. 29 (2006) 516–525.

[367] M. Odievre, et al., Hereditary fructose intolerance: Diagnosis, management and course in 55 patients, Am. J. Dis. Child. 132 (1978) 605.

[368] J. Guerra-Moreno, N. Barrios, P.J. Santiago-Borrero, Severe neutropenia in an infant with methylmalonic acidemia, Bol. Asoc. Med. P. R. 95 (2003) 17.

[369] R.J. Hutchinson, K. Bunnell, J.G. Thoene, Suppression of granulopoietic progenitor cell proliferation by metabolites of the branched-chain amino acids, J. Pediatr. 106 (1985) 62.

[370] V.L. Negre, et al., The siderophore receptor IroN, but not the high-pathogenicity island or the hemin receptor ChuA, contributes to the bacteremic step of *Escherichia coli* neonatal meningitis, Infect. Immun. 72 (2004) 1216–1220.

[371] E.D. Weinberg, Iron and susceptibility to infectious disease, Science 184 (1974) 952.

[372] P. Manzoni, et al., Bovine lactoferrin supplementation for prevention of late-onset sepsis in very low-birth-weight neonates: a randomized trial, JAMA 302 (2009) 1421–1428.

[373] D.M.J. Barry, A.W. Reeve, Increased incidence of gram-negative neonatal sepsis with intramuscular iron administration, Pediatrics 60 (1977) 908.

[374] K. Farmer, The disadvantages of routine administration of intramuscular iron to neonates, N. Z. Med. J. 84 (1976) 286.

[375] C.L. Berseth, et al., Growth, efficacy, and safety of feeding an iron-fortified human milk fortifier, Pediatrics 114 (2004) e699–e706.

[376] I.M. Usta, et al., Comparison of the perinatal morbidity and mortality of the presenting twin and its co-twin, J. Perinatol. 22 (2002) 391.

[377] K. Benirschke, Routes and types of infection in the fetus and newborn, Am. J. Dis. Child. 99 (1960) 714.

[378] J.M. Alexander, et al., The relationship of infection to method of delivery in twin pregnancy, Am. J. Obstet. Gynecol. 177 (1997) 1063–1066.

[379] J.M. Alexander, et al., Cesarean delivery for the second twin, Obstet. Gynecol. 112 (2008) 748–752.

[380] M.A. Pass, S. Khare, H.C. Dillon Jr., Twin pregnancies: incidence of group B streptococcal colonization and disease, J. Pediatr. 97 (1980) 635.

[381] M.S. Edwards, C.V. Jackson, C.J. Baker, Increased risk of group B streptococcal disease in twins, JAMA 245 (1981) 2044.

[382] K.S. Doran, et al., Late-onset group B streptococcal infection in identical twins: insight to disease pathogenesis, J. Perinatol. 22 (2002) 326–330.

[383] K. LaMar, D.A. Dowling, Incidence of infection for preterm twins cared for in cobedding in the neonatal intensive-care unit, J. Obstet. Gynecol. Neonatal. Nurs. 35 (2006) 193–198.

[384a] J.R. Pai, C.H. Tremlett, P. Clarke, Late onset sepsis in a pre-term twin may harbinger life-threatening sepsis for the asymptomatic co-twin, Pediatr Infect Dis J. 29 (2010) 81–382.

[384] P.I. Nieburg, M.L. William, Group A beta-hemolytic streptococcal sepsis in a mother and infant twins, J. Pediatr. 87 (1975) 453.

[385] J.G. Larsen, et al., Multiple antibiotic resistant *Salmonella agora* infection in malnourished neonatal twins, Mt. Sinai J. Med. 46 (1979) 542.

[386] H.R. Devlin, R.M. Bannatyne, Neonatal malaria, Can. Med. Assoc. J. 116 (1977) 20.

[387] S. Romand, et al., Congenital malaria: a case observed in twins born to an asymptomatic mother, Presse Med. 23 (1994) 797.

[388] T. Shafai, Neonatal coccidioidomycosis in premature twins, Am. J. Dis. Child. 132 (1978) 634.

[389] S. Saigal, W.A. Eisele, M.A. Chernesky, Congenital cytomegalovirus infection in a pair of dizygotic twins, Am. J. Dis. Child. 136 (1982) 1094.

[390] J.J. Duvekot, et al., Congenital cytomegalovirus infection in a twin pregnancy: a case report, Eur. J. Pediatr. 149 (1990) 261.

[391] T. Lazzarotto, et al., Congenital cytomegalovirus infection in twin pregnancies: viral load in the amniotic fluid and pregnancy outcome, Pediatrics 112 (2003) e153.

[392] R.C. Montgomery, K. Stockdell, Congenital rubella in twins, J. Pediatr. 76 (1970) 772.

[393] N. Fraser, B.W. Davies, J. Cusack, Neonatal omphalitis: a review of its serious complications, Acta Paediatr. 95 (2006) 519–522.

[394] I. Forshall, Septic umbilical arteritis, Arch. Dis. Child. 32 (1957) 25.

[395] J.N. Cruickshank, Child Life Investigations: The Causes of Neo-natal Death, His Majesty's Stationery Office, London, 1930 Medical Research Council Special Report Series No. 145.

[396] A.H. Cushing, Omphalitis: a review, Pediatr. Infect. Dis. J. 4 (1985) 282.

[397] V.O. Rotimi, B.I. Duerden, The development of the bacterial flora in normal neonates, J. Med. Microbiol. 14 (1981) 51.

[398] W.H. Mason, et al., Omphalitis in the newborn infant, Pediatr. Infect. Dis. J. 8 (1989) 521.

[399] E.A. Ameh, P.T. Nmadu, Major complications of omphalitis in neonates and infants, Pediatr. Surg. Int. 18 (2002) 413.

[400a] L.C. Mullany, G.L. Darmstadt, S.K. Khaty, et al., Topical applications of chlorhexidine to the umbilical cord for prevention of omphalitis and neonatal mortality in southern Nepal; a community-based, cluster-randomised trial, Lancet 367 (2006) 910–918.

[400] W.W. Meyer, J. Lind, The ductus venosus and the mechanism of its closure, Arch. Dis. Child. 41 (1966) 597.

[401] J.E. Morison, Umbilical sepsis and acute interstitial hepatitis, J. Pathol. Bacteriol. 56 (1944) 531.

[402] R.I.K. Elliott, The ductus venosus in neonatal infection, Proc. R. Soc. Med. 62 (1969) 321.

[403] K. Bedtke, H. Richarz, Nabelsepsis mit Pylephlebitis, multiplen Leberabscessen, Lungenabscessen und Osteomyelitis. Ausgang in Heilung, Monatsschr. Kinderheilkd. 105 (1957) 70.

[404] E.N. Thompson, S. Sherlock, The aetiology of portal vein thrombosis with particular reference to the role of infection and exchange transfusion, QJM 33 (1964) 465.

[405] R.W. MacMillan, J.N. Schullinger, T.V. Santulli, Pyourachus: an unusual surgical problem, J. Pediatr. Surg. 8 (1973) 387–389.

[406] C. Navarro, W.A. Blanc, Subacute necrotizing funisitis: a variant of cord inflammation with a high rate of perinatal infection, J. Pediatr. 85 (1974) 689.

[407] A. Ohlsson, Treatment of preterm premature rupture of the membranes: a meta-analysis, Am. J. Obstet. Gynecol. 160 (1989) 890.

[408] P. Crowley, I. Chalmers, M.J. Keirse, The effects of corticosteroid administration before preterm delivery: an overview of the evidence from controlled trials, Br. J. Obstet. Gynaecol. 97 (1990) 11.

[409] S.T. Vermillion, et al., Effectiveness of antenatal corticosteroid administration after preterm premature rupture of the membranes, Am. J. Obstet. Gynecol. 183 (2000) 925.

[410] D. Roberts, S. Dalziel, Antenatal corticosteroids for accelerating fetal lung maturation for women at risk of preterm birth, Cochrane Database Syst. Rev. (3) CD004454, (2006).

[411] Z. Gottesfeld, S.E. Ullrich, Prenatal alcohol exposure selectively suppresses cell-mediated but not humoral immune responsiveness, Int. J. Immunopharmacol. 17 (1995) 247.

[412] S. Johnson, et al., Immune deficiency in fetal alcohol syndrome, Pediatr. Res. 15 (1981) 908.

[413] K.W. Culver, et al., Lymphocyte abnormalities in infants born to drug-abusing mothers, J. Pediatr. 111 (1987) 230.

[414] Chemical dependency and pregnancy, Clin. Perinatol. 18 (1991) 1–191.

[415] J.R. Woods, Drug abuse in pregnancy, Clin. Obstet. Gynecol. 36 (1993) 221.

[416] I.J. Chasnoff, Drug Use in Pregnancy: Mother and Child, MTP Press, Boston, 1986.

[417] R. Ojala, S. Ikonen, O. Tammela, Perinatal indomethacin treatment and neonatal complications in preterm infants, Eur. J. Pediatr. 159 (2000) 153.

[418] C.A. Major, et al., Tocolysis with indomethacin increases the incidence of necrotizing enterocolitis in the low-birth-weight neonate, Am. J. Obstet. Gynecol. 170 (1994) 102.

[419] V.C. Herson, et al., Indomethacin-associated sepsis in very-low-birth-weight infants, Am. J. Dis. Child. 142 (1988) 555.

[420] T.M. O'Shea, et al., Follow-up of preterm infants treated with dexamethasone for chronic lung disease, Am. J. Dis. Child. 147 (1993) 658.

[421] A. Ohlsson, R. Walia, S. Shah, Ibuprofen for the treatment of patent ductus arteriosus in preterm and/or low birth weight infants, Cochrane Database Syst. Rev. CD003481, (2008).

[422] J.L. Tapia, et al., The effect of early dexamethasone administration on bronchopulmonary dysplasia in preterm infants with respiratory distress syndrome, J. Pediatr. 132 (1998) 48–52.

[423] C. Avila-Figueroa, et al., Intravenous lipid emulsions are the major determinant of coagulase-negative staphylococcal bacteremia in very low birth weight newborns, Pediatr. Infect. Dis. J. 17 (1998) 10–17.

[424] A.G. Matlow, et al., A randomized trial of 72- versus 24-hour intravenous tubing set changes in newborns receiving lipid therapy, Infect. Control Hosp. Epidemiol. 20 (1999) 487–493.

[425] S. Bianconi, et al., Ranitidine and late-onset sepsis in the neonatal intensive care unit, J. Perinat. Med. 35 (2007) 147–150.

[426] A.J. Barson, A Postmortem Study of Infection in the Newborn from 1976 to 1988, John Wiley & Sons, New York, 1990.

[427] P.H. Berman, B.Q. Banker, Neonatal meningitis: a clinical and pathological study of 29 cases, Pediatrics 38 (1966) 6.

[428] J.T. Stocker, L.P. Dehner, Pediatric Pathology, JB Lippincott, Philadelphia, 1992.

[429] H.J. Hoffman, E.B. Hendrick, J.L. Hiscox, Cerebral abscesses in early infancy, J. Neurosurg. 33 (1970) 172.

[430] D.G. Watson, Purulent neonatal meningitis: a study of forty-five cases, J. Pediatr. 50 (1957) 352.

[431] J.J. Volpe, Neurology of the Newborn, third ed., WB Saunders, Philadelphia, 1995.

[432] J.M. Perlman, N. Rollins, P.J. Sanchez, Late-onset meningitis in sick, very-low-birth-weight infants: clinical and sonographic observations, Am. J. Dis. Child. 146 (1992) 1297.

[433] F.H. Gilles, J.L. Jammes, W. Berenberg, Neonatal meningitis: the ventricle as a bacterial reservoir, Arch. Neurol. 34 (1977) 560.

[434] M.A. Schiano, J.C. Hauth, L.C. Gilstrap, Second-stage fetal tachycardia and neonatal infection, Am. J. Obstet. Gynecol. 148 (1984) 779.

[435] G.S. Shah, et al., Risk factors in early neonatal sepsis, Kathmandu. Univ. Med. J. (KUMJ) 4 (2006) 187–191.

[436] F. Mwanyumba, et al., Placental inflammation and perinatal outcome, Eur. J. Obstet. Gynecol. Reprod. Biol. 108 (2003) 164–170.

[437] E. Kermorvant-Duchemin, et al., Outcome and prognostic factors in neonates with septic shock, Pediatr. Crit. Care. Med. 9 (2008) 186–191.

[438] M. Soman, B. Green, J. Daling, Risk factors for early neonatal sepsis, Am. J. Epidemiol. 121 (1985) 712.

[439] T. Hegyi, et al., The Apgar score and its components in the preterm infant, Pediatrics 101 (1998) 77.

[440] K.R. Powell, Evaluation and management of febrile infants younger than 60 days of age, Pediatr. Infect. Dis. J. 9 (1990) 153.

[441] W.A. Bonadio, et al., Reliability of observation variables in distinguishing infectious outcome of febrile young infants, Pediatr. Infect. Dis. J. 12 (1993) 111.

[442] M. Kudawla, S. Dutta, A. Narang, Validation of a clinical score for the diagnosis of late onset neonatal septicemia in babies weighing 1000–2500 g, J. Trop. Pediatr. 54 (2008) 66–69.

[443] S. Fielkow, S. Reuter, S.P. Gotoff, Cerebrospinal fluid examination in symptom-free infants with risk factors for infection, J. Pediatr. 119 (1991) 971.

[444] W.H. Albers, C.W. Tyler, B. Boxerbaum, Asymptomatic bacteremia in the newborn infant, J. Pediatr. 69 (1966) 193.

[445] M. Petanovic, Z. Zagar, The significance of asymptomatic bacteremia for the newborn, Acta Obstet. Gynecol. Scand. 80 (2001) 813.

[446] J.B. Howard, G.H. McCracken, The spectrum of group B streptococcal infections in infancy, Am. J. Dis. Child. 128 (1974) 815.

[447] L.E. Weisman, et al., Early-onset group B streptococcal sepsis: a current assessment, J. Pediatr. 121 (1992) 428.

[448] P. Yagupsky, M.A. Menegus, K.R. Powell, The changing spectrum of group B streptococcal disease in infants: an eleven-year experience in a tertiary care hospital, Pediatr. Infect. Dis. J. 10 (1991) 801.

[449] P.G. Ramsey, R. Zwerdling, Asymptomatic neonatal bacteremia, Letter to the editor, N. Engl. J. Med. 295 (1976) 225.

[450] J.S. Yu, A. Grauang, Purulent meningitis in the neonatal period, Arch. Dis. Child. 38 (1963) 391.

[451] S.L. Solomon, E.M. Wallace, E.L. Ford-Jones, et al., Medication errors with inhalant epinephrine mimicking an epidemic of neonatal sepsis, N. Engl. J. Med. 310 (1984) 166.

[452] W.A. Bonadio, M. Hegenbarth, M. Zachariason, Correlating reported fever in young infants with subsequent temperature patterns and rate of serious bacterial infections, Pediatr. Infect. Dis. J. 9 (1990) 158.

[453] J. Messaritakis, et al., Rectal-skin temperature difference in septicaemic newborn infants, Arch. Dis. Child. 65 (1990) 380.

[454] C.A. Dinarello, et al., Production of leukocytic pyrogen from phagocytes of neonates, J. Infect. Dis. 144 (1981) 337.

[455] S.R. Mayfield, et al., Temperature measurement in term and preterm neonates, J. Pediatr. 104 (1984) 271.

[456] K.J. Johnson, P. Bhatia, E.F. Bell, Infrared thermometry of newborn infants, Pediatrics 87 (1991) 34.

[457] A.J. Schuman, The accuracy of infrared auditory canal thermometry in infants and children, Clin. Pediatr. 32 (1993) 347.

[458] D. Anagnostakis, et al., Rectal-axillary difference in febrile and afebrile infants and children, Clin. Pediatr. 32 (1993) 268.

[459] M.E. Weisse, et al., Axillary vs. rectal temperatures in ambulatory and hospitalized children, Pediatr. Infect. Dis. J. 10 (1991) 541.

[460] G.L. Freed, J.K. Fraley, Lack of agreement of tympanic membrane temperature assessments with conventional methods in a private practice setting, Pediatrics 89 (1992) 384.

[461] S. Hutton, et al., Accuracy of different temperature devices in the postpartum population, J. Obstet. Gynecol. Neonatal. Nurs. 38 (2009) 42–49.

[462] S. Voora, et al., Fever in full-term newborns in the first four days of life, Pediatrics 69 (1982) 40.

[463] L.M. Osborn, R. Bolus, Temperature and fever in the full-term newborn, J. Fam. Pract. 20 (1985) 261.

[464] F.J. Garcia, A. Nager, Jaundice as an early diagnostic sign of urinary tract infection in infancy, Pediatrics 109 (2002) 846.

[465] S. Zamora-Castorena, M.T. Murguia-de-Sierra, Five year experience with neonatal sepsis in a pediatric center, Rev. Invest. Clin. 50 (1998) 463.

[466] A.I. Airede, Urinary-tract infections in African neonates, J. Infect. 25 (1992) 55.

[467] R.A. Seeler, Urosepsis with jaundice due to hemolytic Escherichia coli, Am. J. Dis. Child. 126 (1973) 414.

[468] H. Bilgen, et al., Urinary tract infection and hyperbilirubinemia, Turk. J. Pediatr. 48 (2006) 51–55.

[469] S. Ashkenazi, et al., Size of liver edge in full-term, healthy infants, Am. J. Dis. Child. 138 (1984) 377.

[470] M.I. Reiff, L.M. Osborn, Clinical estimation of liver size in newborn infants, Pediatrics 71 (1983) 46.

[471] J. Sfeir, et al., Early onset neonatal septicemia caused by Listeria monocytogenes, Rev. Chil. Pediatr. 61 (1990) 330.

[472] M. Bamji, et al., Palpable lymph nodes in healthy newborns and infants, Pediatrics 78 (1986) 573.

[473] J. Embree, J. Muriithi, Palpable lymph nodes. Letter to the editor, Pediatrics 81 (1988) 598.

[474] R. Monfort Gil, et al., Group B streptococcus late-onset disease presenting as cellulitis-adenitis syndrome, Ann. Pediatr. 60 (2004) 75.

[475] S. Artigas Rodriguez, et al., Group B streptococcus cellulitis-adenitis syndrome in neonates. Is it a marker of bacteremia, An. Esp. Pediatr. 56 (2002) 251.

[476] E.A. Albanyan, C.J. Baker, Is lumbar puncture necessary to exclude meningitis in neonates and young infants: lessons from the group B streptococcus cellulitis-adenitis syndrome, Pediatrics 102 (1998) 985.

[477] A.H. Bell, et al., Meningitis in the newborn: a 14 year review, Arch. Dis. Child. 64 (1989) 873.

[478] M.I. Weintraub, R.N. Otto, Pneumococcal meningitis and endophthalmitis in a newborn, JAMA 219 (1972) 1763.

[479] K. Matasova, J. Hudecova, M. Zibolen, Bilateral endogenous endophthalmitis as a complication of late-onset sepsis in a premature infant, Eur. J. Pediatr. 162 (2003) 346.

[480] F. Nejat, et al., Spinal epidural abscess in a neonate, Pediatr. Infect. Dis. J. 21 (2002) 797.

[481] R.S. Walter, et al., Spinal epidural abscess in infancy: successful percutaneous drainage in a nine-month-old and review of the literature, Pediatr. Infect. Dis. J. 19 (1991) 860.

[482] K. Tang, C. Xenos, S. Sgouros, Spontaneous spinal epidural abscess in a neonate: with a review of the literature, Childs Nerv. Syst. 17 (2001) 629.

[483] R.W. Steele, A revised strategy for the prevention of group B streptococcal infection in pregnant women and their newborns, Medscape Womens Health 1 (1996) 2.

[484] American College of Obstetricians and Gynecologists, ACOG Committee Opinion: no. 279, December 2002. Prevention of early-onset group B streptococcal disease in newborns, Obstet. Gynecol. 100 (2002) 1405.

[485] M.E. Evans, et al., Sensitivity, specificity, and predictive value of body surface cultures in a neonatal intensive care unit, JAMA 259 (1988) 248.

[486] D. Hertz, et al., Comparison of DNA probe technology and automated continuous-monitoring blood culture systems in the detection of neonatal bacteremia, J. Perinatol. 19 (1999) 290.

[487] J.D. Anderson, C. Trombley, N. Cimolai, Assessment of the BACTEC NR660 blood culture system for the detection of bacteremia in young children, J. Clin. Microbiol. 27 (1989) 721.

[488] J.M. Campos, J.R. Spainhour, Rapid detection of bacteremia in children with modified lysis direct plating method, J. Clin. Microbiol. 22 (1985) 674.

[489] J.W. St Geme III, et al., Distinguishing sepsis from blood culture contamination in young infants with blood cultures growing coagulase-negative staphylococci, Pediatrics 86 (1990) 157.

[490] I. Kurlat, B.J. Stoll, J.E. McGowan Jr., Time to positivity for detection of bacteremia in neonates, J. Clin. Microbiol. 27 (1989) 1068.

[491] M.D. Pichichero, J.K. Todd, Detection of neonatal bacteremia, J. Pediatr. 94 (1979) 958.

[492] A.H. Rowley, E.R. Wald, Incubation period necessary to detect bacteremia in neonates, Pediatr. Infect. Dis. J. 5 (1986) 590.

[493] L.A. Jardine, et al., Neonatal blood cultures: effect of delayed entry into the blood culture machine and bacterial concentration on the time to positive growth in a simulated model, J. Paediatr. Child. Health 45 (2009) 210–214.

[494] K. Sprunt, Commentary, Year Book Medical Publishers, Chicago, 1973.

[495] P.R. Neal, et al., Volume of blood submitted for culture from neonates, J. Clin. Microbiol. 24 (1986) 353.

[496] D.E. Dietzman, G.W. Fischer, F.D. Schoenknecht, Neonatal Escherichia coli septicemia—bacterial counts in blood, J. Pediatr. 85 (1974) 128.

[497] J.K. Kennaugh, et al., The effect of dilution during culture on detection of low concentrations of bacteria in blood, Pediatr. Infect. Dis. 3 (1984) 317.

[498] G. Jawaheer, T.J. Neal, N.J. Shaw, Blood culture volume and detection of coagulase negative staphylococcal septicaemia in neonates, Arch. Dis. Child. (1997) 76:57F.

[499] J.A. Kellogg, J.P. Manzella, D.A. Bankert, Frequency of low-level bacteremia in children from birth to fifteen years of age, J. Clin. Microbiol. 28 (2000) 2181.

[500] J.A. Kellogg, et al., Frequency of low-level bacteremia in infants from birth to two months of age, Pediatr. Infect. Dis. J. 16 (1997) 381.

[501] R.L. Schelonka, et al., Volume of blood required to detect common neonatal pathogens, J. Pediatr. 129 (1996) 275.

[502] T.G. Connell, et al., How reliable is a negative blood culture result? Volume of blood submitted for culture in routine practice in a children's hospital, Pediatrics 119 (2007) 891–896.

[503] M. Pourcyrous, et al., Indwelling umbilical arterial catheter: a preferred sampling site for blood cultures, Pediatrics 81 (1988) 621.

[504] V. Bhandari, et al., Nosocomial sepsis in neonates with single lumen vascular catheters, Indian. J. Pediatr. 64 (1997) 529.

[505] D.K. Benjamin Jr., et al., Bacteremia, central catheters, and neonates: when to pull the line, Pediatrics 107 (2001) 1272–1276.

[506] C. Marconi, et al., Usefulness of catheter tip culture in the diagnosis of neonatal infections, J. Pediatr. (Rio J) 85 (2009) 80–83.

[507] T.E. Wiswell, W.E. Hachey, Multiple site blood cultures in the initial evaluation for neonatal sepsis during the first week of life, Pediatr. Infect. Dis. J. 10 (1991) 365.

[508] O. Hammerberg, et al., Comparison of blood cultures with corresponding venipuncture site cultures of specimens from hospitalized premature neonates, J. Pediatr. 120 (1992) 120.

[509] C.M. Healy, et al., Distinctive features of neonatal invasive staphylococcal disease, Pediatrics 114 (2004) 953.

[510] A.A. Humphrey, Use of the buffy layer in the rapid diagnosis of septicemia, Am. J. Clin. Pathol. 14 (1944) 358.

[511] R.J. Boyle, et al., Early identification of sepsis in infants with respiratory distress, Pediatrics 62 (1978) 744.

[512] H.S. Faden, Early diagnosis of neonatal bacteremia by buffy-coat examination, J. Pediatr. 88 (1976) 1032.

[513] W. Storm, Early detection of bacteremia by peripheral smears in critically ill newborns, Acta Paediatr. Scand. 70 (1981) 415.

[514] M.B. Kleiman, et al., Rapid diagnosis of neonatal bacteremia with acridine orange-stained buffy coat smears, J. Pediatr. 105 (1984) 419.

[515] P. Kite, et al., Comparison of five tests used in diagnosis of neonatal bacteremia, Arch. Dis. Child. 63 (1988) 639.

[516] S.K. Tak, P.C. Bhandari, B. Bhandari, Value of buffy coat examination in early diagnosis of neonatal septicemia, Indian Pediatr. 17 (1980) 339.

[517] D.L. Powers, G.L. Mandell, Intraleukocytic bacteria in endocarditis patients, JAMA 227 (1974) 312.

[518] H.E.J. Cattermole, R.P.A. Rivers, Neonatal Candida septicaemia: diagnosis on buffy smear, Arch. Dis. Child. 62 (1987) 302.

[519] R.J. Ascuitto, et al., Buffy coat smears of blood drawn through central venous catheters as an aid to rapid diagnosis of systemic fungal infections, J. Pediatr. 106 (1985) 445.

[520] D.M. Selby, et al., Overwhelming neonatal septicemia diagnosed upon examination of peripheral blood smears, Clin. Pediatr. 29 (1990) 706.

[521] W. Strom, Early detection of bacteremia by peripheral blood smears in critically ill newborns, Acta Paediatr. Scand. 70 (1981) 415.

[522] R.L. Rodwell, A.L. Leslie, D.I. Tudehope, Evaluation of direct and buffy coat films of peripheral blood for the early detection of bacteraemia, Aust. Paediatr. J. 25 (1989) 83.

[523] V.E. Visser, R.T. Hall, Urine culture in the evaluation of suspected neonatal sepsis, J. Pediatr. 94 (1979) 635.

[524] R.J. DiGeronimo, Lack of efficacy of the urine culture as part of the initial workup of suspected neonatal sepsis, Pediatr. Infect. Dis. J. 9 (1992) 764.

[525] B.K. Bonsu, M.B. Harper, Leukocyte counts in urine reflect the risk of concomitant sepsis in bacteriuric infants: a retrospective cohort study, BMC. Pediatr. 7 (2007) 24.

[526] R. Tobiansky, N. Evans, A randomized controlled trial of two methods for collection of sterile urine in neonates, J. Paediatr. Child. Health 34 (1998) 460.

[527] M.T. Garcia Munoz, et al., Suprapubic bladder aspiration: utility and complication, An. Esp. Pediatr. 45 (1996) 377.

[528] J.D. Nelson, P.C. Peters, Suprapubic aspiration of urine in premature and term infants, Pediatrics 36 (1965) 132.

[529] E. Kozer, et al., Pain in infants who are younger than 2 months during suprapubic aspiration and transurethral bladder catheterization: a randomized, controlled study, Pediatrics 118 (2006) e51–e56.

[530] Y.L. Lau, E. Hey, Sensitivity and specificity of daily tracheal aspirate cultures in predicting organisms causing bacteremia in ventilated neonates, Pediatr. Infect. Dis. J. 10 (1991) 290.

[531] L. Finelli, J.R. Livengood, L. Saiman, Surveillance of pharyngeal colonization: detection and control of serious bacterial illness in low birth weight infants, Pediatr. Infect. Dis. J. 13 (1994) 854.

[532] H.B. Srinivasan, D. Vidyasagar, Endotracheal aspirate cultures in predicting sepsis in ventilated neonates, Indian J. Pediatr. 65 (1998) 79–84.

[533] J.O. Klein, S.S. Gellis, Diagnostic needle aspiration in pediatric practice: with special reference to lungs, middle ear, urinary bladder, and amniotic cavity, Pediatr. Clin. North Am. 18 (1971) 219.

[534] L. Eisenfeld, et al., Systemic bacterial infections in neonatal deaths, Am. J. Dis. Child. 137 (1983) 645.

[535] T.M. Minckler, et al., Microbiology experience in human tissue collection, Am. J. Clin. Pathol. 45 (1966) 85.

[536] J.R. Pierce, G.B. Merenstein, J.T. Stocker, Immediate postmortem cultures in an intensive care nursery, Pediatr. Infect. Dis. J. 3 (1984) 510.

[537] J. Levin, et al., Detection of endotoxin in the blood of patients with sepsis due to gram-negative bacteria, N. Engl. J. Med. 283 (1970) 1313.

[538] I. Levin, T.E. Poore, N.S. Young, Gram-negative sepsis: detection of endotoxemia with the limulus test, Ann. Intern. Med. 76 (1972) 1.

[539] R.I. Stumacher, M.J. Kovnat, W.R. McCabe, Limitations of the usefulness of the limulus assay for endotoxin, N. Engl. J. Med. 288 (1973) 1261.

[540] R.J. Elin, et al., Lack of clinical usefulness of the limulus test in the diagnosis of endotoxemia, N. Engl. J. Med. 293 (1975) 521.

[541] G.H. McCracken Jr., L.D. Sarff, Endotoxin in CSF detection in neonates with bacterial meningitis, JAMA 235 (1976) 617.

[542] M.A. Sobanski, et al., Meningitis antigen detection: interpretation of agglutination by ultrasound-enhanced latex immunoassay, Br. J. Biomed. Sci. 56 (1999) 239–246.

[543] K.L. McGowan, Diagnostic value of latex agglutination tests for bacterial infections, Rep. Pediatr. Infect. Dis. 8 (1992) 31.

[544] P.J. Sanchez, et al., Significance of a positive urine group B streptococcal latex agglutination test in neonates, J. Pediatr. 116 (1990) 601.

[545] B.J. Stoll, et al., To tap or not to tap: high likelihood of meningitis without sepsis among very low birth weight infants, Pediatrics 113 (2004) 1181–1186.

[546] M.G. Weiss, S.P. Ionides, C.L. Anderson, Meningitis in premature infants with respiratory distress: role of admission lumbar puncture, J. Pediatr. 119 (1991) 973.

[547] K.D. Hendricks-Munoz, D.L. Shapiro, The role of the lumbar puncture in the admission sepsis evaluation of the premature infant, J. Perinatol. 10 (1990) 60.

[548] M. Eldadah, et al., Evaluation of routine lumbar punctures in newborn infants with respiratory distress syndrome, Pediatr. Infect. Dis. J. 6 (1987) 243.

[549] J. Schwersenski, L. McIntyre, C.R. Bauer, Lumbar puncture frequency and CSF analysis in the neonate, Am. J. Dis. Child. 145 (1991) 54.

[550] S. Fielkow, S. Reuter, S.P. Gotoff, Clinical and laboratory observations: cerebrospinal fluid examination in symptom-free infants with risk factors for infection, J. Pediatr. 119 (1991) 971.

[551] C.A. Gleason, et al., Optimal position for a spinal tap in preterm infants, Pediatrics 71 (1983) 31.

[552] J.M.B. Pinheiro, S. Furdon, L.F. Ochoa, Role of local anesthesia during lumbar puncture in neonates, Pediatrics 91 (1993) 379.

[553] F.L. Porter, et al., A controlled clinical trial of local anesthesia for lumbar punctures in newborns, Pediatrics 88 (1991) 663.

[554] D.H. Fiser, et al., Prevention of hypoxemia during lumbar puncture in infancy with preoxygenation, Pediatr. Emerg. Care 9 (1993) 81.

[555] L.E. Weisman, G.B. Merenstein, J.R. Steenbarger, The effect of lumbar puncture position in sick neonates, Am. J. Dis. Child. 137 (1983) 1077.

[556] V.E. Visser, R.T. Hall, Lumbar puncture in the evaluation of suspected neonatal sepsis, J. Pediatr. 96 (1980) 1063.

[557] S.M. Franco, V.E. Cornelius, B.F. Andrews, Should we perform lumbar punctures on the first day of life? Am. J. Dis. Child. 147 (1993) 133.

[558] H.P. Garges, et al., Neonatal meningitis. What is the correlation among cerebrospinal fluid cultures, blood cultures, and cerebrospinal fluid parameters, Pediatrics 117 (2006) 1094.

[559] B.T. Naidoo, The CSF in the healthy newborn infant, S. Afr. Med. J. 42 (1968) 933.

[560] L.D. Sarff, L.H. Platt, G.H. McCracken Jr., Cerebrospinal fluid evaluation in neonates: comparison of high-risk infants with and without meningitis, J. Pediatr. 88 (1976) 473.

[561] W.A. Bonadio, et al., Reference values of normal CSF composition in infants ages 0 to 8 weeks, Pediatr. Infect. Dis. J. 11 (1992) 589.

[562] A. Ahmed, et al., Cerebrospinal fluid values in the term neonate, Pediatr. Infect. Dis. J. 15 (1996) 298.

[563] H. Wolf, L. Hoepffner, The CSF in the newborn and premature infant, World Neurol. 2 (1961) 871.

[564] E. Otila, Studies on the CSF in premature infants, Acta Paediatr. Scand. 35 (1948) 9.

[565] A. Gyllensward, S. Malmstrom, The CSF in immature infants, Acta Paediatr. Scand. 135 (1962) 54.

[566] S. Widell, On the CSF in normal children and in patients with acute abacterial meningoencephalitis, Acta Pediatr. 47 (1958) 711.

[567] G.H. McCracken Jr., The rate of bacteriologic response to antimicrobial therapy in neonatal meningitis, Am. J. Dis. Child. 123 (1972) 547.

[568] A.F. Rodriguez, S.L. Kaplan, E.O. Mason Jr., Cerebrospinal fluid values in the very low birth weight infant, J. Pediatr. 116 (1990) 971.

[569] M.J. Mhanna, et al., Cerebrospinal fluid values in very low birth weight infants with suspected sepsis at different ages, Pediatr. Crit. Care Med. 9 (2008) 294–298.

[570] A.S. Yeager, F.W. Bruhn, J. Clark, Cerebrospinal fluid: presence of virus unaccompanied by pleocytosis, J. Pediatr. 85 (1974) 578.

[571] C.M. Moore, M. Ross, Acute bacterial meningitis with absent or minimal CSF abnormalities: a report of three cases, Clin. Pediatr. (Phila) 12 (1973) 117.

[572] G. Sarman, A.A. Moise, M.S. Edwards, Meningeal inflammation in neonatal gram-negative bacteremia, Pediatr. Infect. Dis. J. 14 (1995) 701.

[573] P.B. Smith, et al., Meningitis in preterm neonates: importance of cerebrospinal fluid parameters, Am. J. Perinatol. 25 (2008) 421–426.

[574] T. Hedner, K. Iversen, P. Lundborg, Aminobutyric acid concentrations in the CSF of newborn infants, Early. Hum. Dev. 7 (1982) 53.

[575] S. Engelke, et al., Cerebrospinal fluid lactate dehydrogenase in neonatal intracranial hemorrhage, Am. J. Med. Sci. 29 (1986) 391.

[576] G. Worley, et al., Creatine kinase brain isoenzyme: relationship of CSF concentration to the neurologic condition of newborns and cellular localization in the human brain, Pediatrics 76 (1985) 15.

[577] C.Y. Lin, M. Ishida, Elevation of cAMP levels in CSF of patients with neonatal meningitis, Pediatrics 71 (1983) 932.

[578] C.J. Corrall, et al., C-reactive protein in spinal fluid of children with meningitis, J. Pediatr. 99 (1981) 365.

[579] E. BenGershom, G.J. Briggeman-Mol, F. de Zegher, Cerebrospinal fluid C-reactive protein in meningitis: diagnostic value and pathophysiology, Eur. J. Pediatr. 145 (1986) 246.

[580] A.G. Philip, C.J. Baker, Cerebrospinal fluid C-reactive protein in neonatal meningitis, J. Pediatr. 102 (1983) 715.

[581] A. Martin-Ancel, et al., Interleukin-6 in the cerebrospinal fluid after perinatal asphyxia is related to early and late neurological manifestations, Pediatrics 100 (1997) 789.

[582] K. Sayman, et al., Cytokine response in cerebrospinal fluid after birth asphyxia, Pediatr. Res. 43 (1998) 746.

[583] G. Chow, J.W. Schmidley, Lysis of erythrocytes and leukocytes in traumatic lumbar punctures, Arch. Neurol. 41 (1984) 1084.

[584] R.W. Steele, et al., Leukocyte survival in CSF, J. Clin. Microbiol. 23 (1986) 965.

[585] J.P. Osborne, B. Pizer, Effect on the white cell count of contaminating CSF with blood, Arch. Dis. Child. 56 (1981) 400.

[586] R.W. Novak, Lack of validity of standard corrections for white blood cell counts of blood-contaminated CSF in infants, Am. J. Clin. Pathol. 82 (1984) 95.

[587] J.H. Mayefsky, K.J. Roghmann, Determination of leukocytosis in traumatic spinal tap specimens, Am. J. Med. 82 (1987) 1175.

[588] A. Mehl, Interpretation of traumatic lumbar puncture: a prospective experimental model, Clin. Pediatr. 25 (1986) 523.

[589] A. Mehl, Interpretation of traumatic lumbar puncture: predictive value in the presence of meningitis, Clin. Pediatr. 25 (1986) 575.

[590] W.A. Bonadio, et al., Distinguishing CSF abnormalities in children with bacterial meningitis and traumatic lumbar puncture, J. Infect. Dis. 162 (1990) 251.

[591] S.H. Naqvi, et al., Significance of neutrophils in CSF samples processed by cytocentrifugation, Clin. Pediatr. 22 (1983) 608.

[592] W.A. Bonadio, Bacterial meningitis in children whose CSF contains polymorphonuclear leukocytes without pleocytosis, Clin. Pediatr. 27 (1988) 198.

[593] R.G. Greenberg, et al., Traumatic lumbar punctures in neonates: test performance of the cerebrospinal fluid white blood cell count, Pediatr. Infect. Dis. J. 27 (2008) 1047–1051.

[594] E. Weirich, et al., Neutrophil CD11b expression as a diagnostic marker for early-onset neonatal infection, J. Pediatr. 132 (1998) 445.

[595] C. Kennon, et al., Granulocyte colony-stimulating factor as a marker for bacterial infection in neonates, J. Pediatr. 128 (1996) 765.

[596] H. Kuster, et al., Interleukin-1 receptor antagonist and interleukin-6 for early diagnosis of neonatal sepsis 2 days before clinical manifestation, Lancet 352 (1998) 1271.

[597] H. Doellner, et al., Interleukin-6 concentrations in neonates evaluated for sepsis, J. Pediatr. 132 (1998) 295.

[598] A. Panero, et al., Interleukin 6 in neonates with early and late onset infection, Pediatr. Infect. Dis. J. 16 (1997) 370.

[599] D. Harding, et al., Is interleukin-6-174 genotype associated with the development of septicemia in preterm infants? Pediatrics 112 (2003) 800.

[600] B. Resch, W. Gusenleitner, W.D. Muller, Procalcitonin and interleukin-6 in the diagnosis of early-onset sepsis of the neonate, Acta Paediatr. 92 (2003) 243.

[601] A. Kordek, et al., Umbilical cord blood serum procalcitonin concentration in the diagnosis of early neonatal infection, J. Perinatol. 23 (2003) 148.

[602] C. Chiesa, et al., Reliability of procalcitonin concentrations for the diagnosis of sepsis in critically ill neonates, Clin. Infect. Dis. 26 (1998) 664.

[603] M. Cetinkaya, et al., Comparison of serum amyloid A concentrations with those of C-reactive protein and procalcitonin in diagnosis and follow-up of neonatal sepsis in premature infants, J. Perinatol. 29 (2009) 225–231.

[604] E. Yapakci, et al., Serum pro-hepcidin levels in term and preterm newborns with sepsis, Pediatr. Int. 51 (2009) 289–292.

[605] B.H. Yoon, et al., Interleukin-6 concentrations in umbilical cord plasma are elevated in neonates with white matter lesions associated with periventricular leukomalacia, Am. J. Obstet. Gynecol. 174 (1996) 1433.

[606] O. Dammann, A. Leviton, Maternal intrauterine infection, cytokines, and brain damage in the preterm newborn, Pediatr. Res. 42 (1997) 1.

[607] S. Mehr, L.W. Doyle, Cytokines as markers of bacterial sepsis in newborn infants: a review, Pediatr. Infect. Dis. J. 19 (2000) 879.

[608] T. Reier-Nilsen, et al., Comparison of broad range 16S rDNA PCR and conventional blood culture for diagnosis of sepsis in the newborn: a case control study, BMC Pediatr. 9 (2009) 5.

[609] A. Ohlin, et al., Real-time PCR of the 16S-rRNA gene in the diagnosis of neonatal bacteraemia, Acta Paediatr. 97 (2008) 1376–1380.

[610] K.Y. Chan, et al., Rapid identification and differentiation of gram-negative and gram-positive bacterial bloodstream infections by quantitative polymerase chain reaction in preterm infants, Crit. Care Med. 37 (2009) 2441–2447.

[611] L.H. Chen, et al., Rapid diagnosis of sepsis and bacterial meningitis in children with real-time fluorescent quantitative polymerase chain reaction amplification in the bacterial 16S rRNA gene, Clin. Pediatr. (Phila) 48 (2009) 641–647.

[612] M.L. Castor, et al., Antibiotic resistance patterns in invasive group B streptococcal isolates, Infect. Dis. Obstet. Gynecol. 2008 (2008) 2.

[613] S. Dahesh, et al., Point mutation in the group B streptococcal pbp2x gene conferring decreased susceptibility to beta-lactam antibiotics, Antimicrob. Agents Chemother. 52 (2008) 2915–2918.

[614] K. Kimura, et al., First molecular characterization of group B streptococci with reduced penicillin susceptibility, Antimicrob. Agents Chemother. 52 (2008) 2890–2897.

[615] H.M. Swingle, R.L. Bucciarelli, E.M. Ayoub, Synergy between penicillins and low concentrations of gentamicin in the killing of group B streptococci, J. Infect. Dis. 152 (1985) 515.

[616] C.N. Baker, C. Thornsberry, R.R. Facklam, Synergism, killing kinetics, and antimicrobial susceptibility of group A and B streptococci, Antimicrob. Agents Chemother. 19 (1981) 716.

[617] V. Schauf, et al., Antibiotic-killing kinetics of group B streptococci, J. Pediatr. 89 (1976) 194.

[618] A. Deveikis, et al., Antimicrobial therapy of experimental group B streptococcal infection in mice, Antimicrob. Agents Chemother. 11 (1977) 817.

[619] R.J. Backes, et al., Activity of penicillin combined with an aminoglycoside against group B streptococci in vitro and in experimental endocarditis, J. Antimicrob. Chemother. 18 (1986) 491.

[620] C.M. Odio, et al., Comparative efficacy of ceftazidime vs. carbenicillin and amikacin for treatment of neonatal septicemia, Pediatr. Infect. Dis. J. 6 (1987) 371.

[621] P. Begue, et al., Pharmacokinetics and clinical evaluation of cefotaxime in children suffering from purulent meningitis, J. Antimicrob. Chemother. 14 (1984) 161.

[622] C.M. Odio, et al., Cefotaxime vs. conventional therapy for treatment of bacterial meningitis of infants and children, Pediatr. Infect. Dis. J. 5 (1986) 402.

[623] C.M. Odio, Cefotaxime for treatment of neonatal sepsis and meningitis, Diagn. Microbiol. Infect. Dis. 22 (1995) 111.

[624] J.S. Bradley, et al., Meropenem pharmacokinetics, pharmacodynamics, and Monte Carlo simulation in the neonate, Pediatr. Infect. Dis. J. 27 (2008) 794–799.

[625] C.S. Bryan, et al., Gentamicin vs. cefotaxime for therapy of neonatal sepsis, Am. J. Dis. Child. 139 (1985) 1086.

[626] P. Manzoni, et al., Risk factors for progression to invasive fungal infection in preterm neonates with fungal colonization, Pediatrics 118 (2006) 2359–2364.

[627] D.K. Benjamin Jr., et al., Neonatal candidiasis among extremely low birth weight infants: risk factors, mortality rates, and neurodevelopmental outcomes at 18 to 22 months, Pediatrics 117 (2006) 84–92.

[628] P. Man, et al., An antibiotic policy to prevent emergence of resistant bacilli, Lancet 355 (2000) 973.

[629] R.D. Feigin, G.H. McCracken, J.O. Klein, Diagnosis and management of meningitis, Pediatr. Infect. Dis. J. 11 (1992) 785.

[630] J.S. Bradley, et al., Once-daily ceftriaxone to complete therapy of uncomplicated group B streptococcal infection in neonates: a preliminary report, Clin. Pediatr. 31 (1992) 274.

[631] S.L. Kaplan, C.C. Patrick, Cefotaxime and aminoglycoside treatment of meningitis caused by gram-negative enteric organisms, Pediatr. Infect. Dis. J. 9 (1990) 810.

[632] Group B Streptococcal Infections in Pregnancy, American College of Gynecology, Washington, DC, 1996.

[633] American Academy of Pediatrics Committee on Infectious Diseases and Committee on Fetus and Newborn, Guidelines for prevention of group B streptococcal (GBS) infection by chemoprophylaxis, Pediatrics 90 (1992) 775.

[634] Centers for Disease Control and Prevention, Prevention of perinatal group B streptococcal: a public health perspective, MMWR. Morb. Mortal. Wkly. Rep. 45 (1996) 1.

[635] American Academy of Pediatrics, Committee on Infectious Diseases/Committee on Fetus and Newborn. Revised guidelines for prevention of early-onset group B streptococcal infection, Pediatrics 99 (1997) 489.

[636] S. Schrag, et al., Prevention of perinatal group B streptococcal disease: revised guidelines from CDC, MMWR. Morb. Mortal. Wkly. Rep. 51 (2002) 1.

[637] I.P. Uy, et al., Changes in early-onset group B beta hemolytic streptococcus disease with changing recommendations for prophylaxis, J. Perinatol. 22 (2002) 516.

[638] M.A. MacAulay, M. Abou-Sabe, D. Charles, Placental transfer of ampicillin, Am. J. Obstet. Gynecol. 96 (1966) 943.

[639] H. Nau, Clinical pharmacokinetics in pregnancy and perinatology, II: penicillins, Dev. Pharmacol. Ther. 10 (1987) 174.

[640] D.H. Adamkin, E. Marshall, L.B. Weiner, The placental transfer of ampicillin, Am. J. Perinatol. 1 (1984) 310.

[641] B.S. Brozanski, et al., Effect of a screening-based prevention policy on prevalence of early-onset group B streptococcal sepsis, Obstet. Gynecol. 95 (2000) 496.

[642] M.R. Moore, S.J. Schrag, A. Schuchat, Effects of intrapartum antimicrobial prophylaxis for prevention of group-B-streptococcal disease on the incidence and ecology of early-onset neonatal sepsis, Lancet Infect. Dis. 3 (2003) 201.

[643] S.J. Schrag, et al., Group B streptococcal disease in the era of intrapartum antibiotic prophylaxis, N. Engl. J. Med. 342 (2000) 15.

[644] S.P. Gotoff, K.M. Boyer, Prevention of early-onset neonatal group B streptococcal disease, Pediatrics 99 (1997) 866.

[645] E. Squire, B. Favara, J. Todd, Diagnosis of neonatal bacterial infection: hematologic and pathologic findings in fatal and nonfatal cases, Pediatrics 64 (1979) 60.

[646] G.H. McCracken Jr., S.G. Mize, A controlled study of intrathecal antibiotic therapy in gram-negative enteric meningitis of infancy. Report of the Neonatal Meningitis Cooperative Study Group, J. Pediatr. 89 (1976) 66.

[647] G.H. McCracken Jr., S.G. Mize, N. Threlkeld, Intraventricular gentamicin therapy in gram-negative bacillary meningitis of infancy, Lancet 1 (1980) 787.

[648] N. Koksal, et al., Meropenem in neonatal severe infections due to multiresistant gram-negative bacteria, Indian J. Pediatr. 68 (2001) 15.

[649] M. Khaneja, et al., Successful treatment of late-onset infection due to resistant *Klebsiella pneumoniae* in an extremely low birth weight infant using ciprofloxacin, J. Perinatol. 19 (1999) 311.

[650] H.L. van den Oever, et al., Ciprofloxacin in preterm neonates: case report and review of the literature, Eur. J. Pediatr. 157 (1998) 843.

[651] R. Wessalowski, et al., Multiple brain abscesses caused by *Salmonella enteritidis* in a neonate: successful treatment with ciprofloxacin, Pediatr. Infect. Dis. J. 12 (1993) 683.

[652] R.E. Levitz, R. Quintiliani, Trimethoprim-sulfamethoxazole for bacterial meningitis, Ann. Intern. Med. 100 (1984) 881.

[653] Z. Spirer, et al., Complete recovery from an apparent brain abscess treated without neurosurgery: the importance of early CT scanning, Clin. Pediatr. (Phila) 21 (1982) 106.

[654] A.S. Daoud, et al., Lack of effectiveness of dexamethasone in neonatal bacterial meningitis, Eur. J. Pediatr. 158 (1999) 230–233.

[655] M.S. Tekerekoglu, et al., Analysis of an outbreak due to *Chryseobacterium meningosepticum* in a neonatal intensive care unit, New Microbiol. 26 (2003) 57.

[656] R. Lauterbach, M. Zembala, Pentoxifylline reduces plasma tumour necrosis factor-alpha concentration in premature infants with sepsis, Eur. J. Pediatr. 155 (1996) 404.

[657] K.R. Schibler, et al., A randomized, placebo-controlled trial of granulocyte colony-stimulating factor administration to newborn infants with neutropenia and clinical signs of early-onset sepsis, Pediatrics 102 (1998) 6.

[658] P. Kocherlakota, E.F. LaGamma, Preliminary report: rhG-CSF may reduce the incidence of neonatal sepsis in prolonged preeclampsia-associated neutropenia, Pediatrics 102 (1998) 1107.

[659] K. Bilgin, et al., A randomized trial of granulocyte-macrophage colony-stimulating factor in neonates with sepsis and neutropenia, Pediatrics 107 (2001) 36.

[660] A. Ahmad, et al., Comparison of recombinant granulocyte colony-stimulating factor, recombinant human granulocyte-macrophage colony-stimulating factor and placebo for treatment of septic preterm infants, Pediatr. Infect. Dis. J. 21 (2002) 1061.

[661] A. Ohlsson, J.B. Lacy, Intravenous immunoglobulin for suspected or subsequently proven infection in neonates, Cochrane Database Syst. Rev. CD001239, (2004).

[662] INIS Study, International Neonatal Immunotherapy Study: non-specific intravenous immunoglobulin therapy for suspected or proven neonatal sepsis: an international, placebo controlled, multicentre randomised trial, BMC Pregnancy Childbirth 8 (2008) 52.

[663] R. Bennet, et al., The outcome of neonatal septicemia during fifteen years, Acta Paediatr. Scand. 78 (1989) 40.

[664] M.M. Placzek, A. Whitelaw, Early and late neonatal septicaemia, Arch. Dis. Child. 58 (1983) 728.

[665] J. de Louvois, Septicaemia and Meningitis in the Newborn, John Wiley & Sons, New York, 1990.

[666] G. Klinger, et al., Predicting the outcome of neonatal bacterial meningitis, Pediatrics 106 (2000) 477.

[667] E. Wald, et al., Long-term outcome of group B streptococcal meningitis, Pediatrics 77 (1986) 217.

[668] S.M. Franco, V.E. Cornelius, B.F. Andrews, Long-term outcome of neonatal meningitis, Am. J. Dis. Child. 146 (1992) 567.

[669] K.A. Horn, et al., Neurological sequelae of group B streptococcal neonatal infection, Pediatrics 53 (1974) 501.

[670] M.S. Edwards, et al., Long-term sequelae of group B streptococcal meningitis in infants, J. Pediatr. 106 (1985) 717.

[671] G.H. McCracken Jr., et al., Cerebrospinal fluid interleukin-1B and tumor necrosis factor concentrations and outcome from neonatal gram-negative enteric bacillary meningitis, Pediatr. Infect. Dis. J. 8 (1989) 155.

[672] G.H. McCracken Jr., et al., Moxalactam therapy for neonatal meningitis due to gram-negative enteric bacilli: a prospective controlled evaluation, JAMA 252 (1984) 1427.

[673] J. Baier, J.A. Bocchini Jr., E.G. Brown, Selective use of vancomycin to prevent coagulase-negative staphylococcal nosocomial bacteremia in high risk very low birth weight infants, Pediatr. Infect. Dis. J. 17 (1998) 179.

[674] R.W. Cooke, et al., Low-dose vancomycin prophylaxis reduces coagulase-negative staphylococcal bacteraemia in very low birthweight infants, J. Hosp. Infect. 37 (1997) 297–303.

[675] M.A. Kacica, et al., Prevention of gram-positive sepsis in neonates weighing less than 1500 grams, J. Pediatr. 125 (1994) 253–258.

[676] P.S. Spafford, et al., Prevention of central venous catheter-related coagulase-negative staphylococcal sepsis in neonates, J. Pediatr. 125 (1994) 259–263.

[677] A.P. Craft, N.N. Finer, K.J. Barrington, Vancomycin for prophylaxis against sepsis in preterm neonates, Cochrane Database Syst. Rev. CD001971, (2000).

[678] J.S. Garland, et al., A vancomycin-heparin lock solution for prevention of nosocomial bloodstream infection in critically ill neonates with peripherally inserted central venous catheters: a prospective, randomized trial, Pediatrics 116 (2005) e198–e205.

[679] P. Van de Perre, Transfer of antibody via mother's milk, Vaccine 21 (2003) 3374.

[680] In L.A. Hanson, et al., Antiviral and Antibacterial Factors in Human Milk, Raven Press, New York, 1988.

[681] N.B. Mathus, et al., Anti-infective factors in preterm human colostrum, Acta Paediatr. Scand. 79 (1990) 1039.

[682] C.F. Isaacs, et al., Antiviral and antibacterial lipids in human milk and infant formula feeds, Arch. Dis. Child. 65 (1990) 861.

[683] J. Winberg, G. Wessner, Does breast milk protect against septicaemia in the newborn? Lancet 1 (1971) 1091.

[684] R.N. Ashraf, et al., Breast feeding and protection against neonatal sepsis in a high risk population, Arch. Dis. Child. 66 (1991) 488.

[685] M.A. Hylander, D.M. Strobino, R. Dhanireddy, Human milk feedings and infection among very low birth weight infants, Pediatrics 102 (1998) E38.

[686] G.V. Coppa, et al., Preliminary study of breastfeeding and bacterial adhesion to uroepithelial cells, Lancet 1 (1990) 569.

[687] H. Hasselbalch, et al., Decreased thymus size in formula-fed infants compared with breastfed infants, Acta Paediatr. 85 (1996) 1029–1032.

[688] H.F. Pabst, et al., Effect of breast-feeding on immune response to BCG vaccination, Lancet 1 (1989) 295.

[689] S.A. Silfverdal, et al., Long term enhancement of the IgG2 antibody response to Haemophilus influenzae type b by breast-feeding, Pediatr. Infect. Dis. J. 21 (2002) 816–821.

[690] M. Cohen-Wolkowiez, D.K. Benjamin Jr., E. Capparelli, Immunotherapy in neonatal sepsis: advances in treatment and prophylaxis, Curr. Opin. Pediatr. 21 (2009) 177–181.

[691] J.A. Englund, W.P. Glezen, Maternal immunization for the prevention of infection in early infancy, Semin. Pediatr. Infect. Dis. 2 (1991) 225.

[692] M. Vicari, B. Dodet, J. Englund, Protection of newborns through maternal immunization, Vaccine 21 (2003) 3351.

[693] C.J. Baker, M.A. Rench, P. McInnes, Immunization of pregnant women with group B streptococcal type III capsular polysaccharide-tetanus toxoid conjugate vaccine, Vaccine 21 (2003) 3468.

[694] A.A. Fanaroff, et al., A controlled trial of intravenous immune globulin to reduce nosocomial infections in very-low-birth-weight infants. National Institute of Child Health and Human Development Neonatal Research Network, N. Engl. J. Med. 330 (1994) 1107–1113.

[695] M. DeJonge, et al., Clinical trial of safety and efficacy of INH-A21 for the prevention of nosocomial staphylococcal bloodstream infection in premature infants, J. Pediatr. 151 (2007) 260.

[696] D.K. Benjamin, et al., A blinded, randomized, multicenter study of an intravenous Staphylococcus aureus immune globulin, J. Perinatol. 26 (2006) 290–295.

[697] A. Ohlsson, J.B. Lacy, Intravenous immunoglobulin for preventing infection in preterm and/or low-birth-weight infants, Cochrane Database Syst. Rev. CD000361, (2004).

[698] D. Sidiropoulos, et al., Transplacental passage of intravenous immunoglobulin in the last trimester of pregnancy, J. Pediatr. 109 (1986) 505.

[699] E. Roilides, P.A. Pizzo, Modulation of host defenses by cytokines: evolving adjuncts in prevention and treatment of serious infections in immunocompromised patients, Clin. Infect. Dis. 15 (1992) 508.

[700] R.L. Roberts, et al., Neutropenia in an extremely premature infant treated with recombinant human granulocyte colony-stimulating factor, Am. J. Dis. Child. 145 (1991) 808.

[701] M.S. Cairo, et al., A randomized, double-blind, placebo-controlled trial of prophylactic recombinant human granulocyte-macrophage colony-stimulating

[702] K.D. Yang, F.J. Bohnsack, H.R. Hill, Fibronectin in host defense: implications in the diagnosis, prophylaxis and therapy of infectious diseases, Pediatr. Infect. Dis. J. 12 (1993) 234.

[703] M.C. Yoder, Therapeutic administration of fibronectin: current uses and potential applications, Clin. Perinatol. 18 (1991) 325.

[704] R. Carr, et al., Granulocyte-macrophage colony stimulating factor administered as prophylaxis for reduction of sepsis in extremely preterm, small for gestational age neonates (the PROGRAMS trial): a single-blind, multicentre, randomised controlled trial, Lancet 373 (2009) 226–233.

[705] M. Donini, et al., G-CSF treatment of severe congenital neutropenia reverses neutropenia but does not correct the underlying functional deficiency of the neutrophil in defending against microorganisms, Blood 109 (2007) 4716–4723.

[706] B.B. Poindexter, et al., Parenteral glutamine supplementation does not reduce the risk of mortality or late-onset sepsis in extremely low birth weight infants, Pediatrics 113 (2004) 1209–1215.

[707] T.R. Tubman, S.W. Thompson, W. McGuire, Glutamine supplementation to prevent morbidity and mortality in preterm infants, Cochrane Database Syst. Rev. CD001457, (2008).

[708] H.C. Lin, B.H. Su, W. Oh, Oral probiotics prevent necrotizing enterocolitis, J. Pediatr. 148 (2006) 849.

[709] H.C. Lin, et al., Oral probiotics reduce the incidence and severity of necrotizing enterocolitis in very low birth weight infants, Pediatrics 115 (2005) 1–4.

[710] P. Manzoni, et al., Oral supplementation with Lactobacillus casei subspecies rhamnosus prevents enteric colonization by Candida species in preterm neonates: a randomized study, Clin. Infect. Dis. 42 (2006) 1735–1742.

[711] K. Alfaleh, J. Anabrees, D. Bassler, Probiotics reduce the risk of necrotizing enterocolitis in preterm infants: a meta-analysis, Neonatology 97 (2009) 93–99.

[712] N. Orsi, The antimicrobial activity of lactoferrin: current status and perspectives, Biometals 17 (2004) 189–196.

[713] J.J. Damato, D.V. Eitzman, H. Baer, Persistence and dissemination in the community of R-factors of nosocomial origin, J. Infect. Dis. 129 (1974) 205.

[714] J.O. Klein, Family spread of staphylococcal disease following a nursery outbreak, N. Y. State J. Med. 60 (1960) 861.

[715] N. Nakwan, T. Atta, K. Chokephaibulkit, Neonatal pasteurellosis: a review of reported cases, Arch. Dis. Child. Fetal Neonatal Ed. 94 (2009) F373–F376.

[716] S.A. Bhave, L.M. Guy, Pasteurella multocida meningitis in an infant with recovery, BMJ 2 (1977) 741.

[717] C. Guillet, et al., Pasteurella multocida sepsis and meningitis in 2-month-old twin infants after household exposure to a slaughtered sheep, Clin. Infect. Dis. 45 (2007) e80–e81.

[718] T.F. Wolfs, et al., Neonatal sepsis by Campylobacter jejuni: genetically proven transmission from a household puppy, Clin. Infect. Dis. 32 (2001) E97–E99.

[719] L.J. Baraff, et al., Practice guideline for the management of infants and children 0 to 36 months of age with fever without source. Agency for Health Care Policy and Research, Ann. Emerg. Med. 22 (1993) 1198.

[720] M.D. Baker, Evaluation and management of infants with fever, Pediatr. Clin. North. Am. 46 (1999) 1061.

[721] P.C. Ferrera, J.M. Bartfield, H.S. Snyder, Neonatal fever: utility of the Rochester criteria in determining low risk for serious bacterial infections, Am. J. Emerg. Med. 15 (1997) 299.

[722] R. Dagan, et al., Ambulatory care of febrile infants younger than 2 months of age classified as being at low risk for having serious bacterial infections, J. Pediatr. 112 (1988) 355.

[723] J.C. King Jr., E.D. Berman, P.F. Wright, Evaluation of fever in infants less than 8 weeks old, South. Med. J. 80 (1987) 948.

[724] J.O. Klein, P.C. Schlessinger, R.B. Karasic, Management of the febrile infant under three months of age, Pediatr. Infect. Dis. J. 3 (1984) 75.

[725] P. Ishimine, Fever without source in children 0 to 36 months of age, Pediatr. Clin. North Am. 53 (2006) 167–194.

[726] M.D. Baker, L.M. Bell, Unpredictability of serious bacterial illness in febrile infants from birth to 1 month of age, Arch. Pediatr. Adolesc. Med. 153 (1999) 508–511.

[727] H.A. Kadish, et al., Applying outpatient protocols in febrile infants 1-28 days of age: can the threshold be lowered? Clin. Pediatr. (Phila) 39 (2000) 81–88.

[728] M.D. Baker, L.M. Bell, J.R. Avner, Outpatient management without antibiotics of fever in selected infants, N. Engl. J. Med. 329 (1993) 1437–1441.

[729] M.N. Baskin, E.J. O'Rourke, G.R. Fleisher, Outpatient treatment of febrile infants 28 to 89 days of age with intramuscular administration of ceftriaxone, J. Pediatr. 120 (1992) 22–27.

[730] B.K. Bonsu, M. Chb, M.B. Harper, Identifying febrile young infants with bacteremia: is the peripheral white blood cell count an accurate screen? Ann. Emerg. Med. 42 (2003) 216–225.

[731] L. Brown, T. Shaw, W.A. Wittlake, Does leucocytosis identify bacterial infections in febrile neonates presenting to the emergency department? Emerg. Med. J. 22 (2005) 256–259.

[732] D.S. Greenes, M.B. Harper, Low risk of bacteremia in febrile children with recognizable viral syndromes, Pediatr. Infect. Dis. J. 18 (1999) 258–261.

[733] D.A. Levine, et al., Risk of serious bacterial infection in young febrile infants with respiratory syncytial virus infections, Pediatrics 113 (2004) 1728–1734.

[734] W.I. Krief, et al., Influenza virus infection and the risk of serious bacterial infections in young febrile infants, Pediatrics 124 (2009) 30–39.

[735] W.A. Silverman, W.E. Homan, Sepsis of obscure origin in the newborn, Pediatrics 3 (1949) 157.

[736] R.T. Smith, E.S. Platou, R.A. Good, Septicemia of the newborn: current status of the problem, Pediatrics 17 (1956) 549.

[737] R.S. Moorman, S.H. Sell, Neonatal septicemia, South. Med. J. 54 (1962) 137.

[738] K.C. Buetow, S.W. Klein, R.B. Lane, Septicemia in premature infants, Am. J. Dis. Child. 110 (1965) 29.

[739] A. Ronnestad, et al., Blood culture isolates during 6 years in a tertiary neonatal intensive care unit, Scand. J. Infect. Dis. 30 (1998) 245.

[740] B. Ghiorghis, Neonatal sepsis in Addis Ababa, Ethiopia: a review of 151 bacteremic neonates, Ethiop. Med. J. 35 (1997) 169.

[741] H. Saloojee, et al., Changing antibiotic resistance patterns in a neonatal unit and its implications for antibiotic usage, (Abstract) Presented at the International Congress of Pediatric Surgery and Pediatrics, Cape Town, South Africa, (1998) February 1-6.

[742] S. Karan, Purulent meningitis in the newborn, Childs Nerv. Syst. 2 (1986) 26.

[743] K.P. Sanghvi, D.I. Tudehope, Neonatal bacterial sepsis in a neonatal intensive care unit: a 5-year analysis, J. Pediatr. Child. Health 32 (1996) 333.

[744] G.H. McCracken Jr., Personal communication, (1976).

[745] S.S. Namnyak, B. Holmes, S.E. Fathalla, Neonatal meningitis caused by Achromobacter xylosoxidans, J. Clin. Microbiol. 22 (1985) 470–471.

[746] Y.R. Hearn, R.M. Gander, Achromobacter xylosoxidans: An unusual neonatal pathogen, Am. J. Clin. Pathol. 96 (1991) 211–214.

[747] J. Molina-Cabrillana, et al., Outbreak of Achromobacter xylosoxidans pseudo-bacteremia in a neonatal care unit related to contaminated chlorhexidine solution, Eur. J. Clin. Microbiol. Infect. Dis. 26 (2007) 435–437.

[748] G.G. Christo, et al., Acinetobacter sepsis in neonates, Indian Pediatr. 30 (1993) 1413–1416.

[749] A. Mishra, et al., Acinetobacter sepsis in newborns, Indian Pediatr. 35 (1998) 27–32.

[750] N. Mittal, et al., Outbreak of Acinetobacter spp septicemia in a neonatal ICU, Southeast Asian J. Trop. Med. Public Health 34 (2003) 365–366.

[751] A. Kilic, et al., Acinetobacter septicus sp. nov. association with a nosocomial outbreak of bacteremia in a neonatal intensive care unit, J. Clin. Microbiol. 46 (2008) 902–908.

[752] A. Simmonds, et al., Outbreak of Acinetobacter infection in extremely low birth weight neonates, Pediatr. Infect. Dis. J. 28 (2009) 210–214.

[753] A. Kadanali, M.A. Tasyaran, S. Kadanali, Anthrax during pregnancy: case reports and review, Clin. Infect. Dis. 36 (2003) 1343–1346.

[754] N. Manickam, A. Knorr, K.L. Muldrew, Neonatal meningoencephalitis caused by Bacillus cereus, Pediatr. Infect. Dis. J. 27 (2008) 843–846.

[755] C. Larsson, et al., Complications of pregnancy and transplacental transmission of relapsing-fever borreliosis, J. Infect. Dis. 194 (2006) 1367–1374.

[756] P.W. Melkert, H.V. Stel, Neonatal Borrelia infections (relapsing fever): report of 5 cases and review of the literature, East Afr. Med. J. 68 (1991) 999–1005.

[757] S. Chheda, S.M. Lopez, E.P. Sanderson, Congenital brucellosis in a premature infant, Pediatr. Infect. Dis. J. 16 (1997) 81–83.

[758] I. Giannacopoulos, et al., Transplacentally transmitted congenital brucellosis due to Brucella abortus, J. Infect. 45 (2002) 209–210.

[759] J.K. Lee, Two outbreaks of Burkholderia cepacia nosocomial infection in a neonatal intensive care unit, J Paediatr Child Health 44 (2008) 62–66.

[760] O. Kahyaoglu, B. Nolan, A. Kumar, Burkholderia cepacia sepsis in neonates, Pediatr. Infect. Dis. J. 14 (1995) 815–816.

[761] C. Doit, et al., Outbreak of Burkholderia cepacia bacteremia in a pediatric hospital due to contamination of lipid emulsion stoppers, J. Clin. Microbiol. 42 (2004) 2227–2230.

[762] F.C. Abbink, J.M. Orendi, A.J. de Beaufort, Mother-to-child transmission of Burkholderia pseudomallei, N. Engl. J. Med. 344 (2001) 1171–1172.

[763] R. Krishnaswamy, et al., Early onset neonatal sepsis with Campylobacter jejuni: a case report, Eur. J. Pediatr. 150 (1991) 277–278.

[764] J.D. Feldman, E.N. Kontaxis, M.P. Sherman, Congenital bacteremia due to Capnocytophaga, Pediatr. Infect. Dis. 4 (1985) 415–416.

[765] J.R. Rosenman, J.K. Reynolds, M.B. Kleiman, Capnocytophaga canimorsus meningitis in a newborn: an avoidable infection, Pediatr. Infect. Dis. J. 22 (2003) 204–205.

[766] C. Edwards, C.H. Yi, J.L. Currie, Chorioamnionitis caused by Capnocytophaga: case report, Am. J. Obstet. Gynecol. 173 (1995) 244–245.

[767] R. Berner, et al., Fatal sepsis caused by Corynebacterium amycolatum in a premature infant, J. Clin. Microbiol. 35 (1997) 1011–1012.

[768] M.S. Platt, Neonatal Hemophilus vaginalis (Corynebacterium vaginalis) infection, Clin. Pediatr. (Phila) 10 (1971) 513–516.

[769] K. Vohra, et al., Neonatal sepsis and meningitis caused by Edwardsiella tarda, Pediatr. Infect. Dis. J. 7 (1988) 814–815.

[770] O.A. Okubadejo, K.O. Alausa, Neonatal meningitis caused by Edwardsiella tarda, BMJ 3 (1968) 357–358.

[771] E.E. Mowbray, et al., Maternal colonization and neonatal sepsis caused by Edwardsiella tarda, Pediatrics 111 (2003) e296–e298.

[772] K.M. Dahl, J. Barry, R.L. DeBiasi, Escherichia hermannii infection of a cephalohematoma: case report, review of the literature, and description of a novel invasive pathogen, Clin. Infect. Dis. 35 (2002) e96–e98.

[773] H.G. Ginsberg, R.S. Daum, Escherichia hermannii sepsis with duodenal perforation in a neonate, Pediatr. Infect. Dis. J. 6 (1987) 300–302.

[774] M.S. Tekerekoglu, et al., Analysis of an outbreak due to Chryseobacterium meningosepticum in a neonatal intensive care unit, New Microbiol. 26 (2003) 57–63.

[775] T.G. Abrahamsen, P.H. Finne, E. Lingaas, Flavobacterium meningosepticum infections in a neonatal intensive care unit, Acta Paediatr. Scand. 78 (1989) 51–55.

[776] R.A. Amaya, F. Al-Dossary, G.J. Demmler, Gardnerella vaginalis bacteremia in a premature neonate, J. Perinatol. 22 (2002) 585–587.

[777] T.K. Venkataramani, H.K. Rathbun, Corynebacterium vaginale (Hemophilus vaginalis) bacteremia: clinical study of 29 cases, Johns Hopkins Med. J. 139 (1976) 93–97.

[778] S.L. Orlicek, D.F. Welch, T.L. Kuhls, Septicemia and meningitis caused by Helicobacter cinaedi in a neonate, J. Clin. Microbiol. 31 (1993) 569–571.

[779] C. Thompson, et al., Lactobacillus acidophilus sepsis in a neonate, J. Perinatol. 21 (2001) 258–260.

[780] S.M. Cox, et al., Lactobacillemia of amniotic fluid origin, Obstet. Gynecol. 68 (1986) 134–135.

[781] H.O. Gsell Jr., et al., [Intrauterine leptospirosis pomona: 1st reported case of an intrauterine transmitted and cured leptospirosis], Dtsch. Med. Wochenschr. 96 (1971) 1263–1268.

[782] Y. Shaked, et al., Leptospirosis in pregnancy and its effect on the fetus: case report and review, Clin. Infect. Dis. 17 (1993) 241–243.

[783] P. Yossuck, et al., Leuconostoc spp sepsis in an extremely low birth weight infant: a case report and review of the literature, W. V. Med. J. 105 (2009) 24–27.

[784] G. Janow, et al., Leuconostoc septicemia in a preterm neonate on vancomycin therapy: case report and literature review, Am. J. Perinatol. 26 (2009) 89–91.

[785] A.K. Sinha, et al., Early onset Morganella morganii sepsis in a newborn infant with emergence of cephalosporin resistance caused by depression of AMPC beta–lactamase production, Pediatr. Infect. Dis. J. 25 (2006) 376–377.

[786] S. Dutta, A. Narang, Early onset neonatal sepsis due to Morganella morganii, Indian Pediatr. 41 (2004) 1155–1157.

[787] M. Casanova-Roman, A. Sanchez–Porto, M. Casanova–Bellido, Early–onset neonatal sepsis caused by vertical transmission of Morganella morganii, Scand. J. Infect. Dis. 34 (2002) 534–535.

[788] A. Hata, et al., Mycoplasma hominis meningitis in a neonate: case report and review, J. Infect. 57 (2008) 338–343.

[789] R. Duran, et al., Ochrobactrum anthropi bacteremia in a preterm infant with meconium peritonitis, Int. J. Infect. Dis. 13 (2009) e61–e63.

[790] N.Y. Aly, et al., Pantoea agglomerans bloodstream infection in preterm neonates, Med. Princ. Pract. 17 (2008) 500–503.

[791] C.M. Thompson, et al., Neonatal septicemia and meningitis due to Pasteurella multocida, Pediatr. Infect. Dis. J. 3 (1984) 559.

[792] D. Cohen-Adam, et al., Pasteurella multocida septicemia in a newborn without scratches, licks or bites, Isr. Med. Assoc. J. 8 (2006) 657–658.

[793] K. Fujita, et al., Neonatal Plesiomonas shigelloides septicemia and meningitis: a case and review, Acta Paediatr. Jpn. 36 (1994) 450–452.

[794] C. Terpeluk, et al., Plesiomonas shigelloides sepsis and meningoencephalitis in a neonate, Eur. J. Pediatr. 151 (1992) 499–501.

[795] J. Billiet, et al., Plesiomonas shigelloides meningitis and septicaemia in a neonate: report of a case and review of the literature, J. Infect. 19 (1989) 267–271.

[796] Z. Kassim, et al., Isolation of Proteus mirabilis from severe neonatal sepsis and central nervous system infection with extensive pneumocephalus, Eur. J. Pediatr. 162 (2003) 644–645.

[797] C.P. Darby, E. Conner, C.U. Kyong, Proteus mirabilis brain abscess in a neonate, Dev. Med. Child. Neurol. 20 (1978) 366–368.

[798] H. Velvis, N. Carrasco, S. Hetherington, Trimethoprim-sulfamethoxazole therapy of neonatal Proteus mirabilis meningitis unresponsive to cefotaxime, Pediatr. Infect. Dis. 5 (1986) 591–593.

[799] P. Lumbiganon, et al., Neonatal melioidosis: a report of 5 cases, Pediatr. Infect. Dis. J. 7 (1988) 634–636.

[800] M. Lloyd-Puryear, et al., Meningitis caused by Psychrobacter immobilis in an infant, J. Clin. Microbiol. 29 (1991) 2041–2042.

[801] A.C. Kimura, et al., Outbreak of Ralstonia pickettii bacteremia in a neonatal intensive care unit, Pediatr. Infect. Dis. J. 24 (2005) 1099–1103.

[802] J.H. Shin, et al., Rothia dentocariosa septicemia without endocarditis in a neonatal infant with meconium aspiration syndrome, J. Clin. Microbiol. 42 (2004) 4891–4892.

[803] J.W. Ruderman, K.P. Stoller, J.J. Pomerance, Bloodstream invasion with Shigella sonnei in an asymptomatic newborn infant, Pediatr. Infect. Dis. 5 (1986) 379–380.

[804] J.A. Aldrich, R.P. Flowers 3rd, F.K. Hall, Shigella sonnei septicemia in a neonate: a case report, J. Am. Osteopath. Assoc. 79 (1979) 93–98.

[805] E.E. Moore, Shigella sonnei septicaemia in a neonate, BMJ 1 (1974) 22.

[806] C. Gras-Le Guen, et al., Almond oil implicated in a Staphylococcus capitis outbreak in a neonatal intensive care unit, J. Perinatol. 27 (2007) 713–717.

[807] M. Langbaum, F.G. Eyal, Stomatococcus mucilaginosus septicemia and meningitis in a premature infant, Pediatr. Infect. Dis. J. 11 (1992) 334–335.

[808] A. Bose, J.K. Philip, M. Jesudason, Neonatal septicemia caused by Vibrio cholerae O:139, Pediatr. Infect. Dis. J. 19 (2000) 166.

[809] J.A. Kerketta, et al., Non-01 Vibrio cholerae septicemia and meningitis in a neonate, Indian. J. Pediatr. 69 (2002) 909–910.

[810] E.C. Thompson, Yersinia enterocolitica sepsis in a 3-week-old child, J. Natl. Med. Assoc. 86 (1994) 783–785.

[811] M. Challapalli, D.G. Cunningham, Yersinia enterocolitica septicemia in infants younger than three months of age, Pediatr. Infect. Dis. J. 12 (1993) 168–169.

[812] M.E. White, et al., Plague in a neonate, Am. J. Dis. Child. 135 (1981) 418–419.

BACTERIAL INFECTIONS OF THE RESPIRATORY TRACT

Elizabeth D. Barnett ⊛ Jerome O. Klein

CHAPTER OUTLINE

Infections of the Oral Cavity and Nasopharynx 276
    Pharyngitis, Retropharyngeal Cellulitis, and
       Retropharyngeal Abscess 276
    Noma 277
    Epiglottitis 277
    Laryngitis 277
    Infection of the Paranasal Sinuses 277
    Diphtheria 278
    Pertussis 278
Otitis Media 280
    Pathogenesis and Pathology 281
    Epidemiology 282
    Microbiology 282

    Diagnosis 284
    Treatment 285
    Prognosis 285
Mastoiditis 285
Pneumonia 285
    Pathogenesis and Pathology 286
    Microbiology 287
    Epidemiology 288
    Clinical Manifestations 289
    Diagnosis 289
    Differential Diagnosis 291
    Management 292
    Prognosis 292

INFECTIONS OF THE ORAL CAVITY AND NASOPHARYNX

PHARYNGITIS, RETROPHARYNGEAL CELLULITIS, AND RETROPHARYNGEAL ABSCESS

Neonates with bacterial infection of the oropharynx may present with pharyngeal inflammation with or without exudate or with retropharyngeal cellulitis or abscess. Clinical signs and symptoms include respiratory distress, poor feeding, and irritability. Infants may have submandibular swelling, and some may have a weak or hoarse cry. Infection may extend to the surrounding structures, leading to formation of deep neck abscess. Microorganisms identified as the etiologic agents of these infections and their manifestations of disease include the following:

Staphylococcus aureus. Although many children are colonized in the throat and nasopharynx with *S. aureus*, this organism is rarely a primary agent in the etiology of pharyngitis in infants (or adults). There have been reports, however, of localized abscesses in the oral cavity related to *S. aureus*. In 1936, Clark and Barysh [1] reported a case of retropharyngeal abscess in a 6-week-old infant. The infant was critically ill, but recovered after incision and drainage of the abscess. A 6-day-old infant described in a report from India presented with stridor, dysphagia, and lateral cervical swelling. The infant was found to have a retropharyngeal abscess caused by *S. aureus* [2]. Steinhauer [3] reported a case of cellulitis of the floor of the mouth (Ludwig angina) in a 12-day-old infant. The infant was febrile and toxic; examination of the mouth revealed swelling under the tongue. Purulent material was subsequently drained from this lesion, and *S. aureus* was isolated from the pus. A laceration was noted in the floor of the mouth, and the author considered this wound to be the portal of entry of the infection. Increased incidence of methicillin-resistant *S. aureus* has been reflected in two reports of retropharyngeal abscesses caused by methicillin-resistant *S. aureus* in infants 2 to 3 months of age. One case report involved a 2-month-old infant in Japan (who also had evidence of penicillin-resistant pneumococcus) [4], and the second case report involved 3- and 4-month-old infants in the United States, one of whom had extension of the abscess into the mediastinum accompanied by venous thrombosis [5].

Streptococcus pyogenes. Fever and pharyngeal inflammation may result from infection with *S. pyogenes* in the neonate [6].

Streptococcus agalactiae. Retropharyngeal cellulitis has been associated with bacteremia caused by group B streptococci (GBS) [7–9]. Affected neonates presented with poor feeding, noisy breathing, persistent crying, irritability, and widening of the retropharyngeal space on radiographs of the lateral neck. Stridor also may be associated with retropharyngeal abscess, as reported in a 13-day-old infant in Hong Kong [10]. A retropharyngeal abscess caused by GBS occurred in one of three neonates reported in a series of 31 cases of retropharyngeal abscess in children in Camperdown, Australia, during 1954-1990 [11,12]. This infant was found to have a third branchial arch pouch that was subject to recurrent infection until age 5 years.

Listeria monocytogenes. Small focal granulomas on the mucous membrane of the posterior pharynx have been observed in neonates with *L. monocytogenes* infection.

Necrosis of some of the granulomas results in ulcers on the pharynx and tonsils.

Treponema pallidum. Mucous patches occur on the lips, tongue, and palate of infants with congenital *T. pallidum* infection. Rhinitis may appear after the first week of life.

Neisseria gonorrhoeae. A yellow mucoid exudate of the pharynx may be present simultaneously with ophthalmia with *N. gonorrhoeae* infection (Yu A, personal communication, 1981). A case report of in utero gonococcal infection with involvement of multiple tissues included pharyngeal abscess [13].

Enterococcus faecalis. A case of retropharyngeal abscess in which culture of aspirated pus grew *E. faecalis* and two strains of coagulase-negative staphylococci occurred in a 2-week-old full-term infant from Australia [12]. The infant was severely ill and had atlantoaxial dislocation resulting in paraplegia. At autopsy, the findings included bacterial endocarditis, diffuse bilateral pneumonia, and renal infarcts.

Escherichia coli. *E. coli* can be a rare cause of infection of the pharyngeal cavity. Pus from a retropharyngeal abscess in a 1-week-old infant grew two strains of *E. coli* [12]. The infant was afebrile on presentation and had large midline pharyngeal swelling.

Infants may have coryza and other signs of upper respiratory tract disease secondary to infection with respiratory viruses. Infections with respiratory viruses may damage the respiratory mucosa, increasing susceptibility to bacterial infection of the respiratory tract. Eichenwald [14] described an apparent synergy of respiratory viruses and staphylococci that produced an upper respiratory tract infection called the "stuffy nose syndrome." The syndrome occurred only when both organisms were present. Eichenwald and coworkers [15] also documented increased dissemination of bacteria by newborns carrying staphylococci and echovirus 20 or adenovirus type 2 in the nasopharynx and coined the term "cloud babies" for these infants. These studies have not been repeated by other investigators, and the significance of synergy of two or more microorganisms in neonatal respiratory infections is uncertain.

NOMA

Noma (cancrum oris) is a destructive gangrenous process that may affect the nose, lips, and mouth. It occurs almost exclusively in malnourished children in developing countries; nutrient deficiencies have been postulated to play a role in its pathogenesis [16]. Although it is usually a chronic, destructive process in older children, in neonates it may be rapidly fatal. Affected neonates are usually premature and of low birth weight. In older children and adults, noma is caused by fusospirochetes such as *Fusobacterium necrophorum* [17]. The disease in neonates is usually due to *Pseudomonas aeruginosa*. Ghosal and coworkers [18] reported bacteriologic and histologic findings in 35 cases of noma in neonates in Calcutta. *P. aeruginosa* was isolated from blood or the gangrenous area in more than 90% of the cases. In Israel, a full-term infant with bilateral choanal atresia who required an airway developed gangrenous lesions of the cheek on day 11 and palatal lesions that progressed to ulceration and development of an oronasal fistula. Cultures of material from the lesions grew *P. aeruginosa* [19]. Freeman and associates [20] reported the development of noma neonatorum in the 3rd week of life in a 26-week-gestation premature infant; they suggested that this entity represents a neonatal form of ecthyma gangrenosum. Human immunodeficiency virus (HIV) testing has been recommended for infants in whom noma is diagnosed because of the difficulty distinguishing between the early signs of noma and necrotizing diseases of the oral cavity associated with HIV infection [21].

EPIGLOTTITIS

Epiglottitis caused by *S. aureus* in an 8-day-old infant was reported by Baxter [22] in a survey of experience with the disease at Montreal Children's Hospital from 1951-1965. Rosenfeld and associates [23] reported a second case of epiglottitis caused by *S. aureus* in a 5-day-old infant. The infant presented with bradycardia, hoarseness, and inspiratory stridor and had diffuse inflammation of the arytenoids and epiglottis. *S. aureus* was cultured from pus on the epiglottic surface; blood culture was negative. Epiglottitis secondary to *Streptococcus sanguis* in a newborn infant and secondary to GBS in an 11-week-old infant has also been reported [24,25].

LARYNGITIS

Laryngitis in the newborn is rare. A newborn infant with congenital syphilis may have laryngitis and an aphonic cry. Hazard and coworkers [26] described a case of laryngitis caused by *Streptococcus pneumoniae*. A term infant was noted at 12 hours to have a hoarse cry, which progressed to aphonia during the next 3 days. Direct examination of the larynx revealed swelling and redness of the vocal cords. The infant was febrile (38.5° C), but the physical examination was unremarkable. *S. pneumoniae* was isolated from the amniotic fluid, the maternal cervix, and the larynx of the infant. The infant responded rapidly to treatment with parenteral penicillin G. More recently, laryngitis in infants has been linked with acid reflux [27]. Laryngitis may also be a sign of respiratory papillomatosis, usually associated with human papillomavirus.

INFECTION OF THE PARANASAL SINUSES

The paranasal sinuses of the fetus begin to differentiate at about the 4th month of gestation. The sinuses develop by local evagination of nasal mucosa and concurrent resorption of overlying bone. The maxillary and ethmoid sinuses are developed at birth and may be sites for suppurative infection. The sphenoid and frontal sinuses are rudimentary at birth and are not well defined until about 6 years of age [28,29].

Inflammation may occur simultaneously in the paranasal sinuses, the middle ears, and the lungs. Autopsy may reveal that purulent exudate and leukocytic infiltration of the mucosa are present at one or more of these sites. Infection of the ethmoid and maxillary sinuses may be severe and life-threatening in the newborn. Clinical manifestations include general signs of infection, such as fever, lethargy, irritability, and poor feeding, and focal signs indicative of sinus involvement (i.e., nasal congestion, purulent drainage from the nostrils, and periorbital redness and swelling). Proptosis may occur in severely affected children. Although any of the organisms responsible for neonatal sepsis may cause sinusitis, *S. aureus*, group A streptococci, and GBS are responsible for most infections [30–32]. Suppurative infection of the maxillary sinus may progress to osteomyelitis of the superior maxilla (see Chapter 8) [31].

Blood specimens, nasopharyngeal secretions, and purulent drainage material (if present) should be obtained for culture before treatment. Antibacterial therapy must include a penicillinase-resistant penicillin or cephalosporin for activity against *S. aureus*, group A streptococci, and GBS. If no material is available for examination of Gram-stained pus or if results of the preparation are ambiguous, initial therapy should include an aminoglycoside or a third-generation cephalosporin to ensure activity against gram-negative enteric bacilli (see discussion of management in Chapter 6). Surgical drainage of the infected site should be considered. Drainage of the suppurative maxillary sinus should be performed through the nose to avoid scars on the face and damage to the developing teeth [31].

DIPHTHERIA

Neonatal diphtheria, although now extremely rare in the United States, was common before the development and extensive use of immunization with diphtheria toxoid. Outbreaks occurred in hospital nurseries. One of the most striking reports described three separate epidemics in a "foundling hospital" in Tipperary, Ireland, during 1937-1941; 36 infants younger than 1 month of age were affected, and 26 died [33]. Goebel and Stroder [34] described 109 infants younger than 1 year with diphtheria in Germany during the period from the fall of 1945 to the summer of 1947: 59 infants were younger than 1 month of age, and 26 died. In a report from the Communicable Disease Unit of the Los Angeles County Hospital covering a 10-year period ending June 1950, 1433 patients were admitted to the hospital with diphtheria; 19 patients were younger than 1 year, but only 2 patients were younger than 1 month of age [35]. Elsewhere, diphtheria also seems to be declining [35a]; only three cases of neonatal diphtheria were identified in India from 1974-1984 by Mathur and associates [36].

Respiratory diphtheria has been well controlled in the United States since the introduction of diphtheria toxoid in the 1920s, although it remained endemic in some states through the 1970s [37]. The results of a survey of cases of diphtheria reported to the Centers for Disease Control and Prevention (CDC) of the U.S. Public Health Service, Atlanta, Georgia, for the period 1971 to October 1975 showed that no cases involved children younger than 1 month of age and that only six cases occurred in children younger than 1 year (the youngest was 5 months old) (Filice G, personal communication, 1981). During the period 1980-1995, 41 cases of respiratory diphtheria were reported to the CDC; 4 (10%) were fatal, all of which

occurred in unvaccinated children [38]. No cases of diphtheria have been reported in the United States since 2003 [38a]. Importation of diphtheria from countries where diphtheria remains endemic, or where a resurgence of disease occurred such as in the former Soviet Union, accounted for most of the cases in industrialized nations [39]. Reemergence of diphtheria in the newly independent states of the former Soviet Union underscored the need to maintain control measures in the United States, including universal childhood immunization, adult boosters, and maintenance of surveillance activities [40]. Maternal immunization may provide some protection to infants in the neonatal period before diphtheria vaccine is given [41].

A newborn receives antibodies to *Corynebacterium diphtheriae* from the mother if she is immune, and the titers of mother and infant at birth are approximately equivalent [42]. Some degree of protection results in the neonate from this passively transferred antibody. Serologic surveys performed in the United States in the 1970s and 1980s suggested that 20% to 60% of adults older than 20 years may be susceptible to diphtheria [43,44]. Additional data from Europe confirmed that many adults remain susceptible to diphtheria [45,46]. As is the case in general with passively transferred immunity, protection depends on the level of maternal antibody at the time of the infant's birth, and protection decreases during the months after birth unless the infant is immunized [47,48].

Neonatal diphtheria usually is localized to the nares. Diphtheria of the fauces is less common. The skin and mucous membranes may be affected; the two infants in Los Angeles included an 8-day-old neonate with diphtheritic conjunctivitis [35]. Because isolation of *C. diphtheriae* requires inoculation of special culture media, notification of the laboratory about the possibility of diphtheria is important. Specimens of nasal and pharyngeal secretions may improve yield of positive cultures [49]. Infants suspected to have diphtheria should be isolated and receive penicillin or erythromycin to eradicate the organism from the respiratory tract or other foci of infection to terminate toxin production and decrease likelihood of transmission. The mainstay of therapy is diphtheria antitoxin, which should be administered as soon as the diagnosis of diphtheria is considered. This product is available in the United States from the CDC [50].

PERTUSSIS

Infants and young children in the United States are at the highest risk for pertussis and its complications [51]. Although the incidence of pertussis has declined markedly since 1934, when more than 250,000 cases were recorded, resurgence of disease since the early 1980s underscores the need for continued awareness of this disease [52]. There were 29,134 cases of pertussis in the United States in the years 1997-2000; 29% occurred in infants younger than 1 year, representing an 11% increase from surveillance data for 1994-1996 [53]. The number of deaths in infants younger than 4 months increased from 49 (64% of deaths from pertussis) in 1980-1989 to 84 (82% of deaths) in 1990-1999 [54]. In 2000, 17 deaths were attributed to pertussis in the United States; in all cases, onset of symptoms was before 4 months of age [55]. Hospitalization rates for pertussis for infants did not change notably from 1993-2004 in the United States, with rates highest for infants 1 to 2 months of age (293 hospitalizations per 100,000 live births) [56].

Pertussis occurs in exposed and unprotected newborns [57]. From 1959-1977, pertussis was diagnosed in 400 children in Dallas hospitals; 69 patients (17%) were younger than 12 weeks of age. An adult in the household with undiagnosed mild disease was the usual source of infection for these neonates and young infants [58]. A report of a nursery outbreak in Cincinnati highlights the persistent threat of pertussis in young infants and in hospital personnel [59]. Between February and May 1974, pertussis developed in six newborns, eight physicians, and five nurses (documented by isolation of *Bordetella pertussis* from the nasopharynx). Four additional infants had clinical illness, but the organism was not isolated from the upper respiratory tract. Two mothers of uninfected infants became ill. The initial case was a 1-month-old infant managed in a ward whose infection spread to the nursery when house officers became infected and transmitted the organism to other newborns. A 2004 outbreak involved 11 infants exposed to an infected health care worker in a newborn nursery; the attack rate was 9.7%. The median age at diagnosis was 31 days; five infants required admission to the pediatric intensive care unit, four were treated in the general pediatric unit, one was treated in the emergency department, and one was treated as an outpatient [60].

In the United States in the early 1990s, cases of pertussis were reported from every state, and large outbreaks occurred in Cincinnati and Chicago [61]. In the Chicago outbreak, the highest attack rate was in infants younger than 6 months of age; factors associated with transmission of pertussis in this age group included young maternal age and cough lasting 7 days or longer in the mothers [62]. Another risk factor for pertussis may be low birth weight. A study of cases of pertussis in Wisconsin infants and young children concluded that children of low birth weight were more likely than their normal birth weight counterparts to contract pertussis and to be hospitalized with the disease [63]. Fatal pertussis was identified through a pediatric hospital–based active surveillance system in 16 infants in Canada from 1991-2001; 15 of 16 infants were 2 months of age or younger. When fatal cases were matched with 32 nonfatal cases by age, date, and geography, pneumonia and leukocytosis were identified as independent predictors of a fatal outcome in hospitalized infants [64]. A more recent report described the histopathologic findings in the respiratory tracts of 15 infants younger than 4 months of age who died of pertussis. The findings suggested that the organism triggers a cascade of events, including pulmonary vasoconstriction and release of pertussis toxins leading to increased leukocyte mass and refractory pulmonary hypertension [65].

Antibody to *B. pertussis* crosses the placenta, and titers in immune mothers and their newborns are approximately equal [42,43]. If high titers of the passively transferred antibody are present, the antibody is protective for the newborn; this was shown by Cohen and Scadron [66], who observed protection of 6 months' duration in the offspring of recently immunized women. Three cases of clinical pertussis occurred among six infants who were exposed to infection and whose mothers had not been immunized, whereas no cases occurred among eight similarly exposed infants of immunized mothers. In the group of infants 7 to 12 months old, there were two cases of clinical pertussis in offspring of immunized and unimmunized mothers, which suggests that passively transferred immunity was no longer present in the infants whose mothers had been immunized during pregnancy. Many women who were vaccinated during infancy have low levels of antibody when they reach childbearing age, and this concentration of antibody may be insufficient to protect offspring if the infants are exposed to pertussis during the first few months of life (before they are immunized). Older children and adults are important sources of infection for infants [67]. These findings suggest that maternal immunization would provide sufficient antibody to protect infants before durable immunity could be provided by infant immunization. In addition, adolescent and adult immunization could reduce the number of individuals able to contract pertussis and infect infants [68].

Clinical presentation of pertussis in newborns is similar to the presentation in older children, but may lack some features typical of disease in older children. The incubation period ranges from 5 to 10 days. The initial sign usually is mild coughing, which may progress over several days to severe paroxysms with regurgitation and vomiting of food. The characteristic "whoop" may be absent in infants. The clinical picture of the most severely affected infants may be dominated by marked respiratory distress, cyanosis, and apnea, rather than significant cough. Fever is usually absent. Lymphocyte counts are frequently greater than 30,000/mm^3. Cockayne [69] described a case of clinical pertussis in a neonate whose mother and brother were infectious at the time of birth. The infant began to cough on the 5th day of life and had a high white blood cell count (36,000/mm^3), with mostly lymphocytes. Phillips [70] reported two cases of pertussis in newborns who were infected by an obstetric nurse. The infants began to cough on the 8th and 10th days of life. Clinical signs of respiratory infection caused by *Chlamydia trachomatis* are similar to signs of pertussis (see Chapter 19).

Complications of pertussis in young infants include convulsions, bronchopneumonia, and hemorrhage. Bacterial and viral superinfection may occur. In a study of 182 infants and children younger than age 2 hospitalized with pertussis from 1967-1986 in Dallas, apnea and convulsions occurred significantly more frequently in infants younger than 3 months; the three deaths all were in 1-month-old infants with secondary bacterial infection [71]. Mortality among infants younger than 3 months is high; in the earlier Dallas series, 5 of 69 infants (7%) with onset of signs at 2 to 6 weeks died [50]. *B. pertussis* pneumonia may progress rapidly; pulmonary hypertension resulting from difficulty perfusing the congested lung may cause right-sided heart failure or fatal cardiac arrhythmias [72]. Long-term sequelae of whooping cough in infancy and early childhood were studied by Johnston and coworkers [73]; there was a significant reduction in forced vital capacity in adulthood in individuals who had pertussis before age 7 compared with individuals who did not have pertussis. A case of hemolytic uremic syndrome in a neonate has been reported following pertussis [74].

Diagnostic methods for pertussis depend on the age of the patient and the duration of cough. In children younger than 11 years and older patients with cough lasting less than 14 days, nasopharyngeal specimens should be obtained for bacterial culture using Dacron or calcium alginate swabs. Best results are obtained if specimens are inoculated at the bedside or taken immediately to the laboratory in appropriate transport media. It is helpful to inform the laboratory of suspicion of pertussis because specialized agar (Regan-Lowe or Bordet-Gengou) is required. The organism is isolated most easily during the catarrhal or early paroxysmal stage of illness and rarely is found after the 4th week of illness. Direct fluorescent antibody testing of nasopharyngeal secretions has low sensitivity and variable specificity and cannot be relied on to diagnose pertussis. Polymerase chain reaction assay shows promise as a diagnostic tool [75,76], but no FDA-licensed test is available.

Serologic testing is the diagnostic method of choice for patients 11 years old or older in the absence of immunization within 2 years.

Antimicrobial therapy may lessen severity of the disease if it is given in the catarrhal stage, but it has no clinical effect after paroxysms occur. Antibiotic therapy eliminates carriage of organisms from the upper respiratory tract and is valuable in limiting communicability of infection, even if given late in the clinical course. Azithromycin, 10 mg/kg/day orally in one dose for 5 days, with a maximum daily dose of 600 mg, is the drug of choice for infants younger than one month of age [77]. An alternative is erythromycin estolate, 40 mg/kg/day orally in four divided doses for 14 days [77,78].

Resistance of *B. pertussis* to erythromycin has been reported [79], but does not seem to be widespread. Penicillins and first-generation and second-generation cephalosporins are ineffective against *B. pertussis*. One study showed clinical efficacy in treating pertussis with high-dose specific pertussis globulin from donors immunized with acellular pertussis vaccine [80], although efficacy of this regimen on a larger scale has not been proved. One investigator proposed a role for inhaled corticosteroids in the treatment of pertussis [81]. There are no data available to evaluate the role of albuterol or other β-adrenergic agents in the treatment of pertussis.

Erythromycin also is valuable in prevention of pertussis in exposed infants. Granstrom and colleagues [82] described use of erythromycin in 28 newborns of mothers with pertussis. The women had serologic or culture-confirmed pertussis at the time of labor. Mothers and their newborns received a 10-day course of erythromycin. The infected and treated mothers were allowed to nurse their infants. None of the infants developed signs or serologic evidence of pertussis. Erythromycin has also been shown to be effective in preventing secondary spread within households in which infants resided [83]. Azithromycin (10 mg/kg/day as a single dose for 5 days) is currently the preferred macrolide for prevention of pertussis in infants < 1 month of age, with erythromycin (40 mg/kg/day in 4 divided doses for 14 days) available as an alternative. Clarithromycin is not recommended in this age group. Chemoprophylaxis is also recommended for household and other close contacts, such as individuals in the hospital, including medical and surgical personnel [77,82,84].

Reports of clusters of cases of pyloric stenosis among infants given erythromycin for prophylaxis after exposure to pertussis have raised concern about using erythromycin in this setting [85,86]. A study of 469 infants given erythromycin during the first 3 months of life confirmed an association between systemic (but not ophthalmic) erythromycin and pyloric stenosis and identified that risk was highest in the first 2 weeks of life [87]. Because erythromycin is the only medication proven effective for this purpose and the only one approved for this use, and because pertussis can be life-threatening in the neonate, the drug remains one of the recommended agents, with azithromycin an alternative, until other regimens can be shown to be safe and effective. Health care professionals who prescribe erythromycin to newborns should inform parents of the risk of pyloric stenosis and counsel them about signs and symptoms of pyloric stenosis.

Two tetanus toxoid, reduced diphtheria toxoid, and acellular pertussis vaccines (Tdap) were licensed in 2005 to enhance protection against pertussis in adolescents and adults. Data are lacking at this time about safety of these vaccines administered during pregnancy or effectiveness in preventing disease in infants when administered to mothers. These vaccines are not currently recommended during pregnancy, but are recommended in the immediate postpartum period at an interval of at least 2 years from the last tetanus-diphtheria (Td) booster. If a Td booster is due during pregnancy, it is recommended that this be deferred in lieu of giving a dose of Tdap in the immediate postpartum period [88]. The U. S. Advisory Committee on Immunization Practices in 2006 recommended routine administration of Tdap for postpartum women (who were not vaccinated previously with Tdap) to provide personal protection and reduce the risk for transmitting *B. pertussis* to their infants [89]. The American Medical Association and American Academy of Pediatrics have advocated for immunization of parents and close contacts of newborns younger than 6 months of age for influenza and pertussis. These vaccines have also been recommended for health care workers who have direct patient contact [89].

OTITIS MEDIA

Otitis media in the newborn may be an isolated infection, or it may be associated with sepsis, pneumonia, or meningitis. Acute otitis media is defined as the presence of fluid in the middle ear (middle ear effusion) accompanied by an acute sign of illness. Middle ear effusion may be present without other signs of acute illness. Diagnostic criteria for otitis media in newborns are the same as in older children, but the vulnerability of the newborn and potential differences in the microbiology of otitis media in newborns, especially in the first 2 weeks of life, make it necessary to exercise special considerations in choosing antimicrobial therapy.

PATHOGENESIS AND PATHOLOGY

During fetal life, amniotic fluid bathes the entire respiratory tree, including the lungs, paranasal sinuses, and middle ear cleft. Amniotic fluid and cellular debris usually are cleared from the middle ear in most infants within a few days after birth [90]. In term infants, the middle ear usually is well aerated, with normal middle ear pressure and normal tympanic membrane compliance, within the first 24 hours [91]. A study of 68 full-term infants examined by otoscopy, tympanometry, and acoustic reflectometry within the first 3 hours of life revealed the presence of middle ear effusion in all neonates; fluid was absent at 72 hours of life in almost all infants [92].

Studies of the middle ear at autopsy provide important information about the development of otitis media in the neonate. Inflammation in the lungs or paranasal sinuses usually was accompanied by inflammation in the middle ear [30,90–94]. deSa [90] examined 130 infants, including 36 stillborn infants, 74 neonates who died within 7 days of life, and 20 infants who died between 8 and 28 days. In 56 cases, the middle ear was aerated or contained a small amount of clear fluid. In 55 cases, amniotic debris was present; in 2 additional cases, cellular material was mixed with mucus. A purulent exudate was present in the middle ear of 17 infants; these exudates were cultured, and a bacterial pathogen was isolated from 13. Amniotic material was present in specimens obtained from most of the stillborn infants. Purulent exudate was not seen in the stillborns; the frequency of its presence increased with postnatal age at time of death. Of the 20 infants who lived for 7 or more days, 11 had purulent exudate in the middle ear. Each of the 17 infants with otitis media had one or more significant infections elsewhere; 12 had pneumonia, and 6 had meningitis. deSa [95] subsequently identified mucosal metaplasia and chronic inflammation in the middle ears of newborns receiving ventilatory support.

Factors that may affect the development of otitis media in the neonate include the nature of the amniotic fluid, the presence of other infectious processes, the need for resuscitative efforts (especially positive-pressure ventilation), the presence of anatomic defects such as cleft palate, the immunologic status of the infant, and the general state of health of the infant. Aspiration of infected amniotic fluid through the eustachian tube may be one factor in the development of otitis media in the neonate; dysfunction of the eustachian tube, which is shorter, wider, and more horizontal than in the older child, and failure to clear aspirated material from the middle ear probably have etiologic roles as well [96,97]. Piza and associates [98] speculated that infants born through thick meconium fluid may be at greater risk for otitis media because of the inflammatory nature of this fluid. deSa [90] noted that many infants in whom otitis media developed had required assistance in respiration and speculated

that the pressure of ventilation efforts was responsible for propelling infected material into the middle ear. In infants, as in older children, middle ear effusion seems to be frequent in patients with nasotracheal tubes, and the effusion occurs first on the side of intubation [99]. Berman and colleagues [100] described an association between nasotracheal intubation for more than 7 days and the presence of middle ear effusion.

Infants with cleft palate are at high risk for recurrent otitis media and conductive hearing loss owing to the persistence of middle ear effusion. Attempts to reduce the incidence of permanent hearing impairment have included intensive monitoring of children with cleft palate for middle ear effusion and repair of these defects earlier in infancy. One study found, however, that early cleft palate repair did not reduce significantly the subsequent need for ventilating tubes in these children [101].

Breast-fed infants are at lower risk than bottle-fed infants for acute otitis media. Results of studies of Canadian Eskimo infants [102] and of infants in India [103], Finland [104], Denmark [105], and the United States [106] indicate a significant decrease in the incidence of infection of the middle ear in breast-fed infants compared with bottle-fed infants. A study from Cooperstown, New York, identified a significantly lower incidence of acute lower respiratory tract infection in infants who were breast-fed compared with infants who were bottle-fed; the incidence of otitis media was lower in the breast-fed infants, but this difference was not statistically significant [107]. Infants in Boston who were breast-fed had a lower risk for either having had one or more episodes of acute otitis media or having had recurrent acute otitis media (three or more episodes) during the first year of life. The protective association of breast-feeding did not increase with increased duration of breast-feeding; infants who were breast-fed for 3 months had an incidence of otitis media in the first year of life that was as low as infants who were breast-fed for 12 months [108].

The beneficial effects of breast-feeding may be due to immunologic factors in breast milk or to development of musculature in the breast-fed infant that may affect eustachian tube function and assist in promoting drainage of middle ear fluid. Alternatively, the findings could indicate harmful effects of bottle-feeding, including the reclining or horizontal position of the bottle-fed infant that allows fluid to move readily into the middle ear [109,110], allergy to one or more components in cow's milk or formula, or aspiration of fluids into the middle ear during feeding. The hypothesis that breast milk is protective is substantiated by the results of studies of a special feeding bottle for infants with cleft palate. Among infants who were fed by this bottle containing breast milk, the number of days with middle ear effusion was less than in infants fed by this device containing formula, which suggests that protection was more likely to be a quality of the milk, rather than of the mode of feeding [111]. Adherence of *S. pneumoniae* and *Haemophilus influenzae* to buccal epithelial cells was inhibited by human breast milk [112].

Early onset of pneumococcal otitis media has been associated with low levels of cord blood pneumococcal

IgG antibodies. Among a group of infants who had siblings with middle ear disease, low concentrations of cord blood antibody to pneumococcal serotype 14 or 19F were associated with earlier onset of otitis media [113]. Low cord blood antibody concentrations to serotype 19F predicted more episodes of otitis media over the first year of life in a cohort of 415 infants whose mothers enrolled in the study during pregnancy [114]. In these infants, early otitis media was associated significantly with type 14 IgG1 in the lowest quartile, but not with type 19F IgG1 antibody or with either IgG2 antibody [115]. These findings prompted study of maternal immunization to prevent pneumococcal disease in neonates. Immunization of pregnant chinchillas with heptavalent pneumococcal vaccine resulted in reduced incidence and severity of experimental otitis in their infants [116]. Immunization of pregnant women in Bangladesh, the Gambia, the Philippines, and the United States with pneumococcal polysaccharide vaccine resulted in pneumococcal antibody concentrations that were higher at birth in infants of immunized mothers than in controls [117–120]. In addition, pneumococcal IgG antibody acquired by infants of immunized mothers had greater opsonophagocytic activity than that in control infants [119].

Antibody to pneumococci in breast milk has been proposed to have a role in prevention of early otitis media. Early colonization with pneumococci or other bacteria is associated with early otitis media [121]. The role of antibodies to pneumococci in human milk in prevention of nasopharyngeal colonization of infants with pneumococci is controversial. A study in Sweden involving 448 mother-infant pairs failed to show reduction in carriage of pneumococci in neonates fed milk with anticapsular and antiphosphorylcholine activity and showed an increase in colonization when infants were fed milk with anti–cell wall polysaccharide antibody activity [122]. Maternal immunization with pneumococcal polysaccharide vaccine resulted in higher breast milk IgA antibodies to serotype 19F, but not type 6B [117].

EPIDEMIOLOGY

The incidence of acute otitis media or middle ear effusion in the newborn is uncertain because of the paucity of definitive studies. Warren and Stool [123] examined 127 consecutive infants with birth weight less than 2300 g and found 3 with middle ear effusions (at 2, 7, and 26 days of life). Jaffe and coworkers [124] examined 101 Navajo infants within 48 hours of birth and identified 18 with impaired mobility of the tympanic membrane. Berman and colleagues [100] identified effusion in the middle ear of 30% of 125 consecutively examined infants who were admitted to a neonatal intensive care unit. The clinical diagnosis was corroborated by aspiration of middle ear fluid. The basis for the differences in incidence in the various studies is uncertain, but there may be an association with procedures used in the nurseries.

Acute otitis media is common in early infancy. In the prospective study of Boston children, 9% of children had an episode of middle ear infection by 3 months of age [108]. Age at the time of first episode of acute otitis

media seems to be an important predictor for recurrent otitis media [108,124,125]. Children who experience a first episode during the first months of life are more likely to experience repeated infection than children whose first episode occurs after the first birthday. Additional risk factors include parental smoking and low socioeconomic status [126,127].

Some host factors that also are present in infants with neonatal sepsis have been identified in infants with middle ear infection. The incidence of infection is higher in premature infants than in infants delivered at term in some studies [128,129], but not in the prospective study of Boston children [108]. Male infants are more frequently infected than female infants [128]. Otitis media also is associated with a prolonged interval after rupture of maternal membranes and with other obstetric difficulties [90,130]. Middle ear infection is more severe in Native Americans and Canadian Eskimos than in the general population, and it is likely that this is true in neonates and older infants as well [102,124]. Children with cleft palate have a high incidence of otitis media, which may begin soon after birth [131]. Prenatal, innate, and early environmental exposures were assessed in relation to early otitis media in a cohort of 596 infants followed prospectively from birth. In multivariable analysis, prenatal factors were not associated with early onset of otitis media, but environmental (day care, upper respiratory infection, birth in the fall) and innate factors (parental and sibling history of otitis media) were associated with early or recurrent otitis media, or both [132].

MICROBIOLOGY

The bacteriology of otitis media in infants has been studied by investigators in Honolulu [128], Dallas [129], Huntsville [133], Boston [133], Denver [97,100], Milwaukee [134], Tampere Hospital in Finland [135], and Beer-Sheva, Israel (Table 7–1) [136]. *S. pneumoniae* and *H. influenzae* are isolated frequently from fluid aspirated from the middle ear in very young infants, as is the case in older infants and children. Although it has been suggested that otitis media in the youngest neonates (<2 weeks of age) is caused more frequently by organisms associated with neonatal sepsis, such as GBS, *S. aureus*, and gram-negative enteric bacilli, this pattern does not emerge consistently when multiple studies are examined. Pneumococci were isolated from middle ear fluid in the first 2 weeks of life, and otitis associated with gram-negative enteric organisms and GBS occurred in older infants. Microbiology of middle ear disease in infants who are in neonatal intensive care nurseries may be an exception to the pattern associated with otitis media in previously healthy infants and may reflect pathogens present in the neonatal intensive care unit. In a small series of 13 such infants, only gram-negative enteric organisms and staphylococcal species were identified in the 10 samples of middle ear fluid from which bacteria were identified [100]. Table 7–1 shows the microbiology of middle ear isolates from eight studies of otitis media in infants; when possible, data from the youngest neonates have been separated from data from older infants.

TABLE 7-1   Microbiology of Otitis Media in Newborn Infants

Author(s)	Site (Year[s])	Patients		Causative Organism: No. of Cases (%)					Comment
		Age Range	No. in Series	Streptococcus pneumoniae	Haemophilus influenzae	Staphylococcal Species	Enteric Gram-Negative Species	Other	
Bland [128]	Honolulu (1970-1971)	10-14 days	2	1 (50)	—	—	1 (50)	—	Outpatients
		15-42 days	19*	0 (0)	3 (12)	5 (20)	13 (52)	1 (4)	
Tetzlaff et al [129]	Dallas (1974-1976)	0-5 wk	42*	13 (30)	11 (26)	NA†	8 (19)	12 (28)‡	Outpatients
Balkany et al [97]	Denver (1975-1976)	0-4 mo	21	9 (43)	5 (24)	5 (24)	1 (4)	1 (4)	Outpatients
Berman et al [100]	Denver (1975-1976)	0-4 mo	13*	0 (0)	0 (0)	6 (60)	4 (40)	—	NICU patients
Shurin et al [133]	Huntsville, Boston (1976)	0-6 wk	17	4 (24)	2 (12)	—	1 (6)	3 (18)	3 nursery patients ages 4, 4, and 26 days
Karma et al [135]	Finland (1980-1985)	0-1 mo	14	1 (7)	2 (14)	5 (35)	0	2 (14)	
		1-2 mo	93	19 (20)	8 (9)	55 (60)	5 (5)	11 (11)	
Nozicka et al [134]	Milwaukee (1994-1995)	0-2 wk	Unknown*	1 (14)	1 (14)	0	2 (28)	3 (43)	"Nontoxic" outpatients
Turner et al [136]	Israel (1995-1999)	2-8 wk	Unknown*	5 (19)	0	9 (35)	3 (12)	9 (35)	
		0-2 wk	5	2 (40)	—	—	3 (60)	0	Outpatients
		2-8 wk	109*	54 (44)	41 (34)	0	7 (6)	15 (12)	

*In some infants, more than one organism was identified, or cultures of middle ear fluid yielded no growth.
†Nonpathogen in this study (NA, not applicable).
‡Includes group A and group B streptococci, Staphylococcus species, Neisseria species, diphtheroids, and hemolytic streptococci.
NICU, neonatal intensive care unit.

Susceptibility patterns of organisms causing otitis media in newborns reflect local patterns. Generally, trends toward increasing resistance of pneumococci to antibacterial agents and colonization and disease resulting from pneumococcal serotypes not present in the pneumococcal conjugate vaccine used routinely in the United States and other countries have been observed.

Gram-negative enteric bacilli have been the predominant organisms isolated at autopsy from purulent effusions of the middle ear. Of 17 infants studied by deSa [90], 7 were found to have *E. coli*, and 6 had *P. aeruginosa*. β-hemolytic streptococci (not further identified) were isolated from one infant, and no organism was recovered from the remaining three infants. Because pneumonia and meningitis accompanied otitis in all of these cases, the predominance of gram-negative pathogens in this series is not unexpected.

Congenital tuberculosis of the ear [137] and of the ear and parotid gland [138] has been reported in preterm infants from Hong Kong and Turkey. Both cases were notable for significant regional lymphadenopathy, lack of response to antibacterial therapy, and presence of active pulmonary tuberculosis in the mother. Authors of both reports suggest that there is continued need for a high index of suspicion for this disease in appropriate circumstances. Otitis media and bacteremia resulting from *P. aeruginosa* occurring at 19 days of life was thought to occur after inoculation of the organism during a water birth [139]. *B. pertussis* was isolated from middle ear fluid in a 1-month-old infant hospitalized with pertussis; intubation of the infant's airway may have facilitated spread of the organism from the nasopharynx to the middle ear [140].

DIAGNOSIS

During the first few weeks of life, examination of the ear requires patience and careful appraisal of all of the structures of the external canal and the middle ear [141]. The diagnostic criteria for acute otitis media in the neonate are the same as in the older child: presence of fluid in the middle ear accompanied by signs of acute illness. Middle ear effusion and its effect on tympanic membrane mobility are best measured with a pneumatic otoscope. The normal tympanic membrane moves inward with positive pressure and outward with negative pressure. The presence of fluid in the middle ear dampens tympanic membrane mobility.

In the first few days of life, the ear canal is filled with vernix caseosa; this material is readily removed with a small curette or suction tube. The canal walls of the young infant are pliable and tend to expand and collapse with insufflation during pneumatic otoscopy. Continuing pneumatic insufflation as the speculum is advanced is helpful because the positive pressure expands the pliable canal walls. The tympanic membrane often appears thickened and opaque, and mobility may be limited during the first few days of life [142]. In many infants, the membrane is in an extreme oblique position, with the superior aspect proximal to the observer (Fig. 7–1). The tympanic membrane and the superior canal wall may appear to lie almost in the same plane, so it is often difficult to distinguish the point where the canal ends and the pars flaccida of the

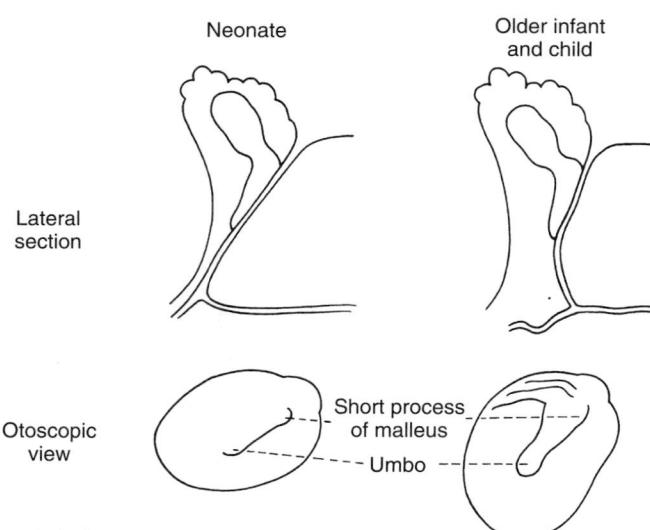

FIGURE 7–1 Lateral section of middle ear and otoscopic view of tympanic membrane in the neonate and older infant and child. *(Courtesy of Charles D. Bluestone, MD.)*

membrane begins. The inferior canal wall may bulge loosely over the inferior position of the tympanic membrane and move with positive pressure, simulating movement of the tympanic membrane. The examiner must distinguish between the movement of the canal walls and the movement of the membrane.

The following considerations are helpful in recognition of these structures: Vessels are seen within the tympanic membrane, but are less apparent in the skin of the ear canal; the tympanic membrane moves during crying or respiration when the middle ear is aerated. The ear canals of most neonates permit entry of only a 2-mm-diameter speculum. Because the entire eardrum cannot be examined at one time, owing to the small diameter of the speculum, quadrants must be examined sequentially. By 1 month of age, the infant's tympanic membrane has assumed an oblique position that is less marked than in the first few weeks of life and is similar to the position in the older child.

Tympanometry is of limited value in diagnosis of middle ear effusion in the neonate. The flat tympanogram indicative of effusion in children 6 months of age or older often is not present in younger infants, even when fluid is documented by aspiration [143]. Acoustic reflectometry may be advantageous compared with tympanometry in the neonate because it does not require insertion into the ear canal or the achievement of a seal within the canal, but there are insufficient data to identify sensitivity and specificity [144].

Culture of the throat or nasopharynx is an imperfect method of identifying the bacterial pathogens responsible for otitis media. Many studies have shown the diagnostic value of needle aspiration of middle ear effusions (tympanocentesis) in acute otitis media. The specific microbiologic diagnosis defines the appropriate antimicrobial therapy and is sufficiently important in the sick neonate to warrant consideration of aspiration of the middle ear fluid. Aspiration of middle ear fluid is more difficult in the neonate than in the older child, and usually the assistance of an otolaryngologist (using an otoscope with a surgical head or an otomicroscope) is required.

When spontaneous perforation has occurred, the fluid exuding into the external canal from the middle ear is contaminated by the microflora from the canal. Appropriate cultures may be obtained by carefully cleaning the canal with 70% alcohol and obtaining cultures from the area of perforation as the fluid emerges or by needle aspiration through the intact membrane.

TREATMENT

Initial therapy for febrile or ill-appearing infants with otitis media during the first 2 weeks of life is similar to therapy for infants with neonatal sepsis. A penicillin and an aminoglycoside or third-generation cephalosporin should be used. Specific therapy can be provided if needle aspiration is performed and the pathogen is identified. Infants who remain in the nursery because of prematurity, low birth weight, or illness require similar management during the first 4 to 6 weeks of life. If the infant was born at term, had a normal delivery and course in the nursery, has been in good health since discharge from the nursery, is not ill-appearing, and is 2 weeks of age or older, the middle ear infection probably is due to *S. pneumoniae* or *H. influenzae* and may be treated with an appropriate oral antimicrobial agent such as amoxicillin or amoxicillin-clavulanate [145]. The infant may be managed outside the hospital if he or she does not seem to have a toxic condition. For infants born at term who have acute otitis media and are in a toxic condition, the physician must consider hospitalization, cultures of blood and cerebrospinal fluid, and use of parenterally administered antimicrobial agents because of possible systemic infection, a focus of infection elsewhere, or presence of a resistant organism.

PROGNOSIS

Infants who have infections of the middle ear in the neonatal period seem to be susceptible to recurrent episodes of otitis media [108,124,125]. The earlier in life an infant has an episode of otitis media, the more likely he or she is to have recurrent infections. It is uncertain whether this means that an early episode of otitis media damages the mucosa of the middle ear and makes the child more prone to subsequent infection, or whether early infection identifies children with dysfunction of the eustachian tube or subtle or undefined immune system abnormalities who have a propensity to infection of the middle ear because of these abnormalities.

MASTOIDITIS

The mastoid air cells are not developed at birth and usually consist of only a single space each. Mastoiditis rarely occurs in neonates. One report cited a case of meningitis and mastoiditis caused by *H. influenzae* in a newborn [146]. Radiographs of the mastoid area showed a cloudy right antrum. At operation, the middle ear was normal, but the antrum was filled with infected mesenchymal tissue.

PNEUMONIA

Pneumonia, inflammation of the lungs, in the fetus and newborn can be classified into four categories according to the time and mode of acquisition of inflammation:

1. *Congenital pneumonia acquired by the transplacental route*: Pneumonia is one component of generalized congenital disease.
2. *Intrauterine pneumonia*: This is an inflammatory disease of the lungs found at autopsy in stillborn or live-born infants who die within the first few days of life, usually associated with fetal asphyxia or intrauterine infection, and includes infectious and noninfectious causes.
3. *Pneumonia acquired during birth*: Signs of pneumonia occur within the first few days of life, and infection is due to microorganisms that colonize the maternal birth canal.
4. *Pneumonia acquired after birth*: The illness manifests during the first month of life, either in the nursery or at home; sources of infection include human contacts and contaminated equipment.

Although helpful as a general framework for understanding neonatal pneumonia, these four categories have clinical features and pathologic characteristics that overlap. Management of pneumonia is essentially the same for all four categories, requiring aggressive supportive measures for the respiratory and circulatory systems along with treatment for the specific underlying infectious disorder.

Pneumonia in the neonate may be caused by viruses, bacteria, or parasitic organisms. Detailed information about causative organisms mentioned in this chapter other than bacteria is found in the appropriate chapters in this book; bacterial disease is covered in detail here.

Pneumonia acquired by the transplacental route may be caused by rubella, cytomegalovirus, herpes simplex virus, adenoviruses [147], mumps virus [148], *Toxoplasma gondii*, *L. monocytogenes*, or *T. pallidum*. Some of these organisms and enteroviruses, genital mycoplasmas, *M. pneumoniae* [148a], *C. trachomatis*, and *Mycobacterium tuberculosis* are also responsible for intrauterine pneumonia resulting from aspiration of infected amniotic fluid. Fatal pneumonitis caused by echovirus has also been reported in newborns (see Chapter 24) [149]. Isolation of *Trichomonas vaginalis* from the tracheal aspirates of infants with pneumonia suggests a possible association of this organism with respiratory tract disease in the neonate [150,151].

GBS is the most frequent cause of bacterial pneumonia acquired at delivery. Pneumonia caused by GBS and other bacteria such as *E. coli* or *L. monocytogenes* may resemble hyaline membrane disease.

Pneumonias acquired after birth, either in the nursery or at home, include those caused by respiratory viruses such as respiratory syncytial virus, influenzavirus, or adenoviruses; gram-positive bacteria such as pneumococci and *S. aureus*; gram-negative enteric bacilli; *Legionella pneumophila* [151a] *C. trachomatis*; *Mycoplasma*; and *Pneumocystis carinii* [152]. A fatal case of adenovirus serotype 14 with pathologic features consistent with bronchiolitis and acute respiratory distress syndrome occurred in a 12-day-old infant in 2006 [153]. Pneumonia caused by nonbacterial microorganisms is discussed in the appropriate chapters. Bacterial pneumonia and neonatal sepsis acquired during or soon after birth share many features of pathogenesis, epidemiology, and management, and these aspects are discussed in Chapter 6. Discussion of pneumonia in the fetus and newborn not presented elsewhere in the text follows.

PATHOGENESIS AND PATHOLOGY
Congenital or Intrauterine Pneumonia

Histologic features of congenital or intrauterine pneumonia have been described from autopsy findings in infants who are stillborn or who die shortly after birth (usually within 24 hours). An inflammatory reaction is found in histologic sections of lung. Polymorphonuclear leukocytes are present in the alveoli and often are mixed with vernix and squamous cells. Infiltrates of round cells may be present in interstitial tissue of small bronchioles and interalveolar septa [154–159]. Alveolar macrophages may be present and have been associated with duration of postnatal life and inflammatory pulmonary lesions [160]. The inflammation is diffuse and usually is uniform throughout the lung. Bacteria are seen infrequently, and cultures for bacteria are often negative. Davies and Aherne [157] noted that the usual characteristics of bacterial pneumonia are missing in congenital pneumonia; among these characteristics are pleural reaction, infiltration or destruction of bronchopulmonary tissue, and fibrinous exudate in the alveoli.

The pathogenesis of congenital pneumonia is not well understood [161]. Asphyxia and intrauterine infection, acting alone or together, seem to be the most important factors [157]. It is thought that microorganisms of the birth canal contaminate the amniotic fluid by ascending infection after early rupture of maternal membranes or through minimal and often unrecognized defects in the membranes. Evidence of aspiration of amniotic fluid is frequent [157]. Naeye and colleagues [162–164] proposed that microbial invasion of the fetal membranes and aspiration of infected amniotic fluid constitute a frequent cause of chorioamnionitis and congenital pneumonia. Bacteriologic studies have produced equivocal results, however. Many infants with congenital pneumonia do not have bacteria in their lungs, yet cultures of the lung of some infants without pneumonia do yield bacteria [165]. Fetal asphyxia or hypoxia seems to be a factor in most cases of congenital pneumonia. The asphyxia may cause death directly or by eliciting a pulmonary response consisting of hemorrhage, edema, and inflammatory cells. From his studies of congenital pneumonia, Barter [166] concluded that hypoxia or infection may produce similar inflammation in the lungs. In addition, Bernstein and Wang [167] found that evidence of fetal asphyxia was frequently present at autopsy in infants with congenital pneumonia who also had generalized petechial hemorrhage, subarachnoid and intracerebral hemorrhage, liver cell necrosis, or ulceration of the gastrointestinal mucosa.

Although it is likely that asphyxia and infection can produce similar inflammatory patterns in lungs of the fetus, available information is insufficient to determine which is more important or more frequent. In a review of fetal and perinatal pneumonia, Finland [168] concluded that "pulmonary lesions certainly play a major role in the deaths of the stillborn and of infants in the early neonatal period. Infection, on the other hand, appears to play only a minor role in what has been called 'congenital pneumonia,' that is, the inflammatory lesion seen in the stillborn or in those dying within the first few hours, or possibly the first day or two; it assumes greater importance in pneumonias that cause death later in the neonatal period." Davies [169] noted that the histologic presentation of congenital pneumonia seems to represent aspiration of materials in amniotic fluid, including maternal leukocytes and amniotic debris, rather than infection originating in the pulmonary air spaces. Evidence of infiltration of alveoli or destruction of bronchopulmonary tissue is rarely present.

Pneumonia Acquired during the Birth Process and in the First Month of Life

The pathology of pneumonia acquired during or after birth is similar to the pathology found in older children or adults. The lung contains areas of densely cellular exudate with vascular congestion, hemorrhage, and pulmonary necrosis [157,167,170]. Bacteria often are seen in sections of the lung. *S. aureus* (see Chapter 14) and *Klebsiella pneumoniae* [171,172] may produce extensive tissue damage, microabscesses, and empyema. Pneumatoceles are a common manifestation of staphylococcal pneumonia, but also may occur in infections with *K. pneumoniae* [171,172] and *E. coli* [173]. Hyaline membranes similar to those seen in respiratory distress syndrome have been observed in the lungs of infants who died with pneumonia caused by GBS. Cocci were present within the membranes, and in some cases, exuberant growth that included masses of organisms was apparent. Although most thoroughly documented in cases of pneumonia caused by GBS, similar membranes have been seen in histologic sections of the lungs of infants who died with pneumonia caused by *H. influenzae* and gram-negative enteric bacilli [174].

The pathogenesis of pneumonia acquired at or immediately after birth is similar to the pathogenesis of neonatal sepsis and is discussed in Chapter 6. Presumably, aspiration of infected amniotic fluid or secretions of the birth canal are responsible for most cases of pneumonia acquired during delivery. After birth, the infant may become infected through human contact or contaminated equipment. Infants who receive assisted ventilation are at risk because of the disruption of the normal barriers to infection owing to the presence of the endotracheal tube and possible irritation of tissues near the tube. Bacteria or other organisms may invade the damaged tissue, which may result in tracheitis or tracheobronchitis [175]. A more recent study identified biofilm formation on endotracheal tubes from infants and hypothesized a relationship between biofilm formation and lower respiratory tract infection in intubated neonates [176].

Ventilator-associated pneumonia may be prevented by reducing bacterial colonization of the aerodigestive tract and decreasing the incidence of aspiration. A review highlighted strategies for prevention of pneumonia in patients receiving mechanical ventilation, including nonpharmacologic strategies such as attention to hand washing and standard precautions, positioning of patients, avoiding abdominal distention, avoiding nasal intubation, and maintaining ventilator circuits and suction catheters and tubing, and pharmacologic strategies such as appropriate use of antimicrobial agents [177]. Newborns with congenital anomalies, such as tracheoesophageal fistula, choanal atresia, and diaphragmatic hernia, have an increased risk of developing pneumonia.

Lung abscess and empyema are uncommon in neonates and usually occur as complications of severe pneumonia. Abscesses also may occur as a result of infection of congenital cysts of the lung.

MICROBIOLOGY

Most information about the bacteriology of fetal and neonatal pneumonia has been derived from studies done at autopsy of stillborn infants and of infants who die during the first month of life. A study reviewing causes of death of infants with very low birth weight concluded, on the basis of histologic studies done at autopsy, that pneumonia was an underrecognized cause of death in these infants [178]. Barter and Hudson [165] reported bacteriologic studies at autopsy of infants with and without pneumonia. The incidence of bacteria in the lungs increased with age in infants dying with and without pneumonia. Among the infants with pneumonia, bacteria were cultured from the lungs of 55% of stillborn infants and infants who died during the first day of life, 70% of infants who died between 24 hours and 7 days of age, and 100% of infants who died between 7 and 28 days of age. Among the infants without pneumonia, bacteria were cultured from the lungs of 36% of stillborn infants and infants who died within the first 24 hours, 53% of infants who died between 24 hours and 7 days of age, and 75% of infants who died between 7 and 28 days of age. The bacterial species were similar in the infants with and without pneumonia, with the exception of GBS, which was found only in infants with pneumonia.

These results were corroborated by Penner and McInnis [159]. Bacteria were cultured from 92% of the lungs of fetuses and neonates with pneumonia and from 40% of the lungs of fetuses and neonates without pneumonia. Davies [179] did lung punctures in stillborn and live-born infants immediately after death, and bacteria were cultured from the lungs of 74% of 93 infants, although pneumonia was diagnosed in only 9 cases. Barson [180] identified bacteria in lung cultures at autopsy of 252 infants dying with bronchopneumonia; positive cultures were obtained in 60% of infants dying on the first day of life and in 78% of infants dying between 8 and 28 days of age. Bacteria were cultured at autopsy from the lungs of many infants with and without pneumonia. Information about bacterial etiology of pneumonia also can be obtained by culturing blood, tracheal aspirates, and pleural fluid and by needle aspiration of the lungs of living children with pneumonia.

The bacterial species responsible for fetal and neonatal pneumonia are those present in the maternal birth canal; included in this flora are gram-positive cocci such as group A, group B, and group F [181] streptococci and gram-negative enteric bacilli, predominantly *E. coli* and,

to a lesser extent, *Proteus, Klebsiella,* and *Enterobacter* species. For infants who remain hospitalized, microorganisms acquired postnatally may reflect the microbial environment of the inpatient setting. For infants who develop pneumonia in the community, typical organisms causing community-acquired pneumonia predominate. In the 1950s and 1960s, *S. aureus* was a common cause of neonatal pneumonia.

Few data exist about relative frequency of specific etiologic agents of neonatal pneumonia or incidence of pneumonia caused by specific organisms. One review of invasive pneumococcal disease monitored prospectively by the U.S. Pediatric Multicenter Pneumococcal Surveillance Group identified 29 cases of pneumococcal infection in infants younger than 30 days of age among 4428 cases in children; 4 of these were bacteremic pneumonia [182]. In addition to *S. pneumoniae* [183–185], *H. influenzae* [174,186] and *Moraxella catarrhalis* [187] also are infrequent causes of pneumonia in newborns. Pneumonia caused by these organisms is frequently associated with bacteremia and sometimes with meningitis [157,183,185,186]. Many other organisms have been reported in association with pneumonia in neonates, including a fatal case of congenital pneumonia caused by *Pasteurella multocida* in a full-term neonate associated with maternal infection and colonization of the family cat with the same organism [188]. A case of pneumonia and sepsis caused by ampicillin-resistant *Morganella morganii* was reported from Texas [189]; the authors speculate about the role of increased use of intrapartum antibiotics in predisposing to colonization and infection with ampicillin-resistant organisms. A case of pneumonia due to *Legionella pneumophila* occurred in a newborn following water birth [189a].

Certain bacteria are associated with a predilection for developing lung abscess or empyema. During the 1950s and 1960s, outbreaks of staphylococcal pneumonia occurred; many times these infections were accompanied by empyemas and pneumatoceles. Although rare in newborns, *H. influenzae* was associated with pneumonia and empyema [190] until its virtual disappearance after initiation of universal immunization in the early 1990s. Single or multiple abscesses may also be caused by GBS, *E. coli,* and *K. pneumoniae* [191,192]. Cavitary lesions may develop in pneumonia caused by *Legionella pneumophila* [193]. Lung abscess and meningitis caused by *Citrobacter koseri* was reported in a previously healthy 1-month-old infant [194]. Nosocomial infection secondary to *L. pneumophila* has been reported, including cases of fatal necrotizing pneumonia and cavitary pneumonia [195]. Reports have identified *Citrobacter diversus* as a cause of lung abscess [196] and *Bacillus cereus* as a cause of a necrotizing pneumonia in premature infants [197].

Empyema can also be associated with extensive pneumonia. Empyema secondary to *E. coli* and *Klebsiella* has been reported in 6- and 8-day-old infants [198], and *Serratia marcescens* was isolated from blood, tracheal aspirate, and empyema fluid in a premature neonate [199]. The past decade was characterized by emergence of increased incidence of invasive disease secondary to group A streptococci. Cases of pleural empyema secondary to group A streptococci have been reported from the United Kingdom and Sweden [200,201].

EPIDEMIOLOGY
Incidence

Table 7–2 presents the incidence of pneumonia at autopsy of stillborn and live-born infants. Pneumonia is a significant cause of death in the neonatal period [202], and infection of amniotic fluid leading to pneumonia may be the most common cause of death in extremely premature infants [203]. The definition of pneumonia in the autopsy studies usually was based on the presence of polymorphonuclear leukocytes in the pulmonary alveoli or interstitium or both. The presence or absence of bacteria was not important in the definition of pneumonia. The incidence rates for congenital and neonatal pneumonia at autopsy are similar despite the different periods of study (1922-1999) and different locations [154–156,158,167,178,201–205] (with the single exception of a report from Helsinki [170]): 15% to 38% of stillborn infants and 20% to 32% of live-born infants had evidence of pneumonia. The incidence rates for pneumonia were similar in premature and in term infants. Rates of pneumonia derived from epidemiologic studies are scarce. Sinha and colleagues [206] reported an attack rate of 0.4 per 100 infants diagnosed during a nursery stay, and 0.03 and 0.01 per 100 infants diagnosed at pediatric office visits and in hospital or emergency department visits. They acknowledged a paucity of data with which to compare their rates, which they derived from retrospective review of data from a large health maintenance organization.

Race and Socioeconomic Status

In two studies, black infants had pneumonia at autopsy significantly more often than white infants. The Collaborative Study of the National Institutes of Health [205] considered the incidence of pneumonia in live-born infants who died within the first 48 hours of life: 27.7% of black infants had evidence of pneumonia, whereas only 11.3% of white infants showed signs of this disease, and this difference was present in every weight group. In New York City, Naeye and coworkers [162] studied 1044 consecutive autopsies of newborn and stillborn infants; black infants had significantly more pneumonia (38%) than Puerto Rican infants (22%) or white infants (20%). The same study showed that the incidence of pneumonia in infants was inversely related to the level of household income. Infants from the families with the lowest income had significantly more pneumonia than infants from the families with the highest income. At comparable levels of household income, black infants had a higher incidence of neonatal pneumonia than Puerto Rican or white infants. These racial and economic differences were not readily explained by the authors or by other investigators.

Epidemic Disease

Pneumonia may be epidemic in a nursery because of a single source of infection, such as a suppurative lesion caused by *S. aureus* in a nursery employee or contamination of a common solution or piece of equipment, usually caused by *Pseudomonas*, *Flavobacterium*, or *S. marcescens*. Infection may also spread by droplet nuclei among infants or between personnel and infants. Epidemics of respiratory infection related to viruses also have been reported (see Chapter 35).

Developing Countries

Pneumonia is a particular threat to neonates in developing countries. A survey of a rural area in central India revealed that the mortality rate for pneumonia in the first 29 days of life was 29 per 1000 live-born children (the rate during the first year was 49.6 per 1000 live-born children) [207]. The aerobic bacteria grown from the vagina of rural women were used as a surrogate for likely pathogens of pneumonia in neonates [208]. Vaginal flora included *E. coli* and other gram-negative enteric bacilli and

TABLE 7–2   Incidence of Congenital and Neonatal Pneumonia Based on Findings at Autopsy

Site (Years) [reference]	No. with Pneumonia/Total No. of Infants (%)						Age or Weight of Infants at Death
	Stillbirths			**Live-Born Infants**			
	Premature	**Term**	**Total**	**Premature**	**Term**	**Total**	
Helsinki (1951) [154]	5/13 (38)	9/32 (28)	14/45 (31)				
Helsinki (1946–1952) [170]				218/361 (60)	210/315 (67)	428/676 (63)	<29 days
Newcastle (1955–956) [155]			13/70 (19)			10/31 (32)	<7 days
Adelaide (1950–1951) [156]	5/44 (11)	10/53 (19)	15/97 (15)	9/32 (28)	3/8 (38)	12/40 (30)	Lived <6 hr after birth
Detroit (1956–1959) [165]						55/231 (24)	<7 days
Winnipeg (1954–1960) [202]	15/46 (33)						<750 g
Winnipeg (1954–1957) [203]						27/110 (25)	<7 days
Edinburgh (1922) [204]						22/80 (26)	8 hr to 5 wk
NIH Collaborative Study (1959–1964) [205]				67/387 (17)	33/125 (26)	100/512 (20)	<48 hr
Manchester (1950–1954) [158]			28/275 (10)			59/219 (27)	<7 days
Los Angeles (1990–1993) [178]				25/111 (23)			<1000 g, <48 hr

staphylococcal species in expected proportions, but a relatively low rate of β-hemolytic streptococci (3.2%). Management of pneumonia cases (the cases that did not necessitate immediate referral to a hospital) included continued breast-feeding and trimethoprim-sulfamethoxazole. Because of the lack of microbiologic information, syndrome-based management of infectious diseases is encouraged in the developing world. A meta-analysis of this approach found a reduction of pneumonia mortality of 42% in neonates managed in this fashion [209].

Singhi and Singhi [210] studied the clinical signs of illness in Chandigarh infants younger than 1 month of age with radiologically confirmed pneumonia to determine how to increase accuracy of diagnosis of pneumonia by health care workers. Rural health care workers (most were illiterate) used revised World Health Organization criteria for pneumonia in infants, including respiratory rate greater than 60 breaths per minute, presence of severe chest indrawing (retraction), or both [211]. Cough and respiratory rate greater than 50 breaths per minute missed 25% of cases; decreasing the threshold respiratory rate to 40 breaths per minute increased the sensitivity. In the absence of cough, chest retraction or respiratory rate greater than 50 breaths per minute or both had maximum accuracy.

CLINICAL MANIFESTATIONS

Onset of respiratory distress at or soon after birth is characteristic of intrauterine or congenital pneumonia. Before delivery, fetal distress may be evident: The infant may be tachycardic, and the fetal tracing may show poor beat-to-beat variability or evidence of deep decelerations. Meconium aspiration may have occurred before delivery, suggesting fetal asphyxia and gasping. The infant may have episodes of apnea or may have difficulty establishing regular respiration. In some cases, severe respiratory distress is delayed, but it may be preceded by increasing tachypnea, apneic episodes, and requirement for increasing amounts of oxygen. The infant may have difficulty feeding, temperature instability, and other signs of generalized sepsis, including poor peripheral perfusion, disseminated intravascular coagulation, and lethargy.

Infants who acquire pneumonia during the birth process or postnatally may have signs of systemic illness, such as lethargy, anorexia, and fever. Signs of respiratory distress, including tachypnea, dyspnea, grunting, coughing, flaring of the alae nasi, irregular respirations, cyanosis, intercostal and supraclavicular retractions, rales, and decreased breath sounds, may be present at the onset of the illness or may develop later. Severe disease may progress to apnea, shock, and respiratory failure. Signs of pleural effusion or empyema may be present in suppurative pneumonias associated with staphylococcal infections, group A [212] and group B streptococcal infections, and *E. coli* infections [213].

In a study of 103 neonates in New Delhi, Mathur and colleagues documented the sensitivity and specificity of signs of neonatal pneumonia: cough (n = 13; 14%; 100%); difficulty in feeding (n = 91; 88%; 6%); chest retractions (n = 96; 93%; 36%); flaring of alae nasi (n = 50; 49%; 70%) [214].

DIAGNOSIS
Clinical Diagnosis

A history of premature delivery, prolonged interval between rupture of maternal membranes and delivery, prolonged labor, excessive obstetric manipulation, and presence of foul-smelling amniotic fluid frequently are associated with neonatal infection, including sepsis and pneumonia. The clinical manifestations of pneumonia may be subtle and nonspecific at the onset, and specific signs of respiratory infection may not be evident until late in the course of illness. Most commonly, pneumonia is associated with evidence of respiratory distress, including tachypnea, retractions, flaring of nasal alae, and increasing requirement for oxygen.

Radiologic Diagnosis

A chest radiograph is the most helpful tool for making the diagnosis of pneumonia. The radiograph of an infant with intrauterine pneumonia may contribute no information, however, or show only the coarse mottling of aspiration. If the radiologic examination is done early in the course of meconium or other aspiration pneumonias, typical radiologic features may not yet have developed. The radiograph of an infant with pneumonia acquired during or after birth may show streaky densities or confluent opacities. Peribronchial thickening, indicating bronchopneumonia, may be present. Pleural effusion, abscess cavities, and pneumatoceles are frequent in infants with staphylococcal infections, but also may occur in pneumonia caused by group A streptococci, *E. coli* [173], or *K. pneumoniae* [172]. Diffuse pulmonary granularity or air bronchograms similar to that seen in respiratory distress syndrome have been observed in infants with pneumonia related to GBS [215]. Computed tomography (CT) with contrast medium enhancement is beneficial in localizing pulmonary lesions such as lung abscess and distinguishing abscess from empyema, pneumatoceles, or bronchopleural fistulas [192]. Ultrasound examination was used to diagnose hydrothorax in utero at 32 weeks of gestation [216].

Although it is impossible to distinguish bacterial from viral pneumonia on the basis of a chest radiograph alone, several features may help distinguish between the two. Findings that are more characteristic of viral pneumonias include hyperexpansion, atelectasis, parahilar peribronchial infiltrates, and hilar adenopathy, which is associated almost exclusively with adenovirus infection. Alveolar disease, consolidation, air bronchograms, pleural effusions, pneumatoceles, and necrotizing pneumonias are more characteristic of bacterial processes [217].

Microbiologic Diagnosis

Because of the difficulty in accessing material from a suppurative focus in the lower respiratory tree, microbiologic diagnosis of pneumonia is problematic. Although cultures of material obtained from lung aspiration have been shown to yield bacterial pathogens in about one third of a group of seriously ill infants with lung lesions accessible to needle aspiration [218], this rate of positive results is unlikely to be obtained in an unselected group of infants with pneumonia. Diagnosis may be based on isolating pathogens from other sites. When generalized systemic infection is present, cultures of blood, urine, or cerebrospinal fluid may yield a pathogen. Bacteremia may be identified in about 10% of febrile children with pneumonia [219]. If a pleural effusion is present and the bacterial diagnosis is not yet evident, pleural fluid biopsy or culture or both may be helpful. Bacterial cultures of the throat and nasopharynx are unrevealing or misleading because of the high numbers of respiratory pathogens present.

Tracheal aspiration through a catheter is frequently valuable when performed by direct laryngoscopy, but the aspirate may be contaminated when the catheter is passed through the nose or mouth. Sherman and colleagues [220] performed a careful study of the use of tracheal aspiration in diagnosis of pneumonia in the first 8 hours of life. Tracheal aspirates were obtained from 320 infants with signs of cardiorespiratory disease and abnormalities on the chest radiograph; 25 infants had bacteria present in the smear of the aspirate, and the same organisms were isolated from cultures of 14 of 25 aspirates. Thureen and colleagues [221] found that tracheal aspirate cultures failed to define an infectious cause of deterioration in ventilated infants. Positive tracheal aspirates were found with equal frequency among infants with clinically suspected lower respiratory tract infection and in "well" controls. Tracheal aspirate cultures may provide useful information about potential pathogens in pneumonia or bacteremia, but rarely indicate the risk or timing of such complications [222]. Often, surveillance cultures of tracheal aspirate material are used to guide empirical therapy when a new illness develops in an infant with a prolonged course on a ventilator.

Bronchoscopy can provide visual, cytologic, and microbiologic evidence of bacterial pneumonia [223]. Aspiration of pulmonary exudate (lung puncture or "lung tap") can be used to provide direct, immediate, and unequivocal information about the causative agent of pneumonia [218]. This procedure is now performed rarely; most reports of its use in infants and young children precede the introduction of antimicrobial agents [224,225].

Open lung biopsy has been used to identify the etiology of lung disease in critically ill infants and seems to have been most helpful at a time when corticosteroids for bronchopulmonary dysplasia were withheld if there was concern about pulmonary infection. Cheu and colleagues [226] identified three infections in 17 infants who had open lung biopsies: respiratory syncytial virus in 1 infant and *Ureaplasma urealyticum* in 2 infants. Although the optimal indications for use of corticosteroids in bronchopulmonary dysplasia are controversial [227,228], generally corticosteroids are not withheld if indicated because of low likelihood of an infectious process [229].

Histologic and Cytologic Diagnosis

The data of Naeye and coworkers [162] indicated that congenital pneumonia or pneumonia acquired during birth is almost always accompanied by chorioamnionitis, although chorioamnionitis may be present in the absence of pneumonia or other neonatal infections. These and other data [230] suggested that the presence of leukocytes in sections of placental membranes and of umbilical

vessels or in Wharton jelly is valuable in diagnosing fetal and neonatal infections, including pneumonia and sepsis. Other investigators were less certain and believed that the presence of inflammation in the placenta or umbilical cord does not distinguish changes caused by hypoxia from those caused by infection [166,167].

Culture of material obtained by aspiration of stomach contents usually is not helpful in diagnosing pneumonia because this material is contaminated by the flora of the upper respiratory tract. In addition, infants with pneumonia may have no evidence of the organism in the gastric aspirate [231]. There is some evidence, however, that microscopic examination of gastric contents may be useful in defining the presence of an inflammatory process in the lung after the first day of life. Because affected infants are unable to expectorate, they swallow bronchial secretions. During the first few hours of life, inflammatory cells present in the gastric aspirate are of maternal origin; however, after the first day, any polymorphonuclear leukocytes present are those of the infant. Tam and Yeung [231] showed that if more than 75% of the cells in the gastric aspirate obtained from infants after the first day of life were polymorphonuclear leukocytes, pneumonia was usually present. A study by Pole and McAllister [232] did not confirm the value of gastric aspirate cytology in the diagnosis of pneumonia, however.

Primary ciliary dyskinesia is congenital and may manifest in the newborn period as respiratory distress. Infants with situs inversus are at risk for this condition. Consultation with a geneticist may be warranted; a biopsy specimen of nasal epithelium may be needed to identify the characteristic abnormal morphology of cilia of the immotile cilia syndrome [233–235].

Immunologic Diagnosis

Immunologic response to various microorganisms responsible for pneumonia is used extensively as an aid to diagnosis with infections caused by GBS, *S. aureus* (see Chapters 12 and 14) and organisms that cause congenital infection (rubella virus, *T. gondii*, herpes simplex virus, cytomegalovirus, and *T. pallidum*). Giacoia and colleagues [236] prepared antigens from microorganisms isolated from bronchial aspirates and correlated specific antibodies and nonspecific IgM antibody with clinical and radiologic evidence of pneumonia. A significant immune response was identified in approximately one fourth of the patients studied. These data are of uncertain significance because of the difficulty of distinguishing immune response to organisms responsible for lower respiratory tract disease from the response to organisms colonizing the respiratory tree [237].

Although controversial, testing of blood, urine, and cerebrospinal fluid for antigens to GBS, pneumococci, *H. influenzae*, and *Neisseria meningitidis* may provide helpful information for selected infants with generalized sepsis and pneumonia [238]. Interpretation of results must take into account possible contamination by organisms colonizing the area around the urethra (in the case of a bag specimen of urine) and possible interference with the test result caused by recent immunization against *H. influenzae* type b or pneumococci or recent infection owing to these organisms. Bedside cold agglutination testing may be helpful in the case of *Mycoplasma* infection, but the test has low sensitivity, so a negative result is not diagnostic. Although polymerase chain reaction testing has provided diagnostic information for many conditions, it does not at present offer any specific advantages in the diagnosis of pneumonia.

DIFFERENTIAL DIAGNOSIS

Various noninfectious diseases and conditions may simulate infectious pneumonia. Respiratory distress syndrome (hyaline membrane disease), atelectasis, aspiration pneumonia, pneumothorax or pneumomediastinum, pulmonary edema and hemorrhage, pleural effusions of the lung (e.g., chylothorax), cystic lung disease, hypoplasia or agenesis, pulmonary infarct, and cystic fibrosis all have some signs and symptoms similar to pneumonia. Meconium aspirated into the distal air passages may produce chemical pneumonitis or segmental atelectasis [239]. Multifocal pulmonary infiltrates have been associated with feeding supplements containing medium-chain triglycerides [240]. Infants with immotile cilia syndrome may present within the first 24 hours of life with tachypnea, chest retraction, and rales. Results of prospective epidemiologic studies of neonatal respiratory diseases from Sweden [241] for the period 1976-1977 and from Lebanon [242] for the period 1976-1984 indicate that infection was second in frequency to hyaline membrane disease in both surveys. Avery and coworkers [243] presented clues to the diagnosis of diseases and conditions producing respiratory distress based on information from the maternal history and signs in the infant (Table 7–3).

Pneumonia may be superimposed on hyaline membrane disease. One survey showed that histologic evidence of pneumonia was present at autopsy in 16% of 1535 infants with hyaline membrane disease [244]. Foote and Stewart [245] showed, by chest radiography, that pneumonia modifies the reticulogranular pattern of hyaline membrane disease by replacing the air in the alveoli with inflammatory exudate. Any modification of the radiographic pattern typical of hyaline membrane disease should lead the physician to consider superinfection.

Ablow and colleagues [246] reported that infants with pneumonia caused by GBS who also showed clinical and radiologic signs of respiratory distress syndrome were easier to ventilate than infants who had hyaline membrane disease with a clinical picture suggestive of respiratory distress syndrome unassociated with infection. These findings are of limited value in identifying infection in individual infants and were not confirmed in a subsequent study by Menke and colleagues [247].

Pleural fluid, usually limited to the lung fissures, occurs in many infants and may be related to slow resorption of fetal lung fluid, to transient tachypnea of the newborn, or to respiratory distress syndrome of noninfectious etiology. Large collections of fluid in the pleural space may represent bacterial empyema; noninfectious causes include chylothorax, hydrothorax (associated with hydrops fetalis, congestive heart failure, or transient tachypnea), meconium aspiration pneumonitis, or hemothorax related to hemorrhagic disease of the newborn.

TABLE 7–3   Clues to Diagnosis of Types of Respiratory Distress

Information from Maternal History	Most Probable Condition in Infant
Peripartum fever	Pneumonia
Foul-smelling amniotic fluid	Pneumonia
Excessive obstetric manipulation at delivery	Pneumonia
Infection	Pneumonia
Premature rupture of membranes	Pneumonia
Prolonged labor	Pneumonia
Prematurity	Hyaline membrane disease
Diabetes	Hyaline membrane disease
Hemorrhage in days before premature delivery	Hyaline membrane disease
Meconium-stained amniotic fluid	Meconium aspiration
Hydramnios	Tracheoesophageal fistula
Pain medications	CNS depression
Use of reserpine	Stuffy nose
Traumatic or breech delivery	CNS hemorrhage; phrenic nerve paralysis
Fetal tachycardia or bradycardia	Asphyxia
Prolapsed cord or cord entanglements	Asphyxia
Postmaturity	Aspiration
Amniotic fluid loss	Hypoplastic lungs

Signs in the Infant	Most Probable Associated Condition
Single umbilical artery	Congenital anomalies
Other congenital anomalies	Associated cardiopulmonary anomalies
Situs inversus	Kartagener syndrome
Scaphoid abdomen	Diaphragmatic hernia
Erb palsy	Phrenic nerve palsy
Inability to breathe with mouth closed	Choanal atresia; stuffy nose
Gasping with little air exchange	Upper airway obstruction
Overdistention of lungs	Aspiration; lobar emphysema or pneumothorax
Shift of apical pulse	Pneumothorax, chylothorax, hypoplastic lung
Fever or increase in body temperature in constant-temperature environment	Pneumonia
Shrill cry, hypertonia or flaccidity	CNS disorder
Atonia	Trauma, myasthenia, poliomyelitis, amyotonia
Frothy blood from larynx	Pulmonary hemorrhage
Head extended in the absence of neurologic findings	Laryngeal obstruction or vascular rings
Choking after feedings	Tracheoesophageal fistula or pharyngeal incoordination
Plethora	Transient tachypnea

CNS, central nervous system.
From Avery ME, Fletcher BD, Williams RG. The Lung and Its Disorders in the Newborn Infant. Philadelphia, WB Saunders, 1981.

The symptoms of cystic fibrosis may begin in early infancy. Of patients with newly diagnosed cases seen in a 5-year period at Children's Hospital Medical Center in Boston, 30% were younger than 1 year of age [248]. The authors described the histories of four children whose respiratory symptoms began before the infants were 1 month of age. The clinical course of the disease in young infants is characterized by a bronchiolitis-like syndrome with secondary chronic obstructive pulmonary disease and respiratory distress, coughing, wheezing, poor exchange of gases, cyanosis, hypoxia, and failure to thrive.

MANAGEMENT

Infants with bacterial pneumonia must receive prompt treatment with appropriate antimicrobial agents. Culture of blood and urine may identify a bacterial pathogen, especially in patients with generalized sepsis. Cerebrospinal fluid culture may be helpful if the infant is not too unstable for lumbar puncture. In intubated infants, tracheal aspirate smears may indicate the presence of inflammatory cells, and cultures may provide information about organisms colonizing the trachea.

Because the microbiology of pneumonia in the newborn is the same as that of sepsis, the guidelines for management discussed in Chapter 6 are applicable. Initial antimicrobial therapy should include a penicillin (penicillin G or ampicillin) or a penicillinase-resistant penicillin (if staphylococcal infection is a possibility) and an aminoglycoside or a third-generation cephalosporin. In situations in which resistant pneumococci or methicillin-resistant *S. aureus* may be the cause of the pneumonia, vancomycin may be used for initial therapy until microbiologic data are available. The oxazolidinone antibiotic linezolid, an agent with a unique mechanism of action with activity against gram-positive organisms, has been studied in neonates. Sixty-three neonates with known or suspected resistant gram-positive infections were randomly assigned to receive linezolid or vancomycin. No difference in efficacy of the two agents was noted, and the authors concluded that linezolid is a safe and effective alternative to vancomycin in treatment of resistant gram-positive infections [249].

Duration of therapy depends on the causative agent: pneumonia caused by gram-negative enteric bacilli or GBS is treated for 10 days; disease caused by *S. aureus* may require 3 to 6 weeks of antimicrobial therapy according to the severity of the pneumonia and the initial response to therapy. Empyema or lung abscesses may also require longer courses of therapy.

When clinical and radiologic signs of hyaline membrane disease are present, infection caused by GBS or gram-negative organisms, including *H. influenzae*, is not readily distinguished from respiratory distress syndrome of noninfectious etiology. Until techniques are developed that can distinguish infectious from noninfectious causes of respiratory distress syndrome, it is reasonable to treat all infants who present with clinical and radiologic signs of the syndrome. Therapy is instituted for sepsis, as outlined earlier, after appropriate cultures have been taken. If the results of cultures are negative and the clinical course subsequently indicates that the illness was not infectious, the antimicrobial regimen is stopped. Because of concern over respiratory signs as a part of the initial presentation of sepsis and the rapid progression of bacterial pneumonia in neonates with associated high mortality rate, particularly pneumonia caused by GBS, early and aggressive therapy is warranted in infants with respiratory distress syndrome.

Antibiotics are only part of the management of the newborn with pneumonia; supportive measures such as maintaining fluid and electrolyte balance, providing oxygen or support of respiration with continuous positive airway pressure, or instituting intubation and ventilation are equally important. Drainage of pleural effusions may be necessary when the accumulation of fluid results in respiratory embarrassment. Single or multiple thoracocenteses may be adequate when the volumes of fluid are small. If larger amounts are present, a closed drainage system with a chest tube may be needed. The tube should be removed as soon as its drainage function is completed because delay may result in injury to local tissues, secondary infection, and sinus formation. Empyema and abscess formation are uncommon but serious complications of pneumonia. They may occur in association with pneumonia caused by *S. aureus* and are discussed in detail in Chapter 14.

PROGNOSIS

Available data on the significance of pneumonia during early life have been obtained in large measure from autopsy studies. There is information about the natural course of pneumonia caused by *S. aureus* in infants (see Chapter 14), but few studies of the sequelae of pneumonia caused by other agents exist. Even autopsy studies are equivocal in determining the importance of pneumonia because respiratory disease may have been the cause of death, a contributing factor in death, or incidental to and apart from the main cause of death [250,251]. Pneumonia was said to be the sole cause of death in about 15% of neonatal deaths studied by Ahvenainen [170]. In the British Perinatal Mortality Study [252], pulmonary infections were considered to be the cause of death in 5.5% of stillborn infants and infants dying in the neonatal period.

Ahvenainen [170] noted that pneumonia often is a fatal complicating factor in infants with certain underlying conditions, such as central nervous system malformations or disease, congenital heart disease, and anomalies of the gastrointestinal tract such as intestinal atresia. A prospective study of premature newborns found ventilator-associated pneumonia to occur frequently and to be significantly associated with death in extremely premature infants who remained in a neonatal intensive care unit for more than 30 days [253].

The presence of pneumonia in the neonatal period has been implicated as a cause of chronic pulmonary disease in infancy and childhood. Pacifico and associates [254] found that isolation of *U. urealyticum* from the respiratory tract of premature low birth weight infants in the first 7 days of life was associated with early development of bronchopulmonary dysplasia and severe pulmonary outcome. Brasfield and colleagues [255] studied a group of 205 infants hospitalized with pneumonitis during the first 3 months of life and identified radiographic and pulmonary function abnormalities that persisted for more than 1 year.

REFERENCES

[1] H. Clark, N. Barysh, Retropharyngeal abscess in an infant of six weeks, complicated by pneumonia and osteomyelitis, with recovery: report of case, Arch. Pediatr. 53 (1936) 417.

[2] C. Ravindra, et al., Retropharyngeal abscesses in infants, Indian J. Pediatr. 50 (1983) 449–450.

[3] P.F. Steinhauer, Ludwig's angina: report of a case in a 12-day-old boy, J. Oral. Surg. 25 (1967) 251.

[4] H. Masaaki, I. Hisashi, T. Kyoko, Retropharyngeal abscess in a 2-month-old infant—a case report, Otolaryngol. Head Neck Surg. (Tokyo) 75 (2003) 651–654.

[5] A.F. Fleisch, et al., Methicillin-resistant *Staphylococcus aureus* as a cause of extensive retropharyngeal abscess in two infants, Pediatr. Infect. Dis. J. 26 (2007) 1161–1163.

[6] W.H. Langewisch, An epidemic of group A, type 1 streptococcal infections in newborn infants, Pediatrics 18 (1956) 438.

[7] B.I. Asmar, Neonatal retropharyngeal cellulitis due to group B streptococcus, Clin. Pediatr. (Phila) 26 (1987) 183.

[8] W.L. Smith, et al., Percutaneous aspiration of retropharyngeal space in neonates, AJR. Am. J. Roentgenol. 139 (1982) 1005.

[9] F.T. Bourgeois, M.W. Shannon, Retropharyngeal cellulitis in a 5-week-old infant, Pediatrics 109 (2002) e51.

[10] V. Abdullah, et al., A case of neonatal stridor, Arch. Dis. Child. Fetal. Neonatal. Ed. 87 (2002) 224.

[11] M. Coulthard, D. Isaacs, Retropharyngeal abscess, Arch. Dis. Child. 66 (1991) 1227.

[12] M. Coulthard, D. Isaacs, Neonatal retropharyngeal abscess, Pediatr. Infect. Dis. J. 10 (1991) 547.

[13] E.H. Oppenheimer, K.J. Winn, Fetal gonorrhea with deep tissue infection occurring in utero, Pediatrics 69 (1982) 74.

[14] H.F. Eichenwald, "Stuffy nose syndrome" of premature infants: an example of bacterial-viral synergism, Am. J. Dis. Child. 96 (1958) 438.

[15] H.F. Eichenwald, O. Kotsevalov, L.A. Fasso, The "cloud baby": an example of bacterial-viral interaction, Am. J. Dis. Child. 100 (1960) 161.

[16] C.O. Enwonwu, et al., Pathogenesis of cancrum oris (noma): confounding interactions of malnutrition with infection, Am. J. Trop. Med. Hyg. 60 (1999) 223.

[17] W.A. Falkler, J.C.O. Enwonwu, E.O. Idigbe, Isolation of *Fusobacterium necrophorum* from cancrum oris (noma), Am. J. Trop. Med. Hyg. 60 (1999) 150.

[18] S.P. Ghosal, et al., Noma neonatorum: its aetiopathogenesis, Lancet 2 (1978) 289.

[19] A. Alkalay, et al., Noma in a full-term neonate, Clin. Pediatr. (Phila) 24 (1985) 528.

[20] A.F. Freeman, A.J. Mancini, R. Yogev, Is noma neonatorum a presentation of ecthyma gangrenosum in the newborn? Pediatr. Infect. Dis. J. 21 (2002) 83.

[21] C.O. Enwonwu, Noma—the ulcer of extreme poverty, N. Engl. J. Med. 354 (2006) 221–224.

[22] J.D. Baxter, Acute epiglottitis in children, Laryngoscope 77 (1967) 1358.

[23] R.M. Rosenfeld, M.A. Fletcher, S.L. Marban, Acute epiglottitis in a newborn infant, Pediatr. Infect. Dis. J. 11 (1992) 594.

[24] N. Young, A. Finn, C. Powell, Group B streptococcal epiglottitis, Pediatr. Infect. Dis. J. 15 (1996) 95.

[25] A.P. Bos, et al., Streptococcal pharyngitis and epiglottitis in a newborn infant, Eur. J. Pediatr. 151 (1992) 874–875.

[26] G.W. Hazard, P.J. Porter, D. Ingall, Pneumococcal laryngitis in the newborn infant: report of a case, N. Engl. J. Med. 271 (1964) 361.

[27] S.O. Ulualp, et al., Pharyngeal pH monitoring in infants with laryngitis, Otolaryngol. Head Neck Surg. 137 (2007) 776–779.

[28] W.B. Davis, Anatomy of the nasal accessory sinuses in infancy and childhood, Ann. Otol. Rhinol. Laryngol. 27 (1918) 940.

[29] W.W. Wasson, Changes in the nasal accessory sinuses after birth, Arch. Otolaryngol. 17 (1933) 197.

[30] M.C. Benner, Congenital infection of the lungs, middle ears and nasal accessory sinuses, Arch. Pathol. 29 (1940) 455.

[31] F. Cavanagh, Osteomyelitis of the superior maxilla in infants: a report on 24 personally treated cases, BMJ 1 (1960) 468.

[32] J.B. Howard, G.H. McCracken Jr., The spectrum of group B streptococcal infections in infancy, Am. J. Dis. Child. 128 (1974) 815.

[33] J.B. O'Regan, M. Heenan, J. Murray, Diphtheria in infants, Ir. J. Med. Sci. 6 (1943) 116.

[34] F. Goebel, J. Stroder, Diphtheria in infants, Dtsch. Med. Wochenschr. 73 (1948) 389.

[35] M.J. Naiditch, A.G. Bower, Diphtheria: a study of 1433 cases observed during a ten-year period at the Los Angeles County Hospital, Am. J. Med. 17 (1954) 229.

[35a] A.M. Galazka, S.E. Robertson, Diphtheria: changing patterns in the developing world and the industrialized world, Eur. J. Epidemiol. 11 (1995) 107–117.

[36] N.B. Mathur, P. Narang, B.D. Bhatia, Neonatal diphtheria, Indian J. Pediatr. 21 (1984) 174.

[37] Centers for Disease Control and Prevention, Toxigenic *Corynebacterium diphtheriae*—Northern Plains Indian Community, August-October 1996, MMWR Morb. Mortal. Wkly. Rep. 46 (1997) 506.

[38] K.M. Bisgard, et al., Virtual elimination of respiratory diphtheria in the United States (abstract no. G12), American Society for Microbiology, Washington, DC, 1995. p 160.

[38a] Centers for Disease Control and Prevention, Notifiable diseases and mortality tables, MMWR 59 (2010) 462–475.

[39] Centers for Disease Control and Prevention, Diphtheria acquired by US citizens in the Russian Federation and Ukraine—1994, MMWR Morb. Mortal. Wkly. Rep. 44 (1995) 237.

[40] A. Golaz, et al., Epidemic diphtheria in the newly independent states of the former Soviet Union: implications for diphtheria control in the United States, J. Infect. Dis. 18 (Suppl 1) (2000) S237.

[41] S. Durbaca, Antitetanus and antidiphtheria immunity in newborns, Rom. Arch. Microbiol. Immunol. 58 (1999) 267.

[42] B. Vahlquist, The transfer of antibodies from mother to offspring, Adv. Pediatr. 10 (1958) 305.

[43] K. Crossley, et al., Tetanus and diphtheria immunity in urban Minnesota adults, JAMA 242 (1979) 2298.

[44] B.A. Koblin, T.R. Townsend, Immunity to diphtheria and tetanus in inner-city women of child-bearing age, Am. J. Public. Health. 79 (1989) 1297.

[45] P.A. Maple, et al., Diphtheria immunity in UK blood donors, Lancet 345 (1995) 963.

[46] A. Galazka, The changing epidemiology of diphtheria in the vaccine era, J. Infect. Dis. 181 (Suppl 1) (2000) S2.

[47] M. Barr, A.T. Glenny, K.J. Randall, Concentration of diphtheria antitoxin in cord blood and rate of loss in babies, Lancet 2 (1949) 324.

[48] P. Cohen, S.J. Scadron, The effects of active immunization of the mother upon the offspring, J. Pediatr. 29 (1946) 609.

[49] K.M. Farizo, et al., Fatal respiratory disease due to *Corynebacterium diphtheriae*: case report and review of guidelines for management, investigation, and control, Clin. Infect. Dis. 16 (1993) 59.

[50] Centers for Disease Control and Prevention. Availability of diphtheria antitoxin through an investigational new drug protocol, MMWR Morb. Mortal. Wkly. Rep. 46 (1997) 380.

[51] Centers for Disease Control and Prevention. Pertussis vaccination: use of acellular pertussis vaccines among infants and young children—recommendations of the Advisory Committee on Immunization Practices (ACIP), MMWR Morb. Mortal. Wkly. Rep. 46 (RR-7) (1997) 2.

[52] Centers for Disease Control and Prevention. Pertussis—United States, January 1992–June 1995, MMWR Morb. Mortal. Wkly. Rep. 44 (1995) 525.

[53] Centers for Disease Control and Prevention. Pertussis—United States, 1997-2000, MMWR Morb. Mortal. Wkly. Rep. 51 (2002) 73.

[54] C.R. Vitek, et al., Increase in deaths from pertussis among young infants in the United States in the 1990s, Pediatr. Infect. Dis. J. 22 (2003) 628.

[55] Centers for Disease Control and Prevention. Pertussis deaths—United States, 2000, MMWR Morb. Mortal. Wkly. Rep. 51 (2002) 616.

[56] M.M. Cortese, et al., Pertussis hospitalizations among infants in the United States, 1993 to 2004, Pediatrics 121 (2008) 484–492.

[57] R.W. Sutter, S.L. Cochi, Pertussis hospitalizations and mortality in the United States, JAMA 267 (1992) 386.

[58] J.D. Nelson, The changing epidemiology of pertussis in young infants, Am. J. Dis. Child. 132 (1978) 371.

[59] C.C. Linnemann Jr., et al., Use of pertussis vaccine in an epidemic involving hospital staff, Lancet 2 (1975) 540.

[60] Centers for Disease Control and Prevention. Hospital-acquired pertussis among newborns—Texas, 2004, MMWR Morb. Mortal. Wkly. Rep. 57 (2008) 600–603.

[61] Centers for Disease Control and Prevention. Resurgence of pertussis—United States, 1993, MMWR Morb. Mortal. Wkly. Rep. 42 (1993) 952.

[62] H.S. Izurieta, et al., Risk factors for pertussis in young infants during an outbreak in Chicago in 1993, Clin. Infect. Dis. 22 (1996) 503.

[63] D.L. Langkamp, J.P. Davis, Increased risk of reported pertussis and hospitalization associated with pertussis in low birth weight children, J. Pediatr. 128 (1996) 654.

[64] L.K. Mikelova, et al., Predictors of death in infants hospitalized with pertussis: a case-control study of 16 pertussis deaths in Canada, J. Pediatr. 143 (2003) 576.

[65] C.D. Paddock, et al., Pathology and pathogenesis of fatal *Bordetella pertussis* infection in infants, Clin. Infect. Dis. 47 (2008) 328–338.

[66] P. Cohen, S.J. Scadron, The placental transmission of protective antibodies against whooping cough by inoculation of the pregnant mother, JAMA 121 (1943) 656.

[67] J.L. Deen, et al., Household contact study of *Bordetella pertussis* infections, Clin. Infect. Dis. 21 (1995) 1211–1219.

[68] J.E. Hoppe, Neonatal pertussis, Pediatr. Infect. Dis. J. 19 (2000) 244.

[68a] K.D. Forsyth, M. Campins-Marti, J. Caro, et al., New pertussis vaccination strategies beyond infancy: recommendations by the Global Pertussis Initiative, Clin. Infect. Dis. J. 39 (2004) 1802–1809.

[69] E.A. Cockayne, Whooping-cough in the first days of life, Br. J. Child. Dis. 10 (1913) 534.

[70] J. Phillips, Whooping-cough contracted at the time of birth, with report of two cases, Am. J. Med. Sci. 161 (1921) 163.

[71] V.N. Gan, T.V. Murphy, Pertussis in hospitalized children, Am. J. Dis. Child. 144 (1990) 1130.

[72] M.A. Lovell, A.M. Miller, O. Hendley, Pathologic case of the month: pertussis pneumonia, Arch. Pediatr. Adolesc. Med. 152 (1998) 925.

[73] I.D.A. Johnston, D.P. Strachan, H.R. Anderson, Effect of pneumonia and whooping cough in childhood on adult lung function, N. Engl. J. Med. 338 (1998) 581.

[74] R. Berner, et al., Hemolytic uremic syndrome due to an altered factor H triggered by neonatal pertussis, Pediatr. Nephrol. 17 (2002) 190.

[75] K. Edelman, et al., Detection of *Bordetella pertussis* by polymerase chain reaction and culture in the nasopharynx of erythromycin-treated infants with pertussis, Pediatr. Infect. Dis. J. 15 (1996) 54.

[76] D.M. Dragsted, et al., Comparison of culture and PCR for detection of *Bordetella pertussis* and *Bordetella parapertussis* under routine laboratory conditions, J. Med. Microbiol. 53 (2004) 749–754.

[77] Pertussis, L.K. Pickering (Ed.), Red Book: Report of the Committee on Infectious Diseases, American Academy of Pediatrics, Elk Grove Village, IL, 2009, pp. 504–519.

[78] M.E. Pichichero, W.J. Hoeger, J.R. Casey, Azithromycin for the treatment of pertussis, Pediatr. Infect. Dis. J. 22 (2003) 847–849.

[79] Centers for Disease Control and Prevention. Erythromycin-resistant *Bordetella pertussis*—Yuma County, Arizona, May-October 1994, MMWR Morb. Mortal. Wkly. Rep. 43 (1994) 807.

[80] M. Granstrom, et al., Specific immunoglobulin for treatment of whooping cough, Lancet 33 (1991) 1230.

[81] A.P. Winrow, Inhaled steroids in the treatment of pertussis, Pediatr. Infect. Dis. J. 14 (1995) 922.

[82] G. Granstrom, et al., Use of erythromycin to prevent pertussis in newborns of mothers with pertussis, J. Infect. Dis. 155 (1987) 1210.

[83] M.A. Sprauer, et al., Prevention of secondary transmission of pertussis in households with early use of erythromycin, Am. J. Dis. Child. 146 (1992) 177.

[84] D.S. Friedman, et al., Surveillance for transmission and antibiotic adverse events among neonates and adults exposed to a healthcare worker with pertussis, Infect. Control. Hosp. Epidemiol. 25 (2004) 967–973.

[85] J. Hoey, Hypertrophic pyloric stenosis caused by erythromycin, Can. Med. Assoc. J. 162 (2000) 1198.

[86] Centers for Disease Control and Prevention. Hypertrophic pyloric stenosis in infants following pertussis prophylaxis with erythromycin—Knoxville, Tennessee, 1999, MMWR Morb. Mortal. Wkly. Rep. 48 (1999) 1117.

[87] B.E. Mahon, M.B. Rosenman, M.B. Kleiman, Maternal and infant use of erythromycin and other macrolide antibiotics as risk factors for infantile hypertrophic pyloric stenosis, J. Pediatr. 139 (2001) 380.

[88] Centers for Disease Control and Prevention. Prevention of pertussis, tetanus, and diphtheria among pregnant and post-partum women and their infants, MMWR Morb. Mortal. Wkly. Rep. 57 (2008) 1–47.

[89] Centers for Disease Control and Prevention. Prevention of tetanus, diphtheria and pertussis among adults: use of tetanus toxoid, reduced diphtheria toxoid, and acellular pertussis vaccine, MMWR Morb. Mortal. Wkly. Rep. 55 (2006) 1–33.

[90] D.J. deSa, Infection and amniotic aspiration of middle ear in stillbirth and neonatal deaths, Arch. Dis. Child. 48 (1973) 872.

[91] R.W. Keith, Middle ear function in neonates, Arch. Otolaryngol. 101 (1975) 376.

[92] D.G. Roberts, et al., Resolution of middle ear effusion in newborns, Arch. Pediatr. Adolesc. Med. 149 (1995) 873.

[93] M.S. McLellan, Otitis media in premature infants: a histopathologic study, J. Pediatr. 61 (1962) 53.

[94] W.W. Johnson, A survey of middle ears: 101 autopsies of infants, Ann. Otol. Rhinol. Laryngol. 70 (1961) 377.

[95] D.J. deSa, Mucosal metaplasia and chronic inflammation in the middle ear of infants receiving intensive care in the neonatal period, Arch. Dis. Child. 158 (1983) 24.

[96] C.D. Bluestone, Pathogenesis of otitis media: role of eustachian tube, Pediatr. Infect. Dis. J. 15 (1996) 281–291.

[97] T.J. Balkany, et al., Middle ear effusions in neonates, Laryngoscope 88 (1978) 398–405.

[98] J. Piza, et al., Meconium contamination of the neonatal middle ear, J. Pediatr. 115 (1989) 910.

[99] M. Persico, G.A. Barker, D.P. Mitchell, Purulent otitis media—a "silent" source of sepsis in the pediatric intensive care unit, Otolaryngol. Head Neck Surg. 93 (1985) 330.

[100] S.A. Berman, T.J. Balkany, M.A. Simmons, Otitis media in neonatal intensive care unit, Pediatrics 62 (1978) 198.

[101] D.R. Nunn, et al., The effect of very early cleft palate closure on the need for ventilation tubes in the first three years of life, Laryngoscope 105 (1995) 905.

[102] O. Schaefer, Otitis media and bottle feeding: an epidemiological study of infant feeding habits and incidence of recurrent and chronic middle ear disease in Canadian Eskimos, Can. J. Public. Health 62 (1971) 478.

[103] R.K. Chandra, Prospective studies of the effect of breast feeding on incidence of infection and allergy, Acta Paediatr. Scand. 68 (1979) 691.

[104] J. Pukander, Acute otitis media among rural children in Finland, Int. J. Pediatr. Otorhinolaryngol. 4 (1982) 325.

[105] U.M. Saarinen, Prolonged breast feeding as prophylaxis for recurrent otitis media, Acta Paediatr. Scand. 71 (1982) 567.

[106] K.G. Dewey, J. Heinig, L.A. Nommsen-Rivers, Differences in morbidity between breast-fed and formula-fed infants, J. Pediatr. 126 (1995) 696.

[107] A.S. Cunningham, Morbidity in breast fed and artificially fed infants, J. Pediatr. 90 (1977) 726.

[108] D.W. Teele, et al., Epidemiology of otitis media during the first seven years of life in children in Greater Boston: a prospective cohort study, J. Infect. Dis. 160 (1989) 83.

[109] R.B. Duncan, Positional otitis media, Arch. Otolaryngol. 72 (1960) 454.

[110] W.G. Beauregard, Positional otitis media, J. Pediatr. 79 (1971) 294.

[111] J.L. Paradise, B.A. Elster, Breast milk protects against otitis media with effusion, Pediatr. Res. 18 (1984) 283a.

[112] B. Andersson, et al., Inhibition of attachment of *Streptococcus pneumoniae* and *Haemophilus influenzae* by human milk and receptor oligosaccharides, J. Infect. Dis. 153 (1986) 232.

[113] J.C. Salazar, et al., Low cord blood pneumococcal immunoglobulin G (IgG antibodies predict early onset acute otitis media in infancy), Am. J. Epidemiol. 145 (1997) 1048.

[114] E.T. Becken, et al., Low cord blood pneumococcal antibody concentrations predict more episodes of otitis media, Arch. Otolaryngol. Head. Neck. Surg. 127 (2001) 517.

[115] N.J. Lockhart, et al., Low cord blood type 14 pneumococcal IgG1 but not IgG2 antibody predicts early infant otitis media, J. Infect. Dis. 181 (2000) 1979.

[116] D.M. Hajek, M. Quartey, G.S. Giebink, Maternal pneumococcal conjugate immunization protects infant chinchillas in the pneumococcal otitis media model, Acta Otolaryngol. 122 (2002) 262.

[117] N.S. Shahid, et al., Serum, breast milk, and infant antibody after maternal immunization with pneumococcal vaccine, Lancet 346 (1995) 1252.

[118] T.J.D. O'Dempsey, et al., Immunization with a pneumococcal capsular polysaccharide vaccine during pregnancy, Vaccine 14 (1996) 963.

[119] F.M. Munoz, et al., Maternal immunization with pneumococcal polysaccharide vaccine in the third trimester of gestation, Vaccine 20 (2001) 826.

[120] B.P. Quimbao, et al., Immunogenicity and reactogenicity of 23-valent pneumococcal polysaccharide vaccine among pregnant Filipino women and placental transfer of antibodies, Vaccine 25 (2007) 4470–4477.

[121] H. Faden, et al., Relationship between nasopharyngeal colonization and the development of otitis media in children, J. Infect. Dis. 175 (1997) 1440.

[122] I.A.V. Rosen, et al., Antibodies to pneumococcal polysaccharides in human milk: lack of relationship to colonization and acute otitis media, Pediatr. Infect. Dis. J. 15 (1996) 498.

[123] W.S. Warren, S.J.E. Stool, Otitis media in low-birth-weight infants, J. Pediatr. 79 (1971) 740.

[124] B.F. Jaffe, F. Hurtado, E. Hurtado, Tympanic membrane mobility in the newborn (with seven months' followup), Laryngoscope 80 (1970) 36.

[125] V.M. Howie, J.H. Ploussard, J. Sloyer, The "otitis-prone" condition, Am. J. Dis. Child. 129 (1975) 676.

[126] J.L. Ey, et al., Passive smoke exposure and otitis media in the first year of life, Pediatrics 95 (1995) 670.

[127] M.R. Stahlberg, O. Ruuskanen, E. Virolainen, Risk factors for recurrent otitis media, Pediatr. Infect. Dis. J. 5 (1986) 30.

[128] R.D. Bland, Otitis media in the first six weeks of life: diagnosis, bacteriology and management, Pediatrics 49 (1972) 187.

[129] T.R. Tetzlaff, C. Ashworth, J.D. Nelson, Otitis media in children less than 12 weeks of age, Pediatrics 59 (1977) 827.

[130] M.S. McLellan, et al., Otitis media in the newborn: relationship to duration of rupture of amniotic membrane, Arch. Otolaryngol. 85 (1967) 380.

[131] J.L. Paradise, C.D. Bluestone, Early treatment of universal otitis media of infants with cleft palate, Pediatrics 53 (1974) 48.

[132] K.A. Daly, et al., Epidemiology of otitis media onset by six months of age, Pediatrics 103 (1999) 1158.

[133] P.A. Shurin, et al., Bacterial etiology of otitis media during the first six weeks of life, J. Pediatr. 92 (1978) 893.

[134] C.A. Nozicka, et al., Otitis media in infants aged 0-8 weeks: frequency of associated serious bacterial disease, Pediatr. Emerg. Care. 15 (1999) 252.

[135] P.H. Karma, et al., Middle ear fluid bacteriology of acute otitis media in neonates and very young infants, Int. J. Pediatr. Otorhinolaryngol. 14 (1987) 141.

[136] D. Turner, et al., Acute otitis media in infants younger than two months of age: microbiology, clinical presentation and therapeutic approach, Pediatr. Infect. Dis. J. 21 (2002) 669.

[137] P.C. Ng, et al., Isolated congenital tuberculosis otitis in a pre-term infant, Acta. Paediatr. 84 (1995) 955.

[138] N. Senbil, et al., Congenital tuberculosis of the ear and parotid gland, Pediatr. Infect. Dis. J. 16 (1997) 1090.

[139] P.C. Parker, R.G. Boles, Pseudomonas otitis media and bacteremia following a water birth, Pediatrics 99 (1997) 653.

[140] M.E. Decherd, et al., *Bordetella pertussis* causing otitis media: a case report, Laryngoscope 113 (2003) 226.

[141] R.D. Eavey, et al., How to examine the ear of the neonate, Clin. Pediatr. 15 (1976) 338.

[142] R.M. Cavanaugh, Pneumatic otoscopy in healthy full-term infants, Pediatrics 79 (1987) 520.

[143] G. Pestalozza, G. Cusmano, Evaluation of tympanometry in diagnosis and treatment of otitis media of the newborn and of the infant, Int. J. Pediatr. Otorhinolaryngol. 2 (1980) 73.

[144] E.D. Barnett, et al., Comparison of spectral gradient acoustic reflectometry and other diagnostic techniques for detection of middle ear effusion in children with middle ear disease, Pediatr. Infect. Dis. J. 17 (1998) 556.

[145] S.F. Dowell, et al., Acute otitis media: management and surveillance in an era of pneumococcal resistance—a report from the Drug-Resistant *Streptococcus pneumoniae* Therapeutic Working Group, Pediatr. Infect. Dis. J. 18 (1999) 1.

[146] B.T. Lee, et al., Neonatal meningitis and mastoiditis caused by *Haemophilus influenzae*, JAMA 235 (1976) 407.

[147] K. Meyer, N. Girgis, V. McGravey, Adenovirus associated with congenital pleural effusion, J. Pediatr. 107 (1985) 433.

[148] O. Reman, et al., Neonatal respiratory distress due to mumps, Arch. Dis. Child. 61 (1986) 80.

[148a] R.M. Srinivasjois, R. Kohan, A.D. Keil, N.M. Smith, Congenital *Mycoplasma pneumoniae* pneumonia in a neonate, Pedi. Infect. Dis. J. 27 (2008) 474–475.

[149] M.T. Boyd, S.W. Jordan, L.E. Davis, Fatal pneumonitis from congenital echovirus type 6 infection, Pediatr. Infect. Dis. J. 6 (1987) 1138.

[150] L.C. McLaren, et al., Isolation of *Trichomonas vaginalis* from the respiratory tract of infants with respiratory disease, Pediatrics 71 (1983) 888.

[151] I. Hiemstra, F. Van Bel, H.M. Berger, Can *Trichomonas vaginalis* cause pneumonia in newborn babies? BMJ 289 (1984) 355.

[151a] Y. Shachor-Meyouhas, I. Kassis, E. Bamberger, et al., Fatal hospital-acquired *Legionella pneumonia* in a neonate, Pedi. Infect. Dis. J. 29 (2010) 280–284.

[152] R.W. Hostoffer, et al., *Pneumocystis carinii* pneumonia in a term newborn infant with a transiently depressed T lymphocyte count, primarily of cells carrying the CD4 antigen, J. Pediatr. 122 (1993) 792.

[153] Centers for Disease Control and Prevention. Acute respiratory disease associated with adenovirus serotype 14—four states, 2006-2007, MMWR Morb. Mortal. Wkly. Rep. 56 (2007) 1181–1184.

[154] E.K. Ahvenainen, On congenital pneumonia, Acta Paediatr. 40 (1951) 1.

[155] G.S. Anderson, et al., Congenital bacterial pneumonia, Lancet 2 (1962) 585.

[156] R. Barter, The histopathology of congenital pneumonia: a clinical and experimental study, J. Pathol. Bacteriol. 66 (1953) 407.

[157] P.A. Davies, W. Aherne, Congenital pneumonia, Arch. Dis. Child. 37 (1962) 598.

[158] F.A. Langley, J.A. McCredie Smith, Perinatal pneumonia: a retrospective study, J. Obstet. Gynaecol. Br. Commonw. 66 (1959) 12.

[159] D.W. Penner, A.C. McInnis, Intrauterine and neonatal pneumonia, Am. J. Obstet. Gynecol. 69 (1955) 147.

[160] E. Alenghat, J.R. Esterly, Alveolar macrophages in perinatal infants, Pediatrics 74 (1984) 221.

[161] A.J. Schaffer, The pathogenesis of intrauterine pneumonia, I: a critical review of the evidence concerning intrauterine respiratory-like movements, Pediatrics 17 (1956) 747.

[162] R.L. Naeye, W.S. Dellinger, W.A. Blanc, Fetal and maternal features of antenatal bacterial infection, J. Pediatr. 79 (1971) 733.

[163] R.L. Naeye, et al., Amniotic fluid infections in an African city, J. Pediatr. 90 (1977) 965.

[164] R.L. Naeye, E.C. Peters, Amniotic fluid infections with intact membranes leading to perinatal death: a prospective study, Pediatrics 61 (1978) 171.

[165] R.A. Barter, J.A. Hudson, Bacteriological findings in perinatal pneumonia, Pathology 6 (1974) 223.

[166] R.A. Barter, Congenital pneumonia, Lancet 1 (1962) 165.

[167] J. Bernstein, J. Wang, The pathology of neonatal pneumonia, Am. J. Dis. Child. 101 (1961) 350.

[168] M. Finland, Fetal and perinatal pneumonia, in: D. Charles, M. Finland (Eds.), Obstetric and Perinatal Infections, Lea & Febiger, Philadelphia, 1973, p. 122.

[169] P.A. Davies, Pathogen or commensal? Arch. Dis. Child. 55 (1980) 169.

[170] E.K. Ahvenainen, Neonatal pneumonia, I: incidence of pneumonia during first month of life, Ann. Med. Intern. Fenn. 42 (Suppl 17) (1953) 1.

[171] M.M. Thaler, *Klebsiella-Aerobacter* pneumonia in infants: a review of the literature and report of a case, Pediatrics 30 (1962) 206.

[172] A. Papageovgiou, et al., *Klebsiella* pneumonia with pneumatocele formation in a newborn infant, Can. Med. Assoc. J. 109 (1973) 1217.

[173] J.P. Kunh, S.B. Lee, Pneumatoceles associated with *Escherichia coli* pneumonias in the newborn, Pediatrics 51 (1973) 1008.

[174] H. Jeffery, et al., Early neonatal bacteraemia: comparison of group B streptococcal, other gram-positive and gram-negative infections, Arch. Dis. Child. 52 (1977) 683.

[175] J. Rojas, T.H. Flanigan, Postintubation tracheitis in the newborn, Pediatr. Infect. Dis. J. 5 (1986) 714.

[176] Y. Jialin, et al., Electron microscopic analysis of bacterial biofilm on tracheal tubes removed from intubated neonates and the relationship between bacterial biofilm and lower respiratory infections, Pediatrics 121 (2008) S121–S122.

[177] M.H. Kollef, The prevention of ventilator-associated pneumonia, N. Engl. J. Med. 340 (1999) 627.

[178] L. Barton, J.E. Hodgman, Z. Pavlova, Causes of death in the extremely low birth weight infant, Pediatrics 103 (1999) 446.

[179] P.A. Davies, Pneumonia in the fetus and newborn, Pediatr. Digest. (1996) 93.

[180] A.F. Barson, A postmortem study of infection in the newborn from 1976 to 1988, in: J. de Louvois, D. Harvey (Eds.), Infection in the Newborn, John Wiley, New York, 1990, p. 13.

[181] D.W. Wells, G.T. Keeney, Group F Streptococcus associated with intrauterine pneumonia. Letter to the editor, Pediatrics 66 (1980) 820.

[182] J.A. Hoffman, et al., *Streptococcus pneumoniae* infections in the neonate, Pediatrics 112 (2003) 1095–2000.

[183] P.G. Rhodes, et al., Pneumococcal septicemia and meningitis in the neonate, J. Pediatr. 86 (1975) 593–595.

[184] R.R. Moriartey, N.N. Finer, Pneumococcal sepsis and pneumonia in the neonate, Am. J. Dis. Child. 133 (1979) 601.

[185] J.C. Naylor, K.R. Wagner, Neonatal sepsis due to *Streptococcus pneumoniae*, Can. Med. Assoc. J. 133 (1985) 1019.

[186] A.M. Collier, J.D. Connor, W.L. Nyhan, Systemic infection with *Haemophilus influenzae* in very young infants, J. Pediatr. 70 (1967) 539.

[187] A. Ohlsson, T. Bailey, Neonatal pneumonia caused by *Branhamella catarrhalis*, Scand. J. Infect. Dis. 17 (1985) 225.

[188] S. Andersson, U. Larinkari, T. Vartia, Fatal congenital pneumonia caused by cat-derived *Pasteurella multocida*, Pediatr. Infect. Dis. J. 13 (1994) 74.

[189] J.L. Rowen, Lopez SM. *Morganella morganii* early onset sepsis, Pediatr. Infect. Dis. J. 17 (1998) 1176.

[189a] L. Franzin, C. Scolfaro, D. Cabodi, M. Valera, P.A. Tovo, *Legionella pneumophila* pneumonia in a newborn after water birth: a new mode of transmission, Clin. Infect. Dis. 33 (2001) e103–e104.

[190] I. Brook, Microbiology of empyema in children and adolescents, Pediatrics 85 (1990) 722.

[191] J.D. Siegel, G.H. McCracken, Neonatal lung abscess, Am. J. Dis. Child. 133 (1979) 947.

[192] T. Mayer, et al., Computed tomographic findings of neonatal lung abscess, Am. J. Dis. Child. 139 (1982) 39.

[193] R.F. Famiglietti, et al., Cavitary legionellosis in two immunocompetent infants, Pediatrics 99 (1997) 899.

[194] S.C. Adler, M.J. Chusid, *Citrobacter koseri* pneumonia and meningitis in an infant, J. Infect. 45 (2002) 65.

[195] R.E. Holmberg, et al., Nosocomial *Legionella* pneumonia in the neonate, Pediatrics 92 (1993) 450.

[196] R. Shamir, et al., *Citrobacter diversus* lung abscess in a preterm infant, Pediatr. Infect. Dis. J. 9 (1990) 221.

[197] G.P. Vevon, et al., *Bacillus cereus* pneumonia in premature neonates: a report of two cases, Pediatr. Infect. Dis. J. 12 (1993) 251.

[198] R. Gupta, M.M. Faridi, P. Gupta, Neonatal empyema thoracis, Indian J. Pediatr. 63 (1996) 704.

[199] E.A. Khan, et al., *Serratia marcescens* pneumonia, empyema and pneumatocele in a preterm neonate, Pediatr. Infect. Dis. J. 16 (1997) 1003.

[200] J. Thaarup, S. Ellermann-Eriksen, J. Sternholm, Neonatal pleural empyema with group A Streptococcus, Acta Paediatr. 86 (1997) 769.

[201] K.A. Nathavitharana, M. Watkinson, Neonatal pleural empyema caused by group A Streptococcus, Pediatr. Infect. Dis. J. 13 (1994) 671.

[202] E.J.N. Briggs, G. Hogg, Pneumonia found at autopsy in infants weighing less than 750 grams, Can. Med. Assoc. J. 85 (1961) 6.

[203] E.J.N. Briggs, G. Hogg, Perinatal pulmonary pathology, Pediatrics 22 (1958) 41.

[204] F.J. Browne, Pneumonia neonatorum, BMJ 1 (1922) 469.

[205] T. Fujikura, L.A. Froehlich, Intrauterine pneumonia in relation to birth weight and race, Am. J. Obstet. Gynecol. 97 (1967) 81.

[206] A. Sinha, D. Yokoe, R. Platt, Epidemiology of neonatal infections: experience during and after hospitalization, Pediatr. Infect. Dis. J. 22 (2003) 244.

[207] A.T. Bang, et al., Pneumonia in neonates. Can it be managed in the community? Arch. Dis. Child. 68 (1993) 550.

[208] K. Kishore, et al., Early onset neonatal sepsis—vertical transmission from maternal genital tract, Indian Pediatr. J. 24 (1987) 45.

[209] S. Sazawal, R.E. Black, Effect of pneumonia case management on mortality in neonates, infants, and preschool children: a meta-analysis of community-based trials, Lancet Infect. Dis. 3 (2003) 547.

[210] S. Singhi, P.D. Singhi, Clinical signs in neonatal pneumonia, Lancet 336 (1990) 1072.

[211] World Health Organization. Acute Respiratory Infections in Children: Case Management in Small Hospitals in Developing Countries, World Health Organization, Geneva, 1990.

[212] S. Petersen, K. Astvad, Pleural empyema in a newborn infant, Acta Paediatr. Scand. 65 (1976) 527.

[213] E.E. Gustavson, *Escherichia coli* empyema in the newborn, Am. J. Dis. Child. 140 (1986) 408.

[214] N.B. Mathur, K. Garg, S. Kumar, Respiratory distress in neonates with special reference to pneumonia, Indian Pediatr. 39 (2002) 529–537.

[215] R.C. Ablow, et al., The radiographic features of early onset group B streptococcal neonatal sepsis, Radiology 124 (1977) 771.

[216] D.B. Thomas, J.C. Anderson, Antenatal detection of fetal pleural effusion and neonatal management, Med. J. Aust. 2 (1979) 435.

[217] R.W. Steele, M.P. Thomas, J.K. Kolls, Current management of community-acquired pneumonia in children: an algorithmic guideline recommendation, Infect. Med. (1999) 46.

[218] J.O. Klein, Diagnostic lung puncture in the pneumonias of infants and children, Pediatrics 44 (1969) 486.

[219] D.W. Teele, et al., Bacteremia in febrile children under 2 years of age: results of cultures of blood of 600 consecutive febrile children seen in a "walk-in" clinic, J. Pediatr. 87 (1975) 227.

[220] M.P. Sherman, et al., Tracheal aspiration and its clinical correlates in the diagnosis of congenital pneumonia, Pediatrics 65 (1980) 258.

[221] P.J. Thureen, et al., Failure of tracheal aspirate cultures to define the cause of respiratory deteriorations in neonates, Pediatr. Infect. Dis. J. 12 (1993) 560.

[222] Y.L. Lau, E. Hey, Sensitivity and specificity of daily tracheal aspirate cultures in predicting organisms causing bacteremia in ventilated neonates, Pediatr. Infect. Dis. J. 10 (1991) 290.

[223] L.L. Fan, L.M. Sparks, J.P. Dulinski, Applications of an ultrathin flexible bronchoscope for neonatal and pediatric airway problems, Chest 89 (1986) 673.

[224] H.E. Alexander, et al., Validity of etiology diagnosis of pneumonia in children by rapid typing from nasopharyngeal mucus, J. Pediatr. 18 (1941) 31.

[225] J.G.M. Bollowa, Primary pneumonias of infants and children, Public. Health. Rep. 51 (1903) 1076.

[226] M.H.W. Cheu, et al., Open lung biopsy in the critically ill newborn, Pediatrics 86 (1990) 561.

[227] A. Greenough, Gains and losses from dexamethasone for neonatal chronic lung disease, Lancet 352 (1998) 835.

[228] T.F. Yeh, et al., Outcomes at school age after postnatal dexamethasone therapy for lung disease of prematurity, N. Engl. J. Med. 350 (2004) 1304–1313.

[229] P. Lister, et al., Inhaled steroids for neonatal chronic lung disease, Cochrane Database Syst. Rev. 4 (2004).

[230] W. Aherne, P.A. Davies, Congenital pneumonia, Lancet 1 (1962) 234.

[231] A.S.Y. Tam, C.Y. Yeung, Gastric aspirate findings in neonatal pneumonia, Arch. Dis. Child. 47 (1972) 735.

[232] V.R.G. Pole, T.A. McAllister, Gastric aspirate analysis in the newborn, Acta. Paediatr. Scand. 64 (1975) 109.

[233] A. Whitelaw, A. Evans, B. Corrin, Immotile cilia syndrome: a new cause of neonatal respiratory distress, Arch. Dis. Child. 56 (1981) 432.

[234] J. Ramet, et al., Neonatal diagnosis of the immotile cilia syndrome, Chest 89 (1986) 138.

[235] Ciliary dyskinesia and ultrastructural abnormalities in respiratory disease, Annotation. Lancet 1 (1988) 1370.

[236] G.P. Giacoia, E. Neter, P. Ogra, Respiratory infections in infants on mechanical ventilation: the immune response as a diagnostic aid, J. Pediatr. 98 (1981) 691.

[237] M.I. Marks, B. Law, Respiratory infections vs. colonization, J. Pediatr. 100 (1982) 508.

[238] L.E. Nigrovic, et al., Cerebrospinal latex agglutination fails to contribute to the microbiologic diagnosis of pre-treated children with meningitis, Pediatr. Infect. Dis. J. 23 (2004) 786–788.

[239] Lung function in children after neonatal meconium aspiration, Annotation. Lancet 2 (1988) 317.

[240] R.M. Smith, G.W. Brumley, M.W. Stannard, Neonatal pneumonia associated with medium-chain triglyceride feeding supplement, J. Pediatr. 92 (1978) 801.

[241] O. Hjalmarson, Epidemiology of classification of acute, neonatal respiratory disorders: a prospective study, Acta Paediatr. Scand. 70 (1981) 773.

[242] N.A. Mounla, Neonatal respiratory disorders, Acta Paediatr. Scand. 76 (1987) 159.

[243] M.E. Avery, B.D. Fletcher, R.E. Williams, The Lung and Its Disorders in the Newborn Infant, WB Saunders, Philadelphia, 1981.

[244] N.R. Butler, E.D. Alberman, Clinicopathological associations of hyaline membranes, intraventricular haemorrhage, massive pulmonary haemorrhage and pulmonary infection, in: British Perinatal Mortality Survey, Second Report: Perinatal Problems, E & S Livingstone, Edinburgh, 1969, p. 184.

[245] G.A. Foote, J.H. Stewart, The coexistence of pneumonia and the idiopathic respiratory distress syndrome in neonates, Br. J. Radiol. 46 (1973) 504.

[246] R.C. Ablow, et al., A comparison of early-onset group B streptococcal infection and the respiratory distress syndrome of the newborn, N. Engl. J. Med. 294 (1976) 65.

[247] J.A. Menke, G.P. Giacoia, H. Jockin, Group B beta hemolytic streptococcal sepsis and the idiopathic respiratory distress syndrome: a comparison, J. Pediatr. 94 (1979) 467.

[248] J.D. Lloyd-Still, K.T. Khaw, H. Schwachman, Severe respiratory disease in infants with cystic fibrosis, Pediatrics 53 (1974) 678.

[249] J.G. Delville, S. Adler, P.H. Azimi, et al., Linezolid versus vancomycin in the treatment of known or suspected resistant gram-positive infections in neonates, Pediatr. Infect. Dis. J. 22 (2003) S158.

[250] E.K. Ahvenainen, A study of causes of neonatal deaths, J. Pediatr. 55 (1959) 691.

[251] G.T. Osborn, Discussion on neonatal deaths, Proc. R. Soc. Med. 51 (1958) 840.

[252] N.R. Butler, D.G. Bonham, Perinatal Mortality, E & S Livingstone, London, 1963.

[253] A. Apisarnthanarak, et al., Ventilator-associated pneumonia in extremely preterm neonates in a neonatal intensive care unit: characteristics, risk factors, and outcomes, Pediatrics 12 (2003) 1283.

[254] L. Pacifico, et al., *Ureaplasma urealyticum* and pulmonary outcome in a neonatal intensive care population, Pediatr. Infect. Dis. J. 16 (1997) 579.

[255] D.M. Brasfield, et al., Infant pneumonitis associated with cytomegalovirus, *Chlamydia*, *Pneumocystis* and *Ureaplasma*: follow-up, Pediatrics 79 (1987) 76.

BACTERIAL INFECTIONS OF THE BONES AND JOINTS

Gary D. Overturf

CHAPTER OUTLINE

Osteomyelitis   296
   Microbiology   297
   Pathogenesis   298
   Clinical Manifestations   300
   Prognosis   301

Diagnosis   302
Differential Diagnosis   304
Therapy   304
Primary Septic Arthritis   305
Osteomyelitis of the Maxilla   306

OSTEOMYELITIS

Osteomyelitis occurring in the first 2 months of life is uncommon. During the worldwide pandemic of staphylococcal disease from the early 1950s to the early 1960s, pediatric centers in Europe [1–5], Australia [6], and North America [6–11] reported the infrequent occurrence of neonatal osteomyelitis, accounting for only one or two admissions per year at each institution. With the introduction of invasive neonatal supportive care and the increased use of diagnostic and therapeutic procedures, there was concern that osteomyelitis and septic arthritis secondary to bacteremia might occur more frequently in the newborn [12]. Yet subsequent experience in Europe [13–15], Canada [16,17], and the United States [11,18,19]

(Nelson JD, personal communication, 1987) during the decade 1970-1979 indicated little or no change in the incidence of this condition. Even in intensive care nurseries, despite an increasing problem with fungal (*Candida*) osteoarthritis [20–24], the overall rate of occurrence of nosocomial bone and joint infections remained low at equal to or less than 2.6 per 1000 admissions [22,25,26]. Infections associated with invasive procedures, such as placement of intravascular catheters, may not appear or be recognized until days or weeks after the perinatal period, however [12,22]. Although the incidence has not changed, causative organisms have become increasingly resistant to antibiotics, as exemplified by the increased incidence of *Staphylococcus aureus* infections resistant to oxacillin (methicillin-resistant *S. aureus* [MRSA]).

Little has been published on the relative incidence of neonatal osteomyelitis during the 1980s and 1990s. An ongoing review of nursery infections at a Kaiser Permanente hospital in southern California revealed only 3 cases of osteomyelitis among 67,000 consecutive live births from 1963-1993, and none occurred in the final years (Miller A, personal communication, 1993). A similar survey performed at two pediatric referral centers in Texas showed no significant variation in the number of annual admissions for this condition from 1964-1986[27] (Nelson JD, personal communication, 1987). Physicians working in intensive care nurseries in Great Britain [28], France [29], Spain [30], and various parts of the United States [31] (Pomerance J [Los Angeles, CA], Bradley JS [Portland, OR], Hall RT [Kansas City, MO], Cashore WJ [Providence, RI], personal communications, 1987) have observed, on average, 1 to 3 cases of bone or joint infection per 1000 admissions, an incidence almost identical to that noted in years past [22,25,26].

In a review of more than 300 cases of neonatal osteomyelitis, male infants predominated over female infants (1.6:1). Premature infants acquire osteomyelitis with relatively greater frequency than term infants [11,13,16,32–41]. In a series of osteomyelitis, 17 of 30 proven cases were in premature infants, 4 occurred in term infants receiving intensive care, and S. aureus was responsible for 23 of the proven cases of osteomyelitis (methicillin-sensitive strains in 16 cases and MRSA in 7 cases) [42]. Escherichia coli and group B streptococci (GBS) caused three and two cases, respectively. Risk factors for osteomyelitis and septic arthritis in premature infants have been mostly iatrogenic, including use of intravenous or intra-arterial catheters, ventilatory support, and bacteremia with nosocomial pathogens.

Although osteomyelitis was rare in the past, more recent series have suggested that the frequency may be increasing in neonates. The spectrum of bacterial and fungal infections in Finland from 1985-1989 was studied in 2836 infections in children [43]. The incidence of osteomyelitis and septic arthritis in children 28 days of age or younger was 67.7 per 100,000 person-years compared with rates of 262.2 and 2013.1 per 100,000 for meningitis and bacteremia; pneumonia (80.4 per 100,000) and pyelonephritis (143.8 per 100,000) also were more frequent than bone or joint infections. Studies from other countries have also suggested an increase in osteomyelitis; among 241 bone infections in Panamanian children, 9 occurred in neonates (3 cases were due to gram-negative bacilli; 3 cases, to S. aureus; 1 case, to GBS; and 2 cases, to other organisms) [44].

MICROBIOLOGY

Because most cases of neonatal osteomyelitis arise as a consequence of bacteremia, the organisms responsible for causing osteomyelitis reflect the changing trends in the etiology of neonatal sepsis. Before 1940, hemolytic streptococci were the predominant organisms responsible for sepsis in newborns [45] and frequently caused osteomyelitis [46,47]. Streptococci were implicated in most cases of osteomyelitis in neonates and infants younger than 6 months of age [48].

After 1950, the incidence of S. aureus osteomyelitis increased. A review of reports from 1952-1972 showed

that 85% of the infections were caused by S. aureus, 6% were caused by hemolytic streptococci (no groups specified), and 2% were due to Streptococcus pneumoniae; either no organisms or miscellaneous organisms (particularly gram-negative bacilli) were isolated in 7% of the cases [2–6,11,35,38,49–56]. MRSA has infected many nurseries and has been associated with disseminated infections of neonates, including endocarditis, skin and soft tissue infections, organ abscesses, and osteomyelitis and septic arthritis. Community-acquired strains of MRSA have become increasingly more common in neonatal units; at the present time, 50% or more of infections are caused by MRSA strains acquired outside of the hospital. Osteomyelitis and septic arthritis have been observed in these outbreaks as part of a general septic dissemination of MRSA to multiple organs and multiple sites (reviewed in Chapters 10 and 14).

Recognition of group B streptococcal sepsis in the 1970s was associated with a concomitant increase in reported frequency of bone and joint infections caused by this organism [20,57]. This change in spectrum was reflected in U.S. reviews of osteomyelitis in infants hospitalized from 1965-1978 showing that GBS had become the most frequent agent [11,19,58]. This experience was not universal, however; newborn centers in Canada [16], Sweden [13], Spain [30], Switzerland [14], Nigeria [59], and sections of the United States [27] continued to find S. aureus as the predominant cause of osteomyelitis, with GBS accounting for only a few cases. Although their relative importance may vary by region or institution, these two organisms have remained the most common cause of neonatal osteomyelitis [31–33,40]. A review of cases of occult bacteremia owing to GBS identified 147 children [60]. Eleven of these children had nonmeningeal foci, including two with septic arthritis and two with osteomyelitis. More recent cases of unusual sites of group B streptococcal osteomyelitis in the iliac wing [61] and the vertebrae [62] emphasize the renewed importance and frequency of this infection.

Osteomyelitis caused by gram-negative enteric bacilli is uncommon despite the frequency of neonatal bacteremia [32,45,63,64]. In Stockholm during 1969-1979, E. coli and Klebsiella-Enterobacter were responsible for about 30% of cases of neonatal septicemia [15], but only 5% of bone infections [13]. S. aureus, although also causing about 30% of neonatal bacteremia cases, was responsible for 75% of cases of osteomyelitis. Several other surveys performed within the past 2 decades show about 10% of cases of neonatal osteomyelitis to be due to gram-negative enteric bacilli,* although rates of 19% [59] and 45% [30,39,40] have been observed. A review of the literature has revealed isolated instances of hematogenous osteomyelitis in newborns caused by E. coli,[†] Proteus species [13,19,28,53,65–69], Klebsiella pneumoniae [13,30,40,41,70–73], Enterobacter [30,66,74,75], Serratia marcescens [19,30], Pseudomonas species,[‡] and Salmonella [16,27,39,77–81].

---

*References [11,14,16,27,31,38].

[†]References [2,8,11,13,14,19,30,34,38–40,47,53,65–70].

[‡]References [19,30,35,38,40,47,76,77].

Although bacteremia from infected invasive devices are a common cause of enteric osteomyelitis, infection may occur directly by translocation from the gut or from urinary tract infection. Studies of neonatal rats have suggested that formula feeding enhances translocation of enteric organisms with subsequent infection of the bone [82], although other organs were infected as well. Although translocation of bacteria occurred in 23% of breast-fed rats, compared with 100% of formula-fed rats, positive bone cultures developed in 77% of the formula-fed rats, whereas none of the breast-fed rats had positive cultures. A single case of a 4-week-old boy with urinary tract infection with *K. pneumoniae* and vesicoureteral reflux suggests that this site also may be a source of gram-negative enteric bone and joint infections [83].

Although suppurative arthritis is the most common manifestation of gonococcal sepsis involving the skeletal system [84], osteomyelitis is associated with sepsis as well and probably represents the site of primary infection in many cases [38,85,86]. Syphilitic osteitis and osteochondritis, although frequent in former years [87], have been largely eliminated through serologic detection of disease during routine antenatal testing and institution of appropriate therapy for infected mothers. An increase in the incidence of syphilis among women of childbearing age has been reflected in a parallel increase in the frequency of neonatal syphilis and attendant problems of treponemal bone infection [88,89].

Mycoplasma and *Ureaplasma* have been reported as rare causes of osteomyelitis in infants. In one infant, bone infection caused by *Mycoplasma hominis* developed in a sternotomy wound after cardiac surgery [90]; in another infant weighing 900 g with osteomyelitis of the hip and femur, the infection was caused by *Ureaplasma urealyticum* [91]. Tuberculous osteomyelitis is extremely rare in neonates, even in the presence of disseminated congenital tuberculosis [92,93]. Among a group of infants with widespread disease acquired in the perinatal or neonatal period, the youngest with skeletal involvement was 3 months of age [86].

PATHOGENESIS

Complications of pregnancy, labor, or delivery may precede the occurrence of neonatal osteomyelitis in one half of patients.* Most bone and joint infections occur in a small or premature infant as a result of prolonged nosocomial exposures and multiple invasive procedures. Although anoxia (as from placenta previa, breech extraction, or fetal distress) or exposure to microorganisms (from premature rupture of membranes) can explain this association in some cases, the means whereby maternal or obstetric problems influence the likelihood of acquiring bone infection is generally unknown.

Microorganisms may reach the skeletal tissues of the fetus and newborn in one of four ways: (1) by direct inoculation, (2) by extension from infection in surrounding soft tissues, (3) as a consequence of maternal bacteremia with transplacental infection and fetal sepsis, and (4) by blood-borne dissemination in the course of neonatal septicemia. Although hematogenous dissemination is responsible for most cases, examples of other routes of infection have appeared occasionally in the literature. As noted previously (see "Microbiology"), other factors, such as preceding urinary tract infection or direct translocation of bacteria across the bowel wall, may explain bone or joint infection in some neonates.

Direct inoculation of bacteria resulting in osteomyelitis has followed femoral venipuncture [36,59,69,94–96], radial artery puncture [30], use of a fetal scalp monitor [14,97–100], great toe [84] or heel [14,30,31,101–105] capillary blood sampling [106], and serial lumbar punctures [107]. Infection after surgical invasion of bony structures (e.g., median sternotomy for cardiac surgery) is uncommon [108]. Nevertheless, trauma has been associated with osteomyelitis of the neonate (an association that has been noted for osteomyelitis in older children); *S. aureus* osteomyelitis has occurred in a neonate at 3 weeks of age at the site of a perinatal fracture of the clavicle [109].

Osteomyelitis caused by extension of infection from surrounding soft tissues usually is associated with organisms from an infected cephalhematoma involving the adjacent parietal bone [98,110–112]. A series of patients with *S. aureus* osteomyelitis of the skull associated with overlying scalp abscesses was reported in 1952 [113]. Predisposing factors in these patients were thought to be prolonged, excessive pressure on the fetal head when it lay against the sacral promontory or symphysis pubis, secondary ischemic necrosis, and localization of infection. Paronychia during the newborn period, although most frequently a source of sepsis and hematogenous dissemination of organisms, may extend into bony structures and cause phalangeal infection [47].

Transplacental bacterial bone infection is most characteristic of syphilis (see Chapter 16). A rare exception, published as a case report in 1933, described a premature infant who died at 19 hours of age with evidence of subacute parietal bone osteomyelitis, meningitis, and cerebritis. Rupture of the amniotic sac immediately before delivery, histopathologic evidence of the prolonged course (at least 2 weeks) of the infection, and the lack of involvement of the overlying scalp epidermis indicate that despite apparent absence of maternal illness, this infant was infected transplacentally. The authors postulated that a primary infection occurred in the parietal bone, with secondary extension to the meninges and brain. Although organisms were not isolated, gram-positive diplococci were identified in infected tissues [114].

Blood-borne dissemination of organisms, with metastatic seeding of the skeletal system through nutrient arteries, is the major cause of neonatal osteomyelitis [48,115]. Before the advent of antibiotics, the long bones reportedly became infected in 10% of infants with bacteremia [47,116]. Since that time, early recognition and effective empirical therapy for bacterial sepsis led to a marked decrease in the incidence of this complication. Candidal invasion of the bloodstream has become a more frequent cause of bone and joint infections in small infants (see Chapter 33).*

---

*References [11,13,16,19,30,38–40].

*References [20,22,23,33,117,118].

The use of intravascular catheters frequently has been associated with bacterial and fungal osteomyelitis in neonates.* Septic embolization occurs from infected catheter-tip thrombi, producing relatively high-grade bacteremias; local hypoxia from partial occlusion of vessels by the catheter may also contribute to bone infections [12,119]. The most common etiologic agent has been *S. aureus*, but other microorganisms, such as *Klebsiella* [73], *Proteus* [64], *Enterobacter* [74,75], and *Candida* [20,22,66,117], have also been implicated. Because the iliac arteries are the most likely pathway for an arterial embolus originating in an aortic catheter tip, the hips or knees or both are involved in more than three fourths of patients.† There is a very close correlation between the site of the catheter and localization of osteomyelitis in the ipsilateral leg [12]. The distribution of infection originating in umbilical vein catheters is less predictable [22,74,117,121–123]. The incidence of osteoarthritis varies greatly, ranging from 1 in 30[119] to less than 1 in 600[12] infants with umbilical artery catheters; it can be reduced significantly by proper attention to aseptic technique and careful monitoring of catheter placement combined with prompt catheter removal whenever possible [12].

The disseminating focus of a bacteremia-producing metastatic abscess in bones is often unknown. Common primary sources include omphalitis,* pustular dermatitis,† purulent rhinitis [5,55,124], paronychia,‡ and mastitis [4,49]. In a few infants, sepsis with subsequent osteomyelitis has arisen from infected circumcisions [8,36], operative sites [8,31,69], intramuscular injections [49,69], or varicella lesions [11]. Although gonococcal osteoarthritis originates most commonly from a purulent conjunctivitis, virtually any orifice may provide a portal of entry [84].

Hematogenous infection of long bones is initiated in dilated capillary loops of the metaphysis, adjacent to the cartilaginous growth plate (physis), where blood flow slows, providing pathogenic bacteria with an ideal environment to multiply, resulting in abscess formation (Fig. 8–1) [115,125,126]. When the infectious process localizes at this site, the following sequence may occur: (1) direct invasion and lysis of the cartilaginous growth plate; (2) spread from metaphyseal vessel loops into transphyseal vessels coursing through the growth plate and into epiphyseal vessels; or (3) rupture occurring laterally, through the cortex into the joint, subperiosteal space, or surrounding soft tissues [125,126]. The large vascular spaces and thin spongy structure of metaphyseal cortex in infants permit early decompression of this primary abscess into the subperiosteal space [48,56]. For this reason, the bone marrow compartment is seldom involved in neonates, and the term osteitis is probably more accurate than osteomyelitis.

After rupture into the subperiosteal space, the abscess dissects rapidly beneath loosely attached periosteum, often involving the entire length and circumference of the bone. As pressure increases from accumulating pus,

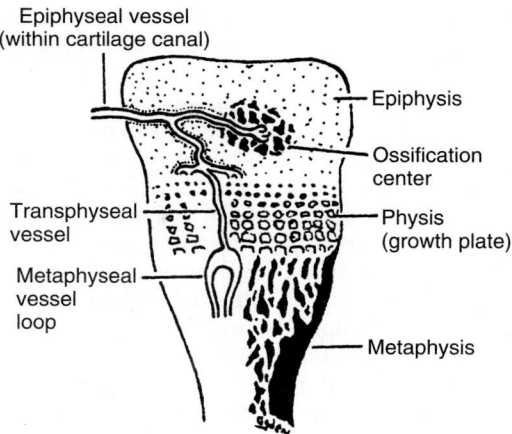

FIGURE 8–1 Schematic depiction of blood supply in the neonatal epiphysis. In children, normally there are two separate circulatory systems: (1) the metaphyseal loops, derived from the diaphyseal nutrient artery, and (2) the epiphyseal vessels, which course through the epiphyseal cartilage within structures termed cartilage canals. In the neonatal period, sinusoidal vessels, termed transphyseal vessels, connect these two systems. With ensuing skeletal maturation, these vessels disappear, and the epiphyseal and metaphyseal systems become totally separated. *(From Ogden JA, Lister G. The pathology of neonatal osteomyelitis. Pediatrics 55:474, 1975.)*

there may be decompression through the thin, periosteal tissue into surrounding soft tissues, and a subcutaneous abscess may form. In the absence of surgical intervention, collected pus "points" and drains spontaneously through the skin, forming a sinus tract. When adequate decompression and drainage have been established, general supportive care often is sufficient to permit complete healing and resolution of osseous and soft tissue foci of infection [46,48,127,128]. Free communication between the original site of osteomyelitis and the subperiosteal space prevents the necrosis and extensive spread of infection through the bone shaft that occurs frequently in older children and adults. Cortical sequestra are less common in infants, and because of the extreme richness of the newborn bone blood supply, sequestra often are completely absorbed if they do form [48]. In addition, the efficient vasculature and fertility of the inner layer of the periosteum encourage early development of profuse new bone formation (involucrum), permitting remodeling of bone within a very short time after the infectious process has been controlled [48,115].

The same characteristics of neonatal bone that serve to prevent many of the features of chronic osteomyelitis seen in older children are also responsible for complications occurring in neonates and young infants, such as epiphysitis and pyarthrosis. A consequence of the excellent bone blood supply in newborns is persistent fetal vessels that penetrate the cartilaginous epiphyseal plate and end in large venous lakes within the epiphysis [115,125,126]. Localization of organisms at these sites early in the course of osteomyelitis leads to an epiphysitis, with resultant severe damage of the cartilage cells on the epiphyseal side of the growth plate. When such damage occurs, it is generally irreparable [70,115] and ultimately results in arrest or disorganization of growth at the ends of the bone. By age 8 to 18 months, the vascular connections between

---

*References [11,13,16,20,22,23,40,78–80,120,122–129].

†References [11,12,73,75,119,120].

*References [4,5,11,32,39,40,49,71,75,119,130–132].

†References [4,11,19,30,33,39,49,53,69].

‡References [4,5,37,52,55,69,124].

metaphysis and epiphysis are obliterated, and the cartilaginous growth plate provides a barrier against the spread of infection that persists throughout childhood and adult life [115,125,126].

Rapid decompression of the primary metaphyseal abscess through the adjacent cortex also permits ready entrance of pus into the articular space of the bones whose metaphyses lie within the articular capsule of the joint. Suppurative arthritis of the hips, shoulders, elbows, and knees is frequently associated with osteomyelitis of the humerus or femur in infants.* When the infection originates in the epiphysis, pyarthrosis also may occur by direct extension of the primary abscess through the articular cartilage and into the joint space. When pus enters the joint, it causes distention of the joint capsule, and the increasing pressure may eventually produce a pathologic dislocation, particularly of the shoulder or hip joint. The lytic action of pyogenic exudate within the joint [129,130] and ischemia produced by the high intra-articular tension often are sufficient to cause dissolution or separation of the entire head of the femur or humerus, both of which are composed almost completely of cartilage during the neonatal period [3,34,35,131–133]. Although serious growth disturbances and deformities may result from septic arthritis at other sites, complete destruction of the joint is rare.

CLINICAL MANIFESTATIONS

Two distinct clinical syndromes that may be associated with suppurative bone involvement in the newborn period are: (1) a benign form, with little or no evidence of infection (other than local swelling) or disability, related to an osteomyelitis involving one or more skeletal sites, and (2) a severe form, with systemic manifestations of sepsis predominating until multiple sites of bone and visceral involvement are noted as manifestations of the infant's underlying condition [3,37,134]. The most likely cause of the benign form of neonatal osteomyelitis is a mild, transient bacteremia that arises peripherally and causes only minimal inflammation and suppuration. The experience of most investigators indicates that this form of illness represents most cases.* The few series in which high fever and evidence of sepsis were noted as common presenting signs probably represent instances in which diagnosis was delayed, resulting in more advanced disease at presentation [2,3,39,49].

Infants with mild illness generally feed well, gain weight, and develop normally. Systemic manifestations are minimal, and the temperature is usually normal or only slightly elevated.* The diagnosis may be missed until 2 to 4 weeks have elapsed, by which time bone destruction may be severe and widespread [47,54,56,136]. Even in intensive care nurseries, where infants are under continuous professional observation, osteomyelitis may be missed for days or weeks. Bone involvement may be discovered during a skeletal survey or computed tomography (CT) or magnetic resonance imaging (MRI) as an unsuspected site or sites of infection in an infant without known bone involvement; osteomyelitis also has been diagnosed as an incidental finding on chest or abdominal radiographs [16,22,137].

The first signs that may be noted by parents or physicians are diffuse edema and swelling of an extremity or joint, usually without discoloration, accompanied by excessive irritability of the infant. Handling the infant causes increased discomfort, and prolonged episodes of crying may be noted during after a diaper change or other physical manipulations of routine care. Examination reveals diminished spontaneous and reflex movement of the affected extremity, either because of pain (pseudoparalysis)* or because of weakness caused by an associated neuropathy [138–141]. Pyarthrosis of the hip joint is characterized by maintenance of the hip in a flexed, abducted, and externally rotated (frog-leg) position [138]. Because the slightest degree of passive motion of an extremity may cause severe pain and prolonged crying, attempts to elicit a point of maximal bone tenderness are often unsuccessful.

As the suppurative process extends through the metaphyseal cortex into the surrounding subperiosteal and subcutaneous tissues, external signs of inflammation become more intense, and points of maximal swelling, redness, and heat are more readily discernible. In most cases, an inflammatory mass is directly adjacent to the involved metaphysis or joint, although when deeper skeletal structures (e.g., vertebrae or pelvis) are involved, the abscess may point in distant sites. Three infants have been described in whom vertebral osteomyelitis was not discovered, or even suspected, until after a large retroperitoneal abscess had developed [6]. An abscess arising from the proximal femur, ilium, or hip joint appears usually in the upper thigh, on the buttocks, or in the groin, but occasionally also in the iliac fossa, where it can be palpated through the abdominal wall or rectum [51]. Even when infection is localized in the distal extremities, it is difficult to determine solely on clinical grounds whether the bone or adjacent joint or both are involved. Radiologic examinations and diagnostic aspiration of suspected joints are generally necessary to establish a diagnosis.

The striking feature of the benign form of neonatal osteomyelitis is the satisfactory general condition of the infant, despite the intensity of the local process; feeding and weight gain are undisturbed, and there is no evidence of involvement of visceral structures. Although deformity and disability may follow such infections, the fatality rate is exceedingly low, and healing is prompt.

By contrast, signs and symptoms of the severe form of neonatal osteomyelitis are predominantly those of a septic process with prolonged and intense bacteremia. Infants with this condition usually exhibit failure to thrive, with associated lethargy, refusal or vomiting of feedings, abdominal distention, jaundice, and other signs characteristic of sepsis in the newborn. Infection of the bones and joints may be noted almost simultaneously with onset of septicemia, or it may appear later, despite administration of antibiotics. The clinical evolution of the osteomyelitic process is identical to that in patients with the benign form of the disease. Early localizing signs and symptoms

---

*References [3,4,6,11,13,16,19,20,35,58,134,137–141].

*References [4,6,11,13,14,16,19,31,32,38,40,51,56,135,136].

*References [4,14,31,32,56,131,135].

---

*References [19,31,32,40,68,72,126].

are frequently overshadowed by the systemic manifestations occurring in the infant. Evidence of a suppurative process in the bone may be discovered accidentally in the course of routine radiographic examinations, or it may not be apparent until formation of a local subcutaneous abscess directs attention to the underlying bone. The prognosis for these infants is guarded; death is generally caused by sepsis, with widespread and multiple foci of infection in the nervous system or viscera. The prognosis for the skeletal lesions among survivors is not different, however, from the prognosis for the benign form.

As group B streptococcal infections have become increasingly prevalent, a distinctive clinical picture associated with osteomyelitis has emerged for GBS [19,31,58,142–146]. Most cases are caused by the type III serotype of streptococci and manifest as a late-onset illness during the 3rd and 4th weeks of life (mean age at diagnosis 25 days). Predisposing factors commonly seen with osteomyelitis caused by other agents, such as maternal obstetric complications, difficulties in the early neonatal period, use of vascular catheters, or other manipulative procedures, are unusual with group B streptococcal disease. The male preponderance usually identified with neonatal osteomyelitis is reversed, with females more affected in a ratio of 1.5:1. In almost 90% of the infants described with this condition, only a single bone has been involved, most commonly the humerus (50%) or femur (33%), affecting the shoulder or knee. In most cases, infants manifest the benign form of osteomyelitis without signs of systemic toxicity or involvement of other organ systems. Nevertheless, most are ill no more than 3 or 4 days before the diagnosis is established. Although affected joints are typically neither warm nor erythematous, local swelling, tenderness, and diminished movement of the affected extremity are usually severe enough for parents to seek early medical attention.

The distribution of bone involvement reported in the literature is shown in Table 8–1, with 741 infected sites among 485 patients. A single bone was involved in 324 patients, and multiple foci were involved in 161 patients (33%) [147,148]. Because radiographic or radionuclide skeletal surveys, which often identify unsuspected foci of osteomyelitis,* were generally not performed, the number of infants reported to have infection in multiple sites is probably falsely low. The high incidence of infections of the femur, humerus, and tibia in neonates has also been noted in adults [150] and older infants and children [8,10,135,151]. The relatively large number of cases of maxillary osteomyelitis is unique, however, to the newborn period; this entity is discussed separately later on.

The exuberant new bone formation associated with osteomyelitis in the newborn period makes it difficult to determine the original foci of infection when radiographs are obtained late in the clinical course. For this reason, either the site of primary metaphyseal abscess was unspecified, or the infection was referred to as a "panosteitis" in many instances. In the femur, proximal, distal, and uncertain sites of early infection are equally distributed, whereas localization in the tibia and humerus occurs most often at proximal ends of bones; in the radius, distal osteomyelitis

TABLE 8–1   Distribution of Bone Involvement in 485 Newborns with Osteomyelitis

Bone	No. Sites*	% of Sites
Femur	287	39
62 Proximal		
91 Distal		
81 Unspecified		
Humerus	134	18
66 Proximal		
16 Distal		
51 Unspecified		
Tibia	102	14
47 Proximal		
11 Distal		
44 Unspecified		
Radius	34	5
5 Proximal		
17 Distal		
12 Unspecified		
Maxilla	30	4
Ulna	22	3
Clavicle	18	2
Tarsal bones	15	2
2 "Tarsus"		
3 Talus		
10 Calcaneus		
Metacarpals	14	2
Phalanges	12	2
Ribs	12	2
Skull	9	1
Fibula	9	1
Ilium	8	1
Metatarsals	7	1
Mandible	7	1
Scapula	7	1
Sternum	6	1
Vertebrae	5	1
Ischium	3	0.4
Patella	1	0.1

*Of infants, 33% had disease in more than one bone.

predominates. The major consequence of these patterns of infection is the high incidence of secondary purulent arthritis of the hips, shoulders, knees, and wrists; this secondary arthritis has been noted in virtually every large series of newborns with bone infection.

PROGNOSIS

From 1920-1940, reports of neonatal osteomyelitis cited mortality rates of 40% in neonates and young infants [48], but stressed an overall benign nature of the disease and the good prognosis for life and function if sepsis was not present [46,48,127,128]. The introduction of antimicrobial agents effective against the common infecting organisms was associated with a considerable

---

*References [13,16,22,32,137,149].

reduction in mortality rates. Only 24 deaths (mortality rate 4.2%) were reported among approximately 575 newborns with osteomyelitis acquired from 1945-1990.*

The improved survival rate directed greater attention to a high incidence of residual joint deformities after neonatal osteomyelitis, particularly with hip and knee involvement or delayed diagnosis for more than 3 or 4 days.* Destruction or separation of the capital femoral epiphysis may result in serious disturbances of growth, usually combined with a marked coxa vara, valga, or magna; an unstable hip joint; flexion contractures; and abnormalities of gait.† Damage to the cartilaginous growth plate in the knees also is often followed by disturbances in longitudinal growth and angulation at the site of infection, leading to genu varum or valgum, restricted motion, and instability of the joint.‡ Although the consequences of shortening of bone and angular deformities are more serious in lower extremities, analogous growth disturbances may follow osteomyelitis of the humerus, radius, or ulna.§ Most of these data have been collected from infants with staphylococcal bone or joint infection; in contrast, the prognosis for full recovery is excellent after group B streptococcal infection [19,58].

Although vertebral osteomyelitis in the newborn is unusual, the consequences can be grave. Collapse or complete destruction of one or more vertebral bodies may occur [13,22,156–160], with severe kyphosis or paralysis caused by spinal cord compression appearing as late complications [13,156,157]. In most cases, vertebral involvement is not recognized until after paraspinal abscesses appear [6,161–163].

The full clinical consequences of osteomyelitis in the newborn period may not be apparent for months to years. Despite a seemingly favorable outcome, even infants with minor bone or joint involvement should be followed to skeletal maturity to observe for the appearance of late deformity, dysfunction, or growth arrest [69,70]. Early evidence of skeletal destruction frequently requires multiple orthopedic procedures to stabilize a joint or to straighten a limb or equalize its length with that of the contralateral arm or leg. Descriptions of late regeneration of femoral epiphyses despite severe injury emphasize the remarkable healing potential and unpredictability of this illness, however [164–170].

Chronic osteomyelitis and sequestration of necrotic bone have been thought to be uncommon complications before and after the availability of antibiotic therapy.* The apparent rarity of these complications in former years should be questioned, however, because in approximately 10% of infants with osteomyelitis who were studied by several groups of investigators, formation of sequestra occurred, and in many cases, sequestrectomy was required for complete cure.† A rare complication of

neonatal osteomyelitis is osteochondroma (or exostosis) at the distal ulna after *S. aureus* osteomyelitis [170].

DIAGNOSIS

Plain film radiographs remain the most useful means of establishing the diagnosis of neonatal osteomyelitis. Experience with CT and MRI in the evaluation of neonatal bone infection is increasing, and use of these modalities is limited only by the ability to transport small neonates to facilities for imaging and the need for monitoring of anesthetized infants. CT and MRI may be used if plain radiographs, ultrasonography (of joints), and bone scans have not yielded a diagnosis [171].

The earliest radiographic sign is swelling of soft tissue around the site of primary infection. Although this finding reflects spreading edema and inflammation that occur as pus breaks through metaphyseal cortex, it is nonspecific and serves only to define an area of inflammation. The first distinct evidence of bone involvement appears as small foci of necrosis and rarefaction, most commonly located in the metaphysis adjoining the epiphyseal growth plate; this may be accompanied by capsular distention or widening of the joint space if inflammatory exudate or pus has entered the articular capsule. In contrast to older children, in whom radiographic changes are commonly delayed for 3 weeks [10,151], neonates almost always show definite signs of bone destruction after only 7 to 10 days.*

Extension of the suppurative process often produces widespread areas of cortical rarefaction, which, despite their appearance, infrequently result in significant bone sequestration. The presence of pus in the hip and shoulder joints may cause progressive lateral and upward displacement of the head of the femur [32,132,133,172] or humerus through stages of subluxation to pathologic dislocation. The absence in the newborn period of ossification centers, with the exception of those at the distal femur and proximal tibia, makes it very difficult to diagnose neonatal epiphysitis in any area but the knees [155]. For similar reasons, epiphyseal separation or destruction of the head of the femur or humerus is difficult to distinguish radiologically from simple dislocation [132,133].

In most infants, the reparative phase begins within 2 weeks after onset of infection. The first sign of healing is the formation of a thin layer of subperiosteal bone, which rapidly enlarges to form a thick involucrum between the raised periosteum and the cortex. Although bone destruction may continue at the same time, necrotic foci are rapidly absorbed and filled in as new bone is deposited. The entire process from the first signs of rarefaction to restoration of the cortical structure may last no longer than 2 months; however, several months usually elapse before minimal deformities disappear and remodeling of the shaft is complete. In some cases, well-circumscribed defects involving the metaphysis and epiphysis may persist for years [155].

The benefit of using radiologic skeletal surveys in newborns with osteomyelitis should be emphasized, particularly because the occurrence of multiple sites of osteomyelitis is much more common in the neonatal period. Clinically unsuspected sites of infection can be discovered

---

*References [2,4–6,11,13,14,16,19,30,31,38–40,54,56,74,129,132].

*References [34–36,38,39,56,69,70,152–154].

†References [35,56,75,90,97,132,143,144,164,165].

‡References [11,33,56,70,124,155].

§References [3,14,37,56,70,156].

*References [6,37,39,48,56,127,128].

†References [2,5,16,50,51,74,116,139,176,177].

*References [5,11,12,19,38,53,55,149,169].

in a significant proportion of infants.* Demonstration of such lesions may be provide therapeutic benefits. In one series [16], 4 of 7 areas of occult infection required aspiration or drainage, whereas in another study [13], 3 of 17 hip joint infections were discovered on routine radiographs taken because the infant had osteomyelitis elsewhere. Plain film skeletal surveys for occult bone and joint infection are recommended in any infant with osteomyelitis.

As mentioned, experience with CT and MRI in the diagnosis of neonatal musculoskeletal infection is limited [174,175]. Although both procedures can be helpful adjuncts to clinical diagnosis and conventional radiography, they are slow and require heavy sedation—usually undesirable in a febrile septic infant—to prevent movement artifact and loss of resolution. CT provides good definition of cortical bone and is sensitive for early detection of bone destruction, periosteal reaction, and formation of sequestra. It has been used to particular advantage in diagnosis of osteomyelitis of the skull associated with infected cephalhematoma [110,111]. Plain radiographs of uninfected cephalhematomas can show soft tissue swelling, periosteal elevation, calcification, and even underlying radiolucency caused by bone resorption [176]—findings also consistent with bone infection. In such cases, CT has been able to define foci of bone destruction more accurately, helping to confirm the presence of osteomyelitis.

MRI is of limited value in defining structural changes in cortical bone, but it provides excellent anatomic detail of muscle and soft tissue, superior to that of any other imaging technique [175]. It is particularly useful in showing the early soft tissue edema seen adjacent to areas of bone involvement before the appearance of any osseous changes. MRI is also helpful in determining the presence of a periosteal abscess and assessing the need for surgical drainage. The major advantage of MRI over CT is the ability to detect inflammatory or destructive intramedullary disease. It is of greater advantage in older children and adults than in neonates, however, because involvement of the marrow compartment is uncommon in neonates. Both modalities provide excellent spatial resolution and anatomic detail; however, CT is best suited to cross-sectional views, whereas MRI can display anatomy with equal clarity in coronal and sagittal planes, permitting visualization in the plane most advantageous for accurate diagnosis. Absence of ionizing radiation is another distinct advantage of MRI over CT.

There has been increasing interest in the use of ultrasonography to detect bone infection and joint effusions [177–181]. Diagnosis of osteomyelitis is based on periosteal thickening or the presence of abscess formation as indicated by periosteal elevation and separation from bone. The exact role of ultrasonography in diagnosis of neonatal osteoarthritis has continued to be defined. It currently seems most useful as a tool for defining the presence of fluid collections in joints or adjacent to bone and as a guide for needle aspiration or surgical drainage of these collections. The occurrence of false-positive or false-negative examinations, although infrequent, requires that infants with conflicting clinical findings be evaluated

further by other techniques. Reports of successful diagnosis of osteomyelitis in neonates with ultrasonography include the diagnosis of rib infection in a 650-g infant with staphylococcal osteomyelitis [182]. Other series have included 2- to 6-week-old infants with osteomyelitis of the costochondral junction and ribs [183,184].

Despite reports emphasizing the reliability of technetium-99m bone imaging in older infants and children [185], experience with the use of this technique in neonates has been far less favorable [16,33,40,149,186–190]. In one study, among 10 newborns subsequently proved to have osteomyelitis involving 20 sites in all, only 8 of these sites were found to be abnormal or equivocal by technetium-99m scan [186]. Of the 12 sites that were normal by technetium-99m scan at 1 to 33 days (mean 8 days) after onset of symptoms, 9 showed destructive changes in the corresponding radiograph. The increased radioactivity in areas of inflammatory hyperemia surrounding an osteomyelitic lesion, usually present in the early "blood-pool" images in children [187], also was not seen, even in infants with ultimately positive delayed bone scans. Although false-negative bone scans also have been described in older infants [191,192], the reason for the excessively high incidence among neonates is unknown. It has been suggested that the discrepancy is due either to differences in the pathophysiology of neonatal disease or to the inability of earlier gamma cameras to separate the increased activity of the growth plate in the first weeks of life from that of infection [137,185].

As indicated by clinical studies, use of newer high-resolution cameras combined with electronic magnification may provide greater diagnostic accuracy [137]. However, In these studies, the investigators also used significantly (fourfold to sixfold) larger doses of technetium-99m, and almost all sites of involvement had radiographically detectable lesions at the time of diagnosis. It seems reasonable at the present time to limit the use of technetium-99m radionuclide scans to evaluation of infants with normal or equivocal radiographs in whom there is a strong clinical suspicion of osteomyelitis.

Among older patients, gallium-67 bone imaging has been shown to be valuable when results of the technetium-99m scan and appearance on plain films are normal and osteomyelitis is strongly suspected [192]. Studies performed in small infants and neonates have shown similar results [191,193]. The radiation burden of this isotope is high, however, and the probability that the results of a scan by themselves would influence therapy is low. The role of gallium-67 bone imaging in the diagnosis of neonatal bone and joint infections is very limited.

Needle aspiration of an inflammatory area may provide a rapid diagnosis [19,31,38,40]. Differentiation of subcutaneous from subperiosteal infection often is difficult; however, significant accumulations of pus aspirated from a periarticular abscess almost invariably are found to originate in bone rather than in the soft tissues [2,126]. Clinical or radiologic evidence of joint space infection, particularly in the hip and shoulder, requires immediate confirmation by needle aspiration. If no effusion is found and clinical signs persist, aspiration should be repeated within 8 to 12 hours. If there is doubt about whether the joint was actually entered, limited arthrography with

---

*References [13,16,22,33,149,173].

small amounts of dye can readily be performed with an aspirating needle [132,133]. Most iodinated contrast materials do not interfere with bacterial growth from aspirated specimens [194]. Inserting a needle into the metaphyseal region or joint 24 hours before scanning does not interfere with the scintigraphic detection of osteomyelitis [188–190].

The total peripheral white blood cell count is of little value in diagnosing neonatal osteomyelitis. In more than 150 cases in which these values were recorded, median peripheral leukocyte count was approximately 17,000 cells/mm^3 (mean 20,000 cells/mm^3, range 4000 to 75,100 cells/mm^3). Polymorphonuclear leukocytes usually represented about 60% of the white blood cells counted; frequently, the number of immature forms was higher than normal. Neonates with osteomyelitis usually have an erythrocyte sedimentation rate higher than 20 mm/hr.* Similar to leukocyte count, erythrocyte sedimentation rate is helpful for diagnosis and follow-up evaluation when elevated, but cannot be used to rule out osteomyelitis when normal [11,13,14,195]. Alternatively, C-reactive protein is more useful than erythrocyte sedimentation rate as an acute-phase reactant in neonates, and most methods for C-reactive protein determination require only 0.1 mL of blood, as opposed to erythrocyte sedimentation rate, which may require 1 to 2 mL of blood.

DIFFERENTIAL DIAGNOSIS

The early descriptions of pyogenic neonatal osteomyelitis emphasized difficulties in distinguishing the pseudoparalysis and irritability that are characteristic of this condition from the symptoms of congenital syphilis and from true paralysis of congenital poliomyelitis [196–198]. The clinical course and radiologic examinations are generally sufficient to rule out polio and other neuroparalytic illnesses; however, the periostitis and metaphyseal bone destruction that accompany congenital syphilis are frequently indistinguishable from bone alterations observed in infants with multicentric pyogenic osteomyelitis (see Chapter 16) [154,156]. Similar osseous changes have been noted at birth in infants with congenital tumors or leukemia [196,199].

Serial radiologic examinations may be necessary to distinguish a superficial cellulitis, subcutaneous abscess, or bursitis [200,201] from a primary bone infection, particularly when these conditions arise in a periarticular location. Similarly, a suppurative arthritis arising in the joint space rather than in the adjacent metaphysis can be defined as such only by determining that no destruction has occurred in bones contiguous to that joint.

The relative lack of any inflammatory sign other than edema is the only clinical feature that helps to differentiate between candidal and bacterial osteomyelitis [20,22]. *Candida* infections have been observed more frequently in recent years, particularly in premature infants, in whom antibiotic therapy, placement of umbilical catheters, and use of parenteral hyperalimentation, together with immature host defense mechanisms, predispose to candidal infection and dissemination.* The lesions of *Candida albicans*

infection typically are seen as well-defined ("punched-out") metaphyseal lucencies on radiographs, but are less aggressive in appearance than the lesions of staphylococcal osteitis and often are surrounded by a slightly sclerotic margin.† Even when characteristic clinical circumstances and radiographic features are present, the diagnosis in almost all cases rests on identification of the organism by Gram stain or culture, although *Candida* organisms are frequently present concomitantly in blood cultures obtained during febrile episodes.

Several congenital viral lesions have also been associated with bone changes. Lesions caused by congenital rubella, although generally seen in the metaphyseal ends of the long bones, are distinct from the lesions of bacterial osteomyelitis during the early stages of pathogenesis and show no evidence of periosteal reaction during the reparative phase [205]. There is little likelihood of confusion of the radiographic features of bone pathology resulting from congenital cytomegalic inclusion disease [206,207] or from herpes simplex virus type 2 infections [208] with those of hematogenous osteomyelitis, particularly when radiographic findings are considered in context with the characteristic clinical signs and symptoms of these infections.

Numerous noninfectious conditions causing bone destruction or periosteal reaction may be confused with osteomyelitis on clinical and radiographic grounds and on the basis of radionuclide scan findings. These conditions include skeletal trauma caused by the birth process or caregiver abuse [137,209–211] or associated with osteogenesis imperfecta; congenital infantile cortical hyperostosis (Caffey disease) [137,210,212]; congenital bone tumors, metastases, and leukemia [134,197]; extravasation of calcium gluconate at an infusion site [213]; and prostaglandin E$_1$ infusion [214]. The periosteal bone growth sometimes seen in normal infants, particularly premature infants, may produce a "double-contour" effect in long bones that appears to be similar to the early involucrum of healing osteomyelitis, but is unassociated with evidence of bone destruction and metaphyseal changes and is never progressive [215].

THERAPY

Successful treatment of osteomyelitis or septic arthritis depends on prompt clinical diagnosis and identification of the infectious agent. Every effort should be made to isolate responsible organisms before therapy is initiated. Pus localized in skin, soft tissues, joint, or bone should be aspirated under strict aseptic conditions and sent to the laboratory for Gram stain, culture, and antibiotic susceptibility testing. Blood specimens for culture should be obtained; such cultures may be the only source of the pathogen.* Because osteomyelitis generally is the consequence of a systemic bacteremia, a lumbar puncture should be considered. Any potential source of infection should be examined, including intravascular catheter tips [217]. Cerebrospinal fluid can occasionally be helpful when direct examination of suppurative material fails to

---

*References [11,31,32,58,119,144].

---

*References [20,22–24,34–37,75,117,202,203].

†References [20,22,34,37,38,75,203,204].

*References [16,27,35,38,52,55,216].

provide an etiologic diagnosis. Choice of therapy should be guided by results of Gram stain, culture, and antibiotic susceptibilities.

When the cause of infection cannot be immediately determined, the initial choice of antimicrobial agents must be based on the presumptive bacteriologic diagnosis. Penicillinase-resistant penicillins (e.g., nafcillin, oxacillin) and vancomycin are active against *S. aureus*, group A streptococci and GBS, and *S. pneumoniae*, which together account for more than 90% of cases of osteoarthritis in neonates. Osteomyelitis caused by enteric organisms is sufficiently common to justify additional therapy with an aminoglycoside such as gentamicin, tobramycin, or amikacin or an extended-spectrum agent (cefotaxime) or the use of an extended-spectrum, *Pseudomonas*-active agent such as cefepime.

MRSA and most strains of coagulase-negative staphylococci are increasingly frequent causes of sepsis and other focal infections in neonates. Numerous outbreaks of nosocomial and community-acquired MRSA infections have been reported. Infants who acquire infection in nurseries where MRSA is prevalent or where community-acquired MRSA infections have occurred should be started on vancomycin, rather than a penicillin antibiotic [149]. Alternative antibiotics approved and licensed for treatment of MRSA infections in older children and adults, including daptomycin, linezolid, and quinupristin-dalfopristin, have not been fully evaluated or approved for use in neonates in the first 2 months of life and should be employed on an individual basis only when the neonate cannot tolerate vancomycin because of acquired toxicity.

When bacterial culture and sensitivity data are available, treatment should be changed to the single safest and most effective drug. If group B streptococcal infection is confirmed, combination therapy with penicillin G (or ampicillin) and gentamicin should be given for 2 to 5 days, after which time penicillin G (or ampicillin) alone is adequate [218]. Standard disk susceptibility tests may falsely indicate sensitivity of MRSA to cephalosporins [219]. Use of β-lactam antibiotics is inappropriate for MRSA infections, and vancomycin should be continued for the full course of therapy. It is controversial whether the synergistic addition of an active aminoglycoside (e.g., gentamicin) to a penicillin antibiotic or vancomycin for a limited period (e.g., 5 days) enhances the clinical outcomes of infants with neonatal osteomyelitis caused by *S. aureus*.

All antibiotics should be given by the parenteral route, usually intravenously. There is no significant clinical advantage to intravenous over intramuscular administration, but the limited number of injection sites available in the newborn makes the intramuscular route impractical for use during prolonged periods. Intra-articular administration of antibiotics is unnecessary in the treatment of suppurative arthritis because adequate levels of activity have been shown in joint fluid after parenteral doses of most drugs that would be used for therapy [216]. Antibiotic therapy for either osteomyelitis or suppurative arthritis should be continued for at least 4 or 6 weeks after defervescence. Monitoring serum acute-phase proteins (particularly C-reactive protein) has been proposed as a useful way to determine resolution of infection and duration of therapy [110,220,221].

There are insufficient data on the absorption and efficacy of orally administered antibiotics in the neonate to recommend their use routinely in this age group for treatment of osteoarthritis. Nevertheless, after an initial course of intravenous therapy, newborns have been treated successfully with oral dicloxacillin [195,222,223], flucloxacillin [32], fusidic acid [32,33], and penicillin V [32,173] for additional periods ranging from 14 to 42 days. If sequential parenteral-oral therapy is used, adequacy of antibiotic absorption and efficacy must be closely monitored with regular clinical evaluation and, possibly, serum bactericidal titers or, preferably, direct measurement of antibiotic agents in blood [173,223,224]. It is likely, but unproved in the neonate, that the traditional antibiotics used for hematogenous osteomyelitis in older children (e.g., amoxicillin or cephalexin, in divided doses totally 100 to 150 mg/kg/day) would be tolerated and effective, but these agents should be used only after successful parenteral therapy has been established and only under the supervision of physicians with adequate training.

To overcome the uncertainties of oral absorption while still allowing discharge of the patient from the hospital, home intravenous antibiotic therapy has been advocated as an alternative form of treatment [21]. Although home management for older children and adults is now widely accepted, experience with newborns is still limited; however, with proper family and medical support, it can be a successful alternative to inpatient treatment. Either carefully monitored oral therapy or, more frequently, the use of intravenous antibiotics given by peripheral intravenous central catheters or surgically implanted central catheters may be used.

Incision and drainage are indicated whenever there is a significant collection of pus in soft tissues. The need for drilling or "windowing" the cortex to drain intramedullary collections of pus is controversial [11,13,14,32]. There is no evidence, based on controlled studies, that these procedures are of any value in either limiting systemic manifestations or decreasing the extent of bone destruction. Open surgical drainage for relief of intra-articular pressure is a critical measure, however, for preserving the viability of the head of the femur or humerus in infants with suppurative arthritis of hip or shoulder joints [6,35,152]. Intermittent needle aspiration with saline irrigation usually is adequate for drainage of other, more readily accessible joints. Lack of improvement after 3 days, rapid reaccumulation of fluid, or loculation of pus and necrotic debris in the joint may indicate the need for open drainage of these joints as well [225].

The affected extremity should be immobilized until inflammation has subsided, and there is radiologic evidence of healing. Prolonged splinting in a brace or cast is necessary when pathologic dislocation of the head of the femur accompanies pyarthrosis of the hip joint. Maintenance of adequate nutrition and fluid requirements is crucial in determining the ultimate course of the illness. Before the advent of antibiotics, attention to these factors alone often was adequate to ensure prompt healing of osseous lesions in infants who survived the initial septic process [48].

PRIMARY SEPTIC ARTHRITIS

Although septic arthritis often is a complication of neonatal osteomyelitis, it also can occur in the absence of demonstrable radiologic changes in adjacent bone.

Infection usually is the result of synovial implantation of organisms in the course of a septicemia. Infrequently, traumatic inoculation of organisms into the articular capsule may occur as a consequence of femoral venipuncture [36,59,94–96]. As in osteomyelitis, there is a strong association between septic arthritis and placement of an umbilical catheter [21]. Whatever the source of infection, the presence of a concurrent osteomyelitis can never be ruled out completely because of the possibility that the original suppurative focus lay in the radiolucent cartilaginous portion of the bone, permitting entry of organisms to the joint by direct extension. The spectrum of agents responsible for primary septic arthritis is similar to that of organisms causing arthritis secondary to a contiguous osteomyelitis. Bacteria that have been isolated from blood or joints of newborns in two series are listed in Table 8–2.

Signs and symptoms of purulent arthritis are virtually identical to the signs and symptoms seen in newborns with osteomyelitis [226,227]. Limitation in use of an extremity progressing to pseudoparalysis is characteristic of both conditions, and although external signs of inflammation tend to be more localized to the periarticular area, recognition of this feature is of little diagnostic value in individual cases. Data are insufficient to provide any meaningful comparison between the skeletal distribution of septic arthritis and that of osteomyelitis. Multiple joint involvement is common to both conditions, however. In one series of 16 consecutive newborns with pyarthrosis, 22 joints were involved; 4 (25%) infants had multifocal infections [27]. A migratory polyarthritis, which may precede localization in a single joint by several days, is particularly characteristic of gonococcal arthritis, as is an extremely high frequency of knee and ankle involvement [84]. In a Malaysian series, the knee, hip, and ankle were involved in 10 cases of septic arthritis, and 9 of the 10 cases were caused by MRSA, exhibiting the frequent occurrence of septic arthritis caused by nosocomial pathogens in premature infants in neonatal intensive care units [228].

The radiologic features, differential diagnosis, and therapy for septic arthritis are discussed in "Osteomyelitis." Studies of long-term evaluations are rare, precluding an accurate assessment of the prognosis for this condition.

TABLE 8–2   Reported Spectrum and Organisms Isolated from Blood or Joints of Neonates with Primary Bacterial Arthritis (1972-1986)

Bacteria	No. Infants
Staphylococcus aureus	9
Group B Streptococci	4
Streptococci, unspecified	2
Staphylococcus epidermidis	1
Haemophilus influenzae type b	0
Escherichia coli	0
Klebsiella pneumoniae	1
Pseudomonas aeruginosa	1
Neisseria gonorrhoeae	1

Data from Nelson JD, personal communication, 1987; Pittard WB III, Thullen JD, Fanaroff AA. Neonatal septic arthritis. J Pediatr 88:621, 1976; and Jackson MA, Nelson JD. Etiology and medical management of acute suppurative bone and joint infections in pediatric patients. J Pediatr Orthop 2:313, 1982.

OSTEOMYELITIS OF THE MAXILLA

Neonatal osteomyelitis of the maxilla is a distinct clinical entity, and early reports of neonatal osteomyelitis frequently focused exclusively on this entity. In terms of total numbers, maxillary osteomyelitis is a rare condition (there are <200 reported cases); yet in earlier surveys of neonatal bone infections, maxillary involvement was noted in approximately 25% of infants.* The far lower incidence in children [8,10] and adults [150] is probably explained by earlier recognition and treatment of sinusitis in these age groups and by the lack of predisposing factors unique to the newborn.

The causative organism is most frequently S. aureus [230–232], although hemolytic streptococci have been isolated on rare occasions from drainage sites [232]. More than 85% of all maxillary infections in infants occur in the first 3 months of life; the incidence is highest during the 2nd to 4th weeks [231–234].

In most cases, the predisposing cause remains obscure. Infants with sources of infection, such as skin abscesses or omphalitis, constitute a small minority [232,233]. It has been postulated that there is a relationship between breast abscess in the nursing mother and maxillary osteomyelitis [232,233,235]; however, it is unclear whether the maternal infection is a source or a result of the infant's condition [236]. The pathogenesis of bone infection after colonization of the infant by staphylococci is equally uncertain. In some cases, osteomyelitis is believed to result from extension from a contiguous focus of infection in the maxillary antrum. Alternatively, organisms may be blood-borne, establishing infection in the rich vascular plexus surrounding tooth buds [234]. Although the hematogenous route may be important in certain cases, particularly cases involving the premaxilla [230], this explanation is incompatible with the fact that mandibular osteomyelitis or associated metastatic involvement of other structures is uncommon [232]. Another theory is that trauma or abrasion of the gum overlying the first molar is the primary route of introduction of organisms [233].

The clinical course of maxillary osteomyelitis begins with acute onset of fever and nonspecific systemic symptoms. Shortly thereafter, redness and swelling of the eyelid appear and are frequently accompanied by conjunctivitis with a purulent discharge. Thrombosis of nutrient vessels and increasing edema may cause a proptosis or chemosis of the affected eye. In most infants, an early and diffuse swelling and inflammation of the cheek may localize to form an abscess or draining fistula below the inner or outer canthus of the eye; this is nearly always followed or accompanied by a purulent unilateral nasal discharge that is increased by pressure on the abscess. The alveolar border of the superior maxilla on the affected side is swollen and soft, as is the adjacent hard palate. Within a few days, abscesses and draining fistulas may form in these areas [237]. Sepsis and death are frequent in untreated cases. In most infants, the illness pursues a relatively chronic course characterized by discharge of premature teeth or numerous small sequestra of necrotic bone through multiple palatal and alveolar sinuses that have formed. The entire course may evolve over several days in severe cases, or it may extend for several weeks in mild or partially treated cases.

*References [3,6,11,48,55,229].

Neonatal maxillary osteomyelitis is frequently confused with either orbital cellulitis or dacryocystitis [13,233,238]. The early edema and redness of the cheeks that accompany acute osteomyelitis constitute an important differentiating feature, which is not observed in orbital cellulitis and occurs only as a late sign in infection of the lacrimal sac. Neither orbital cellulitis nor lacrimal sac infection is associated with a unilateral purulent nasal discharge. The early onset, limited area of involvement, and Gram stain characteristic of ophthalmia neonatorum should be sufficient, in most cases, to permit diagnosis of this condition. CT can be helpful in assessing the extent of infection and evaluating for possible complications, such as cerebral abscess [237].

Therapy for maxillary osteomyelitis should be directed toward early adequate drainage of the maxillary empyema and contiguous abscess and should include appropriate parenterally administered antibiotics. Because most infections are due to *S. aureus* and group A streptococci, systemic use of a penicillinase-resistant penicillin (or vancomycin) alone should be sufficient as initial therapy pending the results of bacterial cultures and sensitivity tests. The need for or desirability of instillation of antibiotics into the maxillary antrum is uncertain.

Before the advent of penicillin therapy, the mortality rate for maxillary osteomyelitis was high, ranging from 15% to 75% in various series [232,233,235,239]. Children who survived often had severe facial and dental deformities. Later studies [232,233,239] showed a mortality rate of closer to 5%, although sequelae such as stenosis of the lacrimal duct, ectropion, permanent loss of teeth, malocclusion, and facial hemiatrophy are still seen [11,231–233]. In many instances, these complications could have been prevented through early recognition of the nature of the illness and prompt institution of appropriate therapy.

REFERENCES

[1] W.S. Craig, Care of the Newly Born Infant, Williams & Wilkins, Baltimore, 1962.

[2] J. Boyes, A.D. Bremner, G.A. Neligan, Haematogenous osteitis in the newborn, Lancet 1 (1957) 544.

[3] W.M. Dennison, Haematogenous osteitis in the newborn, Lancet 2 (1955) 474.

[4] P. Masse, L'ostéomyélité du nouveau-né, Semaine Hôp Paris 34 (1958) 2812.

[5] H. Contzen, Die sogennante Osteomyelitis des Neugeborenen, Dtsch. Med. Wochenschr. 86 (1961) 1221.

[6] A.M. Clarke, Neonatal osteomyelitis: a disease different from osteomyelitis of older children, Med. J. Aust. 1 (1958) 237.

[7] J.E. Hall, E.A. Silverstein, Acute hematogenous osteomyelitis, Pediatrics 31 (1963) 1033.

[8] M. Green, W.L. Nyhan Jr., M.D. Fousek, Acute hematogenous osteomyelitis, Pediatrics 17 (1956) 368.

[9] W. Hung, D.F. McGavisk, Acute hematogenous osteomyelitis: a report of 36 cases seen at Children's Hospital 1950 to 1958, Clin. Proc. Child. Hosp. 16 (1960) 163.

[10] T.S. Morse, C.V. Pryles, Infections of the bones and joints in children, N. Engl. J. Med. 262 (1960) 846.

[11] L. Fox, K. Sprunt, Neonatal osteomyelitis, Pediatrics 62 (1978) 535.

[12] M.O. Lim, et al., Osteomyelitis as a complication of umbilical artery catheterization, Am. J. Dis. Child. 131 (1977) 142.

[13] S. Bergdahl, K. Ekengren, M. Eriksson, Neonatal hematogenous osteomyelitis: risk factors for long-term sequelae, J. Pediatr. Orthop. 5 (1985) 564.

[14] T. Bamberger, E. Gugler, Die akute Osteomyelitis im Kindesalter, Schweiz. Med. Wochenschr. 113 (1983) 1219.

[15] R. Bennett, M. Eriksson, R. Zetterström, Increasing incidence of neonatal septicemia: causative organism and predisposing risk factors, Acta Paediatr. Scand. 70 (1981) 207.

[16] P.M. Mok, B.J. Reilly, J.M. Ash, Osteomyelitis in the neonate with cerebral abscess, Radiology 145 (1982) 677.

[17] M. Dan, Septic arthritis in young infants: clinical and microbiologic correlations and therapeutic implications, Rev. Infect. Dis. 6 (1984) 147.

[18] L.L. Barton, L.M. Dunkle, F.H. Habib, Septic arthritis in childhood: a 13-year review, Am. J. Dis. Child. 141 (1987) 898.

[19] M.S. Edwards, et al., An etiologic shift in infantile osteomyelitis: the emergence of the group B streptococcus, J. Pediatr. 93 (1978) 578.

[20] D.K. Yousefzadeh, J.H. Jackson, Neonatal and infantile candidal arthritis with or without osteomyelitis: a clinical and radiographical review of 21 cases, Skeletal Radiol. 5 (1980) 77.

[21] W.B. Pittard III., J.D. Thullen, A.A. Fanaroff, Neonatal septic arthritis, J. Pediatr. 88 (1976) 621.

[22] P.W. Brill, et al., Osteomyelitis in a neonatal intensive care unit, Radiology 13 (1979) 83.

[23] D.E. Johnson, et al., Systemic candidiasis in very low-birth-weight infants (≤1,500 grams), Pediatrics 73 (1984) 138.

[24] R.B. Turner, L.G. Donowitz, J.O. Hendley, Consequences of candidemia for pediatric patients, Am. J. Dis. Child. 139 (1985) 178.

[25] D.A. Goldmann, W.A. Durbin Jr., J. Freeman, Nosocomial infections in a neonatal intensive care unit, J. Infect. Dis. 144 (1981) 449.

[26] T.R. Townsend, R.P. Wenzel, Nosocomial bloodstream infections in a newborn intensive care unit, Am. J. Epidemiol. 114 (1981) 73.

[27] M.A. Jackson, J.D. Nelson, Etiology and medical management of acute suppurative bone and joint infections in pediatric patients, J. Pediatr. Orthop. 2 (1982) 313.

[28] J.O. Hensey, C.A. Hart, R.W.I. Cooke, Serious infections in a neonatal intensive care unit: a two year survey, J. Hyg. 95 (1985) 289.

[29] C. Lejeune, et al., Fréquence des infections bactériennes néonatales dans les unites de réanimation et/ou néonatologie, Pediatrie 41 (1986) 9.

[30] G.D. Coto-Cotallo, et al., Osteomielitis neonatal: estudio de una serie de 35 casos, Ann. Esp. Pediatr. 33 (1990) 429.

[31] B.I. Asmar, Osteomyelitis in the neonate, Infect. Dis. Clin. North. Am. 6 (1992) 117.

[32] C.J. Knudsen, E.B. Hoffman, Neonatal osteomyelitis, J. Bone. Joint. Surg. Br. 72 (1990) 846.

[33] J.B. Williamson, C.S.B. Galasko, M.J. Robinson, Outcome after acute osteomyelitis in preterm infants, Arch. Dis. Child. 65 (1990) 1060.

[34] A. Baitch, Recent observations of acute suppurative arthritis, Clin. Orthop. 22 (1962) 157.

[35] B.E. Obletz, Suppurative arthritis of the hip joint in premature infants, Clin. Orthop. 22 (1962) 27.

[36] D.W. Ross, Acute suppurative arthritis of the hip in premature infants, JAMA 156 (1954) 303.

[37] J. Thomson, I.C. Lewis, Osteomyelitis in the newborn, Arch. Dis. Child. 25 (1950) 273.

[38] E.D. Weissberg, A.L. Smith, D.H. Smith, Clinical features of neonatal osteomyelitis, Pediatrics 53 (1974) 505.

[39] S. Kumari, et al., Neonatal osteomyelitis: a clinical and follow-up study, Indian. J. Pediatr. 15 (1978) 393.

[40] P.G. Deshpande, et al., Neonatal osteomyelitis and septic arthritis, Indian J. Pediatr. 27 (1990) 453.

[41] P.W. Brill, et al., Osteomyelitis in a neonatal intensive care unit, Radiology 131 (1979) 83.

[42] M. Wong, et al., Clinical and diagnostic features of osteomyelitis in the first three months of life, Pediatr. Infect. Dis. 14 (1995) 1047.

[43] M. Saarinen, et al., Spectrum of 2, 836 cases of invasive bacterial or fungal infections in children: results of prospective nationwide five-year surveillance in Finland, Clin. Infect. Dis. 21 (1995) 1134.

[44] X. Saez-Llorens, J. Velarde, C. Canton, Pediatric osteomyelitis in Panama, Clin. Infect. Dis. 19 (1994) 323.

[45] R.M. Freedman, et al., A half century of neonatal sepsis at Yale: 1928 to 1978, Am. J. Dis. Child. 135 (1981) 140.

[46] R.B. Dillehunt, Osteomyelitis in infants, Surg. Gynecol. Obstet. 61 (1935) 96.

[47] E.C. Dunham, Septicemia in the newborn, Am. J. Dis. Child. 45 (1933) 230.

[48] W.T. Green, J.G. Shannon, Osteomyelitis of infants: a disease different from osteomyelitis of older children, Arch. Surg. 32 (1936) 462.

[49] T.R. Aractingi, Étude de 32 cas d'ostéomyélité du nouveauné, Rev. Chir. Orthop. 47 (1961) 50.

[50] W.M. Dennison, D.A. MacPherson, Haematogenous osteitis of infancy, Arch. Dis. Child. 27 (1952) 375.

[51] I.S. DeWet, Acute osteomyelitis and suppurative arthritis of infants, S. Afr. Med. J. 28 (1954) 81.

[52] C.G. Hutter, New concepts of osteomyelitis in the newborn infant, J. Pediatr. 32 (1948) 522.

[53] L. Lindell, K.V. Parkkulainen, Osteitis in infancy and early childhood: with special reference to neonatal osteitis, Ann. Paediat. Fenn. 6 (1960) 34.

[54] M. Kienitz, M. Schulte, Problematik bakterieller Infectionen des Frühund Neuegeborenen, Munch. Med. Wochenschr. 109 (1967) 70.

[55] G. Wolman, Acute osteomyelitis in infancy, Acta Paediatr. Scand. 45 (1956) 595.

[56] D.W. Blanche, Osteomyelitis in infants, J. Bone. Joint. Surg. Am. 34 (1952) 71.

[57] J.B. Howard, G.H. McCracken Jr., The spectrum of group B streptococcal infections in infancy, Am. J. Dis. Child. 128 (1974) 815.

[58] I.A. Memon, et al., Group B streptococcal osteomyelitis and septic arthritis: its occurrence in infants less than 2 months old, Am. J. Dis. Child. 133 (1979) 921.

[59] J.A. Omene, J.C. Odita, Clinical and radiological features of neonatal septic arthritis, Trop. Geogr. Med. 31 (1979) 207.

[60] B.M. Garcia Pena, M.B. Harper, G.R. Fleisher, Occult bacteremia with group B streptococci in an outpatient setting, Pediatrics 102 (1998) 67.

[61] T.J. Choma, L.B. Davlin, J.S. Wagner, Iliac osteomyelitis in the newborn presenting as nonspecific musculoskeletal sepsis, Orthopedics 17 (1994) 632.

[62] L.L. Barton, R.G. Villar, S.A. Rice, Neonatal group B streptococcal vertebral osteomyelitis, Pediatrics 98 (1996) 459.

[63] C.P. Speer, et al., Neonatal septicemia and meningitis in Göttingen, West Germany, Pediatr. Infect. Dis. 4 (1985) 36.

[64] J. Karpuch, M. Goldberg, D. Kohelet, Neonatal bacteremia: a 4-year prospective study, Isr. J. Med. Sci. 19 (1983) 963.

[65] H.L. Levy, J.F. O'Connor, D. Ingall, Neonatal osteomyelitis due to Proteus mirabilis, JAMA 202 (1967) 582.

[66] W.D. Müller, et al., Septische Arthritis und Osteomyelitis als Komplikation neonataler Intensivpflege, Paediatr. Paedol. 14 (1979) 469.

[67] A. Bogdanovich, Neonatal arthritis due to Proteus vulgaris, Arch. Dis. Child. 23 (1948) 65.

[68] J.A. Omene, J.C. Odita, A.A. Okolo, Neonatal osteomyelitis in Nigerian infants, Pediatr. Radiol. 14 (1984) 318.

[69] I.H. Choi, et al., Sequelae and reconstruction after septic arthritis of the hip in infants, J. Bone. Joint. Surg. Am. 72 (1990) 1150.

[70] W. Peters, J. Irving, M. Letts, Long-term effects of neonatal bone and joint infection on adjacent growth plates, J. Pediatr. Orthop. 12 (1992) 806.

[71] M. Berant, D. Kahana, Klebsiella osteomyelitis in a newborn, Am. J. Dis. Child. 118 (1969) 634.

[72] A.A. White, E.S. Crelin, S. McIntosh, Septic arthritis of the hip joint secondary to umbilical artery catheterization associated with transient femoral and sciatic neuropathy, Clin. Orthop. 100 (1974) 190.

[73] I. Nathanson, G.P. Giacoia, Klebsiella osteoarthritis in prematurity: complication of umbilical artery catheterization, N. Y. State. J. Med. 79 (1979) 2077.

[74] H.V. Voss, et al., Enterobacter-Osteomyelitis bei zwei Säuglingen, Klin. Paediatr. 187 (1975) 465.

[75] S.L. Gordon, M.J. Maisels, W.J. Robbins, Multiple joint infections with Enterobacter cloacae, Clin. Orthop. 125 (1977) 136.

[76] A.S. Bayer, et al., Gram-negative bacillary septic arthritis: clinical, radiographic, therapeutic, and prognostic features, Semin. Arthritis. Rheum. 7 (1977) 123.

[77] D. Gajzago, O. Gottche, Salmonella suipestifer infections in childhood, Am. J. Dis. Child. 63 (1942) 15.

[78] R.J. Levinsky, Two children with Pseudomonas osteomyelitis: the paucity of systemic symptoms may lead to delay in diagnosis, Clin. Pediatr. 14 (1975) 288.

[79] W. Konzert, Über ein Salmonella-Osteomyelitis im Rahmen einer Salmonella-typhimurium Epidemia auf einer Neugeborenen Station, Wien. Klin. Wochenschr. 81 (1969) 713.

[80] A.J. Tur, O.O. Gartoch, Ein Fall von Erkrankung eines frühgeborenen Kindes im ersten Lebensmonate an multiplier Arthritis durch den Bacillus suipestifer, Z. Kinderheilkd. 56 (1934) 696.

[81] A.A. Adeyokunnu, R.G. Hendrickse, Salmonella osteomyelitis in childhood: a report of 63 cases seen in Nigerian children of whom 57 had sickle cell anemia, Arch. Dis. Child. 55 (1980) 175.

[82] G. Steinwender, et al., Gut-derived bone infection in the neonatal rat, Pediatr. Res. 50 (2001) 767.

[83] S. Nair, M.J. Schoeneman, Septic arthritis in an infant with vesicoureteral reflux and urinary tract infection, Pediatrics 111 (2003) e195.

[84] D.P. Kohen, Neonatal gonococcal arthritis: three cases and review of the literature, Pediatrics 53 (1974) 436.

[85] J.E. Gregory, J.L. Chison, A.T. Meadows, Short case report: gonococcal arthritis in an infant, Br. J. Vener. Dis. 48 (1972) 306.

[86] M.B. Cooperman, End results of gonorrheal arthritis: a review of seventy cases, Am. J. Surg. 5 (1928) 241.

[87] D. Nabarro, Congenital Syphilis, Edward Arnold, London, 1954.

[88] P.N. Zenker, S.M. Berman, Congenital syphilis: trends and recommendations for evaluation and management, Pediatr. Infect. Dis. J. 10 (1991) 516.

[89] L.P. Brion, et al., Long-bone radiographic abnormalities as a sign of active congenital syphilis in asymptomatic newborns, Pediatrics 88 (1991) 1037.

[90] L. Lequier, J. Robinson, W. Vaudry, Sternotomy infection with Mycoplasma hominis in a neonate, Pediatr. Infect. Dis. J. 14 (1995) 1010.

[91] G. Gjuric, et al., Ureaplasma urealyticum osteomyelitis in a very low birth weight infant, Perinat. Med. 22 (1994) 79.

[92] M.R. Hughesdon, Congenital tuberculosis, Arch. Dis. Child. 21 (1946) 121.

[93] R. Mallet, et al., Diffuse bony tuberculosis in the newborn (spina ventosa generalisata), Sem. Hôp. Paris. 44 (1968) 36.

[94] D.L. Nelson, K.A. Hable, J.M. Matsen, Proteus mirabilis osteomyelitis in two neonates following needle puncture, Am. J. Dis. Child. 125 (1973) 109.

[95] R.S. Asnes, G.M. Arendar, Septic arthritis of the hip: a complication of femoral venipuncture, Pediatrics 38 (1966) 837.

[96] P.B. Chacha, Suppurative arthritis of the hip joint in infancy: a persistent diagnostic problem and possible complication of femoral venipuncture, J. Bone. Joint. Surg. Am. 53 (1971) 538.

[97] G.D. Overturf, G. Balfour, Osteomyelitis and sepsis: severe complications of fetal monitoring, Pediatrics 55 (1975) 244.

[98] F.J. Plavidal, A. Werch, Fetal scalp abscess secondary to intrauterine monitoring, Am. J. Obstet. Gynecol. 125 (1976) 65.

[99] I. Brook, Osteomyelitis and bacteremia caused by Bacteroides fragilis: a complication of fetal monitoring, Clin. Pediatr. 19 (1980) 639.

[100] J.A. McGregor, T. McFarren, Neonatal cranial osteomyelitis: a complication of fetal monitoring, Obstet. Gynecol. 73 (1989) 490.

[101] L.D. Lilien, et al., Neonatal osteomyelitis of the calcaneus: complication of heel puncture, J. Pediatr. 88 (1976) 478.

[102] M.G. Myers, B.J. McMahon, F.P. Koontz, Neonatal calcaneus osteomyelitis related to contaminated mineral oil, Clin. Microbiol. 6 (1977) 543.

[103] T.A. Blumenfeld, G.K. Turi, W.A. Blanc, Recommended site and depth of newborn heel skin punctures based on anatomical measurements and histopathology, Lancet 1 (1979) 230.

[104] L.C. Borris, H. Helleland, Growth disturbance of the hind part of the foot following osteomyelitis of the calcaneus in the newborn: a report of two cases, J. Bone. Joint. Surg. Am. 68 (1986) 302.

[105] J.L. Fernandez-Fanjul, et al., Osteomyelitis des Calcaneus beim Neugeborenen als Folge diagnostischer Fersenpunktionen, Monatsschr. Kinderheilkd. 127 (1979) 515.

[106] M.S. Puczynski, et al., Osteomyelitis of the great toe secondary to phlebotomy, Clin. Orthop. 190 (1984) 239.

[107] I. Bergman, et al., Epidural abscess and vertebral osteomyelitis following serial lumbar punctures, Pediatrics 72 (1983) 476.

[108] M.S. Edwards, C.J. Baker, Median sternotomy wound infections in children, Pediatr. Infect. Dis. 2 (1983) 105.

[109] P.H. Valerio, Osteomyelitis as a complication of perinatal fracture of the clavicle, Eur. J. Pediatr. 154 (1995) 497.

[110] R.T. Mohon, et al., Infected cephalohematoma and neonatal osteomyelitis of the skull, Pediatr. Infect. Dis. 5 (1986) 253.

[111] L.M. Nightingale, et al., Cephalohematoma complicated by osteomyelitis presumed due to Gardnerella vaginalis, JAMA 256 (1986) 1936.

[112] P.Y.C. Lee, Case report: infected cephalohematoma and neonatal osteomyelitis, J. Infect. 21 (1990) 191.

[113] D. McCarthy, A.H.C. Walker, S. Matthews, Scalp abscesses in the newborn: a discussion of their causation, J. Obstet. Gynaecol. Br. Emp. 59 (1952) 37.

[114] W. Ladewig, Über eine intrauterin entstandene umschriebene Osteomyelitis des Schädeldaches, Virchows Arch. Pathol. Anat. 289 (1933) 395.

[115] J. Trueta, Three types of acute haematogenous osteomyelitis, J. Bone. Joint. Surg. Br. 41 (1959) 671.

[116] R.M. Todd, Septicaemia of the newborn: a clinical study of fifteen cases, Arch. Dis. Child. 23 (1948) 102.

[117] S. Svirsky-Fein, et al., Neonatal osteomyelitis caused by Candida tropicalis: report of two cases and review of the literature, J. Bone. Joint. Surg. Am. 61 (1979) 455.

[118] J.E. Baley, R.M. Kliegman, A.A. Fanaroff, Disseminated fungal infections in very low-birth-weight infants: clinical manifestations and epidemiology, Pediatrics 73 (1984) 144.

[119] F.U. Knudsen, S. Petersen, Neonatal septic osteoarthritis due to umbilical artery catheterisation, Acta Paediatr. Scand. 66 (1977) 225.

[120] P.G. Rhodes, et al., Sepsis and osteomyelitis due to Staphylococcus aureus phage type 94 in a neonatal intensive care unit, J. Pediatr. 88 (1976) 1063.

[121] A.A. deLorimier, D. Haskin, F.S. Massie, Mediastinal mass caused by vertebral osteomyelitis, Am. J. Dis. Child. 111 (1966) 639.

[122] M.E. Qureshi, Osteomyelitis after exchange transfusion, BMJ 1 (1971) 28.

[123] P.B. Simmons, L.E. Harris, A.J. Bianco, Complications of exchange transfusion: report of two cases of septic arthritis and osteomyelitis, Mayo Clin. Proc. 48 (1973) 190.

[124] B. Lindblad, K. Ekingren, G. Aurelius, The prognosis of acute hematogenous osteomyelitis and its complications during early infancy after the advent of antibiotics, Acta Paediatr. Scand. 54 (1965) 24.

[125] S.M.K. Chung, The arterial supply of the developing proximal end of the human femur, J. Bone. Joint. Surg. Am. 58 (1976) 961.

[126] J.A. Ogden, Pediatric osteomyelitis and septic arthritis: the pathology of neonatal disease, Yale J. Biol. Med. 52 (1979) 423.

[127] J.M. Cass, Staphylococcus aureus infection of the long bones in the newly born, Arch. Dis. Child. 15 (1940) 55.

[128] S. Stone, Osteomyelitis of the long bones in the newborn, Am. J. Dis. Child. 64 (1942) 680.

[129] P.H. Curtis, L. Klein, Destruction of articular cartilage in septic arthritis, I: in vitro studies, J. Bone. Joint. Surg. Am. 45 (1963) 797.

[130] P.H. Curtis, L. Klein, Destruction of articular cartilage in septic arthritis, II: in vivo studies, J. Bone. Joint. Surg. Am. 47 (1965) 1595.

[131] B.E. Obletz, Acute suppurative arthritis of the hip in the neonatal period, J. Bone. Joint. Surg. Am. 42 (1960) 23.

[132] G.B. Glassberg, M.B. Ozonoff, Arthrographic findings in septic arthritis of the hip in infants, Radiology 128 (1978) 151.

[133] J.J. Kaye, P.H. Winchester, R.H. Freiberger, Neonatal septic "dislocation" of the hip: true dislocation or pathological epiphyseal separation? Radiology 114 (1975) 671.

[134] J. Greengard, Acute hematogenous osteomyelitis in infancy, Med. Clin. North. Am. 30 (1946) 135.

[135] P. Ingelrans, et al., Les ostéoarthrites du nouveau-né et du nourrison: particuliteés étiologiques, diagnostiques et thérapeutiques: à propos de 35 observations, Lille Med. 13 (1968) 390.

[136] S.M.K. Chung, R.E. Pollis, Diagnostic pitfalls in septic arthritis of the hip in infants and children, Clin. Pediatr. 14 (1975) 758.

[137] E.L. Bressler, J.J. Conway, S.C. Weiss, Neonatal osteomyelitis examined by bone scintigraphy, Radiology 152 (1984) 685.

[138] S.A. Clay, Osteomyelitis as a cause of brachial plexus neuropathy, Am. J. Dis. Child. 136 (1982) 1054.

[139] R.S.K. Young, D.L. Hawkes, Pseudopseudoparalysis. Letter to the editor, Am. J. Dis. Child. 137 (1983) 504.

[140] D. Isaacs, B.D. Bower, E.R. Moxon, Neonatal osteomyelitis presenting as nerve palsy, BMJ 1 (1986) 1071.

[141] I. Obando, et al., Group B streptococcus pelvic osteomyelitis presenting as footdrop in a newborn infant, Pediatr. Infect. Dis. J. 10 (1991) 703.

[142] T.K. Lai, J. Hingston, D. Scheifele, Streptococcal neonatal osteomyelitis, Am. J. Dis. Child. 134 (1980) 711.

[143] R.J. Ancona, et al., Group B streptococcal sepsis with osteomyelitis and arthritis: its occurrence with acute heart failure, Am. J. Dis. Child. 133 (1979) 919.

[144] T.A. McCook, A.H. Felman, E. Ayoub, Streptococcal skeletal infections: observations in four infants, AJR Am. J. Roentgenol. 130 (1978) 465.

[145] S.J. Chilton, S.F. Aftimos, P.W. White, Diffuse skeletal involvement of streptococcal osteomyelitis in a neonate, Radiology 134 (1980) 390.

[146] R.A. Broughton, et al., Unusual manifestations of neonatal group B streptococcal osteomyelitis, Pediatr. Infect. Dis. 1 (1982) 410.

[147] R.A.J. Einstein, C.G. Thomas Jr., Osteomyelitis in infants, AJR Am. J. Roentgenol. 55 (1946) 299.

[148] J.K. Stack, W. Newman, Neonatal osteomyelitis, Q. Bull. Northwes. Univ. Med. Sch. 27 (1953) 69.

[149] M.R. Ish-Horowicz, P. McIntyre, S. Nade, Bone and joint infections caused by multiply resistant *Staphylococcus aureus* in a neonatal intensive care unit, Pediatr. Infect. Dis. J. 11 (1992) 82.

[150] F.A. Waldvogel, G. Medoff, M.N. Swartz, Osteomyelitis: Clinical Features, Therapeutic Considerations, and Unusual Aspects, Charles C Thomas, Springfield, IL, 1971.

[151] V.Q. Dich, J.D. Nelson, K.C. Haltalin, Osteomyelitis in infants and children: a review of 163 cases, Am. J. Dis. Child. 129 (1975) 1273.

[152] R.L. Samilson, F.A. Bersani, M.B. Watkins, Acute suppurative arthritis in infants and children, Pediatrics 21 (1958) 798.

[153] T. Hallel, E.A. Salvati, Septic arthritis of the hip in infancy: end result study, Clin. Orthop. 132 (1978) 115.

[154] O.M. Bennett, S.S. Namyak, Acute septic arthritis of the hip joint in infancy and childhood, Clin. Orthop. 281 (1992) 123.

[155] P.H. Roberts, Disturbed epiphyseal growth at the knee after osteomyelitis in infancy, J. Bone. Joint. Surg. Br. 52 (1970) 692.

[156] K. Ekengren, S. Bergdahl, M. Eriksson, Neonatal osteomyelitis: radiographic findings and prognosis in relation to site of involvement, Acta Radiol. Diagn. 23 (1982) 305.

[157] J.F. Mallet, et al., Les cyphoses par spondylodiscite grave du nourrisson et du jeune enfant, Rev. Chir. Orthop. 70 (1984) 63.

[158] L.K. Ammari, P.A. Offit, A.B. Campbell, Unusual presentation of group B streptococcus osteomyelitis, Pediatr. Infect. Dis. J. 11 (1992) 1066.

[159] N. Altman, et al., Evaluation of the infant spine by direct sagittal computed tomography, AJNR Am. J. Neuroradiol. 6 (1985) 65.

[160] R. Bolivar, S. Kohl, L.K. Pickering, Vertebral osteomyelitis in children: report of 4 cases, Pediatrics 62 (1978) 549.

[161] H. Bode, W. Kunzer, Dornfortsatzosteomyelitis der Brustwirbel 10 und 11 bei einem Neugeborenen, Klin. Paediatr. 197 (1985) 65.

[162] T.A. McCook, A.H. Felman, E. Ayoub, Streptococcal skeletal infections: observations in four infections, AJR Am. J. Roentgenol. 130 (1978) 465.

[163] S.H. Ein, et al., Osteomyelitis of the cervical spine presenting as a neurenteric cyst, J. Pediatr. Surg. 23 (1988) 779.

[164] B.M. Halbstein, Bone regeneration in infantile osteomyelitis: report of a case with 14-year follow-up, J. Bone. Joint. Surg. Am. 49 (1967) 149.

[165] B. Miller, Regeneration of the lateral femoral condyle after osteomyelitis in infancy, Clin. Orthop. 65 (1969) 163.

[166] G.C. Lloyd-Roberts, Suppurative arthritis of infancy: some observations upon prognosis and management, J. Bone. Joint. Surg. Br. 42 (1960) 706.

[167] R.D. Singson, et al., Missing" femoral condyle: an unusual sequela to neonatal osteomyelitis and septic arthritis, Radiology 161 (1986) 359.

[168] C.M.C. Potter, Osteomyelitis in the newborn, J. Bone. Joint. Surg. Br. 36 (1954) 578.

[169] J. Troger, et al., Diagnose und Differentialdiagnose der akuten hämatogenen Osteomyelitis des Säuglings, Radiologe 19 (1979) 99.

[170] A. Vallcanera, et al., Osteochondroma post osteomyelitis, Pediatr. Radiol. 26 (1996) 680.

[171] D. Jaramillo, et al., Osteomyelitis and septic arthritis in children: appropriate use of imaging to guide treatment, Am. J. Radiol. 165 (1995) 399.

[172] F.M. Volberg, et al., Unreliability of radiographic diagnosis of septic hip in children, Pediatrics 74 (1984) 118.

[173] M.D. Perkins, et al., Neonatal group B streptococcal osteomyelitis and suppurative arthritis: outpatient therapy, Clin. Pediatr. 28 (1989) 229.

[174] D.S. Schauwecker, E.M. Braunstein, L.J. Wheat, Diagnostic imaging of osteomyelitis, Infect. Dis. Clin. North Am. 4 (1990) 441.

[175] S.G. Moore, et al., Pediatric musculoskeletal MR imaging, Radiology 179 (1991) 345.

[176] V.J. Harris, W. Meeks, The frequency of radiolucencies underlying cephalohematomas, Pediatr. Radiol. 9 (1970) 391.

[177] M. Einhorn, D.B. Howard, R. Dagan, The use of ultrasound in the diagnosis and management of childhood acute hematogenous osteomyelitis (abstract Pub 77), Thirty-First Interscience Conference on Antimicrobial Agents and Chemotherapy, Anaheim, CA, 1992 October.

[178] S.L. Williamson, et al., Ultrasound in advanced pediatric osteomyelitis: a report of 5 cases, Pediatr. Radiol. 21 (1991) 288.

[179] M.M. Abiri, M. Kirpekar, R.C. Ablow, Osteomyelitis: detection with US, Radiology 172 (1989) 509.

[180] M.M. Zeiger, U. Dorr, R.D. Schulz, Ultrasonography of hip joint effusions, Skeletal Radiol. 16 (1987) 607.

[181] S. Velkes, A. Ganel, A. Chechick, Letter to the editor, Clin. Orthop. 260 (1990) 309.

[182] L.P. Rubin, M.T. Wallach, B.P. Wood, Radiological case of the month, Arch. Pediatr. Adolesc. Med. 150 (1996) 217.

[183] T.W. Riebel, R. Nasir, O. Nazarenko, The value of sonography in the detection of osteomyelitis, Pediatr. Radiol. 26 (1996) 291.

[184] N.B. Wright, G.T. Abbott, H.M.L. Carty, Ultrasound in children with osteomyelitis, Clin. Radiol. 50 (1995) 623.

[185] H.T. Harcke Jr., Bone imaging in infants and children: a review, J. Nucl. Med. 19 (1978) 324.

[186] J.M. Ash, D.L. Gilday, The futility of bone scanning neonatal osteomyelitis: concise communication, J. Nucl. Med. 21 (1980) 417.

[187] D.L. Gilday, D.J. Paul, Diagnosis of osteomyelitis in children by combined blood pool and bone imaging, Radiology 117 (1975) 331.

[188] S.T. Canale, Does aspiration of bones and joints affect results of later bone scanning? J. Pediatr. Orthop. 5 (1985) 23.

[189] P.D. Traughber, et al., Negative bone scans of joints after aspiration or arthrography: experimental studies, AJR Am. J. Roentgenol. 146 (1986) 87.

[190] W.A. Herndon, et al., Nuclear imaging for musculoskeletal infections in children, J. Pediatr. Orthop. 5 (1985) 343.

[191] J.S. Lewin, et al., Acute osteomyelitis in children: combined Tc-99m and Ga-67 imaging, Radiology 158 (1986) 795.

[192] I.D. Berkowitz, W. Wenzel, Normal" technetium bone scans in patients with acute osteomyelitis, Am J. Dis. Child. 134 (1980) 828.

[193] H. Handmaker, S.T. Giammona, Improved early diagnosis of acute inflammatory skeletal-articular diseases in children: a two-radiopharmaceutical approach, Pediatrics 73 (1984) 661.

[194] G.L. Melson, et al., In vitro effects of iodinated arthrographic contrast media on bacterial growth, Radiology 112 (1974) 593.

[195] W.G. Cole, R.E. Dalziel, S. Leitl, Treatment of acute osteomyelitis in childhood, J. Bone. Joint. Surg. Br. 64 (1982) 218.

[196] M.N. Rasool, S. Govender, The skeletal manifestations of congenital syphilis: a review of 197 cases, J. Bone. Joint. Surg. Br. 71 (1989) 752.

[197] S.K. Hiva, J.B. Ganapati, J.B. Patel, Early congenital syphilis: clinicoradiologic features in 202 patients, Sex. Transm. Dis. 12 (1985) 177.

[198] S. McLean, The roentgenographic and pathologic aspects of congenital osseous syphilis, Am. J. Dis. Child. 41 (1931) 130 363, 607, 887, 1128, 1411.

[199] V. Ewerbeck, et al., Knochentumoren und tumorähnliche Veränderungen im Neugeborenen-und Säuglingsalter, Z. Orthop. 123 (1985) 918.

[200] S. Meyers, W. Lonon, K. Shannon, Suppurative bursitis in early childhood, Pediatr. Infect. Dis. 3 (1984) 156.

[201] M.J. Brian, M. O'Ryan, D. Waagner, Prepatellar bursitis in an infant caused by group B streptococcus, Pediatr. Infect. Dis. J. 11 (1992) 502.

[202] M.A. Keller, et al., Systemic candidiasis in infants: a case presentation and literature review, Am J. Dis. Child. 131 (1977) 1260.

[203] V.M. Reiser, N. Rupp, D. Färber, Röntgenologische Befunde bei der septischen Candida-Arthritis, Rofo 129 (1978) 335.

[204] L. Businco, et al., Disseminated arthritis and osteitis by *Candida albicans* in a two month old infant receiving parenteral nutrition, Acta Paediatr. Scand. 66 (1977) 393.

[205] A.J. Rudolph, et al., Osseous manifestations of the congenital rubella syndrome, Am. J. Dis. Child. 110 (1965) 428.

[206] D.F. Merten, C.A. Gooding, Skeletal manifestations of congenital cytomegalic inclusion disease, Radiology 95 (1970) 333.

[207] H.B. Jenson, M.F. Robert, Congenital cytomegalovirus infection with osteolytic lesions: use of DNA hybridization in diagnosis, Clin. Pediatr. 26 (1987) 448.

[208] E.G. Chalhub, et al., Congenital herpes simplex type II infection with extensive hepatic calcification, bone lesions and cataracts: complete postmortem examination, Dev. Med. Child. Neurol. 19 (1977) 527.

[209] E.T. Madsen, Fractures of the extremities in the newborn, Acta Obstet. Gynecol. Scand. 34 (1955) 41.

[210] J. Caffey, Pediatric X-ray Diagnosis, sixth ed., Year Book Medical Publishers, Chicago, 1972.

[211] H.M. Park, C.B. Kernek, J.A. Robb, Early scintigraphic findings of occult femoral and tibial fractures in infants, Clin. Nucl. Med. 13 (1988) 271.

[212] G.S. Marshall, K.M. Edwards, W.B. Wadlington, Sporadic congenital Caffey's disease, Clin. Pediatr. 26 (1987) 177.

[213] S.D. Ravenel, Cellulitis from extravasation of calcium gluconate simulating osteomyelitis, Am. J. Dis. Child. 137 (1983) 402.

[214] R.E. Ringel, et al., Periosteal changes secondary to prostaglandin administration, J. Pediatr. 103 (1983) 251.

[215] S.P. Ditkowsky, et al., Normal periosteal reactions and associated soft-tissue findings, Clin. Pediatr. 9 (1970) 515.

[216] J.D. Nelson, Follow up: the bacterial etiology and antibiotic management of septic arthritis in infants and children, Pediatrics 50 (1972) 437.

[217] G.I. Cooper, C.C. Hopkins, Rapid diagnosis of intravascular catheter-associated infection by direct Gram staining of catheter segments, N. Engl. J. Med. 312 (1985) 1142.

[218] V. Schauf, et al., Antibiotic-killing kinetics of group B streptococci, J. Pediatr. 89 (1976) 194.

[219] H.F. Chambers, et al., Endocarditis due to methicillin-resistant *Staphylococcus aureus* in rabbits: expression of resistance to β-lactam antibiotics in vivo and in vitro, J. Infect. Dis. 149 (1984) 894.

[220] L. Sann, et al., Evolution of serum prealbumin, C-reactive protein, and orosomucoid in neonates with bacterial infection, J. Pediatr. 105 (1984) 977.

[221] A.G.S. Philip, Acute-phase proteins in neonatal infection, J. Pediatr. 105 (1984) 940.

[222] J.E. Fajardo, et al., Oral dicloxacillin for the treatment of neonatal osteomyelitis. Letter to the editor, Am. J. Dis. Child. 138 (1984) 991.

[223] G.J. Schwartz, T. Hegyi, A. Spitzer, Subtherapeutic dicloxacillin levels in a neonate: possible mechanisms, J. Pediatr. 89 (1976) 310.

[224] J.D. Nelson, Options for outpatient management of serious infections, Pediatr. Infect. Dis. J. 11 (1992) 175.

[225] L.M. Dunkle, Towards optimum management of serious focal infections: the model of suppurative arthritis, Pediatr. Infect. Dis. J. 8 (1989) 195.

[226] P.J. Howard, Sepsis in normal and premature infants with localization in the hip joint, Pediatrics 20 (1957) 279.

[227] L. Borella, et al., Septic arthritis in childhood, J. Pediatr. 62 (1963) 742.

[228] D. Halder, et al., Neonatal septic arthritis, Southeast Asian J. Trop. Med. Public Health 27 (1996) 600.

[229] W.N. Gilmour, Acute hematogenous osteomyelitis, J. Bone. Joint. Surg. Br. 44 (1962) 841.

[230] E.C. Allibone, C.P. Mills, Osteomyelitis of the premaxilla, Arch. Dis. Child. 36 (1961) 562.

[231] G. Boete, Zur Frage der Spätschäden nach Kieferosteomyelitis von Säuglingen und Kleinkindern, Arch. Klin. Exp. Ohren. Nasen. Kehlkopfheilkd. 187 (1966) 674.

[232] F. Cavanagh, Osteomyelitis of the superior maxilla in infants: a report on 24 personally treated cases, BMJ 1 (1960) 468.

[233] C.R. McCash, N.L. Rowe, Acute osteomyelitis of the maxilla in infancy, J. Bone. Joint. Surg. Br. 35 (1953) 22.

[234] A.O. Wilensky, The pathogenesis and treatment of acute osteomyelitis of the jaws in nurslings and infants, Am. J. Dis. Child. 43 (1932) 431.

[235] M.H. Bass, Acute osteomyelitis of the superior maxilla in young infants, Am. J. Dis. Child. 35 (1928) 65.

[236] J.F. Webb, Newborn infants and breast abscesses of staphylococcal origin, Can. Med. Assoc. J. 70 (1954) 382.

[237] S.K. Wong, K.R. Wilhelmus, Infantile maxillary osteomyelitis, J. Pediatr. Ophthalmol. Strabismus 23 (1986) 153.

[238] E.D. Burnard, Proptosis as the first sign of orbital sepsis in the newborn, Br. J. Ophthalmol. 43 (1959) 9.

[239] K.H. Hahlbrock, Über die Oberkieferosteomyelitis des Säuglings, Klin. Monatsbl. Augenheilkd. 145 (1964) 744.

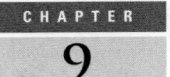

CHAPTER 9

BACTERIAL INFECTIONS OF THE URINARY TRACT

Sarah S. Long ⊕ **Jerome O. Klein**

CHAPTER OUTLINE

Epidemiology 311
Microbiology 311
Pathogenesis 311
Pathology 315
Clinical Manifestations 315
Diagnosis 316
   Culture of Urine 316

   Culture of Blood and Cerebrospinal Fluid 316
   Examination of Urine Sediment 317
   Examination of Blood 318
   Chemical Determinations 318
   Imaging of the Urinary Tract 318
Management and Prevention 319
Prognosis 319

In 1918, Helmholz [1] recognized the cryptogenic nature and underdiagnosis of urinary tract infection (UTI) in the newborn. His observations still hold true today. There are no specific signs of UTI in a newborn; the clinical presentation can vary, ranging from fever with or without other signs of septicemia to minimal changes such as alteration in feeding habits or poor weight gain. The diagnosis of UTI in a neonate is made only by the examination and culture of a properly obtained specimen of urine.

The reported incidence, clinical manifestations, and prognosis of UTI in neonates have varied significantly. There are at least two reasons for discrepant results obtained in studies of UTI: (1) Different criteria have been used to define UTI, and (2) infants with different characteristics have been studied. Before 1960, clean-voided specimens were used almost exclusively for examination and culture of urine. It is now clear that contamination is frequent when this method is used; Schlager and coworkers [2] observed that 16 cultures of urine obtained by bag collection from 98 healthy newborns yielded greater than 10^4 colonies per milliliter of urine, with organisms that were found also on periurethral skin.

The only reliable methods for obtaining urine for bacteriologic study are percutaneous aspiration and urethral catheterization of bladder urine.

Bacterial infections of the kidney and urinary tract in neonates usually are acquired at or after delivery. Fungal infections develop as nosocomial infections in infants with risk factors such as prematurity and use of intravascular catheters, parenteral alimentation, and broad-spectrum antibiotics or after prolonged or intermittent catheterization of the urinary tract [3,4]. Viral infections, including rubella, herpes simplex, and cytomegalovirus infections, are responsible for in utero infection, although the organisms can be excreted in the urine for months after birth. Bacterial infections of the urinary tract (other than those related to *Neisseria gonorrhoeae*, *Staphylococcus aureus*, and group B streptococci) are reviewed here. For information about infection and disease of the kidney and urinary tract caused by other microorganisms, the reader is referred to the chapters on toxoplasmosis, rubella, cytomegalovirus, herpes simplex, syphilis, the mycoplasmas, *Candida*, group B streptococci, gonorrhea, staphylococcal infection, and neonatal diarrhea (*Salmonella*).

EPIDEMIOLOGY

The incidence of UTI in infants in the first month of life varies, ranging from 0.1% to 1% in older studies [5–11]. Using a national database for 2003, rate of hospitalization for UTI was 53.6/100,000 population younger than 1 month of age [12]. Frequency may be 10% in infants of low birth weight [13] and 12% to 25% in infants of very low birth weight evaluated for sepsis (Table 9–1) [14,15]. In contrast to the increased incidence of bacteriuria among females in other age groups, infection of the urinary tract in the first 3 months of life is more frequent in males [2,5–10,15,17].

Infection of the urinary tract is usually sporadic, but clusters of cases, closely related in time, have been reported from nurseries in Cleveland [18] and Baltimore [19]. A nursery epidemic caused by *Serratia marcescens* was responsible for UTI and balanitis. The outbreak was caused by contamination of a solution applied to the umbilical cord [20].

Surveys of infants born in U.S. Army medical centers and subsequently hospitalized for UTI indicate that uncircumcised boys have more UTIs than circumcised boys in the first month and in months 2 to 12 of life (Table 9–2) [11,21,22]. In 1982, Ginsburg and McCracken [23] observed that 95% of 62 infant boys with UTI were uncircumcised. A case-control study performed in 112 infant boys in whom suprapubic aspiration or bladder catheterization had been performed for investigation of acute illness showed that all infants with UTI were uncircumcised compared with 32% of controls [24]. Infection was associated with anatomic abnormalities in 26% of cases. In a meta-analysis of infants younger than 3 months who were evaluated for fever, rates of UTI were 7.5% for girls, 2.4% for circumcised boys, and 20.1% for uncircumcised boys [25]. The records of more than 136,000 boys born in U.S. Army hospitals from 1980-1985 were reviewed through the first month of life to compare clinical courses in uncircumcised and circumcised boys [26]. Of 35,929 uncircumcised boys, 88 (0.24%) had UTI, 33 had concomitant bacteremia, 3 had meningitis, 2 had renal failure, and 2 died. Complications followed 0.19% of 100,157 circumcisions (including 20 UTIs), and all were minor except for three episodes of hemorrhage leading to transfusion. Meta-analysis of nine published studies through 1992 yielded an overall 12-fold increased risk of infection in uncircumcised boys [27].

In 1989, the American Academy of Pediatrics (AAP) rescinded a 1971 position against circumcision, recognizing the relative safety of the procedure and protection against UTI in the first year of life [28]. More recent studies using case-control and cohort design also support an association, with threefold to sevenfold magnitude of risk for uncircumcised boys [29,30]. In 1999, the AAP revised the recommendation, citing that although existing scientific evidence shows potential medical benefits of newborn male circumcision, data are insufficient to recommend its routine performance [31].

Ritual Jewish circumcision performed on the 8th day of life, when periurethral bacterial colonization has been established, seems to have attendant risk for UTI. An epidemiologic study in Israel revealed excessive UTIs in boys only from days 9 to 20 of life (the postcircumcision period) [32]. A case-control study identified performance by a nonphysician (mohel) versus a physician as a risk factor for UTI (odds ratio 4.34); the authors postulate technique of hemostasis and duration of the shaft wrapping as responsible factors [33].

MICROBIOLOGY

Escherichia coli continues to be responsible for most community-acquired infections of the urinary tract in infants younger than 3 months, accounting for 90% or more cases reported through the 1990s [34–36], with lower prevalence since, possibly related to widespread use of intrapartum chemoprophylaxis [4,37]. Many O serotypes of *E. coli* have been associated with UTI. UTI in neonates was associated with a limited number of O:K:H serotypes with P fimbriae, adhesive capacity, hemolysin production, and serum resistance [38,39]. The serotypes of *E. coli* associated with diarrhea rarely cause UTI, however. Cultures of urine can be positive in infants with septicemia caused by group B streptococci, but primary infection of the urinary tract without septicemia is uncommon [17,40]. Community-associated UTI in neonates with or without bloodstream infection has been reported caused by *Staphylococcus aureus* [37,41].

The incidence of neonatal UTI as a complication of intensive care has increased sharply in recent years; intensive care–associated UTI occurs in patients with and without urinary catheters [3]. Microbiology of neonatal nosocomial UTI is dramatically different from that observed in neonatal intensive care units in the 1970s (Table 9–3), with *E. coli* supplanted by other Enterobacteriaceae genera, *Pseudomonas*, *Enterococcus*, *Candida*, and coagulase-negative staphylococci [3,4,14,15,42–44]. Multiple pathogens may be present; Maherzi and colleagues [9] identified more than one bacterial pathogen in 4 of 43 infants with UTI documented by aspiration of bladder urine.

S. aureus and *E. coli* have been responsible for localized suppurative disease of the urinary tract in neonates, including prostatitis, orchitis, and epididymitis [45–49]. Other examples of focal disease in the urinary tract include orchitis caused by *Pseudomonas aeruginosa* [50] and testicular abscess caused by *Salmonella enteritidis* [51]. Blood cultures frequently are positive in affected infants. Bacteria responsible for infections of the circumcision site are discussed in "Infections of the Skin and Subcutaneous Tissue" in Chapter 10.

PATHOGENESIS

In older children and adults, most UTIs are thought to occur by the ascending route after introduction of bacteria through the urethral meatus. Less frequently, blood-borne infection of the kidney occurs. In neonates, it is frequently difficult to know whether UTI was the cause or the result of bacteremia. The predominance of males among infants younger than 3 months with UTI contrasts with the predominance of females in all other age groups. This difference may reflect increased risk of UTI in young uncircumcised boys; increased prevalence of urinary and renal anomalies in boys; transient

TABLE 9-1 Incidence of Urinary Tract Infections in Newborn Infants: Results of Eight Studies

| Study | Methods Used to Obtain Urine | No. Infected/No. Studied (%) | Gender | | | | Birth Weight | | | |
| | | | Male | | Female | | <2500 g | | >2500 g | |
			No. Surveyed	No. Infected	No. Surveyed	No. Infected	No. Surveyed	No. Infected	No. Surveyed	No. Infected
Christchurch, NZ, 1968-1969[5]	CVS, SPA	14/1460 (0.95)	757	11	703	3	NS	—	NS	—
Göteborg, 1960-1966[6]	CVS	75*/57,000 (0.14)	NS	54	NS	21	NS	11	NS	64
New York, 1973[†]	CVS, SPA	12/1042 (1.2)	493	7	549	5	206	6	836	6
Leeds, 1967[8]	CVS, SPA	8/600 (1.3)	309	7	291	1	NS	0	NS	8
Oklahoma City, 1974[13]	SPA	10/102 (10)	NS	NS	NS	NS	102	10	—	—
Lausanne, 1978[9†]	CVS, SPA	43/1762[‡] (2.4)	1006	26	756	7	634[§]	10	1028[¶]	33
Göteborg, 1977-1980[10†]	CVS, SPA	26/198 (0.81)	1502	23	1696	3	—	—	—	—
U.S. Army, 1975-1984[11]**	SPA, Ca	320/422,328 (0.08)	217,116	162	205,212	158	—	—	—	—

*Five male infants with infection and suspected or proven obstruction malformation of urinary tract not included.
†Date of published report; years of study not provided.
‡Includes only infants <28 days of age who were admitted to neonatal intensive care unit.
§Results reported for premature infants (<259 days' gestation).
¶Results reported for term infants (≥259 days' gestation).
¶Results reported for infants 1 wk to 2 mo of age.
**Results reported for infants 1 wk to 2 mo of age who were hospitalized.
Ca, catheter; CVS, clean-voided specimen; NS, not stated; SPA, suprapubic aspiration (of bladder urine).

TABLE 9–2   Incidence of Urinary Tract Infections during the First Year of Life in Infants Born at U.S. Army Hospitals

Study Location and Characteristics	Female Infants	Male Infants	
		Circumcised	Not Circumcised
Tripler Army Hospital (January 1982–June 1983)*			
No. infants	2759	1919	583
No. infants with UTI	13 (0.47%)	4 (0.21%)	24 (4.12%)
Mean age at diagnosis (mo)	2.5	1.4	1.7
Brooke Army Hospital (January 1980–December 1983)†			
No. infants	1905	1575	444
No. infants with UTI	8 (0.42%)	0	8 (1.8%)
Mean age at diagnosis (mo)	4.4	—	1.7
U.S. Army Hospital (January 1975–December 1984)†			
No. infants	205,212	175,317	41,799
No. infants with UTI	1164 (0.57%)	193 (0.11%)	468 (1.12%)
Mean age at diagnosis (mo)	3.9	2.7	2.5

*Data from Wiswell TE, Smith FR, Bass JW. Decreased incidence of urinary tract infection in circumcised males. Pediatrics 75:901, 1985.
†Data from Wiswell TE, Roscelli JD. Corroborative evidence for the decreased incidence of urinary tract infections in circumcised male infants. Pediatrics 78:96, 1986.

TABLE 9–3   Pathogens Responsible for Urinary Tract Infections in Neonatal Intensive Care Units

Organism	Frequency (%) of Isolations of Each Pathogen		
	1969-1978*	1989-1992†	1991-2007‡
Escherichia coli	75.3	10.5	24.8
Klebsiella species	13.4	10.5	25.5
Enterobacter species	1.4	12.3	14.3
Enterococcus species	2.1	14	4.9
Coagulase-negative staphylococci	1.4	31.6	4.3
Candida species	—	12.3	15.5
Other	6.4	8.8	8.7

*Data from 139 patients in nurseries and intensive care nurseries from references [5], [6], [8], and [9].
†Data from 50 patients in neonatal intensive care units from references [42] and [43].
‡Data from 161 patients in neonatal intensive care units from references [4], [14], [15], and [44].

urodynamic dysfunction; vesicoureteral reflux (VUR), which predominantly affects male infants; and the occasional UTI that complicates circumcision. Additionally, bacteremia is more frequent in male infants, and it is likely that hematogenous invasion of the kidney can cause UTI in neonates.

Anatomic or physiologic abnormalities of the urinary tract play a role in the development and consequences of infection in some infants. Obstructive uropathy is the most important. Infection often is the first indication of an abnormality. Infection was the presenting sign in half of 40 infants younger than 2 months of age with anomalies of the kidneys or ureters reported in 1980 [52]. Congenital obstruction of the urinary tract was diagnosed in 5 of 80 children with UTI studied in Göteborg [6] and in 2 of 60 children studied in Leeds [53]; important radiologic abnormalities of the urinary tract were identified in 10 of 46 infant boys and 3 of 13 infant girls younger than 3 months from 1972-1982 in Christchurch, New

Zealand [54]. Increasingly, antenatal ultrasonography identifies fetuses with significant anatomic abnormalities, and early neonatal intervention (with prophylactic use of antibiotics or surgery or both) may decrease likelihood of infection.

VUR is identified in many infants with UTI who are examined by radiologic techniques. It is frequently the result of infection, but also can be a primary defect. VUR is not a prerequisite for upper tract infection (i.e., pyelonephritis); in two studies, less than half of children with pyelonephritis by scintigraphy had VUR [55,56]. Majd and coworkers [57] found that 23 of 29 (79%) children hospitalized for UTI who were found to have reflux had pyelonephritis by scintigraphy; 39 of 65 (60%) children without reflux also were found to have pyelonephritis. VUR can be a congenital abnormality. Fetal ultrasonography showed that 30 of 107 infants with prenatally diagnosed urinary tract abnormalities had reflux, which was the only abnormality found postnatally in 10 infants [58]. Gordon and colleagues [59] observed that 16 of 25 infants with dilation of the fetal urinary tract had reflux, which was of grade 3 to 5 severity in 79%. In Austrian infants, 39 urinary tract abnormalities detected prenatally were compared with 46 urinary tract abnormalities found after first UTI [60]. Obstructive lesions and multicystic dysplastic malformations of the kidneys accounted for 90% of all prenatally diagnosed malformations, and reflux accounted for only 10%. By contrast, reflux accounted for 59% of abnormalities detected after the first UTI.

VUR detected prenatally has a male-to-female distribution of 6:1 (in contrast to VUR detected after UTI, when females predominate) [61], may be determined developmentally by the site of the origin of the ureteral bud from the wolffian duct, and in severe cases can be associated with congenital renal damage consisting of global parenchymal loss (so-called reflux nephropathy) [62]. Gunn and colleagues [63] performed ultrasound examinations of 3228 fetuses; no renal tract abnormalities were detected before 28 weeks of gestation. Subsequently, 3856 fetuses were examined by ultrasonography after

28 weeks of gestation. Urinary tract anomalies were identified in 313 fetuses; 15 had major structural abnormalities, all of which were confirmed postnatally. In 298 (7.7%) of the fetuses, dilated renal pelvis with normal bladder was found; most of the cases resolved spontaneously, but 40 of the cases were confirmed postnatally to be due to serious abnormalities (usually obstruction or VUR) [64]. In one study, preterm infants with nosocomial UTI had a lower incidence of VUR than that noted in term infants with nosocomial UTI [15]; however, in another study comparing 250 neonates (mean gestation age 39 weeks) with community-associated UTI with 51 neonates (mean gestation age 36 weeks) with nosocomial UTI, the neonates with nosocomial infection were more likely to have VUR and abnormal renal ultrasound examination [4].

Isolated mild renal pyelectasis (i.e., <10 mm diameter of the collecting duct and without VUR) in fetuses is likely to be transient, unassociated with pathology or risk for UTI [65,66]. In one study, 54% of such cases had resolved in the first postnatal month, and 85% of the cases of moderate or severe pelviectasis had resolved or improved over the first 2 years of life [67]. In a long-term study performed in the United Kingdom of 425 infants with antenatally detected hydronephrosis, 284 had normal findings on neonatal ultrasound examination; negative predictive value of normal ultrasound findings for subsequent UTI in the first year of life was 99% [68].

In a more recent 5-year retrospective statewide, cohort analysis of 522 Washington infants with birth-hospital discharge diagnosis of antenatal hydronephrosis (not quantified further) and 2610 control infants, hospitalization for UTI in the first year of life was 5% versus 1% (relative risk 11.8, 95% confidence interval 6.8 to 20.5). Relative risk for UTI was higher especially among girls with antenatal hydronephrosis (relative risk 36.3, 95% confidence interval 10.6 to 124.0) [69]. In a 17-year study from a single institution in Seoul of 480 infants with antenatal and postnatal hydronephrosis without VUR, UTI developed in the first year of life in 39% of infants with obstructive uropathy compared with 11% without obstructive uropathy ($P < .001$). Higher grade of hydronephrosis and presence of hydroureteronephrosis were associated with higher incidence of UTI [70].

Results of a long-term outcome study of 125 infants in the Netherlands with antenatal hydronephrosis suggested that a cutoff of less than 15 mm anterior-posterior diameter of the renal pelvis identified infants at low risk for UTI or surgical conditions and low incidence and benign course of VUR [71]. In a long-term study in Toronto of 260 infants with a diagnosis of prenatal hydronephrosis, 25 also had VUR (grade 3 or higher in 73%), received antibiotic prophylaxis, and did not have surgical correction during 4 years of follow-up. Breakthrough infection occurred in only four patients. Improvement was seen in most of the children with VUR, and there was no difference in renal growth in children who had resolved versus unresolved VUR or high-grade versus low-grade VUR [72]. Postnatal management of prenatal hydronephrosis is controversial. Many experts favor evaluation of even mild cases by postnatal ultrasonography and voiding cystourethrography [73].

The outcome of interest for strategies to identify obstructive uropathy, hydronephrosis, VUR, and UTI is to attempt to lessen renal damage. Except for obstructive uropathies, the relative impacts and benefits of special management of hydronephrosis and VUR are increasingly controversial. A National Institutes of Health multicenter, randomized, placebo-controlled, double-blind study has been designed to determine preventive effect of antimicrobial prophylaxis on recurrent UTI and renal scarring in children with primary VUR (i.e., not due to increased bladder pressure as from a neurogenic bladder, outlet obstruction, or other vesicular anomalies) [74]. Chesney and colleagues [75] commented on background knowledge and rationale for the study design. A few relevant points are as follows: (1) The percentage of patients with recurrent UTIs and VUR who develop renal scarring is small. (2) Many children, even those with high-grade VUR, do not develop scars. (3) Patients without VUR who have recurrent UTI can develop scars. (4) Older studies (with poorer outcomes) included patients with secondary VUR (i.e., high-pressure VUR) and genetic renal syndromes. (5) Trials of antimicrobial prophylaxis or surgery or both for VUR generally are underpowered and do not include a nonintervention arm. (6) In a Cochrane analysis using 10 trials involving 964 children, authors could not conclude that identification and treatment of children with VUR conferred a long-term benefit.

In a multicenter, randomized controlled follow-up trial of antimicrobial prophylaxis compared with no prophylaxis in 100 Italian infants with grades II through IV VUR, prophylaxis had no effect on recurrences of UTI, renal scarring, or persistence of VUR. Recurrences in the prophylaxis group were caused by multidrug-resistant bacteria, whereas recurrences in the group not receiving prophylaxis all were due to antibiotic-susceptible *E. coli* [76].

Bacterial virulence factors are likely to play an important role in the pathogenesis of UTIs. Strains of *E. coli* causing UTI are a selected sample of the fecal flora. Pyelonephritic isolates belong to a restricted number of serotypes, are resistant to the bactericidal effect of serum, attach to uroepithelial cells, and produce hemolysins [77]. Pili on the bacterial cell surface that adhere to specific receptors on epithelial cells may play a role in development of UTI [38]. Some of these features of pyelonephritic strains of *E. coli* have been shown in UTIs in newborns [38,39].

The increased rate of UTIs in uncircumcised boys is likely to be associated with periurethral bacterial flora. During the first 6 months of life, uncircumcised boys have significantly higher total urethral bacterial colony counts and more frequent isolation and higher colony counts of uropathogenic organisms such as *E. coli, Klebsiella-Enterobacter* species, *Proteus,* and *Pseudomonas* [78]. With increasing age, the foreskin is more easily retracted, and penile hygiene improves; by 12 months of age, the excessive periurethral flora and UTIs in uncircumcised boys almost disappear [22,78].

Natural defenses in the urinary tract include antibacterial properties of urine, antiadherence mechanisms, mechanical effects of urinary flow and micturition, presence of phagocytic cells, antibacterial properties of the urinary tract mucosa, and immune mechanisms [79]. There is scant knowledge about these mechanisms in the newborn.

PATHOLOGY

The histologic appearance of acute pyelonephritis in newborns is similar to that in the adult [80]. Polymorphonuclear leukocytes are present in the glomeruli, the tubules, and the interstitial tissues. The renal pelvis can show signs of acute inflammation, with loss of the lining epithelium and necrosis. Focal suppuration can be present in the kidney, prostate, or testis. In disease of longer duration, the interstitial tissue is infiltrated with lymphocytes, plasma cells, and eosinophils. The number of glomeruli may be decreased, and some may be hyalinized. The epithelium of tubules is atrophic, and the lumen is filled with colloid casts. Pericapsular fibrosis is present in some infants. If the infant dies within 6 months, there is little scarring or contraction of the kidney. Reversible hydronephrosis and hydroureter are observed manifestations of acute pyelonephritis in the neonate who has no anatomic abnormality or VUR. It is postulated that bacteria and endotoxins inhibit ureteral peristalsis.

Pathologic processes indicative of additional suppurative infections, such as otitis media, pneumonia, and meningitis, also can be seen in infants dying of acute infection of the urinary tract. Hepatocellular damage and bile stasis may be noted in liver sections from jaundiced infants [81].

CLINICAL MANIFESTATIONS

The signs of UTI in neonates are varied and nonspecific. Five patterns are generally observed: (1) septicemia associated with early-onset (within the first 5 days of life) or late-onset (after 5 days of age) disease (see Chapter 21); (2) acute onset of fever without apparent source; (3) insidious illness marked by low-grade fever or failure to gain weight; (4) no apparent signs; and (5) localized signs of infection, including balanitis, prostatitis, urethritis, and orchitis.

The most frequent signs of acute UTI are associated with fever or septicemia or both (see Chapter 21) (Table 9–4) [4–6,8,9]. Less acute and nonspecific manifestations also are common, and the presenting signs include

TABLE 9–4 Clinical Manifestations of Urinary Tract Infections in Newborn Infants

Clinical Manifestations	% of Infants with Manifestations*
Fever	55
Vomiting	27
Failure to thrive	26
Poor feeding	24
Irritability or lethargy	17
Jaundice	10
Diarrhea	8

*When sign was not mentioned in report, the number of infants in the report was removed from the denominator used to determine the percentage of infants with manifestations.
Data from references [4–6], [8], [9].

poor weight gain, vomiting, and poor feeding. Fever was a less common feature of nosocomial UTI in one study compared with community-associated cases [4]. Enlargement of the liver and spleen and distention of the abdomen can be present. The kidneys may be enlarged or abnormal in shape or position, and anomalies of the urethra and penis also can occur. Signs associated with renal anomalies (e.g., a single umbilical artery, supernumerary nipples, spina bifida, low-set ears, and anorectal abnormalities) are seen in some infants.

Jaundice is an important feature of UTI and can be the presenting sign [81,82]; it is frequently sudden in onset and clears rapidly after adequate antimicrobial therapy. Many infants with UTI and jaundice have positive blood cultures [19,82]. Of 306 infants in one study admitted to the hospital within 21 days of birth solely because of indirect hyperbilirubinemia (mean peak serum bilirubin level 18.5 mg/dL), 90% were breast-fed, and none had a positive culture of urine or blood [83]. In another study, 12 of 160 (7.5%) infants younger than 8 weeks of age evaluated solely for jaundice had UTI confirmed by bladder catheterization, however. Renal ultrasound was abnormal in 6 of 11 infants. Infection was especially associated with elevated conjugated bilirubin and age of more than 8 days [84]. In a study of 100 infants whose sole abnormality was jaundice lasting beyond 2 weeks of age, all were breast-fed, and 6 had UTI [85].

A reported case of severe methemoglobinemia observed in a 3-week-old infant with *E. coli* UTI was postulated to be caused by nitrite-forming bacteria, but concurrent diarrhea, dehydration, and acidosis may have been precipitating factors [86]. Hyperammonemic encephalopathy caused by *Proteus* infection in children with urinary tract obstruction or atony also has been described [87]. Bacteriuria without apparent signs of illness also was documented occasionally in screening studies performed in the 1970s and 1980s [5,7,10,13].

Abscesses of the prostate, testis, or epididymis usually manifest as signs of septicemia, including fever, vomiting, and diarrhea [45–51]. Local signs of inflammation, including tenderness and swelling over the surface of the infected organ, may be present. Urinary retention occurs in infants with prostatitis [47]. Renal abscess is rare in neonates; at least one case report in a neonate (with congenital nephrosis) has been published [88].

UTI should be considered in the differential diagnosis for unexplained fever in early infancy. UTI with or without bacteremia is the most common cause of serious bacterial infection in infants younger than 3 months evaluated because of fever; it was responsible for 79% of cases in a Utah study [37]. Presence of UTI has been studied in thousands of infants younger than 3 months who have been evaluated because of fever by practitioners in emergency department and office settings. Rates range from 5% to 13%, depending predominantly on prevalence of circumcision in the population [89–94]. In a New York study, prevalence of UTI in febrile infant boys (82% of whom were not circumcised) was 12.4%. In a Pittsburgh study, prevalence of UTI in febrile infant boys (2% of whom were not circumcised) was only 2.9%. In a multicenter prospective study of febrile infants younger than 2 months, 9% had UTI (21% of uncircumcised boys, 5% of girls, and 2% of circumcised boys) [95]. In a study of 162 febrile Japanese infants younger than 8 weeks, 22 (13.8%) had UTI; 18 were boys, none of whom was circumcised [96].

In a study of 2411 febrile children younger than 24 months evaluated in an emergency department in Philadelphia, history of malodorous urine, prior history of UTI, and presence of abdominal tenderness were significantly associated with the diagnosis of UTI; findings were present in less than 10% of infected infants, however, and only 8% to 13% of infants with findings had UTI confirmed [36]. In a retrospective study of 354 Boston infants younger than 24 months with confirmed UTI, irritability and decreased appetite were each reported in 50% of children; diarrhea, vomiting, lethargy, and congestion were reported in 25%; and malodorous urine, apparent dysuria, frequency of urination, and abdominal pain were reported in less than 10% [17].

DIAGNOSIS

Infection of the urinary tract is defined as the presence of bacteria in urine that was obtained without contamination from the urethra or external genitalia. UTI should be considered in all infants older than 3 days of age who have fever or other signs of septicemia or who have subtle and nonspecific signs of failure to thrive during the first months of life. At present, no clinical finding or simple laboratory test adequately defines the location of infection in the urinary tract of the infant. It is assumed that bacteriuria in the neonate indicates infection throughout the urinary tract (including the kidney).

CULTURE OF URINE

Suprapubic needle aspiration of bladder urine is the most reliable technique for identifying bacteriuria. Although a negative result from culture of bag-collected urine indicates that the urine is sterile, 12% to 21% of bag-collected specimens yield results that are indeterminate or positive (colony count $\geq 10^4$/mL) [2,34], and positive results must be verified by aspiration of bladder urine or by catheterization. There is frequently insufficient time for this stepwise approach before institution of therapy. The technique of needle aspiration of the bladder has been used extensively, is technically simple and safe, and causes minimal discomfort to the infant [97]. Although most infected infants have urine specimens with bacterial colony counts of 10^5/mL or greater, any bacterial growth in urine obtained by suprapubic aspiration is significant.

Morbidity associated with suprapubic aspiration is minimal. Transient gross hematuria has been reported in 0.6% of 654 infants [97]. Gross bleeding that ceased only after cauterization was reported in one case [98]. Perforation of the bowel occurred in two cases, but this complication is avoided if the bladder is defined by palpation or percussion [98]. Hematoma of the anterior wall of the bladder [99], peritonitis [100], and anaerobic bacteremia [101] also have been reported after suprapubic aspiration. These reports warranted publication because the cases are very uncommon. The possibility of these complications should not deter the physician from using this technique for infants with suggested septicemia. Suprapubic

aspiration should not be performed, however, if the infant has recently voided, has abdominal distention, has poorly defined anomalies of the urinary tract, or has a hematologic abnormality that might result in hemorrhage.

Suprapubic aspiration of bladder urine should be performed at least 1 hour after the patient has voided. The infant should lie supine, with the lower extremities held in a frog-leg position. The suprapubic area is cleaned with iodine and alcohol. A 20-gauge, 1½-inch needle attached to a syringe is used to pierce the abdominal wall and bladder approximately 1 inch above the symphysis pubis. The needle is directed caudally toward the fundus of the bladder, and urine is aspirated gently. Vigorous aspiration should be avoided because the mucosa can be drawn in to block the needle opening. The aspirated urine is sent to the laboratory immediately in a sterile tube. If the infant urinates during the procedure, or if the procedure cannot be done properly for other reasons, aspiration should be repeated after 1 to 2 hours. Ultrasound examination may be useful in detecting the presence of urine in the bladder before suprapubic aspiration; with ultrasound-guided aspiration, the success rate for acquisition of an adequate sample of urine improved from 60% to 96.4% [102].

Catheterization of the bladder using sterile technique also is an appropriate sampling method. The incidence of infection related to catheterization in infants is unknown. Urine for culture should be transported to the laboratory as soon as possible, but if a delay is unavoidable, the specimen must be refrigerated. Isolation of 10^3 colonies/mL or greater of urine obtained by catheter may represent significant bacteriuria in this age group [103]. In multiple studies of young children evaluated because of fever (relatively few of whom were neonates), approximately 80% of the children with bacteriuria had colony counts of 10^5/mL or greater. Significant pyuria, elevated serum level of C-reactive protein (CRP), isolation of a single enteric organism, and abnormality on renal scintigraphy were each decreasingly associated with lower colony counts, with only rare positive tests in children with colony counts of less than 10^4/mL [16,17,35,104].

CULTURE OF BLOOD AND CEREBROSPINAL FLUID

Because bacteremia and meningitis can accompany UTI, cultures of the blood and cerebrospinal fluid should be obtained before therapy for UTI is begun if the neonate has fever or any signs of illness. Blood (but not cerebrospinal fluid) for culture also should be obtained from a neonate with UTI, but without specific or nonspecific signs of infection. In a study from Sweden in the 1970s [6], lumbar puncture was performed before therapy in 31 neonates with UTI; 6 infants had purulent meningitis, and in 9 infants the cerebrospinal fluid was sterile but pleocytosis (22 to 200 white blood cells [WBCs]/mm³) also was present. Blood was obtained for culture in 32 infants and was positive in 12 infants. Meningitis accompanied UTI in less than 2% of young Australian infants reported in 2007 [105]. Although sterile cerebrospinal fluid pleocytosis has been reported in association with UTI in young infants, a 2008 report of a multicenter prospective study of 1025 febrile infants younger than 2 months, in which 91 had confirmed UTI, sterile cerebrospinal fluid pleocytosis was uncommon—found in 0% to 8% depending on the definition of pleocytosis. Overinterpretation of pleocytosis resulting from traumatic lumbar puncture may be the explanation for the previously reported association [106].

Bacteremia was present in 11 of 35 (31%) Dallas infants younger than 30 days of age with UTI. The infants had been considered healthy when discharged from the nursery and were evaluated because of fever. Older infants with UTI were less likely to be bacteremic; positive cultures of blood occurred in 5 of 24 infants (21%) with UTI 1 to 2 months of age, 2 of 14 infants (14%) 2 to 3 months of age, and 1 of 18 infants (5.5%) 3 months of age or older [23]. Similarly, in Boston, bacteremia was present in 17 of 80 (21%) febrile infants with UTI younger than 1 month of age, 8 of 59 (13%) 1 to 2 months of age, and 8 of 116 (7%) 2 to 6 months of age; 4 neonates had meningitis [17]. In Pittsburgh, incidence of bacteremia in community-associated UTI was higher in infants younger than 2 months (22%) than in older infants (3%) [107]. No clinical finding or laboratory test discriminated between bacteremic and nonbacteremic infants [17]. In surveillance for UTI among 203,399 infants born in U.S. Army hospitals from 1985-1990, 23% of noncircumcised infant boys younger than 3 months with UTI had concomitant bacteremia; incidence of bacteremia associated with UTI was not different from the incidence in circumcised boys or girls with UTI [27]. Incidence of bacteremia in neonatal nosocomial UTI is higher than in community-associated infection; bacteremia occurred in 38% of cases of nosocomial UTI in one study [14].

EXAMINATION OF URINE SEDIMENT

Many studies and a meta-analysis assessing presence of WBCs in the urine of newborn infants have been performed [5,22,70,108–111]. Healthy infants can have 10 WBCs/mm³ of clean-voided urine [109]. Lincoln and Winberg [110] obtained clean-voided specimens of urine from uninfected infants younger than 1 week of age; boys had up to 25 WBCs/mm³, and girls had up to 50 WBCs/mm³.

Neither presence nor absence of pyuria is completely reliable evidence for or against UTI. Many studies have assessed urine specimens for predictive values for UTI of WBCs or organisms or detection by dipstick of leukocyte esterase or reduction of nitrate. The following results are limited to studies of acutely ill, usually febrile infants whose urine was obtained by catheterization (or suprapubic aspiration where stated). Methods of assessing pyuria and definitions of UTI vary. In 27% of unspun urine samples collected by suprapubic aspiration from Dallas infants with UTI (bacterial colony counts ≥10⁵/mL), less than 10 WBCs per high-power field were present [23]. Landau and coworkers [16] reported that among infants younger than 4 months with positive urine cultures (colony counts ≥10⁴/mL), 4 of 49 (8.2%) with acute pyelonephritis diagnosed on renal scintigraphy had less than 5 WBCs per high-power field (400×) in fresh centrifuged urine compared with 27 of 79 (34.2%) infants with UTI and negative results on scintigraphy.

Quantifying WBCs in uncentrifuged urine using a counting chamber is the most reproducible test for pyuria. Hoberman and colleagues [112] found pyuria (at least 10 WBCs/mm³ of unspun urine) absent in 22 of 190 (20%) febrile infants younger than 24 months with positive urine cultures (colony counts ≥5 × 10⁴/mL) and present in 6.7% with negative cultures; a single patient of 15 cases without pyuria in whom renal scintigraphy was performed under protocol had a positive result. In a study by Hansson and coworkers of 366 infants younger than 1 year with symptomatic UTI (colony counts ≥10³/mL from suprapubic aspirate of urine), 80% had colony counts of 10⁵/mL or greater, 13% had counts of 1 × 10⁴ to 9 × 10⁴/mL, and 7% had counts of 1 × 10³ to 9 × 10³/mL. Pyuria was significantly associated with colony count. In children with UTI with colony counts of less than 10⁵/mL, sensitivity of pyuria (>10 WBCs/mm³) was 69% compared with 88% for children with at least 10⁵ colonies/mL. Nitrate reduction test was highly insensitive; 44% of the patients had a positive result when the colony count was at least 10⁵/mL, and 11% had a positive result with lower counts [35]. Nitrate reduction would be expected to be negative in all cases in which non-Enterobacteriaceae, gram-positive cocci or *Candida* are causative. Renal scintigraphy was not performed in the study by Hansson and coworkers to estimate significance of UTI, but VUR was present equally in infants with high (30%) and low (38%) colony counts.

Dipstick test for leukocyte esterase and nitrite is inadequate to exclude the diagnosis of UTI in infants. In the study by Hoberman and colleagues [104], the test had a sensitivity of 53% and positive predictive value of 82% for detecting 10 or more WBCs/mm³; nitrite determination had a sensitivity of 31% in identifying urine cultures with growth of at least 50,000 colonies/mL. Shaw and coworkers [113] reported dipstick results in 3873 febrile children younger than 2 years evaluated for UTI; sensitivity of a positive result (trace or greater for leukocyte esterase or positive nitrite) was 79%, and positive predictive value was 46% for isolation of at least 10,000 colonies/mL from urine culture.

Microscopic hematuria is present in some infants with UTI [3,44]. Gross hematuria usually is associated with other diseases (e.g., renal vein thrombosis, polycystic disease of the kidney, obstructive uropathy, Wilms tumor) [114].

Usefulness of Gram stain of urine specimens in predicting bacteriuria has been studied prospectively in febrile infants younger than 24 months. Smears were prepared using 2 drops of uncentrifuged urine on a slide within a standardized marked area 1.5 cm in diameter, which was then air dried, fixed, and stained. The presence of at least one organism per 10 high-power fields examined using oil immersion lens was considered a positive result. Sensitivity and positive predictive value were 81% and 43% for isolation of at least 1 × 10⁴ colonies/mL of urine in Shaw and colleagues' study [113] and 93% and 57% for isolation of at least 5 × 10⁴ colonies/mL in Hoberman and coworkers' study [104]. The presence of pyuria and bacteriuria increased positive predictive value for positive cultures in both studies to 85% and 88%.

Studies of neonates with early-onset septicemia indicate that the yield for culture of urine is low [14,15,115,116]. Culture may be eliminated in evaluation of infants younger than 3 days for presumed sepsis. Examination of urine occasionally can aid in microbiologic diagnosis of early-onset septicemia, but initiation of antimicrobial therapy should not be delayed when there is difficulty in obtaining the specimen or narrowed for spectrum of activity.

EXAMINATION OF BLOOD

The peripheral blood leukocyte count varies among infants with UTI. Although significantly higher neutrophil and band counts and band-to-neutrophil ratios are documented in young children with UTI, these do not reliably discriminate among presence, absence, or level of infection in the urinary tract or presence of bacteremia [16,17,112]. In studies from New Zealand [5], half of the neonates had a peripheral blood leukocyte count of greater than 16,000/mm^3, but no information was given about this measure in uninfected infants. Hemolytic anemia frequently accompanies jaundice when the latter is present in infants with UTI. Result of the direct Coombs test usually is negative. The reticulocyte count can be normal or elevated [82].

Although signs of inflammatory response such as elevated erythrocyte sedimentation rate (ESR) or serum CRP or procalcitonin correlate generally with abnormal renal scintigraphy findings suggestive of acute pyelonephritis in children with UTI, standardized cutoff values for stand-alone positive or negative predictive tests have not been possible. In 64 children studied, Majd and colleagues [57] found abnormal scans in 78% of children with ESR of at least 25 mm/hr compared with 33% of children with lower ESR. Benador and coworkers [56] found that ESR greater than 20 mm/hr or CRP level greater than 10 mg/L had a sensitivity of 89% and specificity of 25% for identifying renal lesions among 73 children with UTI. Stokland and colleagues [117] correlated CRP level greater than 20 mg/L at the time of acute infection with resultant renal scar in 157 children reevaluated 1 year later; sensitivity of elevated CRP was 92%, and positive and negative predictive values were 41% and 80%. In 153 children with fever and positive urine culture (colony count ≥5 × 10^4/mL), Hoberman and coworkers [112] reported significant correlations between evidence of pyelonephritis versus cystitis versus asymptomatic bacteriuria with mean peripheral WBC count (22,400/mm^3 versus 14,600/mm^3 versus 11,700/mm^3), ESR (44 mm/hr versus 26.8 mm/hr versus 15.3 mm/hr), and CRP (10.1 mg/L versus 2.7 mg/L versus 1.3 mg/L). In a study using cutoff values of 1 ng/mL for procalcitonin and 20 mg/L for CRP, rates of sensitivity for detection of pyelonephritis in infants with UTI were similar (92%), but specificity of procalcitonin (62%) exceeded that of CRP (34%) [118].

CHEMICAL DETERMINATIONS

Hyperbilirubinemia is present in many infants with UTI; the percentage of conjugated bilirubin often is determined by the age of the infant at the onset of jaundice [81]. During the first week of life, almost all of the bilirubin is unconjugated, but in the second week and thereafter, the fractionation is approximately equivalent. In 80 Boston infants younger than 1 month of age with UTI, 11 (14%) had jaundice and hyperbilirubinemia; only 4 had bacteremia [17]. With the exception of changes in serum bilirubin, the results of serum hepatic enzyme tests generally are normal or only slightly abnormal [81,82]. Azotemia and hyperchloremic acidosis are not unusual; serum bicarbonate measured less than 20 mEq/L in 34.1% of 354 young children with UTI in one study [17].

IMAGING OF THE URINARY TRACT

The major goal of investigation of the urinary tract in infants with UTI (and infants with abnormalities noted prenatally) is to identify important and correctable lesions (including urethral strictures, renal anomalies, obstructive uropathy, urethral valves in boys, and some cases of severe VUR) and to provide the opportunity to begin antibiotic prophylaxis against recurring UTIs in certain infants with reflux or hydronephrosis in whom surgery is not indicated. (See previous discussion of uncertainty of benefit of antibiotic prophylaxis and surgery for primary VUR or hydronephrosis.) Multiple imaging modalities are available, and each modality provides unique evaluations [55,61,117,119–122]. Ultrasonography can delineate the size, shape, and location of kidneys and contributes to the diagnosis of hydronephrosis, hydroureter, ureterocele, bladder distention, and stones, but less so to VUR. Ultrasonography is the most noninvasive study, and its accuracy is dependent on the experience of the interpreter. It is an insensitive test for pyelonephritis, but sometimes shows kidney enlargement with abnormal echogenicity. Renal ultrasonography performed to follow up on fetal studies should be postponed for at least 48 hours after birth to avoid a false-negative result from dehydration or low glomerular filtration rate characteristic of newborns [119].

Renal cortical scintigraphy using technetium-99m–labeled dimercaptosuccinic acid or gluceptate is the most sensitive test for identifying acute pyelonephritis (i.e., focally or diffusely decreased cortical uptake of tracer without evidence of cortical loss, sometimes in an enlarged kidney) or chronic scarring (i.e., decreased uptake with corresponding cortical volume loss); scintigraphy also provides an estimate of renal function. Scintigraphy is the gold standard for diagnosis of acute pyelonephritis; 66% to 75% of children younger than 2 years with febrile UTI in multiple studies have a positive result [56,57]. Renal scintigraphy at the time of UTI was performed in a multicenter study in Spain. In a subset of infants younger than 30 days of age with community-associated UTI (106 cases) and nosocomial UTI (15 cases), cortical defects were present in 31% and 73%. Although abnormal scintigraphy was significantly associated with abnormal ultrasonography and VCUG, 21% of study infants without either finding had abnormal scintigraphy [4].

Voiding cystourethrography using radiographic or radionuclide methodology is the best study to visualize the bladder and urethra and to detect VUR; radionuclide scan is superior to the dye study for detection of intermittent reflux, but is inferior for detection of urethral and bladder wall abnormalities and cannot be used to grade VUR. Both are invasive and associated with discomfort attendant with catheterization. A 24-day-old male infant with ureterovesical junction obstruction was found to have *E. coli* septicemia and UTI 6 days after elective vesicourethrography, which did not show VUR [123]. Toxic reaction to the cystourethrography dye can occur in infants but is rare.

Ultrasonography and cystourethrography have been recommended for all neonates with UTI judged to be other than that secondary to septicemia. Male infants with community-associated first UTI diagnosed before 8 weeks of age have a higher incidence of VUR or anatomic abnormalities (22% of 45 male infants in one Israeli study) than that noted in older children [124]. Ultrasonography is performed at the time of infection to identify major renal and ureteral abnormalities. Cystourethrography sometimes can be delayed to permit resolution of inflammatory VUR; however, in clinical studies, less than 50% of children with acute pyelonephritis proved to have VUR [38,57,120].

Renal scintigraphy is useful in diagnosis and management of selective cases of UTI [125,126]. Computed tomography (CT) is performed infrequently, such as when a mass lesion or abscess is suspected. For infants who have undergone prenatal ultrasonography in an experienced center after 30 to 32 weeks of gestation and whose study findings were normal, repeat ultrasonography at the time of first UTI is not recommended by some experts [110,111].

MANAGEMENT AND PREVENTION

Management of UTI is aimed at halting infection rapidly, reconstituting normal fluid and acid-base status, and assessing medical or surgical interventions required to prevent subsequent episodes of UTI and kidney damage. Antimicrobial agents should be administered as soon as culture specimens of the blood, cerebrospinal fluid (if indicated), and urine have been obtained. The choice of antimicrobial agents for initial therapy and the dosage schedule are the same as outlined in Chapter 6 for septicemia (a penicillin and an aminoglycoside). A penicillinase-resistant penicillin (methicillin or oxacillin) should be used if an abscess of the kidney, prostate, or testis is present, which suggests infection with *S. aureus*. Vancomycin may be appropriate when methicillin-resistant *S. aureus* organisms are prevalent in the community or nursery. Patients who have suspected hospital-acquired infection are frequently given vancomycin and an aminoglycoside as initial therapy because of the significant role of coagulase-negative staphylococci and *Enterococcus* species. The decision to use a third-generation cephalosporin is based on the patient's prior receipt of antibiotics, the patient's clinical state, and the knowledge of bacterial species indigenous in each neonatal intensive care unit.

Extended-spectrum β-lactamase–producing organisms of the family Enterobacteriaceae are increasingly problematic in neonatal nosocomial infections, including UTI. Gram stain of urine sediment is helpful in initiating empirical therapy for UTI, especially when fungal infection is considered. Therapeutic regimens should be reconsidered when the results of cultures and antimicrobial susceptibility tests are available.

Effective antimicrobial agents sterilize the urine within 24 to 48 hours. A second specimen of urine often is obtained for examination and culture at about 48 hours. Persistence of bacteriuria or funguria implies that treatment is ineffective or that a foreign body, fungus ball, or obstruction is present.

The duration of antimicrobial therapy for UTI in neonates usually is 14 days. Longer therapy (up to 3 weeks) is necessary if there is a poor response or if an anatomic or physiologic abnormality suggests that relapse may occur if administration of the drug is not continued. Timing of change from parenterally to orally administered agents depends on rapidity of clinical and microbiologic response and the presence of bacteremia or anatomic, functional, or physiologic abnormalities and availability of a highly active oral agent. Parenteral therapy usually is given for at least 3 to 4 days in uncomplicated cases [127,128]. Clinical vigilance for nonspecific symptoms and signs of illness after conclusion of therapy is important so that recurrent infection can be detected and treated appropriately. Children with certain urinary tract anomalies, functional abnormalities, and higher grades of VUR often are given prophylactic antibiotics continuously for extended periods until the condition improves or surgery is performed [63,119]. (See previous discussion of uncertainty of benefit of standard prophylaxis in primary VUR alone.) A systematic review of randomized controlled trials of prophylaxis revealed limited evidence for its efficacy [129]. A randomized trial in 576 older infants and children in Australia showed statistically significant but modest effect of trimethoprim-sulfamethoxazole over placebo in preventing UTIs (13% measus 19%). [130]. A U.S. multicenter study to test this question is planned [74,75]. Amoxicillin, 20 mg/kg/day divided in doses administered every 12 hours, is the agent most frequently used for prophylaxis in the neonate.

Measures that have been shown to reduce nosocomial UTIs in older children and adults should be applied to newborns. Evidence-based interventions include avoidance of unnecessary urinary catheterization, vigilance in hand hygiene, insertion and maintenance of a catheter in a sterile manner, and discontinuation of catheterization as soon as possible (i.e., daily evaluation of need to continue) [131].

PROGNOSIS

For patients with UTI and underlying genitourinary abnormalities, long-term control of infection is important. After that, prognosis depends on severity of the lesion and associated congenital renal syndromes. The natural history of UTI in the newborn without underlying abnormality is incompletely described. Some infants with asymptomatic bacteriuria have infection that clears without use of antimicrobial agents [5,6,132]. Some infants with symptomatic infection respond readily to therapy and have no subsequent infections, whereas others have recurrences, although the number seems to be smaller than that for older children and adults. In the series from Göteborg [6] and Leeds [8], recurrences occurred in 26% and 19% of infants; the second episode usually occurred during the first few months after the initial infection.

It is possible that inflammatory changes in the kidney early in life may lead to subsequent impairment of growth and development of the kidney and to epithelial damage, fibrosis, and vascular changes, but it is uncertain how frequently these events occur. In a study of 25 children with UTI in whom renal scintigraphy showed evidence of acute pyelonephritis and who underwent repeat scanning an average of 10.5 months later, 16 (64%) had corresponding scars [56]. In another study, 38% of 157 children (with median age 0.4 year at the time of asymptomatic UTI) had renal scars documented 1 year later [117]. Infants do not seem to be at increased risk for scarring; in 50 infants younger than 1 year with UTI and abnormality scintigraphy acutely, repeat scintigraphy after an average of 3 months showed scars in 40% [133].

Obstructive lesions associated with reflux during the neonatal period may be associated with progressive renal damage, whereas children with unobstructive reflux regardless of severity infrequently have progressive renal damage. The hypothesis that outcome depends on prevention of infection has been challenged. [74,75] Repeat ultrasonography for follow-up evaluation after UTI in infants in whom findings on a postnatal ultrasound examination were normal is not indicated [134].

REFERENCES

[1] H.F. Helmholz, Pyelitis in the newborn, Med. Clin. North. Am. 1 (1918) 1451.
[2] T.A. Schlager, et al., Explanation for false-positive urine cultures obtained by bay technique, Arch. Pediatr. Adolesc. Med. 149 (1995) 170.
[3] J.A. Lohr, et al., Hospital-acquired urinary tract infections in the pediatric patient: a prospective study, Pediatr. Infect. Dis. J. 13 (1994) 8.
[4] J.B. Sastre, et al., Urinary tract infection in the newborn: clinical and radio-imaging studies, Pediatr. Nephrol. 22 (2007) 1735.
[5] G.D. Abbott, Neonatal bacteriuria: a prospective study of 1460 infants, BMJ 1 (1972) 267.
[6] T. Bergström, et al., Neonatal urinary tract infections, J. Pediatr. 80 (1972) 859.
[7] C.M. Edelman Jr., et al., The prevalence of bacteriuria in full-term and premature newborn infants, J. Pediatr. 82 (1973) 125.
[8] J.M. Littlewood, P. Kite, B.A. Kite, Incidence of neonatal urinary tract infection, Arch. Dis. Child. 44 (1969) 617.
[9] M. Maherzi, J.P. Guignard, A. Torrado, Urinary tract infection in high-risk newborn infants, Pediatrics 62 (1978) 521.
[10] B. Wettergren, U. Jodal, G. Jonasson, Epidemiology of bacteriuria during the first year of life, Acta. Paediatr. Scand. 74 (1985) 925.
[11] T.E. Wiswell, J.D. Roscelli, Corroborative evidence for the decreased incidence of urinary tract infections in circumcised male infants, Pediatrics 78 (1986) 96.
[12] K.L. Yorita, et al., Infectious disease hospitalizations among infants in the United States, Pediatrics 121 (2008) 244.
[13] B.C. Pendarvis Jr., L.A. Chitwood, J.E. Wenzl, Bacteriuria in the Premature Infant, American Society for Microbiology, Washington, DC, 1969.
[14] M.M. Tamim, H. Alesseh, H. Aziz, Analysis of the efficacy of urine culture as part of sepsis evaluation in the premature infant, Pediatr. Infect. Dis. J. 22 (2003) 805.
[15] S. Bauer, et al., Urinary tract infection in very low birth weight preterm infants, Pediatr. Infect. Dis. J. 22 (2003) 426.
[16] D. Landau, et al., The value of urinalysis in differentiating acute pyelonephritis from lower urinary tract infection in febrile infants, Pediatr. Infect. Dis. J. 13 (1994) 777.
[17] R. Bachur, G.L. Caputo, Bacteremia and meningitis among infants with urinary tract infections, Pediatr. Emerg. Care. 11 (1995) 280.
[18] A.Y. Sweet, E. Wolinsky, An outbreak of urinary tract and other infections due to E. coli, Pediatrics 33 (1964) 865.
[19] J.F. Kenny, et al., An outbreak of urinary tract infections and septicemia due to Escherichia coli in male infants, J. Pediatr. 68 (1966) 530.
[20] R.C. McCormack, C.M. Kunin, Control of a single source nursery epidemic due to Serratia marcescens, Pediatrics 37 (1966) 750.
[21] T.E. Wiswell, F.R. Smith, J.W. Bass, Decreased incidence of urinary tract infections in circumcised male infants, Pediatrics 75 (1985) 901.
[22] T.E. Wiswell, et al., Declining frequency of circumcision: implications for changes in the absolute incidence and male to female sex ratio of urinary tract infections in early infancy, Pediatrics 79 (1987) 338.
[23] C.M. Ginsburg, G.H. McCracken Jr., Urinary tract infections in young infants, Pediatrics 69 (1982) 409.
[24] L.W. Herzog, Urinary tract infections and circumcision: a case-control study, Am. J. Dis. Child. 143 (1989) 348.
[25] N. Shaikh, et al., Prevalence of urinary tract infection in childhood: a meta-analysis, Pediatr. Infect. Dis. J. 27 (2008) 302.
[26] T.E. Wiswell, D.W. Geschke, Risks from circumcision during the first month of life compared with those for uncircumcised boys, Pediatrics 83 (1989) 1011.
[27] T.E. Wiswell, W.E. Hachey, Urinary tract infections and the uncircumcised state: an update, Clin. Pediatr. (1993) 130.
[28] E.J. Schoen, (chairman) American Academy of Pediatrics Task Force Report on Circumcision, Pediatrics 84 (1989) 388.
[29] T. To, et al., Cohort study on circumcision of newborn boys and subsequent risk of urinary-tract infection, Lancet 352 (1998) 1813.
[30] J.C. Craig, et al., Effect of circumcision on incidence of urinary tract infection in preschool boys, J. Pediatr. 128 (1996) 23.
[31] C.M. Lannon, American Academy of Pediatrics Task Force Report on Circumcision, Pediatrics 103 (1999) 686.
[32] H.A. Cohen, et al., Post-circumcision urinary tract infection, Clin. Pediatr. 31 (1992) 322.
[33] L. Harel, et al., Influence of circumcision technique on frequency of urinary tract infections in neonates, Pediatr. Infect. Dis. J. 21 (2002) 879.
[34] E.F. Crain, J.C. Gershel, Urinary tract infections in febrile infants younger than 8 weeks of age, Pediatrics 86 (1990) 363.
[35] A. Hoberman, et al., Oral versus initial intravenous therapy for urinary tract infections in young febrile children, Pediatrics 104 (1999) 79.
[36] K.N. Shaw, et al., Prevalence of urinary tract infection in febrile young children in the emergency department, Pediatrics 102 (1998) 390.
[37] T.S. Glasgow, et al., Association of intrapartum antibiotic exposure and late-onset serious bacterial infections in infants, Pediatrics 116 (2005) 696.
[38] K. Tullus, P. Sjoberg, Epidemiological aspects of P fimbriated E. coli, Acta Paediatr. Scand. 75 (1986) 205.
[39] V. Israele, A. Darabi, G.H. McCracken Jr., The role of bacterial virulence factors and Tamm-Horsfall protein in the pathogenesis of Escherichia coli urinary tract infection in infants, Am. J. Dis. Child. 141 (1987) 1230.
[40] B.M. Pena, M.B. Harper, G.R. Fleisher, Occult bacteremia with group B streptococci in an outpatient setting, Pediatrics 102 (1998) 67.
[41] R.M. Fortunov, et al., Evaluation and treatment of community-acquired Staphylococcus aureus infections in term and late-preterm previously healthy neonates, Pediatrics 120 (2007) 93.
[42] J.A. Lohr, L.G. Donowitz, J.E. Sadler III., Hospital-acquired urinary tract infection, Pediatrics 83 (1989) 193.
[43] H.D. Davies, et al., Nosocomial urinary tract infections at a pediatric hospital, Pediatr. Infect. Dis. J. 11 (1992) 349.
[44] A.H. Sohn, et al., Prevalence of nosocomial infections in neonatal intensive care unit patients: results from the first national point-prevalence survey, J. Pediatr. 139 (2001) 821.
[45] R.C. Giannattasio, Acute suppurative prostatitis in the neonatal period, N. Y. State. J. Med. 60 (1960) 3471.
[46] D.I. Williams, A.G. Martins, Periprostatic haematoma and prostatic abscess in the neonatal period, Arch. Dis. Child. 35 (1960) 177.
[47] S. Mann, Prostatic abscess in the newborn, Arch. Dis. Child. 35 (1960) 396.
[48] W.M. Hendricks, G.N. Kellett, Scrotal mass in a neonate: testicular abscess, Am. J. Dis. Child. 129 (1975) 1361.
[49] V.G. Hemming, Bilateral neonatal group A streptococcal hydrocele infection associated with maternal puerperal sepsis, Pediatr. Infect. Dis. 5 (1986) 107.
[50] E.T. McCartney, I. Stewart, Suppurative orchitis due to Pseudomonas aeruginosa, J. Pediatr. 52 (1958) 451.
[51] R. Foster, et al., Salmonella enteritidis: testicular abscess in a newborn, J. Urol. 130 (1983) 790.
[52] A. Bensman, et al., Uropathies diagnosed in the neonatal period: symptomatology and course, Acta Paediatr. Scand. 69 (1980) 499.
[53] J.M. Littlewood, 66 infants with urinary tract infection in first month of life, Arch. Dis. Child. 57 (1972) 218.
[54] D. Bourcher, E.D. Abbott, T.M.J. Maling, Radiological abnormalities in infants with urinary tract infection, Arch. Dis. Child. 59 (1984) 620.
[55] M.P. Andrich, M. Majd, Diagnostic imaging in the evaluation of the first urinary tract infection in infants and young children, Pediatrics 90 (1992) 436.
[56] D. Benador, et al., Cortical scintigraphy in the evaluation of renal parenchymal changes in children with pyelonephritis, J. Pediatr. 124 (1994) 17.
[57] M. Majd, et al., Relationships among vesicoureteral reflux, P-fimbriated Escherichia coli, and acute pyelonephritis in children with febrile urinary tract infection, J. Pediatr. 119 (1991) 578.
[58] A. Najmaldin, D.M. Burge, J.D. Atwell, Pediatric urology: fetal vesicoureteric reflux, Br. J. Urol. 65 (1990) 403.
[59] A.C. Gordon, et al., Prenatally diagnosed reflux: a follow-up study, Br. J. Urol. 65 (1990) 407.
[60] E. Ring, G. Zobel, Urinary infection and malformations of urinary tract in infancy, Arch. Dis. Child. 63 (1988) 818.
[61] B.T. Steele, J. De Maria, A new perspective on the natural history of vesicoureteric reflux, Pediatrics 90 (1992) 30.
[62] B.M. Assael, et al., Congenital reflux nephropathy: a follow-up of 108 cases diagnosed perinatally, Br. J. Urol. 82 (1998) 252.

[63] T.R. Gunn, J.D. Mora, P. Pease, Outcome after antenatal diagnosis of upper urinary tract dilatation by ultrasonography, Arch. Dis. Child. 63 (1988) 1240.

[64] T.R. Gunn, J.D. Mora, P. Pease, Antenatal diagnosis of urinary tract abnormalities by ultrasonography after 28 weeks' gestation: incidence and outcome, Am. J. Obstet. Gynecol. 172 (1995) 479.

[65] P.A. Dremsek, et al., Renal pyelectasis in fetuses and neonates: diagnostic value of renal pelvis diameter in pre- and postnatal sonographic screening, AJR Am. J. Roentgenol. 168 (1997) 1017.

[66] D.F.M. Thomas, et al., Mild dilatation of the fetal kidney: a follow-up study, Br. J. Urol. 74 (1993) 236.

[67] A.M. Cheng, et al., Outcome of isolated antenatal hydronephrosis, Arch. Pediatr. Adolesc. Med. 158 (2004) 38.

[68] I. Moorthy, et al., Antenatal hydronephrosis: negative predictive value of normal postnatal ultrasound—a 5 year study, Clin. Radiol. 58 (2003) 964.

[69] T.J. Walsh, et al., Antenatal hydronephrosis and the risk of pyelonephritis hospitalization during the first year of life, Pediatr. Urol. 69 (2007) 970.

[70] J.H. Lee, et al., Nonrefluxing neonatal hydronephrosis and the risk of urinary tract infection, J. Urol. 179 (2008) 1524.

[71] E.H. de Kort, S. Oetomo, S.H. Zegers, The long-term outcome of antenatal hydronephrosis up to 15 millimetres justifies a noninvasive postnatal follow-up, Acta Paediatr. 97 (2008) 708.

[72] J. Upadhyay, et al., Natural history of neonatal reflux associated with pre-natal hydronephrosis: long-term results of a prospective study, J. Urol. 169 (2003) 1837.

[73] C.R. Estrada Jr., Prenatal hydronephrosis: early evaluation, Curr. Opin. Urol. 18 (2008) 401.

[74] R. Keren, et al., Rationale and design issues of the randomized intervention for children with vesicoureteral reflux (RIVUR) study, Pediatrics 122 (2008) S241.

[75] R.W. Chesney, et al., Randomized intervention for children with vesicoureteral reflux (RIVUR): Background commentary of RIVUR investigators, Pediatrics 122 (2008) S233.

[76] M. Pennesi, Is antibiotic prophylaxis in children with vesicoureteral reflux effective in preventing pyelonephritis and renal scars? A. randomized, controlled trial, Pediatrics 121 (2008) e1489.

[77] C. Svanborg, et al., Host-parasite interaction in the urinary tract, J. Infect. Dis. 157 (1988) 421.

[78] T.E. Wiswell, et al., Effect of circumcision status on periurethral bacterial flora during the first year of life, J. Pediatr. 113 (1988) 442.

[79] J.D. Sobel, Pathogenesis of urinary tract infections, Infect. Dis. Clin. North. Am. 1 (1987) 751.

[80] K.A. Porter, H.M. Giles, A pathological study of live cases of pyelonephritis in the newborn, Arch. Dis. Child. 31 (1956) 303.

[81] J. Bernstein, A.K. Brown, Sepsis and jaundice in early infancy, Pediatrics 29 (1962) 873.

[82] R.A. Seeler, K. Hahn, Jaundice in urinary tract infection in infancy, Am. J. Dis. Child. 118 (1969) 553.

[83] M.J. Maisels, E. Kring, Risk of sepsis in newborns with severe hyperbilirubinemia, Pediatrics 90 (1992) 741.

[84] F.J. Garcia, A. Nager, Jaundice as an early diagnostic sign of urinary tract infection in infancy, Pediatrics 112 (2003) 1213.

[85] N. Pashapour, A.A. Nikibanhksh, S. Golmohammadlou, Urinary tract infection in term neonates with prolonged jaundice, Urol. J. 4 (2007) 91.

[86] G. Luk, D. Riggs, M. Luque, Severe methemoglobinemia in a 3-week-old infant with a urinary tract infection, Crit. Care. Med. 19 (1992) 1325.

[87] A. Das, D. Henderson, Your diagnosis please, Pediatr. Infect. Dis. J. 15 (1996) 922.

[88] D.B. Crawford, et al., Renal carbuncle in a neonate with congenital nephrotic syndrome, J. Pediatr. 93 (1978) 78.

[89] H. Bauchner, et al., Prevalence of bacteriuria in febrile children, Pediatr. Infect. Dis. J. 6 (1987) 239.

[90] M.S. Krober, et al., Bacterial and viral pathogens causing fever in infants less than 3 months old, Am. J. Dis. Child. 139 (1985) 889.

[91] J. Amir, et al., Fever in the first months of life, Isr. J. Med. Sci. 20 (1984) 447.

[92] A. Hoberman, et al., Prevalence of urinary tract infection in febrile infants, J. Pediatr. 123 (1993) 17.

[93] C.L. Byington, et al., Serious bacterial infections in febrile infants younger than 90 days of age: the importance of ampicillin-resistant pathogens, Pediatrics 111 (2003) 964.

[94] R.H. Pantell, et al., Management and outcomes of care of fever in early infancy, JAMA 10 (2004) 1261.

[95] J.J. Zorc, et al., Clinical and demographic factors associated with urinary tract infection in young febrile infants, Pediatrics 116 (2005) 644.

[96] D.S. Lin, et al., Urinary tract infection in febrile infants younger than eight weeks of age, Pediatrics 105 (2000) 414.

[97] C.V. Pryles, L. Saccharow, Further experience with the use of percutaneous suprapubic aspiration of the urinary bladder: bacteriologic studies in 654 infants and children, Pediatrics 43 (1969) 1018.

[98] W.T. Weathers, J.E. Wenzl, Suprapubic aspiration: perforation of a viscus other than the bladder, Am. J. Dis. Child. 117 (1969) 590.

[99] R.E. Morell, G. Duritz, C. Oltorf, Suprapubic aspiration associated with hematoma, Pediatrics 69 (1982) 455.

[100] R.L. Schreiver, P. Skafish, Complications of suprapubic bladder aspiration, Am. J. Dis. Child. 132 (1978) 98.

[101] R.F. Pass, F.B. Waldo, Anaerobic bacteremia following suprapubic bladder aspiration, J. Pediatr. 94 (1979) 748.

[102] S.C. Kiernan, T.L. Pinckert, M. Kesler, Ultrasound guidance of suprapubic bladder aspiration in neonates, J. Pediatr. 123 (1993) 789.

[103] C.V. Pryles, D. Lüders, M.K. Alkan, A comparative study of bacterial cultures and colony counts in paired specimens of urine obtained by catheter versus voiding from normal infants and infants with urinary tract infection, Pediatrics 27 (1961) 17.

[104] A. Hoberman, et al., Pyuria and bacteriuria in urine specimens obtained by catheter from young children with fever, J. Pediatr. 124 (1994) 513.

[105] P.J. Vuillermin, M. Starr, Investigation of the rate of meningitis in association with urinary tract infection in infants 90 days of age or younger, Emerg. Med. Australas. 19 (2007) 464.

[106] S.S. Shah, et al., Sterile cerebrospinal fluid pleocytosis in young infants with urinary tract infections, J. Pediatr. 153 (2008) 290.

[107] R.D. Pitetti, S. Choi, Utility of blood cultures in febrile children with UTI, Am. J. Emerg. Med. 20 (2002) 271.

[108] A.S. Hewstone, J.S. Lawson, Microscopic appearance of urine in the neonatal period, Arch. Dis. Child. 39 (1964) 287.

[109] J.M. Littlewood, White cells and bacteria in voided urine of healthy newborns, Arch. Dis. Child. 46 (1971) 167.

[110] K. Lincoln, J. Winberg, Studies of urinary tract infection in infancy and childhood, III: quantitative estimation of cellular excretion in unselected neonates, Acta. Paediatr Scand. 53 (1964) 447.

[111] L. Huicho, M. Campos-Sanchez, C. Alamo, Metaanalysis of urine screening tests for determining the risk of urinary tract infection in children, Pediatr. Infect. Dis. J. 21 (2002) 1.

[112] A. Hoberman, et al., Is urine culture necessary to rule out urinary tract infection in young febrile children? Pediatr. Infect. Dis. J. 15 (1996) 304.

[113] K.N. Shaw, et al., Screening for urinary tract infection in infants in the emergency department: which test is best? Pediatrics 101 (1998) 1.

[114] B. Emanuel, N. Aronson, Neonatal hematuria, Am. J. Dis. Child. 128 (1974) 204.

[115] V.E. Visser, R.T. Hall, Urine culture in the evaluation of suspected neonatal sepsis, J. Pediatr. 94 (1979) 635.

[116] R.J. DiGeronimo, Lack of efficacy of the urine culture as part of the initial work up of suspected neonatal sepsis, Pediatr. Infect. Dis. J. 11 (1992) 764.

[117] E. Stokland, et al., Renal damage one year after first urinary tract infection: role of dimercaptosuccinic acid scintigraphy, J. Pediatr. 129 (1996) 815.

[118] C. Prat, et al., Elevated serum procalcitonin values correlate with renal scarring in children with urinary tract infection, Pediatr. Infect. Dis. J. 22 (2003) 438.

[119] R.N. Fine, Diagnosis and treatment of fetal urinary tract abnormalities, J. Pediatr. 121 (1992) 333.

[120] C.F. Strife, M.J. Gelfand, Renal cortical scintigraphy: effect on medical decision making in childhood urinary tract infection, J. Pediatr. 129 (1996) 785.

[121] S. Hellerstein, Evolving concepts in the evaluation of the child with a urinary tract infection, J. Pediatr. 124 (1994) 589.

[122] P.T. Dick, W. Feldman, Routine diagnostic imaging for childhood urinary tract infections: a systematic overview, J. Pediatr. 128 (1996) 15.

[123] A.H. Slyper, J.C. Olson, R.B. Nair, Overwhelming *Escherichia coli* sepsis in ureterovesical junction obstruction without reflux, Arch. Pediatr. Adolesc. Med. 148 (1994) 1102.

[124] M. Goldman, et al., Imaging after urinary tract infection in male neonates, Pediatrics 105 (2000) 1232.

[125] A. Hoberman, et al., Imaging studies after a first febrile urinary tract infection in young children, N. Engl. J. Med. 348 (2003) 195.

[126] F.B. Stapleton, Imaging studies for childhood urinary infections, N. Engl. J. Med. 348 (2003) 251.

[127] S. Hellerstein, Antibiotic treatment for urinary tract infections in pediatric patients, Pediatrics 112 (2003) 1213.

[128] E.C. Magin, et al., Efficacy of short-term intravenous antibiotic in neonates with urinary tract infection, Pediatr. Emerg. Care. 23 (2007) 83.

[129] G. Williams, A. Lee, J. Craig, Antibiotic for the prevention of urinary tract infection in children; a systematic review of randomized controlled trials, J. Pediatr. 138 (2001) 868.

[130] J.C. Craig et al., Antibiotic prophylaxis and recurrent urinary tract infection in children, N. Engl. J. Med. 361 (2009) 1748.

[131] SHEA/IDSA Practice Recommendation, Strategies to prevent catheter-associated urinary tract infections in acute care hospitals, Infect. Control Hosp. Epidemiol. 29 (2008) S41.

[132] C.W. Hoffpauir, D.J. Guidry, Asymptomatic urinary tract infection in premature infants, Pediatrics 45 (1970) 128.

[133] D. Benador, et al., Are younger children at highest risk of renal sequelae after pyelonephritis? Lancet 349 (1997) 17.

[134] L.H. Lowe, et al., Utility of follow-up renal sonography in children with vesicoureteral reflux and normal initial sonogram, Pediatrics 113 (2004) 548.

CHAPTER 10

FOCAL BACTERIAL INFECTIONS

Gary D. Overturf

CHAPTER OUTLINE

Infections of the Liver   322
    Microbiology   322
    Pathogenesis   323
    Clinical Manifestations   324
    Diagnosis   324
    Prognosis   324
    Treatment   325
Splenic Abscess   325
Infections of the Biliary Tract   325
Infections of the Adrenal Glands   326
Appendicitis   327
    Microbiology   327
    Pathogenesis   327
    Clinical Manifestations   327
    Diagnosis   328
    Prognosis   328
    Treatment   329
Peritonitis   329
    Microbiology   329
    Pathogenesis   330
    Clinical Manifestations   331
    Diagnosis   332
    Prognosis   332
    Treatment   333

Necrotizing Enterocolitis   333
    Pathology and Pathogenesis   334
    Microbiology   334
    Clinical Manifestations   335
    Diagnosis   336
    Treatment   337
    Prevention   337
    Prognosis   338
Endocarditis   338
Pericarditis   340
Mediastinitis   341
Esophagitis   342
Infections of Endocrine Organs   342
Infections of the Salivary Glands   342
Infections of the Skin and Subcutaneous Tissue   342
    Pathogenesis   343
    Microbiology   344
    Epidemiology   344
    Clinical Manifestations   344
    Diagnosis   347
    Differential Diagnosis   347
    Treatment   348
    Prevention   348
Conjunctivitis and Other Eye Infections   349

INFECTIONS OF THE LIVER

Bacterial infection of the hepatic parenchyma frequently is recognized as multiple, small inflammatory foci (hepatic microabscesses) observed as an incidental finding in infants dying with sepsis. Diffuse hepatocellular damage, often in conjunction with infection of several organ systems, may be present after transplacental passage of microorganisms to the fetal circulation. Liver involvement rarely may take the form of a solitary purulent abscess. Metastatic focal infections of the liver associated with bacteremia resolve with antimicrobial therapy, are not recognized, or are found only at postmortem examination. Rarely, they are clinically apparent as solitary [1] or multiple [2] large abscesses diagnosed during life.

Although metastatic infections are rare, it is difficult to ascertain their true incidence. In a survey of more than 7500 autopsies of children performed from 1917-1967, Dehner and Kissane [3] found only 3 neonates with multiple, small, pyogenic hepatic abscesses, whereas a review of approximately 4900 autopsies [4] performed at Los Angeles Children's Hospital from 1958-1978 revealed 9 infants with pyogenic hepatic abscesses [5]. Among 175,000 neonates admitted from 1957-1977 to Milwaukee Children's Hospital, 2 died with hepatic microabscesses [6]; 3 patients

with hepatic microabscesses were seen among 83,000 pediatric patients admitted to New York Hospital from 1945-1983 [7]; and one case of hepatic microabscesses was reported at the University of Texas Medical Branch in Galveston from 1963-1984 [8]. Most reviewers who have discussed postmortem observations of infants dying with neonatal sepsis have not described the occurrence of such secondary sites of infection [9–16] or have presented them as an occasional ancillary finding [17,18].

Solitary hepatic abscesses in newborns have also been reported rarely. About 30 such cases have been described [1,3,4,19–41]. These infections frequently are associated with prematurity and umbilical vein catheterization,* whereas solitary abscesses may occur because of bacteremia. Murphy and Baker [42] described a solitary abscess after sepsis caused by *Staphylococcus aureus*.

MICROBIOLOGY

The etiologic agents in the infants described by Dehner and Kissane [3], Moss and Pysher [5], Chusid [6], and included *Escherichia coli*, *S. aureus*, *Pseudomonas aeruginosa*,

---

*References [5,6,21,22,25,28,32,34–41].

Klebsiella species, *Enterobacter* species, and *Listeria monocytogenes*. The causative bacteria of solitary abscesses are generally the bacteria colonizing the umbilical stump [43], including *S. aureus* (11 cases), *E. coli* alone (3 cases), *E. coli* with *S. aureus* (2 cases) or enterococcus (1 case), *Enterobacter* species (3 cases), *Klebsiella pneumoniae* alone (2 cases), *K. pneumoniae* with *Proteus* species (1 case), *P. aeruginosa* (1 case), *Staphylococcus epidermidis* with group F streptococcus (1 case), and *Streptococcus pyogenes* (1 case). In three infants, the abscesses were described as "sterile." [19,28,31] Although one of these infants had received penicillin for 9 days before surgical drainage, it is possible that in all three cases the abscesses were caused by anaerobic bacteria that failed to grow. The presence of gas in seven abscesses [25,28,34,35,39] may indicate infection with anaerobes, a frequent cause of liver abscess in adults [44].

The most common cause of intrauterine bacterial hepatitis, congenital listeriosis, characteristically involves the liver and adrenals (see Chapter 13). Typical lesions are histologically sharply demarcated areas of necrosis (miliary granulomatosis) or microabscesses containing numerous pleomorphic gram-positive bacilli [15]. Descriptions in the early 1900s of miliary necrosis of the liver related to "gram-positive argentophilic rodlike organisms" probably also represented infections with *L. monocytogenes*, which was not isolated and identified until 1926 [26].

Intrauterine tuberculosis results from maternal bacillemia with transplacental dissemination to the fetal bloodstream (see Chapter 18). Because the liver is perfused by blood with a high oxygen content [45] and is the first organ that encounters tubercle bacilli, it is often severely involved [15,44,46]. The presence of primary liver foci is considered evidence for congenital tuberculous infection as a result of hematogenous spread through the umbilical vein [47]. Closed-needle biopsy may be less accurate in the diagnosis of hepatic granulomas, and open biopsy may be required to confirm liver and regional node involvement [48]. Although generalized fetal infection may also arise through aspiration of contaminated amniotic fluid, the lesions acquired in this manner are usually most prominent in the lungs. In addition to hepatomegaly, a clinical picture of fever with elevated serum IgM and chorioretinitis (e.g., choroid tubercles) may be similar to that caused by other congenital infectious agents [49]. In a review by Abughal and coworkers [49], positive sites of culture for tuberculosis included liver (8 of 9), gastric aspirate (18 of 23), tracheal aspirate (7 of 7), ear (5 of 6), and cerebrospinal fluid (3 of 10). Noncaseating granulomatous hepatitis, thought to be caused by a hypersensitivity reaction related to bacille Calmette-Guérin vaccination, has also been described in a neonate [50], but histologic and bacteriologic studies performed on liver biopsy specimens failed to identify the presence of acid-fast bacilli or bacille Calmette-Guérin organisms.

Bacterial infection of the fetal liver rarely has been reported in association with maternal tularemia [51], anthrax [52], typhoid fever [53], and brucellosis [54]. It is uncertain whether the isolation of bacteria from the livers of stillborn fetuses is significantly associated with their clinical course [55,56].

Treponema pallidum is the spirochete most commonly associated with transplacental hepatic infection (see Chapter 16). Pathologic changes in the liver, which may be found in 95% of infants dying with congenital syphilis [57], include diffuse hepatitis or focal areas of inflammation, both frequently accompanied by increased connective tissue and enlargement of the liver [15,57–59]. Involvement of liver has also been documented, on the basis of isolation of organisms or their identification in histologic sections, in newborns with intrauterine infection caused by various *Leptospira* species (*Leptospira icterohaemorrhagiae* [60,61], *Leptospira pomona* [62], *Leptospira canicola* [63], *Leptospira kasman* [64]).

Transplacental infection of the fetus with *Borrelia recurrentis* causes little or no inflammation of liver parenchyma or biliary epithelium despite the presence of numerous spirochetes in the sinusoids [65–68]. Congenital infection has been suggested with *Borrelia burgdorferi* [69] (cause of Lyme disease); hepatic, central nervous system, and cardiac lesions may be observed, and widely disseminated lesions were reported to occur in other tissues. This single case is controversial, however, and the American Academy of Pediatrics does not accept congenital Lyme disease because no "causal relationship between maternal Lyme disease and abnormalities of pregnancy or congenital disease caused by *B. burgdorferi* has been documented conclusively" [68a]; no evidence exists that Lyme disease can be transmitted via human milk.

PATHOGENESIS

Infectious agents may reach the liver of the fetus or newborn by one of several pathways: transplacental or transoral intrauterine infection, extension of thrombophlebitis of the umbilical vein, through the hepatic artery during the course of a systemic bacteremia, pyelophlebitis owing to a focus of infection in the drainage of the portal vein (mesenteric or splenic veins), direct invasion from contiguous structures or because of trauma or surgical inoculation, and extension up the biliary passages in cases of suppurative cholangitis. Abscesses with no apparent focus of infection seem to be common in newborns compared with older children [30]. Three such cases, all in infants with solitary hepatic abscesses, have been described [23,24,31]. Descriptions of the surgical findings, together with the nature of the lesions, suggest that an umbilical vein infection, obscured by the large collection of purulent material in the abscess, was the probable pathogenesis in all infants.

The mode of infection usually determines the pattern of hepatic involvement. Intense and prolonged seeding of the liver parenchyma, such as that which occurs in conjunction with intrauterine infection or neonatal sepsis, almost invariably results in diffuse hepatocellular damage or multiple small inflammatory lesions [3,5,6]. Umbilical vein thrombophlebitis may cause an abscess of the falciform ligament [70] or extend into a single branch of the portal vein to produce a solitary pyogenic abscess,* or it can lead to disseminated foci of infection through dislodgment of septic emboli [6,71–74].

The frequent use of umbilical catheters has been associated with an increase in the numbers of infants

---

*References [6,21,22,26,29,32,33].

with solitary [5,6,20–22,32,34–40] or multiple [5,75,76] hepatic abscesses. In three large series, including almost 500 infants who died after placement of umbilical vein catheters, 29 infants were found to have purulent infections of hepatic vessels or parenchyma [37,75,77]. Use of venous catheters for infusion of hypertonic or acidic solutions may provide a necrotic focus for abscess formation [21,32,34–36,76,77], and prolonged [5,22,32,77] or repeated [63] catheterization of a necrotic umbilical stump provides an ideal pathway for introduction of pathogenic organisms. It has been postulated that some hepatic abscesses have been caused by infusion of contaminated plasma [28] or by the use of nonsterile umbilical catheters [75].

Although neonatal liver abscesses usually are caused by hematogenous dissemination of bacteria through the hepatic artery or umbilical vein, examples of infection arising from various other sources have been described. Solitary abscesses have followed a presumed portal vein bacteremia caused by amebic colitis [19,20]. Direct invasion of adjacent liver parenchyma from purulent cholecystitis [24] or postoperative perihepatic abscesses [5] also has been observed. Ascending cholangitis, the most frequent cause of hepatic purulent infections in adults [30], has not been implicated in the causes of newborn infections.

Disease caused by embryonic anatomic errors is unique to newborns. Shaw and Pierog [78] described a newborn with umbilical herniation of a pedunculated supernumerary lobe of the liver; histologic examination showed numerous small foci of early abscess formation. Although signs and symptoms of sepsis appeared at 18 days of age, possibly the result of bacterial spread from the liver to the umbilical vein, the infant improved and ultimately recovered after removal of the polypoid mass on the 19th day of life.

Descriptions of "umbilical sepsis" and "acute interstitial hepatitis" recorded by Morison [79] seem to indicate that his patients had acquired bacterial infections of umbilical vessels with widespread extension into portal tracts. Although mild periportal parenchymal necrosis was observed in a few infants, hepatocellular damage was minimal or absent in most. Similar lesions have been found in infants dying with sepsis [80] and infantile diarrhea [81].

CLINICAL MANIFESTATIONS

Multiple hepatic abscesses and diffuse hepatitis related to neonatal sepsis or transplacental fetal infection are usually recognized only at autopsy. Very few clinical manifestations referable to hepatocellular damage are evident before death. The signs and symptoms associated with these conditions are those of the underlying sepsis or of secondary metastatic complications, such as meningitis, pneumonitis, or peritonitis.*

Solitary abscesses are indolent in terms of their development and clinical presentation. Although the suppurative umbilical focus or umbilical catheterization responsible for the introduction of microorganisms can usually be traced to the 1st week of life, evidence of hepatic involvement is usually not apparent before the 2nd or 3rd

*References [2,3,29,33,72,75].

week. The abscess frequently becomes a source for the hematogenous dissemination of microorganisms so that most infants have signs and symptoms of a bacteremia. Despite intense infection of the underlying vessels, the umbilical stump usually shows no evidence of inflammation or purulent discharge. The presence of hepatomegaly, a finding commonly associated with neonatal sepsis, also offers little aid in establishing a definitive diagnosis. In one half of infants for whom physical findings are clearly described, a well-delineated, often fluctuant or tender mass could be palpated in the epigastrium or right upper quadrant. On a few occasions, this mass was noticed by the infant's mother several days before the onset of systemic symptoms. Abscesses occur in the right or left lobe of the liver with almost equal frequency and are generally 3 cm or more in diameter at the time of surgical exploration.

DIAGNOSIS

Hematologic studies are of little value in establishing a diagnosis; leukocyte counts and sedimentation rates may be normal or elevated. The serum levels of liver enzymes may also be normal [25,38] or elevated [5,23,36].

Abdominal radiographs are usually normal or show nonspecific displacement of the lower edge of the liver. In five infants, diagnosis was suspected from plain x-ray films by the presence of gas within the hepatic shadow [28,32,34,39]. Radiologic findings that commonly accompany hepatic abscess in older children, such as an altered contour of the diaphragm, right pleural effusion, and platelike atelectasis [82], are rarely present in neonates.

Ultrasonography should be the initial imaging study in newborns with clinical evidence of a hepatic abscess [83–86]. If ultrasound is negative, and the diagnosis is still strongly suspected, more sensitive techniques such as computed tomography (CT) or magnetic resonance imaging (MRI) should be performed [83–88]. Enhancement with contrast agents may increase the definition of smaller abscesses. Because congenital cysts, arteriovenous malformations, and tumors with central necrosis or hemorrhage can mimic hepatic abscess, the diagnosis should always be confirmed by aspiration of purulent material at laparotomy or by means of percutaneous drainage with ultrasound or CT guidance [84,89,90].

PROGNOSIS

The prognosis for infants with diffuse liver involvement related to fetal or neonatal sepsis depends on the underlying condition because hepatic function is rarely compromised sufficiently to determine the outcome. In most cases, pathologic changes in the liver are unsuspected before postmortem examination.

Of 24 infants with solitary hepatic abscesses whose course was described, 8 died. Two infants died before antibiotics were available [26], and the death of another was ascribed to cecal perforation [20]. Four newborns died with sepsis caused by organisms that were identical to the organisms isolated from the abscess [21,25,33,34]. Prematurity was undoubtedly a major contributing factor in two of these deaths [21,25].

TREATMENT

Newborns with a solitary hepatic abscess have traditionally been treated with open surgical drainage in conjunction with antibiotic therapy. Percutaneous catheter drainage is less invasive and often is the preferred first treatment. Several investigators have described the use of percutaneous drainage of intrahepatic abscesses and cysts, guided by CT or ultrasonography, in neonates [41,75,90] and children [7,84,89]. When combined with antibiotic therapy and monitored by ultrasound to ensure resolution, this treatment has been highly effective. It is questionable whether drainage contributed to recovery other than by aiding the selection of antibiotic coverage. Subsequently, patients have been successfully treated with empirical antibiotic therapy alone [91,92]. Conservative medical management in infants has been described in only two neonates and a 5-month-old infant [33,37,78].

The risk of bacteremia and disseminated infection is high in neonates, and the need to identify infecting organisms to guide antibiotic coverage is of greater urgency in the first weeks of life. It is appropriate to ascertain a microbiologic diagnosis with radiographically guided aspiration or drainage of hepatic abscess in a newborn. When proper equipment (e.g., CT, ultrasonography) and experienced personnel are available, this can be attempted percutaneously [89,90]. When they are unavailable, open surgical drainage should be performed. Empirical antibiotic therapy should be reserved only for infants for whom it is believed that the risk of open or closed drainage would exceed the potential benefits.

If purulent material is obtained, initial antibiotic therapy can be selected on the basis of Gram stain. In addition to S. aureus and the aerobic enteric organisms commonly associated with hepatic abscesses, anaerobic bacteria have been suspected as the cause of infection in numerous patients.* If foul-smelling pus is aspirated or if Gram-stained smears show organisms with the characteristic morphology of anaerobes [33], metronidazole, β-lactam and β-lactamase inhibitor combinations (e.g., piperacillin and tazobactam), clindamycin, or imipenem should be included in the initial regimen. Cultures of blood, cerebrospinal fluid, and urine should also be considered before initiation of therapy.

If empirical antibiotic therapy is required, it must be adequate for infections caused by S. aureus, enteric organisms, and anaerobic bacteria. The combination oxacillin, gentamicin, and clindamycin is appropriate. In nurseries where methicillin-resistant S. aureus (MRSA) or methicillin-resistant S. epidermidis infections have been a problem, substitution of vancomycin for oxacillin can provide coverage for these organisms. Gentamicin (and other aminoglycosides) and vancomycin levels must be monitored and dosages adjusted as necessary. Extended-spectrum cephalosporins (e.g., cefotaxime, cefepime, ceftazidime) and carbapenems (e.g., meropenem) may be used for enteric organisms and Pseudomonas species, often obviating the need for aminoglycosides. β-lactam and β-lactamase inhibitor combination drugs (e.g., piperacillin and tazobactam or ampicillin and sulbactam) may provide coverage for many enteric organisms and anaerobic bacteria.

Definitive therapy is based on results of bacteriologic cultures that identify the bacteria and its antibiotic susceptibility. Adequate anaerobic transport and culture techniques must be available if meaningful information is to be obtained. Duration of treatment is based on clinical response, cessation of drainage, and resolution of the abscess cavity as determined by serial ultrasound examinations. Parenteral therapy should be maintained for at least 2 weeks and longer term therapy may be administered when necessary. In older children with multiple abscesses or in children for whom surgery is not feasible, therapy for 6 weeks or more has been recommended.

SPLENIC ABSCESS

Similar to hepatic abscesses, splenic abscesses have been rarely described in infants [93]. Only 1 of 55 splenic abscesses occurred in an infant younger than 6 months. S. aureus, Candida species, and streptococci were the most frequent causes. In 20 of 48 cases, hepatic abscesses coexisted with splenic abscess. In the single infant case, torsion of the splenic vessels was present, whereas in older children, other distant infections of hematologic conditions (e.g., hemoglobinopathy, hematogenous malignancy) were the associated comorbid conditions.

INFECTIONS OF THE BILIARY TRACT

The development of ultrasonography has provided a safe and rapid means for evaluating the neonatal biliary tract. Consequently, an increasing number of reports have appeared describing ultrasound changes seen in the first month of life, with hydrops [94,95], cholelithiasis [95–100], and transient distention of the gallbladder associated [94,95,99,101–104] or unassociated [99,102,103,105–108] with sepsis. Ultrasound criteria for separating normal from pathologically enlarged gallbladders and biliary tracts in neonates have also been described [109,110].

Despite advanced technology and increased surveillance, cholecystitis in the neonate is observed infrequently. The literature has documented about 25 cases, of which 9 were seen in association with an epidemic of neonatal enteritis caused by Salmonella enteritidis [111]. Of the remaining infants, 16 were the subjects of isolated case reports [24,103,112–123], and 3 died of other causes with inflammatory changes in the gallbladder described as an incidental finding at autopsy [81,95,124]. A tissue diagnosis of "chronic cholecystitis" was established in an infant whose biliary disease apparently began at 6 days of age [125].

The pathogenesis of this condition is uncertain; all but three cases [99,118,122] of cholecystitis in the newborn period have been acalculous. It is postulated that sepsis, dehydration, prolonged fasting (e.g., total parenteral nutrition), congenital obstruction, or a stone impacted in the cystic duct leads to biliary stasis and acute distention of the gallbladder. In most cases, resolution of the primary process permits restoration of the flow of bile and relief of distention. In some cases, prolonged obstruction leads to hydrops [94]. Cholecystitis rarely follows, perhaps because of a direct toxic effect of retained bile or because of ischemia related to elevated intraluminal

---

*References [25,28,32,33,35,39].

pressure. Bacterial invasion by fecal flora is probably a secondary phenomenon [114,115,126]. Organisms that have been isolated from gallbladder contents or tissue include *E. coli* [114–116,123], *Serratia marcescens* [103,117], *Pseudomonas* species [115], *Streptococcus faecalis* [123], viridans streptococci [121], *S. aureus* [123], and *Clostridium welchii* [123]. "Gram-positive cocci" were identified by Gram stain in one patient [113].

Infants with cholecystitis may become ill at any time during the first weeks of life; most cases are diagnosed in the 3rd or 4th week. The typical clinical picture is one of sepsis together with signs of peritoneal inflammation and a palpable tender right upper quadrant or epigastric mass. Diarrhea frequently accompanies these findings. Although ultrasonography and radionuclide scintigraphy are helpful in suggesting the presence of gallbladder enlargement or inflammation, diagnosis can be confirmed only by surgical exploration [94,102,103,106,108]. Treatment consists of cholecystectomy or tube cholecystotomy combined with systemic antimicrobial therapy based on Gram stain, culture, and susceptibility studies. If a T tube is placed in the gallbladder, a cholangiogram should be obtained to confirm patency of the biliary system before the tube is removed.

Changes compatible with a diagnosis of ascending cholangitis have been described in histologic sections of liver specimens from infants who died with diarrhea accompanied by hepatocellular injury with cholestasis [91]. Bacteria were also identified in the biliary tree of 2 of 178 premature infants who died after placement of an umbilical venous catheter for an exchange transfusion or for delivery of parenteral fluids [75]. The reasons for this association, if any, are unclear. An infant with spontaneous cholangitis caused by *Enterobacter agglomerans*, presenting as a fever of unknown origin at 3 weeks of age, has also been reported [127].

Severe inflammation and fibrosis of extrahepatic bile ducts and diffuse changes in the portal tracts, resembling changes found in biliary atresia, were found in a premature infant who died 3 hours after birth of listeriosis [128]. The investigator postulated that occult prenatal infections with *L. monocytogenes* might be a rare cause of ascending cholangitis manifesting as idiopathic biliary atresia at birth.

INFECTIONS OF THE ADRENAL GLANDS

Multiple adrenal microabscesses are occasionally found as metastatic lesions associated with neonatal sepsis. These abscesses are particularly characteristic of neonatal listeriosis (see Chapter 13). Solitary adrenal abscesses are rare, however; only about 25 such cases have been described [17,129–150].

The spectrum of organisms responsible for adrenal abscesses is the same as that seen in neonatal sepsis and includes *E. coli* (seven cases) [17,129,130,135–138], group B streptococci (GBS) (four cases) [138–141], *Proteus mirabilis* (three cases) [131,132,144], *S. aureus* [142,143], *Bacteroides* species [133,145], and two cases each of *Streptococcus pneumoniae* with *Bacteroides* species [134]; *Peptostreptococcus* species [146] was recovered from one

case. Drainage of foul-smelling pus at surgery suggests that anaerobic bacteria may have been present in two infants from whom *E. coli* and *S. aureus* were isolated [136,142]. Cultures were not obtained from four patients [147–150].

Fourteen abscesses were located on the right side, seven were located on the left, and three [138,139,147] were bilateral. Three fourths of the infants were male. The same laterality and sex predominance are seen with adrenal hemorrhage in the newborn [147,150–152], and it has been postulated that formation of an adrenal abscess requires a preexisting hematoma as a nidus for bacterial seeding [137,138]. This theory of pathogenesis is supported further by clinical observations[134,135,139,146,147] and by objective evidence (e.g., curvilinear calcifications [130,132] documenting the presence of hemorrhage before development of an abscess [134,138,142,145,150].

Most infants with adrenal abscess have presented in the 3rd or 4th week of life with signs of sepsis and an abdominal or flank mass. A history of difficult delivery or intrapartum asphyxia was observed in about one half of these infants, and significant maternal fever or infection during labor was observed in about one fourth [138,140,141,150]. Although a few infants are afebrile when first evaluated, a palpable mass is almost always present. Abscesses are usually 6 to 8 cm in diameter, with some containing 200 mL of pus [133] and measuring 12 cm in diameter [134] or crossing the midline [146].

Laboratory studies are helpful in the evaluation of a possible adrenal abscess. Most infants exhibit a leukocytosis; about one third are anemic with a history of prolonged neonatal jaundice, both of which are features associated with adrenal hemorrhage. Urinary excretion of catecholamines and their metabolites (particularly vanillylmandelic acid and homovanillic acid), which is usually increased with neuroblastoma, is normal. Because most infants with adrenal abscess are seen for evaluation of possible sepsis, a blood culture, lumbar puncture, urine culture, and chest radiograph should be obtained.

Ultrasonography has become a widely accepted modality for initial evaluation of all neonatal abdominal masses. With the presence of an adrenal abscess, ultrasound examination can help to define the extent and cystic nature of the lesion and often can show movable necrotic debris in the abscess cavity.* With serial examinations, abscesses can be distinguished from masses associated with liquefying hematoma, adrenal cyst, hydronephrosis of an obstructed upper pole duplication, or necrotic neuroblastoma [138,140,150,153,154]. Intravenous pyelography shows downward displacement of the kidney and compression of the upper calyces, which confirms the presence of a suprarenal mass.† A round, suprarenal, radiopaque halo or rim with central lucency, which is characteristic of adrenal abscess, may also be seen on early films [137,139,143], but is not pathognomonic [138]. Intravenous pyelography adds little diagnostic information to that provided by ultrasound studies. Experience with radionuclide scanning [140,142,143], CT [138,144], and

---

*References [132,137,138,141,142,144–148].
†References [130–132,134,136,138,141,142,144–146,149].

MRI [126] in this condition is limited, but these modalities are likely to be as useful as ultrasonography.

Whatever diagnostic methods are used, concern about persisting signs of sepsis and the possible presence of an adrenal neoplasm usually encourage early efforts to establish a diagnosis. In the past, recommended management has been incision and drainage or resection of the abscess [134,138,141,144,150]. Needle aspiration under ultrasound guidance, combined with placement of a catheter for drainage and irrigation, has proved to be a useful alternative method [88,130,131,143] and is likely to supplant open drainage as the preferred method. Antibiotic therapy should be based on Gram stain, culture, and susceptibility studies of abscess fluid and should be continued for 10 to 14 days, provided that drainage can be established.

The adrenals are infected in about 15% of infants with congenital syphilis [57,58]. In addition to the presence of spirochetes, the most frequent and characteristic change is an extraordinary amount of cellular connective tissue in the capsule.

APPENDICITIS

Acute appendicitis is extremely rare in infants younger than 4 weeks of age. Reviews of more than 25,000 cases of appendicitis in infants and children in Great Britain [155], Ireland [156], Norway [157], Germany [158], and the United States [159–164] revealed only 8 infants who presented during the neonatal period. Pediatric surgery centers in Germany [165], Boston [166], Cleveland [167], Chicago [168], and Detroit [169] found only four cases of neonatal appendicitis. Since the condition was first described by Albrecht in 1905 [170,171] and Diess in 1908 [172], approximately 65 cases of neonatal suppurative appendicitis have been reported in the literature with sufficient details to permit characterization of the clinical features [155,160,161,164,173–210]. Infants with appendicitis caused by other conditions, such as Hirschsprung disease [211,212], necrotizing enterocolitis (NEC) [213], or incarceration in an inguinal hernia [214,215], have not been included in this discussion. An additional 25 to 30 cases that have been reported with incomplete clinical observations, listed in series of patients with neonatal peritonitis (see "Peritonitis") or mentioned in other review articles but unavailable for analysis, are also not included.

Inflammation of the appendix is more common in newborn boys than newborn girls. In reports in which the sex was stated, 40 cases occurred in boys, and 17 cases occurred in girls. Prematurity also seems to be a predisposing factor: 23 of the 49 infants whose birth weights were recorded weighed less than 2500 g at birth. The incidence of appendicitis in infants of multiple births (six twins and one triplet) seems to be higher than would be expected on the basis of low birth weight alone.

MICROBIOLOGY

Because obstruction of the appendiceal lumen is responsible for almost all cases of appendicitis [166], it is intuitive that gram-negative enteric organisms resident in the

bowel are usually isolated from the peritoneal fluid or periappendiceal pus of about 75% of infants. Specific etiologic agents include *E. coli*, *Klebsiella* species, *Enterobacter* species, *Pseudomonas* species, *Proteus* species, untyped streptococci, *S. aureus*, and *Bacteroides* species These bacterial species have also been isolated from the peritoneal fluid of older children with appendicitis [163,166,216]. Attempts at isolation of anaerobic bacteria have been rarely described.

A single case of perforated amebic appendicitis with secondary bacterial peritonitis and multiple hepatic abscesses in a premature infant born in Great Britain has been reported. *Entamoeba histolytica* observed in the wall of the necrotic appendix was presumably acquired from the infant's father, who was a carrier [20]. A patient with gangrenous appendicitis associated with *Rhizopus oryzae* has also been reported [217]. It was postulated that the fungus colonized the infant's gut by transfer from an adhesive bandage used to secure an endotracheal tube.

PATHOGENESIS

Obstruction of the appendiceal lumen has been generally accepted as the primary cause of appendicitis in all age groups. The relative rarity of this condition in the first month of life is probably related to factors that serve to decrease the likelihood of obstruction, including a wide-based, funnel-shaped appendix; the predominantly liquid and soft solid diet given to infants; the absence of prolonged periods in the upright position; and the infrequency of infections that cause hyperplasia of the appendiceal lymphoid tissue [163,218,219].

The causes of luminal obstruction in the newborn period, when recognized, are often extrinsic to the appendix itself. Reports of appendicitis caused by the presence of ectopic pancreatic tissue [160], a fecalith [174], or meconium plug [167] are unusual exceptions. In 1911, it was suggested that sharp angulation of the appendix, bent on itself in the narrow retrocolic space, may be an important cause of obstruction [220]; however, this anatomy, found in 11 neonates with inflammatory changes in the appendix and noted among 200 consecutive autopsies in infants younger than 3 months at death, has not been repeated in the past 80 years.

Inflammation of the appendix with perforation has been described as the presenting illness in several infants with neonatal Hirschsprung disease [211,213]. The association of these two conditions has been attributed to functional obstruction, increased intraluminal pressure, and fecal trapping that occur proximal to aganglionic segments. Suppurative appendicitis related to incarceration and strangulation of the cecum within an inguinal or scrotal hernia has been found in numerous infants [214,215].

CLINICAL MANIFESTATIONS

The onset of neonatal appendicitis generally occurs during the first 2 weeks of life. Only 3 of 54 infants with this condition presented between the 1st and 10th day. The reasons for this phenomenon are unclear, particularly in view of the relatively even distribution of cases during the remainder of the 1st year of life [164]. Five cases of "prenatal" appendicitis have been described [221–225]. Of the four available for analysis, only one showed definite evidence of a suppurative process in the appendix and signs of bowel obstruction clearly present at birth [221]; however, cultures and Gram stain of the pus found at surgery were free of bacteria. Poisoning by mercuric chloride was suspected in one [223] of the remaining three cases, and the other two, who were said to have prenatal rupture of the appendix, were asymptomatic until the 2nd [221] and 12th [225] days of life.

The signs of neonatal appendicitis correspond to the signs of any of the various forms of intestinal obstruction that occur during the newborn period (Table 10–1) [225]. Prominent early findings include abdominal distention; progressive and frequently bilious vomiting; and evidence of pain, as manifested by persistent crying, irritability, or "colic." Clinical features such as diarrhea, constipation, lethargy, or refusal to feed may also be evident, but are too nonspecific to be helpful in establishing a diagnosis. The presence or absence of fever is an unreliable sign in appendicitis as in other forms of neonatal infection; temperature has been recorded as normal or subnormal in more than 50% of newborns with this condition. Abdominal tenderness and guarding are inconsistent findings and, when present, are rarely localized to the appendiceal area. Physical signs of sufficient specificity to indicate acute inflammation of the appendix are generally absent until late in the course of the illness, when gangrene and rupture may result in the formation of a localized intra-abdominal abscess or cellulitis of the anterior abdominal wall. Erythema or edema, or both, of the right lower quadrant has been observed in several patients. The presence of this finding, particularly when accompanied by a palpable mass in the right iliac fossa, indicates bowel perforation with peritonitis and should suggest a preoperative diagnosis of NEC or appendicitis (see "Necrotizing Enterocolitis").

DIAGNOSIS

The diagnosis of appendicitis in a neonate is usually determined at surgery performed for evaluation of abdominal distention and suspected peritonitis. With the high incidence of prematurity associated with early appendicitis, bowel perforation from NEC has been a common preoperative consideration [206]. The two conditions can coexist, and in some cases, the appendix may participate in the process of ischemic necrosis and perforation [205,213].

Laboratory studies are of little value in establishing a diagnosis of appendicitis in a newborn. White blood cell counts of less than 10,000/mm^3 were found in 10 of 30 infants. Urinalyses are usually normal, although ketonuria, which reflects diminished caloric intake; hematuria; and proteinuria may be seen. Because bacteremia may accompany appendiceal perforation and peritonitis, a blood culture and evaluation for metastatic infection with lumbar puncture and chest radiography should be performed. The value of paracentesis for diagnosis of bowel perforation and peritoneal infection is discussed later (see "Necrotizing Enterocolitis").

Radiologic examinations are occasionally helpful, but in most cases serve only to confirm a clinical impression of small bowel obstruction. The presence of an increased soft tissue density displacing loops of intestine from the right iliac fossa generally indicates appendiceal perforation with abscess formation and is perhaps the most reliable sign of acute appendicitis in the neonate. Extraluminal gas may be localized briefly to the right lower quadrant after rupture of the appendix [211]. The rapid development of an extensive pneumoperitoneum obscures the site of origin of the escaping gas in most infants within a short time [226]. Ultrasonography may aid in detection of a periappendiceal abscess [83], but is not helpful in establishing an early diagnosis of appendicitis because it lacks sensitivity and specificity.

PROGNOSIS

The overall mortality rate from appendicitis in the newborn is high, but is improving. Eight of the newborns in the last 12 reported cases have survived, whereas of 60 infants with this condition for whom the outcome was recorded, 38 (64%) died. Survival was unrelated to birth weight. Among factors responsible for mortalities, three seem to be of primary importance: delay in diagnosis, a high incidence of perforation, and the rapid onset of diffuse peritonitis after appendiceal rupture.

Perforation has been identified at surgery or autopsy in 70% of newborns with acute appendicitis. The relative frequency of this complication has been attributed to delays in establishing a diagnosis and to certain anatomic features of the appendix in young infants that predispose it to early necrosis and rupture. These features include a meager blood supply that renders the organ more vulnerable to ischemia; a cecum that is relatively smaller and less distensible than that of adults, forcing a greater intraluminal pressure on the appendix; and the presence of a thin muscularis and serosa that readily lose their structural integrity under the combined effects of ischemia and increased internal pressure [163,181,182,191].

After the appendix ruptures, infants are unable to contain infection efficiently at the site of origin. Rapid dissemination of spilled intestinal contents produces a diffuse peritonitis within hours because of the small size

TABLE 10–1   Signs of Intra-abdominal Neonatal Appendicitis in 55 Infants

Sign	Incidence (%)
Abdominal distention	90
Vomiting	60
Refusal of feedings	40
Temperature ≥38° C	40
Temperature 37-38° C	30
Temperature ≤37° C	30
Pain (crying, restlessness)	30
Lethargy	30
Erythema/edema of right lower quadrant	25
Mass in right lower quadrant	20
Diarrhea	20
Passage of bloody stools	20

of the infant's omentum, which fails to provide an efficient envelope for escaping material; the relatively longer and more mobile mesenteries, which favor widespread contamination; and the small size of the peritoneal cavity, which also permits access of infected material to areas distant from the site of perforation [160,166,181,182]. Peritonitis, accompanied by sepsis and by the massive outpouring of fluids, electrolytes, and proteins from inflamed serosal surfaces, is generally the terminal event in neonatal appendicitis. Deterioration of the infant's condition is often extremely rapid; failure to recognize the underlying illness and to institute appropriate therapy promptly is inevitably followed by a fatal outcome.

TREATMENT

Surgical intervention is essential for survival of young infants with appendicitis. Because vomiting, diarrhea, and anorexia frequently accompany this condition, restoration of fluid and electrolyte balance is a major factor in ensuring a favorable outcome. Loss of plasma into the bowel wall and lumen of the dilated intestine may require additional replacement with whole blood, plasma, or an albumin equivalent. Optimal preparation often necessitates a delay of several hours, but is a major determining factor in the success of any surgical procedure done during the neonatal period.

The preoperative use of antibiotics has been recommended in infants with intestinal obstruction to achieve therapeutic blood levels of drug before the time of incision and possible contamination [167,227,228]. Perforation, fecal spillage, and peritonitis occur so early in the course of neonatal appendicitis that almost all infants with this condition require treatment before surgery. After the diagnosis of gangrenous or perforated appendicitis has been established and surgery has been performed, parenteral antibiotic therapy should be continued for a minimum of 10 days. The combination of clindamycin (or metronidazole), gentamicin (or extended-spectrum cephalosporins), and ampicillin provides adequate coverage against most enteric pathogens and can be used for initial empirical therapy. Alternatively, β-lactam and β-lactamase inhibitor combinations such as piperacillin and tazobactam or carbapenem antibiotics (e.g., imipenem or meropenem) can be used alone for broad coverage of enteric bacteria, *Pseudomonas* species, and anaerobic bacteria. Until the infant is able to tolerate alimentation, careful attention to postoperative maintenance of body fluids, electrolyte balance, nutrition, and correction of blood and plasma losses is vital to survival (see "Peritonitis" and "Necrotizing Enterocolitis").

PERITONITIS

Peritonitis in the newborn is most commonly associated with perforation of the gastrointestinal tract, ruptured omphaloceles, or wound infections that follow abdominal surgery [229,230]. It has been estimated that 20% to 40% of gastrointestinal surgical problems in the neonatal period are complicated by bacterial peritonitis (see "Necrotizing Enterocolitis") [185,231]. At pediatric surgical centers in the United States [231–233], Great Britain

[230,234], Hungary [235], Germany [236,237], France [238], and Zimbabwe [239], 1 to 10 cases per year have been reported in retrospective analyses of peritonitis diagnosed during the first month of life. Among almost 3000 infants admitted to a neonatal intensive care unit (NICU) in Liverpool in 1981-1982, there were 6 cases of peritonitis, all from NEC perforation of the gastrointestinal tract [240]. Peritonitis was present in 4 (all of low birth weight) of 501 infants on whom consecutive autopsies were performed from 1960-1966 at St. Christopher's Hospital for Children in Philadelphia. These cases represented approximately 3% of all patients with inflammatory lesions associated with death in this age group [241]. Potter [15] considered the peritoneum "one of the most frequent points of localization" in infants dying with sepsis. Among 121 such infants autopsied from 1976-1988 at St. Mary's Hospital in Manchester, England, generalized peritonitis was found in 9 (7.4%) [230].

A preponderance of boys (2.5:1) [190,239,240] and a high incidence of prematurity (33%)[231,234–236] have been found in unselected series of infants with this condition. These features are probably less a characteristic of bacterial peritonitis in the newborn than of the primary surgical and septic conditions that are responsible for its occurrence (particularly NEC). There seems to be a female preponderance among newborns with primary peritonitis [235,242]. A high incidence of congenital anomalies not involving the intestinal tract has also been observed among neonates with peritonitis [231,236,243,244].

MICROBIOLOGY

The condition that permits bacteria to colonize the peritoneal surface determines the nature of the infecting organisms. Most infants in whom rupture of a viscus and fecal spillage have caused peritonitis are infected by bacteria considered to be part of the normal enteric microflora; however, prior use of antimicrobial agents and colonization patterns within a nursery are important factors in determining which organisms predominate. Although a mixed flora of two to five species can often be recovered [243], single isolates have been reported in a third of infants with peritonitis [245,246]. The predominant aerobic organisms usually include *E. coli*, *Klebsiella* species, *Enterobacter* species, *Pseudomonas* species, *Proteus* species, coagulase-negative and coagulase-positive staphylococci, ungrouped streptococci, *Enterococcus*, and *Candida* [230,231,237,239,246–248].

Techniques adequate for the isolation of anaerobic organisms have been used infrequently. In a series of 43 consecutive infants with gastrointestinal perforation and bacterial growth from peritoneal fluid, a mixed aerobic-anaerobic flora was isolated with *Bacteroides* species as the predominant anaerobes [243]; remaining specimens grew aerobic or facultative organisms alone, and no culture yielded only anaerobes. In that series and others, the same organisms were frequently isolated from the peritoneal cavity and blood [232,243,244,248].

In contrast to fecal flora isolated from infants with gastrointestinal perforation, gram-positive organisms predominated among neonates with "idiopathic primary peritonitis." This condition is caused by sepsis in most cases, but it also has often been associated with omphalitis. Specific organisms in one representative series included *S. pneumoniae* (three cases); ungrouped β-hemolytic streptococcus (three cases); and *S. aureus, Pseudomonas* species, and *E. coli* (one case each) [231]. Gram-positive cocci were also the major isolates in other series of peritonitis associated with hematogenous dissemination of organisms or extension from a peripheral suppurative focus.* Many of the cases caused by *S. aureus* occurred before the advent of antibiotics or during the worldwide pandemic of staphylococcal disease in the late 1950s, whereas streptococci, particularly GBS, have been a prominent cause in recent years [242,249–253].

Rarely, peritonitis may be caused by *Candida albicans* in pure culture or mixed with gram-negative enteric organisms [230,254]. Because clinical findings in this condition are not different from the findings of bacterial peritonitis, the diagnosis is usually established by blood or peritoneal fluid culture. Severe hypothermia has been described as a possible predisposing cause of bowel perforation and peritonitis owing to *Candida* [255]. In addition to well-recognized risk factors, such as prematurity, antibiotic therapy, and parenteral nutrition with deep venous catheters, NEC may be a significant risk factor for systemic candidiasis, in which it was observed in 37% of 30 infants [256]. Only a single infant in this series had a positive culture for *Candida* species from the peritoneum, however. Peritoneal catheters or peritoneal dialysis may also be a risk for direct inoculation of *Candida* organisms into the peritoneal space, which occurred in 1 of 26 children [257] (see Chapter 33).

PATHOGENESIS

Acute bacterial peritonitis may occur whenever bacteria gain access to the peritoneal cavity, through intestinal perforation, by extension from a suppurative focus, or by the hematogenous route. Intrauterine peritonitis owing to *L. monocytogenes* has been reported [230]; however, cases of "fetal peritonitis" described in earlier reports were actually examples of meconium peritonitis caused by intrauterine intestinal perforation [258,259]. Although bacterial colonization of the gastrointestinal tract in the first days of life may lead to infection in this condition, it is an aseptic peritonitis in its initial stages. A similar condition with focal perforation of the ileum or colon occurring postnatally has been described in infants with very low birth weight. Blue-black discoloration of the abdomen, caused by meconium staining of the tissues of the underlying skin, may be the first physical finding in these infants. Clinical, radiographic, and histopathologic evidence of infection or inflammation was notably absent in most cases [228].

Conditions that predispose to neonatal peritonitis are outlined in Table 10–2. Among almost 400 newborns with peritonitis studied from 1959-1978, perforation of the intestinal tract was responsible for 72% of cases, with ruptured omphaloceles or gastroschisis responsible for 12%, hematogenous dissemination or "primary" peritonitis

TABLE 10–2   Etiology of Bacterial Peritonitis in the Neonatal Period

Gastrointestinal perforation [191,231,232,235–240,243,245,249, 262,263]

Necrotizing enterocolitis

Ischemic necrosis

Spontaneous focal gastrointestinal perforation [233,246,249,261, 262,264]

Volvulus

Hirschsprung disease

Meconium ileus (cystic fibrosis) [231,266]

Postoperative complications

Congenital anomalies

Internal hernia

Catheter-associated vascular thrombosis [230]

Indomethacin therapy (enteral or parenteral) [267,268]

Trauma

Feeding tubes [269]

Rectal thermometers, catheters, enema [275–279]

Intrauterine exchange transfusion [231,273]

Paracentesis of ascites fluid

Meconium peritonitis with postnatal bacterial contamination [243,259,260]

Peptic ulcer: stomach, duodenum, ectopic gastric mucosa

Acute suppurative appendicitis

Infection

Shigella or *Salmonella* enterocolitis [274–276]

Congenital luetic enteritis with necrosis [58]

Ruptured omphalocele or gastroschisis

Postoperative: anastomotic leaks, wound dehiscence, wound contamination

Primary peritonitis

Prenatal sepsis: listeriosis, syphilis [58], tuberculosis [46–49]

Neonatal sepsis [10,33,231,232,240,252–254,263,278]

Suppurative omphalitis [26,72,240,244,250,251,263,277]

Transmural migration (theory) [265,279]

responsible for 12%, and omphalitis and postoperative complications responsible for 2% each.* In a comprehensive review of neonatal peritonitis, Bell [229,243] described common sites and causes of gastrointestinal perforation and their relative frequencies (Figs. 10–1 and 10–2).

No cases of neonatal peritonitis in recent years have been attributed to microorganisms entering the peritoneal cavity by traversing the bowel wall through the lymphatics or within macrophages (i.e., transmural migration). Evidence for the existence of this pathway is theoretical and is based primarily on retrospective analyses of pathologic data in humans with supporting observations made on laboratory animals [262,263]. Further confirmation is necessary before the transmural pathway can be accepted as an established source of peritoneal colonization by bacteria.

---

*References [10,26,33,71,242,244–253].

*References [190,229,230,236,260,261].

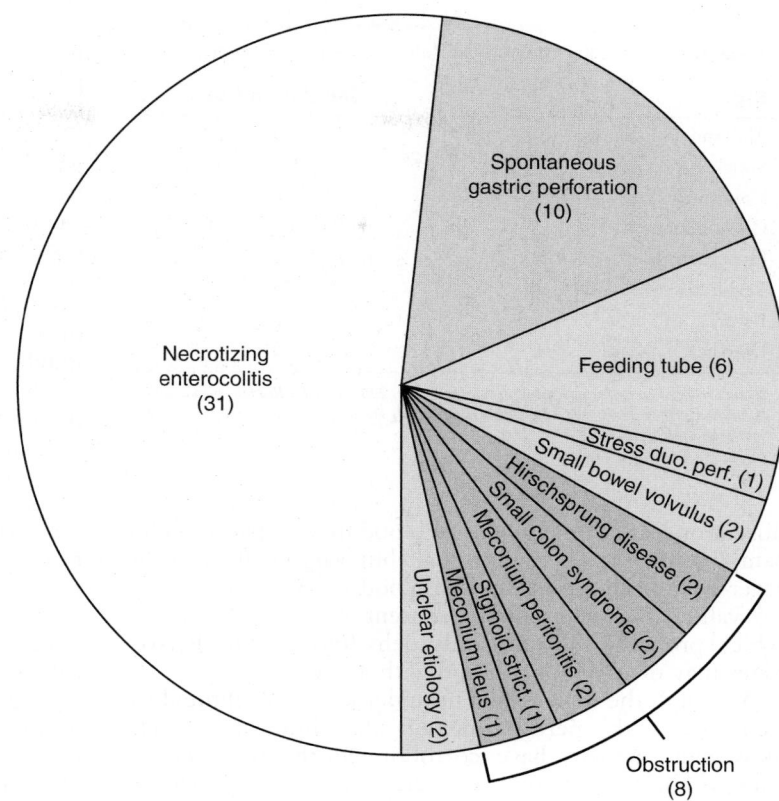

FIGURE 10–1 Causes of perforation in 60 neonates. duo. perf., duodenal perforation; strict., stricture. *(From Bell MJ. Peritonitis in the newborn—current concepts. Pediatr Clin North Am 32:1181, 1985.)*

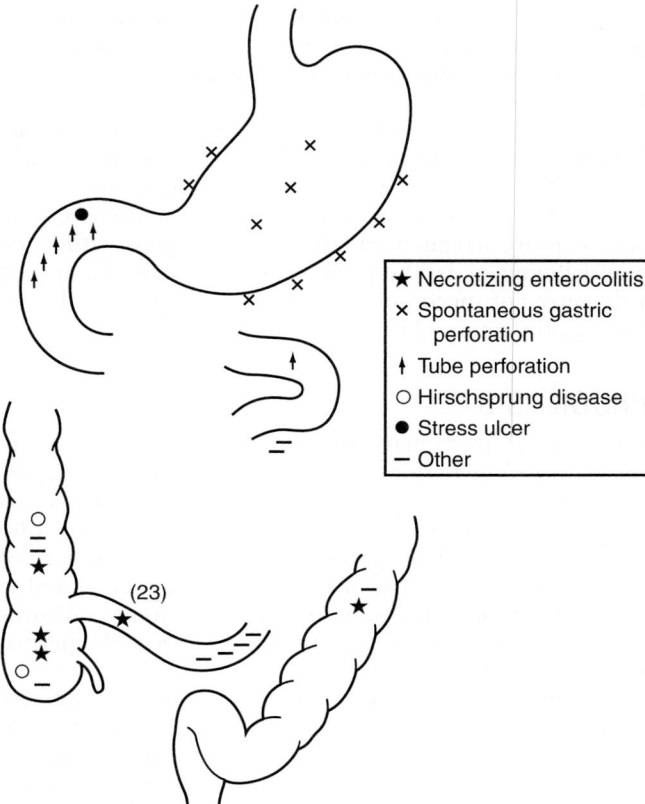

FIGURE 10–2 Sites of perforation in 60 neonates. *(From Bell MJ. Peritonitis in the newborn—current concepts. Pediatr Clin North Am 32:1181, 1985.)*

CLINICAL MANIFESTATIONS

Neonatal peritonitis is a disease primarily of the first 10 days of life; numerous infants have evidence of peritoneal infection within the first 24 hours [231,232,239,244]. An analysis of etiologic factors responsible for peritonitis in the newborn provides a ready explanation for this observation (see Table 10–2). Most cases of NEC [243,264] and spontaneous gastric perforation [232,243,248,260] occur within the 1st week. Ruptured omphaloceles and gastroschisis often develop early infections, and in infants with congenital obstruction, the onset of alimentation during the first 12 to 24 hours accentuates distention and ischemic necrosis of the bowel wall, which leads to early intestinal perforation. Exchange transfusions are performed most frequently within the first 1 or 2 days of life and may be followed by enterocolitis within 4 to 24 hours in infants in whom perforation ultimately occurs [265,266]. Neonatal sepsis, with potential peritoneal seeding of microorganisms, is more frequent during the first 48 hours of life than during any subsequent period [267].

The various signs and symptoms present in a young infant with peritonitis were summarized most succinctly by Thelander [248] in 1939:

"The little patient looks sick. He is cyanotic; the respirations are rapid and grunting; the abdomen is distended, and the abdominal wall, the flanks and the scrotum or vulva are usually edematous. Frequently brawny induration of the edematous area, which may resemble erysipelas, is also present. Food is taken poorly or not at all. Vomiting is frequent and persistent. The vomitus contains bile and may contain blood. The stools are either

TABLE 10–3 Signs of Bacterial Peritonitis in the Neonate*

Sign	Incidence (%)
Abdominal distention	85
Shock	80
Vomiting	70
Constipation	60
Hypothermia	60
Respiratory distress	55
Fever	15
Diarrhea	15

Data are based on patients described in references 232, 240, and 243. Redness, edema, and induration of the anterior abdominal wall, noted in only one series [243], are also recognized as characteristic signs.

absent or scant; some mucus or blood may be passed. The temperature may be subnormal, but varying degrees of fever have been reported. The blood count is of little or no value. The hemoglobin content may be very high, which probably indicates only dehydration. The leukocytes may or may not respond with a rise."

Although the review by Thelander [248] was limited to neonates with perforation of the intestinal tract, subsequent reports have corroborated the presence of these findings in infants with peritonitis resulting from a wide variety of causes.* Not all of the symptoms described may be encountered in any one patient; however, some are always present (Table 10–3).

The large overlap between signs of neonatal peritonitis and sepsis can make it difficult to differentiate the two on the basis of clinical findings. Signs of intestinal obstruction such as abdominal distention and vomiting, which are seen in 10% to 20% of newborns with sepsis [9,17,244], may reflect a coexistent unrecognized peritonitis. Because the early use of antibiotics often cures hematogenous peritonitis in infants with septicemia, the diagnosis may be missed in infants who survive. Peritonitis unassociated with perforation was found at postmortem examination in 4 of 20 infants with sepsis in 1933 [10], 9 of 73 premature infants dying with septicemia from 1959-1964 [9], and 9 of 121 infants with septicemia dying from 1976-1988 [229].

DIAGNOSIS

Ultrasonography [83] or abdominal radiographs taken in the erect and recumbent positions showing free intraperitoneal fluid can be helpful in the diagnosis of peritonitis, and sometimes the only evidence of perforation is apparent on these imaging studies. Absence of definition of the right inferior hepatic margin, increased density of soft tissue, and the presence of "floating" loops of bowel have been recorded as positive signs of ascites [226,268]. Diagnostic paracentesis can be useful in determining whether the fluid is caused by bacterial peritonitis [242,251,269,270], hemoperitoneum, chylous ascites [271], or bile peritonitis [272].

The left lateral ("left-side down") decubitus film is of great value in showing small amounts of intraperitoneal gas [243]. Although pneumoperitoneum can be caused by mediastinal air dissecting from the chest into the abdomen [273,274], free gas in the peritoneal cavity usually indicates intestinal perforation. An associated pneumatosis intestinalis should suggest the diagnosis of NEC, but is not specific for this condition. Several patterns of intraperitoneal gas distribution have been described [83,265–276]: the air-dome sign, falciform ligament sign, football sign, lucent-liver sign, saddlebag sign, and gas in the scrotum. Absence of a gastric air-fluid level on an erect abdominal radiograph, with a normal or decreased amount of gas in the small and large bowel, strongly favors a diagnosis of gastric perforation [276]. This finding is almost always accompanied by pneumoperitoneum.

In equivocal cases, metrizamide contrast studies of the bowel can be helpful in establishing a diagnosis of intestinal perforation [245,273]. Serial abdominal transillumination with a bright fiberoptic light is a useful bedside method for the early detection of ascites or pneumoperitoneum in the newborn [277].

Failure to show free air in the peritoneal cavity does not rule out a diagnosis of perforation, particularly if air swallowing has been reduced or prevented through orotracheal intubation, nasogastric suction, or use of neuromuscular blocking agents [269,273,278]. In some cases, the amount of gas in the bowel lumen is so small that even if perforation occurs, the gas could escape detection. Alternatively, small leaks may become walled off and the free air reabsorbed [273,279,280]. In three large series of infants with peritonitis in whom a patent site of perforation was found at surgery, pneumoperitoneum was absent in 35% to 75% [231,243,244].

Radiographic evidence of intestinal obstruction, although a common cause or consequence of peritonitis, lacks sufficient specificity to be a consistent aid to diagnosis. A diffuse granular appearance of the abdomen, with one or more irregular calcific densities lying within the bowel lumen or in the peritoneal cavity, should suggest a diagnosis of meconium peritonitis with possible bacterial superinfection [259].

PROGNOSIS

Prematurity, pulmonary infections, shock, and hemorrhage related to perforation of the intestinal tract, sepsis, and disseminated intravascular coagulopathy are often the factors responsible for the death of neonates, who may concurrently have peritonitis diagnosed at surgery or at postmortem examination. For this reason, case-fatality rates often represent the mortality rate among newborns dying with, rather than because of, infection of the peritoneal cavity [230,236,243].

Before 1970, the incidence of fatalities was exceedingly high when peritonitis was associated with gastrointestinal perforation; mortality rates of 70% were observed in large series.* Heightened awareness of conditions associated with perforation, more rapid diagnosis, and improved

---

*References [190,231,233–235,239,243,248].

*References [190,231,234,235,237–239,244,280].

surgical management have led to a doubling of survivors in recent years [236,237]. The cause of perforation seems to influence the likelihood of survival, with spontaneous gastric perforation having the lowest mortality rate (10%) and perforation of the duodenum caused by a feeding tube the highest mortality rate (50%); NEC (40%) and all other causes (25%) occupy intermediate positions [243].

As survival rates have improved, the number of nonlethal complications after perforation has increased proportionally. In one review, two thirds of surviving infants had significant postoperative complications pertaining to infection (e.g., bacteremia, wound infection, intra-abdominal abscess) or gastrointestinal tract dysfunction (e.g., esophageal reflux, obstruction, stomal stenosis) [243]. Secondary surgical procedures to correct these problems were required in more than half of the infants. Parenteral hyperalimentation for nutritional support during the recovery period was required in 60% of infants.

The mortality rate among neonates with peritonitis from causes other than perforation of the bowel, such as sepsis [190,231,235,239], omphalitis [239,281], or a ruptured omphalocele [231,236,239], although high in the past, has not been reassessed in recent years [243]. Early diagnosis and institution of appropriate surgical therapy are major factors in reducing the mortality rate [243]. It has been shown that infants operated on within 24 hours after the onset of symptoms have survival rates almost double the rates of infants operated on between 24 and 48 hours and 2½ times higher than the rate for infants whose surgery was delayed more than 48 hours [244]. Factors with an apparent adverse influence on prognosis include low birth weight [231,236,239,243,261], low birth weight for gestational age [229], congenital malformations [236], male sex [230], and initial serum pH of less than 7.30 [230].

TREATMENT

The treatment of bacterial peritonitis is directed primarily toward correction of the causative condition [230]. Careful attention to preoperative preparation of the infant is essential to survival. As soon as bowel obstruction or perforation is diagnosed, continuous nasogastric suction should be instituted for decompression and prevention of aspiration pneumonitis. Diagnostic needle paracentesis is also useful for relief of pneumoperitoneum and may facilitate exchange of gas by reducing the intra-abdominal pressure. Shock, dehydration, and electrolyte disturbances should be corrected through parenteral administration of appropriate electrolyte solutions, plasma, or plasma substitutes. If blood is discovered in fluid recovered by gastric suction or abdominal paracentesis, use of whole blood, packed red blood cells, or other fluids may be necessary to correct hypovolemia. Persistent bleeding must be evaluated for disseminated intravascular coagulation or thrombocytopenia, or both, and treated accordingly. Hypothermia, which frequently accompanies neonatal peritonitis, should be corrected before induction of anesthesia. Infants who are unable to tolerate oral or tube feedings within 2 or 3 postoperative days should be started on parenteral hyperalimentation.

If a diagnosis of peritonitis is established at the time of paracentesis or surgery, aerobic and anaerobic cultures of peritoneal contents should be taken before initiation of antibiotic therapy. Parenteral administration of a combination of gentamicin or an extended-spectrum cephalosporin and clindamycin and ampicillin should be continued for 7 to 10 days [215,228]. Other antibiotics that provide a broad spectrum against enteric organisms, *Pseudomonas* species, enterococci, and anaerobic organisms include β-lactam and β-lactamase inhibitor compounds and carbapenems. In the event of a poor clinical response, culture and susceptibility studies of the infecting organisms should be used as guides for modifying therapy.

Leakage of intestinal contents sometimes results in formation of a localized abscess, rather than contamination of the entire peritoneal cavity. Management of infants with such an abscess should include antimicrobial therapy and surgical drainage of the abscess by the most convenient route.

NECROTIZING ENTEROCOLITIS

NEC with necrosis of the bowel wall is a severe, often fatal disease that has been occurring with increasing frequency in recent years. The average annual NEC mortality rate is 13.1 per 100,000 live births; black infants, particularly boys, are three times more likely to die of NEC than white infants, and mortality rates are highest in the southern United States [280,282–291]. NEC occurs in about 5% of infants admitted to NICUs; however, the incidence varies widely among centers and from year to year at the same institution [292–305]. NEC predominantly affects infants with birth weights less than 2000 g [282,284,298,213,306–312]; in several series, the frequency in infants weighing less than 1500 g was 10% to 15%.* Only 5% to 10% of all cases of classic NEC occur in term infants [291,318–320]. It has been stated that occasional cases of NEC may be the price to be paid for the benefits of modern neonatal intensive care [321].

Although most reports of NEC emanate from the United States, Canada, and Great Britain, the condition occurs worldwide in countries maintaining NICUs. In a review of NEC in two NICUs of academic centers, NEC increased the risk for death (odds ratio 24.5), infections (odds ratio 5.7), and need for central intravenous line placement (odds ratio 14.0) [322]. Infants with surgical and medical NEC had lengths of stay of 60 days and 22 days greater than infants without NEC with additional costs of $186,200 and $73,700, resulting in additional hospital charges of $216,666 per surviving infant.

NEC affects an estimated 7% to 14% of all low birth weight preterm infants [323] and is a leading cause of death and morbidity in the NICU with no change in incidence in the past 20 years [324,325]. More recent reports have estimated that about 9000 cases occur annually in the United States with a case-fatality rate of 15% to 30% [326].

---

*References [282–285,299,300,304,311,313–317].

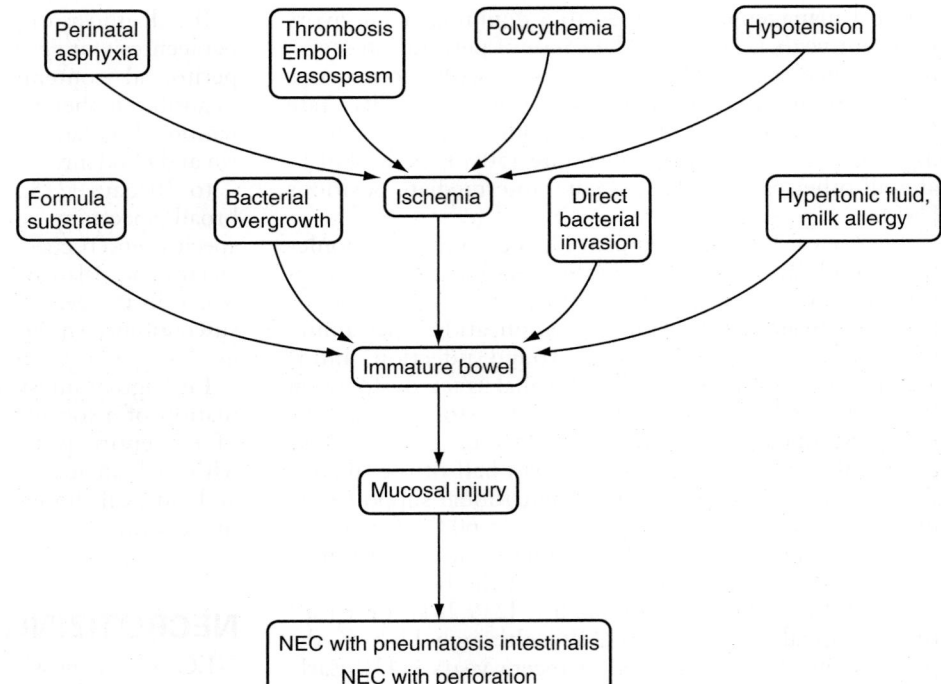

FIGURE 10–3 Pathogenesis of mucosal injury leading to necrotizing enterocolitis (NEC). *(Adapted from Walsh MC, Kliegman RM. Necrotizing enterocolitis. Pediatric Basics 40:5, 1985.)*

PATHOLOGY AND PATHOGENESIS

Bowel wall necrosis of variable length and depth is the characteristic feature of NEC, with perforation in one third of affected infants generally in the terminal ileum or cecum, where microcirculation is poor.* The pathogenesis of NEC is not established, but most investigators agree that the initiating event is some form of stress to the immature gastrointestinal tract, which leads to disruption of the mucosal barrier, bacterial invasion and proliferation, and gas formation within the bowel wall (Fig. 10–3) [213,298,306,330]. Surgical specimens from early stages of the disease show mucosal edema, hemorrhage, and superficial ulceration with very little inflammation or cellular response. By the 2nd or 3rd day, after progression to pneumatosis and transmural necrosis of the bowel wall, bacterial proliferation and the acute inflammatory reaction become more prominent [287,309].

There has been much investigation and little agreement on the importance of various perinatal events in the causation of NEC [213,298,306,331]. Except for immaturity and possibly polycythemia, other factors originally thought to predispose to NEC have been found on further study to occur with equal frequency in control populations of infants.* Maternal complications of pregnancy, labor, and delivery and neonatal respiratory distress syndrome are thought to be unrelated to the development of NEC, whereas evidence linking NEC to birth asphyxia, hypotension, hypothermia, use of vascular catheters, exchange transfusion, feeding history, abnormalities of gut motility, neonatal achlorhydria, and the presence of patent ductus arteriosus is often contradictory. Each of these conditions, singly or together, may act as a stress leading

to mucosal injury, but none has been consistently associated with NEC [334,335]. NEC has occurred among apparently healthy infants with no known predisposing risk factors [282,280,318,330]. Several studies (discussed later) suggest that early feeding of premature neonates may play a causal role in NEC. Dvorak and coworkers [330] showed that maternal milk may be protective compared with artificial formulas in a neonatal rat model of NEC; similar to human NEC, artificial feeding of maternal milk reduced the incidence and severity of NEC injury, and IL-10 expression was significantly increased when neonates were fed maternal milk.

Some epidemiologic observations suggest that NEC is an infectious contagious disease of nosocomial origin. The temporal clustering of cases at institutions, the association of some outbreaks with single infectious agents or alterations in bowel flora, and the possible beneficial effects of breast-feeding, oral nonabsorbable antibiotics, or infection control measures in reducing the incidence of disease suggest a possible nosocomial cause. The evidence linking NEC to a specific infectious agent is often circumstantial or open to alternative interpretation. Evidence suggests that NEC is the end response of the immature gastrointestinal tract to multiple factors acting alone or in concert to produce mucosal injury, with colonization or invasion by the microorganisms representing only one part of the continuum of that disease process [266,272,273,280].

MICROBIOLOGY

Descriptions of sporadic outbreaks of NEC in NICUs have led to a search for transmissible agents, including bacterial, viral, and fungal pathogens [341a].* Predominance

---

*References [243,287,280,309,318,327–329].

*References [213,299,304,310,311,320,332,333].

*References [288,298,306,213,330,336–341].

of a single organism in stool, blood, bowel wall, or peritoneal cavity of infants during epidemics of NEC has implicated numerous agents, including *Klebsiella* species [285,295,312,329,342–344], *Enterobacter* species [345], *E. coli* [346,347], *Pseudomonas* species [348,349], *Salmonella* species [350], *S. epidermidis* and other coagulase-negative staphylococci [351], *S. aureus* [352], rotavirus [353,354], coronavirus [355], coxsackievirus B2 [356], and *Torulopsis glabrata* [357].

The analogous pathology of necrotizing enteritis caused by *Clostridium septicum* [36,72] and *Clostridium perfringens* in domestic animals [297,344,358], older children, and adults [359] favored suggestions that *Clostridium* species might act as a primary pathogen in NEC.* Several reports provided evidence that *C. perfringens* [297,361–364], *Clostridium difficile* [333,365], or *Clostridium butyricum*, acting alone [366,367] or synergistically with *Klebsiella* [368], was able to evoke NEC. Subsequent studies indicated, however, that these species were often acquired from the nursery environment [369,370] and could frequently be recovered from healthy neonates [359,370–376]. Clostridial cytotoxin, which had been recovered from the stool of infants involved in an outbreak of NEC [333,365], has also been found in the stool of 90% of normal infants [333,364,369,375–377]. The role of *Clostridium* species in NEC remains unclear [341,360].

The δ-toxins, hemolysins of coagulase-negative staphylococci [378] and *S. aureus*, have also been proposed as possible primary toxins capable of producing NEC in infants. Frequent colonization by δ-toxin staphylococci and higher levels of toxin production by associated strains causing NEC [379] and one outbreak with δ-toxin–producing *S. aureus* strains have been reported [352]. Prospective studies have documented significant shifts in

---

*References [213,298,306,330,341,360].

aerobic bacterial bowel flora within 72 hours before onset of clinical NEC [380]; the observed shift results from preclinical changes in the intestinal environment. This shift suggests that bacteria isolated at the time of onset were present because of possible intraluminal changes and are not directly involved in NEC.

Pending further experimental or epidemiologic observations, the weight of evidence indicates that although bacteria or bacterial toxins may play a primary or secondary role in the pathogenesis of NEC, the occasional association of this condition with a single organism probably reflects patterns of intestinal colonization prevalent in the nursery at the time of an outbreak [213,298,306,330]. Despite intensive efforts to identify a specific infectious agent or toxin in the cause of NEC, convincing reports implicating the same pathogen in more than one outbreak have not appeared [341].

CLINICAL MANIFESTATIONS

Signs of NEC usually develop in the first 7 days of life [291,318,381], and 50% or more of cases are recognized within 5 days of birth [282,309,312,382,383]. Small immature newborns often develop illness later, during the 2nd to 8th week [314,316], whereas low-risk term infants may become ill shortly after delivery, as early as the first 24 hours [319].

NEC is a disease with a wide spectrum of manifestations, ranging from a mild gastrointestinal disturbance to a fulminant course characterized by early bowel perforation, peritonitis, sepsis, and shock [306,384,385]. A staging system (Table 10–4) taking these clinical variations into account may be useful in guiding patient evaluation and therapy [306,386]. The apparent stage of disease for an individual infant usually can be defined on the 2nd day of illness. An infant who exhibits only mild systemic and

---

TABLE 10–4 Modified Bell Staging Criteria and Recommendations for Therapy for Necrotizing Enterocolitis

| Stage | Signs | | | |
	Systemic	Intestinal	Radiologic	Treatment
IA (suspected)	Temperature instability, apnea, bradycardia, lethargy	Elevated residuals, mild abdominal distention, emesis guaiac-positive stools	Normal, mild ileus	NPO, antibiotics for 3 days
IB (suspected)	Same as IA	Frank rectal blood	Same as IA	Same as IA
IIA (definite), mild	Same as IA and IB	Same as IB plus absent bowel sounds ± abdominal tenderness	Dilation, ileus, pneumatosis intestinalis	NPO, antibiotics for 7-14 days if examination is normal in 24-48 hr
IIB (definite), moderate	Same as IIA with mild metabolic acidosis, mild thrombocytopenia	Same as IIA with definite abdominal tenderness ± abdominal cellulitis or right lower quadrant mass	Same as IIA plus portal gas ± ascites	NPO, antibiotics for 14 days
IIIA (advanced), bowel intact	Same as IIB plus hypotension, bradycardia, severe apnea, respiratory/metabolic acidosis, disseminated intravascular coagulation, neutropenia	Same as IIB plus peritonitis, marked tenderness, abdominal distention	Same as IIB with ascites	Same as IIB plus 200 mL/kg fluid, inotropic agents, assisted ventilation, paracentesis
IIIB (advanced), bowel perforated	Same as IIIA	Same as IIIA	Same as IIIA plus pneumoperitoneum	Same as IIIA plus surgery

NPO, nothing by mouth.
Adapted from Walsh MC, Kliegman RM. Necrotizing enterocolitis: treatment based on staging criteria. Pediatr Clin North Am 33:179, 1986.

intestinal signs 24 to 48 hours after onset is unlikely to develop a more serious illness [306].

The classic presentation of NEC includes a triad of abdominal distention, retention of gastric contents, and gastrointestinal bleeding.* These findings are often preceded or accompanied by signs consistent with sepsis, such as lethargy, poor feeding, temperature instability, apnea, and bradycardia. Diarrhea is variable, rarely observed in some series [306], but common in others [316,347]. Progression of bowel wall necrosis leading to perforation, peritonitis, and sepsis is reflected in deteriorating vital signs accompanied by persistent acidosis [387], clotting disorders, and circulatory collapse. Redness, induration, and edema of the anterior abdominal wall are commonly described in the advanced stages of NEC. In the absence of aggressive medical and surgical intervention, the course is rapidly downhill when late signs appear.

DIAGNOSIS

Radiographic signs of NEC are largely nonspecific [385], and interobserver variability in the interpretation of films is substantial [387]. Radiographic examination of the abdomen remains the most reliable aid, however, in establishing a diagnosis of NEC [282,302,309,387,388]. Ileus with generalized bowel dilation and abdominal distention are the earliest radiologic findings. Increasing distention, separation of loops by peritoneal fluid or edema of the bowel wall, a gasless abdomen, pneumatosis intestinalis, and hepatic or portal air occur as NEC worsens. A persistent single dilated loop of bowel remaining relatively unchanged in shape and position in serial films is strongly suggestive [389–391] but not diagnostic [390,392] of localized bowel ischemia with impending perforation.

If free air or ascites is absent on initial abdominal examination, supine and left lateral decubitus films should be obtained every 6 to 8 hours until improvement or definitive surgery or invasive diagnostic measures have ruled out the presence of perforation. When perforation occurs, it is usually within 1 day after diagnosis [327], but may be delayed for 5 or 6 days [393]. Although the presence of pneumoperitoneum [244,265,275] or intraperitoneal fluid generally indicates perforation, its absence does not exclude perforation [221,243,244]. In one study [327], only 63% of infants with NEC and proven perforation had free air, 21% had ascites, and 16% had neither free air nor ascites.

When plain films are normal or equivocal, other studies may be diagnostic. A metrizamide gastrointestinal series may show intestinal perforation or abnormalities of the bowel wall, mucosa, or lumen [245,273,394]. Real-time ultrasonography may reveal portal venous and hepatic parenchymal gas in standard radiographs [327,395,396]. Serial abdominal transillumination with a fiberoptic light has been described as a bedside method for early detection of ascites or pneumoperitoneum, although its sensitivity compared with standard radiographic methods has not been determined [277].

A rapid and direct means of establishing the presence of intestinal necrosis or perforation is by abdominal paracentesis [269,397,398]. This procedure is unnecessary in

infants to rule out NEC or in infants improving on medical therapy. The procedure is generally reserved for infants suspected, on the basis of clinical, radiographic, and laboratory findings, to have intestinal gangrene. When performed properly, paracentesis is safe and accurate, as described by Kosloske [399]: The abdomen is palpated to locate any masses or enlarged viscera. After an antiseptic skin preparation, a small needle (22-gauge or 25-gauge) is inserted carefully in the flank, at a 45-degree angle. It is advanced slowly and aspirated gently until free flow of 0.5 mL or more of peritoneal fluid is obtained. Any volume less than 0.5 mL is considered a dry tap and cannot be accurately interpreted. The color and appearance of the fluid are noted, and the fluid is transported immediately to the laboratory in an approved anaerobic container for Gram staining and for aerobic and anaerobic cultures. A positive paracentesis consists of brown fluid or bacteria on the unspun fluid.

The accuracy of paracentesis in determining the need for an operation is 90% to 95% [269,398]. False-positive results are rare; false-negative results are quite common. Patients with a dry tap should be closely observed under medical therapy with continuing serial paracenteses until indications for or against surgical intervention are clearly defined. Infants with a positive result should undergo exploratory surgery immediately.

Thrombocytopenia and disseminated intravascular coagulation are the most common hematologic complications [282,312,340,397,399–401], particularly in the presence of bowel gangrene or perforation [287,401,402]. Platelet-activating factor has been used to assist in the staging of NEC [403]; a cutoff level of 10.2 ng/mL had a positive predictive value of 100% in identifying infants with stage II or III NEC. Leukopenia and absolute granulocytopenia, apparently caused by margination of white blood cells rather than bone marrow depletion [404], also have occurred during early stages of the illness [399,400]. A low absolute granulocyte count persisting for 2 to 3 days is associated with a poor prognosis. Hemolytic anemia has been reported in association with NEC related to *C. perfringens* [363]. No consistent urinary abnormalities have been described for NEC, although increased lactate excretion, reflecting heightened enteric bacterial activity, may occur [405]. Increased amounts of fecal-reducing substances have been found in almost three fourths of formula-fed premature infants during early stages of NEC, before the onset of abdominal distention, poor feeding, or emesis [406]. Although not readily available, levels of growth factors in urine have been found to be much higher in children with stage II and III NEC [407]; such an analysis might identify children at higher risk of complications and the need for surgical intervention.

The evaluation of patients with NEC should include culture of blood and, when appropriate and clinically safe, cerebrospinal fluid, urine, and stool. The likelihood of bacteremia accompanying NEC depends on the severity of bowel involvement; the reported incidence has ranged from 10% to 67% among symptomatic infants. Combined data from several large studies showed positive blood cultures in about one third of newborns with NEC [287,288,339,393]. The usual organisms have been *E. coli*, *Klebsiella* species, *S. aureus*, and *Pseudomonas*

---

*References [292,303,316,318,320,329,337,342,391,396].

species, whereas enterococci and anaerobic bacteria were isolated occasionally. A spectrum of organisms similar to those causing sepsis have been isolated from the peritoneal fluid [287,295,316,340,393]. Meningitis may accompany bacteremia, occurring in approximately 1% of NEC cases [319,408].

TREATMENT

Early and aggressive treatment must be initiated for any infant suspected to have NEC [298,306]. The modified Bell staging system of NEC may guide diagnostic studies, management, antibiotics, and surgical consultation and intervention (see Table 10–4). Umbilical catheters should be removed whenever possible, oral feedings should be stopped, and nasogastric tube drainage should be instituted. Fluid and electrolyte deficits and maintenance require rigorous attention; blood, plasma, or colloid infusions are often necessary for volume expansion and maintenance of tissue perfusion.

After appropriate cultures are obtained, parenteral antibiotic therapy should be started with clindamycin and gentamicin or an extended-spectrum cephalosporin and ampicillin. In nurseries where coagulase-negative staphylococcal colonization or infection is prevalent, initial therapy with vancomycin may replace ampicillin [409]. β-lactam and β-lactamase inhibitor combinations (e.g., piperacillin plus tazobactam) can replace gentamicin, ampicillin, and clindamycin, covering anaerobic, gram-negative enteric aerobic, and many gram-positive pathogens. Gentamicin and vancomycin dosages should be modified as necessary on the basis of serum levels. Despite anecdotal evidence that oral nonabsorbable aminoglycosides prevent gastrointestinal perforation in infants with NEC [410], later controlled studies did not corroborate this finding [411]; their use is not routinely recommended. The need for inclusion of clindamycin to provide activity against anaerobic bacteria in the management of NEC has been questioned [412], based on the observation that anaerobic bacteria are late bowel colonizers, present in relatively much lower numbers in infants than in adult subjects, and that anaerobes other than *Clostridium* species have been infrequently identified in NEC.

After immediate treatment has been started, follow-up studies should be instituted. These include serial examinations with measurement of abdominal girth; testing of stools for blood; levels of serum electrolytes, blood glucose, and arterial blood gases; complete blood cell count and platelet count; urine-specific gravity; and supine and left lateral decubitus abdominal radiographs. These tests should be considered every 6 to 8 hours until the infant's clinical condition stabilizes. Attention to vital functions should be provided as necessary on the basis of clinical, laboratory, or radiographic studies. Parenteral nutritional support through a central or peripheral vein must be started as soon as possible.

Early recognition and prompt initiation of medical therapy may reduce the need for surgery. Generally accepted criteria for surgical exploration are a deteriorating clinical condition despite appropriate medical therapy, signs of peritonitis, presence of free air within the abdomen, or a positive paracentesis result. The principles of surgical preparation and management have been discussed by

several investigators [289,398,413,414]. In addition to laparotomy with removal of necrotic bowel, closed peritoneal drainage has been proposed as an alternative in very small infants, with a resultant survival of more than 50% [415].

PREVENTION

The first observations implicating bacterial proliferation as a factor in pathogenesis of NEC prompted efforts at suppression of gut flora with topical antibiotics in the hope of preventing NEC. Attempts to prevent NEC by giving oral kanamycin or gentamicin prophylactically in the first hours of life, before any signs of bowel involvement are recognized, have generated contradictory data. In controlled clinical trials, a significant reduction in the incidence of NEC in treated premature infants was shown in some trials [313,416–419], whereas in others, investigators were unable to show any protective effect [419,420]. Studies of vancomycin [421] have shown a significant reduction in NEC in high-risk infants. Previous studies revealed selective growth of resistant organisms in bowel flora [313,420,422] and evidence of significant systemic absorption of aminoglycoside antibiotics [411,423,424], suggesting that oral aminoglycoside prophylaxis is not free of potential risks. Potential risk factors have not been examined in vancomycin trials, however. Until additional evidence is presented indicating clear-cut benefits from the use of oral aminoglycosides or vancomycin, it does not seem that either agent should be used routinely for prevention of NEC in premature infants. Epidemiologic evidence that early use of parenteral ampicillin and aminoglycoside therapy may delay or decrease the risk of NEC has not been confirmed in controlled studies [329].

Oral probiotics have been suggested to alter the bowel flora of the infant to reduce the incidence and severity of NEC. Infants fed breast milk and a product including *Lactobacillus acidophilus* and *Bifidobacterium infantis* had a reduced incidence and severity of NEC compared with infants fed breast milk alone [335]. A recent metanalysis of 11 trials of probiotics concluded that the risk for NEC and death was significantly lower, but the risk for sepsis did not differ significantly from those neonates not receiving probiotics [335a]. These results seem to confirm the significant benefits of or probiotic oral supplements, with a 30% reduction in the incidence of NEC.

Excessive or accelerated feedings have been associated with increased frequency of endemic NEC [425], and some clinicians have recommended a schedule of slow advancement of daily feeding volumes limited to about 20 mL/kg/day. Infants with NEC are more likely to have been fed earlier, to have received full-strength formulas sooner, and to have received larger feeding volumes and increments, and stress and associated respiratory problems may make such infants more vulnerable to NEC [244,292–297,426]. Prior studies of the use of a feeding regimen employing prolonged periods of bowel rest in high-risk infants showed the regimen to be successful in preventing NEC in some nurseries [298], but totally without value in others [213,300]. Later studies added additional support for standardized feeding schedules in low birth weight infants (500 to 2500 g); all used maximum volumes no greater than 20 mL/kg/day, with feeding beginning at 24 to 72 hours after birth, depending on birth weight and gestational age [307,308]. Synthetic formulas and breast milk have been successful.

Carrion and Egan [427] suggested that relative hypochlorhydria of the neonate may contribute to NEC and found that hydrochloric acid supplements (0.01 to 0.02 1.0 N HCl/mL of formula) significantly reduced NEC rates and lowered gastric pH. Additional studies have shown that standardized feedings begun at a median of 4 days after onset of NEC can be associated with an abbreviated time until institution of full enteral feedings, a reduced incidence of the use of central catheters and catheter infections, and ultimately a shorter hospital stay [428].

Many NEC "epidemics" in NICUs, lasting 2 weeks to 7 months, have been reported from centers worldwide [329,340,341,429,430]. Although the microbiologic agents associated with these outbreaks have varied, institution of strict infection control measures was often useful in bringing about a significant decrease in the incidence of NEC; the reasons for success are less clear. Results have been sufficiently impressive, however, to recommend that enforcement of bedside enteric precautions, together with cohorting of infants and staff, be instituted when two or more cases of NEC occur in a nursery [306,341,431].

The use of human breast milk has been claimed, largely on the basis of experimental evidence, to exert a protective effect against the development of NEC. There are no prospective, controlled studies showing any benefit from the feeding of colostrum or breast milk to human neonates. A study showing the protective effect of an orally administered IgA-IgG preparation suggests a possible way to provide benefits of high levels of functionally active antibodies in the gastrointestinal tract [432]. Orally administered probiotics have been suggested as a possible prophylactic measure in NEC based on an assumption that an accentuated and inappropriate inflammatory response to colonizing pathogenic flora in the premature gut plays a role in the initiation of NEC [433]. Bifidobacteria and lactobacilli are commonly found in breast-fed infants [434] and may be the reason in part for the protective effects of breast milk. A single large, multicenter, randomized controlled trial of *Bifidobacterium bifidum* and *L. acidophilus* was completed and suggested a lower incidence of NEC (stage II or greater) in infants receiving these probiotics [435]. This study showed a lower incidence of death or NEC in recipients of probiotics (4 of 217 probiotic infants versus 20/217 control infants). No adverse effects of the probiotics, such as sepsis, flatulence, or diarrhea, were noted. This large study seems to confirm several smaller studies with similar results [436,437,438].

PROGNOSIS

The mortality rate of NEC is difficult to determine because mild cases of suspected NEC are probably more common than is recognized [306,376,439]. In studies in which analysis has been limited to infants with "definite NEC," mortality figures range from 20% to 40%.* Several longitudinal studies have shown a significant improvement in outcome [291,302,387,440]. A poor prognosis has

been linked with very low birth weight, associated congenital defects, bacterial sepsis, disseminated intravascular coagulation, intestinal perforation, and persistent hemodynamic or respiratory instability [311,336,381,393]. Surgical intervention, generally reserved for the sickest infants with more extensive bowel involvement, is also associated with higher mortality rates [311,381,387,398,439].

Infants who survive the acute phase of illness generally do well, although NEC may recur in 5% to 10% [291,316,440,441]. In addition to surgical complications (e.g., short bowel syndrome, anastomotic leaks, fistula formation), enteric strictures are probably the most common delayed complication in surviving infants, occurring in 4% to 20%. Usually found at sites of ischemia and necrosis in terminal ileum or colon [282,309,442], these strictures often become apparent within a few weeks, but may be delayed 18 months. When multiple strictures occur, the intervening normal bowel may form an enterocyst [388,443]. Clinically, strictures manifest as frequent episodes of abdominal distention, often with vomiting, obstipation, or hematochezia. Diagnosis is confirmed by gastrointestinal contrast studies. Surgery with removal of the stenotic site is necessary to effect a cure.

Long-term follow-up of low birth weight infants with severe NEC (i.e., Bell stages II and III) has documented higher rates of subnormal body weight (15% to 39%) and head circumference (30%) in addition to significant neurodevelopmental impairment (83%) [444]. Clinical observations suggest that infants with bowel resection for NEC are at increased risk of sepsis, occurring 1 week to 3 years (mean 4 months) later. Almost all had had a central venous catheter in place for parenteral nutrition at the time of infection. Enteric bacilli were responsible for more than 40% of bacteremias, whereas only 20% were caused by staphylococcal species, which are the usual causes of catheter sepsis. Several infants had two or more episodes of sepsis, and 2 of 19 died as a direct consequence of infection [427].

ENDOCARDITIS

Neonatal bacterial endocarditis, previously uncommon, has been recognized more frequently in recent years. About 60 cases that meet clinical and bacteriologic criteria sufficient to establish this diagnosis were reported in the literature before the mid-1980s [77,445–472]. The prolonged survival of critically ill infants, including infants with complex congenital heart disease, and the increased use of intravascular catheters, together with advances in the diagnostic sensitivity and availability of echocardiography, may be responsible for an increased recognition of endocarditis. In a 35-year review of 76 cases of endocarditis in children, 10% of patients were younger than 1 year; the youngest patient was 1 month old [473]. Of patients, 62 (83%) had congenital heart disease, and 77% had had prior surgery. Central venous catheters were additional significant risk factors. At the University of New Mexico in a level III nursery with 3200 to 3500 admissions annually, 12 cases of endocarditis occurred in children younger than 3 months [474]. Organisms isolated from these 10 cases included *S. aureus* (6 cases), *K. pneumoniae* (1 case), *Enterobacter cloacae* (2 cases),

---

*References [269,291,298,213,316–320,381,385,387].

Candida species (1 case), α-hemolytic streptococci (1 case), and coagulase-negative staphylococci (1 case). Three patients had congenital heart disease with early surgical intervention; all had surgically implanted catheters or intravenous access devices, one had NEC, and one had an associated osteomyelitis.

Etiologic agents of bacterial endocarditis in newborns have been identified by isolation from blood cultures or morphologic characteristics of organisms entrapped within valvular vegetations examined at autopsy. The causative organisms have included *S. aureus* in 36 infants*; streptococci in 6 infants [425,447,475]; *S. epidermidis* [455,456,476] and GBS [449,459,463] each in 5 infants; *S. pneumoniae* [447,475], *P. aeruginosa* [448,454], and *S. marcescens* [452,464] each in 2 infants; and *Neisseria gonorrhoeae* [447], *S. faecalis* [477], *Streptococcus salivarius* [71], and mixed α-hemolytic streptococcus, *K. pneumoniae*, and *P. mirabilis* [455] each in 1 infant. Despite widespread cardiovascular involvement associated with congenital syphilis, there is no conclusive evidence that this disease produces valvular heart lesions in infected infants [58]. *Candida* endocarditis has become increasingly prevalent, particularly associated with the use of central venous catheters.

Factors that predispose a newborn to endocarditis are not well understood, although intravascular catheters are associated with endocarditis. In contrast to older children, in whom congenital heart disease is often associated with endocarditis [478], cardiac anomalies were found in only nine of the reported cases in neonates in series before 1994.* Bacteremia arising from an infected umbilical stump [446–448], conjunctivitis [447], and skin lesions [447,469] were the presumed sources of valvular involvement in six infants; the invasive organisms associated with these conditions and with neonatal endocarditis in general can infect normal heart valves [480]. Nevertheless, the greater frequency of bacterial and fungal [468,481–488] endocarditis in newborns in recent years, particularly in association with prematurity or placement of central vessel catheters, or both, indicates that other, more complex mechanisms may also be operative in some cases [454–457,471,476,481,489].

Observations in laboratory animals and autopsy studies of adults have shown that damage to the intracardiac endothelium with formation of a sterile platelet-fibrin thrombus at the site of the injury is often the initiating event in a patient with endocarditis [486]. Endocardial trauma caused by placement of cardiac catheters, disseminated intravascular coagulation, and various nonspecific stresses associated with prematurity, such as hypotension and hypoxia, has been implicated in the genesis of thrombi.* Nonbacterial thrombotic endocarditis or verrucous endocarditis usually remains uninfected and is described as an incidental finding at autopsy [454,471,491,492]. With bacteremia, implantation of organisms may lead to valvular infection. Whether this mechanism or direct bacterial invasion is primarily responsible for valvulitis is unknown. A similar pathogenesis has been postulated for formation of mycotic aortic aneurysms in newborns [467,493,494].

Endocarditis should be suspected in any neonate, particularly a premature infant, with an indwelling vascular catheter, evidence of sepsis, and new or changing heart murmurs. When these findings are accompanied by persistent bacteremia or signs of congestive heart failure in the absence of underlying heart disease, the diagnosis must be considered seriously. Although Janeway lesions [471], a generalized petechial rash [466,477,481], and splinter hemorrhages [477] have been seen, murmurs characteristic of semilunar valve insufficiency, Osler nodes, Roth spots, arthritis, and other findings typical of valvular infection in adults and older children have not been observed in neonates. Multiple septic emboli with involvement of the skin, bones, viscera, and central nervous system are common findings, however.*

Two-dimensional echocardiography has proved to be an invaluable rapid, noninvasive method for diagnosing endocarditis [456–459,465,486,495]. Although it cannot differentiate between infected and sterile vegetations and other valvular lesions (discussed later), imaging is quite specific, and false-positive readings are uncommon. Less certainty can be placed on a negative report. Despite detection of vegetations 2 mm in diameter with echocardiography, the number of false-negative examinations is significant [465,471,496]; in one series, two of three infants with thrombotic valvular lesions 3 to 7 mm in diameter had normal two-dimensional echocardiograms [471]. A diagnosis of bacterial endocarditis should be considered in any infant with a compatible history and physical findings regardless of the results obtained by echocardiography. Widespread use of new techniques, such as transesophageal echocardiography, which provides detailed views of the mitral and tricuspid valves, and color flow Doppler imaging, which can identify areas of turbulence as blood passes over vegetations or through narrowed valve leaflets, may greatly improve diagnostic accuracy in the future [495].

When endocarditis is suspected, specimens of blood, cerebrospinal fluid, and urine obtained by catheterization or suprapubic aspiration should be sent for bacterial and fungal culture. Because blood drawn from a central catheter often contains organisms colonizing the line but not present in the systemic circulation, at least two peripheral venous blood cultures should be obtained before antimicrobial therapy is initiated. Volumes of 1 to 5 mL, depending on the infant's size, should be adequate [486].

Routine laboratory studies are helpful in supporting a diagnosis of endocarditis in the newborn. The leukocyte count, differential count, and platelet count are usually indicative of sepsis, rather than cardiac valve infection in particular. Microhematuria has been reported, although rarely [471,477]. A chest radiograph should be obtained to determine signs of cardiac failure or pulmonary or pleural space infection. CT or MRI of the brain can be helpful in an infant with neurologic signs, particularly if left-sided endocarditis or a right-to-left shunt exists. Baseline determinations of inflammatory markers are useful and can be used for assessing the efficacy of the therapy; erythrocyte sedimentation rate and C-reactive protein level have been used.

*References [455–457,460,463–465,467,468,475–487,489–510].
*References [77,450,452,455,459,460,465,479].
*References [455,471,476,480,490,491].

*References [455,457,459,460,464–466,468–474,478,479,481,485,487,489,508–510].

Intravenous therapy with a penicillinase-resistant penicillin and an aminoglycoside should be started after appropriate cultures have been obtained. In nurseries where MRSA or methicillin-resistant *S. epidermidis* infections have been a problem, vancomycin should be substituted initially for the penicillin antibiotic [486,495,496]. If endocarditis caused by *Enterococcus* species is suspected, ampicillin should be added or substituted for the penicillinase-resistant penicillin. After the infecting organism is isolated and antibiotic susceptibilities have been determined, specific antimicrobial therapy can be instituted.

Four to 8 weeks of parenteral treatment is usually adequate, depending on the susceptibility of the organism, response to therapy assessed clinically by reduction or elimination of the observed vegetations, and laboratory response. C-reactive protein level often normalizes 2 to 3 weeks before erythrocyte sedimentation rate, and blood cultures are usually sterile after 3 to 5 days of effective therapy. *Candida* species may persist for weeks, however, despite the use of active antifungal drugs. Dosage and efficacy should be monitored weekly with clinical and bacteriologic response with or without serum antibiotic and bactericidal levels [495,497]. Determination of serum bactericidal titers (Schlichter test) is of uncertain value and has never been validated in neonatal endocarditis [486,495,498]. Efficacy of treatment may also be monitored with serial echocardiograms taken until vegetations remain stable in size or disappear [465,466,468,476,481].

Intravascular catheters must be removed whenever possible, and the tip of the removed catheter should be cultured [486,499]. Extremely large or mobile vegetations occluding an outflow tract or posing a high risk of embolism may have to be removed surgically [463,465,468]. In infants with right-sided endocarditis, demonstration of decreased pulmonary blood flow through the use of ventilation-perfusion scan can be valuable in confirming the presence of emboli, particularly if there is clinical evidence of increasing respiratory effort and diminished peripheral oxygen saturation [463].

With the availability of echocardiography, improved clinical awareness, and early diagnosis, prognosis has improved. Although there were infrequent survivors before 1973 [480], the first survivors with proven endocarditis were reported in 1983 [465,466,471]. Approximately two thirds of subsequent cases have been cured. Death is usually the result of overwhelming sepsis, often in conjunction with cardiac failure. Early reconstructive surgery for infants who fail medical management may be helpful, but has been reported in only a few cases [500,501].

Inspection of the heart at autopsy has shown the mitral valve to be infected, alone or in combination with other valves, in about half of patients. The tricuspid valve was involved in 12 infants, the pulmonary valve in 7, the aortic valve in 6, infected mural thrombi in 12, and an unspecified site in 3. Microscopic examination of valve cusps has revealed the characteristic lesions of endocarditis, with multiple small, confluent, friable vegetations composed principally of bacteria and thrombi surrounded by inflammatory exudate [77,469,471]. On gross inspection, these vegetations are easily confused with noninflammatory lesions, such as those of nonbacterial thrombotic endocarditis, blood cysts [502], developmental valvular defects

[503], or hemangiomas or other vascular anomalies [504]. Cases described as fetal endocarditis in the literature are almost certainly examples of these types of lesions [503,505,506].

PERICARDITIS

Purulent pericarditis is a very unusual complication of neonatal sepsis. Approximately 20 cases of proven bacterial origin have been reported within the past 50 years [18,507–518]. No single causative agent has predominated. *S. aureus* was responsible for seven cases [18,507–509]; *E. coli* was isolated from three patients [509,514,515]; *Haemophilus influenzae* was found in two cases [510,517]; and *Salmonella wichita* [511], *Klebsiella* [518], and *P. aeruginosa* [516] were isolated from single cases. One early review of *Pseudomonas* sepsis described suppurative pericarditis in four neonates [512]. Another report on the recovery of *Pseudomonas* from the pericardium of premature infants dying of septicemia and meningitis during a nursery outbreak is difficult to evaluate because details of clinical and autopsy findings were not provided [519]. Cases caused by *Candida* species and *Mycoplasma hominis* have also been described [481,485,520]. The causes of a pericardial effusion in three fetuses with multiple congenital anomalies, myocardial hypertrophy, and pericarditis are uncertain. Although the inflammatory exudate found at autopsy contained polymorphonuclear leukocytes in addition to lymphocytes, no evidence of bacterial infection was found [521].

Virtually every infant with pericarditis has associated septic foci; pneumonia and multiple pulmonary abscesses are the most common sites. Involvement of pericardium may occur by direct extension from adjoining lung abscesses or by hematogenous spread of bacteria [508]. The presence of infectious processes elsewhere is sufficiently frequent to warrant the suggestion that pericarditis should be suspected in all infants who develop clinical signs of "heart failure" or a sudden increase in the size of the cardiac silhouette during the course of a purulent infection such as meningitis, pneumonia, or omphalitis [510,522].

Neonates with bacterial pericarditis generally present with signs and symptoms suggesting sepsis and respiratory distress. Poor feeding, listlessness, emesis, or abdominal distention may be seen in the presence of tachypnea, tachycardia, and cyanosis of various degrees. More specific signs of cardiac involvement become apparent with the accumulation of increasing amounts of pericardial effusion. The clinical findings of cardiac tamponade are extremely subtle and difficult to differentiate from the findings of myocardial disease with right-sided heart failure. A rapid pulse, quiet precordium, muffled heart sounds, neck vein distention, and hepatomegaly are findings common to both entities. More specific signs of tamponade, such as narrow pulse pressure or respiratory variations in pulse volume of more than 20 mm Hg (i.e., pulsus paradoxus), are technically difficult to obtain in neonates without an arterial catheter in place. A pericardial friction rub is absent in more than 50% of older infants and children and in most neonates with purulent pericarditis.

Rapid enlargement of the cardiac silhouette, a globular heart shape with widening of the base on tilting, and diminished cardiac pulsation on fluoroscopic examination are of little value in differentiating pericardial effusion from cardiac dilation [523]. The early ST segment elevation and subsequent T wave inversion seen on electrocardiogram reflect subepicardial damage or inflammation and are similar to changes seen with primary myocarditis. Diminution in the amplitude of the QRS complex by fluid surrounding the heart is not a constant finding. Confirmation of the presence of a pericardial effusion is usually obtained by two-dimensional echocardiography [507,523]. In some cases, CT or MRI can also be helpful in delineating the extent of a pericardial effusion [524]; occasionally, pericardial fluid is found incidental to the chest or abdominal scanning. Additional causes of neonatal pericardial effusion other than purulent disease include viral pericarditis [525], intrapericardial teratoma [526], maternal lupus [527], immune and nonimmune [528] fetal hydrops, congenital diaphragmatic defects [529], chylopericardium [530], and central venous catheter perforation of the right atrium [531].

A definitive diagnosis of purulent pericarditis can be made only by obtaining fluid at surgery or through needle aspiration. Care and experience are necessary to facilitate aspiration while avoiding the risks of cardiac puncture or laceration [521]. Accurate monitoring of needle position can usually be obtained through CT guidance, with echocardiographic or fluoroscopic imaging, or by attaching the exploring electrode (V lead) of an electrocardiograph to the needle and by looking for injury current if contact is made with the epicardial surface of the heart.

When fluid is obtained, it should be sent for analysis to the laboratory in a laboratory-approved container appropriate for aerobic and anaerobic culture, mycobacteria, and fungi. In addition to cell count and protein and glucose levels, Gram and acid-fast stains should be performed with cultures for bacteria, viruses, mycobacteria, and fungi. Rapid identification of bacterial antigens by latex agglutination or by counterimmunoelectrophoresis of pericardial fluid, urine, or serum may also help to establish an etiologic diagnosis [532]. Specialized testing for rare bacterial, viral, or fungal organisms by molecular methods may be available by request in specialized (research) or reference laboratories.

Purulent pericarditis is a medical and surgical emergency. Therapy must be directed toward relief of the cardiac tamponade through adequate pericardial drainage and toward resolution of the infection. Both modes of treatment are essential for successful therapy for bacterial pericarditis in the newborn. No infant with suppurative pericarditis has recovered when treated by antibiotics alone [508]. Although repeated needle aspirations or catheter drainage [533] may be sufficient, the frequent occurrence of loculations of pus, particularly with staphylococcal infection, suggests that open surgical pericardiostomy is the method of choice to achieve adequate drainage.

Cultures of blood, and, when clinically indicated, cerebrospinal fluid and urine should be obtained before instituting antimicrobial therapy. Initial therapy should be based on results of Gram stain or antigen detection tests of the pericardial fluid. If no organisms can be identified, treatment can be started with penicillinase-resistant penicillin and an aminoglycoside (or extended-spectrum cephalosporin) until definitive culture and susceptibility data are available. In nurseries where MRSA infection has been a problem, vancomycin should be substituted for penicillin [497].

The prognosis of neonatal purulent pericarditis is very poor. Only three survivors had been reported [507,509,518] before the 1990s. Treatment of these patients consisted of needle aspirations, drainage, and systemic antibiotic therapy, and in one case, treatment was combined with local instillation.

MEDIASTINITIS

Purulent mediastinitis has been reported in 11 infants younger than 6 weeks of age, although it is likely that a great many more cases occur than have been reported in the literature, and that it is an occasional complication of cardiothoracic surgery performed in the neonatal period. Six reported patients acquired mediastinal abscess through blood-borne dissemination of organisms [534–536] or by extension from a focus of infection in an adjacent retropharyngeal abscess [537], pleural or pulmonary abscess [508,535], or vertebral osteomyelitis [538]. One infant developed infection as a complication of surgery for esophageal atresia [525]. *S. aureus* was the causative organism in four infants, and *S. pneumoniae*, *Clostridium* species, and mixed *S. aureus* and *E. coli* were causative in one infant each. Organisms were not identified in four cases.

Traumatic perforation of the posterior pharynx or esophagus, often the result of resuscitative efforts in infants involving endotracheal or gastric intubation, produces a potential site for entry of microorganisms [539–546]. Retropharyngeal abscess [547], an infected pseudodiverticulum, or pyopneumothorax may occur as a consequence; purulent mediastinitis has been reported three times as a complication [536,540,541], but it is probably more common than is reported. At least one case of mediastinitis has occurred as the result of overly vigorous passage of a nasogastric tube through an atretic esophageal pouch [540]. Low (intrathoracic) perforations are said to have a higher risk of mediastinitis and abscess formation than perforations in the cervical region [542].

Early symptoms are nonspecific and are similar to symptoms of any septic process in a neonate. As purulent fluid accumulates in the mediastinum, it places increasing pressure on the esophagus, trachea, and tributaries of the superior vena cava and thoracic duct, bringing about rapid development of dysphagia, dyspnea, neck vein distention, and facial cyanosis or edema. To maintain a patent tracheal airway, an affected infant lies in an arched position with head extended in a manner very similar to that seen in neonates with congenital vascular ring. A halting, inspiratory, staccato type of breathing, probably because of pain, is also characteristic. Ultimately, the abscess may point on the anterior chest wall or in the suprasternal notch.

Usually, mediastinitis is first suspected when widening of the mediastinum is observed on a chest radiograph obtained for evaluation of respiratory distress. Forward displacement of the trachea and larynx may accompany these findings when retropharyngeal abscess is associated with mediastinitis. Infection after traumatic perforation of the esophagus or pharynx is often accompanied by pneumomediastinum with or without a pneumothorax [540,542].

Contrast studies performed to define the cause of respiratory or feeding difficulties in infants with mediastinitis may result in flow of radiopaque fluid into an esophageal laceration, mimicking the findings of an atresia, duplication, or diverticulum of the esophagus [542,543]. In such cases, endoscopy often shows a mucosal tear, confirming the diagnosis [543,544].

Treatment should be directed toward establishment of drainage and relief of pressure on vital structures through a mediastinotomy and placement of drainage tubes. A tracheostomy or endotracheal tube may be necessary for maintenance of an adequate airway. Initial empirical antimicrobial therapy with clindamycin (or metronidazole), ampicillin, and an aminoglycoside (or extended-spectrum cephalosporin) and β-lactam and β-lactamase inhibitor combination should be started after cultures of the blood and all other clinically indicated cultures have been obtained. More limited empirical antibiotic therapy can be provided with a β-lactam and β-lactamase inhibitor combination alone, such as piperacillin plus tazobactam, ampicillin plus sulbactam, or ticarcillin plus clavulanate. Specific therapy can subsequently be determined by the results of bacteriologic studies of the cultures or purulent fluid obtained at surgery.

ESOPHAGITIS

The esophagus is infrequently a focus for infection of the fetus or newborn [548]. Esophageal atresia is associated with congenital rubella (see Chapter 28). Severe esophagitis has also been reported in neonates with congenital cytomegalovirus infection [549]. The esophagus may be involved in infants with congenital Chagas disease, identified by signs of dysphagia, regurgitation, and megaesophagus [550]. Esophageal disease may follow mediastinitis in the neonate (discussed earlier). Only occasional cases of bacterial esophagitis in a neonate have been reported; a 940-g infant boy developed signs of sepsis on the 5th day of life and died 5 hours later [551]. Premortem blood cultures were positive for *Bacillus* species. Examination at autopsy revealed histologic evidence of esophagitis with pseudomembranous necrosis of squamous epithelium and many gram-positive bacilli. No other focus of infection was evident.

INFECTIONS OF ENDOCRINE ORGANS

Endocrine glands other than the adrenal are rarely involved in fetal or neonatal infection. Nelson [552] reported neonatal suppurative thyroiditis in a term Laotian infant. The infant presented with a left anterior neck mass at 3 days of age. At surgery, a cystic mass within the left lobe of the thyroid was identified. Purulent material within the mass grew viridans streptococci and nonhemolytic streptococci.

Orchitis caused by *S. enteritidis* was described in a 10-week-old neonate [553]. The infant presented with symptoms of sepsis and diarrhea, subsequently developing unilateral scrotal swelling and erythema on the 5th day after onset of illness. Ultrasound examination of the testis showed a patchy increased echo intensity; the diagnosis

was confirmed at exploratory surgery to rule out testicular torsion. Three other cases of infection of the testes caused by *Salmonella* species in infants younger than 3 months have been described [552].

INFECTIONS OF THE SALIVARY GLANDS

Neonatal infections of salivary glands are uncommon; although rare, involvement of the parotid is the most frequent [554–559], and submandibular gland infection is infrequent [554–556]. Most infections are caused by *S. aureus* [553–556], but *E. coli* [556], *P. aeruginosa* [556], and GBS (see Chapter 12) have also been implicated in suppurative parotitis. Oral anaerobic bacteria, including *Bacteroides* species and *Peptostreptococcus* species, may be found in mixed or isolated infections in more than half of cases [557]. Infections of the salivary glands occur more frequently in premature and male infants [556,559] and most commonly manifest during the 2nd week of life. The oral cavity is the probable portal of entry for the infecting organism. Blood-borne bacteria may invade the salivary glands, however. Dehydration with resultant decreased salivary flow may be a predisposing cause in some infants.

The clinical manifestations of salivary gland infection include fever, anorexia, irritability, and failure to gain weight. There may be swelling, tenderness, or erythema over the involved gland. Purulent material may be expressed from the ductal opening with or without gentle pressure over the gland.

The diagnosis is made by culture, Gram stain, or both of the pus exuding from the duct or by percutaneous aspiration of a fluctuant area. If microscopic examination of the Gram stain does not suggest a responsible pathogen, initial antibiotic therapy should be directed against *S. aureus*, *E. coli*, and *P. aeruginosa* (i.e., penicillinase-resistant penicillin or vancomycin plus an aminoglycoside or extended-spectrum cephalosporin with activity against *Pseudomonas* organisms). If there is a strong suspicion of involvement with anaerobic bacteria (i.e., negative aerobic cultures or failure to respond to therapy directed at aerobic pathogens), consideration should be given to adding or substituting antibiotics appropriate for anaerobic bacteria (e.g., clindamycin, metronidazole in combination with other antibiotics, or a β-lactam and β-lactamase antibiotic alone). The duration of therapy should extend throughout the period of inflammation and 3 to 5 days after signs of local inflammation have disappeared. Incision and drainage often may be required; surgical drainage should be considered if there is not a prompt response to therapy within 72 hours or if the gland becomes fluctuant. When considering incision and drainage, careful attention to preservation of the function of overlying motor branches of cranial nerve VII is important.

INFECTIONS OF THE SKIN AND SUBCUTANEOUS TISSUE

Bacterial infections of the skin of the newborn may manifest as maculopapular rash, vesicles, pustules, bullae, abscesses, cellulitis, impetigo, erythema multiforme, and petechiae or purpura. In a review of 2836 neonatal infections in Finland, only 6 were characterized as cellulitis [561]. Most infections of skin are caused by *S. aureus*, including bullous impetigo, chronic furunculosis, scalded skin syndrome, and breast abscesses (see Chapter 14). Cellulitis frequently accompanied by adenitis and bacteremia may be caused by GBS (see Chapter 12). Cutaneous infections caused by many other bacteria are discussed in this section; however, most microorganisms that cause disease in the neonate may produce cutaneous infections, and those infections are discussed in other chapters when relevant. For additional information on bacterial infections of the skin, the reader is referred to the text by Solomon and Esterly [562] and the reviews by Swartz and Weinberg [563] and Frieden [568]. Excellent color photographs are included in the *Color Atlas of Pediatric Dermatology* by Weinberg and coworkers [569].

Methicillin (oxacillin)-resistant (i.e., MRSA) infection is responsible for about 50% of cutaneous infections and is the frequent portal of entry for cutaneous infections in neonates [564]. MRSA cutaneous infections have included cellulitis and abscess formation, but may progress more frequently and rapidly to septicemia and disseminated infections to involve bones, joints, lung, central nervous system, and the cardiac endothelium [565]. In a 4-year survey (2001-2005) of staphylococcal infections in one center, 89 neonates were infected with staphylococci, and 61 (68.5%) infections were caused by MRSA; 30% of MRSA and methicillin-susceptible *S. aureus* infections manifested with pustular lesions, most often in the groin [566]. Cellulitis or abscess developed with 20% of MRSA and 32% of methicillin-susceptible *S. aureus* lesions, and 13% of lesions developed into an invasive infection (bacteremia, urinary tract infection). Also, infants with MRSA were more likely to have a mother with a history of skin infection (21% versus 4%). Other investigators have attempted to eradicate high colonization and disease rates in neonatal nurseries with the use of bacteriostatic agents applied to the umbilical cord. In one study with a high rate of MRSA impetigo, 0.3% triclosan (Bacti-Stat) was not effective in slowing the progress of the epidemic [567]. In this epidemic, 22 infants were affected, and all but 2 of the affected infants were circumcised, suggesting that the colonization of the surgical site facilitated invasion of the skin.

PATHOGENESIS

The skin of the newborn has unique characteristics, including absent microflora at birth; the presence of vernix caseosa; a less acid pH than that of older children; and often the presence of surgical wounds, including the severed umbilical cord, a circumcision site, and catheter wounds. The infant is immediately exposed to other infants, personnel, and the nosocomial environment. After the staphylococcal pandemic of the 1950s, information on the colonization of the skin, predisposing factors responsible for neonatal skin infection, bacterial transmission in the nursery, the inflammatory response of the skin to bacterial invasion, virulence factors of staphylococci, and methods of prevention of cross-infection became available. These studies are described in part in Chapters 14 and 35 and have been reviewed elsewhere [568,569].

Cutaneous bacterial infection may be a primary event or the result of systemic infection [570]. Septicemic embolic infection may occur at widely separated sites, whereas local infections often occur at a site with an identifiable predisposing cause. Procedures resulting in breaks in the cutaneous continuity, such as forceps abrasions or wounds at fetal electrodes or at venipuncture sites, may be readily identified. The necrotic umbilical cord is a site for proliferation of microorganisms that may invade local tissues.

Infection of the circumcision site remains a concern because it is the most common surgical procedure in infants in the United States. Speert [571] found that cleanliness was frequently disregarded by professional circumcisers in the 19th century. Operators were frequently uneducated, were dirty, and often spat on their instruments. Erysipelas, tetanus, and diphtheria have long been recognized as complications of unsterile surgical technique performed on newborns. In a now obsolete and prohibited part of the Orthodox Jewish circumcision ritual, the operator applied his lips to the fresh circumcision wound and sucked a few drops of blood. Such practices were responsible for transmission of syphilis and tuberculosis in neonates in the past. In one report [570], a 4-month-old infant presented with a penile ulcer, bilateral inguinal adenopathy, and a draining inguinal sinus caused by *Mycobacterium tuberculosis* after the "barber" spat on his razor before circumcision. Reports of 43 cases of tuberculosis associated with circumcision had been published by 1916 [569].

Subsequent case reports of severe infection after circumcision include bacteremia related to GBS [571], local infection and fatal staphylococcal pneumonia [572], staphylococcal scalded skin syndrome [573,574], necrotizing fasciitis [575], and bullous impetigo [576]. Two reports of necrotizing fasciitis after Plastibell circumcision emphasize severe infection as a potential risk of this procedure [577]. One infection caused by *S. aureus* and *Klebsiella* species was associated with prolonged convalescent and multiple surgical repairs, whereas a second infant survived staphylococcal necrotizing fasciitis after 14 days of intravenous antibiotic treatment.

The incidence of infection after elective circumcision was investigated at the University of Washington Hospital [578] from 1963-1972. Infection, defined as the presence of pus or erythema, occurred in 0.41% of 5521 infants and was more frequently associated with the use of a disposable plastic bell (Plastibell, 0.72%) than with the use of a metal clamp (Gomco, 0.14%). Wound cultures were infrequently available, and the microbiologic diagnosis was uncertain for most infants. Circumcision infection is uncommon, but local spread of infection may be devastating and lead to systemic infection.

Intrapartum fetal monitoring with scalp electrodes and intrauterine pressure catheters and measurements of fetal blood gases through scalp punctures have been associated with infections related to herpesvirus (see Chapter 26), *Mycoplasma* (see Chapter 20), and various aerobic and anaerobic bacteria. Bacterial infections have included pustules, abscesses, and fasciitis [579–583]. Infection rates are relatively low (0.1% to 4.5%) [579,580]; however, severe infections, including fasciitis, meningitis, and osteomyelitis, have occurred as severe complications. A review [581] of causative organisms in fetal scalp monitor infections found that 61% of infections were polymicrobial, involving anaerobic bacteria, aerobic gram-positive cocci, and gram-negative bacilli.

A multitude of specific virulence factors may be important determinants of disease. Some phage types of *S. aureus* are responsible for local tissue damage and systemic disease; other staphylococci elaborate toxins that result in bullae and other cutaneous pathology. Groups A and B streptococci are responsible for cellulitis and impetigo in infants. *P. aeruginosa* may invade and proliferate in small blood vessels, causing local necrosis and eschar formation (i.e., ecthyma gangrenosum). Infections with *Clostridium* species cause disease in devitalized tissues such as the umbilical stump [584]. Similarly, organisms usually considered commensals, such as diphtheroids, might be responsible for infection of the cord and fetal membranes [585].

MICROBIOLOGY

The skin of the infant is colonized initially by microorganisms present in the maternal birth canal. The skin of infants delivered by cesarean section is usually sterile at birth. After birth, microorganisms may be transferred to the skin during handling by the parents and nursery personnel. The prevalent organisms on the skin during the first few days of life include coagulase-negative staphylococci, diphtheroids, and gram-negative enteric bacilli (including *E. coli*) [586,587]. The umbilicus, genitalia, and adjacent skin areas (groin and abdomen) are colonized first; organisms then spread to the nose, throat, conjunctivae, and other body sites. Organisms present in the nursery environment colonize neonatal skin after a few days in the nursery. *S. aureus*, GBS, and various species of gram-negative bacilli may be present, but the microbiologic flora differs among nurseries and from time to time in the same nursery. Use of soaps and antiseptic solutions modifies the flora on the skin of the newborn. Hexachlorophene decreases colonization with staphylococci and diphtheroids, but gram-negative organisms are unaffected or may increase after use of this agent [588].

EPIDEMIOLOGY

Infant boys are more susceptible to skin infections caused by *S. aureus* than girls. Thompson and coworkers [589] showed that boys were colonized more frequently in every body site cultured, including the nose, groin, rectum, and umbilicus. Their review of studies indicated that in England, the United States, and Australia, approximately 50% more boys had skin lesions than girls. Although the incidence of breast abscesses is equal in boys and girls during the first 2 weeks of life, such abscesses are more frequent thereafter in girls [590]. The reason for this pattern is unclear, but Rudoy and Nelson [590] hypothesized that physiologic breast enlargement may play a role. Hormone production in the female infant after the 2nd week might account for the increase in abscesses of the breast.

Infections caused by MRSA involving the skin of children and neonates have markedly increased. The *mecA* gene responsible for resistance to oxacillin and nafcillin is often closely linked to a gene responsible for skin invasion. Before 1997, epidemic MRSA infections occurred in neonatal units involving infections of the respiratory tract, nasopharynx, gastrointestinal tract, eye, blood, wounds, or umbilicus [591]; these infections were usually restricted to single nurseries and involved a single genetic variant of MRSA. Since 1990, MRSA infections acquired in the community have been reported with increased frequency [592], including in infants 2 weeks old. Of these infections, 91% have involved the skin and soft tissues. In contrast to typical nosocomial MRSA, community-acquired MRSA organisms have frequently remained susceptible to trimethoprim-sulfamethoxazole and clindamycin. At the University of New Mexico, continued surveillance of MRSA-colonized and MRSA-infected infants in NICUs showed that by 2003, more than half of all isolates were community acquired.

Seasonal variation in the frequency of neonatal skin infections has been reported by Evans and coworkers [593], who conducted a series of studies at Harlem Hospital in New York. The prevalence of *S. aureus*, *E. coli*, and streptococci in the nares and umbilicus of infants was lowest in the autumn and usually highest in the summer or spring. No seasonal variation was observed for *S. epidermidis* or *Enterobacter* species The investigators concluded that seasonal differences must be considered in investigations of bacterial colonization of the newborn skin, and that high humidity may favor gram-negative colonization.

The time of onset of skin lesions associated with sepsis may be early (during the 1st week of life) or late (several weeks or months after birth). Disease acquired in the nursery usually becomes apparent after 5 days of age. Many skin lesions do not appear until after the infant has left the nursery; the observed incidence of skin disease caused by bacteria should include surveillance of infants in the home during the 1st month of life. Physicians responsible for neonatal care must be alert to the unusual occurrence of skin lesions. The introduction of a new and virulent bacterium, an alteration in technique, or the use of contaminated materials must be considered as possible causes of an increased incidence of such infections.

CLINICAL MANIFESTATIONS

Infants who have skin infections that remain localized that are not invasive or part of a systemic infection have few general signs of disease, such as fever, alteration in feeding habits, vomiting, or diarrhea. These signs may be present when significant tissue invasion occurs, as in abscesses or extensive cellulitis. Cutaneous manifestations that result from infectious diseases are listed in Table 10–5.

Among the common and least specific lesions are maculopapular rashes; these rashes may be caused by viruses (measles, rubella, or enteroviruses), fungi (*Candida* species), or bacteria (streptococci or staphylococci), or they may be unassociated with any infectious process. Erythema multiforme lesions have been observed in cases of sepsis related to *S. aureus* [594], streptococci [560], and *P. aeruginosa* [595]. Virtually any rash may be associated with bacterial infection. In an outbreak of sepsis caused by *Achromobacter* in premature infants [596], illness was

TABLE 10–5   Manifestations and Etiologies of Infections of the Skin in Newborns

Clinical Manifestation	Etiologic Agent	
	Bacterial	**Nonbacterial**
Maculopapular rash	*Treponema pallidum*[*,†]	Measles virus*
	Listeria monocytogenes	Rubella virus*
	*Streptococcus**	Enteroviruses*
	Staphylococcus	Molluscum contagiosum [653]
		Candida species*
Cellulitis (erysipelas)	Groups A and B streptococci	
	Achromobacter species [626]	
Impetigo	Groups A and B streptococci [627]*	
	*Staphylococcus aureus**	
	Escherichia coli	
Erythema multiforme	β-hemolytic streptococci [624]	
	*S. aureus**	
	Pseudomonas aeruginosa [625]	
Vesicular or bullous lesions	*S. aureus**	Herpes simplex virus*,†
	P. aeruginosa	Cytomegalovirus*
	T. pallidum	Varicella virus*,†
	Haemophilus influenzae type b [628]	Variola virus†
	L. monocytogenes [629]	Coxsackieviruses*
		Candida species*
		Aspergillus species*
		Drosophila larvae [654]
		Sarcoptes scabiei [655]
Pustular rashes	*S. aureus**	
	*L. monocytogenes**	
	H. influenzae [631]	
Ecthyma gangrenosum	*P. aeruginosa* [632–634]	
Abscesses and wound infections	*S. aureus**	*Mycoplasma hominis**
	*Staphylococcus epidermidis**	*Candida albicans* [656]
	β-hemolytic streptococci [637]	
	Group B streptococci [638]	
	E. coli [639–641]	
	Klebsiella species [642]	
	Proteus mirabilis [643]	
	P. aeruginosa [644]	
	Salmonella species [645]	
	Serratia marcescens [647]	
	H. influenzae [648]	
	Haemophilus parainfluenzae [649]	
	Corynebacterium vaginalis [650]	
	Neisseria gonorrhoeae [658]	
	Gardnerella vaginalis [651]	
	Bacteroides species [652]	
Petechiae, purpura, and ecchymoses	Gram-positive cocci* and gram-negative bacilli* associated with sepsis	Rubella virus*,†
	L. monocytogenes [629]	Cytomegalovirus*,†
	Streptococcus pneumoniae [629]	Herpes simplex virus*,†
	T. pallidum[*,†]	Coxsackievirus B*,†
		Toxoplasma gondii[*,†]

See appropriate chapter for further discussion.
†*Including infections acquired in utero.*

marked by respiratory distress, including apnea and cyanosis, but was characterized by a rash consisting of indurated, erythematous lesions with sharply defined borders that began on the cheeks or chest and spread rapidly to adjacent areas.

Cellulitis, erysipelas, and impetigo are usually associated with streptococcal infection (group A or B) [597], although impetigo caused by *S. aureus* or *E. coli* has also been reported in infants. Vesicles, commonly associated with infections by herpesviruses, also are seen occasionally during early stages of skin lesions caused by *S. aureus, H. influenzae* [598], *L. monocytogenes* [599], and *P. aeruginosa*. GBS [600], *S. aureus, P. aeruginosa*, herpes simplex virus, and *T. pallidum* may also be responsible for bullous lesions. Pustules commonly occur in staphylococcal diseases, but also occur in infections caused by *L. monocytogenes* and, rarely, in skin infections with *H. influenzae* [601].

Ecthyma gangrenosum is a local manifestation of infection with *P. aeruginosa* [602,603]. Lesions begin as a vesicular eruption on a wide erythematous base. Vesicles rupture and form an indurated black eschar followed by larger, sharply demarcated, painless necrotic areas, resulting from a small vessel vasculitis with necrosis of the adjacent tissue. The organisms are present in purulent material underlying the necrotic membrane. These lesions are particularly more common adjacent to nose, lip, ear, mouth, and perineum, resulting in avascular necrosis and loss of tissue. *P. aeruginosa* may be grown in pure culture from blood and lesions. Among 48 infants described in one outbreak, lesions appeared within the first 2 weeks of life; most infants died within 3 days of onset [604]. Ecthyma is relatively specific for *Pseudomonas* infections, but similar or identical lesions have rarely been described in infections owing to *S. aureus, Aeromonas hydrophila, S. marcescens, Aspergillus* species, or *Mucor* species [605]

Many infants with *Candida* infections have cutaneous manifestations. Baley and Silverman [606] described 18 infants with systemic candidiasis; 8 had a burnlike truncal erythema, and 9 other infants had typical candidal diaper rashes or maculopapular rashes of the axillae or neck.

Abscesses of the skin and subcutaneous tissue are usually caused by *S. aureus* and, less frequently, by group A streptococci, GBS [607,608], or gram-negative enteric bacilli [609–617]. Community-acquired MRSA organisms are even more likely to produce skin infections with abscess formation. Organisms that colonize the skin over an area that has been disrupted by an abrasion or other wound may invade the subcutaneous tissue and produce an abscess. *Haemophilus* species [618–620], *Gardnerella vaginalis* [621], *Bacteroides* species [622], molluscum contagiosum [623], *Drosophila* myiasis [624], scabies [625], and *Candida* [626] are examples of diverse causes of cutaneous abscesses; virtually any bacterial, fungal, or parasitic agent that is normally or transiently on skin may become a pathogen. *E. coli, Klebsiella* species, *P. aeruginosa* [605,610,627], *N. gonorrhoeae* [628], and *Bacteroides fragilis* [629] have caused wound infections in infants whose scalps were lacerated by forceps, fetal electrodes, or instruments used for obtaining blood from the scalp in utero. An extensive outbreak of systemic disease caused by *S. marcescens* in an NICU in Puerto Rico included wound infections at the site of intravenous infusions.

A cephalhematoma may become infected during sepsis or from manipulation of the cephalhematoma, such as through diagnostic or therapeutic needle puncture [630] or by puncture from a fetal monitor. Infections may be caused by *Bacteroides* species [622], *E. coli* [609,610], and *P. aeruginosa* [631]. The infection may be associated with meningitis [631] or with osteomyelitis of the underlying skull [609,610].

S. aureus is the most frequent etiologic agent in breast abscess, but gram-negative enteric bacilli may be becoming more common [611,615,616]. Of 36 cases with mastitis seen in Dallas, Texas, during a 16-year period, 32 cases were caused by *S. aureus*, 1 was caused by *E. coli*, and 2 were caused by *Salmonella* species; both *E. coli* and *S. aureus* were isolated from one abscess [632]. At Children's Hospital in Boston from 1947-1983, 41 cases of mastitis in neonates were managed [633]. *S. aureus* was responsible for 29 of 34 cases with an identifiable bacterial pathogen. All cases occurred in term infants during weeks 1 to 5 of life. Bilaterality and extramammary foci were rare. One third of infants were febrile, and most had elevated white blood cell counts (>15,000 cells/mm^3). Other reports have identified GBS [608] and *P. mirabilis* [613] as causes of breast abscesses. Brook [616] found that 5 of 14 breast abscesses contained anaerobic bacteria (i.e., *Bacteroides* species and *Peptostreptococcus*), but *S. aureus*, GBS, or enteric bacteria predominated; anaerobic bacteria occurred alone in only 2 of 14 cases.

Paronychia may occur in neonates after injury to the cuticle. The lesion is usually caused by *S. aureus* or β-hemolytic streptococci [592]. The authors of a report on an outbreak of paronychia in a Kuala Lumpur nursery suggest but do not prove that the lesions were caused by an anaerobic *Veillonella* species [634].

Omphalitis is defined by the presence of erythema or serous or purulent discharge from the umbilical stump or periumbilical tissues. A review by Cushing [635] provided a useful discussion of the pathophysiology, microbiology, diagnosis, and management of omphalitis. The incidence of infection is more frequent in infants with low birth weight and infants with complications of delivery. A survey of infants born at the Royal Woman's Hospital in Brisbane, Australia [636], identified an incidence of approximately 2% among term infants. The mean age of infants at presentation of omphalitis was 3.2 days. Perhaps because hexachlorophene bathing was used, gram-negative bacilli were more frequently associated with infection than gram-positive cocci. Microbiologic results are difficult to interpret, however, because swabs of the site of infection do not exclude surface contaminants, unless cultures are taken with extreme care and precision.

A series from the United States [637] found that periumbilical fasciitis was more frequent in boys, but did not find that umbilical catheterization, low birth weight, or septic delivery was associated with a high risk; overall, the incidence of omphalitis was equal in boys and girls. In this series, omphalitis manifested as discharge, cellulitis, or fasciitis; gram-positive organisms were found in 94% of cultures, and gram-negative bacteria were found in 64%. *S. aureus* was the most frequent isolate, with *E. coli* and *Klebsiella* species the next most common. Group A streptococci have been responsible for nursery outbreaks that may include an indolent form of omphalitis characterized by erythema and oozing of the umbilical stump for days to weeks, accompanied by pustular lesions of the abdominal wall in some cases [638]. Neonatal tetanus usually occurs as a result of contamination of the umbilical wound by *Clostridium tetani* at delivery.

Acute necrotizing fasciitis is a bacterial infection of subcutaneous tissue and fascial sheath [614,639,640]. Infection can arise in an operative wound or in a focal infection, such as a breast abscess, or there may be no apparent predisposing cause. Necrotizing fasciitis has been reported after circumcision [577] and as a complication of insertion of a fetal monitor [641]. The trunk and extremities are the areas most commonly involved; inflammation spreads rapidly along fascial planes, producing thrombosis and extensive necrosis, with infarcts developing in overlying skin. Vesicles and bullae appear, and the skin may become blue-gray or black. Myositis and bacteremia may accompany fasciitis. Staphylococci, GBS [642], *E. coli*, *P. aeruginosa*, anaerobic bacteria [643], and mixtures of gram-positive and gram-negative bacteria have been associated with this disease. The bacteria are present in skin lesions, deep fascia, and, in some cases, blood. The mortality is high despite the use of fasciotomy, wide débridement, and antibiotics.

Perirectal abscesses may occur in newborns. In contrast to older children, most newborns with perirectal abscess do not have underlying immunodeficiency, although infants with acquired or congenital immunodeficiency often present with this condition. The most common causes of perirectal abscess are *S. aureus*, *E. coli*, or other enteric bacilli [644,645]; however, anaerobic bacteria can also be involved. *S. aureus* and enteric bacilli may be more common in infants and newborns [645]. Recent rectal surgery for conditions such as Hirschsprung disease or imperforate anus (myotomy or rectal dilation) may be predisposing causes in infants; as in older children, neutropenia may be associated with an increased risk for perirectal abscess.

Otitis externa is uncommon in newborns. Victorin [646] described an outbreak of neonatal infections in which *P. aeruginosa* was cultured from seven infants with suppuration of the auditory canal. The author suggested that this outbreak was caused by contaminated bath water used in the nursery.

DIAGNOSIS

The appearance of a skin lesion alone may be sufficiently typical to suspect certain etiologic agents (e.g., ecthyma gangrenosum), but more often, the appearance is nonspecific. A microbiologic diagnosis should be sought to provide specific therapy. The lesion and the surrounding tissue should be cleaned with 70% ethanol to prevent contamination from organisms that colonize the surface. If crusts are present, they should be lifted with a sterile swab to provide drainage, and cultures should be obtained from the base of the lesion.

Vesicles and pustules can be aspirated with a needle (20-gauge to 25-gauge) attached to a syringe, or they can be opened and exudate can be collected on a sterile swab. Generally, swabs are not preferred for specimen collection because swab materials bind or inactivate bacterial organisms. Aspiration of abscesses is important; more than one aspiration may be required because the suppurative focus may not be easily distinguished from the surrounding inflammatory tissue. Aspiration of the leading edge or point of maximal inflammation of an area of cellulitis may be valuable and should be performed if no other suppurative or purulent sites are available for culture. A small needle (25-gauge or 26-gauge) should be attached to a tuberculin or other small-volume syringe filled with 0.25 to 0.50 mL of sterile nonbacteriostatic saline; the needle should be inserted into the area of soft tissue to be sampled, with continuous, gentle aspiration applied to the syringe. If no fluid is returned to the syringe, a small amount of fluid should be injected and immediately aspirated back into the syringe. Collected material may be sent to the laboratory in the syringe for Gram stain and culture, or, alternatively, the contents may be washed into a tube of bacteriologic broth medium for transport and subsequent culture.

If swabs are used, care must be taken that the material does not dry before it is plated on bacteriologic media. Swabs preferentially should be directly inoculated or rinsed in bacteriologic media and immediately transported to the microbiology laboratory. Alternatively, they may be refrigerated or placed in appropriate transport media if more than a few hours will elapse before inoculation of media in the laboratory. Whenever sufficient material is available (on swabs or in liquid), several slides should be prepared for Gram staining.

It is often difficult to distinguish petechiae from vascular dilation. Pressure with a glass slide on the border of the lesion is a simple and reliable method for detecting extravasation of red blood cells. If the lesion disappears on pressure, it is probably caused by dilation of small vessels, whereas persistence of the lesion after application of pressure indicates extravasation of red blood cells. Bacteria may be present in petechial lesions that occur in infants with bacterial sepsis. Blood obtained by aspiration or gentle scraping with a scalpel at the center of the petechiae may reveal the causative organism on Gram stain or culture.

DIFFERENTIAL DIAGNOSIS

Sclerema neonatorum, milia, and erythema toxicum are noninfectious lesions that are often confused with infections of the skin [647]. Bullous and purpuric lesions may be caused by noninfectious disorders, including mast cell diseases (e.g., urticaria pigmentosa), histiocytosis X, acrodermatitis enteropathica, dermatitis herpetiformis, epidermolysis bullosa, congenital porphyria [562], and pemphigus vulgaris [648]. A syndrome of generalized erythroderma, failure to thrive, and diarrhea has been associated with various forms of immunodeficiency [649].

Sclerema neonatorum is a diffuse, spreading, waxy hardness of the skin and subcutaneous tissue that occurs during the first weeks of life [628,650]. The subcutaneous tissue seems to be bound to underlying muscle and bone. This condition is usually seen on the thighs, buttocks, and trunk. Although associated with sepsis in some infants, sclerema also affects infants with dehydration, acidosis, and shock. Most evidence supports the hypothesis that sclerema is a manifestation of shock and insufficiency of the peripheral circulation. When it occurs in infants with generalized infection, sclerema is associated with a poor prognosis. In a review of cases of sepsis at The New York Hospital, sclerema was detected in 6 of 71 infants, 5 of whom died [651].

Milia are yellow or pearly white papules that are 1 mm in diameter and usually found scattered over the cheeks, forehead, and nose [647,652]. The lesion is a small cyst formed from retention of sebum in sebaceous glands. Because the cyst is capped by a shiny surface of epidermis, it may be confused with a small pustule. Milia are common; Gordon [652] estimated that 40% of healthy newborns have milia. The lesions are common in the first few weeks of life. These cysts may be distinguished from staphylococcal pustules by aspiration and Gram stain of the material.

Erythema toxicum consists of several types of lesions, including 1- to 3-mm, yellow-white papules or pustules on an erythematous base, erythematous macules, or diffuse erythema. These lesions are usually present on the trunk, but may involve the head and neck and extremities as well. Most lesions appear within the first hours of life and are uncommon after 2 days of age. Erythema toxicum is uncommon in low birth weight or premature infants [653]. Affected infants have no signs of systemic illness or local irritation. A smear of the contents of pustules reveals the presence of eosinophils and an absence of bacteria. Other noninfectious pustular lesions of newborns include neonatal pustular melanosis, which is marked by a mixed infiltrate that has a predominance of neutrophils [654], and infantile acropustulosis, which is characterized by an eosinophilic infiltration of the skin [655,656].

Bullae may occur on the skin of the wrist or forearm and usually are caused by trauma [657]. Sucking of the extremity by the infant is believed to cause the bullae, which contain sterile serous fluid. Purpura may be caused by noninfectious conditions, including trauma; erythroblastosis fetalis; or, less frequently, coagulation disorders, maternal drug ingestion, congenital leukemia, and congenital Letterer-Siwe disease.

Diaper rash is primarily a contact dermatitis associated with soilage of the skin by urine and stool [658–660]. The rash may occur as a mild erythema or scaling, a sharply demarcated and confluent erythema, or discrete shallow ulcerations. A beefy red, confluent rash with raised margins, satellite (e.g., folliculitis) oval lesions, or discrete vesicular-pustular lesions indicates secondary invasion by *C. albicans* or *S. aureus*. Systemic infectious illnesses that manifest as disseminated rashes (e.g., herpes, varicella, syphilis) may be characterized by early typical lesions in the diaper area.

TREATMENT

The treatment of localized skin lesions consists of the use of local antiseptic materials, systemic antimicrobial agents, and appropriate incision and drainage or débridement. Hexachlorophene (3% detergent emulsion) and chlorhexidine (4% solution) are valuable in cleaning small, abraded areas and discrete pustular lesions. Because of concern over its neurotoxicity and cutaneous absorption, hexachlorophene should not be used on large open areas of skin (see Chapter 14).

Systemic antibiotics should be considered for therapy whenever there is significant soft tissue infection with abscess or cellulitis. The specific antibiotic choice should be made on the basis of the microbiology of the lesion; streptococci may be treated effectively with penicillin G, ampicillin, or extended-spectrum cephalosporins (i.e., cefotaxime or ceftriaxone), whereas staphylococci generally must be treated with penicillinase-resistant penicillins or vancomycin. Infections owing to gram-negative enteric bacilli may be treated with aminoglycosides or extended-spectrum cephalosporins based on the results of susceptibility testing. Infections owing to *Pseudomonas* organisms can be effectively treated with aminoglycosides or ceftazidime.

Local heat and moist dressings over areas of abscess formation may facilitate localization or spontaneous drainage. Indications for incision and drainage of abscesses in infants are the same as for the indications in older children and adults.

PREVENTION

Prevention of local skin infections is best provided by appropriate routine hygiene, maintenance of the integrity of skin (i.e., avoidance of drying, trauma, or chemical contact), frequent diaper changes, and hygienic care of the umbilicus or other wounds or noninfectious skin inflammation. The following measures of skin care are recommended by the Committee of the Fetus and Newborn of the American Academy of Pediatrics [660] to prevent infection:

1. The first bath should be postponed until the infant is thermally stable.
2. Nonmedicated soap and water should be used; sterile sponges (not gauze) soaked in warm water may be used.
3. The buttocks and perianal should be cleaned with fresh water and cotton or with mild soap and water at diaper changes.
4. Ideally, agents used on the newborn skin should be dispensed in single-use containers.
5. No single method of cord care has proved to be superior, and none is endorsed [660].

Cord care may include application of alcohol, triple dye (i.e., brilliant green, proflavine hemisulfate, and crystal violet), or antimicrobial agents such as bacitracin. Alcohol hastens drying of the cord, but is probably not effective in preventing cord colonization and omphalitis. A randomized study of triple dye, povidone-iodine, silver sulfadiazine, and bacitracin ointment showed comparability in antimicrobial control [661].

During nursery outbreaks, the Centers for Disease Control and Prevention recommends the judicious use of hexachlorophene bathing [662]. Daily hexachlorophene bathing of the diaper area [663] and umbilical cord care with 4% chlorhexidine solution [664] have shown efficacy for prevention of staphylococcal disease (see Chapter 14).

CONJUNCTIVITIS AND OTHER EYE INFECTIONS

Conjunctivitis in the newborn usually results from one of four causes: infection with *N. gonorrhoeae*, infection with *S. aureus*, inclusion conjunctivitis caused by *Chlamydia trachomatis*, or chemical conjunctivitis caused by silver nitrate solution [665,666]. Less commonly, other microorganisms have been implicated as a cause of conjunctivitis, including group A streptococci, GBS, *S. pneumoniae*, *H. influenzae* (nontypable [591] and group b [667]), *P. aeruginosa*, *Moraxella* (*Neisseria*) *catarrhalis* [668], *Neisseria meningitidis* [669], *Corynebacterium diphtheriae* [670], *Pasteurella multocida* [671], *Clostridium* species [672], herpes simplex virus, echoviruses, *M. hominis*, and *Candida* species. In addition to meningococcal infections, other *Neisseria* species can be confused with gonococcal infections; *Neisseria cinerea* has been reported to cause conjunctivitis that was indistinguishable from gonococcal infection [673].

An epidemic of erythromycin-resistant *S. aureus* conjunctivitis affected 25 of 215 newborns during a 10-month period; control of the epidemic was achieved by identification of staff carriers and substitution of silver nitrate prophylaxis for erythromycin [674]. The major causes of conjunctivitis in neonates are discussed in Chapters 14 and 15. Cultures of the conjunctivae of neonates with purulent conjunctivitis and from the comparable eyes of a similar number of infants chosen as controls revealed significant differences, suggesting causality for viridans streptococci, *S. aureus*, *E. coli*, and *Haemophilus* species [675,676] MRSA infections may have an increased propensity to infect the eye. Conjunctivitis owing to MRSA was reported as the first case in an epidemic that eventually involved 14 neonates in an NICU including multiple invasive infections and two deaths [677]. MRSA has also caused dacrocystitis [678] and keratitis [679] in neonates.

Compared with chemical (e.g., silver nitrate) conjunctivitis, other noninfectious causes for conjunctivitis occur only rarely. Eosinophilic pustular folliculitis has been described since 1970 [680] although this disease usually occurs after 3 months of age, some infants younger than 4 to 6 weeks have been described. These infants present with recurrent crops of pruritic papules primarily affecting the scalp and brow. Biopsy specimens reveal folliculitis with a predominant eosinophilic infiltrate; most infants also have a leukocytosis and eosinophilia. Other acute or chronic cutaneous conditions may also manifest as conjunctival or periorbital inflammation, such as seborrhea, atopic dermatitis, acropustulosis of infancy, and erythema toxicum (see "Infections of the Skin and Subcutaneous Tissue").

In a review by Hammerschlag [681], the incidence of the two major pathogens ranged from 17% to 32% for *C. trachomatis* and 0% to 14.2% for *N. gonorrhoeae* in four U.S. studies. In other developed countries such as England [682], investigators found 8 cases of gonococcal infection and 44 cases of chlamydial infection among 86 newborns with ophthalmia neonatorum; in Denmark [683], investigators found that 72% of infants with conjunctivitis at 4 to 6 days after birth had positive cultures, but 70% were caused by staphylococci (*S. aureus* and *S. epidermidis*), and chlamydiae were isolated from only 2 of 300 newborns.

The incidence and microbiology of neonatal conjunctivitis depend on the incidence of transmissible infections in the maternal genital tract or the nursery and the use and efficacy of chemoprophylaxis. In Nairobi, Kenya, in a hospital where ocular prophylaxis had been discontinued, the incidence of gonococcal and chlamydial ophthalmitis was 3.6 and 8.1 cases per 100 live births [684]; in Harare, Zimbabwe, in a hospital where prophylaxis also was not used, the most common cause of conjunctivitis was *S. aureus* [685]. The introduction of tetracycline ointment for prophylaxis at Bellevue Hospital in New York City led to an overall increase in conjunctivitis associated with an increase in the incidence of gonococcal infection [686] because of the emergence of tetracycline resistance among gonococci.

Infections related to *P. aeruginosa* warrant special attention. Although uncommon, pseudomonal conjunctivitis may be a devastating disease if not recognized and treated appropriately [686]. The infection is usually acquired in the nursery, and the first signs of conjunctivitis appear between the 5th and 18th days of life. At first, the clinical manifestations are localized to the eye and include edema and erythema of the lid and purulent discharge. In some children, the conjunctivitis progresses rapidly, with denuding of the corneal epithelium and infiltration with neutrophils. With extension of the corneal infiltration, perforation of the cornea may occur. The anterior chamber may fill with fibrinous exudate, and the iris can adhere to the cornea. Subsequent invasion of the cornea by small blood vessels (pannus) is characteristic of pseudomonal conjunctivitis. The late ophthalmic complications may be followed by bacteremia and septic foci in other organs [687].

Pseudomonal eye infections in neonates can occur in epidemic form, with subsequent high rates of mortality and ophthalmic morbidity. Burns and Rhodes [687] reported a series of eye infections caused by *P. aeruginosa* in premature infants with purulent conjunctivitis rapidly progressing to septicemia, shock, and death in four infants. Five other children with conjunctivitis alone survived, but one child required enucleation. Drewett and coworkers [688] described a nursery outbreak of pseudomonal conjunctivitis believed to be caused by contaminated resuscitation equipment; of 14 infected infants, 1 became blind, and 1 had severe corneal opacities. Rapidity of the course of this infection is indicated in a case report of a 10-day-old infant who developed a corneal ulcer with perforation within 2 days after first observation of a purulent discharge [689]. An outbreak of four cases of *Pseudomonas* conjunctivitis in premature infants occurred within 2 weeks at the American University of Beirut Medical Center [690]; no cause for the outbreak was found.

A review by Lohrer and Belohradsky [691] of bacterial endophthalmitis in neonates emphasizes the importance of *P. aeruginosa* in invasive bacterial eye infections ranging from keratitis to panophthalmitis. The literature review included 16 cases of invasive eye infections in neonates; 13 were caused by *P. aeruginosa*, and the others were cases of endophthalmitis caused by GBS and *S. pneumoniae*. Other opportunistic gram-negative pathogens associated with outbreaks of infections in nurseries may also include conjunctivitis as a part of the infection syndrome. In a report by Christensen and coworkers [692], multiply antibiotic-resistant *S. marcescens* was responsible for 15 cases of pneumonia, sepsis, and meningitis and for

20 cases of conjunctivitis, cystitis, and wound infection over a 9-month period in an NICU.

Dacryocystitis may complicate a congenital lacrimal sac distention (i.e., dacryocystocele) which may appear as early as the during the first week of life with edema and erythema of the lower lid. Purulent material emerged from the puncta after moderate pressure over the lacrimal sac; *S. marcescens* was grown from the material.

The physician responsible for management of a child with purulent conjunctivitis must consider the major causes of the disease and must be alert to rare pathogens. In hospitals that practice Credé method (i.e., silver nitrate application), purulent conjunctivitis during the first 48 hours of life is almost always caused by chemical toxicity [694]. After the first 2 days, the pus of an exudative conjunctivitis must be carefully examined by Gram stain for the presence of gram-negative intracellular diplococci, gram-positive cocci in clusters, and gram-negative bacilli. Appropriate cultures should be used for isolation of the organisms concerned. If the smears are inconclusive and no pathogens are isolated on appropriate media, and if conjunctivitis persists, a diagnosis of inclusion or chlamydial infection is likely [693,694].

The treatment of staphylococcal and gonococcal conjunctivitis is discussed in Chapters 14 and 15. Chlamydial conjunctivitis is reviewed in Chapter 19.

If infection with *Pseudomonas* species is suspected, treatment should be started at once with an effective parenteral antibiotic, such as an aminoglycoside (e.g., tobramycin, amikacin, or gentamicin) with or without an antipseudomonal penicillin or ceftazidime (see Chapter 35) and with a locally applied ophthalmic ointment. The use of subconjunctival gentamicin or other antipseudomonal aminoglycoside is of uncertain value; however, if the cornea seems to be extensively involved, there is a risk of rapid development of endophthalmitis, and the subconjunctival injection of antibiotics should be considered in consultation with an ophthalmologist. If the diagnosis is confirmed, this regimen is continued until the local signs of *Pseudomonas* infection resolve.

Recommendations for ocular chemoprophylaxis are discussed in Chapters 15 and 19. Additional information is available in the 2009 edition of the *Report of the Committee on Infectious Diseases* published by the American Academy of Pediatrics [695].

REFERENCES

[1] F.M. Murphy, C.J. Baker, Solitary hepatic abscess: a delayed complication of neonatal bacteremia, Pediatr. Infect. Dis. J. 7 (1988) 414.
[2] B. Guillois, et al., Staphylococcie pleuro-pulmonaire néonatale avec abcès hépatiques multiples, Ann. Pediatr. 36 (1989) 681.
[3] L.P. Dehner, J.M. Kissane, Pyogenic hepatic abscesses in infancy and childhood, J. Pediatr. 74 (1969) 763.
[4] H.T. Wright Jr., Personal communication, (1987).
[5] T.J. Moss, T.J. Pysher, Hepatic abscess in neonates, Am. J. Dis. Child. 135 (1981) 726.
[6] M.J. Chusid, Pyogenic hepatic abscess in infancy and childhood, Pediatrics 62 (1978) 554.
[7] P. Dineen, Personal communication, Cornell University Medical College, New York, NY.
[8] T.V. Bilfinger, et al., Pyogenic liver abscesses in nonimmunocompromised children, South. Med. J. 79 (1986) 37.
[9] K.C. Beutow, S.W. Klein, R.B. Lane, Septicemia in premature infants: the characteristics, treatment, and prevention of septicemia in premature infants, Am. J. Dis. Child. 110 (1965) 29.
[10] E.C. Dunham, Septicemia in the newborn, Am. J. Dis. Child. 45 (1933) 229.
[11] W. Nyhan, M.D. Fousek, Septicemia of the newborn, Pediatrics 22 (1958) 268.
[12] S.P. Gotoff, R.E. Behrman, Neonatal septicemia, J. Pediatr. 76 (1970) 142.
[13] J.R. Hamilton, A. Sass-Kortsak, Jaundice associated with severe bacterial infection in young infants, J. Pediatr. 63 (1963) 121.
[14] P. Hänninen, P. Terhe, A. Toivanen, Septicemia in a pediatric unit: a 20-year study, Scand. J. Infect. Dis. 3 (1971) 201.
[15] E. Potter, Pathology of the Fetus and Infant, third ed., Year Book Medical Publishers, Chicago, 1975.
[16] W.A. Silverman, W.E. Homan, Sepsis of obscure origin in the newborn, Pediatrics 3 (1949) 157.
[17] R.T. Smith, E.S. Platau, R.A. Good, Septicemia of the newborn: current status of the problem, Pediatrics 17 (1956) 549.
[18] W.M. Gersony, G.H. McCracken Jr., Purulent pericarditis in infancy, Pediatrics 40 (1967) 224.
[19] J.H.M. Axton, Amoebic proctocolitis and liver abscess in a neonate, S. Afr. Med. J. 46 (1972) 258.
[20] T. Botman, P.J. Ruys, Amoebic appendicitis in newborn infant, Trop. Geogr. Med. 15 (1963) 221.
[21] Y.W. Brans, R. Ceballos, G. Cassady, Umbilical catheters and hepatic abscesses, Pediatrics 53 (1974) 763.
[22] H.J. Cohen, S. Dresner, Liver abscess following exchange transfusion for erythroblastosis fetalis, Q. Rev. Pediatr. 16 (1961) 148.
[23] J. deBeaujeu, et al., Abcès hépatique à forme tumorale chez un nourrisson, Pediatrie 23 (1968) 363.
[24] W. Heck, F. Rehbein, B. Reismann, Pyogene Leberabszesse im Säuglingsalter, Z. Kinderchir. (Suppl. 1) (1966) 49.
[25] S.R. Kandall, A.B. Johnson, L.M. Gartner, Solitary neonatal hepatic abscess, J. Pediatr. 85 (1974) 567.
[26] T. Kutsunai, Abscess of the liver of umbilical origin in infants: report of two cases, Am. J. Dis. Child. 51 (1936) 1385.
[27] C.M. Madsen, N. Secouris, Solitary liver abscess in a newborn, Surgery 47 (1960) 1005.
[28] C. Martin, et al., Abcès gazeux du foie avec coagulopathie chez le nouveau-né: guérison (à propos de 2 observations), Bord. Med. 5 (1972) 1181.
[29] M.D. Pouyanne, Abcès du foie à staphylocoques chez un nouveau-né, compliqué de suppuration sous-phrénique puis de péritonite à évolution subaiguë, Guerison J. Med. Bordeaux 130 (1953) 929.
[30] L.J. Pyrtek, S.A. Bartus, Hepatic pyemia, N. Engl. J. Med. 272 (1965) 551.
[31] K. Sharma, R. Kumar, Solitary abscess of the liver in a newborn infant, Surgery 61 (1967) 812.
[32] J.W. Williams, et al., Liver abscess in newborn: complication of umbilical vein catheterization, Am. J. Dis. Child. 125 (1973) 111.
[33] D.W. Beaven, Staphylococcal peritonitis in the newborn, Lancet 1 (1958) 869.
[34] J.R. Fraga, B.A. Javate, S. Venkatessan, Liver abscess and sepsis due to *Klebsiella pneumoniae* in a newborn, Clin. Pediatr. 13 (1974) 1081.
[35] A.A. Tariq, N.A. Rudolph, E.J. Levin, Solitary hepatic abscess in a newborn infant: a sequel of umbilical vein catheterization and infusion of hypertonic glucose solutions, Clin. Pediatr. 16 (1977) 577.
[36] P. Cushman, O.C. Ward, Solitary liver abscess in a neonate: complication of umbilical vein catheterization, Ir. J. Med. Sci. 147 (1978) 374.
[37] H. Wiedersberg, P. Pawlowski, Pyelophlebitis nach Nabelvenenkatheterismus, Monatsschr. Kinderheilkd. 128 (1980) 128.
[38] F. Gonzalez Rivera, M. Montoro Burgos, A. Cabrera Molina, Absceso hepático en un recién nacido, An. Esp. Pediatr. 23 (1985) 59.
[39] P.W. Nars, L. Klco, C.P. Fliegel, Successful conservative management of a solitary liver abscess in a premature baby, Helv. Paediatr. Acta 38 (1983) 489.
[40] L.R. Larsen, J. Raffensperger, Liver abscess, J. Pediatr. Surg. 14 (1979) 329.
[41] F. Montoya, et al., Abcès du foie chez un nouveau-né guerison après ponction percutanée sous controle échographique, Pediatrie 38 (1983) 547.
[42] S.M. Murphy, C.J. Baker, Solitary hepatic abscess: a delayed complication of neonatal bacteremia, Pediatr. Infect. Dis. J. 7 (1988) 414.
[43] D. Anagnostakis, et al., Risk of infection associated with umbilical vein catheterization: a prospective study in 75 newborn infants, J. Pediatr. 86 (1975) 759.
[44] J. Sabbaj, V. Sutter, S.M. Finegold, Anaerobic pyogenic liver abscess, Ann. Intern. Med. 77 (1972) 629.
[45] W.W. Meyer, J. Lind, Postnatal changes in the portal circulation, Arch. Dis. Child. 41 (1966) 606.
[46] J. Hageman, et al., Congenital tuberculosis: critical reappraisal of clinical findings and diagnostic procedures, Pediatrics 66 (1980) 980.
[47] M.R. Hughesdon, Congenital tuberculosis, Arch. Dis. Child. 21 (1946) 121.
[48] M.F. Cantwell, et al., Brief report: congenital tuberculosis, N. Engl. J. Med. 330 (1994) 1051.
[49] N. Abughali, et al., Congenital tuberculosis, Pediatr. Infect. Dis. J. 13 (1994) 738.
[50] B. Simma, et al., Bacille Calmette-Guérin–associated hepatitis, Eur. J. Pediatr. 150 (1991) 423.
[51] T.N. Lide, Congenital tularemia, Arch. Pathol. 43 (1947) 165.
[52] J.C. Regan, A. Litvak, C. Regan, Intrauterine transmission of anthrax, JAMA 80 (1923) 1769.
[53] H.T. Hicks, H. French, Typhoid fever and pregnancy with special reference to foetal infection, Lancet 1 (1905) 1491.
[54] M. Sarram, et al., Intrauterine fetal infection with *Brucella melitensis* as a possible cause of second-trimester abortion, Am. J. Obstet. Gynecol. 119 (1974) 657.
[55] A. Brim, A bacteriologic study of 100 stillborn and dead newborn infants, J. Pediatr. 15 (1939) 680.

[56] E. Madan, M.P. Meyer, A.J. Amortegui, Isolation of genital mycoplasmas and *Chlamydia trachomatis* in stillborn and neonatal autopsy material, Arch. Pathol. Lab. Med. 112 (1988) 749.

[57] E.H. Oppenheimer, J.B. Hardy, Congenital syphilis in the newborn infant: clinical and pathological observations in recent cases, Johns Hopkins Med. J. 129 (1971) 63.

[58] J.H. Stokes, H. Beerman, N.R. Ingraham, Modern Clinical Syphilology: Diagnosis, Treatment, Case Study, third ed., WB Saunders, Philadelphia, 1944.

[59] A. Venter, et al., Liver function in early congenital syphilis. Does penicillin cause a deterioration? J. Pediatr. Gastroenterol. Nutr. 12 (1991) 310.

[60] S. Lindsay, J.W. Luke, Fetal leptospirosis (Weil's disease) in a newborn infant: case of intrauterine fetal infection with report of an autopsy, J. Pediatr. 34 (1949) 90.

[61] V. Topciu, et al., Voie transplacentaire dans un cas de leptospirose humaine, Gynecol. Obstet. 65 (1966) 617.

[62] H.O. Gsell Jr., et al., Intrauterine leptospirosis pomona: 1st reported case of an intrauterine transmitted and cured leptospirosis, Dtsch. Med. Wochenschr. 96 (1971) 1263.

[63] H.H.W. Cramer, Abortus bein Leptospirosis canicola, Arch. Gynecol. 177 (1950) 167.

[64] H. Chung, et al., Transplacental or congenital infection of leptospirosis: clinical and experimental observations, Chin. Med. J. 82 (1963) 777.

[65] P.C. Fuchs, A.A. Oyama, Neonatal relapsing fever due to transplacental transmission of *Borrelia*, JAMA 208 (1969) 690.

[66] P. Yagupsky, S. Moses, Neonatal *Borrelia* species infection (relapsing fever), Am. J. Dis. Child. 139 (1985) 74.

[67] P.C. Fuchs, Personal communication, 1973.

[68] K. Weber, et al., Borrelia burgdorferi in a newborn despite oral penicillin for Lyme borreliosis during pregnancy, Pediatr. Infect. Dis. J. 7 (1988) 286.

[68a] Lyme disease, in L.K. Pickering et al., (Ed.), Red Book 2006 Report of the Committee on Infectious Diseases, twenty-seventh ed., American Academy of Pediatrics, Elk Grove Village, IL, 2006, pp. 428–433.

[69] A.C. Steere, Lyme disease, N. Engl. J. Med. 321 (1989) 586.

[70] J.K. Lipinski, et al., Falciform ligament abscess in the infant, J. Pediatr. Surg. 20 (1985) 556.

[71] K. Betke, H. Richarz, Nabelsepsis mit Pyelphlebitis, multiplen Leberabscessen, Lungenabscessen, und Osteomyelitis. Ausgang in Heilung, Monatsschr. Kinderheilkd. 105 (1957) 70.

[72] R.I.K. Elliott, The ductus venosus in neonatal infection, Proc. R. Soc. Med. 62 (1969) 321.

[73] C.G. McKenzie, Pyogenic infection of liver secondary to infection in the portal drainage area, BMJ 4 (1964) 1558.

[74] K. Menzel, H. Buttenberg, Pyelophlebitis mit multiplen Leberabszessen als Komplikation mehrfacher Sondierung der Nabelvene, Kinderarztl. Prax. 40 (1972) 14.

[75] S. Sarrut, J. Alain, F. Alison, Les complications précoces de la perfusion par la veine ombilicale chez le premature, Arch. Fr. Pediatr. 26 (1969) 651.

[76] B. Santerne, et al., Diagnostic et traitement d'une abcédation hépatique néo-natale multifocale par l'échographie, Presse. Med. 16 (1987) 12.

[77] J. Scott, Iatrogenic lesions in babies following umbilical vein catheterization, Arch. Dis. Child. 40 (1965) 426.

[78] A. Shaw, S. Pierog, "Ectopic" liver in the umbilicus: an unusual focus of infection in a newborn infant, Pediatrics 44 (1969) 448.

[79] J.E. Morison, Umbilical sepsis and acute interstitial hepatitis, J. Pathol. Bacteriol. 56 (1944) 531.

[80] J. Bernstein, A.K. Brown, Sepsis and jaundice in early infancy, Pediatrics 29 (1962) 873.

[81] R.G.F. Parker, Jaundice and infantile diarrhea, Arch. Dis. Child. 33 (1958) 330.

[82] J.L. Gwinn, F.A. Lee, Radiologic case of the month: pyogenic liver abscess, Am. J. Dis. Child. 123 (1972) 50.

[83] D.J. Martin, Neonatal disorders diagnosed with ultrasound, Clin. Perinatol. 12 (1985) 219.

[84] V.M. Pineiro-Carrero, J.M. Andres, Morbidity and mortality in children with pyogenic liver abscess, Am. J. Dis. Child. 143 (1989) 1424.

[85] K.H. Caron, Magnetic resonance imaging of the pediatric abdomen, Semin. Ultrasound CT MR 12 (1991) 448.

[86] R.A. Halvorsen Jr., et al., Hepatic abscess: sensitivity of imaging tests and clinical findings, Gastrointest. Radiol. 13 (1988) 135.

[87] J.C. Weinreb, et al., Imaging the pediatric liver: MRI and CT, AJR Am. J. Roentgenol. 147 (1986) 785.

[88] M.D. Cohen, Clinical utility of magnetic resonance imaging in pediatrics, Am. J. Dis. Child. 140 (1986) 947.

[89] M.J. Diament, et al., Percutaneous aspiration and catheter drainage of abscesses, J. Pediatr. 108 (1986) 204.

[90] Z. Rubinstein, et al., Ultrasound and computed tomography in the diagnosis and drainage of abscesses and other fluid collections, Isr. J. Med. Sci. 19 (1983) 1050.

[91] T.B. Reynolds, Medical treatment of pyogenic liver abscess, Ann. Intern. Med. 96 (1982) 373.

[92] R. Loh, G. Wallace, Y.H. Thong, Successful non-surgical management of pyogenic liver abscess, Scand. J. Infect. Dis. 19 (1987) 137.

[93] C.M. Keidl, M.J. Chusid, Splenic abscesses in childhood, Pediatr. Infect. Dis. J. 8 (1989) 368.

[94] A. Bowen, Acute gallbladder dilatation in a neonate: emphasis on ultrasonography, J. Pediatr. Gastroenterol. Nutr. 3 (1984) 304.

[95] J.F. Goldthorn, D.W. Thomas, A.D. Ramos, Hydrops of the gallbladder in stressed premature infants, Clin. Res. 28 (1980) 122A.

[96] P.W. Brill, P. Winchester, M.S. Rosen, Neonatal cholelithiasis, Pediatr. Radiol. 12 (1982) 285.

[97] J. Callahan, et al., Cholelithiasis in infants: association with total parenteral nutrition and furosemide, Radiology 143 (1982) 437.

[98] M.S. Keller, et al., Spontaneous resolution of cholelithiasis in infants, Radiology 157 (1985) 345.

[99] W.J. Schirmer, E.R. Grisoni, M.W.L. Gauderer, The spectrum of cholelithiasis in the first year of life, J. Pediatr. Surg. 24 (1989) 1064.

[100] D. Debray, et al., Cholelithiasis in infancy: a study of 40 cases, J. Pediatr. 122 (1993) 38.

[101] J. Neu, A. Arvin, R.L. Ariagno, Hydrops of the gallbladder, Am. J. Dis. Child. 134 (1980) 891.

[102] E.A. Leichty, et al., Normal gallbladder appearing as abdominal mass in neonates, Am. J. Dis. Child. 136 (1982) 468.

[103] K.J. Peevy, H.J. Wiseman, Gallbladder distension in septic neonates, Arch. Dis. Child. 57 (1982) 75.

[104] T. Dutta, et al., Gallbladder disease in infancy and childhood, Prog. Pediatr. Surg. 8 (1975) 109.

[105] R.L. Saldanha, C.A. Stein, A.E. Kopelman, Gallbladder distention in ill preterm infants, Am. J. Dis. Child. 137 (1983) 1179.

[106] M. El-Shafie, C.L. Mah, Transient gallbladder distention in sick premature infants: the value of ultrasonography and radionuclide scintigraphy, Pediatr. Radiol. 16 (1986) 468.

[107] N. Modi, A.J. Keay, Neonatal gallbladder distention, Arch. Dis. Child. 57 (1982) 562.

[108] J.B. Amodio, et al., Neonatal hydrops of the gallbladder: evaluation by cholescintigraphy and ultrasonography, N. Y. State J. Med. 85 (1985) 565.

[109] J.P. McGahan, H.E. Phillips, K.L. Cox, Sonography of the normal pediatric gallbladder and biliary tract, Radiology 144 (1982) 873.

[110] J.O. Haller, Sonography of the biliary tract in infants and children, AJR Am. J. Roentgenol. 157 (1991) 1051.

[111] K.J. Guthrie, G.L. Montgomery, Infections with Bacterium enteritidis in infancy with the triad of enteritis, cholecystitis, and meningitis, J. Pathol. Bacteriol. 49 (1939) 393.

[112] W. Faller, J.E. Berkelhamor, J.R. Esterly, Neonatal biliary tract infection coincident with maternal methadone therapy, Pediatrics 48 (1971) 997.

[113] P.N. Jamieson, D.G. Shaw, Empyema of gallbladder in an infant, Arch. Dis. Child. 50 (1975) 482.

[114] L.A. Arnspiger, J.G. Martin, H.O. Krempin, Acute noncalculous cholecystitis in children: report of a case in a 17-day-old infant, Am. J. Surg. 100 (1960) 103.

[115] J.L. Ternberg, J.P. Keating, Acute acalculous cholecystitis: complication of other illnesses in childhood, Arch. Surg. 110 (1975) 543.

[116] R.F. Crystal, R.L. Fink, Acute acalculous cholecystitis in childhood: a report of two cases, Clin. Pediatr. 10 (1971) 423.

[117] A.E. Robinson, et al., Cholecystitis and hydrops of the gallbladder in the newborn, Radiology 122 (1977) 749.

[118] W.H. Snyder Jr., L. Chaffin, L. Oettinger, Cholelithiasis and perforation of the gallbladder in an infant, with recovery, JAMA 149 (1952) 1645.

[119] M.E. Washburn, P.J. Barcia, Uncommon cause of a right upper quadrant abdominal mass in a newborn: acute cholecystitis, Am. J. Surg. 140 (1980) 704.

[120] W.A. Thurston, E.N. Kelly, M.M. Silver, Acute acalculous cholecystitis in a premature infant treated with parenteral nutrition, Can. Med. Assoc. J. 135 (1986) 332.

[121] R. Pieretti, A.W. Auldist, C.A. Stephens, Acute cholecystitis in children, Surg Obstet. Gynecol. 140 (1975) 16.

[122] B.A. Hanson, G.H. Mahour, M.M. Woolley, Diseases of the gallbladder in infancy and childhood, J. Pediatr. Surg. 6 (1971) 277.

[123] P.A. Dewan, K.B. Stokes, J.R. Solomon, Paediatric acalculous cholecystitis, Pediatr. Surg. Int. 2 (1987) 120.

[124] J. Denes, et al., Die Frühgeborenen-Appendicitis, Z. Kinderchir. 5 (1968) 400.

[125] V.C. Traynelis, E.E. Hrabovsky, Acalculous cholecystitis in the neonate, Am. J. Dis. Child. 139 (1985) 893.

[126] R.D. Aach, Cholecystitis in childhood, in: R.D. Feigin, J.D. Cherry (Eds.), Textbook of Pediatric Infectious Diseases, second ed., WB Saunders, Philadelphia, 1987, pp. 742–743.

[127] R. Wyllie, J.F. Fitzgerald, Bacterial cholangitis in a 10-week-old infant with fever of undetermined origin, Pediatrics 65 (1980) 164.

[128] D.M.O. Becroft, Biliary atresia associated with prenatal infection by *Listeria monocytogenes*, Arch. Dis. Child. 47 (1972) 656.

[129] B.E. Favara, D.R. Akers, R.A. Franciosi, Adrenal abscess in a neonate, J. Pediatr. 77 (1970) 682.

[130] C. Mondor, et al., Nonsurgical management of neonatal adrenal abscess, J. Pediatr. Surg. 23 (1988) 1048.

[131] A. François, et al., Abcès surrénalien neonatal à Proteus mirabilis, Arch. Fr. Pediatr. 48 (1991) 559.

[132] J.R. Lizardo-Barahona, J. Nieto-Zermño, E. Bracho-Blanchet, Absceso adrenal en el recien nacido: informe de un caso y revision de la literatura, Bol. Med. Hosp. Infant. Mex. 47 (1990) 401.

[133] J.M. Torres-Simon, et al., Absceso suprarenal en el recien nacido, An. Esp. Pediatr. 31 (1989) 601.

[134] O. Zamir, et al., Adrenal abscess: a rare complication of neonatal adrenal hemorrhage, Pediatr. Surg. Int. 2 (1987) 117.

[135] J.M. Van de Water, E.W. Fonkalsrud, Adrenal cysts in infancy, Surgery 60 (1966) 1267.

[136] W.J. Blankenship, et al., Suprarenal abscess in the neonate: a case report and review of diagnosis and management, Pediatrics 55 (1975) 239.

[137] D.M. Gibbons, et al., Abdominal flank mass in the neonate, J. Urol. 119 (1978) 671.

[138] G.O. Atkinson Jr., et al., Adrenal abscess in the neonate, Radiology 155 (1985) 101.

[139] A. Carty, P. Stanley, Bilateral adrenal abscesses in a neonate, Pediatr. Radiol. 1 (1973) 63.

[140] K.M. Walker, W.F. Coyer, Suprarenal abscess due to group B Streptococcus, J. Pediatr. 94 (1979) 970.

[141] R. Camilleri, et al., Abcédation d'un hématome surrénal avec hypertension artérielle, Arch. Fr. Pediatr. 41 (1984) 705.

[142] K. Rajani, S.R. Shapiro, B.W. Goetsman, Adrenal abscess: complication of supportive therapy of adrenal hemorrhage in the newborn, J. Pediatr. Surg. 15 (1980) 676.

[143] R.G. Wells, J.R. Sty, N.B. Hodgson, Suprarenal abscess in the neonate: technetium-99m glucoheptonate imaging, Clin. Nucl. Med. 11 (1986) 32.

[144] B.A. Cadarso, A.M.R. Mialdea, Absceso adrenal en la epoca neonatal, An. Esp. Pediatr. 21 (1984) 706.

[145] S. Ohta, et al., Neonatal adrenal abscess due to Bacteroides, J. Pediatr. 93 (1978) 1063.

[146] B.A. Bekdash, M.S. Slim, Adrenal abscess in a neonate due to gas-forming organisms: a diagnostic dilemma, Z. Kinderchir. 32 (1981) 184.

[147] M. Gross, P.K. Kottmeier, K. Waterhouse, Diagnosis and treatment of neonatal adrenal hemorrhage, J. Pediatr. Surg. 2 (1967) 308.

[148] V. Vigi, et al., Suprarenal abscess in a newborn, Helv. Paediatr. Acta 36 (1981) 263.

[149] S. Suri, et al., Adrenal abscess in a neonate presenting as a renal neoplasm, Br. J. Urol. 54 (1982) 565.

[150] C.A. Mittelstaedt, et al., The sonographic diagnosis of neonatal adrenal hemorrhage, Radiology 131 (1979) 453.

[151] A. Rey, et al., Hemorragia suprarenal encapsulada en el recien nacido: estudio de ocho casos, An. Esp. Pediatr. 21 (1984) 238.

[152] J. Black, D.I. Williams, Natural history of adrenal hemorrhage in the newborn, Arch. Dis. Child. 48 (1973) 173.

[153] O. Iklof, W. Mortensson, B. Sandstedt, Suprarenal haematoma versus neuroblastoma complicated by haemorrhage: a diagnostic dilemma in the newborn, Acta Radiol. Diagn. 27 (1986) 3.

[154] S.J. White, et al., Sonography of neuroblastoma, Am. J. Radiol. 141 (1983) 465.

[155] W.E. Etherington-Wilson, Appendicitis in newborn: report of a case 16 days old, Proc. R. Soc. Med. 38 (1945) 186.

[156] P. Puri, B. O'Donnell, Appendicitis in infancy, J. Pediatr. Surg. 13 (1978) 173.

[157] B. Landaas, Diagnosis of appendicitis in young children, Tidsskr. Nor. Laegeforen. 68 (1948) 335.

[158] G. Reuter, I. Krause, Beitrag zur Problematik der Appendizitis des Neugeborenen, Kinderarztl. Prax. 47 (1979) 289.

[159] W.J. Norris, Appendicitis in children, West J Surg Obstet Gynecol 54 (1946) 183.

[160] J.M. Parsons, B.G. Miscall, C.K. McSherry, Appendicitis in the newborn infant, Surgery 67 (1970) 841.

[161] W. Schaupp, E.G. Clausen, P.K. Ferrier, Appendicitis during the first month of life, Surgery 48 (1960) 805.

[162] E.G. Stanley-Brown, Acute appendicitis during the first five years of life, Am. J. Dis. Child. 108 (1964) 134.

[163] W.H. Snyder Jr., L. Chaffin, Appendicitis during the first 2 years of life: report of 21 cases and review of 447 cases from the literature, Arch. Surg. 64 (1952) 549.

[164] I.A. Fields, M.J. Naiditch, P.E. Rothman, Acute appendicitis in infants, Am. J. Dis. Child. 93 (1957) 287.

[165] W. Dick, H.J. Hirt, W. Vogel, Die Appendizitis im Säglings- und Kleinkindesalter, Fortschr. Med. 94 (1976) 125.

[166] R.E. Gross, The Surgery of Infancy and Childhood: Its Principles and Techniques, WB Saunders, Philadelphia, 1953.

[167] J.L. Grosfeld, M. Weinberger, H.W. Clatworthy Jr., Acute appendicitis in the first two years of life, J. Pediatr. Surg. 8 (1973) 285.

[168] J.S. Janik, H.V. Firor, Pediatric appendicitis: a 20-year study of 1, 640 children at Cook County (Illinois) Hospital, Arch. Surg. 114 (1979) 717.

[169] C.D. Benson, J.J. Coury Jr., D.R. Hagge, Acute appendicitis in infants: fifteen-year study, Arch. Surg. 64 (1952) 561.

[170] M. Massad, et al., Neonatal appendicitis: case report and a review of the English literature, Z. Kinderchir. 41 (1986) 241.

[171] G.R. Schorlemmer, C.A. Herbst Jr., Perforated neonatal appendicitis, South. Med J 76 (1983) 536.

[172] F. Diess, Die Appendizitis im Basler Kinderspital. Basle Dissertations, 1908, Case No. 36, p 63. Cited in reference 138 and in Abt IA: Appendicitis in infants, Arch. Pediatr. 34 (1917) 641.

[173] R.H. Bartlett, A.J. Eraklis, R.H. Wilkinson, Appendicitis in infancy, Surg. Gynecol. Obstet. 130 (1970) 99.

[174] N.R.G. Broadbent, J.L. Jardine, Acute appendicitis in a premature infant: a case report, Aust. N. Z. J. Surg. 40 (1971) 362.

[175] L.R. Bryant, et al., Appendicitis and appendiceal perforation in neonates, Am. Surg. 36 (1970) 523.

[176] R.D.G. Creery, Acute appendicitis in the newborn, BMJ 1 (1953) 871.

[177] R.P. Hardman, D. Bowerman, Appendicitis in the newborn, Am. J. Dis. Child. 105 (1963) 99.

[178] F. Klimt, G. Hartmann, Appendicitis perforata mit tiefsitzenden Dündarmverschluss beim Neugeborenen, Paediatr. Prax. 1 (1962) 271.

[179] G. Kolb, E.L. Schaeffer, Über Appendizitis mit Perforation in den ersten Lebenwochen, Kinderarztl. Prax. 1 (1955) 1.

[180] R.E. Liechti, W.H. Snyder Jr., Acute appendicitis under age 2, Am. Surg. 29 (1963) 92.

[181] S.C. Meigher, A.W. Lucas, Appendicitis in the newborn: case report, Ann. Surg. 136 (1952) 1044.

[182] J.F. Meyer, Acute gangrenous appendicitis in a premature infant, J. Pediatr. 41 (1952) 343.

[183] R. Neve, N.F. Quenville, Appendicitis with perforation in a 12-day-old infant, Can. Med. Assoc. J. 94 (1966) 447.

[184] M.A. Nilforoushan, Fever and ascites in a newborn, Clin. Pediatr. 14 (1975) 878.

[185] M. Nuri, W.C. Hecker, W. Duckert, Beitrag zur Appendicitis im Neugeborenenalter, Z. Kinderheilkd. 91 (1964) 1.

[186] G.F. Parkhurst, S.C. Wagoner, Neonatal acute appendicitis, N. Y. State J. Med. 69 (1969) 1929.

[187] S.J. Phillips, B. Cohen, Acute perforated appendicitis in newborn children, N. Y. State J. Med. 71 (1971) 985.

[188] A.L. Smith, R.A. MacMahon, Perforated appendix complicating rhesus immunization in a newborn infant, Med. J. Aust. 2 (1969) 602.

[189] J. Tabrisky, R. Westerfeld, J. Cavanaugh, Appendicitis in the newborn, Am. J. Dis. Child. 111 (1966) 557.

[190] H. Vinz, U. Erben, H. Winkelvoss, Neugeborenen peritonitis, Bruns. Beitr. Klin. Chir. 215 (1967) 321.

[191] R.H. Walker, Appendicitis in the newborn infant, J. Pediatr. 51 (1958) 429.

[192] C.D. Morehead, P.W. Houck, Epidemiology of Pseudomonas infections in a pediatric intensive care unit, Am. J. Dis. Child. 124 (1972) 564.

[193] J.Q. Trojanowski, et al., Fatal postoperative acute appendicitis in a neonate with congenital heart disease, J. Pediatr. Surg. 16 (1981) 85.

[194] A. Ayalon, et al., Acute appendicitis in a premature baby, Acta Chir. Scand. 145 (1979) 285.

[195] W. Schellerer, K. Schwemmle, R. Decker, Perforierte Appendizitis bei einem Frühgeborenen im Alter von 14 Tagen, Z. Kinderchir. 9 (1971) 434.

[196] E.S. Golladay, et al., Intestinal obstruction from appendiceal abscess in a newborn infant, J. Pediatr. Surg. 13 (1978) 175.

[197] V. Hemalatha, L. Spitz, Neonatal appendicitis, Clin. Pediatr. 18 (1979) 621.

[198] P. Tucci, et al., Congenital uretero-pelvic junction obstruction associated with unsuspected acute perforated appendicitis in a neonate, J. Urol. 120 (1978) 247.

[199] G.L. Fowkes, Neonatal appendicitis, BMJ 1 (1978) 997.

[200] M.S. Kwong, M. Dinner, Neonatal appendicitis masquerading as necrotizing enterocolitis, J. Pediatr. 96 (1980) 917.

[201] W.L. Shaul, Clues to the early diagnosis of neonatal appendicitis, J. Pediatr. 98 (1981) 473.

[202] R. Grussner, et al., Appendicitis in childhood, Monatsschr. Kinderheilkd. 133 (1985) 158.

[203] H.A. Lassiter, M.H. Werner, Neonatal appendicitis, South. Med. J. 76 (1983) 1173.

[204] M.J. Carol, et al., Apendicitis neonatal: aportacion de un nuevo caso, An. Esp. Pediatr. 20 (1984) 80.

[205] N.M.A. Bax, et al., Perforation of the appendix in the neonatal period, J. Pediatr. Surg. 15 (1980) 200.

[206] W.L. Buntain, Neonatal appendicitis mistaken for necrotizing enterocolitis, South. Med. J. 75 (1982) 1155.

[207] J.J. Heydenrych, D.F. DuToit, Unusual presentations of acute appendicitis in the neonate: a report of 2 cases, S. Afr. Med. J. 62 (1982) 1003.

[208] Radiological case of the month: neonatal appendicitis with perforation, Am. J. Dis. Child. 145 (1991) 111.

[209] O.P. Pathania, et al., Fatal neonatal perforation of appendix, Indian Pediatr. J. 26 (1989) 1166.

[210] N.K. Arora, et al., Neonatal appendicitis: a rare cause of surgical emergency in preterm babies, Indian Pediatr. J. 28 (1991) 1330.

[211] M.N. Srouji, J. Chatten, C. David, Pseudodiverticulitis of the appendix with neonatal Hirschsprung disease, J. Pediatr. 93 (1978) 988.

[212] J. Arliss, L.O. Holgersen, Neonatal appendiceal perforation and Hirschsprung's disease, J. Pediatr. Surg. 25 (1990) 694.

[213] R.M. Kliegman, A.A. Fanaroff, Necrotizing enterocolitis, N. Engl. J. Med. 310 (1984) 1093.

[214] M.N. Srouji, B.E. Buck, Neonatal appendicitis: ischemic infarction in incarcerated inguinal hernia, J. Pediatr. Surg. 13 (1978) 177.

[215] P. Charif, Perforated appendicitis in premature infants: a case report and review of the literature, Johns Hopkins Med. J. 125 (1969) 92.

[216] H.H. Stone, S.L. Sanders, J.D. Martin Jr., Perforated appendicitis in children, Surgery 69 (1971) 673.

[217] J.E. Dennis, et al., Nosocomial Rhizopus infection (zygomycosis) in children, J. Pediatr. 96 (1980) 824.

[218] K. Buschard, A. Kjaeldgaard, Investigation and analysis of the position, fixation, length, embryology of the vermiform appendix, Acta Chir. Scand. 139 (1973) 293.

[219] W.R. Jones, M.D. Kaye, R.M.Y. Ing, The lymphoid development of the fetal and neonatal appendix, Biol. Neonate 20 (1972) 334.

[220] G.M. Smith, Inflammatory changes in the appendix during early infancy, Am. J. Dis. Child. 1 (1911) 299.

[221] W.B. Hill, C.C. Mason, Prenatal appendicitis with rupture and death, Am. J. Dis. Child. 29 (1925) 86.

[222] W.J. Corcoran, Prenatal rupture of the appendix, Am. J. Dis. Child. 39 (1930) 277.

[223] W.F. Jackson, A case of prenatal appendicitis, Am. J. Med. Sci. 127 (1904) 710.

[224] E.W. Kümmell, Cited in Etherington-Wilson WE. Appendicitis in newborn: report of a case 16 days old, Proc. R. Soc. Med. 38 (1945) 186.

[225] L.W. Martin, P.M. Glen, Prenatal appendiceal perforation: a case report, J. Pediatr. Surg. 21 (1986) 73.

[226] R.H. Wilkinson, R.H. Bartlett, A.J. Eraklis, Diagnosis of appendicitis in infancy: the value of abdominal radiographs, Am. J. Dis. Child. 118 (1969) 687.

[227] T.M. Holder, L.L. Leape, The acute surgical abdomen in the neonate, N. Engl. J. Med. 278 (1968) 605.

[228] J.H.T. Chang, The use of antibiotics in pediatric abdominal surgery, Pediatr. Infect. Dis. 3 (1984) 195.

[229] M.J. Bell, Peritonitis in the newborn—current concepts, Pediatr. Clin. North Am. 32 (1985) 1181.

[230] A.J. Barson, A postmortem study of infection in the newborn from 1976 to 1988, in: J. deLouvois, D. Harvey (Eds.), Infection of the Newborn, John Wiley & Sons, New York, 1990, pp. 13–34.

[231] E.W. Fonkalsrud, D.G. Ellis, H.W. Clatworthy Jr., Neonatal peritonitis, J. Pediatr. Surg. 1 (1966) 227.

[232] J.R. Lloyd, The etiology of gastrointestinal perforations in the newborn, J. Pediatr. Surg. 4 (1969) 77.

[233] W.S. McDougal, R.J. Izant, R.M. Zollinger Jr., Primary peritonitis in infancy and childhood, Ann. Surg. 181 (1975) 310.

[234] P.P. Rickham, Peritonitis in the neonatal period, Arch. Dis. Child. 30 (1955) 23.

[235] J. Denes, J. Leb, Neonatal peritonitis, Acta Paediatr. Acad. Sci. Hung. 10 (1969) 297.

[236] R. Daum, U. Schütze, H. Hoffman, Mortality of preoperative peritonitis in newborn infants without intestinal obstruction, Prog. Pediatr. Surg. 13 (1979) 267.

[237] U. Schütze, K.H. Fey, G. Hess, Die Peritonitis im Neugeborenen-, Säglings-, und Kindesalter, Munch. Med. Wochenschr. 116 (1974) 1201.

[238] J. Prevot, G. Grosdidier, M. Schmitt, Fatal peritonitis, Prog. Pediatr. Surg. 13 (1979) 257.

[239] B. Singer, B. Hammar, Neonatal peritonitis, S. Afr. Med. J. 46 (1972) 987.

[240] O.J. Hensey, C.A. Hart, R.W.I. Cooke, Serious infection in a neonatal intensive care unit: a two-year survey, J. Hyg. (Camb) 95 (1985) 289.

[241] M.A. Valdes-Dapeña, J.B. Arey, The causes of neonatal mortality: an analysis of 501 autopsies on newborn infants, J. Pediatr. 77 (1970) 366.

[242] M.B. Duggan, M.S. Khwaja, Neonatal primary peritonitis in Nigeria, Arch. Dis. Child. 50 (1975) 130.

[243] M.J. Bell, Perforation of the gastrointestinal tract and peritonitis in the neonate, Surg. Gynecol. Obstet. 160 (1985) 20.

[244] A.G. Birtch, A.G. Coran, R.E. Gross, Neonatal peritonitis, Surgery 61 (1967) 305.

[245] M. Lacheretz, et al., Péritonite néo-natale par pérforation gastrique: à propos de 21 observations, Chirurgie 109 (1983) 887.

[246] D.L. Mollitt, J.J. Tepas, J.L. Talbert, The microbiology of neonatal peritonitis, Arch. Surg. 123 (1988) 176.

[247] J.E.S. Scott, Intestinal obstruction in the newborn associated with peritonitis, Arch. Dis. Child. 38 (1963) 120.

[248] H.E. Thelander, Perforation of the gastrointestinal tract of the newborn infant, Am. J. Dis. Child. 58 (1939) 371.

[249] G. Dinari, H. Haimov, M. Geiffman, Umbilical arteritis and phlebitis with scrotal abscess and peritonitis, J. Pediatr. Surg. 6 (1971) 176.

[250] I. Forshall, Septic umbilical arteritis, Arch. Dis. Child. 32 (1957) 25.

[251] E.G. Chadwick, S.T. Shulman, R. Yogev, Peritonitis as a late manifestation of group B streptococcal disease in newborns, Pediatr. Infect. Dis. 2 (1983) 142.

[252] T.M. Reyna, Primary group B streptococcal peritonitis presenting as an incarcerated inguinal hernia in a neonate, Clin. Pediatr. 25 (1987) 422.

[253] W. Serlo, E. Heikkinen, K. Kouvalainen, Group A streptococcal peritonitis in infancy, Ann. Chir. Gynaecol. 74 (1985) 183.

[254] D.E. Johnson, et al., *Candida* peritonitis in a newborn infant, J. Pediatr. 97 (1980) 298.

[255] M. Kaplan, et al., Necrotizing bowel disease with *Candida* peritonitis following severe neonatal hypothermia, Acta Paediatr. Scand. 79 (1990) 876.

[256] K.M. Butler, M.A. Bench, C.J. Baker, Amphotericin B as a single agent in the treatment of systemic candidiasis in neonates, Pediatr. Infect. Dis. J. 9 (1990) 51.

[257] L. MacDonald, C.J. Baker, C. Chenoweth, Risk factors for candidemia in a children's hospital, Clin. Infect. Dis. 26 (1998) 642.

[258] I.A. Abt, Fetal peritonitis, Med. Clin. North Am. 15 (1931) 611.

[259] E.Y. Pan, et al., Radiographic diagnosis of meconium peritonitis: a report of 200 cases including six fetal cases, Pediatr. Radiol. 13 (1983) 199.

[260] L.O. Holgersen, The etiology of spontaneous gastric perforation of the newborn: a reevaluation, J. Pediatr. Surg. 16 (1981) 608.

[261] P.P. Rickham, Neugeborenen-peritonitis, Langenbecks Arch. Klin. Chir. 292 (1959) 427.

[262] R. Fowler, Primary peritonitis: changing aspects 1956–1970, Aust. Paediatr. J. 7 (1971) 73.

[263] C.L. Wells, M.A. Maddaus, R.L. Simmons, Proposed mechanisms for the translocation of intestinal bacteria, Rev. Infect. Dis. 10 (1988) 958.

[264] R. Wilson, et al., Short communication: age at onset of necrotizing enterocolitis: an epidemiologic analysis, Pediatr. Res. 16 (1982) 82.

[265] J.M. Caralaps-Riera, B.D. Cohn, Bowel perforation after exchange transfusion in the neonate: review of the literature and report of a case, Surgery 68 (1970) 895.

[266] R.J. Touloukian, A. Kadar, R.P. Spencer, The gastrointestinal complications of neonatal umbilical venous exchange transfusion: a clinical and experimental study, Pediatrics 51 (1973) 36.

[267] R.M. Freedman, et al., A half century of neonatal sepsis at Yale: 1928 to 1978, Am. J. Dis. Child. 135 (1981) 140.

[268] N.T. Griscom, et al., Diagnostic aspects of neonatal ascites: report of 27 cases, AJR Am. J. Roentgenol. 128 (1977) 961.

[269] A.M. Kosloske, J.R. Lilly, Paracentesis and lavage for diagnosis of intestinal gangrene in neonatal necrotizing enterocolitis, J. Pediatr. Surg. 13 (1978) 315.

[270] U. Töllner, F. Pohlandt, Aszitespunktion zur Differentialdiagnose beim akuten Abdomen des Neugeborenen, Klin. Paediatr. 196 (1984) 319.

[271] J.B.J. McKendry, W.K. Lindsay, M.C. Gerstein, Congenital defects of the lymphatics in infancy, Pediatrics 19 (1959) 21.

[272] W. Lees, J.E. Mitchell, Bile peritonitis in infancy, Arch. Dis. Child. 41 (1966) 188.

[273] M.D. Cohen, T.R. Weber, J.L. Grosfeld, Bowel perforation in the newborn: diagnosis with metrizamide, Radiology 150 (1984) 65.

[274] D.L. Rosenfeld, C.E. Cordell, N. Jadeja, Retrocardiac pneumomediastinum: radiographic finding and clinical implications, Pediatrics 85 (1989) 92.

[275] E.D. Wind, G.P. Pillari, W.J. Lee, Lucent liver in the newborn: a roentgenographic sign of pneumoperitoneum, JAMA 237 (1977) 2218.

[276] R. Pochaczevsky, D. Bryk, New roentgenographic signs of neonatal gastric perforation, Radiology 102 (1972) 145.

[277] S.S. Gellis, M. Finegold, Picture of the month: pneumoperitoneum demonstrated by transillumination, Am. J. Dis. Child. 130 (1976) 1237.

[278] S. Thomas, C. Sainsbury, J.F. Murphy, Pancuronium belly, Lancet 2 (1984) 870.

[279] S.H. Ein, C.A. Stephens, B.J. Reilly, The disappearance of free air after pediatric laparotomy, J. Pediatr. Surg. 20 (1985) 422.

[280] B. Emanuel, P. Zlotnik, J.G. Raffensperger, Perforation of the gastrointestinal tract in infancy and childhood, Surg. Gynecol. Obstet. 146 (1978) 926.

[281] K. Opitz, Beitrag zur Klinik und Pathologie der Nabelschnurinfektionen, Arch. Kinderheilkd. 150 (1955) 174.

[282] V.Y.H. Yu, D.I. Tudehope, G.J. Gill, Neonatal necrotizing enterocolitis. 1. Clinical aspects. 2. Perinatal risk factors, Med. J. Aust. 1 (1977) 685 688.

[283] R.C. Holman, J.K. Stehr-Green, M.T. Zelasky, Necrotizing enterocolitis mortality in the United States, 1979–85, Am. J. Public Health 79 (1989) 987.

[284] N.N. Finer, R.R. Moriartey, Reply, letter to the editor, J. Pediatr. 96 (1980) 170.

[285] L.S. Book, et al., Necrotizing enterocolitis in low-birth-weight infants fed an elemental formula, J. Pediatr. 87 (1975) 602.

[286] J.A. O'Neill Jr., M.T. Stahlman, H.C. Meng, Necrotizing enterocolitis in the newborn: operative indications, Ann. Surg. 182 (1975) 274.

[287] T.D. Moore (Ed.), Necrotizing Enterocolitis in the Newborn Infant: Report of the Sixty-Eighth Ross Conference on Pediatric Research, Ross Laboratories, Columbus, OH, 1975.

[288] N.L. Virnig, J.W. Reynolds, Epidemiological aspects of neonatal necrotizing enterocolitis, Am. J. Dis. Child. 128 (1974) 186.

[289] R.J. Touloukian, Neonatal necrotizing enterocolitis: an update on etiology, diagnosis, and treatment, Surg. Clin. North Am. 56 (1976) 281.

[290] M.J. Bell, J.L. Ternberg, R.J. Bower, The microbial flora and antimicrobial therapy of neonatal peritonitis, J. Pediatr. Surg. 15 (1980) 569.

[291] R.M. Kliegman, A.A. Fanaroff, Neonatal necrotizing enterocolitis: a nine-year experience. I. Epidemiology and uncommon observations, Am. J. Dis. Child. 135 (1981) 603.

[292] H.I. Goldman, Feeding and necrotizing enterocolitis, Am. J. Dis. Child. 134 (1980) 553.

[293] E.G. Brown, A.Y. Sweet, Preventing necrotizing enterocolitis in neonates, JAMA 240 (1978) 2452.

[294] L.S. Book, J.J. Herbst, A. Jung, Comparison of fast- and slow-feeding rate schedules to the development of necrotizing enterocolitis, J. Pediatr. 89 (1976) 463.

[295] M.J. Bell, et al., Epidemiologic and bacteriologic evaluation of neonatal necrotizing enterocolitis, J. Pediatr. Surg. 14 (1979) 1.

[296] A.I. Eidelman, R.J. Inwood, Marginal comments: necrotizing enterocolitis and enteral feeding. Is too much just too much, Am. J. Dis. Child. 134 (1980) 545.

[297] R.M. Kliegman, et al., Clostridia as pathogens in neonatal necrotizing enterocolitis, J. Pediatr. 95 (1979) 287.

[298] E.G. Brown, A.Y. Sweet, Neonatal necrotizing enterocolitis, Pediatr. Clin. North Am. 29 (1982) 1149.

[299] W.P. Kanto Jr., et al., Perinatal events and necrotizing enterocolitis in premature infants, Am. J. Dis. Child. 141 (1987) 167.

[300] S.G. Ostertag, et al., Early enteral feeding does not affect the incidence of necrotizing enterocolitis, Pediatrics 77 (1986) 275.

[301] C.R.B. Merritt, J.P. Goldsmith, M.J. Sharp, Sonographic detection of portal venous gas in infants with necrotizing enterocolitis, AJR Am. J. Roentgenol. 143 (1984) 1059.

[302] D. Cikrit, et al., Significance of portal venous air in necrotizing enterocolitis: analysis of 53 cases, J. Pediatr. Surg. 20 (1985) 425.

[303] G.C. Maguire, et al., Infections acquired by young infants, Am. J. Dis. Child. 135 (1981) 693.

[304] V.Y.H. Yu, et al., Perinatal risk factors for necrotizing enterocolitis, Arch. Dis. Child. 59 (1984) 430.

[305] R.D. Uauy, et al., National Institute of Child Health and Human Development Neonatal Research Network. Necrotizing enterocolitis in very low birth weight infants: biodemographic and clinical correlates, J. Pediatr. 119 (1991) 630.

[306] M.C. Walsh, R.M. Kliegman, Necrotizing enterocolitis: treatment based on staging criteria, Pediatr. Clin. North Am. 33 (1986) 179.

[307] M.D. Kamitsuka, M.K. Horton, M.A. Williams, The incidence of necrotizing enterocolitis after introducing standardized feeding schedules for infants between 1250 and 2500 grams and less than 35 weeks of gestation, Pediatrics 105 (2000) 379.

[308] S.F. Rayyis, et al., Randomized trial of slow versus fast feed advancements on the incidence of necrotizing enterocolitis in very low birth weight infants, J. Pediatr. 134 (1999) 293.

[309] T.V. Santulli, et al., Acute necrotizing enterocolitis in infancy: a review of 64 cases, Pediatrics 55 (1975) 376.

[310] R.M. Kliegman, et al., Epidemiologic study of necrotizing enterocolitis among low-birth-weight infants: absence of identifiable risk factors, J. Pediatr. 100 (1982) 440.

[311] B.J. Stoll, et al., Epidemiology of necrotizing enterocolitis: a case control study, J. Pediatr. 96 (1980) 447.

[312] I.D. Frantz III., et al., Necrotizing enterocolitis, J. Pediatr. 86 (1975) 259.

[313] E.A. Egan, et al., A prospective controlled trial of oral kanamycin in the prevention of neonatal necrotizing enterocolitis, J. Pediatr. 89 (1976) 467.

[314] R. Wilson, et al., Age at onset of necrotizing enterocolitis: an epidemiologic analysis, Pediatr. Res. 16 (1982) 82.

[315] P. Gerard, et al., Mortality in 504 infants weighing less than 1501 g at birth and treated in four neonatal intensive care units of South-Belgium between 1976 and 1980, Eur. J. Pediatr. 144 (1985) 219.

[316] V.Y.H. Yu, et al., Necrotizing enterocolitis in very low birthweight infants: a four-year experience, Aust. Paediatr. J. 20 (1984) 29.

[317] S.R. Palmer, A. Biffin, H.R. Gamsu, Outcome of neonatal necrotising enterocolitis: results of the BAPM/CDSC surveillance study, 1989–84, Arch. Dis. Child. 64 (1989) 388.

[318] E. de Gamarra, et al., Necrotizing enterocolitis in full-term neonates, Biol. Neonate 44 (1983) 185.

[319] E.H. Thilo, R.A. Lazarte, J.A. Hernandez, Necrotizing enterocolitis in the first 24 hours of life, Pediatrics 73 (1984) 476.

[320] R. Wilson, et al., Risk factors for necrotizing enterocolitis in infants weighing more than 2, grams at birth: a case-control study, Pediatrics 71 (1983) 19.

[321] Necrotizing enterocolitis, Editorial, Lancet 1 (1977) 459.

[322] J.A. Bisquera, T.R. Cooper, C.L. Berseth, Impact of necrotizing enterocolitis on length of stay and hospital charges in very low birth weight infants, Pediatrics 109 (2002) 423.

[323] S.R. Hintz, et al., Neurodevelopmental and growth outcomes of extremely low birth weight infants after necrotizing enterocolitis, Pediatrics 115 (2005) 696.

[324] A.A. Fanaroff, M. Hack, M.C. Walsh, The NICHD Neonatal Research Network: changes in practice and outcomes during the first 15 years, Semin. Perinatol. 27 (2003) 281.

[325] R. Holman, et al., Necrotizing enterocolitis hospitalizations among neonates in the United States, Pediatr. Perinatol. Epidemiol. 20 (2006) 498.

[326] P.W. Lin, B.J. Stoll, Necrotising enterocolitis, Lancet 127 (2006) 1271.

[327] E.E. Frey, et al., Analysis of bowel perforation in necrotizing enterocolitis, Pediatr. Radiol. 17 (1987) 380.

[328] R.M. Kliegman, W.B. Pittard, A.A. Fanaroff, Necrotizing enterocolitis in neonates fed human milk, J. Pediatr. 95 (1979) 450.

[329] M. Guinan, et al., Epidemic occurrence of neonatal necrotizing enterocolitis, Am. J. Dis. Child. 133 (1979) 594.

[330] B. Dvorak, et al., Maternal milk reduces the severity of necrotizing enterocolitis and increases intestinal IL-10 in a neonatal rat model, Pediatr Res 55 (2003) 426.

[331] H.C. Lin, et al., Oral probiotics reduce the incidence and severity of necrotizing enterocolitis in very low birthweight infants, Pediatrics 115 (2005) 1–4.

[332] A.M. Kosloske, Pathogenesis and prevention of necrotizing enterocolitis: a hypothesis based on personal observation and a review of the literature, Pediatrics 74 (1984) 1086.

[333] R.P. Gaynes, et al., The role of host factors in an outbreak of necrotizing enterocolitis, Am. J. Dis. Child. 138 (1984) 1118.

[334] V.K.M. Han, et al., An outbreak of *Clostridium difficile* necrotizing enterocolitis: a case for oral vancomycin therapy? Pediatrics 71 (1983) 935.

[335] Neonatal necrotizing enterocolitis: current concepts and controversies, J. Pediatr. 17 (Suppl) (1990) S1.

[335a] G. Deshpande, et al., Updated meta-analysis of probiotics for preventing necrotizing enterocolitis in preterm neonates, Pediatrics 125 (2010) 921.

[336] J.Z. Jona, Advances in neonatal surgery, Pediatr. Clin. North Am. 45 (1998) 605.

[337] M.E. Milner, et al., Risk factors for developing and dying from necrotizing enterocolitis, J. Pediatr. Gastroenterol. Nutr. 5 (1986) 359.

[338] T.E. Wiswell, C.T. Hankins, Twins and triplets with necrotizing enterocolitis, Am. J. Dis. Child. 142 (1988) 1004.

[339] M. DeCurtis, et al., A case control study of necrotizing enterocolitis occurring over 8 years in a neonatal intensive care unit, Eur. J. Pediatr. 146 (1987) 398.

[340] R.M. Kliegman, Neonatal necrotizing enterocolitis: implications for an infectious disease, Pediatr. Clin. North Am. 26 (1979) 327.

[341] L.S. Book, et al., Clustering of necrotizing enterocolitis: interruption by infection-control measures, N. Engl. J. Med. 297 (1977) 984.

[341a] M.J. Morowitz, et al., Redefining the role of intestinal microbes in the pathogenesis of necrotizing enterocolitis, Pediatrics 125 (2010) 777.

[342] H.A. Rotbart, M.J. Levin, How contagious is necrotizing enterocolitis? Pediatr. Infect. Dis. 2 (1983) 406.

[343] S.A. Roback, et al., Necrotizing enterocolitis, Arch. Surg. 109 (1974) 314.

[344] M.D. Stanley, D.M. Null Jr., R.A. deLemos, Relationship between intestinal colonization with specific bacteria and the development of necrotizing enterocolitis, Pediatr. Res. 11 (1977) 543.

[345] H.R. Hill, C.E. Hunt, J.M. Matsen, Nosocomial colonization with *Klebsiella*, type 26, in a neonatal intensive-care unit associated with an outbreak of sepsis, meningitis, and necrotizing enterocolitis, J. Pediatr. 85 (1974) 415.

[346] J. Powell, et al., Necrotizing enterocolitis: epidemic following an outbreak of *Enterobacter cloacae* type 3305573 in a neonatal intensive care unit, Am. J. Dis. Child. 134 (1980) 1152.

[347] M.E. Speer, et al., Fulminant neonatal sepsis and necrotizing enterocolitis associated with a "nonenteropathogenic" strain of *Escherichia coli*, J. Pediatr. 89 (1976) 91.

[348] A.H. Cushing, Necrotizing enterocolitis with *Escherichia coli* heat-labile enterotoxin, Pediatrics 71 (1983) 626.

[349] A. Henderson, J. Maclaurin, J.M. Scott, *Pseudomonas* in a Glasgow baby unit, Lancet 2 (1969) 316.

[350] J.A. Waldhausen, T. Herendeen, H. King, Necrotizing colitis of the newborn: common cause of perforation of the colon, Surgery 54 (1963) 365.

[351] H. Stein, et al., Gastroenteritis with necrotizing enterocolitis in premature babies, BMJ 2 (1972) 616.

[352] J.A. Gruskay, et al., *Staphylococcus epidermidis*-associated enterocolitis, J. Pediatr. 109 (1986) 520.

[353] G.D. Overturf, et al., Neonatal necrotizing enterocolitis associated with delta toxin producing methicillin-resistant *S. aureus*, Pediatr. Infect. Dis. J. 9 (1990) 88.

[354] H.A. Rotbart, et al., Neonatal rotavirus-associated necrotizing enterocolitis: case control study and prospective surveillance during an outbreak, J. Pediatr. 112 (1988) 87.

[355] H.A. Rotbart, et al., Confirmatory testing of Rotazyme results in neonates, J. Pediatr. 107 (1985) 289.

[356] S. Rousset, et al., Intestinal lesions containing coronavirus-like particles in neonatal necrotizing enterocolitis: an ultrastructural analysis, Pediatrics 73 (1984) 218.

[357] F.E. Johnson, et al., Association of fatal coxsackie B2 viral infection and necrotizing enterocolitis, Arch. Dis. Child. 52 (1977) 802.

[358] *Clostridium septicum* and neutropenic enterocolitis. Editorial, Lancet 2 (1987) 608.

[359] S.M. Finegold, Anaerobic Bacteria in Human Diseases, Academic Press, New York, 1977.

[360] G. Lawrence, P.D. Walker, Pathogenesis of enteritis necroticans in Papua New Guinea, Lancet 1 (1976) 125.

[361] R.M. Kliegman, The role of clostridia in the pathogenesis of neonatal necrotizing enterocolitis, in: S.P. Borriello (Ed.), Clostridia in Gastrointestinal Disease, CRC Press, Boca Raton, FL, 1985, pp. 68–92.

[362] P. Volsted-Pedersen, et al., Necrotising enterocolitis of the newborn—is it gas gangrene of the bowels? Lancet 2 (1976) 715.

[363] A.M. Kosloske, J.A. Ulrich, H. Hoffman, Fulminant necrotising enterocolitis associated with clostridia, Lancet 2 (1978) 1014.

[364] S. Warren, J.R. Schreiber, M.F. Epstein, Necrotizing enterocolitis and hemolysis associated with *Clostridium perfringens*, Am. J. Dis. Child. 138 (1984) 686.

[365] J.L. Blakey, et al., Enteric colonization in sporadic neonatal necrotizing enterocolitis, J. Pediatr. Gastroenterol. Nutr. 4 (1985) 591.

[366] W.J. Cashore, et al., Clostridia colonization and clostridial toxin in neonatal necrotizing enterocolitis, J. Pediatr. 98 (1981) 308.

[367] R. Sturm, et al., Neonatal necrotizing enterocolitis associated with penicillin-resistant, toxigenic *Clostridium butyricum*, Pediatrics 66 (1980) 928.

[368] F.M. Howard, et al., Outbreak of necrotising enterocolitis caused by *Clostridium butyricum*, Lancet 2 (1977) 1099.

[369] A.J. Zedd, et al., Nosocomial *Clostridium difficile* reservoir in a neonatal intensive care unit, Pediatr. Infect. Dis. 3 (1984) 429.

[370] I.J. Al-Jumaili, et al., Incidence and origin of *Clostridium difficile* in neonates, J. Clin. Microbiol. 19 (1984) 77.

[371] M.F. Smith, et al., Clinical and bacteriological findings in necrotizing enterocolitis: a controlled study, J. Infect. 2 (1980) 23.

[372] L. Gothefors, I. Blenkharn, *Clostridium butyricum* and necrotising enterocolitis, Lancet 1 (1978) 52.

[373] M. Laverdière, et al., Clostridia in necrotising enterocolitis, Lancet 2 (1978) 377.

[374] M.C. Kelsey, A.J. Vince, Clostridia in neonatal feces, Lancet 2 (1979) 100.

[375] A.D. Kindley, P.J. Roberts, W.H. Tulloch, Neonatal necrotising enterocolitis, Lancet 1 (1977) 649.

[376] A.H. Lishman, et al., *Clostridium difficile* isolation in neonates in a special care unit: lack of correlation with necrotizing enterocolitis, Scand. J. Gastroenterol. 19 (1984) 441.

[377] C.M. Westra-Meijer, et al., Quantitative study of the aerobic and anaerobic faecal flora in neonatal necrotizing enterocolitis, Arch. Dis. Child. 58 (1983) 523.

[378] D.F.M. Thomas, et al., Clostridial toxins in neonatal necrotizing enterocolitis, Arch. Dis. Child. 59 (1984) 270.

[379] D.W. Scheifele, G.L. Bjornson, Delta toxin activity in coagulase-negative staphylococci from the bowel of neonates, J. Clin. Microbiol. 26 (1988) 279.

[380] D.W. Scheifele, Delta-like toxin produced by coagulase-negative staphylococci is associated with neonatal necrotizing enterocolitis, Infect. Immun. 55 (1988) 2268.

[381] C. Hoy, et al., Quantitative changes in faecal microflora preceding necrotizing enterocolitis in premature neonates, Arch. Dis. Child. 65 (1990) 1057.

[382] E.H. Dykes, W.H. Gilmour, A.F. Azmy, Prediction of outcome following necrotizing enterocolitis in a neonatal surgical unit, J. Pediatr. Surg. 20 (1985) 3.

[383] E.R. Wayne, J.D. Burrington, J. Hutter, Neonatal necrotizing enterocolitis: evolution of new principles in management, Arch. Surg. 110 (1975) 476.

[384] R. Wilson, et al., Age at onset of necrotizing enterocolitis, Am. J. Dis. Child. 136 (1982) 814.

[385] J.A. Richmond, V. Mikity, Benign form of necrotizing enterocolitis, AJR Am. J. Roentgenol. 123 (1975) 301.

[386] J.A. Barnard, R.B. Cotton, W. Lutin, Necrotizing enterocolitis: variables associated with the severity of the disease, Am. J. Dis. Child. 139 (1985) 375.

[387] M.J. Bell, et al., Neonatal necrotizing enterocolitis: therapeutic decisions based upon clinical staging, Ann. Surg. 187 (1978) 1.

[388] R. Buras, et al., Acidosis and hepatic portal venous gas: indications for surgery in necrotizing enterocolitis, Pediatrics 78 (1986) 273.

[389] A. Daneman, S. Woodward, M. de Silva, The radiology of neonatal necrotizing enterocolitis (NEC): a review of 47 cases and the literature, Pediatr. Radiol. 7 (1978) 70.

[390] A.G. Mata, R.M. Rosengart, Interobserver variability in the radiographic diagnosis of necrotizing enterocolitis, Pediatrics 66 (1980) 68.

[391] J.F. Johnson, L.H. Robinson, Localized bowel distension in the newborn: a review of the plain film analysis and differential diagnosis, Pediatrics 73 (1984) 206.

[392] T. Leonard Jr., J.F. Johnson, P.G. Pettett, Critical evaluation of the persistent loop sign in necrotizing enterocolitis, Radiology 142 (1982) 385.

[393] M.M. Weinstein, The persistent loop sign in neonatal necrotizing enterocolitis: a new cause, Pediatr. Radiol. 16 (1986) 61.

[394] R.M. Kliegman, A.A. Fanaroff, Neonatal necrotizing enterocolitis: a nine-year experience. II. Outcome assessment, Am. J. Dis. Child. 135 (1981) 608.

[395] M.S. Keller, H.S. Chawla, Neonatal metrizamide gastrointestinal series in suspected necrotizing enterocolitis, Am. J. Dis. Child. 139 (1985) 713.

[396] S. Lindley, et al., Portal vein ultrasonography in the early diagnosis of necrotizing enterocolitis, J. Pediatr. Surg. 21 (1986) 530.

[397] S.W. Malin, et al., Echogenic intravascular and hepatic microbubbles associated with necrotizing enterocolitis, J. Pediatr. 103 (1983) 637.

[398] R.R. Ricketts, The role of paracentesis in the management of infants with necrotizing enterocolitis, Am. Surg. 52 (1986) 61.

[399] A.M. Kosloske, Surgery of necrotizing enterocolitis, World J. Surg. 9 (1985) 277.

[400] C.C. Patel, Hematologic abnormalities in acute necrotizing enterocolitis, Pediatr. Clin. North Am. 24 (1977) 579.

[401] J.J. Hutter Jr., W.E. Hathaway, E.R. Wayne, Hematologic abnormalities in severe neonatal necrotizing enterocolitis, J. Pediatr. 88 (1976) 1026.

[402] P.E. Hyman, C.E. Abrams, R.D. Zipser, Enhanced urinary immunoreactive thromboxane in neonatal necrotizing enterocolitis: a diagnostic indicator of thrombotic activity, Am. J. Dis. Child. 141 (1987) 688.

[403] D.W. Scheifele, E.M. Olson, M.R. Pendray, Endotoxinemia and thrombocytopenia during neonatal necrotizing enterocolitis, Am. J. Clin. Pathol. 83 (1985) 227.

[404] S.S. Rabinowitz, et al., Platelet-activating factor in infants at risk for necrotizing enterocolitis, J. Pediatr. 138 (2001) 81.

[405] R.D. Christensen, et al., Granulocyte transfusion in neonates with bacterial infection, neutropenia, and depletion of mature marrow neutrophils, Pediatrics 70 (1982) 1.

[406] J. Garcia, F.R. Smith, S.A. Cucinell, Urinary d-lactate excretion in infants with necrotizing enterocolitis, J. Pediatr. 104 (1984) 268.

[407] L.S. Book, J.J. Herbst, A. Jung, Carbohydrate malabsorption in necrotizing enterocolitis, Pediatrics 57 (1976) 201.

[408] S. Scott, et al., Effect of necrotizing enterocolitis on urinary epidermal growth factor levels, Am. J. Dis. Child. 145 (1991) 804.

[409] R.M. Kliegman, M.C. Walsh, The incidence of meningitis in neonates with necrotizing enterocolitis, Am. J. Perinatol. 4 (1987) 245.

[410] D.W. Scheifele, et al., Comparison of two antibiotic regimens in neonates with necrotizing enterocolitis, Clin. Invest. Med. 8 (1985) A183.

[411] M.J. Bell, et al., Neonatal necrotizing enterocolitis: prevention of perforation, J. Pediatr. Surg. 8 (1973) 601.

[412] T.N. Hansen, et al., A randomized controlled study of oral gentamicin in the treatment of neonatal necrotizing enterocolitis, J. Pediatr. 97 (1980) 836.

[413] R.B. Faix, T.Z. Polley, T.H. Grasela, A randomized, controlled trial of parenteral clindamycin in neonatal necrotizing enterocolitis, J. Pediatr. 112 (1988) 271.

[414] J.D. Burrington, Necrotizing enterocolitis in the newborn infant, Clin. Perinatol. 5 (1978) 29.

[415] M.J. Ghory, C.A. Sheldon, Newborn surgical emergencies of the gastrointestinal tract, Surg. Clin. North Am. 65 (1985) 1083.

[416] S.H. Ein, et al., A 13-year experience with peritoneal drainage under local anesthesia for necrotizing enterocolitis perforation, J. Pediatr. Surg. 25 (1990) 1034.

[417] L.J. Grylack, J.W. Scanlon, Oral gentamicin therapy in the prevention of neonatal necrotizing enterocolitis: a controlled double-blind trial, Am. J. Dis. Child. 132 (1978) 1192.

[418] E.A. Egan, et al., Additional experience with routine use of oral kanamycin prophylaxis for necrotizing enterocolitis in infants under 1500 grams, J. Pediatr. 90 (1977) 331.

[419] V.E. Brantley, I.M. Hiatt, T. Hegyi, The effectiveness of oral gentamicin in reducing the incidence of necrotizing enterocolitis (NEC) in treated and control infants, Pediatr. Res. 14 (1980) 592.

[420] M.P. Rowley, G.W. Dahlenburg, Gentamicin in prophylaxis of neonatal necrotizing enterocolitis, Lancet 2 (1978) 532.

[421] R. Boyle, et al., Alterations in stool flora resulting from oral kanamycin prophylaxis of necrotizing enterocolitis, J. Pediatr. 93 (1978) 857.

[422] P.R.F. Dear, D.E.M. Thomas, Oral vancomycin in preventing necrotizing enterocolitis, Arch. Dis. Child. 63 (1988) 1390.

[423] M.M. Conroy, R. Anderson, K.L. Cates, Complications associated with prophylactic oral kanamycin in preterm infants, Lancet 1 (1978) 613.

[424] A.M. Bhat, R.G. Meny, Alimentary absorption of gentamicin in preterm infants, Clin. Pediatr. 23 (1984) 683.

[425] L.J. Grylack, J. Boehnert, J.W. Scanlan, Serum concentration of gentamicin following oral administration to preterm newborns, Dev. Pharmacol. Ther. 5 (1982) 47.

[426] D.M. Anderson, R.M. Kleigman, Relationship of neonatal alimentation practices to the occurrence of endemic neonatal necrotizing enterocolitis, Am. J. Perinatol. 8 (1991) 62.

[427] R.E. McKeown, et al., Role of delayed feeding and of feeding increments in necrotizing enterocolitis, J. Pediatr. 121 (1992) 764.

[428] V. Carrion, E.A. Egan, Prevention of neonatal necrotizing enterocolitis, J. Pediatr. Gastroenterol. Nutr. 11 (1990) 317.

[429] B. Bohnhorst, et al., Early feeding after necrotizing enterocolitis in preterm infants, J. Pediatr. 143 (2003) 484.

[430] C.L. Anderson, et al., A widespread epidemic of mild necrotizing enterocolitis of unknown cause, Am. J. Dis. Child. 138 (1984) 979.

[431] A.R. Gerber, et al., Increased risk of illness among nursery staff caring for neonates with necrotizing enterocolitis, Pediatr. Infect. Dis. J. 4 (1985) 246.

[432] G.A. Little (Ed.), American Academy of Pediatrics Committee on the Fetus and Newborn: Guidelines for Perinatal Care, second ed., American Academy of Pediatrics, Elk Grove Village, IL, 1988, pp. 182–183.

[433] E.D. Claud, W.A. Walker, Hypothesis: inappropriate colonization of the premature intestine can cause neonatal necrotizing enterocolitis, FASEB J. 15 (2001) 1398.

[434] M.A. Schell, M. Karmirantzou, B. Snel, et al., The genome sequence of *Bifidobacterium longum* reflects its adaptation to the human gastrointestinal tract, Proc. Natl. Acad. Sci. U. S. A. 99 (2002) 14422.

[435] H.C. Lin, et al., Oral probiotics prevent necrotizing enterocolitis in very low birth weight preterm infants: a multicenter, randomized, controlled trial, Pediatrics 122 (2008) 693.

[436] A. Bin-Nun, et al., Oral probiotics prevent necrotizing enterocolitis in very low birth weight neonates, J. Pediatr. 147 (2005) 192.

[437] C.-H. Lin, et al., Oral probiotics reduce the incidence and severity of necrotizing enterocolitis in very low birth weight infants, Pediatrics 115 (2005) 1.

[438] G. Deshpande, S. Rao, S. Patole, Probiotics for prevention of necrotizing enterocolitis in preterm neonates with very low birthweight: a systematic review of randomised controlled trials, Lancet 369 (2007) 1614.

[439] J.C. Leonidas, R.T. Hall, Neonatal pneumatosis coli: a mild form of neonatal necrotizing enterocolitis, J. Pediatr. 89 (1976) 456.

[440] M.A. Eibl, et al., Prevention of necrotizing enterocolitis in low-birth-weight infants by IgA-IgG feeding, N. Engl. J. Med. 319 (1988) 1.

[441] J.N. Schullinger, et al., Neonatal necrotizing enterocolitis: survival, management, and complications: a 25-year study, Am. J. Dis. Child. 136 (1981) 612.

[442] S. Abbasi, et al., Long-term assessment of growth, nutritional status and gastrointestinal function in survivors of necrotizing enterocolitis, J. Pediatr. 104 (1984) 550.

[443] J.S. Janik, S.H. Ein, K. Mancer, Intestinal structure after necrotizing enterocolitis, J. Pediatr. Surg. 16 (1981) 438.

[444] T.I. Ball, J.B. Wyly, Enterocyst formation: a late complication of neonatal necrotizing enterocolitis, AJR Am. J. Roentgenol. 147 (1986) 806.

[445] M.C. Walsh, R.M. Kliegman, M. Hack, Severity of necrotizing enterocolitis: influence on outcome at 2 years of age, Pediatrics 84 (1989) 808.

[446] L.C. Blieden, et al., Bacterial endocarditis in the neonate, Am. J. Dis. Child. 124 (1972) 747.

[447] I.C. Lewis, Bacterial endocarditis complicating septicemia in an infant, Arch. Dis. Child. 29 (1954) 144.

[448] D. Macaulay, Acute endocarditis in infancy and early childhood, Am. J. Dis. Child. 88 (1954) 715.

[449] D.R. Shanklin, The pathology of prematurity, in: Prematurity and the Obstetrician, Appleton-Century-Crofts, New York, 1969p. 471.

[450] H. Steinitz, L. Schuchmann, G. Wegner, Leberzirrhose, Meningitis, und Endocarditis ulceropolyposa bei einer Neugeborenensepsis durch B-Streptokokken (Streptokokkus agalactiae), Arch. Kinderheilkd. 183 (1971) 382.

[451] D.H. Johnson, A. Rosenthal, A.S. Nadas, Bacterial endocarditis in children under 2 years of age, Am. J. Dis. Child. 129 (1975) 183.

[452] G. Mendelsohn, G.M. Hutchins, Infective endocarditis during the first decade of life: an autopsy review of 33 cases, Am. J. Dis. Child. 133 (1979) 619.

[453] R. Liersch, et al., Gegenwärtige Merkmale der bakteriellen Endokarditis im Kindersalter, Z. Kardiol. 66 (1977) 501.

[454] R. Colville, I. Jeffries, Bilateral acquired neonatal Erb's palsy, Ir. Med. J. 68 (1975) 399.

[455] P.S. Symchych, A.N. Krauss, P. Winchester, Endocarditis following intracardiac placement of umbilical venous catheters in neonates, J. Pediatr. 90 (1977) 287.

[456] K. Edwards, et al., Bacterial endocarditis in 4 young infants: is this complication on the increase? Clin. Pediatr. 16 (1977) 607.

[457] G.A. McGuiness, R.M. Schieken, G.F. Maguire, Endocarditis in the new-born, Am. J. Dis. Child. 134 (1980) 577.

[458] R.L. Bender, et al., Echocardiographic diagnosis of bacterial endocarditis of the mitral valve in a neonate, Am. J. Dis. Child. 131 (1977) 746.

[459] N.R. Lundström, G. Björkhem, Mitral and tricuspid valve vegetations in infancy diagnosed by echocardiography, Acta Paediatr. Scand. 68 (1979) 345.

[460] A.G. Weinberg, W.P. Laird, Group B streptococcal endocarditis detected by echocardiography, J. Pediatr. 92 (1978) 335.

[461] C.W. Barton, et al., A neonatal survivor of group B beta-hemolytic strepto-coccal endocarditis, Am. J. Perinatol. 1 (1984) 214.

[462] B.N. Agarwala, Group B streptococcal endocarditis in a neonate, Pediatr. Cardiol. 9 (1988) 51.

[463] B. Chattapadhyay, Fatal neonatal meningitis due to group B streptococci, Postgrad. Med. J. 51 (1975) 240.

[464] E.T. Cabacungan, G. Tetting, D.Z. Friedberg, Tricuspid valve vegetation caused by group B streptococcal endocarditis: treatment by "vegetectomy.", J. Perinatol. 13 (1993) 398.

[465] H.H. Kramer, et al., Current clinical aspects of bacterial endocarditis in infancy, childhood, and adolescence, Eur. J. Pediatr. 140 (1983) 253.

[466] R.E. Kavey, et al., Two-dimensional echocardiography assessment of infec-tive endocarditis in children, Am. J. Dis. Child. 137 (1983) 851.

[467] K.E. Ward, et al., Successfully treated pulmonary valve endocarditis in a normal neonate, Am. J. Dis. Child. 137 (1983) 913.

[468] D.K. Nakayama, et al., Management of vascular complications of bacterial endocarditis, J. Pediatr. Surg. 21 (1986) 636.

[469] P. Morville, et al., Intérêt de l'échocardiographie dans le diagnostic des endocardités néonatales: à propos de trois observations, Ann. Pediatr. 32 (1985) 389.

[470] J.F. Eliaou, et al., Endocardité infectieuse en période néo-natale, Pediatrie 38 (1983) 561.

[471] J.E. McCartney, A case of acute ulcerative endocarditis in a child aged three and a half weeks, J. Pathol. Bacteriol. 25 (1922) 277.

[472] D.G. Oelberg, et al., Endocarditis in high-risk neonates, Pediatrics 71 (1983) 392.

[473] G. Gossius, P. Gunnes, K. Rasmussen, Ten years of infective endocarditis: a clinicopathologic study, Acta Med. Scand. 217 (1985) 171.

[474] G.J. Noel, J.E. O'Loughlin, P.J. Edelson, Neonatal *Staphylococcus epidermidis* right-sided endocarditis: description of five catheterized infants, Pediatrics 82 (1988) 234.

[475] M.J. Bannon, Infective endocarditis in neonates. Letter to the editor, Arch. Dis. Child. 63 (1998) 112.

[476] Personal communication to Michael Marcy.

[477] E.S. Giddings, Two cases of endocarditis in infants, Can. Med. Assoc. J. 35 (1936) 71.

[478] S.S. Soo, D.L. Boxman, *Streptococcus faecalis* in neonatal infective endocardi-tis, J. Infect. 23 (1991) 209.

[479] C. O'Callaghan, P. McDougall, Infective endocarditis in neonates, Arch. Dis. Child. 63 (1988) 53.

[480] D. Prandstraller, A.M. Marata, F.M. Picchio, *Staphylococcus aureus* endocardi-tis in a newborn with transposition of the great arteries: successful treatment, Int. J. Cardiol. 14 (1987) 355.

[481] T. Zakrzewski, J.D. Keith, Bacterial endocarditis in infants and children, J. Pediatr. 67 (1965) 1179.

[482] L. Weinstein, J.J. Schlesinger, Pathoanatomic, pathophysiologic and clinical correlations in endocarditis, N. Engl. J. Med. 291 (Pt 1) (1974) 832.

[483] P. Morand, et al., Endocardité triscupidienne calcifée du nourisson, Arch. Mal. Coeur 66 (1973) 901.

[484] J.L. Luke, R.P. Bolande, S. Gross, Generalized aspergillosis and *Aspergillus* endocarditis in infancy: report of a case, Pediatrics 31 (1963) 115.

[485] E.L. Wiley, G.M. Hutchins, Superior vena cava syndrome secondary to *Candida* thrombophlebitis complicating parenteral alimentation, J. Pediatr. 91 (1977) 977.

[486] T.J. Walsh, G.M. Hutchins, Postoperative *Candida* infections of the heart in children: clinicopathologic study of a continuing problem of diagnosis and therapy, J. Pediatr. Surg. 15 (1980) 325.

[487] R. Faix, et al., Successful medical treatment of *Candida parapsilosis* endo-carditis in a premature infant, Am. J. Perinatol. 7 (1990) 272.

[488] P.N. Zenker, et al., Successful medical treatment of presumed *Candida* endo-carditis in critically ill infants, J. Pediatr. 119 (1991) 472.

[489] P.J. Sanchez, J.D. Siegel, J. Fishbein, *Candida* endocarditis: successful medi-cal management in three preterm infants and review of the literature, Pediatr. Infect. Dis. J. 10 (1991) 239.

[490] D.D. Millard, S.T. Shulman, The changing spectrum of neonatal endo-carditis, Clin. Perinatol. 15 (1988) 587.

[491] W.R. Morrow, J.E. Haas, D.R. Benjamin, Nonbacterial endocardial thrombosis in neonates: relationship to persistent fetal circulation, J. Pediatr. 100 (1982) 117.

[492] H. Kronsbein, Pathogenesis of endocarditis verrucosa simplex in the new-born, Beitr. Pathol. 161 (1977) 82.

[493] H.F. Krous, Neonatal nonbacterial thrombotic endocarditis, Arch. Pathol. Lab. Med. 103 (1979) 76.

[494] J. Bergsland, et al., Mycotic aortic aneurysms in children, Ann. Thorac. Surg. 37 (1984) 314.

[495] C.A. Bullaboy, et al., Neonatal mitral valve endocarditis: diagnosis and successful management, Clin. Pediatr. 29 (1990) 398.

[496] R.S. Baltimore, Infective endocarditis in children, Pediatr. Infect. Dis. J. 11 (1992) 907.

[497] R.L. Popp, Echocardiography and infectious endocarditis, Curr. Clin. Topics. Infect. Dis. 4 (1983) 98.

[498] C. Watanakunakorn, Treatment of infections due to methicillin-resistant *Staphylococcus aureus*, Ann. Intern. Med. 97 (1982) 376.

[499] J.S. Wolfson, M.N. Swartz, Serum bactericidal activity as a monitor of anti-biotic therapy, N. Engl. J. Med. 312 (1985) 968.

[500] G.I. Cooper, C.C. Hopkins, Rapid diagnosis of intravascular catheter-associated infection by direct Gram staining of catheter segments, N. Engl. J. Med. 312 (1985) 1142.

[501] M.J. Perelman, et al., Aortic root replacement for complicated bacterial endocarditis in an infant, J. Pediatr. Surg. 24 (1989) 1121.

[502] R.M.R. Tulloh, E.D. Silove, L.D. Abrams, Replacement of an aortic valve cusp after neonatal endocarditis, Br. Heart J. 64 (1990) 204.

[503] S.A. Levinson, A. Learner, Blood cysts on the heart valves of newborn infants, Arch. Pathol. 14 (1932) 810.

[504] P. Gross, Concept of fetal endocarditis: a general review with report of an illustrative case, Arch. Pathol. 31 (1941) 163.

[505] B.E. Favara, R.A. Franciosi, L.J. Butterfield, Disseminated intravascular and cardiac thrombosis of the neonate, Am. J. Dis. Child. 127 (1974) 197.

[506] J.G. Begg, Blood-filled cysts in the cardiac valve cusps in foetal life and infancy, J. Pathol. Bacteriol. 87 (1964) 177.

[507] T.R. Thompson, et al., Umbilical artery catheterization complicated by mycotic aortic aneurysm in neonates, Adv. Pediatr. 27 (1980) 275.

[508] L. Charaf, et al., A case of neonatal endocarditis, Acta Pediatr. Scand. 79 (1990) 704.

[509] A.J. Schaffer, M.E. Avery, Diseases of the Newborn, third ed., WB Saunders, Philadelphia, 1971, p. 252.

[510] N. Neimann, et al., Les péricardités purulentes néonatales: à propos du premier cas guéri, Arch. Fr. Pediatr. 22 (1965) 238.

[511] A.M. Collier, J.D. Connor, W.L. Nyhan, Systemic infection with *Hemophilus influenzae* in very young infants, J. Pediatr. 70 (1967) 539.

[512] B. McKinlay, Infectious diarrhea in the newborn caused by an unclassified species of *Salmonella*, Am. J. Dis. Child. 54 (1937) 1252.

[513] H. Chiari, Zur Kenntnis der Pyozyaneus-infektion bei Säuglingen, Zentralb. Allg. Pathol. 38 (1926) 483.

[514] F. Jaiyesimi, A.A. Abioye, A.U. Anita, Infective pericarditis in Nigerian children, Arch. Dis. Child. 54 (1979) 384.

[515] R.J. Wynn, Neonatal *E. coli* pericarditis, J. Perinatol. Med. 7 (1979) 23.

[516] J. Kachaner, J.M. Nouaille, A. Batisse, Les cardiomegalies massives du nouveau-né, Arch. Fr. Pediatr. 34 (1977) 297.

[517] J.P.A. Graham, A. Martin, *B. pyocyaneus* pericarditis occurring four days after birth, Cent. Afr. J. Med. 1 (1955) 101.

[518] W.E. Feldman, Bacterial etiology and mortality of purulent pericarditis in pediatric patients: review of 162 cases, Am. J. Dis. Child. 133 (1979) 641.

[519] R.J. Morgan, et al., Surgical treatment of purulent pericarditis in children, Thorac. Cardiovasc. Surg. 85 (1983) 527.

[520] C.H. Jellard, G.M. Churcher, An outbreak of *Pseudomonas aeruginosa (pyocyanea)* infection in a premature baby unit, with observations on the intestinal carriage of *Pseudomonas aeruginosa* in the newborn, J. Hyg. 65 (1967) 219.

[521] T.C. Miller, S.I. Baman, W.W. Albers, Massive pericardial effusion due to *Mycoplasma hominis* in a newborn, Am. J. Dis. Child. 136 (1982) 271.

[522] L. Shenker, et al., Fetal pericardial effusion, Am. J. Obstet. Gynecol. 160 (1989) 1505.

[523] G.G. Cayler, H. Taybi, H.D. Riley Jr., Pericarditis with effusion in infants and children, J. Pediatr. 63 (1963) 264.

[524] G.R. Noren, E.L. Kaplan, N.A. Staley, Nonrheumatic inflammatory diseases, in: F.H. Adams, G.C. Emmanouilides (Eds.), Moss' Heart Disease in Infants, Children, and Adolescents, third ed., Williams & Wilkins, Baltimore, 1983, pp. 585–594.

[525] K.S. Kanarek, J. Coleman, Purulent pericarditis in a neonate, Pediatr. Infect. Dis. J. 10 (1991) 549.

[526] J.D. Cherry, Enteroviruses, polioviruses (poliomyelitis), coxsackieviruses, echoviruses, and enteroviruses, in: R.D. Feigin, J.D. Cherry (Eds.), Text-book of Pediatric Infectious Diseases, third ed., WB Saunders, Philadelphia, 1992, pp. 1705–1752.

[527] J.T. Zerella, D.C.E. Halpe, Intrapericardial teratoma-neonatal cardiorespi-ratory distress amenable to surgery, J. Pediatr. Surg. 15 (1980) 961.

[528] N. Doshi, B. Smith, B. Klionsky, Congenital pericarditis due to maternal lupus erythematosus, J. Pediatr. 96 (1980) 699.

[529] P. Sasidharan, et al., Nonimmune hydrops fetalis: case reports and brief review, J. Perinatol. 12 (1992) 338.

[530] J.M.B. deFonseca, M.R.Q. Davies, K.D. Bolton, Congenital hydropericar-dium associated with the herniation of part of the liver into the pericardial sac, J. Pediatr. Surg. 22 (1987) 851.

[531] A.J. Jafa, et al., Antenatal diagnosis of bilateral congenital chylothorax with pericardial effusion, Acta Obstet. Gynaecol. Scand. 64 (1985) 455.

[532] R.H. Mupanemunda, H.R. Mackanjee, A life-threatening complication of percutaneous central venous catheters in neonates, Am. J. Dis. Child. 146 (1992) 1414.

[533] P.H. Dennehy, New tests for the rapid diagnosis of infection in children, in: S. Aronoff et al., (Ed.), Advances in Pediatric Infectious Diseases, vol. 8, Mosby-Year Book, St. Louis, 1993, pp. 91–129.

[534] B. Zeevi, et al., Interventional cardiac procedures, Clin. Perinatol. 15 (1988) 633.

[535] S. Achenbach, Mediastinalabszess bei einmen 3 Wochen alten Säugling, Arch. Kinderheilkd. 74 (1924) 193.

[536] H.E. Grewe, M. Martini Pape, Die eitrige Mediastinitis im frühen Saüglingsalter, Kinderarztl. Prax. 32 (1964) 305.

[537] M. Weichsel, Mediastinitis in a newborn, Proc. Rudolf Virchow Med. Soc. City N. Y. 22 (1963) 67.

[538] G. Weber, Retropharyngeal und Mediastinalabszess bei einem 3 Wochen alten Säugling, Chirurg 21 (1950) 308.

[539] A.A. deLorimier, D. Haskin, F.S. Massie, Mediastinal mass caused by vertebral osteomyelitis, Am. J. Dis. Child. 111 (1966) 639.

[540] J.L. Talbert, et al., Traumatic perforation of the hypopharynx in infants, J. Thorac. Cardiovasc. Surg. 74 (1977) 152.

[541] M. Grunebaum, et al., Iatrogenic transmural perforation of the oesophagus in the preterm infant, Clin. Radiol. 31 (1980) 257.

[542] T. Sands, M. Glasson, A. Berry, Hazards of nasogastric tube insertion in the newborn infant, Lancet 2 (1989) 680.

[543] I.H. Krasna, et al., Esophageal perforation in the neonate: an emerging problem in the newborn nursery, J. Pediatr. Surg. 22 (1987) 784.

[544] J. Topsis, H.Y. Kinas, S.R. Kandall, Esophageal perforation—a complication of neonatal resuscitation, Anesth. Analg. 69 (1989) 532.

[545] Y. Vandenplas, et al., Cervical esophageal perforation diagnosed by endoscopy in a premature infant, J. Pediatr. Gastroenterol. Nutr. 8 (1989) 390.

[546] R.J. Touloukian, et al., Traumatic perforation of the pharynx in the newborn, Pediatrics 59 (1977) 1019.

[547] D.E. Johnson, et al., Management of esophageal and pharyngeal perforation in the newborn infant, Pediatrics 70 (1982) 592.

[548] M. Coulthard, D. Isaacs, Neonatal retropharyngeal abscess, Pediatr. Infect. Dis. J. 10 (1991) 547.

[549] A. Bittencourt, Congenital Chagas disease, Am. J. Dis. Child. 130 (1976) 97.

[550] P.H. Azimi, J. Willert, A. Petru, Severe esophagitis in a newborn, Pediatr. Infect. Dis. J. 15 (1966) 385.

[551] T.J. Walsh, N.J. Belitsos, S.R. Hamilton, Bacterial esophagitis in immunocompromised patients, Arch. Intern. Med. 146 (1986) 1345.

[552] A.J. Nelson, Neonatal suppurative thyroiditis, Pediatr. Infect. Dis. 2 (1983) 243.

[553] R. Berner, et al., Salmonella enteritidis orchitis in a 10-week old boy, Acta Pediatr. 83 (1994) 922.

[554] H.N. Sanford, I. Shmigelsky, Purulent parotitis in the newborn, J. Pediatr. 26 (1945) 149.

[555] B.H. Shulman, Acute suppurative infections of the salivary glands in the newborn, Am. J. Dis. Child. 80 (1950) 413.

[556] W.A.B. Campbell, Purulent parotitis in the newborn: report of a case, Lancet 2 (1951) 386.

[557] D. Leake, R. Leake, Neonatal suppurative parotitis, Pediatrics 46 (1970) 203.

[558] I. Brook, E.H. Frazier, D.H. Thompson, Aerobic and anaerobic microbiology of acute suppurative parotitis, Laryngoscope 101 (1991) 170.

[559] R.B. David, E.J. O'Connell, Suppurative parotitis in children, Am. J. Dis. Child. 119 (1970) 332.

[560] W.W. Banks, et al., Neonatal submandibular sialadenitis, Am. J. Otolaryngol. 1 (1980) 261.

[561] M. Saarinen, et al., Spectrum of 2,836 cases of invasive bacterial or fungal infections in children: results of prospective nationwide five-year surveillance in Finland. Finnish Pediatric Invasive Infection Study Group, Clin. Infect. Dis. 21 (1995) 1134–1144.

[562] L.M. Solomon, N.B. Esterly, Neonatal Dermatology, WB Saunders, Philadelphia, 1973.

[563] M.N. Swartz, A.N. Weinberg, Bacterial diseases with cutaneous involvement, in: T.B. Fitzpatrick Jr. (Ed.), Dermatology in General Medicine, McGraw-Hill, New York, 1971.

[564] Personal communication to Michael Marcy.

[565] Personal communication to Michael Marcy.

[566] R.M. Fortunov, et al., Community acquired Staphylococcus aureus infections in term and near-term previously healthy neonates, Pediatrics 118 (2006) 874.

[567] A.B. Zafar, et al., Use of 03.% triclosan (Bacti-Stat) to eradicate an outbreak of methicillin-resistant Staphylococcus aureus in a neonatal nursery, Am J Infect Control 23 (1995) 200.

[568] I.J. Frieden, Blisters and pustules in the newborn, Curr. Probl. Pediatr. 19 (1989) 553.

[569] S. Weinberg, M. Leider, L. Shapiro, Color Atlas of Pediatric Dermatology, McGraw-Hill, New York, 1975.

[570] H.I. Maibach, G. Hildick-Smith (Eds.), Skin Bacteria and Their Role in Infection, McGraw-Hill, New York, 1965.

[571] H. Speert, Circumcision of the newborn: an appraisal of its present status, Obstet. Gynecol. 2 (1953) 164.

[572] S.H. Annabil, A. Al-Hifi, T. Kazi, Primary tuberculosis of the penis in an infant, Tubercle 71 (1990) 229.

[573] T.G. Cleary, S. Kohl, Overwhelming infection with group B beta-hemolytic streptococcus associated with circumcision, Pediatrics 64 (1979) 301.

[574] L. Sauer, Fatal staphylococcal bronchopneumonia following ritual circumcision, Am. J. Obstet. Gynecol. 46 (1943) 583.

[575] D. Annunziato, L.M. Goldblum, Staphylococcal scalded skin syndrome, Am. J. Dis. Child. 132 (1978) 1187.

[576] G.S. Breuer, S. Walfisch, Circumcision complications and indications for ritual recircumcision—clinical experience and review of the literature, Isr. J. Med. Sci. 23 (1987) 252.

[577] J.R. Woodside, Necrotizing fasciitis after neonatal circumcision, Am. J. Dis. Child. 134 (1980) 301.

[578] J. Stranko, M.E. Ryan, A.M. Bowman, Impetigo in newborn infants associated with a plastic bell clamp circumcision, Pediatr. Infect. Dis. 5 (1986) 597.

[579] S.F. Siddiqi, P.M. Taylor, Necrotizing fasciitis of the scalp, Am. J. Dis. Child. 136 (1982) 226.

[580] D.M. Okada, A.W. Chow, V.T. Bruce, Neonatal scalp abscess and fetal monitoring: factors associated with infection, Am. J. Obstet. Gynecol. 129 (1977) 185.

[581] L. Cordero, C.W. Anderson, E.H. Hon, Scalp abscess: a benign and infrequent complication of fetal monitoring, Am. J. Obstet. Gynecol. 146 (1983) 126.

[582] M.M. Wagener, et al., Septic dermatitis of the neonatal scalp and maternal endomyometritis with intrapartum internal fetal monitoring, Pediatrics 74 (1984) 81.

[583] I. Brook, Microbiology of scalp abscesses in newborns, Pediatr. Infect. Dis. J. 11 (1992) 766.

[584] J.C. Bogdan, R.H. Rapkin, Clostridia infection in the newborn, Pediatrics 58 (1976) 120.

[585] W.F. Fitter, D.J. DeSa, H. Richardson, Chorioamnionitis and funisitis due to Corynebacterium kutscheri, Arch. Dis. Child. 55 (1979) 710.

[586] I. Sarkany, C.C. Gaylarde, Skin flora of the newborn, Lancet 1 (1967) 589.

[587] H.E. Evans, S.O. Akpata, A. Baki, Factors influencing the establishment of neonatal bacterial flora. I. The role of host factors, Arch. Environ. Health 21 (1970) 514.

[588] I. Sarkany, L. Arnold, The effect of single and repeated applications of hexachlorophene on the bacterial flora of the skin of the newborn, Br. J. Dermatol. 82 (1970) 261.

[589] D.J. Thompson, et al., Excess risk of staphylococcal infection and disease in newborn males, Am. J. Epidemiol. 84 (1966) 314.

[590] R.C. Rudoy, J.D. Nelson, Breast abscess during the neonatal period: a review, Am. J. Dis. Child. 129 (1975) 1031.

[591] A.C. Reboli, J.F. John, A.H. Levkoff, Epidemic methicillin-gentamicin-resistant Staphylococcus aureus in a neonatal intensive care unit, Am. J. Dis. Child. 143 (1989) 34.

[592] J.E. Fergie, K. Purcell, Community-acquired methicillin-resistant Staphylococcus aureus infection in south Texas children, Pediatr. Infect. Dis. J. 20 (2001) 860.

[593] H.E. Evans, et al., Flora in newborn infants: annual variation in prevalence of Staphylococcus aureus, Escherichia coli, and streptococci, Arch. Environ. Health 26 (1973) 275.

[594] H.J. Starr, P.B. Holliday Jr., Erythema multiforme as a manifestation of neonatal septicemia, J. Pediatr. 38 (1951) 315.

[595] J.L. Washington, R.E.L. Fowler, G.J. Guarino, Erythema multiforme in a premature infant associated with sepsis due to Pseudomonas, Pediatrics 39 (1967) 120.

[596] J.F. Foley, et al., Achromobacter septicemia—fatalities in prematures. I. Clinical and epidemiological study, Am. J. Dis. Child. 101 (1961) 279.

[597] T.K. Belgaumkar, Impetigo neonatorum congenita due to group B beta-hemolytic streptococcus infection. Letter to the editor, J. Pediatr. 86 (1975) 982.

[598] F. Halal, et al., Congenital vesicular eruption caused by Hemophilus influenzae type b, Pediatrics 62 (1978) 494.

[599] M.O. Martin, et al., Les signes cutanés des infections bacteriennes néonatales, Arch. Fr. Pediatr. 42 (1985) 471.

[600] A. Kline, E. O'Connell, Group B streptococcus as a cause of neonatal bullous skin lesions, Pediatr. Infect. Dis. J. 12 (1993) 165.

[601] N. Khuri-Bulos, K. McIntosh, Neonatal Haemophilus influenzae infection: report of eight cases and review of the literature, Am. J. Dis. Child. 129 (1975) 57.

[602] D.A. Bray, Ecthyma gangrenosum: full thickness nasal slough, Arch. Otolaryngol. 98 (1973) 210.

[603] R.W. Heffner, G.F. Smith, Ecthyma gangrenosum in Pseudomonas septicemia, Am. J. Dis. Child. 99 (1960) 524.

[604] S.P. Ghosal, et al., Noma neonatorum: its aetiopathogenesis, Lancet 1 (1978) 289.

[605] G.P. Bodey, et al., Infections caused by Pseudomonas aeruginosa, Rev. Infect. Dis. 5 (1983) 279.

[606] J.E. Baley, R.A. Silverman, Systemic candidiasis: cutaneous manifestations in low birth weight infants, Pediatrics 82 (1988) 211.

[607] L. Cordero Jr., E.H. Hon, Scalp abscess: a rare complication of fetal monitoring, J. Pediatr. 78 (1971) 533.

[608] J.D. Nelson, Bilateral breast abscess due to group B streptococcus, Am. J. Dis. Child. 130 (1976) 567.

[609] H.L. Levy, J.F. O'Connor, D. Ingall, Bacteremia, infected cephalhematoma, and osteomyelitis of the skull in a newborn, Am. J. Dis. Child. 114 (1967) 649.

[610] S.S. Ellis, et al., Osteomyelitis complicating neonatal cephalhematoma, Am. J. Dis. Child. 127 (1974) 100.

[611] H. Stetler, et al., Neonatal mastitis due to Escherichia coli, J. Pediatr. 76 (1970) 611.

[612] H.H. Balfour Jr., et al., Complications of fetal blood sampling, Am. J. Obstet. Gynecol. 107 (1970) 288.

[613] M.A. McGuigan, R.P. Lipman, Neonatal mastitis due to Proteus mirabilis, Am. J. Dis. Child. 130 (1976) 1296.

[614] H.D. Wilson, K.C. Haltalin, Acute necrotizing fasciitis in childhood, Am. J. Dis. Child. 125 (1973) 591.

[615] V.F. Burry, M. Beezley, Infant mastitis due to gram-negative organisms, Am. J. Dis. Child. 124 (1972) 736.

[616] I. Brook, The aerobic and anaerobic microbiology of neonatal breast abscess, Pediatr. Infect. Dis. J. 10 (1991) 785.

[617] Centers for Disease Control, Nosocomial *Serratia marcescens* infections in neonates—Puerto Rico., MMWR Morb. Mortal. Wkly. Rep. 23 (1974) 183.

[618] J.K. Todd, F.W. Bruhn, Severe *Haemophilus influenzae* infections: spectrum of disease, Am. J. Dis. Child. 129 (1975) 607.

[619] S.H. Zinner, et al., Puerperal bacteremia and neonatal sepsis due to *Hemophilus parainfluenzae*: report of a case with antibody titers, Pediatrics 49 (1972) 612.

[620] M.S. Platt, Neonatal *Hemophilus vaginalis* (*Corynebacterium vaginalis*) infection, Clin. Pediatr. 10 (1971) 513.

[621] P.M. Leighton, B. Bulleid, R. Taylor, Neonatal cellulitis due to *Gardnerella vaginalis*, Pediatr. Infect. Dis. 1 (1982) 339.

[622] Y.H. Lee, R.B. Berg, Cephalhematoma infected with *Bacteroides*, Am. J. Dis. Child. 121 (1971) 77.

[623] M.J. Mandel, R.J. Lewis, Molluscum contagiosum of the newborn, Br. J. Dermatol. 84 (1970) 370.

[624] J.M. Clark, W.R. Weeks, J. Tatton, *Drosophila* myiasis mimicking sepsis in a newborn, West. J. Med. 136 (1982) 443.

[625] B.R. Burns, R.M. Lampe, G.H. Hansen, Neonatal scabies, Am. J. Dis. Child. 133 (1979) 1031.

[626] O.J. Hensey, C.A. Hart, R.W.I. Cooke, *Candida albicans* skin abscesses, Arch. Dis. Child. 59 (1984) 479.

[627] D.F. Turbeville, et al., Complications of fetal scalp electrodes: a case report, Am. J. Obstet. Gynecol. 122 (1975) 530.

[628] Centers for Disease Control, Gonococcal scalp-wound infection—New Jersey., MMWR Morb. Mortal. Wkly. Rep. 24 (1975) 115.

[629] I. Brook. Osteomyelitis and bacteremia caused by *Bacteroides fragilis*, Clin. Pediatr. 19 (1980) 639.

[630] R.T. Mohon, et al., Infected cephalhematoma and neonatal osteomyelitis of the skull, Pediatr. Infect. Dis. 5 (1986) 253.

[631] S.M. Cohen, B.W. Miller, H.W. Orris, Meningitis complicating cephalhematoma, J. Pediatr. 30 (1947) 327.

[632] M. Walsh, K. McIntosh, Neonatal mastitis, Clin. Pediatr. 25 (1986) 395.

[633] W.H. Langewisch, An epidemic of group A, type 1 streptococcal infections in newborn infants, Pediatrics 18 (1956) 438.

[634] D. Sinniah, B.R. Sandiford, A.E. Dugdale, Subungual infection in the newborn: an institutional outbreak of unknown etiology, possibly due to *Veillonella*, Clin. Pediatr. 11 (1972) 690.

[635] A.H. Cushing, Omphalitis: a review, Pediatr. Infect. Dis. 4 (1985) 282.

[636] H. McKenna, D. Johnson, Bacteria in neonatal omphalitis, Pathology 7 (1977) 11.

[637] W.H. Mason, et al., Omphalitis in the newborn infant, Pediatr. Infect. Dis. J. 8 (1989) 521.

[638] C.C. Geil, W.K. Castle, E.A. Mortimer Jr., A. Group, streptococcal infections in newborn nurseries, Pediatrics 46 (1970) 849.

[639] D.P. Bliss, P.J. Healey, J.H.T. Waldbraussen, Necrotizing fasciitis after Plastibell circumcision, J. Pediatr. 131 (1997) 459.

[640] A.M. Kosloske, et al., Cellulitis and necrotizing fasciitis of the abdominal wall in pediatric patients, J. Pediatr. Surg. 16 (1981) 246.

[641] W.F. Gee, J.S. Ansell, Neonatal circumcision: a 10-year overview: with comparison of the Gomco clamp and the Plastibell device, Pediatrics 58 (1976) 824.

[642] G.N. Goldberg, R.C. Hansen, P.J. Lynch, Necrotizing fasciitis in infancy: report of three cases and review of the literature, Pediatr. Dermatol. 2 (1984) 55.

[643] R.S. Ramamurthy, G. Srinivasan, N.M. Jacobs, Necrotizing fasciitis and necrotizing cellulitis due to group B streptococcus, Am. J. Dis. Child. 131 (1977) 1169.

[644] R.W. Krieger, M.J. Chusid, Perirectal abscess in childhood, Am. J. Dis. Child. 133 (1979) 411.

[645] M. Arditi, R. Yogev, Perirectal abscess in infants and children: report of 52 cases and review of the literature, Pediatr. Infect. Dis. J. 9 (1990) 411.

[646] L. Victorin, An epidemic of otitis in newborns due to infection with *Pseudomonas aeruginosa*, Acta. Paediatr. Scand. 56 (1967) 344.

[647] E.J. Laubo, A.S. Paller, Common skin problems during the first year of life, Pediatr. Clin. North Am. 41 (1994) 1105.

[648] M.T. Glover, D.J. Atherton, R.J. Levinsky, Syndrome of erythroderma, failure to thrive, and diarrhea in infancy: a manifestation of immunodeficiency, Pediatrics 81 (1988) 66.

[649] L.S. Prod'hom, et al., Care of the seriously ill neonate with hyaline membrane disease and with sepsis (sclerema neonatorum), Pediatrics 53 (1974) 170.

[650] W.E. Hughes, M.L. Hammond, Sclerema neonatorum, J. Pediatr. 32 (1948) 676.

[651] G.H. McCracken Jr., H.R. Shinefield, Changes in the pattern of neonatal septicemia and meningitis, Am. J. Dis. Child. 112 (1966) 33.

[652] I. Gordon, Miliary sebaceous cysts and blisters in the healthy newborn, Arch. Dis. Child. 24 (1949) 286.

[653] J.A. Carr, et al., Relationship between toxic erythema and infant maturity, Am. J. Dis. Child. 112 (1966) 219.

[654] P. Merlob, A. Metzker, S.H. Reisner, Transient neonatal pustular melanosis, Am. J. Dis. Child. 136 (1982) 521.

[655] G. Kahn, A.M. Rywlin, Acropustulosis of infancy, Arch. Dermatol. 115 (1979) 831.

[656] A.W. Lucky, J.S. McGuire, Infantile acropustulosis with eosinophilic pustules, J. Pediatr. 100 (1982) 428.

[657] W.F. Murphy, A. Langley, Common bullous lesions—presumably self-inflicted—occurring in utero in the newborn infant, Pediatrics 32 (1963) 1099.

[658] W.L. Weston, A.T. Lane, J.A. Weston, Diaper dermatitis: current concepts, Pediatrics 66 (1980) 532.

[659] Nappy rashes, Editorial., BMJ 282 (1981) 420.

[660] J.C. Hauth, G.B. Merenstein (Eds.), Guidelines for Perinatal Care, fourth ed., American Academy of Pediatrics and American College of Obstetricians and Gynecologists, Elk Grove Village, IL, 1997.

[661] I.M. Gladstone, et al., Randomized study of six umbilical cord care regimens, Clin. Pediatr. 27 (1988) 127.

[662] Centers for Disease Control, National nosocomial infections study report: nosocomial infections in nurseries and their relationship to hospital infant bathing practices—a preliminary report, Centers for Disease Control, Atlanta, 1974, pp. 9–23.

[663] H.M. Gezon, M.J. Schaberg, J.O. Klein, Concurrent epidemics of Staphylococcus aureus and group A streptococcus disease in a newborn nursery—control with penicillin G and hexachlorophene bathing, Pediatrics 51 (1973) 383.

[664] S. Seeberg, et al., Prevention and control of neonatal pyoderma with chlorhexidine, Acta Paediatr. Scand. 73 (1984) 498.

[665] A.R. de Toledo, J.W. Chandler, Conjunctivitis of the newborn, Infect. Dis. Clin. North Am. 6 (1992) 807.

[666] J.P. Whitcher, Neonatal ophthalmia. Have we advanced in the last 20 years? Int. Ophthalmol. Clin. 30 (1990) 39.

[667] D.D. Millard, R. Yogev, *Haemophilus influenzae* type b: a rare case of congenital conjunctivitis, Pediatr. Infect. Dis. 7 (1988) 363.

[668] D.T. McLeod, F. Ahmad, M.A. Calder, *Branhamella catarrhalis* (beta lactamase positive) ophthalmia neonatorum, Lancet 2 (1984) 647.

[669] M. Ellis, et al., Neonatal conjunctivitis associated with meningococcal meningitis, Arch. Dis. Child. 67 (1992) 1219.

[670] M.J. Naiditch, A.G. Bower, Diphtheria: a study of 1433 cases observed during a ten year period at Los Angeles County Hospital, Am. J. Med. 17 (1954) 229.

[671] M.S. Khan, S.E. Stead, Neonatal *Pasteurella multocida* conjunctivitis following zoonotic infection of mother, J. Infect. Dis. 1 (1979) 289.

[672] I. Brook, W.J. Martin, S.M. Finegold, Effect of silver nitrate application on the conjunctival flora of the newborn, and the occurrence of clostridial conjunctivitis, J. Pediatr. Ophthalmol. Strabismus 15 (1978) 179.

[673] P. Bourbeau, V. Holla, S. Piemontese, Ophthalmia neonatorum caused by *Neisseria cinerea*, J. Clin. Microbiol. 28 (1990) 1640.

[674] K. Hedberg, et al., Outbreak of erythromycin-resistant staphylococcal conjunctivitis in a newborn nursery, Pediatr. Infect. Dis. J. 9 (1990) 268.

[675] M.J. Paentice, G.R. Hutchinson, D. Taylor-Robinson, A microbiological study of neonatal conjunctivitis, Br. J. Ophthalmol. 61 (1977) 9.

[676] K.I. Sandstrom, et al., Microbial causes of neonatal conjunctivitis, J. Pediatr. 105 (1984) 706.

[677] G. Regev-Yochav, et al., Methicillin-resistant *Staphylococcus aureus* in a neonatal intensive care unit, Emerg. Infect. Dis. 11 (2005) 453.

[678] T. Rutar, Vertically acquired community methicillin-resistant *Staphylococcus aureus* dacrocystitis in a neonate, J. AAPOS 13 (2009) 79–81.

[679] J.H. Kim, et al., Outbreak of Gram-positive bacterial keratitis associated with epidemic keratoconjunctivitis in neonates and infants, Eye 23 (2009) 1059–1065.

[680] A.M. Duarte, et al., Eosinophilic pustular folliculitis in infancy and childhood, Am. J. Dis. Child. 147 (1993) 197.

[681] M.R. Hammerschlag, Conjunctivitis in infancy and childhood, Pediatr. Rev. 5 (1984) 285.

[682] J. Wincelaus, et al., Diagnosis of ophthalmia neonatorum, BMJ 295 (1987) 1377.

[683] I.L. Molgaard, P.B. Nielsen, J. Kaern, A study of the incidence of neonatal conjunctivitis and of its bacterial causes including *Chlamydia trachomatis*, Acta Ophthalmol. 62 (1984) 461.

[684] M. Laga, et al., Epidemiology of ophthalmia neonatorum in Kenya, Lancet 2 (1986) 1145.

[685] K.J. Nathoo, A.S. Latif, J.E.S. Trijssenaar, Aetiology of neonatal conjunctivitis in Harare, Cent. Afr. J. Med. 30 (1984) 123.

[686] S. Stenson, R. Newman, H. Fedukowicz, Conjunctivitis in the newborn: observations on incidence, cause, and prophylaxis, Ann. Ophthalmol. 13 (1981) 329.

[687] R.P. Burns, D.H. Rhodes Jr., *Pseudomonas* eye infection as a cause of death in premature infants, Arch. Ophthalmol. 65 (1961) 517.

[688] S.E. Drewett, et al., Eradication of *Pseudomonas aeruginosa* infection from a special-care nursery, Lancet 1 (1972) 946.

[689] G.A. Cole, D.P. Davies, J.A. Austin, *Pseudomonas* ophthalmia neonatorum: a cause of blindness, BMJ 281 (1980) 440.

[690] E.I. Traboulsi, et al., *Pseudomonas aeruginosa* ophthalmia neonatorum, Am. J. Ophthalmol. 98 (1984) 801.

[691] R. Lohrer, B.H. Belohradsky, Bacterial endophthalmitis in neonates, Eur. J. Pediatr. 146 (1987) 354.

[692] G.D. Christensen, et al., Epidemic *Serratia marcescens* in a neonatal intensive care unit: importance of the gastrointestinal tract as a reservoir, Infect. Control 3 (1982) 127.

[693] H. Nishida, H.M. Risemberg, Silver nitrate ophthalmic solution and chemical conjunctivitis, Pediatrics 56 (1975) 3368.

[694] S.S. Kripke, B. Golden, Neonatal inclusion conjunctivitis: a report of three cases and a discussion of differential diagnosis and treatment, Clin. Pediatr. 11 (1972) 261.

[695] L.K. Pickering, et al., Red Book: 2009 Report of the Committee on Infectious Diseases, 28th ed., Elk Grove Village, IL, American Academy of Pediatrics, 2009.

CHAPTER 11

MICROORGANISMS RESPONSIBLE FOR NEONATAL DIARRHEA

Miguel L. O'Ryan ☉ James P. Nataro ☉ Thomas G. Cleary

CHAPTER OUTLINE

Enteric Host Defense Mechanisms   359
Protective Factors in Human Milk   360
Bacterial Pathogens   361
    Escherichia coli   361
    Salmonella   376
    Shigella   381
    Campylobacter   385
    Clostridium difficile   389
    Vibrio cholerae   390
    Yersinia enterocolitica   391
    Aeromonas hydrophila   392

    Plesiomonas shigelloides   392
Other Bacterial Agents and Fungi   393
Parasites   394
    Entamoeba histolytica   394
    Giardia lamblia   394
    Cryptosporidium   395
Viruses   395
    Enteric Viruses   395
    Rotavirus   395
Differential Diagnosis   399

Diarrheal disease continues to be a significant cause of morbidity and mortality worldwide in the 21st century. During the period 1986-2000, an estimated 1.4 billion children younger than 5 years old had an episode of acute diarrhea every year in developing countries; among these, 123.6 million required outpatient medical care, and 9 million required hospitalization. Approximately 2 million diarrhea-associated deaths occurred in this age group annually, primarily in the most impoverished areas of the world [1]. These estimates are decreased from the more than 3 million annual deaths from diarrhea reported in the prior 10 years [2], indicating progress in prevention and treatment of acute diarrhea. In the United States, approximately 400 childhood deaths per year were reported during the late 1980s [3,4], although the actual number may be higher [4].

Nearly 4 million infants die every year in the first 4 weeks of life [5]. Infections account for 36% of these deaths, of which diarrhea causes 3%, accounting for approximately 110,000 deaths (range 80,000 to 410,000) per year [5,6]. These deaths are concentrated in countries with neonatal mortality rates of 30 or more per 1000 live births, mainly in Africa and Southeast Asia. In Haiti, diarrhea was not detected in a small series of 34 cases of neonatal deaths [7]. In India, diarrhea caused 10% of severe illness requiring hospitalization among newborns 7 to 27 days of age [8]. The relative sparing of most newborns probably results from low exposure to enteropathogens and protection associated with breast-feeding [9–13]. After the first few months of life, increasing interaction with other individuals and the environment, including the introduction of artificial feeding, increases the risk of exposure to enteropathogens. For infants with very low birth weight (<1500 g), the death rate from diarrhea is 100-fold greater than for infants with higher birth weight [14].

This chapter discusses the pathogenesis, diagnosis, treatment, and prevention of gastroenteritis based on the available knowledge about pathogens that can cause neonatal diarrhea. Pathogens that rarely or never cause acute diarrhea in neonates are mentioned and discussed briefly. After an overview of host defense mechanisms and protective factors in human milk, the remainder of the chapter is devoted to specific pathogens that cause inflammatory or noninflammatory diarrhea.

ENTERIC HOST DEFENSE MECHANISMS

Significant research, mostly in animal models, has been performed to understand the relationship between the gut and commensal and pathogenic microorganisms. The mechanisms, cells, and molecules involved in microorganism-intestinal interactions are numerous, increasingly complex, and only partially understood. A complete review of this topic is beyond the scope of this chapter; comprehensive reviews on intestinal immunity have been published [15,16], including specific reviews on dendritic cells [17], intestinal IgA [18], intestinal epithelial cells [19], microbial colonization [20], toll-like receptors [21], mast cells [22], and Paneth cells [23]. It is generally accepted that although most of the constituents required for an intestinal immune response against microorganisms are present in the neonatal gut, they are "immature," principally because neonates have not had the opportunity to develop local or systemic immune responses, and in the first few days of life, they have yet to acquire the highly important enteric microflora that protects the normal adult gastrointestinal (GI) tract [9,24–29]. During the early neonatal period, there is a "relative" deficiency in antigen-presenting cell functions and altered cell-mediated immune responses [30]. Little is known about the barrier capabilities of the neonate's gastric acidity [30,31], intestinal mucus [30,32], or motility [33,34], each of which provides protection against GI tract infections in older infants, children, and adults.

The gastric acid barrier seems to be least effective during the first months of life. The average gastric pH level of the newborn is high (pH 4 to 7, mean 6) [35,36]. Although the pH falls to low levels by the end of the first day of life (pH 2 to 3) [35], it subsequently rises again; by 7 to 10 days of life, the hydrochloric acid output of the neonatal stomach is far less than that of older infants and children [36,37]. The buffering action of frequent milk feedings and the short gastric emptying time [38–41] introduce additional factors in the neonate that would be expected to permit viable ingested organisms to reach the small intestine.

Immediately after birth, infants begin to acquire commensal microorganisms from their surroundings. Factors that regulate this acquisition and the degree of variation within and between individuals are only partially understood. Commensal bacteria seem to be acquired as a result of random environmental encounters most likely influenced by feeding patterns (human versus formula milk). The consequences of alterations in the acquisition or composition, or both, of commensal bacterial communities on mammalian development, normal physiology, and susceptibility to disease are an active area of investigation [19,29].

The intestinal epithelium serves as a nutrient absorptive machine, barrier to pathogen entry, regulator of inflammation, and critical element in maintaining immune homeostasis of the gut [19,42]. The thick mucin-rich glycocalix surrounded by mucus forms a physical barrier embedded with antimicrobial peptides and enzymes [30]. The different composition of adult and neonatal glycocalix may influence susceptibility to colonization and infection [30]. Intestinal epithelial cells have receptors for bacterial products and produce chemokines (e.g., interleukin-8, monocyte chemotactic protein type 1, granulocyte-macrophage colony-stimulating factor) and proinflammatory cytokines (e.g., interleukin-6, tumor necrosis factor-α, interleukin-1) in response to invasion by enteropathogens [43]. The gut epithelium orchestrates the immune response. Paneth cells in crypts express toll-like receptors activated by microorganisms leading to release of potent antimicrobial agents including lysozyme and cryptidins [44].

Neonatal B-lymphocyte and T-lymphocyte functions are impaired, resulting in preferential IgM production in response to antigenic stimulation. IgG is actively transferred from mother to infant across the placenta at about 32 weeks of gestation and peaks by about 37 weeks. Premature neonates, especially infants born before 28 weeks' gestation, are deficient in these maternally derived serum antibodies [29,30,44,45].

PROTECTIVE FACTORS IN HUMAN MILK

The importance of breast-feeding to infants for the prevention of diarrheal disease has long been emphasized [9,46–59]. Published studies reporting the association between breast-feeding and diarrhea are extensive and suggest that infants who are breast-fed have fewer episodes of diarrhea than infants who are formula-fed. This protection is greatest during an infant's first 3 months of life and declines with increasing age. During the period of weaning, partial breast-feeding confers protection that is intermediate between the protection gained by infants who are exclusively breast-fed and that by infants who are exclusively formula-fed.

Mata and Urrutia [9] provided a striking demonstration of the protection afforded by breast-feeding of newborns in their studies of a population of infants born in a rural Guatemalan village. Despite extremely poor sanitation and the demonstration of fecal organisms in the colostrum and milk of almost one third of mothers [60], diarrheal disease did not occur in any of the newborns. The incidence of diarrhea increased significantly only after these infants reached 4 to 6 months old, at which time solids and other fluids were used to supplement the human milk feedings. At that time, *Escherichia coli* and gram-negative anaerobes (e.g., *Bacteroides* species) were found to colonize the intestinal tract [9]. In contrast, urban infants of a similar ethnic background who were partly or totally artificially fed frequently acquired diarrheal disease caused by enteropathogenic *E. coli* (EPEC). A more recent study among infants 0 to 3 months old from Bangladesh showed that breast-feeding provided significant protection against diarrheal disease with an adjusted odds ratio of 0.69 (95% confidence interval 0.49-0.98) and respiratory disease with an adjusted odds ratio of 0.69 (95% confidence interval 0.54-0.88) [61]. Protection afforded by breast-feeding against diarrhea during the first months of life has also been observed in more industrialized societies such as the United Kingdom [62].

Multiple mechanisms by which breast-feeding protects against diarrhea have been postulated. Breast-feeding confers protection by active components in milk and by decreased exposure to organisms present on or in contaminated bottles, food, or water. Many protective components have been identified in human milk and generally are classified as belonging to the major categories of cells, antibodies, anti-inflammatory factors, and glycoconjugates and other nonantibody factors [12,63–65]. Examples of milk antibodies are summarized in Table 11–1.

For any given pathogen, multiple milk factors may help protect the infant. Human milk typically targets a major

TABLE 11–1   Association between Antibodies in Human Milk and Protection against Enteropathogens

Organism	Antibody
Vibrio cholerae	Lipopolysaccharide, enterotoxin
Campylobacter jejuni	Surface proteins
Enteropathogenic *Escherichia coli*	Adherence proteins
Enterotoxigenic *E. coli*	Enterotoxin, adherence proteins
Shigatoxin-producing *E. coli*	Adherence proteins
Shigella	Lipopolysaccharide, virulence plasmid–associated antigens
Giardia lamblia	Surface proteins

pathogenic mechanism using multiple, redundant strategies. Redundancy of milk protective factors and targeting of complex virulence machinery have created a formidable barrier to enteropathogens. Despite the fact that pathogens can rapidly divide and mutate, milk continues to protect infants. Human milk has secretory antibodies to *Shigella* virulence antigens and lipopolysaccharides [66,67], neutral glycolipid Gb3 to bind Shiga toxin [68,69], and lactoferrin to disrupt and degrade the surface-expressed virulence antigens. Lactoferrin chelates iron, making it unavailable for bacterial metabolism; stimulates phagocytosis; and inhibits several viruses, such as human immunodeficiency virus (HIV), cytomegalovirus, and herpes simplex virus [30,70–72]. In a similar way, milk contains antibodies directed toward the surface-expressed virulence antigens of EPEC [73], oligosaccharides that block EPEC cell attachment [74], and lactoferrin interference with EPEC surface factors [75]. Human milk can initiate and maintain the growth of *Bifidobacterium* species and low pH in the feces of newborn infants, creating an environment antagonistic to the growth of *E. coli* [9,27,28,76]. Lysozyme in human milk breaks β1,4 bonds between *N*-acetylmuramic acid and *N*-acetylglucosamine, a critical linkage in the peptidoglycans of bacterial cell walls [30].

The protective effect of human milk antibodies against enteropathogen-specific disease has been described for *Vibrio cholerae* [77], *Campylobacter jejuni* [78], EPEC [74], enterotoxigenic *E. coli* (ETEC) [79,80], *Shigella* species [81,82], and *Giardia lamblia* [83,84]. Protective effects for bovine milk concentrate against ETEC [85], rotavirus [86], and *Shigella* species have also been described [87].

In 1933, the nonlactose carbohydrate fraction of human milk was found to consist mainly of oligosaccharides [88]. In 1960, Montreuil and Mullet [89] determined that oligosaccharides constituted 2.4% of colostrum and 1.3% of mature milk. Human milk contains a larger quantity of oligosaccharides than milk from other mammals, and its composition is singularly complex [90]. The metabolic fate of oligosaccharides is of interest. Only water, lactose, and lipids are present in greater amounts than oligosaccharides. Despite the fact that substantial energy must be expended by the mother to synthesize the many hundreds of different milk oligosaccharides, the infant does not use them as food. Most of the oligosaccharides pass through the gut undigested [91,92]. It is thought that they are present primarily to serve as receptor analogues that misdirect enteropathogen attachment factors away from gut epithelial carbohydrate receptors. Likewise, enteropathogens use the oligosaccharide portion of glycolipids and glycoproteins as targets for attachment of whole bacteria and toxins. Evidence is emerging that these glycoconjugates may have an important role in protection of the breast-fed infant from disease [64].

Human milk protects suckling mice from the heat-stable enterotoxin (ST) of *E. coli*; on the basis of its chemical stability and physical properties, the protective factor has been deduced to be a neutral fucosyloligosaccharide [93,94]. Experiments have shown that EPEC attachment to HEp-2 laryngeal epithelial cells and HIV-1 binding to dendritic cell coreceptor DC-SIGN can be inhibited by purified oligosaccharide fractions

from human milk [74].,[93a] Oligosaccharides also may be relevant to protection from Norwalk virus and other caliciviruses because these viruses attach to human ABO, Lewis, and secretor blood group antigens [94,95]. Human milk contains large amounts of these carbohydrates. The ganglioside fraction in human milk has been shown to inhibit the action of heat-labile toxin (LT) and cholera toxin on ileal loops more effectively than secretory IgA [96,97]. Lactadherin in human milk has been shown to bind rotavirus and to inhibit viral replication in vitro and in vivo [98]. A study of infants in Mexico showed that lactadherin in human milk protected infants from symptoms of rotavirus infection [87]. Free fatty acids and monoglyceride products of lingual and gastric lipase activity in human milk triglycerides may have antiviral and antiparasitic activity [30]. Human milk oligosaccharides also inhibit leukocyte endothelial adhesion and help explain the low rate of inflammatory disorders in breast-fed infants [98a].

BACTERIAL PATHOGENS
ESCHERICHIA COLI

E. coli promptly colonize the lower intestinal tracts of healthy infants in the first few days of life [99–102] and constitute the predominant aerobic coliform fecal flora throughout life in humans and in many animals. The concept that this species might cause enteric disease was first suggested in the late 19th and early 20th centuries, when several veterinary workers described the association of diarrhea (i.e., scours) in newborn calves with certain strains of *E. coli* [103–108].

In 1905, Moro [109] observed that *Bacterium* (now *Escherichia*) *coli* was found more often in the small intestines of children with diarrhea than in children without diarrhea. Adam [110,111] confirmed these findings and noted the similarity with Asiatic cholera and calf scours. He extended these observations further by suggesting that *E. coli* strains from patients with diarrhea could be distinguished from normal coliform flora by certain sugar fermentation patterns. Although Adam called these disease-producing organisms "dyspepsicoli" and introduced the important concept that *E. coli* could cause enteric disease, biochemical reactions have not proved to be a reliable means of distinguishing nonpathogenic from pathogenic *E. coli* strains. There are now at least six recognized enteric pathotypes of *E. coli* [112]. The pathotypes can be distinguished clinically, epidemiologically, and pathogenetically (Table 11–2) [112–120].

ETEC organisms are defined by their ability to secrete LT or ST enterotoxin, or both. LT is closely related to cholera toxin and similarly acts by means of intestinal adenylate cyclase [121,122], prostaglandin synthesis [123,124], and possibly platelet-activating factor [125,126]. ST (particularly the variant STa) causes secretion by specifically activating intestinal mucosal guanylate cyclase [127–129]. STb toxin stimulates noncyclic, nucleotide-mediated bicarbonate secretion and seems to be important only in animals [130–132]. Enteroinvasive *E. coli* (EIEC) has the capacity to invade the intestinal mucosa, causing inflammatory enteritis similar to shigellosis [133,134]. EPEC elicits diarrhea by a signal transduction mechanism [112–118,135,136], which

TABLE 11–2 Predominant Serogroups, Mechanisms, and Gene Codes Associated with Enterotoxigenic, Enteroinvasive, Enteropathogenic, Enterohemorrhagic, and Enteroaggregative *Escherichia coli*

ETEC	EIEC	EPEC	EHEC	EAEC
Class I Serogroup				
LT				
O6:K15 O8:K40	O28ac O29, O112 O115, O124 O136, O144	O55:K59 (B5) O111ab:K88 (B4) O119K6a (B14)	O157:H7 O26:H11/H– O128, O103:H2 O39	O3:H2 O44 O78:H33 O15:H11
LT and ST				
O11:H27 O15, O20:K79 O25:K7 O27, O63 O80, O85, O139	O147, O152 O164	O125ac:K70 (B15) O126:K71 (B16) O127a:K63 (B8) O128abc:K67 (B12) O142, O158	O111:K58:H8/H– O113:K75:H7/H21 O121:H–, O145:H– Rough And many others	O77:H18 O51:H11 And many others
Class II Serogroup				
ST				
O groups 78, 115, 128, 148, 149, 153, 159, 166, 167		O44:K74 O86a:K61 (B7) O114:H2		
Mechanisms				
Adenylate or guanylate cyclase activation	Colonic invasiveness (e.g., *Shigella*)	Localized attachment and effacement	Shiga toxins block protein synthesis; attachment and effacement	Aggregative adherence and toxins
Gene Codes				
Plasmid	Chromosomal and plasmid	Chromosomal and plasmid	Phage and chromosomal	Plasmid and chromosomal

EAEC, enteroaggregative E. coli; *EHEC, enterohemorrhagic* E. coli; *EIEC, enteroinvasive* E. coli; *EPEC, enteropathogenic* E. coli; *ETEC, enterotoxigenic* Escherichia coli; *LT, heat-labile toxin; ST, heat-stable toxin.*

is accompanied by a characteristic attaching-and-effacing histopathologic lesion in the small intestine [137]. Enterohemorrhagic *E. coli* (EHEC) also induces an attaching-and-effacing lesion, but in the colon [112]. EHEC secretes Shiga toxin, which gives rise to the dangerous sequela of hemolytic-uremic syndrome (HUS). Diffusely adherent *E. coli* [138] executes a signal transduction effect, which is accompanied by the induction of long cellular processes [139]. Enteroaggregative *E. coli* (EAEC) adheres to the intestinal mucosa and elaborates enterotoxins and cytotoxins [112,119,140].

A major problem in the recognition of ETEC, EIEC, EPEC, and EHEC strains of *E. coli* is that they are indistinguishable from normal coliform flora of the intestinal tract by the usual bacteriologic methods. Serotyping is valuable in recognizing EPEC serotypes [141] and EIEC because these organisms tend to fall into a few specific serogroups (see Table 11–2) [141,142]. EIEC invasiveness is confirmed by inoculating fresh isolates into guinea pig conjunctivae, as described by Sereny [143]. The ability of organisms to produce enterotoxins (LT or ST) is encoded by a transmissible plasmid that can be lost by one strain of *E. coli* or transferred to a previously unrecognized strain [144–146]. Although the

enterotoxin plasmids seem to prefer certain serogroups (different from EPEC or invasive serogroups) [147], ETEC is not expected to be strictly limited to a particular set of serogroups. Instead, these strains can be recognized only by identifying the enterotoxins or the genes encoding them. The toxin can be assayed in ligated animal loops [150], in tissue culture [151,152], or by enzyme-linked immunosorbent assay (ELISA) [153] for LT or in a suckling mouse model for ST [154,155]. Specific DNA probes and, more importantly, polymerase chain reaction (PCR) assays are available to detect LT and ST genes [112–114]. The various *E. coli* pathotypes are generally attended by a broad array of primary and accessory virulence factors, as discussed subsequently [156–158].

Enterotoxigenic *Escherichia coli*

Although early work on the recognition of *E. coli* as a potential enteric pathogen focused on biochemical or serologic distinctions, there followed a shift in emphasis to the enterotoxins produced by previously recognized and entirely "new" strains of *E. coli*. Beginning in the mid-1950s with work by De and colleagues [159,160] in

Calcutta, *E. coli* strains from patients with diarrhea were found to cause a fluid secretory response in ligated rabbit ileal loops analogous to that seen with *V. cholerae*. Work by Taylor and associates [161,162] showed that the viable *E. coli* strains were not required to produce this secretory response and that enterotoxin production correlated poorly with classically recognized EPEC serotypes. In São Paulo, Trabulsi [163] made similar observations with *E. coli* isolated from children with diarrhea, and several veterinary workers showed that ETEC was associated with diarrhea in piglets and calves [164–167]. A similar pattern was described in 1971, when *E. coli* strains were isolated from upper small bowel samples of adults with acute undifferentiated diarrhea in Bengal [168,169]. Such strains of *E. coli* produced a heat-labile nondialyzable ammonium sulfate–precipitable enterotoxin [170].

Analogous to the usually short-lived diarrheal illnesses of *E. coli* reported by several workers, a short-lived course of the secretory response to *E. coli* culture filtrates was described [171]. Similar to responses to cholera toxin, secretory responses to *E. coli* were associated with activation of intestinal mucosal adenylate cyclase that paralleled the fluid secretory response [172,173].

The two types of enterotoxins produced by *E. coli* [174–176] have been found to be plasmid-encoded but genetically unlinked. The plasmids encoding LT and ST also encode the colonization factor antigens (CFAs), adhesins required for intestinal colonization, and the regulator that controls CFA expression [144–146,177].

ST causes an immediate and reversible secretory response [150], whereas the effects of LT (e.g., cholera toxin) follow a lag period necessitated by its intracellular site of action [121,122,151]. LT is internalized into target epithelial cells by retrograde vesicular transport. When inside the cytoplasm, the toxin acts by adenosine diphosphate–ribosylation of the $G_{s\alpha}$ signaling protein [112,121]. The resulting activation of adenylate cyclase leads to accumulation of cyclic adenosine monophosphate (cAMP), which activates the CFTR chloride channel. Activation of adenylate cyclase by LT and by cholera toxin is highly promiscuous, occurring in many cell types and resulting in development of nonintestinal tissue culture assay systems such as the Chinese hamster ovary (CHO) cell assay [151] and Y1 adrenal cell assay [152]. The antigenic similarity of LT and cholera toxin and their apparent binding to the monosialoganglioside GM_1 have enabled development of ELISAs for detection of LT and cholera toxin [155,178–180].

ST is a much smaller molecule and is distinct antigenically from LT and cholera toxin [151,154,155]. Although it fails to alter cAMP levels, ST increases intracellular intestinal mucosal cyclic guanosine monophosphate (cGMP) concentrations and specifically activates apical plasma membrane–associated intestinal guanylate cyclase [127–129]. Similar to cAMP analogues, cGMP analogues cause intestinal secretion that mimics the response to ST [127]. The receptor for STa responds to an endogenous ligand called guanylin, of which STa is a structural homologue [181]. Because the capacity to produce an enterotoxin may be transmissible between different organisms by a plasmid or even a bacteriophage [144–146], interstrain gene transfer is likely to be responsible for occasional toxigenic

non–*E. coli*. Enterotoxigenic *Klebsiella* and *Citrobacter* strains have been associated with diarrhea in a few reports, often in patients coinfected with ETEC [182,183]. Likewise, certain strains of *Salmonella* seem to produce an LT, CHO cell–positive toxin that may play a similar role in the pathogenesis of the watery, noninflammatory diarrhea sometimes seen with *Salmonella enteritidis* infection [184,185].

At least 20 CFAs have been described for human *E. coli* isolates [112,187,188] against which local IgA antibody may be produced. These antigens may potentially be useful in vaccine development. CFAs are proteinaceous hairlike fimbriae that decorate the bacterial surface and serve as a bridge between the bacterium and the epithelial membrane. Veterinary workers first showed that the plasmid-encoded fimbriate K-88 surface antigen was necessary for ETEC to cause disease in piglets [177]. An autosomal dominant allele seems to be responsible for the specific intestinal receptor in piglets. In elegant studies by Gibbons and coworkers [186], the homozygous recessive piglets lacked the receptor for K-88 and were resistant to scours caused by ETEC.

Epidemiology and Transmission

ETEC are important diarrheal pathogens among infants in developing countries. Breast-feeding seems to provide some protection, however, accounting for the classic association of ETEC with weaning diarrhea. Whether or not this epidemiologic pattern still prevails in impoverished countries is not well understood [149]. ETEC have also been recognized among adults with endemic, cholera-like diarrhea in Calcutta, India, and in Dacca, Bangladesh [121,168], and among travelers to areas such as Mexico and Central Africa [189–191].

The isolation of ETEC is uncommon in sporadic diarrheal illnesses in temperate climates where sanitation facilities are good and where winter viral patterns of diarrhea predominate. ETEC is commonly isolated from infants and children with acute watery summer diarrhea in areas where sanitary facilities are suboptimal [49,182, 191–203], such as Africa [182], Brazil [49,191,197,202, 203], Argentina [193], Bengal [194,195], Mexico [196], and Native American reservations in the southwestern United States [198,199]. In a multicenter study of acute diarrhea in 3640 infants and children in China, India, Mexico, Myanmar, and Pakistan, 16% of cases (versus 5% of 3279 controls) had ETEC [200]. A case-control study from northwestern Spain showed a highly significant association of ETEC with 26.5% of neonatal diarrhea, often acquired in the hospital [201]. Although all types of ETEC are associated with cholera-like, noninflammatory, watery diarrhea in adults in these areas, they probably also constitute the major cause (along with rotaviruses) of dehydrating diarrhea in infants and young children in these areas. In this setting, peaks of illnesses tend to occur in the summer or rainy season, and dehydrating illnesses may be life-threatening, especially in infants and young children [49,197,202]. Humans are probably the major reservoirs for the human strains of ETEC, and contaminated food and water probably constitute the principal vectors [204,205]. Although antitoxic immunity to LT and asymptomatic infection with

LT-producing *E. coli* tend to increase with age, ST is poorly immunogenic, and ST-producing *E. coli* continue to be associated with symptomatic illnesses into adulthood in endemic areas [199,203].

The association of ETEC with outbreaks of diarrhea in newborn nurseries is well documented. Ryder and colleagues [206] isolated ST-producing *E. coli* from 72% of infants with diarrhea, from the environment, and in one instance from an infant's formula during a 7-month period in a prolonged outbreak in a special care nursery in Texas. Another ST-producing *E. coli* outbreak was reported in 1976 by Gross and associates [207] from a maternity hospital in Scotland. ETEC and EPEC were significantly associated with diarrhea among infants younger than 1 year in Bangladesh [208].

An outbreak of diarrhea in a newborn special care nursery that was associated with enterotoxigenic organisms that were not limited to the same serotype or even the same species was reported [209]. The short-lived ETEC, *Klebsiella*, and *Citrobacter* species in this outbreak raised the possibility that each infant's indigenous bowel flora might become transiently toxigenic, possibly by receiving the LT gene from a plasmid or even a bacteriophage.

Clinical Manifestations

The clinical manifestations of ETEC diarrhea tend to be mild and self-limited except in small or undernourished infants, in whom dehydration may constitute a major threat to life. In many parts of the developing world, acute diarrheal illnesses are the leading recognized causes of death. There is some suggestion that diarrheal illnesses associated with ST-producing ETEC may be particularly severe [195]. Probably the best definition of the clinical manifestations of ETEC infection comes from volunteer studies with adults. Ingestion of 10^8 to 10^{10} human ETEC isolates that produce LT and ST or ST alone resulted in a 30% to 80% attack rate of mild to moderate diarrheal illnesses within 12 to 56 hours that lasted 1 to 3 days [133]. These illnesses, typical for traveler's diarrhea, were manifested by malaise, anorexia, abdominal cramps, and sometimes explosive diarrhea. Nausea and vomiting occur relatively infrequently, and one third of patients may have a low-grade fever. Although illnesses usually resolve spontaneously within 1 to 5 days, they occasionally may persist for 1 week or longer. The diarrhea is noninflammatory, without fecal leukocytes or blood. In outbreaks in infants and neonates, the duration has been in the same range (1 to 11 days), with a mean of approximately 4 days.

Pathology

As in cholera, the pathologic changes associated with ETEC infection are minimal. From animal experiments in which intestinal loops were infected with these organisms and at a time when the secretory and adenylate cyclase responses were present, there was only a mild discharge of mucus from goblet cells and otherwise no significant pathologic change in the intestinal tract [122]. Unless terminal complications of severe hypotension ensue, ETEC organisms rarely disseminate beyond the intestinal tract. Similar to cholera, ETEC diarrhea is typically limited to being an intraluminal infection.

Diagnosis

The preliminary diagnosis of ETEC diarrhea can be suspected by the epidemiologic setting and the noninflammatory nature of stool specimens, which reveal few or no leukocytes. Although the ability of *E. coli* to produce enterotoxins may be lost or transmitted to other strains, there is a tendency for the enterotoxin-encoding plasmids to occur among certain predominant serotypes, as shown in Table 11–2 [147]. These serotypes differ from EPEC or invasive serotypes, but their demonstration does not prove that they are enterotoxigenic. The traditional way to identify ETEC is to show the enterotoxin itself by a bioassay, such as tissue culture or ileal loop assays for LT or the suckling mouse assay for ST; ELISA is available for LT, and inhibitory ELISA is available for ST [148].

More recently, detection of enterotoxin-encoding genes has superseded detection of the toxins themselves. Gene probe and PCR technologies are available [113,114]. The presence of *E. coli* encoding the enterotoxins in patients with diarrhea is generally considered diagnostic, although asymptomatic carriage is known to occur [149]. In epidemiologic studies, it is common to test only three colonies per stool for the presence of ETEC, but it is generally considered that testing additional colonies increases diagnostic sensitivity [205,210,211]. A novel method of combining immunomagnetic separation (using antibody-coated magnetic beads) followed by DNA or PCR probing may enhance the sensitivity of screening fecal or food specimens for ETEC or other pathogens [212,213].

Therapy and Prevention

The mainstay of treatment of any diarrheal illness is rehydration [214]. This principle especially pertains to ETEC diarrhea, which is an intraluminal infection with high output of fluid and electrolytes. The glucose absorptive mechanism remains intact in *E. coli* enterotoxin–induced secretion, much as it does in cholera, a concept that has resulted in the major advance of oral glucose-electrolyte therapy. This regimen can usually provide fully adequate rehydration in infants and children able to tolerate oral fluids, replacing the need for parenteral rehydration in most cases [215,216]. Use of oral glucose-electrolyte therapy is particularly critical in rural areas and developing nations, where early application before dehydration becomes severe may be lifesaving.

The standard World Health Organization solution contains 3.5 g of NaCl, 2.5 g of $NaHCO_3$, 1.5 g of KCl, and 20 g of glucose per 1 L of clean or boiled drinking water [214]. This corresponds to the following concentrations: 90 mmol/L of sodium, 20 mmol/L of potassium, 30 mmol/L of bicarbonate, 80 mmol/L of chloride, and 110 mmol/L of glucose. Various recipes for homemade preparations have been described [217], but unless the cost is prohibitive, the premade standard solution is preferred. Each 4 oz of this solution should be followed by 2 oz of plain water. If there is concern about hypertonicity, especially in small infants in whom a high intake and constant direct supervision of feeding cannot be ensured, the concentration of salt can be reduced [218]. In a multicenter trial involving 447 children in four countries, a reduced osmolality solution with

60 mmol/L of sodium and 84 mmol/L of glucose and a total osmolality of 224 (instead of 311) mOsm/kg was found to reduce stool output by 28% and illness duration by 18% [219]. Commercially available rehydration solutions are increasingly available worldwide [214].

The role of antimicrobial agents in the treatment or prevention of ETEC is controversial. This infection usually resolves within 3 to 5 days in the absence of antibacterial therapy [214]. There is concern about the potential for coexistence of enterotoxigenicity and antibiotic resistance on the same plasmid, and cotransfer of multiple antibiotic resistance and enterotoxigenicity has been well documented [220]. Widespread use of prophylactic antibiotics in areas where antimicrobial resistance is common has the potential for selecting for rather than against enterotoxigenic organisms. The prevention and control of ETEC infections are similar to those discussed under EPEC serotypes. Breast-feeding infants should be encouraged. When antibiotic therapy is desired, cefixime, azithromycin, and, in adults, ciprofloxacin are recommended [221,222], although infants are generally not treated.

Enteroinvasive *Escherichia coli*

EIEC is similar pathogenetically, epidemiologically, and clinically to shigellosis, although the clinical syndrome associated with EIEC may be milder than that caused by *Shigella* species. EIEC causes diarrhea by means of *Shigella*-like intestinal epithelial invasion (discussed later) [133,134]. The somatic antigens of these invasive strains have been identified and seem to fall into 1 of 10 recognized O groups (see Table 11–2). Most, if not all, of these bacteria share cell wall antigens with one or another of the various *Shigella* serotypes and produce positive reactions with antisera against the cross-reacting antigen [134]. Not all strains of *E. coli* belonging to the 10 serogroups associated with dysentery-like illness are pathogenic, however, because a large (140 MDa) invasive plasmid is also required [223]. Additional biologic tests, including the guinea pig conjunctivitis (Sereny) test or a gene probe for the plasmid, are used to confirm the property of invasiveness [133].

Although an outbreak of food-borne EIEC diarrhea has been well documented among adults who ate an imported cheese [134], little is known about the epidemiology and transmission of this organism, especially in newborns and infants. Whether the infectious dose may be as low as it is for *Shigella* is unknown; however, studies of adult volunteers suggest that attack rates may be lower after ingestion of even larger numbers of EIEC than typical for *Shigella* disease. The outbreak of EIEC diarrhea resulted in a dysentery-like syndrome with an inflammatory exudate in stool and invasion and disruption of colonic mucosa [134].

Descriptions of extensive and severe ileocolitis in infants dying with *E. coli* diarrhea indicate that neonatal disease also can be caused by invasive strains capable of mimicking the pathologic features of shigellosis [224]. The immunofluorescent demonstration of *E. coli* together with an acute inflammatory infiltrate [225] in the intestinal tissue of infants tends to support this impression, although it has been suggested that the organisms may have invaded the bowel wall in the postmortem period [133]. There is still

little direct evidence concerning the role of invasive strains of *E. coli* in the cause of neonatal diarrhea [191]. The infrequency with which newborns manifest a dysentery-like syndrome makes it unlikely that this pathogen is responsible for a very large proportion of the diarrheal disease that occurs during the first month of life.

The diagnosis should be suspected in infants who have an inflammatory diarrhea as evidenced by fecal polymorphonuclear neutrophils or bloody dysenteric syndromes from whom no other invasive pathogens, such as *Campylobacter*, *Shigella*, *Salmonella*, *Vibrio*, or *Yersinia*, can be isolated. In this instance, it may be appropriate to have the fecal *E. coli* isolated and serotyped or tested for invasiveness in the Sereny test. Plasmid pattern analysis and chromosomal restriction endonuclease digestion pattern analysis by pulsed-field gel electrophoresis have been used to evaluate strains involved in outbreaks [226]. The management and prevention of EIEC diarrhea should be similar to management and prevention of acute *Shigella* or other *E. coli* enteric infections.

Enteropathogenic *Escherichia coli*: Classic Serotypes

EPEC is a classic cause of severe infant diarrhea in industrialized countries, although its incidence has diminished dramatically in recent years. The serologic distinction of *E. coli* strains associated with epidemic and sporadic infantile diarrhea was first suggested by Goldschmidt in 1933[227] and confirmed by Dulaney and Michelson in 1935 [351]. These researchers found that certain strains of *E. coli* associated with institutional outbreaks of diarrhea would agglutinate with sera from diarrhea patients in other outbreaks. In 1943, Bray [228] isolated a serologically homogeneous strain of *E. coli* (subsequently identified as serogroup O111) from 95% of infants with summer diarrhea in England. He subsequently summarized a larger experience with this organism, isolated from only 4% of asymptomatic controls, but from 88% of infants with diarrhea, one half of which was hospital acquired [229]. This strain (initially called *E. coli-gomez* by Varela in 1946) also was associated with infantile diarrhea in Mexico [230]. A second type of *E. coli* (called beta by Giles in 1948 and subsequently identified as O55) was associated with an outbreak of infantile diarrhea in Aberdeen, Scotland [231,232].

An elaborate serotyping system for certain *E. coli* strains that were clearly associated with infantile diarrhea developed from this early work primarily with epidemic diarrhea in infants [233–235]. These strains first were called enteropathogenic *E. coli* by Neter and colleagues [236] in 1955, and the association with particular serotypes can still be observed [237]. As shown in Table 11–1, these organisms are distinct from the enterotoxigenic or enteroinvasive organisms or organisms that inhabit the normal GI tract. They exhibit localized adherence to HEp-2 cells, a phenotype that has been suggested to be useful for diagnosis and pathogenesis research [135].

Epidemiology and Transmission

EPEC is now an important cause of diarrhea in infants in developing or transitional countries [112,238–240]. Outbreaks have become rare in the United States and other industrialized countries, but they still occur [241]. Some researchers have attributed the rare recognition of illness in part to the declining severity of diarrheal disease caused by EPEC within the past 30 years, resulting in fewer cultures being obtained from infants with relatively mild symptoms [112,242]. Several other variables influence the apparent incidence of this disease in the community, however. A problem arises with false-positive EPEC identification on the basis of the nonspecific cross-reactions seen with improper shortening of the serotyping procedure [243,244]. Because of their complexity and relatively low yield, neither slide agglutination nor HEp-2 cell adherence or DNA probe tests are provided as part of the routine identification of enteric pathogens by most clinical bacteriology laboratories. Failure to recognize the presence of EPEC in fecal specimens is the inevitable consequence.

The apparent incidence of EPEC gastroenteritis also varies with the epidemiologic circumstances under which stool cultures are obtained. The prevalence of enteropathogenic strains is higher among infants from whom cultures are obtained during a community epidemic compared with cultures obtained during sporadic diarrheal disease. Neither cultures obtained during a community epidemic nor cultures obtained during sporadic diarrheal disease reflect the incidence of EPEC infection among infants involved in a nursery outbreak or hospital epidemic.

EPEC gastroenteritis is a worldwide problem, and socioeconomic conditions play a significant role in determining the incidence of this disease in different populations [245]. It is unusual for newborn infants born in a rural environment to manifest diarrheal disease caused by EPEC; most infections of the GI tract in these infants occur after the first 6 months of life [9,246]. Conversely, among infants born in large cities, the attack rate of EPEC is high during the first 3 months of life. This age distribution reflects in large part the frequency with which EPEC causes cross-infection outbreaks among nursery populations [207,247–254]; however, a predominance of EPEC in infants in the first 3 months of life has also been described in community epidemics [255–257] and among sporadic cases of diarrhea acquired outside the hospital [258–264]. The disparity in the incidence of neonatal EPEC infection between rural and urban populations has been ascribed to two factors: the trend away from breast-feeding among mothers in industrialized societies and the crowding together of susceptible newborns in nurseries in countries in which hospital deliveries predominate over home deliveries [9,246,265]. Although the predominant serogroup can vary from year to year,* the same strains have been prevalent during the past 40 years in Great Britain [268], Puerto Rico [269], Guatemala [9], Panama [223], Israel [264], Newfoundland [257], Indonesia [261], Thailand [270], Uganda [271], and South Africa [272].

When living conditions are poor and overcrowding of susceptible infants exists, there is an increase in the incidence of neonatal diarrhea in general [273] and EPEC gastroenteritis in particular [232,255,274]. A higher incidence of asymptomatic family carriers is likewise found in such situations [255,256].

Newborns can acquire EPEC during the first days of life by one of several routes: (1) organisms from the mother ingested at the time of birth; (2) bacteria from other infants or toddlers with diarrheal disease or from asymptomatic adults colonized with the organism, commonly transmitted on the hands of nursery personnel or parents; (3) airborne or droplet infection; (4) fomites; or (5) organisms present in formulas or solid food supplements [275]. Only the first two routes have been shown conclusively to be of significance in the transmission of disease or the propagation of epidemics.

Most neonates acquire EPEC at the time of delivery through ingestion of organisms residing in the maternal birth canal or rectum. Stool cultures taken from women before, during, or shortly after delivery have shown that 10% to 15% carry EPEC at some time during this period [99,100,102,276,277]. Use of fluorescent antibody techniques [277] or cultures during a community outbreak of EPEC gastroenteritis [102] revealed twice this number of persons excreting the organism. Virtually none of the women carrying pathogenic strains of *E. coli* had symptoms referable to the GI tract.

Many mothers whose stools contain EPEC transmit these organisms to their infants [99,102], resulting in an asymptomatic infection rate of 2% to 5% among newborns cultured at random in nursery surveys [99,100, 207,278]. These results must be considered conservative and are probably an artifact of the sampling technique. One study using 150 O antisera to identify as many *E. coli* as possible in fecal cultures showed a correlation between the coliform flora in 66% of mother-infant pairs [279]. Of particular interest was the observation that the O groups of *E. coli* isolated from the infants' mucus immediately after delivery correlated with those subsequently recovered from their stools, supporting the contention that these organisms were acquired orally at the time of birth. In mothers whose stools contained the same O group as their offspring, the mean time from rupture of membranes to delivery was about 2 hours longer than in mothers whose infants did not acquire the same serogroups, suggesting that ascending colonization before birth also can play a role in determining the newborn's fecal flora.

The contours of the epidemiologic curves in nursery [255,280–285] and community [255–257] outbreaks are in keeping with a contact mode of spread. Transmission of organisms from infant to infant occurs by the fecal-oral route in almost all cases, most likely via the hands of individuals attending to their care [100,283,285,286]. Ill infants represent the greatest risk to individuals around them because of the large numbers of organisms found in their stools [287–290] and vomitus [291–293]. Cross-infection has also been initiated by infants who were healthy at the time of nursery admission [280,288,294–296].

A newborn exposed to EPEC is likely to acquire enteric infection whenever contact with a person excreting the organism is intimate and prolonged, as in a hospital or family setting. Stool culture surveys taken during outbreaks have shown that 20% to 50% of term neonates

---

*References [256,259,260,263,266,267].

residing in the nursery carry EPEC in their intestinal tracts [118,247,248,251]. Despite descriptions of nursery outbreaks in which virtually every neonate or low birth weight infant became infected [278,280,297], there is ample evidence that exposure to pathogenic strains of *E. coli* does not result in greater likelihood of illness for premature infants than for term infants [277,288,295,298]. Any increased prevalence of cross-infections that may exist among premature infants can be explained more readily by their prolonged hospital stays, increased handling, and clustering of infants born in different institutions than by a particular susceptibility to EPEC based on immature defense mechanisms.

The most extensive studies on the epidemiology of gastroenteritis related to *E. coli* have dealt with events that occurred during outbreaks in newborn nurseries. Investigations of this sort frequently regard the epidemic as an isolated phenomenon and ignore the strong interdependence that exists between community-acquired and hospital-acquired illness [296,299,300]. The direction of spread is most often from the reservoir of disease within the community to the hospital. When the original source of a nursery outbreak can be established, frequently it is an infant born of a carrier mother who recently acquired EPEC infection from a toddler living in the home. Cross-infection epidemics also can be initiated by infected newborns that have been admitted directly into a clean nursery unit from the surrounding district [286,288,301] or have been transferred from a nearby hospital [294,296,302].

After a nursery epidemic has begun, it generally follows one of two major patterns. Some epidemics are explosive, with rapid involvement of all susceptible infants and a duration that seldom exceeds 2 or 3 months [280,281,292,303]. The case-fatality rate in these epidemics may be very high. Other nursery outbreaks have an insidious onset with a few mild, unrecognized cases; the patients may not even develop illness until after discharge from the hospital. During the next few days to weeks, neonates with an increased number of loose stools are reported by the nurses; shortly thereafter, the appearance of the first severely ill infants makes it apparent that an epidemic has begun. Unless oral antimicrobial therapy is instituted (see "Therapy"), nursery outbreaks such as these may continue for months [282–285] or years [286], with cycles of illness followed by periods of relative quiescence. This pattern can be caused by multiple strains (of different phage or antibiogram types) sequentially introduced into the nursery [294,304,305].

The nursery can be a source of infection for the community. The release of infants who are in the incubation stages of illness or are convalescent carriers about to relapse may lead to secondary cases of diarrheal disease among young siblings living in widely scattered areas [255,256,260]. These children further disseminate infection to neighboring households, involving playmates of their own age, young infants, and mothers [255,256,259]. As the sickest of these contact cases are admitted to different hospitals, they contaminate new susceptible persons, completing the cycle and compounding the outbreak. This feedback mechanism has proved to be a means of spreading infantile gastroenteritis through entire cities [255,256,259], counties [256,301,306], and provinces [257]. One major

epidemic of diarrhea related to EPEC O111:B4 that occurred in the metropolitan Chicago and northwestern Indiana region during the winter of 1961 involved more than 1300 children and 29 community hospitals during a period of 9 months [257,307]. Almost all of the patients were younger than 2 years, and 10% were younger than 1 month, producing an age-specific attack rate of nearly 4% of neonates in the community. The importance of the hospital as a source of cross-infection in this epidemic was shown through interviews with patients' families, indicating that a minimum of 40% of infants had direct or indirect contact with a hospital shortly before the onset of illness.

It has been suggested, but not proven, that asymptomatic carriers of EPEC in close contact with a newborn infant, such as nursery personnel or family members, might play an important role in the transmission of the bacterium [296,300,308]. Stool culture surveys have shown that at any one time about 1% of adults [259,309] and 1% to 5% of young children [247,255,260] who are free of illness harbor EPEC strains. Higher percentages have been recorded during community epidemics [255,260]. Because this intestinal carriage is transitory [255,296], the number of individuals who excrete EPEC at one time or another during the year is far higher than the 1% figure recorded for single specimens [296,309].

Nursery personnel feed, bathe, and diaper a constantly changing population of newborns, about 2% to 5% of whom excrete EPEC [255,296]. Despite this constant exposure, intestinal carriage among nursery workers is surprisingly low. Even during outbreaks of diarrheal illness, when dissemination of organisms is most intense, less than 5% of the hospital personnel in direct contact with infected neonates are themselves excreting pathogenic strains of *E. coli* [307,310,311].

Although asymptomatic adult carriers generally excrete fewer organisms than patients with acute illness do [288], large numbers of pathogenic bacteria may nevertheless exist in their stools [259,290]. No nursery outbreak and few family cases [257] have been traced to a symptomless carrier, however. Instead, passive transfer of bacteria from infant to infant by the hands of personnel seems to be of primary importance in these outbreaks.

EPEC can be recovered from the throat or nose of 5% to 80% of infants with diarrheal illness [291,310,311] and from about 1% of asymptomatic infants [249,260]. The throat and nasal mucosa may represent a portal of entry or a source of transmission for EPEC. Environmental studies have shown that EPEC is distributed readily and widely in the vicinity of an infant with active diarrheal disease, often within 1 day of admission to the ward [249,312]. Massive numbers of organisms are shed in the diarrheal stool or vomitus of infected infants [266,312]. *E. coli* organisms may survive 2 to 4 weeks in dust [260,312] and can be found in the nursery air when the bedding or diapers of infected infants are disturbed during routine nursing procedures [260,312] or on floors; walls; cupboards; and nursery equipment such as scales, hand towels, bassinets, incubators, and oxygen tents of other infants [102,260,283]. Documentation of the presence of EPEC in nursery air and dust does not by itself establish the importance of this route as a source of cross-infection. One study presented evidence of the respiratory transmission of EPEC; however, even in the cases described, the investigators pointed out that fecal-oral transmission could not be completely ruled out [255]. Additional clinical and experimental data are required to clarify the significance of droplet and environmental infection.

Coliform organisms have also been isolated in significant numbers from human milk [60,313,314], prebottled infant formulas [315], and formulas prepared in the home [308]. EPEC in particular has been found in stool cultures obtained from donors of human milk and workers in a nursery formula room [276]. In one instance, EPEC O111:B4 was isolated from a donor, and subsequently the same serogroup was recovered in massive amounts in almost pure culture from her milk [276]. Pathogenic strains of *E. coli* have also been isolated from raw cow's milk [316] and from drinking water [317]. Likewise, EPEC has been isolated from flies during an epidemic, but this fact has not been shown to be of epidemiologic significance [228,237].

Pathogenesis

Infection of a newborn infant with EPEC occurs exclusively by the oral route. Attempts to induce disease in adult volunteers by rectal instillation of infected material have been unsuccessful [112]. There are no reports of disease occurring after transplacental invasion of the fetal bloodstream by enteropathogenic or nonenteropathogenic strains of *E. coli*. Ascending intrauterine infection after prolonged rupture of the membranes has been reported only once; the neonate in this case had only mild diarrhea [100].

Bacterial cultures of the meconium and feces of newborns indicate that enteropathogenic strains of *E. coli* can effectively colonize the intestinal tract in the first days of life [99–102]. Although *E. coli* may disappear completely from stools of breast-fed infants during the ensuing weeks, this disappearance is believed to be related to factors present in the human milk rather than the gastric secretions [9,318,319]. The use of breast-feeding or expressed human milk has even been effective in terminating nursery epidemics caused by EPEC O111:B4, probably by reducing the incidence of cross-infections among infants [319,320]. Although dose-effect studies have not been performed among newborns, severe diarrhea has occurred after ingestion of 10^8 EPEC organisms by very young infants [321,322]. The high incidence of cross-infection outbreaks in newborn nurseries suggests that a far lower inoculum can often affect spread in this setting.

The role of circulating immunity in the prevention of GI tract disease related to EPEC has not been clearly established. Virtually 100% of maternal sera have been found to contain hemagglutinating [236,323,324], bactericidal [321,325], or bacteriostatic [296,326] antibodies against EPEC. The passive transfer of these antibodies across the placenta is extremely inefficient. Titers in blood of newborn infants are, on average, 4 to 100 times lower than titers in the corresponding maternal sera. Group-specific hemagglutinating antibodies against the O antigen of EPEC are present in 10% to 20% of cord blood samples [236,323,324], whereas bactericidal [323,327] or bacteriostatic [327] activity against these organisms can be found much more frequently. Tests for bacterial agglutination, which are relatively insensitive, are positive in only a small percentage of neonates [236,327].

The importance of circulating antibodies in the susceptibility of infants to EPEC infection is unknown. Experiments with suckling mice have failed to show any effect of humoral immunity on the establishment or course of duration of intestinal colonization with *E. coli* O127 in mothers or their infants [328]. Similar observations have been made in epidemiologic studies among premature human infants using enteropathogenic (O127:B8) [325] and nonenteropathogenic (O4:H5) [285] strains of *E. coli* as the indicator organisms. In a cohort of 63 mothers and their infants followed from birth to 3 months old, Cooper and associates [99] showed a far higher incidence of clinical EPEC disease in infants of EPEC-negative mothers than in infants born of mothers with EPEC isolated from stool cultures. This finding suggests the possibility that mothers harboring EPEC in their GI tracts transfer specific antibodies to their infants that confer some protection during the first weeks of life.

Protection against enteric infections in humans often correlates more closely with levels of local secretory rather than serum antibodies. Although it is known that colonization of newborns with *E. coli* leads to the production of coproantibodies against the ingested organisms [329,330], the clinical significance of this intestinal immunity is uncertain. The previously mentioned experiment with mice showed no effect of active intestinal immunity on enteric colonization [328]. In human infants, the frequency of bacteriologic and clinical relapse related to EPEC of the same serotype [280,281,295] and the capacity of one strain of EPEC to superinfect a patient already harboring a different strain [264,274,284] also cast some doubt on the ability of mucosal antibodies to inhibit or alter the course of intestinal infection. Studies of the protective effects of orally administered EPEC vaccines could help to resolve these questions [265].

The mechanism by which EPEC causes diarrhea involves a complex array of plasmid and chromosomally encoded traits. EPEC serotypes do not make one of the recognized enterotoxins (LT or ST) as usually measured in tissue culture or animal models [331–335], and these serotypes do not cause a typical invasive colitis or produce a positive Sereny test result [330,331]. Only uncommonly do EPEC strains invade the bloodstream or disseminate [304]. Nevertheless, EPEC strains that test negative in these tests are capable of causing diarrhea; inocula of 10^{10} *E. coli* O142 or O127 organisms caused diarrhea in 8 of 10 adult volunteers [335].

Some EPEC strains may secrete weak enterotoxins [336,337], but the consensus opinion is that the attaching-and-effacing lesion constitutes the critical virulence phenotype for secretory disease [112,137]. Clinical pathologic reports reveal the characteristic attaching-and-effacing lesion in the small intestine of infected infants [338]. The lesion is manifested by intimate (about 10 nm) apposition of the EPEC to the plasma membrane of the enterocytes, with dissolution of the normal brush border and rearrangement of the cytoskeleton [137,338].

In some instances, the bacteria are observed to rise up on pedestal-like structures, which are diagnostic of the infection [137]. Villus blunting, crypt hypertrophy, histiocytic infiltration in the lamina propria, and a reduction in the brush border enzymes may also be observed [338,339].

Two major EPEC virulence factors have been described; strains with both factors are designated as typical EPEC [112,115,340]. One such factor is the locus of enterocyte effacement (LEE), a type III secretion system encoded by the LEE chromosomal pathogenicity island [341–343]. The LEE secretion apparatus injects proteins directly from the cytoplasm of the infecting bacterium into the cytoplasm of the target enterocytes [342]. The injected proteins constitute cytoskeletal toxins, which together elicit the close apposition of the bacterium to the cell, cause the effacement of microvilli, and most likely give rise to the net secretory state [112,115,137]. One critical secreted protein, called translocated intimin receptor (Tir) [136], inserts into the plasma membrane of the epithelial cell, where it serves as the receptor for a LEE-encoded EPEC outer membrane protein called intimin [137]. Animals infected with attaching-and-effacing pathogens mount antibody responses to intimin and Tir [344], and both are considered potential vaccine immunogens. The lack of protection from EPEC reinfection suggests that natural antibody responses to Tir and intimin are not protective.

The second major virulence factor of typical EPEC is the bundle-forming pilus (BFP) [345], which is encoded on a partially conserved 60-MDa virulence plasmid called EPEC adherence factor (EAF) [346]. BFP, a member of the type IV pilus family, mediates aggregation of the bacteria to each other and probably to enterocytes themselves, facilitating mucosal colonization [347]. A BFP mutant was shown to be attenuated in adult volunteers [348]. More recent epidemiologic data suggest that some virulent EPEC may lack the BFP; such strains are termed *atypical EPEC* [349,350]. These strains are not of the characteristic EPEC serotypes, and means to distinguish them clinically and microbiologically are unavailable as of this writing.

Pathology

The principal pathologic lesion in EPEC infection is the attaching-and-effacing lesion, manifest by electron microscopy, but not light microscopy. In chronic cases, villus blunting, crypt hypertrophy, histiocytic infiltration of the lamina propria, and reduced brush border enzymes may be seen. Rothbaum and colleagues [338] described similar findings with dissolution of the glycocalyx and flattened microvilli with the nontoxigenic EPEC strain O119:B14. A wide range of pathologic findings has been reported in infants dying with EPEC gastroenteritis. Most newborns dying with diarrheal disease caused by EPEC show no morphologic changes of the GI tract by gross or microscopic examination of tissues [227,351]. Bray [228] described such "meager" changes in the intestinal tract that "the impression received was that the term gastroenteritis is incorrect." At the other extreme, extensive and severe involvement of the intestinal tract, although distinctly unusual among neonates with

EPEC diarrhea, has been discussed in several reviews of the pathologic anatomy of this disease [264,334,352]. Changes virtually identical to the changes found in infants dying with necrotizing enterocolitis have been reported [352]. Drucker and coworkers [334] found that among 17 infants with EPEC diarrhea who were dying, "intestinal gangrene, and/or perforation, and/or peritonitis were present in five, and intestinal pneumatosis in five."

The reasons for such wide discrepancies in EPEC disease pathology are unclear. The severity of intestinal lesions at the time of death does not correlate with the birth weight of the patient, the age of onset of illness, the serogroup of the infecting strain, or the prior administration of oral or systemic antimicrobial agents. The suggestion that the intensity of inflammatory changes may depend on the duration of the diarrhea [334] cannot be corroborated in autopsy studies [232,280,353] or small intestinal biopsy specimens [354,355]. It is difficult to reconcile such a thesis with the observation that a wide range of intestinal findings can be seen at autopsy among newborns infected by a single serotype of EPEC during an epidemic. The nonspecific pathologic picture described by some researchers includes capillary congestion and edema of the bowel wall and an increase in the number of eosinophils, plasma cells, macrophages, and mononuclear cells in the mucosa and submucosa [278,334,353]. Villous patterns are generally well preserved, although some flattening and broadening of the villi are seen in more severe cases. Almost complete absence of villi and failure of regeneration of small bowel mucosa have been reported in an extreme case [356]. Edema in and around the myenteric plexuses of Auerbach, a common associated finding, may cause the GI tract dilation often seen at autopsy in infants with EPEC infections [264,353,357]. Generally, the distal small intestine shows the most marked alterations; however, the reported pathologic findings may be found at all levels of the intestinal tract.

Several complications of EPEC infection have been reported. Candidal esophagitis accounted for significant morbidity in two series collected before [351] and during [264] the antibiotic era. Oral thrush has been seen in 50% of EPEC-infected infants treated with oral or systemic antibiotics [262,280,353]. Some degree of fatty metamorphosis of the liver has been reported by several investigators [232,351,353]; however, these changes are nonspecific and probably result from the poor caloric intake associated with persistent diarrhea or vomiting. Some degree of bronchopneumonia, probably a terminal event in most cases, exists in a large proportion of newborns dying of EPEC infection [232,351,357]. In one reported series of infant cases, EPEC was shown by immunofluorescent staining in the bronchi, alveoli, and interalveolar septa.

Mesenteric lymph nodes are often swollen and congested with reactive germinal centers in the lymphoid follicles [232,278,309]. Severe lymphoid depletion, unrelated to the duration or severity of the antecedent illness, also has been described [301]. The kidneys frequently show tubular epithelial toxic changes. Various degrees of tubular degeneration and cloudy swelling of convoluted tubules are common findings [232,301,353]. Renal vein thrombosis or cortical necrosis may be observed in infants with disseminated intravascular coagulation in the terminal phases of the illness. The heart is grossly normal in most instances, but may show minimal vacuolar changes of nonspecific toxic myocarditis on microscopic examination [353,357]. Candidal abscesses of the heart [357] and kidneys [301,353,357] have been described. With the exception of mild congestion of the pia arachnoid vessels and some edema of the meninges, examination of the central nervous system reveals few changes [232,278].

Clinical Manifestations

Exposure of newborns to EPEC may be followed by one of several possible consequences: no infection, infection without illness, illness with gastroenteritis of variable severity and duration, and, rarely, septicemia with or without metastatic foci of infection accompanying gastroenteritis. When infants are exposed to EPEC, many become colonized as temporary stool [99,102,248] or pharyngeal [255] carriers with no signs of clinical disease. Although Laurell [358] showed that the percentage of asymptomatic infections increases steadily as age increases, this observation has not been confirmed by other investigators [231,359]. Similarly, the suggestion that prematurity per se is associated with a low incidence of inapparent EPEC infection has been documented in several clinical studies [278,280,281], but refuted in others [269,295].

Most neonates who acquire infection with EPEC eventually show some clinical evidence of gastroenteritis. The incubation period is quite variable. Its duration has been calculated mostly from evidence in outbreaks in newborn nurseries, where the time of first exposure can be clearly defined in terms of birth or admission dates. In these circumstances, almost all infants show signs of illness 2 to 12 days after exposure, and most cases show signs within the first 7 days [232,248,280]. In some naturally acquired [99,100] and experimental [322] infections with heavy exposure, the incubation period may be only 24 hours; the stated upper limit is 20 days [249,360]. The first positive stool culture and the earliest recognizable clinical signs of disease occur simultaneously in most infants [280,282], although colonization may precede symptoms by 7 to 14 days [281,282,361].

The gastroenteritis associated with EPEC infection in the newborn is notable for its marked variation in clinical pattern. Clinical manifestations vary from mild illness manifest only by transient anorexia and failure to gain weight to a sudden explosive fulminating diarrhea causing death within 12 hours of onset. Prematurity, underlying disease, and congenital anomalies often are associated with the more severe forms of illness [231,250,362,363]. Experienced clinicians have observed that the severity of EPEC gastroenteritis has declined markedly during the past 3 decades [242]. The onset of illness usually is insidious, with vague signs of reluctance to feed, lethargy, spitting up of formula, mild abdominal distention, or weight loss that may occur for 1 or 2 days before the first loose stool is passed. Diarrhea usually begins abruptly. It may be continuous and violent, or in milder infections, it may run an intermittent course with 1 or more days of

normal stools followed by 1 or more days of diarrhea. Emesis sometimes is a prominent and persistent early finding. Stools are loose and bright yellow initially, later becoming watery, mucoid, and green. Flecks or streaks of blood, which are commonly seen with enterocolitis caused by *Salmonella*, *Campylobacter*, or *Shigella*, are rarely a feature of EPEC diarrheal disease.

A characteristic seminal smell may pervade the environment of infants infected with EPEC O111:B34 [249, 278,364], and an odor variously described as "pungent," "musty," or "fetid" often surrounds patients excreting other strains in their stools [248,272]. Because the buttocks are repeatedly covered with liquid stools, excoriation of the perianal skin can be an early and persistent problem. Fever is an inconstant feature, and when it occurs, the patient's temperature rarely is greater than 39° C (>102.2° F). Convulsions occur infrequently; their occurrence should alert the clinician to the possible presence of electrolyte disturbances, particularly hypernatremia. Prolonged hematochezia, distention, edema, and jaundice are ominous signs and suggest an unfavorable prognosis [232,257,301].

Most infants receiving antimicrobial agents orally show a cessation of diarrhea, tolerate oral feedings, and resume weight gain within 3 to 7 days after therapy has been started [259,262]. Infants with mild illness who receive no treatment can continue to have intermittent loose stools for 1 to 3 weeks. In one outbreak related to EPEC O142:K86, more than one third of untreated or inappropriately treated infants had diarrhea for more than 14 days in the absence of a recognized enteric pathogen on repeated culturing [283]. Recurrence of diarrhea and vomiting after a period of initial improvement is characteristic of EPEC enteritis [207,256,257].

Although seen most often in newborns who have been treated inadequately or not treated at all, clinical relapses also occur after appropriate therapy. Occasionally, the signs of illness during a relapse can be more severe than those accompanying the initial attack of illness [232, 249,301]. Not all clinical relapses result from persistent infection. Many relapses, particularly relapses that consistently follow attempts at reinstitution of formula feedings [278,281], are caused by disaccharide intolerance, rather than bacterial proliferation. Intestinal superinfections, caused by another serotype of EPEC [299,364,365] or by completely different enteric pathogens, such as *Salmonella* or *Shigella* [262], also can delay the resolution of symptoms. Rarely, infants have a "relapse" caused by an organism from the same O group as the original strain but differing in its H antigen. Unless complete serotyping is performed on all EPEC isolates, such an event easily could be dismissed as being a recurrence rather than a superinfection with a new organism [274,284].

Antimicrobial agents to which the infecting organisms are susceptible often may not eradicate EPEC [262, 281,283], which may persist for weeks [280,299,361] or months [366] after the acute illness has subsided. Although reinfection cannot always be excluded, many infants are discharged from the hospital with positive rectal cultures [248,250]. Dehydration is the most common and serious complication of gastroenteritis caused by EPEC or a toxin-producing *E. coli*. Virtually all deaths directly attributable to the intestinal infection are caused by disturbances in fluids and electrolytes. When stools are frequent in number, large in volume, and violent in release, as they often are in severe infections with abrupt onset, a neonate can lose 15% of body weight in a few hours [249,292]. Rarely, fluid excretion into the lumen of the bowel proceeds so rapidly that reduction of circulating blood volume and shock may intervene before passage of a single loose stool [278]. Before the discovery of the etiologic agent, epidemic diarrhea of the newborn was also known by the term *cholera infantum*.

Mild disease, particularly when aggravated by poor fluid intake, can lead to a subtle but serious deterioration of an infant's metabolic status. Sometimes, a week or more of illness elapses before it becomes apparent that an infant with borderline acidosis and dehydration who seemed to be responding to oral fluids alone requires parenteral therapy for improvement [288]. It is incumbent on the clinician caring for small infants with gastroenteritis to follow them closely, with particular attention to serial weights, until full recovery can be confirmed.

Few other complications, with the possible exception of aspiration pneumonia, are directly related to EPEC gastroenteritis. Protracted diarrhea and nutritional failure may occur as a consequence of functional damage to the small intestinal mucosa, with secondary intolerance to dietary sugars [281,356]. Necrotizing enterocolitis, which occasionally results in perforation of the bowel and peritonitis, has not been causally related to infection with EPEC [264,280,282]. A review of most of the large clinical series describing EPEC disease in infants ranging in age from newborn to 2 years revealed only three proven instances of bacteremia [281,294], one possible urinary tract infection [281], and one documented case of meningitis in an infant of unspecified age [367]. Focal infections among neonates were limited to several cases of otitis media [264,278] and a subcutaneous abscess [310] from which EPEC was isolated. Additional complications include interstitial pneumonia [334], GI bleeding with or without disseminated intravascular coagulation [352,368], and methemoglobinemia caused by a mutant of EPEC O127:B8 that was capable of generating large quantities of nitrite from proteins present in the GI tract [369].

Diagnosis

The gold standard of EPEC diagnostics is identification in the stool of *E. coli* carrying genes for BFP and LEE. Identification of these genes can be accomplished by molecular methods (discussed later), but lack of access to these methods has led many laboratories to rely on surrogate markers, such as serotyping [31]. Classic EPEC has been recovered from the vomitus, stool, or bowel contents of infected newborns. Isolation from bile [250] and the upper respiratory tract [99,255,256] has been described in instances in which a specific search has been made. Less commonly, EPEC is isolated from ascitic fluid [269] or purulent exudates [227,232,310]; occasionally, the organism has been recovered from blood cultures [281,294], urine [281], and cerebrospinal fluid.

Stool cultures generally are more reliable than rectal swabs in detecting the presence of enteric pathogens, although a properly obtained swab should be adequate to show EPEC in most cases [234,312,370]. Specimens should be obtained as early in the course of the illness as possible because organisms are present in virtually pure culture during the acute phase of the enteritis, but diminish in numbers during convalescence. Because of the preponderance of EPEC in diarrheal stools, two cultures are adequate for isolation of these pathogens in almost all cases of active disease. Studies using fluorescent antibody methods for identification of EPEC in stool specimens have shown that during the incubation period of the illness, during convalescence, and among asymptomatic carriers of EPEC, organisms can be excreted in such small numbers that they escape detection by standard bacteriologic methods in a significant proportion of infants [262,371,372]. Three to 10 specimens may be required to detect EPEC using methods that identify individual EPEC isolates in the stool [99,363].

After a stool specimen is received, it should be plated as quickly as possible onto noninhibiting media or placed in a preservative medium if it is to be held for longer periods. Deep freezing of specimens preserves viable EPEC when a prolonged delay in isolation is necessary [235]. No selective media, biochemical reactions, or colonial variations permit differentiation of pathogenic and nonpathogenic strains. Certain features may aid in the recognition of two important serogroups. Cultures of serogroups O111:B4 and O55:B5, in contrast to many other coliforms, are sticky or stringy when picked with a wire loop and are rarely hemolytic on blood agar [234,236], whereas O111:B4 colonies emit a distinctive evanescent odor commonly described as "seminal." [231,351] This unusual odor first led Bray [364] to suspect that specific strains of *E. coli* might be responsible for infantile gastroenteritis.

Simpler than molecular detection, serotyping can be used to identify likely EPEC strains, especially in outbreaks [233]. *E. coli*, similar to other Enterobacteriaceae members, possesses cell wall somatic antigens (O), envelope or capsular antigens (K), and, if motile, flagellar antigens (H). Many O groups may be divided further into two or more subgroups (a, b, c), and the K antigens are divisible into at least three varieties (B, L, A) on the basis of their physical behavior. Organisms that do not possess flagellar antigens are nonmotile (designated NM). The EPEC B capsular surface antigen prevents agglutination by antibodies directed against the underlying O antigen. Heating at 100° C for 1 hour inactivates the agglutinability and antigenicity of the B antigen.

Slide agglutination tests with polyvalent O or OB antiserum may be performed on suspensions of colonies typical of *E. coli* that have been isolated from infants with diarrhea, especially in nursery outbreaks. Because of numerous false-positive "cross-reactions," the O and K (or B) type must be confirmed by titration with the specific antisera [244]. Its presence alone does not prove that EPEC is the cause of diarrhea in an individual patient. Mixed cultures with two or three serotypes of EPEC have been shown in 1% to 10% of patients [261,262,368]. This need not mean that both or all three serotypes are causative agents. Secondary infection with hospital-acquired strains can occur during convalescence [189, 297,299,373], and some infants may have been asymptomatic carriers of one serotype at the time that another produced diarrheal disease.

A similar explanation may pertain to mixed infections with EPEC and *Salmonella* or *Shigella* [234,237,374]. Nelson [262] reported the presence of these pathogens in combination with EPEC in 14% of infants who were cultured as part of an antibiotic therapy trial. *Salmonella* and *Shigella* that had not been identified on cultures obtained at admission were isolated only after institution of oral therapy with neomycin. Nelson also [262] postulated that the alteration in bowel flora brought about by the neomycin facilitated the growth of these organisms, which had previously been suppressed and obscured by coliform overgrowth. It is important to seek all enteric pathogens in primary and follow-up cultures of infantile diarrhea, particularly when the specimen originates from a patient in a newborn nursery or infants' ward.

Although EPEC gastroenteritis was previously considered to be synonymous with "summer diarrhea," community outbreaks have occurred as frequently, if not more frequently, in the colder seasons [150,177,375]. It has been suggested that the increased incidence at that time of year might be related to the heightened chance of contact between infants and toddlers that is bound to occur when children remain indoors in close contact [310]. Nursery epidemics, which depend on the chance introduction and dissemination of EPEC within a relatively homogeneous population and stable environment, exhibit no seasonal prevalence. Average relative humidity, temperature, and hours of daylight have no significant effect in determining whether an outbreak follows the introduction of enteropathogenic strains of *E. coli* into a ward of infants [260].

There are no clinical studies of the variations in peripheral leukocyte count, urine, or cerebrospinal fluid in neonatal enteritis caused by EPEC. Microscopic examination of stools of infants with acute diarrheal illness caused by these organisms usually has revealed an absence of fecal polymorphonuclear leukocytes [231,272,335,376], although data on fecal lactoferrin in human volunteers suggest that an inflammatory process may be important in EPEC diarrhea [377,378]. Stool pH can be neutral, acid, or alkaline [76,359]. Serologic methods have not proved to be useful in attempting to establish a retrospective diagnosis of EPEC infection in neonates. Increasing or significantly elevated agglutinin titers rarely could be shown in early investigations [232,248,351]; hemagglutinating antibodies showed a significant response in only 10% to 20% of cases [262,313].

Fluorescent antibody techniques have shown promise for preliminary identification of EPEC in acute infantile diarrhea. This method is specific, with few false-positive results, and it is more sensitive than conventional plating and isolation techniques [298,378,379]. The rapidity with which determinations can be performed makes them ideally suited for screening ill infants and possible carriers in determining the extent and progression of a nursery [288,298] or community [255,307] outbreak. Because immunofluorescence does not depend on the viability of organisms and is not affected by antibiotics that suppress growth on culture plates, it can be used to advantage in following bacteriologic responses and relapses in patients receiving oral therapy [351,380]. The use of fluorescent antibody techniques offers many advantages in the surveillance and epidemiologic control of EPEC gastroenteritis. Immunofluorescent methods should supplement, but not replace, standard bacteriologic and serologic methods for identification of enteric pathogens.

Specific gene probes and PCR primers for the BFP adhesin, for the intimin-encoding gene (*eae*), and for a cryptic plasmid locus (EAF) are available [112]. Detection of BFP or EAF is superior to detection of *eae* because many non-EPEC, including nonpathogens, carry the *eae* gene [112,381]. PCR and gene probe analysis can be performed directly on the stools of suspect infants. Confirmation of infection by the identification of the organism in pure culture should be pursued.

Before widespread use of molecular methods, the HEp-2 cell adherence assay was proposed for EPEC diagnosis [135]. The presence of a focal or localized adherence [135] pattern on the surface of HEp-2 or HeLa cells after 3-hour coincubation is a highly sensitive and specific test for detection of EPEC [382]. The requirement for cell culture and expertise in reading this assay limits its utility to the research setting. An ELISA for BFP has been described, but is not readily available [383]. The capacity of localized adherence plus EPEC to polymerize F-actin can be detected in tissue culture cells stained with rhodamine-labeled phalloidin [384]. This fluorescence-actin staining test is cumbersome and impractical for routine clinical use.

Prognosis

The mortality rate recorded previously in epidemics of EPEC gastroenteritis is impressive for its variability. During the 1930s and 1940s, when organisms later recognized as classic enteropathogenic serotypes were infecting infants, the case-fatality ratio among neonates was about 50% [227,351]. During the 1950s and 1960s, about one of every four infected infants still died in many nursery epidemics, but several outbreaks involving the same serotypes under similar epidemiologic circumstances had fatality rates of less than 3% [251,258,268]. In the 1970s, reports appeared in the literature of a nursery epidemic with a 40% neonatal mortality rate [301] and of an extensive outbreak in a nursery for premature infants with 4% fatalities [281]; another report stated that among "243 consecutive infants admitted to the hospital for EPEC diarrheal disease, none died of diarrheal disease per se." [385].

A significant proportion of the infants who died during or shortly after an episode of gastroenteritis already were compromised by preexisting disease [250,299,345] or by congenital malformations [231,248,257] at the time they acquired gastroenteritis. These underlying pathologic conditions seem to exert a strongly unfavorable influence, probably by reducing the infant's ability to respond to the added stresses imposed by the GI tract infection. Although prematurity is often mentioned as a factor predisposing to a fatal outcome, the overall mortality rate among premature infants with EPEC gastroenteritis has not differed significantly over the years from the mortality recorded for term infants [250,278,280].

Therapy

The management of EPEC gastroenteritis should be directed primarily toward prevention or correction of problems caused by loss of fluids and electrolytes [214]. Most neonates have a relatively mild illness that can be treated with oral rehydration. Infants who appear toxic, infants with voluminous diarrhea and persistent vomiting, and infants with increasing weight loss should be hospitalized for observation and treatment with parenteral fluids and careful maintenance of fluid and electrolyte balance and possibly with antimicrobial therapy. Clinical studies suggest that slow nasogastric infusion of an elemental diet can be valuable in treating infants who have intractable diarrhea that is unresponsive to standard modes of therapy [386].

There is no evidence that the use of proprietary formulas containing kaolin or pectin is effective in reducing the number of diarrheal stools in neonates with gastroenteritis. Attempts to suppress the growth of enteric pathogens by feeding lactobacillus to the infant in the form of yogurt, powder, or granules have not been shown to be valuable [387]. A trial of cholestyramine in 15 newborns with EPEC gastroenteritis had no effect on the duration or severity of diarrhea [281]. The use of atropine-like drugs, paregoric, or loperamide to reduce intestinal motility or cramping should be avoided. Inhibition of peristalsis interferes with an efficient protective mechanism designed to rid the body of intestinal pathogens and may lead to fluid retention in the lumen of the bowel that may be sufficient to mask depletion of extracellular fluid and electrolytes.

The value of antimicrobial therapy in management of neonatal EPEC gastroenteritis, if any, is uncertain. There are no adequately controlled studies defining the benefits of any antibiotic in eliminating EPEC from the GI tract, reducing the risk of cross-infection in community or nursery outbreaks, or modifying the severity of the illness. Proponents of the use of antimicrobial agents have based their claims for efficacy on anecdotal observations or comparative studies [262]. Nonetheless, several clinical investigations have provided sufficient information to guide the physician faced with the dilemma of deciding whether to treat an individual infant or an entire nursery population with EPEC diarrheal disease. These guidelines must be considered tentative, however, until rigidly controlled, double-blind studies have established the efficacy of antibiotics on a more rational and scientific basis.

Oral therapy with neomycin [251,268], colistin [380], or chloramphenicol [361] seems to be effective in rapidly reducing the number of susceptible EPEC organisms in the stool of infected infants. Studies comparing the responses of infants treated orally with neomycin [250], gentamicin [281], polymyxin [259], or kanamycin [388] with the responses of infants receiving supportive therapy alone have shown that complete eradication of EPEC occurs more rapidly in infants receiving an antimicrobial agent. Chloramphenicol is not recommended for use in

neonates. In most cases, stool cultures are free of EPEC 2 to 4 days after the start of therapy [262,380]. Bacteriologic failure, defined as continued isolation of organisms during or after a course of an antimicrobial agent, can be expected to occur in 15% to 30% of patients [262, 281]. Such relapses generally are not associated with a recurrence of symptoms [248,251,262].

The effectiveness of oral antimicrobial therapy in reducing the duration of EPEC excretion serves to diminish environmental contamination and the spread of pathogenic organisms from one infant to another. Breaking the chain of fecal-oral transmission by administering antimicrobial agents simultaneously to all carriers of EPEC and their immediate contacts in the nursery has seemed to be valuable in terminating outbreaks that have failed to respond to more conservative measures [251,280,389]. The apparent reduction in morbidity and mortality associated with oral administration of neomycin [247,250, 251], colistin [263,283,301], polymyxin [259], or gentamicin [263] during nursery epidemics has led to the impression that these drugs also exert a beneficial clinical effect in severely or moderately ill infants. Reports describing clinical [272], bacteriologic [281], or histopathologic [334] evidence of tissue invasion by EPEC have persuaded some investigators to suggest the use of parenteral rather than oral drug therapy in debilitated or malnourished infants. On the basis of these data, there seems to be sufficient evidence to recommend oral administration of nonabsorbable antibiotics in the treatment of severely or moderately ill newborns with EPEC gastroenteritis. The drug most frequently used for initial therapy is neomycin sulfate in a dosage of 100 mg/kg/day administered orally every 8 hours in three divided doses [262]. In communities in which neomycin-resistant EPEC has been prevalent, treatment with colistin sulfate or polymyxin B in a dosage of 15 to 20 mg/kg/day orally and divided into three equal doses may be appropriate. It is rarely necessary to use this approach, however.

Treatment should be continued only until stool cultures become negative for EPEC [262]. Because of the unavoidable delay before cultures can be reported, most infants receive therapy for 3 to 5 days. If fluorescent antibody testing of rectal swab specimens is available, therapy can be discontinued as soon as EPEC no longer is identified in smears; this takes no more than 48 hours in more than 90% of cases [262]. After diarrhea and vomiting have stopped, and the infant tolerates formula feedings, shows a steady weight gain, and appears clinically well, discharge with outpatient follow-up is indicated. Bacteriologic relapses do not require therapy, unless they are associated with illness or high epidemiologic risks to other young infants in the household. Because the infecting organisms in these recurrences generally continue to show in vitro susceptibility to the original drug, it should be reinstituted pending bacteriologic results [262].

When clinical judgment suggests that a neonate may have bacterial sepsis and EPEC diarrheal disease, parenteral antimicrobial therapy is indicated after appropriate cultures have been obtained. The routine use of systemic therapy in severe cases of EPEC enteritis is inappropriate on the basis of current clinical experience.

Antimicrobial susceptibility patterns of EPEC are an important determinant of the success of therapy in infections with these organisms [250,263,264]. These patterns are unpredictable, depending on the ecologic pressures exerted by local antibiotic usage [263,264] and on the incidence of transmissible resistance factors in the enteric flora of the particular population served by an institution [390–395]. For these reasons, variations in susceptibility patterns are apparent in different nurseries [263,393] and even occasionally within the same institution [264,265,267]. Sudden changes in clinical response may occur during the course of a single epidemic as drug-susceptible strains of EPEC are replaced by strains with multidrug resistance [250,307,392]. Because differences can exist in the susceptibilities of different EPEC serogroups to various antimicrobial agents, regional susceptibility patterns should be reported on the basis of OB group or serotype rather than for EPEC as a whole [267]. Knowledge of the resistance pattern in one's area may help in the initial choice of antimicrobial therapy.

Prevention

The prevention of hospital outbreaks of EPEC gastroenteritis is best accomplished by careful attention to infection control policies for a nursery. All infants hospitalized with diarrhea should have a bacteriologic evaluation. If the laboratory is equipped and staffed to perform fluorescent antibody testing, infants transferred from another institution to a newborn, premature, or intensive care nursery and all infants with gastroenteritis on admission during an outbreak of EPEC diarrhea or in a highly endemic area can be held in an observation area for 1 or 2 hours until the results of the fluorescent antibody test or PCR are received. Because of the difficulty in diagnosing EPEC infection, reference laboratories, such as those at the U.S. Centers for Disease Control and Prevention (CDC), should be notified when an outbreak is suspected. Infants suspected to be excreting EPEC, even if healthy in appearance, can be separated from other infants and given oral therapy until the test results are negative.

Some experts have suggested that when the rapid results obtainable with fluorescent antibody procedures are unavailable, all infants admitted with diarrhea in a setting where EPEC is common may be treated as if they were excreting EPEC or some other enteric pathogen until proven otherwise [389]. Stool cultures should be obtained at admission, and contact precautions should be enforced among all individuals who come into contact with the infant. Additional epidemiologic studies are needed to establish the advantages of careful isolation and nursing techniques, particularly in smaller community hospitals in which the number of infants in a "gastroenteritis ward" may be small. The use of prophylactic antibiotics has been shown to be of no value and can select for increased resistance [394–396].

It can be difficult to keep a nursery continuously free of EPEC. Specific procedures have been suggested for handling a suspected outbreak of bacterial enteritis in a newborn nursery or infant care unit [252,371,373]. Evidence indicating that a significant proportion of E. coli

enteritis may be caused by nontypable strains has required some modification of these earlier recommendations. The following infection control measures may be appropriate:

1. The unit is closed, when possible, to all new admissions.
2. Personnel and parents should pay scrupulous attention to hand hygiene when handling infants.
3. Cultures for enteric pathogens are obtained from nursing personnel assigned to the unit at the time of the outbreak.
4. Stool specimens obtained from all infants in the nursery can be screened by the fluorescent antibody or another technique and cultured. Identification of a classic enteropathogenic serotype provides a useful epidemiologic marker; however, failure to isolate one of these strains does not eliminate the possibility of illness caused by nontypable EPEC.
5. Antimicrobial therapy with oral neomycin or colistin can be considered for all infants with a positive fluorescent antibody test or culture result. The initial drug of choice depends on local patterns of susceptibility. Depending on the results of susceptibility tests, subsequent therapy may require modification.
6. If an identifiable EPEC strain is isolated, second and third stool specimens from all infants in the unit are reexamined by the fluorescent antibody technique or culture at 48-hour intervals. If this is impractical, exposed infants should be carefully followed.
7. Early discharge for healthy, mature, uninfected infants is advocated.
8. An epidemiologic investigation should be performed to seek the factor or factors responsible for the outbreak. A surveillance system may be established for all individuals in contact with the nursery, including physicians and other health care personnel, housekeeping personnel, and postpartum mothers with evidence of enteric disease. A telephone, mail, or home survey may be conducted on all infants who were residing in the involved unit during the 2 weeks before the outbreak.
9. When all patients and contacts are discharged and control of the outbreak is achieved, a thorough terminal disinfection of the involved nursery is mandatory [397].

Enterohemorrhagic *Escherichia coli*

Since a multistate outbreak of enterohemorrhagic colitis was associated with *E. coli* O157:H7 [398], Shiga toxin–producing *E. coli* (STEC) have been recognized as emerging GI pathogens in most of the industrialized world. A particularly virulent subset of STEC, EHEC, causes frequent and severe outbreaks of GI disease [112,399]; the most virulent EHEC organisms belong to serotype O157:H7. EHEC has a bovine reservoir and is transmitted by undercooked meat; unpasteurized milk; and contaminated vegetables such as lettuce, alfalfa sprouts, and radish sprouts (as occurred in over 9000 schoolchildren in Japan) [400,401]. It also spreads directly from person to person [401,402]. The clinical syndrome comprises bloody, noninflammatory (sometimes voluminous) diarrhea that is distinct from febrile dysentery with fecal leukocytes seen in shigellosis or EIEC infections [112]. Most cases of EHEC infections have been recognized in outbreaks of bloody diarrhea or HUS in day care centers, schools, nursing homes, and communities [402–404]. Although EHEC infections often involve infants and young children, the frequency of this infection in neonates is unclear; animal studies suggest that receptors for the Shiga toxin may be developmentally regulated and that susceptibility to disease may be age related [405].

The capacity of EHEC to cause disease is related to the phage-encoded capacity of the organism to produce a Vero cell cytotoxin, subsequently shown to be one of the Shiga toxins (first identified in strains of *Shigella dysenteriae* serotype 1) [406–408]. Shiga toxin 1 is neutralized by antiserum against the Shiga toxin of *S. dysenteriae*, whereas Shiga toxin 2, although biologically similar, is not neutralized by anti–Shiga toxin [409,410]. Similar to Shiga toxin made by *S. dysenteriae*, both *E. coli* Shiga toxins act by inhibiting protein synthesis by cleaving an adenosine residue from position 4324 in the 28S ribosomal RNA (rRNA) to prevent elongation factor-1-dependent aminoacyl transfer RNA (tRNA) from binding to the 60S rRNA [406,407]. The virulence of EHEC may also be determined in part by a 60-MDa plasmid that encodes for a fimbrial adhesin in O157 and O26 [411,412]. This phenotype is mediated by the LEE pathogenicity island, which is highly homologous to the island present in EPEC strains [343].

EHEC and other STEC infections should be suspected in neonates who have bloody diarrhea or who may have been exposed in the course of an outbreak among older individuals. Because most cases are caused by ingestion of contaminated food, neonates have a degree of epidemiologic protection from the illness. STEC diarrhea is diagnosed by isolation and identification of the pathogen in the feces. *E. coli* O157:H7 does not ferment sorbitol, and this biochemical trait is commonly used in the detection of this serotype [112,413]. Because some nonpathogenic *E. coli* share this characteristic, confirmation of the serotype by slide agglutination is required. These techniques can be performed in most clinical laboratories. Detection of non-O157 serotypes is problematic, however, and relies on detection of the Shiga toxin; available methods include Shiga toxin ELISA, latex agglutination, and molecular methods [112,413].

Diarrhea-related HUS is almost always caused by STEC; some cases of HUS in infants are not associated with diarrhea or STEC. Even in older patients, the stool is typically negative for STEC at the time that HUS develops [414,415]. Serum and fecal detection of cytotoxin has been performed in such patients, but no diagnostic modality is definitive when HUS has supervened [414,415].

Antimicrobial therapy should not be administered to patients who may have STEC infection, although the role of antimicrobial therapy in inducing HUS is controversial [416,417]. Management of diarrhea and possible sequelae is supportive, with proper emphasis on fluid and electrolyte replacement. Aggressive rehydration is helpful in minimizing the frequency of serious sequelae. Antimotility agents are contraindicated because they may prolong the duration of STEC-associated bloody diarrhea [417a].

Enteroaggregative *Escherichia coli*

The HEp-2 adherence assay is useful for the detection of EPEC organisms, which exhibit a classic localized adherence pattern [135]. Two other adherence patterns can be discerned in this assay: aggregative and diffuse. These two patterns have been suggested to define additional pathotypes of diarrheogenic *E. coli* [112]. Strains exhibiting the aggregative adherence pattern (i.e., EAEC) are common pathogens of infants [140].

EAEC cause diarrhea by colonization of the intestinal mucosa and elaboration of enterotoxins and cytotoxins [140,418]. Many strains can be shown to elicit secretion of inflammatory cytokines in vitro, which may contribute to growth retardation associated with prolonged but otherwise asymptomatic colonization [119]. Several virulence factors in EAEC are under the control of the virulence gene activator AggR [418]. The presence of the AggR regulator or its effector genes has been proposed as a means of detecting truly virulent EAEC strains (called typical EAEC) [418,419], and an empirical gene probe long used for EAEC detection has been shown to correspond to one gene under AggR control [420,421].

Epidemiology and Transmission

The mode of transmission of EAEC has not been well established. In adult volunteer studies, the infectious dose is high ($>10^8$ colony-forming units), suggesting that in adults at least, person-to-person transmission is unlikely [422,423]. Several outbreaks have been linked to consumption of contaminated food [424,425]. The largest of these outbreaks involved almost 2700 schoolchildren in Japan [424]; a contaminated school lunch was the implicated source of the outbreak. Some studies have shown contamination of condiments or milk, which could represent vehicles of food-borne transmission.

Several nursery outbreaks of EAEC have been observed [426,427], although in no case has the mechanism of transmission been established. The first reported nursery outbreak involved 19 infants in Nis, Serbia, in 1995. Because these infants did not ingest milk from a common source, it is presumed that horizontal transmission by environmental contamination or hands of health care personnel was possible. Most of the infants were full term and previously well, and they were housed in two separate nursery rooms.

The earliest epidemiologic studies of EAEC implicated this organism as a cause of endemic diarrhea in developing countries [428–430]. In this setting, EAEC as defined by the aggregative adherence pattern of adherence to HEp-2 cells can be found in upward of 30% of the population at any one time [431]. Newer molecular diagnostic modalities have revised this figure downward, although the organism remains highly prevalent in many areas. Several studies from the Indian subcontinent implicated EAEC among the most frequent enteric pathogens [428,429,432]. Other sites reproducibly reporting high incidence rates include Mexico [430] and Brazil [431,433]. There is evidence that EAEC may be increasing in incidence. A study from São Paulo, Brazil, implicated EAEC as the prevalent *E. coli* pathotypes in infants [433], replacing EPEC in this community. Many other sites in developing countries of Africa [434], Asia [419,435], and South America [436] have described high endemic rates.

Several studies have suggested that EAEC is also a common cause of infant diarrhea in industrialized countries [437–439]. Using molecular diagnostic methods, a large prospective study in the United Kingdom implicated EAEC as the second most common enteric bacterial pathogen after *Campylobacter* [440]. A similar survey from Switzerland found EAEC to be the most common bacterial enteropathogen [437]. Studies from the United States also have shown a high rate of EAEC diarrhea in infants; using molecular diagnostic methods, EAEC was implicated in 11% and 8% of outpatient and inpatient diarrhea cohorts compared with less than 2% of asymptomatic control infants ($P < .05$) [441]. Although epidemiologic studies have shown that EAEC can cause diarrhea in all age groups, several studies suggest that the infection is particularly common in infants younger than 12 months [419,436].

Clinical Manifestations

Descriptions from outbreaks and volunteer studies suggest that EAEC diarrhea is watery in character with mucus, but without blood or frank pus [422,423,426]. Patients typically are afebrile. Several epidemiologic studies have suggested that many infants may have bloody diarrhea [430], but fecal leukocytes are uncommon.

The earliest reports of EAEC infection suggested that this pathogen may be particularly associated with persistent diarrhea (>14 days) [428–430]. Later studies suggest, however, that persistent diarrhea may occur in only a subset of infected infants [424]. In the Serbian outbreak of 19 infected infants, the mean duration of diarrhea was 5.2 days [426]; diarrhea persisted more than 14 days in only 3 patients. Infants in this outbreak had frequent, green, odorless stools. In three cases, the stools had mucus, but none had visible blood. Eleven infants developed temperatures greater than 38° C (>100.4° F); only one had vomiting.

Despite a lack of clinical evidence suggesting inflammatory enteritis, several clinical studies have suggested that EAEC is associated with subclinical inflammation, including the shedding of fecal cytokines and lactoferrin [119,442]. Studies in Fortaleza, Brazil, suggest that children asymptomatically excreting EAEC may exhibit growth shortfalls compared with uninfected peers [119]. A study from Germany reported an association between EAEC isolation and colic in infants without diarrhea [439]. This association was not observed again. EAEC should be considered in the differential diagnosis of persistent diarrhea and failure to thrive in infants.

Diagnosis and Therapy

Diagnosis of EAEC requires identification of the organism in the patient's feces. The HEp-2 adherence assay can be used for this purpose [135]. Some reports suggest that the adherence phenotype can be observed using formalin-fixed cells [443,444], obviating the need to cultivate eukaryotic cells for each assay. PCR for typical EAEC is available and is the preferred diagnostic test [114,445].

Antibiotic therapy using fluoroquinolones in adult patients has been successful [446]. Preliminary studies suggest that azithromycin [447] or rifaximin [448] also may be effective. Therapy in infected infants should be guided by the results of susceptibility testing because EAEC organisms are frequently antibiotic resistant [434].

Other *Escherichia coli* Pathotypes

Additional *E. coli* pathotypes have been described, including diffusely adherent *E. coli* (DAEC) [449], and cyto-detaching *E. coli* [450]. DAEC has been specifically associated with diarrhea after infancy because infants may have some degree of inherent resistance to infection [451]. Cytodetaching *E. coli* represent organisms that secrete the *E. coli* hemolysin [452]. It is unclear whether these latter organisms are true enteric pathogens.

SALMONELLA
Nature of the Organism

Taxonomists classify virtually all pathogenic *Salmonella* strains as a single species, *Salmonella enterica*. Numerous distinct serovars exist within this species, although historically these have been designated as though they were species unto themselves. *Salmonella* strains are correctly designated *S. enterica* serovar Typhi (or simply *S. typhi*) or *S. enterica* serovar Enteritidis. Biochemical and serologic traits are used routinely by hospital laboratories to differentiate *Salmonella* serovars. *S. typhi* is different from other salmonellae because it does not produce gas from glucose [453]. Because there are several thousand serovars designated *S. enteritidis*, serotyping of *S. enteritidis* is usually performed by state health departments rather than by hospital laboratories. The most common serogroups and representative serotypes are listed in Table 11–3. Infection of humans with the other serogroups (e.g., C_3, D_2, E_2, E_3, F, G, H, I) is uncommon.

There are differences in invasiveness of *Salmonella* strains related to serotype. *S. typhi*, *S. choleraesuis*, *Salmonella heidelberg* [454,455], and *Salmonella dublin* [456] are particularly invasive, with bacteremia and extraintestinal focal infections occurring frequently. *Salmonella* species encode injected toxins closely related to the invasion plasmid antigens (Ipa) of *Shigella* species. These proteins mediate invasion of target epithelial cells in *Salmonella* and *Shigella* strains [457]. A common *Salmonella* virulence plasmid confers resistance to complement-mediated bacteriolysis by inhibition of insertion of the terminal C5b-9 membrane attack complex into the outer membrane [458,459]. Laboratory studies have shown dramatic strain-related difference in the ability of *Salmonella typhimurium* to evoke fluid secretion, to invade intestinal mucosa, and to disseminate beyond the gut [460]. The production of an enterotoxin that is immunologically related to cholera toxin by about two thirds of *Salmonella* strains may play a role in the watery diarrhea commonly seen [461]. The significance of protein synthesis–

TABLE 11-3 Common Serotypes and Serogroups of *Salmonella*

Serogroups	Serotypes
A	Paratyphi A
B	Agona
	Derby
	Heidelberg
	Paratyphi B (*schottmuelleri*)
	Saint-paul
	Typhimurium
C_1	Choleraesuis
	Eimsbuettel
	Infantis
	Montevideo
	Oranienburg
	Paratyphi C (*hirschfeldii*)
	Thompson
C_2	Blockley
	Hadar
	Muenchen
	Newport
C_3	Kentucky
D_1	Dublin
	Enteritidis
	Javiana
	Panama
	Typhi
D_2	Maarssen
E_1	Anatum
E_2	London Newington
E_3	Illinois
E_4	Krefeld
	Senftenberg

inhibiting cytotoxins [462] remains to be proved, although such toxins can damage gut epithelium, which could facilitate invasion. The cytotoxins produced by *Salmonella* are not immunologically related to Shiga toxin made by *S. dysenteriae* type 1 [463] or *E. coli* O157:H7.

Salmonellae have the ability to penetrate epithelial cells and reach the submucosa, where they are ingested by phagocytes [464]. In phagocytes, salmonellae are resistant to killing, in part because of the properties of their lipopolysaccharides [465,466] and multiple enzymes for oxidant defense [466a]. Persistence of the organism within phagolysosomes of phagocytic cells may occur with any species of *Salmonella*. It is unclear how the organisms have adapted to survive in the harsh intracellular environment, but their survival has major clinical significance, accounting for relapse after antibiotic therapy and the inadequacy of some antimicrobial agents that do not penetrate phagolysosomes. It is also perhaps the reason for prolonged febrile courses that occur even in the face of appropriate therapy. Although humoral immunity and cell-mediated immunity are stimulated during *Salmonella* infections, it is believed that cell-mediated immunity plays a greater role in eradication of the bacteria [467]. T-cell activation

of macrophages seems to be important in killing intracellular *Salmonella* [468]. Defective interferon-γ production by monocytes of newborns in response to *S. typhimurium* lipopolysaccharide may explain in part the unusual susceptibility of infants to *Salmonella* infection [469]. Studies in mice suggest that T helper type 1 cell responses in Peyer patches and mesenteric lymph nodes may be central to protection of the intestinal mucosa [470]. Humans who lack the interleukin-12 receptor and have impaired T helper type 1 cell responses and interferon-γ production are at increased risk for *Salmonella* infection [471].

S. typhi strains comprise almost entirely a single global clone, recognized by serologic and biochemically distinct characteristics. *S. typhi* does not carry the virulence plasmid of nontyphoid *Salmonella*, but many of the other virulence properties are shared. *S. typhi* alone expressed the Vi antigen, a surface capsule that inhibits phagocytosis. Patients who develop classic enteric fever have positive stool cultures in the first few days after ingestion of the organism and again late in the course after a period of bacteremia. This course reflects early colonization of the gut, penetration of gut epithelium with infection of mesenteric lymph nodes, and reseeding of the gut during a subsequent bacteremic phase [472]. Studies of *S. typhimurium* in monkeys suggest similar initial steps in pathogenesis (e.g., colonization of gut, penetration of gut epithelium, infection of mesenteric lymph nodes), but failure of the organism to cause a detectable level of bacteremia [473].

Although *Salmonella* and *Shigella* invade intestinal mucosa, the resultant pathologic changes are different. *Shigella* multiply within and kill enterocytes with production of ulcerations and a brisk inflammatory response, whereas *Salmonella* pass through the mucosa and multiply within the lamina propria, where the organisms are ingested by phagocytes; consequently, ulcer formation is less striking [460], although villus tip cells are sometimes sloughed. Acute crypt abscesses can be seen in the stomach and small intestine, but the most dramatic changes occur in the colon, where acute diffuse inflammation with mucosal edema and crypt abscesses are the most consistent findings [474,475]. With *S. typhi*, there also is hyperplasia of Peyer patches in the ileum, with ulceration of overlying tissues.

Epidemiology and Transmission

Salmonella strains, with the exception of *S. typhi*, are carried by various vertebrate animal hosts; human infection often can be traced to infected meat, contaminated milk, or contact with a specific animal. Half of commercial poultry samples are contaminated with *Salmonella* [476]. Definition of the serotype causing infection can sometimes suggest the likely source. *S. dublin* is closely associated with cattle; human cases occur with a higher-than-predicted frequency in people who drink raw milk [456]. For *S. typhimurium*, which is the most common serotype and accounts for more than one third of all reported human cases, a single source has not been established, although there is an association with cattle. Despite the 1975 ban by the U.S. Food and Drug Administration (FDA) on interstate commercial distribution of small turtles, these animals continue to be associated with infection, as illustrated by a series of cases in Puerto Rico [477]. Various pet reptiles are an important source of various unusual *Salmonella* serotypes such as *Salmonella marina*, *Salmonella chameleon*, *Salmonella arizonae*, *Salmonella java*, *Salmonella stanley*, *Salmonella poona*, *Salmonella jangwain*, *Salmonella tilene*, and several others [478–480]. *Salmonella* organisms are hardy and capable of prolonged survival; organisms have been documented to survive in flour for nearly a year [481]. *Salmonella tennessee* has been shown to remain viable for many hours on non-nutritive surfaces (i.e., glass, 48 hours; stainless steel, 68 hours; enameled surface, 114 hours; rubber mattress, 119 hours; linen, 192 hours; and rubber tabletop, 192 hours) [482].

Infection with *Salmonella* is, similar to most enteric infections, more common in young children than in adults. The frequency of infection is far greater in the first 4 years of life; roughly equal numbers of cases are reported during each decade beyond 4 years of age. Although the peak incidence occurs in the 2nd through 6th months of life, infection in neonates is relatively common. Researchers at the CDC have estimated the incidence of *Salmonella* infection in the first month of life at nearly 75 cases per 100,000 infants [483].

Adult volunteer studies suggest that large numbers of *Salmonella* (10^5 to 10^9) need to be ingested to cause disease [484]. It is likely, however, that lower doses cause illness in infants. The occurrence of nursery outbreaks [482,485–510] and intrafamilial spread [511] suggests that organisms are easily spread from person to person; this pattern is typical of low-inoculum diseases transmitted by the fecal-oral route. A neonate with *Salmonella* infection infrequently acquires the organism from his or her mother during delivery. Although the index case in an outbreak can often be traced to a mother [488–491,509], subsequent cases result from contaminated objects in the nursery environment [512,513] serving as a reservoir coming in contact with hands of attending personnel [482,497]. The mother of an index case may be symptomatic [493,494,514,515] or asymptomatic with preclinical infection [498], convalescent infection [491,495,516], or chronic carriage [517]. The risk of a newborn becoming infected when *Salmonella* is introduced into a nursery has been reported to be 20% to 27% [501,507], but the frequency of infection may be lower because isolated cases outside the context of a subsequent epidemic are unlikely to be reported.

Gastric acidity is an important barrier to *Salmonella* infection. Patients with anatomic or functional achlorhydria are at increased risk of developing salmonellosis [518,519]. The hypochlorhydria [37] and rapid gastric emptying typical of early life [40] may partly explain the susceptibility of infants to *Salmonella*. Premature and low birth weight infants seem to be at higher risk of acquiring *Salmonella* infection than term neonates [497,499]. Whether this higher risk reflects increased exposure because of prolonged hospital stays or increased susceptibility on the basis of immature intestinal or immune function is unclear.

Contaminated food or water is often the source of *Salmonella* infection in older patients; the limited diet of the infant makes contaminated food a less likely source

of infection. Although human milk [520–522], raw milk [523], powdered milk [524–526], formula [507], and cereal [527] have been implicated in transmission to infants, more often fomites, such as delivery room resuscitators [485], rectal thermometers [500,528], oropharyngeal suction devices [529–531], water baths for heating formula [531], soap dispensers [532], scales [482,486,533], "clean" medicine tables [482], air-conditioning filters [482], mattresses, radiant warmers [512], and dust, serve as reservoirs. One unusual outbreak involving 394 premature and 122 term infants was traced to faulty plumbing, which caused massive contamination of environment and personnel [507]. After *Salmonella* enters a nursery, it is difficult to eradicate. Epidemics lasting 6 to 7 weeks [500,505], 17 weeks [482], 6 months [499,504], 1 year [494], and 27 to 30 months [501,507] have been reported. Spread to nearby pediatric wards has occurred [502,508].

The incubation period in nursery outbreaks has varied widely in several studies where careful attention has been paid to this variable. In one outbreak of *Salmonella oranienburg* involving 35 newborns, 97% of cases occurred within 4 days of birth [501]. In an outbreak of *S. typhimurium*, each of the ill infants presented within 6 days of birth [491]. These incubation periods are similar to those reported for *Salmonella newport* in older children and adults, 95% of whom have been reported to be ill within 8 days of exposure [534,535]. Conversely, one outbreak of *Salmonella nienstedten* involving newborns was characterized by incubation periods of 7 to 18 days [502].

The usual incubation period associated with fecal-oral nursery transmission is not found with congenital typhoid. During pregnancy, typhoid fever is associated with bacteremic infection of the fetus. Congenitally infected infants are symptomatic at birth. They are usually born during the 2nd to 4th week of untreated maternal illness [536]. Usually, the mother is a carrier; fecal-oral transmission of *S. typhi* can occur with delayed illness in the newborn [537].

Clinical Manifestations

Several major clinical syndromes occur with nontyphoidal *Salmonella* infection in young infants. Colonization without illness may be the most common outcome of ingestion of *Salmonella* by the neonate. Colonization usually is detected when an outbreak is under investigation. Most infected infants who become ill have abrupt onset of loose, green, mucus-containing stools, or they have bloody diarrhea; an elevated temperature is also a common finding in *Salmonella* gastroenteritis in the first months of life [455]. Grossly bloody stools are found in a few patients, although grossly bloody stools can occur in the first 24 hours of life. Hematochezia is more typically associated with noninfectious causes (e.g., swallowed maternal blood, intestinal ischemia, hemorrhagic diseases, anorectal fissures) at this early age [538].

There seem to be major differences in presentation related to the serotype of *S. enteritidis* causing infection. In one epidemic of *S. oranienburg* [501] involving 46 newborns, 76% had grossly bloody stools, 11% were febrile, 26% had mucus in their stools, and only 11% were healthy. In a series of *S. newport* infections involving

11 premature infants [488], 90% of infants with gastroenteritis had blood in their stools, 10% had fever, 10% had mucus in their stools, and 9% were asymptomatic. In an outbreak of *S. typhimurium* [491] involving 11 ill and 5 healthy infants, none had bloody stools; all of the symptomatic infants were febrile and usually had loose green stools. Of 26 infants infected by *Salmonella virchow*, 42% were asymptomatic; the rest had mild diarrhea [496]. Seals and colleagues [502] described 12 infants with *S. nienstedten*, all of whom had watery diarrhea and low-grade fever; none had bloody stools. In a large outbreak in Zimbabwe of *S. heidelberg* infection reported by Bannerman [499], 38% of 100 infants were asymptomatic, 42% had diarrhea, 16% had fever, 15% had pneumonia, and 2% developed meningitis. An outbreak of *Salmonella worthington* was characterized primarily by diarrhea, fever, and jaundice, although 3 of 18 infants developed meningitis, and 17% died [529]. In dramatic contrast to these series, none of 27 infants with positive stool cultures for *S. tennessee* had an illness in a nursery found to be contaminated with that organism [483]. A few infants with *Salmonella* gastroenteritis have developed necrotizing enterocolitis [506,539], but it is unclear whether *Salmonella* was the cause.

Although gastroenteritis is usually self-limited, chronic diarrhea has sometimes been attributed to *Salmonella* [517,540]. Whether chronic diarrhea is caused by Salmonella is uncertain. Although some infants develop carbohydrate intolerance after a bout of *Salmonella* enteritis [541,542], and *Salmonella* is typically listed as one of the causes of postinfectious protracted diarrhea [543], it is difficult to be sure that the relationship is causal. The prolonged excretion of *Salmonella* after a bout of gastroenteritis may sometimes cause nonspecific chronic diarrhea to be erroneously attributed to *Salmonella*.

Major extraintestinal complications of *Salmonella* infection may develop in a neonate who becomes bacteremic. Systemic spread may develop in infants who initially present with diarrhea and in some who have no GI tract signs. Bacteremia seems to be more common in neonates than in older children [544]. A study of more than 800 children with *Salmonella* infection showed that extraintestinal infection occurred significantly more often (8.7% versus 3.6%) in the first 3 months of life [545]. Several retrospective studies suggest that infants in the first month of life may have a risk of bacteremia of 30% to 50% [455]. One retrospective study [454] suggested that the risk is not increased in infancy and estimated that the risk of bacteremia in childhood *Salmonella* gastroenteritis is 8.5% to 15.6%. Prospective studies of infants in the first year of life suggest that the risk of bacteremia is 1.8% to 6% [546,547]. Although selection biases in these studies limit the reliability of these estimates, the risk is substantial.

Salmonella species isolated from infants include some serotypes that seem to be more invasive in the first 2 months of life than in older children or healthy adults (*S. newport, Salmonella agona, Salmonella blockley, Salmonella derby, S. enteritidis, S. heidelberg, Salmonella infantis, Salmonella javiana, Salmonella saint-paul*, and *S. typhimurium*) and serotypes that are aggressive in every age group (*S. choleraesuis* and *S. dublin*). Other serotypes seem more

likely to cause bacteremia in adults (*S. typhi, Salmonella paratyphi A*, and *Salmonella paratyphi B*) [544].

Virtually any *Salmonella* serotype can cause bacteremic disease in neonates. A few infants with *Salmonella* gastroenteritis have died with *E. coli* or *Pseudomonas aeruginosa* sepsis [508], and the role of *Salmonella* in these cases is unclear. In contrast to the situation in older children, in whom bacteremic salmonellosis often is associated with underlying medical conditions, bacteremia may occur in infants who have no immunocompromising conditions [548]. *Salmonella* bacteremia is often not suspected clinically because the syndrome is not usually distinctive [454,455]. Even afebrile, well-appearing children with *Salmonella* gastroenteritis have been documented to have bacteremia that persists for several days [549].

Although infants with bacteremia may have spontaneous resolution without therapy [550], a sufficient number develop complications to warrant empirical antimicrobial therapy when bacteremia is suspected. The frequency of complications is highest in the 1st month of life. Meningitis is the most feared complication of bacteremic *Salmonella* disease. Of all cases of nontyphoidal *Salmonella* meningitis, 50% to 75% occur in the first 4 months of life [551]. The serotypes associated with neonatal meningitis (*S. typhimurium, S. heidelberg, S. enteritidis, S. saint-paul, S. newport*, and *Salmonella panama*) [511] are serotypes frequently associated with bacteremia. Meningitis has a high mortality rate, in part because of high relapse rates. Relapse has been reported in 64% of cases [552]. In some studies, more than 90% of patients with meningitis have died [553], although more typically, 30% to 60% of infants die [554,555]. The survivors experience the expected complications of gram-negative neonatal meningitis, including hydrocephalus, seizures, ventriculitis, abscess formation, subdural empyema, and permanent neurologic impairment. Neurologic sequelae have included retardation, hemiparesis, epilepsy, visual impairment, and athetosis [551].

In large nursery outbreaks, it is common to find infants whose course is complicated by pneumonia [499], osteomyelitis [556,557], or septic arthritis [497,499]. Other rare complications of salmonellosis include pericarditis [558], pyelitis [559], peritonitis [491], otitis media [491], mastitis [560], cholecystitis [561], endophthalmitis [562], cutaneous abscesses [506], and infected cephalhematoma [556]. Certain focal infections seen in older children and adults, such as endocarditis and infected aortic aneurysms, rarely or never have been reported in neonates [551,563]. Although the mortality rate in two reviews of nursery outbreaks was 3.7% to 7% [509,510], in some series, the mortality was 18% [499].

Enteric fever, most often related to *S. typhi*, but also occurring with *S. paratyphi A, S. paratyphi B, Salmonella paratyphi C*, and other *Salmonella* species, is reported much less commonly in infants than in older patients. Infected infants develop typical findings of neonatal sepsis and meningitis. Current data suggest that mortality is about 30% [564]. In utero infection with *S. typhi* has been described. Typhoid fever [532,565] and nontyphoidal *Salmonella* infections [566] during pregnancy put women at risk of aborting the fetus. Premature labor usually occurs during the 2nd to 4th week of maternal typhoid if the woman is untreated [536]. In a survey of typhoid fever in pregnancy during the preantibiotic era, 24 of 60 women with well-documented cases delivered prematurely, with resultant fetal death; the rest delivered at term, although only 17 infants survived [567]. The outlook for carrying the pregnancy to term and delivering a healthy infant seems to have improved dramatically during the antibiotic era. One of seven women with typhoid in a series still delivered a dead fetus with extensive liver necrosis, however [568]. In the preantibiotic era, about 14% of pregnant women with typhoid fever died [569]. With appropriate antimicrobial therapy, pregnancy does not seem to put the woman at increased risk of death. Despite these well-described cases, typhoid fever is rare early in life.

Of 1500 cases of typhoid fever that Osler and McCrae [570] reported, only 2 were in the 1st year of life. In areas where typhoid fever is still endemic, systematic search for infants with enteric fever has failed to find many cases. The few infections with *S. typhi* documented in children in the 1st year of life often manifest as a brief nondescript "viral syndrome" or as pneumonitis [571,572]. Fever, diarrhea, cough, vomiting, rash, and splenomegaly may occur. The fever may be high, and the duration of illness may be many weeks [536].

Diagnosis

The current practice of early discharge of newborns, although potentially decreasing the risk of exposure, can make recognition of a nursery outbreak difficult. Diagnosis of neonatal salmonellosis should trigger an investigation for other cases. Other than diarrhea, signs of neonatal *Salmonella* infection are similar to the nonspecific findings seen in most neonatal infections. Lethargy, poor feeding, pallor, jaundice, apnea, respiratory distress, weight loss, and fever are common. Enlarged liver and spleen are common in neonates with positive blood cultures. Laboratory studies are required to establish the diagnosis because the clinical picture is not distinct. The fecal leukocyte examination reveals polymorphonuclear leukocytes in 36% to 82% [376,573] of persons with *Salmonella* infection, but it has not been evaluated in neonates. The presence of fecal leukocytes is consistent with colitis of any cause and is a nonspecific finding. Routine stool cultures usually detect *Salmonella* if two or three different enteric media (i.e., MacConkey, eosin–methylene blue, *Salmonella-Shigella*, Tergitol 7, xylose-lysine-deoxycholate, brilliant green, or bismuth sulfite agar) are used. Stool, rather than rectal swab material, is preferable for culture, particularly if the aim of culture is to detect carriers [574]. On the infrequent occasions when proctoscopy is performed, mucosal edema, hyperemia, friability, and hemorrhages may be seen [475].

Infants who are bacteremic often do not appear sufficiently toxic to raise the suspicion of bacteremia [575]. Blood cultures should be obtained as a routine part of evaluation of neonates with suspected or documented *Salmonella* infection. Ill neonates with *Salmonella* infection should have a cerebrospinal fluid examination performed. Bone marrow cultures also may be indicated when enteric fever is suspected. There are no consistent abnormalities in the white blood cell count. Serologic studies are not helpful in establishing the diagnosis, although antibodies to somatic [576,577] and flagellar antigens [501] develop in many infected newborns.

If an outbreak of salmonellosis is suspected, further characterization of the organism is imperative [478]. Determination of somatic and flagellar antigens to characterize the specific serotype may be crucial to investigate an outbreak. When the serotype found during investigation of an outbreak is a common one (e.g., *S. typhimurium*), antimicrobial resistance testing [489,578] and use of molecular techniques such as plasmid characterization [578] can be helpful in determining whether a single-strain, common-source outbreak is in progress.

Therapy

As in all enteric infections, attention to fluid and electrolyte abnormalities is the first issue that must be addressed by the physician. Specific measures to eradicate *Salmonella* intestinal infection have met with little success. Multiple studies show that antibiotic treatment of *Salmonella* gastroenteritis prolongs the excretion of *Salmonella* [579–586]. Almost half of infected children in the first 5 years of life continue to excrete *Salmonella* 12 weeks after the onset of infection; more than 5% have positive cultures at 1 year [587]. No benefit of therapy has been shown in comparisons of ampicillin or neomycin versus placebo [583], chloramphenicol versus no antibiotic treatment [582], neomycin versus placebo [584], ampicillin or trimethoprim-sulfamethoxazole versus no antibiotic [581], and ampicillin or amoxicillin versus placebo [585]. In contrast to these studies, data suggest that there may be a role for quinolone antibiotics in adults and children [586,588], but these drugs are not approved for use in neonates, and resistance has been encountered [589].

Because these studies have few data regarding the risk-benefit ratio of therapy in the neonate, it is uncertain whether they should influence treatment decisions in neonates. Studies that have included a few neonates suggest little benefit from antimicrobial therapy [491,501,581, 590,591]. Because bacteremia is common in neonates, antimicrobial therapy for infants younger than 3 months who have *Salmonella* gastroenteritis often is recommended [546,547,575], however, especially if the infant appears toxic. Premature infants and infants who have other significant debilitating conditions also should probably be treated. The duration of therapy is debatable, but should probably be no more than 3 to 5 days if the infant is not seriously ill and if blood cultures are sterile. If toxicity, clinical deterioration, or documented bacteremia complicates gastroenteritis, prolonged treatment is indicated. Even with antimicrobial therapy, some infants develop complications. The relatively low risk of extraintestinal dissemination must be balanced against the well-documented risk of prolonging the carrier state. For infants who develop chronic diarrhea and malnutrition, hyperalimentation may be required; the role of antimicrobial agents in this setting is unclear. An infant with typhoid fever should be treated with an appropriate antimicrobial agent; relapses sometimes occur after therapy.

Colonized healthy infants discovered by stool cultures to harbor *Salmonella* during evaluation of an outbreak ought to be isolated, but probably should not receive anti-microbial therapy. These infants should be discharged from the nursery as early as possible and followed carefully as outpatients.

Antimicrobial treatment of neonates who have documented extraintestinal dissemination must be prolonged. *Salmonella* bacteremia without localization is generally treated with at least a 10-day course of therapy. Therapy for meningitis must be given for at least 4 weeks to lessen the risk of relapse. About three fourths of patients who have relapses have been treated for 3 weeks or less [551]. Similar to meningitis, treatment for osteomyelitis must be prolonged to be adequate. Although cures have been reported with 3 weeks of therapy, 4 to 6 weeks of therapy is recommended.

In vitro susceptibility data for *Salmonella* isolates must be interpreted with caution. Aminoglycosides show good in vitro activity but poor clinical efficacy, perhaps because of the low pH of the phagolysosome; aminoglycosides have poor activity in an acid environment. The relative instabilities of some antibiotics in this acid environment also may explain in vitro and in vivo disparities. The intracellular localization and survival of *Salmonella* within phagocytic cells also presumably explains the relapses encountered with virtually every regimen. Resistance to antibiotics has long been a problem with *Salmonella* infection [579,592,593] and has been steadily increasing in the United States [594]. With the emergence of Typhimurium type DT 104, resistance to ampicillin, chloramphenicol, streptomycin, sulfonamides, and tetracycline has increased from 0.6% in 1979 and 1980 to 34% in 1996 [595].

Resistance plasmids have been selected and transmitted partly because therapy has been given for mild illness that should not have been treated [579] and partly because of use of antibiotics in animal feeds. Resistance to chloramphenicol and ampicillin has made trimethoprim-sulfamethoxazole increasingly important for the treatment of *Salmonella* infection in patients who require therapy. With increasing resistance to all three of these agents in Asia [596], the Middle East [597], Africa [598], Europe [599, 600], Argentina [593], and North America [592,601,602], the third-generation cephalosporins and quinolones represent drugs of choice for invasive salmonellosis. The quinolones currently are not approved for patients younger than 18 years. Cefotaxime, ceftriaxone, and cefoperazone represent acceptable alternative drugs for typhoidal and nontyphoidal salmonellosis when resistance is encountered [603,604]. Because second-generation cephalosporins, such as cefuroxime, are less active in vitro than third-generation cephalosporins and are not consistently clinically effective, they should not be used [603,605]. Data suggest that cefoperazone may sterilize blood and cause patients with typhoid fever to become afebrile more rapidly than with chloramphenicol [606], perhaps because cefoperazone is excreted into bile in high concentrations [607]. Third-generation cephalosporins may have higher cure and lower relapse rates than ampicillin or chloramphenicol in children with *Salmonella* meningitis [608].

The doses of ampicillin, chloramphenicol, or cefotaxime used in infants with gastroenteritis pending results of blood cultures are the same as the doses used in treatment of sepsis. Because of the risk of gray baby syndrome, chloramphenicol should not be used in neonates unless other effective agents are unavailable. Trimethoprim-sulfamethoxazole, although useful in older children and adults, is not used in neonates because of the risk of kernicterus. Nosocomial infection with strains of *Salmonella* resistant to multiple antibiotics, including third-generation cephalosporins, has emerged as a problem in South America [593].

Nonantibiotic interventions may be important in the control of *Salmonella* infections. Limited data suggest that intravenous immunoglobulin (500 mg/kg on days 1, 2, 3, and 8 of therapy) coupled with antibiotic therapy may decrease the risk of bacteremia and death in preterm infants with *Salmonella* gastroenteritis [609].

Prevention

Early recognition and intervention in nursery outbreaks of *Salmonella* are crucial to control. When a neonate develops salmonellosis, a search for other infants who have been in the same nursery should be undertaken. When two or more cases are recognized, environmental cultures, cultures of all infants, cohorting and contact isolation of infected infants, rigorous enforcement of hand hygiene, early discharge of infected infants, and thorough cleaning of all possible fomites in the nursery and delivery rooms are important elements of control. If cases continue to occur, the nursery should be closed to further admissions. Cultures of nursery personnel are likely to be helpful in the unusual situation of an *S. typhi* outbreak in which a chronic carrier may be among the caretakers. Whether culture of health care personnel during outbreaks of salmonellosis caused by other *Salmonella* species is helpful is debatable, although it is often recommended. Data suggest that nurses infected with *Salmonella* rarely infect patients in the hospital setting [610]. The fact that nursing personnel are sometimes found to be colonized during nursery outbreaks [482,488,501,503,504] may be a result rather than a cause of the epidemics.

The potential role of vaccines in control of neonatal disease is minimal. For most non–*S. typhi* serotypes, there is no prospect for an immunization strategy. Multiple doses of the commercially available oral live attenuated vaccine (Ty21a; Vivotif, Berna) have been shown in Chilean schoolchildren to reduce typhoid fever cases by more than 70% [611,612]. The vaccine is not recommended, however, for children younger than 6 years, partly because immunogenicity of Ty21a is age dependent; children younger than 24 months fail to respond with development of immunity [613]. Vi capsular polysaccharide vaccine is available for children older than 2 years and is effective in a single dose. Whether some degree of protection of infants could occur if stool carriage were reduced or could be transferred to infants by the milk of vaccinated mothers remains to be studied. Data suggest that breast-feeding may decrease the risk of other *Salmonella* infections [614].

SHIGELLA
Nature of the Organism

On the basis of DNA relatedness, shigellae and *E. coli* organisms belong to the same species [615]. For historical reasons and because of their medical significance,

TABLE 11-4 *Shigella* Serogroups

Serogroups	Species	No. Serotypes
A	*S. dysenteriae*	13
B	*S. flexneri*	15 (including subtypes)
C	*S. boydii*	18
D	*S. sonnei*	1

shigellae have been maintained as separate species, however. Shigellae are gram-negative bacilli that differ from typical *E. coli* because they do not metabolize lactose or do so slowly, are nonmotile, and generally produce no gas during carbohydrate use.

Shigellae are classically divided into four species (serogroups) on the basis of metabolic and antigenic characteristics (Table 11-4). The mannitol nonfermenters usually are classified as *S. dysenteriae*. Although the lipopolysaccharide antigens of the 13 recognized members of this group are not related to each other antigenically, these serotypes are grouped together as serogroup A. Serogroup D (*Shigella sonnei*) are ornithine decarboxylase–positive and slow lactose fermenters. All *S. sonnei* share the same lipopolysaccharide (O antigen). Shigellae that ferment mannitol (in contrast to *S. dysenteriae*), but do not decarboxylate ornithine or ferment lactose (*S. sonnei*) belong to serogroups B and C. Of these, the strains that have lipopolysaccharide antigens immunologically related to each other are grouped together as serogroup B (*Shigella flexneri*), whereas strains whose O antigens are not related to each other or to other shigellae are included in serogroup C (*Shigella boydii*). There are six major serotypes of *S. flexneri* and 13 subserotypes (1a, 1b, 2a, 2b, 3a, 3b, 4a, 4b, 5a, 5b, 6, X, and Y variant). There are 19 antigenically distinct serotypes of *S. boydii*. For *S. dysenteriae* and *S. boydii* serogroup confirmation, pools of polyvalent antisera are used.

The virulence of shigellae has been studied extensively since their recognition as major pathogens at the beginning of the 20th century [616,617]. The major determinants of virulence are encoded by a 120- to 140-MDa plasmid [618,619]. This plasmid, which is found in all virulent shigellae, encodes the synthesis of proteins that are required for invasion of mammalian cells and for the vigorous inflammatory response that is characteristic of the disease [620,621]. Shigellae that have lost this plasmid, have deletions of genetic material from the region involved in synthesis of these proteins, or have the plasmid inserted into the chromosome lose the ability to invade eukaryotic cells and become avirulent [622]; maintenance of the plasmid can be detected in the clinical microbiology laboratory by ability to bind Congo red. The ability to invade cells is the basic pathogenic property shared by all shigellae [623,624] and by *Shigella*-like invasive *E. coli*, which also possesses the *Shigella* virulence plasmid [223,620,621,625,626]. In the laboratory, *Shigella* invasiveness is studied in tissue culture (HeLa cell invasion), in animal intestine, or in rabbit or guinea pig eye, where instillation of the organism causes keratoconjunctivitis (Sereny test) [143]. Animal model studies have shown that bacteria penetrate and kill colonic mucosal cells and then elicit a brisk inflammatory response.

Shigella invasiveness is mediated by a set of toxins injected into host cells by virtue of a type III secretion system, which injects the proteins directly from the bacterial cytoplasm to the host cell cytoplasm. Shigella follows an unusual pathogenetic course. The bacteria invade the epithelial cell via pathogen-directed endocytosis. The bacteria then force lysis of the endocytic vacuole, gaining entry into the host cell cytoplasm. Here, the bacteria nucleate actin proteins into a structure with the appearance of a comet's tail behind the bacterium and use the force of this event to propel them into adjacent cells. This sequence promotes lateral spread through the mucosa. Some organisms pass through the epithelial barrier and are engulfed by macrophages, with subsequent release of proinflammatory cytokines. The release of these cytokines, coupled with the destruction of invaded epithelial cells, gives rise to the inflammatory, destructive nature of shigellosis.

Most key *Shigella* virulence factors are encoded on the virulence plasmid, but several chromosomal loci also enhance virulence [627,628]. This phenomenon has been best studied in *S. flexneri*, in which multiple virulence-enhancing regions of the chromosome have been defined [619,627–629]. The specific gene products of some of the chromosomal loci are unknown; one chromosomal virulence segment encodes for synthesis of the O repeat units of lipopolysaccharide. Intact lipopolysaccharide is necessary but not sufficient to cause virulence [627,630]. At least two cell-damaging cytotoxins that also are chromosomally encoded are produced by shigellae. One of these toxins (Shiga toxin) is made in large quantities by *S. dysenteriae* serotype 1 (the Shiga bacillus) and is made infrequently by other shigellae [631]. Shiga toxin is a major virulence factor in *S. dysenteriae*, enhancing virulence at the colonic mucosa and giving rise to sequelae similar to those caused by STEC (discussed earlier). This toxin kills cells by interfering with peptide elongation during protein synthesis [632–634]. Additional toxins may also be secreted by shigellae, although their roles in virulence are not established [635].

Epidemiology

Although much of the epidemiology of shigellosis is predictable based on its infectious dose, certain elements are unexplained. Shigellae, similar to other organisms transmitted by the fecal-oral route, are commonly spread by food and water, but the low infecting inoculum allows person-to-person spread. Because of this low inoculum, *Shigella* is one of the few enteric pathogens that can infect swimmers [636]. The dose required to cause illness in adult volunteers is 10 organisms for *S. dysenteriae* serotype 1 [637], about 200 organisms for *S. flexneri* [638], and 500 organisms for *S. sonnei* [639]. Person-to-person transmission of infection probably explains the continuing occurrence of *Shigella* in the developed world. Enteropathogens that require large inocula and are best spread by food or drinking water are less common in industrialized societies because of sewage disposal facilities, water treatment, and food-handling practices. In the United States, day care centers currently serve as a major focus for acquisition of shigellosis [640]. Numerous outbreaks of shigellosis related to crowding, poor sanitation, and the low dose required for diseases have occurred in this setting.

Given the ease of transmission, it is not surprising that the peak incidence of disease is in the first 4 years of life. It is, however, paradoxical that symptomatic infection is uncommon in the first year of life [641–644]. The best data on the age-related incidence of shigellosis come from Mata's [641] prospective studies of Guatemalan infants. In these studies, stool cultures were performed weekly on a group of children followed from birth to 3 years old. The rate of infection was more than 60-fold lower in the first 6 months of life than between 2 and 3 years (Fig. 11–1) [641]. The same age-related incidence has been described in the United States [644] and in a rural Egyptian village [643]. This anomaly has been explained by the salutary effects of breast-feeding [645–647]. It is likely, however, that breast-feeding alone does not explain the resistance of infants to shigellosis.

A review of three large case series [648–650] suggests that about 1.6% (35 of 2225) of shigellosis cases occur in infants in the neonatal period. The largest series of neonatal shigellosis [647] suggests that the course, complications, and etiologic serogroups are different in neonates than in older children. Although newborns are routinely contaminated by maternal feces, neonatal shigellosis is rare.

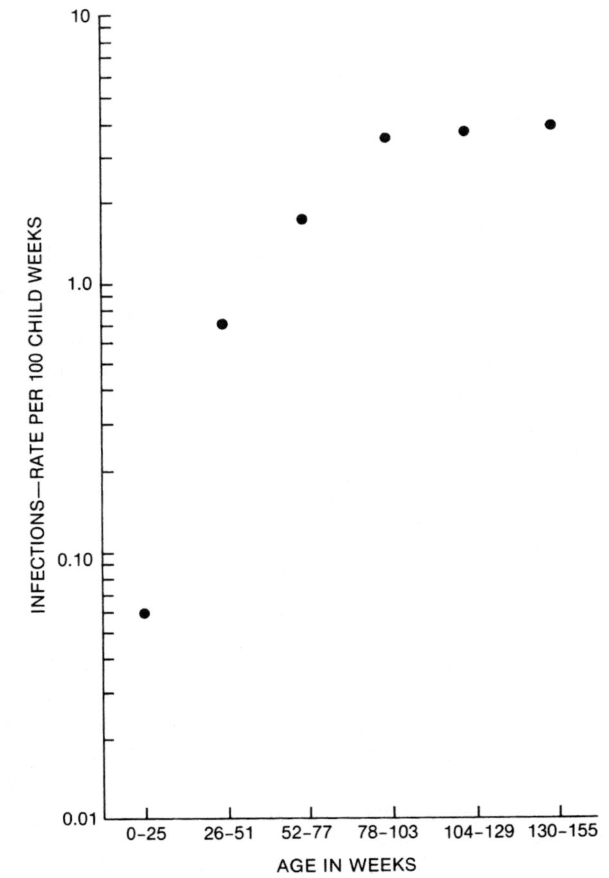

FIGURE 11–1 Age-related incidence of *Shigella* infection. (*Data from Mata LG. The Children of Santa Maria Cauque: A Prospective Field Study of Health and Growth. Cambridge, MA, MIT Press, 1978.*)

Other aspects of the epidemiology of shigellosis elude simple explanation. The seasonality (summer-fall peak in the United States, rainy season peak in the tropics) is not well explained. The geographic variation in species causing infection likewise is not well understood. In the United States, most *Shigella* infections are caused by *S. sonnei* or, less commonly, *S. flexneri*. In most of the developing world, the relative importance of these two species is reversed, and other *Shigella* serotypes, especially *S. dysenteriae* serotype 1, are identified more frequently. As hygiene improves, the proportion of *S. sonnei* increases, and that of *S. flexneri* decreases [651]. Data from Bangladesh suggest that *S. dysenteriae* is less common in neonates, but *S. sonnei* and *S. boydii* are more common [647].

Clinical Manifestations

There seem to be some important differences in the relative frequencies of various complications of *Shigella* infection related to age. Some of these differences and estimates are based on data that are undoubtedly compromised by reporting biases. *S. dysenteriae* serotype 1 characteristically causes a more severe illness than other shigellae with more complications, including pseudomembranous colitis, hemolysis, and HUS. Illnesses caused by various *Shigella* serotypes usually are indistinguishable, however, from each other and conventionally are discussed together.

The incubation period of shigellosis is related to the number of organisms ingested, but in general, it is 12 to 48 hours. Volunteer studies have shown that after ingestion, illness may be delayed for 1 week or more. Neonatal shigellosis seems to have a similar incubation period. More than half of neonatal cases occur within 3 days of birth, consistent with fecal-oral transmission during parturition. Mothers of infected neonates are sometimes carriers, although more typically they are symptomatic during the perinatal period. Intrauterine infection is rare. In an older child, the initial signs are usually high fever, abdominal pain, vomiting, toxicity, and large-volume watery stools; diarrhea may be bloody or may become bloody. Painful defecation and severe, crampy abdominal pain associated with frequent passage of small-volume stools with gross blood and mucus are characteristic findings in older children or adults who develop severe colitis. Many children never develop bloody diarrhea, however. Adult volunteer studies have shown that variations in presentation and course are not related to the dose ingested because some patients develop colitis with dysentery, but others develop only watery diarrhea after ingestion of the same inoculum [638].

The neonate with shigellosis may have a mild diarrheal syndrome or a severe colitis [648,652–660]. Fever in neonates is usually low grade (<38.8° C [<102° F]) if the course is uncomplicated. The neonate has less bloody diarrhea, more dehydration, more bacteremia, and a greater likelihood of death than the older child with shigellosis [647]. Physical examination of the neonate may show signs of toxicity and dehydration, although fever, abdominal tenderness, and rectal findings are less striking than in the older child [649].

Complications of shigellosis are common [661]. Although the illness is self-limited in the normal host, resolution may be delayed for 1 week or more. In neonates and malnourished children, chronic diarrhea may follow a bout of shigellosis [652,660]. Of hospitalized children with *Shigella*, 10% to 35% have convulsions before or during the course of diarrhea [661–663]. Usually, the seizures are brief, generalized, and associated with high fever. Seizures are uncommon in the first 6 months of life, although neonates have been described with seizures [654,664]. The cerebrospinal fluid generally reveals normal values in these children, but a few have mild cerebrospinal fluid pleocytosis. The neurologic outcome generally is good even with focal or prolonged seizures, but fatalities occasionally occur, often associated with toxic encephalopathy [665]. Although the seizures had been postulated to result from the neurotoxicity of Shiga toxin, this explanation was proved to be incorrect because most shigellae make little or no Shiga toxin, and the strains isolated from children with neurologic symptoms do not produce Shiga toxin [631,666]. Hemolysis with or without development of uremia is a complication primarily of *S. dysenteriae* serotype 1 infection [667].

Sepsis during the course of shigellosis may be caused by the *Shigella* itself or by other gut flora that gain access to the bloodstream through damaged mucosa [647,668,669]. The risk of sepsis is higher in the 1st year of life, particularly in neonates [647,652–654,664,670], in malnourished infants, and in infants with *S. dysenteriae* serotype 1 infection [669]. Sepsis may occur in 12% of neonates with shigellosis [646,661,668,671]. Given the infrequency of neonatal shigellosis, it is striking that 9% of reported cases of *Shigella* sepsis have involved infants in the 1st month of life [672]. One of the infants with bacteremia [673] reportedly had no discernible illness. Disseminated intravascular coagulation may develop in patients whose course is complicated by sepsis. Meningitis has been described in a septic neonate. Colonic perforation has occurred in neonates [645,674], older children [675], and adults [676]. Although this complication of toxic megacolon is rare, it seems to be more common in neonates than in older individuals. Bronchopneumonia may complicate the course of shigellosis, but shigellae are rarely isolated from lungs or tracheal secretions [677]. The syndrome of sudden death in the setting of extreme toxicity with hyperpyrexia and convulsions but without dehydration or sepsis (i.e., Ekiri syndrome) [678–680] is rare in neonates. In a nonbacteremic child, other extraintestinal foci of infection, including vagina [681,682] and eye [683], rarely occur. Reiter syndrome, which rarely complicates the illness in children, has not been reported in neonates.

Although infection is less common in infants than in toddlers, case-fatality rates are highest in infants [684,685]. The mortality rate in newborns seems to be about twice that of older children [647]. In industrialized societies, less than 1% of children with shigellosis die, whereas in developing countries, 30% die. These differences in mortality rates are related to nutrition [648], availability of medical care, antibiotic resistance of many shigellae, the frequency of sepsis, and the higher frequency of *S. dysenteriae* serotype 1 infection in the less-developed world [669].

Diagnosis

Although the diagnosis of shigellosis can be suspected on clinical grounds, other enteropathogens can cause illnesses that are impossible to distinguish clinically. Shigellosis in neonates is rare. A neonate with watery diarrhea is more likely to be infected with *E. coli*, *Salmonella*, or rotavirus than *Shigella*. Infants presenting with bloody diarrhea may have necrotizing enterocolitis or infection with *Salmonella*, EIEC, *Yersinia enterocolitica*, *C. jejuni*, or *Entamoeba histolytica*. Before cultures establish a diagnosis, clinical and laboratory data may aid in making a presumptive diagnosis. Abdominal radiographs showing pneumatosis intestinalis suggest the diagnosis of necrotizing enterocolitis. A history of several weeks of illness without fever and with few fecal leukocytes suggests *E. histolytica*, rather than *Shigella* infection [686].

The definitive diagnosis of shigellosis depends on isolation of the organism from stool. Culture may be insensitive, however [687]. In volunteer studies, daily stool cultures failed to detect shigellae in about 20% of symptomatic subjects [638]. Optimal recovery is achieved by immediate inoculation of stool (as opposed to rectal swabs) onto culture media. Use of transport media generally decreases the yield of cultures positive for *Shigella* [688] compared with immediate inoculation.

Examination of stool for leukocytes as an indication of colitis is useful in support of the clinical suspicion of shigellosis. The white blood cell count and differential count also are used as supporting evidence for the diagnosis. Leukemoid reactions (white blood cells $>50,000/mm^3$) occur in almost 15% of children with *S. dysenteriae* serotype 1, but in less than 2% of children with other shigellae [666]. Leukemoid reactions are more frequent in infants than in older children [667]. Even when the total white blood cell count is not dramatically elevated, there may be a striking left shift. Almost 30% of children with shigellosis have greater than 25% bands on the differential cell count [689–691]. Few reports address the white blood cell count in newborns, but those that do suggest that normal or low rather than elevated counts are more common. Although serum and fecal antibodies develop to lipopolysaccharides and virulence plasmid–associated polypeptides [692], serologic studies are not useful in the diagnosis of shigellosis. PCR can identify *Shigella* and EIEC in feces [693]. Colonoscopy typically shows inflammatory changes that are most severe in the distal segments of colon [694].

Therapy

Because dehydration is particularly common in neonatal shigellosis, attention to correction of fluid and electrolyte disturbances is always the first concern when the illness is suspected. Although debate continues over the indications for antimicrobial therapy in patients with shigellosis, the benefits of therapy generally seem to outweigh the risks. The chief disadvantages of antimicrobial therapy include cost, drug toxicity, and emergence of antibiotic-resistant shigellae. Because of the self-limited nature of shigellosis, it has been argued that less severe illness should not be treated. Children can feel quite ill during the typical bout of shigellosis, however, and appropriate antimicrobial therapy shortens the duration of illness and eliminates shigellae from stool, decreasing secondary spread. Complications are probably decreased by antibiotics. Given the high mortality rates of neonatal shigellosis, therapy should not be withheld.

The empirical choice of an antimicrobial agent is dictated by susceptibility data for strains circulating in the community at the time the patient's infection occurs. Multiresistant shigellae complicate the choice of empirical therapy before availability of susceptibility data for the patient's isolate. Plasmid-encoded resistance (R factors) for multiple antibiotics has been observed frequently in *S. dysenteriae* serotype 1 outbreaks [695] and with other shigellae [696–698]. Antimicrobial resistance patterns fluctuate from year to year in a given locale [699]. Despite the guesswork involved, early preemptive therapy is indicated, however, when an illness is strongly suggestive of shigellosis. In vitro susceptibility does not always adequately predict therapeutic responses. Cefaclor [700], furazolidone [701], cephalexin [702], amoxicillin [703], kanamycin [704], and cefamandole [705] all are relatively ineffective agents.

The optimal duration of therapy is debatable. Studies in children older than 2 years and in adults suggest that single-dose regimens may be as effective in relieving symptoms as courses given for 5 days. The single-dose regimens generally are not as effective in eliminating shigellae from the feces as the longer courses. A third-generation cephalosporin, such as ceftriaxone, may be the best empirical choice. Optimal doses for newborns with shigellosis have not been established. Trimethoprim at a dose of 10 mg/kg/day (maximum 160 mg/day) and sulfamethoxazole at a dose of 50 mg/kg/day (maximum 800 mg/day) in two divided doses for a total of 5 days are recommended for older children if the organism is susceptible [706–708]. If the condition of the infant does not permit oral administration of the drug, daily therapy usually is divided into three doses given intravenously over 1 hour [709]. Ampicillin at a dose of 100 mg/kg/day in four divided doses taken orally for 5 days may be used if the strain is susceptible [691].

For the rare newborn who acquires shigellosis, appropriate therapy often is delayed until susceptibility data are available. This delay occurs because shigellosis is so rare in newborns that it is almost never the presumptive diagnosis in a neonate with watery or bloody diarrhea. Although a sulfonamide is as efficacious as ampicillin when the infecting strain is susceptible [690], sulfonamides are avoided in neonates because of concern about the potential risk of kernicterus. The risk of empirical ampicillin therapy is that shigellae are frequently resistant to the drug; 50% of shigellae currently circulating in the United States are ampicillin resistant [709,710].

For the neonate infected with ampicillin-resistant *Shigella*, there are few data on which to base a recommendation. Ceftriaxone is generally active against shigellae, but in the neonate, this drug can displace bilirubin-binding sites and elicit clinically significant cholestasis. Data on children and adults suggest that clinical improvement occurs with ceftriaxone [711,712]. Quinolones, such as ciprofloxacin and ofloxacin, have been shown to be effective agents for treating shigellosis [713,714] in adults,

but they are not approved by the FDA for use in children younger than 18 years. In severe cases of shigellosis, a quinolone may be considered because the fear of quinolone-associated cartilage damage has decreased over time. Other drugs sometimes used to treat diarrhea pose special risks to the infant with shigellosis. The antimotility agents, in addition to their intoxication risk, may pose a special danger in dysentery. In adults, diphenoxylate hydrochloride with atropine has been shown to prolong fever and excretion of the organism [715]. Cefixime may be an effective oral agent in children [221].

The response to appropriate antibiotic therapy is generally gratifying. Improvement is often apparent in less than 24 hours. Complete resolution of diarrhea may not occur until 1 week or more after the start of treatment. In patients who have severe colitis and patients infected by *S. dysenteriae* serotype 1, the response to treatment is delayed.

Prevention

For most of the developing world, the best strategy for prevention of shigellosis during infancy is prolonged breast-feeding. Specific antibodies in milk seem to prevent symptomatic shigellosis [81,83]; nonspecific modification of gut flora and the lack of bacterial contamination of human milk also may be important. Breast-feeding, even when other foods are consumed, decreases the risk of shigellosis; children who continue to consume human milk into the 3rd year of life are still partially protected from illness [716]. In the United States, the best means of preventing infection in the infant is good hand hygiene when an older sibling or parent develops diarrhea. Even in unsanitary environments, secondary spread of shigellae can be dramatically decreased by hand hygiene after defecation and before meals [717]. Spread of shigellae in the hospital nursery can presumably be prevented by the use of contact isolation for infants with diarrhea and attention to thorough hand hygiene. Although nursery personnel have acquired shigellosis from infected newborns [698], further transmission to other infants in the nursery, although described [718], is rare. In contrast to *Salmonella*, large outbreaks of nosocomial shigellosis in neonates are rare.

Good hygiene is a particularly difficult problem in day care centers. The gathering of susceptible children, breakdown in hand hygiene, failure to use different personnel for food preparation and diaper changing, and difficulty controlling the behavior of toddlers all contribute to day care–focused outbreaks of shigellosis.

Immunization strategies have been studied since the turn of the 20th century, but no satisfactory vaccine has been developed. Even if immunizations are improved, a role in managing neonates seems unlikely.

CAMPYLOBACTER
Nature of the Organism

Campylobacter was first recognized in an aborted sheep fetus in the early 1900s [719] and was named *Vibrio fetus* by Smith and Taylor in 1919 [720]. This organism subsequently was identified as a major venereally transmitted cause of abortion and sterility and as a cause of scours in cattle, sheep, and goats [721,722]. It was not until 1947, when it was isolated from the blood culture of a pregnant woman who subsequently aborted at 6 months' gestation, that the significance of *Campylobacter* as a relatively rare cause of bacteremia and perinatal infections in humans was appreciated [723–725]. During the 1970s, *Campylobacter* was recognized to be an opportunistic pathogen in debilitated patients [726,727]. In 1963, *V. fetus* and related organisms were separated from the vibrios (e.g., *V. cholerae* and *Vibrio parahaemolyticus*) and placed in a new genus, *Campylobacter* (Greek word for "curved rod") [729]. Since 1973, several *Campylobacter* species have been recognized as a common cause of enteritis [730–746] and, in some cases, extraintestinal infections.

The genus *Campylobacter* contains 15 species, most of which are recognized as animal and human pathogens. The most commonly considered causes of human disease are *Campylobacter fetus*, *C. jejuni*, *Campylobacter coli*, *Campylobacter lari*, and *Campylobacter upsaliensis* (Table 11-5) [744–746], although *Campylobacter mucosalis* has been isolated from stool of children with diarrhea [747]. DNA hybridization studies have shown that these species are distinct, sharing less than 35% DNA homology under stringent hybridization conditions [748,749].

Strains of *C. fetus* are divided into two subspecies: *C. fetus* subspecies *fetus* and *C. fetus* subspecies *venerealis*. The first subspecies causes sporadic abortion in cattle and sheep [750,751]; in the human fetus and newborn, it causes perinatal and neonatal infections that result in abortion, premature delivery, bacteremia, and meningitis [723–725,750–762]. Outside the newborn period, *Campylobacter* is a relatively infrequent cause of bacteremia, usually infecting patients with impaired host defenses, including elderly or debilitated patients; less frequently, it causes intravascular infection [726–729,763,764].

The most common syndrome caused by a *Campylobacter* species is enteritis. *C. jejuni* and *C. coli* cause gastroenteritis and generally are referred to collectively as *C. jejuni*, although DNA hybridization studies show them to be different. In the laboratory, *C. jejuni* can be differentiated from *C. coli* because it is capable of hydrolyzing hippurate, whereas *C. coli* is not. Most isolates that are associated with diarrhea (61% to 100%) are identified as *C. jejuni* [765–768], and in some cases, individuals have been shown to be simultaneously infected with *C. jejuni* and *C. coli* [766].

Because of the fastidious nature of *C. jejuni*, which is difficult to isolate from fecal flora, its widespread occurrence was not recognized until 1973 [730–746]. Previously called related vibrios by King [763], this organism had been associated with bloody diarrhea and colitis in infants and adults only when it had been associated with a recognized bacteremia [769–771]. In the late 1970s, development of selective fecal culture methods for *C. jejuni* enabled its recognition worldwide as one of the most common causes of enteritis in people of all ages. It is an uncommon infection in neonates, who generally develop gastroenteritis when infected [151,732,772–785]. Bacteremia with *C. jejuni* enteritis also is uncommon [732,773, 778,783,786–792]. Maternal symptoms considered to be related to *C. jejuni* infection generally are mild and include fever (75%) and diarrhea (30%). In contrast to the serious disease in newborns that is caused by *C. fetus*, neonatal infections with *C. jejuni* usually result in a mild illness,* although meningitis occurs rarely [775,783]. Third-trimester infection related to *C. fetus* or *C. jejuni* may result in abortion or stillbirth.

Pathogenesis

C. fetus does not produce recognized enterotoxins or cytotoxins and does not seem to be locally invasive by the Sereny test [727,745]. Instead, these infections may be associated with penetration of the organism through a relatively intact intestinal mucosa to the reticuloendothelial system and bloodstream [727]. Whether this characteristic reflects a capacity to resist serum factors or to multiply intracellularly remains to be determined.

C. jejuni is capable of producing illness by several mechanisms. Increasing laboratory evidence suggests that the organisms are invasive and proinflammatory [728], similar to *Shigella* and *Salmonella*, although the mechanisms of these effects are not well understood. These organisms have been shown to produce an LT enterotoxin and a cytotoxin [793–796]. This enterotoxin is known to be a heat-labile protein with a molecular mass of 60 to 70 MDa [793,796]. It shares functional and immunologic properties with cholera toxin and *E. coli* LT. *C. jejuni* and *C. coli* also elaborate a cytotoxin active against numerous mammalian cells [797–799]. The toxin is heat labile, trypsin sensitive, and not neutralized by immune sera to Shiga toxin or the cytotoxin of *Clostridium difficile*. The role of these toxins as virulence factors in diarrheal disease remains unproved [793,798].

TABLE 11-5   *Campylobacter* Species That Infect Humans

Current Nomenclature	Previous Nomenclature	Usual Disease Produced
C. fetus	*Vibrio fetus*	Bacteremia, meningitis, perinatal infection, intravascular infection
	V. fetus var. *intestinalis*	
	C. fetus subsp. *intestinalis*	
C. jejuni	*Vibrio jejuni*	Diarrhea
C. coli	*C. fetus* subsp. *jejuni*	Diarrhea
C. lari	Grouped with *C. jejuni*, nalidixic acid–resistant, thermophilic *Campylobacter*, *C. laridis* I	Diarrhea, bacteremia
C. upsaliensis	None	Diarrhea, bacteremia
C. hyointestinalis	None	Diarrhea, bacteremia
C. concisus	None	Diarrhea

---

*References [772,774,776,777,779–782,785,792].

Several animal models have been tested for use in the study of this pathogen [800]. Potential models for the study of *C. jejuni* enteritis include dogs, which may acquire symptomatic infection [801]; 3- to 8-day-old chicks [802–804]; chicken embryo cells, which are readily invaded by *C. jejuni* [739]; rhesus monkeys [805]; and rabbits by means of the removable intestinal tie adult rabbit technique. An established small mammal model that mimics human disease in the absence of previous treatment or surgical procedure has not been successful in adult mice [806]. An infant mouse model [807,808] and a hamster model [809] of diarrhea seem promising. *C. jejuni* is negative in the Sereny test for invasiveness [810], and most investigators report no fluid accumulation in ligated rabbit ileal loops.

Pathology

The pathologic findings of *C. fetus* infection in the perinatal period include placental necrosis [724] and, in the neonate, widespread endothelial proliferation, intravascular fibrin deposition, perivascular inflammation, and hemorrhagic necrosis in the brain [811]. A tendency for intravascular location and hepatosplenomegaly in adults infected with *C. fetus* has been shown [727].

The pathologic findings in infants and children infected with *C. fetus* include an acute inflammatory process in the colon or rectum, as evidenced by the tendency for patients to have bloody diarrhea with numerous fecal leukocytes [812]. There also can be crypt abscess formation and an ulcerative colitis or pseudomembranous colitis–like appearance [813,814] or a hemorrhagic jejunitis or ileitis [731,739,815,816]. Mesenteric lymphadenitis, ileocolitis, and acute appendicitis also have been described.

Epidemiology

Infection with *Campylobacter* species occurs after ingestion of contaminated food, including unpasteurized milk, poultry, and contaminated water [740,817–826]. Many farm animals and pets, such as chickens [827], dogs [828,829], and cats (especially young animals), are potential sources. The intrafamilial spread of infection in households [731,830], the occurrence of outbreaks in nurseries [783,784,831], and the apparent laboratory acquisition of *C. jejuni* [832] all suggest that *C. jejuni* infection may occur after person-to-person transmission of the organism. Outbreaks of *C. jejuni* in the child day care setting are uncommon.

Volunteer studies [833] have shown a variable range in the infecting dose, with many volunteers developing no illness. The report of illness after ingestion of 10^6 organisms in a glass of milk [742] and production of illness in a single volunteer by 500 organisms [833] substantiate the variation in individual susceptibility. The potential for low-inoculum disease has significant implications for the importance of strict enteric precautions when infected persons are hospitalized, particularly in maternity and nursery areas. When diarrhea in neonates caused by *C. jejuni* has been reported [772–785], maternal-infant transmission during labor has generally been documented [772–777,779–782,784,785]. The Lior serotyping system, restriction length polymorphism, and pulsed-field gel electrophoresis [834] have been

used to confirm the identity of the infant and maternal isolates. Most mothers gave no history of diarrhea during pregnancy [776,777,779,780]. Outbreaks have occurred in neonatal intensive care units because of person-to-person spread [834].

The frequency of asymptomatic carriage of *C. jejuni* ranges from 0% to 1.3% [730,731] to 13% to 85% [730,731,746,835–837]. In a cohort study in Mexico, 66% of all infections related to *C. jejuni* were asymptomatic [746]. Infected children, if untreated, can be expected to excrete the organisms for 3 or 4 weeks; however, more than 80% are culture-negative after 5 weeks [735,736]. Asymptomatic excreters pose a significant risk in the neonatal period, in which acquisition from an infected mother can be clinically important [732,774,776,780]. *C. jejuni* has increasingly been recognized as a cause of watery and inflammatory diarrhea in temperate and tropical climates throughout the world. It has been isolated from 2% to 11% of all fecal cultures from patients with diarrheal illnesses in various parts of the world [730–738,742,838–843]. There is a tendency for *C. jejuni* enteritis to occur in the summer in countries with temperate climates [839].

The reservoir of *Campylobacter* is the GI tract of domestic and wild birds and animals. It infects sheep, cattle, goats, antelope, swine, chickens, domestic turkeys, and pet dogs. *C. fetus* often is carried asymptomatically in the intestinal or biliary tracts of sheep and cattle. During the course of a bacteremic illness in pregnant animals, *C. fetus* organisms, which have a high affinity for placental tissue, invade the uterus and multiply in the immunologically immature fetus. Infected fetuses generally are aborted. Whether this organism is acquired by humans from animals or is carried asymptomatically for long periods in humans, who may transmit the organism through sexual contact as apparently occurs in animals, is unclear. It is believed that this subspecies rarely is found in the human intestine and that it is not a cause of human enteritis [739].

C. fetus infections predominantly occur in older men with a history of farm or animal exposure and in pregnant women in their third trimester [723,724,730,731]. Symptomatically or asymptomatically infected women may have recurrent abortions or premature deliveries and are the source of organisms associated with life-threatening perinatal infections of the fetus or newborn infant [723,753–762,844]. In several instances of neonatal sepsis and meningitis, *C. fetus* was isolated from culture of maternal cervix or vagina [725,761,809]. A nosocomial nursery outbreak has been associated with carriage in some healthy infants [845]. Other outbreaks have been associated with meningitis [846,847]. Cervical cultures have remained positive in women who have had recurrent abortions and whose husbands have antibody titer elevations [752].

The most commonly incriminated reservoir of *C. jejuni* is poultry [822,826,848,849]. Most chickens in several different geographic locations had numerous (mean 4 × 10^6/g) *C. jejuni* in the lower intestinal tract or feces. This occurred in some instances despite the use of tetracycline, to which *Campylobacter* was susceptible in vitro, in the chicken feed [842]. The internal cavities of chickens remain positive for *Campylobacter* even after they have been cleaned, packaged, and frozen [848]. In contrast to *Salmonella*, *C. jejuni* organisms that survive usually do not multiply to high concentrations [739]. Domestic puppies or kittens with *C. jejuni* diarrhea also can provide a source for spread, especially to infants or small children [731,769,826,850–852].

C. jejuni enteritis also has been associated in numerous outbreaks with consumption of unpasteurized milk [739, 823–825,853–855]. In retrospect, the first reported human cases of *C. jejuni* enteritis were probably in a milk-borne outbreak reported in 1946 [856]. Because *Campylobacter* infections of the udder are not seen, milk is probably contaminated from fecal shedding of the organism. These organisms are killed by adequate heating.

Fecally contaminated water is a potential vehicle for *C. jejuni* infections [857]. Several phenotypic and genotypic methods have been used for distinguishing *C. jejuni* strains from animals and humans involved in epidemics [858]. *C. jejuni* is associated with traveler's diarrhea among people traveling from England or the United States [734].

Clinical Manifestations

Clinical manifestations of infection caused by *Campylobacter* depend on the species involved (see Table 11–5). Human infections with *C. fetus* are rare and generally are limited to bacteremia in patients with predisposing conditions [763,764] or to bacteremia or uterine infections with prolonged fever and pneumonitis that last for several weeks in women during the third trimester of pregnancy. Unless appropriately treated, symptoms usually resolve only after abortion or delivery of an infected infant [723,725,753–762,764]. These infected neonates, who are often premature, develop signs suggesting sepsis, including fever, cough, respiratory distress, vomiting, diarrhea, cyanosis, convulsions, and jaundice. The condition typically progresses to meningitis, which may be rapidly fatal or may result in serious neurologic sequelae [725]. Additional systemic manifestations include pericarditis, pneumonia, peritonitis, salpingitis, septic arthritis, and abscesses [837].

C. jejuni infection typically involves the GI tract, producing watery diarrhea or a dysentery-like illness with fever and abdominal pain and stools that contain blood and mucus [729,746,814]. Older infants and children generally are affected, but neonates with diarrhea have been reported. Infection in neonates generally is not clinically apparent or is mild. Stools can contain blood, mucus, and pus [725,735,776,777]; fever often is absent [735,776]. The illness usually responds to appropriate antimicrobial therapy [774,776,830], which shortens the period of fecal shedding [859]. Extraintestinal infections related to *C. jejuni* other than bacteremia are rare, but include cholecystitis [860], urinary tract infection [861], and meningitis [775]. Bacteremia is a complication of GI infection [862], especially in malnourished children [863]. Meningitis that apparently occurs secondary to intestinal infection also has been reported in premature infants who have had intraventricular needle aspirations for neonatal hydrocephalus [725]. Complications in older children and adults that have been associated with *C. jejuni* enteritis include Reiter syndrome [864], Guillain-Barré syndrome [865,866], and

reactive arthritis [867,868]. Persistent *C. jejuni* infections have been described in patients infected with HIV [869]. Extraintestinal manifestations generally occur in patients who are immunosuppressed or at the extremes of age [727]. *C. lari* has caused chronic diarrhea and bacteremia in a neonate [870].

Diagnosis

Most important in the diagnosis of *Campylobacter* infection is a high index of suspicion based on clinical grounds. *C. fetus* and *C. jejuni* are fastidious and may be overlooked on routine fecal cultures. Isolation of *Campylobacter* from blood or other sterile body sites does not represent the same problem as isolation from stool. Growth occurs with standard blood culture media, but it may be slow. In the case of *C. fetus* infecting the bloodstream or central nervous system, blood culture flasks should be blindly subcultured and held for at least 7 days, or the organism may not be detected because of slow or inapparent growth [756]. The diagnosis of *C. fetus* infection should be considered when there is an unexplained febrile illness in the third trimester of pregnancy or in the event of recurrent abortion, prematurity, or neonatal sepsis with or without meningitis. A high index of suspicion and prompt, appropriate antimicrobial therapy may prevent the potentially serious neonatal complications that may follow maternal *C. fetus* infection.

Campylobacter is distinguished from *Vibrio* organisms by its characteristics of carbohydrate nonfermentation and by its different nucleotide base composition [729,747–749,752]. *Campylobacter* is 0.2 to 0.5 fm wide and 0.5 to 8 fm long. It is a fastidious, microaerophilic, curved, motile gram-negative bacillus that has a single polar flagellum and is oxidase and catalase positive except for *C. upsaliensis*, which is generally catalase negative or weakly positive. *C. jejuni* and *C. fetus* are separated by growth temperature (*C. fetus* grows best at 25° C, but can be cultured at 37° C; *C. jejuni* grows best at 42° C) and by nalidixic acid and cephalosporin susceptibilities because *C. jejuni* is susceptible to nalidixic acid and resistant to cephalosporins.

C. jejuni grows best in a microaerobic environment of 5% oxygen and 10% carbon dioxide at 42° C. It grows on various media, including Brucella and Mueller-Hinton agars, but optimal isolation requires the addition of selective and nutritional supplements. Growth at 42° C in the presence of cephalosporins is used to culture selectively for *C. jejuni* from fecal specimens. In a study of six media, charcoal-based selective media and a modified charcoal cefoperazone deoxycholate agar were the most selective for identification of *Campylobacter* species. Extending the incubation time from 48 to 72 hours led to an increase in the isolation rate regardless of the medium used [871]. Its typical darting motility may provide a clue to identification, even in fresh fecal specimens, when viewed by phase-contrast microscopy [735,872].

When the organism has been cultured, it is presumptively identified by motility and by its curved, sometimes sea gull–like appearance on carbolfuchsin stain. Polymorphonuclear leukocytes are usually found in stools when bloody diarrhea occurs and indicate the occurrence of colitis [776,812]. To avoid potentially serious *C. jejuni* infection in the newborn, careful histories of any diarrheal illnesses in the family should be obtained, and pregnant women with any enteric illness should have cultures for this and other enteric pathogens. Detection of *C. jejuni* and *C. coli* by PCR has been reported [873] and in the future may be useful for the rapid and reliable identification of this organism.

The differential diagnosis of *C. fetus* infections includes the numerous agents that cause neonatal sepsis or meningitis, especially gram-negative bacilli. Diagnostic considerations for inflammatory or bloody enteritis include necrotizing enterocolitis, allergic proctitis, and *Salmonella*; rarely *Shigella* and other infectious agents occur. Agglutination, complement fixation, bactericidal, immunofluorescence, and ELISA tests have been used for serologic diagnosis of *C. jejuni* infection and to study the immune response, but these assays are of limited value in establishing the diagnosis during an acute infection [745].

Therapy

The prognosis is grave in newborns with sepsis or meningitis caused by *C. fetus*. In infants with *C. jejuni* gastroenteritis, limited data suggest that appropriate, early antimicrobial therapy results in improvement and rapid clearance of the organism from stool [859]. *Campylobacter* species are often resistant to β-lactams, including ampicillin and cephalosporins [874,875]. Most strains are susceptible to erythromycin, gentamicin, tetracycline, chloramphenicol, and the newer quinolones, although resistance to these agents has been reported [876,877]. A parenteral aminoglycoside seems to be the drug of choice for *C. fetus* infections, pending in vitro susceptibility studies. In the case of central nervous system involvement, cefotaxime and chloramphenicol are potential alternative drugs. Depending on in vitro susceptibilities, which vary with locale, erythromycin is the drug of choice for treating *C. jejuni* enteritis [731,735,736]. If erythromycin therapy is initiated within the first 4 days of illness, a reduction in excretion of the organism and resolution of symptoms occur [859].

Although data regarding treatment of asymptomatic or convalescent carriers are unavailable, it seems appropriate to treat colonized pregnant women in the third trimester of pregnancy when there is a risk of perinatal or neonatal infection. The failure of prophylactic parenteral gentamicin in a premature infant has been documented, followed by successful resolution of symptoms and fecal shedding with erythromycin. Because there seems to be an increased risk of toxicity with erythromycin estolate during pregnancy and infancy [878], other forms of erythromycin should probably be used in these settings. Azithromycin seems to be effective if the organism is susceptible [879]. Strains that are erythromycin resistant often are resistant to azithromycin [880]. *Campylobacter* tends to have higher minimal inhibitory concentrations for clarithromycin than for azithromycin [881].

Prevention

Contact precautions should be employed during any acute diarrheal illness and until the diarrhea has subsided. Hand hygiene after handling raw poultry and washing cutting boards and utensils with soap and water after contact with raw poultry may decrease risk of infection. Pasteurization of milk and chlorination of water are critical. Infected food handlers and hospital employees who are asymptomatic pose no known hazard for disease transmission if proper personal hygiene measures are maintained. Ingestion of human milk that contains anti–*C. jejuni* antibodies has been shown to protect infants from diarrhea caused by *C. jejuni* [78,882].

CLOSTRIDIUM DIFFICILE
Nature of the Organism and Pathophysiology

C. difficile is a spore-forming, gram-positive, anaerobic bacillus that produces two toxins: enterotoxin that causes fluid secretion (toxin A) and a cytotoxin detectable by its cytopathic effects in tissue culture (toxin B) [151,883]. In the presence of antibiotic pressure, *C. difficile* colonic overgrowth and toxin production occur. Both toxin genes have been cloned and sequenced, revealing that they encode proteins with estimated molecular masses of 308 kDa for toxin A and 270 kDa for toxin B [884].

A wide variety of antibacterial, antifungal, antituberculosis, and antineoplastic agents have been associated with *C. difficile* colitis, although penicillin, clindamycin, and cephalosporins are associated most frequently. Rarely, no precipitating drug has been given [885–889]. *C. difficile* and its toxins can be shown in one third of patients with antibiotic-associated diarrhea and in about 98% of patients with pseudomembranous colitis [890].

Epidemiology

C. difficile can be isolated from soil and frequently exists in the hospital environment. Spores of *C. difficile* are acquired from the environment or by fecal-oral transmission from colonized individuals or from items in the environment, such as thermometers and feeding tubes [891–896]. *C. difficile* has been shown to persist on a contaminated floor for 5 months [892]. Nosocomial spread is related to organisms on the hands of personnel [892,893,897], and to contaminated surfaces, which may serve as reservoirs [898,899]. Although all groups are susceptible to infection, newborns represent a special problem. Less than 5% of healthy children older than 2 years [900] and healthy adults carry *C. difficile* [890], but more than 50% of neonates can be shown to have *C. difficile* and its cytotoxin in their stools, usually in the absence of clinical findings [893,899,901–903].

Infants in neonatal intensive care units have high rates of colonization, in part because of frequent use of antimicrobial agents in these units [902,903]. Clustering of infected infants suggests that much of the colonization of newborn infants represents nosocomial spread [899], rather than acquisition of maternal flora. The number of *C. difficile* organisms present in stools of well infants is similar to that found in older patients with pseudomembranous colitis [903]. The high frequency of colonization has led to justified skepticism about the pathogenic potential of this organism in very young patients [904]. Although some episodes of diarrhea in early infancy may be caused by *C. difficile* [905], the high frequency of asymptomatic carriage in this age group suggests that neither colonization nor detection of toxin production is sufficient to establish the diagnosis of *C. difficile* diarrhea in an infant. Rather, other etiologies should be comprehensively sought, and *C. difficile* should be implicated in the absence of another pathogen.

Clinical Manifestations

The usual manifestations of *C. difficile* disease in older children and adults include watery diarrhea, abdominal pain and tenderness, nausea, vomiting, and low-grade fever. Grossly bloody diarrhea is unusual, although occult fecal blood is common. Leukocytosis is present during severe illness. Diarrhea usually begins 4 to 9 days into a course of antimicrobial therapy, but may be delayed until several weeks after completion of the therapeutic course. Usually, the illness is mild and self-limited if the offending drug is discontinued. Severe colitis with pseudomembranes is less common now than in previous years because the risk of diarrhea developing during antimicrobial therapy is recognized and the antimicrobial agent typically is stopped.

It is unclear whether *C. difficile* causes disease in newborns. One study from a newborn intensive care unit suggested that toxin A in stools is associated with an increased frequency of abnormal stools [906].

Diagnosis

Endoscopic findings of pseudomembranes and hyperemic, friable rectal mucosa suggest the diagnosis of pseudomembranous colitis. Pseudomembranes are not always present in *C. difficile* colitis; mild cases are often described as nonspecific colitis. Several noninvasive techniques are used to establish the diagnosis, including enzyme immunoassay (EIA) for toxin detection and PCR [906–909]. Isolation of *C. difficile* from stool does not distinguish between toxigenic and nontoxigenic isolates. If *C. difficile* is isolated, testing for toxin by cell culture or EIA should be performed to confirm the presence of a toxigenic strain. There are multiple commercially available EIAs that detect either toxin A or both toxins A and B [906–908]. These assays are sensitive and easy to perform. Other assays are available for epidemiologic investigation of outbreaks of disease caused by *C. difficile* [909].

In older children and adults, the diagnosis is confirmed by culture of *C. difficile* and demonstration of toxin in feces. In neonates, these data are inadequate to prove that an illness is related to *C. difficile*. When the clinical picture is consistent, the stool studies are positive for *C. difficile*, and no other cause for illness is found, a diagnosis of "possible" *C. difficile* is made. A favorable response to eradication of *C. difficile* is supportive evidence that the diagnosis is correct [885]. Because of the uncertainty implicit in the ambiguity of neonatal diagnostic criteria, other diagnoses must be considered.

Therapy

When the decision is made that a neonate's illness might be related to *C. difficile*, the initial approach should include fluid and electrolyte therapy and discontinuation of the offending antimicrobial agent. If the illness persists or worsens or if the patient has severe diarrhea, specific therapy with metronidazole [899,910], should be instituted. Metronidazole is considered to be the treatment of choice for most patients with *C. difficile* colitis [911]. Orally administered vancomycin or bacitracin rarely needs to be considered in neonates [912,913].

After initiation of therapy, signs of illness generally resolve within several days, titers decrease, and fecal toxins disappear eventually. Recurrence of colitis after discontinuation of metronidazole or vancomycin has been documented in 10% to 20% of adults [914]. Relapses are treated with a second course of metronidazole or vancomycin. Drugs that decrease intestinal motility should not be administered.

Neutralizing antibody against *C. difficile* cytotoxin has been shown in human colostrum [915]. Secretory component of IgA binds to toxin A to inhibit its binding to receptors [916]. Data show that there are nonantibody factors present in milk that interfere with the action of toxin B in addition to secretory IgA directed at toxin A [917]. Breast-feeding seems to decrease the frequency of colonization by *C. difficile* [918].

Prevention

In addition to standard precautions, contact precautions are recommended for the duration of illness. Meticulous hand hygiene techniques, proper handling of contaminated waste and fomites, and limiting the use of antimicrobial agents are the best available methods for control of *C. difficile* infection.

VIBRIO CHOLERAE
Nature of the Organism

V. cholerae is a gram-negative, curved bacillus with a polar flagellum. Of the many serotypes, only enterotoxin-producing organisms of serotype O1 and O139 cause epidemics. *V. cholerae* O1 is divided into two serotypes, Inaba and Ogawa, and two biotypes, classic and El Tor; the latter is the predominant biotype. Nontoxigenic O1 strains and non-O1 strains of *V. cholerae* can cause diarrhea and sepsis, but do not cause outbreaks [919–921].

Pathogenesis

V. cholerae O group 1 is the classic example of an enteropathogen whose virulence is caused by enterotoxin production. Cholera toxin is an 84-MDa protein whose five B subunits cause toxin binding to the enterocyte membrane ganglioside GM_1 and whose A subunit causes adenosine diphosphate ribosylation of a guanosine triphosphate–binding regulatory subunit of adenylate cyclase [121,921]. The elevated cAMP levels that result from stimulation of enterocytes by cholera toxin cause secretion of salt and water with concomitant inhibition of absorption. Two other toxins are also encoded within the virulence cassette that encodes cholera toxin. These toxins, zona occludens toxin (zot) and accessory cholera toxin (ace), are consistently found in illness-causing strains of O1 and O139, but not usually in *V. cholerae* organisms that are less virulent.

Epidemiology

Since 1960, *V. cholerae* O1, biotype *El Tor*, has spread from India and Southeast Asia to Africa; the Middle East; southern Europe; and the southern, western, and central Pacific islands (Oceania). In late January 1991, toxigenic *V. cholerae* O1, serotype Inaba, biotype *El Tor*, appeared in several coastal cities of Peru [920,921]. It rapidly spread to most countries in South and North America. In reported cases, travel from the United States to Latin America or Asia and ingestion of contaminated food transported from Latin America or Asia have been incriminated. *V. cholerae* O139 (Bengal) arose on the Indian subcontinent as a new cause of epidemic cholera in 1993 [922–927]. It rapidly spread through Asia and continues to reemerge periodically as a cause of epidemic cholera.

In the United States, an endemic focus of a unique strain of toxigenic *V. cholerae* O1 exists on the Gulf Coast of Louisiana and Texas [919,927,928], This strain is different from the one associated with the epidemic in South America. Most cases of disease associated with the strain endemic to the U.S. Gulf Coast have resulted from the consumption of raw or undercooked shellfish. Humans are the only documented natural host, but free-living *V. cholerae* organisms can exist in the aquatic environment. The usual reported vehicles of transmission have included contaminated water or ice; contaminated food, particularly raw or undercooked shellfish; moist grains held at ambient temperature; and raw or partially dried fish. The usual mode of infection is ingestion of contaminated food or water. Boiling water or treating it with chlorine or iodine and adequate cooking of food kill the organism [920]. Asymptomatic infection of family contacts is common, but direct person-to-person transmission of disease has not been documented. Individuals with low gastric acidity are at increased risk for cholera infection.

Clinical Manifestations

Cholera acquired during pregnancy, particularly in the third trimester, is associated with a high incidence of fetal death [929]. Miscarriage can be attributed to fetal acidosis and hypoxemia resulting from the marked metabolic and circulatory changes that this disease induces in the mother. The likelihood of delivering a stillborn infant is closely correlated with the severity of the maternal illness. The inability to culture *V. cholerae* from stillborn infants of infected mothers, together with the usual absence of bacteremia in cholera, suggests that transplacental fetal infection is not a cause of intrauterine death.

Neonatal cholera is a rare disease. This generalization also applies to the new O139 strains, although mild [930] and severe forms of illness have rarely been described in newborns [931]. Among 242 neonates admitted to a cholera research hospital in Dacca, Bangladesh, 25 infants were ill with cholera [932]. Even infants born to mothers with active diarrheal disease may escape infection, despite evidence that rice-water stools, almost certain to be ingested during the birth process, may contain 10^9 organisms/mL [932]. The reason for this apparently low attack rate among newborns is unknown; however,

it probably can be attributed in large part to the protection conferred by breast-feeding [933]. Human milk contains antibodies [77] and receptor-like glycoprotein that inhibit adherence of *V. cholerae* [79] and gangliosides that bind cholera toxin [80]. The role of transplacentally acquired vibriocidal maternal antibodies has not been determined [934]. Because *V. cholerae* causes neither bacteremia nor intestinal invasion, protection against illness is more likely to be a function of mucosal rather than serum antibodies [935,936]. Additional factors that may reduce the incidence of neonatal cholera include the large inoculum required for infection [937] and the limited exposure of the newborn to the contaminated food and water [246].

Diagnosis

Clinicians should request that appropriate cultures be performed for stool specimens from patients suspected to have cholera. The specimen is plated on thiosulfate citrate bile salts sucrose agar directly or after enrichment in alkaline peptone water. Isolates of *V. cholerae* should be confirmed at a state health department and sent to the CDC for testing for production of cholera toxin. A fourfold increase in vibriocidal antibody titers between acute and convalescent serum samples or a fourfold decline in titers between early and late (>2 months) convalescent serum specimens can confirm the diagnosis. Oligonucleotide probes have been developed to test for the cholera toxin gene [938,939],

Therapy and Prevention

The most important modality of therapy is administration of oral or parenteral rehydration therapy to correct dehydration and electrolyte imbalance and maintain hydration [920]. Antimicrobial therapy can eradicate vibrios, reduce the duration of diarrhea, and reduce requirements for fluid replacement. One cholera vaccine, which is administered parenterally, is licensed in the United States, but is of very limited value. Several experimental oral vaccines are being tested [940–942].

YERSINIA ENTEROCOLITICA
Nature of the Organism, Epidemiology, and Pathogenesis

Y. enterocolitica is a major cause of enteritis in much of the industrialized world [943,944], Enteritis caused by this organism primarily occurs in infants and young children, and infections in the United States are reported to be more common in the North than in the South [945–950]. Animals, especially swine, have been shown to serve as the reservoir for *Y. enterocolitica*. A history of recent exposure to chitterlings (i.e., pig intestine) is common. Transmission has also occurred after ingestion of contaminated milk and infusion of contaminated blood products [951,952],

Virulence of *Y. enterocolitica* is related primarily to a virulence plasmid, which is closely related to the virulence plasmids of *Yersinia pseudotuberculosis* and *Yersinia pestis* [953,954]. ST enterotoxin, which is closely related to ST of ETEC [955], may also be important.

Clinical Manifestations

Infection with *Y. enterocolitica* is recognized as one of the causes of bacterial gastroenteritis in young children, but knowledge of neonatal infection with this organism is fragmentary. Even in large series, *Yersinia* is rarely isolated from newborns [943,944,956].

The youngest infants whose clinical course has been described in detail were 11 days to several months old at the onset of illness [944,956–964]. There were no features of the gastroenteritis to distinguish it from gastroenteritis caused by other invasive enteric pathogens, such as *Shigella* or *Salmonella*. Infants presented with watery diarrhea or with stools containing mucus with streaks of blood. Sepsis was common in these infants, particularly in the first 3 months of life when 28% of enteritis was complicated by sepsis [960,961,965,966]. Fever is an inconsistent finding in children with bacteremia, and meningitis is rare. In older children, fever and right lower quadrant pain mimicking appendicitis are often found [952].

Diagnosis

Y. enterocolitica can be recovered from throat swabs, mesenteric lymph nodes, peritoneal fluid, blood, and stool. Because laboratory identification of organisms from stool requires special techniques, laboratory personnel should be notified when *Yersinia* is suspected. Because avirulent environmental isolates occur, biotyping and serotyping are useful in assessing the clinical relevance of isolates. PCR has been used to detect pathogenic strains [967,968].

Therapy

The effect of antimicrobial therapy on the outcome of GI infection is uncertain. It has been recommended that antibiotics be reserved for sepsis or prolonged and severe gastroenteritis [943]; however, there are no prospective studies comparing the efficacy of various antimicrobial agents with each other or with supportive therapy alone. Most strains of *Y. enterocolitica* are susceptible to trimethoprim-sulfamethoxazole, aminoglycosides, piperacillin, imipenem, third-generation cephalosporins, amoxicillin-clavulanate potassium, and chloramphenicol and are resistant to amoxicillin, ampicillin, carbenicillin, ticarcillin, and macrolides [969–971]. Therapy in individual cases should be guided by in vitro susceptibility testing, although cefotaxime has been used successfully in bacteremic infants [966].

AEROMONAS HYDROPHILA
Nature of the Organism, Epidemiology, and Pathogenesis

Aeromonas hydrophila is widely distributed in animals and the environment. Although wound infection, pneumonia, and sepsis (especially in immunocompromised hosts) represent typical *Aeromonas* infections, gastroenteritis increasingly is being recognized. The organism is a gram-negative, oxidase-positive, facultatively anaerobic bacillus belonging to the family Vibrionaceae. Similar to other members of this family, it produces an enterotoxin [972]

that causes fluid secretion in rabbit ileal loops [973]. Some strains cause fluid accumulation in the suckling mouse model [974], whereas other strains are invasive [975] or cytotoxic [976]. The enterotoxin is not immunologically related to cholera toxin or the heat LT of *E. coli* [977].

Although volunteer studies and studies with monkeys have failed to provide supportive evidence for enteropathogenicity [978,979], there is good reason to believe that *A. hydrophila* does cause diarrhea in children. The earliest description of *Aeromonas* causing diarrhea was an outbreak that occurred in a neonatal unit [980]. Although several studies have failed to show an association with diarrhea [981–986], most studies have found more *Aeromonas* isolates among children with gastroenteritis than among controls [986–988]. Part of the controversy may be caused by strain differences; some strains possess virulence traits related to production of gastroenteritis, whereas others do not [982,989].

The diarrhea described in children occurs in summer, primarily affecting children in the first 2 years of life. In one study, 7 (13%) of 55 cases of *Aeromonas* detected during a 20-month period occurred in infants younger than 1 month.

Clinical Manifestations

Typically, watery diarrhea with no fever has been described; although there are descriptions of watery diarrhea with fever [990]. A dysentery-like illness occurred in 22%, however. Dysentery-like illness has been described in neonates [991]. In one third of children, diarrhea has been reported to last for more than 2 weeks [982]. There may be species-related differences in clinical features of Aeromonas-associated gastroenteritis in children [992]. Organisms that were formerly classified as *A. hydrophila* are now sometimes labeled as *Aeromonas sobria* or *Aeromonas caviae* [993, 994], Fever and abdominal pain seem to be particularly common with *A. sobria*. One series of *A. hydrophila* isolates from newborns in Dallas, Texas, showed more blood cultures than stool cultures positive for *Aeromonas* [995].

Diagnosis and Therapy

Enteric infection associated with *Aeromonas* often is not diagnosed because this organism is not routinely sought in stool cultures. When the organism is suspected, the laboratory should be notified so that oxidase testing can be performed. The organism is usually susceptible to aztreonam, imipenem, meropenem, third-generation cephalosporins, trimethoprim-sulfamethoxazole, and chloramphenicol [996–998].

PLESIOMONAS SHIGELLOIDES

Plesiomonas shigelloides is a gram-negative, facultative anaerobic bacillus that, similar to *Aeromonas*, is a member of the Vibrionaceae family. It is widely disseminated in the environment; outbreaks of disease are usually related to ingestion of contaminated water or seafood [999]. Although it has been associated with outbreaks of diarrheal disease [1000] and has been found more commonly in ill than well controls, the role of *P. shigelloides* in diarrheal disease has remained controversial [1001]. If it is a true enteropathogen, the mechanism by which it causes disease is unclear [1002,1003]. The role of this organism in neonatal diarrhea has not been extensively investigated. Infections of neonates have been reported [1004–1007], but most cases of enteric disease currently reported in the United States are in adults [999]. Typical illness consists of watery diarrhea and cramps; sometimes, fever, bloody stools, and emesis occur and last 3 to 42 days.

Diagnosis is not usually made by clinical microbiology laboratory testing because, as with *Aeromonas*, coliforms can be confused with *P. shigelloides* unless an oxidase test is performed [1008]. The true frequency of infection is unknown. The organism has antibiotic susceptibilities similar to *Aeromonas* [1009,1010],

OTHER BACTERIAL AGENTS AND FUNGI

Proving that an organism causes diarrhea is difficult, particularly when it may be present in large numbers in stools of healthy people. Bacteria that have been associated with acute gastroenteritis may be considered causative when the following criteria are met:

1. A single specific strain of the organism should be found as the predominant organism in most affected infants by different investigators in outbreaks of enteric disease in different communities.
2. This strain should be isolated in a significantly lower percentage and in smaller numbers from stool specimens of healthy infants.
3. Available methods must be used to exclude other recognized enteropathogens, including viruses and parasites, enterotoxigenic agents, and fastidious organisms such as *Campylobacter*.
4. Demonstration of effective specific antimicrobial therapy and specific antibody responses and, ultimately, production of experimental disease in volunteers are helpful in establishing the identity of a microorganism as a pathogen.

Optimally, the putative pathogen should have virulence traits that can be shown in model systems. Most bacteria that have been suggested as occasional causes of gastroenteritis in neonates fail to fulfill one or more of these criteria. Their role in the cause of diarrheal disease is questionable. This is particularly true of microorganisms described in early reports in which the possibility of infection with more recently recognized agents could not be excluded. Much of the clinical, bacteriologic, and epidemiologic data collected earlier linking unusual enteropathogens to infantile diarrhea must be reevaluated in light of current knowledge and methodology.

Several reports of acute gastroenteritis believed to have been caused by *Klebsiella* suggest that, rather than playing an etiologic role, these organisms had probably proliferated within an already inflamed bowel [1011–1013]. The recovery of *Klebsiella-Enterobacter* in pure culture from diarrheal stools has led several investigators to suggest that these bacteria may occasionally play a causative role in infantile gastroenteritis and enterocolitis [1014–1019]. Ingestion of infant formula contaminated with

Enterobacter sakazakii has been associated with development of bloody diarrhea and sepsis [1020]. *Klebsiella* species also may be isolated in pure culture from stools of newborns with no enteric symptoms, however [1021–1023]. In one study, certain capsular types of *Klebsiella* were more often isolated from infants with diarrheal disease than from normal infants [1014]. Later work has shown that *Klebsiella pneumoniae*, *Enterobacter cloacae*, and *Citrobacter* species are capable of producing enterotoxins.* Reports of isolation of *Citrobacter* species, describe associations with enteric illnesses in 7% of cases [1026–1028]. There is inadequate evidence to define the roles of *Klebsiella*, *Enterobacter*, and *Citrobacter* species as etiologic agents of enteric illnesses.

Listeria monocytogenes, a classic cause of neonatal sepsis and meningitis (see Chapter 13), has been linked to outbreaks of febrile diarrheal disease in immunocompetent adults and children [1029–1033]. Fever has occurred in 72% of ill individuals [1034]. Outbreaks have been related to ingestion of contaminated foods. *Listeria* has rarely been described as a cause of neonatal gastroenteritis [1035–1038].

Infection with enterotoxin-producing *Bacteroides fragilis* has been associated with mild watery diarrhea [1039]. These infections have a peak incidence in children 2 to 3 years old [1040]. These toxin-producing organisms cannot be detected in routine hospital laboratories.

Various organisms have been isolated from infant stools during episodes of diarrhea. Most of these reports have failed to associate illness with specific organisms in a way that has stood the test of time. *P. aeruginosa* [1041–1046] and *Proteus* [1029,1047–1053], have been associated with diarrhea, but there are few convincing data suggesting that either organism is a true enteropathogen. These organisms generally are recovered as frequently from healthy infants as from infants with diarrheal disease, suggesting that their presence in stool cultures is insignificant [289,1054–1058]. An association between *Providencia* and neonatal enteritis has been substantiated largely by anecdotal reports of nursery outbreaks [232,287,1028,1059]. These bacteria are rarely isolated from infants with sporadic or community-acquired diarrheal disease [1054–1056,1060–1062],

Candida albicans usually is acquired during passage through the birth canal and is considered a normal, although minor, component of the fecal flora of the neonate (see Chapter 33) [1063]. Intestinal overgrowth of these organisms frequently accompanies infantile gastroenteritis [1063,1064], particularly after antimicrobial therapy [1064–1067]. The upper small gut may become colonized with *Candida* in malnourished children with diarrhea [1068]; whether the presence of the organism is cause or effect is unclear. Stool cultures obtained from infants with diarrheal disease are inconclusive, and although *Candida* enteritis has been reported in adults [1069], the importance of this organism as a primary cause of neonatal gastroenteritis has been difficult to prove. Clinical descriptions of nursery epidemics of

*References [156,183,184,191,209,1020,1024,1025].

candidal enteritis are poorly documented, generally preceding the recognition of EPEC and rotaviruses as a cause of neonatal diarrhea. Even well-studied cases of intestinal involvement add little in the way of substantive proof because secondary invasion of *Candida* has been shown to be a complication of coliform enteritis [228,250,264].

Although diarrhea has sometimes been described as a finding in neonatal disseminated candidiasis, more typically, GI tract involvement with disseminated *Candida* is associated with abdominal distention and bloody stools mimicking necrotizing enterocolitis [264,1068–1073]. Typically, affected infants are premature and have courses complicated by antibiotic administration, intravascular catheter use, and surgical procedures during the first several weeks of life. A trial of oral anticandidal therapy may be helpful in neonates with diarrhea in the presence of oral or cutaneous candidiasis. If the therapy is appropriate, a response should be forthcoming within 2 to 5 days.

Diarrhea sometimes occurs as a manifestation of systemic infection. Patients with staphylococcal toxic shock syndrome often have diarrhea. Loose stools sometimes occur in sepsis, but it is unclear whether the diarrhea is a cause or an effect. The organisms isolated from blood cultures in a group of Bangladeshi infants and children with diarrhea included *Staphylococcus aureus*, *Haemophilus influenzae*, *Streptococcus pneumoniae*, *P. aeruginosa*, and various gram-negative enteric bacilli [1074]. It is unknown whether the bacteriology of sepsis associated with diarrhea is similar in the well-nourished infants seen in industrialized countries.

PARASITES

Acute diarrhea associated with intestinal parasites is infrequent during the neonatal period. In areas with high endemicity, infection of the newborn is likely to be associated with inadequate maternal and delivery care, insufficient environmental sanitation, and poor personal hygiene standards. The occurrence of symptomatic intestinal parasitic infection during the first month of life requires acquisition of the parasite during the first days or weeks; the incubation period for *E. histolytica* and *G. lamblia* is 1 to 4 weeks and for *Cryptosporidium parvum* is 7 to 14 days. The newborn can be infected during delivery by contact with maternal feces [1075], in the hospital through contact with the mother or personnel, or in the household through contact with infected individuals in close contact with the infant. Contaminated water can be an important source of infection for *G. lamblia* and *C. parvum*.

ENTAMOEBA HISTOLYTICA

Organisms formerly identified as *E. histolytica* have been reclassified into two species that are morphologically identical but genetically distinct: *E. histolytica* and *E. dispar*. The former can cause acute nonbloody and bloody diarrhea, necrotizing enterocolitis, ameboma, and liver abscess, and the latter is a noninvasive parasite that does not cause disease. Early acquisition of disease tends to be more severe in young infants; rarely, amebic liver abscess and rapidly fatal colitis have been reported in

infants [1076–1084]. A 19-day-old infant from India who presented with 10 to 12 episodes of watery and mucous diarrhea, lethargy, jaundice, and mildly elevated liver enzymes has been described; the child recovered completely after 10 days of intravenous omidazole [1076]. Amebic liver abscess can be preceded by diarrhea or have a clinical presentation of fulminant neonatal sepsis [1077]. Asymptomatic colonization of neonates with various species of amebae is common in areas of high endemicity [1085].

Diagnosis can be established by stool examination for cysts and trophozoites and by serologic studies [1086]. Through the use of PCR, isoenzyme analysis, and antigen detection assays, *E. histolytica* and *E. dispar* can be differentiated [1087,1088], Serum antibody assays may be helpful in establishing the diagnosis of amebic dysentery and extraintestinal amebiasis with liver involvement. The efficacy of treatment with metronidazole for colitis or liver abscess has not been established for the newborn period, although this therapy has been used successfully [1078]. Patients with colitis or liver abscess caused by *E. histolytica* are treated also with iodoquinol, as are asymptomatic carriers.

GIARDIA LAMBLIA

G. lamblia is a binucleate, flagellated protozoan parasite with trophozoite and cyst stages. It is spread by the fecal-oral route through ingestion of cysts. Child care center outbreaks reflecting person-to-person spread have shown its high infectivity potential [1089–1092]. Foodborne transmission and water-borne transmission also occur. Infection is often asymptomatic or mildly symptomatic; cases of severe symptomatic infection during the immediate newborn period have not been reported. Symptoms in giardiasis are related to the age of the patient: Diarrhea, vomiting, anorexia, and failure to thrive are more common in younger children. Seroprevalence studies showed evidence of past or current *G. lamblia* infection in 40% of Peruvian children by the age of 6 months [1093]. In a study of lactating Bangladeshi mothers and their infants, 82% of women and 42% of infants excreted *Giardia* once during the study; in some infants, this occurred before they were 3 months old [1094]. Of these infected infants, 86% had diarrhea, suggesting that the early exposure to the parasite resulted in disease. In a prospective study of diarrhea conducted in Mexico, infants frequently were infected with *Giardia* from birth to 2 months, with a crude incidence rate of first *Giardia* infection of 1.4 infections per child-year in this age group [10]. The symptom status of these children was not reported, but this study strongly suggests that *G. lamblia* may be more common than currently recognized among newborns living in developing areas.

The diagnosis of giardiasis can be made on the basis of demonstration of antigen by EIA or by microscopy of feces, duodenal fluid, or, less frequently, duodenal biopsy specimen [1095,1096], Breast-feeding is believed to protect against symptomatic giardiasis [10,84,1097], This protection may be mediated by cellular and humoral immunity [82,1098,1099], and nonspecifically by the antigiardial effects of unsaturated fatty acids [1100].

Giardia infections causing severe diarrhea may respond to metronidazole or furazolidone [1096].

CRYPTOSPORIDIUM

C. parvum is a coccidian protozoon related to *Toxoplasma gondii*, *Isospora belli*, and *Plasmodium* species [1101,1102], The life cycle involves ingestion of thick-walled oocysts; release of sporozoites, which penetrate intestinal epithelium; and development of merozoites. Asexual reproduction and sexual reproduction occur, with the latter resulting in formation of new oocysts that can be passed in stools.

Cryptosporidium species are ubiquitous. Infection often occurs in people traveling to endemic areas [1103]. Because *Cryptosporidium* infects a wide variety of animal species, there is often a history of animal contact among infected individuals [1104]. Person-to-person spread, particularly in household contacts [1105–1108] and day care centers [1109,1110], is well documented and suggests that the organism is highly infectious. Water-borne outbreaks of cryptosporidiosis occur and can be of massive proportions [1111].

The clinical manifestations of cryptosporidiosis in immunocompetent individuals resemble *Giardia* infection, but are shorter in duration [1112]; asymptomatic carriage is rare. Symptoms and signs include watery diarrhea, abdominal pain, myalgia, fever, and weight loss.* Infection can occur in all age groups, but is largely concentrated in children older than 1 year [1114]. Infection in the first month of life has been described [1115,1116], Because symptoms resolve before excretion of oocysts ceases, a newborn whose mother has been ill with cryptosporidiosis in the month before delivery might be at risk even if the mother is asymptomatic at the time of the child's birth [1117]. With the increasing frequency of HIV infection, it is likely that women with symptomatic cryptosporidiosis may deliver an infant who will become infected. Infants infected early in life may develop chronic diarrhea and malnutrition [1118].

The diagnosis of cryptosporidiosis is most typically made by examination of fecal smears using Giemsa stain, Ziehl-Neelsen stain, auramine-rhodamine stain, Sheather sugar flotation, an immunofluorescence procedure, a modified concentration-sugar flotation method, or EIA [1119,1120], Multiplex real-time PCR for *E. histolytica*, *G. lamblia*, and *C. parvum* and *Cryptosporidium hominis* may prove to be useful in the future [1121]. Nitazoxanide is effective therapy of immunocompetent adults and children with cryptosporidiosis [1122]. Because illness is usually self-limited in the normal host, attention to fluid, electrolyte, and nutritional status is usually sufficient. Enteric isolation of hospitalized infants with this illness is appropriate because of the high infectivity. Several studies suggest that the risk of infection early in life may be decreased by breast-feeding [1116,1123], Using appropriate filtration systems in areas where water treatment is minimal can have a significant impact in decreasing cases of cryptosporidiosis [1124].

_____

*References [1103,1104,1109,1110,1112,1113].

VIRUSES
ENTERIC VIRUSES

Viruses that infect the intestinal mucosa and cause primarily gastroenteritis are referred to as enteric viruses; they should not be confused with enteroviruses, members of Picornaviridae family that are associated primarily with systemic illnesses. Enteric viruses include rotaviruses, enteric adenoviruses, human caliciviruses, and astroviruses. Other viruses such as coronaviruses, Breda viruses, pestiviruses, parvoviruses, toroviruses, and picobirnaviruses have been sporadically associated with acute diarrhea, but are currently considered of uncertain relevance. More recently, Bocaviruses have been postulated as potential respiratory and intestinal pathogens, but the latter seems unclear [1125]. Extensive reviews on the role of enteric viruses in childhood diarrhea can be found elsewhere [1126–1129].

All four enteric viruses could conceivably infect the newborn, but the extent of exposure and clinical manifestations are largely unknown for astrovirus, enteric adenovirus, and human caliciviruses. Rotavirus is the most extensively studied enteric virus. Neonatal rotavirus infections have similar virologic and clinical characteristics to infection in older children, although some differences exist.

ROTAVIRUS

Rotavirus is a 75-nm, nonenveloped virus composed of three concentric protein shells: A segmented genome (11 segments), an RNA-dependent polymerase, and enzymes required for messenger RNA synthesis are located within the inner core. Each segment codes for at least one viral protein (VP). The VP can be part of the structure of the virus, or it may be a nonstructural protein (NSP) required for replication, viral assembly, budding, determination of host range, or viral pathogenesis [1128].

Six distinct rotavirus groups (A through F) have been identified serologically based on common group antigens [1130,1131], of which three (A, B, and C) have been identified in humans [1126]. Because group A rotaviruses represent more than 95% of isolated strains in humans worldwide, further discussion focuses on this group. Group A rotaviruses are subclassified into serotypes based on neutralization epitopes located on the outer capsid. Both rotavirus surface proteins, VP4 and VP7, can induce production of neutralizing antibodies [1132,1133], At least 10 VP7 types (G serotypes: G1 to G6, G8 to G10, and G12) and nine VP4 types (P serotypes: P1A, P1B, P2A, P3, P3B, P4, P5, P8, and P12) have been detected among human rotaviruses [1134,1135]. By sequencing the VP4-coding gene, eight genomic P types (genotypes) have been identified that correspond to one or more of the described P antigenic types (genotype 8 to antigenic type P1A, 4 to P1B, 6 to P2A, 9 to P3, 13 to P3B, 10 to P4, 3 to P5, and 11 to P8) [1128]. Combining G antigenic with P antigenic and genetic typing, a specific rotavirus strain can be identified: P antigenic type (P genetic type), G type. As an example, the human neonatal M37 strain is described as P2A [6], G1.

Five combined GP types—P1A [8], G1; P1B [4], G2; P1A [8], G3; P1A [8], G4; P1A [8], G9—account for more than 95% of the organisms isolated from children, and of these, P1A [8], G1 represents the most common type [1136]. Isolation of less common types seems to be more frequent among neonates with nosocomial rotavirus infections [1137–1143]. Some of these strains seem to be associated with occurrence of asymptomatic infections, although the existence of naturally acquired asymptomatic strains is controversial. Strains P2A [6], G9; P2A [6], G4; P2A [6], G2; P2A [6], G8; and P8 [11], G10 have been reported [1141–1145] from newborn nurseries, some of which seem to be endemic to the newborn units with high rates of asymptomatic infection [1142–1145], and, less commonly, outbreaks of symptomatic infection [1141]. These findings suggest that specific conditions of the newborn environment (e.g., child, nursery, personnel) may increase the possibility of reassortments between human strains; such strains may persist in these settings possibly through constant transmission involving asymptomatic newborns, adults, and contaminated surfaces. Neonates can also be symptomatically infected with unusual animal-human reassortant strains in areas of poor sanitary conditions [1146].

Pathogenesis

Although mechanisms involved in rotavirus pathogenesis have been extensively studied, current understanding of the exact mechanisms involved in human disease is only partial and may be subject to significant conceptual modifications as more knowledge is obtained in the future. Rotavirus primarily infects mature enterocytes located in the mid and upper villous epithelium [1147–1151]. Lactase, which is present only on the brush border of the differentiated epithelial cells at these sites, may act as a combined receptor and uncoating enzyme for the virus, permitting transfer of the particles into the cell [1152]. Perhaps for this reason, infection is limited to the mature columnar enterocytes; crypt cells and crypt-derived cuboidal cells, which lack a brush border, seem to be resistant to rotaviral infection [1152,1153]. This concept also may explain why rotavirus infection is less common in infants younger than 32 weeks' gestational age than in more mature infants [1154]; at 26 to 34 weeks' gestational age, lactase activity is approximately 30% of that found in term infants [1155].

The upper small intestine is most commonly involved in rotavirus enteritis, although lesions may extend to the distal ileum and rarely to the colon [1156,1157], Interaction between intestinal cell and rotavirus structural and nonstructural proteins occurs, resulting in death of infected villous enterocytes [1158]. When infected, the villous enterocyte is sloughed, resulting in an altered mucosal architecture that becomes stunted and flattened. The gross appearance of the bowel is usually normal; however, under the dissecting microscope, scattered focal lesions of the mucosal surface are apparent in most cases. Light microscopy also shows patchy changes in villous morphology, compatible with a process of infection, inflammation, and accelerated mucosal renewal. The villi take on a shortened and blunt appearance as tall columnar cells are shed and replaced by less mature cuboidal enterocytes [1148,1150,1159]. Ischemia may also play a role in

the loss and stunting of villi [1160] and activation of the enteric nervous system; active secretion of fluid and electrolytes may be another pathogenic mechanism [1161].

During the recovery phase, the enteroblastic cells mature and reconstruct the villous structure. Because of the loss of mature enterocytes on the tips of the villi, the surface area of the intestine is reduced. Diarrhea that occurs may be a result of this decrease in surface area, disruption in epithelial integrity, transient disaccharidase deficiency, or altered countercurrent mechanisms and net secretion of water and electrolytes [1148,1155, 1157,1161–1163]. More recent studies suggest that destruction of mature enterocytes does not seem to be a critical element in the pathogenesis of rotavirus infection. The role of NSP4 as a "viral enterotoxin" after the initial report of an age-dependent diarrhea in CD1 mice by triggering calcium-dependent chloride and water secretion [1164] has been supported by new studies [1165]. The exact mechanism of action of this protein at the intestinal level is only partially understood, but known to be different from the action of bacterial enterotoxins. NSP4 does not cause morphologic damage; it impairs glucose absorption and produces moderate calcium-mediated chloride secretion [1165]. The contribution of this "viral enterotoxin" in human rotavirus–associated diarrhea is unclear [1166,1167].

Rotavirus antigenemia and viremia seem to be common events during rotavirus infection, a concept that revolutionized understanding of this infection [1168]. These events could partly explain the sporadic reports of systemic disease associated with rotavirus intestinal infections mentioned further on. An association between viremia and more severe disease has been suggested, but not sufficiently studied to date [1168–1171].

Infection and Immunity

Infants with asymptomatic rotavirus infections in the nursery are less likely than uninfected nursery mates to experience severe rotavirus infection later in life [1172,1173]; this finding suggested protective immunity and supported vaccine development. Most studies have indicated that serum and intestinal antirotavirus antibody levels are correlated with protection against infection [1173–1181], although this correlation has not been universal [1182,1183]. Breast-feeding protects against diarrhea and specifically rotavirus disease during the first year of life [62,72], probably including newborns [1161]. The high prevalence of antirotaviral antibodies in colostrum and human milk has been shown by numerous investigators in widely diverse geographic areas [12]. Maternal rotavirus infection or immunization is accompanied by the appearance of specific antibodies in milk, probably through stimulation of the enteromammary immune system [1184–1189]. Of women examined in London, Bangladesh, Guatemala, Costa Rica, and the United States, 90% to 100% had antirotaviral IgA antibodies in their milk for 2 years of lactation [12,1184–1190]. Rotavirus-specific IgG antibodies have been found during the first few postpartum days in about one third of human milk samples assayed [1184,1187], whereas IgM antibodies were detectable in about half [1187].

Glycoproteins in human milk have been shown to prevent rotavirus infection in vitro and in an animal model [1190]. The concentration of one milk glycoprotein, lactadherin, was found to be significantly higher in human milk ingested by infants who developed asymptomatic rotavirus infection than in milk ingested by infants who developed symptomatic infection [59].

Epidemiology

Rotaviruses probably infect neonates more commonly than previously recognized; most infections seem to be asymptomatic or mildly symptomatic, although symptomatic infections may be more common than previously considered, especially in developing countries [1141–1144,1172,1191–1206]. In a study from India, rotavirus positivity was detected in 56% of symptomatic neonates compared with 45% of asymptomatic neonates [1206]. Rotavirus has a mean incubation period of 2 days, with a range of 1 to 3 days in children and in adults experimentally infected. Fecal excretion of virus often begins a day or so before illness, and maximal excretion usually occurs during the 3rd and 4th days and generally diminishes by the end of the 1st week, although low concentrations of virus have been detected in neonates for 8 weeks [1155,1204–1208].

Rotavirus infections are markedly seasonal (autumn and winter) in many areas of the world, although in some countries seasonality is less striking; the reason for this is unclear [1209–1214]. In nurseries in which persisting endemic infection has permitted long-term surveillance of numerous neonates, rotavirus excretion can follow the seasonal pattern of the community, but can also show no seasonal fluctuation [1215–1217]. It is unclear how units in which infection remains endemic for months or years differ from units with a low incidence of rotavirus. Some nurseries are free of rotavirus infection [1217–1219] or minimally affected [59,1220] whereas others have rotavirus diarrheal disease throughout the year or in outbreaks that involve 10% to 40% of neonates [1141,1154,1196,1197,1221].

Low birth weight does not seem to be an important factor in determining the attack rate among infants at risk, but may be important in mortality [1222]. Infants in premature or special care nurseries, despite their prolonged stays and the increased handling necessary for their care, do not exhibit a higher susceptibility to infection; data regarding shedding of the virus are inconsistent [59,1219].

After infection is introduced into a nursery, rotavirus is likely to spread steadily and remain endemic until the nursery is closed to new admissions or nursing practices permit interruption of the cycle [1223]. Exactly how the virus is introduced and transmitted is uncertain, although limited observations and experience with other types of enteric disease in maternity units suggest several possibilities. The early appearance of virus in stools of some neonates indicates that infection probably was acquired at delivery. Virus particles can be detected on the 1st [59,1204] or 2nd [1217] day of life in many infected infants. By day 3 or 4, most infected infants who will shed virus, with or without signs of illness, are doing so

[1192,1204,1217]. The numerous virus particles excreted [1192,1217] suggest a fairly large and early oral inoculum. It is unlikely that contamination from any source other than maternal feces could provide an inoculum large enough to cause infection by the 2nd day.

Transfer of particles from infant to infant on the hands of nursing and medical staff is probably the most important means of viral spread. With 10^8 to 10^{11} viral particles usually present in 1 g of stool, the hands of personnel easily could become contaminated after infection is introduced into a nursery. There are numerous reports of nosocomial and day care center rotavirus gastroenteritis outbreaks that attest to the ease with which this agent spreads through a hospital or institutional setting [1126]. Admission of a symptomatic infant usually is the initiating event, although transfer of a neonate with inapparent infection from one ward to another also has been incriminated. The most important factors influencing the incidence of rotavirus diarrhea in a nursery are the proximity to other newborns and the frequency of hand washing [1205]. During a 4-month study, infants cared for by nursing staff and kept in communal nurseries experienced three epidemics of diarrhea with attack rates of 20% to 50%. During the same period, only 2% of infants rooming in with their mothers became ill, even though they had frequent contact with adult relatives and siblings.

There is no clear evidence of airborne or droplet infection originating in the upper respiratory tract or spread by aerosolization of diarrheal fluid while diapers are changed. Indirect evidence of airborne transmission includes the high infection rate in closed settings, the isolation of the virus from respiratory secretions [1224], and the experimental observation of transmission by aerosol droplets in mice [1225]. The respiratory isolation achieved by placing an infant in a closed incubator is not fully protective, however [1205]. No evidence indicates that transplacental or ascending intrauterine infection occurs. Transmission of virus through contaminated fomites, formula, or food is possible, but has not been documented in newborns. Rotavirus particles have not been found in human milk or colostrum [1186,1190].

Clinical Manifestations

Exposure of a newborn to rotavirus can result in asymptomatic infection or cause mild or severe gastroenteritis.* Outbreaks with high attack rates as measured by rotavirus excretion have been described, but the extent of symptomatic infection varies.† Severe rotavirus infection is seldom reported during the newborn period [1206,1221], but the extent of underreporting of severe disease, especially in the less developed areas of the world, has not been evaluated.

It has been hypothesized that asymptomatic infections during the newborn period are the result of naturally attenuated strains circulating in this environment. RNA electrophoretic patterns of rotaviruses found in certain

---

*References [1142,1143,1191,1197,1206,1215,1216,1220,1226].
†References [1193,1195,1204,1206,1217,1221].

nurseries have shown uniform patterns [1198,1200, 1202,1226], and it has been suggested that these strains may be attenuated. The presence of unusual antigenic types, such as P2A [6] type, within nurseries also suggests "less virulent strains." At least 10 rotavirus strains were documented to cocirculate in a tertiary care center during a 2-month period [1227], and in a different setting the same rotavirus strains by electropherotype produced asymptomatic infection in neonates and symptomatic infection in older infants [1201]. Newborns within a nursery exposed to a given rotavirus strain can develop symptomatic or asymptomatic infection [1143,1228,1229]. P8 [11], G10 was the most common genotype associated with symptomatic and asymptomatic infections in a tertiary care hospital in India [1206]. Because newborns routinely have frequent relatively loose stools, it is possible that mild diarrhea episodes caused by rotavirus are being wrongly labeled as asymptomatic episodes.

No clinical feature is pathognomonic of rotaviral gastroenteritis. Early signs of illness, such as lethargy, irritability, vomiting, and poor feeding, usually are followed in a few hours by the passage of watery yellow or green stools free of blood but sometimes containing mucus [1205,1230–1232]. Diarrhea usually decreases by the 2nd day of illness and is much improved by the 3rd or 4th day. Occasionally, intestinal fluid loss and poor weight gain may continue for 1 or 2 weeks, particularly in low birth weight infants [1193]. Although reducing substances frequently are present in early fecal samples [191,1154, 1194,1205], this finding is not abnormal in neonates, particularly infants who are breast-fed [1233]. Nevertheless, infants with prolonged diarrhea should be investigated for monosaccharide or disaccharide malabsorption or intolerance to cow's milk protein or both [1234]. In a prospective study [1203], 49% of newborns with GI symptoms in a neonatal intensive care unit had rotavirus detected in their stools. Frequent stooling (present in 60%), bloody mucoid stool (42%), and watery stools (24%) were risk factors for a rotavirus infection. Bloody mucoid stools, intestinal dilation, and abdominal distention were significantly more common in preterm infants, but severe outcomes such as necrotizing enterocolitis and death did not differ among infected term and preterm infants.

Longitudinal studies in newborn nurseries and investigations of outbreaks among neonates rarely describe a severe adverse outcome or death [1154,1188,1205]. Because these infants are under constant observation, early detection of excessive fluid losses and the availability of immediate medical care are probably major factors in determining outcome. Rotavirus gastroenteritis causes almost 400,000 infant deaths every year [1235], concentrated largely in the poorest regions of the world. It is likely that in places where hospital-based care is uncommon, rotavirus causes neonatal deaths secondary to dehydration.

Group A rotavirus has been associated with a wide array of diseases in infants and children; Reye syndromes, encephalitis–aseptic meningitis, sudden infant death syndrome, inflammatory bowel disease, and Kawasaki syndrome have been described, but not systematically studied [1126]. Case reports and small case series have associated neonatal rotavirus infection with necrotizing enterocolitis [1236,1237]. Rotavirus infection may play a role in a small proportion of cases of necrotizing enterocolitis, although it probably represents one of many potential triggering factors [1206]. A significant association between neonatal rotavirus infection and bradycardia-apnea episodes was detected in one prospective study [1238]. The possible association between natural rotavirus infection and intussusception [1239–1241] gained support after the association was made between the human-simian reassortant vaccine and intussusception in infants older than 2 months (attributable risk approximately 1:10,000) [1242]. Epidemiologic studies have not shown a temporal correlation between peaks of rotavirus infection and increase in cases of intussusception [1243]. Intussusception is extremely uncommon in the newborn; it is highly unlikely that rotavirus triggers this disease in neonates.

Diagnosis

There are many methods used for detection of rotavirus in stool specimens, including electron microscopy, immune electron microscopy, ELISA, latex agglutination, gel electrophoresis, culture of the virus, and reverse transcriptase PCR. ELISA and latex agglutination currently are the most widely used diagnostic techniques for detection of rotavirus in clinical samples. Many commercial kits are available that differ in specificity and sensitivity [1244–1248]. Latex agglutination assays generally are more rapid than ELISAs, but are less sensitive. The sensitivity and specificity of commercially available ELISAs surpass 90%. Checking of the ELISA by another method such as gel electrophoresis or PCR amplification may be desirable if there is concern about false-positive results.

Fecal material for detection of rotavirus infection should be obtained during the acute phase of illness. Whole-stool samples are preferred, although suspensions of rectal swab specimens have been adequate for detection of rotavirus by ELISA [1249,1250]. Rotavirus is relatively resistant to environmental temperatures, even tropical temperatures [1251], although 4° C is desirable for short-term storage and −70° C for prolonged storage [1126]. Excretion of viral particles may precede signs of illness by several days [1209]; maximal excretion by older infants and children usually occurs 3 to 4 days after onset of symptoms [1252]. Neonates can shed virus for 1 to 2 weeks after onset of symptoms.

Therapy and Prevention

The primary goal of therapy is restoration and maintenance of fluid and electrolyte balance. Despite the documented defect in carbohydrate digestion with rotavirus diarrhea, rehydration often can be accomplished with glucose-electrolyte or sucrose-electrolyte solutions given orally [215,1253–1255]. Intravenous fluids may be needed in neonates who are severely dehydrated, who have ileus, or who refuse to feed. Persistent or recurrent diarrhea after introduction of milk-based formulas or human milk warrants investigation for secondary carbohydrate or milk protein intolerance [1154,1235]. Disaccharidase levels and xylose absorption return to normal within a few days [1159] to weeks after infection [1148].

Intractable diarrhea related to severe morphologic and enzymatic changes of the bowel mucosa is possible, although rare in the newborn; it may require an elemental diet or parenteral nutrition. Efficacy of antirotavirus antibodies (e.g., hyperimmune colostrum, antibody-supplemented formula, human serum immunoglobulin) and of probiotics has been postulated [1256–1259], although not convincingly shown [1260]; the widespread clinical use of these measures seems remote. One study suggests that use of lactobacillus during the diarrheal episode may decrease the duration of rotavirus-associated hospital stays, especially when used early in the course of the disease, although more studies are needed before recommending widespread use [1259].

Hand hygiene before and after contact with each infant is the most important means of preventing the spread of infection. Because rotavirus is often excreted several days before illness is recognized, isolation of an infant with diarrhea may be too late to prevent cross-infection, unless all nursing personnel and medical staff have adhered to this fundamental precaution. Infants who develop gastroenteritis should be moved out of the nursery area if adequate facilities are available and the infant's condition permits transfer. The use of an incubator is valuable in reducing transmission of disease only by serving as a reminder that proper hand hygiene and glove techniques are required, but is of little value as a physical barrier to the spread of virus [1205]. Encouraging rooming-in of infants with their mothers has been shown to be helpful in preventing or containing nursery epidemics [1261]. Temporary closure of the nursery may be required for clinically significant outbreaks that cannot be controlled with other measures [1141].

Vaccines

Development of rotavirus vaccines began in the early 1980s. Candidate vaccines included bovine and rhesus monkey attenuated strains, human attenuated strains, and bovine-human and rhesus-human reassortant strains [1127]. In August 1998, the first licensed rotavirus vaccine, Rotashield, an oral formulation of a simian-human quadrivalent reassortant vaccine, was recommended for use in children when they were 2, 4, and 6 months old. After approximately 500,000 children were vaccinated with more than 1 million doses, a significantly increased risk of intussusception was observed among vaccinated children, with an overall odds ratio of 1.8 [1262]. Use of this vaccine was terminated. Two new vaccines proved to be safe and effective in large phase III trials: a vaccine including five bovine-human reassortant strains including human G types G1-G4 and P type P1A [8] and a vaccine including one human attenuated P1A [8], G1.

These vaccines have a protective efficacy against moderate to severe rotavirus gastroenteritis leading to hospitalizations that surpasses 85%. Protection is broad against the most common serotypes. Key articles and reviews summarizing the studies that support these vaccines can be found elsewhere [1263–1269]. The epidemiology of rotavirus infection is likely to change significantly as these vaccines become widely available; a significant decrease of rotavirus infection has been reported more recently in the United States where one of the vaccines is being used, but more prolonged surveillance is required [1270]. The impact on neonatal infection will depend on the effect of herd immunity in decreasing circulation of rotavirus strains.

DIFFERENTIAL DIAGNOSIS

Stools from breast-fed neonates are typically watery and yellow, green, or brown. The frequency of stooling can vary from one every other day to eight evacuations per day. In an active, healthy infant who is feeding well, has no vomiting, and has a soft abdomen, these varied patterns of stooling are not a cause for concern. Physicians need to consider the infant's previous frequency and consistency of stools and establish a diagnosis of acute diarrhea on an individual basis. Close follow-up of weight increase in infants with nonformed stools can help confirm the clinical impression. A normal weight gain should direct medical action away from stool examinations or treatment.

Diarrhea during the neonatal period is a clinical manifestation of a wide variety of disorders (Table 11–6). The most common initiating factor is a primary infection of the GI tract that is mild to moderate in severity, self-limited, and responsive to supportive measures. Acute diarrhea can also be an initial manifestation of a systemic infection, including bacterial and viral neonatal sepsis. Infants with moderate to severe diarrhea require close monitoring until the etiologic diagnosis and the clinical evolution are clarified. Noninfectious diseases leading to chronic intractable diarrhea may result in severe nutritional disturbances or even death unless the specific underlying condition is identified and treated appropriately. The differential diagnosis of a diarrheal illness requires a careful clinical examination to determine whether the child has a localized or a systemic process. Lethargy, abnormalities in body temperature, hypothermia or hyperthermia, decreased feeding, abdominal distention, vomiting, pallor, respiratory distress, apnea, cyanosis, hemodynamic instability, hypotension, hepatomegaly or splenomegaly, coagulation or bleeding disorders, petechiae, and exanthemas should lead to an intense laboratory investigation directed at systemic viral or bacterial infection. If the process is deemed a localized intestinal infection, initial evaluation can be focused on differentiating an inflammatory-invasive pathogen from pathogens that cause a noninflammatory process. For this, stool examination for fecal leukocytes, red blood cells, and lactoferrin can be a helpful indicator of the former.

Inflammatory diarrhea can be caused by *Shigella, Salmonella, Campylobacter, V. parahaemolyticus, Y. enterocolitica,* EIEC, EAEC, *C. difficile,* necrotizing enterocolitis, antibiotic-associated colitis, and allergic colitis (i.e., milk or soy intolerance). Noninflammatory causes of diarrhea include ETEC, EPEC, rotaviruses, enteric adenoviruses, calicivirus, astrovirus, *G. lamblia,* and *Cryptosporidium. V. cholerae* can cause severe life-threatening neonatal diarrhea in regions where the infection is endemic [1271]. Cytomegalovirus can cause mild to severe enteritis that may result in ileal stricture [1272]. Enteroviruses can

TABLE 11–6 Differential Diagnosis of Neonatal Diarrhea

Diagnosis	Reference(s)
Anatomic Disorders	
Microvillous inclusion disease	[1274]
Hirschsprung disease	[1275]
Massive intestinal resection (short bowel syndrome)	[1276]
Congenital short bowel syndrome	[1277]
Intestinal lymphangiectasis	[1278]
Metabolic and Enzymatic Disorders	
Congenital disaccharidase deficiency (lactase, sucrase-isomaltase deficiency)	[1279,1280]
Congenital glucose-galactose malabsorption	[1281]
Secondary disaccharide, monosaccharide malabsorption	[1282–1288]
After gastrointestinal surgery	
After infection	
With milk–soy protein sensitivity	
Cystic fibrosis	[1289]
Syndrome of pancreatic insufficiency and bone marrow dysfunction (Shwachman syndrome)	[1290]
Physiologic deficiency of pancreatic amylase	[1291]
Intestinal enterokinase deficiency	[1292]
Congenital bile acid deficiency syndrome	[1293]
α/β-lipoproteinemia	[1294]
Acrodermatitis enteropathica	[1295,1296]
Congenital chloride diarrhea	[1297,1298,1299]
Primary hypomagnesemia	[1300]
Congenital adrenal hyperplasia	[1301]
Intestinal hormone hypersecretion	[1302,1303]
Non-β islet cell hyperplasia (Wolman disease)	[1304]
Transcobalamin II deficiency	[1305]
Congenital iron storage	[1306]
Hartnup disease	[1307]
Congenital Na$^+$ diarrhea	[1308]
Congenital pseudohypoparathyroidism	[1309]
Inflammatory Disorders	
Cow's milk protein intolerance	[1310,1311]
Soy protein intolerance	[1312,1313]
Regional enteritis	[1314]
Ulcerative colitis	[1315,1316]
Primary Immunodeficiency Disorders	
Wiskott-Aldrich syndrome	[1317]
AIDS	[1318]
Miscellaneous	
Irritable colon of childhood (chronic nonspecific diarrhea)	[1319]
Phototherapy for hyperbilirubinemia	[1320]
Neonatal Kawasaki disease	[1321]

[AIDS, acquired immunodeficiency syndrome].

cause outbreaks of fever, diarrhea, and respiratory symptoms in newborn units [1273]. Although supportive fluid therapy is mandatory for all types of diarrhea, the brief examination for fecal leukocytes and red blood cells can direct the diagnostic and therapeutic approach. Pathogens such as *Shigella*, *Salmonella*, and EHEC can cause watery or bloody diarrhea, depending on the specific host-pathogen interaction and the pathogenic mechanisms involved. Some noninfectious diseases responsible for neonatal diarrhea are listed in Table 11–6 [355,542,1274–1319]. The evaluation and management of persistent infantile diarrhea has been reviewed [1320].

REFERENCES

[1] U.D. Prashar, et al., Global illness and deaths caused by rotavirus disease in children, Emerg. Infect. Dis. 9 (2003) 565.

[2] R.L. Guerrant, Lessons from diarrheal diseases: demography to molecular pharmacology, J. Infect. Dis. 169 (1994) 1206.

[3] M.S. Ho, et al., Diarrheal deaths in American children. Are they preventable, JAMA 260 (1988) 3281.

[4] M.L. Cohen, The epidemiology of diarrheal disease in the United States, Infect. Dis. Clin. North. Am. 2 (1988) 557.

[5] J. Lawn, et al., 4 million neonatal deaths. When? Where? Why? Lancet 365 (2005) 891.

[6] J.E. Lawn, K. Wilczynska-Ketende, S. Cousens, Estimating the cause of 4 million neonatal deaths in the year 2000, Int. J. Epidemiol. 35 (2006) 706.

[7] H.B. Perry, A.G. Ross, F. Fernand, Assessing the causes of under-five mortality in the Albert Schweitzer Hospital service area of rural Haiti, Rev. Panam. Salud. Publica. 18 (2005) 178.

[8] A.K. Deorari, et al., Clinicoepidemiological profile and predictors of severe illness in young infants (< 60 days) reporting to a hospital in North India, Indian. Pediatr. 44 (2007) 739.

[9] L.J. Mata, J.J. Urrutia, Intestinal colonization of breastfed children in a rural area of low socioeconomic level, Ann. N. Y. Acad. Sci. 176 (1971) 93.

[10] A.L. Morrow, et al., Protection against infection with *Giardia lamblia* by breast-feeding in a cohort of Mexican infants, J. Pediatr. 121 (1992) 363.

[11] F.R. Velásquez, et al., Serum antibody as a marker of protection against natural rotavirus infection and disease, J. Infect. Dis. 182 (2000) 1602.

[12] A.L. Morrow, L.K. Pickering, Human milk protection against diarrheal disease, Semin. Pediatr. Infect. Dis. 5 (1994) 236.

[13] S. Mihrshahi, N. Ichikawa, M. Shuaib, et al., Prevalence of exclusive breast-feeding in Bangladesh and its association with diarrhoea and acute respiratory infection: results of the multiple indicator cluster survey 2003, J. Health. Popul. Nutr. 25 (2007) 195.

[14] U.D. Parashar, et al., Diarrheal mortality in US infants, Arch. Pediatr. Adolesc. Med. 152 (1998) 47.

[15] E.G. Pamer, Immune responses to commensal and environmental microbes, Nat. Immunol. 8 (2007) 1173.

[16] S.M. Dann, L. Eckmann, Innate immune defenses in the intestinal tract, Curr. Opin. Gastroenterol. 23 (2007) 115.

[17] J.L. Coombes, F. Powrie, Dendritic cells in intestinal immune regulation, Nat. Rev. Immunol. 8 (2008) 435.

[18] A. Cerutti, M. Rescigno, The biology of intestinal immunoglobulin A responses, Immunity 28 (2008) 740.

[19] D. Artis, Epithelial-cell recognition of commensal bacteria and maintenance of immune homeostasis in the gut, Nat. Rev. Immunol. 8 (2008) 411.

[20] D. Kelly, T. King, R. Aminov, Importance of microbial colonization of the gut in early life to the development of immunity, Mutat. Res. 622 (2007) 58.

[21] B. Albiger, et al., Role of the innate immune system in host defence against bacterial infections: focus on the Toll-like receptors, J. Intern. Med. 261 (2007) 511.

[22] S.C. Bischoff, S. Krämer, Human mast cells, bacteria, and intestinal immunity, Immunol. Rev. 217 (2007) 329.

[23] N.H. Salzman, M.A. Underwood, C.L. Bevins, Paneth cells, defensins, and the commensal microbiota: a hypothesis on intimate interplay at the intestinal mucosa, Semin. Immunol. 19 (2007) 70.

[24] L.R. Guerrant, et al., How intestinal bacteria cause disease, J. Infect. Dis. 179 (1999) S331.

[25] L.K. Pickering, T.G. Cleary, Approach to patients with gastrointestinal tract infections and food poisoning, in: R.D. Feigin, J.C. Cherry (Eds.), Textbook of Pediatric Infectious Diseases, fourth ed., WB Saunders, Philadelphia, 1997p. 567.

[26] K.A. Bettelheim, S.M.J. Lennox-King, The acquisition of *Escherichia coli* by newborn babies, Infection 4 (1976) 174.

[27] J. Gorden, P.L.C. Small, Acid resistance in enteric bacteria, Infect. Immun. 61 (1993) 364.

[28] L.K. Pickering, Biotherapeutic agents and disease in infants, Adv. Exp. Med. Biol. 501 (2001) 365.

[29] P. Ogra, R. Welliver, Effects of early environment on mucosal immuno-logic homeostasis, subsequent immune responses and disease outcome, Nestlé. Nutr. Workshop. Ser. Pediatr. Program. 61 (2008) 145.

[30] D.S. Newburg, A. Walker, Protection of the neonate by the innate immune system of developing gut and of human milk, Pediatr. Res. 61 (2007) 2.

[31] R.A. Giannella, S.A. Broitman, N. Zamcheck, Influence of gastric acidity on bacterial and parasitic enteric infections: a perspective, Ann. Intern. Med. 78 (1973) 271.

[32] J. Schrager, The chemical composition and function of gastrointestinal mucus, Gut 11 (1970) 450.

[33] D.N. Challacombe, J.M. Richardson, C.M. Anderson, Bacterial microflora of the upper gastrointestinal tract in infants without diarrhea, Arch. Dis. Child. 49 (1974) 264.

[34] G.T. Furuta, W.A. Walker, Nonimmune defense mechanisms of the gastrointestinal tract, in: M.J. Blaser et al., (Eds.), Infections of the Gastroin-testinal Tract, Raven Press, New York, 1995, pp. 89–97.

[35] G. Avery, J.G. Randolph, T. Weaver, Gastric acidity in the first day of life, Pediatrics 37 (1966) 1005.

[36] J.T. Harries, A.J. Fraser, The acidity of the gastric contents of premature babies during the first fourteen days of life, Biol. Neonate. 12 (1968) 186.

[37] M. Agunod, et al., Correlative study of hydrochloric acid, pepsin, and intrinsic factor secretion in newborns and infants, Am. J. Dig. Dis. 14 (1969) 400.

[38] B. Cavel, Gastric emptying in infants, Acta Paediatr. Scand. 60 (1971) 371.

[39] I. Blumenthal, A. Ebel, R.S. Pildes, Effect of posture on the pattern of stomach emptying in the newborn, Pediatrics 66 (1980) 482.

[40] J. Silverio, Gastric emptying time in the newborn and nursling, Am. J. Med. Sci. 247 (1964) 732.

[41] B. Cavell, Gastric emptying in preterm infants, Acta Paediatr. Scand. 68 (1979) 725.

[42] M. Rimoldi, et al., Intestinal epithelial cells control dendritic cell function, Ann. N. Y. Acad. Sci. 1029 (2004) 66.

[43] L. Eckmann, M. Kagnoff, J. Fierer, Intestinal epithelial cells as watchdogs for the natural immune system, Trends. Microbiol. 3 (1995) 118.

[44] H. Tanabe, et al., Mouse Paneth cell secretory responses to cell surface glycolipids of virulent and attenuated pathogenic bacteria, Infect. Immune. 73 (2005) 2312.

[45] K. Bernt, W. Walker, Human milk as a carrier of biochemical messages, Acta Paediatr. Suppl. 88 (1999) 27.

[46] M.E. Fallot, J.L. Boyd, F.A. Oski, Breast-feeding reduces incidence of hospital admissions for infection in infants, Pediatrics 65 (1980) 1121.

[47] S.A. Larsen, D.R. Homer, Relation of breast versus bottle feeding to hospi-talization for gastroenteritis in a middle-class U.S. population, J. Pediatr. 92 (1978) 417.

[48] A.H. Cushing, L. Anderson, Diarrhea in breast-fed and non-breast-fed infants, Pediatrics 70 (1982) 921.

[49] R.L. Guerrant, et al., Prospective study of diarrheal illnesses in north-eastern Brazil: patterns of disease, nutritional impact, etiologies and risk factors, J. Infect. Dis. 148 (1983) 986.

[50] M.G. Myers, et al., Respiratory and gastrointestinal illnesses in breast- and formula-fed infants, Am. J. Dis. Child. 138 (1984) 629.

[51] M.G. Kovar, et al., Review of the epidemiologic evidence for an association between infant feeding and infant health, Pediatrics 74 (1984) 615.

[52] R.G. Feachem, M.A. Koblinsky, Interventions for the control of diarrhoeal diseases among young children: promotion of breast-feeding, Bull. World Health Organ. 62 (1984) 271.

[53] M.R. Forman, et al., The Pima infant feeding study: breastfeeding and gastroenteritis in the first year of life, Am. J. Epidemiol. 119 (1984) 335.

[54] J.M. Leventhal, et al., Does breastfeeding protect against infections in infants less than 3 months of age? Pediatrics 78 (1986) 8896.

[55] D.H. Rubin, et al., Relationship between infant feeding and infectious illness: a prospective study of infants during the first year of life, Pediatrics 85 (1989) 464.

[56] C.G. Victora, et al., Infant feeding and deaths due to diarrhea, Am. J. Epidemiol. 129 (1989) 1032.

[57] B.M. Popkin, et al., Breast-feeding and diarrheal morbidity, Pediatrics 86 (1990) 874.

[58] A.L. Morrow, L.K. Pickering, Human milk and infectious diseases, in: S.S. Long, L.K. Pickering, C.G. Prober (Eds.), Principles and Practice of Pediatric Infectious Diseases, Churchill-Livingstone, New York, 1997, pp. 87–95.

[59] D.S. Newburg, et al., High levels of lactadherin in human milk are asso-ciated with protection against symptomatic rotavirus infection amongst breast-fed infants, Lancet 351 (1998) 1160.

[60] R.G. Wyatt, L.J. Mata, Bacteria in colostrum and milk in Guatemalan Indian women, J. Trop. Pediatr. 15 (1969) 159.

[61] S. Mirshahi, et al., Prevalence of exclusive breastfeeding in Bangladesh and its association with diarrhoea and acute respiratory infection: results of the multiple indicator cluster survey 2003, J. Health. Popul. Nutr. 25 (2007) 195.

[62] M.A. Quigley, Y.J. Kelly, A. Sacker, Breastfeeding and hospitalization for diarrheal and respiratory infection in the United Kingdom Millennium Cohort Study, Pediatrics 119 (2007) e837.

[63] C.F. Grazioso, et al., Antiinflammatory effects of human milk on chemi-cally induced colitis in rats, Pediatr. Res. 42 (1997) 639.

[64] D.S. Newburg, Oligosaccharides and glycoconjugates in human milk: their role in host defense, J. Mammary. Gland. Biol. Neoplasia. 1 (1996) 271.

[65] L.K. Pickering, et al., Modulation of the immune system by human milk and infant formula containing nucleotides, Pediatrics 101 (1998) 242.

[66] K. Hayani, et al., Concentration of milk secretory immunoglobulin A against *Shigella* virulence plasmid-associated antigens as a predictor of symptom status in *Shigella*-infected breast-fed infants, J. Pediatr. 121 (1992) 852.

[67] K. Hayani, et al., Evidence for long-term memory of the mucosal immune system: milk secretory immunoglobulin A against *Shigella* lipopolysacchar-ides, J. Clin. Microbiol. 29 (1991) 2599.

[68] D. Newburg, S. Ashkenazi, T. Cleary, Human milk contains the Shiga toxin and Shiga-like toxin receptor glycolipid Gb3, J. Infect. Dis. 166 (1992) 832.

[69] I. Herrera-Insua, et al., Human milk lipids bind Shiga toxin, Adv. Exp. Med. Biol. 501 (2001) 333.

[70] H. Gomez, et al., Human lactoferrin impairs virulence of *Shigella flexneri*, J. Infect. Dis. 187 (2003) 87.

[71] H. Gomez, et al., Lactoferrin protects rabbits from *Shigella flexneri*-induced inflammatory enteritis, Infect. Immun. 70 (2002) 7050.

[72] H. Gomez, et al., Protective role of human lactoferrin against invasion of *Shigella flexneri* M90T, Adv. Exp. Med. Biol. 501 (2001) 457.

[73] M. Noguera-Obenza, et al., Human milk secretory antibodies against attach-ing and effacing *Escherichia coli* antigens, Emerg. Infect. Dis. 9 (2003) 545.

[74] A. Cravioto, et al., Inhibition of localized adhesion of enteropathogenic *Escherichia coli* to HEp-2 cells by immunoglobulin and oligosaccharide frac-tions of human colostrum and breast milk, J. Infect. Dis. 163 (1991) 1247.

[75] T. Ochoa, et al., Lactoferrin impairs type III secretory system function in enteropathogenic *Escherichia coli*, Infect. Immun. 71 (2003) 5149.

[76] C.A. Ross, E.A. Dawes, Resistance of the breast fed infant to gastroenteri-tis, Lancet 1 (1954) 994.

[77] R.I. Glass, et al., Milk antibodies protect breastfed children against cholera, N. Engl. J. Med. 308 (1983) 1389.

[78] G.M. Ruiz-Palacios, et al., Protection of breastfed infants against *Campylo-bacter* diarrhea by antibodies in human milk, J. Pediatr. 116 (1990) 707.

[79] J. Holmgren, A.M. Svennerholm, M. Lindblad, Receptor-like glycocom-pounds in human milk that inhibit classical and El Tor *Vibrio cholerae* cell adherence (hemagglutination), Infect. Immun. 39 (1983) 147.

[80] A. Laegreid, A.B.K. Otnaess, J. Fuglesang, Human and bovine milk: com-parison of ganglioside composition and enterotoxin-inhibitory activity, Pediatr. Res. 20 (1986) 416.

[81] K.C. Hayani, et al., Concentration of milk secretory immunoglobulin A against *Shigella* virulence plasmid-associated antigens as a predictor of symptom status in *Shigella*-infected breast-fed infants, J. Pediatr. 121 (1992) 852.

[82] P.G. Miotti, et al., Prevalence of serum and milk antibodies to *Giardia lamblia* in different populations of lactating women, J. Infect. Dis. 152 (1985) 1025.

[83] K.C. Hayani, et al., Evidence for long-term memory of the mucosal immune system: milk secretory immunoglobulin A against *Shigella* lipo-polysaccharides, J. Clin. Microbiol. 29 (1991) 2599.

[84] J.N. Walterspiel, et al., Protective effect of secretory anti-*Giardia lamblia* antibodies in human milk against diarrhea, Pediatrics 93 (1994) 28.

[85] C.O. Tacket, et al., Protection by milk immunoglobulin concentrate against oral challenge with enterotoxigenic *E. coli*, N. Engl. J. Med. 318 (1988) 1240.

[86] G.P. Davidson, et al., Passive immunization of children with bovine colos-trum containing antibodies to human rotavirus, Lancet 2 (1989) 709.

[87] C.O. Tacket, et al., Efficacy of bovine milk immunoglobulin concentrate in preventing illness after *Shigella flexneri* challenge, Am. J. Trop. Med. Hyg. 47 (1992) 276.

[88] M. Polonovsky, A. Lespagnol, Nouvelles acquisitions sur les composés glucidiques du lait de femme, Bull. Soc. Chem. Biol. 15 (1933) 320.

[89] J. Montreuil, S. Mullet, Etude des variations des constituants glucidiques du lait de femme au cours de la lactation, Bull. Soc. Chem. Biol. 42 (1960) 365.

[90] A. Kobata, Milk glycoproteins and oligosaccharides, in: M.I. Horowitz, W. Pigman (Eds.), The Glycoconjugates, I, Academic Press, New York, 1978, p. 423.

[91] M. Gnoth, et al., Human milk oligosaccharides are minimally digested in vitro, J. Nutr. 130 (2000) 3014.

[92] P. Chaturvedi, et al., Survival of human milk oligosaccharides in the intes-tine of infants, Adv. Exp. Med. Biol. 501 (2001) 315.

[93] D.S. Newburg, et al., Fucosylated oligosaccharides of human milk protect suckling mice from heat-stable enterotoxin of *Escherichia coli*, J. Infect. Dis. 162 (1990) 1075.

[93a] P. Hong, et al., Human milk oligosaccharides reduce HIV-1-gp120 bind-ing to dendritic cell-specific ICAM3-grabbing non-integrin (DC-SIGN), Br. J. Nutr. 101 (2009) 482.

[94] P. Huang, et al., Noroviruses bind to human ABO, Lewis, and secretor histo-blood group antigens: identification of 4 distinct strain-specific pat-terns, J. Infect. Dis. 188 (2003) 19.

[95] L. Lindesmith, et al., Human susceptibility and resistance to Norwalk virus infection, Nat. Med. 9 (2003) 548.

[96] A.B. Otnaess, A.M. Svennerholm, Non-immunoglobulin fraction of human milk protects rabbits against enterotoxin-induced intestinal fluid secretion, Infect. Immun. 35 (1982) 738.

[97] A.B. Otnaess, A. Laegreid, K. Ertesvag, Inhibition of enterotoxin from *Escherichia coli* and *Vibrio cholerae* by gangliosides from human milk, Infect. Immun. 40 (1983) 563.

[98] R.H. Yolken, et al., Human milk mucin inhibits rotavirus replication and prevents experimental gastroenteritis, J. Clin. Invest. 90 (1992) 1984.

[98a] L. Bode, et al., Inhibition of monocyte, lymphocyte, and neutrophil adhesion to endothelial cells by human milk oligosaccharides, Thromb Haemost. 92 (2004) 1402.

[99] M.L. Cooper, et al., Isolation of enteropathogenic *Escherichia coli* from mothers and newborn infants, Am. J. Dis. Child. 97 (1959) 255.

[100] H.W. Ocklitz, E.F. Schmidt, Enteropathogenic *Escherichia coli* serotypes: infection of the newborn through mother, BMJ 2 (1957) 1036.

[101] F.E. Gareau, et al., The acquisition of fecal flora by infants from their mothers during birth, J. Pediatr. 54 (1959) 313.

[102] R. Rosner, Antepartum culture findings of mothers in relation to infantile diarrhea, Am. J. Clin. Pathol. 45 (1966) 732.

[103] E. Nocard, E. Leclainche, Les Maladies Microbiennes des Animaux, second ed., Masson, Paris, 1898, p. 106.

[104] E. Joest, Untersuchungen über Kalberruhr, Z. Tiermed. 7 (1903) 377.

[105] C. Titze, A. Weichel, Die Ätiologie der Kalberruhr, Berl. Tierarztl. Wochenschr. 26 (1908) 457.

[106] C.O. Jensen, Handbuch der pathogenen Microorganismen, vol 6, Jena, G Fischer, 1913, p. 131.

[107] T. Smith, M.L. Orcutt, The bacteriology of the intestinal tract of young calves with special reference to the early diarrhea ("scours"), J. Exp. Med. 41 (1925) 89.

[108] Neonatal enteric infections caused by Escherichia coli, Ann. N. Y. Acad. Sci. 176 (1971) 1.

[109] E. Moro, Quoted in Adam A. Über die Biologie der Dyspepsiecoli und ihre Beziehungen zur Pathogenese der Dyspepsie und Intoxikation, Jahrb. Kinderheilkd. 101 (1923) 295.

[110] A. Adam, Über die Biologie der Dyspepsiecoli und ihre Beziehungen zur Pathogenese der Dyspepsie und Intoxikation, Jahrb. Kinderheilkd. 101 (1923) 295.

[111] A. Adam, Zur Frage der bakteriellen Ätiologie der sogenannten alimentaren Intoxikation, Jahrb. Kinderheilkd. 116 (1927) 8.

[112] J.P. Nataro, J.B. Kaper, Diarrheagenic *Escherichia coli*, Clin. Microbiol. Rev. 11 (1998) 142.

[113] U. Reischl, et al., Real-time fluorescence PCR assays for detection and characterization of heat-labile I and heat-stable I enterotoxin genes from enterotoxigenic *Escherichia coli*, J. Clin. Microbiol. 42 (2004) 4092–4100.

[114] K. Kimata, et al., Rapid categorization of pathogenic *Escherichia coli* by multiplex PCR, Microbiol. Immunol. 49 (2005) 485–492.

[115] M.S. Donnenberg, J.B. Kaper, Enteropathogenic *Escherichia coli*, Infect. Immun. 60 (1992) 3953.

[116] M.M. Levine, *Escherichia coli* that cause diarrhea: enterotoxigenic, enteropathogenic, enteroinvasive, enterohemorrhagic, and enteroadherent, J. Infect. Dis. 155 (1987) 377.

[117] R.L. Guerrant, N.M. Thielman, Types of *Escherichia coli* enteropathogens, in: M.J. Blaser (Ed.), Infections of the Gastrointestinal Tract, Raven Press, New York, 1995, p. 687.

[118] T.A. Schlager, R.L. Guerrant, Seven possible mechanisms for *Escherichia coli* diarrhea, Infect. Dis. Clin. North. Am. 2 (1988) 607.

[119] T.S. Steiner, et al., Enteroaggregative *Escherichia coli* produce intestinal inflammation and growth impairment and cause interleukin-8 release from intestinal epithelial cells, J. Infect. Dis. 177 (1998) 88.

[120] R. Guerrant, T. Steiner, Principles and syndromes of enteric infections, in: G.L. Mandell, J. Bennett, R. Dolin (Eds.), Mandell, Douglas, and Bennett's Principles and Practice of Infectious Diseases, fifth ed., WB Saunders, Philadelphia, 1999.

[121] B.D. Spangler, Structure and function of cholera toxin and the related *Escherichia coli* heat-labile enterotoxin, Microbiol. Rev. 56 (1992) 622.

[122] R.L. Guerrant, et al., Effect of *Escherichia coli* on fluid transport across canine small bowel: mechanism and time-course with enterotoxin and whole bacterial cells, J. Clin. Invest. 52 (1973) 1707.

[123] J.W. Peterson, G. Ochoa, Role of prostaglandins and cAMP in the secretory effects of cholera toxin, Science 245 (1989) 857.

[124] J.W. Peterson, et al., Protein synthesis is required for cholera toxin-induced stimulation or arachidonic acid metabolism, Biochim. Biophys. Acta 1092 (1991) 79.

[125] N.M. Thielman, et al., The role of platelet activating factor in Chinese hamster ovary cell responses to cholera toxin, J. Clin. Invest. 99 (1997) 1999.

[126] R.L. Guerrant, et al., Role of platelet activating factor (PAF) in the intestinal epithelial secretory and Chinese hamster ovary (CHO) cell cytoskeletal responses to cholera toxin, Proc. Natl. Acad. Sci. U. S. A. 91 (1994) 9655.

[127] J.M. Hughes, et al., Role of cyclic GMP in the action of heat-stable enterotoxin of *Escherichia coli*. Nature 271 (1978) 755.

[128] M. Field, et al., Heat-stable enterotoxin of *Escherichia coli*: in vitro effects on guanylate cyclase activity, cyclic GMP concentration, and ion transport in small intestine, Proc. Natl. Acad. Sci. U. S. A. 75 (1978) 2800.

[129] R.L. Guerrant, et al., Activation of intestinal guanylate cyclase by heat-stable enterotoxin of *Escherichia coli*: studies of tissue specificity, potential receptors and intermediates, J. Infect. Dis. 142 (1980) 220.

[130] D.J. Kennedy, et al., Effects of *E. coli* heat stable enterotoxin STb on intestines of mice, rats, rabbits, and piglets. Infect. Immun. 46 (1984) 639.

[131] C.S. Weikel, H.N. Nellans, R.L. Guerrant, In vivo and in vitro effects of a novel enterotoxin, STb, produced by *E. coli*, J. Infect. Dis. 153 (1986) 893.

[132] C.S. Weikel, et al., Species specificity and lack of production of STb enterotoxin by *E. coli* strains isolated from humans with diarrheal illness, Infect. Immun. 52 (1986) 323.

[133] H.L. DuPont, et al., Pathogenesis of *Escherichia coli* diarrhea, N. Engl. J. Med. 285 (1971) 1.

[134] E.F. Tulloch, et al., Invasive enteropathic *Escherichia coli* dysentery: an outbreak in 28 adults, Ann. Intern. Med. 79 (1973) 13.

[135] J.P. Nataro, et al., Patterns of adherence of diarrheagenic *E. coli* to HEp-2 cells, Pediatr. Infect. Dis. 6 (1987) 829.

[136] B. Kenny, et al., Enteropathogenic *E. coli* (EPEC) transfers its receptor for intimate adherence into mammalian cells, Cell 91 (1997) 511.

[137] J.P. Nougayrede, P.J. Fernandes, M.S. Donnenberg, Adhesion of enteropathogenic *Escherichia coli* to host cells, Cell. Microbiol. 5 (2003) 359.

[138] J.A. Giron, et al., Diffuse-adhering *Escherichia coli* (DAEC) as a putative cause of diarrhea in Mayan children in Mexico, J. Infect. Dis. 163 (1991) 507.

[139] I. Peiffer, et al., Impairments in enzyme activity and biosynthesis of brush border-associated hydrolases in human intestinal Caco-2/TC7 cells infected by members of the Afa/Dr family of diffusely adhering *Escherichia coli*, Cell. Microbiol. 3 (2001) 341.

[140] I.N. Okeke, J.P. Nataro, Enteroaggregative *Escherichia coli*, Lancet Infect. Dis. 1 (2001) 304.

[141] B. Rowe, S.M. Scotland, R.J. Gross, Enterotoxigenic *Escherichia coli* causing infantile enteritis in Britain, Lancet 1 (1977) 90.

[142] L.R. Trabulsi, M.F.R. Fernandes, M.E. Zuliani, Novas bacterias patogenicas para o intestino do homen, Rev. Inst. Med. Trop. São. Paulo. 9 (1967) 31.

[143] B. Sereny, Experimental *Shigella* keratoconjunctivitis: a preliminary report, Acta Microbiol. Acad. Sci. Hung. 2 (1955) 293.

[144] F.J. Skerman, S.B. Formal, S. Falkow, Plasmid-associated enterotoxin production in a strain of *Escherichia coli* isolated from humans, Infect. Immun. 56 (1972) 22.

[145] Y. Takeda, J. Murphy, Bacteriophage conversion of heat-labile enterotoxin in *Escherichia coli*, J. Bacteriol. 133 (1978) 172.

[146] R. Lathe, P. Hirth, Cell-free synthesis of enterotoxin of *E. coli* from a cloned gene, Nature 284 (1980) 473.

[147] M.H. Merson, et al., Use of antisera for identification of enterotoxigenic *Escherichia coli*, Lancet 2 (1980) 222.

[148] A. Sjöling, et al., Comparative analyses of phenotypic and genotypic methods for detection of enterotoxigenic *Escherichia coli* toxins and colonization factors, J. Clin. Microbiol. 45 (2007) 3295–3301.

[149] F. Qadri, et al., Enterotoxigenic *Escherichia coli* in developing countries: epidemiology, microbiology, clinical features, treatment, and prevention, Clin. Microbiol. Rev. 18 (2005) 465–483.

[150] D.G. Evans, D.J. Evans Jr., N.F. Pierce, Differences in the response of rabbit small intestine to heat-labile and heat-stable enterotoxins of *Escherichia coli*, Infect. Immun. 7 (1973) 873.

[151] C.L. Sears, J.B. Kaper, Enteric bacterial toxins: mechanisms of action and linkage to intestinal secretion, Microbiol. Rev. 60 (1996) 167.

[152] S.T. Donta, H.W. Moon, S.C. Whipp, Detection of heat-labile *Escherichia coli* enterotoxin with the use of adrenal cells in tissue cultures, Science 183 (1974) 334.

[153] R.H. Yolken, et al., Enzyme-linked immunosorbent assay for detection of *Escherichia coli* heat-labile enterotoxin, J. Clin. Microbiol. 6 (1977) 439.

[154] A.G. Dean, et al., Test for *Escherichia coli* enterotoxin using infant mice: application in a study of diarrhea in children in Honolulu, J. Infect. Dis. 125 (1972) 407.

[155] R.A. Giannella, Suckling mouse model for detection of heat-stable *Escherichia coli* enterotoxin: characteristics of the model, Infect. Immun. 14 (1976) 95.

[156] F.A. Klipstein, et al., Enterotoxigenic intestinal bacteria in tropical sprue, Ann. Intern. Med. 79 (1973) 632.

[157] H.W. Smith, S. Halls, Observations by ligated intestinal segment and oral inoculation methods on *Escherichia coli* infections in pigs, calves, lambs and rabbits, J. Pathol. Bacteriol. 93 (1967) 499.

[158] D.G. Evans, et al., Plasmid-controlled colonization factor associated with virulence in *Escherichia coli* enterotoxigenic for humans, Infect. Immun. 12 (1975) 656.

[159] S.N. De, D.N. Chatterjee, An experimental study of the mechanism of action of *Vibrio cholerae* on the intestinal mucous membrane, J. Pathol. Bacteriol. 66 (1953) 559.

[160] S.N. De, K. Bhattachaya, J.K. Sakar, A study of the pathogenicity of strains of *Bacterium coli* from acute and chronic enteritis, J. Pathol. Bacteriol. 71 (1956) 201.

[161] J. Taylor, M.P. Wilkins, J.M. Payne, Relation of rabbit gut reaction to enteropathogenic *Escherichia coli*, Br. J. Exp. Pathol. 42 (1961) 43.

[162] J. Taylor, K.A. Bettelheim, The action of chloroform-killed suspensions of enteropathogenic *Escherichia coli* on ligated rabbit gut segments, J. Gen. Microbiol. 42 (1966) 309.

[163] L.R. Trabulsi, Revelacao de colibacilos associados as diarreias infantis pelo metodo da infeccao experimental de alca ligade do intestino do coehlo, Rev. Inst. Med. Trop. São. Paulo. 6 (1964) 197.

[164] H.W. Moon, et al., Association of *Escherichia coli* with diarrheal disease of the newborn pig, Am. J. Vet. Res. 27 (1966) 1107.

[165] H.W. Smith, S. Halls, Studies on *Escherichia coli* enterotoxin, J. Pathol. Bacteriol. 93 (1967) 531.

[166] M. Truszcynski, J. Pilaszek, Effects of injection of enterotoxin, endotoxin or live culture of *Escherichia coli* into the small intestine of pigs, Res. Vet. Sci. 10 (1969) 469.

[167] C.L. Gyles, D.A. Barnum, A heat-labile enterotoxin from strains of *Escherichia coli* enteropathogenic for pigs, J. Infect. Dis. 120 (1969) 419.

[168] S.L. Gorbach, et al., Acute undifferentiated human diarrhea in the tropics. I. Alterations in intestinal microflora, J Clin Invest 50 (1971) 881.

[169] J.G. Banwell, et al., Acute undifferentiated human diarrhea in the tropics. II. Alterations in intestinal fluid and electrolyte movements, J. Clin. Invest. 50 (1971) 890.

[170] R.B. Sack, et al., Enterotoxigenic *Escherichia coli* isolated from patients with severe cholera-like disease, J. Infect. Dis. 123 (1971) 278.

[171] N.F. Pierce, C.K. Wallace, Stimulation of jejunal secretion by a crude *Escherichia coli* enterotoxin, Gastroenterology 63 (1972) 439.

[172] R.L. Guerrant, C.C.J. Carpenter, N.F. Pierce, Experimental *E. coli* diarrhea: effects of viable bacteria and enterotoxin, Trans. Assoc. Am. Physicians. 86 (1973) 111.

[173] H.S. Kantor, P. Tao, S.L. Gorbach, Stimulation of intestinal adenyl cyclase by *Escherichia coli* enterotoxin: comparison of strains from an infant and an adult with diarrhea, J. Infect. Dis. 129 (1974) 1.

[174] H.W. Smith, C.L. Gyles, The relationship between two apparently different enterotoxins produced by enteropathogenic strains of *Escherichia coli* of porcine origin, J. Med. Microbiol. 3 (1970) 387.

[175] E.M. Kohler, Observations on enterotoxins produced by enteropathogenic *Escherichia coli*, Ann. N. Y. Acad. Sci. 176 (1971) 212.

[176] H.W. Moon, S.C. Whipp, Systems for testing the enteropathogenicity of *Escherichia coli*, Ann. N. Y. Acad. Sci. 176 (1971) 197.

[177] H.W. Smith, M.A. Linggood, Observations on the pathogenic properties of the K88, HLY and ENT plasmids of *Escherichia coli* with particular reference to porcine diarrhea, J. Med. Microbiol. 4 (1971) 467.

[178] J. Holmgren, A.M. Svennerholm, Enzyme-linked immunosorbent assays for cholera serology, Infect. Immun. 7 (1973) 759.

[179] A.M. Svennerholm, J. Holmgren, Identification of *Escherichia coli* heat-labile enterotoxin by means of a ganglioside immunosorbent assay (Gm1 ELISA) procedure, Curr. Microbiol. 1 (1978) 19.

[180] D.A. Sack, et al., Microtiter ganglioside enzyme-linked immunosorbent assay for *Vibrio* and *Escherichia coli* heat-labile enterotoxins and antitoxin, J. Clin. Microbiol. 11 (1980) 35.

[181] M.G. Currie, et al., Guanylin: an endogenous activator of intestinal guanylate cyclase, Proc. Natl. Acad. Sci. U. S. A. 89 (1992) 947.

[182] T. Wadstrom, et al., Enterotoxin-producing bacteria and parasites in stools of Ethiopian children with diarrhoeal disease, Arch. Dis. Child. 51 (1976) 865.

[183] K. Wachsmuth, et al., Heat-labile enterotoxin production in isolates from a shipboard outbreak of human diarrheal illness, Infect. Immun. 24 (1979) 793.

[184] P.D. Sandefur, J.W. Peterson, Isolation of skin permeability factors from culture filtrates of *Salmonella typhimurium*, Infect. Immun. 14 (1976) 671.

[185] P.D. Sandefur, J.W. Peterson, Neutralization of *Salmonella* toxin-induced elongation of Chinese hamster ovary cells by cholera antitoxin, Infect. Immun. 15 (1977) 988.

[186] R.A. Gibbons, et al., Inheritance of resistance to neonatal *E. coli* diarrhea in the pig: examination of the genetic system, Theor. Appl. Genet. 51 (1977) 65.

[187] M.K. Wolf, Occurrence, distribution and associations of O and H serogroups, colonization factor antigens, and toxins of enterotoxigenic *Escherichia coli*, Clin. Microbiol. Rev. 10 (1997) 569.

[188] F.J. Cassels, M.K. Wolf, Colonization factors of diarrheagenic *E. coli* and their intestinal receptors, J. Ind. Microbiol. 15 (1995) 214.

[189] D.A. Sack, et al., Enterotoxigenic *Escherichia coli* diarrhea of travelers: a prospective study of American Peace Corps volunteers, Johns. Hopkins. Med. J. 141 (1977) 63.

[190] R.L. Guerrant, et al., Turista among members of the Yale Glee Club in Latin America, Am. J. Trop. Hyg. 29 (1980) 895.

[191] R.L. Guerrant, et al., Role of toxigenic and invasive bacteria in acute diarrhea of childhood, N. Engl. J. Med. 293 (1975) 567.

[192] P. Echeverria, N.R. Blacklow, D.H. Smith, Role of heat-labile toxigenic *Escherichia coli* and reovirus-like agent in diarrhoea in Boston children, Lancet 2 (1975) 1113.

[193] G.I. Viboud, N. Binsztein, A.M. Svennerholm, Characterization of monoclonal antibodies against putative colonization factors of enterotoxigenic *Escherichia coli* and their use in an epidemiological study? J. Clin. Microbiol. 31 (1993) 558.

[194] R.W. Ryder, et al., Enterotoxigenic *Escherichia coli* and reovirus-like agent in rural Bangladesh, Lancet 1 (1976) 659.

[195] D.R. Nalin, et al., Enterotoxigenic *Escherichia coli* and idiopathic diarrhea in Bangladesh, Lancet 2 (1975) 1116.

[196] Y. Lopez-Vidal, et al., Enterotoxins and adhesins of enterotoxigenic *Escherichia coli*. Are they risk factors for acute diarrhea in the community? J. Infect. Dis. 162 (1990) 442.

[197] M. McLean, et al., Etiology and oral rehydration therapy of childhood diarrhea in northeastern Brazil, Bull. Pan. Am. Health Organ. 15 (1981) 318.

[198] R.B. Sack, et al., Enterotoxigenic *Escherichia coli* associated diarrheal disease in Apache children, N. Engl. J. Med. 292 (1975) 1041.

[199] J.M. Hughes, et al., Etiology of summer diarrhea among the Navajo, Am. J. Trop. Med. Hyg. 29 (1980) 613.

[200] S. Huilan, et al., Etiology of acute diarrhea among children in developing countries: a multicentre study in five countries, Bull. World Health Organ. 69 (1991) 549.

[201] J. Blanco, et al., Enterotoxigenic *Escherichia coli* associated with infant diarrhoea in Galicia, northwestern Spain, J. Med. Microbiol. 35 (1991) 162.

[202] M.K. Nations, et al., Brazilian popular healers as effective promoters of oral rehydration therapy (ORT) and related child survival strategies, Bull. Pan. Am. Health Organ. 22 (1988) 335.

[203] O.M. Korzeniowski, et al., A controlled study of endemic sporadic diarrhea among adult residents of southern Brazil, Trans. R. Soc. Trop. Med. Hyg. 78 (1984) 363.

[204] Y. Kudoh, et al., Outbreaks of acute enteritis due to heat-stable enterotoxin-producing strains of *Escherichia coli*, Microbiol. Immunol. 21 (1977) 175.

[205] M.L. Rosenberg, et al., Epidemic diarrhea at Crater Lake from enterotoxigenic *Escherichia coli*: a large waterborne outbreak, Ann. Intern. Med. 86 (1977) 714.

[206] R.W. Ryder, et al., Infantile diarrhea produced by heat-stable enterotoxigenic *Escherichia coli*, N. Engl. J. Med. 295 (1976) 849.

[207] R.J. Gross, et al., A new *Escherichia coli* O-group, O159, associated with outbreaks of enteritis in infants, Scand. J. Infect. Dis. 8 (1976) 195.

[208] M.J. Albert, et al., Controlled study of *Escherichia coli* diarrheal infections in Bangladeshi children, J. Clin. Microbiol. 33 (1995) 973.

[209] R.L. Guerrant, et al., Toxigenic bacterial diarrhea: nursery outbreak involving multiple bacterial strains, J. Pediatr. 89 (1976) 885.

[210] A. Abe, et al., Trivalent heat-labile- and heat-stable-enterotoxin probe conjugated with horseradish peroxidase for detection of enterotoxigenic *Escherichia coli* by hybridization, J. Clin. Microbiol. 28 (1990) 2616.

[211] H. Sommerfelt, et al., Comparative study of colony hybridization with synthetic oligonucleotide probes and enzyme-linked immunosorbent assay for identification of enterotoxigenic *E. coli*, J. Clin. Microbiol. 26 (1988) 530.

[212] A. Lund, W. Wasteson, O. Olsvik, Immunomagnetic separation and DNA hybridization for detection of enterotoxigenic *Escherichia coli* in a piglet model, J. Clin. Microbiol. 29 (1991) 2259.

[213] E. Hornes, W. Wasteson, O. Olsvik, Detection of *Escherichia coli* heat-stable enterotoxin genes in pig stool specimens by an immobilized, calorimetric, nested polymerase chain reaction, J. Clin. Microbiol. 29 (1991) 2375.

[214] R.L. Guerrant, et al., Practice guidelines for the management of infectious diarrhea, Clin. Infect. Dis. 32 (2001) 331.

[215] D. Pizarro, et al., Oral rehydration of neonates with dehydrating diarrheas, Lancet 2 (1979) 1209.

[216] M. Santosham, et al., Oral rehydration therapy for infantile diarrhea: a controlled study of well nourished children hospitalized in the United States and Panama, N. Engl. J. Med. 306 (1982) 1070.

[217] A.M. Molla, et al., Food based oral rehydration salt solutions for acute childhood diarrhoea, Lancet 2 (1989) 429.

[218] S.H. Walker, V.P. Gahol, B.A. Quintero, Sodium and water content of feedings for use in infants with diarrhea, Clin. Pediatr. 20 (1981) 199.

[219] International Study Group on Reduced Osmolarity ORS Solution, Multi-centre evaluation of reduced-osmolality oral rehydration salts solution, Lancet 345 (1995) 282.

[220] P. Echeverria, et al., Antimicrobial resistance and enterotoxin production among isolates of *Escherichia coli* in the Far East, Lancet 2 (1978) 589.

[221] J.P. Nataro, Treatment of bacterial enteritis, Pediatr. Infect. Dis. J. 17 (1998) 420.

[222] R.L. Guerrant, et al., Infectious Diseases Society of America. Practice guidelines for the management of infectious diarrhea, Clin. Infect. Dis. 32 (2001) 331–351.

[223] J.R. Harris, et al., High-molecular-weight plasmid correlates with *Escherichia coli* invasiveness, Infect. Immun. 37 (1982) 1295.

[224] A. De Assis, *Shigella* guanabara, tipo serologico destacado do group B ceylonensis-dispar, O. Hospital. 33 (1948) 508.

[225] P.D. Lapatsanis, I.M. Irving, A study of specific *E. coli* infections occurring in a unit for surgical neonates, Acta Paediatr. 52 (1963) 416.

[226] M.E. Gordillo, et al., Molecular characterization of strains of enteroinvasive *Escherichia coli* O143, including isolates from a large outbreak in Houston, Texas, J. Clin. Microbiol. 30 (1992) 889.

[227] R. Goldschmidt, Untersuchungen zur Ätiologie der Durchfallserkrankungen des Säuglings, Jahrb. Kinderheilkd. 139 (1933) 318.

[228] J. Bray, Isolation of antigenically homogenous strains of *Bact. coli neopolitanum* from summer diarrhea of infants, J. Pathol. Bacteriol. 57 (1945) 239.

[229] J. Bray, T.E.D. Beaven, Slide agglutination of *Bacterium coli* var. *neopolitanum* in summer diarrhea, J. Pathol. Bacteriol. 60 (1948) 395.

[230] J. Olarte, G. Varela, A complete somatic antigen common to *Salmonella adelaide*, *Escherichia coli-gomez* and *Escherichia coli* O111 B4, J. Lab. Clin. Med. (Lond). 40 (1952) 252.

[231] C. Giles, G. Sangster, An outbreak of infantile gastroenteritis in Aberdeen, J. Hyg. 46 (1948) 1.

[232] C. Giles, G. Sangster, J. Smith, Epidemic gastroenteritis of infants in Aberdeen during 1947, Arch. Dis. Child. 24 (1949) 45.

[233] F. Kaufman, A. Dupont, *Escherichia* strains. from. infantile. epidemic. gastroenteritis, Acta Pathol. Microbiol. Scand. 27 (1950) 552.

[234] P.R. Edwards, W.H. Ewing, Identification of Enterobacteriaceae, third ed., MN, Burgess Publishing, Minneapolis, 1972.

[235] E. Neter, R.F. Korns, R.F. Trussell, Association of *Escherichia coli* serogroup O111 with two hospital outbreaks of epidemic diarrhea of the newborn infant in New York State during 1947, Pediatrics 12 (1953) 377.

[236] E. Neter, et al., Demonstration of antibodies against enteropathogenic *Escherichia coli* in sera of children of various ages, Pediatrics 16 (1955) 801.

[237] J.A. Gronroos, Investigations on certain *Escherichia coli* serotypes, with special reference to infantile diarrhoea, Ann. Med. 32 (1954) 9.

[238] M.S. Donnenberg, T.S. Whittam, Pathogenesis and evolution of virulence in enteropathogenic and enterohemorrhagic *Escherichia coli*, J. Clin. Invest. 107 (2001) 539.

[239] L.R. Trabulsi, R. Keller, T.A. Tardelli Gomes, Typical and atypical enteropathogenic *Escherichia coli*, Emerg. Infect. Dis. 8 (2002) 508.

[240] M. Moyenuddin, K.M. Rahman, Enteropathogenic *Escherichia coli* diarrhea in hospitalized children in Bangladesh, J. Clin. Microbiol. 22 (1985) 838.

[241] J.R. Bower, et al., *Escherichia coli* O114: nonmotile as a pathogen in an outbreak of severe diarrhea associated with a day care center, J. Infect. Dis. 160 (1989) 243.

[242] E. Neter, Discussion, Ann. N. Y. Acad. Sci. 176 (1971) 136.

[243] S.C. Marker, D.J. Blazevic, Enteropathogenic serotypes of *E. coli*, J. Pediatr. 90 (1977) 1037.

[244] J.J. Farmer, et al., Enteropathogenic serotypes" of *Escherichia coli* which really are not, J. Pediatr. 90 (1977) 1047.

[245] J.E. Gordon, Diarrheal disease of early childhood—worldwide scope of the problem, Ann. N. Y. Acad. Sci. 176 (1971) 9.

[246] J.E. Gordon, I.D. Chitkara, J.B. Wyon, Weanling diarrhea, Am. J. Med. Sci. 245 (1963) 345.

[247] C.P. Bernet, C.D. Graber, C.W. Anthony, Association of *Escherichia coli* O127: B8 with an outbreak of infantile gastroenteritis and its concurrent distribution in the pediatric population, J. Pediatr. 47 (1955) 287.

[248] M.L. Cooper, et al., Epidemic diarrhea among infants associated with the isolation of a new serotype of *Escherichia coli*: E. coli O127: B8, Pediatrics 16 (1955) 215.

[249] G. Laurell, et al., Epidemic infantile diarrhea and vomiting, Acta Paediatr. 40 (1951) 302.

[250] B. Martineau, R. Raymond, G. Jeliu, Bacteriological and clinical study of gastroenteritis and enteropathogenic *Escherichia coli* O127: B8, Can. Med. Assoc. J. 79 (1958) 351.

[251] W.E. Wheeler, B. Wainerman, The treatment and prevention of epidemic infantile diarrhea due to E. coli O111 by the use of chloramphenicol and neomycin, Pediatrics 14 (1954) 357.

[252] R.A. Kaslow, et al., Enteropathogenic *Escherichia coli* infection in a newborn nursery, Am. J. Dis. Child. 128 (1974) 797.

[253] K.M. Boyer, et al., An outbreak of gastroenteritis due to E. coli O142 in a neonatal nursery, J. Pediatr. 86 (1975) 919.

[254] R.N. Masembe, The pattern of bacterial diarrhea of the newborn in Mulago Hospital (Kampala), J. Trop. Pediatr. 23 (1977) 61.

[255] M. Boris, et al., A community epidemic of enteropathogenic *Escherichia coli* O126:B16:NM gastroenteritis associated with asymptomatic respiratory infection, Pediatrics 33 (1964) 18.

[256] D.M. Kessner, et al., An extensive community outbreak of diarrhea due to enteropathogenic *Escherichia coli* O111 B4, I. Epidemiologic studies, Am. J. Hyg. 76 (1962) 27.

[257] D. Severs, et al., Epidemic gastroenteritis in Newfoundland during 1963 associated with E. coli O111 B4, Can. Med. Assoc. J. 94 (1966) 373.

[258] M.L. Cooper, H.M. Keller, E.W. Walters, Comparative frequency of detection of enteropathogenic E. coli, Salmonella and Shigella in rectal swab cultures from infants and young children, Pediatrics 19 (1957) 411.

[259] N.A. Hinton, R.R. MacGregor, A study of infections due to pathogenic serogroups of *Escherichia coli*, Can. Med. Assoc. J. 79 (1958) 359.

[260] R.I. Hutchinson, *Escherichia coli* (O-types 111, 55, and 26) and their association with infantile diarrhea: a five-year study, J. Hyg. 55 (1957) 27.

[261] L.K. Joe, et al., Diarrhea among infants and children in Djakarta, Indonesia, with special reference to pathogenic *Escherichia coli*, Am. J. Trop. Med. Hyg. 9 (1960) 626.

[262] J.D. Nelson, Duration of neomycin therapy for enteropathogenic *Escherichia coli* diarrheal disease: a comparative study of 113 cases, Pediatrics 48 (1971) 248.

[263] H.D. Riley Jr., Antibiotic therapy in neonatal enteric disease, Ann. N. Y. Acad. Sci. 176 (1971) 360.

[264] R. Rozansky, et al., Enteropathogenic *Escherichia coli* infections in infants during the period from 1957 to 1962, Pediatrics 64 (1964) 521.

[265] M.A. South, Enteropathogenic *Escherichia coli* disease: new developments and perspectives, J. Pediatr. 79 (1971) 1.

[266] G. Linzenmeier, Wandel im Auftreten und Verhalten enteropathogene Colitypen, Z. Bakteriol. 184 (1962) 74.

[267] D. Nicolopoulos, A. Arseni, Susceptibility of enteropathogenic E. coli to various antibiotics. Letter to the editor, J. Pediatr. 81 (1972) 426.

[268] A.G. Ironside, A.F. Tuxford, B. Heyworth, A survey of infantile gastroenteritis, BMJ 2 (1970) 20.

[269] H.D. Riley Jr., Clinical rounds. Enteropathogenic E. coli gastroenteritis, Clin. Pediatr. 3 (1964) 93.

[270] S. Gaines, et al., Types and distribution of enteropathogenic *Escherichia coli* in Bangkok, Thailand, Am. J. Hyg. 80 (1964) 388.

[271] D.W. Buttner, A. Lado-Kenyi, Prevalence of *Salmonella, Shigella*, and enteropathogenic *Escherichia coli* in young children in Kampala, Uganda, Tropenmed. Parasitol. 24 (1973) 259.

[272] M. Coetzee, P.M. Leary, Gentamicin in *Esch. coli* gastroenteritis, Arch. Dis. Child. 46 (1971) 646.

[273] E. Kahn, The aetiology of summer diarrhoea, S. Afr. Med. J. 31 (1957) 47.

[274] J. Taylor, The diarrhoeal diseases in England and Wales. With special reference to those caused by *Salmonella, Escherichia*, and *Shigella*, Bull. World Health Organ. 23 (1960) 763.

[275] Epidemiological Research Laboratory of the Public Health Laboratory Service, United Kingdom and Republic of Ireland. E. coli gastroenteritis from food, BMJ 1 (1976) 911.

[276] H.W. Ocklitz, E.F. Schmidt, Über das Vorkommen von Dispepsie-Coli bei Erwachsenen, Helv. Paediatr. Acta 10 (1955) 450.

[277] J. Schaffer, et al., Antepartum survey for enteropathogenic *Escherichia coli*: detection by cultural and fluorescent antibody methods, Am. J. Dis. Child. 106 (1963) 170.

[278] A.C. Kirby, E.G. Hall, W. Coackley, Neonatal diarrhoea and vomiting: outbreaks in the same maternity unit, Lancet 2 (1950) 201.

[279] K.A. Bettelheim, et al., The origin of O-serotypes of *Escherichia coli* in babies after normal delivery, J. Hyg. 72 (1974) 67.

[280] C.S. Stulberg, W.W. Zuelzer, A.C. Nolke, An epidemic of diarrhea of the newborn caused by *Escherichia coli* O111 B4, Pediatrics 14 (1954) 133.

[281] K. Farmer, I.B. Hassall, An epidemic of E. coli type O55:K 59(B5) in a neonatal unit, N. Z. Med. J. 77 (1973) 372.

[282] K. Hugh-Jones, G.I.M. Ross, Epidemics of gastroenteritis associated with E. coli O119 infection, Arch. Dis. Child. 33 (1958) 543.

[283] D. Senerwa, et al., Colonization of neonates in a nursery ward with enteropathogenic *Escherichia coli* and correlation to the clinical histories of the children, J. Clin. Microbiol. 27 (1989) 2539.

[284] J. Wright, A.T. Roden, *Escherichia coli* O55B5 infection in a gastroenteritis ward: epidemiological applications of H antigen type determinations, Am. J. Hyg. 58 (1953) 133.

[285] N. Balassanian, E. Wolinsky, Epidemiologic and serologic studies of E. coli O4 115 in a premature nursery, Pediatrics 41 (1968) 463.

[286] J.E. Jameson, T.P. Mann, N.J. Rothfield, Hospital gastroenteritis: an epidemiological survey of infantile diarrhea and vomiting contracted in a children's hospital, Lancet 2 (1954) 459.

[287] S. Thomson, The role of certain varieties of *Bacterium coli* in gastroenteritis in babies, J. Hyg. 53 (1955) 357.

[288] R.H. Page, C.S. Stulberg, Immunofluorescence in epidemiologic control of E. coli diarrhea: incidence, cross-infections, and control in a children's hospital, Am. J. Dis. Child. 104 (1962) 149.

[289] J. Bertrams, et al., Colienteritis des Säuglings. Quantitative und fluoreszenzserologische Verlaufsuntersuchungen, Munch. Med. Wochenschr. 112 (1970) 38.

[290] S. Thomson, The numbers of pathogenic bacilli in faeces in intestinal diseases, J. Hyg. 53 (1955) 217.

[291] J.C. Herweg, J.N. Middlekamp, H.K. Thornton, *Escherichia coli* diarrhea: the relationship of certain serotypes of *Escherichia coli* to sporadic and epidemic cases of infantile diarrhea, J. Pediatr. 49 (1956) 629.

[292] W.D. Belnap, J.J. O'Donnell, Epidemic gastroenteritis due to *Escherichia coli* O-111: a review of the literature, with the epidemiology, bacteriology, and clinical findings of a large outbreak, J. Pediatr. 47 (1955) 178.

[293] K.B. Rogers, S.J. Koegler, Inter-hospital cross-infection epidemic infantile gastroenteritis associated with type strains of *Bacterium coli*, J. Hyg. 49 (1951) 152.

[294] A.H. Stock, M.E. Shuman, Gastroenteritis in infants associated with specific serotypes of *Escherichia coli*. II. An epidemic of *Escherichia coli* O111 B4 gastroenteritis involving multiple institutions, Pediatrics 17 (1956) 196.

[295] C.S. Stulberg, et al., *Escherichia coli* O127 B8, a pathogenic strain causing infantile diarrhea: epidemiology and bacteriology of a prolonged outbreak in a premature nursery, Am. J. Dis. Child. 90 (1955) 125.

[296] S. Thomson, A.G. Watkins, P.O. Grapy, *Escherichia coli* gastroenteritis, Arch. Dis. Child. 31 (1956) 340.

[297] J. Olarte, M. Ramos-Alvarez, Epidemic diarrhea in premature infants: etiological significance of a newly recognized type of *Escherichia coli* (O142:K 86 H6), Am. J. Dis. Child. 109 (1965) 436.

[298] J.D. Nelson, et al., Epidemiological application of the fluorescent antibody technique: study of a diarrhea outbreak in a premature nursery, JAMA 176 (1961) 26.

[299] R. Buttiaux, et al., Etude épidémiologique des gastroentérites à Escherichia coli dans un service hospitalier du nord de la France, Arch. Mal. Appar. Dig. Mal. Nutr. 45 (1956) 225.

[300] A.H. Harris, et al., Control of epidemic diarrhea of the newborn in hospital nurseries and pediatric wards, Ann. N. Y. Acad. Sci. 66 (1956) 118.

[301] S.I. Jacobs, et al., Outbreak of infantile gastroenteritis caused by *Escherichia coli* O114, Arch. Dis. Child. 46 (1970) 656.

[302] M. Curtin, S.H. Clifford, Incidence of pathogenic serologic types of *Escherichia coli* among neonatal patients in the New England area, N. Engl. J. Med. 255 (1956) 1090.

[303] D.C. Greene, R.M. Albrecht, Recent developments in diarrhea of the newborn, N. Y. State. J. Med. 55 (1955) 2764.

[304] W.E. Wheeler, Spread and control of *Escherichia coli* diarrheal disease, Ann. N. Y. Acad. Sci. 66 (1956) 112.

[305] R.R. Buttiaux, et al., Etudes sur les E. coli de gastroentérite infantile, Ann. Inst. Pasteur. 91 (1956) 799.

[306] W.C. Love, et al., Infantile gastroenteritis due to *Escherichia coli* O142, Lancet 2 (1972) 355.

[307] H.J. Shaughnessy, et al., An extensive community outbreak of diarrhea due to enteropathogenic *Escherichia coli* O111 B4, Am. J. Hyg. 76 (1962) 44.

[308] N. Kendall, V.C. Vaughan III., A. Kusakcioglu, A study of preparation of infant formulas: a medical and sociocultural appraisal, Am. J. Dis. Child 122 (1971) 215.

[309] D.R. Gamble, K.E.K. Rowson, The incidence of pathogenic *Escherichia coli* in routine fecal specimens, Lancet 2 (1957) 619.

[310] J. Taylor, B.W. Powell, J. Wright, Infantile diarrhoea and vomiting: a clinical and bacteriological investigation, BMJ 2 (1949) 117.

[311] R.I. Modica, W.W. Ferguson, E.F. Ducey, Epidemic infantile diarrhea associated with *Escherichia coli* O111, B4, J. Lab. Clin. Med. 39 (1952) 122.

[312] K.B. Rogers, The spread of infantile gastroenteritis in a cubicled ward, J. Hyg. 49 (1951) 140.

[313] D.A.A. Mossel, H.A. Weijers, Uitkomsten, verkregen bij bacteriologisch onderzoek van vrouwenmelk van diverse herkomst en de betekenis daarvan de pediatrische praktijk, Maandschr. Kindergeneeskd. 25 (1957) 37.

[314] I. Rantasalo, M.A. Kauppinen, The occurrence of *Staphylococcus aureus* in mother's milk, Ann. Chir. Gynaecol. 48 (1959) 246.

[315] L.D. Edwards, et al., The problem of bacteriologically contaminated infant formulas in a newborn nursery, Clin. Pediatr. 13 (1974) 63.

[316] S. Thomson, Is infantile gastroenteritis fundamentally a milk-borne infection? J. Hyg. 54 (1956) 311.

[317] D. Danielssen, G. Laurell, Fluorescent antibody technique in the diagnosis of enteropathogenic *Escherichia coli*, with special reference to sensitivity and specificity, Acta Pathol. Microbiol. Scand. 76 (1969) 601.

[318] C.L. Bullen, A.T. Willis, Resistance of the breast-fed infant to gastroenteritis, BMJ 3 (1971) 338.

[319] S. Svirsky-Gross, Pathogenic strains of coli (O, 111) among prematures and the use of human milk in controlling the outbreak of diarrhea, Ann. Paediatr. 190 (1958) 109.

[320] B. Tassovatz, A. Kotsitch, Le lait de femme et son action de protection contre les infections intestinales chez le nouveau-né, Ann. Paediatr. 8 (1961) 285.

[321] A. Adam, Fortschritte in der Pathogenese und Therapie der Ernährungsstörungen, Arztl. Forschung. 6 (1952) 59.

[322] E. Neter, C.E. Shumway, Coli serotype D433: occurrence in intestinal and respiratory tracts, cultural characteristics, pathogenicity, sensitivity to antibiotics, Proc. Soc. Exp. Biol. Med. 75 (1950) 504.

[323] H. Arnon, M. Salzberger, A.L. Olitzki, The appearance of antibacterial and antitoxic antibodies in maternal sera, umbilical cord blood and milk: observations on the specificity of antibacterial antibodies in human sera, Pediatrics 23 (1959) 86.

[324] J.F. Kenny, M.I. Boesman, R.H. Michaels, Bacterial and viral coproantibodies in breast-fed infants, Pediatrics 39 (1967) 202.

[325] C.S. Stulberg, W.W. Zuelzer, Infantile diarrhea due to *Escherichia coli*, Ann. N. Y. Acad. Sci. 66 (1956) 90.

[326] J. Dancis, H.W. Kunz, Studies of the immunology of the newborn infant. VI. Bacteriostatic and complement activity of the serum, Pediatrics 13 (1954) 339.

[327] R. Yeivin, M. Salzberger, A.L. Olitzki, Development of antibodies to enteric pathogens: placental transfer of antibodies and development of immunity in childhood, Pediatrics 18 (1956) 19.

[328] J.F. Kenny, D.W. Weinert, J.A. Gray, Enteric infection with *Escherichia coli* O127 in the mouse. II. Failure of specific immunity to alter intestinal colonization of infants and adults, J. Infect. Dis. 129 (1974) 10.

[329] R. Lodinova, V. Jouja, V. Wagner, Serum immunoglobulins and coproantibody formation in infants after artificial intestinal colonization with *Escherichia coli* O83 and oral lysozyme administration, Pediatr. Res. 7 (1973) 659.

[330] A.S. McNeish, H. Gaze, The intestinal antibody response in infants with enteropathic E. coli gastroenteritis, Acta Paediatr. Scand. 63 (1974) 663.

[331] M.C. Goldschmidt, H.L. DuPont, Enteropathogenic *Escherichia coli*: lack of correlation of serotype with pathogenicity, J. Infect. Dis. 133 (1976) 153.

[332] P.D. Echeverria, C.P. Chang, D. Smith, Enterotoxigenicity and invasive capacity of "enteropathogenic" serotypes of *Escherichia coli*, J. Pediatr. 89 (1976) 8.

[333] R.J. Gross, S.M. Scotland, B. Rowe, Enterotoxin testing of *Escherichia coli* causing epidemic infantile enteritis in the U.K, Lancet 1 (1976) 629.

[334] M.M. Drucker, et al., Immunofluorescent demonstration of enteropathogenic *Escherichia coli* in tissues of infants dying with enteritis, Pediatrics 46 (1970) 855.

[335] M.M. Levine, et al., *Escherichia coli* strains that cause diarrhea but do not produce heat-labile or heat-stable enterotoxins and are non-invasive, Lancet 1 (1978) 1119.

[336] W.G. Wade, B.T. Thom, N. Evans, Cytotoxic enteropathogenic *Escherichia coli*, Lancet 2 (1979) 1235.

[337] J.L. Mellies, et al., EspC pathogenicity island of enteropathogenic *Escherichia coli* encodes an enterotoxin, Infect. Immun. 69 (2001) 315.

[338] R.J. Rothbaum, et al., Enterocyte adherent E. coli O119:B 14: a novel mechanism of infant diarrhea, Gastroenterology 80 (1981) 1265.

[339] Y. Polotsky, et al., Pathogenic effect of enterotoxigenic *Escherichia coli* and *Escherichia coli* causing infantile diarrhea, Acta Microbiol. Acad. Sci. Hung. 24 (1977) 221.

[340] B.A. Vallance, et al., Enteropathogenic and enterohemorrhagic *Escherichia coli* infections: emerging themes in pathogenesis and prevention, Can. J. Gastroenterol. 16 (2002) 771.

[341] T.K. McDaniel, et al., A genetic locus of enterocyte effacement conserved among diverse enterobacterial pathogens, Proc. Natl. Acad. Sci. U. S. A. 92 (1995) 1664.

[342] T.K. McDaniel, J.B. Kaper, A cloned pathogenicity island from enteropathogenic *Escherichia coli* confers the attaching and effacing phenotype on E. coli K-12, Mol. Microbiol. 23 (1997) 399.

[343] S.J. Elliott, et al., The complete sequence of the locus of enterocyte effacement (LEE) from enteropathogenic *Escherichia coli* E2348/69, Mol. Microbiol. 28 (1998) 1.

[344] M. Ghaem-Maghami, et al., Intimin-specific immune responses prevent bacterial colonization by the attaching-effacing pathogen *Citrobacter rodentium*, Infect. Immun. 69 (2001) 5597.

[345] J.A. Giron, A.S.Y. Ho, G.K. Schoolnik, An inducible bundle-forming pilus of enteropathogenic *Escherichia coli*, Science 254 (1992) 710.

[346] K.D. Stone, et al., A cluster of fourteen genes from enteropathogenic *Escherichia coli* is sufficient for the biogenesis of a type IV pilus, Mol. Microbiol. 20 (1996) 325.

[347] S. Knutton, et al., The type IV bundle-forming pilus of enteropathogenic *Escherichia coli* undergoes dramatic alterations in structure associated with bacterial adherence, aggregation and dispersal, Mol. Microbiol. 33 (1999) 499.

[348] D. Bieber, et al., Type IV pili, transient bacterial aggregates, and virulence of enteropathogenic *Escherichia coli*, Science 280 (1998) 2114.

[349] J.P. Nataro, Atypical enteropathogenic *Escherichia coli*: typical pathogens? Emerg. Infect. Dis. 12 (2006) 696.

[350] R.N. Nguyen, et al., Atypical enteropathogenic *Escherichia coli* infection and prolonged diarrhea in children, Emerg. Infect. Dis. 12 (2006) 597–603.

[351] A.D. Dulaney, I.D. Michelson, A study of E. coli mutable from an outbreak of diarrhea in the new-born, Am. J. Public Health 25 (1935) 1241.

[352] G.B. Hopkins, et al., Necrotizing enterocolitis in premature infants: a clinical and pathologic evaluation of autopsy material, Am. J. Dis. Child. 120 (1970) 229.

[353] Y. Rho, J.E. Josephson, Epidemic enteropathogenic *Escherichia coli*. Newfoundland, 1963: autopsy study of 16 cases, Can. Med. Assoc. J. 96 (1967) 392.

[354] H. Shwachman, et al., Protracted diarrhea of infancy treated by intravenous alimentation. II. Studies of small intestinal biopsy results, Am. J. Dis. Child. 125 (1973) 365.

[355] T. Lucking, R. Gruttner, Chronic diarrhea and severe malabsorption in infancy following infections with pathogenic E. coli, Acta Paediatr. Scand. 63 (1974) 167.

[356] C.P. Handforth, K. Sorger, Failure of regeneration of small bowel mucosa following epidemic infantile gastroenteritis, Can. Med. Assoc. J. 84 (1961) 425.

[357] D.G. McKay, G.H. Wahle Jr., Epidemic gastroenteritis due to *Escherichia coli* O111 B4. II. Pathologic anatomy (with special reference to the presence of the local and generalized Shwartzman phenomena). Arch. Pathol. 60 (1955) 679.

[358] G. Laurell, Quoted in Ordway NK. Diarrhoeal disease and its control, Bull. World Health Organ. 23 (1960) 93.

[359] O.H. Braun, H. Henckel, Über epidemische Säuglingsenteritis, Z. Kinderheilkd. 70 (1951) 33.

[360] K.B. Rogers, V.M. Cracknell, Epidemic infantile gastroenteritis due to *Escherichia coli* type O, 114, J. Pathol. Bacteriol. 72 (1956) 27.

[361] R.M. Todd, E.G. Hall, Chloramphenicol in prophylaxis of infantile gastroenteritis, BMJ 1 (1953) 1359.

[362] Gastroenteritis due to Escherichia coli, Editorial, Lancet 1 (1968) 32.

[363] D. Senerwa, et al., Enteropathogenic *Escherichia coli* serotype O111:HNT isolated from preterm neonates in Nairobi, Kenya, J. Clin. Microbiol. 27 (1989) 1307.

[364] J. Bray, Bray's discovery of pathogenic Esch. coli as a cause of infantile gastroenteritis, Arch. Dis. Child. 48 (1973) 923.

[365] A.G. Ironside, et al., Cross-infection in infantile gastroenteritis, Arch. Dis. Child. 46 (1971) 815.

[366] E.M. Linetskaya-Novgorodskaya, Acute intestinal infections of nondysenteric etiology, Bull. World Health Organ. 21 (1959) 299.

[367] H. Drimmer-Hernheiser, A.L. Olitzki, The association of *Escherichia coli* (serotypes O111 B4 and O55 B5) with cases of acute infantile gastroenteritis in Jerusalem, Acta Med. Orient. 10 (1951) 219.

[368] K. Linde, H. Kodizt, G. Funk, Die Mehrfachinfektionen mit Dyspepsie-Coli, ihre Beurteilung in statistischer, bakteriologischer und klinischer Sicht, Z. Hyg. 147 (1960) 94.

[369] M. Fandre, et al., Epidemic of infantile gastroenteritis due to *Escherichia coli* O127 B8 with methemoglobinemic cyanosis, Arch. Fr. Pediatr. 19 (1962) 1129.

[370] D. Garcia de Olarte, et al., Treatment of diarrhea in malnourished infants and children: a double-blind study comparing ampicillin and placebo, Am. J. Dis. Child. 127 (1974) 379.

[371] M.D. Yow, Prophylactic antimicrobial agents—panel. Statement of panelist, in: Centers for Disease Control Proceedings of the International

Conference on Nosocomial Infections, August 3–6 1970, American Hospital Association, Chicago, 1971, pp. 315–316.

[372] K.A. Bettelheim, M. Faiers, R.A. Sheeter, Serotypes of *Escherichia coli* in normal stools, Lancet 2 (1972) 1227.

[373] Committee on Fetus and Newborn, Guidelines for Perinatal Care, third ed., American Academy of Pediatrics and American College of Obstetricians and Gynecologists, Elk Grove Village, IL, 1992.

[374] R. Mushin, Multiple intestinal infection, Med. J. Aust. 1 (1953) 807.

[375] D.E. Katz, et al., Oral immunization of adult volunteers with microencapsulated enterotoxigenic *Escherichia coli* (ETEC) CS6 antigen, Vaccine 21 (2003) 341.

[376] J.C. Harris, H.L. DuPont, R.B. Hornick, Fecal leukocytes in diarrheal illness, Ann. Intern. Med. 76 (1972) 697.

[377] R.L. Guerrant, et al., Measurement of fecal lactoferrin as a marker of fecal leukocytes and inflammatory enteritis, J. Clin. Microbiol. 30 (1992) 1238.

[378] J.R. Miller, et al., A rapid test for infectious and inflammatory enteritis, Arch. Intern. Med. 154 (1994) 2660.

[379] W.B. Cherry, B.M. Thomason, Fluorescent antibody techniques for *Salmonella* and other enteric pathogens, Public Health Rep. 84 (1969) 887.

[380] W.A. Murray, J. Kheder, W.E. Wheeler, Colistin suppression of *Escherichia coli* in stools. I. Control of a nosocomial outbreak of diarrhea caused by neomycin-resistant *Escherichia coli* O111 B4, Am. J. Dis. Child. 108 (1964) 274.

[381] T.N. Bokete, et al., Genetic and phenotypic analysis of *Escherichia coli* with enteropathogenic characteristics isolated from Seattle children, J. Infect. Dis. 175 (1997) 1382.

[382] P.A. Vial, et al., Comparison of two assay methods for patterns of adherence to HEp-2 cells of *Escherichia coli* from patients with diarrhea, J. Clin. Microbiol. 28 (1990) 882.

[383] M.J. Albert, et al., An ELISA for the detection of localized adherent classic enteropathogenic *Escherichia coli* serogroups, J. Infect. Dis. 164 (1991) 986.

[384] S. Knutton, et al., Actin accumulation at sites of bacterial adhesion to tissue culture cells: basis of a new diagnostic test for enteropathogenic and enterohemorrhagic *Escherichia coli*, Infect. Immun. 57 (1989) 1290.

[385] J.D. Nelson, Comment, in: S. Gellis (Ed.), Yearbook of Pediatrics, Mosby-Year Book, St Louis, 1973.

[386] J.O. Sherman, C.A. Hamly, A.K. Khachadurian, Use of an oral elemental diet in infants with severe intractable diarrhea, J. Pediatr. 86 (1975) 518.

[387] J.L. Pearce, J.R. Hamilton, Controlled trial of orally administered lactobacilli in acute infantile diarrhea, J. Pediatr. 84 (1974) 261.

[388] J. Marie, A. Hennequet, C. Roux, La kanamycin "per os" dans le traitement des gastroentérites à colibacilles du nourrison, Ann. Paediatr. 9 (1962) 97.

[389] H.B. Valman, M.J. Wilmers, Use of antibiotics in acute gastroenteritis among infants in hospital, Lancet 1 (1969) 1122.

[390] K.M. Dailey, A.B. Sturtevant, T.W. Feary, Incidence of antibiotic resistance and R-factors among gram-negative bacteria isolated from the neonatal intestine, J. Pediatr. 80 (1972) 198.

[391] H.C. Neu, et al., Antibiotic resistance of fecal *Escherichia coli*: a comparison of samples from children of low and high socioeconomic groups, Am. J. Dis. Child. 126 (1973) 174.

[392] T. Watanabe, Transferable antibiotic resistance in Enterobacteriaceae: relationship to the problems of treatment and control of coliform enteritis, Ann. N. Y. Acad. Sci. 176 (1971) 371.

[393] G.H. McCracken, Changing pattern of the antimicrobial susceptibilities of *Escherichia coli* in neonatal infections, J. Pediatr. 78 (1971) 942.

[394] C.M. Kunin, Resistance to antimicrobial drugs—a worldwide calamity, Ann. Intern. Med. 118 (1993) 559.

[395] L.L. Silver, K.A. Bostian, Discovery and development of new antibiotics: the problem of antibiotic resistance, Antimicrob. Agents Chemother. 37 (1993) 377.

[396] J.D. Nelson, Commentary, J. Pediatr. 89 (1976) 471.

[397] K. Sprunt, W. Redman, G. Leidy, Antibacterial effectiveness of routine handwashing, Pediatrics 52 (1973) 264.

[398] Multistate outbreak of *Escherichia coli* O157 H7 infections from hamburgers, MMWR Morb. Wkly. Rep. 42 (1993) 258.

[399] K.L. MacDonald, M.T. Osterholm, The emergence of *Escherichia coli* O157 H7 infection in the United States, JAMA 269 (1993) 2264.

[400] H. Watanabe, et al., Outbreaks of enterohemorrhagic *Escherichia coli* O157 H7 infection by two different genotype strains in Japan, Lancet 348 (1996) 831.

[401] T.J. Ochoa, T.G. Cleary, Epidemiology and spectrum of disease of *Escherichia coli* O157, Curr. Opin. Infect. Dis. 16 (2003) 259.

[402] Hemolytic-uremic syndrome associated with *Escherichia coli* O157 H7 enteric infections—United States, MMWR Morb. Mortal. Wkly. Rep. 34 (1985) 20.

[403] E.A. Belongia, et al., Transmission of *Escherichia coli* O157 H7 infection in Minnesota child day-care facilities, JAMA 269 (1993) 883.

[404] R.E. Besser, et al., An outbreak of diarrhea and hemolytic uremic syndrome from *Escherichia coli* O157 H7 in fresh-pressed apple cider, JAMA 269 (1993) 2217.

[405] M. Mobasellah, et al., Pathogenesis of *Shigella* diarrhea: evidence for a developmentally regulated glycolipid receptor for Shigatoxin involved in the fluid secretory response of rabbit small intestine, J. Infect. Dis. 157 (1988) 1023.

[406] K. Sandvig, Shiga toxins, Toxicon 39 (2001) 1629.

[407] P.E. Ray, X.H. Liu, Pathogenesis of Shiga toxin-induced hemolytic uremic syndrome, Pediatr. Nephrol. 16 (2001) 823.

[408] H. Schmidt, Shiga-toxin-converting bacteriophages, Res. Microbiol. 152 (2001) 687.

[409] S.M. Scotland, H.R. Smith, B. Rowe, Two distinct toxins active on Vero cells from *Escherichia coli* O157, Lancet 2 (1985) 885.

[410] M.A. Karmali, et al., Antigenic heterogeneity of *Escherichia coli* verotoxins, Lancet 1 (1986) 164.

[411] H. Karch, et al., A plasmid of enterohemorrhagic *Escherichia coli* O157 H7 is required for expression of a new fimbrial antigen and for adhesion to epithelial cells, Infect. Immun. 55 (1987) 455.

[412] M.M. Levine, X.U. Jian-guo, J.B. Kaper, A DNA probe to identify enterohemorrhagic *Escherichia coli* of O157 H7 and other serotypes that cause hemorrhagic colitis and hemolytic uremic syndrome, J. Infect. Dis. 156 (1987) 175.

[413] J.C. Paton, A.W. Paton, Methods for detection of STEC in humans: an overview, Methods. Mol. Med. 73 (2003) 9.

[414] E.J. Klein, et al., Shiga toxin-producing *Escherichia coli* in children with diarrhea: a prospective point-of-care study, J Pediatr 141 (2002) 172.

[415] P.I. Tarr, Escherichia coli O157:H7: clinical, diagnostic, and epidemiological aspects of human infection, Clin. Infect. Dis. 20 (1995) 1.

[416] C.S. Wong, et al., The risk of the hemolytic-uremic syndrome after antibiotic treatment of *Escherichia coli* O157 H7 infections, N. Engl. J. Med. 342 (2000) 1930.

[417] N. Safdar, et al., Risk of hemolytic uremic syndrome after antibiotic treatment of *Escherichia coli* O157 H7 enteritis: a meta-analysis, JAMA 288 (2002) 996.

[417a] B.P. Bell, et al., Predictors of hemolytic uremic syndrome in children during a large outbreak of Escherichia coli O157:H7 infections, Pediatrics 100 (1997) E12.

[418] J.P. Nataro, Enteroaggregative *Escherichia coli*, in: J. Hughes (Ed.), Emerging Infections, 6, American Society for Microbiology Press, Washington, DC, 2003.

[419] J. Sarantuya, et al., Typical enteroaggregative *Escherichia coli* are the most prevalent pathotypes causing diarrhea in Mongolian children, J. Clin. Microbiol. 42 (2004) 133.

[420] B. Baudry, et al., A sensitive and specific DNA probe to identify enteroaggregative *Escherichia coli*, a recently discovered diarrheal pathogen, J. Infect. Dis. 161 (1990) 1249.

[421] J. Nishi, et al., The export of coat protein from enteroaggregative *Escherichia coli* by a specific ATP-binding cassette transporter system, J. Biol. Chem. 278 (2003) 45680.

[422] J.J. Mathewson, et al., Pathogenicity of enteroadherent *Escherichia coli* in adult volunteers, J. Infect. Dis. 154 (1986) 524.

[423] J.P. Nataro, et al., Heterogeneity of enteroaggregative *Escherichia coli* virulence demonstrated in volunteers, J. Infect. Dis. 17 (1995) 465.

[424] Y. Itoh, et al., Laboratory investigation of enteroaggregative *Escherichia coli* O untypeable:H10 associated with a massive outbreak of gastrointestinal illness, J. Clin. Microbiol. 35 (1997) 2546.

[425] H.R. Smith, T. Cheasty, B. Rowe, Enteroaggregative *Escherichia coli* and outbreaks of gastroenteritis in UK, Lancet 350 (1997) 814.

[426] M. Cobeljic, et al., Enteroaggregative *E. coli* associated with an outbreak of diarrhea in a neonatal nursery ward, Epidemiol. Infect. 117 (1996) 11.

[427] C.E. Eslava, et al., Identification of a protein with toxigenic activity produced by enteroaggregative Escherichia coli, (1993).

[428] M.K. Bhan, et al., Enteroaggregative *Escherichia coli* associated with persistent diarrhea in a cohort of rural children in India, J. Infect. Dis. 159 (1989) 1061.

[429] M.K. Bhan, et al., Enteroaggregative *Escherichia coli* and *Salmonella* associated with non-dysenteric persistent diarrhea, Pediatr. Infect. Dis. J. 8 (1989) 499.

[430] A. Cravioto, et al., Association of *Escherichia coli* HEp-2 adherence patterns with type and duration of diarrhoea, Lancet 337 (1991) 262.

[431] A.A.M. Lima, et al., Persistent diarrhea in Northeast Brazil: etiologies and interactions with malnutrition, Acta Paediatr. Scand. 381 (1992) 39.

[432] S. Dutta, et al., Use of PCR to identify enteroaggregative *Escherichia coli* as an important cause of acute diarrhoea among children living in Calcutta, India, J. Med. Microbiol. 48 (1999) 1011.

[433] I.C. Scaletsky, et al., HEp-2-adherent *Escherichia coli* strains associated with acute infantile diarrhea, São Paulo, Brazil, Emerg. Infect. Dis. 8 (2002) 855.

[434] I.N. Okeke, et al., Heterogeneous virulence of enteroaggregative *Escherichia coli* strains isolated from children in Southwest Nigeria, J. Infect. Dis. 181 (2000) 252.

[435] S. Bouzari, et al., Adherence of non-enteropathogenic *Escherichia coli* to HeLa cells, J. Med. Microbiol. 40 (1994) 95.

[436] R. Gonzalez, et al., Age-specific prevalence of *Escherichia coli* with localized and aggregative adherence in Venezuelan infants with acute diarrhea, J. Clin. Microbiol. 35 (1997) 1103.

[437] W.L. Pabst, et al., Prevalence of enteroaggregative *Escherichia coli* among children with and without diarrhea in Switzerland, J. Clin. Microbiol. 41 (2003) 2289.

[438] E. Presterl, et al., Enteroaggregative and enterotoxigenic *Escherichia coli* among isolates from patients with diarrhea in Austria, Eur. J. Clin. Microbiol. Infect. Dis. 18 (1999) 209.

[439] H.I. Huppertz, et al., Acute and chronic diarrhoea and abdominal colic associated with enteroaggregative *Escherichia coli* in young children living in western Europe, Lancet 349 (1997) 1660.

[440] D.S. Tompkins, et al., A study of infectious intestinal disease in England: microbiological findings in cases and controls, Commun. Dis. Public Health 2 (1999) 108.

[441] M. Cohen, J.P. Nataro, Unpublished observations, (2005).

[442] A.R. Bouckenooghe, et al., Markers of enteric inflammation in enteroaggregative Escherichia coli diarrhea in travelers, Am. J. Trop. Med. Hyg. 62 (2000) 711.

[443] M.S. Miqdady, et al., Detection of enteroaggregative Escherichia coli with formalin-preserved HEp-2 cells, J. Clin. Microbiol. 40 (2002) 3066.

[444] J. Spencer, et al., Improved detection of enteroaggregative Escherichia coli using formalin-fixed HEp-2 cells, Lett. Appl. Microbiol. 25 (1997) 325.

[445] D.B. Huang, et al., Virulence characteristics and the molecular epidemiology of enteroaggregative Escherichia coli isolates from travellers to developing countries, J. Med. Microbiol. 56. Pt. 10 (2007) 1386–1392.

[446] C.A. Wanke, et al., Successful treatment of diarrheal disease associated with enteroaggregative Escherichia coli in adults infected with human immunodeficiency virus, J. Infect. Dis. 178 (1998) 1369.

[447] J.A. Adachi, et al., Azithromycin found to be comparable to levofloxacin for the treatment of US travelers with acute diarrhea acquired in Mexico, Clin. Infect. Dis. 37 (2003) 1165.

[448] H.L. DuPont, et al., Rifaximin versus ciprofloxacin for the treatment of traveler's diarrhea: a randomized, double-blind clinical trial, Clin. Infect. Dis. 33 (2001) 1807.

[449] S.S. Bilge, et al., Molecular characterization of a fimbrial adhesin, F1845, mediating diffuse adherences of diarrhea-associated Escherichia coli to HEp-2 cells, J. Bacteriol. 171 (1989) 4281.

[450] S.T. Gunzburg, et al., Diffuse and enteroaggregative patterns of adherence of enteric Escherichia coli isolated from aboriginal children from the Kimberley region of western Australia, J. Infect. Dis. 167 (1993) 755.

[451] A.H. Baqui, et al., Enteropathogens associated with acute and persistent diarrhea in Bangladeshi children <5 years of age, J. Infect. Dis. 166 (1992) 792.

[452] S.J. Elliott, et al., Characterization of the roles of hemolysin and other toxins in enteropathy caused by alpha-hemolytic Escherichia coli linked to human diarrhea, Infect. Immun. 66 (1998) 2040.

[453] W.H. Ewing, Edwards and Ewing's Identification of Enterobacteriaceae, fourth ed., Elsevier, New York, 1986.

[454] W.L. Meadow, H. Schneider, M.O. Beem, Salmonella enteritidis bacteremia in childhood, J. Infect. Dis. 152 (1985) 185.

[455] J.S. Hyams, et al., Salmonella bacteremia in the first year of life, J. Pediatr. 96 (1980) 57.

[456] D.N. Taylor, et al., Salmonella dublin infections in the United States, 1979–1980, J. Infect. Dis. 146 (1982) 322.

[457] D. Zhou, J. Galan, Salmonella entry into host cells: the work in concert of type III secreted effector proteins, Microbes. Infect. 3 (2001) 1293.

[458] S.R. Waterman, D.W. Holden, Functions and effectors of the Salmonella pathogenicity island 2 type III secretion system, Cell. Microbiol. 5 (2003) 501.

[459] J. Fierer, et al., Salmonella typhimurium bacteremia: association with the virulence plasmid, J. Infect. Dis. 166 (1992) 639.

[460] R.A. Giannella, et al., Pathogenesis of salmonellosis: studies of fluid secretion, mucosal invasion, and morphologic reaction in the rabbit ileum, J. Clin. Invest. 52 (1973) 441.

[461] S.F. Jiwa, Probing for enterotoxigenicity among the salmonellae: an evaluation of biological assays, J. Clin. Microbiol. 14 (1981) 463.

[462] F.C.W. Koo, et al., Pathogenesis of experimental salmonellosis: inhibition of protein synthesis by cytotoxin, Infect. Immun. 43 (1984) 93.

[463] S. Ashkenazi, et al., Cytotoxin production by Salmonella strains: quantitative analysis and partial characterization, Infect. Immun. 56 (1988) 3089.

[464] A. Takeuchi, Electron microscope studies of experimental Salmonella infection. I. Penetration into the intestinal epithelium by S. typhimurium, Am. J. Pathol. 50 (1967) 109.

[465] M.C. Modrazakowski, J.K. Spitznagel, Bactericidal activity of fractionated granule contents from human polymorphonuclear leukocytes: antagonism of granule cationic proteins by lipopolysaccharide, Infect. Immun. 25 (1979) 597.

[466] J. Weiss, M. Victor, P. Elsbach, Role of charge and hydrophobic interaction in the action of the bactericidal/permeability increasing protein of neutrophils on gram-negative bacteria, J. Clin. Invest. 71 (1983) 540.

[466a] V.J. Cid, Survival of Salmonella inside activated macrophages - why bacteria will not understand the word NO? Microbiology 155 (2009) 2461.

[467] G.V. Mackaness, Resistance to intracellular infection, J. Infect. Dis. 123 (1971) 439.

[468] G.V. Mackaness, R.V. Blander, F.M. Collins, Host parasite relations in mouse typhoid, J. Exp. Med. 124 (1966) 573.

[469] S.E. McKenzie, et al., Enhancement in vitro of the low interferon-gamma production of leukocytes from human newborn infants, J. Leukoc. Biol. 53 (1993) 691.

[470] A. George, Generation of gamma interferon responses in murine Peyer's patches following oral immunization, Infect. Immun. 64 (1996) 4606.

[471] R. de Jong, et al., Severe mycobacterial and Salmonella infections in interleukin-12 receptor-deficient patients, Science 280 (1998) 1435.

[472] R.B. Hornick, et al., Typhoid fever: pathogenesis and immunologic control, N. Engl. J. Med. 283 (1970) 686.

[473] T.H. Kent, S.B. Formal, E.H. LaBrec, Salmonella gastroenteritis in rhesus monkeys, Arch. Pathol. 82 (1966) 272.

[474] J.F. Boyd, Pathology of the alimentary tract of S. typhimurium food poisoning, Gut 26 (1985) 935.

[475] D.W. Day, B.K. Mandel, B.C. Morson, The rectal biopsy appearances in Salmonella colitis, Histopathology 2 (1978) 117.

[476] A.N. Wilder, R.A. MacCready, Isolation of Salmonella from poultry, poultry products and poultry processing plants in Massachusetts, N. Engl. J. Med. 274 (1966) 1453.

[477] Pet turtle-associated salmonellosis—Puerto Rico, MMWR Morb. Mortal. Wkly. Rep. 33 (1984) 141.

[478] D. Sanyal, T. Douglas, R. Roberts, Salmonella infection acquired from reptilian pets, Arch. Dis. Child. 77 (1997) 345.

[479] J. Mermin, B. Hoar, F.J. Angulo, Iguanas and Salmonella marina infection in children: a reflection of the increasing incidence of reptile-associated salmonellosis in the United States, Pediatrics 99 (1997) 399.

[480] D.L. Woodward, R. Khakhria, W.M. Johnson, Human salmonellosis associated with exotic pets, J. Clin. Microbiol. 35 (1997) 2786.

[481] S. Thomson, Paratyphoid fever and Baker's confectionery: analysis of epidemic in South Wales 1952, Monthly Bull Ministry Health Public Health Serv 12 (1953) 187.

[482] J. Watt, et al., Salmonellosis in a premature nursery unaccompanied by diarrheal diseases, Pediatrics 22 (1958) 689.

[483] N.T. Hargrett-Bean, A.T. Pavia, R.V. Tauxe, Salmonella isolates from humans in the United States, 1984-1986, MMWR Morb. Mortal. Wkly. Rep. 37 (1988) 25SS.

[484] M.J. Blaser, L.S. Newman, A review of human salmonellosis. I. Infective dose, Rev. Infect. Dis. 4 (1982) 1096.

[485] A.D. Rubinstein, R.N. Fowler, Salmonellosis of the newborn with transmission by delivery room resuscitators, Am. J. Public Health 45 (1955) 1109.

[486] J.G. Bate, U. James, Salmonella typhimurium infection dustborne in a children's ward, Lancet 2 (1958) 713.

[487] S.D. Rubbo, Cross-infection in hospital due to Salmonella derby, J. Hyg. 46 (1948) 158.

[488] V.A. Lamb, et al., Outbreak of S. typhimurium gastroenteritis due to an imported strain resistant to ampicillin, chloramphenicol, and trimethoprim/sulfamethoxazole in a nursery, J. Clin. Microbiol. 20 (1984) 1076.

[489] I.F. Abramas, et al., A Salmonella newport outbreak in a premature nursery with a one year follow up, Pediatrics 37 (1966) 616.

[490] H.C. Epstein, A. Hochwald, R. Agha, Salmonella infections of the newborn infant, J. Pediatr. 38 (1951) 723.

[491] H. Abramson, Infections with S. typhimurium in the newborn, Am. J. Dis. Child. 74 (1947) 576.

[492] F.S. Leeder, An epidemic of S. panama infections in infants, Ann. N. Y. Acad. Sci. 66 (1956) 54.

[493] J. Watt, E. Carlton, Studies of the acute diarrheal diseases. XVI. An outbreak of S. typhimurium infection among newborn premature infants, Public Health Rep. 60 (Pt 1) (1945) 734.

[494] A.R. Foley, An outbreak of paratyphoid B fever in a nursery of a small hospital, Can. J. Public Health 38 (1947) 73.

[495] E. Seligman, Mass invasion of salmonellae in a babies' ward, Ann. Paediatr. 172 (1949) 406.

[496] B. Rowe, C. Giles, G.L. Brown, Outbreak of gastroenteritis due to S. virchow in a maternity hospital, BMJ 3 (1969) 561.

[497] C.K. Sasidharan, et al., S. typhimurium epidemic in newborn nursery, Indian J. Pediatr. 50 (1983) 599.

[498] J. Borecka, M. Hocmannova, W.J. van Leeuwen, Nosocomial infection of nurslings caused by multiple drug-resistant strain of S. typhimurium—utilization of a new typing method based on lysogeny of strains, Z. Bakteriol. 2336 (1976) 262.

[499] C.H.S. Bannerman, Heidelberg enteritis—an outbreak in the neonatal unit of Harare Central Hospital, Cent. Afr. J. Med. 31 (1985) 1.

[500] T.A. McAllister, et al., Outbreak of S. eimsbuettel in newborn infants spread by rectal thermometers, Lancet 1 (1986) 1262.

[501] V.L. Szanton, Epidemic salmonellosis: a 30-month study of 80 cases of S. oranienburg infection, Pediatrics 20 (1957) 794.

[502] J.E. Seals, et al., Nursery salmonellosis: delayed recognition due to unusually long incubation period, Infect. Control Hosp. Epidemiol. 4 (1983) 205.

[503] E. Hering, et al., Analises clinico-epidemiologica de un brote de infeccion por S. bredeney en recien nacidos, Rev. Clin. Pediatr. 50 (1979) 81.

[504] S. Kumari, R. Gupta, S.K. Bhargava, A nursery outbreak with S. newport, Indian Pediatr. 17 (1980) 11.

[505] T. Omland, O. Gardborg, Salmonella enteritidis infections in infancy with special reference to a small nosocomial epidemic, Acta Paediatr. Belg. 49 (1960) 583.

[506] V. Puri, et al., Nosocomial S. typhimurium epidemic in a neonatal special care unit, Indian Pediatr. 17 (1980) 233.

[507] N.M.P. Mendis, et al., Protracted infection with S. bareilly in a maternity hospital, J. Trop. Med. Hyg. 79 (1976) 142.

[508] G. Marzetti, et al., Salmonella muenchen infections in newborns and small infants, Clin. Pediatr. 12 (1973) 93.

[509] W.B. Baine, et al., Institutional salmonellosis, J. Infect. Dis. 128 (1973) 357.

[510] S.A. Schroeder, B. Aserkoff, P.S. Brachman, Epidemic salmonellosis in hospitals and institutions, N. Engl. J. Med. 279 (1968) 674.

[511] R. Wilson, et al., Salmonellosis in infants: the importance of intrafamilial transmission, Pediatrics 69 (1982) 436.

[512] M.J. Newman, Multiple-resistant *Salmonella* group G outbreak in a neonatal intensive care unit, West Afr. J. Med. 15 (1996) 165.

[513] R. Mahajan, et al., Nosocomial outbreak of *Salmonella typhimurium* infection in a nursery intensive care unit (NICU) and paediatric ward, J. Commun. Dis. 27 (1995) 10.

[514] D.M. Martyn-Jones, G.C. Pantin, Neonatal diarrhea due to *S. paratyphi* B, J. Clin. Pathol. 9 (1956) 128.

[515] A.D. Rubinstein, R.F. Feemster, H.M. Smith, Salmonellosis as a public health problem in wartime, Am. J. Public Health 34 (1944) 841.

[516] E. Neter, Observation on the transmission of salmonellosis in man, Am. J. Public Health 40 (1950) 929.

[517] D.Y. Sanders, S.H. Sinal, L. Morrison, Chronic salmonellosis in infancy, Clin. Pediatr. 13 (1974) 640.

[518] W.R. Waddell, L.J. Kunz, Association of *Salmonella* enteritis with operations on the stomach, N. Engl. J. Med. 255 (1956) 555.

[519] J.A. Gray, A.M. Trueman, Severe *Salmonella* gastroenteritis associated with hypochlorhydria, Scott. Med. J. 16 (1971) 255.

[520] G. Fleischhacker, C. Vutue, H.P. Werner, Infektion eines Neugeborenen durch S. typhimurium-haltige Muttermilch, Wien. Klin. Wochenschr. 24 (1972) 394.

[521] R.W. Ryder, et al., Human milk contaminated with *S. kottbus*: a cause of nosocomial illness in infants, JAMA 238 (1977) 1533.

[522] G. Revathi, et al., Transmission of lethal *Salmonella senftenberg* from mother's breast-milk to her baby, Ann. Trop. Paediatr. 15 (1995) 159.

[523] R.G. Small, J.C.M. Sharp, A milkborne outbreak of *S. dublin*, J. Hyg. 82 (1979) 95.

[524] J.B. Weissman, et al., An island-wide epidemic of salmonellosis in Trinidad traced to contaminated powdered milk, West Indian Med. J. 26 (1977) 135.

[525] *Salmonella anatum* infection in infants linked to dried milk, Commun. Dis. Rep. CDR. Wkly. 7 (1997) 33.

[526] M.A. Usera, et al., Interregional foodborne salmonellosis outbreak due to powdered infant formula contaminated with lactose-fermenting *Salmonella virchow*, Eur. J. Epidemiol. 12 (1996) 377.

[527] L. Silverstope, et al., An epidemic among infants caused by *S. muenchen*, J. Appl. Bacteriol. 24 (1961) 134.

[528] S.W.K. Im, K. Chow, P.Y. Chau, Rectal thermometer-mediated cross-infection with *S. wadsworth* in a pediatric ward, J. Hosp. Infect. 2 (1981) 171.

[529] M.A. Khan, et al., Transmission of *S. worthington* by oropharyngeal suction in hospital neonatal unit, Pediatr. Infect. Dis. J. 10 (1991) 668.

[530] S. Umasankar, et al., An outbreak of *Salmonella enteritidis* in a maternity and neonatal intensive care unit, J. Hosp. Infect. 34 (1996) 117.

[531] L.W. Riley, M.L. Cohen, Plasmid profiles and *Salmonella* epidemiology, Lancet 1 (1982) 573.

[532] J. Michel, et al., Etude clinique et bactériologique d'une épidémie de salmonellose en milieu hospitalier (*S. oranienburg*), Pediatrie 25 (1970) 13.

[533] J.L. Adler, et al., A protracted hospital-associated outbreak of salmonellosis due to a multiple antibiotic-resistant strain of *S. indiana*, J. Pediatr. 77 (1970) 970.

[534] B.O. Bilie, T. Mellbin, F. Nordbring, An extensive outbreak of gastroenteritis caused by *S. newport*, Acta Med. Scand. 175 (1964) 557.

[535] M. Horwitz, et al., A large outbreak of foodborne salmonellosis on the Navajo Nation Indian Reservation: epidemiology and secondary transmission, Am. J. Public Health 67 (1977) 1071.

[536] J.P.C. Griffith, M. Ostheimer, Typhoid fever in children, Am. J. Med. Sci. 124 (1902) 868.

[537] M.L. Freedman, et al., Typhoid carriage in pregnancy with infection of neonate, Lancet 1 (1970) 310.

[538] R.S. Chhabra, J.H. Glaser, *Salmonella* infection presenting as hematochezia on the first day of life, Pediatrics 94 (1994) 739.

[539] H. Stein, et al., Gastroenteritis with necrotizing enterocolitis in premature babies, BMJ 1 (1972) 616.

[540] A. Guarino, et al., Etiology and risk factors of severe and protracted diarrhea, J. Pediatr. Gastroenterol. Nutr. 20 (1995) 173.

[541] F. Lifshitz, et al., Monosaccharide intolerance and hypoglycemia in infants with diarrhea. I. Clinical course of 23 infants, J. Pediatr. 77 (1970) 595.

[542] N. Iyngkaran, et al., Acquired carbohydrate intolerance and cow milk protein-sensitive enteropathy in young infants, J. Pediatr. 95 (1979) 373.

[543] C.W. Lo, W.A. Walker, Chronic protracted diarrhea of infancy: a nutritional disease, Pediatrics 72 (1983) 786.

[544] M.J. Blaser, R.A. Feldman, *Salmonella* bacteremia: reports to the Centers for Disease Control, 1968–1979, J. Infect. Dis. 143 (1981) 743.

[545] G.E. Schutze, S.E. Schutze, R.S. Kirby, Extraintestinal salmonellosis in a children's hospital, Pediatr. Infect. Dis. J. 16 (1997) 482.

[546] R.C. Davis, *Salmonella* sepsis in infancy, Am. J. Dis. Child. 135 (1981) 1096.

[547] S. Torrey, G. Fleisher, D. Jaffe, Incidence of *Salmonella* bacteremia in infants with *Salmonella* gastroenteritis, J. Pediatr. 108 (1986) 718.

[548] S. Sirinavin, et al., Predictors for extraintestinal infection of *Salmonella* enteritis in Thailand, Pediatr. Infect. Dis. J. 7 (1988) 44.

[549] B.Z. Katz, E.D. Shapiro, Predictors of persistently positive blood cultures in children with "occult" *Salmonella* bacteremia, Pediatr. Infect. Dis. J. 5 (1986) 713.

[550] L.G. Yamamoto, M.J. Ashton, *Salmonella* infections in infants in Hawaii, Pediatr. Infect. Dis. J. 7 (1988) 48.

[551] J.I. Cohen, J.A. Bartlett, G.R. Corey, Extraintestinal manifestations of *Salmonella* infections, Medicine (Baltimore) 66 (1987) 349.

[552] S.E. West, R. Goodkin, A.M. Kaplan, Neonatal *Salmonella* meningitis complicated by cerebral abscesses, West. J. Med. 127 (1977) 142.

[553] P.C. Applebaum, J. Scragg, *Salmonella* meningitis in infants, Lancet 1 (1977) 1052.

[554] C.E. Cherubin, et al., *Listeria* and gram-negative bacillary meningitis in New York City 1973–1979, Am. J. Med. 71 (1981) 199.

[555] L.C. Low, et al., *Salmonella* meningitis in infancy, Aust. Paediatr. J. 20 (1984) 225.

[556] N. Diwan, K.B. Sharma, Isolation of *S. typhimurium* from cephalohematoma and osteomyelitis, Indian J. Med. Res. 67 (1978) 27.

[557] W. Konzert, Über eine Salmonella-Osteomyelitis in Rahmen einer S. typhimurium Epidemie auf einer Neugeborenen Station, Wien. Klin. Wochenschr. 81 (1969) 713.

[558] B. McKinlay, Infectious diarrhea of the newborn caused by an unclassified species of *Salmonella*, Am. J. Dis. Child. 54 (1937) 1252.

[559] W. Szumness, et al., The microbiological and epidemiological properties of infections caused by *S. enteritidis*, J. Hyg. 64 (1966) 9.

[560] J.D. Nelson, Suppurative mastitis in infants, Am. J. Dis. Child. 125 (1973) 458.

[561] K.J. Guthrie, G.I. Montgomery, Infections with *Bacterium enteritidis* in infancy with the triad of enteritis, cholecystitis and meningitis, J. Pathol. Bacteriol. 49 (1939) 393.

[562] L.I. Corman, et al., Endophthalmitis due to *S. enteritidis*, J. Pediatr. 95 (1979) 1001.

[563] D.L. Haggman, et al., Nontyphoidal *Salmonella* pericarditis: a case report and review of the literature, Pediatr. Infect. Dis. J. 5 (1986) 259.

[564] R.P. Reed, K.P. Klugman, Neonatal typhoid fever, Pediatr. Infect. Dis. J. 13 (1994) 774.

[565] B.M. Stuart, R.L. Pullen, Typhoid: clinical analysis of 360 cases, Arch. Intern. Med. 78 (1946) 629.

[566] B. Sengupta, N. Ramachander, N. Zamah, *Salmonella* septic abortion, Int. Surg. 65 (1980) 183.

[567] A.W. Diddle, R.L. Stephens, Typhoid fever in pregnancy, Am. J. Obstet. Gynecol. 38 (1939) 300.

[568] F. Riggall, G. Salkind, W. Spellacy, Typhoid fever complicating pregnancy, Obstet. Gynecol. 44 (1974) 117.

[569] H.T. Hicks, H. French, Typhoid fever and pregnancy with special references to fetal infection, Lancet 1 (1905) 1491.

[570] W. Osler, T. McCrae, Typhoid fever, in: W. Osler (Ed.), Principles and Practice of Medicine, eighth ed., D Appleton, New York, 1912, pp. 1–46.

[571] C. Ferreccio, et al., Benign bacteremia caused by *S. typhi* and *S. paratyphi* in children younger than two years, J. Pediatr. 104 (1984) 899.

[572] U. Thisyakorn, P. Mansuwan, D.N. Taylor, Typhoid and paratyphoid fever in 192 hospitalized children in Thailand, Am. J. Dis. Child. 141 (1987) 862.

[573] L.K. Pickering, et al., Fecal leukocytes in enteric infections, Am. J. Clin. Pathol. 68 (1977) 562.

[574] C.E. McCall, W.T. Martin, J.R. Boring, Efficiency of cultures of rectal swabs and fecal specimens in detecting *Salmonella* carriers: correlation with numbers of *Salmonella* excreted, J. Hyg. 64 (1966) 261.

[575] H.S. Raucher, A.H. Eichenfeld, H.L. Hodes, Treatment of *Salmonella* gastroenteritis in infants: the significance of bacteremia, Clin. Pediatr. 22 (1983) 601.

[576] S.P. Gotoff, W.D. Cochran, Antibody response to the somatic antigen of *S. newport* in premature infants, Pediatrics 37 (1966) 610.

[577] H.L. Hodes, H.D. Zepp, E. Ainbender, Production of O and H agglutinins by a newborn infant infected with *S. saint-paul*, J. Pediatr. 68 (1966) 780.

[578] M.J. Rivera, et al., Molecular and epidemiological study of *Salmonella* clinical isolates, J. Clin. Microbiol. 29 (1991) 927.

[579] B. Aserkoff, J.V. Bennett, Effect of antibiotic therapy in acute salmonellosis on the fecal excretion of salmonellae, N. Engl. J. Med. 281 (1969) 636.

[580] J.M.S. Dixon, Effect of antibiotic treatment on duration of excretion of *S. typhimurium* by children, BMW 2 (1965) 1343.

[581] M. Kazemi, T.G. Bumpert, M.I. Marks, A controlled trial comparing trimethoprim/sulfamethoxazole, ampicillin, and no therapy in the treatment of *Salmonella* gastroenteritis in children, J. Pediatr. 83 (1973) 646.

[582] M.A. Neill, et al., Failure of ciprofloxacin to eradicate convalescent fecal excretion after acute salmonellosis: experience during an outbreak in health care workers, Ann. Intern. Med. 114 (1991) 195.

[583] T. Pettersson, E. Klemola, O. Wager, Treatment of acute cases of *Salmonella* infection and *Salmonella* carriers with ampicillin and neomycin, Acta Med. Scand. 175 (1964) 185.

[584] Association for Study of Infectious Diseases, Effect of neomycin in noninvasive *Salmonella* infections of the gastrointestinal tract, Lancet 2 (1970) 1159.

[585] J.D. Nelson, et al., Treatment of *Salmonella* gastroenteritis with ampicillin, amoxicillin, or placebo, Pediatrics 65 (1980) 1125.

[586] M.O. Asperilla, R.A. Smego, L.K. Scott, Quinolone antibiotics in the treatment of *Salmonella* infections, Rev. Infect. Dis. 12 (1990) 873.

[587] D.S. Buchwald, M.J. Blaser, A review of human salmonellosis. II. Duration of excretion following infection with nontyphi *Salmonella*, Rev. Infect. Dis. 6 (1984) 345.

[588] P. Dutta, et al., Ciprofloxacin for treatment of severe typhoid fever in children, Antimicrob. Agents. Chemother. 37 (1993) 1197.

[589] L.J.V. Piddock, et al., Ciprofloxacin resistance in clinical isolates of *Salmonella typhimurium* obtained from two patients, Antimicrob. Agents Chemother. 37 (1993) 662.

[590] W.M. Edgar, B.W. Lacey, Infection with *S. heidelberg*: an outbreak presumably not foodborne, Lancet 1 (1963) 161.

[591] P.A. Rice, P.C. Craven, J.G. Wells, *S. heidelberg* enteritis and bacteremia: an epidemic on two pediatric wards, Am. J. Med. 60 (1976) 509.

[592] K.L. MacDonald, et al., Changes in antimicrobial resistance of *Salmonella* isolated from humans in the United States, JAMA 258 (1987) 1496.

[593] E. Maiorini, et al., Multiply resistant nontyphoidal *Salmonella* gastroenteritis in children, Pediatr. Infect. Dis. J. 12 (1993) 139.

[594] L.A. Lee, et al., Increase in antimicrobial-resistant *Salmonella* infections in the United States, 1989–1990, J. Infect. Dis. 170 (1994) 128.

[595] M.K. Glynn, et al., Emergence of multidrug-resistant *Salmonella enterica* serotype *typhimurium* DT104 infections in the United States, N. Engl. J. Med. 338 (1998) 1333.

[596] G. Koshi, Alarming increases in multi-drug resistant *S. typhimurium* in Southern India, Indian. J. Med. Res. 74 (1981) 635.

[597] E.S. Anderson, et al., Clonal distribution of resistance plasmid carrying *S. typhimurium*, mainly in the Middle East, J. Hyg. 79 (1977) 425.

[598] I.A. Wamola, N.B. Mirza, Problems of *Salmonella* infections in a hospital in Kenya, East. Afr. Med. J. 58 (1981) 677.

[599] V. Falbo, et al., Antimicrobial resistance among *Salmonella* isolates from hospitals in Rome, J. Hyg. 88 (1982) 275.

[600] E.J. Threlfall, et al., Plasmid encoded trimethoprim resistance in multi-resistant epidemic *S. typhimurium* phagotypes 204 and 193 in Britain, BMJ 280 (1980) 1210.

[601] G.I. French, M.F. Lowry, Trimethoprim-resistant *Salmonella*, Lancet 2 (1978) 375.

[602] S.M. Smith, P.E. Palumbo, P.J. Edelson, *Salmonella* strains resistant to multiple antibiotics: therapeutic implications, Pediatr. Infect. Dis. J. 3 (1984) 455.

[603] G.B. Soe, G.D. Overturf, Treatment of typhoid fever and other systemic salmonellosis with cefotaxime, ceftriaxone, cefoperazone, and other newer cephalosporins, Rev. Infect. Dis. 9 (1987) 719.

[604] A. Moosa, C.J. Rubidge, Once daily ceftriaxone vs. chloramphenicol for treatment of typhoid fever in children, Pediatr. Infect. Dis. J. 8 (1989) 696.

[605] E.M. deCarvalho, et al., Cefamandole treatment of *Salmonella* bacteremia, Antimicrob. Agents Chemother. 21 (1982) 334.

[606] J.W. Pape, et al., Typhoid fever: successful therapy with cefoperazone, J. Infect. Dis. 153 (1986) 272.

[607] B. Demmerich, et al., Biliary excretion and pharmacokinetics of cefoperazone in humans, J. Antimicrob. Chemother. 12 (1983) 27.

[608] T.R. Kinsella, et al., Treatment of *Salmonella* meningitis and brain abscess with the new cephalosporins: two case reports and a review of the literature, Pediatr. Infect. Dis. J. 6 (1987) 476.

[609] A.S. Gokalp, et al., Intravenous immunoglobulin in the treatment of *Salmonella typhimurium* infections in preterm neonates, Clin. Pediatr. (Phila). 33 (1994) 349.

[610] R.V. Tauxe, et al., Salmonellosis in nurses: lack of transmission to patients, J. Infect. Dis. 157 (1988) 370.

[611] M.M. Levine, et al., Comparison of enteric coated capsules and liquid formulation of Ty21a typhoid vaccine in randomised controlled field trial, Lancet 336 (1990) 4.

[612] S.J. Cryz Jr., et al., Safety and immunogenicity of *Salmonella typhi* Ty21a vaccine in young Thai children, Infect. Immun. 61 1149.

[613] J.R. Murphy, et al., Immunogenicity of *S. typhi* Ty21a vaccine for young children, Infect. Immun. 59 (1991) 4291.

[614] G.L. France, D.J. Marmer, R.W. Steele, Breast-feeding and *Salmonella* infection, Am. J. Dis. Child. 134 (1980) 147.

[615] D.J. Brenner, et al., Polynucleotide sequence divergence among strains of *E. coli* and closely related organisms, J. Bacteriol. 109 (1972) 953.

[616] A. Phalipon, P.J. Sansonetti, Shigella's ways of manipulating the host intestinal innate and adaptive immune system. A tool box for survival, Immunol. Cell. Biol. 85 (2007) 119–129.

[617] P.J. Sansonetti, The bacterial weaponry: lessons from Shigella, Ann. N. Y. Acad. Sci. 1072 (2006) 307–312.

[618] P.J. Sansonetti, D.J. Kopecko, S.B. Formal, Involvement of a plasmid in the invasive ability of *Shigella flexneri*, Infect. Immun. 35 (1982) 852.

[619] P. Sansonetti, Host-pathogen interactions: the seduction of molecular cross talk, Gut 50 (Suppl. 3) (2002) III2.

[620] M.I. Fernandez, P.J. Sansonetti, Shigella interaction with intestinal epithelial cells determines the innate immune response in shigellosis, Int. J. Med. Microbiol. 293 (2003) 55.

[621] T.L. Hale, E.V. Oaks, S.B. Formal, Identification and characterization of virulence associated, plasmid-coded proteins of *Shigella* spp. and enteroinvasive *E. coli*, Infect. Immun. 50 (1985) 620.

[622] C. Sasakawa, et al., Molecular alteration of the 140-megadalton plasmid associated with the loss of virulence and Congo red binding activity in *Shigella flexneri*, Infect. Immun. 51 (1986) 470.

[623] E.H. LaBrec, et al., Epithelial cell penetration as an essential step in the pathogenesis of bacillary dysentery, J. Bacteriol. 88 (1964) 1503.

[624] H. Ogawa, Experimental approach in studies on pathogenesis of bacillary dysentery—with special reference to the invasion of bacilli into intestinal mucosa, Acta Pathol. Jpn. 20 (1970) 261.

[625] P.J. Sansonetti, et al., Plasmid-mediated invasiveness of "Shigella-like" *Escherichia coli*, Ann. Microbiol. 133A (1982) 351.

[626] P.J. Sansonetti, et al., Molecular comparison of virulence plasmids in *Shigella* and enteroinvasive *Escherichia coli*, Ann. Microbiol. 134A (1983) 295.

[627] P.J. Sansonetti, et al., Alterations in the pathogenicity of *Escherichia coli* K-12 after transfer of plasmids and chromosomal genes from *Shigella flexneri*, Infect. Immun. 39 (1983) 1392.

[628] J. Wei, et al., Complete genome sequence and comparative genomics of *Shigella flexneri* serotype 2a strain 2457T, Infect. Immun. 71 (2003) 2775.

[629] N. Okada, et al., Virulence associated chromosomal loci of *S. flexneri* identified by random Tn5 insertion mutagenesis, Mol. Microbiol. 5 (1991) 187.

[630] N. Okamura, et al., HeLa cell invasiveness and O antigen of *Shigella flexneri* as separate and prerequisite attributes of virulence to evoke keratoconjunctivitis in guinea pigs, Infect. Immun. 39 (1983) 505.

[631] A.V. Bartlett, et al., Production of Shiga toxin and other cytotoxins by serogroups of *Shigella*, J. Infect. Dis. 154 (1986) 996.

[632] J.G. Olenick, A.D. Wolfe, Shigella toxin inhibition of binding and translation of polyuridylic acid by *Escherichia coli* ribosomes, J. Bacteriol. 141 (1980) 1246.

[633] J.E. Brown, S.W. Rothman, B.P. Doctor, Inhibition of protein synthesis in intact HeLa cells by *Shigella dysenteriae* 1 toxin, Infect. Immun. 29 (1980) 98.

[634] K. Al-Hasani, et al., The sigA gene which is borne on the pathogenicity island of *Shigella flexneri* 2a encodes an exported cytopathic protease involved in intestinal fluid accumulation, Infect. Immun. 68 (2000) 2457.

[635] D. Prado, et al., The relation between production of cytotoxin and clinical features in shigellosis, J. Infect. Dis. 154 (1986) 149.

[636] S. Makintubee, J. Mallonee, G.R. Istre, Shigellosis outbreak associated with swimming, Am. J. Public Health 77 (1987) 166.

[637] M.M. Levine, et al., Pathogenesis of *Shigella dysenteriae* 1 (Shiga) dysentery, J. Infect. Dis. 127 (1973) 261.

[638] H.L. DuPont, et al., The response of man to virulent *Shigella flexneri* 2a, J. Infect. Dis. 119 (1969) 296.

[639] M.M. Levine, *Shigella* infections and vaccines: experiences from volunteer and controlled field studies, in: M.M. Rahaman et al., (Eds.), Shigellosis: A Continuing Global Problem, International Centre for Diarrhoeal Disease Research, Dacca, Bangladesh, 1983, p. 208.

[640] L.K. Pickering, S.C. Hadler, Management and prevention of infectious diseases in day care, in: R.D. Feigin, J.C. Cherry (Eds.), Textbook of Pediatric Infectious Diseases, WB Saunders, Philadelphia, 1992, p. 2308.

[641] L.G. Mata, The Children of Santa Maria Cauque: A Prospective Field Study of Health and Growth, MIT Press, Cambridge, MA, 1978.

[642] B.J. Stoll, et al., Surveillance of patients attending a diarrhoeal disease hospital in Bangladesh, BMJ 285 (1982) 1185.

[643] T. Floyd, A.R. Higgins, M.A. Kader, Studies in shigellosis. V. The relationship of age to the incidence of *Shigella* infections in Egyptian children, with special reference to shigellosis in the newborn and infant in the first six months of life, Am. J. Trop. Med. Hyg. 5 (1956) 119.

[644] Summary of notifiable diseases, United States, 1981, MMWR Morb. Mortal. Wkly. Rep. 40 (1992) 10.

[645] J.S. Clemens, et al., Breast-feeding as a determinant of severity in shigellosis, Am. J. Epidemiol. 123 (1986) 710.

[646] L.J. Mata, et al., *Shigella* infections in breast fed Guatemalan Indian neonates, Am. J. Dis. Child. 117 (1969) 142.

[647] W.C. Huskins, et al., Shigellosis in neonates and young infants, J. Pediatr. 125 (1994) 14.

[648] K.C. Haltalin, Neonatal shigellosis, Am. J. Dis. Child. 114 (1967) 603.

[649] J.N. Scragg, C.J. Rubidge, P.C. Appelbaum, *Shigella* infection in African and Indian children with special reference to *Shigella* septicemia, J. Pediatr. 93 (1978) 796.

[650] V.F. Burry, A.N. Thurn, T.G. Co, Shigellosis: an analysis of 239 cases in a pediatric population, Mo. Med. 65 (1968) 671.

[651] Enteric infection due to *Campylobacter, Yersinia, Salmonella* and *Shigella*, Bull. World Health Organ. 58 (1980) 519.

[652] E.N. Kraybill, G. Controni, Septicemia and enterocolitis due to *S. sonnei* in a newborn infant, Pediatrics 42 (1968) 529.

[653] E.E. Moore, *Shigella sonnei* septicemia in a neonate, BMJ 1 (1974) 22.

[654] J.A. Aldrich, R.P. Flowers, F.K. Hall, *S. sonnei* septicemia in a neonate: a case report, J. Am. Osteopath. Assoc. 79 (1979) 93.

[655] L.L. Barton, L.K. Pickering, Shigellosis in the first week of life, Pediatrics 52 (1973) 437.

[656] M. Landsberger, Bacillary dysentery in a newborn infant, Arch. Pediatr. 59 (1942) 330.

[657] E. Neter, *S. sonnei* infection at term and its transfer to the newborn, Obstet. Gynecol. 17 (1961) 517.

[658] M.S. McIntire, H.M. Jahr, An isolated case of shigellosis in the newborn nursery, Nebr. State. Med. J. 39 (1954) 425.

[659] M. Greenberg, S. Frant, R. Shapiro, Bacillary dysentery acquired at birth, J. Pediatr. 17 (1940) 363.

[660] B. Emanuel, J.O. Sherman, Shigellosis in a neonate, Clin. Pediatr. 14 (1975) 725.

[661] E. Barret-Connor, J.D. Connor, Extraintestinal manifestations of shigellosis, Am. J. Gastroenterol. 53 (1970) 234.

[662] E. Fischler, Convulsions as a complication of shigellosis in children, Helv. Paediatr. Acta 4 (1962) 389.

[663] S. Ashkenazi, et al., Convulsions in childhood shigellosis, Am. J. Dis. Child. 141 (1987) 208.

[664] C. Whitfield, J.M. Humphries, Meningitis and septicemia due to *Shigella* in a newborn infant, J. Pediatr. 70 (1967) 805.

[665] A. Goren, S. Freier, J.H. Passwell, Lethal toxic encephalopathy due to childhood shigellosis in a developed country, Pediatrics 89 (1992) 1189.

[666] S. Ashkenazi, et al., The association of Shiga toxin and other cytotoxins with the neurologic manifestations of shigellosis, J. Infect. Dis. 161 (1990) 961.

[667] M.M. Rahaman, et al., Shiga bacillus dysentery associated with marked leukocytosis and erythrocyte fragmentation, Johns. Hopkins. Med. J. 136 (1975) 65.

[668] T.G. Neglia, T.J. Marr, A.T. Davis, *Shigella* dysentery with secondary *Klebsiella* sepsis, J. Pediatr. 63 (1976) 253.

[669] M.J. Struelens, et al., *Shigella* septicemia: prevalence, presentation, risk factors, and outcome, J. Infect. Dis. 152 (1985) 784.

[670] S.E. Levin, *Shigella* septicemia in the newborn infant, J. Pediatr. 71 (1967) 917.

[671] K.C. Haltalin, J.D. Nelson, Coliform septicemia complicating shigellosis in children, JAMA 192 (1965) 441.

[672] T. Martin, B.F. Habbick, J. Nyssen, Shigellosis with bacteremia: a report of two cases and a review of the literature, Pediatr. Infect. Dis. J. 2 (1983) 21.

[673] J.W. Raderman, K.P. Stoller, J.J. Pomerance, Blood-stream invasion with *S. sonnei* in an asymptomatic newborn infant, Pediatr. Infect. Dis. J. 5 (1986) 379.

[674] J.R. Starke, C.J. Baker, Neonatal shigellosis with bowel perforation, Pediatr. Infect. Dis. J. 4 (1985) 405.

[675] M.A.K. Azad, M. Islam, Colonic perforation in *Shigella dysenteriae* 1 infection, Pediatr. Infect. Dis. J. 5 (1986) 103.

[676] J.H. O'Connor, U. O'Callaghan, Fatal *S. sonnei* septicemia in an adult complemented by marrow aplasia and intestinal perforation, J. Infect. 3 (1981) 277.

[677] A.N. Alam, et al., Association of pneumonia with under-nutrition and shigellosis, Indian. Pediatr. 21 (1984) 609.

[678] D. Hoefnagel, Fulminating, rapidly fatal shigellosis in children, N. Engl. J. Med. 258 (1958) 1256.

[679] A. Sakamoto, S. Kamo, Clinical, statistical observations on Ekiri and bacillary dysentery: a study of 785 cases, Ann. Paediatr. 186 (1956) 1.

[680] K. Dodd, J.G. Buddingh, S. Rapoport, The etiology of Ekiri, a highly fatal disease of Japanese children, Pediatrics 3 (1949) 9.

[681] T.C. Davis, Chronic vulvovaginitis in children due to *S. flexneri*, Pediatrics 56 (1975) 41.

[682] T.V. Murphy, J.D. Nelson, *Shigella* vaginitis: report on 38 patients and review of the literature, Pediatrics 63 (1979) 511.

[683] J.D. Tobias, J.R. Starke, M.F. Tosi, *Shigella* keratitis: a report of two cases and a review of the literature, Pediatr. Infect. Dis. J. 6 (1987) 79.

[684] T. Butler, et al., Causes of death and the histopathologic findings in fatal shigellosis, Pediatr. Infect. Dis. J. 8 (1989) 767.

[685] M.L. Bennish, et al., Death in shigellosis: incidence and risk factors in hospitalized patients, J. Infect. Dis. 161 (1990) 500.

[686] P. Speelman, et al., Differential clinical features and stool findings in shigellosis and amoebic dysentery, Trans. R. Soc. Trop. Med. Hyg. 81 (1987) 549.

[687] W.I. Taylor, B. Harris, Isolation of shigellae. II. Comparison of plating media and enrichment broths, Am. J. Clin. Pathol. 44 (1965) 476.

[688] H. Stypulkowska-Misiurewicz, Problems in bacteriological diagnosis of shigellosis, in: M.M. Rahaman et al., (Eds.), Shigellosis: A Continuing Global Problem, International Centre for Diarrhoeal Disease Research, Dacca, Bangladesh, 1983, p. 87.

[689] K.C. Haltalin, et al., Double-blind treatment study of shigellosis comparing ampicillin, sulfadiazine, and placebo, J. Pediatr. 70 (1967) 970.

[690] K.C. Haltalin, et al., Optimal dosage of ampicillin in shigellosis, J. Pediatr. 74 (1969) 626.

[691] K.C. Haltalin, J.D. Nelson, H.T. Kusmiesz, Comparative efficacy of nalidixic acid and ampicillin for severe shigellosis, Arch. Dis. Child. 48 (1973) 305.

[692] E.V. Oaks, T.L. Hale, S.B. Formal, Serum immune response to *Shigella* protein antigens in rhesus monkeys and humans infected with *Shigella* spp, Infect. Immun. 53 (1986) 57.

[693] G. Frankel, et al., Detection of *Shigella* in feces using DNA amplification, J. Infect. Dis. 161 (1990) 1252.

[694] P. Speelman, I. Kabir, M. Islam, Distribution and spread of colonic lesions in shigellosis: a colonoscopic study, J. Infect. Dis. 150 (1984) 899.

[695] J.A. Frost, et al., Plasmid characterization in the investigation of an epidemic caused by multiply resistant *S. dysenteriae* type 1 in Central Africa, Lancet 2 (1981) 1074.

[696] K. Haider, et al., Plasmid characterization of *Shigella* spp. isolated from children with shigellosis and asymptomatic excretors, J. Antimicrob. Chemother. 16 (1985) 691.

[697] R.V. Tauxe, et al., Antimicrobial resistance of *Shigella* isolates in the USA: the importance of international travelers, J. Infect. Dis. 162 (1990) 1107.

[698] T.C. Salzman, C.D. Scher, R. Moss, Shigellae with transferable drug resistance: outbreak in a nursery for premature infants, J. Pediatr. 71 (1967) 21.

[699] M.L. Bennish, et al., Antimicrobial resistance of *Shigella* isolates in Bangladesh, 1983–1990: increasing frequency of strains multiply resistant to ampicillin, trimethoprim/sulfamethoxazole, and nalidixic acid, Clin. Infect. Dis. 14 (1992) 1055.

[700] V.G. Ostrower, Comparison of cefaclor and ampicillin in the treatment of shigellosis, Postgrad. Med. J. 55 (1979) 82.

[701] K.C. Haltalin, J.D. Nelson, Failure of furazolidone therapy on shigellosis, Am. J. Dis. Child. 123 (1972) 40.

[702] J.D. Nelson, K.C. Haltalin, Comparative efficacy of cephalexin and ampicillin for shigellosis and other types of acute diarrhea in infants and children, Antimicrob. Agents Chemother. 7 (1975) 415.

[703] J.D. Nelson, K.C. Haltalin, Amoxicillin less effective than ampicillin against *Shigella* in vitro and in vivo: relationship of efficacy to activity in serum, J. Infect. Dis. 129 (1974) S222.

[704] M.J. Tong, et al., Clinical and bacteriological evaluation of antibiotic treatment in shigellosis, JAMA 214 (1970) 1841.

[705] W.A. Orenstein, et al., Antibiotic treatment of acute shigellosis: failure of cefamandole compared to trimethoprim/sulfamethoxazole and ampicillin, Am. J. Med. Sci. 282 (1981) 27.

[706] M.D. Yunus, et al., Comparative treatment of shigellosis with trimethoprim/sulfamethoxazole and ampicillin, in: M.M. Rahaman et al., (Eds.), Shigellosis: A Continuing Global Problem, International Centre for Diarrhoeal Disease Research, Dacca, Bangladesh, 1983, p. 166.

[707] J.D. Nelson, et al., Trimethoprim/sulfamethoxazole therapy for shigellosis, JAMA 235 (1976) 1239.

[708] J.D. Nelson, H. Kusmiesz, L.H. Jackson, Comparison of trimethoprim/sulfamethoxazole and ampicillin for shigellosis in ambulatory patients, J. Pediatr. 89 (1976) 491.

[709] J.D. Nelson, H. Kusmiesz, S. Shelton, Oral or intravenous trimethoprim/sulfamethoxazole therapy for shigellosis, Rev. Infect. Dis. J. 4 (1982) 546.

[710] R.H. Gilman, et al., Single dose ampicillin therapy for severe shigellosis in Bangladesh, J. Infect. Dis. 143 (1981) 164.

[711] I. Varsano, et al., Comparative efficacy of ceftriaxone and ampicillin for treatment of severe shigellosis in children, J. Pediatr. 118 (1991) 627.

[712] T. Kabir, T. Butler, A. Khanam, Comparative efficacies of single intravenous doses of ceftriaxone and ampicillin for shigellosis in a placebo-controlled trial, Antimicrob. Agents. Chemother. 29 (1986) 645.

[713] M.L. Bennish, et al., Treatment of shigellosis. III. Comparison of one- or two-dose ciprofloxacin with standard 5-day therapy, Ann. Intern. Med. 117 (1992) 727.

[714] J.F. John Jr., et al., Activities of new fluoroquinolones against *Shigella sonnei*, Antimicrob. Agents. Chemother. 36 (1992) 2346.

[715] H.L. DuPont, R.B. Hornick, Adverse effect of Lomotil therapy in shigellosis, JAMA 226 (1973) 1525.

[716] F. Ahmed, et al., Community based evaluation of the effect of breast feeding on the risk of microbiologically confirmed or clinically presumptive shigellosis in Bangladeshi children, Pediatrics 90 (1992) 406.

[717] M.U. Khan, Interruption of shigellosis by handwashing, Trans. R. Soc. Trop. Med. Hyg. 76 (1982) 164.

[718] W.E. Farrar, et al., Interbacterial transfer of R-factor in the human intestine: in vitro acquisition of R-factor mediated kanamycin resistance by a multi-resistant strain of *S. sonnei*, J. Infect. Dis. 126 (1972) 27.

[719] F. McFadyean, S. Stockman, Report of the Departmental Committee Appointed by the Board of Agriculture and Fisheries to Inquire into Epizootic Abortion, vol. 3, His Majesty's Stationery Office, London, 1909.

[720] T. Smith, M.S. Taylor, Some morphological and biochemical characters of the spirilla (*Vibrio fetus*, n. spp.) associated with disease of the fetal membranes in cattle, J. Exp. Med. 30 (1919) 200.

[721] F.S. Jones, M. Orcutt, R.B. Little, Vibrios (*Vibrio jejuni*, n. spp.) associated with intestinal disorders of cows and calves, J. Exp. Med. 53 (1931) 853.

[722] J.H. Bryner, et al., Infectivity of three *Vibrio fetus* biotypes for gallbladder and intestines of cattle, sheep, rabbits, guinea pigs, and mice, Am. J. Vet. Res. 32 (1971) 465.

[723] R. Vinzent, J. Dumas, N. Picard, Septicémie grave au cours de la grossesse due à un vibrion. Avortement consécutif, Bull. Acad. Natl. Med. 131 (1947) 90.

[724] A.N. Eden, Perinatal mortality caused by *Vibrio fetus*: review and analysis, J. Pediatr. 68 (1966) 297.

[725] D.E. Torphy, W.W. Bond, *Campylobacter fetus* infections in children, Pediatrics 64 (1979) 898.

[726] V. Bokkenheuser, *Vibrio fetus* infection in man. I. Ten new cases and some epidemiologic observations, Am. J. Epidemiol. 91 (1970) 400.

[727] R.L. Guerrant, et al., Campylobacteriosis in man: pathogenic mechanisms and review of 91 bloodstream infections, Am. J. Med. 65 (1978) 584.

[728] M. Zilbauer, et al., *Campylobacter jejuni*-mediated disease pathogenesis: an update, Trans. R. Soc. Trop. Med. Hyg. 102 (2008) 123–129.

[729] M. Sebald, M. Veron, Teneur en bases de l'ADN et classification des vibrions, Ann. Inst. Pasteur. 105 (1963) 897.

[730] J.P. Butzler, et al., Related vibrio in stools, J. Pediatr. 82 (1973) 493.

[731] M.B. Skirrow, *Campylobacter* enteritis: a "new" disease, BMJ 2 (1977) 9.

[732] Communicable Disease Surveillance Centre and the Communicable Diseases (Scotland) Unit, *Campylobacter* infections in Britain 1977, BMJ 1 (1978) 1357.

[733] P. De Mol, E. Bosmans, *Campylobacter* enteritis in Central Africa, Lancet 1 (1978) 604.

[734] B. Lindquist, J. Kjellander, T. Kosunen, *Campylobacter* enteritis in Sweden, BMJ 1 (1978) 303.

[735] M.A. Karmali, P.C. Fleming, Campylobacter enteritis in children, J. Pediatr. 94 (1979) 527.

[736] C.M. Pai, et al., Campylobacter gastroenteritis in children, J. Pediatr. 94 (1979) 589.

[737] M.J. Blaser, L.B. Reller, *Campylobacter* enteritis, N. Engl. J. Med. 305 (1981) 1444.

[738] P. Dekeyser, et al., Acute enteritis due to related *Vibrio*: first positive stool cultures, J. Infect. Dis. 125 (1972) 390.

[739] J.P. Butzler, M.B. Skirrow, *Campylobacter* enteritis, Clin. Gastroenterol. 8 (1979) 737.

[740] M.J. Blaser, et al., *Campylobacter* enteritis: clinical and epidemiologic features, Ann. Intern. Med. 91 (1979) 179.

[741] M.A. Karmali, P.C. Fleming, *Campylobacter* enteritis, Can. Med. Assoc. J. 120 (1979) 1525.

[742] T.W. Steele, S. McDermott, *Campylobacter* enteritis in South Australia, Med. J. Aust. 2 (1978) 404.

[743] S. Guandalini, et al., *Campylobacter* colitis in infants, J. Pediatr. 102 (1983) 72.

[744] R.I. Walker, et al., Pathophysiology of *Campylobacter* enteritis, Microbiol. Rev. 50 (1986) 81.

[745] J.L. Penner, The genus *Campylobacter*: a decade of progress, Clin. Microbiol. Rev. 1 (1988) 157.

[746] J.J. Calva, et al., Cohort study of intestinal infection with *Campylobacter* in Mexican children, Lancet 1 (1988) 503.

[747] N. Figura, et al., Two cases of *Campylobacter mucosalis* enteritis in children, J. Clin. Microbiol. 31 (1993) 727.

[748] S.M. Harvey, J.R. Greenwood, Relationships among catalase-positive campylobacters determined by deoxyribonucleic acid-deoxyribonucleic acid hybridization, Int. J. Syst. Bacteriol. 33 (1983) 275.

[749] R.J. Owen, Nucleic acids in the classification of campylobacters, Eur. J. Clin. Microbiol. 2 (1983) 367.

[750] M.A. Hoffer, Bovine campylobacteriosis: a review, Can. Vet. J. 22 (1981) 327.

[751] C.A. Grant, Bovine vibriosis: a brief review, Can. J. Comp. Med. 19 (1955) 156.

[752] R. Vinzent, Une affection méconnue de la grossesse: l'infection placentaire à "*Vibrio fetus*" Presse. Med. 57 (1949) 1230.

[753] S.N. Wong, Y.C. Tam, K.Y. Yeun, *Campylobacter* infection in the neonate: case report and review of the literature, Pediatr. Infect. Dis. J. 9 (1990) 665.

[754] M. Hood, J.M. Todd, *Vibrio fetus*—a cause of human abortion, Am. J. Obstet. Gynecol. 80 (1960) 506.

[755] R.F. van Wering, H. Esseveld, Vibrio fetus, Ned. Tijdschr. Geneeskd. 107 (1963) 119.

[756] W. Burgert Jr., J.W.C. Hagstrom, *Vibrio fetus* meningoencephalitis, Arch. Neurol. 10 (1964) 196.

[757] M.D. Willis, W.J. Austin, Human *Vibrio fetus* infection: report of two dissimilar cases, Am. J. Dis. Child. 112 (1966) 459.

[758] J.P. Smith, J.H. Marymont, J. Schweers Jr., Septicemia due to *Campylobacter fetus* in a newborn infant with gastroenteritis, Am. J. Med. Technol. 43 (1977) 38.

[759] S.E. West, et al., *Campylobacter* spp. isolated from the cervix during septic abortion: case report, Br. J. Obstet. Gynaecol. 89 (1982) 771.

[760] M.M. Lee, R.C. Welliver, L.J. LaScolea, *Campylobacter* meningitis in childhood, Pediatr. Infect. Dis. J. 4 (1985) 544.

[761] A.E. Simor, et al., Abortion and perinatal sepsis associated with *Campylobacter* infection, Rev. Infect. Dis. J. 8 (1986) 397.

[762] J.C. Forbes, D.W. Scheifele, Early onset *Campylobacter* sepsis in a neonate, Pediatr. Infect. Dis. J. 6 (1987) 494.

[763] E.O. King, Human infections with *Vibrio fetus* and a closely related vibrio, J. Infect. Dis. 101 (1957) 119.

[764] P. Francioli, et al., *Campylobacter fetus* subspecies fetus bacteremia, Arch. Intern. Med. 145 (1985) 289.

[765] M.A. Karmali, et al., The biotype and biotype distribution of clinical isolates of *Campylobacter jejuni* and *Campylobacter coli* over a three-year period, J. Infect. Dis. 147 (1983) 243.

[766] M.J. Albert, et al., Serotype distribution of *Campylobacter jejuni* and *Campylobacter coli* isolated from hospitalized patients with diarrhea in Central Australia, J. Clin. Microbiol. 30 (1992) 207.

[767] L.W. Riley, M.J. Finch, Results of the first year of national surveillance of *Campylobacter* infections in the United States, J. Infect. Dis. 151 (1985) 956.

[768] M.C. Georges-Courbot, et al., Distribution and serotypes of *Campylobacter jejuni* and *Campylobacter coli* in enteric *Campylobacter* strains isolated from children in the Central African Republic, J. Clin. Microbiol. 23 (1986) 592.

[769] W.E. Wheeler, J. Borchers, Vibrionic enteritis in infants, Am. J. Dis. Child. 101 (1961) 60.

[770] J.N. Middlekamp, H.A. Wolf, Infection due to a "related" *Vibrio*, J. Pediatr. 59 (1961) 318.

[771] F.L. Ruben, E. Wolinsky, Human infection with *Vibrio fetus*, in: G.L. Hobby (Ed.), Antimicrobial Agents and Chemotherapy, American Society for Microbiology, Bethesda, MD, 1967, p. 143.

[772] S.L. Mawer, B.A.M. Smith, *Campylobacter* infection of premature baby, Lancet 1 (1979) 1041.

[773] *Campylobacter* in a mother and baby, Commun. Dis. Rep. CDR. 7917 (1979) 4.

[774] M.A. Karmali, Y.C. Tan, Neonatal *Campylobacter* enteritis, Can. Med. Assoc. J. 122 (1980) 192.

[775] K. Thomas, K.N. Chan, C.D. Riberiro, *Campylobacter jejuni/coli* meningitis in a neonate, BMJ. 280 (1980) 1301.

[776] B.J. Anders, B.A. Lauer, J.W. Paisley, *Campylobacter* gastroenteritis in neonates, Am. J. Dis. Child. 135 (1981) 900.

[777] T. Vesikari, L. Huttunen, R. Maki, Perinatal *Campylobacter fetus* ss. *jejuni* enteritis, Acta Paediatr. Scand. 70 (1981) 261.

[778] R.C. Miller, R.W. Guard, A case of premature labour due to *Campylobacter jejuni* infection, Aust. N. Z. Obstet. Gynaecol. 22 (1982) 118.

[779] G.E. Buck, et al., *Campylobacter jejuni* in newborns: a cause of asymptomatic bloody diarrhea, Am. J. Dis. Child. 136 (1982) 744.

[780] M.A. Karmali, et al., *Campylobacter* enterocolitis in a neonatal nursery, J. Infect. Dis. 149 (1984) 874.

[781] E.R. Youngs, C. Roberts, D.C. Davidson, *Campylobacter* enteritis and bloody stools in the neonate, Arch. Dis. Child. 60 (1985) 480.

[782] A. Terrier, et al., Hospital epidemic of neonatal *Campylobacter jejuni* infection, Lancet 2 (1985) 1182.

[783] H. Goossens, et al., Nosocomial outbreak of *Campylobacter jejuni* meningitis in newborn infants, Lancet 2 (1986) 146.

[784] A.F. DiNicola, *Campylobacter jejuni* diarrhea in a 3-day old male neonate, Pediatr. Forum. 140 (1986) 191.

[785] S. Hershkowici, et al., An outbreak of *Campylobacter jejuni* infection in a neonatal intensive care unit, J. Hosp. Infect. 9 (1987) 54.

[786] M.J. Gribble, et al., *Campylobacter* infections in pregnancy: case report and literature review, Am. J. Obstet. Gynecol. 140 (1981) 423.

[787] G.L. Gilbert, et al., Midtrimester abortion associated with septicaemia caused by *Campylobacter jejuni*, Med. J. Aust. 1 (1981) 585.

[788] P.M. Jost, et al., *Campylobacter* septic abortion, South. Med. J. 77 (1984) 924.

[789] C.T. Pearce, *Campylobacter jejuni* infection as a cause of septic abortion, Aust. J. Med. Lab. Sci. 2 (1981) 107.

[790] A. Pines, et al., *Campylobacter* enteritis associated with recurrent abortions in agammaglobulinemia, Acta Obstet. Gynecol. Scand. 62 (1983) 279.

[791] M. Kist, et al., *Campylobacter coli* septicaemia associated with septic abortion, Infection 12 (1984) 88.

[792] J. Reina, N. Borrell, M. Fiol, Rectal bleeding caused by *Campylobacter jejuni* in a neonate, Pediatr. Infect. Dis. J. 6 (1992) 500.

[793] G.M. Ruiz-Palacios, J. Torres, N.I. Escamilla, Cholera-like enterotoxin produced by *Campylobacter jejuni*: characterization and clinical significance, Lancet 2 (1983) 250.

[794] W.M. Johnson, H. Lior, Toxins produced by *Campylobacter jejuni* and *Campylobacter coli*, Lancet 1 (1984) 229.

[795] R.L. Guerrant, C.A. Wanke, R.A. Pennie, Production of a unique cytotoxin by *Campylobacter jejuni*, Infect. Immun. 55 (1987) 2526.

[796] B.A. McCardell, J.M. Madden, E.C. Lee, *Campylobacter jejuni* and *Campylobacter coli* production of a cytotonic toxin immunologically similar to cholera toxin, J. Food. Prot. 47 (1984) 943.

[797] F.A. Klipstein, R.F. Engert, Purification of *Campylobacter jejuni* enterotoxin, Lancet 1 (1984) 1123.

[798] F.A. Klipstein, et al., Pathogenic properties of *Campylobacter jejuni*: assay and correlation with clinical manifestations, Infect. Immun. 50 (1985) 43.

[799] A. Lee, S.C. Smith, P.J. Coloe, Detection of a novel *Campylobacter* cytotoxin, J. Appl. Microbiol. 89 (2001) 719.

[800] D.G. Newell, Experimental studies of *Campylobacter* enteritis, in: J.P. Butzler (Ed.), *Campylobacter* Infection in Man and Animals, CRC Press, Boca Raton, FL, 1984, p. 113.

[801] J.F. Prescott, et al., *Campylobacter jejuni* colitis in gnotobiotic dogs, Can. J. Comp. Med. 45 (1981) 377.

[802] G.M. Ruiz-Palacios, E. Escamilla, N. Torres, Experimental *Campylobacter* diarrhea in chickens, Infect. Immun. 34 (1981) 250.

[803] S.C. Sanyal, et al., *Campylobacter jejuni* diarrhea model in infant chickens, Infect. Immun. 43 (1984) 931.

[804] S.L. Welkos, Experimental gastroenteritis in newly hatched chicks infected with *Campylobacter jejuni*, J. Med. Microbiol. 18 (1984) 233.

[805] R.B. Fitzgeorge, A. Baskerville, K.P. Lander, Experimental infection of rhesus monkeys with a human strain of *Campylobacter jejuni*, J. Hyg. 86 (1981) 343.

[806] L.H. Field, J.L. Underwood, L.J. Berry, The role of gut flora and animal passage in the colonization of adult mice with *Campylobacter jejuni*, J. Med. Microbiol. 17 (1984) 59.

[807] M.V. Jesudason, D.J. Hentges, P. Pongpeeh, Colonization of mice by *Campylobacter jejuni*, Infect. Immun. 57 (1989) 2279.

[808] S.U. Kazmi, B.S. Roberson, N.J. Stern, Animal-passed, virulence-enhanced *Campylobacter jejuni* causes enteritis in neonatal mice, Curr. Microbiol. 11 (1984) 159.

[809] C.D. Humphrey, D.M. Montag, F.E. Pittman, Experimental infection of hamsters with *Campylobacter jejuni*, J. Infect. Dis. 151 (1985) 485.

[810] K.I. Manninen, J.F. Prescott, I.R. Dohoo, Pathogenicity of *C. jejuni* isolates from animals and humans, Infect. Immun. 38 (1982) 46.

[811] A.N. Eden, *Vibrio fetus* meningitis in a newborn infant, J. Pediatr. 61 (1962) 33.

[812] M. Maki, R. Maki, T. Vesikari, Fecal leucocytes in *Campylobacter*-associated diarrhoea in infants, Acta Paediatr. Scand. 68 (1979) 271.

[813] M.E. Lambert, et al., *Campylobacter* colitis, BMJ 1 (1979) 857.

[814] M.J. Blaser, R.B. Parsons, W.L. Wang, Acute colitis caused by *Campylobacter fetus* spp. *Jejuni*, Gastroenterology 78 (1980) 448.

[815] E.O. King, The laboratory recognition of *Vibrio fetus* and a closely related *Vibrio* isolated from cases of human vibriosis, Ann. N. Y. Acad. Sci. 78 (1962) 700.

[816] R.G. Evans, J.V. Dadswell, Human vibriosis, BMJ 3 (1967) 240.

[817] J.P. Butzler, J. Oosterom, *Campylobacter*: pathogenicity and significance in foods, Int. J. Food. Microbiol. 12 (1991) 1.

[818] C.O. Gill, L.M. Harris, Contamination of red meat carcasses by *Campylobacter fetus* subsp. *Jejuni*, Appl. Environ. Microbiol. 43 (1982) 977.

[819] S.R. Palmer, et al., Water-borne outbreak of *Campylobacter* gastroenteritis, Lancet 1 (1983) 287.

[820] M. Rogol, et al., Water-borne outbreaks of *Campylobacter* enteritis, Eur. J. Clin. Microbiol. 2 (1983) 588.

[821] S. Shankers, et al., *Campylobacter jejuni*: incidence in processed broilers and biotype distribution in human and broiler isolates, Appl. Environ. Microbiol. 43 (1982) 1219.

[822] A.M. Hood, A.D. Pearson, M. Shahamat, The extent of surface contamination of retailed chickens with *Campylobacter jejuni* serogroups, Epidemiol. Infect. 100 (1988) 17.

[823] N.V. Harris, et al., *Campylobacter jejuni* enteritis associated with raw goat's milk, Am. J. Epidemiol. 126 (1987) 179.

[824] J.A. Korlath, et al., A point-source outbreak of campylobacteriosis associated with consumption of raw milk, J. Infect. Dis. 152 (1985) 592.

[825] B.S. Klein, et al., *Campylobacter* infection associated with raw milk, JAMA 255 (1986) 361.

[826] M.S. Deming, et al., *Campylobacter* enteritis at a university: transmission from eating chicken and from cats, Am. J. Epidemiol. 126 (1987) 526.

[827] T.D. Tenkate, R.J. Stafford, Risk factors for *Campylobacter* infection in infants and young children: a matched case-controlled study, Epidemiol. Infect. 127 (2001) 399.

[828] A.F. Hallett, P.L. Botha, A. Logan, Isolation of *Campylobacter fetus* from recent cases of human vibriosis, J. Hyg. 79 (1977) 381.

[829] T.F. Wolfs, et al., Neonatal sepsis by *Campylobacter jejuni*: genetically proven transmission from a household puppy, Clin. Infect. Dis. 31 (2001) e97.

[830] M.J. Blaser, et al., Outbreaks of *Campylobacter* enteritis in two extended families: evidence for person-to-person transmission, J. Pediatr. 98 (1981) 254.

[831] S. Cadranel, et al., Enteritis due to "related Vibrio" in children, Am. J. Dis. Child. 126 (1973) 152.

[832] J.F. Prescott, M.A. Karmali, Attempts to transmit *Campylobacter enteritis* to dogs and cats, Can. Med. Assoc. J. 119 (1978) 1001.

[833] R.E. Black, et al., Experimental *Campylobacter jejuni* infection in humans, J. Infect. Dis. 157 (1988) 472.

[834] J. Llovo, et al., Molecular typing of *Campylobacter jejuni* isolates involved in a neonatal outbreak indicates nosocomial transmission, J. Clin. Microbiol. 41 (2003) 3926.

[835] V.D. Bokkenheuser, et al., Detection of enteric campylobacteriosis in children, J. Clin. Microbiol. 9 (1979) 227.

[836] M.C. Georges-Courbot, et al., Prospective study of enteric *Campylobacter* infections in children from birth to 6 months in the Central African Republic, J. Clin. Microbiol. 25 (1987) 836.

[837] P.J. Rettig, *Campylobacter* infections in human beings, J. Pediatr. 94 (1979) 855.

[838] M.J. Blaser, et al., *Campylobacter* enteritis: clinical and epidemiological features, Ann. Intern. Med. 91 (1979) 179.

[839] J.P. Butzler, Related vibrios in Africa, Lancet 2 (1973) 858.

[840] S. Lauwers, M. DeBoeck, J.P. Butzler, *Campylobacter* enteritis in Brussels, Lancet 1 (1978) 604.

[841] W.P. Severin, *Campylobacter* en enteritis, Ned. Tijdschr. Geneeskd. 122 (1978) 499.

[842] C.D. Ribeiro, *Campylobacter* enteritis, Lancet 2 (1978) 270.

[843] N.J. Richardson, H.J. Koornhof, *Campylobacter* infections in Soweto, S. Afr. Med. J. 55 (1979) 73.

[844] M.J. Gribble, et al., *Campylobacter* infections in pregnancy: case report and literature review, Am. J. Obstet. Gynecol. 140 (1981) 423.

[845] T. Morooka, et al., Epidemiologic application of pulsed-field gel electrophoresis to an outbreak of *Campylobacter fetus* meningitis in a neonatal intensive care unit, Scand. J. Infect. Dis. 28 (1996) 269.

[846] T. Morooka, et al., Nosocomial meningitis due to *Campylobacter fetus* subspecies *fetus* in a neonatal intensive care unit, Acta Paediatr. Jpn. 34 (1992) 350.

[847] T. Norooka, et al., Nosocomial meningitis due to *Campylobacter fetus* subspecies *fetus* in a neonatal intensive care unit, Acta Paediatr. Jpn. 34 (1992) 530.

[848] M.V. Smith, A.J. Muldoon, *Campylobacter fetus* subspecies *jejuni* (*Vibrio fetus*) from commercially processed poultry, Appl. Microbiol. 27 (1974) 995.

[849] I.H. Grant, N.J. Richardson, V.D. Bokkenheuser, Broiler chickens as potential source of *Campylobacter* infections in humans, J. Clin. Microbiol. 2 (1980) 508.

[850] M.J. Blaser, S.H. Weiss, T.J. Barrett, *Campylobacter* enteritis associated with a healthy cat, JAMA 247 (1982) 816.

[851] M.B. Skirrow, et al., *Campylobacter jejuni* enteritis transmitted from cat to man, Lancet 1 (1980) 1188.

[852] M.J. Blaser, et al., *Campylobacter* enteritis associated with canine infection, Lancet 2 (1978) 979.

[853] P.R. Taylor, W.M. Weinstein, J.H. Bryner, *Campylobacter fetus* infection in human subjects: association with raw milk, Am. J. Med. 66 (1979) 779.

[854] *Campylobacter* enteritis in a household Colorado, MMWR Morb. Mortal. Wkly. Rep. 27 (1979) 273.

[855] D.A. Robinson, et al., *Campylobacter* enteritis associated with the consumption of unpasteurized milk, BMJ 1 (1979) 1171.

[856] A.J. Levy, A gastroenteritis outbreak probably due to bovine strain of *Vibrio*, Yale. J. Biol. Med. 18 (1946) 243.

[857] R.L. Vogt, et al., *Campylobacter* enteritis associated with contaminated water, Ann. Intern. Med. 96 (1982) 292.

[858] C.M. Patton, et al., Evaluation of 10 methods to distinguish epidemic-associated *Campylobacter* strains, J. Clin. Microbiol. 29 (1991) 680.

[859] E. Salazar-Lindo, et al., Early treatment with erythromycin of *Campylobacter jejuni* associated dysentery in children, J. Pediatr. 109 (1986) 355.

[860] W.M. Darling, R.N. Peel, M.B. Skirrow, *Campylobacter* cholecystitis, Lancet 1 (1979) 1302.

[861] J.S. Davis, J.B. Penfold, *Campylobacter* urinary tract infection, Lancet 1 (1979) 1091.

[862] M.A. Hossain, et al., *Campylobacter jejuni* bacteraemia in children with diarrhea in Bangladesh: report of six cases, J. Diarrhoeal. Dis. Res. 10 (1992) 101.

[863] R.P. Reed, et al., *Campylobacter* bacteremia in children, Pediatr. Infect. Dis. J. 15 (1996) 345.

[864] K. Johonsen, et al., HLA-B27-negative arthritis related to *Campylobacter jejuni* enteritis in three children and two adults, Acta Med. Scand. 214 (1983) 165.

[865] J. Kaldor, B.R. Speed, Guillain-Barré syndrome and *Campylobacter jejuni*: a serological study, BMJ 288 (1984) 1867.

[866] S. Kuroki, et al., Guillain-Barré syndrome associated with *Campylobacter* infection, Pediatr. Infect. Dis. J. 10 (1991) 149.

[867] J.R. Ebright, L.M. Ryay, Acute erosive reactive arthritis associated with *Campylobacter jejuni*-induced colitis, Am. J. Med. 76 (1984) 321.

[868] U.B. Schaad, Reactive arthritis associated with *Campylobacter* enteritis, Pediatr. Infect. Dis. J. 1 (1982) 328.

[869] D.M. Perlman, et al., Persistent *Campylobacter jejuni* infections in patients infected with human immunodeficiency virus (HIV), Ann. Intern. Med. 108 (1988) 540.

[870] C.H. Chiu, C.Y. Kuo, J.T. Ou, Chronic diarrhea and bacteremia caused by *Campylobacter lari* in a neonate, Clin. Infect. Dis. 21 (1995) 700.

[871] H.P. Endtz, et al., Comparison of six media, including a semisolid agar for the isolation of various *Campylobacter* species from stool specimens, J. Clin. Microbiol. 29 (1991) 1007.

[872] J.W. Paisley, et al., Darkfield microscopy of human feces for presumptive diagnosis of *Campylobacter fetus* subsp. *jejuni* enteritis, J. Clin. Microbiol. 15 (1982) 61.

[873] B.A. Oyofo, et al., Specific detection of *Campylobacter jejuni* and *Campylobacter coli* by using polymerase chain reaction, J. Clin. Microbiol. 30 (1992) 2613.

[874] J.A. Kiehlbauch, et al., In vitro susceptibilities of aerotolerant *Campylobacter* isolates to 22 antimicrobial agents, Antimicrob. Agents Chemother. 36 (1992) 717.

[875] N. LaChance, et al., Susceptibilities of β-lactamase-positive and -negative strains of *Campylobacter coli* to β-lactam agents, Antimicrob. Agents Chemother. 37 (1993) 1174.

[876] W. Yan, D.E. Taylor, Characterization of erythromycin resistance in *Campylobacter jejuni* and *Campylobacter coli*, Antimicrob. Agents Chemother. 35 (1991) 1989.

[877] J. Segretti, et al., High-level quinolone resistance in clinical isolates of *Campylobacter jejuni*, J. Infect. Dis. 165 (1992) 667.

[878] D. Krowchuk, J.H. Seashore, Complete biliary obstruction due to erythromycin estolate administration in an infant, Pediatrics 64 (1979) 956.

[879] R.A. Kuschner, et al., Use of azithromycin for the treatment of *Campylobacter* enteritis in travelers to Thailand, an area where ciprofloxacin resistance is prevalent, Clin. Infect. Dis. 21 (1995) 536.

[880] H. Rautelin, O.V. Renkonen, T.U. Kosunen, Azithromycin resistance in *Campylobacter jejuni* and *Campylobacter coli*, Eur. J. Clin. Microbiol. Infect. Dis. 12 (1993) 864.

[881] H.P. Endtz, M. Broeren, R.P. Mouton, In vitro susceptibility of quinolone-resistant *Campylobacter jejuni* to new macrolide antibiotics, Eur. J. Clin. Microbiol. Infect. Dis. 12 (1993) 48.

[882] I. Nachamkin, et al., Immunoglobulin A antibodies directed against *Campylobacter jejuni* flagellin present in breast-milk, Epidemiol. Infect. 112 (1994) 359.

[883] S.P. Borriello, et al., Virulence factors of *Clostridium difficile*, Rev. Infect. Dis. 12 (1990) S185.

[884] B.W. Wren, Molecular characterisation of *Clostridium difficile* toxins A and B, Rev. Med. Microbiol. 3 (1992) 21.

[885] J.S. Hyams, M.M. Berman, H. Helgason, Nonantibiotic-associated enterocolitis caused by *Clostridium difficile* in an infant, J. Pediatr. 99 (1981) 750.

[886] H.E. Larson, A.B. Price, Pseudomembranous colitis: presence of clostridial toxin, Lancet 1 (1977) 1312.

[887] S.R. Peikin, J. Galdibin, J.G. Bartlett, Role of *Clostridium difficile* in a case of nonantibiotic-associated pseudomembranous colitis, Gastroenterology 79 (1980) 948.

[888] A. Wald, H. Mendelow, J.G. Bartlett, Nonantibiotic-associated pseudomembranous colitis due to toxin producing clostridia, Ann. Intern. Med. 92 (1980) 798.

[889] S.P. Adler, T. Chandrika, W.F. Berman, *Clostridium difficile* associated with pseudomembranous colitis, Am. J. Dis. Child. 135 (1981) 820.

[890] S. Willey, J.G. Bartlett, Cultures for *C. difficile* in stools containing a cyto-toxin neutralized by *C. sordellii* antitoxin, J. Clin. Microbiol. 10 (1979) 880.

[891] S. Tabaqchali, Epidemiologic markers of *Clostridium difficile*, Rev. Infect. Dis. 12 (1990) S192.

[892] K.H. Kim, et al., Isolation of *C. difficile* from the environment and contacts of patients with antibiotic-associated colitis, J. Infect. Dis. 143 (1981) 42.

[893] R.J. Sheretz, F.A. Sarubb, The prevalence of *C. difficile* and toxin in a nursery population: a comparison between patients with necrotizing enterocolitis and an asymptomatic group, J. Pediatr. 100 (1982) 435.

[894] C.R. Clabots, et al., Acquisition of *Clostridium difficile* by hospitalized patients: evidence for colonized new admissions as a source of infection, J. Infect. Dis. 166 (1992) 561.

[895] D.Z. Bliss, et al., Acquisition of *Clostridium difficile* and *Clostridium difficile*-associated diarrhea in hospitalized patients receiving tube feeding, Ann. Intern. Med. 129 (1998) 1012.

[896] J.A. Jernigan, et al., A randomized crossover study of disposable thermo-meters for prevention of *Clostridium difficile* and other nosocomial infec-tions, Infect. Control. Hosp. Epidemiol. 19 (1998) 494.

[897] S. Johnson, et al., Prospective controlled study of vinyl glove use to inter-rupt *Clostridium difficile* transmission, Am. J. Med. 88 (1990) 137.

[898] A.J. Zedd, et al., Nosocomial *C. difficile* reservoir in a neonatal intensive care unit, Pediatr. Infect. Dis. J. 3 (1984) 429.

[899] S. Johnson, D.N. Gerding, *Clostridium difficile*-associated diarrhea, Clin. Infect. Dis. 26 (1998) 1027.

[900] R. Fekety, A.B. Shah, Diagnosis and treatment of *Clostridium difficile* colitis, JAMA 269 (1993) 71.

[901] M. Kelber, M.E. Ament, *Shigella dysenteriae* 1. A forgotten cause of pseudo-membranous colitis, J. Pediatr. 89 (1976) 595.

[902] S.T. Donta, M.G. Myers, *C. difficile* toxin in asymptomatic neonates, J. Pediatr. 100 (1982) 431.

[903] I. Al-Jumaili, et al., Incidence and origin of *C. difficile* in neonates, J. Clin. Microbiol. 19 (1984) 77.

[904] D.F. Welch, M.T. Marks, Is *C. difficile* pathogenic in infants? J. Pediatr. 100 (1982) 393.

[905] S.T. Donta, M.S. Stuppy, M.G. Myers, Neonatal antibiotic-associated colitis, Am. J. Dis. Child. 135 (1981) 181.

[906] D. Enad, et al., Is *Clostridium difficile* a pathogen in the newborn intensive care unit? A prospective evaluation, J. Perinatol. 17 (1997) 355.

[907] D.M. Lyerly, et al., Multicenter evaluation of the *Clostridium difficile* TOX A/B TEST, J. Clin. Microbiol. 36 (1998) 184.

[908] H. Kato, et al., Identification of toxin A-negative, toxin B-positive *Clostrid-ium difficile* by PCR, J. Clin. Microbiol. 36 (1998) 2178.

[909] M.E. Rafferty, et al., Comparison of restriction enzyme analysis, arbitrarily primed PCR, and protein profile analysis typing for epidemiologic investi-gation of an ongoing *Clostridium difficile* outbreak, J. Clin. Microbiol. 36 (1998) 2957.

[910] D.G. Teasley, et al., Prospective randomized trial of metronidazole vs. vancomycin for *C. difficile* associated diarrhoea and colitis, Lancet 2 (1983) 1043.

[911] C. Wenisch, et al., Comparison of vancomycin, teicoplanin, metronidazole, and fusidic acid for the treatment of *Clostridium difficile*-associated diarrhea, Clin. Infect. Dis. 22 (1996) 813.

[912] G.P. Young, et al., Antibiotic-associated colitis due to *C. difficile*: double-blind comparison of vancomycin with bacitracin, Gastroenterology 89 (1985) 1039.

[913] M.N. Dudley, et al., Oral bacitracin vs. vancomycin therapy for *C. difficile*-induced diarrhea, Arch. Intern. Med. 146 (1986) 1101.

[914] J.G. Bartlett, et al., Relapse following oral vancomycin therapy of antibiotic-associated pseudomembranous colitis, Gastroenterology 78 (1980) 431.

[915] N. Wada, et al., Neutralizing activity against *C. difficile* toxin in the super-natants of cultures of colostral cells, Infect. Immun. 29 (1980) 545.

[916] S. Dallas, R. Rolfe, Binding of *Clostridium difficile* toxin A to human milk secretory component, J. Med. Microbiol. 47 (1998) 879.

[917] K. Kim, et al., In vitro and in vivo neutralizing activity of *C. difficile* purified toxins A and B by human colostrum and milk, J. Infect. Dis. 150 (1984) 57.

[918] M.S. Cooperstock, et al., *C. difficile* in normal infants and sudden death syn-drome: an association with infant formula feeding, Pediatrics 70 (1982) 91.

[919] W.C. Levine, P.M. Griffin, and Gulf Coast Vibrio Working Group, *Vibrio* infections on the Gulf Coast: results of first year of regional surveillance., J. Infect. Dis. 167 (1993) 479.

[920] D.L. Swerdlow, A.A. Ries, Cholera in the Americas: guidelines for the clinician, JAMA 267 (1992) 1495.

[921] R.I. Glass, M. Libel, A.D. Brandling-Bennett, Epidemic cholera in the Americas, Science 256 (1992) 1524.

[922] A.K. Siddique, et al., Emergence of a new epidemic strain of *Vibrio cholerae* in Bangladesh: an epidemiological study, Trop. Geogr. Med. 46 (1994) 147.

[923] S.P. Fisher-Hoch, et al., *Vibrio cholerae* O139 in Karachi, Pakistan, Lancet 342 (1993) 1422.

[924] M. Chongsa-Nguan, et al., *Vibrio cholerae* O139 Bengal in Bangkok, Lancet 342 (1993) 430.

[925] Cholera Working Group, International Centre for Diarrhoeal Diseases Research, Bangladesh, Large epidemic of cholera-like disease in Bangladesh caused by *Vibrio cholerae* O139 synonym Bengal, Lancet 342 (1993) 387.

[926] S.K. Bhattacharya, et al., Clinical profile of acute diarrhoea cases infected with the new epidemic strain of *Vibrio cholerae* O139: designation of the disease as cholera, J. Infect. 27 (1993) 11.

[927] S. Garg, et al., Nationwide prevalence of the new epidemic strain of *Vibrio cholerae* O139 Bengal in India, J. Infect. 27 (1993) 108.

[928] P.A. Blake, et al., Cholera—a possible endemic focus in the United States, N. Engl. J. Med. 302 (1980) 305.

[929] N. Hirschhorn, A. Chowdhury, J. Lindenbaum, Cholera in pregnant women, Lancet 1 (1969) 1230.

[930] A.M. Khan, M.K. Bhattacharyl, M.J. Albert, Neonatal diarrhea caused by *Vibrio cholerae* O139 Bengal, Diagn. Microbiol. Infect. Dis. 23 (1995) 155.

[931] P. Lumbiganon, P. Kosalaraksa, P. Kowsuwan, *Vibrio cholerae* O139 diarrhea and acute renal failure in a three day old infant, Pediatr. Infect. Dis. J. 14 (1995) 1105.

[932] R. Haider, et al., Neonatal diarrhea in a diarrhea treatment center in Bangladesh: clinical presentation, breastfeeding management and outcome, Indian Pediatr. 37 (2000) 37.

[933] R.A. Gunn, et al., Bottle feeding as a risk factor for cholera in infants, Lancet 2 (1979) 730.

[934] A. Ahmed, A.K. Bhattacharjee, W.H. Mosley, Characteristics of the serum vibriocidal and agglutinating antibodies in cholera cases and in normal residents of the endemic and non-endemic cholera areas, J. Immunol. 105 (1970) 431.

[935] M.H. Merson, et al., Maternal cholera immunisation and secretory IgA in breast milk, Lancet 1 (1980) 931.

[936] R.A. Cash, et al., Response of man to infection with *Vibrio cholerae*. I. Clin-ical, serologic and bacteriologic responses to a known inoculum, J. Infect. Dis. 129 (1974) 45.

[937] D.R. Nalin, R.J. Levine, M.M. Levine, Cholera, non-*Vibrio* cholera, and stomach acid, Lancet 2 (1978) 856.

[938] A.C. Wright, et al., Development and testing of a nonradioactive DNA oligonucleotide probe that is specific for *Vibrio cholerae* cholera toxin, J. Clin. Microbiol. 30 (1992) 2302.

[939] M. Yoh, et al., Development of an enzyme-labeled oligonucleotide probe for the cholera toxin gene, J. Clin. Microbiol. 31 (1993) 1312.

[940] K.L. Kotloff, et al., Safety and immunogenicity in North Americans of a single dose of live oral cholera vaccine CVD 103-HgR: results of a rando-mized, placebo-controlled, double-blind crossover trial, Infect. Immun. 60 (1992) 4430.

[941] J.D. Clemens, et al., Evidence that inactivated oral cholera vaccines both prevent and mitigate *Vibrio cholerae* O1 infections in a cholera-endemic area, J. Infect. Dis. 166 (1992) 1029.

[942] M.M. Levine, F. Noriega, A review of the current status of enteric vaccines, P. N. G. Med. J. 38 (1995) 325.

[943] S. Kohl, *Yersinia enterocolitica* infections in children, Pediatr. Clin. North. Am. 26 (1979) 433.

[944] M.I. Marks, et al., *Yersinia enterocolitica* gastroenteritis: a prospective study of clinical, bacteriologic, and epidemiologic features, J. Pediatr. 96 (1980) 26.

[945] L.A. Lee, et al., *Yersinia enterocolitica* 0:3 infections in infants and children, associated with the household preparation of chitterlings, N. Engl. J. Med. 322 (1990) 984.

[946] P. Krogstad, et al., Clinical and microbiologic characteristics of cutaneous infection with *Yersinia enterocolitica*, J. Infect. Dis. 165 (1992) 740.

[947] L.A. Lee, et al., *Yersinia enterocolitica* 0:3: an emerging cause of pediatric gastroenteritis in the United States, J. Infect. Dis. 163 (1991) 660.

[948] J.G. Morris Jr., et al., *Yersinia enterocolitica* isolated from two cohorts of young children in Santiago, Chile: incidence of and lack of correlation between illness and proposed virulence factors, J. Clin. Microbiol. 29 (1991) 2784.

[949] B. Metchock, et al., *Yersinia enterocolitica*: a frequent seasonal stool isolate from children at an urban hospital in the southeast United States, J. Clin. Microbiol. 29 (1991) 2868.

[950] D.R. Kane, P.D. Reuman, *Yersinia enterocolitica* causing pneumonia and empyema in a child and a review of the literature, Pediatr. Infect. Dis. J. 11 (1992) 591.

[951] R.E. Black, et al., Epidemic *Yersinia enterocolitica* infection due to contami-nated chocolate milk, N. Engl. J. Med. 298 (1978) 76.

[952] R.N.I. Pietersz, et al., Prevention of *Yersinia enterocolitica* growth in red blood cell concentrates, Lancet 340 (1992) 755.

[953] G. Kapperud, et al., Plasmid-mediated surface fibrillae of *Y. pseudotuberculosis* and *Y. enterocolitica*: relationship to the outer membrane protein YOP1 and possible importance for pathogenesis, Infect. Immun. 55 (1987) 2247.

[954] R.R. Brubaker, Factors promoting acute and chronic diseases caused by yersiniae, Clin. Microbiol. Rev. 4 (1991) 309.

[955] T. Takao, et al., Primary structure of heat-stable enterotoxin produced by *Y. enterocolitica*, Biochem. Biophys. Res. Commun. 125 (1984) 845.

[956] J.W. Paisley, B.A. Lauer, Neonatal *Yersinia enterocolitica* enteritis, Pediatr. Infect. Dis. J. 11 (1992) 331.

[957] E.D. Shapiro, *Yersinia enterocolitica* septicemia in normal infants, Am. J. Dis. Child. 135 (1981) 477.

[958] B. Chester, et al., Infections due to *Yersinia enterocolitica* serotypes 0:2 3 and 0 4 acquired in South Florida, J. Clin. Microbiol. 13 (1981) 885.

[959] W.J. Rodriguez, et al., *Y. enterocolitica* enteritis in children, JAMA 242 (1978) 1979.

[960] M. Challapalli, D.G. Cunningham, *Yersinia enterocolitica* septicemia in infants younger than three months of age, Pediatr. Infect. Dis. J. 12 (1993) 168.

[961] J.W. Paisley, B.A. Lauer, Neonatal *Yersinia enterocolitica* enteritis, Pediatr. Infect. Dis. J. 11 (1992) 332.

[962] M.T. Antonio-Santiago, et al., *Yersinia enterocolitica* septicemia in an infant presenting as fever of unknown origin, Clin. Pediatr. 25 (1986) 213.

[963] J.M. Sutton, P.S. Pasquariell, *Yersinia enterocolitica* septicemia in a normal child, Am. J. Dis. Child. 137 (1983) 305.

[964] S. Kohl, J.A. Jacobson, A. Nahmias, *Yersinia enterocolitica* infections in children, J. Pediatr. 89 (1976) 77.

[965] S. Naqvi, et al., Presentation of *Yersinia enterocolitica* enteritis in children, Pediatr. Infect. Dis. J. 12 (1993) 386.

[966] N. Abdel-Haq, et al., *Yersinia enterocolitica* infection in children, Pediatr. Infect. Dis. J. 19 (2000) 954.

[967] A. Ibrahim, W. Liesack, E. Stackebrandt, Polymerase chain reaction–gene probe detection system specific for pathogenic strains of *Yersinia enterocolitica*, J. Clin. Microbiol. 30 (1992) 1942.

[968] J. Kwaga, J.O. Iversen, V. Misra, Detection of pathogenic *Yersinia enterocolitica* by polymerase chain reaction and digoxigenin-labeled polynucleotide probes, J. Clin. Microbiol. 30 (1992) 2668.

[969] V.M. Stolk-Engelaar, et al., In-vitro antimicrobial susceptibility of *Yersinia enterocolitica* isolates from stools of patients in the Netherlands from 1982–1991, J. Antimicrob. Chemother. 36 (1995) 839.

[970] R. Alzugaray, et al., *Yersinia enterocolitica* 0:3: antimicrobial resistance patterns, virulence profiles and plasmids, New. Microbiol. 18 (1995) 215.

[971] M.A. Preston, et al., Antimicrobial susceptibility of pathogenic *Yersinia enterocolitica* isolated in Canada from 1972 to 1990, Antimicrob. Agents Chemother. 38 (1994) 2121.

[972] C. James, et al., Immunological cross-reactivity of enterotoxins of *A. hydrophila* and cholera toxin, Clin. Exp. Immunol. 47 (1982) 34.

[973] S.C. Sanyal, S.J. Singh, P.C. Sen, Enteropathogenicity of *A. hydrophila* and *P. shigelloides*, J. Med. Microbiol. 8 (1975) 195.

[974] S.M. Kirov, et al., Virulence characteristics of *Aeromonas* spp. in relation to source and biotype, J. Clin. Microbiol. 24 (1986) 827.

[975] I.M. Watson, et al., Invasiveness of *Aeromonas* spp. in relation to biotype, virulence factors, and clinical features, J. Clin. Microbiol. 22 (1985) 48.

[976] M. Kindshuh, et al., Clinical and biochemical significance of toxin production by A. hydrophila, J. Clin. Microbiol. 25 (1987) 916.

[977] A. Ljungh, P. Eneroth, T. Wadstrom, Cytotonic enterotoxin from *Aeromonas hydrophila*, Toxicon 20 (1982) 787.

[978] D. Morgan, et al., Lack of correlation between known virulence properties of *A. hydrophila* and enteropathogenicity for humans, Infect. Immun. 50 (1985) 62.

[979] C. Pitarangsi, et al., Enteropathogenicity of *A. hydrophila* and *P. shigelloides*: prevalence among individuals with and without diarrhea in Thailand, Infect. Immun. 35 (1982) 666.

[980] R. Martinez-Silva, M. Guzmann-Urrego, F.H. Caselitz, Zur Frage der Bedeutung von Aeromonasstammen bei Saüglingsenteritis, Z. Tropenmed. Parasitol. 12 (1961) 445.

[981] N. Figura, et al., Prevalence, species differentiation, and toxigenicity of *Aeromonas* strains in cases of childhood gastroenteritis and in controls, J. Clin. Microbiol. 23 (1986) 595.

[982] M. Gracey, V. Burke, J. Robinson, *Aeromonas*-associated gastroenteritis, Lancet 2 (1982) 1304.

[983] P. Shread, T.J. Donovan, J.V. Lee, A survey of the incidence of *Aeromonas* in human feces, Soc. Gen. Microbiol. 8 (1981) 184.

[984] P. Escheverria, et al., Travelers' diarrhea among American Peace Corps volunteers in rural Thailand, J. Infect. Dis. 143 (1981) 767.

[985] P. Bhat, S. Shanthakumari, D. Rajan, The characterization and significance of *P. shigelloides* and *A. hydrophila* isolated from an epidemic of diarrhea, Indian. J. Med. Res. 62 (1974) 1051.

[986] W.A. Agger, J.D. McCormick, M.J. Gurwith, Clinical and microbiological features of *A. hydrophila*-associated diarrhea, J. Clin. Microbiol. 21 (1985) 909.

[987] W.A. Agger, Diarrhea associated with *A. hydrophila*, Pediatr. Infect. Dis. J. 5 (1986) S106.

[988] L.P. Deodhar, K. Saraswathi, A. Varudkar, *Aeromonas* spp. and their association with human diarrheal disease, J. Clin. Microbiol. 29 (1991) 853.

[989] H. Santoso, et al., Faecal *Aeromonas* spp. in Balinese children, J. Gastroenterol. Hepatol. 1 (1986) 115.

[990] C.J. Gomez, et al., Gastroenteritis due to *Aeromonas* in pediatrics, An. Esp. Pediatr. 44 (1996) 548.

[991] A. Diaz, et al., *A. hydrophila*-associated diarrhea in a neonate, Pediatr. Infect. Dis. J. 5 (1986) 704.

[992] V.H. San Joaquin, D.A. Pickett, , *Aeromonas*-associated gastroenteritis in children, Pediatr. Infect. Dis. J. 7 (1988) 53.

[993] W.L. George, M.J. Jones, M.M. Nakata, Phenotypic characteristics of *Aeromonas* species isolated from adult humans, J. Clin. Microbiol. 23 (1986) 1026.

[994] J.M. Janda, Recent advances in the study of the taxonomy, pathogenicity, and infectious syndromes associated with the genus *Aeromonas*, Clin. Microbiol. Rev. 4 (1991) 397.

[995] B.J. Freij, Aeromonas: biology of the organism and diseases in children, Pediatr. Infect. Dis. J. 3 (1984) 164.

[996] V. Fainstein, S. Weaver, G.P. Bodey, In vitro susceptibilities of *A. hydrophila* against new antibiotics, Antimicrob. Agents Chemother. 22 (1982) 513.

[997] V.H. San Joaquin, et al., Antimicrobial susceptibility of *Aeromonas* species isolated from patients with diarrhea, Antimicrob. Agents Chemother. 30 (1986) 794.

[998] B.L. Jones, M.H. Wilcox, *Aeromonas* infections and their treatment, J. Antimicrob. Chemother. 35 (1995) 453.

[999] S.D. Holmberg, et al., *Plesiomonas* enteric infections in the United States, Ann. Intern. Med. 105 (1986) 690.

[1000] T. Tsukamoto, et al., Two epidemics of diarrhoeal disease possibly caused by *P. shigelloides*, J. Hyg. 80 (1978) 275.

[1001] S.D. Holmberg, J.J. Farmer, *A. hydrophila* and *P. shigelloides* as causes of intestinal infections, Rev. Infect. Dis. 6 (1984) 633.

[1002] D.A. Herrington, et al., In vitro and in vivo pathogenicity of *P. shigelloides*, Infect. Immun. 55 (1987) 979.

[1003] R.A. Brenden, M.A. Miller, J.M. Janda, Clinical disease spectrum and pathogenic factors associated with *P. shigelloides* infections in humans, Rev. Infect. Dis. 10 (1988) 303.

[1004] A. Pathak, J.R. Custer, J. Levy, Neonatal septicemia and meningitis due to *Plesiomonas shigelloides*, Pediatrics 71 (1983) 389.

[1005] K. Fujita, et al., Neonatal *Plesiomonas shigelloides* septicemia and meningitis: a case review, Acta Paediatr. Jpn. 36 (1994) 450.

[1006] C. Terpeluk, et al., *Plesiomonas shigelloides* sepsis and meningoencephalitis in a neonate, Eur. J. Pediatr. 151 (1992) 499.

[1007] J. Billiet, et al., *Plesiomonas shigelloides* meningitis and septicaemia in a neonate: report of a case and review of the literature, J. Infect. 19 (1989) 267.

[1008] S.A. Alabi, T. Odugbemi, Biochemical characteristics and a simple scheme for the identification of *Aeromonas* species and *Plesiomonas shigelloides*, J. Trop. Med. Hyg. 93 (1990) 166.

[1009] J.F. Reinhardt, W.L. George, Comparative in vitro activities of selected antimicrobial agents against *Aeromonas* species and *P. shigelloides*, Antimicrob. Agents Chemother. 27 (1985) 643.

[1010] N. Visitsunthorn, P. Komolpis, Antimicrobial therapy in *Plesiomonas shigelloides*–associated diarrhea in Thai children, Southeast Asian J. Trop. Med. Public Health 26 (1995) 86.

[1011] M. Jampolis, et al., *Bacillus mucosus* infection of the newborn, Am. J. Dis. Child. 43 (1932) 70.

[1012] J. Olarte, et al., *Klebsiella* strains isolated from diarrheal infants: human volunteer studies, Am. J. Dis. Child. 101 (1961) 763.

[1013] M.M. Murdoch, N.A. Janovski, S. Joseph, , *Klebsiella* pseudomembranous enterocolitis: report of two cases, Med. Ann. Dist. Columbia. 38 (1969) 137.

[1014] G. Ujvary, et al., Beobachtungen Über die Ätiologie der Gastroenterocolitiden des Säuglings- und Kindesalters. II. Untersuchung der Rolle der Klebsiella-Stamme, Acta Microbiol. Acad. Sci. Hung. 10 (1964) 241.

[1015] K. Gergely, Über eine Enteritis-Epidemie bei Frühgeborenen, verursacht durch den Bacillus Klebsiella, Kinderarztl. Prax. 9 (1964) 385.

[1016] D.N. Walcher, *Bacillus mucosus capsulatus*" in infantile diarrhea, J. Clin. Invest. 25 (1946) 103.

[1017] J.M. Cass, *Bacillus lactis aerogenes* infection in the newborn, Lancet 1 (1941) 346.

[1018] S.D. Sternberg, C. Hoffman, B.M. Zweifler, Stomatitis and diarrhea in infants caused by *Bacillus mucosus capsulatus*, J. Pediatr. 38 (1951) 509.

[1019] M.T. Worfel, W.W. Ferguson, A new *Klebsiella* type (capsular type 15) isolated from feces and urine, Am. J. Clin. Pathol. 21 (1951) 1097.

[1020] B.P. Simmons, et al., *Enterobacter sakazakii* infections in neonates associated with intrinsic contamination of a powdered infant formula, Infect. Control. Hosp. Epidemiol. 10 (1989) 398.

[1021] G.A.J. Ayliffe, B.J. Collins, F. Pettit, Contamination of infant feeds in a Milton milk kitchen, Lancet 1 (1970) 559.

[1022] J.L. Adler, et al., Nosocomial colonization with kanamycin-resistant *Klebsiella pneumoniae*, types 2 and 11, in a premature nursery, J. Pediatr. 77 (1970) 376.

[1023] H.R. Hill, C.E. Hunt, J.M. Matsen, Nosocomial colonization with *Klebsiella*, type 16, in a neonatal intensive-care unit associated with an outbreak of sepsis, meningitis, and necrotizing enterocolitis, J. Pediatr. 85 (1974) 415.

[1024] D. Panigrahi, P. Roy, A. Chakrabarti, Enterotoxigenic *Klebsiella pneumoniae* in acute childhood diarrhea, Indian J. Med. Res. 93 (1991) 293.

[1025] A. Guarino, et al., Production of *E. coli* STa-like heat stable enterotoxin by *Citrobacter freundii* isolated from humans, J. Clin. Microbiol. 25 (1987) 110.

[1026] B.A. Lipsky, et al., *Citrobacter* infections in humans: experience at the Seattle Veterans Administration Medical Center and a review of the literature, Rev. Infect. Dis. 2 (1980) 746.

[1027] R. Kahlich, J. Webershinke, A contribution to incidence and evaluation of *Citrobacter* findings in man, Cesk. Epidemiol. Mikrobiol. Imunol. 12 (1963) 55.

[1028] S.N. Parida, et al., An outbreak of diarrhea due to *Citrobacter freundii* in a neonatal special care nursery, Indian J. Pediatr. 47 (1980) 81.

[1029] M. Heitmann, P. Gerner-Smidt, O. Heltberg, Gastroenteritis caused by *Listeria monocytogenes* in a private day-care facility, Pediatr. Infect. Dis. J. 16 (1997) 827.

[1030] J. Sim, et al., Series of incidents of *Listeria monocytogenes* non-invasive febrile gastroenteritis involving ready-to-eat meats, Lett. Appl. Microbiol. 35 (2002) 409.

[1031] W. Schlech, *Listeria* gastroenteritis—old syndrome, new pathogen, N. Engl. J. Med. 336 (1997) 130.

[1032] E. Wing, S. Gregory, *Listeria monocytogenes*: clinical and experimental update, J. Infect. Dis. 185 (2002) S18.

[1033] P. Aureli, et al., An outbreak of febrile gastroenteritis associated with corn contaminated by *Listeria monocytogenes*, N. Engl. J. Med. 342 (2000) 1236.

[1034] C. Dalton, et al., An outbreak of gastroenteritis and fever due to *Listeria monocytogenes* in milk, N. Engl. J. Med. 336 (1997) 100.

[1035] H. Hof, R. Lampidis, J. Bensch, Nosocomial *Listeria* gastroenteritis in a newborn, confirmed by random amplification of polymorphic DNA, Clin. Microbiol. Infect. 6 (2000) 683.

[1036] S. Larsson, et al., *Listeria monocytogenes* causing hospital-acquired enterocolitis and meningitis in newborn infants, BMJ 2 (1978) 473.

[1037] M. Edelbroek, J. De Nef, J. Rajnherc, *Listeria* meningitis presenting as enteritis in a previously healthy infant: a case report, Eur. J. Pediatr. 153 (1994) 179.

[1038] H. Norys, Fetal chronic nonspecific enterocolitis with peritonitis in uniovular twins after *Listeria* infection in the mother, Monatsschr. Kinderheilkd. 108 (1960) 59.

[1039] R. Sack, et al., Isolation of enterotoxigenic *Bacteroides fragilis* from Bangladeshi children with diarrhea: a controlled study, J. Clin. Microbiol. 32 (1994) 960.

[1040] R. Sack, et al., Enterotoxigenic *Bacteroides fragilis*: epidemiologic studies of its role as a human diarrhoeal pathogen, J. Diarrhoeal. Dis. Res. 10 (1992) 4.

[1041] Y. Kubota, P.V. Liu, An enterotoxin of *Pseudomonas aeruginosa*, J. Infect. Dis. 123 (1971) 97.

[1042] D.C.J. Bassett, S.A.S. Thompson, B. Page, Neonatal infections with *Pseudomonas aeruginosa* associated with contaminated resuscitation equipment, Lancet 1 (1965) 781.

[1043] P.R. Ensign, C.A. Hunter, An epidemic of diarrhea in the newborn nursery caused by a milk-borne epidemic in the community, J. Pediatr. 29 (1946) 620.

[1044] D.P. Falcao, et al., Nursery outbreak of severe diarrhoea due to multiple strains of *Pseudomonas aeruginosa*, Lancet 2 (1972) 38.

[1045] A. Henderson, J. Maclaurin, J.M. Scott, *Pseudomonas* in a Glasgow baby unit, Lancet 2 (1969) 316.

[1046] C.H. Jellard, G.M. Churcher, An outbreak of *Pseudomonas aeruginosa* (pyocyanea) infection in a premature baby unit, with observations on the intestinal carriage of *Pseudomonas aeruginosa* in the newborn, J. Hyg. 65 (1967) 219.

[1047] B. Rowe, R.J. Gross, H.A. Allen, *Citrobacter koseri*. II. Serological and biochemical examination of *Citrobacter koseri* strains from clinical specimens, J. Hyg. 75 (1975) 129.

[1048] G.K. Kalashnikova, A.K. Lokosova, R.S. Sorokina, Concerning the etiological role of bacteria belonging to *Citrobacter* and *Hafnia* genera in children suffering from diseases accompanied by diarrhea, and some of their epidemiological peculiarities, Zh. Mikrobiol. Epidemiol. Immunobiol. 6 (1974) 78.

[1049] C.D. Graber, M.C. Dodd, The role of *Paracolobactrum* and *Proteus* in infantile diarrhea, Ann. N. Y. Acad. Sci. 66 (1956) 136.

[1050] E. Neter, M.L. Goodale, Peritonitis due to the *Morgani bacillus*. With a brief review of literature on the pathogenicity of this organism, Am. J. Dis. Child. 56 (1938) 1313.

[1051] E.R. Neter, R.H. Farrar, *Proteus vulgaris* and *Proteus morgani* in diarrheal disease of infants, Am. J. Dig. Dis. 10 (1943) 344.

[1052] E. Neter, N.C. Bender, *Bacillus morgani*, type I, in enterocolitis of infants, J. Pediatr. 19 (1941) 53.

[1053] G. Ujvary, et al., Beobachtungen über die Ätiologie der Gastroenterocolitiden des Säuglings- und Kindesalters. III. Untersuchung der Rolle der Proteus vulgaris- und der Proteus mirabilis-Stamme, Acta Microbiol. Acad. Sci. Hung. 10 (1964) 315.

[1054] H.L. Moffet, H.K. Shulenberger, E.R. Burkholder, Epidemiology and etiology of severe infantile diarrhea, J. Pediatr. 72 (1968) 1.

[1055] M.S. Mohieldin, et al., Bacteriological and clinical studies in infantile diarrhoea. II. Doubtful pathogens: Enterobacteriaceae, *Pseudomonas*, *Alcaligenes* and *Aeromonas*, J. Trop. Pediatr. 11 (1966) 88.

[1056] J.M. Singer, J. Bar-Hay, R. Hoenigsberg, The intestinal flora in the etiology of infantile infectious diarrhea, Am. J. Dis. Child. 89 (1955) 531.

[1057] S. Williams, The bacteriological considerations of infantile enteritis in Sydney, Med. J. Aust. 2 (1951) 107.

[1058] G. Ujvary, et al., Beobachtungen über die Ätiologie der Gastroenterocolitiden des Säuglings- und Kindesalters. IV. Untersuchung der Rolle der Proteus morgani-Stamme, Acta Microbiol. Acad. Sci. Hung. 10 (1964) 327.

[1059] M.E. Sharpe, Group D streptococci in the faeces of healthy infants and of infants with neonatal diarrhea, J. Hyg. 50 (1952) 209.

[1060] H. Kohler, P. Kite, Neonatal enteritis due to *Providencia* organisms, Arch. Dis. Child. 45 (1970) 709.

[1061] L.E.L. Ridge, M.E.M. Thomas, Infection with the Providence type of *Paracolon bacillus* in a residential nursery, J. Pathol. Bacteriol. 69 (1955) 335.

[1062] P. Bhat, R.M. Myers, R.A. Feldman, Providence group of organisms in the aetiology of juvenile diarrhoea, Indian. J. Med. Res. 59 (1971) 1010.

[1063] R.F. Bishop, G.L. Barnes, R.R.W. Townley, Microbial flora of stomach and small intestine in infantile gastroenteritis, Acta Paediatr. Scand. 63 (1974) 418.

[1064] L. Klingspor, et al., Infantile diarrhea and malnutrition associated with *Candida* in a developing community, Mycoses 36 (1993) 19.

[1065] A. Chaudhury, et al., Diarrhoea associated with *Candida* spp.: incidence and seasonal variation, J. Diarrhoeal. Dis. Res. 14 (1996) 110.

[1066] I. Enweani, C. Obi, M. Jokpeyibo, Prevalence of *Candida* species in Nigerian children with diarrhea, J. Diarrhoeal. Dis. Res. 12 (1994) 133.

[1067] K. Ponnuvel, et al., Role of *Candida* in indirect pathogenesis of antibiotic associated diarrhea in infants, Mycopathologia 135 (1996) 145.

[1068] I.U. Omoike, P.O. Abiodun, Upper small intestine microflora in diarrhea and malnutrition in Nigerian children, J. Pediatr. Gastroenterol. Nutr. 9 (1989) 314.

[1069] J.G. Kane, J.H. Chretien, V.F. Garagusi, Diarrhea caused by *Candida*, Lancet 1 (1976) 335.

[1070] F. VonGerloczy, K. Schmidt, M. Scholz, Beiträge zur Frage der Moniliasis in Säuglingsalter, Ann. Pediatr. (Paris). 187 (1956) 119.

[1071] H.R. Hill, et al., Recovery from disseminated candidiasis in a premature neonate, Pediatrics 53 (1974) 748.

[1072] R.G. Faix, Systemic *Candida* infections in infants in intensive care nurseries: high incidence of central nervous system involvement, J. Pediatr. 105 (1984) 616.

[1073] J.E. Baley, R.M. Kliegman, A.A. Fanaroff, Disseminated fungal infections in very low birth weight infants: clinical manifestations and epidemiology, Pediatrics 73 (1984) 144.

[1074] M.J. Struelens, et al., Bacteremia during diarrhea: incidence, etiology, risk factors, and outcome, Am. J. Epidemiol. 133 (1991) 451.

[1075] R. Rodriguez-García, et al., Prevalence and risk factors associated with intestinal parasitoses in pregnant women and their relation to the infant's birth weight, Ginecol. Obstet. Mex. 70 (2002) 338.

[1076] A. Guven, Amebiasis in the newborn, Indian J. Pediatr. 70 (2003) 437.

[1077] Z. Nazir, S.H. Qazi, Amebic liver abscesses among neonates can mimic bacterial sepsis, Pediatr. Infect. Dis. J. 24 (2005) 464.

[1078] J.H.M. Axton, Amoebic proctocolitis and liver abscess in a neonate, S. Afr. Med. J. 46 (1972) 258.

[1079] T. Botman, P.J. Rusy, Amoebic appendicitis in a newborn infant, Trop. Geogr. Med. 15 (1963) 221.

[1080] C.C. Hsiung, Amebiasis of the newborn: report of three cases, Chin. J. Pathol. 4 (1958) 14.

[1081] A.C. Dykes, et al., Extraintestinal amebiasis in infancy: report of three patients and epidemiologic investigations of their families, Pediatrics 65 (1980) 799.

[1082] N.A. Gomez, et al., Amebic liver abscess in newborn: report of a case, Acta Gastroenterol. Latinoam. 29 (1999) 115.

[1083] S. Rao, et al., Hepatic amebiasis: a reminder of the complications, Curr. Opin. Pediatr. 21 (2009) 145.

[1084] W. Rennert, C. Ray, Fulminant amebic colitis in a ten-day-old infant, Arch. Pediatr. 4 (1997) 92.

[1085] E. Kotcher, et al., Acquisition of intestinal parasites in newborn human infants, Fed. Proc. 24 (1965) 442.

[1086] J.I. Ravdin, Amebiasis, Clin. Infect. Dis. 20 (1995) 1453.

[1087] D. Mirelman, Y. Nuchamowitz, T. Stolarsky, Comparison of use of enzyme-linked immunosorbent assay-based kits and PCR amplification of rRNA genes for simultaneous detection of *Entamoeba histolytica* and *E. dispar*, J. Clin. Microbiol. 35 (1997) 2405.

[1088] R. Haque, I.K.M. Ali, W.A. Petri Jr., Comparison of PCR, isoenzyme analysis, and antigen detection for diagnosis of *Entamoeba histolytica* infection, J. Clin. Microbiol. 36 (1998) 449.

[1089] R.E. Black, et al., Giardiasis in day care centers: evidence of person-to-person transmission, Pediatrics 60 (1977) 486.

[1090] L.K. Keystone, S. Krajden, M.R. Warren, Person-to-person transmission of *G. lamblia* in day care nurseries, Can. Med. Assoc. J. 119 (1978) 241.

[1091] L.K. Pickering, et al., Diarrhea caused by *Shigella*, rotavirus, and *Giardia* in day care centers: prospective study, J. Pediatr. 99 (1981) 51.

[1092] L.K. Pickering, et al., Occurrence of *G. lamblia* in children in day care centers, J. Pediatr. 104 (1984) 522.

[1093] P.G. Miotti, et al., Age-related rate of seropositivity and antibody to *Giardia lamblia* in four diverse populations, J. Clin. Microbiol. 24 (1986) 972.

[1094] A. Islam, et al., *Giardia lamblia* infections in a cohort of Bangladeshi mothers and infants followed for one year, J. Pediatr. 103 (1983) 996.

[1095] R.D. Adam, The biology of *Giardia* spp, Microbiol. Rev. 55 (1991) 706.

[1096] L.K. Pickering, P.G. Engelkirk, *Giardia lamblia*, Pediatr. Clin. North. Am. 35 (1988) 565.

[1097] D. Gendrel, et al., Giardiasis and breastfeeding in urban Africa, Pediatr. Infect. Dis. J. 8 (1989) 58.

[1098] D.P. Stevens, D.M. Frank, Local immunity in murine giardiasis: is milk protective at the expense of maternal gut? Trans. Assoc. Am. Physicians 91 (1978) 268.

[1099] J.S. Andrews Jr., E.L. Hewlett, Protection against infection with *Giardia muris* by milk containing antibody to *Giardia*, J. Infect. Dis. 143 (1981) 242.

[1100] L. Rohrer, et al., Killing of *G. lamblia* by human milk mediated by unsaturated fatty acids, Antimicrob. Agents Chemother. 30 (1986) 254.

[1101] W.L. Current, L.S. Garcia, Cryptosporidiosis, Clin. Microbiol. Rev. 4 (1991) 325.

[1102] M.F. Heyworth, Immunology of *Giardia* and *Cryptosporidium* infections, J. Infect. Dis. 166 (1992) 465.

[1103] I.S. Wolfson, et al., Cryptosporidiosis in immunocompetent patients, N. Engl. J. Med. 312 (1985) 1278.

[1104] S. Tzipori, Cryptosporidiosis in animals and humans, Microbiol. Rev. 47 (1983) 84.

[1105] J.K. Stehr-Green, et al., Shedding of oocysts in immunocompetent individuals infected with *Cryptosporidium*, Am. J. Trop. Med. Hyg. 36 (1987) 338.

[1106] R. Soave, P. Ma, Cryptosporidiosis travelers' diarrhea in two families, Arch. Intern. Med. 145 (1985) 70.

[1107] A.C. Collier, R.A. Miller, J.D. Meyers, Cryptosporidiosis after marrow transplantation, person-to-person transmission and treatment with spiramycin, Ann. Intern. Med. 101 (1984) 205.

[1108] T.R. Navin, Cryptosporidiosis in humans: review of recent epidemiologic studies, Eur. J. Epidemiol. 1 (1985) 77.

[1109] G. Alpert, et al., Outbreak of cryptosporidiosis in a day care center, Pediatrics 77 (1986) 152.

[1110] J.P. Taylor, et al., Cryptosporidiosis outbreak in a day care center, Am. J. Dis. Child. 139 (1986) 1023.

[1111] N.J. Hoxie, et al., Cryptosporidiosis-associated mortality following a massive waterborne outbreak in Milwaukee, Wisconsin, Am. J. Public Health 87 (1997) 2032.

[1112] L. Jokipii, S. Pohiola, A.M. Jokipii, *Cryptosporidium*: a frequent finding in patients with gastrointestinal symptoms, Lancet 2 (1983) 358.

[1113] W.L. Current, et al., Human cryptosporidiosis in immunocompetent and immunodeficient persons: studies of an outbreak and experimental transmission, N. Engl. J. Med. 308 (1983) 1252.

[1114] J.S. Yoder, M.J. Beach, Cryptosporidiosis surveillance—United States 2003–2005, MMWR Surveill. Summ. 56 (2007) 1.

[1115] F.J. Enriquez, et al., *Cryptosporidium* infections in Mexican children: clinical, nutritional, enteropathogenic, and diagnostic evaluations, Am. J. Trop. Med. Hyg. 56 (1997) 254.

[1116] L. Mata, et al., Cryptosporidiosis in children from some highland Costa Rican rural and urban areas, Am. J. Trop. Med. Hyg. 33 (1984) 24.

[1117] L. Jokipii, A.M.M. Jokipii, Timing of symptoms and oocyst excretion in human cryptosporidiosis, N. Engl. J. Med. 313 (1986) 1643.

[1118] S. Sallon, et al., *Cryptosporidium*, malnutrition and chronic diarrhea in children, Am. J. Dis. Child. 142 (1988) 312.

[1119] L.S. Garcia, R.Y. Shimizu, Evaluation of nine immunoassay kits (enzyme immunoassay and direct fluorescence) for detection of *Giardia lamblia* and *Cryptosporidium parvum* in human fecal specimens, J. Clin. Microbiol. 35 (1997) 1526.

[1120] D.W. MacPherson, R. McQueen, Cryptosporidiosis: multiattribute evaluation of six diagnostic methods, J. Clin. Microbiol. 31 (1993) 198.

[1121] R. ten Hove, et al., Detection of diarrhoea-causing protozoa in general practice patients in The Netherlands by multiplex real-time PCR, Clin. Microbiol. Infect. 13 (2007) 1001.

[1122] F.J. Rossignol, A. Ayoub, M.S. Ayers, Treatment of diarrhea caused by *Cryptosporidium parvum*: a prospective of randomized, double-blind, placebo-controlled study of nitazoxanide, J. Infect. Dis. 184 (2001) 103.

[1123] D.G. Agnew, et al., Cryptosporidiosis in northeastern Brazilian children: association with increased diarrhea morbidity, J. Infect. Dis. 177 (1998) 754.

[1124] K. Pollock, et al., Cryptosporidiosis and filtration of water from Loch Lomond, Scotland, Emerg. Infect. Dis. 14 (2008) 115.

[1125] W.X. Cheng, et al., Human bocavirus in children hospitalized for acute gastroenteritis: a case-control study, Clin. Infect. Dis. 47 (2008) 161.

[1126] D.O. Matson, et al., Rotavirus, enteric adenoviruses, caliciviruses, astroviruses, and other viruses causing gastroenteritis, in: S. Spector, R.L. Hodinka, S.A. Young (Eds.), Clinical Virology Manual, third ed., ASM Press, Washington, DC, 2000, p. 270.

[1127] A.Z. Kapikian, R.M. Chanock, Rotaviruses, in: B.N. Fields et al., (Eds.), Fields Virology, third ed., Lippincott-Raven Press, Philadelphia, 1996, p. 1657.

[1128] M.K. Estes, Rotaviruses and their replication, in: B.N. Fields et al., (Eds.), Fields Virology, third ed., Lippincott-Raven Press, Philadelphia, 1996, p. 1625.

[1129] I. Wilhelmi, E. Roman, A. Sanchez-Fauquier, Viruses causing gastroenteritis, Clin. Microbiol. Infect. 9 (2003) 247.

[1130] J.C. Bridger, Non-group A rotavirus, in: M. Farthing (Ed.), Viruses in the Gut, Welwyn Garden City, UK, Smith Kline & French, 1988, p. 79.

[1131] U. Desselberger, Molecular epidemiology of rotavirus, in: M. Farthing (Ed.), Viruses in the Gut, Welwyn Garden City, UK, Smith Kline & French, 1988, p. 55.

[1132] Y. Hoshino, L.J. Saif, M.M. Sereno, Infection immunity of piglets to either VP3 or VP7 outer capsid protein confers resistance to challenge with a virulent rotavirus bearing the corresponding antigen, J. Virol. 62 (1988) 74.

[1133] P.A. Offit, H.F. Clark, G. Blavat, Reassortant rotavirus containing structural proteins VP3 and VP7 from different parents are protective against each parental strain, J. Virol. 57 (1986) 376.

[1134] Y. Zhou, et al., Distribution of human rotaviruses, especially G9 strains, in Japan from 1996 to 2000, Microbiol. Immunol. 162 (1990) 810.

[1135] M.L. O'Ryan, et al., Molecular epidemiology of rotavirus in children attending day care centers in Houston, J. Infect. Dis. 162 (1990) 810.

[1136] N. Santos, Y. Hoshino, Global distribution of rotavirus serotypes/genotypes and its implication for the development and implementation of an effective rotavirus vaccine, Rev. Med. Virol. 5 (2005) 29.

[1137] P. Kilgore, et al., Neonatal rotavirus infection in Bangladesh strain characterization and risk factors for nosocomial infection, Pediatr. Infect. Dis. J. 15 (1996) 672.

[1138] J.S. Tam, et al., Distinct populations of rotaviruses circulating among neonates and older infants, J. Clin. Microbiol. 28 (1990) 1033.

[1139] V. Jain, et al., Epidemiology of rotavirus in India, Indian J. Pediatr. 68 (2001) 855.

[1140] J.D. Mascarenhas, et al., Detection and characterization of rotavirus G and P types from children participating in a rotavirus vaccine trial in Belen, Brazil, Mem. Inst. Oswald. Cruz. 97 (2002) 113.

[1141] M.A. Widdowson, et al., An outbreak of diarrhea in a neonatal medium care unit caused by a novel strain of rotavirus: investigation using both epidemiological and microbiological methods, Infect. Control. Hosp. Epidemiol. 23 (2002) 665.

[1142] D. Steele, et al., Characterization of rotavirus infection in a hospital neonatal unit in Pretoria, South Africa, J. Trop. Pediatr. 48 (2002) 161.

[1143] A.C. Linhares, et al., Neonatal rotavirus infection in Belem, northern Brazil: nosocomial transmission of a P[6] G2 strain, J. Med. Virol. 67 (2002) 418.

[1144] N.A. Cunliffe, et al., Detection and characterization of rotaviruses in hospitalized neonates in Blantyre, Malawi, J. Clin. Microbiol. 40 (2002) 1534.

[1145] I. Banerjee, et al., Neonatal infection with G10P[11] rotavirus did not confer protection against subsequent rotavirus infection in a community cohort in Vellore, South India, J. Infect. Dis. 195 (2007) 611.

[1146] J.D. Mascarenhas, et al., Detection of a neonatal human rotavirus strain with VP4 and NSP4 genes of porcine origin, J. Med. Microbiol. 56 (2007) 524.

[1147] G.P. Davidson, et al., Importance of a new virus in acute sporadic enteritis in children, Lancet 1 (1975) 242.

[1148] R.F. Bishop, et al., Virus particles in epithelial cells of duodenal mucosa from children with acute nonbacterial gastroenteritis, Lancet 2 (1973) 1281.

[1149] I.H. Holmes, et al., Infantile enteritis viruses: morphogenesis and morphology, J. Virol. 16 (1975) 937.

[1150] H. Suzuki, T. Konno, Reovirus-like particles in jejunal mucosa of a Japanese infant with acute infectious nonbacterial gastroenteritis, Tohoku. J. Exp. Med. 115 (1975) 199.

[1151] D.Y. Graham, M.K. Estes, Comparison of methods for immunocytochemical detection of rotavirus infections, Infect. Immun. 26 (1979) 686.

[1152] I.H. Holmes, et al., Is lactase the receptor and uncoating enzyme for infantile enteritis (rota) viruses? Lancet 1 (1976) 1387.

[1153] R.W. Shepherd, et al., The mucosal lesion in viral enteritis: extent and dynamics of the epithelial response to virus invasion in transmissible gastroenteritis of piglets, Gastroenterology 76 (1979) 770.

[1154] D.J.S. Cameron, et al., Noncultivable viruses and neonatal diarrhea: fifteen-month survey in a newborn special care nursery, J. Clin. Microbiol. 8 (1978) 93.

[1155] E. Lebenthal, Lactose malabsorption and milk consumption in infants and children, Am. J. Dis. Child. 133 (1979) 21.

[1156] A.D. Philipps, Mechanisms of mucosal injury: human studies, in: M. Farthing (Ed.), Viruses in the Gut, Welwyn Garden City, UK, Smith Kline & French, 1988, p. 30.

[1157] R.W. Shepherd, et al., Determinants of diarrhea in viral enteritis: the role of ion transport and epithelial changes in the ileum in transmissible gastroenteritis in piglets, Gastroenterology 76 (1979) 20.

[1158] Y. Hoshino, et al., Identification of group A rotavirus genes associated with virulence of a porcine rotavirus and host range restriction of a human rotavirus in the gnotobiotic piglet model, Virology 209 (1995) 274.

[1159] F.T. Saulsbury, J.A. Winklestein, R.H. Yolken, Chronic rotavirus infection in immunodeficiency, J. Pediatr. 97 (1980) 61.

[1160] J. Stephen, Functional abnormalities in the intestine, in: M. Farthing (Ed.), Viruses in the Gut, Welwyn Garden City, UK, Smith Kline & French, 1988, p. 41.

[1161] O. Lundgren, et al., Role of the enteric nervous system in the fluid and electrolyte secretion of rotavirus diarrhea, Science 287 (2000) 491.

[1162] B. Kerzner, et al., Transmissible gastroenteritis: sodium transport and the intestinal epithelium during the course of viral gastroenteritis, Gastroenterology 72 (1977) 457.

[1163] D.G. Gall, et al., Na+ transport in jejunal crypt cells, Gastroenterology 72 (1977) 452.

[1164] J.M. Ball, et al., Age-dependent diarrhea induced by a rotaviral nonstructural glycoprotein, Science 272 (1996) 101.

[1165] M. Lorrot, M. Vasseur, How do the rotavirus NSP4 and bacterial enterotoxins lead differently to diarrhea? Virol. J. 4 (2007) 1.

[1166] R.L. Ward, et al., Attenuation of a human rotavirus vaccine candidate did not correlate with mutations in the NSP4 protein gene, J. Virol. 71 (1997) 6267.

[1167] M. Zhang, et al., Mutations in nonstructural glycoprotein NSP4 are associated with altered virus virulence, J. Virol. 72 (1998) 3666.

[1168] S.E. Blutt, et al., Rotavirus antigenemia in children is associated with viremia, PLoS. Med. 4 (2007) e121.

[1169] T.K. Fischer, et al., Rotavirus antigenemia in patients with acute gastroenteritis, J. Infect. Dis. 192 (2005) 913.

[1170] E. Chiappini, et al., Viremia and clinical manifestations in children with rotavirus infection, J. Infect. Dis. 193 (2006) 1333.

[1171] X.L. Huang, et al., Viraemia and extraintestinal involvement after rotavirus infection, Zhejiang. Da. Xue. Xue. Bao. Yi. Xue. Ban. 35 (2006) 69.

[1172] R.F. Bishop, et al., Clinical immunity after neonatal rotavirus infection: a prospective longitudinal study in young children, N. Engl. J. Med. 309 (1983) 72.

[1173] M.K. Bhan, et al., Protection conferred by neonatal rotavirus infection against subsequent rotavirus diarrhea, J. Infect. Dis. 168 (1993) 282.

[1174] S. Chiba, et al., Protective effect of naturally acquired homotypic and heterotypic rotavirus antibodies, Lancet 1 (1986) 417.

[1175] K.Y. Greene, A.Z. Kapikian, Identification of VP7 epitopes associated with protection against human rotavirus illness or shedding in volunteers, J. Virol. 66 (1992) 548.

[1176] K. Hjelt, et al., Protective effect of pre-existing rotavirus-specific immuno-globulin A against naturally acquired rotavirus infection in children, J. Med. Virol. 21 (1987) 39.

[1177] D.O. Matson, et al., Characterization of serum antibody responses to natural rotavirus infections in children by VP7-specific epitope-blocking assays, J. Clin. Microbiol. 30 (1992) 1056.

[1178] R.L. Ward, et al., Relative concentrations of serum neutralizing antibody to VP3 and VP7 protein in adults infected with human rotavirus, J. Virol. 62 (1988) 1543.

[1179] J.D. Clemens, et al., Seroepidemiologic evaluation of antibodies to rotavirus as correlates of the risk of clinically significant rotavirus diarrhea in rural Bangladesh, J. Infect. Dis. 165 (1992) 161.

[1180] D.O. Matson, et al., Fecal antibody responses to symptomatic and asymptomatic rotavirus infections, J. Infect. Dis. 167 (1993) 557.

[1181] M. O'Ryan, et al., Anti-rotavirus G type-specific and isotype-specific antibodies in children with natural rotavirus infections, J. Infect. Dis. 169 (1994) 504.

[1182] B.J. Zheng, et al., Prospective study of community-acquired rotavirus infection, J. Clin. Microbiol. 27 (1989) 2083.

[1183] R.L. Ward, et al., Evidence that protection against rotavirus diarrhea after natural infection is not dependent on serotype-specific neutralizing antibody, J. Infect. Dis. 166 (1992) 1251.

[1184] B.M. Totterdell, I.L. Chrystie, J.E. Banatvala, Cord blood and breast milk antibodies in neonatal rotavirus infection, BMJ 1 (1980) 828.

[1185] R.H. Yolken, et al., Epidemiology of human rotavirus types 1 and 2 as studied by enzyme-linked immunosorbent assay, N. Engl. J. Med. 299 (1978) 1156.

[1186] B. McLean, I.H. Holmes, Transfer of anti-rotaviral antibodies from mothers to their infants, J. Clin. Microbiol. 12 (1980) 320.

[1187] B.S. McLean, I.H. Holmes, Effects of antibodies, trypsin, and trypsin inhibitors on susceptibility of neonates to rotavirus infection, J. Clin. Microbiol. 13 (1981) 22.

[1188] H. Brussow, et al., Antibodies to seven rotavirus serotypes in cord sera, maternal sera, and colostrum of German women, J. Clin. Microbiol. 29 (1991) 2856.

[1189] H. Brussow, et al., Rotavirus-inhibitory activity in serial milk samples from Mexican women and rotavirus infections in their children during their first year of life, J. Clin. Microbiol. 31 (1993) 593.

[1190] R.H. Yolken, et al., Secretory antibody directed against rotavirus in human milk—measurement by means of enzyme-linked immunosorbent assay, J. Pediatr. 93 (1978) 916.

[1191] M. Santosham, et al., Neonatal rotavirus infection, Lancet 1 (1982) 1070.

[1192] C.R. Madeley, B.P. Cosgrove, E.J. Bell, Stool viruses in babies in Glasgow. 2. Investigation of normal newborns in hospital, J. Hyg. 81 (1978) 285.

[1193] J.F.T. Glasgow, et al., Nosocomial rotavirus gastroenteritis in a neonatal nursery, Ulster. Med. J. 47 (1978) 50.

[1194] D.J.S. Cameron, et al., New virus associated with diarrhoea in neonates, Med. J. Aust. 1 (1976) 85.

[1195] A.S. Bryden, et al., Rotavirus infections in a special-care baby unit, J. Infect. 4 (1982) 43.

[1196] L. Grillner, et al., Rotavirus infections in newborns: an epidemiological and clinical study, Scand. J. Infect. Dis. 17 (1985) 349.

[1197] B. Tufvesson, et al., A prospective study of rotavirus infections in neonatal and maternity wards, Acta Paediatr. Scand. 75 (1986) 211.

[1198] Y. Hoshino, et al., Serotypic characterization of rotaviruses derived from asymptomatic human neonatal infections, J. Clin. Microbiol. 21 (1985) 425.

[1199] E. Crewe, A.M. Murphy, Further studies on neonatal rotavirus infection, Med. J. Aust. 1 (1980) 61.

[1200] I. Perez-Schael, et al., Rotavirus shedding by newborn children, J. Med. Virol. 14 (1984) 127.

[1201] P.A. Vial, K.L. Kotloff, G.A. Losonsky, Molecular epidemiology of rotavirus infection in a room for convalescing newborns, J. Infect. Dis. 157 (1988) 668.

[1202] I.E. Haffejee, Neonatal rotavirus infections, Rev. Infect. Dis. 13 (1991) 957.

[1203] W.J. Rodriguez, et al., Rotavirus: a cause of nosocomial infection in a nursery, J. Pediatr. 101 (1982) 274.

[1204] E.S. Jesudoss, et al., Prevalence of rotavirus infection in neonates, Indian. J. Med. Res. 70 (1979) 863.

[1205] R.F. Bishop, et al., Diarrhea and rotavirus infection associated with differing regimens for postnatal care of newborn babies, J. Clin. Microbiol. 9 (1979) 525.

[1206] S. Ramani, et al., Rotavirus infection in the neonatal nurseries of a tertiary care hospital in India, Pediatr. Infect. Dis. J. 27 (2008) 719.

[1207] L.K. Pickering, et al., Asymptomatic rotavirus before and after rotavirus diarrhea in children in day care centers, J. Pediatr. 112 (1988) 361.

[1208] T. Vesikari, H.K. Sarkkinen, M. Maki, Quantitative aspects of rotavirus excretion in childhood diarrhoea, Acta Paediatr. Scand. 70 (1981) 717.

[1209] T. Konno, et al., Influence of temperature and relative humidity on human rotavirus infection in Japan, J. Infect. Dis. 147 (1983) 125.

[1210] A.V. Bartlett III., R.R. Reeves, L.K. Pickering, Rotavirus in infant-toddler day care centers: epidemiology relevant to disease control strategies, J. Pediatr. 113 (1988) 435.

[1211] D.O. Matson, et al., Serotype variation of human group A rotaviruses in two regions of the United States, J. Infect. Dis. 162 (1990) 605.

[1212] M.J. Ryan, et al., Hospital admissions attributable to rotavirus infection in England, J. Infect. Dis. 174 (Suppl. 1) (1996) S12.

[1213] R. Glass, et al., The epidemiology of rotavirus diarrhea in the United States: surveillance and estimates of disease burden, J. Infect. Dis. 74 (Suppl. 1) (1996) S5.

[1214] M. O'Ryan, et al., Rotavirus-associated medical visits and hospitalizations in South America: a prospective study at three large sentinel hospitals, Pediatr. Infect. Dis. J. 20 (2001) 685.

[1215] L.C. Duffy, et al., Modulation of rotavirus enteritis during breast-feeding, Am. J. Dis. Child. 140 (1986) 1164.

[1216] L. van Renterghem, P. Borre, J. Tilleman, Rotavirus and other viruses in the stool of premature babies, J. Med. Virol. 5 (1980) 137.

[1217] A.M. Murphy, M.B. Albrey, E.B. Crewe, Rotavirus infections in neonates, Lancet 2 (1977) 1149.

[1218] Y. Soenarto, et al., Acute diarrhea and rotavirus infection in newborn babies and children in Yogyakarta, Indonesia from June 1978 to June 1979, J. Clin. Microbiol. 14 (1981) 123.

[1219] H. Appleton, et al., A search for faecal viruses in newborn and other infants, J. Hyg. 81 (1978) 279.

[1220] R.D. Schnagl, F. Morey, I.H. Holmes, Rotavirus and coronavirus-like particles in aboriginal and non-aboriginal neonates in Kalgoorlie and Alice Springs, Med. J. Aust. 2 (1979) 178.

[1221] J. Dearlove, et al., Clinical range of neonatal rotavirus gastroenteritis, BMJ 286 (1983) 1473.

[1222] U.D. Parashar, et al., Epidemiology of diarrheal disease among children enrolled in four West Coast health maintenance organizations, Pediatr. Infect. Dis. J. 17 (1998) 605.

[1223] J.C. Leece, M.W. King, W.E. Dorsey, Rearing regimen producing piglet diarrhea (rotavirus) and its relevance to acute infantile diarrhea, Science 199 (1978) 776.

[1224] M. Santosham, et al., Detection of rotavirus in respiratory secretions of children with pneumonia, J. Pediatr. 103 (1983) 583.

[1225] D.S. Prince, et al., Aerosol transmission of experimental rotavirus infection, Pediatr. Infect. Dis. J. 5 (1986) 218.

[1226] A.D. Steele, J.J. Alexander, Molecular epidemiology of rotavirus in black infants in South Africa, J. Clin. Microbiol. 25 (1987) 2384.

[1227] W.J. Rodriguez, et al., Use of electrophoresis of RNA from human rotavirus to establish the identity of stains involved in outbreaks in a tertiary care nursery, J. Infect. Dis. 148 (1983) 34.

[1228] G. Srivinasan, et al., Rotavirus infection in a normal nursery: epidemic and surveillance, Infect. Control. 5 (1984) 478.

[1229] G. Gerna et al., Nosocomial outbreak of neonatal gastroenteritis caused by a new serotype 4, subtype 4B human rotavirus, J. Med. Virol. 31 (1990) 175.

[1230] S. Tallet, et al., Clinical, laboratory, and epidemiologic features of a viral gastroenteritis in infants and children, Pediatrics 60 (1977) 217.

[1231] J.P. Hieber, et al., Comparison of human rotavirus disease in tropical and temperate settings, Am. J. Dis. Child. 132 (1978) 853.

[1232] L.N. Mutanda, Epidemiology of acute gastroenteritis in early childhood in Kenya. VI. Some clinical and laboratory characteristics relative to the aetiological agents, East. Afr. Med. J. 57 (1980) 599.

[1233] R.K. Whyte, R. Homes, C.A. Pennock, Faecal excretion of oligosaccharides and other carbohydrates in normal neonates, Arch. Dis. Child. 53 (1978) 913.

[1234] J.S. Hyams, P.J. Krause, P.A. Gleason, Lactose malabsorption following rotavirus infection in young children, J. Pediatr. 99 (1981) 916.

[1235] U.D. Prashar, et al., Global illness and deaths caused by rotavirus disease in children, Emerg. Infect. Dis. 9 (2003) 565.

[1236] C. Dani, et al., A case of neonatal necrotizing enterocolitis due to rotavirus, Pediatr. Med. Chir. 16 (1994) 185.

[1237] A.R. Goma Brufau, et al., Epidemic outbreak of necrotizing enterocolitis coincident with an epidemic of neonatal rotavirus gastroenteritis, An. Esp. Pediatr. 29 (1988) 307.

[1238] F. Riedel, et al., Rotavirus infection and bradycardia-apnoea-episodes in the neonate, Eur. J. Pediatr. 155 (1996) 36.

[1239] T. Konno, et al., Human rotavirus infection in infants and young children with intussusception, J. Med. Virol. 2 (1978) 265.

[1240] D.L. Mulcahy, et al., A two-part study of the aetiological role of rotavirus in intussusception, J. Med. Virol. 9 (1982) 51.

[1241] J.C. Nicolas, et al., A one-year virological survey of acute intussusception in childhood, J. Med. Virol. 9 (1982) 267.

[1242] T.V. Murphy, et al., Intussusception among infants given an oral rotavirus vaccine, N. Engl. J. Med. 22 (2001) 564.

[1243] M.B. Rennels, et al., Lack of an apparent association between intussusception and wild or vaccine virus rotavirus infection, Pediatr. Infect. Dis. J. 17 (1998) 924.

[1244] P. Dennehy, et al., Evaluation of the inmunocardstat: rotavirus assay for detection of group A rotavirus in fecal specimens, J. Clin. Microbiol. 37 (1999) 1977.

[1245] M.J.R. Gilchrist, et al., Comparison of seven kits for detection of rotavirus in fecal specimens with a sensitive, specific enzyme immunoassay, Diagn. Microbiol. Infect. Dis. 8 (1987) 221.

[1246] C.V. Knisley, A. Bednarz-Prashad, L.K. Pickering, Detection of rotavirus in stool specimens with monoclonal and polyclonal antibody-based assay systems, J. Clin. Microbiol. 23 (1986) 897.

[1247] E.E. Thomas, et al., Evaluation of seven immunoassays for detection of rotavirus in pediatric stool samples, J. Clin. Microbiol. 26 (1988) 1189.

[1248] P.G. Miotti, J. Eiden, R.H. Yolken, Comparative efficacy of commercial immunoassays for the diagnosis of rotavirus gastroenteritis during the course of infection, J. Clin. Microbiol. 22 (1985) 693.

[1249] C.D. Brandt, et al., Comparison of direct electron microscopy, immune electron microscopy, and rotavirus enzyme-linked immunosorbent assay for detection of gastroenteritis viruses in children, J. Clin. Microbiol. 13 (1981) 976.

[1250] R.H. Yolken, et al., Enzyme-linked immunosorbent assay (ELISA) for detection of human reovirus-like agent of infantile gastroenteritis, Lancet 2 (1977) 263.

[1251] T.K. Fischer, H. Steinsland, P. Valentiner-Branth, Rotavirus particles can survive storage in ambient tropical temperatures for more than 2 months, J. Clin. Microbiol. 40 (2002) 4763.

[1252] B. Viera de Torres, R. Mazzali de Ilja, J. Esparza, Epidemiological aspects of rotavirus infection in hospitalized Venezuelan children with gastroenteritis, Am. J. Trop. Med. Hyg. 27 (1978) 567.

[1253] Provisional Committee on Quality Improvement, Subcommittee on Acute Gastroenteritis. Practice parameter: the management of acute gastroenteritis in young children, Pediatrics 97 (1996) 424.

[1254] D.A. Sack, et al., Oral hydration in rotavirus diarrhoea: a double-blind comparison of sucrose with glucose electrolyte solution, Lancet 2 (1978) 280.

[1255] R.E. Black, et al., Glucose vs. sucrose in oral rehydration solutions for infants and young children with rotavirus-associated diarrhea, Pediatrics 67 (1981) 79.

[1256] T. Ebina, et al., Passive immunizations of suckling mice and infants with bovine colostrum containing antibodies to human rotavirus, J. Med. Virol. 38 (1992) 117.

[1257] A. Guarino, et al., Enteral immunoglobulins for treatment of protracted rotaviral diarrhea, Pediatr. Infect. Dis. J. 10 (1991) 612.

[1258] O. Brunser, et al., Field trial of an infant formula containing anti-rotavirus and anti-*Escherichia coli* milk antibodies from hyperimmunized cows, J. Pediatr. Gastroenterol. Nutr. 15 (1992) 63.

[1259] V. Rosenfeldt, et al., Effect of probiotic *Lactobacillus* strains in young children hospitalized with acute diarrhea, Pediatr. Infect. Dis. J. 21 (2002) 411.

[1260] P. Mohan, K. Haque, Oral immunoglobulin for the treatment of rotavirus infection in low birth weight infants, Cochrane Database Syst. Rev. (3) (2003) CD003742.

[1261] C.J. Birch, et al., A study of the prevalence of rotavirus infection in children with gastroenteritis admitted to an infectious disease hospital, J. Med. Virol. 1 (1977) 69.

[1262] L.A. Kombo, et al., Intussusception, infection, and immunization: summary of a workshop on rotavirus, Pediatrics 108 (2001) E37.

[1263] G.M. Ruiz-Palacios, et al., Safety and efficacy of an attenuated vaccine against severe rotavirus gastroenteritis, N. Engl. J. Med. 354 (2006) 11.

[1264] T. Vesikari, et al., Safety and efficacy of a pentavalent human-bovine (WC3) reassortant rotavirus vaccine, N. Engl. J. Med. 354 (2006) 23.

[1265] A.C. Linhares, et al., Efficacy and safety of an oral live attenuated human rotavirus vaccine against rotavirus gastroenteritis during the first 2 years of life in Latin American infants: a randomised, double-blind, placebo-controlled phase III study, Lancet 5 (2008) 1181.

[1266] M. O'Ryan, Rotarix (RIX4414): an oral human rotavirus vaccine, Expert. Rev. Vaccines. 6 (2007) 11.

[1267] M. O'Ryan, D.O. Matson, New rotavirus vaccines: renewed optimism, J. Pediatr. 149 (2006) 448.

[1268] D.O. Matson, The pentavalent rotavirus vaccine, RotaTeq, Semin. Pediatr. Infect. Dis. 17 (2006) 195.

[1269] P.H. Dennehy, Rotavirus vaccines: an overview, Clin. Microbiol. Rev. 21 (2008) 198.

[1270] Centers for Disease Control and Prevention (CDC), Delayed onset and diminished magnitude of rotavirus activity—United States, November 2007–May 2008, MMWR. Morb. Mortal. Wkly. Rep. 57 (2008) 697.

[1271] A.M. Khan, A.S. Faruque, M.S. Hossain, Isolation of *Vibrio cholerae* from neonates admitted to an urban diarrhoeal diseases hospital in Bangladesh, Ann. Trop. Paediatr. 25 (2005) 179.

[1272] R.M. Srinivasjois, et al., Cytomegalovirus-associated ileal stricture in a preterm neonate, J. Pediatr. Child. Health. 44 (2008) 80.

[1273] S. Bina Rai, et al., An outbreak of echovirus 11 amongst neonates in a confinement home in Penang, Malaysia, Med. J. Malaysia. 62 (2007) 223.

[1274] W. Wilson, et al., Intractable diarrhea in a newborn infant: microvillous inclusion disease, Can. J. Gastroenterol. 15 (2001) 61.

[1275] E.M. Stockdale, C.A. Miller, Persistent diarrhea as the predominant symptom of Hirschsprung's disease (congenital dilatation of colon), Pediatrics 19 (1957) 91.

[1276] D.W. Wilmore, Factors correlating with a successful outcome following extensive intestinal resection in newborn infants, J. Pediatr. 80 (1972) 88.

[1277] M. Hasosah, et al., Congenital short bowel syndrome: a case report and review of the literature, Can. J. Gastroenterol. 22 (2008) 71.

[1278] D. Fried, A. Gotlieb, L. Zaidel, Intractable diarrhea of infancy due to lymphangiectasis, Am. J. Dis. Child. 127 (1974) 416.

[1279] E. Lebenthal, Small intestinal disaccharidase deficiency, Pediatr. Clin. North. Am. 22 (1975) 757.

[1280] M.E. Ament, D.R. Perera, L.J. Esther, Sucrase-isomaltose deficiency—a frequently misdiagnosed disease, J. Pediatr. 83 (1973) 721.

[1281] J.F. Marks, J.B. Norton, J.S. Fordtran, Glucose-galactose malabsorption, J. Pediatr. 69 (1969) 225.

[1282] V. Burke, C.M. Anderson, Sugar intolerance as a cause of protracted diarrhea following surgery of the gastrointestinal tract in neonates, Aust. Paediatr. J. 2 (1966) 219.

[1283] R.F. Bishop, et al., Virus particles in epithelial cells of duodenal mucosa from children with acute non-bacterial gastroenteritis, Lancet 2 (1973) 1281.

[1284] P. Coello-Ramirez, F. Lifshitz, V. Zuniga, Enteric microflora and carbohydrate intolerance in infants with diarrhea, Pediatrics 49 (1972) 233.

[1285] F. Akesode, F. Lifshitz, K.M. Hoffman, Transient monosaccharide intolerance in a newborn infant, Pediatrics 51 (1973) 891.

[1286] N. Iyngkaran, et al., Cow's milk protein–sensitive enteropathy: an important contributing cause of secondary sugar intolerance in young infants with acute infective enteritis, Arch. Dis. Child. 54 (1979) 39.

[1287] M.E. Ament, Malabsorption syndromes in infancy and childhood. I, II, J. Pediatr. 81 (1972) 685 867.

[1288] R.K. Whyte, R. Homer, C.A. Pennock, Faecal excretion of oligosaccharides and other carbohydrates in normal neonates, Arch. Dis. Child. 53 (1978) 913.

[1289] H. Schwachman, A. Redmond, K.T. Khaw, Studies in cystic fibrosis: report of 130 patients diagnosed under 3 months of age over a 20 year period, Pediatrics 46 (1970) 335.

[1290] P.J. Aggett, et al., Schwachman's syndrome: a review of 21 cases, Arch. Dis. Child. 55 (1980) 331.

[1291] C.B. Lilibridge, P.L. Townes, Physiologic deficiency of pancreatic amylase in infancy: a factor in iatrogenic diarrhea, J. Pediatr. 82 (1973) 279.

[1292] E. Lebenthal, I. Antonowicz, H. Schwachman, Enterokinase and trypsin activities in pancreatic insufficiency and diseases of the small intestine, Gastroenterology 70 (1979) 508.

[1293] G.K. Powell, L.A. Jones, J. Richardson, A new syndrome of bile acid deficiency—a possible synthetic defect, J. Pediatr. 83 (1973) 758.

[1294] J.K. Lloyd, Disorders of the serum lipoproteins. I. Lipoprotein deficiency states, Arch. Dis. Child. 43 (1968) 393.

[1295] R. Cash, C.K. Berger, Acrodermatitis enteropathica: defective metabolism of unsaturated fatty acids, J. Pediatr. 74 (1969) 717.

[1296] M. Garretts, M. Molokhia, Acrodermatitis enteropathica without hypozincemia, J. Pediatr. 91 (1977) 492.

[1297] E.W. McReynolds, S. Roy III., J.N. Etteldorf, Congenital chloride diarrhea, Am. J. Dis. Child. 127 (1974) 566.

[1298] A.M.B. Minford, D.G.D. Barr, Prostaglandin synthetase inhibitor in an infant with congenital chloride diarrhea, Arch. Dis. Child. 55 (1980) 70.

[1299] S. Hihnala, et al., Long-term clinical outcome in patients with congenital chloride diarrhea, J. Pediatr. Gastroenterol. Nutr. 42 (2006) 369.

[1300] J.C. Woodard, P.D. Webster, A.A. Carr, Primary hypomagnesemia with secondary hypocalcemia, diarrhea and insensitivity to parathyroid hormone, Am. J. Dig. Dis. 17 (1972) 612.

[1301] T. Iversen, Congenital adrenal hyperplasia with disturbed electrolyte regulation, Pediatrics 16 (1955) 875.

[1302] Y. Iida, et al., Watery diarrhoea with a vasoactive intestinal peptide-producing ganglioneuroblastoma, Arch. Dis. Child. 55 (1980) 929.

[1303] F.K. Ghishan, et al., Chronic diarrhea of infancy: nonbeta islet cell hyperplasia, Pediatrics 64 (1979) 46.

[1304] W. Storm, et al., Wolman's disease in an infant, Monatsschr. Kinderheilkd. 138 (1990) 88.

[1305] N. Hakami, et al., Neonatal megaloblastic anemia due to inherited transcobalamin II deficiency in 2 siblings, N. Engl. J. Med. 285 (1971) 1163.

[1306] A. Verloes, et al., Tricho-hepato-enteric syndrome: further delineation of a distinct syndrome with neonatal hemochromatosis phenotype, intractable diarrhea, and hair anomalies, Am. J. Med. Genet. 68 (1997) 391.

[1307] A.J. Jonas, I.J. Butler, Circumvention of defective neutral amino acid transport in Hartnup disease using tryptophan ethyl ester, J. Clin. Invest. 84 (1989) 200.

[1308] C. Holmberg, J. Perheentipa, Congenital Na+ diarrhea: a new type of secretory diarrhea, J. Pediatr. 106 (1985) 56.

[1309] N. Makita, et al., Human G_{ss} mutant causes pseudohypoparathyroidism type Ia/neonatal diarrhea, a potential cell-specific role of the palmitoylation cycle, Proc. Natl. Acad. Sci. U. S. A. 104 (2007) 17424.

[1310] S.L. Bayna, D.C. Heiner, Cow's milk allergy: manifestations, diagnosis and management, Adv. Pediatr. 25 (1978) 1.

[1311] J.B. Hwang, et al., Indexes of suspicion of typical cow's milk protein-induced enterocolitis, J. Korean. Med. Sci. 22 (2007) 993.

[1312] T.C. Halpin, W.J. Byrne, M.E. Ament, Colitis, persistent diarrhea, and soy protein intolerance, J. Pediatr. 91 (1977) 404.

[1313] G.K. Powell, Milk- and soy-induced enterocolitis of infancy: clinical features and standardization of challenge, J. Pediatr. 93 (1978) 553.

[1314] R.C. Miller, E. Larsen, Regional enteritis in early infancy, Am. J. Dis. Child. 122 (1971) 301.

[1315] G.B. Avery, M. Harkness, Bloody diarrhea in the newborn infant of a mother with ulcerative colitis, Pediatrics 34 (1964) 875.

[1316] S.H. Ein, M.J. Lynch, C.A. Stephens, Ulcerative colitis in children under one year: a twenty-year review, J. Pediatr. Surg. 6 (1971) 264.

[1317] P. Sunshine, F.R. Sinatra, C.H. Mitchell, Intractable diarrhoea of infancy, Clin. Gastroenterol. 6 (1977) 445.

[1318] G.B. Scott, et al., Acquired immunodeficiency syndrome in infants, N. Engl. J. Med. 310 (1984) 76.

[1319] M. Davidson, R. Wasserman, The irritable colon of childhood (chronic nonspecific diarrhea syndrome), J. Pediatr. 69 (1966) 1027.

[1320] T.J. Ochoa, E. Salazar-Lindo, T.G. Cleary, Management of children with infection-associated persistent diarrhea, Semin. Pediatr. Infect. Dis. 15 (2004) 229.

[1321] A 9-week-old boy with fever and diarrhoea, Tidsskr. Nor. Laegeforen. 127 (2007) 2386.

GROUP B STREPTOCOCCAL INFECTIONS

Morven S. Edwards ☉ Victor Nizet

CHAPTER OUTLINE

Organism   419
    Colonial Morphology and Identification   420
    Strains of Human and Bovine Origin   420
    Classification   420
    Ultrastructure   421
    Immunochemistry of Polysaccharide Antigens   421
    Growth Requirements and Bacterial Products   422
Epidemiology and Transmission   424
    Asymptomatic Infection (Colonization) in Adults   424
    Asymptomatic Infection in Infants and Children   425
    Transmission of Group B Streptococci to Neonates   426
    Serotype Distribution of Isolates   426
    Molecular Epidemiology   428
    Incidence of Infection in Neonates and Parturients   428
Immunology and Pathogenesis   429
    Host-Bacterial Interactions Related to Pathogenesis   429
    Host Factors Related to Pathogenesis   436
Pathology   439
Clinical Manifestations and Outcome   440
    Early-Onset Infection   440

Late-Onset Infection   442
    Late Late-Onset Infection   442
    Septic Arthritis and Osteomyelitis   443
    Cellulitis or Adenitis   443
    Unusual Manifestations of Infection   444
    Relapse or Recurrence of Infection   446
    Maternal Infections   446
Diagnosis   447
    Isolation and Identification of the Organism   447
    Differential Diagnosis   448
Treatment   448
    In Vitro Susceptibility   448
    Antimicrobial Therapy   449
    Supportive Management   450
    Adjunctive Therapies   451
Prognosis   451
Prevention   452
    Chemoprophylaxis   452
    Immunoprophylaxis   457

Lancefield group B β-hemolytic streptococci were first recorded as a cause of human infection in 1938, when Fry [1] described three patients with fatal puerperal sepsis. Sporadic cases were reported during the next 3 decades, but this microorganism remained unknown to most clinicians until the 1970s, when a dramatic increase in the incidence of septicemia and meningitis in neonates caused by group B streptococci (GBS) was documented from geographically diverse regions. [2–4] Emergence of group B streptococcal infections in neonates was accompanied by an increasing number of these infections in pregnant women and nonpregnant adults. In pregnant women, infection commonly manifested as localized uterine infection or chorioamnionitis, often with bacteremia, and had an almost uniformly good outcome with antimicrobial therapy. In other adults, who typically had underlying medical conditions, infection often resulted in death [5]. The incidence of perinatal infection associated with GBS remained stable through the early 1990s. Case-fatality rates had declined by then, but remained substantial compared with case-fatality rates reported for other invasive bacterial infections in infants.

Several notable events have occurred in recent years. Capsular type IX has been proposed, bringing the number of types causing invasive human disease to 10 [6]. The complete genomes of types III and V GBS have been sequenced, opening new avenues for the identification of novel potential vaccine targets [7,8]. The discovery that surface-associated pili are widely distributed among GBS and that a vaccine based on combinations of the three pilus-island variants protects mice against lethal challenge with a wide variety of group B streptococcal strains paves the way for the design of pilus-based and perhaps other putative surface protein vaccines for testing in humans [9–11].

The implementation of 2002 consensus guidelines to prevent early-onset disease in neonates through universal antenatal culture screening at 35 to 37 weeks' gestation and intrapartum antibiotic prophylaxis (IAP) has been associated with a substantial decline in the incidence of neonatal infection for the first time in 3 decades [12]. Finally, testing of group B streptococcal candidate vaccines in healthy adults has been achieved, offering promise that immunization to prevent maternal and infant and perhaps adult invasive group B streptococcal disease could become a reality.

ORGANISM

Streptococcus agalactiae is the species designation for streptococci belonging to Lancefield group B. This bacterium is a facultative gram-positive diplococcus with an ultrastructure similar to that of other gram-positive cocci. Before Lancefield's classification of hemolytic streptococci in 1933 [13], this microorganism was known to microbiologists by its characteristic colonial morphology,

DOI: 10.1016/B978-1-4160-6400-8.00012-2

its narrow zone of β-hemolysis surrounding colonies on blood agar plates, and its double zone of hemolysis that appeared when plates were refrigerated an additional 18 hours beyond the initial incubation [14]. Occasional strains (approximately 1%) are designated α-hemolytic or nonhemolytic. GBS are readily cultivated in various bacteriologic media. Isolation from certain body sites (respiratory, genital, and gastrointestinal tracts) can be enhanced by use of broth medium containing antimicrobial agents that inhibit growth of other bacterial species indigenous to these sites [15,16].

COLONIAL MORPHOLOGY AND IDENTIFICATION

Colonies of GBS grown on sheep blood agar medium are 3 to 4 mm in diameter, produce a narrow zone of β-hemolysis, are gray-white, and are flat and mucoid. β-hemolysis for some strains is apparent only when colonies are removed from the agar.

Tests for presumptive identification include bacitracin and sulfamethoxazole-trimethoprim disk susceptibility testing (92% to 98% of strains are resistant), hydrolysis of sodium hippurate broth (99% of strains are positive), hydrolysis of bile esculin agar (99% to 100% of strains fail to react), pigment production during anaerobic growth on certain media (96% to 98% of strains produce an orange pigment), and CAMP (Christie-Atkins-Munch-Petersen) testing (98% to 100% of strains are CAMP-positive) [17–19]. The CAMP factor is a thermostable extracellular protein that, in the presence of the β toxin of *Staphylococcus aureus*, produces synergistic hemolysis when grown on sheep blood agar. Hippurate hydrolysis is an accurate method for presumptive identification of GBS, but the requirement for 24 to 48 hours of incubation limits its usefulness. GBS can be differentiated from other streptococci by a combination of the CAMP test, the bile esculin reaction, and bacitracin sensitivity testing [17]. Biochemical micromethods identify GBS with reasonable accuracy after a 4-hour incubation period [20].

Definitive identification of GBS requires detection of the group B–specific antigen common to all strains through use of hyperimmune grouping antiserum. Lancefield's original method required acid treatment of large volumes of broth-grown cells to extract the group B antigen from the cell wall [21]. Supernatants were brought to neutral pH and mixed with hyperimmune rabbit antiserum prepared by immunization with the group B–variant strain (090R) (devoid of type Ia–specific antigen), and precipitins in capillary tubes were recorded. Less time-consuming serologic techniques are now employed, but all use group-specific antiserum to identify the group B antigen in intact cells, broth culture supernatants, or cell extracts. Commercial availability and simplicity make latex agglutination–based assays the most practical and frequently used methods by hospital laboratories [22]. Real time reverse transcriptase polymerase chain reaction (RT-PCR) methods have been developed more recently for grouping of clinical specimens, and PCR has been developed for genotyping of group B streptococcal isolates.

STRAINS OF HUMAN AND BOVINE ORIGIN

GBS were known to cause bovine mastitis before they were appreciated as pathogenic in humans [23]. Modern veterinary practices have largely controlled epidemics of bovine mastitis, but sporadic cases still occur. Substantial biochemical, serologic, and molecular differences exist between human and bovine isolates [24,25]. Among typable bovine strains, patterns of distribution distinct from the patterns of human isolates are noted. Other distinguishing characteristics for bovine strains include their unique fermentation reactions, their decreased frequency of pigment production, and their usual susceptibility to bacitracin. Protein X, rarely found in human strains, is commonly present in pathogenic bovine isolates [26].

CLASSIFICATION

Lancefield defined two cell wall carbohydrate antigens employing hydrochloric acid–extracted cell supernatants and hyperimmune rabbit antisera: the group B–specific or "C" substance common to all strains and the type-specific or "S" substance that allowed classification into types, initially types I, II, and III [27–29]. Strains designated as type I were later shown to have cross-reactive and antigenically distinct polysaccharides, and the antigenically distinct type Ia and type Ib polysaccharides were defined [28]. GBS historically designated type Ic were characterized when strains possessing type Ia capsular polysaccharide (CPS) were shown also to possess a protein antigen common to type Ib, most type II, and rarely type III strains [30]. This protein, originally called the "type Ib/c antigen," now is known as C protein. Rabbit antibodies directed against CPS protected mice against lethal challenge with homologous, but not heterologous, group B streptococcal types, and cross-protection was also afforded when antibodies against C protein were tested.

Current nomenclature designates polysaccharide antigens as type antigens and protein antigens as additional markers for characterization [31,32]. The former type Ic now is designated type Ia/c. Type IV was identified as a new type in 1979, when 62 strains were described that possessed type IV polysaccharide alone or with additional protein antigens [33]. Antigenically distinct types, V through IX, now are characterized. Strains not expressing one of the CPS-specific antigens are designated as nontypable by serologic methods, but often can be characterized by PCR-based methods.

Characterization of C protein showed that it is composed of two unrelated protein components, the trypsin-resistant α C protein and the trypsin-sensitive β C protein [34]. α C protein is expressed on many type Ia, Ib, and II strains [34]. Strains expressing α C protein are less readily opsonized, ingested, and killed by human polymorphonuclear leukocytes in the absence of specific antibody than are α C–negative strains [35]. α C protein consists of a series of tandem repeating units, and in naturally occurring strains, the repeat numbers can vary. The number of repeating units expressed alters antigenicity and influences the repertoires of antibodies elicited [36]. The use of one or two repeat units of α C proteins elicits antibodies that bind all α C proteins with equal affinity, suggesting its potential as a vaccine candidate [37,38].

β C protein is a single protein with a molecular mass of 124 to 134 kDa that is present in about 10% of isolates. β C protein binds the Fc region of human IgA [39–41]. Strains bearing α and β C proteins possess increased resistance to opsonization in vitro.

GBS express numerous additional surface proteins. Designation of additional α-like repetitive proteins (Alp) numerically (e.g., Alp2 and Alp3) is being considered. Most group B streptococcal strains have the gene for just one of the Alp family proteins. Genes encoding Alp1 (also designated "epsilon") are associated with type Ia, and genes encoding Alp3 are associated with type V strains [42]. Alp also are referred to as R proteins, of which R1 and R4 are the major ones found on clinical isolates [42]. Rib protein, expressed by most type III strains, has been shown to have an identical sequence to R4. The gene sequence of a protein initially designated R5 that is expressed by numerous clinically relevant group B streptococcal types has been sequenced and renamed group B protective surface protein [43]. Some GBS contain surface proteins designated as X antigens. These were first described by Pattison and coworkers [44], who introduced reagents for their detection in an attempt to classify nontypable strains further. The X and R antigens are immunologically cross-reactive. A laddering protein from type V GBS shares sequence homology with α C protein [45]. A protein designated Sip (for surface immunogenic protein) is distinct from other known surface proteins. It is produced by all serotypes of GBS and confers protection against experimental infection; its role in human infection is unknown [46].

Genome analysis has revealed that GBS produce long pilus-like structures. These structures extend from the bacterial surface and beyond CPS (Fig. 12–1) [9]. Formed by proteins with adhesive functions, these structures are implicated in host colonization, attachment, and invasion [47]. The pilus-like structures are encoded in genomic pilus islands that have an organization similar to that of pathogenicity islands. Three types of pilus island have been identified through genomic analysis; these are composed of partially homogeneous covalently linked proteins (pilus islands 1, 2a, and 2b). These pili proteins are highly surface-expressed and are involved in paracellular translocation through epithelial cells. At least one of these is present on all group B streptococcal clinical strains tested to date.

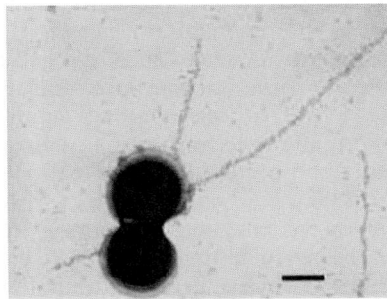

FIGURE 12–1 Immunogold labeling and transmission electron microscopy of group B streptococcal organisms showing long pilus-like structures extending from the cell surface. *(From Lauer P, et al. Genome analysis reveals pili in group B streptococcus. Science 309:105, 2005.).*

ULTRASTRUCTURE

Early concepts suggested a thick, rigid peptidoglycan layer external to the cytoplasmic membrane surrounded by concentric layers of cell wall antigens. The group-specific carbohydrate was thought to be "covered" by a type-specific CPS. Evidence now supports a model in which the group B carbohydrate and the CPS are linked independently to cell wall peptidoglycan [48].

Immunoelectron techniques reveal abundant CPS on Lancefield prototype strains Ia, II, and III, whereas less dense capsules are found on type Ib strains (Fig. 12–2) [49]. Similarly, incubation of the reference strains with homologous type-specific antisera reveals a thick capsular layer on types IV, V, and VI [50,51]. Ultrastructural studies show that the C protein also has a surface location [49]. CPS capsule expression can be regulated by altering cell growth rate [52]. Immunogold labeling and transmission electron microscopy show that the GBS pilus-like structures extend from the bacterial surface [9].

IMMUNOCHEMISTRY OF POLYSACCHARIDE ANTIGENS

Although Lancefield's initial serologic definition was achieved by extraction methods that employed 2N hydrochloric acid and heat treatment, these procedures resulted in degraded antigens of small molecular mass. When more gentle techniques were employed for extraction, large molecular mass or "native" polysaccharides were isolated that contained an additional antigenic determinant, N-acetylneuraminic acid or sialic acid. Human immunity has been shown to correlate with antibody to the sialic acid–containing type III structure [53]. The composition of the group B polysaccharide initially was determined using antigen extracted from whole cells of the Lancefield laboratory–adapted variant strain 090R, devoid of CPS. With the use of contemporary methods for determination, L-rhamnose, D-galactose, 2-acetamido-2-deoxy-D-glucose, and D-glucitol have been identified as its constituent monosaccharides. It is composed of four different oligosaccharides, designated I though IV, and linked by one type of phosphodiester bond to form a complex, highly branched multiantennary structure [54].

The repeating unit structures of the group B streptococcal CPS, determined by methylation analysis combined with gas-liquid chromatography/mass spectrometry, are schematically represented in Figure 12–3. CPS of types Ia, Ib, and III have a five-sugar repeating unit containing galactose, glucose, N-acetylglucosamine, and sialic acid in a ratio of 2:1:1:1 [53,55–57]. The type II and type V polysaccharides have a seven-sugar repeating unit; type IV and type VII polysaccharides have six-sugar repeats; and type VIII polysaccharide has a four-sugar repeating unit [50,58–62]. The molar ratios vary, but the component monosaccharides are the same among the polysaccharide types except that type VI lacks N-acetylglucosamine and type VIII contains rhamnose in the backbone structure [63].

Each antigen has a backbone repeating unit of two (Ia, Ib), four (II), or three (III, IV, V, VII, VIII) monosaccharides to which one or two side chains are linked. Sialic acid is the exclusive terminal side chain sugar except for

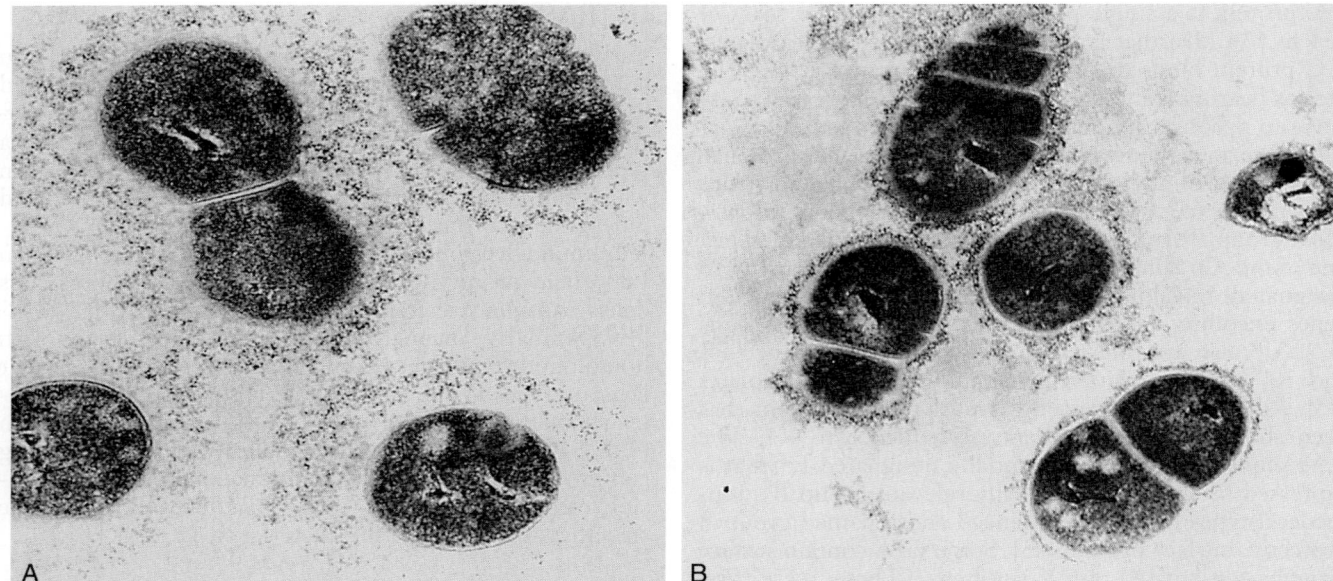

FIGURE 12–2 Electron micrographs of thin sections of type Ia group B streptococcal prototype strains. **A,** Strain 090. **B,** Strain A909. Both are stained with ferritin-conjugated type Ia–specific rabbit antibodies. The larger capsule is representative of those found also in Lancefield prototype II strain (18RS21) and type III isolates from infants with meningitis (M732), whereas the smaller capsule is representative of that also found on Lancefield prototype strain Ib (H36B). *(Micrographs courtesy of Dennis L. Kasper, MD.)*

the type II polysaccharide, which also has a terminal galactose. The structures of the type Ia and type Ib polysaccharides differ only in a single monosaccharide side chain linkage, although there are differences in the tertiary configuration of the molecules [64]. These monosaccharide linkages are critical to their immunologic specificity and explain their immunologic cross-reactivity [28,65]. The desialylated type III polysaccharide is immunologically identical to that of type 14 *Streptococcus pneumoniae* [66]. This observation stimulated investigations concerning the immunodeterminant specificity of human immunity to type III GBS and of antibody recognition of conformational epitopes as a facet of the host immune response [67,68]. The type III polysaccharide also can form extended helices. The position of the conformational epitope along these helices is potentially important to binding site interactions [69,70].

GROWTH REQUIREMENTS AND BACTERIAL PRODUCTS

GBS are quite homogeneous in their amino acid requirements during aerobic or anaerobic growth [71]. A glucose-rich environment enhances the number of viable GBS during stationary phase and the amount of CPS elaborated [72]. In a modified chemically defined medium, the expression of capsule during continuous growth is regulated by the growth rate [52]. Group B streptococcal invasiveness is enhanced by a fast growth rate and is optimal in the presence of at least 5% oxygen [73,74].

GBS elaborate many products during their growth, some of which contribute to virulence of the organism. Among these is the hemolysin that produces the β-hemolysis surrounding group B colonies on blood agar plates. Hemolysin is an extracellular product of almost all strains and is active against the erythrocytes from several mammalian species.

It has been isolated and characterized and is known to function as a virulence factor [75]. Hemolysin is not detected in supernatants of broth cultures, suggesting either that it exists in a cell-bound form, or that it is released by cells and rapidly inactivated.

After growth to stationary phase, GBS produce two types of pigment resembling a β-carotenoid [76]. Pigment, similar to hemolysin, is formed and released by an active metabolic process, retaining its properties only in the presence of a carrier molecule. A potential role for pigment as a virulence factor is proposed, but to date has not been proved.

GBS can hydrolyze hippuric acid to benzoic acid and glycine, and this property has been useful historically to distinguish GBS from other β-hemolytic groups [77]. Ferrieri and coworkers [78] isolated and characterized the hippuricase of GBS. This enzyme is cell associated and is trypsin and heat labile. It is antigenic in rabbits, but its relationship to bacterial virulence, if any, has not been studied.

Most strains of GBS have an enzyme that inactivates complement component C5a by cleaving a peptide at the carboxyl terminus [79]. Group B streptococcal C5a-ase seems to be a serine esterase; it is distinct from the C5a-cleaving enzyme (termed *streptococcal C5a peptidase*) produced by group A streptococci [80], although the genes that encode these enzymes are similar [81]. C5a-ase contributes to the pathogenesis of group B streptococcal disease by rapidly inactivating the neutrophil agonist C5a, preventing the accumulation of neutrophils at the site of infection [82].

Another group of enzymes elaborated by nearly all GBS are the extracellular nucleases [83]. Three distinct nucleases have been physically and immunologically characterized. All are maximally activated by divalent cations of calcium plus manganese. These nucleases are immunogenic in animals, and neutralizing antibodies to them are detectable in sera from pregnant women known to be

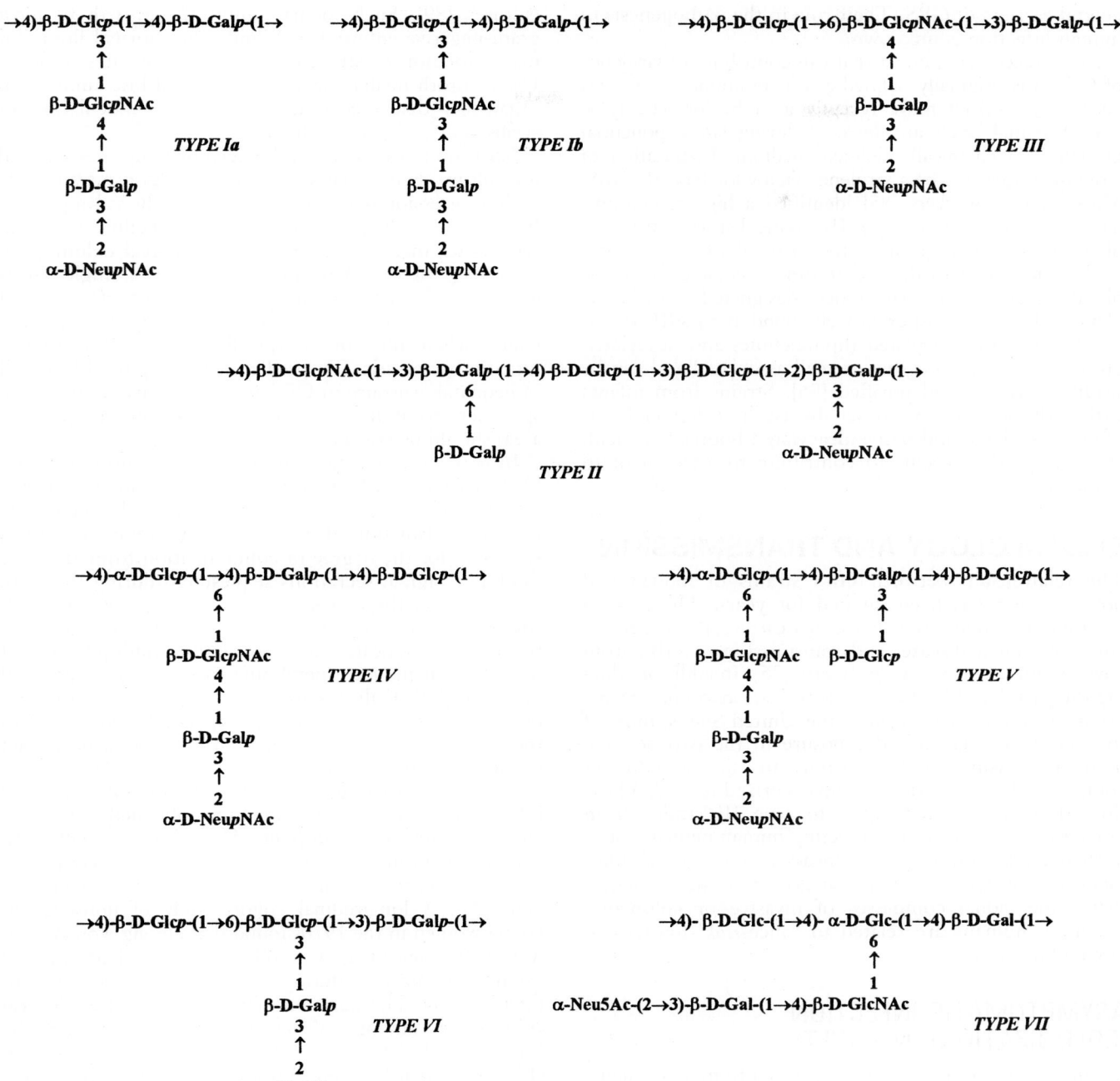

FIGURE 12–3 Repeating unit structures of group B streptococcal capsular polysaccharides type Ia [64], type Ib [64,65], type II [60,62], type III [56,57], type IV [61], type V [58], type VI [730], type VII [59], and type VIII [63].

genital carriers of GBS. Their role in the pathogenesis of human infection is unknown.

An extracellular product that can contribute to virulence of GBS was originally defined as a neuraminidase and has been characterized more recently as a hyaluronate lyase [84]. Maximal levels are detected during late exponential growth in a chemically defined medium. Elaboration of large quantities can be a virulence factor for type III GBS. Musser and coworkers [85] identified a high neuraminidase–producing subset of type III strains that were responsible for most serious group B streptococcal infections. Later studies indicated that these were from a single clonal complex designated ST 17 that has been designated as "hypervirulent." ST 17 is almost exclusively found in type III strains.

GBS synthesize acylated (lipoteichoic) and deacylated glycerol teichoic acids that are cell associated and can be readily extracted and purified [86]. Strains from infants with early-onset or late-onset disease have higher levels of cell-associated and native deacylated lipoteichoic acid, and this product seems to contribute to attachment to human cells [87].

EPIDEMIOLOGY AND TRANSMISSION

The relationship between GBS strains of human and bovine origin has been queried for years. There is no compelling evidence to suggest that cattle serve as a reservoir for human disease, and transmission of GBS from cows to humans is exceedingly rare [25]. In addition, during the past decades when group B *Streptococcus* has been a dominant human pathogen in the United States, most of the population has lacked exposure to the two possible modes of transmission: (1) proximity to dairy cattle (direct contact) and (2) ingestion of unpasteurized milk. Application of molecular techniques to type III strains from bovine sources and strains infecting human neonates supports the assertion that these lineages are unrelated. Phylogenetic lineage determination does indicate, however, that some clonal complexes of invasive or colonizing strains in humans are related to "ancestral" lineages of bovine GBS [88].

ASYMPTOMATIC INFECTION (COLONIZATION) IN ADULTS

Group B streptococcal infection limited to mucous membrane sites is designated as asymptomatic infection, colonization, or carriage. Comparisons of the prevalence of colonization are related to differences in ascertainment techniques. Factors that influence the accuracy of colonization detection include density of colonization, choice of bacteriologic media, body sites sampled, number of culture specimens obtained, and time interval of study.

Isolation rates are higher with use of broth rather than solid agar media, with media containing substances inhibitory for normal flora (usually antimicrobials), and with selective broth rather than selective solid agar media. Among selective broth media, Todd-Hewitt broth with gentamicin (4 to 8 μg/mL) or colistin (or polymyxin B) (10 μg/mL) and nalidixic acid (15 μg/mL) (Lim broth), with or without sheep red blood cells, has been useful for accurate detection of GBS from genital and rectal cultures [89]. Such media inhibit the growth of most gram-negative enteric bacilli and other normal flora that make isolation of streptococci from these sites difficult. Use of broth media enables detection of low numbers of organisms that escape detection when inoculation of swabs is directly onto solid agar.

Isolation rates also are influenced by body sites selected for culture. Female genital culture isolation rates double with progression from the cervical os to the vulva [90,91]. In addition, culture sampling of lower genital tract and rectal sites increases group B streptococcal colonization rates 10% to 15% beyond that found if a single site is cultured [92]. The urinary tract is an important site of group B streptococcal infection, especially during pregnancy, when infection is typically manifested as asymptomatic bacteriuria. To predict accurately the likelihood of neonatal exposure to GBS at delivery, maternal culture specimens from the lower vagina and rectum (not perianal area) should be collected.

In neonates, external auditory canal cultures are more likely to yield GBS than cultures from anterior nares, throat, umbilicus, or rectum in first 24 hours of life [3,93], and isolation of organisms from the ear canal is a surrogate for the degree of contamination from amniotic fluid and vaginal secretions sequestered during the birth process. After the first 48 hours of life, throat and rectal sites are the best sources for detection of GBS, and positive cultures indicate true colonization (multiplication of organisms at mucous membrane sites), not just maternal exposure [94]. Cultures from the throat and rectum are the best sites for detection during childhood and until the start of sexual activity, when the genitourinary tract becomes a common site of colonization [95,96].

The prevalence of group B streptococcal colonization is influenced by the number of cultures obtained from a site and the interval of sampling. Historically, longitudinal assessment during pregnancy defined vaginal colonization patterns as chronic, transient, intermittent, or indeterminant [97]. A longitudinal cohort study of nonpregnant young women in the 1970s found that among women who were culture-negative at enrollment, almost half acquired vaginal colonization during follow-up at three 4-month intervals [98]. The duration of any group B streptococcal colonization among college students was estimated by Foxman and colleagues [99] and is longer for women (14 weeks) than for men (9 weeks). Nearly half of women vaginally colonized at delivery have had negative antenatal culture results. In a more recent longitudinal study of pregnant women, the predictive value of a positive prenatal vaginal or rectal culture from the second trimester for colonization at delivery was 67% [100]. The predictive value of a positive prenatal culture result is highest (73%) in women with vaginal and rectal colonization and lowest (60%) in women with rectal colonization only. Cultures performed 1 to 5 weeks before delivery are fairly accurate in predicting group B streptococcal colonization status at delivery in term parturients. Within this interval, the positive predictive value is 87% (95% confidence interval 83 to 92), and the negative predictive value is 96% (95% confidence interval 95 to 98). Culture specimens collected within this interval perform significantly better than specimens collected 6 or more weeks before delivery [101].

The primary reservoir for GBS is the lower gastrointestinal tract [3,102]. The recovery of GBS from the rectum alone is three to five times more common than recovery from the vagina [92], the rectal-to-vaginal isolation ratio exceeds 1 [100], and the rectal site more accurately predicts persistence [92] or chronicity of carriage [103]. Fecal carriage or rectal colonization with GBS has been documented in individuals ranging in age from 1 day to 80 years [104]. Additional support for the intestine as the primary reservoir of colonization by GBS includes their isolation from the small intestine of adults [105] and their association with infections resulting from surgery of the upper or lower intestinal tract [106]. Rectal colonization also can contribute to the resistance of genital tract colonization to temporary decolonization by antibiotics [107].

Several factors influence genital carriage of GBS. Among healthy young men and women living in a college dormitory, sexually experienced subjects had twice the colonization rates of sexually inexperienced subjects [108]. In a longitudinal cohort study of nonpregnant young women, African American ethnicity, having multiple sex partners during a preceding 4-month interval, having frequent sexual intercourse within the same interval, and having sexual intercourse within the 5 days before a follow-up visit were independently associated with vaginal acquisition of GBS [98]. These findings suggest either that the organism is sexually transmitted or that sexual activity alters the microenvironment to make it more permissive to colonization. In another study of college women, GBS were isolated significantly more often from sexually experienced women, women studied during the first half of the menstrual cycle, women with an intrauterine device, and women 20 years old or younger [109]. Colonization with GBS also occurs at a high rate in healthy college students and is associated with having engaged in sexual activity, tampon use, milk consumption, and hand washing done four times daily or less [110]. Fish consumption increased the risk of acquiring some, but not all, capsular types [111].

A higher prevalence of colonization with GBS has been found among pregnant diabetic patients than among nondiabetic controls [112]. Carriage over a prolonged interval reportedly occurs more often in women who use tampons than women who do not [113]. Colonization is more frequent among teenage women than among women 20 years of age or older [97,109,114] and among women with three or fewer pregnancies than in women with more than three pregnancies [97,114,115]. Genital isolation rates are significantly greater in patients attending sexually transmitted disease clinics than in patients attending other outpatient facilities [90,116]. Ethnicity is related to colonization rates. In one large multicenter U.S. pregnancy study, colonization rates were highest in Hispanic women of Caribbean origin, followed by African Americans, whites, and other Hispanics [115]. In other assessments of geographically and ethnically diverse populations, the rate of colonization at delivery was significantly higher among African American women than in other racial or ethnic groups [98,117,118]. A large inoculum of vaginal group B streptococcal colonization also was more common among African American than among Hispanic or non-Hispanic white women [119].

Factors that do *not* influence the prevalence of genital colonization in nonpregnant women include use of oral contraceptives [109]; marital status; presence of vaginal discharge or other gynecologic signs or symptoms [109]; carriage of *Chlamydia trachomatis*, *Ureaplasma urealyticum*, *Trichomonas vaginalis*, or *Mycoplasma hominis* [115]; and infection with *Neisseria gonorrhoeae* [90,91].

Colonization with GBS can elicit an immune response. In a group of pregnant women evaluated at the time of admission for delivery, vaginal or rectal colonization with serotype Ia, II, III, or V was associated with significantly higher serum concentrations of IgG specific for the colonizing CPS type compared with noncolonized women [117]. Moderate concentrations of Ia, Ib, II, III, and V CPS-specific IgG also were found in association with colonization during pregnancy [120]. Maternal colonization with type III was least likely to be associated with these CPS-specific antibodies. In contrast to infection with organisms such as *N. gonorrhoeae* or genital mycoplasmas, genital infection with GBS is not related to genital symptoms [109,116,121].

GBS have been isolated from vaginal or rectal sites or both in 15% to 40% of pregnant women. These variations in colonization rates relate to intrinsic differences in populations (age, ethnicity, parity, socioeconomic status, geographic location) and to lack of standardization in culture methods employed for ascertainment. True population differences account for some of the disparity in these reported prevalence rates. When selective broth media are used, and vaginal and rectal samples are cultured, the overall prevalence of maternal colonization with GBS by region is 12% in India and Pakistan, 19% in Asia and the Pacific Islands, 19% in sub-Saharan Africa, 22% in the Middle East and North Africa, 14% in Central and South America, and 26% in the United States [117,122]. The reported rates of colonization among pregnant women range from 20% to 29% in eastern Europe, 11% to 21% in western Europe, 21% to 36% in Scandinavia, and 7% to 32% in the southern part of Europe [123]. The rate of persistence of group B streptococcal colonization in a subsequent pregnancy is higher compared with women negative for colonization in their prior pregnancy [124]. The prevalence rates of pharyngeal colonization among pregnant and nonpregnant women and heterosexual men are similar [3,125,126]; however, the rate approaches nearly 20% in men who have sex with men [127]. No definite relationship between isolation of GBS from throat cultures of adults or children and symptoms of pharyngitis has been proved [128], but some investigators have suggested that these organisms can cause acute pharyngitis [126].

ASYMPTOMATIC INFECTION IN INFANTS AND CHILDREN

Sites of colonization with GBS differ in children versus adults. In a study of 100 girls ranging in age from 2 months to 16 years, Hammerschlag and coworkers [95] isolated GBS from lower vaginal, rectal, or pharyngeal sites, or all three, in 20% of children. The prevalence of positive pharyngeal cultures resembled the prevalence of adults in girls 11 years or older (5%), but approached the prevalence reported for neonates in younger girls (15%). Rectal colonization was detected frequently in girls younger than 3 or older than 10 years of age (about 25%), but was uncommon in girls 3 to 10 years of age. Mauer and colleagues [96] isolated GBS from cultures of vaginal, anal, or pharyngeal specimens or all three in 11% of prepubertal boys and girls. Pharyngeal (5% each) and rectal (10% and 7%) isolation rates were similar for boys and for girls. Persson and coworkers [129] detected fecal group B streptococcal carriage in only 4% of healthy boys and girls, and Cummings and Ross [130] found that only 2% of English schoolchildren had pharyngeal carriage. Taken together, these findings indicate that the gastrointestinal tract is a frequent site for carriage during infancy and childhood in boys and girls, and genital colonization in girls is uncommon before puberty [131]. Whether this relates to environmental influences in the prepubertal vagina or to lack of sexual experience before puberty, or both, awaits further study.

TRANSMISSION OF GROUP B STREPTOCOCCI TO NEONATES

The presence of GBS in the maternal genital tract at delivery is the significant determinant of colonization and infection in the neonate. Exposure of the neonate to the organism occurs by the ascending route in utero through translocation through intact membranes, through ruptured membranes, or by contamination during passage via the birth canal. Prospective studies have indicated vertical transmission rates of 29% to 85%, with a mean rate of approximately 50% among neonates born to women from whom GBS were isolated from cultures of vagina or rectum or both at delivery. Conversely, only about 5% of infants delivered to culture-negative women become asymptomatically colonized at one or more sites during the first 48 hours of life.

The risk of a neonate acquiring colonization by the vertical route correlates directly with the density of colonization (inoculum size). Neonates born to heavily colonized women are more likely to acquire carriage at mucous membrane sites than neonates born to women with low colony counts of GBS in vaginal cultures at delivery [132]. Boyer and associates [100] found that rates of vertical transmission were substantially higher in women with heavy than in women with light colonization (65% versus 17%) and that colonization at multiple sites and development of early-onset disease were more likely among infants born to heavily colonized mothers. The likelihood of colonization in a neonate born to a woman who is culture-positive at delivery is unrelated to maternal age, race, parity, or blood type or to duration of labor or method of delivery [100]. It is unclear whether preterm or low birth weight neonates are at higher risk for colonization from maternal sources than term infants.

Most neonates exposed through their mothers to GBS have infection that is limited to surface or mucous membrane sites (colonization) that results from contamination of the oropharynx, gastric contents, or gastrointestinal tract by swallowing of infected amniotic fluid or maternal vaginal secretions. Healthy infants colonized from a maternal source show persistence of infection at mucous membrane sites for weeks [133,134]. The distribution of CPS types in group B streptococcal isolates from mothers is comparable to that in isolates from healthy neonates.

Other sources for group B streptococcal colonization in neonates have been established. Horizontal transmission from hospital or community sources to neonates is an important, albeit less frequently proved, mode for transmission of infection [105,134]. Cross-contamination from maternally infected to uninfected neonates can occur from hands of nursery personnel [135]. In contrast to group A streptococci, which can produce epidemic disease in nurseries, GBS rarely exhibit this potential, and isolation of neonates with a positive culture result from skin, umbilical, throat, or gastric cultures is never indicated. An epidemic cluster of five infants with late-onset bacteremic infection related to type Ib GBS occurred among very low birth weight infants in a neonatal intensive care unit in the 1980s [136]. None of the index cases was colonized at birth, establishing that acquisition during hospitalization had occurred. Phage typing identified two overlapping patterns of susceptibility believed to represent a single epidemic strain. Epidemiologic analysis suggested infant-to-infant spread by means of the hands of personnel, although acquisition from two nurses colonized with the same phage–type Ib strain was not excluded. The infection control measures instituted prevented additional cases. This and other reports [135,137] indicate that cohorting of culture-positive infants during an outbreak coupled with implementation of strict hand hygiene for infant contact significantly diminishes nosocomial acquisition.

Community sources afford potential for transmission of GBS to the neonate. Indirect evidence has suggested that this mode of infection is infrequent [134]. Only 2 of 46 neonates culture-negative for GBS when discharged from the newborn nursery acquired mucous membrane infection at 2 months of age [138]. The mode of transmission likely is fecal-oral. Whether acquired by vertical or horizontal mode, colonization of mucous membrane sites in neonates and young infants usually persists for weeks or months [139].

SEROTYPE DISTRIBUTION OF ISOLATES

The differentiation of GBS into types based on CPS antigens has provided a valuable tool in defining the epidemiology of human infection. In the 1970s and 1980s, virtually all evaluations of GBS isolated from healthy neonates, children, or adults revealed an even distribution into types Ia or Ib, II, and III. This distribution also was reported for isolates from neonates with early-onset infection without meningitis and their mothers [140,141]. In 1990, types other than I, II, or III accounted for less than 5% of all isolates.

Beginning in the early 1990s, reports from diverse geographic regions documented type V as a frequent cause of colonization and invasive disease, first in neonates and later in adults [142–144]. The emergence of type V is not due to a single clone, but most type V isolates do have one pulse-field gel electrophoresis pattern that has been present in the United States since 1975 [145]. Type V now causes a substantial proportion of cases of early-onset disease and of infection among pregnant women. Type Ia has increased in prevalence and a corresponding decline has occurred in type II strains causing perinatal disease [143]. Type III strains, which account for about 70% of isolates from infants with meningitis, continue to be isolated from about two thirds of infants with late-onset disease [146,147]. Types VI, VII, VIII, and IX rarely cause human disease in the United States or the United Kingdom, but types VI and VIII are the most common serotypes isolated from healthy Japanese women [148,149].

The contemporary CPS type distribution of GBS from different patient groups is shown in Figure 12–4. Prospective population-based surveillance through the Active Bacterial Core Surveillance/Emerging Infections Program Network of the U.S. Centers for Disease Control and Prevention (CDC) defined the epidemiology of invasive group B streptococcal disease in the United States from 1999-2005 [150]. Serotyping was performed for greater than 6000 isolates. Among these, the group B streptococcal types represented in 528 early-onset disease cases were Ia (30%), III (28%), V (18%), and II (13%). The distribution for 172 pregnancy-associated cases was similar. The type distribution among 469 late-onset cases was Ia (24%), III (51%), and V (14%). Type V predominated among almost 5000 cases in nonpregnant adults, accounting for 31% of cases, followed by Ia (24%), II (12%), and III (12%).

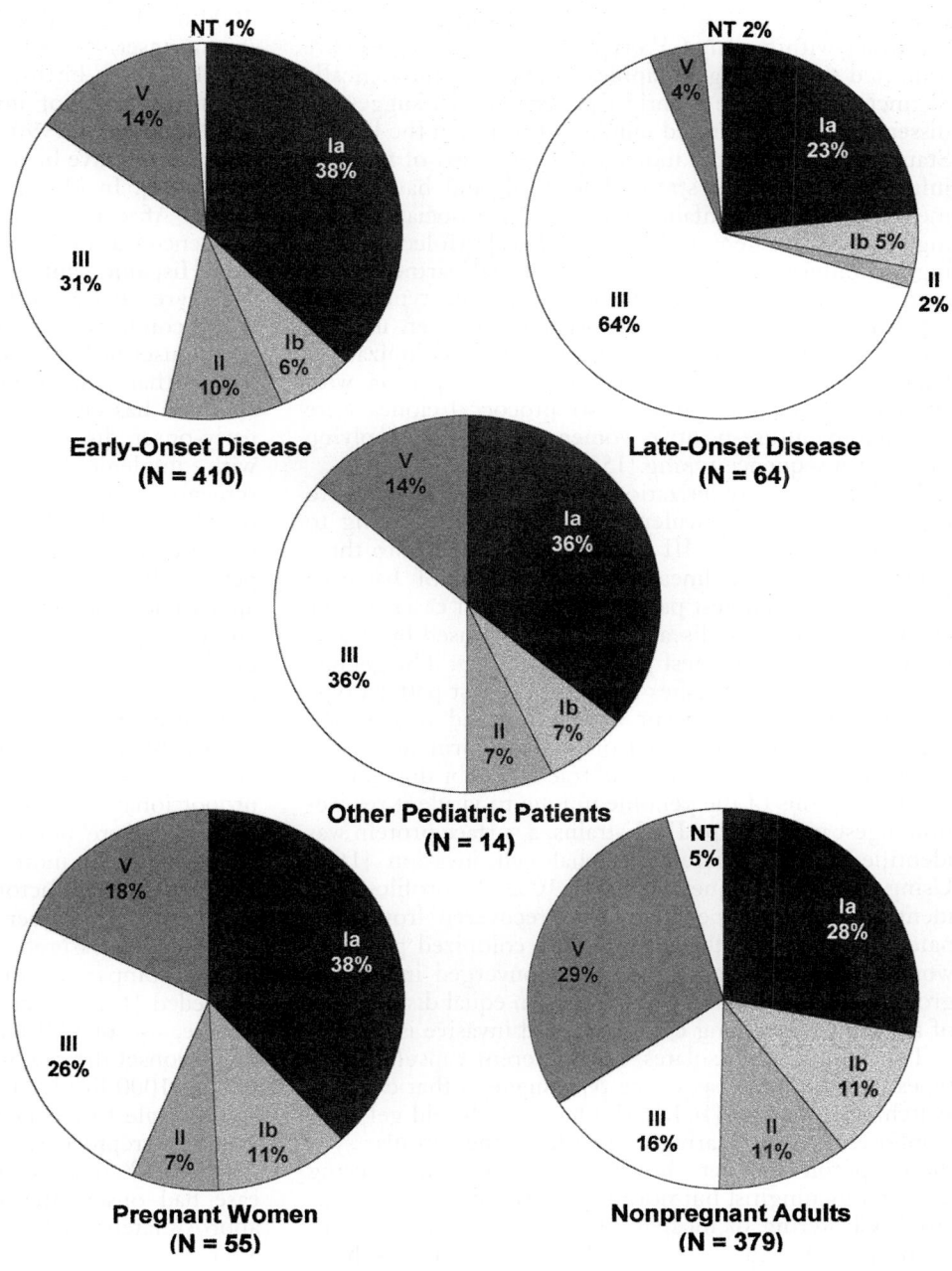

FIGURE 12–4 Schematic representation of group B streptococcal serotypes isolated from various patient groups. N, number of patient isolates studied; NT, nontypable strains. (*Data from references [142,143,699,731].*)

MOLECULAR EPIDEMIOLOGY

In the 1970s and 1980s, epidemiologic investigation of group B streptococcal infections was hampered initially by the lack of a discriminatory typing system. Initial investigations employed phage typing in combination with serologic classification to discriminate between infant acquisition of GBS from maternal or nosocomial sources [151]. Although plasmids have been described in a few GBS [152], their use as epidemiologic markers is complex.

Tools such as multilocus enzyme electrophoresis [85,153,154], restriction enzyme fragment length polymorphism analysis, pulsed-field gel electrophoresis [155], and a random-amplified polymorphic DNA assay [156] have been employed for molecular characterization of group B streptococcal isolates associated with human disease. Restriction enzyme fragment length polymorphism analysis no longer is used because there are allelic variations within some CPS types. These techniques have indicated that some geographically and epidemiologically distinct isolates have identical patterns [157], suggesting dissemination of a limited number of clones in the United States; have shown the molecular relatedness of mother-infant and twin-twin strains [148,156]; and have documented mother-to-infant transmission associated with ingestion of infected mother's milk [157]. Molecular typing techniques have confirmed that sexual partners often carry identical strains. Multilocus sequence typing and capsular gene cluster (*cps*) genotyping has been used to investigate the dynamics of perinatal colonization. Changes in capsule expression and recolonization with antigenically distinct group B streptococcal clones were detected in culture-positive women over time by applying multilocus sequence typing [158].

Molecular characterization has been employed to explore the role of virulence clones in contributing to invasive disease. Type III GBS were classified into three major phylogenetic lineages on the basis of bacterial DNA restriction digest patterns [159]. Most cases of type III neonatal invasive disease seem to be caused by strains with the restriction digest pattern type III-3. The genetic variation that distinguishes restriction digest pattern type III-3 strains seems to occur within localized areas of the genome that contain known or putative virulence genes [160–162]. Using genomic subtractive hybridization to identify regions of the genome unique to virulent restriction digest pattern type III-3 strains, a surface protein was identified that mediates epithelial cell invasion [163]. Using multilocus sequence typing, 10 allelic profiles were identified among type III isolates recovered from neonates with invasive disease and from colonized pregnant women [164]. The allelic profiles converged into three groups on concatenation. There was an equal distribution of these groups among colonizing and invasive isolates.

The finding that isolates with different capsular serotypes have the same sequence type suggests that capsular switching can occur [164,165]. One pulsed-field gel electrophoresis group bearing a gene from the capsular synthesis operon has been shown in type III strains causing neonatal meningitis, but not in type III colonizing strains [166]. Clustering of most invasive neonatal isolates into major pulsed-field gel electrophoresis groups has been noted [167]. Also, among type III strains evaluated by multilocus sequence typing, a single clone, ST 17, also called clonal complex 1 by other investigators, has been reported to be "hypervirulent," but this is controversial. Additional studies are required to elucidate the differences in virulence among clones identified by these techniques [168].

INCIDENCE OF INFECTION IN NEONATES AND PARTURIENTS

Two clinical syndromes occur among young infants with group B streptococcal disease that are epidemiologically distinct and relate to age at onset [2,3]. Historically, the attack rates for the first of these syndromes, designated early-onset because it occurs within the first 6 days of life (mean onset 12 to 18 hours), ranged from 0.7 to 3.7 per 1000 live births. The attack rates for late-onset infection (mean onset 7 to 89 days of age) ranged from 0.5 to 1.8 per 1000 live births. Multistate active surveillance that identified cases of invasive disease in a population of 10.1 million in 1990 reported an incidence of 1.6 and 0.3 per 1000 live births for early-onset and late-onset disease [169]. Incidence of disease was significantly higher among African Americans than among whites. The crude incidence was higher among Hispanic whites than among non-Hispanic whites. These multistate surveillance findings are in accord with findings from a cohort study conducted in Atlanta indicating a higher risk for early-onset or late-onset disease among African American infants than among infants of other ethnic origins [170].

There has been a dramatic decline in the incidence of early-onset disease in the United States in association with implementation of universal antenatal culture screening and use of IAP. From 1993-1998, when risk-based and culture-based methods were in use, incidence of early-onset disease declined by 65%, from 1.7 to 0.6 per 1000 live births [12]. Comparison of the two approaches showed the superiority of the culture-based approach [171]. The incidence of early-onset disease has declined an additional 27% in association with implementation in 2002 of revised consensus guidelines advocating a culture-based approach for prevention of early-onset disease to a rate of 0.34 per 1000 live births in 2007 [150]. The burden of early-onset disease initially was disproportionately high in African American infants for reasons that were not well defined and then decreased in 2003-2005, but more recent data indicate reemergence of this disparity. Factors that might contribute to the disparity include higher maternal colonization rates and higher rates of preterm deliveries in African American women compared with white women, but additional study is needed [172]. In contrast to its impact on early-onset disease, use of IAP has had *no* impact on the incidence of late-onset disease, which has remained stable at 0.3 to 0.4 per 1000 live births since 2002 [150].

The male-to-female ratio for early-onset and late-onset group B streptococcal disease is equal at 1:1. Before 1996, 20% to 25% of all infants with group B streptococcal disease had onset after the first 6 days of life. In 2008, approximately 50% of all infants had disease with onset after 6 days of life [173]. Infants born prematurely constituted 23% of the total with early-onset disease and 52% of the total with late-onset disease.

The importance of group B *Streptococcus* as a common pathogen for the perinatal period relates to the pregnant woman as well as her infant. Postpartum endometritis occurs with a frequency of approximately 2%, and clinically diagnosed intra-amniotic infection occurs in 2.9% of women vaginally colonized with GBS at the time of delivery. The risk of intra-amniotic infection is greater in women with heavy colonization [174]. Implementation of intrapartum chemoprophylaxis has been associated with a significant decline in the incidence of invasive disease in pregnant women, from 0.29 per 1000 live births in 1993 to 0.23 per 1000 live births in 1998 and a further decline to 0.12 per 1000 live births in 1999-2005 [150,171]. Half of these infections were associated with infection of the upper genital tract, placenta, or amniotic sac and resulted in fetal death. Among the other infections, bacteremia without a focus (31%), endometritis without fetal death (8%), and chorioamnionitis without fetal death (4%) were the most common manifestations.

IMMUNOLOGY AND PATHOGENESIS
HOST-BACTERIAL INTERACTIONS RELATED TO PATHOGENESIS

The prevalence and severity of group B streptococcal diseases in neonates have stimulated intensive investigation to elucidate the pathogenesis of infection. The unique epidemiologic and clinical features of group B streptococcal disease pose several basic questions that provide a framework for hypothesis development and experimental testing: How does the organism colonize pregnant women and gain access to the infant before or during delivery? Why are newborns, especially infants born prematurely, uniquely susceptible to infection? What allows GBS to evade host innate immune defenses? How do these organisms gain entry to the bloodstream and then cross the blood-brain barrier to produce meningitis? What specific GBS factors injure host tissues or induce the sepsis syndrome?

Advances in knowledge of pathogenesis have been achieved through development of cell culture systems and animal models. Refinement of molecular genetic techniques has yielded isogenic mutant strains varying solely in the production of a particular component (e.g., CPS). Such mutants are important in establishing the biologic relevance of a given trait and its requirement for virulence in vivo. The sequencing of several complete GBS genomes has provided additional context for interpretation of experimental data and comparison with other well-studied pathogens [7,8].

Although GBS have adapted well to asymptomatic colonization of healthy adults, they remain a potentially devastating pathogen to susceptible infants. This section reviews the current understanding of virulence mechanisms, many of which are revealed or magnified by the unique circumstances of the birth process and the deficiencies of neonatal immune defense. The group B streptococcal virulence factors defined to date, with mode of action and proposed role in pathogenesis, are shown in

Table 12–1. Key stages in the molecular, cellular, and immunologic pathogenesis of newborn infection are summarized schematically in Figure 12–5.

Maternal Colonization

The presence of GBS in the genital tract of the mother at delivery determines whether or not a newborn is at risk for invasive disease. Among infants born to colonized women, the risk of early-onset disease is approximately 30-fold that for infants born to women with a negative result on prenatal cultures [175]. A direct relationship exists between the degree (inoculum size) of group B streptococcal vaginal colonization, the risk of vertical transmission, and the likelihood of serious disease in the newborn [132,176]. Consequently, a crucial step in the pathogenesis of invasive disease in the newborn caused by GBS is colonization of pregnant women.

To establish colonization of the female genital tract, GBS must adhere successfully to the vaginal epithelium. Compared with other microorganisms, GBS bind very efficiently to exfoliated human vaginal cells or vaginal tissue culture cells [177,178], with maximal adherence at the acidic pH characteristic of vaginal mucosa [179,180]. A low-affinity interaction with epithelial cells is mediated by its amphiphilic cell wall–associated lipoteichoic acid, whereas higher affinity interactions with host cells are mediated by hydrophobic surface proteins. Soluble lipoteichoic acid competitively inhibits epithelial cell adherence [181,182] and decreases vaginal colonization of pregnant mice [183].

High-affinity protein-mediated interactions of GBS with epithelium are mediated largely through extracellular matrix components, such as fibronectin, fibrinogen, and laminin, which interact with host cell–anchored proteins such as integrins. Binding occurs to immobilized, but not soluble fibronectin, suggesting that this interaction requires close proximity of multiple fibronectin molecules and group B streptococcal adhesins [184]. More recently, a genome-wide phage display technique revealed a fibronectin-binding property associated with the surface-anchored group B streptococcal C5a peptidase, ScpB [185]. The dual functionality of ScpB was confirmed by decreased fibronectin binding of isogenic ScpB mutants and the direct interaction of recombinant ScpB with solid-phase fibronectin [185,186]. Similar targeted mutagenesis studies showed that adherence of GBS to laminin involves a protein adhesin called Lmb [187], attachment to fibrinogen is mediated by repetitive motifs within the surface-anchored protein FbsA [188], and binding to human keratin 4 is carried out by the serine-rich repeat domain protein Srr-1 [189].

More recently, GBS were revealed to express filamentous cell surface appendages known as pili [9]. Among eight sequenced GBS genomes, two genetic loci encoding pili were identified, although not all genomes contain both loci [190]. One of these islands includes genes encoding PilB, an LP(x)TG motif–containing protein that polymerizes to form a pilus backbone, along with accessory pilus proteins PilA and PilC [47,191]. Epithelial cell adherence was reduced in isogenic GBS mutants lacking PilA or PilC, but not mutants lacking the PilB backbone [191].

TABLE 12-1 Group B Streptococcal Virulence Factors in Pathogenesis of Neonatal Infection

Virulence Factor	Molecular or Cellular Actions	Proposed Role in Pathogenesis
Host Cell Attachment and Invasion		
C surface protein	Binds cervical epithelial cells	Epithelial cell adherence, invasion
Fibrinogen receptor, FbsA	Binds fibrinogen in extracellular matrix	Epithelial cell attachment
Lipoteichoic acid	Binds host cell surfaces	Epithelial cell attachment
C5a peptidase, ScpB	Binds fibronectin in extracellular matrix	Epithelial cell adherence, invasion
Surface protein Lmb	Binds laminin in extracellular matrix	Epithelial cell attachment
Spb1 surface protein	Promotes epithelial cell uptake	Invasion of epithelial barriers
iagA gene	Alteration in bacterial cell surface (?)	Promotes blood-brain barrier invasion
Injury to Host Tissues		
β-Hemolysin/cytolysin	Lyses epithelial and endothelial cells	Damage and spread through tissues
Hyaluronate lyase	Cleaves hyaluronan or chondroitin sulfate	Promotes spread through host tissues
CAMP factor	Lyses host cells (cohemolysin)	Direct tissue injury
Resistance to Immune Clearance		
Exopolysaccharide capsule	Impairs complement C3 deposition and activation	Blocks opsonophagocytic clearance
C5a peptidase, ScpB	Cleaves and inactivates human C5a	Inhibits neutrophil recruitment
CAMP factor	Binds to Fc portion of IgG, IgM	Impairment of antibody function
Serine protease, CspA	Cleaves fibrinogen, coats GBS surface with fibrin	Blocks opsonophagocytosis
Fibrinogen receptor, FbsA	Steric interference with complement function (?)	Blocks opsonophagocytosis
C protein	Nonimmune binding of IgA	Blocks opsonophagocytosis
β-hemolysin/cytolysin	Lyses neutrophils and macrophages, proapoptotic	Impairment of phagocyte killing
Superoxide dismutase	Inactivates superoxide	Impairment of oxidative burst killing
Carotenoid pigment	Antioxidant effect blocks H_2O_2, singlet oxygen	Impairment of oxidative burst killing
Dlt operon genes	Alanylation of lipoteichoic acid	Interferes with antimicrobial peptides
Penicillin-binding protein 1a	Alteration in cell wall composition	Interferes with antimicrobial peptides
Activation of Inflammatory Mediators		
Cell wall lipoteichoic acid	Binds host pattern recognition receptors (TLRs)	Cytokine activation
Cell wall peptidoglycan	Binds host pattern recognition receptors (TLRs)	Cytokine activation
β-Hemolysin/cytolysin	Activation of host cell stress response pathways	Triggers iNOS, cytokine release

GBS, group B streptococci; iNOS, inducible nitric oxide synthase; TLRs, toll-like receptors.

Solution of the crystal structure of PilC reveals a specific IgG-like fold domain (N2) required for epithelial cell binding [192].

Ascending Amniotic Infection

GBS can reach the fetus in utero through ascending infection of the placental membranes and amniotic fluid. Alternatively, the newborn may become contaminated with the organism on passage through the birth canal. Infection by the ascending route plays a pivotal role in early-onset disease. A direct relationship exists between the duration of membrane rupture before delivery and attack rate for early-onset disease [193], whereas an inverse relationship exists between the duration of membrane rupture and the age at which clinical signs of early-onset pneumonia and sepsis first appear [194]. When the duration of membrane rupture was 18 hours or less, the attack rate was 0.7 per 1000 live births; when it was more than 30 hours, the attack rate increased to 18.3 per 1000 [193]. Histologic examination of placentas from women with group B streptococcal chorioamnionitis

showed bacterial infiltration along a choriodecidual course, implying that ascending infection may be a primary trigger in many instances of premature rupture [195].

GBS may promote membrane rupture and premature delivery by several mechanisms. Isolated chorioamniotic membranes exposed to the organism have decreased tensile strength and elasticity and are prone to rupture [196]. The presence of GBS at the cervix activates the maternal decidua cell peroxidase–hydrogen peroxide–halide system, promoting oxidative damage to adjacent fetal membranes [197]. GBS also can modify the arachidonic acid metabolism of cultured human amnion cells, favoring production of prostaglandin E_2 [198,199], which is known to stimulate the onset of labor. Stimulation of chorionic cell release of macrophage inflammatory protein-1α and interleukin (IL)-8 from human chorion cells recruits inflammatory cells that may contribute to infection-associated preterm labor [200].

GBS occasionally seem to penetrate into the amniotic cavity through intact membranes. Clinically, this mechanism of entry is suggested by anecdotal reports of

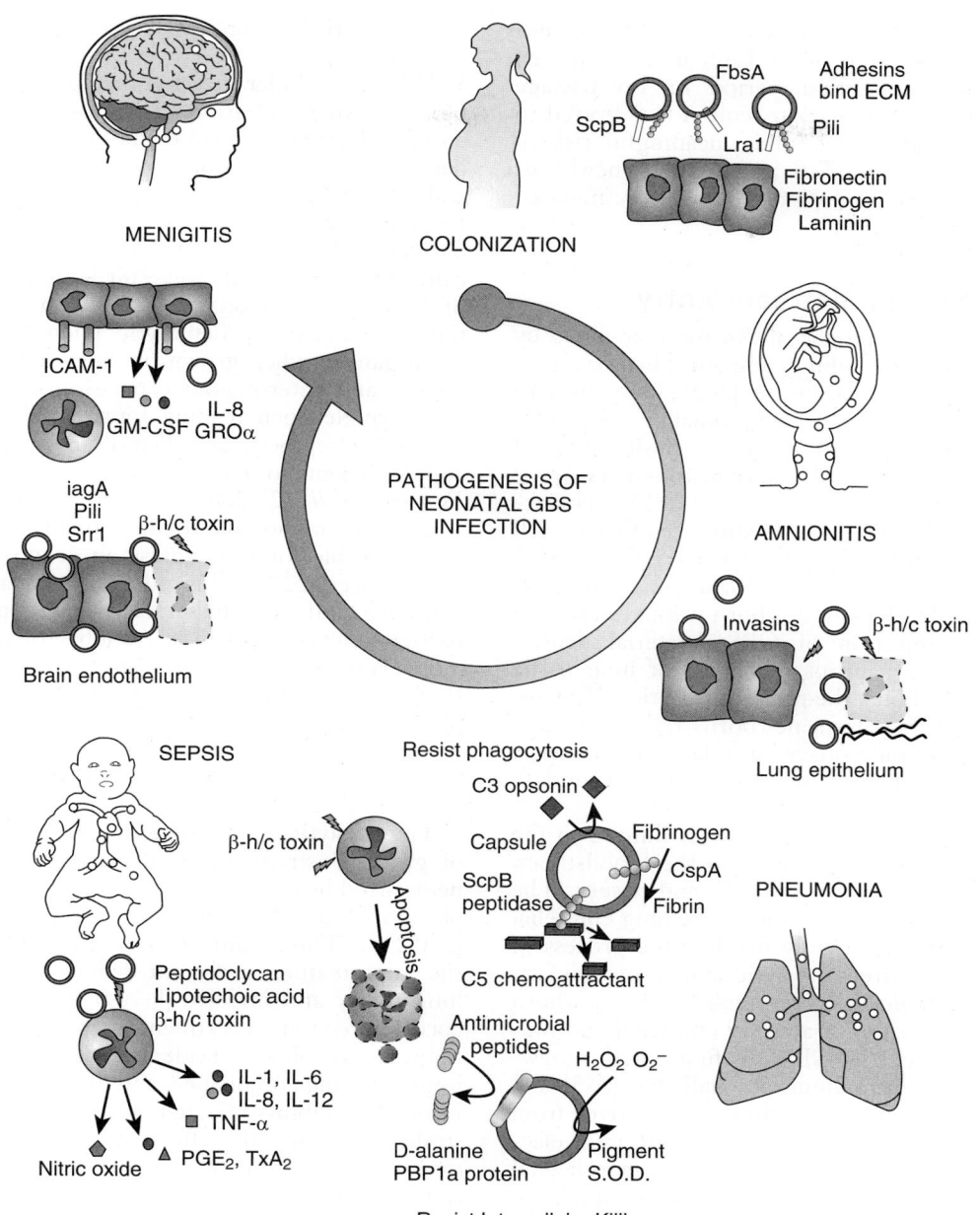

FIGURE 12–5 Pathologic mechanisms for different types of neonatal group B streptococcal (GBS) infection. ECM, extracellular matrix; GM-CSF, granulocyte-macrophage colony-stimulating factor; ICAM, intercellular adhesion molecule; IL-8, interleukin-8; PGE$_2$, prostaglandin E$_2$; SOD, superoxide dismutase; TNF-α, tumor necrosis factor-α; TxA$_2$, thromboxane A$_2$. *(Adapted from Doran KS, Nizet V. Molecular pathogenesis of neonatal group B streptococcal infection: no longer in its infancy. Mol Microbiol 54:23-31, 2004.)*

neonates with fulminant early-onset infection after delivery by cesarean section and no identifiable obstetric risk factors [133,201,202]. Migration of the organism through freshly isolated chorioamniotic membranes has been documented by scanning and transmission electron microscopy [203]. GBS invade primary chorion cells efficiently in vitro and are capable of transcytosing through intact chorion cell monolayers without disruption of intracellular junctions [204]. They also secrete an enzyme that degrades hyaluronic acid, an important component of the extracellular matrix that is abundant

in placental tissues and may facilitate amniotic invasion [84,205].

Amniotic fluid supports the proliferation of GBS [206], such that when the organism gains access to the uterine cavity a large inoculum can be delivered to the fetal lung; this results in a continuum of intrapartum (stillbirth) to early postpartum infant death [176,207–211]. In utero infection probably accounts for the 40% to 60% of newborns with early-onset disease who have poor Apgar scores and in whom pulmonary signs develop within a few hours of birth because these infants almost invariably display clinical or histologic evidence of congenital pneumonia [193,208]. Conversely, when GBS are encountered in the immediate peripartum period or on passage through the birth canal, a lesser inoculum is delivered to the neonate. Although a small but meaningful risk of subsequent invasive disease exists, most of these newborns have asymptomatic colonization limited to mucosal surfaces and remain healthy.

Pulmonary and Bloodstream Entry

Early-onset group B streptococcal disease is heralded by respiratory symptoms, including tachypnea, hypoxia, cyanosis, and pulmonary hypertension [212]. One third to more than half of infants are symptomatic at birth or within 4 to 6 hours after delivery. Autopsies in fatal early-onset cases reveal that 80% have histologic evidence of lobar or multilobar pneumonia [211,213], characterized by dense bacterial infiltration, epithelial cell damage, alveolar hemorrhage, interstitial inflammatory exudate, and hyaline membrane formation [210,214]. When pneumonia develops in newborn primates exposed by intra-amniotic injection of GBS, bacterial density reaches 10^9 to 10^{11} organisms per gram of lung tissue [215]. As shown in rabbits, the poorer resolution of pneumonia in preterm versus term newborns reflects quantitative deficiency of pulmonary alveolar macrophages, mandating the recruitment of neutrophils as a secondary phagocytic defense mechanism [216].

Group B streptococcal disease rarely is limited to the initial pulmonary focus, but spreads to the bloodstream and is circulated through other organs and tissues. The capacity of GBS to cause disruption of the lung epithelial and endothelial barrier evidently involves the process of intracellular invasion, direct cytolytic injury, and damage induced by the inflammatory response of the newborn host. Intracellular invasion of alveolar epithelial and pulmonary endothelial cells by GBS was first noted in newborn macaques after intra-amniotic challenge [215] and later confirmed in human tissue culture lines derived from both cellular barriers [217,218]. In vivo and in vitro electron microscopy studies show that host cytoskeletal changes are triggered that lead to endocytotic uptake of the bacterium within a membrane-bound vacuole. Uptake requires induction of signal transduction pathways in the host cell that are mediated by Rho-family GTPases [219] and phosphatidylinositol-3 kinase [220].

Cellular invasion is correlated with virulence potential. Clinical isolates of GBS from infants with bloodstream infections invade epithelial cells better than strains from the vaginal mucosa of asymptomatic women [221]. FbsA, a group B streptococcal fibrinogen binding protein [222]; Lmb, which mediates laminin binding [223]; and ScpB, which interacts with fibronectin [186], each play a role in promoting efficient epithelial or endothelial cell invasion. Another GBS surface protein, Spb1, was identified by subtractive hybridization to play a specific role in serotype III GBS invasion of epithelial cells [163]. In addition, surface-anchored α C protein specifically interacts with host cell glycosaminoglycan on the epithelial cell surface to promote group B streptococcal internalization [224]. By contrast, CPS decreases intracellular invasion, presumably through steric interference of certain receptor-ligand interactions [225].

Although cellular invasion may play a principal role in bloodstream penetration in late-onset group B streptococcal infection, damage to the lung barrier often is evident in severe early-onset infection. Alveolar exudate and hemorrhage in autopsy studies of infants with group B streptococcal pneumonia attest to significant pulmonary epithelial and endothelial cell injury [210,226]. The cellular damage seems to result largely from the actions of β-hemolysin/cytolysin. This toxin is responsible for the characteristic β-hemolytic phenotype displayed by the organism when grown on sheep's blood agar. Mutagenesis and heterologous expression studies have identified a single open reading frame, *cylE*, as necessary for group B streptococcal β-hemolysin/cytolysin expression and sufficient to confer β-hemolysis when cloned in *Escherichia coli* [227,228]. CylE is a predicted 79-kDa protein sharing no homology to the toxin, streptolysin S, that is responsible for β-hemolysis in group A, C, F, and G streptococci [229]. This pore-forming toxin lyses lung epithelial and endothelial cells and compromises their barrier function [230,231]. At subcytolytic doses, it promotes intracellular invasion and triggers the release of IL-8, the principal chemoattractant for human neutrophils [232]. Mutants lacking hemolysin expression are less virulent than the corresponding wild-type strains in mouse, rat, and rabbit models of group B streptococcal pneumonia [233–235].

The cytolytic, proinvasive, and proinflammatory effects of group B streptococcal β-hemolysin/cytolysin all are neutralized by dipalmitoyl phosphatidylcholine, the major phospholipid constituent of human lung surfactant [230,232]. This finding may partly explain the increased risk in premature, surfactant-deficient neonates for severe lung injury and invasive disease from group B streptococcal infection. Treatment with exogenous surfactant reduces histologic evidence of lung inflammation, improves lung compliance, and mitigates bacterial growth in preterm rabbits infected with GBS [236,237]. Clinical studies exploring the effect of surfactant administration on human infants with group B streptococcal sepsis also suggest a beneficial effect [238,239].

Capsular Polysaccharide and Immune Resistance

On penetration of GBS into the lung tissue or bloodstream of the newborn infant, an immunologic response is recruited to clear the organism. Central to this response are host phagocytic cells including neutrophils and macrophages. Effective uptake and killing by these cells require opsonization of the bacterium by specific antibodies in the presence of complement [240–242]. Neonates are particularly prone to invasive disease because of their quantitative or qualitative deficiencies in phagocytic cell function, specific antibody, or classic and alternate complement pathways. In addition to these newborn host susceptibilities, GBS possess numerous virulence determinants that seek to thwart each of the key components of effective opsonophagocytic killing. Chief among these factors is the sialylated group B streptococcal polysaccharide capsule.

The serotype-specific epitopes of group B streptococcal CPS are created by different arrangements of four monosaccharides (glucose, galactose, N-acetylglucosamine, and sialic acid) into a unique repeating unit (see "Immunochemistry of Polysaccharide Antigens" earlier), but unfailingly these structures contain a terminal sialic acid bound to galactose in an α2→3 linkage. The enzymatic machinery for capsule biosynthesis is encoded in the single long transcript of a 16-gene operon. More recent elegant experiments have shown that the heterologous expression of a single polymerase gene (cpsH) from this operon can cause a group B streptococcal type Ia strain to express type III capsule epitopes, and vice versa [243].

The conserved group B streptococcal terminal α2→3 sialic acid capsular component is identical to a sugar epitope widely displayed on the surface of all mammalian cells [244]. The terminal α2→3-linked sialic acid is overexpressed in humans, who in evolution have lost the genes to produce the alternative sialic acid, Neu5Gc. It is suggested that group B Streptococcus may be a particularly troublesome human pathogen because its sialylated capsule has undergone selection to resemble host "self" and avoid immune recognition. Compared with wild-type strains, isogenic capsule-deficient mutants of GBS elicit greater degrees of proinflammatory cytokine release from human cells [245]. It was shown more recently that GBS can use such molecular mimicry to engage a sialic acid–binding surface receptor, Siglec-9, expressed on human neutrophils, leading to negative cell signaling cascades that dampen the oxidative burst and bactericidal activities of phagocytic cell [246].

The properties of group B streptococcal CPS have been studied most thoroughly in serotype III organisms. Sialic acid is a critical element in the epitope of the type III capsule that confers protective immunity. After treatment with sialidase, the altered CPS fails to elicit protective antibodies against group B streptococcal infection. Protective antibodies derived from native type III capsule do not bind to the altered (asialo) capsule backbone structure [247]. Sialidase-treated type III GBS are opsonized more effectively by complement through the alternative pathway and are more readily phagocytosed by human neutrophils in vitro, and sialidase exhibits diminished lethality of the organism in neonatal rats [248,249].

More definitive evidence for the role of type III capsule in virulence is provided by the construction of isogenic capsule-deficient mutants by transposon mutagenesis or targeted allelic replacement [250–252]. Compared with the parent strains, isogenic capsule mutants are susceptible to opsonophagocytosis in the presence of complement and healthy adult neutrophils [253]. Opsonization by complement is a pivotal element in host defense against invasive infections; however, the extent of C3 deposition on GBS by the alternative complement pathway is inversely related to the size and density of their polysaccharide capsule present [253,254]. C3 fragments bound to the acapsular mutant are predominantly in the active form, C3b, whereas the inactive form, C3bi, is predominantly bound to the surface of the parent strain.

The type III group B streptococcal acapsular mutants also are significantly less virulent in animal models of infection. In a model of pneumonia and bacteremia, neonatal rats were inoculated with either the parent strain or an acapsular mutant by intratracheal injection. In animals that received the acapsular mutant, fewer GBS were recovered per gram of lung, more bacteria were associated with resident alveolar macrophages, and the animals became significantly less bacteremic than animals that received the parent strain [255]. Subcutaneous injection of the acapsular mutants in neonatal rats resulted in LD_{50} values that were at least 100-fold greater than the values obtained with the parent strain [251,256]. Mouse passage of various serotypes of GBS was followed by increases in sialylated capsule content that correlated with increased virulence [257]. Taken together, these data provide compelling evidence that the capsule protects the organism from phagocytic clearance during the initial pulmonary phase and the later bacteremic phase of early-onset infection.

Noncapsular Factors That Interfere with Immune Clearance

The ability of GBS to avoid opsonophagocytosis is enhanced by surface proteins that can act in concert with CPS. Serotype II strains displaying both components of the C protein antigen are more resistant to phagocytic killing than are serotype II strains lacking C protein [258,259]. The b antigen of C protein binds human IgA [260,261], and IgA deposited nonspecifically on the bacterial surface probably inhibits interactions with complement or IgG [262]. A cell surface protease, CspA, targets host fibrinogen, producing adherent fibrin-like cleavage products that coat the bacterial surface and interfere with opsonophagocytic clearance [263]. The group B streptococcal BibA protein binds human C4bp, a component of the classical complement pathway, and increases resistance to phagocytic killing [264]. Finally, certain type Ia group B streptococcal strains can also use the surface anchored b protein to engage Siglec 5 on macrophages and neutrophils and downregulate their innate immune function, a unique example of protein-mediated subversion of a host lectin receptor [265].

After phagocytic uptake of pathogens, neutrophils and macrophages seek to kill the engulfed bacteria by generation of reactive oxygen products and other antimicrobial substances. Streptococci are often thought of as "extracellular pathogens," but these organisms can survive for prolonged periods within the phagolysosome of macrophages [266,267]. Although GBS lack the neutralizing enzyme catalase, they are more than 10 times resistant to killing by hydrogen peroxide than is catalase-positive *S. aureus* [268]. Several mechanisms for enhanced intracellular survival have been identified. The organism possesses an endogenous source of the oxygen metabolite scavenger glutathione [268]. Another defense against oxidative burst killing is the enzyme superoxide dismutase (SodA), as evidenced by the fact that a SodA mutant is highly susceptible to macrophage killing and survives poorly in vivo [269]. Finally, GBS produce an orange carotenoid pigment, a property unique among hemolytic streptococci and genetically linked to the cyl operon encoding β-hemolysin/cytolysin. The free radical scavenging properties of the carotenoid neutralize hydrogen peroxide, superoxide, hypochlorite, and singlet oxygen, providing a shield against several elements of phagocyte oxidative burst killing [270]. The antioxidant effects of glutathione, SodA, and carotenoid pigment apparently compensate for the lack of catalase and explain the unexpected persistence of GBS within host phagolysosomes.

Cationic antimicrobial peptides, such as defensins and cathelicidins produced by host phagocytes, also are an important component of innate immune defense against invasive bacterial infection [271]. The group B streptococcal *ponA* gene codes for an extracytoplasmic penicillin-binding protein (PBP1a) that promotes resistance to phagocytic killing independent of capsule [272]. Group B streptococcal mutants with deletion of the PBP1a gene are less virulent after lung and systemic challenge, and this is correlated to an increased susceptibility to defensins and cathelicidins [272a]. Another way in which the organism avoids antimicrobial peptide clearance is through the D-alanylation of lipoteichoic acid in the bacterial cell wall; this requires activity of gene products that are encoded by the *dlt* operon. A *dlt*A mutant exhibits decreased negative surface charge that impedes cationic host defense peptides from reaching their cell membrane target of action [273]. Similarly, expression of the pilus backbone protein PilB renders GBS more resistant to killing by cathelicidins and is associated with enhanced phagocyte resistance and systemic virulence [274].

Direct cytotoxicity to host phagocytes represents another important virulence mechanism for immune resistance. The group B streptococcal β-hemolysin/cytolysin toxin produces direct cytolytic injury to macrophages and induces macrophage apoptosis over a longer interval. With highly hemolytic strains or with a large bacterial inoculum, killing of the phagocyte seems to outpace the phagocyte's microbicidal mechanisms, allowing bacterial proliferation in vitro in a murine bacteremia model [270]. Addition of an inhibitor of β-hemolysin/cytolysin blocks cytolysis and reduces apoptosis of macrophages, restoring phagocytic killing [270]. GBS-induced macrophage apoptosis can also occur by a β-hemolysin/cytolysin–independent mechanism regulated, at least in part, by glucose [275]. Signaling pathways involved in GBS-induced programmed cell death of macrophages seem to involve either caspase-3 or calpain activation [276,277].

Deficiencies in the neutrophil response to GBS have been documented in newborn infants. Neutropenia and depletion of the marrow neutrophil storage pool are frequent findings in infants with septicemia [278] and are correlated with poor clinical outcome [212]. Although neutrophilia and an increase in granulocytic stem cells develop in adult rats infected with GBS, severe neutropenia without a change in stem cell counts develops in neonatal rats [279]. Fatal infection in neonatal rats is associated with failure of recovery of depleted myeloid storage pools [280]. The explanation for this finding may be that the proliferative rate of neutrophils in noninfected neonatal animals already is maximal or near-maximal and cannot increase further in response to bacterial challenge [281].

GBS actively contribute to poor mobilization of neutrophils by production of an enzyme that cleaves and inactivates human C5a, a complement component that stimulates neutrophil chemotaxis [82]. Expression of C5a peptidase reduces the acute neutrophil response to sites of infection in C5a knockout mice reconstituted with human C5a [282]. Expression of group B streptococcal C5a peptidase is induced in normal human serum [283]; however, its enzymatic activity is often neutralized, in large part because of naturally occurring IgG antibodies present in many adults [82]. IgG also neutralizes C5a peptidase on the surface of a capsule-deficient group B streptococcal mutant, but fails to neutralize the enzyme on the surface of the intact encapsulated type III parent strain. The capsule serves to protect the cell-associated C5a peptidase from inactivation by naturally occurring antibodies.

Inflammatory Mediators and Sepsis

When failures in epithelial barrier function and immunologic clearance allow GBS to establish bacteremia in the neonate, sepsis or septic shock develops. Intravenous infusion of GBS in animal models produces similar pathophysiologic changes to human newborn infection, including hypotension, persistent pulmonary hypertension, tissue hypoxemia and acidosis, temperature instability, disseminated intravascular coagulation, neutropenia, and, ultimately, multiple organ system failure. These similarities have allowed in vivo experiments to elucidate the patterns in which the organism activates host inflammatory mediators to induce sepsis and circulatory shock.

Animal models in which GBS are infused intravenously exhibit a biphasic host inflammatory response [284–286]. The acute phase (≤1 hour after infusion) is manifested by increased pulmonary artery pressure and decreased arterial oxygenation and is associated with an increase in serum levels of thromboxanes. Pulmonary hypertension and hypoxemia persist through the late phase (2 to 4 hours), in which a progressive pattern of systemic hypotension, decreased cardiac output, and metabolic acidosis develops together with hematologic abnormalities; organ system dysfunction; and increase in inflammatory markers, such as thromboxanes, tumor necrosis factor (TNF)-α, and prostacyclins. If production of thromboxane and prostacyclin is blocked by inhibition of the cyclooxygenase pathway in rabbits or lambs infused with GBS, decreased myocardial dysfunction and a significant increase in systemic blood pressure are observed [287–289].

Infusion of GBS produces pulmonary hypertension in piglets and isolated piglet lung preparations, suggesting a direct interaction of the organism with target cells in lung microvasculature [290,291]. GBS induce release of vasoactive eicosanoids prostacyclin and prostaglandin E_2 from lung microvascular cells [292] and stimulate the host inflammatory mediators leukotriene D_4 [293] and thromboxane A_2 [294].

The cytokine IL-12 has an important role in the systemic response to group B streptococcal infection. Elevation of IL-12 occurs 12 to 72 hours after challenge in the neonatal rat. Pretreatment with a monoclonal antibody against IL-12 results in greater mortality and intensity of bacteremia, whereas therapeutic administration of IL-12 is associated with a lower mortality rate and bloodstream replication of the organism [295]. By contrast, IL-1, a known stimulator of cyclooxygenase and lipoxygenase pathways, seems to occupy a proximal position in the deleterious cytokine cascade of septic shock [296]. Treatment with an IL-1 receptor antagonist improves cardiac output and mean arterial pressure, and increases duration of survival in piglets receiving a continuous infusion of GBS [297].

Controversy exists regarding the precise role of TNF-α in neonatal septicemia. TNF-α often is detected in the blood, urine, or cerebrospinal fluid (CSF) of infants with invasive disease [298]. Although infusion of GBS in piglets is associated with TNF-α release during the late phase of hemodynamic response, the TNF-α inhibitor pentoxifylline has only modest effects on pulmonary hypertension, hypoxemia, and systemic hypotension [299]. Marked improvement in these hemodynamic parameters is seen only when pentoxifylline treatment is combined with indomethacin inhibition of thromboxane and prostacyclin synthesis [300]. Serum TNF-α levels in the mouse and rat also increase after challenge; however, administration of polyclonal or monoclonal anti–TNF-α antibody does not affect overall mortality rate in these animal models [300,301].

Studies have sought to establish the components of GBS cell wall that trigger the host cytokine cascade. Host release of IL-l and IL-6 is stimulated by soluble cell wall antigens [302]. Cell wall preparations also cause nuclear factor κB (NF-κB) activation and TNF-α release from human monocytes in a manner requiring CD14 and complement receptor types 3 and 4 [303]. Group B polysaccharide and peptidoglycan are more effective stimulators of TNF-α release from monocytes than lipoteichoic acid or CPS [304]. Knockout mouse studies indicate that cell wall peptidoglycan-induced activation of p38 and NF-κB depends on the cytoplasmic toll-like receptor (TLR) adapter protein MyD88, but does not require the pattern recognition receptor TLR2 or TLR4 [305]. An additional, undefined secreted factor apparently activates phagocytes through TLR2 and TLR6 [306].

Inhibitor studies have shown that the mitogen-activated protein kinase/JNK signaling pathway is required for the NF-κB–dependent inflammatory response of phagocytes to GBS. Because neither phagocytosis nor oxidative killing of bacteria is affected by JNK inhibition, this pathway may represent a viable therapeutic target for group B streptococcal sepsis [307]. The nitric oxide pathway is implicated in overproduction of proinflammatory cytokines such as IL-6 and initiation of cellular injury during group B streptococcal lung infection [308]. Inducible cyclooxygenase-2 is also stimulated on group B streptococcal infection in human monocytes, likely through the mitogen-activated protein kinase pathway [309]. Infection also stimulates cyclooxygenase-2 and prostaglandin E_2 expression in lung tissue in vitro and in vivo. GBS-induced cyclooxygenase-2 and prostaglandin E_2 inflammatory response is reduced on treatment with an inducible nitric oxide synthase inhibitor and restored by addition of a nitric oxide donor, showing at least partial regulation by the nitric oxide pathway [310].

Another proinflammatory molecule contributing to the pathogenesis of group B streptococcal septicemia is β-hemolysin/cytolysin. This potent cytoxin acts to stimulate inducible nitric oxide synthase in macrophages, leading to release of nitric oxide [311]. In a mouse model of bacteremia and arthritis, β-hemolysin/cytolysin expression is associated with higher mortality, increased bacterial loads, greater degrees of joint injury, and release of the proinflammatory cytokines IL-6 and IL-1α systemically and intra-articularly [312]. Challenge of rabbits with isogenic group B streptococcal mutants showed that β-hemolysin/cytolysin production was associated with significantly higher degrees of hypotension, increased mortality, and evidence of liver necrosis with hepatocyte apoptosis [313]. Partially purified β-hemolysin/cytolysin preparations produce significant hypotensive actions when infused in rats and rabbits, including death from shock [314]. β-hemolysin/cytolysin also contributes directly to cardiomyocyte dysfunction and apoptosis, which may magnify its role in the pathophysiology of group B streptococcal sepsis [315].

Blood-Brain Barrier Penetration and Meningitis

The pathophysiology of group B streptococcal meningitis varies according to age at onset. In early-onset disease, autopsy studies show little or no evidence of leptomeningeal inflammation, despite the presence of abundant bacteria, vascular thrombosis, and parenchymal hemorrhage [2,226]. By contrast, infants with late-onset disease usually have diffuse purulent arachnoiditis with prominent involvement of the base of the brain [316]. Similar age-related differences in central nervous system (CNS) pathology are evident in the infant rat model of invasive disease [317]. These histopathologic differences reflect underdevelopment of the host immunologic response in the immediate neonatal period, with a higher proportion of deaths resulting from overwhelming septicemia.

To produce meningitis, GBS must penetrate human brain microvascular endothelial cells, the single-cell layer constituting the blood-brain barrier. Intracellular invasion and transcytosis of human brain microvascular endothelial cell tissue culture monolayers have been shown in vitro [318]. Serotype III strains, which account for most of the isolates causing meningitis, invade more efficiently than strains of other common serotypes. A transposon mutant library of type III GBS was screened in tissue culture assays for alterations in invasiveness. Hypoinvasive mutants were identified with disruptions in *iag*A, sharing homology to genes encoding diglucosyldiacylglycerol synthase. Allelic replacement of *iag*A confirms the in vitro phenotype, and the *iag*A knockout mutant does not produce meningitis in mice [319].

In separate avenues of research, group B streptococcal mutants lacking the fibrinogen receptor FbsA, laminin-binding protein Lmb, or pilus backbone subunit protein PilB also showed reduced adherence or invasion of human brain microvascular endothelial cells in vitro [47,223,320]. More recently, a group B streptococcal mutant lacking the surface-anchored serine-rich repeat motif glycoprotein Srr-1 was attenuated for brain endothelial cell invasion and for production of meningitis in the murine model [321]. At high bacterial densities, invasion by GBS of brain microvascular endothelial cells is accompanied by evidence of β-hemolysin/cytolysin–induced cellular injury [245]. Correspondingly, β-hemolysin/cytolysin knockout mutants show decreased blood-brain barrier penetration and decreased lethality from meningitis in vivo [245].

The host inflammatory response to GBS contributes significantly to the pathogenesis of meningitis and CNS injury. The initiation of the inflammatory response is triggered through the sentinel function of the blood-brain barrier endothelium, which activates a specific pattern of gene transcription for neutrophil recruitment, including production of chemokines (e.g., IL-8, Groα), endothelial receptors (intercellular adhesion molecule-1), and neutrophil activators (granulocyte-macrophage colony-stimulating factor) [245]. A vascular distribution of cortical lesions in neonatal rats with group B streptococcal meningitis indicates that disturbances of cerebral blood flow contribute to neuronal damage [322]. Inflammation of individual brain vessels can lead to focal lesions, whereas diffuse alterations of cerebral blood flow could cause generalized hypoxic-ischemic injury and cerebral edema [322,323]. Arteriolar dysfunction is associated with the presence of oxygen free radicals thought to be a by-product of the phagocytic killing by infiltrating neutrophils [324]. Group B streptococcal β-hemolysin/cytolysin induces IL-8 and the neutrophil receptor intercellular adhesion molecule-1, promoting neutrophil migration across polar brain microvascular endothelial cells (BMEC) monolayers, suggesting that the toxin is crucial to this particular manifestation of CNS disease [245].

TNF-α production by astrocytes, microglial cells, and infiltrating leukocytes seems to contribute to apoptosis of hippocampal neurons [325], further increasing blood-brain barrier permeability during group B streptococcal meningitis [326]. Intraventricular inoculation of newborn piglets with GBS results in an early sharp increase in CSF TNF-α levels, followed shortly by prostaglandin release and neutrophil influx [327]. The magnitude of the observed TNF-α response and inflammatory cascade is markedly increased when an isogenic nonencapsulated mutant is tested in place of the type III parent strain [327], suggesting that a component of the underlying cell wall and not capsule is responsible for inducing the CNS inflammatory response. GBS signal through TLR2 to activate and stimulate nitric oxide production by microglia cells, resulting in neuronal destruction [328]. Simultaneous intracisternal administration of dexamethasone with GBS in the rat model leads to a marked reduction in subarachnoid inflammation, vasculopathy, and neuronal injury [322]. In the course of experimental group B streptococcal meningitis, microglial apoptosis is triggered via the cysteine protease caspase-8 and is hypothesized to represent a self-dampening mechanism that prevents overstimulation of brain inflammation [329].

HOST FACTORS RELATED TO PATHOGENESIS
Risk Factors for Early-Onset Infection

Infant and maternal factors that increase risk for early-onset group B streptococcal infection are listed in Table 12–2. The most obvious risk determinant is exposure through maternal colonization at delivery. Maternal race or ethnicity is correlated significantly with early-

TABLE 12–2   Risk Factors for Early-Onset Group B Streptococcal Disease

Risk Factor	Representative Reference Nos.
Maternal colonization at delivery	3,109,331
High-density maternal colonization	114,132,176
Rupture of membranes before onset of labor	176,330
Preterm delivery <37 wk gestation	330
Prolonged rupture of membranes ≥18 hr	330,706
Chorioamnionitis	679
Intrapartum fever ≥38° C (≥100.4° F)	330
Intrauterine monitoring	330,706
Maternal postpartum bacteremia	334
Multiple pregnancy	332,333
Group B streptococcal bacteriuria or urinary tract infection	330
Cesarean section	3,176
Low level of antibody to infecting CPS type	340
Young maternal age (<20 yr)	330,706
Previous infant with invasive group B streptococcal infection	707
Maternal race/ethnicity	110,170,143

CPS, capsular polysaccharide.

onset group B streptococcal disease, with enhanced risk for infants born to African American and Hispanic mothers compared with infants born to white mothers [117,143,330]. Risk correlates directly with density of maternal genital inoculum [132]. Symptomatic early-onset disease develops in 1% to 2% of infants born to colonized women who do not receive IAP, but this rate is considerably increased if there is premature onset of labor (before 37 weeks of gestation) (15%) [331], chorioamnionitis or interval between rupture of membranes and delivery longer than 18 hours (11%) [176,331], twin pregnancy (35%) [332,333], or maternal postpartum bacteremia (10%) [334].

Maternal group B streptococcal bacteriuria and urinary tract infection are predictive of high-inoculum colonization, which enhances infant risk for invasive infection [335]. Heavy group B streptococcal colonization in the second trimester of pregnancy also is associated with increased risk of delivering a preterm infant with low birth weight [336]. Among infants born to mothers with premature rupture of membranes at term gestation, maternal chorioamnionitis and colonization with GBS are strong predictors of neonatal infection [337]. Vaginal colonization with GBS is an independent risk factor for the development of chorioamnionitis [338].

Prolonged interval after rupture of membranes (>18 hours) before delivery and preterm delivery (<37 weeks' gestation) often are concomitant risk factors in neonates with early-onset group B streptococcal infection. The estimated incidence of early-onset group B streptococcal infection is 10 times higher in preterm than in term neonates [176,193]. Even with correction for preterm delivery, twin pregnancy is an independent risk factor for invasive early-onset group B streptococcal septicemia [332]. The explanation for the increased risk in twins likely relates to genetic factors regulating host susceptibility, lack of specific antibody to the infecting strain in the mother, similar density of maternal colonization, and virulence of disease-producing strains [332,333].

Antibody to Capsular Polysaccharide

Lancefield showed that antibodies directed against capsular type-specific surface antigens of GBS protected mice from lethal challenge [339]. Baker and Kasper [340] showed in 1976 that neonatal risk for type III group B streptococcal disease correlated with a deficiency of antibody to type III CPS in maternal sera. A low concentration of type III CPS-specific antibodies was shown in sera from 32 infants with invasive disease [341]. Women with type III group B streptococcal genital colonization at delivery whose infants remained well more often had antibody concentrations exceeding 2 μg/mL of type III–specific antibodies in their sera than women whose infants developed type III early-onset disease. Quantitative determination of antibodies to type III group B streptococcal polysaccharide by enzyme-linked immunosorbent assay (ELISA) indicated that these antibodies were predominantly IgG [342,343]. Gray and coworkers [344] noted a similar correlation between low concentrations of type II–specific antibodies in maternal delivery sera and susceptibility of infants to invasive infection. Approximately 15% to 20% of pregnant women have a concentration of IgG to CPS in their delivery serum presumed to protect against invasive disease. These higher concentrations are present significantly more often in sera of women colonized with the homologous group B streptococcal type than in noncolonized women [117,120,345].

Attempts have been made to quantify the concentration of antibody to group B streptococcal CPS in maternal serum conferring protection against invasive disease in infants. Using ELISA standardized by quantitative precipitation [346], 1 μg/mL, 0.2 μg/mL, and 1.3 μg/mL of IgG to serotypes Ia, Ib, and III were protective in experimental models of infection [347–350]. A prospective, multicenter, hospital-based, case-control study of mothers delivering infants with type Ia, III, or V early-onset sepsis and matched colonized control mothers delivering healthy infants quantified the maternal serum concentrations of type Ia, III, and V CPS-specific IgG at delivery that protected neonates from early-onset disease. For types Ia and III, maternal IgG concentrations of 0.5 μg/mL or greater corresponded to a 90% risk reduction. For type V, the same antibody concentration corresponded to 70% risk reduction [351]. The findings of Lin and colleagues [352,353] agreed in principle, but described a higher concentration of CPS-specific IgG as the correlate for protection against type Ia or III group B *Streptococcus*. Neonates whose mothers had at least a 5 μg/mL concentration of IgG to type Ia CPS in their sera had an 88% lower risk of developing early-onset disease compared with neonates whose mothers had concentrations less than 0.5 μg/mL. Neonates whose mothers had at least a 10 μg/mL concentration of IgG to type III CPS in their sera by ELISA had a 91% lower risk for early-onset disease compared with neonates whose mothers had concentrations less

than 2 μg/mL. In contrast, antibody to the group B polysaccharide does not confer protection against invasive infant disease [354].

Low concentrations of IgG to type III CPS are uniformly found in acute sera of infants with late-onset type III infection [340,355–357]. In a study of 28 infants with late-onset bacteremia and 51 with meningitis, Baker and coworkers [341] detected low levels of antibodies to type III CPS in acute sera from all infants. These low levels in term infants with late-onset type III group B streptococcal infection correlated with maternal levels at delivery [341,356].

It is important to employ antigens with "native" or intact type III polysaccharide specificity in evaluating human immunity to type III GBS [358,359]. Kasper and colleagues [247] used gently extracted (native) and hydrogen chloride-treated (core) type III group B streptococcal and pneumococcal type 14 antigens to study sera from infants with invasive type III infection and their mothers. Concentrations of type III–specific antibodies in sera of sick infants and their mothers had uniformly low binding to fully sialylated, type III polysaccharide. Opsonic immunity correlated with antibodies to fully sialylated, but not to desialylated type III polysaccharide or to type 14 pneumococcal antigen. Among infants recovering from type III disease in whom a significant increase in antibodies to the fully sialylated polysaccharide developed, no detectable increase in the acid-degraded or core antigen was seen. Human immunity to type III GBS relates to antibodies to capsular type III polysaccharide with an intact protective epitope.

An extension of this concept comes from studies in which adults have been immunized with either type III polysaccharide or pneumococcal polysaccharide vaccine [358]. Adults with low concentrations of type III antibodies in their sera before immunization responded to type III polysaccharide vaccine with a significant increase in type III–specific antibodies. This response was not observed when the structurally related type 14 pneumococcal polysaccharide was used as an immunizing agent. Among adults with moderate to high levels of antibodies to type III polysaccharide, however, significant increases in this antibody developed after pneumococcal polysaccharide vaccine. This finding suggests that the structurally similar antigen could elicit secondary B-cell proliferation in previously primed adults.

Mucosal Immune Response

Genital colonization with GBS may elicit specific antibody responses in cervical secretions. Women with group B streptococcal type Ia, II, or III rectal or cervical colonization have markedly elevated levels of IgA and IgG to the colonizing serotype in their cervical secretions compared with cervical secretions from noncolonized women. Elevated amounts of IgA and IgG to the protein antigen R4 also have been found in women colonized with type III strains (most type III strains contain R4 antigen) compared with noncolonized women [360,361]. These findings suggest that a mucosal immune response occurs in response to colonization with GBS. Induction of mucosal antibodies to surface group B streptococcal polysaccharide or protein antigens may prevent genital colonization, diminishing vertical transmission of infection from mothers to infants.

Complement and Antibody Interactions

Shigeoka and colleagues [240] showed that specific antibody was required and that the classical complement pathway maximized opsonization of types I, II, and III GBS [362]. Capsule-specific antibodies also facilitated alternative complement pathway–mediated opsonization and phagocytosis of type III GBS [248]. The relationship between antibody concentration and the rate constant of killing of type III strains was found to be linear and determined, at least in part, by the number of antibody molecules bound per organism [363,364]. IgG subclasses 1, 2, and 3 and IgM were shown to support opsonic activity in vitro [365–368], and an IgA monoclonal antibody activated C3 and conferred protection against lethal infection [369]. Encapsulated and genetically derived acapsular mutants of type III GBS deposit C3 and support its degradation, but an inverse correlation exists between extent of encapsulation and C3 deposition by the alternative pathway [253,370]. Among infants surviving type III group B streptococcal meningitis, transient development of type-specific antibodies, predominantly IgM, supported opsonophagocytosis during convalescence [371]. When specific IgM concentrations declined, and despite maturation of complement synthesis, opsonophagocytosis of type III organisms by these infant sera remained poor.

In contrast with these findings for type III strains, clinical isolates of type Ia GBS can be efficiently opsonized, phagocytosed, and killed by neutrophils from healthy adults by the classical complement pathway in the absence of antibodies [372]. Surface-bound CPS of type Ia strains mediates C1 binding and activation [373,374]. For type Ib GBS, a role for capsule size and density in modulating C3 deposition has been reported [254]. Variability among these strains in their capacity for C3 deposition by the alternative pathway also has been shown [375].

Type II strains possessing α C and β C proteins are more resistant to opsonization than strains lacking both proteins [258]. Strains lacking type II polysaccharide but having both C proteins are readily opsonized. R protein or an IgA-mediated blocking effect may modulate phagocytosis of some type II strains. Despite the complexity of type II opsonins, it is clear that complement is essential and that integrity of the classical complement pathway is critical. Evaluation of neutrophil-mediated killing of types IV and V GBS also reveals the importance of complement and CPS-specific antibodies [376,377]. When complement is limited, type-specific antibodies facilitate killing. In sufficient concentration, agammaglobulinemic serum promotes opsonization, phagocytosis, and killing of types IV and V GBS.

During the course of septic shock caused by GBS, complement components are consumed. Cairo and associates [378] found a significant association between low levels of total hemolytic complement and fatal outcome from neonatal bacterial sepsis, including GBS. A critical role for C3 activation through the alternative pathway has been shown for potent GBS-induced TNF-α release [379]. This finding and the observation that complement-dependent uptake of CPS by marginal zone B cells seems necessary for an effective immune response to CPS [380] may partially explain this finding. The β component of C protein also can bind human factor F, a negative regulator of complement activation, evading complement attack [381].

Phagocyte Function

Smith and associates [382] examined the role of complement receptors CR1 and CR3 in the opsonic recognition of types Ia and III GBS by neutrophils from healthy neonates and adults. Selective blockade of CR3 or of CR1 and CR3 inhibited killing for each serotype by neutrophils from neonates. These experiments indicated the importance of complement receptor function to opsonization, phagocytosis, and killing of GBS by neutrophils. Whether deficient complement receptor function contributes to susceptibility of neonates to invasive infection is unknown. A role for CR3 also has been shown in nonopsonic recognition of GBS by macrophages [383].

Yang and coworkers [384] performed selective blockade of neutrophil receptors in experiments with type III GBS opsonized with immunoglobulin. Antibodies to neutrophil Fc receptor III (FcR III) inhibited phagocytosis of opsonized bacteria to an extent exceeding that of CR3. Noya and colleagues [385] showed a substantial role for neutrophil FcR II in mediating ingestion of type III GBS opsonized in complement-inactivated serum. When complement receptor function was allowed, FcR II participation no longer was requisite for occurrence of phagocytosis. Participation by FcR and complement receptor in phagocytosis of GBS by peritoneal macrophages also has been reported [386].

Christensen and coworkers [279,281] and others [278] have addressed the explanations for the profound neutropenia often observed in fulminant group B streptococcal infection in neonates. The nearly maximal proliferative rate of granulocytic stem cells in noninfected neonatal animals led to the suggestion that neutrophil transfusion might improve the survival of human neonates with group B streptococcal infection in whom neutrophil storage pool depletion was documented [278,378]. In experimental infection with type III GBS, monoclonal IgM antibody to type III polysaccharide stimulated the release of neutrophils from storage pools into the bloodstream and improved neutrophil migration to the site of infection [387]. This facilitation of neutrophil function by type III–specific antibody improved survival in animals only if the antibody was administered when neutrophil reserves were intact (very early in infection) [388]. Antibody recipients did not become neutropenic and did not experience depletion of their neutrophil reserves. These and similar in vitro and in vivo studies using commercial preparations of immunoglobulin for intravenous administration [389–391] emphasize the importance of IgG in facilitating the neutrophil inflammatory response.

Reticuloendothelial clearance of opsonized GBS also is less efficient in experimental infection of young animals [392,393], as are lung macrophage postphagocytic oxidative metabolic responses [394]. An age-related impairment in clearance of GBS from the lungs has been reported for infant compared with adult rats and for preterm compared with term animals [395,396]. Animal age is a more important determinant of bacterial elimination from the lung than amount of polysaccharide capsule, although encapsulated strains are ingested less efficiently and in fewer numbers in infant rats than in adult rats [255].

Other Factors Related to Pathogenesis

Fibronectin is a high-molecular-weight glycoprotein that participates in adherence and functions as a nonspecific opsonin. The observation that septic neonates have significantly lower fibronectin levels than healthy age-matched controls stimulated evaluation of the possible role of fibronectin in the pathogenesis of group B streptococcal infection [397]. Soluble fibronectin binds poorly to GBS in the absence of other opsonins [398]. GBS do adhere to immobilized fibronectin, however. Fibronectin also enhances ingestion by neutrophils, monocytes, or macrophages of GBS opsonized with type-specific antibody [399–401] and may promote TNF-α production by macrophages [402]. It also has been shown that interaction of type III CPS with the lectin site of CR3 effectively triggers phagocytosis of type III organisms by nonimmune serum. Use of this mechanism provides a potential explanation for the infrequency with which invasive infection develops in susceptible individuals exposed to GBS [403].

It has been hypothesized that some individuals may have a genetically based predisposition to infection with GBS. Among 34 Swedish mothers of infants with group B streptococcal disease, Grubb and coworkers [404] identified a surplus of individuals possessing G3m(5) and a deficit of individuals with G1m(1). Thom and colleagues [405] found deficits of G1m(1) and Km(1) and an increased incidence of G2m(23) among mothers of infected infants. The distribution of allotypic markers may influence responses to protein and polysaccharide antigens. G2m(23) is a marker of IgG$_2$, the subclass most often associated with brisk immune responses to polysaccharide antigens. There could be genetically determined explanations for the deficiency of IgG subclasses [406], high IgM concentration with divergent ratio of IgG to IgM [407,408], and chronic colonization state without immunologic response [409] described in Swedish mothers of infants with group B streptococcal disease. In a study of women in the United States who delivered infants with invasive type III group B streptococcal disease, postpartum immunization with type III group B streptococcal polysaccharide elicited immune responses similar to those in control women [410].

PATHOLOGY

Pathologic findings in early-onset infection depend on the duration of exposure to GBS before or during birth. Intrauterine death has been attributed to group B streptococcal infection [209,409,411] and is considered to be a common cause of mid-gestational fetal loss in women who have experienced either vaginal hemorrhage or septic abortion [411,412]. Fetal membrane infection with GBS can result in spontaneous abortion or premature rupture of membranes or both, as suggested by Hood and associates in 1961 and others [413–415].

Becroft and colleagues [416] noted histologic changes consistent with congenital pneumonia in live-born neonates whose autopsy lung cultures yielded GBS. Numerous placentas showed amnionitis in mothers whose infants had fulminant pneumonia and died within 36 hours after birth. Findings were sufficient in stillborn infants to indicate that death occurred as a direct consequence of group B streptococcal intra-amnionitis infection and intrauterine pneumonia. deSa and Trevenen [412] described pneumonitis with pulmonary interstitial and intra-alveolar inflammatory exudates in 15 infants weighing less than 1000 g who had intra-amniotic infection; 6 infants were stillborn, and 9 died within hours of birth. Placental examination revealed chorioamnionitis. In a primate model of infection, intra-amniotic inoculation of GBS elicited fulminant early-onset neonatal infection [215]. Microscopy of lung tissue revealed organisms within membrane-bound vacuoles of alveolar epithelial cells; interstitial fibroblasts; and organisms present within tissue macrophages of the liver, spleen, and brain, documenting their rapid dissemination.

Amnionitis in association with early-onset group B streptococcal sepsis (1) is more frequently detected when death occurs shortly after birth, (2) is a common finding when membranes have been ruptured 24 hours or longer before delivery [211,412,413], and (3) can be clinically silent in some women. GBS can enter the amniotic fluid cavity through ruptured or intact membranes [417], allowing fetal aspiration of infected fluid and subsequent pulmonary lesions or bacteremia, without eliciting a local inflammatory response or maternal signs of intra-amniotic infection.

Among neonates with fatal early-onset group B streptococcal disease, pulmonary lesions are the predominant pathologic feature. The association between pulmonary inflammation and formation of hyaline membranes was first noted by Franciosi and coworkers [2]. Subsequently, autopsy findings in early-onset disease cases revealed "atypical" pulmonary hyaline membranes in most [2,210,211], and these corresponded with radiographic features consistent with respiratory distress syndrome in some neonates [133]. GBS were frequently present within these membranes, and in some infants these were composed almost entirely of streptococci, rendering them basophilic in hematoxylin and eosin preparations [214]. Katzenstein and colleagues [214] postulated that invasion of alveolar cells and capillary endothelial cells by GBS resulted in exudation of plasma proteins into the alveoli, deposition of fibrin, and hyaline membrane formation. Immune complex–mediated injury to the lung was proposed by Pinnas and associates [418] as a mechanism for this hyaline membrane formation.

Histologic evidence for pneumonia was found historically in approximately 80% of patients with fatal early-onset group B streptococcal pneumonia [210,418,419]. The associated radiographic pattern could be focal, extensive, lobular, or bronchial, involving one or more lobes. The typical histologic features of congenital pneumonia (i.e., alveolar exudates composed of neutrophils, erythrocytes, and aspirated squamous cells, with edema and congestion) were observed either independently or in association with hyaline membrane formation. In neonates with fulminant, rapidly fatal group B streptococcal infection, the cellular inflammatory response was less pronounced. An interstitial inflammatory exudate is a consistent feature of fatal infection, as is pulmonary hemorrhage, which can range from focal interstitial to extensive intra-alveolar bleeding.

In CNS infection, age at onset predicts distinctive morphologic findings in the brain and meninges. In early-onset meningitis, little or no evidence of leptomeningeal inflammation is seen in three quarters of infants [2,176,226], although purulent meningitis can be observed occasionally. This lack of inflammatory response can be the result of rapidly progressive infection, with an interval of only a few hours from onset of clinical illness until death, or can reflect inadequate host response to infection, or both. Bacteria generally are found in large numbers, and perivascular inflammation, thrombosis of small vessels, and parenchymal hemorrhage frequently are noted [226]. In some preterm infants surviving septic shock caused by early-onset group B streptococcal infection, periventricular leukomalacia, a condition characterized by infarction of the white matter surrounding the lateral ventricles, develops [420]. Infants with fatal late-onset meningitis almost always have a diffuse purulent leptomeningitis, especially prominent at the base of the brain, with or without perivascular inflammation and hemorrhage [2,421]. Infants surviving severe meningitis have multiple areas of necrosis, and abscess formation can be found throughout the brain by neuroimaging or later at autopsy.

This age-related inflammatory response in infants with group B streptococcal infection has a parallel in the infant rat model of meningitis [317]. Young infant rats 5 to 10 days of age have numerous bacteria distributed in a perivascular pattern, and organisms can extend transmurally into vessel lumina. These animals generally have no evidence of acute leptomeningeal inflammation or edema. By contrast, 11- to 15-day-old animals have leptomeningitis and cerebritis with a pronounced infiltration of neutrophils and macrophages around meningeal vessels and in perivascular spaces within the cerebral cortex. Because response to infection becomes more efficient within a few weeks after birth, the absence of inflammation in the brain and meninges of infant rats and of human neonates with early-onset group B streptococcal infection

may relate to chemotactic defects [241], exhaustion of neutrophil stores [280,281], reticuloendothelial system immaturity [392], or to other deficits in the host response to infection.

CLINICAL MANIFESTATIONS AND OUTCOME
EARLY-ONSET INFECTION

When the incidence of neonatal infection caused by GBS increased dramatically in the 1970s [422], a bimodal distribution of cases according to age at onset of signs became apparent. Two syndromes related to age were described in 1973 by Franciosi and associates [2] (acute and delayed) and by Baker and colleagues [3] (early and late). Early-onset infection typically manifests within 24 hours of birth (an estimated 85% of cases; median age 12 hours), but it can become evident during the second 24 hours of life (an estimated 10% of cases) or at any time during the subsequent 5 days. Premature infants often experience onset at or within 6 hours of birth; infants with onset after the first 24 hours of life usually are of term gestation [208]. Late-onset infections occur at 7 to 89 days of age (median age 37 days). Classification of syndromes by age at onset is useful, but there also is a continuum in age at onset. A few patients with early-onset disease can present at 5 or 6 days of age, and late late-onset infection can affect 3- to 6-month-old infants, especially infants with gestational age of less than 28 weeks [150]. Onset beyond 6 months of age can herald the presentation of human immunodeficiency virus (HIV) infection or other immune system abnormalities [423].

Early-onset group B streptococcal infection often affects neonates whose mothers have obstetric complications associated with risk for neonatal sepsis (onset of labor before 37 weeks of gestation, prolonged interval at any gestation between rupture of membranes and delivery, rupture of membranes ≥18 hours before delivery, intrapartum fever >38° C [>100.4° F], intra-amniotic infection, early postpartum febrile morbidity, and twin births) (Table 12–3). A nearly threefold risk of early-onset

TABLE 12-3   Features of Group B Streptococcal Disease in Neonates and Infants

Feature	Early-Onset (<7 Days)	Late-Onset (7-89 Days)	Late Late-Onset (>89 Days)
Median age at onset	1 day	37 days	>3 mo
Incidence of prematurity	Increased	Increased	Common
Maternal obstetric complications	Frequent (70%)	Preterm delivery	Varies
Common manifestations	Septicemia (80%-85%)	Meningitis (25%-30%)	Bacteremia without a focus (common)
	Meningitis (5%-10%)	Bacteremia without focus (65%)	Bacteremia with a focus (uncommon)
	Pneumonia (10%-15%)	Soft tissue, bone, or joint pneumonia (5%-10%)	
CPS types isolated	Ia (~30%)	III (~60%)	Several
	II (~15%)	Ia (~25%)	
	III (30%)	V (~15%)	
	V (20%)		
Case-fatality rate	3%-10%	1%-6%	Low

CPS, capsular polysaccharide.

group B streptococcal disease has been observed when six or more vaginal examinations are performed before delivery [424]. The incidence of infection correlates inversely with the degree of preterm birth, and group B *Streptococcus* is the most frequent pathogen associated with early-onset sepsis in neonates with very low birth weight (<1500 g) [425]. One fourth of infants with early-onset disease historically were born before 37 weeks' gestation, but this number has increased since the introduction of routine prenatal culture screening and IAP for women colonized with GBS [150].

Early-onset group B streptococcal infection can occur in term neonates with no defined maternal risk factors other than colonization. In such cases, recognition is often delayed until the appearance of definite signs of sepsis (e.g., tachypnea, apnea, hypotension), but more subtle signs usually precede these overt manifestations. One report found that one third of healthy term neonates with early-onset group B streptococcal infection were identified solely on the basis of evaluation for maternal intrapartum temperature exceeding 38° C (100.4° F) [426].

The three most common expressions of early-onset infection are bacteremia without a defined focus of infection, pneumonia, and meningitis. In the 21st century, bacteremia without a focus occurs in 80% to 85%, pneumonia occurs in 10% to 15%, and meningitis occurs in 5% to 10% of infants [150]. Bacteremia is often detected in neonates with the latter two presentations, but not always. Regardless of site of involvement, respiratory signs (apnea, grunting respirations, tachypnea, or cyanosis) are the initial clinical findings in more than 80% of neonates. Hypotension is an initial finding in approximately 25%. Infants with fetal asphyxia related to group B streptococcal infection in utero can have shock and respiratory failure at delivery [427]. Additional signs include lethargy, poor feeding, hypothermia or fever, abdominal distention, pallor, tachycardia, and jaundice.

Pneumonia occurs in 10% to 15% of infants with early-onset infection, and virtually all of these infants have acute respiratory signs. Most have these respiratory findings in the first few hours of life (many at birth) or within the first 24 hours of life [210]. Among 19 infants with group B streptococcal congenital pneumonia at autopsy, 89% had 1-minute Apgar scores of 4 or less, indicating in utero onset of infection [208]. Radiographic features consistent with and indistinguishable from those of surfactant deficiency are present in more than half of these neonates (Fig. 12–6). Treatment with surfactant improves gas exchange in most, although the response is slower than in noninfected infants, and repeated surfactant doses often are needed [239]. Infiltrates suggesting congenital pneumonia (Fig. 12–7) are present in one third of infants. Increased vascular markings suggesting the diagnosis of transient tachypnea of the newborn or pulmonary edema can occur. Occasionally, respiratory distress is present in the absence of radiographic abnormalities, appearing as persistent fetal circulation and pulmonary hypertension [419,428]. Small pleural effusions and cardiomegaly can occur.

Meningitis occurs in 5% to 10% of neonates with early-onset infection. Neonates with meningitis often have a clinical presentation early in the course that is identical to

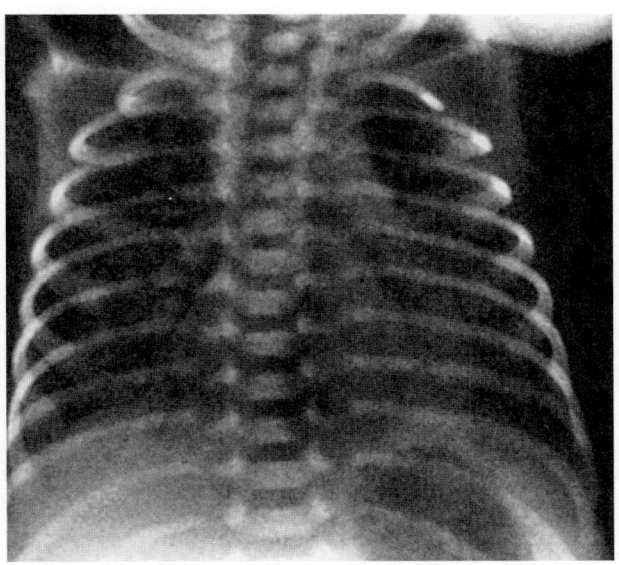

FIGURE 12–6 Chest radiograph from an infant with early-onset group B streptococcal septicemia shows features consistent with respiratory distress syndrome of the newborn.

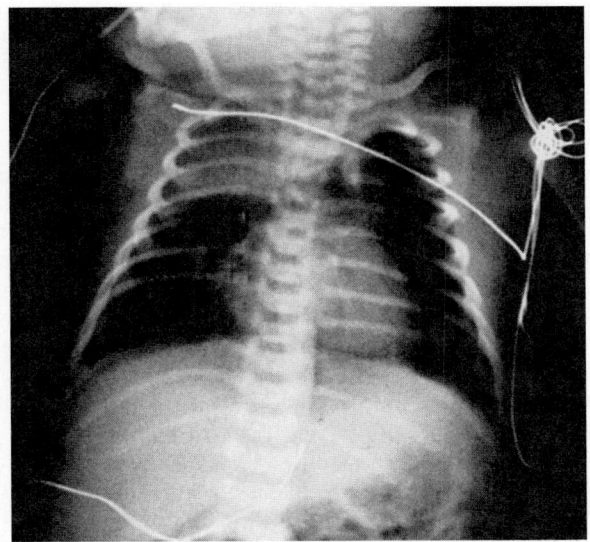

FIGURE 12–7 Chest radiograph shows right upper and lower lobe infiltrates as manifestations of early-onset group B streptococcal pneumonia in an infant.

presentation of neonates without meningeal involvement. Respiratory distress can be the most common initial sign, and in 27 infants with early-onset meningitis, seizures were never a presenting feature [429]. Examination of CSF is the only means to exclude meningitis, a finding that requires modification of supportive and specific chemotherapy (see "Treatment" later on). Seizures occur during the first 24 hours of therapy in nearly 50% of infants with meningitis. Persistent seizures, semicoma or coma, and a CSF protein concentration greater than 300 mg/dL are associated with a poor prognosis [430–432].

TABLE 12-4   Fatality Rates in Early-Onset Group B Streptococcal Infection

Study	Case-Fatality Rate (%) by Birth Weight (g) or Gestational Age (wk)				
	500-1000	**1001-1500**	**1501-2000**	**2001-2500**	**>2500**
Boyer et al [708] (1973-1981)	90	25	29	33	3
Baker [613] (1982-1989)	60	25	26	18	5
Weisman et al [427] (1987-1989)	75	40	20	15	6
Schrag et al [12] (1993-1998)		30 (≤33 wk)		10 (34-36 wk)	2 (≥37 wk)
Phares et al [150] (1999-2005)		20 (<37wk)			3 (≥37 wk)

The case-fatality rate for the nearly 300 neonates with early-onset infection summarized by Anthony and Okada [422] in 1977 was 55%. Current data indicate much lower rates of 2% to 10%. Features associated with fatal outcome include a low 5-minute Apgar score, shock, neutropenia, pleural effusion, apnea, and delay in treatment after onset of symptoms [170,212,427]. Fatal infection also occurs significantly more often among premature than among term neonates (Table 12-4). In 1981, Pyati and colleagues [433] reported a case-fatality rate of 61% among 101 preterm neonates who had early-onset group B streptococcal infection. Infants with a birth weight greater than 1500 g had a fatality rate of 14%, however. Contemporary data document that the risk of death among preterm cases is 20%—nearly 8-fold that of term infants for whom infection was fatal in 3% of cases [150].

LATE-ONSET INFECTION

Late-onset group B streptococcal infection historically affected term infants 7 to 89 days of age who had had an unremarkable maternal obstetric and early neonatal history. Contemporary data indicate that at least half of infants with late-onset disease now are born before 37 weeks of gestation [150]. Late-onset disease has a lower fatality rate (1% to 6%) than early-onset disease. Clinical expressions of late-onset disease include bacteremia without a focus of infection (65% of infants), meningitis (25%), bacteremic cellulitis or osteoarthritis (2% to 3% each), and pneumonia (3%) (see Table 12-3) [150].

Bacteremia without a detectable focus of infection is the most common clinical expression of late-onset group B streptococcal disease [434]. Bacteremia without a focus typically manifests with nonspecific signs (i.e., fever, poor feeding, irritability). Diagnosis results from the practice of obtaining routine blood cultures in febrile infants during the first few weeks of life to exclude serious bacterial infection as an underlying cause. These infants often are mildly ill, but failure to initiate antimicrobial therapy in a timely manner can result in progression to shock, especially in preterm infants, or extension of infection to distant sites such as the CNS. Either transient or persistent bacteremia can occur. Approximately 3% of infants with late-onset bacteremia without a focus die; survivors typically recover without sequelae after treatment.

The presenting signs in infants with late-onset meningitis almost always include fever, irritability or lethargy or both, poor feeding, and tachypnea. Upper respiratory tract infection precedes late-onset meningitis in 20% to 30% of infants, suggesting that alteration of mucosal barrier by respiratory viral illness might facilitate entry of GBS into the bloodstream [2,3,430]. In contrast to early-onset infection, grunting respirations and apnea are less frequent initial findings, and their presence suggests rapidly progressive, fulminant infection. Apnea or hypotension is observed in less than 15% of patients, but there is a spectrum in clinical severity of illness at presentation. Some infants appear clinically well a few hours before initial evaluation and present with seizures, poor perfusion, neutropenia, and large numbers of gram-positive cocci in the CSF. These patients often have a rapidly fatal course, or if they survive, they are left with devastating neurologic sequelae. Leukopenia or neutropenia at the time of diagnosis has been correlated with fatal outcome in these infants [212].

Other initial findings associated with increased risk for fatal outcome or permanent neurologic sequelae include hypotension, coma or semicoma, status epilepticus, absolute neutrophil count less than 1000/mm³, and CSF protein level greater than 300 mg/dL [212,422,430,432]. These findings most likely reflect a high bacterial inoculum in the CSF and cerebritis. Subdural effusions, which usually are small, unilateral, and asymptomatic, are found in 20% of patients with late-onset meningitis. These are not associated with any permanent sequelae. Subdural empyema, obstructive ventriculitis, large infarctions, and encephalomalacia are uncommon complications.

LATE LATE-ONSET INFECTION

Infections in infants older than 89 days of age can account for 20% of cases of late-onset disease [435]. The terms *very late onset*, *late late-onset*, and *beyond early infancy* have been applied to disease in these infants. Most of these infants have a gestational age of less than 35 weeks. The need for prolonged hospitalization and the immature host status in these infants probably contributes to infection beyond the interval for term neonates. Bacteremia without a focus is a common presentation. Occasionally, a focus for infection, such as the CNS, intravascular catheter, or soft tissues, is identified (see Table 12-3). In the outpatient setting, infants older than 89 days of age are likely to have a temperature greater than 39° C (>102.2° F) and a white blood cell count exceeding 15,000/mm³ [434]. A viral infection can precede the onset of bacteremia [436]. When there are no other apparent risk factors for late late-onset infection in a term infant, immunodeficiency including HIV infection should be considered [437,438].

SEPTIC ARTHRITIS AND OSTEOMYELITIS

The clinical features of 20 infants with group B streptococcal septic arthritis alone and 45 infants with osteomyelitis (with or without concomitant septic arthritis) are shown in Table 12–5. The mean age at diagnosis of osteomyelitis (31 days) is greater than that for septic arthritis (20 days). The mean duration of symptoms is shorter for septic arthritis than for osteomyelitis (1.5 days versus 9 days). In some infants with osteomyelitis, failure to move the involved extremity since hospital discharge after birth, or shortly thereafter, may be noted; this lack of movement can persist for 4 weeks before the diagnosis is made [439].

Decreased motion of the involved extremity and evidence of pain with manipulation, such as lifting or diaper changing, are common signs of bone infection. Warmth or erythema can occur occasionally [440,441]; a history of fever is reported in only 20% of infants. The paucity of signs suggesting infection and the finding of pseudoparalysis have led to an initial diagnosis of Erb palsy and to assessment for possible child abuse [439,442,443]. In several infants, osteomyelitis of the proximal humerus has been associated with findings on nerve conduction studies consistent with brachial plexus neuropathy [444,445], and in one infant, sciatic nerve injury at the level of the pelvis caused footdrop in association with iliac osteomyelitis [446].

Physical findings include fixed flexion of the involved extremity, mild swelling, evidence of pain with passive motion, decreased spontaneous movement, and, in a few infants, erythema and warmth. Lack of associated systemic involvement is the rule, although osteomyelitis in association with meningitis, peritonitis, and overwhelming sepsis

with congestive heart failure has been reported [441,442,447–449].

When infants with septic arthritis alone are compared with infants with osteomyelitis, infants with septic arthritis more often have lower extremity involvement, with the hip joint predominating [447,450]. By contrast, more than half of the reported infants with osteomyelitis have had involvement of the humerus, and in infants for whom the location was specified, the proximal humerus predominated [439,442,447,451]. Osteomyelitis involving both proximal humeri has been described [448]. Involvement of the femur, vertebrae, or small bones occurs occasionally [452,453]. Usually, only one bone is affected, although infection involving two adjacent bones or multiple nonadjacent bones can occur rarely [448,454,455]. Although most infants with humeral osteomyelitis have had concomitant infection in the shoulder joint, isolated septic arthritis of the shoulder joint has not been reported.

Group B streptococcal bone and joint infections have a good prognosis. At evaluation 6 months to 4 years after diagnosis, 17 (90%) of 19 infants with osteomyelitis had normal function in the affected extremity.* Residual shortening and limitation of motion of the humerus were noted in a patient who had overwhelming sepsis of acute onset, with congestive heart failure and osteomyelitis involving noncontiguous sites [447]. Growth disturbance can result as a consequence of subluxation of the hip joint after septic arthritis.

Although septic arthritis and osteomyelitis are considered manifestations of late-onset disease, osteomyelitis seems to represent a clinically silent early-onset bacteremia with seeding of a bone and then later onset of clinical expression of infection. An episode of asymptomatic bacteremia with a birth trauma–induced nidus in the proximal humerus could allow localization of bacteria to the bone. Because lytic lesions take more than 10 to 14 days to become radiographically visible, the presence of such lesions on radiographs obtained at hospital admission suggests long-standing infection (Fig. 12–8). Non–type III strains are overrepresented among infants with osteomyelitis, which is consistent with the hypothesis that, in at least some patients, early-onset bacteremia with bony localization of infection may have occurred.

TABLE 12–5   Clinical Features of Group B Streptococcal Bone and Joint Infections*

Feature	Septic Arthritis without Osteomyelitis (20 Patients) [4,447,450,457, 709–711]	Osteomyelitis (45 Patients) [4,439–444,447, 448,451,454–456, 712–715]
Mean age at diagnosis (range)	20 days (5-37)	31 days (8-60)
Mean duration of symptoms (range)	1.5 days (<1-3)	9 days (1-28)
Male-to-female ratio	2:5	2:3
Site (%)	Hip (56)	Humerus (56)
	Knee (38)	Femur (24)
	Ankle (6)	Tibia, talus (4)
		Other† (16)
Group B streptococcal serotype (No. patients)	III (12)	III (15), Ib/c (3), Ia/c (1)
Mean duration of parenteral therapy (range)	2 wk (2-3)	3 wk (2-7)

*Includes authors' unpublished data for seven patients.
†Ilium, acromion, clavicle, skull, digit, vertebrae; ribs—one patient each.

CELLULITIS OR ADENITIS

The manifestation of late-onset group B streptococcal infection designated as facial cellulitis [458], submandibular cellulitis [459], cellulitis/adenitis syndrome [460], or lymphadenitis [461] has been reported in at least 25 infants [462–465]. Presenting signs include poor feeding; irritability; fever; and unilateral facial, preauricular, or submandibular swelling, usually, but not always, accompanied by erythema. The mean age at onset is 5 weeks (range 2 to 11 weeks), and in contrast to all other expressions of late-onset infection, there is a striking male predominance (72%). The most common sites are the submandibular and parotid, and enlarged adjacent nodes become palpable within 2 days after onset of the soft

*References [4,439,440,444,447,448,456,457].

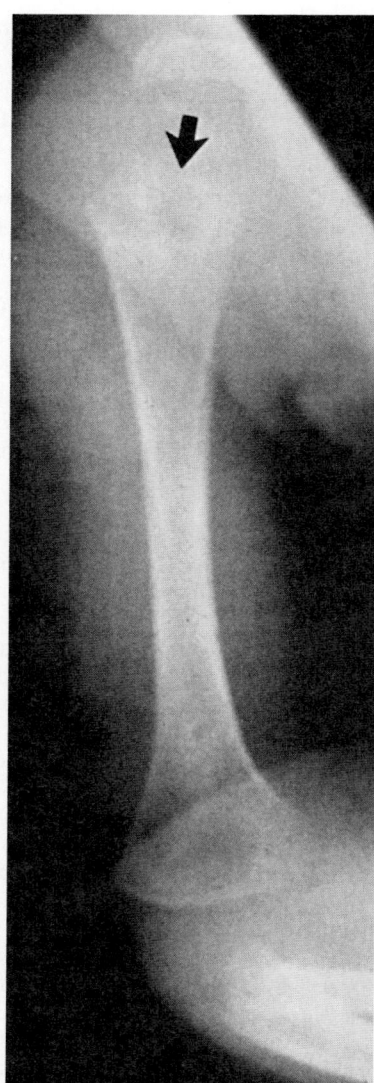

FIGURE 12–8 Radiograph shows lytic lesion (*arrow*) of the proximal humerus in an infant whose bone biopsy showed osteomyelitis caused by type III group B streptococci.

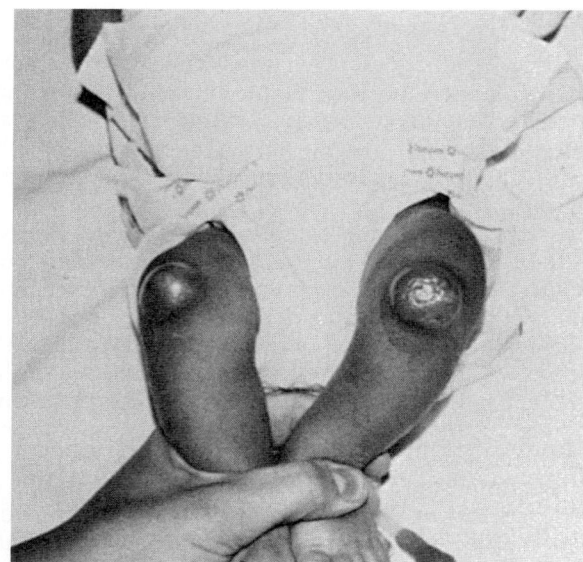

FIGURE 12–9 Prepatellar bursitis of both knees in an infant who had abraded his knees on the bed sheets. Aspiration of purulent material from the prepatellar space yielded type III group B streptococci. The knee joints were not affected.

UNUSUAL MANIFESTATIONS OF INFECTION

Numerous uncommon clinical manifestations of early-onset and late-onset group B streptococcal infection have been recorded (Table 12–6). Peritonitis [467] and adrenal abscess [468–470] have been described as abdominal manifestations of early-onset and late-onset infection. Adrenal abscess is thought to result from bacteremic seeding associated with adrenal hemorrhage and subsequent abscess formation. One neonate thought to have neuroblastoma underwent en bloc resection of a large mass with nephrectomy before the diagnosis of adrenal abscess was established [469]. Gallbladder distention is a nonspecific manifestation of early-onset sepsis that usually resolves with medical management of the infection [471]. Late-onset bacteremia can occur in association with jaundice, elevated levels of liver enzymes, and increased direct-reacting bilirubin fraction. Hemolysis and hepatocellular inflammation possibly contribute to the development of jaundice.

Brain abscess rarely occurs in association with recurrence of group B streptococcal meningitis. One infant recovered after craniotomy and excision of a well-encapsulated frontal mass, but had neurologic sequelae [472]. Sokol and colleagues [473] described a 5-week-old infant with a cerebellar cyst believed to represent an astrocytoma. This infant proved to have obstructive hydrocephalus and chronic group B streptococcal ventriculitis. Rarely, anterior fontanelle herniation can complicate severe meningitis. The presence of a noncystic doughy mass over the fontanelle indicates that brain herniation may have occurred, and cranial ultrasonography or computed tomography (CT) can be obtained to confirm this diagnosis. One patient with cervical myelopathy initially had absence of extremity movement, but made a good recovery and was able to walk at age 3 years [474].

Another unusual complication of group B streptococcal meningitis is subdural empyema, which has been

tissue infection. Four of the five infants with facial or submandibular cellulitis described by Baker [460] had ipsilateral otitis media at the time of diagnosis. Less common sites of involvement with cellulitis are the face, preauricular or inguinal areas, scrotum, anterior neck region, and prepatellar spaces (Fig. 12–9) [460,464,465]. In one patient, cellulitis of the neck occurred in association with an infected thyroglossal duct cyst [460].

Bacteremia almost always is detected in these infants (92%), and cultures of soft tissue or lymph node aspirates have yielded GBS in 83% of the infants in whom this procedure was performed. These infants usually are not seriously ill, few have associated meningitis, and recovery within a few days of initiation of appropriate antimicrobial therapy is the rule. Fulminant and fatal facial cellulitis has been described in a 7-hour-old neonate [4], however, and associated meningitis has been described in two infants [466].

TABLE 12–6 Unusual Clinical Manifestations of Group B Streptococcal Infections

Site and Manifestation	Associated with Early-Onset or Late-Onset Infection	Reference No.
Abdomen		
Peritonitis	Both	467
Adrenal abscess	Both	468–470
Gallbladder distention	Early	471
Brain		
Abscess	Late	472
Anterior fontanelle herniation	Both	716
Chronic meningitis	Late	473
Subdural empyema	Both	475,476
Cerebritis	Late	478
Myelopathy/myelitis	Early	474,717
Ventriculitis complicating myelomeningocele	Both	718
Oculomotor nerve paralysis	Late	719
Ventriculoperitoneal shunt infection	Late	720
Cardiovascular		
Asymptomatic bacteremia	Both	4,721,722
Endocarditis	Both	136,449,479
Pericarditis	Not specified	481
Myocarditis	Late	456
Mycotic aneurysm	Late	482
Ear and sinus		
Ethmoiditis	Late	4
Otitis media/mastoiditis	Both	460,483–486
Eye		
Conjunctivitis/ophthalmia neonatorum	Early	2,487,723
Endophthalmitis	Late	488
Retrobulbar abscess	Early	724
Respiratory tract		
Diaphragmatic hernia	Both	493
Supraglottitis	Late	489
Pleural empyema	Both	4,491,492
Tracheitis	Late	490
Skin and soft tissue		
Abscess of cystic hygroma	Late	506
Breast abscess	Late	509,725
Bursitis	Late	726
Cellulitis/adenitis	Both	4,458–462, 496,727
Dactylitis	Late	728
Fasciitis	Late	499–501
Impetigo neonatorum	Early	502,503
Purpura fulminans	Both	497,498
Omphalitis	Both	421
Rhabdomyolysis	Late	729
Retropharyngeal cellulitis	Late	507,508
Scalp abscess	Both	505
Urinary tract infection	Both	435,510

described in patients with early-onset and late-onset infections [475,476]. The diagnosis was established by needle aspiration of the subdural space at the time of hospital admission [476] or within the first 5 days of treatment. Irritability, vomiting, seizures, increasing head circumference, focal neurologic signs, a tense anterior fontanelle, or a combination of these prompted evaluation [475,477]. Sterilization of the subdural space was accomplished by open or closed drainage in conjunction with antimicrobial therapy. Basal ganglia and massive cerebral infarction also have been described [478].

Cardiovascular manifestations of group B streptococcal infection are rare. Endocarditis [136,449,479,480], pericarditis [481], myocarditis [456], and mycotic aneurysm of the aorta [482] have been documented. Echocardiography can be useful in delineating the nature of cardiac involvement, and this technique was employed successfully to detect a 0.7-cm vegetation on the anterior leaflet of the mitral valve in a 4-week-old infant with endocarditis caused by a type III strain [449]. Paroxysmal atrial tachycardia can be a presenting feature of group B streptococcal septicemia in the absence of focal infection of the heart [133].

GBS are an uncommon cause of otitis media in the first few weeks of life (2% to 3% of cases) [483]. Otitis media is more often associated with late-onset disease manifesting as meningitis or submandibular cellulitis [484–486]. The finding of acute mastoiditis at autopsy in one infant with otitis media and meningitis suggests that the middle ear can serve as a portal of entry in a few patients [486].

Conjunctivitis related to GBS occurs with such rarity that no cases were identified among 302 neonates with ophthalmia neonatorum described by Armstrong and associates [487]. Exudative conjunctivitis has been reported, however, in association with early-onset bacteremia [487]. More severe ocular involvement is rare, but endophthalmitis has been noted in infants with septicemia and meningitis [488]. As is the case for other agents producing endophthalmitis, high-grade bacteremia is a likely prelude to this unusual metastatic focus of group B streptococcal infection.

Supraglottitis was described in a 3-month-old infant with acute onset of stridor [489]. Swelling of the left aryepiglottic fold, but not the epiglottis, was noted at laryngoscopy. An infant with bacterial tracheitis had a similar presentation [490]. Although pulmonary infection caused by GBS is common, pleural involvement is rare, but it has been reported as a complication of early-onset [491] and late-onset [492] pneumonia. An interesting but unexplained association is delayed development of right-sided diaphragmatic hernia and early-onset group B streptococcal sepsis [493]. In affected infants, the onset of respiratory distress invariably occurs at or within 48 hours after birth, whereas the mean age at diagnosis of right-sided diaphragmatic hernia in the 40 reported cases is 11 days (range 4 to 91 days). One speculation is that group B streptococcal pneumonia causes necrosis of the adjacent diaphragm and results in herniation of viscera into the pleural space. Another is that ventilation increases intrathoracic pressure to mask or delay herniation through a congenital diaphragmatic defect. This phenomenon should be a consideration in an infant whose condition deteriorates despite appropriate management for early-onset disease. Radiographic features include increased density in the right lower lung or irregular aeration or both, followed by progression to elevation of right bowel gas and liver shadow.

In addition to cellulitis and adenitis, GBS uncommonly can produce various unusual skin and soft tissue manifestations, including violaceous cellulitis [494], perineal cellulitis and septicemia after circumcision [495], scrotal ecchymosis as a sign of intraperitoneal hemorrhage [496], purpura fulminans [497,498], necrotizing fasciitis [499–501], impetigo neonatorum [502,503], omphalitis [421,504], scalp abscess secondary to fetal scalp electrode [505], abscess complicating cystic hygroma [506], retropharyngeal cellulitis [507,508], and breast abscess [509]. In patients with impetiginous lesions and abscess formation, bacteremia is unusual, but it is a frequent accompaniment to omphalitis and necrotizing fasciitis.

Among infants with early-onset bacteremia, isolation of GBS from the urine is frequent when this body fluid is cultured, but primary urinary tract infection with these organisms is rare. An infant with severe bilateral ureterohydronephrosis and GBS in his urine has been described [510]. The isolation of GBS from a urine culture of a patient without bacteremia is an indication for evaluation for possible structural anomalies of the genitourinary tract.

Sudden death occurred in three infants ranging from 3 to 8 months of age. The deaths were attributed at the time of autopsy to group B streptococcal infection [409].

RELAPSE OR RECURRENCE OF INFECTION

Relapse or recurrence of group B streptococcal infection occurs in an estimated 0.5% to 3% of infants. Signs can develop during treatment for the initial episode or at an interval of 3 days to 3 months after completion of therapy [511–513]. In one review, eight of nine infants with a recurrence were born at 25 to 36 weeks of gestation, and male infants predominated [512]. The first episode occurred at a mean age of 10 days (range 1 to 27 days) and the recurrence at a mean age of 42 days (range 23 to 68 days) of life. In another report that included a set of fraternal twins, seven of eight infants were preterm (mean 30 weeks of gestation), each had a birth weight of less than 2500 g, and all infections were late-onset [513]. The mean age at initial presentation was 38 days (range 13 to 112 days), and at recurrence it was 57 days (range 34 to 130 days). Two relapses in one infant have been documented [514,515].

Relapse or recurrence of infection can be the result of an undrained focus of infection, such as a brain abscess, or can occur in association with congenital heart disease. Identical isolates recovered from maternal genital and breast milk cultures suggest that breast milk can serve as a source of repeated infant exposure [516,517]. Recurrent infection can have a clinical expression similar to that of the initial episode or can involve new sites (meninges, ventricular or subdural fluid, or both; brain parenchyma; and soft tissue). In most instances, the second episode of group B streptococcal disease responds to retreatment with penicillin or ampicillin, but typically the duration

of treatment for the recurrence is extended empirically; evidence for longer duration of therapy in this circumstance is lacking [513].

Because infants who receive treatment for invasive infection often remain colonized with GBS at mucous membrane sites, pharyngeal or gastrointestinal colonization can be the source for recurrence. In addition, infants recovering from invasive infection with type III strains usually lack protective levels of antibody during convalescence. Moylett and colleagues [513] and others [514] used pulsed-field gel electrophoresis to document that isolates from patients with recurrent episodes were identical and were derived from a single clone. Sets of isolates analyzed from first and second episodes and from maternal and infant colonizing and invasive strains were genotypically identical [512,513]. Recurrent infection in most infants likely is a consequence of reinvasion from persistently colonized mucous membrane sites or from reexposure to a household carrier. The timing of the recurrence or relapse in Moylett's series was 4 days after discontinuation of appropriate therapy. Uncommonly, infants have had a second infection with a strain that is genetically unrelated to the original isolate.

MATERNAL INFECTIONS

In 1938, Fry [1] described three fatal cases of endocarditis in postpartum women. This was the initial insight that group B *Streptococcus* was a human pathogen and could cause puerperal infection. Postpartum infections including septic abortion, bacteremia, chorioamnionitis, endometritis, pneumonia, and septic arthritis were recorded sporadically thereafter, but group B streptococcal infections in postpartum women, as in neonates, were uncommonly reported before 1970 [413,518,519]. The dramatic increase in incidence of neonatal infections in the 1970s was paralleled by an increased incidence of infections in pregnant women.

Before the institution of Intrapartum Antibiotic Prophylaxis in the 1990s, GBS accounted for 10% to 20% of blood culture isolates from febrile women on obstetric services [520]. These women had a clinical picture characterized by fever, malaise, uterine tenderness with normal lochia, and occasionally chills. Faro [334] described 40 women with group B streptococcal endometritis and endoparametritis among 3106 women giving birth over a 12-month interval, an incidence of 1.3 per 1000 deliveries. GBS were isolated from the endometrium in pure culture in one third of cases or in addition to other organisms in the remainder; one third of the women had concomitant bacteremia. In most, signs of infection developed within the first 24 hours after cesarean section. Clinical features included chills; tachycardia; abdominal distention; and exquisite uterine, parametrial, or adnexal tenderness. Higher fever correlated with risk for concomitant bacteremia. Recovery was uniform after administration of appropriate antimicrobial agents. Six infants born to these women developed group B streptococcal septicemia, however, and infection was fatal was three. The observation that maternal febrile morbidity could serve as an early clue to bacteremic neonatal infection is important, and infants of such women should be carefully evaluated.

The contemporary incidence of invasive disease in pregnant women is 0.12 per 1000 live births [150]. This incidence has declined significantly in association with implementation of IAP to prevent early-onset neonatal disease [12,143]. Half of the 409 pregnancy-associated disease cases identified in the United States from 1999-2005 by an active population-based surveillance system were associated with infection of the upper genital tract, placenta, or amniotic sac and resulted in fetal death. Among the remainder, manifestations of disease included bacteremia without a focus (31%), endometritis without fetal death (8%), chorioamnionitis without fetal death (4%), pneumonia (2%), and puerperal sepsis (2%). Isolates in pregnancy-associated infections were obtained from blood in 52% of women and from the placenta, amniotic fluid, or conceptus in most of the remainder. When pregnancy outcome was known, most of the women (61%) had a spontaneous abortion or stillborn infant, 5% had infants who developed clinical infection, 4% had induced abortions, and 30% had infants who remained clinically well [150].

Most obstetric patients with group B streptococcal infection, even in the presence of bacteremia, show a rapid response after initiation of antimicrobial therapy. Potentially fatal complications can occur, however, including meningitis [521], ventriculoperitoneal shunt infection [522], abdominal abscess [523], endocarditis [142,524–526], vertebral osteomyelitis [527], epidural abscess [528], or necrotizing fasciitis [529].

Group B streptococcal bacteriuria during pregnancy is a risk factor for intrauterine or neonatal infection. Asymptomatic bacteriuria, cystitis, or pyelonephritis occurs in 6% to 8% of women during pregnancy. In women with asymptomatic bacteriuria, approximately 20% are caused by GBS [530]. Group B streptococcal bacteriuria is a marker for heavy vaginal colonization, so the finding of bacteriuria indicates enhanced risk for maternal and neonatal infection [100]. In the series reported by Moller and associates [414] that predated IAP, a cohort of 68 women with asymptomatic group B streptococcal bacteriuria had significantly increased risk of preterm delivery compared with nonbacteriuric controls. Stillbirth because of congenital group B streptococcal infection can occur even in the current era, and a woman with any quantity of group B streptococcal bacteriuria during pregnancy should receive IAP [531].

DIAGNOSIS
ISOLATION AND IDENTIFICATION OF THE ORGANISM

The definitive diagnosis of invasive group B streptococcal infection is established by isolation of the organism from culture of blood, CSF, or a site of suppurative focus (e.g., bone, joint fluid, empyema fluid). Isolation of GBS from surfaces, such as the skin or umbilicus or from mucous membranes, is of no clinical significance.

Lumbar puncture is required to exclude meningeal involvement in infants with invasive group B streptococcal infection because clinical features cannot reliably distinguish between meningeal and nonmeningeal involvement. GBS often are isolated from blood at the time of initial evaluation of infants with meningitis, but the blood culture is sterile in 20% to 30%. Wiswell and colleagues [532] found that if lumbar puncture were omitted as part of the sepsis evaluation, the diagnosis of meningitis was missed or delayed in more than one third of infants. Infants with late-onset infection can have meningitis even when focal infection, such as cellulitis, is apparent [466]. If lumbar puncture must be deferred because an infant is clinically unstable, penicillin G or ampicillin at the doses recommended for treatment of group B streptococcal meningitis (see "Treatment" later on) should be administered until meningeal involvement can be assessed.

Antigen Detection Methods

Antigen detection is not a substitute for appropriately performed bacterial cultures and now is rarely used to establish a provisional diagnosis of group B streptococcal infection. A positive result indicates that group B streptococcal antigen is detectable, but not that viable organisms are present. Serum and CSF are the only specimens recommended for testing [533]. In neonates with meningitis, the sensitivity of antigen detection is 72% to 89%. The estimated sensitivity for serum is 30% to 40%. False-positive results have been encountered. The estimated specificity of commercial assays ranges from 95% to 98%. Antigen assays should not be employed to assess treatment efficacy.

Real time RT-PCR has been evaluated in a research setting to assess group B streptococcal exposure in infants born to women whose colonization status is unknown at delivery. The rates of colonization detected by culture and PCR were 17% and 51%. The authors suggest that a negative PCR test could be useful in allowing early discharge of infants born to mothers with a negative real time RT-PCR [534]. A fluorescent real time RT-PCR assay was shown to be sensitive and specific for early detection within 4 hours of incubation of GBS in neonatal blood cultures, but at the present time this test is not available commercially [535].

Other Laboratory Tests

Acute-phase reactants, such as C-reactive protein, can be elevated during group B streptococcal infection, but the usefulness for establishing a provisional diagnosis of infection is limited. The return to normal of the C-reactive protein level could be helpful, however, in minimizing antibiotic exposure in the nursery setting [536]. Levels of inflammatory cytokines such as IL-6 are elevated acutely during group B streptococcal sepsis. In one report, production of IL-6 was noted in all 16 neonates with bacteremic early-onset or late-onset group B streptococcal infection when samples were collected within 48 hours of initiation of antimicrobial therapy [537]. These assays generally are not available in clinical laboratories, however.

Abnormalities in the white blood cell count, including leukopenia, neutropenia, leukocytosis, increase in band forms, or decline in the total white blood cell count in the first 24 hours of life, can be suggestive of group B streptococcal infection. Greenberg and Yoder [538] cautioned that repeat testing at 12 to 24 hours of age can enhance sensitivity compared with testing at 1 to 7 hours of age. Fatal early-onset group B streptococcal sepsis can occur with a normal leukocyte count, however [539]. Measurements of peripheral blood leukocytes or inflammatory mediators generally are nonspecific and should be employed only as adjunctive to results from blood and CSF cultures.

DIFFERENTIAL DIAGNOSIS

The clinical features in neonates with early-onset group B streptococcal infection mimic the features in infants with sepsis caused by other etiologic agents and by some noninfectious illnesses. Radiographic findings of pneumonia are present in some neonates with early-onset group B streptococcal sepsis. Neonates with early-onset group B streptococcal pneumonia can have apnea and shock within the first 24 hours of life, a 1-minute Apgar score of 5 or less, and an unusually rapid progression of pulmonary disease [208]. Infection also should be considered in neonates with persistent fetal circulation associated with respiratory distress, neutropenia, and systemic hypotension [212].

The differential diagnosis for late-onset group B streptococcal infection depends on the clinical presentation. For infants with meningitis, the characteristic CSF Gram stain findings can provide a presumptive diagnosis. When this method is inconclusive usually in the setting of partial treatment, other organisms, including viruses, *E. coli*, *Neisseria meningitidis*, *S. pneumoniae*, and nontypable *Haemophilus influenzae*, must be considered. Fever usually is a presenting feature in term infants, and empirical therapy with broad-spectrum antibiotics customarily is employed until results of cultures permitting a specific diagnosis of bacteremia or focal infection are available. The paucity of signs characteristic of group B streptococcal osteomyelitis and the history that signs have been present since birth have caused confusion with Erb palsy and neuromuscular disorders. The characteristic bony lesion; tenderness of the extremity when a careful examination is performed; and isolation of the organism from blood, bone, or joint fluid usually provide a definitive diagnosis [439]. Finally, the lengthy list of uncommon manifestations of infection between 1 week and 3 months of age and beyond indicates that GBS should be suspected as an etiologic agent, regardless of site of infection, for infants in this age group.

TREATMENT

GBS have been a frequent cause of infection in neonates for 4 decades, resulting in increased awareness of associated risk factors and need for prompt and aggressive therapy. Despite striking declines, however, death and disability from these infections still occur. In addition, relapses or reinfections, although uncommon, occur in the face of optimal therapy. These facts should prompt efforts to develop improved treatment modalities.

IN VITRO SUSCEPTIBILITY

Uniform susceptibility of GBS to penicillin G has continued for more than 50 years of usage [540–545]. More recently, reduced susceptibility of certain strains of GBS to penicillin and other β-lactam antibiotics has been documented in the United States [546] and Japan [547] and experimentally traced to point mutations in penicillin-binding proteins reminiscent of first-step mutations in the evolution of pneumococcal penicillin resistance decades ago. The clinical implications of this finding are as yet unclear. Efforts should be continued, however, to monitor clinical isolates for mutations that would suggest the evolution of penicillin-resistant strains. In vitro susceptibility of GBS to ampicillin, semisynthetic penicillins, vancomycin, teicoplanin, linezolid, quinopristin/dalfopristin, gatifloxacin, levofloxacin, and first-generation, second-generation (excluding cefoxitin), and third-generation cephalosporins also is the rule, although the degree of in vitro activity varies [543,544,548–554]. Ceftriaxone is the most active of the cephalosporins in vitro. Imipenem and meropenem are highly active [541,548]. Resistance to quinolones can occur through mutations in the gyrase and topoisomerase IV genes, usually in patients who have received prior quinolone therapy [555].

Resistance to erythromycin and clindamycin is increasing. Contemporary data from multiple studies indicate that 20% to 30% of isolates are erythromycin-resistant, and 10% to 20% are resistant to clindamycin [543,544,556]. Rates of resistance in colonizing isolates can be 40% for erythromycin and clindamycin [557]. These high rates of resistance are reported from geographically diverse regions [558–561].

Macrolide resistance mechanisms include ribosomal modification by a methylase encoded by *erm* genes and drug efflux by a membrane-bound protein encoded by *mef* gene [556]. The presence of *erm* genes results in the macrolide–lincosamide–streptogramin B resistance phenotype [562]. Erythromycin-resistant isolates that are constitutively resistant, inducibly resistant, or susceptible to clindamycin are described [563]. Alone or in combination, *erm*(A), *erm*(B), and *mef*(A) genes are responsible for resistance in GBS. An *erm*(T) gene has been identified in a few strains of GBS inducibly resistant to clindamycin [564]. The presence of a composite transposon in GBS and pneumococci suggests that *erm*(B)-mediated macrolide resistance could be due to the horizontal transfer of a mobile transposable element [565]. A particularly high proportion of strains resistant to erythromycin has been reported for type V [544,566]. Tigecycline and telithromycin are active in vitro against macrolide-resistant GBS, but data confirming their clinical effectiveness are scant [567,568]. The percentage of tetracycline-resistant strains is 75% to nearly 90% [549]. Resistance of GBS to bacitracin, nalidixic acid, trimethoprim-sulfamethoxazole, metronidazole, and aminoglycosides is uniform.

Despite resistance of most group B streptococcal strains to aminoglycosides, synergy often is observed when an aminoglycoside (especially gentamicin) and penicillin or ampicillin are used in combination [553,569]. The best combination theoretically to accelerate the killing of GBS in vivo is penicillin or ampicillin plus gentamicin. Therapeutic concentrations of gentamicin in the serum are not required to achieve synergy. By contrast, the rapid and predictable bactericidal effect of penicillin or ampicillin on GBS in vitro is ablated by the addition of rifampin [570]. Although in vivo data are lacking, the in vitro antagonism of rifampin when combined with penicillins suggests that they should not be employed concurrently in the treatment of proven or suspected group B streptococcal disease.

Among the newer β-lactam antibiotics reputed to attain high concentrations of drug in the CSF, only cefotaxime, ceftriaxone, meropenem, and imipenem achieve minimal bactericidal concentrations (MBCs) comparable with MBCs of penicillin G and ampicillin (0.01 to 0.4 µg/mL) [541,549,553,556], and limited data suggest that their efficacy is equivalent to that of penicillin G [553,571,572]. Despite their uniform susceptibility to penicillin G, GBS require higher concentrations for growth inhibition in vitro than strains belonging to group A. The minimal inhibitory concentration (MIC) of penicillin G to GBS is 4-fold to 10-fold greater than the MIC for group A strains (range 0.003 to 0.4 µg/mL) [540,549,573]. This observation, combined with the observation indicating the significant influence of inoculum size on in vitro susceptibility to penicillin G, may have clinical relevance [540,574].

When the inoculum of group B *Streptococcus* is reduced from 10^5 to 10^4 colony-forming units (CFU)/mL, a two-fold lower concentration of penicillin G is sufficient to inhibit in vitro growth. Similarly, if the inoculum is increased from 10^4 to 10^7 CFU/mL, the MBC of ampicillin is increased from 0.06 to 3.9 µg/mL. Such in vitro observations may have in vivo correlates because some infants with group B streptococcal meningitis have CSF bacterial concentrations of 10^7 to 10^8 CFU/mL [574]. At the initiation of therapy for meningitis, achievable CSF levels of penicillin G or ampicillin may be only one tenth of serum levels. This inoculum effect also has been noted with cefotaxime and imipenem [549]. The dose chosen to treat group B streptococcal meningitis can be crucial to the prompt sterilization of CSF.

Although GBS are susceptible to penicillin G, in vitro tolerance among 4% to 6% of strains has been noted [575]. Defined as MBC in excess of 16 to 32 times the MIC, tolerance in vitro corresponds with delayed bacterial killing, additive rather than synergistic effects when gentamicin is used in combination with penicillin G,

and possibly an autolytic enzyme defect in such strains [576]. Detection of tolerance depends, however, on choice of growth medium, growth phase of bacterial inoculum, and definition of MBC employed for testing.

ANTIMICROBIAL THERAPY

Penicillin G is the drug of choice for treatment of group B streptococcal infections. The recommended dosage for treatment of meningitis is high because of (1) the relatively high MIC of penicillin G for GBS (median 0.06 µg/mL) with respect to attainable levels of this drug in the CSF, (2) the high inoculum in the CSF of some infants [574], (3) reports of relapse in infants with meningitis treated for 14 days with 200,000 U/kg/day of penicillin G, and (4) the safety of high doses of penicillin G in the newborn. To ensure rapid bactericidal effects, particularly in the CSF, we recommend penicillin G (450,000 to 500,000 U/kg/day) or ampicillin (300 to 400 mg/kg/day) for the treatment of meningitis (Table 12-7). There is no evidence to suggest increased risk for adverse reactions at these higher doses even in premature infants.

In the usual clinical setting, antimicrobial therapy is initiated before definitive identification of the organism. Initial therapy should include ampicillin and an aminoglycoside appropriate for the treatment of early-onset neonatal pathogens including GBS. Such a combination is more effective than penicillin G or ampicillin alone for killing of GBS [569,573]. We continue combination therapy until the isolate has been identified as GBS and, in patients with meningitis, until a CSF specimen obtained 24 to 48 hours into therapy is sterile. Kim [576] suggests that MIC and MBC determinations be considered in the following settings: (1) a poor bacteriologic response to antimicrobial therapy, (2) relapse or recurrence of infection without a discernible cause, and (3) infections manifested as meningitis or endocarditis. If tolerance is shown, therapeutic choices include using penicillin G or ampicillin alone or employing cefotaxime. No data are available to indicate the better of these choices [577].

For an infant with late-onset disease in whom CSF reveals gram-positive cocci in pairs or short chains, initial therapy should include ampicillin and gentamicin or

TABLE 12-7   Antimicrobial Regimens Recommended for Treatment of Group B Streptococcal Infections in Infants*

Manifestation of Infection	Drug	Daily Dose (Intravenous)	Duration
Bacteremia without meningitis	Ampicillin plus gentamicin	150-200 mg/kg plus 7.5 mg/kg	Initial treatment before culture results (48-72 hr)
	Penicillin G	200,000 U/kg	Complete a total treatment course of 10 days
Meningitis	Ampicillin plus gentamicin	300-400 mg/kg plus 7.5 mg/kg	Initial treatment (until cerebrospinal fluid is sterile)
	Penicillin G	500,000 U/kg	Complete a minimum total treatment course of 14 days[†]
Septic arthritis	Penicillin G	200,000 U/kg	2-3 wk
Osteomyelitis	Penicillin G	200,000 U/kg	3-4 wk
Endocarditis	Penicillin G	400,000 U/kg	4 wk[‡]

*No modification of dose by postnatal age is recommended. Oral therapy is never indicated.
[†]Longer treatment (up to 4 wk) may be required for ventriculitis.
[‡]In combination with gentamicin for the first 14 days.

ampicillin and cefotaxime, rather than penicillin G alone, because (1) GBS are a frequent cause of meningitis in infants 1 to 8 weeks of age, and combination therapy can improve efficacy early in the course of infection, and (2) *Listeria monocytogenes* can be confused by CSF Gram stain with group B *Streptococcus*, and ampicillin and gentamicin are synergistic in vitro against most strains of *Listeria*. If pneumococcal meningitis is a consideration, cefotaxime and vancomycin would be a reasonable empirical regimen pending culture confirmation. Because group B streptococcal meningitis is uncommon beyond 8 weeks of age, no change is suggested from the use of conventional agents as the initial treatment of meningitis in term infants older than 2 months. For preterm infants remaining hospitalized from birth, empirical therapy can include vancomycin and an aminoglycoside. If meningitis is suspected, ampicillin or cefotaxime should be included in the regimen because vancomycin achieves low CSF concentrations and has a substantially higher MBC against GBS and *L. monocytogenes* than ampicillin.

When the diagnosis of group B streptococcal infection is confirmed, and CSF for patients with meningitis obtained 24 to 48 hours into therapy is sterile, treatment can be completed with penicillin G monotherapy. Good outcomes have been achieved when parenteral therapy is given for 10 days for bacteremia without a focus or with most soft tissue infections, 2 to 3 weeks for meningitis or pyarthrosis, and 3 to 4 weeks for osteomyelitis or endocarditis (see Table 12–7). Limited evidence suggests that a 7-day course of therapy can suffice for uncomplicated bacteremia, but additional data would be required to support a change in current recommendations [578]. For infants with meningitis, failure to achieve CSF sterility suggests an unsuspected suppurative focus (subdural empyema, brain abscess, obstructive ventriculitis, septic thrombophlebitis) or failure to administer an appropriate drug in sufficient dosage.

At the completion of therapy (minimum 14 days), a lumbar puncture should be considered to evaluate whether the CSF findings are compatible with resolution of the inflammatory process or are of sufficient concern to warrant extending treatment or additional diagnostic evaluation. Neutrophils greater than 30% of the total cells or a protein concentration greater than 200 mg/dL warrants consideration for a neuroimaging study of the brain. These findings can be observed in patients with a fulminant course manifested by severe cerebritis, extensive parenchymal destruction with focal suppuration, or severe vasculitis with cerebral infarctions.

Infants with septic arthritis should receive at least 2 weeks of parenteral therapy; infants with bone involvement require 3 to 4 weeks of therapy to optimize an uncomplicated outcome. Drainage of the suppurative focus is an adjunct to antibiotic therapy. In infants with septic arthritis excluding the hip or shoulder, one-time needle aspiration of the involved joint usually achieves adequate drainage. With hip or shoulder involvement, immediate open drainage is warranted. For most infants with osteomyelitis, some type of closed or open drainage procedure is required for diagnosis because blood cultures typically are sterile. These procedures must be performed before or early in the course of therapy to ensure successful isolation of the infecting organism.

With recurrent infection, three points should be considered. First, appropriate antimicrobial therapy fails to eliminate mucous membrane colonization with GBS in 50% of infants [579]. Second, community exposure can result in colonization with a new strain that subsequently invades the bloodstream. Systemic infection in neonates does *not* result in protective levels of CPS type–specific antibodies [341]. Recurrent infections do occur in healthy infants. In this event, an evaluation to exclude an immune abnormality, such as HIV infection or hypogammaglobulinemia, can be considered, but detection of abnormalities is rare. Therapy for recurrent infection need not be extended beyond that appropriate to the clinical expression of the recurrent infection. Finally, although it is desirable to eliminate colonization, an efficacious regimen has not been identified. One small prospective study revealed that administration of oral rifampin (20 mg/kg/day for 4 days) to infants after completion of parenteral therapy eliminated mucous membrane colonization in some subjects [580]. Further study is needed to identify a more reliable approach to eliminating colonization.

SUPPORTIVE MANAGEMENT

Prompt, vigorous, and careful supportive care is important to the successful outcome of most group B streptococcal infections. When early-onset disease is accompanied by respiratory distress, the need for ventilatory assistance should be anticipated before onset of apnea. Early treatment of shock, often not suspected during its initial phase, when systolic pressure is maintained by peripheral vasoconstriction, is crucial. Persistent metabolic acidosis and reasonably normal color are characteristic of this early phase. Persistent perfusion abnormalities after initial attempts to achieve adequate volume expansion warrant placement of a central venous pressure monitoring device and treatment with appropriate inotropic agents. This concept applies also to patients with late-onset meningitis. Fluid management should include packed red blood cell transfusions to optimize oxygen-carrying capacity. In patients with meningitis, effective seizure control is required to achieve proper oxygenation, to decrease metabolic demands, prevent additional cerebral edema, and optimize cerebral blood flow. Monitoring of urine output and attention to electrolyte balance and osmolality are needed to detect and manage the early complications of meningitis, such as inappropriate secretion of antidiuretic hormone and increased intracranial pressure. Such intense and careful supportive management requires treatment in an intensive care unit of a tertiary care facility.

Extracorporeal membrane oxygenation (ECMO) has been suggested as rescue therapy for overwhelming early-onset group B streptococcal sepsis. Hocker and coworkers [581] compared conventional treatment with ECMO for neonates with early-onset disease. Survival was not improved significantly with use of ECMO when all infants or only hypotensive infants were compared. LeBlanc [582] emphasized the difficulty of interpreting this study, citing the retrospective design and the fact that the sickest infants die before ECMO can be initiated. Until a prospective, controlled trial is performed, ECMO therapy should be considered controversial.

ADJUNCTIVE THERAPIES

Despite prompt initiation of antimicrobial therapy and aggressive supportive care, death or sequelae can result from group B streptococcal infection. Considerable investigative efforts have been directed toward adjunctive therapy. High mortality rates for neutropenic neonates prompted clinical evaluation of granulocyte transfusions as adjunctive therapy for early-onset group B streptococcal sepsis. In three trials, 13 infants with neutrophil storage pool depletion were assessed [278,378,583]. The results seemed promising, but the logistics of providing timely transfusion and the concern for adverse effects, such as graft-versus-host reaction, transmission of viral agents, and pulmonary leukocyte sequestration, render this approach to therapy impractical.

Recombinant human cytokine molecules such as granulocyte colony-stimulating factor promote granulocyte proliferation, enhance chemotactic activity and superoxide anion production, and increase expression of neutrophil C3bi receptors. Results in experimental infection suggest that granulocyte colony-stimulating factor might be a useful adjunct in the treatment of group B streptococcal neonatal sepsis, possibly in combination with intravenous immunoglobulin (IVIG) [584–586]. Specific recommendations must await evaluation of their safety and efficacy in controlled clinical trials.

Human immunoglobulin modified for intravenous use could provide specific antibodies to enhance opsonization and phagocytosis of GBS [587–593]. IVIG has been shown in experimental models [594] and septic neonates [595] to improve complement activation and chemotaxis by neonatal sera and to hasten resolution of neutropenia. Administration of sufficient human type-specific antibodies against CPS to animals before lethal challenge with GBS of the homologous serotype is protective [350,587–591]. Despite this sound theoretical rationale, commercial preparations of IVIG contain relatively low concentrations of antibodies to group B streptococcal polysaccharides [590–593,595–600], suggesting that prohibitively large doses would be required and raising concern for reticuloendothelial blockade [589,592]. In addition, functional activity of licensed IVIG preparations can vary by manufacturer and lot [588,589,595–601], and any increase in antibodies after infusion would be transient only [596,602]. Christensen and colleagues [603] administered either IVIG (750 mg/kg) or albumin to 22 neonates with severe, early-onset sepsis, however, and all infants survived. Eleven patients had neutropenia, but in IVIG recipients, this abnormality resolved within 24 hours of infusion, whereas it persisted in placebo recipients.

A hyperimmune group B streptococcal globulin or human-human monoclonal antibodies would theoretically circumvent many potential problems. Raff and coworkers [604] developed a human IgM monoclonal antibody specific for the group B cell wall polysaccharide. This antibody reacted with all group B streptococcal types tested and was shown to be safe and protective in newborn, nonhuman primates [605]. A hyperimmune globulin [599] prepared by vaccinating healthy adults with polysaccharides from types Ia, Ib, II, and III GBS was protective against experimental challenge with types I, II, and III

strains [606]. To date, no commercial preparation of IVIG hyperimmune for IgG directed against type-specific CPS is available, however, for testing in appropriately designed clinical trials.

PROGNOSIS

Several clinical scoring systems have been developed to predict at the time of initial evaluation infants likely to die as a consequence of neonatal group B streptococcal infection [212,432,607]. Payne and colleagues [212] described a score derived from five variables that, together with an initial blood pH less than 7.25, enabled prediction of outcome accurately in 93% of infants with early-onset group B streptococcal infection. These features were birth weight less than 2500 g, absolute neutrophil count less than 1500 cells/mm^3, hypotension, apnea, and pleural effusion seen on the initial chest radiograph.

A fatal outcome can be predicted with reasonable accuracy, but little information is available concerning the long-term prognosis for survivors of neonatal group B streptococcal sepsis. One group at potential risk for sequelae are preterm infants with septic shock, who can develop periventricular leukomalacia. Among these survivors, substantial neurodevelopmental sequelae have been identified at evaluation during the second year of life. The correlates of severity and duration of shock with periventricular leukomalacia and with long-term morbidity from group B streptococcal disease have not been assessed. Prospective, active surveillance of neonatal group B streptococcal infections in Germany conducted from 2001-2003 found that 14% of 347 infants had neurologic sequelae of infection at the time of discharge from the hospital [608].

Long-term outcomes for survivors of group B streptococcal meningitis are guarded. Among 41 survivors from a cohort born in 1996-1997 in England and Wales, 34% had moderate or severe disability, 27% had mild disability, and 39% were functioning normally at 5 years of age [609]. Stoll and colleagues [610] showed for extremely low birth weight infants that meningitis with or without sepsis was associated with poor neurodevelopmental and growth outcomes and impairment of vision and hearing in early childhood.

Among 200 neonates with early-onset or late-onset meningitis cared for in the 1970s and 1980s, one quarter died in the hospital as the direct consequence of meningitis [429,431,432]. Among 112 survivors assessed at mean intervals 2 to 8 years after diagnosis, 20% had major neurologic sequelae. The most serious of these were profound mental retardation, spastic quadriplegia, cortical blindness, deafness, uncontrolled seizures, hydrocephalus, and hypothalamic dysfunction with poor thermal regulation and central diabetes insipidus [429,432,476,611]. Mild or moderate sequelae persisted in an additional 20% of survivors evaluated at a mean of 6 years after diagnosis. These sequelae included profound unilateral sensorineural hearing loss, borderline mental retardation, spastic or flaccid monoparesis, and expressive or receptive speech and language delay.

In a sibling-controlled follow-up study, 12% of survivors had major neurologic sequelae when evaluated at

3 to 18 years of age. When these nine children were excluded, there were no significant differences, as rated by parents, between the children with meningitis and their siblings for academic achievement, measures of intelligence quotient, fine motor dexterity, or behavior difficulties [611]. Meningitis survivors were more likely than siblings to have seizure disorders and hydrocephalus. More subtle deficits, such as delayed language development and mild hearing loss, may not be detected by routine examination [432], and meningitis survivors should undergo audiometric testing during convalescence and careful long-term neurologic and developmental assessments.

PREVENTION

Theoretically, early-onset and late-onset group B streptococcal disease could be prevented if susceptible hosts were not exposed to the microorganism or if exposure occurred in the setting of protective immunity. Several approaches to prevention have been advocated; conceptually, these are directed at eliminating exposure or enhancing host resistance by chemoprophylaxis or immunoprophylaxis. Both strategies have limitations with respect to implementation, but could be targeted for the prevention of maternal and neonatal infections and are theoretically achievable [612,613].

CHEMOPROPHYLAXIS
Historical Precedents

Chemoprophylaxis was suggested as a means to prevent early-onset group B streptococcal infection by Franciosi and coworkers in 1973 [2]. Because maternal genital colonization was recognized to expose infants to the organism, oral penicillin treatment for colonized women was subsequently proposed. Carriers of GBS identified by third-trimester vaginal culture received a course of an oral antimicrobial. Approximately 20% to 30% remained colonized after treatment, and in most of these women, GBS were isolated from vaginal cultures at delivery [614–616]. Reacquisition from colonized sexual partners was suggested as an explanation for these high failure rates, but failure rates remained high when colonized pregnant women and their spouses received concurrent treatment with penicillin by the oral or the parenteral route [2,614,617]. One explanation cited for failure of this approach was the difficulty in eradicating a constituent of the normal bowel flora [614].

Yow and colleagues [618] gave intravenous ampicillin at hospital admission to 34 women in labor and vaginally colonized with GBS and successfully interrupted vertical transmission of colonization in all. Boyer and Gotoff [619,620] provided in 1986 the first documentation that IAP could prevent invasive early-onset neonatal infection. Women colonized with GBS who had risk factors for early-onset infection were randomly assigned to receive routine labor and delivery care or intrapartum ampicillin intravenously until delivery. Group B streptococcal sepsis developed in 5 of 79 neonates in the routine care group, 1 of whom died, whereas 85 infants born to women in the ampicillin treatment group remained well. Intrapartum ampicillin prophylaxis for group B streptococcal carriers also resulted in reduced maternal morbidity

[621]. These data established the efficacy of IAP for prevention of early-onset neonatal disease and reduction of group B Streptococcus–associated febrile maternal morbidity. The cost-effectiveness of this approach subsequently was validated [622,623].

In 1992, the American College of Obstetricians and Gynecologists (ACOG) [624] and the American Academy of Pediatrics (AAP) [625] published separate documents regarding maternal IAP for the prevention of early-onset group B streptococcal infection. The ACOG technical bulletin was educational, whereas the AAP guidelines were directive. The AAP guidelines specified that if culture screening was performed antenatally, specimens should be obtained from lower vaginal and rectal sites, and culture-positive women with one or more risk factors and group B streptococcal colonization should be given intrapartum intravenous penicillin G or ampicillin. The ACOG proposed that culture screening could be avoided by providing treatment for all women with risk factors. Neither the AAP nor ACOG approach was implemented widely, and invasive disease rates remained unacceptably high.

Rapid Assays for Antenatal Detection of Group B Streptococci

There are difficulties inherent to ascertainment of group B streptococcal colonization status rapidly even when assays can be processed 24 hours a day. Latex particle agglutination and enzyme immunoassays for detection of group B streptococcal antigen in cervical or lower vaginal swab specimens are not sufficiently sensitive to determine colonization status accurately at hospital admission, especially for women with a low density of organisms [626]. An optical immunoassay (Strep B OIA test; Biostar, Boulder, CO) was considerably more sensitive than earlier assays for detecting light (13% to 67%) and heavy (42% to 100%) or overall (81%) colonization and has outperformed enzyme immunoassays in direct comparisons [626–630]. Assays using a DNA hybridization methodology have shown variable sensitivity [631,632].

Bergeron and colleagues [633] described a fluorogenic real time RT-PCR technique for rapid identification of women colonized with GBS at admission for delivery. The sensitivity of real time RT-PCR and of conventional PCR was 97%, the negative predictive value was 99%, and the specificity and positive predictive value were 100%. Results were available from real time RT-PCR in 45 minutes; by comparison, conventional PCR required 100 minutes, and conventional cultures required 36 hours minimum. Field testing of commercially available assays such as the Xpert GBS Assay (Cepheid, Sunnyvale, CA) that uses automated rapid real time RT-PCR technology and IDI-StrepB (Infectio Diagnostic, Quebec, Canada) that uses a PCR assay to amplify group B streptococcal target has been conducted [634–636]. The performance of real time RT-PCR and optical immunoassay is sufficiently robust for use in point-of-care settings [637]. A cost-benefit analysis suggests that widespread implementation would afford benefit over the current culture-based strategy, but, to date, these newer methods should be considered as adjunctive tests to antenatal culture-based methods for detection of GBS [638].

Intrapartum Antibiotic Prophylaxis

The current era of IAP dates from 1996, when consensus recommendations for the prevention of early-onset group B streptococcal disease were endorsed by the CDC, AAP, and ACOG [533,639,640]. These recommendations indicated that obstetric care providers and hospitals should adopt a culture-based or a risk-based policy to identify women to receive IAP. The culture-based approach employed lower vaginal and rectal cultures obtained at 35 to 37 weeks of gestation to identify candidates for IAP. The risk-based strategy identified IAP recipients by factors known to increase the likelihood of neonatal group B streptococcal disease: labor onset or membrane rupture before 37 weeks of gestation, intrapartum fever greater than or equal to 38° C (≥100.4° F), or rupture of membranes 18 or more hours before delivery. In both strategies, women with group B streptococcal bacteriuria or previous delivery of an infant with group B streptococcal disease were to receive IAP. These strategies each resulted in the administration of IAP to approximately one in four pregnant women [639].

The incidence of early-onset disease declined by 70% from 1.7 per 1000 live births to 0.5 per 1000 live births by 1999 in association with implementation of one of these two IAP methods (Fig. 12–10) [612,641]. A resulting 3900 to 4500 early-onset infections and 200 to 225 neonatal deaths were estimated to be prevented annually [612,642]. By contrast, the rate of late-onset disease remained constant at 0.5 to 0.6 per 1000 live births. Also, the incidence of invasive group B streptococcal disease, primarily bacteremia with or without intra-amniotic infection or endometritis among pregnant women declined significantly, from 0.29 per 1000 live births in 1993 to 0.23 in 1998 [612,642]. By 1999, two thirds of U.S. hospitals in a multistate survey had a formal prevention policy, and numerous individual practitioners had adopted one of the two strategies proposed in 1996 [612,643].

By 2002, it was evident that further reduction in the incidence of early-onset disease could be accomplished by adoption of universal culture screening. A direct comparison in 5144 births showed that the culture-based strategy was 50% more effective than the risk-based strategy in preventing early-onset disease in neonates [171]. Culture-based screening more often resulted in administration of IAP for at least 4 hours before delivery. The 2002 revised

CDC guidelines recommending a universal culture-based approach to prevention of perinatal group B streptococcal disease are endorsed by the AAP and the ACOG [612,644, 645]. Early-onset disease incidence declined an additional 29% after issuance of the revised guidelines in 2002, to 0.34 cases per 1000 live births from 2003-2007 [172].

Currently, all pregnant women should be screened in each pregnancy for group B streptococcal carriage at 35 to 37 weeks of gestation. The risk-based approach is an acceptable alternative only in circumstances in which the culture has not been performed or results are unavailable before delivery. Culture specimens should be obtained from the lower vagina and the rectum using the same or two different swabs. These swabs should be placed in a non-nutritive transport medium, transferred to and incubated overnight in a selective broth medium, and subcultured onto 5% sheep blood agar medium or colistin–nalidixic acid medium for isolation of GBS. At the time of labor or rupture of membranes, IAP should be given to all pregnant women identified antenatally as carriers of GBS. The indications for IAP are shown in Figure 12–11. Group B streptococcal bacteriuria during the current pregnancy or prior delivery of an infant with invasive group B streptococcal disease always is an indication for IAP, so antenatal screening is unnecessary for these women. If culture results are unknown at the onset of labor or rupture of membranes, the risk factors listed in Figure 12–11 should be used to determine the need to institute IAP. Women who present with preterm labor before antenatal group B streptococcal screening should have cultures obtained and IAP initiated. If labor ceases and cultures are negative, IAP is discontinued, and antenatal screening is performed at 35 to 37 weeks of gestation. If labor ceases and cultures are positive, some experts recommend oral amoxicillin for another 5 to 7 days.

Planned cesarean section before rupture of membranes and onset of labor constitute exceptions to the need for IAP for women colonized with GBS. These women are at extremely low risk for having an infant with early-onset disease. Culture-negative women who are delivered at 37 weeks of gestation or later need not receive IAP routinely, even when a risk factor is present. Therapeutic use of broad spectrum antibiotics in labor should be employed as is appropriate for maternal indications, such as intra-amniotic infection.

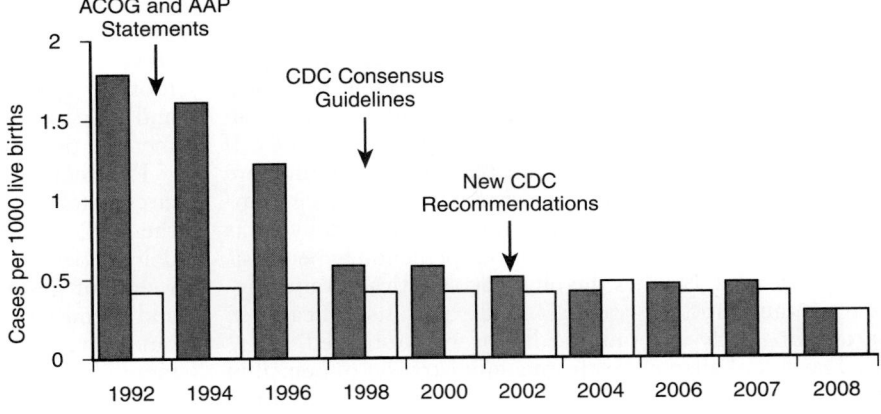

FIGURE 12–10 Incidence of early-onset (*gray bars*) and late-onset (*white bars*) **group B streptococcal disease from 1992-2008.** The dates of the initial prevention statements from the American College of Obstetricians and Gynecologists (ACOG) and the American Academy of Pediatrics (AAP) [624,625], the 1996 consensus guidelines from the Centers for Disease Control and Prevention (CDC) [639], and the revised 2002 CDC guidelines [612] are shown.

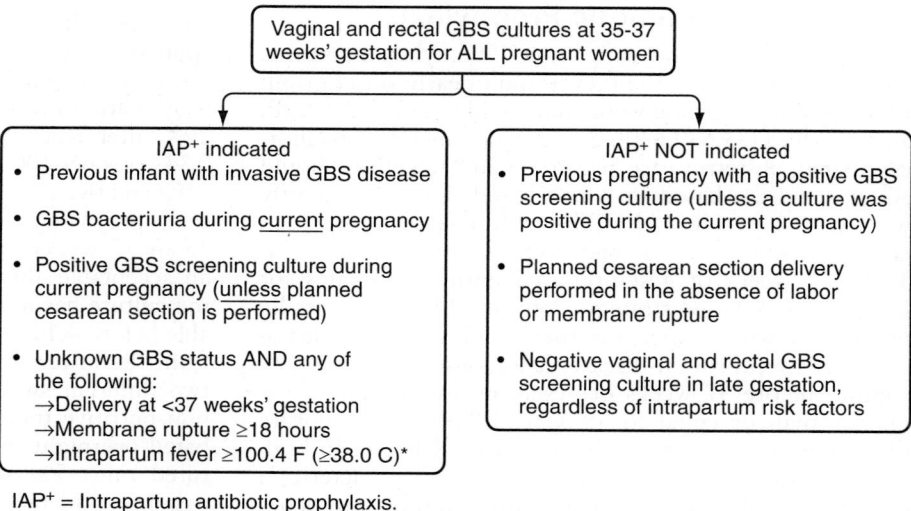

FIGURE 12–11 Revised recommendations for culture-based screening for maternal colonization with group B streptococci (GBS) and administration of intrapartum antibiotic prophylaxis (IAP). *(Adapted from Centers for Disease Control and Prevention. Prevention of perinatal group B streptococcal disease: revised guidelines from CDC. MMWR Morb Mortal Wkly Rep 51[RR-11]:1-22, 2002.)*

The recommended maternal intrapartum chemoprophylaxis regimen consists of penicillin G (5 million U initially and 3 million U every 4 hours thereafter until delivery) [612]. Penicillin or ampicillin given 4 or more hours before delivery reliably prevents vertical transmission and early-onset disease. Ampicillin administered as a 2-g intravenous loading dose and then 1 g every 4 hours until delivery is an alternative to penicillin [612]. The rationale for the high initial dose of the β-lactam antibiotic relates to the desired drug concentrations needed in the amniotic and vaginal fluids (peak approximately 3 hours after completion of the initial dose) to reduce substantially the number of GBS at either site. IAP "failures" typically occur when penicillin or ampicillin has been initiated 2 or less hours before delivery; clindamycin has been given without susceptibility testing, and clindamycin-resistant early-onset group B streptococcal neonatal sepsis ensued; or appropriate IAP is given in the setting of clinically apparent or silent intra-amniotic infection.

Prophylaxis for penicillin-allergic women must take into account increasing resistance among GBS to erythromycin and clindamycin. Women *not* at high risk for anaphylaxis (e.g., a rash without anaphylaxis or respiratory compromise) should receive cefazolin, 2 g intravenously as an initial dose and then 1 g every 8 hours until delivery. Cefazolin has pharmacokinetics similar to penicillin with respect to peak concentrations in serum and amniotic fluid of pregnant women. Women whose group B streptococcal isolates are tested and found to be clindamycin susceptible by D test and who are at high risk for anaphylaxis with penicillin can receive clindamycin at a dose of 900 mg every 8 hours. If susceptibility testing is unavailable or the results are unknown, or when isolates are resistant to clindamycin, vancomycin, 1 g intravenously every 12 hours until delivery, is an alternative for women with serious penicillin hypersensitivity reactions. Neither the pharmacokinetics of vancomycin in amniotic or vaginal fluids nor its efficacy in preventing early-onset disease has been investigated.

The risk of anaphylaxis from administration of penicillin is low. Estimates range from 4 events per 10,000 to 4 per 100,000 patients. Anaphylaxis associated with administration of a β-lactam antibiotic as IAP for the prevention of early-onset group B streptococcal infection has been reported, but is rare [171,646–648]. Most pregnant women reporting a penicillin allergy that is not anaphylaxis have negative skin test on hypersensitivity testing and are able to receive IAP with penicillin safely [649]. A fetal demise in association with new-onset penicillin allergy during IAP has been reported in a woman with rheumatoid arthritis [650]. No adult fatalities in association with IAP are reported, and the risk of a fatal event is low because the antimicrobials are administered in a hospital setting where medical intervention is readily available.

Numerous residual problems, barriers to implementation, and missed opportunities must be overcome to achieve maximal benefit from IAP [651–653]. Procedural issues, such as suboptimal culture processing and collection of cultures earlier than 5 weeks before delivery, constitute one set of problems. Laboratories may not adhere to recommended methods for isolation of GBS, a problem that remains despite the 2002 consensus recommendations and one that results in colonized women delivering infants with early-onset disease. Even optimal antenatal culture methods miss some women who are colonized at delivery, exposing their neonate to GBS and resulting in colonization or illness. Another problem is that women who are not screened adequately more often are medically underserved; women in their teens, blacks, and Hispanics are more likely than whites to receive inadequate prenatal care and prenatal testing, and are less likely to receive recommended prevention interventions.

Problems surround lack of recommended IAP in certain circumstances. The most prominent is lack of adherence to the 2002 recommendation for routine IAP in women who deliver before antenatal screening occurs (i.e., 35 to 37 weeks of gestation). These women should have vaginal and rectal cultures performed and routinely receive IAP, but this recommendation is the one least commonly implemented. Whether this is because delivery ensues too quickly to administer IAP, or the recommendation is unclear to obstetric providers, or both, is unknown. Also, adherence to guidelines in penicillin-allergic women is suboptimal, and cefazolin as the appropriate IAP for women with a nonserious penicillin allergy is administered uncommonly [654]. Reliance on clindamycin as the alternative agent in women without serious penicillin allergy results in inadequate IAP in at least 20% of patients when antimicrobial susceptibility testing of colonizing isolates is not performed antenatally.

A final issue is a need for increased awareness of perinatal group B streptococcal infection. In one report, only 47% of women younger than 50 years of age reported having heard of group B *Streptococcus* [655]. Women with a high school education or less; with low household income; or reporting black, Asian/Pacific Islander, or "other" race had lower awareness than that noted in other women. Efforts to raise awareness should target women from groups that traditionally are medically underserved. Hospital infection control teams can contribute to these efforts by spearheading educational efforts toward effective implementation among hospital obstetric staff and laboratory personnel [642].

Impact of Intrapartum Antibiotic Prophylaxis on Neonatal Sepsis

The efficacy of IAP in preventing early-onset group B streptococcal infection has been shown in numerous observational studies and in countries other than the United States when guidelines have been implemented [171,424,656–658]. The impact of increased use of IAP on the occurrence of sepsis caused by organisms other than GBS is a subject of ongoing evaluation. Concern exists that neonatal sepsis caused by organisms other than group B *Streptococcus* is increasing while group B streptococcal sepsis is decreasing and that the organisms causing non–group B streptococcal sepsis are likely to be ampicillin-resistant [659]. Surveillance trends are insufficient to establish a relationship between IAP for group B *Streptococcus* and *E. coli* sepsis risk, but single hospital–reported increases in *E. coli* sepsis that have occurred in preterm and very low birth weight infants are of concern [660]. A significant increase in the rate of early-onset sepsis caused by *E. coli* has been observed in multicenter studies, but only infants of very low birth weight (<1500 g birth weight) were evaluated [661]. In a multisite surveillance of trends in incidence and antimicrobial resistance of early-onset sepsis, stable rates of sepsis caused by other organisms were found, but an increase in ampicillin-resistant *E. coli* was observed among preterm but not term infants [662].

A relationship between neonatal death caused by ampicillin-resistant *E. coli* and prolonged antepartum exposure to ampicillin was noted by Terrone and colleagues [663]. In another report, the frequency with which ampicillin-resistant Enterobacteriaceae were isolated was similar after exposure to ampicillin or penicillin [664]. Repeat cultures 6 weeks postpartum revealed no increase in antibiotic resistance in either GBS or *E. coli* from women who had received IAP [665]. Ongoing population-based surveillance is required to monitor these trends and to identify possible reasons for the increase

in ampicillin-resistant *E. coli* infections in preterm neonates, in particular, the use of antenatal antimicrobial agents other than IAP [666,667].

Management of Neonates Born to Mothers Receiving Intrapartum Antibiotic Prophylaxis

Management of infants is based on the neonate's clinical status, whether the mother had chorioamnionitis, an indication for IAP, or adequate duration of IAP, and gestation (Fig. 12–12) [612]. If an infant has any signs of sepsis, a full diagnostic evaluation, including complete blood cell count and differential, blood culture, and chest radiograph if the neonate has respiratory signs, and empirical therapy should be initiated pending laboratory results. A lumbar puncture, if feasible, should be performed. Although published reports vary, a minimum of 10% and a maximum of nearly 40% of infants with meningitis have a negative blood culture [532]. If lumbar puncture is deferred and therapy is continued for more than 48 hours because of suspected infection, CSF should be obtained for routine studies and culture. Depending on the CSF results, therapy appropriate for sepsis or presumed meningitis is given.

If a woman receives broad-spectrum antibiotics for suspected chorioamnionitis, her healthy-appearing infant should have a full diagnostic evaluation excluding a lumbar puncture, and most experts would initiate empirical therapy pending culture results regardless of the clinical condition at birth, gestational age, or duration of antibiotics before birth. This approach is based on the infant's exposure to suspected or established infection. The duration of therapy is based on results of cultures and the infant's clinical course (see "Treatment" section). If the infant is healthy-appearing, but has a gestational age of less than 35 weeks, some experts would perform a limited evaluation that includes complete blood count and blood culture, without regard to the duration of maternal IAP. Empirical therapy need not be initiated, unless signs of sepsis develop or the infant is very immature. Healthy-appearing infants with a gestational age of at least 35 weeks whose mothers received intravenous penicillin, ampicillin, or cefazolin less than 4 hours before delivery should be observed closely without a diagnostic evaluation. If the infant is healthy-appearing and has a gestational age of 35 weeks or more, and the mother received penicillin, ampicillin, or cefazolin 4 hours or more before delivery, routine care is advised.

The recommended interval of observation for neonates undergoing a limited evaluation is 48 hours. The approach presented in Figure 12–12 is not to be taken as an exclusive management pathway. Hospital discharge at 24 hours of age can be reasonable under certain circumstances, specifically when the infant is born after the mother has received a β-lactam as IAP for 4 hours or longer before delivery, has a gestational age of 38 weeks or more, and is healthy-appearing. Other discharge criteria should be met, and the infant should be under the care of a person able to comply with instructions for home observation [612,668]. The risk of bacterial infection in healthy-appearing newborns is low. Outcomes

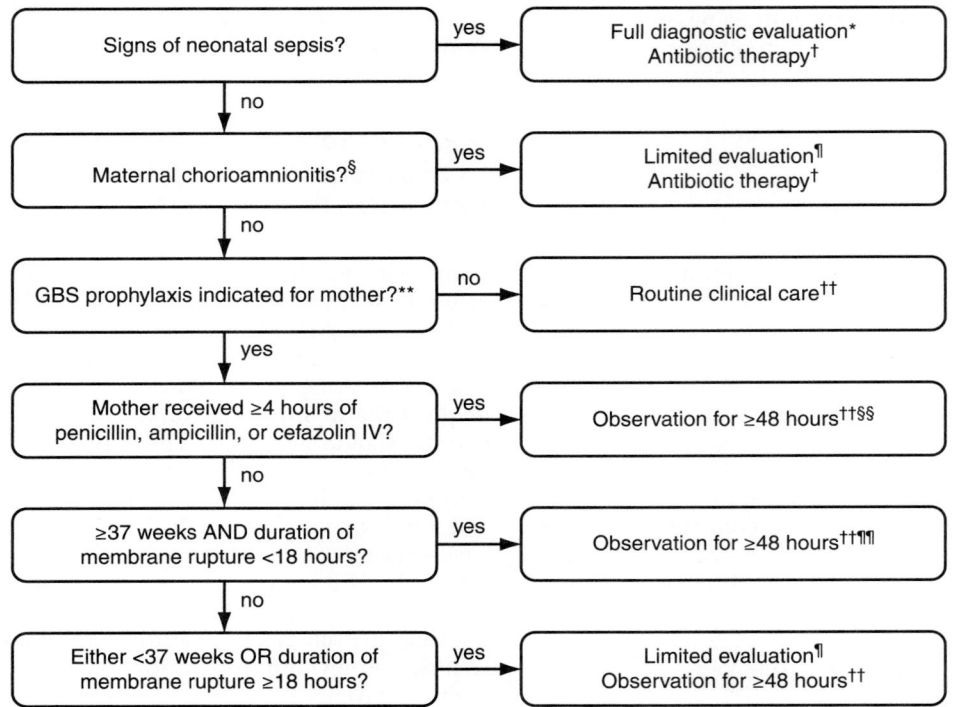

* Full diagnostic evaluation includes CBC with differential, platelets, blood culture, chest radiograph (if respiratory abnormalities are present), and LP (if patient stable enough to tolerate procedure and sepsis is suspected).

† Antibiotic therapy should be directed towards the most common causes of neonatal sepsis including GBS and other organisms (including gram negative pathogens), and should take into account local antibiotic resistance patterns.

§ Consultation with obstetric providers is important to determine the level of clinical suspicion for chorioamnionitis. Chorioamnionitis is diagnosed clinically and some of the signs are non-specific.

¶ Limited evaluation includes blood culture (at birth), and CBC with differential and platelets. Some experts recommend a CBC with differential and platelets at 6-12 hours of age.

** GBS prophylaxis indicated if one or more of the following: (1) mother GBS positive at 35-37 weeks' gestation, (2) GBS status unknown with one or more intrapartum risk factors including <37 weeks' gestation, ROM≥18 hours or T≥100.4°F (38.0°C), (3) GBS bacteriuria during current pregnancy, (4) history of a previous infant with GBS disease.

†† If signs of sepsis develop, a full diagnostic evaluation should be done and antibiotic therapy initiated.

§§ If ≥37 weeks' gestation, observation may occur at home after 24 hours if there is a knowledgeable observer and ready access to medical care.

¶¶ Some experts recommend a CBC with differential and platelets at 6-12 hours of age.

FIGURE 12–12 Algorithm for prevention of early-onset GBS disease among newborns.

among infants whose mothers receive IAP are better than among infants whose mothers do not receive IAP. Rehospitalization is uncommon among these latter infants, however [669].

The influence of maternal IAP on the clinical spectrum of early-onset infection in term infants has been evaluated [669–671]. Exposure to antibiotics in labor does not change the clinical spectrum of disease or the onset of clinical signs of infection within 24 to 48 hours of birth for infants with early-onset group B streptococcal infection. Infants whose mothers have received IAP are less likely to be ill, to require assisted ventilation, or to have proven bacterial infection [669]. These infants are not more likely to undergo invasive procedures or to receive antibiotics [670]. The number of infants undergoing evaluation for sepsis has decreased in association with implementation of IAP guidelines, and among group B *Streptococcus*–negative women, ordering of laboratory tests has diminished by almost 40% [672].

Chemoprophylaxis for the Neonate

Chemoprophylaxis for neonates at birth continues to be advocated by some investigators. Three decades ago, Steigman and colleagues [673] found no cases of early-onset group B streptococcal infection among 130,000 newborns who received a single intramuscular injection of penicillin G (50,000 U) at birth as prophylaxis for gonococcal infection. Neonates with possible in utero acquisition of infection who were ill at birth did not receive prophylaxis and were excluded from the analysis. Pyati and coworkers [674] evaluated more than 1000 neonates with birth weights of less than 2000 g in whom a blood culture was obtained before penicillin was administered. In these high-risk infants, penicillin prophylaxis at birth was ineffective in preventing group B streptococcal bacteremia or in altering the mortality rate associated with infection.

A few centers use a combined maternal and neonatal protocol that advocates a risk-based maternal IAP approach coupled with administration of a single dose of intramuscular penicillin to all infants within 1 hour of birth [675–677]. Observational studies showed a 76% reduction in early-onset infection to 0.47 per 1000 live births when rates for the 5 years from 1986-1994 were compared with rates from 1994-1999.

In the special circumstance of an apparently nonaffected sibling in a twin or multiple birth with early-onset [332,333] or late-onset [333] group B streptococcal disease, the well-appearing sibling of a neonate with invasive infection is at increased risk of developing group B streptococcal disease. At the time of diagnosis of group B streptococcal disease in the index patient of a multiple birth, the other infant or infants should be assessed clinically [333]. If signs of infection are noted, cultures of blood and CSF should be obtained, and empirical antimicrobial treatment should be initiated until laboratory results become available. If cultures yield group B *Streptococcus*, a full course of treatment is appropriate. If findings from the clinical assessment are unremarkable, management should be undertaken on a case-by-case basis. The risk for a poor outcome when the second twin is not evaluated until clinical signs of infection are apparent warrants caution in this circumstance. Even when empirical therapy is given and invasive infection is excluded, later onset is possible [678].

IMMUNOPROPHYLAXIS

The most promising approach to prevention of group B streptococcal disease is immunoprophylaxis [613,679]. The underlying principle is that IgG directed against CPS of GBS, critical for protection against invasive disease, are provided by passive or active immunization. Human sera containing a sufficient concentration of CPS-specific antibody have been shown in animal models of infection to protect against lethal challenge with each of the major group B streptococcal types [350,680]. Provision of protective levels of type-specific immunity to the newborn theoretically can be achieved by passive or active maternal immunization. Passive immunotherapy for the mother would require development of hyperimmune preparations of human immunoglobulin for intravenous use, would be expensive, and would require many hours of infusion before delivery to provide fetal serum levels, but animal studies indicate the potential usefulness of such an approach [681,682].

The first candidate group B streptococcal vaccine, a purified type III CPS, underwent testing in healthy adults in 1978 [359]. Subsequently, types Ia and II CPS vaccines were studied [683]. Although these vaccines were well tolerated and elicited primarily IgG class response within 2 to 4 weeks, the immunogenicity was variable. It was discovered that nearly 90% of adults had very low preimmunization serum concentrations of CPS-specific antibodies in association with presumed immunologic naïvete. These low levels predicted a poor immune response in many, so that only 40% and 60% developed significant type-specific antibody responses after immunization with type Ia and type III CPS vaccines. By contrast, 88% of adults immunized with type II CPS vaccine responded with fourfold or greater increases in type II CPS–specific antibodies.

These early trials verified the feasibility of immunization as an approach to prevent group B streptococcal disease and revealed the need to develop candidate vaccines

with enhanced immunogenicity. The first study conducted in pregnant women was an encouragement to the ultimate potential success of a group B streptococcal vaccine program [410]. Among 25 pregnant responders to a type III CPS group B streptococcal vaccine, 90% delivered infants with substantial levels of specific antibody to the type III CPS in cord sera that promoted functional activity in vitro throughout the first 3 months of life in most instances.

Development of the first group B streptococcal CPS conjugate vaccine, type III CPS–tetanus toxoid, was driven by the prominence of type III among infants with early-onset and late-onset disease and by its dominance as a cause of meningitis. Type III CPS was linked covalently to monomeric tetanus toxoid by reductive amination coupling chemistry [684]. Group B streptococcal CPS–protein conjugate vaccines of all clinically important types subsequently were developed and found to be immunogenic and protective in experimental animals [684–687,689]. The first clinical evaluation of the type III CPS–tetanus toxoid conjugate showed greater than fourfold increases in postimmunization CPS-specific IgG in 90% of healthy nonpregnant women [690]. The vaccine was well tolerated, and the antibodies, predominantly of the IgG class, were functional in vitro and protective in a murine model of infection.

Conjugate vaccines to each of the clinically relevant group B streptococcal CPS types causing invasive disease have been tested in nearly 500 healthy adults 18 to 50 years old [688,690–692]. Systemic responses, such as low-grade fever, chills, headache, or myalgias, always short-lived, were observed in less than 2% of volunteers. Local reactions were frequent but mild, typically consisting of pain without erythema or swelling, and resolved within 48 to 72 hours. Immune responses to each of the conjugate vaccines, with the exception of type V, are dose-dependent. Doses of 4 to 15 μg of the CPS component have elicited greater than fourfold increases in CPS-specific IgG in 80% to 93% of recipients of type Ia, Ib, II, III, and V conjugates at 8 weeks after immunization. Evaluation of a vaccine combining type II and type III CPS, each conjugated to tetanus toxoid, showed no immune interference compared with response after administration of one of the monovalent vaccines [693].

A phase 1 randomized placebo-controlled, double-blinded trial of type III CPS–tetanus toxoid conjugate vaccine was conducted in 30 healthy pregnant women at 30 to 32 weeks of gestation [704]. Immunization was well tolerated. Geometric mean concentrations of IgG to type III CPS from immunized women were significantly increased from preimmunization values and correlated well with infant cord values. Sera from the infants of vaccinated women collected at 1 and 2 months of age promoted in vitro opsonization and killing of type III GBS by human neutrophils.

One alternative strategy for the preparation of group B streptococcal conjugate vaccines is to construct "designer" glycoconjugate vaccines with size-specific antigens and site-controlled coupling that optimizes the magnitude and specificity of the antipolysaccharide response [694]. An oligosaccharide-based tetanus toxoid conjugate vaccine against type III GBS was synthesized to retain the antigenic specificity of the native polysaccharide and has been shown to be immunogenic in mice [695]. Conjugate vaccine size, CPS molecular weight, and the degree of polysaccharide-protein cross-linking all are important considerations in optimizing immunogenicity of candidate vaccines [67].

Use of proteins that are conserved across most group B streptococcal serotypes offers another strategy for vaccine development. The C protein could be an alternative to tetanus toxoid as the protein component of a conjugate vaccine [680,687,696]. Invasive disease, but not colonization, elicits α C–specific and β C–specific IgM and IgG in adults [697,698]. A type III polysaccharide–C protein conjugate vaccine theoretically could prevent most systemic infections [699]. A recombinant β C protein modified to eliminate its IgA-binding site conjugated to type III CSP has been shown to be immunogenic in mice, inducing polysaccharide and protein-specific functional IgG [700]. The group B streptococcal surface proteins, Rib, Sip, and C5a peptidase, each have been shown to elicit antibodies that are protective in experimental models of group B streptococcal infection [701–703]. Their roles in human infection are not established.

The discovery that surface-associated pilus-like islands are distributed widely among group B streptococcal clinical isolates potentially paves the way for the development of pilus island–based vaccines. An entire pilus island has been transferred from group B *Streptococcus* to a non-pathogenic species. Mucosally delivered *Lactococcus*-expressing pilus island 1 protected mice from challenge with pilus 1–containing group B streptococcal strains [10]. Pilus islands 1, 2a, and 2b, alone or in combination, were identified on each of 289 group B streptococcal isolates from infants and adults with invasive disease, and most were highly surface expressed [11]. A combination of the three pilus-island components conferred protection against all tested group B *Streptococcus* challenge strains. A vaccine exclusively constituted by pilus components in concept could be broadly efficacious in preventing infections caused by GBS [11].

Because most pregnant women have low concentrations of type-specific IgG in their sera, a practical approach to immunoprophylaxis would be immunization of women during adolescence, before pregnancy, or late in pregnancy (i.e., early third trimester) [593]. In view of the substantial disease burden in nonpregnant adults, targeted adult immunization (e.g., diabetics or adults ≥65 years old) also is an attractive prevention strategy. Types Ia, III, and V GBS account for 75% to 85% of infections and, together with types Ib and II, for most invasive disease in infants and adults [143,146,699,704]. The production of a trivalent or a pentavalent conjugate vaccine is technically achievable. Physicians and their patients and pharmaceutical industry leaders must perceive this mode of prevention to be of high benefit and negligible risk, especially if pregnant women are to be included in the target population. The cost of developing suitable vaccines, although substantial, is considerably less than the death, disability, and treatment associated with these infections [623,705]. If the prevention of group B streptococcal disease is to become a reality, however, physicians, public health officials, parents, and patients must join together as advocates for pregnant women, neonates and young infants, and at-risk adults.

REFERENCES

[1] R.M. Fry, Fatal infections by haemolytic streptococcus group B, Lancet 1 (1938) 199–201.

[2] R.A. Franciosi, J.D. Knostman, R.A. Zimmerman, Group B streptococcal neonatal and infant infections, J. Pediatr. 82 (1973) 707–718.

[3] C.J. Baker, F.F. Barrett, Transmission of group B streptococci among parturient women and their neonates, J. Pediatr. 83 (1973) 919–925.

[4] J.B. Howard, G.H. McCracken Jr., The spectrum of group B streptococcal infections in infancy, Am. J. Dis. Child. 128 (1974) 815–818.

[5] M.M. Farley, et al., A population-based assessment of invasive disease due to group B *Streptococcus* in nonpregnant adults, N. Engl. J. Med. 328 (1993) 1807–1811.

[6] H.C. Slotved, et al., Serotype IX, a proposed new *Streptococcus agalactiae* serotype, J. Clin. Microbiol. 45 (2007) 2929–2936.

[7] H. Tettelin, et al., Complete genome sequence and comparative genomic analysis of an emerging human pathogen, serotype V *Streptococcus agalactiae*, Proc. Natl. Acad. Sci. U. S. A. 99 (2002) 12391–12396.

[8] P. Glaser, et al., Genome sequence of *Streptococcus agalactiae*, a pathogen causing invasive neonatal disease, Mol. Microbiol. 45 (2002) 1499–1513.

[9] P. Lauer, et al., Genome analysis reveals pili in group B *Streptococcus*, Science 309 (2005) 105.

[10] S. Buccato, et al., Use of *Lactococcus lactis* expressing pili from group B *Streptococcus* as a broad-coverage vaccine against streptococcal disease, J. Infect. Dis. 194 (2006) 331–340.

[11] I. Margarit, et al., Preventing bacterial infections with pilus-based vaccines: the group B streptococcus paradigm, J. Infect. Dis. 199 (2009) 108–115.

[12] S.J. Schrag, et al., Group B streptococcal disease in the era of intrapartum antibiotic prophylaxis, N. Engl. J. Med. 342 (2000) 15–20.

[13] R.C. Lancefield, A serological differentiation of human and other groups of hemolytic streptococci, J. Exp. Med. 57 (1933) 571–595.

[14] J.H. Brown, Appearance of double-zone beta-hemolytic streptococci in blood agar, J. Bacteriol. 34 (1937) 35–48.

[15] C.J. Baker, D.J. Clark, F.F. Barrett, Selective broth medium for isolation of group B streptococci, Appl. Microbiol. 26 (1973) 884–885.

[16] D.V. Lim, W.J. Morales, A.F. Walsh, Lim group B strep broth and coagglutination for rapid identification of group B streptococci in preterm pregnant women, J. Clin. Microbiol. 25 (1987) 452–453.

[17] R.R. Facklam, et al., Presumptive identification of group A, B and D streptococci on agar plate medium, J. Clin. Microbiol. 9 (1979) 665–672.

[18] R. Christie, N.E. Atkins, E. Munch-Petersen, A note on a lytic phenomenon shown by group B streptococci, Aust. J. Exp. Biol. Med. Sci. 22 (1944) 197–200.

[19] J.W. Tapsall, E.A. Phillips, Presumptive identification of group B streptococci by rapid detection of CAMP factor and pigment production, Diagn. Microbiol. Infect. Dis. 7 (1987) 225–228.

[20] R. Facklam, et al., Comparative evaluation of the API 20S and automicrobic gram-positive identification systems for non-beta-hemolytic streptococci and aerococci, J. Clin. Microbiol. 21 (1985) 535–541.

[21] R.C. Lancefield, A microprecipitin technic for classifying hemolytic streptococci, and improved methods for producing antisera, Proc. Soc. Exp. Biol. Med. 38 (1938) 473–478.

[22] J.A. Daly, K.C. Seskin, Evaluation of rapid, commercial latex techniques for serogrouping beta-hemolytic streptococci, J. Clin. Microbiol. 26 (1988) 2429–2431.

[23] A.W. Stableforth, Incidence of various serological types of *Streptococcus agalactiae* in herds of cows in Great Britain, J. Pathol. Bacteriol. 46 (1938) 21–119.

[24] I.H. Pattison, P.R.J. Matthews, W.R. Maxted, Type classification by Lancefield's precipitin method of human and bovine group B streptococci isolated in Britain, J. Pathol. Bacteriol. 70 (1955) 51–60.

[25] L.A. Finch, D.R. Martin, Human and bovine group B streptococci: two distinct populations, J. Appl. Bacteriol. 57 (1984) 273–278.

[26] I.W.T. Wibawan, C. Lämmler, Properties of group B streptococci with protein surface antigens X and R, J. Clin. Microbiol. 28 (1990) 2834–2836.

[27] R.C. Lancefield, R. Hare, The serological differentiation of pathogenic and non-pathogenic strains of hemolytic streptococci from parturient women, J. Exp. Med. 61 (1935) 335–349.

[28] R.C. Lancefield, Two serological types of group B hemolytic streptococci with related, but not identical, type-specific substances, J. Exp. Med. 67 (1938) 25–40.

[29] E.H. Freimer, Type-specific polysaccharide antigens of group B streptococci. II. The chemical basis for serological specificity of the type II HCl antigen, J. Exp. Med. 125 (1967) 381–392.

[30] H.W. Wilkinson, R.G. Eagon, Type-specific antigens of group B type Ic streptococci, Infect. Immun. 4 (1971) 596–604.

[31] J. Jelínková, J. Motlová, The nomenclature of GBS, Antibiot. Chemother. 35 (1985) 49–52.

[32] J. Henrichsen, et al., Nomenclature of antigens of group B streptococci, Int. J. Syst. Bacteriol. 34 (1984) 500.

[33] B. Perch, E. Kjems, J. Henrichsen, New serotypes of group B streptococci isolated from human sources, J. Clin. Microbiol. 10 (1979) 109–110.

[34] D.R. Johnson, P. Ferrieri, Group B streptococcal Ibc protein antigen: distribution of two determinants in wild-type strains of common serotypes, J. Clin. Microbiol. 19 (1984) 506–510.

[35] L.C. Madoff, et al., Phenotypic diversity in the alpha C protein of group B streptococci, Infect. Immun. 59 (1991) 2638–2644.

[36] L.C. Madoff, et al., Group B streptococci escape host immunity by deletion of tandem repeat elements of the alpha C protein, Proc. Natl. Acad. Sci. U. S. A. 93 (1996) 4131–4136.

[37] D.E. Kling, et al., Characterization of two distinct opsonic and protective epitopes within the alpha c protein of the group B Streptococcus, Infect. Immun. 65 (1997) 1462–1467.

[38] C. Gravekamp, et al., Variation in repeat number within the alpha c protein of group B streptococci alters antigenicity and protective epitopes, Infect. Immun. 64 (1996) 3576–3583.

[39] P.G. Jerlström, G.S. Chhatwal, K.N. Timmis, The IgA-binding β antigen of the c protein complex of group B streptococci: sequence determination of its gene and detection of two binding regions, Mol. Microbiol. 54 (1991) 843–849.

[40] L.J. Brady, M.D.P. Boyle, Identification of non-immunoglobulin A-Fc-binding forms and low-molecular-weight secreted forms of the group B streptococcal beta antigen, Infect. Immun. 57 (1989) 1573–1581.

[41] P.G. Jerlström, et al., Identification of an immunoglobulin A binding motif located in the beta-antigen of the c protein complex of group B streptococci, Infect. Immun. 64 (1996) 2787–2793.

[42] P. Ferrieri, et al., Diversity of surface protein expression in group B streptococcal colonizing and invasive isolates, Indian. J. Med. Res. 119 (Suppl.) (2004) 191–196.

[43] S. Erdogan, et al., Molecular analysis of group B protective surface protein, a new cell surface protective antigen of group B streptococci, Infect. Immun. 70 (2002) 803–811.

[44] I.H. Pattison, P.R.J. Matthews, D.G. Howell, The type classification of group B streptococci with special reference to bovine strains apparently lacking in type polysaccharide, J. Pathol. Bacteriol. 69 (1955) 41–50.

[45] C.S. Lachenauer, L.C. Madoff, A protective surface protein from type V group B streptococci shares N-terminal sequence homology with the alpha c protein, Infect. Immun. 64 (1996) 4255–4260.

[46] S. Rioux, et al., Localization of surface immunogenic protein on group B Streptococcus, Infect. Immun. 69 (2001) 5162–5265.

[47] H.C. Maisey, et al., Group B streptococcal pilus proteins contribute to adherence to and invasion of brain microvascular endothelial cells, J. Bacteriol. 189 (2007) 1464–1467.

[48] L. Deng, et al., Characterization of the linkage between the type III capsular polysaccharide and the bacterial cell wall of group B Streptococcus, J. Biol. Chem. 275 (2000) 7497–7504.

[49] D.L. Kasper, C.J. Baker, Electron microscopic definition of surface antigens of group B Streptococcus, J. Infect. Dis. 139 (1979) 147–151.

[50] C. von Hunolstein, et al., Immunochemistry of capsular type polysaccharide and virulence properties of type VI Streptococcus agalactiae (group B streptococci), Infect. Immun. 61 (1993) 1272–1280.

[51] M. Rýc, et al., Immuno-electronmicroscopic demonstration of capsules on group-B streptococci of new serotypes and type candidates, J. Med. Microbiol. 25 (1988) 147–149.

[52] L.C. Paoletti, R.A. Ross, K.D. Johnson, Cell growth rate regulates expression of group B Streptococcus type III capsular polysaccharide, Infect. Immun. 64 (1996) 1220–1226.

[53] C.J. Baker, D.L. Kasper, C.E. Davis, Immunochemical characterization of the native type III polysaccharide of group B Streptococcus, J. Exp. Med. 143 (1976) 258–270.

[54] F. Michon, et al., Multiantennary group-specific polysaccharide of group B Streptococcus, Biochemistry 27 (1988) 5341–5351.

[55] J.Y. Tai, E.C. Gotschlich, R.C. Lancefield, Isolation of type-specific polysaccharide antigen from group B type Ib streptococci, J. Exp. Med. 149 (1979) 58–66.

[56] H.J. Jennings, K.G. Rosell, D.L. Kasper, Structural determination and serology of the native polysaccharide antigen of the type III group B Streptococcus, Can. J. Biochem. 58 (1980) 112–120.

[57] M.R. Wessels, et al., Structure and immunochemistry of an oligosaccharide repeating unit of the capsular polysaccharide of type III group B Streptococcus, J. Biol. Chem. 262 (1987) 8262–8267.

[58] M.R. Wessels, et al., Structural determination and immunochemical characterization of the type V group B Streptococcus capsular polysaccharide, J. Biol. Chem. 266 (1991) 6714–6719.

[59] G. Kogan, et al., Structural elucidation of the novel type VII group B Streptococcus capsular polysaccharide by high resolution NMR spectroscopy, Carbohydr. Res. 277 (1995) 1–9.

[60] D.L. Kasper, et al., Immunochemical analysis and immunogenicity of the type II group B streptococcal capsular polysaccharide, J. Clin. Invest. 72 (1983) 260–269.

[61] M.R. Wessels, et al., Isolation and characterization of type IV group B Streptococcus capsular polysaccharide, Infect. Immun. 57 (1989) 1089–1094.

[62] H.J. Jennings, et al., Structural determination of the capsular polysaccharide antigen of type II group B Streptococcus, J. Biol. Chem. 258 (1983) 1793–1798.

[63] G. Kogan, et al., Structural and immunochemical characterization of the type VIII group B Streptococcus capsular polysaccharide, J. Biol. Chem. 271 (1996) 8786–8790.

[64] H.J. Jennings, et al., Structure of native polysaccharide antigens of type Ia and type Ib group B Streptococcus, Biochemistry 22 (1983) 1258–1264.

[65] R.E. Schifferle, et al., Immunochemical analysis of the types Ia and Ib group B streptococcal polysaccharides, J. Immunol. 135 (1985) 4164–4170.

[66] B. Lindberg, J. Lönngren, D.A. Powell, Structural studies of the specific type 14 pneumococcal polysaccharide, Carbohydr. Res. 58 (1977) 117–186.

[67] M.R. Wessels, et al., Structural properties of group B streptococcal type III polysaccharide conjugate vaccines that influence immunogenicity and efficacy, Infect. Immun. 66 (1998) 2186–2192.

[68] M.R. Wessels, A. Muñoz, D.L. Kasper, A model of high-affinity antibody binding to type III group B Streptococcus capsular polysaccharide, Proc. Natl. Acad. Sci. U. S. A. 84 (1987) 9170–9174.

[69] J.R. Brisson, et al., NMR and molecular dynamics studies of the conformational epitope of the type III group B Streptococcus capsular polysaccharide and derivatives, Biochemistry 36 (1997) 3278–3292.

[70] W. Zou, H.J. Jennings, The conformational epitope of type III group B Streptococcus capsular polysaccharide, Adv. Exp. Med. Biol. 491 (2001) 473–484.

[71] T.W. Milligan, et al., Growth and amino acid requirements of various strains of group B streptococci, J. Clin. Microbiol. 7 (1978) 28–33.

[72] C.J. Baker, D.L. Kasper, Microcapsule of type III strains of group B Streptococcus: production and morphology, Infect. Immun. 13 (1976) 189–194.

[73] G. Malin, L.C. Paoletti, Use of a dynamic in vitro attachment and invasion system (DIVAS) to determine influence of growth rate on invasion of respiratory epithelium by group B Streptococcus, Proc. Natl. Acad. Sci. U. S. A. 98 (2001) 13335–13340.

[74] A.K. Johri, et al., Oxygen regulates invasiveness and virulence of group B Streptococcus, Infect. Immun. 71 (2003) 6707–6711.

[75] J.N. Weiser, C.E. Rubens, Transposon mutagenesis of group B Streptococcus beta-hemolysin biosynthesis, Infect. Immun. 55 (1987) 2314–2316.

[76] J.W. Tapsall, Pigment production by Lancefield-group B streptococci (Streptococcus agalactiae), J. Med. Microbiol. 21 (1986) 75–81.

[77] R.R. Facklam, et al., Presumptive identification of groups A, B and D streptococci, Appl. Microbiol. 27 (1974) 107–113.

[78] P. Ferrieri, L.W. Wannamaker, J. Nelson, Localization and characterization of the hippuricase activity of group B streptococci, Infect. Immun. 7 (1973) 747–752.

[79] J.F. Bohnsack, et al., Group B streptococci inactivate complement component C5a by enzymic cleavage at the C-terminus, Biochem. J. 273 (1991) 635–640.

[80] J.F. Bohnsack, et al., Purification of a protease from group B streptococci that inactivates human C5a, Biochim. Biophys. Acta. 1079 (1991) 222–228.

[81] P.P. Cleary, et al., Similarity between the group B and A streptococcal C5a peptidase genes, Infect. Immun. 60 (1992) 4239–4244.

[82] H.R. Hill, et al., Group B streptococci inhibit the chemotactic activity of the fifth component of complement, J. Immunol. 141 (1988) 3551–3556.

[83] P. Ferrieri, E.D. Gray, L.W. Wannamaker, Biochemical and immunological characterization of the extracellular nucleases of group B streptococci, J. Exp. Med. 151 (1980) 56–68.

[84] D.G. Pritchard, et al., Characterization of the group B streptococcal hyaluronate lyase, Arch. Biochem. Biophys. 315 (1994) 431–437.

[85] J.M. Musser, et al., Identification of a high-virulence clone of type III Streptococcus agalactiae (group B Streptococcus) causing invasive neonatal disease, Proc. Natl. Acad. Sci. U. S. A. 86 (1989) 4731–4735.

[86] T.J. Nealon, S.J. Mattingly, Association of elevated levels of cellular lipoteichoic acids of group B streptococci with human neonatal disease, Infect. Immun. 39 (1983) 1243–1251.

[87] J.C. Goldschmidt Jr., C. Panos, Teichoic acids of Streptococcus agalactiae: chemistry, cytotoxicity, and effect on bacterial adherence to human cells in tissue culture, Infect. Immun. 43 (1984) 670–677.

[88] J.F. Bohnsack, et al., Serotype III Streptococcus agalactiae from bovine milk and human neonatal infections, Emerg. Infect. Dis. 10 (2004) 1412–1419.

[89] C.J. Baker, et al., Comparison of bacteriological methods for the isolation of group B streptococcus from vaginal cultures, J. Clin. Microbiol. 4 (1976) 46–48.

[90] K.K. Christensen, et al., Group B streptococci in human urethral and cervical specimens, Scand. J. Infect. Dis. 8 (1976) 74–78.

[91] S.W. MacDonald, F.R. Manuel, J.A. Embil, Localization of group B beta-hemolytic streptococci in the female urogenital tract, Am. J. Obstet. Gynecol. 133 (1979) 57–59.

[92] H.C. Dillon, et al., Anorectal and vaginal carriage of group B streptococci during pregnancy, J. Infect. Dis. 145 (1982) 794–799.

[93] P. Ferrieri, P.P. Cleary, A.E. Seeds, Epidemiology of group B streptococcal carriage in pregnant women and newborn infants, J. Med. Microbiol. 10 (1976) 103–114.

[94] B.F. Anthony, D.M. Okada, C.J. Hobel, Epidemiology of the group B Streptococcus: maternal and nosocomial sources for infant acquisitions, J. Pediatr. 95 (1979) 431–436.

[95] M.R. Hammerschlag, et al., Colonization with group B streptococci in girls under 16 years of age, Pediatrics 60 (1977) 473–477.

[96] M. Mauer, M.C. Thirumoorthi, A.S. Dajani, Group B streptococcal colonization in prepubertal children, Pediatrics 64 (1979) 65–67.

[97] B.F. Anthony, D.M. Okada, C.J. Hobel, Epidemiology of group B Streptococcus: longitudinal observations during pregnancy, J. Infect. Dis. 137 (1978) 524–530.

[98] L. Meyn, et al., Association of sexual activity with colonization and vaginal acquisition of group B Streptococcus in nonpregnant women, Am. J. Epidemiol. 155 (2002) 949–957.

[99] B. Foxman, et al., Incidence and duration of group B *Streptococcus* by serotype among male and female college students living in a single dormitory, Am. J. Epidemiol. 163 (2006) 544–551.

[100] K.M. Boyer, et al., Selective intrapartum chemoprophylaxis of neonatal group B streptococcal early-onset disease. II. Predictive value of prenatal cultures, J. Infect. Dis. 148 (1983) 802–809.

[101] M.K. Yancey, et al., The accuracy of late antenatal screening cultures in predicting genital group B streptococcal colonization at delivery, Obstet. Gynecol. 88 (1996) 811–815.

[102] M.S. Badri, et al., Rectal colonization with group B *Streptococcus*: relation to vaginal colonization of pregnant women, J. Infect. Dis. 135 (1977) 308–312.

[103] K. Persson, et al., Longitudinal study of group B streptococcal carriage during late pregnancy, Scand. J. Infect. Dis. 19 (1987) 325–329.

[104] E.L. Kaplan, D.R. Johnson, J.N. Kuritsky, Rectal colonization by group B beta-hemolytic streptococci in a geriatric population, J. Infect. Dis. 148 (1983) 1120.

[105] B.F. Anthony, et al., Isolation of group B streptococci from the proximal small intestine of adults, J. Infect. Dis. 147 (1983) 776.

[106] M. Barnham, The gut as a source of the haemolytic streptococci causing infection in surgery of the intestinal and biliary tracts, J. Infect. 6 (1983) 129–139.

[107] C.S.F. Easmon, et al., The carrier state: group B *Streptococcus*, J. Antimicrob. Chemother. 18 (1986) 59–65.

[108] S.D. Manning, et al., Prevalence of group B *Streptococcus* colonization and potential for transmission by casual contact in healthy young men and women, Clin. Infect. Dis. 39 (2004) 380–388.

[109] C.J. Baker, et al., Vaginal colonization with group B *Streptococcus*: a study in college women, J. Infect. Dis. 135 (1977) 392–397.

[110] S.J. Bliss, et al., Group B *Streptococcus* colonization in male and nonpregnant female university students: a cross-sectional prevalence study, Clin. Infect. Dis. 34 (2002) 184–190.

[111] B. Foxman, et al., Risk factors for group B streptococcal colonization: potential for different transmission systems by capsular type, Ann. Epidemiol. 17 (2007) 854–862.

[112] E. Ramos, et al., Group B *Streptococcus* colonization in pregnant diabetic women, Obstet. Gynecol. 89 (1997) 257–260.

[113] K.K. Christensen, A.K. Dykes, P. Christensen, Relation between use of tampons and urogenital carriage of group B streptococci, BMJ 289 (1984) 731–732.

[114] M.D. Yow, et al., The natural history of group B streptococcal colonization in the pregnant woman and her offspring. I. Colonization studies, Am. J. Obstet. Gynecol. 137 (1980) 34–38.

[115] J.A. Regan, et al., The epidemiology of group B streptococcal colonization in pregnancy, Obstet. Gynecol. 77 (1991) 604–610.

[116] J. Wallin, A. Forsgren, Group B streptococci in venereal disease clinic patients, Br. J. Vener. Dis. 51 (1975) 401–404.

[117] J.R. Campbell, et al., Group B streptococcal colonization and serotype-specific immunity in pregnant women at delivery, Obstet. Gynecol. 96 (2000) 498–503.

[118] M.E. Hickman, et al., Changing epidemiology of group B streptococcal (GBS) colonization, Pediatrics 104 (1999) 203–209.

[119] E.R. Newton, M.C. Butler, R.N. Shain, Sexual behavior and vaginal colonization by group B *Streptococcus* among minority women, Obstet. Gynecol. 88 (1996) 577–582.

[120] H.D. Davies, et al., Antibodies to capsular polysaccharides of group B *Streptococcus* in pregnant Canadian women: relationship to colonization status and infection in the neonate, J. Infect. Dis. 184 (2001) 285–291.

[121] P.W. Ross, C.G. Cumming, Group B streptococci in women attending a sexually transmitted diseases clinic, J. Infect. 4 (1982) 161–166.

[122] B.J. Stoll, A. Schuchat, Maternal carriage of group B streptococci in developing countries, Pediatr. Infect. Dis. J. 17 (1998) 499–503.

[123] E. Barcaite, et al., Prevalence of maternal group B streptococcal colonisation in European countries, Acta Obstet. Gynecol. Scand. 87 (2008) 260–271.

[124] M.A. Turrentine, M.M. Ramirez, Recurrence of group B streptococcal colonization in subsequent pregnancy, Obstet. Gynecol. 112 (2008) 259–264.

[125] P. Ferrieri, L.L. Blair, Pharyngeal carriage of group B streptococci: detection by three methods, J. Clin. Microbiol. 6 (1977) 136–139.

[126] J.H. Chretien, et al., Group B beta-hemolytic streptococci causing pharyngitis, J. Clin. Microbiol. 10 (1979) 263–266.

[127] S.G. Sackel, et al., Isolation of group B *Streptococcus* from men, (1978). 18th Interscience Conference on Antimicrobial Agenet and Chemotherapy, 1978 [Abstract 467].

[128] G.F. Hayden, T.F. Murphy, J.O. Hendley, Non-group A streptococci in the pharynx. Pathogens or innocent bystanders? Am. J. Dis. Child. 143 (1989) 794–797.

[129] K.S. Persson, et al., Faecal carriage of group B streptococci, Eur. J. Clin. Microbiol. 5 (1986) 156–159.

[130] C.G. Cummings, P.W. Ross, Group B streptococci (GBS) in the upper respiratory tract of schoolchildren, Health Bull. 40 (1982) 81–86.

[131] M.A. Shafer, et al., Microbiology of the lower genital tract in postmenarchal adolescent girls: differences by sexual activity, contraception, and presence of nonspecific vaginitis, J. Pediatr. 107 (1985) 974–981.

[132] R.J. Ancona, P. Ferrieri, P.P. Williams, Maternal factors that enhance the acquisition of group B streptococci by newborn infants, J. Med. Microbiol. 13 (1980) 273–280.

[133] C.J. Baker, M.S. Edwards, Group B streptococcal infections: perinatal impact and prevention methods, Ann. N. Y. Acad. Sci. 549 (1988) 193–202.

[134] A. Paredes, et al., Nosocomial transmission of group B streptococci in a newborn nursery, Pediatrics 59 (1976) 679–682.

[135] C.S.F. Easmon, et al., Nosocomial transmission of group B streptococci, BMJ 283 (1981) 459–461.

[136] F.J.D. Noya, et al., Unusual occurrence of an epidemic of type Ib/c group B streptococcal sepsis in a neonatal intensive care unit, J. Infect. Dis. 155 (1987) 1135–1144.

[137] J.D. Band, et al., Transmission of group B streptococci, Am. J. Dis. Child. 135 (1981) 355–358.

[138] S.E. Gardner, E.O. Mason Jr., M.D. Yow, Community acquisition of group B *Streptococcus* by infants of colonized mothers, Pediatrics 66 (1980) 873–875.

[139] S.M. Hansen, et al., Dynamics of *Streptococcus agalactiae* colonization in women during and after pregnancy and in their infants, J. Clin. Microbiol. 42 (2004) 83–89.

[140] H.W. Wilkinson, Analysis of group B streptococcal types associated with disease in human infants and adults, J. Clin. Microbiol. 7 (1978) 176–179.

[141] C.J. Baker, F.F. Barrett, Group B streptococcal infection in infants: the importance of the various serotypes, JAMA 230 (1974) 1158–1160.

[142] H.M. Blumberg, et al., Invasive group B streptococcal disease: the emergence of serotype V, J. Infect. Dis. 173 (1996) 365–373.

[143] D.F. Zaleznik, et al., Invasive disease due to group B *Streptococcus* in pregnant women and neonates from diverse population groups, Clin. Infect. Dis. 30 (2000) 276–281.

[144] H.D. Davies, et al., Population-based active surveillance for neonatal group B streptococcal infections in Alberta, Canada: implications for vaccine formulation, Pediatr. Infect. Dis. J. 20 (2001) 879–884.

[145] J.A. Elliott, K.D. Farmer, R.R. Facklam, Sudden increase in isolation of group B streptococci, serotype V, is not due to emergence of a new pulsed-field gel electrophoresis type, J. Clin. Microbiol. 36 (1998) 2115–2116.

[146] A.M. Weisner, et al., Characterization of group B streptococci recovered from infants with invasive disease in England and Wales, Clin. Infect. Dis. 38 (2004) 1203–1208.

[147] K. Fluegge, et al., Serotype distribution of invasive group B streptococcal isolates in infants: results from a nationwide active laboratory surveillance study over 2 years in Germany, Clin. Infect. Dis. 40 (2005) 760–763.

[148] K. Matsubara, et al., Seroepidemiologic studies of serotype VIII group B *Streptococcus* in Japan, J. Infect. Dis. 186 (2002) 855–858.

[149] K. Matsubara, et al., Three fatal cases of invasive serotype VI group B streptococcal infection, J. Infect. 53 (2006) e139–e142.

[150] C.R. Phares, et al., Epidemiology of invasive group B streptococcal disease in the United States, 1999–2005, JAMA 299 (2008) 2056–2065.

[151] J. Stringer, The development of a phage typing system for group-B streptococci, J. Med. Microbiol. 13 (1980) 133–144.

[152] T. Horodniceanu, et al., Conjugative R plasmids in *Streptococcus agalactiae* (group B), Plasmid 2 (1979) 197–206.

[153] S.J. Mattingly, et al., Identification of a high-virulence clone of serotype III *Streptococcus agalactiae* by growth characteristics at 40 C, J. Clin. Microbiol. 28 (1990) 1676–1677.

[154] R. Quentin, et al., Characterization of *Streptococcus agalactiae* strains by multilocus enzyme genotype and serotype: identification of multiple virulent clone families that cause invasive neonatal disease, J. Clin. Microbiol. 33 (1995) 2576–2581.

[155] M.E. Gordillo, et al., Comparison of group B streptococci by pulsed field gel electrophoresis and by conventional electrophoresis, J. Clin. Microbiol. 31 (1993) 1430–1434.

[156] A.S. Limansky, et al., Genomic diversity among *Streptococcus agalactiae* isolates detected by a degenerate oligonucleotide-primed amplification assay, J. Infect. Dis. 177 (1998) 1308–1313.

[157] E. Bingen, et al., Analysis of DNA restriction fragment length polymorphism extends the evidence for breast milk transmission in *Streptococcus agalactiae* late-onset neonatal infection, J. Infect. Dis. 165 (1992) 569–573.

[158] S.L. Luan, et al., Multilocus sequence typing of Swedish invasive group B streptococcus isolates indicates a neonatally associated genetic lineage and capsule switching, J. Clin. Microbiol. 43 (2005) 3727–3733.

[159] E.E. Adderson, S. Takahashi, J.F. Bohnsack, Bacterial genetics and human immunity to group B streptococci, Mol. Genet. Metab. 71 (2000) 451–454.

[160] J.F. Bohnsack, et al., Long-range mapping of the *Streptococcus agalactiae* phylogenetic lineage restriction digest pattern type III-3 reveals clustering of virulence genes, Infect. Immun. 70 (2002) 134–139.

[161] J.F. Bohnsack, et al., Phylogenetic classification of serotype III group B streptococci on the basis of hylB gene analysis and DNA sequences specific to restriction digest pattern type III-3, J. Infect. Dis. 183 (2001) 1694–1697.

[162] S. Takahashi, et al., Correlation of phylogenetic lineages of group B streptococci, identified by analysis of restriction-digestion patterns of genomic DNA, with infB alleles and mobile genetic elements, J. Infect. Dis. 186 (2002) 1034–1038.

[163] E.E. Adderson, et al., Subtractive hybridization identifies a novel predicted protein mediating epithelial cell invasion by virulent serotype III group B *Streptococcus agalactiae*, Infect. Immun. 71 (2003) 6857–6863.

[164] H.D. Davies, et al., Multilocus sequence typing of serotype III group B *Streptococcus* and correlation with pathogenic potential, J. Infect. Dis. 189 (2004) 1097–1102.

[165] N. Jones, et al., Multilocus sequence typing system for group B *Streptococcus*, J. Clin. Microbiol. 41 (2003) 2530–2536.

[166] P. Bidet, et al., Molecular characterization of serotype III group B-*Streptococcus* isolates causing neonatal meningitis, J. Infect. Dis. 188 (2003) 1132–1137.

[167] U. von Both, et al., Molecular epidemiology of invasive neonatal *Streptococcus agalactiae* isolates in Germany, Pediatr. Infect. Dis. J. 27 (2008) 903–906.

[168] N. Dore, et al., Molecular epidemiology of group B streptococci in Ireland: associations between serotype, invasive status and presence of genes encoding putative virulence factors, Epidemiol. Infect. 131 (2003) 823–833.

[169] K.M. Zangwill, A. Schuchat, J.D. Wenger, Group B streptococcal disease in the United States, 1990: report from a multistate active surveillance system, MMWR Morb. Mortal. Wkly. Rep. 41 (1992) 25–32.

[170] A. Schuchat, et al., Population-based risk factors for neonatal group B streptococcal disease: results of a cohort study in metropolitan Atlanta, J. Infect. Dis. 162 (1990) 672–677.

[171] S.J. Schrag, et al., A population-based comparison of strategies to prevent early-onset group B streptococcal disease in neonates, N. Engl. J. Med. 347 (2002) 233–239.

[172] Perinatal group B streptococcal disease after universal screening recommendations—United States, 2003–2005, MMWR Morb. Mortal. Wkly. Rep. 56 (2007) 701–705.

[173] Active Bacterial Core Surveillance (ABCs) Report Emerging Infections Program Network, Group B *Streptococcus*, 2008. Available at http://www.cdc.gov/ncidod/dbmd/abcs/survreports/gbs08.pdf.

[174] J.R. Bobitt, J.D. Damato, J. Sakakini, Perinatal complications in group B streptococcal carriers: a longitudinal study of prenatal patients, Am. J. Obstet. Gynecol. 151 (1985) 711–717.

[175] K.M. Boyer, S.P. Gotoff, Strategies for chemoprophylaxis of GBS early-onset infections, Antibiot. Chemother. 35 (1985) 267–280.

[176] M.A. Pass, et al., Prospective studies of group B streptococcal infections in infants, J. Pediatr. 95 (1979) 437–443.

[177] J.D. Sobel, et al., Comparison of bacterial and fungal adherence to vaginal exfoliated epithelial cells and human vaginal epithelial tissue culture cells, Infect. Immun. 35 (1982) 697–701.

[178] J. Jelínková, et al., Adherence of vaginal and pharyngeal strains of group B streptococci to human vaginal and pharyngeal epithelial cells, Zentralbl. Bakteriol. Mikrobiol. Hyg [A] 262 (1986) 492–499.

[179] S.M. Zawaneh, et al., Factors influencing adherence of group B streptococci to human vaginal epithelial cells, Infect. Immun. 26 (1979) 441–447.

[180] G.S. Tamura, et al., Adherence of group B streptococci to cultured epithelial cells: roles of environmental factors and bacterial surface components, Infect. Immun. 62 (1994) 2450–2458.

[181] T.J. Nealon, S.J. Mattingly, Role of cellular lipoteichoic acids in mediating adherence of serotype III strains of group B streptococci to human embryonic, fetal, and adult epithelial cells, Infect. Immun. 43 (1984) 523–530.

[182] G. Teti, et al., Adherence of group B streptococci to adult and neonatal epithelial cells mediated by lipoteichoic acid, Infect. Immun. 55 (1987) 3057–3064.

[183] F. Cox, Prevention of group B streptococcal colonization with topically applied lipoteichoic acid in a maternal-newborn mouse model, Pediatr. Res. 16 (1982) 816–819.

[184] G.S. Tamura, C.E. Rubens, Group B streptococci adhere to a variant of fibronectin attached to a solid phase, Mol. Microbiol. 15 (1995) 581–589.

[185] C. Beckmann, et al., Identification of novel adhesins from group B streptococci by use of phage display reveals that C5a peptidase mediates fibronectin binding, Infect. Immun. 70 (2002) 2869–2876.

[186] Q. Cheng, et al., The group B streptococcal C5a peptidase is both a specific protease and an invasin, Infect. Immun. 70 (2002) 2408–2413.

[187] B. Spellberg, et al., Lmb, a protein with similarities to the LraI adhesin family, mediates attachment of *Streptococcus agalactiae* to human laminin, Infect. Immun. 67 (1999) 871–878.

[188] A. Schubert, et al., A fibrinogen receptor from group B *Streptococcus* interacts with fibrinogen by repetitive units with novel ligand binding sites, Mol. Microbiol. 46 (2002) 557–569.

[189] U. Samen, et al., The surface protein Srr-1 of *Streptococcus agalactiae* binds human keratin 4 and promotes adherence to epithelial HEp-2 cells, Infect. Immun. 75 (2007) 5405–5414.

[190] R. Rosini, et al., Identification of novel genomic islands coding for antigenic pilus-like structures in *Streptococcus agalactiae*, Mol. Microbiol. 61 (2006) 126–141.

[191] S. Dramsi, et al., Assembly and role of pili in group B streptococci, Mol. Microbiol. 60 (2006) 1401–1413.

[192] V. Krishnan, et al., An IgG-like domain in the minor pilin GBS52 of *Streptococcus agalactiae* mediates lung epithelial cell adhesion, Structure 15 (2007) 893–903.

[193] P.B. Stewardson-Krieger, S.P. Gotoff, Risk factors in early-onset neonatal group B streptococcal infections, Infection 6 (1978) 50–53.

[194] P.I. Tseng, S.R. Kandall, Group B streptococcal disease in neonates and infants, N. Y. State. J. Med. 74 (1974) 2169–2173.

[195] G.R. Evaldson, A.S. Malmborg, C.E. Nord, Premature rupture of the membranes and ascending infection, Br. J. Obstet. Gynaecol. 89 (1982) 793–801.

[196] J.N. Schoonmaker, et al., Bacteria and inflammatory cells reduce chorioamniotic membrane integrity and tensile strength, Obstet. Gynecol. 74 (1989) 590–596.

[197] A.J. Sbarra, et al., Effect of bacterial growth on the bursting pressure of fetal membranes in vitro, Obstet. Gynecol. 70 (1987) 107–110.

[198] R.F. Lamont, M. Rose, M.G. Elder, Effect of bacterial products on prostaglandin E production by amnion cells, Lancet 2 (1985) 1331–1333.

[199] P.R. Bennett, et al., Preterm labor: stimulation of arachidonic acid metabolism in human amnion cells by bacterial products, Am. J. Obstet. Gynecol. 156 (1987) 649–655.

[200] D.J. Dudley, et al., Regulation of decidual cell chemokine production by group B streptococci and purified bacterial cell wall components, Am. J. Obstet. Gynecol. 177 (1997) 666–672.

[201] P. Ferrieri, P.P. Cleary, A.E. Seeds, Epidemiology of group-B streptococcal carriage in pregnant women and newborn infants, J. Med. Microbiol. 10 (1977) 103–114.

[202] T.C. Eickhoff, et al., Neonatal sepsis and other infections due to group B beta-hemolytic streptococci, N. Engl. J. Med. 271 (1964) 1221–1228.

[203] R.P. Galask, et al., Bacterial attachment to the chorioamniotic membranes, Am. J. Obstet. Gynecol. 148 (1984) 915–928.

[204] S.B. Winram, et al., Characterization of group B streptococcal invasion of human chorion and amnion epithelial cells In vitro, Infect. Immun. 66 (1998) 4932–4941.

[205] B. Lin, et al., Cloning and expression of the gene for group B streptococcal hyaluronate lyase, J. Biol. Chem. 269 (1994) 30113–30116.

[206] V.G. Hemming, et al., Rapid in vitro replication of group B *Streptococcus* in term human amniotic fluid, Gynecol. Obstet. Invest. 19 (1985) 124–129.

[207] I.A. Abbasi, et al., Proliferation of group B streptococci in human amniotic fluid in vitro, Am. J. Obstet. Gynecol. 156 (1987) 95–99.

[208] C.J. Baker, Early onset group B streptococcal disease, J. Pediatr. 93 (1978) 124–125.

[209] G. Bergqvist, et al., Intrauterine death due to infection with group B streptococci, Acta Obstet. Gynecol. Scand. 57 (1978) 127–128.

[210] R.C. Ablow, et al., A comparison of early-onset group B streptococcal neonatal infection and the respiratory-distress syndrome of the newborn, N. Engl. J. Med. 294 (1976) 65–70.

[211] J.H. Vollman, et al., Early onset group B streptococcal disease: clinical, roentgenographic, and pathologic features, J. Pediatr. 89 (1976) 199–203.

[212] N.R. Payne, et al., Correlation of clinical and pathologic findings in early onset neonatal group B streptococcal infection with disease severity and prediction of outcome, Pediatr. Infect. Dis. J. 7 (1988) 836–847.

[213] V.G. Hemming, D.W. McCloskey, H.R. Hill, Pneumonia in the neonate associated with group B streptococcal septicemia, Am. J. Dis. Child. 130 (1976) 1231–1233.

[214] A. Katzenstein, C. Davis, A. Braude, Pulmonary changes in neonatal sepsis due to group B beta-hemolytic streptococcus: relation to hyaline membrane disease, J. Infect. Dis. 133 (1976) 430–435.

[215] C.E. Rubens, et al., Pathophysiology and histopathology of group B streptococcal sepsis in *Macaca nemestrina* primates induced after intraamniotic inoculation: evidence for bacterial cellular invasion, J. Infect. Dis. 164 (1991) 320–330.

[216] M.P. Sherman, et al., Role of pulmonary phagocytes in host defense against group B streptococci in preterm versus term rabbit lung, J. Infect. Dis. 166 (1992) 818–826.

[217] C.E. Rubens, et al., Respiratory epithelial cell invasion by group B streptococci, Infect. Immun. 60 (1992) 5157–5163.

[218] R.L. Gibson, et al., Group B streptococci invade endothelial cells: type III capsular polysaccharide attenuates invasion, Infect. Immun. 61 (1993) 478–485.

[219] C.A. Burnham, S.E. Shokoples, G.J. Tyrrell, Rac1, RhoA, and Cdc42 participate in HeLa cell invasion by group B streptococcus, FEMS. Microbiol. Lett. 272 (2007) 8–14.

[220] S. Shin, et al., Focal adhesion kinase is involved in type III group B streptococcal invasion of human brain microvascular endothelial cells, Microb. Pathog. 41 (2006) 168–173.

[221] P. Valentin-Weigand, G.S. Chhatwal, Correlation of epithelial cell invasiveness of group B streptococci with clinical source of isolation, Microb. Pathog. 19 (1995) 83–91.

[222] A. Schubert, et al., The fibrinogen receptor FbsA promotes adherence of *Streptococcus agalactiae* to human epithelial cells, Infect. Immun. 72 (2004) 6197–6205.

[223] T. Tenenbaum, et al., *Streptococcus agalactiae* invasion of human brain microvascular endothelial cells is promoted by the laminin-binding protein Lmb, Microbes. Infect. 9 (2007) 714–720.

[224] M.J. Baron, et al., Alpha C protein of group B *Streptococcus* binds host cell surface glycosaminoglycan and enters cells by an actin-dependent mechanism, J. Biol. Chem. 279 (2004) 24714–24723.

[225] M.L. Hulse, et al., Effect of type III group B streptococcal capsular polysaccharide on invasion of respiratory epithelial cells, Infect. Immun. 61 (1993) 4835–4841.

[226] J. Quirante, R. Ceballos, G. Cassady, Group B beta-hemolytic streptococcal infection in the newborn. I. Early onset infection, Am. J. Dis. Child. 128 (1974) 659–665.

[227] B. Spellberg, et al., Identification of genetic determinants for the hemolytic activity of *Streptococcus agalactiae* by ISS1 transposition, J. Bacteriol. 181 (1999) 3212–3219.

[228] C.A. Pritzlaff, et al., Genetic basis for the beta-haemolytic/cytolytic activity of group B *Streptococcus*, Mol. Microbiol. 39 (2001) 236–247.

[229] V. Nizet, et al., Genetic locus for streptolysin S production by group A *Streptococcus*, Infect. Immun. 68 (2000) 4254.

[230] V. Nizet, et al., Group B streptococcal beta-hemolysin expression is associated with injury of lung epithelial cells, Infect. Immun. 64 (1996) 3818–3826.

[231] R.L. Gibson, V. Nizet, C.E. Rubens, Group B streptococcal beta-hemolysin promotes injury of lung microvascular endothelial cells, Pediatr. Res. 45 (1999) 626–634.

[232] K.S. Doran, et al., Group B streptococcal beta-hemolysin/cytolysin promotes invasion of human lung epithelial cells and the release of interleukin-8, J. Infect. Dis. 185 (2002) 196–203.

[233] D.E. Wennerstrom, J.C. Tsaihong, J.T. Crawford, Evaluation of the role of hemolysin and pigment in the pathogenesis of early onset group B streptococcal infection, Reedbooks, Bracknell, UK, 1985.

[234] V. Nizet, R.L. Gibson, C.E. Rubens, The role of group B streptococci beta-hemolysin expression in newborn lung injury, Adv. Exp. Med. Biol. 418 (1997) 627–630.

[235] M.E. Hensler, G.Y. Liu, S. Sobczak, K. Benirschke, V. Nizet, G.P. Heldt, Virulence role of group B Streptococcus beta-hemolysin/cytolysin in a neonatal rabbit model of early-onset pulmonary infection, J Infect Dis. 191 (8) (2005 Apr 15) 1287–1291. Epub 2005 Mar 10.

[236] E. Herting, et al., Experimental neonatal group B streptococcal pneumonia: effect of a modified porcine surfactant on bacterial proliferation in ventilated near-term rabbits, Pediatr. Res. 36 (1994) 784–791.

[237] E. Herting, et al., Surfactant improves lung function and mitigates bacterial growth in immature ventilated rabbits with experimentally induced neonatal group B streptococcal pneumonia, Arch. Dis. Child. Fetal. Neonatal. Ed. 76 (1997) F3–F8.

[238] R.L. Auten, et al., Surfactant treatment of full-term newborns with respiratory failure, Pediatrics 87 (1991) 101–107.

[239] E. Herting, et al., Surfactant treatment of neonates with respiratory failure and group B streptococcal infection, Pediatrics 106 (2000) 957–964.

[240] A.O. Shigeoka, et al., Role of antibody and complement in opsonization of group B streptococci, Infect. Immun. 21 (1978) 34–40.

[241] D.C. Anderson, et al., Impaired chemotaxigenesis by type III group B streptococci in neonatal sera: relationship to diminished concentration of specific anticapsular antibody and abnormalities of serum complement, Pediatr. Res. 17 (1983) 496–502.

[242] M.S. Edwards, et al., The role of specific antibody in alternative complement pathway-mediated opsonophagocytosis of type III, group B Streptococcus, J. Exp. Med. 151 (1980) 1275–1287.

[243] D.O. Chaffin, et al., The serotype of type Ia and III group B streptococci is determined by the polymerase gene within the polycistronic capsule operon, J. Bacteriol. 182 (2000) 4466–4477.

[244] T. Angata, A. Varki, Chemical diversity in the sialic acids and related alpha-keto acids: an evolutionary perspective, Chem. Rev. 102 (2002) 439–469.

[245] K.S. Doran, G.Y. Liu, V. Nizet, Group B streptococcal beta-hemolysin/cytolysin activates neutrophil signaling pathways in brain endothelium and contributes to development of meningitis, J. Clin. Invest. 112 (2003) 736–744.

[246] A.F. Carlin, et al., Molecular mimicry of host sialylated glycans allows a bacterial pathogen to engage neutrophil Siglec-9 and dampen the innate immune response, Blood 113 (2009) 3333–3336.

[247] D.L. Kasper, et al., Immunodeterminant specificity of human immunity to type III group B streptococcus, J. Exp. Med. 149 (1979) 327–339.

[248] M.S. Edwards, et al., Capsular sialic acid prevents activation of the alternative complement pathway by type III, group B streptococci, J. Immunol. 128 (1982) 1278–1283.

[249] A.O. Shigeoka, et al., Assessment of the virulence factors of group B streptococci: correlation with sialic acid content, J. Infect. Dis. 147 (1983) 857–863.

[250] C.E. Rubens, et al., Molecular analysis of two group B streptococcal virulence factors, Semin. Perinatol. 14 (1990) 22–29.

[251] C.E. Rubens, et al., Transposon mutagenesis of type III group B Streptococcus: correlation of capsule expression with virulence, Proc. Natl. Acad. Sci. U. S. A. 84 (1987) 7208–7212.

[252] H.H. Yim, A. Nittayarin, C.E. Rubens, Analysis of the capsule synthesis locus, a virulence factor in group B streptococci, Adv. Exp. Med. Biol. 418 (1997) 995–997.

[253] M.B. Marques, et al., Prevention of C3 deposition by capsular polysaccharide is a virulence mechanism of type III group B streptococci, Infect. Immun. 60 (1992) 3986–3993.

[254] C.L. Smith, D.G. Pritchard, B.M Gray, Role of polysaccharide capsule in C3 deposition by type Ib group B streptococci (GBS), Thirty-first Interscience Conference on Antimicrobial Agents and Chemotherapy, Washington, DC, (1991).

[255] T.R. Martin, et al., The effect of type-specific polysaccharide capsule on the clearance of group B streptococci from the lungs of infant and adult rats, J. Infect. Dis. 165 (1992) 306–314.

[256] M.R. Wessels, et al., Definition of a bacterial virulence factor: sialylation of the group B streptococcal capsule, Proc. Natl. Acad. Sci. U. S. A. 86 (1989) 8983–8987.

[257] G. Orefici, S. Recchia, L. Galante, Possible virulence marker for Streptococcus agalactiae (Lancefield group B), Eur. J. Clin. Microbiol. Infect. Dis. 7 (1988) 302–305.

[258] N.R. Payne, P. Ferrieri, The relation of the Ibc protein antigen to the opsonization differences between strains of type II group B streptococci, J. Infect. Dis. 151 (1985) 672–681.

[259] C.J. Baker, et al., The role of complement and antibody in opsonophagocytosis of type II group B streptococci, J. Infect. Dis. 154 (1986) 47–54.

[260] G.J. Russell-Jones, E.C. Gotschlich, M.S. Blake, A surface receptor specific for human IgA on group B streptococci possessing the Ibc protein antigen, J. Exp. Med. 160 (1984) 1467–1475.

[261] P.G. Jerlström, G.S. Chhatwal, K.N. Timmis, The IgA-binding beta antigen of the c protein complex of group B streptococci: sequence determination of its gene and detection of two binding regions, Mol. Microbiol. 5 (1991) 843–849.

[262] N.R. Payne, Y.K. Kim, P. Ferrieri, Effect of differences in antibody and complement requirements on phagocytic uptake and intracellular killing of "c" protein-positive and -negative strains of type II group B streptococci, Infect. Immun. 55 (1987) 1243–1251.

[263] T.O. Harris, et al., A novel streptococcal surface protease promotes virulence, resistance to opsonophagocytosis, and cleavage of human fibrinogen, J. Clin. Invest. 111 (2003) 61–70.

[264] I. Santi, et al., BibA: a novel immunogenic bacterial adhesin contributing to group B Streptococcus survival in human blood, Mol. Microbiol. 63 (2007) 754–767.

[265] A.F. Carlin, et al., Group B Streptococcus suppression of phagocyte functions by protein-mediated engagement of human Siglec-5, J. Exp. Med. 206 (2009) 1691–1699.

[266] P. Cornacchione, et al., Group B streptococci persist inside macrophages, Immunology 93 (1998) 86–95.

[267] C.F. Teixeira, et al., Cytochemical study of Streptococcus agalactiae and macrophage interaction, Microsc. Res. Tech. 54 (2001) 254–259.

[268] C.B. Wilson, W.M. Weaver, Comparative susceptibility of group B streptococci and Staphylococcus aureus to killing by oxygen metabolites, J. Infect. Dis. 152 (1985) 323–329.

[269] C. Poyart, et al., Contribution of Mn-cofactored superoxide dismutase (SodA) to the virulence of Streptococcus agalactiae, Infect. Immun. 69 (2001) 5098–5106.

[270] G.Y. Liu, et al., Sword and shield: linked group B streptococcal beta-hemolysin/cytolysin and carotenoid pigment act synergistically to subvert host phagocyte defenses, Proc. Natl. Acad. Sci. U. S. A. 101 (2004) 14491–14496.

[271] V. Nizet, et al., Innate antimicrobial peptide protects the skin from invasive bacterial infection, Nature 414 (2001) 454–457.

[272] A.L. Jones, et al., Penicillin-binding proteins in Streptococcus agalactiae: a novel mechanism for evasion of immune clearance, Mol. Microbiol. 47 (2003) 247–256.

[272a] A. Hamilton, et al., Penicillin-binding protein 1a promotes resistance of group B streptococcus to antimicrobial peptides, Infect. Immun. 74 (2006) 6179–6187.

[273] C. Poyart, et al., Attenuated virulence of Streptococcus agalactiae deficient in d-alanyl-lipoteichoic acid is due to an increased susceptibility to defensins and phagocytic cells, Mol. Microbiol. 49 (2003) 1615–1625.

[274] H.C. Maisey, et al., A group B streptococcal pilus protein promotes phagocyte resistance and systemic virulence, FASEB. J. 6 (2008) 1715–1724.

[275] G.C. Ulett, et al., Beta-hemolysin-independent induction of apoptosis of macrophages infected with serotype III group B streptococcus, J. Infect. Dis. 188 (2003) 1049–1053.

[276] G.C. Ulett, et al., Mechanisms of group B streptococcal-induced apoptosis of murine macrophages, J. Immunol. 175 (2005) 2555–2562.

[277] K. Fettucciari, et al., Group B Streptococcus induces macrophage apoptosis by calpain activation, J. Immunol. 176 (2006) 7542–7556.

[278] J.G. Wheeler, et al., Neutrophil storage pool depletion in septic, neutropenic neonates, Pediatr. Infect. Dis. 3 (1984) 407–409.

[279] R.D. Christensen, et al., Blood and marrow neutrophils during experimental group B streptococcal infection: quantification of the stem cell, proliferative, storage and circulating pools, Pediatr. Res. 16 (1982) 549–553.

[280] B.J. Zeligs, et al., Age-dependent susceptibility of neonatal rats to group B streptococcal type III infection: correlation of severity of infection and response of myeloid pools, Infect. Immun. 37 (1982) 255–263.

[281] R.D. Christensen, H.R. Hill, G. Rothstein, Granulocytic stem cell (CFUc) proliferation in experimental group B streptococcal sepsis, Pediatr. Res. 17 (1983) 278–280.

[282] J.F. Bohnsack, et al., A role for C5 and C5a-ase in the acute neutrophil response to group B streptococcal infections, J. Infect. Dis. 175 (1997) 847–855.

[283] U. Gleich-Theurer, et al., Human serum induces streptococcal c5a peptidase expression, Infect. Immun. 77 (2009) 3817–3825.

[284] J. Rojas, et al., Pulmonary hemodynamic and ultrastructural changes associated with group B streptococcal toxemia in adult sheep and newborn lambs, Pediatr. Res. 17 (1983) 1002–1008.

[285] V.G. Hemming, et al., Studies of short-term pulmonary and peripheral vascular responses induced in oophorectomized sheep by the infusion of a group B streptococcal extract, Pediatr. Res. 18 (1984) 266–269.

[286] R.L. Gibson, et al., Group B streptococcal sepsis in piglets: effect of combined pentoxifylline and indomethacin pretreatment, Pediatr. Res. 31 (1992) 222–227.

[287] K.J. Peevy, et al., Myocardial dysfunction in group B streptococcal shock, Pediatr. Res. 19 (1985) 511–513.

[288] K.J. Peevy, et al., Prostaglandin synthetase inhibition in group B streptococcal shock: hematologic and hemodynamic effects, Pediatr. Res. 20 (1986) 864–866.

[289] W.F. O'Brien, et al., Short-term responses in neonatal lambs after infusion of group B streptococcal extract, Obstet. Gynecol. 65 (1985) 802–806.

[290] R.L. Gibson, et al., Isogenic group B streptococci devoid of capsular polysaccharide or beta-hemolysin: pulmonary hemodynamic and gas exchange effects during bacteremia in piglets, Pediatr. Res. 26 (1989) 241–245.

[291] B.D. Bowdy, et al., Organ-specific disposition of group B streptococci in piglets: evidence for a direct interaction with target cells in the pulmonary circulation, Pediatr. Res. 27 (1990) 344–348.

[292] R.L. Gibson, et al., Group B streptococci (GBS) injure lung endothelium in vitro: GBS invasion and GBS-induced eicosanoid production is greater with microvascular than with pulmonary artery cells, Infect. Immun. 63 (1995) 271–279.

[293] M.D. Schreiber, R.F. Covert, L.J. Torgerson, Hemodynamic effects of heat-killed group B beta-hemolytic streptococcus in newborn lambs: role of leukotriene D4, Pediatr. Res. 31 (1992) 121–126.

[294] J.M. Pinheiro, B.R. Pitt, C.N. Gillis, Roles of platelet-activating factor and thromboxane in group B *Streptococcus*-induced pulmonary hypertension in piglets, Pediatr. Res. 26 (1989) 420–424.

[295] G. Mancuso, et al., Role of interleukin 12 in experimental neonatal sepsis caused by group B streptococci, Infect. Immun. 65 (1997) 3731–3735.

[296] C.A. Dinarello, The role of interleukin-1 in host responses to infectious diseases, Infect. Agents. Dis. 1 (1992) 227–236.

[297] J.D. Vallette, et al., Effect of an interleukin-1 receptor antagonist on the hemodynamic manifestations of group B streptococcal sepsis, Pediatr. Res. 38 (1995) 704–708.

[298] P.A. Williams, et al., Production of tumor necrosis factor by human cells in vitro and in vivo, induced by group B streptococci, J. Pediatr. 123 (1993) 292–300.

[299] R.L. Gibson, et al., Group B streptococcus induces tumor necrosis factor in neonatal piglets: effect of the tumor necrosis factor inhibitor pentoxifylline on hemodynamics and gas exchange, Am. Rev. Respir. Dis. 143 (1991) 598–604.

[300] G. Teti, et al., Production of tumor necrosis factor-alpha and interleukin-6 in mice infected with group B streptococci, Circ. Shock. 38 (1992) 138–144.

[301] G. Teti, G. Mancuso, F. Tomasello, Cytokine appearance and effects of anti-tumor necrosis factor alpha antibodies in a neonatal rat model of group B streptococcal infection, Infect. Immun. 61 (1993) 227–235.

[302] C. von Hunolstein, et al., Soluble antigens from group B streptococci induce cytokine production in human blood cultures, Infect. Immun. 65 (1997) 4017–4021.

[303] A.E. Medvedev, et al., Involvement of CD14 and complement receptors CR3 and CR4 in nuclear factor-kappa B activation and TNF production induced by lipopolysaccharide and group B streptococcal cell walls, J. Immunol. 160 (1998) 4535–4542.

[304] J.G. Vallejo, C.J. Baker, M.S. Edwards, Roles of the bacterial cell wall and capsule in induction of tumor necrosis factor alpha by type III group B streptococci, Infect. Immun. 64 (1996) 5042–5046.

[305] P. Henneke, et al., Cellular activation, phagocytosis, and bactericidal activity against group B streptococcus involve parallel myeloid differentiation factor 88-dependent and independent signaling pathways, J. Immunol. 169 (2002) 3970–3977.

[306] P. Henneke, et al., Novel engagement of CD14 and multiple Toll-like receptors by group B streptococci, J. Immunol. 167 (2001) 7069–7076.

[307] S. Kenzel, et al., c-Jun kinase is a critical signaling molecule in a neonatal model of group B streptococcal sepsis, J. Immunol. 176 (2006) 3181–3188.

[308] V.D. Raykova, et al., Nitric oxide-dependent regulation of pro-inflammatory cytokines in group B streptococcal inflammation of rat lung, Ann. Clin. Lab. Sci. 33 (2003) 62–67.

[309] C.G. Maloney, et al., Induction of cyclooxygenase-2 by human monocytes exposed to group B streptococci, J. Leukoc. Biol. 67 (2000) 615–621.

[310] G. Natarajan, et al., Nitric oxide and prostaglandin response to group B streptococcal infection in the lung, Ann. Clin. Lab. Sci. 37 (2007) 170–176.

[311] A. Ring, et al., Group B streptococcal beta-hemolysin induces nitric oxide production in murine macrophages, J. Infect. Dis. 182 (2000) 150–157.

[312] M. Puliti, et al., Severity of group B streptococcal arthritis is correlated with beta-hemolysin expression, J. Infect. Dis. 182 (2000) 824–832.

[313] A. Ring, et al., Synergistic action of nitric oxide release from murine macrophages caused by group B streptococcal cell wall and beta-hemolysin/cytolysin, J. Infect. Dis. 186 (2002) 1518–1521.

[314] B.B. Griffiths, H. Rhee, Effects of haemolysins of groups A and B streptococci on cardiovascular system, Microbios 69 (1992) 17–27.

[315] M.E. Hensler, S. Miyamoto, V. Nizet, Group B streptococcal beta-hemolysin/cytolysin directly impairs cardiomyocyte viability and function, PLoS One 3 (2008) e2446.

[316] P.H. Berman, B.Q. Banker, Neonatal meningitis: a clinical and pathological study of 29 cases, Pediatrics 38 (1966) 6–24.

[317] P. Ferrieri, B. Burke, J. Nelson, Production of bacteremia and meningitis in infant rats with group B streptococcal serotypes, Infect. Immun. 27 (1980) 1023–1032.

[318] V. Nizet, et al., Invasion of brain microvascular endothelial cells by group B streptococci, Infect. Immun. 65 (1997) 5074–5081.

[319] K.S. Doran, et al., Blood-brain barrier invasion by group B *Streptococcus* depends upon proper cell-surface anchoring of lipoteichoic acid, J. Clin. Invest. 115 (2005) 2499–2507.

[320] T. Tenenbaum, et al., Adherence to and invasion of human brain microvascular endothelial cells are promoted by fibrinogen-binding protein FbsA of *Streptococcus agalactiae*, Infect. Immun. 73 (2005) 4404–4409.

[321] N.M. van Sorge, et al., The group B streptococcal serine-rich repeat 1 glycoprotein mediates penetration of the blood-brain barrier, J. Infect. Dis. 199 (2009) 1479–1487.

[322] Y.S. Kim, et al., Brain injury in experimental neonatal meningitis due to group B streptococci, J. Neuropathol. Exp. Neurol. 54 (1995) 531–539.

[323] M. Wahl, et al., Mediators of blood-brain barrier dysfunction and formation of vasogenic brain edema, J. Cereb. Blood. Flow. Metab. 8 (1988) 621–634.

[324] A.A. McKnight, et al., Oxygen free radicals and the cerebral arteriolar response to group B streptococci, Pediatr. Res. 31 (1992) 640–644.

[325] I. Bogdan, et al., Tumor necrosis factor-alpha contributes to apoptosis in hippocampal neurons during experimental group B streptococcal meningitis, J. Infect. Dis. 176 (1997) 693–697.

[326] K.S. Kim, C.A. Wass, A.S. Cross, Blood-brain barrier permeability during the development of experimental bacterial meningitis in the rat, Exp. Neurol. 145 (1997) 253–257.

[327] E.W. Ling, et al., Biochemical mediators of meningeal inflammatory response to group B streptococcus in the newborn piglet model, Pediatr. Res. 38 (1995) 981–987.

[328] S. Lehnardt, et al., A mechanism for neurodegeneration induced by group B streptococci through activation of the TLR2/MyD88 pathway in microglia, J. Immunol. 177 (2006) 583–592.

[329] S. Lehnardt, et al., TLR2 and caspase-8 are essential for group B *Streptococcus*-induced apoptosis in microglia, J. Immunol. 179 (2007) 6134–6143.

[330] A. Schuchat, et al., Multistate case-control study of maternal risk factors for neonatal group B streptococcal disease, Pediatr. Infect. Dis. J. 13 (1994) 623–629.

[331] H.C. Dillon Jr., S. Khare, B.M. Gray, Group B streptococcal carriage and disease: a 6-year prospective study, J. Pediatr. 110 (1987) 31–36.

[332] M.A. Pass, S. Khare, H.C. Dillon, Twin pregnancies: incidence of group B streptococcal colonization and disease, J. Pediatr. 97 (1980) 635–637.

[333] M.S. Edwards, C.V. Jackson, C.J. Baker, Increased risk of group B streptococcal disease in twins, JAMA 245 (1981) 2044–2046.

[334] S. Faro, Group B beta-hemolytic streptococci and puerperal infections, Am. J. Obstet. Gynecol. 139 (1981) 686–689.

[335] A. Schuchat, Group B *Streptococcus*, Lancet 353 (1999) 51–56.

[336] J.A. Regan, et al., Colonization with group B streptococci in pregnancy and adverse outcome, Am. J. Obstet. Gynecol. 174 (1996) 1354–1360.

[337] P.G. Seaward, et al., International multicenter term PROM study: evaluation of predictors of neonatal infection in infants born to patients with premature rupture of membranes at term, Am. J. Obstet. Gynecol. 179 (1998) 635–639.

[338] M.K. Yancey, et al., Peripartum infection associated with vaginal group B streptococcal colonization, Obstet. Gynecol. 84 (1994) 816–819.

[339] R.C. Lancefield, M. McCarty, W.N. Everly, Multiple mouse-protective antibodies directed against group B streptococci, J. Exp. Med. 142 (1975) 165–179.

[340] C.J. Baker, D.L. Kasper, Correlation of maternal antibody deficiency with susceptibility to neonatal group B streptococcal infection, N. Engl. J. Med. 294 (1976) 753–756.

[341] C.J. Baker, M.S. Edwards, D.L. Kasper, Role of antibody to native type III polysaccharide of group B *Streptococcus* in infant infection, Pediatrics 68 (1981) 544–549.

[342] H.K. Guttormsen, et al., Quantitative determination of antibodies to type III group B streptococcal polysaccharide, J. Infect. Dis. 173 (1996) 142–150.

[343] S. Berg, et al., Antibodies to group B streptococci in neonates and infants, Eur. J. Pediatr. 157 (1998) 221–224.

[344] B.M. Gray, D.G. Pritchard, H.C. Dillon Jr., Seroepidemiological studies of group B *Streptococcus* type II, J. Infect. Dis. 151 (1985) 1073–1080.

[345] S.P. Gotoff, et al., Quantitation of IgG antibody to the type-specific polysaccharide of group B *Streptococcus* type 1b in pregnant women and infected infants, J. Pediatr. 105 (1984) 628–630.

[346] C.K. Papierniak, et al., An enzyme-linked immunosorbent assay (ELISA) for human IgG antibody to the type Ia polysaccharide of group B *Streptococcus*, J. Lab. Clin. Med. 100 (1982) 385–398.

[347] K.M. Boyer, et al., Transplacental passage of IgG antibody to group B *Streptococcus* serotype Ia, J. Pediatr. 104 (1984) 618–620.

[348] M.E. Klegerman, et al., Estimation of the protective level of human IgG antibody to the type-specific polysaccharide of group B *Streptococcus* type Ia, J. Infect. Dis. 148 (1983) 648–655.

[349] K.M. Boyer, et al., Protective levels of human immunoglobulin G antibody to group B streptococcus type Ib, Infect. Immun. 45 (1984) 618–624.

[350] S.P. Gotoff, et al., Human IgG antibody to group B *Streptococcus* type III: comparison of protective levels in a murine model with levels in infected human neonates, J. Infect. Dis. 153 (1986) 511–519.

[351] C.J. Baker, et al., Quantity of maternal antibody at delivery that protects neonates from group B streptococcal disease, Unpublished paper. (2004).

[352] F.Y. Lin, et al., Level of maternal IgG anti-group B streptococcus type III antibody correlated with protection of neonates against early-onset disease caused by this pathogen, J. Infect. Dis. 190 (2004) 928–934.

[353] F.Y. Lin, et al., Level of maternal antibody required to protect neonates against early-onset disease caused by group B *Streptococcus* type Ia: a multicenter, seroepidemiology study, J. Infect. Dis. 184 (2001) 1022–1028.

[354] B.F. Anthony, N.F. Concepcion, K.F. Concepcion, Human antibody to the group-specific polysaccharide of group B *Streptococcus*, J. Infect. Dis. 151 (1985) 221–226.

[355] V.G. Hemming, et al., Assessment of group B streptococcal opsonins in human and rabbit serum by neutrophil chemiluminescence, J. Clin. Invest. 58 (1976) 1379–1387.

[356] C.J. Baker, et al., Quantitative determination of antibody to capsular polysaccharide in infection with type III strains of group B *Streptococcus*, J. Clin. Invest. 59 (1977) 810–818.

[357] L.C. Vogel, et al., Human immunity to group B streptococci measured by indirect immunofluorescence: correlation with protection in chick embryos, J. Infect. Dis. 140 (1979) 682–689.

[358] C.J. Baker, et al., Influence of preimmunization antibody level on the specificity of the immune response to related polysaccharide antigens, N. Engl. J. Med. 303 (1980) 173–178.

[359] C.J. Baker, M.S. Edwards, D.L. Kasper, Immunogenicity of polysaccharides from type III group B *Streptococcus*, J. Clin. Invest. 61 (1978) 1107–1110.

[360] K. Hordnes, et al., Cervical secretions in pregnant women colonized rectally with group B streptococci have high levels of antibodies to serotype III polysaccharide capsular antigen and protein R, Scand. J. Immunol. 47 (1998) 179–188.

[361] K. Hordnes, et al., Colonization in the rectum and uterine cervix with group B streptococci may induce specific antibody responses in cervical secretions of pregnant women, Infect. Immun. 64 (1996) 1643–1652.

[362] H.R. Hill, et al., Neonatal cellular and humoral immunity to group B streptococci, Pediatrics S64 (1979) 787–794.

[363] B.J. De Cueninck, et al., Quantitation of in vitro opsonic activity of human antibody induced by a vaccine consisting of the type III-specific polysaccharide of group B streptococcus, Infect. Immun. 39 (1983) 1155–1160.

[364] S.H. Pincus, et al., Protective efficacy of IgM monoclonal antibodies in experimental group B streptococcal infection is a function of antibody avidity, J. Immunol. 140 (1988) 2779–2785.

[365] L.B. Givner, C.J. Baker, M.S. Edwards, Type III group B *Streptococcus*: functional interaction with IgG subclass antibodies, J. Infect. Dis. 155 (1987) 532–539.

[366] J.S. Kim, et al., A human IgG 3 is opsonic in vitro against type III group B streptococci, J. Clin. Immunol. 10 (1990) 154–159.

[367] B.F. Anthony, N.F. Concepcion, Opsonic activity of human IgG and IgM antibody for type III group B streptococci, Pediatr. Res. 26 (1989) 383–387.

[368] J.R. Campbell, et al., Functional activity of class-specific antibodies to type III, group B *Streptococcus*, Pediatr. Res. 23 (1988) 31–34.

[369] J.F. Bohnsack, et al., An IgA monoclonal antibody directed against type III antigen on group B streptococci acts as an opsonin, J. Immunol. 143 (1989) 3338–3342.

[370] J.R. Campbell, C.J. Baker, M.S. Edwards, Deposition and degradation of C3 on type III group B streptococci, Infect. Immun. 59 (1991) 1978–1983.

[371] M.S. Edwards, et al., Patterns of immune response among survivors of group B streptococcal meningitis, J. Infect. Dis. 161 (1990) 65–70.

[372] C.J. Baker, et al., Antibody-independent classical pathway-mediated opsonophagocytosis of type Ia, group B *Streptococcus*, J. Clin. Invest. 69 (1982) 394–404.

[373] N.J. Levy, D.L. Kasper, Surface-bound capsular polysaccharide of type Ia group B *Streptococcus* mediates C1 binding and activation of the classic complement pathway, J. Immunol. 136 (1986) 4157–4162.

[374] N.J. Levy, D.L. Kasper, Antibody-independent and -dependent opsonization of group B *Streptococcus* requires the first component of complement C1, Infect. Immun. 49 (1985) 19–24.

[375] C.L. Smith, A.H. Smith, Strain variability of type Ib group B streptococci: unique strains are resistant to C3 deposition by the alternate complement pathway, Clin. Res. 40 (1992) 823A.

[376] M.A. Hall, M.S. Edwards, C.J. Baker, Complement and antibody participation in opsonophagocytosis of type IV and V group B streptococci, Infect. Immun. 60 (1992) 5030–5035.

[377] M.A. Hall, et al., Complement and antibody in neutrophil-mediated killing of type V group B *Streptococcus*, J. Infect. Dis. 170 (1994) 88–93.

[378] M.S. Cairo, et al., Role of circulating complement and polymorphonuclear leukocyte transfusion in treatment and outcome in critically ill neonates with sepsis, J. Pediatr. 110 (1987) 935–941.

[379] O. Levy, et al., Critical role of the complement system in group B *Streptococcus*-induced tumor necrosis factor alpha release, Infect. Immun. 71 (2003) 6344–6353.

[380] O. Pozdnyakova, et al., Impaired antibody response to group B streptococcal type III capsular polysaccharide in C3- and complement receptor 2-deficient mice, J. Immunol. 170 (2003) 84–90.

[381] T. Areschoug, et al., Streptococcal beta protein has separate binding sites for human factor H and IgA-Fc, J. Biol. Chem. 277 (2002) 12642–12648.

[382] C.L. Smith, et al., Role of complement receptors in opsonophagocytosis of group B streptococci by adult and neonatal neutrophils, J. Infect. Dis. 162 (1990) 489–495.

[383] J.M. Antal, J.V. Cunningham, K.J. Goodrum, Opsonin-independent phagocytosis of group B streptococci: role of complement receptor type three, Infect. Immun. 60 (1992) 1114–1121.

[384] K.D. Yang, et al., Mechanisms of bacterial opsonization by immune globulin intravenous: correlation of complement consumption with opsonic activity and protective efficacy, J. Infect. Dis. 159 (1989) 701–707.

[385] F.J.D. Noya, C.J. Baker, M.S. Edwards, Neutrophil Fc receptor participation in phagocytosis of type III group B streptococci, Infect. Immun. 61 (1993) 1415–1420.

[386] G.J. Noel, S.L. Katz, P.J. Edelson, The role of C3 in mediating binding and ingestion of group B *Streptococcus* serotype III by murine macrophages, Pediatr. Res. 30 (1991) 118–123.

[387] R.D. Christensen, et al., The effect of hybridoma antibody administration upon neutrophil kinetics during experimental type III group B streptococcal sepsis, Pediatr. Res. 17 (1983) 795–799.

[388] R.D. Christensen, et al., Treatment of experimental group B streptococcal infection with hybridoma antibody, Pediatr. Res. 18 (1984) 1093–1096.

[389] T.E. Harper, et al., Effect of intravenous immunoglobulin G on neutrophil kinetics during experimental group B streptococcal infection in neonatal rats, Rev. Infect. Dis. 8 (1986) S401–S408.

[390] G.W. Fischer, et al., Functional antibacterial activity of a human intravenous immunoglobulin preparation: in vitro and in vivo studies, Vox. Sang. 44 (1983) 296–299.

[391] L.B. Givner, et al., Immune globulin for intravenous use: enhancement of in vitro opsonophagocytic activity of neonatal serum, J. Infect. Dis. 151 (1985) 217–220.

[392] A.O. Shigeoka, et al., Reticuloendothelial clearance of type III group B streptococci opsonized with type III specific monoclonal antibodies of IgM or IgG2a isotypes in an experimental rat model, Pediatr. Res. 21 (1987) 334A.

[393] B. Poutrel, J. Dore, Virulence of human and bovine isolates of group B streptococci (types Ia and III) in experimental pregnant mouse models, Infect. Immun. 47 (1985) 94–97.

[394] M.P. Sherman, R.I. Lehrer, Oxidative metabolism of neonatal and adult rabbit lung macrophages stimulated with opsonized group B streptococci, Infect. Immun. 47 (1985) 26–30.

[395] T.R. Martin, C.E. Rubens, C.B. Wilson, Lung antibacterial defense mechanisms in infant and adult rats: implications for the pathogenesis of group B streptococcal infections in the neonatal lung, J. Infect. Dis. 157 (1988) 91–100.

[396] S.L. Hall, M.P. Sherman, Intrapulmonary bacterial clearance of type III group B *Streptococcus* is reduced in preterm compared with term rabbits and occurs independent of antibody, Am. Rev. Respir. Dis. 145 (1992) 1172–1177.

[397] M. Domula, et al., Plasma fibronectin concentrations in healthy and septic infants, Eur. J. Pediatr. 144 (1985) 49–52.

[398] K.M. Butler, C.J. Baker, M.S. Edwards, Interaction of soluble fibronectin with group B streptococci, Infect. Immun. 55 (1987) 2404–2408.

[399] H.R. Hill, et al., Fibronectin enhances the opsonic and protective activity of monoclonal and polyclonal antibody against group B streptococci, J. Exp. Med. 159 (1984) 1618–1628.

[400] R.F. Jacobs, et al., Phagocytosis of type III group B streptococci by neonatal monocytes: enhancement by fibronectin and gammaglobulin, J. Infect. Dis. 152 (1985) 695–700.

[401] K.D. Yang, et al., Effect of fibronectin on IgA-mediated uptake of type III group B streptococci by phagocytes, J. Infect. Dis. 161 (1990) 236–241.

[402] E.B. Peat, et al., Effects of fibronectin and group B streptococci on tumour necrosis factor-alpha production by human culture-derived macrophages, Immunology 84 (1995) 440–445.

[403] E.A. Albanyan, M.S. Edwards, Lectin site interaction with capsular polysaccharide mediates nonimmune phagocytosis of type III group B streptococci, Infect. Immun. 68 (2000) 5794–5802.

[404] R. Grubb, et al., Association between maternal Gm allotype and neonatal septicaemia with group B streptococci, J. Immunogenet. 9 (1982) 143–147.

[405] H. Thom, D.L. Lloyd, T.M.S. Reid, Maternal immunoglobulin allotype (Gm and Km) and neonatal group B streptococcal infection, J. Immunogenet. 13 (1986) 309–314.

[406] V.A. Oxelius, et al., Deficiency of IgG subclasses in mothers of infants with group B streptococcal septicemia, Int. Arch. Allergy. Appl. Immunol. 72 (1983) 249–252.

[407] K. Rundgren, K.K. Christensen, P. Christensen, Increased frequency of high serum IgM among mothers of infants with neonatal group-B streptococcal septicemia, Int. Arch. Allergy. Appl. Immunol. 77 (1985) 372–373.

[408] K.K. Christensen, et al., Immune response to pneumococcal vaccine in mothers to infants with group B streptococcal septicemia: evidence for a divergent IgG/IgM ratio, Int. Arch. Allergy. Appl. Immunol. 76 (1985) 369–372.

[409] K.K. Christensen, et al., The clinical significance of group B streptococci, J. Perinatol. Med. 10 (1982) 133–146.

[410] C.J. Baker, et al., Immunization of pregnant women with a polysaccharide vaccine of group B *Streptococcus*, N. Engl. J. Med. 319 (1988) 1180–1185.

[411] D.B. Singer, P. Campognone, Perinatal group B streptococcal infection in midgestation, Pediatr. Pathol. 5 (1986) 271–276.

[412] D.J. deSa, C.L. Trevenen, Intrauterine infections with group B beta-haemolytic streptococci, Br. J. Obstet. Gynaecol. 91 (1984) 237–239.

[413] M. Hood, A. Janney, G. Dameron, Beta-hemolytic *Streptococcus* group B associated with problems of perinatal period, Am. J. Obstet. Gynecol. 82 (1961) 809–818.

[414] M. Moller, et al., Rupture of fetal membranes and premature delivery associated with group B streptococci in urine of pregnant women, Lancet 2 (1984) 69–70.

[415] R.W. Novak, M.S. Platt, Significance of placental findings in early-onset group B streptococcal neonatal sepsis, Clin. Pediatr. 24 (1985) 256–258.

[416] D.M.O. Becroft, et al., Perinatal infections by group B 4-hemolytic streptococci, Br. J. Obstet. Gynaecol. 83 (1976) 960–965.

[417] M.W. Varner, et al., Ultrastructural alterations of term human amnionic epithelium following incubation with group B beta-hemolytic streptococci, Am. J. Reprod. Immunol. Microbiol. 9 (1985) 27–32.

[418] J.L. Pinnas, R.C. Strunk, L.J. Fenton, Immunofluorescence in group B streptococcal infection and idiopathic respiratory distress syndrome, Pediatrics 63 (1979) 557–561.

[419] J.C. Leonidas, et al., Radiographic findings of early onset neonatal group B streptococcal septicemia, Pediatrics 59 (1977) S1006–S1011.

[420] R.G. Faix, S.M. Donn, Association of septic shock caused by early-onset group B streptococcal sepsis and periventricular leukomalacia in the preterm infant, Pediatrics 76 (1985) 415–419.

[421] P.F. Van Peenen, R.E. Cannon, D.J. Seibert, Group B beta-hemolytic streptococci causing fatal meningitis, Mil. Med. 130 (1965) 65–67.

[422] B.F. Anthony, D.M. Okada, The emergence of group B streptococci in infections of the newborn infant, Ann. Rev. Med. 28 (1977) 355–369.

[423] D. DiJohn, et al., Very late onset of group B streptococcal disease in infants infected with the human immunodeficiency virus, Pediatr. Infect. Dis. J. 9 (1990) 925–928.

[424] A. Schuchat, et al., Risk factors and opportunities for prevention of early-onset neonatal sepsis: a multicenter case-control study, Pediatrics 105 (2000) 21–26.

[425] B.J. Stoll, et al., Early-onset sepsis in very low birth weight neonates: a report from the National Institute of Child Health and Human Development Neonatal Research Network, J. Pediatr. 129 (1996) 72–80.

[426] K.T. Chen, et al., The role of intrapartum fever in identifying asymptomatic term neonates with early-onset neonatal sepsis, J. Perinatol. 22 (2002) 653–657.

[427] L.E. Weisman, et al., Early-onset group B streptococcal sepsis: a current assessment, J. Pediatr. 121 (1992) 428–433.

[428] C. Hammerman, et al., Prostanoids in neonates with persistent pulmonary hypertension, J. Pediatr. 110 (1987) 470–472.

[429] K.C. Chin, P.M. Fitzhardinge, Sequelae of early-onset group B streptococcal neonatal meningitis, J. Pediatr. 106 (1985) 819–822.

[430] C.J. Baker, et al., Suppurative meningitis due to streptococci of Lancefield group B: a study of 33 infants, J. Pediatr. 82 (1973) 724–729.

[431] R.H.A. Haslam, et al., The sequelae of group B 4-hemolytic streptococcal meningitis in early infancy, Am. J. Dis. Child. 131 (1977) 845–849.

[432] M.S. Edwards, et al., Long-term sequelae of group B streptococcal meningitis in infants, J. Pediatr. 106 (1985) 717–722.

[433] S.P. Pyati, et al., Decreasing mortality in neonates with early-onset group B streptococcal infection: reality or artifact? J. Pediatr. 98 (1981) 625–628.

[434] B.M. Garcia Peña, M.B. Harper, G.R. Fleisher, Occult bacteremia with group B streptococcus in an outpatient setting, Pediatrics 102 (1998) 67–72.

[435] P. Yagupsky, M.A. Menegus, K.R. Powell, The changing spectrum of group B streptococcal disease in infants: an eleven-year experience in a tertiary care hospital, Pediatr. Infect. Dis. J. 10 (1991) 801–808.

[436] J. Raymond, et al., Late-onset neonatal infections caused by group B Streptococcus associated with viral infection, Pediatr. Infect. Dis. J. 26 (2007) 963–1955.

[437] S.M. Hussain, et al., Invasive group B streptococcal disease in children beyond early infancy, Pediatr. Infect. Dis. J. 14 (1995) 278–281.

[438] C.C. De Witt, D.P. Ascher, J. Winkelstein, Group B streptococcal disease in a child beyond early infancy with a deficiency of the second component of complement (C2), Pediatr. Infect. Dis. J. 18 (1999) 77–78.

[439] M.S. Edwards, et al., An etiologic shift in infantile osteomyelitis: the emergence of the group B Streptococcus, J. Pediatr. 93 (1978) 578–583.

[440] E. Ragnhildsreit, L. Ose, Neonatal osteomyelitis caused by group B streptococci, Scand. J. Infect. Dis. 8 (1976) 219–221.

[441] G. Kexel, Occurrence of B streptococci in humans, Z. Hyg. Infektionskr. 151 (1965) 336–348.

[442] L.R. Ashdown, P.H. Hewson, S.K. Suleman, Neonatal osteomyelitis and meningitis caused by group B streptococci, Med. J. Aust. 2 (1977) 500–501.

[443] R.H. Baevsky, Neonatal group B beta-hemolytic Streptococcus osteomyelitis, Am. J. Emerg. Med. 17 (1999) 619–622.

[444] S.A. Clay, Osteomyelitis as a cause of brachial plexus neuropathy, Am. J. Dis. Child. 136 (1982) 1054–1056.

[445] L.G. Sadleir, M.B. Connolly, Acquired brachial-plexus neuropathy in the neonate: a rare presentation of late-onset group-B streptococcal osteomyelitis, Dev. Med. Child. Neurol. 40 (1998) 496–499.

[446] L.K. Ammari, et al., Unusual presentation of group B Streptococcus osteomyelitis, Pediatr. Infect. Dis. J. 11 (1992) 1066–1067.

[447] I.A. Memon, et al., Group B streptococcal osteomyelitis and septic arthritis, Am. J. Dis. Child. 133 (1979) 921–923.

[448] R.A. Broughton, et al., Unusual manifestations of neonatal group B streptococcal osteomyelitis, Pediatr. Infect. Dis. J. 1 (1982) 410–412.

[449] A.G. Weinberg, W.P. Laird, Group B streptococcal endocarditis detected by echocardiography, J. Pediatr. 92 (1978) 335–336.

[450] B.F. Anthony, N.F. Concepcion, Group B Streptococcus in a general hospital, J. Infect. Dis. 132 (1975) 561–567.

[451] J.H. Hutto, E.M. Ayoub, Streptococcal osteomyelitis and arthritis in a neonate, Am. J. Dis. Child. 129 (1975) 1449–1451.

[452] I. Obando, et al., Group B Streptococcus pelvic osteomyelitis presenting as footdrop in a newborn infant, Pediatr. Infect. Dis. J. 10 (1991) 703–705.

[453] L.L. Barton, R.G. Villar, S.A. Rice, Neonatal group B streptococcal vertebral osteomyelitis, Pediatrics 98 (1996) 459–461.

[454] T.A. McCook, A.H. Felman, E.M. Ayoub, Streptococcal skeletal infections: observations in four infants, AJR. Am. J. Roentgenol. 130 (1978) 465–467.

[455] B. Siskind, P. Galliguez, E.R. Wald, Group B beta hemolytic streptococcal osteomyelitis/purulent arthritis in neonates: report of three cases, J. Pediatr. 87 (1975) 659.

[456] R.J. Ancona, et al., Group B streptococcal sepsis with osteomyelitis and arthritis, Am. J. Dis. Child. 133 (1979) 919–920.

[457] G.H. McCracken Jr., Septic arthritis in a neonate, Hosp. Pract. 14 (1979) 158–164.

[458] S.B. Hauger, Facial cellulitis: an early indicator of group B streptococcal bacteremia, Pediatrics 67 (1981) 376–377.

[459] P. Patamasucon, J.D. Siegel, G.H. McCracken Jr., Streptococcal submandibular cellulitis in young infants, Pediatrics 67 (1981) 378–380.

[460] C.J. Baker, Group B streptococcal cellulitis/adenitis in infants, Am. J. Dis. Child. 136 (1982) 631–633.

[461] K. Fluegge, P. Greiner, R. Berner, Late onset group B streptococcal disease manifested by isolated cervical lymphadenitis, Arch. Dis. Child. 88 (2003) 1019–1020.

[462] A. Pathak, H.H. Hwu, Group B streptococcal cellulitis, South. Med. J. 78 (1985) 67–68.

[463] K.N. Haque, O. Bashir, A.M.M. Kambal, Delayed recurrence of group B streptococcal infection in a newborn infant: a case report, Ann. Trop. Paediatr. 6 (1986) 219–220.

[464] T.H. Rand, Group B streptococcal cellulitis in infants: a disease modified by prior antibiotic therapy or hospitalization? Pediatrics 81 (1988) 63–65.

[465] M.T. Brady, Cellulitis of the penis and scrotum due to group B Streptococcus, J. Urol. 137 (1987) 736–737.

[466] E.A. Albanyan, C.J. Baker, Is lumbar puncture necessary to exclude meningitis in neonates and young infants: lessons from group B Streptococcus cellulitis-adenitis syndrome, Pediatrics 102 (1998) 985–986.

[467] E.G. Chadwick, S.T. Shulman, R. Yogev, Peritonitis as a late manifestation of group B streptococcal disease in newborns, Pediatr. Infect. Dis. J. 2 (1983) 142–143.

[468] K.M. Walker, W.F. Coyer, Suprarenal abscess due to group B streptococcus, J. Pediatr. 94 (1979) 970–971.

[469] G.O. Atkinson Jr., et al., Adrenal abscess in the neonate, Radiology 155 (1985) 101–104.

[470] A. Carty, P. Stanley, Bilateral adrenal abscesses in a neonate, Pediatr. Radiol. 1 (1973) 63–64.

[471] K.J. Peevy, H.J. Wiseman, Gallbladder distension in septic neonates, Arch. Dis. Child. 57 (1982) 75–76.

[472] J.D. Siegel, K.M. Shannon, B.M. De Passe, Recurrent infection associated with penicillin-tolerant group B streptococci: a report of two cases, J. Pediatr. 99 (1981) 920–924.

[473] D.M. Sokol, G.J. Demmler, C.J. Baker, Unusual presentation of group B streptococcal ventriculitis, Pediatr. Infect. Dis. J. 9 (1990) 525–527.

[474] S.B. Coker, J.K. Muraskas, C. Thomas, Myelopathy secondary to neonatal bacterial meningitis, Pediatr. Neurol. 10 (1994) 259–261.

[475] L. Ferguson, S.P. Gotoff, Subdural empyema in an infant due to group B beta-hemolytic Streptococcus, Am. J. Dis. Child. 131 (1977) 97.

[476] E.W. McReynolds, R. Shane, Diabetes insipidus secondary to group B beta streptococcal meningitis, J. Tenn. Med. Assoc. 67 (1974) 117–120.

[477] R.D. Dorand, G. Adams, Relapse during penicillin treatment of group B streptococcal meningitis, J. Pediatr. 89 (1976) 188–190.

[478] K.S. Kim, et al., Cerebritis due to group B Streptococcus, Scand. J. Infect. Dis. 14 (1982) 305–308.

[479] C.W. Barton, et al., A neonatal survivor of group B beta-hemolytic streptococcal endocarditis, Am. J. Perinatol. 1 (1984) 214–215.

[480] H. Horigome, et al., Group B streptococcal endocarditis in infancy with a giant vegetation on the pulmonary valve, Eur. J. Pediatr. 153 (1994) 140–142.

[481] I.A. Harper, The importance of group B streptococci as human pathogens in the British Isles, J. Clin. Pathol. 24 (1971) 438–441.

[482] B.N. Agarwala, Group B streptococcal endocarditis in a neonate, Pediatr. Cardiol. 9 (1988) 51–53.

[483] P.A. Shurin, et al., Bacterial etiology of otitis media during the first six weeks of life, J. Pediatr. 92 (1978) 893–896.

[484] S. Sapir-Ellis, A. Johnson, T.L. Austin, Group B streptococcal meningitis associated with otitis media, Am. J. Dis. Child. 130 (1976) 1003–1004.

[485] T.R. Tetzlaff, C. Ashworth, J.D. Nelson, Otitis media in children less than 12 weeks of age, Pediatrics 59 (1977) 827–832.

[486] R. Ermocilla, G. Cassady, R. Ceballos, Otitis media in the pathogenesis of neonatal meningitis with group B beta-hemolytic Streptococcus, Pediatrics 54 (1974) 643–644.

[487] J.H. Armstrong, F. Zacarias, M.F. Rein, Ophthalmia neonatorum: a chart review, Pediatrics 57 (1976) 884–892.

[488] J.R. Sparks, F.M. Recchia, J.H. Weitkamp, Endogenous group B streptococcal endophthalmitis in a preterm infant, J. Perinatol. 27 (2007) 392–394.

[489] A. Lipson, et al., Group B streptococcal supraglottitis in a 3-month-old infant, Am. J. Dis. Child. 140 (1986) 411–412.

[490] J.W. Park, Bacterial tracheitis caused by Streptococcus agalactiae, Pediatr. Infect. Dis. J. 9 (1990) 450–451.

[491] M.M. Sokal, et al., Neonatal empyema caused by group B beta-hemolytic Streptococcus, Chest 81 (1982) 390–391.

[492] Y. LeBovar, P.H. Trung, P. Mozziconacci, Neonatal meningitis due to group B streptococci, Ann. Pediatr. 17 (1970) 207–213.

[493] T. Strunk, et al., Late-onset right-sided diaphragmatic hernia in neonates—case report and review of the literature, Eur. J. Pediatr. 166 (2007) 521–526.

[494] R. Nudelman, et al., Violaceous cellulitis, Pediatrics 70 (1982) 157–158.

[495] L.L. Barton, N.K. Kapoor, Recurrent group B streptococcal infection, Clin. Pediatr. 21 (1982) 100–101.

[496] R.A. Amoury, et al., Scrotal ecchymosis: sign of intraperitoneal hemorrhage in the newborn, South. Med. J. 75 (1982) 1471–1478.

[497] S.H. Isaacman, W.M. Heroman, A. Lightsey, Purpura fulminans following late-onset group B beta-hemolytic streptococcal sepsis, Am. J. Dis. Child. 138 (1984) 915–916.

[498] N.J. Lynn, T.H. Pauly, N.S. Desai, Purpura fulminans in three cases of early-onset neonatal group B streptococcal meningitis, J. Perinatol. 11 (1991) 144–146.

[499] R.S. Ramamurthy, G. Srinivasan, N.M. Jacobs, Necrotizing fasciitis and necrotizing cellulitis due to group B Streptococcus, Am. J. Dis. Child. 131 (1977) 1169–1170.

[500] G.N. Goldberg, R.C. Hansen, P.J. Lynch, Necrotizing fasciitis in infancy: report of three cases and review of the literature, Pediatr. Dermatol. 2 (1984) 55–63.

[501] M.E. Lang, W. Vaudry, J.L. Robinson, Case report and literature review of late-onset group B streptococcal disease manifesting as necrotizing fasciitis in preterm infants. Is this a new syndrome? Clin. Infect. Dis. 37 (2003) e132–e135.

[502] J.B. Lopez, P. Gross, T.R. Boggs, Skin lesions in association with β-hemolytic *Streptococcus* group B, Pediatrics 58 (1976) 859–860.

[503] T.K. Belgaumkar, Impetigo neonatorum congenita due to group B beta-hemolytic *Streptococcus* infection, J. Pediatr. 86 (1975) 982–983.

[504] M.R. Jacobs, H.J. Koornhof, H. Stein, Group B streptococcal infections in neonates and infants, S. Afr. Med. J. 54 (1978) 154–158.

[505] A.M. Feder Jr., W.C. MacLean, R. Moxon, Scalp abscess secondary to fetal scalp electrode, J. Pediatr. 89 (1976) 808–809.

[506] T.E. Wiswell, J.A. Miller, Infections of congenital cervical neck masses associated with bacteremia, J. Pediatr. Surg. 21 (1986) 173–174.

[507] F.T. Bourgeois, M.W. Shannon, Retropharyngeal cellulitis in a 5-week-old infant, Pediatrics 109 (2002) e51–e53.

[508] C.P. Kelly, D.J. Isaacman, Group B streptococcal retropharyngeal cellulitis in a young infant: a case report and review of the literature, J. Emerg. Med. 23 (2002) 179–182.

[509] J.D. Nelson, Bilateral breast abscess due to group B *Streptococcus*, Am. J. Dis. Child. 130 (1976) 567.

[510] T. St. Laurent-Gagnon, M.L. Weber, Urinary tract *Streptococcus* group B infection in a 6-week-old infant, JAMA 240 (1978) 1269.

[511] J.T. Atkins, et al., Recurrent group B streptococcal disease in infants: who should receive rifampin? J. Pediatr. 132 (1998) 537–539.

[512] P.A. Green, et al., Recurrent group B streptococcal infections in infants: clinical and microbiologic aspects, J. Pediatr. 125 (1994) 931–938.

[513] E.H. Moylett, et al., A 5-year review of recurrent group B streptococcal disease: lessons from twin infants, Clin. Infect. Dis. 30 (2000) 282–287.

[514] D.W. Denning, et al., Infant with two relapses of group B streptococcal sepsis documented by DNA restriction enzyme analysis, Pediatr. Infect. Dis. J. 7 (1988) 729–732.

[515] J.L. Simón, et al., Two relapses of group B streptococcal sepsis and transient hypogammaglobulinemia, Pediatr. Infect. Dis. J. 8 (1989) 729–730.

[516] M. Kotiw, et al., Late-onset and recurrent neonatal group B streptococcal disease associated with breast-milk transmission, Pediatr. Dev. Pathol. 6 (2003) 251–256.

[517] L.Y. Wang, et al., Recurrent neonatal group B streptococcal disease associated with infected breast milk, Clin. Pediatr. (Phila). 46 (2007) 547–549.

[518] A.M. Ramsay, M. Gillespie, Puerperal infection associated with haemolytic streptococci other than Lancefield's group A, J. Obstet. Gynaecol. Br. Emp. 48 (1941) 569–585.

[519] M.N.W. Butter, C.E. de Moor, *Streptococcus agalactiae* as a cause of meningitis in the newborn, and of bacteremia in adults, Antonie. van. Leeuwenhoek. 33 (1967) 439–450.

[520] W.J. Ledger, et al., Bacteremia on an obstetric-gynecologic service, Am. J. Obstet. Gynecol. 121 (1975) 205–212.

[521] A. Aharoni, et al., Postpartum maternal group B streptococcal meningitis, Rev. Infect. Dis. 12 (1990) 273–276.

[522] J.M. Kane, K. Jackson, J.H. Conway, Maternal postpartum group B beta-hemolytic streptococcus ventriculoperitoneal shunt infection, Arch. Gynecol. Obstet. 269 (2004) 139–141.

[523] D.J. Sexton, et al., Pregnancy-associated group B streptococcal endocarditis: a report of two fatal cases, Obstet. Gynecol. 66 (1985) 44S–47S.

[524] R.J. Backes, W.R. Wilson, J.E. Geraci, Group B streptococcal infective endocarditis, Arch. Intern. Med. 145 (1985) 693–696.

[525] B.J. Seaworth, D.T. Durack, Infective endocarditis in obstetric and gynecologic practice, Am. J. Obstet. Gynecol. 154 (1986) 180–188.

[526] C.V. Vartian, E.J. Septimus, Tricuspid valve group B streptococcal endocarditis following elective abortion, Rev. Infect. Dis. 13 (1991) 997–998.

[527] J.H. Lischke, P.H.B. McCreight, Maternal group B streptococcal vertebral osteomyelitis: an unusual complication of vaginal delivery, Obstet. Gynecol. 76 (1990) 489–491.

[528] G. Jenkin, et al., Postpartum epidural abscess due to group B Streptococcus, Clin. Infect. Dis. 25 (1997) 1249.

[529] G.P. Sutton, et al., Group B streptococcal necrotizing fasciitis arising from an episiotomy, Obstet. Gynecol. 66 (1985) 733–736.

[530] E.G. Wood, H.C. Dillon, A prospective study of group B streptococcal bacteriuria in pregnancy, Am. J. Obstet. Gynecol. 140 (1981) 515–520.

[531] R.S. Gibbs, D.J. Roberts, Case records of the Massachusetts General Hospital. Case 27-2007. A 30-year-old pregnant woman with intrauterine fetal death, N. Engl. J. Med. 357 (2007) 918–925.

[532] T.E. Wiswell, et al., No lumbar puncture in the evaluation for early neonatal sepsis. Will meningitis be missed? Pediatrics 95 (1995) 803–806.

[533] American Academy of Pediatrics Committee on Infectious Diseases and Committee on Fetus and Newborn. Revised guidelines for prevention of early-onset group B streptococcal (GBS) infection. Pediatrics 99 (1997) 489–496.

[534] G. Natarajan, et al., Real-time polymerase chain reaction for the rapid detection of group B streptococcal colonization in neonates, Pediatrics 118 (2006) 14–22.

[535] S.M. Golden, et al., Evaluation of a real-time fluorescent PCR assay for rapid detection of group B streptococci in neonatal blood, Diagn. Microbiol. Infect. Dis. 50 (2004) 7–13.

[536] A.G. Philip, P.C. Mills, Use of C-reactive protein in minimizing antibiotic exposure: experience with infants initially admitted to a well-baby nursery, Pediatrics 106 (2000) e4.

[537] J.G. Vallejo, C.J. Baker, M.S. Edwards, Interleukin-6 production by human neonatal monocytes stimulated by type III group B streptococci, J. Infect. Dis. 174 (1996) 332–337.

[538] D.N. Greenberg, B.A. Yoder, Changes in the differential white blood cell count in screening for group B streptococcal sepsis, Pediatr. Infect. Dis. J. 9 (1990) 886–889.

[539] R.D. Christensen, et al., Fatal early onset group B streptococcal sepsis with normal leukocyte counts, Pediatr. Infect. Dis. J. 4 (1985) 242–245.

[540] C.J. Baker, B.J. Webb, F.F. Barrett, Antimicrobial susceptibility of group B streptococci isolated from a variety of clinical sources, Antimicrob. Agents Chemother. 10 (1976) 128–131.

[541] M. Fernandez, M.E. Hickman, C.J. Baker, Antimicrobial susceptibilities of group B streptococci isolated between 1992 and 1996 from patients with bacteremia or meningitis, Antimicrob. Agents Chemother. 42 (1998) 1517–1519.

[542] L.A. Meyn, S.L. Hillier, Ampicillin susceptibilities of vaginal and placental isolates of group B *Streptococcus* and *Escherichia coli* obtained between 1992 and 1994, Antimicrob. Agents Chemother. 41 (1997) 1173–1174.

[543] D.J. Biedenbach, J.M. Stephen, R.N. Jones, Antimicrobial susceptibility profile among β-haemolytic *Streptococcus* spp. collected in the SENTRY Antimicrobial Surveillance Program-North America, 2001, Diag. Microbiol. Infect. Dis. 46 (2003) 291–294.

[544] S.D. Manning, et al., Correlates of antibiotic-resistant group B *Streptococcus* isolated from pregnant women, Obstet. Gynecol. 101 (2003) 74–79.

[545] K.T. Chen, et al., No increase in rates of early-onset neonatal sepsis by antibiotic-resistant group B *Streptococcus* in the era of intrapartum antibiotic prophylaxis, Am. J. Obstet. Gynecol. 192 (2005) 1167–1171.

[546] S. Dahesh, et al., Point mutation in the group B streptococcal pbp2x gene conferring decreased susceptibility to beta-lactam antibiotics, Antimicrob. Agents Chemother. 52 (2008) 2915–2918.

[547] N. Nagano, et al., Genetic heterogeneity in pbp genes among clinically isolated group B streptococci with reduced penicillin susceptibility, Antimicrob. Agents Chemother. 52 (2008) 4258–4267.

[548] K.S. Kim, Efficacy of imipenem in experimental group B streptococcal bacteremia and meningitis, Chemotherapy 31 (1985) 304–309.

[549] K.S. Kim, Antimicrobial susceptibility of GBS, Antibiot. Chemother. 35 (1985) 83–89.

[550] K.S. Persson, A. Forsgren, Antimicrobial susceptibility of group B streptococci, Eur. J. Clin. Microbiol. 5 (1986) 165–167.

[551] M.C. Liberto, et al., Cefixime shows good effects on group A and group B beta-hemolytic streptococci, Drugs. Exp. Clin. Res. 17 (1991) 305–308.

[552] M. Sheppard, A. King, I. Phillips, In vitro activity of cefpodoxime, a new oral cephalosporin, compared with that of nine other antimicrobial agents, Eur. J. Clin. Microbiol. Infect. Dis. 10 (1991) 573–581.

[553] K.S. Kim, Effect of antimicrobial therapy for experimental infections due to group B *Streptococcus* on mortality and clearance of bacteria, J. Infect. Dis. 155 (1987) 1233–1241.

[554] S.D. Manning, et al., Frequency of antibiotic resistance among group B *Streptococcus* isolated from healthy college students, Clin. Infect. Dis. 33 (2001) e137–e139.

[555] W. Wehbeh, et al., Fluoroquinolone-resistant *Streptococcus agalactiae*: epidemiology and mechanism of resistance, Antimicrob. Agents Chemother. 49 (2005) 2495–2497.

[556] J.C.S. de Azavedo, et al., Prevalence and mechanisms of macrolide resistance in invasive and noninvasive group B *Streptococcus* isolates from Ontario, Canada, Antimicrob. Agents Chemother. 45 (2001) 3504–3508.

[557] S.M. Borchardt, et al., Frequency of antimicrobial resistance among invasive and colonizing group B streptococcal isolates, BMC. Infect. Dis. 6 (2006) 57.

[558] F. Fitoussi, et al., Mechanisms of macrolide resistance in clinical group B streptococci isolated in France, Antimicrob. Agents Chemother. 45 (2001) 1889–1891.

[559] C. Betriu, et al., Erythromycin and clindamycin resistance and telithromycin susceptibility in *Streptococcus agalactiae*, Antimicrob. Agents Chemother. 47 (2003) 1112–1114.

[560] Z.C. Acikgoz, et al., Macrolide resistance determinants of invasive and noninvasive group B streptococci in a Turkish hospital, Antimicrob. Agents Chemother. 48 (2004) 1410–1412.

[561] P.R. Hsueh, et al., High incidence of erythromycin resistance among clinical isolates of *Streptococcus agalactiae* in Taiwan, Antimicrob. Agents Chemother. 45 (2001) 3205–3208.

[562] J.M. Marimón, et al., Erythromycin resistance and genetic elements carrying macrolide efflux genes in *Streptococcus agalactiae*, Antimicrob. Agents Chemother. 49 (2005) 5069–5074.

[563] J.S. Heelan, M.E. Hasenbein, A.J. McAdam, Resistance of group B *Streptococcus* to selected antibiotics, including erythromycin and clindamycin, J. Clin. Microbiol. 42 (2004) 1263–1264.

[564] L.P. DiPersio, J.R. DiPersio, Identification of an *erm*(T) gene in strains of inducibly clindamycin-resistant group B *Streptococcus*, Diagn. Microbiol. Infect. Dis. 57 (2007) 189–193.

[565] K.M. Puopolo, et al., A composite transposon associated with erythromycin and clindamycin resistance in group B *Streptococcus*, J. Med. Microbiol. 56 (2007) 947–955.

[566] F.Y. Lin, et al., Antibiotic susceptibility profiles for group B streptococci isolated from neonates, 1995–1998, Clin. Infect. Dis. 31 (2000) 76–79.

[567] C. Betriu, et al., In vitro activities of tigecycline against erythromycin-resistant *Streptococcus pyogenes* and *Streptococcus agalactiae*: mechanisms of macrolide and tetracycline resistance, Antimicrob. Agents Chemother. 48 (2004) 323–325.

[568] E. Bingen, et al., Telithromycin susceptibility and genomic diversity of macrolide-resistant serotype III group B streptococci isolated in perinatal infections, Antimicrob. Agents Chemother. 48 (2004) 677–680.

[569] H.M. Swingle, R.L. Bucciarelli, E.M. Ayoub, Synergy between penicillins and low concentrations of gentamicin in the killing of group B streptococci, J. Infect. Dis. 152 (1985) 515–520.

[570] M. Maduri-Traczewski, E.G. Szymczak, D.A. Goldmann, In vitro activity of penicillin and rifampin against group B streptococci, Rev. Infect. Dis. 5 (1983) S586–S592.

[571] M.A. Hall, et al., A randomized prospective comparison of cefotaxime versus netilmicin/penicillin for treatment of suspected neonatal sepsis, Drugs 35 (1988) 169–188.

[572] J.S. Bradley, et al., Once-daily ceftriaxone to complete therapy of uncomplicated group B streptococcal infection in neonates, Clin. Pediatr. 31 (1992) 274–278.

[573] V. Schauf, et al., Antibiotic-killing kinetics of group B streptococci, J. Pediatr. 89 (1976) 194–198.

[574] W.E. Feldman, Concentrations of bacteria in cerebrospinal fluid of patients with bacterial meningitis, J. Pediatr. 88 (1976) 549–552.

[575] K.S. Kim, B.F. Anthony, Penicillin tolerance in group B streptococci isolated from infected neonates, J. Infect. Dis. 144 (1981) 411–419.

[576] K.S. Kim, Clinical perspectives on penicillin tolerance, J. Pediatr. 112 (1988) 509–514.

[577] C.J. Baker, Antibiotic susceptibility testing in the management of an infant with group B streptococcal meningitis, Pediatr. Infect. Dis. J. 6 (1987) 1073–1074.

[578] J.M. Poschl, et al., Six day antimicrobial therapy for early-onset group B streptococcal infection in near-term and term neonates, Scand. J. Infect. Dis. 35 (2003) 302–305.

[579] A. Paredes, P. Wong, M.D. Yow, Failure of penicillin to eradicate the carrier state of group B *Streptococcus* in infants, J. Pediatr. 89 (1976) 191–193.

[580] M. Fernandez, et al., Failure of rifampin to eradicate group B streptococcal colonization in infants, Pediatr. Infect. Dis. J. 20 (2001) 371–376.

[581] J.R. Hocker, et al., Extracorporeal membrane oxygenation and early-onset group B streptococcal sepsis, Pediatrics 89 (1992) 1–4.

[582] M.H. LeBlanc, ECMO and sepsis, Pediatrics 90 (1992) 127.

[583] R.D. Christensen, et al., Granulocyte transfusions in neonates with bacterial infection, neutropenia, and depletion of mature marrow neutrophils, Pediatrics 70 (1982) 1–6.

[584] M.S. Cairo, et al., Prophylactic or simultaneous administration of recombinant human granulocyte colony stimulating factor in the treatment of group B streptococcal sepsis in neonatal rats, Pediatr. Res. 27 (1990) 612–616.

[585] M.S. Cairo, et al., Effect of stem cell factor with and without granulocyte colony-stimulating factor on neonatal hematopoiesis: in vivo induction of newborn myelopoiesis and reduction of mortality during experimental group B streptococcal sepsis, Blood 80 (1992) 96–101.

[586] K. Iguchi, S. Inoue, A. Kumar, Effect of recombinant human granulocyte colony-stimulating factor administration in normal and experimentally infected newborn rats, Exp. Hematol. 19 (1991) 352–358.

[587] H.R. Hill, et al., Intravenous IgG in combination with other modalities in the treatment of neonatal infection, Pediatr. Infect. Dis. J. 5 (1986) S180–S184.

[588] L.B. Givner, Human immunoglobulins for intravenous use: comparison of available preparations for group B streptococcal antibody levels, opsonic activity, and efficacy in animal models, Pediatrics 86 (1990) 955–962.

[589] K.S. Kim, Efficacy of human immunoglobulin and penicillin G in treatment of experimental group B streptococcal infection, Pediatr. Res. 21 (1987) 289–292.

[590] L.B. Givner, C.J. Baker, Pooled human IgG hyperimmune for type III group B streptococci: evaluation against multiple strains in vitro and in experimental disease, J. Infect. Dis. 163 (1991) 1141–1145.

[591] G.W. Fischer, et al., Polyvalent group B streptococcal immune globulin for intravenous administration: overview, Rev. Infect. Dis. 12 (1990) S483–S491.

[592] K.S. Kim, High-dose intravenous immune globulin impairs antibacterial activity of antibiotics, J. Allergy. Clin. Immunol. 84 (1989) 579–588.

[593] C.J. Baker, F.J.D. Noya, Potential use of intravenous immune globulin for group B streptococcal infection, Rev. Infect. Dis. 12 (1990) S476–S482.

[594] H. Redd, R.D. Christensen, G.W. Fischer, Circulating and storage neutrophils in septic neonatal rats treated with immune globulin, J. Infect. Dis. 157 (1988) 705–712.

[595] K.K. Christensen, P. Christensen, Intravenous gamma-globulin in the treatment of neonatal sepsis with special reference to group B streptococci and pharmacokinetics, Pediatr. Infect. Dis. J. 5 (1986) S189–S192.

[596] K.K. Christensen, et al., Intravenous administration of human IgG to newborn infants: changes in serum antibody levels to group B streptococci, Eur. J. Pediatr. 143 (1984) 123–127.

[597] R. van Furth, P.C.J. Leijh, F. Klein, Correlation between opsonic activity for various microorganisms and composition of gammaglobulin preparations for intravenous use, J. Infect. Dis. 149 (1984) 511–517.

[598] K.S. Kim, et al., Functional activities of various preparations of human intravenous immunoglobulin against type III group B *Streptococcus*, J. Infect. Dis. 153 (1986) 1092–1097.

[599] H. Gloser, H. Bachmayer, A. Helm, Intravenous immunoglobulin with high activity against group B streptococci, Pediatr. Infect. Dis. J. 5 (1986) S176–S179.

[600] V. Linden, K.K. Christensen, P. Christensen, Low levels of antibodies to surface antigens of group B streptococci in commercial IgG preparation, Int. Arch. Allergy. Appl. Immunol. 68 (1982) 193–195.

[601] G.W. Fischer, et al., Intravenous immunoglobulin in the treatment of neonatal sepsis: therapeutic strategies and laboratory studies, Pediatr. Infect. Dis. J. 5 (1986) S171–S175.

[602] F.J.D. Noya, et al., Disposition of an immunoglobulin intravenous preparation in very low birth weight neonates, J. Pediatr. 112 (1988) 278–283.

[603] R.D. Christensen, et al., Effect on neutrophil kinetics and serum opsonic capacity of intravenous administration of immune globulin to neonates with clinical signs of early-onset sepsis, J. Pediatr. 118 (1991) 606–614.

[604] H.V. Raff, et al., Human monoclonal antibodies to group B *Streptococcus*: reactivity and in vivo protection against multiple serotypes, J. Exp. Med. 168 (1988) 905–917.

[605] H.V. Raff, et al., Pharmacokinetic and pharmacodynamic analysis of a human immunoglobulin M monoclonal antibody in neonatal *Macaca fascicularis*, Pediatr. Res. 29 (1991) 310–314.

[606] H.R. Hill, et al., Comparative protective activity of human monoclonal and hyperimmune polyclonal antibody against group B streptococci, J. Infect. Dis. 163 (1991) 792–798.

[607] B. Lannering, et al., Early onset group B streptococcal disease: seven year experience and clinical scoring system, Acta Paediatr. Scand. 72 (1983) 597–602.

[608] K. Fluegge, et al., Incidence and clinical presentation of invasive neonatal group B streptococcal infections in Germany, Pediatrics 117 (2006) e1139–e1145.

[609] J. de Louvois, S. Halket, D. Harvey, Neonatal meningitis in England and Wales: sequelae at 5 years of age, Eur. J. Pediatr. 164 (2005) 730–734.

[610] B.J. Stoll, et al., Neurodevelopmental and growth impairment among extremely low-birth-weight infants with neonatal infection, JAMA 292 (2004) 2357–2365.

[611] E.R. Wald, et al., Long-term outcome of group B streptococcal meningitis, Pediatrics 77 (1986) 217–221.

[612] Centers for Disease Control and Prevention, Prevention of perinatal group B streptococcal disease: revised guidelines from CDC, MMWR Morb. Mortal. Wkly. Rep. 51 (2002) 1–22.

[613] C.J. Baker, Immunization to prevent group B streptococcal disease: victories and vexations, J. Infect. Dis. 161 (1990) 917–921.

[614] S.E. Gardner, et al., Failure of penicillin to eradicate group B streptococcal colonization in the pregnant woman, Am. J. Obstet. Gynecol. 135 (1979) 1062–1065.

[615] J.S. Gordon, A.J. Sbara, Incidence, technique of isolation, and treatment of group B streptococci in obstetric patients, Am. J. Obstet. Gynecol. 126 (1976) 1023–1026.

[616] R.T. Hall, et al., Antibiotic treatment of parturient women colonized with group B streptococci, Am. J. Obstet. Gynecol. 124 (1976) 630–634.

[617] E.B. Lewin, M.S. Amstey, Natural history of group B *Streptococcus* colonization and its therapy during pregnancy, Am. J. Obstet. Gynecol. 139 (1981) 512–515.

[618] M.D. Yow, et al., Ampicillin prevents intrapartum transmission of group B *Streptococcus*, JAMA 241 (1979) 1245–1247.

[619] K.M. Boyer, et al., Selective intrapartum chemoprophylaxis of neonatal group B streptococcal early-onset disease. III. Interruption of mother-to-infant transmission, J. Infect. Dis. 148 (1983) 810–816.

[620] K.M. Boyer, S.P. Gotoff, Prevention of early-onset neonatal group B streptococcal disease with selective intrapartum chemoprophylaxis, N. Engl. J. Med. 314 (1986) 1665–1669.

[621] R. Matorras, et al., Maternal colonization by group B streptococci and puerperal infection; analysis of intrapartum chemoprophylaxis, Eur. J. Obstet. Gynecol. Reprod. Biol. 38 (1990) 203–207.

[622] M.K. Yancey, P. Duff, An analysis of the cost-effectiveness of selected protocols for the prevention of neonatal group B streptococcal infection, Obstet. Gynecol. 83 (1994) 367–371.

[623] J.C. Mohle-Boetani, et al., Comparison of prevention strategies for neonatal group B streptococcal infection: an economic analysis, JAMA 270 (1993) 1442–1448.

[624] Group B streptococcal infections in pregnancy, ACOG. Tech. Bull. 170 (1992) 1–5.

[625] Committee on Infectious Diseases and Committee on Fetus and Newborn, Guidelines for prevention of group B streptococcal (GBS) infection by chemoprophylaxis., Pediatrics 90 (1992) 775–778.

[626] C.J. Baker, Inadequacy of rapid immunoassays for intrapartum detection of group B streptococcal carriers, Obstet. Gynecol. 88 (1996) 51–55.

[627] K.C. Carroll, et al., Rapid detection of group B streptococcal colonization of the genital tract by a commercial optical immunoassay, Eur. J. Clin. Microbiol. Infect. Dis. 15 (1996) 206–210.

[628] C.H. Park, et al., Rapid detection of group B streptococcal antigen from vaginal specimens using a new optical immunoassay technique, Diagn. Microbiol. Infect. Dis. 24 (1996) 125–128.

[629] D.P. Reisner, et al., Performance of a group B streptococcal prophylaxis protocol combining high-risk treatment and low-risk screening, Am. J. Obstet. Gynecol. 182 (2000) 1335–1343.

[630] J. Thinkhamrop, et al., Infections in international pregnancy study: performance of the optical immunoassay test for detection of group B *Streptococcus*, J. Clin. Microbiol. 41 (2003) 5288–5290.

[631] C. Rosa, P. Clark, P. Duff, Performance of a new DNA probe for the detection of group B streptococcal colonization of the genital tract, Obstet. Gynecol. 86 (1995) 509–511.

[632] S.M. Kircher, M.P. Meyer, J.A. Jordan, Comparison of a modified DNA hybridization assay with standard culture enrichment for detecting group B streptococci in obstetric patients, J. Clin. Microbiol. 34 (1996) 342–344.

[633] M.G. Bergeron, et al., Rapid detection of group B streptococci in pregnant women at delivery, N. Engl. J. Med. 343 (2000) 175–179.

[634] R.K. Edwards, et al., Rapid group B streptococci screening using a real-time polymerase chain reaction assay, Obstet. Gynecol. 111 (2008) 1335–1341.

[635] H.D. Davies, et al., Multicenter study of a rapid molecular-based assay for the diagnosis of group B *Streptococcus* colonization in pregnant women, Clin. Infect. Dis. 39 (2004) 1129–1135.

[636] M. Gavino, E. Wang, A comparison of a new rapid real-time polymerase chain reaction system to traditional culture in determining group B streptococcus colonization, Am. J. Obstet. Gynecol. 197 (2007) 388e1–e4.

[637] H. Honest, S. Sharma, K.S. Khan, Rapid tests for group B *Streptococcus* colonization in laboring women: a systematic review, Pediatrics 117 (2006) 1055–1066.

[638] C.A. Haberland, et al., Perinatal screening for group B streptococci: cost-benefit analysis of rapid polymerase chain reaction, Pediatrics 110 (2002) 471–480.

[639] Centers for Disease Control and Prevention, Prevention of perinatal group B streptococcal disease: a public health perspective, MMWR Morb. Mortal. Wkly. Rep. 45 (1996) 1–24.

[640] American College of Obstetricians and Gynecologists Committee on Obstetric Practice, Prevention of early-onset group B streptococcal disease in newborns, American College of Obstetricians and Gynecologists, Washington, DC, 1996.

[641] A. Schuchat, Group B streptococcal disease: from trials and tribulations to triumph and trepidation, Clin. Infect. Dis. 33 (2001) 751–756.

[642] S.J. Schrag, C.G. Whitney, A. Schuchat, Neonatal group B streptococcal disease: how infection control teams can contribute to prevention efforts, Infect. Control. Hosp. Epidemiol. 21 (2000) 473–483.

[643] Centers for Disease Control and Prevention, Hospital-based policies for prevention of perinatal group B streptococcal disease—United States, 1999, MMWR Morb. Mortal. Wkly. Rep. 49 (2000) 936–940.

[644] American Academy of Pediatrics, Group B Streptococcal Infections, American Academy of Pediatrics, Elk Grove Village, IL, 2003.

[645] ACOG Committee Opinion No. 279, December 2002, Prevention of early-onset group B streptococcal disease in newborns., Obstet. Gynecol. 100 (2002) 1405–1412.

[646] M. Pylipow, M. Gaddis, J.S. Kinney, Selective intrapartum prophylaxis for group B streptococcus colonization: management and outcome of newborns, Pediatrics 93 (1994) 631–635.

[647] A.B. Dunn, J. Blomquist, V. Khousami, Anaphylaxis in labor secondary to prophylaxis against group B streptococcus: a case report, J. Reprod. Med. 44 (1999) 381–384.

[648] K. Heim, A. Alge, C. Marth, Anaphylactic reaction to ampicillin and severe complication in the fetus, Lancet 337 (1991) 859–860.

[649] E.H. Philipson, et al., Management of group B *Streptococcus* in pregnant women with penicillin allergy, J. Reprod. Med. 52 (2007) 480–484.

[650] J. Sheikh, Intrapartum anaphylaxis to penicillin in a woman with rheumatoid arthritis who had no prior penicillin allergy, Ann. Allergy. Asthma. Immunol. 99 (2007) 287–289.

[651] N.M. Pinto, et al., Neonatal early-onset group B streptococcal disease in the era of intrapartum chemoprophylaxis: residual problems, J. Perinatol. 23 (2003) 265–271.

[652] V. Cárdenas, et al., Barriers to implementing the group B streptococcal prevention guidelines, Birth 29 (2002) 285–290.

[653] S.J. Schrag, et al., Prenatal screening for infectious diseases and opportunities for prevention, Obstet. Gynecol. 102 (2003) 753–760.

[654] K.A. Matteson, et al., Intrapartum group B streptococci prophylaxis in patients reporting a penicillin allergy, Obstet. Gynecol. 111 (2008) 356–364.

[655] K. Cowgill, et al., Report from the CDC: awareness of perinatal group B streptococcal infection among women of childbearing age in the United States, 1999 and 2002, J. Womens Health 12 (2003) 527–532.

[656] A. Schuchat, Impact of intrapartum chemoprophylaxis on neonatal sepsis, Pediatr Infect Dis J 22 (2003) 1087–1088.

[657] D. Isaacs, J.A. Royle, Australasian Study Group for Neonatal I. Intrapartum antibiotics and early onset neonatal sepsis caused by group B *Streptococcus* and by other organisms in Australia, Pediatr. Infect. Dis. J. 18 (1999) 524–528.

[658] F.Y.C. Lin, et al., The effectiveness of risk-based intrapartum chemoprophylaxis for the prevention of early-onset neonatal group B streptococcal disease, Am. J. Obstet. Gynecol. 184 (2001) 1204–1210.

[659] T.A. Joseph, S.P. Pyati, N. Jacobs, Neonatal early-onset *Escherichia coli* disease: the effect of intrapartum ampicillin, Arch. Pediatr. Adolesc. Med. 152 (1998) 35–40.

[660] S.J. Schrag, B.J. Stoll, Early-onset neonatal sepsis in the era of widespread intrapartum chemoprophylaxis, Pediatr. Infect. Dis. J. 25 (2006) 939–940.

[661] B.J. Stoll, et al., Changes in pathogens causing early-onset sepsis in very-low-birth-weight infants, N. Engl. J. Med. 347 (2002) 240–247.

[662] T.B. Hyde, et al., Trends in incidence and antimicrobial resistance of early-onset sepsis: population-based surveillance in San Francisco and Atlanta, Pediatrics 110 (2002) 690–695.

[663] D.A. Terrone, et al., Neonatal sepsis and death caused by resistant *Escherichia coli*: possible consequences of extended maternal ampicillin administration, Am. J. Obstet. Gynecol. 180 (1999) 1345–1348.

[664] R.K. Edwards, et al., Intrapartum antibiotic prophylaxis 1. Relative effects of recommended antibiotics on gram-negative pathogens, Obstet. Gynecol. 100 (2002) 534–539.

[665] R. Spaetgens, et al., Perinatal antibiotic usage and changes in colonization and resistance rates of group B *Streptococcus* and other pathogens, Obstet. Gynecol. 100 (2002) 525–533.

[666] R.S. Baltimore, et al., Early-onset neonatal sepsis in the era of group B streptococcal prevention, Pediatrics 108 (2001) 1094–1098.

[667] C.L. Byington, et al., Serious bacterial infections in febrile infants younger than 90 days of age: the importance of ampicillin-resistant pathogens, Pediatrics 111 (2003) 964–968.

[668] J.C. Mohle-Boetani, et al., Preventing neonatal group B streptococcal disease: cost-effectiveness in a health maintenance organization and the impact of delayed hospital discharge for newborns who received intrapartum antibiotics, Pediatrics 103 (1999) 703–710.

[669] G.J. Escobar, et al., Neonatal sepsis workups in infants greater than or equal to 2000 grams at birth: a population-based study, Pediatrics 106 (2000) 256–263.

[670] S. Balter, et al., Impact of intrapartum antibiotics on the care and evaluation of the neonate, Pediatr. Infect. Dis. J. 22 (2003) 853–857.

[671] P. Bromberger, et al., The influence of intrapartum antibiotics on the clinical spectrum of early-onset group B streptococcal infection in term infants, Pediatrics 106 (2000) 244–250.

[672] R.L. Davis, et al., Introduction of the new Centers for Disease Control and Prevention group B streptococcal prevention guideline at a large West Coast health maintenance organization, Am. J. Obstet. Gynecol. 184 (2001) 603–610.

[673] A.J. Steigman, E.J. Bottone, B.A. Hanna, Control of perinatal group B streptococcal sepsis: efficacy of single injection of aqueous penicillin at birth, Mt. Sinai. J. Med. 45 (1978) 685–693.

[674] S.P. Pyati, et al., Early penicillin in infants <2,000 grams with early onset GBS. Is it effective? Pediatr. Res. 16 (1982) 1019.

[675] S. Velaphi, et al., Early-onset group B streptococcal infection after a combined maternal and neonatal group B streptococcal chemoprophylaxis strategy, Pediatrics 111 (2003) 541–547.

[676] G.D. Wendel Jr., et al., Prevention of neonatal group B streptococcal disease: a combined intrapartum and neonatal protocol, Am. J. Obstet. Gynecol. 186 (2002) 618–626.

[677] J.D. Siegel, N.B. Cushion, Prevention of early-onset group B streptococcal disease: another look at single-dose penicillin at birth, Obstet. Gynecol. 87 (1996) 692–698.

[678] E.E. Rubin, J.C. McDonald, Group B streptococcal disease in twins: failure of empiric therapy to prevent late onset disease in the second twin, Pediatr. Infect. Dis. J. 10 (1991) 921–923.

[679] A. Schuchat, Epidemiology of group B streptococcal disease in the United States: shifting paradigms, Clin. Microbiol. Rev. 11 (1998) 497–513.

[680] L.C. Madoff, et al., Protection of neonatal mice from group B streptococcal infection by maternal immunization with beta C protein, Infect. Immun. 60 (1992) 4989–4994.

[681] L.B. Givner, C.J. Baker, The prevention and treatment of neonatal group B streptococcal infections, Adv. Pediatr. Infect. Dis. 3 (1988) 65–90.

[682] L.C. Paoletti, et al., Therapeutic potential of human antisera to group B streptococcal glycoconjugate vaccines in neonatal mice, J. Infect. Dis. 175 (1997) 1237–1239.

[683] C.J. Baker, D.L. Kasper, Group B streptococcal vaccines, Rev. Infect. Dis. 7 (1985) 458–467.

[684] M.R. Wessels, et al., Immunogenicity in animals of a polysaccharide-protein conjugate vaccine against type III group B *Streptococcus*, J. Clin. Invest. 86 (1990) 1428–1433.

[685] M.R. Wessels, et al., Immunogenicity and protective activity in animals of a type V group B streptococcal polysaccharide-tetanus toxoid conjugate vaccine, J. Infect. Dis. 171 (1995) 879–884.

[686] L.C. Paoletti, et al., Neonatal mouse protection against infection with multiple group B streptococcal (GBS) serotypes by maternal immunization with a tetravalent GBS polysaccharide-tetanus toxoid conjugate vaccine, Infect. Immun. 62 (1994) 3236–3243.

[687] L.C. Madoff, et al., Maternal immunization of mice with group B streptococcal type III polysaccharide-beta C protein conjugate elicits protective antibody to multiple serotypes, J. Clin. Invest. 94 (1994) 286–292.

[688] C.J. Baker, et al., Safety and immunogenicity of capsular polysaccharide-tetanus toxoid conjugate vaccines for group B streptococcal types Ia and Ib, J. Infect. Dis. 179 (1999) 142–150.

[689] L.C. Paoletti, L.C. Madoff, Vaccines to prevent neonatal GBS infection, Semin. Neonatol. 7 (2002) 315–323.

[690] D.L. Kasper, et al., Immune response to type III group B streptococcal polysaccharide-tetanus toxoid conjugate vaccine, J. Clin. Invest. 98 (1996) 2308–2314.

[691] C.J. Baker, et al., Use of capsular polysaccharide-tetanus toxoid conjugate vaccine for type II group B *Streptococcus* in healthy women, J. Infect. Dis. 182 (2000) 1129–1138.

[692] C.J. Baker, et al., Immune response of healthy women to 2 different group B streptococcal type V capsular polysaccharide-protein conjugate vaccines, J. Infect. Dis. 189 (2004) 1103–1112.

[693] C.J. Baker, et al., Safety and immunogenicity of a bivalent group B streptococcal conjugate vaccine for serotypes II and III, J. Infect. Dis. 188 (2003) 66–73.

[694] L.C. Paoletti, et al., An oligosaccharide-tetanus toxoid conjugate vaccine against type III group B *Streptococcus*, J. Biol. Chem. 265 (1990) 18278–18283.

[695] J.Y. Wang, et al., Construction of designer glycoconjugate vaccines with size-specific oligosaccharide antigens and site-controlled coupling, Vaccine 21 (2003) 1112–1117.

[696] J.L. Michel, et al., Cloned alpha and beta C-protein antigens of group B streptococci elicit protective immunity, Infect. Immun. 59 (1991) 2023–2028.

[697] P.S. Pannaraj, et al., Group B *Streptococcus* bacteremia elicits beta C protein-specific IgM and IgG in humans, J. Infect. Dis. 195 (2007) 353–356.

[698] P.S. Pannaraj, et al., Alpha C protein-specific immunity in humans with group B streptococcal colonization and invasive disease, Vaccine 26 (2008) 502–508.

[699] L.H. Harrison, et al., Serotype distribution of invasive group B streptococcal isolates in Maryland: implications for vaccine formulation, J. Infect. Dis. 177 (1998) 998–1002.

[700] H.H. Yang, et al., Recombinant group B streptococcus beta C protein and a variant with the deletion of its immunoglobulin A-binding site are protective mouse maternal vaccines and effective carriers in conjugate vaccines, Infect. Immun. 75 (2007) 3455–3461.

[701] C. Larsson, et al., Intranasal immunization of mice with group B streptococcal protein Rib and cholera toxin B subunit confers protection against lethal infection, Infect. Immun. 72 (2004) 1184–1187.

[702] D. Martin, et al., Protection from group B streptococcal infection in neonatal mice by maternal immunization with recombinant Sip protein, Infect. Immun. 70 (2002) 4897–4901.

[703] Q. Cheng, et al., Immunization with C5a peptidase or peptidase-type III polysaccharide conjugate vaccines enhances clearance of group B streptococci from lungs of infected mice, Infect. Immun. 70 (2002) 6409–6415.

[704] C.J. Baker, M.A. Rench, P. McInnes, Immunization of pregnant women with group B streptococcal type III capsular polysaccharide-tetanus toxoid conjugate vaccine, Vaccine 21 (2003) 3468–3472.

[705] Committee to Study Priorities for Vaccine Development, Division of Health Promotion and Disease Prevention, Institute of Medicine, National Academy of Sciences, Washington, DC, 1999.

[706] C.E. Adair, et al., Risk factors for early-onset group B streptococcal disease in neonates: a population-based case-control study, Can. Med. Assoc. J. 169 (2003) 198–203.

[707] C.J. Baker, et al., The natural history of group B streptococcal colonization in the pregnant woman and her offspring. II. Determination of serum antibody to capsular polysaccharide from type III group B *Streptococcus*, Am. J. Obstet. Gynecol. 137 (1980) 39–42.

[708] K.M. Boyer, et al., Selective intrapartum chemoprophylaxis of neonatal group B streptococcal early-onset disease. I. Epidemiologic rationale, J. Infect. Dis. 148 (1983) 795–801.

[709] W.B. Pittard, J.D. Thullen, A.A. Fanaroff, Neonatal septic arthritis, J. Pediatr. 88 (1976) 621–624.

[710] J.D. Nelson, The bacterial etiology and antibiotic management of septic arthritis in infants and children, Pediatrics 50 (1972) 437–440.

[711] M. Dan, Neonatal septic arthritis, Isr. J. Med. Sci. 19 (1983) 967–971.

[712] L. Fox, K. Sprunt, Neonatal osteomyelitis, Pediatrics 62 (1978) 535–542.

[713] T.K. Lai, J. Hingston, D. Scheifele, Streptococcal neonatal osteomyelitis, Am. J. Dis. Child. 134 (1980) 711.

[714] K.C. Henderson, R.S. Roberts, S.B. Dorsey, Group B 7-hemolytic streptococcal osteomyelitis in a neonate, Pediatrics 59 (1977) 1053–1054.

[715] R.T. Mohon, et al., Infected cephalhematoma and neonatal osteomyelitis of the skull, Pediatr. Infect. Dis. J. 5 (1986) 253–256.

[716] J.P. Cueva, R.T. Egel, Anterior fontanel herniation in group B *Streptococcus* meningitis in newborns, Pediatr. Neurol. 10 (1994) 332–334.

[717] M.S. Schimmel, et al., Transverse myelitis: unusual sequelae of neonatal group B streptococcus disease, J. Perinatol. 22 (2002) 580–581.

[718] R.G. Ellenbogen, D.A. Goldmann, K.R. Winston, Group B streptococcal infections of the central nervous system in infants with myelomeningocele, Surg. Neurol. 29 (1988) 237–242.

[719] S. Mukherjee, J.K. Askwith, Transient isolated oculomotor nerve paralysis in neonatal group B streptococcal meningitis, J. Paediatr. Child. Health. 44 (2008) 231–232.

[720] R.M. McAdams, et al., Ventricular peritoneal shunt infection resulting from group B streptococcus, Pediatr. Crit. Care. Med. 7 (2006) 586–588.

[721] P.G. Ramsey, R. Zwerdling, Asymptomatic neonatal bacteremia, N. Engl. J. Med. 295 (1977) 225.

[722] K.B. Roberts, Persistent group B *Streptococcus* bacteremia without clinical "sepsis" in infants, J. Pediatr. 88 (1976) 1059–1060.

[723] J.M. Poschl, et al., Ophthalmia neonatorum caused by group B *Streptococcus*, Scand. J. Infect. Dis. 34 (2002) 921–922.

[724] A. Klusmann, et al., Retrobulbar abscess in a neonate, Neuropediatrics 32 (2001) 219–220.

[725] M.A. Rench, C.J. Baker, Group B streptococcal breast abscess in a mother and mastitis in her infant, Obstet. Gynecol. 73 (1989) 875–877.

[726] M.J. Brian, M. O'Ryan, D. Waagner, Prepatellar bursitis in an infant caused by group B *Streptococcus*, Pediatr. Infect. Dis. J. 11 (1992) 502–503.

[727] D. Ruiz-Gomez, M.M. Tarpay, H.D. Riley, Recurrent group B streptococcal infections: report of three cases, Scand. J. Infect. Dis. 11 (1979) 35–38.

[728] I.J. Frieden, Blistering dactylitis caused by group B streptococci, Pediatr. Dermatol. 6 (1989) 300–302.

[729] M.C. Turner, E.G. Naumburg, Acute renal failure in the neonate: two fatal cases due to group B streptococci with rhabdomyolysis, Clin. Pediatr. (Phila) 26 (1987) 189–190.

[730] G. Kogan, et al., Structure of the type VI group B *Streptococcus* capsular polysaccharide determined by high resolution NMR spectroscopy, J. Carbohydr. Chem. 13 (1994) 1071–1078.

[731] F.Y. Lin, et al., Capsular polysaccharide types of group B streptococcal isolates from neonates with early-onset systemic infection, J. Infect. Dis. 177 (1998) 790–792.

CHAPTER OUTLINE

Organism **470**
  Morphology 470
  Motility 470
  Culture and Identification 470
  Antigenic Structure and Typing Systems 471
  Virulence Factors 471
Epidemiology and Transmission **472**
  Natural Reservoir and Human Transmission 472
  Occurrence 472
  Nosocomial Transmission 473
Pathogenesis **473**
  Host Response in Normal Adults 473
  Host Response in Neonates 476
Pathology **477**
Clinical Manifestations **478**
  Listeriosis during Pregnancy 478

Early-Onset Neonatal Listeriosis 479
Late-Onset Neonatal Listeriosis 479
Central Nervous System Infection (Adults) 480
Bacteremia 480
Other Clinical Forms of Infection 481
Diagnosis **481**
  Serology 481
  Isolation of the Organism 481
  Molecular Detection 481
Prognosis **481**
Therapy **482**
  In Vitro Studies 482
  In Vivo Studies 482
  Clinical Reports 482
  Suggested Management 483
Prevention and Outbreak Management **483**

Listeria monocytogenes, a gram-positive facultative bacillus, is a frequent veterinary pathogen that causes abortion and meningoencephalitis in sheep and cattle. Infection in a wide variety of other mammals is also recognized. Human disease is uncommon, but is potentially severe and occurs most frequently in neonates, in women during pregnancy, and in elderly or immunosuppressed patients. Nyfeldt [1] described *Listerella hominis* as the cause of human infectious mononucleosis in 1929, but subsequent experience indicates that human infections parallel animal illness, with sepsis and meningoencephalitis as the primary forms of invasive disease.

Murray and coworkers [2] provided the first notable description of the organism in 1926. An epizootic outbreak among laboratory rabbits and guinea pigs provided an isolate, subsequently named *Bacterium monocytogenes*. The greatest incidence and mortality occurred in recently weaned newborn animals. Later, Pirie [3] isolated the organism from South African gerbils and termed it *Listerella hepatolytica*, in honor of Lord Lister. Pirie [4] subsequently revised the name to *Listeria monocytogenes*, the currently accepted species name.

ORGANISM
MORPHOLOGY

The morphology of *L. monocytogenes* varies with the age of the culture. In clinical specimens, Gram stains typically show short intracellular and extracellular gram-positive rods. Careful interpretation of morphology is crucial. Over-decolorized *Listeria* organisms in cerebrospinal fluid have led to a misdiagnosis of *Haemophilus influenzae*

meningitis [5]. Confusion with pneumococcal meningitis is also possible; on primary culture, early bacterial growth may yield coccobacillus morphology in which short chains are occasionally seen. Older cultures may be variable.

MOTILITY

All strains of *L. monocytogenes* are motile, distinguishing the organism from *Erysipelothrix* and most species of *Corynebacterium*. A characteristic "tumbling" motility occurs in hanging drop preparations of primary cultures grown at room temperature [6]. In addition, tubes of semisolid motility medium produce a distinctive "umbrella" pattern at room temperature when inoculated with the stab technique. Electron microscopic studies and protein electrophoresis have shown that *L. monocytogenes* fails to express flagellar protein and loses motility at 37° C [7].

CULTURE AND IDENTIFICATION

L. monocytogenes grows well on common media, including brain-heart infusion, trypticase soy, and thioglycolate broths. Primary isolation from normally sterile sites can be accomplished on blood agar. Growth in ambient air occurs at temperatures of 4° C to 37° C, with fastest growth rates occurring at 30° C to 37° C. Selective media, such as Oxford, modified Oxford, or PALCAM agar (polymyxin B, acriflavine, lithium chloride, ceftazidime, aesculin, and mannitol), should be used for isolation from contaminated specimens and have largely replaced cold enrichment techniques [8,9].

After 48 hours at 37° C on 5% sheep blood agar, colonies are 0.2 to 1.5 mm in diameter. Narrow zones of β-hemolysis may be visualized—often only after moving the colony. Catalase test is positive (rare reports of catalase-negative isolates exist) [10]. *Listeria seeligeri* and *Listeria ivanovii* are also β-hemolytic, but generally are nonpathogenic in humans. Speciation is aided by the Christie-Atkins-Munch-Peterson (CAMP) reaction using *Staphylococcus aureus* for *L. monocytogenes* and *L. seeligeri* and *Rhodococcus equi* for *L. ivanovii* [11].

Discrimination among *Listeria* species is aided by sugar fermentation patterns. *L. monocytogenes* produces acid from L-rhamnose and α-methyl-D-mannoside, but not from xylose. *L. ivanovii* and *L. seeligeri* produce acid from D-xylose only. Automated systems (e.g., Vitek, Microscan Walkway, Siemens, Berlin), commercial biochemical strips (e.g., API Listeria Biomerieux, MICRO-ID Listeria), DNA probes (e.g., AccuProbe Listeria Culture Identification Test, Remel, Kansas City, MO) and home-brew and commercial polymerase chain reaction (PCR, Gen-Probe Life Sciences, Manchester, UK) assays (e.g., LightCycler *Listeria monocytogenes* Detection Kit, Roche, Basel, Switzerland) are now available to aid in the identification of *L. monocytogenes* in clinical microbiology laboratories.

ANTIGENIC STRUCTURE AND TYPING SYSTEMS

There are 13 known serotypes of *Listeria*, distinguished on the basis of somatic (O) and flagellar (H) antigens [12,13]. Serotypes 1/2a, 1/2b, and 4b cause most animal and human disease. Serotyping has little impact on clinical management, but has a role in public health during epidemiologic investigations. Before the 1990s, phage typing was used for epidemiologic investigations—particularly in tracing sources of food-borne *Listeria* outbreaks when serotyping failed to discriminate between epidemic and nonepidemic strains [14–16]. Such strains often remained nontypable.

Molecular typing has provided new levels of discriminatory power. Multilocus enzyme electrophoresis, although not directly DNA based, has proven reliable in distinguishing strains based on electrophoretic mobility of enzymes [17]. Multilocus enzyme electrophoresis is limited, however, by the failure of many nucleotide and amino acid changes to alter net enzyme charge and electrophoretic mobility [18,19].

Analysis of *Listeria* DNA has enhanced the discriminatory power of strain typing [20,21]. Molecular subtyping approaches have been DNA fragment or sequence based. One fragment-based analysis creates microrestriction patterns using high frequency–cutting enzymes (restriction endonucleases). The technique has been used in epidemiologic investigations, but its complex results make strain comparison difficult. Ribotyping simplifies this process by examining only DNA fragments from the ribosomal genes [18]. The automation of ribotyping into commercially available systems has enabled rapid identification of disease clusters and immediate typing of *Listeria* strains.

DNA macrorestriction pattern analysis using pulsed-field gel electrophoresis (PFGE) was adopted by the World Health Organization for typing in 2003 [22]. PFGE is highly discriminating and reproducible—even for serotype 4b strains that are poorly typed by most other methods. The U.S. Centers for Disease Control and Prevention (CDC) created PulseNet, a network of laboratories using standardized PFGE protocols to subtype food-borne bacterial pathogens. Using the Internet for reporting and comparing PFGE patterns, laboratories can now identify regional or national clusters that could be missed with localized reporting.

DNA amplification–based typing methods, such as random amplification of polymorphic DNA, have been shown to have a high degree of discriminatory power as well. The primary drawback at present is the lack of standardization. The combination of DNA amplification with automated sequencing provides ultimate discriminatory power—to the nucleotide level—and is becoming more widely available.

VIRULENCE FACTORS

Food-borne outbreaks of *L. monocytogenes* infections led to intense interest in the characterization of its virulence factors. Similar to *Salmonella typhimurium*, *Yersinia enterocolitica*, and *Legionella pneumophila*, *Listeria* has become a model organism for intracellular parasitism [13,23–25]. In tracing the journey of an organism from ingestion to successful replication in the host, we can appreciate the incredible adaptations that have occurred.

Listeria have the ability to survive environmental change [26]. In response to stressors such as thermal variation, acidic pH, and osmotic challenge, stress response genes—encoding a set of conserved proteins—are upregulated and have roles such as repair and removal of damaged bacterial proteins [27]. Stress response genes are largely regulated by sigma factor B (*sigB* gene), also responsible for stress resistance in other bacterial species [28]. Environmental survival is intricately linked to virulence. In animal models, acid-adapted *Listeria* survive low gastric pH, leading to higher bacterial loads in the intestine and mesenteric lymph nodes after oral infection [29].

Having survived gastric acidity, *Listeria* induce their uptake into host intestinal cells via phagocytic vacuoles. The internalin (Inl) family of bacterial surface proteins mediate attachment to mammalian cells [13,30–32]. InlA and InlB promote engulfment and internalization of bacteria by normally nonphagocytic cells. E-cadherin, the glycoprotein receptor for InlA, is present on the surface of gastrointestinal epithelial cells known to be targets for *Listeria* entry. Lecuit and colleagues [33] identified a single proline residue in E-cadherin that mediates species specificity—the first potential molecular explanation of bacterial–host species specificity. InlB, a 67-kDa protein, has two receptors, Met and gC1q-R (a cellular ligand for the C1q complement fraction), which confer a tropism for hepatocytes and brain microvascular epithelial cells. InlJ, another attachment protein, is expressed only by organisms growing in vivo [32]. A fourth protein, invasion-associated protein (iap or p60), is secreted by invasive *Listeria* strains and is a major antigen for the protective immune response against *L. monocytogenes* [34,35].

Inside the cell, *Listeria* engineers its own escape from the oxidative stress of the phagolysosome [13,36]. Invasive strains of *L. monocytogenes* produce listeriolysin O (LLO) (a sulfhydryl-activated hemolysin similar to streptolysin O). LLO (*hly* gene), which is activated specifically at low pH and disrupts the integrity of phagosome membranes, allows *Listeria* to escape into the cytosol where it begins intracellular replication [37,38]. Here the bacterial surface protein ActA—product of the *actA* gene—triggers polymerization of host cell actin into a "comet tail" that enables intracellular movement and cell-to-cell spread of the pathogen [38–40]. *Listeria* move along these actin filaments to the cell membrane, eventually pushing it outward in a pseudopod-like extension (also termed a *listeriopod*), which is engulfed by neighboring cells as a double-walled secondary phagosome.

Escape from the primary phagosome and the secondary phagosome is also mediated by phospholipase C (*plcA* gene) and a lecithinase (*plcB* gene), which contribute to lysis of phagosomal membranes. Mutations of the *plcA* and *plcB* genes significantly reduce virulence [13,31,41]. A metalloprotease encoded by the gene *mpl* converts lecithinase into its active form [42]. Cell-to-cell spread continues in this cycle with *Listeria* protected the entire time from extracellular host defenses (e.g., antibody, complement, professional phagocytes).

Virulence gene expression is controlled by regulatory genes. The gene, *prfA* (positive regulatory factor A), controls expression of *hly* and *plcB* via PrfA, its protein product [43]. PrfA is the main switch of a regulon containing most virulence genes in *Listeria*. This transcription factor promotes expression of certain genes (*hly*, *plcB*) and downregulates others (the motility-associated genes *motA* and *flaA*) [44], implying a global regulatory role [45]. PrfA/*prfA*–induced regulation is influenced by the bacteria's physicochemical environment. Thermoregulation is one example: PrfA-dependent transcription is minimal at less than 30° C (environmental temperature), but is induced at 37° C (body temperature of mammals) [46,47].

The monocytosis initially observed in animals infected with *L. monocytogenes* has been partially explained. A phospholipid, monocytosis-producing agent, has been isolated that produces monocytosis in rabbits [48]. Monocyte production is stimulated by an endogenous mediator induced by monocytosis-producing agent [49].

EPIDEMIOLOGY AND TRANSMISSION
NATURAL RESERVOIR AND HUMAN TRANSMISSION

Listeria species are ubiquitous in nature, with a natural habitat in decaying plant matter [50]. Spoiled silage seems to be a source of infection for ruminant animals [51]. Fecal carriage of *L. monocytogenes* in animals plays a role in the organism's persistence by providing an enrichment cycle.

Although direct transmission of *L. monocytogenes* to humans from infected animals has been described, [52,53] most human infection is acquired through ingestion of contaminated food [54,55]. The first outbreak confirming an indirect transmission from animals was reported from Canada [16]. In this outbreak, cabbage, stored in the cold over the winter, were contaminated with *Listeria* through infected sheep manure. Clinical disease developed in pregnant women and immunocompromised patients who subsequently consumed the cabbage. Large outbreaks caused by contaminated foods continue to occur in North America and Europe [56–60]. The relative resistance of *Listeria* to high temperatures and its ability to multiply at low temperatures provide opportunities for heavy

contamination of dairy products if pasteurization has been carried out improperly [61,62]. Outbreaks have been commonly associated with prepared meat products, including turkey and deli meats, paté, hot dogs, and seafood products [60,63–68]. *Listeria* has been identified as the leading cause of death from food-borne infection in the United States and France [69,70]. Risk of an outbreak caused by contaminated food seems to be related to a high inoculum of *L. monocytogenes* in the food [71].

The improved ability to detect *L. monocytogenes* by selective culture and molecular methods has provided the opportunity to examine food eaten by patients who have developed sporadic cases of listeriosis [72]. It has been confirmed that most sporadic cases of listeriosis are caused by ingestion of contaminated foods [73–75]. These studies implicated a wide variety of foods, including melons, hummus, undercooked chicken, and soft cheeses, as significant sources of sporadic disease. A review of food-borne listeriosis has been published more recently [76].

OCCURRENCE

L. monocytogenes causes an estimated 2500 serious illnesses and 500 deaths annually in the United States. Active surveillance programs in several countries have suggested an annual incidence of 0.2 to 0.7 cases per 100,000 population [56,57,75,77–80]. With the exception of France and Germany, incidence has been steady or declining [56,59,75]. Countries with active surveillance programs have reported the highest incidence of disease.

L. monocytogenes may cause symptomatic gastroenteritis, a nonreportable condition. Fecal carriage of *Listeria* is uncommon in settings not associated with outbreak [81], but may be 26% in household contacts of patients with listeriosis [55] and 8% in the community during outbreaks [82].

The distribution of serovars causing disease may not be uniform. In North America, serovars 4b and 1/2 account for 95% of strains, with serotype 4b being the most common overall [83]. In Spain and Germany, serovar 4b is predominant [84,85]. whereas in Denmark serovar 1/2 is common [58]. The significance of these geographic differences is unknown.

The incidence of listeriosis is highest among newborn infants. Perinatal and newborn infection represents 30% to 40% of the total caseload in humans [77,78]. The true incidence is probably much higher, however, because spontaneous abortion and stillbirth caused by *Listeria* is largely unrecognized unless bacterial cultures are obtained from tissue. The incidence of perinatal and neonatal listeriosis is 2 to 13 per 100,000 live births [57,84–86]. It is possible that a lower inoculum may cause infection in pregnant women compared with the general population. No differences in carriage rates between pregnant women and nonpregnant individuals have been found in fecal and vaginal specimens [87]. Fecal carriage may lead to vaginal colonization and be responsible for the development of late-onset infection in infants born of healthy mothers.

Most documented human cases of listeriosis occur in high-risk adult populations, including elderly adults and adults with compromised immune function (Table 13–1). Sepsis and meningitis are the most frequent resulting

TABLE 13–1 Individuals at High Risk of Listeriosis

Pregnant Women

Risk of listeriosis is about 20 times higher in pregnant women than in nonpregnant healthy adults

About one third of listeriosis cases are diagnosed in pregnant women

Pregnant women with listeriosis are at increased risk of spontaneous abortion, preterm delivery, or stillbirth

Newborns

Newborns are at greater risk of developing severe infection than pregnant women

Newborns may present clinically with

    Early-onset listeriosis (transmitted via placenta and usually diagnosed as sepsis in the first day of life)

    Late-onset infection ($\geq$7 days of life, high rate of meningitis [>90%])

Elderly Adults and Immunocompromised Patients

About 50% of all cases of listeriosis occur in individuals $\geq$60 yr old

Immunocompromised patients include patients with cancer, diabetes, or kidney disease

Listeriosis is 300 times more likely to occur in patients with HIV/AIDS than in healthy adults

Other immunocompromised patients include

    Patients receiving immunosuppressive drug therapy (e.g., high-dose glucocorticosteroid, tumor necrosis factor inhibitor)

    Transplant patients receiving antirejection drug therapy

---

illness [78]. Louria and coworkers [88] initially described this infection in patients with malignancies, but various other conditions have been reported in association with invasive listeriosis [89,90]. Susceptibility in laboratory animals is increased by the administration of corticosteroids [91], cyclosporine [92], and prostaglandins [93], and the human experience parallels these studies. Renal transplantation seems to be a particularly significant risk factor, and a nosocomial outbreak has been reported in this population [94]. Hemochromatosis with increased iron stores may also predispose to infection. Patients with human immunodeficiency virus (HIV) infection have a 400-fold to 1000-fold increased risk of acquiring invasive listeriosis compared with HIV-negative subjects [95]. Alcoholism, diabetes, and cirrhosis [96] also contribute to infection, although community-acquired listeriosis may occur spontaneously in patients with no underlying predisposing conditions [97]. Animal studies [98] and one outbreak of human listeriosis [99] suggest that decreased gastric acidity may also predispose to invasive infection in patients with immunosuppressive conditions.

NOSOCOMIAL TRANSMISSION

Although most cases of listeriosis occur in the community, nosocomial listeriosis in neonates and adults has been described [100–107]. Person-to-person transmission caused by poor infection control techniques is likely to be responsible for most of these small clusters. Among clusters reported in newborns, the index case may manifest as early-onset infection, and subsequent cases may manifest

as late-onset listeriosis. Multiple cases of early-onset disease in the same unit may suggest the possibility of food-borne disease in the community. Nosocomial infection among adults in one outbreak [99] seemed related to ingestion of contaminated food in the hospital or within 2 weeks of hospitalization. Clear-cut nosocomial infection has been shown in a neonatal outbreak in Costa Rica [108]. In this outbreak, the index case had early-onset disease and was bathed with mineral oil that became contaminated with the epidemic isolate. Subsequent bathing of other infants with the same oil led to late-onset disease in those infants.

PATHOGENESIS
HOST RESPONSE IN NORMAL ADULTS

The pathogenesis of listeriosis in humans is still poorly understood. Because food is the most common source of outbreak and sporadic cases, the gastrointestinal tract is thought to be the usual portal of entry into the host. Although *L. monocytogenes* is probably ingested frequently through contaminated food, the incidence of clinical disease in humans is relatively low [78]. This suggests the organism has relatively low virulence, a concept supported by the high concentration of organisms required to cause infection in the normal host [109].

The entry of *L. monocytogenes* into cells in the intestine is mediated by interaction of an *L. monocytogenes* surface protein, InlA, with its host cell receptor, E-cadherin. The InlA–E-cadherin interaction is species-specific and relies on an amino acid sequence found in only a few animal species, including humans [110]. Translocation of *Listeria* across the intestinal mucosa occurs very rapidly in humans and without histologic evidence of inflammation in the bowel wall [25]. The organism is transported to the liver within minutes of ingestion. This rapid process seems to be independent of the known *Listeria* virulence factors because mutant strains lacking such factors arrive at the liver roughly at the same time as their wild-type parent strains [24].

The first stage of the battle between bacteria and host occurs in the liver [111]. Within hours of ingestion, macrophages of the liver (Kupffer cells) and spleen capture and destroy most of the inoculum. Over the next 3 days, a nonspecific, T cell–independent phase of innate host resistance is operative. Since the 1960s, it was known that *L. monocytogenes* can survive within Kupffer cells that line the hepatic sinusoids. In the late 1980s, it was also appreciated that *Listeria* can infect nonphagocytic cells (e.g., epithelial, hepatocellular, and fibroblast cell lines), providing the organism with an intracellular environment temporarily sheltered from phagocytic cells and soluble effectors of host defense [36,112,113].

Although proteins on the surface of *Listeria*, such as InlA, InlB, and p60, may identify important factors associated with entrance into the cell in vitro [31,34,114], they do not fully explain intracellular spread and multiplication of the organism in vivo [115]. During the early course of infection, *L. monocytogenes* resides within a vacuole (for nonphagocytic cells) or a phagosome (in monocyte/macrophage-derived cells) (Fig. 13–1). Lysis of the

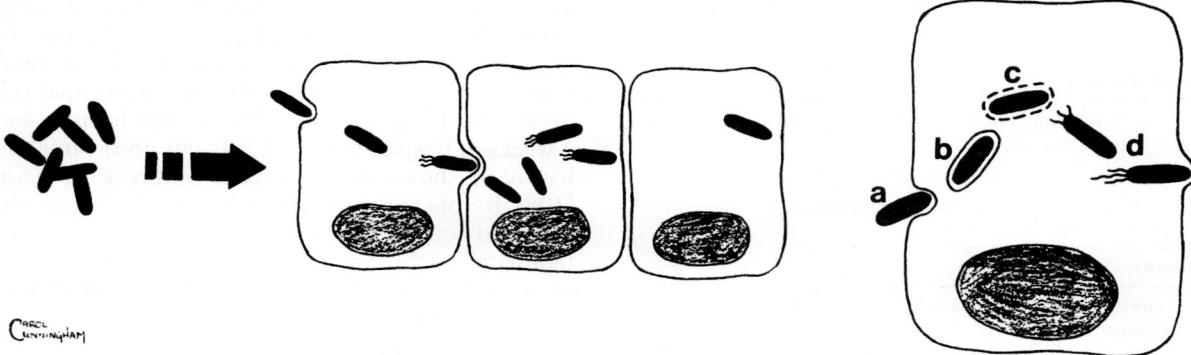

FIGURE 13-1 Cellular invasion by *Listeria monocytogenes.* Attachment of *L. monocytogenes* to the surface of cell membrane (*a*) is determined by a family of bacterial surface proteins including internalins (IntA and IntB). When internalized (*b*) within a vacuole (*c*), listeriolysin O (LLO) can lyse the vacuole membrane, liberating the bacteria into the cytoplasm. Bacterial surface ActA induces polymerization of cellular actin, which concentrates at one end of the bacterium. This "comet tail" (*d*) provides propulsion for the organism to move through the cytoplasm and into adjacent cells where the intracellular process begins again.

phagosome or vacuole is mediated by Listeriolysin O and non-Listeriolysin O proteins [38,116–118]. LLO may also increase the virulence of the organism by contributing to the elimination of immune T cells [119].

Bacterium-derived phospholipase C, a metalloprotease-mediated lysin, and other virulence factors also contribute to escape of *L. monocytogenes* from vacuoles and phagosomes [24,36,120,121]. Release of *L. monocytogenes* from intracellular vacuoles precipitates intracellular growth and actin polymerization [39,122]. Actin polymerization is important in the cell-to-cell transfer of *L. monocytogenes* and is mediated by the ActA product of the *actA* gene [123]. A surface protein, ActA causes host cell actin to assemble into filaments around the bacterium. After 2 or 3 hours, the actin filaments polarize at one end of the organism. This "comet tail" provides propulsive force for the organism to move through the cytoplasm. When the bacterium reaches the cell membrane, it forms a filipod that is ingested by adjacent cells. In the process, the organism avoids exposure to the extracellular environment. In addition to hepatocytes, enterocytes, and phagocytic cells, *Listeria* can grow and spread in fibroblasts, epithelial cells, vascular endothelial cells, and renal tubular epithelial cells [122].

There is normally a decrease in viable bacteria within the monocyte/macrophage phagocytic system 3 to 4 days after infection begins. This decrease heralds the onset of the T cell–dependent stage of anti-*Listeria* defense and the beginning of acquired resistance [124–126]. Development of cellular immunity against *Listeria* peaks at 5 to 8 days of infection and can be shown by adoptive transfer of resistance using immune T cells [126]. At this stage, the number of activated macrophages in infected tissue rapidly increases (Fig. 13–2).

Cellular Response

For adult animals, the process leading to acquired immunity to *Listeria* has been partially elucidated, and the sequence of cell-to-cell interaction resulting in cytolytic activity is becoming clear. In adult immunocompetent animals, *Listeria* are phagocytosed by "professional" phagocytes (macrophages and monocytes) and by "nonprofessional" phagocytic cells (e.g., fibroblasts, hepatocytes) (see Fig. 13–1). When ingested, partial degradation of *Listeria* occurs, and transfer of the *Listeria* protein antigen fragments to the macrophage cell surface takes place [127].

Peptides resulting from digestion of *Listeria* in the cytoplasm are actively processed by the endoplasmic reticulum, where they bind to major histocompatibility complex (MHC) class I molecules (Fig. 13–3) [127]. The *Listeria*-peptide-MHC complex is transported to the cell surface where it can be recognized by cytolytic T lymphocytes (CD8 phenotype).

Bacterial peptides that are digested within phagosomes are transported to the plasma membrane, where they attach to MHC class II molecules. CD4 T lymphocytes recognize specific antigens that are presented by MHC class II membrane receptors [128]. Development of T helper (T_H) subset during an immune response is pivotal because *L. monocytogenes* infection is most effectively controlled through this immune response [128]. *L. monocytogenes* induction of T_H1 development in vitro is mediated by macrophage-produced interleukin (IL)-12. Cells with T_H1 phenotype secrete IL-2 and interferon (IFN)-γ during primary infection [129,130]. Although a few T_H2 cells may develop during *Listeria* infection, they play little role in the clearance of the pathogen [131].

In the presence of *Listeria* antigens and IL-2, T cells divide, producing *Listeria*-specific clones. In vitro evidence shows that immune CD8 T cells are cytolytic for *Listeria*-infected macrophages and hepatocytes (see Fig. 13–3) [132,133]. A robust CD8 T-cell response is induced during *L. monocytogenes* infection. *Listeria*-specific CD8 T cells confer protective immunity to naïve animals in adoptive transfer experiments; however, these T cells lose antibacterial activity within days [134]. Neutrophils and monocytes that migrate to the site of primary infection may participate in the lysis of infected cells, but, more importantly, play a role in the elimination of bacteria that are released to the surrounding tissue. By this stage of infection, phagocytic cells have been primed or activated by IFN-γ or cytokines, making them more effective killers [134–140].

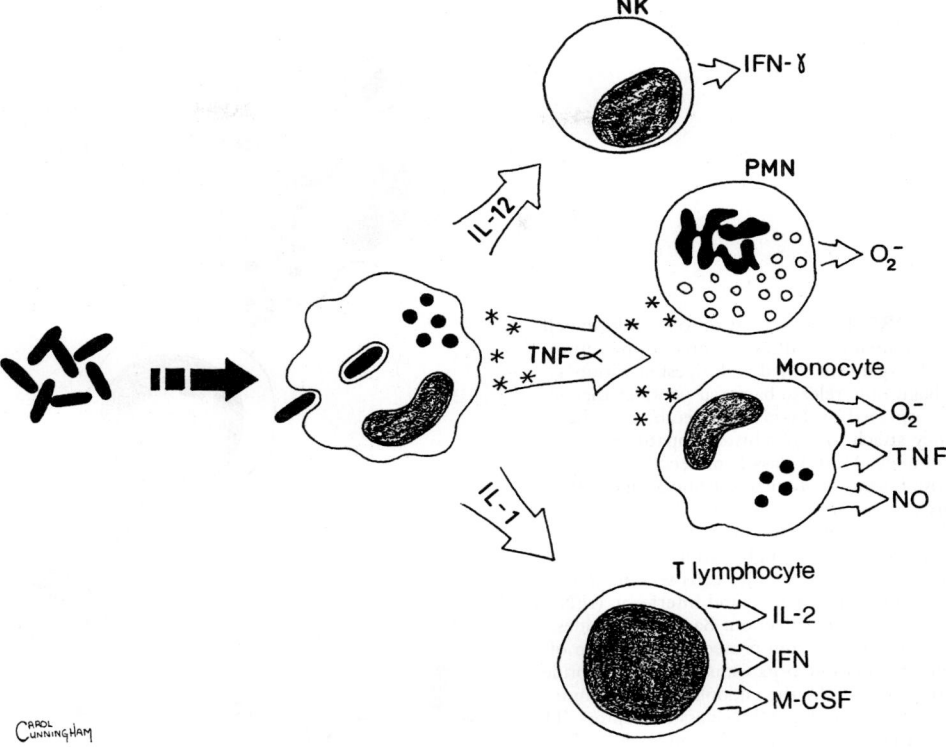

FIGURE 13–2 Interferon (IFN) and cytokine production. Blood monocytes and tissue macrophages produce various cytokines after ingestion of live *Listeria* organisms. Interleukin (IL)-12 causes activation of natural killer (NK) cells, which release high concentrations of IFN-γ. Tumor necrosis factor (TNF)-α is produced in large concentrations by monocytes and macrophages after ingestion of *Listeria* organisms TNF-α leads to priming of polymorphonuclear leukocytes and activation of other macrophage cells, with increased production of superoxide (O_2^-), nitric oxide (NO), and TNF-α. Macrophage-produced IL-1 leads to proliferation of T cells, which produce immunomodulating proteins such as IL-2, macrophage colony-stimulating factor (M-CSF), and IFN-γ.

Role of Toll-like Receptors, Interferon, and Cytokines

Toll-like receptors (TLRs) are conserved primitive membrane proteins found in cells that have been identified more recently as key to initiation of innate immunity [141]. At present, 10 TLRs have been identified. TLR2 and TLR6 are heterodimers for gram-positive peptidoglycan. Surface TLRs stimulate an innate immune response through a signaling pathway involving intracellular kinases and transcription factors. The first intracellular adapter molecule in this cascade is myeloid differentiation antigen 88 (MyD88), which functions as a crucial first adapter protein of several TLRs, including TLR2 and TLR6 [142]. The role of the TLR pathway in innate immunity to *Listeria* has become clear in recent years [36]. TLR2-deficient mice show partial impairment in their resistance to *Listeria* [143]. MyD88 subserves multiple TLRs, however, and has an even more crucial role in early clearance of *Listeria* and cytokine signaling [143–145].

In mature immunocompetent animals, *Listeria* infection induces circulating IFN-γ and IFN-α/β on the 2nd or 3rd day in the acquired phase of immunity. Cytokines such as macrophage colony-stimulating factor (M-CSF) [131] and tumor necrosis factor (TNF)-α also appear during the first 5 days and have been implicated as mediators of *Listeria* clearance [139,146–151]. Peak immunity to *Listeria* is expressed about the 6th day of infection, which coincides with maximal T_H1 cell synthesis of IFN-γ [152,153]. A role for endogenous IFN-γ in resolution of *L. monocytogenes* infection has been shown [154,155]. Adult animals treated with monoclonal antibody directed against IFN-γ

do not develop activated macrophages, and clearance of *Listeria* from liver and spleen is decreased [154].

The cytokine cascade involving various interleukins, IFN, and TNF-α is essential for host response to *Listeria* infection. MyD88-initiated signaling pathways are required for IL-1, IL-12, IL-18, and TNF-α induction in monocytes and other early responsive cells [143,156–159]. All of these cytokines are involved in an early response to *Listeria* infection through their activation of resident macrophage cells, circulating monocytes, and polymorphonuclear neutrophils (PMNs). Activation of dendritic cells in a TLR-dependent fashion leads to early removal of 90% of the bacterial burden in the liver within 6 hours of *Listeria* infection and may represent a critical link between the innate and adaptive immune processes [159,160].

TNF-α is a key cytokine to enhance antibacterial or antiparasitic resistance mechanisms (see Fig. 13–2) [161–164]. Many cell types produce TNF-α, including natural killer (NK) cells [165]; however, monocytes and macrophages are probably the most abundant source. Endotoxin (lipopolysaccharide) and other agents, including mitogens; viruses; protozoa; and cytokines such as M-CSF, IL-1, IL-2, and IFN-γ, have been identified as inducers of TNF-α [166–169]. When administered before infection, TNF-α–inducing agents enhanced resistance of the host to bacterial infection [170].

Endogenously produced TNF-α during sublethal *Listeria* infection in adult animals seems to function as an inducer of resistance [146,148]. Injection of mice with anti–TNF-α immunoglobulin results in a striking proliferation of bacteria during the first 2 to 3 days of infection; however, administration of anti–TNF-α immunoglobulin

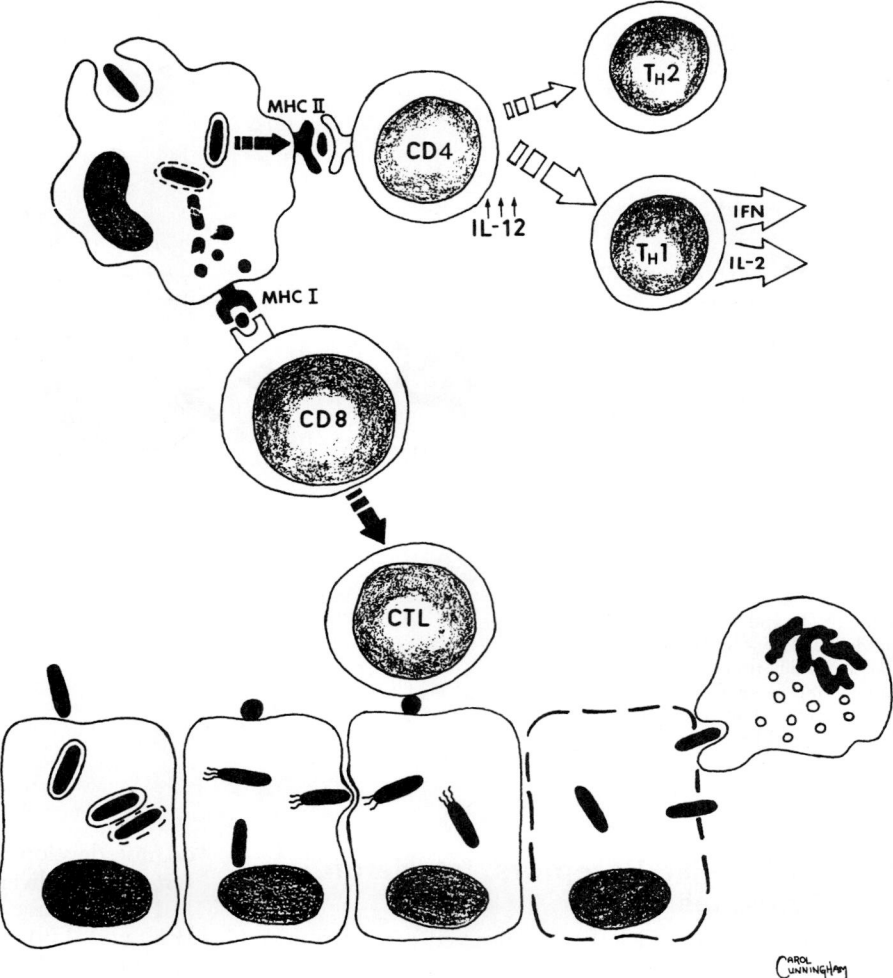

FIGURE 13–3 Activation of cytolytic cell mechanisms. Within an antigen-presenting cell, organisms killed and digested within a phagosome release bacterial peptides that are transported to the plasma membrane, where they attach to major histocompatibility complex (MHC) class II molecules. CD4 T lymphocytes recognize specific antigens that are presented by MHC class II receptors. CD4 T lymphocytes differentiate predominantly into T_H1 cells through stimulation by interleukin (IL)-12. T_H1 cells secrete high concentrations of IL-2 and interferon (IFN)-γ during primary infection. Bacterial peptides may also come from proteolytic digestion of intracytoplasmic organisms. Bacterial peptides are processed by the endoplasmic reticulum where they bind to MHC class I receptors. The bacterial–peptide–MHC I complex is transported to the cell membrane, where it is recognized by cytolytic T lymphocytes (CD8 phenotype). These cells cause lysis of *Listeria*-infected cells, which are recognized by the presence of listerial peptides on their surface. Lysis of *Listeria*-infected cells leaves the organism exposed to phagocytosis and killing by activated phagocytic cells, polymorphonuclear leukocytes, and monocytes.

on day 5 of infection has virtually no effect on *Listeria* replication in the spleen and liver [139,140,148]. These results suggest that TNF-α–dependent mechanisms limit intracellular infection early in the course of infection. Localized production of TNF is shown in supernatants of organ homogenates from the liver or spleen [171].

IL-12 participates in the differentiation of T_H1 cells, IFN-γ production, and NK cell activation [128,151,172]. In the absence of T_H1 activation, animals are more susceptible to *L. monocytogenes* infection [128,172]. IL-1, IL-12, and more recently IL-18, molecules whose receptor signaling requires MyD88, all are required for normal host defense against *Listeria* [144,160,173].

HOST RESPONSE IN NEONATES
Cell Activation

In fetal and newborn animals, susceptibility to *Listeria* seems to be associated with delayed activation of macrophages [174,175]. Studies on the afferent and efferent arms of cell-mediated immunity in fetal and newborn mice have shown that macrophage and T-lymphocyte interaction and macrophage activation is impaired [171,176–181].

Suppression of cell-mediated immunity during pregnancy is necessary to prevent fetal rejection. Cell-mediated immunity is essential, however, to combat intracellular pathogens, and the human placenta is extremely sensitive to microbial invasion by such organisms. After invasion, *Listeria* grows rapidly in the placenta and the fetus. Until more recently, very little was known about the molecular mechanisms responsible for transmission of pathogens across the fetal-placental barrier. A better understanding of species variability in placenta immunology and physiology and cell receptors for *Listeria* has provided insights into the vertical transmission of infection.

Because of similarities between the human and guinea pig placenta, it has been proposed as an animal model to study human fetal infection [182]. The InlA–E-cadherin interaction that facilitates bacteria crossing cellular barriers is exploited by *Listeria* in fetal infection [110]. E-cadherin is present in human and guinea pig placentas. ActA on the surface of *Listeria* is also required to cross the fetal-placental barrier, by enabling cell-to-cell spreading [183]. In the rhesus model, animals exposed to *L. monocytogenes* at the beginning of the third trimester had increased risk of stillbirth delivery and showed pathology similar to

humans [184]. Antibody and *Listeria*-induced cell proliferation was increased in mothers after delivery of stillborn
rhesus monkey infants. The relevance of animal studies to
human infection remains to be determined; however, similar immune responses are found among mothers and
infants surviving natural *Listeria* infection [185].

NK cells also seem to be important in early response to
L. monocytogenes infection. The proportion of mononuclear cells expressing NK cell phenotype and NK cell
activity is decreased at birth, particularly in premature
infants [186,187]. NK cell phenotype and function
increase rapidly in the weeks after birth.

Toll-like Receptors, Interferon, and Cytokines in Newborns

In adult animals and adult-derived cells, *Listeria* infection
induces IL-12 and IL-18 production, which mediates
T_H1 differentiation, NK cell activation, and IFN-α production [114]. The major cellular source of IL-12 and
IL-18 are monocytes, macrophages, and dendritic cells.
After lipopolysaccharide stimulation, IL-12 messenger
RNA (mRNA) expression and protein production in cord
blood mononuclear cells is also greatly decreased compared with adult cells [188]. In addition, the half-life of
IL-12 p40 mRNA is shortened in activated cord blood
cells compared with adult cells [189]. Cord blood mononuclear cells from humans are capable of responding in vitro
to exogenous IL-12 in high concentrations, however.

In adult animals, IFN and agents that induce or augment
IFN production confer protection against lethal listeriosis
[190,191]. Synthesis of IFN-γ, IL-2, and IL-4, all of which
modulate the immune response and macrophage activation,
is deficient in newborns [181,192–194]. Although production of these factors may be defective, newborn animals do
respond to exogenous IFN-γ; pretreatment with IFN-γ or
its inducers [195] protects against subsequent infection.

The ontogeny of cytokine-related host defense mechanisms has not been studied in depth. TNF-α is decreased
in newborn rats infected with *L. monocytogenes* [171]. In
one study of *L. monocytogenes*–infected newborn rats,
TNF-α was detected only in animals older than 8 days of
age. The age at which TNF-α is measurable corresponds
to the approximate age at which increased resistance to
L. monocytogenes is seen. In addition, the study showed that
IFN-γ may enhance resistance to *L. monocytogenes* in newborn animals by permitting them to respond to exogenous
TNF-α.

The pattern of delayed or diminished cytokine
response in human newborns is similar to the response
in animals deficient in TLRs. This possibility has been
explored in human newborns. TLR-2 and TLR-4 expression is normal on mononuclear and PMN cells of
newborns [157]. It is now known that TLRs require
membrane-associated proteins to initiate intracellular
messenger activation and cytokine secretion. Chief among
these proteins is MyD88, an intracellular myeloid differentiating antigen needed for intracellular signaling of all
TLR proteins. In human newborn cells, diminished
TNF-α secretion by stimulated monocytes and diminished superoxide production by PMNs are associated with
diminished intracellular MyD88 [157,196]. The control

of *L. monocytogenes* infection depends on rapid activation
of the innate immune system through TLR-2 and
MyD88, since animals deficient in either succumb to
Listeria infection [315].

Serum Factors

Opsonic activity of newborn serum for *Listeria* is minimal
[197,198]. *Listeria* is opsonized primarily by IgM together
with the classic complement pathway. Because newborn
serum has negligible amounts of IgM and low concentrations of the classic complement pathway, its poor opsonic
activity may contribute to the severity of infection in
newborns. Adult serum may also contain specific antibodies
to inhibit *L. monocytogenes* invasion of brain microvascular
endothelial cells [199]. The inhibitory antibody, which is
absent in newborn cord serum, reacts with the *Listeria* surface protein InlB, described earlier as a key virulence factor.

PATHOLOGY

Histologically, human listeriosis is characterized by miliary granulomas and focal necroses or by suppuration.
The term *listerioma* has been coined for *Listeria*-associated
granulomas. In the newborn, *Listeria* infection of organs
produces multiple, tiny nodules that are visible on
gross examination [200]. Massive involvement of the liver
is typical, reflecting the abundance of internalin receptors
on hepatocytes [201]. Often, as in miliary tuberculosis,
the liver is seeded with grayish yellow nodules. Analogous
findings are observed in the spleen, adrenal glands, lungs,
esophagus, posterior pharyngeal wall, and tonsils. Subepithelial granulomas often undergo necrosis. Focal granulomas may also be detected in the lymph nodes, thymus,
bone marrow, myocardium, testes, and skeletal muscles.
The intestinal tract is affected to a variable degree, with
a preference for the lymphatic structures of the small
intestine and appendix. Cutaneous lesions of neonatal listeriosis were first described by Reiss [202] and occur most
commonly on the back and lumbar region (Fig. 13–4).

Granuloma formation is also typical in listeriosis of the
central nervous system (CNS) [203]. A characteristic histologic picture is seen in *Listeria* encephalitis, consisting
of cerebral tissue necrosis with a loosening of the reticulum and an infiltration of leukocytes and lymphocytes
leading to abscess formation.

Suppurative inflammation is the second form of tissue
reaction to listeriosis. It is predominantly found in the
meninges, conjunctivae, and epithelial linings of the middle ear and nasal sinuses. In meningitis, the subarachnoid
space becomes filled with thick purulent exudate.

The histologic changes in human listeriosis are the
same as the changes observed in animals. The organisms
cause necrosis, followed by a proliferation of reticuloendothelial cells, resulting in the development of granulomas. The center of the granuloma is necrotic, and the
periphery contains an abundance of chronic inflammatory
cells. *Listeria* organisms are present in variable numbers
within these necrotic foci and can be shown with a Gram
stain or Levaditi silver impregnation. Similar changes are
found in all affected organs, independent of the age of the
infected individual.

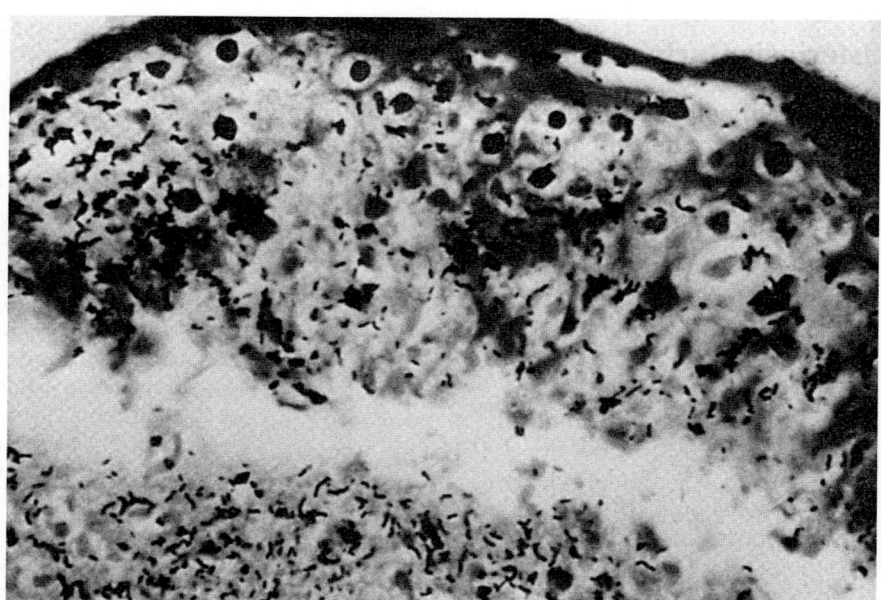

FIGURE 13–4 Cutaneous listeriosis. Note the numerous gram-positive rods that extend from the dermis below into the epidermis above.

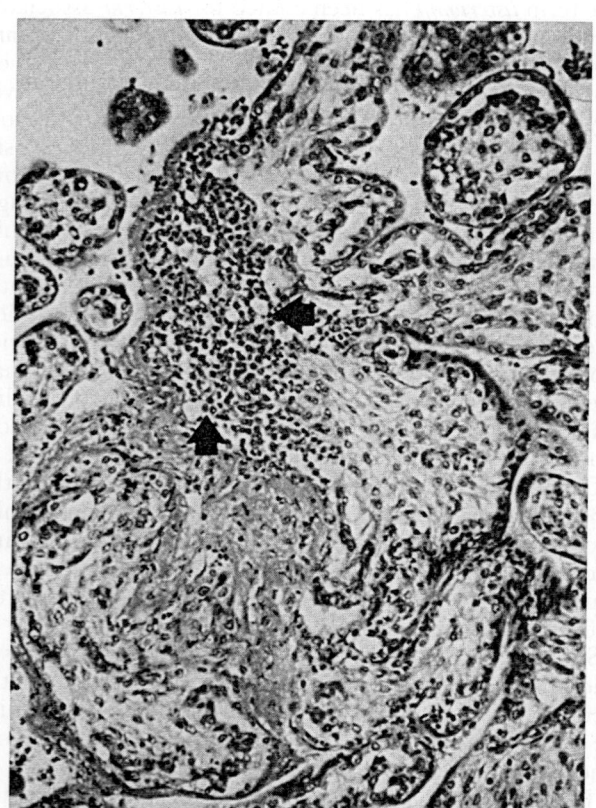

FIGURE 13–5 *Listeria* **placentitis.** Note the microabscess between the necrotic villous trophoblast and the stroma (*arrows*). Chorionic villi are enmeshed by intervillous and inflammatory material.

The gross and microscopic appearance of the placenta in listeriosis, although not pathognomonic, is sufficiently distinct to enable a presumptive diagnosis by an experienced pathologist (Fig. 13–5). *Listeria* placentitis is characterized grossly by multiple minute, white or gray necrotic areas

within the villous parenchyma and decidua; the largest areas tend to occur in basal villi and the decidua basalis [204–206]. These necrotic foci are macroabscesses identical to those described in other fetal organs [200]. Typically, localized collections of PMNs are found between the villous trophoblast and stroma, and inflamed or necrotic chorionic villi are enmeshed in intervillous inflammatory material and fibrin. Chorioamnionitis, deciduitis, villitis, and funisitis (in order of frequency) are seen. Cord lesions may be confined to superficial foci. Gram-positive rods are usually demonstrable within the necrotic centers of villous and decidual microabscesses and within the membranes and umbilical cord. An immunohistochemical stain using polyclonal antibody directed at LLO has also been used for pathologic identification [207].

CLINICAL MANIFESTATIONS

The clinical features of listeriosis are variable and may mimic infection by other organisms or disease states. Five major clinical presentations are distinguishable.

LISTERIOSIS DURING PREGNANCY

The predilection of *Listeria* for the placenta and fetus is well documented in humans [208–212]. Maternal listeriosis is usually transmitted to the fetus by the transplacental route. Although early gestational listeriosis may be undetected [213], clinically identified cases of perinatal listeriosis are easily identifiable after the 5th month of pregnancy, as stillbirth or septic fetuses.

Maternal flulike illness with fever and chills, fatigue, headache, and muscle pains often precedes delivery by 2 to 14 days. Although symptoms in the mother may subside before delivery, infection and fever precipitating delivery are common. Blood cultured from pregnant women can yield *Listeria*. Premature labor in pregnant women with listeriosis is common; length of gestation is less than 35 weeks in approximately 70% of cases. The mortality rate, including stillbirth and abortion, is 40% to 50%. Early treatment of *Listeria* sepsis in pregnancy can prevent infection and sequelae in the fetus and newborn [214,215]. At the time of delivery, maternal symptoms of infection may be pronounced; however, symptoms in the mother usually subside with or without antibiotic treatment soon after delivery.

The pathogenesis of fetal listeriosis is unclear. Because the heaviest foci for neonatal infection are lung and gut, the fetus is probably infected by swallowing contaminated amniotic fluid after placental infection is established. An ascending pathway from the lower genital tract is rare. *L. monocytogenes* chorioamnionitis diagnosed by transabdominal amniocentesis before membrane rupture has been reported and supports a blood-borne route of infection [200,210,215,216]. Placental chorionic vascular thrombi can be associated with maternal coagulopathy. Emboli originating from *Listeria*-infected placental vessels have been described as a cause of congenital stroke in an infant [207].

Susceptibility to *L. monocytogenes* is markedly increased in pregnant animals [181,182,217–219]. Immunoregulation during pregnancy is poorly understood. The placenta constitutes a unique immunologic site because suppression of the local cellular immune response is required to protect the fetus from immunologic rejection [212,220,221]. As a result, infection with intracellular organisms can lead to overwhelming proliferation and disease.

EARLY-ONSET NEONATAL LISTERIOSIS

The first descriptions of neonatal listeriosis were published in the 1930s by Burn [222–224]. Since then, neonatal infection has been recognized as the most common clinical form of human listeriosis. Similar to group B streptococcal infection, neonatal listeriosis is divided into two clinical forms defined by age: early-onset (≤1 week of age) and late-onset (>1 week of age) infection. Clinical and laboratory manifestations of neonatal listeriosis are outlined in Table 13–2, based on clinical cases in which early and late forms of the disease could be differentiated.*

---

*References [78,85,90,102,208,216,225–230].

TABLE 13–2 Clinical and Laboratory Findings of Early-Onset and Late-Onset Neonatal Listeriosis

Feature	Maternal Perinatal Illness (%)	
	Early Onset*	Late Onset[†]
Mortality (%)	25	15
Median age in days (range)	1 (0-6)	14 (7-35)
Male (%)	60	67
Preterm (%)	65	20
Respiratory involvement (%)	50	10
Meningitis (%)	25	95
Blood isolate (%)	75	20
Maternal perinatal illness (%)	50	0

*Data from references [81, 86, 204, 212, 221–225].
[†]Data from references [74, 98, 221, 225, 226].

Classically, early-onset neonatal listeriosis develops within 1 or 2 days of life. Nosocomial transmission is also documented. In one outbreak, nine infants developed nosocomial listeriosis, after being bathed with *L. monocytogenes*–contaminated mineral oil shortly after birth [108]. Contamination of the multidose container occurred with its use on an infant with early-onset listeriosis. Clinical signs of infection developed 4 to 8 days later and were similar to signs seen in late-onset infection (insidious onset of illness with fever and meningitis was common).

Evidence of preceding maternal illness is often described in infants with early-onset disease. Although some maternal symptoms are vague and nonspecific (e.g., malaise, myalgias), others are sufficiently distinctive (i.e., fever, chills) to alert physicians to the risk of prenatally acquired listeriosis. Blood cultures from such mothers are often positive for *Listeria*.

Although early-onset disease may occur in neonates 7 days of age, most cases are clinically apparent at delivery and show meconium staining, cyanosis, apnea, respiratory distress, and pneumonia. Meconium-stained amniotic fluid is a common feature in such infants and may occur at any gestational age. Pneumonia is also common, but radiographic features are nonspecific (peribronchial to widespread infiltration). In long-standing infection, a coarse, mottled, or nodular pattern has been described. Assisted ventilation is frequently necessary in these infants. Persistent hypoxia despite ventilator assistance is seen in severely affected infants.

In severe infection, a granulomatous rash—granulomatosis infantisepticum—has been described (Fig. 13–6). Slightly elevated pale patches (1 to 2 mm in diameter) with a bright erythematous base are seen. Biopsy specimens of these areas show leukocytic infiltrates with multiple bacteria present (see Fig. 13–4).

Laboratory features are nonspecific; a leukocytosis with presence of immature cells may be seen, or neutropenia is noted with severe infection. Thrombocytopenia may also occur [208,226]. Many infants are anemic. These laboratory and clinical features fail to distinguish listeriosis from group B streptococcal or other severe early-onset bacterial infections. The association of early-onset listeriosis with prematurity and maternal infection suggests the presence of intrauterine infection. The frequent presence of chorioamnionitis in the absence of ruptured membranes [85,229] supports the hypothesis of *Listeria* infection occurring by a transplacental route, which differs from the common route of group B streptococcal acquisition via aspiration of contaminated vaginal or amniotic fluids.

LATE-ONSET NEONATAL LISTERIOSIS

Neonatal *Listeria* infection that occurs after 7 days of life is considered late-onset infection. Although there is some overlap between early-onset and late-onset forms of listeriosis, the clinical patterns are usually distinct. Common clinical and laboratory features of late-onset neonatal listeriosis are presented in Table 13–2. The most common form of *Listeria* infection during this period is meningitis, which is present in 94% of late-onset cases. In many centers, *Listeria* ranks second only to group B *Streptococcus* as a cause of bacterial meningitis in this age group, causing approximately 20% of such infection [225].

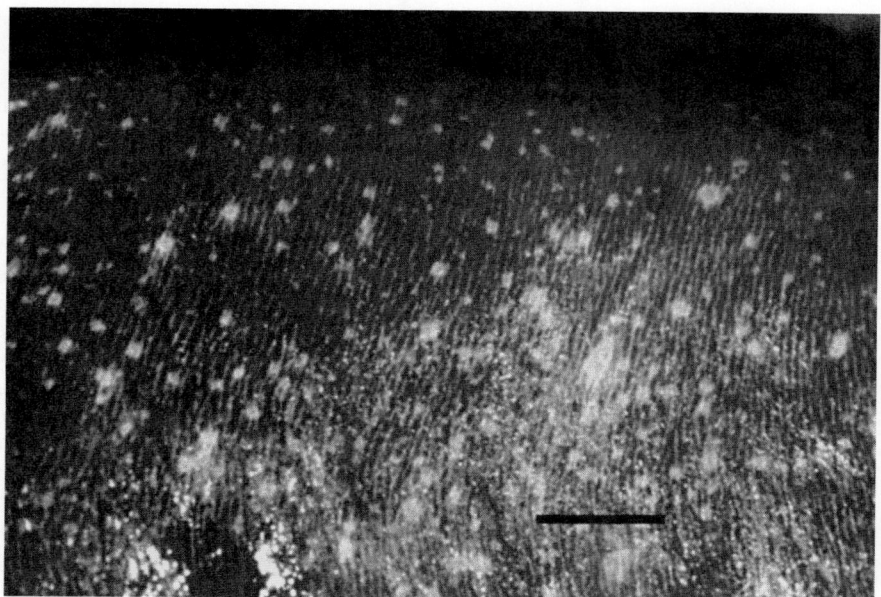

FIGURE 13–6 Rash of neonatal *Listeria monocytogenes* infection. Areas of small, elevated pale pustules surrounded by a deep red erythematous base seen on the abdomen of a premature neonate (*horizontal bar* = approximately 1 cm in length).

Clinical features do not distinguish listerial meningitis in this age group from meningitis with other causes. A striking predominance of boys has been noted in most series. Fever and irritability are predominant clinical features. Often, infants do not appear excessively ill and may elude diagnosis for several days. Other clinical forms of disease at this age are less common, but include *Listeria*-induced colitis with associated diarrhea and sepsis without meningitis [231,232].

Laboratory features of late-onset infection are nonspecific as well. Cell counts in cerebrospinal fluid are usually high, with a predominance of neutrophils and band forms. Occasionally in long-standing disease, numerous monocytes may be seen. Gram stain of cerebrospinal fluid may not always suggest a diagnosis because the organism may be in rare abundance or the morphology can be atypical, or both. Variable decolorization during staining may result in organisms appearing as gram-negative rods or gram-positive cocci. The appearance of organisms as illustrated in Figure 13–7 is characteristic of listeriosis in the early phase of severe meningitis. Mortality of late-onset newborn infection is generally low, unless diagnosis is delayed by more than 3 or 4 days after onset. Long-term sequelae and morbidity are uncommon.

CENTRAL NERVOUS SYSTEM INFECTION (ADULTS)

In many developed countries, *Listeria* has become the third most frequent cause of meningitis in adults, after *Streptococcus pneumoniae* and *Neisseria meningitidis*. A prospective nationwide study examined risk factors and clinical features of *Listeria* meningitis [233]. In 30 cases studied, every patient was either immunocompromised or older than 50 years of age. Clinical features (in contrast to prior atypical descriptions from retrospective studies) were indistinguishable from other causes of community-acquired bacterial meningitis. Almost all patients had at least two of the four classic

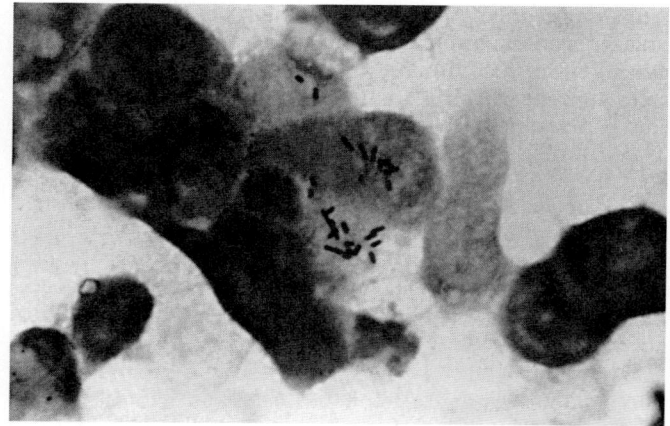

FIGURE 13–7 Short, gram-positive intracellular organisms with variable length and rounded ends are arranged irregularly.

symptoms of fever, headache, neck stiffness, and altered mental status. Congruent with prior reports, onset was subacute in a significant proportion (27%) of cases. Rhombencephalitis with ataxia, cranial nerve palsies, and multiple microabscesses on magnetic resonance imaging (MRI) or computed tomography (CT) is well described as a *Listeria* presentation in humans, as it is in ruminants ("circling disease") [203,234]. Survival of *Listeria* in the CNS is probably helped through cell-to-cell spread of the organism [235]. Morbidity and mortality are high in CNS infection, particularly if brainstem encephalitis is present [90,234,236].

BACTEREMIA

In immunocompromised patients, bacteremia is the most common manifestation of *Listeria* infection, with meningitis second in frequency [77]. Clinical signs are indistinguishable from bacteremia caused by other organisms and typically include fever and myalgias after a prodromal illness of nausea and diarrhea. The risk of invasive listeriosis in patients treated with antibody to TNF-α, with a malignancy, with HIV infection, or after organ transplant may be 1000 times the risk of otherwise healthy persons [85,237,238]. During the bacteremic phase, accompanying conjunctivitis is sometimes observed. Anton eye test [239] actually resulted from a laboratory accident in which a technician contaminated his face.

OTHER CLINICAL FORMS OF INFECTION

A febrile gastroenteritis syndrome is now well recognized in adults and children. Disease appears sporadically, but at least seven outbreaks have been reported [240]. Although symptoms overlap considerably, children are more likely to have fever and vomiting, whereas adults typically have arthromyalgias and nonbloody diarrhea. Other symptoms include sore throat and profound fatigue. After ingestion of contaminated foodstuffs, incubation is usually less than 24 hours, but has ranged from 6 hours to 10 days. Processed meats have been repeatedly implicated [241], but other outbreaks have involved contaminated shrimp salad [242], rice salad [243], and chocolate milk [232]. The largest outbreak, in Italy, affected more than 1500 people [244]. Only a few patients developed invasive disease (sepsis) in these outbreaks, and the level of Listeria contamination apparently was very high [245].

Papular cutaneous lesions are often observed in newborns when listeriosis is disseminated. These lesions are to be distinguished from the primary skin lesions caused by Listeria as observed in adults [52,246], which are the result of direct contact, such as the handling of a cow's placenta after abortion by a veterinarian or farmer [53]. Other unusual forms of listeriosis, such as endocarditis [247,248], endophthalmitis [249,250], liver abscesses [201], peritonitis [251,252], osteomyelitis, and septic arthritis [238], have been described in adults, but are rare in infants.

DIAGNOSIS

The clinical signs and symptoms of listeriosis overlap considerably with other illnesses, making a specific diagnosis difficult, if not impossible, when patients are first seen.

SEROLOGY

The classic agglutination reaction (Widal test) shows antibodies against O and H antigens of the various Listeria serovars. Because of the antigenic complexity of L. monocytogenes, no agreement has been reached on the interpretation of agglutination reactions for diagnostic purposes.

Attempts to show complement-fixing Listeria antibodies date back to the 1930s [253]. In one study, serum samples collected from 32 mothers with perinatal Listeria infection were compared with 128 samples from matched controls [254]. The sensitivity and specificity of the complement fixation test were found to be 78% and 91%; however, the positive predictive value was only 75%. A titer of 1:8 or more is accepted as significant [234,255,256].

Detection of antibodies to LLO has also been used to diagnose human listeriosis [257]. Purified LLO incorporated into nitrocellulose filters is tested with serial dilutions of sera. Absorbed anti-LLO is identified using enzyme-labeled anti–human IgG. Sensitivity and specificity of the test are greater than 90%, and during a febrile gastroenteritis outbreak, it correlated well with clinical illness [232]. Although these results are impressive, the technique is not commercially available. A precipitin test [258], indirect hemagglutination reaction [259], and antigen fixation test [260] have also been described; these showed apparent success, but remain unavailable on a widespread basis.

ISOLATION OF THE ORGANISM

Cultivation of L. monocytogenes is the gold standard of diagnosis. Culture of venous blood, ascitic and other fluids, cervical material, urine, placenta, amniotic fluid, lochia and meconium, and tissues at biopsy or autopsy offers the best chances for identifying Listeria in individuals with disease. Culture of the stool is not done routinely because feces are positive for Listeria in 1% to 5% of healthy women [55,261]. In an outbreak setting, stool culture with selective media may recover organisms for comparative typing (see "Organism").

Microscopic diagnosis may be attempted by use of Gram stain only in normally sterile specimens: cerebrospinal fluid, meconium, and tissue smears. The finding of short, sometimes coccoid, gram-positive rods strongly supports a suspicion of listeriosis and is indicative of this infection in meconium smears. Occasionally, L. monocytogenes may appear Gram positive or Gram negative or even predominantly coccoid. With long-standing disease or when the patient has received antibiotics, Listeria may appear gram-negative and be confused with H. influenzae when observed in the cerebrospinal fluid. In other instances, Listeria has been mistaken for pneumococci and corynebacteria.

MOLECULAR DETECTION

Increasingly, PCR-based methods are used to detect Listeria in clinical samples such as cerebrospinal fluid [262,263]. PCR technology has progressed faster than regulatory standards, however, making quality assurance a significant issue with "home brew" molecular testing. Spurred by the food industry's demand for rapid and sensitive Listeria detection, approved kits for real-time PCR [264] and amplification with sequencing of Listeria 16S ribosomal RNA genes [265] are being adopted for food screening. The infrequent occurrence of clinical Listeria disease and the costly approval process for clinical diagnostic kits have resulted in limited availability of commercial diagnostic kits for clinical specimens.

PROGNOSIS

Neonatal listeriosis accounts for the largest recognizable group of infections caused by L. monocytogenes. Fetal loss with early gestational infection is a recognized complication of maternal infection. In late gestational maternal infection, sparing of the fetus has been reported [266], but it is likely uncommon unless antepartum antibiotic treatment has been given to the mother [267,268].

Although fetal or neonatal infection with L. monocytogenes is known to have a high fatality rate, the long-term morbidity is unclear. Rotheberg and associates [269] found an increased incidence of developmental delay assessed at a mean age of 29.5 months among small (<1250 g at birth), *Listeria*-infected infants who required assisted ventilation. Naege [270], studying children 4 to 7 years after they recovered from early-onset listeriosis, also found increased neurodevelopmental handicaps. Other authors have reported hydrocephalus [271].

In contrast, Evans and coworkers [272] found no evidence of neurodevelopmental sequelae in six of eight survivors studied at a mean age of 15 months and again at 32 months. The two infants with neurodevelopmental sequelae had severe acute perinatal sepsis with meningitis. Both had spastic diplegia. The authors concluded that long-term sequelae after neonatal early-onset listeriosis were uncommon. If meningitis is not present, the outcome may be generally good. The prognosis for infants with late-onset neonatal sepsis and meningitis has not been studied extensively.

THERAPY

Listeria is susceptible to antibiotics commonly used in its treatment [253,273]. The high mortality rate and risk of relapse [254,274] have prompted a search for newer therapeutic regimens, however, including quinolones [275], trimethoprim-sulfamethoxazole [276,277], and rifampin [278]. Transferable plasmid-mediated antibiotic resistance has been reported [279] conferring resistance to chloramphenicol, tetracycline, and erythromycin.

IN VITRO STUDIES

Susceptibility testing for *Listeria* has become more standardized with the publication of guidelines by the Clinical and Laboratory Standards Institute [280]. Until the late 1980s, clinical strains showed nearly universal susceptibility to ampicillin, penicillin, vancomycin, erythromycin, and tetracycline [281–283]. Since then, several reports have documented resistance to non–β-lactam antibiotics such as tetracycline and gentamicin [282,283]. Of more concern, penicillin and gentamicin resistance has been increasingly reported in environmental isolates from farms [284,285]. For many antibiotics, the minimal bactericidal concentration is often higher than clinically attainable levels, making them bacteriostatic, not bactericidal. Bactericidal antibiotics have a potential advantage for patients with impaired host defense mechanisms [286].

Studies with cephalosporin antibiotics have been consistently disappointing: The organism exhibits intrinsic high-level cephalosporin resistance [287]. Cephalosporins are incorporated into selective media (i.e., PALCAM agar) to inhibit other bacteria and enhance *Listeria* recovery [218]. Activity of newer fluoroquinolones against *L. monocytogenes* is promising [288,289]. One study found moxifloxacin to be the most effective antibiotic tested for eradication of the organism from the intracellular compartment [288].

IN VIVO STUDIES

Several combinations of antibiotics [271,289–291] have been compared for their bactericidal activity against *L. monocytogenes* in vivo. Animal models have been a necessary way to assess therapeutic regimens, given the infrequency of human disease. Murine models employing normal adults [277,292], cortisone-treated adults [293], immunodeficient adults [294–296], and animals infected by inhalation of aerosolized *Listeria* [277] have been reported, and a rabbit meningitis model has been described [297,298]. The model most analogous to neonatal disease was described by Hawkins and colleagues [299]. In their study, neonatal rats received intraperitoneal inoculations and were randomly assigned to begin antibiotic regimens 2 days later.

Conflicting results complicate the interpretation of animal models. In addition to variable techniques (e.g., route of injection, bacterial strain, inoculum size), pharmacokinetic differences in various animal species must be considered. Rifampin metabolism differs widely among animal species [297,299,300], and the half-life of ampicillin is longer in human neonates than in most adult animals. In one study of adult mice infected with *L. monocytogenes*, no synergy was shown using ampicillin and gentamicin [301]. In the neonatal listeriosis model of Hawkins and colleagues [299], combining ampicillin and gentamicin was significantly better at eradicating organisms than ampicillin alone. Similarly, the combination trimethoprim-sulfamethoxazole was found to be superior to either drug alone [299]. In vivo studies of other antibiotics are also conflicting: Some authors have found rifampin to be highly active [277,300], whereas others have found it to be ineffective [302]. Strain variation may account for the widely discrepant results. In addition, rifampin monotherapy may lead to development of resistance. The use of ciprofloxacin in animal models has not suggested any therapeutic advantage over ampicillin [293,303]; however, moxifloxacin was equivalent to ampicillin plus gentamicin in an animal model [298].

CLINICAL REPORTS

No prospective clinical trials for *L. monocytogenes* human infection have been reported. Anecdotal case reports or reviews after outbreaks generally support conclusions drawn from in vivo models. In one review of 119 cases of listeriosis from three centers in the United States, excellent therapeutic results were seen for patients treated empirically with penicillin or ampicillin; all had a reduction of fever and clinical improvement. Patients treated initially with cephalosporins had persistent fever and infection, however [303]. In the largest assessment of treatment regimens during a single outbreak [304], a lower mortality was reported for children given ampicillin (16% of 57 children) compared with children treated with chloramphenicol, tetracycline, or streptomycin (33% of 82 children). Trimethoprim-sulfamethoxazole has generally been used as second-line or alternative therapy in patients with significant β-lactam allergy. Case reports have also documented successful therapy of invasive infections with vancomycin [248,249]. Treatment failures and recurrent listeriosis are well described [254]. In some cases, weeks or months elapse between episodes. Two more recent studies looked at susceptibility profiles from clinical isolates over the past 50 years [305,306]. Both studies found that penicillin or ampicillin and gentamicin—the mainstay of therapy—remained predictably effective against *Listeria*.

SUGGESTED MANAGEMENT
Listeriosis during Pregnancy

If amnionitis is present, initial treatment should be given by the intravenous route to ensure adequate tissue levels (ampicillin, 4 to 6 g/day divided into four equal doses plus an aminoglycoside). If amnionitis is not present, or if acute symptoms of amnionitis have subsided, oral antibiotics are an option (amoxicillin, 1 to 2 g/day divided into three equal doses). In both situations, treatment should continue for 14 days. If the patient has a significant β-lactam allergy, therapeutic options are limited. Erythromycin may be given (the estolate form should be avoided because of increased liver toxicity during pregnancy), although there are no universal susceptibility guidelines for erythromycin and *Listeria*. Trimethoprim-sulfamethoxazole is an active agent, but theoretical risks of use in pregnancy must be balanced against potential benefits [307].

Early-Onset Neonatal Listeriosis

Ampicillin in combination with an aminoglycoside is the preferred management for early-onset infection. For infants with body weight less than 2000 g, 100 mg/kg/day divided into two equal doses should be administered for the 1st week of life. For infants with body weight of more than 2000 g, 150 mg/kg/day divided into three equal doses should be administered for the 1st week of life. For the 2nd week of life, the appropriate dosages are 150 mg/kg/day and 200 mg/kg/day for infants weighing less than 2000 g body weight and more than 2000 g body weight respectively. Aminoglycoside doses vary with the agent chosen. For gentamicin, the suggested dosages are 5 mg/kg/day divided into two equal doses for the 1st week of life and 7.5 mg/kg/day divided into three equal doses for the 2nd week of life. For early-onset neonatal sepsis caused by *L. monocytogenes*, 10 to 14 days of treatment is recommended; however, a longer course of treatment should be given in the uncommon event of early-onset neonatal listeriosis with meningitis.

Late-Onset Neonatal Listeriosis

Meningitis is commonly present in late-onset listeriosis. Delayed eradication of the organism may be seen in such cases. Ampicillin (200 to 400 mg/kg/day divided into four to six equal doses) in combination with an aminoglycoside is recommended. Lumbar puncture should be repeated in 48 to 72 hours to assess effectiveness of therapy. In the event of delayed clearance (>2 days), further investigations are indicated, including CT or cranial ultrasound to assess for the presence of cerebritis, brain abscess, or intracranial hemorrhage. If the organism remains present in the cerebrospinal fluid after several days, the addition of vancomycin, rifampin, or trimethoprim-sulfamethoxazole may be considered. Experience with such combination therapy for listeriosis in neonates is limited [308]. Cephalosporin antibiotics are not active against *Listeria*. Length of treatment is generally 14 to 21 days, depending on clinical course.

PREVENTION AND OUTBREAK MANAGEMENT

Food-borne outbreaks of listeriosis are unpredictable and may occur in a wide geographic area. Reporting of all cases of listeriosis to public health authorities is important to identify outbreaks early. Case-control studies and environmental sampling are important aspects of outbreak investigations. Strains of *Listeria* from clinical and environmental isolates should be forwarded to a reference laboratory for appropriate epidemiologic typing. Serotyping and multifocus enzyme electrophoresis typing should be performed to characterize the epidemic strain.

During an outbreak of listeriosis, pregnant women presenting with sepsis syndrome or a flulike illness should be empirically treated with ampicillin and an aminoglycoside after appropriate cultures of blood, rectum, and vagina have been obtained. Amniocentesis for diagnosis of chorioamnionitis may be appropriate [309]. If membranes have ruptured and contamination is suspected, use of selective media may enhance the isolation of *Listeria* from these patients.

The recognition that sporadic cases of listeriosis are food-borne has prompted wide use of preventive guidelines by the CDC (Table 13–3) [60,310]. Guidelines for preventing listeriosis are similar to guidelines for preventing other food-borne illnesses and include thorough cooking of raw food from animals and thorough washing of vegetables and utensils. Persons at high risk, such as pregnant women, should also avoid soft cheeses and prepared salads, meats, and cheeses from deli counters.

TABLE 13–3   Recommendations for Reducing the Risk of Listeriosis

General Recommendations
Thoroughly cook raw food from animal sources (e.g., beef, pork, and poultry)
Wash raw vegetables thoroughly before eating
Keep uncooked meats separate from vegetables and from cooked foods and ready-to-eat foods
Avoid raw (unpasteurized) milk or foods made from unpasteurized milk
Wash hands, knives, and cutting boards after handling uncooked foods
Consume perishable and ready-to-eat foods as soon as possible

Additional Recommendations for High-Risk Groups
Do not eat hot dogs or ready-to-eat foods such as deli meats unless they are reheated until steaming hot
Wash hands after handling hot dogs and ready-to-eat foods
Do not eat soft cheeses (e.g., feta, Brie, and Camembert) or blue-veined cheeses unless they have labels that clearly state they are made from pasteurized milk
Do not eat refrigerated pâtés or meat spreads; canned or "shelf-stable" (pasteurized) pâtés and meat spreads may be eaten
Do not eat refrigerated smoked seafood unless it is contained in a cooked dish, such as a casserole; canned or shelf-stable smoked seafood may be eaten

Data from Lynch M, et al. Surveillance for foodborne-disease outbreaks—United States, 1998-2002. MMWR Surveill Summ 55:1-42, 2006; and Listeria Fact Sheet—Updated. Guelph, Ontario, University of Guelph Food Safety Network, 2003.

One more recent study also implicated hummus and melons as a cause of sporadic *Listeria* illness [74]. Because of the severity of illness, pregnant women and others at risk may wish to add these to the list of foods to avoid. Thoroughly heating leftover foods until they are steaming hot has also been recommended [60]. Appreciation of the food guidelines by pregnant women is limited. Improved education of pregnant women regarding risk of listeriosis in pregnancy is needed [311,312]. A decrease in the rates of listeriosis in some geographic areas in the United States has been temporally associated with the publication of these guidelines and industry efforts directed at removing food-borne pathogens from the food chain [75,310,313].

REFERENCES

[1] A. Nyfeldt, Étiologie de la mononucléose infectieuse, Compt. Rend. Biol. 101 (1929) 590.

[2] E.D.G. Murray, R.A. Webb, M.B.R. Swann, A disease of rabbits characterized by a large mononuclear leucocytosis, caused by a hitherto undescribed *Bacillus: Bacterium monocytogenes*, J. Pathol. Bacteriol. 29 (1926) 407.

[3] J.H.H. Pirie, A new disease of veld rodents, Tiger River disease 3 (1927) 163.

[4] J.H.H. Pirie, Change of name for a genus of bacteria, Nature 145 (1940) 264.

[5] J. Bille, M.P. Doyle, Listeria and Erysipelothrix, in: A. Ballows, et al., (Eds.), Manual of Clinical Microbiology, fifth ed., American Society of Microbiology, Washington, DC, 1991, pp. 287–295.

[6] H.R.P. Seeliger, Listeriosis, S Karger, Basel, 1961.

[7] M. Peel, W. Donachie, A. Shaw, Temperature-dependent expression of flagella of *Listeria monocytogenes* studied by electron microscopy, SDS-PAGE and western blotting, J. Gen. Microbiol. 134 (1988) 2171.

[8] P. van Netten, et al., Liquid and solid selective differential media for the detection and enumeration of *L. monocytogenes* and other *Listeria* species, Int. J. Food. Microbiol. 8 (1989) 299.

[9] M.L. Gray, et al., A new technique for isolating listerellae from the bovine brain, J. Bacteriol. 55 (1948) 471.

[10] J.A. Cepeda, et al., Listeriosis due to infection with a catalase-negative strain of *Listeria monocytogenes*, J. Clin. Microbiol. 44 (2006) 1917–1918.

[11] H.R.P. Seeliger, D. Jones, Genus Listeria, in: P.H.A. Sneeth, et al., (Eds.), Berge's Manual of Systematic Bacteriology, vol. 2, Williams & Wilkins, Baltimore, 1986.

[12] H.R.P. Seeliger, H. Finger, Analytical serology of *Listeria*, in: J.B. G. Kwapinski (Ed.), Analytical Serology of Microorganisms, John Wiley, New York, 1969, p. 549.

[13] D. Liu, Identification, subtyping and virulence determination of *Listeria monocytogenes*, an important foodborne pathogen, J. Med. Microbiol. 55 (Pt 6) (2006) 645–659.

[14] C.P. Sword, M.J. Pickett, The isolation and characterization of bacteriophages from *Listeria monocytogenes*, J. Gen. Microbiol. 25 (1961) 241.

[15] J. McLauchlin, A. Audurier, A.G. Taylor, The evaluation of a phage-typing system for *Listeria monocytogenes* for use in epidemiological studies, J. Med. Microbiol. 22 (1986) 357.

[16] W.F. Schlech 3rd., et al., Epidemic listeriosis—evidence for transmission by food, N. Engl. J. Med. 308 (1983) 203.

[17] J.C. Piffaretti, et al., Genetic characterization of clones of the bacterium *Listeria monocytogenes* causing epidemic disease, Proc. Natl. Acad. Sci. U. S. A. 86 (1989) 3818.

[18] L.M. Graves, et al., Ribosomal DNA fingerprinting of *Listeria monocytogenes* using a digoxigenin-labeled DNA probe, Eur. J. Epidemiol. 7 (1991) 77.

[19] B.P. Richardson, M. Adams, Allozyme Electrophoresis: A Handbook for Animal Systematics and Population Studies, Academic Press, Orlando, FL, 1986.

[20] C. Carriere, et al., DNA polymorphism in strains of *Listeria monocytogenes*, J. Clin. Microbiol. 29 (1991) 1351.

[21] P.J. Slade, D.L. Collins-Thompson, Differentiation of the genus *Listeria* from other gram-positive species based on low molecular weight (LMW) RNA profiles, J. Appl. Bacteriol. 70 (1991) 355.

[22] J.R.J. Bille, B. Swaminathan, *Listeria* and erysipelothrix, in: P.R. Murray (Ed.), Manual of Clinical Microbiology, eighth ed., AMS Press, Washington, DC, 2003, pp. 461–471.

[23] D.A. Portnoy, et al., Molecular determinants of *Listeria monocytogenes* pathogenesis, Infect. Immun. 60 (1992) 1263.

[24] J.A. Vazquez-Boland, et al., Listeria pathogenesis and molecular virulence determinants, Clin. Microbiol. Rev. 14 (2001) 584–640.

[25] V. Ramaswamy, et al., Listeria—review of epidemiology and pathogenesis, J. Microbiol. Immunol. Infect. 40 (2007) 4–13.

[26] M.J. Gray, N.E. Freitag, K.J. Boor, How the bacterial pathogen *Listeria monocytogenes* mediates the switch from environmental Dr. Jekyll to pathogenic Mr. Hyde, Infect. Immun. 74 (2006) 2505–2512.

[27] S. Gottesman, S. Wickner, M.R. Maurizi, Protein quality control: triage by chaperones and proteases, Genes Dev. 11 (1997) 815–823.

[28] W. van Schaik, T. Abee, The role of sigmaB in the stress response of Gram-positive bacteria—targets for food preservation and safety, Curr. Opin. Biotechnol. 16 (2005) 218–224.

[29] H. Saklani-Jusforgues, E. Fontan, P.L. Goossens, Effect of acid-adaptation on *Listeria monocytogenes* survival and translocation in a murine intragastric infection model, FEMS Microbiol. Lett. 193 (2000) 155–159.

[30] J.L. Gaillard, et al., Entry of *L. monocytogenes* into cells is mediated by internalin, a repeat protein reminiscent of surface antigens from gram-positive cocci, Cell 65 (1991) 1127.

[31] K. Ireton, P. Cossart, Host-pathogen interactions during entry and actin-based movement of *Listeria monocytogenes*, Annu. Rev. Genet. 31 (1997) 113–138.

[32] C. Sabet, et al., The *Listeria monocytogenes* virulence factor InlJ is specifically expressed in vivo and behaves as an adhesin, Infect. Immun. 76 (2008) 1368–1378.

[33] M. Lecuit, et al., A single amino acid in E-cadherin responsible for host specificity towards the human pathogen *Listeria monocytogenes*, EMBO J 18 (1999) 3956–3963.

[34] J. Hess, et al., *Listeria monocytogenes* p60 supports host cell invasion by and in vivo survival of attenuated *Salmonella typhimurium*, Infect. Immun. 63 (1995) 2047–2053.

[35] J.T. Harty, E.G. Pamer, CD8 T lymphocytes specific for the secreted p60 antigen protect against *Listeria monocytogenes* infection, J. Immunol. 154 (1995) 4642–4650.

[36] S. Seveau, J. Pizarro-Cerda, P. Cossart, Molecular mechanisms exploited by *Listeria monocytogenes* during host cell invasion, Microbes. Infect. 9 (2007) 1167–1175.

[37] D.A. Portnoy, P.S. Jacks, D.J. Hinrichs, Role of hemolysin for the intracellular growth of *Listeria monocytogenes*, J. Exp. Med. 167 (1988) 1459.

[38] M.A. Moors, et al., Expression of listeriolysin O and ActA by intracellular and extracellular *Listeria monocytogenes*, Infect. Immun. 67 (1999) 131–139.

[39] L.M. Shetron-Rama, et al., Intracellular induction of *Listeria monocytogenes* actA expression, Infect. Immun. 70 (2002) 1087–1096.

[40] C. Kocks, et al., Polarized distribution of *Listeria monocytogenes* surface protein ActA at the site of directional actin assembly, J. Cell. Sci. 105 (Pt 3) (1993) 699–710.

[41] J.A. Vazquez-Boland, et al., Nucleotide sequence of the lecithinase operon of *Listeria monocytogenes* and possible role of lecithinase in cell-to-cell spread, Infect. Immun. 60 (1992) 219.

[42] J. Raveneau, et al., Reduced virulence of a *Listeria monocytogenes* phospholipase-deficient mutant obtained by transposon insertion into the zinc metalloprotease gene, Infect. Immun. 60 (1992) 916.

[43] J. Mengaud, et al., Pleiotropic control of *Listeria monocytogenes* virulence factors by a gene that is autoregulated, Mol. Microbiol. 5 (1991) 2273.

[44] E. Domann, et al., Identification and characterization of a novel PrfA-regulated gene in *Listeria monocytogenes* whose product, IrpA, is highly homologous to internalin proteins, which contain leucine-rich repeats, Infect. Immun. 65 (1997) 101–109.

[45] E. Michel, et al., Characterization of a large motility gene cluster containing the cheR, motAB genes of *Listeria monocytogenes* and evidence that PrfA downregulates motility genes, FEMS. Microbiol. Lett. 169 (1998) 341–347.

[46] P.V. Liu, J.L. Bates, An extracellular haemorrhagic toxin produced by *Listeria monocytogenes*, Can. J. Microbiol. 7 (1961) 107.

[47] M. Leimeister-Wachter, E. Domann, T. Chakraborty, The expression of virulence genes in *Listeria monocytogenes* is thermoregulated, J. Bacteriol. 174 (1992) 947–952.

[48] N.F. Stanley, Studies on *Listeria monocytogenes*. I. Isolation of a monocytosis-producing agent, Aust. J. Exp. Biol. Med. Sci. 27 (1949) 123.

[49] D.T. Shum, S.B. Galsworthy, Stimulation of monocyte production by an endogenous mediator induced by a component from *Listeria monocytogenes*, Immunology 46 (1982) 343.

[50] H.J. Welshimer, Isolation of *Listeria monocytogenes* from vegetation, J. Bacteriol. 95 (1968) 300.

[51] J.C. Low, C.P. Renton, Septicaemia, encephalitis and abortions in a housed flock of sheep caused by *Listeria monocytogenes* type 1/2, Vet. Rec. 114 (1985) 147.

[52] C.R. Owen, et al., A case of primary cutaneous listeriosis, N. Engl. J. Med. 262 (1960) 1026.

[53] J. McLauchlin, J.C. Low, Primary cutaneous listeriosis in adults: an occupational disease of veterinarians and farmers, Vet. Rec. 135 (1994) 615–617.

[54] K. Elischerova, S. Stupalova, Listeriosis in professionally exposed persons, Acta. Microbiol. Acad. Sci. Hung. 19 (1972) 379.

[55] J. Bojsen-Moller, Human listeriosis: Diagnostic, epidemiological and clinical studies, Acta. Pathol. Microbiol. Scand. Suppl. 229 (1972) 1.

[56] V. Goulet, et al., Increasing incidence of listeriosis in France and other European countries, Emerg. Infect. Dis. 14 (2008) 734–740.

[57] Y. Doorduyn, et al., Invasive *Listeria monocytogenes* infections in the Netherlands, 1995–2003, Eur. J. Clin. Microbiol. Infect. Dis. 25 (2006) 433–442.

[58] P. Gerner-Smidt, et al., Invasive listeriosis in Denmark 1994–2003: a review of 299 cases with special emphasis on risk factors for mortality, Clin. Microbiol. Infect. 11 (2005) 618–624.

[59] J. Koch, K. Stark, Significant increase of listeriosis in Germany—epidemiological patterns 2001-2005, Euro. Surveill. 11 (2006) 85–88.

[60] CDC, Outbreak of listeriosis—northeastern United States, 2002, MMWR. Morb. Mortal. Wkly Rep. 51 (2002) 950–951.

[61] W.F. Schlech 3rd., Foodborne listeriosis, Clin. Infect. Dis. 31 (2000) 770–775.

[62] S. Tienungoon, et al., Growth limits of *Listeria monocytogenes* as a function of temperature, pH, NaCl, and lactic acid, Appl. Environ. Microbiol. 66 (2000) 4979–4987.

[63] J. McLauchlin, et al., Human listeriosis and pate: a possible association, BMJ 303 (1991) 773–775.

[64] A. Lepoutre, et al., Epidemie de listerioses en France, Epidemiol. Hebdonv. 25 (1992) 115.

[65] CDC, Multistate outbreak of listeriosis—United States, 2000, MMWR Morb. Mortal. Wkly Rep. 49 (2000) 1129–1130.

[66] L.M. Rorvik, et al., Molecular epidemiological survey of *Listeria monocytogenes* in seafoods and seafood-processing plants, Appl. Environ. Microbiol. 66 (2000) 4779–4784.

[67] S.J. Olsen, et al., Multistate outbreak of *Listeria monocytogenes* infection linked to delicatessen turkey meat, Clin. Infect. Dis. 40 (2005) 962–967.

[68] P.S. Mead, et al., Nationwide outbreak of listeriosis due to contaminated meat, Epidemiol. Infect. 134 (2006) 744–751.

[69] V. Vaillant, et al., Foodborne infections in France, Foodborne Pathog. Dis. 2 (2005) 221–232.

[70] M. Lynch, et al., Surveillance for foodborne-disease outbreaks—United States, 1998–2002, MMWR Surveill. Summ. 55 (2006) 1–42.

[71] J.M. Farber, W.H. Ross, J. Harwig, Health risk assessment of *Listeria monocytogenes* in Canada, Int. J. Food Microbiol. 1–2 (1996) 145–156 30.

[72] J. McLaughlin, M.H. Greenwood, P.M. Pini, The occurrence of *Listeria monocytogenes* in cheese from a manufacturer associated with a case of listeriosis, Int. J. Food Microbiol. 10 (1990) 25.

[73] R.W. Pinner, et al., Role of foods in sporadic listeriosis. II. Microbiologic and epidemiologic investigation, JAMA 267 (1992) 2046.

[74] J.K. Varma, et al., *Listeria monocytogenes* infection from foods prepared in a commercial establishment: a case-control study of potential sources of sporadic illness in the United States, Clin. Infect. Dis. 44 (2007) 521–528.

[75] A.C. Voetsch, et al., Reduction in the incidence of invasive listeriosis in foodborne diseases active surveillance network sites, 1996–2003, Clin. Infect. Dis. 44 (2007) 513–520.

[76] K.C. Klontz, et al., Role of the U.S. Food and Drug Administration in the regulatory management of human listeriosis in the United States, J. Food Prot. 71 (2008) 1277–1286.

[77] B.G. Gellin, et al., The epidemiology of listeriosis in the United States—1986. Listeriosis Study Group, Am. J. Epidemiol. 133 (1991) 392.

[78] Y. Siegman-Igra, et al., *Listeria monocytogenes* infection in Israel and review of cases worldwide, Emerg. Infect. Dis. 8 (2002) 305–310.

[79] M.L. Paul, et al., Listeriosis—a review of eighty-four cases, Med. J. Aust. 160 (1994) 489–493.

[80] L. Newton, et al., Listeriosis surveillance: 1990, CDR (Lond Eng Rev) 1 (1991) R110–R113.

[81] W.F. Schlech 3rd., et al., Does sporadic *Listeria* gastroenteritis exist? A 2-year population-based survey in Nova Scotia, Canada, Clin. Infect. Dis. 41 (2005) 778–784.

[82] L. Mascola, et al., Fecal carriage of *Listeria monocytogenes*: observations during a community-wide, common-source outbreak, Clin. Infect. Dis. 15 (1992) 557–558.

[83] P.V. Varughese, A.O. Carter, Human listeriosis in Canada—1988, Can. Dis. Wkly Rep. 15 (1989) 213.

[84] G. Schmidt-Wolf, H.P. Seeliger, A. Schretten-Brunner, Menschilishe listeroisise-erkrankungen in der Bundesrepublik Deutschland 1969–1985, Zentralbl. Bakteriol. Mikrobiol. Hyg. 265 (1985) 472.

[85] J. Nolla-Salas, et al., Perinatal listeriosis: a population-based multicenter study in Barcelona, Spain (1990–1996), Am. J. Perinatol. 15 (1998) 461–467.

[86] J. McLaughlin, Human listeriosis in Britain, 1967–1985, a summary of 722 cases: 1. Listeriosis during pregnancy and the newborn, Epidemiol. Infect. 104 (1990) 181.

[87] R.J. Lamont, R. Postlethwaite, Carriage of *Listeria monocytogenes* and related species in pregnant and non-pregnant women in Aberdeen, Scotland, J. Infect. 13 (1986) 187.

[88] D.B. Louria, et al., Listeriosis complicating malignant disease: a new association, Ann. Intern. Med. 67 (1967) 261.

[89] A. Schuchat, B. Swaminathan, C.V. Broome, Epidemiology of human listeriosis, Clin. Microbiol. Rev. 4 (1991) 169.

[90] B. Lorber, Listeriosis, Clin. Infect. Dis. 24 (1997) 1–9.

[91] J.K. Miller, M. Hedberg, Effects of cortisone on susceptibility of mice to *Listeria monocytogenes*, Am. J. Clin. Pathol. 43 (1965) 248.

[92] A.W. Hugin, et al., Effect of cyclosporin A on immunity to *Listeria monocytogenes*, Infect. Immun. 52 (1986) 12.

[93] J.C. Petit, et al., Suppression of cellular immunity to *Listeria monocytogenes* by activated macrophages: mediation by prostaglandins, Infect. Immun. 49 (1985) 383.

[94] A.M. Stamm, et al., Listeriosis in renal transplant recipients: report of an outbreak and review of 102 cases, Rev. Infect. Dis. 4 (1982) 665.

[95] B.G. Gellin, C.V. Broome, Listeriosis, JAMA 261 (1989) 1313.

[96] C. Cabellos, et al., Community-acquired bacterial meningitis in cirrhotic patients, Clin. Microbiol. Infect. 14 (2008) 35–40.

[97] R.E. Nieman, B. Lorber, Listeriosis in adults: a changing pattern. Report of eight cases and review of the literature, 1968–1978, Rev. Infect. Dis. 2 (1980) 207.

[98] W.F. Schlech 3rd., D.P. Chase, A. Badley, A model of foodborne *Listeria monocytogenes* infection in the Sprague-Dawley rat using gastric inoculation: development and effect of gastric acidity on infective dose, Int. J. Food. Microbiol. 18 (1993) 15.

[99] J.L. Ho, et al., An outbreak of type 4b *Listeria monocytogenes* infection involving patients from eight Boston hospitals, Arch. Intern. Med. 146 (1986) 520.

[100] A.L. Florman, V. Sundararajan, Listeriosis among nursery mates, Pediatrics 41 (1968) 784.

[101] S. Larson, *Listeria monocytogenes* causing hospital-acquired enterocolitis and meningitis in newborn infants, BMJ 2 (1978) 473.

[102] G.A. Filice, et al., *Listeria monocytogenes* infection in neonates: investigation of an epidemic, J. Infect. Dis. 138 (1978) 17.

[103] A.N. Campbell, P.R. Sill, J.K. Wardle, *Listeria* meningitis acquired by cross infection in a delivery suite, Lancet 2 (1981) 752.

[104] K.E. Nelson, et al., Transmission of neonatal listeriosis in a delivery room, Am. J. Dis. Child. 139 (1985) 903.

[105] M.D. Simmons, P.M. Cockcroft, O.A. Okubadejo, Neonatal listeriosis due to cross-infection in an obstetric theatre, J. Infect. 13 (1986) 235.

[106] J.C. Graham, et al., Hospital-acquired listeriosis, J. Hosp. Infect. 51 (2002) 136–139.

[107] R.E. Guevara, et al., *Listeria monocytogenes* in platelets: a case report, Transfusion 46 (2006) 305–309.

[108] A. Schuchat, et al., Outbreak of neonatal listeriosis associated with mineral oil, Pediatr. Infect. Dis. J. 10 (1991) 183.

[109] M.A. Smith, et al., Dose-response model for *Listeria monocytogenes*-induced stillbirths in nonhuman primates, Infect. Immun. 76 (2008) 726–731.

[110] M. Lecuit, Understanding how *Listeria monocytogenes* targets and crosses host barriers, Clin. Microbiol. Infect. 11 (2005) 430–436.

[111] M. Mitsuyama, et al., Three phases of phagocyte contribution to resistance against *Listeria monocytogenes*, J. Gen. Microbiol. 106 (1978) 165.

[112] P. Cossart, J. Mengaud, *Listeria monocytogenes*: a model system for the molecular study of intracellular parasitism, Mol. Biol. Med. 6 (1989) 463.

[113] M. Denis, Growth of *Listeria monocytogenes* in murine macrophages and its modulation by cytokines: activation of bactericidal activity by interleukin-4 and interleukin-6, Can. J. Microbiol. 37 (1991) 253.

[114] A. Kolb-Maurer, et al., *Listeria monocytogenes*-infected human dendritic cells: uptake and host cell response, Infect. Immun. 68 (2000) 3680–3688.

[115] S.H. Gregory, A.J. Sagnimeni, E.J. Wing, Expression of the inlAB operon by *Listeria monocytogenes* is not required for entry into hepatic cells in vivo, Infect. Immun. 64 (1996) 3983–3986.

[116] H. Marquis, V. Doshi, D.A. Portnoy, The broad-range phospholipase C and a metalloprotease mediate listeriolysin O-independent escape of *Listeria monocytogenes* from a primary vacuole in human epithelial cells, Infect. Immun. 63 (1995) 4531–4534.

[117] H.G. Bouwer, et al., Antilisterial immunity includes specificity to listeriolysin O (LLO) and non-LLO-derived determinants, Infect. Immun. 62 (1994) 1039–1045.

[118] M.M. Gedde, et al., Role of listeriolysin O in cell-to-cell spread of *Listeria monocytogenes*, Infect. Immun. 68 (2000) 999–1003.

[119] J.A. Carrero, H. Vivanco-Cid, E.R. Unanue, Granzymes drive a rapid listeriolysin O-induced T cell apoptosis, J. Immunol. 181 (2008) 1365–1374.

[120] I. Dubail, et al., Functional assembly of two membrane-binding domains in listeriolysin O, the cytolysin of *Listeria monocytogenes*, Microbiology 147 (2001) 2679–2688.

[121] C. Bonnemain, et al., Differential roles of multiple signal peptidases in the virulence of Listeria monocytogenes, Mol. Microbiol. 51 (2004) 1251–1266.

[122] F.S. Southwick, D.L. Purich, Intracellular pathogenesis of listeriosis, N. Engl. J. Med. 334 (1996) 770–776.

[123] C. Kocks, et al., *Listeria monocytogenes* induced actin assembly requires the actA gene product, a surface protein, Cell 68 (1992) 521.

[124] C. de Chastellier, P. Berche, Fate of *Listeria monocytogenes* in murine macrophages: evidence for simultaneous killing and survival of intracellular bacteria, Infect. Immun. 62 (1994) 543–553.

[125] D.D. McGregor, M. Chen-Woan, The cellular response to *Listeria monocytogenes* is mediated by a heterogeneous population of immunospecific T cells, Clin. Invest. Med. 7 (1984) 243.

[126] B.B. Porter, J.T. Harty, The onset of CD8+-T-cell contraction is influenced by the peak of *Listeria monocytogenes* infection and antigen display, Infect. Immun. 74 (2006) 1528–1536.

[127] H. Shen, et al., Compartmentalization of bacterial antigens: differential effects on priming of CD8 T cells and protective immunity, Cell 92 (1998) 535–545.

[128] S.H. Kaufmann, C.H. Ladel, Application of knockout mice to the experimental analysis of infections with bacteria and protozoa, Trends Microbiol. 2 (1994) 235–242.

[129] E.A. Havell, G.L. Spitalny, P.J. Patel, Enhanced production of murine interferon gamma by T cells generated in response to bacterial infection, J. Exp. Med. 156 (1982) 112.

[130] C.S. Hsieh, et al., Development of T$_{H}$1 CD4+ T cells through IL-12 produced by *Listeria*-induced macrophages, Science 260 (1993) 547–549.

[131] J.S. Serody, et al., CD4+ cytolytic effectors are inefficient in the clearance of *Listeria monocytogenes*, Immunology 88 (1996) 544–550.

[132] J.T. Harty, M.J. Bevan, CD8 T-cell recognition of macrophages and hepatocytes results in immunity to *Listeria monocytogenes*, Infect. Immun. 64 (1996) 3632–3640.

[133] J.W. Conlan, R.J. North, Early pathogenesis of infection in the liver with the facultative intracellular bacteria *Listeria monocytogenes, Francisella tularensis,* and *Salmonella typhimurium* involves lysis of infected hepatocytes by leukocytes, Infect. Immun. 60 (1992) 5164–5171.

[134] R.A. Tuma, et al., Rescue of CD8 T cell-mediated antimicrobial immunity with a nonspecific inflammatory stimulus, J. Clin. Invest. 110 (2002) 1493–1501.

[135] M. Chen-Woan, D.D. McGregor, I. Goldschneider, Activation of *Listeria monocytogenes*-induced prekiller T cells by interleukin-2, Clin. Invest. Med. 7 (1984) 287.

[136] S.H. Kaufmann, E. Hug, G. De Libero, *Listeria monocytogenes*-reactive T lymphocyte clones with cytolytic activity against infected target cells, J. Exp. Med. 164 (1986) 363.

[137] Y. Guo, et al., *Listeria monocytogenes* activation of human peripheral blood lymphocytes: induction of non-major histocompatibility complex-restricted cytotoxic activity and cytokine production, Infect. Immun. 60 (1992) 1813.

[138] W. Conlan, R. North, Neutrophil-mediated lysis of infected hepatocytes: selective lysis of permissive host cells is a strategy for controlling intracellular infection in the liver parenchyma, Am. Soc. Microbiol. News 59 (1993) 563–567.

[139] K.S. Boockvar, et al., Nitric oxide produced during murine listeriosis is protective, Infect. Immun. 62 (1994) 1089–1100.

[140] K.P. Beckerman, et al., Release of nitric oxide during the T cell-independent pathway of macrophage activation: its role in resistance to *Listeria monocytogenes*, J. Immunol. 150 (1993) 888–895.

[141] E. Lien, R.R. Ingalls, Toll-like receptors, Crit. Care. Med. 30 (2002) S1–S11.

[142] K.A. Marr, et al., Differential role of MyD88 in macrophage-mediated responses to opportunistic fungal pathogens, Infect. Immun. 71 (2003) 5280–5286.

[143] E. Seki, et al., Critical roles of myeloid differentiation factor 88-dependent proinflammatory cytokine release in early phase clearance of *Listeria monocytogenes* in mice, J. Immunol. 169 (2002) 3863–3883.

[144] B.T. Edelson, E.R. Unanue, MyD88-dependent but Toll-like receptor 2-independent innate immunity to *Listeria*: no role for either in macrophage listericidal activity, J. Immunol. 169 (2002) 3869–3875.

[145] K. Brandl, et al., MyD88-mediated signals induce the bactericidal lectin RegIII gamma and protect mice against intestinal *Listeria monocytogenes* infection, J. Exp. Med. 204 (2007) 1891–1900.

[146] A. Nakane, et al., Interactions between endogenous gamma interferon and tumor necrosis factor in host resistance against primary and secondary *Listeria monocytogenes* infections, Infect. Immun. 57 (1989) 3331.

[147] E.A. Havell, Production of tumor necrosis factor during murine listeriosis, J. Immunol. 139 (1987) 4225.

[148] E.A. Havell, Evidence that tumor necrosis factor has an important role in antibacterial resistance, J. Immunol. 143 (1989) 2894.

[149] A. Nakane, T. Minagawa, K. Kato, Endogenous tumor necrosis factor (cachectin) is essential for host resistance against *Listeria monocytogenes* infection, Infect. Immun. 56 (1988) 2563.

[150] R. van Furth, et al., Anti-tumor necrosis factor antibodies inhibit the influx of granulocytes and monocytes into an inflammatory exudate and enhance the growth of *Listeria monocytogenes* in various organs, J. Infect. Dis. 170 (1994) 234–237.

[151] R.D. Wagner, C.J. Czuprynski, Cytokine mRNA expression in livers of mice infected with *Listeria monocytogenes*, J. Leukoc. Biol. 53 (1993) 525–531.

[152] N.A. Buchmeier, R.D. Schreiber, Requirement of endogenous interferon-gamma production for resolution of *Listeria monocytogenes* infection, Proc. Natl. Acad. Sci. U. S. A. 82 (1985) 7404.

[153] H. Tsukada, et al., Dissociated development of T cells mediating delayed-type hypersensitivity and protective T cells against *Listeria monocytogenes* and their functional difference in lymphokine production, Infect. Immun. 59 (1991) 3589.

[154] E.A. Havell, Augmented induction of interferons during *Listeria monocytogenes* infection, J. Infect. Dis. 153 (1986) 960.

[155] K. Suzue, et al., In vivo role of IFN-gamma produced by antigen-presenting cells in early host defense against intracellular pathogens, Eur. J. Immunol. 33 (2003) 2666–2675.

[156] Q. Wang, et al., Micrococci and peptidoglycan activate TLR2→MyD88→IRAK→TRAF→NIK→IKK→NF-kappaB signal transduction pathway that induces transcription of interleukin-8, Infect. Immun. 69 (2001) 2270–2276.

[157] S.R. Yan, et al., Role of MyD88 in diminished tumor necrosis factor alpha production by newborn mononuclear cells in response to lipopolysaccharide, Infect. Immun. 72 (2004) 1223.

[158] M.A. Miller, et al., IL-12-assisted immunization generates CD4+ T cell-mediated immunity to *Listeria monocytogenes*, Cell. Immunol. 222 (2003) 1–14.

[159] M. Neighbors, et al., A critical role for interleukin 18 in primary and memory effector responses to *Listeria monocytogenes* that extends beyond its effects on interferon gamma production, J. Exp. Med. 194 (2001) 343–354.

[160] C.W. Chan, et al., Interferon-producing killer dendritic cells provide a link between innate and adaptive immunity, Nat. Med. 12 (2006) 207–213.

[161] G.E. Grau, et al., Tumor necrosis factor and disease severity in children with falciparum malaria, N. Engl. J. Med. 320 (1989) 1586.

[162] L.E. Bermudez, L.S. Young, Tumor necrosis factor, alone or in combination with IL-2, but not IFN-gamma, is associated with macrophage killing of *Mycobacterium avium* complex, J. Immunol. 140 (1988) 3006.

[163] I.E. Flesch, S.H. Kaufmann, Activation of tuberculostatic macrophage functions by gamma interferon, interleukin-4, and tumor necrosis factor, Infect. Immun. 58 (1990) 2675.

[164] F. Bazzoni, B. Beutler, The tumor necrosis factor ligand and receptor families, N. Engl. J. Med. 334 (1996) 1717–1725.

[165] S.S. Sung, et al., Production of tumor necrosis factor/cachectin by human B cell lines and tonsillar B cells, J. Exp. Med. 168 (1988) 1539–1551.

[166] W. Cui, et al., Differential modulation of the induction of inflammatory mediators by antibiotics in mouse macrophages in response to viable gram-positive and gram-negative bacteria, J. Endotoxin. Res. 9 (2003) 225–236.

[167] H. Nishimura, et al., The role of gamma delta T cells in priming macrophages to produce tumor necrosis factor-alpha, Eur. J. Immunol. 25 (1995) 1465–1468.

[168] J.P. Mira, et al., Association of TNF2, a TNF-alpha promoter polymorphism, with septic shock susceptibility and mortality: a multicenter study, JAMA 282 (1999) 561–568.

[169] A. Ferrante, et al., Production of tumor necrosis factors alpha and beta by human mononuclear leukocytes stimulated with mitogens, bacteria, and malarial parasites, Infect. Immun. 58 (1990) 3996.

[170] A. Galleli, Y. Le Garrec, L. Chedid, Increased resistance and depressed delayed-type hypersensitivity to *Listeria monocytogenes* induced by pretreatment with lipopolysaccharide, Infect. Immun. 31 (1981) 88.

[171] R. Bortolussi, K. Rajaraman, B. Serushago, Role of tumor necrosis factor-alpha and interferon-gamma in newborn host defense against *Listeria monocytogenes* infection, Pediatr. Res. 32 (1992) 460.

[172] M.J. Brunda, Interleukin-12, J. Leukoc. Biol. 55 (1994) 280–288.

[173] N.V. Serbina, et al., Sequential MyD88-independent and -dependent activation of innate immune responses to intracellular bacterial infection, Immunity 19 (2003) 891–901.

[174] D.B. McKay, C.Y. Lu, Listeriolysin as a virulence factor in *Listeria monocytogenes* infection of neonatal mice and murine decidual tissue, Infect. Immun. 59 (1991) 4286.

[175] R. Bortolussi, Neonatal listeriosis, Semin. Perinatol. 14 (1990) 44.

[176] C.Y. Lu, The delayed ontogenesis of Ia-positive macrophages: implications for host defense and self-tolerance in the neonate, Clin. Invest. Med. 7 (1984) 263.

[177] C.Y. Lu, E.R. Unanue, Ontogeny of murine macrophages: functions related to antigen presentation, Infect. Immun. 36 (1982) 169.

[178] C.Y. Lu, E.G. Calamai, E.R. Unanue, A defect in the antigen-presenting function of macrophages from neonatal mice, Nature 282 (1979) 327.

[179] D. Darmochwal-Kolarz, et al., CD1c(+) immature myeloid dendritic cells are predominant in cord blood of healthy neonates, Immunol. Lett. 91 (2004) 71–74.

[180] T.S. Hamrick, et al., Influence of pregnancy on the pathogenesis of listeriosis in mice inoculated intragastrically, Infect. Immun. 71 (2003) 5202–5209.

[181] C.B. Wilson, The ontogeny of T lymphocyte maturation and function, J. Pediatr. 118 (1991) S4.

[182] A.I. Bakardjiev, et al., Listeriosis in the pregnant guinea pig: a model of vertical transmission, Infect. Immun. 72 (2004) 489–497.

[183] A. Le Monnier, et al., ActA is required for crossing of the fetoplacental barrier by *Listeria monocytogenes*, Infect. Immun. 75 (2007) 950–957.

[184] M.A. Smith, et al., Nonhuman primate model for *Listeria monocytogenes*-induced stillbirths, Infect. Immun. 71 (2003) 1574–1579.

[185] T.B. Issekutz, J. Evans, R. Bortolussi, The immune response of human neonates to *Listeria monocytogenes* infection, Clin. Invest. Med. 7 (1984) 281.

[186] T. McDonald, et al., Natural killer cell activity in very low birth weight infants, Pediatr. Res. 31 (1992) 376.

[187] E. Dominguez, et al., Fetal natural killer cell function is suppressed, Immunology 94 (1998) 109–114.

[188] S.M. Lee, et al., Decreased interleukin-12 (IL-12) from activated cord versus adult peripheral blood mononuclear cells and upregulation of interferon-gamma, natural killer, and lymphokine-activated killer activity by IL-12 in cord blood mononuclear cells, Blood 88 (1996) 945–954.

[189] A.S. Lau, et al., Interleukin-12 induces interferon-gamma expression and natural killer cytotoxicity in cord blood mononuclear cells, Pediatr. Res. 39 (1996) 150–155.

[190] R. Bortolussi, et al., Neonatal host defense mechanisms against *Listeria monocytogenes* infection: the role of lipopolysaccharides and interferons, Pediatr. Res. 25 (1989) 311.

[191] H.W. Murray, Gamma interferon, cytokine-induced macrophage activation, and antimicrobial host defense: in vitro, in animal models, and in humans, Diagn. Microbiol. Infect. Dis. 13 (1990) 411.

[192] B. Cederblad, T. Riesenfeld, G.V. Alm, Deficient herpes simplex virus-induced interferon-alpha production by blood leukocytes of preterm and term newborn infants, Pediatr. Res. 27 (1990) 7.

[193] D.B. Lewis, A. Larsen, C.B. Wilson, Reduced interferon-gamma mRNA levels in human neonates: evidence for an intrinsic T cell deficiency independent of other genes involved in T cell activation, J. Exp. Med. 163 (1986) 1018.

[194] D.B. Lewis, et al., Cellular and molecular mechanisms for reduced interleukin 4 and interferon-gamma production by neonatal T cells, J. Clin. Invest. 87 (1991) 194.

[195] R. Bortolussi, et al., Neonatal *Listeria monocytogenes* infection is refractory to interferon, Pediatr. Res. 29 (1991) 400.

[196] W. Al-Hertani, et al., Human newborn polymorphonuclear neutrophils exhibit decreased levels of MyD88 and attenuated p38 phosphorylation in response to lipopolysaccharide, Clin. Invest. Med. 30 (2007) E44–E53.

[197] R. Bortolussi, *Escherichia coli* infection in neonates: humoral defense mechanisms, Semin. Perinatol. 14 (1990) 40.

[198] R. Bortolussi, A. Issekutz, G. Faulkner, Opsonization of *Listeria monocytogenes* type 4b by human adult and newborn sera, Infect. Immun. 52 (1986) 493.

[199] T. Hertzig, et al., Antibodies present in normal human serum inhibit invasion of human brain microvascular endothelial cells by *Listeria monocytogenes*, Infect. Immun. 71 (2003) 95–100.

[200] E.C. Klatt, et al., Epidemic perinatal listeriosis at autopsy, Hum. Pathol. 17 (1986) 1278.

[201] M. Scholing, et al., Clinical features of liver involvement in adult patients with listeriosis: review of the literature, Infection 35 (2007) 212–218.

[202] H.J. Reiss, Zur patholgischen Anatomie der kindlichen Listeriosis, Kinderarztl Prax Separatum (1953) 92.

[203] R.W. Armstrong, P.C. Fung, Brainstem encephalitis (rhombencephalitis) due to *Listeria monocytogenes*: case report and review, Clin. Infect. Dis. 16 (1993) 689–702.

[204] P.E. Steele, D.S. Jacobs, *Listeria monocytogenes*: macroabscesses of placenta, Obstet. Gynecol. 53 (1979) 124.

[205] M. Topalovski, S.S. Yang, Y. Boonpasat, Listeriosis of the placenta: clinico-pathologic study of seven cases, Am. J. Obstet. Gynecol. 169 (1993) 616–620.

[206] Infections and inflammatory lesions of the placenta, in: H. Fox (Ed.), Pathology of the Placenta, second ed., WB Saunders, Toronto, 1997, pp. 309–311.

[207] Presentation of case 15—1997, N. Engl. J. Med. 336 (1997) 1439–1446.

[208] C.E. Ahlfors, et al., Neonatal listeriosis, Am. J. Dis. Child. 131 (1977) 405.

[209] V.W. Krause, et al., Congenital listeriosis causing early neonatal death, Can. Med. Assoc. J. 127 (1982) 36.

[210] M. Hood, Listeriosis as an infection of pregnancy manifested in the newborn, Pediatrics 27 (1961) 390.

[211] C.S. Kelly, J.L. Gibson, Listeriosis as a cause of fetal wastage, Obstet. Gynecol. 40 (1972) 91.

[212] R.W. Redline, C.Y. Lu, Specific defects in the anti-listerial immune response in discrete regions of the murine uterus and placenta account for susceptibility to infection, J. Immunol. 140 (1988) 3947.

[213] S. Kaur, et al., *Listeria monocytogenes* in spontaneous abortions in humans and its detection by multiplex PCR, J. Appl. Microbiol. 103 (2007) 1889–1896.

[214] C. Kalstone, Successful antepartum treatment of listeriosis, Am. J. Obstet. Gynecol. 164 (1991) 57.

[215] R.I. Liner, Intrauterine *Listeria* infection: prenatal diagnosis by biophysical assessment and amniocentesis, Am. J. Obstet. Gynecol. 163 (1990) 1596.

[216] M.B. Loeb, et al., Perinatal listeriosis, J. Soc. Obstet. Gynecol. Can. 18 (1996) 164–170.

[217] B.J. Luft, J.S. Remington, Effect of pregnancy on resistance to *Listeria monocytogenes* and *Toxoplasma gondii* infections in mice, Infect. Immun. 38 (1982) 1164.

[218] R. Bortolussi, N. Campbell, V. Krause, Dynamics of *Listeria monocytogenes* type 4b infection in pregnant and infant rats, Clin. Invest. Med. 7 (1984) 273.

[219] M. Lecuit, et al., Targeting and crossing of the human maternofetal barrier by *Listeria monocytogenes*: role of internalin interaction with trophoblast E-cadherin, Proc. Natl. Acad. Sci. U. S. A. 101 (2004) 6152–6157.

[220] E. Menu, et al., Immunoactive products of human placenta. IV. Immunoregulatory factors obtained from cultures of human placenta inhibit in vivo local and systemic allogeneic and graft versus-host reactions in mice, J. Reprod. Immunol. 20 (1991) 195.

[221] I. Guleria, J.W. Pollard, The trophoblast is a component of the innate immune system during pregnancy, Nat. Med. 6 (2000) 589–593.

[222] C.G. Burn, Unidentified gram-positive bacillus associated with meningo-encephalitis, Proc. Soc. Exp. Biol. Med. 31 (1934) 1095.

[223] C.G. Burn, Characteristics of a new species of the genus *Listerella* obtained from human sources, J. Bacteriol. 30 (1935) 573.

[224] C.G. Burn, Clinical and pathological features of an infection caused by a new pathogen of the genus *Listerella*, Am. J. Pathol. 13 (1936) 341.

[225] W.L. Albritton, G.L. Wiggins, J.C. Feeley, Neonatal listeriosis: distribution of serotypes in relation to age at onset of disease, J. Pediatr. 88 (1976) 481.

[226] J.R. Evans, et al., Perinatal listeriosis: report of an outbreak, Pediatr. Infect. Dis. 4 (1985) 237.

[227] D. Lennon, et al., Epidemic perinatal listeriosis, Pediatr. Infect. Dis. 3 (1984) 30.

[228] D.M. Becroft, et al., Epidemic listeriosis in the newborn, BMJ 3 (1971) 747.

[229] J. McLauchlin, Human listeriosis in Britain, 1967–85, a summary of 722 cases. 1. Listeriosis during pregnancy and in the newborn, Epidemiol. Infect. 104 (1990) 181–189.

[230] A.M. Visintine, J.M. Oleske, A.J. Nahmias, *Listeria monocytogenes* infection in infants and children, Am. J. Dis. Child. 131 (1977) 339.

[231] B. Pron, et al., Comprehensive study of the intestinal stage of listeriosis in a rat ligated ileal loop system, Infect. Immun. 66 (1998) 747–755.

[232] C.B. Dalton, et al., An outbreak of gastroenteritis and fever due to *Listeria monocytogenes* in milk, N. Engl. J. Med. 336 (1997) 100–105.

[233] M.C. Brouwer, et al., Community-acquired *Listeria monocytogenes* meningitis in adults, Clin. Infect. Dis. 43 (2006) 1233–1238.

[234] E.A. Antal, et al., Brain stem encephalitis in listeriosis, Scand. J. Infect. Dis. 37 (2005) 190–194.

[235] S. Dramsi, et al., Entry of *Listeria monocytogenes* into neurons occurs by cell-to-cell spread: an in vitro study, Infect. Immun. 66 (1998) 4461–4468.

[236] S. Sahin, et al., Brain-stem listeriosis: a comparison of SPECT and MRI findings, Med. Gen. Med. 8 (2006) 47.

[237] R.L. Jurado, et al., Increased risk of meningitis and bacteremia due to *Listeria monocytogenes* in patients with human immunodeficiency virus infection, Clin. Infect. Dis. 17 (1993) 224–227.

[238] K. Nadarajah, C. Pritchard, *Listeria monocytogenes* septic arthritis in a patient treated with etanercept for rheumatoid arthritis, J. Clin. Rheumatol. 11 (2005) 120–122.

[239] W. Anton, Krittisch-experimenteller Beitrag zur Biologie des Bacterium-monocytogens mit besendear Berucksichtigung seiner Bezehung zur infektiosen Mononukleose des Menschen, Zentralbl. Bakteriol. Hyg. 131 (1934) 89.

[240] S.T. Ooi, B. Lorber, Gastroenteritis due to *Listeria monocytogenes*, Clin. Infect. Dis. 40 (2005) 1327–1332.

[241] D.M. Frye, et al., An outbreak of febrile gastroenteritis associated with delicatessen meat contaminated with *Listeria monocytogenes*, Clin. Infect. Dis. 35 (2002) 943–949.

[242] F.X. Riedo, et al., A point-source foodborne listeriosis outbreak: documented incubation period and possible mild illness, J. Infect. Dis. 170 (1994) 693–696.

[243] G. Salamina, et al., A foodborne outbreak of gastroenteritis involving *Listeria monocytogenes*, Epidemiol. Infect. 117 (1996) 429–436.

[244] P. Aureli, et al., An outbreak of febrile gastroenteritis associated with corn contaminated by *Listeria monocytogenes*, N. Engl. J. Med. 342 (2000) 1236–1241.

[245] W.F. Schlech 3rd., *Listeria* gastroenteritis—old syndrome, new pathogen, N. Engl. J. Med. 336 (1997) 130–132.

[246] O. Felsenfeld, Diseases of poultry transmissible to man, Iowa State Coll Vet 13 (1951) 89.

[247] N. Spyrou, M. Anderson, R. Foale, *Listeria* endocarditis: current management and patient outcome—world literature review, Heart 77 (1997) 380–383.

[248] J.M. Miguel-Yanes, V.J. Gonzalez-Ramallo, L. Pastor, Outcome of *Listeria monocytogenes* prosthetic valve endocarditis. As bad as it looks? Scand. J. Infect. Dis. 36 (2004) 709–711.

[249] T.L. Jackson, et al., Endogenous bacterial endophthalmitis: a 17-year prospective series and review of 267 reported cases, Surv. Ophthalmol. 48 (2003) 403–423.

[250] C. Betriu, et al., Endophthalmitis caused by *Listeria monocytogenes*, J. Clin. Microbiol. 39 (2001) 2742–2744.

[251] J.J. Sivalingam, et al., *Listeria monocytogenes* peritonitis: case report and literature review, Am. J. Gastroenterol. 87 (1992) 1839–1845.

[252] J.S. Dylewski, Bacterial peritonitis caused by *Listeria monocytogenes*: case report and review of the literature, Can. J. Infect. 7 (1996) 59–62.

[253] H. Hof, Therapeutic activities of antibiotics in listeriosis, Infection 19 (1991) S229.

[254] J. McLauchlin, A. Audurier, A.G. Taylor, Treatment failure and recurrent human listeriosis, J. Antimicrob. Chemother. 27 (1991) 851.

[255] A.P. Hudak, et al., Comparison of three serological methods—enzyme-linked immunosorbent assay, complement fixation, and microagglutination—in the diagnosis of human perinatal *Listeria monocytogenes* infection, Clin. Invest. Med. 7 (1984) 349.

[256] S. Winblad, Studies of antibodies in human listeriosis, Acta. Pathol. Microbiol. Scand. 58 (1963) 123.

[257] P. Berche, et al., Detection of anti-listeriolysin O for serodiagnosis of human listeriosis, Lancet 335 (1990) 624.

[258] R.M. Drew, Occurrence of two immunological groups within the genus *Listeria*: studies based upon precipitation reactions, Proc. Soc. Exp. Biol. Med. 61 (1946) 30.

[259] G. Schierz, A. Burger, The detection of *Listeria* antibodies by passive hemagglutination, Proceedings of the Third International Symposium on Listeriosis, Bilthoven, 1966, p. 77.

[260] A.N. Njoku-Obi, An antigen-fixation test for the serodiagnosis of *Listeria monocytogenes* infections, Cornell. Vet. 52 (1962) 415.

[261] E.H. Kampelmacher, W.T. Huysinga, L.M. van Noorle Jansen, Het voorkomen van *Listeria monocytogenes* in faeces van gravidae en pasgeborenen, Ned. Tijdschr. Geneeskd. 116 (1972) 1685.

[262] A. Backman, et al., Evaluation of an extended diagnostic PCR assay for detection and verification of the common causes of bacterial meningitis in CSF and other biological samples, Mol. Cell. Probes 13 (1999) 49–60.

[263] C.P. Lohmann, et al., *Listeria monocytogenes*-induced endogenous endophthalmitis in an otherwise healthy individual: rapid PCR-diagnosis as the basis for effective treatment, Eur. J. Ophthalmol. 9 (1999) 53–57.

[264] X.W. Huijsdens, et al., *Listeria monocytogenes* and inflammatory bowel disease: detection of *Listeria* species in intestinal mucosal biopsies by real-time PCR, Scand. J. Gastroenterol. 38 (2003) 332–333.

[265] M. Chiba, et al., Presence of bacterial 16S ribosomal RNA gene segments in human intestinal lymph follicles, Scand. J. Gastroenterol. 35 (2000) 824–831.

[266] O.S. Hune, Maternal *Listeria monocytogenes* septicemia with sparing of the fetus, Obstet. Gynecol. 48 (1976) 335.

[267] V.L. Katz, L. Weinstein, Antepartum treatment of *Listeria monocytogenes* septicemia, South. Med. J. 75 (1982) 1353.

[268] S. Fuchs, D. Hochner-Celnikier, O. Shalev, First trimester listeriosis with normal fetal outcome, Eur. J. Clin. Microbiol. Infect. Dis. 13 (1994) 656–658.

[269] A.D. Rotheberg, et al., Outcome for survivors of mechanical ventilation weighing less than 1200 gm at birth, J. Pediatr. 98 (1981) 106.

[270] R.L. Naege, Amnionic fluid infections, neonatal hyperbilirubinemia and psychomotor impairment, Pediatrics 62 (1978) 497.

[271] F.G. Line, F.G. Appleton, *Listeria* meningitis in a premature infant, J. Pediatr. 41 (1952) 97.

[272] J.R. Evans, et al., Follow-up study of survivors of fetal and early onset neonatal listeriosis, Clin. Invest. Med. 7 (1984) 329.

[273] E.P. Espaze, et al., In vitro susceptibility of *Listeria monocytogenes* to some antibiotics and their combinations, Zentralbl. Bakteriol. [Orig. A] 240 (1978) 76.

[274] G.W. Watson, et al., *Listeria* cerebritis: relapse of infection in renal transplant patients, Arch. Intern. Med. 138 (1978) 83.

[275] H. Hof, Treatment of experimental listeriosis by CI 934, a new quinolone, J. Antimicrob. Chemother. 25 (1990) 121.

[276] P.G. Spitzer, S.M. Hammer, A.W. Karchmer, Treatment of *Listeria monocytogenes* infection with trimethoprim-sulfamethoxazole: case report and review of the literature, Rev. Infect. Dis. 8 (1986) 427.

[277] R.W. Armstrong, B. Slater, *Listeria monocytogenes* meningitis treated with trimethoprim-sulfamethoxazole, Pediatr. Infect. Dis. 5 (1986) 712.

[278] W.A. Vischer, C. Rominger, Rifampicin against experimental listeriosis in the mouse, Chemotherapy 24 (1978) 104.

[279] C. Poyart-Salmeron, et al., Transferable plasmid-mediated antibiotic resistance in *Listeria monocytogenes*, Lancet 335 (1990) 1422.

[280] Clinical and Laboratory Standards Institute Methods for Antimicrobial Dilution and Disk Susceptibility Testing of Infrequently Isolated or Fastidious Bacteria: Approved Guideline, Approved Standard 26 (2006) 27.

[281] A.P. MacGowan, et al., In vitro antimicrobial susceptibility of *Listeria monocytogenes* isolated in the UK and other *Listeria* species, Eur. J. Clin. Microbiol. Infect. Dis. 9 (1990) 767.

[282] F. Soriano, J. Zapardiel, E. Nieto, Antimicrobial susceptibilities of *Corynebacterium* species and other non-spore-forming gram-positive bacilli to 18 antimicrobial agents, Antimicrob. Agents Chemother. 39 (1995) 208–214.

[283] E. Charpentier, et al., Incidence of antibiotic resistance in *Listeria* species, J. Infect. Dis. 172 (1995) 277–281.

[284] V. Srinivasan, et al., Prevalence of antimicrobial resistance genes in *Listeria monocytogenes* isolated from dairy farms, Foodborne Pathog. Dis. 2 (2005) 201–211.

[285] M.A. Prazak, et al., Antimicrobial resistance of *Listeria monocytogenes* isolated from various cabbage farms and packing sheds in Texas, J. Food Prot. 65 (2002) 1796–1799.

[286] H. Hof, T. Nichterlein, M. Kretschmar, Management of listeriosis, Clin. Microbiol. Rev. 10 (1997) 345–357.

[287] W.H. Traub, Perinatal listeriosis: Tolerance of a clinical isolate of *Listeria monocytogenes* for ampicillin and resistance against cefotaxime, Chemotherapy 27 (1981) 423.

[288] S. Carryn, et al., Comparative intracellular (THP-1 macrophage) and extracellular activities of beta-lactams, azithromycin, gentamicin, and fluoroquinolones against *Listeria monocytogenes* at clinically relevant concentrations, Antimicrob. Agents Chemother. 46 (2002) 2095–2103.

[289] L. Martinez-Martinez, et al., Activities of gemifloxacin and five other antimicrobial agents against *Listeria monocytogenes* and coryneform bacteria isolated from clinical samples, Antimicrob. Agents Chemother. 45 (2001) 2390–2392.

[290] A. Lavetter, et al., Meningitis due to *Listeria monocytogenes*: a review of 25 cases, N. Engl. J. Med. 285 (1971) 598.

[291] G.M. Eliopoulos, R.C. Moellering Jr, Susceptibility of enterococci and *Listeria monocytogenes* to N-formimidoyl thienamycin alone and in combination with an aminoglycoside, Antimicrob. Agents Chemother. 19 (1981) 789.

[292] C.E. Edmiston, R.C. Gordon, Evaluation of gentamicin and penicillin as a synergistic combination in experimental murine listeriosis, Antimicrob. Agents Chemother. 16 (1979) 862.

[293] M.L. van Ogtrop, et al., Comparison of the antibacterial efficacies of ampicillin and ciprofloxacin against experimental infections with *Listeria monocytogenes* in hydrocortisone-treated mice, Antimicrob. Agents Chemother. 36 (1992) 2375.

[294] H. Hof, P. Emmerling, H.P. Seeliger, Murine model for therapy of listeriosis in the compromised host, Chemotherapy 27 (1981) 214.

[295] I.A. Bakker-Woudenberg, et al., Efficacy of ampicillin therapy in experimental listeriosis in mice with impaired T-cell-mediated immune response, Antimicrob. Agents Chemother. 19 (1981) 76.

[296] I.A. Bakker-Woudenberg, et al., Free versus liposome-entrapped ampicillin in treatment of infection due to *Listeria monocytogenes* in normal and athymic (nude) mice, J. Infect. Dis. 151 (1985) 917.

[297] W.M. Scheld, et al., Response to therapy in an experimental rabbit model of meningitis due to *Listeria monocytogenes*, J. Infect. Dis. 140 (1979) 287.

[298] O.R. Sipahi, et al., Moxifloxacin versus ampicillin + gentamicin in the therapy of experimental *Listeria monocytogenes* meningitis, J. Antimicrob. Chemother. 61 (2008) 670–673.

[299] A.E. Hawkins, R. Bortolussi, A.C. Issekutz, In vitro and in vivo activity of various antibiotics against *Listeria monocytogenes* type 4b, Clin. Invest. Med. 7 (1984) 335.

[300] P.E. Dans, et al., Rifampin: antibacterial activity in vitro and absorption and excretion in normal young men, Am. J. Med. Sci. 259 (1970) 120.

[301] H. Hof, H. Guckel, Lack of synergism of ampicillin and gentamicin in experimental listeriosis, Infection 15 (1987) 40.

[302] W.M. Scheld, Evaluation of rifampin and other antibiotics against *Listeria monocytogenes* in vitro and in vivo, Rev. Infect. Dis. 5 (1983) S593.

[303] C.E. Cherubin, et al., Epidemiological spectrum and current treatment of listeriosis, Rev. Infect. Dis. 13 (1991) 1108.

[304] L. Weingartner, S. Ortel, Zur Behandlung der Listeriose mit Ampicillin, Dtsch. Med. Wochenschr. 92 (1967) 1098.

[305] A. Safdar, D. Armstrong, Antimicrobial activities against 84 *Listeria monocytogenes* isolates from patients with systemic listeriosis at a comprehensive cancer center (1955–1997), J. Clin. Microbiol. 41 (2003) 483–485.

[306] J.M. Hansen, P. Gerner-Smidt, B. Bruun, Antibiotic susceptibility of *Listeria monocytogenes* in Denmark 1958–2001, APMIS 113 (2005) 31–36.

[307] F. Forna, et al., Systematic review of the safety of trimethoprim-sulfamethoxazole for prophylaxis in HIV-infected pregnant women: implications for resource-limited settings, AIDS Rev. 8 (2006) 24–36.

[308] V. Fanos, A. Dall'Agnola, Antibiotics in neonatal infections: a review, Drugs 58 (1999) 405–427.

[309] E.S. Petrilli, G. D'Ablaing, W.J. Ledger, *Listeria monocytogenes* chorioamnionitis: diagnosis by transabdominal amniocentesis, Obstet. Gynecol. 55 (1980) 5S.

[310] CDC, Update: foodborne listeriosis—United States, 1988–1990, MMWR Morbid. Mortal. Wkly Rep. 41 (1992) 251.

[311] F. Ogunmodede, et al., Listeriosis prevention knowledge among pregnant women in the USA, Infect. Dis. Obstet. Gynecol. 13 (2005) 11–15.

[312] D. Bondarianzadeh, H. Yeatman, D. Condon-Paoloni, *Listeria* education in pregnancy: lost opportunity for health professionals, Aust. N. Z. J. Public Health 31 (2007) 468–474.

[313] J.W. Tappero, et al., Reduction in the incidence of human listeriosis in the United States. Effectiveness of prevention efforts? The Listeriosis Study Group, JAMA 273 (1995) 1118–1122.

[314] Listeria Fact Sheet—Updated, University of Guelph Food Safety Network, Guelph, Ontario, 2003.

[315] D. Torres, M. Barrier, F. Bihl, et al., Toll-like receptor 2 is required for optimal control of *Listeria monocytogenes* infection, Infection and Immunity. 72 (2004) 2131–2139.

STAPHYLOCOCCAL INFECTIONS

Victor Nizet ☉ John S. Bradley

CHAPTER OUTLINE

Epidemiology and Transmission 489
   Staphylococcus aureus 489
   Coagulase-Negative Staphylococci 490
Microbiology 491
   Staphylococcus aureus 491
   Coagulase-Negative Staphylococci 492
Pathogenesis of Disease 492
   Virulence Mechanisms of *Staphylococcus aureus* 492
   Epithelial Attachment and Invasion 492
   Innate Immune Resistance 493
   Secreted Toxins 494
   Quorum Sensing and Regulation of Virulence Factor
      Expression 495
   Virulence Mechanisms of Coagulase-Negative
      Staphylococci 495
   Role of the Host Defenses 496
Pathology 497
Clinical Manifestations 497
   Bacteremia and Sepsis 497
   Toxic Shock Syndromes 499
   Endocarditis 499
   Pustulosis, Cutaneous Abscess, and Cellulitis 500
   Adenitis and Parotitis 500
   Breast Infection 500

Funisitis, Omphalitis, and Necrotizing Fasciitis 500
Staphylococcal Scalded Skin Syndrome and Bullous
   Impetigo 502
Pneumonia 502
Meningitis 504
Brain Abscess 504
Osteoarticular Infection 504
Infections of the Gastrointestinal Tract 505
Diagnosis 505
Antibiotic Treatment 506
   General Principles 506
   Vancomycin 506
   Clindamycin and Erythromycin 507
   Linezolid 507
   Daptomycin 508
   Quinupristin-Dalfopristin 508
   Combination Antimicrobial Therapy 508
   Catheter Removal 508
Prevention 509
   Hygienic Measures 509
   Antibiotic Prophylaxis 509
   Immunoprophylaxis 509
Conclusion 510

Staphylococcal disease has been recognized in neonates for centuries; it was reported in 1773, when pemphigus neonatorum was described [1]. Outbreaks of staphylococcal disease in nurseries were first noted in the late 1920s [2], and the memorable term "cloud baby" was subsequently coined to describe index cases, often asymptomatic, who contaminated the nursery atmosphere with *Staphylococcus aureus* colonizing their respiratory tract, skin, or umbilical cord [3]. Until the late 1970s, staphylococcal disease in newborn infants was caused most often by *S. aureus* [4]. In recent decades, coagulase-negative staphylococci (CoNS) have assumed an equally important role, especially in premature infants in neonatal intensive care units (NICUs) [5–7], often responsible for 50% or more of all cases of clinically significant bacterial disease. Management of staphylococcal disease in infants has become increasingly more complicated, reflecting the increasing incidence of methicillin resistance and the threat of vancomycin resistance among isolates of *S. aureus* and CoNS. This chapter summarizes current information about *S. aureus* and CoNS and the diseases these organisms produce in newborns and young infants.

EPIDEMIOLOGY AND TRANSMISSION
STAPHYLOCOCCUS AUREUS

Many factors influence transmission of staphylococci among newborns, including nursery design, density of infant population, and obstetric and nursery practices. Other factors certain to influence transmission include virulence properties of the individual *S. aureus* strains and often poorly defined immunogenetic host factors. The complexity of isolating and investigating each variable in the epidemiologic equation accounts for the disagreement in the literature about which factors predominate in transmission and prevention of staphylococcal disease. A particular factor that is critical in one epidemic may not be a driving factor under different circumstances.

Quantitative culture studies show that very few *S. aureus* organisms are capable of initiating colonization in the newborn. Less than 10 bacteria can establish umbilical colonization in 50% of newborns, whereas approximately 250 organisms can achieve a similar effect on the nasal mucosa [8]. Colonization of the newborn umbilicus, nares, and skin occurs early in life. By the 5th day in the nursery, the colonization rate among nursery inhabitants

DOI: 10.1016/B978-1-4160-6400-8.00014-6

may be 90% [9]. The umbilicus or rectum usually is colonized before the nares [10,11].

These findings provide a plausible explanation for the challenge of defining any single factor in the environment (e.g., fomites, hands, clothes) as the ultimate source of infection. Nevertheless, most evidence indicates that the initial and perhaps major source of infection is medical and nursing personnel [8]. A strain of *S. aureus* common among medical attendants is far more likely than a maternal strain to colonize a given infant in the nursery [12]; in 85% of cases, infant colonization with *S. aureus* is likely to originate from an attendant's touch [13]. Persons with overt cutaneous lesions or disease often are highly infectious, but asymptomatic carriers can be infectious also [14], and carriage on the skin, in the anterior nares, and in the perineal area is relevant [15,16]. The frequency of intestinal carriage of the pathogen may be greatly underestimated as well [17].

Soon after the introduction of methicillin in 1960, methicillin-resistant *S. aureus* (MRSA) emerged as an important nosocomial pathogen [18]. For MRSA, resistance is mediated through the *mecA* gene, which codes for an altered penicillin-binding protein (called PBP2a) that has a dramatically reduced affinity for β-lactam antibiotics [19]. Beyond possessing *mecA*, MRSA isolates frequently harbor other antibiotic resistance determinants as well, limiting treatment options further. Risk factors for infection with MRSA include treatment with antimicrobials, prolonged hospitalization, and stay within an intensive care unit [20]. Since the mid-1990s, infection with community-acquired MRSA (CA-MRSA) isolates has been reported increasingly in patients without hospital contact or traditional risk factors for MRSA [21,22]. CA-MRSA strains typically have a distinct antibiotic susceptibility pattern and more frequently cause skin and soft tissue infections and necrotizing pneumonias compared with methicillin-sensitive *S. aureus* (MSSA). These isolates are readily transmitted between family members and close contacts [22].

The National Institute of Child Health and Human Development (NICHD) Neonatal Research Network reported that from 1998-2000, approximately 8% of initial episodes of late-onset sepsis among infants with very low birth weight (<1500 g) were caused by *S. aureus* [6]. More recently, Carey and colleagues [23] reported the epidemiology of MSSA and MRSA infections in the NICU at Columbia University Medical Center. During the study period, there were 123 infections caused by MSSA and 49 infections caused by MRSA. Overall, the clinical presentations and the crude mortality rates (16% to 17%) were similar in both groups, although infants with MRSA infections were significantly younger at clinical presentation than infants with MSSA infections. The most common manifestations were bacteremia (36%); skin, soft tissue, wound (31%); bacteremia plus skin and soft tissue (15%); endocarditis (7%); and rare cases of tracheitis, osteomyelitis, meningitis, or mediastinitis. The risk of developing MSSA or MRSA infection was inversely related to birth weight, with 53% of infections occurring in very low birth weight infants; most infections in infants weighing more than 2500 g were associated with surgical procedures. Reports of small outbreaks of

CA-MRSA in NICUs and well-infant nurseries are appearing with increasing frequency [24–26].

When clusters of staphylococcal disease associated with hospital exposure occur, temporal clustering of cases suggests the possibility of an outbreak caused by a single strain [27]. In these situations, identity of the strain requires characterization based on a molecular technique, such as pulsed-field gel electrophoresis (PFGE) or multilocus sequence typing (MLST). MLST is a sequence-based typing system that uses the sequence of seven or more housekeeping genes to evaluate the genetic relatedness of strains of staphylococci [28]. The discriminatory power of this approach is less than that of PFGE, so the usefulness for the evaluation of local outbreaks is less [29]. Nevertheless, MLST allows the user to compare sequences from isolates of various locations through a central database (http://www.mlst.net).

COAGULASE-NEGATIVE STAPHYLOCOCCI

CoNS are common inhabitants of human skin and mucous membranes. *Staphylococcus epidermidis* is the species found most commonly as a member of the normal flora of the nasal mucosa and the umbilicus of the newborn [30]. With sensitive culture techniques, the nose, umbilicus, and chest skin are found to be colonized with CoNS in 83% of neonates by 4 days of age [31]. Rates of colonization with *S. epidermidis* in one study of infants in a NICU were as follows: nose, 89%; throat, 84%; umbilicus, 90%; and stool, 86%; simultaneous percentages for *S. aureus* were 17%, 17%, 21%, and 10% [30]. Although most infants acquire CoNS from environmental sources, including hospital personnel, a small percentage are colonized by vertical transmission [32,33]. Isolates of *S. epidermidis* and other CoNS resistant to multiple antibiotic agents are common. In a study involving premature neonates, D'Angio and associates showed that the incidence of strains resistant to multiple antibiotics increased from 32% to 82% by the end of the 1st week of life [34].

The observation that CoNS are important nosocomial pathogens among newborns, especially low birth weight infants in NICUs, is explained by the prevalence of colonization with these organisms at multiple sites and the widespread use of invasive therapeutic modalities that subvert normal host epithelial barrier defenses. Examples of invasive treatments include endotracheal intubation, mechanical ventilation, placement of umbilical and other central venous catheters and ventriculoperitoneal shunts, and use of feeding tubes. In more recent epidemiology, CoNS account for more than half of bloodstream isolates obtained from neonates with late-onset sepsis [5–7].

An inverse relationship exists between the rate of infection with CoNS and birth weight and gestational age. Additional risk factors that are associated with CoNS bacteremia among very low birth weight neonates include respiratory distress syndrome, bronchopulmonary dysplasia, patent ductus arteriosus, severe intraventricular hemorrhage, and necrotizing enterocolitis [6].

Certain nutritional factors are associated with the development of late-onset sepsis, including delayed initiation of enteral feeding, prolonged period to reach full enteral feeding status, delayed reattainment of birth weight, and prolonged parenteral hyperalimentation [6]. In a case-control study, administration of intralipids through a polytetrafluoroethylene (Teflon) catheter was also shown to be associated with an increased risk of bacteremia caused by CoNS [35]. Most experts believe the clinical and experimental data suggest that CoNS have not become more virulent over time. Rather, these ubiquitous organisms have become more common pathogens because therapeutic approaches have become increasingly invasive, and because very low birth weight premature infants, with compromised immunity, are surviving for longer periods.

MICROBIOLOGY

Staphylococci are members of the family Staphylococcaceae and are nonmotile, non–spore-forming bacteria that are catalase-negative. Species of staphylococci are separated into two large groups on the basis of ability to produce the extracellular enzyme coagulase. Organisms that produce coagulase are known as coagulase-positive staphylococci, or *S. aureus* [36], and organisms that produce no coagulase are referred to as CoNS. The presence of coagulase can be evaluated either by assessing broth medium for secreted enzyme, which reacts with coagulase-reacting factor in plasma and results in formation of a fibrin clot, or by testing for cell-bound enzyme, which results in clumping when a suspension of organisms is incubated with plasma.

Staphylococci grow best in an aerobic environment, but are capable of growing under anaerobic conditions as well. They grow readily on most routine laboratory media, including Luria broth, and usually are isolated from clinical specimens using sheep blood agar. Gram staining reveals gram-positive cocci 0.7 to 1.2 mM in diameter that are usually visible in irregular grapelike clusters (Fig. 14–1A). Growth in liquid culture often results in a predominance of single cocci, pairs, tetrads, and chains of three or four cells. Dying organisms and bacteria in stationary phase or ingested by phagocytes may appear to be gram-negative. Growth on blood agar

results in round, convex, shiny opaque colonies that are 1 to 2 mm in diameter after 24 hours of incubation. Colonies of *S. aureus* often are deep yellow or golden in color and typically are surrounded by a zone of β-hemolysis (Fig. 14–1B). By contrast, colonies of CoNS usually are chalk-white, often lacking surrounding hemolysis.

STAPHYLOCOCCUS AUREUS

For clinical purposes, many of the key characteristics of *S. aureus* can be determined by simple procedures performed with commercial rapid identification kits and automated systems [36]. Historically, phage typing and serologic typing were the most common systems for differentiating strains of *S. aureus* for epidemiologic purposes [37]. In contemporary analysis, molecular approaches such as PFGE and MSLT have become the standard for defining strain identity in a patient with multiple isolates or in a possible outbreak involving multiple patients [38,39].

The staphylococcal cell wall is composed of two major components, peptidoglycan and teichoic acid [40,41]. *S. aureus* peptidoglycan is composed of chains of acetylglucosamine, acetylmuramic acid, alanine, glutamic acid, and lysine or diaminopimelic acid, with pentaglycine bridges that cross-link these chains. Four penicillin-binding proteins called PBP1, PBP2, PBP3, and PBP4 play an important role in peptidoglycan biosynthesis and are inactivated by β-lactams [42]. A mutated form of PBP2 (PBP2a) encoded by the *mecA* gene is the basis of methicillin resistance in the current epidemic of hospital-acquired MRSA (HA-MRSA) and CA-MRSA disease. Teichoic acid is a polymer of ribitol phosphate that is held in the cell wall by covalent attachment to the insoluble peptidoglycan. Staphylococcal teichoic acid is antigenic, and antibodies to this substance cause agglutination of isolated staphylococcal cell walls [43]. Antibodies to teichoic acid enhance opsonophagocytic killing of nonencapsulated strains of *S. aureus*, but have little effect on encapsulated isolates [44]. In contrast, antibodies to peptidoglycan play a key role in the opsonization of encapsulated *S. aureus* [45].

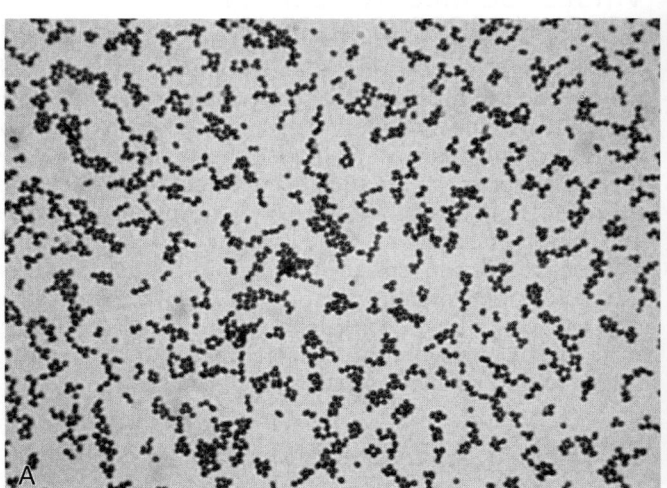
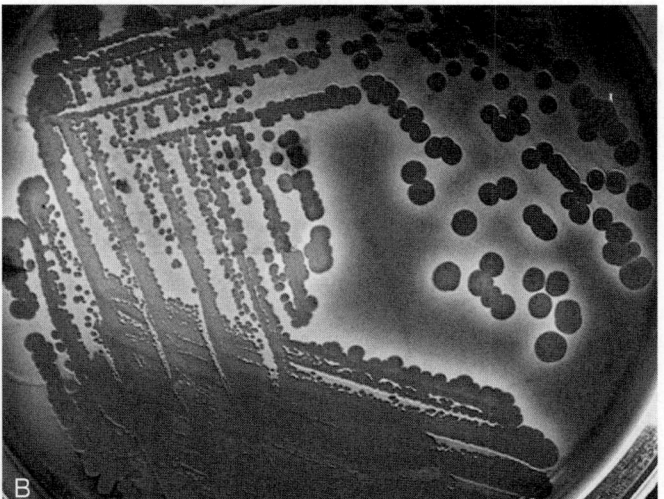

FIGURE 14–1 A, Gram stain of *Staphylococcus aureus* showing characteristic clusters. **B,** Blood agar plate showing growth of *S. aureus* with zone of β-hemolysis surrounding colonies.

Antibodies to *S. aureus* teichoic acid and peptidoglycan are widespread in screens of the human population [45].

In addition to peptidoglycan and teichoic acid, other components of the *S. aureus* cell wall include the group antigen known as protein A, an immunoglobulin Fc binding protein, and numerous other surface-expressed proteins. Similar to the situation with other gram-positive bacteria, many *S. aureus* proteins anchored in the cell wall possess a carboxy-terminal LP(X)TG motif, which serves as a sorting signal for a membrane enzyme called sortase (SrtA) [46,47]. This enzyme cleaves polypeptides between the threonine and the glycine of the LP(X)TG motif and catalyzes formation of an amide bond between the carboxy group of threonine and the amino group of peptidoglycan cross-bridges [47]. These include several proteins involved in extracellular matrix binding and promoting *S. aureus* adherence to host epithelium [48].

S. aureus produces a polysaccharide capsular layer external to the cell wall. Capsular antigens are limited in antigenic specificity and highly conserved among clinical isolates, where the predominant capsules identified are serotype 5 and serotype 8 [49]. The serotype 5 *S. aureus* capsule has the structure $(\rightarrow 4)$-3-O-Ac-β-d-ManNAcA-$(1\rightarrow 4)$-α-l-FucNAc-$(1\rightarrow 3)$-β-d-FucNAc-$(1\rightarrow)_n$, whereas the serotype 8 capsule has the structure $(\rightarrow 3)$-4-O-Ac-β-d-ManNAcA-$(1\rightarrow 3)$-α-l-FucNAc-$(1\rightarrow 3)$-β-d-FucNAc-$(1\rightarrow)_n$ [50,51]. Although these two capsular polysaccharides differ only in the sugar linkages at the sites of *O*-acetylation of the mannosaminuronic acid residues, they remain serologically distinct. Capsule plays a role in the pathogen's resistance to phagocyte clearance.

Small colony variants of *S. aureus* isolated from clinical specimens have been recognized for nearly a century. Small colony variants have now been linked to persistent and relapsing *S. aureus* infections, including chronic osteomyelitis and soft tissue abscesses [52,53]. These phenotypes can be traced to biochemical defects in electron transport, which are associated with slow growth and reduced α-toxin production that promote survival and persistence within endothelial cells. It is hypothesized that the intercellular location represents a privileged niche against the actions of host innate defense molecules and antibiotics. Because they can be overlooked in the laboratory owing to their fastidious growth, extra efforts to identify small colony variants should be undertaken in the setting of persistent or relapsing *S. aureus* infection despite antibiotic therapy [52,53].

Nucleotide sequencing of the whole genome for several isolates of *S. aureus* [54,55], including MRSA strains [56,57], has established that the genome is 2.8 to 2.9 Mb in size, with approximately 2600 to 2700 open reading frames and an overall guanine-to-cytosine content of approximately 33% [54,55]. Much of the *S. aureus* genome seems to have been acquired by lateral gene transfer [56]. Most antibiotic resistance genes are carried on mobile genetic elements, including a unique resistance island. Pathogenicity islands belonging to at least three different classes have been identified, including toxic shock syndrome (TSS) toxin islands, exotoxin islands, and enterotoxin islands. The exotoxin and enterotoxin islands are closely linked to other gene clusters encoding putative virulence factors.

COAGULASE-NEGATIVE STAPHYLOCOCCI

CoNS are a heterogeneous group of organisms that have been divided into 32 species [36]. The following 15 species of CoNS are found as members of the normal human flora: *S. epidermidis*, *Staphylococcus haemolyticus*, *Staphylococcus saprophyticus*, *Staphylococcus capitis*, *Staphylococcus warneri*, *Staphylococcus hominis*, *Staphylococcus xylosus*, *Staphylococcus cohnii*, *Staphylococcus simulans*, *Staphylococcus auricularis*, *Staphylococcus saccharolyticus*, *Staphylococcus caprae*, *Staphylococcus pasteuri*, *Staphylococcus lugdunensis*, and *Staphylococcus schleiferi* [36,58]. Among these species, several occupy very specific niches on the skin. *S. capitis* is most abundant on the head, where sebaceous glands are plentiful. *S. auricularis* has a striking predilection for the external auditory canal. *S. hominis* and *S. haemolyticus* are most common in the axillae and the pubic area, where apocrine glands are numerous.

Speciation of CoNS is accomplished on the basis of a series of biochemical characteristics, simplified in recent years by the commercial availability of miniaturized kits [36]. Differentiation of two strains belonging to the same species (subspeciation) represents a more difficult problem, however. Analogous to the situation with *S. aureus*, contemporary techniques for distinguishing strains of a given species include PFGE and MLST [59]. The composition of CoNS is quite similar to the makeup of *S. aureus* except that the teichoic acid contains glycerol in place of ribose, and the cell wall lacks protein A. Determination of the genome of *S. epidermidis* strain ATCC 12228 (a commensal isolate not associated with disease) revealed a genome approximately 2.5 Mb in size with 2419 open reading frames, greater than 10% smaller than the published genomes of *S. aureus* isolates [60]. Compared with the available *S. aureus* genomes, ATCC 12228 contains fewer antibiotic resistance genes and lacks pathogenicity islands and a capsule locus. A homologue of the *S. aureus srtA* gene is present, along with nine proteins predicted to contain an LP(X)TG motif.

PATHOGENESIS OF DISEASE
VIRULENCE MECHANISMS OF *STAPHYLOCOCCUS AUREUS*

The pathogenic process of *S. aureus* infection begins with colonization of host skin or mucosal surfaces and involves bacterial attachment to host cells often via components of the extracellular matrix. To persist, the organism produces molecules that decrease the effectiveness of complement-mediated and antibody-mediated opsonophagocytosis and block effectors of host immune cell killing, such as reactive oxygen species and antimicrobial peptides. Ultimately, the organism expresses specific factors that damage host cells and degrade components of the extracellular matrix, contributing to persistence and facilitating spread within normally sterile sites of the host.

EPITHELIAL ATTACHMENT AND INVASION

S. aureus initiates adherence by binding to components of the extracellular matrix of the host. This adherence is mediated by protein adhesins known as MSCRAMMs (*m*icrobial *s*urface *c*omponents *r*ecognizing *a*dhesive *m*atrix *m*olecules), which are typically covalently anchored to the cell wall peptidoglycan through the action of sortase enzymes that recognize an LP(X)TG motif in the C-terminal region of the protein [48]. *S. aureus* MSCRAMMs can promote binding to fibronectin, fibrinogen, and collagen. Most strains express two related fibronectin-binding proteins, FnBPA and FnBPB, which mediate bacterial attachment to immobilized fibronectin in vitro and contribute to *S. aureus* binding to plasma clots and foreign bodies. *S. aureus* also expresses the fibrinogen-binding proteins, or "clumping factors," ClfA and ClfB [61,62]. Each Clf protein recognizes a different part of the fibrinogen model and could synergize to allow *S. aureus* to attach more firmly to vascular thrombi under flow stress within the bloodstream. A fibronectin bridge from surface-anchored *S. aureus* ClfA to integrins in the epithelial cell surface promotes intracellular invasion by the pathogen [63]. In rat endocarditis studies, ClfA mutant *S. aureus* have reduced virulence [64]. Finally, the collagen-binding MSCRAMM Cna allows *S. aureus* to adhere to collagenous tissues such as cartilage [65]. In a murine septic arthritis model, a Cna-null mutant strain of *S. aureus* was significantly attenuated for

virulence [66]. The *ica*ADBC-encoded polysaccharide intercellular adhesin (PIA) and polymeric *N*-acetylglucosamine contribute to *S. aureus* biofilm development [67]; these genes and resultant phenotype shared by *S. epidermidis* are discussed in more detail subsequently.

INNATE IMMUNE RESISTANCE

The propensity of *S. aureus* to produce systemic infections, even in otherwise healthy infants, children, and adults, reflects the capacity of this pathogen to resist host innate immune clearance mechanisms that normally function to prevent microbial dissemination beyond epithelial surfaces. The multiple mechanisms used by this preeminent disease agent are summarized schematically in Figure 14–2.

Cationic antimicrobial peptides, such as cathelicidins and defensins produced by epithelial cells and phagocytes, are an important first line of defense against invasive bacterial infection. By incorporating positively charged residues into its cell wall lipoteichoic and teichoic acid, *S. aureus* increases electrostatic repulsion of these defense peptides. D-alanylation of teichoic acids mediated by the *dlt* operon is present in both pathogens, promoting resistance to antimicrobial peptides and neutrophil killing [68,69].

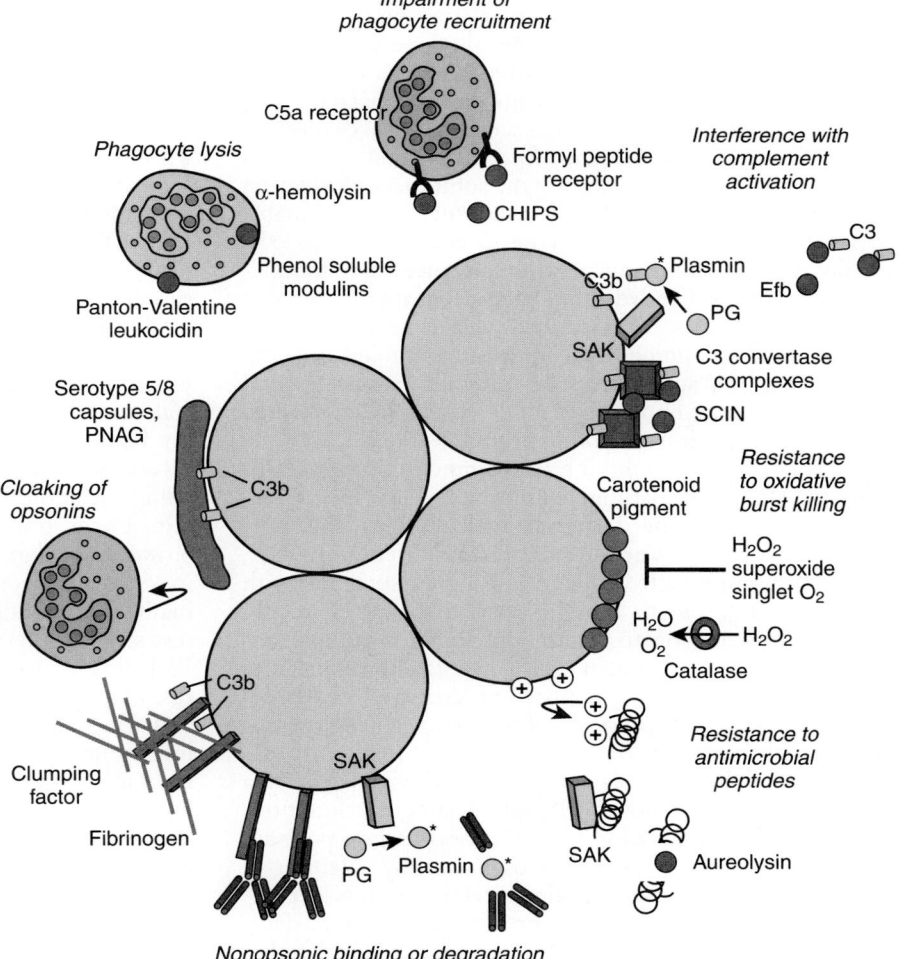

FIGURE 14–2 *Staphylococcus aureus* **possesses multiple virulence mechanisms to resist clearance by host phagocytic cells.** Phagocyte recruitment is restricted by "chemotaxis inhibitory protein of staphylococci" (CHIPS) binding to chemokine receptors. Complement activation is blocked by protein Efb binding of soluble C3 and inhibition of the classical/lectin and alternative C3 convertases by staphylococcal complement inhibitor (SCIN). Carotenoid pigment provides an antioxidant shield, whereas catalase detoxifies hydrogen peroxide (H₂O₂). Resistance to cationic antimicrobial peptides is afforded by positive charge modifications of the cell wall, aureolysin-mediated proteolysis, and binding and inactivation by staphylokinase (SAK). Protein A binds Fc domains of immunoglobulins in a nonopsonic manner, whereas fibrinogen-binding clumping factor and the surface polysaccharide capsule and polymeric *N*-acetylglucosamine (PNAG) cloak surface-bound opsonins from phagocyte recognition. The heptameric pore-forming toxins α-hemolysin and Panton-Valentine leukocidin and phenol-soluble modulins target leukocyte membranes. The plasminogen (PG) binding protein (SAK) activates the zymogen to the active protease plasmin, which can degrade complement opsonin C3b and the immunoglobulin Fc domain.

Additionally, positively charged lysyl-phosphatidylglycerol modifications of teichoic acids are encoded in the functions the *S. aureus* *mpr*F or *lys*C genes and contribute to human antimicrobial peptide resistance [70,71]. *S. aureus* mutants defective in Dlt or MprF show reduced virulence in small animal infection models [69,72]. The secreted proteases V8 and aureolysin of *S. aureus* function to degrade antimicrobial peptides, which could contribute further to *S. aureus* resistance to this important branch of the innate defense system [73,74].

Many *S. aureus* strains produce the "chemotaxis inhibitory protein of staphylococci" that binds with high avidity to the leukocyte receptors for C5a and *N*-formyl peptides, blocking functional engagement of the respective chemoattractants and delaying neutrophil recruitment to the site of infection [75]. *S. aureus* also expresses the extracellular adherence protein that binds and inhibits intracellular adhesion molecule 1, the endothelial receptor required to initiate leukocyte adhesion and diapedesis [76].

S. aureus expresses multiple factors to interfere with host complement-mediated clearance [77]. Cleavage of C3 to opsonically active C3b is accomplished after assembly of C3 convertase complex C4bC2a (classic/lectin pathways) or C3bBb (alternative pathway) on the bacterial surface. The secreted approximately 10 kDa *S. aureus* protein known as staphylococcal complement inhibitor binds and stabilizes both convertases on the bacterial surface, preventing generation of additional convertases, impairing their enzymatic activities, and effectively inhibiting all three complement pathways [78]. The surface-anchored *S. aureus* fibrinogen-binding protein ClfA recruits fibrinogen to the bacterial surface in a fashion that impairs complement deposition [79,80]. The secreted *S. aureus* fibrinogen-binding protein Efb-C can bind free C3, altering the solution conformation of this crucial complement component such that it is unable to participate in its downstream opsonization functions [81]. Finally, another mechanism of interference with complement opsonization derives from bacterial coaptation of host proteolytic activities. The *S. aureus* surface receptor staphylokinase binds plasminogen from host serum and converts zymogen to the active protease, plasmin. Surface bound plasmin can cleave human C3b and C3bi from the bacterial cell wall and impair neutrophil phagocytosis [82].

S. aureus is able to inhibit effector function of immunoglobulin when the pathogen binds its Fc region, effectively decorating the bacterial surface with the host molecule in a "backwards," nonopsonic orientation [83]. This Fc-binding activity is classically associated with protein A of *S. aureus*, which serves to block Fc receptor–mediated phagocytosis and contributes to animal virulence [84]. In addition, most *S. aureus* clinical isolates express surface capsules composed of serotype 5 or 8 polysaccharide [49]. The presence of *S. aureus* capsule is associated with reduced opsonophagocytic uptake of the pathogen by neutrophils and increased virulence in a mouse bacteremia model [85,86]. Analogous functions can be ascribed to an additional *S. aureus* surface polysaccharide, polymeric *N*-acetylglucosamine [87]. Neither of the *S. aureus* exopolysaccharides directly inhibits deposition of complement factors on the bacterial surface; rather, they seem to serve as a superficial "cloak" that restricts access of phagocytes to the opsonins [83].

Catalase production is a diagnostic tool to distinguish staphylococci from streptococci in the clinical laboratory, and the ability of staphylococcal catalase to detoxify hydrogen peroxide generated during oxidative burst may promote phagocyte resistance and virulence [88]. The golden pigment for which *S. aureus* is named is a carotenoid molecule with potent antioxidant properties that is necessary and sufficient to promote bacterial neutrophil resistance and virulence in subcutaneous infection models [89,90]. *S. aureus* also resists oxidative stress through superoxide dismutases, as confirmed by diminished in vivo survival of mutants lacking these enzymes [91].

SECRETED TOXINS

Numerous toxins secreted by *S. aureus* possess cytolytic activity against host cells and can facilitate tissue spread; promote inflammatory responses; and, especially when the target is a phagocytic cell, promote bacterial innate immune evasion. Perhaps the best-studied toxin is *S. aureus* α-toxin (also referred to as α-hemolysin), which forms heptamers in the membranes of various cell types, creating large pores [92,93]. Pore formation induced by *S. aureus* α-toxin is associated with release of nitric oxide from endothelial cells and stimulation of apoptosis in lymphocytes [94,95]. *S. aureus* production of α-toxin may also promote escape from the phagolysosome after macrophage engulfment [96]. MRSA production of α-toxin is essential for virulence of the pathogen in the mouse model of pneumonia [97]. The level of α-toxin expression by differing *S. aureus* strains directly correlates with their virulence. Immunization with an inactivated form of α-toxin, which cannot form pores, generates antigen-specific IgG responses and provides protection against MRSA pneumonia [98].

S. aureus also produces an additional family of two-subunit heteroheptameric toxins capable of oligomerizing in the membrane of target leukocytes to produce pores and promote hypo-osmotic cell lysis. These include γ-hemolysin and the bacteriophage encoded Panton-Valentine leukocidin (PVL) [99]. PVL has gained notoriety because of its strong epidemiologic association with severe cases of CA-MRSA infections [100]. The true contribution of the PVL toxin to *S. aureus* virulence is uncertain. Phage transduction of PVL into a previously naïve *S. aureus* background was reported to increase virulence in a murine necrotizing pneumonia model [101], but an inadvertent mutation in the *agr* regulatory locus of the test strain probably led to spurious interpretations of the PVL linkage to disease pathogenesis [102]. A more direct test of isogenic deletion of PVL in the epidemic USA300 and USA400 clones associated with severe CA-MRSA infections had no effect on neutrophil lysis or virulence in murine skin abscess and systemic infection models [103], but did contribute to proinflammatory cytokine release and muscle necrosis at higher inocula and in certain mouse genetic backgrounds [104]. PVL is much more active against human neutrophils than murine neutrophils, explaining some of the limitations of this animal species as a model for analysis of the virulence functions of the cytotoxin.

Other toxins secreted by *S. aureus* include β-hemolysin, a sphingomyelinase enzyme [105]. Through targeted mutagenesis, β-hemolysin more recently was found to contribute to *S. aureus*–induced lung injury, neutrophilic inflammation, and vascular leakage of serum proteins into the alveolar spaces, in part mediated by the ability of the toxin to promote ectodomain shedding of syndecan-1, a major proteoglycan coating lung epithelial cells [106]. Phenol-soluble modulins are a novel family of small, amphipathic, α-helical cytolytic peptides with in vitro and in vivo leukocidal and proinflammatory activities [107]. Phenol-soluble modulins are produced at high levels by CA-MRSA compared with HA-MRSA and contribute to virulence in necrotizing skin and bacteremia mouse models of infection [108].

S. aureus elaborates numerous toxins with superantigenic capacity, able to promote aberrant interaction between MHC class II on the surface of antigen-presenting cells (e.g., macrophages) with the β-chain of the T-cell receptor, leading to polyclonal T-cell activation and potentially staphylococcal TSS [109]. Twenty distinct *S. aureus* superantigens are known, prominently including TSS toxin-1 and staphylococcal enterotoxins A through E and G through J. The genes encoding the *S. aureus* superantigens are present on accessory genetic elements such as prophages, transposons, plasmids, and chromosomal pathogenicity islands. The contribution of the superantigens to the severe disease manifestations of *S. aureus* are well shown, but the potential evolutionary advantage of superantigen production to the pathogen is unclear. One possible advantage of T-cell activation at the site of infection might be dysregulated cytokine expression patterns that suppress effective local inflammatory responses [109].

Certain strains of *S. aureus* express the exfoliative (epidermolytic) toxins ETA, ETB, ETC, or ETD. These toxins have been identified as glutamate-specific serine proteases that specifically and efficiently cleave a single peptide bond in the extracellular region of human and mouse desmoglein 1, a desmosomal intercellular adhesion molecule, leading to the exfoliative phenotype of scalded skin syndrome and bullous impetigo [110,111].

QUORUM SENSING AND REGULATION OF VIRULENCE FACTOR EXPRESSION

S. aureus seems to impose tight regulation on the differential expression of specific sets of virulence determinants at different stages of growth or the pathogenic process. Cell wall–associated adhesive factors that facilitate the initial stages of infection are selectively produced during the exponential phase of in vitro growth [112]. Conversely, almost all *S. aureus* extracellular proteins and secreted toxins presumed to play a greater role in evasion of the immune system and tissue spread are synthesized predominantly in the postexponential phase of growth [112]. These processes are under the cell density (quorum sensing)–dependent control of the accessory gene regulator (*agr*) locus [113,114]. Similar to other bacterial quorum sensing systems, *agr* encodes an autoactivating peptide (AIP) that is the inducing ligand for a signal receptor (AgrC), the *agr* signal receptor. The unique effector of

global gene regulation in the *agr* system is the regulatory RNA molecule, RNAIII [114]. *agr* mutants show decreased virulence in murine infection models [115].

VIRULENCE MECHANISMS OF COAGULASE-NEGATIVE STAPHYLOCOCCI

Until more recently, the pathogenic potential of CoNS received little attention. With the emergence of these organisms as prominent pathogens in neonates and hospitalized patients with intravascular devices, investigation has intensified in an effort to identify important virulence factors and to inform new approaches to treatment and prevention [116]. Two main reasons for the increasing rate of CoNS infections are spreading antibiotic resistance among CoNS and the ever-increasing development and use of medical devices [117]. Attention has centered primarily on *S. epidermidis*, the species most commonly associated with clinical disease, usually in association with central intravenous catheters. Other species that have been examined, although to a lesser extent, include *S. saprophyticus*, *S. lugdunensis*, and *S. schleiferi*.

When CoNS infections are initiated on intravascular catheters and other prosthetic devices, the ability of the bacterium to adhere to the hydrophobic surface of the foreign body is a first critical step in the pathogenic process (Fig. 14–3). CoNS are able to colonize virtually any plastic surface [118]. In addition, plastic objects in the human body soon become coated with host extracellular matrix proteins [119], such that CoNS can colonize the devices either by directly attaching to the plastic or by binding to the host extracellular matrix, and both processes are likely to play a role in the initial establishment of infection. Overall surface hydrophobicity varies among CoNS strains, and increased hydrophobicity can be correlated to better plastic binding [120]; however, no linkage between surface hydrophobicity and clinical infectivity has been established [117].

Transposon mutagenesis identified AltE, a putative CoNS autolysin protein, as promoting adherence to plastic surfaces [121]; in a rat model of catheter-associated infection, *S. epidermidis* AltE mutant shows diminished pathogenicity [122]. Two large surface proteins present in some *S. epidermidis* strains—SSP-1 and SSP-2, one likely a degradation product of the other—are present in fibrillar structures on the bacterial surface and promote binding to polystyrene [123].

Following in the pattern of *S. aureus*, extracellular matrix binding surface components or MSCRAMMs are beginning to be well characterized in CoNS. The fibrinogen-binding protein Fbe (also known as SdrG) of *S. epidermidis* resembles *S. aureus* clumping factor with the presence of

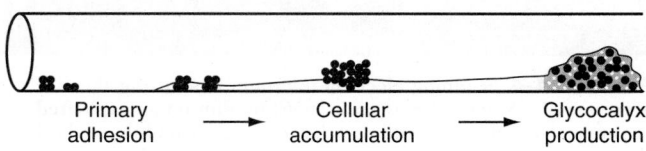

FIGURE 14–3 Schematic model of phases involved in *Staphylococcus epidermidis* biofilm formation.

multiple serine/aspartic repeat domains and a capacity to bind to the β-chain of the host matrix protein [124–126]. *S. epidermidis* cell wall teichoic acid enhances overall adherence to fibronectin, perhaps serving as a bridging molecule between bacterial MSCRAMMs and fibronectin-coated surfaces [127]. Phage-display technology was used to identify *S. epidermidis* protein, EmbP, capable of mediating binding to fibronectin, whereas *S. epidermidis* lipase enzyme, GehD, seems to promote collagen attachment [128]. Finally, the above-mentioned AltE also contains a domain with vitronectin-binding capacity that may contribute to its virulence phenotype in the rat model [121].

After initial attachment to a biomaterial, organisms multiply and form complex multilayered aggregates that involve intercellular adhesion and are referred to as biofilms (Fig. 14–4; see also Fig. 14–3). Historically, isolates of CoNS were often described as elaborating "slime" and "slime-associated antigen," terms that we now realize refer to biofilms and the presence of abundant quantities of a specific polysaccharide molecule. Significant degrees of slime production were reported in more than 80% of CoNS isolates from infants with invasive disease [129,130]. The main virulence factor responsible for the formation of these cellular aggregates in certain *S. epidermidis* strains is now recognized to be a secreted exopolysaccharide, PIA [131,132]. PIA is an unbranched β-1, 6-linked *N*-acetylglucosaminic acid polymer, produced by the enzymes of the four-gene *ica* operon [133]. An *ica* knockout mutant shows reduced virulence in a rat model of catheter infection [122], and *S. epidermidis* strains isolated from patients with foreign infections were more likely to possess the *ica* genes and form robust biofilms in vitro than strains from asymptomatic individuals [134]. Expression of PIA is subject to on-off phase-switching that may be attributable to reversible insertion and excision of mobile genetic element (IS256) in the *ica*

operon [135]. A 140-kDa CoNS extracellular protein known as accumulation-associated protein apparently cooperates with PIA in promoting biofilm growth [136].

CoNS biofilm provides a nonspecific physical barrier to cellular and humoral defense mechanisms [132,137]. The formation of CoNS biofilms depends on the regulatory control exerted by a homologue of the *S. aureus agr* locus [138]. *S. epidermidis* organisms embedded within biofilms bind less complement C3b and IgG and are less susceptible to neutrophil killing [139]. CoNS biofilm–associated polysaccharide also is capable of inhibiting the antimicrobial action of vancomycin and teicoplanin [140]. In the clinical setting, formation of biofilms on the catheter surface has been shown to make eradication of CoNS infection more problematic [141,142].

S. epidermidis expresses a 27-kDa serine protease called GluSE that is expressed during biofilm formation and has been shown to degrade fibrinogen and the complement-derived chemoattractant C5, suggesting a potential role in immune evasion [143]. *S. epidermidis* also expresses a group of secreted amphiphilic peptides called phenol-soluble modulins that have neutrophil chemotactic ability and generate other proinflammatory effects including activating neutrophil oxidative burst and degranulation [144].

ROLE OF THE HOST DEFENSES

Even under the most ideal conditions, infants in the hospital are surrounded by staphylococci. Physical barriers such as the skin and mucous membranes represent a major defense against staphylococcal disease. Bacteremic disease most often develops when organisms colonizing the skin gain access to the bloodstream through the portal created by an intravascular catheter. Other routes for entry into the bloodstream include the intestinal tract after injury to the epithelial barrier, the respiratory tract in patients receiving mechanical ventilation, and the umbilicus when the umbilical cord remains in place. Localized disease occurs when colonizing organisms are implanted into deeper tissues, often related to a break in skin or mucous membrane integrity and sometimes during placement of a foreign body.

As with other pathogenic bacteria, the presence of intact neutrophil phagocytic function is probably the most important factor involved in controlling replication and spread of staphylococci [145]. The ability of the newborn's bone marrow to respond to infection with rapidly enhanced production and maturation of neutrophil precursors is limited compared with adults [146]. Neutrophils from newborns have relatively diminished motility toward chemoattractants compared with cells from older children and adults [147]; this is partly the result of diminished chemotactic factors such as the complement-derived C5a and the CXC chemokine interleukin (IL)-8 [148,149]. Neutrophils from young infants also exhibit decreased diapedesis across endothelium, possibly because of impaired capacity to upregulate endothelial cell expression of the CR3 receptor [150]. Beyond decreases in neutrophil number, chemotaxis, and trans-epithelial migration, the capacity for neutrophil adherence and phagocytosis is reduced in neonates, largely

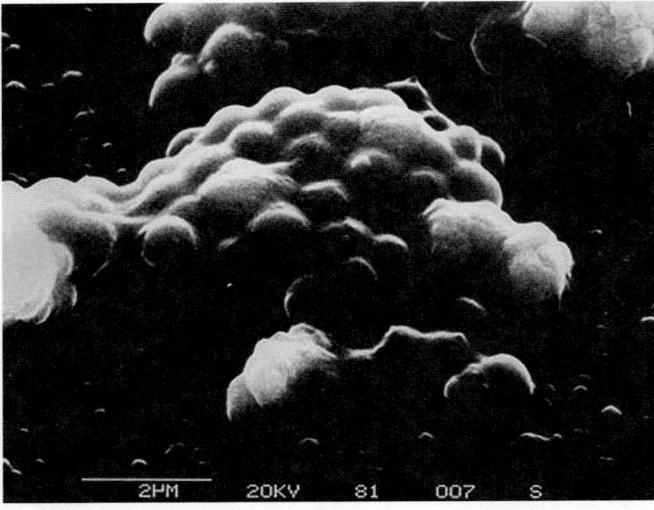

FIGURE 14–4 Scanning electron micrograph showing the presence of a *Staphylococcus epidermidis* biofilm on an explanted intravascular catheter. Biofilm is characterized by multilayered cell clusters embedded in an extracellular polysaccharide. *(From von Eiff C, Peters G, Heilmann C. Pathogenesis of infections due to coagulase-negative staphylococci. Lancet Infect Dis 2:677-685, 2002.)*

owing to deficiencies in opsonins, including complement and specific antibody [145].

Phagocytic killing seems to be intact in normal newborns, but may be compromised in stressed infants, at least in part because of reduced production of reactive oxygen species [151,152]. The multifaceted antioxidant capacities of *S. aureus*, including catalase and the carotenoid pigment, likely support its prominent role as an opportunistic pathogen in stressed infants and in patients with chronic granulomatous disease, where defects in reduced nicotinamide adenine dinucleotide phosphate oxidase lead to marginal oxidative burst function. Chronic granulomatous disease may occasionally present with *S. aureus*, *Serratia*, or *Aspergillus* infection in the neonatal period [153].

Specific antibody is less important than complement in opsonization of *S. aureus* and plays a limited role in defense against neonatal staphylococcal disease [154]. In general, there is no correlation between antibody titers against *S. aureus* and the likelihood of asymptomatic carriage versus clinical disease [155,156]. Consistent with this information, an attempt to protect the newborn from staphylococcal disease by immunizing the mother near term was unsuccessful [157].

In most cases of neonatal staphylococcal disease, the role of T cells is unclear. In animal models, T cells are found to contribute to the development of abscesses during *S. aureus* infection [158]. T cells are centrally involved, however, in the immune response to several *S. aureus* toxins, including TSST-1, the staphylococcal enterotoxins, and the staphylococcal exfoliative toxins (ETA, ETB, ETC, and ETD), and in associated pathogenesis. The consequence of this dysregulated T-cell overactivation is proliferation of a large proportion of T cells and release of numerous cytokines, including tumor necrosis factor (TNF)-α, IL-1, and interferon-γ [159]. These molecules are major contributors to the systemic manifestations of staphylococcal scalded skin syndrome (SSSS), TSS, and food poisoning.

PATHOLOGY

The most characteristic pathologic lesion associated with *S. aureus* infection is a local abscess, consisting of necrotic tissue, fibrin, and numerous live and dead neutrophils. Similarly, CoNS infection is characterized by infiltration of neutrophils, usually with moderate necrosis. Other pathologic findings are described next in the sections on clinical manifestations.

CLINICAL MANIFESTATIONS

Staphylococci are capable of producing a wide variety of clinical syndromes in the newborn infant, including syndromes with high mortality rates, as was reviewed almost 50 years ago [160]. The clinical manifestations of staphylococcal infection are most prominently a function of two factors: the gestational age of the infant, with extremely low birth weight infants at highest risk of infection and subsequent complications, and the strain of *Staphylococcus* causing the infection, with CoNS generally causing more mild infection compared with *S. aureus*, particularly

relevant to more recent CA-MRSA. As noted earlier, staphylococci are armed with an impressive array of virulence factors. They may merely colonize skin or respiratory or gastrointestinal tract mucosa without apparent harm to the host or cause invasive, lethal disease. CoNS are most often benign colonizers of skin and gastrointestinal tract in newborns, causing frequent but relatively mild infections in hospitalized premature infants. In contrast, coagulase-positive strains (*S. aureus*) are more commonly associated with clinically aggressive, invasive infections. The subsequent sections provide a general overview of clinical manifestations and organ-specific manifestations.

BACTEREMIA AND SEPSIS

The most common manifestations of invasive staphylococcal infection are bacteremia and sepsis. Studies describing symptomatic community-acquired and hospital-acquired bacteremia in neonates provide an overall framework in which CoNS and *S. aureus* infection can be defined and include early-onset sepsis and late-onset sepsis syndromes [6,25,161–175].

Early-onset sepsis is most often related to acute infectious complications of late pregnancy and delivery or colonization of the infant at birth and subsequent development of clinical symptoms within the first 48 to 72 hours of life [176]. The signs and symptoms associated with staphylococcal septicemia usually are nonspecific and include disturbances of temperature regulation, respiration, circulation, gastrointestinal function, and central nervous system activity. Hypothermia is more common than fever and often is observed as the initial sign. Respiratory distress frequently manifests as episodes of apnea and bradycardia, particularly in infants who weigh less than 1500 g. Other abnormalities related to respiration include tachypnea, retractions, and cyanosis. In 20% to 30% of infants, gastrointestinal abnormalities develop, including poor feeding, regurgitation, abdominal distention, diarrhea, and bloody stools. Evidence of poor perfusion includes mottling and poor capillary refill. In some infants, lethargy, irritability, or poor suck may also be noted.

The incidence of early-onset sepsis caused by *S. aureus* seems to reflect the characteristics of circulating strains and varies by year and region of the world (see "Epidemiology and Transmission"). Clinical descriptions of staphylococcal sepsis include a positive blood culture, usually in the context of nonspecific clinical signs and symptoms that may include apnea, bradycardia, irritability, poor feeding, abdominal distention, lethargy, hypotonia, hypothermia or hyperthermia, hypotension with poor tissue perfusion, cyanosis, and increased oxygen requirement with respiratory distress. In an ongoing 75-year collection of data from Yale–New Haven Hospital [7], *S. aureus* represented the etiology of early-onset sepsis from 28% (1928-1932) to 3% (1979-1988), with a current rate (1989-2003) of 7%. Mortality from all causes of early-onset sepsis declined from about 90% with the earliest data set to approximately 5% of all newborn infants in 1989-2003.

A report from Finland documented *S. aureus* as an etiology of sepsis from 1976-1980 in 22% of all infants with positive blood cultures [177], with an overall mortality rate of 31%, although for infants with birth weight 1500 g or less, the mortality rate was 44%. Published data from centers in Australia and New Zealand from 1992-1999 documented *S. aureus* rates that varied considerably by year and by institution, with differences in rates even noted within different hospitals in the same city [163], resulting in an overall rate of 19 cases out of 244,718 births (0.008%). In this report, MRSA accounted for only 8% of cases from 1992-1994, but 34% of cases from 1995-1998. Of 26 cases of *S. aureus* sepsis documented in 1999, none were caused by MRSA. The overall mortality rate from MRSA was 25% compared with 10% for MSSA.

Early-onset sepsis caused by CoNS is reported extremely infrequently, likely because of the noninvasive nature of most strains. These reports may reflect true infection, particularly in very low birth weight infants [167,178], although the extent of symptoms attributable to infection in these infants is difficult to assess. Otherwise, particularly for term infants, a positive culture of blood for CoNS may represent a contaminant, unrelated to the underlying illness.

When considering late-onset neonatal sepsis syndrome, occurring after the 5th day of life in hospitalized infants, *S. aureus* and CoNS are well-documented pathogens. In the NICHD Neonatal Research Network, *S. aureus* was the second most common pathogen to cause late-onset sepsis in very low birth weight (401 to 1500 g) infants [6]. CA-MRSA produces particularly devastating infection, with seven of eight infants hospitalized in the NICU of Texas Children's Hospital in Houston presenting in septic shock; the case-fatality ratio was 38% in this series, despite appropriate support and antimicrobial therapy [179]. In a maternity hospital in Houston during the same period, mortality attributable to the invasive *S. aureus* infection was 6%, with late sequelae attributable to infection of 12% [179]. In this report, only 3 of 39 *S. aureus* infections were caused by MRSA; all 3 infants recovered without sequelae.

In a retrospective review of 12 neonates with bacteremia caused by MSSA compared with 11 neonates infected by CA-MRSA, collected during 1993-2003 in Tel Aviv, Israel, mortality rates were virtually identical, 25% versus 27% [172]. In a larger series of 90 infants from Taiwan with bacteremia caused by MRSA, 75% of infants were premature, 54% of infections were believed to be catheter-related, 21% were associated with skin and soft tissue infections, 17% were associated with pneumonia, 8% were associated with bone and joint infection, 3% were associated with meningitis, and 3% were associated with peritonitis [180]. This rate of metastatic infection attributed to MRSA seems greater than that noted with MSSA and is clearly greater than rates seen with CoNS bacteremia. Of infants with resolved MRSA infection, 10% had at least one recurrence. At Duke University Medical Center, mortality and neurodevelopmental outcomes in infants with bacteremia caused by MSSA (median age 26.5 days) were compared with MRSA (median age 26 days) [181]. Although the duration of staphylococcal bacteremia was shorter in neonates with MSSA (1 day versus 4.5 days), the mortality and neurodevelopmental outcomes were statistically similar to infants infected with MRSA.

The largest burden of disease in late-onset sepsis caused by staphylococci is catheter-related CoNS bacteremia in premature infants. In the NICU, CoNS cause 40% to 60% of all documented bacteremia [6,162,182,183]. Rates of catheter-associated bacteremia have been tracked by the U.S. Centers for Disease Control and Prevention [184] and other collaborative groups, including the Pediatric Prevention Network [161] and the Vermont Oxford National Evidence-Based Quality Improvement Collaborative for Neonatology [185]. Clinical manifestations of infection are frequently related to the gestational and chronologic age of the newborn, but are most often nonspecific. In a retrospective review of invasive staphylococcal infections in a maternity hospital in Houston, Texas, during 2000-2002, bacteremia was present in 94% of 108 infants with invasive CoNS infection, resulting in a wide range of nonspecific symptoms, including apnea and bradycardia in 52%, an increased oxygen requirement in 90%, lethargy in 31%, abdominal distention in 30%, increased blood pressure support requirement in 22%, and temperature instability in 18% [178]. Similar findings were published by investigators in the Neonatal Research Network, sponsored by the NICHD [186], highlighting the burden of disease in very low birth weight infants.

CoNS infections have often been associated with many risk factors (see "Epidemiology and Transmission"), but the ultimate outcome of infants infected with CoNS may more closely follow their comorbidities than be linked to bacterial pathogenicity. In a review of data collected by the Pediatrix Medical Group, Benjamin and colleagues [165] noted that the survival of low birth weight infants ($\leq$1250 g) after a positive blood culture for CoNS was virtually identical (8%) to survival of infants evaluated for sepsis yielding sterile blood cultures, in contrast to much higher rates of mortality with gram-negative organisms or *Candida*. Similar findings suggesting lack of attributable mortality to CoNS bacteremia documented that for infants who ultimately died of any cause, death occurred more than 7 days after the positive blood culture for CoNS in 75% of infants [6]. These findings were also confirmed in very low birth weight infants in Israel, reporting on 3462 episodes of late-onset sepsis, documenting a mortality within 72 hours of CoNS bacteremia of only 1.8% [187]. Other authors have suggested that persisting positive blood cultures for CoNS, despite appropriate antibiotic coverage, are associated with an increase in overall complications, with a mortality of 7% [164].

Treatment of catheter-associated CoNS infections is controversial. Karlowicz and colleagues [188] prospectively evaluated treatment with vancomycin versus catheter removal. In neonates treated with vancomycin who experienced clearing of bacteremia within 1 to 2 days, success without catheter removal occurred in 79%, whereas in neonates with persisting bacteremia of 3 to 4 days, the success rate declined to 44%, and in neonates with bacteremia persisting beyond 4 days, none were successfully treated with medical therapy alone, a finding similar to that reported by Benjamin and associates [189] in a retrospective review, in which the rate of metastatic infection increased significantly after four or more positive cultures. Other authors have attempted to limit the empirical use of vancomycin in the NICU by comparing outcomes using vancomycin-containing empirical regimens during one period of study with cloxacillin-containing regimens during another period. When all-cause mortality was assessed at 14 days after positive blood culture, 0 of 45 infants receiving vancomycin versus 4 of 37 infants not receiving vancomycin had died. When examined on a individual case basis, only one of the deaths was possibly attributed to CoNS sepsis [190].

TOXIC SHOCK SYNDROMES

In addition to clinical manifestations related to bacteremia, toxin-mediated clinical disease may occur, including SSSS (see later), TSS [191], and neonatal TSS-like exanthematous disease [192]. TSS is caused by pyrogenic toxin superantigens produced by *S. aureus*. These superantigens include TSST-1 and several enterotoxins, most commonly staphylococcal enterotoxin serotype B or C [193,194]. TSS has been described in a 4-day-old term infant boy, with poor feeding and vomiting at 3 days of age, followed by hypotension, respiratory distress, and multiorgan failure on day 4 of life. Generalized erythema developed at 6 days of age. This infant was colonized on the umbilicus with a methicillin-susceptible strain that produced staphylococcal enterotoxins C, G and I [191].

A similar disease has been described in Japan, caused by MRSA, producing erythema in association with thrombocytopenia, elevated C-reactive protein, or fever [195]; this presentation has been termed neonatal TSS-like exanthematous disease (Fig. 14–5) [196]. Since the time of the first description, surveys in Japan have shown that 70% of Japanese hospitals have reported a similar illness in neonates [197]. The causative strains all carried the TSST-1 gene and the staphylococcal enterotoxin C gene [192]. The pathophysiology of neonatal TSS-like exanthematous disease begins with colonization with MRSA, a common occurrence among Japanese newborns. Typically, the colonizing strain of MRSA produces TSST-1 [192], and the symptoms of the disease are related to the overactivation of TSST-1–reactive T cells [196]. Neonatal TSS-like exanthematous disease does not develop in all infants who are colonized with TSST-1–producing MRSA, suggesting that protection from this illness may be mediated by the transplacental transfer of maternal antibody directed against TSST-1 [197].

ENDOCARDITIS

Although infective endocarditis in neonates is rare, autopsy studies from the 1970s revealed unsuspected endocarditis in 0.2% to 3% of neonates who were examined post-mortem [198,199]. Historically, *S. aureus* has been the predominant bacterial pathogen among neonates with endocarditis [200], but more recent reports indicate that CoNS is now most common [201–204]. Premature infants with prolonged central catheter bacteremia and infants with congenital heart disease are most likely to develop *S. aureus* endocarditis in association with bacteremia [202,204–208]. Endocarditis has also been described in infants infected by CA-MRSA [209].

The signs and symptoms of infective endocarditis in neonates often are nonspecific and similar to signs and symptoms of other conditions such as sepsis or congenital heart disease, including poor feeding, tachycardia, and respiratory distress [200]. Clinical features in general may be unable to distinguish bacteremia with endocarditis from infants with bacteremia without endocarditis [204]. Murmurs can be appreciated in 75% of neonates with endocarditis, with hepatosplenomegaly present in 50%, skin abscesses in 44%, arthritis in 12%, and petechiae in 12%. Blood cultures and echocardiography are the most important diagnostic tests, although urine cultures may be positive in 38% [202,207]. The yield of a single blood culture has been reported to be 77% to 97%. When three blood cultures are obtained, the yield approaches 100% [207].

All neonates with *S. aureus* bacteremia should be evaluated by echocardiogram. The thin chest wall of the neonate makes echocardiography a highly sensitive tool for diagnosis of endocarditis in this age group. Limitations of this technique include the inability to detect lesions less than 2 mm in diameter and to differentiate between vegetations and other masses such as thrombi [202]. In all age groups of children, 12% of children with bacteremia with *S. aureus* may have clear evidence of endocarditis; children with underlying congenital heart disease and *S. aureus* bacteremia have a much greater risk of endocarditis compared with children with no cardiac malformations (53% versus 3%) [205]. Mortality in children with *S. aureus* bacteremia and endocarditis has been reported to be 40% [205].

In the Australasian Study Group for Neonatal Infections, bacteremia caused by CoNS in 1281 infants during 1991-2000 was associated with endocarditis in 3 (0.2%); in infants with bacteremia caused by *S. aureus*, endocarditis occurred in 3 of 223 (1.3%) infected with MSSA strains and in 1 of 65 (2%) infected with CA-MRSA strains. Historically, the prognosis for neonates with endocarditis has been grave. Numerous series published in recent years report disease-specific survival rates ranging from 40% to 70% [202,204,207]. Survival of neonates with infective endocarditis is likely to be improved with early diagnosis and aggressive management [200].

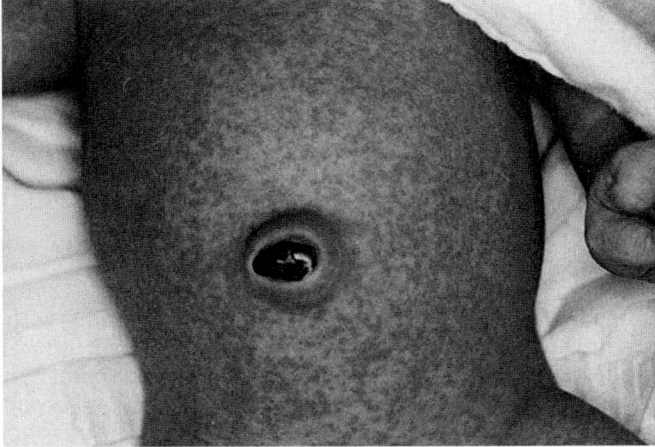

FIGURE 14–5 Typical exanthem in full-term infant with neonatal toxic shock syndrome–like exanthematous disease. *(From Takahashi N, et al. Exanthematous disease induced by toxic shock syndrome toxin 1 in the early neonatal period. Lancet 351:1614-1619, 1998.)*

PUSTULOSIS, CUTANEOUS ABSCESS, AND CELLULITIS

For infants presenting to Texas Children's Hospital in Houston, skin infection was the most common manifestation of staphylococcal disease (88%) in term or late preterm infants (≥36 weeks of gestation). Of infants with skin infection, about two thirds presented with cellulitis or abscess, whereas one third presented with pustulosis, a localized, nonsystemic, invasive cutaneous form of infection [210]. Two thirds of all *S. aureus* infections were caused by CA-MRSA, with CA-MRSA and MSSA manifesting with skin or invasive infection in roughly equal percentages; the proportion of infections caused by CA-MRSA increased over the period of observation from 2001-2006 [210,211]. A similar experience was reported from Chicago, in which 11 infants less than 1 month of age were culture-positive for CA-MRSA, with cutaneous lesions consisting of pustules and vesicles, most commonly present in the diaper area. Resolution of cutaneous infection occurred with the use of mupirocin ointment. No infant required surgical drainage, and no infant developed systemic manifestations of disease or required hospitalization with intravenous antibiotic therapy [212]. Similar clusters of skin-only pustules and vesicles have been reported from other centers [213].

Evaluation of newborn infants discharged from the hospital, but readmitted within 30 days of age, provided a different profile of clinical disease caused by staphylococci [210]. Infants infected with MRSA presented at 7 to 12 days of age, in contrast to infants infected with MSSA, whose presentations occurred evenly spaced over the 1st month of life. Most of these infants (87% for MRSA and 86% for MSSA) presented with skin and soft tissue infection. Cellulitis with or without abscess was responsible for about two thirds of hospitalizations. Pustulosis, primarily involving skin covered by a diaper, was the most prominent sign in approximately one third of infections. Invasive disease occurred in about 10% of infants, including bacteremia, urinary tract infection, osteomyelitis, myositis, and empyema. A study of the clinical characteristics of neonates hospitalized in a level III (40-bed) NICU and cultured weekly from the nose and inguinal areas to assess ongoing colonization status showed that of 152 infants known to be colonized over the study period 2002-2004, 6 (3.9%) developed MRSA sepsis, 3 (2%) developed conjunctivitis, 2 (1.3%) developed chest tube site wound infections, and 2 (1.3%) developed cellulitis [214].

ADENITIS AND PAROTITIS

S. aureus cervical adenitis can be another manifestation of nursery colonization in newborns. At least two outbreaks of cervical adenitis resulting from nurseries were reported in 1972. One outbreak involving 25 infants had an attack rate of 1.9%, and another involving 9 infants had an attack rate of 5.6% [215,216]. As with other manifestations of nursery-associated *S. aureus* disease, illness usually appears after discharge from the hospital. The mean incubation periods in the two outbreaks in England were 86 days and 72 days. Because of the delay in onset of disease, confirmation of a nursery as the source of the infection may be difficult and necessitates careful epidemiologic investigation. Neonatal suppurative parotitis is an uncommon infection among newborns, occurring with an incidence of 13.8 per 10,000 admissions [217]. Premature neonates and boys seem to be at highest risk for suppurative parotitis, which is most frequently caused by *S. aureus* [218,219]. Diagnosis of suppurative parotitis relies on the clinical findings of parotid swelling and purulent exudate from Stensen duct on compression of the parotid gland [220].

BREAST INFECTION

A series of 39 neonatal breast abscesses caused by *S. aureus* were reported by Rudoy and Nelson [221] from Dallas, Texas, in 1975. These infants developed infection most commonly during the 2nd week of life, when neonatal breast tissue is still enlarged in response to transplacental estrogens. The infection is clinically easy to detect, with acute onset of swelling, erythema, and tenderness of the affected breast, with progression of the infection over several hours, occasionally spreading to surrounding tissues (Fig. 14–6). Spontaneous drainage of purulent material from the infant's breast may or may not occur. Culture and Gram stain of purulent discharge is diagnostic. Management includes systemic antistaphylococcal antimicrobials and careful surgical drainage of abscessed tissue within the breast, particularly in female infants. In the report from Dallas, one third of infant girls followed into early adolescence were documented to have decreased breast size as a complication of the infection [221].

In other series of cases in which follow-up histories were obtained, a decrease in breast size was noted in two of six individuals who were examined at ages 8 and 15 years [221,222]. A series of three female neonates with necrotizing fasciitis as a complication of breast infection and abscess was collected from the Hôpital Necker in Paris over a 30-year period, all caused by MSSA, with no infant having a concurrently positive blood culture. All infants survived after extensive surgery and prolonged antibiotic therapy. In one of three cases followed through puberty, breast development did not occur on the affected side [223]. Antimicrobial therapy should be provided intravenously until a clear, substantial response can be documented. In locations with a high prevalence of CA-MRSA, therapy should include clindamycin or vancomycin.

FUNISITIS, OMPHALITIS, AND NECROTIZING FASCIITIS

Funisitis, mild inflammation of the umbilical stump with minimal drainage and minimal erythema in the surrounding tissue, is a local, noninvasive entity. Infections of the umbilical stump may become invasive, however, and occur in a full spectrum of clinical presentations from funisitis to massive abdominal wall inflammation with erythema and indurative edema associated with necrotizing fasciitis. In an attempt to define the stages of the spectrum of infection, some experts have separated the infection into

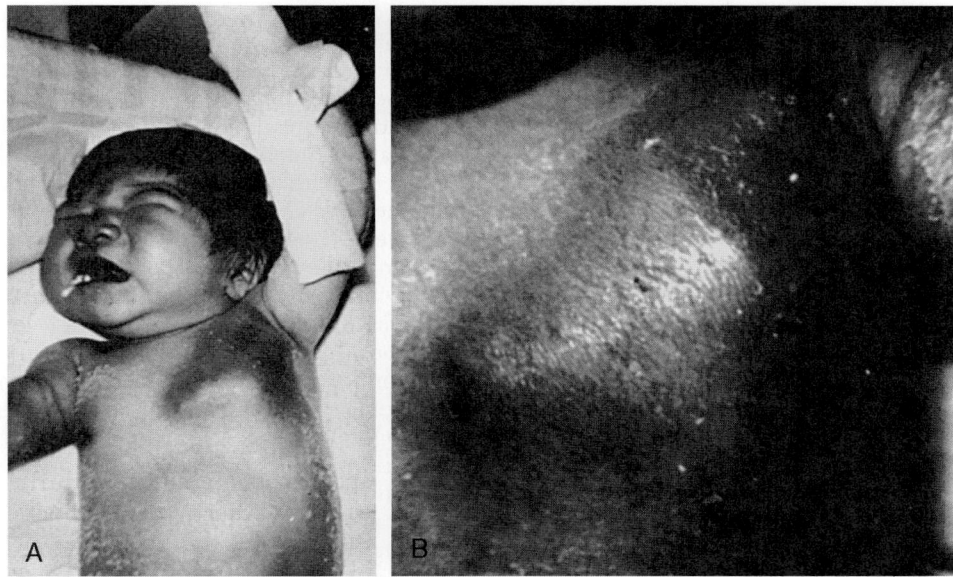

FIGURE 14–6 **A** and **B**, Left breast abscess in a 12-day-old infant. Abscess extends toward the right side of chest and up over the arm. The infant responded well to incision and drainage and antibiotic treatment.

distinct categories: category 1, funisitis and umbilical discharge (shaggy unhealthy umbilical stump, malodorous or purulent discharge); category 2, omphalitis with abdominal wall cellulitis (periumbilical erythema and superficial tenderness in addition to findings in category 1); category 3, omphalitis with systemic sepsis; and category 4, omphalitis with fasciitis (umbilical necrosis with extensive local disease, periumbilical ecchymosis, crepitus bullae, and evidence of involvement of superficial and deep fascia) [224].

Cultures of umbilical tissue in all categories of infection often yield several organisms, including *S. aureus* and CA-MRSA [211,225]. Management of categories 1 through 3 is usually with aggressive local care and systemic, broad-spectrum antibiotic therapy active against enteric bacilli, anaerobes, and *S. aureus*, with an option to provide oral therapy only for infants in category 1 if close observation and frequent reexamination can be arranged.

The most life-threatening entity, necrotizing fasciitis, requires immediate administration of broad-spectrum antibiotics and supportive care, with aggressive surgical débridement. Because *S. aureus* may be just one of several pathogens cultured, the exact role of *S. aureus* in the overall clinical disease process cannot be accurately assessed. Of seven infants presenting at 4 to 14 days of age with necrotizing fasciitis in Los Angeles, California, four were culture-positive for *S. aureus* in a mixed infection [226]. In Muscat, Oman, 10 of 14 neonates had *S. aureus* cultured from umbilical tissue, including 1 infant positive for MRSA, with 3 of the 10 infants having concurrent staphylococcal bacteremia [227]. Despite aggressive management, the mortality rates of polymicrobial necrotizing fasciitis have been 60% to 70% from sites in the United States [226,227], suggesting that earlier recognition with aggressive surgical management, critical care support, and antimicrobial therapy that includes activity against

S. aureus or CA-MRSA if appropriate may be necessary to improve outcomes.

Necrotizing fasciitis caused solely by MRSA in the newborn is extremely unusual. The report of the first three cases from the Chang Gung Children's Hospital in Taiwan in 1999 [228] did not include information on the molecular characterization of these strains, raising the possibility that these MRSA strains may not be similar to the currently prevalent USA300 pulsotype, PVL-positive CA-MRSA strains. The clinical course of extensive soft tissue necrosis with relatively mild systemic symptoms, no mortality, and hospital discharge after 3 to 4 weeks of hospitalization is consistent, however, with current reports of CA-MRSA necrotizing fasciitis in 14 adults in Los Angeles and reports of single cases in neonates from San Diego, California, and Chicago, Illinois [229–231].

These neonates present for medical attention at 5 to 16 days of age with acute development of symptoms over 24 to 48 hours and rapid spread of erythema with indurative edema of infected tissues that have not been known to be previously traumatized. The infants may appear systemically ill with fever, irritability, and a laboratory evaluation suggesting acute inflammation with elevated peripheral white blood cell count, C-reactive protein, and frequently blood culture that is positive for *S. aureus*. Although imaging should not delay emergent surgical débridement, magnetic resonance imaging (MRI) is the preferred modality in adults, and presumably infants, to define the soft tissue characteristics of necrotizing fasciitis [232,233]. In addition to broad-spectrum antimicrobials outlined previously and surgical débridement, hyperbaric oxygen treatment has been used, but its role is poorly defined, with no prospective, randomized clinical trial data and only single cases or small case series that may or may not support adjunctive hyperbaric oxygen therapy [228,233,234].

STAPHYLOCOCCAL SCALDED SKIN SYNDROME AND BULLOUS IMPETIGO

SSSS has been reported in full-term and premature infants [235–239]. The first series of patients in 1878 from Prague by Ritter von Rittershain [240] described clinical infection that is likely to have included patients with SSSS. Clinical characteristics in neonates are similar to characteristics in infants and older children [241] with acute onset of infection associated with macular or generalized erythema usually starting on the face and moving to the trunk within 24 hours. Erythema is accentuated in the flexor creases of the extremities, similar to streptococcal toxin disease, but with minimal mucous membrane erythema. Within 48 hours, the involved tender skin, primarily on the face, diaper area, and extremities, begins to form superficial, clear, flaccid bullae that subsequently break, revealing bright red, moist skin. These lesions show a separation of tissue layers within the epidermis, at the junction of the stratum spinosum and stratum granulosum, owing to the effect of staphylococcal exfoliative toxins A and B on desmoglein-1 (see "Pathogenesis of Disease").

The characteristic histologic feature of SSSS is intraepidermal cleavage through the granular layer, without evidence of epidermal necrosis or inflammatory cell infiltrate (Fig. 14–7) [242]. This appearance is distinct from the appearance in toxic epidermal necrolysis, which is characterized by a subepidermal split-thickness and full-thickness necrosis of the epidermis. Desquamation may be local, under the bullae, or generalized (Fig. 14–8). Before formation of bullae, erythematous skin shows intraepidermal separation when gentle tangential pressure is applied (Nikolsky sign), resulting in blister formation. These cutaneous findings may occur in the context of low-grade fever in about 20% of infants. Given the relatively high layer of epidermis involved, no major clinical sequelae occur because there are no substantial fluid, electrolyte, or protein losses, in contrast to erythema

multiforme involving the dermal-epidermal junction. After appropriate antimicrobial therapy, the denuded skin dries within the subsequent few days and, in the absence of superinfection, heals completely within a few weeks with no scar formation.

Localized staphylococcal infection leading to SSSS may also occur with wound infections, cutaneous abscesses, or conjunctivitis [237,239]. Bacteremia is rare with SSSS, but has been reported [243,244]. Although infection is most commonly described in full-term neonates during the first few months of life, infections in premature infants, including infants with extremely low birth weight, have also been described [235–238]. Scarlatina, as the only clinical manifestation of infection caused by an epidemic strain of SSSS-causing *S. aureus*, has also been observed [239].

Congenital SSSS infection, acquired before delivery as a function of maternal amnionitis, has also been reported in term [244,245] and preterm [246] infants, with a mortality rate that may be higher than the extremely low rate documented for disease acquired postnatally. Outbreaks of disease among hospitalized infants in nurseries have occurred, but most have been effectively stopped with standard infection control practices [239,247].

PNEUMONIA

Neonatal pneumonia caused by *S. aureus* has been described for decades, often reported to occur in community epidemics in infants during the first month of life. These infections, even before the advent of CA-MRSA, have been known to cause severe disease with a high mortality rate that may reflect virulence of strains circulating at that time [160,248,249].

In the current era, staphylococcal pulmonary infections produce many different clinical syndromes, depending on the pathogen and presence or absence of underlying lung disease and other comorbidities. The severity of infection caused by CoNS, as with all staphylococcal site-specific infections, is less than that caused by MSSA or CA-MRSA. A lower respiratory tract infection may occur as a primary pneumonia as the sole clinical manifestation of infection caused by *S. aureus*, with acquisition of the organism after contact with family members or hospital staff. Pneumonia may also occur as part of more generalized, invasive, disseminated staphylococcal infection. In large series of neonatal sepsis and bacteremia cases, pneumonia caused by either CoNS or *S. aureus* is only rarely listed as a primary diagnosis, or a complication, without details provided about the clinical presentation of lower respiratory tract disease [6,161–163,175]. The infection is often hospital-acquired in a neonate with underlying lung disease, most commonly chronic lung disease (bronchopulmonary dysplasia), especially in infants receiving concurrent mechanical ventilation.

An early study of staphylococcal pneumonia in the first month of life was reported from New Zealand in 1956 during an epidemic that primarily caused cutaneous infection. The eight infants who died of pneumonia in this epidemic presented at 2 to 3 weeks of age with irritability and poor feeding noted for a few days, followed by dyspnea, cough, and fever [248]. Death occurred in these infants 1 to 5 days

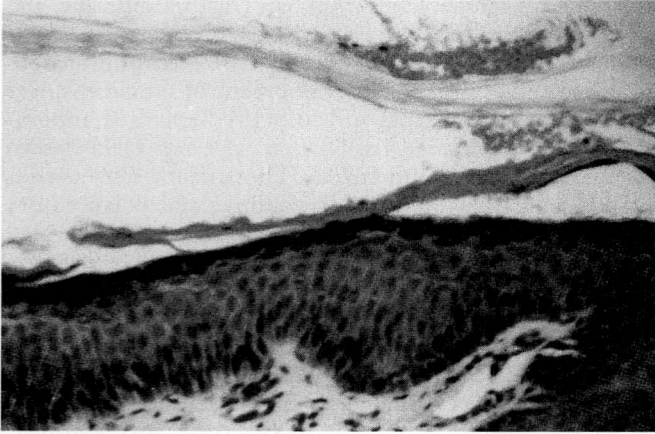

FIGURE 14–7 **Photomicrograph of skin biopsy specimen from a patient with staphylococcal scalded skin syndrome, stained with hematoxylin and eosin.** Histologic appearance is characterized by epidermal splitting at the granular layer of the epidermis. (Magnification approximately 200×.) *(From Hardwick N, Parry CM, Sharpe GR. Staphylococcal scalded skin syndrome in an adult: influence of immune and renal factors. Br J Dermatol 132:468-471, 1995.)*

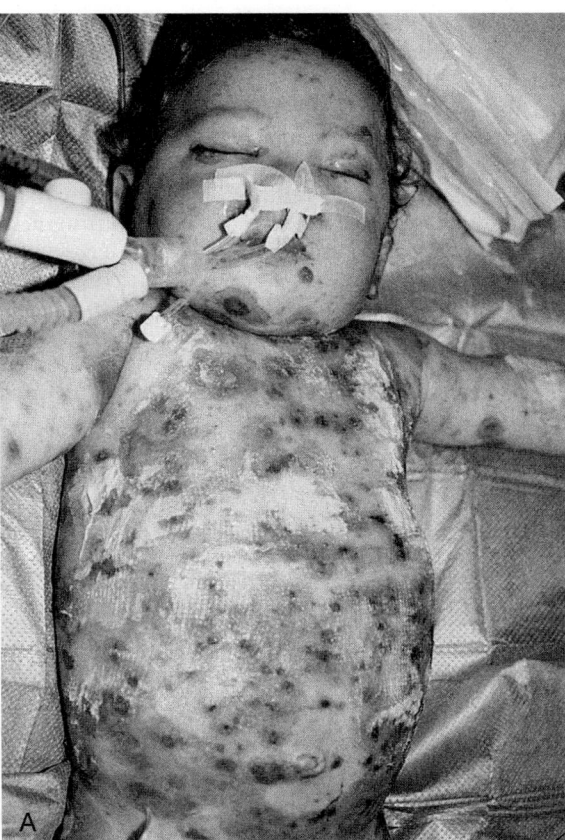
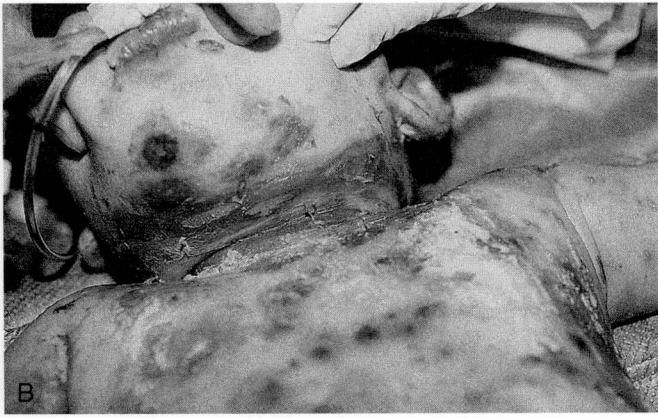

FIGURE 14–8 **Generalized staphylococcal scalded skin syndrome in previously well newborn infant. A** and **B,** Characteristic well-demarcated erythematous superficial exfoliation, with areas of skin sparing, can be seen. *(From Ladhani S, et al. Clinical, microbial, and biochemical aspects of the exfoliative toxins causing staphylococcal scalded-skin syndrome. Clin Microbiol Rev 12:224-242, 1999.)*

after admission, with autopsy findings documenting empyema, consolidation, and abscess formation. In a study of community-acquired *S. aureus* infection in neonates from Houston, Texas, from 2001-2005, infants were described who had no underlying disease, no indwelling catheters, and no previous hospitalization. Of 89 neonates identified with *S. aureus* infection, only 1 had a primary lung infection, caused by CA-MRSA, producing a necrotizing pneumonia complicated by pneumothorax and empyema and requiring video-assisted thoracoscopic surgery and chest tube drainage.

Other cases of severe CA-MRSA neonatal pneumonia have been reported, including hospital-acquired infections in premature neonates [25,168,250]. In hospitalized neonates with bacteremia with CA-MRSA in Houston, two of eight had lung involvement: a 24-week gestation 14-day-old infant with empyema, pneumatoceles, and concurrent endocarditis and a 28-week gestation infant with multiple comorbidities including bronchopulmonary dysplasia with infection acquired at 411 days of age, characterized by lung abscess. Both infants died. At present, these cases are uncommon, but they seem to be increasing. The striking severity of CA-MRSA pulmonary disease in the neonate with an extremely high mortality rate despite adequate antimicrobial therapy and supportive care is of great concern. Accurate data on the population-based rates of *S. aureus* pneumonia in neonates are currently unavailable.

In a point-prevalence survey of neonatal infections in 29 Pediatric Prevention Network NICUs in the United States and Canada, 116 NICU-acquired infections were reported: 15 (13%) were respiratory associated, virtually all in infants with birth weights of 501 to 1500 g; only 2 were associated with CoNS, and only 1 was associated with *S. aureus* [161]. In a review of invasive staphylococcal infections of hospitalized neonates admitted to level II or level III nurseries in Houston, 3 of 41 infants with *S. aureus* infection and 14 of 108 with CoNS infection were documented to have pneumonia. In this population, many had comorbidities, including respiratory distress syndrome in 85% of neonates ultimately diagnosed with any invasive *S. aureus* infection and in 95% of neonates with CoNS. Similarly, bronchopulmonary dysplasia was documented in 65% of *S. aureus*–infected infants and 75% of infants infected by CoNS. In this series, no infant with *S. aureus* pneumonia was documented to develop pneumatoceles or empyemas in the course of infection [178]. The Australasian Study Group for Neonatal Infections collected data on infants with documented bacteremia, occurring at 48 hours to 30 days of age. Of 1281 episodes of CoNS bacteremia, only 6 (0.5%) were documented to have pneumonia [162], in contrast to 223 with MSSA bacteremia associated with 9 (4%) cases of pneumonia and 65 cases of MRSA bacteremia associated with 8 (12%) cases of pneumonia [163].

MENINGITIS

Meningitis is infrequently encountered in neonates with *S. aureus* bacteremia [178,210,211], but may be found when a lumbar puncture is performed even after empirical antibiotic therapy has been started. In a large series of 90 episodes of MRSA bacteremia in neonates in a Taiwanese NICU, 2 were noted to have meningitis [180]. In a report from Australia and New Zealand, meningitis was reported in 5 of 223 infants with MSSA bacteremia (2.2%) and 3 of 65 infants with MRSA bacteremia (5%) [162]. In most reports in which cerebrospinal fluid white blood cell counts are provided, they are often less than 200 cells/mm^3, however, suggesting that these infants with a cerebrospinal fluid pleocytosis and negative cerebrospinal fluid cultures may not have true staphylococcal bacterial meningitis. Virtually no infant from any series had a positive cerebrospinal fluid culture for *S. aureus*, including 12 infants with bacteremia with a documented pleocytosis from Texas Children's Hospital [211]. It is possible that the pleocytosis represents the entry of staphylococcal cell wall components or inflammatory mediators into cerebrospinal fluid during bacteremia, perhaps facilitated by capillary leak that often accompanies staphylococcal sepsis. Other possibilities include very early bacterial meningitis or a staphylococcal parameningeal focus of infection that was not identified in infants or included in the reports.

In a report from the Australasia Study Group data, of 1281 episodes of CoNS sepsis, 5 (0.4%) were reported to be associated with meningitis [162]. An additional two cases were reported in premature infants from another institution, born at 24 weeks and 25 weeks of gestation, one with a grade IV intraventricular hemorrhage. Multiple cultures in both infants confirmed infection caused by *S. epidermidis* in one infant and *S. capitis* and *S. warneri* in the other infant [251].

BRAIN ABSCESS

Brain abscesses caused by *S. aureus* have been described in neonates, most often as a complication of sepsis [252–254]. Clinical presentation includes nonspecific symptoms of systemic infection and a bulging fontanelle; focal neurologic deficits may not occur. The key to diagnosis includes ultrasound or computed tomography (CT) of the head with administration of an intravenous contrast agent and, if not contraindicated, an evaluation of lumbar cerebrospinal fluid. Surgical drainage of the abscess is usually done followed by prolonged antistaphylococcal therapy. Long-term outcome has included neurologic deficits of varying degrees.

Neonates with intraventricular hemorrhage, acute hydrocephalus, congenital malformation, or central nervous system parenchymal injury often require management of increased intracranial pressure by repeated lumbar puncture or by placement of a shunt originating in the cerebrospinal fluid ventricles [255,256]. CoNS are the most common organisms to infect shunt material, producing mild to moderate inflammation and systemic signs and symptoms of infection [255–259]; occasional infection caused by *S. aureus* has also been reported [256,259]. Shunt removal is the preferred method of treatment because sterilization of in situ shunt material is often quite difficult [257]. Treatment with high-dose systemic antimicrobials active against the isolated pathogens, usually vancomycin, 3 to 10 days after shunt removal is recommended, depending on the clinical status and the microbiologic response to treatment. Some authors also recommend using intraventricular vancomycin therapy if therapeutic ventricular cerebrospinal fluid concentrations cannot be achieved with systemic therapy [257,260,261]. The role of linezolid in the treatment of shunt infections remains to be defined, but may represent an option for CA-MRSA strains that are not fully susceptible to vancomycin [262]. Although CoNS infections are seldom associated with acute toxicity or mortality, management with long-term antibiotic therapy and repeated surgical interventions for removal and placement of shunts each carry risks to the neonate.

OSTEOARTICULAR INFECTION

Bone and joint infection has long been known to occur with invasive staphylococcal infection in the neonate, with rates of late sequelae of 50% [263–268]. In contrast to infections in older children, the usual distinction between infection of the bone and infection of the joint in a neonate is not as easily made because of the unique neonatal anatomy, with easy spread of organisms initially inoculated into metaphyseal bone through transphyseal vessels into the epiphysis and subsequently into the joint [269,270]. In addition to decompression of metaphyseal bone infection into the adjacent joint, erosion through the thin cortical bone may also occur, creating subperiosteal abscesses and subsequent involvement of the soft tissues of the extremity [263,269,271]. Virtually all reported cases have been caused by *S. aureus*, although more recent reports document the occurrence of CA-MRSA as a cause of neonatal osteomyelitis [268,272].

The clinical presentation of neonatal bone and joint infections seems to take three general forms. First, the infection may be secondary to staphylococcal sepsis with bacteremia in which case the focal bone and joint findings may not be the most prominent presenting symptom, but bone and joint sequelae of bacteremia become more apparent as the systemic infection is treated [163,268]. Second, and probably most common, an occult bacteremic inoculation of bone may occur, leading to either a single site or, in up to 50% of infants, multiple sites of infection [267,268,272]. In these infants, the clinical findings may be subtle and include signs of irritability, swelling around the affected bone or joint or both, and occasionally failure to move the limb (pseudoparalysis); fever may or may not be present [268,273,274]. Risk factors for bacteremia in these infants include umbilical artery catheterization and prematurity [266–268,275]. In bacteremic disease, the femur and tibia are the most prominently involved bones, infected in approximately 80% of all cases of osteomyelitis [266–268]. Adjacent joints may be involved clinically in 25% to 50% of cases, although in an autopsy review of staphylococcal osteomyelitis, all infants with bone infection were documented on pathology to have adjacent arthritis [266,268–270]. Because most data are from small case series, accurate data on the presenting signs and symptoms may reflect strains circulating in a region at a particular point in time or may be related to outbreaks of specific strains [163]. Because of delays in diagnosis of osteomyelitis, the location of the infection that often involves bone on both sides of the physis, and frequent involvement of the adjacent joint, late sequelae are common after bacteremic infection; 50% of infants may have long-term sequelae, including limb shortening and decreased range of motion [265–267].

A third clinical scenario leading to a bone or joint infection may be specifically linked to trauma. Osteomyelitis of the calcaneus has been documented to occur as a complication of heel-stick blood sampling, most often manifesting with focal swelling, erythema, and drainage [276]. More recent reports cite continuing problems secondary to a single heel-stick that is used for metabolic screening in all newborns [277]. Fetal scalp monitoring has been associated with skull osteomyelitis [278]. Pyogenic arthritis of the hip is a reported complication of femoral vein venipuncture [279].

Bone radiographs can show destructive changes in the bone becoming apparent in the 2nd week of infection. In the case of arthritis, widening of the joint space and bulging of the soft tissues may be seen as a clue to diagnosis. Ultrasound may identify collections of pus that are subperiosteal or in the soft tissues. Although radionuclide bone scanning with technetium-99m may provide additional useful information regarding the involvement of multiple bones, the normal increased vascularity of the neonatal metaphysis may blur the differentiation between infection and increased uptake that is commonly seen in osteomyelitis in older children. Decreased blood flow from necrotic injury to the bone may lead to false negative test results in the newborn. MRI is becoming the preferred imaging modality, based on excellent visualization of soft tissues and bone with a lack of ionizing radiation. MRI may be too sensitive, however, in assessment of tissue inflammation in bones and soft tissues adjacent to the infected site, suggesting a greater extent of infection than is actually present. MRI with contrast agent provides additional information on inflammation in bones and soft tissues and may be particularly helpful when imaging the spine to detect vertebral osteomyelitis or diskitis. CT of neonatal bones and joints has a more limited role in diagnosis of acute infection.

INFECTIONS OF THE GASTROINTESTINAL TRACT

S. aureus is a common colonizer of the gastrointestinal tract of newborns, present in up to 93% of asymptomatic infants [280]. The prevalence of colonization is not surprising, considering that *S. aureus* organisms can be recovered from samples of breast milk [281].

Infections of the gastrointestinal tract can be caused by one of the enterotoxins produced by *S. aureus* or can be a manifestation of invasion of the mucosa resulting in enterocolitis [282]. Although *S. aureus* has been described to colonize the gastrointestinal tract in the absence of clinical disease [280], certain poorly defined risk factors may place colonized infants at risk of invasive disease, including feeding tubes and previous antibiotic therapy that may have facilitated colonization with *S. aureus* [283]. Clinical presentation includes signs and symptoms of generalized sepsis in association with frequent, blood-tinged, thin, mucus-containing diarrheal stools. A report of neonatal staphylococcal enterocolitis caused by MRSA described a need for therapy with intravenous and oral vancomycin to establish a microbiologic cure for the systemic infection and colonization; the infant ultimately developed colonic stricture as a late complication of infection [284]. Delta toxin–producing-CoNS [285] and MRSA [286] have not been confirmed to have a major role in the pathogenesis of neonatal necrotizing enterocolitis, although they may have a supporting role in the disease process in some infants.

DIAGNOSIS

In the previously cited reports on clinical manifestations of staphylococcal infection, diagnosis has most often been made by direct culture of the infected tissues or abscesses if the disease is focal or by cultures of blood, urine, or cerebrospinal fluid for diagnosis of sepsis and bacteremia, pyelonephritis, or meningitis and shunt infection. Organism identification and susceptibility testing are essential in understanding the organism-specific severity of disease and provide information on appropriate antimicrobial therapy. In addition, having the laboratory save the neonate's isolate allows one to compare subsequent episodes of infection by that organism in that infant or compare episodes of infection by the organism that may have spread to or from other neonates.

The diagnosis of infection by nonspecific laboratory tests that assess inflammation in the infant being evaluated can provide supportive evidence for infection. A detailed evaluation of specific tests, such as total white blood cell count, immature neutrophil (band-form) count, mature-to-immature white blood cell ratio, C-reactive protein, procalcitonin, cytokines (IL-6, IL-8, IL-10, TNF-α) [287–291], and chemokines [292,293] (interferon-γ-inducible protein-10, monocyte chemoattractant protein-1, RANTES, epithelial neutrophil activating peptide-78), is beyond the scope of this chapter. The sensitivity, specificity, and positive predictive values vary with the investigating institution and the population of neonates studied; some laboratory test results become abnormal within a few hours of the onset of infection, whereas others may not increase for 1 to 2 days.

Rather than a single test, a set of tests may offer the best hope for diagnosing early infection and tracking the response to therapy [293,294]. At the present time, C-reactive protein and procalcitonin seem to be among the most useful and the most widely available tests for assessment of neonatal sepsis. Some studies have suggested the usefulness of an elevated immature-to-total neutrophil ratio in identifying infants with CoNS septicemia [295–297]. No test has the ability to identify all infected infants, with decisions on further investigation and empirical antimicrobial therapy still requiring clinical judgment. With more premature and younger infants, the interval is greater from the time of infection to the time of a positive nonspecific test for inflammation. MSSA and MRSA *S. aureus* seem to generate far more vigorous responses than CoNS. These nonspecific tests of inflammation should not play a decisive role in the determination of whether a single positive blood culture for CoNS represents a true positive culture or a contaminant.

Multiple positive blood cultures for the same strain of CoNS in a relatively asymptomatic infant may provide evidence of true infection that is more reliable than the white blood cell count or any inflammatory marker. Polymerase chain reaction techniques to detect 16S-rRNA in plasma followed by specific probes for *S. aureus* and CoNS show promise, but cannot currently be used as the sole diagnostic test for staphylococcal infection [298]. Emerging non–culture-based diagnostic methodologies for neonatal infection are evaluated in detail in Chapter 36.

ANTIBIOTIC TREATMENT
See also Chapter 37.

GENERAL PRINCIPLES
Optimal treatment for staphylococcal infections in neonates is designed to achieve an appropriate antimicrobial exposure at the site of infection and surgical control of the infection by drainage of any abscess and removal of any potentially infected foreign material. As with all neonatal bacterial infections, cultures of appropriate samples, based on signs and symptoms of infection, physical examination, and imaging, should provide the necessary information regarding the identity and susceptibility pattern of the pathogen. The choice of empirical therapy, before susceptibility test results are known, depends on the local antibiotic resistance patterns for coagulase-positive and coagulase-negative staphylococci, the severity of infection, and the toxicity profile of the antibiotic for that infant.

For CoNS, susceptibility patterns are quite varied and are often based on the particular species isolated. For coagulase-positive strains, it is essential to know the susceptibility to β-lactamase–stable penicillins. Culture and susceptibility information has a direct impact on selection of definitive therapy, allowing the use of the most narrow-spectrum, least toxic antimicrobial regimens.

Although β-lactam agents are preferred for treatment of infections with MSSA in the neonate because of their bactericidal activity and overall safety, several other clinically useful classes may also show in vitro activity, including glycopeptides, aminoglycosides, lipopeptides, oxazolidinones, lincosamides, rifamycins, and trimethoprim-sulfamethoxazole. As with so many other drugs for neonates, adequate prospective data on the safety and efficacy of these antimicrobials for the various tissue sites of infection caused by CoNS, MSSA, and MRSA are unavailable. Extrapolation from other pediatric and adult data is necessary, with cautions for the neonate on outcomes at dosages suggested and on the safety of these antimicrobials.

For antimicrobial therapy of *S. aureus* infections, infections should be separated into MSSA and MRSA. Among MRSA, further differentiation should be made between the more antibiotic-resistant hospital-acquired strains (HA-MRSA) and community-acquired strains (CA-MRSA).

No MRSA strains can be killed by penicillin or ampicillin, β-lactamase–stable antistaphylococcal penicillins (methicillin, nafcillin, oxacillin, dicloxacillin), currently available cephalosporins (cephalexin, cephalothin, cefazolin, cefuroxime, cefotaxime, ceftriaxone), or carbapenems (meropenem, imipenem, ertapenem, doripenem). HA-MRSA strains carry relatively large antibiotic resistance gene cassettes with concurrent resistance to clindamycin, macrolides (erythromycin, clarithromycin, and azithromycin), and aminoglycosides, a resistance profile that is usually not seen in CA-MRSA strains.

For mild to moderate invasive staphylococcal infections in neonates in areas of the world where methicillin resistance is still minimal, empirical therapy with first-generation cephalosporins (parenteral cefazolin, oral cephalexin) or antistaphylococcal penicillins (parenteral methicillin, oxacillin, or nafcillin) is preferred. In some cases of mild skin infection, topical antibiotic therapy with mupirocin may suffice. For mild to moderate infections in areas where CA-MRSA occurs at substantial rates ($\geq$5% to 10%), clindamycin or vancomycin intravenously should be used empirically until susceptibility data are available. If clindamycin is used, caution should be exercised in treating erythromycin-resistant, clindamycin-susceptible strains of *S. aureus* with clindamycin because those strains may display inducible clindamycin resistance (see "Clindamycin and Erythromycin" subsequently). The role of oral therapy for neonatal staphylococcal infections is not yet well defined. For MRSA strains that are susceptible, erythromycin, azithromycin, and clindamycin may be considered for mild infections, or step-down therapy may be considered in newborns who have responded well initially to intravenous therapy. Trimethoprim-sulfamethoxazole may be considered for mild infections in infants who no longer exhibit physiologic jaundice.

For serious infections in neonates in regions of the world in which CA-MRSA is routinely isolated, empirical therapy with vancomycin is preferred over clindamycin, given the bactericidal nature of killing and extensive experience with vancomycin in newborns. For suspected *S. aureus* infections that are nosocomially acquired within institutions in which MRSA is present in other neonates, empirical therapy with vancomycin for presumed MRSA is also recommended. With data suggesting that the most common pathogen responsible for bloodstream infections in late-onset sepsis in hospitalized neonates is CoNS, most often resistant to β-lactam antibiotics, vancomycin is likely to provide effective therapy. For situations in which cultures show MSSA or methicillin-susceptible or penicillin-susceptible CoNS, it is imperative that therapy be switched back to traditional β-lactam antibiotics to minimize antibiotic pressure on staphylococcal species from vancomycin or clindamycin, to delay the emergence of resistance to these antibiotics. β-lactam antibiotics are generally less toxic to the neonate compared with vancomycin and clindamycin and are better tolerated.

VANCOMYCIN
Vancomycin is a first-generation bactericidal glycopeptide antibiotic. Vancomycin normally inhibits growth of the organism by binding to cell wall precursors, inhibiting

transglycosylase function and cell wall synthesis. Complete resistance to vancomycin is relatively recent and quite limited, with the first cases of complete resistance having been reported in 2002. Within every population of *S. aureus*, a very low frequency of organisms with intermediate resistance to vancomycin exists, however, and these organisms may become selected out in infants with prolonged exposure to vancomycin. By contrast, complete vancomycin resistance is still exceedingly rare and created by a different mechanism that parallels vancomycin resistance in enterococci.

Dosing of vancomycin is designed to achieve an area under the curve-to-minimal inhibitory concentration ratio (AUC:MIC) of approximately 250 and is associated with microbiologic cure in experimental in vitro and in vivo animal models and in retrospective analyses of infections in adults [299]. In neonates, many dosing recommendations exist, including intermittent dosing and continuous infusion, primarily based on chronologic and gestational age and based on serum creatinine [300–304]. An initial loading dose of 15 mg/kg is most often recommended, followed by repeated dosing every 8 to 24 hours, reflecting longer dosing intervals for the youngest, most premature infants. Each dose should be administered over 60 minutes. Close monitoring of renal function and serum concentrations of vancomycin are recommended in all neonates receiving therapy, allowing for adjustment of vancomycin dosing regardless of the initial empirical dosing regimen chosen. Intraventricular vancomycin has been used to treat central nervous system infections, primarily ventriculoperitoneal shunt infections caused by CoNS [260,261], although cerebrospinal fluid concentrations may be therapeutic after intravenous administration [301].

CLINDAMYCIN AND ERYTHROMYCIN

Clindamycin, a lincosamide, and erythromycin, a macrolide, inhibit ribosomal function and produce a primarily bacteriostatic effect by binding to sites on the ribosome. Most strains of MSSA remain susceptible to clindamycin and erythromycin. Many strains of CA-MRSA remain susceptible, but most strains of HA-MRSA and CoNS are resistant to these antibiotics. Staphylococcal resistance to erythromycin may occur by two mechanisms: by methylase-mediated dimethylation of the 23S ribosomal binding site of the macrolides and by the presence of an efflux pump that expels the macrolide from the intracellular environment of the pathogen. The methylase gene, *erm*, is usually inducible, but in any large population of organisms, mutants occur that constitutively produce methylase, providing complete resistance to all macrolides (erythromycin, azithromycin, clarithromycin), clindamycin, and streptogramins (quinupristin-dalfopristin).

By contrast, the most prevalent macrolide efflux pump for staphylococci, *msrA*, does not recognize, bind to, or eliminate clindamycin from within the bacteria, allowing these strains to remain susceptible to clindamycin. Any strain that shows in vitro erythromycin resistance and clindamycin susceptibility must also be tested for methylase-mediated clindamycin resistance by an additional assay, the D-test. Current laboratory reporting guidelines suggest that hospitals report erythromycin-resistant,

D-test–positive strains as clindamycin-resistant, on the basis of reported clinical failures of clindamycin in treating infections caused by inducible organisms. Because the true clinical significance of inducible *erm*-mediated resistance for clindamycin is not well defined at present, it is prudent to use other antibiotic options for a seriously ill neonate with infection caused by a D-test–positive strain.

Erythromycin is associated with the occurrence of pyloric stenosis in the newborn infant, a side effect that is likely to be less prevalent in clarithromycin and azithromycin. Clindamycin, erythromycin, and azithromycin are available in oral and intravenous formulations, but little prospective, comparative data exist for their use in neonates.

LINEZOLID

Of the antibiotics approved during the past decade with activity against MRSA, linezolid is the only one currently approved by the U.S. Food and Drug Administration (FDA) for use in neonates. As might be predicted, resistance to linezolid has been documented to develop in adults receiving therapy for a bacteremic MRSA infection, although to date resistance remains rare [305]. Linezolid is an oxazolidinone-class protein synthesis inhibitor, the first of this new class of antibiotics. Linezolid is a ribosome-inhibiting, bacteriostatic agent, active against coagulase-positive and coagulase-negative staphylococci. Data on pharmacokinetics are available for all pediatric age groups, including premature neonates less than 34 weeks' gestational age.

Linezolid can be administered intravenously and orally, with virtually 100% of the agent absorbed by the oral route. Protein binding in plasma is approximately 30%, and the drug is well distributed into tissues. Linezolid is cleared by the kidneys, unchanged and after oxidation of the parent compound. Because oxidation of linezolid does not depend on renal function, no dose reduction is needed for renal insufficiency. Linezolid has been studied in neonates and older children for nosocomial and community-acquired pneumonia and for complicated and uncomplicated skin and skin structure infections [306,307]. The clinical response rates for each of these tissue-specific infections were equivalent to comparator agents, usually vancomycin. The pathogen-specific response rates for infections caused by *S. aureus*, including MSSA and MRSA strains, and response rates for infections caused by CoNS were also statistically equivalent to vancomycin. Similarly, the rates for clinical and laboratory adverse events were equivalent to adverse events in vancomycin-treated control patients. In neonates and children enrolled in these registration trials, the hematologic toxicity profiles for neutropenia and thrombocytopenia were equivalent to vancomycin. These data suggest that hematologic toxicity of thrombocytopenia and neutropenia seen in adults may not be seen as frequently in neonates and children.

Recommendations for the dosage regimen for preterm neonates less than 7 days of age (gestational age <34 weeks) are based on data from registration trials involving very few neonates. Preterm neonates should be initially given 10 mg/kg every 12 hours. For neonates with a poor response to infection caused by a susceptible organism, an increased dose of 10 mg/kg every 8 hours can be provided. By 7 days of age, all neonates, regardless of gestational age, should receive 10 mg/kg every 8 hours. The interpatient variability in neonates was noted to be greater than that seen in adults and may reflect variation in the rate of maturation of mechanisms of elimination.

In studies of cerebrospinal fluid linezolid concentrations in infants with ventriculoperitoneal shunts receiving systemic therapeutic dosing, adequate concentrations were not consistently achieved. Although a case report exists for the treatment of a staphylococcal central nervous system infection in a neonate [262], the routine use of linezolid for the treatment of central nervous system infections cannot be recommended at this time. Similarly, case reports on the treatment of neonatal endocarditis caused by MRSA exist, but the safety and efficacy of linezolid for this indication remain to be defined. The role of combination therapy using linezolid is also not defined.

DAPTOMYCIN

An antibiotic approved only for use in adults, daptomycin is a novel lipopeptide bactericidal agent for gram-positive organisms, including S. aureus and CoNS. Structurally, daptomycin is a 13-amino acid cyclic peptide with a lipophilic tail that inserts into the cell membrane, leading to depolarization of the membrane, inhibition of protein, DNA, and RNA synthesis, and cell death. Daptomycin shows concentration-dependent killing pharmacodynamics. It is available only in an intravenous formulation. Pharmacokinetic studies are ongoing in older children, but no data exist for neonates. The prolonged half-life in adults of 8 to 9 hours allows for once-daily dosing. The antibiotic is highly protein bound (90%) and is excreted primarily by the kidney with little degradation of the parent compound. In renal insufficiency, the dose is decreased according to the degree of renal failure.

In adults, daptomycin is approved by the FDA for the treatment of complicated skin and skin structure infections (caused by S. aureus, including MRSA) and for bacteremia and endocarditis. Daptomycin also shows in vitro activity against vancomycin-resistant S. aureus and should represent an effective agent if these strains become more widespread. Daptomycin is not indicated for the treatment of pneumonia because surfactant binding to the antibiotic is associated with inactivation. Myopathy is a potential adverse event, which was noted in early phase 1 studies, but with once-daily dosing in adults, no muscle toxicity was documented. Current guidelines suggest monitoring serum creatine phosphokinase concentrations weekly.

QUINUPRISTIN-DALFOPRISTIN

Streptogramins are antibiotic derivatives of natural products of Streptomyces pristinaespiralis. Two streptogramins, quinupristin and dalfopristin, when used together in a fixed combination have been shown to be bactericidal against many gram-positive organisms, including staphylococci and certain enterococci. Each antibiotic is bacteriostatic, but when used together in a 30:70 ratio, the combination is bactericidal. The combination is approved by the FDA for adults as Synercid, for the treatment of vancomycin-resistant Enterococcus faecium infections and for the treatment of skin and skin structure infections caused by S. aureus (only MSSA strains were isolated from study patients). In vitro, quinupristin-dalfopristin is also active against MRSA and vancomycin-resistant S. aureus, although no clinical data are available for treatment of these infections. Quinupristin-dalfopristin is available only in an intravenous preparation. Both drugs are primarily eliminated through biliary excretion, with minimal metabolism. Inflammation and pain at the infusion site are substantial problems. Many mechanisms of bacterial resistance have been documented, ultimately limiting the clinical usefulness of this combination.

COMBINATION ANTIMICROBIAL THERAPY

Although many combinations of antibiotics have been used in adults, few have been studied prospectively, with virtually no prospective comparative evaluations available for children and neonates. For invasive S. aureus disease, infective endocarditis in adults has resulted in some of the highest mortality rates, resulting in guidelines that recommend aggressive combination therapy based on animal model data, in vitro data, and data from CoNS infections [308]. For MSSA endocarditis, combination therapy with a β-lactam penicillin (oxacillin or nafcillin) and rifampin, plus the addition of gentamicin for the first 2 weeks of therapy, is believed to result in optimal microbiologic efficacy. For MRSA, vancomycin plus rifampin, with gentamicin for the first 2 weeks of therapy, should be considered [308]. A report on vancomycin plus rifampin combination therapy of persisting CoNS bacteremia after removal of a central catheter provides some support to this approach [309].

A Cochrane review of intravenous immunoglobulin therapy of suspected or documented neonatal sepsis evaluated nine clinical trials. Although substantial heterogeneity existed across studies in immunoglobulin preparations, dosing regimens, and populations studied, no substantial benefit was derived from treatment, particularly with respect to mortality in infants with either suspected infection or subsequently proven infection [310].

CATHETER REMOVAL

The decision to remove an indwelling catheter from a neonate with bacteremia often is difficult, especially when securing subsequent intravascular access may be challenging. Delayed removal of a central catheter in the setting of bacteremia may be associated with an increased risk of infection-related complications [189]. For infants with CoNS bacteremia, successful treatment of bacteremia may be possible with the central venous catheter in situ [189]. If bacteremia persists for longer than 4 days, the chance for subsequent clearance is reduced [188], however, and the risk of end-organ damage may be increased [164,189]. The presence of a ventricular reservoir or ventriculoperitoneal shunt increases the chance of the development of meningitis in the setting of prolonged catheter-related bacteremia. Prompt removal of an indwelling central venous catheter should be considered in infants with central nervous system hardware [188].

PREVENTION
HYGIENIC MEASURES

Major efforts to prevent staphylococcal infections in neonates, rather than being required to treat them, are of great value. General principles underlying nosocomial infection in the NICU and measures to reduce occurrence of infections that apply broadly to staphylococcal infections are discussed in detail in Chapter 35. Some specific considerations relevant to staphylococci are discussed briefly here.

Staphylococci may be spread through fomites; overcrowding of infants in the NICU may increase the risk of colonization and the potential for disease. In an outbreak situation, attempts to control the spread of staphylococci through remediation of overcrowding and isolation of infected or colonized patients have been shown to be effective in helping to curtail the outbreak, even in the case of MRSA [311].

A primary determinant of infant colonization is nursing care. Maintaining an appropriate nurse-to-infant ratio is an important factor in reducing disease when a disease-associated S. aureus strain gains entrance to a nursery, especially in the NICU [312]. In addition, various preventive maneuvers are directed at persons with direct infant contact, including frequent mask, gown, and glove changes before handling of infants [313,314]; application of antimicrobial or antiseptic ointment or spray [315,316]; and elimination of carriers from the nursery area [317,318]. In some situations, control of an epidemic requires removal of the nurse carrier from the nursery [319].

Currently, the U.S. Centers for Disease Control and Prevention recommends contact isolation for patients colonized or infected with MRSA [320]. This practice was shown to reduce nosocomial transmission of MRSA by 16-fold during an outbreak of MRSA in an NICU [321]. Several more recent publications have focused on nursery infection control measures, documented to be effective in preventing the entry of CA-MRSA into a nursery and its spread within the nursery [322–325].

In the early 1960s, attempts were made to stop virulent S. aureus epidemics in 10 NICUs throughout the United States using the technique of bacterial interference [326,327]. This technique involved deliberate implantation of S. aureus of low virulence (502A) on the nasal mucosa and umbilicus of newborns to prevent colonization with the virulent S. aureus strain. Although this procedure was successful in curtailing epidemics [328], it is not widely used or recommended currently.

Proper hand hygiene among nursery health care providers is a fundamental factor in reducing colonization rates. Mortimer and associates [329] achieved a reduction in infant colonization from 92% to 53% by insisting that attendants wash their hands. Proper education and monitoring of hand hygiene practices are critical to the effectiveness of this intervention [330,331]. Hands must be cleaned before and after patient contact or contact with equipment that is used for patient care. Hands also should be cleaned after glove removal. Proper hand hygiene involves applying alcohol-based waterless rubs if hands are not soiled [332] or washing the hands for at least 10 to 15 seconds with either chlorhexidine gluconate or triclosan hand-washing agents [333].

With the increase in prominence of CoNS as nosocomial pathogens, strategies for disease prevention have become increasingly important. As with S. aureus, strict hand hygiene is of primary importance in minimizing staff-to-patient and patient-to-patient spread of CoNS. In addition, meticulous surgical technique to limit intraoperative bacterial contamination is critical in minimizing infection related to foreign bodies. Strict attention to protocols for the insertion and management of intravenous and intra-arterial catheters may decrease the risk of catheter-related infections [334]. In patients who require intravenous access for prolonged periods, percutaneous placement of a small-diameter Silastic catheter is preferred when possible. In one study, these catheters were maintained for 80 days, with an infection rate of less than 10% in infants weighing less than 1500 g [335].

ANTIBIOTIC PROPHYLAXIS

Investigational therapies to reduce neonatal bacteremia caused by staphylococci have been directed at the use of antibiotic prophylaxis and antibiotic-impregnated devices. Given the large burden of CoNS catheter infections in premature infants, investigations of prophylactic antibiotics to prevent infection were undertaken by many institutions, as reviewed more recently [336–340]. Vancomycin was documented to be successful in significantly decreasing the rate of suspected or documented sepsis caused by CoNS. Antibiotic-based methods to prevent bacteremic infection have included the use of a vancomycin solution (25 μg/mL) to dwell inside the infant's central venous catheter two to three times daily for up to 60 minutes [339]; the administration of low-dose vancomycin at 5 mg/kg twice daily [338]; or the addition of vancomycin to hyperalimentation solutions to a concentration of 25 μg/mL for routine administration. Although all three methods were successful at decreasing episodes of sepsis, the overall mortality in treatment versus control groups was not affected. Because of concerns for the emergence of vancomycin-resistant organisms, routine use of prophylactic vancomycin for all neonates at risk of CoNS bacteremia is not currently recommended. Potential risks associated with prophylactic vancomycin, including ototoxicity, nephrotoxicity, and selection for resistant bacteria, have not been well evaluated.

IMMUNOPROPHYLAXIS

Studies evaluating the effectiveness of immunoglobulin preparations generally have not documented convincing, substantial benefits for the populations of premature infants studied [310]. These studies may reflect the lack of effectiveness of a specific biologic preparation, however, or suggest that particular subpopulations may benefit more from treatment than others, rather than proving that immunoglobulins have no potential role in prophylaxis or treatment. Other polyclonal antibody approaches to prophylaxis in premature infants have used high-titer anti–*S. aureus* immunoglobulin (Altastaph), prepared from adult volunteers immunized with a staphylococcal vaccine. Pharmacokinetic, safety, and clinical outcome data in neonates randomly assigned to receive either immunoglobulin or placebo did not show benefit in early, limited trials [341].

Studies of monoclonal antibodies directed against specific staphylococcal epitopes are ongoing. A randomized, placebo-controlled trial was conducted in premature infants to prevent staphylococcal infection, using an intravenous immunoglobulin preparation selected from donors with high activity against specific staphylococcal fibrinogen-binding protein, ClfA, and Ser-Asp dipeptide repeat G (INH-A00021, Veronate). No benefit to prophylaxis was noted in the recipients of this staphylococcus-specific immunoglobulin [342,343]. An anti-staphylococcal monoclonal antibody, BSYX-A110, has been developed for the prevention of CoNS sepsis. This antibody targets staphylococcal lipoteichoic acid and has been shown to be safe and well tolerated when administered by intravenous infusion to high-risk neonates [344]. The efficacy of the antibody in preventing CoNS infections and related morbidity and mortality remains to be established.

Lactoferrin is an iron-binding glycoprotein present in breast milk that is believed to contribute to innate antibacterial immunity of the intestinal barrier, through a combination of restricting pathogen access to iron, cell wall lytic activity of its component peptides, and promotion of epithelial barrier maturation [345]. A randomized study of bovine lactoferrin supplementation in very low birth weight premature infants showed a promising reduction in the rate of late-onset sepsis in the treatment group (risk ratio 0.34, 95% confidence interval 0.17 to 0.70) [346].

CONCLUSION

Staphylococcal infections result in significant morbidity and mortality in neonates. Although CoNS are frequent causes of less severe infections, the continuing relatively high rate of community-associated and hospital-associated infections caused by more aggressive *S. aureus* and the emergence of CA-MRSA with exceptionally high mortality rates have created an unprecedented need to understand the biology and mechanisms of virulence of staphylococci. With this understanding, we can generate improved approaches to prevent and treat infections. A profound need exists to develop more safe and effective antimicrobials and immunotherapies to mitigate the substantial morbidity and mortality caused by these pathogens.

ACKNOWLEDGMENTS

The authors are indebted to Rachel C. Orscheln, Henry R. Shinefield, and Joseph W. St. Geme III, whose previous contributions to this chapter and clinical images provided the strong baseline framework and inspiration for the current version.

REFERENCES

[1] T. Fox, Epidemic pemphigus of newly born (impetigo contagiosa et bullosa neonatorum), Lancet 1 (1935) 1323.

[2] E.T. Rulison, Control of impetigo neonatorum: advisability of a radical departure in obstetrical care, JAMA 93 (1929) 903.

[3] H.F. Eichenwald, O. Kotsevalov, L.A. Fasso, The "cloud baby": an example of bacterial-viral interaction, Am. J. Dis. Child. 100 (1960) 161–173.

[4] R.E. Dixon, et al., Staphylococcal disease outbreaks in hospital nurseries in the United States—December 1971 through March 1972, Pediatrics 51 (1973) 413.

[5] R.P. Gaynes, et al., Nosocomial infections among neonates in high-risk nurseries in the United States. National Nosocomial Infections Surveillance System, Pediatrics 98 (1996) 357.

[6] B.J. Stoll, et al., Late-onset sepsis in very low birth weight neonates: the experience of the NICHD Neonatal Research Network, Pediatrics 110 (2002) 285–291.

[7] M.J. Bizzarro, et al., Seventy-five years of neonatal sepsis at Yale: 1928–2003, Pediatrics 116 (2005) 595–602.

[8] H.R. Shinefield, et al., Bacterial interference: its effect on nursery-acquired infection with *Staphylococcus aureus*. I. Preliminary observations, Am. J. Dis. Child. 105 (1963) 646.

[9] J.P. Fairchild, et al., Flora of the umbilical stump: 2479 cultures, J. Pediatr. 53 (1958) 538.

[10] W.A. Gillespie, K. Simpson, R.C. Tozer, Staphylococcal infection in a maternity hospital: epidemiology and control, Lancet 2 (1958) 1075.

[11] V. Hurst, Transmission of hospital staphylococci among newborn infants. II. Colonization of the skin and mucous membranes of the infants, Pediatrics 25 (1960) 204.

[12] T.E. Schaffer, et al., Staphylococcal infections in newborn infants. II. Report of 19 epidemics caused by an identical strain of *Staphylococcus pyogenes*, Am. J. Public Health 47 (1957) 990.

[13] E. Wolinsky, P.J. Lipsitz, E.A. Mortimer Jr., Acquisition of staphylococci by newborns: direct versus indirect transmission, Lancet 2 (1960) 620.

[14] H.R. Shinefield, et al., Bacterial interference: its effect on nursery-acquired infection with *Staphylococcus aureus*. II. The Ohio epidemic, Am. J. Dis. Child. 105 (1963) 655.

[15] R. Hare, C.G.A. Thomas, The transmission of *Staphylococcus aureus*, BMJ 2 (1956) 840.

[16] M. Ridely, Perineal carriage of *Staphylococcus aureus*, BMJ 1 (1959) 270.

[17] D.S. Acton, et al., Intestinal carriage of *Staphylococcus aureus*. How does its frequency compare with that of nasal carriage and what is its clinical impact? Eur. J. Clin. Microbiol. Infect. Dis. 28 (2009) 115–127.

[18] R.L. Thompson, I. Cabezudo, R.P. Wenzel, Epidemiology of nosocomial infections caused by methicillin-resistant *Staphylococcus aureus*, Ann. Intern. Med. 97 (1982) 309.

[19] K. Hiramatsu, et al., The emergence and evolution of methicillin-resistant *Staphylococcus aureus*, Trends Microbiol. 9 (2001) 486.

[20] J.M. Boyce, Methicillin-resistant *Staphylococcus aureus*: detection, epidemiology, and control measures, Infect. Dis. Clin. North Am. 3 (1989) 901.

[21] C.D. Salgado, B.M. Farr, D.P. Calfee, Community-acquired methicillin-resistant *Staphylococcus aureus*: a meta-analysis of prevalence and risk factors, Clin. Infect. Dis. 36 (2003) 131.

[22] E.A. Eady, J.H. Cove, Staphylococcal resistance revisited: community-acquired methicillin resistant *Staphylococcus aureus*—an emerging problem for the management of skin and soft tissue infections, Curr. Opin. Infect. Dis. 16 (2003) 103.

[23] A.J. Carey, et al., The epidemiology of methicillin-susceptible and methicillin-resistant *Staphylococcus aureus* in a neonatal intensive care unit, 2000-2007, J. Perinatol. 30 (2009) 135–139.

[24] I.M. Gould, et al., Report of a hospital neonatal unit outbreak of community-associated methicillin-resistant *Staphylococcus aureus*, Epidemiol. Infect. 137 (2009) 1242–1248.

[25] R.M. McAdams, et al., Spread of methicillin-resistant *Staphylococcus aureus* USA300 in a neonatal intensive care unit, Pediatr. Int. 50 (2008) 810–815.

[26] Community-associated methicillin-resistant *Staphylococcus aureus* infection among healthy newborns—Chicago and Los Angeles County, 2004, MMWR Morb. Mortal. Wkly Rep. 55 (2006) 329–332.

[27] L. Saiman, et al., Molecular epidemiology of staphylococcal scalded skin syndrome in premature infants, Pediatr. Infect. Dis. J. 17 (1998) 329.

[28] M.C. Enright, et al., Multilocus sequence typing for characterization of methicillin-resistant and methicillin-susceptible clones of *Staphylococcus aureus*, J. Clin. Microbiol. 38 (2000) 1008.

[29] B.A. Diep, F. Perdreau-Remington, G.F. Sensabaugh, Clonal characterization of *Staphylococcus aureus* by multilocus restriction fragment typing, a rapid screening approach for molecular epidemiology, J. Clin. Microbiol. 41 (2003) 4559.

[30] D.A. Goldmann, Bacterial colonization and infection in the neonate, Am. J. Med. 70 (1981) 417.

[31] R.A. Simpson, et al., Colonization by gentamicin-resistant *Staphylococcus epidermidis* in a special care baby unit, J. Hosp. Infect. 7 (1986) 108.

[32] S.L. Hall, et al., Evaluation of coagulase-negative staphylococcal isolates from serial nasopharyngeal cultures of premature infants, Diagn. Microbiol. Infect. Dis. 13 (1990) 17.

[33] C.H. Patrick, et al., Relatedness of strains of methicillin-resistant coagulase-negative *Staphylococcus* colonizing hospital personnel and producing bacteremias in a neonatal intensive care unit, Pediatr. Infect. Dis. J. 11 (1992) 935.

[34] C.T. D'Angio, et al., Surface colonization with coagulase-negative staphylococci in premature neonates, J. Pediatr. 114 (1989) 1029.

[35] J. Freeman, et al., Association of intravenous lipid emulsion and coagulase negative staphylococcal bacteremia in neonatal intensive care units, N. Engl. J. Med. 323 (1990) 301.

[36] W. Kloos, Taxonomy and Systemics of Staphylococci Indigenous to Humans, Churchill Livingstone, New York, 1997.

[37] M.T. Parker, P.M. Roundtree, Report (1966B1970) of the Subcommittee on Phage Typing of Staphylococci to the International Committee on Nomenclature of Bacteria, Int. J. Syst. Bacteriol. 21 (1971) 167.

[38] G. Prevost, B. Jaulhoc, Y. Piedmont, DNA fingerprinting of pulsed-field gel electrophoresis is more effective than ribotyping in distinguishing among methicillin-resistant *Staphylococcus aureus* isolates, J. Clin. Microbiol. 30 (1992) 967.

[39] F.C. Tenover, et al., Comparison of traditional and molecular methods of typing isolates of *Staphylococcus aureus*, J. Clin. Microbiol. 32 (1994) 407.

[40] P. Giesbrecht, J. Wecke, B. Reinicke, On the morphogenesis of the cell wall of staphylococci, Int. Rev. Cytol. 44 (1976) 225–318.

[41] J. Braddiley, et al., The wall composition of micrococci, J. Gen. Microbiol. 54 (1968) 393.

[42] H. Labischinski, Consequences of interaction of β-lactam antibiotics with penicillin binding proteins from sensitive and resistant *Staphylococcus aureus* strains, Med. Microbiol. Immunol. (Berl.) 181 (1992) 241.

[43] W.G. Juergens, A.R. Sanderson, J.L. Strominger, Chemical basis for the immunological specificity of a strain of *Staphylococcus aureus*, Bull. Soc. Chim. Biol. (Paris) 42 (1960) 110.

[44] J.C. Lee, G.B. Pier, Vaccine-based Strategies for Prevention of Staphylococcal Diseases, Churchill Livingstone, New York, 1997.

[45] H.A. Verburgh, et al., Antibodies to cell wall peptidoglycan of *Staphylococcus aureus* in patients with serious staphylococcal infections, J. Infect. Dis. 144 (1981) 1.

[46] V.A. Fischetti, V. Pancholi, O. Schneewind, Conservation of a hexapeptide sequence in the anchor region of surface proteins from gram-positive cocci, Mol. Microbiol. 4 (1990) 1603.

[47] S.K. Mazmanian, H. Ton-That, O. Schneewind, Sortase-catalysed anchoring of surface proteins to the cell wall of *Staphylococcus aureus*, Mol. Microbiol. 40 (2001) 1049.

[48] T.J. Foster, M. Hook, Surface protein adhesins of *Staphylococcus aureus*, Trends Microbiol. 6 (1998) 484–488.

[49] K. O'Riordan, J.C. Lee, *Staphylococcus aureus* capsular polysaccharides, Clin. Microbiol. Rev. 17 (2004) 218–234.

[50] M. Moreau, et al., Structure of the type 5 capsular polysaccharide of *Staphylococcus aureus*, Carbohydr. Res. 201 (1990) 285–297.

[51] J.M. Fournier, W.F. Vann, W.W. Karakawa, Purification and characterization of *Staphylococcus aureus* type 8 capsular polysaccharide, Infect. Immun. 45 (1984) 87–93.

[52] C. von Eiff, G. Peters, K. Becker, The small colony variant (SCV) concept—the role of staphylococcal SCVs in persistent infections, Injury 37 (Suppl. 2) (2006) S26–S33.

[53] R.A. Proctor, J.M. Balwit, O. Vesga, Variant subpopulations of *Staphylococcus aureus* as cause of persistent and recurrent infections, Infect. Agents Dis. 3 (1994) 302–312.

[54] T. Baba, et al., Genome and virulence determinants of high virulence community-acquired MRSA, Lancet 359 (2002) 1819.

[55] M. Kuroda, et al., Whole genome sequencing of methicillin-resistant *Staphylococcus aureus*, Lancet 357 (2001) 1225.

[56] M.T. Holden, et al., Complete genomes of two clinical *Staphylococcus aureus* strains: evidence for the rapid evolution of virulence and drug resistance, Proc. Natl. Acad. Sci. U. S. A. 101 (2004) 9786–9791.

[57] B.A. Diep, et al., Complete genome sequence of USA300, an epidemic clone of community-acquired methicillin-resistant *Staphylococcus aureus*, Lancet 367 (2006) 731–739.

[58] M.A. Pfaller, L.A. Herwaldt, Laboratory, clinical and epidemiological aspects of coagulase-negative staphylococci, Clin. Microbiol. Rev. 1 (1988) 281.

[59] F. Wu, P. Della-Latta, Molecular typing strategies, Semin. Perinatol. 26 (2002) 357.

[60] Y.Q. Zhang, et al., Genome-based analysis of virulence genes in a non-biofilm-forming *Staphylococcus epidermidis* strain (ATCC 12228), Mol. Microbiol. 49 (2003) 1577.

[61] D. Ni Eidhin, et al., Clumping factor B (ClfB), a new surface-located fibrinogen-binding adhesin of *Staphylococcus aureus*, Mol. Microbiol. 30 (1998) 245–257.

[62] D.P. O'Connell, et al., The fibrinogen-binding MSCRAMM (clumping factor) of *Staphylococcus aureus* has a Ca2+-dependent inhibitory site, J. Biol. Chem. 273 (1998) 6821–6829.

[63] T. Fowler, et al., Cellular invasion by *Staphylococcus aureus* involves a fibronectin bridge between the bacterial fibronectin-binding MSCRAMMs and host cell beta1 integrins, Eur. J. Cell. Biol. 79 (2000) 672–679.

[64] P. Moreillon, et al., Role of *Staphylococcus aureus* coagulase and clumping factor in pathogenesis of experimental endocarditis, Infect. Immun. 63 (1995) 4738–4743.

[65] J.M. Patti, et al., Molecular characterization and expression of a gene encoding a *Staphylococcus aureus* collagen adhesin, J. Biol. Chem. 267 (1992) 4766–4772.

[66] J.M. Patti, et al., The *Staphylococcus aureus* collagen adhesin is a virulence determinant in experimental septic arthritis, Infect. Immun. 62 (1994) 152–161.

[67] J.P. O'Gara, ica and beyond: biofilm mechanisms and regulation in *Staphylococcus epidermidis* and *Staphylococcus aureus*, FEMS Microbiol. Lett. 270 (2007) 179–188.

[68] A. Peschel, et al., Inactivation of the dlt operon in *Staphylococcus aureus* confers sensitivity to defensins, protegrins, and other antimicrobial peptides, J. Biol. Chem. 274 (1999) 8405–8410.

[69] L.V. Collins, et al., *Staphylococcus aureus* strains lacking D-alanine modifications of teichoic acids are highly susceptible to human neutrophil killing and are virulence attenuated in mice, J. Infect. Dis. 186 (2002) 214–219.

[70] P. Staubitz, et al., MprF-mediated biosynthesis of lysylphosphatidylglycerol, an important determinant in staphylococcal defensin resistance, FEMS Microbiol. Lett. 231 (2004) 67–71.

[71] H. Nishi, et al., Reduced content of lysyl-phosphatidylglycerol in the cytoplasmic membrane affects susceptibility to moenomycin, as well as vancomycin, gentamicin, and antimicrobial peptides, in *Staphylococcus aureus*, Antimicrob. Agents Chemother. 48 (2004) 4800–4807.

[72] C. Weidenmaier, et al., DltABCD- and MprF-mediated cell envelope modifications of *Staphylococcus aureus* confer resistance to platelet microbicidal proteins and contribute to virulence in a rabbit endocarditis model, Infect. Immun. 73 (2005) 8033–8038.

[73] M.E. Selsted, et al., Purification, primary structures, and antibacterial activities of beta-defensins, a new family of antimicrobial peptides from bovine neutrophils, J. Biol. Chem. 268 (1993) 6641.

[74] M. Sieprawska-Lupa, et al., Degradation of human antimicrobial peptide LL-37 by *Staphylococcus aureus*-derived proteinases, Antimicrob. Agents Chemother. 48 (2004) 4673–4679.

[75] B. Postma, et al., Chemotaxis inhibitory protein of *Staphylococcus aureus* binds specifically to the C5a and formylated peptide receptor, J. Immunol. 172 (2004) 6994–7001.

[76] A. Haggar, et al., The extracellular adherence protein from *Staphylococcus aureus* inhibits neutrophil binding to endothelial cells, Infect. Immun. 72 (2004) 6164–6167.

[77] S.H. Rooijakkers, K.P. van Kessel, J.A. van Strijp, Staphylococcal innate immune evasion, Trends Microbiol. 13 (2005) 596–601.

[78] S.H. Rooijakkers, et al., Immune evasion by a staphylococcal complement inhibitor that acts on C3 convertases, Nat. Immunol. 6 (2005) 920–927.

[79] N. Palmqvist, et al., Expression of staphylococcal clumping factor A impedes macrophage phagocytosis, Microbes Infect. 6 (2004) 188–195.

[80] J. Higgins, et al., Clumping factor A of *Staphylococcus aureus* inhibits phagocytosis by human polymorphonuclear leucocytes, FEMS Microbiol. Lett. 258 (2006) 290–296.

[81] M. Hammel, et al., A structural basis for complement inhibition by *Staphylococcus aureus*, Nat. Immunol. 8 (2007) 430–437.

[82] T. Jin, et al., *Staphylococcus aureus* resists human defensins by production of staphylokinase, a novel bacterial evasion mechanism, J. Immunol. 172 (2004) 1169–1176.

[83] T.J. Foster, Immune evasion by staphylococci, Nat. Rev. Microbiol. 3 (2005) 948–958.

[84] N. Palmqvist, et al., Protein A is a virulence factor in *Staphylococcus aureus* arthritis and septic death, Microb. Pathog. 33 (2002) 239–249.

[85] M. Thakker, et al., *Staphylococcus aureus* serotype 5 capsular polysaccharide is antiphagocytic and enhances bacterial virulence in a murine bacteremia model, Infect. Immun. 66 (1998) 5183–5189.

[86] T.T. Luong, C.Y. Lee, Overproduction of type 8 capsular polysaccharide augments *Staphylococcus aureus* virulence, Infect. Immun. 70 (2002) 3389–3395.

[87] A. Kropec, et al., Poly-N-acetylglucosamine production in *Staphylococcus aureus* is essential for virulence in murine models of systemic infection, Infect. Immun. 73 (2005) 6868–6876.

[88] G.L. Mandell, Catalase, superoxide dismutase, and virulence of *Staphylococcus aureus*: in vitro and in vivo studies with emphasis on staphylococcal-leukocyte interaction, J. Clin. Invest. 55 (1975) 561–566.

[89] G.Y. Liu, et al., *Staphylococcus aureus* golden pigment impairs neutrophil killing and promotes virulence through its antioxidant activity, J. Exp. Med. 202 (2005) 209–215.

[90] A. Clauditz, et al., Staphyloxanthin plays a role in the fitness of *Staphylococcus aureus* and its ability to cope with oxidative stress, Infect. Immun. 74 (2006) 4950–4953.

[91] M.H. Karavolos, et al., Role and regulation of the superoxide dismutases of *Staphylococcus aureus*, Microbiology 149 (2003) 2749–2758.

[92] J.E. Gouaux, et al., Subunit stoichiometry of staphylococcal alpha-hemolysin in crystals and on membranes: a heptameric transmembrane pore, Proc. Natl. Acad. Sci. U. S. A. 91 (1994) 12828.

[93] S. Bhakdi, J. Tranum-Jensen, Alpha-toxin of *Staphylococcus aureus*, Microbiol. Rev. 55 (1991) 733.

[94] N. Suttorp, et al., Pore-forming bacterial toxins potently induce release of nitric oxide in porcine endothelial cells, J. Exp. Med. 178 (1993) 337.

[95] D. Jonas, et al., Novel path to apoptosis: small transmembrane pores created by staphylococcal alpha-toxin in T lymphocytes evoke internucleosomal DNA degradation, Infect. Immun. 62 (1994) 1304.

[96] T.M. Jarry, G. Memmi, A.L. Cheung, The expression of alpha-haemolysin is required for *Staphylococcus aureus* phagosomal escape after internalization in CFT-1 cells, Cell. Microbiol. 10 (2008) 1801–1814.

[97] J. Bubeck Wardenburg, et al., Poring over pores: alpha-hemolysin and Panton-Valentine leukocidin in *Staphylococcus aureus* pneumonia, Nat. Med. 13 (2007) 1405–1406.

[98] J. Bubeck Wardenburg, O. Schneewind, Vaccine protection against *Staphylococcus aureus* pneumonia, J. Exp. Med. 205 (2008) 287–294.

[99] J. Kaneko, Y. Kamio, Bacterial two-component and hetero-heptameric pore-forming cytolytic toxins: structures, pore-forming mechanism, and organization of the genes, Biosci. Biotechnol. Biochem. 68 (2004) 981–1003.

[100] Y. Gillet, et al., Association between *Staphylococcus aureus* strains carrying gene for Panton-Valentine leukocidin and highly lethal necrotising pneumonia in young immunocompetent patients, Lancet 359 (2002) 753–759.

[101] M. Labandeira-Rey, et al., *Staphylococcus aureus* Panton-Valentine leukocidin causes necrotizing pneumonia, Science 315 (2007) 1130–1133.

[102] A.E. Villaruz, et al., A point mutation in the agr locus rather than expression of the Panton-Valentine leukocidin caused previously reported phenotypes in *Staphylococcus aureus* pneumonia and gene regulation, J. Infect. Dis. 200 (2009) 724–734.

[103] J. Bubeck Wardenburg, et al., Panton-Valentine leukocidin is not a virulence determinant in murine models of community-associated methicillin-resistant *Staphylococcus aureus* disease, J. Infect. Dis. 198 (2008) 1166–1170.

[104] C.W. Tseng, et al., *Staphylococcus aureus* Panton-Valentine leukocidin contributes to inflammation and muscle tissue injury, PLoS One 4 (2009) e6387.

[105] T. Wadstrom, R. Mollby, Studies on extracellular proteins from *Staphylococcus aureus*. VII. Studies on beta-hemolysin, Biochim. Biophys. Acta 242 (1972) 308.

[106] A. Hayashida, et al., *Staphylococcus aureus* beta-toxin induces lung injury through syndecan-1, Am. J. Pathol. 174 (2009) 509–518.

[107] B.A. Diep, M. Otto, The role of virulence determinants in community-associated MRSA pathogenesis, Trends Microbiol. 16 (2008) 361–369.

[108] R. Wang, et al., Identification of novel cytolytic peptides as key virulence determinants for community-associated MRSA, Nat. Med. 13 (2007) 1510–1514.

[109] J.D. Fraser, T. Proft, The bacterial superantigen and superantigen-like proteins, Immunol. Rev. 225 (2008) 226–243.

[110] K. Nishifuji, M. Sugai, M. Amagai, Staphylococcal exfoliative toxins: "molecular scissors" of bacteria that attack the cutaneous defense barrier in mammals, J. Dermatol. Sci. 49 (2008) 21–31.

[111] L.R. Plano, *Staphylococcus aureus* exfoliative toxins: how they cause disease, J. Invest. Dermatol. 122 (2004) 1070–1077.

[112] A. Bjorklind, S. Arvidson, Mutants of *Staphylococcus aureus* affected in the regulation of exoprotein synthesis, FEMS Microbiol. Lett. 7 (1980) 203.

[113] R.P. Novick, Autoinduction and signal transduction in the regulation of staphylococcal virulence, Mol. Microbiol. 48 (2003) 1429.

[114] R.P. Novick, E. Geisinger, Quorum sensing in staphylococci, Annu. Rev. Genet. 42 (2008) 541–564.

[115] A. Abdelnour, et al., The accessory gene regulator (agr) controls *Staphylococcus aureus* virulence in a murine arthritis model, Infect. Immun. 61 (1993) 3879–3885.

[116] K.L. Rogers, P.D. Fey, M.E. Rupp, Coagulase-negative staphylococcal infections, Infect. Dis. Clin. North. Am. 23 (2009) 73–98.

[117] M. Otto, Virulence factors of the coagulase-negative staphylococci, Front. Biosci. 9 (2004) 841–863.

[118] A. Ludwicka, et al., Microbial colonization of prosthetic devices. V. Attachment of coagulase-negative staphylococci and "slime"-production on chemically pure synthetic polymers, Zentralbl. Bakteriol. Mikrobiol. Hyg. B 177 (1983) 527–532.

[119] A. Gristina, Biomaterial-centered infection: microbial adhesion versus tissue integration. 1987, Clin. Orthop. Relat. Res. (427) (2004) 4–12.

[120] K.G. Kristinsson, Adherence of staphylococci to intravascular catheters, J. Med. Microbiol. 28 (1989) 249–257.

[121] C. Heilman, et al., Evidence for autolysin-mediated primary attachment of *Staphylococcus epidermidis* to a polystyrene surface, Mol. Microbiol. 24 (1997) 1013.

[122] M.E. Rupp, et al., Characterization of the importance of *Staphylococcus epidermidis* autolysin and polysaccharide intercellular adhesin in the pathogenesis of intravascular catheter-associated infection in a rat model, J. Infect. Dis. 183 (2001) 1038.

[123] C.P. Timmerman, et al., Characterization of a proteinaceous adhesion of *Staphylococcus epidermidis* which mediates attachment to polystyrene, Infect. Immun. 59 (1991) 4187.

[124] K.W. McCrea, et al., The serine-aspartate repeat (Sdr) protein family in *Staphylococcus epidermidis*, Microbiology 146 (2000) 1535.

[125] L. Pei, J.I. Flock, Lack of fbe, the gene for a fibrinogen-binding protein from *Staphylococcus epidermidis*, reduces its adherence to fibrinogen coated surfaces, Microb. Pathog. 31 (2001) 185.

[126] M. Nilsson, et al., A fibrinogen-binding protein of *Staphylococcus epidermidis*, Infect. Immun. 66 (1998) 2666.

[127] M. Hussain, et al., Teichoic acid enhances adhesion of *Staphylococcus epidermidis* to immobilized fibronectin, Microb. Pathog. 31 (2001) 261.

[128] M.G. Bowden, et al., Is the GehD lipase from *Staphylococcus epidermidis* a collagen binding adhesin? J. Biol. Chem. 277 (2002) 43017–43023.

[129] R.T. Hall, et al., Characteristics of coagulase-negative staphylococci from infants with bacteremia, Pediatr. Infect. Dis. J. 6 (1987) 377.

[130] J.A. Gruskay, et al., Predicting the pathogenicity of coagulase-negative *Staphylococcus* in the neonate: slime production, antibiotic resistance, and predominance of *Staphylococcus epidermidis* species, Pediatrics 20 (1986) 397A.

[131] D. Mack, et al., Characterization of transposon mutants of biofilm-producing *Staphylococcus epidermidis* impaired in the accumulative phase of biofilm production: genetic identification of a hexosamine-containing polysaccharide intercellular adhesion, Infect. Immun. 62 (1994) 3244.

[132] H. Rohde, et al., Structure, function and contribution of polysaccharide intercellular adhesin (PIA) to *Staphylococcus epidermidis* biofilm formation and pathogenesis of biomaterial-associated infections, Eur. J. Cell. Biol. 89 (2010) 103–111.

[133] D. McKenney, et al., The ica locus of *Staphylococcus epidermidis* encodes production of the capsular polysaccharide/adhesin, Infect. Immun. 66 (1998) 4711.

[134] J.O. Galdbart, et al., Screening for *Staphylococcus epidermidis* markers discriminating between skin-flora strains and those responsible for infections of joint prostheses, J. Infect. Dis. 182 (2000) 351–355.

[135] W. Ziebuhr, et al., A novel mechanism of phase variation of virulence in *Staphylococcus epidermidis*: evidence for control of the polysaccharide intercellular adhesin synthesis by alternating insertion and excision of the insertion sequence element IS256, Mol. Microbiol. 32 (1999) 345.

[136] M. Hussain, et al., A 140-kilodalton extracellular protein is essential for the accumulation of *Staphylococcus epidermidis* strains on surfaces, Infect. Immun. 65 (1997) 519.

[137] S. Kocianova, et al., Key role of poly-gamma-DL-glutamic acid in immune evasion and virulence of *Staphylococcus epidermidis*, J. Clin. Invest. 115 (2005) 688–694.

[138] C. Vuong, F. Götz, M. Otto, Construction and characterization of an agr deletion mutant of *Staphylococcus epidermidis*, Infect. Immun. 68 (2000) 1048.

[139] S.A. Kristian, et al., Biofilm formation induces C3a release and protects *Staphylococcus epidermidis* from IgG and complement deposition and from neutrophil-dependent killing, J. Infect. Dis. 197 (2008) 1028–1035.

[140] B.F. Farber, M.H. Kaplan, A.G. Clogston, *Staphylococcus epidermidis* extracted slime inhibits the antimicrobial action of glycopeptide antibodies, J. Infect. Dis. 161 (1990) 37.

[141] K.G. Kristinsson, R.C. Spencer, Slime production as a marker for clinically significant infection with coagulase-negative staphylococci, J. Infect. Dis. 154 (1986) 728.

[142] J.J. Younger, et al., Coagulase-negative staphylococci isolated from cerebrospinal fluid shunts: importance of slime production, species identification, and shunt removal to clinical outcome, J. Infect. Dis. 156 (1987) 548.

[143] Y. Ohara-Nemoto, et al., Characterization and molecular cloning of a glutamyl endopeptidase from *Staphylococcus epidermidis*, Microb. Pathog. 33 (2002) 33–41.

[144] W.C. Liles, et al., Stimulation of human neutrophils and monocytes by staphylococcal phenol-soluble modulin, J. Leukoc. Biol. 70 (2001) 96–102.

[145] J.M. Koenig, M.C. Yoder, Neonatal neutrophils: the good, the bad, and the ugly, Clin. Perinatol. 31 (2004) 39–51.

[146] A.D. Mease, Tissue neutropenia: the newborn neutrophil in perspective, J. Perinatol. 10 (1990) 55.

[147] D.C. Anderson, B. Hughes, C.W. Smith, Abnormality motility of neonatal polymorphonuclear leukocytes, J. Clin. Invest. 68 (1981) 863.

[148] K.R. Schibler, et al., Diminished transcription of interleukin-8 by monocytes from preterm neonates, J. Leukoc. Biol. 53 (1993) 399.

[149] T.K. Yoshimura, et al., Purification of a human monocyte derived neutrophil chemotactic factor that shares sequence homology with other host defense cytokinase, Proc. Natl. Acad. Sci. U. S. A. 84 (1987) 9233.

[150] G.A. Zimmerman, S.M. Prescott, T.M. McIntyre, Endothelial cell, interactions with granulocytes: tethering and signaling molecules, Immunol. Today 13 (1992) 93.

[151] A.O. Shigeoka, et al., Defective oxidative metabolic responses of neutrophils from stressed infants, J. Pediatr. 98 (1981) 392.

[152] R.G. Strauss, E.L. Snyder, Activation and activity of the superoxide-generating system of neutrophils from human infants, Pediatr. Res. 17 (1983) 662.

[153] T.E. Herman, M.J. Siegel, Chronic granulomatous disease of childhood: neonatal serratia, hepatic abscesses, and pulmonary aspergillosis, J. Perinatol. 22 (2002) 255–256.

[154] J.R.J. Banffer, J.F. Franken, Immunization with leucocidin toxoid against staphylococcal infection, Pathol. Microbiol. (Basel) 30 (1967) 166.

[155] C.H. Lack, A.G. Towers, Serological tests for staphylococcal infection, BMJ 2 (1962) 1227.

[156] A.L. Florman, et al., Relation of 7S and 19S staphylococcal hemagglutinating antibody to age of individual, Pediatrics 32 (1963) 501.

[157] G.J. Lavoipierre, et al., A vaccine trial for neonatal staphylococcal disease, Am. J. Dis. Child. 122 (1971) 377.

[158] R.M. McLoughlin, et al., CD4+ T cells and CXC chemokines modulate the pathogenesis of Staphylococcus aureus wound infections, Proc. Natl. Acad. Sci. U. S. A. 103 (2006) 10408–10413.

[159] P. Marrach, J. Kappler, The staphylococcal enterotoxin and their relatives, Science 248 (1990) 705.

[160] H.F. Eichenwald, H.R. Shinefield, The problem of staphylococcal infection in newborn infants, J. Pediatr. 56 (1960) 665–674.

[161] A.H. Sohn, et al., Prevalence of nosocomial infections in neonatal intensive care unit patients: results from the first national point-prevalence survey, J. Pediatr. 139 (2001) 821–827.

[162] D. Isaacs, A ten year, multicentre study of coagulase negative staphylococcal infections in Australasian neonatal units, Arch. Dis. Child. Fetal Neonatal Ed. 88 (2003) F89–F93.

[163] D. Isaacs, S. Fraser, G. Hogg, et al., *Staphylococcus aureus* infections in Australasian neonatal nurseries, Arch. Dis. Child. Fetal Neonatal Ed. 89 (2004) F331–F335.

[164] R.L. Chapman, R.G. Faix, Persistent bacteremia and outcome in late onset infection among infants in a neonatal intensive care unit, Pediatr. Infect. Dis. J. 22 (2003) 17–21.

[165] D.K. Benjamin, et al., Mortality following blood culture in premature infants: increased with Gram-negative bacteremia and candidemia, but not Gram-positive bacteremia, J. Perinatol. 24 (2004) 175–180.

[166] A. Ronnestad, et al., Septicemia in the first week of life in a Norwegian national cohort of extremely premature infants, Pediatrics 115 (2005) e262–e268.

[167] B.J. Stoll, et al., Very low birth weight preterm infants with early onset neonatal sepsis: the predominance of gram-negative infections continues in the National Institute of Child Health and Human Development Neonatal Research Network, 2002–2003, Pediatr. Infect. Dis. J. 24 (2005) 635–639.

[168] G. Regev-Yochay, et al., Methicillin-resistant *Staphylococcus aureus* in neonatal intensive care unit, Emerg. Infect. Dis. 11 (2005) 453–456.

[169] Y.C. Huang, et al., Methicillin-resistant *Staphylococcus aureus* colonization and its association with infection among infants hospitalized in neonatal intensive care units, Pediatrics 118 (2006) 469–474.

[170] M. Khashu, et al., Persistent bacteremia and severe thrombocytopenia caused by coagulase-negative *Staphylococcus* in a neonatal intensive care unit, Pediatrics 117 (2006) 340–348.

[171] C. Gomez-Gonzalez, et al., Long persistence of methicillin-susceptible strains of *Staphylococcus aureus* causing sepsis in a neonatal intensive care unit, J. Clin. Microbiol. 45 (2007) 2301–2304.

[172] J. Kuint, et al., Comparison of community-acquired methicillin-resistant *Staphylococcus aureus* bacteremia to other staphylococcal species in a neonatal intensive care unit, Eur. J. Pediatr. 166 (2007) 319–325.

[173] V. Hira, et al., Clinical and molecular epidemiologic characteristics of coagulase-negative staphylococcal bloodstream infections in intensive care neonates, Pediatr. Infect. Dis. J. 26 (2007) 607–612.

[174] U. Seybold, et al., Emergence of and risk factors for methicillin-resistant *Staphylococcus aureus* of community origin in intensive care nurseries, Pediatrics 122 (2008) 1039–1046.

[175] A.J. Carey, L. Saiman, R.A. Polin, Hospital-acquired infections in the NICU: epidemiology for the new millennium, Clin. Perinatol. 35 (2008) 223–249.

[176] D.L. Palazzi, J.O. Klein, C.J. Baker, Bacterial sepsis and meningitis, in: J.S. Remington et al., (Eds.), Infectious Diseases of the Fetus and Newborn Infant, sixth ed., Saunders, Philadelphia, 2006, pp. 247–296.

[177] T. Vesikari, et al., Neonatal septicaemia, Arch. Dis. Child. 60 (1985) 542–546.

[178] C.M. Healy, et al., Features of invasive staphylococcal disease in neonates, Pediatrics 114 (2004) 953–961.

[179] C.M. Healy, et al., Emergence of new strains of methicillin-resistant *Staphylococcus aureus* in a neonatal intensive care unit, Clin. Infect. Dis. 39 (2004) 1460–1466.

[180] Y.Y. Chuang, et al., Methicillin-resistant *Staphylococcus aureus* bacteraemia in neonatal intensive care units: an analysis of 90 episodes, Acta Paediatr. 93 (2004) 786–790.

[181] M. Cohen-Wolkowiez, et al., Mortality and neurodevelopmental outcome after *Staphylococcus aureus* bacteremia in infants, Pediatr. Infect. Dis. J. 26 (2007) 1159–1161.

[182] K.P. Sanghvi, D.I. Tudehope, Neonatal bacterial sepsis in a neonatal intensive care unit: a 5 year analysis, J. Paediatr. Child Health 32 (1996) 333.

[183] C.M. Beck-Sague, et al., Bloodstream infections in neonatal intensive care unit patients: results of a multicenter study, Pediatr. Infect. Dis. J. 13 (1994) 1110.

[184] J.R. Edwards, et al., National Healthcare Safety Network (NHSN) Report, data summary for 2006 through 2007, issued November 2008, Am. J. Infect. Control. 36 (2008) 609–626.

[185] H.W. Kilbride, et al., Evaluation and development of potentially better practices to prevent neonatal nosocomial bacteremia, Pediatrics 111 (2003) e504–e518.

[186] A.A. Fanaroff, et al., Incidence, presenting features, risk factors and significance of late onset septicemia in very low birth weight infants. The National Institute of Child Health and Human Development Neonatal Research Network, Pediatr. Infect. Dis. J. 17 (1998) 593–598.

[187] I.R. Makhoul, et al., Pathogen-specific early mortality in very low birth weight infants with late-onset sepsis: a national survey, Clin. Infect. Dis. 40 (2005) 218–224.

[188] M.G. Karlowicz, et al., Central venous catheter removal versus in situ treatment in neonates with coagulase-negative staphylococcal bacteremia, Pediatr. Infect. Dis. J. 21 (2002) 22–27.

[189] D.K. Benjamin Jr., et al., Bacteremia, central catheters, and neonates: when to pull the line, Pediatrics 107 (2001) 1272–1276.

[190] S.L. Lawrence, et al., Cloxacillin versus vancomycin for presumed late-onset sepsis in the Neonatal Intensive Care Unit and the impact upon outcome of coagulase negative staphylococcal bacteremia: a retrospective cohort study, BMC Pediatr. 5 (2005) 49.

[191] C. Powell, S. Bubb, J. Clark, Toxic shock syndrome in a neonate, Pediatr. Infect. Dis. J. 26 (2007) 759–760.

[192] K. Kikuchi, et al., Molecular epidemiology of methicillin-resistant *Staphylococcus aureus* strains causing neonatal toxic shock syndrome-like exanthematous disease in neonatal and perinatal wards, J. Clin. Microbiol. 41 (2003) 3001–3006.

[193] P.M. Schlievert, Alteration of immune function by staphylococcal pyrogenic exotoxin type C: possible role in toxic-shock syndrome, J. Infect. Dis. 147 (1983) 391.

[194] P.M. Schlievert, Staphylococcal enterotoxin B and toxic-shock syndrome toxin-1 are significantly associated with non-menstrual TSS, Lancet 1 (1986) 1149.

[195] N. Takahashi, H. Nishida, New exanthematous disease with thrombocytopenia in neonates, Arch. Dis. Child. Fetal Neonatal Ed. 77 (1997) F79.

[196] N. Takahashi, et al., Exanthematous disease induced by toxic shock syndrome toxin 1 in the early neonatal period, Lancet 351 (1998) 1614.

[197] N. Takahashi, et al., Immunopathophysiological aspects of an emerging neonatal infectious disease induced by a bacterial superantigen, J. Clin. Invest. 106 (2000) 1409.

[198] P.S. Symchych, A.N. Krauss, P. Winchester, Endocarditis following intracardiac placement of umbilical venous catheters in neonates, J. Pediatr. 90 (1977) 287.

[199] D.H. Johnson, A. Rosenthal, A.S. Nadas, A forty-year review of bacterial endocarditis in infancy and childhood, Circulation 51 (1975) 581.

[200] D.D. Millard, S.T. Shulman, The changing spectrum of neonatal endocarditis, Clin. Perinatol. 15 (1988) 587.

[201] I.K. Mecrow, E.J. Ladusans, Infective endocarditis in newborn infants with structurally normal hearts, Acta Paediatr. 83 (1994) 35.

[202] A.H. Daher, F.E. Berkowitz, Infective endocarditis in neonates, Clin. Pediatr. (Phila) 34 (1995) 198–206.

[203] S.A. Pearlman, et al., Infective endocarditis in the premature neonate, Clin. Pediatr. (Phila) 37 (1998) 741.

[204] G.F. Opie, et al., Bacterial endocarditis in neonatal intensive care, J. Paediatr. Child Health 35 (1999) 545–548.

[205] A.M. Valente, et al., Frequency of infective endocarditis among infants and children with *Staphylococcus aureus* bacteremia, Pediatrics 115 (2005) e15–e19.

[206] A.S. Milazzo Jr., J.S. Li, Bacterial endocarditis in infants and children, Pediatr. Infect. Dis. J. 20 (2001) 799–801.

[207] C. O'Callaghan, P. McDougall, Infective endocarditis in neonates, Arch. Dis. Child. 63 (1988) 53–57.

[208] D. Armstrong, et al., *Staphylococcus aureus* endocarditis in preterm neonates, Am. J. Perinatol. 19 (2002) 247–251.

[209] T.J. Sung, H.M. Kim, M.J. Kim, Methicillin-resistant *Staphylococcus aureus* endocarditis in an extremely low-birth-weight infant treated with linezolid, Clin. Pediatr. (Phila) 47 (2008) 504–506.

[210] R.M. Fortunov, et al., Community-acquired *Staphylococcus aureus* infections in term and near-term previously healthy neonates, Pediatrics 118 (2006) 874–881.

[211] R.M. Fortunov, et al., Evaluation and treatment of community-acquired *Staphylococcus aureus* infections in term and late-preterm previously healthy neonates, Pediatrics 120 (2007) 937–945.

[212] L. James, et al., Methicillin-resistant *Staphylococcus aureus* infections among healthy full-term newborns, Arch. Dis. Child. Fetal Neonatal Ed. 93 (2008) F40–F44.

[213] D.M. Nguyen, et al., Risk factors for neonatal methicillin-resistant *Staphylococcus aureus* infection in a well-infant nursery, Infect. Control. Hosp. Epidemiol. 28 (2007) 406–411.

[214] Y.H. Kim, et al., Clinical outcomes in methicillin-resistant *Staphylococcus aureus*-colonized neonates in the neonatal intensive care unit, Neonatology 91 (2007) 241–247.

[215] G.A. Ayliffe, et al., Staphylococcal infection in cervical glands of infants, Lancet 2 (1972) 479.

[216] J. Dewar, I.A. Porter, G.H. Smylie, Staphylococcal infection in cervical glands of infants, Lancet 2 (1972) 712.

[217] G. Sabatino, et al., Neonatal suppurative parotitis: a study of five cases, Eur. J. Pediatr. 158 (1999) 312.

[218] R. Spiegel, et al., Acute neonatal suppurative parotitis: case reports and review, Pediatr. Infect. Dis. J. 23 (2004) 76.

[219] I.I. Raad, M.F. Sabbagh, G.J. Caranasos, Acute bacterial sialadenitis: a study of 29 cases and review, Rev. Infect. Dis. 12 (1990) 591.

[220] R.B. David, E.J. O'Connel, Suppurative parotitis in children, Am. J. Dis. Child. 119 (1970) 332.

[221] R.C. Rudoy, J.D. Nelson, Breast abscess during the neonatal period: a review, Am. J. Dis. Child. 129 (1975) 1031–1034.

[222] H. Kalwbow, Über Mastitis neonatorum und ihre Folgen, Zentralbl. Gynakol. 60 (1936) 1821.

[223] C. Bodemer, et al., Staphylococcal necrotizing fasciitis in the mammary region in childhood: a report of five cases, J. Pediatr. 131 (1997) 466–469.

[224] K.P. Sawardekar, Changing spectrum of neonatal omphalitis, Pediatr. Infect. Dis. J. 23 (2004) 22–26.

[225] W.H. Mason, et al., Omphalitis in the newborn infant, Pediatr. Infect. Dis. J. 8 (1989) 521–525.

[226] K.P. Lally, et al., Necrotizing fasciitis: a serious sequela of omphalitis in the newborn, Ann. Surg. 199 (1984) 101–103.

[227] M. Samuel, et al., Necrotizing fasciitis: a serious complication of omphalitis in neonates, J. Pediatr. Surg. 29 (1994) 1414–1416.

[228] W.S. Hsieh, et al., Neonatal necrotizing fasciitis: a report of three cases and review of the literature, Pediatrics 103 (1999) e53.

[229] L.G. Miller, et al., Necrotizing fasciitis caused by community-associated methicillin-resistant *Staphylococcus aureus* in Los Angeles, N. Engl. J. Med. 352 (2005) 1445–1453.

[230] W. Dehority, et al., Community-associated methicillin-resistant *Staphylococcus aureus* necrotizing fasciitis in a neonate, Pediatr. Infect. Dis. J. 25 (2006) 1080–1081.

[231] K.C. Hayani, et al., Neonatal necrotizing fasciitis due to community-acquired methicillin resistant *Staphylococcus aureus*, Pediatr. Infect. Dis. J. 27 (2008) 480–481.

[232] J.S. Yu, P. Habib, MR imaging of urgent inflammatory and infectious conditions affecting the soft tissues of the musculoskeletal system, Emerg. Radiol. 16 (2009) 267–276.

[233] R.F. Edlich, et al., Modern concepts of the diagnosis and treatment of necrotizing fasciitis, J. Emerg. Med. (2008) in press.

[234] D.R. Brown, et al., A multicenter review of the treatment of major truncal necrotizing infections with and without hyperbaric oxygen therapy, Am. J. Surg. 167 (1994) 485–489.

[235] V. Kapoor, J. Travadi, S. Braye, Staphylococcal scalded skin syndrome in an extremely premature neonate: a case report with a brief review of literature, J. Paediatr. Child Health 44 (2008) 374–376.

[236] I.R. Makhoul, et al., Staphylococcal scalded-skin syndrome in a very low birth weight premature infant, Pediatrics 108 (2001) E16.

[237] B. Peters, et al., Staphylococcal scalded-skin syndrome complicating wound infection in a preterm infant with postoperative chylothorax, J. Clin. Microbiol. 36 (1998) 3057–3059.

[238] E. Rieger-Fackeldey, et al., Staphylococcal scalded skin syndrome related to an exfoliative toxin A- and B-producing strain in preterm infants, Eur. J. Pediatr. 161 (2002) 649–652.

[239] J.P. Curran, F.L. Al-Salihi, Neonatal staphylococcal scalded skin syndrome: massive outbreak due to an unusual phage type, Pediatrics 66 (1980) 285–290.

[240] G. Ritter von Rittershain, Die exfoliative Dermatitis jüngerer Säuglinge, Zentralztg. Kinderheilkd. 2 (1878) 3–23.

[241] M.E. Melish, L.A. Glasgow, Staphylococcal scalded skin syndrome: the expanded clinical syndrome, J. Pediatr. 78 (1971) 958–967.

[242] A.M. Farrell, Staphylococcal scalded-skin syndrome, Lancet 354 (1999) 880–881.

[243] R. Hoffmann, et al., Staphylococcal scalded skin syndrome (SSSS) and consecutive septicaemia in a preterm infant, Pathol. Res. Pract. 190 (1994) 77–81.

[244] W.T. Lo, C.C. Wang, M.L. Chu, Intrauterine staphylococcal scalded skin syndrome: report of a case, Pediatr. Infect. Dis. J. 19 (2000) 481–482.

[245] J.L. Loughead, Congenital staphylococcal scaled skin syndrome: report of a case, Pediatr. Infect. Dis. J. 11 (1992) 413–414.

[246] L.M. Haveman, et al., Congenital staphylococcal scalded skin syndrome in a premature infant, Acta Paediatr. 93 (2004) 1661–1662.

[247] S.J. Dancer, et al., Outbreak of staphylococcal scalded skin syndrome among neonates, J. Infect. 16 (1988) 87–103.

[248] D.W. Beaven, A.F. Burry, Staphylococcal pneumonia in the newborn: an epidemic with 8 fatal cases, Lancet 271 (1956) 211–215.

[249] H.R. Shinefield, N.L. Ruff, Staphylococcal infections: a historical perspective, Infect. Dis. Clin. North Am. 23 (2009) 1–15.

[250] S. Yee-Guardino, et al., Recognition and treatment of neonatal community-associated MRSA pneumonia and bacteremia, Pediatr. Pulmonol. 43 (2008) 203–205.

[251] D. Drinkovic, et al., Neonatal coagulase-negative staphylococcal meningitis: a report of two cases, Pathology 34 (2002) 586–588.

[252] R.S. de Oliveira, et al., Brain abscess in a neonate: an unusual presentation, Childs Nerv. Syst. 23 (2007) 139–142.

[253] R.H. Regev, T.Z. Dolfin, C. Zamir, Multiple brain abscesses in a premature infant: complication of Staphylococcus aureus sepsis, Acta Paediatr. 84 (1995) 585–587.

[254] G. Vartzelis, et al., Brain abscesses complicating Staphylococcus aureus sepsis in a premature infant, Infection 33 (2005) 36–38.

[255] M. Vinchon, P. Dhellemmes, Cerebrospinal fluid shunt infection: risk factors and long-term follow-up, Childs Nerv. Syst. 22 (2006) 692–697.

[256] A. Reinprecht, et al., Posthemorrhagic hydrocephalus in preterm infants: long-term follow-up and shunt-related complications, Childs Nerv. Syst. 17 (2001) 663–669.

[257] E.J. Anderson, R. Yogev, A rational approach to the management of ventricular shunt infections, Pediatr. Infect. Dis. J. 24 (2005) 557–558.

[258] D.M. Sciubba, et al., Antibiotic-impregnated shunt catheters for the treatment of infantile hydrocephalus, Pediatr. Neurosurg. 44 (2008) 91–96.

[259] J. Filka, et al., Nosocomial meningitis in children after ventriculoperitoneal shunt insertion, Acta Paediatr. 88 (1999) 576–578.

[260] H.E. James, J.S. Bradley, Aggressive management of shunt infection: combined intravenous and intraventricular antibiotic therapy for twelve or less days, Pediatr. Neurosurg. 44 (2008) 104–111.

[261] A.A. Nava-Ocampo, et al., Antimicrobial therapy and local toxicity of intraventricular administration of vancomycin in a neonate with ventriculitis, Ther. Drug Monit. 28 (2006) 474–476.

[262] A.M. Cook, et al., Linezolid for the treatment of a heteroresistant Staphylococcus aureus shunt infection, Pediatr. Neurosurg. 41 (2005) 102–104.

[263] C.M. Potter, Osteomyelitis in the newborn, J. Bone Joint Surg. Br. 36 (1954) 578–583.

[264] S.Z. Walsh, J.D. Craig, Generalized osteomyelitis in a newborn infant, J. Pediatr. 52 (1958) 313–318.

[265] S. Bergdahl, K. Ekengren, M. Eriksson, Neonatal hematogenous osteomyelitis: risk factors for long-term sequelae, J. Pediatr. Orthop. 5 (1985) 564–568.

[266] B. Frederiksen, P. Christiansen, F.U. Knudsen, Acute osteomyelitis and septic arthritis in the neonate, risk factors and outcome, Eur. J. Pediatr. 152 (1993) 577–580.

[267] J.B. Williamson, C.S. Galasko, M.J. Robinson, Outcome after acute osteomyelitis in preterm infants, Arch. Dis. Child. 65 (1990) 1060–1062.

[268] M. Wong, et al., Clinical and diagnostic features of osteomyelitis occurring in the first three months of life, Pediatr. Infect. Dis. J. 14 (1995) 1047–1053.

[269] J.A. Ogden, Pediatric osteomyelitis and septic arthritis: the pathology of neonatal disease, Yale J. Biol. Med. 52 (1979) 423–448.

[270] J.A. Ogden, G. Lister, The pathology of neonatal osteomyelitis, Pediatrics 55 (1975) 474–478.

[271] A.C. Offiah, Acute osteomyelitis, septic arthritis and discitis: differences between neonates and older children, Eur. J. Radiol. 60 (2006) 221–232.

[272] E. Korakaki, et al., Methicillin-resistant Staphylococcus aureus osteomyelitis and septic arthritis in neonates: diagnosis and management, Jpn. J. Infect. Dis. 60 (2007) 129–131.

[273] M. Waseem, G. Devas, E. Laureta, A neonate with asymmetric arm movements, Pediatr. Emerg. Care 25 (2009) 98–99.

[274] J. Parmar, Case report: septic arthritis of the temporomandibular joint in a neonate, Br. J. Oral. Maxillofac. Surg. 46 (2008) 505–506.

[275] M.O. Lim, et al., Osteomyelitis as a complication of umbilical artery catheterization, Am. J. Dis. Child. 131 (1977) 142–144.

[276] L.D. Lilien, et al., Neonatal osteomyelitis of the calcaneus: complication of heel puncture, J. Pediatr. 88 (1976) 478–480.

[277] S. Yuksel, et al., Osteomyelitis of the calcaneus in the newborn: an ongoing complication of Guthrie test, Eur. J. Pediatr. 166 (2007) 503–504.

[278] G.D. Overturf, G. Balfour, Osteomyelitis and sepsis: severe complications of fetal monitoring, Pediatrics 55 (1975) 244–247.

[279] R.S. Asnes, G.M. Arendar, Septic arthritis of the hip: a complication of femoral venipuncture, Pediatrics 38 (1966) 837–841.

[280] D. Barrie, Staphylococcal colonization of the rectum in the newborn, BMJ 1 (1966) 1574–1576.

[281] E.J. Ottenheimer, et al., Studies of the epidemiology of staphylococcal infection, Bull. Johns Hopkins Hosp. 109 (1961) 114.

[282] C.D. Christie, E. Lynch-Ballard, W.A. Andiman, Staphylococcal enterocolitis revisited: cytotoxic properties of Staphylococcus aureus from a neonate with enterocolitis, Pediatr. Infect. Dis. J. 7 (1988) 791–795.

[283] L.T. Gutman, et al., Neonatal staphylococcal enterocolitis: association with indwelling feeding catheters and S. aureus colonization, J. Pediatr. 88 (1976) 836–839.

[284] K. Masunaga, et al., Colonic stenosis after severe methicillin-resistant Staphylococcus aureus enterocolitis in a newborn, Pediatr. Infect. Dis. J. 18 (1999) 169–171.

[285] D.W. Scheifele, et al., Delta-like toxin produced by coagulase-negative staphylococci is associated with neonatal necrotizing enterocolitis, Infect. Immun. 55 (1987) 2268–2273.

[286] G.D. Overturf, et al., Neonatal necrotizing enterocolitis associated with delta toxin-producing methicillin-resistant Staphylococcus aureus, Pediatr. Infect. Dis. J. 9 (1990) 88–91.

[287] S. Mehr, L.W. Doyle, Cytokines as markers of bacterial sepsis in newborn infants: a review, Pediatr. Infect. Dis. J. 19 (2000) 879–887.

[288] U.K. Mishra, et al., Newer approaches to the diagnosis of early onset neonatal sepsis, Arch. Dis. Child. Fetal Neonatal Ed. 91 (2006) F208–F212.

[289] I.R. Makhoul, et al., Values of C-reactive protein, procalcitonin, and Staphylococcus-specific PCR in neonatal late-onset sepsis, Acta Paediatr. 95 (2006) 1218–1223.

[290] R. Vazzalwar, et al., Procalcitonin as a screening test for late-onset sepsis in preterm very low birth weight infants, J. Perinatol. 25 (2005) 397–402.

[291] C. Sherwin, et al., Utility of interleukin-12 and interleukin-10 in comparison with other cytokines and acute-phase reactants in the diagnosis of neonatal sepsis, Am. J. Perinatol. 25 (2008) 629–636.

[292] M.C. Harris, et al., Cytokine elaboration in critically ill infants with bacterial sepsis, necrotizing enterocolitis, or sepsis syndrome: correlation with clinical parameters of inflammation and mortality, J. Pediatr. 147 (2005) 462–468.

[293] H.S. Lam, P.C. Ng, Biochemical markers of neonatal sepsis, Pathology 40 (2008) 141–148.

[294] J.B. Lopez Sastre, et al., Procalcitonin is not sufficiently reliable to be the sole marker of neonatal sepsis of nosocomial origin, BMC Pediatr. 6 (2006) 16.

[295] C.C. Patrick, et al., Persistent bacteremia due to coagulase-negative staphylococci in low birthweight neonates, Pediatrics 84 (1989) 977.

[296] S. Baumgart, et al., Sepsis with coagulase-negative staphylococci in critically ill newborns, Am. J. Dis. Child. 137 (1983) 461.

[297] B.K. Schmidt, et al., Coagulase-negative staphylococci as true pathogens in newborn infants: a cohort study, Pediatr. Infect. Dis. J. 6 (1987) 1026.

[298] A. Ohlin, et al., Real-time PCR of the 16S-rRNA gene in the diagnosis of neonatal bacteraemia, Acta Paediatr. 97 (2008) 1376–1380.

[299] M. Rybak, et al., Therapeutic monitoring of vancomycin in adult patients: a consensus review of the American Society of Health-System Pharmacists, the Infectious Diseases Society of America, and the Society of Infectious Diseases Pharmacists, Am. J. Health Syst. Pharm. 66 (2009) 82–98.

[300] E.V. Capparelli, et al., The influences of renal function and maturation on vancomycin elimination in newborns and infants, J. Clin. Pharmacol. 41 (2001) 927–934.

[301] P.D. Reiter, M.W. Doron, Vancomycin cerebrospinal fluid concentrations after intravenous administration in premature infants, J. Perinatol. 16 (1996) 331–335.

[302] M. de Hoog, J.W. Mouton, J.N. van den Anker, Vancomycin: pharmacokinetics and administration regimens in neonates, Clin. Pharmacokinet. 43 (2004) 417–440.

[303] O. Plan, et al., Continuous-infusion vancomycin therapy for preterm neonates with suspected or documented Gram-positive infections: a new dosage schedule, Arch. Dis. Child. Fetal Neonatal Ed. 93 (2008) F418–F421.

[304] P. Sanchez, J.S. Bradley, J.D. Nelson, Antiinfective therapy for newborns, in: J.S. Bradley, J.D. Nelson (Eds.), 2008-2009 Nelson's Pocket Book of

Pediatric Antimicrobial Therapy, seventeenth ed., American Academy of Pediatrics, Chicago, 2008, pp. 16–29.

[305] V.G. Meka, H.S. Gold, Antimicrobial resistance to linezolid, Clin. Infect. Dis. 39 (2004) 1010–1015.

[306] J.G. Deville, et al., Linezolid versus vancomycin in the treatment of known or suspected resistant gram-positive infections in neonates, Pediatr. Infect. Dis. J. 22 (2003) S158–S163.

[307] G.L. Jungbluth, I.R. Welshman, N.K. Hopkins, Linezolid pharmacokinetics in pediatric patients: an overview, Pediatr. Infect. Dis. J. 22 (2003) S153–S157.

[308] L.M. Baddour, W.R. Wilson, A.S. Bayer, et al., Infective endocarditis: diagnosis, antimicrobial therapy, and management of complications: a statement for healthcare professionals from the Committee on Rheumatic Fever, Endocarditis, and Kawasaki Disease, Council on Cardiovascular Disease in the Young, and the Councils on Clinical Cardiology, Stroke, and Cardiovascular Surgery and Anesthesia, American Heart Association: endorsed by the Infectious Diseases Society of America, Circulation 111 (2005) e394–e434.

[309] A.S. Soraisham, M.Y. Al-Hindi, Intravenous rifampicin for persistent staphylococcal bacteremia in premature infants, Pediatr. Int. 50 (2008) 124–126.

[310] A. Ohlsson, J.B. Lacy, Intravenous immunoglobulin for suspected or subsequently proven infection in neonates, Cochrane Database Syst. Rev. (2004) CD001239.

[311] B.M. Andersen, et al., Spread of methicillin-resistant *Staphylococcus aureus* in a neonatal intensive unit associated with understaffing, overcrowding and mixing of patients, J. Hosp. Infect. 50 (2002) 18.

[312] R.W. Haley, et al., Eradication of endemic methicillin-resistant *Staphylococcus aureus* infections from a neonatal intensive care unit, J. Infect. Dis. 171 (1995) 614.

[313] P.M. Rountree, et al., Control of staphylococcal infection of newborn by treatment of nasal carriers in staff, Med. J. Aust. 1 (1956) 528.

[314] W.A. Gillespie, V.G. Adler, Control of an outbreak of staphylococcal infection in a hospital, Lancet 1 (1957) 632.

[315] W.J. Martin, D.R. Nichols, E.D. Henderson, The problem of management of nasal carriers of staphylococci, Proc. Mayo Clin. 35 (1960) 282.

[316] J.D. Williams, et al., Trials of five antibacterial creams in the control of nasal carriage of *Staphylococcus aureus*, Lancet 2 (1967) 390.

[317] R.T. Smith, The role of the chronic carrier in an epidemic of staphylococcal disease in a newborn nursery, Am. J. Dis. Child. 95 (1958) 461.

[318] D.N. Wysham, et al., Staphylococcal infections in an obstetric unit. I. Epidemiologic studies of pyoderma neonatorum, N. Engl. J. Med. 257 (1957) 295.

[319] A. Belani, et al., Outbreak of staphylococcal infection in two hospital nurseries traced to a single nasal carrier, Infect. Control. 7 (1986) 487.

[320] J.S. Garner, Guideline for isolation precautions in hospitals. The Hospital Infection Control Practices Advisory Committee, [erratum appears in Infect. Control. Hosp. Epidemiol. 17 (1996) 214], Infect. Control. Hosp. Epidemiol. 17 (1996) 5.

[321] J.A. Jernigan, et al., Effectiveness of contact isolation during a hospital outbreak of methicillin-resistant *Staphylococcus aureus*, [erratum appears in Am. J. Epidemiol.], Am. J. Epidemiol. 143 (1996) 496.

[322] S.I. Gerber, et al., Management of outbreaks of methicillin-resistant *Staphylococcus aureus* infection in the neonatal intensive care unit: a consensus statement, Infect. Control. Hosp. Epidemiol. 27 (2006) 139–145.

[323] M.L. Bertin, et al., Outbreak of methicillin-resistant *Staphylococcus aureus* colonization and infection in a neonatal intensive care unit epidemiologically linked to a healthcare worker with chronic otitis, Infect. Control. Hosp. Epidemiol. 27 (2006) 581–585.

[324] J.A. Otter, et al., Identification and control of an outbreak of ciprofloxacin-susceptible EMRSA-15 on a neonatal unit, J. Hosp. Infect. 67 (2007) 232–239.

[325] J.R. McDonald, et al., Methicillin-resistant *Staphylococcus aureus* outbreak in an intensive care nursery: potential for interinstitutional spread, Pediatr. Infect. Dis. J. 26 (2007) 678–683.

[326] H.R. Shinefield, J.C. Ribble, M. Boris, Bacterial interference between strains of *Staphylococcus aureus*, 1960 to 1970, Am. J. Dis. Child. 121 (1971) 148.

[327] I.J. Light, J.M. Sutherland, J.E. Schott, Control of a staphylococcal outbreak in a nursery—use of bacterial interference, JAMA 193 (1965) 699.

[328] H.R. Shinefield, Bacterial interference, Ann. N. Y. Acad. Sci. 236 (1974) 444.

[329] E.A. Mortimer Jr., et al., Transmission of staphylococci between newborns: importance of the hands of personnel, Am. J. Dis. Child. 104 (1962) 289.

[330] E.K. Kretzer, E.L. Larson, Behavioral interventions to improve infection control practices, Am. J. Infect. Control 26 (1998) 245.

[331] J. Tibballs, Teaching hospital medical staff to handwash, Med. J. Aust. 164 (1996) 395.

[332] D. Pittet, Improving compliance with hand hygiene in hospitals, Infect. Control Hosp. Epidemiol. 21 (2000) 381.

[333] N.J. Ehrenkranz, B.C. Alfonso, Failure of bland soap handwash to prevent hand transfer of patient bacteria to urethral catheters, Infect. Control Hosp. Epidemiol. 12 (1991) 654.

[334] H. Aly, et al., Is bloodstream infection preventable among premature infants? A tale of two cities, Pediatrics 115 (2005) 1513–1518.

[335] M. Durand, et al., Prospective evaluation of percutaneous central venous Silastic catheters in newborn infants with birth weights of 510 to 3, 920 grams, Pediatrics 78 (1986) 245.

[336] A. Lodha, et al., Prophylactic antibiotics in the prevention of catheter-associated bloodstream bacterial infection in preterm neonates: a systematic review, J. Perinatol. 28 (2008) 526–533.

[337] P.S. Spafford, et al., Prevention of central venous catheter-related coagulase-negative staphylococcal sepsis in neonates, J. Pediatr. 125 (1994) 259–263.

[338] R.W. Cooke, et al., Low-dose vancomycin prophylaxis reduces coagulase-negative staphylococcal bacteraemia in very low birthweight infants, J. Hosp. Infect. 37 (1997) 297–303.

[339] J.S. Garland, et al., A vancomycin-heparin lock solution for prevention of nosocomial bloodstream infection in critically ill neonates with peripherally inserted central venous catheters: a prospective, randomized trial, Pediatrics 116 (2005) e198–e205.

[340] L.A. Jardine, G.D. Inglis, M.W. Davies, Prophylactic systemic antibiotics to reduce morbidity and mortality in neonates with central venous catheters, Cochrane Database Syst. Rev. (2008) CD006179.

[341] D.K. Benjamin, et al., A blinded, randomized, multicenter study of an intravenous *Staphylococcus aureus* immune globulin, J. Perinatol. 26 (2006) 290–295.

[342] M. DeJonge, et al., Clinical trial of safety and efficacy of INH-A21 for the prevention of nosocomial staphylococcal bloodstream infection in premature infants, J. Pediatr. 151 (2007) 260–265.

[343] M.T. de la Morena, Specific immune globulin therapy for prevention of nosocomial staphylococcal bloodstream infection in premature infants: not what we hoped for!, J. Pediatr. 151 (2007) 232–234.

[344] L.E. Weisman, H.M. Thackray, J.A. Cracia-Prats, Phase I/II double blind, placebo controlled, dose escalation, safety and pharmacokinetics study in very low birth weight neonates of BSYX-a110, an anti-staphylococcal monoclonal antibody for the prevention of staphylococcal bloodstream infections, PAS Late-Breaker Abstract Presentations, San Francisco, 2004.

[345] N. Orsi, The antimicrobial activity of lactoferrin: current status and perspectives, Biometals 17 (2004) 189–196.

[346] P. Manzoni, et al., Bovine lactoferrin supplementation for prevention of late-onset sepsis in very-low-birth-weight neonates: a randomized trial, JAMA 302 (2009) 1421–1428.

Joanne E. Embree

CHAPTER OUTLINE

Epidemiology and Transmission   516
Microbiology   518
Pathogenesis   518
Pathology   519
Clinical Manifestations   519

Diagnosis   519
Differential Diagnosis   520
Treatment   520
Prognosis   521
Prevention   521

Infections of the fetus and newborn infant caused by *Neisseria gonorrhoeae* are restricted primarily to mucosal surfaces of the newborn infant. The most common condition related to infection by this organism during the neonatal period is ophthalmia neonatorum, or neonatal conjunctivitis. *N. gonorrhoeae* produces purulent conjunctivitis in the newborn that may lead to blindness if untreated. Ophthalmia neonatorum is the primary disease entity discussed in this chapter.

Ophthalmia neonatorum had been a well-recognized entity, affecting 1% to 15% of newborns, in Europe and North America when Hirschberg and Krause [1] first described neonatal infection caused by *N. gonorrhoeae* in an infant with purulent conjunctivitis in 1881. Shortly thereafter, the topical instillation of silver nitrate into the newborn's eyes immediately after birth dramatically reduced the incidence of this disease caused by *N. gonorrhoeae*, albeit with the complication in most infants of milder conjunctivitis, limited to the first 24 hours of life, owing to the silver nitrate itself [2,3]. Use of erythromycin or tetracycline ointments for this purpose has proved to be efficacious for preventing gonococcal ophthalmia, with markedly reduced problems related to the chemical conjunctivitis seen with silver nitrate [4–6]. Systemic neonatal infection is unusual, but infants may present with various clinical syndromes (in particular, arthritis), which implies that dissemination of the bacteria does occur [7,8].

Maternal systemic infection during pregnancy also is rare, and transplacental congenital infection of the fetus has not been described. Maternal genital mucosal infection may result in an ascending infection, however, with chorioamnionitis leading to premature rupture of the placental membranes and preterm delivery [9]. In developed countries, screening and treatment of pregnant women for gonococcal infections with tracing of named contacts, along with the use of neonatal ophthalmic prophylaxis, have substantially reduced the incidence of gonococcal ophthalmia neonatorum. In developing countries, improvements in access to medical care and aggressive pilot programs for prevention and treatment of sexually transmitted diseases (STDs) are additional public health measures of direct relevance. In conjunction with prevention strategies for human immunodeficiency virus (HIV)

infection and acquired immunodeficiency syndrome (AIDS), such programs have continued to decrease the incidence of gonococcal infection and its complications, such as ophthalmia neonatorum, in areas where these interventions have been introduced [10]. Despite the overall decreasing prevalence of *N. gonorrhoeae* infection worldwide, however, gonococcal ophthalmia neonatorum remains a significant illness.

EPIDEMIOLOGY AND TRANSMISSION

The incidence of neonatal gonococcal illness is related to the prevalence of *N. gonorrhoeae* colonization among women of childbearing age and to the rates of acute gonococcal infection during pregnancy. These numbers are quite variable worldwide and now are heavily influenced by the HIV-1 epidemic. Generally, when antibiotic treatment for gonorrhea became available in the mid-20th century, rates of infection among women decreased worldwide as these agents became more readily accessible and heath care programs improved. With the emergence of penicillin chromosomal resistance, the development of penicillinase production by some strains, and the expansion of the AIDS epidemic in the 1990s, however, rates began to increase again during that decade. In response, efforts to control this infection—which some authorities had hoped could ultimately be eliminated by the middle of the 21st century—have been increased.

Estimates by the World Health Organization of the burden of gonorrheal disease in various regions at the end of the 20th century are presented in Table 15–1 [11]. These estimates have not changed appreciably over the past decade, and although they are useful in indicating areas of high burden of disease, considerable variation within regions exists. This variation is reflected in the differences seen in the number of reported cases of gonorrhea among women in North America. In the United States during 2006, 358,366 cases of gonorrhea were tallied, resulting in a reported prevalence of 120.9 cases per 100,000 population, which was an increase of 5.5% over that reported in 2005 [12]. Previously, no significant changes had been noted in the prevalence rate among women in the United States during the past decade.

TABLE 15–1   World Health Organization Estimated Numbers of Cases of Gonorrhea in Adults, 1999

Geographic Location	Estimated No. Cases
North America	1.5 million
Latin America	7.5 million
Western Europe	1 million
Eastern Europe and Central Asia	3.5 million
East Asia	3 million
South and Southeast Asia	27 million
North Africa and the Middle East	1.5 million
Sub-Saharan Africa	17 million
New Zealand and Australia	120,000

Data from World Health Organization. Global prevalence and incidence of selected curable sexually transmitted infections: overview and estimates. WHO/CDS/CSR/EDC/2001 10:1–50, 2001.

The prevalence among women has equaled that among men since 1998. Infection rates have decreased since 1986, when the prevalence among women was approximately 310 cases per 100,000 population. Further significant differences are noted among specific populations in the United States, however, when rates are compared for groups of different races or ethnicity and for location. The prevalence among blacks in the United States is still considerably higher than in other ethnic groups—at around 720 per 100,000 in 2006. The background prevalence also differs significantly among various regions of the United States, with higher rates of reported infections in the South and Midwest compared with the Northeast and West.

The United States has set a goal of reducing the national prevalence of gonorrhea to less than 19 cases per 100,000 among adults; however, that goal is unlikely to be met. Canada has placed an emphasis on STD control as well, but has an exclusively publicly funded health care system. Gonorrhea prevalence rates have decreased from 1980, when the prevalence among women was 166 per 100,000 population. The highest rates at that time were among women 15 to 19 years old and 20 to 24 years old, which were extremely high at 510 and 598 per 100,000. In 2007, the prevalence among women was approximately 28.6 per 100,000, which represents a significant increase from 1997, when rates were a low of 11 per 100,000. The increase has occurred primarily among women 15 to 19 years old and 20 to 24 years old; in these age groups, rates increased from 69 and 60 per 100,000 in 1997 to 167 and 148 per 100,000. In 1997, Canada had set as its goal the elimination of endemic transmission of *N. gonorrhoeae* by 2010 [13]. Similar to the United States, Canada is not expected to meet its elimination goals. The reasons for the rate increases are complex, but a proportion of the increase is likely related to the almost universal change in diagnostic procedures in Canada from culture to nucleic acid–based testing which is considerably more sensitive.

Factors that increase a pregnant woman's risk of acquiring *N. gonorrhoeae* infection are similar to the factors that increase the risk of acquisition of any other sexually transmitted infection [14]. The prevalence of *N. gonorrhoeae* in

the population or network in which a woman socializes and chooses her sexual partners determines the likelihood of exposure to this pathogen. Women who have multiple sexual partners or whose partners have multiple sexual contacts increase their risk of exposure to *N. gonorrhoeae*. Women who do not use condoms or other barrier protection increase their risk of acquisition of *N. gonorrhoeae* infection on exposure to the organism. It is unknown whether women who are HIV-positive have an increased risk of infection by *N. gonorrhoeae* on exposure to it. Factors associated with an increased likelihood of at-risk behavior that results in an increased risk of gonococcal infection among pregnant women include younger age, unmarried status, homelessness, problems with drug or alcohol abuse, prostitution, low-income professions, and, in the United States, being black. Gonococcal infections are diagnosed more frequently in the summer months in the United States, probably reflecting transient changes in social behavior during vacations [15].

Varying gonococcal rates reported in various studies worldwide reflect the differences in risk among the populations studied. In a study in Brazil, involving a cross-sectional study of 200 women 14 to 29 years old who attended an HIV testing site in central Rio de Janeiro, the prevalence of gonorrhea was high at 9.5%. Of the 200 women surveyed, 8% were HIV-infected, confirming that the population studied had a high risk of STD exposure [16]. The prevalence of gonorrhea among 547 pregnant women attending a first-visit antenatal hospital clinic during 1999 and 2000 in Vila, Vanuatu, was 5.9%, but no women were found to be HIV-infected at that time [17]. The occurrence rates of gonorrhea were quite high among this population, reflecting the prevalence in the general population. A study in Thailand in 1996 that investigated the prevalence of STDs among pregnant women, where case reporting suggested a marked decrease in STDs after a campaign promoting condom use during commercial sex, showed that the prevalence of gonorrhea was extremely low at 0.2% [18]. By contrast, in a population in Nairobi, where condom use was advocated for commercial sex workers but not promoted to the same extent as in Thailand and not routinely practiced by the at-risk general population, in a cross-sectional study of 520 women seeking treatment at an STD clinic, 4% were infected with gonorrhea, and 29% were HIV-positive [19]. In Nigeria, where the prevalence of HIV infection is low, the rate of gonorrhea also is lower among pregnant women. In a cross-sectional study, 230 pregnant women attending the antenatal clinic of a teaching hospital in Nigeria from January 2000 to December 2000 were screened randomly to determine the prevalence of common STDs; 1.3% were found to have gonorrhea [20].

N. gonorrhoeae usually is transmitted from the infected maternal cervix during vaginal delivery. Ascending infection does occur, however, in the instance of prolonged rupture of the membranes and has been observed after cesarean delivery following ruptured membranes [21–24]. It has been estimated that colonization and infection of the neonate occur in only one third of instances in which the mother is infected [25]. The infant's mucous membranes become colonized on swallowing contaminated fluid during labor and delivery.

In instances of congenital infection, it is speculated that the chorioamnion is infected through an ascending infection [26]. Premature rupture of membranes then occurs, with early onset of labor and premature delivery or septic abortion [9,27–29]. This association was dramatically shown in one study in which premature rupture of membranes occurred in 6 (43%) of 14 women with untreated gonococcal infection during pregnancy compared with 4 (3%) of 144 women whose infection had been treated [29]. Screening and treatment programs for gonococcal infections during pregnancy are appropriate to reduce the risk of adverse pregnancy outcomes related to maternal infection.

MICROBIOLOGY

N. gonorrhoeae is a gram-negative diplococcus. It uses glucose for growth, but not maltose, sucrose, or lactose. This is one of the characteristics used to distinguish *N. gonorrhoeae* isolates from *Neisseria meningitidis* and other colonizing *Neisseria* species, such as *Neisseria cinerea*, *Neisseria flava*, *Neisseria subflava*, *Neisseria lactamica*, *Neisseria mucosa*, and *Neisseria sicca*. *N. gonorrhoeae* produces acid only when grown in glucose. In addition, the organism is oxidase positive, hydroxyprolyl aminopeptidase positive, nitrate negative, DNase negative, catalase positive, strongly superoxol positive, and colistin resistant [30]. *N. gonorrhoeae* is an obligate aerobe, but lacks superoxide dismutase, which moderates the effects of oxygen radicals in most other aerobic bacteria. When grown in anaerobic conditions, virulent strains express a lipoprotein called Pan 1. Its function is unknown, but it elicits an IgM antibody response in acute infection.

When cultured in the laboratory, *N. gonorrhoeae* forms four different colony types. Pinpoint colonies, classified as type 1 and type 2, usually are seen only on primary isolation. These colony types are distinguished from the large granular colonies classified as type 3 and type 4 by the presence of pili, which are thin bacterial appendages on the cell surface that are involved in attachment to mammalian cells. *N. gonorrhoeae* has the genetic capacity to turn on and turn off the expression of pili [31]. With repeated subculturing at 37 ° C, the genes are no longer expressed, and the pili disappear, resulting in colonial-type changes, with type 1 colonies shifting to type 4 and type 2 colonies shifting to type 3. Associated with this change is a reduction in virulence [32]. *N. gonorrhoeae* also may form colonies that are either opaque or clear. This characteristic is related to the presence of a specific surface protein called outer membrane protein II. Transparent colonies lack outer membrane protein II and are more resistant to phagocytosis. Individual strains can also phase shift from forming opaque to forming clear colonies [33].

Colonial morphology is of no use in differentiating gonococcal types or strains. Strains can be differentiated by auxotyping. Different strains have differing stable auxotrophic requirements for amino acids, purines, pyrimidines, or vitamins. Typing based on these requirements has been useful in some epidemiologic surveys. Additionally, enzyme-linked immunosorbent typing, based on differences in protein I, can be done. Nine distinct strains are detectable with this typing system. It is clinically relevant in that type 1 and type 2 strains are more likely to disseminate in adult patients. Use of serologic typing schemes can detect three serogroups: WI, WII, and WIII. Strains 1 to 3 are usually found in serogroup WI, strains 4 to 8 are found in serogroup WII, and strain 9 is found in serogroup WIII [34]. Finally, strains also are typed by coagulation testing after exposure to monoclonal antibodies made against the outer membrane protein I. Two major serogroups exist: 1A, which has 26 subgroups, and 1B, which has 32 subgroups [35]. The combination of auxotyping and serologic typing is now used in most epidemiologic studies to determine the linkages among infected persons [36].

PATHOGENESIS

To produce infection, *N. gonorrhoeae* first attaches to epithelial cells, penetrates into them, and then destroys the infected cells. Attachment to epithelial cells is related to the presence of pili and the outer membrane protein II [37]. Penetration of the gonococcus into cells occurs through either phagocytosis or endocytosis [38–40]. Several bacteria usually are found within each infected cell, but whether this represents invasion of the cell by multiple organisms or growth and multiplication of organisms within the infected cell is unknown. Gonococci possess a cytotoxic lipopolysaccharide and produce proteases, phospholipases, and elastases that ultimately destroy the infected cells. Some strains of gonococci seem to be relatively less susceptible to phagocytosis and are thought to be more capable of causing disseminated infection. Gonococci are found in the subepithelial connective tissue very quickly after infection. This dissemination may be due to the disruption of the integrity of the epidermal surface with cell death, or the gonococci may migrate into this area by moving between cells. Epithelial cell death triggers a vigorous inflammatory response, initially with neutrophils and then macrophages and lymphocytes in untreated patients.

Human serum contains IgM antibody directed against lipopolysaccharide antigens on the gonococcus, which inhibits invasion. An IgG antibody against a surface protein antigen also is normally present on some gonococci that are classified as serum-resistant gonococci; this antibody blocks the bactericidal action of the antilipopolysaccharide IgM antibody [41,42]. These serum-resistant strains are the most common ones involved in systemic infections in adults and probably in neonates as well [43]. Infants' sera, in which maternal IgM antibody is absent, do not show serum bactericidal activity against *N. gonorrhoeae* [44]; in theory, infants should be highly susceptible to invasive infection. Because such infection does not occur frequently, additional protective factors must function to prevent it.

N. gonorrhoeae produces an IgA1 protease, which inactivates secretory IgA by cleaving it at the hinge region. This inactivation facilitates mucosal colonization and probably plays a role in the poor mucosal protection seen against subsequent gonococcal reinfection. IgA1 protease is also a proinflammatory factor and can trigger the release of proinflammatory cytokines from human monocytic subpopulations and a dose-dependent T helper type 1 T-cell response [45]. Although symptomatic gonococcal infection stimulates a brisk inflammatory response, it does not produce a significant immunologic response [46]. There is very little immunologic memory; as a result, recurrent infections occur easily on reexposure. Epidemiologic evidence suggests that at least partial protection is obtained against subsequent infection with the same serotype [47]. Generally, antibody responses are modest after initial infection, however, and no evidence of a boosting effect has been found when antibody levels are studied in response to subsequent infections. Also, adults with mucosal gonococcal infections have a discernible decreased CD4$^+$ count, which recovers with treatment or clearance of the infection.

It has been speculated that the gonococci actually have a suppressive effect on the host immune response. In support of this theory, *N. gonorrhoeae* Opa proteins more recently were shown to be able to bind CEACAM1 expressed by primary CD4$^+$ T lymphocytes and to suppress their activation and proliferation [48]. This immunosuppressive effect may have significant consequences in populations with coexisting epidemics of gonorrhea and HIV/AIDS. In a study of prostitutes in Nairobi, the presence of gonococcal cervicitis was shown to reduce interferon-γ production by HIV-1 epitope–specific CD8$^+$ T-lymphocyte populations, showing a deleterious effect of gonococcal cervicitis on HIV-1 immune control and susceptibility [49].

Because only approximately one third of neonates exposed to *N. gonorrhoeae* during vaginal delivery become colonized and infected, additional protective innate factors are in effect. Significant antibacterial polypeptide activity has been shown in human amniotic fluid and within the vernix caseosa [50,51]. The presence of numerous antibacterial polypeptides in the vernix may be important for surface defense against gonococcal infection, but specific studies have not yet been done.

Antibiotic resistance to penicillin, tetracycline, quinolones, and spectinomycin has become problematic in many regions [52]. Penicillin resistance can be a result of either alterations in the penicillin-binding protein or the production of penicillinase [53–55]. By 1991, 11% of all strains of *N. gonorrhoeae* in the United States were penicillinase-producing, and 32% of all strains were resistant to at least one antimicrobial agent. As a result, penicillin is no longer recommended for primary therapy for gonococcal disease in the United States and in other regions where these strains are commonly found.

PATHOLOGY

In most affected infants, gonococcal disease manifests as infection of mucosal membranes. The eye is most frequently involved, but funisitis and infant vaginitis, rhinitis, and urethritis also have been observed [56–59]. Primary mucosal infection by *N. gonorrhoeae* involves the columnar and transitional epithelia. When pharyngeal colonization is looked for, it is found in 35% of ophthalmia neonatorum cases [60]. Systemic infection is rarely observed among neonates, but cases of meningitis and arthritis have been described [7,8,61–68]. Gonococcal scalp abscesses attributed to intrauterine fetal monitoring,

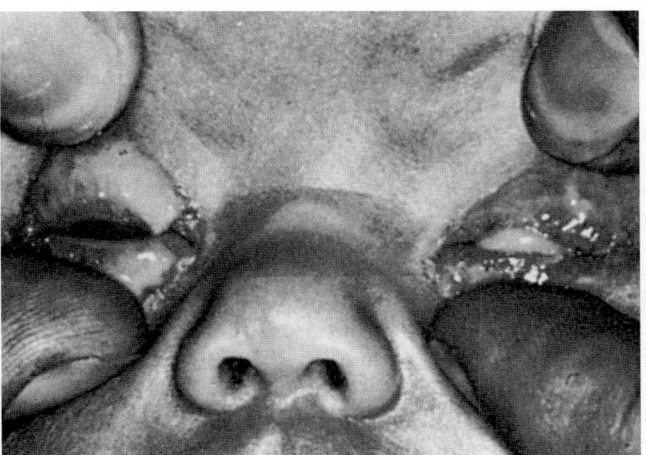

FIGURE 15–1 **Bilateral acute gonococcal ophthalmia neonatorum.** Appearance after inappropriate topical therapy for 2 weeks with neomycin–polymyxin B–bacitracin (Neosporin), sulfonamide, and chloramphenicol ophthalmic ointments.

omphalitis, and gingival abscess also have been reported [69–75]. One case of gonococcal ventriculitis has been reported in an infant who received a ventriculoamniotic shunt in utero [76].

CLINICAL MANIFESTATIONS

Ophthalmia neonatorum caused by *N. gonorrhoeae* is classically an acute purulent conjunctivitis that appears 2 to 5 days after birth. Occasionally, the initial presentation is more subacute, or the onset may be delayed beyond 5 days of life [77,78]. Asymptomatic colonization has been documented [79]. Infants who become infected in utero may have symptoms at or shortly after birth [21,22,77]. Typically, early in the illness, tense edema of both lids develops, followed by profuse purulent conjunctival exudates (Fig. 15–1). If treatment is delayed, the infection progresses beyond the superficial epithelial layers of the eye to involve the subconjunctival connective tissue of the palpebral conjunctivae and the cornea. Infection of the cornea can lead to ulcerations, perforation, or rarely panophthalmitis. In some instances, it may result in loss of the eye [80]. Neonatal sepsis, arthritis, and skin abscesses caused by *N. gonorrhoeae* are not clinically distinguishable from conditions caused by other bacterial pathogens more commonly associated with these syndromes in this age group.

DIAGNOSIS

Clinicians should suspect gonococcal ophthalmia neonatorum in an infant in whom purulent conjunctivitis develops during the first week of life or if what was thought to be chemical conjunctivitis is prolonged beyond 24 to 48 hours. Gram stain of the exudate usually reveals the gram-negative intracellular bean-shaped diplococci typical of *N. gonorrhoeae*, which provide a presumptive diagnosis. Other *Neisseria* species—in particular, *N. meningitidis*—cannot be distinguished from the gonococcus by Gram stain appearance. *N. gonorrhoeae* must be isolated and tested for antibiotic susceptibility before a definitive diagnosis is made. A definitive diagnosis is important because of the public health and social consequences of the diagnosis of gonorrhea in an infant. If gonococcal ophthalmia neonatorum is suspected on the basis of the Gram stain appearance, cultures should be obtained from additional mucosal sites in the infant. The mother and her sexual partner or partners also should be tested for gonorrhea. Additional testing of the infant, mother, and sexual partners for other sexually transmitted infections, including HIV infection, is strongly recommended [81,82].

Isolation of *N. gonorrhoeae* from the exudate by culture is the diagnostic gold standard. Samples of the exudate should be collected by swabbing and should be inoculated directly onto blood agar, MacConkey's agar, and chocolate agar or chocolate-inhibitory media. The inhibitory medium should be placed in a commercial carbon dioxide incubator or candle jar to provide an adequate concentration of carbon dioxide and should be incubated at 36° C. Cultures are examined daily for the presence of typical colonies. Colonies resembling *N. gonorrhoeae* are identified further by Gram stain, by a positive oxidase test, and by use of glucose, but not maltose, sucrose, or lactose. Antibiotic sensitivity and penicillinase production should be tested.

Further testing to confirm the identification of the isolate may be done in a reference laboratory if desired. DNA-based and polymerase chain reaction–based technologies have replaced gonococcal cultures in many laboratories [81–85]. These assays have a high degree of sensitivity and detect more true cases of gonorrheal infection in adults than can be achieved by current culture methods. When correctly used, they also are very specific. Their suitability for diagnosis of gonorrheal infections in children without the additional use of culture methods, with the associated legal implications in older children, has not been extensively studied, however. Additionally, extensive use of these methods for primary diagnosis impairs the tracking of antimicrobial resistance patterns.

If gonococcal ophthalmia neonatorum is presumptively or definitively diagnosed, testing also should be conducted for other sexually transmitted pathogens, in particular, *Chlamydia trachomatis* because the two organisms frequently are found to coinfect pregnant women [86]. Also, the diagnosis of gonococccal infection in the neonate should trigger an investigation of the infant's mother and her sexual partner or partners for STDs.

DIFFERENTIAL DIAGNOSIS

At the present time, *N. gonorrhoeae* causes less than 1% of cases of ophthalmia neonatorum in North America, western Europe, Australia, and New Zealand and in areas and communities elsewhere where there is access to prenatal care and STD prevention programs. In other areas, the risk of gonococcal ophthalmia is higher depending on the prevalence of gonococcal infection among the pregnant women in the population. Even in areas with high prevalence rates, however, ophthalmia caused by *N. gonorrhoeae* accounts for less than 5% of cases of neonatal conjunctivitis. Other organisms that can produce conjunctivitis in the newborn period and the relative overall frequency of

TABLE 15–2   Differential Diagnosis of Ophthalmia Neonatorum

Etiologic Condition/Agent	Percentage of Cases	Relative Severity	Usual Time of Onset after Delivery
Chemical conjunctivitis	Dependent on use	+	6-24 hr
Neisseria gonorrhoeae	<1	+++	2-5 days
Neisseria meningitidis	<1	++	2 days–2 wk
Neisseria cinerea	<1	+	2 days–2 wk
Herpes simplex virus	<1	++	2-14 days
Chlamydia trachomatis	2-40	+	5 days–2 wk
Other bacteria	30-50	++	2 days–2 wk
Group A and B streptococci			
Staphylococcus aureus			
Haemophilus species			
Klebsiella pneumoniae			
Escherichia coli			
Pseudomonas aeruginosa			
Enterococcus			
Pneumococcus			

resultant infections, the usual time of presentation since birth relative severity, and are shown in Table 15–2.

Generally, conjunctivitis seen within 24 hours of birth usually is assumed to be a reaction to silver nitrate, if this has been used for prophylaxis. As described previously, however, in the instance of prolonged rupture of membranes and premature delivery, symptomatic gonococcal ophthalmia may be observed during this period as well. Also, some infants have a less acute course, with appearance of symptoms after 5 days of age. Reliance on the timing between 2 and 5 days after delivery of the onset of symptoms may be an unreliable clinically distinguishing feature. The possibility of gonococcal infection should be considered in every neonate with conjunctivitis present after 24 hours of birth, and appropriate diagnostic testing to detect the organism should be done. In some instances, neonates with gonococcal ophthalmia neonatorum may be infected by additional pathogens, in particular, *C. trachomatis*. The differential diagnosis of cutaneous or systemic gonococcal infection of the neonate includes the bacterial or fungal pathogens that are frequently involved in these types of infections during this time period and are discussed in more detail in Chapters 6, 10, 33, and 34.

TREATMENT

The principles of management of STDs in any age group apply when a neonate is determined to have a suspected or confirmed gonococcal infection. As stated previously, investigation and treatment of the mother and her sexual contacts for *N. gonorrhoeae* are essential, as is the investigation of the infant, the mother, and her sexual contacts for other sexually transmitted infections. STDs are like wolves—they travel in packs.

TABLE 15–3 Recommended Treatment for Neonatal Gonococcal Infections

Condition	Recommended Therapy
Ophthalmia neonatorum	Ceftriaxone 25-50 mg/kg IV or IM in a single dose, not to exceed 125 mg; topical antibiotic therapy alone is inadequate and is unnecessary if systemic treatment is administered
Gonococcal meningitis, arthritis, or scalp lesions	Ceftriaxone 25-50 mg/kg/day IV or IM in a single daily dose for 7 days *or* cefotaxime 25 mg/kg IV or IM every 12 hours for 7 days, with a duration of 10-14 days if meningitis is documented or 14 days if arthritis is documented
Known exposure at birth but asymptomatic	Ceftriaxone 25-50 mg/kg IV or IM in a single dose, not to exceed 125 mg

IM, intramuscularly; IV, intravenously.

As discussed previously, because a significant proportion of gonococci worldwide is resistant to penicillin, either by decreased penicillin binding or by penicillinase production, this antibiotic is no longer recommended for therapy, unless the infecting isolate has been tested and found to be sensitive. Most recommendations and guidelines for the treatment of gonococcal ophthalmia neonatorum identify ceftriaxone as the agent of choice (Table 15–3) [81,82]. Regimens using this drug have been studied and shown to be effective [87–89]. Kanamycin is an alternative, but is not as effective, with a failure rate of approximately 5% [90]. Ceftriaxone should be administered cautiously to infants with hyperbilirubinemia, especially infants born prematurely. Infants who have gonococcal ophthalmia should be hospitalized and evaluated for signs of disseminated infection (e.g., sepsis, arthritis, meningitis). One dose of ceftriaxone is adequate therapy for gonococcal conjunctivitis. Disseminated infection in the neonate should be treated in consultation with an expert in infectious diseases. Infants born to mothers who have documented untreated infection are at high risk of acquiring *N. gonorrhoeae*. If the membranes have been ruptured, if the infant is premature, or if close follow-up cannot be ensured, treatment for ophthalmia neonatorum, rather than use of eye prophylaxis, is recommended.

PROGNOSIS

With early recognition and appropriate treatment, cure rates for gonococcal ophthalmia and other neonatal manifestations of gonococcal infection in the newborn are close to 100%. By contrast, permanent corneal damage after gonococcal ophthalmia neonatorum was the usual clinical outcome in the preantibiotic era.

PREVENTION

Prevention of gonococcal infection of the fetus and neonate is best done by preventing gonococcal infection of the mother. One way to accomplish this goal is by the reduction of the prevalence of *N. gonorrhoeae* in the core high-risk populations that serve as its reservoir for pregnant women. Targeted treatment and prevention campaigns among commercial sex workers, sexually active adolescents and young adults who have multiple partners, and groups with other risk factors that result in increased high-risk sexual activity such as individuals with street drug and alcohol abuse problems and homosexual men who have multiple contacts would reduce the prevalence in the general population. Education of youth before sexual maturity about the risks of STDs and about ways in which they can protect themselves from acquiring these diseases does not increase the rates of sexual activity among adolescents and should be encouraged as a joint responsibility of parents or primary care providers and the schools. Provision of accessible health care with readily available antibiotics that are appropriate and effective against circulating strains of *N. gonorrhoeae* also is imperative for this purpose. Finally, to support optimal health behaviors, persons of all ages need to be able to feel confident that they will not be stigmatized for seeking health care for an STD.

Because infection with *N. gonorrhoeae* during pregnancy may result in adverse pregnancy outcomes, such as premature rupture of membranes and preterm delivery, screening of pregnant women for infection in early pregnancy is advisable. Women identified as having gonococcal infection should receive prompt treatment [81,82]. Recommended treatment includes the use of cefixime, 400 mg orally, in a single dose if available, or ceftriaxone, 125 mg intramuscularly in a single dose. Women for whom a third-generation cephalosporin is contraindicated should receive spectinomycin, 2 g intramuscularly as a single dose. Either erythromycin or amoxicillin is recommended for treatment of presumptive or diagnosed coinfection with *C. trachomatis*. Follow-up cultures to ensure eradication of the infection are imperative.

Testing for other STDs should be done, and the mother should be offered HIV testing. In addition, counseling related to avoidance of further infection is an important component of management. Tracing and treatment of sexual contacts are necessary to reduce the risk of subsequent infection. In one study in Louisiana of 751 pregnant women whose charts were reviewed retrospectively, 5.1% were diagnosed with gonorrhea at the first prenatal visit, and 2.5% acquired the infection during their pregnancy [91]. Women whose sexual behavior or social circumstances place them at risk of acquiring sexually transmitted infection during pregnancy should be retested for gonorrhea (and other STDs) in the third trimester. Retesting is most conveniently done at the time of screening for group B streptococci.

Since the late 1800s, eye prophylaxis has been the hallmark of prevention of gonococcal ophthalmia neonatorum. Currently, many jurisdictions mandate the use of ocular prophylaxis for newborns through legislation. Most others recommend and encourage its use. The issue is controversial in areas of low prevalence of *N. gonorrhoeae* infection and among populations with extremely low risk of the disease. In these situations, the concerns regarding the complications of the use of the prophylactic agents must be balanced against the actual risk of the disease and the ability, or the wish, to provide an alternative management approach involving close observation of the infant with early therapy if necessary.

At the present time, data from clinical trials support the use of 1% silver nitrate, 0.5% erythromycin, 1% tetracycline, or 2.5% povidone-iodine for prophylaxis against gonococcal ophthalmia neonatorum [4–6,81,82,92–96]. All of these agents are less effective against chlamydial conjunctivitis, however, and to date, there is no truly effective ocular agent to prevent this infection. Most agents are well tolerated, although a chemical conjunctivitis commonly is seen after instillation of silver nitrate. This reaction involves epithelial desquamation and a polymorphonuclear leukocytic exudate [97] and usually appears within 6 to 8 hours and disappears within 24 to 48 hours. A mild chemical conjunctivitis may be seen in 10% to 20% of infants who received povidone-iodine prophylaxis as well. Use of antibiotic agents has the potential to lead to increased antibiotic resistance in other colonizing bacteria, which could lead to outbreaks of infection in the nursery [98].

Failure of prophylaxis can occur. If the illness is established by the time of delivery, ocular prophylaxis is ineffective. Irrigation of the eyes with saline too soon after the application of silver nitrate has been suggested by some experts to be the cause of such failure. In extremely rare instances, infection may be acquired after prophylaxis had been provided. Occasionally, the erythromycin eye ointment may not have penetrated to the eye itself as a result of difficulties in keeping the infant's eye exposed during application of the ointment.

At the present time, specific prophylaxis given immediately (minimum delay of 1 hour) after birth, using any of the following regimens, is recommended by most professional societies and government bodies: (1) 1% silver nitrate in single-dose ampules, (2) 0.5% erythromycin ophthalmic ointment in single-use tubes, or (3) 1% tetracycline ophthalmic ointment in single-use tubes. Povidone-iodine also is a safe and effective alternative in resource-poor countries.

REFERENCES

[1] J. Hirschberg, F. Krause, Zentralbl. Prakt. Augen. 5 (1881) 39.
[2] L. Howe, Credé's method for prevention of purulent ophthalmia in infancy in public institutions, Trans. Am. Ophthalmol. Soc. 8 (1897) 52–57.
[3] G. Forbes, G.M. Forbes, Silver nitrate and the eyes of the newborn, Am. J. Dis. Child. 121 (1971) 1–3.
[4] M. Laga, et al., Prophylaxis of gonococcal and chlamydial ophthalmia neonatorum: a comparison of silver nitrate and tetracycline, N. Engl. J. Med. 17 (1988) 653–657.
[5] M.R. Hammerschlag, et al., Efficacy of neonatal ocular prophylaxis for the prevention of chlamydial and gonococcal conjunctivitis, N. Engl. J. Med. 320 (1989) 769–772.
[6] J.Y. Chen, Prophylaxis of ophthalmia neonatorum: comparison of silver nitrate, tetracycline, erythromycin and no prophylaxis, Pediatr. Infect. Dis. J. 11 (1992) 1026–1030.
[7] D.P. Kohen, Neonatal gonococcal arthritis: three cases and review of the literature, Pediatrics 53 (1974) 436–440.
[8] F.E. Babl, et al., Neonatal gonococcal arthritis after negative prenatal screening and despite conjunctival prophylaxis, Pediatr. Infect. Dis. J. 19 (2000) 346–349.
[9] B. Elliott, et al., Maternal gonococcal infection as a preventable risk factor for low birth weight, J. Infect. Dis. 161 (1990) 531–553.
[10] S. Moses, et al., Response of a sexually transmitted infection epidemic to a treatment and prevention programme in Nairobi, Kenya, Sex. Transm. Infect. 78 (2002) 114–120.
[11] World Health Organization, Global prevalence and incidence of selected curable sexually transmitted infections: overview and estimates, WHO/CDS/CSR/EDC/2001 10 (2001) 1–50.
[12] CDC, Sexually Transmitted Disease Surveillance 2006 Supplement. Gonococcal Isolate Surveillance Project (GISP) Annual Report 2006, U.S. Department of Health and Human Services, Atlanta, GA, 2008.
[13] A Brief Report on Sexually Transmitted Diseases in Canada, (2007) http://www.phac-aspc.gc.ca/publicat/sti-its/index-eng.php.
[14] J.D. Klausner, et al., Risk factors for repeated gonococcal infections: San Francisco, 1990–1992, J. Infect. Dis. 177 (1998) 1766–1769.
[15] C.E. Cornelius III, Seasonality of gonorrhea in the United States, HSMHA Health Rep. 86 (1971) 157–160.
[16] R.L. Cook, et al., High prevalence of sexually transmitted diseases in young women seeking HIV testing in Rio de Janeiro, Brazil, Sex. Transm. Dis. 31 (2004) 67–72.
[17] E.A. Sullivan, et al., Prevalence of sexually transmitted infections among antenatal women in Vanuatu, 1999–2000, Sex. Transm. Dis. 30 (2003) 362–366.
[18] P.H. Kilmarx, et al., Rapid assessment of sexually transmitted diseases in a sentinel population in Thailand: prevalence of chlamydial infection, gonorrhoea, and syphilis among pregnant women—1996, Sex. Transm. Infect. 74 (1998) 189–193.
[19] K. Fonck, et al., Pattern of sexually transmitted diseases and risk factors among women attending an STD referral clinic in Nairobi, Kenya, Sex. Transm. Dis. 27 (2000) 417–423.
[20] A.P. Aboyeji, C. Nwabuisi, Prevalence of sexually transmitted diseases among pregnant women in Ilorin, Nigeria, J. Obstet. Gynecol. 23 (2003) 637–639.
[21] T.R. Thompson, R.E. Swanson, P.J. Wiesner, Gonococcal ophthalmia neonatorum: relationship of time of infection to relevant control measures, JAMA 228 (1974) 186–188.
[22] B. Diener, Cesarean section complicated by gonococcal ophthalmia neonatorum, J. Fam. Pract. 13 (1981) 739–744.
[23] C.W. Nickerson, Gonorrhea amnionitis, Obstet. Gynecol. 48 (1973) 815–817.
[24] E. Varady, H. Nsanze, T. Slattery, Gonococcal scalp abscess in a neonate delivered by caesarean section, Sex. Transm. Infect. 74 (1998) 451.
[25] R. Rothenberg, Ophthalmic neonatorum due to Neisseria gonorrhoeae: prevention and treatment, Sex. Transm. Dis. 6 (1979) 187–191.
[26] M.J. Rothbard, T. Gregory, L.J. Salerno, Intrapartum gonococcal amnionitis, Am. J. Obstet. Gynecol. 121 (1975) 565–566.
[27] P.M. Sarrell, K.A. Pruett, Symptomatic gonorrhea during pregnancy, Obstet. Gynecol. 32 (1968) 670–673.
[28] M.S. Amstey, K.T. Steadman, Symptomatic gonorrhea and pregnancy, J. Am. Vener. Dis. Assoc. 3 (1976) 14–16.
[29] A.G. Charles, et al., Asymptomatic gonorrhea in prenatal patients, Am. J. Obstet. Gynecol. 108 (1970) 595–599.
[30] H.H. Handsfield, P.F. Sparling, Neisseria gonorrhoeae, in: G.L. Mandell, J.E. Bennett, R. Dolin (Eds.), Principles and Practice of Infectious Diseases, fourth ed., Churchill Livingstone, New York, 1995, pp. 1909–1926.
[31] E. Juni, G.A. Heym, Simple method for distinguishing gonococcal colony types, J. Clin. Microbiol. 6 (1977) 511–517.
[32] J. Swanson, Studies on gonococcus infection, IV. Pili: their role in attachment of gonococci to tissue culture cells, J. Exp. Med. 137 (1973) 571–589.
[33] P.F. Sparling, J.G. Cannon, M. So, Phase and antigenic variation of pili and outer membrane protein II of Neisseria gonorrhoeae, J. Infect. Dis. 153 (1986) 196–201.
[34] E.G. Sandstrom, S. Bygdeman, Serological classification of Neisseria gonorrhoeae: clinical and epidemiological applications, in: J.T. Poolman (Ed.), Gonococci and Meningococci, Kluwer Academic Publishers, Dordrecht, The Netherlands, 1986, pp. 45–50.
[35] J.S. Knapp, et al., Serological classification of Neisseria gonorrhoeae with use of monoclonal antibodies to gonococcal outer membrane protein I, J. Infect. Dis. 150 (1984) 44–48.
[36] H.H. Handsfield, et al., Epidemiology of penicillinase-producing Neisseria gonorrhoeae infections: analysis by auxotyping and serogrouping, N. Engl. J. Med. 306 (1982) 950–954.
[37] D. Bessen, E.C. Gotschlich, Interactions of gonococci with HeLa cells: attachment, detachment, replication, penetration, and the role of protein II, Infect. Immun. 54 (1986) 154–160.
[38] M.E. Ward, P.J. Watt, Adherence of Neisseria gonorrhoeae to urethral mucosal cells: an electron microscopic study of human gonorrhea, J. Infect. Dis. 126 (1972) 601–605.
[39] Z.A. McGee, A.P. Jolinson, D. Taylor-Robinson, Pathogenic mechanisms of Neisseria gonorrhoeae: observations on damage to human fallopian tubes in organ culture by gonococci of colony type 1 and type 4, J. Infect. Dis. 143 (1981) 413–422.
[40] M.E. Ward, A.A. Glynn, P.J. Watt, The fate of gonococci in polymorphonuclear leukocytes: an electron microscopic study of the natural disease, Br. J. Exp. Pathol. 53 (1972) 289–294.
[41] P.A. Rice, D.L. Kasper, Characterization of serum resistance of gonococci that disseminate, J. Clin. Invest. 70 (1982) 157–167.
[42] K.A. Joiner, et al., Mechanism of action of blocking immunoglobulin G for Neisseria gonorrhoeae, J. Clin. Invest. 76 (1985) 1765–1772.
[43] G.K. Schoolnik, T.M. Buchanan, K.K. Holmes, Gonococci causing disseminated gonococcal infection are resistant to the bactericidal action of normal human sera, J. Clin. Invest. 58 (1976) 1163–1173.
[44] G.K. Schoolnik, H.D. Ochs, T.M. Buchanan, Immunoglobulin class responsible for bactericidal activity of normal human sera, J. Immunol. 122 (1979) 1771–1779.
[45] A. Tsirpouchtsidis, et al., Neisserial immunoglobulin A1 protease induces specific T-cell responses in humans, Infect. Immunol. 70 (2002) 335–344.

[46] S.R. Hedges, et al., Limited local and systemic antibody responses to *Neisseria gonorrhoeae* during uncomplicated genital infections, Infect. Immun. 67 (1999) 3937–3946.

[47] T.M. Buchanan, et al., Gonococcal salpingitis is less likely to recur with *Neisseria gonorrhoeae* of the same principal outer membrane protein (POMP) antigenic type, Am. J. Obstet. Gynecol. 135 (1980) 978–980.

[48] I.C. Boulton, S.D. Gray-Owen, Neisserial binding to CEACAM1 arrests the activation and proliferation of CD4+ T lymphocytes, Nat. Immunol. 3 (2002) 229–236.

[49] R. Kaul, et al., Gonococcal cervicitis is associated with reduced systemic CD8+ T cell responses in human immunodeficiency virus type-1-infected and exposed, uninfected sex workers, J. Infect. Dis. 185 (2002) 1525–1529.

[50] H. Yoshio, et al., Antimicrobial polypeptides of human vernix caseosa and amniotic fluid: implications for newborn innate defense, Pediatr. Res. 53 (2003) 211–216.

[51] G. Marchini, et al., The newborn infant is protected by an innate antimicrobial barrier: peptide antibiotics are present in the skin and vernix caseosa, Br. J. Dermatol. 147 (2002) 127–134.

[52] T.J. Dougherty, Genetic analysis and penicillin-binding protein alterations in *Neisseria gonorrhoeae* with chromosomally mediated resistance, Antimicrob. Agents Chemother. 30 (1986) 649–652.

[53] T. Thirumoorthy, V.S. Rajan, C.L. Goh, Penicillinase-producing *Neisseria gonorrhoeae* ophthalmia neonatorum in Singapore, Br. J. Vener. Dis. 58 (1982) 308–310.

[54] R. Pang, et al., Gonococcal ophthalmia neonatorum caused by beta-lactamase-producing *Neisseria gonorrhoeae*, BMJ 1 (1979) 380.

[55] B. Doraiswamy, et al., Ophthalmia neonatorum caused by β-lactamase-producing *Neisseria gonorrhoeae*, JAMA 250 (1983) 790–791.

[56] G.W. Hunter, N.D. Fargo, Specific urethritis (gonorrhea) in a male newborn, Am. J. Obstet. Gynecol. 38 (1939) 520–521.

[57] A.R. Stark, M.P. Glode, Gonococcal vaginitis in a neonate, J. Pediatr. 94 (1979) 298–299.

[58] L.L. Barton, M. Shuja, Neonatal gonococcal vaginitis, J. Pediatr. 98 (1981) 171–172.

[59] H. Kirkland, R.V. Storer, Gonococcal rhinitis in an infant, BMJ 1 (1931) 263–267.

[60] L. Fransen, et al., Ophthalmia neonatorum in Nairobi, Kenya: the roles of *Neisseria gonorrhoeae* and *Chlamydia trachomatis*, J. Infect. Dis. 153 (1986) 862–869.

[61] W.L. Bradford, H.W. Kelley, Gonococcal meningitis in a newborn infant, Am. J. Dis. Child. 46 (1933) 543–549.

[62] L.E. Holt, Gonococcus infections in children with especial reference to their prevalence in institutions and means of prevention, N. Y. Med. J. 81 (1905) 521–527.

[63] M.B. Cooperman, Gonococcus arthritis in infancy, Am. J. Dis. Child. 33 (1927) 932–948.

[64] P.P. Parrish, W.A. Console, J. Battaglia, Gonococcic arthritis of a newborn treated with sulfonamide, JAMA 114 (1940) 241–242.

[65] J.B. Jones, R.C. Ramsey, Acute suppurative arthritis of hip in children, U. S. Armed Forces Med. J. 7 (1956) 1621–1628.

[66] E.E. Soonzilli, J.J. Calabro, Gonococcal arthritis in the newborn, JAMA 177 (1961) 919–921.

[67] S. Glaser, B. Boxerbaum, J.H. Kennell, Gonococcal arthritis in the newborn, Am. J. Dis. Child. 112 (1966) 185–188.

[68] J.E. Gregory, J.L. Chisom, A.T. Meadows, Gonococcal arthritis in an infant, Br. J. Vener. Dis. 48 (1972) 306–307.

[69] M.B. Kleiman, G.A. Lamb, Gonococcal arthritis in a newborn infant, Pediatrics 52 (1973) 285–287.

[70] A. D'Auria, et al., Gonococcal scalp wound infection, MMWR Morb. Mortal. Wkly Rep. 24 (1975) 115–116.

[71] H. Thadepalli, et al., Gonococcal sepsis secondary to fetal monitoring, Am. J. Obstet. Gynecol. 126 (1976) 510–512.

[72] F.J. Plavidal, A. Werch, Gonococcal fetal scalp abscess: a case report, Am. J. Obstet. Gynecol. 127 (1977) 437–438.

[73] M. Reveri, C. Krishnamurthy, Gonococcal scalp abscess, J. Pediatr. 94 (1979) 819–820.

[74] I. Brook, et al., Gonococcal scalp abscess in a newborn, South. Med. J. 73 (1980) 396–397.

[75] M.N. Urban, A.R. Heruada, Gonococcal gum abscess in a 10-week-old infant, Clin. Pediatr. 16 (1977) 193–194.

[76] R.S. Bland, et al., Gonococcal ventriculitis associated with ventriculoamniotic shunt placement, Pediatr. Res. 17 (1983) 265A.

[77] J.H. Armstrong, F. Zacarias, M.F. Rein, Ophthalmia neonatorum: a chart review, Pediatrics 57 (1976) 884–892.

[78] W.M. Brown, H.H. Cowper, J.E. Hodgman, Gonococcal ophthalmia among newborn infants at Los Angeles County General Hospital, 1957–1963, Public Health Rep. 81 (1966) 926–928.

[79] E.R. Wald, et al., Gonorrheal disease among children in a university hospital, Sex. Transm. Dis. 7 (1980) 41–43.

[80] H.E. Pearson, Failure of silver nitrate prophylaxis for gonococcal ophthalmia neonatorum, Am. J. Obstet. Gynecol. 73 (1957) 805–807.

[81] Centers for Disease Control and Prevention, Sexually transmitted diseases treatment guidelines—2006, MMWR Morb. Mortal. Wkly Rep. 55 (2006) 1–94.

[82] LCDC Expert Working Group on Canadian Guidelines for Sexually Transmitted Diseases, Canadian STD Guidelines, 2006 edition, Ottawa, Health, Canada, 2006.

[83] B. Van Der Pol, et al., Multicenter evaluation of the BDProbeTec ET System for detection of *Chlamydia trachomatis* and *Neisseria gonorrhoeae* in urine specimens, female endocervical swabs, and male urethral swabs, J. Clin. Microbiol. 39 (2001) 1008–1016.

[84] G.J. van Doornum, et al., Comparison between the LCx Probe system and the COBAS AMPLICOR system for detection of *Chlamydia trachomatis* and *Neisseria gonorrhoeae* infections in patients attending a clinic for treatment of sexually transmitted diseases in Amsterdam, The Netherlands, J. Clin. Microbiol. 39 (2001) 829–835.

[85] K.C. Carroll, et al., Evaluation of the Abbott LCx ligase chain reaction assay for detection of *Chlamydia trachomatis* and *Neisseria gonorrhoeae* in urine and genital swab specimens from a sexually transmitted disease clinic population, J. Clin. Microbiol. 36 (1998) 1630–1633.

[86] L. Fransen, et al., Parents of infants with ophthalmia neonatorum: a high-risk group for sexually transmitted diseases, Sex. Transm. Dis. 12 (1985) 150–154.

[87] D.A. Haase, et al., Single-dose ceftriaxone therapy for gonococcal ophthalmia neonatorum, Sex. Transm. Dis. 13 (1986) 53–55.

[88] S.A. Rawston, et al., Ceftriaxone treatment of penicillinase-producing *Neisseria gonorrhoeae* infections in children, Pediatr. Infect. Dis. J. 8 (1989) 445–448.

[89] M. Laga, et al., Single-dose therapy of gonococcal ophthalmia neonatorum with ceftriaxone, N. Engl. J. Med. 315 (1986) 1382–1385.

[90] L. Fransen, et al., Single dose kanamycin therapy of gonococcal ophthalmia neonatorum, Lancet 2 (1984) 1234–1236.

[91] J.M. Miller Jr., et al., Initial and repeated screening for gonorrhea during pregnancy, Sex. Transm. Dis. 30 (2003) 728–730.

[92] American Academy of Pediatrics, Prevention of neonatal ophthalmia, in: L.K. Pickering et al., (Ed.), Redbook 2006, Report of the Committee on Infectious Diseases, twentyseventh ed., American Academy of Pediatrics, Elk Grove Village, IL, 2006, pp. 828–838.

[93] S.J. Isenberg, et al., A double application approach to ophthalmia neonatorum prophylaxis, Br. J. Ophthalmol. 87 (2003) 1449–1452.

[94] S.J. Isenberg, L. Apt, M. Wood, A controlled trial of povidone-iodine as prophylaxis against ophthalmia neonatorum, N. Engl. J. Med. 332 (1995) 562–566.

[95] W.J. Benevento, et al., The sensitivity of *Neisseria gonorrhoeae*, *Chlamydia trachomatis*, and herpes simplex type II to disinfection with povidone-iodine, Am. J. Ophthalmol. 109 (1990) 329–333.

[96] D. Zanoni, S.J. Isenberg, L. Apt, A comparison of silver nitrate with erythromycin for prophylaxis against ophthalmia neonatorum, Clin. Pediatr. 31 (1992) 295–298.

[97] M.S. Norn, Cytology of the conjunctival fluid in newborn with references to Credé's prophylaxis, Acta Ophthalmol. 38 (1960) 491–495.

[98] K. Hedberg, et al., Outbreak of erythromycin-resistant staphylococcal conjunctivitis in a newborn nursery, Pediatr. Infect. Dis. J. 9 (1990) 268–273.

SYPHILIS

Tobias R. Kollmann ⊛ Simon Dobson

CHAPTER OUTLINE

Organism 525
Transmission 526
    Acquired Syphilis 526
    Congenital Syphilis 526
    Syphilis and Human Immunodeficiency Virus 526
    Syphilis in Sexually Abused Children 527
    Infection Control 527
Epidemiology 527
    Acquired Syphilis 527
    Congenital Syphilis 528
    Global Perspective 528
Pathogenesis 529
    Treponemal Virulence–Associated Factors 529
    Host Response 529
    Immune-Mediated Protection 531
Pathology 532
Clinical Manifestations 534
    Syphilis in Pregnancy 534
    Acquired Syphilis in Children 535
    Congenital Syphilis 535
Diagnosis 542
    Direct Identification 542
    Indirect, Serologic Identification 543

    Approach to Diagnosis of Acquired Syphilis in Pregnancy 545
    Approach to Diagnosis of Congenital Syphilis 546
Differential Diagnosis 548
    Dermatologic Manifestations 548
    Snuffles 549
    Lymphadenopathy 549
    Hepatosplenomegaly 549
    Hydrops Fetalis 549
    Renal Disease 549
    Ophthalmologic Involvement 550
    Bony Involvement 550
Therapy 550
    Treatment of Acquired Syphilis in Pregnancy 550
    Treatment of Congenital Syphilis 551
    Follow-up for a Pregnant Woman Infected with Syphilis 552
    Follow-up for an Infant Infected with Syphilis 552
    Problems Associated with Penicillin Therapy 553
Prevention 554
    Prenatal Screening 554
    Contact Investigation 556
    Mass Treatment Programs 556
    Education 556
    Advocacy 556

Syphilis is a sexually transmitted disease caused by infection with the bacterium *Treponema pallidum*. Congenital syphilis results when the infection is transmitted from a pregnant mother to her fetus. Although some evidence suggests syphilis was present in Africa and China centuries earlier, the first European epidemic coincided with the return of Columbus from the New World in 1493. It was speculated that Columbus' crew might have contracted the "serpentine disease of Hispaniola" from the island where Haiti and the Dominican Republic are situated today. Another theory is that syphilis entered into a susceptible European population around that time from endemic yaws or bejel of African peoples [1]. Regardless of its origins, syphilis affected Europeans over many centuries, rapidly sweeping through the continent. The first major publication on syphilis was written by Francisco Lopez de Villalobos and appeared in 1498 [2,3]. In 1530, Hieronymus Fracastorius wrote a poem describing an Italian shepherd boy named Syphilus, who contracted the "French disease" sweeping through Europe in the early 16th century [4]. A generation later, Gale introduced the word *syphilis* into the English language [5]. The subsequent spread of syphilis throughout the rest of the world was facilitated largely by wars with associated large troop and population movements and general social disarray [6,7].

The venereal transmission of syphilis was not recognized until the 18th century [1]. Delineation of the characteristics of syphilis was hindered further by the confusion of its symptoms with symptoms of gonorrhea: In 1767, John Hunter, an English experimental biologist and physician, inoculated himself with urethral exudate from a patient with gonorrhea. The patient also had syphilis, however, and the subsequent symptoms experienced by Hunter convinced two generations of physicians of the unity of gonorrhea and syphilis. The separate nature of gonorrhea and syphilis was shown in 1838 by Ricord, who reported his observations on more than 2500 human inoculations. Recognition of the stages of syphilis followed, and in 1905, Schaudinn and Hoffman discovered the causative agent. The following year, Wassermann introduced the diagnostic blood test that bears his name [1].

Lopez and Fracastorius had already mentioned syphilis of the newborn, but they and others thought that infants became infected through contact at delivery or postpartum by ingestion of infected breast milk [2,5,8]. Because many mothers of infants with congenital syphilis had no obvious signs of infection, some investigators believed that congenital disease was transmitted by the father [1]. A lengthy account of the signs of syphilis in infants was published in 1854 by Diday [5], but he failed to recognize

DOI: 10.1016/B978-1-4160-6400-8.00016-X

that infants who were without symptoms by 6 months of age could still have been infected at or before birth. In 1858, Sir Jonathan Hutchinson described the famous triad of late congenital syphilis: notched incisor teeth, interstitial keratitis, and eighth cranial nerve deafness [9]. Myriad further presenting signs and symptoms have earned syphilis the title of "the great imitator" [10,11].

The horror syphilis causes is best encapsulated in its other old name *lues*, which means "plague" in Latin. This is still the most appropriate name because a staggering number of adults and newborn infants in developed and developing countries are suffering and dying as a consequence of infection with *T. pallidum*. The most shocking aspect of this plague is that hundreds of thousands are newly infected every year despite the availability of feasible, cost-effective interventions to detect, treat, and prevent syphilis [12,13]. The World Health Organization (WHO) estimates that globally every year 1 million pregnancies are complicated by syphilis, with approximately half resulting in early abortion or perinatal death, a quarter resulting in infants with low birth weight or premature birth, and a final quarter resulting in infants with overt congenital syphilis [13]. The 2000 Report on Global Burden of Disease estimated that congenital syphilis is responsible for 1.3% of deaths among live-born children younger than 5 years [14]. The annual number of children born with congenital syphilis has now exceeded the number of newborns with human immunodeficiency virus (HIV) [12,15]. Consequently, the elimination of congenital syphilis is an important global objective [12,15,16].

ORGANISM

Syphilis is caused by *T. pallidum*. The name *Treponema* (Greek, meaning "turning thread") is based on its twisting motion, and *pallidum* (Latin) is derived from its pale, yellow color. *T. pallidum* belongs to the order Spirochaetales, family Spirochaetaceae, and genus *Treponema*. *Borrelia*, *Spirochaeta*, *Leptospira*, and *Cristispira* are other genera of this order, grouped together primarily based on their morphologic characteristics (i.e., helix-shaped) (Fig. 16–1). *T. pallidum* has approximately 8 to 14 helices per cell [17]. Despite greater than 95% sequence homology,

complete DNA sequencing has allowed the human disease–causing *Treponema* to be identified as subspecies— *T. pallidum* subspecies *pallidum* (syphilis), *T. pallidum* subspecies *pertenue* (yaws), *Treponema* subspecies *carateum* (pinta), and *T. pallidum* subspecies *endemicum* (Bejel) [18–23]. Only *T. pallidum* and possibly *T. pertenue* [24] can cause congenital infection [25–27]. Several nonpathogenic treponemes also inhabit the oral cavity and intestinal tract of humans [28]. *T. pallidum* has finely tapered ends, lacking the hook shape found in several human commensal spirochetes [18,19]. An outer membrane consisting of a lipid bilayer surrounds the endoflagella, cytoplasmic membrane, and protoplasmic cylinder. The spirochete's corkscrew motility results from the action of these endoflagella and can be observed in fresh preparations examined with the dark-field microscope [29–32].

The genome of *T. pallidum* subspecies *pallidum* (Nichols strain; maintained in rabbits since 1912) has been sequenced in its entire length. It represents an approximately 1-Mb circular chromosome with slightly more than 1000 predicted open reading frames (ORFs) encoding all factors necessary for replication, transcription, translation, and mobility, but only a minimal number of genes encoding molecules important in metabolism, indicating a necessary close interaction with the host cell [23,33–36]. In contrast to many bacterial pathogens, *T. pallidum* does not seem to rely on iron acquisition from the host [34,36,37]. Biologic functions have so far been predicted for only about 55% of *T. pallidum* ORFs, and a further 17% show homology with proteins from other species; a high proportion of *T. pallidum* ORFs are still uncharacterized and presumably contribute to its distinctive and complex parasitic strategy, including immune evasion, latency, and a feature unique to *T. pallidum* subspecies *pallidum*—neuroinvasion. The genome sequence contains ORFs encoding for putative virulence factors similar to known bacterial hemolysins and cytotoxins, but does not seem to have the mechanism for secreting them into the host. Genetic polymorphisms more recently identified at two loci have enabled strain typing of clinical isolates of *T. pallidum*, providing new tools for the investigation of syphilis transmission and epidemiology [10,38].

T. pallidum is a macroaerophilic gram-negative bacterium that depends primarily on glycolysis for energy production. It is highly sensitive to oxygen and temperature and is not readily maintained in culture [26,39–41]. It can be passaged for a limited number of replicative cycles with a generation time of 30 to 33 hours using rabbit epithelial cell monolayers under microaerobic conditions at 33° C to 35° C [10]. *T. pallidum* can be propagated by intratesticular inoculation of rabbits, where it displays a slow replicative cycle of approximately 30 hours. From infected rabbit testes, *T. pallidum* can be purified through density centrifugation. Such purified organisms retain their antigenicity, but not their motility or their virulence. Outside of humans, only rabbits and primates infected with *T. pallidum* develop primary and secondary, but not tertiary, syphilis, and neither rabbits nor primates have been shown to pass *T. pallidum* on vertically [25,42,43]. Although *T. pallidum* can be passed on vertically in pigs, no good animal model for congenital syphilis exists that

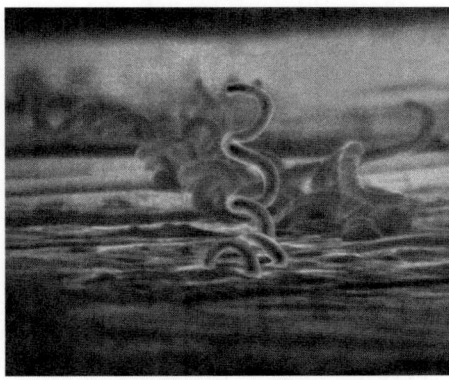

FIGURE 16–1 Electron micrograph of *Treponema pallidum* on cultures of cotton-tail rabbit epithelium cells, displaying the characteristic helical structure of treponemes. *(Courtesy of CDC/Dr. David Cox; Public Health Image Library #1977.)*

recapitulates the clinical findings in humans transplacentally infected [44–47]. This lack of a good animal model and the inability to culture and manipulate these organisms in vitro have prevented a detailed mechanistic understanding of virulence mechanisms or host-pathogen interactions in congenital syphilis [48,49].

TRANSMISSION

Syphilis can be passed horizontally from person to person through direct contact, such as during sexual activity resulting in acquired syphilis, or vertically from mother to infant, resulting in congenital syphilis. The organism does not survive outside of its human host and is easily killed by heat, drying, soap, and water. Syphilis is not known to be spread through casual contact or through contact with fomites [50].

ACQUIRED SYPHILIS

Humans are the only known natural host of *T. pallidum*. Horizontal transmission results primarily from sexual activity, although anecdotal reports cite kissing as a potential route as well [51]. Because of the low survival rate of *T. pallidum* outside of its host, direct contact with an infected person's bodily secretions containing spirochetes is necessary for transmission. Although sexual transmission depends on many factors, such as stage of the disease, overall around half of individuals who have sexual contact with an infected partner acquire the disease, with an estimated median infective dose of 50 bacteria [52–54]. Because sexual contact is the most common mode of transmission for acquired disease, the sites of inoculation usually are the genital organs, but lips, tongue, and abraded areas of the skin have been described as well. Such an entry point is identified as the site of the initial ulcerating sore, or chancre [51]. Health care providers or laboratory workers have apparently become infected with *T. pallidum* through accidental contact with infected secretions, when appropriate protection gear (gloves) was not worn [51].

CONGENITAL SYPHILIS

Vertical transmission from infected mother to child most often occurs prenatally, but perinatal and postnatal transmission have been described. Although transmission of syphilis to the fetus can occur throughout pregnancy (spirochetes have been visualized in tissue at gestational age of 9 weeks) [55–57], the likelihood of vertical transmission increases with advancing gestation. The organism is isolated with increasing frequency during gestation from umbilical cord blood, amniotic fluid [58–62], and placenta [63–65]. A newborn occasionally may be infected perinatally (i.e., at delivery by contact with an infectious lesion present in the birth canal or perineum). Postnatal transmission from mother to child is exceedingly rare. Centuries ago, when it was more common for infants to be fed by a wet nurse, small epidemics of syphilis were caused by an infectious lesion on the nipple of a wet nurse, but no data indicate that breast milk itself is associated with mother-to-child transmission [66,67].

The likelihood of vertical transmission is directly related to the maternal stage of syphilis, with early primary syphilis resulting in significantly higher transmission rates than late latent infection (known as Kassowitz's law) [68,69]. This transmission pattern may relate to maternal spirochetemia in early syphilis [70]. Among women with untreated primary or secondary early syphilis, the rate of transmission is 60% to 100% and slowly decreases with later stages of maternal infection to approximately 40% with early latent infection and 8% with late latent infection. In one study, in which *T. pallidum* was passed on from mother to fetus during early primary or secondary (<4 years' duration) untreated syphilis, approximately half of the infants were born prematurely, stillborn, or died as neonates, and congenital syphilis developed in the other half (i.e., 100% were affected). In contrast, in women with early latent syphilis, 20% to 60% of their infants were healthy at birth, 20% were premature, and only 16% were stillborn; 4% died as neonates, and 40% of infants appearing healthy at birth developed the stigmata of congenital syphilis later in life. In the case of untreated late syphilis, about 70% of newborns appeared healthy, 10% were stillborn, and approximately 9% were premature; about 1% died as neonates, and about 10% of infants appearing healthy at birth developed signs of congenital syphilis later in life [68,69,71]. A family study illustrating Kassowitz's law described a syphilitic mother who had five pregnancies resulting in eight children: [72] The first pregnancy produced a stillborn infant; the second produced a full-term infant with congenital syphilis; the third produced triplets, two of whom had congenital syphilis; the fourth produced twins, one of whom had congenital syphilis; and the fifth produced a healthy full-term infant.

SYPHILIS AND HUMAN IMMUNODEFICIENCY VIRUS

Despite the recognition that syphilis and HIV are a dangerous combination, limited conclusive data exist to describe the interaction between the two infections or their impact on vertical transmission [73,74]. Potential interactions include acceleration of the natural history of either disease, alterations in the clinical or laboratory manifestations, increased risk for syphilitic complications, and diminished response to syphilis therapy [10,51,75,76]. Genital sores (i.e., chancres) caused by syphilis make it easier to transmit sexually and acquire HIV infection, with an estimated twofold to fivefold increased risk of acquiring HIV if exposed to that infection when a syphilitic chancre is present [50]. This increased risk is likely caused by the breaks in the skin or mucous membranes in a syphilitic chancre, which bleed easily and, when they come into contact with oral, genital, and rectal mucosa, increase the infectiousness of and susceptibility to HIV.

Virulent *T. pallidum* can promote the induction of HIV gene expression in infected cells, possibly resulting in increased systemic HIV levels and more rapid progression of HIV infection [77]. Increasing proportions of newborns with congenital syphilis also are born to mothers with HIV, and vice versa. One study noted higher rates of congenital syphilis in infants born to coinfected mothers, but the diagnosis of congenital syphilis was based on the older surveillance definition used by the U.S. Centers for Disease Control and Prevention (CDC) [78] and not on strict diagnostic criteria [79]. Immune dysfunction associated with HIV infection may also permit a greater degree of treponemal proliferation and lead to a higher rate of fetal infection. HIV-infected women who acquire syphilis during pregnancy also may not respond adequately to currently recommended penicillin therapy, increasing the risk of fetal infection with *T. pallidum* [80]. Available data suggest, however, that if the natural history of acquired syphilis is modified by HIV, the difference shows considerable overlap with the course of syphilitic disease progression in persons without HIV [10].

SYPHILIS IN SEXUALLY ABUSED CHILDREN

Identification of syphilis in young children raises the question of possible sexual abuse [81]. It is an uncommon complication among sexually abused children, found in 1% or less in a case series from the United States. The frequency of syphilis transmission to sexually abused children may be higher, however, in regions with higher adult prevalence of the disease. The clinical manifestations may provide insight into the timing of acquisition of infection. This information may not always help to resolve the potential dilemma of whether the clinical findings are those of previously unrecognized congenital syphilis versus postnatally acquired syphilis. Also, some experts have postulated that antibiotics commonly prescribed for common childhood illnesses may partially treat congenital syphilis and alter the nature of late clinical manifestations. Evaluation of children by specialists in the area of child sexual abuse is recommended. Children diagnosed with syphilis also should be evaluated for HIV infection and other sexually transmitted diseases as clinically indicated.

INFECTION CONTROL

Standard precautions are recommended for all patients, including infants with suspected or proven congenital syphilis. Infected infants and adults with infectious lesions should be placed in contact isolation for the first 24 hours of therapy, and appropriate protective gear (e.g., gloves) should be worn by staff members for all patient contact during this period. When antimicrobial therapy has been initiated, the risk of transmission is virtually nonexistent because penicillin in sufficient dosage causes a complete disappearance of viable treponemes from syphilitic lesions within a few hours [82]. All people, including hospital personnel, who have had unprotected close contact with a patient with early congenital syphilis before identification of the disease or within the first 24 hours of therapy should be examined clinically for the presence of lesions 2 to 3 weeks after contact. Close unprotected contact is defined as skin (intact or abraded) contact with infectious bodily fluids. Serology in the exposed individual should be assessed at time 0 and again at 1 month and 3 to 6 months postexposure, or sooner if symptoms occur. If the degree of exposure is considered substantial, immediate treatment should be considered, as outlined

subsequently under postexposure prophylaxis in "Therapy." [81,83]. All exposures should also be reported to the occupational health office.

EPIDEMIOLOGY

The epidemiologic curve of syphilis has consistently reflected social trends, with an upward swing during stressful societal transitions [84]. After major public health successes in the early 1990s, the incidence of acquired syphilis showed an alarming resurgence throughout the world. The trends for congenital syphilis follow trends of acquired syphilis in women.

ACQUIRED SYPHILIS

Because of the exquisite susceptibility of *T. pallidum* to penicillin, it was believed that use of this antimicrobial agent would lead to the virtual disappearance of acquired syphilis. A dramatic decline in the number of cases did occur after the introduction of penicillin, with the incidence reaching a low point in the United States in the mid-1950s. When a disease approaches eradication, however, often the control program rather than the disease is eradicated. As a result of reduction in funds in the early 1960s, syphilis resurged. More resources were again committed to control efforts, and the incidence of syphilis promptly declined in the 1970s, only to increase dramatically again in the 1980s [85,86]. The impact of illegal drugs, particularly crack cocaine, seems to have played a major role in that resurgence [85–88], but a reduction in resources for syphilis control programs can be implicated as well [85,89].

Secondary to increased funding and focus on public health intervention, from 1990–2000, the incidence of primary and secondary syphilis in the United States decreased by 90% [50,85,90–92]. The reasons for this dramatic success were many, but likely include the following: (1) wider screening practices secondary to medical and public awareness of the syphilis epidemic of the late 1980s, which led to identification and treatment of infected individuals; (2) increased state and local funding for syphilis control programs such as partner notification, community-based screening and presumptive treatment strategies, and risk reduction counseling; (3) introduction of HIV prevention programs that target prevention of other sexually transmitted diseases; (4) decrease in crack cocaine use and sex-for-drug behaviors; and possibly (5) development of acquired immunity to syphilis among high-risk populations, which may have resulted in less reacquisition of infectious syphilis. These trends did not continue, and the upward swing is becoming evident once more (Fig. 16–2).

In the United States in 2005–2006, the total number of cases of syphilis (all stages—primary and secondary, early latent, late, late latent, and congenital syphilis) increased 11% (from 33,288 to 36,935). The rate of primary and secondary syphilis in 2006 (3.3 cases per 100,000 population) was 13.8% higher than the rate in 2005—far greater than the Healthy People 2010 target of 0.2 cases per 100,000 population. The rate increased in all racial and ethnic groups (5.6% among non-Hispanic whites

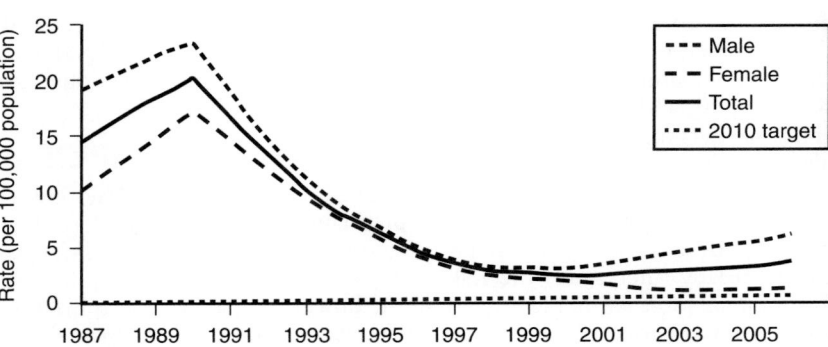

FIGURE 16–2 Primary and secondary syphilis rates, total and by sex, United States, 1987–2006, and the Healthy People 2010 target. The Healthy People 2010 target for primary and secondary syphilis is 0.2 case per 100,000 population. *(From Division of STD Prevention. National Center for HIV/AIDS, Viral Hepatitis, STD, and TB Prevention. Last updated November 13, 2007. Available at http://cdc.gov/std/stats/figures/figure27.htm.)*

[from 1.8 to 1.9 cases per 100,000 population], 16.5% among African Americans [from 9.7 to 11.3 cases per 100,000 population], 12.5% among Hispanics [from 3.2 to 3.6 cases per 100,000 population], 18.2% among Asian/Pacific Islanders [from 1.1 to 1.3 cases per 100,000 population], and 37.5% among American Indian/Alaska Natives [from 2.4 to 3.3 cases per 100,000 population]). Most primary and secondary syphilis cases occurred in persons 20 to 39 years old; rates were highest in women 20 to 24 years old and in men 35 to 39 years old. Rates have increased in men each year from 2000–2006 from 2.6 to 5.7, with 65% of cases in 2006 occurring among men who have sex with men (it is only since 2005 that the CDC requested that all state health departments report gender of sex partners for persons with syphilis). After persistent declines since 1990, the rate of primary and secondary syphilis among women increased from 0.8 case per 100,000 population in 2004 to 0.9 case per 100,000 population in 2005 to 1 case per 100,000 population in 2006 [85].

Similar trends have been observed in Canada. Just when Canadian public health officials aimed at possibly eliminating syphilis entirely, Alberta and British Columbia reported outbreaks of syphilis: From 1996–1999, the rate of infectious syphilis in British Columbia increased from 0.5 to 7.7 cases per 100,000 population, with incidence peaks of 150 cases per 100,000 among sex trade workers and their clients [93–95].

Local outbreaks of primary and secondary syphilis have occurred in North America in almost cyclic patterns roughly every 7 to 10 years [96–98]. These cycles underscore the need for syphilis elimination rather than merely control. The idea for a comprehensive approach to eliminate endemic syphilis in the United States had been raised several years back, with the CDC [78] developing a National Plan for Elimination of Syphilis from the United States [50,85]. The plan did not succeed, however, and had to be revised in 2006 in the face of resurgent rates [85].

CONGENITAL SYPHILIS

The incidence of congenital syphilis closely mimics the incidence of primary and secondary disease in women of childbearing age: The incidence of congenital syphilis increased dramatically in the late 1980s, then declined, but again has increased after 2005. The dramatic increase in the number of cases of congenital syphilis in 1990–1991 was due to an increase in actual cases and to the use of revised reporting guidelines beginning in 1989 [96,99,100]. Previous criteria for reporting cases of congenital syphilis had been based on a clinical case definition [101]. Because of the high incidence of congenital disease in infants born to inadequately treated mothers, current definitions of congenital syphilis for a probable case (which should be reported and treated) require only (1) that the infant be born to a mother with untreated or inadequately treated syphilis or (2) that the infant has physical or laboratory signs of congenital syphilis. Use of these guidelines increased the number of reported cases of congenital syphilis almost fourfold in the 1990s [102,103].

The current definition by the CDC acknowledges the public health burden of the disease because these infants require medical and public health interventions. Using this new surveillance-based case definition, up until 2005, the rate of congenital syphilis in the United States had declined every year over 14 consecutive years, with an overall reduction of 74.2%. From 2005–2006 for the first time, the rate of congenital syphilis increased again (3.7%, from 8.2 to 8.5 cases per 100,000 live births). In 2006, 349 cases were reported in the United States compared with 339 cases in 2005. In 2006, 26 states, the District of Columbia, and one outlying area had rates of congenital syphilis that exceeded the Healthy People 2010 target of 1 case per 100,000 live births [85], indicating how widespread the resurgence of congenital syphilis is in the United States. In Canada, the rates of congenital syphilis followed a similar trend [104]. Delayed access to prenatal care has been identified as the main issue, and nearly all mothers in the outbreak in downtown Vancouver who delivered an infant with congenital syphilis had histories of substance abuse or street involvement [84].

GLOBAL PERSPECTIVE

Worldwide, syphilis has grown into a staggering public health problem. According to a WHO estimate, 12 million people are infected with syphilis each year, and 90% of these infections occur in developing countries [105]. In Europe, the emerging resurgence has brought about great concern. In the United Kingdom, the highest number of congenital syphilis cases in 10 years were identified in 2005 [106], raising doubts that existing antenatal programs are adequate for the identification and treatment of women at risk [11,107]. Outbreaks have also been registered in Ireland, France, Holland, Norway, Germany, and Switzerland [108–110]. Congenital syphilis was very rare before 1990 in Eastern Europe and the former Soviet Union, but the number of infants born with syphilis in the Russian Federation increased from 29 in 1991 to 743 in 1999, an increase from 0.9 to 8.5 cases per 100,000 live births. Overall, 1% to 2% of all pregnancies in Russia and other countries of the former Soviet Union now occur in women with syphilis.

In sub-Saharan Africa, syphilis is common among women of childbearing age, with more recent national surveys reporting rates of 3.1% in Uganda, 4.2% in Madagascar, 6.6% in Ghana, and 8.3% in Zambia [111,112]. In Burkina Faso, 2.5% of all pregnancies occur in women with syphilis, and in Cameroon, 17.4% of pregnancies occur in women with syphilis. In southern Africa, an estimated 25% of all stillbirths and 10% of all neonatal deaths are due to congenital syphilis [113]. In South America, the problem of syphilis and congenital syphilis is recognized as well. In Buenos Aires, 10% of women with reactive serologic tests for syphilis had a history of stillbirth that was believed to be caused by syphilis. In Bolivia, 26% of women who were delivered of stillborn infants had syphilis compared with only 4% of mothers of live-born infants [114]. The highest documented increase in acquired and congenital syphilis has been noted in China, where congenital syphilis has had an average yearly increase of 71.9%, from 0.01 cases per 100,000 live births in 1991 to 19.68 cases in 2005 [115]. These statistics likely still underestimate the total burden of congenital syphilis in China because they do not take into account stillbirths.

More recent data from the WHO indicate that only 68% of women in the world currently receive antenatal care. Even if perfectly executed, existing prenatal programs would not be able to prevent transmission of syphilis in the one third of pregnant women not seen early enough to be tested and treated [116]. The global toll of congenital syphilis is severe: Every year, about 1 million pregnancies globally are adversely affected by syphilis (about 270,000 infants are born with congenital syphilis, 460,000 pregnancies end in abortion or perinatal death, and 270,000 infants are born prematurely or with low birth weight). This represents a higher impact than any other major neonatal infection, including HIV infection and tetanus [117,118]. With that, considerable burden is placed on the already limited health services in many developing countries [119,120]. Newborns with congenital syphilis are more likely to be admitted to a neonatal intensive care unit, to stay longer in the hospital, and to receive care costing three times more than newborns without the disease. In one large South African referral hospital, on average 1 neonatal intensive care unit bed out of a total of 12 is occupied by an infant with syphilis [15]. In most countries, more attention has been given to screening for HIV, for which, at present, no cure is available; this has led to the situation where infants are "avoiding HIV but dying of syphilis" [16].

PATHOGENESIS

In an infected pregnant woman, the parasite encounters a host environment that is altered to favor the development of the fetus [10]. Understanding the pathogenesis of

T. pallidum in pregnancy relies on understanding the complex relationships between the unique ability of this particular treponeme to cross the placental barrier and its ability to cause fetal demise or the many early and late manifestations of congenital syphilis in a live-born infant. These complex and changing relationships are superimposed on the genetic background of the mother and the fetus, which together govern the host response to infection during the different stages of pregnancy and development [10]. The complexity of these host-pathogen relationships has made gathering mechanistic insights into the molecular, cellular, and organism pathogenesis extremely difficult.

TREPONEMAL VIRULENCE–ASSOCIATED FACTORS

As reviewed by Woods [121], congenital syphilis starts with *T. pallidum* bacteria crossing from mother to fetus. Transplacental transmission during maternal spirochetemia can occur at 9 to 10 weeks of gestation and at any subsequent time during pregnancy. Viable spirochetes in amniotic fluid obtained by amniocentesis from a woman with early syphilis have been reported at 14 weeks of gestation, proving that the fetus can sustain replication of viable treponemes after infection with *T. pallidum* very early in pregnancy [60]. Transmission in utero causes the wide dissemination of the organism in the fetus (analogous to secondary acquired syphilis). Untreated congenital syphilis can progress through the same stages as postnatally acquired syphilis. Infection begins when virulent *T. pallidum* attach to host cells via the proximal hook. A ligand-receptor adherence mechanism involving the treponemal outer membrane proteins seems to be present. Virulent strains attach to metabolically active mammalian cells, and treponemes are capable of multiplication only during attachment. Highly replicative fetal and infant cells seem to support treponemal growth maximally, and endothelial cells seem to be the prime target. Virulent treponemal strains produce hyaluronidase, which may facilitate the perivascular infiltration that is apparent by histopathologic study. Virulent *T. pallidum* is coated with fibronectin of host origin. This coating seems to protect the organism from antibody-mediated phagocytosis; allows the organism to adhere to the surface of host phagocytes with only limited ingestion; may block complement-mediated lysis of the coated treponemes; and, finally, may allow the treponemes to acquire host proteins, such as ceruloplasmin and transferrin, on which they are dependent [121,122].

HOST RESPONSE

Pathologic changes in congenital syphilis are similar to changes that occur in acquired syphilis except for the absence of a primary or chancre stage. Because infection involves the placenta [55] and spreads hematogenously to the fetus, widespread involvement is characteristic. No matter which organ is involved, the essential microscopic appearance of lesions is that of perivascular infiltration of lymphocytes, plasma cells, and histiocytes, with obliterative endarteritis and extensive fibrosis [25,123]. These typical histopathologic features of the inflammatory response to invasion by *T. pallidum* suggest an important role for immune-mediated injury in the pathogenesis of congenital syphilis [124]. Harter and Benirschke [125] showed spirochetes in fetal tissue from spontaneous abortions at 9 and 10 weeks of gestation. The apparent lack of pathologic changes in fetal tissues earlier than the 5th month of gestation could be a result of lower fetal immune function during early gestation [57].

T. pallidum infection simultaneously elicits local and systemic innate and adaptive immune responses [126,127]. It is generally believed that a strong T helper type 1 (T_H1) response to any infection during pregnancy may compromise pregnancy outcome. In pregnancy, a gradual dampening of the intensity of the innate and cell-mediated immune responses to favor the maintenance and growth of the fetus may result in incomplete clearance of *T. pallidum* from lesions, allowing the development of a chronic infection and the resulting multitude of clinical findings in congenital syphilis [128]. The increased production of inflammatory cytokines interleukin-2, interferon-γ, tumor necrosis factor-α, and prostaglandins induced by fetal infection together with the intense inflammatory responses associated with activation of macrophages by treponemal lipoproteins may be responsible for fetal death or preterm delivery in a mother with primary or early secondary syphilis and severe growth restriction or some of the manifestations of congenital syphilis in the infant [36]. The resolution of the primary and the secondary manifestations of infection correlate with the development of cellular immune responses [10].

Host Innate Immune Response

Although *T. pallidum* does not contain lipopolysaccharide, the lipoproteins and glycolipids present under the outer membrane have been shown to activate the innate inflammatory response via toll-like receptor 4 (TLR4) [129]. These lipoproteins are not surface-exposed; live *T. pallidum* elicits a lower inflammatory response than with *T. pallidum* lysates [10,124,130]. This feature may explain how live treponemes can persist in extracellular loci, yet elicit little or no inflammatory response, and may account for the pronounced systemic (Jarisch-Herxheimer) reaction observed soon after the initiation of penicillin therapy, in which dying treponemes release proinflammatory mediators in large quantities. Polymorphonuclear leukocytes ingest *T. pallidum*, incorporating them into phagocytic vacuoles where they are killed and digested. Overall, phagocytosis occurs relatively slowly and is facilitated by the presence of immune serum [131].

Numerous treponemes are needed to activate the phagocytic response, and small numbers of treponemes may escape recognition [132]. Lipoproteins of *T. pallidum* are thought to gain access to toll-like receptors on the surface of macrophages only after degradation of organisms in phagolysosomal vacuoles [10,124,130]. When this degradation occurs, macrophages are induced to produce tumor necrosis factor [132,133] and messenger RNA for interleukin-12 [134], which favors the development of T_H1-type immunity. The spirochete also has been shown to activate human promyelomonocytic cell line THP-1 cells in a CD14-dependent manner [135]. These findings support the concept that lipoproteins are the principal components of spirochetes responsible for innate immune activation. The direct interaction of *T. pallidum* with vascular endothelium also seems to be an important early event in the initiation of the host innate immune response to syphilitic infection [133]. A purified 47-kDa treponemal lipoprotein can activate human vascular endothelial cells to upregulate cell surface expression of intercellular adhesion molecule-1 and procoagulant activity [136]. These actions may contribute to the fibrin deposition and perivasculitis that are characteristic histopathologic findings in syphilis [10].

Host Adaptive Immune Response

In acquired syphilis, IgM and IgG antibodies are detectable by the time the primary chancre appears, but humoral immunity is insufficient to control the infection. T cell–mediated immunity seems to be suppressed during the primary and secondary stages of infection [121]. Nevertheless, ultimate eradication of acute infection occurs only when T cells infiltrate syphilitic lesions, which leads to activation of macrophages and phagocytosis of antibody-opsonized treponemes.

Host Cell–Mediated Immune Response

The lack of outer membrane immune targets has led *T. pallidum* to be labeled a "stealth pathogen." [10] The importance of cellular immunity in containing the infection and in its immunopathology is shown by the presence of granulomata, which, in the case of gummatous disease (see later), assume a necrotizing character [121]. T lymphocytes responsive to *T. pallidum* appear in syphilitic lesions as the number of treponemes decreases, suggesting a role of cellular immunity in controlling infection. In primary chancres, CD4+ T cells and macrophages predominate, whereas in the lesions of secondary syphilis, most of the cellular infiltrate is composed of CD8+ T cells; this is surprising because *T. pallidum* is believed to be mostly an extracellular pathogen. Increased expression of the T_H1 cytokines interleukin-2 and interferon-γ are seen in lesions of primary and secondary syphilis, in humans and in the rabbit model [130,137,138]. Circulating T lymphocytes responsive to treponemal antigens can already be detected in late primary syphilis, but cell-mediated immune responses peak in the secondary stage. Clinically measurable delayed-type hypersensitivity to treponemal antigens appears only late in secondary syphilis and may be related to the onset of latency. Increased apoptosis of peripheral blood lymphocytes and CD4+ T cells by a Fas-mediated pathway in patients with secondary early syphilis could account for the incomplete clearance of *T. pallidum* from the lesions, leading to the establishment of chronic infection [139]. Overall, however, the mechanisms that lead to latency are not understood [10].

Host Antibody–Mediated Humoral Immune Response

Humoral immunity has been a subject of study in syphilis since the serendipitous discovery of antibody to cardiolipin by Wassermann early in the 19th century. Circulating

IgG and IgM antibodies to *T. pallidum* are detectable by the time the chancre appears (i.e., with the onset of primary syphilis), with antibodies to *T. pallidum* detected in 90% and antibody to cardiolipin detected in 75% of cases [140]. Antibodies to *T. pallidum* recognize a wide range of proteins [141], with the 47-kDa antigen being the most immunogenic [142]. Higher titers are reached as the infection disseminates in the secondary stage [143,144]. In primary syphilis, the main IgG subclass is IgG1, whereas in secondary syphilis, IgG1 and IgG3 predominate [145]. If the patient is treated adequately, IgM antibody declines during the next 1 to 2 years, but IgG antibody usually persists through the lifetime of the patient. The stages of syphilis evolve, despite the treponeme-specific antibody response [10].

The overall antibody response of congenitally infected infants parallels the response in acquired syphilis. IgM antibodies to specific *T. pallidum* proteins can often be detected in neonatal serum obtained at birth [146–149]. The range of IgM antibody responses to the proteins of *T. pallidum* in the sera of overtly infected newborns is comparable to that for disseminated (secondary) infection in adults [150]. The IgM response of the infant is distinct, however, from that of the mother and is uniformly directed against the 47-kDa immunodominant membrane lipoprotein antigen. As would be expected based on the transplacental transfer of IgG, the IgG levels and antigen specificity of infected infants largely match those of their mothers [148–150].

Human sera containing antibodies can immobilize *T. pallidum* in the presence of complement—the basis of the old *T. pallidum* immobilization test for diagnosing syphilis—and can block attachment of the organism to eukaryotic cells. Human immune serum facilitates uptake of *T. pallidum* by human polymorphonuclear leukocytes [132]. The antigens to which these immobilizing antibodies are directed are unknown. Only a small percentage of patients with primary syphilis have immobilizing antibodies [25,151]. *T. pallidum*–immobilizing antibody is also present in most patients who have active secondary syphilis [27]. Passive immunization of rabbits with large amounts of serum from rabbits that have recovered from experimental *T. pallidum* infection and are immune to rechallenge delays and attenuates infection, but does not prevent the development of syphilitic lesions [27,152,153]. Why the disease progresses despite abundant and even neutralizing antibody responses is unclear, but suggests that humoral immunity is insufficient to clear active infection and that cellular immunity is required [10].

T. pallidum contains a family of repeat genes, the *tpr* genes [10], which encode proteins homologous to the major surface proteins of *T. denticola* that mediate attachment to host tissue and function as porins [154]. Tpr proteins are immunogenic in rabbits, and one of them, TprK, has been shown to be a target for opsonic antibody. TprK differs in seven discrete variable regions, and in a rabbit model, antibodies to these variable regions offer protection against homologous, but not heterologous strains [147,155]. With successive passage, diversity is observed in the TprK V region genes [156]. Antigenic variation through gene conversion in infection has been hypothesized to be another mechanism by which the organism evades the host immune response, allowing for prolonged infection and persistence in the presence of a robust host response. The immune response to TprK seems to be a primary means of killing treponemes. T-cell responses apparently are directed against conserved epitopes of TprK, whereas opsonic antibodies are directed against variable region epitopes. This factor may account for the common clinical scenario of reinfection with syphilis. Similar mechanisms have been described for spirochetes of the genus *Borrelia*, which cause relapsing fever [124].

Secondary syphilis and congenital infection sometimes are accompanied by an immune-mediated nephrotic syndrome. This nephrosis characteristically responds rapidly to penicillin, and light microscopy reveals membranous glomerulonephritis with glomerular mesangial cell proliferation. The subendothelial basement membrane deposits contain IgG and C3 or only globulin. Acute syphilitic glomerulonephritis seems to be an immune complex disease in acquired [157–159] and congenital syphilis [160]. Similar immune complex–mediated processes may underlie other clinically apparent signs of congenital syphilis as well [161].

IMMUNE-MEDIATED PROTECTION

Although patients who have been previously treated for syphilis can be reinfected, untreated patients seem to have at least a degree of immunity to repeated infection. In the 19th century in Dublin, Colles observed that wet nurses who breast-fed infants with congenital syphilis often developed chancres of the nipple, whereas the mothers of such infants did not, implying that they were somehow protected from repeated infection; this has become known as Colles' law [162,163]. Subsequent studies in which prisoner volunteers in the United States were inoculated with *T. pallidum* likewise showed that men with untreated syphilis did not develop chancres at the site of cutaneous inoculation, whereas men who had been treated for syphilis in the past (especially men who had been treated early during primary or secondary stages) and men who had not had the infection did develop infection [52].

Persons with untreated secondary syphilis or true latent infection are resistant to rechallenge with *T. pallidum*, as are individuals with untreated congenital syphilis [52]. This state has been referred to as "chancre immunity" or "chancre fast." Such protection from untreated previous disease represents only a relative resistance to reinfection, such that the development of a chancre with reinfection is unusual, but may simply depend on the challenge inoculum. This state of relative resistance applies to persons who maintain a reactive nontreponemal antibody test (serofast) and to individuals whose sera become nonreactive [164,165].

Physicians in the 19th century knew that a degree of maternal immunity is acquired during infection. In 1846, Kassowitz observed that the longer syphilis exists untreated in a woman before pregnancy occurs, the more likely it is that when she does become pregnant, her treponemes will be held in check, and the less likely it is that her fetus will die in utero or be born with congenital syphilis (Kassowitz's law) [1,162]. It remains unclear what factors determine which mothers, particularly in the latent stage of infection, pass disease to their fetuses. It also is unclear why some infants who are infected in utero are born without any clinical manifestations, with the subsequent development of overt disease in the first weeks or months of life or even later at puberty.

Although active or prior syphilis modifies the response of the patient to subsequent reinfection, protection is only relative and is unreliable [10]. Rabbits immunized with irradiated *T. pallidum* display complete protective immunity to challenge [166]. Together, these findings argue that it should be possible to achieve protective immunity, possibly through vaccination [10].

PATHOLOGY

Although there are many similarities in the pathology of acquired and congenital syphilis, there also are some key differences. Acquired syphilis is a lifelong infection that progresses in three clear characteristic stages [121,167]. After initial invasion through mucous membranes or skin, the organism undergoes rapid multiplication and is disseminated widely. Spread through the perivascular lymphatics and then through the systemic circulation probably occurs even before the clinical development of the primary lesion.

The patient manifests an inflammatory response to the infection at the site of the inoculation 10 to 90 days later, usually within 3 to 4 weeks. The resulting lesion, the chancre, is characterized by the profuse discharge of spirochetes, accumulation of mononuclear leukocytes, and swelling of capillary endothelia. The regional lymph nodes become enlarged as well, with the cellular infiltrate in the lymph node resembling that of the primary chancre lesions. Resolution of the primary lesion eventually occurs via fibrosis (scarring) at the primary chancre site and reconstruction of the normal architecture in the lymph node. Secondary lesions develop when tissues of ectodermal origin, such as skin, mucous membranes, and central nervous system (CNS), become infected with resulting vasculitis. The cellular infiltrate resembles that of the primary lesion, with the predominance of plasma cells, but CD8 T cells instead of CD4 T cells. There is little or no necrosis, and healing of secondary lesions occurs without scarring.

Tertiary syphilis seems to occur from chronic swelling of the capillary endothelium resulting in tissue fibrosis or necrosis and may involve any organ system. It often is asymmetric. Gummata are lesions typified by extensive necrosis, a few giant cells, and a paucity of organisms. They commonly occur in internal organs, bone, and skin. The other major form of tertiary lesion is a diffuse chronic perivascular inflammation, with plasma cells and lymphocytes but without caseation, which may result in an aortic aneurysm, paralytic dementia, or tabes dorsalis.

Congenital syphilis cannot be divided neatly into these three stages [168]. Because it is a result of hematogenous infection, dissemination is wide resulting in involvement of almost all viscera. Most pathologic studies were done on stillborn infants or infants who died early in life, producing significant heterogeneity in the findings secondary to varying length of infection before pathologic

examination. Similar to the acquired form, in congenital syphilis an intense inflammatory response is also focused on the perivascular environment, rather than distributed throughout the parenchyma [162]. Bone, liver, pancreas, intestine, kidney, and spleen are involved most reproducibly and severely. Other tissues, such as the brain, pituitary gland, lymph nodes, and lungs, may be infected as well [169].

The grossly apparent clinical findings of a live-born infant with congenital syphilis are described later in this chapter. A stillborn infant with syphilis often has a macerated appearance, with a collapsed skull and protuberant abdomen. Erythroblastosis involving the placenta has been seen more commonly among stillborn infants with congenital syphilis than in infected live-born infants with or without clinical findings of syphilis at birth [170]. Live-born or stillborn, the placenta of infants with congenital syphilis is often large, thick, and pale. Spirochetes may be identified in placental tissue using conventional staining, although they may be difficult to visualize [55,63,171]. Nucleic acid amplification methods have successfully identified *T. pallidum* genome in involved placental specimens [172]. Three histopathologic features commonly are seen (Fig. 16–3): enlarged and hypercellular villi, proliferative fetal vascular changes, and acute and chronic inflammation of the villi [173,174]. The inflamed villi become enlarged and hypercellular and often have bullous projections [63,171]; these larger villi, with respect to the amount of blood in the capillaries, are the cause of the pallor [174]. In addition, an increased amount of connective tissue surrounds the capillaries and makes up the stroma.

The umbilical cord may exhibit significant inflammation with abscess-like foci of necrosis located within Wharton jelly, centered around the umbilical vessels resulting in what is termed *necrotizing funisitis* [175]. Macroscopically, the umbilical cord resembles a "barber's pole"; the edematous portions have a spiral striped zone of red and pale blue discoloration, interspersed with

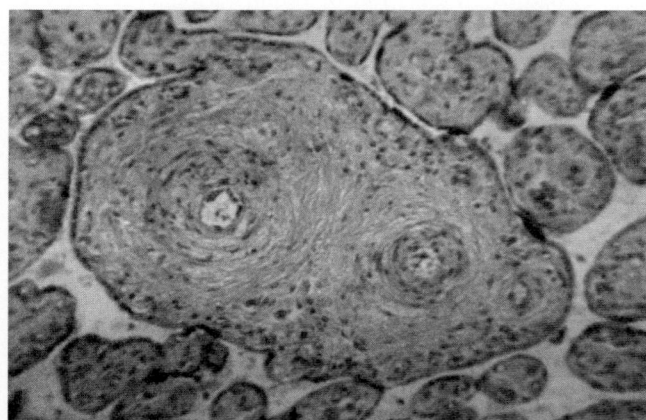

FIGURE 16–3 Photomicrograph revealing cytoarchitectural changes seen in congenital syphilis of the placenta. The chorionic villi are enlarged and contain dense laminated connective tissue, and the capillaries distributed throughout the villi are compressed by this connective tissue proliferation. (Hematoxylin and eosin stain; magnification 450×.) *(Courtesy of CDC/Susan Lindsley; 1971; Public Health Image Library #2347.)*

streaks of chalky white [174,176,177]. Histochemical staining and nucleic acid amplification approaches have shown spirochetes within the wall of the umbilical vessels [178]. Given these typical findings, placental and umbilical cord histopathology should be performed on every case of suspected syphilis, especially if the placenta is unexpectedly large.* Sheffield and colleagues [174] showed that the addition of histologic evaluation to conventional diagnostic evaluations improved the detection rate for congenital syphilis from 67% to 89% in live-born infants and 91% to 97% in stillborn infants.

The basic architecture of the fetal and infant tissue involved influences the ultimate pattern of macropathologic and micropathologic findings. The deposition of collagen around arteries of the spleen produces a typical onion-skin appearance, and liver and spleen are enlarged secondary to fibrosis [180].

A divergence of opinion still exists regarding the nature and precise extent of hepatic involvement in congenital syphilis. The traditional view has been that diffuse interstitial inflammation is present and can progress to disrupt the normal hepatic architecture by extensive scarring. Oppenheimer and Hardy [180] found that 15 of 16 livers from infants who died before 9 weeks of age were abnormal; lesions varied considerably in severity, but included inflammation in the interstitial stroma and perivascular network, especially in the area of the portal triads, with diffuse hepatitis and excessive extramedullary hematopoiesis [180]. Wright and Berry [181] found that 50 of 59 sections of livers from stillborn infants stained with hematoxylin and eosin were histologically normal, although silver stains revealed heavy infiltration with treponemes. The discrepancies in the observations of these studies may be related to the different ages of the patients and the severity of the infections. The patients described by Wright and Berry [181] were up to 1 year old. Gummata have rarely been described in the liver of infants with congenital syphilis; cirrhosis also seems to be uncommon [180]. As a result of liver and spleen fibrosis, extensive extramedullary hematopoiesis often accompanies congenital syphilis.

The gastrointestinal tract shows a pattern of mononuclear cell infiltration in the mucosa and submucosa, with subsequent thickening owing to the ensuing fibrosis. This pattern is most prominent in the small bowel [180,182,183]. An intense pancreatitis is often present, with a perivascular inflammatory infiltrate, obliteration of ductules and acini, reduction in the number of islets, and extensive fibrosis [180].

Renal involvement seems to be the consequence of injury to the glomeruli by immune complex deposition [159], just as has been described for the glomerulitis of secondary syphilis in adults [158]. An epimembranous glomerulopathy [184] is common and is associated with two different forms of immune complex injury, one involving complement deposition in addition to IgA, IgM, and IgG and the other involving immune complexes without complement deposition along the basement membrane [159]. A perivascular inflammatory infiltrate, consisting of plasma cells and lymphocytes involving the interstitial tissues, is prominent. The visceral and parietal epithelial cells of the glomeruli are swollen and increased in number. Increased matrix, collagen, and cells broaden axial regions in each tuft. Numerous electron-dense nodular deposits are noted on the epithelial aspect of the thickened glomerular basement membrane [159,184]. Elution studies have shown the presence of antitreponemal antibodies in the eluate and of treponemal antigen in the eluted sections [185]. A seemingly more rare proliferative glomerulonephritis also has been described, with mesangioendothelial proliferation and crescent formation [186].

Pneumonia alba of congenital syphilis is characterized by yellow-white, heavy, firm, and grossly enlarged lungs [123]. A marked increase in the amount of connective tissue in the interalveolar septa and the interstitium associated with collapse and loss of alveolar spaces explains the increased weight and density of the lung. This obliterative fibrosis of the lung is now reported only rarely [180].

Widespread involvement of bones is characteristic of congenital syphilis. Radiographs of long bones show evidence of osteochondritis and periostitis, especially in the long bones and ribs. Osteochondritis is recognized grossly by the presence of a moderate and irregular yellow line in the zone of provisional calcification. The trabeculae are irregular, discontinuous, and variable in size and shape. The excessive fibrosis occurring at the osseous-cartilaginous junction is termed *syphilitic granulation tissue* and contains numerous blood vessels surrounded by the inflammatory infiltrate [123]. The characteristic saw-toothed appearance, produced by irregularity in the provisional zone of calcification, corresponding to an irregularity in growth of capillaries, has been described historically, but is now uncommonly found in radiographs [187]. Small islands of cartilage may persist in the ossified bone [180]. A subperiosteal deposit of osteoid, which can completely encircle the shaft of the long bone, is a feature of periostitis [162]. An associated osteomyelitis (osteitis) usually is present and when it involves the long bones is called *diaphysitis* [188]. Microscopically, an inflammatory infiltrate with erosion of the trabeculae and prominent fibrosis is seen [187]. In the skull, the periosteal reaction eventually can lead to the radiographic feature of frontal bossing. The basic process of the osseous disturbance seems to involve a failure to convert cartilage in the normal sequence to mature bone. Controversy about the pathogenesis of these bone changes has been ongoing for years. One view is that the changes are specific results of local infection by the spirochete; the other is that they represent nonspecific trophic changes on endochondral bone formation caused by severe generalized disease. The fact that they heal without specific antibiotic therapy tends to favor the latter view [158].

The skin shows vesicular or bullous lesions, which have fluid rich in treponemes. Guarner and associates [182] reported that a constant feature throughout the dermal tissues was concentric macrophage infiltrate around vessels, giving an onion-skin appearance.

The neuropathologic features of congenital syphilis are comparable with those of acquired syphilis except that the parenchymatous processes (general paresis, tabes dorsalis) that were infrequently described in the older literature

---

now are extremely rare. Meningeal involvement is apparent as a discoloration and thickening of the basilar meninges [123], especially around the brainstem and the optic chiasm. Microscopically, endarteritis typically is present, depending on the severity and chronicity of the infection and on the blood vessels involved. Various degrees of neuronal injury can ensue. As the infection resolves, fibrosis can occur, with formation of adhesions that obliterate the subarachnoid space, leading to an obstructive hydrocephalus or to various cranial nerve palsies. Interstitial inflammation and fibrosis of the anterior lobe of the pituitary gland, sometimes accompanied by focal necrosis, also have been reported among infants with congenital syphilis [189]. The posterior lobe remains unaffected. An evolving anterior pituitary gumma was noted at autopsy in a 3-day-old infant with congenital syphilis that did not respond to treatment [169].

CLINICAL MANIFESTATIONS

Because of its protean clinical manifestations, syphilis, whether acquired or congenital, has been described as the "great imitator" [10,11]. A high index of suspicion is needed for the clinician to consider syphilis in the pregnant woman and the newborn infant.

SYPHILIS IN PREGNANCY

Two caveats should be heeded by the clinician caring for pregnant women: (1) Any ulcer, regardless of location, that is indurated and indolent and fails to heal within 2 weeks warrants exclusion of syphilis as a diagnosis. (2) Any generalized skin eruption, regardless of its morphology, should be viewed as secondary (disseminated) syphilis until proved otherwise [190].

Pregnancy has no known effect on the clinical course of acquired syphilis. Untreated syphilis can profoundly affect pregnancy outcome, however [175,178,191–193]. One of the most common sequelae of untreated syphilis during pregnancy is spontaneous abortion during the second and early third trimesters [194]. Untreated maternal syphilis can result in preterm delivery, perinatal death, and congenital infection (see later). Antenatal ultrasonography can be a helpful adjunct in the diagnosis of fetal syphilis; hydramnios, fetal hydrops, enlarged placenta, hepatosplenomegaly, and bowel dilation have been described [190,195]. Ultrasonography performed in pregnant women with early syphilis has suggested that fetal hepatosplenomegaly can be an important early indicator of congenital infection.

Whether the patient is pregnant or not, it is characteristic for the course of untreated acquired syphilis to progress through three or four stages over many years. Most clinical definitions of acquired *T. pallidum* infection categorize early syphilis as including primary and secondary syphilis and early latent syphilis with a latency of less than 1 year [78] or less than 2 years (WHO) after infection. Late syphilis consists of late latent, tertiary, and—depending on nomenclature—quaternary syphilis (or metalues). This classification is an oversimplification and does not take into account the many variations in signs and symptoms in relation to timing of infection in any particular individual [196].

Primary Syphilis in Pregnancy

The time between infection with syphilis and the start of the first symptom ranges from 10 to 90 days (average 21 days), at which point a dark red macule or papule develops at the site of inoculation and rapidly progresses to an erosion called a *chancre*. It usually occurs as a single lesion, but there may be multiple lesions [197]. The chancre increases in size to 0.5 to 2 cm over 1 to 2 weeks until a typical, indolent, well-circumscribed, flat ulcer with a yellow-coated base and an indurated, non-undermined wall results. Edema and bilateral painless lymphadenopathy follow. Chancres often are unrecognized in women because they cause no symptoms and because their location on the labia minora, within the vagina, or on the cervix or perineum makes detection difficult. As a result, only 30% to 40% of infected women are diagnosed in the primary stage [73,110]. Two thirds of extragenital chancres occur orally or periorally; most of the rest occur perianally. Chancres rarely occur on the lips, tongue, tonsil, nipple, or fingers. Because a chancre can appear 1 to 3 weeks before a serologic response, direct detection of the pathogen (e.g., by dark-field microscope) is vital in this phase of the disease [198]. The chancre lasts 3 to 8 weeks, and then heals without treatment. The mechanism for healing is obscure; it is believed that local immunity is partly responsible because secondary lesions appear during or after the regression of the primary one. If adequate treatment is not administered, however, the infection progresses to the secondary stage.

Secondary Syphilis in Pregnancy

An infected woman may experience secondary disease, characterized by fever, fatigue, weight loss, anorexia, pharyngitis, myalgia, arthralgia, and generalized lymphadenopathy 2 to 10 weeks after the primary lesions. These constitutional symptoms are accompanied by various exanthems and alopecia. Because of the protean clinical manifestations, secondary syphilis is often misdiagnosed [199–201]. Lesions of secondary syphilis result from the dissemination of *T. pallidum* from syphilitic chancres, and the term *disseminated syphilis* probably would be more appropriate [202].

The rash of secondary syphilis [196], often the first clinical manifestation noticed, develops symmetrically in approximately 75% of untreated subjects and appears as rough, red, or reddish brown spots (syphilids); they occur most often on the palms, soles, and trunk, where they tend to follow skin lines. Rashes with a different appearance may occur on any part of the body, however, and pustular, papular, lichenoid, nodular, ulcerative, plaquelike, annular, and even urticarial and granulomatous forms can occur. The vesiculobullous eruption that is common in congenital syphilis rarely occurs in adults. Contrary to a widely held belief, the exanthema can itch, especially in dark-skinned patients. Often the rash is very faint and not recognized at all. Rashes associated with secondary syphilis can already appear as the chancre is healing (the chancre is still present in approximately 15%) or several weeks after the chancre has healed.

Various mucosal manifestations can be of diagnostic importance and are present in one third to one half of patients. Mucosal plaques (representing superficial mucosal erosions) and syphilitic angina are the most frequent and can involve the oral cavity, vulva, vagina, or cervix. Localized enanthems or perlèche-like lesions are also possible. Expansive, smooth lesions and gray-white plaques are rare. Erythematous, moist plaques can occur in warm, moist intertriginous regions where initial papules enlarge and become exuberant, raised, wartlike lesions termed *condylomata lata* (often confused with condyloma acuminata, which are caused by human papillomavirus infection). Papules of the scalp can lead to "moth-eaten" alopecia. This hair loss can occasionally also affect eyebrows and eyelashes. All secondary lesions of the skin and mucous membranes are highly infectious [196].

Generalized lymphadenopathy, fever, malaise, splenomegaly, sore throat, headache, and arthralgia (with a noticeable nocturnal pattern) can be present [198]. Other organ involvement may include gastritis, hepatitis [203,204], glomerulonephritis or nephrotic syndrome [157,205], periostitis [206–208], uveitis, iritis, and meningitis [202]. *T. pallidum* has been isolated from the cerebrospinal fluid (CSF) of 30% of adults with untreated secondary syphilis [80]. The signs and symptoms of secondary syphilis usually resolve with or without treatment. Without treatment, however, the infection progresses to the latent and possibly late stages of disease [70].

Latent Syphilis in Pregnancy

Subclinical or latent syphilis is defined as the period after infection when patients are seroreactive, but show no clinical manifestations of disease. This latent phase can last for years [193,209]. This latent period is sometimes interrupted during the first few (<4) years by recurrences of symptoms of secondary syphilis. Treponemes can still be present in the blood intermittently and be passed across the placenta to the fetus during latent syphilis in a pregnant woman. The first year after infection is considered early latent, and the subsequent period is late latent syphilis. This classification is based on the time period of communicability (not just to the fetus), which is higher in the first year after infection compared with later time points [50]. If the duration of syphilis infection cannot be determined, the disease is classified as latent syphilis of unknown duration. Approximately 60% of untreated patients in the late latent stage continue to have an asymptomatic course, whereas 30% to 40% develop symptoms of late or tertiary disease. Progression of disease from late latent to late symptomatic syphilis usually is prevented if appropriate antimicrobial therapy is given at this stage [50].

Late Stages (Tertiary Disease) in Pregnancy

Knowledge about the clinical appearances of late stages of acquired syphilis comes from two prospective studies and one retrospective study [10]. Initiated in 1891, a Swedish study explored the hypothesis that the therapy of that time (mercury-containing antimicrobials and other heavy metals) caused more illness than the untreated infection [162]. This study followed approximately 2000 patients with early syphilis for more than 20 years and concluded that about one third of the patients developed tertiary complications if untreated. Mortality from untreated

syphilis was 8% to 14%. In 1932, the U.S. Public Health Service initiated the infamous Tuskegee study, in which 412 African-American men with latent syphilis were monitored without treatment for 40 years, with 204 matched uninfected control subjects. After 15 years, three quarters of the infected men showed evidence of tertiary syphilis, 50% of which were cardiovascular complications [210]. A single retrospective study examined autopsy records of 77 patients with untreated tertiary syphilis. Of these, 83% had cardiovascular complications, 9% had gummatous involvement, and 8% had neurosyphilis [211].

The gummata of tertiary disease are nonprogressive, localized nodules that can have central necrosis. Because these lesions are relatively quiescent, the term *benign tertiary syphilis* often is used. Spirochetes are extremely sparse or absent. The gummatous reaction primarily is a pronounced immunologic reaction of the host.

Approximately 15% of untreated infected subjects develop neurosyphilis in the tertiary stage, but in persons infected with HIV manifestations of neurosyphilis can occur at any stage. Neurosyphilis may be asymptomatic or, if symptomatic, may have various manifestations. Classic manifestations include paralytic dementia, tabes dorsalis, amyotrophic lateral sclerosis, meningovascular syphilis, seizures, optic atrophy, and gummatous changes of the spinal cord. Neurosyphilis may resemble virtually any other neurologic disease. Cardiovascular involvement of tertiary syphilis most commonly involves the great vessels of the heart, in which syphilitic aortic and pulmonary arteritis develop. One of the complications of this involvement is aortic regurgitation. The inflammatory reaction also may cause stenosis of the coronary ostia, with resulting angina, myocardial insufficiency, and death [212].

ACQUIRED SYPHILIS IN CHILDREN

Most recognized syphilitic disease in children is congenital (see next). Acquired syphilis in prepubertal children seldom is reported and is assumed to resemble the clinical course of acquired syphilis in adulthood. Children with acquired syphilis should be assumed to have been infected through sexual abuse, unless another method of transmission can clearly be identified [213–217].

CONGENITAL SYPHILIS

The spectrum of congenital syphilis is similar in many ways to the spectrum of other congenital infections in which the infecting organism spreads hematogenously from the pregnant woman to involve the placenta and infect the fetus [168]. The extent of damage to the fetus presumably depends on the stage of development when infection occurs and the elapsed time before treatment is initiated. With infection early in pregnancy and in the absence of therapy, fetal demise with spontaneous abortion (often after the first trimester) or late-term stillbirth occurs in approximately 30% to 40% of cases, but premature delivery or neonatal death also can occur.* In liveborn infants, infection can be clinically recognizable or silent at birth (approximately two thirds of infected

---

*References 55, 72, 83, 162, 192, 218.

live-born infants are asymptomatic at birth, but then develop signs and symptoms sometimes decades later) [121].

The postnatal clinical course of congenitally acquired syphilis has been divided arbitrarily into early and late stages [10,121]. Clinical manifestations appearing within the first 2 years of life are designated early congenital syphilis, and manifestations occurring after this time are considered late congenital syphilis. The clinical manifestations of early congenital syphilis appear as a direct result of active infection with resulting inflammation. Infants can have hepatosplenomegaly, snuffles, lymphadenopathy, mucocutaneous lesions, osteochondritis and pseudoparalysis, edema, rash, hemolytic anemia, or thrombocytopenia, all of which usually appear within the first 2 to 8 weeks of life (Table 16–1). The clinical manifestations of late congenital syphilis represent the scars induced by initial lesions of early congenital syphilis or reactions to persistent and ongoing inflammation. These so-called stigmata of late congenital syphilis reflect the delayed expression of a prenatal insult in a fashion comparable with the occurrence of deafness beyond infancy that is related to congenital rubella. Manifestations of late congenital syphilis may involve the CNS, bones and joints, teeth, eyes, and skin; these manifestations may not become apparent until many years after birth (Table 16–2) [219–221].

Early Congenital Syphilis

After fetal infection occurs, any organ system can be affected because of widespread spirochetal dissemination. The diagnosis of early congenital syphilis should be considered in any infant who is born at less than 37 weeks of gestation with no other apparent explanation or if unexplained hydrops fetalis or an enlarged placenta is present.

TABLE 16–1   Clinical Manifestations of Early Congenital Syphilis*

Osteochondritis, periostitis
Snuffles, hemorrhagic rhinitis
Condylomata lata
Bullous lesions, palmar and plantar rash
Mucous patches
Hepatomegaly, splenomegaly
Jaundice
Nonimmune hydrops fetalis
Generalized lymphadenopathy
Central nervous system signs
Elevated cell count or protein in cerebrospinal fluid
Hematologic findings
Hemolytic anemia
Diffuse intravascular coagulation
Thrombocytopenia
Pneumonitis
Nephrotic syndrome
Placental villitis or vasculitis (unexplained enlarged placenta)
Intrauterine growth restriction

*Arranged in decreasing order of importance.
Data from Rathbun KC. Congenital syphilis: a proposal for improved surveillance, diagnosis and treatment. Sex Transm Dis 10:102, 1983.

TABLE 16–2   Clinical Manifestations of Late Congenital Syphilis

Dentition	Hutchinson teeth, mulberry molars (Moon, Fournier)
Eye	Interstitial keratitis, healed chorioretinitis, secondary glaucoma (uveitis), corneal scarring
Ear	Eighth nerve deafness
Nose and face	"Saddle nose," protuberant mandible
Skin	Rhagades
Central nervous system	Mental retardation, arrested hydrocephalus, convulsive disorders, optic nerve atrophy, juvenile general paresis, cranial nerve palsies
Bones and joints	"Saber shins," Higouménakis sign, Clutton joints

In infancy, failure to move an extremity (pseudoparalysis of Parrot), persistent rhinitis (snuffles), a maculopapular or papulosquamous rash (especially in the diaper area), unexplained jaundice, hepatosplenomegaly or generalized lymphadenopathy, or anemia or thrombocytopenia of uncertain cause should raise suspicion of congenital syphilis (see Table 16–1). The abnormal physical and laboratory findings in early congenital syphilis are varied and unpredictable. The onset of most clinical findings of early congenital syphilis is between birth and about 3 months of age, with most cases occurring within the first 8 weeks of age [159,178,180,187,222–225].

Intrauterine Growth Restriction

Intrauterine growth restriction may be present at birth [211]. The effect of syphilis on the growth of the fetus in utero is likely to be related to the timing and severity of the fetal infection. In a carefully performed quantitative morphologic study, Naeye [226] showed that syphilitic infection in utero did not seem to have a significant effect on the growth of the fetus, as manifested by a study of 36 perinatal deaths associated with congenital syphilis. Naeye's findings were similar to his previous results that showed a relative lack of effect on fetal growth from toxoplasmosis, contrasting with the intrauterine growth restriction associated with rubella and cytomegalovirus infections [226]. Case reports have indicated, however, that newborns with congenital syphilis were small for their gestational age [227]. Whether small size for gestational age is the result of syphilitic infection or other cofactors (e.g., use of illicit intravenous drugs by the mother) [228] that affect fetal growth is unknown. Historically, a severely infected infant with congenital syphilis has been described as a premature infant with marasmus, a pot belly, "old man" facies, and withered skin [162]. The degree of such extreme early-onset failure to thrive has been correlated with the frequently encountered pathologic finding of intense pancreatitis and inflammation of the gastrointestinal tract [180]. Rectal bleeding resulting from syphilitic ileitis with ulcer formation and associated intestinal obstruction has also been reported to be linked to this appearance [159]. Finally, involvement of the anterior pituitary gland in congenital syphilis can manifest as persistent hypoglycemia beyond the early neonatal period and, through such endocrine abnormalities, contribute to the failure to thrive [189].

Mucocutaneous Manifestations

Mucous patches may be seen in the mouth and genitalia [211,229]. Mucous patches in the mouth are more prevalent in infants with severe systemic disease [230]. After the first 2 or 3 months of life, condylomata can arise on such affected mucous membranes or other areas of skin affected by moisture or friction (e.g., the perioral area, especially the nares and the angles of the mouth, and the perianal area) [231,232]. These highly infective areas are flat or wartlike and moist. Condylomata can be single or multiple and frequently occur in the absence of other signs of infection. Rhinitis, coryza, or snuffles (Fig. 16–4) indicates involvement of the upper respiratory tract mucosa. This manifestation usually appears in the 1st week of life and seldom later than the 3rd month. It was reported in two thirds of patients in the early literature [233], but now seems to be less common [229]. A mucus discharge develops, with character similar to that of discharge in upper respiratory tract infections, but is more severe and persists longer than in the common cold. The discharge can become progressively more profuse and occasionally is blood-tinged. Secondary bacterial infection can occur, causing the discharge to become purulent. If ulceration of the nasal mucosa is sufficiently deep and involves the nasal cartilage, a saddle-nose deformity, one of the later stigmata of congenital syphilis, can result. Snuffles also has been associated with laryngitis and an aphonic cry [229,234].

A syphilitic rash appears in 70% of infected infants [235]. It may be apparent at birth or develop during the first few weeks of life, usually 1 to 2 weeks after the onset of rhinitis [229,234]. The typical skin eruption consists of small, oval, copper-red maculopapular lesions (reminiscent of secondary acquired syphilitic lesions) that subsequently become coppery brown [232]. The hands and

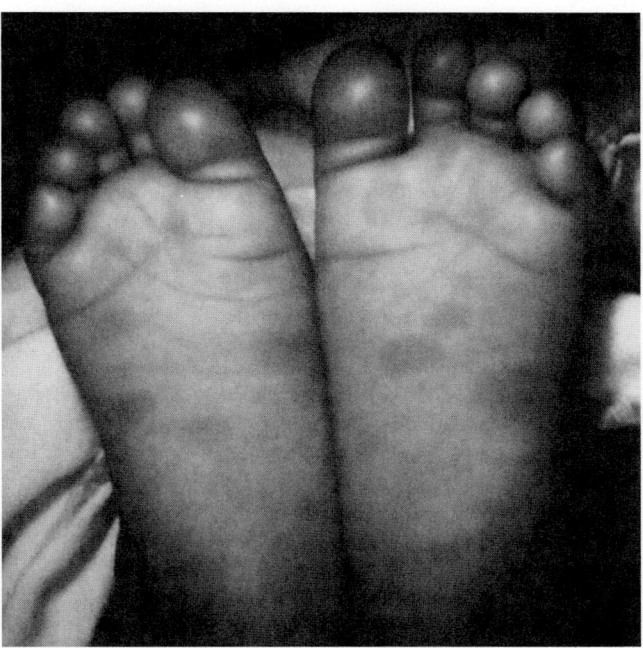

FIGURE 16–5 This newborn presented with symptoms of congenital syphilis that included lesions on the soles of both feet. *(Courtesy of CDC; 1970; Public Health Image Library #4148.)*

feet often are most severely affected. As the rash changes color, very fine superficial desquamation or scaling can occur, particularly on the palms and soles (Fig. 16–5). If the rash is present at birth, it often is widely disseminated and bullous and is called *pemphigus syphiliticus*; it typically involves the palms and soles (Fig. 16–6) [232]. The lesions vary in size and can contain a cloudy hemorrhagic fluid that teems with treponemes. When these bullae rupture,

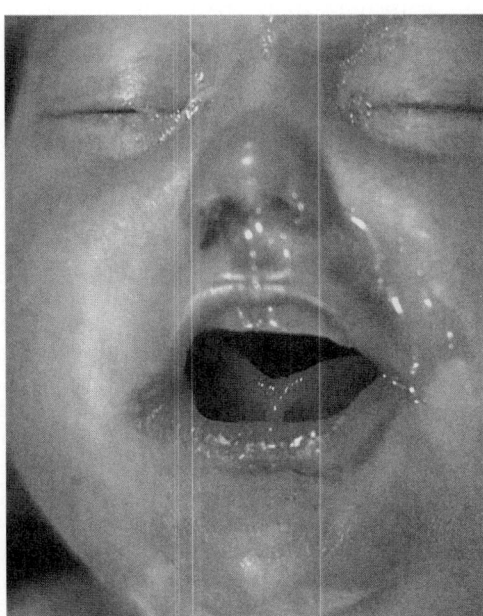

FIGURE 16–4 The face of a newborn infant with congenital syphilis displaying snuffles. *(Courtesy of CDC/Dr. Norman Cole; 1963; Public Health Image library #2246.)*

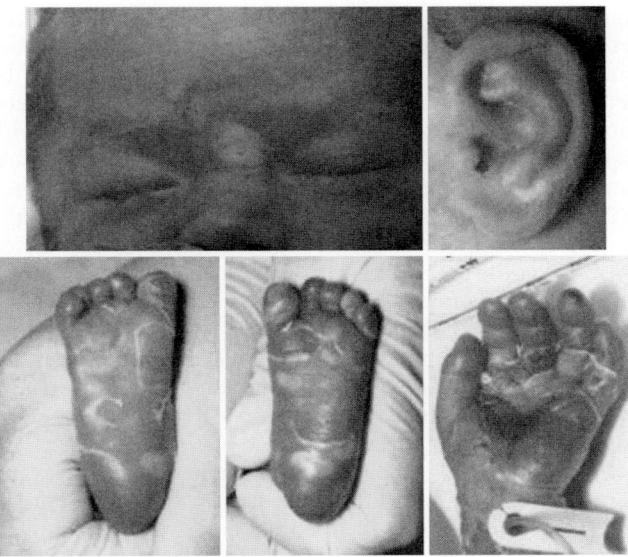

FIGURE 16–6 This newborn infant with congenital syphilis displays multiple, punched-out, pale, blistered lesions on the ear and the bridge of the nose; also shown is an associated desquamation of palms and plantar surfaces of the feet. *(From Battin M, Voss L. Beware of infants with respiratory distress, rash, and hepatomegaly at birth: a case of congenital syphilis. N Z Med J 120:U2448, 2007.)*

they leave a denuded area that can undergo extensive maceration and crusting. Pemphigus syphiliticus evolves over 1 to 3 weeks and is followed by desquamation and crusting. As the rash fades, the lesions become coppery or dusky red, and pigmentation may persist.

Other maculopapular types of eruptions are also found in early congenital syphilis. The lesions can be annular or circinate or can have the appearance of any other kind of lesion seen in acquired secondary syphilis. Petechial lesions can result from thrombocytopenia. Generalized edema can also be present [229,236] as a result of hypoproteinemia related to renal or hepatic disease. Ectodermal changes in syphilitic infants include suppuration and exfoliation of the nails, loss of hair and eyebrows, choroiditis, and iritis [237]. Fissures develop around the lips, nares, and anus. They bleed readily and heal with scarring. A cluster of scars radiating around the mouth is termed *rhagades* and is a characteristic of late congenital syphilis. Comparable eruptions also can be found in other body folds or intertriginous areas, but are considered to be more characteristic of the later stage of early congenital syphilis. Healing, with possible desquamation and crusting of the various skin lesions, occurs over 1 to 3 weeks [238,239]. All mucocutaneous lesions and discharges contain abundant spirochetes and are contagious via direct contact [233].

Hepatomegaly, Hepatitis, Splenomegaly, and Lymphadenopathy

Hepatomegaly is present in nearly all infants with congenital syphilis and may occur in the absence of splenomegaly, although the reverse is not true (in contrast to congenital cytomegalovirus infection) [229]. Hepatomegaly and ascites are attributed largely to heart failure, but may be caused in part by hepatic infection and extramedullary hematopoiesis. Maternal treatment can interrupt this progression, but is less likely to be successful when fetal hepatomegaly and ascites have developed [240]. Hepatitis seems to be an early manifestation and can be detected as elevation of transaminase levels even in fetal blood. Neonatal syphilitic hepatitis is associated with visible spirochetes on biopsy specimen of liver tissue. Jaundice, which has been recorded in 33% of patients [229], can be caused by syphilitic hepatitis or by the hemolytic component of the disease and can be associated with elevation predominantly of direct or indirect bilirubin levels. Jaundice may be the only manifestation of the disease. The prothrombin time may be delayed [241]. Hepatic dysfunction in the form of elevated serum aminotransferases, alkaline phosphatase, and direct bilirubin initially can worsen with initiation of penicillin therapy and can persist for several weeks [241–243].

Splenomegaly is present in half of cases, and generalized nonsuppurative adenopathy, including epitrochlear sites, is present in some cases [211,229]. The lymph nodes themselves can be 1 cm in diameter and typically are nontender and firm. If an infant has palpable epitrochlear nodes, the diagnosis of syphilis is highly probable [121]. Generalized enlargement of the lymph nodes is rare in neonates and young infants with congenital syphilis.

Hematologic Manifestations

Anemia, thrombocytopenia, leukopenia, or leukocytosis are common findings in congenital syphilis [222]. A characteristic feature in the immediate newborn period is that of a Coombs-negative hemolytic anemia. The hemolytic process is often accompanied by cryoglobulinemia, immune complex formation, and macroglobulinemia. The hemolysis, similar to the liver disease, is refractory to therapy and may persist for weeks. After the neonatal period, chronic nonhemolytic anemia can develop, accentuated by the usual physiologic anemia of infancy [236,244]. Other findings include polychromasia and erythroblastemia. This pattern of anemia and erythropoietic response historically led to confusion with erythroblastosis fetalis [162]. Although the leukocyte count usually falls within the normal range [236], leukopenia, leukocytosis, and a leukemoid reaction all can occur [229]. Lymphocytosis and monocytosis may be features. Thrombocytopenia, related to decreased platelet survival rather than to insufficient production of platelets, often is present and can be the only manifestation of congenital infection. Hemophagocytosis has been described and may play an important role in the pathogenesis of anemia and thrombocytopenia [245]. Hydrops fetalis also is a manifestation of congenital syphilis in newborns [246]. Paroxysmal nocturnal hemoglobinuria is a late manifestation of congenital syphilis [247,248]. Hydrops fetalis, or diffuse edema, results from anemia-related congestive heart failure, and a negative Coombs test in the setting of hydrops strongly suggests congenital syphilis [246].

Bone Involvement

Bone findings [249] are a frequent manifestation of early congenital syphilis and occur in 60% to 80% of untreated cases. It may be the only abnormality seen in infants born to mothers with untreated syphilis and usually occurs as multiple and symmetric lesions. Overall, bone abnormalities are due to periostitis and cortical demineralization mostly in the metaphyseal and diaphyseal portions of long bones and osteochondritis, which affects the joints, primarily knees, ankles, wrists, and elbows. Characteristically, bone involvement in periostitis is widespread; the femur and humerus are affected most often, but the cranium, spine, and ribs also are affected [249]. The earliest and most characteristic changes are found in the metaphysis, with sparing of the epiphysis [249]. The changes are nonspecific and variable, ranging from radiopaque bands to actual fragmentation and apparent destruction with mottled areas of radiolucency.

Frequently, an enhanced zone of provisional calcification (radiopaque band) is associated with osteoporosis immediately beneath the dense zone. Variations of these paretic changes are seen, including peripheral (lateral) paresis only and alternating bands of density sandwiching a paretic zone [188]; this may appear smooth or serrated. The serrated appearance is known as *Wegner sign* and represents points of calcified cartilage along the nutrient cartilage canal. Although this sign now is uncommon, it can still be seen on radiographs of stillborn infants with congenital syphilis. A zone of rarefaction at the metaphysis may also be seen, which represents syphilitic granulation tissue containing a few scattered calcified remnants and a mass of connective tissue displaying areas of perivascular infiltration of small round cells. Irregular areas of increased density and rarefaction produce the moth-eaten appearance on the radiograph.

The demineralization and osseous destruction of the upper medial tibial metaphysis is called Wimberger sign (Fig. 16–7) [234]. Rarely, similar changes may occur at the upper ends of the humeri. Epiphyseal separation may occur as a result of a fracture of the brittle layer of calcified cartilage. Irregular periosteal thickening also is common. The changes usually are present at birth, but may appear in the first few weeks of life. Focal areas of patchy cortical radiolucency with spreading of the medullary canal and irregularity of the endosteal and periosteal aspects of the cortex can be seen on radiographs. In severe cases, the radiolucent areas that probably represent a growth arrest abnormality can appear as columns, giving a "celery stick" appearance of alternating bands of longitudinal translucency and relative density [234]. The inflammatory reaction in the diaphysis stimulates the periosteum to lay down new bone. The single or multiple layers of periosteal new bone extend along the cortex of the entire diaphysis. In contrast to the other two forms of osseous involvement (metaphyseal dystrophy and

osteitis-like dystrophy), diaphyseal abnormalities are less often present at birth. Single bone involvement is unique, but solitary involvement of the radius has been described [250].

Solomon and Rosen [251,252] reported that in more than one third of 112 infants with congenital syphilis, radiographic findings were consistent with trauma of bone made more fragile by syphilitic infection. Although the above-described findings of periostitis require about 16 weeks for radiographic diagnosis, osteochondritic events in the major joints can be evident radiographically 5 weeks after fetal infection has occurred [253]. Involvement of the metacarpals, metatarsals, or proximal phalanges of the hand is rare. Dactylitis appears radiologically as a spindle-shaped enlargement of the bone and can occur from the ages of 3 to 24 months [254]. Unusual manifestations also have been reported. A case of syphilitic arthritis of the hip and elbow in association with osteomyelitis of the femur and humerus has been described in the immediate newborn period [255,256].

Obstetric radiography allows for in utero diagnosis of fetal syphilis by showing periosteal cloaking [257]. Maternal treatment has been associated with radiologic resolution of these lesions. Bone scans have been performed in very few patients; they reveal diffuse abnormalities when performed, but such scans are neither helpful nor recommended [258–260]. Because of their frequency and early appearance, the radiographic changes in the bones of osteochondritis and periostitis are of diagnostic value [187]. The correlation between the clinical and the radiologic findings is poor, however, inasmuch as other areas of bone involvement can look more severely affected on radiographs even though no clinical signs suggest their presence.

Most bone lesions are not clinically discernible except in pseudoparalysis of Parrot [261,262], in which the bony changes or a superimposed fracture, or both, lead to pain, causing the infant to refuse to move the involved extremity. Clinically, it can manifest as irritability in an infant a few weeks old who does not move one of the limbs [227]. Upper extremities are affected more frequently than lower extremities, and unilateral involvement predominates. This clinical picture can mimic Erb palsy, but rarely is present at birth. Cases where pseudoparalysis of Parrot has been the only presenting symptom in a newborn with congenital syphilis have been described and should not be missed [263]. Bony involvement usually resolves spontaneously (i.e., even without therapy) during the first 6 months of life [211,227,261,264].

Nervous System and Ocular Manifestations

Neurologic manifestations, although well documented in the earlier literature, are now less frequently reported [265]. Without therapy, approximately 15% of infants with congenital syphilis develop findings such as meningitis, meningeal irritation, bulging fontanelles, cranial nerve palsies, seizures, hydrocephalus, or abnormal pituitary function [211].

There are two primary clinical presentations of neurosyphilis, although overlap may be considerable. Acute syphilitic leptomeningitis appears during the first year of

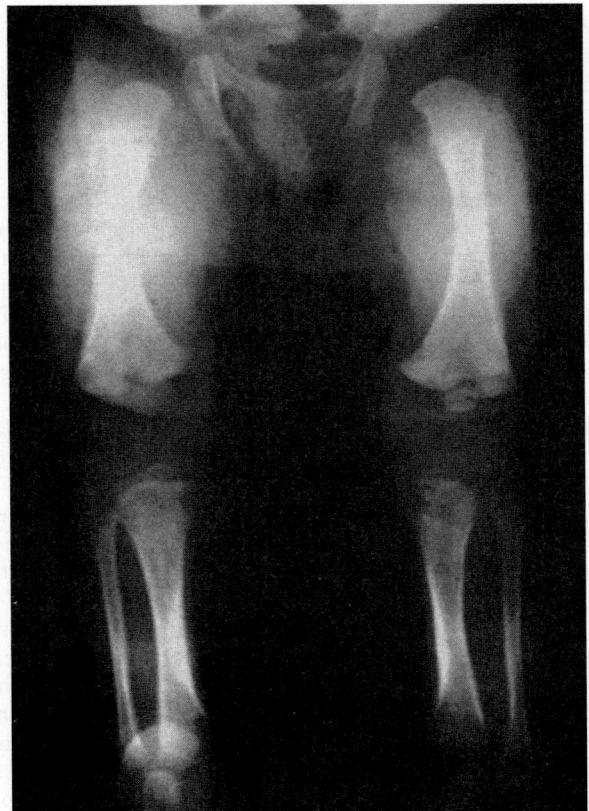

FIGURE 16–7 Anteroposterior film of both lower extremities of a 1-month-old infant with congenital syphilis, showing demineralization and osseous destruction of the proximal medial tibial metaphysis bilaterally (Wimberger sign).

life, usually between 3 and 6 months of age. Signs can suggest acute bacterial meningitis, including a stiff neck, progressive vomiting, Kernig sign, bulging fontanelles, separation of the suture, and hydrocephalus [265]. In contrast to this clinical picture, CSF reveals abnormalities consistent with an aseptic meningitis, with approximately 200 mononuclear cells/mm^3, a modest increase in protein (50 to 200 mg/dL), and a normal glucose value. The CSF Venereal Disease Research Laboratory (VDRL) test is positive. This is the one form of CNS involvement that responds to specific therapy [211,234,265].

Chronic meningovascular syphilis generally manifests toward the end of the 1st year of life and can have a protracted course, resulting in progressive hydrocephalus, cranial nerve palsies or vascular lesions of the brain, and gradual intellectual deterioration [265]. The hydrocephalus is of low grade, progressive, and communicating as a result of obstruction in the basilar cisternae. Cranial nerve palsies and seizures can complicate the picture. The seventh cranial nerve most often is involved, but cranial nerves III, IV, and VI also can be affected. Optic atrophy can be preceded by papilledema.

Various cerebrovascular syndromes have been described, but they are rare. Cerebral infarction results from syphilitic endarteritis and can occur between the 1st and 2nd years of life, commonly manifesting as acute hemiplegia. Convulsions frequently complicate this clinical picture. In addition, involvement of the pituitary gland in congenital syphilis is common, occurring in approximately 40% of autopsy cases, and consists of interstitial inflammation and fibrosis with gumma formation in the anterior lobe. Clinical disease in affected infants is manifested by persistent hypoglycemia and diabetes insipidus [189,266].

Because of the wide range of normal values for CSF protein, red blood cells, and white blood cells (WBCs) in the neonatal period, it has been difficult to define unequivocally the proportion of infants with congenital syphilis who have abnormalities of these laboratory values. Current consensus [83] identifies an abnormal CSF WBC count in infants being evaluated for possible congenital syphilis as greater than 25 cells/mm^3 and abnormal protein as greater than 150 mg/dL (>170 mg/dL if the infant is premature).

A reactive CSF VDRL test is considered to be specific for neurosyphilis in older children and adults. In neonates, the significance of a reactive CSF VDRL test is suspect, however, because maternal nontreponemal IgG antibodies can pass from maternal serum to fetal and neonatal serum and then diffuse into the CSF. Children may fail to have a reactive VDRL test on initial examination and still develop signs of neurosyphilis later. Using rabbit infectivity testing, which involves the inoculation of CSF into rabbits to determine the presence of the spirochete in the CSF specimen, Michelow and coworkers [267] found that CNS invasion with *T. pallidum* occurs in 41% of infants who have clinical, laboratory, or radiographic abnormalities of congenital syphilis. None of these infants had clinical signs of neurologic disease. When compared with isolation of spirochetes in CSF by rabbit inoculation, the sensitivity and specificity in CSF of a reactive VDRL test, elevated WBC count, and elevated protein were 54% and 90%

for reactive VDRL test, 38% and 88% for elevated WBC count, and 56% and 78% for elevated protein. CSF findings consistent with neurosyphilis are very common findings among infants with other clinical signs of congenital syphilis and are present in approximately 8% of asymptomatic infants born to mothers with untreated early syphilis [190,211,267].

Involvement of the eye in early congenital syphilis is rare. Chorioretinitis, salt-and-pepper fundus, glaucoma, uveitis, cataract [268], and chancres of the eyelid have been described [162]. Involvement by syphilis leads to a granular appearance of the fundus; pigmentary patches of various shapes and colors are seen in the periphery of the retina [162]. Young infants rarely manifest the signs of photophobia and diminution in vision that occur in older patients. Congenital glaucoma can occur and should be a diagnostic consideration in the presence of blepharospasm, cloudy cornea, enlarged cornea (diameter >12 mm), and excessive tearing. Inflammation of the uveal tract (including the iris and ciliary body anteriorly and the choroid posteriorly) affects the retina because of the close anatomic relationship of the cornea to the structures of the uveal tract [162]. Consequently, chorioretinitis rather than uveitis is the more commonly diagnosed ocular problem in infancy [268]. Rarely, a chancre of the eyelid appears 4 weeks after birth, presumably resulting from recently developed syphilitic lesions of the maternal genitalia [162].

Other Findings

Fever has been reported to accompany other signs of congenital syphilis in infants beyond the immediate newborn period [242,269]. Pneumonia alba, a fibrosing pneumonitis, occurs in a few cases in the developed world, but still represents a frequent finding in developing countries [121]. The classic radiographic appearance is one of complete opacification of both lung fields. More commonly, a diffuse infiltrate involving all lung areas is seen on chest radiograph. At autopsy, pneumonia alba consists of a focal obliterative fibrosis with scarring and thickening of alveolar walls with loss of alveolar spaces. Follow-up evaluation of children who have recovered from congenital syphilis has shown that at least 10% may develop chronic pulmonary disease, particularly if they were premature and required mechanical ventilation [121].

The clinical picture of nephrotic syndrome may appear at 2 or 3 months of age, the predominant manifestation being generalized edema, including pretibial, scrotal, and periorbital areas, together with ascites [270–274]. Rarely, the infant can have hematuria with less severe proteinuria, but more profound azotemia, which suggests that a glomerulitis predominates. Myocarditis [180] has been found at autopsy in approximately 10% of infants who die, although the clinical significance of this finding is unclear. Gastrointestinal presentations include rectal bleeding owing to syphilitic ileitis, necrotizing enterocolitis, malabsorption secondary to fibrosis of the gastrointestinal tract, and fetal bowel dilation seen on antenatal ultrasonography. Some children with symptomatic congenital syphilis also may present with sepsis resulting from other bacteria, including *Escherichia coli*, group B streptococci, and *Yersinia* species, presumed to be secondary to the breakdown of the gastrointestinal mucosal barrier [223,275].

Late Congenital Syphilis

As noted earlier, the clinical manifestations of late congenital syphilis are stigmata that represent scars induced by the initial lesions of early congenital syphilis or reactions to persistent and ongoing inflammation (see Table 16–2). In patients older than 2 years, late congenital syphilis can be manifested by (1) the stigmata of the disorder that represent the scars of initial lesions or developmental changes induced by the early infection; (2) ongoing inflammation, although *T. pallidum* is not demonstrable; or (3) a persistently positive result on treponemal serologic tests for syphilis in the absence of apparent disease [78,83]. Treatment of neonates with congenital syphilis has nearly eliminated these consequences in developed countries, but late manifestations occur in approximately 40% of untreated survivors. Many of these manifestations do not seem to be reversible with antibiotic treatment [121,276].

Mucocutaneous Manifestations

An infrequent sign of late congenital syphilis is linear scars that become fissured or ulcerated, resulting in deeper scars called rhagades. These scars are located around body orifices, including the mouth, nostrils, genitalia, and anus [162]. The sequelae of syphilitic rhinitis include failure of the maxilla to grow fully, resulting in a concave configuration in the middle section of the face with relative protuberance of the mandible and an associated high palatal arch. Inflammation of the nasal mucosa can affect the cartilage, leading to destruction of the underlying bone and perforation of the nasal septum. The resulting depression of the roof of the septum gives the appearance of a saddle nose [162].

Bone and Joint Findings

Bone involvement in late congenital syphilis is infrequent compared with the frequent occurrence of abnormalities in early congenital syphilis [66,162]. The sequelae of prolonged periosteal reactions can involve the skull, resulting in frontal bossing ("Olympian brow"); anterior bowing of the mid-tibia, resulting in "saber shin"; or thickening of the sternoclavicular portion of the clavicle, resulting in a deformity called Higouménakis sign [219]. For unknown reasons, the last-named finding tends to occur only on the side of dominant handedness. Joint involvement is rare. Clutton joints are symmetric, painless, sterile, synovial effusions, usually localized to the knees. Radiographs do not show involvement of the bones, and examination of the joint fluid reveals a few mononuclear cells [277,278]. Perforation of the hard palate almost is pathognomonic of congenital syphilis [162,279].

Dental Involvement

Syphilitic vasculitis around the time of birth can damage the developing tooth buds and lead to dental anomalies. Hutchinson teeth are abnormal permanent upper central

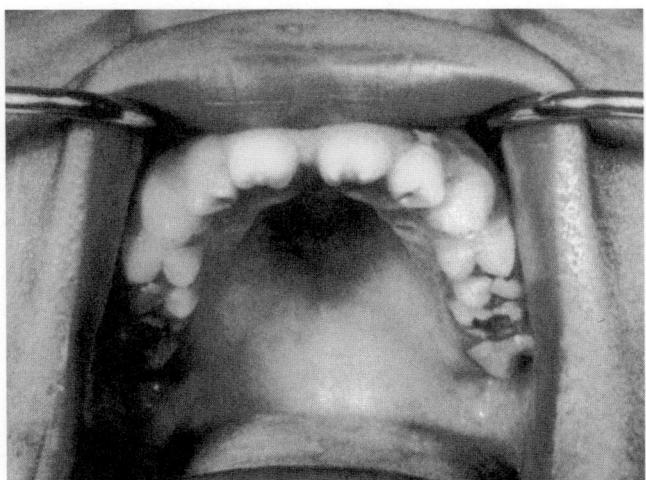

FIGURE 16–8 **Photograph of Hutchinson teeth resulting from congenital syphilis.** Hutchinson teeth are a congenital anomaly in which the permanent incisor teeth are narrow and notched. Note the notched edges and "screwdriver" shape of the central incisors. *(Courtesy of CDC/Susan Lindsley; 1971; Public Health Image Library #2385.)*

incisors that are peg-shaped and notched, usually with obvious thinning and discoloration of enamel in the area of the notching; they are widely spaced and shorter than the lateral incisors; the width of the biting surface is less than that of the gingival margin (Fig. 16–8) [280]. Mulberry molars (also known as Moon or Fournier molars) are multicuspid first molars in which the tooth's grinding surface, which is narrower than that at the gingival margin, has many small cusps instead of the usual four well-formed cusps (Fig. 16–9). The enamel itself tends to be poorly developed [162,219]. X-ray studies can lead to the diagnosis, even while deciduous teeth are in place. Deciduous teeth are largely unaffected except for a possible predisposition to dental caries [162].

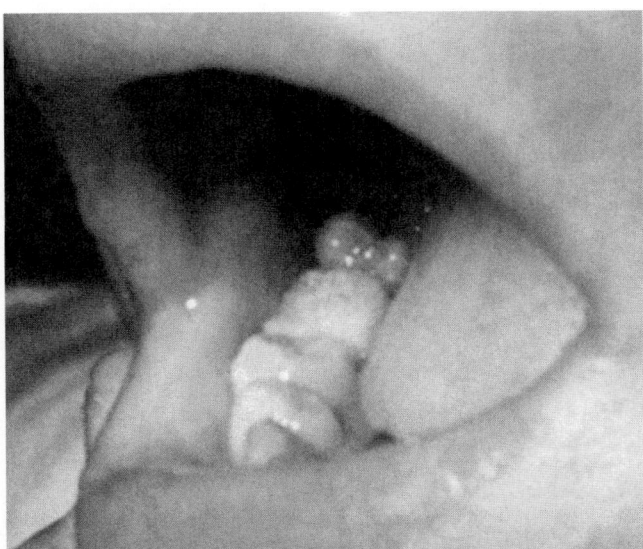

FIGURE 16–9 **Photograph of mulberry molar resulting from congenital syphilis.** Mulberry molar is a condition where the first lower molar tooth has become dome-shaped because of malformation caused by congenital syphilis. *(Courtesy of CDC/Susan Lindsley; 1971; Public Health Image Library #2386.)*

Putkonen [276] examined 30 children whose infected mothers had received penicillin during the latter half of pregnancy and an additional 36 children whose initial therapy for congenital syphilis was initiated during the first few months of life. He noted distinct syphilitic dental changes in 7 of 15 children whose treatment began at age 4 months or later, but in none of the children whose mothers had received treatment during the last half of pregnancy or before age 3 months. He concluded that early treatment prevented the dental changes of syphilis.

Nervous System, Ear, and Ocular Manifestations

The same manifestations of neurosyphilis seen in acquired syphilis may occur in congenital syphilis and can include mental retardation; arrested hydrocephalus; convulsive disorders; juvenile general paresis; and cranial nerve abnormalities, including deafness and blindness, which is due to optic nerve atrophy [265]. Paresis is seen more frequently and tabes dorsalis is seen less frequently in the congenital form than in the acquired form of the disease [102,162,233]. Overall, these findings are uncommon in cases described during the last 50 years [281].

Eighth cranial nerve deafness develops in approximately 3% of untreated cases. The Hutchinson triad comprises Hutchinson teeth, interstitial keratitis, and eighth nerve deafness [102], with eighth nerve deafness the least common component of the triad. The histopathologic features of luetic involvement of the temporal bone include mononuclear leukocytic infiltration and obliterative endarteritis, with involvement of the periosteal, endochondral, and endosteal layers of bone. Osteochondritis affecting the otic capsule can lead to cochlear degeneration and fibrous adhesions, resulting in eighth nerve deafness and vertigo. Although deafness usually occurs in the first decade, it may not appear until the third or fourth decade of life. It often starts with sudden loss of high-frequency hearing, with normal conversational tones affected later. It may respond to long-term corticosteroid therapy [219,282,283].

Eye involvement can lead to interstitial keratitis, secondary glaucoma, or corneal scarring. In keratitis, a severe inflammatory reaction begins in one eye, detectable as ground-glass appearance of the cornea (Fig. 16–10), accompanied by vascularization of the adjacent sclera; this generally becomes bilateral during the ensuing weeks or months. Spirochetes have not been detected [284]. Symptoms include photophobia, pain, excessive lacrimation, and blurred vision. Patients can have conjunctival injection, miosis, keratitis, anterior uveitis, or a combination of these findings. Interstitial keratitis is considered preventable if treatment is given before age 3 months [276]. Interstitial keratitis usually appears at puberty and is not affected by penicillin therapy, but responds transiently to corticosteroid treatment [285]. It often has a relapsing course that can result in secondary glaucoma or corneal clouding. Early retinal involvement or hydrocephalous can lead to optic atrophy [102].

DIAGNOSIS

The diagnosis of congenital or acquired syphilis is usually suspected based on clinical and epidemiologic findings and ideally is confirmed by direct identification of treponemes in clinical specimens, supported by positive serologic findings. In clinical practice, diagnosis is most often made, however, by clinical findings supported by serologic methods alone [286,287].

DIRECT IDENTIFICATION

Currently available methods to identify *T. pallidum* in clinical specimens obtained from a primary chancre or active secondary lesions in the mother or any lesion, body fluid, or tissue biopsy specimen in an infant are (1) dark-field microscopy, (2) direct fluorescent antibody staining, (3) demonstration of the organism by special stains on histopathologic examination, (4) the rabbit infectivity test, and (5) detection of *T. pallidum* DNA [50,58,121,211,288]. (*Note*: Gloves should be worn when examining suspected syphilitic lesions and when performing dark-field examinations). Ideal starting material is lesion exudate or tissue material, including placenta or umbilical cord. Specimens can also be scraped from moist mucocutaneous lesions or aspirated from a regional lymph node. The scaly eruption of syphilis is not a good source of material for dark-field microscopy. Bullae should be aspirated with a sterile syringe and needle. Papules or condylomata should be cleaned thoroughly with physiologic saline solution with no additives, then abraded with a gauze until oozing occurs, and scraped firmly to collect serum rather than blood.

For dark-field microscopy, a sterile glass slide is applied to the exudate, which is covered by a drop of normal saline and placed under a coverslip. Evaluation of these slides requires much experience and must be done immediately (within 5 to 10 minutes) on freshly obtained tissue because these corkscrew-shaped organisms are identified by their characteristic movements. Because about 10^5 organisms/mL are required for visualization, a negative dark-field examination does not rule out syphilis. Nonpathogenic commensal spirochetes (e.g., of the oral flora) can be confused with *T. pallidum* even by experienced examiners. Examination of oral lesions with the dark-field microscope should not be done for this reason, unless direct fluorescent antibody techniques are employed that allow the examiner to distinguish *T. pallidum* from

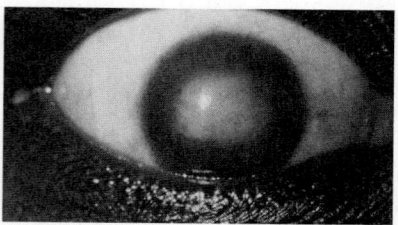

FIGURE 16–10 Photograph depicts the presence of a diffuse stromal haze in the cornea of a child, known as interstitial keratitis, which was due to late-stage congenital syphilis. Interstitial keratitis, which is an inflammation of the connective tissue structure of the cornea, usually affects both eyes and can occur as a complication to congenital or acquired syphilis. Interstitial keratitis usually occurs in children older than 2 years. (*Courtesy of CDC/Susan Lindsley; 1973; Public Health Image Library #6837.*)

nonpathogenic treponemes. For experienced examiners, the sensitivity of the dark-field microscope is 79% to 97%, and specificity is 77% to 100%. If the result of the initial dark-field examination is negative, it should be repeated on at least 2 successive days to confirm a negative result. Although not evaluated for use in specimens from newborns, a modification called the "dark ground" microscopy method has been used in adults with primary and secondary syphilis, with sensitivities of 97% and 84% and with good specificity [289]. This rapid and sensitive test also requires a dark-field microscope and trained personnel.

If a dark-field microscope is unavailable, a direct fluorescent antibody stain for *T. pallidum* can be employed [178]. Exudate is collected in capillary tubes or slides and stained with specific antibody in a direct or indirect fluorescent antibody test for *T. pallidum*. These tests use either monoclonal or polyclonal antibodies against *T. pallidum* that are directly fluorescein-tagged or use a second fluorescein-tagged antibody (indirect fluorescent antibody) to detect the primary antibody-antigen complex [290]. The advantage of immunofluorescent methods over dark-field microscopy is that slides are more permanent and can be mailed to reference laboratories for review by experts [178,291,292].

The rabbit infectivity test is still the gold standard for the identification of viable *T. pallidum* in clinical specimens, having a sensitivity of less than 10 organisms [52,62,80,149,293]. It involves intratesticular inoculation of the specimen into a rabbit and awaiting serologic seroconversion and orchitis with subsequent visualization of motile spirochetes by dark-field microscope in testicular tissue. The rabbit infectivity test is performed only in research laboratories, however, and may take several months for identification of the organism.

Polymerase chain reaction (PCR)–based tests eventually may replace the rabbit infectivity test as the reference standard for syphilis diagnostic tests [45,58,294–296]. The PCR assay is said to be capable of detecting an amount of purified treponemal DNA equivalent to that of only a few organisms (about 0.01 pg) [58]. Compared with isolation of the organism by rabbit infectivity testing, the sensitivity of PCR on CSF was 65% to 71%, and specificity was 97% to 100% [149,267,296–299]. *T. pallidum* DNA has been detected by PCR in body fluids such as amniotic fluid and infant blood, CSF, and endotracheal aspirate [149,267,296]. PCR tests are not yet clinically validated, for now precluding routine use [297,298]. The lack of access to PCR, the time required for the rabbit infectivity test, and the frequent false-negative microscopic results clearly indicate that serologic testing often is necessary.

INDIRECT, SEROLOGIC IDENTIFICATION

Serologic assays have played a prominent role in the clinical diagnosis of syphilis since the early 1900s [300]. Nontreponemal antibody tests detect a nonspecific immune reaction and consist of the rapid plasma reagin (RPR) and VDRL assays. Serologic tests detect a specific interaction between serum immunoglobulins and surface antigens of *T. pallidum* and are called treponemal antibody tests. Nontreponemal and treponemal tests have their advantages and disadvantages. In most circumstances, both tests need to be employed in conjunction to make the serodiagnosis of infection with syphilis.

Nontreponemal tests for syphilis are believed to detect antibodies to cardiolipin (diphosphatidylglycerol), a component of normal cell membranes in mammalian tissue. The original test as described by Wassermann used syphilitic tissue as complement-fixing antigen to detect the presence of antibody (*reagin*, a term that should not be used anymore because it is easily confused with IgE) that is induced by *T. pallidum*. Extracts of other normal tissue, such as beef heart, had similar properties, and purification and standardization of these materials led to their use as antigen of preparations containing cardiolipin [300]. Diphosphatidylglycerol constitutes only a small proportion of the lipids of *T. pallidum*, and these organisms may be unable to synthesize this substance at all; it is possible that they incorporate it from damaged host tissues [301]. Production of anticardiolipin antibody could reflect an autoimmune host response to a slightly altered or a differently presented cardiolipin. In this context, it is interesting that anticardiolipin antibody reflects ongoing tissue damage, its detection correlating closely with the amount of activity in the early stages of syphilis infection. These observations may explain why patients with autoimmune diseases, such as systemic lupus erythematosus, characteristically have positive nontreponemal test results as well [300].

The currently available nontreponemal tests, RPR and the automated reagin test, and VDRL slide test, use purified cardiolipin in lecithin-cholesterol liposomes. The nontreponemal tests measure IgG and IgM antibodies [141,302,303]. RPR is positive in approximately 85% of cases of primary syphilis and in 98% of cases of secondary syphilis. VDRL is positive in approximately 80% of primary cases and in 95% of secondary cases (Table 16–3). VDRL is the only serologic assay approved for testing reactivity of spinal fluid [140,279]. RPR and VDRL

TABLE 16–3   Seroreactivity of Common Tests for Untreated Syphilis

Test	% Positive			
	Primary Stage	**Secondary Stage**	**Latent Stage**	**Tertiary Stage**
VDRL or RPR	80-85	95-98	75	<66
FTA-ABS, TP-PA	75-85	100	100	100

FTA-ABS, fluorescent treponemal antibody, absorbed with non-T. pallidum treponemes; RPR, rapid plasma reagin; TP-PA, T. pallidum particle agglutination; VDRL, Venereal Disease Research Laboratory.

results are reported as dilutions or titers so that a relative degree of reactivity can be determined. Changes of two dilutions (e.g., a fourfold change from 1:2 to 1:8) are considered significant when assessing disease activity. The RPR titer is often one to two dilutions higher than that obtained using VDRL, so caution must be exercised when comparing results [78].

These quantitative titers help define disease activity and monitor response to therapy: A fourfold decrease suggests adequate therapy, whereas a fourfold increase indicates active disease (treatment failure or reinfection). The quantitative nontreponemal test usually decreases fourfold within 6 months after adequate therapy for primary or secondary syphilis and usually becomes nonreactive within 1 year after successful therapy if the infection was treated during the early stages (primary or secondary syphilis). The patient usually becomes seronegative within 2 years even if the initial titer was high or the infection was congenital [78,304,305]. Even without treatment, the VDRL titer slowly declines and is negative in one third of patients with late syphilis [140]. A few patients remain serofast, with persisting low positive titers despite receiving adequate therapy. This serofast state is more common in patients treated for latent or tertiary syphilis. When nontreponemal tests are used to monitor treatment response, the same specific test (e.g., VDRL or RPR or automated reagin test) must be used throughout the follow-up period, preferably by the same laboratory, to ensure comparability of results [198].

These tests occasionally produce positive results in patients for whom there is no evidence of syphilitic infection, called *biologic false-positive* (BFP); this term is meant to distinguish BFP results from positive reactions owing to technical errors (e.g., Wharton jelly contamination in cord blood specimens leads to technical false-positive reactions) [279,306]. Nontreponemal antibody cross-reacts with more than 200 non–*T. pallidum* spirochetal antigens (although not with the agents of Lyme disease) and can produce false-positive results. Usually, BFP test results have titers less than 1:8 and negative confirmatory test, but they are reported with a frequency of 1% to 20% [198,300,307]. They are classified as either acute (<6 months) or chronic BFP results. Acute BFP reactions can be associated with other infections (e.g., Epstein-Barr virus, varicella, measles, malaria, tuberculosis, brucellosis, mumps, lymphogranuloma venereum, and hepatitis). Chronic BFP reactions are often associated with old age, autoimmune diseases and chronic inflammatory processes (e.g., systemic lupus erythematosus, polyarteritis nodosa, antiphospholipid syndrome, chronic liver disease, endocarditis), malignancy (especially if associated with production of excess IgM), and, rarely, with pregnancy itself [198,300,304,307–313]. Among HIV-positive patients, 10% to 30% have false-positive nonspecific reactions [314]. The antibody detected by VDRL in chronic BFP reactions predominantly is IgM, whereas in syphilis it is mainly IgG; patients with chronic BFP reactions and systemic lupus erythematosus commonly also have a reactive fluorescent treponemal antibody absorption (FTA-ABS) test (see subsequently).

False-negative results can occur when a high concentration of antibody inhibits agglutination (the prozone

phenomenon), which can be avoided with serial dilutions of the serum; this occurs in approximately 1% to 2% of individuals, usually with secondary syphilis [247,315,316]. Failure to recognize a prozone effect in maternal serum tested during pregnancy has resulted in failure to diagnose congenital syphilis [247]. Nontreponemal test results may also be falsely negative (i.e., nonreactive) in early (prechancre state) primary syphilis, latent acquired syphilis of long duration, and late congenital syphilis because over the course of time even some untreated patients may revert to seronegative nontreponemal status [198,317–319]. Nontreponemal tests are used primarily for screening (i.e., to establish a "presumptive" diagnosis) and monitoring of therapy [320]. In most instances, a nontreponemal positive reaction is followed up with a treponeme-specific test for confirmation.

Treponeme-Specific Serologic Tests

Infection with *T. pallidum* causes the host to produce antitreponemal antibodies, which are detected by specific assays, including FTA-ABS and treponeme-specific microhemagglutination test (microhemagglutination–*T. pallidum* [MHA-TP]), now replaced by *T. pallidum* particle agglutination test (TP-PA). FTA-ABS and TP-PA tests measure IgG and IgM antibodies directed against lyophilized Nichols strain antigen. For FTA-ABS, antigen is fixed on a slide, the patient's serum is allowed to react with antigen, and the bound antibody is detected with fluorescently labeled antihuman immunoglobulin antibody, identified by fluorescent microscopy. Test sera are usually preabsorbed with extracts from nonpathogenic *Treponema phagedenis* to eliminate group-reactive antibody, rendering FTA-ABS relatively specific for disease with virulent treponemal species. FTA-ABS is expensive, is time-consuming, and requires a fluorescence microscope and a highly trained technician. It is recommended only for confirmation of positive nontreponemal tests and the diagnosis of later stages of syphilis in which the results of nontreponemal tests may be negative.

Microhemagglutination tests, specifically TP-PA, depend on the passive hemagglutination of erythrocytes or latex particles that have been coated with Nichols strain *T. pallidum* antigen. These tests have been automated, are easy to perform, and are relatively inexpensive. They have largely replaced FTA-ABS [145,305,313,321–327]. MHA-TP is no longer commercially available. TP-PA uses the same treponemal antigen as MHA-TP, but uses gelatin particles rather than sheep red blood cells, which eliminates some nonspecific reactions [328]. Both of the treponeme-specific tests are positive in 75% (TP-PA) to 85% (FTA-ABS) of patients with primary syphilis and in 100% of patients with secondary syphilis (see Table 16–3).* In contrast to nontreponemal tests, titers of the treponemal tests are irrelevant because they do not correlate with disease activity.

False-positive results of specific treponemal tests rarely occur, but may occur in patients with other spirochetal diseases, including Lyme disease, leptospirosis, rat-bite fever, relapsing fever, and diseases caused by other

---

*References 145, 305, 313, 321, 323–327, 329, 330.

pathogenic *Treponema* species (e.g., yaws, pinta) [121]. A few disease states, such as systemic lupus erythematosus, polyarteritis, or related conditions, and, in one report, even pregnancy are said to cause a false-positive FTA-ABS result [308]. Nontreponemal tests can be used to differentiate Lyme disease from syphilis because VDRL is nonreactive in Lyme disease. Treponemal specific tests are unlikely to revert to a nonreactive state after treatment of the patient, unless treatment was given very early. In one study, however, 24% of patients with a first episode of primary syphilis exhibited a nonreactive result on FTA-ABS testing, and 13% had a nonreactive result on MHA-TP testing at 36 months after treatment [331]. Positive nontreponemal reactions are not helpful in determining whether active infection is present, but a negative result excludes a diagnosis of all but early primary infection and the rare subject who converted back to a serologically negative state.

Other Serologic Tests

Specific treponemal IgM tests have been developed and have shown great promise in small studies. In contrast to IgG, IgM does not cross the placenta, and detection of specific IgM in an infant would be a strong indication of infection. At this time, these tests are not yet commercially available [121]. Efforts to produce a more sensitive and more specific test are ongoing (e.g., using recombinant *T. pallidum* antigens) [149,332,333]. Some clinical laboratories and blood banks are using treponemal enzyme immunoassay tests [333–339] as initial screening tests. Such reactive screening tests need to be confirmed with another treponemal test different from the one used for screening, such as TP-HA if an enzyme immunoassay is used for screening, and a quantitative test to assess disease activity (RPR or VDRL). These treponemal enzyme immunoassays have advantages such as automation, lack of prozone phenomenon, and increased sensitivity in late stages of disease [340–342].

Several developments in diagnostic tests for syphilis promise to make screening and diagnosis of syphilis infection in pregnant women easier for antenatal clinics, particularly in developing countries. The WHO Sexually Transmitted Diseases Diagnostics Initiative (SDI) developed the *ASSURED* criteria as a benchmark to determine whether tests address disease control needs: *a*ffordable, *s*ensitive, *s*pecific, *u*ser-friendly, *r*apid and robust, *e*quipment-free, and *d*eliverable to end-users [111]. Numerous rapid, low-cost specific antibody detection tests based on immunochromatography or latex particle agglutination have already been developed [336,343]. New RPR reagents that are stable at room temperature and simple, rapid treponemal tests that do not require electricity or other equipment are now available with sensitivities, specificities, and costs similar to TP-PA. Some of them require only a finger-prick for venous blood, can use whole blood, do not require refrigeration, and take only 10 to 15 minutes before they can be read. A field trial in Mozambique found that the diagnostic accuracy of some of these newer tests compared favorably with RPR and standards consisting of TP-HA, RPR, and direct immunofluorescence stain undertaken in a reference laboratory

[111]. The tests that have been evaluated and found to have acceptable performance characteristics are likely to have a significant impact on the control of syphilis globally [288,344].

Nontreponemal antibody tests (VDRL and RPR and automated reagin test) are best used for screening, and treponemal tests (FTA-ABS and TP-PA) are useful to establish the diagnosis. Nontreponemal antibody tests are also useful in assessing the adequacy of therapy and in detecting reinfection and relapse.

Cerebrospinal Fluid Tests

For evaluation of possible neurosyphilis, VDRL should be performed on CSF. In addition to VDRL testing of CSF, evaluation of CSF protein and WBC count is used to assess the likelihood of CNS involvement [345]. FTA-ABS testing of CSF is less specific than VDRL, but some experts recommend using FTA-ABS, believing it to be more sensitive. Fewer data exist for TP-PA for CSF, and none exist for RPR; these two tests should not be used for CSF evaluation. Only VDRL is recommended by the CDC for use in CSF evaluation [346–348]. Results from VDRL should be interpreted cautiously because a negative result on VDRL of CSF does not exclude a diagnosis of neurosyphilis. As in evaluating a patient for neurosyphilis, a CSF specimen without contamination by peripheral blood is needed [349].

APPROACH TO DIAGNOSIS OF ACQUIRED SYPHILIS IN PREGNANCY

All women should be screened serologically for syphilis early in pregnancy with a nontreponemal test (e.g., VDRL or RPR) and preferably again at delivery. In areas of high prevalence of syphilis and in patients considered at high risk of syphilis, nontreponemal serum testing at the beginning of the third trimester (28 weeks of gestation) and at delivery is also indicated [78,175,350,351]. RPR is most commonly used to screen pregnant women for possible infection with *T. pallidum* [224,352].

A definitive laboratory diagnosis of syphilis in pregnancy can be made when the presence of *T. pallidum* is confirmed by direct tests of clinical specimens. A probable or presumptive diagnosis of syphilis can be made when (1) specific or nonspecific serologic tests are reactive in the presence of clinical findings compatible with syphilis, (2) CSF is reactive by VDRL testing, or (3) a specific treponemal antibody test is reactive [78]. Specific treponemal serologic tests should be used to confirm diagnoses suspected on the basis of clinical findings or positive nontreponemal tests. Use of only one type of serologic test is insufficient for a probable diagnosis because false-positive nontreponemal test results occur with various medical conditions, and false-positive treponemal test results occur with other spirochetal diseases (see earlier). Low-titer false-positive nontreponemal antibody test results occasionally occur even in pregnancy. When a pregnant woman has a reactive nontreponemal test result and a persistently negative treponemal test result, a false-positive test result is confirmed. The probability of syphilis is high in a sexually active pregnant woman whose serum is newly reactive on nontreponemal and treponemal tests, whether the woman is symptomatic or not. Some laboratories now screen pregnant women using an enzyme immunoassay treponemal test; pregnant women with reactive treponemal screening tests should have confirmatory testing with a nontreponemal test with quantitative titers.

Differentiating syphilis treated in the past from reinfection often is difficult unless the nontreponemal titer is increasing. For women who tested positive and were treated during pregnancy, follow-up serologic testing is necessary to assess the efficacy of therapy. A woman who had been adequately treated with penicillin and followed with quantitative serologic testing and who has no evidence of reinfection does not need retreatment with each subsequent pregnancy. One third of congenital syphilis infections seem to be due to repeat infections [353], however, indicating that any pregnant woman with syphilis, past or present, should be reevaluated carefully, and if any doubt exists about the adequacy of previous treatment or the presence of active infection or risk for reinfection, a course of treatment should be given to prevent congenital syphilis. All pregnant women who have syphilis should also be tested for other sexually transmitted diseases, including HIV infection. Any woman who delivers a stillborn infant after 20 weeks' gestation should also be tested for syphilis [78,83].

The above-described approach of serologic screening is a poor diagnostic approach during the incubation or early primary stage of syphilis, and cases of congenital syphilis have occurred in women who were incubating syphilis at the time of delivery (i.e., at a time their screening serologic tests were still negative). During those times, results of nontreponemal (RPR or VDRL) tests may not show reactivity because reactivity occurs 4 to 8 weeks after the infection is acquired and several days to 1 week after the development of a chancre [309]. In primary syphilis during pregnancy, nonreactivity on nontreponemal testing is reported to occur in one fourth to one third of cases [247,316]. Nonreactivity on the specific TP-PA and FTA test occurs in 36% and 18% of cases of primary syphilis [300]. The clinician caring for a pregnant woman has to maintain a high level of suspicion in cases of a sexually active pregnant woman. Detection of the spirochete from active lesions is the only means to establish the diagnosis in this scenario; this requires careful physical examination at multiple time points during pregnancy [78].

Usually, HIV infection in women does not alter serology, but atypical results must be expected [198]. Frequent false-negative serology in primary and secondary syphilis [354,355], prozone phenomenon [356], serofast reactions [357], and specific antibodies becoming negative after therapy [358] all have been reported. False-positive nonspecific reactions are observed in 11% of patients [359]. Sometimes there is a false-negative FTA-ABS test. A delayed decline in titer can occur and apparently is of no clinical relevance. Despite such varying serologic responses, work-up for syphilis in HIV-infected women should not be different from that of HIV-negative cases [354]. However, the possibility of negative serology in early syphilis must be considered, and detection of the pathogen must be attempted in such cases [73].

APPROACH TO DIAGNOSIS OF CONGENITAL SYPHILIS

Several diagnostic categories for congenital syphilis have been proposed, and minor differences among case definitions formulated by several agencies and experts still exist [78,89,360,361]. In Table 16–4, we have attempted to reconcile several of these diagnostic categories with the CDC guidelines from 2006. A *definitive* diagnosis of congenital syphilis can be made in the rare situation in which the organism can be identified directly in the infant. A *highly probable* diagnosis is suggested if there are clinical findings consistent with congenital syphilis (see Tables 16–1 and 16–2), if the infant has a fourfold higher nontreponemal serologic titer than the mother, or if the infant has a positive CSF VDRL result. The diagnostic category of *probable* describes clinically asymptomatic infants who have a nontreponemal serologic titer that is equal to or less than that of the mother, but where maternal treatment did not occur at all, was inadequate, was not documented, or failed (i.e., did not lead to a sufficient decline in maternal nontreponemal titers).

The diagnosis of *possible* congenital syphilis is made when the nontreponemal serologic test result of an asymptomatic infant is reactive, but equal to or less than that of the mother who did receive adequate treatment either during or before this pregnancy. The diagnosis of congenital syphilis is *unlikely* if the nontreponemal serologic test result of an asymptomatic infant born to an

TABLE 16–4   Modified Diagnostic Categories of Infants Born to Mothers with Clinical or Serologic Evidence of Syphilis

Definite Diagnosis (CDC Scenario 1)

1. Confirmation of presence of *T. pallidum* by dark-field microscopic or histologic examination or RIT; positive PCR

Highly Probable Diagnosis (CDC Scenario 1)

1. STS (RPR, VDRL) titer 4-fold greater than maternal STS titer
2. STS (RPR, VDRL) reactive in presence of clinical findings consistent with syphilis
3. STS (VDRL) reactive in cerebrospinal fluid
4. Reactive treponemal antibody test after age 15 mo

Probable Diagnosis (CDC Scenario 2)

1. Infant STS (RPR, VDRL) titer reactive, but same or less than 4-fold maternal titer in absence of clinical disease, but in the face of inadequate* maternal therapy

Possible Diagnosis (CDC Scenario 3 and 4)

1. Asymptomatic infant STS (RPR, VDRL) reactive, but adequate maternal therapy

Unlikely Diagnosis

1. Asymptomatic infant STS (RPR, VDRL) nonreactive and adequate maternal therapy
2. STS nonreactive before age 6 mo

*Mother was not treated, inadequately treated (i.e., was treated with a nonpenicillin regimen, or was treated <30 days before delivery, or titers did not fall appropriately), or has no documentation of having received treatment.
CDC, Centers for Disease Control and Prevention; PCR, polymerase chain reaction; RIT, rabbit infectivity test; RPR, rapid plasma reagin (test); STS, serologic test for syphilis; VDRL, Venereal Disease Research Laboratory (test).
Modified from Centers for Disease Control and Prevention. Available at http://www.cdc.gov/std/treatment/2006/congenital-syphilis.htm. Accessed January 21 2008.

adequately treated mother is nonreactive. The "unlikely" label does not exclude the possibility of congenital infection, however, in cases where the mother is seronegative at the time of testing because she is in the incubation period of early syphilis [78,101,242,362–365]. Given the difficulty of diagnosis and the severity of untreated congenital syphilis, the "evaluate and treat when uncertain" approach to congenital syphilis is the most prudent (see "Therapy").

Overall, the decision to evaluate and ultimately to treat an infant for congenital syphilis is largely based on clinical, serologic, and epidemiologic considerations. The evaluation includes an assessment of the mother for general risk factors, followed by an evaluation of the mother's current known serologic status. No newborn infant should be discharged from the hospital without determination of the mother's serologic status for syphilis, regardless of whether the mother and the infant are asymptomatic [366]. Cord blood should not be tested because it frequently yields false-positive or false-negative results, and tests of postnatal infant serum can be nonreactive if maternal titers are low or the mother was infected late in pregnancy. Conversely, transplacental transmission of nontreponemal and treponemal antibodies to the fetus can occur in a mother who has been treated appropriately for syphilis during pregnancy, resulting in positive test results in the uninfected newborn infant (the neonate's nontreponemal test titer in these circumstances usually reverts to negative in 4 to 6 months, whereas a positive FTA-ABS or TP-PA result from passively acquired antibody may not become negative for ≥ 1 year).

Taking the aforementioned considerations together, the optimal starting point for the serologic evaluation of a suspected case of congenital syphilis is maternal serum [78,179,275]. An infant's serologic titer often is one to two dilutions less than that of the mother's titer; an infant may have a nonreactive umbilical cord VDRL, but have a mother with a reactive serologic test for syphilis at delivery. From 1987–1990, Sanchez and coworkers [362] compared results of maternal serologic studies at delivery with results obtained from VDRL testing of umbilical cord blood and documented 534 cases with reactive maternal serologic tests at delivery, but negative umbilical cord blood VDRL results. Of these infants, 87 (16%) were born to mothers with untreated syphilis at delivery and were at risk for infection if treatment were not given. These infants would not have been identified if only the umbilical cord blood had been screened. When the only evidence of congenital syphilis is a newly positive maternal nontreponemal test, the maternal diagnosis should be confirmed with a treponemal test before an otherwise well, asymptomatic infant undergoes further evaluation and treatment for congenital syphilis, unless the wait for results would unduly delay providing appropriate care for the infant, or there is significant risk for loss to follow-up [83,121].

All infants born to seropositive mothers require a careful examination and a quantitative nontreponemal syphilis test. The test performed on the infant should be the same as the test performed on the mother to enable comparison of titer results. It is generally agreed that an infant should be evaluated further for congenital syphilis if the maternal titer has increased fourfold, if the infant titer is fourfold greater than the mother's titer, or if the infant has clinical manifestations of syphilis [149]. Infant nontreponemal titers fourfold higher than maternal titers are uncommon even in symptomatic cases, however, and infant-to-mother ratios less than fourfold do not exclude congenital infection. High nontreponemal titers at the time of maternal treatment during pregnancy and at delivery and gestational age less than 37 weeks at delivery are risk factors for the acquisition of congenital syphilis in the neonate even when maternal treatment was adequate [367].

Assessment of maternal treatment for syphilis, in terms of the regimen used, timing of therapy relative to delivery (<30 days versus ≥ 30 days), and maternal follow-up and results of serial nontreponemal antibody titers, is key in determining the extent of evaluation and treatment needed for an infant at risk for congenital syphilis. The only maternal treatment considered effective (see "Therapy") is benzathine penicillin G, 2.4 million U intramuscularly; a single dose is deemed sufficient when the mother has primary, secondary, or early latent syphilis. Three doses administered at 1-week intervals are required for late latent or tertiary syphilis [78,121].

Infants born to women who have had syphilis in the past, received therapy, and remained seroreactive also are seroreactive. Ensuring that such an infant does not have congenital disease in the immediate newborn period may be impossible. If the infant's reactive RPR is caused by passively transferred antibody from a previously infected mother, the reactivity in the infant progressively declines as time passes and should disappear by 6 months of age. A persistently reactive RPR in the infant beyond 12 to 15 months of age suggests an active infection, and an increasing titer makes this diagnosis certain [279,368]. Infants who have (1) normal physical findings *and* (2) a serum quantitative nontreponemal antibody titer that is fourfold or less than the maternal titer do not require further laboratory or clinical evaluation *if* (1) maternal treatment adequate for the stage of syphilis was administered more than 4 weeks before delivery (including before pregnancy), *and* either (2a) the mother had early syphilis at the time of treatment and her nontreponemal titers decreased at least fourfold and have remained low and stable through the time of delivery, or (2b) the mother had late syphilis at the time of treatment, her nontreponemal titers have remained low and stable, and there is no evidence of relapse and no risk for reinfection [121,352].

If these requirements are not completely met, or even the slightest doubt exists, evaluation for syphilis in an infant should occur and include the following: [50,83]

1. Physical examination.
2. A quantitative nontreponemal serologic test for syphilis using serum from the infant (not cord blood because false-positive and false-negative results can occur). A specific treponemal test such as FTA-ABS is unnecessary in the newborn period if the mother is known to have a reactive result.
3. Long bone radiographs, unless the diagnosis has been established otherwise. Long bone radiographs are one of the most sensitive clinical studies for detection of physical evidence of congenital

syphilis in otherwise asymptomatic infants [369]. They are abnormal in approximately 65% of infants with clinical findings of syphilis, but only in a few asymptomatic infants (i.e., if osteochondritis or periostitis is found in an infant born to a mother with a reactive serologic test for syphilis, this is indicative of congenital syphilis, and the infant requires a full course of intravenous penicillin therapy). The value of long bone radiographs and CSF examinations in the diagnosis of congenital syphilis has been questioned during a time when syphilis was of low prevalence in the study population [370,371], but the recommendations for long bone radiographs and CSF VDRL determinations are based on their sensitivity and specificity from previous epidemics [369] and are most relevant today.

4. Complete blood cell count including hematocrit and hemoglobin, red blood cell count, reticulocyte count, platelet count, WBC count with differential, and direct Coombs test.
5. Other clinically indicated tests (e.g., chest radiograph, liver function tests, cranial ultrasound, ophthalmologic examination, and auditory brainstem response).
6. Pathologic examination of the placenta or umbilical cord using specific fluorescent antitreponemal antibody staining.
7. VDRL of CSF and analysis of CSF for cells and protein concentration (specific indications are explained subsequently).

CSF should be examined in an infant who is evaluated for congenital syphilis if the infant has any of the following: (1) abnormal physical examination findings consistent with congenital syphilis, (2) a serum quantitative nontreponemal titer that is fourfold greater than the mother's titer, or (3) positive dark-field microscopy or fluorescent antibody test result on body fluid [78,83,149,372]. Infants with these findings are considered to have proven disease, and spirochetemia with invasion of the CNS occurs in approximately 40% to 50% of these infants, so they must receive a full 10-day course of intravenous penicillin therapy [149,267]. Leukocytosis ($\geq$25 WBCs/mm^3) and elevated protein content (>150 mg/dL in full-term infants and >170 mg/dL in preterm infants) in the CSF in an infant who exhibits any features suggestive of congenital syphilis should be regarded as supportive of the diagnosis. Also, an infant with reactive CSF on VDRL testing should receive presumptive treatment for neurosyphilis [345].

Specific treponemal tests should not be done using CSF in infants suspected to have congenital syphilis because the results cannot be interpreted properly [346–348]. Given that the diagnosis of congenital neurosyphilis is difficult to establish without a positive direct test, and because findings such as the presence of red blood cells in the CSF owing to a traumatic lumbar puncture can produce a false-positive serologic reaction, and other markers in the CSF of newborns and infants (CSF WBC counts and protein concentrations) vary widely as well, it is generally agreed that any infant with proven or probable congenital syphilis requires 10 days of parenteral treatment with penicillin G regardless of CSF test results [78,83]. The problem of unequivocally identifying an infected infant underscores the need for an "evaluate and treat when uncertain" approach to congenital syphilis in general and to congenital neurosyphilis in particular. Given this paradigm, although a complete evaluation is preferred for optimal planning of care, it may be unnecessary if a full 10-day course of parenteral penicillin is provided because such therapy would treat congenital CNS infection [369,370].

In settings with poor resources, the major difficulties in making a diagnosis of congenital syphilis are identifying the potentially large number of infants who have congenital syphilis as their mother's infection has remained undetected during pregnancy and confirming clinical suspicion without sophisticated laboratory tests. In these situations, confirmation of clinical suspicion is restricted to VDRL or RPR. The results in the mother and infant using the same test should be compared, and a fourfold higher titer in the infant should be accepted as probable infection. The value of performing a lumbar puncture or bone radiographs in asymptomatic infants in settings with poor resources in an attempt to confirm the diagnosis is of questionable value. In instances where infection is probable or suspected, the infant should be treated for congenital syphilis with a full 10-day course of intravenous penicillin G [111].

DIFFERENTIAL DIAGNOSIS

The typical findings of congenital syphilis, such as snuffles, vesiculobullous eruption, hepatosplenomegaly, generalized lymphadenopathy, and symmetric bony lesions, closely resemble features of other diseases in neonates that are unrelated to syphilis. The numerous neonatal conditions that have to be considered in the differential diagnosis include congenital infections caused by cytomegalovirus, *Toxoplasma gondii*, herpes simplex virus, rubella virus, and bacterial sepsis; blood group incompatibility; battered child syndrome; and periostitis of prematurity. Most findings in syphilis are due to the inflammatory reaction to a widely disseminated pathogen, and this pathogenesis unites many of the above-listed entities [121,373–375].

DERMATOLOGIC MANIFESTATIONS

The vesiculobullous manifestations of congenital syphilis may be confused with other infections or with congenital disorders of the skin that can manifest as vesiculobullous eruptions [376]. Infection caused by *Staphylococcus aureus* can produce vesicles or bullae on any part of the body. Severe infection may result in confluent bullae with erythema and desquamation (Ritter's disease). Examination of aspirated fluid reveals many polymorphonuclear leukocytes and occasionally gram-positive cocci in clusters, and culture yields the organism. *Pseudomonas aeruginosa* septicemia can be accompanied by a cutaneous eruption consisting of clustered pearly vesicles on an erythematous background, which rapidly becomes purulent green or hemorrhagic [377]. When the lesion ruptures, a circumscribed ulcer with a necrotic base appears and may persist, surrounded by a purplish cellulitis. Culture of the lesion and the blood confirms the diagnosis. In the septicemic early-onset form of listeriosis, a cutaneous eruption consisting of miliary lesions resembling papules, pustules, or papulopustules can occur over the entire body, with a predilection for the back [378]. Culture of these lesions and blood usually reveals *Listeria monocytogenes* as the etiologic agent. Additional infectious causes of vesicular or bullous lesions of the skin of the newborn include group B streptococci [379], *Haemophilus influenzae* type b [380], *Mycobacterium tuberculosis* [381], and cytomegalovirus [382].

In virus-induced eruptions, the vesicles are located in the mid-epidermis. In herpesvirus infection, vesicles are the most common dermatologic manifestation. They tend to be sparsely disseminated throughout the body, or they may occur in crops or clusters. Involvement of the palms and soles has been recorded, as has the formation of bullae. Recurrence of these skin lesions is not unusual. Culture, fluorescent staining, or PCR on scrapings from the base of these lesions reveals herpes simplex virus. Varicella-zoster infection seems to have a similar pattern, but rarely occurs in the newborn period, and the diagnosis may be discarded on epidemiologic or clinical grounds. Variola and vaccinia can affect the fetus or newborn and cause vesicular eruptions. Appropriate epidemiologic evidence should be sought to exclude these diagnoses.

Mucocutaneous candidiasis may manifest as a vesicular dermatitis at the end of the 1st week of life. The vesicles usually become confluent and rupture, leaving a denuded area surrounded by satellite vesicles or pustules. Congenital candidiasis with skin manifestations also has been described, and severe systemic involvement may accompany this intrauterine infection [383].

Various hereditary disorders of the skin appear at birth or in early infancy as vesiculobullous eruptions [376]. Epidermolysis bullosa is a group of specific genetic disorders. Erythema toxicum, miliaria rubra, incontinentia pigmenti, urticaria pigmentosa, epidermolytic hyperkeratosis, acrodermatitis enteropathica, Langerhans cell histiocytosis (histiocytosis X), transient neonatal pustular melanosis, infantile acropustulosis, and aplasia cutis congenita all should be included in the differential diagnosis [376].

SNUFFLES

Increased neonatal nasal discharge is a common phenomenon, but has not been well studied. It is described as mucoid rhinorrhea with nasal mucosal edema in an afebrile newborn that results in stertor, poor feeding, and respiratory distress. The etiology is most often not identified, but is presumed to be allergic in nature. The recognition and treatment of this condition is important because neonates are obligate nasal breathers. A diagnostic-therapeutic trial consisting of conservative therapy (suctioning) and corticosteroid is recommended. An important alternative consideration not to be missed is infection with *Chlamydia trachomatis*, but this entity should be recognized by the associated clinical findings [387].

LYMPHADENOPATHY

Lymph node size varies with age and the location, but in neonates, lymph nodes are normally barely palpable. Localized lymphadenopathy can be found in one third of neonates and infants, usually in nodes that drain areas with skin irritation or localized infections. Generalized adenopathy is rare in the neonate and if present can be seen with other congenital infections such as cytomegalovirus [384].

HEPATOSPLENOMEGALY

When the clinical presentation includes hepatosplenomegaly with or without jaundice, the list of possibilities in the differential diagnosis is extensive and includes all causes of elevated direct and indirect bilirubin. The physician should consider isoimmunization (e.g., Rh incompatibility, ABO incompatibility); other infectious diseases, such as early-onset sepsis, cytomegalovirus infection congenital rubella, herpes simplex infection, coxsackievirus B or other enteroviral infections, and toxoplasmosis; neonatal hepatitis; diseases of the biliary tract (e.g., extrahepatic biliary atresia, choledochal cyst); and genetic and metabolic disorders (e.g., cystic fibrosis, galactosemia, α_1-antitrypsin deficiency) [384].

HYDROPS FETALIS

Hydrops fetalis can be caused by chronic anemia (isoimmunization disorder, homozygous α-thalassemia, fetal-maternal or fetal-fetal transfusions); cardiac or pulmonary failure from causes other than anemia (large arteriovenous malformations, premature closure of the foramen ovale, cystic adenomatoid malformation, pulmonary lymphangiectasia); perinatal tumors (neuroblastoma, chorioangioma); achondroplasia; renal disorders (congenital nephrosis, renal vein thrombosis); and infections, such as congenital cytomegalovirus infection, toxoplasmosis, parvovirus B19 infection [385], and congenital hepatitis [384]. Most cases of hydrops are caused by isoimmunization disorders, which can be excluded as a cause by a negative direct Coombs test result. A normal hemoglobin electrophoresis pattern excludes the diagnosis of α-thalassemia. The Kleihauer-Betke technique of acid elution for identifying fetal cells in the maternal circulation can aid in ruling out the diagnosis of fetal-maternal transfusion. Other diagnostic considerations can be discarded on the basis of appropriate radiographic studies, placental examination, urinalysis with microscopy, biopsy, and immunologic studies [384].

RENAL DISEASE

In neonates and young infants, nephrotic syndrome and acute nephritis occur infrequently. The former more often is associated with infantile microcystic disease, minimal-lesion nephrotic syndrome, or renal vein thrombosis than with congenital syphilis [384]. Neonatal nephritis can occur as a manifestation of congenital syphilis, hereditary nephritis, hemolytic-uremic syndrome, and, rarely, pyelonephritis. The clinical signs that distinguish syphilitic renal involvement from the other conditions mentioned include the presence of other manifestations of early congenital syphilis, a positive result on serologic tests for syphilis, elevated levels of IgG (in infantile microcystic disease, the levels of IgG are low), and the response to specific therapy for syphilis [279].

OPHTHALMOLOGIC INVOLVEMENT

Neonatal glaucoma, an uncommon finding in syphilis, occurs as an isolated genetic disorder and may be associated with various syndromes, such as aniridia, Hallermann-Streiff syndrome, Rieger anomaly, Lowe syndrome, Sturge-Weber syndrome, oculodentodigital syndrome, and Pierre Robin syndrome; it also is associated with congenital rubella [386]. Nasolacrimal duct obstruction is a more frequent cause of excessive lacrimation in the newborn period and early infancy.

BONY INVOLVEMENT

Periostitis of congenital syphilis usually occurs during the early months of life and must be distinguished from periostitis seen in healing rickets, battered child syndrome, infantile cortical hyperostosis, various poorly understood disorders presumed to be related to nutritional deficiencies, occasionally pyogenic osteomyelitis [187], and prostaglandin-induced periostitis [387]. Although Wimberger sign formerly was thought to be pathognomonic of congenital syphilis, it has been described in other disease states, including osteomyelitis, hyperparathyroidism, and infantile generalized fibromatosis [234]. The "celery stick" appearance of alternating bands of longitudinal translucency and relative density is a finding also seen in congenital rubella and cytomegalovirus infection [187].

THERAPY

Early treatments for syphilis included mercury (first used in 1497), arsphenamine, other heavy metals, and malaria inoculation for paretic cases [388]. The breakthrough in treatment came in 1943 when Mahoney [389] successfully used penicillin to treat primary syphilis in four patients. Parenteral penicillin has since remained the preferred drug for treatment of syphilis at any stage [50]. Recommendations for specific types of penicillin and duration of therapy vary, depending on the stage of disease and clinical manifestations. However, parenteral penicillin G is the only documented effective therapy for patients who have neurosyphilis, congenital syphilis, or syphilis during pregnancy and is recommended for HIV-infected patients. Such patients always should be treated with penicillin, even if desensitization for penicillin allergy is necessary [50,390]. Penicillin resistance has not been described in *T. pallidum*, which is exquisitely sensitive with a penicillin minimal inhibitory concentration of 0.004 U (or 0.0025 µg/mL) [391–393]. Effective therapy for syphilis has to be maintained for at least 7 to 10 days, however, because of the slow replication of *T. pallidum* (every 30 hours) [394]. Therapy is designed to achieve and maintain several times the necessary inhibitory levels [50].

TREATMENT OF ACQUIRED SYPHILIS IN PREGNANCY

A serologic test for syphilis should be performed on all pregnant women at the first prenatal visit or not later than the time a pregnancy is confirmed [50]. Pregnant women with any reactive serologic tests for syphilis should be considered infected unless an adequate treatment history is documented and sequential nontreponemal antibody titers have declined [78,372]. A pregnant woman with a negative RPR screening test should still receive immediate therapy if the following conditions are present: (1) She has a suspicious lesion, and a negative RPR result may reflect the early stage of her infection; detection of treponemes by dark-field microscope should lead to therapy without regard to results of serologic tests; RPR should be repeated in 3 to 6 weeks in all of these cases. (2) She has neither lesions nor positive results of serologic studies, but has been exposed sexually to a person who has or may have syphilis; in this case she should receive treatment for the chance that she has acquired syphilis and is in the early phase of the infection and might transmit infection to her fetus [242,362].

Regardless of the stage of pregnancy, patients should be treated with penicillin according to the dosage schedules appropriate for the stage of syphilis [50,287]. Early syphilis—primary, secondary, and early latent infection—is treated with benzathine penicillin G, 50,000 U/kg up to the maximal dose of 2.4 million U intramuscularly in a single dose [50,394–396]. Many experts recommend that an additional dose of benzathine penicillin G be provided 1 week after the initial dose [50]. Late latent syphilis requires benzathine penicillin administered as 50,000 U/kg up to the adult dose of 2.4 million U at 1-week intervals for 3 consecutive weeks (i.e., total combined dose of 150,000 U/kg up to the maximal dose of 7.2 million U), but only if the CSF examination has excluded neurosyphilis. When the duration of infection is unknown, the patient should be treated as for late latent disease. Management and treatment decisions may be guided further by the use of fetal ultrasonography. Evidence of fetal infection may require additional doses of benzathine penicillin G until resolution of fetal abnormalities can be documented [279].

A pregnant woman with a history of penicillin allergy should be treated with penicillin after desensitization (see subsequently for instructions) because no proven alternative therapy has been established. In some patients, skin testing may be helpful. In pregnant women, desensitization should be performed in consultation with a specialist and only in facilities in which emergency assistance is available [397]. Pregnant women who received therapy for gonorrhea with ceftriaxone have a high rate of cure of primary syphilis, but failures have occurred, and efficacy in pregnancy is not well studied [398]. This regimen cannot be assumed to provide adequate therapy for syphilis in pregnancy. Any therapy other than penicillin is considered to be inadequate therapy during pregnancy [65,399]. Nonetheless, failure rates of penicillin for prevention of fetal infection ranging from 2% to 14% have been reported [400]. Most fetal treatment failures seem to occur after maternal treatment for secondary syphilis [401]. Treatment failure in such cases may be explained partly by the marked spirochetemia that occurs during secondary syphilitic infection. Other reasons for the presumptive treatment failures have been related to possibly altered penicillin pharmacokinetics in pregnancy [402] or to advanced fetal disease [403].

Neurosyphilis

Invasion of the CNS by *T. pallidum* can occur during any stage of syphilis [80]. During early syphilis, evaluation of CSF in a pregnant adolescent or adult is necessary only if clinical signs or symptoms of neurologic or ophthalmic involvement are present [50,404]. A lumbar puncture in a pregnant adolescent or adult in the late stages of syphilis is indicated if there are findings on neurologic or ophthalmic examination of active tertiary syphilis (e.g., aortitis, gumma), the patient has had previous treatment failure, or the patient was treated with an antimicrobial agent other than penicillin [89]. Some experts also recommend performing a CSF examination on all patients who have latent syphilis and a nontreponemal serologic test result of 1:32 or greater. All HIV-infected pregnant women with late latent syphilis or syphilis of unknown duration should have a lumbar puncture and CSF examined [80,395,405].

Benzathine penicillin does not reliably produce inhibitory CSF levels of penicillin [406], and numerous reports describe the persistence of treponemes in the CSF after therapy for syphilis [57,407–413]. Shorter acting penicillins must be employed for neurosyphilis. The recommended regimen for pregnant adults with neurosyphilis is aqueous crystalline penicillin G, 18 to 24 million U/day, administered as 3 to 4 million U intravenously every 4 hours or continuous infusion for 10 to 14 days. If adherence to therapy can be ensured, patients may be treated with an alternative regimen of intramuscular penicillin G, 2.4 million U intramuscularly once daily, plus probenecid, 500 mg orally four times per day, for 10 to 14 days. Because these regimens are shorter than the regimen used for late latent syphilis, some experts recommend following both of these regimens with benzathine penicillin G, 2.4 million U (or 50,000 U/kg per dose) intramuscularly weekly for one to three doses [78].

Human Immunodeficiency Virus

For HIV-infected pregnant women with primary or secondary syphilis, some authorities recommend up to three weekly doses of 2.4 million U of benzathine penicillin G in addition to the single intramuscular dose of benzathine penicillin G. HIV-infected patients who have either late latent syphilis or syphilis of unknown duration require a CSF examination before treatment. If nontreponemal antibody titers have not declined fourfold by 6 months in primary or secondary syphilis or by 6 to 12 months in early latent syphilis, or if the titer has increased fourfold at any time, a CSF examination should be performed, and the patient should be retreated with 7.2 million U of benzathine penicillin G (administered as three weekly doses of 2.4 million U each) if CSF examination findings are normal. HIV-infected pregnant patients who have CSF abnormalities consistent with neurosyphilis should receive treatment for neurosyphilis as described earlier [73,78].

Postexposure Prophylaxis

Recommendations for postexposure prophylaxis for syphilis for exposed or possibly exposed health care providers are benzathine penicillin G, 2.4 million U intramuscularly × 1 dose or doxycycline, 100 mg orally twice daily × 2 weeks, as an alternative for nonpregnant health care providers. These recommendations are largely based on guidelines for the epidemiologic treatment of suspected sexual contacts [414–417].

TREATMENT OF CONGENITAL SYPHILIS

Infants should be treated for congenital syphilis if they have *definite*, *highly probable*, *probable*, or *possible* disease. Infants in the *unlikely* category (for definitions of these terms, see Table 16–4) are recommended to receive therapy, as are infants born to mothers with either clinical or serologic evidence of syphilis infection for whom test results cannot exclude infection, who cannot be evaluated completely, or for whom adequate follow-up cannot be ensured [78,390]. The difference between these categories is only the type of therapy that is recommended. Infants in the *definite* and *highly probable* categories (i.e., clinically symptomatic infants) should be treated with intravenous aqueous crystalline penicillin G for 10 to 14 days at 50,000 U/kg per dose every 12 hours (100,000 U/kg/d) during the first 7 days of life and every 8 hours during days 8 to 30 (150,000 U/kg/d). Intramuscular procaine penicillin G, 50,000 U/kg/d as a single daily dose for 10 to 14 days, has also been proposed by some experts as an alternative [78,369,390]. Adequate CSF concentrations may not be achieved with intramuscular procaine penicillin; if intramuscular procaine penicillin is chosen, an unequivocally negative CSF examination must be available before initiating this form of therapy [418]. A full 10-day course of penicillin is preferred even if the infant received ampicillin initially for possible sepsis. Also, if more than 1 day of therapy is missed, the entire course needs to be restarted [78].

Clinically Asymptomatic Infants

Treatment decisions of clinically "asymptomatic" infants (i.e., in the probable, possible, or unlikely category) are based on (1) the maternal history of syphilis and past treatment and (2) the infant serologic evaluation. Maternal treatment for syphilis is deemed inadequate if (1) the mother's penicillin dose is unknown, undocumented, or inadequate; (2) the mother received a treatment regimen not including penicillin during pregnancy for syphilis; (3) treatment was given within less than 30 days of the infant's birth; or (4) mother has early syphilis and has a nontreponemal titer that either has not decreased fourfold or has increased fourfold [364,419]. For an asymptomatic infant of a mother with a positive serologic screen, three possible scenarios need to be considered: [78,149,390]

1. If the mother's treatment was inadequate, and an asymptomatic infant's nontreponemal test is reactive, the infant is deemed to have *probable* congenital syphilis [78]. If medical follow-up is certain, the infant may be treated with a single intramuscular dose of benzathine penicillin G, 50,000 U/kg. Single-dose benzathine penicillin therapy has been widely used in the past, and its use allows for earlier hospital discharge of the infant with subsequent improved maternal-infant interaction and decrease in hospitalization costs [420]. This regimen has also

been supported by two small clinical studies [421,422]. If the infant is to receive a single intramuscular injection of benzathine penicillin G, a complete evaluation—including a lumbar puncture—is mandatory [78,279,390,421,422]. Given the difficulty of ruling out neurosyphilis unequivocally, many experts prefer the 10-day intravenous course with aqueous crystalline penicillin G for all infants in this category [267,287,397]. If any part of the evaluation is abnormal, unavailable, or uninterpretable (e.g., CSF contaminated by blood), a full 10- to 14-day regimen is recommended [390]. If the meaning of a positive RPR result in an otherwise normal infant is in doubt, and the results of all other tests are negative, repeat quantitative RPR testing should be undertaken [78,390].

2. If the mother's treatment was adequate, but an asymptomatic infant's nontreponemal serum test is reactive, the infant is said to have *possible* congenital syphilis. Some experts recommend that a single dose of benzathine penicillin be administered as described previously [78,121,390,421,422]. Failure of such therapy in three infants has been reported [406,423,424]. Given these concerns, most experts suggest that all infants with possible congenital syphilis receive parenteral penicillin therapy for 10 days, especially if the mother had secondary syphilis at delivery or seroconverted during the pregnancy [60,170,402].

3. If the mother was treated adequately during the pregnancy, and the serologic assessment is non-reactive in an asymptomatic infant, the infant is *unlikely* to have congenital syphilis. Because of the inability to rule out possible transmission to the fetus in these cases, we recommend a single intramuscular dose of benzathine penicillin even for infants falling into this *unlikely* group. If the choice is made not to treat an infant in this category, close follow-up has to be ensured, and such an infant needs to undergo a second RPR test within 3 to 4 weeks of birth. Finally, the appearance of secondary or tertiary syphilis in a mother within 1 year after delivery should prompt a thorough reevaluation of the infant [242,362].

Internationally Adopted Children

Congenital syphilis sometimes is undiagnosed and often inadequately treated in developing countries. Syphilis testing is recommended as part of the evaluation of internationally adopted children, regardless of history or report of evaluation and treatment abroad [121,425]. When congenital syphilis of any stage and site is identified beyond the neonatal period, the treatment regimen for acquired neurosyphilis should be used: 200,000 to 300,000 U/kg/d of aqueous crystalline penicillin G, given as 50,000 U/kg every 4 to 6 hours for a minimum of 10 to 14 days. Some experts follow this regimen with intramuscular doses of benzathine penicillin G, 50,000 U/kg weekly for 3 weeks. If the patient has no clinical manifestations of disease, CSF examination is normal, and the result of VDRL of CSF is negative, some experts treat

only with three weekly doses of benzathine penicillin G (50,000 U/kg intramuscularly). When intravenous or intramuscular penicillin preparations are unavailable (see later) or cannot be tolerated, intravenous ampicillin or parenteral ceftriaxone can be considered as alternative therapy, but careful clinical and serologic follow-up is essential when these regimens are used because data for efficacy are insufficient [78,121,390].

FOLLOW-UP FOR A PREGNANT WOMAN INFECTED WITH SYPHILIS

Treated pregnant women with syphilis should have quantitative nontreponemal serologic tests repeated at 28 to 32 weeks of gestation, at delivery, and following the recommendations for the stage of disease. Serologic titers may be repeated monthly in women at high risk of reinfection or in geographic areas where the prevalence of syphilis is high. The clinical and antibody response should be appropriate for stage of disease. In practice, however, most women deliver before their serologic response to treatment can be assessed definitively. All pregnant women with acquired syphilis and all of their recent sexual contacts should be evaluated for syphilis and other sexually transmitted infections. For pregnant HIV-infected women with syphilis, careful follow-up is essential because higher rates of treatment failure have been reported [78,390].

In a pregnant woman with primary or secondary syphilis, retreatment should be considered necessary if clinical signs or symptoms persist or recur, if a fourfold increase in titer of a nontreponemal test occurs (also evaluate CSF and HIV status), or if the nontreponemal titer fails to decrease fourfold within 6 months after therapy (the woman also should be evaluated for HIV and retreated, unless follow-up for continued clinical and serologic assessment can be ensured). In a pregnant woman with latent syphilis, a CSF evaluation should be performed, and the woman should be retreated if titers increase fourfold, if an initially high titer (>1:32) fails to decrease at least fourfold within 12 to 24 months, or if signs or symptoms attributable to syphilis develop at anytime. In all these instances, retreatment should be with three weekly injections of benzathine penicillin G, 2.4 million U intramuscularly, unless CSF examination indicates that neurosyphilis is present, at which time treatment for neurosyphilis should be initiated. Generally, only one retreatment course is indicated. The possibility of reinfection or concurrent HIV infection always should be considered when retreating pregnant patients with syphilis. Pregnant patients with neurosyphilis must have periodic serologic testing, clinical evaluation at 6-month intervals, and repeated CSF examinations. If the CSF cell count has not decreased after 6 months, or CSF is not entirely normal after 2 years of therapy, retreatment should be considered [78,390].

FOLLOW-UP FOR AN INFANT INFECTED WITH SYPHILIS

Infants should be reevaluated after treatment for definite, probable, or possible congenital syphilis at 1, 2, 3, 6, and 12 months of age [426]. Nontreponemal serologic tests should be performed 2 to 4, 6, and 12 months (i.e., incorporated into routine pediatric care) after conclusion of treatment, or until results become nonreactive or the titer has decreased fourfold [233,279]. When nontreponemal antibodies are of maternal origin, titers usually become negative within 3 months and should be negative by 6 months of age if the infant was not infected [427]. The serologic response after therapy may decline more slowly for infants treated after the neonatal period.

If the choice was made not to treat an infant in the *unlikely* category, a nontreponemal test has to be performed at 3 to 4 weeks of age; untreated infants who are not seronegative by 6 months of age should be fully reevaluated clinically and treated. If titers of nontreponemal antibodies remain stable or increase after age 6 to 12 months in any infant, he or she should be reevaluated (including CSF analysis) and treated with a 10-day parenteral course of penicillin G, even if the infant had been treated previously [78,390]. Treponeme-specific antibodies of maternal origin may persist for 12 to 15 months in 15% of uninfected infants [428], rendering these tests of little help during infancy. Reactivity at 18 months or beyond is indicative of congenital infection [429,430]. The recommendation of a second treponemal test beyond 15 months as a way of retrospectively diagnosing congenital syphilis is not merely for epidemiologic use—an established diagnosis can help in medical and developmental follow-up evaluation of the child [224,431].

All infants and children should be evaluated thoroughly for the extent of disease if there is serologic evidence of treatment failure or of recurrent disease. Such evaluation at a minimum should consist of CSF examination and complete blood count and platelet count. Other tests, such as long bone radiographs, liver function tests, hearing evaluation, and ophthalmologic evaluation, should be performed as clinically indicated. Infants with congenital neurosyphilis (or unavailable, abnormal, or uninterpretable CSF WBC count or protein concentration or positive CSF VDRL) should have repeat clinical and CSF evaluations every 6 months until CSF indices are normal. A reactive CSF VDRL test at any time represents an indication for retreatment with a full 10- to 14-day course. If CSF WBC counts do not steadily decline at each examination or remain abnormal at 2 years, retreatment also is indicated [78,121,390].

Although treatment can cure the infection, the prognosis in treated congenital syphilis depends on the degree of damage before the initiation of therapy. Generally, the earlier treatment is initiated, the more likely it is that a satisfactory response can be obtained [225]. If marked damage to the fetus has occurred, treatment in utero may not prevent abortion, stillbirth, or neonatal death, and even if treatment keeps the newborn infant alive, stigmata can remain. If treatment is provided prenatally or within the first 3 months of life, and such stigmata have not yet become apparent, they generally can be prevented [276]. Interstitial keratitis is an exception; this complication does not seem to be responsive to specific antibiotic therapy. Occasionally, dramatic relief has been afforded by the use of corticosteroids and mydriatics, although relapses have occurred with cessation of corticosteroid therapy. Osseous lesions seem to heal independently of specific therapy. Treatment of congenital syphilis in the late stage does not reverse the stigmata [432].

PROBLEMS ASSOCIATED WITH PENICILLIN THERAPY

Penicillin Hypersensitivity

Skin testing for penicillin hypersensitivity with the major and minor determinants can reliably identify people at high risk of reacting to penicillin; currently, only the major determinant (benzylpenicilloyl poly-L-lysine) and penicillin G skin tests are available commercially. Testing with the major determinant of penicillin G is estimated to miss 3% to 6% of penicillin-allergic patients, who are at risk of serious or fatal reactions. A cautious approach (i.e., hospitalization) to penicillin therapy is advised when a patient cannot be tested with all of the penicillin skin test reagents. An oral or intravenous desensitization protocol for patients with a positive skin test result is available (www.cdc.gov/nchstp/dstd/penicillinG.htm) and should be performed in a hospital setting [390,433]. Oral desensitization is regarded as safer and easier to perform. Desensitization usually can be completed in approximately 4 hours, after which the first therapeutic dose of penicillin can be given [78,433].

Jarisch-Herxheimer Reaction

Jarisch-Herxheimer reaction, a common occurrence in the treatment of acquired early syphilis in adults [434], consists of chills, fever ($\geq$38° C [$\geq$100.4° F]), generalized malaise, hypotension, tachycardia, tachypnea, accentuation of cutaneous lesions, leukocytosis, and, exceedingly rarely, death. The reaction begins within 2 hours of treatment, peaks at approximately 8 hours, and disappears in 24 to 36 hours. The cause of Jarisch-Herxheimer reaction is unknown [435], although release of *T. pallidum* membrane lipoproteins that stimulate proinflammatory cytokines likely explains this clinical phenomenon [436]. Approximately 40% of pregnant women who receive treatment for syphilis exhibit a Jarisch-Herxheimer reaction [437,438]. In addition, these women may experience the onset of uterine contractions and preterm labor, with decreased fetal activity and fetal heart rate changes, including late decelerations, which last 24 to 48 hours and may lead to fetal death. No prophylactic measure or treatment is currently available. Abnormal ultrasound findings in the fetus and fetal monitoring for 24 hours may identify pregnancies at highest risk, but concern for occurrence of Jarisch-Herxheimer reaction should not delay treatment [438,439].

In congenital syphilis, the incidence of Jarisch-Herxheimer reaction is low, although it may be more common when treatment occurs later in infancy [242]; when it does occur, it varies in severity, ranging from fever to cardiovascular collapse and seizures [149]. In the series by Platou and Kometani [233], almost half of the infants sustained a febrile reaction during the first 36 hours after initiation of penicillin therapy. No relationship was observed between the severity or the outcome of the infection and this temperature elevation.

Penicillin Shortage

During periods of penicillin shortage, see http://www.cdc.gov/nchstp/dstd/penicillinG.htm for updates. Currently, the following is recommended: [50]

1. For infants with clinical *definitive* or *highly probable* congenital syphilis, check local sources for aqueous crystalline penicillin G (potassium or sodium). If intravenous penicillin G is limited, substitute some or all daily doses with procaine penicillin G (50,000 U/kg/dose intramuscularly a day in a single daily dose for 10 days). If aqueous or procaine penicillin G is unavailable, ceftriaxone (in doses according to age and weight) may be considered with careful clinical and serologic follow-up. Ceftriaxone must be used with caution in infants with jaundice. For infants 30 days or more of age, use 75 mg/kg intravenously or intramuscularly a day in a single daily dose for 10 to 14 days; dose adjustment might be necessary based on birth weight. For older infants, the dose should be 100 mg/kg/d in a single dose. Studies that strongly support ceftriaxone for the treatment of congenital syphilis have not been conducted. Ceftriaxone should be used in consultation with a specialist in the treatment of infants with congenital syphilis. Management may include a repeat CSF examination at age 6 months if the initial examination was abnormal.

2. For infants at risk with probable or possible congenital syphilis, use procaine penicillin G, 50,000 U/kg/dose intramuscularly a day in a single dose for 10 days, or benzathine penicillin G, 50,000 U/kg intramuscularly as a single dose. If any part of the evaluation for congenital syphilis is abnormal, CSF examination is not interpretable, CSF examination was not performed, or follow-up is uncertain, procaine penicillin G is recommended. A single dose of ceftriaxone is not considered adequate therapy.

3. For premature infants with probable or possible congenital syphilis and who might not tolerate intramuscular injections because of decreased muscle mass, intravenous ceftriaxone may be considered with careful clinical and serologic follow-up. Ceftriaxone dosing must be adjusted to age and birth weight [50].

PREVENTION

The history of syphilis prevention, reviewed by Hossain and colleagues [12], holds important lessons for prevention of congenital syphilis. Reports of attempts to understand and control syphilis in the 15th century can be found. Throughout Europe, legislation previously penalized infected individuals who knowingly infected others or did not complete treatment. The introduction of the Wassermann test in 1907 helped to increase the momentum of "venereal disease" control efforts, and public health efforts began to adapt to the changing epidemiologic nature and social perception of a stigmatized infection. By 1943, "rapid treatment centers" were available

in the United States with 5 to 10 days of arsenical therapy; in Europe, venereal disease clinics opened providing free and confidential treatment with Ehrlich's salvarsan.

Europe and the United States saw a 90% decline in congenital syphilis from 1941–1972 with the widespread availability of screening and penicillin, the promotion of treatment of sexual partners, and blood donor screening. This success was attributed to policies providing free treatment, case finding and control, public education, a high degree of political will, and cooperation between medical professionals and the national health department. Initial public health efforts to combat this preventable infection in pregnancy arose in the 1940s in the form of antenatal syphilis screening and surveillance programs. Concepts developed by these early syphilis control strategies provided the model used by current sexually transmitted infection control programs, including HIV/AIDS: early identification, effective treatment of the index case and partner, intense follow-up, and behavioral modification of high-risk sexual practices.

Out of these historical lessons, concrete suggestions to halt the current increase in congenital syphilis have been extracted and have been summarized by Walker and Walker [111] and Schmid [16]. The cornerstone of immediate congenital syphilis control is antenatal screening and treatment of infected mothers with penicillin, which is a cost-effective intervention across the globe. In affluent countries, screening needs to be strengthened among people at high risk, who are most often society's marginalized groups [84,440], and clinicians need to be ever more vigilant for the possibility of infants born with congenital syphilis. In less developed countries, high priority needs to be given to improving the efficiency of antenatal screening and the treatment and management of infected neonates. This management includes promoting early attendance for antenatal care and educating women (and men) about the benefits of syphilis screening and treatment; promoting modification of high-risk sexual behavior and use of condoms; implementing decentralized same-day screening and treatment, and using more recently developed rapid heat-stable point-of-care screening tests; performing a second test late in pregnancy to manage reinfections; testing all women at delivery; and prompt treatment of all infants who have confirmed, probable, or suspected congenital syphilis. Where health infrastructures are weak and syphilis prevalence is high, total reliance on a complex system of antenatal screening and treatment is unrealistic, and alternative strategies, such as mass treatment, might offer a more cost-effective initial approach for controlling congenital syphilis. Because of lack of commitment of politicians and public health officials in charge, funds for the control—much less the elimination—of congenital syphilis are inadequate. This situation allows syphilis to increase once more [111].

PRENATAL SCREENING

Although the concept of screening every pregnant woman for syphilis is simple, implementing the program may not be [16]. Screening of pregnant mothers for syphilis ranges from 17% to 88% in Bolivia, 63.6% to 79% in Brazil,

51% to 81% in Kenya, 43.2% in Malawi, less than 5% to 40% in Mozambique, 83.2% in Tanzania, and 32% to 83.2% in the United States. Despite these disparities in screening, in every society, the main cause of congenital syphilis is similar: lack of appropriate antenatal care [118]. In the industrialized world, failure to attend antenatal care is the most common cause of congenital syphilis with late care (too late to prevent stillbirth) a major contributing factor [353,441]. In the developing world, only an estimated 68% of pregnant women receive prenatal care, and the average time of first attendance is late—5 to 6 months [16]. For antenatal care to work, testing must be available and accessible. Availability can be addressed by decentralization of testing [442,443]. Accessibility argues that testing and treatment should be free of charge; cost to the patient has been identified as the greatest impediment to syphilis testing in sub-Saharan Africa [113]. Ideally, every woman who becomes pregnant should undergo at least one serologic test for syphilis during the first trimester [179,306,350,444]. For communities and populations in which the prevalence of syphilis is high or for women in high-risk groups, repeated testing at the beginning of the third trimester (at 28 weeks of gestation) [114] and at delivery is recommended [50].

It is a national policy in the United States that no infant should be discharged from the nursery before results of maternal serologic screening have been documented [50]. Laws pertaining to prenatal syphilis screening exist in 46 of the 50 U.S. states and the District of Columbia. Of these, 34 state laws mandate at least one prenatal serology, and 12 include a third-trimester test for either all or high-risk women [445]. The presence of state laws tends to correlate with the burden of congenital syphilis among the states [121]. With the practice of early discharge at 48 hours or less, it becomes the responsibility of the health care provider to arrange for adequate follow-up in infants who are discharged before the result of the maternal serologic test is known. The alternative to prenatal screening, targeted testing, is impractical to implement and would save little money, even if rates of syphilis were to decline in women and infants [287].

Prenatal testing systems do not help women who do not enter the medical care system until the moment before delivery. Lack of prenatal care, as already mentioned, is the most important cause for the persistence of congenital syphilis despite the wide availability of effective penicillin therapy [16,111]. Congenital syphilis is preventable, but only if prenatal care is available to and sought by the often hard-to-reach groups that are most at risk, such as teenage mothers, drug users, sex trade workers [446], and members of disadvantaged minority groups.

Several investigators have called attention to problems with antenatal management and communication crucial to the prevention of congenital syphilis [117,447–449]. These problems include failure to (1) obtain an appropriate and complete maternal history, (2) perform routine screening at appropriate times during the pregnancy, (3) interpret serologic results correctly, (4) recognize signs of maternal syphilis, (5) provide treatment for the pregnant sexual partner of an acutely infected man, and

(6) communicate pertinent maternal history and results of screening tests to the infant's health care practitioner. Local health departments and clinicians must improve the exchange of information between obstetric and pediatric services. These issues underscore further the need for education of health care providers on the management of sexually transmitted diseases. Given the limitation of current screening serologic tests to detect early cases of syphilis, even a perfectly executed prenatal prevention strategy would not eliminate all congenital syphilis [300]. Other measures are needed in conjunction with optimal prenatal screening policies. Contact tracing of sexual partners, careful physical examination of women in labor for evidence of primary syphilis, and additional testing of postpartum women at 4 to 6 weeks after delivery represent steps that would potentially be helpful [60,92,242,362].

Beyond the obvious medical and ethical advantages, universal screening of every pregnant woman for syphilis would save more money than it costs. As reviewed by Walker and Walker [111] and Schmid [16], economic evaluations of antenatal syphilis screening programs have been conducted in developed and developing countries and shown significant cost-effectiveness in either setting [450]. In the developed world and some middle-income countries where the prevalence of syphilis is lower, studies have shown universal screening of pregnant women to be cost-effective because treatment and support for the cases of missed congenital syphilis in such settings are extremely expensive. In the United States, an infant with congenital syphilis is hospitalized, on average, for 7.5 days longer than other infants and costs, on average, an additional US$5253 (2001 prices). The inclusion of indirect costs sharply increases the cost per case of congenital syphilis. Compared with these costs, syphilis screening is inexpensive. Where syphilis prevalence is extremely low, targeted screening might be marginally more cost-effective, but the political cost and practical difficulties of implementing this are considered to be unacceptably high.

In low-income countries, where the prevalence of syphilis remains high, fewer economic evaluations have been performed. In contrast to developed countries, the direct costs of congenital syphilis are relatively modest. Nevertheless, studies have found that screening is an efficient use of scarce resources. Terris-Prestholt and associates [451] estimated the cost per disability adjusted life year (DALY) averted in Tanzania and compared this with other studies from Zambia and Kenya in terms of the cost per DALY averted, which included all fetal consequences of maternal syphilis (i.e., abortions, stillbirths, low birth weight, and congenital syphilis). The cost per DALY averted was estimated to be US$3.97 to US$18.73 (2001 prices). Based on the recommendation of the Commission on Macroeconomics and Health, the WHO classifies interventions as "highly cost-effective" for a given country if results show that they avert a DALY for less than the per capita national gross domestic product, so antenatal syphilis screening is highly cost-effective in most developing countries. These calculations do not take into account the additional benefit of detecting and treating infection in the woman and her partner or partners [118]. As health care systems increasingly concentrate on preventing HIV infection in infants born to mothers with HIV infection, it is inexplicable that they do not do the same for syphilis because prevention of one DALY owing to congenital syphilis in a screening program for maternal syphilis using traditional testing methods is about 25 times more cost-effective as preventing one DALY among infants born to women who are HIV-positive [451,452].

CONTACT INVESTIGATION

Mothers of infants with congenital syphilis should be evaluated for gonorrhea, *C. trachomatis*, HIV, hepatitis B, and potentially hepatitis C infections. All cases should be reported to local public health authorities, who should undertake evaluation of recent sexual contacts for possible sexually transmitted diseases [50,85]. Patients who have had sexual contact with an untreated person should have a full clinical evaluation, serologic testing, and treatment. The time periods before treatment used for identifying at-risk sexual partners are (1) 3 months plus duration of symptoms for primary syphilis, (2) 6 months plus duration of symptoms for secondary syphilis, and (3) 1 year for early latent syphilis [50]. Persons who were exposed within 90 days preceding the diagnosis of primary, secondary, or early latent syphilis in a sexual partner might be infected even if seronegative and should receive presumptive treatment.

As partner notification has become more challenging because of anonymous sex and the inability to locate sexual partners, attention has focused on identifying core environments and populations in which syphilis transmission is occurring at a high rate [453]. Such knowledge has resulted in provision of prophylactic syphilis treatment to groups of people in high-risk populations (see subsequent section). The CDC has designed a strategy to assist public health providers at state and local levels to design interventions for targeted at-risk populations. Called the rapid ethnographic community assessment process (RECAP), the assessment is a package of activities and tools designed to use ethnographic methods for improving community involvement and developing interventions that fit a population's social and behavioral context [85].

MASS TREATMENT PROGRAMS

When enhancements of standard public health measures, such as contact tracing, education of at-risk groups and physicians, increased diagnostic and treatment services, and intensified screening, cannot control outbreaks, an alternative employed in developing and developed countries with some success is targeted mass treatment. The British Columbia Centre for Disease Control implemented a mass treatment and prophylaxis program with good short-term success, delivering more than 7000 treatment doses of azithromycin (1.8 g orally in a single dose) in two rounds over 5 weeks for syphilis to adults at high risk [93–95]. A later rebound in numbers of cases occurred, however, which is presumed to have been due to incomplete coverage of "high-frequency transmitters." [94,454] A similar program in Rinakai, Uganda, delivered more than 20,000 1-g treatment doses of azithromycin

[455–457]. The use of azithromycin and oral forms of penicillin offers advantages over the traditional use of injectable penicillin in terms of compliance [287,458]. More recent reports of azithromycin-resistant *T. pallidum* in the United States, where the use of azithromycin is far higher than in sub-Saharan Africa, indicate the potential problems associated with its use for syphilis [459,460]. Two smaller scale mass treatment programs in North America had been conducted using benzathine penicillin G, and both were judged successful [461,462]. There currently is no evidence to suggest that oral treatment is sufficient for the treatment of syphilis in pregnancy [458,463].

EDUCATION

Despite great progress in recent years, the prevention, control, and elimination of endemic syphilis in North America and other developed countries remains an elusive goal in public health policy. This is also true on a global scale in countries where resources may be limited and, as explained earlier, the practicalities of serologic screening and treatment in prenatal care settings are challenging. Another way to counteract the spread of syphilis and other sexually transmitted infections is through sexual education. The surest way to avoid transmission of sexually transmitted diseases, including syphilis, is to abstain from sexual contact or to be in a long-term, mutually monogamous relationship with a partner who has been tested and is known to be uninfected [50,85].

As outlined by the CDC, syphilis occurs in male and female genital areas that are covered or protected by a latex condom. The chancres also occur in areas that are not covered, and a substantial proportion (13.7%) of syphilis cases are attributed to oral sex [50,85]. Correct and consistent use of latex condoms can reduce the risk of syphilis, but does not eliminate the risk of transmission. Condoms lubricated with spermicides (especially nonoxynol 9) are no more effective than other lubricated condoms and are not recommended for sexually transmitted disease and HIV prevention. Persons who are not in a long-term monogamous relationship and who engage in oral sex should use appropriate barrier protection to reduce the risk for transmission of syphilis or other sexually transmitted infections. Just as important as it is that sex partners talk to each other about their HIV status and history of other sexually transmitted infections so that preventive action can be taken, it is equally important for the physician to educate sexually active patients continually [50,85].

ADVOCACY

The World Health Assembly stated in May 2006 in its "Strategy for the Prevention and Control of Sexually Transmitted Infections" that elimination of congenital syphilis is a global priority and emphasized the importance of incorporating this fight against congenital syphilis into wider initiatives that deal with the spread of sexually transmitted infections and HIV in general [111]. The Department of Reproductive Health and Research (RHR) at WHO published a series of "state-of-the-art" reviews on maternal and congenital syphilis in the *Bulletin of the World Health Organization* to advocate for action for the elimination of congenital syphilis worldwide [16]. The Scientific Technical Advisory Group of RHR in WHO endorsed a strategy for the global elimination of congenital syphilis, and elimination of congenital syphilis was included in its 2004–2009 work plan [16,111].

The broad goal of the WHO Strategy is the elimination of congenital syphilis as a public health problem, with the specific goals of prevention of mother-to-child transmission of syphilis through early antenatal care for all women, treatment of all sexual partners of infected women, and prophylactic treatment with a single dose of penicillin of all neonates born to RPR-positive mothers. These goals, together with the reduction of prevalence of syphilis in pregnant women as stated in the WHO Strategy, would ensure sustainability of the elimination goal of congenital syphilis. The WHO Strategy at country level consists of four pillars: to ensure sustained political commitment and advocacy; to increase access to, and quality of, maternal and newborn health services; to screen and treat all pregnant women; and to establish surveillance, monitoring, and evaluation systems. In its report, the WHO promised to assume the necessary leadership role, ensuring that the elimination of congenital syphilis becomes an institutional priority.

No date has been set as a target for eliminating congenital syphilis. Rather, interim goals have been set to introduce operationally programs into countries to eliminate congenital syphilis. The WHO points out that countries do not face insurmountable obstacles in attempts to achieve elimination of congenital syphilis, but lack political commitment, evidence-based priority setting, and advocacy at all levels [16,111]. There is little reason why the elimination of congenital syphilis is not a priority for every nation, and many reasons why it should be.

ACKNOWLEDGMENT

Drs. Ingall, Sanchez and Baker were co-authors of this chapter in previous editions.

REFERENCES

[1] T. Rosebury, Microbes and Morals: The Strange Story of Venereal Disease, Viking Press, New York, 1971.
[2] H. Goodman, Notable Contributions to the Knowledge of Syphilis, Froben Press, New York, 1943.
[3] C.C. Dennie, A History of Syphilis, Charles C Thomas, Springfield, IL, 1962.
[4] M. Truffi, Hieronymous Fracastor's Syphilis: A Translation in Prose, Urologic and Cutaneous Press, St. Louis, 1931.
[5] W.A. Pusey, The History and Epidemiology of Syphilis, Charles C Thomas, Springfield, IL, 1933.
[6] B.M. Rothschild, et al., First European exposure to syphilis: the Dominican Republic at the time of Columbian contact, Clin. Infect. Dis. 31 (2000) 936–941.
[7] P.F. Sparling, Natural History of Syphilis, McGraw-Hill, New York, 1999.
[8] W.J. Brown, Syphilis and Other Venereal Diseases, Harvard University Press, Cambridge, MA, 1970.
[9] J. Hutchinson, On the different forms of the inflammation of the eye consequent on inherited syphilis, Ophthalmol. Hosp. Rev. 1 (1858) 191.
[10] R.W. Peeling, E.W. Hook 3rd, The pathogenesis of syphilis: the Great Mimicker, revisited, J. Pathol. 208 (2006) 224–232.
[11] R. Chakraborty, S. Luck, Syphilis is on the increase: the implications for child health, Arch. Dis. Child. 93 (2008) 105–109.
[12] M. Hossain, N. Broutet, S. Hawkes, The elimination of congenital syphilis: a comparison of the proposed World Health Organization action plan for the elimination of congenital syphilis with existing national maternal and congenital syphilis policies, Sex. Transm. Dis. 34 (2007) S22–S30.
[13] D.G. Walker, G.J. Walker, Prevention of congenital syphilis—time for action, Bull. World Health Organ. 82 (2004).
[14] C.J. Murray, et al., The Global Burden of Disease 2000 project: aims, methods and data sources, in: Global Programme on Evidence for Health Policy Discussion Paper No. 36, World Health Organization, Geneva, 2001.
[15] H. Saloojee, et al., The prevention and management of congenital syphilis: an overview and recommendations, Bull. World Health Organ. 82 (2004) 424–430.
[16] G.P. Schmid, et al., The need and plan for global elimination of congenital syphilis, Sex. Transm. Dis. 34 (2007) S5–S10.
[17] R.E. Lafond, S.A. Lukehart, Biological basis for syphilis, Clin. Microbiol. Rev. 19 (2006) 29–49.
[18] K. Hovind-Hougen, Determination by means of electron microscopy of morphological criteria of value for classification of some spirochetes in particular treponemes, Acta Pathol. Microbiol. Scand. B Suppl. 225 (1976).
[19] E. Canale-Parola, Physiology and evolution of spirochetes: treponemal infection, Bacteriol. Rev. 157 (1977) 32.
[20] M.J. Fohn, et al., Specificity of antibodies from patients with pinta for antigens of Treponema pallidum subspecies pallidum, J. Infect. Dis. 157 (1988) 32–37.
[21] D.H. Bergey, Manual of Systematic Bacteriology, Williams & Wilkins, Baltimore, 1984.
[22] A. Centurion-Lara, et al., Conservation of the 15-kilodalton lipoprotein among Treponema pallidum subspecies and strains and other pathogenic treponemes: genetic and antigenic analyses, Infect. Immun. 65 (1997) 1440–1444.
[23] C.M. Fraser, S.J. Morris, G.M. Weinstock, Complete genome sequence of Treponema pallidum, the syphilis spirochete, Science 281 (1998) 375.
[24] G.C. Roman, L.N. Roman, Occurrence of congenital, cardiovascular, visceral, neurologic and neuro-ophthalmologic complications in late yaws: a theme for future research, Rev. Infect. Dis. 8 (1986) 760–770.
[25] T.B. Turner, D.H. Hollander, Biology of the treponematoses, WHO Monogr. Ser. 35 (1957) 1.
[26] R.R. Wilcox, T. Guthe, Treponema pallidum: a bibliographical review of the morphology, culture and survival of T. pallidum and associated organisms, Bull. World Health Organ. 35 (1966) 1.
[27] T.B. Turner, Syphilis and the treponematoses, in: S. Mudd (Ed.), Infectious Agents and Host Reactions, Saunders, Philadelphia, 1970.
[28] D.A. Bruckner, Nomenclature for aerobic and anaerobic bacteria, in: R.D. Feigin (Ed.), Textbook of Pediatric Infectious Diseases, fifth ed., Saunders, Philadelphia, 2004, pp. 1082–1099.
[29] S.C. Holt, Anatomy and chemistry of spirochetes, Microbiol. Rev. 42 (1978) 114–160.
[30] A.H. Johnson, Treatment of venereal diseases. II. Syphilis, Semin. Drug. Treat. 2 (1972) 289–293.
[31] A.N. Walker, Rapid plasma reagin (RPR) card test: a screening method for treponemal disease, Br. J. Vener. Dis. 47 (1971) 259–262.
[32] J.D. Radolf, et al., Serodiagnosis of syphilis by enzyme-linked immunosorbent assay with purified recombinant Treponema pallidum antigen 4D, J. Infect. Dis. 153 (1986) 1023–1027.
[33] E. Pennisi, Genome reveals wiles and weak points of syphilis, Science 281 (1998) 324–325.
[34] G.M. Weinstock, et al., From microbial genome sequence to applications, Res. Microbiol. 151 (2000) 151–158.
[35] S.J. Norris, C.M. Fraser, G.M. Weinstock, Illuminating the agent of syphilis: the Treponema pallidum genome project, Electrophoresis 19 (1998) 551–553.
[36] J.D. Radolf, B. Steiner, D. Shevchenko, Treponema pallidum: doing a remarkable job with what it's got, Trends Microbiol. 7 (1999) 7–9.
[37] J.M. Flood, et al., Neurosyphilis during the AIDS epidemic, San Francisco, 1985–1992, J. Infect. Dis. 177 (1998) 931–940.
[38] A. Pillay, et al., Molecular subtyping of Treponema pallidum subspecies pallidum, Sex. Transm. Dis. 25 (1998) 408–414.
[39] J.B. Baseman, Summary of the workshop on the biology of Treponema pallidum: cultivation and vaccine development, J. Infect. Dis. 136 (1977) 308–311.
[40] P.G. Lysko, C.D. Cox, Terminal electron transport in Treponema pallidum, Infect. Immun. 16 (1977) 885–890.
[41] P.G. Lysko, C.D. Cox, Respiration and oxidative phosphorylation in Treponema pallidum, Infect. Immun. 21 (1978) 462–473.
[42] J.O. Klein, Current concepts of infectious diseases in the newborn infant, Adv. Pediatr. 31 (1984) 405–446.
[43] E.W. Hook 3rd, C.M. Marra, Acquired syphilis in adults, N. Engl. J. Med. 326 (1992) 1060–1069.
[44] T.J. Fitzgerald, Experimental congenital syphilis in rabbits, Can. J. Microbiol. 31 (1985) 757–762.
[45] K. Wicher, et al., Experimental congenital syphilis: guinea pig model, Infect. Immun. 60 (1992) 271–277.
[46] A. Kajdacsy-Balla, A. Howeedy, O. Bagasra, Experimental model of congenital syphilis, Infect. Immun. 61 (1993) 3559–3561.
[47] K. Wicher, et al., Vertical transmission of Treponema pallidum to various litters and generations of guinea pigs, J. Infect. Dis. 179 (1999) 1206–1212.
[48] A.H. Fieldsteel, F.A. Becker, J.G. Stout, Prolonged survival of virulent Treponema pallidum (Nichols strain) in cell-free and tissue culture systems, Infect. Immun. 18 (1977) 173–182.

[49] A.H. Fieldsteel, D.L. Cox, R.A. Moeckli, Cultivation of virulent *Treponema pallidum* in tissue culture, Infect. Immun. 32 (1981) 908–915.

[50] Centers for Disease Control, Sexually transmitted diseases treatment guidelines, 2006, [erratum appears in MMWR Recomm. Rep. 55(36) (2006) 997] Morb. Mortal. Wkly Recomm. Rep. 55 (2006) 1–94.

[51] A.E. Singh, B. Romanowski, Syphilis: review with emphasis on clinical, epidemiologic, and some biologic features, Clin. Microbiol. Rev. 12 (1999) 187–209.

[52] H.J. Magnuson, H. Eagle, R. Fleischman, The minimal infectious inoculum of *Spirochaeta pallida* (Nichols strain), and a consideration of its rate of multiplication in vivo, Am. J. Syph. Gonorrhea Vener. Dis. 32 (1948).

[53] W. Cates Jr., R.B. Rothenberg, J.H. Blount, Syphilis control. The historic context and epidemiologic basis for interrupting sexual transmission of *Treponema pallidum*, Sex. Transm. Dis. 23 (1996) 68–75.

[54] H.J. Magnuson, E.W. Thomas, S. Orlansky, Inoculation syphilis in human volunteers, Medicine (Baltimore) 35 (1956) 33–82.

[55] H.G. Dorman, B.F. Sahyun, Identification and significance of spirochetes in placenta: report of 105 cases with positive findings, Am. J. Obstet. Gynecol. 33 (1937) 954–967.

[56] C.A. Harter, K. Benirschke, Fetal syphilis in the first trimester, Am. J. Obstet. Gynecol. 124 (1976) 705–711.

[57] A.M. Silverstein, Congenital syphilis and the timing of immunogenesis in the human foetus, Nature 194 (1962) 196–197.

[58] J.M. Burstain, E. Grimprel, S.A. Lukehart, M.V. Norgard, J.D. Radolf, Sensitive detection of *Treponema pallidum* by using the polymerase chain reaction, J. Clin. Microbiol. 29 (1991) 62–69.

[59] L. Nathan, D.M. Twickler, M.T. Peters, Fetal syphilis: correlation of sonographic findings and rabbit infectivity testing of amniotic fluid, J. Ultrasound Med. 12 (1993) 97–101.

[60] L. Nathan, et al., In utero infection with *Treponema pallidum* in early pregnancy, Prenat. Diagn. 17 (1997) 119–123.

[61] P.J. Sanchez, G.D. Wendel, E. Grimprel, Evaluation of molecular methodologies and rabbit infectivity testing for the diagnosis of congenital syphilis and central nervous system invasion by *Treponema pallidum*, J. Infect. Dis. 167 (1993) 148–157.

[62] G.D. Wendel Jr., et al., Identification of *Treponema pallidum* in amniotic fluid and fetal blood from pregnancies complicated by congenital syphilis, Obstet. Gynecol. 78 (1991) 890–895.

[63] F. Qureshi, S.M. Jacques, M.P. Reyes, Placental histopathology in syphilis, Hum. Pathol. 24 (1993) 779–784.

[64] R.M. Fojaca, G.T. Hensely, L. Moskowitz, Congenital syphilis and necrotizing funisitis, JAMA 12 (1989) 1788–1792.

[65] L.J. Fenton, I.J. Light, Congenital syphilis after maternal treatment with erythromycin, Obstet. Gynecol. 47 (1976) 492–494.

[66] J.N.D. Nabarro, Congenital Syphilis, Williams & Wilkins, Baltimore, 1954.

[67] J.W. Ballantyne, Manual of Antenatal Pathology and Hygiene, William Green & Son, Edinburgh, 1902.

[68] N.J. Fiumara, The incidence of prenatal syphilis at the Boston City Hospital, N. Engl. J. Med. 247 (1952) 48.

[69] N.R. Ingraham, The value of penicillin alone in the prevention and treatment of congenital syphilis, Acta Derm. Venereol. 31 (1951).

[70] R.E. Baughn, D.M. Musher, Secondary syphilitic lesions, Clin. Microbiol. Rev. 18 (2005) 205–216.

[71] J.S. Sheffield, G.D. Wendel, F. Zeray, Congenital syphilis: The influence of maternal stage of syphilis on vertical transmission, Am. J. Obstet. Gynecol. 180 (1999) (Supplement) 85–88.

[72] N.J. Fiumara, A legacy of syphilis, Arch. Dermatol. 92 (1965) 676–678.

[73] W.A. Lynn, S. Lightman, Syphilis and HIV: a dangerous combination, Lancet Infect. Dis. 4 (2004) 456–466.

[74] E.J. Erbelding, Syphilis rates climb again, Hopkins HIV Rep. 16 (2004) 8–9.

[75] M.R. Golden, C.M. Marra, K.K. Holmes, Update on syphilis: resurgence of an old problem, JAMA 290 (2003) 1510–1514.

[76] M. Poulton, et al., Syphilis: mimicking yet another disease!, Sex. Transm. Infect. 77 (2001) 325.

[77] S.A. Theus, D.A. Harrich, R. Gaynor, *Treponema pallidum*, lipoproteins, and synthetic lipoprotein analogues induce human immuno-deficiency virus type 1 gene expression in monocytes via NF- B activation, J. Infect. Dis. 177 (1998) 941–950.

[78] CDC, 2006. Available at http://www.cdc.gov/std/syphilis. Accessed November 2008.

[79] J.M. Schulte, et al., Syphilis among HIV-infected mothers and their infants in Texas from 1988 to 1994, Sex. Transm. Dis. 28 (2001) 315–320.

[80] S.A. Lukehart, et al., Invasion of the central nervous system by *Treponema pallidum*: implications for diagnosis and treatment, Ann. Intern. Med. 109 (1988) 855–862.

[81] C.R. Woods, Syphilis in children: congenital and acquired, Semin. Pediatr. Infect. Dis. 16 (2005) 245–257.

[82] H.A. Tucker, R.C.V. Robinson, Disappearance time of *T. pallidum* from lesions of early syphilis following administration of crystalline penicillin G, Bull. Johns. Hopkins. Hosp. 80 (1947) 169.

[83] American Academy of Pediatrics, Syphilis, in: L.K. Pickering (Ed.), Red Book: Report of the Committee on Infectious Diseases, twentyseventh ed., American Academy of Pediatrics, Elk Grove Village, IL, 2006, pp. 631–634.

[84] J.M. Zenilman, Congenital syphilis in immigrants—are politics and nativism driving us in reverse? Sex. Transm. Dis. 35 (2008) 344–345.

[85] Centers for Disease Control and Prevention, Sexually Transmitted Disease Surveillance 2006 Supplement, Syphilis Surveillance Report, U.S. Department of Health and Human Services, Centers for Disease Control and Prevention, Atlanta, GA, 2007 Available at http://www.cdc.gov/std/Syphilis2006/Syphilis2006Short.pdf. Accessed March 13, 2008.

[86] R.T. Rolfs, A.K. Nakashima, Epidemiology of primary and secondary syphilis in the United States, 1981 through 1989, JAMA 264 (1990) 1432–1437.

[87] J.M. Ricci, R.M. Fojaco, M.J. O'Sullivan, Congenital syphilis: the University of Miami/Jackson Memorial Medical Center experience, 1986–1988, Obstet. Gynecol. 74 (1989) 687–693.

[88] P.E. Klass, E.R. Brown, S.I. Pelton, The incidence of prenatal syphilis at the Boston City Hospital: a comparison across four decades, Pediatrics 94 (1994) 24–28.

[89] K.C. Rathbun, Congenital syphilis, Sex. Transm. Dis. 10 (1983) 93–99.

[90] L.A. Webster, et al., Regional and temporal trends in the surveillance of syphilis, United States, 1986–1990, MMWR CDC Surveill. Summ. 40 (1991) 29–33.

[91] L.A. Webster, R.T. Rolfs, Surveillance for primary and secondary syphilis—United States, 1991, MMWR CDC Surveill. Summ. 42 (1993) 13–19.

[92] A.K. Nakashima, et al., Epidemiology of syphilis in the United States, 1941–1993, Sex. Transm. Dis. 23 (1996) 16–23.

[93] M. Rekart, et al., Mass treatment/prophylaxis during an outbreak of infectious syphilis in Vancouver, British Columbia, Can. Commun. Dis. Rep. 26 (2000) 101–105.

[94] M.L. Rekart, et al., Targeted mass treatment for syphilis with oral azithromycin, Lancet 361 (2003) 313–314.

[95] M.L. Rekart, et al., The impact of syphilis mass treatment one year later: self-reported behaviour change among participants, Int. J. STD AIDS 16 (2005) 571–578.

[96] R.A. Dunn, et al., Surveillance for geographic and secular trends in congenital syphilis—United States, 1983–1991, MMWR CDC Surveill. Summ. 42 (1993) 59–71.

[97] St.M.E. Louis, J.M. Wasserheit, Elimination of syphilis in the United States, Science 281 (1998) 353.

[98] R.A. Hahn, et al., Race and the prevalence of syphilis seroreactivity in the United States population: a national sero-epidemiologic study, Am. J. Public Health 79 (1989) 467–470.

[99] P. Zenker, New case definition for congenital syphilis reporting, Sex. Transm. Dis. 18 (1991) 44–45.

[100] M.K. Ikeda, H.B. Jenson, Evaluation and treatment of congenital syphilis, J. Pediatr. 117 (1990) 843–852.

[101] L. Mascola, R. Pelosi, J.H. Blount, Congenital syphilis revisited, Am. J. Dis. Child. 139 (1985) 575–580.

[102] P.J. Sanchez, Congenital syphilis, Adv. Pediatr. Infect. Dis. 7 (1992) 161–180.

[103] D.A. Cohen, et al., The effects of case definition in maternal screening and reporting criteria on rates of congenital syphilis, Am. J. Public Health 80 (1990) 316–317.

[104] A.E. Singh, et al., Resurgence of early congenital syphilis in Alberta, Can. Med. Assoc. J. 177 (2007) 33–36.

[105] World Health Organization, Global Prevalence and Incidence of Curable STIs, World Health Organization, Geneva, 2001.

[106] Health Protection Agency, All new diagnoses made at GUM clinics: 1996–2005 United Kingdom and country specific tables, (2005) Available at http://www.hpa.org.uk/infections/topics_az/hiv_and_sti/epidemiology/datatables2005.htm. Accessed October 30, 2007.

[107] A. Doroshenko, J. Sherrard, A.J. Pollard, Syphilis in pregnancy and the neonatal period, Int. J. STD AIDS 17 (2006) 221–227.

[108] A. Nicoll, F.F. Hamers, Are trends in HIV, gonorrhoea, and syphilis worsening in western Europe? BMJ 324 (2002) 1324–1327.

[109] U. Marcus, O. Hamouda, Syphilis in Germany, 2004: diagnoses increasing, particularly in smaller cities and rural areas, Eur. Surveill. 10 (2005) E050728.

[110] S. Lautenschlager, Sexually transmitted infections in Switzerland: return of the classics, Dermatology 210 (2005) 134–142.

[111] G.J. Walker, D.G. Walker, Congenital syphilis: a continuing but neglected problem, Semin. Fetal. Neonatal. Med. 12 (2007) 198–206.

[112] B.H. Chi, et al., Predictors of stillbirth in sub-Saharan Africa, Obstet. Gynecol. 110 (2007) 989–997.

[113] S. Gloyd, S. Chai, M.A. Mercer, Antenatal syphilis in sub-Saharan Africa: missed opportunities for mortality reduction, Health Policy Plan. 16 (2001) 29–34.

[114] K.L. Southwick, et al., Maternal and congenital syphilis in Bolivia, 1996: prevalence and risk factors, Bull. World Health Organ. 79 (2001) 33–42.

[115] Z.Q. Chen, et al., Syphilis in China: results of a national surveillance programme, Lancet 369 (2007) 132–138.

[116] S. Hawkes, et al., Antenatal syphilis control: people, programmes, policies and politics, Bull. World Health Organ. 82 (2004) 417–423.

[117] L. Finelli, et al., Congenital syphilis, Bull. World Health Organ. 76 (Suppl. 2) (1998) 126–128.

[118] G. Schmid, Economic and programmatic aspects of congenital syphilis prevention, Bull. World Health Organ. 82 (2004) 402–409.

[119] F.X. Mbopi Keou, et al., Antenatal HIV prevalence in Yaounde, Cameroon, Int. J. STD AIDS 9 (1998) 400–402.

[120] P. Gichangi, et al., Congenital syphilis in a Nairobi maternity hospital, East Afr. Med. J. 81 (2004) 589–593.

[121] C.R. Woods, Syphilis in children: congenital and acquired, Semin. Pediatr. Infect. Dis. 16 (2005) 245–257.

[122] K. Peterson, J.B. Baseman, J.F. Alderete, *Treponema pallidum* receptor binding proteins interact with fibronectin, J. Exp. Med. 157 (1983) 1958–1970.

[123] S.L. Robbins, Pathologic Basis of Disease, Saunders, Philadelphia, 1974.

[124] J.D. Radolf, Role of outer membrane architecture in immune evasion by *Treponema pallidum* and *Borrelia burgdorferi*, Trends Microbiol. 2 (1994) 307–311.

[125] C. Harter, K. Benirschke, Fetal syphilis in the first trimester, Am. J. Obstet. Gynecol. 124 (1976) 705–711.

[126] J.C. Salazar, et al., *Treponema pallidum* elicits innate and adaptive cellular immune responses in skin and blood during secondary syphilis: a flow-cytometric analysis, J. Infect. Dis. 195 (2007) 879–887.

[127] T.J. Sellati, et al., The cutaneous response in humans to *Treponema pallidum* lipoprotein analogues involves cellular elements of both innate and adaptive immunity, J. Immunol. 166 (2001) 4131–4140.

[128] V. Wicher, K. Wicher, Pathogenesis of maternal-fetal syphilis revisited, Clin. Infect. Dis. 33 (2001) 354–363.

[129] N.W. Schroder, et al., Immune responses induced by spirochetal outer membrane lipoproteins and glycolipids, Immunobiology 213 (2008) 329–340.

[130] J.C. Salazar, K.R.O. Hazlett, J.D. Radolf, The immune response to infection with *Treponema pallidum*, the stealth pathogen, Microbes Infect. 4 (2002) 1133–1140.

[131] J.D. Alder, L. Friess, M. Tengowski, R.F. Schell, Phagocytosis of opsonized Treponema pallidum subsp. pallidum proceeds slowly, Infect. Immun. 58 (1990) 1167–1173.

[132] D.M. Musher, et al., The interaction between *Treponema pallidum* and human polymorphonuclear leukocytes, J. Infect. Dis. 147 (1983) 77–86.

[133] D.D. Thomas, et al., *Treponema pallidum* invades intercellular junctions of endothelial cell monolayers, Proc. Natl. Acad. Sci. U. S. A. 85 (1988) 3608–3612.

[134] H.D. Brightbill, et al., Host defense mechanisms triggered by microbial lipoproteins through toll-like receptors, Science 285 (1999) 732–736.

[135] T.J. Sellati, et al., Virulent *Treponema pallidum*, lipoprotein, and synthetic lipopeptides induce CCR5 on human monocytes and enhance their susceptibility to infection by human immunodeficiency virus type 1, J. Infect. Dis. 181 (2000) 283–293.

[136] B.S. Riley, et al., Virulent *Treponema pallidum* activates human vascular endothelial cells, J. Infect. Dis. 165 (1992) 484–493.

[137] J. Podwinska, et al., The pattern and level of cytokines secreted by Th1 and Th2 lymphocytes of syphilitic patients correlate to the progression of the disease, FEMS Immunol. Med. Microbiol. 28 (2000) 1–14.

[138] W.C. Van Voorhis, et al., Primary and secondary syphilis lesions contain mRNA for Th1 cytokines, J. Infect. Dis. 173 (1996) 491–495.

[139] Y.M. Fan, et al., Immunophenotypes, apoptosis, and expression of Fas and Bcl-2 from peripheral blood lymphocytes in patients with secondary early syphilis, Sex. Transm. Dis. 31 (2004) 221–224.

[140] S. Olansky, Serodiagnosis of syphilis, Med. Clin. North Am. 56 (1972) 1145–1150.

[141] M.A. Swancott, J.D. Radolf, M.V. Norgard, The 34-kilodalton membrane immunogen of *Treponema pallidum* is a lipoprotein, Infect. Immun. 58 (1990) 384–392.

[142] R.R. Willcox, Changing patterns of treponemal disease, Br. J. Vener. Dis. 50 (1974) 169–178.

[143] S.A. Baker-Zander, et al., Antigens of *Treponema pallidum* recognized by IgG and IgM antibodies during syphilis in humans, J. Infect. Dis. 151 (1985) 264–272.

[144] A. Gerber, S. Krell, J. Morenz, Recombinant *Treponema pallidum* antigens in syphilis serology, Immunobiology 196 (1996) 535–549.

[145] R.E. Baughn, et al., Ig class and IgG subclass responses to *Treponema pallidum* in patients with syphilis, J. Clin. Immunol. 8 (1988) 128–139.

[146] L.L. Lewis, L.H. Taber, R.E. Baughn, Evaluation of immunoglobulin M western blot analysis in the diagnosis of congenital syphilis, J. Clin. Microbiol. 28 (1990) 296–302.

[147] C.A. Morgan, S.A. Lukehart, W.C. Van Voorhis, Protection against syphilis correlates with specificity of antibodies to the variable regions of *Treponema pallidum* repeat protein K, Infect. Immun. 71 (2003) 5605–5612.

[148] P.J. Sanchez, et al., Molecular analysis of the fetal IgM response to *Treponema pallidum* antigens: implications for improved serodiagnosis of congenital syphilis, J. Infect. Dis. 159 (1989) 508–517.

[149] P.J. Sanchez, et al., Evaluation of molecular methodologies and rabbit infectivity testing for the diagnosis of congenital syphilis and neonatal central nervous system invasion by Treponema pallidum, J. Infect. Dis. 167 (1993) 148–157.

[150] S.R. Dobson, L.H. Taber, R.E. Baughn, Recognition of *Treponema pallidum* antigens by IgM and IgG antibodies in congenitally infected newborns and their mothers, J. Infect. Dis. 157 (1988) 903–910.

[151] M.F. Garner, et al., *Treponema pallidum* haemagglutination test for syphilis: comparison with TPI and FTA-ABS tests, Br. J. Vener. Dis. 48 (1972) 470–473.

[152] R.J. Weisser Jr., R.J. Marshall, Syphilitic aneurysms with bone erosion and rupture, W. V. Med. J. 72 (1976) 1–4.

[153] S. Graves, J. Downes, Experimental infection of man with rabbit-virulent *Treponema paraluis-cuniculi*, Br. J. Vener. Dis. 57 (1981) 7–10.

[154] A. Centurion-Lara, et al., *Treponema pallidum* major sheath protein homologue Tpr K is a target of opsonic antibody and the protective immune response, [erratum appears in J. Exp. Med. 189(11) (1999) following 1852], J. Exp. Med. 189 (1999) 647–656.

[155] B.T. Leader, et al., Antibody responses elicited against the *Treponema pallidum* repeat proteins differ during infection with different isolates of *Treponema pallidum* subsp. *Pallidum*, Infect. Immun. 71 (2003) 6054–6057.

[156] A. Centurion-Lara, et al., Gene conversion: a mechanism for generation of heterogeneity in the tprK gene of *Treponema pallidum* during infection, Mol. Microbiol. 52 (2004) 1579–1596.

[157] G.D. Braunstein, et al., The nephrotic syndrome associated with secondary syphilis: an immune deposit disease, Am. J. Med. 48 (1970) 643–648.

[158] C.N. Gamble, J.B. Reardan, Immunopathogenesis of syphilitic glomerulonephritis: elution of antitreponemal antibody from glomerular immune-complex deposits, N. Engl. J. Med. 292 (1975) 449–454.

[159] B.S. Kaplan, et al., The glomerulopathy of congenital syphilis—an immune deposit disease, J. Pediatr. 81 (1972) 1154–1156.

[160] S.R. Dobson, L.H. Taber, R.E. Baughn, Characterization of the components in circulating immune complexes from infants with congenital syphilis, J. Infect. Dis. 158 (1988) 940–947.

[161] O. Vasquez-Manzanilla, S.M. Dickson-Gonzalez, A.J. Rodriguez-Morales, Congenital syphilis and ventricular septal defect, J. Trop. Pediatr. 55 (2008) 63.

[162] D. Nabarro, Congenital Syphilis, E Arnold, London, 1954.

[163] C.C. Dennie, The dying syphilologist, AMA Arch. Derm. Syphilol. 62 (1950) 615–621.

[164] N.J. Fiumara, Acquired syphilis in three patients with congenital syphilis, N. Engl. J. Med. 290 (1974) 1119–1120.

[165] K. Pavithran, Acquired syphilis in a patient with late congenital syphilis, Sex. Transm. Dis. 14 (1987) 119–121.

[166] J.N. Miller, Value and limitations of nontreponemal and treponemal tests in the laboratory diagnosis of syphilis, Clin. Obstet. Gynecol. 18 (1975) 191–203.

[167] R.W. Peeling, E.W. Hook, The pathogenesis of syphilis: the great mimicker, revisited, J. Pathol. 208 (2006) 224–232.

[168] S. Dobson, Congenital syphilis resurgent, Adv. Exp. Med. Biol. 549 (2004) 35–40.

[169] A.E. Benzick, et al., Pituitary gland gumma in congenital syphilis after failed maternal treatment: a case report, Pediatrics 104 (1999) e4.

[170] J.S. Sheffield, et al., Congenital syphilis after maternal treatment for syphilis during pregnancy, *Am J Obstet Gynecol* 186 (2002) 569–573.

[171] P. Russell, G. Altshuler, Placental abnormalities of congenital syphilis: a neglected aid to diagnosis, Am. J. Dis. Child. 128 (1974) 160–163.

[172] D.R. Genest, S.R. Choi-Hong, J.E. Tate, F. Qureschi, S.M. Jacques, C. Crum, Diagnosis of congenital syphilis from placental examination: Comparison of histopathology, Steiner stain, and polymerase chain reaction for Treponema pallidum DNA, Hum. Pathol. 27 (1996) 366–372.

[173] D.R. Genest, et al., Diagnosis of congenital syphilis from placental examination: comparison of histopathology, Steiner stain, and polymerase chain reaction for *Treponema pallidum* DNA, Hum. Pathol. 27 (1996) 366–372.

[174] J.S. Sheffield, et al., Placental histopathology of congenital syphilis, Obstet. Gynecol. 100 (2002) 126–133.

[175] G.D. Wendel, Gestational and congenital syphilis, Clin. Perinatol. 15 (1988) 287–303.

[176] R.M. Fojaco, G.T. Hensley, L. Moskowitz, Congenital syphilis and necrotizing funisitis, JAMA 261 (1989) 1788–1790.

[177] S.M. Jacques, F. Qureshi, Necrotizing funisitis: a study of 45 cases, Hum. Pathol. 23 (1992) 1278–1283.

[178] K. Bromberg, S. Rawstron, G. Tannis, Diagnosis of congenital syphilis by combining *Treponema pallidum*-specific IgM detection with immunofluorescent antigen detection for *T. pallidum*, J. Infect. Dis. 168 (1993) 238–242.

[179] M.P. Reyes, et al., Maternal/congenital syphilis in a large tertiary-care urban hospital, Clin. Infect. Dis. 17 (1993) 1041–1046.

[180] E.H. Oppenheimer, J.B. Hardy, Congenital syphilis in the newborn infant: clinical and pathological observations in recent cases, Johns Hopkins Med. J. 129 (1971) 63–82.

[181] D.J. Wright, C.L. Berry, Letter: Liver involvement in congenital syphilis, Br. J. Vener. Dis. 50 (1974) 241.

[182] J. Guarner, et al., Congenital syphilis in a newborn: an immunopathologic study, Mod. Pathol. 12 (1999) 82–87.

[183] N.A. Ajayi, et al., Intestinal ulceration, obstruction, and haemorrhage in congenital syphilis, Pediatr. Surg. Int. 15 (1999) 391–393.

[184] L.L. Hill, et al., The nephrotic syndrome in congenital syphilis: an immunopathy, Pediatrics 49 (1972) 260–266.

[185] A. Losito, et al., Membranous glomerulonephritis in congenital syphilis, Clin. Nephrol. 12 (1979) 32–37.

[186] J. Wiggelinkhuizen, et al., Congenital syphilis and glomerulonephritis with evidence for immune pathogenesis, Arch. Dis. Child. 48 (1973) 375–381.

[187] B.J. Cremin, R.M. Fisher, The lesions of congenital syphilis, Br. J. Radiol. 43 (1970) 333–341.

[188] B.J. Cremin, R. Draper, The value of radiography in perinatal deaths, Pediatr. Radiol. 11 (1981) 143–146.

[189] J.J. Daaboul, W. Kartchner, K.L. Jones, Neonatal hypoglycemia caused by hypopituitarism in infants with congenital syphilis, J. Pediatr. 123 (1993) 983–985.

[190] L. Nathan, et al., Fetal syphilis: correlation of sonographic findings and rabbit infectivity testing of amniotic fluid, J. Ultrasound Med. 12 (1993) 97–101.

[191] J.R. Barton, et al., Nonimmune hydrops fetalis associated with maternal infection with syphilis, Am. J. Obstet. Gynecol. 167 (1992) 56–58.

[192] D.A. Gust, et al., Mortality associated with congenital syphilis in the United States, 1992–1998, Pediatrics 109 (2002) E79–90.

[193] P.J. Sanchez, G.D. Wendel, Syphilis in pregnancy, Clin. Perinatol. 24 (1997) 71–90.

[194] S.A. Rawstron, et al., Congenital syphilis: detection of *Treponema pallidum* in stillborns, Clin. Infect. Dis. 24 (1997) 24–27.

[195] L.M. Hill, J.B. Maloney, An unusual constellation of sonographic findings associated with congenital syphilis, Obstet. Gynecol. 78 (1991) 895–897.

[196] S. Lautenschlager, Cutaneous manifestations of syphilis: recognition and management, Am. J. Clin. Dermatol. 7 (2006) 291–304.

[197] T.A. Chapel, The variability of syphilitic chancres, Sex. Transm. Dis. 5 (1978) 68–70.

[198] S. Lautenschlager, Diagnosis of syphilis: clinical and laboratory problems, J. Dtsch. Dermatol. Ges. 4 (2006) 1058–1075.

[199] E.K. Blair, et al., Unsuspected syphilitic hepatitis in a patient with low-grade proteinuria and abnormal liver function, Mayo Clin. Proc. 65 (1990) 1365–1367.

[200] L.M. Drusin, B. Topf-Olstein, E. Levy-Zombek, Epidemiology of infectious syphilis at a tertiary hospital, Arch. Intern. Med. 139 (1979) 901–904.

[201] S.L. Manton, et al., Oral presentation of secondary syphilis, Br. Dent. J. 160 (1986) 237–238.

[202] D.M. Musher, Syphilis, Infect. Dis. Clin. North Am. 1 (1987) 83–95.

[203] J. Feher, et al., Syphilitic hepatitis: clinical, immunological and morphological aspects, Acta. Med. Acad. Sci. Hung. 32 (1975) 155–161.

[204] L. Jozsa, et al., Hepatitis syphilitica: a clinico-pathological study of 25 cases, Acta Hepatogastroenterol. (Stuttg.) 24 (1977) 344–347.

[205] M.S. Bhorade, et al., Nephropathy of secondary syphilis: a clinical and pathological spectrum, JAMA 216 (1971) 1159–1166.

[206] W.E. Dismukes, et al., Destructive bone disease in early syphilis, JAMA 236 (1976) 2646–2648.

[207] R.R. Tight, J.F. Warner, Skeletal involvement in secondary syphilis detected by bone scanning, JAMA 235 (1976) 2326.

[208] R.N. Shore, H.A. Kiesel, H.D. Bennett, Osteolytic lesions in secondary syphilis, Arch. Intern. Med. 137 (1977) 1465–1467.

[209] W.R. Holder, J.M. Knox, Syphilis in pregnancy, Med. Clin. North. Am. 56 (1972) 1151–1160.

[210] B. Roy, The Tuskegee Syphilis Experiment: biotechnology and the administrative state, J. Natl. Med. Assoc. 87 (1995) 56–67.

[211] D. Ingall, P.J. Sanchez, Syphilis, in: J.S. Remington, J.O. Klein (Eds.), Infectious Diseases of the Fetus and Newborn Infant, fifth ed., Saunders, Philadelphia, 2001, pp. 643–681.

[212] B.T. Goh, Syphilis in adults, Sex. Transm. Infect. 81 (2005) 448–452.

[213] J. Bays, D. Chadwick, The serologic test for syphilis in sexually abused children and adolescents, Adolesc. Pediatr. Gynecol. 4 (1991) 148–151.

[214] J. Knight, A.C. Richardson, K.C. White, The role of syphilis serology in the evaluation of suspected sexual abuse, Pediatr. Infect. Dis. 11 (1992) 125–127.

[215] M.B. Lande, A.C. Richardson, K.C. White, The role of syphilis serology in the evaluation of suspected sexual abuse, Pediatr. Infect. Dis. J. 11 (1992) 125–127.

[216] M.L. Shew, J.D. Fortenberry, Syphilis screening in adolescents, J. Adolesc. Health 13 (1992) 303–305.

[217] T.J. Silber, N.F. Niland, The clinical spectrum of syphilis in adolescence, J. Adolesc. Health Care 5 (1984) 112–116.

[218] N.R. Ingraham, The value of penicillin alone in the prevention and treatment of congenital syphilis, Acta Derm. Venereol. 31 (1951) 60.

[219] N.J. Fiumara, S. Lessell, Manifestations of late congenital syphilis, Arch. Dermatol. 102 (1970) 78–83.

[220] W.J. Brown, M.B. Moore Jr., Congenital syphilis in the United States, Clin. Pediatr. (Phila) 2 (1963) 220–222.

[221] J.L. Sever, Effects of infections on pregnancy risk, Clin. Obstet. Gynecol. 16 (1973) 225–234.

[222] A.D. Lascari, J. Diamond, B.E. Nolan, Anemia as the only presenting manifestation of congenital syphilis, Clin. Pediatr. (Phila) 15 (1976) 90–91.

[223] J.M. Ricci, R.M. Fojaco, M.J. O'Sullivan, Congenital syphilis: the University of Miami/Jackson Memorial Medical Center experience, 1986–1988, Obstet. Gynecol. 74 (1989) 687–693.

[224] L.H. Taber, T.W. Huber, Congenital syphilis, Prog. Clin. Biol. Res. 3 (1975) 183–190.

[225] K.L. Tan, The re-emergence of early congenital syphilis, Acta Paediatr. Scand. 62 (1973) 601–607.

[226] R.L. Naeye, Fetal growth with congenital syphilis: a quantitative study, Am. J. Clin. Pathol. 55 (1971) 228–231.

[227] A. Teberg, J.E. Hodgman, Congenital syphilis in newborn, Calif. Med. 118 (1973) 5–10.

[228] M.P. Webber, et al., Maternal risk factors for congenital syphilis: a case-control study, Am. J. Epidemiol. 137 (1993) 415–422.

[229] F. Saxoni, P. Lapaanis, S.N. Pantelakis, Congenital syphilis: a description of 18 cases and re-examination of an old but ever-present disease, Clin. Pediatr. (Phila) 6 (1967) 687–691.

[230] J.C. Leao, L.A. Gueiros, S.R. Porter, Oral manifestations of syphilis, Clinics 61 (2006) 161–166.

[231] R.R. Willcox, Venereal diseases in the newborn; some recent developments, Br. J. Clin. Pract. 11 (1957) 868–870.

[232] A.J. King, Advances in the study of venereal disease, Br. J. Clin. Pract. 25 (1971) 295–301.

[233] R.V. Platou, J.T. Kometani, Penicillin therapy of late congenital syphilis, Pediatrics 1 (1948) 601–616.

[234] N.C. Woody, W.F. Sistrunk, R.V. Platou, Congenital syphilis: a laid ghost walks, J. Pediatr. 64 (1964) 63–67.

[235] A. Lugo, S. Sanchez, J.L. Sanchez, Congenital syphilis, Pediatr. Dermatol. 23 (2006) 121–123.

[236] J.A. Whitaker, P. Sartain, M. Shaheedy, Hematological aspects of congenital syphilis, J. Pediatr. 66 (1965) 629–636.

[237] S. Reddy, et al., Early diffuse alopecia in a neonate with congenital syphilis, Pediatr. Dermatol. 23 (2006) 564–566.

[238] S. Olansky, W.G. Rogers, W.C. Anthony, Diagnosis of anogenital ulcers, Cutis 17 (1976) 705–708.

[239] L.T. Gutman, Congenital syphilis, in: G.L. Mandell (Ed.), Atlas of Infectious Disease, Current Medicine, Philadelphia, 1996.

[240] L.M. Hollier, et al., Fetal syphilis: clinical and laboratory characteristics, Obstet. Gynecol. 97 (2001) 947–953.

[241] M.C. Shah, L.L. Barton, Congenital syphilitic hepatitis, Pediatr. Infect. Dis. J. 8 (1989) 891–892.

[242] D.H. Dorfman, J.H. Glaser, Congenital syphilis presenting in infants after the newborn period, N. Engl. J. Med. 323 (1990) 1299–1302.

[243] W.A. Long, M.H. Ulshen, E.E. Lawson, Clinical manifestations of congenital syphilitic hepatitis: implications for pathogenesis, J. Pediatr. Gastroenterol. Nutr. 3 (1984) 551–555.

[244] P. Sartain, The anemia of congenital syphilis, South. Med. J. 58 (1965) 27–31.

[245] M. Pohl, et al., Haemophagocytosis in early congenital syphilis, Eur. J. Pediatr. 158 (1999) 553–555.

[246] S.I. Bulova, E. Schwartz, W.V. Harrer, Hydrops fetalis and congenital syphilis, Pediatrics 49 (1972) 285–287.

[247] Z. Levine, et al., Nonimmune hydrops fetalis due to congenital syphilis associated with negative intrapartum maternal serology screening, Am. J. Perinatol. 15 (1998) 233–236.

[248] A.A. Shah, A.B. Desai, Paroxysmal cold hemoglobinuria (case report), Indian Pediatr. 14 (1977) 219–221.

[249] J.S. Toohey, Skeletal presentation of congenital syphilis: case report and review of the literature, J. Pediatr. Orthop. 5 (1985) 104–106.

[250] B.E. Chipps, L.E. Swischuk, W.W. Voelter, Single bone involvement in congenital syphilis, Pediatr. Radiol. 5 (1976) 50–52.

[251] A. Solomon, E. Rosen, The aspect of trauma in the bone changes of congenital lues, Pediatr. Radiol. 3 (1975) 176–178.

[252] A. Solomon, E. Rosen, Focal osseous lesions in congenital lues, Pediatr. Radiol. 7 (1978) 36–39.

[253] E.K. Rose, P. Gyorgy, N.R. Ingraham Jr., Treatment of infantile congenital syphilis: results with aqueous penicillin alone in 60 infants followed for an average of 2 years after treatment, Am. J. Dis. Child. 77 (1949) 729–735.

[254] J.W. Rethmeier, Infantile cortical hyperostosis (Caffey's disease): two case reports, Radiol. Clin. (Basel) 45 (1976) 251–257.

[255] V.J. Harris, C.A. Jimenez, D. Vidyasagar, Congenital syphilis with syphilitic arthritis. Radiological quiz, Radiology 123 (1977) 416 518.

[256] L.D. Lilien, V.J. Harris, R.S. Pildes, Congenital syphilitic osteitis of scapulae and ribs, Pediatr. Radiol. 6 (1977) 183–185.

[257] B.J. Cremin, M.I. Shaff, Congenital syphilis diagnosed in utero, Br. J. Radiol. 48 (1975) 939–941.

[258] S. Heyman, G.A. Mandell, Skeletal scintigraphy in congenital syphilis, Clin. Nucl. Med. 8 (1983) 531–534.

[259] A. Wolpowitz, Osseous manifestations of congenital syphilis, S. Afr. Med. J. 50 (1976) 675–676.

[260] D. Siegel, S.Z. Hirschman, Syphilitic osteomyelitis with diffusely abnormal bone scan, Mt. Sinai J. Med. 46 (1979) 320–322.

[261] R.H. Wilkinson, R.M. Heller, Congenital syphilis: resurgence of an old problem, Pediatrics 47 (1971) 27–30.

[262] L.P. Brion, et al., Long-bone radiographic abnormalities as a sign of active congenital syphilis in asymptomatic newborns, Pediatrics 88 (1991) 1037–1040.

[263] P. Fan, et al., Early congenital syphilis presented with exclusive bending pain of extremity: case report, J. Dermatol. 34 (2007) 214–216.

[264] G.C. Szalay, A. Teberg, Congenital syphilis in newborn, Calif. Med. 119 (1973) 75.

[265] B. Wolf, K. Kalangu, Congenital neurosyphilis revisited, Eur. J. Pediatr. 152 (1993) 493–495.

[266] D. Nolt, et al., Survival with hypopituitarism from congenital syphilis, Pediatrics 109 (2002) e63.

[267] I.C. Michelow, et al., Central nervous system infection in congenital syphilis, N. Engl. J. Med. 346 (2002) 1792–1798.

[268] F. Contreras, J. Pereda, Congenital syphilis of the eye with lens involvement, Arch. Ophthalmol. 96 (1978) 1052–1053.

[269] M.C. Berry, A.S. Dajani, Resurgence of congenital syphilis, Infect. Dis. Clin. North Am. 6 (1992) 19–29.

[270] A.C. Papaioannou, G.G. Asrow, N.H. Schuckmell, Nephrotic syndrome in early infancy as a manifestation of congenital syphilis, Pediatrics 27 (1961) 636–641.

[271] P. Pollner, Nephrotic syndrome associated with congenital syphilis, JAMA 198 (1966) 263–266.

[272] E.U. Rosen, C. Abrahams, L. Rabinowitz, Nephropathy of congenital syphilis, S. Afr. Med. J. 47 (1973) 1606–1609.

[273] A.M. Yuceoglu, et al., The glomerulopathy of congenital syphilis: a curable immune-deposit disease, JAMA 229 (1974) 1085–1089.

[274] R. McDonald, J. Wiggelinkhuizen, R.O. Kaschula, The nephrotic syndrome in very young infants, Am. J. Dis. Child. 122 (1971) 507–512.

[275] S.A. Rawstron, K. Bromberg, Comparison of maternal and newborn serologic tests for syphilis, Am. J. Dis. Child. 145 (1991) 1383–1388.

[276] T. Putkonen, Does early treatment prevent dental changes in congenital syphilis? Acta Derm. Venereol. 43 (1963) 240–249.

[277] N.J. Fiumara, S. Lessell, Manifestations of late congenital syphilis: an analysis of 271 patients, Arch. Dermatol. 102 (1970) 78–83.

[278] L. Borella, J.E. Goobar, G.M. Clark, Synovitis of the knee joints in late congenital syphilis: Clutton's joints, JAMA 180 (1962) 190–192.

[279] M.R. Sanchez, Infectious syphilis, Semin. Dermatol. 13 (1994) 234–242.

[280] N.J. Fiumara, A retrospective approach to syphilis in the 1970s, Int. J. Dermatol. 21 (1982) 400–403.

[281] N.J. Fiumara, W.L. Fleming, J.G. Downing, F.L. Good, The incidence of prenatal syphilis at the Boston City Hospital, N. Engl. J. Med. 247 (1970) 48–52.

[282] E.L. Hendershot, Luetic deafness, Otolaryngol. Clin. North Am. 11 (1978) 43–47.

[283] R. Rothenberg, G. Becker, R. Wiet, Syphilitic hearing loss, South. Med. J. 72 (1979) 118–120.

[284] D. Ashley, et al., Medical conditions present during pregnancy and risk of perinatal death in Jamaica, Paediatr. Perinat. Epidemiol. 8 (Suppl. 1) (1994) 66–85.

[285] P.H. Azimi, Interstitial keratitis in a five-year-old, Pediatr. Infect. Dis. J. 18 (1999) 299–311.

[286] L.L. Lewis, Congenital syphilis: serologic diagnosis in the young infant, Infect. Dis. Clin. North Am. 6 (1992) 31–39.

[287] G.D. Wendel, et al., Treatment of syphilis in pregnancy and prevention of congenital syphilis, Clin. Infect. Dis. 35 (2002) s200–s209.

[288] R.W. Peeling, et al., Rapid tests for sexually transmitted infections (STIs): the way forward, Sex. Transm. Infect. 82 (Suppl. 5) (2006) v1–v6.

[289] H.L. Wheeler, S. Agarwal, B.T. Goh, Dark ground microscopy and treponemal serological tests in the diagnosis of early syphilis, Sex. Transm. Infect. 80 (2004) 411–414.

[290] A.R. Yobs, D.H. Rockwell, J.W. Clark Jr., Treponemal survival in humans after penicillin therapy: a preliminary report, Br. J. Vener. Dis. 40 (1964) 248–253.

[291] D.D. Glover, et al., Diagnostic considerations in intra-amniotic syphilis, Sex. Transm. Dis. 12 (1985) 145–149.

[292] G.D. Wendel, et al., Examination of amniotic fluid in diagnosing congenital syphilis with fetal death, Obstet. Gynecol. 74 (1989) 967–970.

[293] T.B. Turner, P.H. Hardy, B. Newman, Infectivity tests in syphilis, 1969, Sex. Transm. Infect. 76 (Suppl. 1) (2000) S7.

[294] P.E. Hay, et al., Detection of treponemal DNA in the CSF of patients with syphilis and HIV infection using the polymerase chain reaction, Genitourin. Med. 66 (1990) 428–432.

[295] G.T. Noordhoek, et al., Detection by polymerase chain reaction of Treponema pallidum DNA in cerebrospinal fluid from neurosyphilis patients before and after antibiotic treatment, J. Clin. Microbiol. 29 (1991) 1976–1984.

[296] E. Grimprel, et al., Use of polymerase chain reaction and rabbit infectivity testing to detect Treponema pallidum in amniotic fluid, fetal and neonatal sera, and cerebrospinal fluid, J. Clin. Microbiol. 29 (1991) 1711–1718.

[297] H.M. Palmer, et al., Use of PCR in the diagnosis of early syphilis in the United Kingdom, Sex. Transm. Infect. 79 (2003) 479–483.

[298] H. Liu, et al., New tests for syphilis: rational design of a PCR method for detection of Treponema pallidum in clinical specimens using unique regions of the DNA polymerase I gene, J. Clin. Microbiol. 39 (2001) 1941–1946.

[299] C.M. Marra, Neurosyphilis, Curr. Neurol. Neurosci. Rep. 4 (2004) 435–440.

[300] S.A. Larsen, B.M. Steiner, A.H. Rudolph, Laboratory diagnosis and interpretation of tests for syphilis, Clin. Microbiol. Rev. 8 (1995) 1–21.

[301] T.G. Matthews, C. O'Herlihy, Significance of raised immunoglobulin M levels in cord blood of small-for-gestational-age infants, Arch. Dis. Child. 53 (1978) 895–898.

[302] M. Moskophidis, F. Muller, Molecular analysis of immunoglobulins M and G immune response to protein antigens of Treponema pallidum in human syphilis, Infect. Immun. 43 (1984) 127–132.

[303] F. Muller, Specific immunoglobulin M and G antibodies in the rapid diagnosis of human treponemal infections, Diagn. Immunol. 4 (1986) 1–9.

[304] A.L. Schroeter, et al., Treatment for early syphilis and reactivity of serologic tests, JAMA 221 (1972) 471–476.

[305] N.J. Fiumara, Reinfection primary, secondary, and latent syphilis: the serologic response after treatment, Sex. Transm. Dis. 7 (1980) 111–115.

[306] R.S. Chhabra, et al., Comparison of maternal sera, cord blood, and neonatal sera for detecting presumptive congenital syphilis: relationship with maternal treatment, Pediatrics 91 (1993) 88–91.

[307] R. Nandwani, D.T. Evans, Are you sure it's syphilis? A review of false positive serology, Int. J. STD AIDS 6 (1995) 241–248.

[308] D. Musher, An unusual cause of FUO, Hosp. Pract. 13 (1978) 134–135.

[309] Y. Felman, How useful are the serologic tests for syphilis? Int. J. Dermatol. 21 (1982) 79–81.

[310] G.H. Kostant, Familial chronic biologic false-positive seroreactions for syphilis: report of two families, one with three generations affected, JAMA 219 (1972) 45–48.

[311] C.S. Buchanan, J.R. Haserick, FTA-ABS test in pregnancy: a probable false-positive reaction, Arch. Dermatol. 102 (1970) 322–325.

[312] W.C. Duncan, J.M. Knox, R.D. Wende, The FTA-ABS test in dark-field-positive primary syphilis, JAMA 228 (1974) 859–860.

[313] A.H. Rudolph, Serologic diagnosis of syphilis: an update, South Med. J. 69 (1976) 1196–1197 1203.

[314] A.V. Kuznetsov, W.H. Burgdorf, J.C. Prinz, Latent syphilis confirmed by polymerase chain reaction in 2 HIV-positive patients with inconclusive serologic test results, Arch. Dermatol. 141 (2005) 1169–1170.

[315] Y.M. Felman, J.A. Nikitas, Sexually transmitted diseases: secondary syphilis, Cutis 29 (1982) 322–324 326–328, 334.

[316] P.F. Sparling, Diagnosis and treatment of syphilis, N. Engl. J. Med. 284 (1971) 642–653.

[317] G. Smith, R.P. Holman, The prozone phenomenon with syphilis and HIV-1 co-infection, South Med. J. 97 (2004) 379–382.

[318] S. Taniguchi, K. Osato, T. Hamada, The prozone phenomenon in secondary syphilis, Acta Derm. Venereol. 75 (1995) 153–154.

[319] Y. Taniguchi, et al., Syphilis in old age, Int. J. Dermatol. 34 (1995) 38–39.

[320] P.J. Sanchez, Laboratory tests for congenital syphilis, Pediatr. Infect. Dis. J. 17 (1998) 70–71.

[321] M.F. Garner, The IgM FTA test for syphilis in the newborn, Aust. N. Z. J. Obstet. Gynaecol. 12 (1972) 179–181.

[322] A.H. Rudolph, The microhemagglutination assay for Treponema pallidum antibodies (MHA-TP), a new treponemal test for syphilis. Where does it fit? J. Am. Vener. Dis. Assoc. 3 (1976) 3–8.

[323] S.A. Larsen, et al., Specificity, sensitivity, and reproducibility among the fluorescent treponemal antibody-absorption test, the microhemagglutination assay for Treponema pallidum antibodies, and the hemagglutination treponemal test for syphilis, J. Clin. Microbiol. 14 (1981) 441–445.

[324] N.J. Fiumara, Treatment of primary and secondary syphilis: serological response, JAMA 243 (1980) 2500–2502.

[325] P. O'Neill, R.W. Warner, C.S. Nicol, Treponema pallidum haemagglutination assay in the routine serodiagnosis of treponemal disease, Br. J. Vener. Dis. 49 (1973) 427–431.

[326] J. Lesinski, J. Krach, E. Kadziewicz, Specificity, sensitivity, and diagnostic value of the TPHA test, Br. J. Vener. Dis. 50 (1974) 334–340.

[327] S.A. Larsen, et al., Staining intensities in the fluorescent treponemal antibody-absorption (FTA-Abs) test: association with the diagnosis of syphilis, Sex. Transm. Dis. 13 (1986) 221–227.

[328] N. Yoshioka, et al., Evaluation of a chemiluminescent microparticle immunoassay for determination of Treponema pallidum antibodies, Clin. Lab. 53 (2007) 597–603.

[329] M.F. Garner, The serological diagnosis of treponemal infection, N. Z. Med. J. 75 (1972) 353–355.

[330] F. Ito, et al., Specific immunofluorescence staining of Treponema pallidum in smears and tissues, J. Clin. Microbiol. 29 (1991) 444–448.

[331] B. Romanowski, et al., Serologic response to treatment of infectious syphilis, Ann. Intern. Med. 114 (1991) 1005–1009.

[332] R.D. Isaacs, J.D. Radolf, Molecular approaches to improved syphilis serodiagnosis, Serodiagn. Immunother. Infect. Dis. 3 (1989) 299–306.

[333] W.C. Van Voorhis, et al., Serodiagnosis of syphilis: antibodies to recombinant Tp0453, Tp92, and Gpd proteins are sensitive and specific indicators of infection by Treponema pallidum, J. Clin. Microbiol. 41 (2003) 3668–3674.

[334] P.E. Brentlinger, et al., Intermittent preventive treatment of malaria during pregnancy in central Mozambique, Bull. World Health Organ. 85 (2007) 873–879.

[335] T. Adam, et al., Cost effectiveness analysis of strategies for maternal and neonatal health in developing countries, BMJ 331 (2005) 1107.

[336] M.V. Norgard, et al., Sensitivity and specificity of monoclonal antibodies directed against antigenic determinants of Treponema pallidum Nichols in the diagnosis of syphilis, J. Clin. Microbiol. 20 (1984) 711–717.

[337] J.C. Lefevre, M.A. Bertrand, R. Bauriaud, Evaluation of the Captia enzyme immunoassays for detection of immunoglobulins G and M to Treponema pallidum in syphilis, J. Clin. Microbiol. 28 (1990) 1704–1707.

[338] H. Young, et al., Enzyme immunoassay for anti-treponemal IgG: screening or confirmatory test? J. Clin. Pathol. 45 (1992) 37–41.

[339] J. Ross, et al., An analysis of false positive reactions occurring with the Captia Syph G EIA, Genitourin. Med. 67 (1991) 408–410.

[340] S.I. Egglestone, A.J. Turner, Serological diagnosis of syphilis. PHLS Syphilis Serology Working Group, Commun. Dis. Public Health 3 (2000) 158–162.

[341] H. Young, Guidelines for serological testing for syphilis, Sex. Transm. Infect. 76 (2000) 403–405.

[342] H. Young, G. Aktas, A. Moyes, Enzywell recombinant enzyme immunoassay for the serological diagnosis of syphilis, Int. J. STD AIDS 11 (2000) 288–291.

[343] P. Zarakolu, et al., Preliminary evaluation of an immunochromatographic strip test for specific *Treponema pallidum* antibodies, J. Clin. Microbiol. 40 (2002) 3064–3065.

[344] A. Herring, et al., Evaluation of rapid diagnostic tests: syphilis, Nat. Rev. Microbiol. 4 (2006) S33–S40.

[345] J.D. Thorley, et al., Passive transfer of antibodies of maternal origin from blood to cerebrospinal fluid in infants, Lancet 1 (1975) 651–653.

[346] G. Leclerc, et al., Study of fluorescent treponemal antibody test on cerebrospinal fluid using monospecific anti-immunoglobulin conjugates IgG, IgM, and IgA, Br. J. Vener. Dis. 54 (1978) 303–308.

[347] F. Muller, Immunological and laboratory aspects of treponematoses, Dermatol. Monatsschr. 170 (1984) 357–366.

[348] J.B. Lee, et al., Detection of immunoglobulin M in cerebrospinal fluid from syphilis patients by enzyme-linked immunosorbent assay, J. Clin. Microbiol. 24 (1986) 736–740.

[349] N.N. Izzat, et al., Validity of the VDRL test on cerebrospinal fluid contaminated by blood, Br. J. Vener. Dis. 47 (1971) 162–164.

[350] G.R. Monif, et al., The problem of maternal syphilis after serologic surveillance during pregnancy, Am. J. Obstet. Gynecol. 117 (1973) 268–270.

[351] F.R. Bellingham, Syphilis in pregnancy: transplacental infection, Med. J. Aust. 2 (1973) 647–648.

[352] B.J. Stoll, et al., Clinical and serologic evaluation of neonates for congenital syphilis: a continuing diagnostic dilemma, J. Infect. Dis. 167 (1993) 1093–1099.

[353] L. Warner, et al., Missed opportunities for congenital syphilis prevention in an urban southeastern hospital, Sex. Transm. Dis. 28 (2001) 92–98.

[354] M. Augenbraun, et al., Treponemal specific tests for the serodiagnosis of syphilis. Syphilis and HIV Study Group, Sex. Transm. Dis. 25 (1998) 549–552.

[355] C.B. Hicks, et al., Seronegative secondary syphilis in a patient infected with the human immunodeficiency virus (HIV) with Kaposi sarcoma: a diagnostic dilemma, Ann. Intern. Med. 107 (1987) 492–495.

[356] P. Haslett, M. Laverty, The prozone phenomenon in syphilis associated with HIV infection, Arch. Intern. Med. 154 (1994) 1643–1644.

[357] J.L. Malone, et al., Syphilis and neurosyphilis in a human immunodeficiency virus type-1 seropositive population: evidence for frequent serologic relapse after therapy, Am. J. Med. 99 (1995) 55–63.

[358] M. Janier, et al., A prospective study of the influence of HIV status on the seroreversion of serological tests for syphilis, Dermatology 198 (1999) 362–369.

[359] A.M. Rompalo, et al., Association of biologic false-positive reactions for syphilis with human immunodeficiency virus infection, J. Infect. Dis. 165 (1992) 1124–1126.

[360] W.L. Risser, L.Y. Hwang, Problems in the current case definitions of congenital syphilis, J. Pediatr 129 (1996) 499–505.

[361] K.C. Rathbun, Congenital syphilis: a proposal for improved surveillance, diagnosis, and treatment, Sex. Transm. Dis. 10 (1983) 102–107.

[362] P.J. Sanchez, G.D. Wendel, M.V. Norgard, Congenital syphilis associated with negative results of maternal serologic tests at delivery, Am. J. Dis. Child. 145 (1991) 967–969.

[363] C. Beck-Sague, R. Alexander, Failure of benzathine penicillin G treatment in early congenital syphilis, Pediatr. Infect. Dis. 6 (1987) 1061–1064.

[364] A.E. Benzick, D.P. Wirthwein, A. Weinberg, G.D. Wendel, R. Alsaadi, N.K. Leos, F. Zeray, P.J. Sánchez, Pituitary gland gumma in congenital syphilis after failed maternal treatment: a case report, Pediatrics 104 (1999) e1–e4.

[365] L. Mascola, R. Pelosi, C.E. Alexander, Inadequate treatment of syphilis in pregnancy, Am. J. Obstet. Gynecol. 150 (1984) 945–947.

[366] N.M. Zetola, et al., Syphilis in the United States: an update for clinicians with an emphasis on HIV coinfection, Mayo Clin. Proc. 82 (2007) 1091–1102.

[367] J.S. Sheffield, et al., Congenital syphilis after maternal treatment for syphilis during pregnancy, Am. J. Obstet. Gynecol. 186 (2002) 569–573.

[368] L.H. Taber, Interview with Larry H. Taber: Evaluation and management of syphilis in pregnant women and newborn infants. Interview by John D. Nelson, Pediatr. Infect. Dis. 1 (1982) 224–227.

[369] V.A. Moyer, et al., Contribution of long-bone radiographs to the management of congenital syphilis in the newborn infant, Arch. Pediatr. Adolesc. Med. 152 (1998) 353–357.

[370] M.R. Beeram, et al., Lumbar puncture in the evaluation of possible asymptomatic congenital syphilis in neonates, J. Pediatr. 128 (1996) 125–129.

[371] W.L. Risser, L.Y. Hwang, Problems in the current case definitions of congenital syphilis, J. Pediatr. 129 (1996) 499–505.

[372] F.B. Coles, et al., Congenital syphilis surveillance in upstate New York, 1989–1992: implications for prevention and clinical management, J. Infect. Dis. 171 (1995) 732–735.

[373] G. Lee, et al., Congenital syphilis as a differential diagnosis of non-accidental injury, Eur. J. Pediatr. 167 (2008) 1071–1072.

[374] M.C. Lee, et al., An infant with seizures, rash, and hepatosplenomegaly, Clin. Infect. Dis. 46 (2008) 451–452, 472–453.

[375] V. Lee, G. Kinghorn, Syphilis: an update, Clin. Med. 8 (2008) 330–333.

[376] N.B. Esterly, L.M. Solomon, Neonatal dermatology. II. Blistering and scaling dermatoses, J. Pediatr. 77 (1970) 1075–1088.

[377] L.J. Geppert, et al., *Pseudomonas* infections in infants and children, J. Pediatr. 41 (1952) 555–561.

[378] C.G. Ray, R.J. Wedgwood, Neonatal listeriosis: six case reports and a review of the literature, Pediatrics 34 (1964) 378–392.

[379] J.B. Lopez, P. Gross, T.R. Boggs, Skin lesions in association with beta-hemolytic *Streptococcus* group B, Pediatrics 58 (1976) 859–861.

[380] F. Halal, et al., Congenital vesicular eruption caused by *Haemophilus influenzae* type b, Pediatrics 62 (1978) 494–496.

[381] J. Hageman, et al., Congenital tuberculosis: critical reappraisal of clinical findings and diagnostic procedures, Pediatrics 66 (1980) 980–984.

[382] J. Blatt, O. Kastner, D.S. Hodes, Cutaneous vesicles in congenital cytomegalovirus infection, J. Pediatr. 92 (1978) 509.

[383] A.M. Dvorak, B. Gavaller, Congenital systemic candidiasis: report of a case, N. Engl. J. Med. 274 (1966) 540–543.

[384] F.A. Oski, J.L. Naiman, Hematologic Problems in the Newborn, Saunders, Philadelphia, 1972.

[385] A. Anand, et al., Human parvovirus infection in pregnancy and hydrops fetalis, N. Engl. J. Med. 316 (1987) 183–186.

[386] D.I. Weiss, L.Z. Cooper, R.H. Green, Infantile glaucoma: a manifestation of congenital rubella, JAMA 195 (1966) 725–727.

[387] C.O. Nathan, A.B. Seid, Neonatal rhinitis, Int. J. Pediatr. Otorhinolaryngol. 39 (1997) 59–65.

[388] S. Prabhakar, et al., Non-compressive myelopathy: clinical and radiological study, Neurol. India 47 (1999) 294–299.

[389] J.K. Mahoney, Penicillin treatment of early syphilis, Am. J. Public Health 33 (1943).

[390] M. Sivakumaran, et al., Paroxysmal cold haemoglobinuria caused by non-Hodgkin's lymphoma, Br. J. Haematol. 105 (1999) 278–279.

[391] H. Eagle, R. Fleischman, A.D. Musselman, Effect of schedule of administration on the therapeutic efficacy of penicillin: importance of the aggregate time penicillin remains at effectively bactericidal levels, Am. J. Med. 9 (1950) 280–299.

[392] H. Eagle, R. Fleischman, A.D. Musselman, The effective concentrations of penicillin in vitro and in vivo for streptococci, pneumococci, and *Treponema pallidum*, J. Bacteriol. 59 (1950) 625–643.

[393] H. Eagle, R. Fleischman, A.D. Musselman, The bactericidal action of penicillin in vivo: the participation of the host, and the slow recovery of the surviving organisms, Ann. Intern. Med. 33 (1950) 544–571.

[394] O. Idsoe, T. Guthe, R.R. Willcox, Penicillin in the treatment of syphilis. The experience of three decades, Bull. World Health Organ. 47 (1972) 1–68.

[395] M.H. Augenbraun, R. Rolfs, Treatment of syphilis, 1998: nonpregnant adults, Clin. Infect. Dis. 28 (Suppl. 1) (1999) S21–S28.

[396] D.M. Musher, How much penicillin cures early syphilis? Ann. Intern. Med. 109 (1988) 849–851.

[397] G.D. Wendel, J.S. Sheffield, L.M. Hollier, Penicillin allergy and desensitization in serious infections during pregnancy, N. Engl. J. Med. 312 (1985) 1229–1232.

[398] E.W. Hook, R.E. Roddy, H.H. Hardsfield, Ceftriaxone therapy for incubating and early syphilis, J. Infect. Dis. 158 (2001) 881–884.

[399] A. Philipson, L.D. Sabeth, D. Charles, Transplacental passage of erythromycin and clindamycin, N. Engl. J. Med. 288 (1973) 1219–1221.

[400] V.J. Harris, C.A. Jimenez, D. Vidyasagar, Value of bone roentgenograms in diagnosis: congenital syphilis with unusual clinical presentations, IMJ Ill. Med. J. 151 (1977) 371–374.

[401] J.M. Alexander, et al., Efficacy of treatment for syphilis in pregnancy, Obstet. Gynecol. 93 (1999) 5–8.

[402] C.S. Conover, et al., Congenital syphilis after treatment of maternal syphilis with a penicillin regimen exceeding CDC guidelines, Infect. Dis. Obstet. Gynecol. 6 (1998) 134–137.

[403] L. Nathan, R.E. Bawdon, E. Sidawi, Penicillin levels following administration of benzathine penicillin G in pregnancy, Obstet. Gynecol. 82 (1993) 338–420.

[404] L.K. Pickering (Ed.), Red Book: Report of the Committee on Infectious Diseases, American Academy of Pediatrics, Elk Grove Village, IL, 2003.

[405] R.T. Rolfs, et al., A randomized trial of enhanced therapy for early syphilis in patients with and without human immunodeficiency virus infection. The Syphilis and HIV Study Group, N. Engl. J. Med. 337 (1997) 307–314.

[406] M.E. Speer, et al., Cerebrospinal fluid levels of benzathine penicillin G in the neonate, J. Pediatr. 91 (1977) 996–997.

[407] J.N. Goldman, K.F. Girard, Intraocular treponemes in treated congenital syphilis, Arch. Ophthalmol. 78 (1967) 47–50.

[408] E.M. Dunlop, A.J. King, A.E. Wilkinson, Study of late ocular syphilis. Demonstration of treponemes in aqueous humour and cerebrospinal fluid. 3. General and serological findings, Trans. Ophthalmol. Soc. U. K. 88 (1969) 275–294.

[409] S.J. Ryan, et al., Persistence of virulent *Treponema pallidum* despite penicillin therapy in congenital syphilis, Am. J. Ophthalmol. 73 (1972) 258–261.

[410] J.B. Hardy, et al., Failure of penicillin in a newborn with congenital syphilis, JAMA 212 (1970) 1345–1349.

[411] L.L. Bayne, J.W. Schmidley, D.S. Goodin, Acute syphilitic meningitis: its occurrence after clinical and serologic cure of secondary syphilis with penicillin G, Arch. Neurol. 43 (1986) 137–138.

[412] J. Jorgensen, G. Tikjob, K. Weismann, Neurosyphilis after treatment of latent syphilis with benzathine penicillin, Genitourin. Med. 62 (1986) 129–131.

[413] D.M. Markovitz, et al., Failure of recommended treatment for secondary syphilis, JAMA 255 (1986) 1767–1768.

[414] A. Franco, et al., Clinical case of seroconversion for syphilis following a needlestick injury: why not take a prophylaxis? Infez. Med. 15 (2007) 187–190.

[415] A.J. De Baets, S. Sifovo, I.E. Pazvakavambwa, Access to occupational post-exposure prophylaxis for primary health care workers in rural Africa: a cross-sectional study, Am. J. Infect. Control 35 (2007) 545–551.

[416] G.S. Meyer, Occupational infection in health care: the century-old lessons from syphilis, Arch. Intern. Med. 153 (1993) 2439–2447.

[417] G. Hart, Epidemiologic treatment for syphilis and gonorrhea, Sex. Transm. Dis. 7 (1980) 149–152.

[418] P.H. Azimi, et al., Concentrations of procaine and aqueous penicillin in the cerebrospinal fluid of infants treated for congenital syphilis, J. Pediatr. 124 (1994) 649–653.

[419] M. Radcliffe, et al., Single-dose benzathine penicillin in infants at risk of congenital syphilis—results of a randomised study, S. Afr. Med. J. 87 (1997) 62–65.

[420] D.A. Bateman, et al., The hospital cost of congenital syphilis, J. Pediatr. 130 (1997) 752–758.

[421] S.G. Paryani, et al., Treatment of asymptomatic congenital syphilis: benzathine versus procaine penicillin G therapy, J. Pediatr. 125 (1994) 471–475.

[422] M. Radcliffe, et al., Single-dose benzathine penicillin in infants at risk of congenital syphilis—results of a randomised study, S. Afr. Med. J. 87 (1997) 62–65.

[423] C. Beck-Sague, E.R. Alexander, Failure of benzathine penicillin G treatment in early congenital syphilis, Pediatr. Infect. Dis. J. 6 (1987) 1061–1064.

[424] A. Woolf, C.M. Wilfert, D.B. Kelsey, Childhood syphilis in North Carolina, N. C. Med. J. 41 (1980) 443–449.

[425] M.A. Staat, Infectious disease issues in internationally adopted children, Pediatr. Infect. Dis. J. 21 (2002) 257–258.

[426] U. Sothinathan, et al., Detection and follow up of infants at risk of congenital syphilis, Arch. Dis. Child. 91 (2006) 620.

[427] S.N. Chang, et al., Seroreversion of the serological tests for syphilis in the newborns born to treated syphilitic mothers, Genitourin. Med. 71 (1995) 68–70.

[428] S.A. Rawstron, et al., Congenital syphilis and fluorescent treponemal antibody test reactivity after the age of 1 year, Sex. Transm. Dis. 28 (2001) 412–416.

[429] M.K. Ikeda, H.B. Jenson, Evaluation and treatment of congenital syphilis, J. Pediatr. 117 (1990) 843–852.

[430] K.C. Rathbun, Congenital syphilis, Sex. Transm. Dis. 10 (1983) 93–99.

[431] L.H. Taber, R.D. Feigin, Spirochetal infections, Pediatr. Clin. North. Am. 26 (1979) 377–413.

[432] E.P. Pendergrass, R.S. Bromer, Congenital bone syphilis: preliminary report: roentgenologic study with notes on the histology and pathology of the condition, AJR Am. J. Roentgenol. 22 (1929) p. 1.

[433] G.D. Wendel Jr., et al., Penicillin allergy and desensitization in serious infections during pregnancy, N. Engl. J. Med. 312 (1985) 1229–1232.

[434] J.A. Gelfand, et al., Endotoxemia associated with the Jarisch-Herxheimer reaction, N. Engl. J. Med. 295 (1976) 211–213.

[435] E.J. Young, et al., Studies on the pathogenesis of the Jarisch-Herxheimer reaction: development of an animal model and evidence against a role for classical endotoxin, J. Infect. Dis. 146 (1982) 606–615.

[436] J.D. Radolf, et al., *Treponema pallidum* and *Borrelia burgdorferi* lipoproteins and synthetic lipopeptides activate monocytes/macrophages, J. Immunol. 154 (1995) 2866–2877.

[437] V.R. Klein, et al., The Jarisch-Herxheimer reaction complicating syphilotherapy in pregnancy, Obstet. Gynecol. 75 (1990) 375–380.

[438] T.D. Myles, et al., The Jarisch-Herxheimer reaction and fetal monitoring changes in pregnant women treated for syphilis, Obstet. Gynecol. 92 (1998) 859–864.

[439] V.R. Klein, et al., The Jarisch-Herxheimer reaction complicating syphilotherapy in pregnancy, Obstet. Gynecol. 92 (1990) 375–380.

[440] P.J. Hotez, Neglected infections of poverty in the United States of America, PLoS Negl. Trop. Dis. 2 (2008) e256.

[441] L. Tikhonova, et al., Congenital syphilis in the Russian Federation: magnitude, determinants, and consequences, Sex. Transm. Infect. 79 (2003) 106–110.

[442] P.J. Montoya, et al., Comparison of the diagnostic accuracy of a rapid immunochromatographic test and the rapid plasma reagin test for antenatal syphilis screening in Mozambique, Bull. World Health Organ. 84 (2006) 97–104.

[443] K. Fonck, et al., Syphilis control during pregnancy: effectiveness and sustainability of a decentralized program, Am. J. Public Health 91 (2001) 705–707.

[444] A.K. Hurtig, et al., Syphilis in pregnant women and their children in the United Kingdom: results from national clinician reporting surveys 1994–7, BMJ 317 (1998) 1617–1619.

[445] L.M. Hollier, et al., State laws regarding prenatal syphilis screening in the United States, Am. J. Obstet. Gynecol. 189 (2003) 1178–1183.

[446] L.M. Hollier, et al., State laws regarding prenatal syphilis screening in the United States, Am. J. Obstet. Gynecol. 189 (2003) 1178–1183.

[447] J. Knight, et al., Contributions of suboptimal antenatal care and poor communication to the diagnosis of congenital syphilis, Pediatr. Infect. Dis. J. 14 (1995) 237–240.

[448] L. Finelli, E.M. Crayne, K.C. Spitalny, Treatment of infants with reactive syphilis serology, New Jersey: 1992 to 1996, Pediatrics 102 (1998) e27.

[449] L. Finelli, et al., Syphilis outbreak assessment, Sex. Transm. Dis. 28 (2001) 131–135.

[450] C.E. Rydzak, S.J. Goldie, Cost-effectiveness of rapid point-of-care prenatal syphilis screening in sub-Saharan Africa, Sex. Transm. Dis. 35 (2008) 775–784.

[451] F. Terris-Prestholt, et al., Is antenatal syphilis screening still cost effective in sub-Saharan Africa, Sex. Transm. Infect. 79 (2003) 375–381.

[452] D.G. Walker, G.J. Walker, Forgotten but not gone: the continuing scourge of congenital syphilis, Lancet Infect. Dis. 2 (2002) 432–436.

[453] L.A. Williams, et al., Elimination and reintroduction of primary and secondary syphilis, Am. J. Public Health 89 (1999) 1093–1097.

[454] B. Pourbohloul, M.L. Rekart, R.C. Brunham, Impact of mass treatment on syphilis transmission: a mathematical modeling approach, Sex. Transm. Dis. 30 (2003) 297–305.

[455] M.J. Wawer, et al., Control of sexually transmitted diseases for AIDS prevention in Uganda: a randomised community trial. Rakai Project Study Group, Lancet 353 (1999) 525–535.

[456] M.G. Kiddugavu, et al., Effectiveness of syphilis treatment using azithromycin and/or benzathine penicillin in Rakai, Uganda, Sex. Transm. Dis. 32 (2005) 1–6.

[457] G. Riedner, et al., Single-dose azithromycin versus penicillin G benzathine for the treatment of early syphilis, N. Engl. J. Med. 353 (2005) 1236–1244.

[458] G. Riedner, et al., Decline in sexually transmitted infection prevalence and HIV incidence in female barworkers attending prevention and care services in Mbeya Region, Tanzania, AIDS 20 (2006) 609–615.

[459] K.K. Holmes, Azithromycin versus penicillin G benzathine for early syphilis, N. Engl. J. Med. 353 (2005) 1291–1293.

[460] R.C. Ballard, S.M. Berman, K.A. Fenton, Azithromycin versus penicillin for early syphilis, N. Engl. J. Med. 354 (2006) 203–205 author reply 203–205.

[461] H.W. Jaffe, et al., Selective mass treatment in a venereal disease control program, Am. J. Public Health 69 (1979) 1181–1182.

[462] J.R. Hibbs, R.A. Gunn, Public health intervention in a cocaine-related syphilis outbreak, Am. J. Public Health 81 (1991) 1259–1262.

[463] P. Zhou, et al., Occurrence of congenital syphilis after maternal treatment with azithromycin during pregnancy, Sex. Transm. Dis. 34 (2007) 472–474.

BORRELIA INFECTIONS: LYME DISEASE AND RELAPSING FEVER

Eugene D. Shapiro ☼ Michael A. Gerber

CHAPTER OUTLINE

Lyme Disease   564
    Epidemiology and Transmission   564
    Microbiology   566
    Pathogenesis and Pathology   566
    Clinical Manifestations   568

Diagnosis   569
Management and Treatment   571
Prognosis   573
Prevention   573
Relapsing Fever   574

LYME DISEASE

Lyme disease, caused by the spirochete *Borrelia burgdorferi*, is the most common vector-borne illness in the United States. Although, in retrospect, a form of the illness had been recognized in Scandinavia in the early 1900s, modern awareness of Lyme disease began after a cluster of cases of "juvenile rheumatoid arthritis" in children living on one small street was reported by their parents in the mid-1970s. Investigation of this unexplained "epidemic" of arthritis led to the description of "Lyme arthritis" in 1976 and, ultimately, to the discovery of its bacterial etiology [1–3]. The reported incidence of Lyme disease and its geographic range have increased dramatically in recent years [4].

Several spirochetes are known to cause transplacental infections in various animals and in humans [5–17]. *Treponema pallidum* has been the most thoroughly investigated spirochete with respect to transplacental transmission in humans [5]. Infection of the mother with *T. pallidum* during pregnancy frequently is associated with transplacental infection, resulting in congenital syphilis in the offspring. Congenital syphilis often is associated with clinically significant neurologic disease, such as hydrocephalus, cerebral palsy, deafness, blindness, convulsive disorders, and mental retardation [5]. Adverse fetal outcomes also have been documented in gestational infections with *Leptospira canicola*, the etiologic agent of leptospirosis, and with other *Borrelia* species, including the etiologic agents of relapsing fever (discussed later) [7–17]. Because *B. burgdorferi* is a spirochete, whether it too can cause congenital infection naturally is of considerable interest.

EPIDEMIOLOGY AND TRANSMISSION

B. burgdorferi is transmitted by species of ticks of the *Ixodes* genus. In the United States, the usual vector in the Northeast and the upper Midwest is *Ixodes scapularis* (the black-legged tick), commonly called the deer tick, whereas *Ixodes pacificus* (the Western black-legged tick) is the usual vector on the Pacific Coast [18]. In Europe, the most important vector for the spirochete is *Ixodes ricinus*, which commonly feeds on sheep and cattle.

The life cycle of *I. scapularis* consists of three stages—larva, nymph, and adult—that develop during a 2-year period [18]. Ticks feed once during each stage of the life cycle. The larvae emerge in the early summer from eggs laid in the spring by the adult female tick. More than 95% of the larvae are born uninfected with *B. burgdorferi* because transovarial transmission rarely occurs. The larvae feed on a wide variety of small mammals, such as the white-footed mouse, which are natural reservoirs for *B. burgdorferi*. Larvae become infected by feeding on animals that are infected with the spirochete. The tick emerges the following spring in the nymphal stage. This stage of the tick is most likely to transmit infections to humans [19], presumably because it is active at times during which humans are most likely to be in tick-infested areas and because it is very small and difficult to see. Consequently, it is more likely to be able to feed for a relatively long time, which increases the likelihood of transmission. If the nymphal tick is not infected with *B. burgdorferi*, it may subsequently become infected if it feeds on an infected animal in this stage of its development. The nymphs molt in the late summer or early fall and reemerge as adults. If the adult is infected, it also may transmit *B. burgdorferi* to humans. The adult deer tick may spend the winter on an animal host, a favorite being white-tailed deer (hence its name, the deer tick). In the spring, the females lay their eggs and die, completing the 2-year life cycle.

Numerous factors are associated with the risk of transmission of *B. burgdorferi* from infected ticks to humans. The proportion of infected ticks varies greatly by geographic area and by the stage of the tick in its life cycle. *I. pacificus* often feeds on lizards, which are not a competent reservoir for *B. burgdorferi*. Consequently, less than 5% of these ticks are infected with *B. burgdorferi*, so Lyme disease is rare in the Pacific states. By contrast, *I. scapularis* feeds on small mammals, which are competent reservoirs for *B. burgdorferi*. As a result, in highly endemic areas the rates of infection for different stages of deer ticks are, approximately, 2% for larvae, 15% to 30% for nymphs, and 30% to 50% for adults.

B. burgdorferi is transmitted when an infected tick inoculates saliva into the blood vessels of the skin of its host. The risk of transmission of *B. burgdorferi* from infected deer ticks has been shown to be related to the duration of feeding. It takes hours for the mouth parts of ticks to implant in the host, and much longer (days) for the tick to become fully engorged from feeding. *B. burgdorferi* is found primarily in the midgut of the tick, but as the tick feeds and becomes engorged, the bacteria migrate to the salivary glands, from which they can be transmitted. Experiments with animals have shown that infected nymph-stage ticks must feed for 48 hours or longer and infected adult ticks must feed for 72 hours or longer before the risk of transmission of *B. burgdorferi* becomes substantial [20–22]. Results of a study of transmission of Lyme disease to humans are consistent with these experimental results [19]. Among persons bitten by nymph-stage ticks for which the duration of feeding could be estimated, the risk of Lyme disease was zero among persons bitten by nymphs that had fed for less than 72 hours, but was 25% among persons bitten by nymphs that had fed for 72 hours or more. Approximately 75% of persons who recognize that they have been bitten by a deer tick remove the tick within 48 hours after it has begun to feed [23], which may explain why only a small proportion of persons who recognize that they have been bitten by deer ticks subsequently develop Lyme disease. The risk of Lyme disease probably is greater from unrecognized bites because in such instances the tick is able to feed for a longer time.

Substantial evidence indicates that the risk of Lyme disease after a recognized deer tick bite, even in hyperendemic areas, is only 1% to 3% [19,24,25]. The expertise to identify the species, stage, and degree of engorgement of a tick—and to assess the degree of risk—is rarely available to individuals who are bitten. Many "ticks" submitted for identification by physicians turned out actually to be spiders, lice, scabs, or dirt, none of which can transmit Lyme disease. In addition, estimates by patients of the duration for which the tick fed are unreliable [26].

Lyme disease occurs throughout the world (Fig. 17–1). In the United States, most cases occur in a few highly endemic areas—southern New England, New York, New Jersey, Pennsylvania, Minnesota, and Wisconsin (Fig. 17–2) [4]. In Europe, most cases occur in the Scandinavian countries and in central Europe (especially in Germany, Austria, and Switzerland), although cases have been reported from throughout the region.

Although an increase in frequency and an expansion of the geographic distribution of Lyme disease in the United States have occurred in recent years, the incidence of Lyme disease even in endemic areas varies substantially—from region to region and within local areas. Information about the incidence of the disease is complicated by reliance, in most instances, on passive reporting of cases and by the high frequency of misdiagnosis of the disease.

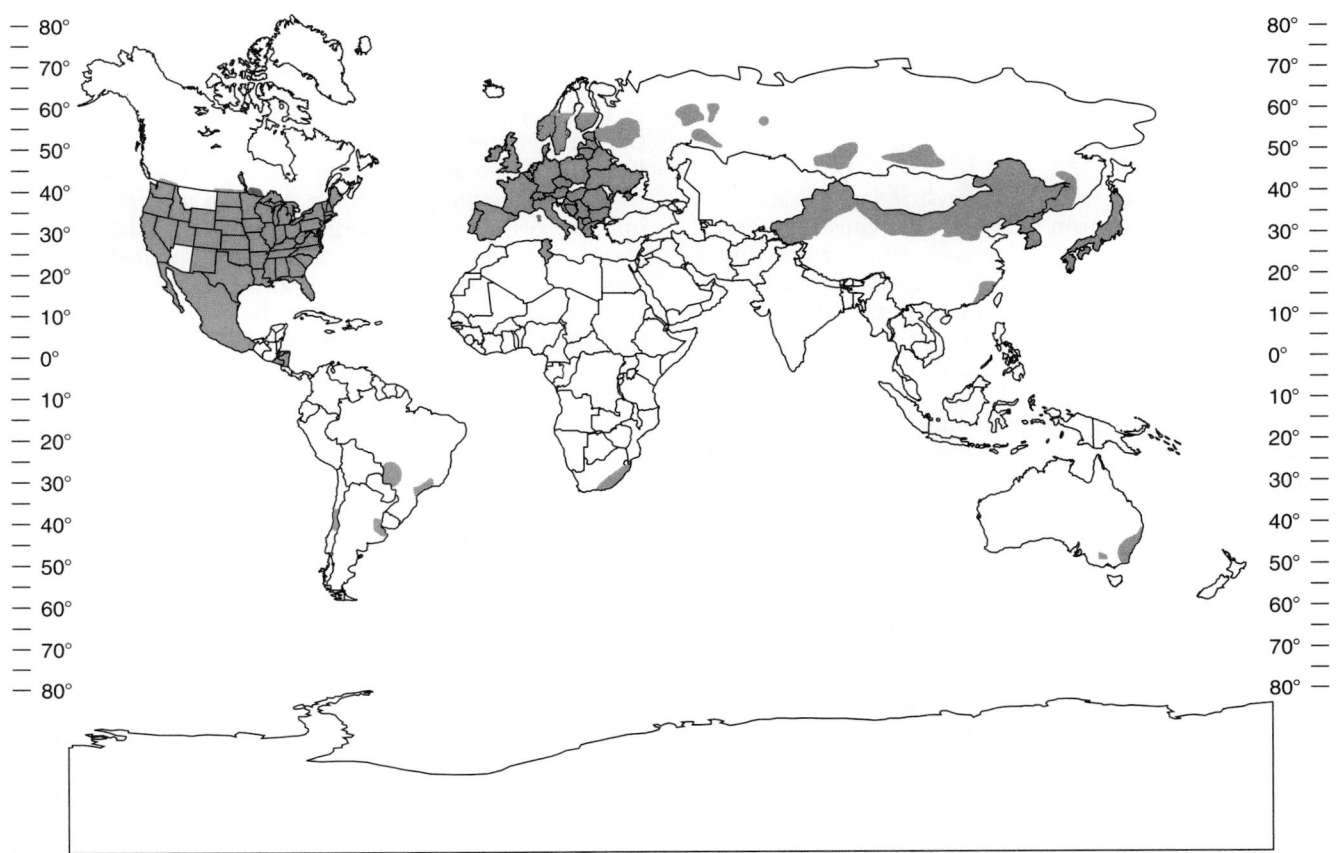

FIGURE 17–1 Worldwide geographic distribution of reported Lyme disease.

NUMBER* OF NEWLY REPORTED LYME DISEASE CASES, BY COUNTY† — UNITED STATES, 2005

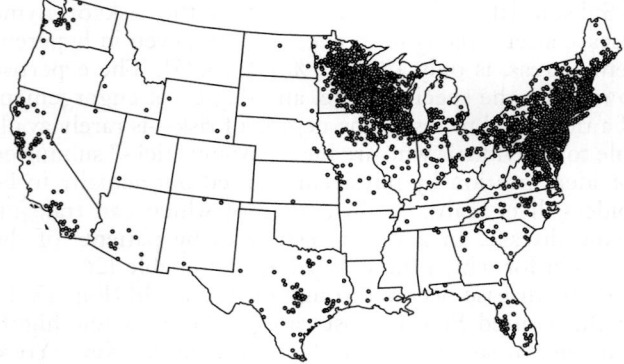

*N = 23,174; county not available for 131 other cases.
†One dot was placed randomly within the county of patient residence for each reported case.

FIGURE 17–2 Number of cases of Lyme disease, by county in the United States, 2005. *(From CDC. Lyme disease—United States, 2003-2005. MMWR Morb Mortal Wkly Rep 56:573-576, 2007. Available at http://www.cdc.gov/mmwr/preview/mmwrhtml/mm5623a1.htm.)*

Studies have indicated that some patients in whom serologic evidence of recent infection with *B. burgdorferi* develops are asymptomatic [27,28].

From 2003-2005, 64,382 cases of Lyme disease were reported to the U.S. Centers for Disease Control and Prevention (CDC) (an average of 21,460 cases/yr) [4]. Of the cases, 93% (29.2 cases per 100,000 population) were reported in just 10 states (Connecticut, Delaware, Maryland, Massachusetts, Minnesota, New Jersey, New York, Pennsylvania, Rhode Island, and Wisconsin) (see Fig. 17–2).

MICROBIOLOGY

The spirochetal bacterium *B. burgdorferi* is a fastidious, microaerophilic organism that in vitro must be grown on special media. It is a slow-growing bacterium with a cell membrane that is covered by flagella and a loosely associated outer membrane. Major antigens of the bacteria include the outer surface lipoproteins OspA, OspB, and OspC (highly charged basic proteins of molecular masses of about 31 kDa, 34 kDa, and 23 kDa) and the 41-kDa flagellar protein. The organism is more properly classified as the *Borrelia burgdorferi sensu lato* ("in the broad sense") species complex, which has been subclassified into several genomospecies, among which the major ones that cause human diseases are *Borrelia burgdorferi sensu stricto* ("in the strict sense"), *Borrelia garinii*, and *Borrelia afzelii*. In the United States, only *B. burgdorferi sensu stricto* has been isolated from humans. By contrast, substantial variability exists in the species of *B. burgdorferi* isolated from humans in Europe, most of which are either *B. garinii* or *B. afzelii*. The complete genome of the organism has been sequenced [29]. The biology of *B. burgdorferi* is complex, as might be expected in view of the complicated life cycle of this vector-borne bacterium, part of which is spent in ticks (with a primitive immune system) and part of which is spent in mammals, which have a highly evolved immune system. The reader

is referred to other sources for detailed discussion of the biology of this organism [30].

PATHOGENESIS AND PATHOLOGY

In approximately 90% of patients in the United States, Lyme disease begins with the characteristic expanding skin lesion, erythema migrans, at the site of the tick bite [31,32]. The spirochete subsequently disseminates via the bloodstream, producing the malaise, fatigue, headache, arthralgia, myalgia, fever, and regional lymphadenopathy that may be associated with early Lyme disease and the clinical manifestations of early disseminated and, ultimately, of late Lyme disease. The ability of the spirochete to spread through skin and other tissues may be facilitated by the binding of human plasminogen and its activators to the surface of the organism [33]. During dissemination, *B. burgdorferi* attaches to certain host integrins [34,35], matrix glycosaminoglycans [36], and extracellular matrix proteins [37], which may explain the organism's particular tissue tropisms (e.g., collagen fibrils in the extracellular matrix in the heart, nervous system, and joints) [36]. In addition, the sequences of OspC vary considerably among strains, and only a few groups of sequences are associated with disseminated disease [38].

Studies in mice have shown the importance of inflammatory innate immune responses in controlling early disseminated Lyme disease [39,40]. In humans with erythema migrans, infiltrates of macrophages and T cells produce inflammatory and anti-inflammatory cytokines [41]. In addition, evidence suggests that in disseminated infections, adaptive T-cell and B-cell responses in lymph nodes produce antibodies against many components of the spirochete [42,43].

The mechanism by which *B. burgdorferi* interacts with the host immune responses to produce Lyme neuroborreliosis or Lyme arthritis is not fully understood [44–47]. In the initial attempt to eliminate *B. burgdorferi*, the innate immune response to the organism results in the release of cytokines, chemokines, and other immune mediators that produce an inflammatory response. This inflammatory response damages host tissues in the process of attempting to eradicate the *Borrelia* organisms. Subsequently, an adaptive immune response is initiated through the processing and presentation of *B. burgdorferi* antigens by macrophages and dendritic cells. This response results in the release of additional immune mediators, which exacerbate further the damage produced by the inflammatory response [44–47].

Several spirochetes have exhibited the ability to cause transplacental infections in various animals and in humans [5–17]. Transplacental transmission of *B. burgdorferi* has been documented in several animal studies, including case reports, case series, and transmission studies. *B. burgdorferi* has been cultured from fetal tissues of a coyote and a white-footed mouse and from the blood of a newborn calf [48–50]. The presence of *B. burgdorferi* in fetal tissues of a white-footed mouse and a house mouse also has been shown by polymerase chain reaction (PCR) assay [51]. Serologic evaluations also have been used to document in utero fetal infection with *B. burgdorferi* in an aborted calf, a newborn foal, and four beagle pups [49,50,52].

Several animal studies have linked infection with *B. burgdorferi* during pregnancy with fetal wastage and reproductive failure in cows and beagles [50,52]. Infection with *B. burgdorferi* during pregnancy also has been associated with reproductive failure and severe fetal infection in horses [53] and with increased fetal loss in mice [54].

In animal experiments, transplacental transmission of *B. burgdorferi* was documented by PCR assay in 19 of 40 pups born to female beagles that had been intradermally inoculated with this spirochete multiple times during pregnancy [52]. Only 4 of the 19 pups had culture-positive tissues, and none of the pups had any evidence of inflammation. In other studies, female rats inoculated with *B. burgdorferi* intraperitoneally at 4 days of gestation and pregnant hamsters infected by tick bite just before gestation showed no evidence by culture of transplacental transmission of *B. burgdorferi* to their offspring [55,56]. In another study, offspring of naturally infected white-footed mice were unable to transmit *B. burgdorferi* to spirochete-free deer ticks allowed to feed on them [57].

Transplacental transmission of *B. burgdorferi* in humans has been shown in association with adverse fetal outcome in several case reports. The first was a report by Schlesinger and coworkers in 1985 [58] that described a 28-year-old woman with untreated Lyme disease during the first trimester of pregnancy, who gave birth, at 35 weeks of gestation, to an infant with widespread cardiovascular abnormalities. The infant died during the first week of life, and postmortem examination showed spirochetes morphologically compatible with *B. burgdorferi* in the infant's spleen, kidneys, and bone marrow, but not in the heart. In contrast with the mononuclear cell infiltrate and proliferation of fibroblasts usually seen with congenital syphilis [59], there was no evidence of inflammation, necrosis, or granuloma formation in the infant's heart or other organs. In 1987, MacDonald and coworkers [60] described a 24-year-old woman with untreated Lyme disease in the first trimester of pregnancy who gave birth at term to a stillborn infant weighing 2500 g. *B. burgdorferi* was cultured from the liver, and spirochetes were seen in the heart, adrenal glands, liver, brain, and placenta with immunofluorescence and silver staining techniques. No evidence of inflammation was seen, however, and no abnormalities were noted except for a small ventricular septal defect.

Weber and colleagues in 1988 [61] described a 37-year-old woman who received penicillin orally for 1 week for erythema migrans during the first trimester of pregnancy. She subsequently gave birth to a 3400-g infant at term who died at 23 hours of age, of what was believed to be "perinatal brain damage." *B. burgdorferi* was identified in the newborn's brain using immunochromogenic staining with monoclonal antibodies. No significant inflammation or other abnormalities were found, however, in any organ, including the brain, on postmortem examination. In 1997, Trevisan and associates [62] described an otherwise healthy infant who presented with multiple annular erythematous lesions, fever, and generalized lymphadenopathy at 3 weeks of age. These clinical abnormalities recurred throughout the first 3 years of life despite oral therapy with amoxicillin and josamycin. A skin biopsy specimen revealed spirochetes by silver stain and was

positive for *B. burgdorferi* by PCR assay. In addition, serologic studies were positive for infection with *B. burgdorferi*. The patient's mother had no history of either a tick bite or Lyme disease, but she had been involved in outdoor activities in an endemic area and had a weakly positive serologic test for Lyme disease.

Several case reports have described pregnant women with either erythema migrans or neuroborreliosis who received appropriate antimicrobial therapy at different stages of their pregnancies [63–67]. In none of these reports was there an association between Lyme disease in the mother and an adverse outcome of the pregnancy.

Transplacental transmission of *B. burgdorferi* also has been investigated in a study of 60 placentas from asymptomatic women who lived in an area endemic for Lyme disease and whose results on serologic testing by enzyme-linked immunosorbent assay (ELISA) were either positive or equivocal for antibodies to *B. burgdorferi* [68]. All 60 placentas were examined with a Warthin-Starry silver stain for evidence of infection with *B. burgdorferi*; 3 (5%) were positive for spirochetes. PCR assays for *B. burgdorferi* nucleotide sequences were performed on two of these three placentas and were positive in both. The women from whom these three placentas were obtained all had equivocal results on ELISAs and negative results on Western blot analysis for Lyme disease and negative results on serologic tests for syphilis. In addition, none of these women had a history of either a tick bite or a clinical course consistent with Lyme disease. All of these pregnancies had entirely normal outcomes.

In addition to the individual case reports, several published case series have assessed the relationship between Lyme disease in pregnant women and fetal outcomes. Two of these case studies were conducted by the CDC. The first was a retrospective investigation conducted in 19 women with Lyme disease during pregnancy who were identified by the investigators without knowing the fetal outcomes [69]. The adverse outcomes included prematurity, cortical blindness, intrauterine fetal death, syndactyly, and a generalized neonatal rash. Infection with *B. burgdorferi* could not be directly implicated as the cause of any of these outcomes, however. The second case series included 17 women who acquired Lyme disease during pregnancy and were evaluated prospectively [70]. One woman had a spontaneous abortion with no evidence of an infection with *B. burgdorferi* on either stains or cultures of the fetal tissue, 1 woman had an infant with isolated syndactyly, and 15 women were delivered of normal infants with no clinical or serologic evidence of infection with *B. burgdorferi*.

In 1999, Maraspin and coworkers [71] reported a series of 105 women with erythema migrans during pregnancy. Ninety-three (88.6%) of the 105 women had healthy infants delivered at term, 2 (1.9%) pregnancies ended with a miscarriage, and 6 (5.7%) ended with a preterm birth. One of the preterm infants had cardiac abnormalities, and two died shortly after birth. Four (3.8%) infants born at term had congenital anomalies (one with syndactyly and three with urologic abnormalities). As with a previous study, infection with *B. burgdorferi* could not be directly implicated as the cause of any of these adverse outcomes.

Several epidemiologic studies of Lyme disease during pregnancy also have been conducted. In the first, Williams and coworkers [72] examined 421 serum specimens obtained from cord blood and found no association between the presence of IgG antibodies to *B. burgdorferi* and congenital malformations. In another study, Nadal and associates [73] investigated outcomes in 1434 infants of 1416 women for the presence of antibodies to *B. burgdorferi* at the time of delivery. Of the women, 12 (0.85%) were found to be seropositive, but only 1 woman had a history consistent with Lyme disease during pregnancy. Of the infants born to the 12 seropositive women, 2 had transient hyperbilirubinemia; 1 had transient hypotonia; 1 was post-term and small for gestational age, with evidence of chronic placental insufficiency; 1 had transient macrocephaly; and 1 had transient supraventricular extra beats. The infant born to the woman with a clinical history of Lyme disease during pregnancy had a ventricular septal defect. At follow-up evaluations approximately 9 to 17 months later, all of the children except for the child with the cardiac defect were entirely well, and none had serologic evidence of infection with *B. burgdorferi*.

In 1994, Gerber and Zalneraitis [74] surveyed neurologists in areas of the United States in which Lyme disease was endemic at that time to determine how many had seen a child with clinically significant neurologic disease whose mother had been diagnosed as having Lyme disease during pregnancy. None of the 162 pediatric and 37 adult neurologists who responded to the survey had ever seen a child whose mother had been diagnosed with Lyme disease during pregnancy. The investigators concluded that congenital neuroborreliosis was either not occurring or occurring at an extremely low frequency in areas endemic for Lyme disease. In a retrospective case-control study carried out in an area endemic for Lyme disease, 796 "case" children with congenital cardiac anomalies were compared with 704 "control" children without cardiac defects with respect to Lyme disease in their mothers either during or before the pregnancy [75]. No association was found between congenital heart defects and either a tick bite or Lyme disease in the mothers either within 3 months of conception or during pregnancy.

Investigators in New York performed two studies of the relationship between Lyme disease in pregnant women and adverse outcomes of the pregnancies. The first was an unselected, prospective, population-based investigation in an area endemic for Lyme disease in which approximately 2000 women in Westchester County, New York, were evaluated for clinical and serologic evidence of Lyme disease at the first prenatal visit and again at delivery [76]. Of these women, 11 (0.7%) were seropositive, and 79 (4%) reported at the first prenatal visit that they had had Lyme disease sometime in the past. One woman with an untreated influenza-like illness in the second trimester had a negative result on serologic testing for Lyme disease at the prenatal visit, but a positive result at delivery. In addition, during the study period, clinical Lyme disease was diagnosed in 15 pregnant women. No association was found between exposure of the mother to *B. burgdorferi* either before conception or during pregnancy and fetal death, prematurity, or congenital

malformations. In the second study, the researchers compared 5000 infants, half from an area in which Lyme disease was endemic and half from an area without Lyme disease, who served as controls. The researchers found no significant difference in the overall incidence of congenital malformations between the two groups [77]. Although there was a statistically significant higher rate of cardiac malformations in the endemic area compared with that in the control area, no relationship was noted between a cardiac malformation and either a clinical history or serologic evidence of Lyme disease. The researchers concluded from the findings of these two studies that a pregnant woman with a past infection with *B. burgdorferi*, either treated or untreated, did not have an increased risk of early fetal loss or of having a low birth weight infant or an infant with congenital malformations [77].

Two reports have documented the presence of *B. burgdorferi* in cow's milk. In 1988, Burgess [50] cultured *B. burgdorferi* from 1 of 3 samples of colostrum from cows, but from none of 44 samples of cow's milk. Lischer and colleagues [78] used a PCR assay to identify nucleotide sequences of *B. burgdorferi* in the milk of a cow with clinical Lyme disease. In a similar investigation of human milk, Schmidt and coworkers [79] examined breast milk from two lactating women with erythema migrans and from three lactating women with no clinical evidence of Lyme disease. The breast milk samples from both women with erythema migrans tested positive for *B. burgdorferi* by PCR assay, whereas the breast milk samples from all three healthy women tested negative. No other reports have corroborated these findings in human milk, however, and transmission of Lyme disease through breast-feeding has never been documented.

CLINICAL MANIFESTATIONS

The clinical manifestations of Lyme disease depend on the stage of the illness—early localized disease, early disseminated disease, or late disease [31,80]. Erythema migrans, the manifestation of early localized Lyme disease, appears at the site of the tick bite, 3 to 30 days (typically 7 to 10 days) after the bite. Erythema migrans is found in about 90% of patients with objective evidence of infection with *B. burgdorferi* [31,32,81]. Erythema migrans begins as a red macule or papule and expands for days to weeks to form a large, annular erythematous lesion that ranges from 5 to 70 cm in diameter (median 15 cm). This rash may be uniformly erythematous, or it may appear as a target lesion with a variable degree of central clearing. It can vary greatly in shape and, occasionally, may have vesicular or necrotic areas in the center. Erythema migrans is usually asymptomatic, but may be pruritic or painful, and it may be accompanied by systemic findings, such as fever, malaise, headache, regional lymphadenopathy, stiff neck, myalgia, or arthralgia.

The most common manifestation of early disseminated Lyme disease in the United States is multiple erythema migrans. The secondary skin lesions, which usually appear 3 to 5 weeks after the tick bite, consist of multiple annular erythematous lesions similar to, but usually smaller than, the primary lesion. Other common manifestations of early disseminated Lyme disease are cranial nerve palsies, especially facial nerve palsy, and meningitis. Systemic symptoms such as fever, myalgia, arthralgia, headache, and fatigue also are common in this stage of Lyme disease. Carditis, which usually is manifested by various degrees of heart block, is a rare manifestation of early disseminated disease [32].

The most common manifestation of late Lyme disease, which occurs weeks to months after the initial infection, is arthritis. The arthritis is usually monarticular or oligoarticular and affects the large joints, particularly the knee. Although the affected joint often is swollen and tender, the intense pain associated with a septic arthritis usually is not present; frequently, the swollen joint is only mildly symptomatic. Encephalitis, encephalopathy, and polyneuropathy also are manifestations of late Lyme disease, but they are rare.

The clinical manifestations of Lyme disease also may depend on which subspecies of *B. burgdorferi* is causing the infection [31]. The differences in subspecies found in Europe and in North America may account for differences in the frequencies of certain clinical manifestations of Lyme disease in these areas. Neurologic manifestations of Lyme disease are more common in Europe, whereas rheumatologic manifestations are more common in North America. In addition, certain skin and soft tissue manifestations of Lyme disease, such as acrodermatitis chronica atrophicans and lymphocytomas, occur in Europe, but are extremely rare in the United States.

There has been substantial controversy about an entity that has been called "chronic Lyme disease." There is no evidence that such a condition exists [82]. Nonspecific symptoms (e.g., fatigue, arthralgia, or myalgia) may persist for several weeks, even in patients who are successfully treated for early Lyme disease; their presence should not be regarded as an indication for additional treatment with antimicrobials. These symptoms usually respond to nonsteroidal anti-inflammatory drugs. Within 6 months of completion of the initial course of antimicrobial therapy, these nonspecific symptoms usually resolve without additional antimicrobial therapy. For the unusual patients who have symptoms that persist longer than 6 months after the completion of antimicrobial therapy, an attempt should be made to determine whether these symptoms are the result of a postinfectious phenomenon or have another etiology [82].

Most patients with "chronic Lyme disease" have no evidence of either current or past infection with *B. burgdorferi*. There have been four double-blind randomized clinical trials of long-term antibiotic treatment for patients with at least some evidence of past infection with *B. burgdorferi* and subsequent symptoms that persist for at least 6 months after conventional (or longer) treatment with antibiotics [83–85]. The results of all of these studies showed that long-term treatment provided little or no benefit, but was associated with substantial risks to the patient [86]. In addition, prolonged use of antibiotics encourages selection of antibiotic-resistant bacteria that pose risks to the patients and to the community. These results add to the already substantial data that "chronic Lyme disease" is not a persistent infection, but more likely should be classified as a syndrome of medically unexplained symptoms [87].

Ixodes ticks may transmit other pathogens in addition to *B. burgdorferi*, including *Babesia, Anaplasma*, other *Borrelia* species, and viruses. These agents may be transmitted either separately from or simultaneously with *B. burgdorferi*. The frequency with which coinfection occurs is unknown. The impact of coinfection on the clinical presentation and the response to treatment of Lyme disease, although well documented and important in rare selected cases, seems to be of minor significance in most instances. In the south-central United States, in areas such as Missouri, another tick-borne infection that causes erythema migrans has been recognized: [88,89] Southern tick-associated rash illness (STARI) is transmitted by the tick *Amblyomma americanum*, the Lone Star tick. The organism that causes STARI, originally thought to be *Borrelia lonestari*, has not been identified, however. In contrast to Lyme disease, it does not seem to cause systemic disease. Similar to Lyme disease, there is no evidence that STARI is associated with congenital disease in children.

DIAGNOSIS

The CDC clinical case definition for Lyme disease initially was intended for epidemiologic surveillance purposes [90]. When used in conjunction with CDC and U.S. Food and Drug Administration (FDA) guidelines for diagnostic tests [90–92], however, this case definition has been widely accepted as a means to standardize the clinical diagnosis of Lyme disease (Table 17–1).

TABLE 17–1 CDC Lyme Disease Case Definition for Public Health Surveillance Purposes

Erythema migrans: Single primary red macule or papule, expanding over days to weeks to large round lesion ≥5 cm diameter (physician-confirmed), ± central clearing, ± secondary lesions, ± systemic symptoms (fever, fatigue, headache, mild neck stiffness, arthralgia, myalgia)

Plus

Known exposure ≤30 days before onset to endemic area (in which ≥2 confirmed cases have been acquired, or in which *Borrelia burgdorferi*-infected tick vectors are established)

Or

One or more late manifestations without other etiology

1. Musculoskeletal: Recurrent brief episodes of monarticular or pauciarticular arthritis with objective joint swelling, ± chronic arthritis
2. Neurologic: Lymphocytic meningitis, facial palsy, other cranial neuritis, radiculoneuropathy, encephalomyelitis (confirmed by CSF *B. burgdorferi* antibody > serum *B. burgdorferi* antibody)
3. Cardiovascular: Acute second-degree or third-degree atrioventricular conduction defects, lasting days to weeks, ± myocarditis

Plus

Laboratory confirmation by either

1. Isolation of *B. burgdorferi* from patient specimen
2. Diagnostic levels of *B. burgdorferi* IgM or IgG antibodies in serum or CSF (initial ELISA or IFA screen followed by Western blot of positive or equivocal results)

CDC, Centers for Disease Control and Prevention; CSF, cerebrospinal fluid; ELISA, enzyme-linked immunosorbent assay; IFA, immunofluorescence assay.
Adapted from CDC. Case definitions for infectious conditions under public health surveillance. MMWR 1997;46(No. RR-10) 20-21, 1997.

For patients in locations endemic for Lyme disease who present with the characteristic lesion of erythema migrans, the diagnosis of Lyme disease should be based on the clinical presentation alone. In such situations, laboratory testing is neither necessary nor recommended. With the exception of erythema migrans, however, the clinical manifestations of Lyme disease are nonspecific. For patients who do not have erythema migrans, the diagnosis of Lyme disease should be based on clinical findings supported by results of laboratory tests. These laboratory tests may consist of either direct identification of *B. burgdorferi* in the patient or demonstration of a serologic response to the organism.

Methods for identifying the presence of *B. burgdorferi* in a patient (e.g., culture, histopathologic examination, antigen detection) generally have poor sensitivity or specificity or both and may require invasive procedures (e.g., a biopsy of the skin) to obtain an appropriate specimen for testing. Isolation of *B. burgdorferi* from a symptomatic patient should be considered diagnostic of Lyme disease. *B. burgdorferi* has been isolated from blood, skin biopsy specimens, cerebrospinal fluid (CSF), myocardial biopsy specimens, and the synovium of patients with Lyme disease. The medium in which *B. burgdorferi* is cultured is expensive, however, and it can take 6 weeks for the spirochete to grow in culture. The best chance of culturing *B. burgdorferi* from a patient is when erythema migrans is present [93], although at this stage of the disease, the diagnosis should be largely clinical. During the later stages of Lyme disease, culture is much less sensitive. In addition, it is necessary for patients to undergo an invasive procedure, such as a biopsy, to obtain appropriate tissue or fluid for culture. Culture is indicated only in rare circumstances.

B. burgdorferi has been identified with silver stains (Warthin-Starry or modified Dieterle) and with immunohistochemical stains (with monoclonal or polyclonal antibodies) in skin, synovial, and myocardial biopsy specimens. *B. burgdorferi* can be confused with normal tissue structures, however, or it may be missed because it often is present in low concentrations. Considerable training and experience are needed for skill in identifying spirochetes in tissues. Direct detection of *B. burgdorferi* in tissue is of limited practical value.

Attempts have been made to develop antigen-based diagnostic tests for Lyme disease, but no convincing data indicating the accuracy of any of these tests are available. All of these tests should be considered experimental until additional studies confirm their validity and reproducibility. Assays to detect *B. burgdorferi* antigens in CSF or urine, including the Lyme urine antigen test based on the procedure of Hyde and colleagues [94,95], have poor specificity and poor sensitivity and are not recommended [96].

Tests that use PCR techniques to identify *B. burgdorferi* may be helpful. Results of such tests may be positive for some time after the spirochetes are no longer viable, however. In addition, the risk of false-positive results on PCR assays is great, especially when they are performed in commercial laboratories. If a PCR test is done, it should be performed in a reference laboratory that meets the highest standards of quality control for diagnostic PCR assays [95]. Because of its limited availability, expense, and insufficient evidence of its value in the management of most patients, PCR is at present reserved for special situations [97]. Use of PCR assay may be appropriate in testing of specimens such as synovial tissue or fluid from patients with persistent arthritis after a course of appropriate antibiotic therapy for late Lyme disease; samples of abnormal CSF from patients who are seropositive for antibodies to *B. burgdorferi* and have a neurologic illness that is compatible with, but not typical of, Lyme disease; and skin biopsy specimens from patients who have a localized rash that is consistent with erythema migrans, but have no history of possible exposure or residence in or travel to areas where Lyme disease is endemic [97]. At present, there is insufficient evidence of the accuracy, predictive value, or clinical significance of a PCR test of urine for *B. burgdorferi*, and its use for decisions regarding the management of patients has been strongly discouraged [97].

Because of the limitations of laboratory tests designed to identify directly the presence of *B. burgdorferi* in a patient, the confirmation of Lyme disease in patients without erythema migrans usually is based on the demonstration of antibodies to *B. burgdorferi* in the serum. The normal antibody response to acute infection with *B. burgdorferi* is well described [98]. Specific IgM antibodies appear first, usually 3 to 4 weeks after the infection begins. These antibodies peak after 6 to 8 weeks and subsequently decline. A prolonged elevation of IgM antibodies sometimes is seen, however, even after effective antimicrobial treatment [99]. Consequently, the results of serologic tests for specific IgM antibodies should not be used as the sole indicator of the timing of an infection. Specific IgG antibodies usually appear 6 to 8 weeks after the onset of the infection. These antibodies peak in 4 to 6 months. The IgG antibody titer may decline after treatment, but even after the patient is clinically cured, these antibodies usually remain detectable for many years [100,101].

The immunofluorescent antibody test was the initial serologic test for diagnosing Lyme disease. It requires subjective interpretation and is time-consuming to perform, however, and has largely been replaced by ELISA. The ELISA method may give false-positive results because of cross-reactive antibodies in patients with other spirochetal infections (e.g., syphilis, leptospirosis, relapsing fever), certain viral infections (e.g., varicella), and certain autoimmune diseases (e.g., systemic lupus erythematosus). In contrast to patients with syphilis, patients with Lyme disease do not have positive results on nontreponemal tests for syphilis, such as the Venereal Disease Research Laboratory or rapid plasma reagin. In addition, antibodies directed against bacteria in the normal oral flora may cross-react with antigens of *B. burgdorferi* to produce a false-positive ELISA result.

The first-generation ELISA method uses either whole cells of *B. burgdorferi* or the supernatant of sonicated spirochetes as the antigen. To improve the specificity of the ELISA, new assays have been developed that use less complex fractions of the spirochetes, such as the bacterial membrane, or purified native or recombinant proteins, alone or in combination [97].

Immunoblot (Western blot) analysis for serum antibodies to *B. burgdorferi* also is used as a serologic test for Lyme disease. Although some investigators have suggested that immunoblot is more sensitive and more specific than ELISA, there is still some debate about its interpretation. Immunoblot is most useful for validating a positive or equivocal ELISA result, especially in patients with a low clinical likelihood of having Lyme disease. For serologic testing for Lyme disease, it is recommended that a sensitive ELISA be performed, and, if results are either positive or equivocal, that a Western blot analysis be done to confirm the specificity of the result [88]. Specimens that give a negative result on a sensitive ELISA do not require immunoblot.

One reason for the poor sensitivity of serologic tests for Lyme disease is that erythema migrans, which is the clinical finding that usually brings patients to medical attention, usually appears within 2 to 3 weeks of onset of infection with *B. burgdorferi*. Antibodies to *B. burgdorferi* often are not detected at this early stage of the disease. The antibody response to *B. burgdorferi* also may be abrogated in patients with early Lyme disease who receive prompt treatment with an effective antimicrobial agent; in these patients, antibodies against *B. burgdorferi* may never develop, at least as a result of that exposure. Most patients with early, disseminated Lyme disease and virtually all patients with late Lyme disease have serum antibodies to *B. burgdorferi*, however. Seropositivity may persist for years even after successful antimicrobial therapy. Ongoing seropositivity, even persistence of IgM, is not a marker of active infection. Likewise, serologic tests should not be used to assess the adequacy of antimicrobial therapy.

Serologic tests for Lyme disease have not been adequately standardized. The accuracy and the reproducibility of currently available serologic tests, especially widely used, commercially produced kits, are poor [102–106]. Use of these commercial diagnostic test kits for Lyme disease would result in a high rate of misdiagnosis. As with any diagnostic test, the predictive value of serologic tests for Lyme disease depends primarily on the probability that the patient has Lyme disease based on the clinical and epidemiologic history and the physical examination (the "pretest probability" of Lyme disease). Use of serologic tests to "rule out" Lyme disease in patients with a low probability of the illness would result in a very high proportion of test results that are falsely positive [107]. Antibody tests for Lyme disease should not be used as screening tests [92,107,108].

With few exceptions, the probability that a patient has Lyme disease would be very low in areas in which Lyme disease is rare. Even in areas with a high prevalence of Lyme disease, patients with only nonspecific signs and symptoms, such as fatigue, headache, and arthralgia, are not likely to have Lyme disease [107,108]. Although such nonspecific symptoms are common in patients with Lyme disease, they are almost always accompanied by more specific objective findings, such as erythema migrans, facial nerve palsy, or arthritis. Even when more accurate tests performed by reference laboratories are available, clinicians should order serologic tests for Lyme disease selectively, reserving them for patients from populations with a relatively high prevalence of Lyme disease who have specific objective clinical findings that are suggestive of Lyme disease, so that the predictive value of a positive result is high [107–109].

Clinicians should realize that even though a symptomatic patient has a positive result on serologic testing for antibodies to *B. burgdorferi*, Lyme disease may not be the cause of that patient's symptoms. In addition to the possibility that it is a false-positive result (a common occurrence), the patient may have been infected with *B. burgdorferi* previously, and the patient's symptoms may be unrelated to that previous infection. As noted earlier, when serum antibodies to *B. burgdorferi* do develop, they may persist for many years despite adequate treatment and clinical cure of the illness [100,101]. In addition, because symptoms never develop in some people who become infected with *B. burgdorferi*, in endemic areas there is a background rate of seropositivity among patients who have never had clinically apparent Lyme disease.

The diagnosis of an infection of the central nervous system (CNS) with *B. burgdorferi* is made by showing the presence of inflammation in the CSF and *Borrelia*-specific intrathecal antibodies [95,110]. Most patients with typical cases of Lyme neuroborreliosis have antibodies to *B. burgdorferi* in serum, and testing for the presence of antibodies in the CSF usually is unnecessary [97]. In some instances, examination of the CSF for antibodies to *B. burgdorferi* may be indicated. Because antibodies to *B. burgdorferi* may be present in the CSF as the result of passive transit through a leaky blood-brain barrier, detection of antibodies in the CSF is not proof of infection of the CNS by the organism. Better evidence of CNS disease is the demonstration of intrathecal production of antibodies; this is accomplished by simultaneously measuring the antibodies in the serum and CSF by ELISA and calculating the "CSF index" [97]. As noted previously, a PCR test of the CSF may be helpful in confirming the diagnosis of CNS Lyme disease [95,97].

A lymphoproliferative assay that assesses the cell-mediated immune response to *B. burgdorferi* has been developed and used as a diagnostic test for Lyme disease. This assay has not been standardized, however, and is not approved by the FDA. The indications for this lymphoproliferative assay are few, if any [97].

The diagnosis of Lyme disease in a pregnant woman should be made in accordance with the currently accepted CDC case definition (see Table 17–1). There is no indication for routine prenatal serologic screening of asymptomatic healthy women. Serosurveys have shown that the seroprevalence rates among pregnant women were comparable with those in the general population [76,77,111] and that asymptomatic seroconversion during pregnancy was unusual [76].

MANAGEMENT AND TREATMENT

Pediatricians are sometimes confronted with the challenge of how to manage an infant born to a woman who was diagnosed with Lyme disease during her pregnancy. The difficulty arises because of the paucity of evidence that congenital Lyme disease is a clinical problem. In addition, for reasons cited earlier, the diagnosis in the mother often is inaccurate. First, parents should be reassured that there is no evidence that the infant is at increased risk of any problem from maternal Lyme disease. Next, an attempt should be made to ascertain the accuracy of the diagnosis in the mother; if the mother did not have objective signs of Lyme disease (e.g., erythema migrans) or if the diagnosis was based on nonspecific symptoms (e.g., fatigue, myalgia) and a positive serologic test result, it is likely that the diagnosis is inaccurate.

There is no reason to order serologic tests for Lyme disease in infants who are asymptomatic (even if diagnosis of Lyme disease in the mother is accurate). If such tests are ordered, it is important to remember that if the mother did have Lyme disease and is seropositive, the infant may have passively acquired antibodies from the mother and so may remain seropositive for many months even in the absence of infection. Because of the high frequency of false-positive test results, a positive test result for IgM antibodies against *B. burgdorferi* in an asymptomatic child should be interpreted with a high degree of skepticism.

The choice of antibiotic and the duration of treatment for Lyme disease depend on the stage of the disease that is being treated (Table 17–2). Generally, pregnant women should receive the same treatment as other patients except that use of doxycycline is not recommended during pregnancy [112–114].

Early Localized Disease

Doxycycline is the drug of choice for children 8 years and older with early localized Lyme disease [112]. Exposure to the sun should be avoided by individuals who are taking doxycycline because a rash develops in sun-exposed areas 20% to 30% of the time. Use of sunscreen may decrease this risk. Amoxicillin is recommended for children younger than 8 years, for pregnant women, and for patients who cannot tolerate doxycycline. For patients allergic to penicillin, alternative drugs are cefuroxime axetil, erythromycin, and azithromycin. Erythromycin and azithromycin may be less effective than other agents. Most experts recommend a 14- to 21-day course of therapy for early localized Lyme disease, although evidence indicates that 10 days of doxycycline constitutes adequate treatment in adults with uncomplicated infection [115].

A prompt clinical response to treatment is usual, with resolution of erythema migrans within several days of initiating therapy. Occasionally, a Jarisch-Herxheimer reaction, which usually consists of an elevated temperature and worsening myalgia, develops shortly after antimicrobial treatment is initiated. These reactions typically last 1 to 2 days and do not constitute an indication to discontinue antimicrobial therapy, and symptoms respond to nonsteroidal anti-inflammatory drugs. Appropriate treatment of erythema migrans almost always prevents development of the later stages of Lyme disease.

Early Disseminated and Late Disease

Multiple erythema migrans and initial episodes of arthritis should be treated with orally administered antimicrobial agents. If peripheral facial nerve palsy is the only neurologic manifestation of Lyme disease, the patient can be given an oral regimen of antimicrobials. If the facial nerve palsy is accompanied by clinical evidence of CNS involvement (e.g., severe headache, nuchal rigidity), a lumbar puncture should be performed. If there is pleocytosis, parenterally administered antimicrobials should

---

TABLE 17–2   Antimicrobial Treatment of Lyme Disease

Early Disease
Localized Erythema Migrans
Doxycycline, 2-4 mg/kg/d twice daily (maximum 100 mg/dose) for 14-21 days (do not use in children <8 yr old), or amoxicillin, 50 mg/kg/d three times a day (maximum 500 mg/dose) for 14-21 days. Preferred alternative agent for patients who cannot take either amoxicillin or doxycycline is cefuroxime axetil, 30 mg/kg/d twice daily (maximum 500 mg/dose) for 14-21 days. Erythromycin and azithromycin are less effective alternatives for patients who cannot take other recommended agents
Neurologic Disease
Isolated seventh cranial nerve or other cranial nerve palsy: Treat as for localized erythema migrans, but for 14-21 days (doxycycline preferred if possible)
Meningitis (with or without encephalitis or radiculoneuritis): Ceftriaxone, 50-75 mg/kg once daily (maximum 2 g/dose) for 14-28 days. Alternatives include penicillin G, 200,000-400,000 U/kg/d (maximum 18-24 million U/d) every 4 hr, or cefotaxime 150 mg/kg/d (maximum 2 g/dose) divided every 8 hr for 14-28 days, and oral doxycycline, 4 mg/kg/d twice daily (maximum 200 mg/dose) for 14-21 days
Carditis
First-degree or second-degree heart block: Treat as for localized erythema migrans
Third-degree heart block or other evidence of severe carditis: Treat as for meningitis
Late Disease
Arthritis
Doxycycline, 2-4 mg/kg/d twice daily (maximum 100 mg/dose) for 28 days (do not use in children <8 yr old), or amoxicillin, 50 mg/kg/d twice daily (maximum 500 mg/dose) for 28 days. Preferred alternative agent for patients who cannot take either amoxicillin or doxycycline is cefuroxime axetil, 30 mg/kg/d twice daily (maximum 500 mg/dose) for 28 days. For recurrent or persistent arthritis for which oral treatment has failed, either a second course of one of the orally administered agents for 28 days or a course of parenteral treatment for 14-28 days (as for meningitis) is indicated
Neurologic Disease
Treat as for meningitis above for 14-28 days

be prescribed. Meningitis and recurrent or persistent arthritis also should be treated with parenterally administered antimicrobial agents. Some experts prescribe a second course of an orally administered antimicrobial agent for recurrent or persistent arthritis, however, before using a parenterally administered agent. Nonsteroidal anti-inflammatory drugs are a useful adjunct to antimicrobial therapy for patients with arthritis. Although mild carditis is usually treated orally with either doxycycline or amoxicillin, most experts recommend parenterally administered therapy for severe carditis. Other neurologic manifestations of late Lyme disease (e.g., encephalitis, encephalopathy, polyneuropathy) should be treated with antimicrobials administered parenterally.

The optimal duration of antimicrobial therapy for the various stages of Lyme disease is not well established, but there is no evidence that children with any manifestation of Lyme disease benefit from prolonged (>4 weeks) courses of either orally or parenterally administered antimicrobial agents. Lyme disease, similar to other infections, may trigger a fibromyalgia syndrome that does not respond to additional courses of antimicrobials, but may be managed with symptomatic therapy.

PROGNOSIS

Attempts to determine the potential impact of gestational Lyme disease on the outcome of the pregnancy have been limited for several reasons [116]. First, the prevalence of Lyme disease among pregnant women, even in highly endemic areas, is low, making it difficult to perform studies with sufficient statistical power. Second, diagnoses of gestational Lyme disease that are based on seropositivity, a history of a tick bite, or even a retrospective clinical history are often unreliable. Finally, because of increased awareness and concern about Lyme disease, it is difficult to find women with suspected gestational Lyme disease who did not receive antimicrobial treatment.

Despite these limitations, *B. burgdorferi* can cross the placenta, presumably during a period of spirochetemia. The frequency and clinical significance of transplacental transmission of *B. burgdorferi* are unclear, however. Although a temporal relationship between Lyme disease during pregnancy and adverse outcomes has been documented, a causal relationship has not been established. The claims for the existence of a congenital Lyme disease syndrome are undermined by the absence of an inflammatory response in fetal tissue, absence of a fetal immunologic response, and lack of a consistent clinical outcome in affected pregnancies. Analysis of the current data indicates that there is no evidence of increased risk of abnormal outcomes with Lyme disease during pregnancy.

It is difficult to conduct high-quality studies of clinical outcome in patients with Lyme disease. On the basis of the available data, the long-term prognosis for adults or children who receive appropriate antimicrobial therapy for Lyme disease, regardless of the stage of the disease, seems to be excellent [117]. The most common reason for a lack of response to appropriate antimicrobial therapy for Lyme disease is misdiagnosis (i.e., the patient actually does not have Lyme disease). In approximately 10% of adults and less than 5% of children with Lyme arthritis,

inflammatory joint disease develops that typically affects one knee for months to years and does not respond to antimicrobial therapy. An increased frequency of certain HLA-DR4 alleles has been noted among these patients, and more recent findings suggest that an autoimmune process is involved [118].

PREVENTION

Reducing the risk of tick bites is one strategy to prevent Lyme disease. In endemic areas, clearing brush and trees, removing leaf litter and woodpiles, and keeping grass mowed may reduce exposure to ticks. Application of pesticides to residential properties is effective in suppressing populations of ticks, but may be harmful to other wildlife and to people. Erecting fences to exclude deer from residential yards and maintaining tick-free pets also may reduce exposure to ticks.

Tick and insect repellents that contain N,N-diethyl-m-toluamide (DEET) applied to the skin provide additional protection, but most preparations require reapplication every 1 to 2 hours for maximum effectiveness. Serious neurologic complications in children from frequent or excessive application of DEET-containing repellents have been reported, but they are rare, and the risk is low when these products are used according to instructions on the label. Use of products with concentrations of DEET greater than 30% is unnecessary and increases the risk of adverse effects. DEET should be applied sparingly only to exposed skin, but not to a child's face, hands, or skin that is either irritated or abraded. After the child returns indoors, skin that was treated should be washed with soap and water. Permethrin (a synthetic pyrethroid) is available in a spray for application to clothing only and is particularly effective because it kills ticks on contact.

Because most people (approximately 75%) who recognize that they were bitten by a tick remove the tick within 48 hours [23], the risk of Lyme disease from recognized deer tick bites is low—approximately 1% to 3% in areas with a high incidence of Lyme disease. The risk of Lyme disease probably is higher from unrecognized bites (because in those cases the tick feeds for a longer time). A large study of antimicrobial prophylaxis after tick bites among adults found that a single, 200-mg dose of doxycycline was 87% effective in preventing Lyme disease, although the 95% confidence interval around this estimate of efficacy was wide (the lower bound was ≤25%, depending on the method used) [19]. In that study, the only persons in whom Lyme disease developed had been bitten by nymph-stage ticks that were at least partially engorged; the risk of Lyme disease in this group was 9.9% (among recipients of placebo), whereas it was zero for bites by all larval and adult deer ticks.

The expertise to identify the species, stage, and degree of engorgement of a tick—and to assess the degree of risk—is rarely available to people who are bitten. Consequently, routine use of antimicrobial agents to prevent Lyme disease in people who are bitten by a deer tick, even in highly endemic areas, generally is not recommended because the overall risk of Lyme disease is low. Only doxycycline (which is not recommended for children <8 years old) has been shown to be effective in prophylaxis of Lyme disease [25]. In the unusual instance in which doxycycline prophylaxis is used (e.g., in a non-pregnant patient >8 years old who removes a fully engorged nymph-stage deer tick in an endemic area), only a single dose of doxycycline (200 mg) should be pre-scribed, and it should be taken with food to minimize nausea.

There is no evidence that pregnant women are at increased risk of Lyme disease after a deer tick bite. The only drug that has been shown to be effective in prevent-ing Lyme disease after a tick bite, doxycycline, is not recommended for use during pregnancy because of its possible effect on the developing fetus. Consequently, antimicrobial prophylaxis is not recommended for pregnant women.

Serologic testing for Lyme disease after a recognized tick bite also is not recommended. Antibodies to *B. burg-dorferi* that are present at the time that the tick is removed likely would be due either to a false-positive test result or to an earlier infection with *B. burgdorferi*, rather than to a new infection from the recent bite. Likewise, in this setting the predictive value of a positive result is very low.

Ascertainment of whether the tick is infected, using tests such as PCR, is also not recommended. Although testing ticks with PCR may provide important epidemio-logic information, the predictive values for infection of humans of either a positive or a negative PCR test result is unknown. The result may be positive even if only very few organisms are present, and it provides no information about the duration of feeding, a key determinant of the risk of transmission. In addition, the problems of false-positive results owing to contamination with amplifica-tion products and false-negative results owing to inhibi-tion of PCR by substances in the sample (e.g., blood) limit the test's validity.

People should be taught to inspect themselves and their children's bodies and clothing daily after possible expo-sure to ixodid ticks. An attached tick should be grasped with medium-tipped tweezers as close to the skin as pos-sible and removed by gently pulling the tick straight out. If some of the mouth parts remain embedded in the skin, they should be left alone because they usually are extruded eventually; additional attempts to remove them often result in unnecessary damage to tissue and may increase the risk of local bacterial infection.

RELAPSING FEVER

Relapsing fever is an arthropod-borne zoonosis caused by various *Borrelia* species [10]. There are two forms of relapsing fever. Tick-borne relapsing fever (TBRF), or endemic relapsing fever, is caused by various *Borrelia* spe-cies associated with soft ticks of the genus *Ornithodoros*. Louse-borne relapsing fever (LBRF), or epidemic relaps-ing fever, is caused by *B. recurrentis*, which is associated with the human body louse (*Pediculus humanus*) [10].

The distribution and occurrence of TBRF depend on the enzootic cycle of the transmitting tick vector. In contrast, the distribution and occurrence of LBRF depend on socio-economic and ecologic factors. LBRF usually occurs in epi-demics that are associated with catastrophic events (e.g., war, famine, natural disasters) that result in overcrowding

and dissemination of body lice [10]. LBRF is endemic in the highlands of East Africa (Ethiopia, Sudan, Somalia, Chad) and in the South American Andes (Bolivia, Peru). TBRF has been reported worldwide, with the exception of a few areas in the South Pacific. In North America, *B. hermsii* and *B. turicatae* are the major causes of TBRF [11].

LBRF is transmitted when there is contamination of abraded or normal skin with hemolymph of an infected crushed louse. In TBRF, human infection occurs when saliva or coxal fluid containing the *Borrelia* organisms are released in the feeding puncture.

After an incubation period of approximately 7 days (range 4 to ≥18 days), the onset of disease is signaled by fever [10]. The fever coincides with large numbers of *Bor-relia* organisms in the blood. The relapsing pattern is due to variation of lipoproteins that results in new antigenic variants of major surface lipoproteins and the recurrence of large numbers of *Borrelia* organisms in the blood [11,12]. The most common clinical manifestations of relapsing fever are splenomegaly (41% to 77%), hepato-megaly (17% to 66%), jaundice (7% to 36%), rash (8% to 28%), respiratory symptoms (16% to 34%), and CNS involvement (9% to 30%) [10]. Other complaints include nausea, vomiting, cough, dizziness, and epistaxis [13]. The findings on physical examination may be normal, but tachycardia, tachypnea, jaundice, purpura, or hepato-splenomegaly may be present. The clinical manifestations of LBRF and TBRF are similar, although LBRF is usually associated with a single relapse, whereas multiple relapses are more common with TBRF.

The definitive diagnosis of relapsing fever is established by the demonstration of *Borrelia* organisms in the periph-eral blood of febrile patients. In approximately 70% of cases, spirochetes can be seen in the initial blood smear, and the yield increases with multiple smears [14]. Sero-logic tests are not generally available and, if performed, are of limited diagnostic value because of antigenic varia-tion of strains and the complexity of the relapsing phe-nomenon. Where available, molecular methods are highly effective in detecting and identifying *Borrelia* species [15].

Several antibiotics, including, tetracyclines, penicillin, ampicillin, erythromycin, and chloramphenicol, are known to be effective for treating relapsing fever [10]. TBRF has an overall case-fatality rate of 2% to 5%, but the rate is greater than 20% in infants younger than 1 year of age [9,10].

In some areas of Africa, relapsing fever during preg-nancy is associated with a 30% risk of pregnancy loss and fetal and infant mortality rates of 15% and 44% [12,13]. Common complications of relapsing fever during pregnancy are low birth weight, preterm delivery, sponta-neous abortion, and neonatal death. Most pregnancy and perinatal complications have been reported from sub-Saharan Africa, although there are reports from devel-oped countries as well [12]. Pregnant women showed significantly higher densities of spirochetes than nonpreg-nant women, and a correlation has been seen between density of spirochetes and risk of birth during the attack and risk of complications [16,17].

Maternal-infant transmission of relapsing fever has been reported primarily from sub-Saharan Africa, but cases from developed countries such as the United States and Israel have also been reported [12]. Transplacental transmission in humans has been established and seems to be the most likely explanation for most of the neonatal cases. In many of these neonatal cases, infections after or during the birth could not be definitively excluded, however [12].

The clinical signs of relapsing fever in the newborn are those of neonatal sepsis and are nonspecific—apathy, vomiting, tachypnea, acidosis, and bleeding tendency. An unusually high concentration of *Borrelia* organisms is found in the peripheral blood smears in affected neonates. The overall mortality in this age group is higher (>40%) than in any other age group [9,12].

REFERENCES

[1] A.C. Steere, et al., Lyme arthritis: an epidemic of oligoarticular arthritis in children and adults in three Connecticut communities, Arthritis Rheum. 20 (1977) 7–17.

[2] W. Burgdorfer, et al., Lyme disease: a tick-borne spirochetosis? Science 216 (1982) 1317–1319.

[3] A.C. Steere, et al., The spirochetal etiology of Lyme disease, N. Engl. J. Med. 308 (1983) 733–740.

[4] CDC, Lyme, disease—United States, 2003-2005, MMWR Morb. Mortal. Wkly Rep. 56 (2007) 573–576.

[5] D. Kollmann, S. Dobson, Treponema pallidum, in: J.S. Remington, et al. (Ed.), Infectious Diseases of the Fetus and Newborn Infant, seventh ed., Saunders, Philadelphia, 2010.

[6] R.S. Lane, et al., Isolation of a spirochete from the soft tick, *Ornithodoros coriaceus*: a possible agent of epizootic bovine abortion, Science 230 (1985) 85–87.

[7] J.D. Coghlan, A.D. Bain, Leptospirosis in human pregnancy followed by death of the foetus, BMJ 1 (1969) 228–230.

[8] S. Lindsay, I.W. Luke, Fatal leptospirosis (Weil's disease) in a newborn infant, J. Pediatr. 34 (1949) 90–94.

[9] P. Yagupsky, S. Moses, Neonatal *Borrelia* species infection (relapsing fever), Am. J. Dis. Child. 139 (1985) 74–76.

[10] P.M. Southern, J.P. Sanford, Relapsing fever: a clinical and microbiological review, Medicine 48 (1969) 129–149.

[11] A. Nordstrand, et al., Tickborne relapsing fever diagnosis obscured by malaria, Togo Emerg. Infect. Dis. 13 (2007) 117–123.

[12] C. Larsson, et al., Complications of relapsing fever and transplacental transmission of relapsing-fever borreliosis, J. Infect. Dis. 194 (2006) 1367–1374.

[13] H.T. Dupont, et al., A focus of tick-borne relapsing fever in southern Zaire, Clin. Infect. Dis. 25 (1997) 139–144.

[14] C.T. Le, Tick-borne relapsing fever in children, Pediatrics 66 (1980) 963–966.

[15] B. Wyplosz, et al., Imported tickborne relapsing fever, France, Emerg. Infect. Dis. 11 (2005) 1801–1803.

[16] V.H. Jongen, et al., Tick-borne relapsing fever and pregnancy outcome in rural Tanzania, Acta. Obstet. Gynecol. Scand. 76 (1997) 834–838.

[17] P.W.J. Melkert, et al., Relapsing fever in pregnancy: analysis of high-risk factors, Br. J. Obstet. Gynaecol. 95 (1988) 1070–1072.

[18] R.S. Lane, J. Piesman, W. Burgdorfer, Lyme borreliosis: relation of its causative agent to its vectors and hosts in North America and Europe, Annu. Rev. Entomol. 36 (1991) 587–609.

[19] R.B. Nadelman, et al., Prophylaxis with single-dose doxycycline for the prevention of Lyme disease after an Ixodes scapularis tick bite, N. Engl. J. Med. 345 (2001) 79–84.

[20] J. Piesman, T.N. Mather, R. Sinsky, Duration of tick attachment and *Borrelia burgdorferi* transmission, J. Clin. Microbiol. 25 (1987) 557–558.

[21] J. Piesman, et al., Duration of adult female *Ixodes dammini* attachment and transmission of *Borrelia burgdorferi*, description of a needle aspiration isolation method, J. Infect. Dis. 163 (1991) 895–897.

[22] J. Piesman, Dynamics of *Borrelia burgdorferi* transmission by nymphal *Ixodes dammini* ticks, J. Infect. Dis. 167 (1993) 1082–1085.

[23] R.C. Falco, D. Fish, J. Piesman, Duration of tick bites in a Lyme disease-endemic area, Am. J. Epidemiol. 143 (1996) 187–192.

[24] E.D. Shapiro, et al., A controlled trial of antimicrobial prophylaxis for Lyme disease after deer-tick bites, N. Engl. J. Med. 327 (1992) 1769–1773.

[25] E.D. Shapiro, Doxycycline for tick bites—not for everyone, N. Engl. J. Med. 345 (2001) 133–134.

[26] B. Schwartz, et al., Entomologic and demographic correlates of anti-tick saliva antibody in a prospective study of tick bite subjects in Westchester County, New York, Am. J. Trop. Med. Hyg. 48 (1993) 50–57.

[27] J.P. Hanrahan, et al., Incidence and cumulative frequency of endemic Lyme disease in a community, J. Infect. Dis. 150 (1984) 489–496.

[28] A.C. Steere, et al., Longitudinal assessment of the clinical and epidemiological features of Lyme disease in a defined population, J. Infect. Dis. 154 (1986) 295–300.

[29] C.M. Fraser, et al., Genomic sequence of a Lyme disease spirochaete, *Borrelia burgdorferi*, Nature 390 (1997) 580–586.

[30] S. Bergstrom, et al., In: Molecular and cellular biology of Borrelia burgdorferi sensu lato. J.S. Gray, O. Kahl, R.S. Lane, G. Stanek (Eds.), CABI Publishing, Wallingford, UK, 2002, pp. 47–90.

[31] R.B. Nadelman, G.P. Wormser, Lyme borreliosis, Lancet 352 (1998) 557–565.

[32] M.A. Gerber, et al., Lyme disease in children in southeastern Connecticut. Pediatric Lyme Disease Study Group, N. Engl. J. Med. 335 (1996) 1270–1274.

[33] J.L. Coleman, et al., Plasminogen is required for efficient dissemination of B. burgdorferi in ticks and for enhancement of spirochetemia in mice, Cell 89 (1997) 1111–1119.

[34] J. Coburn, J.M. Leong, J.K. Erban, Integrin alpha IIb beta 3 mediates binding of the Lyme disease agent *Borrelia burgdorferi* to human platelets, Proc. Natl. Acad. Sci. U. S. A. 90 (1993) 7059–7063.

[35] J. Coburn, et al., Integrins alpha(v)beta3 and alpha5beta1 mediate attachment of Lyme disease spirochetes to human cells, Infect. Immun. 66 (1998) 1946–1952.

[36] B.P. Guo, E.L. Brown, D.W. Dorward, Decorin-binding adhesins from *Borrelia burgdorferi*, Mol. Microbiol. 30 (1998) 711–723.

[37] W.S. Probert, B.J. Johnson, Identification of a 47 kDa fibronectin-binding protein expressed by *Borrelia burgdorferi* isolate B31, Mol. Microbiol. 30 (1998) 1003–1015.

[38] G. Seinost, et al., Four clones of *Borrelia burgdorferi sensu stricto* cause invasive infection in humans, Infect. Immun. 67 (1999) 3518–3524.

[39] J.J. Weiss, et al., Identification of quantitative trait loci governing arthritis severity and humoral responses in the murine model of Lyme disease, J. Immunol. 162 (1999) 948–956.

[40] S.W. Barthold, M. de Souza, Exacerbation of Lyme arthritis in beige mice, J. Infect. Dis. 172 (1995) 778–784.

[41] R.R. Mullegger, et al., Differential expression of cytokine mRNA in skin specimens from patients with erythema migrans or acrodermatitis chronica atrophicans, J. Invest. Dermatol. 115 (2000) 1115–1123.

[42] A. Krause, et al., T cell proliferation induced by *Borrelia burgdorferi* in patients with Lyme borreliosis: autologous serum required for optimum stimulation, Arthritis Rheum. 34 (1991) 393–402.

[43] E. Akin, et al., The immunoglobulin (IgG) antibody response to OspA and OspB correlates with severe and prolonged Lyme arthritis and the IgG response to P35 correlates with mild and brief arthritis, Infect. Immun. 67 (1999) 173–181.

[44] D.T. Nardelli, et al., Lyme arthritis: current concepts and a change in paradigm, Clin. Vaccine Immunol. 15 (2008) 21–34.

[45] L. Hu, Lyme arthritis, Infect. Dis. Clin. North Am. 19 (2005) 947–961.

[46] A.R. Pachner, Lyme neuroborreliosis: infection, immunity, and inflammation, Lancet Neurol. 6 (2007) 544–552.

[47] T.A. Rupprecht, et al., The pathogenesis of Lyme neuroborreliosis: from infection to inflammation, Mol. Med. 14 (2008) 205–212.

[48] J.F. Anderson, R.C. Johnson, L.A. Margnarelli, Seasonal prevalence of *Borrelia burgdorferi* in natural populations of white-footed mice, *Peromyscus leucopus*, J. Clin. Microbiol. 25 (1987) 1564–1566.

[49] E.C. Burgess, L.A. Windberg, *Borrelia* sp. infection in coyotes, black-tailed jack rabbits and desert cottontails in southern Texas, J Wildl Dis 25 (1989) 47–51.

[50] E.C. Burgess, *Borrelia burgdorferi* infection in Wisconsin horses and cows, Ann. N. Y. Acad. Sci. 539 (1988) 235–243.

[51] E.C. Burgess, M.D. Wachal, T.D. Cleven, *Borrelia burgdorferi* infection in dairy cows, rodents, and birds from four Wisconsin dairy farms, Vet. Microbiol. 35 (1993) 61–77.

[52] J.M. Gustafson, et al., Intrauterine transmission of *Borrelia burgdorferi* in dogs, Am. J. Vet. Res. 54 (1993) 882–890.

[53] E.C. Burgess, A. Gendron-Fitzpatrick, M. Mattison, Foal mortality associated with natural infection of pregnant mares with *Borrelia burgdorferi*. Proceedings of the 5th International Conference on Equine Infectious Diseases, 1989, pp. 217–220.

[54] R.M. Silver, et al., Fetal outcome in murine Lyme disease, Infect. Immun. 63 (1995) 66–72.

[55] K.D. Moody, S.W. Barthold, Relative infectivity of *Borrelia burgdorferi* in Lewis rats by various routes of inoculation, Am. J. Trop. Med. Hyg. 44 (1991) 135–139.

[56] J.E. Woodrum, J.H. Oliver Jr., Investigation of venereal, transplacental, and contact transmission of the Lyme disease spirochete, *Borrelia burgdorferi*, in Syrian hamsters, J. Parasitol. 85 (1999) 426–430.

[57] T.N. Mather, S.R. Telford III., G.H. Adler, Absence of transplacental transmission of Lyme disease spirochetes from reservoir mice (*Peromyscus leucopus*) to their offspring, J. Infect. Dis. 164 (1991) 564–567.

[58] P.A. Schlesinger, et al., Maternal-fetal transmission of the Lyme disease spirochete, *Borrelia burgdorferi*, Ann. Intern. Med. 103 (1985) 67–68.

[59] E.H. Oppenheimer, J.B. Hardy, Congenital syphilis in the newborn infant: clinical and pathological observations in recent cases, Johns Hopkins Med. J. 129 (1971) 63–82.

[60] A.B. MacDonald, J.L. Benach, W. Burgdorfer, Stillbirth following maternal Lyme disease, N. Y. State. J. Med. 87 (1987) 615–616.

[61] K. Weber, et al., *Borrelia burgdorferi* in a newborn despite oral penicillin for Lyme borreliosis during pregnancy, Pediatr. Infect. Dis. J. 7 (1988) 286–289.

[62] G. Trevisan, G. Stinco, M. Cinco, Neonatal skin lesions due to a spirochetal infection: a case of congenital Lyme borreliosis? Int. J. Dermatol. 36 (1997) 677–680.

[63] M.J. Grandsaerd, Lyme borreliosis as a cause of facial palsy during pregnancy, Eur. J. Obstet. Gynecol. Reprod. Biol. 91 (2000) 99–101.

[64] A.L. Mikkelson, C. Palle, Lyme disease during pregnancy, Acta Obstet. Gynecol. Scand. 6 (1987) 477–478.

[65] R. Schaumann, Facial palsy caused by *Borrelia* infection in a twin pregnancy in an area of nonendemicity, Clin. Infect. Dis. 29 (1999) 955–956.

[66] S.E. Schutzer, C.K. Janniger, R.A. Schwartz, Lyme disease during pregnancy, Cutis 47 (1991) 267–268.

[67] G. Stiernstedt, Lyme borreliosis during pregnancy, Scand. J. Infect. Dis. 71 (1990) 99–100.

[68] R. Figueroa, et al., Confirmation of *Borrelia burgdorferi* spirochetes by polymerase chain reaction in placentas of women with reactive serology for Lyme antibodies, Gynecol. Obstet. Invest. 41 (1996) 240–243.

[69] L.E. Markowitz, et al., Lyme disease during pregnancy, JAMA 255 (1986) 3394–3396.

[70] C.A. Ciesielski, et al., Prospective study of pregnancy outcome in women with Lyme disease. Program and Abstracts of Twenty-Seventh International Conference of Antimicrobial Agents and Chemotherapy., New York, 1987 Abstract 39.

[71] V. Maraspin, et al., Erythema migrans in pregnancy, Wien. Klin. Wochenschr. 111 (1999) 933–940.

[72] C.L. Williams, et al., Lyme disease during pregnancy: a cord blood serosurvey, Ann. N. Y. Acad. Sci. 539 (1988) 504–506.

[73] D. Nadal, et al., Infants born to mothers with antibodies against *Borrelia burgdorferi* at delivery, Eur. J. Pediatr. 148 (1989) 426–427.

[74] M.A. Gerber, E.L. Zalneraitis, Childhood neurologic disorders and Lyme disease during pregnancy, Pediatr. Neurol. 11 (1994) 41–43.

[75] B. Strobino, S. Abid, M. Gewitz, Maternal Lyme disease and congenital heart disease: a case-control study in an endemic area, Am. J. Obstet. Gynecol. 180 (1999) 711–716.

[76] B.A. Strobino, et al., Lyme disease and pregnancy outcome: a prospective study of two thousand prenatal patients, Am. J. Obstet. Gynecol. 169 (1993) 367–374.

[77] C.L. Williams, et al., Maternal Lyme disease and congenital malformations: a cord blood serosurvey in endemic and control areas, Paediatr. Perinat. Epidemiol. 9 (1995) 320–330.

[78] C.J. Lischer, C.M. Leutenegger, B.H. Lutz, Diagnosis of Lyme disease in two cows by the detection of *Borrelia burgdorferi* DNA, Vet. Rec. 146 (2000) 497–499.

[79] B.L. Schmidt, et al., Detection of *Borrelia burgdorferi* DNA by polymerase chain reaction in the urine and breast milk of patients with Lyme borreliosis, Diagn. Microbiol. Infect. Dis. 21 (1995) 121–128.

[80] E.D. Shapiro, M.A. Gerber, Lyme disease, Clin. Infect. Dis. 31 (2000) 533–542.

[81] A.C. Steere, et al., Vaccination against Lyme disease with recombinant *Borrelia burgdorferi* outer-surface lipoprotein A with adjuvant, N. Engl. J. Med. 339 (1998) 209–216.

[82] H.M. Feder Jr., et al., A critical appraisal of "chronic Lyme disease", N. Engl. J. Med. 357 (2007) 1422–1430.

[83] M. Klempner, et al., Two controlled trials of antibiotic treatment in patients with persistent symptoms and a history of Lyme disease, N. Engl. J. Med. 345 (2001) 85–92.

[84] L.B. Krupp, et al., Study and treatment of post Lyme disease (STOP-LD): a randomized double masked clinical trial, Neurology 60 (2003) 1923–1930.

[85] B. Fallon, et al., A randomized, placebo-controlled trial of repeated IV antibiotic therapy for Lyme encephalopathy, Neurology 70 (2008) 992–1003.

[86] J.J. Halperin, Prolonged Lyme disease treatment: enough is enough, Neurology 70 (2008) 986–987.

[87] S. Hatcher, B. Arroll, Assessment and management of medically unexplained symptoms, BMJ 336 (2008) 1124–1128.

[88] E.J. Masters, et al., STARI, or Masters disease: Lone Star tick-vectored Lyme-like illness, Infect. Dis. Clin. North Am. 22 (2008) 361–376.

[89] G.P. Wormser, et al., Prospective clinical evaluation of patients from Missouri and New York with erythema migrans-like skin lesions, Clin. Infect. Dis. 41 (2005) 958–965.

[90] Case definitions for public health surveillance, MMWR Morb. Mortal. Wkly Rep. 39 (1990) 1–43.

[91] Centers for Disease Control and Prevention, Recommendations for test performance and interpretation from the Second National Conference on Serologic Diagnosis of Lyme Disease, MMWR Morb. Mortal. Wkly Rep. 44 (1995) 590–591.

[92] Food and Drug Administration, FDA Public Health Advisory: assays for antibodies to *Borrelia burgdorferi*, Limitations, use, and interpretation for supporting a clinical diagnosis of Lyme disease. July 7, 1997.

[93] G.P. Wormser, et al., Use of a novel technique of cutaneous lavage for diagnosis of Lyme disease associated with erythema migrans, JAMA 268 (1992) 1311–1313.

[94] F.W. Hyde, et al., Detection of antigens in urine of mice and humans infected with *Borrelia burgdorferi*, etiologic agent of Lyme disease, J. Clin. Microbiol. 27 (1989) 58–61.

[95] U.R. Hengge, et al., Lyme borreliosis, Lancet Infect. Dis. 3 (2003) 489–500.

[96] M.S. Klempner, et al., Intralaboratory reliability of serologic and urine testing for Lyme disease, Am. J. Med. 110 (2001) 217–219.

[97] J. Bunikis, A.G. Barbour, Laboratory testing for suspected Lyme disease, Med. Clin. North Am. 86 (2002) 311–340.

[98] J.E. Craft, R.L. Grodzicki, A.C. Steere, Antibody response in Lyme disease: evaluation of diagnostic tests, J. Infect. Dis. 149 (1984) 789–795.

[99] E. Hilton, et al., Temporal study of immunoglobulin M seroreactivity to *Borrelia burgdorferi* in patients treated for Lyme borreliosis, J. Clin. Microbiol. 35 (1997) 774–776.

[100] H.M. Feder Jr., et al., Persistence of serum antibodies to *Borrelia burgdorferi* in patients treated for Lyme disease, Clin. Infect. Dis. 15 (1992) 788–793.

[101] R.A. Kalish, et al., Evaluation of study patients with Lyme disease, 10–20-year follow-up, J. Infect. Dis. 183 (2001) 453–460.

[102] Bacterial Zoonoses Branch, Centers for Disease Control and Prevention, Evaluation of serologic tests for Lyme disease: report of a national evaluation, Lyme Dis Surveill. Summ. 1 (1991) 1–8.

[103] L.L. Bakken, et al., Interlaboratory comparison of test results for detection of Lyme disease by 516 participants in the Wisconsin State Laboratory of Hygiene/College of American Pathologists Proficiency Testing Program, J. Clin. Microbiol. 35 (1997) 537–543.

[104] B.S. Schwartz, et al., Antibody testing in Lyme disease: a comparison of results in four laboratories, JAMA 262 (1989) 3431–3434.

[105] L.L. Bakken, et al., Performance of 45 laboratories participating in a proficiency testing program for Lyme disease serology, JAMA 268 (1992) 891–895.

[106] S.W. Luger, E. Krauss, Serologic tests for Lyme disease: interlaboratory variability, Arch. Intern. Med. 150 (1990) 761–776.

[107] E.G. Seltzer, E.D. Shapiro, Misdiagnosis of Lyme disease: when not to order serologic tests, Pediatr. Infect. Dis. J. 15 (1996) 762–763.

[108] P. Tugwell, et al., Laboratory evaluation in the diagnosis of Lyme disease, Ann. Intern. Med. 127 (1997) 1109–1123.

[109] G. Nichol, et al., Test-treatment strategies for patients suspected of having Lyme disease: a cost-effectiveness analysis, Ann. Intern. Med. 128 (1998) 37–48.

[110] A.C. Steere, et al., Evaluation of the intrathecal antibody response to *Borrelia burgdorferi* as a diagnostic test for Lyme neuroborreliosis, J. Infect. Dis. 161 (1990) 1203–1209.

[111] L.A. Bracero, et al., Prevalence of seropositivity to the Lyme disease spirochete during pregnancy in an epidemic area: a preliminary report, J. Matern. Fetal. Invest. 2 (1992) 265–268.

[112] G.P. Wormser, et al., The clinical assessment, treatment, and prevention of Lyme disease, human granulocytic anaplasmosis, and babesiosis: clinical practice guidelines by the Infectious Diseases Society of America, Clin. Infect. Dis. 43 (2006) 1089–1134.

[113] J.J. Halperin, et al., Practice parameter: treatment of nervous system Lyme disease, Neurology 69 (2007) 91–102.

[114] J. Oksi, et al., Duration of antibiotic treatment in disseminated Lyme borreliosis: a double-blind, randomized, placebo-controlled, multicenter clinical study, Eur. J. Clin. Microbiol. Infect. Dis. 26 (2007) 571–581.

[115] G.P. Wormser, et al., Duration of antibiotic therapy for early Lyme disease: a randomized, double-blind, placebo-controlled trial, Ann. Intern. Med. 138 (2003) 697–704.

[116] D.J. Elliott, S.C. Eppes, J.D. Klein, Teratogen update: Lyme disease, Teratology 64 (2001) 276–281.

[117] E.D. Shapiro, Long-term outcomes of persons with Lyme disease, Vector Borne Zoonotic. Dis. 2 (2002) 279–281.

[118] D.M. Gross, et al., Identification of LFA-1 as a candidate autoantigen in treatment-resistant Lyme arthritis, Science 281 (1998) 703–706.

TUBERCULOSIS

Jeffrey R. Starke ☉ Andrea T. Cruz

CHAPTER OUTLINE

Terminology   577
Mycobacteriology   578
Epidemiology   579
Tuberculosis in Pregnancy   580
    Pathogenesis   580
    Effect of Pregnancy on Tuberculosis   581
    Effect of Tuberculosis on Pregnancy   582
    Screening for Tuberculosis in Pregnancy   582
Congenital Tuberculosis   583
    Tuberculosis in the Mother   583
    Routes of Transmission   584
    Criteria for Diagnosis of Congenital Tuberculosis   585
    Clinical Features and Diagnosis of Congenital Tuberculosis   585
Treatment of Tuberculosis   586
    General Principles   588
    Pregnant Women   588

Neonates and Infants   590
Following the Infant on Therapy   590
Prognosis   590
Vaccination against Tuberculosis—Bacille Calmette-Guérin   591
    History and Development of Bacille Calmette-Guérin Vaccines   591
    Vaccine Preparation and Administration   591
    Adverse Reactions to Bacille Calmette-Guérin Vaccination   592
    Effect of Bacille Calmette-Guérin Vaccination on Tuberculin Skin Test Results   592
    Effectiveness of Bacille Calmette-Guérin Vaccines   593
Management of a Neonate Born to a Mother with a Positive Tuberculin Skin Test   593
Management of Neonates after Postnatal Exposure   594
Conclusion   595

Tuberculosis is a classic familial disease [1]. The household is the main setting throughout the world for the person-to-person spread of *Mycobacterium tuberculosis*. With the resurgence of tuberculosis in many industrialized nations, issues concerning pregnant women and their children have been reexamined by practitioners of tuberculosis control.

Before 1985, tuberculosis in pregnant women and newborns had become uncommon in the United States. Although specific statistics concerning tuberculosis in pregnancy are not reported, the increase in total tuberculosis cases in the late 1980s and 1990s and the shift in numbers to young adults and children suggested that tuberculosis in pregnancy may become a more prevalent problem [2,3]. In the United States, 6% of cases occur in persons younger than 15 years of age, and almost 40% occur in persons 15 to 44 years old [4,5]. Tuberculosis disproportionately affects minority urban populations because they have very high tuberculosis case rates, a greater relative shift in cases to adults of childbearing age, and generally less access to prenatal care and screening for disease and infection caused by *M. tuberculosis*.

The influence of pregnancy on the occurrence and prognosis of tuberculosis has been discussed and debated for centuries. At various times, pregnancy has been thought to improve, worsen, or have no effect on the prognosis of tuberculosis. This controversy has lost much of its importance since the advent of effective antituberculosis chemotherapy. The greatest areas of debate at present concern the use of chemotherapy to prevent the progression of *M. tuberculosis* infection to tuberculosis during pregnancy and the postpartum period and

treatment of exposed infants to prevent the development of serious tuberculosis [6].

TERMINOLOGY

A practical approach to tuberculosis terminology is to follow the natural history of the disease, which can be divided into three stages: exposure, infection, and disease [7]. *Exposure* implies that the patient has had recent (<3 months) and significant contact with an adult with suspected or confirmed contagious pulmonary tuberculosis. An infant born into a family in which an adult has active tuberculosis would be in the exposure stage. In this stage, the infant's tuberculin skin test is negative, the chest radiograph result is normal, and the infant is free of signs and symptoms of tuberculosis. It is impossible to know whether a young child in the exposure stage is truly infected with *M. tuberculosis* because the development of delayed-type hypersensitivity to a tuberculin skin test may take 3 months after the organisms have been inhaled.

Infection with *M. tuberculosis* is present if an individual has a positive tuberculin skin test or interferon-γ release assay result, but lacks signs or symptoms of tuberculosis. In this stage, findings on the chest radiograph either are normal or reveal only granuloma or calcification in the lung parenchyma or regional lymph nodes. The purpose of treating *M. tuberculosis* infection is to prevent future disease. In newborns, the progression from infection to disease can occur very rapidly—within several weeks to months. Of untreated infants with a positive tuberculin skin test, 40% progress to disease.

Tuberculosis *disease* occurs if signs or symptoms or radiographic manifestations caused by *M. tuberculosis* become apparent. Because 25% to 35% of children with tuberculosis have extrapulmonary involvement, a thorough physical examination, in addition to a high-quality chest radiograph, is essential to rule out disease [7]. Genitourinary tuberculosis in women often causes only subtle symptoms until it is far advanced. Initially, 10% to 20% of immunocompetent adults and children with the disease have a negative tuberculin skin test result, usually because of immunosuppression from tuberculosis itself. The rate of negative skin test results with disease from *M. tuberculosis* is much higher in newborns and small infants, however, especially if they have life-threatening forms of tuberculosis, such as disseminated (miliary) disease or meningitis.

MYCOBACTERIOLOGY

Mycobacteria are nonmotile, non–spore-forming pleomorphic, weakly gram-positive rods that are 1 to 5 μm long, usually slender, and slightly curved. *M. tuberculosis* may appear beaded or clumped. The cell wall constituents of mycobacteria determine their most striking biologic properties. The cell wall is composed of 20% to 60% lipids bound to proteins and carbohydrates. These and other properties make mycobacteria more resistant than most other bacteria to light, alkali, acid, and bactericidal activity of antibodies. Growth of *M. tuberculosis* is slow, with a generation time of 12 to 24 hours on solid media.

The hallmark of mycobacteria is acid-fastness, the capacity to form stable mycolate complexes with certain aryl methane dyes that are not removed even by rinsing with 95% ethanol plus hydrochloric acid. The cells appear red when stained with carbol fuchsin (Ziehl-Neelsen or Kinyoun stains) or purple when stained with crystal violet or exhibit yellow-green fluorescence under ultraviolet light when stained with Truant auramine-rhodamine stain. Truant auramine-rhodamine stain is considered the most sensitive stain, especially when small numbers of organisms are present. Approximately 10,000 cells/mm³ must be present in a sample for them to be seen in an acid-fast stained smear.

Identification of mycobacteria depends on their staining properties and their biochemical, metabolic, and growth characteristics. *M. tuberculosis* also can be distinguished from nontuberculous mycobacteria by high-power liquid chromatography. Mycobacteria are obligate aerobes with simple growth requirements. *M. tuberculosis* can grow in classic media whose essential ingredients are egg yolk and glycerin (Löwenstein-Jensen or Dorset media) or simple synthetic media (Middlebrook 7H10 agar, Tween-albumin). Isolation on solid media takes 2 to 6 weeks, followed by another 2 to 4 weeks for drug-susceptibility testing.

More rapid isolation (7 to 21 days) can be achieved using synthetic liquid medium in an automated radiometric system; the most common is BACTEC (Becton-Dickinson, Towson, MD). A specimen is inoculated into a bottle of medium containing carbon-14–labeled palmitic acid as a substrate. As mycobacteria metabolize the

palmitic acid, carbon dioxide-14 accumulates in the head space of the bottle, where radioactivity can be measured. Because bottles are often analyzed in series by repetitive needle aspiration in an automated, single-needle system, cross-contamination leading to a false-positive culture can occur. Drug susceptibility testing can be performed on the same system using bottles with antimicrobial agents added to the medium. In this radiometric system, identification and drug-susceptibility testing often can be completed in 2 to 3 weeks, depending on the concentration of organisms in the patient sample.

More recently, a novel system has been developed wherein the culture and susceptibility are performed simultaneously in liquid media. This system—microscopic-observed drug susceptibility (MODS)—can provide results in 7 days [8,9]. MODS methodology also has been effective for children, showing increased yield over traditional culture techniques (87% versus 55%) and decreased time to positive cultures (10 days versus 24 days) [10].

It is often difficult to isolate *M. tuberculosis* from infants and toddlers with tuberculosis [11,12]. Infants and children with pulmonary tuberculosis rarely produce sputum, the usual culture material for adults. The preferred source of culture for children is a gastric aspirate, performed early in the morning before the stomach has been emptied of the respiratory secretions swallowed overnight. For older children, the culture yield from gastric aspirates obtained on 3 consecutive mornings is 20% to 40% [13]. The yield from infants is usually higher, up to 75% [14]. For many infants with congenital pulmonary tuberculosis, *M. tuberculosis* can be cultured from a tracheal aspirate because of the numerous organisms in the lungs. Induced sputum cultures, obtained by nasopharyngeal suctioning after administration of albuterol, nebulized oxygen, and chest percussion, are safe and effective in infants 1 month old. The yield for one induced sputum culture is similar to the yield of three gastric aspirate specimens, specimens obtained by induced sputum collection are more likely to be acid-fast positive, and the specimens may be obtained more readily in the outpatient setting [15].

Several types of nucleic acid amplification have been developed to detect *M. tuberculosis* in patient samples. The main form of nucleic acid amplification studied in children with tuberculosis is polymerase chain reaction (PCR), which uses specific DNA sequences as markers for microorganisms. Various PCR techniques, most using the mycobacterial insertion element IS6110 as the DNA marker for *M. tuberculosis* complex organisms, have a sensitivity and specificity of greater than 90% compared with sputum culture for detecting pulmonary tuberculosis in adults. Test performance varies, however, even among reference laboratories. The test is expensive and requires fairly sophisticated equipment and scrupulous technique to avoid cross-contamination of specimens.

Use of PCR in childhood tuberculosis has been limited. Compared with a clinical diagnosis of pulmonary tuberculosis in children, sensitivity of PCR ranges from 25% to 83%, and specificity ranges from 80% to 100% [16]. PCR detection rates are higher for specimens positive for acid-fast bacilli smear (100% versus 76%) [17,18]. PCR of gastric aspirates may be positive in a recently infected child even when the chest radiograph is normal, showing the occasional arbitrariness of the distinction between *M. tuberculosis* infection and disease in children. PCR may have a useful but limited role in evaluating children for tuberculosis. A negative PCR never eliminates tuberculosis as a diagnostic possibility, and a positive result does not confirm it. The major use of PCR would be in evaluating children with significant pulmonary disease when the diagnosis is not established readily on clinical or epidemiologic grounds.

PCR may be particularly helpful in evaluating immunocompromised children with pulmonary disease, especially children with human immunodeficiency virus (HIV) infection, although published reports of its performance in such children are lacking. PCR also may aid in confirming the diagnosis of extrapulmonary tuberculosis, although few data have been published. In one study, PCR of cerebrospinal fluid in children with suspected tuberculous meningitis showed a sensitivity of 76% and a specificity of 89% [19]. Finally, PCR assays are now being designed to amplify regions of the bacterial genome where mutations are known to confer resistance to commonly used medications; this has the potential to provide drug-resistance profiles even on patients whose cultures remain negative [20]. There is concern, however, that genotypes and phenotypes may not overlap entirely [21]. No information has been published concerning the accuracy of PCR or other techniques of nucleic acid amplification in samples from pregnant women or neonates with congenital or postnatally acquired tuberculosis.

Relatedness of strains of *M. tuberculosis* was determined in the past by analysis of bacteriophages, a cumbersome and difficult task. A newer technique, restriction fragment length polymorphism analysis of mycobacterial DNA, has become an accurate and powerful tool for determining strain relatedness [22,23]. It is used frequently in some communities and may help determine if an infant with tuberculosis has true congenital infection or was infected by another source.

EPIDEMIOLOGY

Tuberculosis is the leading infectious disease in the world [24]. It is estimated that 2 billion persons are infected with *M. tuberculosis*, 9 million develop tuberculosis disease annually, and 2 million die with tuberculosis each year [24]. In the developing world, the World Health Organization (WHO) estimates that there are 1.3 million cases of tuberculosis and 400,000 tuberculosis-related deaths annually among children younger than 15 years of age. In most developing countries, the highest rates of tuberculosis occur among young adults. Although much attention has been given more recently to the growing number of children orphaned in developing countries by their parents' deaths from HIV-related illnesses, many orphans also are being created by tuberculosis.

In the United States from 1953-1984, the incidence of tuberculosis disease declined an average of 5% per year. From 1985-1992, there was a 20% increase in total cases of tuberculosis in the United States and a 40% increase in tuberculosis cases among children [25]. Most experts cite four major factors contributing to this increase: (1) the coepidemic of HIV infection [26], which is the strongest

risk factor known for development of tuberculosis disease in an adult infected with *M. tuberculosis* [27]; (2) the increase in immigration of people to the United States from countries with a high prevalence of tuberculosis, enlarging the pool of infected individuals [28,29]; (3) the increased transmission of *M. tuberculosis* in congregate settings, such as jails, prisons, hospitals, nursing homes, and homeless shelters; and (4) the general decline in tuberculosis-related public health services and access to medical care for the indigent in many communities [30]. In 2007, the approximately 13,300 cases of tuberculosis in the United States represented a 50% decline from the peak number of cases in 1992 [31]. The average annual percent decline has slowed, however, from 7.3% per year in 1993-2000 to 3.8% per year in 2000-2007 [31].

In the early 20th century in the United States, when tuberculosis was more prevalent, the risk of becoming infected with *M. tuberculosis* was high across the entire population. Currently, tuberculosis has retreated into fairly well-defined pockets of high-risk individuals, such as foreign-born persons from high-prevalence countries, persons who travel to high-prevalence countries, inmates of correctional institutions, illicit drug users, unprotected health care workers who care for high-risk patients, migrant families, homeless persons, and anyone likely to encounter people with contagious tuberculosis. One must distinguish the risk factors for becoming infected with *M. tuberculosis* from factors that increase the likelihood that an infected individual will develop disease. Age, immunocompromised status, and recent infection with *M. tuberculosis* are the major risk factors for progression of infection to disease.

Although tuberculosis occurs throughout the United States, cases are disproportionately reported from large urban areas. Cities with populations exceeding 250,000 account for only 18% of the U.S. population, but almost 50% of tuberculosis cases in the United States. Among U.S.-born persons, tuberculosis disproportionately affects African Americans, whose rates of tuberculosis disease remain 8.5 times the rates seen in whites born in the United States [31,32].

The number of tuberculosis cases in the United States is increasing among foreign-born persons from countries with a high prevalence of tuberculosis. The percentage of total cases of tuberculosis in the United States that occurs in foreign-born individuals increased from 22% in 1986 to 59% in 2007, and foreign-born individuals have a 9.7 times higher rate of tuberculosis than individuals born in the United States [31]. In addition, 85% of cases of multidrug-resistant (MDR) tuberculosis are seen in foreign-born individuals [31]. In previous estimates, two thirds of foreign-born individuals with tuberculosis were younger than 35 years when entering the United States, and in many cases, their disease could have been prevented if they had been identified as infected after immigration and given appropriate treatment for *M. tuberculosis* infection.

Until very recently, new immigrants to the United States older than 15 years of age were required to have a chest radiograph but no tuberculin skin test to detect asymptomatic infection; children younger than 15 years old received no tuberculosis testing as part of immigration

[33]. This policy ignored a huge reservoir of future tuberculosis cases. Studies have estimated that 30% to 50% of the almost 1 million annual new immigrants to the United States are infected with *M. tuberculosis* [29]. Foreign-born women and adolescents of childbearing age should be one group targeted for appropriate tuberculosis screening and prevention [34]. There are data suggesting that the current U.S. Centers for Disease Control and Prevention (CDC) and American Thoracic Society (ATS) policies on targeted screening of immigrants [35] would fail to prevent most cases [36]. A more effective strategy to decrease tuberculosis in the United States may be to expand treatment programs in countries from which immigrants originate [37].

Another factor that has had a great impact on tuberculosis case rates in the United States has been the epidemic of HIV infection [27]. The proportion of women with HIV infection is increasing; the population demographic in which HIV is most rapidly spreading is persons of reproductive age (13 to 44 years old), who accounted for 73% of newly diagnosed cases in 2006 [38]. Because the risk factors for HIV infection intersect with risk factors for tuberculosis, the number of coinfected women is expected to increase [39–41]. Approximately 16% of tuberculosis patients 25 to 44 years old in the United States are also HIV-seropositive [42]. In most locales experiencing increases in tuberculosis cases, the demographic groups with the greatest tuberculosis morbidity rates are the same as those with high morbidity rates from HIV infection. HIV-infected persons with a reactive tuberculin skin test develop tuberculosis at a rate of 5% to 10% per year compared with a historical average of 5% to 10% for the lifetime of an immunocompetent adult. There is controversy concerning the infectiousness of adults with HIV-associated pulmonary tuberculosis. Although some studies have indicated dually infected adults are as likely as non–HIV-infected adults with tuberculosis to infect others, some studies have shown less transmission from HIV-infected adults [43].

The current epidemiology of tuberculosis in pregnancy is unknown. From 1966-1972, the incidence of tuberculosis during pregnancy at New York Lying-In Hospital ranged from 0.6% to 1% [44]. During this time, 3.2% of the patients with culture-proven pulmonary tuberculosis were first diagnosed during pregnancy, a rate equal to that of nonpregnant women of comparable age. Only two series of pregnant women with tuberculosis have been reported from the United States in the past 2 decades [45,46], and two series have been reported from the United Kingdom [47,48]. In the latter two series, diagnosis was delayed in many women with extrapulmonary manifestations of tuberculosis. Increased risk of tuberculosis is most striking for foreign-born women, who have high rates of tuberculosis infection, and poor minority women.

In the United States, almost 40% of tuberculosis cases in minority women occur in women younger than 35 years. Approximately 80% of cases of tuberculosis infection and disease among children in the United States occur in minority populations [25,49]. Most of these cases occur after exposure to an ill family member. In all populations, whether the disease incidence is high or low,

tuberculosis infection and disease tend to occur in clusters, often centered on the close or extended family, meaning that minority newborns are at greatly increased risk of congenital and postnatally acquired tuberculosis infection and disease.

TUBERCULOSIS IN PREGNANCY
PATHOGENESIS

The pathogenesis of tuberculosis infection and disease during pregnancy is similar to the pathogenesis for non-pregnant individuals [50,51]. The usual portal of entry for *M. tuberculosis* is the lung through inhalation of infected droplet nuclei discharged by an infectious individual. The inoculum of organisms necessary to establish infection is unknown, but is probably less than 10 [52]. When tubercle bacilli are deposited in the lung, they multiply in the nonimmune host for several weeks. This uninhibited replication usually produces no symptoms, but a patient may experience low-grade fever, cough, or mild pleuritic pain.

Shortly after infection, some organisms are carried from the initial pulmonary focus within macrophages to the regional lymph nodes [53]. From there, organisms enter lymphatic and blood vessels and disseminate throughout the body; the genitalia, the endometrium, and, if the woman is pregnant, the placenta may be seeded [54]. By 1 to 3 months after infection, the host usually develops cell-mediated immunity and hypersensitivity to the tubercle bacillus, reflected by the development of a reactive tuberculin skin test [55]. As immunity develops, the primary infection in the lung and foci in other organs begin to heal through a combination of resolution, fibrosis, and calcification [56]. Although walling-off of these foci occurs, viable tubercle bacilli persist. If the host later becomes immunosuppressed, these dormant bacilli may become active, leading to "reactivation" tuberculosis [57].

There are two major ways that tuberculosis infection in the mother can lead to infection of the fetus in utero. If dissemination of organisms through the blood and lymphatic channels occurs during pregnancy, the placenta may be infected directly. This can occur either during the asymptomatic dissemination that is part of the mother's initial infection or during pulmonary, miliary, or disseminated tuberculosis disease in the mother [58–72]. Miliary tuberculosis in women can arise from a long-standing dormant infection, but more often complicates a recent infection (Fig. 18–1). Infection with *M. tuberculosis* that occurs during pregnancy, as opposed to dormant infection that occurred before the pregnancy, probably poses a greater risk to the fetus. This is a major reason why pregnant women with new onset of *M. tuberculosis* infection usually should be treated carefully during the pregnancy; delay could result in disease in the mother, the infant, or both.

The second mechanism by which a fetus can become infected with *M. tuberculosis* is directly from established genitourinary tuberculosis in the mother. Genital tuberculosis is most likely to start around the time of menarche and can have a very long and relatively asymptomatic course. The fallopian tubes most often are involved

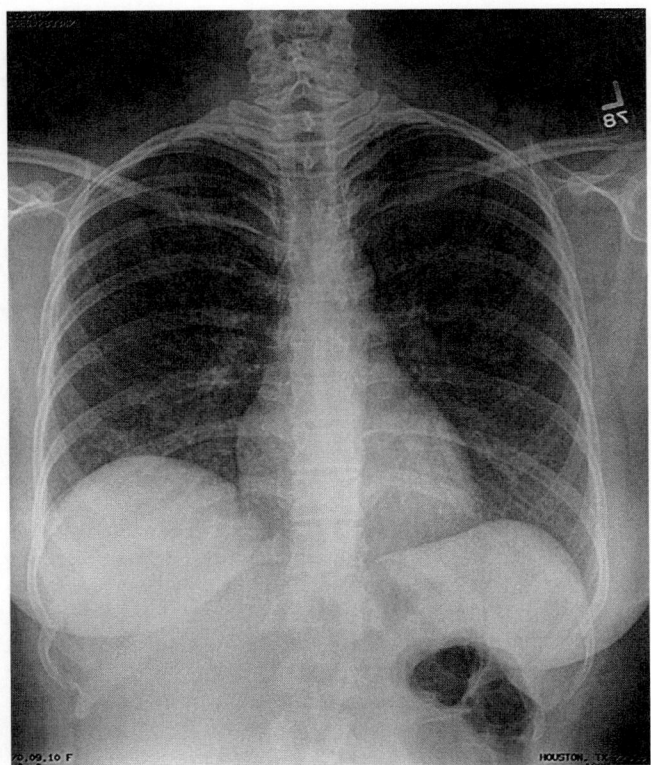

FIGURE 18–1 Chest radiograph from the mother of the infant shown in Figure 18–2. This radiograph reveals early miliary tuberculosis.

(in 90% to 100% of women), followed by the uterus (50% to 60%), ovaries (20% to 30%), and cervix (5% to 15%) [44,54]. Sterility often is the presenting complaint of tuberculosis endometritis, which diminishes the likelihood of congenital tuberculosis occurring [73,74]. One series from India reported that 28% of women seeking therapy for infertility had genital tuberculosis [75]. Findings on hysterosalpingography of beaded or non-patent fallopian tubes or irregular uterine filling defects may suggest the diagnosis [75a]. If infection of the placenta occurs, it results more frequently from disseminated tuberculosis in the mother than from a local endometritis. Tuberculous endometritis can lead to congenital infection of the newborn, however [54,76–79]. Tuberculosis in the mother as a complication of in vitro fertilization has been described [80].

EFFECT OF PREGNANCY ON TUBERCULOSIS

Over the past 2 millennia, medical opinions regarding the interaction of pregnancy and tuberculosis have varied considerably. Hippocrates believed that pregnancy had a beneficial effect on tuberculosis, a view that persisted virtually unchallenged well into the 19th century [81]. In 1850, Grisolle reported 24 cases of tuberculosis that developed during pregnancy [82]. In all patients, the progression of tuberculosis during pregnancy was more severe than that usually seen in nonpregnant women of the same age. Shortly thereafter, several other articles were published that implied that pregnancy had a deleterious effect on tuberculosis. This view gained so much

support that by the early 20th century, the practice of induced abortion to deal with the consequences of tuberculosis during pregnancy became widely accepted.

The opinion that pregnancy had a deleterious effect on tuberculosis predominated until the late 1940s. In 1943, Cohen [83] detected no increased rate of progression of tuberculosis among 100 pregnant women with abnormal chest radiograph results. In 1953, Hedvall [82] presented a comprehensive review of published studies concerning tuberculosis in pregnancy. He cited studies totaling more than 1000 cases that reported deleterious effects of pregnancy on tuberculosis. He discovered a nearly equal number of reported cases, however, in which a neutral or favorable relationship between pregnancy and tuberculosis was observed. In his own study of 250 pregnant women with abnormal chest radiograph results thought to be due to tuberculosis, he noted that 9% improved, 7% worsened, and 84% remained unchanged during pregnancy. During the first postpartum year, 9% improved, 15% worsened, and 76% were stable. Cromie [84] noted that 31 of 101 pregnant women with quiescent tuberculosis experienced relapse after delivery. Of the 31 relapses, 20 occurred in the 1st postpartum year.

Several other investigators observed the higher risk of relapse during the puerperium. Several theories were proposed to explain this phenomenon, including postpartum descent of the diaphragm, nutritional stress of pregnancy and lactation, insufficient sleep for the new mother, rapid hormonal changes, and depression in immunity in late pregnancy and postpartum. A similar number of other studies failed to support an increased risk of progression of tuberculosis in the postpartum period, however [85–89].

Cohen's study [85] failed to show an increase in activity of tuberculosis during pregnancy or any postpartum interval. Rosenbach and Gangemi [87] and Cohen and colleagues [85] showed that only 9% to 13% of women with long-standing tuberculosis had progression of disease during the pregnancy or first postpartum year, a rate thought to be comparable to that in nonpregnant women. Few of these studies had adequate control populations. From all the studies reported, it became clear that the anatomic extent of disease, the radiographic pattern, and the susceptibility of the individual patient to tuberculosis were more important than pregnancy itself in determining the course and prognosis of the pregnant woman with tuberculosis.

The controversy concerning the effect of pregnancy or the postpartum period on tuberculosis has lost most of its importance with the advent of effective chemotherapy [90,91]. With adequate treatment, pregnant women with tuberculosis have the same excellent prognosis as nonpregnant women. Several studies documented no adverse effects of pregnancy, birth, postpartum period, or lactation on the course of tuberculosis in women receiving chemotherapy [92,93].

Most studies have dealt with the risk of reactivation of tuberculosis among women with abnormal chest radiograph results but no evidence of active tuberculous lesions. It is unclear if women with asymptomatic *M. tuberculosis* infection but no radiographic findings are at increased risk of developing tuberculosis during pregnancy or the postpartum period. In 1961, Pridie and Stradling [94] found that the incidence of pulmonary tuberculosis among pregnant women was the same as in the nonpregnant female population of the area. From 1966-1972, Schaefer and associates [44] found that the annual pulmonary tuberculosis case rate among pregnant women in New York Lying-In Hospital was 18 to 29 per 100,000 population, comparable to the incidence of tuberculosis during the same period in women of childbearing age in all of New York City. Although no definitive study has been reported, it seems unlikely that progression from asymptomatic *M. tuberculosis* infection to tuberculosis disease is accelerated during pregnancy or the postpartum period.

EFFECT OF TUBERCULOSIS ON PREGNANCY

In the prechemotherapy era, active tuberculosis at an advanced stage carried a poor prognosis for the mother and the child. Schaefer and associates [44] reported that the infant and maternal mortality rates from untreated tuberculosis were 30% to 40%. Mortality rates for infants with congenital tuberculosis remain greater than 20% in some more recent series [95], and all-cause mortality is threefold higher in infants born to HIV-infected mothers with tuberculosis [96]. The incidence of congenital tuberculosis parallels the incidence in childbearing women, and increased rates of tuberculosis in infants have been noted in many regions [97].

One study from Norway showed a higher incidence of toxemia, postpartum hemorrhage, and difficult labor in mothers with untreated tuberculosis compared with control subjects [98]. The incidence of miscarriage was almost 10 times higher in the tuberculous mothers, but there was no significant difference in the rate of congenital malformations for children born to mothers with and without tuberculosis. Another study reported an incidence of prematurity ranging from 23% to 64%, depending on the severity of tuberculosis in the mother, for infants born to untreated mothers in a tuberculosis sanitarium [99].

One series compared the clinical courses of 111 pregnant women with treated pulmonary tuberculosis with controls who either had tuberculosis and were not pregnant or were pregnant and did not have tuberculosis. There were no differences in gestational duration, preterm labor, or other pregnancy complications between cases and controls if the women received adequate therapy [100]. Another series reported that maternal extrapulmonary tuberculosis, aside from cervical lymphadenopathy, was associated with higher rates of prenatal hospitalization and lower infant birth weights [101]. Most experts now believe, however, that with proper treatment of a pregnant woman with tuberculosis, the prognosis of the pregnancy should not be affected adversely by the presence of tuberculosis. Because of the excellent prognosis for the mother and the child, the recommendation for therapeutic abortion has been abandoned.

SCREENING FOR TUBERCULOSIS IN PREGNANCY

For all pregnant women, the history obtained at an early prenatal visit should include questions about a previously positive tuberculin skin test or interferon-γ release assay

result, previous treatment for *M. tuberculosis* infection or disease, current symptoms compatible with tuberculosis, and known exposure to other adults with the disease [35,102]. Membership in a high-risk group is a sufficient reason for a tuberculin skin test. For many high-risk women, prenatal or peripartum care represents their only contact with the health care system, and the opportunity to test them for tuberculosis infection or disease should not be lost. Some experts believe that all pregnant women should receive a tuberculin skin test [103]. Most experts believe, however, that only women with specific risk factors for *M. tuberculosis* infection or disease should be tested [35]. Women coinfected with HIV and *M. tuberculosis* may show no reaction to a tuberculin skin test. Pregnant women with high risk for or with known HIV infection should have a thorough investigation for tuberculosis.

Changes in the interpretation of the Mantoux tuberculin skin test have been promoted by the CDC, ATS, and American Academy of Pediatrics [35]. The rationale for using different sizes of induration as representing a positive result in different populations has been discussed thoroughly in many publications. The current recommendation is that for individuals at the highest risk of having *M. tuberculosis* infection progress to tuberculosis—contacts to adults with infectious tuberculosis, patients with an abnormal chest radiograph or clinical evidence of tuberculosis, or persons with HIV infection or other condition associated with an immunocompromised state—a Mantoux tuberculin skin test reaction of at least 5 mm is classified as positive, indicating infection with *M. tuberculosis*. For other high-risk groups, a reaction of at least 10 mm is positive. For all other persons deemed at low risk for tuberculosis, a reaction of at least 15 mm is positive.

This classification scheme depends on the ability and willingness of the family and health care provider to develop a thorough epidemiologic history for tuberculosis exposures and risk. It also depends on accurate interpretation of the skin test. One study implied that pediatricians tend to underread induration in tuberculin skin tests [104], and there is much variability in skin test interpretation by patients and health care workers [105].

There have been no studies to verify whether the classification scheme for the Mantoux tuberculin skin test is valid in pregnant women, but there is no reason to suspect otherwise [106,107]. The effect of pregnancy on tuberculin hypersensitivity as measured by the tuberculin skin test is controversial [108]. Some studies have shown a decrease in in vitro lymphocyte reactivity to purified protein derivative during pregnancy [109]. In vivo studies using patients as their own controls have shown no effect of pregnancy on cutaneous delayed hypersensitivity to tuberculin [110,111]. Most experts believe the tuberculin skin test by the Mantoux technique is valid throughout pregnancy. There is no evidence that the tuberculin skin test has adverse effects on the pregnant mother or fetus or that skin testing reactivates quiescent foci of tuberculosis infection [112].

Whole-blood interferon-γ release assays have been introduced in an attempt to address some of the limitations of the Mantoux tuberculin skin test. Interferon-γ release assay measures interferon-γ response after challenge with antigens that are not shared with antigens in *Mycobacterium avium* complex and the bacille Calmette-Guérin (BCG) vaccine. The advantages are that the test should theoretically be more specific to tuberculosis than the tuberculin skin test; it requires only one health care encounter; and because the test is done in vitro, there is no risk of the boosting phenomenon [113]. No controlled studies to date have evaluated the efficacy of interferon-γ release assays in pregnancy or in infants.

One of the most difficult problems in the interaction of tuberculosis and pregnancy is deciding whether a pregnant woman with *M. tuberculosis* infection should receive immediate treatment, or whether the treatment should be postponed until after the infant is delivered [114]. Not all infected individuals have the same chance of developing tuberculosis during a short period of time. Individuals who were infected remotely (>2 years previously) have a low chance of developing tuberculosis during a given 9-month period. Individuals who have been infected more recently, particularly if their infection is discovered during a contact investigation of an adult with active tuberculosis, are at much higher risk; about half of the lifetime risk of progression of infection to disease occurs during the first 1 to 2 years after infection. Other vulnerable adults, particularly adults coinfected with HIV, also are at greatly increased risk of having progression of infection to disease.

Treatment for tuberculosis infection should be initiated during pregnancy if the woman likely has been infected recently (especially in the setting of a contact investigation of a recently diagnosed case) or she is at increased risk of rapid development of tuberculosis. Although isoniazid (INH) is not thought to be teratogenic, some experts recommend waiting until the second trimester of pregnancy to begin treatment. Patient adherence to INH treatment for tuberculosis infection seems to be very low if the initiation of treatment is delayed until after the child is delivered. The reason for this low adherence is unclear, but several problems include the perception of nonimportance because a treatment delay of many months is allowed, transfer of care from one segment of the health care system to another, and, perhaps, the lack of reinforcement by health care professionals concerning the importance of the treatment.

One retrospective series indicated that women who were newly diagnosed with tuberculosis infection were more likely to be referred to specialty clinics and start therapy, but completion rates for the cohort as a whole were less than 10% [115]. Although screening and treatment of high-risk pregnant women may seem to be an effective strategy to prevent future cases of tuberculosis, it has not yet been shown that this strategy is successful in the U.S. health care system [116].

Routine chest radiography is not advisable as a screening tool for pregnant women because the prevalence of tuberculosis disease remains fairly low [117,118]. With appropriate shielding, pregnant women with positive tuberculin skin test results should have chest radiographs to rule out tuberculosis [119]. In addition, a thorough review of systems and physical examination should be done to exclude extrapulmonary tuberculosis.

CONGENITAL TUBERCULOSIS
TUBERCULOSIS IN THE MOTHER

The clinical manifestations of tuberculosis in a pregnant woman generally are the same as the manifestations in nonpregnant individuals. The most important determinants of the clinical presentation are the extent and anatomic location of disease. In one series of 27 pregnant and postpartum women with pulmonary tuberculosis, the most common clinical findings were cough (74%), weight loss (41%), fever (30%), malaise and fatigue (30%), and hemoptysis (19%) [46]. Almost 20% of patients had no significant symptoms; other studies also have found less significant symptoms in pregnant women with tuberculosis [45]. The tuberculin skin test result was positive in 26 of 27 patients. The diagnosis was established in all cases by culture of sputum for *M. tuberculosis*. Sixteen of the patients in this series had drug-resistant tuberculosis; their clinical course was marked by more extensive pulmonary involvement, a higher incidence of pulmonary complications, longer sputum conversion times, and a higher incidence of death.

In other series, 5% to 10% of pregnant women with tuberculosis have had extrapulmonary disease, a rate comparable with nonpregnant women of the same age [45]. Delay in diagnosis has been associated with extrapulmonary forms of tuberculosis or nonspecific symptoms [48]. In some regions of the developing world, tuberculosis (often with HIV coinfection) accounts for 25% of nonobstetric maternal mortality, and mothers coinfected with HIV and tuberculosis have a twofold increased risk of postpartum death compared with mothers without coinfection [120]. In one series of pregnant women coinfected with HIV and tuberculosis, 29% of postpartum cases were diagnosed in the first 2 weeks after delivery [96], indicating that these women likely had subclinical disease late in pregnancy.

Although the female genital tract may be the portal of entry for a primary tuberculosis infection, more often infection at this site originates by continuity from an adjacent focus of disease or by blood-borne seeding of the fallopian tubes [73]. Progression of disease usually is by descent in the genital tract. Mucosal ulceration within the fallopian tube develops, and pelvic adhesions occur frequently. Many patients are asymptomatic. The most common complaints are sterility and menstrual irregularity with menorrhagia or amenorrhea. These findings greatly diminish the likelihood of congenital tuberculosis. Other, less frequent signs and symptoms include lower abdominal pain and tenderness, weight loss, fever, and night sweats. Diagnosis in a nonpregnant woman is usually established by culture and histologic examination of tissue recovered after uterine curettage. The highest recovery rates of *M. tuberculosis* are obtained from scrapings obtained just before or during menstruation.

Tuberculosis mastitis is very rare in the United States, but occurs almost exclusively in women of childbearing age [121–123]. The most common finding is a single breast mass, with or without a draining sinus. Nipple retraction and peau d'orange skin changes suggestive of carcinoma also may be present. The ipsilateral axillary lymph nodes usually are enlarged. Diagnosis is confirmed by biopsy of the mass or axillary node and culture of the tissue for *M. tuberculosis*. Radiographic findings are often nonspecific [124]. Transmission of *M. tuberculosis* to the infant through breast milk is exceedingly rare, if it occurs at all.

ROUTES OF TRANSMISSION

Tuberculosis in the neonate can be either truly congenital (i.e., acquired in utero) or truly neonatal (i.e., acquired early in life from the mother, members of the family, friends, or caretakers). Each of these two kinds of perinatal tuberculosis may be subdivided. *Congenital tuberculosis* can be acquired in three ways: (1) from the infected placenta via the umbilical vein, (2) by inhalation of infected amniotic fluid, and (3) by ingestion of infected amniotic fluid. *Neonatal tuberculosis* can be acquired in four ways: (1) by inhalation of infected droplets, (2) by ingestion of infected droplets, (3) by ingestion of infected milk (theoretical), and (4) by contamination of traumatized skin or mucous membranes.

It is not always possible to ascertain the route of infection in a particular neonate, and with effective chemotherapy at hand, it is not essential for the care of the infant. It is important, however, to try to identify the source of infection so that the person infecting the infant can be treated, and further transmission can be prevented [125].

The potential modes of inoculation of the fetus or newborn with *M. tuberculosis* from the mother are shown in Table 18–1 [126]. Infection of the fetus through the umbilical cord has been rare, with less than 350 cases reported in the English-language literature [127]. Mothers of these infants frequently have tuberculous pleural effusion, meningitis, or disseminated disease during pregnancy or soon after [61,64,66,69,128]. In some series of congenital tuberculosis, fewer than 50% of the mothers were known to have tuberculosis at the time of delivery and beginning of symptoms in the newborn [129,130]. In most of these cases, diagnosis of the child led to the discovery of the mother's tuberculosis.

The intensity of lymphohematogenous spread during pregnancy is one of the factors that determines if congenital tuberculosis will occur. Hematogenous dissemination in the mother leads to infection of the placenta with subsequent transmission of organisms to the fetus. *M. tuberculosis* has been shown in the decidua, amnion, and chorionic villi of the placenta. The organisms also have been shown to reach the placenta through direct extension from a tuberculous salpingeal tube. Even

massive involvement of the placenta with tuberculosis does not always give rise to congenital tuberculosis, however [131]. It is unclear if the fetus can be infected directly from the mother's bloodstream without a caseous lesion forming first in the placenta, although this phenomenon has been shown in experimental animal models [132].

In hematogenous congenital tuberculosis, the organisms reach the fetus through the umbilical vein. If bacilli infect the liver, a primary focus develops with involvement of the periportal lymph nodes. The bacilli can pass through the liver, however, into the main circulation through the patent foramen ovale. Alternatively, they can pass through the right ventricle into the pulmonary circulation, leading to a primary focus in the lung. The organisms in the lung often remain dormant until after birth when oxygenation and circulation increase significantly, leading to growth of organisms and pulmonary tuberculosis in young infants. In many children with congenital tuberculosis, multiple lesions occur throughout the body; it is impossible to determine if they represent multiple primary foci or if some occur secondary to primary lesions in the lung or liver. The only lesion of the neonate that is unquestionably associated with congenital infection is a primary complex in the liver with caseating hepatic granulomas [127,133].

Congenital infection of the infant also can occur through aspiration or ingestion of infected amniotic fluid [134]. If the caseous lesion in the placenta ruptures directly into the amniotic cavity, the fetus can inhale or ingest the bacilli. Inhalation or ingestion of infected amniotic fluid is the most likely cause of congenital tuberculosis if the infant has multiple primary foci in the lung, gut, or middle ear [135]. In congenital tuberculosis caused by aspiration, the primary complex can be in the liver, the lung, or both organs.

The pathology of congenital tuberculosis in the fetus and newborn usually shows the predisposition to dissemination ensured by the modes of transmission, particularly through the umbilical vein. The liver and lungs are the primary involved organs with bone marrow, bone, gastrointestinal tract, adrenal glands, spleen, kidney, abdominal lymph nodes, and skin also involved frequently [136,137]. The histologic patterns of involvement are similar to the patterns in adults; tubercles and granulomas are common. Central nervous system involvement occurs in fewer than 50% of cases [129,137]. In most more recent series, the mortality rate of congenital tuberculosis has been close to 50%, primarily because of the failure to suspect the correct diagnosis. Most fatal cases are diagnosed at autopsy [129,130].

Postnatal acquisition of *M. tuberculosis* through airborne inoculation is the most common route of infection of the neonate [138–140]. It may be impossible to differentiate postnatal infection from prenatal acquisition on clinical grounds alone [141]. Any adult in the neonate's environment can be a source of airborne tuberculosis, including health care workers [142,143]. Of infants with untreated *M. tuberculosis* infection, 40% develop tuberculosis disease within 1 to 2 years. There are few data concerning the time of onset of tuberculosis when the infection is acquired at or shortly after birth. It is estimated that 9% to 15% of mothers with tuberculosis transmit infection

TABLE 18–1   Modes of Inoculation of the Fetus or Newborn with *Mycobacterium tuberculosis*

Maternal Focus	Mode of Spread
Placentitis	Hematogenous (umbilical vessel)
Amniotic fluid	Aspiration
Cervicitis	Direct contact
Pneumonitis	Airborne (postnatal)

to their infants in the postpartum period. Higher transmission rates are seen in mothers who are untreated or diagnosed late in pregnancy [97]. In one series of 48 infants exposed postnatally to mothers with pulmonary tuberculosis in the prechemotherapy era, 21 became infected; of infants who became ill, signs such as fever, tachypnea, weight loss, and hepatosplenomegaly developed in 4 to 8 weeks [144]. Because newborns infected with the organism are at extremely high risk of developing severe forms of disease, investigation of an adult with tuberculosis whose household contacts include a pregnant woman or newborn should be considered a public health emergency. In addition, all adults in contact with an infant suspected to have *M. tuberculosis* infection or disease should undergo a thorough investigation for disease.

The skin and mucous membranes are rare portals of entry for *M. tuberculosis* in neonates. Infection through the skin has been mentioned several times in association with lesions of the head and face, very likely related to minor traumatic lesions being infected by kissing. Primary lesions of the mucous membranes of the mouth also have been recognized, although usually in infants beyond the newborn period. In both of these situations, the primary lesion was insignificant, but the enlarged regional lymph nodes called attention to the problem [145].

A previously well-known form of skin and mucous membrane infection was tuberculosis of the male genitalia after circumcision in the years when it was customary for the individual performing the circumcision to suck the blood around the incision. This procedure was obviously dangerous if that individual happened to have bacilli in the sputum. The primary focus of inoculation on the penis was often inconspicuous, but within 1 to 4 weeks ulceration, suppuration, and bilateral inguinal lymphadenopathy would develop. At first firm and nontender, the nodes might later break down with sinus formation to the exterior. In his review of circumcision tuberculosis, Holt [146] described a case with extensive ulceration of the penis and scrotum, greatly swollen lymph nodes, a generalized rash resembling varicella, hepatosplenomegaly, fever, cough, rales, and a positive tuberculin test, with recovery of tubercle bacilli from sputum and penile discharge. Of the 41 patients described by Holt [146], 16 died and 6 recovered, with the outcome of the others unknown.

CRITERIA FOR DIAGNOSIS OF CONGENITAL TUBERCULOSIS

In 1935, Beitzke [133] suggested the following criteria for diagnosis of congenital tuberculosis in a thoughtful, detailed, and often-quoted review of the reported cases up to that time:

1. Tuberculosis in the child must be firmly established.
2. A primary complex in the liver is proof of congenital tuberculosis because this complex could arise only through perfusion of the liver with tubercle bacilli contained in umbilical cord blood.
3. If a primary complex is lacking in the liver, tuberculosis can be considered to be congenital only if

tuberculous lesions are present in a fetus or in a newborn only a few days old, *or*, in an older infant, extrauterine infection can be excluded with certainty—that is, if the infant was removed from the tuberculous mother at birth to a tuberculosis-free environment.

Cantwell and coworkers [127], based on a review of cases of congenital tuberculosis published before and after 1980, proposed a modification of Beitzke's criteria. The infant must have proven tuberculous lesions and at least one of the following: (1) lesions in the first week of life, (2) a primary hepatic complex or caseating hepatic granulomas, (3) tuberculosis infection of the placenta or maternal genital tract or both, or (4) exclusion of postnatal transmission by a thorough contact investigation. Although Beitzke's criteria are fully met by many of the approximately 350 reported cases of congenital tuberculosis, in other cases it is impossible to ascertain whether infection was transmitted in utero or was acquired during the early days or weeks of life. In many cases of true congenital tuberculosis, the mother was not known to have active tuberculosis.

Two articles contain tables with detailed information on 26 cases and 15 cases [129,130]. In only 10 of the 26 cases was tuberculosis diagnosed in the mother antepartum, although it became apparent in another 15 after diagnosis in the infant [129]. Five of the 26 mothers died of tuberculosis, an indirect confirmation of the fact that the diagnosis was made very late. In the series of 15 cases, 7 mothers were thought to be well at the time of delivery, but all 15 were subsequently found either to have had pleural effusion antepartum (four cases) or to have developed endometrial, miliary, or meningeal tuberculosis postpartum [130].

CLINICAL FEATURES AND DIAGNOSIS OF CONGENITAL TUBERCULOSIS

The clinical manifestations of tuberculosis in the fetus and newborn vary in relation to the site and size of the caseous lesions. Symptoms may be present at birth, but more commonly begin by the 2nd or 3rd week of life. The most frequent signs or symptoms of true congenital tuberculosis are listed in Table 18–2 [127,129,147–177]. Most infants have an abnormal chest radiograph, with about half having a miliary pattern [178]. Some infants with a normal chest radiograph early in the course develop profound radiographic abnormalities as the disease progresses (Fig. 18–2). The most common abnormalities are adenopathy and parenchymal infiltrates. Occasionally, pulmonary involvement progresses very rapidly, leading to cavitation [179–181]. Tuberculosis of the middle ear in children with congenital tuberculosis has often been described [129,139,179,182–186]. The eustachian tube in newborns permits ready access to infected pharyngeal fluids or vomitus. Multiple perforations or total destruction of the tympanic membrane, otorrhea, enlarged cervical lymph nodes, and facial paralysis all are possible sequelae.

The clinical presentation of tuberculosis in a newborn is similar to bacterial sepsis [169–171] and congenital infections with syphilis and cytomegalovirus [14].

TABLE 18–2   Most Frequent Signs and Symptoms of Congenital Tuberculosis

Symptom or Sign	Frequency (%)
Hepatosplenomegaly	76
Respiratory distress	72
Fever	48
Lymphadenopathy	38
Abdominal distention	24
Lethargy or irritability	21
Ear discharge	17
Papular skin lesions	14
Vomiting, apnea, cyanosis, jaundice, seizures, petechiae	<10 each

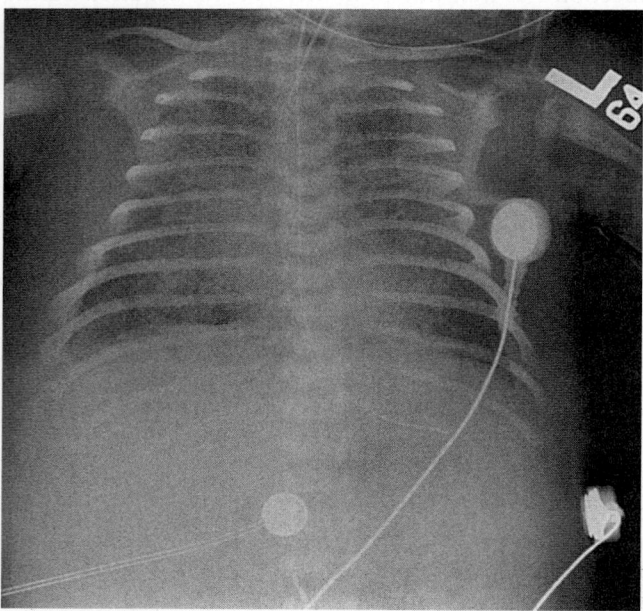

FIGURE 18–2   Chest radiograph from a 1-month-old infant with congenital tuberculosis.

Abnormalities of liver function are common [172,174]. The diagnosis of congenital tuberculosis should be suspected in any infant with signs and symptoms of sepsis or viral infection who does not respond to vigorous antibiotic therapy and whose evaluation for other congenital infections is unrevealing. Suspicion also should be high if the mother has or has had tuberculosis, or if she is in a high-risk group for tuberculosis. The importance of obtaining an adequate history for the presence of risk factors for tuberculosis in the mother cannot be overemphasized. Suspicion should increase if the mother has had unexplained pneumonia, bronchitis, pleural effusion, meningeal disease, or endometritis during, shortly before, or even after pregnancy.

Evaluation of both parents and other family members can yield important clues about the presence of tuberculosis within the family. One study screened adult caregivers of children with suspected tuberculosis by chest radiograph and found that 15% of the screened adults had previously undetected pulmonary tuberculosis [187].

The timely diagnosis of congenital or neonatal tuberculosis is often difficult [125,188,189]. Whenever possible, the placenta should be examined and cultured for *M. tuberculosis*. The tuberculin skin test result is negative initially, although it may become positive after 1 to 3 months of treatment. There are no controlled trial data on the utility of interferon-γ release assays in infants. Two case reports in three infants with negative skin tests whose mothers had tuberculosis showed that the infants had positive interferon-γ release assays, facilitating appropriate therapy [190,191].

The diagnosis must be established by finding acid-fast bacilli in body fluids or tissue or by culturing *M. tuberculosis*. A positive acid-fast bacilli smear of an early morning gastric aspirate obtained from a newborn should be considered indicative of tuberculosis, although false-positive results can occur [13]. Direct acid-fast bacilli smears from middle ear fluid, bone marrow, tracheal aspirate, or biopsy tissue can be useful and should be obtained more often [174,192]. Hageman and colleagues [129] found positive cultures for *M. tuberculosis* in 10 of 12 gastric aspirates, 3 of 3 liver biopsy specimens, 3 of 3 lymph node biopsy specimens, and 2 of 4 bone marrow aspirations from children with congenital tuberculosis. Open lung biopsy also has been used to establish the diagnosis [193]. The cerebrospinal fluid should be examined and cultured, although the yield for isolating *M. tuberculosis* is less than 20%, and meningitis occurs in only one third of cases of congenital tuberculosis. There are no data addressing the utility of PCR for infants with tuberculous meningitis.

TREATMENT OF TUBERCULOSIS

The drugs used most commonly to treat *M. tuberculosis* infection and disease, their dosage forms, and doses are listed in Table 18–3 [194]. Detailed discussion of the pharmacokinetics of each drug is beyond the scope of this chapter. No published study has examined in detail the pharmacokinetics of drugs used as antituberculosis agents in premature or term neonates [195].

INH is the mainstay of treatment for tuberculosis infection and disease in infants, children, and adults. It is inexpensive, highly effective in preventing the multiplication of tubercle bacilli, of low molecular weight and readily diffusible to all tissues in the body, and relatively nontoxic to children. It can be administered orally or intramuscularly. When INH is taken orally, high plasma, sputum, and cerebrospinal fluid levels are reached within a few hours and persist at least 6 to 8 hours. Because of the slow multiplication of *M. tuberculosis*, the total daily dose can be given at one time.

The principal toxic effects of INH are peripheral neuritis and hepatitis. Peripheral neuritis, resulting from competitive inhibition of pyridoxine, is almost unknown in North American children because cow's milk (and formula) and meat are the main dietary sources of pyridoxine. In some well-nourished children, serum

TABLE 18–3   Antituberculosis Drugs in Children

Drugs	Dosage Forms	Daily Dose (mg/kg)	Twice-Weekly Dose (mg/kg per dose)	Maximum Dose
Isoniazid	Scored tablets: 100, 300 mg	10-15	20-30	Daily: 300 mg
	Syrup: 10 mg/mL			Twice weekly: 900 mg
Rifampin	Capsules: 150, 300 mg	10-20	10-20	600 mg
	Syrup: formulated in syrup from capsules			
Pyrazinamide	Scored tablets: 500 mg	30-40	50	2 g
Streptomycin	Vials: 1, 4 g	20-40 (IM)	20-40 (IM)	1 g
Ethambutol	Scored tablets: 100, 400 mg	20	50	2.5 g

IM, intramuscular.

pyridoxine concentrations are mildly depressed by INH, but clinical signs are not apparent. For most children, it is not necessary to use supplementary pyridoxine. In pregnant women, HIV-infected children and adolescents, teenagers whose diets may be inadequate, children from ethnic groups with a low milk and meat intake, and breast-fed infants, pyridoxine supplementation (25 to 50 mg/day) is important. Hepatotoxicity from INH is rare in children, increases in frequency with age, and is not preventable with pyridoxine supplementation. Monitoring serum aspartate aminotransferase and serum alanine aminotransferase sometimes reveals transient increases during treatment with INH, but the levels usually return spontaneously to normal without interruption of treatment. Liver enzyme abnormalities in adolescents receiving INH likewise are common and usually disappear spontaneously, but severe hepatitis can occur. Although neonates usually tolerate INH well, some experts recommend routine biochemical monitoring in the first several months of therapy.

The usual dosage of INH in children is 10 to 15 mg/kg daily (maximum dose 300 mg) or 20 to 30 mg/kg (maximum dose 900 mg) two or three times weekly (called intermittent). INH is available in scored tablets of 100 mg and 300 mg. A syrup of INH in sorbitol (10 mg/mL) seems to be satisfactory; however, it is unstable at room temperature and should be kept cool. Many children develop significant gastrointestinal intolerance (nausea, vomiting, diarrhea) while taking the INH suspension, but neonates and infants tolerate the lower required volume of suspension well. Changing from daily to intermittent therapy in young children should be carefully considered, however, because the incremental increase in medication volume may cause emesis. If tablets are used, they are easily crushed in a dessert spoon and given with some soft food such as mashed banana, thawed undiluted frozen orange juice, or another palatable medium. The crushed tablets should not be added to the nursing bottle or offered in milk or water because they would be ingested only partially.

Rifampin (RIF) is a semisynthetic drug derived from *Streptomyces mediterranei.* The drug is absorbed readily from the gastrointestinal tract in the fasting state. Excretion mainly is through the biliary tract; however, effective levels are achieved in the kidneys and urine. In many patients receiving RIF treatment, the tears, saliva, urine, and stool turn orange as a result of a harmless metabolite, and the patient and parents always must be warned of this in advance. RIF can be made into a suspension easily for use in children. RIF is very well tolerated by neonates and infants. The incidences of hepatitis, leukopenia, and thrombocytopenia are extremely low. RIF should be used alone only when treating *M. tuberculosis* infection caused by an INH-resistant organism. If one uses INH, 20 mg/kg, and RIF, 10 to 20 mg/kg (maximum daily dose 600 mg), there is an appreciable incidence of hepatotoxicity. When using the two together, one should approximate dosages of INH, 10 mg/kg, and RIF, 10 to 20 mg/kg.

Pyrazinamide (PZA) contributes to the killing of *M. tuberculosis,* particularly at a low pH such as that within macrophages. The exact mechanism of action of PZA is controversial. PZA has no effect on extracellular tubercle bacilli in vitro, but contributes to the killing of intracellular bacilli. Primary resistance is very rare except that *Mycobacterium bovis* is intrinsically resistant. The drug diffuses readily into all areas, including the cerebrospinal fluid. The usual pediatric daily dose is 30 to 40 mg/kg (maximum daily dose 2 g) or 50 mg/kg intermittently. The optimal dose for infants and children has not been established firmly; however, young children (<5 years old) have lower serum concentrations of PZA than older children given the same per-kilogram dose [196]. The adult dose is tolerated well by infants and children, results in high cerebrospinal fluid concentrations, and is effective in therapy trials for active tuberculosis in children. PZA seems to exert its maximum effect during the first 2 months of therapy. Hepatotoxicity can occur at high doses, but is rare at the usual dose. PZA routinely causes an increase in the serum uric acid concentration by inhibiting its excretion through the kidneys. Toxic reactions in adults include flushing, cutaneous hypersensitivity, arthralgia, and overt gout; however, the considerable experience with this drug in children in Latin American countries, Hong Kong, and the United States has revealed few problems.

Ethambutol (EMB) has been used for many years as a companion drug for INH in adults. The usual pediatric oral dose is 20 mg/kg/day or 50 mg/kg intermittently (maximum dose 2.5 g). At this dose, the drug primarily is bacteriostatic, its major role being to prevent emergence of resistance to other drugs. At doses greater than 30 mg/kg/day or 50 mg/kg given intermittently, EMB has some bactericidal action. At these higher doses, optic neuritis or red-green color blindness has occurred in some adults. The incidence of ophthalmologic toxicity in children is extremely low; this may be due in part to children having lower serum levels of EMB than adults who receive the same dose per kilogram [196,197]. EMB is safe in children at recommended doses and is recommended for children of all ages by the WHO [198]. EMB is used frequently and safely in children with life-threatening forms of tuberculosis or with drug-resistant tuberculosis.

Streptomycin (STM) is a valuable drug used in conjunction with INH and RIF in life-threatening forms of tuberculosis. It is bactericidal and tolerated well by children in the usual dose of 20 to 40 mg/kg/day intramuscularly up to 1 g. Usually, STM can be discontinued within 1 to 3 months if clinical improvement is definite, whereas the other two or three drugs are continued with oral administration. Other aminoglycosides, such as amikacin, have broader therapeutic windows and do not show cross-resistance in STM-resistant strains of *M. tuberculosis*.

GENERAL PRINCIPLES

The tubercle bacillus can be killed only during replication, which occurs among organisms that are active metabolically. In one model, bacilli in a host exist in different populations [7]. They are active metabolically and replicate freely where oxygen tension is high and the pH is neutral or alkaline. Environmental conditions for growth are best within cavities, leading to a large bacterial population. Older children with pulmonary tuberculosis and patients of all ages with only extrapulmonary tuberculosis are infected with a much smaller number of tubercle bacilli because the cavitary population is not present. Neonates with congenital tuberculosis tend to have a large burden of organisms at diagnosis, however.

Naturally occurring drug-resistant mutant organisms occur within large populations of tubercle bacilli even before chemotherapy is started. All known genetic loci for drug resistance in *M. tuberculosis* are located on the chromosome; no plasmid-mediated resistance is known. The rate of resistance within populations of organisms is related to the rate of mutations at these loci. Although a large population of bacilli as a whole may be considered drug-susceptible, a subpopulation of drug-resistant organisms occurs at a fairly predictable rate. The mean frequency of these drug-resistant mutations is about 10^{-6}, but varies among drugs: STM, 10^{-5}; INH, 10^{-6}; and RIF, 10^{-7} [199]. A cavity containing 10^9 tubercle bacilli has thousands of single drug-resistant mutant organisms, whereas a closed caseous lesion contains few, if any, resistant mutants.

The population size of tubercle bacilli within a patient determines the appropriate therapy. For patients with a large bacterial population (adults with cavities or extensive infiltrates), many single drug-resistant mutants are present, and at least two antituberculosis drugs must be used. Conversely, for patients with *M. tuberculosis* infection but no disease, the bacterial population is very small (about 10^3 to 10^4 organisms), drug-resistant mutants are rare, and a single drug can be used. Older children with pulmonary tuberculosis and patients of all ages with

extrapulmonary tuberculosis have medium-sized populations in which drug-resistant mutants may or may not be present. Generally, these patients should be treated with at least two drugs. Neonates and infants with tuberculosis disease have large mycobacterial populations, and several drugs are required to effect a cure.

PREGNANT WOMEN

The only drug with well-documented efficacy against *M. tuberculosis* infection in pregnant women is INH. Infants and children tolerate INH very well, and adverse reactions are rare. Adverse reactions are more common in adults. Of young adults taking INH, 7% to 20% have an asymptomatic increase in serum liver transaminase levels; 1% to 2% have symptomatic hepatitis, which is reversible if the medication is stopped immediately [200]. For most young adults, monitoring for hepatitis is done clinically. Routine or periodic evaluation of serum liver enzyme tests is reserved for adults with underlying liver disease or adults taking other potentially hepatotoxic drugs.

Many experts recommend obtaining baseline aspartate aminotransferase, bilirubin, alkaline phosphatase, creatinine, and platelet count [201], and some experts think all pregnant women taking INH should have routine biochemical monitoring for hepatitis. Serum liver enzyme elevations of three to four times normal are common and do not necessitate discontinuation of the drug. There is no evidence that giving INH to a pregnant woman adversely affects the liver of the fetus. The other important adverse reaction of INH is peripheral neuritis caused by inhibition of pyridoxine metabolism. Pyridoxine (25 to 50 mg daily) should be given to pregnant women and breast-feeding infants because breast milk has low concentrations of pyridoxine, even if the mother is receiving vitamin supplements [202].

The current recommendation of the CDC is to treat adults and children infected with *M. tuberculosis* with INH for 9 months [201]. The medication usually is taken daily under self-supervision. If poor patient adherence is likely and resources are available, INH can be given twice weekly using directly observed therapy [203]. Directly observed therapy requires that a health care worker, often from the local health department, observe the patient take antituberculosis medications. Generally, directly observed therapy should be used for all patients with tuberculosis disease because of the difficulty in predicting patient adherence and the consequences of poor adherence (relapse and development of drug resistance). Directly observed therapy is often used for high-risk newborns with tuberculosis exposure or infants with *M. tuberculosis* infection.

For adult patients who cannot take INH for treatment of *M. tuberculosis* infection because of side effects of the medication or because they are infected with an INH-resistant but RIF-susceptible strain of *M. tuberculosis*, the treatment of choice for *M. tuberculosis* infection is RIF for 4 months, which also can be given daily or twice a week under directly observed therapy [204]. If the mother is known to be infected with a strain of tuberculosis that is resistant to INH and RIF (MDR tuberculosis), an expert should be consulted for the management of the mother and the child after delivery [205].

Although treatment of active tuberculosis during pregnancy is unquestioned, the treatment of a pregnant woman who has asymptomatic *M. tuberculosis* infection is more controversial. Some clinicians prefer to delay therapy until after delivery because pregnancy does not seem to increase the risk of developing active tuberculosis. Others believe that because recent infection can be accompanied by hematogenous spread to the placenta, it is preferable to treat without delay or to wait until the second trimester to start chemotherapy. Some reports suggest that the risk of INH-associated hepatitis and death is higher in women than in men [206] and that women in the postpartum period are slightly more vulnerable to INH hepatotoxicity [207]. These authors suggest that it might be prudent to avoid INH during the postpartum period or at least to monitor postpartum women taking INH within 3 months of delivery with frequent examinations and laboratory studies [200]. The possible increased risk of INH hepatotoxicity must be weighed against the risk of developing active tuberculosis and the consequences to the mother and the infant if active tuberculosis develops.

The indications for treatment and the basic principles of management for the pregnant woman with tuberculosis disease are no different from those in nonpregnant patients. The recommendations for which drugs to use and how long to give them are slightly different, however, mostly because of possible effects of several of the drugs on the developing fetus.

The currently recommended treatment for drug-susceptible pulmonary tuberculosis in the United States in nonpregnant individuals is 6 months of INH and RIF, supplemented during the first 2 months with PZA and EMB [201,208]. With any of the regimens, the drugs usually are given every day for the first 2 weeks to 2 months; then they can be given daily or intermittently (under directly observed therapy) for the remainder of therapy with equal effectiveness and rates of adverse reactions [209].

Untreated tuberculosis represents a far greater risk to a woman and her fetus than appropriate treatment of the disease [91,210–214]. Extensive experience with the use of INH in pregnancy has been reported. Although it crosses the placenta, it is not teratogenic even when given during the first 4 months of gestation [215]. EMB also seems to be safe during pregnancy. In 650 cases in which pregnant women were treated with EMB, no evidence of fetal malformations, including eye abnormalities, was found [112,216–218].

The action of RIF to inhibit DNA-dependent RNA polymerase combined with its ability to cross the placental barrier has created some concern about its use in pregnancy [219]. Only 3% of 446 fetuses exposed in utero to RIF had abnormalities, however, compared with 2% for EMB and 1% for INH [112]. The noted abnormalities included limb reductions, central nervous system abnormalities, and hypoprothrombinemia. Hemorrhagic disease of the newborn also has been described after the use of RIF in the mother. The incidence of abnormalities in fetuses not exposed to antituberculosis

medications ranges from 1% to 6%. Generally, the powerful antituberculosis effect of RIF outweighs concern about its effect on the fetus. Nonpregnant women receiving RIF should receive contraception counseling because receiving RIF can impair the efficacy of oral contraceptives, leading to unintended pregnancy in a tuberculous woman [220].

Several antituberculosis drugs generally are not used in pregnant women because of possible toxicity to the fetus [221–223]. STM has variable passage across the placental barrier. Its use in pregnancy is now limited by the availability of better drugs and its effect on the fetus [224–226]. In a review of 206 infants exposed in utero to STM, 34 (17%) had significant eighth cranial nerve damage; abnormalities ranged from mild vestibular damage to profound bilateral deafness [112]. The deleterious effects of STM are independent of the critical periods earlier in embryogenesis, and it is potentially hazardous throughout gestation. It is assumed that capreomycin, kanamycin, and amikacin, other aminoglycosides with antituberculosis activity, could have the same toxic potential as STM. One review of intravenous gentamicin and oral neomycin did not show teratogenicity, however, in a population-based cohort of pregnant women in Hungary [227].

Little is known about the specific effects of PZA on the fetus. Current ATS guidelines recommend avoiding PZA during pregnancy; this strategy would increase length of therapy to 9 months [201]. Although there are no data, an increasing number of experts are using PZA during pregnancy with no reported adverse reactions, and WHO guidelines do not recommend PZA avoidance in pregnancy [228]. Nonspecific teratogenic effects have been attributed to ethionamide [229]. The central nervous system effects of cycloserine and the gastrointestinal effects of para-aminosalicylic acid in adults make their use in pregnancy undesirable.

Fluoroquinolone use is not currently recommended by the ATS during pregnancy because there is concern for arthropathy, and one Danish study showed a higher rate of bone malformations in the offspring of women who received fluoroquinolones in the first trimester [230]. For adults with MDR tuberculosis, fluoroquinolones may be essential components of the therapeutic regimen, however, and risk-benefit analysis must be considered carefully. Fluoroquinolone use is not recommended for breast-feeding mothers [201]; however, there have been no reports of arthropathy in children under these conditions. Numerous second-line agents (e.g., aminoglycosides, cycloserine, ethionamide, fluoroquinolones, para-aminosalicylic acid) have been used successfully to treat pregnant women with MDR tuberculosis, and short follow-up analyses have shown no evidence of teratogenicity in the children of these patients [231,232].

The currently recommended initial treatment of drug-susceptible tuberculosis disease in pregnancy is INH and RIF daily, with the addition of EMB initially, under directly observed therapy [233,234]. Pyridoxine (50 mg daily) always should be given with INH during pregnancy because of the increased requirements for this vitamin in pregnant women. After drug susceptibility testing of the isolate of *M. tuberculosis* reveals it to be susceptible to INH and RIF, EMB can be discontinued. If PZA is not used in the initial regimen, INH and RIF must be given for 9 months instead of 6 months. After the first 2 weeks to 2 months of daily treatment, the drugs can be given twice a week under directly observed therapy, which is the preferred method of treatment by most experts. The treatment of any form of drug-resistant tuberculosis during pregnancy is extraordinarily difficult and should be handled by an expert with great experience with the disease [235].

Because treatment of tuberculosis in pregnant women often continues after delivery, there is concern as to whether it is safe for the mother to breast-feed her infant. Snider and Powell [236] concluded that a breast-feeding infant would have serum levels of no more than 20% of the usual therapeutic levels of INH for infants and less than 11% of other antituberculosis drugs. Potential toxic effects of drugs delivered in breast milk have not been reported. Because pyridoxine deficiency in neonates can cause seizures, and because breast milk has relatively low levels of pyridoxine, infants who are taking INH or whose breast-feeding mothers are taking INH should receive supplemental pyridoxine [237].

Pregnant women coinfected with HIV and tuberculosis present multiple treatment challenges because each disease potentiates the other, and there are often interactions between RIF and antiretroviral therapy [238]. Additionally, patients who are coinfected are at risk for paradoxical disease worsening after starting antimycobacterial therapy—immune reconstitution inflammatory syndrome (IRIS)—which occasionally can be fatal [239]. Maternal mortality rates are higher for coinfected women than for women with either infection alone, and much of the excess mortality is due to tuberculosis [96,238].

NEONATES AND INFANTS

The optimal treatment of congenital tuberculosis has not been established because the rarity of this condition precludes formal treatment trials. The basic principles for treatment of other children and adults seem also to apply to the treatment of congenital tuberculosis [193,240]. All children with suspected congenital tuberculosis should be started on four antituberculosis medications (INH, RIF, PZA, plus either EMB or an aminoglycoside) until the diagnostic evaluation and susceptibility testing of isolated organisms are concluded. Although the optimal duration of therapy has not been established, many experts treat infants with congenital or postnatally acquired tuberculosis for 9 to 12 months because of the decreased immunologic capability of the young infant.

INH given alone is known to be safe in neonates, including premature infants. There are no comparable data for INH given in combination with other drugs or for other drugs alone. Several studies have shown that RIF can be given safely to premature infants for indications other than tuberculosis. In addition, anecdotal information supports the notion that PZA, STM, amikacin, and kanamycin are safe in neonates. Young infants taking these drugs should have biochemical monitoring of serum liver enzymes and uric acid (for PZA) performed on a regular basis. Hearing screens and evaluation of renal function should be considered for children taking aminoglycosides. Although the pharmacokinetics of antituberculosis drugs in neonates are essentially unknown, extensive clinical experience suggests that the doses listed in Table 18–3 are effective and safe. All neonates and infants with tuberculosis should be treated by directly observed therapy.

FOLLOWING THE INFANT ON THERAPY

Follow-up of children treated with antituberculosis drugs has become more streamlined in recent years. While receiving chemotherapy, patients should be seen monthly to encourage regular taking of the prescribed drugs and to check, by a few simple questions (e.g., concerning appetite, well-being) and a few observations (e.g., weight gain; appearance of skin and sclerae; palpation of liver, spleen, and lymph nodes), that the disease is not spreading and that toxic effects of the drugs are not appearing. Repeat chest radiographs probably should be obtained 1 to 2 months after the onset of chemotherapy to ascertain the maximal extent of disease before chemotherapy takes effect; thereafter, radiographs rarely are necessary.

Chemotherapy has been so successful that follow-up beyond its termination is not usually necessary except for children with serious disease, such as congenital tuberculosis or meningitis, or children with extensive residual chest radiographic findings at the end of chemotherapy. By law, every case of definite or suspected tuberculosis must be reported immediately by telephone to the health department to ensure (1) prompt contact investigation [241–247]; (2) free antituberculosis drugs, which are available for diagnosed cases and for intimate contacts in almost every state of the United States; and (3) provision of directly observed therapy.

PROGNOSIS

The prognosis for congenital tuberculosis was dismal in the prechemotherapy era [248]. In Hughesdon's report [135], 3 infants died on the first day of life, 8 died between 18 and 30 days, 15 died between 31 and 60 days, and 3 died between 65 and 112 days. Hageman and associates [129] reviewed 26 patients born since the introduction of INH in 1952: 12 died, and 9 of these were untreated, the diagnosis being established only at autopsy. The results in survivors were good, but the follow-up was usually short [182,249]. A child reported by Nemir and O'Hare [130], who was treated intensively with INH, STM, and aminosalicylic acid in the 1950s, recovered, was followed for 27 years, and is herself the mother of two tuberculin-negative children.

In the modern era, mortality rates of 38% have been reported in some series [238]. All-cause mortality rates are 3.4-fold higher in children born to mothers with tuberculosis [96]. Children of mothers coinfected with untreated HIV and tuberculosis have a high rate of HIV acquisition [96], and in one series, almost two thirds of children died before 1 year of age [97]. There is little question that today's multidrug, short-course chemotherapeutic regimens should be extremely effective in bringing the disease under rapid and permanent control, if the disease is due to drug-susceptible organisms. Experience with treatment of tuberculosis disease that is due to drug-resistant organisms is so limited as to preclude prognosis.

VACCINATION AGAINST TUBERCULOSIS—BACILLE CALMETTE-GUÉRIN

The BCG vaccines are the oldest of the vaccines used throughout the world. They have been given to 4 billion people and have been used routinely since the 1960s in every country of the world except the United States and the Netherlands [250]. Despite their widespread use, tuberculosis remains among the most destructive infectious diseases in the world, however, indicating that the BCG vaccines alone are not sufficient to eliminate or even control the disease. The vaccine is generally administered during the newborn period. In some countries, children receive a booster of BCG during adolescence [251,252].

HISTORY AND DEVELOPMENT OF BACILLE CALMETTE-GUÉRIN VACCINES

The BCG vaccines are attenuated strains of *M. bovis*. Starting in 1908, the original strain was subcultured every 3 weeks for 13 years [253]. The genotype changes that resulted at various stages cannot be determined because none of the original cultures or subcultures were preserved. This long process was marked by a loss of virulence first for calves, then for guinea pigs. In 1948, despite the complete lack of reported controlled trials or case-control studies, the First International BCG Congress stated that the BCG vaccines were effective and safe. After World War II, the WHO and UNICEF organized campaigns to promote vaccination with BCG in several countries. The seed lot system for BCG was established in 1956 [253], and the WHO developed requirements for freeze-dried BCG in 1966 [254]. By the end of 1974, more than 1.5 billion individuals had received a BCG vaccination. Since 1977, BCG vaccination has been included in the WHO Expanded Programme on Immunization. Approximately 100 million children receive a BCG vaccination each year, expanding the total number of individuals who have received it to more than 4 billion.

The original strain of *M. bovis* used to make BCG was maintained by serial passage at the Pasteur Institute until it was lost or discarded. It previously was distributed to dozens of laboratories, each of which produced and maintained its own BCG stain. It soon became apparent that the conditions for culture used in the various laboratories resulted in the production of many "daughter" BCG strains that differed widely in growth characteristics, biochemical activity, ability to induce delayed hypersensitivity, and animal virulence [255–258]. The patterns of large restriction fragments created by the digestion of BCG DNA vary among strains [259]. In the 1960s, the WHO recommended stabilization of the biologic characteristics of the derivative strains by lyophilization and storage at low temperatures [260].

Interlaboratory studies and genomic evaluation have shown that the BCG strains in use today vary widely in many characteristics [261,262]. Different strains of BCG can activate different immune pathways and incite varying proinflammatory cascades [263]. The possible consequences on vaccine efficacy and adverse effects are unknown, however. When comparing the various published clinical trials and case-control series, it is difficult to show that one strain of BCG is superior to another in the protection of humans against tuberculosis. Some laboratory and clinical observations have suggested that BCG strains can be separated into "strong" (Pasteur 1173 P2, Danish 1331) and "weak" (Glaxo 1077, Tokyo 172) groups. Although the relative efficacy of these two groups has been inconsistent, the strong strains have been associated with a higher rate of adverse reactions in neonates, including lymphadenitis and osteitis [264–267]. One South African study showed that after a change from the Tokyo 172 BCG to the Danish 1331 BCG, the rates of disseminated tuberculosis disease declined [268].

There is no consensus about which strain of BCG is optimal for general use. It has been postulated that investigators and public health authorities have selected BCG strains by their desire to maximize tuberculin reactivity and minimize adenitis, which may create strains that are the inverse of the ideal vaccine. It also seems that some BCG strains have lost efficacy over time [269].

VACCINE PREPARATION AND ADMINISTRATION

Seed lots are lyophilized bacilli that are part of the original harvest of the various BCG strains. The bacilli usually are grown in Sauton medium and are harvested early (day 6 to 9) to ensure good survival of organisms after lyophilization. The mass of mycobacterial cells is filtered, pressed, homogenized, diluted, and then freeze-dried. Reconstituted vaccines contain live bacilli and dead bacteria. Regulating the ratio of live to dead organisms is an important aspect of quality control and can affect efficacy and rates of adverse reactions.

Most BCG vaccine programs use the intradermal route of administration employing a syringe and needle; the dose is 0.05 mL for children in the first year of life and 0.1 mL for children older than 12 months of age. Japan and most of South Africa use percutaneous administration with a multipuncture device. It is generally accepted that the intradermal method is more accurate and consistent because the dose is measured precisely, and the administration is controlled. The deltoid region of the arm is the most common injection site, although many other body sites are used in individual patients.

Greater than 90% of patients receiving their first BCG vaccination develop a local reaction (e.g., erythema, induration, tenderness) followed by healing and scar formation within 3 months. One West African study showed that BCG-vaccinated children who had a BCG scar had significantly lower all-cause mortality rates than vaccinated children who did not develop a scar [270]. Possible explanations are that the development of a BCG scar is a marker of cell-mediated immunity, that infants who are premature or of low birth weight are less likely to develop scars [271], that the BCG vaccine may have nonspecific activity against unrelated bacterial pathogens, or that vaccine failure may play a role in the failure to develop a scar.

Other methods of administration were developed to try to address problems of local reactions created by intradermal administration. Subcutaneous injection seems to be effective, but often produces retracted scars. Other techniques, such as scarification, jet injection, and use of bifurcated needles, have yielded highly variable and, in some cases, inadequate results [272]. There have been no conclusive reported trials that compared the various techniques of BCG administration for protection against tuberculosis, but local complication rates generally are lowest with the multipuncture devices.

ADVERSE REACTIONS TO BACILLE CALMETTE-GUÉRIN VACCINATION

Local ulceration and regional lymphadenitis are the most common complications, occurring in less than 1% of immunocompetent recipients after intradermal administration of BCG [273,274]. These lesions usually occur within a few weeks to months after vaccination, but can be delayed for months in immunocompetent persons and for years in immunocompromised hosts [275]. Axillary, cervical, or supraclavicular nodes may be involved on the ipsilateral side of vaccination. Outbreaks of lymphadenitis after BCG vaccination have followed the introduction of a new BCG strain into the vaccination program [276,277]. There is no evidence that children who experience local complications are more likely to have immune deficits or to have enhanced or diminished protection against tuberculosis [276,277]. Because the risk of lymphadenitis is significantly higher when newborns are given a full dose of BCG, the WHO recommends using a reduced dose in children younger than 30 days of age.

The treatment of local adenitis as a complication of BCG vaccination is controversial, with suggestions ranging from observation to surgical drainage to administration of antituberculosis chemotherapy to a combination of surgery and chemotherapy [278]. Nonsuppurative lymph nodes usually resolve spontaneously, although resolution may take several months [279,280]. The WHO recommends drainage and direct installation of an antituberculosis drug into the lesion for adherent or fistulated lymph nodes [281]. One study of 120 patients with BCG-induced lymphadenitis treated for 6 months with an oral antituberculosis drug showed, however, that medical therapy was no better than observation, and that the rate of spontaneous drainage of lymph nodes was higher among children who received INH than children who were observed only [282]. Most experts now agree that nonsuppurative adenitis associated with BCG vaccination should be managed by observation only.

Other complications of BCG vaccination are far less frequent. The mean risk of osteitis after BCG vaccination has varied from 0.01 per 1 million in Japan to 300 per 1 million in Finland [283–285]. As with lymphadenitis, osteitis rates occasionally have increased dramatically after introduction of a new vaccine strain into a vaccination program. Other very rare complications of BCG vaccination include lupus vulgaris, erythema nodosum, iritis, and osteomyelitis. Generally, these complications should

be treated with antituberculosis medications (except PZA, to which *M. bovis* is intrinsically resistant).

Generalized BCG infection is extremely rare in immunocompetent hosts [286–288]. Overall rates of fatal disseminated BCG disease in recently vaccinated persons have been reported at 0.19 to 1.56 cases per 1 million vaccinated, most cases occurring in children with severe defects in cellular immunity, such as severe combined immunodeficiency, malnutrition, cancer, DiGeorge syndrome, interferon-γ receptor deficiency, or symptomatic HIV infection [273,289–295]. It is likely that the actual incidence of disseminated BCG infection is higher because some cases undoubtedly are misdiagnosed as disseminated tuberculosis.

The exact safety of BCG vaccination in children and adults with HIV infection is unknown. Disseminated BCG infection was described in an HIV-infected adult 30 years after he received BCG [296]. BCG can also be associated with immune reconstitution syndrome in children, generally within 10 weeks of initiating antiretroviral therapy [297]. One French study showed that 9 of 68 HIV-infected children given BCG vaccine developed complications: 7 had large satellite adenitis, and 2 developed disseminated lesions [298]. A retrospective review of BCG disease cases in the Western Cape Province of South Africa found 25 cases in a 2.5-year period, or 1 in every 240 HIV-infected vaccinees. Seventeen (68%) patients were HIV-infected; immunocompetent children were more likely to have regional disease at the inoculation site, whereas immunocompromised hosts were at risk for disseminated disease [299].

Because many HIV-infected children were asymptomatic before presentation, and disease was severe in nature, new WHO guidelines (2007) modified recommendations for BCG vaccination in HIV-infected children. Prior WHO guidelines recommended giving BCG vaccination to asymptomatic HIV-infected infants who live in high-risk areas for tuberculosis. Current guidelines recommend avoiding BCG vaccination in two groups: (1) children known to be HIV-infected, regardless of symptomatic categorization, and (2) children of uncertain HIV infection status with signs or symptoms of HIV infection born to HIV-infected mothers [300]. Asymptomatic children of uncertain HIV infection status born to HIV-infected mothers should receive the BCG vaccine if the perceived benefits outweigh the risk of disseminated BCG infection. Despite the presence of live BCG organisms in ulcerated vaccination sites, person-to-person transmission of BCG has never been documented.

EFFECT OF BACILLE CALMETTE-GUÉRIN VACCINATION ON TUBERCULIN SKIN TEST RESULTS

Although the BCG vaccines have an effect on the result of the tuberculin skin test, the effect is variable, and no reliable method can distinguish tuberculin reactions caused by BCG vaccination from reactions caused by infection with *M. tuberculosis*. In various studies with different populations, the proportion of previously BCG-vaccinated individuals with significant skin test reactions has ranged from 0% to 90% [301–305]. The size of the skin test reaction after BCG vaccination varies with the strain and dose of the vaccine [303,306], the route of administration [305,307], the age at vaccination [271,302,308], the child's nutritional status, the time interval since vaccination [251,302,308], and the frequency of skin testing [309].

Several studies have shown that when newborns are given a BCG vaccination, 50% may have a negative tuberculin skin test reaction at 6 months of age, and most have a negative reaction by 2 to 5 years of age [302,310,311]. Interpretation of the skin test in BCG-vaccinated children may be complicated, however, by the booster phenomenon. The booster effect is the increase in reaction size caused by repetitive testing in a person sensitized to mycobacterial antigens [312]. Skin test reactions can be boosted in children who previously received a BCG vaccination, giving the false impression of "conversion" of a skin test from negative to positive, which usually indicates a new tuberculosis infection [313].

Strong or severe reactions to a tuberculin skin test are rare in previously BCG-vaccinated individuals who are *not* also infected with *M. tuberculosis*. Prior receipt of a BCG vaccine is never a contraindication for tuberculin skin testing. Most skin reactions caused by BCG vaccination are less than 10 mm in size. Generally, the tuberculin skin test should be interpreted in the same manner for an adult or child who has received a BCG vaccination as it is for a person with similar epidemiologic characteristics who has not received BCG vaccination.

EFFECTIVENESS OF BACILLE CALMETTE-GUÉRIN VACCINES

A detailed discussion of the effectiveness of the BCG vaccines and the variables which may have an impact on effectiveness is beyond the scope of this chapter. There have been eight major controlled trials conducted in various populations and many published case-control and cohort studies of various BCG preparations [314,315]. Investigators at the Harvard School of Health found 15 prospective trials and 12 case-control studies that met their criteria for adequacy in study design and controls against potential bias. In the prospective trials, the protective effect of BCG vaccines against tuberculosis disease was 51% [315]. Analysis of eight studies involving only vaccination of newborns revealed a protective effect of 55% [314]. For trials that measured these outcomes, BCG vaccines showed 71% protection against death from tuberculosis, 64% protection against tuberculosis meningitis, and 72% protection against disseminated tuberculosis. Another meta-analysis estimated that the approximately 100 million BCG vaccinations administered in 2002 would prevent almost 30,000 cases of meningitis and more than 11,000 cases of miliary tuberculosis, with highest numbers of cases prevented in Southeast Asia and sub-Saharan Africa [316].

Different BCG preparations and strains used in the same population gave similar levels of protection, whereas genetically identical BCG strains gave different levels of protection in different populations [314,315]. The duration of any protective effect is poorly studied and unknown, but probably short-lived (<10 years at best). There are no data on the efficacy of BCG vaccines in HIV-infected children, and given the risk of disseminated BCG disease and severe local reactions, HIV seropositivity is a contraindication to receipt of the BCG vaccine [300].

It seems that BCG vaccines have worked well in some circumstances, but poorly in others. Because only a small percentage of infectious cases of tuberculosis in adults are prevented by childhood BCG vaccination, BCG vaccination as currently practiced is not an effective instrument of disease control. The best use of BCG is the prevention of life-threatening forms of tuberculosis—meningitis, disseminated, severe pulmonary disease—in infants and young children.

MANAGEMENT OF A NEONATE BORN TO A MOTHER WITH A POSITIVE TUBERCULIN SKIN TEST

If a mother with a positive tuberculin skin test is well and her chest radiograph result is normal, no separation of the mother and infant is required. Although the mother is a candidate for treatment of *M. tuberculosis* infection, the infant does not need special evaluation or therapy. Other family members should have a tuberculin skin test and further evaluation, if indicated. The local health department often does not have the resources to do this testing, however, which should be performed by the treating physicians. There is no need to delay discharge of the infant from the newborn nursery pending the results of this family investigation. The need for further evaluation of the infant depends on whether disease is found in the family or cannot be excluded within the family's environment.

If the radiograph is abnormal, the mother and infant should be separated until the mother has been evaluated thoroughly. If active tuberculosis is present in the mother, she should be started on effective antituberculosis medications right away. Examination of the mother's sputum for acid-fast organisms always is necessary even if obtaining a sample requires vigorous measures. All other household members and frequent visitors should be investigated for *M. tuberculosis* infection and disease.

If the mother's chest radiograph is abnormal, but the history, physical examination, sputum smear, and interpretation of the radiograph suggest no evidence of active tuberculosis, it is reasonable to assume that the infant is at low risk for infection. The radiographic abnormality is due to another cause or a quiescent focus of previous infection with *M. tuberculosis*. If the mother remains untreated, however, she may develop reactivation tuberculosis and subsequently expose her infant. If not previously treated, the mother should receive appropriate therapy, and she and her infant should receive frequent follow-up care. In this situation, the infant does not need chemotherapy. All household members should be evaluated for tuberculosis by a clinician.

If the mother has clinical and radiographic evidence of active, possibly contagious tuberculosis, the local health department should be informed immediately about the mother so that a contact investigation can be performed. The infant should be evaluated for congenital tuberculosis with a physical examination and high-quality posteroanterior and lateral chest radiographs. If possible, serologic testing for HIV should be performed on the mother and her infant. The mother and infant should be separated until the infant is receiving chemotherapy or the mother is judged to be noncontagious [317]. Prophylactic INH (10–15 mg/kg/day) for newborns born to mothers with tuberculosis has been so efficacious that separation of the mother and infant is no longer considered mandatory when therapy is started [318–320]. Separation should occur only if the mother is ill enough to require hospitalization, if she has been or is expected to become nonadherent to her treatment, or if she is thought to be infected with a drug-resistant strain of *M. tuberculosis*.

INH therapy should be continued in the infant at least until the mother has been shown to be culture-negative for 3 months. At that time, a Mantoux tuberculin skin test is done on the infant. If it is positive, the infant should be investigated for the presence of tuberculosis with a physical examination and chest radiograph and further appropriate work-up if disease is suggested. If disease is absent, the infant should continue INH for 9 months. If the follow-up skin test is negative, and the mother or contact with tuberculosis has good adherence and response to treatment, INH many be discontinued in the infant. The infant needs close follow-up, and it is prudent to repeat a tuberculin skin test after 6 to 12 months.

If the mother or other family member with contagious tuberculosis has disease caused by an MDR strain of *M. tuberculosis* or has poor adherence to treatment, and better supervision of therapy for the adult and infant is impossible, the CDC recommends that the infant be separated from the contagious adult. Vaccination with BCG may be considered, as long as the infant is not HIV-infected [300,321,322]. Vaccination with BCG seems to decrease the risk of tuberculosis in exposed infants, but the effect is variable [323,324].

Kendig [325] reported 117 infants born to mothers with active tuberculosis around the time of delivery; none of the 30 BCG-vaccinated infants developed tuberculosis, and 38 cases of tuberculosis and 3 deaths occurred among the 75 infants who received neither BCG vaccine nor INH therapy. Twenty-four of the 30 infants who received BCG vaccine also were separated from their mother for at least 6 weeks; it is impossible to determine what degree of protection was conferred by this separation. Similar studies in England and Canada also describe the apparent efficacy of BCG given to neonates [326]. Usually, the infant must be kept out of the household, away from the contagious case, until the skin test result becomes reactive (marking protection from infection). Some infants who receive a BCG vaccination do not develop a reactive tuberculin skin test, however.

It is unknown if developing a reactive skin test correlates with protection. It is also unknown if a second BCG vaccination given to a child who maintains a negative tuberculin skin test reaction after the first BCG vaccination would cause an enhanced level of protection. Although BCG vaccines have some protective effect for the exposed newborn, most experts in the United States believe that appropriate separation and taking whatever steps are necessary to provide adequate chemotherapy for the child and the contagious adult is a superior approach to BCG vaccination. The use of directly observed therapy has made the need for BCG vaccination of infants in the United States almost nonexistent.

MANAGEMENT OF NEONATES AFTER POSTNATAL EXPOSURE

Occasionally, workers in nurseries have been found to have infectious tuberculosis [143,327–329]. These experiments of nature provide useful data on the risk to the infants. Generally, risk of infection of neonates in a modern hospital nursery seems to be low. Most nurseries have large air volumes, flows, and adequate air exchanges to decrease risk of infection. Also, the minute volume of neonates is low, diminishing the risk of infection after a brief time of exposure. Light and coworkers [319] followed 437 infants exposed to a nurse with a cough and a sputum smear that was positive for tuberculosis. Of these infants, 160 were considered to be at greatest risk and received daily INH for 3 months; all infants remained tuberculin-negative. Nania and colleagues [328] investigated exposures in a neonatal intensive care unit after a respiratory therapist was diagnosed with acid-fast bacilli smear-positive tuberculosis. Over a 1-month period, 180 infants were potentially exposed, as were 240 coworkers. No cases of tuberculosis infection or disease were identified. Steiner and colleagues [143] observed development of miliary tuberculosis in 2 of 1647 infants exposed in a nursery.

Infection is rare under nursery conditions, but it can and does occur. Strict control measures should prevent such episodes. Nursery personnel should undergo Mantoux testing or whole-blood interferon-γ release assays before starting work and, if the result is negative, yearly thereafter. If the skin test is positive, a prospective employee should have a chest radiograph. If the radiograph is normal, appropriate therapy for *M. tuberculosis* infection should be given, accompanied by careful medical follow-up. Prospective employees with positive skin tests and abnormal chest radiographs must be carefully and thoroughly evaluated. Many require antituberculosis therapy. Theoretically, these same guidelines apply to workers in licensed and unlicensed day care facilities, but in many cases they have not yet been implemented.

The decision to administer chemoprophylaxis to infants exposed in nurseries is controversial. In cases in which the source case is deemed not to be highly contagious through evaluation of the close adult contacts, and where contact between the source case and child was minimal, the infant usually can be managed without antituberculosis chemotherapy. One decision analysis evaluated whether INH prophylaxis was preferable, given the low risk of exposure, risk of INH-induced hepatotoxicity, and risk of severe disease in affected neonates. The model suggested that prophylaxis was preferable, unless the probability of infection was extremely low. The incremental cost-effectiveness was greater than $21 million per death prevented, however [330].

Children with primary tuberculosis are rarely contagious because of the nature of their pulmonary disease, absence of forceful cough, and small number of organisms in the diseased tissue [331,332]. Infants with congenital tuberculosis often have extensive pulmonary involvement with positive acid-fast stains of tracheal aspirates and numerous tubercle bacilli in the lungs and airways [333,334]. In several cases, there has been evidence of transmission of *M. tuberculosis* from congenitally infected infants to health care workers [335–340]; transmission to other infants has not been reported except in one neonate likely infected because of transmission from contaminated respiratory equipment [341]. Neonates with suspected congenital tuberculosis should be placed in appropriate isolation until it can be determined that they are not infectious, by acid-fast stain and culture of respiratory secretions.

If a member of the household other than the mother is found to have or to have had tuberculosis recently, chemotherapy and BCG vaccine for the infant remain controversial. If the tuberculous family member has completed treatment in the past, that individual should undergo a checkup before the infant enters the home. If the family member is still being treated, he or she should have been sputum culture-negative for at least 3 months before contact with the infant. If the infant must return to a home in which one of the family members has only recently started treatment, he or she should receive daily INH for at least 3 to 4 months, which Dormer and associates [318] showed to be very effective in preventing the development of tuberculosis in infants born to mothers in a sanatorium. If the family cannot be relied on to administer daily medication, if directly observed therapy is impossible, or if there are numerous household members suspected to have tuberculosis, BCG vaccination of the neonate should be considered.

CONCLUSION

Perinatal tuberculosis, although rare, will continue to occur, particularly among high-risk groups such as blacks, Hispanics, Asian/Pacific Islanders, and Native American/ Alaskan natives, and particularly among recent immigrants to the United States. Intrauterine transmission to the fetus occurs particularly in pregnant women experiencing initial *M. tuberculosis* infection and disease such as pleural effusion or miliary tuberculosis; less often, it is a complication of endometrial tuberculosis. Postnatal tuberculosis is usually acquired from a mother, other close family member, or caregiver with cavitary tuberculosis. Only by keeping the possibility of tuberculosis in mind and by carrying out appropriate history taking and tuberculin testing of pregnant patients, particularly pregnant women from high-risk groups, can tuberculosis be diagnosed and treated in time in the mother and newborn. If it does occur and is diagnosed in time, intensive treatment should result in an excellent outcome.

REFERENCES

[1] R. Dubos, J. Dubos, The White Plague: Tuberculosis, Man and Society, Little, Brown, Boston, 1952.
[2] M. Adhikari, T. Pillay, D.G. Pillay, Tuberculosis in the newborn: an emerging disease, Pediatr. Infect. Dis. J. 16 (1997) 1108–1121.
[3] E. Margono, et al., Resurgence of active tuberculosis among pregnant women, Obstet. Gynecol. 83 (1994) 911–914.
[4] L.J. Nelson, et al., Epidemiology of childhood tuberculosis in the United States, 1993–2001: the need for continued vigilance, Pediatrics 114 (2004) 333–341.
[5] M.H. Baumann, et al., Pleural tuberculosis in the United States: incidence and drug resistance, Chest 131 (2007) 1125–1132.
[6] J.R. Starke, Pediatric tuberculosis: a time for a new approach, Tuberculosis 83 (2002) 208–212.
[7] J.R. Starke, R. Jacobs, J. Jereb, Resurgence of tuberculosis in children, J. Pediatr. 120 (1992) 839–855.
[8] D.A.J. Moore, et al., Microscopic-observation drug-susceptibility assay for the diagnosis of TB, N. Engl. J. Med. 355 (2006) 1539–1550.
[9] M. Tovar, et al., Improved diagnosis of pleural tuberculosis using the microscopic-observation drug-susceptibility technique, Clin. Infect. Dis. 46 (2008) 909–912.
[10] R.A. Oberhelman, et al., Improved recovery of *Mycobacterium tuberculosis* from children using the microscopic observation drug susceptibility method, Pediatrics 118 (2006) e100–e106.
[11] P. Eamranond, E. Jaramillo, Tuberculosis in children: reassessing the need for improved diagnosis in global control strategies, Int. J. Tuberc. Lung Dis. 5 (2001) 544–603.
[12] B. Balaka, et al., Tuberculosis in newborns in a tropical neonatology unit, Arch. Pediatr. 9 (2002) 1156–1159.
[13] W.F. Pomputius III., et al., Standardization of gastric aspirate technique improves yield in the diagnosis of tuberculosis in children, Pediatr. Infect. Dis. J. 16 (1997) 222–226.
[14] J. Vallejo, L. Ong, J. Starke, Clinical features, diagnosis and treatment of tuberculosis in infants, Pediatrics 94 (1994) 1–7.
[15] H.J. Zar, et al., Induced sputum versus gastric lavage for microbiological confirmation of pulmonary tuberculosis in infants and young children: a prospective study, Lancet 365 (2005) 130–134.
[16] K.C. Smith, et al., Detection of *Mycobacterium tuberculosis* in clinical specimens from children using a polymerase chain reaction, Pediatrics 97 (1996) 155–690.
[17] S.H. Montenegro, et al., Improved detection of *Mycobacterium tuberculosis* in Peruvian children by use of a heminested IS6110 polymerase chain reaction assay, Clin. Infect. Dis. 36 (2003) 16–23.
[18] B.J. Marais, M. Pai, Recent advances in the diagnosis of childhood tuberculosis, Arch. Dis. Child. 92 (2007) 446–452.
[19] W. Rafi, et al., Role of IS6110 uniplex PCR in the diagnosis of tuberculous meningitis: experience at a tertiary neurocentre, Int. J. Tuberc. Lung Dis. 11 (2007) 209–214.
[20] S.L. Zhang, et al., A novel genotypic test for rapid detection of multidrug-resistant *Mycobacterium tuberculosis* isolates by a multiplex probe array, J. Appl. Microbiol. 103 (2007) 1262–1271.
[21] M.H. Hazbon, et al., Population genetics study of isoniazid resistance mutations and evolution of multidrug-resistant *Mycobacterium tuberculosis*, Antimicrob. Agents Chemother. 50 (2006) 2640–2649.
[22] P.F. Barnes, M.D. Cave, Molecular epidemiology of tuberculosis, N. Engl. J. Med. 349 (2003) 1149–1156.
[23] S.H. Wootton, et al., Epidemiology of pediatric tuberculosis using traditional and molecular techniques: Houston, Texas, Pediatrics 116 (2005) 1141–1147.
[24] C. Dye, Global epidemiology of tuberculosis, Lancet 367 (2006) 938–940.
[25] X.T. Ussery, et al., Epidemiology of tuberculosis among children in the United States: 1985 to 1994, Pediatr. Infect. Dis. J. 15 (1996) 697–704.
[26] I.B. Palme, et al., Impact of human immunodeficiency virus 1 infection on clinical presentation, treatment outcome and survival in a cohort of Ethiopian children with tuberculosis, Pediatr. Infect. Dis. J. 21 (2002) 1053–1061.
[27] P.F. Barnes, et al., Tuberculosis in persons with human immunodeficiency virus infection, N. Engl. J. Med. 324 (1991) 1644–1650.
[28] M.F. Cantwell, et al., Tuberculosis and race/ethnicity in the United States: impact of socioeconomic status, Am. J. Respir. Crit. Care. Med. 157 (1997) 1016–1020.
[29] M.T. McKenna, E. McCray, I.M. Onorato, The epidemiology of tuberculosis among foreign-born persons in the United States, 1986 to 1993, N. Engl. J. Med. 332 (1995) 1071–1076.
[30] S. Asch, et al., Why do symptomatic patients delay obtaining care for tuberculosis? Am. J. Respir. Crit. Care Med. 157 (1998) 1244–1248.
[31] Centers for Disease Control and Prevention, Trends in tuberculosis— United States, 2007, MMWR Morb. Mortal. Wkly Rep. 57 (2008) 281–285.
[32] K.G. Keppel, Ten largest racial and ethnic health disparities in the United States based on Healthy People 2010 objectives, Am. J. Epidemiol. 166 (2007) 97–103.
[33] D.P. Chin, et al., Differences in contributing factors to tuberculosis incidence in U.S.-born and foreign-born persons, Am. J. Respir. Crit. Care Med. 158 (1998) 1797–1803.
[34] M.N. Lobato, P.C. Hopewell, *Mycobacterium tuberculosis* infection after travel to or contact with visitors from countries with a high prevalence of tuberculosis, Am. J. Respir. Crit. Care Med. 158 (1998) 1871–1875.
[35] American Thoracic Society, Targeted tuberculin testing and treatment of latent tuberculosis infection, Am. J. Resp. Crit. Care Med. 161 (2000) 1376–1395.
[36] N.D. Walter, et al., Reaching the limits of tuberculosis prevention among foreign-born individuals: a tuberculosis-control program perspective, Clin. Infect. Dis. 46 (2008) 103–106.
[37] K. Schwartzman, et al., Domestic returns from investment in the control of tuberculosis in other countries, N. Engl. J. Med. 353 (2005) 1008–1020.

[38] Centers for Disease Control and Prevention, HIV/AIDS Surveillance Report, 2006, vol. 18, U.S. Department of Health and Human Services, CDC, Atlanta, GA, 2008.

[39] H.M. Coovadia, D. Wilkinson, Childhood human immunodeficiency virus and tuberculosis co-infections: reconciling conflicting data, Int. J. Tuberc. Lung Dis. 2 (1998) 844–851.

[40] P.M. Jeena, et al., Effects of the human immunodeficiency virus on tuberculosis in children, Tuber. Lung Dis. 77 (1996) 437–443.

[41] L.M. Mofenson, et al., *Mycobacterium tuberculosis* infection in pregnant and nonpregnant women infected with HIV in the women and infants transmission study, Arch. Intern. Med. 155 (1995) 1066–1072.

[42] Centers for Disease Control and Prevention, Reported HIV status of tuberculosis patients—United States, 1993-2005, MMWR Morb. Mortal. Wkly Rep. 56 (2007) 1103–1106.

[43] A.C.C. Carvallo, et al., Transmission of *Mycobacterium tuberculosis* to contacts of HIV-infected tuberculosis patients, Am. J. Respir. Crit. Care Med. 164 (2001) 2166–2171.

[44] G. Schaefer, et al., Pregnancy and pulmonary tuberculosis, Obstet. Gynecol. 46 (1975) 706–715.

[45] E.J. Carter, S. Mates, Tuberculosis during pregnancy: the Rhode Island experience, 1987 to 1991, Chest 106 (1994) 1466–1470.

[46] J.T. Good Jr., et al., Tuberculosis in association with pregnancy, Am. J. Obstet. Gynecol. 140 (1981) 492–498.

[47] M. Llewelyn, et al., Tuberculosis diagnosed during pregnancy: a prospective study from London, Thorax 55 (2000) 129–132.

[48] A. Kothari, N. Mahadevan, A. Girling, Tuberculosis and pregnancy—results of a study in a high prevalence area in London, Eur. J. Obstet. Gynecol. Reprod. Biol. 1236 (2006) 48–55.

[49] D.E. Bennett, et al., Prevalence of tuberculosis infection in the United States population, Am. J. Respir. Crit. Care Med. 177 (2008) 348–355.

[50] R. Debré, M. Lelong, quoted by Rich AR, Pathogenesis of Tuberculosis, second ed., Charles C Thomas, Springfield, IL, 1951, p. 72.

[51] S.E. Weinberger, et al., Pregnancy and the lung, Am. Rev. Respir. Dis. 121 (1980) 559–1581.

[52] D. Van Zwanenberg, Influence of the number of bacilli on the development of tuberculous disease in children, Am. Rev. Respir. Dis. 83 (1960) 31–44.

[53] A.R. Rich, The Pathogenesis of Tuberculosis, second ed., Charles C Thomas, Springfield, III, 1951.

[54] P.G. Kini, Congenital tuberculosis associated with maternal asymptomatic endometrial tuberculosis, Ann. Trop. Paediatr. 22 (2002) 179–181.

[55] N.W. Schluger, W.H. Rom, The host immune response to tuberculosis, Am. J. Respir. Crit. Care Med. 157 (1998) 679–691.

[56] A. Wallgren, The "time-table" of tuberculosis, Tubercle 29 (1948) 245–251.

[57] S. Smith, R.F. Jacobs, C.B. Wilson, Immunobiology of childhood tuberculosis: a window on the ontogeny of cellular immunity, J. Pediatr. 131 (1997) 16–26.

[58] G. Abraham, B. Teklu, Miliary tuberculosis in pregnancy and puerperium: analysis of eight cases, Ethiop. Med. J. 19 (1981) 87–90.

[59] H.S. Brar, S.H. Golde, J.E. Egan, Tuberculosis presenting as puerperal fever, Obstet. Gynecol. 70 (1987) 488–491.

[60] J.H. Brooks, G.M. Stirrat, Tuberculous peritonitis in pregnancy: case report, Br. J. Obstet. Gynaecol. 93 (1986) 1009–1010.

[61] R.S. Centeno, J. Winter, J.R. Bentson, Central nervous system tuberculosis related to pregnancy, J. Comput. Tomogr. 6 (1982) 141–145.

[62] D. Freeman, Abdominal tuberculosis in pregnancy, Tubercle 70 (1989) 143–145.

[63] D.B. Garrioch, Puerperal tuberculosis, Br. J. Clin. Pract. 29 (1975) 280–281.

[64] I.M. Golditch, Tuberculous meningitis and pregnancy, Am. J. Obstet. Gynecol. 10 (1971) 1144–1146.

[65] S. Govender, S.C. Moodley, M.J. Grootboom, Tuberculous paraplegia during pregnancy: a report of 4 cases, S. Afr. Med. J. 75 (1989) 190–192.

[66] R. Grenville-Mathers, W.C. Harris, H.J. Trenchard, Tuberculous primary infection in pregnancy and its relation to congenital tuberculosis, Tubercle 41 (1960) 181–185.

[67] J.C.P. Kingdom, D.H. Kennedy, Tuberculous meningitis in pregnancy, Br. J. Obstet. Gynaecol. 96 (1989) 233–235.

[68] C. Maheswaran, R.S. Neuwirth, An unusual cause of postpartum fever: acute hematogenous tuberculosis, Obstet. Gynecol. 41 (1973) 765–769.

[69] J.P. Myers, et al., Tuberculosis in pregnancy with fatal congenital infection, Pediatrics 67 (1981) 89–94.

[70] B.I. Nsofor, O.N. Trivedi, Postpartum paraplegia due to spinal tuberculosis, Trop. Doc. 18 (1988) 52–53.

[71] B. Petrini, et al., Perinatal transmission of tuberculosis: meningitis in mother, disseminated disease in child, Scand. J. Infect. Dis. 15 (1983) 403–405.

[72] T. Suvonnakote, D. Obst, Pulmonary tuberculosis with pregnancy, J. Med. Assoc. Thor. 64 (1981) 26–30.

[73] G. Bazaz-Malik, B. Maheshwari, N. Lal, Tuberculosis endometritis: a clinicopathological study of 1000 cases, Br. J. Obstet. Gynaecol. 90 (1983) 84–86.

[74] R. Punnonen, P. Kiilholma, L. Meurman, Female genital tuberculosis and consequent infertility, Int. J. Fertil. 28 (1983) 235–238.

[75] N. Singh, S. Gumana, S. Mittal, Genital tuberculosis: a leading cause of infertility in women seeking assisted contraception in North India, Arch. Gynecol. Obstet. 278 (2008) 325–327.

[75a] J.B. Sharma, et al., Hysterosalpingographic findings in infertile women with genital tuberculosis, Int. J. Gynaecol. Obstet. 101:150–155, 2008.

[76] W. Baumgartner, H. Van Calker, W. Eisenberger, Congenital tuberculosis, Monatschr. Kinderheilkd. 128 (1980) 563–566.

[77] A.R. Cooper, W. Heneghan, J.D. Mathew, Tuberculosis in a mother and her infant, Pediatr. Infect. Dis. J. 4 (1985) 181–183.

[78] J.L. Hallum, H.E. Thomas, Full term pregnancy after proved endometrial tuberculosis, J. Obstet. Gynaecol. Br. Emp. 62 (1955) 548–550.

[79] C. Kaplan, K. Benirschke, B. Tarzy, Placental tuberculosis in early and late pregnancy, Am. J. Obstet. Gynecol. 137 (1980) 858–860.

[80] G.M. Addis, et al., Miliary tuberculosis in an in-vitro fertilization pregnancy: a case report, Eur. J. Obstet. Gynecol. Reprod. Biol. 27 (1988) 351–353.

[81] D.E. Snider Jr., Pregnancy and tuberculosis, Chest 86 (Suppl) (1984) 10S–13S.

[82] E. Hedvall, Pregnancy and tuberculosis, Acta Med. Scand. 147 (Suppl. 286) (1953) 1–101.

[83] R.C. Cohen, Effect of pregnancy and parturition on pulmonary tuberculosis, BMJ 2 (1943) 775–776.

[84] J.B. Cromie, Pregnancy and pulmonary tuberculosis, Br. J. Tuberc. 48 (1954) 97–101.

[85] J.D. Cohen, E.A. Patton, T.L. Badger, The tuberculous mother, Am. Rev. Tuberc. 65 (1952) 1–23.

[86] J.R. Edge, Pulmonary tuberculosis and pregnancy, Br. J. Med. 2 (1952) 845–846.

[87] L.M. Rosenbach, C.R. Gangemi, Tuberculosis and pregnancy, JAMA 161 (1956) 1035–1037.

[88] C.J. Stewart, F.A.H. Simmonds, Child-bearing and pulmonary tuberculosis, BMJ 2 (1947) 726–729.

[89] C.J. Stewart, F.A.H. Simmonds, Prognosis of pulmonary tuberculosis in married women, Tubercle 35 (1954) 28–30.

[90] E.A. Wilson, T.J. Thelin, P.V. Dilts Jr., Tuberculosis complicated by pregnancy, Am. J. Obstet. Gynecol. 115 (1973) 526–529.

[91] A.E. Cziezel, et al., A population-based case control study of the safety of oral anti-tuberculosis drug treatment during pregnancy, Int. J. Tuberc. Lung Dis. 5 (2001) 564–568.

[92] A.P. de March, Tuberculosis and pregnancy: five to ten-year review of 215 patients in their fertile age, Chest 68 (1975) 800–804.

[93] B.R. Mehta, Pregnancy and tuberculosis, Dis. Chest 39 (1961) 505–511.

[94] R.B. Pridie, P. Stradling, Management of pulmonary tuberculosis during pregnancy, Br Med J. 2 (1961) 78–79.

[95] R. Figueroa-Damián, J.L. Arredondo-García, Neonatal outcome of children born to women with tuberculosis, Arch. Med. Res. 32 (2001) 66–69.

[96] A. Gupta, et al., Postpartum tuberculosis incidence and mortality among HIV-infected women and their infants in Pune, India, 2002–2005, Clin. Infect. Dis. 45 (2007) 241–249.

[97] T. Pillay, et al., Vertical transmission of *Mycobacterium tuberculosis* in KwaZulu Natal: impact of HIV-1 co-infection, Int. J. Tuberc. Lung Dis. 8 (2004) 59–69.

[98] T. Bjerkedal, S.L. Bahna, E.H. Lehmann, Course and outcome of pregnancy in women with pulmonary tuberculosis, Scand. J. Respir. Dis. 56 (1975) 245–250.

[99] B. Ratner, A.E. Rostler, P.S. Salgado, Care, feeding and fate of premature and full term infants born of tuberculous mothers, Am. J. Dis. Child. 81 (1951) 471–482.

[100] S.N. Tripathy, S.N. Tripathy, Tuberculosis and pregnancy, Int. J. Gynecol. Obstet. 80 (2003) 247–253.

[101] N. Jana, et al., Obstetrical outcomes among women with extrapulmonary tuberculosis, N. Engl. J. Med. 341 (1999) 645–649.

[102] J.J. Bernsee Rush, Protocol for tuberculosis screening in pregnancy, J. Obstet. Gynecol. Neonat. Nurs. 14 (1986) 225–230.

[103] P.B. McIntyre, J.G. McCormack, A. Vacca, Tuberculosis in pregnancy—implications for antenatal screening in Australia, Med. J. Aust. 146 (1987) 42–44.

[104] E.L. Kendig, et al., Underreading of the tuberculin skin test reaction, Chest 113 (1998) 1175–1177.

[105] P.O. Ozuah, et al., Assessing the validity of tuberculin skin test readings by trained health professionals and patients, Chest 116 (1999) 104–106.

[106] H.D. Covelli, R.T. Wilson, Immunologic and medical consideration in tuberculin-sensitized pregnant patients, Am. J. Obstet. Gynecol. 132 (1978) 256–259.

[107] M.A. Keller, et al., Transfer of tuberculin immunity from mother to infant, Pediatr. Res. 22 (1987) 277–281.

[108] M.D. Gillum, D.G. Maki, Brief report: tuberculin testing, BCG in pregnancy, Infect. Cont. Hosp. Epidemiol. 9 (1988) 119–121.

[109] J.K. Smith, E.A. Caspary, E.J. Field, Lymphocyte reactivity to antigen pregnancy, Am. J. Obstet. Gynecol. 113 (1972) 602–606.

[110] W.P. Montgomery, et al., The tuberculin test in pregnancy, Am. J. Obstet. Gynecol. 100 (1968) 829–831.

[111] P.A. Present, G.W. Comstock, Tuberculin sensitivity in pregnancy, Am. Rev. Respir. Dis. 112 (1975) 413–416.

[112] D.E. Snider Jr., et al., Treatment of tuberculosis during pregnancy, Am. Rev. Respir. Dis. 122 (1980) 65–78.

[113] G.H. Mazurek, et al., Prospective comparison of the tuberculin skin test and two whole-blood interferon-gamma release assays in persons with suspected tuberculosis, Clin. Infect. Dis. 45 (2007) 837–845.

[114] J.G. Vallejo, J.R. Starke, Tuberculosis and pregnancy, Clin. Chest. Med. 13 (1992) 693–707.
[115] J.E. Sackoff, et al., Tuberculosis prevention for non-US-born pregnant women, Am. J. Obstet. Gynecol. 194 (2006) 451–456.
[116] J.R. Starke, Tuberculosis: an old disease but a new threat to the mother, fetus and neonate, Clin. Perinatol. 24 (1997) 107–128.
[117] C.R. Bonebrake, et al., Routine chest roentgenography in pregnancy, JAMA 240 (1978) 2747–2748.
[118] M.L. Maccato, Pneumonia and pulmonary tuberculosis in pregnancy, Obstet. Gynecol. Clin. North Am. 16 (1989) 417–430.
[119] L. Weinstein, T. Murphy, The management of tuberculosis during pregnancy, Clin. Perinatol. 1 (1974) 395–405.
[120] Y. Ahmed, et al., A study of maternal mortality at the University Teaching Hospital, Lusaka, Zambia: the emergence of tuberculosis as a major non-obstetric cause of maternal death, Int. J. Tuberc. Lung Dis. 3 (1999) 675–680.
[121] J.A. Hale, G.N. Peters, J.H. Cheek, Tuberculosis of the breast: rare but still extant, Am. J. Surg. 150 (1985) 620–624.
[122] R.F. Jacobs, R.S. Abernathy, Management of tuberculosis in pregnancy and the newborn, Clin. Perinatol. 15 (1988) 305–319.
[123] I.L. Wapnir, et al., Latent mammary tuberculosis: a case report, Surgery 98 (1985) 976–978.
[124] K.E. Bani-Hani, et al., Tuberculous mastitis: a disease not to be forgotten, Int. J. Tuberc. Lung Dis. 9 (2005) 920–925.
[125] J.R. Hageman, Congenital and perinatal tuberculosis: discussion of difficult issues in diagnosis and management, J. Perinatol. 18 (1998) 389–394.
[126] K.C. Smith, Congenital tuberculosis: a rare manifestation of a common infection, Curr. Opin. Infect. Dis. 15 (2002) 269–274.
[127] M.F. Cantwell, et al., Brief report: congenital tuberculosis, N. Engl. J. Med. 330 (1994) 1051–1054.
[128] M.S. Micozzi, Skeletal tuberculosis, pelvic contraction and parturition, Am. J. Phys. Anthropol. 58 (1982) 441–445.
[129] J. Hageman, et al., Congenital tuberculosis: critical reappraisal of clinical findings and diagnostic procedures, Pediatrics 66 (1980) 980–984.
[130] R.L. Nemir, D. O'Hare, Congenital tuberculosis: review and guidelines, Am. J. Dis. Child. 139 (1985) 284–287.
[131] A.R. Rich, R.H. Follis Jr., Effect of low oxygen tension upon the development of experimental tuberculosis, Bull. Johns Hopkins Hosp. 71 (1942) 345–357.
[132] A.J. Vorwald, Experimental tuberculous infection in the guinea-pig foetus compared with that in the adult, Am. Rev. Tuberc. 35 (1937) 260–295.
[133] H. Beitzke, Uber die angeborene tuberkulose infektion, Ergeb. Ges. Tuberk. 7 (1935) 1–30.
[134] A.J. Hertzog, S. Chapman, J. Herring, Congenital pulmonary aspiration tuberculosis, Am. J. Clin. Pathol. 19 (1949) 1139–1142.
[135] M.R. Hughesdon, Congenital tuberculosis, Arch. Dis. Child. 21 (1946) 121–139.
[136] B.D. Corner, N.J. Brown, Congenital tuberculosis: report of a case with necropsy findings in mother and child, Thorax 10 (1955) 99–103.
[137] M. Siegel, Pathological findings and pathogenesis of congenital tuberculosis, Am. Rev. Tuberc. 29 (1934) 297–309.
[138] T.W.P. Bate, R.E. Sinclair, M.J. Robinson, Neonatal tuberculosis, Arch. Dis. Child. 61 (1986) 512–514.
[139] P.K. Devi, et al., Pregnancy and pulmonary tuberculosis: observations on the domiciliary management of 238 patients in India, Tubercle 45 (1964) 211–216.
[140] E.L. Kendig Jr., Tuberculosis in the very young: report of three cases in infants less than one month of age, Am. Rev. Respir. Dis. 70 (1954) 161–165.
[141] R. Watchi, et al., Tuberculous meningitis in a five-week-old child, Int. J. Tuberc. Lung Dis. 2 (1998) 255–257.
[142] J.R. Burk, et al., Nursery exposure of 528 newborns to a nurse with pulmonary tuberculosis, South. Med. J. 71 (1978) 7–10.
[143] P. Steiner, et al., Miliary tuberculosis in two infants after nursery exposure: epidemiologic, clinical and laboratory findings, Am. Rev. Respir. Dis. 113 (1976) 267–271.
[144] E.L. Kendig Jr., W.L. Rodgers, Tuberculosis in the neonatal period, Am. Rev. Tuberc. Pulm. Dis. 77 (1958) 418–422.
[145] M.K. McCray, N.B. Esterly, Cutaneous eruptions in congenital tuberculosis, Arch. Dermatol. 117 (1981) 460–464.
[146] L.E. Holt, Tuberculosis acquired through ritual circumcision, JAMA 61 (1913) 99–102.
[147] N. Abughali, et al., Congenital tuberculosis, Pediatr. Infect. Dis. J. 13 (1994) 738–741.
[148] L. Arthur, Congenital tuberculosis, Proc. R. Soc. Med. 60 (1967) 19–20.
[149] F. Asensi, et al., Congenital tuberculosis, still a problem, Pediatr. Infect. Dis. J. 9 (1990) 223–224.
[150] P.B. Blackall, Tuberculosis: maternal infection of the newborn, Med. J. Aust. 42 (1969) 1055–1058.
[151] A.L. Foo, K.K. Tan, D.M. Chay, Congenital tuberculosis, Tuber. Lung Dis. 74 (1993) 59–61.
[152] J.B. Hardy, J.R. Hartman, Tuberculous dactilitis in childhood, J. Pediatr. 30 (1947) 146–156.
[153] R. Hopkins, R. Ermocilla, G. Cassady, Congenital tuberculosis, South. Med. J. 69 (1976) 1156.
[154] K. Koutsoulieris, E. Kaslaris, Congenital tuberculosis, Arch. Dis. Child. 45 (1970) 584–586.
[155] L. Krishnan, et al., Neonatal tuberculosis: a case report, Ann. Trop. Paediatr. 14 (1994) 333–335.
[156] D.H. Morens, J.V. Baublis, K.P. Heidelberger, Congenital tuberculosis and associated hypoadrenocorticism, South. Med. J. 72 (1979) 160–165.
[157] R.A. Niles, Puerperal tuberculosis with death of infant, Am. J. Obstet. Gynecol. 144 (1982) 131–132.
[158] P.M. Pai, P.R. Parikh, Congenital miliary tuberculosis: case report, Clin. Pediatr. 15 (1976) 376–378.
[159] S.M. Polansky, et al., Congenital tuberculosis, AJR Am. J. Roentgenol. 130 (1978) 994–996.
[160] A.D. Ramos, L.T. Hibbard, J.R. Graig, Congenital tuberculosis, Obstet. Gynecol. 43 (1974) 61–64.
[161] K.S. Reisinger, et al., Congenital tuberculosis: report of case, Pediatrics 54 (1974) 74–76.
[162] P. Sauer, et al., La tuberculose congénitale, Pédiatrie 36 (1981) 217–224.
[163] A. Soeiro, Congenital tuberculosis in a small premature baby, S. Afr. Med. J. 45 (1971) 1025–1026.
[164] R.M. Todd, Congenital tuberculosis: report of a case with unusual features, Tubercle 41 (1960) 71–73.
[165] M.A. Voyce, A.C. Hunt, Congenital tuberculosis, Arch. Dis. Child. 41 (1966) 299–300.
[166] Z. Vucicevic, T. Suskovic, Z. Ferencic, A female patient with tuberculous polyserositis and congenital tuberculosis in her new-born child, Tuber. Lung Dis. 76 (1995) 460–462.
[167] A. Chen, S.L. Shih, Congenital tuberculosis in two infants, AJR Am. J. Roentgenol. 182 (2004) 253–256.
[168] S.B. Grover, et al., Sonographic diagnosis of congenital tuberculosis: an experience with four cases, Abdom. Imaging 25 (2000) 622–626.
[169] D.L. Weisoly, et al., Congenital tuberculosis regarding extracorporeal membrane oxygenation, Pediatr. Pulmonol. 37 (2004) 470–473.
[170] K. Kobayashi, et al., Cerebral hemorrhage associated with vitamin K deficiency in congenital tuberculosis treated with isoniazid and rifampin, Pediatr. Infect. Dis. J. 21 (2002) 1088–1089.
[171] M.A. Mazade, et al., Congenital tuberculosis presenting an sepsis syndrome: case report and review of the literature, Pediatr. Infect. Dis. J. 20 (2001) 439–442.
[172] D.R. Berk, K.G. Sylvester, Congenital tuberculosis presenting as progressive liver dysfunction, Pediatr. Infect. Dis. J. 23 (2004) 78–80.
[173] M. Sood, et al., Congenital tuberculosis manifesting as cutaneous disease, Pediatr. Infect. Dis. J. 19 (2000) 1109–1111.
[174] Y.H. Chou, Congenital tuberculosis proven by percutaneous liver biopsy: report of a case, J. Perinat. Med. 30 (2002) 423–425.
[175] S. Pejham, et al., Congenital tuberculosis with facial nerve palsy, Pediatr. Infect. Dis. J. 21 (2002) 1085–1086.
[176] Z. Hatzistamatiou, et al., Congenital tuberculous lymphadenitis in a preterm infant in Greece, Acta Paediatr. 92 (2003) 392–394.
[177] S.B. Grover, et al., Congenital spine tuberculosis: early diagnosis by imaging studies, Am. J. Perinatol. 20 (2003) 147–152.
[178] M.R. Dische, et al., Congenital tuberculosis in a twin of immigrant parentage, Can. Med. Assoc. J. 119 (1978) 1068–1070.
[179] D.G. Cunningham, et al., Neonatal tuberculosis with pulmonary cavitation, Tubercle 63 (1982) 217–219.
[180] J. Teeratkulpisarn, et al., Cavitary tuberculosis in a young infant, Pediatr. Infect. Dis. J. 13 (1994) 545–546.
[181] S.B. Griffith-Richards, et al., Cavitating pulmonary tuberculosis in children: correlating radiology with pathogenesis, Pediatr. Radiol. 37 (2007) 798–804.
[182] P. De Angelis, et al., Congenital tuberculosis in twins, Pediatrics 69 (1981) 402–416.
[183] D.C. Gordon-Nesbitt, G. Rajan, Congenital tuberculosis successfully treated. Letter to the editor, BMJ 1 (1972) 233–234.
[184] R.C. Naranbai, W. Mathiassen, A.F. Malan, Congenital tuberculosis localized to the ear, Arch. Dis. Child. 63 (1989) 738–740.
[185] N. Senbil, et al., Congenital tuberculosis of the ear and parotid gland, Pediatr. Infect. Dis. J. 16 (1997) 1090.
[186] Y. Nicolau, C. Northrop, R. Eavey, Tuberculous otitis in infants: temporal bone histopathology and clinical extrapolation, Otol. Neurotol. 27 (2006) 667–671.
[187] F.M. Muñoz, et al., Tuberculosis among adult visitors of children with suspected tuberculosis and employees at a children's hospital, Infect. Control Hosp. Epidemiol. 23 (2002) 568–572.
[188] H.S. Schaaf, et al., Tuberculosis presenting in the neonatal period, Clin. Pediatr. 28 (1989) 474–475.
[189] H.S. Schaaf, et al., Tuberculosis in infants less than 3 months of age, Arch. Dis. Child. 69 (1993) 371–374.
[190] L. Richeldi, et al., T-cell-based diagnosis of neonatal multidrug-resistant latent tuberculosis infection, Pediatrics 119 (2007) e1–e5.
[191] T. Connell, N. Bar-Zeev, N. Curtis, Early detection of perinatal tuberculosis using a whole blood interferon-1 release assay, Clin. Infect. Dis. 42 (2006) e82–e85.
[192] E.A. Khan, J.R. Starke, Diagnosis of tuberculosis in children: increased need for better methods, Emerg. Infect. Dis. 1 (1995) 115–123.

[193] J.R. Stallworth, D.M. Brasfield, R.E. Tiller, Congenital miliary tuberculosis proved by open lung biopsy specimen and successfully treated, Am. J. Dis. Child. 14 (1980) 320–321.

[194] American Thoracic Society/Centers for Disease Control and Prevention/ Infectious Disease Society of America, Treatment of tuberculosis, Am. J. Respir. Crit. Care Med. 167 (2003) 603–662.

[195] J.N. Mieeli, W.A. Olson, S.N. Cohen, Elimination kinetics of isoniazid in the newborn infant, Dev. Pharmacol. Ther. 2 (1981) 235–239.

[196] S.M. Graham, et al., Low levels of pyrazinamide and ethambutol in children with tuberculosis and the impact of age, nutritional status, and human immuno- deficiency virus infection, Antimicrob. Agents Chemother. 50 (2006) 407–413.

[197] P.R. Donald, et al., Ethambutol dosage for the treatment of children: litera- ture review and recommendations, Int. J. Tuberc. Lung Dis. 10 (2006) 1318–1330.

[198] World Health Organization, Ethambutol efficacy and toxicity: literature review and recommendations for daily and intermittent dosage in children, World Health Organization, Geneva..

[199] H.L. David, Probability distribution of drug-resistant mutants in unselected populations of *Mycobacterium tuberculosis*, Appl. Microbiol. 20 (1970) 810–814.

[200] American Thoracic Society, Hepatotoxicity of antituberculosis therapy, Am. J. Respir. Crit. Care Med. 174 (2006) 935–952.

[201] Centers for Disease Control and Prevention, Treatment of tuberculosis, American Thoracic Society, CDC, and Infectious Diseases Society of America, MMWR Morb. Mortal. Wkly Rep. 52 (No. RR-11) 2003.

[202] J.N. Atkins, Maternal plasma concentration of pyridoxal phosphate during pregnancy: adequacy of vitamin B_6 supplementation during isoniazid ther- apy, Am. Rev. Respir. Dis. 126 (1982) 714–717.

[203] E. Sumartojo, When tuberculosis treatment fails: a social behavior account of patient adherence, Am. Rev. Respir. Dis. 147 (1993) 1311–1320.

[204] M.E. Villarino, et al., Rifampin preventive therapy for tuberculosis infection: experience with 157 adolescents, Am. J. Respir. Crit. Care Med. 155 (1997) 1735–1738.

[205] Centers for Disease Control, Management of persons exposed to multidrug- resistant tuberculosis, MMWR Morb. Mortal. Wkly Rep. 41 (RR-11) (1992) 1–8.

[206] M. Døssing, et al., Liver injury during antituberculosis treatment: an 11-year study, Tuberc. Lung Dis. 77 (1996) 335–340.

[207] A.L. Franks, et al., Isoniazid hepatitis among pregnancy and postpartum Hispanic patients, Public Health Rep. 104 (1989) 151–155.

[208] F.S. Al-Dossary, et al., Treatment of childhood tuberculosis with a six month directly observed regimen of only two weeks of daily therapy, Pediatr. Infect. Dis. J. 21 (2002) 91–97.

[209] D. Shingadia, V. Novelli, Diagnosis and treatment of tuberculosis in chil- dren, Lancet 3 (2003) 624–632.

[210] P. Flanagan, N.M. Hensler, The course of active tuberculosis complicated by pregnancy, JAMA 170 (1959) 783–787.

[211] G. Schaeffer, R.G. Douglas, F. Silverman, A re-evaluation of the manage- ment of pregnancy and tuberculosis, J. Obstet. Gynecol. Br. Emp. 66 (1959) 990–997.

[212] G. Schaeffer, S.J. Birnbaum, Present-day treatment of tuberculosis and preg- nancy, JAMA 165 (1957) 2163–2167.

[213] E. Varpela, On the effect exerted by first-line tuberculosis medicines on the foetus, Acta Tuberc. Scand. 35 (1964) 53–69.

[214] M.A. Wall, Treatment of tuberculosis during pregnancy, Am. Rev. Respir. Dis. 122 (1980) 989–993.

[215] D.J. Scheinhorn, V.A. Angelillo, Antituberculous therapy in pregnancy: risks to the fetus, West. J. Med. 127 (1977) 195–198.

[216] I.D. Bobrowitz, Ethambutol in pregnancy, Chest 66 (1974) 20–24.

[217] T. Lewit, et al., Ethambutol in pregnancy: observations on embryogenesis, Chest 68 (1974) 25–27.

[218] V.A. Place, Ethambutol administration during pregnancy: a case report, J. New Drugs 4 (1964) 206–208.

[219] J.S.M. Steen, D.M. Stainton-Ellis, Rifampin in pregnancy, Lancet 2 (1977) 604–605.

[220] J.L. Skolnick, et al., Rifampin, oral contraceptives, and pregnancy, JAMA 236 (1976) 1382.

[221] P.G. Brock, M. Rooch, Antituberculosis drugs in pregnancy, Lancet 1 (1981) 43–44.

[222] R.B. Byrd, Treating the pregnant tuberculous patient: curing the mother without harming the fetus, J. Respir. Dis. 3 (1982) 27–32.

[223] C.R. Lowe, Congenital defects among children born to women under super- vision or treatment for pulmonary tuberculosis, Br. J. Prev. Soc. Med. 18 (1964) 14–16.

[224] P.R. Donald, S.L. Sellars, Streptomycin ototoxicity in the unborn child, S. Afr. Med. J. 60 (1981) 316–318.

[225] G.C. Robinson, K.G. Cambon, Hearing loss in infants of tuberculous mothers treated with streptomycin during pregnancy, N. Engl. J. Med. 271 (1964) 949–951.

[226] E. Varpela, J. Hietalahti, M.J.T. Aro, Streptomycin and dihydrostrepto- mycin medication during pregnancy and their effect on the child's inner ear, Scand. J. Respir. Dis. 50 (1969) 101–109.

[227] A.E. Czeizel, et al., A teratological study of aminoglycoside antibiotic treat- ment during pregnancy, Scand. J. Infect. Dis. 32 (2000) 309–313.

[228] World Health Organization, Guidance for national tuberculosis pro- grammes on the management of tuberculosis in children, World Health Organization, Geneva, 2006.

[229] M. Potworowska, E. Sianozecka, R. Szufladowicz, Ethionamide treatment and pregnancy, Pol. Med. J. 5 (1966) 1152–1158.

[230] P. Wogelius, et al., Further analysis of adverse birth outcome after maternal use of fluoroquinolones, Int. J. Antimicrob. Agents 26 (2005) 323–326.

[231] S. Shin, et al., Treatment of multidrug-resistant tuberculosis during preg- nancy: a report of 7 cases, Clin. Infect. Dis. 36 (2003) 996–1003.

[232] P.C. Drobac, et al., Treatment of multidrug-resistant tuberculosis during pregnancy: long-term follow-up of 6 children, Clin. Infect. Dis. 40 (2005) 1689–1692.

[233] P.T. Davidson, Managing tuberculosis during pregnancy, Lancet 346 (1995) 199–200.

[234] M.T. Medchill, M. Gillum, Diagnosis and management of tuberculosis during pregnancy, Obstet. Gynecol. Rev. 44 (1989) 81–91.

[235] M.A. Aziz, et al., Epidemiology of antituberculosis drug resistance (the Global Project on Anti-tuberculosis Drug Resistance Surveillance): an updated analysis, Lancet 368 (2006) 2142–2154.

[236] D.E. Snider Jr., K.E. Powell, Should women taking antituberculosis drugs breast-feed? Arch. Intern. Med. 144 (1984) 589–590.

[237] S.A. McKenzie, A.J. Macnab, G. Katz, Neonatal pyridoxine responsive convulsions due to isoniazid therapy, Arch. Dis. Child. 51 (1976) 567–569.

[238] L.M. Mofenson, B.E. Laughon, Human immunodeficiency virus, *Mycobacte- rium tuberculosis*, and pregnancy: a deadly combination, Clin. Infect. Dis. 45 (2007) 250–253.

[239] H. McIlleron, et al., Complications of antiretroviral therapy in patients with tuberculosis: drug interactions, toxicity, and immune reconstitution inflam- matory syndrome, J. Infect. Dis. 196 (2007) S63–S75.

[240] M.C. Steinhoff, J. Lionel, Treatment of tuberculosis in newborn infants and their mothers, Indian J. Pediatr. 55 (1988) 240–245.

[241] C.A. Doerr, J.R. Starke, L.T. Ong, Clinical and public health aspects of tuberculous meningitis in children, J. Pediatr. 127 (1995) 27–33.

[242] B.D. Gessner, N.S. Weiss, C.M. Nolan, Risk factors for pediatric tuberculo- sis infection and disease after household exposure to adult index cases in Alaska, J. Pediatr. 132 (1998) 509–513.

[243] C.R. MacIntyre, A.J. Plant, Preventability of incident cases of tuberculosis in recently exposed contacts, Int. J. Tuberc. Lung Dis. 2 (1998) 56–61.

[244] J.B. Mehta, S. Bentley, Prevention of tuberculosis in children: missed oppor- tunities, Am. J. Prev. Med. 8 (1992) 283–286.

[245] R. Nolan Jr., Childhood tuberculosis in North Carolina: a study of the opportunities for intervention in the transmission of tuberculosis in children, Am. J. Public Health 76 (1986) 26–30.

[246] T. Rodrigo, et al., Characteristics of tuberculosis patients who generate secondary cases, Int. J. Tuberc. Lung Dis 1 (1997) 352–357.

[247] R.P. Spark, et al., Perinatal tuberculosis and its public health impact: a case report, Tex. Med. 92 (1996) 50–53.

[248] E.L. Kendig, Prognosis of infants born of tuberculous mothers, Pediatrics 26 (1960) 97–100.

[249] B.M. Laurance, Congenital tuberculosis successfully treated. Letter to the editor, BMJ 2 (1973) 55.

[250] World Health Organization, Immunization surveillance, assessment, and monitoring, 2006. Available at www.who.int/vaccines/globalsummary/ immunizations. Accessed May 6, 2008.

[251] R.E. Weir, et al., Persistence of the immune response induced by BCG vaccination, BCM Infect. Dis. 8 (2008) 9–18.

[252] L.C. Rodrigues, et al., Effect of BCG revaccination on incidence of tubercu- losis in school-aged children in Brazil: the BCG-REVAC cluster- randomized trial, Lancet 366 (2005) 1290–1295.

[253] International Union Against Tuberculosis, Phenotypes of BCG vaccine seed lot strains: results of an international cooperative study, Tubercle 59 (1978) 139–142.

[254] J.B. Milstein, J.J. Gibson, Quality control of BCG vaccines by WHO: a review of factors that may influence vaccine effectiveness and safety, Bull. World Health Org. 68 (1990) 93–108.

[255] T.W. Osborn, Changes in BCG strains, Tubercle 64 (1983) 1–13.

[256] R.F. Jacox, G.M. Meade, Variation in the duration of tuberculin skin test sensitivity produced by two strains of BCG, Am. Rev. Tuberc. 60 (1949) 541–546.

[257] R.J. Dubos, C.H. Pierce, Differential characteristics in vitro and in vivo of several substrains of BCG. I. Multiplication and survival in vitro, Am. Rev. Tuber. Pulm Dis 74 (1956) 655–666.

[258] R.J. Dubos, C.H. Pierce, Differential characteristics in vitro and in vivo of several substrains of BCG. IV. Immunizing effectiveness, Am. Rev. Tuberc. Pulm Dis 74 (1956) 699–717.

[259] Y. Zhang, R.J. Wallace Jr., G.H. Mazurek, Genetic differences between BCG substrains, Tuberc. Lung Dis. 76 (1995) 43–50.

[260] M. Gheorghiu, The present and future role of BCG vaccine in tuberculosis control, Biologicals 18 (1990) 135–141.

[261] M. Gheorghiu, P.H. Lagrange, Viability, heat stability and immunogenicity of four BCG vaccines prepared from four different BCG strains, Ann. Immunol. 134C (1983) 124–147.

[262] M.A. Behr, Correlation between BCG genomics and protective efficacy, Scand. J. Infect. Dis. 33 (2001) 249–252.

[263] B. Wu, et al., Unique gene expression profiles in infants vaccinated with different strains of *Mycobacterium bovis* Bacille Calmette-Guérin, Infect. Immun. 75 (2007) 3658–3664.

[264] HG. Lehman, et al., BCG vaccination of neonates, infants, school children and adolescents. II. Safety of vaccine with strain 1331 Copenhagen, Dev. Biol. Stand. 43 (1979) 133–135.

[265] Expanded Programme on Immunization/Biologicals Unit, Lymphadenitis associated with BCG immunization, Wkly Epidemiol. Rec. 63 (1988) 381–388.

[266] Expanded Programme on Immunization/Biologicals Unit, BCG associated lymphadenitis in infants, Wkly Epidemiol. Rec. 30 (1989) 231–323.

[267] L. Kroger, et al., Osteitis after newborn vaccination with three different bacillus Calmette-Guérin vaccines: twenty-nine years of experience, Pediatr. Infect. Dis. J. 12 (1994) 113–116.

[268] H. Mahomed, et al., The impact of a change in Bacille Calmette-Guérin vaccine policy on tuberculosis incidence in children in Cape Town, South Africa, Pediatr. Infect. Dis. J. 25 (2006) 1167–1172.

[269] M.A. Behr, P.M. Small, Declining efficacy of BCG strains over time? A new hypothesis for an old controversy (abstract), Am. J. Respir. Crit. Care Med. 155 (1997) A222.

[270] M.L. Garly, et al., BCG scar and positive tuberculin reaction associated with reduced child mortality in West Africa: a non-specific beneficial effect of BCG? Vaccine 21 (2003) 2782–2790.

[271] A. Roth, et al., Low birth weight infants and Calmette-Guérin bacillus vaccination at birth: community study from Guinea-Bissau, Pediatr. Infect. Dis. J. 23 (2004) 544–550.

[272] H.G. Ten Dam, Research on BCG vaccination, Adv. Tuberc. Res. 21 (1984) 79–106.

[273] A. Lotte, et al., Second IUATLD study on complications induced by intradermal BCG-vaccination, Bull. Int. Union Tuberc. 63 (1988) 47–59.

[274] F.M. Turnbull, et al., National study of adverse reactions after vaccination with bacilli Calmette-Guérin, Clin. Infect. Dis. 34 (2002) 447–453.

[275] J. Reynes, et al., Bacille-Calmette-Guérin adenitis 30 years after immunization in a patient with AIDS (letter), J. Infect. Dis. 160 (1989) 727.

[276] C.G. Helmick, A.J. D'Souza, N. Goddard, An outbreak of severe BCG axillary lymphadenitis in Saint Lucia, 1982–83, West. Indies, Med. J. 35 (1986) 12–17.

[277] K.N. Praveen, et al., Outbreak of bacillus Calmette-Guérin-associated lymphadenitis and abscesses in Jamaican children, Pediatr. Infect. Dis. J. 9 (1990) 890–893.

[278] J.S. Goraya, V.S. Virdi, Treatment of Calmette-Guérin bacillus adenitis: a metaanalysis, Pediatr. Infect. Dis. J. 20 (2001) 632–634.

[279] A. Singla, et al., The natural course of nonsuppurative Calmette-Guérin bacillus lymphadenitis, Pediatr. Infect. Dis. J. 21 (2002) 446–448.

[280] F. Oguz, et al., Treatment of bacillus Calmette-Guérin associated lymphadenitis, Pediatr. Infect. Dis. J. 11 (1992) 887–888.

[281] World Health Organization, BCG Vaccination of the Newborn: Rationale and Guidelines for Country Programs, World Health Organization, Geneva, 1986.

[282] I. Micheli, et al., Evaluation of the effectiveness of BCG vaccination using the case control method in Buenos Aires, Argentina, Int. J. Epidemiol. 17 (1988) 629–634.

[283] A. Lotte, et al., BCG complication: estimates of the risks among vaccinated subjects and statistical analysis of their main characteristics, Adv. Tuberc. Res. 21 (1984) 107–193.

[284] L. Kroger, et al., Osteitis caused by bacillus Calmette-Guérin vaccination: a retrospective analysis of 222 cases, J. Infect. Dis. 172 (1995) 574–576.

[285] M. Bottiger, Osteitis and other complications caused by generalized BCGitis, Acta Paediatr. Scand. 71 (1982) 471–478.

[286] F.K. Pederson, et al., Fatal BCG infection in an immunocompetent girl, Acta Paediatr. Scand. 67 (1978) 519–523.

[287] C.L. Trevenen, R.D. Pagtakhan, Disseminated tuberculoid lesions in infants following BCG, Can. Med. J. 15 (1982) 502–504.

[288] M. Tardieu, et al., Tuberculosis meningitis due to BCG in two previously healthy children, Lancet 1 (1988) 440–441.

[289] A.C. Hesseling, et al., Danish bacilli Calmette-Guérin vaccine-induced disease in human immunodeficiency virus-infected children, Clin. Infect. Dis. 37 (2003) 1226–1233.

[290] J.L. Casanova, et al., Idiopathic disseminated bacilli Calmette-Guérin infection: a French national retrospective study, Pediatrics 98 (1996) 774–778.

[291] B. Gonzalez, et al., Clinical presentation of bacillus Calmette-Guérin infections in patients with immunodeficiency syndromes, Pediatr. Infect. Dis. J. 8 (1989) 201–206.

[292] C. Houde, P. Dery, *Mycobacterium bovis* sepsis in an infant with human immunodeficiency virus infection, Pediatr. Infect. Dis. J. 11 (1988) 810–811.

[293] E.A. Talbot, et al., Disseminated bacilli Calmette-Guérin disease after vaccination: case report and review, Clin. Infect. Dis. 24 (1997) 1139–1146.

[294] E. Jovanguy, et al., Interferon-ChrW(61543)-receptor deficiency in an infant with fatal bacille Calmette-Guérin infection, N. Engl. J. Med. 335 (1996) 1956–1961.

[295] H. Elloumi-Zghal, et al., Clinical and genetic heterogeneity of inherited autosomal recessive susceptibility to disseminated *Mycobacterium bovis* bacilli Calmette-Guérin infection, J. Infect. Dis. 185 (2002) 1468–1475.

[296] C. Armbruster, et al., Disseminated bacilli Calmette-Guérin infection in AIDS patient 30 years after BCG vaccination (letter), J. Infect. Dis. 162 (1990) 1216.

[297] T. Puthanakit, et al., Immune reconstitution syndrome due to bacillus Calmette-Guérin after initiation of antiretroviral therapy in children with HIV infection, Clin. Infect. Dis. 41 (2005) 1049–1052.

[298] M. Besnard, et al., Bacillus Calmette-Guérin infection after vaccination of human immunodeficiency virus-infected children, Pediatr. Infect. Dis. J. 12 (1993) 993–997.

[299] A.C. Hesseling, et al., Bacille Calmette- Guérin vaccine-induced disease in HIV-infected and HIV-uninfected children, Clin. Infect. Dis. 42 (2006) 548–558.

[300] World Health Organization, Revised BCG vaccination guidelines for infants at risk for HIV infection, Wkly Epidemiol. Rec. 21 (2007) 193–196.

[301] R. Menzies, B. Vissandjee, Effect of bacille Calmette-Guérin vaccination on tuberculin reactivity, Am. Rev. Respir. Dis. 145 (1992) 621–625.

[302] M. Lifschitz, The value of the tuberculin skin test as a screening test for tuberculosis among BCG vaccinated children, Pediatrics 36 (1965) 624–627.

[303] O. Horwitz, K. Bunch-Christensen, Correlation between tuberculin sensitivity after 2 months and 5 years among BCG-vaccinated subjects, Bull. World Health Organ. 47 (1972) 49–58.

[304] G.W. Comstock, L.B. Edwards, H. Nabangxang, Tuberculin sensitivity eight to fifteen years after BCG vaccination, Am. Rev. Respir. Dis. 103 (1971) 572–575.

[305] S. Landi, M.J. Ashley, S. Grzybowski, Tuberculin skin sensitivity following the intradermal and multiple puncture methods of BCG vaccination, Can. Med. Assoc. J. 97 (1967) 222–225.

[306] M.J. Ashley, C.O. Seibenmann, Tuberculin skin sensitivity following BCG vaccination with vaccines of high and low viable counts, Can. Med. Assoc. J. 97 (1967) 1335–1338.

[307] E.B. Kemp, R.B. Belshe, D.F. Hoft, Immune responses stimulated by percutaneous and intradermal bacilli Calmette-Guérin, J. Infect. Dis. 174 (1996) 113–119.

[308] J.H. Joncas, R. Robitaille, T. Gauthier, Interpretation of the PPD skin test in BCG-vaccinated children, Can. Med. Assoc. J. 113 (1975) 127–128.

[309] K. Mangus, L.B. Edwards, The effect of repeated tuberculin testing on post-vaccination allergy, Lancet 1 (1955) 643–644.

[310] S. Karalliede, L.P. Katugha, C.G. Uragoda, The tuberculin response of Sri Lankan children after BCG vaccination at birth, Tubercle 68 (1987) 33–38.

[311] R. Sleiman, et al., Interpretation of the tuberculin skin test in bacille Calmette-Guérin vaccinated and nonvaccinated school children, Pediatr. Infect. Dis. J. 26 (2007) 134–138.

[312] N.J. Thompson, et al., The booster phenomenon in serial tuberculin testing, Am. Rev. Respir. Dis. 119 (1979) 587–597.

[313] R.L. Sepulveda, et al., Booster effect of tuberculin testing in healthy 6-year-old school children vaccinated with bacillus Calmette-Guérin at birth in Santiago, Chile, Pediatr. Infect. Dis. J. 7 (1988) 578–581.

[314] G. Colditz, et al., The efficacy of bacillus Calmette-Guérin vaccination of newborns and infants in the prevention of tuberculosis: meta-analysis of the published literature, Pediatrics 96 (1995) 29–35.

[315] G.A. Colditz, et al., Efficacy of BCG vaccine in the prevention of tuberculosis: meta-analysis of the published literature, JAMA 271 (1994) 698–702.

[316] B.B. Trunz, P.E.M. Fine, C. Dye, Effect of BCG vaccination on childhood tuberculosis meningitis and miliary tuberculosis worldwide: a meta-analysis and assessment of cost-effectiveness, Lancet 367 (2006) 1173–1180.

[317] M.E. Avery, J. Wolfsdorf, Diagnosis and treatment: approaches to newborn infants of tuberculous mothers, Pediatrics 42 (1968) 519–521.

[318] B.A. Dormer, et al., Prophylactic isoniazid protection of infants in a tuberculosis hospital, Lancet 2 (1959) 902–903.

[319] I.J. Light, M. Saidleman, J.M. Sutherland, Management of newborns after nursery exposure to tuberculosis, Am. Rev. Respir. Dis. 109 (1974) 415–419.

[320] H.S. Raucher, I. Grimbetz, Care of the pregnant woman with tuberculosis and her newborn infant: a pediatrician's perspective, Mt. Sinai J. Med. 53 (1986) 70–75.

[321] Centers for Disease Control and Prevention, The role of BCG vaccine in the prevention and control of tuberculosis in the United States: a joint statement by the Advisory Council for the Elimination of Tuberculosis and the Advisory Committee on Immunization Practices, MMWR Morb. Mortal. Wkly Rep. 45 (RR-4) (1996) 1–18.

[322] M.R. Sedaghatian, F. Hashem, M.M. Hossain, Bacille Calmette Guérin vaccination in pre-term infants, Int. J. Tuberc. Lung Dis. 2 (1998) 679–682.

[323] J. Lorber, P.C. Menneer, Long-term effectiveness of B.C.G. vaccination of infants in close contact with infectious tuberculosis, BMJ 1 (1959) 1430–1433.

[324] H.F. Pabst, et al., Effect of breastfeeding on immune response to BCG vaccination, Lancet 1 (1989) 295–297.

[325] E.L. Kendig Jr., The place of BCG vaccine in the management of infants born to tuberculous mothers, N. Engl. J. Med. 281 (1969) 520–523.

[326] H.M. Curtis, F.N. Bamford, I. Leck, Incidence of childhood tuberculosis after neonatal BCG vaccination, Lancet 1 (1984) 145–148.

[327] B. Nivin, et al., A continuing outbreak of multidrug-resistant tuberculosis with transmission in a hospital nursery, Clin. Infect. Dis. 26 (1998) 303–307.

[328] J.J. Nania, et al., Exposure to pulmonary tuberculosis in a neonatal intensive care unit: unique aspects of contact investigation and management of hospitalized neonates, Infect. Control Hosp. Epidemiol. 28 (2007) 661–665.

[329] H. Ohno, et al., A contact investigation of the transmission of *Mycobacterium tuberculosis* from a nurse working in a newborn nursery and maternity ward, J. Infect. Chemother. 14 (2008) 66–71.

[330] F.E. Berkowitz, J.L. Severens, H.M. Blumberg, Exposure to tuberculosis among newborns in a nursery: decision analysis for initiation of prophylaxis, Infect. Control Hosp. Epidemiol. 27 (2006) 604–611.

[331] Centers for Disease Control and Prevention, Guidelines for preventing the transmission of *Mycobacterium tuberculosis* in health-care facilities, MMWR Morb. Mortal. Wkly Rep. 43 (RR-13):1–133, 1994.

[332] J.R. Starke, Transmission of *Mycobacterium tuberculosis* to and from children and adolescents, Semin. Pediatr. Infect. Dis. 12 (2001) 115–123.

[333] H.L. Lee, C.M. LeVea, P.S. Graman, Congenital tuberculosis in a neonatal intensive care unit: case report, epidemiological investigation, and management of exposures, Clin. Infect. Dis. 27 (1998) 474–477.

[334] K.P. Manji, et al., Tuberculosis (presumed congenital) in a neonatal unit in Dar-es-Salaam, Tanzania, J. Trop. Pediatr. 47 (2001) 15–155.

[335] T. Pillay, M. Adhikari, Congenital tuberculosis in a neonatal intensive care unit, Clin. Infect. Dis. 29 (1999) 467–468.

[336] G.A. Machin, et al., Perinatally acquired neonatal tuberculosis: report of two cases, Pediatr. Pathol. 12 (1992) 707–716.

[337] G. Rabalais, G. Adams, B. Stover, PPD skin test conversion in healthcare workers after exposure to *Mycobacterium tuberculosis* infection in infants, Lancet 338 (1991) 826.

[338] M. Saitoh, et al., Connatal tuberculosis in an extremely low birth weight infant: case report and management of exposure to tuberculosis in a neonatal intensive care nursery, Eur. J. Pediatr. 160 (2001) 88–90.

[339] B.W. Laartz, et al., Congenital tuberculosis and management of exposures in a neonatal intensive care unit, Infect. Control Hosp. Epidemiol. 23 (2002) 573–579.

[340] F. Mouchet, et al., Tuberculosis in healthcare workers caring for a congenitally infected infant, Infect. Control Hosp. Epidemiol. 35 (2004) 1062–1066.

[341] M. Crockett, et al., Nosocomial transmission of congenital tuberculosis in a neonatal intensive care unit, Clin. Infect. Dis. 39 (2004) 1719–1723.

CHLAMYDIA INFECTIONS

Toni Darville

CHAPTER OUTLINE

Epidemiology and Transmission   601
Microbiology   601
    Pathogen   601
    Chlamydial Developmental Cycle   602
Pathogenesis   602
    Conjunctivitis   602
    Pneumonia   603
Pathology   603
Clinical Manifestations   603
    Conjunctivitis   603
    Pneumonia   603
    Perinatal Infections at Other Sites   603

Diagnosis   604
    Conjunctivitis   604
    Pneumonia   604
Differential Diagnosis   604
    Conjunctivitis   604
    Pneumonia   604
Prognosis   605
    Conjunctivitis   605
    Pneumonia   605
Therapy   605
Prevention   605

In 1911, Lindner and colleagues [1] identified typical intracytoplasmic inclusions in infants with a nongonococcal form of ophthalmia neonatorum called *inclusion conjunctivitis of the newborn* (ICN) or inclusion blennorrhea, leading to the elucidation of the epidemiology of sexually transmitted chlamydial infections. Mothers of affected infants were found to have inclusions in their cervical epithelial cells, and fathers of affected infants had inclusions in their urethral cells. For 50 years, cytologic demonstration of chlamydial inclusions in epithelial cells was the only diagnostic procedure available. When chlamydial isolation procedures were developed, first in the yolk sac of the embryonated hen's egg and later in tissue culture, studies again showed *Chlamydia trachomatis* as the etiology of conjunctivitis in the index case and then confirmed the genital tract reservoir of the agent [2]. Although ICN was studied for 60 years, an appreciation of the importance of chlamydial infection of the respiratory tract in infants did not evolve until the late 1970s, with the impetus of the report by Beem and Saxon [3].

C. trachomatis is now recognized as the most common sexually transmitted pathogen in Western industrialized society. Although most *C. trachomatis* infections in men and women are asymptomatic, infection can lead to severe reproductive complications in women. The infection can be transmitted from an infected mother to her newborn during delivery, producing conjunctivitis or pneumonia or both. *C. trachomatis* is likely the most common cause of conjunctivitis in infants younger than 1 month of age and is a common cause of afebrile pneumonia in infants younger than 3 months.

EPIDEMIOLOGY AND TRANSMISSION

C. trachomatis is the most common bacterial cause of sexually transmitted infections in the United States. Reported prevalence rates in the United States include 2% to 7% among female college students, 4% to 12% among women attending a family planning clinic, and 6% to 20% among men and women attending a clinic for sexually transmitted diseases or persons entering correctional facilities [4,5]. In the United Kingdom, data suggest that the rate of infection among young women exceeds 10% [6]. Prevalence rates have declined in areas where screening and treatment programs have been implemented [7]. Many men and most women infected with *C. trachomatis* are either asymptomatic or minimally symptomatic, and presentation for diagnosis is a result of screening or referral after a contact develops symptoms. This is in contrast to gonococcal infections, in which most infected individuals are symptomatic and present acutely for care. Regional estimates are hampered by underdiagnosis and underreporting of cases. Because symptoms are absent or minimal in most women and many men, a large reservoir of asymptomatic infection is present that can sustain the pathogen within a community.

Young age (<20 years) is the sociodemographic factor most strongly associated with chlamydial infection (relative risk among women <25 years old compared with older women is 2 to 3.5) [8]. Although the prevalence of chlamydial infection is increased in black or socioeconomically disadvantaged individuals, there is broad socioeconomic and geographic distribution of infection [9,10]. Other risk factors for cervical chlamydial infection in women are anatomic or hormonal (i.e., use of depot-medroxyprogesterone acetate injections [11] or ectopy after use of oral contraceptives), behavioral (i.e., number of sexual partners), or microbiologic (i.e., concurrent gonorrhea) [12].

For purposes relevant to this chapter, the major method of transmission of *C. trachomatis* is sexual. The child-to-child and intrafamilial infecting patterns that predominate in trachoma endemic areas have not been proven to cause disease in newborns [13]. Chlamydiae cause one-third to one half of nongonococcal urethritis in men, and concomitant infections with gonococci are common in both men and women [14,15].

An infant born to a mother with a chlamydial infection of the cervix is at 60% to 70% risk of acquiring the infection during passage through the birth canal [16]. Of exposed infants, 20% to 50% develop conjunctivitis, and 10% to 20% develop pneumonia. The rectum and vagina of infants exposed during delivery may also be infected, but a clear-cut relationship with disease in these sites has not yet been elucidated [17]. In utero transmission is not known to occur. Infection after cesarean section is seen rarely, usually after premature rupture of the membranes. No evidence supports postnatal transmission from the mother or other family members.

Studies in the 1980s identified *C. trachomatis* in 14% to 46% of infants younger than 1 month of age with conjunctivitis [18]. The prevalence of neonatal chlamydial inclusion conjunctivitis has decreased in recent years in areas where screening and treatment of chlamydial infection in pregnant women is a regular practice [19]. In the Netherlands, prenatal screening for *C. trachomatis* is not routine.

Evaluation of infants younger than 3 months of age referred to a Dutch children's hospital or to an ophthalmologist for evaluation of persistent conjunctivitis from 1996-2002 revealed *C. trachomatis* infection in 63% [20].

There is no evidence to suggest that infants with chlamydial infections should be isolated. Transmission of the organism to other infants in nurseries or intensive care units has not been reported. Standard precautions consisting of hand hygiene between patient contacts is recommended. Use of protective gloves, masks or face shields, and nonsterile gowns is recommended when performing procedures likely to generate splashes of body fluids, secretions, or excretions.

MICROBIOLOGY
PATHOGEN

Chlamydiae are obligate intracellular parasites that cause various diseases in animal species at virtually all phylogenetic levels. Traditionally, the order Chlamydiales has contained one genus with four recognized species: *C. trachomatis*, *Chlamydia psittaci*, *Chlamydia pneumoniae*, and *Chlamydia pecorum*. More recent taxonomic analysis involving the 16S and 23S rRNA genes have found that the order Chlamydiales contains at least four distinct groups at the family level and provides a potential rationale for splitting the genus *Chlamydia* into two genera, *Chlamydia* and *Chlamydophila* [21]. The genus *Chlamydophila* would contain *C. pneumoniae*, *C. pecorum*, and *C. psittaci*. This new classification continues to be controversial, and for the purposes of this chapter these organisms are referred to as *Chlamydia*.

C. psittaci is responsible for psittacosis, a chlamydial infection contracted by humans from infected birds and characterized by interstitial pneumonitis. This infection should be suspected in any patient with atypical pneumonia who has contact with birds. *C. pneumoniae* causes pneumonia, pharyngitis, and bronchitis in humans and may accelerate atherosclerosis. Epidemiologic studies have revealed that *C. pneumoniae* is a common cause of infection in school-age children and young adults; along with *Mycoplasma*, it is probably the most common cause of community-acquired pneumonia in this age group. It is not known to cause disease in newborns and is not discussed further. *C. trachomatis* is associated with a spectrum of diseases. The species *C. trachomatis* contains 18 serologically distinct variants known as serovars. Serovars A, B, Ba, and C cause ocular trachoma, a major cause of blindness in many developing countries, particularly in Africa, Asia, and the Middle East. Ocular trachoma is considered the most common cause of preventable blindness in the world. Three serovars, L_1, L_2, and L_3, are associated with lymphogranuloma venereum, a sexually transmitted disease that is rare in the United States, but is still quite prevalent in many developing countries, and are particularly prevalent in tropical and subtropical areas. Perinatal transmission is rare with lymphogranuloma venereum. Serovars D through K produce infections of the genital tract—urethritis and epididymitis in men and cervicitis and salpingitis in women—the most prevalent chlamydial diseases. Major complications of female genital tract disease include acute pelvic inflammatory disease, ectopic pregnancy, infertility, and infant pneumonia and conjunctivitis.

Similar to gram-negative bacteria, chlamydiae have an outer membrane that contains lipopolysaccharide and membrane proteins, but their outer membrane contains no detectable peptidoglycan, despite the presence of genes encoding proteins for its synthesis [22]. This more recent genomic finding is the basis for the so-called chlamydial peptidoglycan paradox, for it has been known for years that chlamydial development is inhibited by β-lactam antibiotics. Although chlamydiae contain DNA, RNA, and ribosomes, during growth and replication they obtain high-energy phosphate compounds from the host cell. Consequently, they are considered energy parasites. The chlamydial genome size is only 660 kDa, which is smaller than that of any other prokaryote except *Mycoplasma* species. All chlamydiae encode an abundant protein, the major outer membrane protein (MOMP) that is surface exposed in *C. trachomatis* and *C. psittaci*, but not in *C. pneumoniae* [23]. MOMP is the major determinant of the serologic classification of *C. trachomatis* and *C. psittaci* isolates.

CHLAMYDIAL DEVELOPMENTAL CYCLE

The biphasic developmental cycle of chlamydiae is unique among microorganisms and involves two highly specialized morphologic forms, as shown in Figure 19–1. The extracellular form or elementary body (EB) contains extensive disulfide cross-links within and between outer membrane proteins giving it an almost sporelike structure that is stable outside of the cell. The small (350 nm in diameter) infectious EB is inactive metabolically. The developmental cycle is initiated when an EB attaches to a susceptible epithelial cell. Numerous candidate adhesins have been proposed, but their identity and that of associated epithelial cell receptors remain uncertain. One documented mechanism of entry into the epithelial cell is by receptor-mediated endocytosis via clathrin-coated pits [24], but evidence exists that chlamydiae may exploit multiple mechanisms of entry. The process of EB internalization is very efficient, suggesting that EBs trigger their own internalization by cells that are not considered professional phagocytes.

When inside the cell, surface antigens of the EB seem to prevent fusion of the endosome with lysosomes, protecting itself from enzymatic destruction. Hiding from host attack by antibody or cell mediated defenses, the EB reorganizes into the replicative form, the reticulate body (RB). RBs successfully parasitize the host cell and divide and multiply. As the RB divides by binary fission, it fills the endosome, now a cytoplasmic inclusion, with its progeny. After 48 to 72 hours, multiplication ceases, and nucleoid condensation occurs as the RBs transform to new infectious EBs. The EBs are released from the cell by cytolysis [25]; by a process of exocytosis [26]; or by extrusion of the whole inclusion [26], leaving the host cell intact. The last-mentioned process may explain the frequency of asymptomatic or subclinical chlamydial infections. Release of the infectious EBs allows infection of new host cells to occur.

PATHOGENESIS
CONJUNCTIVITIS

Chlamydiae replicate extensively in epithelial cells of the conjunctiva and cause considerable cell damage. The inflammatory reaction consists mostly of polymorphonuclear leukocytes. Conjunctivitis in most untreated patients resolves spontaneously during the first few months of life. Occasionally, infants maintain persistent conjunctivitis, and pannus formation (neovascularization of the cornea) and scarring typical of trachoma have been reported [2,27]. Loss of vision is rare. Micropannus and some scarring may occur in infants if they are not treated within the first 2 weeks of the disease [28]. If treated early, no ocular sequelae develop.

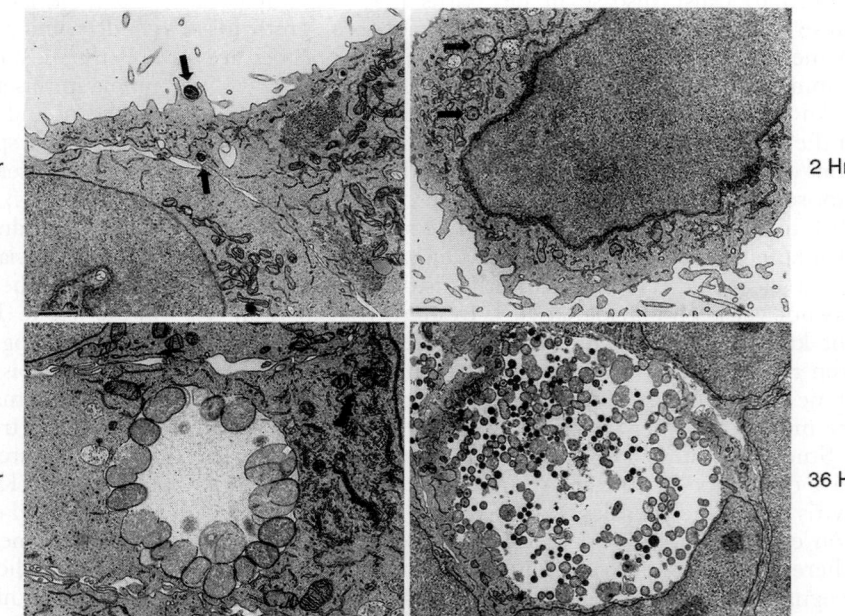

FIGURE 19–1 *Chlamydia trachomatis developmental cycle.* Infection is initiated by elementary bodies (EBs). *0 Hr,* Immediately after endocytosis. EBs are found within tightly associated membrane vesicles. *2 Hr,* Within a few hours, EBs differentiate into larger, metabolically active reticulate bodies (RBs). *18 Hr,* As RBs multiply, inclusion increases in size to accommodate bacterial progeny. RBs are typically observed juxtaposed to inclusion membrane. *36 Hr,* As infection progresses, increasing numbers of chlamydiae are observed unattached in interior of inclusion. These unattached organisms are, for the most part, EBs and intermediate developmental forms. EBs accumulate within inclusion even as RBs, still associated with inclusion membrane, continue to multiply, until cell undergoes lysis at 40 to 48 hours after infection. *(From Stephens RS [ed]. Chlamydia: Intracellular Biology, Pathogenesis, and Immunity. Washington, DC, ASM Press, 1999, p 102.)*

PNEUMONIA

The nasopharynx is the most frequent site of perinatally acquired chlamydial infection, with approximately 70% of infected infants having positive cultures at that site [29]. Most of these infections are asymptomatic and may persist for 29 months [30]. Chlamydial pneumonia develops in only about 30% of infants with nasopharyngeal infection. Conjunctivitis is not a prerequisite for development of pneumonia.

PATHOLOGY

In ICN, the affected conjunctiva is highly vascularized and edematous. Inclusions are found in the conjunctival epithelial cells. There is a massive infiltration of polymorphonuclear leukocytes, and pseudomembrane formation may occur. Lymphoid follicles, such as are seen in adults or older children with chlamydial infection of the conjunctiva, are not usually observed until the disease has been active for 1 or 2 months. Because ICN spontaneously resolves by that time in most infants, lymphoid follicles are not commonly observed.

Because pneumonia is rarely fatal, and in most infants the course is relatively benign, there has been little occasion to obtain lung specimens. When lung specimens have been obtained, no characteristic features have been described. Biopsy material has shown pleural congestion and alveolar and bronchiolar mononuclear cell infiltrates with eosinophils and focal aggregations of neutrophils [31,32].

CLINICAL MANIFESTATIONS

The principal clinical manifestations in infants are ICN, occurring in the first 3 weeks of life, and pneumonia, which occurs within the first 3 months.

CONJUNCTIVITIS

ICN usually has an incubation period of 5 to 14 days after delivery or earlier if amniotic membranes ruptured prematurely. Approximately one third of infants exposed to chlamydiae during vaginal delivery develop conjunctivitis [33]. Disease manifestations vary widely and range from mild conjunctival injection with scant mucoid discharge to severe mucopurulent conjunctivitis with chemosis and pseudomembrane formation. The eyelids swell, and the conjunctivae become injected and swollen (Fig. 19–2). The "pseudomembrane" consists of inflammatory exudate that adheres to the inflamed surface of the conjunctiva. Except for micropannus formation, the cornea is usually spared. Evaluation of 37 Dutch infants who tested positive for *Chlamydia* revealed mucopurulent eye discharge as the presenting symptom for 35 (95%), swelling of the eyelids for 27 (73%), and conjunctival erythema for 24 (65%); bilateral eye involvement was observed in 27 infants (73%). Presenting symptoms were similar in a group of 22 infants diagnosed with other bacterial pathogens [20].

PNEUMONIA

Neonatal chlamydial pneumonia was first reported in 1975, and the characteristic clinical picture was described in 1977 [3,34]. Most infants with chlamydial pneumonia

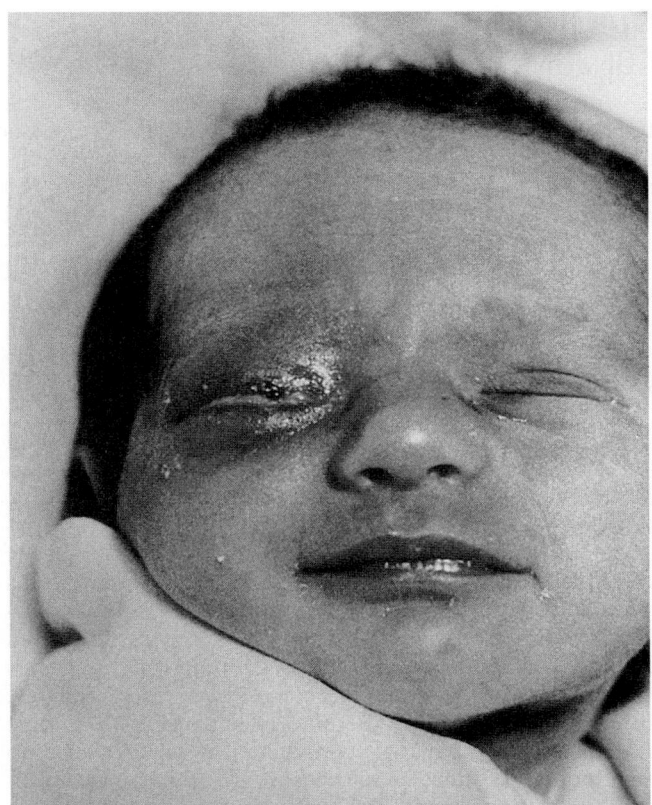

FIGURE 19–2 Infant with chlamydial conjunctivitis. *(From Long S, Pickering LK, Prober CG [eds]. Principles and Practice of Pediatric Infectious Diseases. New York, Churchill Livingstone, 2003, p 904.)*

are symptomatic before the 8th week of life with the insidious development of nasal obstruction or discharge or both, tachypnea, and a repetitive staccato cough. Some infants may have symptoms the 2nd week of life, initially involving the upper respiratory tract. Characteristically, infants have been symptomatic for 3 or more weeks before presentation. Most are only moderately ill and are afebrile. A history or presence of conjunctivitis can be elicited in half the cases [35]. Some infants may develop apnea. Crepitant inspiratory rales are commonly heard. Expiratory wheezes are distinctly uncommon.

Hyperinflation of the lungs usually accompanies the infiltrates seen on chest radiographs. Infiltrates are most commonly bilateral and interstitial; reticulonodular patterns and atelectasis have also been described [36]. Possible laboratory findings include a distinctive peripheral eosinophilia (>400 cells/mm^3), mild arterial hypoxemia, and elevated serum immunoglobulins. Untreated disease can linger or recur. In very young infants, infection may be more severe and associated with apnea.

PERINATAL INFECTIONS AT OTHER SITES

Infants born to mothers infected with *C. trachomatis* may also become infected in the rectum and urogenital tract [37]. Although these infections are generally asymptomatic, they may persist for 3 years [37]. Consequently, differentiating infection acquired perinatally from infection resulting from sexual abuse can be particularly difficult in young children.

DIAGNOSIS

CONJUNCTIVITIS

Several nonculture methods are approved by the U.S. Food and Drug Administration (FDA) for the diagnosis of ICN. These include enzyme immunoassays, specifically, Chlamydiazyme (Abbott Diagnostics, Chicago, IL) and MicroTrak EIA (Genetic Systems, Seattle, WA) and direct fluorescent antibody assays using fluorescein-conjugated monoclonal antibodies to stain chlamydial EBs in a smear, including Syva MicroTrak (Genetic Systems) and Pathfinder (Sanofi-Pasteur, Chaska, MN). These tests perform well on conjunctival specimens, with sensitivities of greater than 90% and specificities of 95% or greater compared with culture [38–40].

For resource-poor settings, a useful diagnostic method is examination of Giemsa-stained conjunctival scrapings for the presence of blue-stained intracytoplasmic inclusions within epithelial cells. The sensitivity of the test varies from 22% to 95% depending on the technique of specimen collection and the examiner's expertise. This method also allows visualization of bacteria, such as gonococci, and of cytologic findings suggesting viral infection. Isolation of chlamydiae from conjunctival scrapings inoculated into tissue cell culture is a more reliable, although more costly, method of diagnosis. Serologic diagnosis of chlamydial conjunctivitis (in contrast to pneumonia) is unreliable because of the presence of maternally transmitted IgG antibody and the unreliable appearance of IgM antibody in this infection.

Even if a firm diagnosis of chlamydial conjunctivitis is established, one must be mindful of the possibility of a dual infection, particularly with *Neisseria gonorrhoeae*. For this reason, appropriate stain and culture of the conjunctival exudate should be obtained.

Highly sensitive nucleic acid amplification tests (NAATs) are commercially available for diagnosis of genital chlamydial infection in adolescents and adults [41,42]. NAATs have FDA approval for cervical swabs from women, urethral swabs from men, and urine from men and women. These tests have high sensitivity, perhaps even detecting 10% to 20% more cases of genital chlamydial infection than possible with culture, while retaining high specificity [43]. Information on the use of NAATs in children is limited, but preliminary data suggest that PCR is equivalent to culture for the detection of *C. trachomatis* in the conjunctiva and nasopharynx of infants with conjunctivitis [44]. More recent data indicate NAATs are significantly more sensitive than cell culture for diagnosis of *C. trachomatis* from genital and nongenital specimens [45].

PNEUMONIA

Enzyme immunoassays and direct fluorescent antibody assays for *Chlamydia* do not perform well with nasopharyngeal specimens and are not approved for this purpose. The definitive diagnosis of pneumonia can be made by culture of the organism from the respiratory tract. *Chlamydia* culture has been defined by the U.S. Centers for Disease Control and Prevention (CDC) as isolation of the organism in tissue culture and confirmation by microscopic identification of the characteristic inclusions by fluorescent antibody staining [46]. The likelihood of obtaining a positive culture is enhanced by deep suction of the trachea or by collecting a nasopharyngeal aspirate, rather than obtaining a specimen with a swab [3,47]. An acute microimmunofluorescence serum titer of *C. trachomatis*–specific IgM of 1:32 or greater is also diagnostic. In contrast, IgG is not diagnostic because passively transferred maternal antibody may persist at high titers for months. The serologic test of choice is the microimmunofluorescent procedure of Wang and colleagues [48], in which EBs are used as antigen. Only a few clinical reference laboratories perform this test.

Indirect evidence of chlamydial pneumonia includes hyperinflation and bilateral diffuse infiltrates on chest radiographs, eosinophilia of 0.3 to 0.4 × 10^9/L (300 to 400/μL) or more in peripheral blood counts, and increased total serum IgG (>5 g/L [>500 mg/dL]) and IgM (>1.1 g/L [>110 mg/dL]) concentrations. The absence of any or all of these findings does not exclude the diagnosis, however.

DIFFERENTIAL DIAGNOSIS

CONJUNCTIVITIS

ICN must be distinguished from conjunctivitis produced by pyogenic bacteria, particularly *N. gonorrhoeae*. Gonococcal ophthalmia usually occurs earlier, about 2 to 5 days after birth, although overlap in age at onset can occur. Gonococcal disease is usually more rapidly progressive than disease caused by *C. trachomatis*. Gonococcal infection can be diagnosed presumptively by examination of the Gram-stained smear of the exudate and confirmed by culture of the exudate. Staphylococcal conjunctivitis is usually acquired nosocomially from the nursery environment. It is characterized more by purulent discharge than by redness. This and other forms of pyogenic conjunctivitis—which may be due to *S. pneumoniae*, *Haemophilus* species, or gram-negative bacteria such as *Pseudomonas aeruginosa*—can be appropriately diagnosed by Gram stain and culture of the exudate.

Of viral infections, neonatal herpes simplex (see Chapter 26) is the most important. This disease is characterized by involvement of the skin and the eye, vesicle formation, and sometimes corneal involvement. Adenovirus infection of the newborn is very rare, but has been described.

Chemical conjunctivitis related to instillation of silver nitrate at birth may also produce marked redness and a purulent discharge. These symptoms start on the first day of life and disappear after a few days, however, distinguishing this entity from a chlamydial infection.

PNEUMONIA

An afebrile, tachypneic infant presenting with a staccato cough in the first 3 months of life is very likely to have chlamydial disease. Cytomegalovirus may produce an interstitial pneumonia in preterm newborns who receive transfusions from cytomegalovirus-positive donors; however, it often produces signs and symptoms in other organ systems. Congenital infections with the rubella virus and

Toxoplasma gondii also produce multiorgan involvement, as does perinatal infection with herpes simplex virus. Adenovirus or parainfluenza virus infection may produce an interstitial pneumonia, but without the characteristic staccato cough or eosinophilia. Respiratory syncytial virus is a common cause of pneumonia in early infancy, but it often produces fever in the early stages, and wheezing because of airway obstruction is common with this illness. Respiratory syncytial virus is not associated with eosinophilia. Respiratory syncytial virus infection can be rapidly diagnosed by performing an enzyme immunoassay on a nasopharyngeal wash specimen.

Many pyogenic bacteria may produce lower respiratory tract infections in infancy. Group B streptococci, *Streptococcus pneumoniae*, *Staphylococcus aureus*, *Haemophilus influenzae*, and coliform bacteria are the most common. These patients are generally much sicker, are more toxic and febrile, and have pulmonary consolidation rather than an interstitial infiltrate. *Bordetella pertussis* classically causes a paroxysmal cough with an inspiratory whoop and post-tussive emesis. Lymphocytosis is seen with whooping cough, and apnea occurs in infants younger than 6 months of age. Infants with *Pneumocystis jiroveci* pneumonia develop a characteristic syndrome of subacute diffuse pneumonitis with dyspnea at rest, tachypnea, oxygen desaturation, nonproductive cough, and fever.

PROGNOSIS
CONJUNCTIVITIS

If untreated, ICN may persist for many weeks, but it usually resolves spontaneously without complications. The scarring that occurs in trachoma that leads to lid deformities is not seen. Superficial corneal vascularization and conjunctival scar formation can occur, however [27,28,49].

PNEUMONIA

Untreated infants are usually ill for several weeks, with frequent cough, poor feeding, and poor weight gain. A few infants require oxygen, and fewer require ventilatory support. Beem and colleagues [50] found in a series of 11 infants that the total course of illness is 24 to 61 days, with an average of 43 days; mortality is exceptionally rare. Follow-up evaluation of a small cohort of children who had *C. trachomatis* pneumonia in infancy showed an increased prevalence of chronic cough and abnormal lung function compared with age-matched controls [51].

THERAPY

Topical treatment of inclusion conjunctivitis is not recommended primarily because of failure to eliminate concurrent nasopharyngeal infection. Recommended therapy for conjunctivitis is oral erythromycin, 50 mg/kg/day in four divided doses for 14 days. Topical treatment of conjunctivitis is ineffective and unnecessary. The failure rate is around 20%, and a second course of therapy may be required [29,52]. Problems with compliance and tolerance are frequent. Oral sulfonamides may

be used after the immediate neonatal period for infants who do not tolerate erythromycin.

Chlamydial pneumonia is treated with oral azithromycin, 20 mg/kg, once daily for 3 days, or erythromycin, 50 mg/kg/day in four divided doses for 14 days. An oral sulfonamide is an alternative for infants who do not tolerate macrolides. There is convincing evidence that this treatment shortens the clinical course of pneumonia and eliminates the organism from the respiratory tract. Beyond specific antimicrobial therapy, infants require standard support measures, with attention to nutrition and to fluid status. Oxygen and ventilatory therapy may be required in a few cases. A specific diagnosis of *C. trachomatis* infection in an infant should prompt treatment of the mother and sexual partners.

An association between orally administered erythromycin and infantile hypertrophic pyloric stenosis (IHPS) has been reported in infants younger than 6 weeks of age who were given the drug for prophylaxis after nursery exposure to pertussis [53,54]. The risk of IHPS after treatment with other macrolides (e.g., azithromycin dihydrate and clarithromycin) is unknown. Because confirmation of erythromycin as a contributor to cases of IHPS requires additional investigation and because alternative therapies are not as well studied, the American Academy of Pediatrics continues to recommend use of erythromycin for treatment of *C. trachomatis* in infants. Parents of infants treated with erythromycin should be informed about the signs and potential risks of developing IHPS. Cases of pyloric stenosis after use of oral erythromycin should be reported to the FDA as an adverse drug reaction. One small study suggests that a short course of orally administered azithromycin, 20 mg/kg/day, one dose daily for 3 days, may be effective [19].

Prophylactic therapy of infants born to mothers known to have untreated chlamydial infection is not indicated because the efficacy of such prophylaxis is unknown. Infants should be monitored for signs of infection and to ensure appropriate treatment if infection develops. If adequate follow-up cannot be ensured, prophylaxis may be considered.

PREVENTION

Because *C. trachomatis* infections are transmitted vertically from mother to infant during delivery, an effective prevention measure is screening and treatment of pregnant women for *C. trachomatis* infection before delivery. The CDC currently recommends screening all pregnant women during their first prenatal visit and during the third trimester if high risk (<25 years old or other risk factors such as new or multiple sexual partners) [46]. Erythromycin base (2 g/day in four divided doses) and amoxicillin (1.5 g/day in three divided doses) for 7 days are recommended treatment regimens for pregnant women. Half doses of erythromycin daily for 14 days may be given in pregnant women who are intolerant of the full dose regimen. Because these regimens are not highly efficacious, a second course of therapy may be needed. Azithromycin (1 g orally as a single dose) is an alternative; preliminary data suggest it is safe and effective [55]. Doxycycline and ofloxacin are contraindicated during pregnancy.

Ocular prophylaxis with topical erythromycin or tetracycline has reduced the incidence of gonococcal ophthalmia, but does not seem to be effective against *C. trachomatis* [56]. The only means of preventing chlamydial infection of the newborn is treatment of infected mothers before delivery.

Ongoing efforts to develop a *C. trachomatis* vaccine to protect persons from genital tract infection have concentrated primarily on the use of peptides derived from MOMP or recombinant synthetic MOMP polypeptides as immunogens. Future work may incorporate molecular technology and our increasing understanding of the host response to chlamydiae to develop one or more new vaccines. Stimulation of long-term mucosal immunity in the genital tract is a challenge; it is unclear whether all genital infections could be prevented, or whether only more invasive disease, such as salpingitis, might be preventable using vaccine technology.

REFERENCES

[1] K. Lindner, Gonoblennorrhoe, einschlussblennorrhoe und trachoma, Albrecht Von Graefes Arch. Ophthalmol. 78 (1911) 380.

[2] B.R. Jones, M.K. Al-Hussaini, E.M.C. Dunlop, Genital infection in association with TRIC virus infection of the eye. I. Isolation of virus from urethra, cervix, and eye: preliminary report, Br. J. Vener. Dis. 40 (1964) 19–24.

[3] M.O. Beem, E.M. Saxon, Respiratory tract colonization and a distinctive pneumonia syndrome in infants infected with *Chlamydia trachomatis*, N. Engl. J. Med. 296 (1977) 306–310.

[4] W.E. Stamm, *Chlamydia trachomatis* infections of the adult, in: K.K. Holmes, P.A. Mardh, P.F. Sparling (Eds.), Sexually Transmitted Diseases, third ed., McGraw-Hill, New York, 1999, pp. 407–422.

[5] J. Hardick, et al., Surveillance of *Chlamydia trachomatis* and *Neisseria gonorrhoeae* infections in women in detention in Baltimore, Maryland, Sex. Transm. Dis. 30 (2003) 64–70.

[6] JM. Tobin, Chlamydia screening in primary care. Is it useful, affordable and universal? Curr. Opin. Infect. Dis. 15 (2002) 31–36.

[7] B. Herrmann, M. Egger, Genital *Chlamydia trachomatis* infections in Uppsala County, Sweden, 1985–1993. Declining rates for how much longer? Sex. Transm. Dis. 22 (1995) 253–260.

[8] C.A. Gaydos, et al., Sustained high prevalence of *Chlamydia trachomatis* infections in female army recruits, Sex. Transm. Dis. 30 (2003) 539–544.

[9] G.R. Burstein, et al., Incident *Chlamydia trachomatis* infections among inner-city adolescent females, JAMA 280 (1998) 521–526.

[10] C.A. Gaydos, et al., *Chlamydia trachomatis* infections in female military recruits, N. Engl. J. Med. 339 (1998) 739–744.

[11] D.L. Jacobson, et al., Relationship of hormonal contraception and cervical ectopy as measured by computerized planimetry to chlamydial infection in adolescents, Sex. Transm. Dis. 27 (2000) 313–319.

[12] M.R. Chacko, J.C. Lovchik, *Chlamydia trachomatis* infection in sexually active adolescents: prevalence and risk factors, Pediatrics 73 (1984) 836–840.

[13] B.R. Jones, The prevention of blindness from trachoma, Trans. Ophthalmol. Soc. U.K. 95 (1975) 16–33.

[14] K.K. Holmes, et al., Etiology of nongonococcal urethritis, N. Engl. J. Med. 292 (1975) 1199–1204.

[15] CDC, Sexually Transmitted Disease Surveillance. 2001, Centers for Disease Control and Prevention, Atlanta, GA, 2002.

[16] M.R. Hammerschlag, et al., Prospective study of maternal and infantile infection with *Chlamydia trachomatis*, Pediatrics 64 (1979) 142–148.

[17] J. Schachter, et al., Infection with *Chlamydia trachomatis*: involvement of multiple anatomic sites in neonates, J. Infect. Dis. 139 (1979) 232–234.

[18] P.A. Rapoza, et al., Assessment of neonatal conjunctivitis with a direct immunofluorescent monoclonal antibody stain for *Chlamydia*, JAMA 255 (1986) 3369–3373.

[19] M.R. Hammerschlag, et al., Treatment of neonatal chlamydial conjunctivitis with azithromycin, Pediatr. Infect. Dis. J. 17 (1998) 1049–1050.

[20] I.G. Rours, et al., *Chlamydia trachomatis* as a cause of neonatal conjunctivitis in Dutch infants, Pediatrics 121 (2008) e321–e326.

[21] K.D. Everett, R.M. Bush, A.A. Andersen, Emended description of the order Chlamydiales, proposal of Parachlamydiaceae fam. nov. and Simkaniaceae fam. nov., each containing one monotypic genus, revised taxonomy of the family Chlamydiaceae, including a new genus and five new species, and standards for the identification of organisms, Int. J. Syst. Bacteriol. 49 (Pt 2) (1999) 415–440.

[22] S. Kalman, et al., Comparative genomes of *Chlamydia pneumoniae* and *C. trachomatis*, Nat. Genet. 21 (1999) 385–389.

[23] D.D. Rockey, J. Lenart, R.S. Stephens, Genome sequencing and our understanding of chlamydiae, Infect. Immun. 68 (2000) 5473–5479.

[24] P.B. Wyrick, et al., Entry of genital *Chlamydia trachomatis* into polarized human epithelial cells, Infect. Immun. 57 (1989) 2378–2389.

[25] L.M. De La Maza, E.M. Peterson, Scanning electron microscopy of McCoy cells infected with *Chlamydia trachomatis*, Exp. Mol. Pathol. 36 (1982) 217–226.

[26] W.J. Todd, H.D. Caldwell, The interaction of *Chlamydia trachomatis* with host cells: ultrastructural studies of the mechanism of release of a biovar II strain from HeLa 229 cells, J. Infect. Dis. 151 (1985) 1037–1044.

[27] C.H. Mordhorst, S.P. Wang, J.T. Grayston, Childhood trachoma in a nonendemic area: Danish trachoma patients and their close contacts, 1963 to 1973, JAMA 239 (1978) 1765–1771.

[28] C.H. Mordhorst, C. Dawson, Sequelae of neonatal inclusion conjunctivitis and associated disease in parents, Am. J. Ophthalmol. 71 (1971) 861–867.

[29] M.R. Hammerschlag, et al., Longitudinal studies on chlamydial infections in the first year of life, Pediatr. Infect. Dis. 1 (1982) 395–401.

[30] T.A. Bell, et al., Chronic *Chlamydia trachomatis* infections in infants, JAMA 267 (1992) 400–402.

[31] G.T. Frommell, F.W. Bruhn, J.D. Schwartzman, Isolation of *Chlamydia trachomatis* from infant lung tissue, N. Engl. J. Med. 296 (1977) 1150–1152.

[32] C. Arth, et al., Chlamydial pneumonitis, J. Pediatr. 93 (1978) 447–449.

[33] J. Schachter, Chlamydial infections (third of three parts), N. Engl. J. Med. 298 (1978) 540–549.

[34] J. Schachter, et al., Pneumonitis following inclusion blennorrhea, J. Pediatr. 87 (1975) 779–780.

[35] M.A. Tipple, M.O. Beem, E.M. Saxon, Clinical characteristics of the afebrile pneumonia associated with *Chlamydia trachomatis* infection in infants less than 6 months of age, Pediatrics 63 (1979) 192–197.

[36] M.A. Radkowski, et al., *Chlamydia* pneumonia in infants: radiography in 125 cases, AJR Am. J. Roentgenol. 137 (1981) 703–706.

[37] J. Schachter, et al., Prospective study of perinatal transmission of *Chlamydia trachomatis*, JAMA 255 (1986) 3374–3377.

[38] M.R. Hammerschlag, et al., Comparison of enzyme immunoassay and culture for diagnosis of chlamydial conjunctivitis and respiratory infections in infants, J. Clin. Microbiol. 25 (1987) 2306–2308.

[39] M.R. Hammerschlag, et al., Enzyme immunoassay for diagnosis of neonatal chlamydial conjunctivitis, J. Pediatr. 107 (1985) 741–743.

[40] B.A. Judson, P.P. Lambert, Improved Syva MicroTrak *Chlamydia trachomatis* direct test method, J. Clin. Microbiol. 26 (1988) 2657–2658.

[41] J. Schachter, et al., Ligase chain reaction to detect *Chlamydia trachomatis* infection of the cervix, J. Clin. Microbiol. 32 (1994) 2540–2543.

[42] G. Jaschek, et al., Direct detection of *Chlamydia trachomatis* in urine specimens from symptomatic and asymptomatic men by using a rapid polymerase chain reaction assay, J. Clin. Microbiol. 31 (1993) 1209–1212.

[43] C.M. Black, Current methods of laboratory diagnosis of *Chlamydia trachomatis* infections, Clin. Microbiol. Rev. 10 (1997) 160–184.

[44] M.R. Hammerschlag, et al., Use of polymerase chain reaction for the detection of *Chlamydia trachomatis* in ocular and nasopharyngeal specimens from infants with conjunctivitis, Pediatr. Infect. Dis. J. 16 (1997) 293–297.

[45] D.J. Jespersen, et al., Prospective comparison of cell cultures and nucleic acid amplification tests for laboratory diagnosis of *Chlamydia trachomatis* infections, J. Clin. Microbiol. 43 (2005) 5324–5326.

[46] Centers for Disease Control and Prevention, Sexually transmitted diseases treatment guidelines 2002, MMWR Recomm. Rep. 51 (RR-6) (2002) 30–36.

[47] H.R. Harrison, et al., *Chlamydia trachomatis* infant pneumonitis: comparison with matched controls and other infant pneumonitis, N. Engl. J. Med. 298 (1978) 702–708.

[48] S.P. Wang, et al., Simplified microimmunofluorescence test with trachoma-lymphogranuloma venereum (*Chlamydia trachomatis*) antigens for use as a screening test for antibody, J. Clin. Microbiol. 1 (1975) 250–255.

[49] J. Schachter, C.R. Dawson, Human Chlamydial Infections, PSG Publishing Company, Littleton, MA, 1978.

[50] M.O. Beem, E. Saxon, M.A. Tipple, Treatment of chlamydial pneumonia of infancy, Pediatrics 63 (1979) 198–203.

[51] H.R. Harrison, L.M. Taussig, V.A. Fulginiti, *Chlamydia trachomatis* and chronic respiratory disease in childhood, Pediatr. Infect. Dis. 1 (1982) 29–33.

[52] P. Patamasucon, et al., Oral v topical erythromycin therapies for chlamydial conjunctivitis, Am. J. Dis. Child. 136 (1982) 817–821.

[53] CDC, Hypertrophic pyloric stenosis in infants following pertussis prophylaxis with erythromycin—Knoxville, Tennessee, 1999, MMWR Morb. Mortal. Wkly Rep. 48 (1999) 1117–1120.

[54] From the Centers for Disease Control and Prevention, Hypertrophic pyloric stenosis in infants following pertussis prophylaxis with erythromycin—Knoxville, Tennessee, 1999, JAMA 283 (2000) 471–472.

[55] J.M. Miller, D.H. Martin, Treatment of *Chlamydia trachomatis* infections in pregnant women, Drugs 60 (2000) 597–605.

[56] M.R. Hammerschlag, et al., Efficacy of neonatal ocular prophylaxis for the prevention of chlamydial and gonococcal conjunctivitis, N. Engl. J. Med. 320 (1989) 769–772.

MYCOPLASMAL INFECTIONS

R. Doug Hardy ☉ **Octavio Ramilo**

CHAPTER OUTLINE

Ureaplasma and *Mycoplasma hominis*: Colonization and Diseases of the Urinary and Reproductive Tracts in Adults **607**
    Colonization **607**
    Urinary Tract **608**
    Reproductive Tract **608**
Chorioamnionitis, Clinical Amnionitis, and Maternal Septicemia **608**
    Histologic Chorioamnionitis **608**
    Infection of the Amniotic Fluid and Clinical Amnionitis **608**
    Postpartum and Postabortal Fever **609**
Adverse Pregnancy Outcome **610**
    Fetal Loss **610**
    Preterm Birth **610**

Transmission of *Ureaplasma* and *Mycoplasma hominis* to the Fetus and Newborn **611**
Perinatal *Ureaplasma* and *Mycoplasma hominis* Infection **611**
    Pneumonia **612**
    Chronic Lung Disease **612**
    Bloodstream Infections **614**
    Central Nervous System Infections **614**
    Other Sites of Infection in the Neonate **615**
Other Mycoplasmas **615**
Diagnosis **616**
Treatment of Neonatal Infections **617**

Mycoplasmas are prokaryotes of the class Mollicutes and represent the smallest known free-living organisms. Their small size of 150 to 350 nm is more on the order of viruses than of bacteria. They lack a cell wall and are bound by a cell membrane. Many of the biologic properties of mycoplasmas are due to the absence of a rigid cell wall, including resistance to β-lactam antibiotics and marked pleomorphism among individual cells. The mycoplasmal cell membrane contains phospholipids, glycolipids, sterols, and various proteins. Mycoplasmas are able to grow in cell-free media and possess RNA and DNA. The entire genomes of many of the *Mycoplasma* species have been sequenced and have been found to be among the smallest of prokaryotic genomes; the *Mycoplasma genitalium* genome consists of only 580,070 DNA base pairs. The elimination of genes related to synthesis of amino acids, fatty acid metabolism, and cholesterol necessitates a parasitic dependence on their host for exogenous nutrients, such as nucleic acid precursors, amino acids, fatty acids, and sterols. In mammals, *Mycoplasma* species most commonly colonize mucosal surfaces, such as the respiratory and genital tracts. At least 16 different species of Mollicutes colonize the mucosa of humans.

Ureaplasma species and *Mycoplasma hominis* are the mycoplasmas most commonly isolated from the genital tract of women and are associated with maternal and fetal infection. This chapter focuses on these two species in the maternal and fetal, neonatal, and very young infant populations. Mycoplasmal illnesses in other populations, such as immunocompromised older children and nonpregnant adults, are not discussed. *Mycoplasma pneumoniae*, *M. genitalium*, and *Mycoplasma fermentans* are mentioned briefly.

The originally identified species *Ureaplasma urealyticum* has been divided into two species, *Ureaplasma parvum* and *Ureaplasma urealyticum*, based on 16S rRNA sequences; the 14 described serovars were reassigned, with *U. parvum* containing 4 serovars (1, 3, 6, and 14) and *U. urealyticum* containing the remaining 10 serovars (2, 4, 5, 7, 8, 9, 10, 11, 12, and 13). Most of the available literature simply refers to *U. urealyticum* without differentiation into *U. parvum* or *U. urealyticum*. A few more recent investigations distinguish between *U. parvum* and *U. urealyticum* in their results, but not enough data are available to determine if the two species or 14 serovars differ in pathogenicity. In this chapter, *Ureaplasma* is used to refer to *U. parvum* and *U. urealyticum* without differentiation.

UREAPLASMA AND MYCOPLASMA HOMINIS: COLONIZATION AND DISEASES OF THE URINARY AND REPRODUCTIVE TRACTS IN ADULTS

COLONIZATION

Ureaplasma and *M. hominis* are commensal organisms in the lower female genital tract. Colonization of the female lower urogenital tract by *Ureaplasma* and *M. hominis* generally occurs as a result of sexual activity. Sexual contact is the major mode of transmission of these organisms, and colonization increases dramatically with increasing numbers of sexual partners [1–3].

In an asymptomatic woman, these mycoplasmas may be found throughout the lower urogenital tract, including the external cervical os, vagina, labia, and urethra [4,5]. The vagina yields the largest number of organisms, followed by the periurethral area and the cervix [5]. *Ureaplasma* is isolated less often from urine than from the cervix, but *M. hominis* is present in the urine and in the cervix with approximately the same frequency. In asymptomatic men, mycoplasmas also have been isolated from urine, semen, and the distal urethra [6].

Ureaplasma can be isolated from the vagina of 40% to 80% of sexually active, asymptomatic women; *M. hominis* is found in 21% to 70%. Both microorganisms can be found concurrently in 31% to 60% of women [7,8]. In men, colonization with each is less prevalent. In women, colonization has been linked to younger age, lower socioeconomic status, multiple sexual partners, black ethnicity, oral contraceptive use, and recent antimicrobial therapy [3,9]. Additionally, mycoplasmas are prevalent in the lower genital tract of pregnant women [7,10,11]. When genital mycoplasmas are present at the first prenatal visit, usually they persist throughout the pregnancy. Studies suggest that postmenopausal women are infrequently colonized with genital mycoplasmas [12].

URINARY TRACT

Three disease associations have been established for *Ureaplasma* and *M. hominis* in the urinary tract: urethritis in men caused by *Ureaplasma*, urinary calculi caused by *Ureaplasma*, and pyelonephritis caused by *M. hominis* [13]. Intraurethral inoculation of human volunteers and nonhuman primates with *Ureaplasma* produces urethritis [13]. Serologic studies and clinical responsiveness in antimicrobial treatment trials also support a causative role of this organism in urethritis [13]. The common presence of ureaplasmas in the urethra of asymptomatic men suggests either that only certain serovars of ureaplasmas are pathogenic or that predisposing factors, such as lack of mucosal immunity, must exist in individuals in whom symptomatic infection develops. Alternatively, disease may develop only on initial exposure to ureaplasmas. *Ureaplasma* also has been implicated in urethroprostatitis and epididymitis [14].

Ureaplasma has been shown to have a limited role in the production of urinary calculi. *Ureaplasma* produces urease, which splits urea into ammonia and carbon dioxide, and has been shown to induce crystallization of struvite and calcium phosphates in artificial urine in vitro, showing the capacity of the pathogen to induce stone formation [15,16]. Renal calculi have been induced experimentally by inoculation of pure cultures of *Ureaplasma* directly into the bladder and renal pelvis of rats. *Ureaplasma* has been isolated from stones recovered by surgery in 6 of 15 patients. In four of the six patients, no other urease-producing organisms were isolated either in the stone or in urine sampled from the renal pelvis. *Proteus mirabilis* is the most common infectious cause of similar stones in humans. The frequency with which *Ureaplasma* reaches the kidney, the predisposing factors that allow this to occur, and the relative frequency of renal calculi induced by this organism compared with that of calculi induced by other organisms is unknown.

Even with the high incidence of *M. hominis* in the lower urogenital tract, this organism has been isolated from the upper urinary tract only in patients with symptoms of acute infection [17]. In one study, *M. hominis* was recovered from samples of ureteral urine collected during surgery from 7 of 80 patients (4 in pure culture) with acute pyelonephritis, and in a second study from 3 of 18 patients with acute exacerbation of chronic pyelonephritis. *M. hominis* was not found in the upper urinary tract of 22 patients with chronic pyelonephritis without acute exacerbation or in 60 patients with noninfectious urinary tract disease.

REPRODUCTIVE TRACT

M. hominis is considered an etiologic agent of pelvic inflammatory disease [18–21]. Inoculation of *M. hominis* into fallopian tubes of primates induces parametritis and salpingitis within 3 days [22], whereas inoculation of human fallopian tube explants produces ciliostasis [23]. The organism has been isolated in pure cultures from the fallopian tubes of approximately 8% of women with salpingitis diagnosed by laparoscopy, but not in any women without salpingitis [18]. The organism also can be isolated from the endometrium. A role for this organism in cases of pelvic inflammatory disease not associated with either *Neisseria gonorrhoeae* or *Chlamydia trachomatis* is supported by significant increases in specific antibodies to *M. hominis* [20]. *Ureaplasma* is not considered to be a cause of pelvic inflammatory disease [14].

CHORIOAMNIONITIS, CLINICAL AMNIONITIS, AND MATERNAL SEPTICEMIA
HISTOLOGIC CHORIOAMNIONITIS

Isolation of *Ureaplasma*, but not *M. hominis*, from the chorioamnion uniformly has shown a significant association with histologic chorioamnionitis [24–30]. Studies in which extensive culture for other agents was performed reported that women whose amniotic membranes contained *Ureaplasma* were more likely to have histologic evidence of chorioamnionitis than women without *Ureaplasma*, even after adjusting for duration of labor, premature rupture of membranes, duration of membrane rupture, and presence of other bacteria [27]. *Ureaplasma* in the chorioamnion was found to be significantly associated with histologic chorioamnionitis in the presence of intact membranes when delivery was by cesarean section [31]. In some cases, *Ureaplasma* was the only organism isolated. Case reports [25,32,33] indicate that *Ureaplasma* can persist in the amniotic fluid for 7 weeks in the presence of an intense inflammatory response and in the absence of ruptured membranes or labor and can be isolated as a single microorganism when cultures for multiple agents are performed. These findings show that ureaplasmas can produce histologic evidence of chorioamnionitis.

INFECTION OF THE AMNIOTIC FLUID AND CLINICAL AMNIONITIS

Although *Ureaplasma* and *M. hominis* can invade the amniotic fluid at 16 to 20 weeks of gestation in the presence of intact membranes and in the absence of other microorganisms, these infections tend to be clinically silent and chronic (Fig. 20–1) [25,32]. *Ureaplasma* and *M. hominis* have been isolated more frequently from the chorioamnion than from the amniotic fluid. Isolation of organisms from the chorioamnion or amniotic fluid has been

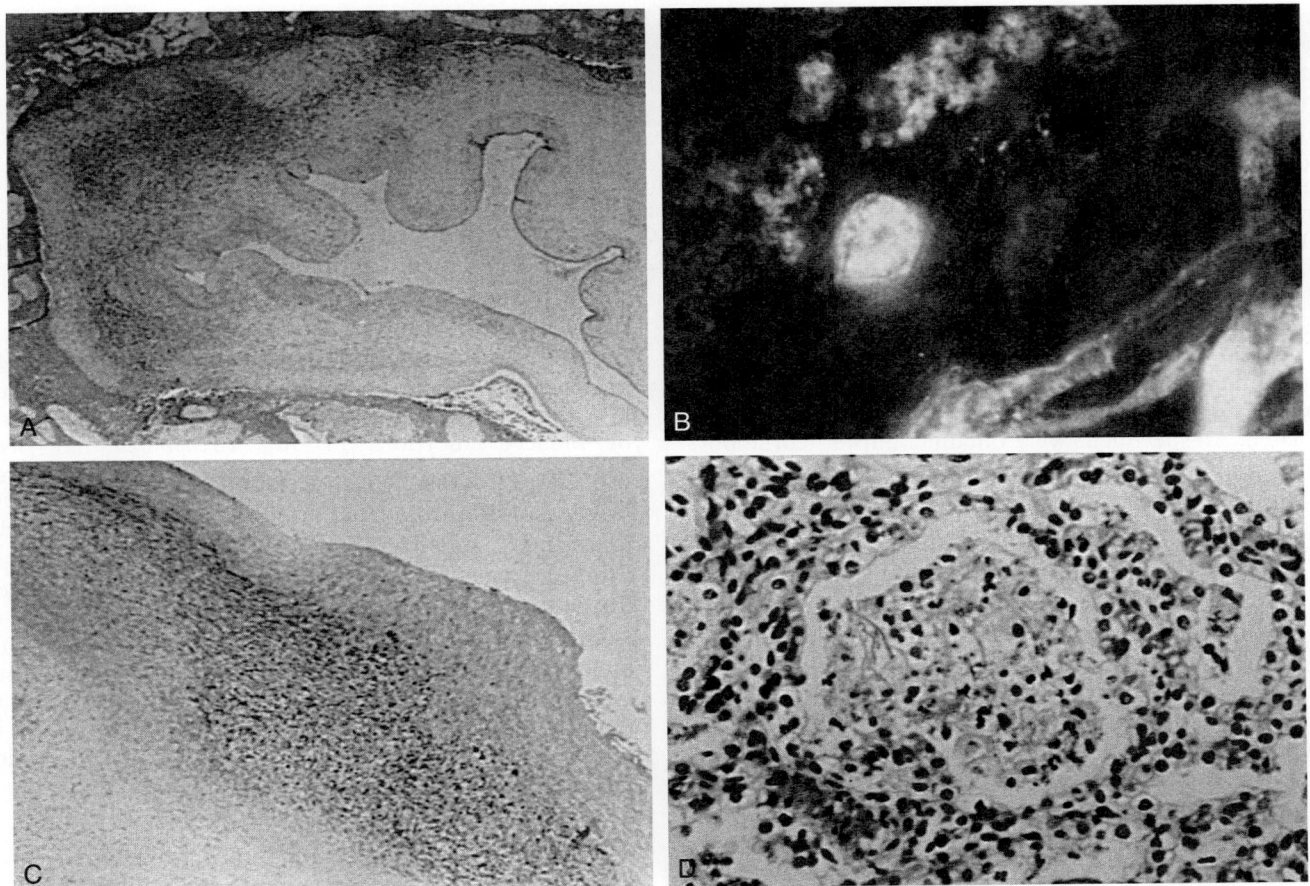

FIGURE 20–1 A, Section of placenta at 24 weeks of gestation showing extensive inflammation in amnion and chorion. (Magnification 25×.) *Ureaplasma* was isolated from amniotic fluid 7 weeks before delivery and from multiple fetal organs at postmortem examination. **B,** Adjacent section of placenta stained with rabbit anti-*Ureaplasma* serovar 1 serum and reacted with fluorescein-labeled goat anti-rabbit IgG. (Magnification 750×.) **C,** Photomicrograph of umbilical cord from same case as in **A** and **B** shows extensive inflammation. (Magnification 25×.) **D,** Photomicrograph of lung tissue shows histologic evidence of pneumonia. (Magnification 50×.)

significantly associated with histologic evidence of chorioamnionitis, but not with clinical amnionitis [31]. Ureaplasmas can be detected in the amniotic fluid in 50% of asymptomatic and symptomatic individuals [34]. These reports indicate that the role of *Ureaplasma* in clinical amnionitis is unclear.

In an investigation by Yoon and colleagues [35], amniocentesis was performed in 154 patients with preterm premature rupture of membranes. Amniotic fluid was cultured for aerobic and anaerobic bacteria and for mycoplasmas. Polymerase chain reaction (PCR) assay for *Ureaplasma* also was performed on the fluid. These investigators found that amniotic fluid culture for mycoplasmas missed 42% of cases identified as positive by *Ureaplasma* PCR assay. Patients with a negative result on amniotic fluid culture for *Ureaplasma* but a positive result on PCR assay had a significantly shorter interval from amniocentesis to delivery, higher amniotic fluid interleukin-6 concentrations, and higher white blood cell counts compared with patients without detection of *Ureaplasma* by culture or PCR assay. Subsequently, in a similar investigation by the same group [36] in 257 patients with

preterm labor and intact membranes, significant findings were similar except that the prevalence of *Ureaplasma* was lower.

The detection of *M. hominis* does not correlate with clinical symptoms. *M. hominis* commonly invades the chorioamnion and amniotic fluid, but such invasion rarely occurs in the absence of other organisms, particularly ureaplasmas. It is unclear whether this organism alone is a cause of histologic chorioamnionitis or clinical amnionitis [31].

POSTPARTUM AND POSTABORTAL FEVER

M. hominis [37–40] and *Ureaplasma* [41,42] have been isolated from blood cultures from women with postpartum fever and septic abortion. Serologic investigations indicate that *M. hominis* is a common cause of postpartum fever, as shown by a fourfold or greater increase in mycoplasmacidal antibody titer [43]. In a study at Boston City Hospital [44], blood was obtained from 327 women shortly after vaginal delivery. Of these 327 women, 10 had blood cultures that grew *M. hominis, Ureaplasma* grew in 15, and *M. hominis* and *Ureaplasma* were isolated in 1 woman. The frequency of isolation of mycoplasmas was inversely related to the interval between delivery and the time at which the blood was obtained for culture. Twenty women whose blood culture grew mycoplasmas at the time of delivery were reevaluated with a second culture 1 or more days later; a positive result was obtained on the second blood culture in only 1 of the 20 women. Pathogenic bacteria were cultured from the blood of 16 of the 327 women, including 4 of the 11 women with *M. hominis*, but none from the women with *Ureaplasma*.

In a prospective study of 620 blood cultures from febrile obstetric patients [45], *Ureaplasma* was the second and *M. hominis* the third most common microorganism isolated. All specimens were obtained during febrile postpartum or postabortum episodes. Mycoplasmas were isolated on numerous occasions from blood drawn more than 2 days after the procedure. Endometritis or histologically documented chorioamnionitis was present in half of the patients, and fever persisted after delivery or abortion in many of the cases despite administration of antimicrobial agents directed at organisms other than mycoplasmas. Fever resolved after tetracycline therapy.

It has been shown that colonization of the chorioamnion with ureaplasmas in women with intact membranes undergoing cesarean delivery is a significant and independent predictor of ensuing endometritis [46]. Endometritis occurred in 28% of women with ureaplasmas isolated from the chorioamnion at cesarean delivery compared with only 8.4% if the culture result was negative and 8.8% if only bacteria but no ureaplasmas were isolated.

Roberts and associates [47] found ureaplasmas to be the most common microorganism isolated from postcesarean wound infections. Of 47 cultures with a positive result from 939 wounds, ureaplasmas were recovered from 29. Additionally, one third of the cultures positive for ureaplasmas yielded no other microorganisms. *M. hominis* has been recovered from the joint fluid of women postpartum. These women had been febrile during the immediate postpartum period, and signs of arthritis developed 7 days to 3 weeks after delivery [48]. Cases of postpartum pneumonia with isolation of *M. hominis* from pleural fluid and cases of *M. hominis* wound infections after cesarean section also have been reported [49–52].

Andrews and coworkers [53] performed a randomized, double-blind, placebo-controlled trial in 597 women to compare rates of postcesarean endometritis after prophylaxis with cefotetan versus cefotetan plus doxycycline and azithromycin. The frequency of postcesarean endometritis and wound infection was significantly lower in the group that received cefotetan plus doxycycline and azithromycin. The investigators concluded that this extended-spectrum antibiotic prophylaxis regimen, with activity against mycoplasmas, reduced the frequency of postcesarean endometritis and wound infection. *Mycoplasma* cultures were not obtained in this investigation, however, so it is unclear that the improved outcome was specifically due to the addition of doxycycline and azithromycin prophylaxis aimed at *Mycoplasma* infections versus other synergistic antibacterial or immunomodulatory effects of these agents.

ADVERSE PREGNANCY OUTCOME
FETAL LOSS

Although studies have found the presence of *Ureaplasma* and *M. hominis* in the genital tract to be significantly associated with spontaneous abortion and early pregnancy loss [54], their actual role in these events is uncertain. Both organisms have been isolated from the lungs, brain, heart, and viscera of aborted fetuses and stillborn infants, in some cases in the presence of an inflammatory response and in the absence of other organisms [25,29,55,56]. In these cases, it was unclear whether death of the fetus occurred before these organisms "invaded." *Ureaplasma* has been found more frequently in the products of early abortions and mid-trimester fetal losses than in products of induced abortions [57,58]. *Ureaplasma* has been isolated more frequently from the placentas of aborted fetuses than from controls [26,29].

Although rates of isolation of ureaplasmas from the lower genital tract of women with habitual abortion are not different from those of normal controls, ureaplasmas are isolated more frequently from the endometrium of women with habitual abortion [57,58]. When only patients with a positive result on cervical culture are considered, no higher endometrial colonization rates are found [59]. Antibody titers to *Ureaplasma* are higher in mothers with a history of fetal loss [60]. These epidemiologic studies are difficult to interpret, however, because the comparability of the various groups of women is uncertain, and the role of other potential infectious agents was not always taken into account.

Isolation of *Ureaplasma* from amniotic fluid in pure culture from women with intact membranes and subsequent fetal loss in the presence of histologic chorioamnionitis has been reported [25,32,33]. Berg and associates [61] performed a retrospective analysis of 2718 amniocentesis specimens obtained for genetic indications and cultured for *Ureaplasma* and *M. hominis*. Of the 2718 patients, 49 (1.8%) patients were found to be positive for one or both organisms. Of 43 patients who could be evaluated, 35 were given oral erythromycin at the discretion of the physician caring for the patient. Rates of mid-trimester loss were 11.4% and 44.4% ($P = .04$) in the treated and untreated groups. This study showed that treatment of amniotic mycoplasmal colonization with erythromycin may decrease mid-trimester losses. Prospective controlled trials are necessary to validate this hypothesis.

PRETERM BIRTH

Multiple studies involving almost 12,000 patients have been conducted to evaluate the association of cervical ureaplasmal infection with prematurity [62,63]. The evidence suggests no consistent relationship between the presence of *Ureaplasma* in the lower genital tract of the mother and prematurity or low birth weight in the infant.

At least six prospective studies have evaluated the role of ureaplasmal infection of the amniotic fluid in the etiology of prematurity. Three of these studies investigated the outcome of pregnancy when ureaplasmas were detected at the time of genetic amniocentesis at 12 to 20 weeks of gestation, when membranes were intact and when labor had not begun [25,32,64]. In an investigation by Cassell and colleagues [25], two infants with *Ureaplasma* isolated from amniotic fluid were born preterm; both infants died, and both had evidence of pneumonia. *Ureaplasma* was isolated in pure culture at postmortem examination in both cases. In a study by Gray and associates [32], 7 of 10 patients from whom ureaplasmas were isolated by culture of the amniotic fluid subsequently aborted within 4 to 7 weeks after amniocentesis and at less than 25 weeks of gestation. The three remaining infants were born at less than 37 weeks of gestation, and two of these died. Histologic evidence of chorioamnionitis was present in all 10 placentas, and histologic evidence of pneumonia was present in all eight fetuses. Placentas grew *Ureaplasma*, but results were negative for cultures of all other microorganisms in six of seven evaluated at delivery and in four of the six fetal lungs that were evaluated.

The third and largest investigation by Gerber and co-workers [64] used PCR assay and detected *Ureaplasma* in 29 of 254 (11.4%) amniotic fluid specimens. As might be expected, a higher percentage of *Ureaplasma*-positive amniotic fluid samples were found in this study that used PCR than in previous investigations that relied solely on culture. Subsequent preterm labor occurred in 17 (58.6%) *Ureaplasma*-positive women compared with 10 (4.4%) women whose cultures were *Ureaplasma*-negative ($P < .0001$). Preterm birth occurred in seven (24.1%) *Ureaplasma*-positive women compared with one (0.4%) *Ureaplasma*-negative woman ($P < .0001$). *Ureaplasma*-positive women had a higher prevalence of preterm labor in a prior pregnancy (20.7%) than the *Ureaplasma*-negative women (2.7%; $P < .0008$).

In contrast to the above-mentioned studies, in the remaining three studies culture of amniotic fluid was performed on women hospitalized with preterm labor and intact membranes. *Ureaplasma* in the amniotic fluid was not consistently associated with preterm birth in these studies [65–67]. In these later studies of women with preterm labor, the mean gestation was 31.5 weeks compared with 12 to 20 weeks of gestation in the previous studies of women with no labor.

A significant relationship between isolation of *Ureaplasma* from the chorioamnion and preterm birth has been documented in three of six prospective studies [26–28, 68–70]. In most patients in these investigations, membrane rupture had occurred, however, which could have led to intrapartum microbial invasion of the chorioamnion, potentially confounding the results even if the duration of membrane rupture is taken into account.

As noted previously, Berg and associates [61] performed a retrospective analysis of 2718 genetic amniocentesis specimens cultured for *Ureaplasma* and *M. hominis*. Of the 2718 specimens, 49 (1.8%) were found to be positive for either organism. Of 43 patients who could be evaluated in this study, 35 received treatment with oral erythromycin. Preterm delivery rates were similar in the treated and untreated groups (19.4% and 20%). The investigators speculated that the lack of a treatment effect may have been due to recolonization with mycoplasmas.

The sum of the evidence suggests that the risk of preterm labor and delivery is increased when ureaplasmas are detected at amniocentesis at 12 to 20 weeks of gestation in women with intact membranes before onset of labor. Otherwise, the association between preterm birth and ureaplasmas is uncertain.

TRANSMISSION OF *UREAPLASMA* AND *MYCOPLASMA HOMINIS* TO THE FETUS AND NEWBORN

Ureaplasma and *M. hominis* can be transmitted to a fetus from an infected woman either in utero or at the time of delivery by passage through a colonized birth canal. The isolation of *Ureaplasma* in pure culture from the chorioamnion, amniotic fluid, and internal fetal organs in the presence of funisitis and pneumonia [25] and a specific IgM response [71] can be taken as evidence that fetal infection can occur in utero. Investigators [72,73] also have found that *Ureaplasma* and *M. hominis* can be isolated from endotracheal specimens collected within 30 minutes to 24 hours after birth from infants who were delivered by cesarean section with intact membranes. It is thought that the acquisition of *Ureaplasma* and *M. hominis* can occur in utero either by an ascending route secondary to colonization of the mother's genital tract or transplacentally from the mother's blood. Each of these organisms has been isolated from maternal and umbilical cord blood at the time of delivery [74,75].

The rate of vertical transmission of *Ureaplasma* and *M. hominis* ranges from 18% to 88% [75–79]. Chua and colleagues [79] prospectively investigated the transmission and colonization of *Ureaplasma* and *M. hominis* from mothers to term and preterm newborns delivered by the vaginal route. The rates of maternal cervical colonization with *Ureaplasma* and *M. hominis* were 57.5% and 15.8%, whereas the rates for isolation of *Ureaplasma* and *M. hominis* from nasopharyngeal secretions of the newborns were 50.8% and 6.6%. The vertical transmission rates were 88.4% for *Ureaplasma* and 42.1% for *M. hominis*. Maternal transmission was not associated with gestational age. In preterm neonates, the isolation of mycoplasmas was not associated with gestational age or birth weight. There was a tendency for *Ureaplasma* to persist in preterm newborns, especially in neonates with birth weight less than 2 kg. Colonization of full-term infants seems to be transient, with a sharp decrease in isolation rates after 3 months of age [80]. In premature infants with ureaplasmal infection, persistence of the organism in the lower respiratory tract and cerebrospinal fluid (CSF) has been documented for weeks to months [72,81].

PERINATAL *UREAPLASMA* AND *MYCOPLASMA HOMINIS* INFECTION

Many prospective studies based on direct culture of the affected site indicate that *Ureaplasma* and *M. hominis* can cause invasive disease in infants, particularly in infants born prematurely. The presence of mycoplasmas in the chorioamnion or amniotic fluid does not always result in infection of the fetus, however. Similarly, the isolation of mycoplasmas from surface cultures (e.g., eyes, ears, nose, throat, gastric aspirates, vagina) is not indicative of invasive disease.

PNEUMONIA

Case reports [32,82,83], retrospective studies [84], and prospective studies [25,29,32] indicate an association of *Ureaplasma* with congenital and neonatal pneumonia. The organism has been isolated from affected lungs in the absence of other pathogens, such as chlamydiae, viruses, fungi, and bacteria, in the presence of chorioamnionitis and funisitis [25] and has been shown within fetal membranes by immunofluorescence [25] and in lung lesions by electron and immunofluorescent microscopy [71]. A specific IgM response has been shown in some cases of neonatal pneumonia [71].

In a study of 98 infants [72], respiratory distress syndrome, the need for assisted ventilation, severe respiratory insufficiency, and death were significantly more common in infants born at less than 34 weeks of gestation from whom *Ureaplasma* was recovered from endotracheal aspirates at delivery than in infants with a negative culture result. In another series of 292 infants with birth weights less than 2500 g who were studied by follow-up evaluation for 4 weeks after birth, isolation of *Ureaplasma* from the endotracheal aspirate within 1 week of birth (mean age 1.3 days) was significantly associated with radiographic pneumonia, whereas no such association was found for uninfected infants [85]. *Ureaplasma* was the most common organism isolated (15% of infants) among these 292 patients, and it was isolated in pure culture in 71%.

Cultrera and colleagues [86] investigated for molecular evidence of *U. urealyticum* or *U. parvum* respiratory colonization in preterm infants with or without respiratory distress syndrome. Significantly, 15 of 24 preterm neonates with respiratory distress syndrome and 4 of 26 without respiratory distress syndrome were PCR-positive for *Ureaplasma* ($P < .001$). Of the 15 preterm infants PCR-positive for *Ureaplasma*, 5 had *U. urealyticum* and 10 had *U. parvum* isolated. In this investigation, *Ureaplasma* culture was positive in 5 of 50 subjects compared with 19 of 50 subjects by PCR method ($P < .05$).

Conversely, other investigators have found a possibly protective effect associated with the isolation of *Ureaplasma* from preterm infants. In a prospective consecutive investigation of 143 ventilated newborns born at less than 28 weeks of gestation, Hannaford and coworkers [87] isolated *Ureaplasma* from endotracheal aspirates of 39 (27%) infants. Respiratory distress syndrome occurred significantly less often in infants from whom *Ureaplasma* was isolated than in infants from whom it was not isolated ($P = .002$). In addition, a trend for lower mortality rates in the first 28 days of life was identified among *Ureaplasma*-positive infants. Berger and associates [88] also found an apparently protective effect of *Ureaplasma* isolated from the amniotic cavity at the time of delivery against hyaline membrane disease in infants with a mean gestational age of 29 to 30 weeks, although this was nonsignificant. No increase in acute morbidity or mortality was found to be associated with *Ureaplasma* isolation.

The baboon model of prematurity has been employed to investigate the pathogenicity of *Ureaplasma*. At age 140 days, baboons show physiologic and pathologic characteristics similar to those of human neonates of 30 to 32 weeks of gestation (e.g., they have hyaline membrane disease) [89]. Endotracheal inoculation of premature baboons with *Ureaplasma* isolated from human infants results in histologic pulmonary lesions, including acute bronchiolitis with epithelial ulceration and polymorphonuclear infiltration, that are indistinguishable from those of hyaline membrane disease [90].

Yoder and colleagues [91] performed an investigation in premature baboons that offers an explanation for the divergent findings in human studies of *Ureaplasma* and respiratory status in preterm infants. Premature baboon infants were delivered 48 to 72 hours after maternal intra-amniotic inoculation with *Ureaplasma*. Two distinct patterns of disease were observed in the baboon infants. Baboons with persistent *Ureaplasma* tracheal colonization manifested worse lung function and prolonged elevated tracheal cytokines. Conversely, colonized baboons that subsequently cleared *Ureaplasma* from tracheal cultures showed improved lung function compared with unexposed control animals.

In addition, pneumonia with persistent pulmonary hypertension has been described in newborn infants with *Ureaplasma* isolated from the lower respiratory tract [82,83]. Although cases of ureaplasmal pneumonia have been documented in full-term infants, pneumonia resulting from this agent is thought to occur much less frequently than in premature neonates. Case reports indicate that *M. hominis* can be a cause of pneumonia in newborns, but it has not been implicated as a common etiologic agent in prospective studies. These mycoplasmas are not thought to be a significant cause of acute respiratory disease in otherwise healthy infants after the first month of life [31].

CHRONIC LUNG DISEASE

Ureaplasma frequently colonizes the neonatal respiratory tract. Although most investigations support a significant association between ureaplasmas and chronic lung disease (CLD) in preterm infants, its role in causation of CLD is uncertain. CLD is most often defined as a requirement for supplemental oxygen at 28 days of age or at 36 weeks of postconceptional age. Presence of concurrent chest radiographic changes compatible with CLD sometimes is included in this definition.

In a meta-analysis of 17 investigations published before 1995, Wang and coworkers [92] explored the association between *Ureaplasma* and CLD. The studies in this analysis included preterm and term neonates. CLD was defined as a requirement for oxygen at 28 to 30 days of age, and diagnosis of *Ureaplasma* colonization required the recovery of *Ureaplasma* from a respiratory or surface specimen. The estimates of relative risk exceeded 1 in all of the investigations; however, the lower confidence interval included 1 in 7 (41%). The meta-analysis concluded that the relative risk for the development of CLD in colonized infants was 1.72 (95% confidence interval 1.5 to 1.96) times that for noncolonized infants. In the analysis, investigations that focused on extremely premature, very low birth weight (VLBW) neonates did not identify a significantly different relative risk from that for investigations that included all neonates. Also, the relative risk did not differ significantly between studies in which only endotracheal aspirates were used to define colonization and other studies.

Subsequent to this meta-analysis, the association of *Ureaplasma* with chronic pulmonary disease, including bronchopulmonary dysplasia (or CLD), has been confirmed in multiple studies [87,88,93–101], but not in others [102–108]. Perzigian and colleagues [94] prospectively investigated a cohort of 105 VLBW (<1500 g) infants; in 22 (21%) infants, results of tracheal aspirate cultures were positive for *Ureaplasma* at birth. At 28 days of age, *Ureaplasma*-positive patients were significantly more likely to have CLD than were *Ureaplasma*-negative patients, despite routine use of exogenous surfactant. *Ureaplasma*-positive infants also required significantly longer duration of oxygen therapy and of mechanical ventilation. No significant differences were found for CLD at 36 weeks of postconceptional age or for duration of hospitalization.

Another meta-analysis appraisal of the association between *Ureaplasma* and CLD was undertaken by Schelonka and coworkers [109] with investigations published before 2005. This analysis included 23 studies of infants colonized or infected with *Ureaplasma* with an aggregate of 2216 infants in whom CLD was defined as persisting oxygen requirement at 28 days of age and included 8 studies of 751 infants in whom CLD was defined at 36 weeks of postconceptional age. A significant association between respiratory *Ureaplasma* and CLD was shown at 28 days of age (odds ratio 2.8; 95% confidence interval 2.3 to 3.5) and 36 weeks of postconceptional age (odds ratio 1.6; 95% confidence interval 1.1 to 2.3).

Because neither the relationship of *Ureaplasma* species nor the concentration of ureaplasmas with the development of CLD had yet been investigated, a prospective study was designed to look for such an association. In 175 VLBW infants, endotracheal aspirates were obtained at birth for quantitative culture; the results were analyzed for correlation with the development of CLD [106]. Ureaplasmas were isolated from 66 (38%) of the 175 infants. No statistically significant associations were identified between the development of CLD and the *Ureaplasma* species isolated (*U. urealyticum* or *U. parvum*) or the concentration of ureaplasmas in the lower respiratory tract secretions.

Because the observed disparities in these studies might be explained in part by the variable persistence of *Ureaplasma* colonization of the infant respiratory tract, a prospective longitudinal study was performed to investigate this possibility. In 125 VLBW infants, culture and PCR assay were used to sample for *Ureaplasma* in the respiratory tract frequently over the course of their neonatal intensive care unit stay. It was found that the pattern of colonization was predictive for the development of CLD [95]. In this study, 40 (32%) of 125 infants had at least one specimen positive for *Ureaplasma*; however, only 18 (45%) of the 40 had persistent colonization throughout their hospitalization. Only persistent *Ureaplasma* colonization was associated with a significantly increased risk of development of CLD at 28 days of age and at 36 weeks after conception. Neither early transient colonization nor late acquisition of *Ureaplasma* was associated with CLD.

The study by Yoder and colleagues [91] in premature baboons similarly found that the pattern of tracheal colonization was important in the manifestations of respiratory disease.

Inadequate detection of *Ureaplasma* in neonates can be another confounding factor in CLD research. False-negative results for isolation of *Ureaplasma* from respiratory specimens could weaken the calculated association with CLD. Using in situ hybridization for *Ureaplasma* on lung autopsy tissue from seven infants with positive cultures and seven infants with negative cultures for *Ureaplasma* from the lower respiratory tract, Benstein and coworkers [93] found all seven culture-positive infants were positive for *Ureaplasma* by in situ hybridization; two of the culture-negative infants were positive by in situ hybridization. The in situ hybridization results had 100% correlation with the presence of histopathologic evidence of bronchopulmonary dysplasia at autopsy of these 14 infants.

Although properly conducted antimicrobial agent trials showing reduction in CLD incidence and severity in neonates with *Ureaplasma* would support a causal role for this microorganism, failure of amelioration with effective therapy does not indicate that *Ureaplasma* does not have some role in the development of CLD. Small trials of therapy with erythromycin or clarithromycin have failed to provide evidence that therapy, predicted by in vitro testing to be effective, decreases CLD severity or produces clinical improvement in neonates with *Ureaplasma* [88,98,107,110–113]. Only two randomized, controlled trials have been conducted, together involving 37 VLBW infants with *Ureaplasma* isolated from the respiratory tract; each failed to show a reduction in the incidence of CLD after 7 to 10 days of erythromycin therapy [110]. In one of these trials, erythromycin treatment significantly reduced the isolation of *Ureaplasma* from the respiratory tract, but it did not significantly alter required length of time with supplemental oxygen [107]. A large, definitive, well-controlled trial is needed, perhaps with more prolonged antimicrobial therapy.

Debate over the concept that initiating therapy after birth may be too late to influence the outcome of an inflammatory process with possible onset in utero was partially addressed in the ORACLE (Overview of Role of Antibiotics in the Curtailment of Labour and Early Delivery) I and ORACLE II prenatal trials (erythromycin or amoxicillin-clavulanic acid or both in a randomized double-blind, placebo-controlled design) involving a combined total of 11,121 women with preterm, prelabor rupture of fetal membranes or spontaneous preterm labor [114,115]. One of the primary outcomes of these trials was CLD, defined as the need for daily supplementary oxygen at age 36 weeks after conception; the other primary outcomes were neonatal death and major cerebral abnormality. ORACLE I and ORACLE II revealed no statistically significant reduction in any primary outcome. *Ureaplasma* colonization was not specifically addressed in these trials, however, so the results should not be generalized to address *Ureaplasma* and CLD directly.

To investigate for the presence of a long-term detrimental effect of perinatal *Ureaplasma* infection, a cohort of 40 preterm infants was prospectively followed for

12 months [116]. In 22 (55%) infants, *Ureaplasma* was present in samples obtained from the trachea or blood or both at birth. Infants with perinatal *Ureaplasma* required significantly more days of hospitalization than infants without *Ureaplasma*. The difference was attributed to an increase in respiratory tract disease among the infants with perinatal *Ureaplasma*. In addition, CLD was associated with significantly more admissions in infants with perinatal *Ureaplasma* than in infants without it. Syrogiannopoulos and associates [75] monitored 108 full-term infants during the first 3 months of life. These researchers were unable to show an increased risk of lower respiratory illness during this period of observation in 51 of 108 infants with persistent pharyngeal *Ureaplasma* colonization compared with infants who were not pharyngeally colonized at 3 months of life.

Although *Ureaplasma* has not been definitively shown to cause CLD, investigations have identified possible pathogenic mechanisms through which it may contribute to CLD. *Ureaplasma* has been hypothesized to induce lung injury through immunopathogenic mechanisms involving the release of pulmonary cytokines and chemokines after exposure to this microorganism either in utero or postnatally. It also has been proposed that *Ureaplasma* infection potentiates oxygen-induced lung injury [93,95,117].

Although much effort has been expended to define the role of *Ureaplasma* in CLD, no clear conclusions can be made at the present time, although most of the investigations seem to indicate a significant association. Novel strategies need to be instituted to explore the link between these entities further.

BLOODSTREAM INFECTIONS

Ureaplasmas have been isolated from blood cultures from neonates [45,73,74,81,118–121]. Case reports also have described the isolation of ureaplasmas from the bloodstream of neonates with pneumonia [72,83]. Cassell and associates [73] found that 26% of preterm infants with endotracheal aspirates that grew *Ureaplasma* also had a positive result on blood cultures for this organism, suggesting that bacteremia with ureaplasmas can be common in preterm infants. Cases of *M. hominis* bacteremia with systemic symptoms accompanied by an antibody response also have been reported [122,123].

Not all investigations have been successful in recovering mycoplasmas from the blood of infants [118,124,125]. Mycoplasmas were not isolated from blood cultures obtained within 30 minutes of birth from 146 preterm infants in Israel [118]. In addition, investigators did not isolate mycoplasmas from the 191 blood cultures in a prospective study of older infants hospitalized for possible sepsis [125].

Goldenberg and coworkers [126] evaluated the frequency of umbilical cord blood infections with *Ureaplasma* and *M. hominis* in 351 mother-infant pairs with deliveries between 23 and 32 weeks' gestational age to determine their association with various obstetric conditions, markers of placental inflammation, and newborn outcomes. *Ureaplasma* or *M. hominis* or both were present in 82 (23%) cord blood cultures. Of the women with a positive cord blood culture for *Ureaplasma* or *M. hominis* or both, 43 (52%) had *Ureaplasma* only, 21 (26%) had *M. hominis* only, and 18 (22%) had *Ureaplasma* and *M. hominis*. Positive cultures for *Ureaplasma* or *M. hominis* or both were more common in infants of nonwhite women (27.9% versus 16.8%; $P = .016$), in women younger than 20 years of age, in women undergoing a spontaneous compared with an indicated preterm delivery (34.7% versus 3.2%; $P = .0001$), and in women delivering at earlier gestational ages. Intrauterine infection and inflammation were more common among infants with a positive cord blood culture for *Ureaplasma* or *M. hominis* or both, as evidenced by positive placental cultures for these and other bacteria, elevated cord blood interleukin-6 levels, and placental histology. Infants with positive cord blood cultures for *Ureaplasma* or *M. hominis* or both were more likely to have neonatal systemic inflammatory response syndrome (41.3% versus 25.7%; adjusted odds ratio 1.86; 95% confidence interval 1.08 to 3.21), but were not significantly different for other neonatal outcomes, including CLD (26.8% versus 10.1%; adjusted odds ratio 1.99; 95% confidence interval 0.91 to 4.37), respiratory distress syndrome, intraventricular hemorrhage, or death.

CENTRAL NERVOUS SYSTEM INFECTIONS

Generally, the clinical significance of recovering *Ureaplasma* or *M. hominis* from a central nervous system (CNS) specimen from a neonate is uncertain. In some situations, an association with a disease process seems plausible, whereas in others, no corresponding disease state is apparent. Multiple cases of *M. hominis* CNS infection (meningitis, brain abscess) have been described in full-term and preterm infants [127–137]. *Ureaplasma* also has been isolated from the CSF of infants with suspected sepsis and meningitis [3,72,81,124,138–140].

In a prospective trial in 100 mostly premature infants, *Ureaplasma* was isolated from the CSF of 8 and *M. hominis* was isolated from the CSF of 5 who were undergoing investigation for suspected sepsis or treatment of hydrocephalus [81]. Of the eight neonates with *Ureaplasma*, six had severe intraventricular hemorrhage, three had hydrocephalus, and four had ureaplasmas isolated several times in the CSF. *Ureaplasma* infection was significantly associated with severe intraventricular hemorrhage ($P < .001$). *Ureaplasma* was isolated from the respiratory tract of four of the eight infants with CSF infections. Five infants received treatment with erythromycin or doxycycline. Three infants with *Ureaplasma* infection died. All five of the neonates from whom *M. hominis* was isolated from the CSF were being investigated for suspected sepsis; prominent neurologic signs and CSF pleocytosis were noted in only one neonate. This infant received doxycycline treatment and improved, but had substantial neurologic sequelae (Fig. 20–2) [81]. No infants infected with *M. hominis* died. A subsequent study by the same group of investigators in 318 infants isolated *Ureaplasma* from the CSF of 5 and *M. hominis* from the CSF of 9. Spontaneous clearance of the organisms was documented in 5 of the infants, and 12 infants had a good outcome [141].

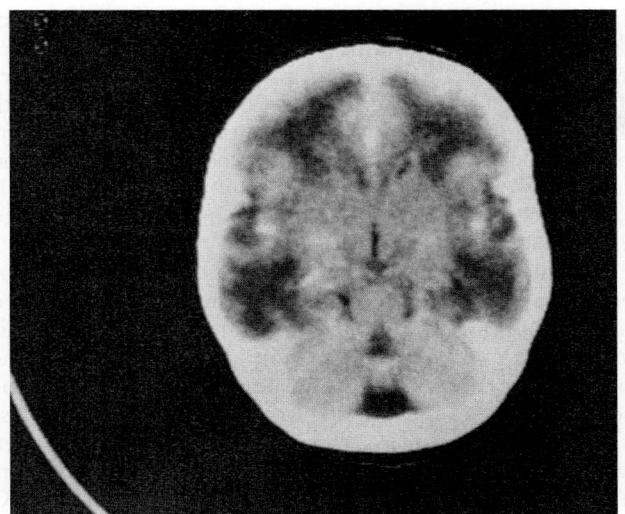

FIGURE 20–2 A 37-week gestation newborn who had
hypothermia, hypotonia, and lethargy noted at age 3 days.
Computed tomography (CT) showed decreased attenuation
predominantly of supratentorial white matter symmetrically with
punctate early calcified lesions. Examination of cerebrospinal fluid
showed mononuclear pleocytosis, and *Mycoplasma hominis* was isolated.
Cerebrospinal fluid culture was sterile after 5 days of doxycycline
treatment, but the infant had spastic quadriplegia at 6 months of age.

Shaw and colleagues [142] performed a prospective
study of 135 preterm infants undergoing lumbar puncture
and found *Ureaplasma* in the CSF of 1 neonate and
M. hominis in none. *Ureaplasma* continued to be isolated
from this one infant over the course of 16 weeks, despite
treatment with erythromycin. The organism maintained
in vitro susceptibility to erythromycin. Doxycycline treatment was associated with the disappearance of the
organism.

In a prospective study by Ollikainen and coworkers
[72], *Ureaplasma* was isolated from the CSF of four
of six infants born at less than 34 weeks of gestation.
None had pleocytosis or hypoglycorrhachia in the CSF.
Three had the organism also isolated from blood, and
one had *Ureaplasma* isolated from a tracheal sample.
One infant died and had a postmortem brain culture positive for *Ureaplasma*. None had intracranial hemorrhage.

Valencia and associates [124] isolated *M. hominis* from
9 and *Ureaplasma* from 1 of 69 consecutive infants in
whom CSF was cultured within the first 3 months of life
for suspected sepsis. The CSF indices except for bloody
specimens were considered to be normal for newborns.
Only one of the infants whose CSF culture grew *M. hominis* had clinical signs compatible with systemic infection.
The other infants were healthy, but were evaluated secondary to maternal fever and prolonged rupture of membranes. All 10 infants received ampicillin and gentamicin,
antimicrobial agents without good activity against these
organisms, and had a good clinical outcome.

In cultures of CSF from 920 infants in a neonatal intensive care unit, *Ureaplasma* was isolated from 2 (0.2%),
and *M. hominis* was isolated from none [111]. Likitnukul
and colleagues [125] and Mardh [127] failed to recover
mycoplasmas from CSF of infants in prospective

investigations. The study by Likitnukul's group [125]
involved infants who had been previously discharged from
the hospital and had returned because of suspected sepsis.
No mycoplasmas were recovered from the CSF of 47
preterm infants cultured within the 1st week of life by
Izraeli and coworkers [118]. The reason for the frequent
isolation of mycoplasmas in some studies but not in
others is uncertain. Possible technical reasons are discussed by Waites and colleagues [143] and Heggie and
associates [144].

The question of whether mycoplasmas are linked to
abnormalities on CNS imaging also has been investigated, although in an indirect manner. Perzigian and
associates [94] prospectively investigated a cohort of 105
VLBW infants in whom 22 (21%) results of tracheal
aspirate culture were positive for *Ureaplasma* at birth.
No differences were found between the groups for intraventricular hemorrhage or cystic periventricular leukomalacia. Similarly, in a study of 464 VLBW infants,
Dammann and coworkers [145] addressed the question
of whether *Ureaplasma* or *M. hominis* cultured from the
placenta was associated with an increased risk of cerebral
white matter echolucency on ultrasonography as a measure of white matter damage. The cranial ultrasound
studies were performed up to a median of 22 days of life.
Culture results were as follows: 139 of 464 (30%) were
positive for *Ureaplasma*, 27 (6%) were positive for
M. hominis, and 21 (5%) were positive for *Ureaplasma*
and *M. hominis*. It was found that with a positive result
on culture for *Ureaplasma*, the infants were not at
increased risk of cerebral white matter damage. The presence of *M. hominis* was associated with a trend toward an
increased risk of echolucency ($P = .08$).

The clinical findings in newborns with *Ureaplasma* and
M. hominis isolated from the CSF are variable. *Ureaplasma*
and *M. hominis* may produce abnormal CSF indices with
pleocytosis, or an inflammatory reaction in CSF may be
absent [72,81,124,127]. In some infants, mycoplasmas
are cleared spontaneously from the CSF, whereas in
others, the organisms have been shown to persist for
weeks to months even after appropriate treatment
[31,134,146–148].

OTHER SITES OF INFECTION IN THE NEONATE

M. hominis also has been isolated from pericardial fluid
[149], subcutaneous abscesses [150–152], and the submandibular lymph node of neonates [153]. The first
reported case of *M. hominis* endocarditis in a child was
published more recently [154]. *Ureaplasma* and *M. hominis*
have been isolated from the urine, but the clinical significance was uncertain [125].

OTHER MYCOPLASMAS

The role of other mycoplasmas, such as *M. genitalium*,
M. fermentans, and *M. pneumoniae*, in maternal and fetal
and neonatal infections is not thought to be prominent,
although investigations are limited. *M. genitalium* was
not isolated by culture of the chorioamnion of 609
women or by culture or PCR assay of 232 amniotic
fluid samples tested [155]. To evaluate the impact of

M. genitalium on the outcome of pregnancy, cervical samples from 1014 women were assayed by PCR techniques for the presence of *M. genitalium* [156]. Among those women, *M. genitalium* was isolated in 6.2%, but its isolation was not significantly associated with adverse outcomes of pregnancy (preterm delivery, small for gestational age, spontaneous abortion, stillbirth). Taylor-Robinson [157] more recently reviewed disease associations with *M. genitalium*.

M. fermentans was detected in amniotic fluid collected at the time of cesarean section from 4 of 232 women with intact membranes [155]. Placental tissue also was positive for *M. fermentans* on PCR assay in three women. Villitis and chorioamnionitis were present in two of the four positive specimens, and no other organisms were detected.

DIAGNOSIS

Culture and PCR assay are appropriate methods for the diagnosis of *Mycoplasma* and *Ureaplasma* infections. Culture of *Ureaplasma* and *M. hominis* requires special handling, however, with techniques and media generally unavailable outside major medical centers or reference laboratories. Detailed laboratory techniques for culture and identification of mycoplasmas and ureaplasmas have been reviewed by others [31,158].

Ureaplasmas and mycoplasmas are extremely susceptible to adverse environmental conditions. Correct methods of collecting, processing, and transporting specimens are important for reliable and interpretable culture results. A specific ureaplasmal transport medium, such as Shepard's 10B broth [159,160], for *Ureaplasma* and *M. hominis* should be available for direct inoculation of clinical specimens and swabs at the time of collection. If specimens are allowed to sit at room temperature and are not inoculated into appropriate media, the recovery of these organisms is unlikely. Only swabs tipped with calcium alginate or Dacron with plastic or wire shafts should be used for sampling of mucosal surfaces. Blood should be collected free of anticoagulants and immediately inoculated into the transport medium in a 1:5 to 1:10 ratio [31].

Specimens should be refrigerated at 4° C and protected from drying in a sealed container until transported to the laboratory. If transport to a suitable laboratory is not possible within 6 to 12 hours after collection, the specimen in appropriate transport medium should be stored at −70° C and shipped frozen on dry ice. Ureaplasmas and mycoplasmas are stable for long periods when kept frozen at −70° C in a protein-containing support medium such as Shepard's 10B broth. Storage at −20° C is less reliable and results in a significant loss in number of organisms in a relatively short time [31]. Before collecting a clinical sample for culture, it is appropriate to arrange processing of samples with the microbiology laboratory.

Ureaplasma and *M. hominis* grow within 2 to 5 days. Broth cultures are incubated at 37° C under atmospheric conditions; agar plates are incubated under 95% nitrogen and 5% carbon dioxide. Colonies of *Ureaplasma* can be identified on A8 agar by urease production. The colonies often are amorphous. Colonies of other mycoplasmas are urease-negative and have a typical "fried egg" appearance (Fig. 20–3).

PCR assays for the detection of *Ureaplasma* and *M. hominis* [104,161–163] have been developed. These

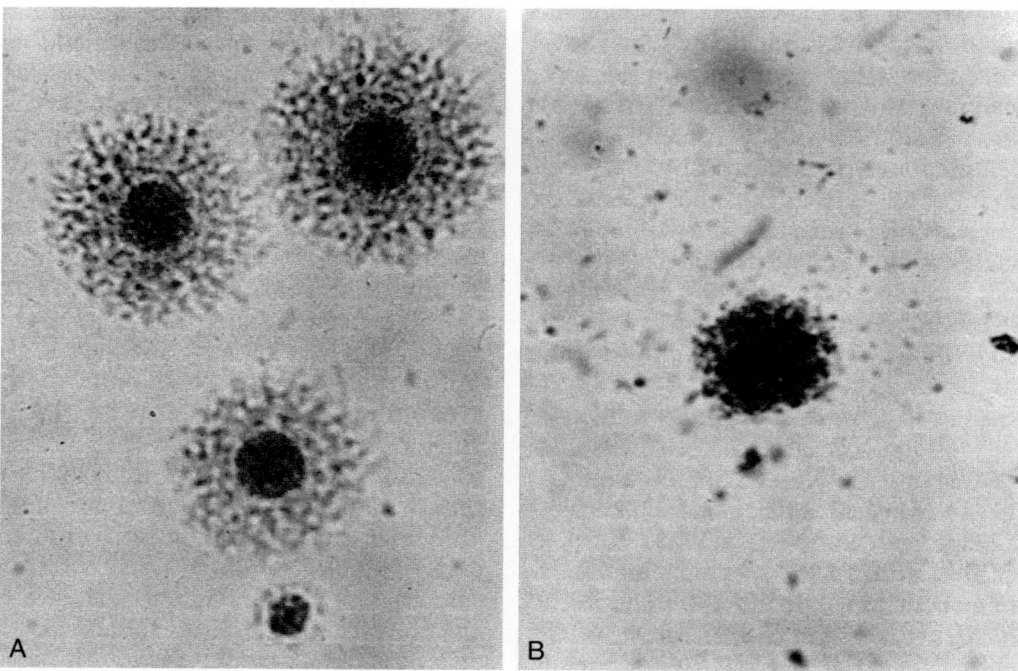

FIGURE 20–3 A, *Mycoplasma hominis*. (Original magnification 100×.) **B**, *Ureaplasma*. (Original magnification 1000×.) *(Adapted from Klein JO. Mycoplasmas, genitourinary tract infection, and reproductive failure. Hosp Pract 6:127-133, 1971.)*

assays seem to have greater sensitivity than culture in most studies [35,36,95,164,165]. A combination of PCR assay and culture should give the most reliable results. Although enzyme-linked immunosorbent assays have been developed to detect *Ureaplasma*-specific and *M. hominis*–specific antibodies in sera, serologic testing is not recommended for the routine diagnosis of *Ureaplasma* and *M. hominis* infections. The use of these assays is limited to the research setting. Owing to the fastidiousness and slow growth of *M. genitalium* and *M. fermentans*, PCR assay, in situ hybridization, and immunohistochemistry are recommended for detection of these mycoplasmas [155,166,167].

TREATMENT OF NEONATAL INFECTIONS

A positive result on culture or PCR assay for *Ureaplasma* or *M. hominis* from a normally sterile site, particularly in the absence of other microorganisms, is justification to consider treatment for infants with evidence of infectious inflammation. On the basis of the current understanding of these organisms, however, the isolation of *Ureaplasma* or *M. hominis* in the absence of disease generally does not warrant treatment.

Formulation of guidelines for treatment when these organisms are isolated from a maternal or fetal or neonatal specimen is difficult, in view of the following considerations as reviewed in this chapter:

- Causation has not been clearly established for many conditions associated with *Ureaplasma* and *M. hominis* (all maternal and fetal and neonatal associations except postpartum and postabortal fever).
- Organisms often are present (e.g., in CSF, bloodstream, respiratory tract, amniotic fluid, or lower genital tract) with little or no adverse clinical outcome.
- Organisms often are spontaneously cleared (e.g., from CSF, bloodstream, or respiratory tract) without treatment.
- No definitive controlled trials have been performed for many sites of infection (e.g., CSF, bloodstream, amniotic fluid, lung in acute pneumonia).
- Small randomized, controlled trials have not shown benefit of treatment for CLD.
- Evidence that treatment can be useful comes from uncontrolled case reports for which the outcome without treatment is unknown.
- Comparative clinical trials among antimicrobials have not been performed to assess their relative efficacy.
- Often the clinical indication for culture or PCR assay has resolved before the positive result is reported.

Treatment may be warranted in some situations, so decisions must be made on a case-by-case basis, to ensure full consideration of the risk-benefit ratio related to disease and treatment. The relative contribution of *Ureaplasma* and *M. hominis* infection to morbidity and mortality is difficult to establish because most cases have been reported in VLBW preterm infants with multiple complications or in infants with clinical problems that probably contribute to the poor outcome. An authoritative reference states that antimicrobial therapy for *Ureaplasma* cannot be recommended for pregnant women to prevent preterm delivery or for preterm infants to prevent pulmonary disease because trials of antimicrobial therapy for these indications generally have not shown efficacy [168]. It also suggests that definitive efficacy of antimicrobial agents in the treatment of CNS *Ureaplasma* infections in infants is lacking [168].

The treatment of some non-neonatal *Ureaplasma* and *M. hominis* infections is better established. *Ureaplasma* urethritis and *M. hominis* pyelonephritis, pelvic inflammatory disease, postabortal fever, and postpartum fever and infections with either organism in immunocompromised patients (especially patients with hypogammaglobulinemia) generally are considered to warrant treatment.

Erythromycin generally has been considered the antimicrobial agent of choice for neonatal ureaplasmal infections (not involving the CNS), although clinical superiority over other agents has not been investigated [169]. Erythromycin has been employed in most clinical trials in infants with *Ureaplasma* [98,107,110–113]. Other agents with in vitro activity against *Ureaplasma* and variable clinical experience include clarithromycin, azithromycin, doxycycline, and chloramphenicol [88,170–173]. In vitro activities of newer agents, such as quinolones and ketolides, against *Ureaplasma* have been reported; clinical experience is largely lacking [169,174–177]. Resistance to macrolides, doxycycline, fluoroquinolones, and chloramphenicol has been reported [169,178–180]. *M. hominis* is resistant to erythromycin and to other macrolides and azolides [169–172]. Doxycycline is the drug of choice for treatment of *M. hominis* infections, although resistance has been reported [13,134,181–183]. Clindamycin and chloramphenicol also are generally active in vitro against *M. hominis* [169]. In vitro activity of newer antimicrobials against *M. hominis* has been reported; clinical experience is lacking, however [169,174–177].

Antimicrobial susceptibility testing should be considered when it is deemed necessary to treat *Ureaplasma* or *M. hominis* infection in a neonate, especially for the persistent isolation of either organism from a normally sterile site, because resistance to commonly used antibiotics is not rare. Some tetracycline-resistant strains of *Ureaplasma* can be erythromycin resistant, but high-level erythromycin resistance in *Ureaplasma* is uncommon [164]. Penetration of the blood-brain barrier by antimicrobials should be considered in treating a CNS infection, as should the safety and pharmacokinetics of antimicrobials in newborns in making treatment decisions.

REFERENCES

[1] W.M. McCormack, Y.H. Lee, S.H. Zinner, Sexual experience and urethral colonization with genital mycoplasmas, Ann. Intern. Med. 78 (1973) 696–698.

[2] W.M. McCormack, et al., Sexual activity and vaginal colonization with genital mycoplasmas, JAMA 221 (1972) 1375–1377.

[3] W.M. McCormack, *Ureaplasma urealyticum*: ecologic niche and epidemiologic considerations, Pediatr. Infect. Dis. 5 (1986) S232–S233.

[4] W.M. McCormack, J.S. Rankin, Y.H. Lee, Localization of genital mycoplasmas in women, Am. J. Obstet. Gynecol. 112 (1972) 920–923.

[5] P. Braun, et al., Methodologic investigations and prevalence of genital mycoplasmas in pregnancy, J. Infect. Dis. 121 (1970) 391–400.

[6] D. Taylor-Robinson, W.M. McCormack, The genital mycoplasmas, N. Engl. J. Med. 302 (1980) 1003–1010.

[7] H. Faye-Kette, et al., Genital mycoplasmas among pregnant women in Cote d'Ivoire, West Africa: prevalence and risk factors, Int. J. STD AIDS 11 (2000) 599–602.

[8] A. Clegg, et al., High rates of genital *Mycoplasma* infection in the highlands of Papua New Guinea determined both by culture and by a commercial detection kit, J. Clin. Microbiol. 35 (1997) 197–200.

[9] W.M. McCormack, et al., Vaginal colonization with *Mycoplasma hominis* and *Ureaplasma urealyticum*, Sex. Transm. Dis. 134 (1986) 67–70.

[10] W.M. McCormack, B. Rosner, Y.H. Lee, Colonization with genital mycoplasmas in women, Am. J. Epidemiol. 97 (1973) 240–245.

[11] P. Braun, et al., Birth weight and genital mycoplasmas in pregnancy, N. Engl. J. Med. 284 (1971) 167–171.

[12] P.A. Mardh, L. Westrom, T-mycoplasmas in the genitourinary tract of the female, Acta Pathol. Microbiol. Scand. 78B (1970) 367–374.

[13] G.H. Cassell, et al., Pathogenesis and significance of urogenital mycoplasmal infections, in: A. Bondi et al., (Ed.), Urogenital Infections: New Developments in Laboratory Diagnosis and Treatment, Plenum Publishing, New York, 1987, pp. 93–115.

[14] D. Taylor-Robinson, *Ureaplasma urealyticum*, *Mycoplasma hominis*, and *Mycoplasma genitalium*, in: G.L. Mandell, J.E. Bennett, R. Dolan (Eds.), Principles and Practice of Infectious Diseases, Churchill Livingstone, Philadelphia, 2000, pp. 2027–2032.

[15] T. Becopoulos, et al., *Ureaplasma urealyticum* and infected renal calculi, J. Chemother. 3 (1991) 39–41.

[16] L. Grenabo, H. Hedelin, S. Pettersson, Urinary stones caused by *Ureaplasma urealyticum*: a review, Scand. J. Infect. Dis. Suppl. 53 (1988) 46–49.

[17] A.C. Thomsen, et al., The infrequent occurrence of mycoplasmas in amniotic fluid from women with intact fetal membranes, Acta Obstet. Gynecol. Scand. 3 (1983) 425–429.

[18] P.A. Mardh, L. Westrom, Tubal and cervical cultures in acute salpingitis with special reference to *Mycoplasma hominis* and T-strain mycoplasmas, Br. J. Vener. Dis. 46 (1970) 179–186.

[19] P.A. Mardh, Mycoplasmal PID: a review of natural and experimental infections, Yale J. Biol. Med. 56 (1983) 529.

[20] A. Miettinen, et al., Enzyme immunoassay for serum antibody to *Mycoplasma hominis* in women with acute pelvic inflammatory disease, Sex. Transm. Dis. 10 (Suppl.) (1983) 289.

[21] J. Henry-Suchet, et al., Microbiology of specimens obtained by laparoscopy from controls and from patients with pelvic inflammatory disease or infertility with tubal obstruction: *Chlamydia trachomatis* and *Ureaplasma urealyticum*, Am. J. Obstet. Gynecol. 138 (1980) 1022.

[22] B.R. Moller, et al., Experimental infection of the genital tract of female grivet monkeys by *Mycoplasma hominis*, Infect. Immun. 20 (1978) 248.

[23] P.A. Mardh, L. Westrom, C. Mecklenburg, Studies on ciliated epithelia of the human genital tract. I. Swelling of the cilia of fallopian tube epithelium in organ cultures infected with *Mycoplasma hominis*, Br. J. Vener. Dis. 52 (1976) 52.

[24] Proceedings of the International Symposium, Ureaplasmas of humans with emphasis on maternal and neonatal infections, Pediatr. Infect. Dis. 5 (Suppl. 6) (1986).

[25] G.H. Cassell, et al., Isolation of *Mycoplasma hominis* and *Ureaplasma urealyticum* from amniotic fluid at 16–20 weeks gestation: potential effect on pregnancy outcome, Sex. Transm. Dis. 10 (1983) 294–302.

[26] J.E. Embree, et al., Placental infection with *Mycoplasma hominis* and *Ureaplasma urealyticum*: clinical correlation, Obstet. Gynecol. 56 (1980) 475–481.

[27] S.L. Hillier, et al., A case-control study of chorioamnionic infection and histologic chorioamnionitis in prematurity, N. Engl. J. Med. 319 (1988) 972–978.

[28] R.B. Kundsin, et al., Association of *Ureaplasma urealyticum* in the placenta with perinatal morbidity and mortality, N. Engl. J. Med. 310 (1984) 941–945.

[29] P.A. Quinn, et al., A prospective study of microbial infection in stillbirths and early neonatal death, Am. J. Obstet. Gynecol. 151 (1985) 238–249.

[30] P.A. Quinn, et al., Chorioamnionitis: its association with pregnancy outcome and microbial infection, Am. J. Obstet. Gynecol. 156 (1987) 379–387.

[31] G.H. Cassell, K.B. Waites, D.T. Crouse, Mycoplasmal infections, in: J.S. Remington, J.O. Klein (Eds.), Infectious Diseases of the Fetus and Newborn Infant, fifth ed., Saunders, Philadelphia, 2001, pp. 733–767.

[32] D.J. Gray, et al., Adverse effect on pregnancy following amniotic fluid isolation of *Ureaplasma urealyticum*, Prenat. Diagn. 12 (1992) 111–117.

[33] W. Foulon, et al., Chronic *Ureaplasma urealyticum* amnionitis associated with abruptio placentae, Obstet. Gynecol. 68 (1986) 280.

[34] G.H. Cassell, et al., The role of *Ureaplasma urealyticum* in amnionitis, Pediatr. Infect. Dis. J. 5 (1986) 247–252.

[35] B.H. Yoon, et al., Clinical implications of detection of *Ureaplasma urealyticum* in the amniotic cavity with the polymerase chain reaction, Am. J. Obstet. Gynecol. 183 (2000) 1130–1137.

[36] B.H. Yoon, et al., The clinical significance of detecting *Ureaplasma urealyticum* by the polymerase chain reaction in the amniotic fluid of patients with preterm labor, Am. J. Obstet. Gynecol. 189 (2003) 919–924.

[37] E.J. Stokes, Human infection with pleuropneumonia-like organisms, Lancet 1 (1955) 276–279.

[38] H.J. Harwick, et al., *Mycoplasma hominis* and abortion, J. Infect. Dis. 121 (1970) 260–268.

[39] H.J. Harwick, et al., *Mycoplasma hominis* septicemia associated with abortion, Am. J. Obstet. Gynecol. 99 (1967) 725–727.

[40] J.G. Tully, et al., Septicemia due to *Mycoplasma hominis* type 1, N. Engl. J. Med. 273 (1965) 648–650.

[41] E. Caspi, et al., Amnionitis and T strain mycoplasmemia, Am. J. Obstet. Gynecol. 111 (1971) 1102–1106.

[42] D. Sompolinsky, et al., Puerperal sepsis due to T-strain *Mycoplasma*, Isr. J. Med. Sci. 7 (1971) 745–748.

[43] K.C. Edelin, W.M. McCormack, Infection with *Mycoplasma hominis* in postpartum fever, Lancet 2 (1980) 1217–1221.

[44] W.M. McCormack, et al., Isolation of genital mycoplasmas from blood obtained shortly after vaginal delivery, Lancet 1 (1975) 596–599.

[45] V. Neman-Simha, et al., Isolation of genital mycoplasmas from blood of febrile obstetrical-gynecologic patients and neonates, Scand. J. Infect. Dis. 24 (1992) 317–321.

[46] W. Andrews, et al., Post-cesarean endometritis: role of asymptomatic antenatal colonization of the chorioamnion with *Ureaplasma urealyticum*, Am. J. Obstet. Gynecol. 170 (1994) 416.

[47] S. Roberts, et al., The microbiology of post-cesarean wound morbidity, Obstet. Gynecol. 81 (1993) 383–386.

[48] *Mycoplasma hominis*. Newsnotes. BMJ 2 (1974) 816.

[49] B.M. Word, A. Baldridge, *Mycoplasma hominis* pneumonia and pleural effusion in a postpartum adolescent, Pediatr. Infect. Dis. J. 9 (1990) 295–296.

[50] M.J. Young, R.A. Cox, Near fatal puerperal fever due to *Mycoplasma hominis*, Postgrad. Med. J. 66 (1990) 147–149.

[51] L.E. Phillips, et al., Postcesarean wound infection by *Mycoplasma hominis* in a patient with persistent postpartum fever, Diagn. Microbiol. Infect. Dis. 7 (1987) 193–197.

[52] M. Maccato, S. Faro, K.L. Summers, Wound infections after cesarean section with *Mycoplasma hominis* and *Ureaplasma urealyticum*: a report of three cases, Diagn. Microbiol. Infect. Dis. 13 (1990) 363–365.

[53] W.W. Andrews, et al., Randomized clinical trial of extended spectrum antibiotic prophylaxis with coverage for *Ureaplasma urealyticum* to reduce post-cesarean delivery endometritis, Obstet. Gynecol. 101 (2003) 1183–1189.

[54] G.G. Donders, et al., Relationship of bacterial vaginosis and mycoplasmas to the risk of spontaneous abortion, Am. J. Obstet. Gynecol. 183 (2000) 431–437.

[55] G.H. Cassell, B.C. Cole, Mycoplasmas as agents of human disease, N. Engl. J. Med. 304 (1981) 80–89.

[56] W.M. McCormack, D. Taylor-Robinson, The genital mycoplasmas, in: K.K. Holmes et al., (Eds.), Sexually Transmitted Diseases, McGraw-Hill, New York, 1984, pp. 408–419.

[57] D. Sompolinsky, et al., Infections with *Mycoplasma* and bacteria in induced midtrimester abortion and fetal loss, Am. J. Obstet. Gynecol. 121 (1975) 610–616.

[58] B. Stray-Pederson, J. Engard, T.M. Reikvam, Uterine T-Mycoplasma colonization in reproductive failure, Am. J. Obstet. Gynecol. 130 (1978) 307.

[59] A. Naessens, et al., Epidemiology and pathogenesis of *Ureaplasma urealyticum* in spontaneous abortion and early preterm labor, Acta. Obstet. Gynecol. Scand. 66 (1987) 513–516.

[60] P.A. Quinn, et al., Serologic evidence of *Ureaplasma urealyticum* infection in women with spontaneous pregnancy loss, Am. J. Obstet. Gynecol. 145 (1983) 245–250.

[61] T.G. Berg, et al., *Ureaplasma/Mycoplasma*-infected amniotic fluid: pregnancy outcome in treated and nontreated patients, J. Perinatol. 19 (1999) 275–277.

[62] G.H. Cassell, et al., *Ureaplasma urealyticum* intrauterine infection: role in prematurity and disease in newborns, Clin. Microbiol. Rev. 6 (1993) 69–87.

[63] R. Romero, et al., Is genital colonization with *Mycoplasma hominis* or *Ureaplasma urealyticum* associated with prematurity/low birth weight? Obstet. Gynecol. 73 (1989) 532–536.

[64] S. Gerber, et al., Detection of *Ureaplasma urealyticum* in second-trimester amniotic fluid by polymerase chain reaction correlates with subsequent preterm labor and delivery, J. Infect. Dis. 187 (2003) 518–521.

[65] M.G. Gravett, et al., Preterm labor associated with subclinical amniotic fluid infection and with bacterial vaginosis, Obstet. Gynecol. 67 (1986) 229–237.

[66] R. Romero, et al., Infection and labor. V. Prevalence, microbiology, and clinical significance of intraamniotic infection in women with preterm labor and intact membranes, Am. J. Obstet. Gynecol. 161 (1989) 817–824.

[67] D.H. Watts, et al., The association of occult amniotic fluid infection with gestational age and neonatal outcome among women in preterm labor, Obstet. Gynecol. 79 (1992) 351–357.

[68] S.L. Hillier, et al., Microbiologic causes and neonatal outcomes associated with chorioamnion infection, Obstet. Gynecol. 165 (1991) 955–961.

[69] A. Naessens, et al., Postpartum bacteremia and placental colonization with genital mycoplasmas and pregnancy outcome, Am. J. Obstet. Gynecol. 160 (1989) 647–650.

[70] F.J. Zlatnik, et al., Histologic chorioamnionitis, microbial infection, and prematurity, J. Obstet. Gynaecol. 76 (1990) 355–359.

[71] P.A. Quinn, et al., Intrauterine infection with *Ureaplasma urealyticum* as a cause of fatal neonatal pneumonia, Pediatr. Infect. Dis. J. 4 (1985) 538–543.

[72] J. Ollikainen, et al., *Ureaplasma urealyticum* infection associated with acute respiratory insufficiency and death in premature infants, J. Pediatr. 122 (1993) 756–760.

[73] G.H. Cassell, et al., Association of *Ureaplasma urealyticum* infection of the lower respiratory tract with chronic lung disease and death in very low birthweight infants, Lancet 2 (1988) 240–245.

[74] V.N. Kelly, S.M. Garland, G.L. Gilbert, Isolation of genital mycoplasmas from the blood of neonates and women with pelvic infection using conventional SPS-free blood culture media, Pathology 19 (1987) 277–280.

[75] G.A. Syrogiannopoulos, et al., *Ureaplasma urealyticum* colonization of full term infants: perinatal acquisition and persistence during early infancy, Pediatr. Infect. Dis. J. 9 (1990) 236–240.

[76] P. Sanchez, J.A. Regan, Vertical transmission of *Ureaplasma urealyticum* in full term infants, Pediatr. Infect. Dis. J. 6 (1988) 825–828.

[77] P. Sanchez, J.A. Regan, Vertical transmission of *Ureaplasma urealyticum* from mothers to preterm infants, Pediatr. Infect. Dis. J. 9 (1990) 398–401.

[78] M.J. Dinsmoor, R.S. Ramamurthy, R.S. Gibbs, Transmission of genital mycoplasmas from mother to neonate in women with prolonged membrane rupture, Pediatr. Infect. Dis. J. 8 (1989) 483–487.

[79] K.B. Chua, et al., Colonization and transmission of *Ureaplasma urealyticum* and *Mycoplasma hominis* from mothers to full and preterm babies by normal vaginal delivery, Med. J. Malaysia 54 (1999) 242–246.

[80] H.M. Foy, et al., Acquisition of mycoplasmata and T-strains during infancy, J. Infect. Dis. 121 (1970) 579–587.

[81] K.B. Waites, et al., Chronic *Ureaplasma urealyticum* and *Mycoplasma hominis* infections of central nervous systems in preterm infants, Lancet 2 (1988) 17–21.

[82] K.B. Waites, et al., *Ureaplasma* pneumonia and sepsis associated with persistent pulmonary hypertension of the newborn, Pediatrics 83 (1991) 84–89.

[83] F. Brus, et al., Fatal ureaplasmal pneumonia and sepsis in a newborn infant, Eur. J. Pediatr. 150 (1991) 782–783.

[84] N. Tafari, et al., Mycoplasma "T" strains and perinatal death, Lancet 1 (1976) 108–109.

[85] D.T. Crouse, et al., Radiographic changes associated with tracheal isolation of *Ureaplasma urealyticum* from neonates, Clin. Infect. Dis. 17 (Suppl. 1) (1993) S122–S130.

[86] R. Cultrera, et al., Molecular evidence of *Ureaplasma urealyticum* and *Ureaplasma parvum* colonization in preterm infants during respiratory distress syndrome, BMC Infect. Dis. 6 (2006) 166.

[87] K. Hannaford, et al., Role of *Ureaplasma urealyticum* in lung disease of prematurity, Arch. Dis. Child. Fetal. Neonatal. Ed. 81 (1999) F162–F167.

[88] A. Berger, et al., Microbial invasion of the amniotic cavity at birth is associated with adverse short-term outcome of preterm infants, J. Perinat. Med. 31 (2003) 115–121.

[89] M.B. Escobedo, et al., A baboon model of bronchopulmonary dysplasia, Exp. Mol. Pathol. 37 (1982) 323–324.

[90] W.F. Walsh, et al., A primate model of *Ureaplasma urealyticum* infection in the premature infant with hyaline membrane disease, Clin. Infect. Dis. 17 (1993) S158–S162.

[91] B.A. Yoder, et al., Effects of antenatal colonization with *Ureaplasma urealyticum* on pulmonary disease in the immature baboon, Pediatr. Res. 54 (2003) 797–807.

[92] E.E.L. Wang, A. Ohlsson, J.D. Kellner, Association of *Ureaplasma urealyticum* colonization with chronic lung disease of prematurity: results of a metaanalysis, J. Pediatr. 127 (1995) 640–644.

[93] B.D. Benstein, et al., *Ureaplasma* in lung. 2. Association with bronchopulmonary dysplasia in premature newborns, Exp. Mol. Pathol. 75 (2003) 171–177.

[94] R.W. Perzigian, et al., *Ureaplasma urealyticum* and chronic lung disease in very low birth weight infants during the exogenous surfactant era, Pediatr. Infect. Dis. J. 17 (1998) 620–625.

[95] S. Castro-Alcaraz, et al., Patterns of colonization with *Ureaplasma urealyticum* during neonatal intensive care unit hospitalizations of very low birth weight infants and the development of chronic lung disease, Pediatrics 110 (2002) e45.

[96] S.M. Garland, E.D. Bowman, Role of *Ureaplasma urealyticum* and *Chlamydia trachomatis* in lung disease in low birth weight infants, Pathology 28 (1996) 266–269.

[97] R. Iles, et al., Infection with *Ureaplasma urealyticum* and *Mycoplasma hominis* and the development of chronic lung disease in pre-term infants, Acta Paediatr. 85 (1996) 482–484.

[98] L. Pacifico, et al., *Ureaplasma urealyticum* and pulmonary outcome in a neonatal intensive care population, Pediatr. Infect. Dis. J. 16 (1997) 579–586.

[99] D.A. Kafetzis, et al., Maternal genital colonization with *Ureaplasma urealyticum* promotes preterm delivery: association of the respiratory colonization of premature infants with chronic lung disease and increased mortality, Clin. Infect. Dis. 39 (2004) 1113–1122.

[100] M. Abele-Horn, et al., *Ureaplasma urealyticum* colonization and bronchopulmonary dysplasia: a comparative prospective multicentre study, Eur. J. Pediatr. 157 (1998) 1004–1011.

[101] P. Agarwal, et al., *Ureaplasma urealyticum* and its association with chronic lung disease in Asian neonates, J. Paediatr. Child Health 36 (2000) 487–490.

[102] O. Da Silva, D. Gregson, O. Hammerberg, Role of *Ureaplasma urealyticum* and *Chlamydia trachomatis* in development of bronchopulmonary dysplasia in very low birth weight infants, Pediatr. Infect. Dis. J. 16 (1997) 364–369.

[103] W.M. Van Waarde, et al., *Ureaplasma urealyticum* colonization, prematurity and bronchopulmonary dysplasia, Eur. Respir. J. 10 (1997) 886–890.

[104] X.I. Couroucli, et al., Detection of microorganisms in the tracheal aspirates of preterm infants by polymerase chain reaction: association of adenovirus infection with bronchopulmonary dysplasia, Pediatr. Res. 47 (2000) 225–232.

[105] L. Cordero, et al., Bacterial and *Ureaplasma* colonization of the airway: radiologic findings in infants with bronchopulmonary dysplasia, J. Perinatol. 17 (1997) 428–433.

[106] A.D. Heggie, et al., Identification and quantification of ureaplasmas colonizing the respiratory tract and assessment of their role in the development of chronic lung disease in preterm infants, Pediatr. Infect. Dis. J. 20 (2001) 854–859.

[107] B. Jonsson, M. Rylander, G. Faxelius, *Ureaplasma urealyticum*, erythromycin and respiratory morbidity in high-risk preterm neonates, Acta Paediatr. 87 (1998) 1079–1084.

[108] J. Ollikainen, et al., Chronic lung disease of the newborn is not associated with *Ureaplasma urealyticum*, Pediatr. Pulmonol. 32 (2001) 303–307.

[109] R.L. Schelonka, et al., Critical appraisal of the role of *Ureaplasma* in the development of bronchopulmonary dysplasia with metaanalytic techniques, Pediatr. Infect. Dis. J. 24 (2005) 1033–1039.

[110] C. Buhrer, T. Hoehn, J. Hentschel, Role of erythromycin for treatment of incipient chronic lung disease in preterm infants colonised with *Ureaplasma urealyticum*, Drugs 61 (2001) 1893–1899.

[111] A.D. Heggie, et al., Frequency and significance of isolation of *Ureaplasma urealyticum* and *Mycoplasma hominis* from cerebrospinal fluid and tracheal aspirate specimens from low birth weight infants, J. Pediatr. 124 (1994) 956–961.

[112] A.J. Lyon, et al., Randomised trial of erythromycin on the development of chronic lung disease in preterm infants, Arch. Dis. Child. Fetal. Neonatal. Ed. 78 (1998) F10–F14.

[113] E.D. Bowman, et al., Impact of erythromycin on respiratory colonization of *Ureaplasma urealyticum* and the development of chronic lung disease in extremely low birth weight infants, Pediatr. Infect. Dis. J. 17 (1998) 615–620.

[114] S.L. Kenyon, D.J. Taylor, W. Tarnow-Mordi, Broad-spectrum antibiotics for preterm, prelabour rupture of fetal membranes: the ORACLE I randomised trial. ORACLE Collaborative Group, Lancet 357 (2001) 979–988.

[115] S.L. Kenyon, D.J. Taylor, W. Tarnow-Mordi, Broad-spectrum antibiotics for spontaneous preterm labour: the ORACLE II randomised trial. ORACLE Collaborative Group, Lancet 357 (2001) 989–994.

[116] J. Ollikainen, Perinatal Ureaplasma urealyticum infection increases the need for hospital treatment during the first year of life in preterm infants, Pediatr Pulmonol 30 (2000) 402–405.

[117] R.M. Viscardi, et al., Antenatal *Ureaplasma urealyticum* respiratory tract infection stimulates proinflammatory, profibrotic responses in the preterm baboon lung, Pediatr. Res. 60 (2006) 141–146.

[118] S. Izraeli, et al., Genital mycoplasmas in preterm infants: prevalence and clinical significance, Eur. J. Pediatr. 150 (1991) 804–807.

[119] D. Taylor-Robinson, P.M. Furr, M.M. Liberman, The occurrence of genital mycoplasmas in babies with and without respiratory diseases, Acta Paediatr. Scand. 73 (1984) 383–386.

[120] J.G. Steytler, Statistical studies on mycoplasma-positive human umbilical cord blood cultures, S. Afr. J. Obstet. Gynecol. 8 (1970) 10–13.

[121] J. Ollikainen, et al., *Ureaplasma urealyticum* cultured from brain tissue of preterm twins who died of intraventricular hemorrhage, Scand. J. Infect. Dis. 25 (1993) 529–531.

[122] M. Dan, et al., *Mycoplasma hominis* septicemia in a burned infant, J. Pediatr. 99 (1981) 743–744.

[123] P.F. Unsworth, et al., Neonatal mycoplasmemia. *Mycoplasma hominis* as a significant cause of disease? J. Infect. 10 (1985) 163–168.

[124] G.B. Valencia, et al., *Mycoplasma hominis* and *Ureaplasma urealyticum* in neonates with suspected infection, Pediatr. Infect. Dis. J. 12 (1993) 571–573.

[125] S. Likitnukul, et al., Role of genital mycoplasmas in young infants with suspected sepsis, J. Pediatr. 109 (1986) 971–974.

[126] R.L. Goldenberg, et al., The Alabama preterm birth study: Umbilical cord blood *Ureaplasma urealyticum* and *Mycoplasma hominis* cultures in very preterm newborn infants, Am. J. Obstet. Gynecol. 198 (2008) 43.e1–43.e5.

[127] P.A. Mardh, *Mycoplasma hominis* infections of the central nervous system in newborn infants, Sex. Transm. Dis. 10 (1983) 331–334.

[128] J.C. McDonald, *Mycoplasma hominis* meningitis in a premature infant, Pediatr. Infect. Dis. J. 7 (1988) 795–798.

[129] S.R. Wealthall, *Mycoplasma* meningitis in infants with spina bifida, Dev. Med. Child. Neurol. 17 (1975) 117–122.

[130] G.R. Siber, et al., Neonatal central nervous system infection due to *Mycoplasma hominis*, J. Pediatr. 90 (1977) 625–627.

[131] N. Kirk, I. Kovar, *Mycoplasma hominis* meningitis in a preterm infant, J. Infect. 15 (1987) 109–110.

[132] E. Hjelm, et al., Meningitis in a newborn infant caused by *Mycoplasma hominis*, Acta Paediatr. Scand. 69 (1980) 415–418.

[133] M. Gewitz, et al., *Mycoplasma hominis*: a cause of neonatal meningitis, Arch. Dis. Child. 54 (1979) 231–233.

[134] G.L. Gilbert, F. Law, S.J. Macinnes, Chronic *Mycoplasma hominis* infection complicating severe intraventricular hemorrhage, in a premature neonate, Pediatr. Infect. Dis. J. 7 (1988) 817–818.

[135] O. Boe, J. Diderichsen, R. Matre, Isolation of *Mycoplasma hominis* from cerebrospinal fluid, Scand. J. Infect. Dis. 5 (1973) 285–288.

[136] R.P. Rao, et al., *Mycoplasma hominis* and *Ureaplasma* species brain abscess in a neonate, Pediatr. Infect. Dis. J. 21 (2002) 1083–1085.

[137] M. Knausz, et al., Meningo-encephalitis in a neonate caused by maternal *Mycoplasma hominis* treated successfully with chloramphenicol, J. Med. Microbiol. 51 (2002) 187–188.

[138] K.B. Waites, et al., *Mycoplasma* infection of the central nervous system in humans and animals, Int. J. Med. Microbiol. 20 (1990) 379–386.

[139] K.B. Waites, et al., Mycoplasmal infection of cerebrospinal fluid in newborn infants from a community hospital population, Pediatr. Infect. Dis. J. 9 (1990) 241–245.

[140] K.B. Waites, D.T. Crouse, G.H. Cassell, Systemic neonatal infection due to *Ureaplasma urealyticum*, Clin. Infect. Dis. 17 (Suppl. 1) (1993) S131–S135.

[141] K.B. Waites, et al., Mycoplasmal infections of cerebrospinal fluid in newborn infants from a community hospital population, Pediatr. Infect. Dis. J. 9 (1990) 241–245.

[142] N.J. Shaw, B.C. Pratt, A.M. Weindling, *Ureaplasma* and *Mycoplasma* infections of central nervous systems in preterm infants, Lancet 2 (1989) 1530–1531.

[143] K.B. Waites, et al., Isolation of *Ureaplasma urealyticum* from low birth weight infants, J. Pediatr. 126 (1995) 502.

[144] A.D. Heggie, et al., Isolation of *Ureaplasma urealyticum* from low birth weight infants, J. Pediatr. 126 (1995) 503–504.

[145] O. Dammann, et al., Antenatal *Mycoplasma* infection, the fetal inflammatory response and cerebral white matter damage in very-low-birthweight infants, Paediatr. Perinat. Epidemiol. 17 (2003) 49–57.

[146] N.J. Shaw, B.C. Pratt, A.M. Weindling, *Ureaplasma* and *Mycoplasma* infections of the central nervous system in preterm infants, Lancet 23 (1989) 1530–1531.

[147] K.B. Waites, et al., Association of genital mycoplasmas with exudative vaginitis in a 10 year old: a case of misdiagnosis, Pediatrics 71 (1983) 250–252.

[148] S.M. Garland, L.J. Murton, Neonatal meningitis caused by *Ureaplasma urealyticum*, Pediatr. Infect. Dis. J. 6 (1987) 868–870.

[149] T.C. Miller, S.I. Baman, W.H. Albers, Massive pericardial effusion due to *Mycoplasma hominis* in a newborn, Am. J. Dis. Child. 136 (1982) 271–272.

[150] J.B. Glaser, M. Engelbert, M. Hamerschlag, Scalp abscess associated with *Mycoplasma hominis* infection complicating intrapartum monitoring, Pediatr. Infect. Dis. J. 2 (1983) 468–470.

[151] I. Sacker, P.A. Brunell, Abscess in newborn infants caused by *Mycoplasma*, Pediatrics 46 (1970) 303–304.

[152] N. Abdel-Haq, B. Asmar, W. Brown, *Mycoplasma hominis* scalp abscess in the newborn, Pediatr. Infect. Dis. J. 21 (2002) 1171–1173.

[153] D.A. Powell, K. Miller, W.A. Clyde Jr., Submandibular adenitis in a newborn caused by *Mycoplasma hominis*, Pediatrics 63 (1979) 789–799.

[154] S.R. Dominguez, C. Littlehorn, A.C. Nyquist, *Mycoplasma hominis* endocarditis in a child with a complex congenital heart defect, Pediatr. Infect. Dis. J. 25 (2006) 851–852.

[155] A. Blanchard, et al., Use of the polymerase chain reaction for detection of *Mycoplasma fermentans* and *Mycoplasma genitalium* in the urogenital tract and amniotic fluid, Clin. Infect. Dis. 17 (Suppl. 1) (1993) S272–S279.

[156] A.C. Labbe, et al., *Mycoplasma genitalium* is not associated with adverse outcomes of pregnancy in Guinea-Bissau, Sex. Transm. Infect. 78 (2002) 289–291.

[157] D. Taylor-Robinson, *Mycoplasma genitalium*—an up-date, Int. J. STD AIDS 13 (2002) 145–151.

[158] G.H. Cassell, et al., Mycoplasmas, in: B.J. Howard, et al. (Eds.), Clinical and Pathogenic Microbiology, Mosby-Year Book, St. Louis, 1994, pp. 491–502.

[159] M.C. Shepard, G.K. Masover, Special features of ureaplasmas, in: M.F. Barile, S. Razin (Eds.), The Mycoplasmas. I. Cell Biology, Academic Press, New York, 1979, pp. 452–494.

[160] M.C. Shepard, Culture media for ureaplasmas, in: S. Razin, J.G. Tully (Eds.), Methods in Mycoplasmology, Academic Press, New York, 1983.

[161] A. Blanchard, et al., Detection of *Ureaplasma urealyticum* by polymerase chain reaction in the urogenital tract of adults, in amniotic fluid, and in the respiratory tract of newborns, Clin. Infect. Dis. 17 (Suppl. 1) (1993) S148–S153.

[162] A. Blanchard, et al., Evaluation of intraspecies genetic variation within the 16S rRNA gene of *Mycoplasma hominis* and detection by polymerase chain reaction, J. Clin. Microbiol. 31 (1993) 1358–1361.

[163] N. Luki, et al., Comparison of polymerase chain reaction assay with culture for detection of genital mycoplasmas in perinatal infections, Eur. J. Clin. Microbiol. Infect. Dis. 17 (1998) 255–263.

[164] M. Abele-Horn, et al., Polymerase chain reaction versus culture for detection of *Ureaplasma urealyticum* and *Mycoplasma hominis* in the urogenital tract of adults and the respiratory tract of newborns, Eur. J. Clin. Microbiol. Infect. Dis. 15 (1996) 595–598.

[165] N.A. Cunliffe, et al., Comparison of culture with the polymerase chain reaction for detection of *Ureaplasma urealyticum* in endotracheal aspirates of preterm infants, J. Med. Microbiol. 45 (1996) 27–30.

[166] B. de Barbeyrac, et al., Detection of *Mycoplasma pneumoniae* and *Mycoplasma genitalium* in clinical samples by polymerase chain reaction, Clin. Infect. Dis. 17 (Suppl. 1) (1993) S83–S89.

[167] S.C. Lo, et al., Identification of *Mycoplasma incognitus* infection in patients with AIDS: an immunohistochemistry, in situ hybridization and ultrastructural study, Am. J. Trop. Med. Hyg. 41 (1989) 601–616.

[168] American Academy of Pediatrics, *Ureaplasma urealyticum* infections, in: L.K. Pickering (Ed.), Red Book: Report of the Committee on Infectious Diseases, American Academy of Pediatrics, Elk Grove Village, IL, 2006, pp. 709–710.

[169] D. Taylor-Robinson, C. Bebear, Antibiotic susceptibilities of mycoplasmas and treatment of *Mycoplasma* infections, J. Antimicrob. Chemother. 40 (1997) 622–630.

[170] K.B. Waites, D.T. Crouse, G.H. Cassell, Antibiotic susceptibilities and therapeutic options for *Ureaplasma urealyticum* infections in neonates, Pediatr. Infect. Dis. J. 11 (1992) 23–29.

[171] K.B. Waites, D.T. Crouse, G.H. Cassell, Therapeutic consideration for *Ureaplasma urealyticum* infections in neonates, Clin. Infect. Dis. 17 (Suppl. 1) (1993) S208–S214.

[172] K.B. Waites, et al., In vitro susceptibilities of mycoplasmas and ureaplasmas to new macrolides and aryl-fluoroquinolones, Antimicrob. Agents Chemother. 32 (1988) 1500–1502.

[173] M.B. Kober, B.A. Mason, Colonization of the female genital tract by resistant *Ureaplasma urealyticum* treated successfully with azithromycin, Clin. Infect. Dis. 278 (1998) 401–402.

[174] K.B. Waites, et al., In vitro susceptibilities to and bactericidal activities of garenoxacin (BMS-284756) and other antimicrobial agents against human mycoplasmas and ureaplasmas, Antimicrob. Agents Chemother. 47 (2003) 161–165.

[175] G.E. Kenny, F.D. Cartwright, Susceptibilities of *Mycoplasma hominis*, *M. pneumoniae*, and *Ureaplasma urealyticum* to GAR-936, dalfopristin, dirithromycin, evernimicin, gatifloxacin, linezolid, moxifloxacin, quinupristin-dalfopristin, and telithromycin compared to their susceptibilities to reference macrolides, tetracyclines, and quinolones, Antimicrob. Agents Chemother. 45 (2001) 2604–2608.

[176] K.B. Waites, D.M. Crabb, L.B. Duffy, In vitro activities of ABT-773 and other antimicrobials against human mycoplasmas, Antimicrob. Agents Chemother. 47 (2003) 39–42.

[177] C.M. Bebear, et al., In vitro activity of trovafloxacin compared to those of five antimicrobials against mycoplasmas including *Mycoplasma hominis* and *Ureaplasma urealyticum* fluoroquinolone-resistant isolates that have been genetically characterized, Antimicrob. Agents Chemother. 44 (2000) 2557–2560.

[178] P. Braun, J.O. Klein, E.H. Kass, Susceptibility of *Mycoplasma hominis* and T-strains to 14 antimicrobial agents, Appl. Microbiol. 19 (1970) 62–70.

[179] C. Thornsberry, A.J. Barry, Methods for dilution-anti-microbial susceptibility tests for bacteria that grow aerobically, in: Tentative Standards, 2nd ed., National Committee for Clinical Laboratory Standards, Villanova, PA, 1988.

[180] L. Duffy, et al., Fluoroquinolone resistance in *Ureaplasma parvum* in the United States, J. Clin. Microbiol. 44 (2006) 1590–1591.

[181] P.A. Mardh, *Mycoplasma hominis* infection of the central nervous system in newborn infants, Sex. Transm. Dis. 10 (1983) 332–334.

[182] L.A. Koutsky, et al., Persistence of *Mycoplasma hominis* after therapy: importance of tetracycline resistance and of co-existing vaginal flora, Sex. Transm. Dis. 10 (1983) 374–381.

[183] M.C. Cummings, W.M. McCormack, Increase in resistance of *Mycoplasma hominis* to tetracyclines, Antimicrob. Agents Chemother. 34 (1990) 2297–2299.

VIRAL INFECTIONS

SECTION OUTLINE

21 Human Immunodeficiency Virus/Acquired Immunodeficiency Syndrome in the Infant   622

22 Chickenpox, Measles, and Mumps   661

23 Cytomegalovirus   706

24 Enterovirus and Parechovirus Infections   756

25 Hepatitis   800

26 Herpes Simplex Virus Infections   813

27 Human Parvovirus   834

28 Rubella   861

29 Smallpox and Vaccinia   899

30 Less Common Viral Infections   905

HUMAN IMMUNODEFICIENCY VIRUS/ACQUIRED IMMUNODEFICIENCY SYNDROME IN THE INFANT

Avinash K. Shetty ☉ Yvonne A. Maldonado

CHAPTER OUTLINE

Epidemiology 623
Transmission 623
   Intrauterine Transmission 623
   Intrapartum Infection 624
   Postpartum Infection 624
Molecular Biology 625
Pathogenesis of Early Infant Infection 626
   Viral Pathogenesis 626
   Immune Abnormalities in Human Immunodeficiency
   Virus Infection 626
   Human Immunodeficiency Virus–Specific Immune Control 626
Diagnosis 627
   Human Immunodeficiency Virus Testing of Pregnant
   Women 627
   Early Infant Diagnosis 627
Classification of Human Immunodeficiency Virus Infection
in Children 628
Clinical Manifestations and Pathology 632
   Infectious Complications 632
   Encephalopathy 634
   Ophthalmologic Pathology 635

Interstitial Lung Disease 635
Cardiovascular Complications 636
Pathology of the Gastrointestinal Tract 636
Nephropathy 636
Pathology of Endocrine Organs 637
Involvement of Lymphoid Organs and Thymus 637
Hematologic Problems 637
Skin 637
Malignancies 637
Morbidity, Mortality, and Prognosis 637
Prevention 638
   Experience in Perinatal Human Immunodeficiency Virus Prevention
   in the United States 638
   International Experience in Perinatal Human Immunodeficiency
   Virus Prevention 640
   Safety and Toxicity of Antiretroviral Prophylaxis 645
   Antiretroviral Resistance 646
Treatment 646
   Supportive Care and General Management 646
   Antiretroviral Therapy 648
Future Goals 651

Since the first descriptions of acquired immunodeficiency syndrome (AIDS) in infants and children in the early 1980s [1–4] the epidemiology of pediatric human immunodeficiency virus (HIV) infection has changed significantly in the United States [5–7]. Perinatal transmission is the most common source of HIV infection among infants and children [8]. Although HIV infection in children has been acquired in the past by the transfusion of contaminated blood or coagulation products, this route has been virtually eliminated in the United States. Remarkable progress has been made in prevention of perinatal transmission of HIV during the last decade in developed nations [9]. Dramatic declines in the number of HIV-infected children who acquired the infection perinatally have been reported in the United States because of prompt implementation of effective, cost-saving strategies to prevent mother-to-child transmission of HIV [10–13].

Rates of perinatal HIV transmission in the United States and Europe have decreased to 2% or less because of widespread implementation of universal antenatal HIV testing, combination antiretroviral treatment during pregnancy, elective cesarean section, and avoidance of breast-feeding [14–17]. Currently, less than 200 infants acquire HIV from their mothers in the United States annually primarily because of missed prevention opportunities [18]. Availability of highly active antiretroviral therapy (HAART) has led to improved survival of HIV-infected children into adolescence and adulthood changing most HIV infections into a treatable chronic disease rather than a fatal disease [19–25].

In contrast, prevention of mother-to-child transmission of HIV is a major public health challenge in resource-limited nations [9,26]. More than 90% of these affected children reside in sub-Saharan Africa [27]. Although several effective, simple, and less expensive prophylactic antiretroviral regimens are available to prevent perinatal HIV transmission, less than 10% of HIV-infected pregnant women have access to these preventive interventions in the developing world [28]. In addition, progress has been slow in scaling-up HAART in sub-Saharan Africa; only 23% of HIV-infected individuals who need HAART are receiving it [28], and only 5% to 7% of the individuals receiving treatment are children [29,30]. This chapter reviews advances in the prevention of perinatal HIV transmission; discusses evaluation and management of HIV-exposed infants in the United States; and highlights certain unique features of HIV infection in infants, with a focus on early diagnosis, clinical manifestations, treatment, and prognosis.

EPIDEMIOLOGY

HIV infection is a pandemic with cases reported to the World Health Organization (WHO) from virtually every country. At the end of December 2007, an estimated 33 million people were living with HIV, including 13 million women of childbearing age and 2.5 million children younger than 15 years [28]. Resource-limited settings bear the brunt of the epidemic with 22.5 million HIV-infected people living in sub-Saharan Africa [28]. It has been estimated that in 2007, 420,000 children were newly infected with HIV [28], primarily through mother-to-child transmission of HIV; 70% of infants were born in sub-Saharan Africa, 25% in Southeast Asia, and the remainder in Latin America and the Carribean [28]. In 2007, 330,000 children younger than 15 years died of HIV-related complications [28]. In developing nations, children constitute 14% of new HIV infections worldwide and nearly one fifth of annual HIV deaths [28].

Primary HIV infection among women of childbearing age fuels the perinatal HIV epidemic. In some countries in sub-Saharan Africa, antenatal HIV prevalence can reach 40% [28]. Approximately 3.28 million pregnant women infected with HIV give birth annually primarily in resource-limited settings, where approximately 1800 HIV-infected infants are born each day. More than 50% of HIV-infected children in sub-Saharan Africa die by 2 years of age [31]. The Joint United Nations Program on HIV/AIDS (UNAIDS) estimates that 15 million children have been orphaned by the AIDS epidemic [28].

The average HIV seroprevalence among women in the United States has been estimated at 1.5 to 1.7 in 1000 women of childbearing age [32]. Characteristics of the HIV epidemic among women of reproductive age affect the pediatric HIV epidemic [32]. Regional HIV seroprevalence rates vary, with the highest rates found among women residing in the Northeast and in the South, especially in New York, Florida, Texas, and New Jersey [32]. Based on these rates, it is estimated that around 6000 to 7000 HIV-infected women give birth in the United States each year [32,33]. Of the estimated 123,405 women and adolescent girls living with HIV/AIDS at the end of 2004, 71% contracted infection through heterosexual contact, and 27% had been exposed through injection drug use [34]. Although the association of intravenous drug use as a risk factor for HIV infection among women has been relatively constant, HIV-infected women with heterosexual contact as the only risk factor for HIV infection increased from 14% in 1982 to 40% of all HIV-infected women in 2000 [35]. Heterosexual transmission of HIV to women of childbearing age is likely to continue to account for most perinatal HIV infection in the United States.

The rate of HIV infection among women of childbearing age has continued to increase. Of reported AIDS cases in adults, women accounted for 7% in 1985, 13% in 1993, and 23% in 1999 [33]. In 2004, 27% of 44,615 reported AIDS cases among adults and adolescents were in women and adolescent girls [34]. African American and Hispanic women are disproportionately affected by the HIV epidemic. More than 75% of women with AIDS are in the reproductive age group at the time of diagnosis. Despite improved survival because of effective HAART regimens, transmission is ongoing, and young women are at highest risk [36].

Adolescents represent a growing population of HIV infection, with at least 5000 individuals 13 to 19 years old living with HIV. Many HIV-infected adolescents acquired their infection perinatally. In the United States, HIV-infected children younger than 13 years account for only 1% of all AIDS cases [37]. Since the beginning of the epidemic, 9441 cases of AIDS in children younger than 13 years have been reported in the United States [36]. Perinatal transmission is the most common source of pediatric HIV infection, accounting for 91% of cases; 4% acquired infection through receipt of blood or blood products, and another 2% acquired HIV-1 from transfusion because of hemophilia. Approximately 2% of cases have been reported to have no identifiable risk factor [36,38]. The number of infants born with HIV-1 has decreased from a high of 2000 per year in the early 1990s to less than 150 [10]. At the same time, new pediatric AIDS cases and AIDS deaths also have dramatically declined, primarily because of availability of HAART.

In 2005, 93 AIDS cases were reported in children younger than 13 years compared with 122 cases in 2004 and 858 cases in 1992. New York and Florida reported the highest number of cases. The racial and ethnic and geographic distribution of AIDS cases in children parallels that of women with AIDS. Minority groups are disproportionately affected, with 59% of cases occurring among African American, non-Hispanic children (who account for only 14% of the U.S. pediatric population) and 23% occurring in Hispanics (17% of the U.S. pediatric population) compared with 17% occurring in white, non-Hispanic children (64% of the U.S. pediatric population) [36].

TRANSMISSION

Mother-to-child transmission of HIV-1 can occur in utero, during labor and delivery, or postnatally through breast-feeding [6–8] Data suggest that most children are infected during the immediate peripartum period [6]. In the United States, the transmission rate without intervention is estimated to be 25% to 30%; in Europe, it is lower at 15% to 20%. A transmission rate of 25% to 45% has been observed among breast-feeding populations in Africa [39,40]. These variations in transmission rates likely reflect differences in infant feeding patterns, maternal and obstetric risk factors, viral factors, and methodologic differences among studies. Maternal disease status, especially a high viral load or a CD4$^+$ count less than 200 cells/mm^3, is highly correlated, however, with the risk for vertical transmission [39,41–45]

Knowledge about the precise timing of transmission is crucial for the design of potential preventive strategies [46]. In non–breast-fed infants, about one third of transmissions occur during late gestation, and the remaining two thirds occur during delivery [47]. In breast-fed infants, one third to one half of overall transmission may occur after delivery during lactation [48,49].

INTRAUTERINE TRANSMISSION

In utero transmission may occur through HIV infection in the placenta or fetal exposure to cell-free or cell-associated HIV in the amniotic fluid. Virus has been detected in some aborted fetuses of 8 to 20 weeks' gestational age and in amniotic fluid [50–53]. Maternal decidual leukocytes, villous macrophages (Hofbauer cells), and endothelial cells stain positive for gp41 antigen and HIV nucleic acids [54]. The placenta can be infected through CD4$^+$ trophoblasts or through the occasional occurrence of chorioamnionitis [55,56]. There is not a clear predictive value for the identification of HIV in the placenta and the infection of the fetus or newborn [57]. There are important technical limitations to studies of fetal or placenta tissues, particularly because of the difficulty in excluding contamination with maternal blood.

INTRAPARTUM INFECTION

Intrapartum transmission may occur in various ways, including direct exposure of the fetus or infant with infected maternal secretions during birth, ascending infection after rupture of membranes, or maternal-to-fetal microtransfusions during uterine contractions [58]. The bimodal course of disease in HIV-infected children and the fact that at the time of birth virus can be recovered from less than 25% of the infants who are subsequently shown to be infected suggest that a large proportion of perinatal infections occur late during pregnancy or during delivery [58]. An infant is considered to have been infected in utero if the HIV-1 genome can be detected by polymerase chain reaction (PCR) or be cultured from blood within 48 hours of birth [59].

In contrast, an infant is considered to have intrapartum infection if diagnostic assays such as culture, PCR, and serum p24 antigen were negative in blood samples obtained during the first week of life, but became positive during the period from day 7 to day 90, and the infant had not been breast-fed [59]. Intrapartum transmission is supported by studies failing to detect HIV in infants born to HIV-infected women in the first month of life but with subsequent detection of virus after 1 to 3 months of life [60–64]. In a study by the French Collaborative Study Group, timing of transmission was estimated with a mathematical model [65]. Data for the 95 infected infants (infants seropositive at 18 months and infants who died of HIV disease before this age and who were exclusively bottle-fed) were used in the model, which indicated that one third of the infants were infected in utero less than 2 months before delivery (95th percentile). In the remaining 65% of cases (95% confidence interval [CI] 22% to 92%), the date of infection was estimated as the day of birth. The estimated median period between birth and the positivity of viral markers (HIV PCR or HIV culture) was 10 days (95% CI 6% to 14%), and the 95th percentile was estimated at 56 days [65].

Discordance of infection has been described among the progeny of different pregnancies and even among twins [66–69] Retrospective studies of twins born to HIV-infected women found a higher HIV transmission rate among twins born by vaginal delivery compared with twins born by cesarean delivery and among first-born compared with second-born twins. In a large multinational study, data were collected on 100 sets of twins and one set of triplets born to HIV-seropositive mothers [68]. HIV-1 infection was more common in first-born than in second-born twins ($P = .004$), with 50% of first-born twins delivered vaginally and 38% of first-born twins delivered by cesarean section being infected compared with 19% of second-born twins delivered by either route. These data support exposure to maternal virus during delivery as a likely route of transmission.

Although numerous maternal, obstetric, infant, and viral factors may modify perinatal HIV transmission risk [70,71], the strongest predictor of intrauterine and intrapartum transmission is the maternal serum HIV RNA level [43,72–79]. Transmission can occur rarely, however, among pregnant women with low or undetectable serum levels of HIV around the time of labor and delivery [41].

Other maternal risk factors associated with higher rates of perinatal HIV infection include women with progressive symptoms of AIDS, acute HIV infection during pregnancy, and low CD4$^+$ counts [80–84]. HIV viral load in cervicovaginal secretions is an independent risk factor for perinatal HIV transmission [85]. Obstetric risk factors associated with increased risk of transmission include vaginal delivery, rupture of membranes for more than 4 hours, chorioamnionitis, and invasive obstetric procedures [84,86,87]. Premature infants born to HIV-infected women have a higher rate of perinatal HIV infection than full-term infants [88–90] Data from a large international meta-analysis of 15 prospective cohort studies and a randomized controlled trial from Europe have shown that cesarean section performed before labor and rupture of membranes reduces perinatal transmission of HIV-1 by 50% to 87% independent of the use of antiretroviral therapy or zidovudine prophylaxis [91,92]. Other risk factors reported include viral subtype and host genetic factors [6,47]. High viral heterogeneity in the mother is a risk factor for vertical transmission [93,94]. Increased transmission of HIV strains that are fetotropic is reported; isolation of HIV strains with highly conserved gene sequences from HIV-infected infants has been shown, despite the numerous genetically diverse strains isolated from their mothers [93]. Maternal-fetal HLA concordance and maternal HLA homozygosity increase the risk of perinatal transmission [94], whereas CCR5 haplotype may be permissive or protective, depending on the specific mutation [95].

POSTPARTUM INFECTION

In resource-poor settings, where breast-feeding is the cultural norm and safe replacement feeding is not affordable, feasible, sustainable, or safe, postnatal transmission of HIV through breast milk remains a significant challenge [48,49]. Transmission of HIV through breast-feeding can account for one third to one half of all HIV infections globally and carries an estimated transmission risk of about 15% when prolonged and continued into the 2nd year of life [48,49,96–100]. HIV has been isolated from cellular and cell-free fractions of human breast milk from HIV-infected women [101,102]. HIV has been shown by culture or PCR in varying frequencies (39% to 89%) in breast milk specimens from HIV-seropositive women [103–105]. More recent studies indicate that cell-associated virus is a stronger predictor for transmission of HIV to the infant than cell-free virus [106,107].

More recent data also indicate that HAART administered during pregnancy or postpartum suppresses HIV RNA, but not HIV DNA, in breast milk [108].

A meta-analysis estimated the overall additional risk of breast milk transmission as 14% (95% CI 7% to 22%) for established maternal infection to 29% (95% CI 16% to 42%) for primary infection [109]. Some studies show that the highest risk of breast milk HIV transmission occurs during the first few months of life, with a lower but continued risk thereafter [98,110]. In a randomized controlled trial of breast-feeding versus formula-feeding on HIV-1 transmission in Kenya, investigators found that formula-feeding reduced transmission by 44% at age 2 years and that 75% of infections were acquired during the first 6 months of life [110]. Studies from Malawi report a risk of 0.6% to 0.7% per month in the 1st year of life from 1 month through 12 months and 0.3% per month in the 2nd year of breast-feeding [98,111].

In an international multicenter pooled meta-analysis of greater than 900 mother-infant pairs, the risk of late postnatal transmission (>4 months of age) was 3.2 cases (CI 3.1 to 3.8) per year per 100 breast-fed infants [112]. Data from a more recent meta-analysis suggest that the risk of postnatal HIV transmission is constant (approximately 0.9% per month) between 1 and 18 months of age [113]. Risk factors for breast milk HIV transmission include women seroconverting during lactation, high HIV DNA or RNA level in plasma and breast milk, decreased maternal CD4+ cell count, maternal symptomatic disease or AIDS, prolonged breast-feeding, mixed infant feeding, thrush and other infant coinfections, bleeding or cracked nipples, subclinical and clinical mastitis, and breast abscesses [48,49,96,114–117].

Several large studies have shown a lack of transmission of HIV infection to household contacts through casual interactions [118–121]. The American Academy of Pediatrics (AAP) does not place any special restrictions on day care or school attendance of HIV-infected children, but recommends observance of universal precaution measures for all handling of blood and body fluids, regardless of the infection status of the child [122,123]. The same guidelines apply to the handling of all newborns during or after birth. Gloves should be worn when handling body fluids, including amniotic fluid, and only bulb or wall suction devices should be used to avoid exposure of medical personnel [124].

MOLECULAR BIOLOGY

HIV-1 is an enveloped virus with a diameter of approximately 110 nm and a cylindrical, electrodense core. HIV-1 and its close relative HIV-2 are members of the Lentiviridae family of retroviruses, which have a complex genomic structure [125,126]. HIV-1 variants are classified into three major groups: group M (main), group O (outlier), and group N (non-M/non-O). Group M accounts for most HIV-1 infections globally and is divided further into 10 subtypes or clades (A to K). Individuals who acquire HIV-1 infection in the United States, Western Europe, and Australia are most frequently infected with subtype B [125,126]. Other HIV-1 subtypes circulate

globally. Subtypes C and D predominate in southern and eastern Africa, subtype C predominates on the Indian subcontinent, and subtype E is common in Southeast Asia [125,126].

Similar to all retroviruses, HIV-1 contains the genes for *gag*, which encodes the core nucleocapsid polypeptides (gp24, p17, p9); *env*, which encodes for the surface-coated proteins of the virus (gp120 and gp41), and *pol*, which encodes for the viral reverse transcriptase and other enzymatic activities (i.e., integrase and protease). There are two regulatory (*tat* and *rev*) and four accessory proteins (*vif*, *vpr*, *vpu*, and *nef*) that are essential for viral replication and pathogenicity [127]. The retroviral core also contains two copies of the viral single-stranded RNA associated with enzymes such as the reverse transcriptase, RNase H, integrase, and protease [128].

The life cycle of HIV-1 is characterized by several distinct stages [128]. The first step in the entry process of HIV into a cell is the binding of the virion envelope glycoproteins (gp120 and gp41) to CD4 on resting or activated T cells. This binding results in conformational change in the envelope, interaction with a coreceptor, and fusion of the viral and cell membranes, allowing the viral genome to gain entry into the cell [129–135]. Members of the chemokine receptor family are coreceptors for HIV. Human cord blood mononuclear cells are preferentially infected by macrophage-tropic (M-tropic) strains of HIV-1 using the CC chemokine receptor CCR5 [133,135,136]. T cell–tropic strains replicate in CD4+ T cells and macrophages. They use the chemokine receptor CXCR4, a member of the CXC chemokine family [129,132,133,135].

HIV virions enter the cell and are rapidly uncoated. The viral reverse transcriptase transforms the single-stranded viral RNA into linear double-stranded DNA, whereas the less specific ribonuclease H degrades and removes the RNA template [137]. This viral DNA is circularized and transferred to the nucleus, where it is inserted by the viral integrase at random sites as a provirus [138,139]. It is also a common feature of all retroviruses to accumulate large amounts of unintegrated viral DNA that are fully competent templates for HIV-1 core and envelope antigen production [140]. The inactive provirus in the form of HIV-1 DNA has been found in 0.1% to 13.5% of peripheral blood mononuclear cells compared with viral mRNA, which is found in 0.002% to 0.25% of these cells [141–143]. The latent provirus is activated by host cell responses to antigens, mitogens, cytokines such as tumor necrosis factor, and different gene products of other viruses [143–146].

HIV gene expression follows by using host cell RNA polymerase II (among other factors), forming a ribonucleoprotein core containing *gag* and *pol* gene products. The 53-kDa precursor of the *gag* protein is cleaved by the HIV-1–derived protease into p24, p17, p9, and p7 proteins [147–149]. The assembly of new virions consists of the formation of the critical viral enzymes, including reverse transcriptase, integrase, ribonuclease, and a protease, and the aggregation into a ribonucleoprotein core [150,151]. The core subsequently moves to the cell surface and buds as mature virions through the plasma membrane.

The exact molecular mechanisms of vertical transmission are unclear, but studies analyzing the *env* gene have shown that the minor genotypes of HIV-1 with macrophage tropic and non–syncytium-inducing phenotypes (R5 viruses) are transmitted from mother to infant [152–155]. Studies have shown that HIV-1 replicates more efficiently in neonatal (cord blood) cells compared with adult cells because of increased HIV-1 gene expression [156], resulting in high viral load and rapid disease progression [157,158]. Analysis of many HIV-1 regulatory and accessory genes, including *vif, vpr, vpu, nef, tat,* and *rev,* has revealed conservation of functional domains of these genes during vertical transmission [159,160]. In addition, the *vif* and *vpr* sequences of transmitting mothers were more heterogeneous and more functional than sequences of nontransmitting mothers [153,160]. Other HIV-1 genes may also play a crucial role in virus transmission and pathogenesis. A more recent study showed that functional domains in the HIV-1 functional long terminal repeat (LTR) were conserved during vertical transmission, suggesting that a functional LTR sequence is crucial in viral gene expression, transmission, and pathogenesis [161].

PATHOGENESIS OF EARLY INFANT INFECTION
VIRAL PATHOGENESIS
Research conducted over the past 2 decades has yielded significant insights into understanding of the viral and immunopathogenesis of vertical HIV infection [153,162]. Although the exact mechanism of vertical transmission is unknown, intrapartum transmission probably results from infant mucosal exposure to maternal blood or cervicovaginal tract secretions during delivery [58]. Dendritic cells or macrophages are initially targeted by HIV, which transmit the virus to CD4+ T cells [162]. The activation and direct infection of CD4+ T cells result in high rates of viral production and dissemination throughout the body [163,164]. In individuals receiving suppressive antiretroviral therapy, HIV can establish a state of latent infection in resting memory CD4+ T cells [165]. Viruses isolated in early vertical infection predominantly use the CCR5 coreceptor, although use of other receptors has been reported [166]. Regardless of the route of infection, the gastrointestinal lymphoid tissues are a major site of viral replication and persistence and loss of CD4+ T lymphocytes throughout infection [167,168].

Perinatal HIV infection is characterized by plasma RNA levels that rapidly reach very high levels often exceeding 10^5 to 10^7 copies/mL [42,169–171]. In a study of 106 HIV-infected infants, the median plasma HIV RNA value at 1 month old was 318,000 copies/mL, and it was common to see viral levels that exceeded 10^6 copies/mL. In the absence of antiretroviral therapy, the levels decrease only gradually over the first 24 to 36 months of life [172]. A continued decrease in plasma HIV-1 RNA levels (mean −0.2 to −0.3 log decline/yr) has been noted in vertically infected children through 5 to 6 years of age [171,172]. As in adults, higher viral loads correlate with a more rapid disease progression [169,173–176] whereas lower levels of plasma HIV RNA with HAART are

associated with clinical benefit [177,178]. These data indicate that high viral load is a critical determinant of pediatric disease progression and provides a strong argument for early and aggressive intervention with antiretroviral therapy. The persistently high levels of plasma HIV RNA observed in vertically infected infants may be related to many factors, including the kinetics of viral replication, a large and renewable CD4+ cell pool size, presence of an active thymus, and delayed or ineffective HIV-specific immune responses [166].

IMMUNE ABNORMALITIES IN HUMAN IMMUNODEFICIENCY VIRUS INFECTION
Infection with HIV results in profound deficiencies in cell-mediated and humoral immunity caused by quantitative and qualitative defects, leading to a progressive dysfunction of the immune system with depletion of CD4+ T cells. Compared with adults, CD4+ T–cell depletion may be less striking in children because of their relative lymphocytosis. Flow cytometric analysis of lymphocyte subpopulations in healthy children revealed age-related changes in many of the different subgroups [179–181]. Comparison of lymphocyte subsets in HIV-infected versus noninfected children younger than 2 years showed no difference for absolute CD8+ counts, but clearly decreased levels of CD4+ cells [182]. In the absence of early antiretroviral therapy, an abnormal CD4+ count (<10th percentile for uninfected children) was found in 83% of the infected children, and an abnormally low absolute CD4+ count was observed in 67%. As in adults, the relative risks of death or disease progression are inversely related to the CD4+ cell count, which is closely related to the viral load [171,176,183]. A rapid increase in HIV RNA levels correlates with early disease progression and loss of CD4+ cells in vertically infected infants [183], suggesting that antiretroviral therapy should be started in early infection to preserve immune function.

Other immune abnormalities include decreased lymphocyte proliferation in response to an antigen, polyclonal B-cell activation resulting in hypergammaglobulinemia, and altered function of monocytes and neutrophils [184–187]. In the European Collaborative Study, hypergammaglobulinemia (IgG, IgM, and IgA) identified 77% of infected infants at age 6 months with 97% specificity [188]. In a group of 47 HIV-infected children (17 asymptomatic and 30 symptomatic), Roilides and coworkers [184] found an abnormality of at least one IgG subclass in 83%, including some patients who had IgG2, IgG4, or combined IgG2-IgG4 deficiencies. There was no clear correlation of the incidence of bacterial infections with specific subclass deficiencies.

HUMAN IMMUNODEFICIENCY VIRUS–SPECIFIC IMMUNE CONTROL
Vertically infected infants face many challenges in mounting a specific immune response to HIV [5]. First, HIV transmission occurs before the immune system is fully developed in an infant allowing for more efficient viral replication and less efficient immunologic containment of the virus [5]. Second, infected infants carry a high frequency of

maternally inherited HLA class I alleles (e.g., HLA-B*1801 and HLA-B*5802) associated with poor control of HIV [189]. Third, transmitted maternal escape mutants are adapted to maternal HLA alleles and preadapted to the infant's HLA [190,191]. Finally, passive transfer of maternal, non-neutralizing antibodies could inhibit development of HIV-specific immune responses [192].

It is well established that the CD8$^+$ cytotoxic T lymphocytes (CTL) play a crucial role in generation of HIV-specific immune response in acute adult infection [192–195]. Although, HIV-1–specific CTL activity can be shown at a very early age, even in the fetus, the response is weak and less broad compared with adults with primary infection [196–200]. Because infants share at least three HLA class I alleles with their mothers, vertical transmission of maternal CTL escape mutants could affect the infant's ability to mount an early CTL response restricted by shared HLA alleles [191,201,202]. HIV-specific CTL responses become more frequent and broad in infected infants after 6 months of life [198,203]. More recent reports indicate that some CTL responses in infants can select for viral escape variants very early in life [204–206]. In addition, disease progression is slower in children who express HLA-B*27 or HLA-B*57 [206,207], indicating that CTL responses can have an important role in suppression of HIV in pediatric infection [5].

In neonates, defective, antibody-dependent, cell-mediated cytotoxicity of HIV-infected cells by natural killer cells has been reported [208]. After the decline of passively transferred maternal antibody-dependent, cell-mediated cytotoxicity antibodies, the production of HIV-envelope cytotoxic antibodies is delayed in vertically infected infants [209]. Although neutralizing antibodies can be generated during early infection [210–212] the precise role of neutralizing antibodies in limiting mother-to-child transmission of HIV is unclear [5].

Several studies indicate that HIV-infected children have reduced antibody responses to certain childhood vaccines (e.g., diphtheria, acellular pertussis vaccine) [209,213–215]. Reduced antibody responses after immunization and vaccine failures in HIV-infected infants may result from a poor primary immune response, failure to generate memory responses, or loss of memory cells [209]. Most vertically infected infants who receive HAART before 3 months of age develop antibody and lymphoproliferative responses to routine infant vaccines, although persistent HIV-specific immune responses are not detected [192,196,199,209]. More recent studies have reported a sustained increase in peripheral blood CD5 cell counts and robust immune reconstitution among HIV-infected children after prolonged HAART [216,217], permitting discontinuation of prophylactic therapy for opportunistic infections [218].

DIAGNOSIS
HUMAN IMMUNODEFICIENCY VIRUS TESTING OF PREGNANT WOMEN

Diagnosis of HIV infection as part of routine prenatal care of pregnant women is very important because preventive therapies are now widely available, even in developing countries [26]. The U.S. Centers of Disease Control and Prevention (CDC), the AAP, and the American College of Obstetricians and Gynecologists recommend documented, routine antenatal HIV testing for all women in the United States after notifying the patient that testing will be done unless the patient refuses HIV testing ("opt-out" approach with right of refusal) [219–221]. Repeat HIV testing is recommended in the third trimester for women at high risk of acquiring HIV infection [219–221]. Physicians should be aware of state and local laws, regulations, and policies related to rapid HIV testing of pregnant women and newborns.

Most commercially available enzyme immunoassays measure IgG antibodies to HIV. A positive enzyme immunoassay must be confirmed by a secondary test, typically a Western blot. Several rapid tests detect HIV antibodies, and most are highly sensitive and specific (99% to 100%). Rapid HIV testing is recommended for women presenting in labor with unknown HIV status so that intrapartum antiretroviral prophylaxis can be administered to the mother in a timely fashion [219–221]. All positive rapid tests must be confirmed by another test. Early identification of HIV infection in pregnant women is crucial to prevent perinatal HIV transmission and provides an opportunity to evaluate the infected woman's health and begin HAART if indicated [222,223]. Rapid HIV antibody testing should be performed on the infant if the mother's HIV status is unknown. If the infant's rapid HIV antibody test result is positive, antiretroviral prophylaxis should be administered to the infant as soon as possible after birth but certainly within 12 hours of life [220,224]. Rapid HIV antibody testing should be available at all health care facilities with maternity and neonatal units.

EARLY INFANT DIAGNOSIS

Prenatal diagnosis in the fetus is difficult because of the risk for bleeding and contamination of the sample with maternal blood or the possibility for accidental iatrogenic infection of the fetus. Amniotic fluid has been found to be positive for p24 antigen and HIV reverse transcriptase [50,51]. Chorionic villus sampling and percutaneous umbilical blood sampling are associated with a higher risk for the fetus. Noninvasive techniques such as fetal ultrasonography or the clinical assessment of the mother give unspecific and not very predictive information.

Many advances have been made in the area of laboratory diagnosis of HIV infection [220,224–226]. Routine HIV antibody testing cannot be used in infants for the diagnosis of HIV infection because of transplacental passage of maternal IgG antibodies to the virus that are present in infants up to 18 months of age. The diagnosis of HIV infection has advanced from antibody and antigen detection to PCR-based DNA or RNA assays (referred to as HIV nucleic acid amplification tests) that are highly sensitive and specific [227,228] and now widely available in industrialized countries [220].

HIV-1 DNA PCR assay detects viral DNA in peripheral blood mononuclear cells and is frequently used in the United States for diagnosis of HIV in infants and children younger than 18 months; the sensitivity and specificity of HIV-1 DNA PCR assays are 96% and 99% by 1 month of age for detection of HIV-1 subtype B [227,228]. HIV-1 DNA PCR assays are less sensitive for identifying non–B subtype virus, however, and have been associated with false-negative tests in patients with non–B subtype HIV-1 infection [229,230].

Plasma HIV-1 RNA PCR assay can also be used for early diagnosis of HIV-1 infection in infancy [220]. The HIV-1 RNA assay is as sensitive or more sensitive and as specific for detection of HIV-1 subtype B compared with HIV-1 DNA PCR [228,231–234]. False-positive results can occur, however [232,234,235]. Any positive test should be repeated for confirmation [236]. HIV-1 RNA PCR may be more sensitive than HIV-1 DNA PCR for detection of non–B subtype virus [234]. It is prudent to use HIV RNA PCR for diagnosis of infants born to women known or suspected to have non–B subtype HIV infection [220]. The sensitivity of HIV-1 RNA PCR is not affected by the presence of maternal or infant zidovudine prophylaxis [236].

HIV-1 DNA or RNA PCR testing is recommended at birth and 14 to 21 days of age, and if test results are negative, repeat testing is recommended at 1 to 2 months and at 4 to 6 months [220]. A cord blood specimen should not be used because of possible contamination with maternal blood. It is assumed that infants who have a positive HIV PCR result within the first 48 hours after birth were infected in utero, whereas infants who are infected during the intrapartum period might become positive 2 to 6 weeks after birth [59,237]. Testing HIV-exposed infants at birth with HIV DNA or RNA PCR may be considered if mothers did not receive antiretroviral drugs during pregnancy or in other high-risk scenarios [224]. Two separate positive HIV-1 DNA or RNA PCR tests are needed for diagnosis of HIV-1 infection in infants [220].

If infection is confirmed, the infant should be promptly referred to a pediatric HIV specialist for consideration of HAART and care [220] to prevent rapid disease progression noted in some vertically infected infants [238]. HIV-1 infection can be *presumptively excluded* in non–breast-feeding, HIV-exposed infants and children younger than 18 months with (1) two negative HIV-1 DNA or RNA PCR test results from separate specimens, both of which were obtained at 2 weeks or more of age and one of which was obtained at 4 weeks or more of age; or (2) one negative HIV-1 RNA or DNA PCR test result from a specimen obtained at 8 weeks or more of age; or (3) one negative HIV-1 antibody test obtained at 6 months or more of age [224]. HIV-1 infection can be *definitively excluded* in non–breast-feeding, HIV-exposed infants and children younger than 18 months with (1) two negative HIV-1 DNA or RNA PCR test results from separate specimens, both of which were obtained at 1 month or more of age and one of which was obtained at 4 months or more of age, or (2) two negative HIV-1 antibody tests from separate specimens, both of which were obtained at 6 months or more of age [220].

Many physicians confirm the absence of HIV infection by documenting a negative HIV-1 antibody test result at 12 to 18 months of age [220]. These laboratory tests can be used to exclude HIV-1 infection only if there is no other laboratory (e.g., no subsequent positive PCR test results if performed) or clinical (e.g., no AIDS-defining illness) evidence of HIV-1 infection.

Virtually all infants born to seropositive mothers are positive for HIV antibodies at birth, even though only a few are infected. Of uninfected infants, 75% lose these passively transferred antibodies between 6 and 12 months of age, but persistence of maternal antibodies has been documented in 2% up to 18 months of age [239]. Many physicians confirm the absence of HIV infection by documenting a negative HIV-1 antibody test result at 12 to 18 months of age [220]. If HIV-1 antibody testing is performed at 12 months of age in an infant exposed to HIV but not known to be infected, and if still antibody positive, repeat testing at 18 months of age is recommended [220]. Detection of HIV-1 antibody in a child 18 months of age or older is diagnostic of HIV-1 infection. Documentation of seroreversion may be more important when non–subtype B HIV-1 is possible or present.

HIV-1 culture is as sensitive as HIV-1 DNA PCR assay, but it is more expensive and needs a specialized laboratory, and results are unavailable for 2 to 3 weeks [240]. Use of HIV-1 p24 antigen detection is not recommended for diagnosis of infant HIV-1 because of its poor sensitivity [241].

Clinical and nonspecific laboratory parameters may also suggest HIV infection. Hypergammaglobulinemia is a nonspecific but early finding of HIV infection, and CD4+ counts must be interpreted within the bounds of the age-dependent normal range [179–181,242] In 1994, the CDC published revised guidelines for the diagnosis of HIV infection in infants and children younger than 13 years (Table 21–1) [243]. No changes have been made to the AIDS surveillance case definition for children younger than 18 months [244]. Table 21–2 provides a diagram outlining the initial evaluation and the necessary follow-up tests for an asymptomatic infant born to an HIV-positive mother, as recommended by the AAP [220].

CLASSIFICATION OF HUMAN IMMUNODEFICIENCY VIRUS INFECTION IN CHILDREN

In 1994, the CDC published a revised pediatric classification system for HIV infection in children younger than 13 years based on clinical disease and immunologic status (Table 21–3) [243]. Clinical categories range from N, indicating no signs or symptoms, through A, B, and C, for mild, moderate, and severe (AIDS-defining) symptoms and signs. Diagnosis is established if an AIDS-defining disease occurs (Table 21–4) [246]. In the pre-HAART era, *Pneumocystis jiroveci* (formerly *carinii*) pneumonia (PCP) pneumonia was the leading AIDS-defining illness diagnosed during the first year of life and associated with a high mortality rate [245]. Other common AIDS-defining conditions in U.S. children with vertically acquired infection include lymphoid interstitial pneumonitis, multiple or recurrent serious bacterial infections, HIV encephalopathy, wasting syndrome, *Candida* esophagitis, cytomegalovirus disease, and *Mycobacterium avium-intracellulare* complex infection (see Table 21–4) [246].

The immunologic categories place an emphasis on the CD4+ T-lymphocyte count and percentages for age and

TABLE 21–1   Centers for Disease Control and Prevention Definition of Human Immunodeficiency Virus Infection in Children Younger than 13 Years of Age

HIV Infected

A. Child <18 mo old who is known to be HIV-seropositive or born to HIV-infected mother

 and

 Has positive results on two separate determinations (excluding cord blood) from one or more of the following HIV detection tests:

   HIV polymerase chain reaction
   HIV culture
   HIV antigen (p24)

 or

 Meets criteria for AIDS diagnosis based on 1987 AIDS surveillance case definition

B. Child >18 mo old born to HIV-infected mother or any child infected by blood, blood products, or other known modes of infection who

 Is HIV antibody–positive by repeatedly reactive EIA and confirmatory test (e.g., Western blot or immunofluorescence assay)

 or

 Meets any of the criteria in A

Perinatally Exposed (Prefix E)

A child who does not meet the above-listed criteria and who

 Is HIV-seropositive by EIA and confirmatory test and is <18 mo old

 or

 Has unknown antibody status, but was born to a mother known to be HIV infected

Seroreverter (SR)

Child who is born to HIV-infected mother and who

 Has been documented as HIV antibody–negative (i.e., two or more negative EIA tests performed at age 6-18 mo or one negative EIA test performed after age 18 mo)

 or

 Has had no laboratory evidence of infection

 and

 Has not had an AIDS-defining condition

EIA, enzyme immunoassay.
Adapted from 1994 Revised classification system for human immunodeficiency virus infection in children less than 13 years of age. MMWR Morb Mortal Wkly Rep 431:1-10, 1994.

TABLE 21–2   Evaluation and Management of Infants Exposed to Human Immunodeficiency Virus

Test	Birth	2 wk	4 wk	6 wk	2 mo	4 mo	12-18 mo
History and physical examination (including weight, height, head circumference)*	+	+	+				
Assess risk of other infections	+						
Antiretroviral prophylaxis	+			+†			
Formula feeding	+	+	+	+	+	+	+
Complete blood cell count	+		+		+‡		
HIV-1 DNA or RNA PCR§	+¶	+		+		+	
PCP prophylaxis				+#			
HIV-1 antibody testing							+**

Review maternal history for possible exposure to coinfections (e.g., tuberculosis, syphilis, herpes simplex virus, cytomegalovirus, or hepatitis B virus).
†*Zidovudine to prevent perinatal transmission should be started soon after birth but certainly within 12 hr. Zidovudine is discontinued at 6 wk of age; however, other antiretroviral therapy should be started in a child who is proved to be infected according to pediatric treatment guidelines with close laboratory monitoring.*
‡*Complete blood cell count is measured at 4 wk and rechecked at 8 wk if severe anemia was noted at the 4-wk visit.*
§*Repeat polymerase chain reaction (PCR) immediately if positive to confirm infection. If the initial test is negative, repeat test at 4 wk to 2 mo and 4-6 mo of age to identify or exclude HIV-1 infection as early as possible.*
¶*Consider obtaining birth HIV DNA or RNA PCR test to exclude intrauterine HIV infection if the mother did not receive highly active antiretroviral therapy during pregnancy or in other high-risk situations.*
#*Pneumocystis jiroveci (formerly carinii) pneumonia (PCP) prophylaxis should be continued for 1 year if infant is diagnosed with HIV.*
**HIV-1 antibody testing is performed to confirm the absence of HIV infection.*

TABLE 21–3   1994 Centers for Disease Control and Prevention Revised Classification System for Human Immunodeficiency Virus Infection in Children Younger than 13 Years of Age

Using this system, children are classified according to three parameters: infection status, clinical status, and immunologic status. The categories are mutually exclusive. When classified in a more severe category, a child is not reclassified in a less severe category even if the clinical or immunologic status improves.*

Pediatric HIV Classification

Immune Categories	Clinical Categories			
	No Symptoms (N)	Mild Symptoms (A)	Moderate Symptoms (B)[†]	Severe Symptoms (C)[†]
No suppression (1)	N1	A1	B1	C1
Moderate suppression (2)	N2	A2	B2	C2
Severe suppression (3)	N3	A3	B3	C3

Immunologic Categories Based on Age-Specific CD4+ T Lymphocyte Counts and Percent of Total Lymphocytes

The immunologic category classification is based on age-specific CD4+ T lymphocyte count or percent of total lymphocytes and is designed to determine severity of immunosuppression attributable to HIV for age. If either CD4+ count or percent results in classification into a different category, the child should be classified into the more severe category. A value should be confirmed before the child is reclassified into a less severe category.

Immunologic Category	Age Groups		
	0-11 mo	1-5 yr	>6 yr
No suppression (1)	>1500 cells/μL (>25%)	>1000 cells/μL (>25%)	>500 cells/μL (>25%)
Moderate suppression (2)	750-1499 cells/μL (15%-24%)	500-999 cells/μL (15%-24%)	200-499 cells/μL (15%-24%)
Severe suppression (3)	<750 cells/μL (<15%)	<500 cells/μL (<15%)	<200 cells/μL (<15%)

Clinical Categories for Children with HIV Infection

Category N: Not Symptomatic

Children who have no signs or symptoms considered to be the result of HIV infection or who have only one of the conditions listed in category A

Category A: Mildly Symptomatic

Children with two or more of the following conditions, but none of the conditions listed in categories B and C:
- Lymphadenopathy (>0.5 cm at more than two sites; bilateral = one site)
- Hepatomegaly
- Splenomegaly
- Dermatitis
- Parotitis
- Recurrent or persistent respiratory infection, sinusitis, or otitis media

Category B: Moderately Symptomatic

Children who have symptomatic conditions other than those listed for category A or C that are attributed to HIV infection
Examples of conditions in clinical category B include but are not limited to:
- Anemia (<8 g/dL), neutropenia (<1000/mm³), or thrombocytopenia (<100,000/mm³) persisting >30 days
- Bacterial meningitis, pneumonia, or sepsis (single episode)
- Candidiasis, oropharyngeal thrush, persisting for >2 mo in children >6 mo old
- Cardiomyopathy
- Cytomegalovirus infection, with onset before 1 mo of age
- Diarrhea, recurrent or chronic
- Hepatitis
- Herpes simplex virus stomatitis, recurrent (more than two episodes within 1 yr)
- Herpes simplex virus bronchitis, pneumonitis, or esophagitis with onset before 1 mo of age
- Herpes zoster (shingles) involving at least two distinct episodes or more than one dermatome
- Leiomyosarcoma
- Lymphoid interstitial pneumonia or pulmonary lymphoid hyperplasia complex
- Nephropathy
- Nocardiosis
- Persistent fever (lasting >1 mo)
- Toxoplasmosis, onset before 1 mo of age
- Varicella, disseminated (complicated chickenpox)

Continued

TABLE 21–3   1994 Centers for Disease Control and Prevention Revised Classification System for Human Immunodeficiency Virus Infection in Children Younger than 13 Years of Age—cont'd

	Age Groups		
Immunologic Category	**0-11 mo**	**1-5 yr**	**>6 yr**
Category C: Severely Symptomatic[†]			

Children who have any condition listed in the 1987 surveillance case definition for AIDS, with the exception of lymphoid interstitial pneumonia

Serious bacterial infections, multiple or recurrent (i.e., any combination of at least two culture-confirmed infections within a 2-yr period of the following types: septicemia, pneumonia, meningitis, bone or joint infection, or abscess of an internal body organ or body cavity, excluding otitis media, superficial skin or mucosal abscesses, and indwelling catheter-related infections)

Candidiasis, esophageal or pulmonary (bronchi, trachea, lungs)

Coccidioidomycosis, disseminated (at site other than or in addition to lungs or cervical or hilar nodes)

Cryptosporidiosis or isosporidiosis with diarrhea persisting >1 mo

Cytomegalovirus disease with onset of symptoms at age >1 mo (other than liver, spleen, or lymph nodes)

Encephalopathy (at least one of the following progressive findings present for at least 2 mo in the absence of a concurrent illness other than HIV infection that could explain the findings): (1) failure to attain or loss of developmental milestones or loss of intellectual ability verified by standard developmental scale or neuropsychologic tests; (2) impaired brain growth or acquired microcephaly shown by head circumference measurements or brain atrophy shown by CT or MRI (serial imaging is required for children <2 yr old); (3) acquired symmetric motor deficit manifested by two or more of the following: paresis, pathologic reflexes, ataxia, or gait disturbance

Herpes simplex virus infection causing a mucocutaneous ulcer that persists for >1 mo or bronchitis, pneumonitis, or esophagitis for any duration affecting a child >1 mo old

Histoplasmosis, disseminated (other than or in addition to lungs or cervical lymph nodes)

Kaposi sarcoma

Lymphoma, primary, in brain

Lymphoma, small, noncleaved cell (Burkitt), or immunoblastic or large cell lymphoma of B cell or unknown immunologic phenotype

Mycobacterium tuberculosis, disseminated or extrapulmonary

Mycobacterium, other species or unidentified species, disseminated (other than or in addition to lungs, skin, or cervical or hilar lymph nodes)

Mycobacterium avium-intracellulare complex or *Mycobacterium kansasii*, disseminated (other than or in addition to lungs, skin, or cervical or hilar lymph nodes)

Pneumocystis jiroveci (formerly *carinii*) pneumonia

Progressive multifocal leukoencephalopathy

Salmonella (nontyphoid) septicemia, recurrent

Toxoplasmosis of the brain with onset >1 mo of age

Wasting syndrome in the absence of a concurrent illness other than HIV infection that could explain the following findings: persistent weight loss >10% of baseline *or* downward crossing of at least two of the following percentiles on weight-for-height chart on two consecutive measurements >30 days apart *plus* chronic diarrhea (i.e., at least two loose stools per day for >30 days) *or* documented fever (for >30 days, intermittent or constant)

Children whose HIV infection status is not confirmed are classified by using the grid with a letter E (for vertically exposed) placed before the appropriate classification code (e.g., EN2).
[†]*Category C and lymphoid interstitial pneumonitis in category B are reportable to state and local health departments as AIDS.*
From Centers for Disease Control and Prevention. Recommendations of the U.S. Public Health Service Task Force on the use of zidovudine to reduce perinatal transmission of human immunodeficiency virus. MMWR Morb Mortal Wkly Rep 43:1-20, 1994.

include stage 1, no evidence of immunosuppression; stage 2, moderate immunosuppression; and stage 3, severe immunosuppression [243]. After being classified, a child cannot be reclassified into a less severe category, even if the child's clinical status or immune function improves in response to antiretroviral treatment or resolution of clinical events. HIV-exposed infants whose HIV infection status is indeterminate (unconfirmed) are classified by placing a prefix *E* (for perinatally exposed) before the appropriate classification code (e.g., EN2) [243].

The current AIDS case definitions devised by the CDC for surveillance and reporting purposes are similar with some important exceptions [247]. Lymphoid interstitial pneumonitis and multiple or recurrent serious bacterial infections are AIDS-defining illnesses only for children. Also, certain herpesvirus infections (cytomegalovirus, herpes simplex virus) and toxoplasmosis of the central nervous system are AIDS-defining conditions only for adults and children older than 1 month. In 1994, the CDC published

a revised pediatric classification system for HIV infection in children younger than 13 years according to the following parameters: (1) HIV infection status, (2) clinical disease, and (3) immunologic status [243].

HIV infection in infants and children has a different presentation from that in adults [5]. Children are more likely than adults to have serious bacterial infections, and lymphocytic interstitial pneumonitis is almost entirely restricted to the pediatric age group. Opportunistic infections such as PCP often manifest as primary diseases with a more aggressive course because of lack of prior immunity [245]. Toxoplasmosis; cryptococcal infection; and the occurrence of cancer, especially Kaposi sarcoma, are less common in HIV-infected children [5,246].

In developing countries with limited diagnostic resources, the diagnosis often has to be based on clinical symptoms, and a modified provisional definition for pediatric cases of AIDS has been issued by the WHO [248]. Evaluations of clinical staging systems for the diagnosis

TABLE 21–4 AIDS Indicator Diseases Diagnosed in 8086 Children Younger than Age 13 Years Reported to the Centers for Disease Control and Prevention through 1997

Disease	No. Children Diagnosed	Percent of Total*
Pneumocystis jiroveci (formerly *carinii*) pneumonia	2700	33
Lymphocytic interstitial pneumonitis	1942	24
Recurrent bacterial infections	1619	20
Wasting syndrome	1419	18
Encephalopathy	1322	16
Candida esophagitis	1266	16
Cytomegalovirus disease	658	8
Mycobacterium avium infection	639	8
Severe herpes simplex infection	370	5
Pulmonary candidiasis	307	4
Cryptosporidiosis	291	4
Cancer	162	2

The sum of percentages is greater than 100 because some patients have more than one disease. From Centers for Disease Control and Prevention (CDC). U.S. HIV and AIDS cases reported through December 1997. HIV/AIDS Surveillance report: year-end edition. MMWR Morb Mortal Wkly Rep 9:1-44, 1997.

of HIV in early infancy have reported limited sensitivity in sub-Saharan Africa, however [249–251]. The WHO has published revised case definitions of HIV infection for surveillance and a revised clinical staging and immunologic classification of HIV disease in adults and children [252].

CLINICAL MANIFESTATIONS AND PATHOLOGY

The clinical manifestations of HIV infection in infants are highly variable and often nonspecific [253]. Infants with perinatally acquired HIV infection are often asymptomatic, and physical examination is usually normal in the neonatal period. Although a distinctive craniofacial dysmorphism characterized by a prominent boxlike forehead, hypertelorism, flattened nasal bridge, triangular philtrum, and patulous lips was suggested as a possible congenital HIV syndrome [254], these findings have not been confirmed in subsequent reports [255]. In a prospective cohort study of 200 perinatally acquired HIV-1 infections, the median age of onset of any HIV-related symptom or sign was 5.2 months; the probability of remaining asymptomatic was 19% at 1 year and 6.1% at 5 years [256]. In another large prospective cohort study, AIDS-defining conditions developed in approximately 23% and 40% of perinatally infected infants by 1 and 4 years [246,257].

The initial symptoms of HIV infection in infants may be subtle and sometimes difficult to distinguish from manifestations caused by drug use during pregnancy, from problems associated with prematurity, or from congenital infections other than HIV. Premature birth has been reported in 19%, with no difference between children born to drug-using mothers and children of mothers who were infected through other routes [188,258]. Children of drug-addicted mothers had significantly lower birth weights and smaller head circumferences, however.

Growth delay is an early and frequent finding of untreated perinatal HIV infection, and linear growth is most severely affected in children with high viral loads [259]. Common clinical features seen during the first year of life include lymphadenopathy and hepatosplenomegaly. Other manifestations noted during the course of HIV infection in children are failure to thrive, unexplained persistent fevers, developmental delay, encephalopathy, recurrent and chronic otitis media and sinusitis, recurrent invasive bacterial infections, opportunistic infections, chronic diarrhea, presence and persistence of oral candidiasis, parotitis, cardiomyopathy, nephropathy, and many nonspecific cutaneous manifestations [260].

INFECTIOUS COMPLICATIONS

Infections in HIV-infected infants not receiving antiretroviral therapy can be serious or life-threatening. The difficulty in treating these infectious episodes, their chronicity, and their tendency to recur distinguish them from the normal infections of early infancy. It is helpful to document each episode and to evaluate the course and frequency of their recurrences. With early diagnosis and access to antiretroviral treatment, opportunistic infections rarely develop in HIV-infected children living in the United States.

Bacterial Infections

Recurrent serious bacterial infections, such as meningitis, sepsis, and pneumonia, are so typical of HIV infection in children that they were included in the revised CDC definition of 1987 [247,261]. Recurrent bacterial infections accounted for 18% of all pediatric AIDS-defining conditions reported to the CDC in 1997. *Streptococcus pneumoniae* is the most frequent cause of serious bacterial infection in children infected with HIV. In a study of 42 vertically infected children, a mean of 1.8 febrile visits per child-year of observation was reported [262]. Eleven of the 27 positive blood cultures grew *S. pneumoniae*, and 16 grew organisms that were considered central venous line–related (coagulase-negative staphylococci, gram-negative enterics, *Staphylococcus aureus*, *Pseudomonas aeruginosa*, and *Candida* species). This increased incidence of pneumococcal infections has been confirmed by other studies [263,264].

Infections in HIV-infected newborns have the same pattern as seen commonly in the neonatal period. A syndrome of very-late-onset group B streptococcal disease (at 3½ to 5 months of age) has been described in HIV-infected children [265]. Other rare infections, such as congenital syphilis or neonatal gonococcal disease, may become more frequent in the future as the incidence increases among pregnant women [266–269]. Congenital syphilis may be missed if serologic tests are not performed on the mother and child at the time of delivery and repeated later if indicated.

Mycobacterial infections have assumed an increasingly important role in the pathology of HIV-infected infants and children. Although the number of HIV-infected children with *Mycobacterium tuberculosis* infection is still small, organisms resistant to multiple antituberculosis drugs cultured from adults and children pose a threat not only to other immunocompromised patients, but also to health care providers [270–273]. An important issue for the neonatologist is whether the mother is infected with M. tuberculosis and may transmit the disease to her child. The diagnosis of *M. tuberculosis* infection is complicated in HIV-infected patients because of the frequent anergy leading to a negative Mantoux test result even in the presence of infection. To diagnose anergy, a control (e.g., for mumps, *Candida*, or tetanus) should always be placed simultaneously with the Mantoux test [274]. Treatment of *M. tuberculosis* infection in children is complicated by the lack of pediatric formulations, but usually includes isoniazid, rifampin, and, during the first 2 months, pyrazinamide [275].

Infection with *M. avium-intracellulare* complex occurs in almost 20% of HIV-infected children with advanced disease and manifests as nonspecific symptoms such as night sweats, weight loss, and low-grade fevers [276,277]. Treatment usually consists of three or more drugs (e.g., clarithromycin, ethambutol, rifampin or amikacin or both, ciprofloxacin, clofazimine), but commonly provides only temporary symptomatic relief and not eradication of the infection. Prophylaxis with clarithromycin or azithromycin should be initiated in infants younger than 1 year with a $CD4^+$ count less than 750 cells/mm^3, in children 1 to 2 years old with a $CD4^+$ count less than 500 cells/mm^3, and in children 2 to 6 years old with a $CD4^+$ count less than 75 cells/mm^3. In children older than 6 years, the adult threshold of 50 cells/mm^3 can be used [278].

Viral Infections

Viral infections are important causes for morbidity and mortality in HIV-infected children. Primary varicella can be unusually severe and can recur as zoster, often manifesting with very few, atypical lesions. The virus may become resistant to standard treatment with acyclovir [279–281]. Cytomegalovirus infection can result in esophagitis, hepatitis, enterocolitis, or retinitis [282–285]. Cytomegalovirus can become resistant to treatment with ganciclovir, necessitating the use of foscarnet or combination regimens [286,287].

Other commonly encountered viruses in HIV-infected infants and children are hepatitis A, B, and C, often associated with a more fulminant or chronic aggressive course than in non–HIV-infected patients [288–290]. Hepatitis C infection has been shown to be more common in children born to HIV-infected mothers in some studies [290], but others have found no association between maternal HIV status and perinatal hepatitis C transmission [291,292].

Infection with the measles virus is associated with a high mortality in HIV-infected children and often manifests without the typical rash and can result in fatal giant cell pneumonia [293–296]. Infection with respiratory syncytial virus or adenovirus, alone or in combination, can also result in rapid and sometimes fatal respiratory compromise and in chronic or persistent viral shedding or infection [297–299].

The occurrence of a polyclonal lymphoproliferative syndrome is often associated with evidence of primary or reactivated Epstein-Barr virus infection. These patients develop impressive lymphadenopathy and sometimes have concurrent lymphocytic interstitial pneumonitis or parotitis [300]. The distinction between a self-limited, benign hyperproliferation and the development of a monoclonal lymphoid malignancy is crucial for determining treatment and prognosis.

Fungal and Protozoal Infections

Oral candidiasis is common even in healthy, non–HIV-infected newborns and infants. Infection beyond infancy, involvement of pharynx and esophagus, and persistence despite treatment with antifungal agents are more typical for immunocompromised children. Disseminated candidiasis is uncommon, however, in the absence of predisposing factors, such as central venous catheters or total parenteral nutrition [301].

Although infection with *Cryptococcus neoformans* is common in adults with HIV infection, it is less common in children [302,303]. Colonization with *Aspergillus* species and invasive disease has been described in adult patients with HIV infection, and we have observed at least one infant with perinatally acquired HIV infection and associated myelodysplastic syndrome who developed fatal pulmonary aspergillosis [304–306]. The incidence of other fungal infections varies with the prevalence of the organism in the specific geographic area. Disseminated histoplasmosis as the AIDS-defining illness has been described in a few infants [307–309].

Early in the HIV epidemic, PCP was the AIDS indicator disease in almost 40% of the pediatric cases reported to the CDC [245]. This situation has changed dramatically, however, since the introduction of guidelines for PCP prophylaxis in HIV-exposed infants and HIV-infected children, and PCP accounted for only 25% of the AIDS cases in 1997 [310,311]. The peak incidence of PCP in infancy occurs during the first 3 to 6 months of life, often as the first symptom of HIV infection. Presumably, PCP represents primary infection in these infants. At least one case of maternal-to-fetal transmission of PCP has also been documented [312].

Most children with PCP present with an acute illness, with hypoxemia, and without a typical radiographic picture [313,314]. The diagnosis is usually made by obtaining an induced sputum (which can be done by experienced therapists even in very young children) or by performing a bronchoalveolar lavage, and an open lung biopsy is only rarely necessary [315,316]. Treatment options are high-dose intravenous trimethoprim-sulfamethoxazole (TMP-SMX) and pentamidine as first-line drugs [317]. Early adjunctive treatment with corticosteroids has been beneficial in adults and children with moderate to severe PCP and is commonly recommended for patients with an initial arterial oxygen pressure of less than 70 mm Hg or an arterial-alveolar gradient of more than 35 mm Hg [318–321].

PCP has been associated with a mortality of 39% to 65% in infants despite improved diagnosis and treatment [322,323]. In 1991, the CDC issued guidelines for PCP prophylaxis in children, taking into account the age-dependent levels of normal $CD4^+$ cell numbers [324]. These recommendations were applicable, however, only if a child was known to be HIV infected. A survey published in 1995 revealed basically no change between 1988 and 1992 in the incidence of PCP among infants born to HIV-infected mothers [325]. Two thirds of these infants had never received PCP prophylaxis, and 59% were recognized as having been exposed to HIV infection within 30 days or less of PCP diagnosis. Among the infants known to be HIV infected who had a CD4$^+$ count performed within 1 month of PCP diagnosis, 18% had a CD4$^+$ count greater than 1500 cells/mm^3, the recommended threshold for initiation of PCP prophylaxis [325]. At the same time, it was shown that primary prophylaxis during the first year of life was highly effective in the prevention of PCP [326]. These pivotal studies led to revised guidelines in 1995 [310]. The major new recommendation was that all infants born to HIV-infected women should be started on PCP prophylaxis at 4 to 6 weeks of age, regardless of their CD4$^+$ counts (Table 21–5) [218].

The recommended prophylactic regimen is TMP-SMX with 150 mg/m^2/day of TMP and 750 mg/m^2/day of SMX given orally in divided doses twice each day during 3 consecutive days per week. The alternative regimen is TMP-SMX given once daily for 3 days per week or twice daily 7 days per week [220]. If TMP-SMX is not tolerated, alternative regimens are dapsone taken orally (2 mg/kg once daily or 4 mg/kg once weekly) or intravenous pentamidine (4 mg/kg every 2 to 4 weeks) or atovaquone (30 mg/kg once daily for infants 1 to 3 months of age and 45 mg/kg once daily for infants 4 to 24 months) [220]. Breakthrough infections can occur with every regimen, however, and seem to be most frequent with intravenous pentamidine and least common with TMP-SMX [327,328].

Encephalitis caused by *Toxoplasma gondii* is common in adults with HIV infection, but only rarely seen in children [218]. Several case reports of *T. gondii* encephalitis in infants between 5 weeks and 18 months old have been published, however. Some of these infants probably acquired *Toxoplasma* infection in utero [329,330]. Toxoplasmosis is an important differential diagnosis in a patient with an intracerebral mass.

Protozoal infections of the gastrointestinal tract often represent difficult diagnostic and therapeutic problems and can be associated with an intractable diarrhea. Infection with *Cryptosporidium* has a prevalence of 3% to 3.6% among children with diarrhea [331]. HIV-infected children are at risk for prolonged diarrheal disease with often severe wasting.

ENCEPHALOPATHY

Encephalopathy, often with early onset, was a frequent and typical manifestation of HIV infection in children before the introduction of antiretroviral therapy. Symptoms of encephalopathy in the newborn or young infant initially include delayed head control or delayed acquisition of a social smile and variable degrees of truncal hypotonia [332–334]. Subsequently, impairment of cognitive, behavioral, and motor functions becomes apparent. Typical findings include a loss of or failure to attain normal developmental milestones; weakness; intellectual deficits; or neurologic symptoms such as ataxia and pyramidal tract signs, including spasticity or rigidity [335]. Seizures are rare, but have been described, and cerebrovascular disease resulting in strokes or the formation of giant aneurysms at the base of the brain has been reported [336,337].

The course can be static, wherein the child attains milestones, albeit at a slower rate than normal for age, or the development can reach a plateau and then the child ceases to acquire new milestones. The most severe form is manifested by a subacute-progressive course in which the

---

TABLE 21–5 Recommendations for *Pneumocystis jiroveci* (formerly *carinii*) Pneumonia (PCP) Prophylaxis and CD4$^+$ Monitoring in HIV-Exposed Infants and HIV-Infected Children

Age/HIV Infection Status	PCP Prophylaxis	CD4$^+$ Monitoring
Birth to 4-6 wk, HIV exposed or infected	No prophylaxis (because PCP is rare and because of concerns regarding kernicterus with TMP-SMX)	1 mo
4-6 wk to 4 mo, HIV exposed or infected	Prophylaxis*	3 mo
4-12 mo		
HIV infection presumptively excluded†	No prophylaxis	None
HIV infection indeterminate	Prophylaxis	6, 9, 12 mo
HIV infected	Prophylaxis	6, 9, 12 mo
1-5 yr, HIV infected	Prophylaxis if	Every 3-4 mo (more frequently if indicated)
	CD4$^+$ count is <500 cells/mm^3 *or*	
	CD4$^+$ percentage is <15%	
>6 yr, HIV infected	Prophylaxis if	Every 3-4 yr
	CD4$^+$ count <200 cells/mm^3 *or*	
	CD4$^+$ percentage is <15%	

*PCP prophylaxis is not needed if HIV RNA or DNA polymerase chain reaction (PCR) result is negative at 14 days and 4 wk of age. If no testing was performed before this, or only a single test was performed between 14 days and 6 weeks of age, PCP prophylaxis is started at this point until HIV infection is presumptively excluded.
†HIV-1 infection can be presumptively excluded in non–breast-feeding HIV-exposed infants and children <18 mo old if (1) two negative HIV-1 DNA or RNA PCR test results from separate specimens, both of which were obtained at ≥2 wk of age and one of which was obtained at ≥4 wk of age, or (2) one negative HIV-1 RNA or DNA PCR test result from a specimen obtained at ≥8 wk of age, or (3) one negative HIV-1 antibody test obtained ≥6 mo of age[224].
TMP-SMX, trimethoprim-sulfamethoxazole.
From Centers from Disease Control and Prevention. 1995 Revised guidelines for prophylaxis against Pneumocystis carinii pneumonia for children infected with or perinatally exposed to human immunodeficiency virus. MMWR Morb Mortal Wkly Rep 44:1-12, 1995.

child loses previously acquired capabilities [338,339]. Older children have impaired expressive language function, whereas receptive language seems to be slightly less affected [340,341]. Physical examination can reveal hypotonia or spasticity, and microencephaly may be present. Radiologic examination can suggest cerebral atrophy, calcifications in the basal ganglia and periventricular frontal white matter, and decreased attenuation in the white matter (Fig. 21–1) [342–346].

HIV-1 can be found in brain monocytes, macrophages, and microglia, and limited expression of the regulatory gene *nef*, but not of structural gene products, has been shown in astrocytes [347–350]. Analysis of cerebrospinal fluid revealed HIV RNA in 90% of samples, and more than 10,000 copies/mL were associated with severe neurodevelopmental delay [351,352]. It is likely that immune-mediated mechanisms or the secretion of toxic cytokines by infected cells contributes to the pathogenesis of central nervous system disease in AIDS patients [353]. The level of quinolinic acid, a neurotoxin that has been implicated in the development of HIV-related encephalopathy, is elevated in children with symptomatic central nervous system disease and decreased during treatment with zidovudine [354,355].

Postmortem examination shows variable degrees of white matter abnormalities, calcific deposits in the wall of blood vessels of the basal ganglia and the frontal white matter, and subacute encephalitis. At least one report described HIV-related meningoencephalitis in a newborn, supporting the assumption of an intrauterine infection [356]. Spinal cord disease, manifested by vacuolar myelopathy, has been described in children, but is less common than in adults [357].

Dramatic improvements in the degree of encephalopathy have been achieved by treating children with zidovudine, especially when given as a continuous intravenous infusion (see later) [358]. Therapy with corticosteroids has also been shown to be beneficial in some patients [359].

OPHTHALMOLOGIC PATHOLOGY

Ophthalmologic complications associated with HIV infection can be particularly devastating. HIV-1 can infect the retina and manifest as cotton-wool spots on examination, but it rarely leads to impaired vision [360,361]. Several other pathogens, some of them acquired in utero, can affect the eye, however, and affect visual acuity. The incidence of blindness remains low in pediatric AIDS patients, but infections caused by herpesviruses and especially cytomegalovirus retinitis can be difficult to control and require intensive intravenous treatment [282,284,285]. A few children have been described with congenital toxoplasmosis and associated chorioretinitis, and an extrapulmonary manifestation of *P. jiroveci* infection is involvement of the retina [362–364]. Early recognition and aggressive intervention are crucial to prevent progression of visual impairment, and routine ophthalmologic examinations should be part of the care of all HIV-infected children.

INTERSTITIAL LUNG DISEASE

Lymphocytic interstitial pneumonitis, or pulmonary lymphoid hyperplasia, is seen almost exclusively in the pediatric patient with HIV infection and is still included into the CDC definition of AIDS-defining diseases for children younger than 13 years (see Table 21–3). The incidence of lymphocytic interstitial pneumonitis is difficult to assess, but may affect 50% of HIV-infected children [365]. Clinically, there is a wide spectrum in the severity of this disease; a child may be asymptomatic with only radiologic changes, or he or she can become severely compromised with exercise intolerance or with oxygen dependency and the need for high-dose corticosteroid therapy. Children with lymphocytic interstitial pneumonitis are at higher risk to develop frequent bacterial and viral infections [366].

A diffuse, interstitial, often reticulonodular infiltrative process is typically observed on radiologic examination and is sometimes associated with hilar or mediastinal

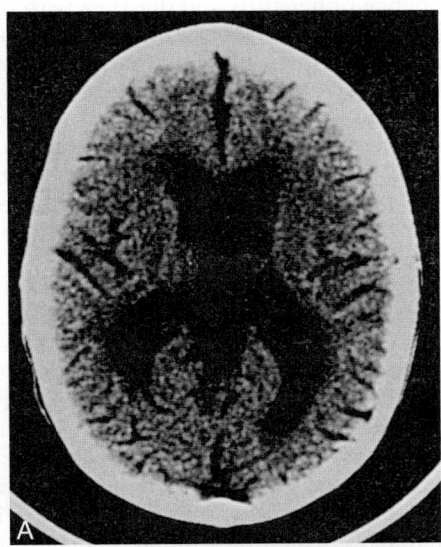

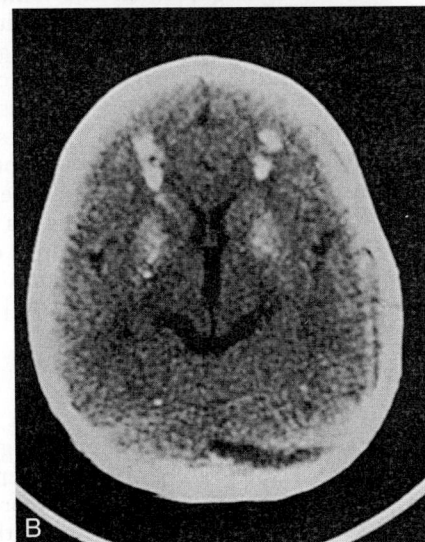

FIGURE 21–1 CT scans of the brains of two infants with HIV-associated encephalopathy. **A,** Cerebral atrophy with enlarged ventricles and widened sulci. **B,** Calcifications in basal ganglia and frontal white matter.

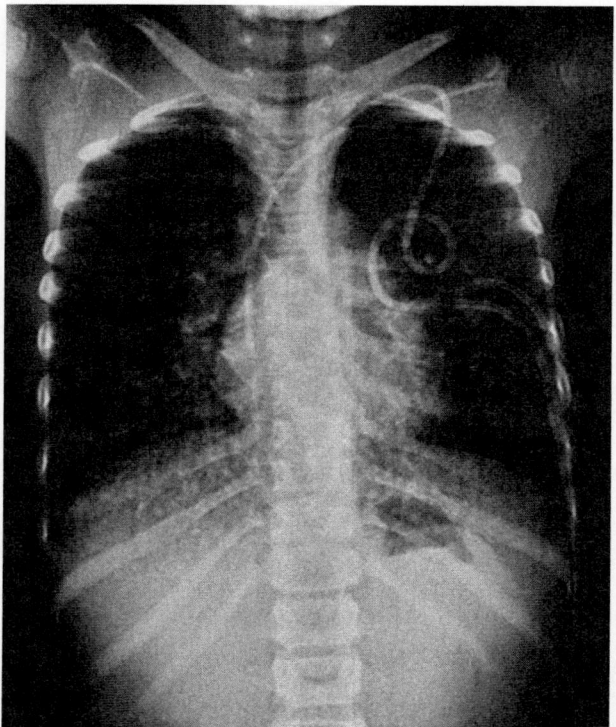

FIGURE 21–2 Chest radiograph of an 8-year-old girl with severe lymphocytic interstitial pneumonitis who is oxygen and steroid dependent.

lymphadenopathy (Fig. 21–2) [365]. On biopsy, peribronchiolar lymphoid aggregates or a diffuse lymphoid infiltration of the alveolar septa and peribronchiolar areas is seen [300]. Treatment of lymphocytic interstitial pneumonitis is indicated only in a symptomatic child with hypoxia and consists of oral therapy with corticosteroids to suppress the lymphocytic proliferation [365]. Lymphocytic interstitial pneumonitis has been associated in some studies with a better prognosis than other HIV-related manifestations such as encephalopathy or PCP, with a median survival of 72 months after diagnosis compared with 1 month for encephalopathy and 11 months for PCP [367].

CARDIOVASCULAR COMPLICATIONS

Cardiovascular abnormalities are seen in more than 50% of HIV-infected adults and have been described in children [368,369]. A progressive left ventricular dilation and an increase in ventricular afterload were shown in a group of 51 children with symptomatic HIV disease but with a normal initial echocardiogram [369]. Clinical manifestations include hepatosplenomegaly, tachypnea, and tachycardia, often with an S_3 gallop or another arrhythmia. Postmortem examination is remarkable for biventricular dilation with grossly unremarkable valves and coronary arteries and, less frequently, a pericardial effusion. Cardiomyopathy is more commonly found in children with HIV-related encephalopathy (30%) than in children without this manifestation (2%) [334].

Microscopically, hypertrophy of the myocardium with only rare foci of inflammatory lymphocytic infiltrates is usually present [370,371]. HIV RNA can be shown in only a few cells, probably representing macrophages, monocytes, or endothelial cells, but the distribution does not correlate with the structural damage [372,373].

Another poorly understood phenomenon is the formation of aneurysms of the cerebral and coronary arteries in association with HIV infection [337,374,375]. A child who developed large cerebral aneurysms, leading to hypothalamic dysfunction and neurologic impairment, has been described [376].

PATHOLOGY OF THE GASTROINTESTINAL TRACT

Dysfunction of the digestive tract is a frequent problem in children with AIDS. In an Italian study of 200 HIV-infected children, Galli and colleagues [377] observed a higher incidence of hepatitis and diarrhea with onset during the first year of life (occurring in 20% to 50% of cases) than at any later time. Commonly encountered pathogens that may cause severe diarrhea are *Cryptosporidium*, *M. avium-intracellulare* complex, *Microsporidium*, *Salmonella*, and *Shigella* [378]. HIV nucleic acids have been found in the feces of children with persistent diarrheal disease [379]. Many HIV-infected children have a gastrointestinal dysfunction owing to disaccharide intolerance, however [379].

Progressive weight loss, anorexia, and sometimes pathogen-negative diarrhea characterize the wasting syndrome often seen in association with HIV disease [380–383]. The cause is unclear, but probably represents a combination of a metabolic imbalance with hypermetabolism, disturbed nitrogen balance, and increased cytokine levels. No specific treatment is available, but individual patients may benefit from appetite stimulants, dietary supplements, or parenteral nutrition [384].

Liver dysfunction resulting from an infection, including cytomegalovirus, Epstein-Barr virus, the hepatitis viruses, *M. avium-intracellulare* complex, or HIV-1, is a common feature and can evolve into a chronic hepatitis or cholangitis [385,386]. *Candida albicans* and the herpesviruses are often the cause of infections of the oral cavity and of esophagitis. Esophagitis in the HIV-infected child does not manifest with typical symptoms or dysphagia, but may be the cause of poor appetite and weight loss. Pancreatitis is a rare complication of HIV infection in children and may occur as a result of opportunistic infections such as cytomegalovirus or as a side effect of therapeutic agents [387,388].

NEPHROPATHY

Renal disease in children with HIV infection manifests most often as focal glomerulosclerosis or mesangial hyperplasia. In one study, 12 of 155 children between the ages of 7 months and 8 years were found to have proteinuria, and 5 of them developed severe renal failure within 1 year of diagnosis [389,390]. This nephrotic syndrome is often resistant to treatment with corticosteroids, but cyclosporine may induce a remission [391]. IgA nephritis has been observed in a few HIV-infected children and adults, clinically manifesting as recurrent gross hematuria [392,393]. An infection with cytomegalovirus or treatment with the protease inhibitor indinavir can also cause hematuria [394,395]. Immune complex disease may be involved in the pathogenesis of HIV-related nephropathy.

PATHOLOGY OF ENDOCRINE ORGANS

Failure to thrive or grow is commonly seen in children with HIV infection. In a study of 35 HIV-positive hemophiliacs, a decrease of more than 15 percentile points in height or weight for age was a predictive marker for children who became symptomatic for AIDS [396–398]. Although a few patients may have some dysregulation of thyroid function or a lack of growth hormone, often no definable endocrine cause is recognizable [399,400]. The exception is a child with adrenal insufficiency, which may be caused by cytomegalovirus infection of the adrenal gland [401]. One child with severe salt craving was described who required therapy with fluorocortisol. In a study of 167 HIV-infected children, Hirschfeld and associates [402] found decreased levels of free thyroxine in 18% and increased thyrotropin or thyroid-binding globulin levels in 30% of children.

INVOLVEMENT OF LYMPHOID ORGANS AND THYMUS

Thymic abnormalities have been found in 3 of 37 fetuses aborted between 20 and 27 weeks' gestation [403]. Thymic abnormality may represent the initial injury to the lymphoid system. In children with AIDS, the thymus can show precocious involution, with marked depletion of lymphocytes and loss of corticomedullary differentiation, or thymitis, characterized by the presence of lymphoid follicles with germinal centers or a diffuse lymphomononuclear infiltration [404]. Multilocular thymic cysts can occur, often detected as an incidental finding [404]. Lymphadenopathy is common among infected children and adults, and lymphoid organs function as reservoirs for HIV-1 [405–408].

HEMATOLOGIC PROBLEMS

Anemia is the most common hematologic disorder observed in HIV-infected children, with incidence depending on the severity of HIV disease, the age group, and the use of antiretroviral therapy [409–411]. In a retrospective study of 75 HIV-infected children, 19.7% had anemia at age 6 months, 32.9% at 9 months, and 37.3% at 12 months [412]. Bone marrow aspirate or biopsy specimens may show lymphoid aggregates, some degree of dysplasia, or an ineffective erythropoiesis [413]. Pure red blood cell aplasia from acute or persistent B19 parvovirus infection has been described in some HIV-infected children and adults and should be considered when the red blood cell production rate is less than expected for the degree of anemia [414–416].

A white blood cell count of less than 3000 cells/mm³ has been observed in 26% to 38% of untreated pediatric patients, and neutropenia, defined as an absolute neutrophil count of less than 1500 cells/mm³, has been found in 43% [409–411]. This neutropenia can result from HIV infection, infection with opportunistic pathogens such as *M. avium-intracellulare* complex or cytomegalovirus, or therapy with a myelotoxic drug, including zidovudine.

In the patient population at the National Cancer Institute, a platelet count of less than 50,000 cells/mm³ was found in 19% of the children; thrombocytopenia has also been described in HIV-infected infants [417–419]. Treatment options are similar to those of noninfected children and include intravenous gamma globulins, corticosteroids, and WinRho (anti-D immunoglobulin). Improvement is often best achieved, however, by optimizing the antiretroviral therapy and decreasing the circulating viral load.

Deficiency of vitamin K–dependent factors II, VII, IX, and X is common in HIV-infected children and can result in a coagulopathy that is relatively easy to correct. Also commonly seen are autoimmune phenomena, such as lupus anticoagulants and antiphospholipid or anticardiolipid antibodies [420–422]. Disseminated intravascular coagulopathy has been described as a complication of fulminant infectious conditions, but there are no data to indicate that this complication occurs more frequently in HIV-infected individuals.

SKIN

Mucocutaneous disease is very common in pediatric HIV infection, but often manifests in an unusual or atypical form [423,424]. The most common lesions with an infectious cause are oral thrush and diaper rash (*C. albicans*), chickenpox (acute or chronic), recurrent shingles (varicella-zoster virus), and molluscum contagiosum [425]. Bacterial infections and a highly contagious form of scabies have also been reported with some frequency. Severe seborrheic dermatitis or a nonspecific, intensely pruritic eczematous dermatitis can pose difficult and frustrating clinical problems, necessitating prolonged therapy. Because of the atypical presentations and wide variety of possible causes, it is often prudent to culture lesions for bacteria or for varicella-zoster virus or to perform a scraping or biopsy. Drug eruptions seem to be more common in HIV-infected patients and can develop into a toxic epidermal necrolysis [423]. Most drug-related rashes resolve after stopping the causative agent, however.

MALIGNANCIES

Several case reports of malignancies associated with HIV infection in infants and children have been published; however, cancer is the AIDS-defining illness in only 2% of children compared with 14% of adults [426]. The most common cancer in HIV-infected children is non-Hodgkin lymphoma as a systemic disease or as a primary central nervous system tumor [427–429]. Kaposi sarcoma has been described in a few children, including a 6-day-old infant, but is relatively uncommon [430–432]. Leiomyomas and leiomyosarcomas, soft tissue tumors associated with Epstein-Barr virus infection in immunocompromised patients, are increasingly common [433,434].

MORBIDITY, MORTALITY, AND PROGNOSIS

The natural history of HIV infection in children has changed significantly in the United States and Europe since the introduction of antiretroviral therapy [5,19–25]. As a result of more effective treatment of HIV infection and associated complications and improved guidelines for prophylaxis of opportunistic infections, major decreases in the morbidity and mortality rates of HIV-infected children and adults have occurred in developed countries [5,19–25]. HIV-infected infants with unknown status or infants not receiving antiretroviral treatment are still at high risk for early and severe morbidity, however, and continue to have a high mortality rate [237,435,436]. Without treatment, the risk of mortality in HIV-infected children living in the United States and Europe is approximately 10% to 20% [5,258]. In contrast, HIV-associated morbidity and mortality are very high in African cohorts; results of a pooled analysis showed that about one third of children with HIV infection die by 1 year of age, and more than half die by age 2 years [31]. Infants with intrauterine or intrapartum acquisition of infection have the fastest disease progression [31].

The clinical course of HIV infection in children differs greatly from infected adults [5]. Studies from developed countries and sub-Saharan Africa indicate that HIV disease often progresses more rapidly in infants than in adults [31,437]. Infants with perinatally acquired HIV-1 infection have widely variable clinical courses and durations of survival. Although the course of HIV infection in children is generally more accelerated than in adults, distinct subgroups are noticeable. Early reports suggest a bimodal disease expression with 20% to 25% of untreated HIV-1–infected infants rapidly progressing to AIDS or death during the 1st year of life, and others having a better prognosis, with some now surviving into young adulthood [237,253,258].

These studies of the natural history of perinatal HIV infection were performed before the routine use of antiretroviral therapy in pregnant women and their infants. In a European study of 392 HIV-infected children, Blanche and colleagues [237] found that 20% of children died or developed an AIDS-defining symptom (CDC category C; see Table 21–3) within the 1st year of life and 4.7% per year thereafter, reaching a cumulative incidence of 36% by 6 years of age. Two thirds of the children alive at 6 years of age had only minor symptoms, and one third had well-preserved $CD4^+$ counts (<25%) despite prior clinical manifestations. Children with HIV infection acquired through a transfusion during the neonatal period tend to have a prolonged asymptomatic period [438].

Clinical and laboratory factors have been evaluated in regard to their prognostic value. Children born to mothers with advanced disease, low $CD4^+$ counts, and high viral load tend to progress more rapidly to category C disease or death, emphasizing the importance of diagnosis and adequate treatment of HIV-infected pregnant women [176,323,439,440]. Early clinical manifestations of HIV infection in the infant, especially development of AIDS-defining conditions such as PCP and HIV encephalopathy or hepatosplenomegaly, has repeatedly been associated with a poor prognosis [253,258,441,442]. In contrast, slow depletion of $CD4^+$ T-lymphocyte count, late onset of clinical symptoms, and occurrence of lymphocytic interstitial pneumonitis are associated with improved survival [253,258].

A high virus copy number in the blood has been shown to be a strong predictor for progression of HIV disease [171,443,444]. Infants with very high HIV RNA copy numbers shortly after birth are presumed to have been infected in utero and tend to have early onset of symptoms [444]. Dickover and associates [444], when calculating HIV-infected infants followed for up to 8 years, found that a 1-log higher HIV-1 RNA copy number at birth increased the relative hazard of developing CDC class A or B symptoms by 40% (P = .004), of developing AIDS by 60% (P = .01), and of the risk of death by 80% (P = .023). The peak HIV-1 RNA copy number during the period of primary viremia was also predictive of progression to AIDS (relative hazard 9.9, 95% CI 1.8% to 541%, P = .008) and death (relative hazard 6.9, 95% CI 1.1% to 43.8%, P = .04) [444].

PREVENTION

An important goal in the care of HIV-infected individuals is the prevention of further infections and especially the transmission of HIV from mother to infant. Many countries have initiated large educational programs to halt the spread of the epidemic in the heterosexual community. The prevalence of HIV infection is so high in certain populations, especially in developing countries, that a change in behavior results in only a very slow decrease in the number of new infections. Identifying pregnant women who are HIV infected is essential for the potential initiation of combination antiretroviral therapy for maternal health and to prevent mother-to-child transmission of HIV [222,223].

EXPERIENCE IN PERINATAL HUMAN IMMUNODEFICIENCY VIRUS PREVENTION IN THE UNITED STATES

Major advances have been made in prevention of perinatal transmission of HIV during the last decade in the United States and Europe [6–13]. Perinatal HIV transmission rates has decreased to less than 2% as a result of widespread implementation of routine antenatal HIV testing ("opt-out" approach), use of antiretroviral prophylaxis and HAART, elective cesarean delivery, and avoidance of breast-feeding [15,16]. Efforts to prevent perinatal HIV transmission have been pursued since the discovery of the virus in 1983 [1–4]. In 1985, the CDC issued guidelines recommending that HIV-infected women in the United States should not breast-feed [445]. The success of the Pediatric AIDS Clinical Trials Group (PACTG) 076 protocol in 1994 has had a major impact on the prevention of perinatal transmission of HIV-1 and has resulted in guidelines issued by the CDC [222,223,446,447]. In that landmark study, pregnant HIV-infected women received oral zidovudine starting at 14 to 34 weeks of gestation and intravenous zidovudine during labor and delivery, and the infants were treated with 6 weeks of oral zidovudine during the postpartum period (Table 21–6). This regimen resulted in a 67% reduction in the perinatal transmission rate, from 25% to 8.3% (P = .00006) [446]. It has also been shown that a high maternal plasma concentration of HIV-1 is a risk factor for transmission to the infant [41]. The mechanism of action of zidovudine is not fully understood. In the

TABLE 21–6   Pediatric AIDS Clinical Trials Group 076 Zidovudine Regimen

Time of Zidovudine Administration	Route	Regimen
Antepartum	Oral	100 mg zidovudine five times daily, initiated at 14-34 wk of gestation and continued throughout pregnancy
Intrapartum	Intravenous	During labor and delivery, intravenous administration of zidovudine in a 1-hr initial dose of 2 mg/kg, followed by continuous infusion of 1 mg/kg/hr until delivery
Postpartum	Oral	Oral zidovudine to newborn (zidovudine syrup at 2 mg/kg per dose every 6 hr) for the first 6 wk of life, beginning at 8-12 hr after birth; if infant cannot tolerate oral zidovudine, it can be given intravenously at a dosage of 1.5 mg/kg every 6 hr

From Centers for Disease Control and Prevention. Public Health Service task force recommendations for the use of antiretroviral drugs in pregnant women infected with HIV-1 for maternal health and for reducing perinatal HIV-1 transmission in the United States. MMWR Morb Mortal Wkly Rep 47:1-31, 1998.

PACTG 076 study, zidovudine reduced maternal HIV-1 RNA only modestly, and change in maternal HIV-1 RNA levels accounted for only 17% of the reported efficacy of zidovudine [41]. In addition, zidovudine reduced transmission at all levels of maternal HIV-1 RNA levels. The continued efficacy of zidovudine in reducing transmission even in women with low viral loads suggests that preexposure and postexposure prophylaxis of the infant during labor and delivery may be a substantial component of protection [8].

After the publication of PACTG 076 study results in 1994, the CDC issued guidelines that all pregnant women should be offered HIV testing and recommended zidovudine for all pregnant HIV-infected women according to the PACTG regimen [222]. In 1998, the Institute of Medicine released a report recommending universal HIV screening with right of refusal for all pregnant women [448]. In 1999, the U.S. Congress provided target funding for prevention of perinatal HIV infection in states with high prevalence. In 2001, the CDC issued revised HIV counseling and testing guidelines for pregnant women, recommending strategies to reduce barriers to offering antenatal HIV testing to ensure routine HIV testing and offering rapid HIV testing during the labor and delivery period for women with unknown HIV status [449].

In 2003-2006, the CDC reported high uptake of screening of pregnant women using the "opt-out" strategy. In 2006, the CDC expanded the use of the "opt-out" strategy to include routine HIV testing in health care facilities to all patients 13 to 64 years old and all pregnant women as part of the routine panel of antenatal tests, a second HIV test in the third trimester for women living in areas with high incidence of HIV or women at high risk, and rapid testing for women with unknown status at the time of labor and delivery [219]. Widespread implementation of these

recommendations and the introduction of combination antiretroviral therapy since the late 1990s has led to a marked decrease in the number of newly HIV-infected infants in industrialized countries [10–13]. In 1992, approximately 2000 infants in the United States acquired perinatal HIV infection, whereas currently less than 200 infants acquire HIV infection [10,18].

Because maternal plasma viral load is a critical predictor of perinatal HIV transmission [43,72–77] the effect of maternal HAART and combination antiretroviral regimens on transmission has been studied in open-label and epidemiologic studies. Combination antiretroviral regimens are more effective for prevention of perinatal HIV transmission than single-drug regimens alone. Investigators from France and Thailand reported that zidovudine and lamivudine prophylaxis is more effective than zidovudine alone in reducing mother-to-child transmission of HIV [450,451].

In the United States, a large multicenter prospective cohort study of 1542 HIV-1–infected, non–breast-feeding pregnant women and their infants (Women and Infant Transmission Study) found that HIV-1 transmission was 20% (95% CI 16.1% to 23.9%) for 396 women with no prenatal antiretroviral therapy, 10.4% (95% CI 8.2% to 12.6%) for 710 women receiving zidovudine monotherapy, 3.8% (95% CI 1.1% to 6.5%) for 186 women receiving dual therapy without protease inhibitors, and 1.2% (95% CI 0 to 2.5%) for 250 women receiving combination antiretroviral therapy with protease inhibitors [16]. Transmission also varied by maternal HIV-1 RNA level at delivery: 1% for less than 400 copies/mL, 5.3% for 400 to 3499 copies/mL, 9.3% for 3500 to 9999 copies/mL, 14.7% for 10,000 to 29,999 copies/mL, and 23.4% for greater than 30,000 copies/mL. The odds of transmission increased 2.4-fold (95% CI 1.7 to 3.5) for every log [10] increase in delivery viral load. In multivariate analyses adjusting for maternal viral load, duration of therapy, and other factors, the odds ratio for transmission for women receiving combination therapy with or without protease inhibitors compared with women receiving zidovudine monotherapy was 0.30 (95% CI 0.09 to 1.02) and 0.27 (95% CI 0.08 to 0.94) [16].

Levels of maternal viral load at delivery and antenatal antiretroviral therapy were independently associated with transmission. The protective effect of therapy increased with the complexity and duration of the regimen, and maternal HAART was associated with the lowest rates of transmission [16].

Current perinatal HIV prevention guidelines issued by the CDC recommend combination antiretroviral therapy with at least three antiretroviral drugs during pregnancy if maternal viral load is 1000 copies/mL or greater (Table 21–7) [223]. In addition, elective cesarean delivery is recommended if maternal viral load is 1000 copies/mL or greater near delivery. Because of the proven benefit of antiretroviral prophylaxis in preventing perinatal HIV-1 transmission in women, including women with viral load less than 1000 copies/mL [74], all HIV-infected women should receive prophylaxis using the PACTG zidovudine regimen alone or combination antiretroviral therapy. Zidovudine monotherapy administered to HIV-infected women with viral load less than 1000 copies/mL has been

TABLE 21-7   Guidelines for Preventing Perinatal HIV-1 Transmission*

Maternal HIV-1 RNA Level >1000 copies/mL
Combination ART (ideally including zidovudine after first trimester), intravenous zidovudine infusion during labor, followed by oral zidovudine for 6 wk to infant
Elective cesarean section if maternal HIV-1 RNA level >1000 copies near delivery
Maternal HIV-1 RNA Level <1000 copies/mL
Zidovudine alone after first trimester (controversial) or combination ART (ideally including zidovudine after first trimester), intravenous zidovudine infusion during labor, followed by oral zidovudine for 6 wk to infant
HIV-1-Infected Women Who Have Had No ART before Labor
When woman has not received any therapy during pregnancy, several efficacious intrapartum and postpartum regimens are available
Intravenous zidovudine infusion during labor followed by oral zidovudine for 6 wk to infant OR
Intravenous zidovudine infusion plus single-dose nevirapine at onset of labor. To reduce the development of nevirapine resistance, add lamivudine during labor and maternal zidovudine/lamivudine for 7 days postpartum. Infant should receive single-dose nevirapine plus zidovudine for 6 weeks.
HIV-1-Infected Women Who Have Had No ART before or during Labor
Oral zidovudine should be prescribed to neonate as soon as possible after delivery (preferably within 6-12 hr of birth) and continued for 6 wk
Some experts advocate use of postnatal zidovudine regimen in conjunction with other antiretroviral agents

ART, antiretroviral therapy.
*From Centers for Disease Control and Prevention. U.S. Public Health Service task force recommendations for use of antiretroviral drugs in pregnant HIV-infected women for maternal health and interventions to reduce perinatal HIV-1 transmission in the United States. Available at http://aidsinfo.nih.gov/contentfiles/PerinatalGL001020.pdf. 8 July 2008, posting date.

shown to reduce perinatal HIV transmission to 1% [74]. In addition, no long-term effects on women's health have been noted among U.S. women enrolled in the PACTG 076 trial in terms of disease progression, mortality, viral load, or zidovudine resistance between randomized treatment and placebo arms [452].

When the mother has not received any therapy during pregnancy or during the labor and delivery period because of detection of HIV in the mother or infant after delivery, observational data suggest that administration of oral zidovudine for 6 weeks to the infant started within 24 hours after birth may provide some benefit against transmission [453]. In such instances, other antiretroviral agents could be added to the postnatal zidovudine regimen [220].

The role of elective cesarean section delivery in reducing perinatal HIV-1 transmission was recognized before the advent of combination antiretroviral therapy during pregnancy [91,92]. Data from a large international meta-analysis of 15 prospective cohort studies and a randomized controlled trial from Europe showed that cesarean section performed before labor and rupture of membranes is associated with at least a 50% decrease in the risk of perinatal HIV transmission independent of the use of antiretroviral

therapy or zidovudine prophylaxis [91,92]. Both these studies were done before the advent of HAART during pregnancy, and there was no information on maternal serum HIV-1 RNA level. Because the level of maternal serum HIV RNA level is an important predictor of perinatal HIV-1 transmission [43,72-77] it is unclear if elective cesarean section would offer any additional benefit in women successfully treated with HAART who have a very low or undetectable viral load [454].

The risk of postnatal HIV-1 transmission through breast-feeding has been documented [48,49]. In resource-rich countries where infant formulas are safe and readily available, HIV-infected mothers should be advised not to breast-feed their infants [113,455].

Despite significant advances in prevention of maternal-to-child transmission of HIV, approximately 150 HIV-infected infants are born annually in the United States, primarily because of missed prevention opportunities, including inadequate prenatal care, lack of antenatal HIV testing, and clinicians offering prenatal HIV testing only to women they consider high risk [9,456]. Knowledge of HIV status during labor is crucial for providing zidovudine prophylaxis for women who test positive and their infants to prevent perinatal transmission [457]. The Mother-Infant Rapid Intervention at Delivery (MIRIAD) study showed the feasibility of rapid HIV-1 testing of women with unknown HIV status during labor [457]. The MIRIAD study results have important implications for populations in developed countries, but may have a greater impact in sub-Saharan Africa, where approximately 29% of women do not receive prenatal care [458]. Other challenges include preventing new HIV infections in women of childbearing age, especially adolescent girls of minority race or ethnicity, and preventing unplanned pregnancy in adolescent girls [9,456].

INTERNATIONAL EXPERIENCE IN PERINATAL HUMAN IMMUNODEFICIENCY VIRUS PREVENTION

Although the PACTG 076 regimen is very effective, it is not feasible to implement this intervention in resource-limited countries where 1800 new perinatal infections occur per day [28]. In addition, most transmission occurs late in pregnancy or at the time of delivery [6,47]. Shorter, less expensive regimens that are more applicable to resource-limited countries were studied in trials. The results of major studies on antiretroviral prophylaxis to prevent perinatal HIV transmission in breast-feeding and non–breast-feeding populations are presented in Tables 21–8 and 21–9. Initial studies focused on regimens that were modifications of zidovudine monotherapy.

The efficacy of short-course prophylaxis regimens of zidovudine, started at 36 weeks of gestation with no infant prophylaxis, in reducing perinatal HIV transmission was studied among non–breast-feeding populations in Thailand (see Table 21–8) [459]. Results from this study, performed in Thailand as a collaboration between the Thailand Ministry of Health and the CDC, showed a 50% reduction in perinatal HIV transmission in a non–breast-feeding population [22]. This trial enrolled non–breast-feeding women who were treated with zidovudine

TABLE 21-8   Antiretroviral (ARV) Prophylaxis Regimens to Reduce Perinatal HIV-1 Transmission in Non–Breast-feeding Infants

Study	Schedule of ARV Prophylaxis	Transmission Rate and Relative Efficacy
ZDV/Placebo[446] PACTG 076; $N = 477$; U.S., France (formula feeding)	AP+IP+PP AP = oral ZDV 100 mg 5 times per day starting at 14 wk of gestation IP = 2 mg/kg, then 1 mg/kg/hr IV PP (mother) = none PP (infant) = oral ZDV 2 mg/kg q6h for 6 wk	At 18 mo: 8.3% ZDV versus 25.5% placebo; 68% efficacy
ZDV/Placebo[459]; $N = 392$; Thailand/CDC (formula feeding)	AP+IP AP = oral ZDV 300 mg q12h starting at 36 wk of gestation IP = oral ZDV 300 mg q3h PP = None	At 6 mo: 9.4% ZDV versus 18.9% placebo; 50% efficacy
ZDV/Comparative[462]; $N = 1437$; Thailand Perinatal HIV Prevention Trial (PHPT) PHPT/Harvard (formula feeding)	AP+IP+PP ZDV (LL) AP = oral ZDV 300 mg q12h starting at 28 wk of gestation IP = oral ZDV 300 mg q3h PP (mother) = none PP (infant) = oral ZDV 2 mg/kg q6h for 6 wk ZDV (LS) AP = oral ZDV 300 mg q12h starting at 28 wk of gestation IP = oral ZDV 300 mg q3h PP (mother) = none PP (infant) = oral ZDV 2 mg/kg q6h for 3 days ZDV (SL) AP = oral ZDV 300 mg q12h starting at 36 wk of gestation IP = oral ZDV 300 mg q3h PP (mother): none PP (infant) = oral ZDV 2 mg/kg q6h for 6 wk ZDV (SS) AP = oral ZDV 300 mg q12h starting at 36 wk of gestation IP = oral ZDV 300 mg q3h PP (mother): none PP (infant) = oral ZDV 2 mg/kg q6h for 3 days	At 6 mo final analysis: 6.5% LL versus 4.7% LS versus 8.6% SL In utero transmission: 1.6% (LL + LS) versus 5.1% (SL + SS) At 6 mo interim analysis: 4.1% (LL) versus 10.5% (SS) (SS arm stopped)
NVP/Placebo[473]/PACTG 316; $N = 1248$; U.S., Europe, Brazil, Bahamas (formula feeding)	AP+IP+PP NVP arm: AP = standard ART starting from 14 wk of gestation (77% combination, 23% ZDV alone) IP = ZDV 2 mg/kg, then 1 mg/kg/hr IV plus NVP 200 mg × 1 PP (mother) = ART if needed PP (infant) = ZDV 2 mg/kg for 6 wk plus NVP 2 mg/kg × 1 at birth Placebo arm: AP = standard ART starting from 14 wk of gestation (77% combination, 23% ZDV alone) IP = ZDV 2 mg/kg, then 1 mg/kg/hr IV plus NVP placebo PP (mother) = ART if needed PP (infant) = ZDV 2 mg/kg q6h for 6 wk plus NVP placebo at birth	At 6 mo: 1.4% NVP versus 1.6% placebo

AP, antepartum; ART, antiretroviral therapy; CDC, Centers for Disease Control and Prevention; IP, intrapartum; LL, long-long; LS, long-short; NVP, nevirapine; PACTG, Pediatric AIDS Clinical Trials Group; PP, postpartum; SL, short-long; SS, short-short; ZDV, zidovudine.

TABLE 21–9   Antiretroviral (ARV) Prophylaxis Regimens to Reduce Perinatal HIV-1 Transmission in Breast-feeding Infants

Study	Schedule of ARV Prophylaxis	Mother-to-Child HIV Transmission (MTCT) Rate and Relative Efficacy
ZDV/Placebo[460]; $N = 280$; Ivory Coast (breast-feeding)	AP+IP AP = oral ZDV 300 mg q12h starting at 36 wk of gestation IP = oral ZDV 300 mg q3h PP (mother) = none PP (infant) = none	At 3 mo: 16.5% ZDV versus 26.1 placebo; 37% efficacy
ZDV/Placebo[461,463] DITRAME (ANRS 049a); $N = 400$; Ivory Coast, Burkina Faso (breast-feeding)	AP+IP+PP AP = oral ZDV 300 mg q12h starting at 36 wk of gestation IP = oral ZDV 600 mg × 1 PP (mother) = 300 mg q12h for 1 wk PP (infant) = none	At 6 mo: 18% ZDV versus 27.5 placebo; 38% efficacy At 15 mo: 21.5% ZDV versus 30.6% placebo; 30% efficacy At 24 mo (pooled analysis): 22.5% ZDV versus 30.2% placebo; 26% efficacy
ZDV-3TC/Placebo (PETRA)[466]; $N = 1797$; South Africa, Uganda, and Tanzania (breast-feeding and formula feeding)	AP+IP+PP; IP+PP; IP only ZDV/3TC (Arm 1) AP = oral ZDV 300 mg q12h plus 3TC 150 mg q12h starting at 36 wk of gestation IP = oral ZDV 300 mg q3h plus 3TC 150 mg q12h PP (mother): oral ZDV 300 mg q12h plus 3TC 150 mg q12h for 1 wk PP (infant) = oral ZDV 4 mg/kg q12h plus 3TC 2 mg/kg q12h for 1 wk ZDV/3TC (Arm 2) AP = none IP = oral ZDV 300 mg q3h plus 3TC 150 mg q12h PP (mother): oral ZDV 300 mg q12h plus 3TC 150 mg q12h for 1 wk PP (infant) = oral ZDV 4 mg/kg q12h plus 3TC 2 mg/kg q12h for 1 wk ZDV/3TC (Arm 3) AP = none IP = oral ZDV 300 mg q3h plus 3TC 150 mg q12h PP (mother) = none PP (infant) = none	At 6 wk: Arm 1, 5.7%; Arm 2, 8.9%; Arm 3, 14.2%; placebo, 15.3%; efficacy: Arm 1, 63%; Arm 2, 42%; Arm 3, not significant At 18 mo: Arm 1, 14.9%; Arm 2, 18.1%; Arm 3, 20%; placebo, 22.2%; efficacy: Arm 1, 33%; Arm 2, not significant; Arm 3, not significant
NVP/ZDV (HIVNET 012)[467,468]; $N = 626$; Uganda (breast-feeding)	IP+PP NVP arm: AP = none IP = NVP 200 mg × 1 PP (mother) = none PP (infant) = NVP 2 mg/kg × 1 at birth ZDV arm: AP = none IP = ZDV 600 mg, then 300 mg q3h PP (mother) = none PP (infant) = ZDV 4 mg/kg q12h for 1 wk	At 14-16 wk: 13.1% NVP versus 25.1% ZDV; 47% efficacy At 18 mo: 15.7% NVP versus 25.8 ZDV; 41% efficacy
NVP/ZDV-3TC[470]; $N = 1331$; South Africa (breast-feeding and formula feeding)	IP+PP NVP arm: AP = none IP = NVP 200 mg × 1 PP (mother) = NVP 200 mg × 1 PP (infant) = NVP 2 mg/kg × 1 at birth	At 8 wk: 12.3% NVP versus 9.3% ZDV/3TC; not statistically significant ($P = .11$)

Continued

TABLE 21–9 Antiretroviral (ARV) Prophylaxis Regimens to Reduce Perinatal HIV-1 Transmission in Breast-feeding Infants—cont'd

Study	Schedule of ARV Prophylaxis	Mother-to-Child HIV Transmission (MTCT) Rate and Relative Efficacy
	ZDV/3TC arm: AP = none IP = ZDV 300 mg q3h plus 3TC 150 mg q12h PP (mother) = ZDV 300 mg q12h plus 3TC 150 mg q12h for 1 wk PP (infant) = ZDV 4 mg/kg q12h plus 3TC 2 mg/kg q12h for 1 wk	
Open-label study: ZDV + SD NVP[472] DITRAME (ANRS 1201.0); N = 420; Abidjan (breast-feeding and formula feeding)	AP+IP+PP AP = oral ZDV 300 mg q12h starting at 36 wk of gestation IP = oral ZDV 600 mg × 1 + NVP 200 mg × 1 PP (mother) = none PP (infant) = ZDV syrup (2 mg/kg q6h) for 7 days + SD NVP syrup (2 mg/kg) on day 2	At 6 wk: transmission was 6.5% (95% confidence interval 3.9%-9.1%) with ZDV + SD NVP; 12.8% transmission in historical control group receiving short-course ZDV alone (98% breast-fed in historical control group)
Open-label study: ZDV+3TC+SD NVP[472] DITRAME (ANRS 1201.1); N = 373; Abidjan (breast-feeding and formula feeding)	AP+IP+PP AP = oral ZDV 300 mg q12h + 3TC 150 mg q12h starting at 32 wk of gestation IP = oral ZDV 600 mg × 1 + 3TC 300 mg + NVP 200 mg × 1 PP (mother) = oral ZDV 300 mg q12h + 3TC 150 mg q12h for 3 days only PP (infant) = ZDV syrup (2 mg/kg q6h) for 7 days + SD NVP syrup (2 mg/kg) on day 2	At 6 wk: transmission was 4.7% (95% confidence interval 2.4%-7.0%) with ZDV + 3TC + SD NVP; 12.8% transmission in historical control group receiving short-course ZDV alone (98% breast-fed in historical control group)
Neonatal SD NVP/SD NVP plus ZDV (NVAZ trial)[475]; N = 484; Malawi (breast-feeding)	PP (infant only) SD NVP plus ZDV arm: AP = none (late presenters) IP = None (late presenters) PP (mother) = none PP (infant) = SD NVP syrup (2 mg/kg) + ZDV syrup (4 mg/kg q12h) given immediately after birth for 7 days SD NVP arm: AP = none (late presenters) IP = none (late presenters) PP (mother) = none PP (infant) = SD NVP syrup (2 mg/kg) only	At 6-8 wk: 15.3% SD NVP + ZDV arm versus 20.9% SD NVP–only arm; MTCT rate among infants who were HIV uninfected at birth was 7.7% and 12.1% (36% efficacy)
Postnatal NVP plus ZDV trial[476]; N = 894; Malawi (breast-feeding)	PP (infant only) SD NVP plus ZDV arm: AP = none IP = SD NVP PP (mother) = none PP (infant) = SD NVP syrup (2 mg/kg) + ZDV syrup (4 mg/kg q12h) given immediately after birth for 7 days SD NVP arm: AP = none IP = SD NVP PP (mother) = none PP (infant) = SD NVP syrup (2 mg/kg) only	At 6-8 wk: 16.3% SD NVP + ZDV arm versus 14.1% SD NVP–only arm (difference not statistically significant); MTCT rate among infants who were HIV uninfected at birth was 6.5% and 16.9%

AP, antepartum; IP, intrapartum; NVP, nevirapine; SD, single-dose; PP, postpartum; 3TC, lamivudine; ZDV, zidovudine.

(300 mg twice daily) beginning by 36 weeks of gestation with no infant prophylaxis component. During labor and delivery, the oral dose of maternal zidovudine was increased to 300 mg every 3 hours. The estimated efficacy of this therapy was 51% (decrease from 18.6% transmission rate in placebo group to 9.2% in treated group) [459].

The identical short-course zidovudine antepartum and intrapartum regimen used in Thailand [459], when evaluated in a placebo-controlled trial in Abidjan, Cote d'Ivoire, involving breast-feeding populations, showed an efficacy of 37% reduction in transmission to infants compared with placebo at 3 months of age [460]. Another placebo-controlled trial in West Africa studied a similar antepartum and intrapartum short-course zidovudine prophylaxis regimen with the addition of a 1-week course of zidovudine to mothers during the postpartum period and reported an efficacy of 38% at 6 months of age in predominantly breast-fed infants [461]. An additional week of postpartum maternal zidovudine therapy did not confer any additional benefit over the antepartum and intrapartum zidovudine-alone prophylaxis regimen. A study in Thailand showed that longer duration of zidovudine prophylaxis (starting at 28 weeks of gestation) is more effective than shorter duration regimens (starting at 36 weeks) [462]. In addition, if the duration of the maternal antepartum regimen is short (<4 weeks), longer infant prophylaxis (4 to 6 weeks) is more effective than shorter infant prophylaxis (3 days to 1 week) [460].

The efficacy of antiretroviral regimens in reducing antepartum and intrapartum transmission is diminished over time in breast-feeding populations. Long-term pooled analysis showed an efficacy of 26% by 24 months of age compared with 37% to 38% efficacy noted in infants at 3 months and 6 months of age in this population with long-term breast-feeding [463]. The overall efficacy of short-course zidovudine is less in breast-feeding populations in sub-Saharan Africa than in formula-fed populations [460,461], and the early efficacy seems to diminish with prolonged breast-feeding [463].

When the efficacy of short-course zidovudine was established, studies explored whether combination antiretroviral regimens are more effective than single-drug prophylaxis. Investigators from the United States and France and Thailand evaluated whether combining a second antiretroviral agent such as lamivudine would enhance further the efficacy of short-course zidovudine in reducing transmission in non–breast-feeding populations [464,465]. The French open-label, nonrandomized study assessed the safety of perinatal lamivudine-zidovudine combination prophylaxis in infants and its effects on perinatal transmission of HIV in a non–breast-feeding population [464]. The study enrolled 445 HIV-1–infected pregnant women, who received lamivudine at 32 weeks' gestation through delivery in addition to the standard PACTG 076 zidovudine prophylaxis regimen. Infants received lamivudine for 6 weeks in addition to the standard 6-week course of zidovudine. The transmission rate in the study group was 1.6% compared with 6.8% in a historical control group of HIV-infected mother-infant pairs in France who had received only zidovudine [464].

The Thailand open-label, nonrandomized trial studied the efficacy of lamivudine added to short-course zidovudine prophylaxis. This study enrolled 106 HIV-1–infected pregnant women, and lamivudine and zidovudine were begun at 34 weeks' gestation and given orally during labor. Infants received a 4-week course of zidovudine alone. The transmission rate in the study group was 2.8% compared with 11.7% in a historical control group of HIV-infected women in Thailand who had received only short-course zidovudine [465]. A WHO/UNAIDS multicenter, placebo-controlled trial involving breast-feeding populations in Africa to prevent mother-to-child transmission of HIV by short-course antiretroviral regimen (PETRA trial) showed an efficacy of 63% at 6 weeks for zidovudine and lamivudine given from 36 weeks' gestation, intrapartum, and for 1 week postpartum to mothers and infants; 42% efficacy for intrapartum-postpartum zidovudine and lamivudine; and no efficacy for intrapartum treatment only (see Table 21–9) [466].

When the woman has not received any therapy during pregnancy, several efficacious intrapartum and postpartum regimens are available based on data from several international clinical trials. Shorter antepartum and intrapartum regimens are not as effective for preventing perinatal HIV transmission, however, as regimens that include longer three-part antepartum, intrapartum, and postpartum prophylaxis. In a study in Uganda (HIVNET 012), a single dose of nevirapine given to the mother at onset of labor and a single oral dose of 2 mg/kg given to the infant at 48 to 72 hours of life were safe and reduced perinatal HIV transmission by 47% at 14 to 16 weeks of life and by 41% at 18 months in breast-feeding infants (see Table 21–9) [467,468]. Nevirapine is a very potent non-nucleoside analogue with a long half-life and excellent penetration across the placenta [469]. The single-dose nevirapine regimen is simple, inexpensive, and feasible to implement in resource-limited settings. Another trial conducted in South Africa comparing the efficacy of nevirapine (intrapartum and a single dose postpartum to mothers and to infants) versus zidovudine and lamivudine (intrapartum and for 1 week postpartum to mothers and infants) showed that the risk of infant HIV-1 infection at 8 weeks of age was similar in the two groups (see Table 21–9) [470].

Addition of single-dose nevirapine can significantly improve the efficacy of other short-course antiretroviral regimens [471,472]. Two trials conducted in Thailand (non–breast-feeding women) and West Africa (partly breast-feeding population) showed that addition of single maternal intrapartum and neonatal nevirapine doses to short-course maternal zidovudine (with oral zidovudine during labor and either no infant prophylaxis or 1 week of infant zidovudine prophylaxis) may provide increased efficacy for reducing perinatal HIV-1 transmission compared with short-course maternal zidovudine prophylaxis alone or short-course zidovudine and lamivudine [471,472]. The combined two-drug regimen study from Thailand conducted in a non–breast-feeding population showed equivalent efficacy in reducing perinatal HIV transmission as HAART regimens used in developed countries [471].

In contrast, an international, blinded, placebo-controlled phase 3 trial conducted in non–breast-feeding populations in the United States, Europe, Brazil, and the Bahamas (PACTG 316) found no additional benefit from two intrapartum and newborn nevirapine doses when women received prenatal care and standard antenatal antiretroviral therapy and elective cesarean section was made available. All neonates in this study received the standard 6-week zidovudine course, and the overall risk of perinatal HIV transmission was very low (1.5%) [473]. In this study, nevirapine resistance developed in 15% of the women who received single-dose intrapartum nevirapine [473,474]; addition of intrapartum and newborn nevirapine doses is not recommended in HIV-infected women who have received HAART during pregnancy [16].

In resource-limited settings, women often present in late labor and do not receive intrapartum antiretroviral prophylaxis in a timely fashion. A study conducted in a breast-feeding population in Malawi evaluated the efficacy of infant antiretroviral prophylaxis when no antepartum or intrapartum maternal antiretroviral therapy was received. This trial compared the efficacy of single-dose infant nevirapine versus single-dose infant nevirapine plus 1-week infant zidovudine; results showed that the combined regimen had a superior efficacy (7.7% transmission) compared with single-dose infant nevirapine alone (12.1% transmission) at 6 to 8 weeks of age [475]. When mothers received intrapartum nevirapine as preexposure prophylaxis, transmission rates were similar, however, for infants who received combined single-dose nevirapine plus zidovudine (6.9%) and for infants who received single-dose nevirapine only (6.5%) [476]. A future clinical trial is currently ongoing in non–breast-fed populations in the United States and Brazil to assess the efficacy of the standard 6-week infant zidovudine regimen when compared with two combination regimens (nevirapine dose at birth and 3 and 7 days of life and 2-week course of lamivudine and nelfinavir) [8].

The WHO recommends a tiered approach for the use of antiretroviral drugs for treatment of HIV-infected women and prevention of perinatal HIV transmission in resource-limited settings [477]. The revised recommendations include provision of triple-drug antiretroviral treatment for HIV-infected pregnant women who are eligible for treatment (CD4 count < 350 cells per cubic millimeter or WHO stage 3 or 4 disease). For pregnant women who are not eligible for HAART or where antiretroviral therapy is unavailable, the WHO recommends a combination antiretroviral prophylaxis regimen, preferably zidovudine from 28 weeks of gestation; zidovudine, lamivudine, and single-dose nevirapine during delivery; and zidovudine and lamivudine for 7 days postpartum to reduce the development of nevirapine resistance. Newborn infants who are breastfeeding should receive daily nevirapine prophylaxis until the cessation of breast-feeding [477]. Provision of antepartum and postpartum maternal triple-drug prophylaxis which is continued until the cessation of breast-feeding is another option for women who do not need HAART for their own health. Although efforts are ongoing to provide more effective regimens, the single-dose nevirapine regimen alone should still be used in settings where it is not feasible to implement more effective regimens or where these regimens are unavailable [477].

Despite the use of simple, efficacious prophylactic antiretroviral regimens worldwide, in resource-limited countries, less than 10% of HIV-infected pregnant women receive antiretroviral drugs to prevent mother-to-child transmission of HIV [28]. There are major barriers to implementation of perinatal HIV prevention programs in resource-poor countries [9,26]. Challenges include weak health care systems, limited resources, no stock of antiretroviral drugs and HIV test kits, lack of integration of perinatal HIV prevention programs into existing maternal-child services, limited prenatal care services, and limited HIV counseling and testing centers [9]. Other challenges include lack of male involvement, issues of disclosure, and lack of family planning services [9,26]. Social, cultural, and gender issues and divergent political agendas compound the dilemma further [9].

Transmission of HIV through breast-feeding is a major public health challenge in settings where replacement feeding is not feasible [48,49,97]. The risks of acquiring HIV infection through breast-feeding may be lower than the risk of death from diarrheal diseases and malnutrition in areas where replacement feeding is unavailable or unsafe. Decision models to determine the optimal choice of interventions to reduce breast-feeding transmission have been proposed [478]. For developing areas of the world, the WHO recommends exclusive breast-feeding through the first 6 months of life, introduce complementary foods thereafter, and continue breast-feeding for the first 6 months of life. Commercial infant formula milk as a replacement feed is acceptable only in countries where replacement feeding is "acceptable, feasible, affordable, sustainable, and safe" [479].

There is an urgent need to make breast-feeding by HIV-1–infected women safer to prevent postnatal transmission of the virus [480]. Innovative strategies have been proposed for prevention of HIV-1 transmission via breast milk in resource-poor settings, including maternal or infant, or both, postpartum antiretroviral prophylaxis for 6 months during breast-feeding; provision of combination antiretroviral therapy during lactation; active (infant vaccines) and passive (antibodies) immunoprophylaxis that boost infant immune responses during the period of breast-feeding; and exclusive breast-feeding with or without early weaning [48,49,117]. Early infant weaning, at or before age 6 months, may be associated with increased risk of morbidity and mortality owing to malnutrition, gastroenteritis, and other infectious diseases [97,480]. More recent observational studies indicate that infant prophylaxis is safe and may reduce transmission of HIV through breast-feeding [480]. International readers should refer to the WHO guidelines for updates regarding recent clinical trials of antiretroviral interventions to reduce postnatal transmission of HIV during breastfeeding [477].

SAFETY AND TOXICITY OF ANTIRETROVIRAL PROPHYLAXIS

With widespread use of antiretroviral prophylaxis to prevent perinatal HIV transmission in resource-poor countries and the availability of combination antiretroviral therapy for HIV-infected mothers during pregnancy, an increasing number of infants are being exposed to antiretroviral agents in utero and during the postnatal period [33,481]. Animal data have shown that nucleoside analogues may be carcinogenic and can cause mitochondrial dysfunction [223]. An extensive review of short-term and medium-term data from several studies indicates, however, that antiretroviral therapy during pregnancy has been well tolerated by mothers and infants [33,481]. Except for mild, transient anemia [8], no serious short-term maternal or infant adverse effects have been noted with prophylactic zidovudine regimens [482,483].

A European study reported an association between low birth weight or preterm delivery with the use of combination antiretroviral agents during pregnancy [484]. Data from a large meta-analysis of seven studies performed in the United States found no association, however, between increased rates of low birth weight, preterm delivery, low Apgar scores, or stillbirths and the use of combination antiretroviral therapy [485].

Current data indicate that infants exposed to commonly used antiretroviral agents such as zidovudine, lamivudine, stavudine, nevirapine, and nelfinavir during early pregnancy are no more likely to have a congenital anomaly than infants in the general population [484,486]. The French perinatal cohort study group reported possible mitochondrial abnormalities resulting in fatal outcomes in a large cohort of uninfected infants exposed to zidovudine alone or zidovudine and lamivudine during pregnancy or in the neonatal period [487]. Another study from France suggested a possible association of early febrile seizure with perinatal exposure to nucleoside analogues [488].

In contrast, a retrospective review of 16,000 uninfected U.S. children born to HIV-infected mothers, with and without antiretroviral exposure, failed to identify any deaths related to mitochondrial dysfunction [489]. Short-term to medium-term follow-up data from the European Collaborative Study involving 2414 uninfected children born to HIV-infected mothers and exposed to antiretroviral agents in utero or early life did not show any serious adverse events, including febrile seizures and clinical manifestations suggestive of mitochondrial abnormalities [490]. The long-term outcomes of infants exposed to combination antiretroviral therapy in utero are unknown. Long-term follow-up of all infants born to mothers exposed to antiretroviral therapy is recommended [223].

ANTIRETROVIRAL RESISTANCE

Emergence of viral resistance is a concern with global use of antiretroviral prophylaxis to prevent perinatal HIV transmission [491]. Nevirapine resistance has been a topic of major interest because the WHO recommends nevirapine-based treatment regimens as the first-line therapy in resource-limited nations [492]. A single gene mutation in HIV-1 reverse transcriptase can confer rapid resistance to commonly used antiretroviral agents such as lamivudine and nevirapine [491]. In an open-label study from France, addition of lamivudine to zidovudine after 32 weeks of gestation was associated with lamivudine resistance (M184V mutation) in 39% of women postpartum [464].

In the HIVNET 012 study, 19% of women exposed to the single intrapartum nevirapine dose acquired nevirapine-resistant mutations (predominantly K103N mutation); however, resistance was transient and no longer detectable 12 to 24 months after delivery [493]. In the same study, nevirapine-induced genotypic resistance was detected in 46% of nevirapine-exposed infants who subsequently became infected, but the mutations faded by 12 months of age [493]. The mutations were different in mothers and infants, and no resistant virus was transmitted from mother to infant. In the absence of continued drug exposure, these resistance mutations fade from detection in women and infants over time, and transmission of nevirapine-resistant virus seems less likely [491]. In a more recent study, nevirapine resistance mutations were detected 10 days after delivery in 32% of women who had received intrapartum nevirapine; women who received intrapartum nevirapine were less likely to have virologic suppression after 6 months of postpartum treatment with a nevirapine-based regimen [494]. The long-term clinical consequences of nevirapine-induced genotypic resistance on future treatment options are unknown and warrant future study [495].

With the use of more sensitive techniques, nevirapine resistance can be found in 60% to 89% of women after early exposure [496–499]. Emergence of nevirapine-resistant HIV-1 in this setting is more common among women who have a high viral load, low CD4+ count, and subtype C and D rather than A [500]. This subset of women should be considered for HAART to improve their own health and to reduce the risk of perinatal and possibly postnatal HIV-1 transmission [491,501]. In contrast, nevirapine resistance is less likely to emerge in healthy women who do not require HAART during pregnancy and could benefit from single-dose nevirapine prophylaxis to prevent perinatal HIV-1 transmission [491,501].

TREATMENT
SUPPORTIVE CARE AND GENERAL MANAGEMENT

Optimizing prenatal care, including nutrition, avoidance of drugs and other harmful substances, and recognition and treatment of concurrent infections, is crucial to prevent the premature delivery of infants with low birth weight. The general care of the newborn and infant is not different for infants born to HIV-seropositive mothers, but special attention should be given to the documentation of developmental milestones, frequency and course of infections, and nutritional status.

HIV-infected children are at higher risk for developing vaccine-preventable diseases than HIV-uninfected children. The AAP recommends routine immunizations with some modifications for all HIV-exposed infants, whether they are infected or not [38,124,226]. Similar to other newborns, infants born to HIV-infected mothers should receive hepatitis B vaccinations, but if the mother is positive for hepatitis B surface antigen, the infant should also receive hepatitis immune globulin within 12 hours after birth. Readers are referred to the 2006 edition of the *Red Book* for guidance regarding immunization practices in HIV-infected children [38].

Infants infected with HIV should be vaccinated at the appropriate age with inactivated vaccines (diphtheria, tetanus toxoids, and acellular pertussis; *Haemophilus influenzae* type b; hepatitis B; hepatitis A; and pneumococcal conjugate vaccine) and the influenza vaccine annually.

The current recommendation is that live virus vaccine (oral poliovirus) or live bacterial vaccines (bacillus Calmette-Guérin) should not be given to patients with HIV infection. The exception is measles-mumps-rubella (MMR) vaccine because of the high risk of mortality noted among HIV-infected children who develop wild-type measles, although only children with mild to moderate immunosuppression should have the MMR vaccine [38]. Children may receive the second dose of MMR vaccine 4 weeks after the first dose rather than waiting until school entry.

Varicella-zoster immunization is contraindicated in HIV-infected children and adults with severe immunosuppression. Data regarding varicella vaccine in HIV-infected children are limited, and physicians should examine the potential risks and benefits. The AAP recommends that varicella vaccine should be administered to HIV-infected children 12 months or older in CDC categories N1 and A1 (i.e., asymptomatic or mild signs and symptoms of disease and CD4$^+$ lymphocyte percentage ≥15% and no evidence of varicella immunity) [38]. The CDC recommends that two doses of varicella vaccine should be given, with a 3-month interval between doses [502]. Some experts consider varicella vaccination for asymptomatic HIV-infected patients receiving HAART with normal immune function (CD4$^+$ lymphocyte percentage >25%) for more than 6 months, even if they previously exhibited symptoms or had severe immunosuppression (CDC category C) [38]. Household contacts of HIV-infected infants can receive varicella vaccine because transmission of vaccine-type varicella-zoster virus is unusual. More recently, the Advisory Committee on Infectious Diseases has recommended the oral rotavirus vaccine for HIV-infected infants.

Immunization with the conjugated pneumococcal vaccine (PCV7) series is recommended as a four-dose series for infants at 2, 4, 6, and 12 to 15 months of age. PCV7 induces protective antibody responses in infants 2 months of age. Alternatively, children older than 2 years with HIV infection who previously have not received PCV7 should be administered a series of two doses of PCV7 and one dose of the 23-valent polysaccharide pneumococcal vaccine (PPV23) given at an 8-week interval between doses, followed by another dose of PPV23 3 to 5 years after the first dose [38].

Passive immunization of children with HIV infection is recommended in certain circumstances, especially after exposure to measles, varicella, or tetanus. A recommended prophylaxis regimen in HIV-infected infants after exposure to wild-type measles is the administration of intramuscular immunoglobulin (0.5 mL/kg, maximum dose 15 mL) regardless of their measles immunization status. Likewise, HIV-infected children exposed to varicella or shingles should receive intravenous immunoglobulin (IVIG) or specific hyperimmune globulin (if available) within 96 hours after exposure to varicella-zoster virus

regardless of their immunization status [38]. Children who have received IVIG within 2 weeks of exposure to measles or varicella do not need additional prophylaxis. Children with HIV infection with tetanus-prone wounds should receive tetanus immune globulin regardless of immunization status.

The monthly administration of IVIG has been studied in asymptomatic and symptomatic children with HIV infection. IVIG has been shown to prevent serious bacterial infections in patients with congenital immunodeficiencies. In a group of children who did not receive any antiretroviral treatment, only children with a CD4$^+$ count of 200 cells/mm^3 or greater seemed to benefit from monthly IVIG administration [503]. A study evaluating children receiving antiretroviral therapy did not find a statistically significant difference between children who received IVIG and children treated with placebo (albumin), as long as they were also receiving PCP prophylaxis with TMP-SMX. The current recommendation is to use prophylactic IVIG (400 mg/kg per dose every 28 days) in HIV-infected children with hypogammaglobulinemia (IgG <400 mg/dL) [38]. IVIG should be considered for HIV-infected children who develop recurrent serious infections such as bacteremia, meningitis, or pneumonia during a 1-year period [38].

The evaluation and therapy for infectious complications in HIV-infected children mandate a high level of suspicion for unusual presentations; an aggressive approach to establish the diagnosis; and the use of intravenous antibiotics, at least during the initial days. Chronic and recurrent infections can compromise the nutritional status of the child and influence the neurodevelopmental state. These symptoms are also typical for progressive HIV infection and should be monitored carefully.

The CDC has published guidelines for prevention and treatment of opportunistic infections among HIV-infected infants and children [218,278,504]. Prophylactic measures for the prevention of PCP have been discussed previously. Prophylaxis for *M. tuberculosis* exposure follows the guidelines used for immunocompetent children, but all children born to HIV-infected mothers should have a purified protein derivative test placed at or before 9 to 12 months of age and should be retested every 2 to 3 years [159]. Prophylaxis with clarithromycin or azithromycin for *M. avium-intracellulare* complex infection should be offered to infants younger than 12 months with CD4$^+$ counts less than 750 cells/µL, children 1 to 2 years old with CD4$^+$ counts less than 500 cells/µL, children 2 to 6 years old with CD4$^+$ counts less than 75 µL, and children older than 6 years with CD4$^+$ counts less than 50 cells/µL [218,278,504].

Data are limited regarding the safety of discontinuing prophylaxis in HIV-infected children receiving antiretroviral therapy. Many experts recommend stopping primary prophylaxis for PCP, however, in children older than 1 year receiving HAART and with CD4$^+$ percentage greater than 25%. Other aspects of HIV management include assessment of organ system involvement, development and psychosocial assessments, and intervention [38,504]. A family-centered approach involving a multidisciplinary team to integrate medical, social, and psychosocial support is crucial.

ANTIRETROVIRAL THERAPY

Early Treatment

HAART is the standard of care for pediatric HIV infection in the United States and other developed countries to improve growth and development, reduce risk of opportunistic infections and other complications, reduce hospitalizations, and prevent development of encephalopathy [18–25]. HAART has evolved from simple nucleoside reverse transcriptase inhibitor (NRTI) regimens of the 1980s and early 1990s to current complex regimens of NRTI in combination with protease inhibitors or non-nucleoside reverse transcriptase inhibitors (NNRTIs) or both [505]. The introduction of combination antiretroviral therapy has resulted in dramatic reductions in mortality and morbidity by greater than 80% to 90% in children in the United States and Europe [18–25,178].

As knowledge about the dynamics of viral replication and its implications for disease progression and prognosis has evolved, it has become clear that early and aggressive therapy offers the potential benefit of a prolonged asymptomatic period. The consideration of treatment initiation for asymptomatic infants is based on the rationale that infants are at highest risk of rapid disease progression to AIDS or death, even when immune degradation and virus replication are moderately well contained, and that there are no reliable clinical or laboratory markers to distinguish infants who will progress from infants who will not progress [506–509]. Studies have shown that the initiation of combination antiretroviral therapy within the first 3 months of life can result in complete cessation of viral replication and preservation of normal immune function [192,510,511]. Studies suggest that several regimens of antiretroviral therapy are safe, effective, and well tolerated for long periods when started in early infancy [510,512].

Treatment Recommendations

Panels of experts have developed guidelines for the use of antiretroviral agents in children, adolescents, and adults including pregnant women with HIV infection [513]. Indications for the initiation of antiretroviral therapy include clinical, immunologic, and virologic parameters (Table 21–10). Pediatric HIV experts agree that infected infants with clinical symptoms of HIV disease or with evidence of immune compromise should be treated, but controversy remains regarding treatment of asymptomatic infants with normal immunologic status [506]. A study from a South African clinical trial (Children with HIV Early Antiretroviral Therapy [CHER] study) addressed the critical question of when to begin combination antiretroviral therapy in asymptomatic HIV-1–infected infants who are diagnosed early in life [514]. CHER found that initiation of therapy at less than 12 weeks of age in asymptomatic infants with normal immune function resulted in 76% reduction in mortality and 75% reduction in HIV disease progression compared with waiting to initiate treatment in such infants until they met standard criteria for initiation of therapy [514]. Based on the results of CHER, current U.S. guidelines from the

TABLE 21–10 Indications for Initiation of Antiretroviral Therapy

Infants <12 mo old

All HIV-infected infants <12 mo old regardless of clinical symptoms, immune status, or HIV RNA level should be treated

Children >12 mo old to <5 yr old

Therapy should be *started* for all children >12 mo old with AIDS (clinical category C [see Table 21–3]) *or* CD4$^+$ <25%, regardless of symptoms or HIV RNA level

Therapy should be *considered* for children who are asymptomatic or have mild clinical symptoms *and* CD4$^+$ ≥25% *and* HIV RNA ≥100,000 copies/mL

Therapy may be *deferred* for children who are asymptomatic or have mild symptoms *and* CD4$^+$ ≥25% *and* HIV RNA <100,000 copies/mL

Children >5 yr old

Therapy should be *started* for all children with AIDS or significant HIV-related symptoms (clinical category C [see Table 21–3]) *or* CD4$^+$ <350 cells/mm^3

Therapy should be *considered* for children who are asymptomatic or have mild clinical symptoms *and* CD4 ≥350 cells/mm^3 *and* HIV RNA ≥100,000 copies/mL

Therapy may be *deferred* for children who are asymptomatic or have mild symptoms *and* CD4$^+$ ≥350 cells/mm^3 *and* HIV RNA <100,000 copies/mL

From Working Group for Antiretroviral Therapy and Medical Management of HIV-infected Children. Guidelines for the use of antiretroviral agents in pediatric HIV infection. February 24, 2009. Available at http://aidsinfo.nih.gov/contentfiles/PediatricGuidelines.pdf.

Working Group on Antiretroviral Therapy and Medical Management of HIV-Infected Children recommend initiation of antiretroviral therapy for all HIV-infected infants younger than 12 months regardless of clinical status, CD4$^+$ percentage, or HIV RNA level (see Table 21–10) [513].

The Working Group recommends that treatment should be started for all children older than 12 months with AIDS (clinical category C) or significant symptoms (clinical category C) or most clinical category B conditions, regardless of CD4$^+$ percentage or count or plasma HIV RNA level [513]. Treatment with antiretroviral therapy is also recommended for children older than 12 months who have severe immunosuppression (immune category 3), for children 1 year to younger than 5 years who have CD4$^+$ less than 25% and less than 350 cells/mm^3 for children 5 years or older regardless of symptoms or plasma HIV RNA level [513].

Initiation of antiretroviral therapy should be *considered* for children older than 1 year who are asymptomatic or have mild symptoms (clinical category N and A) or moderate clinical symptoms (clinical category B—single episode of serious bacterial infection or lymphoid interstitial pneumonitis), *and* have CD4$^+$ percentage 25% or for children aged 1 year to younger than 5 years 350 cells/mm^3 or greater for children 5 years or older associated with plasma HIV RNA level greater than 100,000 copies/mL (see Table 21–10) [513]. Many experts would *defer* treatment in asymptomatic or mildly symptomatic children older than 1 year in situations in which the risk for clinical disease progression is low (e.g., CD4$^+$ percentage ≥25%

aged 1 to <5 years and ≥350 cell/mm³ for children >5 years and have HIV RNA <100,000 copies/mL for children >5 years) and when other factors (i.e., concern for adherence, safety, and persistence of antiretroviral response) favor postponing treatment [513]. In such cases, the health care provider should monitor virologic, immunologic, and clinical status closely.

Choice of Initial Antiretroviral Therapy

Monotherapy is no longer considered appropriate treatment for HIV-infected children and adults. The only exception is the use of zidovudine monotherapy in infants with indeterminate HIV status during the first 6 weeks of life as part of the regimen to prevent perinatal transmission. As soon as an infant is proved to be infected while on zidovudine prophylaxis, therapy should be changed to a combination of agents [513]. Because of adverse effects and drug interactions, not all agents can be paired in the regimens [513]. Based on results from data from clinical trials, a recommended three-drug combination provides the best opportunity to preserve immune function and to prevent disease progression. This therapy should include a highly active protease inhibitor plus two NRTIs as the initial therapeutic regimen or two NRTIs and one NNRTI [513].

Suppression of virus to undetectable levels and long-term preservation of immune function are the goals. Resistance testing should be considered before starting antiretroviral therapy in newly diagnosed infants younger than age 12 months, especially if the mother has known or suspected infection with drug-resistant virus [513]. A change in HAART regimen should be considered if there is evidence of disease progression (clinical, immunologic, or virologic), adverse effects related to antiretroviral therapy occur, or a new superior regimen becomes available [513].

Antiretroviral Drug Classes

As of July 2008, 25 antiretroviral drugs were approved for use in the United States in HIV-infected adolescents and adults; of those, 16 have approved pediatric indications, and 15 are available as a pediatric formulation or capsule [505,509,513]. Therapeutic drugs fall into four major classes based on mechanism of action: nucleoside analogues or NRTIs, NNRTIs, protease inhibitors, and fusion inhibitors [505,509,513]. More detailed information about these agents can be obtained at the U.S. federal AIDS information website (http://aidsinfo.nih.gov/guidelines).

The most pediatric experience with NRTIs is with zidovudine, lamivudine, didanosine, and stavudine. All are available in a liquid formulation. Dual NRTI combinations are the backbone of HAART in children. The combinations of NRTIs with the most data available include zidovudine and lamivudine, zidovudine and didanosine, and stavudine and lamivudine. The zidovudine-lamivudine combination is the most widely used because of its extensive safety data in children [505,513]. Added to this dual NRTI backbone is an NNRTI or a protease inhibitor. The acceptable NNRTIs for pediatric use are nevirapine and efavirenz (approved for children >3 years old); efavirenz is not available in a liquid formulation. Delavirdine is the other available NNRTI, but it is not approved for pediatric use. The one available nucleotide reverse transcriptase inhibitor, tenofovir, is approved only for adult use and is not approved for use in children younger than 18 years [513].

Protease inhibitors recommended for pediatric use are nelfinavir, ritonavir, and lopinavir plus ritonavir. These are available in powder or liquid formulations. Other protease inhibitors available for pediatric use are available in capsule formulation only and include indinavir, saquinavir, and amprenavir. These agents are not recommended, however, because no data are available for long-term tolerance and efficacy of any of these combinations in children. Certain combinations are not recommended because of overlapping toxicities, including zalcitabine and didanosine, zalcitabine and stavudine, and zalcitabine and lamivudine. The combination of stavudine and zidovudine is not recommended because of their antagonism [38,509,513].

The most commonly used antiretroviral agents in newborns and infants—the NRTIs zidovudine, lamivudine, and didanosine; the NNRTI nevirapine; and the protease inhibitors lopinavir-ritonavir combination and ritonavir—are briefly reviewed in Table 21–11. More extensive reviews are available in specific textbooks or the current recommendations from the CDC and the federal guidelines website (http://aidsinfo.nih.gov) [505,513]. Because the standards of care are still evolving, collaboration between the child's primary health care provider and an HIV treatment center is strongly suggested. Whenever possible, children should be enrolled in clinical trials; access and information can be obtained by calling 1-800-TRIALS-A (AIDS Clinical Trials Group [ACTG]), or 301-402-0696 (HIV & AIDS Malignancy Branch, National Cancer Institute).

Challenges

Treatment of infected infants with combination antiretroviral therapy is complex, and high rates of virologic failure have been noted [515,516]. Many practical difficulties in administering drugs to young children compound the problem further. Challenges include issues of medication compliance to complex and demanding regimens, difficulties in developing pediatric formulations, need for refrigeration (e.g., lopinavir), drugs not palatable (e.g., ritonavir), drugs with short shelf life (e.g., didanosine), immature drug metabolism, and lack of age-specific pharmacokinetic data to guide pediatric dosing [517,518]. Toxicity and development of drug resistance are other serious concerns [519].

Resistance is common when a single-dose nevirapine regimen is used for perinatal HIV prevention [493,520]. In one study, an adverse effect on subsequent treatment response was reported in a few infants who started an NNRTI-containing HAART regimen [520]. The WHO still recommends that children should begin on a nevirapine-based HAART regimen pending further studies [521]. Several promising second-generation agents and new classes of antiretroviral agents are currently being

TABLE 21–11 Antiretroviral Drugs and Recommended Dosages in Neonates and Infants <3 Months of Age

Drug	Preparations	Dosage	Adverse Effects
Nucleoside Reverse Transcriptase Inhibitors			
Zidovudine	Syrup: 10 mg/mL	*Premature infants*: 1.5 mg/kg body weight (IV) or 2 mg/kg body weight (oral) q12h, increased to q8h at 2 wk of age (neonates ≥30 wk of gestational age) or at 4 wk (neonates <30 wk of gestational age)	*More frequent*: anemia, neutropenia
		Neonatal/infant dose (<6 wk old): 1.5 mg/kg of body weight (IV) q6h or 2 mg/kg of body weight (oral) q6h	*Less frequent*: hepatotoxicity, myopathy
		Pediatric dose (6 wk to <18 yr old): 240 mg/m^2 q12h *or* 160 mg/m^2 q8h; twice-daily dosing preferred in clinical practice	*Rare*: lactic acidosis, hepatomegaly with steatosis
Lamivudine	Solution: 10 mg/mL	*Neonatal/infant dose (infants <30 days old)*: 2 mg/kg body weight q12h	*More frequent*: headache, fatigue, reduced appetite, nausea, diarrhea, rash
		Pediatric dose: 4 mg/kg body weight q12h	*Less frequent*: pancreatitis, peripheral neuropathy, anemia, neutropenia, lactic acidosis, hepatomegaly with steatosis
Didanosine	Pediatric powder for oral solution: 10 mg/mL	*Premature infants*: no data	*More frequent*: diarrhea, vomiting
		Neonatal/infant dose (2 wk to 8 mo old): 100 mg/m^2 q12h	*Less frequent*: peripheral neuropathy, electrolyte abnormalities, lactic acidosis, hepatomegaly with steatosis. Combination of stavudine with didanosine may result in enhanced toxicity (fatal and nonfatal cases of lactic acidosis and pancreatitis)
		Pediatric dose (>8 mo old): 120 mg/m^2 q12h	*Rare*: pancreatitis, retinitis
Stavudine	Solution: 1 mg/mL	*Neonatal/infant dose (birth to 13 days)*: 0.5 mg/kg q12h	*More frequent*: headache, gastrointestinal upsets, rash, lipoatrophy
		Pediatric dose (age 14 days up to weight of 30 kg): 1 mg/kg of body weight q12h	*Less frequent*: peripheral neuropathy, pancreatitis, lactic acidosis, hepatomegaly with steatosis. Combination of stavudine with didanosine may result in enhanced toxicity (fatal and nonfatal cases of lactic acidosis and pancreatitis)
			Rare: increased liver enzymes, ascending neuromuscular weakness
Non-nucleoside Reverse Transcriptase Inhibitors			
Nevirapine	Suspension: 10 mg/mL	*Neonatal/infant dose (<14 days old)*: treatment dose not defined	*More frequent*: skin rash including Stevens-Johnson syndrome and toxic epidermal necrolysis, fever, headache, nausea, abnormal liver enzymes
		Pediatric dose (≥15 days old): start treatment with 150 mg/m^2 (maximum dose 200 mg) given once daily for the first 14 days. If no rash or adverse effects, 150 mg/m^2 given twice daily (maximum 200 mg twice daily); higher dosing (i.e., 200 mg/m^2 twice daily, not exceeding total daily dose of 400 mg) may be needed for younger children (≤8 yr old)	*Less frequent*: severe life-threatening hepatotoxicity, hypersensitivity reactions
Protease Inhibitors			
Ritonavir	Oral solution: 80 mg/mL	*Neonatal/infant dose*: not approved for use in neonates/infants ≤1 mo old	*More frequent*: nausea, vomiting, diarrhea, abdominal pain, anorexia, circumoral paresthesias, lipid abnormalities
		Pediatric dose (>1 mo old): 350-450 mg per m^2 body surface area twice daily (maximum dose 600 mg). Dose escalation over several days to reduce gastrointestinal adverse effects	*Less frequent*: fat redistribution, exacerbation of chronic liver disease
			Rare: new-onset diabetes mellitus, hyperglycemia, ketoacidosis, hemolytic anemia, pancreatitis, life-threatening hepatitis, allergic reactions, prolongation of P–R interval and second-degree or third-degree atrioventricular block
Lopinavir-ritonavir	Pediatric oral solution: 80 mg lopinavir/20 mg ritonavir per mL)	*Neonatal/infant dose (14 days to 6 mo old)*: 300 mg lopinavir per m^2 body surface area/75 mg ritonavir per m^2 body surface area, *or* 16 mg lopinavir per kg body weight/4 mg ritonavir per kg body weight twice daily. Because dosage data are unavailable for lopinavir-ritonavir administered with nevirapine in infants <6 mo old, lopinavir-ritonavir should not be administered in combination with nevirapine in these infants	*More frequent*: diarrhea, nausea, vomiting, headache, skin rash in patients receiving other antiretroviral agents, lipid abnormalities
			Less frequent: fat redistribution
			Rare: new-onset diabetes mellitus, hyperglycemia, ketoacidosis, hemolytic anemia, pancreatitis, life-threatening hepatitis cardiac toxicity (heart blocks) in newborns, particularly in preterm infants.

evaluated in adult clinical trials, but pharmacokinetic and safety data are limited in children [522]. These agents include darunavir (protease inhibitor), maraviroc (CCR5 antagonist), raltegravir (integrase inhibitor), and etravirine (new NNRTI) [505]. Data are insufficient to recommend these agents as initial therapy of children [513].

Access to antiretroviral therapy for HIV-infected children is a major challenge in resource-limited settings [523]. Of the estimated 600,000 children who need HAART in sub-Saharan Africa, less than 5% are receiving treatment [29]. Funding from the WHO, the U.S. President's Emergency Plan for AIDS Relief (PEPFAR), and the Global Funds has resulted in significantly increased access to antiretroviral treatment for adults in resource-limited countries; however, implementation of a pediatric HAART program has been very slow. Barriers to treatment include lack of diagnostic testing for early diagnosis of HIV infection in infants, lack of availability of appropriate pediatric antiretroviral drugs, limited infrastructure and health care personnel, and lack of prioritization and advocacy for pediatric treatment [29].

In developing countries, antiretroviral therapy is initiated, if available, with CD4$^+$ percentage less than 20% for children younger than 18 months and with CD4$^+$ percentage less than 15% for older children. HAART generally is initiated at older ages and with advanced immunosuppression compared with in developed countries [524,525]. More recent studies indicate that good clinical and virologic outcomes can be achieved using combination antiretroviral therapy in HIV-infected children living in sub-Saharan Africa and other resource-limited countries [526–528].

FUTURE GOALS

Major advances in the understanding, prevention, and treatment of HIV disease have occurred in recent years. Dramatic declines in the number of perinatally HIV-1–infected children have been reported in developed countries because of prompt implementation of strategies to prevent mother-to-child transmission of HIV-1. Better understanding of the interactions between viral load and immunologic status and their implications for prognosis has prompted earlier and more aggressive antiretroviral therapy. The advent of the protease inhibitors and the accelerated approval of antiretroviral drugs for children and adults have broadened the therapeutic armamentarium. Availability of HAART has led to improved survival of HIV-1–infected children into adolescence and adulthood, changing most HIV-1 infections into a chronic rather than a fatal disease.

The most urgent need continues to be the prevention of further spread of HIV infection among adults and from a mother to her unborn child. Almost 2 decades after the description of the clinical syndrome of AIDS, we are still dealing with an ever-growing pandemic, affecting certain minorities, both sexes, and all age groups and social levels, but targeting mainly the developing countries with already limited resources. The staggering demands put on public health systems and their financial resources could easily create tensions regarding the distribution of available funds. Before the widespread use of combination

therapy and protease inhibitors, the estimated lifetime cost of hospital-based care for children with HIV infection was $408,307 [529]. Assuming that hospital-based care represents 83% of the total charges, the mean overall lifetime cost would be about $500,000. The cost of current antiretroviral therapy is even higher, and life expectancy is longer, although this is partially offset by fewer hospitalizations. Major efforts are needed to make prevention and therapy for HIV infection feasible and affordable for developing nations because they have the highest numbers of infected people with the fewest financial and organizational resources.

New and different antiretroviral agents are needed because of toxicities and emergence of resistance to provide more effective or even permanent inhibition of viral replication. We need to know the pharmacokinetic properties of drugs when given to the pregnant mother, the neonate, or the very young infant. Progress has been made in the early recognition and prophylaxis of opportunistic infections. As patients with HIV infection survive longer, problems with resistant organisms, multidrug allergies, altered organ function, and long-term side effects of medications emerge and complicate adequate therapy.

Advocacy for children and pregnant women, ensuring equal access to new drugs and providing sound data regarding dosing and potential toxicities, continues to be important. The U.S. Food and Drug Administration (FDA) allows the approval of drugs for use in children based on efficacy data gathered in adults if the disease in children and adults is reasonably similar and if the pharmaceutical companies provide dosing (pharmacokinetic) and safety (toxicity) data from controlled trials performed in an adequate number of children. The treatment and care of HIV-infected children and adults has become increasingly complex, and close collaboration with physicians and centers specialized in their care is highly recommended.

Despite successes in developed countries, many serious challenges remain for resource-limited countries. There is a clear need to bridge the gap in perinatal HIV prevention and treatment programs between resource-rich and resource-limited countries [8,9]. Future efforts must focus on rapid scale-up and sustaining effective, simpler, and low-cost prevention of mother-to-child transmission of HIV programs worldwide and developing innovative strategies to prevent transmission of HIV via breast-feeding [117]. Developing a safe, effective preventive infant HIV vaccine would be an optimal strategy to reduce transmission of HIV via breast-feeding [49,166]. Increased public health and political will is needed to reduce the number of pediatric HIV infections worldwide.

REFERENCES

[1] Centers for Disease Control, Unexplained immunodeficiency and opportunistic infections in infants—New York, New Jersey, California, MMWR Morb. Mortal. Wkly Rep. 31 (1982) 665–667.
[2] A.J. Ammann, et al., Acquired immunodeficiency in an infant: possible transmission by means of blood products, Lancet 1 (1983) 956–958.
[3] J. Oleske, et al., Immune deficiency syndrome in children, JAMA 249 (1983) 2345–2349.
[4] A. Rubinstein, et al., Acquired immunodeficiency with reversed T4/T8 ratios in infants born to promiscuous and drug-addicted mothers, JAMA 249 (1983) 2350–2356.

[5] A. Prendergast, et al., International perspectives, progress, and future challenges of paediatric HIV infection, Lancet 370 (2007) 68–80.

[6] C. Thorne, M.L. Newell, HIV, Semin. Fetal Neonatal Med. 12 (2007) 174–181.

[7] A.K. Shetty, Y. Maldonado, Advances in the prevention of perinatal HIV-1 transmission, NeoReviews 6 (2005) 12–25.

[8] L.M. Mofenson, Advances in the prevention of vertical transmission of human immunodeficiency virus, Semin. Pediatr. Infect. Dis. 14 (2003) 295–308.

[9] M.G. Fowler, et al., Reducing the risk of mother-to-child immunodeficiency virus transmission: past successes, current progress and challenges, and future directions, Am. J. Obstet. Gynecol. 197 (Suppl. 3) (2007) S3–S9.

[10] Centers for Disease Control and Prevention, Achievements in public health: reduction in perinatal transmission of HIV Infection—United States, 1985–2005, MMWR Morb. Mortal. Wkly Rep. 55 (2006) 592–597.

[11] G.D. Sanders, et al., Cost-effectiveness of screening for HIV in the era of highly active antiretroviral therapy, N. Engl. J. Med. 352 (2005) 570–585.

[12] L.C. Immergluck, et al., Cost-effectiveness of universal compared with voluntary screening for human immunodeficiency virus among pregnant women in Chicago, Pediatrics 105 (4) (2000).

[13] R.D. Gorsky, et al., Preventing perinatal transmission of HIV: costs and effectiveness of a recommended intervention, Public Health Rep. 111 (1996) 335–341.

[14] M.L. Newell, Current issues in the prevention of mother-to-child transmission of HIV-1 infection, Trans. R. Soc. Trop. Med. Hyg. 100 (2006) 1–5.

[15] European Collaborative Study, Mother-to-child transmission of HIV infection in the era of highly active antiretroviral therapy, Clin. Infect. Dis. 40 (2005) 458–465.

[16] E.R. Cooper, et al., Combination antiretroviral strategies for the treatment of pregnant HIV-1 infected women and prevention of perinatal HIV-1 transmission, J. Acquir. Immune Defic. Syndr. Hum. Retroviral. 29 (2002) 484–494.

[17] J. McIntyre, Strategies to prevent mother-to-child transmission of HIV, Curr. Opin. Infect. Dis. 19 (2006) 33–38.

[18] M.T. McKenna, et al., Recent trends in the incidence and morbidity that are associated with perinatal human immunodeficiency virus infection in the United States, Am. J. Obstet. Gynecol. 197 (Suppl. 3) (2007) S3–S9.

[19] C.A. Chiriboga, et al., Incidence and prevalence of HIV encephalopathy in children receiving highly active antiretroviral therapy (HAART), J. Pediatr. 146 (2005) 402–407.

[20] D.M. Gibb, et al., Decline in mortality, AIDS, and hospital admissions in perinatally HIV-1 infected in the United Kingdom and Ireland, BMJ 327 (2003) 1019.

[21] P. Gona, et al., Incidence of opportunistic and other infections in HIV-infected children in the HAART era, JAMA 296 (2006) 292–300.

[22] A. Judd, et al., Morbidity, mortality, and response to treatment by children in the United Kingdom and Ireland with perinatally acquired HIV infection during 1996–2006: planning for teenage and adult care, Clin. Infect. Dis. 45 (2007) 918–924.

[23] M.S. McConnell, et al., Trends in antiretroviral therapy use and survival rates for a large cohort of HIV-infected children and adolescents in the United States, 1998–2001, J. Acquir. Immune Defic. Syndr. 38 (2005) 488–494.

[24] S.A. Nachman, et al., Growth of human immunodeficiency virus-infected children receiving highly active antiretroviral therapy, Pediatr. Infect. Dis. J. 24 (2005) 352–357.

[25] K. Patel, et al., Long-term effectiveness of highly active antiretroviral therapy on the survival of children and adolescents with HIV infection: a 10-year follow-up study, Clin. Infect. Dis. 46 (2008) 507–515.

[26] T. Sripipatana, et al., Site-specific interventions to improve prevention of mother-to-child transmission of human immunodeficiency virus programs in less developed countries, Am. J. Obstet. Gynecol. 197 (Suppl. 3) (2007) S107–S112.

[27] UNAIDS, UNAIDS Fact Sheet: Sub Saharan Africa, UNAIDS, Geneva, 2006.

[28] UNAIDS & WHO, AIDS epidemic update. Available at http://data.unaids.org/pub/EPISlides/2007/2007_epiupdate_en.pdf. December 2007.

[29] J.T. Boerma, et al., Monitoring the scale-up of antiretroviral therapy programmes: methods to estimate coverage, Bull. World Health Organ. 84 (2006) 145–150.

[30] F. Dabis, et al., Preventing mother-to-child transmission of HIV-1 in Africa in the year 2000, AIDS 14 (2000) 1017–1026.

[31] M.L. Newell, et al., Ghent International AIDS Society (IAS) Working Group on HIV Infection in Women and Children. Mortality of infected and uninfected infants born to HIV-infected mothers in Africa: a pooled analysis, Lancet 364 (2004) 1236–1243.

[32] M.L. Lindegren, R.H. Byers Jr, P. Thomas, Trends in perinatal HIV/AIDS in the United States, JAMA 282 (1999) 531–538.

[33] L.M. Mofenson, American Academy of Pediatrics, Committee on Pediatric AIDS, Technical report: perinatal human immunodeficiency virus testing and prevention of transmission, Pediatrics 106 (6) (2000).

[34] Centers for Disease Control and Prevention, HIV AIDS Surveill. Rep. 16 (2004) 1–45.

[35] Centers for Disease Control and Prevention, HIV AIDS Surveill. Rep. 12 (2000) 1–45.

[36] M.L. Lindegren, S. Steinberg, R.H. Byers, Epidemiology of HIV/AIDS in children, Pediatr. Clin. North Am. 47 (2004) 1–20.

[37] Centers for Disease Control and Prevention, HIV AIDS Surveill. Rep. 14 (2002) 1–48.

[38] American Academy of Pediatrics. Human immunodeficiency virus infection, L.K. Pickering (Ed.), Red Book: Report of the Committee on Infectious Diseases, twentysixth ed., American Academy of Pediatrics, Elk Grove Village, IL, 2003, pp. 360–382.

[39] The European Collaborative Study, Vertical transmission of HIV-1: maternal immune status and obstetric factors, AIDS 10 (1996) 1675–1681.

[40] The Working Group on Mother-to-Child Transmission of HIV, Rates of mother-to-child transmission of HIV-1 in Africa, America, and Europe: results from 13 perinatal studies, J. Acquir. Immune Defic. Syndr. Hum. Retrovirol. 8 (1995) 506–510.

[41] R.S. Sperling, et al., Maternal viral load, zidovudine treatment, and the risk of transmission of human immunodeficiency virus type 1 from mother to infant. Pediatric AIDS Clinical Trials Group Protocol 076 Study Group, N. Engl. J. Med. 335 (1996) 1621–1629.

[42] E.J. Abrams, et al., Association of human immunodeficiency virus (HIV) load early in life with disease progression among HIV-infected infants. New York City Perinatal HIV Transmission Collaborative Study Group, J. Infect. Dis. 178 (1998) 101–108.

[43] P.M. Garcia, et al., Maternal levels of plasma human immunodeficiency virus type 1 RNA and the risk of perinatal transmission. Women and Infants Transmission Study Group, N. Engl. J. Med. 341 (1999) 394–402.

[44] G.C. John, et al., Correlates of mother-to-child human immunodeficiency virus type 1 (HIV-1) transmission: association with maternal plasma HIV-1 RNA load, genital HIV-1 DNA shedding, and breast infections, J. Infect. Dis. 183 (2001) 206–212.

[45] M. Montano, et al., Comparative prediction of perinatal human immunodeficiency virus type 1 transmission, using multiple virus load markers, J. Infect. Dis. 188 (2003) 406–413.

[46] A.P. Kourtis, et al., Mother-to-child transmission of HIV-1: timing and implications for prevention, Lancet Infect. Dis. 6 (2006) 726–732.

[47] C. Thorne, M.L. Newell, Prevention of mother-to-child transmission of HIV infection, Curr. Opin. Infect. Dis. 17 (2004) 247–252.

[48] M.G. Fowler, M.L. Newell, Breastfeeding and HIV-1 transmission in resource-limited settings, J. Acquir. Immune Defic. Syndr. 30 (2002) 230–239.

[49] A.P. Kourtis, et al., Prevention of human immunodeficiency virus-1 to the infant through breastfeeding: new developments, Am. J. Obstet. Gynecol. 197 (Suppl. 3) (2007) S113–S122.

[50] S. Sprecher, et al., Vertical transmission of HIV in 15-week fetus, Lancet 2 (1986) 288–289.

[51] E. Jovaisas, et al., LAV/HTLV-III in 20-week fetus, Lancet 2 (1985) 1129.

[52] H. Mano, J.C. Chermann, Fetal human immunodeficiency virus type 1 infection of different organs in the second trimester, AIDS Res. Hum. Retroviruses 7 (1991) 83–88.

[53] D.C. Mundy, et al., Human immunodeficiency virus isolated from amniotic fluid, Lancet 2 (1987) 459–460.

[54] S.H. Lewis, et al., HIV-1 in trophoblastic and villous Hofbauer cells, and haematological precursors in eight-week fetuses, Lancet 335 (1990) 565–568.

[55] N. Amirhessami-Aghili, S.A. Spector, Human immunodeficiency virus type 1 infection of human placenta: potential route for fetal infection, J. Virol. 65 (1991) 2231–2236.

[56] V. Zachar, et al., Vertical transmission of HIV: detection of proviral DNA in placental trophoblasts, AIDS 8 (1994) 129–130.

[57] C.F.T. Mattern, et al., Localization of human immunodeficiency virus core antigen in term human placentas, Pediatrics 89 (1992) 207–209.

[58] C. Peckham, D. Gibb, Mother-to-child transmission of the human immunodeficiency virus, N. Engl. J. Med. 333 (1995) 298–302.

[59] Y.J. Bryson, et al., Proposed definitions for in utero versus intrapartum transmission of HIV-1, N. Engl. J. Med. 327 (1992) 1246–1247.

[60] A. Krivine, et al., A comparative study of virus isolation, polymerase chain reaction, and antigen detection in children of mothers infected with human immunodeficiency virus, J. Pediatr. 116 (1990) 372–376.

[61] M.F. Rogers, et al., Use of the polymerase chain reaction for early detection of the proviral sequences of human immunodeficiency virus in infants born to seropositive mothers, N. Engl. J. Med. 320 (1989) 1649–1654.

[62] B.J. Weiblen, et al., Early diagnosis of HIV infection in infants by detection of IgA HIV antibodies, Lancet 335 (1990) 988–990.

[63] T.C. Quinn, et al., Early diagnosis of perinatal HIV infection by detection of viral-specific IgA antibodies, JAMA 266 (1991) 3439–3942.

[64] A. Krivine, et al., HIV replication during the first weeks of life, Lancet 339 (1992) 1187–1189.

[65] C. Rouzioux, et al., Estimated timing of mother-to-child human immunodeficiency virus type 1 (HIV-1) transmission by use of a Markov model. The HIV Infection in Newborns French Collaborative Study Group, Am. J. Epidemiol. 142 (1995) 1330–1337.

[66] S.R. Nesheim, et al., Lack of increased risk for perinatal human immunodeficiency virus transmission to subsequent children born to infected women, Pediatr. Infect. Dis. J. 15 (1996) 886–890.

[67] K.Y. Young, R.P. Nelson, Discordant human immunodeficiency virus infection in dizygotic twins detected by polymerase chain reaction, Pediatr. Infect. Dis. J. 9 (1990) 454–456.

[68] J.J. Goedert, et al., High risk of HIV-1 infection for first-born twins, Lancet 338 (1991) 1471–1475.

[69] A.M. Duliege, et al., Birth order, delivery route, and concordance in the transmission of human immunodeficiency virus type 1 from mothers to twins, J. Pediatr. 126 (1995) 625–632.

[70] P.L. Havens, D. Waters, Management of the infant born to a mother with HIV infection, Pediatr. Clin. North Am. 51 (2004) 909–937.

[71] C. Thorne, M.L. Newell, Mother-to-child transmission of HIV infection and its preventions, Curr. HIV Res. 1 (2003) 447–462.

[72] L.M. Mofenson, et al., Risk factors for perinatal transmission of human immunodeficiency virus type 1 in women treated with zidovudine, N. Engl. J. Med. 341 (1999) 385–393.

[73] L.S. Magder, et al., Risk factors for in utero and intrapartum transmission of HIV, J. Acquir. Immune Defic. Syndr. 38 (2005) 87–95.

[74] J.P.A. Ioannidis, et al., Perinatal transmission of human immunodeficiency virus type 1 by pregnant women with RNA virus loads < 1000 copies/ml, J. Infect. Dis. 183 (2001) 539–545.

[75] S. O'Shea, et al., Maternal viral load, CD4 cell count and vertical transmission of HIV-1, J. Med. Virol. 54 (1998) 113–117.

[76] P. Mock, et al., Maternal viral load and timing of mother-to-child HIV transmission, Bangkok, Thailand, AIDS 13 (1999) 407–414.

[77] M.E. St Louis, et al., Risk for perinatal HIV-1 transmission according to maternal immunologic, virologic, and placental factors, JAMA 269 (1993) 2853–2859.

[78] W. Borkowsky, et al., Correlation of perinatal transmission of human immunodeficiency virus type 1 with maternal viremia and lymphocyte phenotypes, J. Pediatr. 125 (1994) 345–351.

[79] D.M. Thea, et al., The effect of maternal viral load on the risk of perinatal transmission of HIV-1. New York City Perinatal HIV Transmission Collaborative Study Group, AIDS 11 (1997) 437–444.

[80] M.L. Newell, C. Peckham, Risk factors for vertical transmission of HIV-1 and early markers of HIV-1 infection in children, AIDS 7 (Suppl. 1) (1993) S591–S597.

[81] C. Gabiano, et al., Mother-to-child transmission of human immunodeficiency virus type 1: risk of infection and correlates of transmission, Pediatrics 90 (1992) 369–374.

[82] P.A. Thomas, et al., Maternal predictors of perinatal human immunodeficiency virus transmission, Pediatr. Infect. Dis. J. 13 (1994) 489–495.

[83] M.M. Mayers, et al., A prospective study of infants of human immunodeficiency virus seropositive and seronegative women with a history of intravenous drug use or of intravenous drug-using sex partners, in the Bronx, New York City, Pediatrics 88 (1991) 1248–1256.

[84] European Collaborative Study, Risk factors for mother-to-child transmission of HIV-1, Lancet 339 (1992) 1007–1012.

[85] R. Chuachoowong, et al., Short-course antenatal zidovudine reduces both cervicovaginal human immunodeficiency virus type 1 RNA levels and risk of perinatal transmission. Bangkok Collaborative Perinatal HIV Transmission Study Group, J. Infect. Dis. 181 (2000) 99–106.

[86] S.H. Landesman, et al., Obstetrical factors and the transmission of human immunodeficiency virus type 1 from mother-to-child, N. Engl. J. Med. 334 (1996) 1617–1623.

[87] European Collaborative Study, Vertical transmission of HIV-1: maternal immune status and obstetric factors, AIDS 10 (1996) 1675–1681.

[88] J.J. Goedert, et al., Mother-to-infant transmission of human immunodeficiency virus type 1: association with prematurity or low antigp120, Lancet 2 (1989) 1351–1354.

[89] P.A. Tovo, et al., Mode of delivery and gestational age influence perinatal HIV-1 transmission, J. Acquir. Immune Defic. Syndr. Hum. Retrovirol. 11 (1996) 88–94.

[90] L.S. Magder, et al., Risk factors for in utero and intrapartum transmission of HIV, J. Acquir. Immune Defic. Syndr. 38 (2005) 87–95.

[91] The International Perinatal HIV Group, The mode of delivery and the risk of vertical transmission of human immunodeficiency virus type 11: a meta-analysis of 15 prospective studies, N. Engl. J. Med. 340 (1999) 977–987.

[92] The European Mode of Delivery Collaboration, Elective cesarean section versus vaginal delivery in prevention of vertical HIV-1 transmission: a randomized clinical trial, Lancet 353 (1999) 1035–1039.

[93] S.M. Wolinsky, et al., Selective transmission of human immunodeficiency virus type-1 variants from mothers to infants, Science 255 (1992) 1134–1137.

[94] R.D. Mackelprang, et al., Maternal HLA homozygosity and mother-child HLA concordance increase the risk of vertical transmission of HIV-1, J. Infect. Dis. 197 (2008) 1156–1161.

[95] L.G. Kostrikis, Impact of natural chemokine receptor polymorphisms on perinatal transmission of human immunodeficiency virus type 1, Teratology 61 (2000) 387–390.

[96] G. John-Stewart, et al., Breast-feeding and transmission of HIV-1, J. Acquir. Immune Defic. Syndr. 35 (2004) 196–202.

[97] H.M. Coovadia, A. Coutsoudis, HIV, infant feeding, and survival: old wine in new bottles, but brimming with promise, AIDS 21 (2007) 1837–1840.

[98] P.G. Miotti, et al., HIV transmission through breastfeeding: a study in Malawi, JAMA 282 (1999) 744–749.

[99] K.M. De Cock, et al., Prevention of mother-to-child HIV transmission in resource-poor countries: translating research into policy and practice, JAMA 283 (2000) 1175–1182.

[100] W. Fawzi, et al., Transmission of HIV-1 through breastfeeding among women in Dar es Salaam, Tanzania, J. Acquir. Immune Defic. Syndr. 31 (2002) 331–338.

[101] P. Lewis, et al., Cell-free HIV type 1 in breast milk, J. Infect. Dis. 177 (1998) 34–39.

[102] I.N. Koulinska, et al., Transmission of cell-free and cell-associated HIV-1 through breastfeeding, J. Acquir. Immune Defic. Syndr. 41 (2006) 93–99.

[103] A.J. Ruff, et al., Breast-feeding and maternal-infant transmission of human immunodeficiency virus type 1, J. Pediatr. 121 (1992) 325–329.

[104] L. Thiry, et al., Isolation of AIDS virus from cell-free breast milk of three healthy virus carriers, Lancet 2 (1985) 891–892.

[105] P. Lewis, et al., Cell-free human immunodeficiency virus type 1 in breast milk, J. Infect. Dis. 177 (1998) 34–39.

[106] C.M. Rousseau, et al., Longitudinal analysis of HIV-1 RNA in breast milk and its relationship to infant infection and maternal disease, J. Infect. Dis. 187 (2003) 741–747.

[107] I.N. Koulinska, et al., Transmission of cell-free and cell-associated HIV-1 through breastfeeding, Virus Res. 120 (2006) 191–198.

[108] R.L. Shapiro, et al., Highly active antiretroviral therapy started during pregnancy or postpartum suppresses HIV-1 RNA, but not DNA, in breast milk, J. Infect. Dis. 192 (2005) 713–719.

[109] D.T. Dunn, et al., Risk of human immunodeficiency virus type 1 transmission through breastfeeding, Lancet 340 (1992) 585–588.

[110] R. Nduati, et al., Effect of breastfeeding and formula feeding on transmission of HIV-1: a randomized controlled trial, JAMA 283 (2000) 1167–1174.

[111] J.E. Embree, et al., Risk factors for postnatal mother to child transmission of HIV-1, AIDS 14 (2000) 2535–2541.

[112] V. Leroy, et al., International multicenter pooled analysis of late postnatal mother-to-child transmission of HIV-1 infection, Lancet 352 (1998) 597–600.

[113] A. Coutsoudis, et al., Late postnatal transmission of HIV-1 in breastfed children: an individual patient data meta-analysis, J. Infect. Dis. 189 (2004) 2154–2166.

[114] T.E. Taha, et al., Late postnatal transmission of HIV-1 and associated risk factors, J. Infect. Dis. 196 (2007) 10–14.

[115] P.J. Iliff, et al., Early exclusive breastfeeding reduces the risk of postnatal HIV-1 transmission and increases HIV-free survival, AIDS 19 (2005) 699–708.

[116] H.M. Coovadia, et al., Mother-to-child transmission of HIV-1 infection during exclusive breastfeeding in the first 6 months of life: an intervention cohort study, Lancet 369 (2007) 1107–1116.

[117] J.S. Read, Prevention of mother-to-child transmission of HIV through breastmilk, Pediatr. Infect. Dis. J. 27 (2008) 649–650.

[118] G.H. Friedland, et al., Lack of transmission of HTLV-III/LAV infection to household contacts of patients with AIDS or AIDS-related complex with oral candidiasis, N. Engl. J. Med. 314 (1986) 334–339.

[119] J.M. Mann, et al., Prevalence of HTLV-III/LAV in household contacts of patients with confirmed AIDS and controls in Kinshasa, Zaire, JAMA 256 (1986) 721–724.

[120] Centers for Disease Control and Prevention, Human immunodeficiency virus transmission in household settings—United States, MMWR Morb. Mortal. Wkly. Rep. 43 (1994) 347–356.

[121] M.N. Lobato, et al., Infection control practices in the home: a survey of households of HIV-infected persons with hemophilia, Infect. Control. Hosp. Epidemiol. 17 (1996) 721–725.

[122] American Academy of Pediatrics Task Force of Pediatric AIDS, Education of children with human immunodeficiency virus infection, Pediatrics 88 (1991) 645–648.

[123] Committee on Infectious Diseases, Health guidelines for the attendance in day-care and foster care settings of children infected with human immunodeficiency virus, Pediatrics 79 (1987) 466–470.

[124] American Academy of Pediatrics, Evaluation and medical treatment of the HIV-exposed infant, Pediatrics 99 (1997) 909–917.

[125] L. Buonaguro, et al., Human immunodeficiency virus type 1 subtype distribution in the worldwide epidemic: pathogenetic and therapeutic implications, J. Virol. 81 (2007) 10209–10219.

[126] A.M. Geretti, HIV-subtypes: epidemiology and significance for HIV management, Curr. Opin. Infect. Dis. 19 (2006) 1–7.

[127] B.R. Cullen, HIV-1 auxiliary proteins: making connections in a dying cell, Cell 93 (1998) 685–692.

[128] A.S. Fauci, et al., Immunopathogenic mechanisms of HIV infection, Ann. Intern. Med. 124 (1996) 654–663.

[129] Y. Feng, et al., HIV-1 entry cofactor: functional cDNA cloning of a seven-transmembrane G protein-coupled receptor, Science 272 (1996) 872–877.

[130] F. Cocchi, et al., The V3 domain of the HIV-1 gp120 envelope glycoprotein is critical for chemokine-mediated blockade of infection, Nat. Med. 2 (1996) 1244–1247.

[131] A.L. Kinter, et al., HIV replication in CD4+ T cells of HIV-infected individuals is regulated by a balance between viral suppressive effects of endogenous β-chemokines and the viral inductive effects of other endogenous cytokines, Proc. Natl. Acad. Sci. U. S. A. 93 (1996) 14076–14081.

[132] C.K. Lapham, et al., Evidence for cell-surface association between fusin and the CD4-gp120 complex in human cell lines, Science 274 (1996) 602–605.

[133] L. Wu, et al., CD4-induced interaction of primary HIV-1 gp120 glycoproteins with the chemokine receptor CCR-5, Nature 384 (1996) 179–183.

[134] A.T. Hasse, Perils at mucosal front lines for HIV and SIV and their hosts, Nat. Rev. Immunol. 5 (2005) 783–792.

[135] J.S. Cairns, M.P. D'Souza, Chemokines and HIV-1 second receptors: the therapeutic connection, Nat. Med. 4 (1998) 563–568.

[136] P.P. Reinhardt, et al., Human cord blood mononuclear cells are preferentially infected by non-syncytium-inducing, macrophage-tropic human immunodeficiency virus type 1 isolates, J. Clin. Microbiol. 33 (1995) 292–297.

[137] A.T. Panganiban, Retroviral reverse transcription and DNA integration, Virology 1 (1990) 187–194.

[138] F.D. Bushman, T. Fujiwara, R. Craigie, Retroviral DNA integration directed by HIV integration protein in vitro, Science 249 (1990) 1555–1558.

[139] P.O. Brown, et al., Retroviral integration: structure of the initial covalent product and its precursor, and a role for the viral IN protein, Proc. Natl. Acad. Sci. U. S. A. 86 (1989) 2525–2529.

[140] M. Stevenson, et al., Integration is not necessary for expression of human immunodeficiency virus type 1 protein products, J. Virol. 64 (1990) 2421–2425.

[141] O. Bagasra, et al., Detection of human immunodeficiency virus type 1 provirus in mononuclear cells by in situ polymerase chain reaction, N. Engl. J. Med. 326 (1992) 1385–1391.

[142] S. Chevret, et al., Provirus copy number to predict disease progression in asymptomatic human immunodeficiency virus type 1 infection, J. Infect. Dis. 169 (1994) 882–885.

[143] D.D. Ho, Dynamics of HIV-1 replication in vivo, J. Clin. Invest. 99 (1997) 2565–2567.

[144] D.D. Ho, et al., Rapid turnover of plasma virions and CD4 lymphocytes in HIV-1 infection, Nature 373 (1995) 123–126.

[145] A.S. Perelson, et al., HIV-1 dynamics in vivo: clearance rate, infected cell life-span, and viral generation time, Science 271 (1996) 1582–1586.

[146] A.S. Perelson, et al., Decay characteristics of HIV-1-infected compartments during combination therapy, Nature 387 (1997) 188–191.

[147] N.E. Kohl, et al., Active human immunodeficiency virus protease is required for viral infectivity, Proc. Natl. Acad. Sci. U. S. A. 85 (1988) 4686–4690.

[148] R. Swanstrom, A.H. Kaplan, M. Manchester, The aspartic proteinase of HIV-1, Semin. Virol. 17 (1997) 175–186.

[149] C.F. Perno, et al., Inhibition of the protease of human immunodeficiency virus blocks replication and infectivity of the virus in chronically infected macrophages, J. Infect. Dis. 168 (1993) 1148–1156.

[150] J. Smith, R. Daniel, Following the path of the virus: the exploitation of host DNA repair mechanisms by retroviruses, ACS Chem. Biol. 1 (2006) 217–226.

[151] O. Jegede, et al., HIV type 1 integrate inhibitors: from basic research to clinical applications, AIDS Rev. 10 (2008) 172–189.

[152] N. Ahmad, The vertical transmission of human immunodeficiency virus type 1: molecular and biological properties of the virus, Crit. Rev. Clin. Lab. Sci. 42 (2005) 1–34.

[153] N. Ahmad, Molecular mechanisms of HIV-1 vertical transmission and pathogenesis in infants, Adv. Pharmacol. 56 (2008) 453–508.

[154] N. Ahmad, et al., Genetic analysis of human immunodeficiency virus type 1 envelope V3 region isolates from mothers and infants after perinatal transmission, J. Virol. 69 (1995) 1001–1012.

[155] F. Salvatori, G. Scarlatti, HIV type 1 chemokine receptor usage in mother-to-child transmission, AIDS Res. Hum. Retroviruses 17 (2001) 925–935.

[156] V. Sundaravaradan, et al., Differential HIV-1 replication in neonatal and adult blood mononuclear cells is influenced at the level of HIV-1 gene expression, Proc. Natl. Acad. Sci. U. S. A. 103 (2006) 11701–11706.

[157] E.J. Abrams, et al., Association of human immunodeficiency virus (HIV) load early in life with disease progression among HIV-infected infants. New York City Perinatal HIV Transmission Collaborative Study Group, J. Infect. Dis. 178 (1998) 101–108.

[158] P.A. Tovo, et al., Prognostic factors and survival in children with perinatal HIV-1 infection. The Italian Register for HIV Infections in Children, Lancet 339 (1992) 1249–1253.

[159] T. Hahn, R. Ramakrishnan, N. Ahmad, Evaluation of genetic diversity of human immunodeficiency virus type 1 NEF gene associated with vertical transmission, J. Biomed. Sci. 10 (2003) 436–450.

[160] R. Ramakrishnan, et al., Evaluations of HIV type 1 rev gene diversity and functional domains following perinatal transmission, AIDS Res. Hum. Retroviruses 21 (2005) 1035–1045.

[161] R. Mehta, et al., Mutations generated in human immunodeficiency virus type 1 long terminal repeat during vertical transmission correlate with viral gene expression, Virology 375 (2008) 170–181.

[162] L.I. Wu, Biology of HIV mucosal transmission, Curr. Opin. Infect. Dis. 5 (2008) 534–540.

[163] A.S. Perelson, et al., Decay characteristics of HIV-1 infected compartments during combination therapy, Nature 387 (1997) 188–191.

[164] K. Luzuriaga, et al., Dynamics of HIV-1 replication in vertically-infected infants, J. Virol. 73 (1999) 362–367.

[165] T.W. Chun, et al., HIV-infected individuals receiving effective antiviral therapy for extended periods of time continually replenish their viral reservoir, J. Clin. Invest. 115 (2005) 3250–3255.

[166] K. Luzuriaga, et al., Vaccines to prevent transmission of HIV-1 via breast-milk: scientific and logistical priorities, Lancet 368 (2006) 511–521.

[167] S. Mehandru, et al., Primary HIV-1 infection is associated with preferential depletion of CD4+ T lymphocytes from effector sites in the gastrointestinal tract, J. Exp. Med. 200 (2004) 761–770.

[168] R.S. Veazey, A.A. Lackner, HIV swiftly guts the immune system, Nat. Med. 11 (2005) 469–470.

[169] W.T. Shearer, et al., Viral load and disease progression in infants infected with human immunodeficiency virus type 1, N. Engl. J. Med. 336 (1997) 1337–1342.

[170] P.E. Palumbo, et al., Viral measurement by polymerase chain reaction-based assays in human immunodeficiency virus-infected infants, J. Pediatr. 126 (1995) 592–595.

[171] L.M. Mofenson, et al., The relationship between serum human immunodeficiency virus type 1 (HIV-1) RNA level, CD4 lymphocyte percent, and long-term mortality risk in HIV-1-infected children. National Institute of Child Health and Human Development Intravenous Immunoglobulin Clinical Trial Study Group, J. Infect. Dis. 175 (1997) 1029–1038.

[172] K. McIntosh, et al., Age- and time-related changes in extracellular viral load in children vertically infected by human immunodeficiency virus, Pediatr. Infect. Dis. J. 15 (1996) 1087–1091.

[173] C. Balotta, et al., Plasma viremia and virus phenotype are correlates of disease progression in vertically human immunodeficiency virus type 1-infected children, Pediatr. Infect. Dis. J. 16 (1997) 205–211.

[174] J.W. Mellors, et al., Quantitation of HIV-1 RNA in plasma predicts outcome after seroconversion, Ann. Intern. Med. 122 (1995) 573–579.

[175] J.W. Mellors, et al., Prognosis of HIV-1 infection predicted by the quantity of virus in plasma, Science 272 (1996) 1167–1170.

[176] K.C. Rich, et al., Maternal and infant factors predicting disease progression in human immunodeficiency virus type 1-infected infants. Women and Infants Transmission Study Group, Pediatrics 105 (2000) e8.

[177] P.E. Palumbo, et al., Predictive value of quantitative plasma HIV RNA and CD4 lymphocyte count in HIV-infected infants and children, JAMA 279 (1998) 756–761.

[178] S.L. Gortmaker, et al., Effect of combination therapy including protease inhibitors on mortality among children and adolescents infected with HIV-1, N. Engl. J. Med. 345 (2001) 1522–1528.

[179] F.M. Erkeller-Yuksel, et al., Age-related changes in human blood lymphocyte subpopulations, J. Pediatr. 120 (1992) 216–222.

[180] European Collaborative Study, Age-related standards for T lymphocyte subsets based on uninfected children born to human immunodeficiency virus 1-infected mothers, Pediatr. Infect. Dis. J. 11 (1992) 1018–1026.

[181] W.M. Comans-Bitter, et al., Immunophenotyping of blood lymphocytes in childhood: reference values for lymphocyte subpopulations, J. Pediatr. 130 (1997) 388–393.

[182] R.E. McKinney, C.M. Wilfert, Lymphocyte subsets in children younger than 2 years old: normal values in a population at risk for human immunodeficiency virus infection and diagnostic and prognostic application to infected children, Pediatr. Infect. Dis. J. 11 (1992) 639–644.

[183] R.E. Dickover, et al., Rapid increases in load of human immunodeficiency virus correlate with early disease progression and loss of CD4 cells in vertically infected infants, J. Infect. Dis. 170 (1994) 1279–1284.

[184] E. Roilides, et al., Serum immunoglobulin G subclasses in children infected with human immunodeficiency virus type 1, Pediatr. Infect. Dis. J. 10 (1991) 134–139.

[185] K. Luzuriaga, et al., Deficient human immunodeficiency virus type 1-specific cytotoxic T cell responses in vertically infected children, J. Pediatr. 119 (1991) 230–236.

[186] A.D.A. Monforte, et al., T-cell subsets and serum immunoglobulin levels in infants born to HIV-seropositive mothers: a longitudinal evaluation, AIDS 4 (1990) 1141–1144.

[187] W. Borkowsky, et al., Cell-mediated and humoral immune responses in children infected with human immunodeficiency virus during the first four years of life, J. Pediatr. 120 (1992) 371–375.

[188] European Collaborative Study, Children born to women with HIV-1 infection: natural history and risk of transmission, Lancet 337 (1991) 253–260.

[189] P. Kiepiela, et al., Dominant influence of HLA-B in mediating the potential co-evolution of HIV and HLA, Nature 432 (2004) 769–775.

[190] L. Kuhn, et al., Maternal versus paternal inheritance of HLA class I alleles among HIV-infected children: consequences for clinical disease progression, AIDS 18 (2004) 1281–1289.

[191] B.J. Goulder, et al., Evolution and transmission of stable CTL escape mutations in HIV infection, Nature 412 (2001) 334–338.

[192] K. Luzuriaga, et al., Early therapy of vertical human immunodeficiency virus type 1 (HIV-1) infection: control of viral replication and absence of persistent HIV-1-specific immune responses, J. Virol. 74 (2000) 6984–6991.

[193] P. Borrow, et al., Virus-specific CD8+ cytotoxic T-lymphocyte activity associated with control of viremia in primary human immunodeficiency virus type 1 infection, J. Virol. 68 (1994) 6103–6110.

[194] P.J. Goulder, D.I. Watkins, HIV and SIV CTL escape: implications for vaccine design, Nat. Rev. Immunol. 4 (2004) 630–640.

[195] R.A. Koup, et al., Temporal association of cellular immune responses with the initial control of viremia in primary human immunodeficiency virus type 1 syndrome, J. Virol. 68 (1994) 4650.

[196] K. Luzuriaga, et al., HIV-1-specific cytotoxic T lymphocyte responses in the first year of life, J. Immunol. 154 (1995) 433–443.

[197] C.A. Pikora, et al., Early HIV-1 envelope-specific cytotoxic T lymphocyte responses in vertically infected children, J. Exp. Med. 185 (1997) 1153–1161.

[198] B.L. Lohman, et al., Longitudinal assessment of human immunodeficiency virus type-1 (HIV-1)-specific γ interferon responses during the first year of life in HIV-1 infected infants, J. Virol. 79 (2005) 8121–8130.

[199] K. Luzuriaga, J.L. Sullivan, HIV-1 specific cytotoxic T lymphocyte (CTL) responses in pediatric infection, in: B. Korber et al., (Ed.), HIV Molecular Immunology Database 1997, Los Alamos National Laboratory, Theoretical Biology and Biophysics, Los Alamos, 1997, pp. IV–12-8.

[200] S. Huang, et al., Deficiency of HIV-gag-specific T cells in early childhood correlates with poor viral containment, J. Immunol. 181 (2008) 8103–8111.

[201] T. Pillay, et al., Unique acquisition of cytotoxic T-lymphocyte escape mutants in infant human immunodeficiency virus type 1 infection, J. Virol. 79 (2005) 12100–12105.

[202] V. Sanchez-Merino, et al., HIV-1-specific CD8 T cell responses and viral evolution in women and infants, J. Immunol. 175 (2005) 6976–6986.

[203] E. Leal, et al., Selective pressures of human immunodeficiency virus tupe-1 (HIV-1) during pediatric infection, Infect. Genet. Evol. 7 (2007) 694–707.

[204] A. Leslie, et al., Transmission and accumulation of CTL escape variants drive negative associations between HIV polymorphisms and HLA, J. Exp. Med. 201 (2005) 891–902.

[205] M.E. Feeney, et al., HIV-1 viral escape in infancy followed by emergence of a variant-specific CTL response, J. Immunol. 174 (2005) 7524–7530.

[206] M.E. Feeney, et al., Immune escape precedes breakthrough human immunodeficiency virus type 1 viremia and broadening of the cytotoxic T-lymphocyte response in an HLA-B27-positive long-term-nonprogressing child, J. Virol. 78 (2004) 8927–8930.

[207] M. Jenkins, et al., Natural killer cytotoxicity and antibody-dependent cellular cytotoxicity of human immunodeficiency virus-infected cells by leukocytes from human neonates and adults, Pediatr. Res. 33 (1993) 469–474.

[208] D. Pugatch, et al., Delayed generation of antibodies mediating HIV-1 specific antibody-dependent cellular cytotoxicity in vertically-infected infants, J. Infect. Dis. 176 (1997) 643–648.

[209] S.K. Obaro, et al., Immunogenicity and efficacy of childhood vaccines in HIV-infected children, Lancet Infect. Dis. 4 (2004) 510–518.

[210] X. Wei, et al., Antibody neutralization and escape by HIV-1, Nature 422 (2003) 307–312.

[211] X. Wu, et al., Neutralization escape variants of human immunodeficiency virus type 1 are transmitted from mother to infant, J. Virol. 80 (2006) 835–844.

[212] R. Geffin, et al., A longitudinal assessment of autologous neutralizing antibodies in children perinatally infected with human immunodeficiency virus type 1, Virology 310 (2003) 207–215.

[213] N. Ching, et al., Cellular and humoral immune responses to a tetanus toxoid booster in perinatally HIV-1-infected children and adolescents receiving highly active antiretroviral therapy (HAART), Eur. J. Pediatr. 166 (2007) 51–56.

[214] A.J. Melvin, K.M. Mohan, Response to immunization with measles, tetanus, and *Haemophilus influenzae* type b vaccines in children who have human immunodeficiency virus type 1 infection and are treated with highly active antiretroviral therapy, Pediatrics 111 (6) (2003).

[215] M. De Martino, et al., Acellular pertussis vaccine in children with perinatal human immunodeficiency virus-type 1 infection, Vaccine 15 (1997) 1235–1238.

[216] K. Patel, et al., Long-term effects of highly active antiretroviral therapy on CD4 cell evolution among children and adolescents infected with HIV: 5 years and counting, Clin. Infect. Dis. 46 (2008) 1751–1760.

[217] A. Weinberg, et al., Continuous improvement in the immune system of HIV-infected children on prolonged antiretroviral therapy, AIDS 22 (2008) 2267–2277.

[218] Centers for Disease Control and Prevention, Guidelines for the prevention and treatment of opportunistic infections among HIV-exposed and HIV-infected children: recommendations from the Centers for Disease Control and Prevention, the HIV Medicine Association of the National Institutes of Health, Infectious Disease Society of America, MMWR Recomm. Rep. 55 (RR-14) (2008) 1–17.

[219] Centers for Disease Control and Prevention, Revised recommendations for HIV testing of adults, adolescents, and pregnant women in health-care settings, MMWR Recomm. Rep. 55 (RR-14) (2006) 1–17.

[220] P.L. Havens, L.M. Mofenson, American Academy of Pediatrics, Committee on Pediatric AIDS. HIV testing and prophylaxis to prevent mother-to-child transmission in the United States, Pediatrics 122 (2008) 1127–1134.

[221] American College of Obstetricians and Gynecologists, Committee on Obstetric Practice. Prenatal and perinatal human immunodeficiency virus testing: expanded recommendations. ACOG Committee Opinion No, 304, Obstet. Gynecol. 104 (5 Pt 1) (2004) 119–1124.

[222] Centers for Disease Control and Prevention, Recommendations of the U.S. Public Health Service Task Force on the use of zidovudine to reduce perinatal transmission of human immunodeficiency virus, MMWR Morb. Mortal. Wkly Rep. 43 (1994) 1–20.

[223] Centers for Disease Control and Prevention, U.S. Public Health Service Task Force recommendations for use of antiretroviral drugs in pregnant HIV-infected women for maternal health and interventions to reduce perinatal HIV-1 transmission in the United States. Available at http://aidsinfo.nih.gov/contentfiles/PerinatalGL001020.pdf. 8 July 2008, posting date.

[224] E.P. Paintsil, et al., Care and management of the infant of the HIV-1 infected mother, Semin. Perinatol. 31 (2007) 112–123.

[225] J.S. Read, American Academy of Pediatrics, Committee on Pediatric AIDS. Diagnosis of HIV infection in children younger than 18 months in the United States, Pediatrics 120 (6) (2007).

[226] S.M. King, American Academy of Pediatrics, Committee on Pediatric AIDS. Evaluation and treatment of the human immunodeficiency virus-1-exposed infant, Pediatrics 114 (2004) 497–505.

[227] A.M. Comeau, et al., Early detection of human immunodeficiency virus on dried blood spot specimens: sensitivity across serial specimens, J. Pediatr. 129 (1996) 111–118.

[228] J.S. Lambert, et al., Performance characteristics of HIV-1 culture and HIV-1 DNA and RNA amplification assays for early diagnosis of perinatal HIV-1 infection, J. Acquir. Immune Defic. Syndr. 34 (2003) 512–519.

[229] N.E. Kline, H. Schwarzwald, M.W. Kline, False negative DNA polymerase chain reaction in an infant with subtype C human immunodeficiency virus 1 infection, Pediatr. Infect. Dis. J. 21 (2002) 885–886.

[230] J. Haas, et al., Infection with non-B subtype HIV type 1 complicates management of established infection in adult patients and diagnosis of infection in infant infants, Clin. Infect. Dis. 34 (2002) 417–418.

[231] C. Delamare, et al., HIV-1 RNA detection in plasma for the diagnosis of infection in neonates. The French Pediatric HIV Infection Study Group, J. Acquir. Immune Defic. Syndr. 15 (1997) 121–125.

[232] C.K. Cunningham, et al., Comparison of human immunodeficiency virus 1 DNA polymerase chain reaction and qualitative and quantitative RNA polymerase chain reaction in human immunodeficiency virus 1-exposed infants, Pediatr. Infect. Dis. J. 18 (1999) 30–35.

[233] R.J. Simonds, et al., Sensitivity and specificity of a qualitative RNA detection assay to diagnose HIV infection in young infants. Perinatal AIDS Collaborative Transmission Study, AIDS 12 (1998) 1545–1549.

[234] F. Rouet, et al., Early diagnosis of paediatric HIV-1 infection among African breast-fed children using a quantitative plasma HIV RNA assay, AIDS 15 (2001) 1849–1856.

[235] S. Nesheim, et al., Quantitative RNA testing for diagnosis of HIV-infected infants, J. Acquir. Immune Defic. Syndr. 32 (2003) 192–195.

[236] N.L. Young, et al., Early diagnosis of HIV-1-infected infants in Thailand using RNA and DNA PCR assays sensitive to non-B subtypes, J. Acquir. Immune Defic. Syndr. 24 (2000) 401–407.

[237] S. Blanche, et al., Morbidity and mortality in European children vertically infected by HIV-1. The French Pediatric HIV Infection Study Group and European Collaborative Study, J. Acquir. Immune Defic. Syndr. Hum. Retrovirol. 14 (1997) 442–450.

[238] K. Luzuriaga, J.L. Sullivan, DNA polymerase chain reaction for the diagnosis of vertical HIV infection, JAMA 275 (1996) 1360–1361.

[239] C.J. Chantry, et al., Seroreversion in human immunodeficiency virus-exposed but uninfected infants, Pediatr. Infect. Dis. J. 14 (1995) 382–387.

[240] K. McIntosh, et al., Blood culture in the first 6 months of life for the diagnosis of vertically transmitted human immunodeficiency virus infection. The Women and Infants Transmission Study Group, J. Infect. Dis. 170 (1994) 996–1000.

[241] A. Krivine, et al., A comparative study of virus isolation, polymerase chain reaction, and antigen detection in perinatally acquired human immunodeficiency virus, J. Pediatr. 116 (1990) 372–376.

[242] Y. Yanase, et al., Lymphocyte subsets identified by monoclonal antibodies in healthy children, Pediatr. Res. 20 (1986) 1147–1151.

[243] CDC, Revised classification system for human immunodeficiency virus infection in children less than 13 years of age, MMWR Recomm. Rep. 43 (No. RR-12) (1994) 1–7.

[244] CDC, Revised surveillance case definitions for HIV infection among adults, adolescents, and children aged <18 months and for HIV infection and AIDS among children aged 18 months to <13 years—United States, 2008, MMWR Recomm. Rep. 57 (No. RR-10) (2008) 1–8.

[245] R.J. Simonds, et al., *Pneumocystis carinii* pneumonia among US children with perinatally acquired human immunodeficiency virus, JAMA 270 (1993) 470–473.

[246] L.M. Mofenson, et al., Treating opportunistic infections among HIV-exposed and infected children: recommendations from CDC, the National Institutes of Health, and the Infectious Diseases Society of America, MMWR Recomm. Rep. 53 (RR-14) (2004) 1–92.

[247] Centers for Disease Control, Revision of the CDC surveillance case definition for acquired immune deficiency syndrome, MMWR Morb. Mortal. Wkly Rep. 36 (Suppl. 1S) (1987) 1S–15S.

[248] T.C. Quinn, A. Ruff, N. Halsey, Pediatric acquired immunodeficiency syndrome: special considerations for developing nations, Pediatr. Infect. Dis. J. 11 (1992) 558–568.

[249] S.A. Jones, G.G. Sherman, A.H. Coovadia, Can clinical algorithms deliver an accurate diagnosis of HIV infection in infancy? Bull. World Health Organ. 83 (2005) 559–560.

[250] P. Lepage, et al., Evaluation and simplification of the World Health Organization clinical case definition for paediatric AIDS, AIDS 3 (1989) 221–225.

[251] C. Horwood, et al., Diagnosis of paediatric HIV infection in a primary health care setting with a clinical algorithm, Bull. World Health Organ. 81 (2003) 858–866.

[252] World Health Organization, WHO case definitions of HIV for surveillance and revised clinical staging and immunological classification of HIV-related disease in adults and children, World Health Organization, Geneva, 2006.

Available at www.who.int/hiv/pub/guidelines/hivstaging/en. Accessed February 2, 2008.

[253] G.B. Scott, et al., Survival in children with perinatally acquired human immunodeficiency virus type 1 infection, N. Engl. J. Med. 321 (1989) 1791–1796.

[254] R.W. Marion, et al., Human T-cell lymphotropic virus type III (HTLV-III) embryopathy: a new dysmorphic syndrome associated with intrauterine HTLV-III infection, Am. J. Dis. Child. 140 (1986) 638–640.

[255] Q.H. Qazi, et al., Lack of evidence for craniofacial dysmorphism in perinatal human immunodeficiency virus infection, J. Pediatr. 112 (1998) 7–11.

[256] L. Galli, et al., Italian Register for HIV Infection in Children. Onset of clinical signs with HIV-1 perinatal infection, AIDS 9 (1995) 455–461.

[257] M.L. Newell, et al., Natural history of vertically-acquired human immunodeficiency virus-1 infection. The European Collaborative Study, Pediatrics 94 (1994) 815–819.

[258] S. Blanche, et al., Longitudinal study of 94 symptomatic infants with perinatally acquired human immunodeficiency virus infection, Am. J. Dis. Child. 144 (1990) 1210–1215.

[259] H. Pollack, et al., Impaired early growth of infants perinatally infected with human immunodeficiency virus: correlation with viral load, J. Pediatr. 130 (1997) 915–922.

[260] M.W. Kline, Vertically acquired human immunodeficiency virus infection, Semin. Pediatr. Infect. Dis. 10 (1999) 147–153.

[261] W.A. Andiman, J. Mezger, E. Shapiro, Invasive bacterial infections in children born to women infected with human immunodeficiency virus type 1, J. Pediatr. 124 (1994) 846–852.

[262] R. Lichenstein, et al., Bacteremia in febrile human immunodeficiency virus-infected children presenting to ambulatory care settings, Pediatr. Infect. Dis. J. 17 (1998) 381–385.

[263] E.N. Janoff, et al., Pneumococcal disease during HIV infection: epidemiology, clinical, and immunologic perspectives, Ann. Intern. Med. 117 (1992) 314–324.

[264] J.J. Farley, et al., Invasive pneumococcal disease among infected and uninfected children of mothers with human immunodeficiency virus infection, J. Pediatr. 124 (1994) 853–858.

[265] D. Di John, et al., Very late onset of group B streptococcal disease in infants infected with the human immunodeficiency virus, Pediatr. Infect. Dis. J. 9 (1990) 925–928.

[266] D.H. Dorfman, J.H. Glaser, Congenital syphilis presenting in infants after the newborn period, N. Engl. J. Med. 323 (1990) 1299–1302.

[267] J.A. Dumois, Potential problems with the diagnosis and treatment of syphilis in HIV-infected pregnant women, Pediatr. AIDS HIV Infect. Fetus Adolesc. 3 (1992) 22–24.

[268] K. McIntosh, Congenital syphilis—breaking through the safety net, N. Engl. J. Med. 323 (1990) 1339–1341.

[269] Centers for Disease Control, Screening for tuberculosis and tuberculous infection in high-risk populations and the use of preventive therapy for tuberculous infections in the United States, MMWR Morb. Mortal. Wkly Rep. 39 (1990) 1–12.

[270] Y.F. Khoury, et al., *Mycobacterium tuberculosis* in children with human immunodeficiency virus type 1 infection, Pediatr. Infect. Dis. J. 11 (1992) 950–955.

[271] L.T. Gutman, et al., Tuberculosis in human immunodeficiency virus-exposed or -infected United States children, Pediatr. Infect. Dis. J. 13 (1994) 963–968.

[272] Committee on Infectious Diseases, Screening for tuberculosis in infants and children, Pediatrics 93 (1994) 131–134.

[273] M. Adhikari, T. Pillay, D.G. Pillay, Tuberculosis in the newborn: an emerging disease, Pediatr. Infect. Dis. J. 16 (1997) 1108–1112.

[274] Committee on Infectious Diseases, Update on tuberculosis skin testing of children, Pediatrics 97 (1996) 282–284.

[275] J.R. Starke, A.G. Correa, Management of mycobacterial infection and disease in children, Pediatr. Infect. Dis. J. 14 (1995) 455–470.

[276] L.L. Lewis, et al., Defining the population of human immunodeficiency virus-infected children at risk for *Mycobacterium avium-intracellulare* infection, J. Pediatr. 121 (1992) 677–683.

[277] R.M. Rutstein, et al., *Mycobacterium avium intracellulare* complex infection in HIV-infected children, AIDS 7 (1993) 507–512.

[278] USPHS/IDSA Prevention of Opportunistic Infections Working Group, USPHS/IDSA guidelines for the prevention of opportunistic infections in persons infected with human immunodeficiency virus, MMWR Morb. Mortal. Wkly Rep. 46 (1997) 1–46.

[279] E. Jura, et al., Varicella-zoster virus infections in children infected with human immunodeficiency virus, Pediatr. Infect. Dis. J. 8 (1989) 586–590.

[280] C.C. Silliman, et al., Unsuspected varicella-zoster virus encephalitis in a child with acquired immunodeficiency syndrome, J. Pediatr. 123 (1993) 418–422.

[281] E.G. Lyall, et al., Acyclovir resistant varicella zoster and HIV infection, Arch. Dis. Child. 70 (1994) 133–135.

[282] S. Chandwani, et al., Cytomegalovirus infection in human immunodeficiency virus type 1-infected children, Pediatr. Infect. Dis. J. 15 (1996) 310–314.

[283] G. Nigro, et al., Rapid progression of HIV disease in children with cytomegalovirus DNAemia, AIDS 10 (1996) 1127–1133.

[284] M. Doyle, J.T. Atkins, I.R. Rivera-Matos, Congenital cytomegalovirus infection in infants infected with human immunodeficiency virus type 1, Pediatr. Infect. Dis. J. 15 (1996) 1102–1106.

[285] B.J. Kitchen, et al., Cytomegalovirus infection in children with human immunodeficiency virus infection, Pediatr. Infect. Dis. J. 16 (1997) 358–363.

[286] D. Zaknun, et al., Concurrent ganciclovir and foscarnet treatment for cytomegalovirus encephalitis and retinitis in an infant with acquired immunodeficiency syndrome: case report and review, Pediatr. Infect. Dis. J. 16 (1997) 807–811.

[287] R.C. Walton, et al., Combined intravenous ganciclovir and foscarnet for children with recurrent cytomegalovirus retinitis, Ophthalmology 102 (1995) 1865–1870.

[288] N.J. Bodsworth, D.A. Cooper, B. Donovan, The influence of human immunodeficiency virus type 1 infection on the development of the hepatitis B virus carrier state, J. Infect. Dis. 163 (1991) 1138–1140.

[289] M.E. Eyster, et al., Natural history of hepatitis C virus infection in multitransfused hemophiliacs: effect of co-infection with human immunodeficiency virus, J. Acquir. Immune Defic. Syndr. 6 (1993) 602–610.

[290] S. Paccagnini, et al., Perinatal transmission and manifestation of hepatitis C virus infection in a high risk population, Pediatr. Infect. Dis. J. 14 (1995) 195–199.

[291] D. Conte, et al., Prevalence and clinical course of chronic hepatitis C virus (HCV) infection and rate of HCV vertical transmission in a cohort of 15,250 pregnant women, Hepatology 31 (2000) 751–755.

[292] M. Resti, et al., Maternal drug use is a preeminent risk factor for mother-to-child hepatitis C virus transmission: results from a multicenter study of 1372 mother-infant pairs, J. Infect. Dis. 185 (2002) 567–572.

[293] L.J. Kaplan, et al., Severe measles in immunocompromised patients, JAMA 267 (1992) 1237–1241.

[294] P. Palumbo, et al., Population-based study of measles and measles immunization in human immunodeficiency virus-infected children, Pediatr. Infect. Dis. J. 11 (1992) 1008–1014.

[295] S. Nadel, et al., Measles giant cell pneumonia in a child with human immunodeficiency virus infection, Pediatr. Infect. Dis. J. 10 (1991) 542–544.

[296] K. Krasinski, W. Borkowsky, Measles and measles immunity in children infected with human immunodeficiency virus, JAMA 261 (1989) 2512–2516.

[297] S. Chandwani, et al., Respiratory syncytial virus infection in human immunodeficiency virus-infected children, J. Pediatr. 117 (1990) 251–254.

[298] M. Ellaurie, et al., Spectrum of adenovirus infection in pediatric HIV infection, Pediatr. AIDS HIV Infect. 4 (1993) 211–214.

[299] J.C. King, et al., Respiratory syncytial virus illnesses in human immunodeficiency virus- and noninfected children, Pediatr. Infect. Dis. J. 12 (1993) 733–739.

[300] V.V. Joshi, et al., Polyclonal polymorphic B-cell lymphoproliferative disorder with prominent pulmonary involvement in children with acquired immune deficiency syndrome, Cancer 59 (1987) 1455–1462.

[301] C.E. Gonzales, et al., Risk factors for fungemia in children infected with human immunodeficiency virus: a case control study, Clin. Infect. Dis. 23 (1996) 515–521.

[302] R.J. Leggiadro, M.W. Kline, W.T. Hughes, Extrapulmonary cryptococcosis in children with acquired immunodeficiency syndrome, Pediatr. Infect. Dis. J. 10 (1991) 658–662.

[303] G.E. Gonzales, et al., Cryptococcosis in human immunodeficiency virus-infected children, Pediatr. Infect. Dis. J. 15 (1996) 796–800.

[304] G.Y. Minamoto, T.F. Barlam, N.J. Vander Els, Invasive aspergillosis in patients with AIDS, Clin. Infect. Dis. 14 (1992) 66–74.

[305] D.W. Denning, et al., Pulmonary aspergillosis in the acquired immunodeficiency syndrome, N. Engl. J. Med. 324 (1991) 654–662.

[306] D. Shetty, et al., Invasive aspergillosis in human immunodeficiency virus-infected children, Pediatr. Infect. Dis. 16 (1997) 216–221.

[307] G.A. Sarosi, P.C. Johnson, Disseminated histoplasmosis in patients infected with human immunodeficiency virus, Clin. Infect. Dis. 14 (Suppl. 1) (1992) S60–S67.

[308] P.G. Pappas, et al., Blastomycosis in patients with the acquired immunodeficiency syndrome, Ann. Intern. Med. 116 (1992) 847–853.

[309] M. Byers, S. Feldman, J. Edwards, Disseminated histoplasmosis as the acquired immunodeficiency syndrome-defining illness in an infant, Pediatr. Infect. Dis. J. 11 (1992) 127–128.

[310] Centers for Disease Control and Prevention, Revised guidelines for prophylaxis against *Pneumocystis carinii* pneumonia for children infected with or perinatally exposed to human immunodeficiency virus, MMWR Morb. Mortal. Wkly Rep. 44 (1995) 1–12.

[311] Centers for Disease Control and Prevention, HIV AIDS Surveill. Rep. 9 (1997) 1–43.

[312] E. Mortier, et al., Maternal-fetal transmission of *Pneumocystis carinii* in human immunodeficiency virus infection, N. Engl. J. Med. 332 (1995) 825–826.

[313] M.R. Bye, et al., *Pneumocystis carinii* pneumonia in young children with AIDS, Pediatr. Pulmonol. 9 (1990) 251–253.

[314] E. Connor, et al., Clinical and laboratory correlates of *Pneumocystis carinii* pneumonia in children infected with HIV, JAMA 265 (1991) 1693–1697.

[315] L.L. Gosey, et al., Advantages of a modified toluidine blue O stain and bronchoalveolar lavage for the diagnosis of *Pneumocystis carinii* pneumonia, J. Clin. Microbiol. 22 (1985) 803–807.

[316] F.P. Ognibene, et al., Induced sputum to diagnose *Pneumocystis carinii* pneumonia in immunosuppressed pediatric patients, J. Pediatr. 115 (1989) 430–433.

[317] F.R. Sattler, et al., Trimethoprim-sulfamethoxazole compared with pentamidine for treatment of *Pneumocystis carinii* pneumonia in the acquired immunodeficiency syndrome: a prospective, noncrossover study, Ann. Intern. Med. 109 (1988) 280–287.

[318] S. Gagnon, et al., Corticosteroids as adjunctive therapy for severe *Pneumocystis carinii* pneumonia in the acquired immunodeficiency syndrome, N. Engl. J. Med. 323 (1990) 1444–1450.

[319] S.A. Bozzette, et al., A controlled trial of early adjunctive treatment with corticosteroids for *Pneumocystis carinii* pneumonia in the acquired immunodeficiency syndrome, N. Engl. J. Med. 1323 (1990) 1451–1457.

[320] The National Institutes of Health–University of California Expert Panel for Corticosteroids as Adjunctive Therapy for Pneumocystis Pneumonia, Consensus statement on the use of corticosteroids as adjunctive therapy for *Pneumocystis* pneumonia in the acquired immunodeficiency syndrome, N. Engl. J. Med. 323 (1990) 1500–1504.

[321] G.E. McLaughlin, et al., Effect of corticosteroids on survival of children with acquired immunodeficiency syndrome and *Pneumocystis carinii*-related respiratory failure, J. Pediatr. 126 (1995) 821–824.

[322] L.J. Bernstein, M.R. Bye, A. Rubinstein, Prognostic factors and life expectancy in children with acquired immunodeficiency syndrome and *Pneumocystis carinii* pneumonia, Am. J. Dis. Child. 143 (1989) 775–778.

[323] A. Kovacs, et al., CD4 T-lymphocyte counts and *Pneumocystis carinii* pneumonia in pediatric HIV infection, JAMA 265 (1991) 1698–1703.

[324] Centers for Disease Control, Guidelines for prophylaxis against *Pneumocystis carinii* pneumonia for children infected with human immunodeficiency virus, MMWR Morb. Mortal. Wkly Rep. 40 (1991) 1–13.

[325] R.J. Simonds, et al., Prophylaxis against *Pneumocystis carinii* pneumonia among children with perinatally acquired human immunodeficiency virus infection in the United States, N. Engl. J. Med. 332 (1995) 786–790.

[326] D.M. Thea, et al., Benefit of primary prophylaxis before 18 months of age in reducing the incidence of *Pneumocystis carinii* pneumonia and early death in a cohort of 112 human immunodeficiency virus-infected infants, Pediatrics 97 (1996) 59–64.

[327] B.U. Mueller, et al., *Pneumocystis carinii* pneumonia despite prophylaxis in children with human immunodeficiency virus infection, J. Pediatr. 119 (1991) 992–994.

[328] S.A. Nachman, et al., High failure rate of dapsone and pentamidine as *Pneumocystis carinii* pneumonia prophylaxis in human immunodeficiency virus-infected children, Pediatr. Infect. Dis. J. 13 (1994) 1004–1006.

[329] C.D. Mitchell, et al., Congenital toxoplasmosis occurring in infants infected with human immunodeficiency virus 1, Pediatr. Infect. Dis. J. 9 (1990) 512–518.

[330] M.D. Medlock, J.T. Tilleli, G.S. Pearl, Congenital cardiac toxoplasmosis in a newborn with acquired immunodeficiency syndrome, Pediatr. Infect. Dis. J. 9 (1990) 129–132.

[331] R.L. Cordell, D.G. Addiss, Cryptosporidiosis in child care settings: a review of the literature and recommendations for prevention and control, Pediatr. Infect. Dis. J. 13 (1994) 310–317.

[332] M.N. Lobato, et al., Encephalopathy in children with perinatally acquired human immunodeficiency virus infection, J. Pediatr. 126 (1995) 710–715.

[333] C. Diaz, et al., Disease progression in a cohort of infants with vertically acquired HIV infection observed from birth. The Women and Infants Transmission Study (WITS), J. Acquir. Immune Defic. Syndr. Hum. Retrovirol. 18 (1998) 221–228.

[334] E.R. Cooper, et al., Encephalopathy and progression of human immunodeficiency virus disease in a cohort of children with perinatally acquired human immunodeficiency virus infection. Women and Infants Transmission Study Group, J. Pediatr. 132 (1998) 808–812.

[335] European Collaborative Study, Neurologic signs in young children with human immunodeficiency virus infection, Pediatr. Infect. Dis. J. 9 (1990) 402–406.

[336] Y.D. Park, et al., Stroke in pediatric acquired immunodeficiency syndrome, Ann. Neurol. 28 (1990) 303–311.

[337] C. Lang, et al., Rapid development of giant aneurysm at the base of the brain in an 8-year-old boy with perinatal HIV infection, Acta Histochem. Suppl 42 (1992) S83–S90.

[338] A.L. Belman, et al., Pediatric acquired immunodeficiency syndrome: neurologic symptoms, Am. J. Dis. Child. 142 (1988) 29–35.

[339] L.G. Epstein, L.R. Sharer, J. Goudsmit, Neurological and neuropathological features of human immunodeficiency virus infection in children, Ann. Neurol. 23 (Suppl.) (1988) S19–S23.

[340] G.L. Gay, et al., The effects of HIV on cognitive and motor development in children born to HIV-seropositive women with no reported drug use: birth to 24 months, Pediatrics 96 (1995) 1078–1082.

[341] P.L. Wolters, et al., Differential receptive and expressive language functioning of children with symptomatic HIV disease and relation to CT scan brain abnormalities, Pediatrics 95 (1995) 112–119.

[342] P. Brouwers, A. Belman, L. Epstein, Central nervous system involvement: manifestations, evaluation, and pathogenesis, in: P.A. Pizzo, C.A. Wilfert (Eds.), Pediatric AIDS. The Challenge of HIV Infection in Infants, Children, and Adolescents, Williams & Wilkins, Baltimore, 1994, pp. 433–455.

[343] P. Brouwers, et al., Correlation between computed tomographic brain scan abnormalities and neuropsychological function in children with symptomatic human immunodeficiency virus disease, Arch. Neurol. 52 (1995) 39–44.

[344] P. Brouwers, et al., Interrelations among patterns of change in neurocognitive, CT brain imaging and CD4 measures associated with anti-retroviral therapy in children with symptomatic HIV infection, Adv. Neuroimmunol. 4 (1994) 223–231.

[345] C. DeCarli, et al., The prevalence of computed tomographic abnormalities of the cerebrum in 100 consecutive children symptomatic with the human immunodeficiency virus, Ann. Neurol. 34 (1993) 198–205.

[346] C. DeCarli, et al., Brain growth and cognitive improvement in children with human immunodeficiency virus-induced encephalopathy after 6 months of continuous infusion zidovudine therapy, J. Acquir. Immune Defic. Syndr. 4 (1991) 585–592.

[347] L.R. Sharer, et al., Detection of HIV-1 DNA in pediatric AIDS brain tissue by two-step ISPCR, Adv. Neuroimmunol. 4 (1994) 283–285.

[348] L.R. Sharer, Neuropathological aspects of HIV-1 infection in children, in: H.E. Gendelman et al., (Ed.), The Neurology of AIDS, Chapman & Hall, New York, 1998, pp. 408–418.

[349] Y. Saito, et al., Overexpression of nef as a marker for restricted HIV-1 infection of astrocytes in postmortem pediatric central nervous tissues, Neurology 44 (1994) 474–481.

[350] T.W. Baba, V. Liska, R.M. Ruprecht, HIV-1/SIV infection of the fetal and neonatal nervous system, in: H.E. Gendelman et al., (Ed.), The Neurology of AIDS, Chapman & Hall, New York, 1998, pp. 443–456.

[351] R.D. Pratt, et al., Virologic markers of human immunodeficiency virus type 1 in cerebrospinal fluid of infected children, J. Infect. Dis. 174 (1996) 288–293.

[352] S. Sei, et al., Evaluation of HIV-1 RNA levels in cerebrospinal fluid and viral resistance to zidovudine in children with HIV encephalopathy, J. Infect. Dis. 174 (1996) 1200–1206.

[353] H.A. Gelbard, HIV-1-induced neurotoxicity in the developing central nervous system, in: H.E. Gendelman et al., (Ed.), The Neurology of AIDS, Chapman & Hall, New York, 1998, pp. 419–424.

[354] P. Brouwers, et al., Quinolinic acid in the cerebrospinal fluid of children with symptomatic human immunodeficiency virus type 1 disease: relationships to clinical status and therapeutic response, J. Infect. Dis. 168 (1993) 1380–1386.

[355] S. Sei, et al., Increased human immunodeficiency virus (HIV) type 1 DNA content and quinolinic acid concentration in brain tissues from patients with HIV encephalopathy, J. Infect. Dis. 172 (1995) 638–647.

[356] I. Srugo, et al., Meningoencephalitis in a neonate congenitally infected with human immunodeficiency virus type 1, J. Pediatr. 120 (1992) 93–95.

[357] L.R. Sharer, et al., Spinal cord disease in children with HIV-1 infection: a combined molecular biological and neuropathological study, Neuropathol. Appl. Neurobiol. 16 (1990) 317–331.

[358] P. Brouwers, et al., Effect of continuous-infusion zidovudine therapy on neuropsychologic functioning in children with symptomatic human immunodeficiency virus infection, J. Pediatr. 117 (1990) 980–985.

[359] E.R. Stiehm, et al., Prednisone improves human immunodeficiency virus encephalopathy in children, Pediatr. Infect. Dis. J. 11 (1992) 49–50.

[360] E.T. Cunningham, T.P. Margolis, Ocular manifestations of HIV infection, N. Engl. J. Med. 339 (1998) 236–244.

[361] M.D. de Smet, R.B. Nussenblatt, Ocular manifestations of HIV in pediatric populations, in: P.A. Pizzo, C.A. Wilfert (Eds.), Pediatric AIDS. The Challenge of HIV Infection in Infants, Children, and Adolescents, Williams & Wilkins, Baltimore, 1994, pp. 457–466.

[362] F. Bottoni, et al., Diffuse necrotizing retinochoroiditis in a child with AIDS and toxoplasmic encephalitis, Graefes Arch. Clin. Exp. Ophthalmol. 228 (1990) 36–39.

[363] J.S. Lopez, et al., Orally administered 566C80 for treatment of ocular toxoplasmosis in a patient with the acquired immunodeficiency syndrome, Am. J. Ophthalmol. 113 (1992) 331–333.

[364] E.E. Telzak, et al., Extrapulmonary *Pneumocystis carinii* infections, Rev. Infect. Dis. 12 (1990) 380–386.

[365] E.M. Connor, W.A. Andiman, Lymphoid interstitial pneumonitis, in: P.A. Pizzo, C.A. Wilfert (Eds.), Pediatric AIDS. The Challenge of HIV Infection in Infants, Children, and Adolescents, Williams & Wilkins, Baltimore, 1994, pp. 467–482.

[366] M. Sharland, D.M. Gibb, F. Holland, Respiratory morbidity from lymphocytic interstitial pneumonitis (LIP) in vertically acquired HIV infection, Arch. Dis. Child. 76 (1997) 334–336.

[367] G.B. Scott, et al., Survival in children with perinatally acquired human immunodeficiency virus type 1 infection, N. Engl. J. Med. 321 (1989) 1791–1796.

[368] L.M. Luginbuhl, et al., Cardiac morbidity and related mortality in children with HIV infection, JAMA 269 (1993) 2869–2875.

[369] S.E. Lipshultz, et al., Cardiac structure and function in children with human immunodeficiency virus infection treated with zidovudine, N. Engl. J. Med. 327 (1992) 1260–1265.

[370] S.E. Lipshultz, et al., Identification of human immunodeficiency virus-1 RNA and DNA in the heart of a child with cardiovascular abnormalities and congenital acquired immune deficiency syndrome, Am. J. Cardiol. 66 (1990) 246–250.

[371] V.V. Joshi, et al., Dilated cardiomyopathy in children with acquired immunodeficiency syndrome: a pathologic study of five cases, Hum. Pathol. 19 (1988) 69–73.

[372] W. Lewis, AIDS: cardiac findings from 115 autopsies, Prog. Cardiovasc. Dis. 32 (1989) 207–215.

[373] W.W. Grody, L. Cheng, W. Lewis, Infection of the heart by the human immunodeficiency virus, Am. J. Cardiol. 66 (1990) 203–206.

[374] V.V. Joshi, et al., Arteriopathy in children with acquired immune deficiency syndrome, Pediatr. Pathol. 7 (1987) 261–275.

[375] K. Kure, et al., Immunohistochemical localization of an HIV epitope in cerebral aneurysmal arteriopathy in pediatric acquired immunodeficiency syndrome (AIDS), Pediatr. Pathol. 9 (1989) 655–667.

[376] R.N. Husson, et al., Cerebral artery aneurysms in children infected with human immunodeficiency virus, J. Pediatr. 121 (1992) 927–930.

[377] L. Galli, et al., Onset of clinical signs in children with HIV-1 perinatal infection, AIDS 9 (1995) 455–461.

[378] L.K. Pickering, Infections of the gastrointestinal tract, in: P.A. Pizzo, C.A. Wilfert (Eds.), Pediatric AIDS. The Challenge of HIV Infection in Infants, Children, and Adolescents, Williams & Wilkins, Baltimore, 1994, pp. 377–404.

[379] R.H. Yolken, et al., Persistent diarrhea and fecal shedding of retroviral nucleic acids in children infected with human immunodeficiency virus, J. Infect. Dis. 164 (1991) 61–66.

[380] C. Grunfeld, K.R. Feingold, Metabolic disturbances and wasting in the acquired immunodeficiency syndrome, N. Engl. J. Med. 327 (1992) 329–337.

[381] J.D. Lewis, H.S. Winter, Intestinal and hepatobiliary diseases in HIV-infected children, Gastroenterol. Clin. North Am. 24 (1995) 119–132.

[382] K.L. Kotloff, et al., Diarrheal morbidity during the first 2 years of life among HIV-infected infants, JAMA 271 (1994) 448–452.

[383] D.M. Thea, et al., A prospective study of diarrhea and HIV-1 infection among 429 Zairian infants, N. Engl. J. Med. 329 (1993) 1696–1702.

[384] T.L. Miller, Nutritional assessment and its clinical application in children infected with the human immunodeficiency virus, J. Pediatr. 129 (1996) 633–636.

[385] G. Maggiore, Chronic hepatitis in children, Curr Opin Pediatr. 7 (1995) 539–546.

[386] D. Persaud, et al., Cholestatic hepatitis in children infected with the human immunodeficiency virus, Pediatr. Infect. Dis. J. 12 (1993) 492–498.

[387] T.L. Miller, et al., Pancreatitis in pediatric human immunodeficiency virus infection, J. Pediatr. 120 (1992) 223–227.

[388] K.M. Butler, et al., Pancreatitis in human immunodeficiency virus-infected children receiving dideoxyinosine, Pediatrics 91 (1993) 747–751.

[389] J. Strauss, et al., Renal disease in children with the acquired immunodeficiency syndrome, N. Engl. J. Med. 321 (1989) 625–630.

[390] J. Strauss, et al., Human immunodeficiency virus nephropathy, Pediatr. Nephrol. 7 (1993) 220–225.

[391] E. Ingulli, et al., Nephrotic syndrome associated with acquired immunodeficiency syndrome in children, J. Pediatr. 119 (1991) 710–716.

[392] M.J. Schoeneman, et al., IgA nephritis in a child with human immunodeficiency virus. A unique form of human immunodeficiency virus-associated nephropathy, Pediatr. Nephrol. 6 (1992) 46–49.

[393] P.L. Kimmel, et al., Brief report: idiotypic IgA nephropathy in patients with human immunodeficiency virus infection, N. Engl. J. Med. 327 (1992) 702–706.

[394] B.U. Mueller, et al., A phase I/II study of the protease inhibitor indinavir in children with HIV infection, Pediatrics 102 (1998) 101–109.

[395] R.G. Bruce, et al., Urolithiasis associated with the protease inhibitor indinavir, Urology 50 (1997) 513–518.

[396] J.M. Gertner, et al., Delayed somatic growth and pubertal development in human immunodeficiency virus-infected hemophiliac boys. Hemophilia Growth and Development Study, J. Pediatr. 124 (1994) 896–902.

[397] G.D. Fisher, et al., Seroprevalence of HIV-1 and HIV-2 infection among children diagnosed with protein-calorie malnutrition in Nigeria, Epidemiol. Infect. 110 (1993) 373–379.

[398] D.B. Brettler, et al., Growth failure as a prognostic indicator for progression to acquired immunodeficiency syndrome in children with hemophilia, J. Pediatr. 117 (1990) 584–588.

[399] L. Laue, et al., Growth and neuroendocrine dysfunction in children with acquired immunodeficiency syndrome, J. Pediatr. 117 (1990) 541–545.

[400] L.J. Schwartz, et al., Endocrine function in children with human immunodeficiency virus infection, Am. J. Dis. Child. 145 (1991) 330–333.

[401] S.K. Grinspoon, J.P. Bilezikian, HIV disease and the endocrine system, N. Engl. J. Med. 327 (1992) 1360–1365.

[402] S. Hirschfeld, et al., Thyroid abnormalities in children infected with human immunodeficiency virus, J. Pediatr. 128 (1996) 70–74.

[403] M. Papiernik, et al., Thymic abnormalities in fetuses aborted from human immunodeficiency virus type 1 seropositive women, Pediatrics 89 (1992) 297–301.

[404] V.V. Joshi, et al., Thymus biopsy in children with acquired immunodeficiency syndrome, Arch. Pathol. Med. 110 (1986) 837–842.

[405] S. Sei, et al., Quantitative analysis of viral burden in tissues from adults and children with symptomatic human immunodeficiency virus type 1 infection assessed by polymerase chain reaction, J. Infect. Dis. 170 (1994) 325–333.

[406] G. Pantaleo, et al., Evolutionary pattern of human immunodeficiency virus (HIV) replication and distribution in lymph nodes following primary infection: implications for antiviral therapy, Nat. Med. 4 (1998) 341–345.

[407] G. Pantaleo, A.S. Fauci, HIV-1 infection in the lymphoid organs: a model of disease development, J. Natl. Inst. Health Res 5 (1993) 68–72.

[408] B.U. Mueller, et al., Comparison of virus burden in blood and sequential lymph node biopsy specimens from children infected with human immunodeficiency virus, J. Pediatr. 129 (1996) 410–418.

[409] G.B. Scott, et al., Acquired immunodeficiency syndrome in infants, N. Engl. J. Med. 310 (1984) 76–81.

[410] M. Ellaurie, E.R. Burns, A. Rubinstein, Hematologic manifestations in pediatric HIV infection: severe anemia as a prognostic factor, Am. J. Pediatr. Hematol. Oncol. 12 (1990) 449–453.

[411] B.U. Mueller, Hematological problems and their management in children with HIV infection, in: P.A. Pizzo, C.A. Wilfert (Eds.), Pediatric AIDS. The Challenge of HIV Infection in Infants, Children, and Adolescents, Williams & Wilkins, Baltimore, 1994, pp. 591–602.

[412] B.W. Forsyth, W.A. Andiman, T. O'Connor, Development of a prognosis-based clinical staging system for infants infected with human immunodeficiency virus, J. Pediatr. 129 (1996) 648–655.

[413] B.U. Mueller, S. Tannenbaum, P.A. Pizzo, Bone marrow aspirates and biopsies in children with human immunodeficiency virus infection, J. Pediatr. Hematol. Oncol. 18 (1996) 266–271.

[414] L. Parmentier, D. Boucary, D. Salmon, Pure red cell aplasia in an HIV-infected patient, AIDS 6 (1992) 234–235.

[415] G. Nigro, et al., Parvovirus-B19-related pancytopenia in children with HIV infection, Lancet 340 (1992) 115.

[416] J.L. Abkowitz, et al., Clinical relevance of parvovirus B19 as a cause of anemia in patients with human immunodeficiency virus infection, J. Infect. Dis. 176 (1997) 269–273.

[417] M. Holodniy, et al., Quantitative relationship between platelet count and plasma virion HIV RNA, AIDS 10 (1996) 232–233.

[418] P.J. Ballem, et al., Kinetic studies of the mechanism of thrombocytopenia in patients with human immunodeficiency virus infection, N. Engl. J. Med. 327 (1992) 1779–1789.

[419] M. Rigaud, et al., Thrombocytopenia in children infected with human immunodeficiency virus: long-term follow-up and therapeutic considerations, J. Acquir. Immune Syndr. 5 (1992) 450–455.

[420] N. Abuaf, et al., Autoantibodies to phospholipids and the coagulation proteins in AIDS, Thromb. Haemost. 77 (1997) 856–861.

[421] M. Sorice, et al., Protein S and HIV infection: the role of anticardiolipin and anti-protein S antibodies, Thromb. Res. 73 (1994) 165–175.

[422] M. Rodriguez-Mahou, et al., Autoimmune phenomena in children with human immunodeficiency virus infection and acquired immunodeficiency syndrome, Acta Paediatr. Suppl. 400 (1994) 31–34.

[423] S.A. Coopman, et al., Cutaneous disease and drug reactions in HIV infection, N. Engl. J. Med. 328 (1993) 1670–1674.

[424] N.S. Prose, Skin problems, in: P.A. Pizzo, C.A. Wilfert (Eds.), Pediatric AIDS. The Challenge of HIV Infection in Infants, Children, and Adolescents, Williams & Wilkins, Baltimore, 1994, pp. 535–546.

[425] L. von Seidlein, et al., Frequent recurrence and persistence of varicella-zoster virus infections in children infected with human immunodeficiency virus type 1, J. Pediatr. 128 (1996) 52–57.

[426] B.U. Mueller, Cancers in human immunodeficiency virus-infected children, J. Natl. Cancer Inst. Monogr. 23 (1998) 31–35.

[427] G.P. Siskin, et al., AIDS-related lymphoma: radiologic features in pediatric patients, Radiology 196 (1995) 63–66.

[428] D. Nadal, et al., Non-Hodgkin's lymphoma in four children infected with the human immunodeficiency virus, Cancer 73 (1994) 224–230.

[429] M.O. Granovsky, et al., HIV-associated tumors in children: a case series from the Children's Cancer Group and National Cancer Institute, J Clin Oncol. 16 (1998) 1729–1735.

[430] E. Connor, et al., Cutaneous acquired immunodeficiency syndrome-associated Kaposi's sarcoma in pediatric patients, Arch. Dermatol. 126 (1990) 791–793.

[431] B.E. Buck, et al., Kaposi sarcoma in two infants with acquired immune deficiency syndrome, J. Pediatr. 103 (1983) 911–913.

[432] P. Gutierrez-Ortega, et al., Kaposi's sarcoma in a 6-day-old infant with human immunodeficiency virus, Arch. Dermatol. 125 (1989) 432–433.

[433] K.L. McClain, et al., Association of Epstein-Barr virus with leiomyosarcomas in young people with AIDS, N. Engl. J. Med. 332 (1995) 12–18.

[434] H.B. Jenson, et al., Benign and malignant smooth muscle tumors containing Epstein-Barr virus in children with AIDS, J. Acquir. Immune Defic. Syndr. Hum. Retrovirol. 14 (1997) A49.

[435] F.J. Palella, et al., Declining morbidity and mortality among patients with advanced human immunodeficiency virus infection, N. Engl. J. Med. 338 (1998) 853–860.

[436] S.S. Jean, et al., Clinical manifestations of human immunodeficiency virus infection in Haitian children, Pediatr. Infect. Dis. J. 16 (1997) 600–606.

[437] L. Gray, et al., Fluctuations in symptoms in human immunodeficiency virus-infected children: the first 10 years of life, Pediatrics 108 (2001) 116–122.

[438] T. Frederick, et al., Progression of human immunodeficiency virus disease among infants and children infected perinatally with human immunodeficiency virus or through neonatal blood transfusion, Pediatr. Infect. Dis. J. 13 (1994) 1091–1097.

[439] G. Lambert, et al., Effect of maternal CD4+ cell count, acquired immunodeficiency syndrome, and viral load on disease progression in infants with perinatally acquired human immunodeficiency virus type 1 infection, J. Pediatr. 130 (1997) 890–897.

[440] E.J. Abrams, et al., Maternal health factors and early pediatric antiretroviral therapy influence the rate of perinatal HIV-1 disease progression in children, AIDS 17 (2003) 867–877.

[441] S. Blanche, et al., A prospective study of infants born to women seropositive for human immunodeficiency virus type 1, N. Engl. J. Med. 320 (1989) 1643–1648.

[442] M.J. Mayaux, et al., Neonatal characteristics in rapidly progressive perinatally acquired HIV-1 disease, JAMA 275 (1996) 606–610.

[443] D. Zaknun, et al., Correlation of ribonucleic acid polymerase chain reaction, acid dissociated p24 antigen, and neopterin with progression of disease, J. Pediatr. 130 (1997) 898–905.

[444] R.E. Dickover, et al., Early prognostic indicators in primary perinatal human immunodeficiency virus type 1 infection: importance of viral RNA and the timing of transmission on long-term outcome, J. Infect. Dis. 178 (1998) 375–387.

[445] Centers for Disease Control and Prevention, Recommendations for assisting in the prevention of perinatal transmission of human T-lymphotrophic virus type III/lymphadenopathy-associated virus and acquired immunodeficiency, MMWR Morb. Mortal. Wkly Rep. 34 (1985) 721–732.

[446] E.M. Connor, et al., Reduction of maternal-infant transmission of immunodeficiency virus type 1 with zidovudine treatment, N. Engl. J. Med. 331 (1994) 1173–1180.

[447] E.M. Connor, L.K. Mofenson, Zidovudine for the reduction of perinatal human immunodeficiency virus transmission. Pediatric AIDS Clinical Trials Group protocol 076—results and treatment recommendations, Pediatr. Infect. Dis. J. 14 (1995) 536–541.

[448] Institute of Medicine, National Research Council, Reducing the Odds: Preventing Perinatal Transmission of HIV in the United States, National Academy Press, Washington, DC, 1999.

[449] Centers for Disease Control and Prevention, Revised guidelines for HIV counseling, testing, and referral and revised recommendations for HIV screening of pregnant women, MMWR Morb. Mortal. Wkly Rep. 50 (RR-19) (2001) 1–110.

[450] L. Mandelbrot, et al., Lamivudine-zidovudine combination for prevention of maternal-infant transmission of HIV-1, JAMA 285 (2001) 2083–2093.

[451] P. Chaisilwattana, et al., Short-course therapy with zidovudine plus lamivudine for prevention of mother-to-child transmission of human immunodeficiency virus type 1 in Thailand, Clin. Infect. Dis. 335 (2002) 1405–1413.

[452] A.D. Bardeguez, et al., Effect of cessation of zidovudine prophylaxis to reduce vertical transmission on maternal HIV disease progression and survival, J. Acquir. Immune Defic. Syndr. 32 (2003) 170–181.

[453] N.A. Wade, et al., Abbreviated regimens of zidovudine prophylaxis and perinatal transmission of the human immunodeficiency virus, N. Engl. J. Med. 339 (1998) 1409–1414.

[454] J. Read, M.K. Newell, Efficacy and safety of cesarean delivery for prevention of mother-to-child transmission of HIV-1, Cochrane Database Syst. Rev. 4 (2005) CD005479.

[455] J.S. Read, American Academy of Pediatrics, Committee on Pediatric AIDS. Human milk, breastfeeding, and transmission of human immunodeficiency virus type1 in the United States, Pediatrics 112 (2003) 1196–1205.

[456] L.M. Mofenson, Successes and challenges in the perinatal HIV-1 epidemic in the United States as illustrated by the HIV-1 serosurvey of childbearing women, Arch. Pediatr. Adolesc. Med. 158 (2004) 422–425.

[457] M. Bulterys, et al., Rapid HIV-1 testing during labor: a multicenter study, JAMA 292 (2004) 219–233.

[458] C.M. Wilfert, J.S. Stringer, Prevention of pediatric human immunodeficiency virus, Semin. Pediatr. Infect. Dis. 15 (2004) 190–198.

[459] N. Shaffer, et al., Short-course zidovudine for perinatal HIV-1 transmission in Bangkok, Thailand: a randomized controlled trial, Lancet 353 (1999) 773–780.

[460] S.Z. Wiktor, et al., Short-course zidovudine for prevention of mother-to-child transmission of HIV-1 in Abidjan, Cote d'Ivoire: a randomized trial, Lancet 353 (1999) 781–785.

[461] F. Dabis, et al., 6-month efficacy, tolerance, and acceptability of a short regimen of oral zidovudine to reduce transmission of HIV in breastfed children in Cote d'Ivoire and Burkina Faso: a double-blind placebo-controlled multicentre trial, Lancet 353 (1999) 786–792.

[462] M. Lallemant, et al., A trial of shortened zidovudine regimens to prevent mother-to-child transmission of human immunodeficiency virus type 1, N. Engl. J. Med. 343 (2000) 982–991.

[463] V. Leroy, et al., Twenty-four month efficacy of a maternal short-course zidovudine regimen to prevent mother to child transmission of HIV-1 in West Africa, AIDS 16 (2002) 631–641.

[464] L. Mandelbrot, et al., Lamivudine-zidovudine combination for prevention of maternal-infant transmission of HIV-1, JAMA 285 (2001) 2083–2093.

[465] P. Chaisilwattana, et al., Short-course therapy with zidovudine plus lamivudine for prevention of mother-to-child transmission of human immunodeficiency virus type 1 in Thailand, Clin. Infect. Dis. 335 (2002) 1405–1413.

[466] PETRA Study Team, Efficacy of three short-course regimens of zidovudine and lamivudine in preventing early and late transmission of HIV-1 from mother to child in Tanzania, South Africa, and Uganda (Petra study): a randomised, double-blind, placebo-controlled trial, Lancet 359 (2002) 1178–1186.

[467] L.A. Guay, et al., Intrapartum and neonatal single-dose nevirapine compared with zidovudine for prevention of mother-to-child transmission of HIV-1 Kampala, Uganda: HIVNET 012 randomized trial, Lancet 354 (1999) 795–802.

[468] J.B. Jackson, et al., Intrapartum and neonatal single-dose nevirapine compared with zidovudine for prevention of mother-to-child transmission of HIV-1 Kampala, Uganda: 18 month follow-up of the HIVNET 012 randomized trial, Lancet 362 (2003) 859–868.

[469] M. Mirochnick, et al., Pharmacokinetics of nevirapine in human immunodeficiency virus type 1-infected pregnant women and their neonates, J. Infect. Dis. 178 (1998) 368–374.

[470] D. Moodley, et al., A multicenter randomized trial of nevirapine versus a combination of zidovudine and lamivudine to reduce intrapartum and early postpartum mother-to-child transmission of HIV-1, J. Infect. Dis. 187 (2003) 725–735.

[471] M. Lallemant, et al., Single-dose perinatal nevirapine plus standard zidovudine to prevent mother-to-child transmission of HIV-1 in Thailand, N. Engl. J. Med. 351 (2004) 217–228.

[472] F. Dabis, et al., Field efficacy of zidovudine, lamivudine and single-dose nevirapine to prevent peripartum HIV transmission, AIDS 19 (2005) 309–318.

[473] A. Dorenbaum, et al., Two-dose intrapartum/newborn nevirapine and standard antiretroviral therapy to reduce perinatal HIV transmission: a randomized trial, JAMA 288 (2002) 189–198.

[474] C.K. Cunningham, et al., Development of resistance mutations in women receiving standard antiretroviral therapy who received intrapartum nevirapine to prevent perinatal human immunodeficiency virus type 1 transmission. A substudy of Pediatric AIDS Clinical Trials Group Protocol 316, J. Infect. Dis. 186 (2002) 181–188.

[475] T.E. Taha, et al., Short postexposure prophylaxis in newborn babies to reduce mother-to-child transmission of HIV-1: NVAZ randomized clinical trial, Lancet 362 (2003) 1171–1177.

[476] T.E. Taha, N. Kumwenda, D.R. Hoover, Nevirapine and zidovudine at birth to reduce perinatal transmission of HIV in an African setting: a randomized controlled trial, JAMA 292 (2004) 202–209.

[477] World Health Organization, Antiretroviral Drugs for Treating Pregnant Women and Preventing HIV Infection in Infants in Resource-Limited Settings: Towards Universal Access. Recommendations for a Public Health Approach, World Health Organization, Geneva, 2009.

[478] R. Shapiro, et al., Infant morbidity, mortality, and breast milk immunologic profiles among breastfeeding HIV-infected and uninfected women in Botswana, J. Infect. Dis. 196 (2007) 562–569.

[479] World Health Organization. HIV and Infant Feeding, Revised principles and recommendations, World Health Organization, Geneva, 2009. Available at www.who.int (accessed June 16, 2010).

[480] L.M. Mofenson, et al., Antiretroviral prophylaxis to reduce breast milk transmission of HIV type 1: new data but still questions, J. Acquir. Immune Defic. Syndr. 48 (2008) 237–240.

[481] L.M. Mofenson, P. Munderi, Safety of antiretroviral prophylaxis of perinatal transmission for HIV-infected pregnant women and their infants, J. Acquir. Immune Defic. Syndr. 30 (2002) 200–215.

[482] R.S. Sperling, et al., Safety of the maternal-infant zidovudine utilized in the Pediatric AIDS Clinical Trial Group 076 Study, AIDS. 12 (1998) 1805–1813.

[483] M. Culnane, et al., Lack of long-term effects of in-utero exposure to zidovudine among uninfected children born to HIV-infected women, JAMA 281 (1999) 151–157.

[484] European Collaborative Study and the Swiss Mother + Child HIV Cohort Study, Combination antiretroviral therapy and duration of pregnancy, AIDS 14 (2000) 2913–2920.

[485] R.E. Tuomala, et al., Antiretroviral therapy during pregnancy and the risk of an adverse outcome, N. Engl. J. Med. 354 (2002) 1084–1089.

[486] Antiretroviral Pregnancy Registry Steering Committee, Antiretroviral Pregnancy Registry interim report for 1 January 1989 through 31 January 2002, Registry Coordinating Center, Wilmington, NC, 2002.

[487] S. Blanche, et al., Persistent mitochondrial dysfunction and perinatal exposure to antiretroviral nucleoside analogues, Lancet 354 (1999) 1084–1089.

[488] French Perinatal Study Group, Risk of early febrile seizure with perinatal exposure to nucleoside analogues, Lancet 359 (2002) 583–584.

[489] Perinatal Safety Review Working Group, Nucleoside exposure in the children of HIV-infected women receiving antiretroviral drugs: absence of clear evidence for mitochondrial disease in children who died before 5 years of age in five United States cohort, J. Acquir. Immune Defic. Syndr. 25 (2000) 261–268.

[490] European Collaborative Study, Exposure to antiretroviral therapy in utero or early life: the health of uninfected children born to HIV-infected women, J. Acquir. Immune Defic. Syndr. 32 (2003) 380–387.

[491] M. Nolan, M.G. Fowler, L.M. Mofenson, Antiretroviral prophylaxis of perinatal HIV-1 transmission and the potential impact of antiretroviral resistance, J. Acquir. Immune Defic. Syndr. 30 (2002) 216–229.

[492] Treat 3 Million by 2005 Initiative, Treating 3 million by 2005: making it happenthe WHO and UNAIDS global initiative to provide antiretroviral therapy to 3 million people with HIV/AIDS in developing countries by the end of 2005. Available at http://www.who.int/3by5/publications/documents/en/3by5StrategyMakingItHappen.pdf (accessed June 22, 2004).

[493] S.H. Eshleman, et al., Selection and fading of resistance mutations in women and infants receiving nevirapine to prevent HIV-1 vertical transmission (HIVNET 012), AIDS 15 (2001) 1951–1957.

[494] G. Jourdain, et al., Intrapartum exposure to nevirapine and subsequent maternal responses to nevirapine-based antiretroviral therapy, N. Engl. J. Med. 351 (2004) 229–240.

[495] H. Coovadia, Antiretroviral agents—how best to protect infants from HIV and save their mothers from AIDS, N. Engl. J. Med. 351 (2004) 289–292.

[496] S. Loubser, et al., Decay of K103N mutants in cellular DNA and plasma RNA after single-dose nevirapine to reduce mother-to-child HIV transmission, AIDS 20 (2006) 995–1002.

[497] S. Palmer, et al., Persistence of nevirapine-resistant HIV-1 in women after single-dose nevirapine therapy for prevention of maternal-to-fetal HIV-1 transmission, Proc. Natl. Acad. Sci. U. S. A. 103 (2006) 7094–7099.

[498] J.A. Johnson, et al., Emergence of drug-resistant HIV-1 after intrapartum administration of single-dose nevirapine is substantially underestimated, J. Infect. Dis. 192 (2005) 16–23.

[499] T. Flys, et al., Sensitive drug-resistance assays reveal long-term persistence of HIV-1 variants with the K103N nevirapine (NVP) resistance mutation in some women and infants after the administration of single-dose NVP. HIVNET 012, J. Infect. Dis. 192 (2005) 24–29.

[500] S.H. Eshleman, et al., Characterization of nevirapine resistance mutations in women with subtype A vs. D HIV-1 6-8 weeks after single-dose nevirapine (HIVNET 012), J. Acquir. Immune Defic. Syndr. 35 (2004) 126–130.

[501] H. Dao, et al., International recommendations on antiretroviral drugs for treatment of HIV infected women and prevention of mother-to-child HIV transmission in resource-limited settings: 2006 update, Am. J. Obstet. Gynecol. 197 (Suppl. 3) (2007) S42–S55.

[502] Centers for Disease Control and Prevention. Prevention of varicella: updated recommendations of the Advisory Committee on Immunization Practices. (ACIP), MMWR Recomm. Rep. 48 (RR-6) (1999) 1–5.

[503] National Institute of Child Health and Human Development Intravenous Immunoglobulin Study Group, Intravenous immune globulin for the prevention of bacterial infections in children with symptomatic human immunodeficiency virus infection, N. Engl. J. Med. 325 (1991) 73–80.

[504] Centers for Disease Control and Prevention. Treating opportunistic infections among HIV-exposed and infected children: recommendations from the CDC, the National Institutes of Health, and the Infectious Disease Society of America, MMWR Recomm. Rep. (RR-14) (2004) 1–92.

[505] M.S. McKellar, et al., Pediatric HIV infection: the state of antiretroviral therapy, Exp. Rev. Infect. Ther. 6 (2008) 167–180.

[506] E.J. Abrams, L. Kuhn, Should treatment be started among all HIV-infected children and then stopped? Lancet 362 (2003) 1595–1596.

[507] L. Gray, et al., Fluctuations in symptoms in human immunodeficiency virus-infected children: the first 10 years of life, Pediatrics 108 (2001) 116–122.

[508] C. Diaz, et al., Disease progression in a cohort of infants with vertically acquired HIV infection observed from birth. The Women and Infants Transmission Study (WITS), J. Acquir. Immune Defic. Syndr. Hum. Retrovirol. 18 (1998) 221–228.

[509] G.M. Anabwani, E.A. Woldetsadik, M.W. Kline, Treatment of human immunodeficiency virus (HIV) in children using antiretroviral drugs, Semin. Pediatr. Infect. Dis. 16 (2005) 116–124.

[510] K. Luzuriaga, et al., A trial of three antiretroviral regimens in HIV-1 infected children, N. Engl. J. Med. 350 (2004) 2471–2480.

[511] K. Luzuriaga, et al., Combination treatment with zidovudine, didanosine, and nevirapine in infants with human immunodeficiency virus type 1 infection, N. Engl. J. Med. 336 (1997) 1343–1349.

[512] M. Hainaut, et al., Effectiveness of antiretroviral therapy initiated before the age of 2 months in infants vertically infected with human immunodeficiency virus type 1, Eur. J. Pediatr. 159 (2000) 778–782.

[513] Working Group for Antiretroviral Therapy and Medical Management of HIV-Infected Children, Guidelines for the use of antiretroviral agents in pediatric HIV infection. Available at http://aidsinfo.nih.gov/contentfiles/PediatricGuidelines.pdf (accessed February 28, 2008).

[514] A. Violari, et al., Early antiretroviral therapy and mortality among HIV-infected infants, N. Eng. J. Med. 359 (2008) 2233–2244.

[515] A. Faye, et al., Early multitherapy including a protease inhibitor for human immunodeficiency virus type 1 infected infants, Pediatr. Infect. Dis. J. 21 (2002) 518–525.

[516] Paediatric European Network for Treatment of AIDS (PENTA), Highly active antiretroviral therapy started in infants under 3 months of age: 72 week follow-up for CD4 cell count, viral load and drug resistance outcome, AIDS 18 (2004) 237–245.

[517] C. Litalien, et al., Pharmacokinetics of nelfinavir and its active metabolite, hydroxyl-tert-butylamide, in infants less than 1 year old perinatally infected with HIV-1, Pediatr. Infect. Dis. J. 22 (2003) 48–56.

[518] L.V. Adams, The time to treat the children is now, J. Infect. Dis. 195 (2007) 1396–1398.

[519] D.W. Hoody, C.V. Fletcher, Pharmacology considerations for antiretroviral therapy in human immunodeficiency virus (HIV)-infected children, Semin. Pediatr. Infect. Dis. 14 (2003) 286–294.

[520] S. Lockman, et al., Response to antiretroviral therapy after a single, peripartum dose of nevirapine, N. Engl. J. Med. 356 (2007) 135–147.

[521] World Health Organization, Antiretroviral Therapy of HIV Infection in Infants and Children in Resource-Limited Settings: Towards Universal Access. Recommendations for a Public Health Approach, WHO, Geneva, 2006. Available at http://www.who.int/hiv/pub/guidelines/WHPpaediatric.pdf (accessed February 14, 2008).

[522] R.E. McKinney, C.K. Cunningham, Newer treatment for HIV in children, Curr. Opin. Pediatr. 16 (2004) 76–79.

[523] L.M. Mofenson, R. Becquet, Early antiretroviral therapy of HIV-infected infants in resource-limited countries: possible, feasible, effective and challenging, AIDS 22 (2008) 1365–1368.

[524] E. George, et al., Early response to highly active antiretroviral therapy in HIV-1 infected Kenyan children, J. Acquir. Immune Defic. Syndr. 45 (2007) 311–317.

[525] C. Bolton-Moore, et al., Clinical outcomes and CD4-cell response in children receiving antiretroviral therapy at primary healthcare facilities in Zambia, JAMA 298 (2007) 1888–1899.

[526] A. Prendergast, et al., Early virologic suppression with three-class antiretroviral therapy in HIV-infected African infants, AIDS 22 (2008) 1333–1343.

[527] E. George, et al., Antiretroviral therapy for HIV-1 infected children in Haiti, J. Infect. Dis. 195 (2007) 1411–1418.

[528] B. Janssens, et al., Effectiveness of highly active antiretroviral therapy in HIV-positive children: evaluation at 12 months in a routine program in Cambodia, Pediatrics 120 (2007) e1134–e1140.

[529] P.L. Havens, B.E. Cuene, D.R. Holtgrave, Lifetime cost of care for children with human immunodeficiency virus infection, Pediatr. Infect. Dis. J. 16 (1997) 607–610.

CHICKENPOX, MEASLES, AND MUMPS

Anne A. Gershon

CHAPTER OUTLINE

Chickenpox and Zoster   661
    Organism   662
    Epidemiology and Transmission   662
    Pathogenesis of Varicella and Zoster   666
    Pathology   667
    Clinical Manifestations   668
    Diagnosis and Differential Diagnosis   678
    Therapy   679
    Prevention   680
Measles   685
    Organism   685
    Transmission and Epidemiology   686
    Pathogenesis   686
    Pathology   687

Clinical Manifestations   688
Diagnosis and Differential Diagnosis   692
Therapy   693
Prevention   693
Mumps   695
    Organism   695
    Epidemiology and Transmission   695
    Pathogenesis   696
    Pathology   696
    Clinical Manifestations   696
    Diagnosis and Differential Diagnosis   698
    Therapy   698
    Prevention   698

The viruses that cause varicella, zoster, measles, and mumps may complicate the management of a mother, fetus, or newborn when maternal infection with one of these agents occurs during pregnancy or at term. In the United States, most women of childbearing years are immune to measles and mumps, and there is little opportunity for exposure to these infections because the current population is highly immunized. These diseases posed more problems during pregnancy during the first half of the 20th century than they do now.

Because a licensed varicella vaccine has routinely been used in the United States since 1995, the incidence of varicella among women of childbearing age has also declined owing to personal and herd immunity with decreased transmission of virus. Varicella-zoster virus (VZV) may still inflict significant fetal damage as the cause of congenital varicella syndrome, especially in locations where the vaccine is not being used. Improved methods for control, including better diagnostic methods, antiviral therapy with acyclovir, passive immunization with varicella-zoster immunoglobulin (VZIG), and use of live-attenuated varicella vaccine, have decreased prenatal and postnatal morbidity from this virus, however. Understanding of this viral infection at the molecular level including clarification of the cause of zoster by studies of viral DNA, RNA, and proteins in latency and study of specific viral glycoproteins and their importance in the immune response have advanced our knowledge and can be expected to lead to further improved therapeutic modalities.

CHICKENPOX AND ZOSTER

Chickenpox (i.e., varicella) is an acute, highly contagious disease that most commonly occurs in childhood. It is characterized by a generalized exanthem consisting of vesicles that develop in successive crops and that rapidly evolve to pustules, crusts, and scabs. Zoster (i.e., herpes zoster, shingles) occurs in persons who have previously had chickenpox. It is typified by a painful or pruritic (or both) vesicular eruption usually restricted to one or more segmental dermatomes. An abundance of virologic, epidemiologic, and immunologic evidence has been amassed indicating that these two illnesses are caused by the same etiologic agent [1], which was designated VZV. Chickenpox is a manifestation of primary infection with VZV. After the acute infection subsides, VZV, similar to other herpesviruses, persists in a latent form. For VZV, the site of latent infection is in the dorsal root and cranial nerve ganglia and intestinal ganglia where certain early viral genes and proteins are expressed in latency [2–5]. VZV may subsequently be reactivated with expression of all of its genes as immunity wanes with time. The reactivated infection assumes the segmental distribution of the nerve cells in which latent virus resided, giving rise to zoster. A description of the historical recognition of disease caused by VZV follows.

Varicella is a modernized Latin word used since at least 1764 and intended to connote a diminutive of the more serious variola (i.e., smallpox) [6]. The etymology of "chicken" in chickenpox is less clear. It may also be a diminutive derived from the French *pois chiche*, or "chick pea," a dwarf species of pea (*Cicer arietinum*) [6]. Other authors doubt this Latin origin and conjecture that the word originated from the farmyard fowl, in which case it has a Teutonic ancestry in the Old English *cicen* and the Middle High German *kuchen* [7]. *Herpes* has been used to designate a malady since 1398 ("this euyll callyd Herpes") [8] and derives from the Greek word meaning "to creep"; *zoster* is the Greek and Latin word meaning "girdle" or "belt." Shingles, from the Latin *cingulus* (meaning "girdle"), was also used in the 14th century as *schingles* to describe "icchynge and scabs wett and drye" [8].

ORGANISM
Classification and Morphology

VZV (Herpesvirus varicellae) is a member of the herpesvirus family. In addition to a burgeoning number of animal herpesviruses, this group includes seven additional, closely related viruses that infect humans: herpes simplex viruses (HSV) types 1 and 2 (Herpesvirus hominis), cytomegalovirus (CMV), Epstein-Barr virus, and human herpesviruses 6, 7, and 8. Only one antigenic type of VZV has been identified, but molecular studies have revealed some minor differences in VZV that have proved useful for epidemiologic studies [9,10].

Common properties of the family include a DNA genome and enveloped virions exhibiting icosahedral symmetry with a diameter of 180 to 200 nm [1]. Nucleocapsids, which are assembled in the nucleus, have a diameter of about 100 nm and consist of a DNA core surrounded by 162 identical subunits, or capsomeres. Nucleocapsids acquire a temporary envelope at the nuclear membrane; they are transported further via the endoplasmic reticulum to the Golgi, where they receive a final envelope. In cell cultures, virions are packaged in vesicles identified as endosomes, which are acidic [11,12]. Virus particles are released from these structures at the cell surface by exocytosis. Extracellular virions are extremely pleomorphic compared with virions of HSV. This pleomorphism, presumably reflecting injury to the envelope possibly caused by exposure to acid or enzymes in endosomes, is believed to account for the lability and lack of cell-free virus that characterizes VZV in tissue culture and in its spread through the body during varicella infection, and it distinguishes VZV from HSV [11–13]. In vivo, enveloped and well-formed VZV is released from cells of the superficial epidermis (strateum corneum), yielding highly infectious virions capable of airborne spread and with a great degree of communicability [14].

Molecular studies have elucidated some details concerning how latent VZV infection is established, maintained, and reactivated. Latent infection probably comes from virions present in skin during varicella. It is unlikely, however, that complete viral replication occurs in the neuron during establishment of latency because the neuron must survive, and replication would be expected to cause cell death. The replication process of VZV is begun during latent infection, but a block in the cascade of viral gene expression probably occurs. About six viral genes and their protein gene products are expressed in latently infected neurons. These proteins are confined to the cell cytoplasm. It seems that when these proteins are transduced into the nucleus by factors still to be determined, reactivation occurs, with formation of all 70 VZV gene products and synthesis of infectious, enveloped virions in the nerve and skin [4].

Propagation

VZV grows readily in diploid human fibroblasts such as WI 38 cells, the most commonly used cell type for virus isolation. VZV also can be propagated in certain epithelial cells, such as human embryonic kidney, primary human amnion cells, primary human thyroid cells, and Vero (African green monkey kidney) cells. Similar to CMV, the cytopathic effect of VZV is focal in cell culture because of its cell-associated character, and cytopathic effects develop more slowly (3 to 7 days) than with HSV. Animal models for varicella (guinea pigs) [15] and for zoster (rats) [16] have been described. An in vitro model of latency and reactivation in guinea pig enteric neurons has also been developed and provides a setting in which to study factors that influence latency and reactivation [4].

Serologic Tests and Antigenic Properties of Varicella-Zoster Virus

Several serologic tests are available to measure antibodies to VZV, including indirect immunofluorescence, often called fluorescent antibody to membrane antigen (FAMA) [17,18]; latex agglutination [19]; enzyme-linked immunosorbent assay (ELISA) [20–23]; radioimmunoassay [24]; immune adherence hemagglutination [25]; neutralization [20,26]; and complement-enhanced neutralization [27]. All of these methods are more sensitive than the complement fixation assay [28]. Data gathered from these assays show that antibody to VZV develops within a few days after the onset of varicella, persists for many years, and is present before the onset of zoster.

Serologic cross-reactions between HSV and VZV have been described [29,30]. HSV and VZV share common antigens, and similar polypeptides and glycoproteins have been identified for both viruses, but cross-protection has not been observed [31–33]. Rare simultaneous infections with one or more human herpesviruses have been reported [34,35]. Elevations in heterologous antibody titers in apparent HSV or VZV infections may result from cross-reactions of the viruses, but also may indicate simultaneous infection by both viruses.

VZV produces at least eight major glycoprotein antigens—B, C, E, H, I, K, L, and M—all of which are on the envelope of the virus and on the surface of infected cells. The glycoproteins and internal antigens, such as the capsid and tegument, stimulate production of neutralizing and other types of antibodies and cellular immunity [36–38]. The most prominent glycoprotein of VZV is glycoprotein E. Antibodies elaborated in varicella and zoster are of the IgG, IgA, and IgM classes [39,40].

EPIDEMIOLOGY AND TRANSMISSION

Chickenpox ranks as one of the most communicable of human diseases. No extrahuman reservoir of VZV is known. Because the supply of susceptible persons, especially in the era before the urbanization of society, would be rapidly exhausted by so contagious a disease, virus latency may have adaptive evolutionary significance in perpetuating infection. In isolated communities, cases of zoster would be responsible for the reintroduction of VZV and its transmission as varicella to new generations of susceptible individuals [1,41].

Communicability by Droplets and Contact

Historically, transfer of VZV was believed to occur via respiratory droplets, and epidemiologic evidence suggests that transmission can occur before the onset of rash [42–44]. It is rare, however, to isolate VZV from the pharynx of infected patients. A study using polymerase chain reaction (PCR) methods showed that VZV DNA is present in the nasopharynx of a high percentage of children during the early stages of clinical varicella [45], but PCR does not indicate the presence of infectious virus. In contrast, the vesicular lesions in varicella and zoster are full of infectious VZV that can readily be cultured. In a study of leukemic recipients of live-attenuated varicella vaccine, only individuals with skin lesions as a side effect of varicella vaccination spread vaccine-type virus to varicella-susceptible close contacts [46]. Similarly, the rare instances of transmission of vaccine virus from healthy vaccinees to other susceptible individuals occurred only when the vaccinee had a rash [47]. Cell-free VZV virions are known to be copiously produced in skin lesions and are the type of particle that could be aerosolized and involved in viral transmission. The major source of infectious VZV seems to be the skin, although it is possible that transmission from the respiratory tract can also occur.

Airborne spread of varicella has been documented [48,49], but indirect transfer by fomites has not. VZV DNA has been detected in air samples for many hours in hospitals [50], but the relationship to infectivity of the virus is unclear. Varicella is most contagious at the time of onset of rash and for 1 to 2 days afterward [51], but the period of infectivity probably encompasses 1 to 2 days before the rash is noticed until 5 days after onset of the rash.

Incubation Period

The usual incubation period for chickenpox is 13 to 17 days (mean 15 days). The range is 10 to 21 days, unless passive immunization has been given, in which case the incubation period may be prolonged [44,52].

Relationship between Varicella and Zoster

It is amply documented that exposure of susceptible persons to zoster may result in chickenpox. Vesicular fluid from patients with zoster produced chickenpox when inoculated into susceptible children [53,54]. Other studies have confirmed that a similar relationship exists under conditions of natural exposure [55]. Claims to the contrary notwithstanding [56,57], it has not been documented that zoster is acquired from other patients with zoster or chickenpox. Instances that have been reported do not exclude the chance sporadic occurrence of zoster in persons who happen to have been exposed to chickenpox or zoster. It is difficult to reconcile this postulated mode of transmission with current concepts of the pathogenesis of zoster, particularly the strict segmental distribution of lesions and the demonstrated presence of VZV DNA, RNA, and certain viral proteins in ganglia during latency [2,3,58]. Studies have also determined that VZV DNA from zoster isolates is identical to that which caused the primary infection, proving that zoster is caused by reactivation of latent VZV [59–61].

Transplacental Transmission

In pregnancy, VZV may be transmitted across the placenta, resulting in congenital or neonatal chickenpox [62]. The consequences of transplacental infection are discussed in a later section.

Incidence and Distribution of Chickenpox

There is worldwide distribution of chickenpox. Because vaccination is now routine for children in the United States, significant changes in the epidemiology of varicella have occurred, with evidence of personal and herd immunity [63]. Before the vaccine era in the United States, which began in 1995 with vaccine licensure, outbreaks of varicella occurred each year without major fluctuations between years [64]. Although the disease was seen in all months, more cases occurred in the winter and early spring. This seasonal variation was attributed primarily to the gathering of children in school, but also may be related to changes in environmental temperature. With introduction of the vaccine, there is less varicella disease occurring in all age groups, and the seasonality of the disease is blurred [63].

Chickenpox is more contagious than mumps, but less so than measles [5,65]. After exposure within households, 61% of susceptible persons of all age groups (without a history of previous disease) developed chickenpox compared with 76% for measles and 31% for mumps [52]. Compared with measles, chickenpox is about 80% as infectious in the household, but only 35% to 65% as infectious in society. The reason probably is that chickenpox requires relatively intimate contact for transmission, such as that occurring in the household, whereas in society, there are more casual contacts. Measles may infect efficiently even through casual contacts [65].

An estimated 4 million cases of chickenpox used to occur annually in the United States. Varicella remains a nonreportable disease, but this is expected to change as more and more vaccine is used, and there are fewer and fewer cases of varicella each year. The disease affects both sexes equally and is most commonly seen in children of early school age. Increasing urbanization was associated with acquisition of the disease at younger ages. In Massachusetts from 1952–1961, 29% of children reported with chickenpox were younger than 4 years old, 62% were 5 to 9 years old, 7% were 10 to 14 years old, and less than 3% were older than 15 years old [66]. Later data also indicated that varicella is primarily a disease of young children [67]. A history of varicella is reported by 70% to 80% of young American adults [66,68]. This compares with histories in the same age group in the prevaccine era of 92% for measles, 45% for mumps, and 31% for rubella. Subclinical varicella is uncommon. Data from family studies indicate that only 8% of adults without a history of varicella develop clinical disease when exposed to their own infected children [69]. The relative importance of faulty memory or past subclinical infection in this secondary attack rate is uncertain.

With the use of sensitive assays for the measurement of antibodies to VZV, less than 25% of adults with no history of chickenpox seem to be susceptible [70]. Based on a population of adults in which 90% are immune, this finding suggests a subclinical attack rate of varicella of approximately 7%.

Incidence of Chickenpox, Mumps, and Measles in Pregnancy

Only a few studies have addressed the incidence of chickenpox, mumps, and measles during pregnancy. In these studies, two questions are posed. First, of all pregnancies, how many are complicated by measles, mumps, or chickenpox? Second, among all reported cases of those diseases, how many occur in pregnant women? In a prospective study of clinically recognized infections that occurred during 30,059 pregnancies in 1958–1964, approximately 1600 women with presumed measles, varicella, and mumps were identified [71]. Taking into account the many possible inaccuracies in such a study, the minimum frequency per 10,000 pregnancies was 0.6 case for measles, 5 cases for varicella, and 10 cases for mumps. In another study of maternal virus diseases in New York City in 1957–1964, Siegel and Fuerst [72] followed pregnant women: 417 were infected with rubella (50.5%), 150 with chickenpox (18.1%), 128 with mumps (15.5%), and 66 with measles (8%).

The data in these studies are undoubtedly flawed because of lack of proven diagnoses and, more importantly, reflect findings in the prevaccine era and cannot be considered as representative today. Today, measles and mumps are rare in the United States, and varicella is becoming less and less common. In highly immunized populations such as exist in the United States, an even lower incidence of infection during pregnancy is predicted for measles, mumps, and varicella. It is possible that the incidence of varicella in pregnant women in the United States is affected by the influx of varicella-susceptible immigrants from countries with tropical climates. A calculation in 1992 projected an incidence of 7 cases of varicella per 10,000 pregnancies, the same as reported earlier in the prevaccine era [73] Given the success of their vaccines, however, one assumes that varicella, mumps, and measles all are now unusual during pregnancy.

Incidence and Distribution of Zoster

In contrast to chickenpox, zoster is primarily a disease of adults, especially older adults or immunosuppressed patients. Hope-Simpson [41], describing patients of all ages in a general practice observed during a 16-year period, found an incidence of 3.4 cases per 1000 otherwise healthy people per year.

Adults and children older than 2 years who have zoster usually give a history of a previous attack of varicella; in younger infants, a history of intrauterine exposure to VZV can often be elicited [41]. The latency period between primary infection and zoster is shorter if varicella occurs in prenatal rather than in postnatal life [74]. Chickenpox in the 1st year of life also increases the risk of childhood zoster, with a relative risk roughly between 3 and 21 [75,76]. Possibly, this phenomenon is caused by immaturity of the immune response to chickenpox in young infants, permitting early viral reactivation [77].

After infancy, the incidence of zoster increases progressively with age. The attack rate in octogenarians was 14 times that of children in the series by Hope-Simpson [41]. Second attacks of zoster are unusual; 8 were

observed in 192 cases in the previously cited series [41]. Four of those attacks involved the same dermatome as the first attack, suggesting a tendency for reactivation of VZV from the same ganglion cells in which the virus was dormant. Some of these cases might have been caused by reactivation of HSV, however; in one study, HSV was isolated from 13% of a series of 47 immunocompetent patients with clinically diagnosed zoster [78]. Zoster in adults and children occurs with increased frequency in patients with malignant hematopoietic neoplasms (especially Hodgkin disease), patients after organ transplantation, and patients infected with human immunodeficiency virus (HIV) [79–81]. Spinal trauma, irradiation, and corticosteroid therapy may also be precipitating factors. The distribution of lesions in chickenpox, which primarily affects the trunk, head, and neck, is reflected in a proportionately greater representation of these regions in the segmental lesions of zoster [41].

Incidence of Zoster in Pregnancy

More recent studies on the incidence of zoster in pregnancy are lacking. Brazin and associates [82] projected an incidence of 6000 cases annually in pregnant women, which suggests that gestational zoster might be more common than gestational chickenpox, particularly in the vaccine era. Assuming that there are 3.5 million pregnant women yearly in the United States, this calculates to a rate of 20 cases per 10,000 pregnant women per year. Nevertheless, zoster, similar to varicella, seems to be rare or uncommon in pregnancy. The severity or natural history of zoster does not seem to be worse in pregnant women than in the population at large. Implications of gestational zoster for the fetus are discussed in a subsequent section.

Nosocomial Chickenpox in the Nursery

The precise risk of horizontal transmission in maternity wards or the newborn nursery after VZV has been introduced is unclear, but based on experience, it is very low. This low risk is in part because maternal immunity plays a role in protection of the infant. About 70% of persons give a history of chickenpox by age 20 years, and still others are immune in the absence of a positive history, so that most mothers and hospital personnel are not at risk. Many hospital workers require proof of immunity to varicella (or vaccination) for employment. Only 5% to 10% of women born in the United States seem to be susceptible to varicella, and more than 75% of women with no history of chickenpox seem to be immune [70,83–86]. The percentage of susceptible women among persons raised in tropical climates is higher, probably because viral spread is impeded by high temperatures and the lack of urbanization [83,87–90].

Because IgG antibodies to VZV cross the placenta [83,91], full-term newborns of immune mothers should be at least partially protected from chickenpox. Using the sensitive FAMA assay to measure antibodies to VZV, in a study of 67 infants during the 1st year of life, 50% still had detectable VZV antibodies by age 5 months [83]. Even in premature infants and infants with low birth weight, antibodies to VZV are likely to be detectable [92–94]. Nevertheless, perinatal chickenpox has been reported rarely in infants born to women with positive histories of chickenpox [95–99]. In the study by Newman [98], varicella developed in a mother and her infant after exposure to a student midwife with chickenpox. The mother had experienced varicella as a child and had a few remaining skin scars; apparently, she had developed a second attack as an adult. Readett and McGibbon [99] reported two cases of extrauterine infection in neonates whose mothers had histories of chickenpox. After delivery at home, each of these infants was exposed within 24 hours of birth to a sibling with chickenpox and subsequently developed skin lesions when 12 and 14 days old. Their mothers did not develop chickenpox in the perinatal period and were found to have serum-neutralizing antibodies to VZV.

In the literature before 1975, VZV antibody titers were not often reported because sensitive tests for measuring these antibodies were not readily available. Since that time, infection of a few seropositive infants after postnatal exposure to VZV has been documented [95,96]. These infants had mothers with a history of varicella, and the VZV antibody in the infants' blood was transplacentally acquired. In one instance, mild varicella developed in a 2-week-old, 1040-g infant who was seropositive at exposure and was passively immunized with VZIG 72 hours after the exposure [96]. In another study, five infants younger than 2 months old, all of whom were seropositive at exposure, developed varicella in a children's custodial institution [95]. Even when varicella develops in the presence of maternal antibodies, it seems to be modified. Although complete protection of every neonate against chickenpox is not guaranteed by immunity in the mother, protection is the exception rather than the rule.

Horizontal transmission of chickenpox in maternity wards and newborn nurseries is uncommon. In some reports, lack of transmission is difficult to explain. In 1965, Newman [98] reported two cases of varicella that occurred in mothers in the same prenatal ward 18 to 19 days after exposure to the index-infected infant and its mother. One mother developed chickenpox 7 days antepartum, and the other developed the disease 3 days postpartum. Each mother was immediately isolated from the ward, but not from her own infant; neither of the infants developed chickenpox. In all, 139 mothers, excluding the index case, were exposed, and 8 developed infection. Three of 42 staff members also became infected. The index infant was the only neonate infected; all other infants, including those born to the eight infected mothers, remained free of disease. Gershon and coworkers [83] described an outbreak in which a woman developed varicella postpartum and exposed 10 mothers and their infants, 1 antepartum woman, and approximately 25 staff members during a brief period while she was waiting in the hospital corridor. Her infant developed varicella 10 days afterward. About 2 weeks later, three cases of varicella developed in the exposed persons: a hospital employee and a postpartum woman and her infant. Gustafson and colleagues [96] described another mini-outbreak that occurred during a 2-month period in a neonatal intensive care unit in which 29 infants were exposed.

Two of these infants, whose mothers gave a history of previous varicella, developed chickenpox after exposure to two hospital employees who had been infected nosocomially.

Other reports largely confirm the low rate of transmissibility of chickenpox in neonates. Freud [100] described an infant who had transplacentally acquired disease and developed lesions on the 2nd day of life. None of the other 17 neonates in the nursery became infected, but the index infant had been isolated immediately, so exposure had been very brief. When transferred to another ward, this same infant transmitted the disease to two older children, who were 4 and 7 years old. Odessky and associates [101] reported three instances of congenital varicella: Two infants were immediately isolated, but the third was not recognized as having chickenpox and exposed other neonates for 4 days. The number at risk is not stated, but no instances of transmission were observed. In a report by Harris [102], 35 infants were exposed to 2 infants with congenital chickenpox for periods of 18 and 10 hours before isolation. None subsequently became infected, possibly because all the mothers had positive histories of chickenpox. In an additional case described by Matseoane and Abler [103], an infant developed transplacentally acquired chickenpox at 9 days of age and exposed 13 other neonates in the nursery for periods of 2 to 10 hours before isolation. Six mothers had a positive history of varicella, three did not, and four did not know. None of the exposed mothers or infants developed chickenpox. Lack of transmission despite hospital exposure to an adult with varicella in neonatal intensive care nurseries was also reported by Wang and associates [94] (32 infants), Lipton and Brunell [104] (22 infants), Patou and coworkers [105] (15 infants), Mendez and associates [92] (16 infants), and Gold and coworkers [106] (29 infants).

One experience in a neonatal intensive care unit in Mississippi is illustrative [107]. After the development of hemorrhagic varicella in a 25-week-gestation infant whose mother had varicella 2 weeks previously, 14 infants in the unit were exposed over several days. None of the infants in isolettes became ill, but four who were in open warming units at exposure developed varicella 10 days later. All had received VZIG, and in each instance, the mother gave a history of varicella. The illnesses were mild with only a few papular skin lesions, but three of the four infants were positive for VZV on immunofluorescence testing of skin scrapings. Each infant with varicella was treated with intravenous acyclovir. The incidence of disease was higher in infants of less than 29 weeks' gestation than in infants of longer gestation.

An extensive epidemic lasting 5 months described by Apert [108] in 1895 is of historical interest. Two infants in a newborn nursery developed chickenpox on January 7 and 8. They were immediately transferred with their mothers to another ward, where they were isolated, but a third infant (second generation of chickenpox) developed disease on January 24 and was likewise isolated with his or her mother. A fourth infant (third generation) developed varicella on February 7, but was not isolated until February 13 because the mother deliberately obscured the fact that the infant had lesions. Subsequently, a fifth infant (fourth generation) developed chickenpox on February 21. Because the number of infants exposed and the maternal histories of varicella are not stated, the attack rates are unclear. Although this was the last case of chickenpox in the newborn nursery, one of the infected neonates introduced the virus to another ward of 40 to 45 debilitated infants. Before the epidemic was over in May, nine generations of chickenpox separated with mathematical precision by 14 days had occurred. In all, 19 infants (12 <6 months old) were infected along with two mothers.

These experiences with nosocomial chickenpox in the newborn nursery are summarized in Table 22–1. In the 20th century, in reports in which the number of neonates exposed is explicitly stated, 218 exposures resulted in only 8 instances of transmission to infants. Most of the mothers had histories of varicella, although in many the history was unknown. Several factors undoubtedly contribute to the low rate of transmission of disease to neonates, including passive immunity in most; relatively brief exposure compared with the household setting, where 80% to 90% of susceptible persons become clinically infected [41,69]; and relative lack of intimacy of contact in the nursery, particularly for infants in isolettes.

PATHOGENESIS OF VARICELLA AND ZOSTER

In the usual case of chickenpox, the portal of entry and initial site of virus replication is probably the oropharynx, specifically the tonsil [108a]. Attempts to show this directly have been unrewarding, however. In five patients whose blood, throat secretions, and skin were cultured repeatedly during the prodromal period and after the appearance of cutaneous lesions, VZV was recovered from a throat swab in only one instance and from the blood in none. In contrast, vesicle fluid from these patients yielded VZV in all instances [109]. Attempts to isolate the virus from the blood of six additional patients were positive in only one instance: on the 2nd day of rash in an immunosuppressed host. Other, more extensive searches for VZV in throat secretions of patients with varicella, even during the incubation period, proved essentially negative [110,111]. In one report, VZV was isolated from nasal swabs in 4 of 11 children on days 2 through 4 after onset of the rash. VZV could not be isolated during the incubation period or even during the first day of the rash. It was unclear whether the virus was multiplying in the nasal mucosa [112].

VZV has been isolated from blood obtained from patients with varicella. Ozaki and colleagues [113] cultured blood from seven immunocompetent children;

TABLE 22–1   Nosocomial Chickenpox Infections in the Nursery

Year	Case No.	Period Others Exposed after Onset of Rash	Prior History of Varicella in Mothers of Infants Exposed			No. Persons Exposed	No. Subsequently Infected
			Yes	No	Unknown		
1895 [108]	1	Variable		No data		<40 young infants	19
1954 [101]	2	4 days		No data		Not stated	0
	3	0 (immediate isolation)		No data		Not stated	0
	4	0 (immediate isolation)		No data		Not stated	0
1958 [100]	5	0 (immediate isolation in nursery)	0	0	17	17 neonates	0
		3 days (other ward)		No data		Not stated	2*
1963 [102]	6	18 hr					
	7	10 hr	35	0	0	35 neonates	0
1965 [103]	8	2, 3, 8, 10 hr in susceptible neonates	6	3	4	13 neonates	0
1965 [98]	9	Variable	1	7	132	139 mothers	8
						?139 neonates	0†
1976 [83]	10	Brief	0	2	9	11 mothers	2
						10 infants	1 infant
						25 staff	1
1983 [94]	11	Brief		No data		32 infants	0
1984 [96]	12	Variable	8	0	21	29 infants	2 infants‡
1989 [104]	13	Brief, intimate	22			22 infants	0
1990 [105]	14	Brief‡,§	13	1	1	15 infants	0
1992 [92]	15	Brief‡,§		No data		16 infants	0
1993 [106]	16	1 hr on each of 3 days		No data		29 infants	0
1994 [107]	17	Intimate	10		4	14 infants	4 infants
Total reported						218 infants	7 infants

*Infected infant transferred to another ward, where two older children (4 and 7 years old) later developed chickenpox.
†No cases of chickenpox in neonates, despite appearance of chickenpox in eight mothers from 34 days antepartum to 14 days postpartum.
‡In neonatal intensive care unit.
§Exposure 1–2 days before rash in index case.

VZV was isolated a few days before the onset of rash or within 1 day after onset. Asano and coworkers [114] similarly isolated VZV from the blood of 7 of 12 otherwise healthy patients with early varicella. The patients from whom virus could not be isolated had been studied after they had the rash for more than 4 days. Both groups of investigators introduced an additional technical step into the blood culture process that might explain why they were successful in isolating VZV when many others before them had not been. The white blood cells were separated on Ficoll-Hypaque gradients and added to cell cultures. Although there was no evidence of viral growth in these cultures, they were blindly passaged onto new cell cultures. Evidence of growth of VZV was present in these second cultures after the blind passage within 2 to 5 days. Before these studies, VZV had been isolated only from blood obtained from immunocompromised patients with varicella or zoster [110,115,116]. The white blood cell infected with VZV is a mononuclear cell, but it is uncertain whether monocytes or lymphocytes, or both, are involved [113,114]. Experiments in the SCID-hu mouse model have shown that VZV is lymphotropic for human CD4$^+$ and CD8$^+$ T lymphocytes and that human T cells release some infectious virus [117].

Data from PCR studies of patients with varicella have yielded various results. In the study by Koropchak and colleagues [118], performed 24 hours after rash onset in 12 patients, 3.3% of oropharyngeal samples, 67% of mononuclear cells, and 75% of skin vesicles were positive for VZV DNA. In the study by Ozaki and coworkers [119] of pharyngeal secretions of chickenpox patients, 26% were positive during the incubation period, and 90% were positive after clinical onset.

Virus is readily recovered from cutaneous lesions soon after the onset of chickenpox. Isolation of VZV was successful in 23 of 25 cases in which vesicle fluid was cultured within 3 days after the onset of the rash, but was successful in only 1 of 7 specimens collected 4 to 8 days after onset [109]. In contrast, the virus apparently persists longer in vesicles of zoster patients, in whom 7 of 10 specimens collected later than 3 days after onset were positive [104]. PCR is more sensitive than virus culture. In the study by Koropchak and colleagues [118], VZV was recovered from only 21% of skin lesions, but 75% were positive by PCR. In contrast to smallpox, chickenpox is no longer communicable by the time the lesions have crusted and scabbed.

The pathogenesis of chickenpox seems to be as follows: Transmission is probably effected by airborne spread of virus from cutaneous vesicles and to a lesser extent by respiratory droplets from patients with varicella or zoster. After an initial period of virus replication in the oropharynx in the susceptible individual, there is invasion of the local lymph nodes and a primary viremia of low magnitude, delivering virus to the viscera [120]. After several more days of virus multiplication, a secondary viremia of greater magnitude occurs, resulting in widespread cutaneous dissemination of virus and rash. Data in SCID-hu mouse model alternatively suggest that VZV is targeted to the skin early in varicella and is initially controlled to a great extent by innate immunity [120a]. Cropping of the vesicles is thought to represent several viremic phases.

In the body, the virus spreads by cell-to-cell contact; viremia also is cell associated. Enveloped, cell-free infectious VZV is present, however, in the vesicular skin vesicles. Crusting and scabbing of the vesicles and pustules occur as host defense mechanisms, particularly as various forms of cell-mediated immunity become active. Latency is achieved from the cell-free VZV particles in the skin that are in proximity to sensory nerve endings.

The pathogenesis of zoster differs from that of varicella. Before development of zoster, latent VZV begins to reactivate and multiply in the sensory ganglion (or ganglia) because of unknown local factors [2]. The virus travels down the axon to the skin supplied by that nerve. Development of a localized rash occurs if there is a deficiency in cell-mediated immunity to VZV [121–124]. This compromise in cell-mediated immunity may be obvious, as in patients who have had transplantation, therapy for malignant disease, or HIV infection [125], or, presumably, it may be transient, as in healthy persons who develop zoster for no apparent reason. In immunosuppressed patients, a viremic phase with zoster has been documented occasionally [126,127], and this probably happens after skin involvement has occurred, especially if there continues to be an inadequate immune response to VZV after the virus has reached the skin. The clinical manifestation of this viremia is disseminated zoster, in which vesicular lesions develop outside the original dermatome. A viremic phase in pregnant patients with disseminated zoster has not been documented, but it seems logical to assume that viremia would be a prerequisite for dissemination.

PATHOLOGY
Cutaneous Lesions

Histologic changes in the skin leading to the formation of vesicles are essentially identical for chickenpox, zoster, and HSV infection. The hallmark of each is the presence of multinucleated giant cells and intranuclear inclusions, changes that are not found in the vesicular lesions caused by vaccinia virus and coxsackieviruses. The lesion is primarily localized in the epidermis, where ballooning degeneration of cells in the deeper layers is accompanied by intercellular edema. As edema progresses, the cornified layers are separated from the more basal layers to form a delicate vesicle with a thin roof. An exudate consisting primarily of mononuclear cells is seen in the dermis, but the characteristic nuclear changes of epithelial cells are absent in this region.

The predominant cells in vesicular lesions are polymorphonuclear leukocytes. These cells may play a role in generating interferon in vesicular lesions, which may be important in recovery from the disease [128]. In vitro data also suggest that the polymorphonuclear leukocyte plays a role in host defense against VZV, possibly by mediating antibody-dependent cell-mediated cytotoxicity [129–131].

Visceral Lesions in the Fetus and Placenta

Few reports describe the appearance of the placenta in cases of congenital chickenpox with or without survival. Garcia [132] observed grossly visible necrotic lesions of the placenta in a case of chickenpox occurring in the 4th month of pregnancy that resulted in spontaneous abortion. Microscopically, central areas of necrosis were surrounded by epithelioid cells and rare giant cells of the foreign body type, giving a granulomatous appearance. Some decidual cells had typical intranuclear inclusions.

Descriptions of the pathology of visceral lesions in fetal or neonatal chickenpox are restricted to autopsies in fatal cases [132–137]. Grossly, the lesions are small, punctate, and white or yellow and resemble miliary tuberculosis. Microscopically, their appearance resembles the lesions of the placenta: central necrotic areas, often resembling fibrinoid necrosis, surrounded by a few epithelioid cells and a scant infiltrate of mononuclear cells. Intranuclear inclusions are present. The skin, lungs, and liver are uniformly involved (Table 22–2) [132]. In the case described by Garcia [132], the cortical, subependymal, and basilar structures of the cerebrum were totally destroyed and accompanied by extensive calcification. Although a search for *Toxoplasma* was negative, serologic data to rule out dual infection are lacking in the report. The gross and microscopic lesions of fatal perinatal chickenpox resemble lesions of disseminated HSV infection, including a preference for the liver and adrenal gland, but the provided data suggest that involvement of the brain is more common in neonatal HSV infection than it is in fatal neonatal chickenpox. A neonate with fatal hemorrhagic varicella with pneumonia and hepatitis is shown in Figure 22–1.

Visceral Lesions in the Mother

In fatal cases of chickenpox in pregnant women, maternal death is usually caused by pulmonary involvement. The pathologic course of chickenpox pneumonia in pregnant women is identical to the course in nonpregnant women and in children [138,139]. Interstitial pneumonitis may

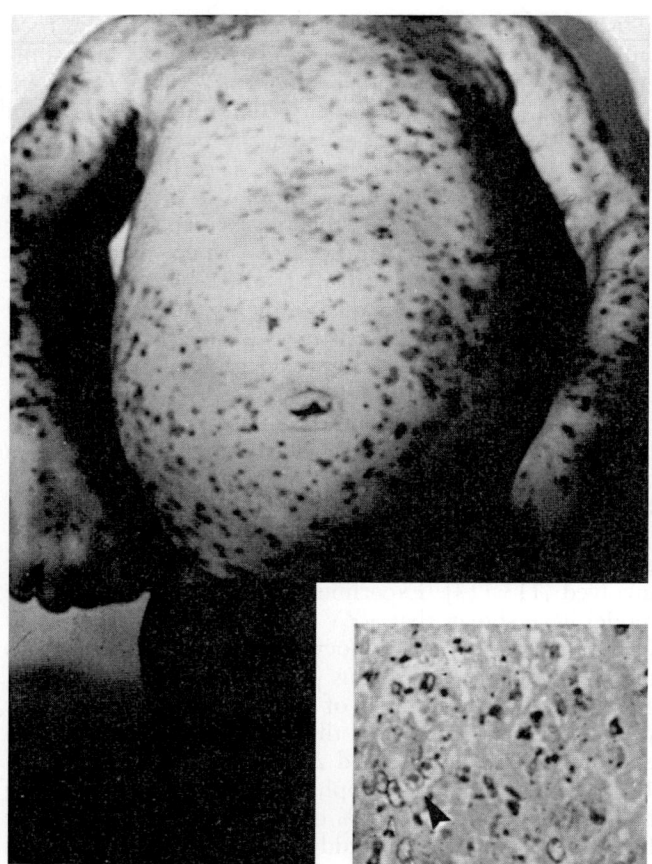

FIGURE 22–1 Congenital hemorrhagic varicella complicated by pneumonia and hepatitis. The mother of this infant developed varicella a few days before delivery. Zoster immunoglobulin was unavailable at that time. *Inset* shows section of liver with intranuclear inclusion bodies obtained at autopsy.

follow a peribronchiolar distribution of disease. Intranuclear inclusions may be found in alveolar lining cells, macrophages, capillary endothelium, and tracheobronchial mucosa. Necrotic foci may be accompanied by hemorrhage, and hyaline membranes lining the alveoli are often prominent.

Zoster

The pathologic picture of cutaneous lesions in zoster is indistinguishable from chickenpox lesions. The dorsal root ganglion of the affected dermatome exhibits a mononuclear inflammatory infiltrate. There may also be necrosis of ganglion cells and demyelination of the corresponding axon. There are no descriptions of these lesions in pregnant women or in neonates specifically.

CLINICAL MANIFESTATIONS
Chickenpox Rash

After an incubation period of usually 13 to 17 days [41,66], chickenpox is heralded by the approximately simultaneous occurrence of fever and rash. In adults, the exanthem is often preceded by a prodromal fever and constitutional symptoms lasting 2 or 3 days [7]. Occasionally, one or more isolated vesicles may precede a generalized

TABLE 22–2 Frequency of Gross and Microscopic Lesions in Seven Autopsied Cases of Fetal and Neonatal Chickenpox

Organ	No. Cases/No. Examined (%)	References
Skin	7/7 (100)	[132–137]
Lungs	7/7 (100)	[132–137]
Liver	7/7 (100)	[132–137]
Adrenals	6/7 (86)	[132, 133, 135–137]
Esophagus or intestines	5/6 (83)	[127–132]
	4/5 (80)	
Thymus	5/7 (71)	[132, 133, 135, 137]
Kidneys	4/7 (56)	[132, 133, 135, 137]
Spleen	3/7 (43)	[132, 135–137]
Pancreas	2/7 (29)	[132, 133, 135]
Heart	1/5 (20)	[132, 136]
Brain*		[132]
Miscellaneous		
Ovaries	1	[133]
Bone marrow	1	[135]
Placenta	1	[132]

Not well documented; possibility of concomitant toxoplasmosis not definitely excluded.

exanthem by 1 or 2 days. The rash is characteristically centripetal, beginning on the face or scalp and spreading rapidly to the trunk, but with relative sparing of the extremities. The lesions begin as red macules, but progress quickly to vesicles and crusts. Itching is the rule. There is a tendency for new lesions to occur in crops. In contrast to smallpox, all stages of lesions—vesicles, pustules, and scabs—may occur simultaneously in the same anatomic region. New crops often continue to appear over a 2- to 5-day period. Lesions may be more numerous in skin folds or in the diaper area. The total number of vesicles varies from only two or three in very mild cases, especially in infants, to thousands of lesions that border on confluence, especially in adults [7]. In many cases, one or two mucosal lesions may occur in the mouth or, less commonly, on the vulva. Occasionally, the lesions may be bullous or hemorrhagic. Residual scarring is exceptional. Constitutional symptoms tend to be mild even in the presence of an extensive exanthem.

Complications of Chickenpox

The most common complication is secondary bacterial infection, usually caused by group A β-hemolytic streptococci or staphylococci. Skin infections may lead to severe sequelae, such as toxic shock syndrome and necrotizing fasciitis [140–148]. Central nervous system complications, which are uncommon, include encephalitis, cerebellar ataxia, aseptic meningitis, and myelitis [149,150]. Glomerulonephritis [151,152], myocarditis [153,154], and arthritis [155,156] have also been reported.

Chickenpox in Immunocompromised Children

It is widely appreciated that varicella may be severe and even fatal in children with an underlying malignancy, children with congenital deficits in cellular immunity, children receiving high doses of corticosteroids for any reason [157], and children with underlying infection with HIV and acquired immunodeficiency syndrome (AIDS) [81,158]. Historically, children with leukemia had a mortality rate approaching 10% if untreated [159] and sometimes developed what has been called progressive varicella. Instead of developing new vesicular lesions for several days, they continued to have fever and new lesions for 2 weeks after the onset of illness. Frequently, their skin lesions become hemorrhagic, large, and umbilicated. Varicella pneumonia often ensued and was a major factor contributing to the death of a child. It is believed that this abnormal response to VZV represents a failure of the normal cell-mediated immunity response to eliminate the virus [159]. The cell-mediated immunity response to VZV includes antibody-dependent cell-mediated cytotoxicity, natural killer cells, and cytotoxic T cells including CD4 and CD8 cells [36,129–131,160–162]. Today, in the vaccine era, severe or fatal pneumonia in immunocompromised children has become rare or unusual.

Chickenpox Pneumonia

Primary varicella pneumonia is a dreaded complication of chickenpox and is responsible for most fatalities. It is most common in immunocompromised patients, in adults, and in most fatal cases of neonatal chickenpox [132–134,163], but it is rarely seen in otherwise healthy children. It has been suggested that the incidence is about 15% in adults and that 90% of cases have occurred in persons older than 19 years [163,164]. The true incidence is difficult to determine because chest radiographs are not performed in most cases of chickenpox, and extensive radiographic evidence of disease may be present when pulmonary symptoms are only minimal. In male military recruits with varicella, virtually all of whom had been hospitalized and had chest radiographs, radiographic evidence of pneumonia was found in 16.3% of 110 cases [165].

Two reviews of chickenpox pneumonia in adults outline the major features [139,166]. The onset of pneumonia usually occurs in 2 to 4 days, but sometimes occurs 10 days after the appearance of the exanthem. Fever and cough are present in 87% to 100% of cases, and dyspnea occurs in 70% to 80%. Other symptoms and signs include cyanosis (42% to 55%), rales (55%), hemoptysis (35% to 38%), and chest pain (21%). Radiographic changes seem to correlate best with the severity of the rash rather than with the physical examination of the lungs. The radiograph typically reveals a diffuse nodular or miliary pattern, most pronounced in the perihilar regions. The radiographic appearance changes rapidly. The white blood cell count ranges from 5000 to 20,000 cells/mm^3 and is of little help in differentiating viral from secondary bacterial pneumonia. Pneumonia is usually self-limiting, and recovery is temporally correlated with clearing of skin lesions. The fatality rate has been variously estimated at 10% to 30%, but it probably approximates the lower of these values if immunocompromised hosts are excluded [139,166]. Blood gas analyses and pulmonary function tests indicate a significant diffusion defect that may persist in some cases for months after clinical recovery [167]. The introduction of antiviral chemotherapy has greatly improved the outcome in this disease.

Maternal Effects of Chickenpox

Reports from the mid-20th century suggested that when chickenpox occurred during pregnancy, it was a highly lethal disease. Deaths usually resulted from varicella pneumonia, in some cases accompanied by glomerulitis and renal failure or myocarditis, occurring after the 4th month of gestation [168,169]. Harris and Rhoades [170] reviewed the literature to 1963 and found a reported mortality of 41% for 17 pregnant women with chickenpox pneumonia compared with 11% for 236 nonpregnant adults with chickenpox pneumonia. Other reports question, however, whether varicella, especially in the absence of pneumonia, is more serious in pregnant women than in the adult population at large [136,171,172]. Because most cases of gestational varicella with an uncomplicated course are undoubtedly not reported, the denominator of the case-fatality ratio is unknown. In a prospective study of 150 cases of chickenpox in pregnancy in 1966, only one maternal death related to chickenpox pneumonia was recorded [173].

In a very large, collaborative, prospective study published in 2002, there were no fatalities in 347 consecutive pregnant women with varicella, although 18 (5.2%) had radiologic evidence of pneumonia [174,175]. Although the data did not reach statistical significance in this study, it seems striking that 16 (89%) of 18 reported cases of pneumonia occurred in women who developed varicella after the 16th week of pregnancy.

Table 22–3 adds data from subsequent case reports of gestational varicella, with and without pneumonia, and reports of perinatal varicella in which the outcome in the mother is described to a review of the literature on varicella pneumonia in pregnancy before 1964 [170]. Among 545 cases of chickenpox in pregnant women, there were 16 deaths (3%). All of the deaths occurred among the 75 women who had chickenpox pneumonia (21% fatality rate for pneumonia). Deaths occurred in 1 (<1%) of 166 women whose disease occurred during the first trimester, 4 (2%) of 168 women whose disease occurred during the second trimester, and 11 (5%) of 208 women whose disease occurred during the third trimester. No deaths occurred among eight women who were exposed to chickenpox in late pregnancy, but did not develop an exanthem until the first few days postpartum.

It remains uncertain whether chickenpox pneumonia has a graver prognosis when it occurs during pregnancy. There is no definitive evidence that chickenpox in the absence of pneumonia is a more serious illness in pregnant women than in other adults; however, the risk of developing pneumonia may be increased after the 16th week of pregnancy. It seems likely that older mortality information on varicella in pregnancy reflected the pre-antiviral therapy era and was biased by selective reporting of fatal cases.

Some patients with varicella during pregnancy who were treated with acyclovir have been reported [172,174–188]. These reports suggest that acyclovir has improved the outcome of this complication of varicella, although controlled studies have not been performed. Although various dosages have been used, the standard dosage of 30 mg/kg/day given intravenously would seem appropriate for treatment of pregnant women with varicella pneumonia. Congenital abnormalities from administration of acyclovir to women during pregnancy have not been observed [189,190].

Controlled studies of the value of corticosteroids in pregnant women with varicella pneumonia have not been performed. Several reports indicate that 2 of 6 pregnant women treated with corticosteroids died, whereas 8 of 17 pregnant women given supportive therapy without corticosteroids died [170,191–194]. It seems that administration of an antiviral drug is of greater importance than administration of corticosteroids. Passive immunization

TABLE 22–3 Maternal Mortality Associated with Gestational Varicella*

Year	No. Cases	No. with Varicella Pneumonia	No. Deaths	Onset of Rash[†]			Immediately Postpartum
				0–3 mo	4–6 mo	7–9 mo	
1963 [132]	2	0	0	0	1	1	0
1964 [532]	18	0	0	0	0	15	3
1964 [136]	16	1	1	0	0	16 (1)[‡]	0
1965 [98]	9	0	0	0	0	5	4
1966 [207]	11[§]	0	0	0	4	7	0
1965 [170][¶]	17	17	7	2 (1)[‡]	3 (2)	11 (4)	1 (0)
1968 [191]	1	1	1	0	1 (1)	0	0
1969 [192]	2	2	1	0	0	2 (1)	0
1971 [193]	1	1	0	0	0	1	1
1986 [208]	43	4	1	11	11 (1)	21	0
1989 [176]	3	3	1	0	1	2 (1)	0
1990 [177]	5	5	1	3	0	2 (1)	0
1991 [187]	1	1	0	0	2	0	0
1991 [178][¶¶]	21	21	3	0	7	14 (3)	0
1996 [172][**]	28	1	0	7	7	11	0
1997 [533]	22	0	0	3	9	0	0
2002 [175,176][††]	347	18	0	140	122	100	0
Totals	545	75 (14%)	16 (3%)	166 (<1%)	168 (2%)	208 (5%)	

*The antiviral therapy era is considered to have begun after 1985.
[†]If specified.
[‡]Numbers in parentheses give deaths at indicated gestational periods.
[§]Includes one patient with zoster whose gestational dates were not given.
[¶]Includes review of the literature before 1963.
[¶¶]Reports five new cases with a review of additional case reports in the literature.
[**]In a series of 28 pregnant women with varicella, 1 (3.6%) had pneumonia.
[††]In a series of 347 pregnant women with varicella, 18 (5.2%) had pneumonia.

may be administered to seronegative women after close exposure to VZV to attempt to modify the infection; although uncertain, this approach may prevent fetal infection [195–197]. In a study from 1994, among 97 women who developed varicella after passive immunization with VZIG, there were no observed cases of congenital varicella syndrome [196]. About two abnormal infants could be expected in a series of this magnitude, but the number of women followed is too low to achieve statistical significance.

Effects of Gestational Varicella on the Fetus
Chromosomal Aberrations
Available data on chromosomal aberrations are often difficult to interpret, particularly in the absence of controls, which is often the case. VZV can induce chromosomal abnormalities in vitro and in vivo. When human diploid fibroblasts were infected with the virus, a high proportion of cells observed were in metaphase arrest, as if they were under the influence of colchicine [198]. The incidence of chromatid and chromosomal breaks ranged from 26% to 45% 24 hours after infection compared with 2% for control cultures. In the acute phase of chickenpox, up to the 5th day of rash, peripheral blood leukocytes show a 17% to 28% incidence of chromosomal breaks compared with 6% in controls, but 1 month after infection, these abnormalities disappeared [199]. A single case report suggested the possibility that chromosomal damage may be more lasting when chickenpox is acquired in utero. A boy with bird-headed dwarfism, born to a mother who contracted chickenpox in the 6th month of pregnancy, had a 26% incidence of chromosomal breakage in peripheral blood leukocytes when he was examined at 2 years of age [200]. Chromosomal analyses in four infants with congenital varicella syndrome, whose mothers had chickenpox at the 8th, 14th, 16th, and 20th week of gestation, were reported as normal [201–204].

Information on chromosomal aberrations in infants who have no congenital anomalies and are the offspring of mothers with gestational varicella is lacking. Further concern about the possibility of persistent chromosomal abnormalities after intrauterine exposure to VZV is suggested by a prospective survey of deaths among children born in England and Wales from 1950–1952 whose

mothers had chickenpox in pregnancy. Two deaths, both from acute leukemia, were reported among the offspring of 270 women; the two children developed acute leukemia at the ages of 3 and 4 years after intrauterine exposure at 25 and 23 weeks of gestation [205]. In the absence of confirmation, it remains questionable whether exposure to chickenpox in utero is a risk factor for leukemia or other malignancies.

Abortion and Prematurity
Several studies have addressed the question of whether gestational chickenpox and other viral diseases result in an increased incidence of spontaneous abortion or prematurity. In a retrospective study in 1948, only 4 cases of chickenpox were identified among 26,353 pregnant women [206]. No stillbirths occurred in these cases. Prospective studies have tended to confirm that maternal chickenpox during pregnancy is not associated with a significant excess of prematurity [173] or fetal death [207]. Among 826 virus-infected pregnant subjects observed in New York City from 1957–1964, 150 women with chickenpox were followed to term. After exclusion of fetal deaths and multiple births, 5 of 135 live-born infants were found to have birth weights of less than 2500 g. This incidence of prematurity was lower than in the control group of non–virus-infected pregnant women (Table 22–4). Similarly, in the study by Paryani and Arvin [208], premature delivery occurred in 2 (5%) of 42 pregnancies, with delivery at 31 and 35 weeks of gestation.

In a prospective study involving 194 women with gestational varicella and 194 control women, the rate of spontaneous abortion was 3% and 7% in the first 20 weeks [209]. In the large prospective series of Enders and associates [196] of 1330 women in England and Germany who developed varicella, 36 (3%) experienced spontaneous abortions after varicella in the first 16 weeks. In the prospective study of Pastuszak and coworkers [210] involving 106 women with varicella in the first 20 weeks of pregnancy, there were more premature births (14.3%) among women with varicella than among controls (5.6%; $P = .05$). There is no question, however, that the congenital varicella syndrome is associated with low birth weight. Approximately one third of reported cases of the syndrome have been premature, had low birth weight, or were small for gestational age.

TABLE 22–4 Frequency of Low Birth Weight among Infants Born to Mothers with Selected Viral Infections during Pregnancy

	Virus-Infected Group			Control Group*		
Disease	No. Live Births	No. with Low Birth Weight[†]	%	No. Live Births	No. with Low Birth Weight[†]	%
Rubella	359	50	13.9	402	21	5.2
Chickenpox	135	5	3.7	146	13	8.9
Mumps	117	9	7.7	122	4	3.3
Measles	60	10	16.7	62	2	3.3

Note: *Fetal deaths and multiple births were excluded from the analysis.*
Control group was matched for age, race, and parity of mother and type of obstetric service.
[†]*Low birth weight was defined as <2500 g.*
Modified from data of Siegel M, Fuerst HT. Low birth weight and maternal virus diseases: a prospective study of rubella, measles, mumps, chickenpox, and hepatitis. JAMA 197:88, 1966.

An accurate assessment of the incidence of fetal mortality after maternal chickenpox is difficult to obtain. Fetal wastage is probably underreported, in part because some spontaneous abortions occur before prenatal care is sought. In the prospective study of maternal viral diseases in New York City referred to earlier [207], nine fetal deaths were observed among 144 instances of maternal chickenpox. Five fetal deaths occurred among 32 pregnancies in the first trimester, four among 60 second-trimester pregnancies, and none among 52 third-trimester pregnancies (Table 22–5). These deaths do not represent significant increases in fetal wastage associated with chickenpox infection compared with control groups in which no maternal viral infection occurred. There was a significant excess of fetal deaths only for mumps, and these occurred primarily in the first trimester. Only three of the nine fetal deaths associated with maternal chickenpox occurred within 2 weeks of the onset of the mother's illness, and two of these were in the first trimester. Two additional deaths occurred 2 to 4 weeks after the onset of maternal chickenpox, two occurred 5 to 9 weeks after the onset of maternal illness, and two occurred 10 or more weeks after the onset of maternal illness. The absence of a close temporal relationship between most fetal deaths and maternal disease provides further support for the concept that maternal chickenpox during pregnancy does not commonly result in fetal mortality.

Although the incidence of fetal death is not increased by maternal varicella, fetal deaths have been associated with maternal varicella. Deaths in utero may result from direct invasion of the fetus by VZV [132,196,211–213] or from the presumed toxic effects of high fever, anoxia, or metabolic changes caused by maternal disease [207].

TABLE 22–5 Fetal Deaths in Relation to Gestational Age after Selected Virus Infections during Pregnancy

Infection Groups	Weeks of Gestation		
	0–11	12–27	>28
Mumps			
No. cases	33	51	43
No. fetal deaths	9	1	0
%	27.3	2	—
Measles			
No. cases	19	29	17
No. fetal deaths	3	1	1.9
%	15.8	3.4	5.9
Chickenpox			
No. cases	32	60	52
No. fetal deaths	5	4	0
%	15.6	4.7	—
Controls			
No. cases	1010*	392†	152†
No. fetal deaths	131	15	1
%	13	3.8	0.7

*Subjects were attending prenatal clinic in first trimester without virus infections.
†Controls were matched for age, race, and parity of the mother and type of obstetric service.
Modified from Siegel M, Fuerst HT, Peress NS. Comparative fetal mortality in maternal virus diseases: a prospective study on rubella, measles, mumps, chickenpox, and hepatitis. N Engl J Med 274:768, 1966.

The precise mechanisms of these toxic effects have not been elucidated. When maternal disease is unusually severe, particularly in cases of chickenpox pneumonia, fetal death may also result from premature onset of labor or death in utero caused by maternal death.*

Congenital Malformations

For many years, there was uncertainty about whether gestational varicella led to a symptomatic congenital infection. Intensive investigation from the mid-1970s until the end of the 20th century led to the recognition that VZV can cause fetal malformations. Two types of investigations were done to determine whether chickenpox during pregnancy leads to a congenital syndrome. The first investigations were retrospective analyses or case reports describing specific anomalies that occurred in the offspring of mothers who had gestational varicella. These reports were necessarily highly selective and did not define the incidence of such anomalies. They consistently described a syndrome of skin scarring, eye and brain damage, and limb hypoplasia, however, that might follow intrauterine varicella.

The second type of analysis consisted of prospective studies of pregnant women followed throughout pregnancy and afterward. The problem was to delineate the coincidence of two events, each of which is itself uncommon—gestational chickenpox and congenital malformations—to determine the magnitude of risk to the fetus. Siegel [72], despite an 8-year observation period encompassing approximately 190,000 pregnancies annually in New York City, was able to identify only four malformations among infants born to 135 mothers who had chickenpox during pregnancy compared with five malformations among 146 matched controls. The follow-up period was 5 years and included psychomotor and audiometric tests. Chickenpox occurred during the first trimester in only 27 of the pregnancies complicated by chickenpox, and of these, 2 (7.4%) were associated with congenital anomalies compared with anomalies in 3 (3.4%) of 87 pregnancies in the control population.

The largest single prospective series is that of Enders and associates [196]. In a joint prospective study in Germany and the United Kingdom from 1980–1993, Enders and associates [196] followed 1373 women with varicella and 366 with zoster during pregnancy. Of the women with varicella, 1285 continued to term, and 9 had defects attributed to congenital varicella syndrome. The incidence was 2 (0.4%) of 472 for infections between 0 and 12 weeks and 7 (2%) of 351 for infections between 13 and 20 weeks. In a collaborative prospective study in the United States, 347 women with gestational varicella were reported, and adequate follow-up of their infants was available in 231 [175]. In this cohort, there was one case (0.4%) of the congenital syndrome and two cases of fetal death, including one case of hydrops. If these cases are included, the rate of congenital varicella was 1.3%. The mother of the one child with the syndrome had varicella at 24 weeks; the child had skin, eye, and central nervous system involvement.

---

*References [136,170,177,191,192,212].

That congenital varicella syndrome is a reality is now widely appreciated. It has become possible to make a tissue diagnosis of congenital varicella syndrome only more recently because affected infants do not chronically shed virus as is seen in congenital infections with rubella virus and CMV [196,211,213–215]. Congenital varicella syndrome may be prevented in the future by widespread use of varicella vaccine, analogous to the situation for congenital rubella.

The constellation of developmental abnormalities described in individual case reports of infants born to mothers who had varicella in early pregnancy and in prospective series is sufficiently distinctive to indicate that VZV is a teratogen. In 1947, LaForet and Lynch [216] described an infant with multiple congenital anomalies after maternal chickenpox in early pregnancy. The infant had hypoplasia of the entire right lower extremity, talipes equinovarus, and absent deep tendon reflexes on the right. Cerebral cortical atrophy, cerebellar aplasia, chorioretinitis, right torticollis, insufficiency of the anal and vesical sphincters, and cicatricial cutaneous lesions of the left lower extremity were present. The syndrome then seemed to be all but forgotten until 1974, when Srabstein and coworkers [217] rekindled interest in the subject by reporting another case and reviewed the literature, concluding that although the virus could not be isolated from the infants, congenital varicella syndrome typically consisted of some combination of cicatricial skin lesions, ocular abnormalities, limb deformities, mental retardation, and early death after maternal varicella in early pregnancy (Figs. 22–2 to 22–4). Numerous additional reports in the literature of the syndrome, encompassing more than 100 cases, indicate there is a wide spectrum of manifestations (Table 22–6).*

Although at one time it was thought that congenital varicella syndrome occurred after maternal VZV infection in the first trimester of pregnancy, current evaluation of

*References [74,191,196,201–206,208–283].

the data indicates that cases also occur in the second trimester. Of 82 cases for which data are available, 32 (39%) occurred after maternal varicella that developed before the 13th week, 47 (59%) occurred after maternal varicella that developed between weeks 13 and 26, and 1 (1%) [247] occurred after maternal varicella that developed during the 28th week. The average gestation when maternal varicella occurred was 15 weeks. Only six cases occurring after maternal zoster have been reported [248,249,278,279,284]; not all of these are well documented virologically. Four occurred after maternal zoster in the first trimester, one followed zoster in the second trimester [278], and one followed zoster in the third trimester [284]. Of 109 reported affected infants, 103 (95%) cases followed maternal varicella, and 6 (5%) followed maternal zoster (disseminated in one instance).

Scars of the skin, usually cicatricial lesions, are the most prominent stigmata, although a few patients have had no rash at all [265,268,269,285]. Eye abnormalities (i.e., chorioretinitis, microphthalmia, Horner syndrome, cataract, and nystagmus) and neurologic damage are almost as common; other features include a hypoplastic limb, prematurity, and early death. The features of the syndrome are summarized in Table 22–6.

Cutaneous scars were usually observed overlying a hypoplastic limb, but also have been seen in the contralateral limb [216]. Characteristically, the skin scars are cicatricial, depressed, and pigmented and often have a zigzag configuration. Such scars are thought to be the result of zoster that occurred before birth. In some patients, large areas of scarred skin have required skin grafting [229,237]. In other patients, the rash was bullous [236] or consisted of multiple, scattered, depressed, white scars [240,244,257]. In one infant, healing zoster was present at the T11 dermatome at birth; there was also spinal cord atrophy at the same level and aganglionosis of the intestine [256].

Ocular abnormalities include chorioretinitis, Horner syndrome or anisocoria, microphthalmia, cataract, and

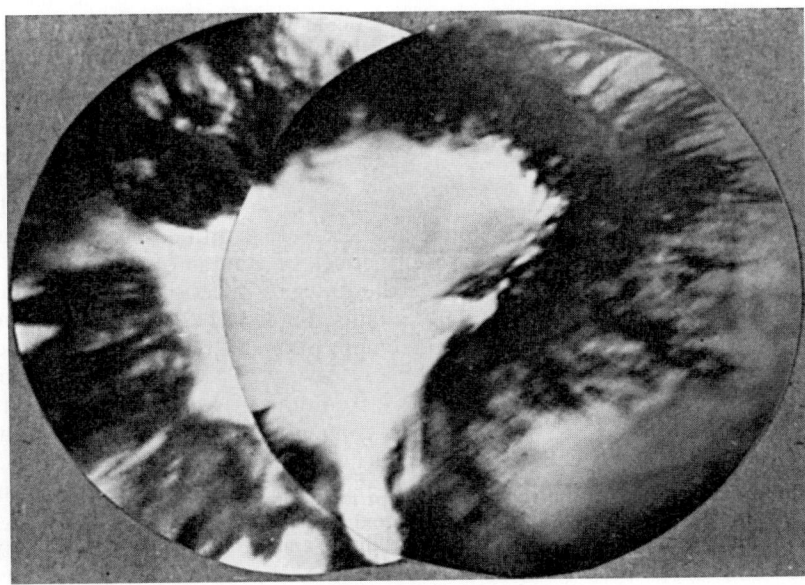

FIGURE 22–2 **Fundus photograph of right eye of a 13-month-old patient shows central gliosis with surrounding ring of black pigment.** The child's mother had varicella during the early 4th month of pregnancy. *(Adapted from Charles N, Bennett TW, Margolis S. Ocular pathology of the congenital varicella syndrome. Arch Ophthalmol 95:2034, 1977.)*

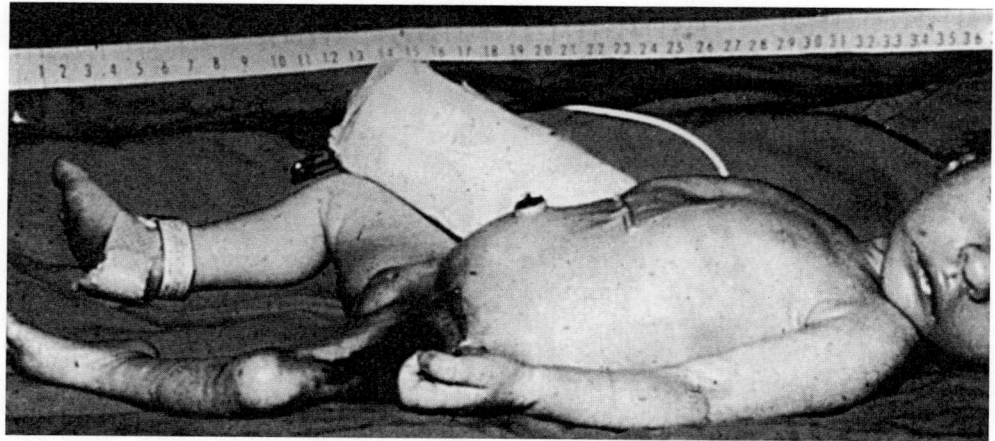

FIGURE 22–3 This infant, whose mother had varicella during the 13th to 15th weeks of pregnancy, had bilateral microphthalmia with cataracts and an atrophic left leg. The infant died of bronchopneumonia at age 6½ months. *(From Srabstein JC, et al. Is there a congenital varicella syndrome? J Pediatr 84:239, 1974.)*

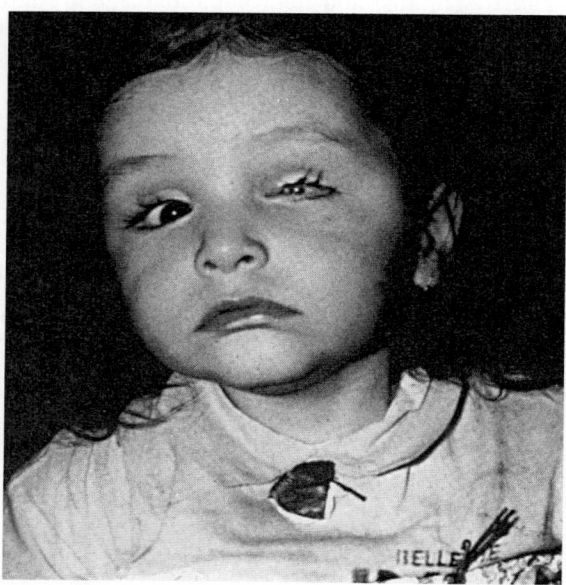

FIGURE 22–4 A child, whose mother had varicella during the 16th week of pregnancy, had atrophy of the left orbit, with blindness that required cosmetic enucleation. Severe chorioretinitis occurred in the right eye. Except for blindness, the child developed normally. She died of pneumonia when approximately 4 years old. *(Adapted from Frey HM, Bialkin G, Gershon A. Congenital varicella: case report of a serologically proved long-term survivor. Pediatrics 59:110, 1977.)*

TABLE 22–6   Reported Symptoms and Signs in Infants with Congenital Varicella Syndrome, 1947–2002

Symptom	Estimated Incidence (%)
Skin lesions (cicatricial scars, skin loss)	60–70
Ocular abnormalities (chorioretinitis, Horner syndrome, anisocoria, microphthalmia, cataract, nystagmus)	60
Neurologic abnormalities (cortical atrophy, mental retardation, microcephaly, seizures, dysphagia, limb paresis)	60
Abnormal limbs (hypoplasia, equinovarus, abnormal or absent digits)	50
Prematurity, low birth weight	35
Death in early infancy	25
Abnormalities of gastrointestinal tract	10
Urinary tract abnormalities	10
Zoster in infancy	20

See references [72, 201–284].

nystagmus.* Rarely, major abnormalities were confined to the eye. There was no apparent effect of timing of maternal varicella during gestation; the times of infection varied from 9 to 23 weeks in these infants. Figure 22–2 is a photograph showing retinal involvement in one of these patients [240,251].

Neurologic involvement is about as common as skin and eye abnormalities in infants with congenital varicella syndrome. Patients with cerebral cortical atrophy, diffuse brain involvement, or mental retardation (frequently accompanied by abnormal electroencephalograms and seizures or myoclonic jerks) have been described [216,217,224–226,259]. In a few patients, cerebrospinal fluid findings were normal [74,217,226,253]; in others, there were increased numbers of leukocytes or protein levels [216,223,225]. Bulbar palsy is suspected to result in dysphagia and bouts of aspiration pneumonia in some of these children.* Deep tendon reflexes were reported as normal in one infant [225] and diminished to absent in six,† and they were in some cases accompanied by sensory deficits [74,217,222,226,253]. Electromyography in some patients revealed a denervation pattern with loss of motor units [217,226,227,249,253]. A biopsy specimen in one instance showed replacement of muscle bundles by fat [217]. At least five children with vocal cord paralysis have been reported [259,267,270–272].

Abnormalities of the limbs can be extremely dramatic in presentation and are seen in about half of affected infants. The most common limb abnormality, which first called attention to this congenital syndrome, is hypoplasia of a limb, most commonly unilateral involvement of a leg or arm (see Table 22–6). Hypoplasia or absence of digits has also been observed [216,218,221,222,225–227]. Talipes equinovarus or a calcaneovalgus deformity has also occurred.* This complex of abnormalities in the limbs, including the bony abnormalities, is probably attributable to a neuropathy caused by direct viral invasion of the ganglia and spinal cord [268].

About one fourth of these infants died within the first 14 months of life. One infant with the obvious syndrome was stillborn [213]. In one infant who died at 6 months, autopsy revealed a necrotizing encephalitis with various degrees of gliosis and inflammatory infiltrates. Focal calcification was observed in white and gray matter of the cerebrum, brainstem, and cerebellum. Atrophy of the anterior columns of the spinal cord and scarring in the ganglion corresponding to the distribution of the skin lesions and an atrophic limb were also present. No inclusion bodies were identified [217]. Among infants with a hypoplastic limb, 40% had evidence of mental retardation or died early. The presence of a hypoplastic limb on an ultrasound examination suggests a poor outcome.

About one third of affected infants were premature or had low birth weight for their gestational ages, and about 10% had various abnormalities of the gastrointestinal tract, including reflux, duodenal stenosis, jejunal dilation, microcolon, atresia of the sigmoid colon, and sphincter malfunction.* A similar percentage had abnormalities of the urinary tract, often caused by poor or absent bladder sphincter function.† Involvement of the cervical or lumbar spinal cord and the autonomic nervous system is thought to account for the observed hypoplasia or aplasia of limbs and digits, motor and sensory defects, decrease or absence of deep tendon reflexes, Horner syndrome, and gastrointestinal and urinary tract abnormalities [280].

Figures 22–3 and 22–4 depict two children with stigmata of congenital varicella syndrome. One has severe [217] and one has relatively mild involvement [240,251].

Zoster after Congenital Varicella Syndrome

Of children with congenital varicella syndrome, 15% develop clinical zoster in infancy or early childhood, almost all in the 1st year of life.* This finding is of particular interest because cell-mediated immunity to VZV in 2 of 10 of children with the syndrome has been reported to be absent as determined by lymphocyte transformation [202,208]. In the series by Enders and associates [196] of 1291 live births (without congenital varicella syndrome), of whom conservatively perhaps 25% were infected with VZV (the attack rate could be as high as 50%), the rate

of zoster in childhood was 3%. Zoster seems to be more common in children with congenital varicella syndrome than in infants who were infected with VZV in utero, but were asymptomatic at birth.

Diagnosis of Congenital Varicella Syndrome

During the neonatal period or infancy, attempts to isolate VZV from the skin, cerebrospinal fluid, eye, and other tissues in infants with developmental defects were negative.* Although rubella virus and CMV are commonly isolated from young infants affected by these viruses, failure to isolate VZV in these cases is probably explained by the fact that the period of viral replication occurred during early gestation, and no replicating virus persisted by the time of birth. In children who developed zoster at an early age, it has been possible to isolate VZV from the rash [206,227,252]. In seven infants who died, autopsy results showed apparent dissemination of VZV with varicella-like involvement of the lungs, liver, spleen, adrenals, or pancreas [202–204,210,226–229].

Total IgM concentrations in the serum or cord blood of six infants were measured [201,217,226,238–240]. In three instances, the levels were clearly increased, with values of 48 to 100 mg/dL found when the infants were 1.5 to 6 weeks old. Specific VZV antibodies in the IgM fraction were not detected in seven cases in which they were sought [208,226,240,246,280], but they were detectable in six other cases [196,202,203,230,238]. In one of these cases, VZV IgM was detected prenatally by obtaining blood by cordocentesis [280]. In most infants, a decline of antibodies in the serum was observed, a finding compatible with a fetal or a maternal origin. In 10 instances, persistence of or an increase in antibodies in the infant supported a presumption of intrauterine infection.*

It has been possible to document some reported cases of congenital varicella syndrome, but not all of them, because antibody titers may be inconclusive even in children with the apparent full-blown and distinctive constellation of abnormalities. Some children were diagnosed even before it was possible to measure antibody titers to VZV. The development of zoster at an early age can be interpreted as substantiating VZV infection in utero. Although many of the cases reported as congenital varicella syndrome lack proof, it has been possible to show that some infants with characteristic stigmata were infected in utero with VZV, although an active, chronic infection does not exist. Modern molecular methods such as PCR and in situ hybridization have been useful for proving congenital varicella syndrome in a few reported infants and will undoubtedly be used to prove future cases [196,211,213–215,259]. In the future, it is expected that these will become the methods of choice rather than antibody testing. It is also predicted that with widespread use of varicella vaccine, the incidence of this unusual cause of congenital disease will become rare.

---

*References [203,204,210,214,216,225,233,247,249,253,278].

*References [215,216,223,237,251,252,255,256,258].

†References [208,216,217,220,235,248,253,256].

*References [196,214,215,220,234,239,244,245,253,257,259,260,264].

---

*References [201,217,225,233,234,239,240].

*References [201,219,224,239–241,251,253].

Fetal Malformations and Management of Pregnant Women with Varicella-Zoster Virus Infection

In the 1990s, the incidence of fetal malformations after maternal VZV infection was clarified. Varicella is a significantly greater threat than zoster; 95% of reported cases of congenital varicella syndrome have followed maternal chickenpox. In the series by Enders and associates [196] of 366 women with zoster in pregnancy, there were no cases of congenital varicella syndrome. This outcome is not unexpected because zoster is probably less likely to be accompanied by a viremia than is varicella; many fetuses may escape VZV infection from maternal zoster. Because zoster is a secondary infection, residual maternal immunity to VZV may at least partially protect the fetus from damage, analogous to that seen when congenital CMV infection is caused by reactivation rather than primary CMV infection [285]. As with CMV infection, however, it is possible, although rare, for fetal stigmata to follow secondary maternal infection.

The time at which maternal VZV infection occurs during gestation also influences whether the infant is likely to be severely damaged. Infection during the first and early second trimesters seems to be the most critical. Most reported cases of congenital varicella syndrome have occurred when the onset of maternal infection was before the 20th week of pregnancy. Only seven infants with some of the stigmata have been recorded as the result of maternal varicella after the 20th week [175,211, 245–247,255,284]. When maternal varicella occurs after the 20th week, the infant may be infected, but usually the only evidence is a positive VZV antibody titer when the infant is older than 1 year and, in some cases, development of zoster at an early age.

Eleven prospective studies of the incidence of congenital varicella syndrome have been published. Data from these studies are presented in Table 22–7. There are 14 cases of congenital varicella syndrome in 858 (1.6%) women who developed varicella in the first 20 weeks of pregnancy. If the entire gestational period is considered, 2245 women who had varicella during pregnancy were delivered of live-born infants; the overall incidence of congenital varicella syndrome was 0.6%. These data indicate that the risk for development of congenital varicella syndrome is mostly confined to the first 20 weeks of pregnancy, and the risk after maternal varicella in the first 20 weeks of pregnancy is extremely low, on the order of 1% to 2%. Weeks 7 to 20 are the time of the greatest risk [196]. The tendency to develop overwhelming forms of VZV infection in the fetus indicates the increased ability of VZV to multiply in fetal tissues, which is similar to that of other viruses such as rubella virus and CMV.

Counseling of pregnant women who have acquired varicella during pregnancy can be very difficult. Because the congenital syndrome is rare, termination of pregnancy is not routinely recommended, in contrast to recommendations for gestational rubella. When the syndrome does occur, however, it is likely to be severe. It would be helpful if prenatal diagnoses were available, but diagnostic attempts such as measurement of maternal antibody titers and amniocentesis have not proved useful. Although

TABLE 22–7 Incidence of Congenital Varicella Syndrome: Results of Prospective Studies 1960–1997

| Year | Incidence of Syndrome | |
	First Trimester/ First 20 Weeks	Total Gestation
1960 [508]	0/70	0/288
1973 [72]	2/27	2/135
1984 [231]	0/23	
1986 [182]	1/11	1/38
1992 [72]	0/40	
1994 [212]	1/49	
1994 [201]	7/351	7/1291
1994 [211]	2/99	2/146
1996 [173]	0/26	
1997 [184]	0/22	
2002 [176]	0/140	1/347
Total reported	13/858 (1.6%)	14/2245 (0.6%)

blood may be obtained by cordocentesis for antibody testing, the presence of fetal VZV IgM does not mean that the infant has congenital varicella syndrome, but only that infection with VZV has occurred. Similarly, PCR may identify an infected fetus, but not one with malformations [283,286].

Ultrasonography has been used successfully to identify the following fetal abnormalities after maternal varicella: hydrocephalus 12 weeks later [202]; clubfeet and hydrocephalus 13 weeks later [233]; a large, bullous skin lesion originally believed to be a meningocele 15 weeks later [236]; calcifications in the liver and other organs 9, 15, and 18 weeks later [214,234,261]; a hypoplastic limb and clubfoot 11 and 16 weeks later [196,214]; and a lacuna of the skull 25 weeks later [230]. Successful use of ultrasound as a diagnostic tool to identify this syndrome prenatally has also been reported in cases with evidence of widespread infection [273–276]. Three published reports indicate, however, that ultrasound is not infallible. In two infants, ultrasound scans were normal 3 weeks after maternal varicella, but the fetuses were later diagnosed as having congenital varicella syndrome [203,233]. One infant was diagnosed with liver calcifications by ultrasonography at 27 weeks and a positive PCR for VZV; his mother had varicella at 12.5 weeks. At birth, no obvious anomalies were present, and the infant did well except for development of zoster at age 8 months [283]. Even defects detected by ultrasonography must be interpreted with some caution.

Because about 40% of reported patients with a hypoplastic limb also sustained brain damage or died in early infancy, the presence of a limb abnormality on ultrasound seems to suggest a poor overall prognosis for the fetus. Two women were reported to have terminated their pregnancies after the diagnosis of congenital varicella syndrome was made based on abnormal limbs on ultrasound scan. At autopsy, the fetuses were found to be severely affected [196,283]. Because abnormalities may not be detected by ultrasound immediately after maternal varicella, by the time any is noticed, it may be too late to consider interruption of pregnancy, depending on the time of onset of maternal varicella.

Although congenital varicella syndrome varies in severity, most cases are severe. It would be helpful if maternal infection could be identified and appropriate management initiated as early as possible. It is unknown whether administration of VZIG or acyclovir to a pregnant woman can prevent her fetus from developing congenital varicella syndrome. In the study by Enders and associates [196], there were no cases of the congenital syndrome in 97 women who were given VZIG on exposure; it is unknown how many of these women were in the first 20 weeks of pregnancy.

Perinatal Chickenpox

Perinatal chickenpox includes disease that is acquired postnatally by droplet infection and that is transplacentally transmitted or congenital. Chickenpox is considered to be transplacentally transmitted when it occurs within 10 days of birth.

Postnatally Acquired Chickenpox

Postnatally acquired chickenpox, which begins 10 to 28 days after birth, is generally mild [287]. The experiences with nosocomial chickenpox infections in the newborn nursery that were described in a previous section further corroborate the benign nature of the disease and the fact that transmission to neonates in this environment is inefficient and rarely reaches epidemic proportions.

Deaths among neonates caused by postnatally acquired disease are rare, but some data indicate an appreciably higher incidence of complications or deaths in neonates than in older children [96,101–103,108,287,288]. Preblud and associates [287] found that of 92 reported deaths caused by varicella from 1968–1978 in children younger than 1 year, only 5 occurred in newborns (8 hours to 19 days old). Although mortality was increased by a factor of 4 for infants younger than 1 year compared with older children, there was a low calculated death rate for varicella throughout childhood (8 in 100,000 patients if <1 year and 2 in 100,000 patients 1 to 14 years old) [287]. One 15-day-old infant with severe disseminated chickenpox born to a woman who developed varicella 7 days after delivery has been described [288]. The child survived; acyclovir was administered for 10 days. The only other report in the English literature of severe postnatally acquired varicella in an infant younger than 1 month is that of Gustafson and colleagues [96]. The term infant with Turner syndrome was exposed to varicella when 7 days old, developed more than 200 vesicles, and died of pneumonia; however, the role of VZV in this infant's death was unclear because no autopsy was performed.

Congenital Chickenpox: Maternal Infection Near Term

Congenital chickenpox is not inevitable when maternal chickenpox occurs in the 21 days preceding parturition. In only 8 (24%) of 34 reported cases of maternal disease with onset during this period did chickenpox

develop in the neonate within the first 10 days of life [98,136,171,173]. An identical attack rate of 24% for congenital varicella after the occurrence of maternal varicella within 17 days preceding delivery was arrived at by Meyers [289], who reviewed many cases in the literature and 14 examples reported to the U.S. Centers for Disease Control and Prevention (CDC) in 1972–1973. Attack rates on the order of 50% were reported, however, in two studies on the efficacy of passive immunization to prevent severe neonatal varicella [290,291]. In Meyers' study [289], there was no statistically significant relationship between day of onset of the rash in the mother and subsequent attack rates of congenital varicella. Seven of 22 neonates born to mothers whose rash appeared less than 5 days antepartum ultimately developed congenital chickenpox, whereas 4 of 24 infants born to mothers whose rash began 5 to 14 days antepartum had congenital disease [289]. These data indicate that the attack rate in congenital varicella (25% to 50%) is lower than after household exposure to VZV (80% to 90%) and suggest that blood-borne transmission may be less efficient than transmission by the skin and respiratory routes.

The incubation period in congenital varicella, defined as the interval between the onset of rash in the mother and onset in the fetus or neonate, is usually 9 to 15 days [292]. This interval is slightly shorter than the normal postnatal incubation period, possibly because fetal tissues are more susceptible to VZV than more mature tissues. Rarely, presumably when fetal infection is caused by the primary maternal viremia, the exanthem appears in the mother and neonate within 3 days of each other [101] or even simultaneously [292]. The average incubation period in 36 cases reported in the literature was 11 days, with a maximum of 16 days. In only three instances was the incubation period less than 6 days [289].

In contrast to postnatally acquired neonatal chickenpox, congenital chickenpox can be associated with significant mortality. Severe cases clinically resemble varicella in the immunocompromised host. An infant who died of hemorrhagic varicella with pulmonary and liver involvement is shown in Figure 22–1. The spectrum of illness also includes extremely mild infections with only a handful of vesicles. Erlich and coworkers [133] first observed that infants born with the rash or who had an early onset of rash survived, whereas infants who died had a relatively late onset of rash. It was hypothesized that for neonates with early onset, maternal illness had occurred long enough before parturition to allow antibodies to be elaborated by the mother and to cross the placenta. Subsequent reports offer strong confirmation of these observations. There were no deaths among 22 infants with congenital chickenpox (reviewed by Meyers [289] whose onset of rash occurred between birth and 4 days of age. In contrast, 4 (21%) of 19 neonates in whom the rash began when they were 5 to 10 days old died (Table 22–8) [289]. These four deaths occurred among 13 neonates (31%) whose mothers' exanthems developed within 4 days before birth, but no deaths were observed among 23 neonates with congenital chickenpox whose mothers developed a rash 5 or more days before birth.

Further support for the protective or modifying effect of maternal antibody has come from measurements of

TABLE 22–8 Deaths from Congenital Varicella in Relation to Date of Onset of Rash in Mother or Neonate

Onset	Neonatal Deaths	Neonatal Cases	%
Day of onset of rash in neonate			
0–4	0	22	0
5–10	4	19	21
Onset of maternal rash, days antepartum			
≥5	0	23	0
0–4	4	13	31

Data from Meyers JD. Congenital varicella in term infants: risk reconsidered. J Infect Dis 129:215, 1974; with permission from the University of Chicago.

placental transfer of IgG to VZV [91]. When varicella occurred more than 1 week before delivery, complement-fixing antibody titers in maternal and cord blood were similar. In contrast, when infection occurred 3 to 5 days before delivery, maternal antibody was present at parturition, and antibodies to VZV in the neonate were absent or at least eightfold lower. These data suggest that a lag of several days occurs before IgG antibodies to VZV cross the placenta and equilibrate with the fetal circulation. The development of mild congenital varicella in the presence of placentally transferred maternal antibody has also been shown using the more sensitive FAMA test [62]. The neonate may be at risk for developing severe varicella because the immune system is immature, as has been shown by Kohl [293] with regard to host defense against HSV.

Zoster in Neonates and Older Children

The most characteristic feature of zoster is the localization of the rash. It is nearly always unilateral, does not cross the midline, and is typically limited to an area of skin served by one to three sensory ganglia. In children, prodromes of malaise, fever, headache, and nausea may be observed. Pain and paresthesias in the involved dermatome may precede the exanthem by 4 or 5 days. Involvement of the dermatomes of the head, neck, and trunk is more common than involvement of the extremities, a distribution that also reflects the density of lesions in chickenpox [41]. Erythematous papules give rise to grouped vesicles, which progress to pustules in 2 to 4 days. New crops of vesicles may keep appearing for 1 week. Pain may be associated with the exanthem and usually abates as the skin lesions scab; in elderly adults, severe and incapacitating neuralgia of the involved nerve may persist for months. Cutaneous dissemination of vesicles to sites distant from the involved dermatome is observed uncommonly and is more frequent in compromised hosts, such as patients with lymphoma or immunologic deficiencies.

Zoster occurs as host defense mechanisms against VZV wane in a person who has previously experienced chickenpox. Because immunity is relatively durable, this hypothesis presumes that zoster occurs predominantly in older persons and is rare in neonates. Among 192 patients

with zoster in a general practice, the attack rate increased progressively with age [41]. Only six patients were younger than 10 years; the youngest was 2 years old. In two reported series describing zoster in a total of 22 children, only two cases occurred in children younger than 2 years old [171,294]. These reports confirm the rarity of zoster among infants. When zoster occurs in children who have not previously had chickenpox, there is often a history of intrauterine exposure to VZV. In these reports, the mothers contracted chickenpox during gestation, but gave birth to normal infants who, without ever developing chickenpox despite frequent childhood exposure, developed typical zoster at a young age, many in the first few months of life [74,260,295–299]. In most of these infants, the course of zoster was benign. One infant developed a second attack of zoster when 10 months old; the first occurred when the infant was 4 months old [295].

Although there are six reports of zoster during the neonatal period [300–305], it is doubtful whether any of these cases diagnosed on clinical grounds is an authentic example of zoster. HSV may produce a vesicular exanthem in the newborn that appears to have a dermatomal distribution. Virus isolation (or demonstration of VZV DNA or antigen from skin lesions) is required before a diagnosis of zoster can be accepted. Serologic studies are not useful in differentiating these diseases.

DIAGNOSIS AND DIFFERENTIAL DIAGNOSIS
Chickenpox

In a neonate with a widespread, generalized vesicular exanthem and a history of recent maternal varicella or postnatal exposure, a diagnosis of chickenpox can usually be made with confidence on clinical grounds alone. Greater difficulty is encountered when lesions are few, or when there is no history of exposure.

Diagnostic Techniques

If laboratory diagnosis is required, it is best accomplished by showing VZV antigen or DNA in skin lesions or isolating virus from vesicular fluid. VZV antigen may be shown by using immunofluorescence, employing a monoclonal antibody to VZV that is conjugated to fluorescein and is commercially available [306–308]. For virus isolation, fluid should be promptly inoculated onto tissue cultures because VZV is labile. PCR has proved extremely sensitive and accurate for diagnosis of VZV infections [118,309–315]. In situ hybridization is also a useful diagnostic technique [215,316,317].

VZV infections may be documented by demonstration of a fourfold or greater increase in VZV antibody titer by using a sensitive test such as FAMA or ELISA. The presence of specific IgM in one serum specimen suggests recent VZV infection [39,40,318]. Persistence of VZV antibody beyond the age of 8 months is highly suggestive of intrauterine varicella, provided that there is no history of clinical varicella after birth [25]. Persistence of VZV antibody with no decrease in titer over several months in a young infant (as long as all sera are tested simultaneously) is highly suggestive of intrauterine infection. A FAMA or latex agglutination antibody titer of

1:4 or greater beyond 8 months of life is suggestive of immunity to varicella, provided that the patient has not received γ-globulin or other blood products in the previous 3 to 4 months. Physicians should be aware that no serologic test is 100% accurate for identifying individuals immune to varicella, although these antibody tests are generally reliable [319].

Differential Diagnosis

Several diseases may be considered in the differential diagnosis of varicella in the newborn, including neonatal HSV, contact dermatitis, hand-foot-and-mouth syndrome and other enterovirus infections, and impetigo. In neonatal HSV, cutaneous lesions may be relatively sparse and may be absent altogether despite widespread visceral dissemination. Vesicles tend to occur in clusters, rather than in the more even distribution seen in chickenpox. Fever, marked toxicity, and encephalitis are more common in neonates with HSV. Stained smears of vesicle fluid (i.e., Tzanck preparation) are not helpful in differentiating HSV from varicella because both are characterized by multinucleated giant cells and intranuclear inclusion bodies. In cell cultures, HSV typically produces a widespread cytopathic effect in 24 to 48 hours, whereas the cytopathic effect caused by VZV is cell associated and focal and develops more slowly. Indirect immunofluorescence using monoclonal antibodies conjugated to fluorescein can be performed on smears of skin scrapings; if positive, the assay can identify VZV, HSV-1, and HSV-2 within several hours. Paired serum samples can be examined for increasing antibody titers to HSV and VZV antigens. It is exceedingly rare for varicella to develop in a newborn in the absence of any (i.e., infant or mother) exposure to varicella or zoster. In contrast, most infants with neonatal HSV have no recognized exposure to the virus.

Although 95% of cases of perinatal HSV are transmitted during delivery, a syndrome similar to congenital varicella syndrome, with limb and eye abnormalities, skin scarring, and zosteriform rashes, has rarely been observed after the unusual occurrence of intrauterine transmission of HSV [320,321]. In an infant with stigmata of congenital varicella syndrome whose mother has no history of varicella during pregnancy, congenital HSV should be considered. It may be impossible to make a definitive diagnosis immediately, unless the infant develops a vesicular rash from which the causative virus can be identified. Determination of antibody titers to HSV and VZV at presentation and when infants are 8 to 12 months old may be useful to establish a diagnosis.

In some cases of contact dermatitis, papules and vesicles may appear after exposure to specific chemical irritants. Typically, they appear on exposed body surfaces and do not have the characteristic distribution of chickenpox or smallpox.

In patients with hand-foot-and-mouth syndrome, a vesicular exanthem usually caused by coxsackievirus A16 or A5 may be observed during the enterovirus season (i.e., summer or early autumn). There are rarely more than a dozen vesicles, and they typically occur on the distal extremities, especially the palms and soles. Vesicular lesions that ulcerate quickly may also be seen in the oropharynx. The causative virus is readily isolated from vesicle fluid or from feces.

Impetigo may occur in neonates. In bullous impetigo (i.e., pemphigus neonatorum), large blebs are present instead of the smaller vesicles of chickenpox. This disease, which is caused by *Staphylococcus aureus*, may be associated with high fever, toxicity, septicemia, and death. Alternative diagnoses include syphilis, group B streptococcal infection, and incontinentia pigmenti, which may cause vesiculobullous lesions in a neonate.

Smallpox is traditionally part of the differential diagnosis of vesicular lesions in neonates. Although smallpox was eradicated, there is concern that the disease may reemerge because of bioterrorism. Classically, the vesicles of smallpox appear to be at the same stage of development instead of showing the pattern of crops over several days. A centrifugal distribution of the skin rash is prominent. The best approach in a suspicious situation is to rule out the possibility of VZV or HSV infection as described previously, preferably by immunofluorescence testing. If the test results are negative, a search for smallpox may be indicated, especially if the history of the patient warrants it. Accurate diagnosis may be achieved in hours by electron microscopy of the vesicle fluid or crusts; such microscopic examination reveals virus particles whose morphology is very different from that of viruses of the herpes family. Smallpox modified by exposure to vaccinia in the distant past and alastrim (i.e., variola minor) may be particularly difficult to distinguish from chickenpox. In suspicious cases, the CDC and local health department should be promptly involved.

Disseminated vaccinia is rare today because smallpox vaccine (i.e., vaccinia virus) is not routinely used, although a bioterrorism attack could change the scenario. Vaccinia can be considered in a neonate exposed postnatally to a person who has been recently vaccinated. The lesions resemble those of smallpox. Impression smears of vesicle fluid do not show intranuclear inclusions or giant cells. Laboratory diagnosis may be achieved by electron microscopy and immunofluorescence.

Zoster

Zoster usually is easily recognized by the typical dermatomal distribution of the vesicular lesions. In the differential diagnosis, the main entity to be distinguished in the neonatal period is HSV appearing in a linear pattern. Identification of VZV or HSV DNA by PCR, antigen by immunofluorescence or virus isolation is the only reliable means of differentiating these entities when the distribution of the exanthem is linear. Contact dermatitis should also be considered in the differential diagnosis of zosteriform lesions in the neonatal period.

THERAPY
Treatment of the Mother

Acyclovir is the antiviral drug of choice for treatment of potentially severe or severe VZV infections [322,323]. Acyclovir itself has no antiviral action, but when it is phosphorylated by enzymes produced by cells infected with VZV, it is incorporated as a DNA chain terminator, and it inhibits viral DNA polymerase. Because these actions occur only in virus-infected cells, acyclovir is well tolerated and associated with little toxicity. The drug is available in topical, oral, and intravenous formulations.

The safety of acyclovir has been shown in the past 35 years, and there is good reason to use this drug liberally in clinical situations for which it is indicated, even during pregnancy. Although most VZV infections in normal hosts are self-limited, there is a low but real fatality rate from varicella in adults. For this reason and because long-term toxicity of acyclovir in the fetus seems unlikely, acyclovir is recommended more often for use during pregnancy in women with varicella than previously. A registry of patients (and their offspring) who have received acyclovir during pregnancy has been established [189,190]. Generally, pregnant women who develop varicella should be treated with orally administered acyclovir and observed carefully. Pregnant women who develop severe varicella while receiving oral therapy, especially patients who develop pneumonia, should be promptly treated with intravenous acyclovir [324]. Supportive respiratory therapy (e.g., nasal oxygen, tracheostomy, ventilatory assistance) should be used as needed. Controlled studies of corticosteroids for varicella pneumonia are unavailable; steroids are not recommended. Antibiotics should be given if there is evidence of bacterial superinfection.

Anecdotal reports on the apparently successful use of acyclovir in pregnant women with varicella have been published, although controlled studies have not been performed. The data suggest that most women who develop varicella in pregnancy ultimately survive without sequelae [174]. This is undoubtedly the result of increasing awareness of the potential seriousness of the illness on the part of medical providers and the more liberal use of acyclovir today.

There is little information on the use of acyclovir for pregnant women with zoster. Presumably, because zoster would be expected to be self-limited in most women of childbearing age, there would be little need for antiviral therapy in this situation. Especially in the setting of an extensive rash or severe pain, use of acyclovir, particularly as oral therapy, should be strongly considered. Alternatively, one of the newer drugs, such as famciclovir or valacyclovir, can be used to treat pregnant women who develop severe zoster. The dose of famciclovir is 500 mg taken orally three times daily; the dose of valacyclovir is 1 g taken orally three times daily. Both medications are administered for 7 days. There is no information on the use of famciclovir or valacyclovir in pregnancy. Although famciclovir and valacyclovir are converted to acyclovir, and acyclovir is the active drug in the blood, there is more safety information on use of acyclovir in pregnancy, and for that reason it is probably preferable.

Acyclovir has been most effective when it is administered within 1 day after the onset of varicella and 3 days after onset of zoster. The usual adult dose for intravenous acyclovir is 10 mg/kg, given three times per day. Orally administered acyclovir has been found to have a modest effect on the fever and rash of varicella in otherwise healthy populations. A multicenter, double-blind, placebo-controlled, collaborative study involving 815 similarly treated children, who were given 20 mg/kg of acyclovir orally four times per day, shortened the course of illness by about 1 day [325]. The benefit to secondary household cases was not increased beyond that of primary cases. Similar results emerged from a study involving adolescents with varicella [326]. The modest benefit conferred by oral acyclovir therapy is not surprising in view of the self-limited nature of chickenpox in children and the poor oral absorption of acyclovir. There is a similar benefit for adults with varicella who were given oral acyclovir (800 mg taken five times each day for 5 days) within 24 hours of onset of rash [327,328].

In the double-blind, placebo-controlled study of Wallace and associates [328], involving 76 military recruits, the duration of illness was shortened by about 1 day, and the personnel were able to return to work 1 day sooner on average, if they received acyclovir. There is no information regarding treatment of pregnant women, and physicians are reluctant to extrapolate to them from studies involving mainly healthy young men. Given the possibility that acyclovir will help and is unlikely to harm, however, the drug should be strongly considered for most adults today with early varicella, pregnant or not.

Treatment of the Newborn Infant

Although there is little information on the use of acyclovir in newborns for varicella, it has been used to treat many infants with neonatal HSV infection. In a study in which 95 infants received acyclovir (30 mg/kg/day given intravenously), no short-term or long-term toxicity was observed [323–325]. Pharmacokinetic studies have indicated that dose adjustments for acyclovir may be necessary in premature infants and infants with hepatic or renal dysfunction [329–331]. There are no data about the use of oral acyclovir for severe neonatal infections caused by VZV, and acyclovir is poorly absorbed when given by the gastrointestinal route. A dose of 1500 mg/m² of acyclovir, given intravenously in three divided daily doses, is recommended for infants with severe or rapidly progressing varicella. It is not recommended that infants with congenital varicella syndrome receive treatment with acyclovir except in the unusual setting of active zoster.

PREVENTION

Immunity to Varicella-Zoster Virus

Immunity to VZV may be incomplete in some persons. It was recognized years ago that waning of immunity to VZV might predispose a person to zoster [41]. That immunity to varicella might wane occasionally and result in a second case of chickenpox has been recognized only more recently. Immunologic evidence consistent with asymptomatic reinfection with VZV, manifested by an increase in VZV-specific IgG or IgA or the production of IgM and an increase in the cell-mediated immune response to VZV, has been documented in adults with a household exposure to varicella [332,333]. Symptomatic reactivation with subsequent boosting of immunity is also possible, but is difficult to substantiate.

Clinical reinfection with VZV has been observed in some persons despite a positive antibody titer at exposure [334–337]. Most clinical reinfections are mild, however, which suggests that partial immunity to the virus may be present. Cellular immunity and antibodies may play a role in protection. In a study by Bogger-Goren and co-workers [338], children with positive cellular immune responses were likely to be protected against varicella after household exposure even if they were seronegative; in contrast, children with negative responses became infected. Secretory IgA against VZV has also been shown after chickenpox [339]. Although it has not been shown, it is hypothesized that cellular immunity at the mucosal level may play a role in protection against clinical varicella.

In addition to predisposing to reinfection with the virus, incomplete immunity to VZV is associated with development of zoster. In addition to clinical zoster, silent reactivation of latent VZV in persons who have had previous varicella probably occurs; this may be detected immunologically by an increase in antibody titer or the transient appearance of specific IgM, although it is difficult to rule out the possibility of an exogenous exposure [40,340–342]. Sometimes, clinical manifestations of zoster such as pain may occur in the absence of a rash—so-called zoster sine herpete. Silent reactivation of VZV in bone marrow transplant patients has been shown by PCR [343]. Zoster results in patients who have latent VZV infection when specific cell-mediated immunity is depressed [121,122,124,344]. Defective antibody responses to VZV glycoproteins have not been associated with development of zoster in immunocompromised persons [345]. Similarly, the increased incidence of zoster in elderly adults has been associated with loss of cell-mediated immunity to VZV [346,347], whereas antibody to VZV does not wane with age but tends to increase [348]. Immunity to VZV may be seen as a complex interaction between humoral and cell-mediated immunity responses, with the possibility of partial and complete immunity to the virus.

It is possible to provide humoral immunity to persons at high risk for developing severe varicella by passive immunization. Until more recently, this was done with VZIG. Although used successfully to prevent severe varicella, passive immunization has not prevented zoster in persons at high risk for it [349], and it is not believed to be useful to treat patients with varicella or zoster [350]. Passive immunization should not be employed to try to prevent development of varicella pneumonia in the pregnant woman with chickenpox or dissemination in an already infected infant. It is uncertain whether passive immunization of a woman with varicella can prevent infection of her fetus or development of congenital varicella syndrome. It is possible to increase cell-mediated immunity to VZV by immunization, and this approach was explored in several studies [351–353]. Results of a large, double-blind, controlled study in healthy vaccinees older than 60 years indicated that approximately half of more than 15,000 vaccinated individuals were protected

from developing zoster [354]. This study by Oxman and colleagues also indicated that there are currently about 1 million annual cases of zoster in the United States.

Passive Immunization against Varicella

Controlled studies have indicated that pooled immunoglobulin attenuates, but does not prevent, chickenpox when administered to susceptible family contacts [64] and that zoster immunoglobulin (ZIG) prevents clinical chickenpox when given to susceptible healthy children within 72 hours of household exposure [355]. Additional uncontrolled studies of immunocompromised children, such as children with leukemia receiving maintenance chemotherapy, at high risk for developing severe or fatal varicella have indicated that ZIG administered within 3 to 5 days of a household exposure usually modifies varicella so that the infection is mild or subclinical [356–358]. VZIG under the trade name VariZIG is manufactured in Canada and is available under an investigational new drug application expanded access protocol (telephone number for requests: 800 843-7477). The dose is 1.25 mL (1 vial or 125 U) for each 10 kg of body weight, with a maximum dosage of 6 mL (5 vials or 625 U) intramuscularly [197,359].

Passive immunization may prolong the incubation period of varicella [357]. Passive immunization has also been studied for its possible efficacy in modifying severe congenital varicella that may occur in the infant of a woman who develops chickenpox close to term. Infants born to women with the onset of varicella more than 5 days before delivery can be expected to have mild infection [62,133,289,360,361], and these infants do not require passive immunization. In contrast, infants born to women who develop varicella 5 days or less before delivery are at risk for developing disseminated or fatal varicella, and these infants can be expected to benefit from passive immunization. In an uncontrolled study by Hanngren and coworkers [290] of 41 neonates born to women who developed varicella between 4 days before and 2 days after delivery, the illness seemed to be modified. These infants received 1 mL of ZIG. Although the attack rate was 51%, and the incubation period averaged 11 days, there were no fatalities instead of the expected mortality rate of about 30%, and 13 (62%) of 21 had fewer than 20 vesicles with no fever. Two (10%) had severe infections, and one was treated with interferon.

In a similar study of VZIG by Preblud and colleagues [291], a similar varicella attack rate of 45% was observed in 132 infants. In this study, a dose of 125 U (1.25 mL) of VZIG was administered. The illness also seemed to be modified because of 53 infants with varicella, 74% had less than 50 vesicles, and only 10% had more than 100 vesicles. No antiviral therapy was given; there was one death in the group, but it was unclear that it was caused by varicella. The high attack rates of varicella in these studies compared with historical data have not been explained. In previous studies, infant attack rates of 24% in late [289] and overall [208] pregnancy have been reported. Successful passive immunization would, if anything, be expected to decrease the attack rate, rather than increase it. Nevertheless, the mildness of the illness and absence of mortality in these two studies are suggestive, if not proof positive, of successful passive immunization of infants born to women with varicella at term. Since the introduction of ZIG and VZIG for use in appropriate neonates, fatalities from neonatal varicella have become rare.

It is recommended that VZIG or VariZIG be administered to infants whose mothers have the onset of varicella 5 days or less before delivery or in the first 48 hours after delivery [195,362,363]. A dose of 125 U (1.25 mL or one vial) should be administered intramuscularly as soon as possible after birth. Administration of VZIG to the mother before delivery of the infant is not recommended because a larger dose would be required to provide passive immunization to the infant, and no benefit to the mother would result. Early delivery of the infant of a mother with active varicella is also not recommended; the longer the infant remains in utero, the more likely there will be transplacental transfer of maternal antibody. A diagram of the relationship between maternal and infant varicella, development of maternal antibodies, and transplacental transfer of these antibodies is shown in Figure 22–5. Because women with zoster near term have high antibody titers to VZV, it is unnecessary to administer VZIG to their infants.

A few infants have developed severe or fatal congenital varicella despite prompt administration of VZIG in adequate dosage [364–369]. The reason for the severity of these cases is not fully understood, but they seem to be unusual or rare. Presumably, they were immunologically normal infants. Many of these children were reported from the United Kingdom, and the VZIG used there might have been less potent than that produced in the United States. The antibody titers of the two preparations were never compared. Passively immunized infants should be observed carefully, however, for the rare instance in which antiviral therapy may also be required. Rapid evolution of large numbers of vesicles, hemorrhagic manifestations, and respiratory involvement are indications for the use of intravenous acyclovir. Some investigators have recommended prophylactic use of intravenously administered acyclovir in any infant who develops varicella despite passive immunization [365,366,370,371], but this strategy has not been formally studied.

Based on the studies cited previously, most passively immunized infants who develop clinical illness have mild or moderate infections. Administration of intravenous acyclovir to all such infants who develop clinical illness

would result in needless hospitalization of many infants and potential iatrogenic problems and would not be cost-effective. Unless additional data become available, intravenous acyclovir should be given only to infants who manifest early signs of potentially severe varicella. Infants who develop varicella despite passive immunization may be given a trial of orally administered acyclovir and observed carefully for the remote possibility of development of severe varicella, at which point intravenous acyclovir may be given.

Although it is recommended that VZIG or VariZIG be administered to infants born to women who develop varicella in the first 2 days after delivery, few reports indicate that this timing of birth at onset of maternal varicella is associated with increased risk to the infant. One of the reported infants with fatal varicella despite passive immunization was born to a woman who developed chickenpox on the 2nd postpartum day [367]. A child with severe varicella whose mother developed chickenpox 3 days after delivery has also been reported [372]. This child was treated with a leukocyte transfusion from her mother and thymic hormone and survived. In view of the absence of data indicating efficacy and the potential danger of graft-versus-host reaction after leukocyte transfusion in immunocompromised patients [373], this therapy cannot be recommended.

To minimize the possibility of infection of the infant, mother and infant should be separated until the mother's chickenpox vesicles have dried, even if the infant has been passively immunized. Normally, this would be 5 to 7 days after the onset of maternal rash. If the infant develops clinical varicella, the mother may care for the infant.

Pregnant women who are closely exposed to persons with varicella or zoster and who have no history of varicella and are seronegative may be passively immunized with VZIG [195]. Although precise information regarding dosage is unavailable, a dose of 5 mL (625 U) is usually recommended for adults. The rationale for passive immunization of the mother is to protect her from developing severe chickenpox.

Because some low birth weight infants may have low or absent levels of transplacentally acquired maternal VZV antibody, it is recommended that infants of less than 28 weeks' gestation or who weighed less than 1000 g at birth be passively immunized after close exposure

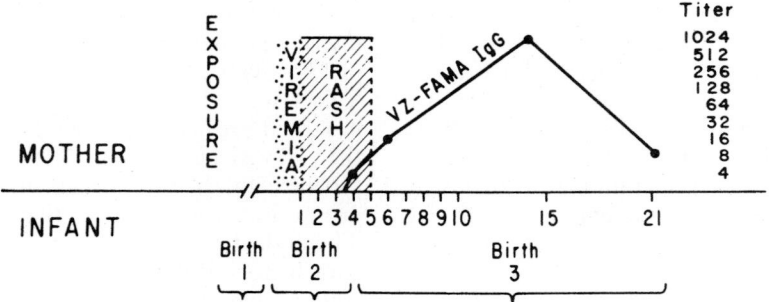

FIGURE 22–5 **Diagrammatic representation of transmission of varicella-zoster virus (VZV) and VZV antibody to a fetus in maternal varicella near term.** When the infant is born during the maternal incubation period (*1*), no varicella occurs unless the infant is exposed postnatally to the infection. When the infant is born 0 to 4 days after onset of maternal varicella (*2*), disseminated varicella may develop because the infection is not modified by maternal antibody. The onset of varicella occurs when the infant is 5 to 10 days old. Infants born 5 days or more after maternal varicella (*3*) receive maternal antibody, which leads to mild infection. This diagram is based on data for 50 newborn infants with varicella. (*Adapted from Gershon A. Varicella in mother and infant: problems old and new.* In *Krugman S, Gershon A [eds]. Infection of the Fetus and Newborn Infant. New York, Alan R Liss, 1975, pp 79–95.*)

[195,362,363]. There is no recognized age at which passive immunization is no longer recommended for these infants, but presumably it would be unnecessary in an infant more than several weeks old. Administration of passive immunization to term infants who are 2 to 7 days old at the time of exposure is not recommended, but it may be done optionally to decrease morbidity from varicella in this age group [374]. Passive immunization should not be used to try to control nosocomial varicella because it does not prevent varicella, but rather modifies it.

Guidelines for Preventive Measures and Isolation Procedures in the Nursery

In contrast to transplacentally transmitted chickenpox, there is little evidence that postnatally acquired chickenpox (defined as disease beginning after the infant is 10 days old) is significantly more serious in infants than in older children (discussed in the preceding section). Nevertheless, despite the evidence cited previously indicating that nosocomial chickenpox among infants in the nursery is uncommon, it is desirable to institute preventive measures to minimize the possibility of transmission of infection to other neonates, mothers, and hospital personnel.

Any hospital patient isolated because of chickenpox or zoster should be in a separate room with the door closed, preferably in a room with air pressure negative compared with that in the corridor. Visitors and staff should be limited to persons immune to varicella. They should wear a new gown for each entry and wash their hands when leaving. Bedding and tissues soiled with respiratory excreta of the patient should be bagged and autoclaved. Special precautions for feces, urine, and needles or blood products are not required. Terminal disinfection of the room is likewise unnecessary.

Guidelines for isolation procedures and other measures are summarized in Table 22–9. In the vaccine era, these options rarely need to be considered because the incidence of varicella in children is rapidly decreasing. If there are siblings or others at home with active VZV infections at the time mother and infant are ready for discharge from the hospital, one of the following alternatives is recommended:

1. The mother and neonate may be sent home after boarding the older siblings with immune relatives until they are no longer infectious, generally when no new vesicles have appeared for 72 hours and all lesions have progressed to the stage of crusts.
2. The mother can return home while the neonate remains in the nursery.
3. The neonate can be boarded with a surrogate mother until the siblings are no longer infectious.
4. VZIG may be given to the newborn.

If siblings at home develop chickenpox at the time of delivery or shortly after birth, and the mother lacks a definite history of previous chickenpox, the first or last alternative is recommended. Serologic determination of the mother's immune status to varicella is recommended. Women with detectable VZV antibodies may be discharged home. Women who are seronegative should be offered varicella vaccine. Theoretically, if a woman has

a history of varicella, her newborn should be at least partially protected from varicella. It seems prudent, however, to use a conservative approach, such as outlined here, because the real risk of varicella to the newborn is unknown.

When a mother with a negative history is exposed to chickenpox or zoster 6 to 20 days antepartum, she may become infectious before the onset of exanthem, during hospitalization for labor and the puerperium, assuming an average stay of 72 hours. This calculation is based on a minimum incubation period (exposure until onset of rash) of 10 days and a period of communicability preceding the exanthem by 3 days. When maternal exposure occurs less than 6 days before the onset of labor, the mother is unlikely to become infectious until after she has returned home. In either case, if the mother is exposed to chickenpox during the 20-day period antepartum, it is advisable to send the mother and infant home at the earliest possible date.

No special management is necessary for other mothers and infants in the nursery or for physicians and nurses potentially exposed in the delivery room or the nursery if they have previously had chickenpox. In the absence of a positive history, immediate serologic testing to determine the immune status of exposed hospital personnel may be performed when diagnostic facilities are available. Exposed personnel with negative histories may continue to work in the nursery for 8 days after exposure pending serologic results because they are not potentially infectious during this period. Personnel with positive VZV antibody titers in serum are probably immune. Nonimmune (seronegative) nursery and delivery personnel should be excluded from patient care activities between days 8 and 21 after exposure. Subsequently, they should be strongly encouraged to be immunized against varicella, and they may be given postexposure prophylaxis with varicella vaccine (discussed later).

The greatest risk of nosocomial chickenpox exists when a mother develops chickenpox lesions less than 5 days before delivery or in the immediate postpartum period. If the neonate is born with lesions (i.e., congenital chickenpox), the mother and her newborn should be isolated together and sent home as soon as they are clinically stable. Other exposed mothers and infants in the nursery may also be sent home at the earliest date possible. Restriction of patient care activities and serologic testing of exposed delivery and nursery personnel as described earlier should be instituted. Passive immunization of exposed infants is optional considering the usually benign course of postnatally acquired chickenpox.

When maternal chickenpox occurs within approximately 5 days of delivery or immediately postpartum and no lesions are present in the neonate, the mother and the infant should be isolated separately. Transplacentally acquired chickenpox, beginning 7 to 15 days after disease appears in the mother, ultimately develops in about one half of these neonates despite administration of passive immunization. The remainder are at risk for postnatally acquired chickenpox unless isolated from their mothers. If no lesions develop in the neonate by the time the mother is noninfectious, both may be sent home. Guidelines for exposed hospital personnel and patients are similar to those described previously.

TABLE 22–9   Guidelines for Preventive Measures after Exposure to Chickenpox in the Nursery or Maternity Ward

Type of Exposure or Disease	Chickenpox Lesions Present		Disposition
	Mother	**Neonate**	
A. Siblings at home have active chickenpox when neonate and mother are ready for discharge from hospital	No	No	1. *Mother*: If she has history of chickenpox, she may return home. Without a history, she should be tested for VZV antibody titer.* If test is positive, she may return home. If test is negative, VZIG† may be administered, and she may be discharged home. If she is antibody negative, 3 mo after VZIG she may also be immunized and sent home. A second vaccine dose should be given 4-8 weeks after the first
			2. *Neonate*: Neonate may be discharged home with mother if mother has history of varicella or is VZV antibody positive. If mother is susceptible, administer VZIG or VariZIG to infant and discharge home or place in protective isolation
B. Mother with no history of chickenpox; exposed during period 6–20 days antepartum‡	No	No	1. *Exposed mother and infant*: Send home at earliest date unless siblings at home have communicable chickenpox.§ If so, may administer VZIG or VariZIG and/or vaccinate mother and discharge home, as above
			2. *Other mothers and infants*: No special management is indicated
			3. *Hospital personnel*: No precautions are indicated if there is history of previous chickenpox or zoster. In absence of history, immediate serologic testing is indicated to determine immune status.* Nonimmune personnel should be excluded from patient contact until 21 days after intimate exposure. Vaccination of nonimmune personnel should be encouraged. Immunized personnel who develop vaccine-associated rash should be excluded from work until rash has healed
			4. If mother develops varicella 1–2 days postpartum, infant should be given VZIG or VariZIG
C. Onset of maternal chickenpox antepartum‡ or postpartum	Yes	No	1. *Infected mother*: Isolate mother until no longer clinically infectious. If seriously ill, treat with acyclovir
			2. *Infected mother's infant*: Administer VZIG† or VariZIG to neonates born to mothers with onset of chickenpox <5 days before delivery and isolate separately from mother. Send home with mother if no lesions develop by the time mother is noninfectious
			3. *Other mothers and infants*: Send home at earliest date. VZIG or VariZIG may be given optionally to exposed neonates
			4. *Hospital personnel*: Follow same recommendations as B-3
D. Onset of maternal chickenpox antepartum§			1. *Mother*: Isolation is unnecessary if mother is no longer infectious
			2. *Infant*: Isolate from other infants, but not from mother
			3. *Other mothers and infants*: Follow same recommendations as C-3 (if exposed)
			4. *Hospital personnel*: Follow same recommendations as B-3
E. Congenital chickenpox	No	Yes	1. *Infected infant and mother*: Follow same recommendations as D-1 and D-2
			2. *Other mothers and infants*: Follow same recommendations as C-3
			3. *Hospital personnel*: Follow same recommendations as B-3

Send serum to virus diagnostic laboratory for determination of antibodies to VZV by a sensitive technique such as fluorescent antibody to membrane antigen, latex agglutination, or enzyme-linked immunosorbent assay. Personnel may continue to work for 8 days after exposure pending serologic results because they are not potentially infectious during this period. Antibodies to VZV >1:4 probably are indicative of immunity.

†*VariZIG is available from Canada. Telephone number for requests is 800 843-7477. The dose for a newborn is 1.25 mL (1 vial). The dose for a pregnant woman is conventionally 6.25 mL (5 vials).*

‡*If exposure occurred <6 days antepartum, mother would not be potentially infectious until at least 72 hr postpartum.*

§*Considered noninfectious when no new vesicles have appeared for 72 hours, and all lesions have crusted.*

VZIG, varicella-zoster immunoglobulin; VZV, varicella-zoster virus.

In congenital chickenpox, lesions may be absent in the mother at the time of delivery, but present in the neonate. This may occur after rare subclinical infection in the mother [98] or because the onset of the exanthem in the infant occurs after the lesions in the mother have already healed. In either circumstance, the mother is not at risk and may be isolated with her newborn.

Active Immunization against Chickenpox

A live-attenuated varicella vaccine was developed in Japan by Takahashi and colleagues [375]. This vaccine was licensed in 1995 by the U.S. Food and Drug Administration (FDA) for varicella-susceptible healthy children older than 1 year, adolescents, and adults. The vaccine is also licensed for routine use in many countries in Europe and in Asia, including Japan. The vaccine has proved to be safe and highly effective [47,376,377], and it is recommended for routine use by the American Academy of Pediatrics [362,378] and the CDC [195,363].

The vaccine protects against varicella in about 85% of individuals vaccinated and decreases the incidence of zoster in immunocompromised patients and presumably in healthy vaccinees [122,359,376,377,379]. Since vaccine licensure, the incidence and complications of varicella have decreased by about 80% in the United States [359].

The major adverse effect of vaccination is development of a very mild transient rash about 1 month (ranging from a few days to 6 weeks) after immunization. Originally, there was concern that the vaccine virus could spread to others, but spread is extremely rare (1 instance per 10 million doses distributed). Contagion has not been reported in the absence of rash, and contact cases have uniformly been mild. There is no evidence of clinical reversion to wild-type VZV [46,157,359,376]. One instance of spread occurred when a healthy child was immunized and his pregnant mother developed mild varicella, from which the vaccine-type virus was identified by PCR [380]. The mother terminated the pregnancy; the products of conception were negative for VZV by PCR. There is no record of the Oka vaccine strain causing congenital varicella syndrome. It is important, nevertheless, to immunize susceptible women of childbearing age before they become pregnant.

The risk of immunizing healthy toddlers is calculated to be lower than not immunizing them and risking their development of natural varicella that would expose a varicella-susceptible pregnant mother to the fully virulent virus [381]. Widespread use of vaccine in the United States may decrease or even eliminate the problems of congenital malformations and severe varicella in the neonatal period, as has occurred with rubella. Although varicella vaccine–type virus has not been shown to cause congenital varicella syndrome, immunization during pregnancy is contraindicated. It is also recommended that immunized women refrain from becoming pregnant for at least 3 months after receipt of vaccine [195,362,363,378].

In 2006, it was recommended that all vaccinees receive two doses of vaccine at least 4 weeks apart [363]. The reported seroconversion rate after two doses of vaccine in healthy adults is about 90% [157,376]. Ideally, women should have serologic testing for immunity after immunization, but this is not recommended because negative antibody titer after immunization does not indicate vaccine failure, as commercially available ELISA antibody tests often fail to identify individuals who have responded to the vaccine [382]. The vaccine program in the United States has been highly successful; the vaccine is extremely safe. There is evidence of herd immunity with this vaccine [359].

The vaccine is under some scrutiny for one particular reason. The question has been raised whether widespread vaccination would lead to a significant increase in the incidence of zoster in unvaccinated persons. Zoster is less common in vaccinate persons than in persons who have had natural infection. After natural infection, reexposure to wild-type VZV can boost immunity to the virus, resulting in protection against zoster, presumably caused by control of reactivating virus before it results in illness [359]. The important question is how significant an increase in zoster is likely to be in the vaccine era. Based mainly on epidemiologic evidence and computer modeling, some studies predict a serious increase in zoster with accompanying fatalities [383,384]. The incidence of zoster is roughly 2 to 4 cases per 1000 person-years of observation [385]. If this incidence doubles as a result of routine vaccination, it is unlikely to represent an epidemic of zoster. Zoster is rarely fatal even in immunocompromised patients, in contrast to varicella, which continues to cause fatalities and has a higher mortality rate than zoster [386–389].

MEASLES

Measles (i.e., rubeola) is a highly communicable childhood disease whose hallmarks are fever, coryza, conjunctivitis, cough, and a generalized maculopapular rash that usually appears 1 to 2 days after a specific enanthem (i.e., Koplik spots). The word *measles* means "little spots" and is derived from the Dutch word for the disease, *maeselen*, a diminutive of *maese*, meaning "spot" or "stain" [390]. Although measles was described in medieval times, it was not until the 17th century that Sydenham differentiated the disease from smallpox and scarlet fever.

ORGANISM
Classification and Morphology

Measles virus is a paramyxovirus, but some of its properties, such as the lack of neuraminidase, are distinct from properties of other members of this family. Similar to paramyxoviruses, measles virions have a diameter of 100 to 250 nm and consist of a helical ribonucleoprotein core surrounded by a lipid envelope.

In cell culture, virions replicate predominantly in the cytoplasm and are released from the cell surface by budding. The envelope of the virion is composed of at least two glycoproteins: F, which causes membrane fusion and is crucial for infectivity, and H, the hemagglutinin. A nonglycosylated matrix protein, M, also exists on the envelope. Antibodies to glycoprotein F inhibit viral infectivity [391]. Other internal structural proteins are the large protein (L), the phosphoprotein or polymerase (P), and the nucleocapsid protein (N). C and V proteins interact with cellular proteins and play roles in regulation of transcription and replication. The cellular receptors for measles virus are the complement regulatory protein CD46 expressed on human lymphocytes and many other human cell types and the signaling lymphocyte activation molecule (SLAM) CDw150 molecule [392–394].

Measles virus has been fully sequenced. Genomic data indicate that the viruses that caused the resurgence of measles in 1989–1992 were not new strains, that most of the reported cases in 1994–1995 were the result of international importation of virus, and that aggressive control measures in 1992 resulted in control of the viruses circulating at that time [395]. The latest data support this contention and indicate that there is no endemic measles in the United States; the few circulating viruses identified are imported from other countries [393,396].

Propagation of Measles Virus

Primary cultures of human embryonic kidney and rhesus monkey kidney cells have proved to be superior to all others for the isolation of measles virus, although the agent has been adapted after several passages to numerous continuous cell lines [392,394]. Cytopathic effect on primary isolation is not generally detected before 5 to 10 days. Rapid identification may be accomplished by use of immunofluorescent staining using monoclonal antibodies [392,394].

Antigenic Properties and Serologic Tests

Measles virus isolates are antigenically homogeneous, although there are numerous genotypes. Some cross-reactivity of soluble ribonucleoprotein antigens and hemagglutinins has been observed among measles and the related viruses of rinderpest and canine distemper, but not with other paramyxoviruses. The hemagglutination inhibition test has essentially been replaced with more modern assays for antibodies [394].

ELISA presently is the most useful and sensitive method for measuring antibodies to measles virus [392,397]. A similar test that identifies specific IgM antibody and is useful diagnostically when only one serum specimen is available has also been developed [392,394,398,399].

TRANSMISSION AND EPIDEMIOLOGY
Transmission by Droplets and Fomites

Measles is the most communicable of the childhood exanthems [52,65]. The virus is spread chiefly by droplets expectorated by an infected subject in proximity to susceptible persons. Rarely, transmission may occur by means of articles soiled by respiratory secretions. There is some uncertainty concerning the precise portal of entry of the virus. Although the virus may gain access through the nose or the oropharynx, the work of Papp [400] suggests that the conjunctival mucosa is at least a possible portal of entry. Others have proposed viral entry at the tonsils [401].

Measles occurs worldwide in temperate, tropical, and arctic climates. Before the introduction of live measles vaccines, urban areas of the United States typically experienced epidemics at intervals of 2 to 3 years. In interepidemic years, few cases of measles occur, probably because the supply of susceptible persons has been exhausted. Additional births add to this pool, permitting epidemic transmission when the pool is sufficiently large. In the United States, the disease had a peak incidence between March and May. Seasonal variation is attributed to the crowding of children indoors and in schools in the winter, resulting in increased transmission. Amplification of each cycle leads to a progressively larger number of cases of measles by the end of the winter. Attack rates are highest among the lowest socioeconomic populations.

Patterns of disease vary strikingly with respect to age, incidence, and severity in different geographic regions. In urban areas of industrialized countries, measles infects predominantly children 2 to 6 years old, and the disease is relatively mild. In rural areas of the same countries, children are characteristically older when they contract the disease and may reach adulthood without becoming infected. For this reason, measles in pregnant women may be observed more often among women from rural or otherwise geographically isolated localities (see later discussion). A different pattern of disease is seen in less

developed areas, such as equatorial Africa, where measles occurs predominantly in children younger than 2 years and has a high fatality rate [402]. Protein deficiency is associated with an increased incidence of complications, such as bronchopneumonia and death. Still another pattern of infection has been observed in extremely isolated regions of the world, where whole populations may never have experienced measles before its exogenous introduction. In a classic description of such an epidemic in the Faroe Islands in 1846, measles was observed to spread rapidly through an entire population, regardless of age, with an attack rate of virtually 100% [403]. Mortality rates tend to be higher in populations having little experience with measles. An extreme example is the Fiji Islands epidemic of 1875, in which 20,000 people, or about one fourth of the population, are said to have died [403].

The use of live-attenuated measles vaccine in the United States since 1963 has decreased the incidence of measles to less than 1% of its former incidence. Before 1963, there were about 400,000 reported cases of measles annually; a record low of 1497 cases was reported in 1983, but in the late 1980s and early 1990s, there was an increase in the incidence of measles that eventually came under control [371]. From 1989–1991, there were more than 55,000 reported cases with more than 120 measles-associated deaths reported to the CDC, but after 1991, the number of reported cases decreased significantly [404]. Measles occurring despite vaccination may be the result of primary vaccine failure, a "no take" for the vaccine, or secondary vaccine failure because of loss of immunity to measles after vaccination [405,406]. There is little evidence, however, that secondary immune failure (i.e., that protective immunity induced by measles wanes with time) is significant [405–408].

Since the requirement for two doses of measles vaccine in childhood was instituted in 1993, the number of annual cases of measles has declined to an all-time low. In 1995, 309 cases were reported, and in 1996, 508 cases were reported to the CDC [404]. Measles has become a rare disease in the United States; from 2000–2007, 63 annual cases were reported on average [409]. In the first 6 months of 2008, 131 cases of measles were reported to the CDC, however; 76% were ascribed to importations from Europe, Asia, and the Middle East. About 85% of cases were eligible for immunization [410]. The current vaccine coverage in the United States is greater than 90%, which is sufficient to prevent sustained transmission, although it does not prevent imported cases (http://www.cdc.gov/media/pressrel/2008/r080821.htm) [411].

Incidence of Measles in Pregnant Women

Because measles is well controlled in the United States by immunization, it occurs less frequently during pregnancy than chickenpox.

PATHOGENESIS

By analogy with other viral infections whose pathogenesis has been better delineated, the initial multiplication of measles virus is believed to occur in epithelial and lymphoid cells near the portal of entry. A transient viremia delivers virus to the reticuloendothelial system, where further replication occurs. A second viremia, more severe and more sustained, disseminates virus to the skin, gut, respiratory tract, and other affected organs. In monkeys, this viremia may occur over 1 week before the appearance of the prodrome or exanthem. Measles virus replicates in and probably destroys lymphocytes in the peripheral blood [412], giving rise to a circulating lymphopenia. The symptoms of measles are probably attributable to inflammation accompanying necrosis of cells in which the virus is replicating. By the time the exanthem appears, 13 to 14 days after infection, measles virus is actively replicating in the skin, gut, and respiratory mucosa.

Electron microscopy of biopsy specimens of Koplik spots and cutaneous lesions reveals syncytial giant cells whose nuclear and cytoplasmic inclusions contain aggregates of microtubules that are 15 to 20 nm in diameter and characteristic of paramyxovirus infection [413]. This finding and the observation that convalescent measles serum injected into the skin can prevent the local development of the exanthem [414] suggest that replication of virus per se is directly responsible for the lesions. Nevertheless, it is possible that an interaction between viral antigen and antibody is required. The latter hypothesis is supported by the observation that immunosuppressed children who develop giant cell pneumonia caused by measles virus do not develop a rash and do not elaborate antibodies [396,415]. Virus titers in the viscera have already diminished considerably by the time the exanthem appears, and serum antibodies are readily detectable within 24 hours. There is also experimental evidence that T lymphocytes are important in the development of some symptoms of measles such as the rash and in recovery from the disease [416].

Incubation Period for Measles Acquired by Droplet Infection

The usual interval between exposure to measles and onset of first symptoms (i.e., prodrome) is about 10 days; 12 to 14 days usually elapse before the onset of rash. Considerable variation may be observed, however [381]. The incubation period in modified measles (see "Clinical Manifestations") may last 17 to 21 days because of the presence of low levels of measles antibodies [417].

Incubation Period for Hematogenously Acquired Measles

It has been claimed that infantile measles may be acquired by transfusion of maternal blood presumably containing measles virus [418]. Two infants developed typical enanthems and exanthems 13 and 14 days after transfusion, and their mothers developed measles exanthems 4 and 2 days after blood donation. The infants had not been visited by their mothers for 4 days and 1 day before transfusion. Hematogenous transmission may not have occurred, however, because the mothers may have been shedding virus from the respiratory tract at the time they last handled their infants.

Intrauterine hematogenous transmission is well documented (discussed later). In these cases, the onset of disease in the infant may occur almost simultaneously with that in the mother or after a variable interval that is less than the minimum time required for extrauterine infection by the respiratory route.

Period of Communicability

Measles is more communicable during the prodrome and catarrhal stage of infection than during the period of the exanthem. Dramatic corroboration of this observation was provided during an epidemic in Greenland in 1962 [419]. Deliberate exposure of 400 susceptible persons to disease was achieved by having a patient on the first day of appearance of the exanthem cough twice in the face of each. Not a single transmission resulted. When the experiment was repeated with a patient during the preexanthematous period, measles was readily transmitted.

Patients with measles should be considered infectious from the onset of the prodrome (about 4 days before the appearance of the exanthem) until 3 days after the onset of the exanthem, although the risk of contagion abruptly diminishes 48 hours after the rash appears, concomitant with the appearance of circulating neutralizing antibodies. Measles virus is most readily recovered from respiratory secretions from 2 days before until 1 or 2 days after the onset of the rash.

PATHOLOGY

The replication of measles virus in epithelial cells of the mucous membranes and skin leads to the formation of intranuclear inclusions and syncytial giant cells, which can contain 100 nuclei per cell (i.e., Warthin-Finkeldey cells) [420]. Focal hyaline necrosis of epithelial cells is accompanied by a subepithelial exudate containing predominantly mononuclear leukocytes. The pathology of cutaneous lesions and Koplik spots is essentially similar [413]. It is likely that virus replicates simultaneously in the skin and mucous membranes, but Koplik spots are detected earlier than the exanthem, probably because the epithelium that forms the roof of the lesions is thinner and more translucent in the mucous membranes.

Similar lesions containing the characteristic multinucleated giant cells may be widespread throughout the respiratory and gastrointestinal tracts. The pharynx, tonsils, bronchial epithelium, appendix, colon, and lymph nodes have been involved. Viral bronchitis occurs in most cases of measles. Necrotic columnar epithelial cells and giant cells are sloughed into the lumen of the bronchi and bronchioles. When this damage is extensive, the regenerating epithelium frequently undergoes squamous metaplasia and is accompanied by bronchial and peribronchial inflammation. Extension of the process into the alveolar septa results in interstitial pneumonitis. Secondary bacterial infection commonly supervenes, leading to a bronchopneumonia with purulent exudate.

Using immunofluorescence and immunoperoxidase methodology, measles virus has been shown in the placental syncytial trophoblastic cells and decidua in a 25-week fetus of a woman who developed gestational measles. The fetus was spared. It is postulated that placental damage induced by the virus, leading to hypoxia, is responsible for fetal death during maternal measles [421].

The pathologic signs of measles encephalitis are not readily distinguishable from signs of other postinfectious encephalitides, such as those caused by vaccinia, chickenpox, and rubella. The characteristic lesion is perivenous demyelination, often accompanied by mild perivascular infiltrates of mononuclear leukocytes, petechial hemorrhages, and microglial proliferation. Neuronal damage and meningeal inflammation are not prominent. Nuclear or cytoplasmic inclusions and giant cells are inconstant. Measles virus has been isolated infrequently from the brain or spinal cord, and it is unclear whether the pathologic changes in the brain are a direct result of measles virus or an allergic response to a virus-induced product or antigen-antibody complexes [422,423].

Because of the spectrum of pathology, including acute demyelinating encephalitis and acute hemorrhagic leukoencephalitis, it has been postulated that measles encephalitis is an autoimmune process. Myelin basic protein has been shown in the cerebrospinal fluid of patients with measles encephalitis, and the pathologic process has been likened to experimental allergic encephalitis as produced in animal models [424]. One theory regarding pathogenesis is that measles virus has an epitope similar to the epitope of the encephalitogenic sequence in central nervous system myelin (i.e., an instance of molecular mimicry leading to disease) [425]. A second form of encephalitis is caused by continued replication of measles virus in the brains of immunocompromised patients [426].

CLINICAL MANIFESTATIONS
Prodrome and Rash

The prodrome typically begins 10 to 11 days after exposure, with fever and malaise, followed within 24 hours by coryza, sneezing, conjunctivitis, and cough. During the next 2 to 3 days, this catarrhal phase is accentuated, with markedly infected conjunctivae and photophobia. Toward the end of the prodrome, Koplik spots appear. They are tiny (no larger than a pinhead), granular, slightly raised white lesions surrounded by a halo of erythema. Beginning with less than a dozen specks on the lateral buccal mucosa, Koplik spots may multiply during a 24-hour period to affect virtually all the mucous membranes of the cheeks and may extend to the lips and eyelids. Hundreds of spots may be present. At this stage, the lesions may be said to resemble grains of salt on a wet background. Koplik spots appear 1 to 2 days before the exanthem.

The rash, which appears 12 to 14 days after exposure, begins on the head and neck, especially behind the ears and on the forehead. At first, the lesions are red macules 1 to 2 mm in diameter, but over 2 or 3 days, they enlarge and coalesce. By the 2nd day, the exanthem has spread to the trunk and upper extremities. The lower extremities are involved by the 3rd day. The lesions are most prominent in regions where the exanthem appears first—the face and upper trunk. By the 3rd or 4th day, the exanthem begins to fade in the order of its appearance. A brown staining of the lesions often persists for 7 to 10 days and is followed by fine desquamation.

The clinical course of measles may be greatly altered by administration of immunoglobulin during the incubation period. In modified measles, the catarrhal phase may be completely suppressed, and the exanthem may be limited to a few macules on the trunk.

Complications and Mortality

The most frequent complications of measles involve the respiratory tract. Otitis media and mild croup are common in young children during the catarrhal phase, but bacterial pneumonia is the complication that results in death most frequently. If carefully sought, fine rales and radiologic evidence of bronchopneumonia can be found during the early exanthematous phase in most patients. Cough may persist beyond the peak of the exanthem in uncomplicated measles, but when the fever fails to decline or recurs as the rash is fading, a bacterial superinfection is usually present. The chest radiograph may show consolidation. A peripheral blood polymorphonuclear leukocytosis is present. When bacterial superinfection occurs, antimicrobial therapy is indicated and should be directed against the most likely etiologic agents—*Streptococcus pneumoniae*, *S. aureus*, and *Streptococcus pyogenes*. Smears and cultures of sputum should be obtained, but in young infants it may be necessary to treat bacterial superinfection without a specific etiologic diagnosis because of the difficulty in obtaining adequate sputum and the potential gravity of the illness (see "Therapy").

After otitis and pneumonia, encephalitis is the most frequent serious complication of measles. It is far less common than pneumonia. Encephalitis, including coma and gross cerebral dysfunction, is estimated to occur with a frequency of 1 per 1000 cases [422], but is probably more common if drowsiness, irritability, and transient electroencephalographic changes are accepted as evidence of encephalitis. This complication occurs in all age groups, including the neonatal period. A fatal outcome has been recorded in an infant, born in the hospital, who developed measles with encephalitis when 27 days old [423]. Measles encephalitis may occur at any stage of the illness, but appears most commonly 3 to 7 days after the onset of the exanthem. The initial symptoms are drowsiness and irritability, followed by lethargy, convulsions, and coma. The cerebrospinal fluid changes are those of a mild aseptic meningitis. Mental obtundation may clear over 1 to 4 days or may assume a more protracted course that is associated with a higher incidence of such sequelae as severe behavioral abnormalities and mental retardation. Death occurs in about 11% of cases [422].

Other complications of measles that have been described include thrombocytopenic purpura, appendicitis, myocarditis, subacute sclerosing panencephalitis, and reactivation or exacerbation of previously acquired tuberculosis. In a study of 3220 U.S. Air Force recruits with measles, whose mean age was 19 years, in 1976–1979, bacterial superinfection and elevated serum transaminase levels were observed in 30%, otitis was seen in 29%, sinusitis was seen in 25%, bronchospasm was seen in 17%, and pneumonia was seen in 3% [427].

The precise case-fatality ratio in measles is highly variable among different populations and at different periods in the history of the same population. From 1920–1950 in Massachusetts, deaths caused by measles declined progressively during each successive 5-year period from 7.6 to 0.28 per 100,000 people, despite an approximately constant morbidity related to measles [403]. Because the decline preceded the widespread use of antibiotics, much of the change is attributed to improved social conditions: less crowding, improved nutrition, and medical care. In the United States since 1963, the case-fatality ratio has averaged about 0.1% based on reported cases, but it may be closer to 0.01% if estimated unreported cases of measles are included in the calculation [428]. The risk is considerably greater, however, in children younger than 1 year old.

The age-specific death rates for measles in the United States reported in 1949 (per 100,000 people) were 7.8 at younger than 1 year old, 2.8 at 1 to 4 years old, 1.3 at 5 to 9 years old, and 0.4 at 10 to 14 years old. Data obtained during an epidemic in Greenland in 1951 confirmed that death rates are higher for infants. The age-specific death rates (per 1000 people) were 26 for infants younger than 1 year and 15 for infants 1 to 2 years old; no deaths were recorded in children 2 to 14 years old [429]. In cases for which adequate information was available, all deaths of children younger than 1 year old apparently were caused by pneumonia, which occurred during the prodrome or shortly after the onset of the exanthem.

Children with underlying infection with HIV have been reported to be at risk for developing severe measles, and fatalities have been reported, especially in children who have developed AIDS [430]. In Africa, it has also been observed that infants born to HIV-infected women have lower titers of measles antibodies in cord sera than infants from women not infected with HIV. The outcome has been that these infants are at greater risk for developing measles early in infancy [431]. One adolescent with HIV infection who had previously received measles vaccine developed fatal measles pneumonia after the second dose [432]. Because the infection was proved to be from the vaccine virus, measles vaccine is no longer recommended for HIV-infected children who have developed AIDS or evidence of severe immunosuppression [404]. Immunocompromised children with underlying malignant diseases who have not been immunized are also at risk for developing severe and fatal measles [433–435].

Maternal Effects of Measles

A pregnant woman with measles likely is at greater risk of serious complications and death than other adults with this disease. Some of the published experiences leading to this conclusion are summarized in the following paragraphs.

In the early part of the 20th century, fatality rates for pregnant women with measles were reported to be approximately 15%, mostly caused by pneumonia in the puerperium [436,437]. In the 1951 Greenland epidemic, 4 deaths (4.9%) occurred among 83 women who had measles during pregnancy or the puerperium. In contrast, 19 deaths (1.7%) occurred among 1099 nonpregnant women between the ages of 15 and 54 [429]. This difference is probably significant ($\chi^2 = 3.9$, $P = .05$). There was no significant difference in the frequency of pneumonia as a complication of measles among pregnant and nonpregnant women in the same age group, but heart failure was observed far more often in pregnant women with measles. Heart failure was observed in seven patients with gestational measles. Of these, three were in the second half of pregnancy, and four were in the puerperium. Although in some patients heart failure occurred during the prodrome, it occurred within 2 weeks after onset of the exanthem in most women.

Additional experience in the United States and Australia since 1940 supports the concept that measles during pregnancy is only rarely catastrophic. Among 24 women with gestational measles in an outbreak in rural Oklahoma, no deaths occurred, and serious morbidity was likewise not increased [438]. In another epidemic, reported in 1950 from Australia, 18 cases of gestational measles were observed. Complications were reported in only one case—a woman in the third trimester with measles pneumonia [439].

From 1988–1992 in the United States, when there was a resurgence of measles, numerous pregnant women developed this infection. Thirteen such women who were hospitalized in Houston, Texas, were reported because 7 (54%) had respiratory complications that were the basis for their hospitalization. They required supplemental oxygen and monitoring in the intensive care unit, and one woman died [440]. These women seemed to have primary measles pneumonia, rather than bacterial superinfection. Nine of these 13 women were treated with aerosolized ribavirin administered by facemask. Hepatitis, shown by elevations of transaminases, also occurred frequently in these women, but this is a common finding in nonpregnant adults that seems to be of little clinical importance. During this same period, medical records from 58 pregnant women from Los Angeles with measles were reviewed. Of these women, 35 (60%) were hospitalized for measles, 15 (26%) developed pneumonia, and 2 (3%) died [441]. Although it is difficult to prove that measles is more severe in pregnant than nonpregnant women, it seems likely to be so.

Effects of Gestational Measles on the Fetus
Chromosomal Aberrations

The possibility that measles occurring in pregnancy may damage the fetus is suggested by the observation that there is a high frequency of chromosomal breaks in leukocyte metaphase preparations between the 2nd and 5th day of the exanthem [442]. Other reports have not fully confirmed the preceding observations, however. Miller [443] found no chromosomal breaks in leukocytes of patients with measles who were examined 1 to 12 days after onset of the rash, but he attributed this discrepancy to methodologic differences involving more gentle treatment of the leukocytes. A report from Japan [444] also failed to show an increased frequency of chromosomal breaks per cell in patients with measles compared with those in normal subjects. A significant increase in chromosomal breaks was observed, however, in patients with Down syndrome who had measles, and it was inferred that their chromosomes were more sensitive to measles infection [444].

These chromosomal abnormalities are transient and disappear during convalescence. No studies have examined whether intrauterine exposure of the fetus to measles results in more lasting chromosomal aberrations.

Abortion and Prematurity

The consensus of several reports dealing with the frequency of premature births is that this untoward event occurs more often in association with measles during pregnancy than in the pregnant population at large. In contrast to rubella, in which there is retarded intrauterine development, prematurity caused by measles is associated with normal intrauterine development, but premature expulsion of the fetus. Although there is no statistically valid proof that gestational measles also causes a higher rate of abortion, it seems probable that measles is responsible for some instances of abortion.

Among the retrospective studies is that of Dyer [438], who reported 24 cases of gestational measles from rural Oklahoma in 1938–1939. Uterine contractions, which typically occurred during the illness, were identified in 11 of the 24 women and caused premature delivery of the fetus in 9 (38%). In one woman in whom measles occurred at 18 weeks of gestation, the exanthem was followed by spontaneous abortion 7 days later. Two additional pregnancies were associated with premature births at 33 weeks of gestation. No abortions were associated with eight cases of measles occurring in the first trimester.

Adverse outcomes of gestational measles on the fetus involving 18 pregnant women with measles were reported in the epidemic in South Australia in 1950 [439]. There were three spontaneous abortions (17%), which occurred in one of seven women who had measles in the first trimester, one of eight women who had measles in the second trimester, and one of three women who had measles in the third trimester. Abortions followed the onset of the exanthem by 2 to 3 weeks in the patients who became ill in the first and second trimesters. The patient with measles in the third trimester had severe measles pneumonia and expelled a macerated fetus 7 weeks later. One live premature birth was recorded in the third trimester.

In the 1951 Greenland epidemic, birth or abortion occurred in 26 of the 76 pregnant women while they had measles [429]. Thirteen were term pregnancies. Of the remainder, spontaneous abortion at 3 to 5 months of gestation occurred in seven women (9%). There were six instances of premature delivery (8%), and perinatal death ensued in three. A retrospective analysis of 51 women in Greenland who developed measles during the first 3 months of pregnancy from 1951–1962 also suggested a high fetal death rate. One half with measles in the first 2 months and one fifth with measles in the 3rd month had spontaneous abortions [445]. Five infants born to women with measles during an outbreak in 1981–1982 in Israel were reported [446]. All were born prematurely (range 28 to 34 weeks) with a mean duration between maternal onset of illness and delivery of 3.5 days and a mean birth weight of 1496 g. None had any signs of measles at birth or in the neonatal period.

Controlled, prospective studies done in New York City during 1957–1964 showed a significant association between maternal measles and prematurity, but not between maternal measles and abortion. Low birth weight (<2500 g) was identified in 10 (16.7%) of 60 infants born to measles-infected mothers compared with 2 (3.3%) of 62 matched controls ($\chi^2 = 6.2$; $P < .025$) (see Table 22–4) [207]. When fetal mortality was examined in relation to gestational age (see Table 22–5), it was found that 3 deaths (15.8%) occurred in 19 cases of measles in the first trimester, 1 (3.4%) occurred in 29 in the second trimester, and 1 (5.9%) occurred in 17 in the third trimester [207]. These figures were not significantly different from those for fetal deaths in control pregnancies not involving measles. Of the five fetal deaths that occurred in pregnant women with measles, two of the deaths occurred within 2 weeks of maternal disease.

The resurgence of measles from 1989–1991 resulted in measles in numerous pregnant women. In the experience of Atmar and associates [440], there was an adverse fetal outcome in 4 (31%) of 13 pregnancies complicated by maternal measles. Two women gave birth in the 34th and 35th weeks, and one spontaneously aborted at 16 weeks during measles. One additional woman and her fetus died at 20 weeks. In a report from Los Angeles of 58 women, the incidence of abortion was 5 (9%), and the incidence of prematurity was 13 (22%) [441].

Congenital Defects

The teratogenic potential of gestational measles for the fetus has been neither proved nor refuted because of the rarity of the infection during pregnancy, particularly during the first trimester when the process of organogenesis is most active. It seems clear, however, that if measles causes congenital malformations, it does so far less frequently than rubella. In contrast to gestational chickenpox, no particular constellation of abnormalities has been found among the sporadic instances of congenital defects that have occurred because of measles in the mother during pregnancy.

Isolated instances of buphthalmos [447], congenital heart disease [448], cleft lip [206], pyloric stenosis [448], genu valgum [447], cerebral leukodystrophy [445], and cyclopia [445] have been reported in infants born to mothers with measles diagnosed during the organogenic period. In these and other cases, documentation that the maternal illness was measles and not rubella or other exanthems is often lacking.

No congenital malformations were observed in four infants born to mothers who had measles during the first 4 months of pregnancy in the Oklahoma outbreak [438]. Similarly, in the 1951 Greenland epidemic, there were no congenital malformations among the infants of 76 mothers with gestational measles, although the number of cases that occurred in the first trimester is unclear [429]. After the epidemic in South Australia [439], two infants with congenital defects (one with Down syndrome and one with partial deafness) were recorded among infants whose mothers had measles during the first trimester. No birth defects occurred in infants born to eight mothers with measles in the second trimester and three mothers who had been ill in the third trimester. Although one of the five infants born during the outbreak in 1981–1982 in Israel was severely malformed, this was not caused by maternal measles, which had begun only a few days before birth. Five additional reported Israeli infants had no congenital anomalies, but all their mothers had measles just before delivery [446]. In the Houston report of 13 pregnant women, the fetal gestational age at onset of maternal measles ranged from 16 to 35 weeks (mean 27 weeks). Follow-up of eight of these infants, delivered a mean of 12 weeks later (range 1 to 24 weeks), revealed that no infants had congenital malformations [440].

These analyses are incapable of establishing whether the incidence of congenital defects is increased as a result of gestational measles because they were uncontrolled. One controlled prospective study is inconclusive because only small numbers of pregnant women with measles could be studied. Among 60 children who were born to mothers who had gestational measles and were followed to the age of 5 years, only one congenital malformation was identified compared with a virtually identical incidence of one defect among 62 controls [173]. The defect in the infected group was bilateral deafness in an infant weighing 1990 g born to a mother who had measles at 6 weeks of gestation. If there is any increased risk of malformations from gestational measles, this risk seems to be small if it exists at all.

Perinatal Measles

As in chickenpox, perinatal measles includes transplacental infection and disease acquired postnatally by the respiratory route. Because the usual incubation period from infection to the first appearance of the exanthem is 13 to 14 days, measles exanthems acquired in the first 10 days of life may be considered transplacental in origin, whereas disease appearing at 14 days or later is probably acquired outside the uterus.

Postnatally Acquired Measles

Several reports describe cases of measles in which the onset of the exanthem occurred in infants 14 to 30 days old. The course of the disease in these cases was generally mild [438,449,450]. In one infant with notably mild illness and little fever, the illness began at 14 days of age. This neonate had been nursed by the mother, in whom the prodrome of measles developed on the 1st postpartum day. Because circulating and presumably also secretory antibodies appear within 48 hours of the onset of the exanthem, it is possible that the neonate's illness was modified by measles-specific IgA antibodies present in the mother's milk [438,449,450]. A report from Japan in 1997 described seven cases of measles in infants during the 1st month of life. No case was believed to be severe, although there were three infants with pneumonia, two of whom had received immunoglobulin at exposure [451].

Measles acquired postnatally may also cause more severe illness; when a mother developed the disease 20 days postpartum, her infant was quite sick with measles 10 days later, but complications such as pneumonia or otitis apparently did not develop [452]. There are reports of infants with prolonged presence of the measles genome in their mononuclear cells after vertical transmission of measles [453,454]. Rapidly progressive subacute sclerosing panencephalitis has also been reported after vertically acquired measles infection [455–460].

Outbreaks of nosocomial measles in the newborn nursery apparently have not been recorded in the 20th century. This is probably because of the low incidence of measles in the United States and other developed countries, nearly universal immunity in mothers in urban areas, and corresponding protection of the newborn by passive antibodies.

Congenital Measles

Congenital measles includes cases in which the exanthem is present at birth and infections acquired in utero in which the rash appears during the first 10 days of life. In congenital measles, the incubation period, defined as the interval between onset of exanthem in the mother and in the infant, ranges from 2 [438] to 10 days [461] (mean 6 days). A nearly simultaneous onset in the mother and neonate implies that measles virus in the maternal bloodstream may sometimes cross the placenta in sufficient quantity to cause disease in the fetus without the need for many additional cycles of replication. The placenta may act as a barrier of limited effectiveness, however, as suggested by instances in which disease does not appear in the fetus until 10 days after its appearance in the mother. Even more cogent is the fact that maternal measles immediately preceding parturition by no means invariably involves the fetus. Of 44 pregnancies in which a maternal rash was present at delivery, exanthematous measles was reported in only 13 neonates (30%) [437].

Later reports include 13 instances in which maternal rashes with onsets ranging from 7 days antepartum to 3 days postpartum were associated with clinically apparent measles in the infant in only 3 cases (23%) [438,446,452,462]. Eight of these infants received immunoglobulin (0.25 mL/kg) at birth, however, including the three who developed measles [446,462]. During the Greenland epidemic of 1951, no examples of congenital measles were observed among infants born to 13 women who had measles at parturition [429]. It seems that most of these neonates do not experience subclinical measles without exanthem, but simply are not infected. This conclusion is supported by the observation that infants whose mothers had measles late in the third trimester are fully susceptible to infection later in childhood [437]. During the Faroe Islands epidemic of 1846, many pregnant women had measles, and 36 years later, their infants were infected as adults in a new epidemic in 1882 [452].

As in congenital chickenpox, the spectrum of illness in congenital measles varies from a mild illness, in which the rash is transient and Koplik spots may be absent, to rapidly fatal disease. The precise case-fatality ratio is uncertain because the course of measles in different populations has been so variable, even in older children and adults. Among 22 cases of congenital measles culled from the literature in which immunoglobulin prophylaxis was not given, there were seven deaths (Table 22–10) [437,438,452,461]. Approximately the same case-fatality ratio (30% to 33%) was observed whether the rash was present at birth or appeared subsequently. Although the number of observations is small, it seems that for premature infants with congenital measles, the death rate is higher (5 of 9) than for infants with congenital measles delivered at term (2 of 10). The death rate has also been high among premature infants born to women who had measles at parturition even when the infant never developed clinically apparent measles (see Table 22–10) [429,437].

TABLE 22–10 Deaths in Neonates Whose Mothers Had Measles at Parturition

Exanthem in Neonate	Neonatal Deaths*	Neonatal Cases	%
Present at birth	4	12	33
Appeared after birth	3	10	30
Did not appear	7[†]	16	44

*Stillborns excluded.
[†]All of these were premature infants reported in a single series [441].

TABLE 22–11 Deaths from Congenital Measles in Relation to Date of Onset of Rash in Mothers

Onset of Maternal Rash	Neonatal Deaths	Neonatal Cases	%
Antepartum	4	15	27
Postpartum	3	11	27

Insufficient data are available to evaluate whether transplacentally acquired antibodies to measles virus may diminish the case-fatality ratio in congenital measles when the mother's exanthem appears more than 48 hours antepartum. The death rate from congenital measles does not seem to differ appreciably whether the maternal rash appears antepartum or postpartum (Table 22–11), but more precise information on the time of appearance of the maternal rash is needed to answer this question definitively. Although firm data are unavailable, administration of immunoglobulin at birth may also decrease mortality [440,446,462].

Most reports of death related to congenital measles do not specify the immediate cause, but pneumonia is among the leading complications.* Because nearly all reports of deaths preceded the antibiotic era, the current case-fatality ratio may be significantly lower than it was previously because of improved supportive care and appropriate antimicrobial therapy of bacterial superinfections.

DIAGNOSIS AND DIFFERENTIAL DIAGNOSIS

The diagnosis of measles is easy when there is a history of recent exposure, and the typical catarrhal phase is followed by Koplik spots and a maculopapular exanthem in the characteristic distribution. Koplik spots are pathognomonic. The diagnosis is more difficult, however, during the prodrome (when the illness is maximally communicable) or when the illness and the exanthem are attenuated by passively acquired measles antibodies. Measles antibodies may be contained in transfused plasma or immunoglobulin, or they may cross the placenta to the neonate if the mother develops measles shortly before parturition. The atypical exanthem of measles in subjects who have been previously immunized with inactivated measles vaccine may potentially also cause diagnostic difficulties.

When the diagnosis cannot be made confidently on clinical and epidemiologic grounds, laboratory confirmation is

*References [437,438,440,446,462,463].

indicated so that appropriate measures can be taken to prevent the occurrence of nosocomial measles among susceptible persons. Aids to rapid diagnosis include examination of exfoliated cells from the pharynx, nasal and buccal mucosa, conjunctiva, or urinary tract by direct staining for epithelial giant cells [464,465] or identification of measles antigens by direct immunofluorescence [466–468]. PCR assays can diagnose acute measles [392]. These tests are positive in more than 90% of patients during the prodrome and the period of the early exanthem. At later stages of the illness, the diagnosis may be confirmed by detecting measles-specific IgM antibodies in serum or increasing antibody titers in acute and convalescent sera [397,398,469]. Because serum antibodies appear within 48 hours of the exanthem, it is important that the acute-phase serum be collected at the onset of the rash or earlier.

The following diseases and conditions are to be considered in the differential diagnosis of measles. None is likely to occur in the newborn.

1. *Drug eruptions and other allergies.* Maculopapular exanthems may be caused by various drugs and chemicals in susceptible persons. A history of exposure is of paramount importance in distinguishing these causes from measles. An urticarial component may be seen in some instances of drug hypersensitivity, but is not present in measles.

2. *Kawasaki disease.* This illness is often confused with measles and vice versa in children younger than 5 years. Classic signs include conjunctivitis, red cracked lips, strawberry tongue, morbilliform or scarlatiniform rash, induration of the hands and feet, and usually a solitary enlarged cervical lymph node. In confusing cases, viral diagnostic procedures may be necessary to rule measles in or out.

3. *Rubella.* The maculopapular exanthem of rubella is finer and more transient. It undergoes a more rapid evolution and does not assume the blotchy configuration often seen in measles. The posterior cervical and postauricular lymphadenopathies of rubella are not present in measles, and conversely the prominent catarrhal symptoms in the prodrome of measles are not a feature of rubella.

4. *Scarlet fever.* The rash of scarlet fever is punctate and extremely fine rather than papular. It blanches on pressure and is accentuated in skin folds. The onset is typically abrupt without a prodrome. There is an accompanying sore throat, and the cheeks are flushed. Peripheral blood leukocytosis is usual, in contrast to the leukopenia of measles.

5. *Meningococcemia.* When the early rash of meningococcemia is maculopapular rather than petechial, it may be confused with measles. In contrast to measles, it has no characteristic distribution.

6. *Roseola.* The exanthem of roseola, which usually appears when the patient's temperature decreases to normal, typically appears on the trunk before it is evident on the head. It lasts only 1 or 2 days. Roseola, which is caused by human herpesvirus type 6, is seen most often in children younger than 3 years and is almost never seen in adults.

7. *Atypical measles*. This hypersensitivity disease is related to infection with measles virus in persons who received killed measles vaccine years ago. Killed measles vaccine was removed from the U.S. market in 1968. Extremely high measles hemagglutination inhibition antibody titers (e.g., 1:1 million) have been observed in patients with this disease.

8. *Other infections*. Rocky Mountain spotted fever, toxoplasmosis, enterovirus infections, parvovirus infection, and infectious mononucleosis may cause maculopapular exanthems resembling measles.

THERAPY

The treatment of uncomplicated measles is symptomatic. Immunoglobulin has no proven value in established disease. Antibiotics are not indicated for prophylaxis of bacterial superinfections (i.e., otitis and pneumonia). When these complications develop, antimicrobial therapy should be selected on the basis of Gram stain and culture of appropriate body fluids, such as sputum. If culture specimens cannot be obtained or if the illness is grave, broad-spectrum antibiotics may be selected on the basis of the most likely offending pathogens. The antibiotic regimen for pneumonia, most commonly caused by *S. pneumoniae* or *S. aureus*, should include a penicillinase-resistant penicillin; the drug of choice for otitis media, which is usually caused by *S. pneumoniae* or *Haemophilus influenzae*, is amoxicillin. Vitamin A (200,000 IU orally once daily for 2 days for infants 12 months of age and older, 100,000 IU orally once daily for 2 days for infants 6 through 11 months of age, and 50,000 IU orally once daily for 2 days for infants less than 6 months of age) has been used to tread infants with measles and seems to decrease the severity of the infection [470–472]. The drug ribavirin has been used experimentally to treat severe measles in immunocompromised and other high-risk patients [473,474].

PREVENTION

Passive Immunization

Passive immunization is recommended for the prevention of measles in exposed, susceptible pregnant women, neonates, and their contacts in the delivery room or newborn nursery (see "Nosocomial Measles in the Nursery"). Therapy with intramuscularly administered immunoglobulin should be given as soon as possible after exposure. A dose of 0.25 mL/kg given within 72 hours of exposure to healthy children (0.5mL/kg for immunocompromised children; maximum 15 mL) is a reliable means of prevention of clinical measles, although immunoglobulin given later (7 days after exposure) or in smaller doses (0.04 mL/kg) may also prevent or at least modify the infection. It is recommended that passive prophylaxis be followed in 5 months or more by administration of live measles vaccine in patients old enough to receive it [362].

Active Immunization

The currently recommended live measles vaccines are derivatives of the Edmonston B strain that have been further attenuated. They produce a noncommunicable infection, which is mild or inapparent. Fever occurs in about 5% of susceptible recipients. A mild rash is observed in 10% to 20% of susceptible recipients 5 to 10 days after administration. The vaccines induce seroconversion in 95% and prevent clinical disease in more than 90% of exposed susceptible recipients. Live-attenuated measles vaccines are contraindicated in pregnant women [362]. In one small series, Edmonston B measles vaccine and γ-globulin were administered to seven pregnant women, 18 to 34 years old, who were in the 2nd to 8th months of pregnancy. There were no serologic data. Three of the seven developed fever (>38.5° C) and rash. All were delivered of healthy infants at term [475]. Vaccination is likewise not usually recommended for infants younger than 12 months because the induction of immunity and the elaboration of antibodies may be suppressed by residual transplacentally acquired antibodies in the fetal circulation or other mechanisms. A single fatality in a young adult with HIV infection resulting from pneumonia after reimmunization has been reported [432].

In exposed populations having little experience with measles or in populations in which the incidence of natural measles before the age of 1 year is high, live vaccines may be given when infants are 6 to 9 months old, but should be followed by a second dose at 15 months to increase the seroconversion rate [362]. Data indicate that measles antibody titers are lower in women vaccinated as children than in women who have previously had natural measles and that the offspring of vaccinated women lose transplacentally acquired measles antibodies before they are 1 year old [476,477]. It is predicted that routine vaccination against measles may be recommended at 12 months rather than 15 months. Nevertheless, passive immunization should be given to protect young infants exposed during an epidemic.

Although the measles, mumps, and rubella (MMR) vaccine had an excellent safety record in 2000, the question was raised about whether this vaccine might result in autism in previously healthy children antepartum or postpartum [478]. The public in the United Kingdom became so fearful of this possibility that use of measles vaccine has decreased significantly, leading to reported outbreaks [479]. Potentially this development could lead to an increase in measles in pregnant women in the United Kingdom and other countries such as the United States where MMR coverage might decline.

Nosocomial Measles in the Nursery: Guidelines for Prevention

Most women of childbearing age in urban areas are immune to measles because of previous natural infection or vaccination. Because it is amply documented that infants born to immune mothers are usually protected by transplacentally acquired antibodies, measles outbreaks in newborn nurseries are extraordinarily rare. Studies by Krugman and colleagues [480] indicated that before the introduction of live-attenuated measles vaccine, 94% of infants had passive hemagglutination inhibition antibodies when 1 month old, 47% had antibodies at 4 months, and 26% had antibodies at 6 months. The rarity of measles among mothers, newborns, and hospital staff in the newborn nursery makes it difficult to assess the precise risk when the virus has been introduced. Nonetheless, the fact that age-specific mortality rates related to measles are highest in the first year of life (see previous discussion) justifies instituting measures designed to prevent disease in individuals exposed and the spread of infection to neonates of uncertain immune status (Table 22–12).

Infants born to mothers with an unequivocal history of previous natural measles or vaccination with live-attenuated measles virus are assumed not to be at risk when exposed to measles in the neonatal period. If siblings at home have measles in a communicable stage, neonates born to immune mothers may be discharged from the hospital with no treatment. In the absence of a maternal history of measles or measles vaccine, the mother's serum should be tested for the presence of antibodies to measles. If the mother's serum contains detectable levels of measles antibodies by a reliable method, the mother and neonate may be sent home. If specific antibodies are not detected in the mother's serum, the neonate and mother should not have contact with the older siblings until they are no

longer infectious. The mother and neonate and any non-immune older siblings without disease should receive immunoglobulin (0.25 mg/kg given intramuscularly) to prevent or modify subsequent measles infection that might have been incubating at the time of delivery.

If a mother without a history of previous measles or measles vaccination is exposed 6 to 15 days antepartum, she may be in the incubation period and capable of transmitting measles infection during the postpartum period before discharge from the hospital. In such a situation, it is optimal to test the mother for measles antibodies. If no antibodies are detected (or the test cannot be performed), and if she had been exposed less than 6 days antepartum, she could not transmit measles by the respiratory route until at least 72 hours postpartum. By this time in most instances, the mother would have been discharged from the hospital, and potential nosocomial transmission would not be a problem. In either event (exposure from 0 to 5 days or from 6 to 15 days antepartum), the exposed susceptible mother and her neonate

TABLE 22–12 Guidelines for Preventive Measures after Exposure to Measles in the Nursery or Maternity Ward

Type of Disease or Disease	Measles Present (Prodrome or Rash)*		Disposition
	Mother	Neonate	
A. Siblings at home with measles* when neonate and mother are ready for discharge from hospital	No	No	1. *Neonate*: Protective isolation and IG are indicated unless mother had unequivocal history of previous measles or measles vaccination[†]
			2. *Mother*: With history of previous measles or measles vaccination, she may remain with neonate or return to older children. Without previous history, she may remain with neonate until older siblings are no longer infectious, or she may receive IG prophylactically and return to older children
B. Mother without history of measles or measles vaccination exposed during period 6–15 days antepartum[‡]	No	No	1. *Exposed mother and infant*: Administer IG to each and send home at earliest date unless there are siblings at home with communicable measles. Test mother for susceptibility if possible. If susceptible, administer live measles vaccine 5 mo after IG
			2. *Other mothers and infants*: Follow the same recommendations, unless clear history of previous measles or measles vaccination in mother
			3. *Hospital personnel*: Unless clear history of previous measles or measles vaccination, administer IG within 72 hr of exposure. Vaccinate ≥5 mo later
C. Onset of maternal measles antepartum or postpartum[§]	Yes	Yes	1. *Infected mother and infant*: Isolate mother and infant together until clinically stable, then send home
			2. *Other mothers and infants*: Follow same recommendations as B-3 except infants should be vaccinated at 15 mo old
			3. *Hospital personnel*: Follow same recommendations as B-3
D. Onset of maternal measles antepartum or postpartum[§]	Yes	No	1. *Infected mother*: Isolate until no longer infectious[§]
			2. *Infected mother's infant*: Isolate infant separately from mother. Administer IG immediately. Send infant home when mother is no longer infectious. Alternatively, observe in isolation for 18 days for modified measles,[¶] especially if IG administration was delayed >4 days
			3. *Other mothers and infants*: Follow same recommendations as C-2
			4. *Hospital personnel*: Follow same recommendations as B-3

*Catarrhal stage or <72 hr after onset of exanthem.
[†]Vaccination with live-attenuated measles virus (see text).
[‡]With exposure <6 days antepartum, mother would not be potentially infectious until at least 72 hr postpartum.
[§]Considered infectious from onset of prodrome until 72 hr after onset of exanthem.
[¶]Incubation period for modified measles may be prolonged beyond usual 10–14 days.
IG, immunoglobulin.

should receive immunoglobulin and be sent home as soon as possible unless siblings at home have measles in a communicable stage.

If the mother's exposure occurred 6 to 15 days antepartum, prophylaxis with immunoglobulin should also be administered to the other mothers, neonates, and hospital personnel in the delivery room and nursery except those with a history of natural measles or vaccination with live-attenuated measles virus or who have detectable antibodies to measles virus. Globulin prophylaxis given within 72 hours of exposure prevents infection in nearly all instances, and in many cases it is effective for 7 days [403,481]. Immunoglobulin given after this period but before the prodrome usually results in modified measles infection with diminished morbidity [403,481]. Patients to whom immunoglobulin had to be given should later be vaccinated, after allowing an interval of at least 5 months so that residual measles antibody does not interfere with the immune response to the vaccine [403].

If a mother develops measles immediately antepartum or postpartum and her infant is born with congenital measles, the mother and infant should be isolated together until 72 hours after the appearance of the exanthem. Close observation of the neonate for signs of bronchopneumonia and other complications is warranted. Other susceptible mothers, neonates, and hospital personnel should receive immediate prophylaxis with immunoglobulin as outlined previously, followed by vaccination at a later date.

If a mother develops perinatal measles, but her infant is born without signs of infection, each should be isolated separately. The infant may be incubating transplacentally acquired measles or may be at risk for postnatally acquired droplet infection. In either case, the infant should receive immunoglobulin. The mother may be discharged with her infant after the 3rd day of exanthem. The neonate should be followed closely and observed for signs of modified measles, which may require 18 days of observation because of the abnormally long incubation period of modified measles [403].

The availability of virus diagnostic facilities varies, and the approach to potential nosocomial spread of measles may differ from place to place. If serologic testing is expensive or unavailable, it may be simpler to administer immunoglobulin to all exposed persons who do not have an unequivocal history of previous measles or previous vaccination with live-attenuated measles virus vaccine. Serologic testing of persons exposed who are thought possibly to be susceptible to measles, with administration of immunoglobulin to persons exposed who are truly susceptible, would seem to be the ideal management for prevention of nosocomial measles.

Neonates or mothers isolated because of measles require a separate room with the door closed and negative pressure ventilation. Only immune visitors and staff should enter the room. Gown and hand-washing precautions must be observed, and containment of bedding and tissues soiled with respiratory excreta by double bagging and autoclaving is indicated. Because measles virus is excreted in the urine during the early exanthematous phase, it is also advisable to treat the urine as potentially infectious and to disinfect bedpans. Terminal disinfection of the room is recommended.

MUMPS

Mumps is an acute, generalized, communicable disease whose most distinctive feature is swelling of one or both parotid glands. Involvement of other salivary glands, the meninges, the pancreas, and the testes of postpubertal males is also common. The origin of the name is obscure, but probably is related to the Old English verb *to mump*, meaning "to sulk," or to the Scottish verb meaning "to speak indistinctly."

ORGANISM
Properties and Propagation

Mumps virus is a member of the paramyxovirus family and has most of the morphologic and physicochemical properties described for measles. Five antigens have been described: two envelope glycoproteins, a hemagglutinin-neuraminidase (H-N), a hemolysis cell fusion (F) glycoprotein antigen, and a matrix envelope protein. There are two internal antigens: a nucleocapsid protein (NP) and an RNA polymerase protein (P) [482].

Mumps virus is readily isolated after inoculation of appropriate clinical specimens into various host systems. Rapid identification may be accomplished by use of cells grown in shell vials and use of fluorescein-labeled monoclonal antibodies and molecular methods such as reverse transcriptase PCR [483–485]. The virus may be recovered during the first few days of illness from saliva, throat washings, and urine and from the cerebrospinal fluid of patients with mumps meningitis. Shedding of virus in the urine may persist longer, sometimes 2 weeks. Less commonly, the virus is present in blood, milk, and testicular tissue [482,484].

A highly sensitive ELISA useful for diagnosing and determining susceptibility to mumps has been described. This assay has also been used to diagnose acute mumps in one serum specimen by the presence of specific IgM [482]. The diagnosis may also be established by showing an increasing antibody titer in paired acute and convalescent sera.

EPIDEMIOLOGY AND TRANSMISSION
Period of Communicability

Mumps occurs worldwide and is endemic in most urban areas where routine vaccination is not practiced. In the United States, before widespread vaccination against mumps, the incidence was highest in the winter, reaching a peak in March and April. Mumps was principally a disease of childhood, with most infections occurring between the ages of 5 and 15 years. Mumps in infancy is very uncommon (discussed later). In the prevaccine era, approximately one third of infections were subclinical. Epidemics tended to occur in confined populations, such as those in boarding schools, the military, and other institutions. Since the introduction of live-attenuated mumps vaccine in 1967, the incidence of clinical mumps has declined dramatically in the United States, and mumps remains an extremely uncommon disease. In 2006, there was a resurgence of mumps, however, with 6584 cases reported to the CDC. Many occurred on college campuses, and disease occurred in individuals who had received the recommended two doses of vaccine [486,487]. Mumps outbreaks are continuing to be problematic among young adults in the U.S. in 2010. Administration of a 3rd routine dose is being explored as a possible means of control.

Incubation Period

The usual incubation period, measured between exposure to infection and onset of parotitis, is 14 to 18 days (range 7 to 23 days). Because the contact may be shedding virus before the onset of clinical disease or may have subclinical infection and be unrecognizable, the incubation period in individual cases is often uncertain.

Incidence of Mumps in Pregnancy

The incidence of mumps in pregnancy is unknown. Because there is now little opportunity for exposure to mumps and many women are immune, the incidence is expected to be low. The incidence in prospective studies in the prevaccine era was variously estimated as between 0.8 and 10 cases per 10,000 pregnancies [71,173].

PATHOGENESIS

Mumps is transmitted by droplet nuclei, saliva, and fomites. The precise pathogenesis of infection has not been established; although experimentally infected monkeys may develop parotitis, no animal model closely resembles human disease. After entry into the host, the virus initially replicates in the epithelium of the upper respiratory tract. A viremia ensues, after which there is localization in glandular or central nervous system tissues. Parotitis is believed to occur as a result of viremia, rather than the reverse, because in many instances generalized disease precedes involvement of the parotid gland, which may not be involved at all.

PATHOLOGY

Studies of the pathology of mumps are few because the disease is rarely fatal. The histologic changes that have been observed in the parotid gland and the testis are similar. The inflammatory exudate consists of perivascular and interstitial infiltrates of mononuclear cells accompanied by prominent edema. There is necrosis of acinar and duct epithelial cells in the salivary glands and of the germinal epithelium of the seminiferous tubules.

There are few reports of placental pathology in gestational mumps. Garcia and associates [488] described a 29-year-old Brazilian woman with a history of two bleeding episodes during pregnancy who developed mumps in her 5th month. A hysterotomy was subsequently performed, yielding a macerated 90-g fetus. Necrotizing villitis and accumulation of necrotic material, mononuclear cells, and nuclear fragments were found in the intervillous spaces of the placenta. Necrotizing granulomas and cytoplasmic inclusions consistent with mumps virus infection were also identified. Two additional women with mumps in the 10th week and 2nd month of pregnancy underwent therapeutic abortions. Typical inclusion bodies were identified in both placentas and in the adrenal cortex of one fetus [488]. No serologic data were available on these

three women, however, so it is possible that their parotitis was caused by an agent other than mumps virus.

CLINICAL MANIFESTATIONS

The prodrome of mumps consists of fever, malaise, myalgia, and anorexia. Parotitis, when present, usually appears within the next 24 hours, but may be delayed for 1 week or more. Swelling of the gland is accompanied by tenderness to palpation and obliteration of the space between the earlobe and the angle of the mandible. The swelling progresses for 2 to 3 days, then gradually subsides, and disappears in 1 week or less. The orifice of Stensen duct is commonly red and swollen. In most cases, parotitis is bilateral, although the onset in each gland may be asynchronous by 1 or more days. The submaxillary glands are involved less often than the parotid and almost never by themselves. The sublingual glands are only rarely affected.

Orchitis is the most common manifestation other than parotitis in postpubertal males; it affects about 20% of this group of patients. Orchitis in infancy has been described, but is not well documented [489]. Oophoritis is far less common. It is associated with lower abdominal pain, and the ovaries rarely may be palpable. Oophoritis does not lead to sterility.

Aseptic meningitis may occur in children and adults of either sex, but is more common in males. Although pleocytosis of the cerebrospinal fluid may occur in 50% of cases of clinical mumps, signs of meningeal irritation occur in a smaller proportion of cases, variably estimated at 5% to 25%. The cerebrospinal fluid may contain 1000 cells/mm³. Within the first 24 hours, polymorphonuclear leukocytes may predominate, but by the 2nd day, most cells are lymphocytes. In the absence of parotitis, the syndrome of aseptic meningitis in mumps is indistinguishable clinically from meningitis caused by enteroviruses and other viruses. The course is almost invariably self-limited. Rarely, cranial nerve palsies have led to permanent sequelae, of which deafness is the most common.

Mumps pancreatitis may cause abdominal pain. The incidence of this manifestation is unclear because reliable diagnostic criteria are difficult to obtain. An elevated serum amylase level may be present in parotitis or pancreatitis. The character of the abdominal pain is rarely sufficiently distinctive to permit unequivocal diagnosis. Other complications of mumps include mastitis, thyroiditis, myocarditis, nephritis, and arthritis.

The peripheral blood cell count in mumps is not characteristic. The white blood cell count may be elevated, normal, or depressed, and the differential count may reveal a mild lymphocytosis or a polymorphonuclear leukocytosis.

Maternal Effects of Mumps

In contrast to varicella and measles, when mumps occurs in pregnant women, the illness is generally benign and is not appreciably more severe than it is in other women [489–498]. In a 1957 "virgin soil" epidemic of mumps among the Inuit, 20 infections occurred in pregnant women. Of these, only 8 (40%) were clinically apparent compared with an incidence of 57 clinically apparent cases (62%) among 92 nonpregnant women. Overt disease does not seem to be more common during pregnancy

[495]. Some complications, such as mastitis and perhaps thyroiditis, are more frequent in postpubertal women than in men, but probably do not occur more commonly in pregnant women than in other women [495]. Mumps virus has been isolated on the 3rd postpartum day from the milk of a woman who developed parotitis 2 days antepartum [499]. Her infant, who was not breast-fed, did not develop clinically apparent mumps. Aseptic meningitis, apparently without unduly high incidence or severity, has also been reported in pregnant women [500]. Deaths from mumps are exceedingly rare in pregnant women and in the population as a whole. One death has been reported in a woman who developed mumps complicated by glomerulonephritis at 8 months' gestation [500].

Effects of Gestational Mumps on the Fetus
Abortion

An excessive number of abortions is associated with gestational mumps when the disease occurs during the first trimester. In prospective studies of fetal mortality in virus diseases, Siegel and associates [207] observed 9 fetal deaths (27%) among 33 first-trimester pregnancies complicated by mumps compared with 131 (13%) of 1010 matched uninfected controls (see Table 22–5). This difference is significant ($\chi^2 = 5.6$; $P < .02$). Mumps-associated fetal deaths occurred in only 1 of 51 second-trimester pregnancies and none of 43 third-trimester pregnancies. In contrast to fetal deaths associated with measles, fetal deaths associated with mumps were closely related temporally to maternal infection: 6 of the 10 deaths occurred within 2 weeks after the onset of maternal mumps [207].

Many other reports describe isolated cases of abortion associated with gestational mumps. Most cases occurred in the first 4 months of pregnancy [490,495,496,498, 501–503]. In one instance, mumps virus was isolated from a 10-week fetus spontaneously aborted 4 days after the mother developed clinical mumps [503].

Prematurity

In the only prospective study of low birth weight in relation to maternal mumps infection, no significant association was found [207]. Nine (7.7%) of 117 pregnant women with mumps gave birth to infants with birth weights of less than 2500 g compared with 4 (3.3%) of 122 uninfected pregnant women in a control group (see Table 22–4).

Congenital Malformations

In experimentally infected animals, mumps virus may induce congenital malformations [504–506]. Definitive evidence of a teratogenic potential for mumps virus in humans has not been shown, however. Many reports describe the occurrence of congenital malformations after gestational mumps, but no data are available in most of these studies regarding the incidence of anomalies in uninfected matched control pregnancies. Swan [501] reviewed the literature in 1951 and found 18 anomalies in the offspring of 93 pregnancies complicated by mumps. These included four malformations originating in the first trimester (i.e., cutaneous nevus, imperforate anus, spina bifida, and Down syndrome) and nine originating in the

second trimester (i.e., four cases of Down syndrome and miscellaneous other malformations). Other reports have described malformation of the external ear [491], intestinal atresia [498], chorioretinitis and optic atrophy in the absence of evidence of congenital toxoplasmosis [507], corneal cataracts [448], and urogenital abnormalities [508]. One case of hydrocephalus caused by obstruction of the foramen of Monro in an infant whose mother had serologically proven mumps during the 5th month of pregnancy has been described [509]. A similar phenomenon has been seen after extrauterine mumps with encephalitis [510] and in an animal model [506]. In the only controlled, prospective study, the rate of congenital malformations in children whose mothers had mumps during pregnancy (2 of 117) was essentially identical to the rate in infants born to uninfected mothers (2 of 123) [72]. The two affected infants, both of whom were mentally retarded, were not born to any of the 24 pregnant women who had mumps in the first trimester. Similarly, no association between gestational mumps and fetal malformations was reported by British investigators, who evaluated the outcomes of 501 pregnancies complicated by maternal mumps and found no significant differences compared with a control series [511].

Endocardial Fibroelastosis

A postulated association between gestational mumps infection and endocardial fibroelastosis in the offspring was at one time the subject of much debate [512]. An extensive review of evidence for and against an etiologic role for mumps virus in this condition by Finland [513] in the 1970s was inconclusive, and there was little more information in the literature for the next 30 years. The issue remains unresolved. The rarity of mumps during pregnancy and the rarity of endocardial fibroelastosis as a possible sequela in the fetus make it unlikely that conclusive data will ever be obtained.

Molecular approaches seem to have shed new light on the issue. Using PCR, mumps virus genome was detected in two of two fatal cases of fibroelastosis [514]. In another study of 29 fatal cases of mumps, fragments of the mumps genome were identified in 20 cases [515]. Adenovirus was identified in the remainder. It was hypothesized that endocardial fibroelastosis is the end result of myocarditis. As mumps has become rare because of vaccination, endocardial fibroelastosis has also become rare [515]. The possible role of intrauterine mumps was not addressed in these two modern studies and may be impossible to evaluate further given the rarity of mumps in developed countries today.

Perinatal Mumps

In contrast to congenital chickenpox and measles, congenital mumps or even postnatally acquired perinatal mumps has rarely been documented virologically or serologically. Although several cases of parotitis have been reported in women near delivery and their neonates and infants [495,516–519], the significance of these reports is often uncertain, especially when clinically apparent mumps only is present in the mother. Other viral, bacterial, and noninfectious causes are difficult to exclude without laboratory evidence of mumps infection. Among the possible explanations for the rarity of transplacental and postnatally acquired mumps in neonates are the rarity of mumps today, protection of the neonate by passive maternal antibodies, exclusion of mumps virus from the fetus by a hypothetical placental barrier, relative insusceptibility of fetal and neonatal tissues to infection by mumps virus, and occurrence of infections that are predominantly subclinical.

Passage of mumps virus across the human placenta has occasionally been reported. Live-attenuated mumps virus has been recovered from the placenta of pregnant women (but not from fetal tissues) who were vaccinated 10 days before undergoing saline-induced abortion [520]. Mumps virus was isolated from two infants whose mothers had mumps at delivery. One infant had parotitis, and the other had pneumonia; presumably, transplacental transmission had occurred [518]. Mumps virus was also isolated from a fetus spontaneously aborted on the 4th day after the onset of maternal mumps [488]. Transplacental passage of virus should not be assumed to occur invariably, however, because in several instances passage could not be documented [488,521,522].

A differentiation between lack of susceptibility and subclinical infection as explanations for failure of the neonate to develop parotitis or other manifestations of mumps can be made only by adequate serologic investigations and viral isolation attempts. These data are unavailable. Several investigators have observed that clinically apparent mumps with parotitis [523,524] or orchitis [489] during the 1st year of life tends to be a very mild disease and that age-specific attack rates for manifest disease related to mumps increase progressively until age 5 years [525]. Antibodies to mumps virus are known to cross the placenta and to persist for several months [526].

DIAGNOSIS AND DIFFERENTIAL DIAGNOSIS

The diagnosis of mumps is easy when there is acute, bilateral, painful parotitis with a history of recent exposure. More difficulty is encountered when the disease is unilateral or when the manifestations are confined to organs other than the parotid gland. In these cases, laboratory confirmation may be obtained by virus isolation or demonstration of an increasing antibody titer.

Among neonates, few conditions need be considered in the differential diagnosis. Clinical parotitis in this age group is rare. Suppurative parotitis of the newborn, usually caused by *S. aureus,* is most often unilateral [527]. Pus can be expressed from the parotid duct, and there is a polymorphonuclear leukocytosis of the peripheral blood. Other diagnostic considerations in neonates include infection with parainfluenza viruses and coxsackieviruses, drug-induced parotitis, and facial cellulitis. In addition to these conditions in neonates, the differential diagnosis in pregnant women includes anterior cervical lymphadenitis, idiopathic recurrent parotitis, salivary gland calculus with obstruction, sarcoidosis with uveoparotid fever, and salivary gland tumors.

Other entities should be considered when the manifestations appear in organs other than the parotid. Testicular torsion in infancy may produce a painful scrotal mass resembling mumps orchitis [489]. Aseptic meningitis

related to mumps typically occurs in the winter and early spring, and enterovirus aseptic meningitis is most common in the summer and early autumn. Other viruses may also cause aseptic meningitis that is clinically indistinguishable from mumps.

THERAPY

Treatment of parotitis is symptomatic. Analgesics and application of heat or cold to the parotid area may be helpful. Mumps immunoglobulin has no proven value in the prevention or treatment of mumps. Mastitis may be managed by the application of ice packs and breast binders. Testicular pain may be minimized by the local application of cold and gentle support for the scrotum. In some instances, severe cases of orchitis have seemed to respond to systemic administration of corticosteroids.

PREVENTION

Active Immunization

Live-attenuated mumps virus vaccine induces antibodies that protect against infection in more than 95% of recipients. The subcutaneously administered vaccine may be given to children older than 1 year, but its use in infants younger than this is not recommended because of possible interference by passive maternal antibodies. Usually, it is administered simultaneously with measles and rubella vaccines when children are 15 months old, with a second dose later in childhood. The vaccine is highly recommended for older children and adolescents who have not been immunized or had mumps; it is not recommended for pregnant women, for patients receiving corticosteroids, or for other immunocompromised hosts. Because of the resurgence of mumps beginning in 2006, in which vaccine failure after two doses was documented, needs for booster immunization are being explored, although no new policies have yet been implemented [486,487,528].

Passive Immunization

Passive immunization for mumps is ineffective and unavailable.

Prevention of Nosocomial Mumps in the Newborn Nursery

In contrast to chickenpox and measles, mumps does not seem to be a potentially serious hazard in the newborn nursery. No outbreaks of nosocomial mumps have been described in this setting, and transmission of mumps in a hospital setting is highly unusual [529]. Most mothers are immune, and neonates born to nonimmune mothers rarely develop clinically apparent mumps. Prudence dictates that mothers who develop parotitis or other manifestations of mumps in the period immediately antepartum or postpartum should be isolated from other mothers and neonates. The case is less strong for isolating a mother with mumps in the puerperium from her own newborn. In the hospital setting, isolation of patients with mumps from the time of onset of parotitis has proved to be ineffective in preventing the spread of disease [530]. Infected subjects shed mumps virus in respiratory secretions for several days before the onset of parotitis or other manifestations recognizable as mumps.

At one time, exposed hospital personnel, particularly postpubertal males, and mothers with a negative history of mumps could be given mumps immunoglobulin, although the prophylactic effectiveness of this product was never established. This preparation is no longer available. Live-attenuated mumps virus vaccine has not been evaluated for protection after exposure, but may theoretically modify or prevent disease by inducing neutralizing antibodies before the onset of illness because of the long incubation period of mumps. It should be considered for exposed susceptible hospital personnel and puerperal mothers. Some hospitals have the facilities to test for susceptibility to mumps by measurement of antibody titers, whereas others do not. Testing for susceptibility could eliminate some use of vaccine for the previously described situation.

Isolation procedures for mumps include the use of a single room for a patient with the door closed at all times except to enter. Immune personnel caring for the patient should exercise gown and hand-washing precautions. Isolation is continued until parotid swelling has subsided. Terminal disinfection of the room is desirable. Updated CDC policy concerning persons with mumps recommends that patients with parotitis be isolated for 5 days after onset [531].

REFERENCES

[1] T.H. Weller, Varicella and herpes zoster: changing concepts of the natural history, control, and importance of a not-so-benign virus, N. Engl. J. Med. 309 (1983) 1362.
[2] O. Lungu, et al., Reactivated and latent varicella-zoster virus in human dorsal root ganglia, Proc. Natl. Acad. Sci. U. S. A. 92 (1995) 10980.
[3] O. Lungu, et al., Aberrant intracellular localization of varicella-zoster virus regulatory proteins during latency, Proc. Natl. Acad. Sci. U. S. A. 95 (1998) 780.
[4] J. Chen, et al., Latent and lytic infection of isolated guinea pig enteric and dorsal root ganglia by varicella zoster virus, J. Med. Virol. 70 (2003) S71.
[5] R. Mahalingam, et al., Expression of protein encoded by varicella-zoster virus open reading frame 63 in latently infected human ganglionic neurons, Proc. Natl. Acad. Sci. U. S. A. 93 (1996) 2122.
[6] Old English Dictionary, Oxford University Press, London, 1933.
[7] A.B. Christie, Chickenpox, in: Infectious Diseases: Epidemiology and Clinical Practice, E & S Livingstone, Edinburgh, 1969.
[8] B. Angelicus, De Propreitatibus Rerum, Liber septimus, vol xciii, Trevisa John, London, 1398.
[9] W.B. Muir, R. Nichols, J. Breuer, Phylogenetic analysis of varicella-zoster virus: evidence of intercontinental spread of genotypes and recombination, J. Virol. 76 (2002) 1971.
[10] N. Sengupta, et al., Varicella-zoster-virus genotypes in East London: a prospective study in patients with herpes zoster, J. Infect. Dis. 196 (2007) 1014–1020.
[11] C. Gabel, et al., Varicella-zoster virus glycoproteins are phosphorylated during posttranslational maturation, J. Virol. 63 (1989) 4264.
[12] A. Gershon, L. Cosio, P.A. Brunell, Observations on the growth of varicella-zoster virus in human diploid cells, J. Gen. Virol. 18 (1973) 21.
[13] M.L. Cook, J. Stevens, Labile coat: reason for noninfectious cell-free varicella zoster virus in culture, J. Virol. 2 (1968) 1458.
[14] J.J. Chen, et al., Mannose 6-phosphate receptor dependence of varicella zoster virus infection in vitro and in the epidermis during varicella and zoster, Cell 119 (2004) 915–926.
[15] M. Myers, B.L. Connelly, Animal models of varicella, J. Infect. Dis. 166 (1992) S48.
[16] C. Sadzot-Delvaux, et al., An in vivo model of varicella-zoster virus latent infection of dorsal root ganglia, J. Neurosci. Res. 26 (1990) 83.
[17] V. Williams, A. Gershon, P. Brunell, Serologic response to varicella-zoster membrane antigens measured by indirect immunofluorescence, J. Infect. Dis. 130 (1974) 669.
[18] J. Zaia, M. Oxman, Antibody to varicella-zoster virus-induced membrane antigen: immunofluorescence assay using monodisperse glutaraldehyde-fixed target cells, J. Infect. Dis. 136 (1977) 519.
[19] A. Gershon, S. Steinberg, P. LaRussa, Measurement of Antibodies to VZV by Latex Agglutination, Society for Pediatric Research, Anaheim, CA, 1992.
[20] B. Forghani, N. Schmidt, J. Dennis, Antibody assays for varicella-zoster virus: comparison of enzyme immunoassay with neutralization, immune adherence hemagglutination, and complement fixation, J. Clin. Microbiol. 8 (1978) 545.
[21] A. Gershon, et al., Enzyme-linked immunosorbent assay for measurement of antibody to varicella-zoster virus, Arch. Virol. 70 (1981) 169.
[22] P. LaRussa, et al., Comparison of five assays for antibody to varicella-zoster virus and the fluorescent-antibody-to-membrane-antigen test, J. Clin. Microbiol. 25 (1987) 2059.
[23] Z. Shehab, P. Brunell, Enzyme-linked immunosorbent assay for susceptibility to varicella, J. Infect. Dis. 148 (1983) 472.
[24] M.G. Friedman, S. Leventon-Kriss, I. Sarov, Sensitive solid-phase radioimmunoassay for detection of human immunoglobulin G antibodies to varicella-zoster virus, J. Clin. Microbiol. 9 (1979) 1.
[25] A. Gershon, Z. Kalter, S. Steinberg, Detection of antibody to varicella-zoster virus by immune adherence hemagglutination, Proc. Soc. Exp. Biol. Med. 151 (1976) 762.
[26] A.E. Caunt, D.G. Shaw, Neutralization tests with varicella-zoster virus, J. Hyg. (Lond) 67 (1969) 343.
[27] C. Grose, B.J. Edmond, P.A. Brunell, Complement-enhanced neutralizing antibody response to varicella-zoster virus, J. Infect. Dis. 139 (1979) 432.
[28] E. Gold, G. Godek, Complement fixation studies with a varicella-zoster antigen, J. Immunol. 95 (1965) 692.
[29] N.J. Schmidt, E.H. Lennette, R.L. Magoffin, Immunological relationship between herpes simplex and varicella-zoster viruses demonstrated by complement-fixation, neutralization and fluorescent antibody tests, J. Gen. Virol. 4 (1969) 321.
[30] G.J.P. Schaap, J. Huisman, Simultaneous rise in complement-fixing antibodies against herpesvirus hominis and varicella-zoster virus in patients with chickenpox and shingles, Arch. Gesamte Virusforsch. 25 (1968) 52.
[31] N.J. Schmidt, Further evidence for common antigens in herpes simplex and varicella-zoster virus, J. Med. Virol. 9 (1982) 27.
[32] K. Shiraki, et al., Polypeptides of varicella-zoster virus (VZV) and immunological relationship of VZV and herpes simplex virus (HSV), J. Gen. Virol. 61 (1982) 255.
[33] K. Kitamura, et al., Induction of neutralizing antibody against varicella-zoster virus (VZV) by gp 2 and cross-reactivity between VZV gp 2 and herpes simplex viruses gB, Virology 149 (1986) 74.
[34] S.M. Lemon, et al., Simultaneous infection with multiple herpesviruses, Am. J. Med. 66 (1979) 270.
[35] M.L. Landry, G.D. Hsiung, Diagnosis of dual herpesvirus infection: varicella-zoster virus (VZV) and herpes simplex viruses, in: A.J. Nahmias, W.R. Dowdle, R.F. Schinazi (Eds.), The Human Herpesviruses, Elsevier, New York, 1981.
[36] A.M. Arvin, Cell-mediated immunity to varicella-zoster virus, J. Infect. Dis. 166 (1992) S35.
[37] A. Davison, et al., New common nomenclature for glycoprotein genes of varicella-zoster virus and their products, J. Virol. 57 (1986) 1195.
[38] A.M. Arvin, et al., Memory cytotoxic T cell responses to viral tegument and regulatory proteins encoded by open reading frames 4, 10, 29, and 62 of varicella-zoster virus, Viral. Immunol. 15 (2002) 507.
[39] P. Brunell, Varicella-zoster immunoglobulins during varicella, latency, and zoster, J. Infect. Dis. 132 (1975) 49.
[40] A. Gershon, et al., IgM to varicella-zoster virus: demonstration in patients with and without clinical zoster, Pediatr. Infect. Dis. 1 (1979) 164.
[41] R.E. Hope-Simpson, The nature of herpes zoster: a long-term study and a new hypothesis, Proc. R. Soc. Med. 58 (1965) 9.
[42] P.A. Brunell, Transmission of chickenpox in a school setting prior to the observed exanthem, Am. J. Dis. Child. 143 (1989) 1451.
[43] P. Evans, An epidemic of chickenpox, Lancet 2 (1940) 339.
[44] J.E. Gordon, F.M. Meader, The period of infectivity and serum prevention of chickenpox, JAMA 93 (1929) 2013.
[45] S. Kido, et al., Detection of varicella-zoster virus (VZV) DNA in clinical samples from patients with VZV by the polymerase chain reaction, J. Clin. Microbiol. 29 (1991) 76.
[46] M. Tsolia, et al., Live attenuated varicella vaccine: evidence that the virus is attenuated and the importance of skin lesions in transmission of varicella-zoster virus, J. Pediatr. 116 (1990) 184.
[47] R.G. Sharrar, et al., The postmarketing safety profile of varicella vaccine, Vaccine 19 (2000) 916.
[48] T.L. Gustafson, et al., An outbreak of nosocomial varicella, Pediatrics 70 (1982) 550.
[49] J.M. Leclair, et al., Airborne transmission of chickenpox in a hospital, N. Engl. J. Med. 302 (1980) 450.
[50] M. Sawyer, et al., Detection of varicella-zoster virus DNA in air samples from hospital rooms, J. Infect. Dis. 169 (1993) 91.
[51] D.A. Moore, R.S. Hopkins, Assessment of a school exclusion policy during a chickenpox outbreak, Am. J. Epidemiol. 133 (1991) 1161.
[52] R.E. Hope-Simpson, Infectiousness of communicable diseases in the household (measles, mumps, and chickenpox), Lancet 2 (1952) 549.
[53] K. Kundratitz, Experimentelle Übertragung von Herpes Zoster auf den Menschen und die Beziehungen von Herpes Zoster zu Varicellen, Monatsschr. Kinderheilkd. 29 (1925) 516.
[54] E. Bruusgaard, The mutual relation between zoster and varicella, Br. J. Dermatol. Syphilis 44 (1932) 1.
[55] H.E. Seiler, A study of herpes zoster particularly in its relationship to chickenpox, J. Hyg. (Lond) 47 (1949) 253.
[56] S. Schimpff, et al., Varicella-zoster infection in patients with cancer, Ann. Intern. Med. 76 (1972) 241.
[57] B.S. Berlin, T. Campbell, Hospital-acquired herpes zoster following exposure to chickenpox, JAMA 211 (1970) 1831.

[58] R. Mahalingham, et al., Latent varicella-zoster viral DNA in human trigeminal and thoracic ganglia, N. Engl. J. Med. 323 (1990) 627.

[59] Y. Hayakawa, et al., Biologic and biophysical markers of a live varicella vaccine strain (Oka): identification of clinical isolates from vaccine recipients, J. Infect. Dis. 149 (1984) 956.

[60] S.E. Straus, et al., Endonuclease analysis of viral DNA from varicella and subsequent zoster infections in the same patient, N. Engl. J. Med. 311 (1984) 1362.

[61] D.L. Williams, et al., Herpes zoster following varicella vaccine in a child with acute lymphocytic leukemia, J. Pediatr. 106 (1985) 259.

[62] A. Gershon, Varicella in mother and infant: problems old and new, in: S. Krugman, A. Gershon (Eds.), Infections of the Fetus and Newborn Infant, Alan R Liss, New York, 1975.

[63] J.F. Seward, et al., Varicella disease after introduction of varicella vaccine in the United States, 1995–2000, JAMA 287 (2002) 606.

[64] W.P. London, J.A. Yorke, Recurrent outbreaks of measles, chickenpox and mumps. I. Seasonal variation in contact rates, Am. J. Epidemiol. 98 (1973) 453.

[65] J.A. Yorke, W.P. London, Recurrent outbreaks of measles, chickenpox and mumps: II. Systematic differences in contact rates and stochastic effects, Am. J. Epidemiol. 98 (1973) 469.

[66] J.E. Gordon, Chickenpox: an epidemiologic review, Am. J. Med. Sci. 244 (1962) 362.

[67] S. Preblud, W. Orenstein, K. Bart, Varicella: clinical manifestations, epidemiology, and health impact on children, Pediatr. Infect. Dis. 3 (1984) 505.

[68] S.R. Preblud, L.J. D'Angelo, Chickenpox in the United States, 1972–1977, J. Infect. Dis. 140 (1979) 257.

[69] A.H. Ross, E. Lencher, G. Reitman, Modification of chickenpox in family contacts by administration of gamma globulin, N. Engl. J. Med. 267 (1962) 369.

[70] P. LaRussa, et al., Determination of immunity to varicella by means of an intradermal skin test, J. Infect. Dis. 152 (1985) 869.

[71] J. Sever, L.R. White, Intrauterine viral infections, Annu. Rev. Med. 19 (1968) 471.

[72] M. Siegel, Congenital malformations following chickenpox, measles, mumps, and hepatitis: results of a cohort study, JAMA 226 (1973) 1521.

[73] J. Balducci, et al., Pregnancy outcome following first-trimester varicella infection, Obstet. Gynecol. 79 (1992) 5.

[74] P.A. Brunell, G.S.J. Kotchmar, Zoster in infancy: failure to maintain virus latency following intrauterine infection, J. Pediatr. 98 (1981) 71.

[75] K. Baba, et al., Increased incidence of herpes zoster in normal children infected with varicella-zoster virus during infancy: community-based follow up study, J. Pediatr. 108 (1986) 372.

[76] H. Guess, et al., Epidemiology of herpes zoster in children and adolescents: a population-based study, Pediatrics 76 (1985) 512.

[77] K. Terada, et al., Varicella-zoster virus (VZV) reactivation is related to the low response of VZV-specific immunity after chickenpox in infancy, J. Infect. Dis. 169 (1994) 650.

[78] C.M. Kalman, O.L. Laskin, Herpes zoster and zosteriform herpes simplex virus infections in immunocompetent adults, Am. J. Med. 81 (1986) 775.

[79] R.M. Locksley, et al., Infection with varicella-zoster virus after marrow transplantation, J. Infect. Dis. 152 (1985) 1172.

[80] J. Veenstra, et al., Herpes zoster, immunological deterioration and disease progression in HIV-1 infection, AIDS 9 (1995) 1153.

[81] A. Gershon, et al., Varicella-zoster virus infection in children with underlying HIV infection, J. Infect. Dis. 175 (1997) 1496.

[82] S.A. Brazin, J.W. Simkovich, W.T. Johnson, Herpes zoster during pregnancy, Obstet. Gynecol. 53 (1979) 175.

[83] A. Gershon, et al., Antibody to varicella-zoster virus in parturient women and their offspring during the first year of life, Pediatrics 58 (1976) 692.

[84] Z. Shehab, P. Brunell, E. Cobb, Epidemiological standardization of a test for susceptibility to mumps, J. Infect. Dis. 149 (1984) 810.

[85] S.P. Sirpenski, T. Brennan, D. Mayo, Determination of infection and immunity to varicella-zoster virus with an enzyme-linked immunosorbent assay, J. Infect. Dis. 152 (1985) 1349.

[86] R. Steele, et al., Varicella-zoster in hospital personnel: skin test reactivity to monitor susceptibility, Pediatrics 70 (1982) 604.

[87] H. Kjersem, S. Jepsen, Varicella among immigrants from the tropics, a health problem, Scand. J. Soc. Med. 18 (1990) 171.

[88] J.N. Longfield, et al., Varicella outbreaks in army recruits from Puerto Rico, Arch. Intern. Med. 150 (1990) 970.

[89] Z. Maretic, M.P.M. Cooray, Comparisons between chickenpox in a tropical and a European country, J. Trop. Med. Hyg. 66 (1963) 311.

[90] D.P. Sinha, Chickenpox—a disease predominantly affecting adults in rural west Bengal, India, Int. J. Epidemiol. 5 (1976) 367.

[91] P. Brunell, Placental transfer of varicella-zoster antibody, Pediatrics 38 (1966) 1034.

[92] D. Mendez, et al., Transplacental immunity to varicella-zoster virus in extremely low birthweight infants, Am. J. Perinatol. 9 (1992) 236.

[93] R. Raker, et al., Antibody to varicella-zoster virus in low birth weight infants, J. Pediatr. 93 (1978) 505.

[94] E. Wang, C. Prober, A.M. Arvin, Varicella-zoster virus antibody titers before and after administration of zoster immune globulin to neonates in an intensive care nursery, J. Pediatr. 103 (1983) 113.

[95] K. Baba, et al., Immunologic and epidemiological aspects of varicella infection acquired during infancy and early childhood, J. Pediatr. 100 (1982) 881.

[96] T.L. Gustafson, Z. Shehab, P. Brunell, Outbreak of varicella in a newborn intensive care nursery, Am. Dis. Child. 138 (1984) 548.

[97] H.W. Hyatt, Neonatal varicella, J. Natl. Med. Assoc. 59 (1967) 32.

[98] C.G.H. Newman, Perinatal varicella, Lancet 2 (1965) 1159.

[99] M.D. Readett, C. McGibbon, Neonatal varicella, Lancet 1 (1961) 644.

[100] P. Freud, Congenital varicella, Am. J. Dis. Child. 96 (1958) 730.

[101] L. Odessky, B. Newman, G.B. Wein, Congenital varicella, N. Y. State J. Med. 54 (1954) 2849.

[102] L.E. Harris, Spread of varicella in nurseries, Am. J. Dis. Child. 105 (1963) 315.

[103] S.L. Matseoane, C. Abler, Occurrence of neonatal varicella in a hospital nursery, Am. J. Obstet. Gynecol. 92 (1965) 575.

[104] S. Lipton, P.A. Brunell, Management of varicella exposure in a neonatal intensive care unit, JAMA 261 (1989) 1782.

[105] G. Patou, et al., Immunoglobulin prophylaxis for infants exposed to varicella in a neonatal unit, J. Infect. 20 (1990) 207.

[106] W.L. Gold, et al., Management of varicella exposures in the neonatal intensive care unit, Pediatr. Infect. Dis. J. 12 (1993) 954.

[107] C.A. Friedman, et al., Outbreak and control of varicella in a neonatal intensive care unit, Pediatr. Infect. Dis. J. 13 (1994) 152.

[108] M.E. Apert, Une epidemic de varicelle dans une maternite, Bull. Med. (Paris) 9 (1985) 827.

[108a] C.C. Ku, J.A. Padilla, C. Grose, E.C. Butcher, A.M. Arvin, Tropism of Varicella-Zoster Virus for Human Tonsillar CD4(+) T Lymphocytes That Express Activation, Memory, and Skin Homing Markers, J Virol 76 (2002) 11425–11433.

[109] E. Gold, Serologic and virus-isolation studies of patients with varicella or herpes zoster infection, N. Engl. J. Med. 274 (1966) 181.

[110] M.G. Myers, Viremia caused by varicella-zoster virus: association with malignant progressive varicella, J. Infect. Dis. 140 (1979) 229.

[111] A. Nelson, J. Geme St., On the respiratory spread of varicella-zoster virus, Pediatrics 37 (1966) 1007.

[112] J. Trlifajova, D. Bryndova, M. Ryc, Isolation of varicella-zoster virus from pharyngeal and nasal swabs in varicella patients, J. Hyg. Epidemiol. Microbiol. Immunol. 28 (1984) 201.

[113] T. Ozaki, et al., Lymphocyte-associated viremia in varicella, J. Med. Virol. 19 (1986) 249.

[114] Y. Asano, et al., Viremia is present in incubation period in nonimmunocompromised children with varicella, J. Pediatr. 106 (1985) 69.

[115] S. Feldman, E. Epp, Isolation of varicella-zoster virus from blood, J. Pediatr. 88 (1976) 265.

[116] S. Feldman, E. Epp, Detection of viremia during incubation period of varicella, J. Pediatr. 94 (1979) 746.

[117] J.F. Moffat, et al., Tropism of varicella-zoster virus for human CD4+ and CD8+ T lymphocytes and epidermal cells in SCID-hu mice, J. Virol. 69 (1995) 5236.

[118] C. Koropchak, et al., Investigation of varicella-zoster virus infection by polymerase chain reaction in the immunocompetent host with acute varicella, J. Infect. Dis. 163 (1991) 1016.

[119] T. Ozaki, et al., Varicella-zoster virus DNA in throat swabs of vaccinees, Arch. Dis. Child. 267 (1993) 328.

[120] C.H. Grose, Variation on a theme by Fenner, Pediatrics 68 (1981) 735.

[120a] C.C. Ku, L. Zerboni, H. Ito, B.S. Graham, M. Wallace, A.M. Arvin, Varicella-Zoster Virus Transfer to Skin by T Cells and Modulation of Viral Replication by Epidermal Cell Interferon-α, J Exp Med 200 (2004) 917–925.

[121] A.M. Arvin, et al., Selective impairment in lymphocyte reactivity to varicella-zoster antigen among untreated lymphoma patients, J. Infect. Dis. 137 (1978) 531.

[122] I.B. Hardy, et al., The incidence of zoster after immunization with live attenuated varicella vaccine: a study in children with leukemia, N. Engl. J. Med. 325 (1991) 1545.

[123] K.H. Rand, et al., Cellular immunity and herpesvirus infections in cardiac transplant patients, N. Engl. J. Med. 296 (1977) 1372.

[124] J.C. Ruckdeschel, et al., Herpes zoster and impaired cell-associated immunity to the varicella-zoster virus in patients with Hodgkin's disease, Am. J. Med. 62 (1977) 77.

[125] A. Friedman-Kien, et al., Herpes zoster: a possible early clinical sign for development of acquired immunodeficiency syndrome in high-risk individuals, J. Am. Acad. Dermatol. 14 (1988) 1023.

[126] S. Feldman, et al., A viremic phase for herpes zoster in children with cancer, J. Pediatr. 91 (1977) 597.

[127] A. Gershon, S. Steinberg, R. Silber, Varicella-zoster viremia, J. Pediatr. 92 (1978) 1033.

[128] D. Stevens, et al., Cellular events in zoster vesicles: relation to clinical course and immune parameters, J. Infect. Dis. 131 (1975) 509.

[129] E. Szanton, I. Sarov, Interaction between polymorphonuclear leukocytes and varicella-zoster infected cells, Intervirology 24 (1985) 119.

[130] T. Ihara, et al., Human polymorphonuclear leukocyte-mediated cytotoxicity against varicella-zoster virus-infected fibroblasts, J. Virol. 51 (1984) 110.

[131] T. Ihara, M. Ito, S.E. Starr, Human lymphocyte, monocyte and polymorphonuclear leucocyte mediated antibody-dependent cellular cytotoxicity against varicella-zoster virus-infected targets, Clin. Exp. Immunol. 63 (1986) 179.

[132] A.G.P. Garcia, Fetal infection in chickenpox and alastrim, with histopathologic study of the placenta, Pediatrics 32 (1963) 895.

[133] R.M. Erlich, J.A.P. Turner, M. Clarke, Neonatal varicella, J. Pediatr. 53 (1958) 139.

[134] P.F. Lucchesi, A.C. LaBoccetta, A.R. Peale, Varicella neonatorum, Am. J. Dis. Child. 73 (1947) 44.

[135] E.H. Oppenheimer, Congenital chickenpox with disseminated visceral lesions, Bull. Johns Hopkins Hosp. 74 (1944) 240.

[136] H.E. Pearson, Parturition varicella-zoster, Obstet. Gynecol. 23 (1964) 21.

[137] J. Steen, R.V. Pederson, Varicella in a newborn girl, J. Oslo. City Hosp. 9 (1959) 36.

[138] E.K. Ranney, M.G. Norman, M.D. Silver, Varicella pneumonitis, Can. Med. Assoc. J. 96 (1967) 445.

[139] J.H. Triebwasser, et al., Varicella pneumonia in adults: report of seven cases and a review of the literature, Medicine (Baltimore) 46 (1967) 409.

[140] J.S. Bradley, P.M. Schlievert, T.G. Sample, Streptococcal toxic shock-like syndrome as a complication of varicella, Pediatr. Infect. Dis. J. 10 (1991) 77.

[141] T.V. Brogan, et al., Group A streptococcal necrotizing fasciitis complicating primary varicella: a series of fourteen patients, Pediatr. Infect. Dis. J. 14 (1995) 588.

[142] Centers for Disease Control, Outbreak of invasive group A streptococcus associated with varicella in a childcare center—Boston, MA, 1997, MMWR Morb. Mortal. Wkly. Rep. 46 (1997) 944.

[143] H.D. Davies, et al., Invasive group A streptococcal infections in Ontario, Canada, N. Engl. J. Med. 335 (1996) 547.

[144] A. Doctor, M.B. Harper, G.R. Fleischer, Group A beta-hemolytic streptococcal bacteremia: historical review, changing incidence, and recent association with varicella, Pediatrics 96 (1995) 428.

[145] A. Gonzalez-Ruiz, et al., Varicella gangrenosa with toxic shock-like syndrome due to group A streptococcus infection in an adult, Clin. Infect. Dis. 20 (1995) 1058.

[146] W.J. Mills, et al., Invasive group A streptococcal infections complicating primary varicella, J. Pediatr. Orthop. 16 (1996) 522.

[147] C.L. Peterson, et al., Risk factors for invasive group A streptococcal infections in children with varicella: a case-control study, Pediatr. Infect. Dis. J. 15 (1996) 151.

[148] G. Wilson, et al., Group A streptococcal necrotizing fasciitis following varicella in children: case reports and review, Clin. Infect. Dis. 20 (1995) 1333.

[149] R. Johnson, P.E. Milbourn, Central nervous system manifestations of chickenpox, Can. Med. Assoc. J. 102 (1970) 831.

[150] R.B. Jenkins, Severe chickenpox encephalopathy, Am. J. Dis. Child. 110 (1965) 137.

[151] S. Minkowitz, et al., Acute glomerulonephritis associated with varicella infection, Am. J. Med. 44 (1968) 489.

[152] A.M. Yuceoglu, S. Berkovich, S. Minkowitz, Acute glomerular nephritis as a complication of varicella, JAMA 202 (1967) 113.

[153] A. Morales, S. Adelman, G. Fine, Varicella myocarditis, Arch. Pathol. 91 (1971) 29.

[154] C.M. Moore, et al., Varicella myocarditis, Am. J. Dis. Child. 118 (1969) 899.

[155] J.R. Priest, K.E. Groth, H.H. Balfour, Varicella arthritis documented by isolation of virus from joint fluid, J. Pediatr. 93 (1978) 990.

[156] J.R. Ward, B. Bishop, Varicella arthritis, JAMA 212 (1970) 1954.

[157] A. Gershon, Varicella-zoster virus: prospects for control, Adv. Pediatr. Infect. Dis. 10 (1995) 93.

[158] E. Jura, et al., Varicella-zoster virus infections in children infected with human immunodeficiency virus, Pediatr. Infect. Dis. J. 8 (1989) 586.

[159] S. Feldman, W. Hughes, C. Daniel, Varicella in children with cancer: 77 cases, Pediatrics 80 (1975) 388.

[160] T. Ihara, et al., Natural killing of varicella-zoster virus (VZV)-infected fibroblasts in normal children, children with VZV infections, and children with Hodgkin's disease, Acta. Pediatr. Jpn. 31 (1989) 523.

[161] A. Arvin, et al., Equivalent recognition of a varicella-zoster virus immediate early protein (IE62) and glycoprotein I by cytotoxic T lymphocytes of either CD4+ or CD8+ phenotype, J. Immunol. 146 (1991) 257.

[162] E. Cooper, L. Vujcic, G. Quinnan, Varicella-zoster virus-specific HLA-restricted cytotoxicity of normal immune adult lymphocytes after in vitro stimulation, J. Infect. Dis. 158 (1988) 780.

[163] S. Krugman, C. Goodrich, R. Ward, Primary varicella pneumonia, N. Engl. J. Med. 257 (1957) 843.

[164] R.H. Mermelstein, A.W. Freireich, Varicella pneumonia, Ann. Intern. Med. 55 (1961) 456.

[165] D.M. Weber, J.A. Pellecchia, Varicella pneumonia: study of prevalence in adult men, JAMA 192 (1965) 572.

[166] E.N. Sargent, M.J. Carson, E.D. Reilly, Varicella pneumonia: a report of 20 cases with postmortem examination in 6, Calif. Med. 107 (1967) 141.

[167] J.S. Bocles, N.J. Ehrenkranz, A. Marks, Abnormalities of respiratory function in varicella pneumonia, Ann. Intern. Med. 60 (1964) 183.

[168] S.A. Fish, Maternal death due to disseminated varicella, JAMA 173 (1960) 978.

[169] D.B. Hackel, Myocarditis in association with varicella, Am. J. Pathol. 29 (1953) 369.

[170] R.E. Harris, E.R. Rhoades, Varicella pneumonia complicating pregnancy: report of a case and review of the literature, Obstet. Gynecol. 25 (1965) 734.

[171] P.A. Brunell, Varicella-zoster infections in pregnancy, JAMA 199 (1967) 315.

[172] J. Baren, P. Henneman, R. Lewis, Primary varicella in adults: pneumonia, pregnancy, and hospital admission, Ann. Emerg. Med. 28 (1996) 165.

[173] M. Siegel, H.T. Fuerst, Low birth weight and maternal virus diseases: a prospective study of rubella, measles, mumps, chickenpox, and hepatitis, JAMA 197 (1966) 88.

[174] J.H. Harger, et al., Risk factors and outcome of varicella-zoster virus pneumonia in pregnant women, J. Infect. Dis. 185 (2002) 422.

[175] J.H. Harger, et al., Frequency of congenital varicella syndrome in a prospective cohort of 347 pregnant women, Obstet. Gynecol. 100 (2002) 260.

[176] T.F. Esmonde, G. Herdman, G. Anderson, Chickenpox pneumonia: an association with pregnancy, Thorax 44 (1989) 812.

[177] S.M. Cox, F.G. Cunningham, J. Luby, Management of varicella pneumonia complicating pregnancy, Am. J. Perinatol. 7 (1990) 300.

[178] R.A. Smego, M.O. Asperilla, Use of acyclovir for varicella pneumonia during pregnancy, Obstet. Gynecol. 78 (1991) 1112.

[179] E.J. Landsberger, W.D. Hager, J.H. Grossman, Successful management of varicella pneumonia complicating pregnancy: a report of 3 cases, J. Reprod. Med. 31 (1986) 311.

[180] R.R. Lotshaw, J.M. Keegan, H.R. Gordon, Parenteral and oral acyclovir for management of varicella pneumonia in pregnancy: a case report with review of literature, W. V. Med. J. 87 (1991) 204.

[181] R.S. Hockberger, R.J. Rothstein, Varicella pneumonia in adults: a spectrum of disease, Ann. Emerg. Med. 115 (1986) 931.

[182] H.M. Hollingsworth, M.R. Pratter, R.S. Irwin, Acute respiratory failure in pregnancy, J. Intensive Care Med. 4 (1989) 11.

[183] G.D.V. Hankins, L.C. Gilstrap, A.R. Patterson, Acyclovir treatment of varicella pneumonia in pregnancy (letter), Crit. Care Med. 15 (1987) 336.

[184] J.B. Glaser, et al., Varicella in pregnancy (letter), N. Engl. J. Med. 315 (1986) 1416.

[185] K. Boyd, E. Walker, Use of acyclovir to treat chickenpox in pregnancy, BMJ 296 (1988) 393.

[186] R.G. White, Chickenpox in pregnancy (letter), BMJ 196 (1988) 864.

[187] O.F. Broussard, D.K. Payne, R.B. George, Treatment with acyclovir of varicella pneumonia in pregnancy, Chest 99 (1991) 1045.

[188] S.E. Eder, J.A. Apuzzio, G. Weiss, Varicella pneumonia during pregnancy: treatment of 2 cases with acyclovir, Am. J. Perinatol. 5 (1988) 16.

[189] E.B. Andrews, et al., Acyclovir in pregnancy registry, Am. J. Med. 85 (1988) 123.

[190] Centers for Disease Control, Acyclovir registry, MMWR Morb. Mortal. Wkly. Rep. 42 (1993) 806.

[191] R.E. Pickard, Varicella pneumonia in pregnancy, Am. J. Obstet. Gynecol. 101 (1968) 504.

[192] D.A. Mendelow, G.C. Lewis, Varicella pneumonia during pregnancy, Obstet. Gynecol. 33 (1969) 98.

[193] R.B. Geeves, D.A. Lindsay, T.I. Robertson, Varicella pneumonia in pregnancy with varicella neonatorum: report of a case followed by severe digital clubbing, Aust. N. Z. J. Med. 1 (1971) 63.

[194] B.M. Pearse, Characterization of coated-vesicle adaptors: their reassembly with clathrin and with recycling receptors, Methods Cell Biol. 31 (1989) 229.

[195] Centers for Disease Control, Prevention of varicella: recommendations of the Advisory Committee on Immunization Practices (ACIP), MMWR Morb. Mortal. Wkly. Rep. 45 (1996) 1.

[196] G. Enders, et al., Consequences of varicella and herpes zoster in pregnancy: prospective study of 1739 cases, Lancet 343 (1994) 1548.

[197] Centers for Disease Control, A new product (VariZIG) for postexposure prophylaxis of varicella available under an investigational new drug application expanded access protocol, MMWR Morb. Mortal. Wkly. Rep. 55 (2006) 209–210.

[198] M. Benyesh-Melnick, et al., Viruses and mammalian chromosomes. III. Effect of herpes zoster virus on human embryonal lung cultures, Proc. Soc. Exp. Biol. Med. 117 (1964) 546.

[199] P. Aula, Chromosomes and virus infections, Lancet 1 (1964) 720.

[200] I. Massimo, et al., Chickenpox and chromosome aberrations, BMJ 2 (1965) 172.

[201] E. Collier, Congenital varicella cataract, Am. J. Ophthalmol. 86 (1978) 627.

[202] G. Cuthbertson, et al., Prenatal diagnosis of second-trimester congenital varicella syndrome by virus-specific immunoglobulin M, J. Pediatr. 111 (1987) 592.

[203] B. Harding, J.A. Bonner, Congenital varicella-zoster: a serologically proven case with necrotizing encephalitis and malformations, Acta Neuropathol. 76 (1988) 311.

[204] E. Hammad, I. Helin, A. Pasca, Early pregnancy varicella and associated congenital anomalies, Acta Paediatr. Scand. 78 (1989) 963.

[205] A.M. Adelstein, J.W. Donovan, Malignant disease in children whose mothers had chickenpox, mumps, or rubella in pregnancy, BMJ 2 (1972) 629.

[206] M.J. Fox, E.R. Krumpiegel, J.L. Teresi, Maternal measles, mumps, and chickenpox as a cause of congenital anomalies, Lancet 1 (1948) 746.

[207] M. Siegel, H.T. Fuerst, N.S. Peress, Comparative fetal mortality in maternal virus diseases: a prospective study on rubella, measles, mumps, chickenpox, and hepatitis, N. Engl. J. Med. 274 (1966) 768.

[208] S.G. Paryani, A.M. Arvin, Intrauterine infection with varicella-zoster virus after maternal varicella, N. Engl. J. Med. 314 (1986) 1542.

[209] K.L. Jones, K.A. Johnson, C.D. Chambers, Offspring of women infected with varicella during pregnancy: a prospective study, Teratology 49 (1994) 29.

[210] A. Pastuszak, et al., Outcome after maternal varicella infection in the first 20 weeks of pregnancy, N. Engl. J. Med. 330 (1994) 901.

[211] C.A. Michie, et al., Varicella-zoster contracted in the second trimester of pregnancy, Pediatr. Infect. Dis. J. 10 (1992) 1050.

[212] L. Connan, et al., Intra-uterine fetal death following maternal varicella infection, Eur. J. Obstet. Gynecol. 68 (1996) 205.

[213] A. Sauerbrai, et al., Detection of varicella-zoster virus in congenital varicella syndrome: a case report, Obstet. Gynecol. 88 (1996) 687.

[214] F. Mouly, et al., Prenatal diagnosis of fetal varicella-zoster virus infection with polymerase chain reaction of amniotic fluid in 107 cases, Am. J. Obstet. Gynecol. 177 (1997) 894.

[215] X.T. Ussery, et al., Congenital varicella-zoster infection and Barrett's esophagus, J. Infect. Dis. 178 (1998) 539.

[216] E.G. LaForet, L.L. Lynch, Multiple congenital defects following maternal varicella, N. Engl. J. Med. 236 (1947) 534.

[217] J.C. Srabstein, et al., Is there a congenital varicella syndrome? J. Pediatr. 84 (1974) 239.

[218] I. Alfonso, et al., Picture of the month: congenital varicella syndrome, Am. J. Dis. Child. 138 (1984) 603.

[219] A.L. Alkalay, et al., Congenital anomalies associated with maternal varicella infections during early pregnancy, J. Perinatol. 7 (1987) 69.

[220] M. Borzykowski, R.F. Harris, R.W.A. Jones, The congenital varicella syndrome, Eur. J. Pediatr. 137 (1981) 335.

[221] H. Dietzsch, P. Rabenalt, J. Trlifajova, Varizellen-Embryopathie: kliniche und serologische Verlaufsbeobachtungen, Kinderarztl. Prax. 3 (1980) 139.

[222] D.A. Fuccillo, Congenital varicella, Teratology 15 (1977) 329.

[223] G. Hajdi, et al., Congenital varicella syndrome, Infection 14 (1986) 177.

[224] J.B.J. McKendry, Congenital varicella associated with multiple defects, Can. Med. Assoc. J. 108 (1973) 66.

[225] R. Rinvik, Congenital varicella encephalomyelitis in surviving newborn, Am. J. Dis. Child. 117 (1969) 231.

[226] M.O. Savage, A. Moosa, R.R. Gordon, Maternal varicella infection as a cause of fetal malformations, Lancet 1 (1973) 352.

[227] I. Schlotfeld-Schafer, et al., Congenitales Varicellensyndrom, Monatsschr. Kinderheilkd. 131 (1983) 106.

[228] Broomhead, Cited in: H.A. Dudgeon (Ed.), Viral Diseases of the Fetus and Newborn, Saunders, Philadelphia, 1982, p. 161.

[229] G. Enders, Varicella-zoster virus infection in pregnancy, Prog. Med. Virol. 29 (1984) 166.

[230] A. Essex-Cater, H. Heggarty, Fatal congenital varicella syndrome, J. Infect. 7 (1983) 77.

[231] M. Lamy, A. Minkowski, J. Choucroun, Embryopathie d'origine infectieuse, Semaine Med. (1951) 72.

[232] R. Konig, et al., Konnatale varizellen-embryo-fetopathy, Helv. Paediatr. Acta 40 (1985) 391.

[233] A. Scharf, et al., Virus detection in the fetal tissue of a premature delivery with a congenital varicella syndrome, J. Perinat. Med. 18 (1990) 317.

[234] O. DaSilva, O. Hammerberg, G.W. Chance, Fetal varicella syndrome, Pediatr. Infect. Dis. J. 9 (1990) 854.

[235] A.M. Magliocco, et al., Varicella embryopathy, Arch. Pathol. Lab. Med. 116 (1992) 181.

[236] I. Alexander, Congenital varicella, BMJ 2 (1979) 1074.

[237] F.B. Bailie, Aplasia cutis congenita of neck and shoulder requiring a skin graft: a case report, Br. J. Plast. Surg. 36 (1983) 72.

[238] J.E.H. Brice, Congenital varicella resulting from infection during second trimester at pregnancy, Arch. Dis. Child. 51 (1976) 474.

[239] J. Dodion-Fransen, D. Dekegel, L. Thiry, Maternal varicella infection as a cause of fetal malformations, Scand. J. Infect. Dis. 5 (1973) 149.

[240] H. Frey, G. Bialkin, A. Gershon, Congenital varicella: case report of a serologically proved long-term survivor, Pediatrics 59 (1977) 110.

[241] O. Pettay, Intrauterine and perinatal viral infections, Ann. Clin. Res. 11 (1979) 258.

[242] J. Taranger, J. Blomberg, O. Strannegard, Intrauterine varicella: a report of two cases associated with hyper-A-immunoglobulinemia, Scand. J. Infect. Dis. 13 (1981) 297.

[243] J. Unger-Koppel, P. Kilcher, O. Tonz, Varizellenfetopathie, Helv. Paediatr. Acta 40 (1985) 399.

[244] M.I. White, et al., Connective tissue naevi in a child with intra-uterine varicella infection, Clin. Exp. Dermatol. 15 (1990) 149.

[245] C.G.S. Palmer, R.M. Pauli, Intrauterine varicella infection, J. Pediatr. 112 (1988) 506.

[246] S.R. Lambert, et al., Ocular manifestations of the congenital varicella syndrome, Arch. Ophthalmol. 107 (1989) 52.

[247] P.V.A. Bai, T.J. John, Congenital skin ulcers following varicella in late pregnancy, J. Pediatr. 94 (1979) 65.

[248] G.T. Klauber, F.J. Flynn, B.D. Altman, Congenital varicella syndrome with genitourinary anomalies, Urology 8 (1976) 153.

[249] L. Michon, D. Aubertin, G. Jager-Schmidt, Deux observations de malformations congenitales paraissant relever d'embryopathies zosteriennes, Arch. Fr. Pediatr. 16 (1959) 695.

[250] G. Enders, Serodiagnosis of varicella-zoster virus infection in pregnancy and standardisation of the ELISA IgG and IgM antibody tests, Dev. Biol. Stand. 52 (1982) 221.

[251] N. Charles, T.W. Bennett, S. Margolis, Ocular pathology of the congenital varicella syndrome, Arch. Ophthalmol. 95 (1977) 2034.

[252] A. Andreou, et al., Fetal varicella syndrome with manifestations limited to the eye, Am. J. Perinatol. 12 (1995) 347.

[253] G. Kotchmar, C. Grose, P. Brunell, Complete spectrum of the varicella congenital defects syndrome in 5-year-old child, Pediatr. Infect. Dis. 3 (1984) 142.

[254] C. Grose, Congenital varicella-zoster virus infection and the failure to establish virus-specific cell-mediated immunity, Mol. Biol. Med. 6 (1989) 453.

[255] M.B. Salzman, S.K. Sood, Congenital anomalies resulting from maternal at 25 and a half weeks of gestation, Pediatr. Infect. Dis. J. 11 (1992) 504.

[256] R. Hitchcock, et al., Colonic atresia and spinal cord atrophy associated with a case of fetal varicella syndrome, J. Pediatr. Surg. 30 (1995) 1344.

[257] K.M. Lloyd, J.L. Dunne, Skin lesions as the sole manifestation of the fetal varicella syndrome, Clin. Exp. Dermatol. 15 (1990) 149.

[258] I.E. Scheffer, M. Baraitser, E.M. Brett, Severe microcephaly associated with congenital varicella infection, Dev. Med. Child. Neurol. 33 (1991) 916.

[259] R. Randel, D.B. Kearns, M.H. Sawyer, Vocal cord paralysis as a presentation of intrauterine infection with varicella-zoster virus, Pediatrics 97 (1996) 127.

[260] R. Bennet, M. Forsgren, P. Herin, Herpes zoster in a 2-week-old premature infant with possible congenital varicella encephalitis, Acta Pediatr. Scand. 74 (1985) 979.

[261] J.L.B. Byrne, et al., Prenatal sonographic diagnosis of fetal varicella syndrome, Am. J. Hum. Genet. 47 (1990) A470.

[262] A. Sauerbrai, et al., Detection of varicella-zoster virus in congenital varicella syndrome: a case report, Obstet. Gynecol. 88 (1996) 687.

[263] M. Mazzella, et al., Severe hydrocephalus associated with congenital varicella syndrome, Can. Med. Assoc. J. 168 (2003) 561.

[264] C.S. Huang, et al., Congenital varicella syndrome as an unusual cause of congenital malformation: report of one case, Acta Paediatr. Taiwan. 42 (2001) 239.

[265] P.S. Dimova, A.A. Karparov, Congenital varicella syndrome: case with isolated brain damage, J. Child. Neurol. 16 (2001) 595.

[266] A. Kent, B. Paes, Congenital varicella syndrome: a rare case of central nervous system involvement without dermatological features, Am. J. Perinatol. 17 (2000) 253.

[267] C.D. Liang, T.J. Yu, S.F. Ko, Ipsilateral renal dysplasia with hypertensive heart disease in an infant with cutaneous varicella lesions: an unusual presentation of congenital varicella syndrome, J. Am. Acad. Dermatol. 43 (2000) 864.

[268] C. Cooper, et al., Congenital varicella syndrome diagnosed by polymerase chain reaction—scarring of the spinal cord, not the skin, J. Paediatr. Child Health 36 (2000) 186.

[269] C.S. Choong, S. Patole, J. Whitehall, Congenital varicella syndrome in the absence of cutaneous lesions, J. Paediatr. Child Health 36 (2000) 184.

[270] J. Forrest, S. Mego, M. Burgess, Congenital and neonatal varicella in Australia, J. Paediatr. Child Health 36 (2000) 108.

[271] E.B. Gaynor, Congenital varicella and the newborn cry, Otolaryngol. Head Neck Surg. 104 (1991) 541.

[272] W.G. Taylor, S.A. Walkinshaw, M.A. Thompson, Antenatal assessment of neurological impairment, Arch. Dis. Child. 68 (1993) 604.

[273] K.W. Kerkering, Abnormal cry and intracranial calcifications: clues to the diagnosis of fetal varicella-zoster syndrome, J. Perinatol. 21 (2001) 131.

[274] J. Hartung, et al., Prenatal diagnosis of congenital varicella syndrome and detection of varicella-zoster virus in the fetus: a case report, Prenat. Diagn. 19 (1999) 163.

[275] G.J. Hofmeyr, S. Moolla, T. Lawrie, Prenatal sonographic diagnosis of congenital varicella infection—a case report, Prenat. Diagn. 16 (1996) 1148.

[276] P. Petignat, et al., Fetal varicella-herpes zoster syndrome in early pregnancy: ultrasonographic and morphological correlation, Prenat. Diagn. 21 (2001) 121.

[277] H. Verstraelen, et al., Prenatal ultrasound and magnetic resonance imaging in fetal varicella syndrome: correlation with pathology findings, Prenat. Diagn. 23 (2003) 705.

[278] P.A. Duehr, Herpes zoster as a cause of congenital cataract, Am. J. Ophthalmol. 39 (1955) 157.

[279] M.H. Webster, C.S. Smith, Congenital abnormalities and maternal herpes zoster, BMJ 4 (1977) 1193.

[280] C. Grose, O. Itani, C. Weiner, Prenatal diagnosis of fetal infection: advances from amniocentesis to cordocentesis—congenital toxoplasmosis, rubella, cytomegalovirus, varicella virus, parvovirus and human immunodeficiency virus, Pediatr. Infect. Dis. J. 8 (1989) 459.

[281] A.L. Alkalay, J.J. Pomerance, D. Rimoin, Fetal varicella syndrome, J. Pediatr. 111 (1987) 320.

[282] G.J. Hofmeyer, S. Moolla, T. Lawrie, Prenatal sonographic diagnosis of congenital varicella infection—a case report, Prenat. Diagn. 16 (1996) 1148.

[283] F. Leicuru, et al., Varicella-zoster virus infection during pregnancy: the limits of prenatal diagnosis, Eur. J. Obstet. Gynecol. Reprod. Biol. 56 (1994) 67.

[284] S.L. West, et al., Recurrent hemiplegia associated with cerebral vasculopathy following third trimester maternal herpes zoster infection, Dev. Med. Child Neurol. 48 (2006) 991–993.

[285] K.B. Fowler, et al., The outcome of congenital cytomegalovirus infection in relation to maternal antibody status, N. Engl. J. Med. 326 (1992) 663.

[286] N.B. Isada, et al., In utero diagnosis of congenital varicella zoster infection by chorionic villus sampling and polymerase chain reaction, Am. J. Obstet. Gynecol. 165 (1991) 1727.

[287] S. Preblud, D.J. Bregman, L.L. Vernon, Deaths from varicella in infants, Pediatr. Infect. Dis. 4 (1985) 503.

[288] L. Rubin, et al., Disseminated varicella in a neonate: implications for immunoprophylaxis of neonates postnatally exposed to varicella, Pediatr. Infect. Dis. 5 (1986) 100.

[289] J. Meyers, Congenital varicella in term infants: risk reconsidered, J. Infect. Dis. 129 (1974) 215.

[290] K. Hanngren, M. Grandien, G. Granstrom, Effect of zoster immunoglobulin for varicella prophylaxis in the newborn, Scand. J. Infect. Dis. 17 (1985) 343.

[291] S. Preblud, et al., Modification of congenital varicella infection with VZIG, Interscience Conference on Antimicrobial Agents and Chemotherapy, New Orleans, 1986.

[292] G.A. Nankervis, E. Gold, Varicella-zoster viruses, in: A.S. Kaplan (Ed.), The Herpesviruses, Academic Press, New York, 1973.

[293] S. Kohl, The neonatal human's immune response to herpes simplex virus infection: a critical review, Pediatr. Infect. Dis. J. 8 (1989) 67.

[294] R.K. Winkelman, H.O. Perry, Herpes zoster in children, JAMA 171 (1959) 876.

[295] T. David, M. Williams, Herpes zoster in infancy, Scand. J. Infect. Dis. 11 (1979) 185.

[296] M. Dworsky, R. Whitely, C. Alford, Herpes zoster in early infancy, Am. J. Dis. Child. 134 (1980) 618.

[297] I. Helander, P. Arstila, P. Terho, Herpes zoster in a 6 month old infant, Acta Dermatol. 63 (1982) 180.

[298] I.K. Lewkonia, A.A. Jackson, Infantile herpes zoster after intrauterine exposure to varicella, BMJ 3 (1973) 149.

[299] J.H. Lyday, Report of severe herpes zoster in a 13 and one-half-year-old boy whose chickenpox infection may have been acquired in utero, Pediatrics 50 (1972) 930.

[300] M.A. Adkisson, Herpes zoster in a newborn premature infant, J. Pediatr. 66 (1965) 956.

[301] B.E. Bonar, C.J. Pearsall, Herpes zoster in the newborn, Am. J. Dis. Child. 44 (1932) 398.

[302] C.E. Counter, B.J. Korn, Herpes zoster in the newborn associated with congenital blindness: report of a case, Arch. Pediatr. 67 (1950) 397.

[303] G.V. Feldman, Herpes zoster neonatorum, Arch. Dis. Child. 27 (1952) 126.

[304] P. Freud, G.D. Rook, S. Gurian, Herpes zoster in the newborn, Am. J. Dis. Child. 64 (1942) 895.

[305] S.I. Music, E.M. Fine, Y. Togo, Zoster-like disease in the newborn due to herpes-simplex virus, N. Engl. J. Med. 284 (1971) 24.

[306] A. Gershon, S. Steinberg, P. LaRussa, Varicella-zoster virus, in: E.H. Lennette (Ed.), Laboratory Diagnosis of Viral Infections, Marcel Dekker, New York, 1992.

[307] W.D. Rawlinson, et al., Rapid diagnosis of varicella-zoster virus infection with a monoclonal antibody based direct immunofluorescence technique, J. Virol. Methods 23 (1989) 13.

[308] M. Vazquez, et al., The effectiveness of the varicella vaccine in clinical practice, N. Engl. J. Med. 344 (2001) 955.

[309] P. Hughes, et al., Transmission of varicella-zoster virus from a vaccinee with underlying leukemia, demonstrated by polymerase chain reaction, J. Pediatr. 124 (1994) 932.

[310] M. Ito, et al., Detection of varicella zoster virus (VZV) DNA in throat swabs and peripheral blood mononuclear cells of immunocompromised patients with herpes zoster by polymerase chain reaction, Clin. Diagn. Virol. 4 (1995) 105.

[311] P. LaRussa, et al., Restriction fragment length polymorphism of polymerase chain reaction products from vaccine and wild-type varicella-zoster virus isolates, J. Virol. 66 (1992) 1016.

[312] P. LaRussa, S. Steinberg, A. Gershon, Diagnosis and typing of varicella-zoster virus (VZV) in clinical specimens by polymerase chain reaction (PCR), Thirty-fourth International Conference on Antimicrobial Agents and Chemotherapy, Orlando, FL, September 1994.

[313] R. Mahalingham, et al., Polymerase chain reaction diagnosis of varicella-zoster virus, in: Y. Becker, G. Darai (Eds.), Diagnosis of Human Viruses by Polymerase Chain Reaction Technology, vol. 1, Springer-Verlag, New York, 1992.

[314] E. Puchhammer-Stockl, et al., Detection of varicella zoster virus (VZV) in fetal tissue by polymerase chain reaction, J. Perinat. Med. 22 (1994) 65.

[315] M. Sawyer, Y.N. Wu, Detection of varicella-zoster virus DNA by polymerase chain reaction in CSF of patients with VZV-related central nervous system complications, International Conference on Antimicrobial Agents and Chemotherapy, New Orleans, September 1993.

[316] P. Annunziato, et al., In situ hybridization detection of varicella zoster virus in paraffin-embedded skin biopsy specimens, Clin. Diagn. Virol. 7 (1997) 69.

[317] C.C. Silliman, et al., Unsuspected varicella-zoster virus encephalitis in a child with acquired immunodeficiency syndrome, J. Pediatr. 123 (1993) 418.

[318] A.A. Gershon, P. LaRussa, Varicella-zoster virus, in: L.G. Donowitz (Ed.), Hospital-Acquired Infection in the Pediatric Patient, Williams & Wilkins, Baltimore, 1988.

[319] C.T. Le, M. Lipson, Difficulty in determining varicella-zoster immune status in pregnant women, Pediatr. Infect. Dis. J. 8 (1989) 650.

[320] G.T. Vasileiadis, et al., Intrauterine herpes simplex infection, Am. J. Perinatol. 20 (2003) 55.

[321] C. Grose, Congenital infections caused by varicella zoster virus and herpes simplex virus, Semin. Pediatr. Neurol. 1 (1994) 43.

[322] R.J. Whitley, S. Straus, Therapy for varicella-zoster virus infections. Where do we stand? Infect. Dis. Clin. Pract. 2 (1993) 100.

[323] R.J. Whitley, J.W. Gnann, Acyclovir: a decade later, N. Engl. J. Med. 327 (1992) 782.

[324] B.S. Greffe, et al., Transplacental passage of acyclovir, J. Pediatr. 108 (1986) 1020.

[325] L. Dunkel, et al., A controlled trial of oral acyclovir for chickenpox in normal children, N. Engl. J. Med. 325 (1991) 1539.

[326] H.H. Balfour, et al., Acyclovir treatment of varicella in otherwise healthy adolescents, J. Pediatr. 120 (1992) 627.

[327] H. Feder, Treatment of adult chickenpox with oral acyclovir, Arch. Intern. Med. 150 (1990) 2061.

[328] M.R. Wallace, et al., Treatment of adult varicella with oral acyclovir: a randomized, placebo-controlled trial, Ann. Intern. Med. 117 (1992) 358.

[329] R.J. Whitley, M. Middlebrooks, J.W. Gnann, Acyclovir: the past ten years, Adv. Exp. Med. Biol. 278 (1990) 243.

[330] R. Whitley, et al., A controlled trial comparing vidarabine with acyclovir in neonatal herpes simplex virus infection, N. Engl. J. Med. 324 (1991) 444.

[331] J. Englund, C.V. Fletcher, H.H. Balfour, Acyclovir therapy in neonates, J. Pediatr. 119 (1991) 129.

[332] A.A. Gershon, S. Steinberg, NIAID Collaborative Varicella Vaccine Study Group, Live attenuated varicella vaccine: protection in healthy adults in comparison to leukemic children, J. Infect. Dis. 161 (1990) 661.

[333] A. Arvin, C.M. Koropchak, A.E. Wittek, Immunologic evidence of reinfection with varicella-zoster virus, J. Infect. Dis. 148 (1983) 200.

[334] A.A. Gershon, et al., Clinical reinfection with varicella-zoster virus, J. Infect. Dis. 149 (1984) 137.

[335] A.K. Junker, E. Angus, E. Thomas, Recurrent varicella-zoster virus infections in apparently immunocompetent children, Pediatr. Infect. Dis. J. 10 (1991) 569.

[336] A.K. Junker, P. Tilley, Varicella-zoster virus antibody avidity and IgG-subclass patterns in children with recurrent chickenpox, J. Med. Virol. 43 (1994) 119.

[337] K.A. Martin, et al., Occurrence of chickenpox during pregnancy in women seropositive for varicella-zoster virus, J. Infect. Dis. 170 (1994) 991.

[338] S. Bogger-Goren, et al., Mucosal cell mediated immunity to varicella zoster virus: role in protection against disease, J. Pediatr. 105 (1984) 195.

[339] S. Bogger-Goren, et al., Antibody response to varicella-zoster virus after natural or vaccine-induced infection, J. Infect. Dis. 146 (1982) 260.

[340] P. Ljungman, et al., Clinical and subclinical reactivations of varicella-zoster virus in immunocompromised patients, J. Infect. Dis. 153 (1986) 840.

[341] K. Weigle, C. Grose, Molecular dissection of the humoral immune response to individual varicella-zoster viral proteins during chickenpox, quiescence, reinfection, and reactivation, J. Infect. Dis. 149 (1984) 741.

[342] D.H. Gilden, et al., Zoster sine herpete, a clinical variant, Ann. Neurol. 35 (1994) 530.

[343] A. Wilson, et al., Subclinical varicella-zoster virus viremia, herpes zoster, and T lymphocyte immunity to varicella-zoster viral antigens after bone marrow transplantation, J. Infect. Dis. 165 (1992) 119.

[344] I.B. Hardy, et al., Incidence of zoster after live attenuated varicella vaccine, International Conference on Antimicrobial Agents and Chemotherapy, Chicago, September 1991.

[345] P.L. LaRussa, et al., Antibodies to varicella-zoster virus glycoproteins I, II, and III in leukemic and healthy children, J. Infect. Dis. 162 (1990) 627.

[346] B.L. Burke, et al., Immune responses to varicella-zoster in the aged, Arch. Intern. Med. 142 (1982) 291.

[347] A.E. Miller, Selective decline in cellular immune response to varicella-zoster in the elderly, Neurology 30 (1980) 582.

[348] A. Gershon, S. Steinberg, Antibody responses to varicella-zoster virus and the role of antibody in host defense, Am. J. Med. Sci. 282 (1981) 12.

[349] D. Stevens, T. Merigan, Zoster immune globulin prophylaxis of disseminated zoster in compromised hosts, Arch. Intern. Med. 140 (1980) 52.

[350] A. Gershon, Immunoprophylaxis of varicella-zoster infections, Am. J. Med. 76 (1984) 672.

[351] M. Levin, Can herpes zoster be prevented? Eur. J. Clin. Microbiol. Infect. Dis. 15 (1996) 1.

[352] M. Levin, et al., Immune response of elderly individuals to a live attenuated varicella vaccine, J. Infect. Dis. 166 (1992) 253.

[353] M. Levin, et al., Immune responses of elderly persons 4 years after receiving a live attenuated varicella vaccine, J. Infect. Dis. 170 (1994) 522.

[354] M.N. Oxman, et al., A vaccine to prevent herpes zoster and postherpetic neuralgia in older adults, N. Engl. J. Med. 352 (2005) 2271–2284.

[355] P. Brunell, et al., Prevention of varicella by zoster immune globulin, N. Engl. J. Med. 280 (1969) 1191.

[356] P. Brunell, et al., Prevention of varicella in high-risk children: a collaborative study, Pediatrics 50 (1972) 718.

[357] A. Gershon, S. Steinberg, P. Brunell, Zoster immune globulin: a further assessment, N. Engl. J. Med. 290 (1974) 243.

[358] W. Orenstein, et al., Prophylaxis of varicella in high risk children: response effect of zoster immune globulin, J. Pediatr. 98 (1981) 368.

[359] A. Gershon, M. Takahashi, J. Seward, Live attenuated varicella vaccine, in: S. Plotkin, W. Orenstein, P. Offit (Eds.), Vaccines, Saunders, Philadelphia, 2008.

[360] A. Neustadt, Congenital varicella, Am. J. Dis. Child. 106 (1963) 96.

[361] R.R. O'Neill, Congenital varicella, Am. J. Dis. Child. 104 (1962) 391.

[362] L.K. Pickering (Ed.), Red Book: Report of the Committee on Infectious Diseases, twenty sixth ed., American Academy of Pediatrics, Elk Grove Village, IL, 2003.

[363] Centers for Disease Control, Prevention of varicella: recommendations of the Advisory Committee on Immunization Practices (ACIP), MMWR Morb. Mortal. Wkly. Rep. 56 (2007) 1–40.

[364] S. Bakshi, et al., Failure of VZIG in modification of severe congenital varicella, Pediatr. Infect. Dis. 5 (1986) 699.

[365] J. Haddad, U. Simeoni, D. Willard, Perinatal varicella, Lancet 1 (1986) 494.

[366] P. Holland, D. Isaacs, E.R. Moxon, Fatal neonatal varicella infection, Lancet 2 (1986) 1156.

[367] S. King, et al., Fatal varicella-zoster infection in a newborn treated with varicella-zoster immunoglobulin, Pediatr. Infect. Dis. 5 (1986) 588.

[368] M.M. Oglivie, J.R.D. Stephens, M. Larkin, Chickenpox in pregnancy, Lancet 1 (1986) 915.

[369] H. Williams, et al., Acyclovir in the treatment of neonatal varicella, J. Infect. 15 (1987) 65.

[370] J. Haddad, et al., Acyclovir in prophylaxis and perinatal varicella, Lancet 1 (1987) 161.

[371] J. Sills, et al., Acyclovir in prophylaxis and perinatal varicella, Lancet 1 (1987) 161.

[372] D. Fried, A. Hanukoglu, O. Birk, Leukocyte transfusion in severe neonatal varicella, Acta Pediatr. Scand. 71 (1982) 147.

[373] J. Betzhold, R. Hong, Fatal graft versus host reaction in a small leucocyte transfusion in a patient with lymphoma and varicella, Pediatrics 60 (1978) 62.

[374] A. Gershon, Commentary on VZIG in infants, Pediatr. Infect. Dis. J. 6 (1987) 469.

[375] M. Takahashi, et al., Live vaccine used to prevent the spread of varicella in children in hospital, Lancet 2 (1974) 1288.

[376] A. Arvin, A. Gershon, Live attenuated varicella vaccine, Annu. Rev. Microbiol. 50 (1996) 59.

[377] C.J. White, Varicella-zoster virus vaccine, Clin. Infect. Dis. 24 (1997) 753.

[378] Committee on Infectious Diseases, Live attenuated varicella vaccine, Pediatrics 95 (1995) 791.

[379] M. Broyer, et al., Varicella and zoster in children after kidney transplantation: long term results of vaccination, Pediatrics 99 (1997) 35.

[380] M.B. Salzman, et al., Transmission of varicella-vaccine virus from a healthy 12 month old child to his pregnant mother, J. Pediatr. 131 (1997) 151.

[381] S. Long, Toddler-to-mother transmission of varicella-vaccine virus. How bad is that? J. Pediatr. 131 (1997) 10.

[382] L. Saiman, K. Crowley, A. Gershon, Control of varicella-zoster infections in hospitals, in: E. Abrutyn et al., (Eds.), Infection Control Reference Service, Saunders, Philadelphia, 1997.

[383] M. Brisson, et al., Varicella vaccine and shingles, JAMA 287 (2002) 2211.

[384] M. Brisson, et al., Exposure to varicella boosts immunity to herpes-zoster: implications for mass vaccination against chickenpox, Vaccine 20 (2002) 2500.

[385] J.G. Donahue, et al., The incidence of herpes zoster, Arch. Intern. Med. 155 (1995) 1605.

[386] Centers for Disease Control, Varicella-related deaths among children—United States, 1997, MMWR Morb. Mortal. Wkly. Rep. 279 (1998) 1773.

[387] Centers for Disease Control, Varicella-related deaths—Florida, MMWR Morb. Mortal. Wkly. Rep. 48 (1999) 379.

[388] S. Feldman, L. Lott, Varicella in children with cancer: impact of antiviral therapy and prophylaxis, Pediatrics 80 (1987) 465.

[389] R. Whitley, et al., Early vidarabine to control the complications of herpes zoster in immunosuppressed patients, N. Engl. J. Med. 307 (1982) 971.

[390] H. Wain, The Story Behind the Word, Charles C Thomas, Springfield, IL, 1958.

[391] P. Choppin, et al., The functions and inhibition of the membrane glycoproteins of paramyxoviruses and myxoviruses and the role of the measles virus M protein in subacute sclerosing panencephalitis, J. Infect. Dis. 143 (1981) 352.

[392] W.J. Bellini, J. Icenogle, Measles and rubella virus, in: P.R. Murray et al., (Eds.), Manual of Clinical Microbiology, ASM Press, Washington, DC, 2003.

[393] P.A. Rota, et al., Molecular epidemiology of measles viruses in the United States, 1997–2001, Emerg. Infect. Dis. 8 (2002) 902.

[394] W.J. Bellini, J. Icenogle, Measles and rubella virus, in: P.R. Murray et al. (Eds.), Manual of Clinical Microbiology, ASM Press, Washington, DC, 2007.

[395] P.A. Rota, J.S. Rota, W.J. Bellini, Molecular epidemiology of measles virus, Semin. Virol. 6 (1995) 379.

[396] J. Enders, et al., Isolation of measles virus at autopsy in cases of giant cell pneumonia without rash, N. Engl. J. Med. 261 (1959) 875.

[397] K. Weigle, D. Murphy, P. Brunell, Enzyme-linked immunosorbent assay for evaluation of immunity to measles virus, J. Clin. Microbiol. 19 (1984) 376.

[398] D.R. Mayo, et al., Evaluation of a commercial measles virus immunoglobulin M enzyme immunoassay, J. Clin. Microbiol. 29 (1991) 2865.

[399] A. Lievens, P.A. Brunell, Specific immunoglobulin M enzyme-linked immunosorbent assay for confirming the diagnosis of measles, J. Clin. Microbiol. 24 (1986) 391.

[400] K. Papp, Experiences prouvant que la voie d'infection de la rougeole est la contamination de la musqueuse conjunctivale, Rev. Immunol. 20 (1956) 27.

[401] V.H. Leonard, et al., Measles virus blind to its epithelial cell receptor remains virulent in rhesus monkeys but cannot cross the airway epithelium and is not shed, J. Clin. Invest. 118 (2008) 2448–2458.

[402] D.C. Morley, M. Woodland, W.J. Martin, Measles in Nigerian children: a study of the disease in West Africa, and its manifestations in England and other countries during different epochs, J. Hyg. (Lond) 61 (1963) 113.

[403] F.L. Babbott Jr., J.E. Gordon, Modern measles, Am. J. Med. Sci. 225 (1954) 334.

[404] Centers for Disease Control, Measles, mumps, and rubella-vaccine use and strategies for elimination of measles, rubella, and congenital rubella syndrome and control of mumps, MMWR Morb. Mortal. Wkly. Rep. 47 (1998) 1.

[405] J. Frank, et al., Major impediments to measles elimination, Am. J. Dis. Child. 139 (1985) 881.

[406] L.E. Markowitz, et al., Duration of live measles vaccine-induced immunity, Pediatr. Infect. Dis. J. 9 (1990) 101.

[407] S. Krugman, Further-attenuated measles vaccine: characteristics and use, Rev. Infect. Dis. 5 (1983) 477.

[408] R.G. Mathias, et al., The role of secondary vaccine failures in measles outbreaks, Am. J. Public Health 79 (1989) 475.

[409] Measles—United States, 2000, MMWR Morb. Mortal. Wkly. Rep. 51 (2002) 120–123.

[410] Update: measles—United States, January-July 2008. MMWR Morb. Mortal. Wkly. Rep. 57 (2008) 893–896.

[411] Centers for Disease Control, National, state, and local area vaccination coverage among children aged 19–35 months—United States, 2007, MMWR Morb. Mortal. Wkly. Rep. 57 (2008) 961–966.

[412] R.B. Berg, M.S. Rosenthal, Propagation of measles virus in suspensions of human and monkey leukocytes, Proc. Soc. Exp. Biol. Med. 106 (1961) 581.

[413] D.W.R. Suringa, L.J. Bank, A.B. Ackerman, Role of measles virus in skin lesions and Koplik's spots, N. Engl. J. Med. 283 (1970) 1139.

[414] R. Debre, J. Celers, Measles: pathogenicity and epidemiology, in: R. Debre, J. Celers (Eds.), Clinical Virology, Saunders, Philadelphia, 1970.

[415] A. Mitus, et al., Persistence of measles virus and depression of antibody formation in patients with giant cell pneumonia after measles, N. Engl. J. Med. 261 (1959) 882.

[416] P. Lachmann, Immunopathology of measles, Proc. R. Soc. Med. 67 (1974) 12.

[417] M. Stillerman, W. Thalhimer, Attack rate and incubation period of measles, Am. J. Dis. Child. 67 (1944) 15.

[418] H. Baugess, Measles transmitted by blood transfusion, Am. J. Dis. Child. 27 (1924) 256.

[419] J. Littauer, K. Sorensen, The measles epidemic at Umanak in Greenland in 1962, Dan. Med. Bull. 12 (1965) 43.

[420] A.S. Warthin, Occurrence of numerous large giant cells in tonsils and pharyngeal mucosa in prodromal stage of measles: report of four cases, Arch. Pathol. 11 (1932) 864.

[421] K. Moroi, et al., Fetal death associated with measles virus infection of the placenta, Am. J. Obstet. Gynecol. 164 (1991) 1107.

[422] A.C. La Boccetta, A.S. Tornay, Measles encephalitis: report of 61 cases, Am. J. Dis. Child. 107 (1964) 247.

[423] J.H. Musser, G.H. Hauser, Encephalitis as a complication of measles, JAMA 90 (1928) 1267.

[424] P.L. Pearl, et al., Neuropathology of two fatal cases of measles in the 1988–1989 Houston epidemic, Pediatr. Neurol. 6 (1990) 126.

[425] U. Jahnke, E.H. Fischer, E.C. Alvord, Hypothesis—certain viral proteins contain encephalitogenic and/or neuritogenic sequences, J. Neuropathol. Exp. Neurol. 44 (1985) 320.

[426] A. Kipps, G. Dick, J.W. Moodie, Measles and the central nervous system, Lancet 2 (1983) 1406.

[427] D.H. Gremillion, G.E. Crawford, Measles pneumonia in young adults: an analysis of 106 cases, Am. J. Med. 71 (1981) 539.

[428] Centers for Disease Control, Measles surveillance, MMWR Morb. Mortal. Wkly. Rep. (1973) 9.

[429] P.E. Christensen, et al., An epidemic of measles in southern Greenland, 1951, Acta Med. Scand. 144 (1953) 430.

[430] K. Krasinski, W. Borkowsky, Measles and measles immunity in children infected with human immunodeficiency virus, JAMA 261 (1989) 2512.

[431] J.E. Embree, et al., Increased risk of early measles in infants of human immunodeficiency type 1-seropositive mothers, J. Infect. Dis. 165 (1992) 262.

[432] J.B. Angel, et al., Vaccine-associated measles pneumonitis in an adult with AIDS, Ann. Intern. Med. 129 (1998) 104.

[433] L.J. Kaplan, et al., Severe measles in immunocompromised patients, JAMA 267 (1992) 1237.

[434] J. Kernahan, J. McQuillin, A. Craft, Measles in children who have malignant disease, BMJ 295 (1987) 15.

[435] V. Breitfeld, et al., Fatal measles infection in children with leukemia, Lab. Invest. 28 (1973) 279.

[436] J.P. Greenhill, Acute (extragenital) infections in pregnancy, labor, and the puerperium, Am. J. Obstet. Gynecol. 25 (1933) 760.

[437] J.R. Nouvat, Rougeole et Grossesse, Bordeaux, 1904.

[438] I. Dyer, Measles complicating pregnancy: report of 24 cases with three instances of congenital measles, South Med. J. 33 (1940) 601.

[439] A.D. Packer, The influence of maternal measles (morbilli) on the newborn child, Med. J. Aust. 1 (1950) 835.

[440] R.L. Atmar, J.A. Englund, H. Hammill, Complications of measles during pregnancy, Clin. Infect. Dis. 14 (1992) 217.

[441] J.E. Eberhart-Phillips, et al., Measles in pregnancy: a descriptive study of 58 cases, Obstet. Gynecol. 82 (1993) 797.

[442] W.W. Nichols, et al., Measles-associated chromosome breakage. Preliminary communication, Hereditas 48 (1962) 367.

[443] Z.B. Miller, Chromosome abnormalities in measles, Lancet 2 (1963) 1070.

[444] M. Higurashi, T. Tamura, T. Nakatake, Cytogenic observations in cultured lymphocytes from patients with Down's syndrome and measles, Pediatr. Res. 7 (1973) 582.

[445] C.S. Jespersen, J. Littauer, U. Sigild, Measles as a cause of fetal defects, Acta Pediatr. Scand. 66 (1977) 367.

[446] E. Gazala, M. Karplus, I. Sarov, The effect of maternal measles on the fetus, Pediatr. Infect. Dis. 4 (1985) 202.

[447] B. Rones, The relationship of German measles during pregnancy to congenital ocular defects, Med. Ann. DC 13 (1944) 285.

[448] C. Swan, et al., Congenital defects in infants following infectious diseases during pregnancy, with special reference to relationship between German measles and cataract, deaf mutism, heart disease and microcephaly, and to period in pregnancy in which occurrence of rubella was followed by congenital abnormalities, Med. J. Aust. 2 (1943) 201.

[449] A.F. Canelli, Sur le comportement normal et pathologique de l'immunity antimorbilleuse chez le nourison jeune, Rev. Fr. Pediatr. 5 (1929) 668.

[450] G.W. Ronaldson, Measles at confinement with subsequent modified attack in the child, Br. J. Child Dis. 23 (1926) 192.

[451] M. Narita, T. Togashi, H. Kikuta, Neonatal measles in Hokkaido, Japan, Pediatr. Infect. Dis. J. 16 (1997) 908.

[452] J.L. Kohn, Measles in newborn infants (maternal infection), J. Pediatr. 23 (1933) 192.

[453] S.L. Betta Ragazzi, et al., Congenital and neonatal measles during an epidemic in Sao Paulo, Brazil in 1997, Pediatr. Infect. Dis. J. 24 (2005) 377–378.

[454] Y. Nakata, et al., Measles virus genome detected up to four months in a case of congenital measles, Acta Paediatr. 91 (2002) 1263–1265.

[455] A. Catanzaro, M. Jackson, Rapidly progressive subacute sclerosing panence-phalitis in perinatally acquired measles virus infection, Lancet 345 (1995) 8957.

[456] D. Cruzado, et al., Early onset and rapidly progressive subacute sclerosing panencephalitis after congenital measles infection, Eur. J. Pediatr. 161 (2002) 438–441.

[457] M. Dasopoulou, A. Covanis, Subacute sclerosing panencephalitis after intra-uterine infection, Acta Paediatr. 93 (2004) 1251–1253.

[458] E. Simsek, et al., Subacute sclerosing panencephalitis (SSPE) associated with congenital measles infection, Turk. J. Pediatr. 47 (2005) 58–62.

[459] Y. Sawaishi, et al., SSPE following neonatal measles infection, Pediatr. Neurol. 20 (1999) 63–65.

[460] K. Zwiauer, et al., Rapid progressive subacute sclerosing panencephalitis after perinatally acquired measles virus infection, Lancet 345 (1995) 1124.

[461] D.L. Richardson, Measles contracted in utero, R. I. Med. J. 3 (1920) 13.

[462] B. Muhlbauer, L.M. Berns, A. Singer, Congenital measles—1982, Isr. J. Med. Sci. 19 (1983) 987.

[463] G.R. Noren, P. Adams Jr., R.C. Anderson, Positive skin reactivity to mumps virus antigen in endocardial fibroelastosis, J. Pediatr. 62 (1963) 604.

[464] F. Abreo, J. Bagby, Sputum cytology in measles infection: a case report, Acta Cytol. 35 (1991) 719.

[465] R. Lightwood, R. Nolan, Epithelial giant cells in measles as an aid in diag-nosis, J. Pediatr. 77 (1970) 59.

[466] R. Llanes-Rodas, C. Liu, Rapid diagnosis of measles from urinary sediments stained with fluorescent antibody, N. Engl. J. Med. 275 (1966) 516.

[467] L.L. Minnich, F. Goodenough, C.G. Ray, Use of immunofluorescence to identify measles virus infections, J. Clin. Microbiol. 29 (1991) 1148.

[468] M.F. Smaron, et al., Diagnosis of measles by fluorescent antibody and culture of nasopharyngeal secretions, J. Virol. Methods 33 (1991) 223.

[469] E. Rossier, et al., Comparison of immunofluorescence and enzyme immuno-assay for detection of measles-specific immunoglobulin M antibody, J. Clin. Microbiol. 29 (1991) 1069.

[470] C. Arrieta, et al., Vitamin A levels in children with measles in Long Beach, California, J. Pediatr. 121 (1992) 75.

[471] T.R. Frieden, et al., Vitamin A levels and severity of measles, Am. J. Dis. Child. 146 (1992) 182.

[472] G.D. Hussey, M. Klein, A randomized, controlled trial of vitamin A in chil-dren with severe measles, N. Engl. J. Med. 323 (1990) 160.

[473] A.L. Forni, N.W. Schluger, R.B. Roberts, Severe measles pneumonitis in adults: evaluation of clinical characteristics and therapy with intravenous ribavirin, Clin. Infect. Dis. 19 (1994) 454.

[474] M.M. Mustafa, et al., Subacute measles encephalitis in the young immuno-compromised host: report of two cases diagnosed by polymerase chain reac-tion and treated with ribavirin and review of the literature, Clin. Infect. Dis. 16 (1993) 654.

[475] M. Gudnadottir, F.L. Black, Measles vaccination in adults with and without complicating conditions, Arch. Gesamte Virusforsch. 16 (1965) 521.

[476] L.L. Chui, R.G. Marusyk, H.F. Pabst, Measles virus specific antibody in infants in a highly vaccinated society, J. Med. Virol. 33 (1991) 199.

[477] J. Lennon, F. Black, Maternally derived measles immunity in sera of vaccine-protected mothers, J. Pediatr. 108 (1986) 671.

[478] M. Hornig, et al., Lack of association between measles virus vaccine and autism with enteropathy: a case-control study, PLoS ONE 3 (2008) e3140.

[479] S. Coughlan, et al., Suboptimal measles-mumps-rubella vaccination coverage facilitates an imported measles outbreak in Ireland, Clin. Infect. Dis. 35 (2002) 84.

[480] S. Krugman, J.P. Giles, H. Friedman, Studies on immunity to measles, J. Pediatr. 66 (1965) 471.

[481] M. Stillerman, H.H. Marks, W. Thalhimer, Prophylaxis of measles with convalescent serum, Am. J. Dis. Child. 67 (1944) 1.

[482] C. Orvell, The reactions of monoclonal antibodies with structural proteins of mumps virus, J. Immunol. 132 (1984) 2622.

[483] E. Lennette, Laboratory Diagnosis of Viral Infections, Marcel Dekker, New York, 1992.

[484] J.D. Boddicker, et al., Real-time reverse transcription-PCR assay for detec-tion of mumps virus RNA in clinical specimens, J. Clin. Microbiol. 45 (2007) 2902–2908.

[485] F. Reid, et al., Epidemiologic and diagnostic evaluation of a recent mumps outbreak using oral fluid samples, J. Clin. Virol. 41 (2008) 134–137.

[486] L.J. Anderson, J.F. Seward, Mumps epidemiology and immunity: the anatomy of a modern epidemic, Pediatr. Infect. Dis. J. 27 (Suppl. 10) (2008) S75–S79.

[487] G.H. Dayan, et al., Recent resurgence of mumps in the United States, N. Engl. J. Med. 358 (2008) 1580–1589.

[488] A. Garcia, et al., Intrauterine infection with mumps virus, Obstet. Gynecol. 56 (1980) 756.

[489] N.K. Connolly, Mumps orchitis without parotitis in infants, Lancet 1 (1953) 69.

[490] D. Bowers, Mumps during pregnancy, West J. Surg. Obstet. Gynecol. 61 (1953) 72.

[491] M.W. Greenberg, J.S. Beilly, Congenital defects in the infant following mumps during pregnancy, Am. J. Obstet. Gynecol. 57 (1949) 805.

[492] J.B. Hardy, Viral infection in pregnancy: a review, Am. J. Obstet. Gynecol. 93 (1965) 1052.

[493] A. Homans, Mumps in a pregnant woman: premature labor, followed by the appearance of the same disease in the infant, twenty-four hours after its birth, Am. J. Med. Sci. 29 (1855) 56.

[494] J.H. Moore, Epidemic parotitis complicating late pregnancy: report of a case, JAMA 97 (1931) 1625.

[495] R.N. Philip, K.R. Reinhard, D.B. Lackman, Observations on a mumps epi-demic in a "virgin" population, Am. J. Epidemiol. 69 (1959) 91.

[496] H.A. Schwartz, Mumps in pregnancy, Am. J. Obstet. Gynecol. 60 (1950) 875.

[497] R.S. Siddall, Epidemic parotitis in late pregnancy, Am. J. Obstet. Gynecol. 33 (1937) 524.

[498] O. Ylinen, P.A. Jervinen, Parotitis during pregnancy, Acta. Obstet. Gynecol. Scand. 32 (1953) 121.

[499] L. Kilham, Mumps virus in human milk and in milk of infected monkey, Am. J. Obstet. Gynecol. 33 (1951) 524.

[500] P.C. Dutta, A fatal case of pregnancy complicated with mumps, J. Obstet. Gynaecol. Br. Emp. 42 (1935) 869.

[501] C. Swan, Congenital malformations associated with rubella and other virus infections, in: H.S. Banks (Ed.), Modern Practice in Infectious Fevers, PB Hoeber, New York, 1951.

[502] H. Hyatt, Relationship of maternal mumps to congenital defects and fetal deaths, and to maternal morbidity and mortality, Am. Pract. Dig. Treat. 12 (1961) 359.

[503] J. Kurtz, A. Tomlinson, J. Pearson, Mumps virus isolated from a fetus, BMJ 284 (1982) 471.

[504] G.G. Robertson, A.P. Williamson, R.J. Blattner, Origin and development of lens cataracts in mumps-infected chick embryos, Am. J. Anat. 115 (1964) 473.

[505] J.W. Geme St. Jr., et al., The biologic perturbations of persistent embryonic mumps virus infection, Pediatr. Res. 7 (1973) 541.

[506] R.T. Johnson, K.P. Johnson, C.J. Edmonds, Virus-induced hydrocephalus: development of aqueductal stenosis in hamsters after mumps infection, Sci-ence 157 (1967) 1066.

[507] J. Holowach, D.L. Thurston, B. Becker, Congenital defects in infants fol-lowing mumps during pregnancy: a review of the literature and a report of chorioretinitis due to fetal infection, J. Pediatr. 50 (1957) 689.

[508] H. Grenvall, P. Selander, Some virus diseases during pregnancy and their effect on the fetus, Nord. Med. 37 (1948) 409.

[509] B. Baumann, et al., Unilateral hydrocephalus due to obstruction of the fora-men of Monro. Another complication of intrauterine mumps infection, Eur. J. Pediatr. 139 (1982) 158.

[510] G. Timmons, K. Johnson, Aqueductal stenosis and hydrocephalus after mumps encephalitis, N. Engl. J. Med. 283 (1970) 1505.

[511] M.M. Manson, W.P.D. Logan, R.M. Loy, Rubella and Other Virus Infec-tions During Pregnancy, Her Majesty's Stationery Office, London, 1960.

[512] J.W. Geme St. Jr., G.R. Noren, P. Adams, Proposed embryopathic relation between mumps virus and primary endocardial fibroelastosis, N. Engl. J. Med. 275 (1966) 339.

[513] M. Finland, Mumps, in: D. Charles, M. Finland (Eds.), Obstetric and Peri-natal Infections, Lea & Febiger, Philadelphia, 1973.

[514] F. Calabrese, et al., Molecular diagnosis of myocarditis and dilated cardio-myopathy in children: clinicopathologic features and prognostic implica-tions, Diagn. Mol. Pathol. 11 (2002) 212.

[515] J. Ni, et al., Viral infection of the myocardium in endocardial fibroelastosis: molecular evidence for the role of mumps virus as an etiologic agent, Circu-lation 95 (1997) 133.

[516] V. Zardini, Eccezionale casso di parotite epidemica in neonato da madre convalescente della stessa malattia, Lattante 33 (1962) 767.

[517] D. Shouldice, S. Mintz, Mumps in utero, Can. Nurse 51 (1955) 454.

[518] J.F. Jones, G. Ray, V.A. Fulginiti, Perinatal mumps infection, J. Pediatr. 96 (1980) 912.

[519] O. Reman, et al., Neonatal respiratory distress due to mumps, Arch. Dis. Child. 61 (1986) 80.

[520] T. Yamauchi, C. Wilson, J.W. Geme St. Jr., Transmission of live, attenuated mumps virus to the human placenta, N. Engl. J. Med. 290 (1974) 710.

[521] Y. Chiba, P.A. Ogra, T. Nakao, Transplacental mumps infection, Am. J. Obstet. Gynecol. 122 (1975) 904.

[522] G.R. Monif, Maternal mumps infection during gestation: observations on the progeny, Am. J. Obstet. Gynecol. 121 (1974) 549.

[523] M.B. Meyer, An epidemiologic study of mumps: its spread in schools and families, Am. J. Hyg. 75 (1962) 259.

[524] E. Hoen, Mumpsinfektion beim jungen Sugling, Kinderprtzl 36 (1968) 27.

[525] R.W. Harris, et al., Mumps in a Northeast metropolitan community: epide-miology of clinical mumps, Am. J. Epidemiol. 88 (1968) 224.

[526] D. Hodes, P. Brunell, Mumps antibody: placental transfer and disappearance during the first year of life, Pediatrics 45 (1970) 99.

[527] H.N. Sanford, I.I. Shmigelsky, Purulent parotitis in the newborn, J. Pediatr. 26 (1945) 149.

[528] H. Peltola, et al., Measles, mumps, and rubella in Finland: 25 years of an ationwide elimination programme, Lancet Infect. Dis. 8 (2008) 796–803.

[529] M. Wharton, et al., Mumps transmission in hospitals, Arch. Intern. Med. 150 (1990) 47.

[530] P.A. Brunell, et al., Ineffectiveness of isolation of patients as a method of preventing the spread of mumps, N. Engl. J. Med. 279 (1968) 1357.

[531] Updated recommendations for isolation of persons with mumps, MMWR Morb. Mortal. Wkly. Rep. 57 (2008) 1103–1105.

[532] C. Maiter, Neonatal varicella, Am. J. Dis. Child. 107 (1964) 492.

[533] R. Figueroa-Damian, J.L. Arrendondo-Garcia, Perinatal outcome of preg-nancies complicated with varicella infection during the first 20 weeks of gestation, Am. J. Perinatol. 14 (1997) 411–414.

CHAPTER OUTLINE

Virus   707
   Cytomegalovirus Replication   709
   Cytomegalovirus Cellular Tropism   711
Epidemiology   711
   Overview   711
   Breast-feeding   712
   Young Children as a Source of Cytomegalovirus   713
   Maternal Infection and Vertical Transmission   714
   Sexual Transmission   717
   Nosocomial Transmission   717
   Transmission to Hospital Workers   718
Pathogenesis   719
   Cytomegalovirus Infection and Cell-Associated Viremia   719
   Virus-Encoded Pathogenic Functions   720
   Host Immunity and Pathogenesis of Cytomegalovirus Infections   722
   Modulation of Host Immune Response to Cytomegalovirus   723
   Pathogenesis of Acute Infections   724
   Pathogenesis of Central Nervous System Infections in Congenitally Infected Infants   724
   Pathogenesis of Hearing Loss Associated with Congenital Cytomegalovirus Infection   725
   Nature of Maternal Infection   726
   Perinatal Infection   727
   Persistent Viral Excretion   727
Pathology   728
   Commonly Involved Organ Systems   728
Clinical Manifestations   730
   Congenital Infection   730
   Perinatal Infection   736
Diagnosis   737
   Detection of Virus   737
   Tissue Culture   738
   DNA Hybridization   738
   Polymerase Chain Reaction Amplification   738
   Antigenemia   739
   Detection of Immune Response   739
   Diagnosis of Cytomegalovirus Infection during Pregnancy   740
   Prenatal Diagnosis   741
   Diagnosis of Perinatally Acquired Infections   742
Differential Diagnosis   742
   Congenital Rubella Syndrome   742
   Congenital Toxoplasmosis   742
   Congenital Syphilis   742
   Neonatal Herpes Simplex Virus Infections   742
Treatment   743
   Chemotherapy   743
   Passive Immunization   743
   Vaccines   743
Prevention   744
   Pregnant Women   744
   Nosocomial Infection   745

Human cytomegaloviruses (CMVs) constitute a group of agents in the herpesvirus family known for their ubiquitous distribution in humans and in numerous other mammals. In vivo and in vitro infections with CMV are highly species specific and result in a characteristic cytopathology of greatly enlarged (cytomegalic) cells containing intranuclear and cytoplasmic inclusions [1]. The strikingly large, inclusion-bearing cells with a typical owl's eye appearance were first reported by Ribbert [2] in 1881 from the kidneys of a stillborn infant with congenital syphilis. Subsequently, Jesionek and Kiolemenoglou [3] reported similar findings in another stillborn infant with congenital syphilis. In 1907, Lowenstein [4] described inclusions in 4 of 30 parotid glands obtained from children 2 months to 2 years of age. Subsequently, Goodpasture and Talbot [5] noted the similarity of these cells to the inclusion-bearing cells (giant cells) found in cutaneous lesions caused by varicella virus, and they postulated that cytomegaly was the result of a similar agent.

The observation of a similar cytopathic effect after infection with herpes simplex virus (HSV) led Lipschutz [6] and then others to suggest that these characteristic cellular changes were a specific reaction of the host to infection with a virus. The observation by Cole and Kuttner [7] that inclusion-bearing salivary glands from older guinea pigs were infectious for younger animals after being passed through a filter in a highly species-specific manner led to the denomination of these agents as salivary gland viruses. The cellular changes observed in tissue sections from patients with a fatal infection led to the use of the term *cytomegalic inclusion disease* (CID) years before the causative agent was identified.

In 1954, Smith [8] succeeded in propagating murine CMV in explant cultures of mouse embryonic fibroblasts. Use of similar techniques led to the independent isolation of human CMV shortly thereafter by Smith [8], Rowe and coworkers [9], and Weller and colleagues [10]. Smith [8] isolated the agent from two infants with CID. Rowe and coworkers [9] isolated three strains of CMV from adenoidal tissue of children undergoing adenoidectomy, including the commonly used laboratory-adapted strain of CMV, AD169. Weller and colleagues [10] isolated the virus from the urine and liver of living infants with generalized CID. The term *cytomegalovirus* was proposed in 1960 by Weller and colleagues [11] to replace the names CID and salivary gland virus, which were misleading because the virus usually infected other organs and because the name *salivary gland virus* had been used to designate unrelated agents obtained from bats.

The propagation of CMV in vitro led to the rapid development of serologic methods. Using such antibody assays and viral isolation, several investigators quickly established that human CMV was a significant pathogen in humans. This ancient virus, similar to other members of the herpesvirus family, infects almost all humans at some time during their lives [12,13]. Evidence of infection has been found in all populations tested. The age at acquisition of infection differs in various geographic groups and socioeconomic settings, which results in major differences in prevalence among groups. The natural history of human CMV infection is complex. After a primary infection, viral excretion, occasionally from several sites, persists for weeks, months, or years. Episodes of recurrent infection with renewed viral shedding are common years after the primary infection. These episodes of recurrent infection are thought to be due to reactivation of latent viruses, increased levels of virus production from a source of persistent infection, or reinfections with a genetically different strain of CMV.

In immunocompetent hosts, CMV infections are generally subclinical. Infection can occur during pregnancy without consequences for the mother; however, it can have serious repercussions for the fetus. Although most immunocompromised hosts tolerate CMV infections without overt clinical symptoms, in some instances, such as in patients with acquired immunodeficiency syndrome (AIDS) and allograft recipients who have received immunosuppressive agents, CMV can cause disease of diverse severity, and the infection can be life-threatening. As a result of a long-standing and close host-parasite relationship, many—probably thousands—genetically different strains of CMV have evolved and circulate in the general population [14,15].

VIRUS

CMV is the largest and structurally most complex member of the family of human herpesviruses. It has been classified as a beta-herpesvirus based on several biochemical criteria, such as the genome size, guanosine and cytosine content, slow replicative cycle, and restricted in vivo and in vitro tropism. Other members of this subfamily of herpesviruses include other mammalian CMVs and human herpesviruses 6 and 7, the agents associated with the exanthem roseola [16–18]. Early estimates of its size based on electron microscopic studies indicated that the CMV particle was approximately 200 nm in diameter, a finding consistent with measurements obtained by more contemporary techniques [19,20]. Intracellular and extracellular particles are heterogeneous in size, which is likely a reflection of the variability of envelope glycoprotein content.

The virus genome consists of more than 230 kilobase pairs of linear double-stranded DNA, making CMV nearly 50% larger than the alpha-herpesviruses with HSV and varicella-zoster virus [21]. In contrast to other beta-herpesviruses, including other CMVs, CMV contains terminal and internal repeated nucleotide sequences that enable the genome to exist in four isomeric forms, similar to HSV and other alpha-herpesviruses [22]. The biologic advantages that favor four isomeric forms of the genome of this virus have not been determined, but clearly depend on replication of the genome in a permissive cell [23].

The nucleotide sequence of several clinical isolates of CMV has been determined, and from analysis of these strains it is estimated that CMVs can encode more than 200 open reading frames (ORFs). Individual viral genes and ORFs are designated by their location in the unique long region (UL), unique short region (US), or internal or terminal repeat regions (IRS, IRL, TRS, TRL) of the prototypic genome of CMV [22,24]. In addition to the massive size of the genome, other post-transcriptional modifications can also increase the complexity of the coding sequence of CMV. A few CMV genes represent spliced transcripts, primarily those encoding immediate and early gene products. In some cases, multiple proteins can arise from a single gene by use of internal translation initiation sites.

Although in many cases experimental verification of viral specific proteins arising from predicted ORFs has not been accomplished, it is nevertheless obvious that the proteome of virus-encoded proteins within the virus-infected cell is exceedingly complex. Consistent with this postulate has been the complexity of the proteome of the virion revealed by mass spectrometry. This study indicated that the extracellular particle contained more than 100 unique virus-encoded proteins and an indeterminate number of host cell proteins [25]. Also, the organization of the CMV genome is similar to other herpesviruses in that conserved gene blocks encoding replicative and virion structural proteins can be found in similar locations [22,24]. The organization of the genome has allowed the assignment of positional homologues between members for different subfamilies of herpesviruses, an approach that has been instrumental in the identification of genomic coding sequences of CMV proteins. Outside of these conserved gene blocks are genes or gene families that are unique to individual betaherpesviruses. These genes are thought to impart specific in vivo tropism and the species-restricted growth characteristic of these viruses [22,26].

The CMV virion consists of three identifiable regions: the capsid containing the dsDNA viral genome, the tegument, and the envelope (Fig. 23–1A). The capsid of CMV consists of six proteins that have functional and structural homologues in other herpesviruses [27,28].

The capsid of CMV has been studied by high-resolution cryoelectron microscopy, and its structure is nearly identical to HSV except that it has slightly different internal dimensions secondary to the requirement that it must incorporate a genome that is about 60% larger than HSV. The capsid consists of 162 capsomere subunits consisting of 150 hexons and 12 pentons arranged in iscosahedral symmetry [19]. The subunits of the capsid are thought to be partially assembled in the cytoplasm of the infected cell followed by self-assembly using products of the viral

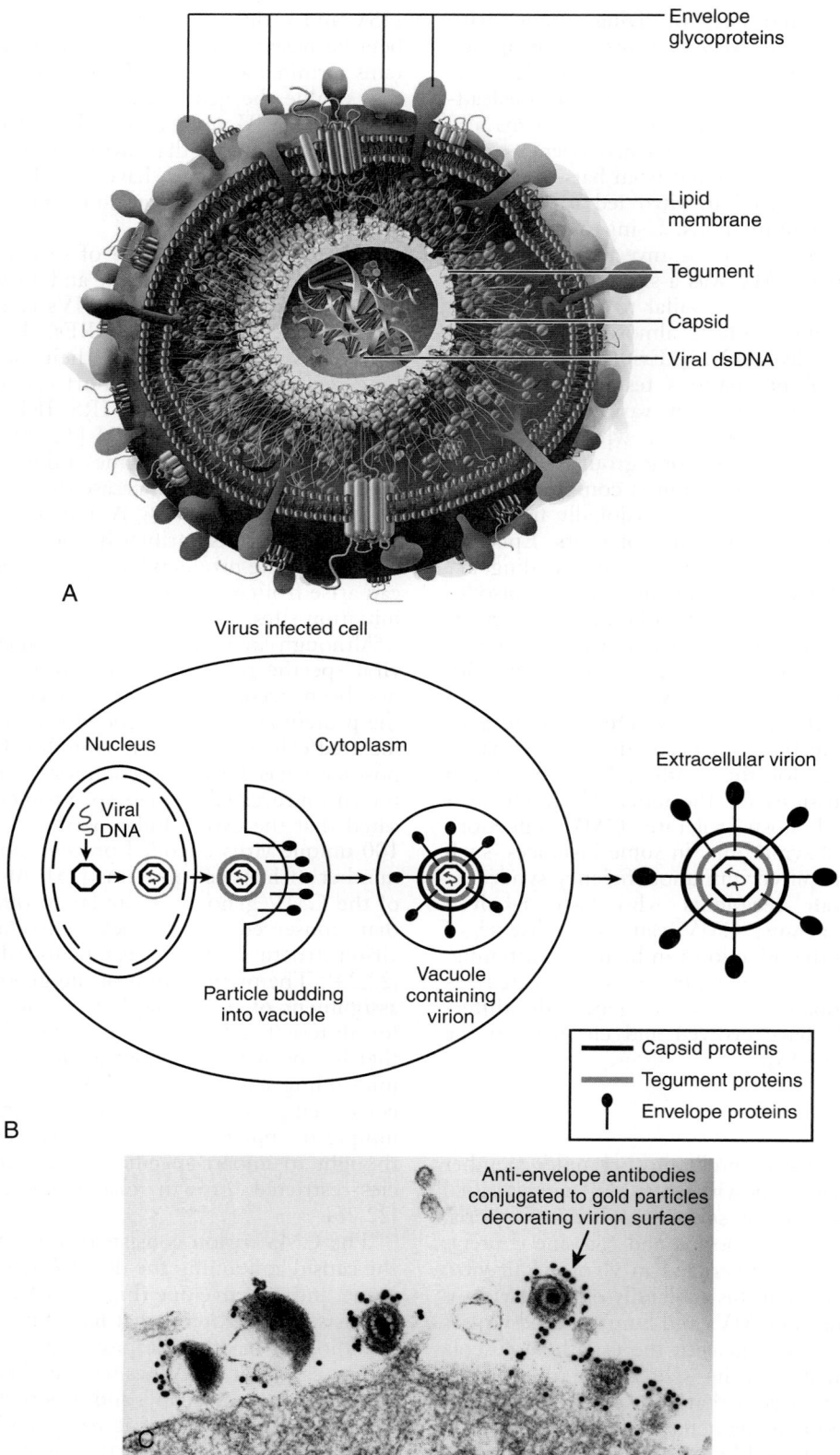

FIGURE 23–1 A, Schematic representation of human cytomegalovirus virion. Viral double-stranded DNA (dsDNA) is shown encapsulated in protein capsid, which is surrounded by amorphous layer designated the tegument. Surrounding these structures is a lipid envelope into which glycoproteins are embedded. **B,** Proposed pathways of human cytomegalovirus assembly within infected cells. Note tegument particle budding into cytoplasmic vacuoles where it acquires its final envelope. Virus leaves cells by exocytic mechanism. **C,** Electron microscopic analysis of extracellular virus with envelope glycoprotein gN decorated with gold particles (*dark spheres*). *Schematic of virus (A) modified from original figure that was kindly provided by Jay Nelson, Daniel Streblow, and Andrew Townsend, Vaccine and Gene Therapy Institute, OHSU, Portland, OR.*

UL80a ORF [28]. Proteins encoded by this ORF serve as a scaffold for the assembly of the individual capsomeres [28]. When the shell is assembled, newly replicated concatemeric viral DNA enters the capsid shell through a portal generated by the portal protein and the action of virus-encoded protein complex termed the *terminase complex* generating the intranuclear capsid [27–31]. This replication strategy is very similar to that for generating double-stranded DNA bacteriophages.

Several steps in the assembly of the viral DNA–containing capsid are unique to CMV, including the cleavage of unit length DNA and the formation of the capsid portal. At least one of these steps in virus replication has been shown to be the target of antiviral drugs [31]. Capsids containing infectious DNA leave the nucleus by as yet poorly understood pathways and are enveloped in the cytoplasm. Evidence has been presented to suggest that CMVs could leave the nucleus by focal disruption of the nuclear membrane, whereas investigators have presented data suggesting that HSV can exit the nucleus through a similar mechanism or possibly through budding into the lumen of the endoplasmic reticulum [32–35]. A mechanism that is consistent with available evidence remains to be presented, although an operational pathway of virus assembly has been suggested by several lines of evidence (see Fig. 23–1B).

The tegument of CMV is the most structurally complex and heterogeneous structure in the virion. An undetermined number of viral proteins and, as was shown more recently, viral RNAs can be found in the tegument of infectious particles [36]. Although it is generally argued that the tegument has no identifiable structure and is usually described as an amorphous layer between the envelope and the capsid, more recent studies have argued that at least the innermost region of the tegument assumes the structure of the underlying icosahedral capsid [19].

Proteins within the tegument are characteristically phosphorylated and in many cases serve regulatory functions for virus replication. In addition, some tegument proteins seem to have a primary role in maintenance of the structural integrity of the virion. Tegument proteins have various functions in the infected cell ranging from blocking intrinsic cellular responses that degrade incoming DNA to directly stimulating cell cycle progression from G_0 to G_1 by degradation of the product of the retinoblastoma gene, *Rb*, and blocking progression at the G_1-S junction of the cell cycle [37–42]. In addition, other tegument proteins have been shown to enhance transcription from the IE genes and to accelerate the replication of viral DNA [43]. Other tegument proteins have been proposed to modify critical cellular responses to stress, such as through the mammalian target of rapamycin (mTOR) pathway, and to alter cellular structures, such as the infected cell nucleus, to facilitate nuclear egress of capsids containing viral DNA [44–49].

These examples illustrate the functional complexity of CMV tegument proteins and suggest that it would be difficult in some cases to assign a unique function to an individual protein in the replicative cycle of CMV. Finally, the tegument contains the most immunogenic proteins of the virions, including the immunodominant targets of T-lymphocyte responses and antibody responses

[50–53]. In the case of one of the most abundant tegument proteins, pp65 (UL83 ORF), studies have shown that 2% to 5% of peripheral blood $CD8^+$ lymphocytes from CMV-infected hosts are specific for this single protein [52,54,55]. More recent studies have identified numerous CMV-encoded targets of $CD8^+$ and CD4+ responses and have provided evidence that in some individuals 15% of total T-cell reactivity is directed at antigens encoded by CMV [52]. It is unclear why the normal host has devoted such a large percentage of peripheral CD8+ lymphocyte reactivity to CMV, although persistence of the virus, which is facilitated by immune evasion functions, has been offered as an explanation.

The envelope of CMV rivals the tegument in terms of the number of unidentified proteins and the limited amount of information on the function of many envelope proteins. Sequence analysis of the CMV genome indicates that greater than 50 viral ORFs exhibit predicted amino acid motifs found in glycoproteins [14,21,56]. The number of glycoproteins that are present in the envelope of CMV is unknown, but at least 12 different glycoproteins have been defined experimentally [57–59].

More recent studies have suggested that the gM/gN complex represents the most abundant protein in the virion envelope, with gB and the gH/gL/gO complex being the second and third most abundant groups of glycoproteins in the envelope of laboratory strains of CMV [25]. The abundance of these different glycoproteins in the envelope of recent clinical isolates of CMV has not been studied, but the gH/gL/gO complex has been replaced with gH/gL/gUL128-131 complex in some of these viruses [60–62]. There seems to be a redundancy in function for several of these glycoproteins such that several are thought to be responsible for attachment and fusion; however, it also likely that these redundancies are a reflection of in vitro assays and that in vivo each of these proposed functions could be essential for virus infectivity, particularly in different cell types.

The envelope glycoproteins induce a readily detectable antibody response in the infected hosts, and neutralizing antibodies directed against gB, gH, gM/gN, and gH/gL/gUL128-131 complex can be shown in human CMV immune serum [63–68]. Considerable data from human and animal studies have indicated that antiviral antibodies directed at proteins of the envelope are a major component of the host protective response to this virus, such as illustrated by the decoration of the viral envelope with antibodies directed at specific glycoproteins (see Fig. 23–1C). These and other findings further show that envelope glycoproteins play a key role in the early steps of viral infection and represent a logical target for the development of prophylactic vaccines.

CYTOMEGALOVIRUS REPLICATION

Virus replication begins when CMV attaches to the cell surface. Early studies suggested that the initial engagement of virion glycoproteins with cell surface proteoglycans was followed by more specific receptor interactions and fusion with the plasma membrane [69,70]. The cellular receptor for CMV was initially proposed to be epidermal growth factor receptor, and then later integrins were proposed as receptors [71–73]. More recent findings have argued against the role of epidermal growth factor receptor as a receptor for CMV and have suggested that platelet-derived growth factor receptor can function at least as a signaling receptor for CMV [74,75].

Regardless of the specific receptor used by CMV, several studies have shown that CMV attachment and possibly fusion with the host cell membrane results in a cascade of cellular responses mediated by signaling pathways [70,76–79]. Signaling pathways can be activated by the attachment of ultraviolet (UV) light-inactivated, noninfectious virus and a single envelope glycoprotein indicating that the process of binding and fusion with the cell membrane is sufficient to induce these cellular responses. After infection with CMV, greater than 1400 cellular genes are either induced or repressed suggesting that infection with this virus elicits myriad host cell responses [78]. Included in these early responses are activation of transcription factors such as nuclear factor κB (NF-κB), increases in second messengers such as phosphoinositide-3 (PI3) kinase activity, increased expression of type I interferons and interferon-stimulated genes, and induction of responses that inhibit cellular innate responses that block virus infection (RNA-activated protein kinase [PKR]) or lead to apoptosis of the infected cell [80–84]. CMV infection prepares the host cell for virus replication and inhibits host cellular responses that could attenuate virus infection.

After attachment and penetration, the DNA-containing viral capsid is rapidly transported to the nucleus, likely using the microtubular network of the cell [85–87]. When in the nucleus, the immediate-early (IE) genes of the virus are expressed in the absence of any de novo viral protein synthesis, suggesting that either host or virion proteins are responsible for their induction. These genes include the abundant IE-1 and IE-2 genes. Both gene products arise from the same region of the genome and share some amino acid sequences secondary to RNA splicing the primary transcripts. The IE-1 gene product is a 72-kDa phosphoprotein (pp72, or IE-1) that is readily detectable throughout infection in permissive cells and is the target of antibody assays for detection of CMV-infected cells. The IE-2 gene product is a promiscuous transactivating protein and likely is responsible for activating many of the early and late genes of CMV and some cellular genes [24,88].

Additional IE genes include virus-encoded inhibitors of cellular apoptotic responses [89]. The remaining replication program of CMV is similar to that initially described for bacteriophages and for HSV and involves the coordinated and sequential temporal expression of viral genes and the coordinated inhibition of viral gene expression [24]. The regulation of CMV transcription, translation, and replication is exceedingly complex and beyond the scope of this chapter. It includes conventional modes of regulation including transactivation or silencing, or both, of promoter elements and splicing and regulation of spliced message transport from the nucleus; more recently, a role for virus-encoded micro-RNAs has been identified as a mechanism of viral gene regulation in infected cells [90–96]. A major goal of virus control of replication is to permit regulated expression of the viral genome.

The next set of viral genes expressed during infection are early or β genes. These genes are primarily composed of genes encoding viral proteins that are required for replication of viral DNA or alteration of cellular responses such as progression through the cell cycle or cellular apoptotic responses [24,97]. Examples of these genes are the viral DNA polymerase, alkaline exonuclease, ribonucleotide reductase, and other replicative enzymes. Some virion structural proteins are also made during this interval. The final set of viral genes that are expressed are the late or γ genes. These genes encode virion structural proteins and are required for the assembly of an infectious particle. The entire replicative cycle is estimated to take 36 to 48 hours in permissive human fibroblast cells. Abortive infections in nonpermissive cells have also been characterized, and viral gene expression generally is limited to the IE genes and possibly to a few early genes.

After viral DNA replication in the nucleus of infected cells, concatameric DNA is cleaved during packaging into the procapsid by mechanisms that closely resemble the pathway of bacteriophage assembly. More recent studies in the assembly of alphaherpesviruses have provided a much greater understanding of the mechanisms and pathways of viral capsid assembly and DNA packaging during herpesvirus replication. Interested readers are referred to these studies [98,99]. The viral capsid leaves the nucleus by as-yet-undetermined mechanisms and enters the cytoplasm as a partially tegumented, subviral particle. Assembly of the mature particle occurs in the cytoplasm of the infected cell in a specialized compartment that has been termed the *assembly compartment* [100]. It is believed that this is a modified cellular compartment of the distal secretory pathway [58,58–102]. Virion structural proteins are transported to this compartment, and presumably through a series of protein interactions, the virus is assembled and finally enveloped. This latter step is considerably complex because of the numerous virion glycoproteins that compose the envelope of infectious virion. Virus is presumably released by cell lysis in cells such as fibroblasts and by poorly defined exocytic pathways in certain other cell types.

Latency is a common theme of herpesviruses, particularly of the alphaherpesviruses such as HSV. The concept of latency with CMV in the human host and not at a single cell level is more controversial in that virus persistence in the host is more likely associated with chronic low-level productive infection and intermittent excretion. Latent CMV infection has been shown in macrophages obtained from infected nonimmunocompromised donors, however, and in in vitro models of infection with CMV [103–107]. The mechanisms that favor the establishment of latent infections are unknown, and the viral genome in latently infected cells is thought to be maintained as closed circular viral DNA that persists as an episome in latently infected cells and not by integration into the host DNA [108].

More definitive information is available on the signals that induce reactivation from latent infection. These signals include proinflammatory cytokines such as tumor necrosis factor-α and, possibly, interferon-γ [106,109]. It has been argued that in latently infected cells of the monocytic lineage, human CMV can become activated and replicate CMV after exposure to these cytokines in vivo, such as in the setting of rejection of an allograft. This mechanism could explain aspects of the pathogenesis of CMV infection in uninfected allograft recipients transplanted with an organ from a CMV-infected donor [110–112]. It is also likely that such latently infected cells could account for the transmission of CMV from blood products from a seronegative host [113]. More recently, arguments for a role of host and viral micro-RNAs in maintenance of herpesvirus latency have been put forth, raising the possibility for even more complexity in the relationship between these large DNA viruses and their persistently infected host [90–96].

CYTOMEGALOVIRUS CELLULAR TROPISM

CMV can be detected in a wide variety of cell types in vivo [114–116]. Studies using tissue from autopsies or biopsies have shown virus in almost every cell type, including epithelial cells, endothelial cells, smooth muscle cells, neuronal cells and supporting cells in the central nervous system (CNS), retinal epithelium, dermal fibroblasts, and cells of the monocyte/macrophage lineage. There seems to be a very limited restriction of the host cellular tropism in vivo. Routine virus isolation and propagation in vitro requires that the host cell be permissive for CMV replication. Although transformed cells are generally not susceptible to CMV infection, primary cells such as astrocytes, endothelial cells, smooth muscle cells, macrophages, and fibroblasts all have been shown to be permissive for CMV replication in vitro. The yield of infectious virus from these various cell types is highly variable, however, ranging from very low (macrophages) to high (fibroblasts).

Primary human fibroblasts are the most commonly employed cells for the recovery and propagation of CMV and if adequately maintained can yield 10^6 to 10^7 infectious particles/mL of supernatant from cultures infected with laboratory strains of CMV. In contrast, more recent clinical viral isolates often yield a fraction of this amount of virus, and almost all of the progeny virions are cell-associated. The explanation for the differences in replication phenotype is not completely understood, but more recent studies have suggested that it is the presence of a complex of glycoproteins in the envelope of recent clinical isolates, the gH/gL/gpUL128-131 complex, that not only allows extended cellular tropism of recent clinical isolates, but also results in increased cell fusion of primary fibroblasts and concomitant reduction in virus production [60]. Because the gH/gL/gpUL128-131 complex is not required for in vitro replication in fibroblasts and perhaps even inhibits replication, particularly the production of extracellular virus, viruses with mutations within genomic sequences encoding these proteins are selected against during prolonged in vitro culture. The expression of this glycoprotein complex by recent clinical isolates is required for their extended tropism, and these viruses infect primary endothelial cells, macrophages, and primary smooth muscle cells, whereas commonly used laboratory strains of CMV do not infect these cell types.

Although not understood, studies have provided some inkling as to possible mechanisms that lead to extended cellular tropisms of some recent clinical viral isolates. Assays of virus entry into cells have indicated that CMV can enter cells by direct fusion with the plasma membrane after engagement with a cell surface receptor by a pH-independent mechanism or, alternatively, after attachment to a receptor, internalization by endocytosis, and low pH fusion with the limiting membrane of the endocytic vesicle [117]. It has been shown that that the gH/gL/gpUL128-131 complex is required for the latter mechanism of entry, suggesting that cellular receptors on permissive cells other than human fibroblasts may dictate the cellular tropism of CMV.

EPIDEMIOLOGY
OVERVIEW

CMV is highly species specific, and humans are believed to be the only reservoir. CMV infection is endemic and without seasonal variation. Seroepidemiologic surveys have found CMV infection in every human population that has been tested [13]. The prevalence of antibody to CMV increases with age, but according to geographic and ethnic and socioeconomic backgrounds, the patterns of acquisition of infection vary widely among populations depending on the racial makeup of each population (Fig. 23–2) [118,119].

Seroprevalence based on testing of specimens from the Third National Health and Nutrition Examination Survey (NHANES III) ranged from 36% in individuals 6 to 11 years old to 88.8% in individuals 70 to 79 years old, showing the lifelong risk of acquiring CMV infection [118,119]. Overall in the United States, CMV seroprevalence was reported to be 58.9% [118,119]. Racial differences were apparent from this study with higher seroprevalence seen in African Americans and Hispanics than in whites [118,119]. A more recent study raised the possibility that the seroprevalence in urban African Americans in the United States may be decreasing such that an increasing number of individuals reach early adulthood without evidence of CMV infection [120]. This observation has not been confirmed in other populations, however. In addition to age and race, other risk factors for CMV infection included fewer years of formal education, government-sponsored insurance, and being born in another country [118,119].

Generally, the prevalence of CMV infection is higher in developing countries and among persons of lower socioeconomic status in developed nations. These differences are particularly striking during childhood. In sub-Saharan Africa, South America, and Asia, the rate of seropositivity was 95% to 100% among preschool children studied, whereas surveys in Great Britain and in certain populations in the United States have generally found that less than 20% of children of similar ages are seropositive.

The level of immunity among women of childbearing age, which is an important factor in determining the incidence and significance of congenital and perinatal CMV infections, also varies widely among different populations. Past reports indicated that seropositivity rates in young women in the United States and Western Europe range

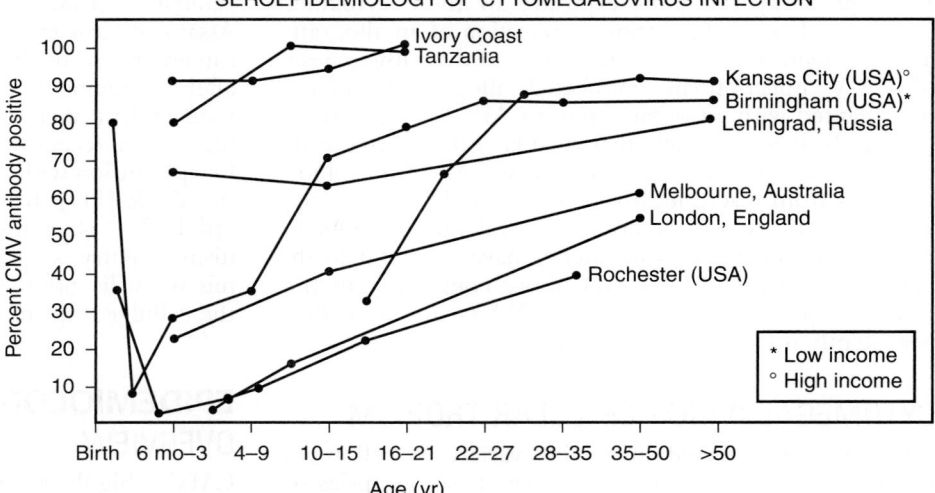

SEROEPIDEMIOLOGY OF CYTOMEGALOVIRUS INFECTION

FIGURE 23–2 Age-related prevalence of antibody to cytomegalovirus in various populations. *(From Alford CA, et al. Epidemiology of cytomegalovirus. In Nahmias AJ, Dowdle WR, Schinazi RE [eds]. The Human Herpesviruses. New York, Elsevier, 1981, p 161, with permission.)*

from less than 50% to 85%. In contrast, in sub-Saharan Africa, Central and South America, India, and the Far East, the rate of seropositivity is greater than 90% by the end of the 2nd decade of life. More importantly from the point of view of congenital infection, prospective studies of pregnant women in the United States indicate that the rate of CMV acquisition for women of childbearing age of middle to higher socioeconomic background is approximately 2% per year, whereas it is 6% per year among women of childbearing age of lower socioeconomic background, a finding that argues for the relationship between risks of exposure and rates of congenital CMV infection [121,122].

The modes of transmission from person to person are incompletely understood. The following features of CMV infection make it difficult to study the modes of acquisition. In most individuals, CMV infections are subclinical, including infections acquired in utero and during the perinatal period. Infected persons continue to expose other susceptible persons. Virus excretion persists for years after congenital, perinatal, and early postnatal infections. Prolonged viral shedding lasting more than 6 months in most individuals is also a feature of primary infection in older children and adults. Because recurrent infections are common, intermittent excretion of virus can be anticipated in a significant proportion of seropositive adults. Regardless of whether or not CMV is maintained as a latent infection with periodic reactivation or as a chronic persistent infection yielding low titers of infectivity, the virus continually spreads within a population.

A large reservoir of CMV exists in the population at all times. Transmission occurs by direct or indirect person-to-person contact. Sources of virus include urine, oropharyngeal secretions, cervical and vaginal secretions, semen, milk, tears, blood products, and organ allografts.

CMV is thought to have limited capacity to infect populations because the spread of infection seems to require close or intimate contact with infected secretions. Although at first glance this type of contact would seem to result in the limited exposure of most individuals to

CMV, the unremitting nature of exposure to individuals persistently excreting virus could result in frequent infection, a finding consistent with seroprevalence to CMV exceeding 90% in most populations in the world. The prevalence of CMV infection is higher for populations of low socioeconomic status, possibly a reflection of factors that account for increased exposure to CMV such as crowding, sexual practices, and increased exposure to infants and toddlers. Sexual contact also contributes to the spread of CMV. Higher rates of seropositivity have been observed among men and women with multiple sex partners and histories of sexually transmitted diseases [123–127].

BREAST-FEEDING

CMV is commonly excreted in milk collected postpartum from seropositive women [128–131]; the rates of excretion range from 13% to 32% by isolation of virus in tissue cultures to greater than 70% when tested by PCR. The peak of excretion is between 2 weeks and 2 months postpartum. The risk of transmission of CMV infection to infants ranges from 39% to 59%. The risk of transmission by lactating mothers correlates with viral loads of 7×10^3 genome equivalents/mL. CMV can be detected in different components of breast milk. There is consensus that milk whey is the material of choice to detect the virus during lactation. Fractions of milk containing milk cells are less likely to have detectable virus by either culture or PCR methods; this may explain why rates of viral isolation are lower in colostrum compared with mature milk. Most infants infected after ingestion of virus containing breast milk begin to excrete CMV between 3 weeks and 3 months of age.

Conservatively, it is estimated that nearly 40% of all infants nursed for at least 1 month by CMV-seropositive mothers become infected postnatally. Most of these infants chronically excrete CMV in urine and saliva, creating a large pool of infected infants. Because in most populations of the world the seroprevalence of CMV

TABLE 23–1 Breast-Feeding Patterns and Prevalence of Cytomegalovirus Infections in Young Children

Nation	Breast-Feeding Rate		Percent Seropositive	
	Ever	At 3 Months	Mothers	Children (Age)
Solomon Islands	100	97	100	100 (5 mo–4 yr)
India				
Vellore	96	64	98	80 (1 yr)
Pondicherry	?	?	97	67 (1-5 yr)
Barbados	96	?	77	62 (1-5 yr)
Guatemala	95	?	98	47 (6 mo–1 yr)
Chile	89	?	92	42 (1-2 yr)
Japan				
Sapporo	?	56	67	42 (6 mo–2 yr)
Sendai			85	38 (1 yr)
Finland (Helsinki)	95	50	55	28 (1 yr)
United States				
Houston, Texas	46	?	48	15 (1 yr)
Birmingham, Alabama	8	?	85	8 (1 yr)
France (Paris)	85	?	56	10 (10 mo)
Canada (Nova Scotia)	49	26	34	12 (6 mo–1 yr)
United Kingdom (Manchester)	51	13	59	12 (3-11 mo)

Modified from Pass RF. Transmission of viruses through human milk. In Howell RR, Morris FH Jr, Pickering K (eds). Role of Human Milk in Infant Nutrition and Health. Springfield, IL, Charles C Thomas, 1986, pp 205-224.

infection in women of childbearing age is high (80% to 100%), and most women breast-feed their infants for more than 1 month, acquisition of CMV through ingestion of breast milk from a seropositive woman is quite high (Table 23–1).

YOUNG CHILDREN AS A SOURCE OF CYTOMEGALOVIRUS

Certain child-rearing practices influence the spread of CMV among children. In 1971, Weller [1] suggested that the high rate of seropositivity among Swedish children was probably due to the frequent use of day care centers. Swedish children had a rate of infection that was three to four times higher than that observed in London or in Rochester, New York. As shown in Table 23–2, high rates of CMV infection among children attending day care centers were later confirmed in Sweden and have been reported in several studies in the United States [132–136].

The studies, which included a control group of children, confirmed that the rate of CMV infection was substantially higher among children in day care centers than in children who stayed at home [132–136]. In a study of 70 children of middle- to upperincome background in day care whose ages ranged from 3 to 65 months, the rate of CMV excretion in urine and saliva was 51% [132]. The lowest rate of excretion (9%) occurred in infants younger than 1 year, and the highest rate (88%) was among toddlers 2 years old. Twelve infants whose mothers were seronegative excreted CMV, which indicated that their infection was not congenitally or perinatally acquired. These findings have been corroborated by other investigators.

Similar results were reported by Adler [133], who also noted that greater than 50% of initially seronegative

TABLE 23–2 Prevalence of Cytomegalovirus Excretion among Children in Day Care Centers

Investigator	Year	Location	% Infected (No.)
Stangert	1976	Stockholm	35 (7/20)
Strom	1979	Stockholm	72 (13/18)
Pass	1982	Birmingham, Alabama	51 (36/70)
Adler	1985	Richmond, Virginia	24 (16/66)
Hutto	1985	Birmingham, Alabama	41 (77/188)
MMWR	1985	Birmingham, Alabama	29 (66/231)
Jones	1985	San Francisco, California	22 (31/140)
Murph	1986	Iowa City, Iowa	22 (9/41)
Adler	1987	Richmond, Virginia	53 (55/104)

MMWR, Morbidity and Mortality Weekly Report.
Data from Adler SP. Cytomegalovirus transmission among children in day care, their mothers, and caretakers. Pediatr Infect Dis J 7:279-285, 1988.

children acquired day care–associated strains of CMV as determined by restriction fragment polymorphism of viral DNA. The findings of Adler [133], which have been confirmed by others, showed that CMV is efficiently transmitted from child to child in the day care setting and that it was not unusual to find excretion rates of 20% to 40% in young toddlers [137]. In many instances, these rates of infection are substantially higher than the seroprevalence rates for the parents of the children and young adults in the cities where the studies were done [138]. Evidence strongly suggests that the high rate of CMV infection among children in group day care is caused by horizontal transmission from child to child. The route of transmission that seems most likely is the transfer of virus through saliva on hands and toys [139,140]. CMV has been shown to retain infectivity for hours on plastic surfaces and has been isolated from randomly selected toys and surfaces in a day care center. No studies have shown CMV transmission through respiratory droplets.

These observations in day care centers indicate that transmission of CMV among young children is very efficient. When infected, these children excrete CMV in large quantities and for extended periods. With the changes in child-rearing practices now occurring in the United States and the resurgence of breast-feeding, significant changes in the epidemiology of CMV can be expected within the coming decades [138].

An important issue is whether children excreting CMV can become a source of infection for susceptible child-care personnel and parents, particularly women who may become pregnant. This type of transmission has been confirmed by genetic analysis of CMV DNA [141–144]. Seroepidemiologic studies suggest that parents often acquire CMV from their children who became infected outside the family. Yeager [145] first reported that 7 of 15 (47%) seronegative mothers of premature infants who acquired CMV in a nursery seroconverted within 1 year. Dworsky and colleagues [146] reported that the rate of seroconversion for women with at least one child living at home was 5.5%, significantly higher than the 2.3% rate for women from the same clinic who were pregnant for the first time or the rates for susceptible nursery nurses and for physicians in training. Taber and associates showed a significant association between seroconversion among children and seroconversion among susceptible parents and that in most cases the infection in a child preceded seroconversion in the parents [147].

There is also compelling evidence linking the acquisition of CMV by children in day care with subsequent infection in their mothers and caregivers [148–152].

Several studies have shown that CMV-seronegative parents have a significant risk of acquiring CMV infection if their infants and children attend day care. The highest risk of seroconversion is approximately 20% to 45% in parents with a child shedding CMV at 18 months of age. On average, parents acquired infection within 4.2 months (range 3 to 7 months) after their children became infected. Genetic analysis of viral DNA indicated that many of the strains isolated from the children, their parents, and their caretakers were related by epidemiologic characteristics. For caretakers working with young children in day care centers, the annual rate of seroconversion is approximately 10%, which is significantly higher than the 2% annual rate occurring in hospital employees matched for age, race, and marital status. These observations provided evidence that parents and women who work with children in day care centers have an occupational risk of acquiring CMV. It is reasonable to expect that 50% of susceptible children between the age of 1 and 3 years who attend day care will acquire CMV from their classmates and will become an important source of infection for susceptible parents and caregivers.

MATERNAL INFECTION AND VERTICAL TRANSMISSION

Because maternal CMV infection is the origin of congenital infections and of most perinatal infections, it is important to review the relevant issues that pertain to vertical transmission. As used here, the term *vertical transmission* implies transmission from mother to infant.

Congenital Infection

Congenital infection is assumed to be the result of transplacental transmission. In the United States, congenital CMV infection occurs in 0.2% to 2.2% (average 1%) of all newborns [121]. As shown in Table 23–3, the incidence of congenital infection is quite variable, however, among different populations.

TABLE 23–3   Rate of Congenital Cytomegalovirus (CMV) Infection in Relation to Rate of Maternal Immunity in Various Locales

Location and Date	No. Infants	% Congenital CMV Infection	% Maternal Seropositive
Manchester, England, 1978	6051	0.24	25
Aarhus-Viborg, Denmark, 1979	3060	0.4	52
Hamilton, Canada, 1980	15,212	0.42	44
Halifax, Canada, 1975	542	0.55	37
Birmingham, Alabama (upper SES), 1981	2698	0.6	60
Houston, Texas (upper SES), 1980	461	0.6	50
London, England, 1973	720	0.69	58
Houston, Texas (low SES), 1980	493	1.2	83
Abidjan, Ivory Coast, 1978	2032	1.38	100
Sendai, Japan, 1970	132	1.4	83
Santiago, Chile, 1978	118	1.7	98
Helsinki, Finland, 1977	200	2	85
Birmingham, Alabama (low SES), 1980	1412	2.2	85

SES, socioeconomic status.
Data from Stagno S, et al. Maternal cytomegalovirus infection and perinatal transmission. Clin Obstet Gynecol 25:564, 1982.

The natural history of CMV during pregnancy is particularly complex and dependent on several characteristics of the population. Infections such as rubella and toxoplasmosis cannot serve as models, and in some aspects, the natural history of congenital CMV infections more closely resembles the natural history of congenital syphilis. In the case of rubella and toxoplasmosis, in utero transmission occurs only as a result of a primary infection acquired during pregnancy, whereas in utero transmission of CMV can occur as a consequence of primary and recurrent infections (reinfection or reactivation) [153,154].

Far from being a rare event, congenital infection resulting from recurrent CMV infection has been shown to be common, especially in highly immune populations. The initial clue was provided by three independent reports of congenital CMV infections that occurred in consecutive pregnancies [12,155]. In all three instances, the first infant was severely affected or died, and the second born in each case was subclinically infected. More convincing evidence came from a prospective study of women known to be seroimmune before conception [154]. As shown in Table 23-4, the rate of congenital CMV infection was 1.9% among 541 infants born to these seropositive women. The 10 congenitally infected infants were not infected as a result of primary maternal CMV infection because all mothers were known to have been infected with CMV 1 to several years before the onset of pregnancy.

Shortly after these studies were published, Schopfer and associates [153] found that in an Ivory Coast population in which virtually all inhabitants are infected in childhood, the prevalence of congenital CMV infection was 1.4%. More recent studies from Brazil and India have confirmed these early reports and shown again that the rate of congenital CMV infection is directly related to the CMV seroprevalence of the maternal population. In these populations, maternal seroprevalence is nearly 100%, yet the rate of congenital CMV infection was approximately 1% [156–158].

This phenomenon of intrauterine transmission in the presence of substantial maternal immunity has been attributed to reactivation of endogenous virus in some

cases and to reinfection with different strains of CMV in other instances. Initially, support for a mechanism of reactivation as an explanation for recurrent infection came from the observation that the viruses isolated from each of three pairs of congenitally infected siblings were identical when examined by restriction endonuclease analysis [159]. In two of these three pairs, the first-born infant was severely affected, whereas the second-born sibling was subclinically infected, which suggested that virulence of infection was not related to strain and that maternal immunity in some way attenuated the fetal infection. Closer examination of these early data suggested, however, that in at least one of these cases, reinfection with a new strain of virus that differed genetically from the previous maternal isolate could explain the recurrent congenital infection.

More recent studies indicate that women who are CMV-seropositive can become reinfected with a different strain of CMV, leading to intrauterine transmission and symptomatic congenital infection [160]. This study assessed maternal humoral immunity to strain-specific epitopes of CMV glycoprotein H in serum specimens from women with preconceptional immunity who were sampled during a previous pregnancy and the current pregnancy. Of the 16 mothers with congenitally infected infants, 10 had acquired new antibody specificities against glycoprotein H compared with only 4 of the 30 mothers of uninfected infants. The women participating in this study were predominantly of low socioeconomic status; young; with a high seroprevalence of CMV; unmarried; and with a strong background of sexually transmitted diseases, including high rates of CMV excretion. The observations from this study have been confirmed in other populations, most recently in Brazil, in which reinfection occurred at an annualized rate of nearly 35% in a maternal population with near-universal seroimmunity to CMV (Yamamoto A, manuscript submitted for publication).

Intrauterine transmission of CMV in immune women explains the direct relationship between the incidence of congenital CMV infection and the rate of seropositivity as shown in Table 23-4. At present, it is extremely difficult to define by virologic or serologic markers which

TABLE 23-4 Rate of Congenital Cytomegalovirus (CMV) Infection in Relation to Rate of Maternal Seroimmunity

Location	No. Studied	% Congenital CMV Infection	% Seroimmune
Manchester, England	6051	1.38	100
Aarhus-Viborg, Denmark	3060	0.4	52
Hamilton, Canada	15,212	0.42	44
Birmingham, Alabama (upper SES)	2698	0.6	60
Birmingham, Alabama (low SES)	1412	2.2	85
Houston, Texas (low SES)	461	1.2	83
Abidjan, Ivory Coast	2032	0.24	25
Santiago, Chile	118	1.7	98
Ribeirao Preto, Brazil	451	2	96
Ballabhgarh, India	272	2.2	100
Sukuta, The Gambia	741	5.4	96

SES, socioeconomic status.
Data from Stagno S, et al. Maternal cytomegalovirus infection and perinatal transmission. Clin Obstet Gynecol 25:564, 1982.

patient may undergo a reactivation of CMV or reinfection with a new strain of virus, and it is nearly impossible to define the timing of intrauterine transmission with such reactivations or reinfections during pregnancy. The sites from which CMV reactivates to produce congenital infection are unknown and are likely inaccessible to sampling during pregnancy. Although CMV excretion is a common event during and after pregnancy, the simple isolation of virus during pregnancy is a poor indicator of the risk of intrauterine infection.

Virus can be shed at variable rates from single or multiple sites after primary or recurrent infections in women whether pregnant or not. Sites of excretion include the genital tract, cervix, urinary tract, pharynx, and breast. In pregnant women, virus is excreted most commonly from the cervix and, in decreasing order, the urinary tract and the oropharynx. In the immediate postpartum period, the frequency of viral shedding into breast milk is quite high and can reach 40% among seropositive women when assayed by conventional virus isolation and on the order of 70% to 90% when analyzed by PCR techniques. The rates of cervical and urinary tract shedding in nonpregnant women are comparable to rates found in pregnant cohorts with similar demographic and socioeconomic characteristics. Generally, rates of cervical shedding range from 5.2% for nonpregnant women enrolled in private obstetric practice or family planning clinics to 24.5% among women attending a sexually transmitted disease clinic [124,126]. Pregnancy per se has no discernible effect on the overall prevalence of viral shedding. The prevalence of excretion is lower (2.6%) in the first trimester, however, than near term (7.6%) [159]. This rate is comparable to the prevalence of genital excretion in nonpregnant women.

The rates of CMV excretion in the genital and urinary tracts of women are inversely related to age after puberty. In one study, the rate of genital CMV excretion decreased from 15% in girls 11 to 14 years of age to undetectable levels in women age 31 years and older [159]. From a peak of 8% in the younger group, urinary excretion fell to zero in women age 26 years and older. No CMV excretion occurred from either site in postmenopausal women.

A transient depression of cellular immune responses to CMV antigens during the second and third trimesters was reported in early studies, suggesting a role for altered immunity during pregnancy and CMV replication [161]. Other studies suggested that there was no generalized depression of cellular immunity based on the numbers of T lymphocytes, T-cell proliferative responses to other mitogens, and serum antibody titers. None of these mothers shed virus during the period of depressed cellular immune response, and they did not transmit the infection to their infants.

More recently, Lilleri and coworkers [162] identified a cohort of pregnant women with primary CMV infection and analyzed their virus specific T-cell responses. Several findings of this study are directly relevant to role of T lymphocytes in the natural history of congenital CMV. First, there was no difference in the kinetics of $CD4^+$ and $CD8^+$ CMV-specific responses between pregnant and nonpregnant women, a finding that argues against a virus-specific immunodeficiency during pregnancy that

could increase CVM transmission to the fetus [162]. The duration of viremia was similar in women who transmitted virus to their fetuses and in women who failed to transmit virus, suggesting that obvious defects in control of virus replication cannot readily explain intrauterine transmission [162]. Women with primary infection who did not transmit virus to their offspring developed quantitatively higher CMV-specific $CD4^+$ T lymphocytes demonstrated responses, however, and developed these responses sooner than women who transmitted virus to their offspring [162]. This finding is provocative and suggested that the more rapid development of T-cell responses to CMV could in some way alter parameters of the maternal infection and lessen the risk of transmission to the fetus.

It has also been shown that antibody responses to glycoprotein B are significantly higher at the time of delivery in women with primary CMV infection who transmitted the infection in utero compared with women who did not, suggesting that the amount of antiviral antibody is not reflective of protection from transmission [163]. Analysis of the qualitative antibody response revealed lower neutralizing antibody titers in transmitters, however, suggesting an association between neutralizing activity and intrauterine transmission. In this study, a significant correlation was found between neutralizing titers and antibody avidity, indicating that antibody avidity maturation is crucial for production of high levels of neutralizing antibodies during primary CMV infection, a finding that at least on a superficial level parallels the findings of Lilleri and coworkers [162].

In a separate study, higher levels of transplacentally acquired maternal antibodies against glycoprotein B and neutralizing antibodies were observed in infants with symptomatic infection at birth who went on to develop sequelae [164]. These and other studies have limitations associated with measurement of immunologic functions in specimens from patients in which the timing of maternal infection, placental infection, or fetal transmission cannot be ascertained but only defined within large time intervals such as trimesters of pregnancy. Critical features of protective responses, such as the level of protective immune responses at the time of virus dissemination to the placenta and fetus, cannot be defined by such studies, and only correlations or associations can be inferred from existing data.

Perinatal Infection

In contrast with the poor correlation that exists between CMV excretion during pregnancy and congenital infection, there is a good correlation between maternal shedding in the genital tract and milk and perinatal acquisition. As shown in Table 23–5, the two most efficient sources of transmission in the perinatal period were infected breast milk, which resulted in a 63% rate of perinatal infection, and the infected genital tract, particularly in late gestation, which was associated with transmission in 26% and 57% of the cases (natal infection). Viral shedding from the pharynx and urinary tract of the mother late in gestation and during the first months postpartum has not been associated with perinatal transmission.

TABLE 23–5 Association between maternal excretion of CMV from various sites and subsequent infection of the infant

Only Site of Maternal Excretion	No. Infants Infected/ No. Exposed (%)
Breast milk	
Breast-fed infant	19/30 (63)
Bottle-fed infant	0/9 (0)
Cervix	
Third trimester and postpartum	8/14 (57)
Third trimester	18/68 (26)
First and second trimester	1/8 (12)
Urine*	0/11 (0)
Saliva[†]	0/15 (0)
Nonexcreting women	
Bottle-fed infant	0/125 (0)
Breast-fed infant	0/11 (9)

*Late third trimester.
[†]Excretion 1 day postpartum.
From Stagno S, et al. Breast milk and the risk of cytomegalovirus infection. N Engl J Med 302:1073, 1980.

There is considerable variability in perinatal transmission of CMV throughout the world [165]. The age of the mother and her prior experience with CMV, which influence the frequency of viral excretion into the genital tract and breast milk, are important factors. Younger seropositive women who breast-feed have an increased risk for transmitting virus to their infants, especially women from lower socioeconomic groups [138]. In Japan, Guatemala, Finland, and India, where the rates of CMV excretion within the 1st year of life are extremely high (39% to 56%), the practice of breast-feeding is almost universal, and most women of childbearing age are sero-immune for CMV likely secondary to perinatal acquisition of CMV.

SEXUAL TRANSMISSION

Numerous epidemiologic studies support the classification of CMV as a sexually transmitted infection, consistent with excretion of this virus in cervical secretions, vaginal fluid, and semen. In developing areas of the world, 90% to 100% of the population is infected during childhood, some by 5 years of age, providing an large reservoir for virus transmission. Sexual transmission in these populations could play a minor role as a source of primary CMV infection, but its importance in reinfection is suspected, although unproven. In developed countries, the infection is acquired at a lower rate in childhood, resulting in a burst in the prevalence of infection after puberty in some populations, an observation that parallels the acquisition of other herpesviruses such as Epstein-Barr virus. Several lines of evidence indicate that sexual transmission of CMV is at least partly responsible for this increase in seroprevalence.

As noted previously, an increased seroprevalence of CMV and excretion of virus has been found in women attending sexually transmitted disease clinics and in young homosexual men. Handsfield and colleagues [166]

showed that previously infected individuals could be reinfected by a different strain of CMV. More recently, an association between CMV excretion and bacterial vaginosis has been described together with findings that argued that infection with multiple strains of CMV could be correlated with the presence of bacterial vaginosis, a sexually transmitted infection [127]. Evidence has also been provided for sexual transmission in general populations [167]. Among the many variables investigated, significant correlations were found among seropositivity to CMV, greater numbers of lifetime sexual partners, and past or present infection with other sexually transmitted infections.

NOSOCOMIAL TRANSMISSION

Nosocomial CMV infection is an important hazard of blood transfusion and organ transplantation. In immunocompromised hosts, such as small premature newborns and bone marrow transplant recipients, transfusion-acquired CMV infection has been associated with serious morbidity and even fatal infection. The association between the acquisition of CMV infection and blood transfusion was first suggested in 1960 by Kreel and co-workers [168], who described a syndrome characterized by fever and leukocytosis occurring 3 to 8 weeks after open heart surgery. The reports that followed soon after expanded the syndrome to include fever, atypical lymphocytosis, splenomegaly, rash, and lymphadenopathy [169–172]. The term *postperfusion mononucleosis* was then proposed. Prospective studies incriminated blood transfusion as the major risk factor and showed that although the clinical syndrome occurred in approximately 3% of the patients undergoing transfusion, inapparent acquisition of CMV infection ranged from 9% to 58% as determined by seroconversion, a fourfold increase in complement-fixing antibody titers, or viral excretion occurring 3 to 12 weeks after surgery.

It has been estimated that the percentage of blood donors capable of transmitting CMV ranges from 2.5% to 12%. In a study of seronegative children receiving blood for cardiac surgery, the risk of acquiring CMV was calculated to be 2.7% per unit of blood [170]. A significant correlation between the risk of acquisition of CMV by patients labeled seronegative and the number of units of blood (total volume) transfused was noted early on [171]. Under conditions found in blood banks, CMV inoculated in whole blood persisted for 28 days, and CMV inoculated in freshly frozen plasma persisted for 97 days. More recent modifications of blood banking practices have greatly reduced the risk of CMV infection after blood transfusion; however, studies from Europe have shown that 15% of serologically negative blood donors as detected by commercial antibody assays may harbor CMV DNA in their peripheral blood and potentially transmit virus to a donor, a finding that may also explain that approximately 1% to 2% of recipients of blood transfusions from CMV-seronegative donors develop CMV infections [113].

The observation that two newborns who received large volumes of fresh blood subsequently developed symptomatic CMV infections led McCracken and associates [173] to suggest an association between blood transfusion and clinically apparent postnatal CMV infection. Subsequent reports indicated an association between postnatal CMV infection and exchange transfusions [174]. Intrauterine transfusions have also been implicated in CMV infection of mothers and their infants and transmission from cord blood–derived stem cells.

CMV infections resulting from transfusion of blood products have also been shown to cause significant disease in newborn infants, particularly premature infants and infants born to women without immunity to CMV. Extremely premature infants born to seropositive mothers are also at increased risk because the transplacental transfer of specific antibodies does not occur until the later stages of gestation. Infected infants with passively acquired anti-CMV antibodies develop milder disease than infected infants without passively acquired antibodies [175]. This observation is a compelling argument for the role of antiviral antibodies in protecting the host against severe disease.

Transmission of CMV by transplantation of an allograft from donors previously infected with CMV represents a major clinical problem in allograft transplantation. Transplantation of a kidney from a seropositive donor into a seronegative recipient results in primary CMV infection in 80% of patients. The clinical manifestations of the infection vary widely, depending principally on immunosuppressive regimens. Most investigators have found that CMV infection has an adverse effect on the survival of the allograft. CMV was recognized as a major cause of morbidity and mortality in recipients of hematopoietic allografts and autografts and continues to represent an important opportunistic infection in these populations [176–179]. Interstitial pneumonitis is the most significant manifestation of the infection; mortality approached 100% before the availability of antiviral agents. CMV is excreted by 70% to 100% of recipients of heart transplants [180–183]. Severe disease has traditionally been thought to be associated more often with primary than with reactivated infection. Studies in several transplant populations have documented significant disease after superinfection with strains of CMV derived from the allograft [184–187]. These early findings and subsequent findings argue for a complex relationship between host immunity, infection with new strains of virus, and protective responses. The demonstration of CMV nucleic acid in kidneys of infected donors and of latent CMV in cells of macrophage/monocyte lineage showed that the transplanted organs and hematopoietic allografts can serve as the source of virus in transplant recipients [110].

Nosocomial transmission is possible in the nursery setting, which suggests that workers' hands or contaminated fomites might be involved. The very low rate of CMV infection in newborn infants of seronegative mothers who are not exposed to other important sources such as seropositive blood products indicates that transmission of CMV via fomites or workers' hands is uncommon.

TRANSMISSION TO HOSPITAL WORKERS

Because hospital workers are often women of childbearing age, there has been concern about occupational risk through contact with patients shedding CMV. As illustrated in Table 23–6, most older studies indicated that

TABLE 23–6   Rates of Primary CMV Infection Among Health Care Workers and Others

Study	Group	Numbers	Seroconversion (%/yr)
Yeager, 1975	Non-nurses	27	0
	Neonatal nurses	34	4.1
	Pediatric nurses	31	7.7
Dworsky et al, 1983	Medical students	89	0.6
	Pediatric residents	25	2.7
	Neonatal nurses	61	3.3
Friedman et al, 1984*	"High risk": pediatric intensive care unit, blood intravenous team	57	12.3
	"Low risk": pediatric ward nurses, noncontact	151	3.3
Brady et al, 1985	Pediatric residents	122	3.8
Adler et al, 1986	Pediatric nurses	31	4.4
	Neonatal nurses	40	1.8
Demmler et al, 1986	Pediatric nurses	43	0
	Pediatric "therapists"	76	0
Balfour and Balfour, 1986	Transplant/dialysis nurses	117	1.04
	Neonatal intensive care unit nurses	96	2.28
	Nursing students	139	2.25
	Blood donors	167	1.57
Stagno et al, 1986	Middle-income pregnant women	4692	2.5
	Low-income pregnant women	507	6.8

Only study in a children's hospital reporting a statistically significant difference in relation to occupational contact.
Modified from Pass RF, Stagno S. Cytomegalovirus. In Donowitz LG (ed). Hospital Acquired Infection in the Pediatric Patient. Baltimore, Williams & Wilkins, 1988.

the risk was not significantly different from the general population.

The risk for CMV seroconversion among hospital personnel is a function of the prevalence of CMV excretion among patients, the prevalence of susceptible health care workers, and the degree of their exposure to infected patients. Generally, among hospitalized infants and children, viruria occurs in approximately 1% of newborns and 5% to 10% of older infants and toddlers.

Working with hospitalized children inevitably leads to contact with a child shedding CMV; however, it is important that workers who develop a primary infection not assume that their occupational exposure or contact with a specific patient is the source of infection. Three old reports illustrate this point. Yow and coworkers [188], Wilfert and associates [189], and Adler and associates [149] described health care workers who acquired CMV while pregnant and after attending patients known to be excreting CMV. In each of these reports, the source of CMV for hospital workers was not from patients. With the implementation of universal precautions in the care of hospitalized patients, the risk of nosocomial transmission of CMV to health care workers is expected to be much lower than the risk of acquiring the infection in the community.

PATHOGENESIS

The disease manifestations of CMV infections can be conveniently divided into manifestations associated with acute infection and virus replication and manifestations associated with chronic infections in which the relationship between disease and virus replication is not easily defined. Considerably more is known about acute infectious syndromes because acute CMV infections can be temporally related to specific symptoms and specific laboratory abnormalities. Infrequently, acute CMV syndromes can occur in presumably normal individuals and in these cases manifest as an infectious mononucleosis that is indistinguishable clinically from the infectious mononucleosis associated with Epstein-Barr virus infection [190,191]. Normal individuals with symptomatic infections often have increased viral burdens as measured by serologic responses compared with individuals with asymptomatic infections [53]. More commonly, acute CMV infections that result in symptomatic disease occur in immunocompromised hosts.

Generally, acute CMV syndromes that are associated with clinical disease often share several common characteristics, including (1) occurrence in hosts with altered cellular immunity, (2) poorly controlled virus replication, (3) multiorgan involvement, (4) end-organ disease secondary to direct viral cytopathic effects, and (5) clinical manifestations of disease correlated with virus burden. In patients with invasive CMV infections, such as those in allograft recipients, organ dysfunction and often disease course can be correlated with increasing virus burden [192–196]. There is usually not an absolute level of viral replication as measured by viral genome copy number in the peripheral blood that is predictive of the onset of an invasive infection and end-organ disease in all individuals. Rather, increasing levels of virus replication (genome copy number) seem more useful in the identification of individuals at risk for invasive disease and presumably reflect ongoing viral replication in the absence of efficient host control with an increasing risk of dissemination.

Chronic disease syndromes that have been associated with CMV include various chronic inflammatory diseases of older populations such as atherosclerotic vascular disease and vascular processes associated with chronic allograft rejection [197–206]. In addition, the progressive and late-onset hearing loss associated with congenital CMV infection could be considered in this same category [207–212]. The characteristics of populations experiencing these manifestations of CMV infection differ from the populations described previously and do not include hosts with obvious immune dysfunction. Most individuals have normal immunity, and allograft recipients experiencing chronic graft rejection may have increased immune responsiveness within the allograft.

Viral replication may be a prerequisite for disease, but the level of virus replication has not been correlated with disease. The course of the disease in animal models of CMV-associated vascular disease is ongoing inflammation that is enhanced and prolonged by the presence of CMV [213–217]. Inhibition of virus replication early in the course of infection in animal models has been shown to alter the course of disease dramatically, suggesting that virus must seed these areas and establish a persistent infection [215]. The presence of the virus in areas of inflammation increases the expression of soluble mediators of inflammation such as cytokines and chemokines, and in some cases, virus-infected cells actively recruit inflammatory cells including monocytes into the area of disease [218–220]. The bidirectional interactions between CMV and the host inflammatory response are unique and seem to favor virus persistence, viral gene expression, and probably virus dissemination.

CYTOMEGALOVIRUS INFECTION AND CELL-ASSOCIATED VIREMIA

An important aspect of the pathogenesis of CMV infection is the route of infection and spread within the host. It is generally believed that virus is acquired either at mucosal sites (community exposures) or by blood-borne transmission, such as after blood transfusion or transplantation of an infected allograft. Understanding the pathogenesis of these types of infections requires an understanding of the mode of virus transmission and virus dissemination. It is believed that cell-free virus is responsible for community-acquired CMV infection based on recovery of virus from saliva and from cell-free genital tract secretions, but only limited data directly support this claim. More convincing evidence comes from studies in breast-feeding women, which have shown that infectious virus is present in the cell-free fraction of breast milk [130]. This finding suggests that cell-free virus can infect a mucosal surface. Animal models of CMV infection have most commonly used either intraperitoneal or subcutaneous inoculations; however, oral infection with cell-free murine CMV has been accomplished (Jonjic S, University of Rijeka, Rijeka, Croatia, personal communication).

After infection and local replication and amplification of virus titer in regional sites, the spread of CMV within an infected host is likely to be cell-associated based on findings from immunocompromised patients and studies in experimental animal models [103,221–225]. During infections of mucosal surfaces that occur after exposures in the community and blood-borne infections in transplant patients, the mode of spread and dissemination of the virus is likely the same, albeit with different kinetics and quantity of infected cells in the vasculature and infected organs. In all but the most severely immunocompromised patients, infectivity that can be shown in the blood compartment is most frequently associated with endothelial cells and polymorphonuclear leukocytes from the buffy coat fraction of peripheral blood [226–228].

Polymorphonuclear neutrophils (PMNs) cannot support virus replication, but have been shown to carry infectious virus and viral gene products [229,230]. It has been proposed that CMV-infected endothelial cells or fibroblasts can transfer infectious virus to PMNs, and these cells can transmit virus by a microfusion event between virus-containing vesicles and susceptible cells [229]. This mechanism has not been experimentally verified in animal models of CMV infection, but the role of PMNs in transmission of infectious CMV in vivo is consistent with clinical observations, and the correlation between CMV antigen-positive PMNs (antigenemia assay) and disseminated infection has been shown to be a diagnostic tool for the identification of patients at risk for invasive infection with CMV [231–236]. In addition, antigen-positive PMNs can be detected in normal hosts infected with CMV, but with a drastically reduced frequency compared with immunocompromised patients, suggesting that even in normal hosts PMNs may be a common mode of virus dissemination.

Other cells within the leukocyte fraction of peripheral blood cells support CMV persistence and transmit infectious virus, including monocyte/macrophages derived by differentiation of blood monocytes [223,237–239]. Granulocyte-monocyte progenitor cells have been proposed as sites of latency based on in vitro infections and can be detected as antigen-containing cells in immunocompromised patients with disseminated CMV infection [104–106,223,224,239–241]. In animal models of human CMV infection, an important role of myeloid precursors in the spread of murine CMV has been shown, including the role of virus-encoded chemokine-like molecules in chemoattraction of myeloid progenitor cells leading to dissemination of the virus from local sites of replication (see following section).

Macrophages derived from peripheral blood monocytes have been shown to harbor infectious CMV on stimulation with specific cytokines, including tumor necrosis factor-α [103,109,111]. Viral replication and expression of various early and late proteins can be shown in macrophages after infection with recently derived CMV clinical isolates. Together, these data have argued for a mechanism of in vivo spread that includes infection of circulating monocytes, which on entry into an organ undergo differentiation into a tissue macrophage that can support productive CMV infection [109].

Another cell lineage believed to be crucial for in vivo spread of CMV is endothelial cells in various microvascular beds. Endothelial cells have been shown to support CMV replication in vitro, and infection of these cells results in various cellular responses, including the release of cytokines and chemokines [237,242–249]. Lytic and nonlytic productive infections have been described suggesting that endothelial cells can respond very differently to infection [242,245,250,251]. Virus infection of endothelial cells is thought to be an initial step for infection of various tissues during CMV dissemination, and, likewise, endothelial cell infection seems to be crucial for hematogenous spread from infected tissue [229,237,249]. Early studies in transplant populations described viral antigen–containing endothelial cells circulating in the blood of viremic transplant patients [246,252,253]. These cells are believed to be infected endothelial cells that slough into the circulation, presumably secondary to local infection or inflammation or both. A similar role for endothelial cells in spread of CMV in the murine model and guinea pig CMV model has also been proposed [254]. Finally, in an elegant series of experiments, Sacher and coworkers [225] showed that replication of murine CMV within endothelial cells was essential for dissemination of this virus from sites such as the liver.

VIRUS-ENCODED PATHOGENIC FUNCTIONS

To date, specific CMV-encoded virulence factors have not been identified. Early studies attempted to correlate differences in restriction fragment lengths of endonuclease-digested DNA of viral isolates from congenitally infected infants with clinical outcome. This genetic analysis proved too crude to allow identification of subtle changes in the viral genome. More recently, numerous studies have reported a possible linkage between polymorphisms in a gene encoding the major envelope glycoprotein gB and disease [255–258]. Almost all of these studies have failed to show any specific linkage between different gB genotypes and disease, and most recently, studies using other polymorphisms in several viral genes (UL11, UL18, UL40, UL73, UL74, UL144) have failed to establish a specific genetic linkage between a unique genotype and disease [259–267].

Although the explanation for the vast polymorphisms in CMV is unclear, several characteristics of CMV infections, including frequent reinfections with new strains of virus in exposed populations and recombination between strains of virus, are likely reasons for the variability in the nucleotide sequences of different viral isolates [160,187,257,268]. Differences in biologic behavior of CMVs exist, however, such that some strains exhibit extended tropism and can infect endothelial cells, macrophages, and epithelial cells in addition to permissive primary fibroblast cells. This extended tropism is a property of recently derived isolates of CMV, and after these viruses are repeatedly passaged through fibroblast cells, their extended tropism is quickly lost. It is believed that one or more viral genes are responsible for their extended tropism in vivo, and that without the selective pressure of replication in vivo, these genes are lost or mutated under in vitro conditions.

Specific genes that permit extended tropism in vitro have been identified and include the most well-characterized group encoded by the ORFs UL128 through UL131 [61,269,270]. In addition, the presence of numerous genes that modify the immune response to CMV raises the possibility that these genes encode a function that inhibits an innate response from cells such as macrophages that could also contribute to the extended tropism of some isolates. Other viral genes encode functional chemokine receptors (US28), viral cytokine-like molecules (vIL10, vIL-8), and viral antiapoptotic functions (vICA, UL37), all of which have been proposed to contribute to in vivo replication and virulence of CMV infections [271–280]. An observation suggested that different viral genotypes could be found in different tissues from infants with symptomatic congenital CMV infections who died in early infancy, a provocative finding that raises the possibility of as-yet-undefined viral functions that target different viruses to different tissues in vivo [281].

Although defining the function of viral genes in in vivo replication and spread of CMV has been difficult because of the restricted tropism of CMV to cells of human origin, much information has been gathered from studies in animal models. Using the mouse model of CMV infection, several laboratories identified specific viral genes that seemed to be required for efficient replication and spread in vivo [221,282–288]. Three viral genes encoded by m139, m140, and m141 ORFs of murine CMV have been shown to play a crucial role in viral replication in monocyte/macrophages, but have little to no effects on the replication of the virus in mouse fibroblasts [222,283,289–291]. The in vivo phenotype of viruses that lacked these genes indicated these genes were required for in vivo dissemination and spread of murine CMV [274,290]. To date, the mechanism that accounts for restricted replication in monocytes of murine CMV with deletions in these specific genes is unknown. The CMV gene that permits replication in monocyte/macrophages has not been definitively identified, but the murine CMV genes m139, m140, and m141 are homologous to a family of CMV genes (US22 gene family).

Another example of a viral gene that directly influences in vivo tropism and replication of CMV is the murine CMV gene M45. Endothelial cell tropism of murine CMV can be linked to the single viral gene M45, and it is believed that expression of this gene limits resistance of endothelial cells to murine CMV–induced apoptosis [254]. The deletion of the homologous reading frame in CMV (UL45) was not associated with the loss of endothelial tropism [292]. As noted earlier, the more recent findings that murine CMV dissemination required replication in endothelial cells provides additional evidence for the requirement of specific cellular tropism and in vivo behavior of CMVs.

Other genes in murine CMV encode functional chemokines, such as MCK-1, which exhibits activity similar to that of interleukin (IL)-8 in humans [222,274,289]. Studies in mice have suggested that the capacity of this gene product to recruit inflammatory cells into a site of virus replication is important for cell-associated virus spread within infected animals [222,274]. In the absence of this virus-encoded function, virus replication remains localized to the site of infection secondary to a failure to recruit and infect infiltrating inflammatory cells, limiting viral dissemination [222,274]. A functionally homologous viral gene in CMV, UL146, could influence the spread of CMV in vivo [293]. The protein encoded by UL146 is a secreted protein that seems to function as a CXCL chemokine (v-CXCL1) and can induce chemotaxis and degranulation of PMNs [293]. It has been postulated that this viral chemokine can recruit PMNs in vivo and promote CMV dissemination [274].

In severely immunocompromised hosts, such as AIDS patients with gastrointestinal and retinal disease secondary to disseminated CMV infection, neutrophil infiltration can be observed in the lamina propria and in the retina [294–296]. Infection of lamina propria macrophages with CMV in vitro results in the induction of IL-8 release from these cells, suggesting that CMV can induce IL-8 release and encode a viral IL-8-like molecule [274,297]. Such findings are consistent with the proposed mechanism of chemokine expression and CMV dissemination from sites of virus replication. This mechanism of dissemination is consistent with the histopathologic findings noted in severely immunocompromised patients; however, a neutrophil infiltrate is not an invariant feature of the histopathology of naturally acquired CMV infections, and interactions between other virus-encoded chemokines and chemokine receptors and peripheral blood leukocytes could contribute to virus dissemination.

Finally, more recent findings have shown that CMV engages toll-like receptors with resultant induction of proinflammatory cytokines and chemokine cascades [298]. This observation raises the possibility that virus infection alone can recruit cells such as monocytes and PMNs to sites of infection without the requirement of a specific viral chemokine [298]. Other viral genes likely induce host cell genes, which facilitate virus replication. Microarray and differential display experiments have shown that CMV infection induces the expression of cyclooxygenase-2, an enzyme required for prostaglandin synthesis and initiation of early steps of inflammation. Subsequent experiments have shown that if cyclooxygenase-2 activity is blocked, CMV replication is blocked [299]. Together, these experiments showed that a CMV-encoded gene could induce a cellular enzyme, which facilitated its replication possibly by increasing the inflammatory response to the infection. This host response presumably leads to the recruitment of inflammatory cells into the site of virus replication, promoting infection of infiltrating cells and virus spread.

CMV encodes four G-coupled protein receptor–like molecules in ORFs UL33, UL78, US27, and US28 [218,300–303]. The US28 gene encodes a G-coupled protein receptor that is constitutively activated and that can signal after interaction with chemokines, including RANTES, MCP-1, and fractalkine [218,303–305]. Reports have detailed possible roles for this molecule in the spread of CMV in vivo, including (1) as a chemokine sink to limit host cell chemotaxis to CMV-infected cells, (2) providing an antiapoptotic function, (3) recruitment of infected mononuclear cells to the sites of inflammation leading to dissemination of virus, and (4) perhaps even by binding of virus or virus-infected cells to chemokine-expressing endothelial cells [303–307]. Arterial smooth muscle cells expressing US28 have been shown to migrate down chemokine gradients, providing a mechanism for the localization of CMV-infected cells to sites containing inflammatory cellular infiltrates [218].

Although the role of US28 in CMV-induced vascular disease has been well described and supported by in vitro models of smooth muscle cell migration, the importance of US28 in virus dissemination from local site of infection remains to be more completely defined. A more recent report has also provided evidence that US28 can respond to different chemokines depending on the resident cell infected by CMV, a finding that shows the adaptation of this virus to different host cells [305]. Together, these and other studies suggest that the large coding sequence of CMV encodes proteins that are essential for efficient replication and for spread within the infected animal, but probably has little, if any, function in in vitro replication of virus.

HOST IMMUNITY AND PATHOGENESIS OF CYTOMEGALOVIRUS INFECTIONS

In normal hosts, innate and adaptive cellular immune responses can limit, but not prevent, the spread of CMV from secondary sites such as the liver and spleen. The roles of innate and adaptive cellular immune responses in the control of virus replication and spread to other sites have been extensively investigated in experimental animal models of CMV infection [308,309]. Increased levels of virus replication follow the loss of either group of cellular immune responses [309–313]. The importance of innate immunity, including natural killer (NK) cell responses and interferon responses, has been repeatedly shown in small animal models of human CMV infections [309,314]. The loss of virus-specific CD4+ or CD8+ cytotoxic T lymphocyte (CTL) responses is associated with uncontrolled virus replication and lethal disease in these models [310,312,313,315]. The role of virus-specific antibodies has also been defined in these models; these antibodies seem to contribute minimally to control of local virus replication, but play a key role in limiting blood-borne dissemination of the virus [316,317].

Antiviral antibody responses can control virus replication even in animals devoid of T lymphocytes, suggesting a critical role of this adaptive response to protective immunity to this virus [318]. A more recent study described the role of antiviral antibodies in limiting spread of murine CMV to specific organs, providing additional evidence for an important function of antiviral antibodies in control of virus dissemination [317]. These findings are of interest because in this model of CMV infection, virus spread is almost entirely by cell-associated virus and not cell-free virus, raising several questions, including regarding the mechanism by which antiviral antibodies restrict virus dissemination [221,284].

Consistent with the findings in experimental animal models, studies in immunocompromised human hosts have repeatedly shown that deficits in innate immunity and the loss of adaptive immune responses predispose the host to CMV infections and, depending on the severity of the immune deficit, can lead to invasive

disease resulting in significant morbidity and mortality [178,319–326]. Several striking examples of the relationship between deficits in adaptive immunity and invasive CMV disease have been documented, including the development of pneumonitis in bone marrow and cardiac allograft recipients, prolonged CMV viremia and end-organ disease such as retinitis in AIDS patients with high viral (human immunodeficiency virus [HIV]) burdens and low CD4+ lymphocyte counts, and in fetuses infected in utero.

Perhaps the most convincing evidence for the critical role of T-lymphocyte responses in host resistance to invasive CMV infection was provided in studies in bone marrow allograft recipients who received ex vivo expanded CMV-specific CD8+ CTLs and were transiently protected from invasive CMV infection compared with a group of historical control patients, a finding that suggested that in this case CMV-specific CD8+ effector cells served only to control virus replication, but not eliminate virus infection [321]. Another interesting finding from this study was that patients who failed to generate CMV-specific CD4+ lymphocyte responses failed to generate long-term protection from CMV and developed invasive infections late in the course of their transplant [178,321]. This observation predated more recent studies that have shown that a CD4+ response is required for maintenance of long-term immunity to infectious agents [327–331].

Effector cells and mediators of the innate immune response have also been shown to be critical for control of CMV infections. Although most studies have been done in murine models of CMV infections, loss of NK cell activity and invasive CMV infection has been reported [332–336]. More recent studies have also suggested that individuals with specific defects in innate immune responses, such as those associated with interferon responses, may be at increased risk for herpesvirus infections, although CMV infections have not been identified in these individuals [337,338]. As noted earlier, in murine models, NK cells and interferons have been shown to play a critical role in resistance to murine CMV infection and seem to represent an initial host response that can limit virus replication and spread during the development of more efficient effector functions of the adaptive immune system [339,340].

In contrast to the role of antiviral antibodies in limiting dissemination of murine CMV, the importance of antiviral antibodies in protective responses to human CMV infections remains controversial. Numerous studies have shown a correlation between antiviral antibody responses, particularly virus-neutralizing antibodies, and patient outcome [175,341–344]. In addition, studies in solid organ transplant patients given intravenous immunoglobulins containing anti-CMV antibodies have suggested that virus-specific antibodies can provide some degree of protection from invasive infections [345–350]. In other transplant populations, such as bone marrow allograft recipients, the efficacy of anti-CMV immunoglobulins remains unproven, and their use varies among different transplant centers [179,194,351–357]. Animal models other than mice have also indicated that antiviral antibodies could provide some degree of protection. In a guinea pig model of congenital CMV infection, passive transfer of anti–guinea pig CMV (gpCMV) antibodies limited maternal disease and disease in infected offspring [317,358,359].

A study in pregnant women suggested that passive transfer of antibodies could limit intrauterine transmission of CMV, reduce the incidence of significant disease, and lead to resolution of existing CNS defects [360]. The results of this study were provocative and have stirred considerable debate in this field of investigation. Aspects of the study design, clinical outcome measures, and uncertainty surrounding mechanisms of action of the immunoglobulin preparations all have contributed to the lack of a consensus on the validity of the results of this study; however, these results have increased interest in similar therapeutic approaches. Available data would argue for a role of antiviral antibodies in limiting disease caused by CMV, and in the case of intrauterine infections, antiviral antibodies could freely pass into the fetal circulation and, if protective, could alter the outcome of intrauterine infections. The ramifications for the mode of action of antiviral antibodies can be readily appreciated when the design of prophylactic vaccines is undertaken.

MODULATION OF HOST IMMUNE RESPONSE TO CYTOMEGALOVIRUS

Numerous laboratories have identified multiple viral genes whose products interfere with immune recognition and clearance of virus-infected cells. Table 23–7 describes some of these genes and their modes of action. The importance of these genes in the biology of CMV in vivo is not completely understood; however, animal models of CMV infection have allowed investigators to determine the importance of homologous genes during virus replication. The results from these studies have indicated that viral functions can actively interfere with virus

clearance during acute infection in experimental animals [361–365]. Although a complete discussion of these viral genes and their mechanisms of immune evasion is beyond the scope of this chapter, several pertinent observations can be made regarding the importance of these viral genes in the pathogenesis of CMV infections.

First, these genes do not prevent recognition and control of CMV infections in normal hosts, as evidenced by the limited pathogenicity of this virus in normal individuals and in experimental animal models. Some investigators have argued that the phenotype of these viral genes can be appreciated only in immunocompromised hosts. The vast amount of literature describing the function of immune evasion genes has described studies carried out in experimental animals and during acute infection. In most studies, the function of these viral genes has been evaluated only in a few target organs, raising the question of whether some of these genes could be tissue-specific. Finally, other investigators have raised the question of whether these genes function to focus the immune response to a few viral antigens, restricting the available antigens for immune recognition. These viruses have committed a large amount of their genome to immune evasion functions (an estimated 20 genes in the genome of CMV), however, and many of these genes are conserved in animal and human CMVs. Studies in experimental animals have shown that immune evasion functions facilitate tissue-specific virus replication advantage in vivo [362,364,365]. These observations suggest that these genes almost certainly play a critical role in the biology of these viruses.

Immune evasion functions encoded by CMVs have been shown to interfere with innate immune responses and adaptive immune responses to virus-infected cells. In addition, mutations that result in mutation in viral structural proteins and in viral proteins recognized by the immune system also seem to allow escape from

TABLE 23–7 Mechanisms of Cytomegalovirus Modulation of Host Immune Responses

	Viral Gene	Mechanism
Innate Immune Responses		
↓ Intrinsic cellular response to virus infection	UL82	Inhibits function of cellular Daxx function (degradation)
↓ Interferon responses	UL83 (pp65)	↓ IRFs, ↓ NF-κB
	TRS1	↓ PKR activity
↓ NK cell activity	UL18	MHC class I decoy
	UL40	↑ HLA-E expression
Adaptive Immune Responses		
↓ CD8+, MHC restricted CTL	US2, US3, US11	↓ Class I expression
↓ CD4+ responses	US2	HLA-DR degradation
	US6	Blocks TAP transport
↓ Antibody activity	TRL11	Viral Fc receptor
Antigenic variation	UL73, UL55, UL75	Loss of antibody binding
Cytokines, Chemokine Responses		
Chemokine receptors (GPCRs)	US28, US27	GPCR acts a sink for extracellular chemokines
Chemokines	UL21.5	Chemokine receptor decoy inhibits RANTES
Cytokine	UL111a	Viral IL-10

immunologic control. Mutations in CMV viral genes encoding targets of dominant CD8$^+$ CTL responses have been reported [366]. One murine CMV gene, m157, previously shown to activate NK responses through NK receptor Ly49H in strains of mice that were genetically resistant to murine CMV infection, acquired mutations within weeks of infection [367,368]. Viruses with mutations in m157 were shown to replicate to higher titers in strains of resistant mice. This mutational event seems to be secondary to immune selection because genetically susceptible strains of mice that do not use this NK cell activation pathway do not generate viruses with mutations in the m157 gene [368].

Antigenic variation in virion envelope glycoproteins that are targets of virus-neutralizing antibodies have been well described. Strain-specific neutralizing antibody responses to the envelope glycoprotein B have been described [369,370]. In addition, a study of the polymorphic envelope glycoprotein N suggested that immune selection was responsible for the variation in amino acid sequence of gN derived from different virus isolates [266,371]. CMVs, including human CMV, can evade immune recognition by various active mechanisms, such as immune evasion genes, and by more conventional strategies, such as loss of antigenic determinants or loss of key antigens required for activation and recognition by immune cells.

PATHOGENESIS OF ACUTE INFECTIONS

Very early in the study of CMV infections, disease manifestations associated with congenital and perinatal CMV infections were related to the level of virus excretion, a marker for virus replication [372]. Subsequent studies in allograft recipients and in patients with AIDS have confirmed these findings and have consistently shown that increased levels of CMV replication in these patients was a key predictor of invasive disease. Unchecked virus replication and dissemination leads to multiorgan disease as illustrated by autopsy studies of neonates with congenital CMV infections, allograft recipients, and AIDS patients.

Studies in rhesus macaques infected with rhesus CMV have yielded results consistent with the proposed pathogenesis of human infection and provided a more detailed view of infection with this virus [373]. In these studies, virus given either intravenously or by a mucosal route resulted in blood-borne dissemination and widespread infection of numerous organs, including the liver and spleen [373]. The kinetics of the virus replication were different within the two groups with a lag in peak virus titers and liver infection noted in animals inoculated by a mucosal route. This result suggested that a local or regional amplification of virus was required after mucosal infection before blood-borne dissemination to the liver and spleen. This finding is consistent with experimental findings in guinea pigs and mice infected with CMVs [287,374–376].

The rhesus macaques that were inoculated by mucosal exposure remained asymptomatic and failed to exhibit clinical and laboratory abnormalities observed in animals given virus intravenously [373]. Together, these findings

parallel clinical and laboratory findings in humans with infections from community exposures versus infections derived from blood products. Human infections after parenteral exposure to virus often exhibit similar clinical and laboratory abnormalities as described in these experimental animal models.

The dissemination of CMV from the liver and spleen to distal sites likely occurs in normal immunocompetent individuals and in immunocompromised hosts. It is also quite likely, however, that the quantity and duration of the viral dissemination are different in these two populations. In contrast to community-acquired CMV infections in normal adults, persistent viral DNAemia as detected by PCR is characteristic of populations with disseminated CMV infections, such as AIDS patients or infants with symptomatic congenital CMV infection [195,377–382]. It seems that the natural history of CMV infection includes local replication at mucosal sites followed by amplification of virus locally and possibly in regional lymphoid tissue and spread to the viscera such as liver and spleen. Virus replication in these organs further increases the quantity of viruses, and virus then spreads to distal organs and sites of persistence, such as the salivary glands and renal tubules.

From observations in humans and in experimental models of infection, symptomatic infection seems to be related to the level of virus replication in sites seeded by the primary viremia, such as the liver and spleen. It follows that parenteral exposure from sources such as contaminated blood is associated with symptomatic infections because a larger viral inoculum is delivered to organs such as the liver, often in the absence of a developing immune response that would normally be present after infection of a mucosal surface. The duration of virus replication is likely represents a composite of the level of dissemination and the efficiency of the host immune response in the control of replicating CMV.

PATHOGENESIS OF CENTRAL NERVOUS SYSTEM INFECTIONS IN CONGENITALLY INFECTED INFANTS

The disease manifestations of congenital CMV infections include manifestations seen in adult immunocompromised hosts with disseminated CMV infections, such as hepatitis and, infrequently, pneumonitis and adrenalitis [383–385]. Unique to congenital CMV infection is the presence of CNS disease, a manifestation rarely seen even in the most immunocompromised allograft recipients. CMV encephalitis has been reported in patients with AIDS, but this disease can be distinctly different clinically and pathologically from CMV infection of the CNS associated with intrauterine infection [383,386]. CNS involvement in infants with congenital CMV infections often is associated with ongoing disease, such as progressive hearing loss during the first few years of life, at a time when there is no apparent progression of structural damage in the CNS [207–211, 387–393].

The pathogenesis of CMV CNS infection in the developing fetus is poorly understood for several reasons, including the lack of a sufficiently large number of cases from autopsy studies. In addition, there are no well-developed animal models of CNS infection associated with congenital CMV infection. The murine CMV model is useful for the study of many aspects of CMV infection, but congenital infection with murine CMV does not occur in mice. The other widely employed small animal model, the guinea pig, can be used to study intrauterine infections, and early reports suggested that CNS infections developed in these animals [394,395]. The usefulness of this model for studying CNS infection has not been defined, however, and because only a few observational studies have been reported, it has been difficult to assess its value as an informative model. The rhesus macaque offers perhaps the most relevant model for the study of CMV CNS infections for several obvious reasons, including the similarities in brain development shared between macaques and humans. In addition, rhesus CMV is more closely related to CMV than the rodent and guinea pig CMVs. This model is expensive, however, and these experimental animals are in limited supply secondary to their use in studies of HIV. For these reasons, our understanding of CNS infection with CMV remains limited.

Infection of the developing CNS is associated with many structural abnormalities that are dependent on the age of fetus at the time of CNS infection. Imaging studies of living infants and children with congenital CMV infections and clinical findings consistent with CNS disease have been informative. Commonly noted abnormalities include periventricular calcifications, ventriculomegaly, and loss of white-gray matter demarcation [396–398]. More refined imaging studies have detailed loss of normal brain architecture with loss of normal radial neuronal migration and cerebellar hypoplasia [399–408]. Limited autopsy studies have confirmed these imaging abnormalities and have shown the presence of inflammatory infiltrates in the parenchyma of the brain [397]. This latter finding is consistent with the presence of increased protein and inflammatory cells in spinal fluid obtained from congenitally infected infants with CNS disease. Together, these findings argue for a pathogenic spectrum that likely includes lytic infection of neuronal progenitor cells in the subventricular gray area, vasculitis with loss of supporting vessels in the developing brain, and meningoencephalitis with release of inflammatory mediators.

It is unclear why the fetal and newborn brain are susceptible to CMV infection in contrast to the adult brain; however, findings from experimental models suggest that the developing cells of the CNS are particularly susceptible to the lytic or possibly the apoptotic effects of CMVs [409–411]. In animal models, including mice and rhesus macaques, infection of the developing CNS results in widespread lytic virus replication, including neuronal progenitor cells of the subventricular gray area and endothelium [412–414]. Lytic virus replication in this area would lead to loss of normal neuronal development, radial migration, and vascularity of the developing brain. Extravasation of blood from damaged microvasculature would lead to calcifications that are prominent findings in imaging studies of CMV-infected newborn infants. Virus could spread through the ventricular system and infect additional areas of the subventricular germinal zone.

The more severe manifestations of CMV CNS infection can be explained by lytic virus infection of neuronal progenitor cells, glial cells in the CNS, and destruction of supporting vasculature. As indicated previously, intracerebral inoculation of fetal rhesus macaques with rhesus CMV results in similar findings as described in severely affected human infants and suggests that if CMV enters the CNS early in development, significant structural damage ensues.

Other infants infected in utero with CMV exhibit clinical findings consistent with CNS involvement, including developmental delays and loss of perceptual functions, but do not have structural damage of the brain that can be detected by routine imaging techniques. At least one autopsy series suggested that affected infants without calcifications can have neuronal migration deficits manifest as pachygyria and other abnormalities such as cerebellar hypoplasia [397,404,408]. The mechanisms leading to loss of normal architecture are unknown, but could be related to ongoing inflammation in the CNS secondary to intrauterine meningoencephalitis. Various inflammatory mediators have been shown to cause loss of neuron and supporting cell function and can modify vascular permeability and endothelial function. Evidence from experimental animal models has suggested that cytokines and chemokines may directly influence neuronal radial migration [415,416]. Ongoing inflammation may result in loss of normal brain architecture secondary to delayed or absent radial migration of neurons destined for the cerebral cortex [417].

PATHOGENESIS OF HEARING LOSS ASSOCIATED WITH CONGENITAL CYTOMEGALOVIRUS INFECTION

Hearing loss is one of the most common long-term sequelae of congenital CMV infection, and its pathogenesis is perhaps the least understood of any manifestation of CMV infection. As discussed in preceding sections, hearing loss can range from mild to profound, can be unilateral or bilateral, and can develop or progress after the perinatal period. It is possible that hearing impairment may represent a common outcome resulting from CMV infections in different parts of the auditory apparatus or, alternatively, resulting from infection in different stages in the development of the auditory system.

Besides the potential complexity of the disease, several other reasons likely contribute to the lack of understanding of the pathogenesis of hearing loss that follows congenital CMV infection. One of the most apparent is the lack of adequate histopathologic examinations of affected tissue from infected infants. A literature review revealed that only 12 temporal bones from congenitally infected infants have been studied and described in the medical literature [418]. In addition, most of the studies were done without the aid of modern techniques of virus and viral antigen detection and relied almost entirely on conventional histologic examinations. These limitations together with the lack of adequate information on the maternal and fetal infection have resulted in the lack of solid clues to the possible mechanisms of virus-induced damage to the auditory system.

Hearing loss in CNS infections in adults with AIDS or transplant infections is rare and not well described, presumably because these infections differ significantly from congenital CMV infection in the extent of CNS involvement and the underlying diseases and treatment that lead to CNS infection in these immunocompromised patients, and perhaps most importantly, congenital CMV infections occur during development. Finally, animal models of CMV hearing loss have been developed and have provided some information regarding selected aspects of the hearing loss associated with CMV. They have generally failed to recapitulate the disease, however, and in some cases early findings have been difficult to reproduce. More recently, a murine model of perinatal (congenital?) CMV infection and hearing loss has been developed that could provide some insight into the pathogenesis of the human disease (Bradford R, Britt W, unpublished).

Strauss [419,420] provided a comprehensive review of temporal bone pathology in infants with congenital CMV infection. The specimens in this series were from infants who died between 3 weeks and 5 months of age. A single case report of a 14-year-old patient with severe neuromuscular sequelae resulting from congenital CMV was described [421]. Findings in the inner ear, cochlea, vestibular system, and auditory and vestibular neural structures were described in all patients. Five of the original nine specimens had evidence of endolabyrinthitis, and virus was isolated from the endolymph in three of the nine specimens [420]. Viral antigen was detected by immunofluorescence in two cases in which routine histology failed to show viral inclusions [207]. Cochlear and vestibular findings were variable and ranged from rare inclusion-bearing cells in or adjacent to the sensory neuroepithelium of the cochlea or vestibular system to more extensive involvement of the nonsensory epithelium. Routine histology failed to detect viral inclusions in the auditory and vestibular neural structures, but viral antigens were detected in the spiral ganglion when specimens were examined by immunofluorescence [207]. Inflammatory infiltrates were minimal and reported in only three patients in this series [420]. Perhaps the most interesting results were those reported in the examination of tissue from the 14-year-old patient with extensive sequelae from congenital CMV infection. In this patient, extensive cellular degeneration, fibrosis, and calcifications were observed in the cochlea and vestibular systems [421].

Several generalizations can be made from these limited data. First, in all but two of these cases, virus, viral antigens, or histopathologic findings consistent with virus infection were present in the cochlea or vestibular apparatus. These findings indicate that virus replication could have occurred in the sensory neuroepithelium and nonsensory epithelium and that cellular damage could be explained by a direct viral cytopathic effect. In addition, viral-induced damage can also result from bystander effects secondary to immune-mediated cytopathology. CMV could induce loss of sensory neuroepithelium in the absence of direct infection of the sensory neuroepithelium, but secondary to infection of supporting epithelium followed by host immunopathologic responses. An inflammatory infiltrate was seen in only three of nine specimens, however, an unexpected finding based on the role that the inflammatory response is thought to play in CMV end-organ disease in other patient populations.

It is well documented that infants with congenital CMV have a delay in the development of immunologic responses to CMV, and it could be argued that findings in the cochlea and vestibular apparatus are consistent with the ineffectual immune responses of congenitally infected infants. An alternative and not exclusive possibility is that infection of the inner ear structures is a late, and in some cases a postnatal, event. The relationship between susceptibility of cells of the sensory neuroepithelium and supporting epithelium to infection with CMV and their developmental status is unknown. These cells could be resistant to CMV infection until late in development. In this case, findings from specimens of the above-described autopsy series may reflect recent infection before host inflammatory responses. Such an explanation is inconsistent, however, with the course of fetal CMV infection in other parts of the CNS in most of the patients included in autopsy studies. A third possibility is that hearing loss in some infected infants is related to alterations in the neural networks leading from the cochlea to the eighth cranial nerve. Finally, the finding of extensive degenerative changes together with fibrosis and calcifications in the temporal bones from the oldest patient presumably reflects the natural history of CMV labyrinthitis and, depending on the rate at which these changes develop, could also explain the progressive nature of hearing loss associated with congenital CMV infection.

The loss of neuroepithelium, secondary to either direct virus-mediated damage or host-derived inflammation followed by fibrosis, would be consistent with the profound hearing impairment that develops in some children with congenital CMV infection. Findings in experimental animal models have indicated that exaggerated deposition of extracellular matrix is part of the inflammatory response in the inner ear, and this host response possibly leads to the ossification that is observed in animals inoculated directly into the labyrinth with CMV [422,423].

Studies in animal models have provided limited insight into the pathogenesis of hearing loss after congenital CMV infection. Small animal models have provided some information and have mirrored findings in humans. Virus and inflammation are required for the development of pathology in the inner ear. A study in guinea pigs showed that virus infection in immunocompromised animals was not associated with the typical pathologic findings of virus infection in normal animals [422]. Similarly, blocking virus replication with antiviral compounds or pretreating animals with virus-neutralizing antibodies limited the development of inner ear pathology [424–429]. From the available studies, the pathogenesis of hearing loss associated with congenital CMV infection requires virus replication and a host immune response. Interrupting either virus replication or the local host inflammatory response could offer some therapeutic benefit to these patients.

NATURE OF MATERNAL INFECTION

The nature of the maternal infection is a major pathogenetic factor for congenital CMV infection. Primary infections are more likely to be transmitted to the fetus and are thought to be more frequently associated with fetal damage than recurrent infections [430]. With primary CMV infection, as in other infections during pregnancy, there seems to be some innate barrier against vertical transmission [121,122,212,431,432]. Intrauterine transmission after primary infection occurs in 30% to 40% of cases [121,212]. Current information suggests that gestational age has no apparent influence on the risk of transmission of CMV in utero [121,122,212,431,433]. With regard to the role of gestational age on the expression of disease in the fetus and offspring, infection at an earlier gestational age has been associated with more severe disease and worse outcome [122,212,431,432,434]. Definition of the interval in pregnancy in which maternal seroconversion occurred does not define a similar time of fetal infection, however.

Congenital infection may also result from recurrences of infection [121,153–155,157,158,435–440]. The term *recurrence* is used here to represent either reactivation of infection or reinfection with the same or a different strain of CMV during pregnancy. Despite the inability of maternal immunity to prevent transmission of this virus to the fetus, congenital infections that result from recurrent infections are thought to be less likely to produce clinical evidence of disease in infected offspring than those resulting from primary infections [121,430]. The relationship between primary infection and clinically apparent congenital infection in offspring was challenged initially by studies from Sweden and more recently in the United States and other regions of the world [157,158,436–444]. These studies have shown that clinically apparent congenital infections are frequently observed in infants infected after a recurrent maternal infection and that long-term sequelae such as hearing loss can be present in such infants. Clinical experience continues to suggest, however, that severe multiorgan disease in congenitally infected infants should suggest the possibility of primary maternal infection.

The risk of congenital CMV infection resulting from a recurrence of infection during pregnancy ranges from 1.5% for a U.S. population of low socioeconomic background to 0.19% for women of middle or upper socioeconomic background from the United States, Great Britain, or Sweden [121,212,441,445]. In the developing world, studies in maternal populations with near-universal seroimmunity have shown congenital infection rates of 1% to 2%, and infants with clinically apparent infections and infants who develop long-term sequelae from congenital CMV infections have been described in these populations [153,157,158,439,446].

In recurrent infection, it is likely that preexisting maternal immunity could alter the parameters of CMV in the mother and developing fetus at least to some extent. It is unknown if preexisting cellular immunity is more important than humoral immunity; however, maternal IgG antibodies are transmitted to the fetus and at a first approximation could alter the virologic parameters of fetal infection. Several cases of symptomatic congenital infection have been reported in offspring of women after therapeutic immunosuppression, women with lupus or AIDS, and women with intact immune systems, suggesting that altered maternal immunity either from immunosuppression or from an inability to recognize a recurrent

maternal infection (reinfection) can lead to fetal infection and disease [441,447–452].

In the rhesus macaque model of CMV neuropathogenesis, a direct infection of the developing rhesus fetus can lead to disease even in the presence of maternal T-lymphocyte and antiviral antibody immunity to the virus [413]. This result would argue that when virus enters the fetus, a critical balance between fetal immunity, maternal immunity that can be transferred to the fetus, and viral inoculum determines the extent and severity of fetal infection. Such a complex relationship between virus and immunity suggests that analysis of specimens derived from human natural history studies would likely provide only a limited insight into this intrauterine infection.

PERINATAL INFECTION

Naturally acquired perinatal CMV infections result from exposure to infected maternal genital secretions at birth or to breast milk during the first months of postnatal life [130,131,453,454]. The presence of CMV at these two sites may be the result of either primary or recurrent maternal infection. Iatrogenic CMV infections are acquired predominantly from transfusions of blood or blood products and, in the past, banked breast milk from CMV-infected donors. Exposure to CMV in the maternal genital tract can result in a 30% to 50% rate of perinatal infection. The transmission from mother to infant through breast milk occurs in 30% to 70% if nursing lasts for more than 1 month [130,131,165,455–459]. After ingestion of the virus, CMV infection is presumably established at a mucosal surface (buccal, pharyngeal, or esophageal mucosa) or in the salivary glands, for which CMV is known to have a special tropism. Perinatal CMV infections occasionally and congenital CMV infections rarely have been associated with pneumonitis; in early reports, CMV pneumonia was reported to account for significant mortality in congenitally infected infants [173].

Transmission of CMV by blood transfusion is more likely to occur when large quantities of blood are transfused, providing some clues as to the nature of persistence of CMV in cells of the blood and an indirect assessment of the frequency of CMV-infected cells in the blood. The failure to isolate CMV from the blood or blood elements of healthy seropositive blood donors suggests that the virus exists in a latent state, presumably within leukocytes. It has been suggested that CMV reactivates after transfusion when infected cells encounter the allogeneic stimulus. CMV genomes are activated when transfused to a recipient, particularly if immunologically immature or deficient.

PERSISTENT VIRAL EXCRETION

Congenitally and perinatally acquired CMV infections are characterized by chronic viral excretion [384]. Virus is consistently shed into the urine for 6 years or longer and into saliva for 2 to 4 years. Not only does excretion persist much longer in congenitally infected infants than in infected older children and adults, but also the quantity of virus excreted is much greater. Even asymptomatic, congenitally or perinatally infected infants excrete quantities of virus that usually exceed quantities detectable in seriously ill

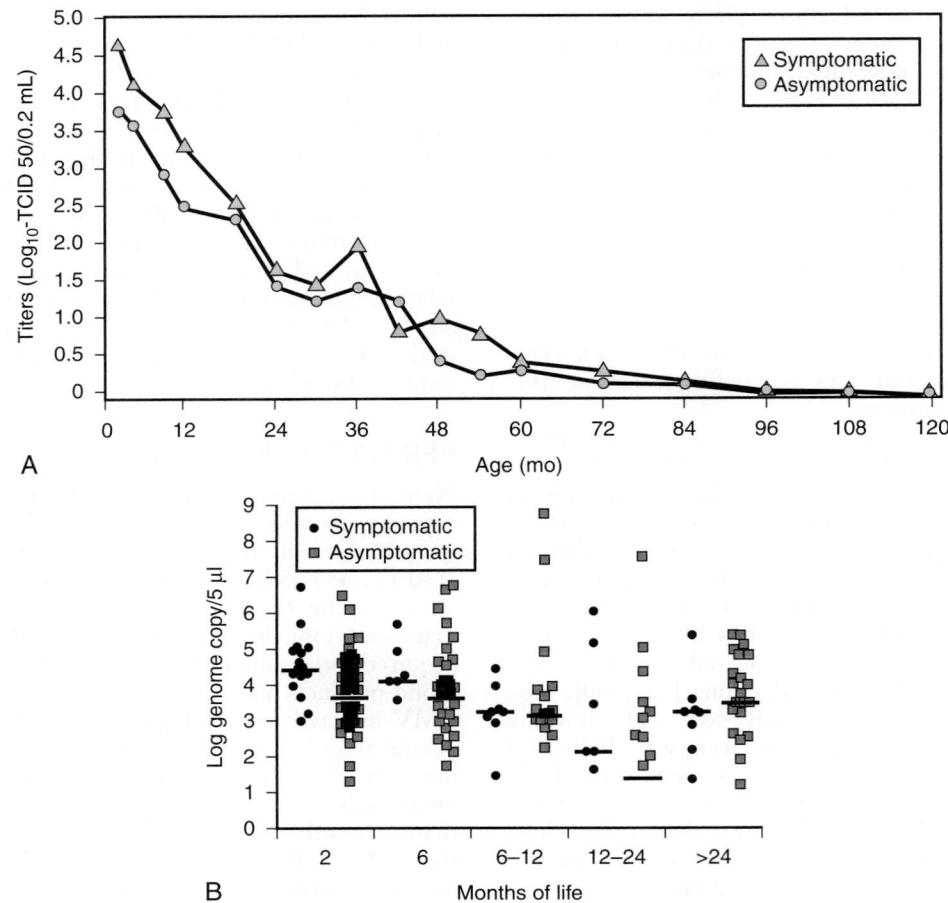

FIGURE 23–3 **A,** Viral load detected by urine excretion of infectious virus in infants with symptomatic and asymptomatic congenital human cytomegalovirus infection as a function of age. Titers are expressed as log of tissue culture infectious doses (TCID) in which 50% of wells contained virus. **B,** Genomic copies of human cytomegalovirus in blood from congenitally infected infants with symptomatic (●) and asymptomatic (■) infections. Median values are designated by *red horizontal bars.*

immunocompromised older patients by 1 to 2 logs. As illustrated in Figure 23–3A, the highest quantities of virus are excreted during the first 6 months of life. Infants with symptomatic congenital CMV infection excrete significantly larger amounts than infants with asymptomatic congenitally or perinatally acquired infections. Similar results have been obtained when peripheral blood of congenitally infected infants has been analyzed by quantitative polymerase chain reaction (PCR) (Fig. 23–3B) [460]. A relationship has been identified between the viral DNA copy number in peripheral blood and long-term outcome suggesting that monitoring congenitally infected infants by this assay could identify infants at risk for sequelae and select a population of congenitally infected infants that could be considered as potential candidates for treatment with antiviral agents (see following sections) [460,461].

PATHOLOGY

Early reports of histopathologic changes associated with CMV infections relied on a demonstration of classic changes characterized by cytomegaly and nuclear and cytoplasmic inclusions. The distinctive features include large cells 20 to 35 mm in diameter with a large nucleus containing round, oval, or reniform inclusions. These large inclusions are separated from the nuclear membrane by a clear zone, which gives the inclusion the so-called owl's eye appearance. The inclusions within the nucleus show DNA positivity by histochemical staining, whereas the cytoplasmic inclusions contain carbohydrates, as evidenced by periodic acid–Schiff positivity. The cytoplasmic inclusions vary from minute dots to distinct rounded bodies 3 to 4 mm in diameter. The cytoplasmic inclusions are usually aggregated opposite to the eccentrically placed inclusion-bearing nucleus and seem to represent a cytoplasmic site of virus assembly [462]. The classic CMV inclusion-bearing cell may be only scattered throughout involved tissue and missed by routine sectioning. This finding has been confirmed when more refined techniques, such as in situ DNA hybridization and immunofluorescence using CMV-specific monoclonal antibodies, have been used to define the extent of infection with CMV in immunocompromised patients.

COMMONLY INVOLVED ORGAN SYSTEMS

Disseminated disease can occur in the infected fetus and the congenitally infected infant. CMV can cause a multisystem disease in which almost all major organ systems are involved [383].

Central Nervous System

Involvement of the CNS is perhaps the most important consequence of fetal infection with CMV. Most descriptions of the pathology of CNS infection are relevant only to infants with severe CID, which is occasionally fatal [383,397,463–465]. In most infected infants, the infection can be described grossly as focal encephalitis and periependymitis. Encephalitis can involve cells of the gray and the white matter and cells within the choroid plexus. Inclusion-bearing cells have been identified in neurons, glia, ependyma, choroid plexus, meninges, and vascular endothelium and in cells lying free in the ventricles. Rarely, inclusion-bearing cells have been identified in the cerebrospinal fluid [466]. Resolution of acute encephalitis leads to gliosis and calcification. Previous descriptions have emphasized the periventricular location of calcifications; however, these lesions can be located anywhere in the brain [398,404,408].

CMV has been isolated on a few occasions from cerebrospinal fluid, and PCR has been used more recently to show CMV in the cerebrospinal fluid [467,468]. The only other patients with a significant incidence of CMV encephalitis are individuals with HIV/AIDS. Infection of the CNS by CMV is well described in these patients and has been characterized as ventriculoencephalitis in which the virus is thought to spread through the ventricular system and result in widespread disease in the periventricular neuroepithelium and a second more common form described as a focal encephalitis [386].

CMV infection of structures of the hearing apparatus has been described as noted in the previous sections. Viral inclusion-bearing cells and viral antigen–containing cells can also be found within structures of the inner ear, including the organ of Corti, and in epithelial cells of striae vascularis of the cochleae [207,469–471]. Finally, involvement of the eye, including chorioretinitis, optic neuritis, cataract formation, colobomas, and microphthalmos, has been shown [207,472–474]. The histopathologic changes associated with retinitis begin as an acute vasculitis that spreads into the choroid through the vascular basement membrane. CMV has been isolated from fluid of the anterior chamber of the eye [475]. Anecdotal cases of cataracts have been described in congenitally infected infants. Finally, the clinical findings of infants with CMV chorioretinitis differ from the clinical findings of HIV/AIDS patients with retinitis in that level of retinal involvement is often less; the cellular infiltrate and retinal edema are also limited when the findings in these patients are compared with patients with HIV/AIDS. Chorioretinitis in congenitally infected infants has been associated with an increased risk of long-term cognitive disorders in congenitally infected infants [476].

Liver

Involvement of the liver is common in congenital CMV infections. Clinical evidence of hepatitis as manifested by hepatomegaly, elevated levels of serum transaminases, and direct hyperbilirubinemia is frequently seen in infants with symptomatic congenital infections. Pathologic descriptions of hepatic involvement include mild cholangitis with CMV infections of bile duct cells, intralobular

cholestasis, and obstructive cholestasis secondary to extramedullary hematopoiesis [383]. Liver calcifications have been detected radiologically in infants with congenital infections [477,478]. Clinical and laboratory evidence of liver disease eventually subsides in surviving infants, and only anecdotal cases of cirrhosis have been reported.

Hematopoietic System

Hematologic abnormalities, including thrombocytopenia, anemia, and extramedullary hematopoiesis, are common in symptomatically infected infants, but these abnormalities almost invariably resolve within the 1st year of life. The exact mechanism accounting for these disturbances is uncertain, although congestive splenomegaly resulting in platelet and red blood cell trapping must play some part in the overall process. Significant splenomegaly is common, and congestion, extramedullary hematopoiesis, and diminished size of lymphoid follicles can be seen histologically.

In congenital CMV infections, thrombocytopenia may persist for several months or years, with or without petechiae. Anemia is another feature of symptomatic congenital CMV infection. The presence of indirect hyperbilirubinemia, extramedullary hematopoiesis, and erythroblastemia indicates active hemolysis, but mechanisms that account for these findings have not been well described.

Kidneys

Macroscopically, the kidneys show no alterations. Microscopically, inclusion-bearing cells are commonly seen, especially in the cells lining the distal convoluted tubules and collecting ducts [383,479]. Affected cells may desquamate into the lumens of the tubules and appear in the urine sediment. Inclusions can be found occasionally in Bowman capsules and proximal tubules. Mononuclear cell infiltration may be present in the peritubular zones of the kidney.

Endocrine Glands

Secretory cells of endocrine glands commonly contain typical CMV inclusions. In the pancreas, the endocrine and the exocrine cells are affected [383]. Some reports describe intralobular or periductal mononuclear infiltration, suggesting focal pancreatitis. There is no credible association between congenital CMV infection and the development of diabetes mellitus. CMV inclusion-bearing cells have been documented in follicular cells of the thyroid, the adrenal cortex, and the anterior pituitary.

Gastrointestinal Tract

The salivary glands are commonly involved in congenital and perinatal CMV infections. There are no reliable figures, however, on the frequency of involvement because the examination of the salivary glands is not always part of autopsies [383]. CMV inclusions have also been described in the mucosal surfaces of the esophagus, stomach, and intestine and in the vessels of ulcerative intestinal lesions [383,480].

Lungs

Pulmonary CMV lesions are similar in newborn and adults. Microscopically, most inclusion-bearing cells are alveolar cells that lay free in terminal air spaces. Generally, there is little inflammatory reaction; however, in the more severe cases, focal interstitial infiltration by lymphocytes and plasma cells can be found.

Placenta

Abnormalities are present in the placentas of most patients with symptomatic CMV infection and are infrequent with subclinical infections [481–485]. CMV DNA can be detected frequently in the decidua and placenta of seropositive women, even though the rate of congenital infection in this population is on the order of 1%, a finding that supported the hypothesis that the placenta represents a barrier for fetal infection [486–488]. Previous studies have suggested that placentas are not remarkable in size or macroscopic appearance; however, a more recent study suggested placenta enlargement in some women who delivered infected infants [489].

The most specific feature histologically is the presence of inclusion-bearing cells, which may be found in endothelial cells, in cells attached to the capillary walls, or in Hofbauer or stromal cells [482,484]. Other lesions include focal necrosis, which in early gestation shows sparse infiltration by lymphocytes, macrophages, and a few plasma cells. The early lesions manifest as foci of necrosis of the stroma and occasionally of the vessels of the villi. The focus of necrosis is later invaded by inflammatory cells, histiocytes, and fibroblasts. At later gestational ages, these focal lesions become densely cellular, with plasma cells predominating over lymphocytes. Deposition of intracellular and extracellular hemosiderin can be found in stem and terminal villi and is presumably the result of fetal hemorrhage during the necrotizing phase or of maternal intervillous thrombosis. Calcification within villi or on basement membranes has also been described as a late manifestation of placental CMV infection.

In recent years, there has been increased interest in understanding the role the placenta plays in congenital CMV infection [481,490]. In vitro systems have been developed to examine interactions between CMV and the placenta. Studies from these systems have uncovered a complex relationship between maternal immunity and the likelihood of CMV replication in distinct areas of the placenta and the decidua [249,481,491]. In addition, other investigators have noted that the immune tolerance of the placenta could limit efficient clearance of virus. The placenta produces the immunosuppressive chemokine IL-10, and expression of HLA-G in the placenta is thought to limit NK cell activity [492–497].

These findings have led investigators to suggest that CMV replication in the placenta is poorly controlled and that transmission to the fetus occurs after infection of cytotrophoblasts [491]. More recent studies have suggested that CMV can dysregulate the expression of proteins essential for normal placentation and that CMV infection of the placenta can lead to placental insufficiency and intrauterine growth restriction and potentially

other effects on the fetus [481]. This proposed mechanism of disease is consistent with a potential immunomodulatory role of passively transferred intravenous immunoglobulin in pregnant women [360]. A study in the guinea pig model of congenital infection that showed the protection from perinatal CMV disease by a recombinant virus expressing a guinea pig CMV envelope glycoprotein could be interpreted as reflecting the capacity of antiviral immunity to limit the placental insufficiency induced by guinea pig CMV infection in these pregnant animals [498].

CLINICAL MANIFESTATIONS
CONGENITAL INFECTION

Approximately 10% of the estimated 44,000 infants (1% of all live births) born annually with congenital CMV infection in the United States have signs and symptoms at birth that are consistent with the diagnosis of a congenital infection. Only half of these symptomatic infants have typical generalized CID, characterized mainly by the clinical manifestations listed in Table 23–8 [212,385,430,499,500]. Another 5% of these infants present with milder or atypical involvement, and 90% are born with subclinical congenital infection. Because early studies emphasized only symptomatic infections, congenital CMV was considered a rare and often fatal disease. In the early reports, many patients were referred to the investigators because of

TABLE 23–8   Clinical and Laboratory Findings in 106 Infants with Symptomatic Congenital Cytomegalovirus Infection in the Newborn Period

Clinical/Laboratory Abnormality	Positive/Total Examined (%)
Prematurity (<38 wk)	36/106 (34)
Small for gestational age	53/106 (50)
Petechiae	80/106 (76)
Jaundice	69/103 (67)
Hepatosplenomegaly	63/105 (60)
Purpura	14/105 (13)
Neurologic findings (one or more of the following)	72/106 (68)
Microcephaly	54/102 (53)
Lethargy/hypotonia	28/104 (27)
Poor suck	20/103 (19)
Seizures	7/105 (7)
Elevated alanine aminotransferase (>80 U/L)	46/58 (83)
Thrombocytopenia	
<100 × 10³/mm³	62/81 (77)
<50 × 10³/mm³	43/81 (53)
Conjugated hyperbilirubinemia	
Direct serum bilirubin >4 mg/dL	47/68 (69)
Hemolysis	37/72 (51)
Increased cerebrospinal fluid protein (>120 mg/dL)*	24/52 (46)

*Determinations in the 1st wk of life.
From Boppana S, et al. Symptomatic congenital cytomegalovirus infection: neonatal morbidity and mortality. Pediatr Infect Dis J 11:93-99, 1992.

abnormalities in normal development; this led to a selection bias of a group of patients at a higher risk for persistent abnormalities and neurologic damage. The use of more sensitive and specific methods of diagnosis, particularly viral isolation and newer methods of rapid virus detection, has allowed prospective longitudinal studies of newborns with symptomatic and asymptomatic congenital CMV infections. These studies have resulted in a more accurate understanding of the infection and its clinical spectrum.

Symptomatic Infection
Acute Manifestations

Clinically apparent infections or CID is characterized by involvement of multiple organs, in particular, the reticuloendothelial system and CNS, with or without ocular and auditory damage. Weller and Hanshaw [501] defined the abnormalities found most frequently in infants with symptomatic congenital infection as hepatomegaly, splenomegaly, microcephaly, jaundice, and petechiae. As shown in Table 23–8, petechiae, hepatosplenomegaly, and jaundice are the most frequently noted presenting signs.

In addition, the magnitude of the prenatal insult is reflected by the occurrence of microcephaly with or without cerebral calcification, intrauterine growth restriction, and prematurity.* Inguinal hernia in boys and chorioretinitis with or without optic atrophy are less common. Clinical findings occasionally include hydrocephalus, hemolytic anemia, and pneumonitis. Among the most severely affected infants, mortality rates may be 10% to 30% [173,385]. Most deaths occur in the neonatal period and are usually due to multiorgan disease with severe hepatic dysfunction, bleeding, disseminated intravascular coagulation, and secondary bacterial infections. When death occurs after the 1st month but during the 1st year, it is usually secondary to severe failure to thrive, possibly owing to ongoing liver disease and dysfunction. Death after the 1st year is usually restricted to severely neurologically damaged children and is due to malnutrition, aspiration pneumonia, and infections associated with neurologically impaired infants.

Hepatomegaly

Hepatomegaly, along with splenomegaly, is probably the most common abnormality found in the newborn period in infants born with a symptomatic congenital CMV infection [503]. The liver edge is smooth and nontender and usually measures 4 to 7 cm below the right costal margin. Liver function tests are often abnormal and reflect hepatocellular dysfunction and cholestasis. The persistence of hepatomegaly is variable. In some infants, liver enlargement disappears by age 2 months. In others, significant enlargement persists throughout the 1st year of life. Hepatomegaly extending beyond the first 12 months of life is an uncommon finding in infants with CID.

Splenomegaly

Enlargement of the spleen exists to a greater or lesser degree in all the common human congenital infections and is especially frequent in congenital CMV infections [385]. Splenomegaly may be the only abnormality present at birth. In some instances, splenomegaly and a petechial rash coexist as the only manifestations of disease. Occasionally, the enlargement is such that the spleen may be felt 10 to 15 cm below the costal margin. Splenomegaly usually persists longer than hepatomegaly.

Jaundice

Jaundice is a common manifestation of congenital CID. The pattern of hyperbilirubinemia may take several forms, ranging from high levels on the 1st day to undetectable jaundice on the 1st day with gradual elevation of the bilirubin level to clinically apparent jaundice. The level of jaundice in the early weeks of life may fluctuate considerably [385]. In some instances, jaundice is transient, beginning on the 1st day and disappearing by the end of the 1st week. More often, jaundice tends to persist beyond the time of physiologic jaundice. Transient jaundice may occasionally occur in early infancy with pronounced elevation of bilirubin levels during the 3rd month. Bilirubin levels are elevated in the direct and the indirect components. Characteristically, the direct component increases after the first few days of life and may constitute 50% of the total bilirubin level. Hepatic transaminases are elevated, but abnormalities in coagulation secondary to liver disease are infrequently observed.

Petechiae and Purpura

There is evidence from experimental animal models that CMV has a direct effect on the megakaryocytes of the bone marrow that results in a depression of the platelets and a localized or generalized petechial rash, although similar studies have not been done in humans infected with CMV. In some patients, the rash is purpuric (Fig. 23–4), similar to that observed in the expanded rubella syndrome.

In contrast to rubella, pinpoint petechiae are a more common manifestation. These petechiae are rarely present at birth, but often appear within a few hours thereafter; they may be transient, disappearing within 48 hours. The petechiae may be the only clinical manifestation of CMV infection. More often, enlargement of the spleen and liver is associated with the finding of petechiae. The petechiae may persist for weeks after birth. Crying, coughing, the application of a tourniquet, performance of a lumbar puncture, or application of restraints of any kind may result in the appearance of petechiae months after birth. Platelet counts in the 1st week of life range from less than 10,000/μL to 125,000/μL, with most in the range of 20,000/μL to 60,000/μL. Some infants with petechial rashes do not have associated thrombocytopenia. Significant bleeding is rarely, if ever, associated with the thrombocytopenia of congenital CMV infection.

Microcephaly

Microcephaly, currently defined in epidemiologic studies as a head circumference of less than the third percentile, was found to be present in 14 of 17 patients with CID

---

*References [86,368–371,385,396,398,404,408,431,444,502].

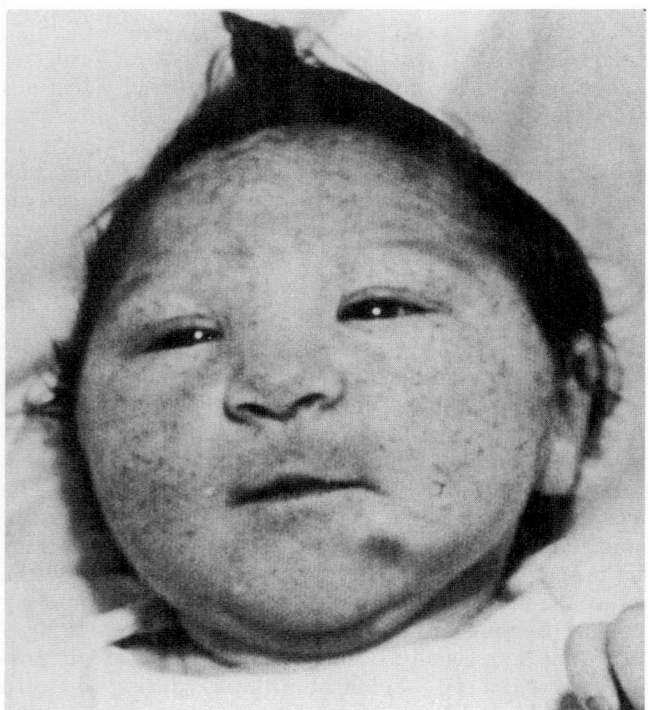

FIGURE 23–4 Symptomatic congenital cytomegalovirus infection manifested by microcephaly and petechiae.

in the early studies of Medearis [504] in 1964. As tissue culture methods became more widely used, and clinical awareness of the infection increased, microcephaly became a less prominent symptom in subsequent series that included mainly infants born with less severe disease. In a more recent examination of 106 surviving patients who were born with symptomatic CMV infection, 53% were microcephalic [385]. Not all infants who are microcephalic in the perinatal period continue to have head circumferences of less than the third percentile later in infancy. Microcephaly is the most specific predictor of future cognitive impairment in congenitally infected infants (this is especially true if the head measurement is close to the fifth percentile in an infant with low birth weight). Intracranial calcifications suggest that the infant will have at least moderate and probably severe delays in cognitive development [398,505].

Ocular Defects

The principal abnormality related to the eye in CMV infection is chorioretinitis, with strabismus and optic atrophy [207,398,473]. Microphthalmos, cataracts, retinal necrosis and calcification, blindness, anterior chamber and optic disk malformations, and pupillary membrane vestige have also been described in association with generalized congenital CID. Despite the aforementioned, the presence of abnormalities such as microphthalmos and cataracts is strong presumptive evidence that the disease process is not caused by CMV. Chorioretinitis has been reported to occur in approximately 14% of infants born with symptomatic congenital infection [398,473]. Although chorioretinitis occurs less frequently in

symptomatic congenital CMV than in congenital toxoplasmosis, lesions caused by CMV and *Toxoplasma* cannot be differentiated on the basis of location or appearance [207,473]. *Toxoplasma gondii* and CMV can induce central retinal lesions. Occasionally, the appearance of strabismus with subsequent referral to an ophthalmologist results in the diagnosis of chorioretinitis. Any infant with suspected CMV infection or strabismus in early life should be examined carefully for retinal lesions. Chorioretinitis caused by CMV differs, however, from that caused by *Toxoplasma* in that postnatal progression is uncommon.

Fetal Growth Restriction

Intrauterine growth restriction, occasionally severe, was reported in 50% of 106 patients with symptomatic congenital CMV infection, whereas prematurity occurred in 34% (see Table 23–8) [398]. Infants with asymptomatic congenital infection generally do not exhibit intrauterine growth restriction or prematurity, and CMV has not been considered a common cause of either condition in infants without overt clinical findings of congenital CMV infections.

Pneumonitis

Pneumonitis, a common clinical manifestation of CMV infection after hematopoietic and solid organ transplantation in adults, is not usually a part of the clinical presentation of congenital CMV infection in newborns. Diffuse interstitial pneumonitis occurs in less than 1% of congenitally infected infants, even when the most severely affected cases are considered. CMV-associated pneumonitis has been described in infants with perinatally acquired CMV infections [506].

Dental Defects

Congenital CMV infection is also associated with a distinct defect of enamel, which so far seems to affect mainly primary dentition [507]. This defect is more severe in children with the symptomatic form of the infection than in children born with asymptomatic infections (Fig. 23–5). The mechanism leading to enamel dysplasia in infants with congenital CMV is unknown.

Clinically, this defect appears on all or nearly all of the teeth and is characterized by generalized yellowish discoloration. The enamel is opaque and moderately soft and tends to chip away from dentin. Affected teeth tend to be susceptible to mechanical trauma leading to dental caries that are frequently seen in these children. In our longitudinal studies, this defect of enamel was documented in 27% of 92 children born with symptomatic congenital CMV infection and in 4% of 267 children who were born with the subclinical form and who were observed for at least 2 years. These patients usually require extensive orthodontic therapy. It is evident that these defects do not involve permanent teeth to the same degree.

Deafness

Sensorineural deafness is the most common handicap caused by congenital CMV infection. Medearis [504] was the first investigator to call attention to the presence

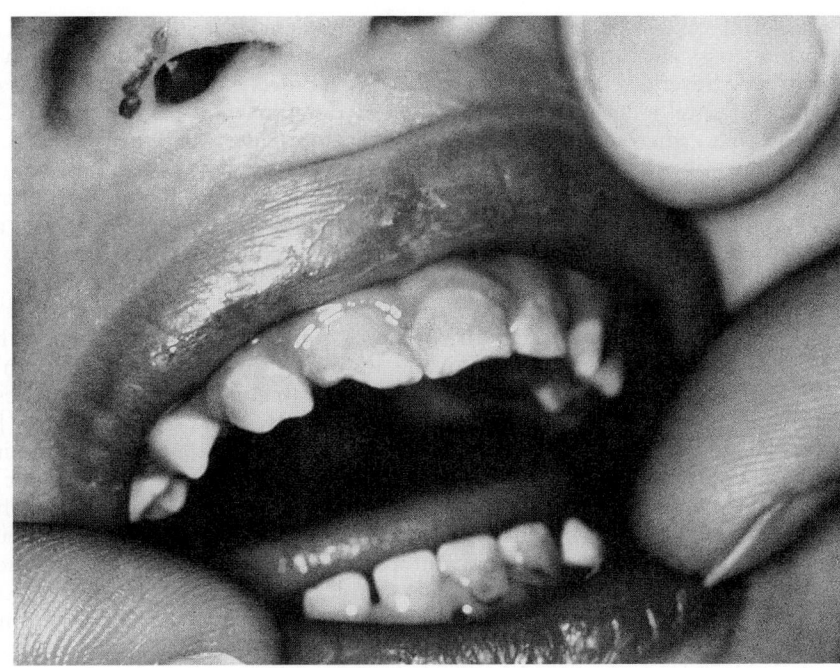

FIGURE 23–5 Cytomegalovirus-affected teeth. This patient had a clinically severe congenital cytomegalovirus infection. Note fractured borders and opaque and hypocalcified enamel.

TABLE 23–9 Sequelae in Children after Congenital Cytomegalovirus Infection

Sequelae	% Symptomatic (No.)	% Asymptomatic (No.)
Sensorineural hearing loss	58 (58/100)	7.4 (22/299)
Bilateral hearing loss	37 (37/100)	2.7 (8/299)
Speech threshold moderate to profound (60-90 dB)*	27 (27/100)	1.7 (5/299)
Chorioretinitis	20.4 (19/93)	2.5 (7/281)
IQ <70	55 (33/60)	3.7 (6/159)
Microcephaly, seizures, or paresis/paralysis	51.9 (54/104)	2.7 (9/330)
Microcephaly	37.5 (39/104)	1.8 (6/330)
Seizures	23.1 (24/104)	0.9 (3/330)
Paresis/paralysis	12.5 (13/104)	0 (0/330)
Death†	5.8 (6/104)	0.3 (1/330)

*For the ear with better hearing.
†After newborn period.
Adapted from Pass RF, Fowler KB, Boppana S. Progress in cytomegalovirus research. In *Landini MP (ed). Proceedings of the Third International Cytomegalovirus Workshop, Bologna, Italy, June 1991. London, Excerpta Medica, 1991, pp 3-10.*

of deafness in symptomatic congenitally infected infants. Subsequent reports confirmed this association and provided evidence that CMV can also cause sensorineural hearing loss in children with clinically inapparent congenital infection (Table 23–9).* CMV is now considered one of the most important causes of deafness in childhood and in the United States is thought to be the most common

*References [173,207–209,211,387,398,508–512].

etiology of nonfamilial sensorimotor hearing loss [211,513].

The frequency and severity of hearing impairment are increased in patients with symptomatic infection (58%) compared with asymptomatic infection at birth (7.4%). Generally, hearing loss is progressive in 50% of cases, bilateral in 50%, and of late onset in 20%. The predictors of hearing loss in children with symptomatic congenital CMV infection are intrauterine growth restriction, petechiae, hepatosplenomegaly, thrombocytopenia, and intracerebral calcifications. These are similarly the predictors of significantly higher viral loads in newborn infants [460,461,514,515]. The presence of microcephaly and other neurologic abnormalities in one study failed to predict hearing loss, however [514]. Using logistic regression analysis, only petechiae and intrauterine growth restriction were shown to be independent predictors of hearing loss. As noted previously, the viral load measured in peripheral blood predicts the hearing outcome of infants with congenital infection [460,461,515].

Long-Term Outcome

The likelihood of survival with normal intellect and hearing after symptomatic congenital CMV infection is small [173,385,473,516–521]. As shown in Table 23–9, in our prospective studies, one or more sequelae have occurred in nearly 90% of the patients with symptomatic congenital infection who survived [385].

Psychomotor retardation, usually combined with neurologic complications and microcephaly, occurred in nearly 70% of infants. Sensorineural hearing loss was seen in 50%. The hearing loss is bilateral in 67% of patients with hearing loss and is progressive in 54%. A more recent study from Europe reported a significant incidence of vestibular dysfunction in infants with congenital CMV [522]. Chorioretinitis or optic atrophy occurred in 20%

of cases. Expressive language delays independent from hearing loss and mental impairment have also been described. Several studies have searched for clinical predictors of intelligence and developmental outcome and found that microcephaly at birth, development of neurologic abnormalities during the 1st year of life, ocular lesions (chorioretinitis), and microcephaly that became apparent after birth were significantly associated with a low performance on cognitive and developmental testing [476].

A consistent predictor of adverse neurodevelopmental outcome is the presence of cranial computed tomography (CT) abnormalities detected within the 1st month of life [398,505,523]. In infants with symptomatic congenital CMV infection, abnormal CT findings, particularly intracerebral calcifications, are common (70%). Nearly 90% of children with abnormal newborn CT scans develop at least one sequela compared with 29% of children with a normal study [398]. In this particular study, which included 56 children with symptomatic congenital CMV, only 1 child with a normal CT scan had an IQ of less than 70, in contrast to 59% of children with imaging abnormalities. Newborn CT abnormalities were also associated with an abnormal hearing screen at birth and hearing loss on follow-up. None of the neonatal neurologic findings was predictive of an abnormal CT scan [398]. Overall, it can be anticipated that 90% to 95% of infants with symptomatic congenital infections who survive will exhibit mild to severe long-term sequelae.

Asymptomatic Infection

As indicated in the previous section, nearly 90% of infants with congenital CMV infections have no early clinical manifestations, and their long-term outcome seems to be much better than infants with clinically apparent infections. Nevertheless, there is now solid evidence derived from controlled prospective studies that 10% to 15% of these infants are at risk of developing numerous developmental abnormalities, such as sensorineural hearing loss, microcephaly, motor defects (e.g., spastic diplegia or quadriplegia), mental retardation, chorioretinitis, dental defects, and others that were once thought to be limited to infants with symptomatic congenital infections. These abnormalities usually become apparent within the first 2 years of life [207,210,508,517,524]. Table 23–9 shows results based on a prospective longitudinal study of 330 patients with asymptomatic congenital infection who were followed by using serial clinical, psychometric, audiometric, and visual assessments. Follow-up studies of patients with inapparent congenital CMV infection have also been reported [210,505,521,525–530]. Generally, the findings are consistent with the results of studies from this institution that are presented in Table 23–9.

Most of the patients in these various studies and their controls were from a low socioeconomic background. The most significant abnormality in children born with subclinical congenital CMV infection is hearing loss. Fowler and associates [210] evaluated 307 children with documented asymptomatic congenital CMV infection and compared their audiometric assessments with 76 uninfected siblings of children with asymptomatic

congenital CMV infection and 201 children whose neonatal screen for this infection showed negative results. Sensorineural hearing loss occurred only in children with congenital CMV infection. Among them, 22 (7.2%) had hearing loss. The hearing loss was bilateral in 11 of the 22 children (50%). Among the children with hearing loss, further deterioration of hearing occurred in 50% with a median age at first progression of 18 months (range 2 to 70 months). Delayed onset of sensorineural hearing loss occurred in 18% of the children with the median age of detection at 27 months (range 25 to 62 months). Also, fluctuating hearing loss was documented in 22.7% of the children with hearing loss. These results are very similar to results obtained by Williamson and coworkers in Houston [527].

A study in Sweden of more than 10,000 newborns screened for hearing loss and congenital CMV infection found that this congenital infection was the leading cause of sensorineural hearing loss, accounting for 40% of the cases with hearing loss [508]. Hicks and colleagues [513] found 14 cases of congenital CMV infection with sensorineural hearing loss in 12,371 neonates screened for CMV, a rate of approximately 1.1 per 1000 live births. The rate was 0.6 per 1000 when only cases with bilateral loss of 50 dB or greater were considered. These results suggest that CMV infection could account for at least one third of sensorineural hearing loss in young children in the U.S. population [513]. Similar results have been obtained in populations outside of the United States and northern Europe. In a study from Brazil derived from a population of women with greater than 96% seroprevalence for CMV, congenital infection was detected in 1% of newborn infants, and hearing loss (>60 dB) was present in approximately 8% of infected infants [158].

Taken together, these studies indicate that universal screening for hearing loss would detect less than half of all the cases of sensorineural hearing loss caused by congenital CMV infection. Because most of these infants are asymptomatic at birth, they are not recognized as being at high risk for hearing loss and perhaps more importantly are not being tested further to detect late-onset hearing loss. The universal screening of neonates for hearing loss should be combined with screening for congenital CMV infections.

Prospective studies of children with subclinical congenital CMV infections have also revealed a wide but significant spectrum of neurologic complications [527]. It has been estimated that within the first 2 years of life, 2% to 7% of the infants in this group develop microcephaly with various degrees of mental retardation and neuromuscular defects. How often milder forms of brain damage, such as learning or behavioral difficulties, occur as these patients grow older is unknown and not being investigated. Studies of the intellectual development of children with asymptomatic congenital CMV infections have shown conflicting results. One study evaluated 204 prospectively followed children with asymptomatic congenital CMV infections and 177 uninfected siblings ranging in age from 6 to 203 months [531]. Parents were administered a developmental profile, and the children were administered an objective intelligence measure. Results showed that children with asymptomatic congenital

CMV infection did not exhibit intellectual impairment, and they performed similarly to uninfected siblings.

Children with asymptomatic congenital CMV infections have a low risk of chorioretinitis. The current estimate is that it occurs in 2% of these children and, similar to hearing loss, may not be present at birth.

These observations underscore the need for longitudinal follow-up of patients with congenital CMV infection regardless of the initial clinical presentation. Careful assessments of perceptual functions (hearing, visual acuity), psychomotor development, and learning abilities must be made to recognize the full impact of CMV. With early identification of a problem, corrective measures can be instituted to reduce psychosocial and learning problems.

Effect of Type of Maternal Infection on Symptoms and Long-Term Outcome

Studies have shown that preexisting maternal immunity does not prevent CMV from reactivating during pregnancy and cannot reliably prevent transmission in utero or symptomatic congenital infections.* A prospective study of young, predominantly African American women with one or more previous deliveries was done to estimate the protection conferred by preconception maternal immunity [532]. In the nearly 3500 multiparous women who had previously delivered newborns screened for congenital CMV infection and who subsequently enrolled in this study, the overall rate of congenital CMV infection was 1.3%. Congenital infection occurred in 18 of 604 newborns (3%; 95% confidence interval 1.8% to 4.7%) born to initially seronegative mothers compared with 29 of 2857 newborns (1%; 95% confidence interval 0.7% to 1.4%) born to immune mothers. Of the initially seronegative women, 23.5% seroconverted for an annualized seroconversion rate of 7.8% per year with 12.7% of these seroconversions resulting in congenital CMV infection. Of infants born to mothers immune to CMV before conception, 1% had congenital infection.

These results show that young women who have immunity to CMV from naturally acquired infections have about 60% lower relative risk of delivering an infant with congenital CMV infections within a 3-year period compared with women who were initially seronegative. Although this study confirmed a relative protective effect of preexisting immunity that was first reported nearly 3 decades ago, the absolute protective effect was modest if one considers that nearly twofold more infants with congenital infection were born to women with preexisting serologic immunity than women with primary infection during pregnancy in this same population [532]. This study, together with studies from maternal populations with high seroprevalence for CMV, suggested that although maternal immunity to CMV can limit the incidence of congenital infections presumably by decreasing the rate of transmission, most infants with congenital CMV are born to women with serologic immunity before conception in maternal populations of high CMV seroprevalence.

It is generally recognized that primary infection has a higher risk of causing symptomatic infection; however, data that have emerged in recent years, including our own prospective studies, raise the possibility that recurrent maternal infection may result in adverse outcome more frequently than previously thought. In 1999, prospective studies done in Sweden and the United States reported the presence of symptoms at birth and the development of long-term sequelae in children born with congenital CMV infection after a recurrence of maternal infection (Table 23–10) [442,533].

Our study included 246 children with congenital CMV infection from the screening of 20,885 neonates (1.18%) [442]. Of the 246 infants, 47 were symptomatic at birth, and 8 of the 47 (17%) were born to mothers with recurrent CMV infection as defined by seropositive status at the time of a previous pregnancy. Demographically, the women in this study have been characterized as predominantly black (93%), single (96%), and young (46% ≤20 years of age), with no private insurance. More recently, a summary of the outcome of congenital CMV infection as a function of the type of maternal infection from a screened population has been tabulated, and from this study it is apparent that damaging congenital infections are frequent after nonprimary maternal infections (Table 23–11) [212].

A more recent study in this population concluded that in women who are seropositive for CMV, reinfection with different strains of CMV rather than reactivation of the endogenous strain can lead to intrauterine transmission and symptomatic congenital infection [160]. In contrast, the study of women who are predominantly white, married, of middle to high socioeconomic background, and older has not revealed the occurrence of symptomatic

TABLE 23–10   Classification of Maternal Infection and Outcome of Infants with Congenital Cytomegalovirus Infection

Maternal Infection	% Symptomatic at Birth (No.)	% Central Nervous System Sequelae (No.)
Primary	30 (9/30)	22 (5/23)
Nonprimary	28 (9/32)	35 (8/23)

From Ahlfors K, Ivarsson SA, Harris S. Report on a long-term study of maternal and congenital cytomegalovirus infection in Sweden: review of prospective studies available in the literature. Scand J Infect Dis 31:443-457, 1999.

TABLE 23–11   Outcome of Congenital Cytomegalovirus Infection in Relation to Classification of Maternal Infection

Sequelae	Primary (n = 76)	Nonprimary (n = 75)	Unknown (n = 136)
Hearing loss	9 (12%)	10 (13%)	22 (16%)
IQ <70	4/37 (11%)	3/33 (9%)	13/76 (17%)
Motor deficits	2	3	5
Seizures	5	1	5
Chorioretinitis	2	1	1
Any sequela	13 (17%)	12 (16%)	31 (23%)

Adapted from references 441-443.

*References [12,153,154,157,158,160].

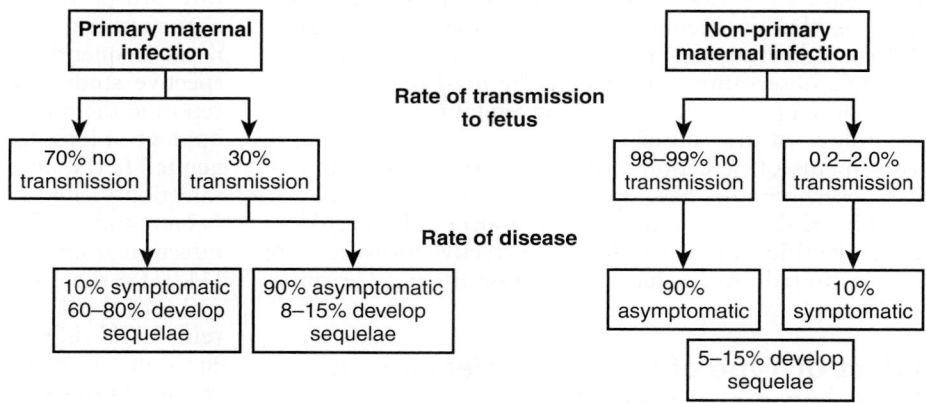

NATURAL HISTORY OF CONGENITAL HCMV
INFECTIONS: 1975–1998

Classification of maternal infection

FIGURE 23–6 Natural history of congenital human cytomegalovirus (HCMV) infection.

* The transmission rate varies depending on the population. Women of lower socioeconomic status have rates reported as high as 2.0%, whereas women from middle and upper middle class socioeconomic groups have rates less than 0.2%.

congenital CMV infection as a result of a recurrence of maternal infection. A summary of available data from nearly 4 decades of study of congenital CMV infections from a single institution has been presented as a schematic of the natural history of congenital CMV infections (Fig. 23–6).

Public Health Significance

The public health impact of congenital CMV infection in the United States is significant, as shown in Table 23–12. Using models of congenital CMV infection with the average rate of 1% and a birth rate of 4 million per annum, approximately 40,000 infants are born each year with congenital CMV infections. Of these, 2800 infants present with signs and symptoms of infection (CID). About 336 of these infants can be expected to die within the 1st year, and nearly 2160 of the survivors develop handicaps. Another 5580 or so of subclinically infected (asymptomatic infections) infants develop significant hearing and

mental deficits. In addition to the personal and family suffering associated with these conditions, the cost to society for caring for these children has been estimated to amount to more than $1 billion each year [534].

PERINATAL INFECTION

As discussed in previous sections, perinatal infections can be acquired from exposure to virus in the maternal genital tract at delivery, from breast milk, or through multiple blood transfusions [131,453–455,459,535–543]. To establish the diagnosis of perinatal CMV infection, one must first exclude congenital infection by showing an absence of viral excretion during the first 2 weeks of life. Findings suggest that PCR assays can detect viral DNA in saliva or blood specimens from infants exposed to CMV after delivery but not congenitally infected, further indicating that confirmation of congenital CMV infections requires isolation of virus within 2 weeks of birth. The incubation period of perinatal CMV infection is 4 to 12 weeks. Although the quantity of virus excreted by infants with perinatal infection is less than that seen with intrauterine acquisition, the infection is also chronic, with viral excretion persisting for years [544].

Most infants with naturally acquired perinatal infections remain asymptomatic. Most of these infections result from recurrent maternal infections, and infants are born with variable levels of maternal antibody. Asymptomatic perinatal CMV infection in full-term and otherwise healthy infants does not seem to have an adverse effect on growth, perceptual functions, or motor or psychosocial development. CMV has been incriminated as a cause of pneumonitis in infants younger than 4 months [506]. In a study undertaken to define the possible association of CMV and other respiratory pathogens with pneumonitis in young infants, CMV was isolated in 21 of 104 patients (21%) enrolled [506]. Only 3% of 97 hospitalized controls were infected. CMV-associated pneumonitis occurs throughout the year, in contrast with

TABLE 23–12   Public Health Impact of Congenital CMV Infection in the United States

Parameter	Estimated Figure
No. live births per year	4 million
Rate of congenital CMV infection (average)	1%
No. infected infants	40,000
No. infants symptomatic at birth (5%-7%)	2800
No. with fatal disease (± 12%)	336
No. with sequelae (90% of survivors)	2160
No. infants asymptomatic at birth (93%-95%)	37,200
No. with late sequelae (15%)	5580
Total no. with sequelae or fatal outcome	8076

Adapted from Fowler KB, et al. The outcome of congenital cytomegalovirus infection in relation to maternal antibody status. N Engl J Med 326:663-667, 1992.

the common respiratory virus infections, which occur most often in winter and early spring.

In premature and ill full-term infants, Yeager and colleagues [545] originally reported that naturally acquired CMV infection may pose a greater risk. They found that premature infants weighing less than 1500 g at birth who acquired CMV from a maternal source often developed hepatosplenomegaly, neutropenia, lymphocytosis, and thrombocytopenia, coinciding with the onset of virus excretion. Infected newborns required longer treatment with oxygen than uninfected patients. In a later study, Paryani and coworkers [546] from the same group reported a prospective study of 55 premature infants including controls and suggested that there may be a propensity for an increased incidence of neuromuscular impairments, particularly in premature infants with the onset of CMV excretion during the first 2 months of life. Sensorineural hearing loss, chorioretinitis, and microcephaly occurred with similar frequency in both groups. Similar findings were reported by Vochem and colleagues [455] and Maschmann and coworkers [547,646].

In the past, transfusion-acquired perinatal CMV infection was associated with significant morbidity and mortality, particularly in premature infants with a birth weight of less than 1500 g born to CMV-seronegative mothers [174,548]. The syndrome of post-transfusion CMV infection in premature newborns was characterized by Ballard and coworkers [549]. They isolated CMV from 16 of 51 preterm infants of a mean birth weight of 1000 g and found that 14 of the 16 virus-positive infants had a constellation of symptoms that resembled CID. This recognizable, self-limited syndrome consisted of deterioration of respiratory function, hepatosplenomegaly, unusual gray pallor with disturbing septic appearance, an atypical and an absolute lymphocytosis, thrombocytopenia, and hemolytic anemia. The syndrome was more severe in infants with low birth weight and occurred 4 to 12 weeks after the transfusion, when the infants were progressing satisfactorily. Although the course of the disease was generally self-limited (lasting 2 to 3 weeks), death occurred in 20% of the ill infants. Subsequent work by Yeager and

associates [545,548] and Adler and colleagues [550] confirmed these observations.

DIAGNOSIS
DETECTION OF VIRUS

The diagnosis of congenital CMV infection should be considered in any newborn with signs of congenital infection, if there is a history of maternal seroconversion or a mononucleosis-like illness during pregnancy, or if an infant fails a newborn screening examination. The most reliable method for the diagnosis of congenital infection is virus isolation in tissue culture, which is generally accomplished with urine or saliva or demonstration of CMV DNA by PCR (Table 23–13) [378,551–555].

CMV IgM serology has never been shown to have adequate sensitivity or specificity for the diagnosis of congenital CMV infection. With diagnostic methods that detect the virus, viral antigens, and nucleic acids, it is possible to confirm the diagnosis from blood, cerebrospinal fluid, and biopsy material. Of particular interest is the possibility of diagnosis by PCR on blood stored on filter paper [555,556]. This approach is being studied by many laboratories, and numerous reports have suggested its potential value [515,556–561]. Representative studies include those from Sweden in which CMV DNA was detected in dried blood specimens of 13 of 16 (81%) infants with congenital CMV infection [555]. Italian investigators using a similar method obtained a sensitivity of 100% and a specificity of 98.5% in a study of 205 neonates including 14 with congenital infections [562]. Both groups of investigators used a nested PCR method to detect CMV DNA in dried blood specimens, which added complexity to this assay, reducing its potential use as a screening assay. Large prospective studies have not adequately evaluated the sensitivity and specificity of this approach in screening populations. More recent results from a large ongoing study of greater than 20,000 specimens from screened populations have suggested that dried blood spot testing using PCR is inferior in terms of sensitivity to conventional methodology using inoculation of

TABLE 23–13 Summary of Available Diagnostic Methods for Identification of Infants with Congenital Cytomegalovirus (CMV) Infection

Method	Advantages	Disadvantages
Detection of Virus or Viral Antigens		
Standard tube culture method	Standard reference method	Takes 2-4 wk, not suitable for screening
Shell vial assay	Rapid, sensitive, and commercially available	Expensive, not suitable for screening
Microtiter plate immunofluorescent antibody assay	Rapid, sensitive, reliable, simple, inexpensive	Cell culture–based, not commercially available
CMV antigenemia	Rapid and simple	Sensitivity and utility for screening newborns unknown, expensive
Nucleic Acid Amplification Methods		
DNA hybridization assay	Sensitive and reliable	Complicated, need for a radiolabeled probe
Polymerase chain reaction amplification methods	Simple and can be used to screen large numbers	Utility as a screening assay has not been proved
Serologic Methods		
Anti-CMV IgM antibody assay	Simple and widely available	Low sensitivity and unreliable for screening

saliva or urine on permissive human fibroblasts followed by detection of immediate early protein by immunologic approaches [563].

To confirm congenital CMV infection, demonstration of virus must be attempted in the first 2 weeks of life because viral excretion after that time may represent an infection acquired at birth (natal) by exposure to an infected birth canal or one acquired in the neonatal period by exposure to breast milk or blood products. In the previous section, it was noted that viral nucleic acid detection by PCR in specimens from saliva or blood within the first 2 weeks of life should be confirmed by detection of viral nucleic acids in urine or virus isolation from urine or both. Although isolation of CMV during the first 2 weeks of life proves a congenital CMV infection, it does not confirm an etiologic relationship with an existing disease. Urine and saliva are the preferred specimens for culture because they contain larger amounts of virus. The viability of CMV is good when specimens are properly stored. When positive urine specimens (without preservatives) are stored at 4° C for 7 days, the rate of isolation decreases to only 93%; it decreases to only 50% after 1 month of storage [564]. Storage and transport at ambient temperature or freezing should never be used because infectivity is rapidly lost.

TISSUE CULTURE

Standard tissue culture based viral isolation requires inoculation of specimen into monolayers of primary human fibroblasts. Typically, 2 to 4 weeks may be required for the appearance of the characteristic cytopathic effect. Methods for rapid viral diagnosis became available in 1980. Several modifications of the standard tissue culture method combined with immunologic detection of IE CMV-induced antigens have maintained high specificity and sensitivity, yet allowed the confirmation of diagnosis within 24 hours of inoculation of the clinical specimen [565–567].

Typically, this test includes the use of monoclonal antibodies to CMV-specific early antigens with low-speed centrifugation of the clinical specimens onto the monolayer of fibroblasts growing on coverslips inside shell vials [565–567]. When this method was evaluated with clinical specimens (e.g., blood; urine; bronchoscopy lavage; lung, liver, and kidney biopsy samples; sputum), obtained primarily from immunosuppressed patients, the sensitivity approached 80%, and the specificity ranged from 80% to 100%. Subsequently, another adaptation of this rapid immunofluorescent assay used 96-well microtiter plates and a monoclonal antibody that is reactive with the major IE human CMV protein that is expressed in the nucleus of infected cells within hours of virus entry [566]. This rapid assay detected all but 1 of 19 specimens identified by standard virus isolation method from 1676 newborn urine specimens, achieving a sensitivity of 94.5% and a specificity of 100%. This test retained high sensitivity and specificity when saliva instead of urine was tested [568].

To date, the microtiter plate method using either saliva or urine samples is the most rapid, simple to perform, and inexpensive alternative to the standard virus isolation method. It is perfectly suitable for mass screening, and there is no decline in sensitivity for specimens at 4° C for up to 3 days. This study also showed that the sensitivity of the microtiter plate method declined rapidly for specimens from older infants and children with congenital CMV infection and from virus-infected children attending day care centers. It is not recommended for either screening or diagnosing CMV infections in older infants and children.

DNA HYBRIDIZATION

Rapid diagnosis of CMV has been accomplished by DNA hybridization [569–572]. The sensitivity and specificity of this method is good when the specimens contain 103 or more tissue culture infective doses per milliliter. The methodology is rarely, if ever, used in routine settings, however, and has largely been replaced with PCR-based technologies.

POLYMERASE CHAIN REACTION AMPLIFICATION

Detection of viral DNA by PCR amplification has proved extremely sensitive and versatile for the detection of CMV genetic material in various clinical samples, including urine, cerebrospinal fluid, blood, plasma, saliva, and biopsy material. In one of the earliest applications of this technology for the diagnosis of congenital CMV, Demmler and associates [553] identified 41 urine specimens positive by PCR from a total of 44 specimens positive by tissue culture. No positive PCR results were found in 27 urine specimens that were negative by tissue culture. In another early study, Warren and coworkers [554] used the PCR technique to detect CMV in saliva from children who were between the ages of 1 month and 14 years and who had either congenital or perinatal CMV infection and compared the results with a standard tissue culture method and microtiter plate detection of immediate early antigen with tissue culture results as a reference. The sensitivity of PCR was 89.2%, and the specificity was 95.8%. Reproducibility was excellent.

If primer selection and amplification conditions are carefully chosen, PCR results are comparable to standard tissue culture isolation of virus except in extreme cases of very low levels of virus infectivity. Some advantages include the minute amount of specimen and the fact that infectious virus is not required, allowing for retrospective diagnosis of CMV infection if the appropriate specimens are available. Nelson and colleagues [551] showed that PCR detection of CMV DNA in serum is a sensitive, specific, and rapid method for diagnosis of infants with symptomatic congenital CMV infection. PCR detected CMV DNA in the serum of 18 infants with symptomatic infection, 1 of 2 infants with asymptomatic infection, and 0 of 32 controls.

Virus isolation from blood specimens is often difficult and insensitive compared with PCR detection of viremia. The use of quantitative PCR (real-time PCR) to detect and quantitate CMV DNA in various clinical specimens, including dried blood spots obtained from a drop of neonatal blood applied to a solid support such as a Guthrie card at the time of the newborn metabolic screen, could offer diagnostic and prognostic information from a single test. Advantages of PCR-based methods to screen newborn infants include the following: (1) no need for tissue culture facilities; (2) minute amount of specimens; (3) when dried, samples on filter paper are no longer infectious reducing the biohazard risk; (4) easy to ship and transport without occupational exposure to infectious material; (5) possibility to quantify CMV DNA in PCR-positive samples; (6) adaptation of robotic automation; (7) retrospective diagnosis when appropriate specimens are available; and (8) simplified storage at room temperature for many years.

As an example of the value of such an approach that could lead to identification of infants at risk for hearing loss, Boppana and colleagues [460] determined virus burden in the peripheral blood of a group of congenitally infected infants with and without hearing loss. Their findings indicated that it is possible to identify infected infants at higher risk for the development of hearing loss (Fig. 23–7).

ANTIGENEMIA

An assay to detect CMV antigenemia by means of monoclonal antibodies to the tegument protein pp65 encoded by CMV in polymorphonuclear leukocytes has shown good sensitivity and, perhaps more importantly, good predictive value of the risk of disease compared with conventional methods (serology, culture) for the diagnosis of CMV disease in immunocompromised adults [231, 573–577]. Revello and Gerna [378] assayed pp65 antigenemia, viremia, and DNAemia in peripheral blood leukocytes from 75 infants born to mothers who had primary CMV infection during pregnancy. The results of this study revealed that compared with the technique of virus isolation from urine, the sensitivity of PCR, antigenemia, and viremia were 100%, 42.5%, and 28%. The specificity of the three assays was 100%.

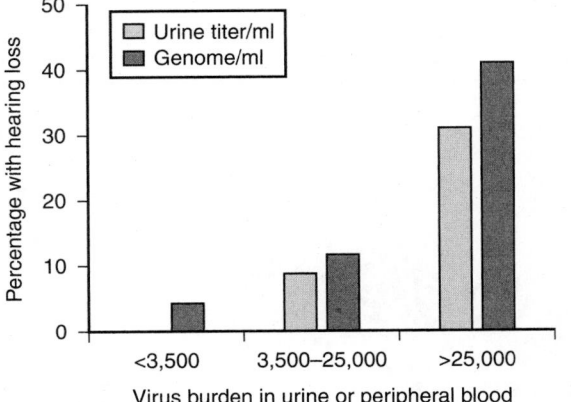

FIGURE 23–7 Hearing loss in infants with human cytomegalovirus congenital infection as a function of viral genome copy number in urine and blood. Note increasing incidence of hearing loss with increasing genome copy number. *(Primary data courtesy Dr. Suresh Boppana, University of Alabama, Birmingham.)*

DETECTION OF IMMUNE RESPONSE

With congenital CMV infection, antibody production begins in utero and is continued probably during the life span of the host.

Detection of IgG Antibodies

Serologic tests that measure IgG antibody are readily available, easier to perform, and more readily automated than most virologic methods. Their correct interpretation is complicated, however, by the presence of antibodies (IgG class) that are normally transmitted from the mother to the fetus [372]. A negative antibody titer in cord and maternal sera is sufficient evidence in almost all cases to exclude the diagnosis of congenital CMV infection. In uninfected infants born to seropositive mothers, IgG antibodies decrease with a half-life of approximately 1 month and become undetectable by most routine assays by 4 to 9 months of age. In contrast, in infected infants, IgG antibody levels persist for long periods at comparable or sometimes higher levels than in their mothers. CMV infections are commonly acquired during the neonatal period mostly from maternal sources (milk, genital secretions) and blood or blood products, and the distinction from congenital infection is impossible by routine serologic means. In both situations, IgG antibody titers tend to remain stable for many months. A neonatal infection in the face of a negative maternal IgG antibody titer should point to transmission from other sources (e.g., blood transfusion or nosocomial).

Many serologic assays have been described and evaluated for the detection of CMV IgG antibodies. Among these, enzyme-linked immunosorbent assays (ELISAs) are most commonly employed.

Detection of IgM Antibodies

Infected fetuses usually produce specific IgM antibodies. IgM antibodies are not transferred by the placenta, and their detection in cord or neonatal blood represents a fetal antibody response. There are many different assays for IgM antibodies, but before deciding on the use of any particular test it is important to know its specificity, sensitivity, and reproducibility. No test has so far reached a level of specificity and sensitivity to match the virologic assays described in the previous section.

The solid-phase radioimmunoassay described by Griffiths and Kangro [578] remains among the best, with a reported sensitivity of 89% and a specificity of 100% for diagnosis of congenital CMV infections. With the first generation of commercially available IgM ELISAs, the specificity was nearly 95% with a sensitivity of approximately 70% when evaluating congenitally infected infants [579]. The IgM capture ELISA and other immunoassays have not fared much better when testing for congenital CMV infection. A Western blot format has been used in the study of IgM antibodies in patients with active CMV infection and was based on antibodies reactive with the viral structural polypeptides pp150 and pp52 [580]. Clinicians should not rely on IgM assays to diagnose congenital CMV infection. Continued research in this area may provide a simple and generally available method for rapid, definitive diagnosis of congenital infections in ill and asymptomatic neonates.

DIAGNOSIS OF CYTOMEGALOVIRUS INFECTION DURING PREGNANCY
Clinical Signs and Symptoms

Most primary CMV infections in immunocompetent hosts are subclinical, and infections occurring in pregnant women are no exception. Less than 5% of pregnant women with proven primary CMV infections are symptomatic with an even smaller percentage manifesting mononucleosis-like syndrome. Clinical manifestations have not been reported with recurrent infections (reactivations or reinfections).

Laboratory Markers

The diagnosis of primary CMV infection can be easily confirmed by documenting seroconversion (i.e., de novo appearance of virus-specific IgG antibodies in a pregnant woman who was seronegative). In the absence of serologic screening, this confirmation is seldom available in clinical practice. The presence of IgG antibodies denotes past infection from 2 weeks to years in duration.

IgM Assays

Of the several IgM assays commercially available, most perform reasonably well with excellent specificity (95%) and sensitivity (100%) [581–583]. The IgM antibody response varies widely from one patient to another. Seropositivity can be detected for up to 16 weeks, but it is unusual to last more than 1 year. It is typical to see sharp declines in titers within the first 2 to 3 months of infection. More sensitive assays of IgM antibodies have detected maternal CMV specific IgM antibodies 1 year from enrollment in clinical studies [163].

IgM assays have been developed based on recombinant CMV proteins and peptides. Structural and nonstructural CMV-encoded proteins react with IgM antibodies. The detection of specific IgM antibodies can be accomplished by Western blot, immunoblot, or microparticle enzyme immunoassay [580–583]. As noted earlier, sensitivities

approaching 98% and specificities of 98% have been claimed with commercially available assays.

IgG Avidity Assay

The IgG avidity assay is based on the observation that IgG antibodies of low avidity are present during the first months after onset of infection. With time, IgG antibodies of increasingly higher avidity are produced, and eventually only IgG of high avidity is detected in individuals with long-standing CMV infection. An application of this approach was first used to define differences in avidity in women with primary infection who transmitted virus to their offspring [163]. This study showed differences in the avidity of CMV anti-IgG responses that were correlated with the development of virus-neutralizing antibodies, suggesting that maturation of the virus-neutralizing antibody response was linked to avidity maturation of IgG antibody responses [163].

The results of the currently available avidity test are reported as an index representing the percentage of IgG antibody bound to the antigen after denaturation treatment with 6M urea [378,552,583–588]. Similar approaches have been reported for other infectious agents, including rubella. In one study, an avidity index value of approximately 20% was obtained in serum samples collected within 3 months after onset of primary infection, in contrast to an avidity index of 78% in sera from individuals with remote infection (Fig. 23–8) [589].

In determining the risk of congenital CMV, a moderate to high avidity index obtained before the 18th week of gestation has a negative predictive value of 100%. When the avidity index is determined at 21 to 23 weeks of gestation, the negative predictive value decreases to 91% [552,590]. The explanation for this observation is that some women who transmitted the infection in utero had acquired the infection at a very early gestational age. One important limitation of early studies using the IgG avidity test was the lack of standardization. In one study, the ability of these IgG avidity assays to identify primary CMV infection almost reached 100%, whereas the ability to exclude a recent infection ranged from 20% to 96%. When coupled with the detection of CMV-specific IgM antibodies, the avidity test has been used to estimate risk

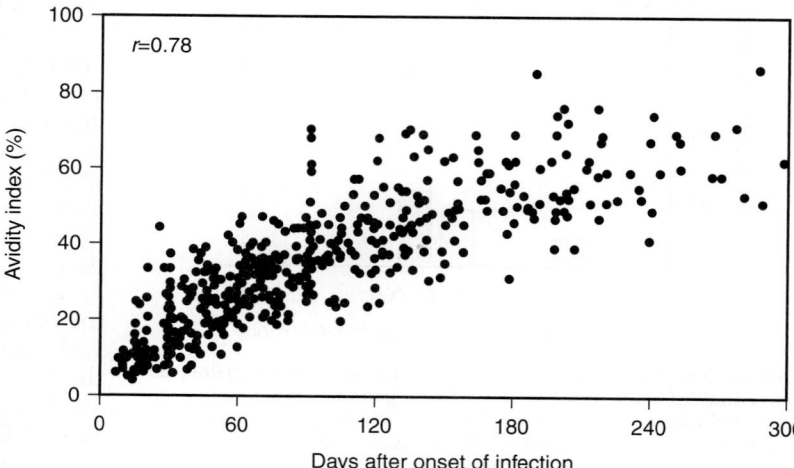

FIGURE 23–8 Kinetics of IgG avidity index. *(From Revello MG, Gerna G. Diagnosis and management of human cytomegalovirus infection in the mother, fetus, and newborn infant. Clin Microbiol Rev 15:680-715, 2002.)*

of primary infection and damaging congenital infection [552,583,586]. Although this approach has been extensively used in Europe, it is not widely used in the United States presumably because of the lack of widespread screening for CMV infections in pregnant women.

Viral Cultures

CMV excretion from multiple sites, such as urine, saliva, and genital secretions, is common and can last weeks to several months after a primary infection. The same occurs with reinfections and reactivations, making viral culture as a diagnostic approach of limited value. Viremia, as determined by conventional tissue culture methods, is too insensitive to confirm the diagnosis of primary infection in immunocompetent hosts.

Other Tests

Other diagnostic methods with greater sensitivity and specificity include the determination of antigenemia (number of pp65-positive peripheral blood leukocytes); PCR quantification of CMV DNA in whole blood (DNAemia), leukocytes (leuko-DNAemia), or plasma; and determination of IE and late messenger RNA (mRNA) in blood (RNAemia). Some of these assays are commercially available. The data supporting their diagnostic value derive largely from studies in immunosuppressed patients with primary CMV infections, reactivations, and dissemination of infection and evaluation of antiviral treatments.

In many cases, individual assays are center specific, and results from one center are often difficult to standardize within other centers. One study of immunocompetent adults including a large proportion of pregnant women with primary CMV infection showed that pp65 antigenemia was detected in 57% of patients examined within the 1st month after the onset of primary infection [591]. The percent of positive results decreased to 25% 1 month later and to 0% 5 months later. Viremia was detected in 26% of patients during the 1st month only. DNAemia (by PCR test) was detected in 100% of patients tested during the first month, in 89% of patients tested during the 2nd month, and in 47% of patients tested 3 months after the onset of primary infection. DNAemia lasted 4 to 6 months in 26% of patients; no patient remained positive beyond 6 months from the onset of infection.

None of the three assays were positive in patients with remote CMV infection, including nine subjects with proven recurrences. The results of this study indicated that antigenemia and DNAemia when run on blood specimens rapidly and specifically diagnosed CMV infection, and it was argued that these assays could provide an estimate of the onset for primary infection in pregnant women [591]. The detection of IE mRNA was also proposed as a diagnostic tool for primary CMV infection in healthy individuals [229,592]. This test was consistently negative in all subjects with old or recurrent CMV infection. In contrast, all subjects within the 1st month of a primary infection tested positive. The proportion of positive results declined over time with all patients testing negative after 6 months of the onset of CMV infection. The kinetics of this test resembled that of DNA

detection, and in at least one comparison, the IE mRNA test was slightly more sensitive in the early phase of primary CMV infection [229].

Maternal Laboratory Tests of Fetal Infection

In utero transmission of CMV infection occurs in approximately 30% to 40% of primary infections acquired during pregnancy [121]. No reliable tests are available so far to identify transmission of infection to the fetus. There are no maternal prognostic markers of fetal infection with recurrent maternal infections. A more recent study has shown that reinfection with a different strain of CMV, as measured by new antibody specificity against epitopes of the virion envelope glycoprotein H, can be associated with symptomatic congenital CMV infection [160]. The methodology used in this study is far from a standard laboratory assay and can identify only maternal reinfections and does not define the risk of a damaging fetal infection.

PRENATAL DIAGNOSIS

The prenatal diagnosis of CMV is possible by testing fetal blood obtained by cordocentesis and amniotic fluid obtained by amniocentesis. Fetal blood can be used for determination of specific IgM antibodies and direct viral markers. IgM antibodies have been reported to be detectable after 20 weeks of gestation. Because of low sensitivity (approximately 50%), however, it has limited diagnostic value [593–595]. Studies of viral load in fetal blood show that the sensitivity of antigenemia was approximately 58%; of viremia, 55%;, and of DNAemia 82%. The specificity was 100% for the three assays [378]. In one study, PCR in fetal blood had a sensitivity of 41%, whereas viral culture had a sensitivity of only 7%. With the use of fetal blood, even the most sensitive assays miss nearly 15% to 20% of infected fetuses. In addition, the risk of fetal loss after fetal blood sampling must be considered.

Results in amniotic fluid are far better, and this method can be viewed as the current standard for prenatal diagnosis. Viral isolation in tissue culture has a sensitivity of approximately 60%, whereas the sensitivity of PCR can reach 100%. The specificity of both assays is excellent [378,552,593,596,597]. Quantitative PCR has shown that when the amniotic fluid contains 10^5 or more genome equivalents of CMV DNA, the risk of symptomatic congenital CMV infection is significantly higher than when the viral load is 10^3 genome equivalents or less [552,598–600].

A confounding factor that remains in prenatal diagnosis of congenital CMV is the gestational age at the time of amniocentesis or cordocentesis. After a primary maternal infection, it may take weeks to months for transplacental transmission of CMV to occur. An interval of 7 weeks between maternal onset of infection and diagnostic tests for fetal infection has been proposed as a reasonable interval by some investigators [596,601–603]. Gestational age at the time of testing is also important because the sensitivity can be only 30% when amniotic fluid is obtained before the 21st week of gestation, whereas it can be 100% if the test is performed after 21 weeks of gestation

[552,594–596,601,602,604–606]. More recently, imaging techniques have been applied to the prenatal diagnosis of congenital CMV infections. The improved specificity for the diagnosis of CNS abnormalities as detected by ultrasound and more recently by magnetic resonance imaging (MRI) suggests that these techniques could contribute significantly to the diagnosis of this intrauterine infection [440,607].

To counsel pregnant women, it is important to remember that most (80% to 90%) children with congenital CMV infection do not have clinically definable CNS sequelae. In the absence of specific antiviral treatment for prenatal therapy, the only options available after a prenatal diagnosis of congenital CMV infection are to terminate the pregnancy and do nothing. The presence or absence of ultrasound evidence of fetal abnormalities should be taken into consideration during counseling of women at risk.

DIAGNOSIS OF PERINATALLY ACQUIRED INFECTIONS

For perinatally acquired infections, viral culture or CMV DNA detection by PCR from urine and saliva are the preferred diagnostic methods, but CMV excretion usually does not begin until 3 to 12 weeks after exposure. For diagnostic specificity, it is imperative to have a negative result from urine or saliva specimens collected within the first 2 weeks of life. In early infancy, antibody assays have the same limitations described earlier for infants with congenital CMV infection. Differentiation between congenital and perinatal CMV infections is important because the risks of long-term sequelae are very different.

DIFFERENTIAL DIAGNOSIS

During the newborn period, the constellation of hepatosplenomegaly, petechiae, and direct hyperbilirubinemia with or without pneumonitis, microcephaly, and ocular and neurologic abnormalities that characterizes CID is common to several disease entities, including other congenital infections, such as congenital rubella syndrome, toxoplasmosis, syphilis, neonatal HSV infections, and, less likely, hepatitis B and varicella virus infections. The differential diagnosis of symptomatic congenital CMV infection also includes bacterial sepsis, noninfectious disorders such as hemolytic diseases related to Rh or ABO incompatibilities or red blood cell defects, metabolic disorders such as galactosemia and tyrosinemia, immune thrombocytopenia, histiocytosis X, congenital leukemia, and other diseases in which hepatosplenomegaly is a prominent clinical component. The list of diseases that must be considered in the differential diagnosis becomes broader as the clinical manifestations diminish in severity.

In addition, multiple infections may coexist in the same patient. Consequently, the laboratory work-up for the differential diagnosis must be complete.

CONGENITAL RUBELLA SYNDROME

Congenital rubella has been virtually eliminated in the United States after the successful immunization program adopted years ago. Although symptomatic congenital rubella and CMV infections share many signs and symptoms, central cataracts, congenital heart defects, raised purpuric rather than petechial rash, salt-and-pepper lesions as opposed to chorioretinitis, and absence of cerebral calcifications are more likely to occur with congenital rubella syndrome than with CID.

CONGENITAL TOXOPLASMOSIS

Almost all of the manifestations observed in CID have been described for symptomatic congenital toxoplasmosis. Some differences are worth noting. The calcifications of toxoplasmosis are generally scattered throughout the cerebral cortex, whereas the calcifications of CID tend to occur in the periventricular areas. The rash associated with toxoplasmosis is usually maculopapular, but is not petechial or purpuric. Chorioretinitis in the two diseases cannot be differentiated on the basis of appearance or distribution. It is more likely, however, that chorioretinitis related to CMV is associated with other major clinical manifestations, such as microcephaly. The chorioretinitis of toxoplasmosis commonly is an isolated finding.

CONGENITAL SYPHILIS

The most consistent signs of early congenital syphilis are osteochondritis and epiphysitis on the radiograph of the long bones. These occur in approximately 90% of infected patients and are more likely to appear in patients who become symptomatic in the 1st week of life. Rhinitis, sometimes associated with laryngitis, is another common manifestation of congenital syphilis; it is often followed by a dark red maculopapular rash. Lesions of the skin and mucous membranes are also seen. Hepatosplenomegaly and hepatocellular damage with cholestatic jaundice occur, but are less common in early syphilis than in CID. Calcifications of the brain are not characteristic of congenital syphilis. Choroiditis may be seen.

NEONATAL HERPES SIMPLEX VIRUS INFECTIONS

Congenital HSV infections are less common than neonatal HSV infections and likely account for approximately 5% of cases of perinatal herpes simplex infections, yet they are more likely to pose a diagnostic dilemma because they may resemble CID. Microcephaly, intracranial calcifications, chorioretinitis with and without optic atrophy, and hepatosplenomegaly are common clinical manifestations of intrauterine HSV infections. The presence of skin vesicles or scarring at birth is valuable for the differential diagnosis. The more common form of HSV infection, neonatal infection, is acquired during parturition and does not usually manifest as an acute disease until 5 to 21 days of age. In contrast to the situation in typical CID, the infant is well during most of the 1st week of life. When illness does occur, it may be accompanied by seizures, encephalitis, respiratory distress, bleeding disorders, and small vesicular lesions that tend to cluster into crops.

TREATMENT
CHEMOTHERAPY

A few systemically administered antiviral agents have been used in therapeutic trials of serious, life-threatening or sight-threatening CMV disease. Currently, two antiviral agents, ganciclovir and foscarnet, are licensed for this purpose in immunocompromised patients. Foscarnet inhibits viral replication by inhibiting viral DNA polymerase, and ganciclovir acts as a chain terminator during elongation of the newly synthesized viral DNA.

The Collaborative Antiviral Study Group (CASG) under the auspices of the National Institute of Allergy and Infectious Diseases first conducted a phase II pharmacokinetic and pharmacodynamic study that established the safe dose of ganciclovir to be used in young infants [608]. A phase III randomized, controlled study followed newborn infants with symptomatic congenital infection involving the CNS [609]. The study enrolled 100 patients. Patients in the ganciclovir treatment arm received 6 mg/kg/dose administered intravenously every 12 hours for 6 weeks of treatment. The primary end point was improved hearing (as assessed by brainstem evoked response) between baseline and 6 months of follow-up or, for patients with normal hearing at enrollment, preservation of normal hearing at follow-up. At 6 months, 21 (84%) of 25 ganciclovir-treated patients had hearing improvement or maintained normal hearing compared with 10 of 17 (59%) patients in the no-treatment group ($P = .06$). At 6 months of follow-up, none of the ganciclovir-treated infants had hearing deterioration (0 of 25) compared with 7 of 17 (41%) in the no-treatment group ($P < .01$). Alternatively, 5 of 24 (21%) ganciclovir recipients had worsening in hearing in their best ear between baseline and 1 year or longer compared with 13 of 19 (68%) in the no-treatment group ($P < .01$).

This study was viewed as evidence of the feasibility of treatment of selected cases of congenital CMV infections with an antiviral agent. There were limitations in this study, including a significant number of patients not included in the final analysis and the requirement to treat each ear as a separate data point, a statistically justifiable method, but one that may have uncertain rationale from a standpoint of CNS plasticity and neural development. Regardless of these limitations, the information from this study suggested that at least in some patients, treatment of congenital CMV in the perinatal period could alter the long-term morbidity of this infection.

The most significant toxicity in the treated group was neutropenia with 29 of 46 (63%) patients developing moderate to severe neutropenia compared with 9 of 43 (21%) of the no-treatment group ($P < .01$). Half of the patients with neutropenia required dosage adjustment, and 12% had discontinuation of therapy. This study shows that 6 weeks of intravenous ganciclovir in symptomatic infants with congenital CMV infection prevents worsening of hearing loss at 6 months and 1 year of follow-up. In addition, treated patients had a more rapid resolution of liver function abnormalities and improvements in short-term growth and head circumference compared with controls. There are no reports on the therapeutic efficacy of combined therapy (i.e., foscarnet-

ganciclovir). CASG is currently conducting a similar study of valganciclovir, the orally bioavailable prodrug of ganciclovir, to determine if similar results can be obtained using a more convenient alternative to intravenous ganciclovir. So far, anecdotal reports have not supported the use of hyperimmune immunoglobulin or antiviral treatment for the purpose of treating the fetus in utero [360,610].

PASSIVE IMMUNIZATION

Hyperimmune plasma and immunoglobulin have been used with some success as prophylaxis for primary CMV infections in immunosuppressed transplant patients. A meta-analysis of randomized, controlled trials of immunoglobulin as prophylaxis for CMV disease in adult transplant recipients found a significant beneficial effect [459].

It is unclear if the effect of CMV immunoglobulins on the improved outcome in transplant patients is directly related to their antiviral effects. Some authors have argued that at least in the case of hematopoietic allograft recipients, any benefit from passive transfer of immunoglobulins is secondary to immunomodulatory activities of these biologics.

It has been argued for many years that passive immunoprophylaxis would not work for treatment of congenital infections because the cases are identified weeks and months after infection occurred in utero. An uncontrolled trial performed in Italy in 2005 provided data, however, that raise the possibility that such an approach could limit diseases in the infected fetus and perhaps lessen the risk of transmission from an infected woman.

The study used a commercial source of CMV immunoglobulin to treat women with primary CMV during pregnancy. The passive transfer of antibody reduced the frequency of virus transmission to the offspring and reduced the incidence of disease in infected infants [360]. In addition to being an uncontrolled study, the use of clinical end points that were controversial (i.e., head ultrasound) led to considerable skepticism of the validity of the findings by many investigators. This study raised several provocative questions, however, including the possibility that the beneficial effect of immunoglobulin treatment in this study could be related more to its anti-inflammatory effects on the placenta, rather than a direct antiviral effect within the infected fetus. More questions were generated by this study than addressed; however, this study has increased interest in passive prophylaxis and therapy with biologics as an alternative to vaccines for the prevention of damaging congenital CMV infections.

VACCINES

In the United States, congenital CMV infection is a significant public health problem. It is the leading cause of sensorineural hearing loss and the leading infectious cause of brain damage in children [611,612]. The Institute of Medicine of the National Academy of Sciences concluded that a vaccine to prevent congenital CMV infection should be a top priority. Despite 30 years of research efforts, no such vaccine is available. The prevailing thought is that neutralizing antibodies and cell-mediated immunity are necessary for prevention. Of the CMV proteins, gB, gM/gN, pp65, and pp150 can induce neutralizing antibodies and CTL responses [55,613–616]. A major hurdle for the design and testing of vaccines is the lack of a relevant animal model. Each model has drawbacks, perhaps the most significant being that human CMV has unique characteristics in terms of its replication, cellular tropism, and pathogenesis in humans that are not precisely recapitulated in any animal model. Each animal model can study aspects of human CMV infections, but cannot fully reproduce the human disease.

The strategies for vaccine development have included live attenuated vaccine (Towne strain). This vaccine induces a significant antibody response and cell-mediated immunity, as determined by lymphoproliferative response. In CMV-seronegative recipients of kidneys from seropositive donors, this vaccine reduced disease severity, but did not prevent infection [617]. It also protected against a very-low-dose virulent CMV challenge in normal volunteers [618]. In a more recent trial, this vaccine failed to decrease the rate of acquisition of CMV in parents of children in day care centers. The magnitude of the induced immune response was 10-fold lower than that generated by natural infection [619]. The Towne vaccine was not excreted by vaccinees.

Recombinant Virus Vaccine

The genome of the virulent Toledo strain of CMV, divided into four fragments, was inserted in the genetic background of the attenuated Towne strain gene creating four chimeras. The ability of these four recombinant virus strains to generate antibody and cell-mediated immune responses in the absence of clinical side effects has been evaluated in a phase I study [620].

Subunit Vaccines

A CMV vaccine based on the envelope glycoprotein gB combined with a novel adjuvant (MF59) was tested in a double-blind, placebo-controlled trial of seronegative adult volunteers [613]. Results showed that after three doses, the antibody responses to gB and neutralizing antibodies exceeded the levels in seropositive control subjects. Cell-mediated immunity as measured by lymphocyte proliferation was generated in vaccinees. A study done in seronegative women suggested that gB subunit vaccine prevented maternal infection as measured by seroconversion in about 50% of vaccinated women, a surprising finding that must be confirmed, but one that does suggest that vaccine immunity against CMV is feasible [621].

A major target of the cell-mediated immune response is pp65. In an effort to elicit this response, a more recent study used the nonreplicating canarypox expression vector in which CMV pp65 has been inserted. A phase I trial on seronegative volunteers found that pp65-specific CTLs were elicited after only two vaccinations. An antibody response to pp65 was also shown. In this preliminary study, the canarypox CMV pp65 recombinant vaccine seems to generate an immune response similar to that provided by natural infection [615]. A canarypox CMV recombinant vaccine that contained gB did not induce neutralizing antibodies. Other approaches have included recombinant alphavirus vectored CMV gB and fusion protein between pp65 and

IE-1 [622,623]. This vectored subunit vaccine induced significant neutralizing antibody and interferon-γ responses to T lymphocytes in immunized adult volunteers [624].

Another approach has been the use of the DNA vaccine platform. A clinical trial using a bivalent DNA vaccine (DNA encoding gB and pp65) induced antibodies and cellular immune responses in adult volunteers that included long-term T-lymphocyte memory [625]. Finally, the capacity of CMV to reinfect immune individuals has led several investigators to propose CMV as a vaccine vector for other agents. Findings in rhesus macaques have validated this strategy and have shown not only reinfection of previously immune animals, but also induction of immunity against simian immunodeficiency virus, a model of HIV infection in humans [626]. Together with findings in other animal models of CMV infection and the reported frequency of reinfections in immunocompetent humans, these results suggest that the prevention of infection by this virus is a difficult goal for any vaccine that can induce natural levels of immunity.

PREVENTION

Generally, CMV is not very contagious, and its horizontal transmission requires close direct contact with infected material—secretions that contain the virus and, less likely, fomites. With the exception of studies that were designed to prevent infection through blood and blood products and grafted organs, no broad-based strategies for preventing the transmission of CMV have been tested. Education of susceptible individuals has been shown to reduce significantly the incidence of infection, a finding that must be incorporated into any vaccine or biologic trial with an end point for preventing maternal infection or limiting congenital infection or both [627].

PREGNANT WOMEN

An average of 2% of susceptible pregnant women acquire CMV infection during pregnancy in the United States; most of these individuals have no symptoms, and only 40% of the episodes result in fetal infection (see Fig. 23–6) [152,628]. Because there is no proven prenatal therapy, and the risk of fetal morbidity is low, several investigators have concluded that routine serologic screening of pregnant women for primary CMV infections during pregnancy is of limited value. Reliable and inexpensive serologic tests are now available, however, so that women of childbearing age can be informed of their immune status. Because of the risk of congenital infection in offspring of immune women, seroimmune women should also be counseled as to risks of virus exposure and routes of virus acquisition.

Primary CMV infection should be suspected in pregnant women with symptoms compatible with a heterophil-negative, mononucleosis-like syndrome. To define more precisely a recent asymptomatic primary CMV infection, serologic tests such as IgM capture ELISA, IgG avidity index, and DNAemia (PCR) could be used. At present, there are no reliable means to determine whether intrauterine transmission has occurred after symptomatic or subclinical primary infection in early gestation or to assess the relatively few fetuses at risk for disease. The sensitivity and specificity of prenatal diagnosis by testing fetal blood obtained by cordocentesis or amniotic fluid PCR and viral culture are good after 20 weeks of gestation. There is still limited information to serve as a basis for recommendations regarding termination of pregnancy after a primary CMV infection acquired in early gestation. Similarly, there is no definitive information regarding how long conception should be delayed after documented primary infection is acquired in a woman of childbearing age. Viral excretion is not a sensitive and specific indicator because virus is shed into saliva for weeks or months after infection and into urine and the cervix for months or years.

The data on which to base recommendations for prevention of congenital CMV infection after recurrent maternal infection are even more incomplete. Preexisting immunity does not prevent the virus from reactivating or reinfection, and it does not effectively control the occasional spread to the fetus. Preexisting maternal immunity affords significant protection to the fetus. Evidence that in some high-risk populations reinfections with antigenically different virus can cause fetal disease and long-term sequelae may temper this statement, however. At present, there are no techniques for identifying women with reactivation of CMV that results in intrauterine transmission.

The principal sources of CMV infection among women of childbearing age are exposure to children excreting CMV and sexual contacts. Recommendations for prevention of sexual transmission of CMV are beyond the scope of this chapter. Suffice it to say that they are similar to practices advocated for the prevention of other sexually transmitted infections. As for the risk from exposure to children, susceptible pregnant mothers of CMV-infected children who attend day care centers are at greater risk. Hand washing and simple hygienic measures that are routine for hospital care can be recommended, but it is unrealistic to expect all mothers to comply.

Because CMV has been found to be endemic in the day care setting and is found everywhere in hospitals, questions often arise about the occupational risks to pregnant personnel in these facilities. Although hospital workers do not seem to be at increased risk for CMV infection, personnel who work in day care centers are at increased risk.* In the hospital, universal precautions and routine procedures for hand washing and infection control should make nonparenteral acquisition of CMV infections less likely than in the community. Although most patients who shed CMV are asymptomatic and go unrecognized, when caring for known CMV-excreting patients, these routine measures should be combined with a special recommendation that pregnant caretakers be especially careful in handling such patients [629].

In the day care setting, where hygiene is difficult at best, these preventive measures may be more difficult to implement. Although there is still debate about the need for routine serologic screening of female personnel and day care workers, some investigators believe that it should be recommended for potentially childbearing women whose occupation exposes them to CMV. Knowing their immune status can be helpful in counseling pregnant women at risk. All personnel should be provided with information on prevention measures and reassured that commonsense steps such as hand washing and avoiding contact with secretions should prevent acquisition of infection [627,629]. Attempts to identify all children with congenital CMV infection and children excreting this virus in the workplace so that seronegative workers and parents can avoid contact with them pose serious logistic problems and would require frequent periodic testing.

NOSOCOMIAL INFECTION

Hospitalized patients who receive blood products and organ transplants are at risk for nosocomial CMV infection. Transfusion of blood products can be an important source of perinatal CMV infections. Early studies showed that the use of blood products from seronegative donors prevents the transmission of CMV and the subsequent risk of disease [175,632–634]. This approach has obvious drawbacks, however, in areas where a large percentage of the donor population is seropositive. The availability of seronegative donors and the additional cost involved in serologic screening and processing the blood must be evaluated by regional blood banks.

Use of filters to remove leukocytes also is an effective means of eliminating post-transfusion CMV infection in adult patients and in newborns, even in low birth weight infants [635–640]. Filtration results in a significant disruption and depletion of leukocytes and is thought to provide a similar reduction in the rate of CMV transmission after transfusion. Studies have shown a 1% to 2% transmission rate of CMV when exclusively CMV-seronegative donor blood has been used, a finding that is in agreement with a more recent finding that 15% of antibody-negative individuals have CMV circulating in peripheral blood mononuclear cells as detected by PCR [113,641]. Many hospitals are using one of these approaches to prevent transfusion-acquired perinatal CMV infections. It is a local hospital and blood bank policy to determine whether transfusion-associated CMV disease is a problem and which method to choose based on their donor populations. Individual nurseries have adopted the policy that all transfusions of blood or blood products should be with seronegative blood, regardless of the infant's birth weight and maternal immune status.

The absence of CMV infection in premature infants born to seronegative mothers and who receive only seronegative blood products suggests that spread of CMV from hands of personnel or from fomites must be rare. Until more information is available, the only logical recommendation is hand washing and routine infection control measures.

Perinatal infection through breast milk is rarely a cause for concern, at least for full-term newborns who receive their mother's milk [454]. Premature infants, who generally do not receive sufficient quantities of specific transplacental antibodies, are at higher risk for morbidity.*

---

*References [132,137,139,146,149,150,629–631].

*References [454,455,457,535–537,542,543,547,642,643].

Storage of naturally infected breast milk at −20° C (freezer temperature) significantly reduces, but does not eliminate, infectivity [644,645]. Heat treatment of breast milk at 72° C for 10 seconds eliminates all infectious viruses without affecting the nutritional and immunologic properties of milk [455,537,646].

REFERENCES

[1] T.H. Weller, The cytomegaloviruses: ubiquitous agents with protean clinical manifestations, N. Engl. J. Med. 285 (1971) 203–214.

[2] D. Ribbert, Uber protozoenartige zellen in der niere eines syphilitischen neugoborenen und in der parotis von kindern, Zentralbl. Allg. Pathol. 15 (1904) 945–948.

[3] A. Jesionek, B. Kiolemenoglou, Uber einen befund von protozoenartigen gebilden in den organen eines heriditarluetischen fotus, Munch. Med. Wochenschr. 51 (1904) 1905–1907.

[4] C. Lowenstein, Uber protozoenartigen Gebilden in de Organen von Dindern, Zentralbl. Allg. Pathol. 18 (1907) 513–518.

[5] E.W. Goodpasture, F.B. Talbot, Concerning the nature of "proteozoan-like" cells in certain lesions of infancy, Am. J. Dis. Child. 21 (1921) 415–421.

[6] B. Lipschutz, Untersuchungen uber die atiologie der krankheiten der herpesgruppe (herpes zoster, herpes genitalis, herpes febrilis), Arch. Derm. Syph. (Berl) 136 (1921) 428–482.

[7] R. Cole, A.G. Kuttner, A filtrable virus present in the submaxillary glands of guinea pigs, J. Exp. Med. 44 (1926) 855–873.

[8] M.G. Smith, Propagation in tissue cultures of a cytopathogenic virus from human salivary gland virus disease, Proc. Soc. Exp. Biol. (NY) 92 (1956) 424–430.

[9] W.P. Rowe, et al., Cytopathogenic agents resembling human salivary gland virus recovered from tissue cultures of human adenoids, Proc. Soc. Exp. Biol. (NY) 92 (1956) 418–424.

[10] T.H. Weller, et al., Isolation of intranuclear inclusion producing agents from infants with illnesses resembling cytomegalic inclusion disease, Proc. Soc. Exp. Biol. Med. 94 (1957) 4–12.

[11] T.H. Weller, J.B. Hanshaw, D.E. Scott, Serologic differentiation of viruses responsible for cytomegalic inclusion disease, Virology 12 (1960) 130–132.

[12] U. Krech, Z. Konjajev, M. Jung, Congenital cytomegalovirus infection in siblings from consecutive pregnancies, Helv. Paediatr. Acta. 26 (1971) 355–362.

[13] E. Gold, G.A. Nankervis, Cytomegalovirus, in: A.S. Evans (Ed.), Viral Infections of Humans: Epidemiology and Control, second ed., Plenum Press, New York, 1982, pp. 167–186.

[14] A.J. Davison, et al., The human cytomegalovirus genome revisited: comparison with the chimpanzee cytomegalovirus genome [erratum appears in J Gen Virol 84(Pt 4):1053, 2003], J. Gen. Virol. 84 (2003) 17–28.

[15] A.J. Bradley, et al., Genotypic analysis of two hypervariable human cytomegalovirus genes, J. Med. Virol. 80 (2008) 1615–1623.

[16] J.B. Black, P.E. Pellett, Human herpesvirus 7, Rev. Med. Virol. 9 (1999) 245–262.

[17] G. Campadelli-Fiume, P. Mirandola, L. Menotti, Human herpesvirus 6: an emerging pathogen, Emerg. Infect. Dis. 5 (1999) 353–366.

[18] D.A. Clark, Human herpesvirus 6, Rev. Med. Virol. 10 (2000) 155–173.

[19] D.H. Chen, et al., Three-dimensional visualization of tegument/capsid interactions in the intact human cytomegalovirus, Virology 260 (1999) 10–16.

[20] B.L. Trus, et al., Capsid structure of simian cytomegalovirus from cryoelectron microscopy: evidence for tegument attachment sites [erratum appears in J Virol 73(5):4540, 1999], J. Virol. 73 (1999) 2181–2192.

[21] E. Murphy, et al., Coding capacity of laboratory and clinical strains of human cytomegalovirus, Proc. Natl. Acad. Sci. U. S. A. 100 (2003) 14976–14981.

[22] E.S. Mocarski, C. Tan Courcelle, Cytomegaloviruses and their replication, in: B.N. Fields et al., (Eds.), Virology, fourth ed., Lippincott Williams & Wilkins, Philadelphia, 2001, pp. 2629–2673.

[23] E.M. Borst, et al., Cloning of the human cytomegalovirus (HCMV) genome as an infectious bacterial artificial chromosome in *Escherichia coli*: a new approach for construction of HCMV mutants, J. Virol. 73 (1999) 8320–8329.

[24] E. Mocarski, Betaherpes viral genes and their function, in: A. Arvin (Ed.), Human Herpesviruses: Biology, Therapy, and Immunoprophylaxis, Cambridge University Press, Cambridge, 2007, pp. 204–230.

[25] S.M. Varnum, et al., Identification of proteins in human cytomegalovirus (HCMV) particles: The HCMV proteome [erratum appears in J Virol 78(23):13395, 2004], J. Virol. 78 (2004) 10960–10966.

[26] E. Murphy, T. Shenk, Human cytomegalovirus genome, in: T. Shenk, M.F. Stinski (Eds.), Human Cytomegalovirus, Springer-Verlag, Berlin, 2008, pp. 1–20.

[27] W. Britt, Maturation and egress, in: A. Arvin (Ed.), Human Herpesviruses: Biology, Therapy, and Immunoprophylaxis, Cambridge University Press, Cambridge, 2007, pp. 311–323.

[28] W. Gibson, Structure and function of the cytomegalovirus virion, in: T. Shenk, M.F. Stinski (Eds.), Human Cytomegalovirus, Springer-Verlag, Berlin, 2008, pp. 187–204.

[29] E. Bogner, K. Radsak, M.F. Stinski, The gene product of human cytomegalovirus open reading frame UL56 binds the pac motif and has specific nuclease activity, J. Virol. 72 (1998) 2259–2264.

[30] H. Scheffczik, et al., The terminase subunits pUL56 and pUL89 of human cytomegalovirus are DNA-metabolizing proteins with toroidal structure, Nucl. Acids Res. 30 (2002) 1695–1703.

[31] P.M. Krosky, et al., Resistance of human cytomegalovirus to benzimidazole ribonucleosides maps to two open reading frames: UL89 and UL56, J. Virol. 72 (1998) 4721–4728.

[32] F. Mou, et al., Effects of lamin A/C, lamin B1, and viral US3 kinase activity on viral infectivity, virion egress, and the targeting of herpes simplex virus U(L)34-encoded protein to the inner nuclear membrane, J. Virol. 82 (2008) 8094–8104.

[33] A.E. Reynolds, et al., Ultrastructural localization of the herpes simplex virus type 1 UL31, UL34, and US3 proteins suggests specific roles in primary envelopment and egress of nucleocapsids, J. Virol. 76 (2002) 8939–8952.

[34] P.M. Krosky, M.C. Baek, D.M. Coen, The human cytomegalovirus UL97 protein kinase, an antiviral drug target, is required at the stage of nuclear egress, J. Virol. 77 (2003) 905–914.

[35] S. Hamirally, et al., Viral mimicry of Cdc2/cyclin-dependent kinase 1 mediates disruption of nuclear lamina during human cytomegalovirus nuclear egress, PLoS Pathog. 5 (2009) e1000275.

[36] W.A. Bresnahan, T. Shenk, A subset of viral transcripts packaged within human cytomegalovirus particles, Science 288 (2000) 2373–2376.

[37] A.J. Hume, R.F. Kalejta, Regulation of the retinoblastoma proteins by the human herpesviruses, Cell Div. 4 (2009) 1.

[38] R.F. Kalejta, Functions of human cytomegalovirus tegument proteins prior to immediate early gene expression, Curr. Top. Microbiol. Immunol. 325 (2008) 101–115.

[39] A.J. Hume, et al., Phosphorylation of retinoblastoma protein by viral protein with cyclin-dependent kinase function, Science 320 (2008) 797–799.

[40] E.A. Fortunato, D.H. Spector, p53 and RPA are sequestered in viral replication centers in the nuclei of cells infected with human cytomegalovirus, J. Virol. 72 (1998) 2033–2039.

[41] B.S. Salvant, E.A. Fortunato, D.H. Spector, Cell cycle dysregulation by human cytomegalovirus: influence of the cell cycle phase at the time of infection and effects on cyclin transcription, J. Virol. 72 (1998) 3729–3741.

[42] M.L. Hayashi, C. Blankenship, T. Shenk, Human cytomegalovirus UL69 protein is required for efficient accumulation of infected cells in the G1 phase of the cell cycle, Proc. Natl. Acad. Sci. U. S. A. 97 (2000) 2692–2696.

[43] C.J. Baldick Jr., et al., Human cytomegalovirus tegument protein pp 71 (ppUL82) enhances the infectivity of viral DNA and accelerates the infectious cycle, J. Virol. 71 (1997) 4400–4408.

[44] N.J. Buchkovich, et al., The TORrid affairs of viruses: effects of mammalian DNA viruses on the PI3K-Akt-mTOR signalling pathway, Nat. Rev. Microbiol. 6 (2008) 266–275.

[45] J.C. Alwine, Modulation of host cell stress responses by human cytomegalovirus, Curr. Top. Microbiol. Immunol. 325 (2008) 263–279.

[46] N.J. Buchkovich, et al., Human cytomegalovirus specifically controls the levels of the endoplasmic reticulum chaperone BiP/GRP78, which is required for virion assembly, J. Virol. 82 (2008) 31–39.

[47] S.B. Kudchodkar, et al., Human cytomegalovirus infection alters the substrate specificities and rapamycin sensitivities of raptor- and rictor-containing complexes, Proc. Natl. Acad. Sci. U. S. A. 103 (2006) 14182–14187.

[48] J. Munger, et al., Systems-level metabolic flux profiling identifies fatty acid synthesis as a target for antiviral therapy, Nat. Biotechnol. 26 (2008) 1179–1186.

[49] N.J. Moorman, et al., Human cytomegalovirus protein UL38 inhibits host cell stress responses by antagonizing the tuberous sclerosis protein complex, Cell Host Microbe 3 (2008) 253–262.

[50] M.P. Landini, M. LaPlaca, Humoral immune response to human cytomegalovirus proteins: a brief review, Comp. Immunol. Microbiol. Infect. Dis. 14 (1991) 97–105.

[51] J.A. Zaia, et al., Polypeptide-specific antibody response to human cytomegalovirus after infection in bone marrow transplant recipients, J. Infect. Dis. 153 (1986) 780–787.

[52] A.W. Sylwester, et al., Broadly targeted human cytomegalovirus-specific CD4+ and CD8+ T cells dominate the memory compartments of exposed subjects, J. Exp. Med. 202 (2005) 673–685.

[53] K. Hayes, C.A. Alford, W.J. Britt, Antibody response to virus-encoded proteins after cytomegalovirus mononucleosis, J. Infect. Dis. 156 (1987) 615–621.

[54] F. Kern, et al., Cytomegalovirus (CMV) phosphoprotein 65 makes a large contribution to shaping the T cell repertoire in CMV-exposed individuals, J. Infect. Dis. 185 (2002) 1709–1716.

[55] S.B. Boppana, W.J. Britt, Recognition of human cytomegalovirus gene products by HCMV-specific cytotoxic T cells, Virology 222 (1996) 293–296.

[56] M.S. Chee, et al., Analysis of the protein-coding content of the sequence of human cytomegalovirus strain AD169, Curr. Top. Microbiol. Immunol. 154 (1990) 125–170.

[57] W.J. Britt, S. Boppana, Human cytomegalovirus virion proteins, Hum. Immunol. 65 (2004) 395–402.

[58] M. Eickmann, D. Glickhorn, K. Radsak, Glycoprotein trafficking in virion morphogenesis, in: M.J. Reddehase (Ed.), Cytomegaloviruses: Molecular Biology and Immunology, Casiter, Norfolk, UK, 2006, pp. 245–264.

[59] M. Mach, Antibody-mediated neutralization of infectivity, in: M.J. Reddehase (Ed.), Cytomegaloviruses: Molecular Biology and Immunology, Caister, Norfolk, UK, 2006, pp. 265–283.

[60] D. Wang, et al., Human cytomegalovirus uses two distinct pathways to enter retinal pigmented epithelial cells, Proc. Natl. Acad. Sci. U. S. A. 104 (2007) 20037–20042.

[61] G. Hahn, et al., Human cytomegalovirus UL131–128 genes are indispensable for virus growth in endothelial cells and virus transfer to leukocytes, J. Virol. 78 (2004) 10023–10033.

[62] B.J. Ryckman, M.C. Chase, D.C. Johnson, HCMV gH/gL/UL128–131 interferes with virus entry into epithelial cells: evidence for cell type-specific receptors, Proc. Natl. Acad. Sci. U. S. A. 105 (2008) 14118–14123.

[63] X. Cui, et al., Cytomegalovirus vaccines fail to induce epithelial entry neutralizing antibodies comparable to natural infection, Vaccine 26 (2008) 5760–5766.

[64] W.J. Britt, et al., Cell surface expression of human cytomegalovirus (HCMV) gp55–116 (gB): use of HCMV-vaccinia recombinant virus infected cells in analysis of the human neutralizing antibody response, J. Virol. 64 (1990) 1079–1085.

[65] H. Meyer, Y. Masuho, M. Mach, The gp116 of the gp58/116 complex of human cytomegalovirus represents the amino-terminal part of the precursor molecule and contains a neutralizing epitope, J. Gen. Virol. 71 (1990) 2443–2450.

[66] L. Rasmussen, et al., Antibody response to human cytomegalovirus glycoproteins gB and gH after natural infection in humans, J. Infect. Dis. 164 (1991) 835–842.

[67] G.S. Marshall, et al., Antibodies to recombinant-derived glycoprotein B after natural human cytomegalovirus infection correlate with neutralizing activity, J. Infect. Dis. 165 (1992) 381–384.

[68] M. Urban, et al., Glycoprotein H of human cytomegalovirus is a major antigen for the neutralizing humoral immune response, J. Gen. Virol. 77 (1996) 1537–1547.

[69] T. Compton, Receptors and immune sensors: the complex entry path of human cytomegalovirus, Trends Cell Biol. 14 (2004) 5–8.

[70] K.W. Boehme, T. Compton, Virus entry and activation of innate immunity, in: M.J. Reddehase (Ed.), Cytomegaloviruses: Molecular Biology and Immunology, Caister, Norfolk, UK, 2006, pp. 111–130.

[71] X. Wang, et al., Epidermal growth factor receptor is a cellular receptor for human cytomegalovirus, Nature 424 (2003) 456–461.

[72] X. Wang, et al., Integrin αvβ3 is a coreceptor for human cytomegalovirus, Nat. Med. 11 (2005) 515–521.

[73] A.L. Feire, H. Koss, T. Compton, Cellular integrins function as entry receptors for human cytomegalovirus via a highly conserved disintegrin-like domain, Proc. Natl. Acad. Sci. U. S. A. 101 (2004) 15470–15475.

[74] L. Soroceanu, A. Akhavan, C.S. Cobbs, Platelet-derived growth factor-alpha receptor activation is required for human cytomegalovirus infection, Nature 455 (2008) 391–395.

[75] C.S. Cobbs, et al., Human cytomegalovirus induces cellular tyrosine kinase signaling and promotes glioma cell invasiveness, J. Neurooncol. 85 (2007) 271–280.

[76] H. Zhu, et al., Cellular gene expression altered by human cytomegalovirus: global monitoring with oligonucleotide arrays, Proc. Natl. Acad. Sci. U. S. A. 95 (1998) 14470–14475.

[77] H. Zhu, J.P. Cong, T. Shenk, Use of differential display analysis to assess the effect of human cytomegalovirus infection on the accumulation of cellular RNAs: induction of interferon-responsive RNAs, Proc. Natl. Acad. Sci. U. S. A. 94 (1997) 13985–13990.

[78] E.P. Browne, et al., Altered cellular mRNA levels in human cytomegalovirus-infected fibroblasts: viral block to the accumulation of antiviral mRNAs, J. Virol. 75 (2001) 12319–12330.

[79] K.A. Simmen, et al., Global modulation of cellular transcription by human cytomegalovirus is initiated by viral glycoprotein B, Proc. Natl. Acad. Sci. U. S. A. 98 (2001) 7140–7145.

[80] Y. Yu, J.C. Alwine, Human cytomegalovirus major immediate-early proteins and simian virus 40 large T antigen can inhibit apoptosis through activation of the phosphatidylinositide 3p-OH kinase pathway and the cellular kinase Akt, J. Virol. 76 (2002) 3731–3738.

[81] L.C. Sambucetti, et al., NF-kappa B activation of the cytomegalovirus enhancer is mediated by a viral transactivator and by T cell stimulation, EMBO J. 8 (1989) 4251–4258.

[82] S. Child, et al., Complementation of vaccinia virus lacking the double stranded RNA-binding protein gene E3L by human cytomegalovirus, J. Virol. 76 (2002) 4912–4918.

[83] M. Hakki, A.P. Geballe, Double-stranded RNA binding by human cytomegalovirus pTRS1, J. Virol. 79 (2005) 7311–7318.

[84] A. Zimmerman, H. Hengel, Cytomegalovirus interference with interferons, in: M.J. Reddehase (Ed.), Cytomegaloviruses: Molecular Biology and Immunology, Caister, Norfolk, UK, 2006, pp. 321–339.

[85] K. Ogawa-Goto, et al., Microtubule network facilitates nuclear targeting of human cytomegalovirus capsid, J. Virol. 77 (2003) 8541–8547.

[86] K. Radtke, K. Dohner, B. Sodeik, Viral interactions with the cytoskeleton: a hitchhiker's guide to the cell, Cell. Microbiol. 8 (2006) 387–400.

[87] A. Wolfstein, et al., The inner tegument promotes herpes simplex virus capsid motility along microtubules in vitro, Traffic 7 (2006) 227–237.

[88] M.F. Stinski, T. Shenk, Functional roles of the human cytomegalovirus essential IE86 protein, in: T. Shenk, M.F. Stinski (Eds.), Human Cytomegalovirus, Springer-Verlag, Berlin, 2008, pp. 133–152.

[89] A.L. McCormick, Control of apoptosis by human cytomegalovirus, in: T. Shenk, M.F. Stinski (Eds.), Human Cytomegalovirus, Springer-Verlag, Berlin, 2008, pp. 281–294.

[90] B.R. Cullen, Viral and cellular messenger RNA targets of viral microRNAs, Nature 457 (2009) 421–425.

[91] E. Gottwein, B.R. Cullen, Viral and cellular microRNAs as determinants of viral pathogenesis and immunity, Cell Host Microbe 3 (2008) 375–387.

[92] F. Grey, J. Nelson, Identification and function of human cytomegalovirus microRNAs, J. Clin. Virol. 41 (2008) 186–191.

[93] F. Grey, et al., A human cytomegalovirus-encoded microRNA regulates expression of multiple viral genes involved in replication, PLoS Pathog. 3 (2007) e163.

[94] J.A. Nelson, Small RNAs and large DNA viruses, N. Engl. J. Med. 357 (2007) 2630–2632.

[95] F. Grey, et al., Identification and characterization of human cytomegalovirus-encoded microRNAs, J. Virol. 79 (2005) 12095–12099.

[96] E. Murphy, et al., Suppression of immediate-early viral gene expression by herpesvirus-coded microRNAs: implications for latency, Proc. Natl. Acad. Sci. U. S. A. 105 (2008) 5453–5458.

[97] G. Pari, Nuts and bolts of human cytomegalovirus lytic DNA replication, in: T. Shenk, M.F. Stinski (Eds.), Human Cytomegalovirus, Springer-Verlag, Berlin, 2008, pp. 153–166.

[98] W.W. Newcomb, et al., In vitro assembly of the herpes simplex virus procapsid: formation of small procapsids at reduced scaffolding protein concentration, J. Struct. Biol. 133 (2001) 23–31.

[99] J.B. Heymann, et al., Dynamics of herpes simplex virus capsid maturation visualized by time-lapse cryo-electron microscopy, Nat. Struct. Biol. 10 (2003) 334–341.

[100] V. Sanchez, et al., Accumulation of virion tegument and envelope proteins in a stable cytoplasmic compartment during human cytomegalovirus replication: characterization of a potential site of virus assembly, J. Virol. 74 (2000) 975–986.

[101] M. Homman-Loudiyi, et al., Envelopment of human cytomegalovirus occurs by budding into Golgi-derived vacuole compartments positive for gB, Rab 3, trans-Golgi network 46, and mannosidase II [erratum appears in J Virol 77(14):8179, 2003], J. Virol. 77 (2003) 3191–3203.

[102] S. Das, A. Vasanji, P.E. Pellett, Three-dimensional structure of the human cytomegalovirus cytoplasmic virion assembly complex includes a reoriented secretory apparatus, J. Virol. 81 (2007) 11861–11869.

[103] J. Taylor-Wiedeman, P. Sissons, J. Sinclair, Induction of endogenous human cytomegalovirus gene expression after differentiation of monocytes from healthy carriers, J. Virol. 68 (1994) 1597–1604.

[104] K. Kondo, J. Xu, E.S. Mocarski, Human cytomegalovirus latent gene expression in granulocyte-macrophage progenitors in culture and in seropositive individuals, Proc. Natl. Acad. Sci. U. S. A. 93 (1996) 11137–11142.

[105] C. Soderberg-Naucler, K.N. Fish, J.A. Nelson, Reactivation of latent human cytomegalovirus by allogeneic stimulation of blood cells from healthy donors, Cell 91 (1997) 119–126.

[106] C. Soderberg-Naucler, K.N. Fish, J.A. Nelson, Interferon-gamma and tumor necrosis factor-alpha specifically induce formation of cytomegalovirus-permissive monocyte-derived macrophages that are refractory to the antiviral activity of these cytokines, J. Clin. Invest. 100 (1997) 3154–3163.

[107] M. Reeves, J. Sinclair, Aspects of human cytomegalovirus latency and reactivation, in: T. Shenk, M.F. Stinski (Eds.), Human Cytomegalovirus, Springer-Verlag, Berlin, 2008, pp. 297–313.

[108] C.A. Bolovan-Fritts, E.S. Mocarski, J.A. Wiedeman, Peripheral blood CD14 (+) cells from healthy subjects carry a circular conformation of latent cytomegalovirus genome, Blood 93 (1999) 394–398.

[109] C. Soderberg-Naucler, et al., Reactivation of latent human cytomegalovirus in CD14(+) monocytes is differentiation dependent, J. Virol. 75 (2001) 7543–7554.

[110] J.W. Gnann, et al., Inflammatory cells in transplanted kidneys are infected by human cytomegalovirus, Am. J. Pathol. 132 (1988) 239–248.

[111] M. Hummel, et al., Allogeneic transplantation induces expression of cytomegalovirus immediate-early genes in vivo: a model for reactivation from latency, J. Virol. 75 (2001) 4814–4822.

[112] M. Hummel, M.M. Abecassis, A model for reactivation of CMV from latency, J. Clin. Virol. 25 (Suppl. 2) (2002) S123–S136.

[113] J.D. Roback, et al., Multicenter evaluation of PCR methods for detecting CMV DNA in blood donors, Transfusion 41 (2001) 1249–1257.

[114] C. Sinzger, et al., Cell types infected in human cytomegalovirus placentitis identified by immunohistochemical double staining, Virchows Arch A. Pathol. Anat. Histopathol. 423 (1993) 249–256.

[115] C. Sinzger, et al., Immunohistochemical detection of viral antigens in smooth muscle, stromal, and epithelial cells from acute human cytomegalovirus gastritis, J. Infect. Dis. 167 (1993) 1427–1432.

[116] C. Sinzger, M. Digel, G. Jahn, Cytomegalovirus cell tropism, in: T. Shenk, M.F. Stinski (Eds.), Human Cytomegalovirus, Springer-Verlag, Berlin, 2008, pp. 63–84.

[117] B.J. Ryckman, et al., Human cytomegalovirus entry into epithelial and endothelial cells depends on genes UL128 to UL150 and occurs by endocytosis and low-pH fusion, J. Virol. 80 (2006) 710–722.

[118] F.A. Colugnati, et al., Incidence of cytomegalovirus infection among the general population and pregnant women in the United States, BMC Infect. Dis. 7 (2007) 71.

[119] S.A. Staras, et al., Seroprevalence of cytomegalovirus infection in the United States, 1988–1994, Clin. Infect. Dis. 43 (2006) 1143–1151.

[120] I.R. Wilms, A.M. Best, S.P. Adler, Cytomegalovirus infections among African-Americans, BMC Infect. Dis. 8 (2008) 107.

[121] A. Kenneson, M.J. Cannon, Review and meta-analysis of the epidemiology of congenital cytomegalovirus (CMV) infection, Rev. Med. Virol. 17 (2007) 253–276.

[122] S. Stagno, et al., Primary cytomegalovirus infection in pregnancy: incidence, transmission to fetus, and clinical outcome, JAMA 256 (1986) 1904–1908.

[123] M.C. Jordan, et al., Association of cervical cytomegaloviruses with venereal disease, N. Engl. J. Med. 288 (1973) 932–934.

[124] D. Coonrod, et al., Association between cytomegalovirus seroconversion and upper genital tract infection among women attending a sexually transmitted disease clinic: a prospective study, J. Infect. Dis. 177 (1998) 1188–1193.

[125] W.L. Drew, et al., Prevalence of cytomegalovirus infection in homosexual men, J. Infect. Dis. 143 (1981) 188–192.

[126] S.H. Chandler, et al., The epidemiology of cytomegaloviral infection in women attending a sexually transmitted disease clinic, J. Infect. Dis. 152 (1985) 597–605.

[127] S.A. Ross, et al., Association between genital tract cytomegalovirus infection and bacterial vaginosis, J. Infect. Dis. 192 (2005) 1727–1730.

[128] D. Hayes, et al., Cytomegalovirus in human milk, N. Engl. J. Med. 287 (1972) 177.

[129] M. Dworsky, et al., Cytomegalovirus infection of breast milk and transmission in infancy, Pediatrics 72 (1983) 295–299.

[130] K. Hamprecht, et al., Detection of cytomegaloviral DNA in human milk cells and cell free milk whey by nested PCR, J. Virol. Method. 70 (1998) 167–176.

[131] K. Hamprecht, et al., Epidemiology of transmission of cytomegalovirus from mother to preterm infant by breastfeeding, Lancet 357 (2001) 513–518.

[132] R.F. Pass, et al., Cytomegalovirus infection in a day care center, N. Engl. J. Med. 307 (1982) 477–479.

[133] S.P. Adler, The molecular epidemiology of cytomegalovirus transmission among children attending a day care center, J. Infect. Dis. 152 (1985) 760–768.

[134] J.R. Murph, et al., Cytomegalovirus transmission in a Midwest day care center: possible relationship to child care practices, J. Pediatr. 109 (1986) 35–39.

[135] J.R. Murph, J.F. Bale Jr., The natural history of acquired cytomegalovirus infection among children in group day care, Am. J. Dis. Child. 142 (1988) 843–846.

[136] S.C. Hutto, et al., Epidemiology of cytomegalovirus infections in young children: day care vs home care, Pediatr. Infect. Dis. 4 (1985) 149–152.

[137] R.F. Pass, et al., Young children as a probable source of maternal and congenital cytomegalovirus infection, N. Engl. J. Med. 316 (1987) 1366–1370.

[138] S. Stagno, G.A. Cloud, Working parents: the impact of day care and breast-feeding on cytomegalovirus infections in offspring, Proc. Natl. Acad. Sci. U. S. A. 91 (1994) 2384–2389.

[139] C. Hutto, et al., Isolation of cytomegalovirus from toys and hands in a day care center, J. Infect. Dis. 154 (1986) 527–530.

[140] R.G. Faix, Survival of cytomegalovirus on environmental surfaces, J. Pediatr. 106 (1985) 649–652.

[141] M. Dworsky, A. Lakeman, S. Stagno, Cytomegalovirus transmission within a family, Pediatr. Infect. Dis. 3 (1984) 236–238.

[142] J.R. Murph, et al., Epidemiology of congenital cytomegalovirus infection: maternal risk factors and molecular analysis of cytomegalovirus strains, Am. J. Epidemiol. 147 (1998) 940–947.

[143] J.R. Murph, et al., The occupational risk of cytomegalovirus infection among day-care providers, JAMA 265 (1991) 603–608.

[144] S.A. Spector, D.H. Spector, Molecular epidemiology of cytomegalovirus infections in premature twin infants and their mother, Pediatr. Infect. Dis. J. 1 (1982) 405–409.

[145] A.S. Yeager, Transmission of cytomegalovirus to mothers by infected infants: another reason to prevent transfusion-acquired infections, Pediatr. Infect. Dis. 2 (1983) 295.

[146] M. Dworsky, et al., Occupational risk for primary cytomegalovirus infection among pediatric health care workers, N. Engl. J. Med. 309 (1983) 950–953.

[147] L.H. Taber, A.L. Frank, M.D. Yow, A. Bagley, Acquisition of cytomegaloviral infections in families with young children: a serological study, J Infect Dis 151 (1985) 948–952.

[148] S.P. Adler, Cytomegalovirus and child day care: evidence for an increased infection rate among day-care workers, N. Engl. J. Med. 321 (1989) 1290–1296.

[149] S.P. Adler, Molecular epidemiology of cytomegalovirus: viral transmission among children attending a day care center, their parents, and caretakers, J. Pediatr. 112 (1988) 366–372.

[150] S.P. Adler, et al., Molecular epidemiology of cytomegalovirus in a nursery: lack of evidence for nosocomial transmission, J. Pediatr. 108 (1986) 117–123.

[151] R.F. Pass, et al., Increased rate of cytomegalovirus infection among parents of children attending day care centers, N. Engl. J. Med. 314 (1986) 1414–1418.

[152] B.C. Marshall, S.P. Adler, The frequency of pregnancy and exposure to cytomegalovirus infections among women with a young child in day care, Am. J. Obstet. Gynecol. 200 (163) (2009) e1–e5.

[153] K. Schopfer, E. Lauber, U. Krech, Congenital cytomegalovirus infection in newborn infants of mothers infected before pregnancy, Arch. Dis. Child. 53 (1978) 536–539.

[154] S. Stagno, et al., Congenital cytomegalovirus infection: occurrence in an immune population, N. Engl. J. Med. 296 (1977) 1254–1258.

[155] J.A. Embil, R.J. Ozere, E.V. Haldane, Congenital cytomegalovirus infection in two siblings from consecutive pregnancies, J. Pediatr. 77 (1970) 417–421.

[156] A.Y. Yamamoto, et al., Congenital cytomegalovirus infection in preterm and full-term newborn infants from a population with a high seroprevalence rate, Pediatr. Infect. Dis. J. 20 (2001) 188–192.

[157] L. Dar, et al., Congenital cytomegalovirus infection in a highly seropositive semi-urban population in India, Pediatr. Infect. Dis. J. 27 (2008) 841–843.

[158] M.M. Mussi-Pinhata, et al., Birth prevalence and natural history of congenital cytomegalovirus (CMV) infection in highly seroimmune population, Clin. Infect. Dis. 49 (2009) 522–528.

[159] S. Stagno, et al., Maternal cytomegalovirus infection and perinatal transmission, Clin. Obstet. Gynecol. 25 (1982) 563–576.

[160] S.B. Boppana, et al., Intrauterine transmission of cytomegalovirus to infants of women with preconceptional immunity, N. Engl. J. Med. 344 (2001) 1366–1371.

[161] R.C. Gehrz, et al., Cytomegalovirus specific humoral and cellular immune responses in human pregnancy, J. Infect. Dis. 143 (1981) 391–395.

[162] D. Lilleri, et al., Development of human cytomegalovirus-specific T cell immunity during primary infection of pregnant women and its correlation with virus transmission to the fetus, J. Infect. Dis. 195 (2007) 1062–1070.

[163] S.B. Boppana, W.J. Britt, Antiviral antibody responses and intrauterine transmission after primary maternal cytomegalovirus infection, J. Infect. Dis. 171 (1995) 1115–1121.

[164] S.B. Boppana, J. Miller, W.J. Britt, Transplacentally acquired antiviral antibodies and outcome in congenital human cytomegalovirus infection, Viral Immunol. 9 (1996) 211–218.

[165] R.F. Pass, Transmission of viruses through human milk, in: R.R. Howell, F.H. Morriss, L.K. Pickering (Eds.), Role of Human Milk in Infant Nutrition and Health, Charles C Thomas, Springfield, IL, 1986, pp. 205–224.

[166] H.H. Handsfield, et al., Cytomegalovirus infection in sex partners: evidence for sexual transmission, J. Infect. Dis. 151 (1985) 344–348.

[167] S.A. Staras, et al., Influence of sexual activity on cytomegalovirus seroprevalence in the United States, 1988–1994, Sex. Transm. Dis. 35 (2008) 472–479.

[168] I. Kreel, et al., A syndrome following total body perfusion, Surg. Gynecol. Obstet. 111 (1960) 317–321.

[169] A.J. Seaman, A. Starr, Febrile post-cariotomy lymphocytic splenomegaly: a new entity, Ann. Surg. 156 (1962) 956–960.

[170] J.A. Armstrong, et al., Cytomegalovirus infection in children undergoing open heart surgery, Yale J. Biol. Med. 49 (1976) 83–91.

[171] A.M. Prince, et al., A serologic study of cytomegalovirus infections associated with blood transfusions, N. Engl. J. Med. 284 (1971) 1125–1131.

[172] D.P. Stevens, et al., Asymptomatic cytomegalovirus infection following blood transfusion in tumor patients, JAMA 211 (1970) 1341–1344.

[173] G.J. McCracken, et al., Congenital cytomegalic inclusion disease: a longitudinal study of 20 patients, Am. J. Dis. Child. 117 (1969) 522–539.

[174] A. Kumar, et al., Acquisition of cytomegalovirus infection in infants following exchange transfusion: a prospective study, Transfusion 20 (1980) 327–331.

[175] A.S. Yeager, Prevention of transfusion-acquired cytomegalovirus infections in newborn infants, J. Pediatr. 98 (1981) 281–287.

[176] J.D. Meyers, N. Flournoy, E.D. Thomas, Nonbacterial pneumonia after allogeneic marrow transplantation: a review of ten years' experience, Rev. Infect. Dis. 4 (1982) 1119–1132.

[177] R. Rubin, Clinical approach to infection in the compromised host, in: R. Rubin, L.S. Young (Eds.), Infection in the Organ Transplant Recipient, Kluwer Academic Press, New York, 2002, pp. 573–679.

[178] M. Boeckh, et al., Late cytomegalovirus disease and mortality in recipients of allogeneic hematopoietic stem cell transplants: importance of viral load and T-cell immunity, Blood 101 (2003) 407–414.

[179] M. Boeckh, Management of cytomegalovirus infections in blood and marrow transplant recipients, Adv. Exp. Med. Biol. 458 (1999) 89–109.

[180] H.A. Valantine, et al., Impact of cytomegalovirus hyperimmune globulin on outcome after cardiothoracic transplantation: a comparative study of combined prophylaxis with CMV hyperimmune globulin plus ganciclovir versus ganciclovir alone, Transplantation 72 (2001) 1647–1652.

[181] H.A. Valantine, Role of CMV in transplant coronary artery disease and survival after heart transplantation, Transpl. Infect. Dis. 1 (Suppl. 1) (1999) 25–30.

[182] N. Singh, Cytomegalovirus infection in solid organ transplant recipients: new challenges and their implications for preventive strategies, J. Clin. Virol. 35 (2006) 474–477.

[183] P.D. Griffiths, D.A. Clark, V.C. Emery, Betaherpesviruses in transplant recipients, J. Antimicrob. Chemother. 45 (2000) 29–34.

[184] J.E. Grundy, et al., The source of cytomegalovirus infection in seropositive renal allograft recipients is frequently the donor kidney, Transplant. Proc. 19 (1987) 2126–2128.

[185] J.E. Grundy, et al., Symptomatic cytomegalovirus infection in seropositive kidney recipients: reinfection with donor virus rather than reactivation of recipient virus, Lancet 16 (1988) 132–135.

[186] S.W. Chou, Acquisition of donor strains of cytomegalovirus by renal-transplant recipients, N. Engl. J. Med. 314 (1986) 1418–1423.

[187] S.W. Chou, Cytomegalovirus infection and reinfection transmitted by heart transplantation, J. Infect. Dis. 155 (1987) 1054–1056.

[188] M.D. Yow, et al., Use of restriction enzymes to investigate the source of a primary cytomegalovirus infection in a pediatric nurse, Pediatrics 70 (1982) 713–716.

[189] C.M. Wilfert, E.S. Huang, S. Stagno, Restriction endonuclease analysis of cytomegalovirus deoxyribonucleic acid as an epidemiologic tool, Pediatrics 70 (1982) 717–721.

[190] E. Klemola, L. Kaariainen, Cytomegalovirus as a possible cause of a disease resembling infectious mononucleosis, BMJ 2 (1965) 1099–1102.

[191] J. Andersson, H. Stern, Cytomegalovirus as a possible cause of a disease resembling infectious mononucleosis, BMJ 1 (1966) 672.

[192] A.F. Hassan-Walker, et al., Quantity of human cytomegalovirus (CMV) DNAemia as a risk factor for CMV disease in renal allograft recipients: relationship with donor/recipient CMV serostatus, receipt of augmented methylprednisolone and antithymocyte globulin (ATG), J. Med. Virol. 58 (1999) 182–187.

[193] J.A. Zaia, et al., Prolonged human cytomegalovirus viremia following bone marrow transplantation, Transplantation 37 (1984) 315–317.

[194] J.A. Zaia, Prevention and management of CMV-related problems after hematopoietic stem cell transplantation, Bone Marrow Transplant. 29 (2002) 633–638.

[195] S.A. Spector, et al., Cytomegalovirus (CMV) DNA load is an independent predictor of CMV disease and survival in advanced AIDS, J. Virol. 73 (1999) 7027–7030.

[196] V.C. Emery, et al., Application of viral-load kinetics to identify patients who develop cytomegalovirus disease after transplantation, Lancet 355 (2000) 2032–2036.

[197] M.T. Grattan, et al., Cytomegalovirus infection is associated with cardiac allograft rejection and atherosclerosis, JAMA 261 (1989) 3561–3566.

[198] J.L. Melnick, et al., Cytomegalovirus antigen within human arterial smooth muscle cells, Lancet 2 (1983) 644–647.

[199] F.J. Nieto, M. Szklo, P.D. Sorlie, Cytomegalovirus infection and coronary heart disease, Circulation 100 (1999) e139.

[200] F.J. Nieto, et al., Cohort study of cytomegalovirus infection as a risk factor for carotid intimal-medial thickening, a measure of subclinical atherosclerosis, Circulation 94 (1996) 922–927.

[201] J.D. Hosenpud, Coronary artery disease after heart transplantation and its relation to cytomegalovirus, Am. Heart. J. 138 (1999) S469–S472.

[202] P.K. Koskinen, et al., Cytomegalovirus infection and cardiac allograft vasculopathy, Transplant. Infect. Dis. 1 (1999) 115–126.

[203] H.A. Valantine, et al., Impact on prophylactic immediate posttransplant ganciclovir on development of transplant atherosclerosis: a post host analysis of a randomized, placebo-controlled study, Circulation 100 (1999) 61–66.

[204] J. Zhu, et al., Cytomegalovirus in the pathogenesis of atherosclerosis: the role of inflammation as reflected by elevated C-reactive protein levels, J. Am. Coll. Cardiol. 34 (1999) 1738–1743.

[205] P.C. Evans, et al., An association between cytomegalovirus infection and chronic rejection after liver transplantation, Transplantation 69 (2000) 30–35.

[206] C. Soderberg-Naucler, V.C. Emery, Viral infections and their impact on chronic renal allograft dysfunction, Transplantation 71 (2001) SS24–SS30.

[207] S. Stagno, et al., Auditory and visual defects resulting from symptomatic and subclinical congenital cytomegaloviral and toxoplasma infections, Pediatrics 59 (1977) 669–678.

[208] A.J. Dahle, et al., Progressive hearing impairment in children with congenital cytomegalovirus infection, J. Speech. Hear. Disord. 44 (1979) 220–229.

[209] A. Dahle, et al., Longitudinal investigation of hearing disorders in children with congenital cytomegalovirus, J. Am. Acad. Audiol. 11 (2000) 283–290.

[210] K.B. Fowler, et al., Progressive and fluctuating sensorineural hearing loss in children with asymptomatic congenital cytomegalovirus infection, J. Pediatr. 130 (1997) 624–630.

[211] K.B. Fowler, S.B. Boppana, Congenital cytomegalovirus (CMV) infection and hearing deficit, J. Clin. Virol. 35 (2006) 226–231.

[212] S. Boppana, K.B. Fowler, Persistence in the population: epidemiology and transmission, in: A. Arvin (Ed.), Human Herpesviruses: Biology, Therapy, and Immunoprophylaxis, Cambridge University Press, Cambridge, 2007, pp. 795–813.

[213] P. Koskinen, et al., Acute cytomegalovirus infection induces a subendothelial inflammation (endotheliaitis) in the allograft vascular wall: a possible linkage with enhanced allograft arteriosclerosis, Am. J. Pathol. 144 (1994) 41–50.

[214] K. Lemstrom, et al., Cytomegalovirus antigen expression, endothelial cell proliferation, and intimal thickening in rat cardiac allografts after cytomegalovirus infection, Circulation 92 (1995) 2594–2604.

[215] K.B. Lemstrom, et al., Triple drug immunosuppression significantly reduces immune activation and allograft arteriosclerosis in cytomegalovirus-infected rat aortic allografts and induces early latency of viral infection, Am. J. Pathol. 144 (1994) 1334–1347.

[216] F. Li, et al., Cytomegalovirus infection enhances the neointima formation in rat aortic allografts: effect of major histocompatibility complex class I and class II antigen differences, Transplantation 65 (1998) 1298–1304.

[217] Y.F. Zhou, et al., Cytomegalovirus infection of rats increases the neointimal response to vascular injury without consistent evidence of direct infection of the vascular wall, Circulation 100 (1999) 1569–1575.

[218] D.N. Streblow, et al., The human cytomegalovirus chemokine receptor US28 mediates vascular smooth muscle cell migration, Cell 99 (1999) 511–520.

[219] D.N. Streblow, et al., Mechanisms of cytomegalovirus-accelerated vascular disease: induction of paracrine factors that promote angiogenesis and wound healing, Curr. Top. Microbiol. Immunol. 325 (2008) 397–415.

[220] D.N. Streblow, et al., The role of angiogenic and wound repair factors during CMV-accelerated transplant vascular sclerosis in rat cardiac transplants, Am. J. Transplant. 8 (2008) 277–287.

[221] C.A. Stoddart, et al., Peripheral blood mononuclear phagocytes mediate dissemination of murine cytomegalovirus, J. Virol. 68 (1994) 6243–6253.

[222] S. Noda, et al., Cytomegalovirus MCK-2 controls mobilization and recruitment of myeloid progenitor cells to facilitate dissemination, Blood 107 (2006) 30–38.

[223] J. Taylor-Wiedeman, et al., Monocytes are a major site of persistence of human cytomegalovirus in peripheral blood mononuclear cells, J. Gen. Virol. 72 (1991) 2059–2064.

[224] J. Sinclair, P. Sissons, Latent and persistent infections of monocytes and macrophages, Intervirology 39 (1996) 293–301.

[225] T. Sacher, et al., Conditional gene expression systems to study herpesvirus biology in vivo, Med. Microbiol. Immunol. 197 (2008) 269–276.

[226] G. Gerna, et al., Human cytomegalovirus infection of the major leukocyte subpopulations and evidence for initial viral replication in polymorphonuclear leukocytes from viremic patients, J. Infect. Dis. 166 (1992) 1236–1244.

[227] P. Schafer, et al., Cytomegalovirus cultured from different major leukocyte subpopulations: association with clinical features in CMV immunoglobulin G-positive renal allograft recipients, J. Med. Virol. 61 (2000) 488–496.

[228] H. Liapis, et al., CMV infection of the renal allograft is much more common than the pathology indicates: a retrospective analysis of qualitative and quantitative buffy coat CMV-PCR, renal biopsy pathology and tissue CMV-PCR, Nephrol. Dial. Transplant. 18 (2003) 397–402.

[229] G. Gerna, et al., Human cytomegalovirus replicates abortively in polymorphonuclear leukocytes after transfer from infected endothelial cells via transient microfusion events, J. Virol. 74 (2000) 5629–5638.

[230] A.M. Kas-Deelen, et al., Uptake of pp 65 in in vitro generated pp65-positive polymorphonuclear cells mediated by phagocytosis and cell fusion? Intervirology 44 (2001) 8–13.

[231] T.H. The, et al., Cytomegalovirus antigenemia, Rev. Infect. Dis. 12 (S) (1990) 734–744.

[232] W. van der Bij, R. Speich, Management of cytomegalovirus infection and disease after solid-organ transplantation, Clin. Infect. Dis. 33 (2001) 1.

[233] N. Singh, et al., Cytomegalovirus antigenemia directed pre-emptive prophylaxis with oral versus I.V. ganciclovir for the prevention of cytomegalovirus disease in liver transplant recipients: a randomized, controlled trial, Transplantation 70 (2000) 717–722.

[234] W.G. Nichols, M. Boeckh, Recent advances in the therapy and prevention of CMV infections, J. Clin. Virol. 16 (2000) 25–40.

[235] M. Boeckh, et al., Cytomegalovirus pp 65 antigenemia-guided early treatment with ganciclovir versus ganciclovir at engraftment after allogeneic marrow transplantation: a randomized double-blind study, Blood 88 (1996) 4063–4071.

[236] W.G. Nichols, et al., Rising pp 65 antigenemia during preemptive anticytomegalovirus therapy after allogeneic hematopoietic stem cell transplantation: risk factors, correlation with DNA load, and outcomes, Blood 97 (2001) 867–874.

[237] W.J. Waldman, et al., Bidirectional transmission of infectious cytomegalovirus between monocytes and vascular endothelial cells: an in vitro model, J. Infect. Dis. 171 (1995) 263–272.

[238] S. Riegler, et al., Monocyte-derived dendritic cells are permissive to the complete replicative cycle of human cytomegalovirus, J. Gen. Virol. 81 (2000) 393–399.

[239] K.N. Fish, et al., Cytomegalovirus persistence in macrophages and endothelial cells, Scand. J. Infect. Dis. Suppl. 99 (1995) 34–40.

[240] G. Hahn, R. Jores, E.S. Mocarski, Cytomegalovirus remains latent in a common precursor of dendritic and myeloid cells, Proc. Natl. Acad. Sci. U. S. A. 95 (1998) 3937–3942.

[241] J. Sinclair, Human cytomegalovirus: latency and reactivation in the myeloid lineage, J. Clin. Virol. 41 (2008) 180–185.

[242] K.N. Fish, et al., Human cytomegalovirus persistently infects aortic endothelial cells, J. Virol. 72 (1998) 5661–5668.

[243] C. Sinzger, et al., Fibroblasts, epithelial cells, endothelial cells and smooth muscle cells are major targets of human cytomegalovirus infection in lung and gastrointestinal tissues, J. Gen. Virol. 76 (1995) 741–750.

[244] B. Plachter, C. Sinzger, G. Jahn, Cell types involved in replication and distribution of human cytomegalovirus, Adv. Virus. Res. 46 (1996) 195–261.

[245] C. Sinzger, et al., Quantification of replication of clinical cytomegalovirus isolates in cultured endothelial cells and fibroblasts by a focus expansion assay, J. Virol. Method. 63 (1997) 103–112.

[246] G. Gerna, et al., Circulating cytomegalic endothelial cells are associated with high human cytomegalovirus (HCMV) load in AIDS patients with late-stage disseminated HCMV disease, J. Med. Virol. 55 (1998) 64–74.

[247] P.C. Evans, et al., Cytomegalovirus infection of bile duct epithelial cells, hepatic artery and portal venous endothelium in relation to chronic rejection of liver grafts, J. Hepatol. 31 (1999) 913–920.

[248] A.M. Kas-Deelen, et al., Uninfected and cytomegalic endothelial cells in blood during cytomegalovirus infection: effect of acute rejection, J. Infect. Dis. 181 (2000) 721–724.

[249] E. Maidji, et al., Transmission of human cytomegalovirus from infected uterine microvascular endothelial cells to differentiating/invasive placental cytotrophoblasts, Virology 304 (2002) 53–69.

[250] C. Sinzger, et al., Tropism of human cytomegalovirus for endothelial cells is determined by a post-entry step dependent on efficient translocation to the nucleus, J. Gen. Virol. 81 (2000) 3021–3035.

[251] M. Kahl, et al., Efficient lytic infection of human arterial endothelial cells by human cytomegalovirus strains, J. Virol. 74 (2000) 7628–7635.

[252] E. Percivalle, et al., Circulating endothelial giant cells permissive for human cytomegalovirus (HCMV) are detected in disseminated HCMV infections with organ involvement, J. Clin. Invest. 92 (1993) 663–670.

[253] A. Grefte, et al., Circulating cytomegalovirus (CMV)-infected endothelial cells in patients with an active CMV infection, J. Infect. Dis. 167 (1993) 270–277.

[254] W. Brune, et al., A ribonucleotide reductase homolog of cytomegalovirus and endothelial cell tropism, Science 291 (2001) 303–305.

[255] B.C. Fries, et al., Frequency distribution of cytomegalovirus envelope glycoprotein genotypes in bone marrow transplant recipients, J. Infect. Dis. 169 (1994) 769–774.

[256] L. Rasmussen, et al., Cytomegalovirus gB genotype distribution differs in human immunodeficiency virus-infected patients and immunocompromised allograft recipients, J. Infect. Dis. 175 (1997) 179–184.

[257] M. Haberland, U. Meyer-Konig, F.T. Hufert, Variation within the glycoprotein B gene of human cytomegalovirus is due to homologous recombination, J. Gen. Virol. 80 (1999) 1495–1500.

[258] J.F. Bale Jr., et al., Intrauterine cytomegalovirus infection and glycoprotein B genotypes, J. Infect. Dis. 182 (2000) 933–936.

[259] N.S. Lurain, et al., Human cytomegalovirus UL144 open reading frame: sequence hypervariability in low-passage clinical isolates, J. Virol. 73 (1999) 10040–10050.

[260] J.F. Bale Jr., et al., Human cytomegalovirus a sequence and UL144 variability in strains from infected children, J. Med. Virol. 65 (2001) 90–96.

[261] L. Rasmussen, A. Geissler, M. Winters, Inter- and intragenic variations complicate the molecular epidemiology of human cytomegalovirus, J. Infect. Dis. 187 (2003) 809–819.

[262] L. Rasmussen, et al., The genes encoding the gCIII complex of human cytomegalovirus exist in highly diverse combinations in clinical isolates, J. Virol. 76 (2002) 10841–10848.

[263] I. Garrigue, et al., Variability of UL18, UL40, UL111a and US3 immunomodulatory genes among human cytomegalovirus clinical isolates from renal transplant recipients, J. Clin. Virol. 40 (2007) 120–128.

[264] I. Garrigue, et al., UL40 human cytomegalovirus variability evolution patterns over time in renal transplant recipients, Transplantation 86 (2008) 826–835.

[265] S. Hitomi, et al., Human cytomegalovirus open reading frame UL11 encodes a highly polymorphic protein expressed on the infected cell surface, Arch. Virol. 142 (1997) 1407–1427.

[266] S. Pignatelli, et al., Human cytomegalovirus glycoprotein N (gpUL73-gN) genomic variants: identification of a novel subgroup, geographical distribution and evidence of positive selective pressure, J. Gen. Virol. 84 (2003) 647–655.

[267] S. Pignatelli, P. Dal Monte, M.P. Landini, gpUL73 (gN) genomic variants of human cytomegalovirus isolates are clustered into four distinct genotypes, J. Gen. Virol. 82 (2001) 2777–2784.

[268] S.W. Chou, Reactivation and recombination of multiple cytomegalovirus strains from individual organ donors, J. Infect. Dis. 160 (1989) 11–15.

[269] B.J. Ryckman, et al., Characterization of the human cytomegalovirus gH/gL/UL128-131 complex that mediates entry into epithelial and endothelial cells, J. Virol. 82 (2008) 60–70.

[270] D. Wang, T. Shenk, Human cytomegalovirus virion protein complex required for epithelial and endothelial cell tropism, Proc. Natl. Acad. Sci. U. S. A. 102 (2005) 18153–18158.

[271] W.A. Hayajneh, et al., The sequence and antiapoptotic functional domains of the human cytomegalovirus UL37 exon 1 immediate early protein are conserved in multiple primary strains, Virology 279 (2001) 233–240.

[272] A. Skaletskaya, et al., A cytomegalovirus-encoded inhibitor of apoptosis that suppresses caspase-8 activation, Proc. Natl. Acad. Sci. U. S. A. 98 (2001) 7829–7834.

[273] V.S. Goldmacher, vMIA, a viral inhibitor of apoptosis targeting mitochondria, Biochimie 84 (2002) 177–185.

[274] E.S. Mocarski Jr., Immunomodulation by cytomegaloviruses: manipulative strategies beyond evasion, Trends Microbiol. 10 (2002) 332–339.

[275] N. Saederup, E.S. Mocarski Jr., Fatal attraction: cytomegalovirus-encoded chemokine homologs, Curr. Top. Microbiol. Immunol. 269 (2002) 235–256.

[276] J.V. Spencer, et al., Potent immunosuppressive activities of cytomegalovirus-encoded interleukin-10, J. Virol. 76 (2002) 1285–1292.

[277] C. Jenkins, et al., Immunomodulatory properties of a viral homolog of human interleukin-10 expressed by human cytomegalovirus during the latent phase of infection, J. Virol. 82 (2008) 3736–3750.

[278] A.L. McCormick, Control of apoptosis by human cytomegalovirus, Curr. Top. Microbiol. Immunol. 325 (2008) 281–295.

[279] V.S. Goldmacher, Cell death suppression by cytomegaloviruses, Apoptosis 10 (2005) 251–265.

[280] K.M. Lockridge, et al., Primate cytomegaloviruses encode and express an IL-10-like protein, Virology 268 (2000) 272–280.

[281] R. Arav-Boger, et al., Human cytomegalovirus-encoded alpha-chemokines exhibit high sequence variability in congenitally infected newborns, J. Infect. Dis. 193 (2006) 788–791.

[282] L.K. Hanson, et al., Replication of murine cytomegalovirus in differentiated macrophages as a determinant of viral pathogenicity, J. Virol. 73 (1999) 5970–5980.

[283] L.K. Hanson, et al., Products of US22 genes M140 and M141 confer efficient replication of murine cytomegalovirus in macrophages and spleen, J. Virol. 75 (2001) 6292–6302.

[284] J.F. Bale, M.E. O'Neil, Detection of murine cytomegalovirus DNA in circulating leukocytes harvested during acute infection of mice [erratum appears in J Virol 63(9):4120, 1989], J. Virol. 63 (1989) 2667–2673.

[285] T.M. Collins, M.R. Quirk, M.C. Jordan, Biphasic viremia and viral gene expression in leukocytes during acute cytomegalovirus infection of mice, J. Virol. 68 (1994) 6305–6311.

[286] B.M. Mitchell, A. Leung, J.G. Stevens, Murine cytomegalovirus DNA in peripheral blood of latently infected mice is detectable only in monocytes and polymorphonuclear leukocytes, Virology 223 (1996) 198–207.

[287] E.R. Kern, Animal models for cytomegalovirus infection: murine CMV, in: O. Zak, M. Sande (Eds.), Handbook of Animal Models of Infection, Academic Press, London, 1999, pp. 927–934.

[288] M.J. Reddehase, J. Podlech, N.K. Grzimek, Mouse models of cytomegalovirus latency: overview, J. Clin. Virol. 25 (2002) S23–S36.

[289] N. Saederup, et al., Cytomegalovirus-encoded beta chemokine promotes monocyte-associated viremia in the host, Proc. Natl. Acad. Sci. U. S. A. 96 (1999) 10881–10886.

[290] N. Saederup, et al., Murine cytomegalovirus CC chemokine homolog MCK-2 (m131–129) is a determinant of dissemination that increases inflammation at initial sites of infection, J. Virol. 75 (2001) 9966–9976.

[291] C. Menard, et al., Role of murine cytomegalovirus US22 gene family members in replication in macrophages, J. Virol. 77 (2003) 5557–5570.

[292] G. Hahn, et al., The human cytomegalovirus ribonucleotide reductase homolog UL45 is dispensable for growth in endothelial cells, as determined by a BAC-cloned clinical isolate of human cytomegalovirus with preserved wild-type characteristics, J. Virol. 76 (2002) 9551–9555.

[293] M.E. Penfold, et al., Cytomegalovirus encodes a potent alpha chemokine, Proc. Natl. Acad. Sci. U. S. A. 96 (1999) 9839–9844.

[294] J.S. Pepose, et al., Acquired immune deficiency syndrome: pathogenic mechanisms of ocular disease, Ophthalmology 92 (1985) 472–484.

[295] M.A. Jacobson, et al., Retinal and gastrointestinal disease due to cytomegalovirus in patients with the acquired immune deficiency syndrome: prevalence, natural history and response to ganciclovir therapy, QJM 67 (1988) 473.

[296] C.M. Wilcox, et al., Cytomegalovirus colitis in acquired immunodeficiency syndrome: a clinical and endoscopic study, Gastrointest. Endosc. 48 (1998) 39–43.

[297] T.K. Redman, et al., Human cytomegalovirus enhances chemokine production by lipopolysaccharide-stimulated lamina propria macrophages, J. Infect. Dis. 185 (2002) 584–590.

[298] T. Compton, et al., Human cytomegalovirus activates inflammatory cytokine responses via CD14 and Toll-like receptor 2, J. Virol. 77 (2003) 4588–4596.

[299] H. Zhu, et al., Inhibition of cyclooxygenase 2 blocks human cytomegalovirus replication, Proc. Natl. Acad. Sci. U. S. A. 99 (2002) 3932–3937.

[300] B.J. Margulies, H. Browne, W. Gibson, Identification of the human cytomegalovirus G protein-coupled receptor homologue encoded by UL33 in infected cells and enveloped virus particles, Virology 225 (1996) 111–125.

[301] M.M. Rosenkilde, et al., Virally encoded 7TM receptors, Oncogene 20 (2001) 1582–1593.

[302] P.S. Beisser, et al., Viral chemokine receptors and chemokines in human cytomegalovirus trafficking and interaction with the immune system, CMV chemokine receptors, Curr. Top. Microbiol. Immunol. 269 (2002) 203–234.

[303] P. Beisser, et al., Chemokines and chemokine receptors encoded by cytomegaloviruses, in: T. Shenk, M.F. Stinski (Eds.), Human Cytomegalovirus, Springer-Verlag, Berlin, 2008.

[304] M. Billstrom Schroeder, G.S. Worthen, Viral regulation of RANTES expression during human cytomegalovirus infection of endothelial cells, J. Virol. 75 (2001) 3383–3390.

[305] J. Vomaske, et al., Differential ligand binding to a human cytomegalovirus chemokine receptor determines cell type-specific motility, PLoS. Pathog. 5 (2009) e1000304.

[306] M. Billstrom Schroeder, R. Christensen, G.S. Worthen, Human cytomegalovirus protects endothelial cells from apoptosis induced by growth factor withdrawal, J. Clin. Virol. 25 (2002) S149–S157.

[307] J.R. Randolph-Habecker, et al., The expression of the cytomegalovirus chemokine receptor homolog US28 sequesters biologically active CC chemokines and alters IL-8 production, Cytokine 19 (2002) 37–46.

[308] M.R. Wills, A. Carmichael, J.G. Sissons, Adaptive cellular immunity of human cytomegalovirus, in: M.J. Reddehase (Ed.), Cytomegaloviruses: Molecular Biology and Immunology, Casiter, Norfolk, UK, 2006, pp. 341–367.

[309] S. Jonjic, I. Bubic, A. Krmpotic, Innate immunity to cytomegaloviruses, in: M.J. Reddehase (Ed.), Cytomegaloviruses: Molecular Biology and Immunology, Casiter, Norfolk, UK, 2006, pp. 285–321.

[310] R. Holtappels, et al., CD8 T-cell-based immunotherapy of cytomegalovirus disease in the mouse model of the immunocompromised bone marrow transplantation recipient, in: M.J. Reddehase (Ed.), Cytomegaloviruses: Molecular Biology and Immunology, Casiter, Norfolk, UK, 2006, pp. 383–419.

[311] H.P. Steffens, et al., Preemptive CD8 T-cell immunotherapy of acute cytomegalovirus infection prevents lethal disease, limits the burden of latent viral genomes, and reduces the risk of virus recurrence, J. Virol. 72 (1998) 1797–1804.

[312] B. Polic, et al., Hierarchical and redundant lymphocyte subset control precludes cytomegalovirus replication during latent infection, J. Exp. Med. 188 (1998) 1047–1054.

[313] A. Krmpotic, et al., Pathogenesis of murine cytomegalovirus infection, Microbes Infect. 5 (2003) 1263–1277.

[314] P. Lucin, et al., Gamma interferon-dependent clearance of cytomegalovirus infection in salivary glands, J. Virol. 66 (1992) 1977–1984.

[315] G.R. Bantug, et al., CD8+ T lymphocytes control murine cytomegalovirus replication in the central nervous system of newborn animals, J. Immunol. 181 (2008) 2111–2123.

[316] S. Jonjic, et al., Antibodies are not essential for the resolution of primary cytomegalovirus infection but limit dissemination of recurrent virus, J. Exp. Med. 179 (1994) 1713–1717.

[317] D. Cekinovic, et al., Passive immunization reduces murine cytomegalovirus-induced brain pathology in newborn mice, J. Virol. 82 (2008) 12172–12180.

[318] K. Klenovsek, et al., Protection from CMV infection in immunodeficient hosts by adoptive transfer of memory B cells, Blood 110 (2007) 3472–3479.

[319] P. Reusser, et al., Cytotoxic T-lymphocyte response to cytomegalovirus after human allogeneic bone marrow transplantation: pattern of recovery and correlation with cytomegalovirus infection and disease, Blood 78 (1991) 1373–1380.

[320] S.R. Riddell, et al., Reconstitution of protective CD8+ cytotoxic T lymphocyte responses to human cytomegalovirus in immunodeficient humans by the adoptive transfer of T cell clones, in: S. Michelson, S.A. Plotkin (Eds.), Multidisciplinary Approach to Understanding Cytomegalovirus Disease, Elsevier Science, Amsterdam, 1993, pp. 155–164.

[321] E.A. Walter, et al., Reconstitution of cellular immunity against cytomegalovirus in recipients of allogeneic bone marrow by transfer of T-cell clones from the donor, N. Engl. J. Med. 333 (1995) 1038–1044.

[322] C.R. Li, et al., Recovery of HLA-restricted cytomegalovirus (CMV)-specific T-cell responses after allogeneic bone marrow transplant: correlation with CMV disease and effect of ganciclovir prophylaxis, Blood 83 (1994) 1971–1979.

[323] S.F. Lacey, et al., Characterization of cytotoxic function of CMV-pp 65-specific CD8+ T-lymphocytes identified by HLA tetramers in recipients and donors of stem-cell transplants, Transplantation 74 (2002) 722–732.

[324] B. Horn, et al., Infusion of cytomegalovirus specific cytotoxic T lymphocytes from a sero-negative donor can facilitate resolution of infection and immune reconstitution, Pediatr. Infect. Dis. J. 28 (2009) 65–67.

[325] M. Cobbold, et al., Adoptive transfer of cytomegalovirus-specific CTL to stem cell transplant patients after selection by HLA-peptide tetramers, J. Exp. Med. 202 (2005) 379–386.

[326] P. Reusser, et al., Cytomegalovirus (CMV)-specific T cell immunity after renal transplantation mediates protection from CMV disease by limiting the systemic virus load, J. Infect. Dis. 180 (1999) 247–253.

[327] M. Matloubian, R.J. Concepcion, R. Ahmed, CD4+ T cells are required to sustain CD8+ cytotoxic T-cell responses during chronic viral infection, J. Virol. 68 (1994) 8056–8063.

[328] A. Grakoui, et al., Turning on the off switch: regulation of anti-viral T cell responses in the liver by the PD-1/PD-L1 pathway, J. Hepatol. 45 (2006) 468–472.

[329] D.L. Barber, et al., Restoring function in exhausted CD8 T cells during chronic viral infection, Nature 439 (2006) 682–687.

[330] H. Shin, et al., Viral antigen and extensive division maintain virus-specific CD8 T cells during chronic infection, J. Exp. Med. 204 (2007) 941–949.

[331] J.C. Sun, M.J. Bevan, Defective CD8 T cell memory following acute infection without CD4 T cell help, Science 300 (2003) 339–342.

[332] C.A. Biron, K.S. Byron, J.L. Sullivan, Severe herpesvirus infections in an adolescent without natural killer cells, N. Engl. J. Med. 320 (1989) 1731–1735.

[333] K. Hadaya, et al., Natural killer cell receptor repertoire and their ligands, and the risk of CMV infection after kidney transplantation, Am. J. Transplant. 8 (2008) 2674–2683.

[334] C.A. Biron, L. Brossay, NK cells and NKT cells in innate defense against viral infections, Curr. Opin. Immunol. 13 (2001) 458–464.

[335] T.W. Kuijpers, et al., Human NK cells can control CMV infection in the absence of T cells, Blood 112 (2008) 914–915.

[336] M. Stern, et al., The number of activating KIR genes inversely correlates with the rate of CMV infection/reactivation in kidney transplant recipients, Am. J. Transplant. 8 (2008) 1312–1317.

[337] S.Y. Zhang, et al., Inborn errors of interferon (IFN)-mediated immunity in humans: insights into the respective roles of IFN-alpha/beta, IFN-gamma, and IFN-lambda in host defense, Immunol. Rev. 226 (2008) 29–40.

[338] S.Y. Zhang, et al., TLR3 deficiency in patients with herpes simplex encephalitis, Science 317 (2007) 1522–1527.

[339] S.H. Robbins, et al., Natural killer cells promote early CD8 T cell responses against cytomegalovirus, PLoS Pathog. 3 (2007) e123.

[340] R.M. Presti, et al., Interferon gamma regulates acute and latent murine cytomegalovirus infection and chronic disease of the great vessels, J. Exp. Med. 188 (1998) 577–588.

[341] L. Rasmussen, et al., Deficiency in antibody response to human cytomegalovirus glycoprotein gH in human immunodeficiency virus-infected patients at risk for cytomegalovirus retinitis, J. Infect. Dis. 170 (1994) 673–677.

[342] S.B. Boppana, et al., Virus specific antibody responses to human cytomegalovirus (HCMV) in human immunodeficiency virus type 1-infected individuals with HCMV retinitis, J. Infect. Dis. 171 (1995) 182–185.

[343] K. Schoppel, et al., The humoral immune response against human cytomegalovirus is characterized by a delayed synthesis of glycoprotein-specific antibodies, J. Infect. Dis. 175 (1997) 533–544.

[344] K. Schoppel, et al., Kinetics of the antibody response against human cytomegalovirus-specific proteins in allogeneic bone marrow transplant recipients, J. Infect. Dis. 178 (1998) 1233–1243.

[345] D.R. Snydman, et al., Use of cytomegalovirus immune globulin to prevent cytomegalovirus disease in renal transplant recipients, N. Engl. J. Med. 317 (1987) 1049–1054.

[346] D.R. Snydman, et al., Cytomegalovirus immune globulin prophylaxis in liver transplantation: a randomized, double-blind placebo-controlled trial, Ann. Intern. Med. 119 (1993) 984–991.

[347] N.E. Bonaros, et al., Comparison of combined prophylaxis of cytomegalovirus hyperimmune globulin plus ganciclovir versus cytomegalovirus hyperimmune globulin alone in high-risk heart transplant recipients, Transplantation 77 (2004) 890–897.

[348] N. Bonaros, et al., CMV-hyperimmune globulin for preventing cytomegalovirus infection and disease in solid organ transplant recipients: a meta-analysis, Clin. Transplant. 22 (2008) 89–97.

[349] K. Hoetzenecker, et al., Cytomegalovirus hyperimmunoglobulin: mechanisms in allo-immune response in vitro, Eur. J. Clin. Invest. 37 (2007) 978–986.

[350] F. Leroy, et al., Cytomegalovirus prophylaxis with intravenous polyvalent immunoglobulin in high-risk renal transplant recipients, Transplant. Proc. 38 (2006) 2324–2326.

[351] P. Raanani, et al., Immunoglobulin prophylaxis in hematopoietic stem cell transplantation: systematic review and meta-analysis, J. Clin. Oncol. 27 (2009) 770–781.

[352] D.J. Winston, et al., Intravenous immune globulin for prevention of cytomegalovirus infection and interstitial pneumonia after bone marrow transplantation, Ann. Intern. Med. 106 (1987) 12–18.

[353] D. Emanuel, et al., Cytomegalovirus pneumonia after bone marrow transplantation successfully treated with the combination of ganciclovir and high-dose intravenous immune globulin, Ann. Intern. Med. 109 (1988) 777–782.

[354] G.M. Schmidt, et al., Ganciclovir/immunoglobulin combination therapy for the treatment of human cytomegalovirus-associated interstitial pneumonia in bone marrow allograft recipients, Transplantation 46 (1988) 905–907.

[355] M. Boeckh, et al., Cytomegalovirus in hematopoietic stem cell transplant recipients: current status, known challenges, and future strategies, Biol. Blood Marrow Transplant. 9 (2003) 543–558.

[356] R.A. Bowden, et al., Cytomegalovirus immune globulin and seronegative blood products to prevent primary cytomegalovirus infection after marrow transplantation, N. Engl. J. Med. 314 (1986) 1006–1010.

[357] R.A. Bowden, et al., Cytomegalovirus (CMV)-specific intravenous immunoglobulin for the prevention of primary CMV infection and disease after marrow transplantation, J. Infect. Dis. 164 (1991) 483–487.

[358] D.F. Bratcher, et al., Effect of passive antibody on congenital cytomegalovirus infection in guinea pigs, J. Infect. Dis. 172 (1995) 944–950.

[359] A. Chatterjee, et al., Modification of maternal and congenital cytomegalovirus infection by anti-glycoprotein b antibody transfer in guinea pigs, J. Infect. Dis. 183 (2001) 1547–1553.

[360] G. Nigro, et al., Passive immunization during pregnancy for congenital cytomegalovirus infection, N. Engl. J. Med. 353 (2005) 1350–1362.

[361] A. Krmpotic, et al., The immunoevasive function encoded by the mouse cytomegalovirus gene m152 protects the virus against T cell control in vivo, J. Exp. Med. 190 (2001) 1285–1296.

[362] S. Jonjic, et al., Immune evasion of natural killer cells by viruses, Curr. Opin. Immunol. 20 (2008) 30–38.

[363] M.J. Reddehase, Antigens and immunoevasins: opponents in cytomegalovirus immune surveillance, Nat. Rev. Immunol. 2 (2002) 831–844.

[364] M.J. Reddehase, et al., Murine model of cytomegalovirus latency and reactivation, Curr. Top. Microbiol. Immunol. 325 (2008) 315–331.

[365] R. Holtappels, et al., Cytomegalovirus misleads its host by priming of CD8 T cells specific for an epitope not presented in infected tissues, J. Exp. Med. 199 (2004) 131–136.

[366] J.A. Zaia, et al., Infrequent occurrence of natural mutations in the pp 65 (495–503) epitope sequence presented by the HLA A*0201 allele among human cytomegalovirus isolates, J. Virol. 75 (2001) 2472–2474.

[367] A.A. Scalzo, W.M. Yokoyama, Cmv1 and natural killer cell responses to murine cytomegalovirus infection, Curr. Top. Microbiol. Immunol. 321 (2008) 101–122.

[368] V. Voigt, et al., Murine cytomegalovirus m157 mutation and variation leads to immune evasion of natural killer cells, Proc. Natl. Acad. Sci. U. S. A. 100 (2003) 13483–13488.

[369] M. Klein, et al., Strain-specific neutralization of human cytomegalovirus isolates by human sera, J. Virol. 73 (1999) 878–886.

[370] W.J. Britt, Recent advances in the identification of significant human cytomegalovirus-encoded proteins, Transplant. Proc. 23 (1991) 64–69.

[371] C. Burkhardt, et al., The glycoprotein N of human cytomegalovirus induce a strain specific antibody response during natural infection, J. Gen. Virol. 90 (2009) 1951–1961.

[372] S. Stagno, et al., Comparative, serial virologic and serologic studies of symptomatic and subclinical congenital and natally acquired cytomegalovirus infection, J. Infect. Dis. 132 (1975) 568–577.

[373] K.M. Lockridge, et al., Pathogenesis of experimental rhesus cytomegalovirus infection, J. Virol. 73 (1999) 9576–9583.

[374] B.P. Griffith, et al., Inbred guinea pig model of intrauterine infection with cytomegalovirus, Am. J. Pathol. 122 (1986) 112–119.

[375] B.P. Griffith, et al., Cytomegalovirus-induced mononucleosis in guinea pigs, Infect. Immun. 32 (1981) 857–863.

[376] B.P. Griffith, M.J. Aquino-de Jesus, Guinea pig model of congenital cytomegalovirus infection, Transplant. Proc. 23 (1991) 29–31.

[377] E.F. Bowen, et al., Cytomegalovirus (CMV) viraemia detected by polymerase chain reaction identifies a group of HIV-positive patients at high risk of CMV disease, AIDS 11 (1997) 889–893.

[378] M.G. Revello, G. Gerna, Diagnosis and management of human cytomegalovirus infection in the mother, fetus, and newborn infant, Clin. Microbiol. Rev. 15 (2002) 680–715.

[379] M. Boeckh, G. Boivin, Quantitation of cytomegalovirus: methodologic aspects and clinical applications, Clin. Microbiol. Rev. 11 (1998) 533–554.

[380] X.L. Pang, et al., Interlaboratory comparison of cytomegalovirus viral load assays, Am. J. Transplant. 9 (2009) 258–268.

[381] W.L. Drew, Laboratory diagnosis of cytomegalovirus infection and disease in immunocompromised patients, Curr. Opin. Infect. Dis. 20 (2007) 408–411.

[382] S.A. Spector, et al., Detection of human cytomegalovirus in plasma of AIDS patients during acute visceral disease by DNA amplification, J. Clin. Microbiol. 30 (1992) 2359–2365.

[383] D.M.O. Becroft, Prenatal cytomegalovirus infection: epidemiology, pathology, and pathogenesis, in: H.S. Rosenberg, J. Bernstein (Eds.), Perspective in Pediatric Pathology, Masson Press, New York, 1981, pp. 203–241.

[384] S. Stagno, et al., Congenital and perinatal cytomegaloviral infections, Semin. Perinatol. 7 (1983) 31–42.

[385] S.B. Boppana, et al., Symptomatic congenital cytomegalovirus infection: neonatal morbidity and mortality, Pediatr. Infect. Dis. J. 11 (1992) 93–99.

[386] J.R. Arribas, et al., Cytomegalovirus encephalitis, Ann. Intern. Med. 125 (1996) 577–587.

[387] W.D. Williamson, et al., Progressive hearing loss in infants with asymptomatic congenital cytomegalovirus infection, Pediatrics 90 (1992) 862–866.

[388] A. Ludwig, H. Hengel, Epidemiological impact and disease burden of congenital cytomegalovirus infection in Europe, Euro. Surveill. 14 (2009) 26–32.

[389] H. Ogawa, et al., Etiology of severe sensorineural hearing loss in children: independent impact of congenital cytomegalovirus infection and GJB2 mutations, J. Infect. Dis. 195 (2007) 782–788.

[390] M.L. Engman, et al., Congenital CMV infection: prevalence in newborns and the impact on hearing deficit, Scand. J. Infect. Dis. 40 (2008) 935–942.

[391] M. Barbi, et al., Multicity Italian study of congenital cytomegalovirus infection, Pediatr. Infect. Dis. J. 25 (2006) 156–159.

[392] S. Iwasaki, et al., Audiological outcome of infants with congenital cytomegalovirus infection in a prospective study, Audiol. Neurootol. 12 (2007) 31–36.

[393] S.D. Grosse, D.S. Ross, S.C. Dollard, Congenital cytomegalovirus (CMV) infection as a cause of permanent bilateral hearing loss: a quantitative assessment, J. Clin. Virol. 41 (2008) 57–62.

[394] B.P. Griffith, H.L. Lucia, G.D. Hsiung, Brain and visceral involvement during congenital cytomegalovirus infection of guinea pigs, Pediatr. Res. 16 (1982) 455–459.

[395] F.J. Bia, et al., Cytomegalovirus infections in the guinea pig: experimental models for human disease, Rev. Infect. Dis. 5 (1983) 177–195.

[396] J.F. Bale, P.F. Bray, W.E. Bell, Neuroradiographic abnormalities in congenital cytomegalovirus infection, Pediatr. Neurol. 1 (1985) 42–47.

[397] J.M. Perlman, C. Argyle, Lethal cytomegalovirus infection in preterm infants: clinical, radiological, and neuropathological findings, Ann. Neurol. 31 (1992) 64–68.

[398] S.B. Boppana, et al., Neuroradiographic findings in the newborn period and long-term outcome in children with symptomatic congenital cytomegalovirus infection, Pediatrics 99 (1997) 409–414.

[399] C. Boesch, et al., Magnetic resonance imaging of the brain in congenital cytomegalovirus infection, Pediatr. Radiol. 19 (1989) 91–93.

[400] A.J. Barkovich, C.E. Lindan, Congenital cytomegalovirus infection of the brain: imaging analysis and embryologic considerations, AJNR Am. J. Neuroradiol. 15 (1994) 703–715.

[401] M.I. Steinlin, et al., Late intrauterine cytomegalovirus infection: clinical and neuroimaging findings, Pediatr. Neurol. 15 (1996) 249–253.

[402] O. Picone, et al., Comparison between ultrasound and magnetic resonance imaging in assessment of fetal cytomegalovirus infection, Prenat. Diagn. 28 (2008) 753–758.

[403] H.J. Baskin, G. Hedlund, Neuroimaging of herpesvirus infections in children, Pediatr. Radiol. 37 (2007) 949–963.

[404] L.S. de Vries, et al., The spectrum of cranial ultrasound and magnetic resonance imaging abnormalities in congenital cytomegalovirus infection, Neuropediatrics 35 (2004) 113–119.

[405] J.C. Hayward, et al., Lissencephaly-pachygyria associated with congenital cytomegalovirus infection, J. Child. Neurol. 6 (1991) 109–114.

[406] V. Mejaski-Bosnjak, Congenital CMV infection: a common cause of childhood disability, Dev. Med. Child. Neurol. 50 (2008) 403.

[407] Y. Suzuki, et al., Epilepsy in patients with congenital cytomegalovirus infection, Brain. Dev. 30 (2008) 420–424.

[408] K. Sugita, et al., Magnetic resonance imaging of the brain in congenital rubella virus and cytomegalovirus infections, Neuroradiology 33 (1991) 239–242.

[409] Y. Tsutsui, I. Kosugi, H. Kawasaki, Neuropathogenesis in cytomegalovirus infection: indication of the mechanisms using mouse models, Rev. Med. Virol. 15 (2005) 327–345.

[410] M.C. Cheeran, et al., Neural precursor cell susceptibility to human cytomegalovirus diverges along glial or neuronal differentiation pathways, J. Neurosci. Res. 82 (2005) 839–850.

[411] M.H. Luo, P.H. Schwartz, E.A. Fortunato, Neonatal neural progenitor cells and their neuronal and glial cell derivatives are fully permissive for human cytomegalovirus infection, J. Virol. 82 (2008) 9994–10007.

[412] A.F. Tarantal, et al., Neuropathogenesis induced by rhesus cytomegalovirus in fetal rhesus monkeys (Macaca mulatta), J. Infect. Dis. 177 (1998) 446–450.

[413] W.L. Chang, et al., A recombinant rhesus cytomegalovirus expressing enhanced green fluorescent protein retains the wild-type phenotype and pathogenicity in fetal macaques, J. Virol. 76 (2002) 9493–9504.

[414] A.N. van den Pol, J.D. Reuter, J.G. Santarelli, Enhanced cytomegalovirus infection of developing brain independent of the adaptive immune system, J. Virol. 76 (2002) 8842–8854.

[415] Y.R. Zou, et al., Function of the chemokine receptor CXCR4 in haematopoiesis and in cerebellar development, Nature 393 (1998) 595–599.

[416] Y. Zhu, et al., Role of the chemokine SDF-1 as the meningeal attractant for embryonic cerebellar neurons, Nat. Neurosci. 5 (2002) 719–720.

[417] T. Koontz, et al., Altered development of the brain after focal herpesvirus infection of the central nervous system, J. Exp. Med. 205 (2008) 423–435.

[418] S. Boppana, W. Britt, Cytomegalovirus, in: V.E. Newton, P.J. Vallely (Eds.), Infection and Hearing Impairment, John Wiley & Sons, Sussex, UK, 2006, pp. 67–93.

[419] M. Strauss, A clinical pathologic study of hearing loss in congenital cytomegalovirus infection, Laryngoscope 95 (1985) 951–962.

[420] M. Strauss, Human cytomegalovirus labyrinthitis, Am. J. Otolaryngol. 11 (1990) 292–298.

[421] K.E. Rarey, L.E. Davis, Temporal bone histopathology 14 years after cytomegalic inclusion disease: a case study, Laryngoscope 103 (1993) 904–909.

[422] J.P. Harris, J.T. Fan, E.M. Keithley, Immunologic responses in experimental cytomegalovirus labyrinthitis, Am. J. Otolaryngol. 11 (1990) 304–308.

[423] M.C. Chen, J.P. Harris, E.M. Keithley, Immunohistochemical analysis of proliferating cells in a sterile labyrinthitis animal model, Laryngoscope 108 (1998) 651–656.

[424] J.P. Harris, et al., Immunologic and electrophysiological response to cytomegaloviral inner ear infection in the guinea pig, J. Infect. Dis. 150 (1984) 523–530.

[425] S. Harris, et al., Congenital cytomegalovirus infection and sensorineural hearing loss, Ear Hearing. 5 (1984) 352–355.

[426] N.K. Woolf, et al., Congenital cytomegalovirus labyrinthitis and sensorineural hearing loss in guinea pigs, J. Infect. Dis. 160 (1989) 929–937.

[427] N.K. Woolf, Guinea pig model of congenital CMV-induced hearing loss: a review, Transplant. Proc. 23 (1991) 32–34.

[428] N.K. Woolf, et al., Ganciclovir prophylaxis for cochlear pathophysiology during experimental guinea pig cytomegalovirus labyrinthitis, Antimicrob. Agents Chemother. 32 (1988) 865–872.

[429] S. Fukuda, E.M. Keithley, J.P. Harris, Experimental cytomegalovirus infection: viremic spread to the inner ear, Am. J. Otolaryngol. 9 (1988) 135–141.

[430] K.B. Fowler, et al., The outcome of congenital cytomegalovirus infection in relation to maternal antibody status, N. Engl. J. Med. 326 (1992) 663–667.

[431] G.J. Demmler, Infectious Diseases Society of America and Centers for Disease Control, Summary of a workshop on surveillance for congenital cytomegalovirus disease, Rev. Infect. Dis. 13 (1991) 315–329.

[432] G.R.G. Monif, et al., The correlation of maternal cytomegalovirus infection during varying stages in gestation with neonatal involvement, J. Pediatr. 80 (1972) 17–20.

[433] M.D. Yow, et al., Epidemiologic characteristics of cytomegalovirus infection in mothers and their infants, Am. J. Obstet. Gynecol. 158 (1988) 1189–1195.

[434] R.F. Pass, et al., Congenital cytomegalovirus infection following first trimester maternal infection: symptoms at birth and outcome, J. Clin. Virol. 35 (2006) 216–220.

[435] K. Ahlfors, et al., Secondary maternal cytomegalovirus infection causing symptomatic congenital infection, N. Engl. J. Med. 305 (1981) 284.

[436] K. Ahlfors, S.A. Ivarsson, S. Harris, Report on a long-term study of maternal and congenital cytomegalovirus infection in Sweden: review of prospective studies available in the literature, Scand. J. Infect. Dis. 31 (1999) 443–457.

[437] K. Ahlfors, S.A. Ivarsson, S. Harris, Secondary maternal cytomegalovirus infection—a significant cause of congenital disease, Pediatrics 107 (2001) 1227–1228.

[438] G. Rahav, et al., Primary versus nonprimary cytomegalovirus infection during pregnancy, Israel. Emerg. Infect. Dis. 13 (2007) 1791–1793.

[439] S. Kaye, et al., Virological and immunological correlates of mother-to-child transmission of cytomegalovirus in The Gambia, J. Infect. Dis. 197 (2008) 1307–1314.

[440] Y. Zalel, et al., Secondary cytomegalovirus infection can cause severe fetal sequelae despite maternal preconceptional immunity, Ultrasound Obstet. Gynecol. 31 (2008) 417–420.

[441] K. Ahlfors, et al., Congenital cytomegalovirus infection and disease in Sweden and the relative importance of primary and secondary maternal infections, Scand. J. Infect. Dis. 16 (1984) 129–137.

[442] S.B. Boppana, et al., Symptomatic congenital cytomegalovirus infection in infants born to mothers with preexisting immunity to cytomegalovirus, Pediatrics 104 (1999) 55–60.

[443] S.A. Ross, et al., Hearing loss in children with congenital cytomegalovirus infection born to mothers with preexisting immunity, J. Pediatr. 148 (2006) 332–336.

[444] S.A. Ross, S.B. Boppana, Congenital cytomegalovirus infection: outcome and diagnosis, Semin. Pediatr. Infect. Dis. 16 (2005) 44–49.

[445] P.D. Griffiths, C. Baboonian, A prospective study of primary cytomegalovirus infection during pregnancy: final report, Br. J. Obstet. Gynaecol. 91 (1984) 307–315.

[446] A.P. Yamamoto, et al., Congenital cytomegalovirus infection in preterm and full-term newborn infants from a population with a high seroprevalence rate, Pediatr. Infect. Dis. J. 20 (2001) 188–192.

[447] D. Rutter, P. Griffiths, R.S. Trompeter, Cytomegalic inclusion disease after recurrent maternal infection, Lancet 2 (1985) 1182.

[448] T.J. Evans, J.P.K. McCollum, H. Valdimarsson, Congenital cytomegalovirus infection after maternal renal transplantation, Lancet 1 (1975) 1359–1360.

[449] S.A. Laifer, et al., Congenital cytomegalovirus infection in offspring of liver transplant recipients, Clin. Infect. Dis. 20 (1995) 52–55.

[450] M.M. Mussi-Pinhata, et al., Congenital and perinatal cytomegalovirus infection in infants born to mothers infected with human immunodeficiency virus, J. Pediatr. 132 (1998) 285–290.

[451] M. Doyle, J.T. Atkins, I.R. Rivera-Matos, Congenital cytomegalovirus infection in infants infected with human immunodeficiency virus type 1, Pediatr. Infect. Dis. J. 15 (1996) 1102–1106.

[452] M.M. Jones, et al., Congenital cytomegalovirus infection and maternal systemic lupus erythematosus: a case report, Arthritis Rheum. 29 (1986) 1402–1404.

[453] D.W. Reynolds, et al., Maternal cytomegalovirus excretion and perinatal infection, N. Engl. J. Med. 289 (1973) 1–5.

[454] S. Stagno, et al., Breast milk and the risk of cytomegalovirus infection, N. Engl. J. Med. 302 (1980) 1073–1076.

[455] M. Vochem, et al., Transmission of cytomegalovirus to preterm infants through breast milk, Pediatr. Infect. Dis. J. 17 (1998) 53–58.

[456] M. Stronati, et al., Breastfeeding and cytomegalovirus infections, J. Chemother. 19 (Suppl. 2) (2007) 49–51.

[457] R. Takahashi, et al., Severe postnatal cytomegalovirus infection in a very premature infant, Neonatology 92 (2007) 236–239.

[458] A. Yasuda, et al., Evaluation of cytomegalovirus infections transmitted via breast milk in preterm infants with a real-time polymerase chain reaction assay, Pediatrics 111 (2003) 1333–1336.

[459] C. Alford, Breast milk transmission of cytomegalovirus (CMV) infection, Adv. Exp. Med. Biol. 310 (1991) 293–299.

[460] S.B. Boppana, et al., Congenital cytomegalovirus infection: association between virus burden in infancy and hearing loss, J. Pediatr. 146 (2005) 817–823.

[461] M. Lanari, et al., Neonatal cytomegalovirus blood load and risk of sequelae in symptomatic and asymptomatic congenitally infected newborns, Pediatrics 117 (2006) e76–e83.

[462] V. Sanchez, et al., Localization of human cytomegalovirus structural proteins to the nuclear matrix of infected human fibroblasts, J. Virol. 72 (1998) 3321–3329.

[463] A. Wolf, D. Cowden, Perinatal infections of the central nervous system, J. Neurol. Pathol. Exp. Neurol. 18 (1959) 191–243.

[464] R.L. Naeye, Cytomegalic inclusion disease, the fetal disorder, Am. J. Clin. Pathol. 47 (1967) 738–744.

[465] M.J. Marques Dias, et al., Prenatal cytomegalovirus disease and cerebral microgyria: evidence for perfusion failure, not disturbance of histogenesis, as the major cause of fetal cytomegalovirus encephalopathy, Neuropediatrics 15 (1984) 18–24.

[466] L.B. Arey, Cytomegalic inclusion disease in infancy, Am. J. Dis. Child. 88 (1954) 525–526.

[467] J. Troendle Atkins, et al., Polymerase chain reaction to detect cytomegalovirus DNA in the cerebrospinal fluid of neonates with congenital infection, J. Infect. Dis. 169 (1994) 1334–1337.

[468] K.B. Balcarek, M.K. Oh, R.F. Pass, Maternal viremia and congenital CMV infection, in: S. Michelson, S.A. Plotkin (Eds.), Multidisciplinary Approach to Understanding Cytomegalovirus Disease, Elsevier Science, Amsterdam, 1993, pp. 169–173.

[469] E.M. Keithley, N.K. Woolf, J.P. Harris, Development of morphological and physiological changes in the cochlear induced by cytomegalovirus, Laryngoscope 99 (1989) 409–414.

[470] E.N. Myers, S. Stool, Cytomegalic inclusion disease of the inner ear, Laryngoscope 78 (1968) 1904–1915.

[471] G.L. Davis, Cytomegalovirus in the inner ear: case report and electron microscopic study, Ann. Otol. Rhinol. Laryngol. 78 (1969) 1179–1188.

[472] S. Boppana, et al., Late onset and reactivation of chorioretinitis in children with congenital cytomegalovirus infection, Pediatr. Infect. Dis. J. 13 (1994) 1139–1142.

[473] K.S. Anderson, et al., Ocular abnormalities in congenital cytomegalovirus infection, J. Am. Optom. Assoc. 67 (1996) 273–278.

[474] M.B. Mets, Eye manifestations of intrauterine infections, Ophthalmol. Clin. North Am. 14 (2001) 521–531.

[475] T.B. Guyton, et al., New observations in generalized cytomegalic-inclusion disease of the newborn: report of a case with chorioretinitis, N. Engl. J. Med. 257 (1957) 803–807.

[476] T.J. Conboy, et al., Early clinical manifestations and intellectual outcome in children with symptomatic congenital cytomegalovirus infection, J. Pediatr. 111 (1987) 343–348.

[477] B.M. Ansari, D.B. Davies, M.R. Jones, Calcification in liver associated with congenital cytomegalic inclusion disease, J. Pediatr. 90 (1977) 661–662.

[478] D. Alix, Y. Castel, H. Gouedard, Hepatic calcification in congenital cytomegalic inclusion disease, J. Pediatr. 92 (1978) 856.

[479] G.H. Fetterman, et al., Generalized cytomegalic inclusion disease of the newborn: localization of inclusions in the kidney, Arch. Pathol. 86 (1968) 86–94.

[480] C. Reyes, et al., Cytomegalovirus enteritis in a premature infant, J. Pediatr. Surg. 32 (1997) 1545–1547.

[481] L. Pereira, E. Maidji, Cytomegalovirus infection in the human placenta: maternal immunity and developmentally regulated receptors on trophoblasts converge, Curr. Top. Microbiol. Immunol. 325 (2008) 383–395.

[482] K. Muhlemann, M.A. Menegus, R.K. Miller, Cytomegalovirus in the perfused human term placenta in vitro, Placenta 16 (1995) 367–373.

[483] R. Sachdev, et al., In situ hybridization analysis for cytomegalovirus in chronic villitis, Pediatr. Pathol. 10 (1990) 909–917.

[484] K. Benirschke, G.R. Mendoza, P.L. Bazeley, Placental and fetal manifestations of cytomegalovirus infection, Virchows Arch. 16 (1974) 121–139.

[485] K. Benirschke, P. Kaufmann, Pathology of the Human Placenta, Springer-Verlag, New York, 1990.

[486] S. McDonagh, et al., Patterns of human cytomegalovirus infection in term placentas: a preliminary analysis, J. Clin. Virol. 35 (2006) 210–215.

[487] W.M. Dankner, et al., Polymerase chain reaction for the detection of cytomegalovirus in placentas from congenitally infected infants, Pediatr. Res. 31 (1992) 160A.

[488] D.E. Trincado, et al., Highly sensitive detection and localization of maternally acquired human cytomegalovirus in placental tissue by in situ polymerase chain reaction, J. Infect. Dis. 192 (2005) 650–657.

[489] R. La Torre, et al., Placental enlargement in women with primary maternal cytomegalovirus infection is associated with fetal and neonatal disease, Clin. Infect. Dis. 43 (2006) 994–1000.

[490] L. Pereira, et al., Insights into viral transmission at the uterine-placental interface, Trends Microbiol. 13 (2005) 164–174.

[491] S. Fisher, et al., Human cytomegalovirus infection of placental cytotrophoblasts in vitro and in utero: implications for transmission and pathogenesis, J. Virol. 74 (2000) 6808–6820.

[492] I. Roth, et al., Human placental cytotrophoblasts produce the immunosuppressive cytokine interleukin 10, J. Exp. Med. 184 (1996) 539–548.

[493] O. Blanco, et al., Human decidual stromal cells express HLA-G: effects of cytokines and decidualization, Hum. Reprod. 23 (2008) 144–152.

[494] K. Kuroki, K. Maenaka, Immune modulation of HLA-G dimer in maternal-fetal interface, Eur. J. Immunol. 37 (2007) 1727–1729.

[495] J.S. Hunt, et al., The role of HLA-G in human pregnancy, Reprod. Biol. Endocrinol. 4 (Suppl. 1) (2006) S10.

[496] A. Ishitani, N. Sageshima, K. Hatake, The involvement of HLA-E and -F in pregnancy, J. Reprod. Immunol. 69 (2006) 101–113.

[497] R.H. McIntire, J.S. Hunt, Antigen presenting cells and HLA-G—a review, Placenta 26 (Suppl. A) (2005) S104–S109.

[498] M.R. Schleiss, et al., Preconceptual administration of an alphavirus replicon UL83 (pp 65 homolog) vaccine induces humoral and cellular immunity and improves pregnancy outcome in the guinea pig model of congenital cytomegalovirus infection, J. Infect. Dis. 195 (2007) 789–798.

[499] T.H. Weller, The cytomegaloviruses: ubiquitous agents with protean clinical manifestations, II. N. Engl. J. Med. 285 (1971) 267–274.

[500] T.H. Weller, The cytomegaloviruses: ubiquitous agents with protean clinical manifestations, I. N. Engl. J. Med. 285 (1971) 203–214.

[501] T.H. Weller, J.B. Hanshaw, Virologic and clinical observations on cytomegalic inclusion disease, N. Engl. J. Med. 266 (1962) 1233–1244.

[502] G. Malm, M.L. Engman, Congenital cytomegalovirus infections, Semin. Fetal Neonatal Med. 12 (2007) 154–159.

[503] J.B. Hanshaw, Cytomegalovirus infections, Pediatr. Rev. 4 (1983) 332.

[504] D.N. Medearis, Observations concerning human cytomegalovirus infection and disease, Bull. Johns Hopkins Med. J. 114 (1964) 181–211.

[505] D.E. Noyola, et al., Early predictors of neurodevelopmental outcome in symptomatic congenital cytomegalovirus infection, J. Pediatr. 138 (2001) 325–331.

[506] S. Stagno, et al., Infant pneumonitis associated with cytomegalovirus, chlamydia, pneumocystis, and ureaplasma: a prospective study, Pediatrics 68 (1981) 322–329.

[507] S. Stagno, et al., Defects of tooth structure in congenital cytomegalovirus infection, Pediatrics 69 (1982) 646–648.

[508] S. Harris, et al., Congenital cytomegalovirus infection and sensorineural hearing loss, Ear Hear. 5 (1984) 352–355.

[509] L.M.H. Hickson, D. Alcock, Progressive hearing loss in children with congenital cytomegalovirus, J. Paediatr. Child. Health 27 (1991) 105–107.

[510] I. Foulon, et al., A 10-year prospective study of sensorineural hearing loss in children with congenital cytomegalovirus infection, J. Pediatr. 153 (2008) 84–88.

[511] M. Barbi, et al., Neonatal screening for congenital cytomegalovirus infection and hearing loss, J. Clin. Virol. 35 (2006) 206–209.

[512] W.E. Nance, B.G. Lim, K.M. Dodson, Importance of congenital cytomegalovirus infections as a cause for pre-lingual hearing loss, J. Clin. Virol. 35 (2006) 221–225.

[513] T. Hicks, et al., Congenital cytomegalovirus infection and neonatal auditory screening, J. Pediatr. 123 (1993) 779–782.

[514] L.B. Rivera, et al., Predictors of hearing loss in children with symptomatic congenital cytomegalovirus infection, Pediatrics 110 (2002) 762–767.

[515] S. Walter, et al., Congenital cytomegalovirus: association between dried blood spot viral load and hearing loss, Arch. Dis. Child. Fetal Neonatal Ed. 93 (2008) F280–F285.

[516] W.D. Williamson, et al., Symptomatic congenital cytomegalovirus: disorders of language, learning and hearing, Am. J. Dis. Child. 136 (1982) 902–905.

[517] S. Saigal, et al., The outcome in children with congenital cytomegalovirus infection: a longitudinal follow-up study, Am. J. Dis. Child. 136 (1982) 896–901.

[518] W. Berenberg, G. Nankervis, Long-term follow-up of cytomegalic inclusion disease of infancy, Pediatrics 37 (1970) 403.

[519] R.F. Pass, et al., Outcome of symptomatic congenital CMV infection: results of long-term longitudinal follow-up, Pediatrics 66 (1980) 758–762.

[520] M.E. Ramsay, E. Miller, C.S. Peckham, Outcome of confirmed symptomatic congenital cytomegalovirus infection, Arch. Dis. Child. 66 (1991) 1068–1069.

[521] S.A. Ivarsson, B. Lernmark, L. Svanberg, Ten-year clinical, developmental and intellectual follow-up of children with congenital cytomegalovirus infection without neurologic symptoms at one year of age, Pediatrics 99 (1997) 800–803.

[522] O. Zagolski, Vestibular-evoked myogenic potentials and caloric stimulation in infants with congenital cytomegalovirus infection, J. Laryngol. Otol. (2007) 1–6.

[523] R.I. Kylat, E.N. Kelly, E.L. Ford-Jones, Clinical findings and adverse outcome in neonates with symptomatic congenital cytomegalovirus (SCCMV) infection, Eur. J. Pediatr. 165 (2006) 773–778.

[524] M.E. Melish, J.B. Hanshaw, Congenital cytomegalovirus infection: developmental progress of infants detected by routine screening, Am. J. Dis. Child. 126 (1973) 190–194.

[525] M.L. Kumar, G.A. Nankervis, E. Gold, Inapparent congenital cytomegalovirus infection: a follow-up study, N. Engl. J. Med. 288 (1973) 1370–1377.

[526] D.W. Reynolds, et al., Inapparent congenital cytomegalovirus infection with elevated cord IgM levels: causal relationship with auditory and mental deficiency, N. Engl. J. Med. 209 (1974) 291–296.

[527] W.D. Williamson, et al., Asymptomatic congenital cytomegalovirus infection, Am. J. Dis. Child. 144 (1990) 1365–1368.

[528] J. Kashden, et al., Intellectual assessment of children with asymptomatic congenital cytomegalovirus infection, J. Dev. Behav. Pediatr. 19 (1998) 254–259.

[529] P.M. Preece, K.N. Pearl, C.S. Peckham, Congenital cytomegalovirus infection, Arch. Dis. Child. 59 (1984) 1120–1126.

[530] K.N. Pearl, et al., Neurodevelopmental assessment after congenital cytomegalovirus infection, Arch. Dis. Child. 62 (1986) 323–326.

[531] T.J. Conboy, et al., Intellectual development in school-aged children with asymptomatic congenital cytomegalovirus infection, Pediatrics 77 (1986) 801–806.

[532] K.B. Fowler, S. Stagno, R.F. Pass, Maternal immunity and prevention of congenital cytomegalovirus infection, JAMA 289 (2003) 1008–1011.

[533] K. Ahlfors, S.A. Ivarsson, S. Harris, Report on a long-term study of maternal and congenital cytomegalovirus infection in Sweden: review of prospective studies available in the literature, Scand. J. Infect. Dis. 31 (1999) 443–457.

[534] A.M. Arvin, et al., Vaccine development to prevent cytomegalovirus disease, Report from the National Vaccine Advisory Committee, Clin. Infect. Dis. 39 (2004) 233–239.

[535] M.G. Capretti, et al., Very low birth weight infants born to cytomegalovirus-seropositive mothers fed with their mother's milk: a prospective study, J. Pediatr. 154 (2009) 842–848.

[536] P. Neuberger, et al., Case-control study of symptoms and neonatal outcome of human milk-transmitted cytomegalovirus infection in premature infants, J. Pediatr. 148 (2006) 326–331.

[537] K. Hamprecht, et al., Cytomegalovirus transmission to preterm infants during lactation, J. Clin. Virol. 41 (2008) 198–205.

[538] A. Kothari, V.G. Ramachandran, P. Gupta, Cytomegalovirus infection in neonates following exchange transfusion, Indian J. Pediatr. 73 (2006) 519–521.

[539] G.A. Nankervis, N.A. Bhumbra, Cytomegalovirus infections of the neonate and infant, Adv. Pediatr. Infect. Dis. 1 (1986) 61–74.

[540] N.A. Bhumbra, et al., Evaluation of a prescreening blood donor program for prevention of perinatal transfusion-acquired cytomegalovirus (CMV) infection, J. Perinat. Med. 16 (1988) 127–131.

[541] D. Miron, et al., Incidence and clinical manifestations of breast milk-acquired cytomegalovirus infection in low birth weight infants, J. Perinatol. 25 (2005) 299–303.

[542] M.M. Mussi-Pinhata, et al., Perinatal or early-postnatal cytomegalovirus infection in preterm infants under 34 weeks gestation born to CMV-seropositive mothers within a high-seroprevalence population, J. Pediatr. 145 (2004) 685–688.

[543] S. Doctor, et al., Cytomegalovirus transmission to extremely low-birthweight infants through breast milk, Acta Paediatr. 94 (2005) 53–58.

[544] S. Stagno, et al., Congenital and perinatal cytomegalovirus infections, Semin. Perinatol. 7 (1983) 31–42.

[545] A.S. Yeager, et al., Sequelae of maternally derived cytomegalovirus infections in premature infants, J. Pediatr. 102 (1983) 918–922.

[546] S.G. Paryani, et al., Sequelae of acquired cytomegalovirus infection in premature and sick term infants, J. Pediatr. 107 (1985) 451–456.

[547] J. Maschmann, et al., Cytomegalovirus infection of extremely low-birth weight infants via breast milk, Clin. Infect. Dis. 33 (2001) 1998–2003.

[548] A.S. Yeager, Transfusion-acquired cytomegalovirus infection in newborn infants, Am. J. Dis. Child. 128 (1974) 478–483.

[549] R.B. Ballard, et al., Acquired cytomegalovirus infection in pre-term infants, Am. J. Dis. Child. 133 (1979) 482–485.

[550] S.P. Adler, et al., Cytomegalovirus infections in neonates acquired by blood transfusions, Pediatr. Infect. Dis. 2 (1983) 114–118.

[551] C.T. Nelson, et al., PCR detection of cytomegalovirus DNA in serum as a diagnostic test for congenital cytomegalovirus infection, J. Clin. Microbiol. 33 (1995) 3317–3318.

[552] T. Lazzarotto, et al., New advances in the diagnosis of congenital cytomegalovirus infection, J. Clin. Virol. 41 (2008) 192–197.

[553] G.J. Demmler, et al., Detection of cytomegalovirus in urine from newborns by using polymerase chain reaction DNA amplification, J. Infect. Dis. 158 (1988) 1177–1184.

[554] W.P. Warren, et al., Comparison of rapid methods of detection of cytomegalovirus in saliva with virus isolation in tissue culture, J. Clin. Microbiol. 30 (1992) 786–789.

[555] P.J. Johansson, et al., Retrospective diagnostics of congenital cytomegalovirus infection performed by polymerase chain reaction in blood stored on filter paper, Scand. J. Infect. Dis. 29 (1997) 465–468.

[556] M. Barbi, et al., Diagnosis of congenital cytomegalovirus infection by detection of viral DNA in dried blood spots, Clin. Diagn. Virol. 6 (1996) 27–32.

[557] A.Y. Yamamoto, et al., Usefulness of blood and urine samples collected on filter paper in detecting cytomegalovirus by the polymerase chain reaction technique, J. Virol. Methods 97 (2001) 159–164.

[558] O. Soetens, et al., Evaluation of different cytomegalovirus (CMV) DNA PCR protocols for analysis of dried blood spots from consecutive cases of neonates with congenital CMV infections, J. Clin. Microbiol. 46 (2008) 943–946.

[559] Y. Yamagishi, et al., CMV DNA detection in dried blood spots for diagnosing congenital CMV infection in Japan, J. Med. Virol. 78 (2006) 923–925.

[560] M. Barbi, S. Binda, S. Caroppo, Diagnosis of congenital CMV infection via dried blood spots, Rev. Med. Virol. 16 (2006) 385–392.

[561] M. Barbi, et al., Cytomegalovirus DNA detection in Guthrie cards: a powerful tool for diagnosing congenital infection, J. Clin. Virol. 17 (2000) 159–165.

[562] M. Barbi, et al., Congenital cytomegalovirus infection in a northern Italian region, NEOCMV Group, Eur. J. Epidemiol. 14 (1998) 791–796.

[563] S.B. Boppana, S.A. Ross, Z. Novak, et al., Dried blood spot real-time polymerase chain reaction assays to screen newborns for congenital cytomegalovirus infection, Jama 303 (2010) 1375–1382.

[564] D.W. Reynolds, S. Stagno, C. Alford, Laboratory diagnosis of cytomegalovirus infections, in: E. Lennette, N.J. Schmidt (Eds.), Diagnostic Procedures for Viral, Rickettsial, and Chlamydial Infections, fifth ed., American Public Health Association, Washington, DC, 1979, pp. 399–439.

[565] E.A. Shuster, et al., Monoclonal antibody for rapid laboratory detection of cytomegalovirus infections: characterization and diagnostic application, Mayo Clin. Proc. 60 (1985) 577–585.

[566] S.B. Boppana, et al., Evaluation of a microtiter plate fluorescent antibody assay for rapid detection of human cytomegalovirus infections, J. Clin. Microbiol. 30 (1992) 721–723.

[567] P.R. Stirk, P.D. Griffiths, Use of monoclonal antibodies for the diagnosis of cytomegalovirus infection by the detection of early antigen fluorescent foci (DEAFF) in cell culture, J. Med. Virol. 21 (1987) 329–337.

[568] K.B. Balcarek, et al., Neonatal screening for congenital cytomegalovirus infection by detection of virus in saliva, J. Infect. Dis. 167 (1993) 1433–1436.

[569] S. Chou, T.C. Merigan, Rapid detection and quantitation of human cytomegalovirus in urine through DNA hybridization, N. Engl. J. Med. 308 (1983) 921–925.

[570] S.A. Spector, et al., Detection of human cytomegalovirus in clinical specimens by DNA-DNA hybridization, J. Infect. Dis. 150 (1984) 121–126.

[571] N.S. Lurain, K.D. Thompson, S.K. Farrand, Rapid detection of cytomegalovirus in clinical specimens by using biotinylated DNA probes and analysis of cross-reactivity with herpes simplex virus, J. Clin. Microbiol. 24 (1986) 724–730.

[572] V. Schuster, et al., Detection of human cytomegalovirus in urine by DNA-DNA and RNA-DNA hybridization, J. Infect. Dis. 154 (1986) 309–314.

[573] A. Erice, et al., Cytomegalovirus (CMV) antigenemia assay is more sensitive than shell vial cultures for rapid detection of CMV in polymorphonuclear blood leukocytes, J. Clin. Microbiol. 30 (1992) 2822–2825.

[574] E. Percivalle, et al., Comparison of a new Light Diagnostics and the CMV Brite to an in-house developed human cytomegalovirus antigenemia assay, J. Clin. Virol. 43 (2008) 13–17.

[575] S. Hernando, et al., Comparison of cytomegalovirus viral load measure by real-time PCR with pp 65 antigenemia for the diagnosis of cytomegalovirus disease in solid organ transplant patients, Transplant. Proc. 37 (2005) 4094–4096.

[576] M. Boeckh, Rising CMV PP65 antigenemia and DNA levels during preemptive antiviral therapy, Haematologica 90 (2005) 439.

[577] K.M. Sullivan, et al., Preventing opportunistic infections after hematopoietic stem cell transplantation: the Centers for Disease Control and Prevention, Infectious Diseases Society of America, and American Society for Blood and Marrow Transplantation Practice Guidelines and beyond, Hematology. Am. Soc. Hematol. Educ. Program (2001) 392–421.

[578] P.D. Griffiths, H.O. Kangro, A user's guide to the indirect solid-phase radioimmunoassay for the detection of cytomegalovirus-specific IgM antibodies, J. Virol. Methods 8 (1984) 271–282.

[579] S. Stagno, et al., Immunoglobulin M antibodies detected by enzyme-linked immunosorbent assay and radioimmunoassay in the diagnosis of cytomegalovirus infections in pregnant women and newborn infants, J. Clin. Microbiol. 21 (1985) 930–935.

[580] T. Lazzarotto, et al., Development of a new cytomegalovirus (CMV) immunoglobulin M (IgM) immunoblot for detection of CMV-specific IGM, J. Clin. Microbiol. 36 (1998) 3337–3341.

[581] M. Gentile, et al., Measurement of the sensitivity of different commercial assays in the diagnosis of CMV infection in pregnancy, Eur. J. Clin. Microbiol. Infect. Dis. 28 (2009) 977–981.

[582] C. Busse, A. Strubel, P. Schnitzler, Combination of native and recombinant cytomegalovirus antigens in a new ELISA for detection of CMV-specific antibodies, J. Clin. Virol. 43 (2008) 137–141.

[583] K. Lagrou, et al., Evaluation of the new ARCHITECT CMV IgM, IgG and IgG avidity assays, J. Clin. Microbiol. 47 (2009) 1695–1699.

[584] T. Lazzarotto, et al., Anticytomegalovirus (anti-CMV) immunoglobulin G avidity in identification of pregnant women at risk of transmitting congenital CMV infection, Clin. Diagn. Lab. Immunol. 6 (1999) 127–129.

[585] T. Lazzarotto, et al., Avidity of immunoglobulin G directed against human cytomegalovirus during primary and secondary infections in immunocompetent and immunocompromised subjects, Clin. Diagn. Lab. Immunol. 4 (1997) 469–473.

[586] M. Bodeus, et al., Anticytomegalovirus IgG avidity in pregnancy: a 2-year prospective study, Fetal. Diagn. Ther. 17 (2002) 362–366.

[587] M. Bodeus, D. Beulne, P. Goubau, Ability of three IgG-avidity assays to exclude recent cytomegalovirus infection, Eur. J. Clin. Microbiol. Infect. Dis. 20 (2001) 248–252.

[588] B. Kanengisser-Pines, et al., High cytomegalovirus IgG avidity is a reliable indicator of past infection in patients with positive IgM detected during the first trimester of pregnancy, J. Perinat. Med. 37 (2009) 15–18.

[589] M.G. Revello, G. Gerna, Diagnosis and implications of human cytomegalovirus infection in pregnancy, Fetal Matern. Med. Rev. 11 (1999) 117–134.

[590] G.T. Maine, T. Lazzarotto, M.P. Landini, New developments in the diagnosis of maternal and congenital CMV infection, Expert Rev. Mol. Diagn. 1 (2001) 19–29.

[591] M.G. Revello, et al., Human cytomegalovirus in blood of immunocompetent persons during primary infection: prognostic implications for pregnancy, J. Infect. Dis. 177 (1998) 1170–1175.

[592] M.G. Revello, et al., Human cytomegalovirus immediate-early messenger RNA in blood of pregnant women with primary infection and of congenitally infected newborns, J. Infect. Dis. 184 (2001) 1078–1081.

[593] C. Donner, et al., Prenatal diagnosis of 52 pregnancies at risk for congenital cytomegalovirus infection, Obstet. Gynecol. 82 (1993) 481–486.

[594] M.E. Lamy, et al., Prenatal diagnosis of fetal cytomegalovirus infection, Am. J. Obstet. Gynecol. 166 (1992) 91–94.

[595] L. Lynch, et al., Prenatal diagnosis of fetal cytomegalovirus infection, Am. J. Obstet. Gynecol. 165 (1991) 714–718.

[596] S. Lipitz, et al., Prenatal diagnosis of fetal primary cytomegalovirus infection, Obstet. Gynecol. 89 (1997) 763–767.

[597] C.A. Liesnard, P. Revelard, Y. Englert, Is matching between women and donors feasible to avoid cytomegalovirus infection in artificial insemination with donor semen? Hum. Reprod. 13 (1998) 25–31 discussion 2-4.

[598] T. Lazzarotto, et al., Prenatal indicators of congenital cytomegalovirus infection, J. Pediatr. 137 (2000) 90–95.

[599] T. Lazzarotto, et al., Congenital cytomegalovirus infection in twin pregnancies: viral load in the amniotic fluid and pregnancy outcome, Pediatrics 112 (2003) 153–157.

[600] B. Guerra, et al., Prenatal diagnosis of symptomatic congenital cytomegalovirus infection, Am. J. Obstet. Gynecol. 183 (2000) 476–482.

[601] C. Liesnard, et al., Prenatal diagnosis of congenital cytomegalovirus infection: prospective study of 237 pregnancies at risk, Obstet. Gynecol. 95 (2000) 881–888.

[602] C. Donner, et al., Accuracy of amniotic fluid testing before 21 weeks' gestation in prenatal diagnosis of congenital cytomegalovirus infection, Prenat. Diagn. 14 (1994) 1055–1059.

[603] M. Bodeus, et al., Prenatal diagnosis of human cytomegalovirus by culture and polymerase chain reaction: 98 pregnancies leading to congenital infection, Prenat. Diagn. 19 (1999) 314–317.

[604] C. Grose, T. Meehan, C.P. Weiner, Prenatal diagnosis of congenital cytomegalovirus infection by virus isolation after amniocentesis, Pediatr. Infect. Dis. J. 11 (1992) 605–607.

[605] R.F. Pass, Commentary: Is there a role for prenatal diagnosis of congenital cytomegalovirus infection? Pediatr. Infect. Dis. J. 11 (1992) 608–609.

[606] C.P. Weiner, C. Grose, Prenatal diagnosis of congenital cytomegalovirus infection by virus isolation from amniotic fluid, Am. J. Obstet. Gynecol. 163 (1990) 1253–1255.

[607] G. Benoist, et al., Cytomegalovirus-related fetal brain lesions: comparison between targeted ultrasound examination and magnetic resonance imaging, Ultrasound Obstet. Gynecol. 32 (2008) 900–905.

[608] R.J. Whitley, et al., A pharmacokinetic and pharmacodynamic evaluation of ganciclovir for the treatment of symptomatic congenital cytomegalovirus infection: results of a phase II study, J. Infect. Dis. 175 (1997) 1080–1086.

[609] D.W. Kimberlin, et al., Effect of ganciclovir therapy on hearing in symptomatic congenital cytomegalovirus disease involving the central nervous system: a randomized, controlled trial, J. Pediatr. 143 (2003) 16–25.

[610] G. Nigro, et al., Regression of fetal cerebral abnormalities by primary cytomegalovirus infection following hyperimmunoglobulin therapy, Prenat. Diagn. 28 (2008) 512–517.

[611] M.R. Schleiss, Prospects for development and potential impact of a vaccine against congenital cytomegalovirus (CMV) infection, J. Pediatr. 151 (2007) 564–570.

[612] R.F. Pass, R.L. Burke, Development of cytomegalovirus vaccines: prospects for prevention of congenital CMV infection, Semin. Pediatr. Infect. Dis. 13 (2002) 196–204.

[613] R.F. Pass, et al., A subunit cytomegalovirus vaccine based on recombinant envelope glycoprotein B and a new adjuvant, J. Infect. Dis. 180 (1999) 970–975.

[614] S.P. Adler, et al., A canarypox vector expressing cytomegalovirus (CMV) glycoprotein B primes for antibody responses to a live attenuated CMV vaccine (Towne), J. Infect. Dis. 180 (1999) 843–846.

[615] K. Berencsi, et al., A canarypox vector-expressing cytomegalovirus (CMV) phosphoprotein 65 induces long-lasting cytotoxic T cell responses in human CMV-seronegative subjects, J. Infect. Dis. 183 (2001) 1171–1179.

[616] M. Shimamura, M. Mach, W.J. Britt, Human cytomegalovirus infection elicits a glycoprotein M (gM)/gN-specific virus-neutralizing antibody response, J. Virol. 80 (2006) 4591–4600.

[617] E. Gonczol, S. Plotkin, Development of a cytomegalovirus vaccine: lessons from recent clinical trials, Expert Opin. Biol. Ther. 1 (2001) 401–412.

[618] S.A. Plotkin, et al., Protective effects of Towne cytomegalovirus vaccine against low-passage cytomegalovirus administered as a challenge, J. Infect. Dis. 159 (1989) 860–865.

[619] S.P. Adler, et al., Immunity induced by primary human cytomegalovirus infection protects against secondary infection among women of childbearing age, J. Infect. Dis. 171 (1995) 26–32.

[620] T.C. Heineman, et al., A phase 1 study of 4 live, recombinant human cytomegalovirus Towne/Toledo chimeric vaccines, J. Infect. Dis. 193 (2006) 1350–1360.

[621] R.F. Pass, et al., Vaccine prevention of maternal cytomegalovirus infection, N. Engl. J. Med. 360 (2009) 1191–1199.

[622] E.A. Reap, et al., Cellular and humoral immune responses to alphavirus replicon vaccines expressing cytomegalovirus pp 65, IE1, and gB proteins, Clin. Vaccine Immunol. 14 (2007) 748–755.

[623] E.A. Reap, et al., Development and preclinical evaluation of an alphavirus replicon particle vaccine for cytomegalovirus, Vaccine 25 (2007) 7441–7449.

[624] D.I. Bernstein, E.A. Reap, K. Katen, et al., Randomized, double-blind, Phase 1 trial of an alphavirus replicon vaccine for cytomegalovirus in CMV seronegative adult volunteers, Vaccine 28 (2009) 484–493.

[625] M.K. Wloch, et al., Safety and immunogenicity of a bivalent cytomegalovirus DNA vaccine in healthy adult subjects, J. Infect. Dis. 197 (2008) 1634–1642.

[626] S.G. Hansen, et al., Effector memory T cell responses are associated with protection of rhesus monkeys from mucosal simian immunodeficiency virus challenge, Nat. Med. 15 (2009) 293–299.

[627] M.J. Cannon, K.F. Davis, Washing our hands of the congenital cytomegalovirus disease epidemic, BMC Public Health 5 (2005) 70.

[628] S. Stagno, R.J. Whitley, Herpesvirus infections of pregnancy, Part I: Cytomegalovirus and Epstein-Barr virus infections, N. Engl. J. Med. 313 (1985) 1270–1274.

[629] R. Pass, S. Stagno, Cytomegalovirus, in: L. Donowitz (Ed.), Hospital Acquired Infection in the Pediatric Patient, Williams & Wilkins, Baltimore, 1988.

[630] H.M. Friedman, et al., Acquisition of cytomegalovirus infection among female employees at a pediatric hospital, Pediatr. Infect. Dis. J. 3 (1984) 233–235.

[631] J.R. Murph, et al., The occupational risk of cytomegalovirus infection among day care providers, JAMA 265 (1991) 603–608.

[632] R.A. Bowden, Cytomegalovirus infections in transplant patients: methods of prevention of primary cytomegalovirus, Transplant. Proc. 23 (1991) 136–138.

[633] R.A. Bowden, Transfusion-transmitted cytomegalovirus infection, Hematol. Oncol. Clin. North Am. 9 (1995) 155–166.

[634] S.P. Adler, Transfusion-associated cytomegalovirus infections, Rev. Infect. Dis. 5 (1983) 977–993.

[635] S.M. Lipson, et al., Cytomegalovirus infectivity in whole blood following leukocyte reduction by filtration, Am. J. Clin. Pathol. 116 (2001) 52–55.

[636] R.N. Pietersz, P.F. van der Meer, M.J. Seghatchian, Update on leucocyte depletion of blood components by filtration, Transfus. Sci. 19 (1998) 321–328.

[637] D. Xu, et al., Acquired cytomegalovirus infection and blood transfusion in preterm infants, Acta Paediatr. Jpn. 37 (1995) 444–449.

[638] G.L. Gilbert, et al., Prevention of transfusion-acquired cytomegalovirus infection in infants by blood filtration to remove leucocytes, Neonatal Cytomegalovirus Infection Study Group, Lancet 1 (1989) 1228–1231.

[639] J.M. Fisk, E.L. Snyder, Universal pre-storage leukoreduction—a defensible use of hospital resources: the Yale-New Haven Hospital experience, Dev. Biol. (Basel) 120 (2005) 39–44.

[640] M.A. Blajchman, et al., Proceedings of a consensus conference: prevention of post-transfusion CMV in the era of universal leukoreduction, Transfus. Med. Rev. 15 (2001) 1–20.

[641] S. Larsson, et al., Cytomegalovirus DNA can be detected in peripheral blood mononuclear cells from all seropositive and most seronegative healthy blood donors over time, Transfusion 38 (1998) 271–278.

[642] R. Goelz, et al., Effects of different CMV-heat-inactivation-methods on growth factors in human breast milk, Pediatr. Res. 65 (2009) 458–461.

[643] B. Knorr, et al., A haemophagocytic lymphohistiocytosis (HLH)-like picture following breastmilk transmitted cytomegalovirus infection in a preterm infant, Scand. J. Infect. Dis. 39 (2007) 173–176.

[644] M. Dworsky, et al., Persistence of cytomegalovirus in human milk after storage, J. Pediatr. 101 (1982) 440–443.

[645] J. Maschmann, et al., Freeze-thawing of breast milk does not prevent cytomegalovirus transmission to a preterm infant, Arch. Dis. Child. Fetal Neonatal Ed. 91 (2006) F288–F290.

[646] K. Hamprecht, et al., Cytomegalovirus (CMV) inactivation in breast milk: reassessment of pasteurization and freeze-thawing, Pediatr. Res. 56 (2004) 529–535.

CHAPTER 24
ENTEROVIRUS AND PARECHOVIRUS INFECTIONS

James D. Cherry ⊕ Paul Krogstad

CHAPTER OUTLINE

Viruses   757
    Classification   757
    Morphology and Replication   758
    Replication Characteristics and Host Systems   759
    Antigenic Characteristics   759
    Host Range   761
Epidemiology and Transmission   761
    General Considerations   761
    Transplacental Transmission   761
    Ascending Infection and Contact Infection during Birth   762
    Neonatal Infection   762
    Host Range   764
    Geographic Distribution and Season   764
Pathogenesis   765
    Events during Pathogenesis   765
    Factors That Affect Pathogenesis   767
Pathology   768
    General Considerations   768
    Polioviruses   768
    Coxsackievirus A Strains   768

Coxsackievirus B Strains   768
Echoviruses   769
Clinical Manifestations   769
    Abortion   770
    Congenital Malformations   770
    Prematurity and Stillbirth   771
    Neonatal Infection   772
Diagnosis and Differential Diagnosis   787
    Clinical Diagnosis   787
    Laboratory Diagnosis   788
    Differential Diagnosis   789
Prognosis   789
    Polioviruses   789
    Nonpolio Enteroviruses and Parechoviruses   790
Therapy   790
    Specific Therapy   790
    Nonspecific Therapy   791
Prevention   791
    Immunization   791
    Other Measures   792

Enteroviruses (i.e., coxsackieviruses, echoviruses, newer enteroviruses, and polioviruses) and parechoviruses are responsible for significant and frequent human illnesses, with protean clinical manifestations [1–14]. *Enterovirus* and *Parechovirus* are two genera of the family Picornaviridae [11,13,15,16]. Enteroviruses were first categorized together and named in 1957 by a committee sponsored by the National Foundation for Infantile Paralysis [17]; the human alimentary tract was believed to be the natural habitat of these agents. Enteroviruses and parechoviruses are grouped together because of similarities in physical, biochemical, and molecular properties and shared features in epidemiology and pathogenesis and the many disease syndromes that they cause. Congenital and neonatal infections have been linked with many different enteroviruses and parechoviruses. Representatives of all four major enterovirus groups and parechoviruses have been associated with disease in neonates [1–14,18–35].

Poliomyelitis, the first enterovirus disease to be recognized and the most important one, has had a long history [36]. The earliest record is an Egyptian stele of the 18th dynasty (1580-1350 BC), which shows a young man with a withered, shortened leg, the characteristic deformity of paralytic poliomyelitis [37,38]. Underwood [39], a London pediatrician, published the first medical description in 1789 in his *Treatise on Diseases of Children*. During the 19th century, many reports appeared in Europe and the United States describing small clusters of cases of "infantile paralysis." The authors were greatly puzzled about the nature of the affliction; not until the 1860s and 1870s was the spinal cord firmly established as the seat of the pathologic process. The contagious nature of poliomyelitis was not appreciated until the latter part of the 19th century. Medin, a Swedish pediatrician, was the first to describe the epidemic nature of poliomyelitis (1890), and his pupil Wickman [40] worked out the basic principles of the epidemiology.

The virus was first isolated in monkeys by Landsteiner and Popper in 1908 [41]. The availability of a laboratory animal assay system opened up many avenues of research that in the ensuing 40 years led to the demonstration that an unrecognized intestinal infection was common and that paralytic disease was a relatively uncommon event.

Coxsackieviruses and echoviruses have had a shorter history. Epidemic pleurodynia was first clinically described in northern Germany in 1735 by Hannaeus [3,42] more than 200 years before coxsackievirus as the cause of this disease was discovered. In 1948, Dalldorf and Sickles [43] first reported the isolation of a coxsackievirus by using suckling mouse inoculation.

In 1949, Enders and associates [44] reported the growth of poliovirus type 2 in tissue culture, and their techniques paved the way for the recovery of numerous other cytopathic viruses. Most of these "new" viruses failed to produce illness in laboratory animals. Because the relationships of many of these newly recovered agents to human disease were unknown, they were called *orphan viruses* [5]. Later, several agents were grouped together and termed *enteric cytopathogenic human orphan viruses*, or *echoviruses*. Some studies [13–16] of the viral genome of echoviruses 22 and 23 found that they were distinctly different from other enteroviruses, and they have been placed in the new genus, *Parechovirus*.

Live-attenuated oral poliovirus vaccines (OPV) became available in the 1960s, and the most notable advance during recent decades has been the dramatic reduction in worldwide poliomyelitis because of immunization with OPV and efforts of the global immunization initiative [45–50]. The last case of confirmed paralytic polio in the Western Hemisphere, caused by a nonvaccine type, occurred in 1991 [50].

Aside from the polio immunization successes, there have been few major advances or new modes of treatment for enterovirus diseases. The use of nucleic acid detection systems for enterovirus and parechovirus diagnosis has progressed over the past 2 decades, however, and rapid diagnosis of meningitis and other enterovirus and parechovirus illnesses has become possible [19,51–67]. There has been progress in the development of specific anti-enterovirus drugs [68–71].

VIRUSES
CLASSIFICATION

Enteroviruses and parechoviruses are RNA viruses belonging to the family Picornaviridae (*pico* means "small"). They are grouped together because they share certain physical, biochemical, and molecular properties. On electron microscopy, the viruses are seen as 30-nm particles that consist of naked (nonenveloped) protein capsids constituting approximately 70% to 75% of the mass of particles and dense central cores (nucleoid) of the genomic RNA [9,11,15,72–86].

The original classification of human enteroviruses is presented in Table 24–1. The enteroviruses were originally distributed into four groups based on their different effects in tissue culture and pattern of disease in experimentally infected animals: polioviruses (causal agents of poliomyelitis in humans and nonhuman primates), coxsackie A viruses (associated with herpangina, human central nervous system [CNS] disease, and flaccid paralysis in

suckling mice), coxsackie B viruses (human CNS and cardiac disease, spastic paralysis in mice), and echoviruses (nonpathogenic in mice, not initially linked to human disease).

Although this scheme was initially useful, many strains were subsequently isolated that do not conform to such rigid specificities. Several coxsackievirus A strains replicate and have a cytopathic effect in monkey kidney tissue cultures, and some echovirus strains cause paralysis in mice. For this reason, and to simplify the nomenclature, subsequent enteroviruses were assigned sequential numbers. Following this convention, the prototype enterovirus strains Fermon, Toluca-1, J 670/71, and BrCr (identified 1959-1973) were designated enterovirus 68 through 71. Additional enteroviruses continued to be identified that could not be identified using antisera specific for the classic serotypes. More than 30 additional such enterovirus types have been provisionally assigned, although many have not been linked to human disease.

Complicating matters, studies of echoviruses 22 and 23 found that they exhibited genomic and proteomic differences from other enteroviruses, and they were reclassified in the new genus *Parechovirus* as parechoviruses 1 and 2 [13,15,16]. Similarly, hepatitis A virus was initially assigned the designation of enterovirus 72, but was reclassified as the sole member of the *Hepatovirus* genus within the Picornaviridae family because of marked genetic and biologic distinctions from the enteroviruses.

In recent years, genetic, biologic, and molecular properties have been employed to revise picornavirus taxonomy, leading to a reorganization of human enteroviruses into five groups: the polioviruses and four alphabetically designated human enterovirus species (HEV-A, HEV-B, HEV-C, and HEV-D) (Table 24–2). Determining the nucleotide sequence encoding the viral VP1 capsid protein is important in the approach to taxonomy and predictably identifies viruses originally classified by serologic means, leading to the term *molecular serotyping* [82,84,87,88].

This approach is likely to dominate future phylogenetic studies. Additional reclassification of enteroviruses is likely to occur. It has been proposed that the polioviruses be included as members of the HEV-C species because there does not seem to be any poliovirus-specific nucleotides, amino acid sequence, or motif that allows the three polioviruses to be distinguished from the current HEV-C

TABLE 24–1 Original Classification of Human Enteroviruses: Animal and Tissue Culture Spectrum*

Virus	Antigenic Types[†]	Cytopathic Effect		Illness and Pathology	
		Monkey Kidney Tissue Culture	Human Tissue Culture	Suckling Mouse	Monkey
Polioviruses	1-3	+	+	−	+
Coxsackieviruses A	1-24[‡]	−	−	+	−
Coxsackieviruses B	1-6	+	+	+	−
Echoviruses	1-34[§]	+	±	−	−

*Many enterovirus strains have been isolated that do not conform to these categories, leading to the revised classification scheme shown in Table 24–2.
[†]New types, beginning with type 68, were assigned enterovirus type numbers instead of coxsackievirus or echovirus numbers. Types 68-71 were identified.
[‡]Type 23 was found to be the same as echovirus 9.
[§]Echovirus 10 was reclassified as a reovirus, echoviruses 22 and 23 were made the first members of the parechovirus genus of picornaviridae, and echovirus 28 was reclassified as a rhinovirus.

TABLE 24-2 Genomic Classification of Enteroviruses

Species Designation	Original Enterovirus*
Poliovirus	Poliovirus types 1-3
Human enterovirus A (HEV-A)	Coxsackievirus A2-8, A10, A12, A14, A16
	Enterovirus 71, 76, 89-92
Human enterovirus B (HEV-B)	Coxsackievirus A9
	Coxsackievirus B1-6
	Echovirus 1-9, 11-21, 24-27, 29-33
	Enterovirus 69, 73-75, 77-78, 93, 97, 98, 100, 101
Human enterovirus C (HEV-C)	Coxsackievirus A1, A11, A13, A17, A19-22, A24
	Enterovirus 95, 96, 99, 102
Human enterovirus D (HEV-D)	Enterovirus 68, 70, 94

*Coxsackievirus A15 has been reclassified as a strain of coxsackievirus A11, and coxsackievirus A18 has been reclassified as a strain of coxsackievirus A13.
From Fauquet CM, Mayo MA, Maniloff J, Desselberger U, and Ball LA (Eds). Virus Taxonomy. Eighth Report of the International Committee on Taxonomy of Viruses. Elsevier Academic Press, 2005.

members [89]. The application of molecular phylogenetic approaches has also revealed that recombination between circulating enteroviruses is a frequent event and is likely to increase their genetic diversity [90–98]. This propensity for recombination has played a role in more recent outbreaks of paralytic diseases involving vaccine-derived strains [15].

MORPHOLOGY AND REPLICATION

The genome of enteroviruses and parechoviruses is a single-stranded, positive-sense RNA molecule approximately 7.4 kilobases in length [83]. It consists of a 5′ noncoding region followed by a single long open-reading frame, a short 3′ noncoding region, and a polyA tail. The 5′ noncoding region contains an internal ribosome entry site, which is essential for the initiation of translation. The 3′ noncoding region folds into highly conserved secondary and tertiary structures that are thought to play a role in the initiation of the replication of the viral genome. This genome is packaged into naked capsids that exhibit icosahedral symmetry with 20 triangular faces and 12 vertices.

Enterovirus replication begins with the adsorption of virions to cell surface receptors, which, for the most part, are integrins or immunoglobulin-like proteins (Table 24–3). The virions penetrate the cell surface, uncoat, and the viral genome functions as messenger RNA for the viral polyprotein. This polypeptide contains three domains, P1 to P3, which are cleaved into three to four proteins each. The P1 region is liberated from the polyprotein by the viral 2A protein, a chymotrypsin-like protease. P1 is initially split into three proteins, VP0, VP1, and VP3, by the viral 3C protease. VP0 is processed further into two smaller proteins, VP4 and VP2. Portions of VP1, VP2, and VP3 are exposed at the surface of the virion, whereas VP4 is entirely internal. VP1, VP2, and VP3 have no sequence homology, but they share the same topology [15]. Specifically, they form an eight-stranded antiparallel β-barrel that is wedge-shaped and composed of two antiparallel β-sheets. The amino acid sequences in the loops that connect the β-strands and the N-terminal and C-terminal sequences that extend from the β-barrel domain of VP1, VP2, and VP3 give each enterovirus its distinct antigenicity.

In contrast to the enteroviruses, the parechovirus 2A protein does not function as a protease. Viral capsids are composed of three proteins: VP2, VP3, and an uncleaved VP0 protein. Although parechoviruses appear structurally similar to other picornaviruses on electron microscopy, the structural arrangement of the three capsid proteins has not been established.

The replication of enteroviruses typically occurs in the cytoplasm in membrane-associated replication complexes and is completed rapidly (5 to 10 hours). Studies of polioviruses and coxsackieviruses have shown that enterovirus replication is associated with disruption of cellular protein secretion, and host-cell protein synthesis is suppressed because of cleavage of eIF4G by the enterovirus 2A protein. The coxsackievirus 2A protein also cleaves dystrophin, a cytoskeletal protein; this activity has been hypothesized to play a role in damage to the myocardium [99,100].

Parechoviruses replicate in a similar fashion [101]. Integrins, $\alpha_v\beta_3$ and perhaps $\alpha_v\beta_1$, are used as receptors, and replication occurs in cytoplasmic structures. As noted previously, the P1 portion of the viral polyprotein is processed into only three capsid proteins, however, and one only protease has been identified in parechoviruses. In addition, parechovirus replication occurs in small, discrete foci in the cytoplasm, rather than in large accumulations

TABLE 24-3 Cellular Receptors and Cofactors for Infection of Representative Human Enteroviruses (HEV)

Virus	HEV Species	Receptor	Cofactor for Infection*
Polioviruses 1-3	Poliovirus	CD155; Pvr (poliovirus receptor)	
Coxsackieviruses B1-6	HEV-B	CAR (coxsackievirus-adenovirus receptor)	CVB 1, 3, 5 may use CD 55 (DAF [decay accelerating factor])
Coxsackievirus A9	HEV-B	$\alpha_v\beta_3$ integrin (vitronectin receptor)	MAP-70
Echovirus 1, 8	HEV-B	VLA-2 ($\alpha_2\beta_1$ integrin)	Heparin sulfate
Coxsackievirus A13, A17, A20, A21, A24	HEV-C	ICAM-1 (intercelluar adhesion molecule 1)	
Enterovirus 70	HEV-D	CD55 (DAF)	

*The cofactors generally facilitate adhesion to cells, but their sole expression is insufficient to permit infection to occur.

of membranous vesicles as in enteroviruses. Transcription and translation do not seem to be disrupted by parechoviruses, perhaps explaining their relatively mild and delayed cytopathic effect when grown in tissue culture [13].

REPLICATION CHARACTERISTICS AND HOST SYSTEMS

Enteroviruses and parechoviruses are relatively stable viruses in that they retain activity for several days at room temperature and can be stored indefinitely at ordinary freezer temperatures ($-20°$ C). They are inactivated quickly by heat ($>56°$ C), formaldehyde, chlorination, and ultraviolet light, but are refractory to ether, ethanol, and isopropanol [11,80,102,103].

Enterovirus strains grow rapidly when adapted to susceptible host systems and cause cytopathology in 2 to 7 days. The typical tissue culture cytopathic effect is shown in Figure 24–1; characteristic pathologic findings in mice are shown in Figures 24–2 and 24–3. Final titers of virus recovered in the laboratory vary markedly among different viral strains and the host system used; typically, concentrations of 10^3 to 10^7 infectious doses per 0.1 mL of tissue culture fluid or tissue homogenate are obtained. Unadapted viral strains frequently require long periods of incubation. In tissue culture and suckling mice, evidence of growth usually is visible. Blind passage occasionally is necessary for the cytopathology to become apparent.

Although many different primary and secondary tissue culture systems support the growth of various enteroviruses, primary rhesus monkey kidney cultures generally are accepted to have the most inclusive spectrum. Other simian kidney tissue cultures also have the same broad spectrum [104]. Tissue cultures of human origin have a more limited spectrum, but several echovirus types have shown more consistent primary isolation in human than in monkey kidney culture [105–107]. A satisfactory system for the primary recovery of enteroviruses from clinical specimens would include primary rhesus, cynomolgus, or African green monkey kidney; a diploid, human embryonic lung fibroblast cell strain; rhabdomyosarcoma cell line tissue cultures; and intraperitoneal and intracerebral inoculation of suckling mice younger than 24 hours.*

ANTIGENIC CHARACTERISTICS

Although some minor cross-reactions exist among several coxsackievirus and echovirus types, common group antigens of diagnostic importance have not been defined well. Heat treatment of virions and the use of synthetic peptides have produced antigens with broad enterovirus reactivity [110,111]. These antigens have been used in enzyme-linked immunosorbent assay (ELISA) and complement fixation tests to determine IgG and IgM enterovirus antibodies and for antigen detection. In one study, Terletskaia-Ladwig and colleagues [110] reported the identification of patients infected with enteroviruses by the use of an IgM enzyme immunoassay. This test used heat-treated coxsackievirus B5 and echovirus 9 as antigens, and it identified patients infected with echoviruses 4, 11, and 30. The sensitivity of the test was 35%. In another study involving heat-treated virus and synthetic peptides, the sensitivities were 67% and 62% [111]. Both tests lacked specificity, however. Intratypic strain differences are common findings, and some strains (prime strains) are neutralized poorly by antisera to prototype viruses. In animals, these prime strains induce antibodies that neutralize the specific prototype viruses [9,11,38, 77,80].

The identification of poliovirus, coxsackievirus, and echovirus types by neutralization in suckling mice or tissue culture with antiserum pools is relatively well defined.

---

*References 77,80,103,106,108,109.

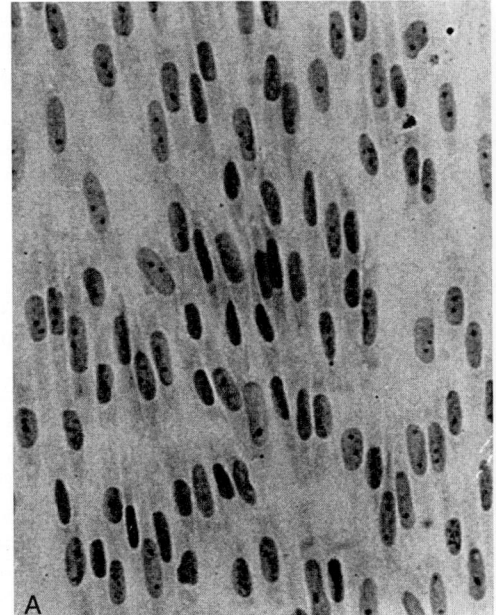 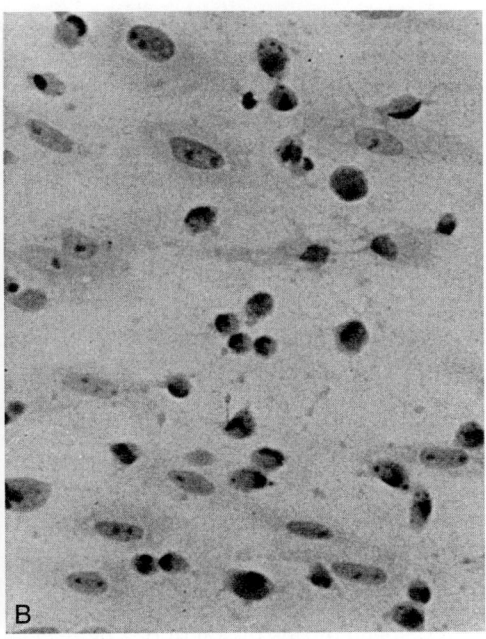

FIGURE 24–1 **Fetal rhesus monkey kidney tissue culture (HL-8). A,** Uninoculated tissue culture. **B,** Echovirus 11 cytopathic effect.

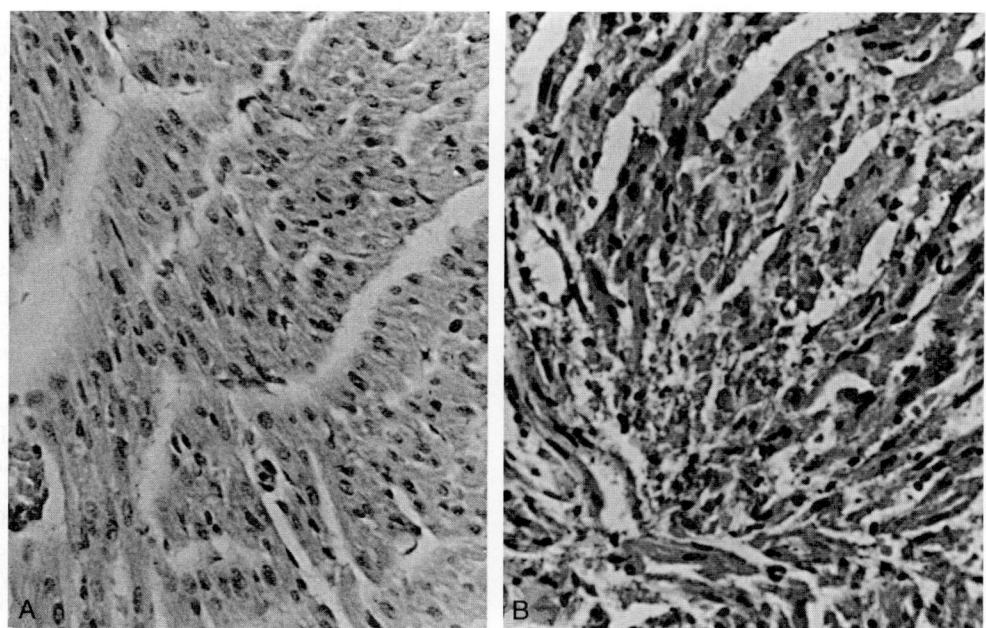

FIGURE 24–2 **Suckling mouse myocardium. A,** Normal suckling mouse myocardium. **B,** Myocardium of suckling mouse infected with coxsackievirus B1.

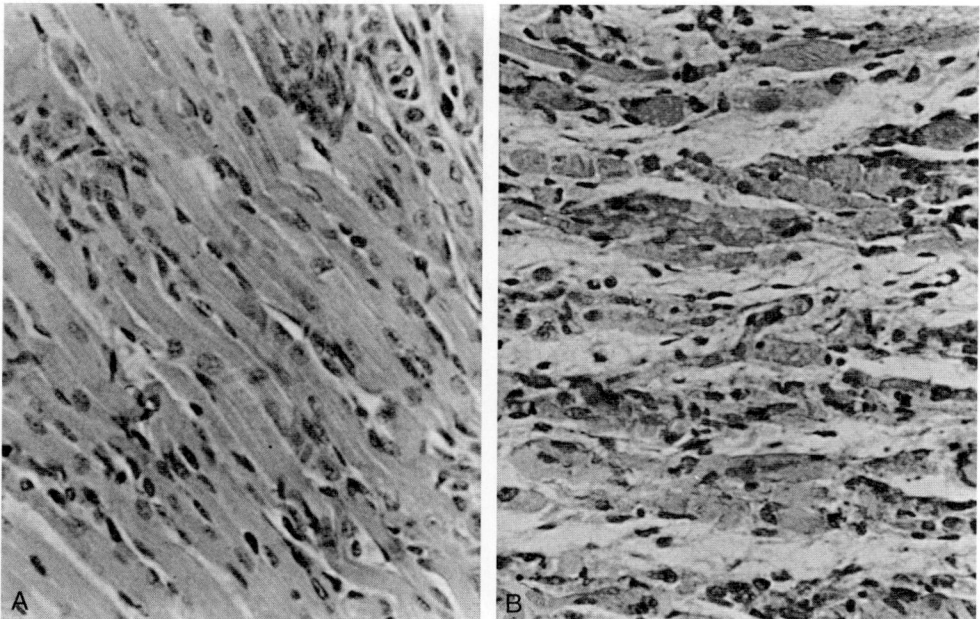

FIGURE 24–3 **Suckling mouse skeletal muscle. A,** Normal suckling mouse skeletal muscle. **B,** Skeletal muscle of suckling mouse infected with coxsackievirus A16.

Neutralization is induced by the epitopes on structural proteins VP1, VP2, and VP3; in particular, several epitopes are clustered on VP1. Prime strains do cause diagnostic difficulty because frequently they are not neutralized by the reference antisera, which is a particular problem with echoviruses 4, 9, and 11 and enterovirus 71. If these types are suspected, this problem can be overcome in some instances by using antisera in less diluted concentrations or antisera prepared against several different strains of problem viruses. Kubo and associates [76] were able to type enterovirus isolates not identified through neutralization by nucleotide sequence analysis of the VP4 gene. They specifically identified prime strains of echovirus 18 and enterovirus 71. Sequence analysis of the VP1 gene also is useful for typing enterovirus prime strains not identified by neutralization [81].

HOST RANGE

Humans are the only natural hosts of polioviruses, coxsackieviruses, and echoviruses [3–5,12,14,112]. However a total of 18 genetically distinct enteroviruses have been isolated from nonhuman primates [71]. Of 10 of these strains, 7 were related closely genetically to human enteroviruses, whereas the other 3 were related only distantly.

EPIDEMIOLOGY AND TRANSMISSION
GENERAL CONSIDERATIONS

Enteroviruses and parechoviruses are spread from person to person by fecal-oral and possibly by oral-oral (respiratory) routes.* Swimming and wading pools may serve as a means of spread of enteroviruses during the summer [114]. Oral-oral transmission via contaminated hands of health care personnel and transmission by fomites have been documented on a long-term care pediatric ward [115]. Echovirus 18 was isolated from human breast milk, and it was possible that enterovirus transmission to the infant occurred through the breast milk [116]. Chang and colleagues [117] detected coxsackievirus B3 in breast milk of two symptomatic mothers, and their infants experienced severe illnesses with hepatic necrosis and meningitis owing to coxsackievirus B3. Enteroviruses have been recovered from trapped flies, and this carriage probably contributes to the spread of human infections, particularly in lower socioeconomic populations that have poor sanitary facilities [118–120].

Children are the main susceptible cohort; they are immunologically susceptible, and their unhygienic habits facilitate spread. Spread is from child to child (by feces to skin to mouth) and then within family groups. Recovery of enteroviruses is inversely related to age; the prevalence of specific antibodies is directly related to age. The incidence of infections and the prevalence of antibodies do not differ between boys and girls.

TRANSPLACENTAL TRANSMISSION
Polioviruses

Poliovirus infections in pregnancy can result in abortion, stillbirth, neonatal disease, or no evidence of fetal involvement [121]. Gresser and associates [122] showed that the human amniotic membrane in organ culture can be infected, resulting in a persistent low-grade infection. On many occasions, maternal poliomyelitis occurring late in pregnancy has resulted in transplacental transmission of the virus to the fetus in utero [123–144]. The evidence that transplacental passage of virus occurs in early pregnancy is meager. Schaeffer and colleagues [136] were able to recover virus from the placenta and the fetus after a spontaneous abortion in a 24-year-old woman with poliomyelitis.

Although attenuated poliovirus vaccines have been given to pregnant women, there has never been a search for the transplacental passage of vaccine virus [145–147].

---

*References 1–5,8–10,12,14,112,113.

Viremia occurs after oral administration of polio vaccine, and this virus probably is occasionally passed transplacentally to the fetus [148–155].

Coxsackieviruses

Several investigators have studied coxsackievirus infections in pregnant animals and the transplacental passage of virus to the fetus. Dalldorf and Gifford [156] studied two strains of coxsackievirus B1 and one strain of coxsackievirus A8 in gravid mice. In only one instance (coxsackievirus B1) were they able to recover virus from a fetus. They thought that this result was inconclusive because they were unable to recover virus in five other instances. Berger and Roulet [157] observed muscle lesions in the young of gravid mice infected with coxsackieviruses A1 and B1. Selzer [158] studied several viruses in gravid mice; coxsackievirus A9 was found in the placentas of two mice, but in no fetuses, and coxsackievirus A18 was not recovered from fetuses or placentas. Selzer [158] found that coxsackieviruses B3 and B4 passed the placental barrier. Soike [159] also observed that in the last week of pregnancy, coxsackievirus B3 reached fetal mice transplacentally. Modlin and Crumpacker [160] reported that infection in late gestational mice was more severe than infection occurring in early pregnancy and that transplacental infection of the fetus occurred transiently during the maternal infection. Flamm [161] observed that coxsackievirus A9, when injected intravenously in rabbits, reached the blastocyst early in pregnancy and the amniotic fluid later in pregnancy. He also showed congenital infection in mice with coxsackievirus A1 [162].

Palmer and coworkers [163] studied the gestational outcome in pregnant mice inoculated intravenously with Theiler murine encephalomyelitis virus, a murine enterovirus. In early gestational infections, they found a high rate of placental and fetal abnormalities. The rates of fetal abnormalities and placental infection were greater than the rate of fetal viral infection, suggesting that the adverse effects of the viral infections were direct and indirect. Gestational infection could result in virus passage to the fetus and fetal damage or in placental compromise with indirect fetal damage. In another study using the same murine model with Theiler murine encephalomyelitis virus, Abzug [164] found that maternal factors (i.e., compromised uteroplacental blood flow, concomitant infection, and advanced age) increased the risk of transplacental fetal infection.

In humans, the transplacental passage of coxsackieviruses at term has been documented on several occasions. Benirschke [165] studied the placentas in three cases of congenital coxsackievirus B disease and could find no histologic evidence of infection. In 1956, Kibrick and Benirschke [166] reported the first case of intrauterine infection with coxsackievirus B3. In this instance, the infant was delivered by cesarean section and had clinical evidence of infection several hours after birth. Brightman and colleagues [167] recovered coxsackievirus B5 from the placenta and rectum of a premature infant. No histologic abnormalities of the placenta were identified. Konstantinidou and associates [168] confirmed transplacental infection with coxsackievirus B3 using molecular techniques. At fetal autopsy, they found mild arthrogryposis, necrotic meningoencephalitis with vascular calcifications, interstitial pneumonitis, mild myocardial hypertrophy, and chronic monocytic placental villitis. Coxsackievirus RNA was detected in placental tissue of six infants who had severe respiratory failure and subsequent CNS sequelae [169]. Other evidence of intrauterine infection has been presented for coxsackieviruses A4 and B2 through B6 [170–178].

Evidence for intrauterine infection during the first and second trimesters of pregnancy with coxsackieviruses is less clear. Burch and coworkers [179] reported the results of immunofluorescent studies of two fetuses of 5 months' gestation and one fetus of 6 months' gestation. The 6-month fetus had evidence of coxsackievirus B4 myocarditis; one 5-month fetus showed signs of coxsackievirus B3 infection; and the other 5-month fetus showed evidence of coxsackievirus B2, B3, and B4 infections. Basso and associates [170] recovered coxsackievirus B2 from the placenta, liver, and brain of a fetus after a spontaneous abortion at 3 months' gestation. Plager and coworkers [180] found no evidence of intrauterine viral transmission of coxsackievirus B5 infections during the first and second trimesters of pregnancy.

Euscher and associates [181] detected coxsackievirus RNA in placental tissue from six of seven newborn infants with respiratory difficulties and other manifestations at birth. One of these infants died shortly after birth, and the other six had neurodevelopmental delays. The placentas of 10 normal infants were examined for coxsackievirus RNA, and results of these studies were negative. Three of the placentas from the affected infants showed focal chronic villitis, two showed focal hemorrhagic endovasculitis, and one showed focal calcifications. In addition to respiratory distress, two neonates had rashes, two had seizures, two had thrombocytopenia, and one had intraventricular hemorrhage.

Echoviruses, Enteroviruses, and Parechoviruses

Less is known about transplacental passage of echoviruses compared with coxsackieviruses and polioviruses. Echovirus infections are regular occurrences in all populations. Women in all stages of pregnancy are frequently infected, and viremia is commonly seen in these infections [182]. In particular, epidemic disease related to echovirus 9 has been studied epidemiologically and serologically [183–185]. In these studies, a search for teratogenesis has been made, but no definitive virologic investigations have been done; asymptomatic transplacental infection might have occurred.

Cherry and colleagues [174] cultured samples from 590 newborns during a period of enterovirus prevalence without isolating an echovirus. Antepartum serologic study of 55 mothers in this study showed that 5 (9%) were actively infected with echovirus 17 during the 6-week period before delivery. In two other large nursery studies, there was no suggestion of intrauterine echovirus infections [186,187].

Berkovich and Smithwick [188] described a newborn without clinical illness who had specific IgM parechovirus 1 antibody in the cord blood, suggesting intrauterine infection with this virus. Hughes and colleagues [189] reported a newborn with echovirus 14 infection who had a markedly elevated level of IgM (190 mg/dL) on the 6th day of life. It seems likely that this infant was also infected in utero. Echoviruses 6, 7, 9, 11, 19, 27, and 33 have been identified in cases of transplacentally acquired infections [143,160–168].

Chow and associates [190] described a 1300-g fetus, which was stillborn after 26 weeks' gestation, with unilateral hydrocephalus, hepatosplenomegaly, fibrotic peritonitis, and meconium staining. Enterovirus 71 was isolated from the amniotic fluid, and the same virus was identified by polymerase chain reaction (PCR) in the cord blood and by immunohistochemical staining in the fetal midbrain and liver. Otonkoski and coworkers [191] reported the occurrence of neonatal type 1 diabetes after possible maternal echovirus 6 infection.

ASCENDING INFECTION AND CONTACT INFECTION DURING BIRTH

Definitive evidence is lacking for ascending infection or contact infection with enteroviruses during birth. In prospective studies of genital herpes simplex and cytomegalovirus infections, there have been no isolations of enterovirus [192,193]. These results suggest that ascending infections with enteroviruses, if they occur at all, are rare. Reyes and associates [194] recovered coxsackievirus B5 from the cervix of four women in their third trimester, however. Three of the four positive cultures were obtained 3 weeks or more before delivery. In the fourth case, the cervical culture was obtained the day before delivery, and the infant was delivered by cesarean section. All of the infants were healthy, but culture for virus was possible only from the infant delivered by cesarean section; the result was negative. In an earlier study, Reyes and associates [195] reported a child who died of a disseminated echovirus 11 infection. The illness had its onset on the 3rd day of life, and the virus was recovered from the mother's cervix at that time.

Infection with enteroviruses during the birth process seems probable [25,174,196]. The fecal carriage rate of enteroviruses in asymptomatic adults ranges from 0% to 6% or greater in different population groups [197–199]. Cherry and associates [174] found that in 2 (4%) of 55 mothers, enteroviruses were present in the feces shortly after delivery. Katz [200], in a discussion of an infant with neonatal coxsackievirus B4 infection, suggested that the infant might have inhaled maternally excreted organisms during birth. The fact that this infant had pneumonia tends to support the contention. Infections occurring 2 to 7 days after birth could have been acquired during passage through the birth canal.

NEONATAL INFECTION

Neonatal infections and illnesses from enteroviruses are common [201]. Transmission of enteroviruses to newborns is similar to populations of older people. The main factor in the spread of virus is human-to-human contact.

During the summer and fall of 1981 in Rochester, New York, 666 neonates were cultured for enteroviruses within 24 hours of birth and then weekly for 1 month [195]. The incidence of acquisition of nonpolio enterovirus infections during this period was 12.8%. Two risk factors were identified: lower socioeconomic status and lack of breast-feeding.

Polioviruses

Clinical poliomyelitis is rare in neonates, but the infection rate before the vaccine era was never determined. It is probable that the rarity of neonatal poliomyelitis was not related to lack of viral transmission, but reflected the protection from disease offered by specific, transplacentally transmitted poliovirus antibodies. From experience gained in vaccine studies, it is apparent that infants with passively acquired antibody can be regularly infected [202–214].

In 1955, Bates [127] reviewed the literature on poliomyelitis in infants younger than 1 month. He described six infants who apparently were not infected by their mothers and who had had other likely contacts. A neighbor was the contact in one case, siblings in two cases, nursery nurses in two cases, and an uncle in the sixth case. In most other infants, the mother had had poliomyelitis shortly before the infant was born and probably was the contact. The mode of transmission—intrauterine, during birth, or postnatal contact—is unknown.

Bergeisen and colleagues [215] reported a case of paralytic poliomyelitis from a type 3 vaccine viral strain. They suggested that the source of this virus might have been the child of the neonate's babysitter, who was vaccinated about 2 weeks before the onset of the illness.

Coxsackieviruses

Several epidemics with strains of coxsackievirus B in newborn nurseries have been studied. Brightman and coworkers [167] observed an epidemic of coxsackievirus B5 in a premature newborn nursery. Their data suggested that the virus was introduced into the nursery by an infant with a clinically inapparent infection who had been infected in utero. Secondary infections occurred in 12 infants and 2 nurses. The timing of the secondary cases suggested that three generations of infection had occurred and that the nurses had been infected during the second generation. The investigators suggested that the infection had spread from infant to infant and from infant to nurse.

Javett and colleagues [216] documented an acute epidemic of myocarditis associated with coxsackievirus B3 infection in a Johannesburg maternity home. No epidemiologic investigation or search for asymptomatic infected infants was performed. Analysis of the onset dates of the illnesses indicated, however, that single infections occurred for five generations, and then five children became ill within a 3-day period.

Kipps and colleagues [217] performed epidemiologic investigations in two coxsackievirus B3 nursery epidemics. In the first epidemic, the initial infection was probably transmitted from a mother to her child; this infant was the source of five secondary cases in newborns and one

illness in a nurse. Infants with four of the five secondary cases were located on one side of the nursery, but only one cot was close to the cot of the index patient, and this cot did not adjoin the cots of the three other infants with contact cases. In the second outbreak, an infant who also was infected by his mother probably introduced the virus into the nursery. Infants with the three secondary cases were geographically far removed from the infant with the primary case of infection.

There have been many other instances of isolated nursery infections and small outbreaks with coxsackieviruses, and it seems that the most consistent source of original nursery infection is transmission from a mother to her child [216–256]. Introduction of virus into the nursery by personnel also occurs, however [232,257].

Echoviruses and Parechoviruses

Although many outbreaks of echovirus infections have been observed in newborn nurseries, information on viral transmission is incomplete [28,258–286]. Cramblett and coworkers [261] reported an outbreak of echovirus 11 disease in four infants in an intensive care nursery. All infants were in enclosed incubators, and three patients became ill within 24 hours; the fourth child became ill 4 days later. Echovirus 11 was recovered from two members of the nursery staff. These data suggest that transmission from personnel to infants occurred because of inadequate hand washing. In another outbreak in an intensive care unit, the initial patient was transferred to the nursery because of severe echovirus 11 disease [279]. After transfer, infection occurred in the senior house officer and a psychologist in the unit. It was inferred by the investigators that spread by respiratory droplets to nine other infants occurred from these infected personnel.

In a maternity unit outbreak of echovirus 11 involving six secondary cases [275], infection spread through close contact between the infected newborns and the nurses. In another reported nosocomial echovirus 11 outbreak, infants in an intermediate care unit for more than 2 days were more likely to become infected than infants who were there for less than 2 days. Illness was also associated with gavage feeding, mouth care, and being a twin [272].

Modlin [28] reviewed reports of 16 nursery outbreaks involving 206 ill infants. The source was identified in only 4 of the 16 outbreaks, and the primary case in all 4 was an infant who acquired infection vertically from his or her mother. After introduction of an infected newborn into a nursery, spread to other infants by personnel is common [278,282,285,286]. Risk factors for nursery transmission as described by Rabkin and coworkers [282] were "lower gestational age or birth weight; antibiotic or transfusion therapy; nasogastric intubation or feeding; proximity in the nursery to the index patient; and care by the same nurse during the same shift as the index patient."

Wilson and associates [285] reported an intensive care nursery epidemic in which respiratory syncytial virus and echovirus 7 infections occurred concurrently. This epidemic persisted from January to June 1984 despite an aggressive isolation cohorting program. A major factor in persistence was asymptomatic infections with both viruses.

Sato and associates [287] reported a point-source outbreak of echovirus 33 infection in nine newborns related to one nursery over a 10-day period. The primary case was born to a mother who was febrile and who had a high echovirus 33 neutralizing antibody titer in a convalescent-phase serum specimen.

Jack and colleagues [270] observed the endemic occurrence of asymptomatic infection with parechovirus 1 in a nursery during an 8-month period. During this time, 44 infants were infected, and nursery infection occurred when there was no known activity of parechovirus 1 in the community at large. The investigators believed that the endemic viral infection was spread by fecal contamination of hands of nursery personnel. Nakao and colleagues [280] and Berkovich and Pangan [259] also documented parechovirus 1 infections in nurseries. Similar to Jack and colleagues [270], they observed that the infections seemed to be endemic to the nurseries, rather than related to community epidemics.

HOST RANGE

It is the general opinion that humans are the only natural hosts of enteroviruses [112]. Enteroviruses have been recovered, however, in nature from sewage [119], flies [118–120], swine [288,289], dogs [290,291], a calf [292], a budgerigar [293], a fox [294], mussels [295], and oysters [296]. Serologic evidence of infection with enteroviruses similar to human strains has been found in chimpanzees [297], cattle [298], rabbits [299], a fox [300], a chipmunk [301], and a marmot [262]. It is probable that infection of these animals was the result of their direct contact with an infected human or infected human excreta. Although enteroviruses do not multiply in flies, flies seem to be a possible significant vector in situations of poor sanitation and heavy human infection. The contamination of shellfish is also intriguing [294,295,299–304] because in addition to their possible role in human infection, they offer a source of enterovirus storage during cold weather. Contaminated foods are another possible source of human infection [305].

GEOGRAPHIC DISTRIBUTION AND SEASON

Enteroviruses and parechoviruses have a worldwide distribution [2,9,112,305,306]. Neutralizing antibodies for specific viral types have been found in serologic surveys throughout the world, and most strains have been recovered in worldwide isolation studies. In any one area, there are frequent fluctuations in predominant types. Epidemics probably depend on new susceptible persons in the population rather than on reinfections; they may be localized and sporadic and may vary in cause from place to place in the same year. Pandemic waves of infection also occur.

In temperate climates, enterovirus infections occur primarily in the summer and fall, but in the tropics, they are prevalent all year [9,112,307]. A basic concept in understanding their epidemiology is the far greater frequency of unrecognized infection than that of clinical disease. This concept is illustrated by poliomyelitis, which remained

an epidemiologic mystery until it was appreciated that unrecognized infections were the main source of contagion. Serologic surveys were instrumental in elucidating the problem. In populations living in conditions of poor sanitation and hygiene, epidemics do not occur; but wide dissemination of polioviruses has been confirmed by showing the presence of specific antibodies to all three types in nearly 100% of children by age 5 years.

Epidemics of poliomyelitis first began to appear in Europe and the United States during the latter part of the 19th century; they continued with increasing frequency in economically advanced countries until the introduction of effective vaccines in the 1950s and 1960s [36,37,307,308]. The evolution from endemic to epidemic follows a characteristic pattern, beginning with collections of a few cases, then endemic rates that are higher than usual, followed by severe epidemics with high attack rates.

The age group attacked in endemic areas and in early epidemics is the youngest one; more than 90% of paralytic cases begin in children younger than 5 years. After a pattern of epidemicity begins, it is irreversible unless preventive vaccination is carried out. Because epidemics recur over years, there is a shift in age incidence such that relatively fewer cases are in the youngest children; the peak often occurs in the 5- to 14-year-old group, and an increasing proportion is in young adults. These changes are correlated with socioeconomic factors and improved standards of hygiene; when children are protected from immunizing infections in the first few years of life, the pool of susceptible persons builds up, and introduction of a virulent strain often is followed by an epidemic [309].

Extensive use of vaccines in the past 5 decades has resulted in elimination of paralytic poliomyelitis from large geographic areas, but the disease remains endemic in various parts of the world. Although seasonal periodicity is distinct in temperate climates, some viral activity does occur during the winter [310]. Infection and acquisition of postinfection immunity occur with greater intensity and at earlier ages among crowded, economically deprived populations with less efficient sanitation facilities.

Molecular techniques have allowed the study of genotypes of specific viral types in populations over time [310–313]. Mulders and colleagues [314] studied the molecular epidemiology of wild poliovirus type 1 in Europe, the Middle East, and the Indian subcontinent. They found four major genotypes circulating. Two genotypes were found predominantly in Eastern Europe, a third genotype was circulating mainly in Egypt, and the fourth genotype was widely dispersed. All four genotypes were found in Pakistan.

The epidemiologic behavior of coxsackieviruses and echoviruses parallels that of polioviruses; unrecognized infections far outnumber infections with distinctive symptoms. The agents are disseminated widely throughout the world, and outbreaks related to one or another type of virus occur regularly. These outbreaks tend to be localized, with different agents being prevalent in different years. In the late 1950s, echovirus 9 had a far wider circulation, however, sweeping through a large part of the world and infecting children and young adults. This behavior has been repeated occasionally with other enteroviruses; after a long absence, a particular agent returns and circulates among susceptible persons of different ages who have been born since the previous epidemic occurred. Other agents remain endemic in a given area, surfacing as sporadic cases and occasionally as small outbreaks. Multiple types are frequently active at the same time, although one agent commonly predominates in a given locality.

There are no available data on the incidence of symptomatic congenital and neonatal enterovirus infections. From the frequency of reports in the literature, it seems that severe neonatal disease caused by enteroviruses decreased slightly during the late 1960s and early 1970s and then became more common again. In 2007, there was an increase in the detection of severe neonatal disease owing to coxsackievirus B1 infection [315].

The five most prevalent nonpolio enterovirus isolations per year in the United States from 1961–2005 are shown in Table 24–4 [6,316–323]. Most patients from whom viruses were isolated had neurologic illnesses. It is possible that other enteroviruses were also prevalent, but did not produce clinical disease severe enough to cause physicians to submit specimens for study. Many coxsackievirus A infections, even in epidemic situations, probably went undiagnosed because suckling mouse inoculation was not performed. Although more than 62 nonpolio enterovirus types and 6 parechovirus types have been identified, only 24 different virus types have been noted in the 45 years covered in Table 24–4.

Khetsuriani and associates [33] at the Centers for Disease Control and Prevention (CDC) presented an extensive report on enterovirus surveillance in the United States for the period 1970-2005. During this period, the five most common enterovirus isolates in order have been echovirus 9, echovirus 11, echovirus 30, coxsackievirus B5, and echovirus 6. During the most recent period (2000-2005), the most common isolates in order have been echovirus 9, echovirus 30, echovirus 18, echovirus 13 and coxsackievirus B5. Similar data are available for the most common enterovirus isolates in Spain from 1988-1997 and Belgium from 1980-1994 [324,325]. The most common enterovirus isolated in both countries was echovirus 30. In 1997 and 1998, major epidemic disease caused by enterovirus 71 occurred in Taiwan, Malaysia, Australia, and Japan [325–329].

An analysis of the CDC nonpolio enterovirus data for 14 years found that early isolates in a particular year were predictive of isolates for the remainder of that year [323]. The six most common isolates during March, April, and May were predictive of 59% of the total isolates during July through December of the same year.

Although the use of live poliovirus vaccine has eliminated epidemic poliomyelitis in the United States, it is hard to determine what effect poliovirus vaccine has had on enterovirus ecology. In 1970, polioviruses accounted for only 6% of the total enterovirus isolations from patients with neurologic illnesses [330]. Although the figures are not directly comparable, more than one third of the enterovirus isolations in 1962 from similar patients were polioviruses [331]. Horstmann and associates [332]

studied specimens from sewage and asymptomatic children during the vaccine era and found that the number of yearly poliovirus isolations (presumably vaccine strains) was greater than the number of nonpolio enteroviruses. The prevalence of vaccine viruses did not seem to affect the seasonal epidemiology of other enteroviruses.

PATHOGENESIS
EVENTS DURING PATHOGENESIS
Congenital infections with enteroviruses result from transplacental passage of virus to fetus. The method of transport from mother to fetus is poorly understood. Maternal viremia during enterovirus infections is common, and because virus has been recovered from the placenta on several occasions, it is probable that active infection of the placenta also occurs. Benirschke [165] found no histologic evidence of placental disease in three cases of established transplacentally acquired coxsackievirus B infections. Batcup and associates [333] found diffuse perivillous fibrin deposition with villous necrosis and inflammatory cell infiltration of the placenta in a woman who 2 weeks previously, at 33 weeks' gestation, had coxsackievirus A9 meningitis. The woman was delivered of a macerated, stillborn infant. At birth, virus was recovered from the placenta, but not from the stillborn infant.

It is assumed that infection in the fetus results from hematogenous dissemination initiated in the involved placenta. It is also possible that some in utero infection results from the ingestion of virus contained in amniotic fluid; in this situation, primary fetal infection involves the pharynx and lower alimentary tract. The portal of entry of infection during the birth process and the neonatal period is similar to that for older children and adults.

Figure 24–4 shows a schematic diagram of the events of pathogenesis. After initial acquisition of virus by the oral or respiratory route, implantation occurs in the pharynx and the lower alimentary tract. Within 1 day, the infection extends to the regional lymph nodes. On about the 3rd day, minor viremia occurs, resulting in involvement of many secondary infection sites. In congenital infections, infection is initiated during the minor viremia phase. Multiplication of virus in secondary sites coincides with the onset of clinical symptoms. Illness can vary from minor to fatal infections. Major viremia occurs during the period of multiplication of virus in the secondary infection sites; this period usually lasts from the 3rd to the 7th days of infection. In many echovirus and coxsackievirus infections, CNS involvement apparently occurs at the same time as other secondary organ involvement. This occasionally seems to happen with poliovirus infections; however, more commonly, the CNS symptoms of poliomyelitis are delayed, suggesting that seeding occurred later in association with the major viremia.

Cessation of viremia correlates with the appearance of serum antibody. The viral concentration in secondary infection sites begins to diminish on about the 7th day. Infection continues in the lower intestinal tract for prolonged periods, however.

TABLE 24–4 Predominant Types of Nonpolio Enterovirus Isolations in the United States: 1961-2005*

Year	First	Second	Third	Fourth	Fifth
			Five Most Common Viral Types per Year		
1961	Coxsackievirus B5	Coxsackievirus B2	Coxsackievirus B4	Echovirus 11	Echovirus 9
1962	Coxsackievirus B3	Echovirus 9	Coxsackievirus B2	Echovirus 4	Coxsackievirus B5
1963	Coxsackievirus B1	Coxsackievirus A9	Echovirus 9	Echovirus 4	Coxsackievirus B4
1964	Coxsackievirus B4	Coxsackievirus B2	Coxsackievirus A9	Echovirus 4	Echovirus 6, coxsackievirus B1
1965	Echovirus 9	Echovirus 6	Coxsackievirus B2	Coxsackievirus B5	Coxsackievirus B4
1966	Echovirus 9	Coxsackievirus B2	Echovirus 6	Coxsackievirus B5	Coxsackievirus A9, A16
1967	Coxsackievirus B5	Echovirus 9	Coxsackievirus A9	Echovirus 6	Coxsackievirus B2
1968	Echovirus 9	Echovirus 30	Coxsackievirus A16	Coxsackievirus B3	Coxsackievirus B4
1969	Echovirus 30	Echovirus 9	Echovirus 18	Echovirus 6	Coxsackievirus B4
1970	Echovirus 3	Echovirus 9	Echovirus 6	Echovirus 4	Coxsackievirus B4
1971	Echovirus 4	Echovirus 9	Echovirus 6	Coxsackievirus B4	Coxsackievirus B2
1972	Coxsackievirus B5	Echovirus 4	Echovirus 6	Echovirus 9	Coxsackievirus B3
1973	Coxsackievirus A9	Echovirus 9	Echovirus 6	Coxsackievirus B2	Coxsackievirus B5, echovirus 5
1974	Echovirus 11	Echovirus 4	Echovirus 6	Echovirus 9	Echovirus 18
1975	Echovirus 9	Echovirus 4	Echovirus 6	Coxsackievirus A9	Coxsackievirus B4
1976	Coxsackievirus B2	Echovirus 4	Coxsackievirus B4	Coxsackievirus A9	Coxsackievirus B3, echovirus 6
1977	Echovirus 6	Coxsackievirus B1	Coxsackievirus B3	Echovirus 9	Coxsackievirus A9
1978	Echovirus 9	Echovirus 4	Coxsackievirus A9	Echovirus 30	Coxsackievirus B4
1979	Echovirus 11	Echovirus 7	Echovirus 30	Coxsackievirus B2	Coxsackievirus B4
1980	Echovirus 11	Coxsackievirus B3	Echovirus 30	Coxsackievirus B2	Coxsackievirus A9
1981	Echovirus 30	Echovirus 9	Echovirus 11	Echovirus 3	Coxsackievirus A9, echovirus 5
1982	Echovirus 11	Echovirus 30	Echovirus 5	Echovirus 9	Coxsackievirus B5
1983	Coxsackievirus B5	Echovirus 30	Echovirus 20	Echovirus 11	Echovirus 24
1984	Echovirus 9	Echovirus 11	Coxsackievirus B5	Echovirus 30	Coxsackievirus B2, A9
1985	Echovirus 11	Echovirus 21	Echovirus 6, 7†		Coxsackievirus B2
1986	Echovirus 11	Echovirus 4	Echovirus 7	Echovirus 18	Coxsackievirus B5
1987	Echovirus 6	Echovirus 18	Echovirus 11	Coxsackievirus A9	Coxsackievirus B2
1988	Echovirus 11	Echovirus 9	Coxsackievirus B4	Coxsackievirus B2	Echovirus 6
1989	Coxsackievirus B5	Echovirus 9	Echovirus 11	Coxsackievirus B2	Echovirus 6
1990	Echovirus 30	Echovirus 6	Coxsackievirus B2	Coxsackievirus A9	Echovirus 11
1991	Echovirus 30	Echovirus 11	Coxsackievirus B1	Coxsackievirus B2	Echovirus 7
1992	Echovirus 11	Echovirus 30	Echovirus 9	Coxsackievirus B1	Coxsackievirus A9
1993	Echovirus 30	Coxsackievirus B5	Coxsackievirus A9	Echovirus 7	Coxsackievirus B1
1994	Coxsackievirus B2	Coxsackievirus B3	Echovirus 6	Echovirus 30	Enterovirus 71
1995	Echovirus 9	Echovirus 11	Coxsackievirus A9	Coxsackievirus B2	Echovirus 30, coxsackievirus B5
1996	Coxsackievirus B5	Echovirus 17	Echovirus 6	Coxsackievirus A9	Coxsackievirus B4
1997	Echovirus 30	Echovirus 6	Echovirus 7	Echovirus 11	Echovirus 18
1998	Echovirus 30	Echovirus 9	Echovirus 11	Coxsackievirus B3	Echovirus 6
1999	Echovirus 11	Echovirus 16	Echovirus 9	Echovirus 14	Echovirus 25
2000	Coxsackievirus B2	Echovirus 6	Coxsackievirus A9	Coxsackievirus B4	Echovirus 11
2001	Echovirus 18	Echovirus 13	Coxsackievirus B2	Echovirus 6	Echovirus 4
2002	Echovirus 7	Echovirus 9	Coxsackievirus B1	Echovirus 11	Coxsackievirus B5
2003	Echovirus 9	Echovirus 30	Coxsackievirus B1	Coxsackievirus B4	Coxsackievirus A9
2004	Echovirus 30	Echovirus 9	Coxsackievirus A9	Coxsackievirus B5	Coxsackievirus B4
2005	Coxsackievirus B5	Echovirus 6	Echovirus 30	Echovirus 18	Coxsackievirus B3

Most patients from whom viruses were isolated had neurologic illnesses.
†*Third and fourth place tie.*
Data from references 6,316–323, and 547 and personal communication from LaMonte-Fowlkes A, Epidemiology Branch, Division of Viral Diseases, NCIRD, CDC (2005 data).

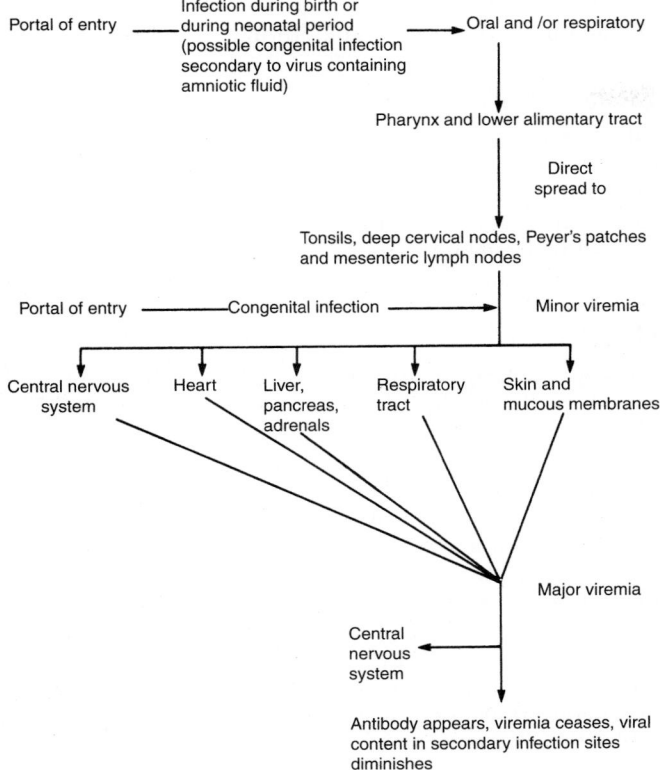

FIGURE 24–4 Pathogenesis of congenital and neonatal enterovirus infections.

FACTORS THAT AFFECT PATHOGENESIS

The pathogenesis and pathology of enterovirus and parechovirus infections depend on the virulence, tropism, and inoculum concentration of virus and on many specific host factors. Enteroviruses have marked differences in tropism and virulence. Although some generalizations can be made in regard to tropism, there are marked differences even among strains of specific viral types. Differences in virulence of specific enterovirus types may be the result of recombination among enteroviruses or point mutations [333–335].

Enterovirus infections of the fetus and neonate are thought to be more severe than similar infections in older individuals. This is undoubtedly true for coxsackievirus B infections and probably for coxsackievirus A, echovirus, and poliovirus infections as well. Although the reasons for this increased severity are largely unknown, several aspects of neonatal immune mechanisms offer clues. The similarity of coxsackievirus B infections in suckling mice to infections in human neonates has provided a useful animal model. Heineberg and coworkers [336] compared coxsackievirus B1 infections in 24-hour-old suckling mice with similar infections in older mice. They observed that adult mice produced interferon in all infected tissues, whereas only small amounts of interferon were identified in the liver in suckling mice. The investigators thought that the difference in outcome of coxsackievirus B1 infections in suckling and older mice could be explained by the inability of the cells of the

immature animal to elaborate interferon. Additional studies of abnormalities of innate immunity in neonates may enhance our understanding of the severity of enterovirus infections in newborns [337].

Other investigators thought that the increased susceptibility of suckling mice to severe coxsackievirus infections was related to the transplacentally acquired, increased concentrations of adrenocortical hormones [338,339]. Kunin [340] suggested that the difference in age-specific susceptibility might be explained at the cellular level. He showed that various tissues of newborn mice bound coxsackievirus B3, whereas tissues of adult mice were virtually inactive in this regard [340,341]. It has been suggested that the progressive loss of receptor-containing cells or of receptor sites on persisting cells with increasing age might be the mechanism that accounts for infections of lesser severity in older animals. Supporting this suggestion, Ito and colleagues [342] showed that coxsackievirus-adenovirus receptor expression decreases with increasing age in rats. Teisner and Haahr [343] suggested that the increased susceptibility of suckling mice to severe and fatal coxsackievirus infections might be from physiologic hypothermia and poikilothermia during the 1st week of life.

In the past, it was assumed that specific pathology in various organs and tissues in enterovirus infections was caused by the direct cytopathic effect and tropism of a particular virus. Numerous studies using murine myocarditis model systems have suggested, however, that host immune responses contribute to the pathology [13,307,316–331]. These studies suggest that T cell–mediated processes and virus-induced autoimmunity cause acute and chronic tissue damage. Other studies suggest that the primary viral cytopathic effect is responsible for tissue damage and that various T-cell responses are a response to the damage, not the cause [344].

From our review of various murine myocarditis model systems, it is apparent that the genetics of the hosts and of the viral strains determine the likelihood of autoimmune, cell-mediated cellular damage [333,343,345–354]. None of the model systems is appropriate, however, for the evaluation of the pathogenesis of neonatal myocarditis. Although available studies suggest that enterovirus-induced myocarditis in older children and adults occasionally may have a delayed cell-mediated component, the short incubation period and fulminant nature of neonatal disease and the similar infection in suckling mice suggest that autoimmune factors are not of major importance in the pathogenesis of myocarditis in neonates.

During the last 45 years, the clinical manifestations caused by several enterovirus serotypes have changed. Echovirus 11 infection initially was noted in association with an outbreak of upper respiratory infection in a day-nursery more than 50 years ago [355]. In the 1960s, it was found to be related to exanthem and aseptic meningitis [221,356]. Following this and occurring presently is the association of echovirus infection and severe sepsis-like illnesses with hepatitis in neonates.*

---

*References 195,262,277,279,282,284,357–364.

Another example relates to enterovirus 71 infections. Initially, this virus was noted in association with aseptic meningitis with only a few cases also having exanthem [365,366]. During the last decade, severe epidemic disease with enterovirus 71 occurred in Taiwan, Singapore, Australia, Malaysia, and Japan. In these epidemics, hand-foot-and-mouth syndrome was a major finding, and neurologic disease was more severe than in the past [367–374].

These phenotypic changes could be the result of point mutations or the result of recombination among enteroviruses.* Chan and AbuBakar [91] presented evidence indicating that a recombination event occurred between enterovirus 71 and coxsackievirus A16.

PATHOLOGY
GENERAL CONSIDERATIONS

Great variations in the clinical signs of congenital and neonatal enterovirus infections are paralleled by wide variations in pathology. Because pathologic material usually is available only from patients with fatal illnesses, the discussion in this section considers only the more severe enterovirus manifestations. These fatal infections account for only a small portion of all congenital and neonatal enterovirus infections, however. The pathologic findings in infants with milder infections, such as nonspecific febrile illness, have not been described.

POLIOVIRUSES

The pathologic findings in fatal neonatal poliomyelitis are similar to findings in disease of older children and adults [29,123,126,130,141]. The major findings have involved the CNS, specifically the anterior horns of the spinal cord and the motor nuclei of the cranial nerves. Involvement is usually irregularly distributed and asymmetric. Microscopically, the anterior horn cells show neuronal destruction, gliosis, and perivascular small round cell infiltration. Myocarditis has also been observed [126], characterized by focal necrosis of muscle fibers and various degrees of cellular infiltration.

COXSACKIEVIRUS A STRAINS

Records of neonatal illnesses associated with coxsackievirus A strains are rare [378–380]. In a study of sudden unexpected death in infants, Gold and coworkers [380], recovered coxsackievirus A4 from the brains of three children. Histologic abnormalities were not identified in the brains or spinal cords of these patients. Baker and Phillips [378] reported the death of twins in association with coxsackievirus A3 intrauterine infections; the first twin was stillborn, and the second twin died when 2 days old of viral pneumonia. Eisenhut and associates [381] described a full-term neonate with coxsackievirus A9 infection with

meningitis, myocarditis, and disseminated intravascular coagulation who died on the 7th day of life.

COXSACKIEVIRUS B STRAINS

Of the enteroviruses, coxsackievirus B strains have been most frequently associated with severe and catastrophic neonatal disease. The most common findings in these cases have been myocarditis or meningoencephalitis or both. Involvement of the adrenals, pancreas, liver, and lungs has occurred.

Heart

Grossly, the heart is usually enlarged, with dilation of the chambers and flabby musculature [166,177,216,226,229]. Microscopically, the pericardium frequently contains some inflammatory cells, and thickening, edema, and focal infiltrations of inflammatory cells may be found in the endocardium. The myocardium (Fig. 24–5) is congested and contains infiltrations of inflammatory cells (i.e., lymphocytes, mononuclear cells, reticulum cells, histiocytes, plasma cells, and polymorphonuclear and eosinophil leukocytes). Involvement of the myocardium is often patchy and focal, but occasionally is diffuse. The muscle shows loss of striation, edema, and eosinophilic degeneration. Muscle necrosis without extensive cellular infiltration is common.

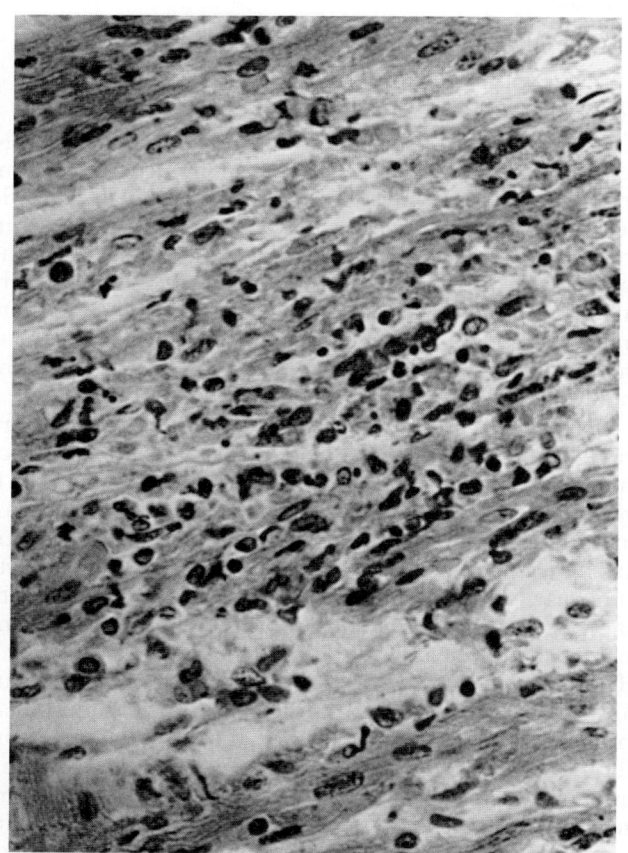

FIGURE 24–5 **Coxsackievirus B4 myocarditis in a 9-day-old infant.** Notice myocardial necrosis and mononuclear cellular infiltration.

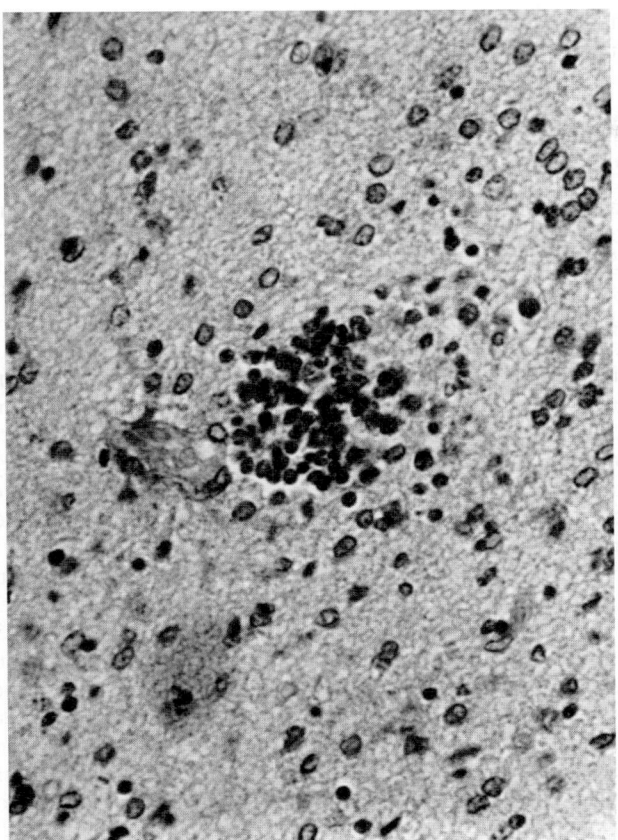

FIGURE 24–6 Coxsackievirus B4 encephalitis in a 9-day-old infant. Notice focal infiltrate of mononuclear and glial cells.

Brain and Spinal Cord

The meninges are congested, edematous, and occasionally mildly infiltrated with inflammatory cells.* Lesions in the brain and spinal cord are focal rather than diffuse, but frequently involve many different areas. The lesions consist of areas of eosinophilic degeneration of cortical cells, clusters of mononuclear and glial cells (Fig. 24–6), and perivascular cuffing. Occasionally, areas of liquefaction necrosis unassociated with inflammation are seen.

Other Organs

The lungs commonly have areas of mild focal pneumonitis with peribronchiolar mononuclear cellular infiltrations [166,200,229,242]. Massive pulmonary hemorrhage has been observed. The liver is frequently engorged and occasionally contains isolated foci of liver cell necrosis and mononuclear cell infiltrations. A neonate with a coxsackievirus B1 infection developed a sepsis-like illness on the 4th day of life with severe hepatitis and subsequently developed progressive liver calcifications [382]. In the pancreas, infiltration of mononuclear cells, lymphocytes, and plasma cells has been observed, and occasional

focal degeneration of the islet cells occurs. Congestion has been observed in the adrenal glands, with mild to severe cortical necrosis and infiltration of inflammatory cells.

ECHOVIRUSES

In an earlier period, although frequently responsible for neonatal illnesses, echoviruses were rarely associated with fatal infections. During the past 30 years, however, there have been many reports of fatal illnesses in newborns from echovirus type 11.* In virtually all cases, the major pathologic finding was massive hepatic necrosis; other findings included hemorrhagic necrosis of the adrenal glands, hemorrhage in other organs, myocardial necrosis, and acute tubular necrosis of the kidneys. Wang and colleagues [364] studied four neonates (three with echovirus 11 infections and one with echovirus 5 infection) with fulminant hepatic failure and observed two histopathologic patterns associated with minimal inflammation, but extensive hemorrhagic necrosis. One pattern showed ongoing endothelial injury with endotheliitis and fibrinoid necrosis. The second pattern, which was seen in the two neonates who initially survived, showed veno-occlusive disease.

Virus has not been identified in hepatocytes. Extensive myositis of the strap muscles of the neck occurred in one case [360]. Massive hepatic necrosis has also occurred in infections with echoviruses 3, 5, 6, 7, 9, 14, 19, 20, and 21.† Wreghitt and associates [389] described a neonate with a fatal echovirus 7 infection. This infant was found to have massive disseminated intravascular coagulation, with bleeding in the adrenal glands, renal medulla, liver, and cerebellum.

At autopsy, one infant with echovirus 6 infection was found to have cloudy and thickened leptomeninges, liver necrosis, adrenal and renal hemorrhage, and mild interstitial pneumonitis [363]. One infant with echovirus 9 infection had an enlarged and congested liver with marked central necrosis [387], and another with this virus had interstitial pneumonitis without liver involvement [390]. Three infants with echovirus 11 infections had renal and adrenal hemorrhage and small-vessel thrombi in the renal medulla and in the medulla and the inner cortex of the adrenal glands [279]. In these patients, the livers were normal. Two infants, one with echovirus 6 and the other with echovirus 31 infection, had only extensive pneumonias [274,391]. Willems and colleagues [392] described an infant with echovirus 11 infection who had pneumonia, persistent pulmonary hypertension and purpura fulminans.

CLINICAL MANIFESTATIONS

In this section we present clinical manifestations by the specific viral agents and by serotypes of the specific viruses. Many infections with enteroviruses and parechoviruses are

---

*References 166,177,200,226,229,242.

*References 28,275,357,359–363,382,383.
†References 21,189,277,364,382,384–388.

now diagnosed by PCR, however, and serotype information is unavailable. Because of this, much of the specific information in this section was determined more than 2 decades ago. In recent years, phenotypic presentations have been altered by recombination between different enteroviruses, and clinical characteristics of specific enterovirus types today may be different from the findings identified 4 or 5 decades ago.

ABORTION
Polioviruses
Poliomyelitis is associated with an increased incidence of abortion. Horn [121] reported 43 abortions in 325 pregnancies complicated by maternal poliomyelitis. Abortion was directly related to the severity of the maternal illness, including the degree of fever during the acute phase of illness. Abortion also was associated with mild, nonparalytic poliomyelitis, however. Schaeffer and colleagues [136] studied the placenta and abortus 12 days after the onset of illness in a mother. Poliovirus type 1 was isolated from the placenta and the fetal tissues.

Other investigators [391,393–396] have reported an increased incidence of abortions in cases of maternal poliomyelitis. Siegel and Greenberg [140] noticed that fetal death occurred in 14 (46.7%) of 30 instances of maternal poliomyelitis during the first trimester. Kaye and colleagues [397] reviewed the literature in 1953 and found 19 abortions in 101 cases of poliomyelitis in pregnancy. In a small study in Evanston Hospital in Illinois, the abortion rate associated with maternal poliomyelitis was similar to the expected rate [395]. In a study of 310 pregnant women who received trivalent oral poliovirus vaccine, there was no increase in abortions beyond the expected rate [146]. In a later study in Finland that involved about 9000 pregnant women immunized with oral poliovirus vaccine, there was no evidence of an increase in stillbirths [398].

Coxsackieviruses
Although in the late 1950s and early 1960s there were extensive outbreaks of illness caused by coxsackievirus A16, there was no evidence of adverse outcomes of pregnancy related to this virus. Because infections with other coxsackieviruses rarely involve large segments of the population, rate studies have not been performed.

Frisk and Diderholm [399] found that 33% of women with abortions had IgM antibody to coxsackievirus B strains, whereas only 8% of controls had similar antibody. In a second, larger study, the same research group confirmed their original findings [400].

Echoviruses
There is no available evidence suggesting that echovirus infections during pregnancy are a cause of spontaneous abortion. Landsman and associates [184] studied 2631 pregnancies during an epidemic of echovirus 9 and could find no difference in antibody to echovirus 9 between mothers who aborted and mothers who delivered term infants. A similar study in Finland revealed no increase

in the abortion rate among mothers infected in early pregnancy with echovirus 9 [185].

CONGENITAL MALFORMATIONS
Polioviruses
In the Collaborative Perinatal Research Project sponsored by the National Institutes of Health comprising 45,000 pregnancies, the congenital malformation rate associated with poliovirus infection was 4.1% [401]. Although isolated instances of congenital malformation and maternal poliomyelitis have been reported, there is little statistical evidence showing that polioviruses are teratogens. In their review of the literature, Kaye and colleagues [397] identified six anomalies in 101 infants born to mothers with poliomyelitis during pregnancy. In the reviews of Horn [121], Bates [127], and Siegel and Greenberg [140] there was no evidence of anomalies induced by maternal poliovirus infection.

The possibility of congenital anomalies associated with attenuated oral poliovirus vaccine has also been studied [145,146,397,401–403]. Pearson and coworkers [145] studied the fetal malformation rate in a community in which a large vaccine field trial had been done; although it is probable that pregnant women became infected with vaccine virus by secondary spread, there was no community increase in fetal malformations. Prem and associates [146] studied the infants of 69 women who received attenuated vaccine before 20 weeks of gestation and found that none had anomalies. In contrast, the rate of congenital defects in Blackburn, England, increased coincident with mass vaccination with trivalent poliomyelitis vaccine [402]. There is no evidence of cause and effect related to this observation, however. Connelly and colleagues [403] commented on a child with a unique renal disease acquired in utero. The child's mother had received oral polio vaccine during the 2nd month of pregnancy.

In February 1985, a mass vaccination program with live oral poliovirus vaccine was carried out in Finland [404]. Although pregnant women received vaccine, there was no evidence that vaccine virus had a harmful effect on developing fetuses.

Coxsackieviruses
In large prospective studies, Brown [405–407] and others [408–410] made a serologic search for selected maternal enterovirus infections in association with congenital malformations. In one study, serum samples from 22,935 women had been collected [410]. From this group, serum samples from 630 mothers of infants with anomalies and from 1164 mothers of infants without defects were carefully studied. Specifically, serologic evidence was sought for infection during the first trimester and last 6 months of pregnancy with coxsackieviruses B1 through B5 and A9 and with echoviruses 6 and 9. In this study, infants were examined for 113 specific abnormalities; these anomalies were grouped into 12 categories for analysis.

The investigators showed a positive correlation between maternal infection and infant anomaly with coxsackieviruses B2 through B4 and A9. The overall first-trimester infection rate with coxsackievirus B4 was significantly higher in patients with anomalies than in controls. Maternal coxsackievirus B2 infection throughout pregnancy, coxsackievirus B4 infections during the first trimester of pregnancy, and infection with at least one of the five coxsackievirus B strains during pregnancy all were associated with urogenital anomalies. Coxsackievirus A9 infection was associated with digestive anomalies, and coxsackieviruses B3 and B4 were associated with cardiovascular defects. When coxsackievirus B strains were analyzed as a group (B1 to B5), there was an overall association with congenital heart disease; the likelihood of cardiovascular anomalies was increased when maternal infection with two or more coxsackievirus B strains occurred.

In this study, the mothers had been instructed to keep illness diary sheets. There was no correlation between reported maternal clinical illnesses and serologic evidence of infection with the selected enteroviruses. This lack of correlation suggests that many infections that may have been causally related to the anomalies were asymptomatic. A disturbing finding in this study was the lack of seasonal occurrence of the births of children with specific defects. Because enterovirus transmission is most common in the summer and fall, the birth rate of children with malformations should have been greatest in the spring and summer if coxsackieviruses were a major cause of malformation.

In the Collaborative Perinatal Research Project sponsored by the National Institutes of Health, Elizan and coworkers [411] were unable to find any relationships between maternal infections with coxsackievirus B strains and congenital CNS malformations. Scattered case reports in the literature describe congenital anomalies associated with maternal coxsackievirus infections. Makower and colleagues [176] reported a child with congenital malformations who was born at 32 weeks' gestation and from whom a coxsackievirus A4 strain was recovered from the meconium. The child's mother had been well throughout pregnancy except for a febrile illness during the 1st month. The relationship of the viral infection to the congenital malformations or to the prematurity is uncertain.

Gauntt and associates [412] studied ventricular fluids from 28 newborn infants with severe congenital anatomic defects of the CNS. In four infants (two with hydranencephaly, one with an occipital meningocele, and one with aqueductal stenosis), neutralizing antibody to one or more coxsackievirus B types was found in the fluid. In one case, IgM-neutralizing antibody to coxsackievirus B6 was found. The investigators concluded that their data suggested the possibility of an association between congenital infections with coxsackievirus B strains and severe CNS defects.

Echoviruses

In the large prospective study of Brown and Karunas [410], the possible association of maternal infections with echoviruses 6 and 9 and congenital malformations was examined. Maternal infection with these selected echoviruses apparently was not associated with any anomaly.

In three other studies [183–185], no association was found between maternal echovirus 9 infection and congenital malformation.

PREMATURITY AND STILLBIRTH
Polioviruses

In the study by Horn [121] of 325 pregnancies, nine infants died in utero. In each instance, the mother was critically ill with poliomyelitis. Horn [121] also observed that 45 infants weighed less than 6 lb, and 17 of these had a birth weight of less than 5 lb. These low birth weight infants were born predominantly to mothers who had had poliomyelitis early in pregnancy. Aycock [124,413] reported a similar finding. In New York City, Siegel and Greenberg [140] also documented an increase in prematurity after maternal poliomyelitis infection. This increase was specifically related to maternal paralytic poliomyelitis. There has been no observation of stillbirth or prematurity in relation to vaccine administration [398].

Coxsackieviruses

Bates [171] reported a fetus of 8 months' gestational age who was stillborn and had calcific pancarditis and hydrops fetalis at autopsy. Fluorescent antibody study revealed coxsackievirus B3 antigen in the myocardium. Burch and colleagues [179] described three stillborn infants who had fluorescent antibody evidence of coxsackievirus B myocarditis, one each with coxsackieviruses B2, B3, or B4. They also reported a premature boy who had histologic and immunofluorescent evidence of cardiac infection with coxsackieviruses B2 through B4; he lived only 24 hours. A macerated stillborn girl was delivered 2 weeks after the occurrence of aseptic meningitis caused by coxsackievirus A9 in a 27-year-old woman [333]. Virus was recovered from the placenta, but not from the infant. Coxsackievirus B6 has been recovered from the brain, liver, and placenta of a stillborn infant [170]. An infant of 26 weeks' gestation with nonimmune hydrops fetalis with an intrauterine infection with coxsackievirus B3 was reported by Ouellet and coworkers [414].

Echoviruses and Enteroviruses

Freedman [415] reported the occurrence of a full-term, fresh stillbirth in a woman infected with echovirus 11. Because the infant had no pathologic or virologic evidence of infection, the stillbirth was attributed to a secondary consequence of maternal infection from fever and dehydration, rather than primary transplacental infection. Echovirus 27 has been associated with intrauterine death on two occasions [170,416].

In an extensive study of neonatal enterovirus infections in Milwaukee in 1979, Piraino and associates [383] found that 12 of 19 stillbirths occurred from July through October coincident with a major outbreak of enterovirus disease. Echovirus 11 was the main agent isolated during this period. A 1300-g fetus, stillborn after 26 weeks' gestation, had hydrocephalus, fibrotic peritonitis, and hepatosplenomegaly and was found to have enterovirus 71 infection by PCR and immunohistochemical study [190].

NEONATAL INFECTION
Nonpolio Enteroviruses and Parechoviruses

Illnesses caused by nonpolio enteroviruses and parechoviruses are discussed by clinical classification (Table 24–5) in the following sections.

Inapparent Infection

Although it is probable that inapparent infections in neonates occasionally occur with many different enteroviruses, and parechoviruses, there is little documentation of this assumption. Cherry and coworkers [174] studied 590 normal newborns during a 6-month period and found only one infection without clinical signs of illness. This was a child infected in utero or immediately thereafter with coxsackievirus B2. The mother had an upper respiratory illness 10 days before delivery. In a similar but more comprehensive study, Jenista and associates [201] failed to isolate any enteroviruses from cultures from 666 newborns on the 1st postpartum day. During weekly cultures during the month after birth, 75 enteroviruses were isolated, however. Symptomatic enterovirus disease occurred in 21% (16 of 75).

During a survey of perinatal virus infections, 44 infants were found to be infected with parechovirus 1 during the study period May to December 1966 [270]. The virus prevalence and the incidence of new infections during this period were fairly uniform. No illness was attributed to parechovirus 1 infection, and the virus disappeared from the nursery in mid-December 1966. Inapparent infections with parechovirus 1 have been reported on two other occasions [259,280]. Infections without evidence of illness have occurred with coxsackieviruses A9, B1, B4, and B5 and with echoviruses 3, 5, 9, 11, 13, 14, 20, 30, and 31.*

Mild, Nonspecific Febrile Illness

In a review of 338 enterovirus infections in early infancy, 9% were classified as nonspecific febrile illnesses [420]. Illness may be sporadic in nature or part of an outbreak with a specific viral type. In the latter situation, clinical manifestations vary depending on the viral type; some infants have aseptic meningitis and other signs and symptoms, and some have only nonspecific fever. Viral types most commonly found in nonspecific fevers were coxsackievirus B5 and echoviruses 5, 11, and 33; other agents identified have included coxsackieviruses A9, A16, and B1 through B4 and echoviruses 4, 7, 9, and 17.† A 6-day-old infant with parechovirus 4 and fever and poor feeding has been described [424].

Mild, nonspecific febrile illness occurs most commonly in full-term infants after uneventful pregnancies and deliveries without complications. Illness can occur at any time during the 1st month of life. When the onset occurs after the infant is 7 days old, a careful history frequently reveals a trivial illness in a family member. The onset of illness is characterized by mild irritability and fever

(usually 38° C to 39° C, but higher temperatures occasionally occur). Poor feeding is frequently observed. One or two episodes of vomiting or diarrhea or both may occur in some infants. The usual duration of illness is 2 to 4 days.

Routine laboratory study is not helpful, but cerebrospinal fluid (CSF) examination may reveal an increased protein concentration and leukocyte count indicative of aseptic meningitis. Although illness in this category is mild by definition, the degree of viral infection may be extensive. When looked for, virus may be isolated from the blood, urine, and CSF of infants with mild illnesses [234,417].

Sepsis-like Illness

The major diagnostic problem in neonatal enterovirus infections is differentiation of bacterial from viral disease. Even in an infant with mild, nonspecific fever, bacterial disease must be strongly considered. The sepsis-like illness described here is always alarming. This illness is characterized by fever, poor feeding, abdominal distention, irritability, rash, lethargy, and hypotonia [339, 381–383]. Other findings include diarrhea, vomiting, seizures, shock, disseminated intravascular coagulation, thrombocytopenia, hepatomegaly, jaundice, and apnea. The onset of illness is heralded by irritability, poor feeding, and fever; other manifestations follow within 24 hours. In a group of 27 neonates, Lake and associates [427] observed that 54% had temperatures of 39° C or greater. The duration of fever varies from 1 to 8 days (most commonly 3 to 4 days). Barre and colleagues [426] reported a 3-day-old boy with an enterovirus-associated hemophagocytic syndrome. This neonate presented with a typical sepsis-like picture with fever, hepatosplenomegaly, coagulopathy, thrombocytopenia, and anemia. The child recovered and had no hemophagocytic relapses.

Sepsis-like illness is common. Morens [420] described its occurrence in one fifth of 338 enterovirus infections in infants. In an attempt to differentiate bacterial from viral disease, Lake and associates [427] studied 27 infants with enterovirus infections. White blood cell counts were not helpful because the total count, the number of neutrophils, and the number of band form neutrophils were elevated in most instances. Historical data were most important. Most mothers had evidence of a recent febrile, viral-like illness. Other factors often associated with bacterial sepsis, such as prolonged rupture of membranes, prematurity, and low Apgar scores, were unusual in the enterovirus infection group.

Sepsis-like illness has been identified most often with coxsackieviruses B2 through B5; echovirus types 5, 11, and 16; and parechovirus 3. Other viruses detected include coxsackieviruses A9 and B1; echoviruses 2, 3, 4, 6, 9, 14, 19, and 21; and parechovirus 1.* Since the early 1980s, echovirus 11 has been associated most frequently with fatal septic events, hepatic necrosis, and disseminated intravascular coagulation.†

---

*References 113,186,187,201,233,274,279,415,417–420.

†References 25,174,218,234,241,247,250,258,262,266,267,271,276,279,383,417, 421–425.

---

*References 25,27,28,34,35,169,195,240,257,261,262,265,275,279,283,357–359, 361,364,381–383,385–387,389,390,427–442.

†References 28,195,275,357–361,363,383,443.

TABLE 24–5   Major Manifestations of Neonatal Nonpolio Enterovirus and Parechovirus Infections

Specific Involvement	Common	Rare
Inapparent infection	Parechovirus 1	Coxsackievirus A9, B1, B2, B4, B5
		Echovirus 3, 5, 9, 11, 13, 14, 20, 30, 31
Mild, nonspecific, febrile illness	Coxsackievirus B5	Coxsackievirus B1, B2, B3, B4, A9, A16
	Echovirus 5, 11, 33	Echovirus 4, 7, 9, 17
Sepsis-like illness	Coxsackievirus B2, B3, B4, B5	Coxsackievirus B1, A9
	Echovirus 5, 11, 15	Echovirus 2, 3, 4, 6, 9, 14, 19, 21
		Parechovirus 1, 3
Respiratory illness (general)	Echovirus 11	Coxsackievirus B1, B4, B5, A9
	Parechovirus 1	Echovirus 9, 17
Herpangina		Coxsackievirus A5
Coryza		Coxsackievirus A9
		Echovirus 11, 17, 19
		Parechovirus 1
Pharyngitis		Coxsackievirus B4
		Echovirus 11, 17, 18
Laryngotracheitis or bronchitis		Coxsackievirus B1, B4
		Echovirus 11
Pneumonia		Coxsackievirus B4, A9
		Echovirus 6, 9, 11, 17, 31
		Parechovirus 1
Cloud baby		Echovirus 20
Gastrointestinal		
Vomiting or diarrhea	Echovirus 5, 17, 18	Coxsackievirus B1, B2, B5
		Echovirus 4, 6, 8, 9, 11, 16, 19, 21
		Parechovirus 1
		Enterovirus 71
Hepatitis	Echovirus 11, 19	Coxsackievirus B1, B3, B4, A9
		Echovirus 5, 6, 7, 9, 14, 20, 21
Pancreatitis		Coxsackievirus B3, B4, B5
Necrotizing enterocolitis		Coxsackievirus B2, B3
		Parechovirus 1
Cardiovascular		
Myocarditis and pericarditis	Coxsackievirus B1, B2, B3, B4	Coxsackievirus B5, A9
		Echovirus 11, 19
Skin	Coxsackievirus B5	Coxsackievirus B1
	Echovirus 5, 17	Echovirus 4, 7, 9, 11, 18
	Parechovirus 1	Enterovirus 71
Neurologic		
Aseptic meningitis	Coxsackievirus B2, B3, B4, B5	Coxsackievirus B1, A9, A14
	Echovirus 3, 9, 11, 17	Echovirus 1, 5, 13, 14, 21, 30
		Enterovirus 71
		Parechovirus 3
Encephalitis	Coxsackievirus B1, B2, B3, B4	Coxsackievirus B5
		Echovirus 6, 9, 23
		Parechovirus 2, 3
		Enterovirus 71
Paralysis		Coxsackievirus B2
Sudden infant death		Coxsackievirus B1, B3, B4, A4, A5, A8
		Parechovirus 1

Data from Cherry JD, Krogstad P. Enteroviruses and parechoviruses. In Feigin RD, et al (eds). Textbook of Pediatric Infectious Diseases, 6th ed. Philadelphia, Saunders, 2009.

Respiratory Illness

Respiratory complaints are generally overshadowed by other manifestations of neonatal disease caused by enteroviruses and parechoviruses. Only 7% of 338 enterovirus infections in early infancy were classified as respiratory illness [420]. Respiratory illness associated with enteroviruses has been sporadic except for illnesses associated with echovirus 11 and parechovirus 1 [259,269].

Hercík and coworkers [269] reported an epidemic of respiratory illness in 22 newborns associated with echovirus 11 infection. All of these infants had rhinitis and pharyngitis, 50% had laryngitis, and 32% had interstitial pneumonitis. Berkovich and Pangan [259] studied respiratory illnesses in premature infants and reported 64 with illness, 18 of whom had virologic or serologic evidence of parechovirus 1 infection. Many other infants had high but constant levels of serum antibody to parechovirus 1. The infants with proven parechovirus 1 infections could not be clinically differentiated from infants without evidence of parechovirus 1 infection. Of the infants, 90% had coryza, and 39% had radiographic evidence of pneumonia. Respiratory tract symptoms were noted in about half of the neonates in two parechovirus studies in the Netherlands [429,444].

Herpangina

Chawareewong and associates [445] described several infants with herpangina and coxsackievirus A5 infection. A vesicular lesion on an erythematous base on a tonsillar pillar in a 6-day-old infant with coxsackievirus B2 meningitis has also been reported [446]. Two 1-month-old infants were described in an outbreak of herpangina owing to coxsackievirus B3 in a welfare home in Japan [447].

Coryza

Several agents have been associated with coryza: coxsackievirus A9; echoviruses 11, 17, and 19; and parechoviruses 1 and 3 [188,269,280,283,426].

Pharyngitis

Pharyngitis is uncommon in neonatal enterovirus infections. In more than 50 infants with enterovirus infections studied by Linnemann and colleagues [437] and Lake and associates [427], pharyngitis did not occur. Suzuki and coworkers [448] observed pharyngitis in 3 of 42 neonates with echovirus 11 infections. In contrast, in the same study, 67% of children 1 month to 4 years old had pharyngitis. Pharyngitis has been associated with coxsackievirus B4 and with echoviruses 11, 17, and 18 [247,269,273,434,438].

Laryngotracheobronchitis or Bronchitis

A few enteroviruses have been identified in cases of laryngotracheobronchitis or bronchitis: coxsackieviruses B1 and B4 and echovirus 11 [269,449]. Specific clinical descriptions of laryngotracheobronchitis or bronchitis associated with enterovirus infections are scarce. Hercík and coworkers [269] observed laryngitis in 11 and croup in 4 of 22 neonates during an echovirus 11 outbreak. All

of the affected infants had upper respiratory tract findings, vomiting, and lethargy. Many were also cyanotic and had hepatosplenomegaly.

Pneumonia

Pneumonia as the main manifestation of neonatal enterovirus and parechovirus infections is rare. Morens [420] documented only seven instances of pneumonia in 338 neonatal enterovirus infections. Outbreaks of pneumonia in neonates have been reported with echovirus 11 and parechovirus 1 [259,269]. Pneumonia resulting from other enteroviruses is a sporadic event and has been reported for the following nonpolio enteroviruses: coxsackieviruses A9 and B4 and echoviruses 9, 17, and 31.

During a nursery outbreak of echovirus 11, 7 of 22 neonates had pneumonia [269]. All infants had signs of upper respiratory infection and general signs of sepsis-like illness. In infants with pneumonia associated with a nursery epidemic of parechovirus 1, coryza, cough, and dyspnea were early signs [259]. The illnesses tended to be protracted, with radiographic changes persisting for 10 to 100 days.

Cloud Baby

Eichenwald and associates [264] recovered echovirus 20 from four full-term infants younger than 8 days. Although these infants apparently were well, it was found that they were extensively colonized with staphylococci and that they disseminated these organisms into the air around them. Because of this ability to disseminate staphylococci, they were called "cloud babies." The investigators believed that these cloud babies contributed to the epidemic spread of staphylococci in the nursery. Because active staphylococcal dissemination occurred only during the time that echovirus 20 could be recovered from the nasopharynx, it was theorized that viral-bacterial synergism occurred.

Gastrointestinal Manifestations

Vomiting or Diarrhea

Vomiting and diarrhea are common but usually just part of the overall illness complex and not major manifestations. In 1958, Eichenwald and colleagues [263] described epidemic diarrhea associated with echovirus 18 infections.

In 22 infants with epidemic respiratory disease caused by echovirus 11, all had vomiting as a manifestation of the illness [269]. Linnemann and colleagues [437] reported vomiting in 36% and diarrhea in 7% of neonates with echovirus infections. In another study, Lake and associates [427] found diarrhea in 81% and vomiting in 33% of neonates with nonpolio enterovirus infections. Vomiting and diarrhea in neonates have been associated with coxsackieviruses B1, B2, and B5; echoviruses 4 through 6, 8, 9, 11, 16 through 19, and 21; parechoviruses 1 and 3; and enterovirus 71.*

---

*References 187,234,240,257,258,263,265,266,269,276,283,436,437,450–452.

Hepatitis

Morens [420] observed that 2% of neonates with clinically severe enterovirus disease had hepatitis. Lake and associates [427] found that 37% of neonates with enterovirus infections had hepatomegaly, and hepatosplenomegaly was observed by Hercík and coworkers [269] in 12 of 22 newborns with echovirus 11 respiratory illnesses.

Severe hepatitis, frequently with hepatic necrosis, has been associated with echoviruses 5, 6, 7, 9, 11, 14, 19, 20, 21, and 30.* In 1980, Modlin [277] reported four fatal echovirus 11 illnesses in premature infants. All had hepatitis, disseminated intravascular coagulation, thrombocytopenia, lethargy, poor feeding, and jaundice. Since 1980, there have been many reports of sepsis-like illness with fatal hepatitis related to echovirus 11.[†] Coxsackieviruses B1, B3, and B4 and other B types have been associated with neonatal hepatitis.[‡] Abzug [455] reviewed medical records of 16 neonates with hepatitis and coagulopathy and found a case-fatality rate of 31%. All of the five patients who died had myocarditis, and three had encephalitis. Although sepsis-like illness frequently occurs in infections with parechovirus, hepatitis is relatively uncommon [34,35,424].

Pancreatitis

Pancreatitis was recognized in three of four newborns with coxsackievirus B5 meningitis [238] and in coxsackieviruses B3 and B4 infections at autopsy [254]. In other fatal coxsackievirus B infections, pancreatic involvement has been identified, but clinical manifestations have rarely been observed.

Necrotizing Enterocolitis

Lake and associates [427] described three infants with necrotizing enterocolitis. Coxsackievirus B3 was recovered from two of these infants, and coxsackievirus B2 was recovered from the third. Parechovirus 1 was associated with an outbreak of necrotizing enterocolitis [456].

Cardiovascular Manifestations

In contrast with enterovirus cardiac disease in children and adults, in which pericarditis is common, neonatal disease virtually always involves the heart muscle.[§] Most cases of neonatal myocarditis are related to coxsackievirus B infections, and nursery outbreaks have occurred on several occasions. In 1961, Kibrick [26] reviewed the clinical findings in 45 cases of neonatal myocarditis; his findings are summarized in Table 24–6. Many early experiences, particularly in South Africa, involved catastrophic nursery epidemics. Since the observation in 1972 of five newborns with echovirus 11 infections and myocarditis, there have been no further reports of nursery epidemics [459].

---

*References 189,282,360,361,363,364,382,384,386,388,435,441.

[†]References 28,275,357,358,360,361,383,387.

[‡]References 7,25,230,256,445,446,453,454.

[§]References 7,10,25,27,34,35,166,171,172,177,179,216,217,220,223,224,226, 228–230,233,237,241,242,245,246,248–253,255,358,359,361,383,429,435,441, 453,454,457–464.

TABLE 24–6   Findings in Neonatal Coxsackievirus B Myocarditis

Finding	Frequency (%)
Feeding difficulty	84
Listlessness	81
Cardiac signs	81
Respiratory distress	75
Cyanosis	72
Fever	70
Pharyngitis	64
Hepatosplenomegaly	53
Biphasic course	35
Central nervous system signs	27
Hemorrhage	13
Jaundice	13
Diarrhea	8

Modified from Kibrick S. Viral infections of the fetus and newborn. Perspect Virol 2:140, 1961.

The illness as described by Kibrick [26] most commonly had an abrupt onset and was characterized by listlessness, anorexia, and fever. A biphasic pattern was observed in about one third of the patients. Progression was rapid, and signs of circulatory failure appeared within 2 days. If death did not occur, recovery was occasionally rapid, but usually occurred gradually during an extended period. Most patients had cardiac findings, such as tachycardia, cardiomegaly, electrocardiogram (ECG) changes, and transitory systolic murmurs. Many patients showed signs of respiratory distress and cyanosis. About one third of infants had signs suggesting neurologic involvement. Of the 45 patients analyzed by Kibrick [26], only 12 survived.

In the nursery outbreak of echovirus 11 reported by Drew [460], 5 of 10 infants had tachycardia out of proportion to fevers. Three of these infants had ECGs; supraventricular tachycardia occurred in all, and ST segment depression was observed in two. Supraventricular tachycardia has also been seen in patients with coxsackievirus B infections [233]. Echovirus 19 has been associated with myocarditis [465].

Until more recently, neonatal myocarditis related to enteroviruses was less common than it was 5 decades ago. In his review in 1978, Morens [420] reported only two instances among 248 severe neonatal enterovirus illnesses. In 2007, severe neonatal disease associated with coxsackievirus B1 infection was noted in several areas of the United States [315]. In Los Angeles County, California, 12 neonates had myocarditis. Similarly, in Chicago, Illinois, 11 neonates ranging in age from less than 1 to 12 days had myocarditis. Other cases with coxsackievirus B1 myocarditis occurred in Alaska and Colorado.

Exanthem

Exanthem as a manifestation of neonatal infections with enteroviruses and parechoviruses has occurred with coxsackieviruses B1, B3, and B5; echoviruses 4, 5, 7, 9, 11,

16, 17, 18, and 21; and parechoviruses 1 and 3.* In most instances, rash is just a minor manifestation of moderate to severe neonatal disease. Of 27 infants studied by Lake and associates [427], 41% had exanthem. Similarly, Linnemann and colleagues [437] reported exanthem in 4 of 14 neonates with echovirus infections.

Cutaneous manifestations usually occur between the 3rd and 5th days of illness. The rash is usually macular or maculopapular, and petechial lesions occasionally are seen. Vesicular lesions have been reported only once with coxsackievirus B3 infection and once with enterovirus 71 infection in neonates. Theodoridou and associates [470] described a full-term newborn boy with vesicular lesions at birth. PCR revealed coxsackievirus B3. A 1-month-old infant with enterovirus 71 infection and hand-foot-and-mouth syndrome has been reported [471]. Hall and associates [436] reported two neonates with echovirus 16 infections in which the illnesses were similar to roseola. The patients had fevers for 2 and 3 days, defervescence, and then the appearance of maculopapular rashes.

Neurologic Manifestations
Meningitis and Meningoencephalitis
As shown in Table 24–5, meningitis and meningoencephalitis have been associated with coxsackieviruses B1 through B5, many echoviruses, and parechoviruses.† In most instances, the differentiation of meningitis from meningoencephalitis is difficult in neonates. Meningoencephalitis is common in infants with sepsis-like illness, and autopsy studies reveal many infants with disseminated viral disease (e.g., heart, liver, adrenals) in addition to CNS involvement. In the review of Morens [420], 50% of the neonates with enterovirus infections had encephalitis or meningitis.

The initial clinical findings in neonatal meningitis or meningoencephalitis are similar to findings in nonspecific febrile illness or sepsis-like illness. Most often, the child is normal and then becomes febrile, anorectic, and lethargic. Jaundice frequently affects newborns, and vomiting occurs in neonates of all ages. Less common findings include apnea, tremulousness, and general increased tonicity. Seizures occasionally occur.

CSF examination reveals considerable variation in protein, glucose, and cellular values. In seven newborns with meningitis related to coxsackievirus B5 studied by Swender and associates [257], the mean CSF protein value was 244 mg/dL, and the highest value was 480 mg/dL. The mean CSF glucose value was 57 mg/dL, and one of the seven newborns had pronounced hypoglycorrhachia (12 mg/dL). The mean CSF leukocyte count for the seven infants was 1069 cells/mm^3, with 67% polymorphonuclear cells. The highest cell count was 4526 cells/mm^3, with 85% polymorphonuclear cells. In another study involving 28 children younger than 2 months in whom coxsackievirus B5 was the implicated pathogen,

36% of the infants had CSF leukocyte counts of 500 cells/mm^3 or greater [438]. In this same study, only 13% of the infants had CSF protein values of 120 mg/dL or greater; 12% of the infants had glucose values of less than 40 mg/dL.

The CSF findings in cases of neonatal nonpolio enterovirus and parechovirus infections are frequently similar to CSF findings in bacterial disease. In particular, the most consistent finding in bacterial disease, hypoglycorrhachia, affects about 10% of newborns with enterovirus meningitis [257,418,450,452,493].

Paralysis
Johnson and associates [484] reported a 1-month-old boy with right facial paralysis and loss of abdominal reflexes. The facial paralysis persisted through convalescence; the reflexes returned to normal within 2 weeks. The boy was infected with coxsackievirus B2. A 1-month-old boy with hand-foot-and-mouth syndrome and bilateral lower limb weakness owing to enterovirus 71 infection has been described [471].

Sudden Infant Death
Balduzzi and Greendyke [379] recovered coxsackievirus A5 from the stool of a 1-month-old infant after sudden infant death. In a similar investigation of sudden infant death, Gold and coworkers [380] recovered coxsackievirus A4 from the brains of three infants. Coxsackievirus A8 was recovered from the stool of a child in whom anorexia was diagnosed on the day before death. Coxsackievirus B3 was recovered at autopsy from an infant who died suddenly on the 8th day of life [379]. Morens and associates [10] reported eight cases of sudden infant death associated with enterovirus infection; parechovirus 1 was found on two occasions. In five instances of cot death in one study, echovirus 11 was isolated from the lungs in two infants, from the myocardium in one, and from the nose or feces in the other two [357].

Grangeot-Keros and coworkers [494] looked for evidence of enterovirus infections using PCR and an IgM immunoassay in cases of sudden and unexplained infant deaths. They divided their infant death population into two groups. One group had clinical, biologic, or histologic signs of viral infection, and the other group had no indicators of an antecedent infection. Of infants with evidence of a preceding infection, 54% had PCR evidence of an enterovirus in samples from the respiratory tract or lung or both, whereas none of the infants without evidence of a prior infection had similar positive PCR findings. Their IgM antibody studies supported their PCR findings.

Manifestations of Polioviruses
General Considerations
Infection with poliovirus in children classically results in a spectrum of clinical illness. As described by Paul [495] and accepted by others, 90% to 95% of infections in children after the neonatal period are inapparent, 4% to 8% are abortive, and 1% to 2% are frank cases of poliomyelitis. Whether neonatal poliovirus infection is acquired in

---

*References 25,27,34,35,177,188,219,221,243,261,266,276,283,356,383,390,430, 435–437,459,465–470.

†References 25,27,28,34,35,179,187,224,243,258,261,265,275,276,284,315,321, 361,366,381, 383,418,419,429,438,440,446,450,451,453,456,458,459,466,468, 471–491.

utero, during birth, or after birth, the more severe manifestations of clinical illness seem to be similar to those of older children. Available reports in the literature suggest, however, that the frequencies of occurrence of inapparent, abortive, and frank cases are quite different from older children. Most reports describe severely affected infants [123,125–137,139–141,143,144]. Asymptomatic infection does occur, however [124,138].

In the excellent review by Bates [127] in 1955, 58 cases of clinically overt poliomyelitis in infants younger than 1 month were described. Although complete data were unavailable on many of the cases, 51 had paralysis or died from their disease, or both. Of the total number of infants for whom there were clinical data, only one had nonparalytic disease. Because follow-up observation was recorded for only a short time in many infants, the evaluation of residual paralysis (presence or absence) may be unreliable. Pertinent clinical data from the study by Bates are presented in Table 24–7; these data show that more than half of the cases resulted from maternal disease. Because others have identified congenital infection without symptomatic maternal infection, it is probable that infection in the mothers was the source for an even greater percentage of the neonatal illnesses. Because the incubation period of neonatal poliomyelitis has not been determined, it is difficult to know how many infants were infected in utero. Most illnesses occurring within the first 5 days of life probably were congenital. Most neonates had symptoms of fever, anorexia or dysphagia, and listlessness. Almost half of the infants described in this review died, and of those surviving, 48% had residual paralysis.

TABLE 24–7   Clinical Findings in 58 Cases of Neonatal Poliomyelitis

Finding	No. Cases with Particular Finding/ No. Cases Evaluated (%)
Time of Onset after Birth	
≤5 days	13/55 (24)
6-14 days	25/55 (45)
≥15 days	17/55 (31)
Infection Source for Symptomatic Illness	
Mother	22/42 (52)
Other contact	6/42 (14)
Unknown	14/42 (34)
Acute Illness	
Fever	17/29 (59)
Anorexia or dysphagia	16/24 (67)
Listlessness	24/33 (73)
Irritability	3/33 (9)
Diarrhea	2/11 (18)
Paralysis	43/44 (98)
Outcome	
Death	21/44 (48)
Residual paralysis	12/44 (27)
Recovery without paralysis	11/44 (25)

Adapted from Bates T. Poliomyelitis in pregnancy, fetus, and newborn. Am J Dis Child 90:189, 1955.

Inapparent Infection

Shelokov and Habel [138] followed a virologically proven infected newborn without signs of illness. The infant was normal when 1 year old. Wingate and coworkers [142] studied an infant delivered by cesarean section from a woman with poliomyelitis who died 1 hour after delivery. Her infant was treated with gamma globulin intramuscularly at the postnatal age of 21 hours. The infant boy remained asymptomatic; poliovirus 1 was recovered from a stool specimen on the 5th day of life.

Infection Acquired In Utero

Elliott and colleagues [130] described an infant girl in whom "complete flaccidity" was observed at birth. The infant's mother had had mild paralytic poliomyelitis, with the onset of minor illness occurring 19 days before the infant's birth. Fetal movements had ceased 6 days before delivery, suggesting that paralysis had occurred at this time. On examination, the infant was severely atonic; when supported under the back, she was passively opisthotonic. Respiratory efforts were abortive and confined to accessory muscles, and laryngoscopy revealed complete flaccidity in the larynx.

Johnson and Stimson [132] reported a case in which the mother's probable abortive infection occurred 6 weeks before the birth of the infant. The newborn was initially thought to be normal, but apparently had no medical examination until the 4th day of life. At that time, the physician diagnosed a right hemiplegia. The next day, a more complete examination revealed lateral bulging of the right abdomen accompanied by crying and the maintenance of the lower extremities in a frog-leg position. Adduction and flexion at the hips were weak, and knee and ankle jerks were absent. Laboratory studies were unremarkable except for the examination of the CSF, which revealed 20 lymphocytes/mm^3 and a protein concentration of 169 mg/dL. During a 6-month period, the child's paralysis gradually improved and resulted in only residual weakness of the left lower extremity.

Paresis of the left arm occurred in another child with apparent transplacentally acquired poliomyelitis shortly after birth [135]. The 2-day-old infant was quadriplegic, but patellar reflexes were present, and there were no respiratory or swallowing difficulties. This child had pneumonia when 3 weeks old, but general neurologic improvement occurred. Examination when the infant was 8 weeks old revealed bilateral atrophy of the shoulder girdle muscles. The CSF in this case revealed 63 leukocytes/mm^3, with 29% polymorphonuclear cells, and a protein value of 128 mg/dL. All three of the above-described infants were apparently infected in utero several days before birth. Their symptoms were exclusively neurologic; fever, irritability, and vomiting did not occur.

Postnatally Acquired Infection

In contrast to infections acquired in utero, infections that are acquired postnatally are more typical of classic poliomyelitis. Shelokov and Weinstein [139] described an infant who was asymptomatic at birth. Onset of minor symptoms in the mother occurred 3 weeks before delivery, and major symptoms occurred 1 day before delivery. On the 6th day of life, the infant became suddenly ill with watery diarrhea. He looked grayish and pale. The next day, he was irritable, lethargic, and limp and had a temperature of 38° C. Mild opisthotonos and weakness of both lower extremities developed. He was responsive to sound, light, and touch. The CSF had an elevated protein level and an increased number of leukocytes. His condition worsened over 3 days, and then gradual improvement began. At 1 year, he had severe residual paralysis of the right leg and moderate weakness in the left leg.

Baskin and associates [126] described two infants with neonatal poliomyelitis. The first infant, whose mother had severe poliomyelitis at the time of delivery, was well for 3 days and then developed a temperature of 38.3° C. On the 5th day of life, the boy became listless and cyanotic. CSF examination revealed a protein level of 300 mg/dL and 108 leukocytes/mm³. His condition worsened, and extreme flaccidity, irregular respiration, and progressive cyanosis developed; he died on the 7th day of life. The second infant was a boy who was well until he was 8 days old; he then became listless and developed a temperature of 38.3° C. During the next 5 days, he developed flaccid quadriplegia; irregular, rapid, and shallow respirations; and an inability to swallow. He died on the 14th day of life. His mother had developed acute poliomyelitis 6 days before the onset of his symptoms.

Abramson and colleagues [123] reported four children with neonatal poliomyelitis, two of whom died. In three of the children, the illnesses were typical of acute poliomyelitis seen in older children; they were similar to the cases of Baskin and associates [126] described previously. The fourth child died at 13 days of age with generalized paralysis. The onset of his illness was difficult to define, and he was never febrile. Swarts and Kercher [141] also described an infant whose illness had an insidious onset. When 10 days old, the infant gradually became lethargic and anorectic and regurgitated formula through his nose. On the next day, flaccid quadriplegia developed. Winsser and associates [143] and Bates [127] reported infants with acute poliomyelitis with clinical illnesses similar to illnesses that occur in older individuals.

Vaccine Viral Infections

Oral polio vaccines have been administered to newborns in numerous studies [146,202–214]. Vaccine viral infection occurs in newborns with all three types of poliovirus, although the rate of infection is less than for immunized older children. This rate is governed by the dose of virus, transplacentally acquired maternal antibody, and antibody acquired from colostrum and breast milk. Although clinical illness rarely has resulted from attenuated poliovirus in older children and adults, there is only one specific report of paralytic poliomyelitis in a newborn associated with infection with a vaccine viral strain [215]. In that case, the possible source for the infection was the recently vaccinated child of the babysitter. In a review of 118 cases of vaccine-associated paralytic poliomyelitis in the United States from 1980–1992, the age of patients ranged from 1 month to 69 years, but details about neonates were not presented [496].

Manifestations of Specific Nonpolio Enteroviruses
Coxsackieviruses
Coxsackievirus A

There have been few reports of neonatal coxsackievirus A infections. Baker and Phillips [378] reported an infant small for gestational age with pneumonia and a sepsis-like illness with disseminated intravascular coagulation. This newborn died on the 2nd day of life, and culture of CSF grew coxsackievirus A3. Balduzzi and Greendyke [379] recovered coxsackievirus A5 from the stool of a 1-month-old infant with sudden infant death. In a similar investigation of sudden infant death, Gold and coworkers [380] recovered coxsackievirus A4 from the brains of three infants. Coxsackievirus A8 was also recovered from the stool of a child in whom anorexia was observed on the day before death. Berkovich and Kibrick [258] reported a 3-day-old neonate with nonspecific febrile illness (38.3° C) who was infected with coxsackievirus A9. Coxsackievirus A9 was also recovered from an 11-day-old infant with rhinitis, lethargy, anorexia, and fever [283]. This illness lasted 3 days. Jack and associates [270] described a 3-day-old newborn with fever, cyanosis, and respiratory distress who died on the 7th day of life; an autopsy revealed bronchopneumonia. Coxsackievirus A9 was isolated from the feces on the 4th and 6th days of life.

Lake and associates [427] reported two neonates with coxsackievirus A9 infections, but no clinical details were presented. Jenista and coworkers [201] recovered coxsackievirus A9 strains from seven nonhospitalized neonates who were thought to be well. In the Netherlands, a neonate with coxsackievirus A9 illness had pericarditis, meningitis, pneumonitis, and hepatitis; he recovered completely [464]. Krajden and Middleton [27] described a neonate with a sepsis-like illness who died. Coxsackievirus A9 was recovered from the liver and lung. Morens [420] also reported a death associated with this same virus type. Eisenhut and associates [381] reported an outbreak that included four neonates with coxsackievirus A9 infections. One infant who had meningitis, myocarditis, and disseminated intravascular coagulation died. A second neonate had vomiting, rhinitis, and abdominal distention, and two neonates had asymptomatic infections.

Of 598 neonates admitted to a regular nursery in Bangkok, Thailand, in spring 1977, 48 had herpangina [381]. Coxsackievirus A5 was isolated from nine specimens from the affected infants, and an increase in the serum antibody titer was identified in 10 instances. Helin and colleagues [483] described 16 newborns with aseptic meningitis caused by coxsackievirus A14. During a 2.5-year follow-up period, they all developed normally, and no sequelae were identified. Coxsackievirus A16 was recovered from one newborn with nonspecific illness; his mother had had hand-foot-and-mouth syndrome 4 days previously [483].

Coxsackievirus B1

Until more recently, coxsackievirus B1 was only occasionally recovered from newborns (Table 24–8). Eckert and coworkers [449] recovered a coxsackievirus B1 strain from the stool of a 1-month-old boy with bronchitis. Jahn and

TABLE 24–8 Clinical and Pathologic Findings in Coxsackievirus B Infection of Newborns

Finding	References for Coxsackievirus				
	B1	**B2**	**B3**	**B4**	**B5**
Exanthem	221,435		172		177,219,243,477
Nonspecific febrile illness		178	250	241,247	421
Sepsis-like illness	25,232,245,435, 441,453	25	27,232	358,378	25
Paralysis	441	484			
Diarrhea		452			
Sudden infant death	494		379,494	494	
Pneumothorax					270
Aseptic meningitis, meningoencephalitis, encephalomyelitis	234,240,256,315, 453,476	179,225,231,246, 378,418,423, 446,472,486	25,27,166,175,242, 243,248,414	25,219,223,226, 230,243,418	27,167,177,179,233, 238,239,244,249,257, 419,438,461,480,498
Myocarditis	227,232,240,253, 256,315,382, 435,441	25,179,222,225, 228,233,246, 378,423,473	25,27,93,166,172, 220,231,245,247, 265,283,413,463	27,179,219,223, 226,230,237,241, 251,378,383,457, 458,473	27,177,249, 419,480
Hepatitis	232,256,315, 382,435,445		196,232	230,237	
Pancreatitis				254	238
Adrenocortical necrosis			242		
Bronchitis				449	

Cherry [234] described a 4-day-old infant who became febrile and lethargic. This illness persisted for 5 days without other signs or symptoms. An examination of the CSF showed a slight increase in the number of leukocytes, and most were mononuclear cells. Coxsackievirus B1 was recovered from the throat, stool, urine, and serum.

Wright and colleagues [256] reported an infant fatality associated with coxsackievirus B1 infection. This premature boy was well until he was 4 days old, when he had two episodes of cyanosis and apnea. He then became anorexic and listless and lost the Moro reflex. On the 9th day of life, he had shallow respirations, hepatomegaly, jaundice, petechiae, and thrombocytopenia. He was edematous and lethargic, and he had a temperature of 34.5° C, a pulse rate of 130 beats/min, and a respiratory rate of 20 breaths/min. He became weaker, unresponsive, and apneic and died. Positive laboratory findings included the following values: platelets, less than $10,000 /mm^3$; CSF protein, 283 mg/dL; serum bilirubin, 20.5 mg/dL; and serum aspartate aminotransferase, 100 U. Autopsy revealed hepatic necrosis, meningoencephalitis, and myocarditis. Coxsackievirus B1 was recovered from the throat, urine, liver, lung, kidney, and brain.

Twin boys with a sepsis-like illness with hepatitis and disseminated intravascular coagulation have been reported [25]. The first twin died on the 16th day of life, and the second twin survived. Another set of twins had coxsackievirus B1 infections shortly after birth; one twin had myocarditis, and the other had hepatitis with subsequent progressive liver calcifications [382]. A third set of twins had coxsackievirus B1 infections with illness that began when they were 5 days old [453]. One twin had

disseminated intravascular coagulation, and the other twin had meningitis. Three other newborns with fatal sepsis-like illnesses with hepatitis have been described [435,441].

Isacsohn and colleagues [232] described four severe cases of neonatal illnesses owing to coxsackievirus B1; three of the four neonates died. One neonate died of myocarditis, and the other two died of multiorgan dysfunction. The surviving infant had hepatitis, congestive heart failure, thrombocytopenia, and residual neurologic damage.

McLean and colleagues [240] described a newborn boy who had a temperature of 39° C, vomiting, and diarrhea on the 4th day of life. When 6 days old, he appeared gray and mottled and developed shallow respirations. He died on the 7th day of life after increased respiratory distress (90 breaths/min), hepatomegaly, generalized edema, and cardiac enlargement. Coxsackievirus B1 was recovered from the heart and brain.

Gear [227] studied an extensive epidemic of Bornholm disease related to coxsackievirus B1 in Johannesburg in summer 1960 through summer 1961. After the first coxsackievirus B1 isolations, the medical officers of the area were on the alert for nursery infections and the prevention of nursery epidemics. Despite careful isolation procedures, Gear [227] reported that infection "was introduced into all the large maternity homes in Johannesburg." About 20 cases of neonatal myocarditis and three deaths were documented. The isolation procedures apparently prevented secondary nursery cases.

Volakova and Jandasek [253] reported epidemic myocarditis related to coxsackievirus B1. Cherry and Jahn [221] described a child with a mild febrile exanthematous illness, which had its onset within 10 minutes of birth.

In 2007, coxsackievirus B1 was the predominant enterovirus in the United States [315]. An increased detection of severe neonatal disease owing to coxsackievirus B1 occurred in association with this predominance. Five fatal cases were noted. Manifestations included myocarditis, meningitis/meningoencephalitis, sepsis-like illness, hepatitis and coagulopathy.

Coxsackievirus B2

The reported instances of coxsackievirus B2 infections in neonates are listed in Table 24–8. In most instances, the infants had myocarditis or neurologic manifestations. Of the 12 infants with myocarditis, 11 died. The one child with myocarditis who survived was reexamined when 2 years old and was found to be normal [222]. The child's mother became ill with sore throat, coryza, and malaise on the day after delivery. When 3 days old, the child became febrile (38.9° C) and had periods of apnea and cardiac irregularities. The cry was "pained." ECG showed a left-sided heart pattern in the V leads and T wave abnormalities. The infant's symptoms lasted less than 48 hours. Coxsackievirus B2 was isolated from the nose, urine, throat, and CSF of the child and from the mother's stool. The mother breast-fed the infant (while she wore a mask) during her illness. A later specimen of breast milk was cultured for virus without successful recovery of an agent.

Puschak [178] reported a child who became febrile (39.5° C) 8 hours after birth. During the next 9 days, the infant's temperature fluctuated between 36.7° C and 38.9° C. The infant had no other symptoms. Serologic evidence of coxsackievirus B2 infection was found.

Johnson and associates [484] described a 1-month-old infant with aseptic meningitis who developed a persistent right facial paralysis. In a study of undifferentiated diarrheal syndromes, Ramos-Alvarez [452] observed a child with coxsackievirus B2 infection. Eilard and associates [423] reported a nursery outbreak in which 12 infants were infected. All had aseptic meningitis, and two also had myocarditis. One of the two infants died on the 13th day of life. One child with thrombocytopenia and respiratory failure died [427].

Coxsackievirus B3

Instances of neonatal infections with coxsackievirus B3 are listed in Table 24–8. Most reported cases have been severe illnesses with myocarditis or meningoencephalitis or both. One case involved sudden infant death [379], in which coxsackievirus B3 was recovered from a pool of organs from an infant who died on the 8th day of life.

Tuuteri and coworkers [250] studied a nursery outbreak of coxsackievirus B3 infection. Seven infants had mild disease characterized by anorexia, listlessness, and fever, and two infants had fatal myocarditis. Of the 57 infants with reported neonatal infections with coxsackievirus B3, 30 died; most deaths were associated with myocarditis and sepsis-like illness. Three infants had febrile illnesses with meningitis and were reported to have had no residual effects; long-term follow-up is unavailable, however [175,243].

Isacsohn and colleagues [232] reported two neonates with multiorgan dysfunction who survived. A full-term boy delivered by cesarean section had scattered vesicular lesions at birth [470]. New lesions appeared over a 5-day period, and the rash lasted for 10 days. The infant had no other symptoms, and the mother had no febrile illness during pregnancy.

Chesney and associates [478] studied a 3-week-old girl with meningoencephalitis. This infant had hypoglycorrhachia; the CSF glucose value on the 6th day of illness was 23 mg/dL, with a corresponding blood glucose level of 78 mg/dL. As described in another review [427], two infants who died had thrombocytopenia and respiratory failure; a clinical picture suggestive of necrotizing enterocolitis also was observed.

During a 5-year period in Toronto, Krajden and Middleton [27] assessed 24 neonates with enterovirus infections who were admitted to the Hospital for Sick Children. Nine infants were infected with coxsackievirus B3; of these, two infants had meningitis, three had myocarditis, and four had a sepsis-like illness. Of this group, one infant with meningitis, one with myocarditis, and all with sepsis-like illness died. All the neonates with sepsis-like illness had clinical evidence of multiorgan involvement; they had respiratory distress, hepatomegaly, hemorrhagic manifestations, and congestive heart failure. Two neonates with herpangina and coxsackievirus B3 infections were described in an outbreak involving 25 infants [447]. Fatal myocarditis has been noted in two more recent cases [93,463]. In one case, the infecting virus was found to be a recombinant human enterovirus B variant [93]. The genomic chimera arose from recombination between coxsackievirus B3 and enteroviruses 86 and 87.

Coxsackievirus B4

Table 24–8 summarizes listings of coxsackievirus B4 neonatal infections. Most were severe and frequently were fatal illnesses with neurologic and cardiac involvement. Sieber and associates [247] described an infant with less severe disease. This infant was well until 6 days after delivery, when he developed pharyngitis, diarrhea, and gradually increasing lethargy; this was followed by fever for 36 hours. No other signs or symptoms were observed, and the infant was well when 11 days old. He had virologic and serologic evidence of coxsackievirus B4 infection.

Winsser and Altieri [254] studied an infant who suddenly became cyanotic and convulsed and died at 2 days of age. At autopsy, the only findings were bronchopneumonia, congestive splenomegaly, and chronic interstitial pancreatitis. Coxsackievirus B4 was isolated from the spleen.

Barson and associates [457] reported the survival of an infant with myocarditis. Cardiac calcification was revealed on radiographs when the infant was 4 weeks old, and ECG revealed a left bundle branch block. When the infant was 7 months old, the conduction defect remained, but the myocardial calcification had resolved.

Coxsackievirus B5

The spectrum of neonatal infection with coxsackievirus B5 is greater than with the other coxsackievirus B strains. Studies are listed in Table 24–8. Meningitis and encephalitis are common neonatal manifestations of coxsackievirus B5 infection.* Nursery epidemics have been observed. Rantakallio and associates [244] studied 17 infants with aseptic meningitis in one nursery. None of the infants was severely ill. All had fever, with a temperature of 38° C to 40° C. Eleven of the 17 neonates were boys. Signs included irritability, nuchal rigidity, increased tone, anorexia, opisthotonos, whimpering, loose stools, and diminution of alertness. In another nursery outbreak, Farmer and Patten [419] found 28 infected infants; 15 had aseptic meningitis, 4 had diarrhea, and 9 had no signs of illness. The 15 children who had had meningitis were studied 6 years later; 13 were found to be physically normal and to have normal intelligence. Two children had intelligence levels below the mean for the group and had residual spasticity. At the time of the initial illness, these two infants and one additional child were twitching, irritable, or jittery.

Swender and associates [257] studied seven cases of aseptic meningitis in an intensive care nursery during a 6-week period during the summer of 1972. Two of the infants had apnea. One of the infants had a CSF glucose level of 12 mg/dL. During a community outbreak of coxsackievirus B5 infections, Marier and colleagues [438] studied 32 infants with aseptic meningitis. In this group, 36% had CSF leukocyte counts of 500 cells/mm³ or greater, and neutrophils accounted for 50% or more of the count in 19% of these infants. In 12% of patients, the CSF glucose level was less than 40 mg/dL. Blood leukocyte counts of 15,000 cells/mm³ or greater were detected in 38% of the infants.

Of particular interest is the observation of exanthem in four reports. Cherry and coworkers [477] described a 3-week-old boy with fever, maculopapular rash, and enlarged cervical and postauricular lymph nodes. Examination of the CSF revealed 141 leukocytes/mm³, of which 84% were lymphocytes, and a protein value of 100 mg/dL. ECG was normal. In this infant, the rash appeared before the fever. Coxsackievirus B5 was isolated from the pharynx and the CSF. Nogen and Lepow [243] reported an infant with a similar illness. This infant had a nonspecific erythematous papular rash on the face and scalp. He became febrile and irritable 1 week later. The CSF contained 440 white blood cells/mm³, and 96% of them were mononuclear. Virus was isolated from the feces, throat, and CSF.

Artenstein and associates [219] reported a 23-day-old girl with fever and erythematous macular rash that spread from the scalp to the entire body except the palms and soles and lasted 4 days. Coxsackievirus B5 was recovered from the stool, but no evidence of serum antibody to this virus was found. McLean and coworkers [177] also described an infant with a papular rash on the trunk and limbs that was present at birth. On the 4th day of life, the rash had disappeared, but the patient then developed a temperature of 39.4° C. Irritability, twitching, and fullness of the anterior fontanelle were observed, and CSF examination showed meningitis. During an 8-day period,

the infant had repeated episodes of vomiting and diarrhea. On the 11th day of life, the infant had hyperpnea, tachycardia, and an enlarging liver. The infant died on the 13th day of life. Autopsy revealed extensive encephalitis and focal myocardial necrosis. Virus was recovered from the brain, heart, lungs, and liver.

Neonatal infection with coxsackievirus B5 seems less likely to be fatal than infection with other strains of coxsackievirus B. Only 6 of 36 infants presented in Table 24–8 died. In contrast to coxsackieviruses B2, B3, and B4, coxsackievirus B5 seems to be more neurotropic than cardiotropic.

Echoviruses

Echovirus 1

Dömök and Molnár [224] described aseptic meningitis related to echovirus 1.

Echovirus 2

Krajden and Middleton [27] described three infants with echovirus 2 infections. Two of the neonates had meningitis and recovered. The third infant, who died, had a sepsis-like illness. Virus was isolated from the CSF, lung, liver, and urine. One other neonate with echovirus 2 infection has been observed, but no details are available [427].

Echovirus 3

In summer 1970, Haynes and coworkers [481] studied an epidemic of infection caused by echovirus 3. Three infected neonates were observed, all of whom had meningitis. One child, a full-term girl, developed tonic seizures and an inability to suck on the 3rd day of life. The serum bilirubin level was 28 mg/dL. Shortly thereafter, the infant became cyanotic, flaccid, and apneic and developed a bulging anterior fontanelle; she was in shock. She received assisted ventilation with a respirator for 3 days. When the child was 1 month old, severe neurologic damage with developing hydrocephalus was obvious. Echovirus 3 was recovered from the CSF, and the CSF protein level was 880 mg/dL on the 6th day of life. The other two infants in this study apparently had uncomplicated aseptic meningitis. The CSF findings in one infant revealed 1826 white blood cells/mm³, 91% of which were polymorphonuclear cells. The other infant had 320 cells/mm³, 98% of which were polymorphonuclear cells.

A 4-day-old infant from whom echovirus 3 was recovered from the CSF has been reported [27]. This child had less than 3 white blood cells/mm³ in the CSF. Other neonates with echovirus 3 infection have been observed, but no details are available [201,427].

Echovirus 4

Linnemann and colleagues [437] studied 11 infants with echovirus 4 infections. All infants had fevers, and most were irritable. Four infants had a fine maculopapular rash, which was located on the face or abdomen or both. In two infants, the extremities were also involved. Other neonates with echovirus 4 infections have been reported, but details of their illness are unavailable [201,427].

*References 27,167,177,179,238,239,244,249,257,419,438,480.

Echovirus 5

There have been six reports of neonatal illnesses associated with echovirus 5 infections [360,418,420,470]. In one nursery epidemic, six infants were involved [267]. All infants had fever (38.3° C to 39.7° C) that lasted 4 to 8 days. Two neonates had tachycardia that was disproportionately rapid compared with the degree of fever, but there was no evidence of myocarditis in either infant. Four infants had splenomegaly and enlarged lymph nodes; these findings persisted for several weeks.

In 1966 (July to October), an epidemic of echovirus 5 infection involved 23% of the infants in the maternity unit at the Royal Air Force Hospital in Chargi, Singapore [266]. Of the infants, 56 had symptomatic infection, and 10 had asymptomatic infection. Infants who were ill were 2 to 12 days old at the onset of disease. All 56 symptomatic infants had fever; 87% of them had a temperature of 38.3° C or greater. The mean duration of fever was 3.5 days (range 2 to 7 days). In 20 infants, a faint erythematous macular rash occurred that was most prominent on the limbs and buttocks, but also appeared on the trunk and face. The rash, which began 24 to 36 hours after the beginning of fever, lasted 48 hours. Diarrhea occurred in 17 infants, 4 of whom passed blood and mucus. Vomiting was observed in about half of the neonates. All infants apparently recovered completely.

A newborn girl had a nonspecific, biphasic febrile illness [497]. Echovirus 5 was recovered from the CSF, but the cell count, protein level, and glucose value were normal. Another study included a 9-day-old infant with aseptic meningitis [498]. During an epidemiologic investigation in Rochester, New York, 13 of 75 enterovirus isolates were echovirus 5 [201]. Six of the infants were asymptomatic; no clinical details of the other seven patients were presented. A neonate with sepsis-like illness and hepatic failure died 9 days after birth [364].

Echovirus 6

Sanders and Cramblett [283] reported a boy who was well until 9 days of age, when he developed a fever (38° C), severe diarrhea, and dehydration. His white blood cell count was 27,900 cells/mm³, and virologic and serologic evidence of echovirus 6 infection was found. Treatment consisted of intravenous hydration, to which there was a good response. Krous and colleagues [363] described an infant who died on the 9th day of life with a sepsis-like illness. The infant had meningitis, disseminated intravascular coagulation, hepatic necrosis, and adrenal and renal hemorrhage. Ventura and associates [388] reported the death of a full-term neonate with sepsis-like syndrome who at postmortem examination had massive hepatic necrosis, adrenal hemorrhagic necrosis, renal medullary hemorrhage, hemorrhagic noninflammatory pneumonia, and severe encephalomalacia.

Yen and coworkers [442,499] reported a premature boy who developed a sepsis-like illness on the 5th day of life. This infant had hepatic failure and was treated with intravenous immunoglobulin. He recovered gradually, but at 62 days of life, he died of a nosocomial *Enterobacter cloacae* infection. Echovirus type 6 has been associated with

neonatal illness on two other occasions, but no clinical details are available [427,437].

Echovirus 7

Piraino and colleagues [383] reported three infants with echovirus 7 infections. All three had fever, one had respiratory distress and exanthem, and one had irritability and loose stools. Two neonates with fatal sepsis-like illnesses with massive disseminated intravascular coagulation have been reported [286,389]. One neonate with severe hepatitis was treated with pleconaril and survived [500]. Daboval and colleagues [467] described an outbreak of echovirus 7 infection in 6 newborns over 12 days. The index case was the mother of one of the infants. The infant of the index case developed fever on the 6th day of life. The subsequent five infants all had illnesses suggestive of sepsis. Five of the infants had macular rashes. All six of the infants had high C-reactive protein levels, but none had evidence of bacterial infection.

Echovirus 8

In a search for etiologic associations in infantile diarrhea, Ramos-Alvarez [452] identified one neonate from whom echovirus 8 was recovered from the stool. The antibody titer to this virus increased fourfold.

Echovirus 9

Echovirus 9 is the most prevalent of all the enteroviruses (see Table 24–4). From 1955-1958, epidemic waves of infection spread throughout the world [501]. Since that time, echovirus 9 has been a common cause of human illness. Despite its prevalence and its frequent association with epidemic disease, descriptions of neonatal illness are uncommon. In contrast to experiences with several other enteroviruses, newborn nursery epidemics caused by echovirus 9 have been described rarely.

Neonatal echovirus 9 data are provided in Table 24–9. Moscovici and Maisel [186] described an asymptomatic infant with echovirus 9 infection. When echovirus 9 was

TABLE 24–9 Neonatal Infection with Echovirus 9

Study	Finding
Moscovici and Maisel [186]	Asymptomatic infection
Mirani et al [451]	Meningitis (4 cases)
	Gastroenteritis (2 cases)
	Pneumonia (1 case)
Rawls et al [387]	Hepatic necrosis
Cho et al [433]	Severe, generalized disease
Jahn and Cherry [234]	Mild febrile illness
Eichenwald and Kostevalov [187]	Aseptic meningitis
	Gastroenteritis (2 cases)
Haynes et al [482]	Meningoencephalitis
Cheeseman et al [390]	Fatal interstitial pneumonia
Krajden and Middleton [27]	Meningitis

prevalent in Erie County, New York, during the summer of 1971, seven neonatal cases were observed [451]. Four children had aseptic meningitis, but only moderate elevations of CSF protein values and white blood cells were observed. A 15-day-old infant had radiologic evidence of bronchopneumonia, and two infants had gastroenteritis. Rawls and coworkers [387] described an infant who was well until the 7th day of life, when progressive lethargy, anorexia, and irritability developed. The child became moribund, and jaundice, scattered petechiae, and hypothermia were observed. The pulse rate was 90 beats/min, the respiratory rate was 40 breaths/min, and the liver was enlarged. The infant died 3 days after the onset of symptoms. Echovirus 9 was recovered from the lung, brain, and CSF. Cho and colleagues [433] described a similar severe neonatal illness in an infant boy from whom echovirus 9 was recovered from the CSF. This infant was hypothermic and hypotonic on the 3rd day of life. He had bilateral pneumonia and leukopenia. After a stormy course, which included an exchange transfusion for suspected sepsis and mechanical ventilation for apnea, he eventually recovered.

Jahn and Cherry [234] described an infant who became febrile (38.3° C), irritable, and anorectic on the 6th day of life. This infant became asymptomatic within 2 days; echovirus 9 was recovered from the throat, feces, serum, and CSF. Eichenwald and Kostevalov [187] reported two children with mild irritability, fever, and diarrhea and a third child with diarrhea and convulsions in whom laboratory findings showed aseptic meningitis. Haynes and colleagues [482] studied a large outbreak of meningo-encephalitis caused by echovirus 9 and described nine infants who were 2 weeks to 2 months old. Cheeseman and associates [390] studied a neonate with fatal interstitial pneumonia, and Krajden and Middleton [27] reported a 4-day-old infant from whom echovirus 9 was recovered from the CSF. This infant had less than 3 white blood cells/mm³ in the CSF.

TABLE 24–10   Neonatal Infection with Echovirus 11

Study	Finding
Miller et al [276]	Exanthem and pneumonia (1 case)
	Nonspecific febrile illness (1 case)
	Aseptic meningitis (1 case)
Sanders and Cramblett [283]	Gastroenteritis (2 cases)
Berkovich and Kibrick [258]	Gastroenteritis (1 case)
	Meningitis (1 case)
Cramblett et al [261]	Meningitis (3 cases, 1 with rash)
	Severe, nonspecific febrile illness (1 case)
Hercík et al [269]	Respiratory illness (22 cases)
Hasegawa [268]	Fever (31 cases)
	Stomatitis (4 cases)
	Fever and stomatitis (6 cases)
Davies et al [262]	Encephalopathy (1 case)
	Nonspecific febrile illness (1 case)
	Sepsis-like illness with cardiac failure (1 death)
	Lower respiratory infection (1 case)
Jones et al [362]	Sepsis-like illness with hepatitis and rash (1 case)
Lapinleimu and Hakulinen [273]	Aseptic meningitis (4 cases)
	Gastroenteritis or respiratory distress or both (3 cases)
Nagington et al [279]	Sepsis-like illness with shock, diffuse bleeding, and renal hemorrhage (3 deaths)
Suzuki et al [448]	Fever (100%); pharyngitis (7%) (42 cases)
Krous et al [363]	Sepsis-like illness with disseminated intravascular coagulation, and hepatic necrosis (1 death)
Modlin [277]	Sepsis-like illness with apnea, lethargy, poor feeding, jaundice, hepatitis, and disseminated intravascular coagulation (4 deaths)
Drew [460]	Myocarditis (5 cases)
Piraino et al [383]	Meningitis and rash (2 cases)
	Meningitis (4 cases)
	Fatal case with cardiac failure, interstitial pneumonia, and interventricular cerebral hemorrhage
Krajden and Middleton [27]	Meningitis
Mertens et al [275]	Fever (2 cases)
	Meningitis (4 cases)
Reyes et al [195]	Fatal sepsis-like illness

Continued

TABLE 24–10 Neonatal Infection with Echovirus 11—cont'd

Study	Finding
Berry and Nagington [357]	Sepsis-like illness (11 deaths)
	Sudden death
Gh et al [359]	Sepsis-like illness (5 deaths)
Bose et al [358]	Sepsis-like illness (1 death, 1 survived)
Bowen et al [475]	Meningitis (34 infants ≤4 mo old)
Halfon and Spector [361]	Sepsis-like illness (2 deaths)
Steinmann and Albrecht [284]	Sepsis-like illness with meningitis and apnea (5 cases)
	Meningitis (4 cases)
	Gastroenteritis (3 cases)
Gitlin et al [360]	Sepsis-like illness with hepatic necrosis (4 deaths)
Kinney et al [272]	Meningitis (8 cases with 1 death)
	Mild illness (4 cases)
	Inapparent infection (2 cases)
Rabkin et al [282]	Sepsis-like illness (9 cases, 5 with meningitis)
	Inapparent infection (1 case)
Isaacs et al [548]	Meningitis (2 cases, 1 with myocarditis)
	Pneumonia (1 case)
	Inapparent infection (7 cases)
	Apnea (1 case)
Wang et al [364]	Sepsis-like illness with hepatic failure
Tarcan et al [503]	Bone marrow failure
Bina Rai et al [422]	Fever (11 cases), diarrhea (5 cases), coryza (3 cases), breathing difficulty (2 cases), jaundice (1 case)
Tang et al [440]	Pleurodynia (mother), and aseptic meningitis (newborn)
Chen et al [432]	Fever (10 cases), sepsis-like illnesses with DIC (2 cases), asymptomatic (1 case)
Willems et al [392]	Fatal sepsis-like illness with pulmonary hypertension

Echovirus 11

Neonatal illness associated with echovirus 11 infection has been varied. Reported cases are listed in Table 24–10. Eleven of the reports involved nursery outbreaks; in five reports, the neonatal cases were part of a larger community epidemic. Miller and associates [276] studied an epidemic of aseptic meningitis and other acute febrile illnesses in New Haven, Connecticut, in summer 1965. This epidemic was unique in that half of the patients with meningitis from whom virus was isolated were younger than 6 months. The echovirus 11 in this epidemic was a prime strain. Three neonatal illnesses were reported. One of the patients, a 1-month-old infant, was initially irritable and feverish and had diarrhea. Chest radiographs revealed bilateral pneumonitis. A generalized, discrete maculopapular rash, which lasted 24 hours, was seen on the 3rd day of illness. Fever persisted for 6 days. A 12-day-old girl had fever (39.4° C) lasting 1 day, but no other findings. Echovirus 11 was recovered from her throat. Another 1-month-old infant had aseptic meningitis.

Sanders and Cramblett [283] described two infants with diarrhea. Both infants were acutely ill; one was jaundiced and irritable and had feeding difficulty. In another study, two infants with echovirus 11 infections had diarrhea [258]. One infant had a temperature of 39.3° C and a "stuffy nose," and the other had a temperature of 39.8° C and aseptic meningitis. Cramblett and coworkers

[261] observed an outbreak of nosocomial infections caused by echovirus 11 in a neonatal intensive care unit. In a 1-month-old premature infant with frequent apneic episodes, the CSF contained 2200 white blood cells/mm³, 89% of which were polymorphonuclear cells, and the protein level was 280 mg/dL. The infant made a gradual recovery. Echovirus 11 was isolated from the CSF and stool. In another premature infant, apneic episodes and bradycardia suddenly began on the 20th day of life. Fever developed, the apneic spells continued, and digitalis therapy was necessary because of congestive heart failure. Examination of the CSF revealed aseptic meningitis, and echovirus 11 was recovered from the CSF, throat, and stool. A third child with aseptic meningitis had an exanthem. The disease began suddenly, and the child had shallow respirations and poor skin color. On the next day, generalized seizures occurred, and a maculopapular rash developed on the trunk, extremities, and face. The child made a gradual recovery. A fourth child had a severe, nonspecific febrile illness.

A particularly noteworthy finding in neonatal echovirus 11 infection has been severe sepsis-like illness with hepatitis or hepatic necrosis, disseminated intravascular coagulation, and extensive hemorrhagic manifestations.*

---

*References 195,262,277,279,357–363,382,387.

During the past 15 years, more than 40 such cases have been described, and most of the illnesses have been fatal.

Hercík and coworkers [269] reported an epidemic of respiratory illness in 22 newborns. Six of the infants were severely ill, and one subsequently died. The incubation period varied from 17 hours to 9 days (average 3 days). Seven infants had interstitial pneumonia, and all had rhinitis, pharyngitis, and vomiting. Toce and Keenan [502] reported two newborns with respiratory distress and pneumonia at birth. Both infants died of echovirus 11 infection. Tarcan and colleagues [503] described a 5-day-old boy who developed fever and diarrhea. He developed a maculopapular rash on the face, generalized petechiae and hemorrhagic bullae, and pancytopenia owing to bone marrow failure. This infant was treated with intravenous immunoglobulin and recovered.

An outbreak of echovirus 11 infections in neonates in a confinement home in Penaug, Malaysia, was noted in September and October 2004 [422]. Of the two primary cases from a hospital nursery, one went to the confinement home and became symptomatic there. Of the 13 infants in the confinement home, 11 developed febrile illnesses. In addition, five infants had diarrhea, three infants had coryza, two infants had difficulty breathing, and one infant had jaundice.

An infant in a neonatal unit in London, England, developed lethargy and fed poorly 3 days after birth [440]. The neonate had temperature fluctuations and recurrent hypoglycemia and aseptic meningitis. The mother of the infant had pleurodynia at the time of delivery. An echovirus 11 outbreak occurred in a nursery in Taipei, Taiwan, in November 2003 [504]. Symptomatic illness developed in 12 neonates; 3 infants had asymptomatic infection. One infant developed respiratory failure, hypotonia, disseminated intravascular coagulopathy, and bacterial grade IV intraventricular hemorrhage and died at a referral center from extensive pulmonary hemorrhage 6 days after admission. A second infant had fulminant hepatitis, anemia, aseptic meningitis, and disseminated intravascular coagulopathy, but survived after a lengthy hospital stay. The other 10 infants who were referred because of fever all recovered without sequelae. The source of infection in the index patient was the mother.

Echovirus 13

Before 2000, infection with echovirus 13 was rare in neonates. The virus was isolated from one asymptomatic infant in a neonatal surveillance study [201]. In 2001 in the United States, echovirus 13 was the leading cause of aseptic meningitis, and during 2001-2002, aseptic meningitis outbreaks with this agent occurred in many countries [366,480,483,505]. Many cases were infants who were 3 months or younger [506]. A 28-day-old boy in Tennessee had aseptic meningitis and hepatitis [507]. Neonatal cases were reported in Israel and Spain, but details were not presented [508,509].

Echovirus 14

Hughes and colleagues [189] reported an infant boy who became febrile (38° C) and had cyanotic episodes on the 3rd day of life. When 4 days old, his temperature was 38.9° C, and he experienced recurrent apneic spells. Liver enlargement, hypothermia, bradycardia, periodic breathing, and spontaneous ecchymoses developed, and the infant died on the 7th day of life. Laboratory studies revealed the presence of leukopenia and thrombocytopenia, and autopsy showed severe hepatic necrosis. Drouhet [510] described a child with aseptic meningitis and echovirus 14 infection, and Hinuma and associates [511] reported four newborns with apparent asymptomatic echovirus 14 infections.

Echovirus 16

In 1974, Hall and colleagues [436] studied five neonates with echovirus 16 infections. All five infants were admitted to the hospital because sepsis was suspected. Four of five were febrile, all were lethargic and irritable, and two had abdominal distention. Three of the neonates had erythematous maculopapular exanthems, and in two, the rash appeared after or with defervescence. Leukocyte counts in four infants revealed an increased percentage of band form neutrophils. Two neonates had aseptic meningitis. Lake and associates [427] observed three infants with echovirus 16 infections. In their study, clinical findings were not itemized by virus type, but it is inferred that sepsis-like illnesses occurred.

Echovirus 17

Neonatal infection with echovirus 17 has been observed by three investigators. Cherry and coworkers [174] reported two ill infants. A 19-day-old infant developed otitis media 5 days after his mother had a flulike illness. Echovirus 17 was isolated from his feces, and serologic evidence of echovirus 17 infection was found in the infant and the mother. The second infant had a nonspecific febrile illness at the age of 4 weeks, which was severe enough to require hospitalization. Virus was isolated from the infant's throat, feces, and serum.

Sanders and Cramblett [283] described two neonates with exanthem associated with echovirus 17. The first infant, a 3-week-old girl, became drowsy, anorectic, and febrile. She had a fine maculopapular rash on the trunk, a slightly injected pharynx, and a few petechiae on the soft palate. She remained febrile for 5 days. Echovirus 17 was recovered from the CSF and the feces. The second infant became ill at 3 weeks of age. His symptoms were mild rhinitis and cough followed by lethargy and refusal to eat. His temperature was 39° C 4 days after the onset of symptoms, and his respiratory rate was 60 breaths/min. A fine maculopapular rash appeared on the trunk, and radiographs revealed an infiltrate in the right lung. The infant's course was uneventful, and he was much improved 12 days after the onset of symptoms.

Faulkner and van Rooyen [265] described an outbreak of echovirus 17 infection with illness in a nursery in mid-August 1971. Seven infants were involved, including one with aseptic meningitis who was 7 weeks old. All the infants had fever, four had CNS signs, three had abdominal distention, four had diarrhea, and three had a rash. One other infant from another community was also studied by the investigators. This infant had febrile pneumonitis when 3.5 weeks old. The findings abated in 5 days, but the infant suddenly died 6 days later. Autopsy revealed interstitial pneumonitis with extensive edema and scattered petechial hemorrhages of the viscera. Echovirus 17 was isolated from the liver, lung, spleen, and kidney.

Echovirus 18

In 1958, Eichenwald and colleagues [263] described epidemic diarrhea associated with echovirus 18 infections. In a nursery unit of premature infants, 12 of 21 infants were mildly ill. Neither temperature elevation nor hypothermia occurred. Six infants were lethargic and listless, and two developed moderate abdominal distention. The diarrhea lasted 1 to 5 days; there were five or six watery, greenish stools per day, occasionally expelled explosively. In two infants, a small amount of blood was seen in the stools, but there was no mucus or pus cells. Five other infants in another nursery had similar diarrheal illness. Echovirus 18 was recovered from all ill infants.

Medearis and Kramer [512] reported a 3-week-old girl with fever, irritability, lethargy, pharyngitis, and postnasal drainage. She was admitted to the hospital because of apneic spells and developed a generalized erythematous blotchy macular rash and had frequent stools. The illness lasted about 7 days. Echovirus 18 was recovered from the blood, throat, and feces. Berkovich and Kibrick [258] found echovirus 18 in the stool of a 12-day-old twin infant with fever and a red throat. The relationship of echovirus 18 to the illness is uncertain because the patient's twin was infected with echovirus 11, and the patient also had serologic evidence of echovirus 11 infection. The fever and red throat may have been caused by echovirus 11, rather than echovirus 18 infection. Wilfert and associates [505] observed a 9-day-old infant with aseptic meningitis.

Kusuhara and coworkers [469] described an outbreak of echovirus 18 infection in a neonatal intensive care unit involving 20 patients. This outbreak occurred between November 3 and November 24, 2003, and involved patients 1 week to 6 months old. Of the infants, 8 had acute exanthematous diseases, 1 had transient fever, and the other 11 were asymptomatic.

Echovirus 19

Cramblett and coworkers [465] described two neonates with echovirus 19 infections. One infant had an upper respiratory infection, cough, and paroxysmal atrial tachycardia. The other infant also had an upper respiratory infection, but in addition to echovirus 19 infection, coxsackievirus B4 was recovered from the throat of this infant. Butterfield and associates [260] isolated echovirus 19 post mortem from the brain, lung, heart, liver, spleen, lymph nodes, and intestine of a premature infant who had cystic emphysema. The relationship between the generalized viral infection and the pulmonary disease is not understood.

Philip and Larson [386] reported three catastrophic neonatal echovirus 19 infections, which resulted in hepatic necrosis and massive terminal hemorrhage. One infant, infected in utero, was symptomatic at birth. The Apgar score was 3, and multiple petechiae were observed. The infant had generalized ecchymoses and apneic episodes and died when 3.5 hours old. Thrombocytopenia was identified, and echovirus 19 was isolated from the brain, liver, spleen, and lymph nodes. The other two infants who died of echovirus 19 infection were twins. They were normal during the first 3 days of life, but then became mildly cyanotic and lethargic. Shortly thereafter, apneic episodes occurred, and jaundice and petechiae developed. Both twins became oliguric, and they died on the 8th and 9th days of life, with severe gastrointestinal bleeding. Both twins were thrombocytopenic, and virus was recovered from systemic sites in both. Two similar catastrophic cases have been described [493].

Purdham and associates [281] reported an outbreak of echovirus 19 in a neonatal unit in which 12 infants were affected; 11 infants were febrile, 10 were irritable, 7 had marked abdominal distention with decreased bowel sounds, and 5 had apneic episodes. Bacon and Sims [428] described two neonates with sepsis-like illness. The infants were cyanotic with peripheral circulatory failure. In another study involving the same echovirus 19 epidemic, five infants younger than 3 months were reported [434]. All had sepsis-like illness with hypotonia and peripheral circulatory failure. Two infants had aseptic meningitis, and two others had diarrhea.

Echovirus 20

Eichenwald and Kostevalov [187] recovered echovirus 20 from four asymptomatic infants younger than 8 days (see "Cloud Baby"). Five neonates with severe illness owing to echovirus 20 have also been described [384,443]. All had hepatitis, and two died.

Echovirus 21

Jack and coworkers [270] recovered echovirus 21 from the feces of a 7-day-old infant with jaundice and diarrhea. No other details of the infant's illness are available. Chonmaitree and associates [459] studied a 19-day-old infant with aseptic meningitis and rash, and Georgieff and colleagues [385] reported a newborn with fulminant hepatitis. Lake and colleagues [427] also mentioned one infected infant, but presented no specific details.

Echovirus 25

Linnemann and colleagues [437] reported one neonate with echovirus 25 infection. They gave no virus-specific details except that fever and irritability occurred.

Echovirus 30

Matsumoto and associates [485] described a nursery outbreak involving 11 infants during a 2-week period. All the neonates had aseptic meningitis, and all recovered. Two symptomatic and six asymptomatic neonates were reported in the Rochester, New York, surveillance study [201]. Chen and associates [431] described twin neonates who had fever followed by thrombocytopenia, coagulopathy, and hepatic failure. One of the neonates died, and the other survived and had no obvious sequelae at 1 year of age. In another study, twins had a sepsis-like illness with hepatitis [439]. These twins survived and had normal development and normal liver function at 1 year of age.

Echovirus 31

McDonald and associates [274] described three neonates in an intensive care nursery with echovirus 31 infections. One infant had a fatal encephalitis-like illness, with hypertonicity, hyperreflexia, and apneic spells. The other two infants also experienced apneic spells, and one also had pneumonia and meningitis.

Echovirus 33

In a study of epidemic illness related to echovirus 33 disease in the Netherlands, Kapsenberg [271] stated that 7- to 8-day-old neonates in a maternity ward had a febrile illness. No further data were presented.

Enterovirus 71

Schmidt and colleagues [366] mentioned one 3-week-old infant with meningitis and enterovirus 71 infection. Chonmaitree and colleagues [450] described one 9-day-old neonate with aseptic meningitis and one 14-day-old infant with gastroenteritis from enterovirus 71. Chen and associates [471] reported a child with bilateral lower limbs weakness in association with the hand-foot-and-mouth syndrome.

Parechoviruses

Parechovirus 1

Parechovirus 1 has been associated with three epidemics of nursery infections. During a survey of perinatal virus infections by Jack and coworkers [270], 44 infants were found to be infected with parechovirus 1 during a study period from May to December 1966. The virus prevalence and the incidence of new infections during this period were fairly uniform. No illness was attributed to parechovirus 1 infection, and the virus disappeared from the nursery in mid-December 1966. Berkovich and Pangan [259] studied respiratory illnesses in premature infants and reported 64 infants with illness, 18 of whom had virologic or serologic evidence of parechovirus 1 infection. Many other infants had high but constant levels of serum antibody to parechovirus 1. Some of these infants were probably also infected with parechovirus 1. The children with proven parechovirus 1 infections could not be clinically differentiated from children without evidence of parechovirus 1 infection.

Of 18 infants with documented parechovirus 1 infections, 90% had coryza, 39% had pneumonia, and 11% had morbilliform rash or conjunctivitis or both. In contrast to the studies of Jack and coworkers [270], only 3 of 35 asymptomatic infants were found to be infected with parechovirus 1. Nakao and associates [280] recovered parechovirus 1 from 29 premature infants. Many of the infected infants were asymptomatic, and infants who were ill had only mild symptoms of coryza, cough, and diarrhea. Jenista and colleagues [201] described 17 parechovirus 1 infections in nonhospitalized neonates. Clinical details were not presented, but it seems that all of these infants were asymptomatic. Parechovirus 1 infection was associated with a nosocomial necrotizing enterocolitis outbreak [456].

In a study in Dutch children, Benschop and colleagues [429] compared the clinical findings in 27 children with parechovirus 1 with 10 children with parechovirus 3. They identified only the median ages of the children, so we do not know the number of neonates with illnesses. The investigators found that sepsis-like illness and CNS symptoms were more common in the parechovirus 3 cases compared with parechovirus 1 cases.

Parechovirus 2

Ehrnst and Eriksson [479] reported a 1-month-old girl with encephalopathy resulting from a nosocomial parechovirus 2 infection. No further details of this case were provided.

Parechovirus 3

Many more recent studies of illness with parechovirus 3 infections in neonates and young infants have been presented [34,35,429,430,491]. Four of five studies occurred in the Netherlands. In one study of 10 neonates and young infants, 90% had fever, 70% had sepsis-like illness, 70% had gastrointestinal tract symptoms, 50% had CNS symptoms, and 30% had respiratory tract symptoms [429]. In a subsequent study of 29 young children (median age 1.2 months) by members of the same group, the following findings were noted: fever 97%, irritability 86%, sepsis-like illness 75%, meningitis 12%, seizures 7%, encephalitis 4%, paralysis 4%, rash 17%, gastrointestinal tract symptoms 39%, and respiratory tract symptoms 36%.

Boivin and associates [430] in Quebec, Canada, reported three neonates with high fever, erythematous rash, and tachypnea. Verboon-Maciolak and coworkers [34] compared neonatal illness with parechovirus 3 with illness owing to enteroviruses; the only differences noted were that gastrointestinal tract symptoms were more common in the parechovirus 3 group, and C-reactive protein and CSF protein were higher in the enterovirus group [491]. Members of the same group carefully studied encephalitis in 10 neonates. All had white matter injury. Six of the 10 neonates were normal on later follow-up. One child had cerebral palsy with epilepsy, one child had learning disabilities, one child had epilepsy but normal cognitive outcome at 3 years of age, and one child had mild distal hypertonia at 18 months of age.

Parechovirus 4

A neonate with fever and poor feeding was found to be infected with parechovirus 4 [424].

DIAGNOSIS AND DIFFERENTIAL DIAGNOSIS

CLINICAL DIAGNOSIS

The clinical differentiation of neonatal infectious diseases frequently seems to be an impossible task. Although treatable bacterial and viral illnesses should always be considered and treated first, when all the circumstances of a particular neonatal illness are considered, enterovirus and parechovirus diseases can be suspected on clinical grounds. The most important factors in clinical diagnosis are season of the year, geographic location, exposure, incubation period, and clinical symptoms.

In temperate climates, enterovirus and parechovirus prevalence is distinctly seasonal, and disease is usually seen in the summer and fall. Neonatal enterovirus disease is unlikely in the winter. In the tropics, enteroviruses are prevalent throughout the year, and the season is not helpful diagnostically.

As with all infectious illnesses, knowledge of exposure and incubation time is important. A careful history of maternal illness is vital, particularly the symptoms of maternal illness. Nonspecific mild febrile illness in the mother that occurs in the summer and fall should warn of the possibility of more severe neonatal illness. More specific findings in the mother (e.g., aseptic meningitis, pleurodynia, herpangina, pericarditis, myocarditis) should alert the clinician to look for more specific enterovirus illnesses. Minor illness in nursery personnel during enterovirus seasons and the short incubation period of enterovirus and parechovirus infections should be taken into consideration. Manifestations of neonatal nonpolio enterovirus and parechovirus infections are listed in Table 24–5.

LABORATORY DIAGNOSIS

Virus Isolation

Most viral diagnostic laboratories have facilities for the recovery of most enteroviruses and parechoviruses that cause congenital and neonatal illness. Three tissue culture systems—primary rhesus, cynomolgus, or African green monkey kidney tissue culture; a diploid, human embryonic lung fibroblast cell strain; and the RD cell line—allow the isolation of all polioviruses, coxsackievirus B strains, echoviruses, newer enteroviruses, parechoviruses, and many coxsackievirus A strains. In a 1988 study in which Buffalo green monkey kidney cells and subpassages of primary human embryonic kidney cells were used in addition to primary monkey kidney and human diploid fibroblast (MRC-5) cells, the enterovirus recovery rate was increased by 11% [513]. For a complete diagnostic isolation spectrum, suckling mouse inoculation should also be performed. Optimally, at least one blind passage should be done in each of the culture systems.

Proper selection and handling of specimens are most important in the isolation of viruses from ill neonates. Because infection in neonates tends to be generalized, collection of material from multiple sites is important. Specimens should be taken from any or all of the following: nasopharynx, throat, stool, blood, urine, CSF, and any other body fluids that are available. Swabs from the nose, throat, and rectum should be placed in a transport medium.

Transport medium provides a protective protein, neutral pH, and antibiotics for control of microbial contamination and, most importantly, prevents desiccation. Many viral transport and storage media are commercially available or are prepared readily in the laboratory; their utility has been reviewed elsewhere [514]. Convenient and practical collection devices, such as the Culturette (Becton-Dickinson, Cockeysville, MD) or Virocult (Medical Wire

and Equipment Co, Victory Gardens, NY), consist of a swab, usually Dacron or rayon, on a plastic or aluminum shaft accompanied by a self-contained transport medium (Stuart or Amies) and are routinely available in most hospitals for bacteriologic culture. Calcium alginate swabs, which are toxic to herpes simplex virus, and wooden shafts, which may be toxic for viruses and the cell culture system itself, should not be used. Saline or holding media that contain serum also should be avoided. Useful liquid transport media (2-mL aliquots in screw-capped vials) consist of tryptase phosphate broth with 0.5% bovine albumin; Hanks balanced salt solution with 5% gelatin or 10% bovine albumin; or buffered sucrose phosphate (0.2M, 2-SP) [514,515], which has been used as a combined transport for viral, chlamydial, and mycoplasmal culture requests and is appropriate for long-term frozen storage of specimens and isolates [516].

Fluid specimens should be collected in sterile vials. Specimens of autopsy material are best collected in vials that contain transport medium. Generally, specimens should be refrigerated immediately after collection and during transportation to the laboratory. Specimens should not be exposed to sunlight during transportation. If an extended period is likely to elapse before a specimen can be processed in the laboratory, it is advisable to ship and store it frozen.

Evidence of enterovirus growth from tissue cultures takes only a few days in many cases and less than 1 week in most [109]. The use of the spin amplification, shell vial technique, and monoclonal antibodies has significantly reduced the time for detection of enterovirus cultures [55,517]. After isolation of an enterovirus, identification of its type is conventionally done by neutralization, which is an expensive and lengthy process.

Rapid Virus Identification

Because of the many different serotypes of enteroviruses and parechoviruses, immunofluorescence, agglutination, counterimmunoelectrophoresis, and ELISA techniques for the direct detection of antigen in suspected enterovirus infections have not been useful. Nucleic acid techniques with cDNA and RNA probes have been useful for the direct identification of enteroviruses [74,496,507–509]. The development of numerous PCR techniques has been most important. Since 1990, innumerable reports have described enterovirus and more recently parechovirus PCR methods and their use in identifying enterovirus and parechovirus RNA in clinical specimens.* PCR has proved most useful for the direct identification of enteroviruses and parechoviruses in the CSF of patients with meningitis. Compared with culture of CSF specimens, PCR is more rapid and sensitive, and the specificity is equal.

PCR also has proved useful in the identification of enteroviruses in blood, urine, and throat specimens.† Particularly impressive are the findings of Byington and associates [19]. Using PCR on specimens of blood and CSF, these investigators found that more than 25% of

---

*References 51–53,55–58,61–67,109,501,510,513–518.
†References 19,51,58,64,513,514,519.

infants admitted to the hospital for suspected sepsis in 1997 had nonpolio enterovirus infections. Based on this study and a subsequent study in Utah and the work of Adréoletti and coworkers and others [52,520], the general work-up for febrile neonates hospitalized for possible sepsis should include PCR for enteroviruses in blood and CSF. This is most important during enterovirus and parechovirus season (summer and fall in temperate climates), but because enterovirus circulation continues all year, it is reasonable to perform PCR in the off seasons. Although PCR detects enterovirus RNA, the specific enterovirus type is not identified. Because of this shortcoming, conventional culture should be performed along with PCR.

PCR has also identified enteroviruses in frozen and formalin-fixed biopsy and autopsy specimens of myocardium [51,58,64,513,514]. In one study, enteroviruses were identified in myocardial tissue from four neonates who died of myocarditis [521]. In one case, the specimen was obtained during life by a right ventricular endomyocardial biopsy, and in the other three, frozen or formalin-fixed autopsy samples were used. Most PCR methods can detect one tissue culture infective dose of enterovirus in CSF, stool, or throat specimen [522]. Polioviruses can be separated from other enteroviruses, and poliovirus vaccine strains can be rapidly identified by PCR [109,492,515–518,523].

Enterovirus RNA has been identified in numerous tissue specimens from patients with chronic medical conditions, such as idiopathic dilated cardiomyopathy. The possibility of lack of specificity (false-positive results) is a concern, however.

Serology

Except in special circumstances, the use of serologic techniques in the primary diagnosis of suspected neonatal enterovirus infections is impractical. Standard serologic study depends on the demonstration of an increase in antibody titer in response to a specific virus as an indication of infection with that agent. Although hemagglutination inhibition, ELISA, and complement fixation tests take only a short time to perform, these tests can be done only after the collection of a second, convalescent-phase blood specimen. These tests are also impractical in searching for the cause of a specific illness in a child because there are so many antigenically different enteroviruses. As discussed in "Antigenic Characteristics," group antigens can be produced that allow serologic diagnosis by IgM enzyme immunoassay and complement fixation, but these tests lack specificity [110,111,524].

In the evaluation of an infant with a suspected enterovirus infection, serum should be collected as soon as possible after the onset of illness and again 2 to 4 weeks later. This serum should be stored frozen. In most clinical situations, it is unnecessary to perform serologic tests on the collected serum because demonstration of an antibody titer increase in the serum of an infant from whom a specific virus has been isolated from a body fluid is superfluous. Collected serum can be useful diagnostically, however, if the prevalence of specific enteroviruses or parechoviruses in a community is known. In this situation,

it is easy to look for antibody titer changes to a selected number of viral types. More rapid diagnosis using a single serum sample is possible if a search for specific IgM enterovirus antibody is made [247,519,521,522,525–530].

Enterovirus IgM antibody tests are not commercially available. Commercial laboratories offer enterovirus complement fixation antibody panels. These tests are expensive, however, and their results in the clinical setting are almost always meaningless unless acute phase and convalescent phase sera are analyzed.

Histology

There are no specific histologic findings in enterovirus infections, such as seen in cytomegalovirus or herpes simplex virus infections. Tissues can be examined, however, for specific enterovirus antigens by immunofluorescent study and by PCR [179,501,531,532].

DIFFERENTIAL DIAGNOSIS

The differential diagnosis of congenital and neonatal enterovirus infections depends on the clinical manifestations. Generally, the most important illness categories are generalized bacterial sepsis or meningitis, congenital heart disease, and congenital and neonatal infections with other viruses.

Hypothermia and hyperthermia associated with nonspecific signs, such as lethargy and poor appetite, are common in neonatal enterovirus infections; they are also the presenting manifestations in bacterial sepsis. Proper bacterial cultures are essential. Differentiation between congenital heart disease and neonatal myocarditis is frequently difficult. The occurrence of fever or hypothermia, generalized lethargy and weakness, and characteristic ECG changes should suggest a viral cause.

Congenital infections with rubella virus, cytomegalovirus, *Toxoplasma gondii*, or *Treponema pallidum* are frequently associated with intrauterine growth restriction; this is not usual with enterovirus infections. Generalized herpes simplex virus infections are clinically similar to severe infections with several enteroviruses; in herpes infections, skin lesions are common, and a scraping of a lesion and a culture should allow a rapid diagnosis. In infants with signs of CNS involvement, it is particularly important to consider herpes simplex virus infection as a possible cause because infection with this agent is treatable, and early treatment is essential. In infants with meningitis, proper cultures and PCR testing are essential because the CSF findings in bacterial and viral illnesses are frequently similar.

PROGNOSIS
POLIOVIRUSES

As substantiated in the review by Bates [127] and the summary in Table 24–7, poliovirus infections in neonates are generally severe. Of the 44 cases with available follow-up data, there were 21 deaths; of the survivors, 12 had residual paralyses. Because infant survivors of poliomyelitis are susceptible to infection by the other two types of poliovirus, they should receive polio vaccine.

NONPOLIO ENTEROVIRUSES AND PARECHOVIRUSES

The immediate prognosis for patients with coxsackievirus and echovirus infections is related to the specific manifestations. Mortality rates are highest for infants with myocarditis, encephalitis, or sepsis-like illness with liver involvement. Differences in the severity of illness depend on viral type and strain variations. Generally, infections with coxsackieviruses B1 to B4 and with echovirus 11 seem to carry the most ominous initial prognoses. Also of concern are CNS infections with parechovirus 3.

Information related to long-term sequelae of neonatal coxsackievirus and echovirus infections is sparse. In a 4-year follow-up study, Gear [229] found no evidence of permanent cardiac damage in several children who had coxsackievirus B myocarditis. For children with aseptic meningitis, there is little available evidence of neurologic damage. One of five infants studied by Nogen and Lepow [243] from whom virus was recovered from the CSF was suspected to have brain damage. Cho and colleagues [433] reported that a child who had had severe neonatal echovirus 9 disease was developing normally at 1 year of age. Tuuteri and associates [250] reported that two children who had had clinically mild neonatal coxsackievirus B3 infections were thriving when seen at 1 year of age. After an epidemic of mild febrile disease related to echovirus 5, 51 children were examined at 1 year of age and found to be normal [266].

Farmer and colleagues [480] did a careful follow-up study of 15 children who had meningoencephalitis related to coxsackievirus B5 during the neonatal period. When 6 years old, two of the children were found to have developed spasticity, and their intelligence was below the mean for the study group as a whole and below the mean of a carefully selected control group. Three children who had myocarditis and meningoencephalitis had no cardiac sequelae at the age of 6 years. Sells and associates [487] described neurologic impairment at later follow-up of some children who had CNS enterovirus infections during the 1st year of life.

In a study in which nine children with enterovirus meningitis during the first 3 months of life were compared with nine matched control children, Wilfert and associates [498] found that the receptive language functioning of patients was significantly less than that of the controls. Head circumference, hearing, and intellectual function were similar for patients and controls. Bergman and colleagues [473] reported an extensive study in which 33 survivors of enterovirus meningitis during infancy were compared with their siblings. In this comprehensive study, none of the survivors had major neurologic sequelae, and they performed as well as their siblings on numerous cognitive, achievement, perceptual motor skills, and language tests. Rantakallio and coworkers [461] found that 16 of 17 patients with neonatal meningitis related to coxsackievirus B5 had normal neurologic development on follow-up. The one exception was a child with suspected intrauterine myocarditis. In another study, 16 newborns with meningitis related to coxsackievirus A14 were normal 2.5 years later.

The most alarming report is that of Eichenwald [533], who gave details of a 5-year follow-up study of infants who had had neonatal diarrhea associated with echovirus 18 infection [263]. Thirteen of 16 infants who had had an echovirus 18 infection during the neonatal period showed neurologic damage; these children had an IQ of less than 70, spasticity, deafness, blindness, or a combination of these effects.

In most instances, the antibody response of neonates after enterovirus infection is good. It is to be expected that one attack of infection with a particular viral type provides immunity to the specific agent in the future. From the evidence derived from polio vaccine studies, it is probable that reinfection with all enteroviruses is common, but that after an initial antibody response, a secondary inapparent infection occurs and is confined to the gastrointestinal tract.

THERAPY
SPECIFIC THERAPY

No specific therapy for any enterovirus infection is approved for use in the United States. In severe, catastrophic, and generalized neonatal infection, it is likely that the infant received no specific antibody for the particular virus from the mother. In this situation, it is probably advisable to administer human immune serum globulin to the infant. Dagan and associates [534] examined three lots of human serum globulin and found the presence of neutralizing antibodies to several commonly circulating and infrequently circulating enteroviruses. Although there is no evidence that this therapy is beneficial in treating acute neonatal infections, there is evidence of some success in the treatment of chronic enterovirus infections in agammaglobulinemic patients [535]. Because it was found by Hammond and coworkers [536] that a single dose of intramuscular immunoglobulin resulted in little change in circulating neutralizing antibodies to coxsackievirus B4 and echovirus 11 in seven infants, it seems advisable when therapy is decided on to use high-dose intravenous immunoglobulin. One neonate with disseminated echovirus 11 infection with hepatitis, pneumonitis, meningitis, disseminated intravascular coagulation, decreased renal function, and anemia survived after receiving a large dose of intravenous immunoglobulin and supportive care [537].

Abzug and colleagues [538] performed a small controlled study in which nine enterovirus-infected neonates received intravenous immunoglobulin, and seven similarly infected infants received supportive care. In this study, there was no significant difference in clinical scores, antibody values, or magnitude of viremia and viruria in infants treated compared with the control infants. Five infants received intravenous immunoglobulin with a high neutralizing antibody titer ($\geq$1:800) to their individual viral isolates, however, and they had a more rapid cessation of viremia and viruria.

Jantausch and associates [539] reported an infant with a disseminated echovirus 11 infection who survived after maternal plasma transfusions. The role, if any, of these transfusions in the infant's recovery is unknown, and this form of therapy cannot be recommended. A neonate with fulminant hepatitis caused by echovirus 11 infection survived after orthotopic liver transplantation [540].

Many antipicornavirus drugs and biologicals have been studied during the past 30 years [68,69]. The antiviral drug pleconaril offers promise for the treatment of enterovirus infections.* This drug is a novel compound that integrates into the capsid of enteroviruses. It prevents the virus from attaching to cellular receptors and prevents uncoating and subsequent release of viral RNA into the host cell. In a double-blinded, placebo-controlled study of 39 patients with enterovirus meningitis, a statistically significant shortening of the disease duration was noted from 9.5 days in controls to 4 days in drug recipients [68]. Pleconaril also has been used on a compassionate-release basis in the treatment of patients with life-threatening infection [542]. Several categories of enterovirus illnesses have been treated: chronic meningoencephalitis in patients with agammaglobulinemia or hypogammaglobulinemia, neonatal sepsis, myocarditis, poliomyelitis (wild-type or vaccine associated), encephalitis, and bone marrow transplant patients. Favorable clinical responses were observed in 22 of 36 treated patients, including 12 of 18 patients with chronic meningoencephalitis. In the absence of controls, the extent to which the favorable outcomes can be attributed to pleconaril is unknown. At the present time, pleconaril is unavailable in the United States.

In severe illnesses, such as neonatal myocarditis or encephalitis, it is frequently tempting to administer corticosteroids. Although some investigators thought this approach was beneficial in treating coxsackievirus myocarditis, we believe that corticosteroids should not be given during acute enterovirus infections. The deleterious effects of these agents in coxsackievirus infections of mice [543] are particularly persuasive. Immunosuppressive therapy for myocarditis of unknown origin with prednisone and cyclosporine or azathioprine was evaluated in a controlled trial of 111 adults, and no beneficial effect was observed [544].

Because the possibility of bacterial sepsis cannot be ruled out in most instances of neonatal enterovirus infections, antibiotics should be administered for the most likely potential pathogens. Care in antibiotic selection and administration is urged so that drug toxicity is not added to the problems of the patient. In neonates with meningitis or meningoencephalitis and in some infants with sepsis-like illnesses, the possibility of herpes simplex virus infections should be strongly considered, and empirical treatment with intravenous acyclovir should be instituted after obtaining appropriate herpesvirus studies.

NONSPECIFIC THERAPY
Mild, Nonspecific Febrile Illness

In infants in whom fever is the only symptom, careful observation is most important. Many infants who eventually become severely ill have 2 to 3 days of fever initially without other localized findings. Care should be taken to administer adequate fluids to febrile infants, and excessive elevation of temperature should be prevented, if possible.

Sepsis-like Illness

In infants with severe sepsis-like illness, the major problems are shock, hepatitis and hepatic necrosis, and disseminated intravascular coagulation. For shock, attention should be directed toward treating hypotension and acidosis and ensuring adequate oxygenation.

For hepatitis, oral neomycin (25 mg/kg every 6 hours) or other nonabsorbable antibiotics to suppress intestinal bacterial flora may be helpful. The administration of blood (i.e., exchange transfusion) and vitamin K may be useful when bleeding occurs because of liver dysfunction. Heparin therapy should be considered when disseminated intravascular coagulation occurs.

Myocarditis

There is no specific therapy for myocarditis. Congestive heart failure and arrhythmias should be treated by the usual methods. In administering digitalis preparations to infants with enterovirus myocarditis, careful attention to the initial dosage is most important because the heart is often extremely sensitive; frequently, only small amounts of digoxin are necessary.

Meningoencephalitis

In patients with meningoencephalitis, convulsions, cerebral edema, and disturbances of fluid and electrolyte balance occur frequently and respond to treatment. Seizures are best treated with phenobarbital, phenytoin (Dilantin), or lorazepam. Cerebral edema can be treated with urea, mannitol, or large doses of corticosteroids. It seems unwise to use corticosteroids in active enterovirus infections, however, because the potential benefits may be outweighed by deleterious effects. Fluids should be monitored closely, and serum electrolyte levels should be assessed frequently because inappropriate antidiuretic hormone secretion is common.

Paralytic Poliomyelitis

Infants should be observed carefully for evidence of respiratory paralysis. If respiratory failure occurs, the early use of a positive-pressure ventilator is essential. In newborns, this is better performed without tracheotomy. Careful attention to pooling of secretions is important. Blood gas levels should be monitored frequently. Passive exercises of all involved extremities should be started if the infant has been afebrile for 3 days.

PREVENTION
IMMUNIZATION

Congenital and neonatal poliomyelitis should be illnesses of historical interest only. Because segments of populations in a few regions of the world have not been

---

*References 68,71,441,446,533–535,541.

adequately immunized with poliovirus vaccines, however, clinical poliomyelitis continues to occur. In adequately immunized populations, congenital and neonatal poliomyelitis have been eliminated.

Attenuated viral vaccines for other enteroviruses are unavailable. If a virulent enterovirus type became prevalent, however, it is probable that a specific vaccine for active immunization could be developed.

Passive protection with intramuscular immunoglobulin (0.15 to 0.5 mL/kg) or perhaps intravenous immunoglobulin can be useful in preventing disease [538–540, 545–548]. In practice, this approach seems to be worthwhile only in sudden and virulent nursery outbreaks. If several cases of myocarditis occurred in a nursery, it would seem wise to administer immunoglobulin to all infants in the nursery. Pooled human immunoglobulin in most instances can be expected to contain antibodies against coxsackieviruses B1 through B5 and echovirus 11. This procedure could offer protection to infants without transplacentally acquired specific antibody who had not yet become infected.

OTHER MEASURES

Breast-feeding should be encouraged in all newborns. Sadeharju and associates [546] found that infants exclusively breast-fed for longer than 2 weeks had fewer enterovirus infections by the age of 1 year compared with infants exclusively breast-fed for 2 weeks or less.

Careful attention to routine nursery infection control procedures is important in preventing and controlling epidemics of enterovirus diseases. Nursery personnel should exercise strict care in washing their hands after handling each infant. It is also important to restrict the nursery area to personnel who are free of even minor illnesses. Nursery infection, when it occurs, is best controlled in units that follow a cohort system. When illness occurs, the infant in question should be immediately isolated, and the nursery should be closed to all new admissions.

REFERENCES

[1] D. Bodian, D.M. Horstmann, Polioviruses, Lippincott, Philadelphia, 1965.
[2] J.D. Cherry, D.B. Nelson, Enterovirus infections: their epidemiology and pathogenesis, Clin. Pediatr. 5 (1966) 659.
[3] G. Dalldorf, J.L. Melnick, Coxsackie Viruses, Lippincott, Philadelphia, 1965.
[4] S. Kibrick, Current status of Coxsackie and ECHO viruses in human disease, Prog. Med. Virol. 6 (1964) 27.
[5] J.L. Melnick, Echoviruses, Lippincott, Philadelphia, 1965.
[6] J.D. Cherry, P. Krogstad, Enteroviruses and parechoviruses. In: R. Feigin, J.D. Cherry (Eds.), Textbook of Pediatric Infectious Diseases, sixth ed., Saunders, Philadelphia, 2009.
[7] J.H.S. Gear, V. Measroch, Coxsackievirus infections of the newborn, Prog. Med. Virol. 15 (1973) 42.
[8] N.R. Grist, E.J. Bell, F. Assaad, Enteroviruses in human disease, Prog. Med. Virol. 24 (1978) 114.
[9] J.L. Melnick, Enteroviruses, Plenum Publishing, New York, 1989.
[10] D.M. Morens, R.M. Zweighaft, J.M. Bryan, Nonpolio enterovirus disease in the United States, 1971–1975, Int. J. Epidemiol. 8 (1979) 49.
[11] M.A. Pallansch, R.P. Roos, Enteroviruses: Polioviruses, Coxsackieviruses, Echoviruses, and Newer Enteroviruses, Lippincott Williams & Wilkins, Philadelphia, 2001.
[12] T.F.M. Scott, Clinical syndromes associated with entero virus and REO virus infections, Adv Virus Res. 8 (1961) 165.
[13] G. Stanway, T. Hyypiä, Parechoviruses, J. Virol. 73 (1999) 5249.
[14] H.A. Wenner, A.M. Behbehani, Echoviruses, Springer-Verlag, New York, 1968.
[15] V.R. Racaniello, Picornaviridae: The Viruses and Their Replication, Lippincott Williams & Wilkins, Philadelphia, 2001.
[16] G. Stanway, P. Joki-Korpela, T. Hyypiä, Human parechoviruses—biology and clinical significance, Rev. Med. Virol. 10 (2000) 57.
[17] J.L. Melnick, et al., The enteroviruses, Am. J. Public Health 47 (1957) 1556.
[18] R.J. Blattner, F.M. Heys, Role of viruses in the etiology of congenital malformations, Prog. Med. Virol. 3 (1961) 311.
[19] C.L. Byington, et al., A polymerase chain reaction-based epidemiologic investigation of the incidence of nonpolio enteroviral infections in febrile and afebrile infants 90 days and younger, Pediatrics 103 (1999) E27.
[20] H.F. Eichenwald, G.H. McCracken, S.J. Kindberg, Virus infections of the newborn, Prog. Med. Virol. 9 (1967) 35.
[21] J.B. Hanshaw, J.A. Dudgeon, Viral Diseases of the Fetus and Newborn, Saunders, Philadelphia, 1978.
[22] J.B. Hardy, Viral infection in pregnancy: a review, Am. J. Obstet. Gynecol. 93 (1965) 1052.
[23] J.B. Hardy, Viruses and the fetus, Postgrad. Med. 43 (1968) 156.
[24] D.M. Horstmann, Viral infections in pregnancy, Yale J. Biol. Med. 42 (1969) 99.
[25] M.H. Kaplan, et al., Group B coxsackievirus infections in infants younger than three months of age: a serious childhood illness, Rev. Infect. Dis. 5 (1983) 1019.
[26] S. Kibrick, Viral infections of the fetus and newborn, Perspect. Med. Virol. 2 (1961) 140.
[27] S. Krajden, P.J. Middleton, Enterovirus infections in the neonate, Clin. Pediatr. 22 (1983) 87.
[28] J.F. Modlin, Perinatal echovirus infection: insights from a literature review of 61 cases of serious infection and 16 outbreaks in nurseries, Rev. Infect. Dis. 8 (1986) 918.
[29] G.R.G. Monif, Viral Infections of the Human Fetus, Macmillan, Toronto, 1969.
[30] J.C. Overall Jr., L.A. Glasgow, Virus infections of the fetus and newborn infant, J. Pediatr. 77 (1970) 315.
[31] E.J. Plotz, Virus disease in pregnancy, N. Y. J. Med. 65 (1965) 1239.
[32] S.M. Wang, et al., Fatal coxsackievirus B infection in early infancy characterized by fulminant hepatitis, J. Infect. 37 (1998) 270.
[33] N. Khetsuriani, et al., Neonatal enterovirus infections reported to the national enterovirus surveillance system in the United States, 1983–2003, Pediatr. Infect. Dis. J. 25 (2006) 889–893.
[34] M.A. Verboon-Maciolek, et al., Severe neonatal parechovirus infection and similarity with enterovirus infection, Pediatr. Infect. Dis. J. 27 (2008) 241–245.
[35] K.C. Wolthers, et al., Human parechoviruses as an important viral cause of sepsislike illness and meningitis in young children, Clin. Infect. Dis. 47 (2008) 358–363.
[36] J.R. Paul, A History of Poliomyelitis, Yale University Press, New Haven, CT, 1971.
[37] D.M. Horstmann, The poliomyelitis story: a scientific hegira, Yale. J. Biol. Med. 58 (1985) 79.
[38] J.L. Melnick, Portraits of viruses: the picornaviruses, Intervirology 20 (1983) 61.
[39] M. Underwood, A Treatise on the Diseases of Children, second ed., J Mathews, London, 1789.
[40] I. Wickman, On the epidemiology of Heine-Medin's disease, Rev. Infect. Dis. 2 (1980) 319.
[41] K. Landsteiner, E. Popper, Übertragung der Poliomyelitis acuta auf Affen, Z. Immun. Forsch. 2 (1909) 377.
[42] G. Hannaeus, Dissertation, Copenhagen, (1735).
[43] G. Dalldorf, G.M. Sickles, An unidentified, filtrable agent isolated from the feces of children with paralysis, Science 108 (1948) 61.
[44] J.F. Enders, T.H. Weller, F.C. Robbins, Cultivation of the Lansing strain of poliomyelitis virus in cultures of various human embryonic tissues, Science 109 (1949) 85.
[45] Centers for Disease Control and Prevention, Progress toward global poliomyelitis eradication, 1985-1994, MMWR Morb. Mortal. Wkly Rep. 44 (1995) 273.
[46] World Health Organization, Poliomyelitis, Fact Sheet No. 114, 2003. Available at http://www.who.int/mediacentre/factsheets/fs114/en/print.html.
[47] Centers for Disease Control and Prevention, Progress toward global eradication of poliomyelitis, 2002, MMWR Morb. Mort. Wkly Rep. 52 (2003) 366.
[48] S.L. Cochi, et al., Commentary: the unfolding story of global poliomyelitis eradication, J. Infect. Dis. 175 (1997) S1.
[49] H.F. Hull, et al., Paralytic poliomyelitis: seasoned strategies, disappearing disease, Lancet 343 (1994) 1331.
[50] F.C. Robbins, C.A. de Quadros, Certification of the eradication of indigenous transmission of wild poliovirus in the Americas, J. Infect. Dis. 175 (1997) S281.
[51] M.J. Abzug, M. Loeffelholz, H.A. Rotbart, Clinical and laboratory observations, J. Pediatr. 126 (1995) 447.
[52] L. Andréoletti, et al., Comparison of use of cerebrospinal fluid, serum, and throat swab specimens in the diagnosis of enteroviral acute neurological infection by a rapid RNA detection PCR assay, J. Clin. Microbiol. 36 (1998) 589.

[53] L. Andréoletti, et al., Rapid detection of enterovirus in clinical specimens using PCR and microwell capture hybridization assay, J. Virol. Methods 62 (1996) 1.

[54] H. Ishiko, et al., Molecular diagnosis of human enteroviruses by phylogeny-based classification by use of the VP4 sequence, J. Infect. Dis. 185 (2002) 744.

[55] S.L. Klespies, et al., Detection of enterovirus from clinical specimens by spin amplification shell vial culture and monoclonal antibody assay, J. Clin. Microbiol. 34 (1996) 1465.

[56] B. Lina, et al., Multicenter evaluation of a commercially available PCR assay for diagnosing enterovirus infection in a panel of cerebrospinal fluid specimens, J. Clin. Microbiol. 34 (1996) 3002.

[57] G.S. Marshall, et al., Potential cost savings through rapid diagnosis of enteroviral meningitis, Pediatr. Infect. Dis. J. 16 (1997) 1086.

[58] L.P. Nielsen, J.F. Modlin, H.A. Rotbart, Detection of enteroviruses by polymerase chain reaction in urine samples of patients with aseptic meningitis, Pediatr. Infect. Dis. J. 15 (1996) 125.

[59] M.S. Oberste, et al., Improved molecular identification of enteroviruses by RT-PCR and amplicon sequencing, J. Clin. Virol. 26 (2003) 375.

[60] J.R. Romero, H.A. Rotbart, Sequence diversity among echoviruses with different neurovirulence phenotypes, Pediatr. Res. 33 (1993) 181A.

[61] H.A. Rotbart, Reproducibility of AMPLICOR enterovirus PCR test results, J. Clin. Microbiol. 35 (1997) 3301.

[62] M.H. Sawyer, et al., Diagnosis of enteroviral central nervous system infection by polymerase chain reaction during a large community outbreak, Pediatr. Infect. Dis. J. 13 (1994) 177.

[63] Y. Schlesinger, M.H. Sawyer, G.A. Storch, Enteroviral meningitis in infancy: potential role for polymerase chain reaction in patient management, Pediatrics 94 (1994) 157.

[64] M. Sharland, et al., Enteroviral pharyngitis diagnosed by reverse transcriptase-polymerase chain reaction, Arch. Dis. Child. 74 (1996) 462.

[65] R.E. Tanel, et al., Prospective comparison of culture vs genome detection for diagnosis of enteroviral meningitis in childhood, Arch. Pediatr. Adolesc. Med. 150 (1996) 919.

[66] E. Uchio, et al., Detection of enterovirus 70 by polymerase chain reaction in acute hemorrhagic conjunctivitis, Am. J. Ophthalmol. 122 (1996) 273.

[67] S. Yerly, et al., Rapid and sensitive detection of enteroviruses in specimens from patients with aseptic meningitis, J. Clin. Microbiol. 34 (1996) 199.

[68] H.A. Rotbart, J.F. O'Connel, M.A. McKinlay, Treatment of human enterovirus infections, Antiviral. Res. 38 (1998) 1.

[69] G.D. Diana, D.C. Pevear, Antipicornavirus drugs: current status, Antivir. Chem. Chemother. 8 (1997) 401.

[70] H.A. Rotbart, A.D. Webster, Treatment of potentially life-threatening enterovirus infections with pleconaril, Clin. Infect. Dis. 32 (2001) 228.

[71] R.A. Desmond, et al., Enteroviral meningitis: natural history and outcome of pleconaril therapy, Antimicrob. Agents Chemother. 50 (2006) 2409–2414.

[72] S. Diedrich, G. Driesel, E. Schreier, Sequence comparison of echovirus type 30 isolates to other enteroviruses in the 5vr noncoding region, J. Med. Virol. 46 (1995) 148.

[73] F. Fenner, Classification and nomenclature of viruses: second report of the International Committee on Taxonomy of Viruses, Intervirology 7 (1976) 1.

[74] T. Hyypiä, et al., Classification of enteroviruses based on molecular and biological properties, J. Gen. Virol. 78 (1997) 1.

[75] O.M. Kew, et al., Molecular epidemiology of polioviruses, Virology 6 (1995) 401.

[76] H. Kubo, N. Iritani, Y. Seto, Molecular classification of enteroviruses not identified by neutralization tests, Emerg. Infect. Dis. 8 (2002) 298.

[77] J.L. Melnick, Enteroviruses: polioviruses, coxsackieviruses, echoviruses and newer enteroviruses, in: B.N. Fields, D.M. Knipe (Eds.), Virology, second ed., Raven Press, New York, 1990, pp. 549–605.

[78] J.L. Melnick, My role in the discovery and classification of the enteroviruses, Annu. Rev. Microbiol. 50 (1996) 1–24.

[79] J.L. Melnick, et al., Picornavirus group, Virology 19 (1963) 114–116.

[80] J.L. Melnick, H.A. Wenner, Enteroviruses, American Public Health Association, New York, 1969.

[81] H. Norder, et al., Sequencing of 'untypable' enteroviruses reveals two new types, EV-77 and EV-78, within human enterovirus type B and substitutions in the BC loop of the VP1 protein for known types, J. Gen. Virol. 84 (2003) 827.

[82] T. Pöyry, et al., Molecular analysis of coxsackievirus A16 reveals a new genetic group of enteroviruses, Virology 202 (1994) 962.

[83] T. Pöyry, et al., Genetic and phylogenetic clustering of enteroviruses, J. Gen. Virol. 77 (1996) 1699.

[84] T. Pulli, P. Koskimies, T. Hyypiä, Molecular comparison of coxsackie A virus serotypes, Virology 212 (1995) 30.

[85] R.R. Rueckert, Picornaviridae and Their Replication, Raven Press, New York, 1990.

[86] G. Stanway, et al., Family picornaviridae, in: C.M. Fauquet (Ed.), Virus Taxonomy, Eighth Report of the International Committee on Taxonomy of Viruses, Elsevier/Academic Press, London, 2005, pp. 757–778.

[87] M.S. Oberste, et al., Typing of human enteroviruses by partial sequencing of VP1, J. Clin. Virol. 37 (1999) 1288–1293.

[88] M.S. Oberste, et al., Molecular identification of 13 new enterovirus types, EV79–88, EV97, and EV100–101, members of the species human enterovirus B, Virus. Res. 128 (2007) 34–42.

[89] B. Brown, et al., Complete genomic sequencing shows that polioviruses and members of human enterovirus species C are closely related in the noncapsid coding region, J. Virol. 77 (2003) 8973–8984.

[90] K.S. Benschop, et al., Widespread recombination within human parechoviruses: analysis of temporal dynamics and constraints, J. Gen. Virol. 89 (Pt 4) (2008) 1030–1035.

[91] Y.F. Chan, S. AbuBakar, Recombinant human enterovirus 71 in hand, foot and mouth disease patients, Emerg. Infect. Dis. 10 (2004) 1468–1470.

[92] S. Chevaliez, et al., Molecular comparison of echovirus 11 strains circulating in Europe during an epidemic of multisystem hemorrhagic disease of infants indicates that evolution generally occurs by recombination, Virology 325 (2004) 56–70.

[93] P. Krogstad, et al., Fatal neonatal myocarditis caused by a recombinant human enterovirus-B variant, Pediatr. Infect. Dis. J. 27 (2008) 668–669.

[94] A.N. Lukashev, Role of recombination in evolution of enteroviruses, Rev. Med. Virol. 15 (2005) 157–167.

[95] A.N. Lukashev, et al., Recombination in circulating enteroviruses, J. Virol. 77 (2003) 10423–10431.

[96] A.N. Lukashev, et al., Recombination in circulating human enterovirus B: independent evolution of structural and non-structural genome regions, J. Gen. Virol. 86 (Pt. 12) (2005) 3281–3290.

[97] M.S. Oberste, K. Maher, M.A. Pallansch, Evidence for frequent recombination within species human enterovirus B based on complete genomic sequences of all thirty-seven serotypes, J. Virol. 78 (2004) 855–867.

[98] M.S. Oberste, S. Penaranda, M.A. Pallansch, RNA recombination plays a major role in genomic change during circulation of coxsackie B viruses, J. Virol. 78 (2004) 2948–2955.

[99] C. Badorff, et al., Enteroviral protease 2A cleaves dystrophin: evidence of cytoskeletal disruption in an acquired cardiomyopathy, Nat. Med. 5 (1999) 320–326.

[100] J.R. Doedens, K. Kirkegaard, Inhibition of cellular protein secretion by poliovirus proteins 2B and 3A, Embo. J. 14 (1995) 894–907.

[101] C. Krogerus, et al., Replication complex of human parechovirus 1, J. Virol. 77 (2003) 8512–8523.

[102] G.T. Noordhoek, et al., Clinical validation of a new real-time PCR assay for detection of enteroviruses and parechoviruses, and implications for diagnostic procedures, J. Clin. Virol. 41 (2008) 75–80.

[103] J.R. Romero, Enteroviruses and parechoviruses, in: P.R. Murray (Ed.), Manual of Clinical Microbiology, nineth ed., ASM Press, Washington, DC, 2007, pp. 1392–1404.

[104] A.S. Bryden, Isolation of enteroviruses and adenoviruses in continuous simian cell lines, Med. Lab. Sci. 49 (1992) 60.

[105] J.D. Cherry, et al., Acute hemangiomalike lesions associated with ECHO viral infections, Pediatrics 44 (1969) 498.

[106] M.H. Hatch, G.E. Marchetti, Isolation of echoviruses with human embryonic lung fibroblast cells, Appl. Microbiol. 22 (1971) 736.

[107] A.E. Kelen, J.M. Lesiak, N.A. Labzoffsky, An outbreak of aseptic meningitis due to ECHO 25 virus, Can. Med. Assoc. J. 90 (1964) 1349.

[108] E.J. Bell, B.P. Cosgrove, Routine enterovirus diagnosis in a human rhabdomyosarcoma cell line, Bull. World Health Organ. 58 (1980) 423.

[109] E.C. Herrmann Jr., Experience in providing a viral diagnostic laboratory compatible with medical practice, Mayo Clin. Proc. 42 (1967) 112.

[110] E. Terletskaia-Ladwig, et al., Evaluation of enterovirus serological tests IgM-EIA and complement fixation in patients with meningitis, confirmed by detection of enteroviral RNA by RT-PCR in cerebrospinal fluid, J. Med. Virol. 61 (2000) 221.

[111] E. Terletskaia-Ladwig, et al., A new enzyme immunoassay for the detection of enteroviruses in faecal specimens, J. Med. Virol. 60 (2000) 439.

[112] H.M. Gelfand, The occurrence in nature of the Coxsackie and ECHO viruses, Prog. Med. Virol. 3 (1961) 193.

[113] J.D. Cherry, Enteroviruses and Parechoviruses, Saunders, Philadelphia, 2003.

[114] B.H. Keswick, C.P. Gerba, S.M. Goyal, Occurrence of enteroviruses in community swimming pools, Am. J. Public Health 71 (1981) 1026.

[115] I. Johnson, G.W. Hammond, M.R. Verma, Nosocomial Coxsackie B4 virus infections in two chronic-care pediatric neurological wards, J. Infect. Dis. 151 (1985) 1153.

[116] M.V. Maus, et al., Detection of echovirus 18 in human breast milk, J. Clin. Microbiol. 46 (2008) 1137–1140.

[117] M.L. Chang, et al., Coxsackievirus B3 in human milk, Pediatr. Infect. Dis. J. 25 (2006) 955–957.

[118] T.W. Downey, Polioviruses and flies: studies on the epidemiology of enteroviruses in an urban area, Yale J. Biol. Med. 35 (1963) 341.

[119] J.L. Melnick, et al., Seasonal distribution of Coxsackie viruses in urban sewage and flies, Am. J. Hyg. 59 (1954) 164.

[120] J.L. Melnick, R.P. Dow, Poliomyelitis in Hidalgo County, Texas 1948: poliomyelitis and Coxsackie viruses from flies, Am. J. Hyg. 58 (1953) 288.

[121] P. Horn, Poliomyelitis in pregnancy: a twenty-year report from Los Angeles County, California, Obstet. Gynecol. 6 (1955) 121.

[122] I. Gresser, C. Chany, J.F. Enders, Persistent poliovirus infection of intact human amniotic membrane without apparent cytopathic effect, J. Bacteriol. 89 (1965) 470.

[123] H. Abramson, M. Greenberg, M.C. Magee, Poliomyelitis in the newborn infant, J. Pediatr. 43 (1953) 167.

[124] W.L. Aycock, The frequency of poliomyelitis in pregnancy, N. Engl. J. Med. 225 (1941) 405.

[125] P. Barsky, A.J. Beale, The transplacental transmission of poliomyelitis, J. Pediatr. 51 (1957) 207.

[126] J.L. Baskin, E.H. Soule, S.D. Mills, Poliomyelitis of the newborn: pathologic changes in two cases, Am. J. Dis. Child. 80 (1950) 10.

[127] T. Bates, Poliomyelitis in pregnancy, fetus, and newborn, Am. J. Dis. Child. 90 (1955) 189.

[128] R.J. Blattner, Intrauterine infection with poliovirus, type I, J. Pediatr. 62 (1963) 625.

[129] H.M. Carter, Congenital poliomyelitis, Obstet. Gynecol. 8 (1956) 373.

[130] G.B. Elliott, J.E. McAllister, C. Alberta, Fetal poliomyelitis, Am. J. Obstet. Gynecol. 72 (1956) 896.

[131] A.L. Jackson, J.X. Louw, Poliomyelitis at birth due to transplacental infection, S. Afr. Med. J. 33 (1959) 357.

[132] J.F. Johnson, P.M. Stimson, Clinical poliomyelitis in the early neonatal period, J. Pediatr. 40 (1956) 733.

[133] H. Kreibich, W. Wold, Ueber einen Fall von diaplazenter poliomyelitis Infektion des Feten in 9 Schwangerschaftsmonat, Zentralbl. Gynaekol. 72 (1950) 694.

[134] M. Lance, Paralysie infantile (poliomyelité) constatée des la naissance, Bull. Soc. Pediatr. (Paris) 31 (1933) 2297.

[135] E. Lycke, L.R. Nilsson, Poliomyelitis in a newborn due to intrauterine infection, Acta Paediatr. 51 (1962) 661.

[136] M. Schaeffer, M.J. Fox, C.P. Li, Intrauterine poliomyelitis infection, JAMA 155 (1954) 248.

[137] G. Severin, Case of poliomyelitis in newborn, Nord. Med. 1 (1939) 55.

[138] A. Shelokov, K. Habel, Subclinical poliomyelitis in a newborn infant due to intrauterine infection, JAMA 160 (1956) 465.

[139] A. Shelokov, L. Weinstein, Poliomyelitis in the early neonatal period: report of a case of possible intrauterine infection, J. Pediatr. 38 (1951) 80.

[140] M. Siegel, M. Greenberg, Poliomyelitis in pregnancy: effect on fetus and newborn infant, J. Pediatr. 49 (1956) 280.

[141] C.L. Swarts, E.F. Kercher, A fatal case of poliomyelitis in a newborn infant delivered by cesarean section following maternal death due to poliomyelitis, Pediatrics 14 (1954) 235.

[142] M.B. Wingate, H.K. Meller, G. Ormiston, Acute bulbar poliomyelitis in late pregnancy, BMJ 1 (1961) 407.

[143] J. Winsser, M.L. Pfaff, H.E. Seanor, Poliomyelitis viremia in a newborn infant, Pediatrics 20 (1957) 458.

[144] H.V. Wyatt, Poliomyelitis in the fetus and the newborn: a comment on the new understanding of the pathogenesis, Clin. Pediatr. 18 (1979) 33.

[145] R.J.C. Pearson, D.G. Miller, M.L. Palmier, Reactions to the oral vaccine, Yale J. Biol. Med. 34 (1962) 498.

[146] K.A. Prem, et al., Vaccination of Pregnant Women and Young Infants with Trivalent Oral Attenuated Live Poliomyelitis Vaccine, Pan American Sanitary Bureau, Washington, DC, 1960.

[147] K.A. Prem, J.L. McKelvey, Immunologic Response of Pregnant Women to Oral Trivalent Poliomyelitis Vaccine, Pan American Sanitary Bureau, Washington, DC, 1959.

[148] V.J. Cabasso, et al., Oral poliomyelitis vaccine, Lederle: thirteen years of laboratory and field investigation, N. Engl. J. Med. 263 (1960) 1321.

[149] D.M. Horstmann, Epidemiology of poliomyelitis and allied diseases—1963, Yale J. Biol. Med. 36 (1954) 5.

[150] D.M. Horstmann, et al., Viremia in infants vaccinated with oral poliovirus vaccine (Sabin), Am. J. Hyg. 79 (1964) 47.

[151] S.L. Katz, Efficacy, potential and hazards of vaccines, N. Engl. J. Med. 270 (1964) 884.

[152] H.W. McKay, A.R. Fodor, U.P. Kokko, Viremia following the administration of live poliovirus vaccines, Am. J. Public Health 53 (1963) 274.

[153] J.L. Melnick, et al., Free and bound virus in serum after administration of oral poliovirus vaccine, Am. J. Epidemiol. 84 (1966) 329.

[154] A.M.M. Payne, Summary of the Conference, Pan American Sanitary Bureau, Washington, DC, 1960.

[155] L.R. White, Comment, in: Viral Etiology of Congenital Malformations, May 19-20, 1967, U.S. Government Printing Office, Washington, DC, 1968.

[156] G. Dalldorf, R. Gifford, Susceptibility of gravid mice to Coxsackie virus infection, J. Exp. Med. 99 (1954) 21.

[157] E. Berger, F. Roulet, Beitrage zur Ausscheidung und Tierpathogenität des Coxsackie-virus, Schweiz. Z. Allg. Pathol. 15 (1952) 462.

[158] G. Selzer, Transplacental infection of the mouse fetus by Coxsackie viruses, Isr. J. Med. Sci. 5 (1969) 221.

[159] K. Soike, Coxsackie B-3 virus infection in the pregnant mouse, J. Infect. Dis. 117 (1967) 203.

[160] J.F. Modlin, C.S. Crumpacker, B. Coxsackievirus, infection in pregnant mice and transplacental infection of the fetus, Infect. Immun. 37 (1982) 222.

[161] H. Flamm, Some Considerations Concerning the Pathogenesis of Prenatal Infections, U.S. Government Printing Office, Washington, DC, 1966.

[162] H. Flamm, Untersuchungen über die diaplazentare Übertragung des Coxsackievirus, Schweiz. Z. Allg. Pathol. 18 (1955) 16.

[163] A.L. Palmer, et al., Adverse effects of maternal enterovirus infection on the fetus and placenta, J. Infect. Dis. 176 (1997) 1437.

[164] M.J. Abzug, Maternal factors affecting the integrity of the late gestation placental barrier to murine enterovirus infection, J. Infect. Dis. 176 (1997) 41.

[165] K. Benirschke, Viral Infection of the Placenta, U.S. Government Printing Office, Washington, DC, 1968.

[166] S. Kibrick, K. Benirschke, Acute aseptic myocarditis and meningoencephalitis in the newborn child infected with Coxsackie virus group B, type 3, N. Engl. J. Med. 255 (1956) 883.

[167] V.J. Brightman, et al., An outbreak of Coxsackie B-5 virus infection in a newborn nursery, J. Pediatr. 69 (1966) 179.

[168] A. Konstantinidou, et al., Transplacental infection of coxsackievirus B3 pathological findings in the fetus, J. Med. Virol. 79 (2007) 754–757.

[169] E. Euscher, et al., Coxsackie virus infection of the placenta associated with neurodevelopmental delays in the newborn, Obstet. Gynecol. 98 (2001) 1019–1026.

[170] N.G.S. Basso, et al., Enterovirus isolation from foetal and placental tissues, Acta Virol. 34 (1990) 49.

[171] H.R. Bates, Coxsackie virus B3 calcific pancarditis and hydrops fetalis, Am. J. Obstet. Gynecol. 106 (1970) 629.

[172] J. Bendig, et al., Coxsackievirus B3 sequences in the blood of a neonate with congenital myocarditis, plus serological evidence of maternal infection, J. Med. Virol. 70 (2003) 606.

[173] K. Benirschke, M.E. Pendleton, Coxsackie virus infection: an important complication of pregnancy, Obstet. Gynecol. 12 (1958) 305.

[174] J.D. Cherry, F. Soriano, C.L. Jahn, Search for perinatal viral infection: a prospective, clinical, virologic and serologic study, Am. J. Dis. Child. 116 (1968) 245.

[175] L. Hanson, et al., Clinical and serological observations in cases of Coxsackie B3 infections in early infancy, Acta Paediatr. Scand. 55 (1966) 577.

[176] H. Makower, Z. Skurska, L. Halazinska, On transplacental infection with Coxsackie virus, Texas Rep. Biol. Med. 16 (1958) 346.

[177] D.M. McLean, et al., Coxsackie B5 virus as a cause of neonatal encephalitis and myocarditis, Can. Med. Assoc. J. 85 (1961) 1046.

[178] R.B. Puschak, Coxsackie virus infection in the newborn with case report, Harrisburg Polyclinic Hosp. J. (1962) 14.

[179] G.E. Burch, et al., Interstitial and coxsackievirus B myocarditis in infants and children, JAMA 203 (1968) 1.

[180] H. Plager, R. Beeve, J.K. Miller, Coxsackie B-5 pericarditis in pregnancy, Arch. Intern. Med. 110 (1962) 735.

[181] E. Euscher, et al., Coxsackievirus virus infection of the placenta associated with neurodevelopmental delays in the newborn, Obstet. Gynecol. 98 (2001) 1019.

[182] I. Yoshioka, D.M. Horstmann, Viremia in infection due to ECHO virus type 9, N. Engl. J. Med. 262 (1960) 224.

[183] H. Kleinman, et al., ECHO 9 virus infection and congenital abnormalities: a negative report, Pediatrics 29 (1962) 261.

[184] J.B. Landsman, N.R. Grist, C.A.C. Ross, Echo 9 virus infection and congenital malformations, Br. J. Prev. Soc. Med. 18 (1964) 152.

[185] I. Rantasalo, et al., ECHO 9 virus antibody status after an epidemic period and the possible teratogenic effect of the infection, Ann. Paediatr. Fenn. 6 (1960) 175.

[186] C. Moscovici, J. Maisel, Intestinal viruses of newborn and older prematures, Am. J. Dis. Child. 101 (1961) 771.

[187] H.F. Eichenwald, O. Kostevalov, Immunologic responses of premature and full-term infants to infection with certain viruses, Pediatrics 25 (1960) 829.

[188] S. Berkovich, E.M. Smithwick, Transplacental infection due to ECHO virus type 22, J. Pediatr. 72 (1968) 94.

[189] J.R. Hughes, et al., Echovirus 14 infection associated with fatal neonatal hepatic necrosis, Am. J. Dis. Child. 123 (1972) 61.

[190] K. Chow, et al., Congenital enterovirus 71 infection: a case study with virology and immunochemistry, Clin. Infect. Dis. 31 (2000) 509.

[191] T. Otonkoski, et al., Neonatal type I diabetes associated with maternal echovirus 6 infection: a case report, Diabetologia 43 (2000) 1235.

[192] B. Kleger, Herpes simplex infection of the female genital tract, I. Incidence of infection, Am. J. Obstet. Gynecol. 102 (1968) 745.

[193] R. Montgomery, L. Youngblood, D.N. Medearis Jr., Recovery of cytomegalovirus from the cervix in pregnancy, Pediatrics 49 (1972) 524.

[194] M.P. Reyes, et al., Coxsackievirus-positive cervices in women with febrile illnesses during the third trimester in pregnancy, Am. J. Obstet. Gynecol. 155 (1986) 159.

[195] M.P. Reyes, et al., Disseminated neonatal echovirus 11 disease following antenatal maternal infection with a virus-positive cervix and virus-negative gastrointestinal tract, J. Med. Virol. 12 (1983) 155.

[196] L.L. Cheng, et al., Probable intrafamilial transmission of coxsackievirus b3 with vertical transmission, severe early-onset neonatal hepatitis, and prolonged viral RNA shedding, Pediatrics 118 (2006) e929–e933.

[197] R.M. Cole, et al., Studies of Coxsackie viruses: observations on epidemiologic aspects of group A viruses, Am. J. Public Health 41 (1951) 1342.

[198] M. Ramos-Alvarez, A.B. Sabin, Intestinal viral flora of healthy children demonstrable by monkey kidney tissue culture, Am. J. Public Health 46 (1956) 295.

[199] M. Vandeputte, L'endémicité des virus entériques à Léopoldville, Congo, Bull. WHO/OMS 22 (1960) 313.

[200] S.L. Katz, Case records of the Massachusetts General Hospital. Case 20-1965, N. Engl. J. Med. 272 (1965) 907.

[201] J.A. Jenista, K.R. Powell, M.A. Menegus, Epidemiology of neonatal enterovirus infection, J. Pediatr. 104 (1984) 685.

[202] P. Földes, et al., Vaccination of newborn children with live poliovirus vaccine, Acta Microbiol. Acad. Sci. Hung. 9 (1962) 305.

[203] M. Katz, S.A. Plotkin, Oral polio immunization of the newborn infant: a possible method of overcoming interference by ingested antibodies, J. Pediatr. 73 (1968) 267.

[204] R. Keller, et al., Intestinal IgA neutralizing antibodies in newborn infants following poliovirus immunization, Pediatrics 43 (1969) 330.

[205] M.L. Lepow, et al., Effect of Sabin type 1 poliomyelitis vaccine administered by mouth to newborn infants, N. Engl. J. Med. 264 (1961) 1071.

[206] M.L. Lepow, et al., Sabin type 1 (LSc2ab) oral poliomyelitis vaccine, Am. J. Dis. Child. 104 (1962) 67.

[207] W. Murphy, Response of infants to trivalent poliovirus vaccine (Sabin strains), Pediatrics 40 (1967) 980.

[208] J.S. Pagano, S.A. Plotkin, D. Cornely, The response of premature infants to infection with type 3 attenuated poliovirus, J. Pediatr. 65 (1964) 165.

[209] J.S. Pagano, et al., The response of premature infants to infection with attenuated poliovirus, Pediatrics 29 (1962) 794.

[210] J.S. Pagano, S.A. Plotkin, H. Koprowski, Variations in the response of infants to living attenuated poliovirus vaccines, N. Engl. J. Med. 264 (1961) 155.

[211] S.A. Plotkin, et al., Oral poliovirus vaccination in newborn African infants, Am. J. Dis. Child. 111 (1966) 27.

[212] A.B. Sabin, et al., Effect of oral poliovirus vaccine in newborn children. I. Excretion of virus after ingestion of large doses of type 1 or of mixture of all three types, in relation to level of placentally transmitted antibody, Pediatrics 31 (1963) 623.

[213] A.B. Sabin, et al., Effect of oral poliovirus vaccine in newborn children. II. Intestinal resistance and antibody response at 6 months in children fed type 1 vaccine at birth, Pediatrics 31 (1963) 641.

[214] R.J. Warren, et al., The relationship of maternal antibody, breast feeding, and age to the susceptibility of newborn infants to infection with attenuated polioviruses, Pediatrics 34 (1964) 4.

[215] G.H. Bergeisen, R.J. Bauman, R.L. Gilmore, Neonatal paralytic poliomyelitis: a case report, Arch. Neurol. 43 (1986) 192.

[216] S.N. Javett, et al., Myocarditis in the newborn infant, J. Pediatr. 48 (1956) 1.

[217] A. Kipps, et al., Coxsackie virus myocarditis of the newborn, Med. Proc. 4 (1958) 401.

[218] E. Archibald, D.R. Purdham, Coxsackievirus type A16 infection in a neonate, Arch. Dis. Child. 54 (1979) 649.

[219] M.S. Artenstein, F.C. Cadigan, E.L. Buescher, Epidemic Coxsackie virus infection with mixed clinical manifestations, Ann. Intern. Med. 60 (1964) 196.

[220] N. Butler, et al., Fatal Coxsackie B3 myocarditis in a newborn infant, BMJ 1 (1962) 1251.

[221] J.D. Cherry, C.L. Jahn, Virologic studies of exanthems, J. Pediatr. 68 (1966) 204.

[222] J.D. Cherry, et al., Unpublished data (1962).

[223] T.B. Delaney, F.H. Fakunaga, Myocarditis in a newborn with encephalomeningitis due to Coxsackie virus group B, type 5, N. Engl. J. Med. 259 (1958) 234.

[224] I. Dömök, E. Molnár, An outbreak of meningoencephalomyocarditis among newborn infants during the epidemic of Bornholm disease of 1958 in Hungary, II. Aetiological findings, Ann. Pediatr. 194 (1959) 102.

[225] S. Farber, G.F. Vawter, Clinical pathological conference, J. Pediatr. 62 (1963) 786.

[226] R.E. Fechner, M.G. Smith, J.N. Middelkamp, Coxsackie B virus infection of the newborn, Am. J. Pathol. 42 (1963) 493.

[227] J. Gear, Coxsackie virus infections in Southern Africa, Yale J. Biol. Med. 34 (1961) 289.

[228] J. Gear, V. Measroch, F.R. Prinsloo, The medical and public health importance of the Coxsackie viruses, S. Afr. Med. J. 30 (1956) 806.

[229] J.H.S. Gear, Coxsackie virus infection of the newborn, Prog. Med. Virol. 1 (1958) 106.

[230] D.M. Hosier, W.A. Newton, Serious Coxsackie infection in infants and children, Am. J. Dis. Child. 96 (1958) 251.

[231] R. Hurley, A.P. Norman, J. Pryse-Davies, Massive pulmonary hemorrhage in the newborn associated with Coxsackie B virus infection, BMJ 3 (1969) 636.

[232] M. Isacsohn, et al., Neonatal coxsackievirus group B infections: experience of a single department of neonatology, Isr. J. Med. Sci. 30 (1994) 371.

[233] I. Jack, R.R.W. Townley, Acute myocarditis of newborn infants, due to Coxsackie viruses, Med. J. Aust. 2 (1961) 265.

[234] C.L. Jahn, J.D. Cherry, Mild neonatal illness associated with heavy enterovirus infection, N. Engl. J. Med. 274 (1966) 394.

[235] R.C. Jennings, Coxsackie group B fatal neonatal myocarditis associated with cardiomegaly, J. Clin. Pathol. 19 (1966) 325.

[236] W.R. Johnson, Manifestations of Coxsackie group B infections in children, Del. Med. J. 32 (1960) 72.

[237] S. Kibrick, K. Benirschke, Severe generalized disease (encephalohepatomyocarditis) occurring in the newborn period and due to infection with Coxsackie virus, group B, Pediatrics 22 (1958) 857.

[238] V.F. Koch, G. Enders-Ruckle, E. Wokittel, Coxsackie B5-Infektionen mit signifikanter Antikörperentwicklung bei Neugeborenen, Arch. Kinderheilkd. 165 (1962) 245.

[239] K. Lapinleimu, U. Kaski, An outbreak caused by coxsackievirus B5 among newborn infants, Scand. J. Infect. Dis. 4 (1972) 27.

[240] D.M. McLean, et al., Viral infections of Toronto children during 1965, I. Enteroviral disease, Can. Med. Assoc. J. 94 (1966) 839.

[241] J. Montgomery, et al., Myocarditis of the newborn: an outbreak in a maternity home in Southern Rhodesia associated with Coxsackie group-B virus infection, S. Afr. Med. J. 29 (1955) 608.

[242] J. Moossy, J.C. Geer, Encephalomyelitis, myocarditis and adrenal cortical necrosis in Coxsackie B3 virus infection, Arch. Pathol. 70 (1960) 614.

[243] A.G. Nogen, M.L. Lepow, Enteroviral meningitis in very young infants, Pediatrics 40 (1967) 617.

[244] P. Rantakallio, K. Lapinleimu, R. Mäntyjärvi, Coxsackie B5 outbreak in a newborn nursery with 17 cases of serious meningitis, Scand. J. Infect. Dis. 2 (1970) 17.

[245] G. Rapmund, et al., Neonatal myocarditis and meningoencephalitis due to Coxsackie virus group B, type 4: virologic study of a fatal case with simultaneous aseptic meningitis in the mother, N. Engl. J. Med. 260 (1959) 819.

[246] G. Robino, et al., Fatal neonatal infection due to Coxsackie B2 virus, J. Pediatr. 61 (1962) 911.

[247] O.F. Sieber, et al., Immunological response of the newborn infant to Coxsackie B-4 infection, Pediatrics 40 (1967) 444.

[248] P.V. Suckling, L. Vogelpoel, Coxsackie myocarditis of the newborn, Med. Proc. 4 (1958) 372.

[249] M.L. Sussman, L. Strauss, H.L. Hodes, Fatal Coxsackie group B infection in the newborn, Am. J. Dis. Child. 97 (1959) 483.

[250] L. Tuuteri, K. Lapinleimu, L. Meurman, Fatal myocarditis associated with Coxsackie B3 infection in the newborn, Ann. Paediat. Fenn. 9 (1963) 56.

[251] S. Van Creveld, H. De Jager, Myocarditis in newborns, caused by Coxsackie virus: clinical and pathological data, Ann. Pediatr. 187 (1956) 100.

[252] J.D. Verlinde, H.A.E. Van Tongeren, A. Kret, Myocarditis in newborns due to group B Coxsackie virus: virus studies, Ann. Pediatr. 187 (1956) 113.

[253] N. Volakova, L. Jandasek, Epidemic of myocarditis in newborn infants caused by Coxsackie B1 virus, Cesk. Epidemiol. 13 (1963) 88.

[254] J. Winsser, R.H. Altieri, A three-year study of Coxsackie virus, group B, infection in Nassau County, Am. J. Med. Sci. 247 (1964) 269.

[255] T.E. Woodward, et al., Viral and rickettsial causes of cardiac disease, including the Coxsackie virus etiology of pericarditis and myocarditis, Ann. Intern. Med. 53 (1960) 1130.

[256] H.T. Wright Jr., K. Okuyama, R.M. McAllister, An infant fatality associated with Coxsackie B1 virus, J. Pediatr. 63 (1963) 428.

[257] P.T. Swender, R.J. Shott, M.L. Williams, A community and intensive care nursery outbreak of coxsackievirus B5 meningitis, Am. J. Dis. Child. 127 (1974) 42.

[258] S. Berkovich, S. Kibrick, ECHO 11 outbreak in newborn infants and mothers, Pediatrics 33 (1964) 534.

[259] S. Berkovich, J. Pangan, Recoveries of virus from premature infants during outbreaks of respiratory disease: the relation of ECHO virus type 22 to disease of the upper and lower respiratory tract in the premature infant, Bull. N. Y. Acad. Med. 44 (1968) 377.

[260] J. Butterfield, et al., Cystic emphysema in premature infants: a report of an outbreak with the isolation of type 19 ECHO virus in one case, N. Engl. J. Med. 268 (1963) 18.

[261] H.G. Cramblett, et al., Nosocomial infection with echovirus type 11 in handicapped and premature infants, Pediatrics 51 (1973) 603.

[262] D.P. Davies, et al., Echovirus-11 infection in a special-care baby unit, Lancet 1 (1979) 96.

[263] H.F. Eichenwald, et al., Epidemic diarrhea in premature and older infants caused by ECHO virus type 18, JAMA 166 (1958) 1563.

[264] H.F. Eichenwald, O. Kostevalov, L.A. Fasso, The "cloud baby": an example of bacterial-viral interaction, Am. J. Dis. Child. 100 (1960) 161.

[265] R.S. Faulkner, C.E. van Rooyen, Echovirus type 17 in the neonate, Can. Med. Assoc. J. 108 (1973) 878.

[266] L.J. German, A.W. McCracken, K.M. Wilkie, Outbreak of febrile illness associated with ECHO virus type 5 in a maternity unit in Singapore, BMJ 1 (1968) 742.

[267] E.W. Hart, et al., Infection of newborn babies with ECHO virus type 5, Lancet 2 (1962) 402.

[268] A. Hasegawa, Virologic and serologic studies on an outbreak of echovirus type 11 infection in a hospital maternity unit, Jpn. J. Med. Sci. Biol. 28 (1975) 179.

[269] L. Hercík, et al., Epidemien der Respirationstrakterkrankunger bei Neugeborenen durch ECHO 11-Virus, Zentrabl. Bakteriol. 213 (1970) 18.

[270] I. Jack, et al., A survey of prenatal virus disease in Melbourne. Personal communication, July (1967) 21.

[271] J.G. Kapsenberg, ECHO virus type 33 as a cause of meningitis, Arch. Gesamte Virusforsch. 23 (1968) 144.

[272] J.S. Kinney, et al., Risk factors associated with echovirus 11 infection in a hospital nursery, Pediatr. Infect. Dis. 5 (1986) 192.

[273] K. Lapinleimu, A. Hakulinen, A hospital outbreak caused by ECHO virus type 11 among newborn infants, Ann. Clin. Res. 4 (1972) 183.

[274] L.L. McDonald, St. Geme JW, Arnold BH. Nosocomial infection with ECHO virus type 31 in a neonatal intensive care unit, Pediatrics 47 (1971) 995.

[275] T. Mertens, H. Hager, H.J. Eggers, Epidemiology of an outbreak in a maternity unit of infections with an antigenic variant of echovirus 11, J. Med. Virol. 9 (1982) 81.

[276] D.G. Miller, et al., An epidemic of aseptic meningitis, primarily among infants, caused by echovirus 11-prime, Pediatrics 41 (1968) 77.

[277] J.F. Modlin, Fatal echovirus 11 disease in premature neonates, Pediatrics 66 (1980) 775.

[278] J.F. Modlin, Echovirus infections of newborn infants, Pediatr. Infect. Dis. 7 (1988) 311.

[279] J. Nagington, et al., Fatal echovirus 11 infections in outbreak in special-care baby unit, Lancet 2 (1978) 725.

[280] T. Nakao, R. Miura, M. Sato, ECHO virus type 22 in a premature infant, Tohoku, J. Exp. Med. 102 (1970) 61.

[281] D.R. Purdham, et al., Severe ECHO 19 virus infection in a neonatal unit, Arch. Dis. Child. 51 (1976) 634.

[282] C.S. Rabkin, et al., Outbreak of echovirus 11 infection in hospitalized neonates, Pediatr. Infect. Dis. J. 7 (1988) 186.

[283] D.Y. Sanders, H.G. Cramblett, Viral infections in hospitalized neonates, Am. J. Dis. Child. 116 (1968) 251.

[284] J. Steinmann, K. Albrecht, Echovirus 11 epidemic among premature newborns in a neonatal intensive care unit, Zentralbl. Bakteriol. Mikrobiol. Hyg. 259 (1985) 284.

[285] C.W. Wilson, D.K. Stevenson, A.M. Arvin, A concurrent epidemic of respiratory syncytial virus and echovirus 7 infections in an intensive care nursery, Pediatr. Infect. Dis. J. 8 (1989) 24.

[286] T.G. Wreghitt, et al., Fatal echovirus 7 infection during an outbreak in a special care baby unit, J. Infect. 19 (1989) 229.

[287] K. Sato, et al., A new-born baby outbreak of echovirus type 33 infection, J. Infect. 37 (1998) 123.

[288] J.D. Verlinde, J. Versteeg, H. Beeuwkes, Mogelijkheid van een besmetting van de mens door varkens lijdende aan een Coxsackievirus pneumonie, Ned. Tijdschr. Geneeskd. 102 (1958) 1445.

[289] C. Moscovici, et al., Virus 1956 R.C., Ann. Ist. Super. Sanita. 20 (1957) 1137.

[290] D.L. Lundgren, W.E. Clapper, A. Sanchez, Isolation of human enteroviruses from beagle dogs, Proc. Soc. Exp. Biol. Med. 128 (1968) 463.

[291] D.L. Lundgren, et al., A survey for human enteroviruses in dogs and man, Arch. Gesamte. Virusforsch. 32 (1970) 229.

[292] H. Koprowski, Counterparts of human viral disease in animals, Ann. N. Y. Acad. Sci. 70 (1958) 369.

[293] R.G. Sommerville, I. Type, poliovirus isolated from a budgerigar, Lancet 1 (1959) 495.

[294] H. Makower, Z. Skurska, Badania nad wirusami Coxsackie, Doniesienie III. Izolacja wirusa Coxsackie z mózgu lisa, Arch. Immunol. Ter. Dosw. 5 (1957) 219.

[295] M. Bendinelli, A. Ruschi, Isolation of human enterovirus from mussels, Appl. Microbiol. 18 (1969) 531.

[296] T.G. Metcalf, W.C. Stiles, Enterovirus within an estuarine environment, Am. J. Epidemiol. 88 (1968) 379.

[297] D.M. Horstmann, E.E. Manuelidis, Russian Coxsackie A-7 virus ("AB IV" strain)—neuropathogenicity and comparison with poliovirus, J. Immunol. 81 (1958) 32.

[298] P. Bartell, M. Klein, Neutralizing antibody to viruses of poliomyelitis in sera of domestic animals, Proc. Soc. Exp. Biol. Med. 90 (1955) 597.

[299] J.A. Morris, J.R. O'Connor, Neutralization of the viruses of the Coxsackie group by sera of wild rabbits, Cornell Vet. 42 (1952) 56.

[300] P.W. Chang, et al., Multiplication of human enteroviruses in northern quahogs, Proc. Soc. Exp. Biol. Med. 136 (1971) 1380.

[301] T.G. Metcalf, W.C. Stiles, Accumulation of enteric viruses by the oyster, Crassostrea. virginica, J. Infect. Dis. 115 (1965) 68.

[302] R.P. Atwood, J.D. Cherry, J.O. Klein, Clams and viruses, Hepat. Surveill. Rep. 20 (1964) 26.

[303] M.F. Duff, The uptake of enteroviruses by the New Zealand marine blue mussel *Mytilus edulis aoteanus*, Am. J. Epidemiol. 85 (1967) 486.

[304] O.C. Liu, H.R. Seraichekas, B.L. Murphy, Viral depuration of the Northern quahaug, Appl. Microbiol. 15 (1967) 307.

[305] R.K. Lynt, Survival and recovery of enterovirus from foods, Appl. Microbiol. 14 (1966) 218.

[306] S.S. Kalter, A serological survey of antibodies to selected enteroviruses, Bull. World Health Organ. 26 (1962) 759.

[307] Centers for Disease Control, Enterovirus Surveillance, Summary 1970-1979, (1981) November.

[308] D. Bodian, D.M. Horstmann, Poliomyelitis, Lippincott, Philadelphia, 1965.

[309] F. Assaad, K. Ljungars-Esteves, World overview of poliomyelitis: regional patterns and trends, Rev. Infect. Dis. 6 (1984) S302.

[310] C.A. Phillips, et al., Enteroviruses in Vermont, 1969–1978: an important cause of illness throughout the year, J. Infect. Dis. 141 (1980) 162.

[311] M.A. Drebit, et al., Molecular epidemiology of enterovirus outbreaks in Canada during 1991–1992: identification of echovirus 30 and coxsackievirus B1 strains by amplicon sequencing, J. Med. Virol. 44 (1994) 340.

[312] H. Ishiko, et al., Phylogenetic analysis of a coxsackievirus A24 variant: the most recent worldwide pandemic was caused by progenies of a virus prevalent around 1981, Virology 187 (1992) 748.

[313] K.H. Lin, et al., Molecular epidemiology of a variant of coxsackievirus A24 in Taiwan: two epidemics caused by phylogenetically distinct viruses from 1985 to 1989, J. Clin. Microbiol. 31 (1993) 1160.

[314] M.N. Mulders, et al., Molecular epidemiology of wild poliovirus type 1 in Europe, the Middle East, and the Indian subcontinent, J. Infect. Dis. 171 (1995) 1399.

[315] Increased detections and severe neonatal disease associated with coxsackievirus B1 infection—United States, 2007, MMWR Morb. Mortal. Wkly Rep. 57 (2008) 553–556.

[316] Enterovirus surveillance—United States, 1985, MMWR Morb. Mortal. Wkly Rep. 34 (1985) 494–495.

[317] From the Centers for Disease Control and Prevention, Nonpolio enterovirus surveillance—United States, 1993-1996, JAMA 278 (1997) 975.

[318] Enterovirus surveillance—United States, 1997–1999, MMWR Morb. Mortal. Wkly Rep. 49 (2000) 913–916.

[319] Enterovirus surveillance—United States, 2000-2001, MMWR Morb. Mortal. Wkly Rep. 51 (2002) 1047–1049.

[320] Enterovirus surveillance—United States, 2002-2004, MMWR Morb. Mortal. Wkly Rep. 55 (2006) 153–156.

[321] J.P. Alexander, L.J. Anderson, Respiratory and Enterovirus Branch, Centers for Disease Control and Prevention, Personal communication (1990).

[322] H. Gary, Respiratory and Enteric Viruses Branch, Centers for Disease Control and Prevention, Personal communication (1996).

[323] R.A. Strikas, L.J. Anderson, R.A. Parker, Temporal and geographic patterns of isolates of nonpolio enterovirus in the United States, 1970–1983, J. Infect. Dis. 153 (1986) 346.

[324] E. Druyts-Voets, Epidemiological features of entero non-poliovirus isolations in Belgium 1980–94, Epidemiol. Infect. 119 (1997) 71.

[325] G. Trallero, et al., Enteroviruses in Spain: virological and epidemiological studies over 10 years (1988–97), Epidemiol. Infect. 124 (2000) 497.

[326] B.A. Brown, et al., Molecular epidemiology and evolution of enterovirus 71 strains isolated from 1970 to 1998, J. Virol. 73 (1999) 9969.

[327] L.G. Chan, et al., Deaths of children during an outbreak of hand, foot, and mouth disease in Sarawak, Malaysia: clinical and pathological characteristics of the disease, Clin. Infect. Dis. 31 (2000) 678.

[328] M. Ho, et al., An epidemic of enterovirus 71 infection in Taiwan, N. Engl. J. Med. 341 (1999) 929.

[329] H. Komatsu, et al., Outbreak of severe neurologic involvement associated with enterovirus 71 infection, Pediatr. Neurol. 20 (1999) 17.

[330] Center for Disease Control, Neurotropic Diseases Surveillance, No. 3. Annual Summary, U.S. Department of Health, Education, and Welfare, Washington, DC, 1970.

[331] Communicable Disease Center, Poliomyelitis Surveillance, No. 274, U.S. Department of Health, Education, and Welfare, Washington, DC, 1963.

[332] D.B. Horstmann, et al., Enterovirus surveillance following a community-wide oral poliovirus vaccination program: a seven-year study, Am. J. Epidemiol. 97 (1973) 173.

[333] G. Batcup, et al., Placental and fetal pathology in coxsackie virus A9 infection: a case report, Histopathology 9 (1985) 1227.

[334] A.I. Ramsingh, D.N. Collins, A point mutation in the VP4 coding sequence of coxsackievirus B4 influences virulence, J. Virol. 69 (1995) 7278.

[335] J.E. Rinehart, R.M. Gomez, R.P. Roos, Molecular determinants for virulence in coxsackievirus B1 infection, J. Virol. 71 (1997) 3986.

[336] H. Heineberg, E. Gold, F.C. Robbins, Differences in interferon content in tissues of mice of various ages infected with coxsackie B1 virus, Proc. Soc. Exp. Biol. Med. 115 (1964) 947.

[337] O. Levy, Innate immunity of the newborn: basic mechanisms and clinical correlates, Nat. Rev. Immunol. 7 (2007) 379–390.

[338] A.M. Behbehani, S.E. Sulkin, C. Wallis, Factors influencing susceptibility of mice to coxsackie virus infection, J. Infect. Dis. 110 (1962) 147.

[339] W.D. Boring, D.M. Angevine, D.L. Walker, Factors influencing host-virus interactions. I. A comparison of viral multiplication and histopathology in infant, adult, and cortisone-treated adult mice infected with the Conn-5 strain of coxsackie virus, J. Exp. Med. 102 (1955) 753.

[340] C.W. Kunin, Cellular susceptibility to enteroviruses, Bacteriol. Rev. 28 (1964) 382.

[341] C.M. Kunin, Virus-tissue union and the pathogenesis of enterovirus infections, J. Immunol. 88 (1962) 556.

[342] M. Ito, et al., Expression of coxsackievirus and adenovirus receptor in hearts of rats with experimental autoimmune myocarditis, Circ. Res. 86 (2000) 275–280.

[343] B. Teisner, S. Haahr, Poikilothermia and susceptibility of suckling mice to coxsackie B1 virus, Nature 247 (1974) 568.

[344] B.M. McManus, et al., Direct myocardial injury by enterovirus: a central role in the evolution of murine myocarditis, Clin. Immunol. Immunopath. 68 (1993) 159.

[345] A. Arola, et al., Experimental myocarditis induced by two different coxsackievirus B3 variants: aspects of pathogenesis and comparison of diagnostic methods, J. Med. Virol. 47 (1995) 251.

[346] W. Chehadeh, et al., Increased level of interferon-alpha in blood of patients with insulin-dependent diabetes mellitus: relationship with coxsackievirus B infection, J. Infect. Dis. 181 (2000) 1929.

[347] C.J. Gauntt, et al., Molecular mimicry, anti-coxsackievirus B3 neutralizing monoclonal antibodies, and myocarditis, J. Immunol. 154 (1995) 2983.

[348] C.J. Gauntt, et al., Epitopes shared between coxsackievirus B3 (CVB3) and normal heart tissue contribute to CVB3-induced murine myocarditis, Clin. Immunol. Immunopath. 68 (1993) 129.

[349] A. Herskowitz, et al., Coxsackievirus B3 murine myocarditis: wide pathologic spectrum in genetically defined inbred strains, Hum. Pathol. 16 (1985) 671.

[350] D.M. Hosier, W.A. Newton Jr., Serious coxsackie infection in infants and children: myocarditis, meningoencephalitis, and hepatitis, Am. J. Dis. Child. 96 (1958) 251.

[351] S. Juhela, et al., T-cell responses to enterovirus antigens in children with type 1 diabetes, Diabetes 49 (2000) 1308.

[352] R.E. Pague, Role of anti-idiotypic antibodies in induction, regulation, and expression of coxsackievirus-induced myocarditis, Prog. Med. Virol. 39 (1992) 204.

[353] I. Rabausch-Starz, et al., Persistence of virus and viral genome in myocardium after coxsackievirus B3-induced murine myocarditis, Clin. Exp. Immunol. 96 (1994) 69.

[354] Y. Seko, et al., Restricted usage of T-cell receptor Va genes in infiltrating cells in murine hearts with acute myocarditis caused by coxsackie virus B3, J. Pathol. 178 (1996) 330.

[355] L. Philipson, Association between a recently isolated virus and an epidemic of upper respiratory disease in a day nursery, Arch. Gesamte Virusforsch. 8 (1958) 204–215.

[356] J.D. Cherry, et al., Echo 11 virus infections associated with exanthems, Pediatrics 32 (1963) 509–516.

[357] P.J. Berry, J. Nagington, Fatal infection with echovirus 11, Arch. Dis. Child. 57 (1982) 22.

[358] C.L. Bose, et al., Dissimilar manifestations of intrauterine infection with echovirus 11 in premature twins, Arch. Pathol. Lab. Med. 107 (1983) 361.

[359] M.M. Gh, et al., Postmortem manifestations of echovirus 11 sepsis in five newborn infants, Hum. Pathol. 14 (1983) 818.

[360] N. Gitlin, et al., Fulminant neonatal hepatic necrosis associated with echovirus type 11 infection, West. J. Med. 138 (1983) 260.

[361] N. Halfon, S.A. Spector, Fatal echovirus type 11 infections, Am. J. Dis. Child. 135 (1981) 1017.

[362] M.J. Jones, et al., Intrauterine echovirus type 11 infection, Mayo Clin. Proc. 55 (1980) 509.

[363] H.F. Krous, D. Dietzman, C.G. Ray, Fatal infections with echovirus types 6 and 11 in early infancy, Am. J. Dis. Child. 126 (1973) 842.

[364] J. Wang, et al., Echovirus hepatic failure in infancy: report of four cases with speculation on the pathogenesis, Pediatr. Dev. Pathol. 4 (2001) 454.

[365] M.L. Kennett, et al., Enterovirus type 71 infection in Melbourne, Bull. World Health Organ. 51 (1974) 609–615.

[366] N.J. Schmidt, E.H. Lennette, H.H. Ho, An apparently new enterovirus isolated from patients with disease of the central nervous system, J. Infect. Dis. 129 (1974) 304.

[367] M.J. Cardosa, et al., Molecular epidemiology of human enterovirus 71 strains and recent outbreaks in the Asia-Pacific region: comparative analysis of the VP1 and VP4 genes, Emerg. Infect. Dis. 9 (2003) 461–468.

[368] K.P. Chan, et al., Epidemic hand, foot and mouth disease caused by human enterovirus 71, Singapore, Emerg. Infect. Dis. 9 (2003) 78–85.

[369] L.G. Chan, et al., Deaths of children during an outbreak of hand, foot, and mouth disease in sarawak, malaysia: clinical and pathological characteristics of the disease, For the Outbreak Study Group, Clin. Infect. Dis. 31 (2000) 678–683.

[370] L.Y. Chang, et al., Transmission and clinical features of enterovirus 71 infections in household contacts in Taiwan, JAMA 291 (2004) 222–227.

[371] C.Y. Chong, et al., Hand, foot and mouth disease in Singapore: a comparison of fatal and non-fatal cases, Acta Paediatr. 92 (2003) 1163–1169.

[372] M. Hosoya, et al., Genetic diversity of enterovirus 71 associated with hand, foot and mouth disease epidemics in Japan from 1983 to 2003, Pediatr. Infect. Dis. J. 25 (2006) 691–694.

[373] C.C. Li, et al., Clinical manifestations and laboratory assessment in an enterovirus 71 outbreak in southern Taiwan, Scand. J. Infect. Dis. 34 (2002) 104–109.

[374] C.Y. Lu, et al., Incidence and case-fatality rates resulting from the 1998 enterovirus 71 outbreak in Taiwan, J. Med. Virol. 67 (2002) 217–223.

[375] O. Kew, et al., Outbreak of poliomyelitis in Hispaniola associated with circulating type 1 vaccine-derived poliovirus, Science 296 (2002) 356–359.

[376] J. Santti, et al., Evidence of recombination among enteroviruses, J. Virol. 73 (1999) 8741–8749.

[377] P. Simmonds, J. Welch, Frequency and dynamics of recombination within different species of human enteroviruses, J. Virol. 80 (2006) 483–493.

[378] D.A. Baker, C.A. Phillips, Maternal and neonatal infection with coxsackievirus, Obstet. Gynecol. 55 (1980) 12S.

[379] P.C. Balduzzi, R.M. Greendyke, Sudden unexpected death in infancy and viral infection, Pediatrics 38 (1966) 201.

[380] E. Gold, et al., Viral infection: a possible cause of sudden, unexpected death in infants, N. Engl. J. Med. 264 (1961) 53.

[381] M. Eisenhut, et al., Fatal coxsackie A9 virus infection during an outbreak in a neonatal unit, J. Infect. 40 (2000) 297.

[382] O. Konen, et al., Progressive liver calcifications in neonatal coxsackievirus infection, Pediatr. Radiol. 30 (2000) 343.

[383] F.F. Piraino, G. Sedmak, K. Raab, Echovirus 11 infections of newborns with mortality during the 1979 enterovirus season in Milwaukee, Wisc, Public Health Rep. 97 (1982) 346.

[384] M. Chambon, et al., Fatal hepatitis necrosis in a neonate with echovirus 20 infection: use of the polymerase chain reaction to detect enterovirus in the liver tissue, Clin. Infect. Dis. 24 (1997) 523.

[385] M.K. Georgieff, et al., Fulminant hepatic necrosis in an infant with perinatally acquired echovirus 21 infection, Pediatr. Infect. Dis. 6 (1987) 71.

[386] A.G.S. Philip, E.J. Larson, Overwhelming neonatal infection with ECHO 19 virus, J. Pediatr. 82 (1973) 391.

[387] W.E. Rawls, R.G. Shorter, E.C. Herrmann Jr., Fatal neonatal illness associated with ECHO 9 (coxsackie A-23) virus, Pediatrics 33 (1964) 278.

[388] K. Ventura, et al., Fatal neonatal echovirus 6 infection: autopsy case report and review of the literature, Mod. Pathol. 14 (2001) 85.

[389] T.G. Wreghitt, et al., Fatal neonatal echo 7 virus infection, Lancet 2 (1984) 465.

[390] S.H. Cheeseman, et al., Fatal neonatal pneumonia caused by echovirus type 9, Am. J. Dis. Child. 131 (1977) 1169.

[391] M.T. Boyd, S.W. Jordan, L.E. Davis, Fatal pneumonitis from congenital echovirus type 6 infection, Pediatr. Infect. Dis. J. 6 (1987) 1138.

[392] A. Willems, et al., Fatal illness associated with pulmonary hypertension in a neonate caused by intrauterine echovirus 11 infection, Am. J. Perinatol. 23 (2006) 59–61.

[393] G.W. Anderson, et al., Poliomyelitis in pregnancy, Am. J. Hyg. 55 (1952) 127.

[394] W.L. Aycock, T.H. Ingalls, Maternal disease as a principle in the epidemiology of congenital anomalies, Am. J. Med. Sci. 212 (1946) 366.

[395] V.M. Bowers Jr., D.N. Danforth, The significance of poliomyelitis during pregnancy—an analysis of the literature and presentation of twenty-four new cases, Am. J. Obstet. Gynecol. 65 (1953) 34.

[396] J. Schaefer, E.B. Shaw, Poliomyelitis in pregnancy, Calif. Med. 70 (1949) 16.

[397] B.M. Kaye, D.C. Rosner, I. Stein Sr., Viral diseases in pregnancy and their effect upon the embryo and fetus, Am. J. Obstet. Gynecol. 65 (1953) 109.

[398] T. Harjulehto-Mervaala, et al., Oral polio vaccination during pregnancy: lack of impact on fetal development and perinatal outcome, Clin. Infect. Dis. 18 (1994) 414.

[399] G. Frisk, H. Diderholm, Increased frequency of coxsackie B virus IgM in women with spontaneous abortion, J. Infect. 24 (1992) 141.

[400] C. Axelsson, et al., Coxsackie B virus infections in women with miscarriage, J. Med. Virol. 39 (1993) 282.

[401] H.W. Berendes, et al., The NIH collaborative study. A progress report, Presented at Third International Conference on Congenital Malformations, The Hague, Netherlands, 1969.

[402] News and Notes, Polio vaccine and congenital defects, BMJ 1 (1967) 510.

[403] J.P. Connelly, et al., Viral and drug hazards in pregnancy, Clin. Pediatr. 3 (1964) 587.

[404] T. Harjulehto, et al., Congenital malformations and oral poliovirus vaccination during pregnancy, Lancet 1 (1989) 771.

[405] G.C. Brown, Maternal virus infection and congenital anomalies, Arch. Environ. Health 21 (1970) 362.

[406] G.C. Brown, Recent advances in the viral aetiology of congenital anomalies, Adv. Teratol. 1 (1966) 55.

[407] G.C. Brown, Coxsackie virus infections and heart disease, Am. Heart J. 75 (1968) 145.

[408] T.N. Evans, G.C. Brown, Congenital anomalies and virus infections, Am. J. Obstet. Gynecol. 87 (1963) 749.

[409] G.C. Brown, T.N. Evans, Serologic evidence of coxsackievirus etiology of congenital heart disease, JAMA 199 (1967) 183.

[410] G.C. Brown, R.S. Karunas, Relationship of congenital anomalies and maternal infection with selected enteroviruses, Am. J. Epidemiol. 95 (1972) 207.

[411] T.S. Elizan, et al., Viral infection in pregnancy and congenital CNS malformations in man, Arch. Neurol. 20 (1969) 115.

[412] C.J. Gauntt, et al., Coxsackievirus group B antibodies in the ventricular fluid of infants with severe anatomic defects in the central nervous system, Pediatrics 76 (1985) 64.

[413] W.L. Aycock, Acute poliomyelitis in pregnancy: its occurrence according to month of pregnancy and sex of fetus, N. Engl. J. Med. 235 (1946) 160.

[414] A. Ouellet, et al., Antenatal diagnosis of intrauterine infection with coxsackievirus B3 associated with live birth, Infect. Dis. Obstet. Gynecol. 12 (2004) 23–26.

[415] P.S. Freedman, Echovirus 11 infection and intrauterine death, Lancet 1 (1979) 96.

[416] J.L. Nielsen, G.K. Berryman, G.D. Hankins, Intrauterine fetal death and the isolation of echovirus 27 from amniotic fluid, J. Infect. Dis. 158 (1988) 501.

[417] L.L. Barton, Febrile neonatal illness associated with echo virus type 5 in the cerebrospinal fluid, Clin. Pediatr. 16 (1977) 383.

[418] M.L. Estes, L.B. Rorke, Liquefactive necrosis in coxsackie B encephalitis, Arch. Pathol. Lab. Med. 110 (1986) 1090.

[419] K. Farmer, P.T. Patten, An outbreak of coxsackie B5 infection in a special care unit for newborn infants, N. Z. Med. J. 68 (1968) 86.

[420] D.M. Morens, Enteroviral disease in early infancy, J. Pediatr. 92 (1978) 374.

[421] News and Notes, Coxsackie B virus infections in 1971, BMJ 1 (1972) 453.

[422] S. Bina Rai, et al., An outbreak of echovirus 11 amongst neonates in a confinement home in Penang, Malaysia, Med. J. Malaysia 62 (2007) 223–226.

[423] T. Eilard, et al., An outbreak of coxsackie virus type B2 among neonates in an obstetrical ward, Acta Paediatr. Scand. 63 (1974) 103.

[424] K.S. Benschop, et al., Fourth human parechovirus serotype, Emerg. Infect. Dis. 12 (2006) 1572–1575.

[425] J.P. Fox, Epidemiological aspects of coxsackie and ECHO virus infections in tropical areas, Am. J. Public Health 54 (1964) 1134.

[426] V. Barre, et al., Enterovirus-associated haemophagocytic syndrome in a neonate, Acta Paediatr. 87 (1998) 467.

[427] A.M. Lake, et al., Enterovirus infections in neonates, J. Pediatr. 89 (1976) 787.

[428] C.J. Bacon, D.G. Sims, Echovirus 19 infection in infants under six months, Arch. Dis. Child. 51 (1976) 631.

[429] K.S. Benschop, et al., Human parechovirus infections in Dutch children and the association between serotype and disease severity, Clin. Infect. Dis. 42 (2006) 204–210.

[430] G. Boivin, Y. Abed, F.D. Boucher, Human parechovirus 3 and neonatal infections, Emerg. Infect. Dis. 11 (2005) 103–105.

[431] C.A. Chen, et al., Severe echovirus 30 infection in twin neonates, J. Formos. Med. Assoc. 102 (2003) 59–61.

[432] J.H. Chen, et al., A neonatal echovirus 11 outbreak in an obstetric clinic, J. Microbiol. Immunol. Infect. 38 (2005) 332–337.

[433] C.T. Cho, J.G. Janelle, A. Behbehani, Severe neonatal illness associated with ECHO 9 virus infection, Clin. Pediatr. 12 (1973) 304.

[434] A.A. Codd, et al., Epidemic of echovirus 19 in the northeast of England, J. Hyg. (Lond.) 76 (1976) 307.

[435] M. Grossman, P. Azimi, Fever, hepatitis and coagulopathy in a newborn infant, Pediatr. Infect. Dis. J. 11 (1992) 1069.

[436] C.B. Hall, et al., The return of Boston exanthem, Am. J. Dis. Child. 131 (1977) 323.

[437] C.C. Linnemann Jr., et al., Febrile illness in early infancy associated with ECHO virus infection, J. Pediatr. 84 (1974) 49.

[438] R. Marier, et al., Coxsackievirus B5 infection and aseptic meningitis in neonates and children, Am. J. Dis. Child. 129 (1975) 321.

[439] R.M. Pino-Ramirez, et al., Neonatal echovirus 30 infection associated with severe hepatitis in twin neonates, Pediatr. Infect. Dis. J. 27 (2008) 88.

[440] J.W. Tang, J.W. Bendig, I. Ossuetta, Vertical transmission of human echovirus 11 at the time of Bornholm disease in late pregnancy, Pediatr. Infect. Dis. J. 24 (2005) 88–89.

[441] S.N. Wong, et al., Fatal coxsackie B1 virus infection in neonates, Pediatr. Infect. Dis. J. 8 (1989) 638.

[442] H. Yen, et al., Hepatic failure in a newborn with maternal peripartum exposure to echovirus 6 and enterovirus 71, Eur. J. Pediatr. 162 (2003) 648.

[443] M.A. Verboon-Maciolek, et al., Severe neonatal echovirus 20 infection characterized by hepatic failure, Pediatr. Infect. Dis. J. 16 (1997) 524.

[444] D. Hober, et al., Coxsackievirus B3-induced chronic myocarditis in mouse: use of whole blood culture to study the activation of TNF alpha-producing cells, Microbiol. Immunol. 40 (1996) 837.

[445] S. Chawareewong, et al., Neonatal herpangina caused by coxsackie A-5 virus, J. Pediatr. 93 (1978) 492.

[446] D. Murray, M. Altschul, J. Dyke, Aseptic meningitis in a neonate with an oral vesicular lesion, Diagn. Microbiol. Infect. Dis. 3 (1985) 77.

[447] T. Nakayama, et al., Outbreak of herpangina associated with coxsackievirus B3 infection, Pediatr. Infect. Dis. J. 8 (1989) 495.

[448] N. Suzuki, et al., Age-related symptomatology of ECHO 11 virus infection in children, Pediatrics 65 (1980) 284.

[449] H.L. Eckert, et al., Group B Coxsackie virus infection in infants with acute lower respiratory disease, Pediatrics 39 (1967) 526.

[450] T. Chonmaitree, et al., Enterovirus 71 infection: report of an outbreak with two cases of paralysis and a review of the literature, Pediatrics 67 (1981) 489.

[451] M. Mirani, P.L. Ogra, A. Barron, Epidemic of echovirus type 9 infection: certain clinical and epidemiologic features, N. Y. J. Med. 73 (1973) 403.

[452] M. Ramos-Alvarez, Cytopathogenic enteric viruses associated with undifferentiated diarrheal syndromes in early childhood, Ann. N. Y. Acad. Sci. 67 (1957) 326.

[453] S. Bauer, et al., Severe coxsackie virus B infection in preterm newborns treated with pleconaril, Eur. J. Pediatr. 161 (2002) 491.

[454] T. Iwasaki, et al., An immunofluorescent study of generalized coxsackie virus B3 infection in a newborn infant, Acta Pathol. Jpn. 35 (1985) 741.

[455] M.J. Abzug, Prognosis for neonates with enterovirus hepatitis and coagulopathy, Pediatr. Infect. Dis. J. 20 (2001) 758.

[456] D. Boccia, et al., Nosocomial necrotising enterocolitis outbreaks: epidemiology and control measures, Eur. J. Pediatr. 160 (2001) 385.

[457] W.J. Barson, et al., Survival following myocarditis and myocardial calcification associated with infection by coxsackie virus B4, Pediatrics 68 (1981) 79.

[458] S.H. Chan, K.S. Lun, Ventricular aneurysm complicating neonatal coxsackie B4 myocarditis, Pediatr. Cardiol. 22 (2001) 247.

[459] T. Chonmaitree, M.A. Menegus, K.R. Powell, The clinical relevance of "CSF viral culture." A two-year experience with aseptic meningitis in Rochester, N.Y, JAMA 247 (1982) 1843.

[460] J.H. Drew, ECHO 11 virus outbreak in a nursery associated with myocarditis, Aust. Paediatr. J. 9 (1973) 90.

[461] P. Rantakallio, et al., Follow-up study of 17 cases of neonatal coxsackie B5 meningitis and one with suspected myocarditis, Scand. J. Infect. Dis. 2 (1970) 25.

[462] J. Simmonds, et al., Successful heart transplantation following neonatal necrotic enterovirus myocarditis, Pediatr. Cardiol. 29 (2008) 834–837.

[463] K. Smets, et al., Detection of enteroviral RNA on Guthrie card dried blood of a neonate with fatal Coxsackie B3 myocarditis on day 17, J. Clin. Virol. 42 (2008) 207–210.

[464] M. Talsma, M. Vegting, J. Hess, Generalised coxsackie A9 infection in a neonate presenting with pericarditis, Br. Heart J. 52 (1984) 683.

[465] H.G. Cramblett, et al., ECHO 19 virus infections, Arch. Intern. Med. 110 (1962) 574.

[466] M.J. Abzug, M.J. Levin, H.A. Rotbart, Profile of enterovirus disease in the first two weeks of life, Pediatr. Infect. Dis. J. 12 (1993) 820.

[467] T. Daboval, E. Ferretti, R. Duperval, High C-reactive protein levels during a benign neonatal outbreak of echovirus type 7, Am. J. Perinatol. 23 (2006) 299–304.

[468] J. Haddad, et al., Enterovirus infections in neonates: a retrospective study of 21 cases, Eur. J. Med. 2 (1993) 209.

[469] K. Kusuhara, et al., An echovirus type 18 outbreak in a neonatal intensive care unit, Eur. J. Pediatr. 167 (2008) 587–589.

[470] M. Theodoridou, et al., Vesiculopapular rash as a single presentation in intrauterine coxsackie virus infection, Eur. J. Pediatr. 161 (2002) 412.

[471] C.Y. Chen, et al., Acute flaccid paralysis in infants and young children with enterovirus 71 infection: MR imaging findings and clinical correlates, AJNR Am. J. Neuroradiol. 22 (2001) 200.

[472] W.J. Barson, C.B. Reiner, Coxsackievirus B2 infection in a neonate with incontinentia pigmenti, Pediatrics 77 (1986) 897.

[473] I. Bergman, et al., Outcome in children with enteroviral meningitis during the first year of life, J. Pediatr. 110 (1987) 705.

[474] M.L. Blokziji, M. Koskiniemi, Echovirus 6 encephalitis in a preterm baby, Lancet 2 (1989) 164.

[475] G.S. Bowen, et al., Epidemic of meningitis and febrile illness in neonates caused by echo type 11 virus in Philadelphia, Pediatr. Infect. Dis. 2 (1983) 359.

[476] J. Callen, B.A. Paes, A case report of a premature infant with coxsackie B1 meningitis, Adv. Neonatal. Care 7 (2007) 238–247.

[477] J.D. Cherry, et al., Coxsackie B5 infections with exanthems, Pediatrics 31 (1963) 445.

[478] P.J. Chesney, P. Quennec, C. Clark, Hypoglycorrhachia and coxsackie B3 meningoencephalitis, Am. J. Clin. Pathol. 70 (1978) 947.

[479] A. Ehrnst, M. Eriksson, Coxsackie type 23 observed as a nosocomial infection in infants, Scand. J. Dis. 28 (1996) 205.

[480] K. Farmer, B.A. MacArthur, M.M. Clay, A follow-up study of 15 cases of neonatal meningoencephalitis due to coxsackie virus B5, J. Pediatr. 87 (1975) 568.

[481] R.E. Haynes, et al., ECHO virus type 3 infections in children: clinical and laboratory studies, J. Pediatr. 80 (1972) 589.

[482] R.E. Haynes, H.G. Cramblett, H.J. Kronfol, Echovirus 9 meningoencephalitis in infants and children, JAMA 208 (1969) 1657.

[483] I. Helin, et al., Outbreak of coxsackievirus A-14 meningitis among newborns in a maternity hospital ward, Acta Paediatr. Scand. 76 (1987) 234.

[484] R.T. Johnson, H.E. Shuey, E.L. Buescher, Epidemic central nervous system disease of mixed enterovirus etiology, I. Clinical and epidemiologic description, Am. J. Hyg. 71 (1960) 321.

[485] K. Matsumoto, et al., Characterization of an echovirus type 30 variant isolated from patients with aseptic meningitis, Microbiol. Immunol. 30 (1986) 333.

[486] W. Schurmann, et al., Two cases of coxsackie B2 infection in neonates: clinical, virological, and epidemiological aspects, Eur. J. Pediatr. 140 (1983) 59.

[487] C.J. Sells, R.L. Carpenter, C.G. Ray, Sequelae of central-nervous-system enterovirus infections, N. Engl. J. Med. 293 (1975) 1.

[488] C.V. Sumaya, L.I. Corman, Enteroviral meningitis in early infancy: significance in community outbreaks, Pediatr. Infect. Dis. 1 (1982) 151.

[489] R.L. King, et al., Routine cerebrospinal fluid enterovirus polymerase chain reaction testing reduces hospitalization and antibiotic use for infants 90 days of age or younger, Pediatrics 120 (2007) 489–496.

[490] N.P. Tavakoli, et al., Detection and typing of enteroviruses from CSF specimens from patients diagnosed with meningitis/encephalitis, J. Clin. Virol. 43 (2008) 207–211.

[491] M.A. Verboon-Maciolek, et al., Human parechovirus causes encephalitis with white matter injury in neonates, Ann. Neurol. 64 (2008) 266–273.

[492] O. Kew, et al., Outbreak of poliomyelitis in Hispaniola associated with circulating type 1 vaccine-derived poliovirus, Science 296 (2002) 356.

[493] R. Arnon, et al., Fatal outcome of neonatal echovirus 19 infection, Pediatr. Infect. Dis. J. 10 (1991) 788.

[494] L. Grangeot-Keros, et al., Enterovirus in sudden unexpected deaths in infants, Pediatr. Infect. Dis. J. 15 (1996) 123.

[495] J.R. Paul, Epidemiology of poliomyelitis, Monogr. Ser. World Health Organ 26 (1955) 9.

[496] R.E. Weibel, D.E. Benor, Reporting vaccine-associated paralytic poliomyelitis: concordance between the CDC and the National Vaccine Injury Compensation Program, Am. J. Public Health 86 (1996) 734.

[497] L.J. Wolfgram, N.R. Rose, Coxsackievirus infection as a trigger of cardiac autoimmunity, Immunol. Res. 8 (1989) 61.

[498] C.M. Wilfert, et al., Longitudinal assessment of children with enteroviral meningitis during the first three months of life, Pediatrics 67 (1981) 811.

[499] H.R. Yen, et al., Hepatic failure in a newborn with maternal peripartum exposure to echovirus 6 and enterovirus 71, Eur. J. Pediatr. 162 (2003) 648–649.

[500] E. Aradottir, E. Alonso, S. Shulman, Severe neonatal enteroviral hepatitis treated with pleconaril, Pediatr. Infect. Dis. J. 20 (2001) e457.

[501] A.B. Sabin, E.R. Krumbiegel, R. Wigand, ECHO type 9 virus disease, Am. J. Dis. Child. 96 (1958) 197.

[502] S.S. Toce, W.J. Keenan, Congenital echovirus 11 pneumonia in association with pulmonary hypertension, Pediatr. Infect. Dis. J. 7 (1988) 360.

[503] A. Tarcan, N. Özbek, B. Gürakan, Bone marrow failure with concurrent enteroviral infection in a newborn, Pediatr. Infect. Dis. J. 20 (2001) e719.

[504] K.T. Chen, et al., Epidemiologic features of hand-foot-mouth disease and herpangina caused by enterovirus 71 in Taiwan, 1998–2005, Pediatrics 120 (2007) e244–e252.

[505] C.M. Wilfert, et al., An epidemic of echovirus 18 meningitis, J. Infect. Dis. 131 (1975) 75.

[506] J.A. Mullins, et al., Emergence of echovirus type 13 as a prominent enterovirus, Clin. Infect. Dis. 38 (2004) 70.

[507] D.L. Kirschke, et al., Outbreak of aseptic meningitis associated with echovirus 13, Pediatr. Infect. Dis. J. 21 (2002) 1034.

[508] E. Somekh, et al., An outbreak of echovirus 13 meningitis in central Israel, Epidemiol. Infect. 130 (2003) 257.

[509] G. Trallero, et al., First epidemic of aseptic meningitis due to echovirus type 13 among Spanish children, Epidemiol. Infect. 130 (2003) 251.

[510] V. Drouhet, Enterovirus infection and associated clinical symptoms in children, Ann. Inst. Pasteur. 98 (1960) 562.

[511] Y. Hinuma, Y. Murai, T. Nakao, Two outbreaks of echovirus 14 infection: a possible interference with oral poliovirus vaccine and a probable association with aseptic meningitis, J. Hyg. (Lond). 63 (1965) 277.

[512] D.N. Medearis Jr., R.A. Kramer, Exanthem associated with ECHO virus type 18 viremia, J. Pediatr. 55 (1959) 367.

[513] T. Chonmaitree, et al., Comparison of cell cultures for rapid isolation of enteroviruses, J. Clin. Microbiol. 26 (1988) 2576.

[514] F.B. Johnson, Transport of viral specimens, Clin. Microbiol. Rev. 3 (1990) 120.

[515] C.L. Howell, M.J. Miller, Effect of sucrose phosphate and sorbitol on infectivity of enveloped viruses during storage, J. Clin. Microbiol. 18 (1983) 658.

[516] M.J. August, A. Warford, Evaluation of a commercial monoclonal antibody for detection of adenovirus antigen, J. Clin. Microbiol. 25 (1987) 2233.

[517] A. Trabelsi, et al., Evaluation of an enterovirus group-specific anti-VPI monoclonal antibody, 5–D8/1, in comparison with neutralization and PCR for rapid identification of enteroviruses in cell culture, J. Clin. Microbiol. 33 (1995) 2454.

[518] J.M. Carstens, et al., Detection of enteroviruses in cell cultures by using in situ transcription, J. Clin. Microbiol. 30 (1992) 25.

[519] R. Abraham, et al., Rapid detection of poliovirus by reverse transcription and polymerase chain amplification: application for the differentiation between poliovirus and nonpoliovirus enteroviruses, J. Clin. Microbiol. 31 (1993) 295.

[520] K.R. Rittichier, et al., Diagnosis and outcomes of enterovirus infections in young infants, Pediatr. Infect. Dis. J. 24 (2005) 546–550.

[521] A.B. Martin, et al., Acute myocarditis: rapid diagnosis by PCR in children, Circulation 90 (1994) 330.

[522] P. Muir, et al., Multicenter quality assessment of PCR methods for detection of enteroviruses, J. Clin. Microbiol. 37 (1999) 1409.

[523] L. De, et al., Identification of vaccine-related polioviruses by hybridization with specific RNA probes, J. Clin. Microbiol. 33 (1995) 562.

[524] H.A. Rotbart, Nucleic acid detection systems for enteroviruses, Clin. Microbiol. Rev. 4 (1991) 156.

[525] C. Chezzi, Rapid diagnosis of poliovirus infection by PCR amplification, J. Clin. Microbiol. 34 (1996) 1722.

[526] D. Egger, et al., Reverse transcription multiplex PCR for differentiation between polio and enteroviruses from clinical and environmental samples, J. Clin. Microbiol. 33 (1995) 1442.

[527] M. Gorgievski-Hrisoho, et al., Detection by PCR of enteroviruses in cerebrospinal fluid during a summer outbreak of aseptic meningitis in Switzerland, J. Clin. Microbiol. 36 (1998) 2408.

[528] P. Muir, et al., Rapid diagnosis of enterovirus infection by magnetic bead extraction and polymerase chain reaction detection of enterovirus RNA in clinical specimens, J. Clin. Microbiol. 31 (1993) 31.

[529] J. Petitjean, et al., Detection of enteroviruses in cerebrospinal fluids: enzymatic amplification and hybridization with a biotinylated riboprobe, Mol. Cell. Probes 8 (15) (1994) B22.

[530] R.W. Redline, D.R. Genest, B. Tycko, Detection of enteroviral infection in paraffin-embedded tissue by the RNA polymerase chain reaction technique, Am. J. Clin. Pathol. 96 (1991) 568.

[531] C. Ramers, et al., Impact of a diagnostic cerebrospinal fluid enterovirus polymerase chain reaction test on patient management, JAMA 283 (2000) 2680.

[532] C.F. Yang, et al., Detection and identification of vaccine-related polioviruses by the polymerase chain reaction, Viral Res. 20 (159) (1991) B79.

[533] The Prevention of Mental Retardation Through Control of Infectious Diseases, U.S. Government Printing Office, Washington, DC, 1966.

[534] R. Dagan, et al., Neutralizing antibodies to non-polio enteroviruses in human immune serum globulin, Pediatr. Infect. Dis. 2 (1983) 454.

[535] R.E. McKinney Jr., S.L. Katz, C.M. Wilfert, Chronic enteroviral meningoencephalitis in agammaglobulinemic patients, Rev. Infect. Dis. 9 (1987) 334.

[536] G.W. Hammond, et al., Maternal and neonatal neutralizing antibody titers to selected enteroviruses, Pediatr. Infect. Dis. 4 (1985) 32.

[537] J.M. Johnston, J.C. Overall Jr., Intravenous immunoglobulin in disseminated neonatal echovirus 11 infection, Pediatr. Infect. Dis. J. 8 (1989) 254.

[538] M.J. Abzug, et al., Neonatal enterovirus infection: virology, serology, and effects of intravenous immune globulin, Clin. Infect. Dis. 20 (1995) 1201.

[539] B.A. Jantausch, et al., Maternal plasma transfusion in the treatment of disseminated neonatal echovirus 11 infection, Pediatr. Infect. Dis. J. 14 (1995) 154.

[540] E. Chuang, et al., Successful treatment of fulminant echovirus 11 infection in a neonate by orthotopic liver transplantation, J. Pediatr. Gastroenterol. Nutr. 17 (1993) 211.

[541] P.A. Bryant, et al., Neonatal coxsackie B virus infection—a treatable disease? Eur. J. Pediatr. 163 (2004) 223–228.

[542] H.A. Rotbart, M.J. Abzug, M.J. Levin, Development and application of RNA probes for the study of picornaviruses, Mol. Cell. Probes 2 (1988) 65.

[543] E.D. Kilbourne, C.B. Wilson, D. Perrier, The induction of gross myocardial lesions by a Coxsackie (pleurodynia) virus and cortisone, J. Clin. Invest. 35 (1956) 367.

[544] J.W. Mason, et al., A clinical trial of immunosuppressive therapy for myocarditis, N. Engl. J. Med. 333 (1995) 269.

[545] E.J. Bell, et al., Mu-antibody capture ELISA for the rapid diagnosis of enterovirus infections in patients with aseptic meningitis, J. Med. Virol. 19 (1986) 213.

[546] K. Sadeharju, et al., Maternal antibodies in breast milk protect the child from enterovirus infections, Pediatrics 119 (2007) 941–946.

[547] J.D. Cherry, Enteroviruses: polioviruses (poliomyelitis), coxsackieviruses, echoviruses, and enteroviruses, in: R.D. Feigin, J.D. Cherry (Eds.), Textbook of Pediatric Infectious Diseases, second ed., Saunders, Philadelphia, 1987, pp. 1729–1790.

[548] D. Isaacs, et al., Conservative management of an echovirus 11 outbreak in a neonatal unit, Lancet 1 (1989) 543.

HEPATITIS

Wikrom Karnsakul ☉ Kathleen B. Schwarz

CHAPTER OUTLINE

Hepatitis A Virus   800
  Epidemiology and Transmission   800
  Microbiology   801
  Pathogenesis   801
  Pathology   802
  Clinical Manifestations   802
  Diagnosis   802
  Treatment   802
  Prevention   802
Hepatitis B Virus and Hepatitis D Virus   803
  Epidemiology and Transmission   803
  Microbiology   803
  Pathogenesis   804
  Pathology   804
  Clinical Manifestations   804
  Diagnosis   804
  Treatment   804
  Prevention   805
Hepatitis C Virus   806
  Epidemiology and Transmission   806

  Microbiology   806
  Pathogenesis   806
  Pathology   807
  Clinical Manifestations   807
  Diagnosis   807
  Treatment   807
  Prevention   807
Hepatitis E Virus   807
  Epidemiology and Transmission   807
  Microbiology   808
  Pathogenesis   808
  Pathology   808
  Clinical Manifestations   808
  Diagnosis   809
  Treatment   809
  Prevention   809
Other Hepatotropic Viruses   809
  GB Virus Type C/Hepatitis G Virus   809
  Transfusion-Transmitted Virus   810
Conclusion   811

Knowledge about the hepatotropic viruses has grown dramatically in the past century, with contributions from clinicians, molecular virologists, immunologists, and pharmacologists. For the last decade, several government and nongovernment organizations have held consensus conferences on the management of acute and chronic viral hepatitis to update previous management recommendations. This chapter reviews updated information on the hepatotropic viruses (hepatitis A through G viruses and transfusion-transmitted virus [TTV]), with a particular focus on pregnant women and young infants and breakthroughs in vaccine development and global preventive measures (Table 25–1).

HEPATITIS A VIRUS

Hepatitis A virus (HAV) is one of the most common communicable diseases and has a worldwide distribution, with estimated recognized cases of 1.5 million annually [1]. The rate of HAV in the United States has declined by 89% since the first availability of hepatitis A vaccine in 1995 [2,3]. In May 2006, the Advisory Committee on Immunization Practices recommended routine HAV vaccination for all children beginning at 12 months of age [4]. The same year, the lowest incidence of HAV ever was recorded at 1.2 per 100,000 [5]. Routine HAV immunization is close to cost-neutral on a cost-per-quality-adjusted-life-year basis [6].

EPIDEMIOLOGY AND TRANSMISSION

In the United States, person-to-person transmission through the fecal-oral route is the primary mode of HAV transmission [7]. Infections usually result from a contact from a family member or a sex partner. In most infected individuals, the stool contains a higher concentration of virus and is likely highly contagious during the 1 to 2 weeks before the illness compared with later in the course [1]. The risk of transmission subsequently diminishes by 1 week after onset of jaundice [8]. HAV can be detected in stool for longer periods, however, especially in neonates and young children [9]. Most index cases who are usually unaware of this risk are international travelers to developing countries, regardless of travel budget, who account for 11% of documented cases of infection without a known source [10].

In one study, 84% of all known reported cases of HAV were travelers from Mexico [11]. Other risk groups for transmission are people who live with or have sex with an infected person, people living in areas where children are not routinely vaccinated against HAV (where outbreaks are more likely in children attending day care and day care employees), men who have sex with men, and illicit drug users. Water-borne outbreaks can occur, but are uncommon in developed countries with well-maintained sanitation and water supply systems.

Cooked foods also can transmit HAV if the temperature during food preparation is inadequate to kill the

TABLE 25-1   Hepatitis Viruses

Virus	Virus Structure	Primary Route of Neonatal Infection	Transmission in Children and Adults
HAV (picornavirus)	SS RNA, nonenveloped	Perinatal	Fecal-oral
HBV (*Hepadnavirus*)	DS circular DNA, enveloped	Perinatal	Blood-borne
HCV (*Flavivirus*)	SS RNA, enveloped	Perinatal	Blood-borne
HDV (*Deltavirus*)	SS, circular RNA (HBV envelope)	Not reported	Blood-borne
HEV (*Calicivirus*)	SS RNA, nonenveloped	In utero; perinatal	Fecal-oral
HGV (*Flavivirus*)	SS RNA, nonenveloped	In utero; perinatal	Blood-borne, sexual
TTV (*Circovirus*)	SS, circular DNA, nonenveloped	Perinatal	Fecal-oral, blood-borne, sexual contact

DS, double-stranded; HAV, hepatitis A virus; HBV, hepatitis B virus; HCV, hepatitis C virus; HDV, hepatitis D virus; HEV, hepatitis E virus; HGV, hepatitis G virus (GB virus type C); SS, single-stranded; TTV, TT virus.
Adapted from Bradley JS. Hepatitis. In Remington JS, et al (eds). Infectious Diseases of the Fetus and Newborn Infant, 6th ed. Philadelphia, Saunders, 2006, p 824.

virus, or if food is contaminated after cooking, as occurs in outbreaks associated with infected food handlers [1]. Foods such as lettuce, tomatoes, green onions, strawberries, raspberries, and shellfish have been associated with the outbreaks. Contamination can occur during growing, processing, or food preparation. In November 2003, a large unprecedented HAV outbreak was identified among patrons of a single Pennsylvania restaurant where mild salsa containing green onions grown in Mexico was prepared and was the source of HAV in these cases [7]. An extended study using biomarkers placed on the soil showed that HAV can contaminate the inside of the growing onion and can be taken up intracellularly through the roots [12].

The age at infection varies with socioeconomic status and associated living conditions. In developing countries particularly of high endemicity, infection usually occurs during the 1st decade of life. In the United States, the rate of HAV declined after vaccine introduction in 2002 [13]. Pockets of high prevalence still remain, however, emphasizing the importance of adhering to the recommendation for universal childhood vaccination.

Maternal-to-fetal transmission has been reported in mothers with acute icteric HAV 1 week to several weeks before delivery [14–17]. Nosocomial transmission is unusual, but outbreaks caused by transmission from hospitalized patients to health care staff have been reported [9,18]. In addition, outbreaks have occurred in neonatal intensive care units from neonates receiving infected transfused blood and subsequently transmitting HAV to other neonates and health care staff [9,18].

MICROBIOLOGY

HAV is a single-stranded RNA virus classified as a member of the picornavirus group (Fig. 25-1). Most human strains belong to genotype I or III [8]. The three major proteins of viral capsid—VP1, VP2, and VP3 (structural proteins)—are encoded by P1 region on viral genome. The structural arrangement of capsid proteins VP1 and VP3 forms a single, dominant, serologic epitope on the virus capsid and accounts for a neutralizing antibody response. The virus can be stable in the environment for several months. HAV can live outside the body for months, which is likely explained by the slow translation rate, depending on the environmental conditions [19].

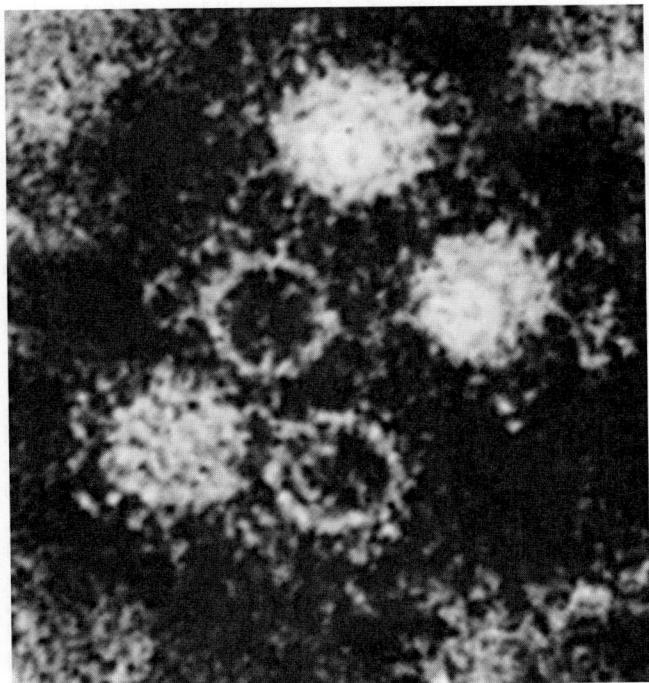

FIGURE 25-1 Hepatitis A virus (HAV) particles. Electron micrograph of the 27-nm HAV virions in a stool specimen. *(Reprinted with permission from Feinstone SM, Kapikian AZ, Purcell RH. Hepatitis A: detection by immune electron microscopy of a viruslike antigen associated with acute illness. Science 182:1026. Copyright 1973 by the American Association for the Advancement of Science.)*

PATHOGENESIS

HAV crosses through the gastrointestinal tract by an uncharacterized mechanism to the liver, where it solely replicates in hepatocytes [20]. The pathogenetic mechanism leading to liver tissue injury by HAV is not a viral cytopathogenic effect. Rather, it is suggested to be an immunopathologic reaction of sensitized cytotoxic T lymphocytes against infected hepatocytes where these T lymphocytes are present as an antiviral reaction similar to that directed against hepatitis B virus (HBV) [8,21]. A low translation rate and RNA replication rate may play a role in escaping host cell defenses [19]. Almost all individuals infected with HAV develop IgG and IgM antibodies to VP1 [8].

PATHOLOGY

After the availability of serology to confirm HAV, a liver histopathology study was performed in patients with acute viral hepatitis caused by HAV (n = 86) or HBV (n = 78). The liver parenchymal changes in patients with HAV, including focal necrosis, hepatocellular ballooning, and acidophilic degeneration, were milder than changes seen in patients with HBV, but the degree of portal inflammation seemed similar in these two groups [22].

CLINICAL MANIFESTATIONS

HAV typically is an acute, self-limited illness associated with fever, malaise, jaundice, anorexia, nausea, and abdominal discomfort after an incubation period of approximately 28 days (range 15–50 days) [1]. The appearance of jaundice usually leads to further investigation and the diagnosis of HAV; however, 70% of infected children younger than 6 years are anicteric or have a mild flulike illness. Jaundice is observed in only 7% of children younger than 4 years old [23]. In contrast, older children and adults usually are symptomatic, with jaundice occurring in 70% or more, and infection typically lasts several weeks. Symptoms usually last less than 2 months, although 10% to 15% of individuals with HAV have prolonged or relapsing hepatitis for up to 6 months.

A significant number (69%) of pregnant women with acute HAV infection during the second and third trimesters of pregnancy have gestational complications leading to preterm labor, including premature contractions, placental separation, and premature rupture of membranes [24,25]. Although uncommon, neonatal cholestasis resulting from maternal-to-fetal transmission has been reported [26,27]. Four cases of intrauterine infection have been reported. Two mothers had symptomatic HAV at 20 and 13 weeks of gestation. The fetuses developed ascites, meconium peritonitis, and perforation of the distal ileum in utero, requiring surgery after birth. The newborn infants subsequently recovered. In two other mothers with HAV at 20 days before delivery, infants developed neonatal icteric hepatitis A on day 3 of life and had a full recovery [27,28]. Mild acute hepatitis in newborn infants followed the onset of hepatitis in their mothers developing in the late third trimester (gestational week >33) probably resulting from a perinatal contact with infected blood or feces [14–17].

Although typically self-limited, HAV can be potentially life-threatening, with an estimated fatality rate of 0.3% to 0.6% reaching 1.8% among adults older than 50 years [7]. Fulminant hepatitis is rare, but is more common in people with underlying liver disease [29]. Chronic infection does not occur with HAV [23]. Rare extrahepatic manifestations include pancreatitis, renal failure, arthritis, vasculitis, thrombocytopenia, aplastic anemia, red blood cell aplasia, transverse myelitis, and toxic epidermal necrolysis [5].

DIAGNOSIS

Serologic tests for HAV-specific total and IgM antibody are available commercially [1]. Serum IgM is present at the onset of illness and usually disappears within 4 months, but may persist for 6 months or longer [1]. The presence of serum IgM may indicate current infection, recent infection, or HAV vaccination, although false-positive results can occur. Anti-HAV IgG is detectable shortly after the appearance of IgM. The presence of anti-HAV IgG alone indicates past infection and immunity.

TREATMENT

Treatment generally is supportive. In addition to standard precautions, contact precautions are recommended for diapered and incontinent patients for at least 1 week after onset of symptoms [1]. One of the most important aspects of management of infected individuals is active and passive immunization of close contacts (see "Prevention" next). Some patients with cholestasis may not tolerate a fatty diet. In individuals with fulminant hepatitis or liver failure, specific management is determined by the complications, and evaluation for liver transplant may be required [8].

PREVENTION

HAV vaccination is recommended and licensed for all children 1 to 18 years old, for adults who are at increased risk for infection, for adults who are at increased risk for complications from HAV such as persons with underlying liver disease, and for any person wishing to obtain immunity to HAV. Although the vaccine is well tolerated even in studies of the safety and immunogenicity in young infants 2 to 6 months of age, the presence of passive maternal HAV antibody during the first 6 to 12 months of life interferes with vaccine immunogenicity [30–34].

HAV vaccines are given intramuscularly in a two-dose schedule with a 6- to 12-month interval [1]. Doses and schedules for HAV vaccines and formulations produced by different manufacturers are recommended by the American Academy of Pediatrics (AAP) [1]. Current HAV vaccines have been shown to be safe, to be highly immunogenic, and to confer long-lasting protection. Vaccine-induced antibodies persist for longer than 12 years in vaccinated adults, and mathematical modeling predicts antibody persistence for longer than 25 years in greater than 95% of vaccine recipients [35].

Intramuscular immunoglobulin is more than 85% effective in preventing symptomatic infection when given within 2 weeks after the most recent exposure to HAV in a household or sexual contact [1]. Immunoglobulin and the first dose of vaccine can be administered simultaneously when travel plans are imminent. Acute HAV infection during pregnancy and perinatal transmission seem to be rare, especially at the time of delivery. There have been no data to suggest cesarean infection as a mode of delivery for HAV-infected pregnant women; infants born via vaginal delivery to mothers with acute HAV infection have a favorable outcome [24]. The infant usually has exposure to HAV before the diagnosis is made in the mother. HAV has been shown in breast milk, but only one newborn case of HAV transmission in breast milk has been reported [14]. Although the efficacy has not yet been established, immunoglobulin (0.02 mL/kg) is advised to be administered to the infant if the mother's symptoms of HAV began between 2 weeks before and 1 week after delivery [1]. To prevent nosocomial transmission, particularly in the neonatal intensive care unit or newborn nursery, the infected mother and the neonate should be isolated, and careful hygiene practices should be emphasized [36].

Because acute HAV infection during pregnancy is associated with a high risk of maternal complications and preterm labor, HAV serology and maternal immunization during prenatal or prepregnancy evaluation could be considered in areas in which adult populations are susceptible to HAV. As the prevalence of early HAV infection seems to be decreasing in countries that are moving from high to intermediate endemicity, it is expected that an increased number of adolescents and adults susceptible to symptomatic disease may be associated with greater morbidity, mortality, and treatment costs [35].

HEPATITIS B VIRUS AND HEPATITIS D VIRUS

HBV is believed to have infected 2 billion persons worldwide; more than 350 million individuals are currently infected [37]. The maternal-to-fetal route of transmission is responsible for most infections. Past efforts to prevent this route of transmission resulted in the strategy of providing a combination of passive and active immunization within 24 hours of birth. Although this strategy is 90% to 95% effective when properly administered, remaining areas of concern are the need to disseminate this practice for all high-risk infants and to achieve universal vaccination of all infants, as recommended by the World Health Organization. In addition there is a need to develop effective measures to prevent transmission in 100% of newborns born to infected mothers. Such measures would be highly cost-effective given the ongoing morbidity and mortality from HBV, which accounts for 500,000 to 1 million deaths from cirrhosis, liver failure, and hepatocellular carcinoma worldwide per year [38].

The delta virus (hepatitis D virus [HDV]) is always linked to HBV because it requires the surface coat of HBV for replication. Little information exists regarding perinatal transmission of HDV; even in highly endemic areas, infection with HDV is infrequent in infants and is mainly acquired during the 2nd and 3rd decades of life, suggesting a horizontal rather than vertical transmission of the virus [39].

EPIDEMIOLOGY AND TRANSMISSION

Before the development of the combination vaccination strategy (hepatitis B immunoglobulin [HBIG] plus vaccine) for high-risk neonates, most neonates born to HBV-infected mothers were infected with HBV. Chen and colleagues [40]. reported that the presence of HBV surface antigen (HBsAg) in gastric aspirates of newborns was strongly associated with the acquisition of HBsAg by the infants; there was no correlation between the rate of infant antigenemia and the duration of the first stage of labor, and cesarean section did not decrease the rate of vertical HBV transmission.

Sexual intercourse in the second trimester of pregnancy has also been implicated in HBV intrauterine transmission [41]. Mothers positive for hepatitis B early antigen

(HBeAg) and mothers with very high serum DNA levels (e.g., $\geq 10^9$ copies/mL) have the greatest risk of transferring HBV to their offspring despite adherence to the recommended combination of active and passive immunization of newborns within 24 hours of birth [42]. In one Chinese study, 7.4% of infants born to HBV-infected mothers were infected with HBV during the 1st year of life, despite receiving passive and active immunoprophylaxis in the immediate newborn period [43]. Even in countries such as Canada, where the government mandates screening of all pregnant women for HBV and provides prophylaxis to infants born to HBV-infected women, less than 85% complete prophylaxis and serologic follow-up was documented, suggesting that there is a need for public health programs with more effective universal neonatal immunization for infants at highest risk of HBV acquisition [44]. Although HBsAg can be detected in the breast milk of HBV-infected mothers, several studies have shown there is no additional risk of transmission of HBV to breast-fed infants of infected mothers, provided that proper active and passive immunoprophylaxis is carried out [45].

MICROBIOLOGY

HBV is a well-characterized, partially double-stranded DNA virus (Fig. 25–2). HBsAg is the hallmark of chronic infection. This marker is the first to appear in acute infection. The presence of HBsAg for 6 months or more connotes chronic infection. HBeAg is associated with infectivity and indicates active replication of HBV.

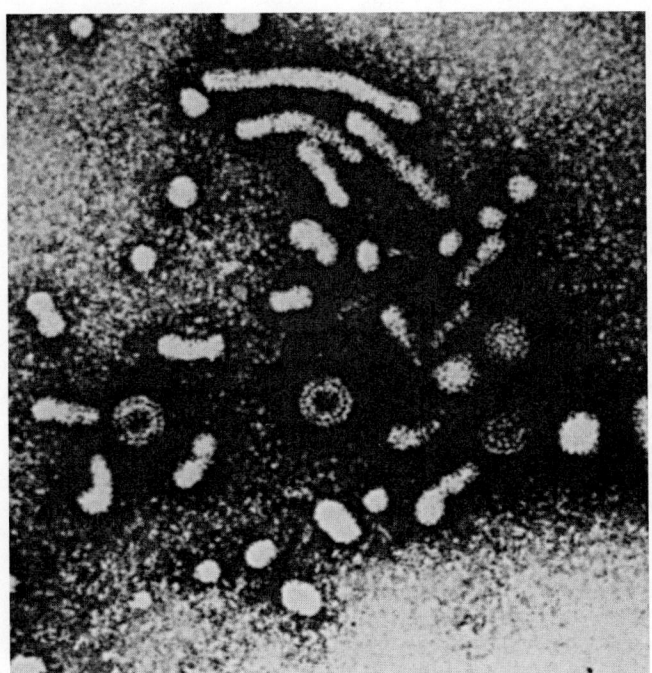

FIGURE 25–2 Hepatitis B virus (HBV) particles. Electron micrograph from a patient with acute HBV infection demonstrates three circulating particles: 20-nm structures and filamentous structures containing HBsAg envelope proteins (primarily the S, or major protein, but no HBV viral genome); and the 47-nm infectious virion structures containing both envelope proteins and a nucleocapsid containing genomic HBV DNA. HBSAg, hepatitis B surface antigen. *(Courtesy of Dr. June Almeida.)*

More recent reports have described "occult HBV," as defined by the presence of HBV DNA in serum or tissue in the absence of other markers. There are now several HBV genotypes, and knowledge is emerging regarding their clinical significance. It is recognized that HBV genotype C is associated with an increased risk of development of hepatocellular carcinoma as are the basal core promoter mutant and the pre-S deletion mutant [46]. Whether or not there is a role for quantification of HBV antigens or intrahepatic HBV covalently closed circular DNA, or both, is currently under investigation.

PATHOGENESIS

HBV is thought to cause liver injury in immunocompetent subjects via cytotoxic T cells directed to the infected hepatocyte. Functionally impaired dendritic cells may play a role in viral persistence [47], and B and T cells are involved in viral clearance. In immunocompromised subjects, such as individuals who have undergone liver transplantation, the virus itself may be hepatotoxic because HBV recurrence in the allograft is associated with poor patient and graft survival. The HB-X protein is a transcriptional activator of cellular genes and may play a role in the hepatocarcinogenesis of HBV via effects on apoptosis, DNA repair, mitogen-activated protein kinase, and JAK/STAT pathways [48].

PATHOLOGY

There are few reports of HBV hepatic histopathology in young infants, although hepatocellular carcinoma has been reported at 8 months of age [49]. In case series of children with active HBV hepatitis enrolled in antiviral trials, liver biopsy specimens generally show mild to moderate inflammation and mild to moderate fibrosis [50]. HBV infection has been associated with immune complex disease in nonhepatic organs. Clinical manifestations include membranoproliferative glomerulonephritis, cryoglobulinemia, Gianotti-Crosti papular acrodermatitis of childhood, and arthritis.

CLINICAL MANIFESTATIONS

The clinical manifestations of HBV infection depend on the age of acquisition. Neonates have a greater than 90% risk of chronic infection, and children and adolescents have a 25% to 50% risk; chronic infection is observed in only 5% of adults exposed to HBV [51]. Most newborns who acquire HBV remain in the immunotolerant stage for 1 or 2 decades. This stage is characterized by HBsAg and HBeAg antigenemia, high levels of HBV DNA, normal or minimally elevated serum aminotransferases, and minimal inflammation in the liver biopsy specimen. Approximately 6% of infants born to mothers who are positive for anti–hepatitis B early antibody develop acute hepatitis at 2 months of age [52]. Infants are ill with fever, jaundice, and hepatic tenderness. Serum aminotransferases are elevated, and there is active inflammation in the liver biopsy specimen. About one third of older children and adolescents with acute HBV develop these classic symptoms [53].

Most infants, children, and adolescents have chronic infection (lasting >6 months) of the asymptomatic immunotolerant type. In infants who are perinatally infected, the estimated spontaneous clearance of HBV is 0.6% per year over the 1st decade of life, but in subjects infected as adolescents and adults, the rate of clearance is 1.8% per year [54]. A few young subjects have active hepatitis with elevation of serum aminotransferases and active inflammation in the liver biopsy specimen. These subjects are most likely to respond to antiviral treatment. Inactive carriers are characterized by HBsAg positivity, seroconversion of HBeAg to anti–hepatitis B early antibody, undetectable HBV DNA, and normal serum aminotransferases.

Individuals with active hepatitis are at greatest risk for developing cirrhosis and hepatocellular carcinoma, but there is a growing concern that persistently high levels of HBV DNA for decades, even in immunotolerant subjects, are associated with an increased risk of hepatocellular carcinoma [55]. In one Chinese study, HBV infection in pregnancy was associated with high rates of complications (abortion, 16.7%; preterm births, 43%; neonatal asphyxia, 15.6%; and fetal death, 4.5%) [56].

DIAGNOSIS

The diagnosis of HBV is most commonly made by the presence of HBsAg in the circulation. Other studies commonly performed include HBeAg, HBV DNA, and anti–core antibody (Fig. 25–3). IgM anti–core antibody is indicative of recent exposure to HBV, whereas IgG core antibody is positive in individuals with chronic infection and in individuals who have cleared infection. Subjects who have been successfully immunized with HBV vaccine exhibit anti-HBsAg positivity. If a liver biopsy specimen is obtained, immunohistochemistry can be performed using an antibody against the surface antigen. Screening has been recommended for all pregnant women and for newly arrived immigrants to the United States from countries where HBV prevalence rate is 2% or greater [57]. Whether or not there should be screening of pregnant women living in areas of high HBV endemicity for occult HBV infection using sensitive assays for HBV DNA, is a matter of current study.

TREATMENT

There are currently two treatments for chronic HBV infection in children 2 to 18 years old approved by the U.S. Food and Drug Administration (FDA): standard α-interferon, which is given parenterally three times a week for 16 to 24 weeks, and lamivudine, which is given via the oral route. Interferon therapy should not be given to infants younger than 1 year because of the risk of spastic diplegia; in older children, side effects are common and are usually flulike in nature. Drug resistance has not been a problem. When interferon is administered to children with active hepatitis B, 20% to 58% show undetectable HBV DNA or HBeAg, or both, in serum [58]. Lamivudine is much better tolerated by children than interferon, but drug resistance is common—approximately 20% per year of administration. Currently complete and ongoing

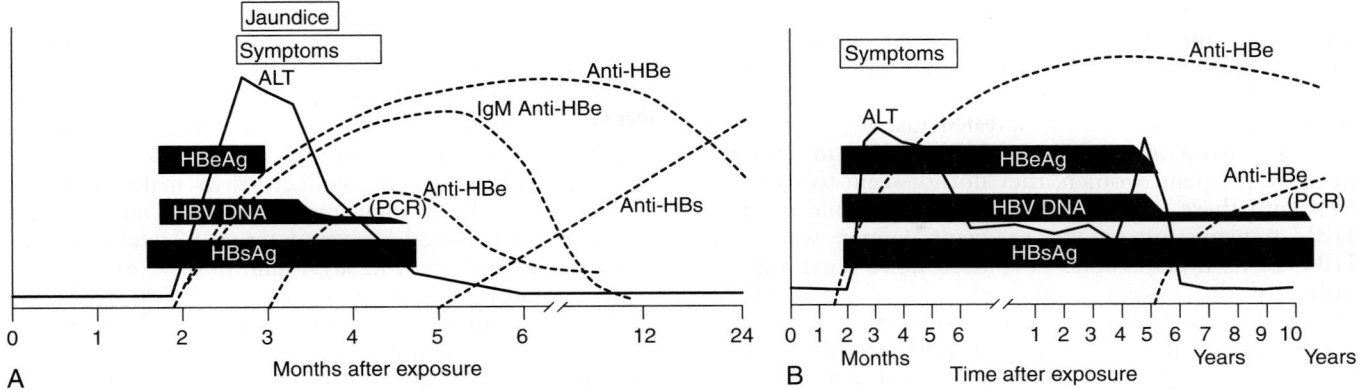

FIGURE 25–3 Viral and host serologic markers and clinical correlates of hepatitis B virus (HBV) infection. **A,** Acute infection with appropriate host response and resolution of infection. **B,** Chronic infection. (*Data from Servoss JC, Friedman LS. Serologic and molecular diagnosis of hepatitis B virus. Clin Liver Dis 2004;8[2]:267-81.*)

pediatric trials of more potent nucleoside/nucleotide analogues include adefovir dipivoxil and entecavir [59].

PREVENTION

Detailed HBV vaccine schedules are available from the AAP *Red Book* [1]. Schedules are provided for the various pediatric age groups, for vaccination of preterm infants, and for newborns depending on maternal HBsAg status (Table 25–2). Systematic HBV vaccination has markedly decreased the incidence of new HBV infections in the pediatric age group over the last 2 decades. Although

much less is known about the impact of HBV vaccine programs on HDV incidence, one Italian study showed the incidence decreased from 1.7 to 0.5 cases per 1 million population after introduction of the universal anti-HBV campaign [60]. Efforts have been made to assess the impact of maternal HBV screening on perinatal HBV vaccination. In a U.S. study, to assess the completeness of maternal screening for newborn prophylaxis, the mother's HBsAg status was known within 12 hours of delivery for 84% of mothers screened; however, of the infants whose mothers' HBsAg status was unknown, only 28% were vaccinated the 1st day of life [61].

TABLE 25–2 Hepatitis B Neonatal Intervention Strategies Based on Maternal Hepatitis B Virus (HBV) Screening Status*

Maternal HBV Status	Interpretation	Laboratory Evaluation at Birth and during Infancy	Infant Treatment
HBsAg-positive	Mother is infectious; significant risk of neonatal infection	HBsAg on peripheral venous blood sampling to diagnose intrauterine infection; check infant after age 9 mo for anti-HBs and HBsAg	*All infants*: HBIG 0.5 mL ≤12 hr after birth; in addition, 12 hr after birth, second and third doses of vaccine for infants with birth weight ≥2000 g as for HBsAg-negative status *Preterm infants <2000 g birth weight*: Initial birth dose should not be counted as one of immunizing series because of immature response to vaccine; subsequent 3 immunizations in primary immunizing series for these infants should start at age 1–2 mo
HBsAg status unknown	Mother's infectious status should be determined by HBsAg testing as soon as possible	None required at birth; in infants whose mothers are subsequently found to be HBsAg-positive, check infant after age 9 mo for anti-HBs and HBsAg	*Full-term infants*: Give first dose of hepatitis B vaccine ≤12 hr of birth; if maternal HBsAg is positive, give HBIG 0.5 mL as soon as possible, ≤7 days of age; if maternal HBsAg is negative, HBIG is not needed; subsequent doses as for HBsAg-negative status *Preterm infants <2000 g birth weight*: If maternal HBsAg status cannot be determined ≤12 hr of birth, give HBIG in addition to hepatitis vaccine ≤12 hr of birth; provide subsequent 3 hepatitis B immunizations for primary series, starting at 1 mo of age, as above for preterm infants
HBsAg-negative	Mother is not considered infectious; no risk to neonate	None required	*All newborn infants*: Standard 3-dose immunization regimen with hepatitis B vaccine recommended: dose 1 given soon after birth before discharge, dose 2 given at 1–2 mo of age at least 4 wk after dose 1; dose 3 given at 6–18 mo, at least 16 wk after dose 1, and at least 8 wk after dose 2, with last dose not before 24 wk of age

*This table recommends only single-antigen vaccine; for single-antigen vaccine combination, refer to Red Book 2006 recommendation [1].
HBIG, hepatitis B immunoglobulin; HBsAg, hepatitis B surface antigen.
Adapted from Bradley JS. Hepatitis. In Remington JS, et al (eds). Infectious Diseases of the Fetus and Newborn Infant, 6th ed. Philadelphia, Saunders, 2006, p 833.

HBV DNA virus levels increase during the last trimester of pregnancy and early in the postpartum period; the value of assessing these levels to modify immunoprophylaxis of the newborn is a matter of current study [62]. Although serum alanine aminotransferase levels are often used as surrogate markers of HBV DNA in HBeAg-negative pregnant women, they do not seem to correlate well with these levels [63]. Because of possible in utero HBV transmission among pregnant women with high HBV DNA titers, studies have been done regarding the utility of the possible added efficacy of using HBIG during the third trimester of pregnancy to prevent maternal-to-fetal transmission of HBV; results to date have been conflicting. One study reported that protective anti-HBsAg rates at 6 months were higher in infants born to either HBeAg-positive or HBeAg-negative mothers who had received three doses of HBIG in late pregnancy along with infant passive and active immunization [64]. Another study showed no difference in the protective efficacy rates assessed at 12 months of age in infants of mothers receiving HBIG or not receiving HBIG [65].

Although the high efficacy of neonatal HBV vaccination suggests that most cases are transmitted perinatally, some neonates who have failed vaccine have been found to be positive for HBsAg or HBeAg at birth, suggesting intrauterine transmission [66]. There is a need to elucidate the role of nucleoside/nucleotide agents in treating chronic HBV in the last part of pregnancy in women with high HBV DNA levels who are positive for HBeAg and who are most likely to infect their newborns [67,68].

HEPATITIS C VIRUS

Since the discovery of hepatitis C virus (HCV) in 1989, HCV has become a global public health problem, infecting approximately 170 million individuals. Although transfusion-transmitted HCV was the major form of HCV in the pediatric age group when the virus was first described [69], since 1992, when most blood units transfused have been free of HCV, the maternal-to-fetal route of transmission of this virus has become the dominant route for new cases of HCV. Jhaveri and colleagues [70]. estimated the direct medical costs related to HCV in childhood projected for the next decade. Expressed as U.S. dollars, these include $26 million for screening, $117 to $206 million for monitoring, and $56 to $104 million for treatment costs.

There are currently two FDA-approved treatments for HCV in children starting at age 3 years [58]. No strategy to date has been shown to be effective in interrupting maternal-to-fetal transmission, so this is a major research goal in the future.

EPIDEMIOLOGY AND TRANSMISSION

Maternal-to-fetal transmission has been studied extensively. The prevalence of anti-HCV antibody in pregnant women is 0.1% to 2.4%, and 60% to 70% are viremic. Transmission rates are 4% to 7% when the mother is viremic, and mothers with HCV RNA greater than 10^6 copies/mL are more likely to transmit the infection to the fetus compared with mothers with lower levels of viremia [71]. Coinfection with human immunodeficiency virus (HIV) increases the risk of transmission fourfold to fivefold, but highly active retroviral therapy may significantly decrease this risk [72]. In the setting of coinfection with HCV and HIV, there is no evidence that HCV neutralizing antibodies are associated with the prevention of maternal-to-fetal transmission of HCV [73].

Female infants are more likely than male infants to acquire HCV from their mothers [74]. One Japanese study, which reported higher maternal-to-fetal transmission rates than most (14.2%), found positive associations between transmission rate and maternal viral load, liver dysfunction, and blood loss of >500 mL at delivery [75]. Although it is unknown when during pregnancy and delivery HCV transmission occurs, one study suggested that one third to one half of infants acquiring HCV from their mothers were infected in utero [76].

MICROBIOLOGY

HCV is a well-characterized, single-stranded enveloped RNA virus 10 kb in length and 30 to 60 nm in diameter. It contains a single open reading frame that encodes a polyprotein of approximately 3000 amino acids. There are three structural proteins—one core and two envelope (E1 and E2)—and five nonstructural proteins (NS2, NS3, NS4A, NSB, and NS5B). The related genes encode the NS2-3 protease, the NS3/NS4A serine protease, and the NS5B RNA-dependent RNA polymerase [77]. The polyprotein undergoes cleavage by cellular and viral proteases to yield functional proteins. Tissue culture studies in the past had employed replicon systems that produced viral proteins but not infectious virions. In 2005, Kato and Wakita [78] reported a major breakthrough when they were able to culture the JFH-1 HCV virus in Huh 7 cells to produce infectious virions. There are at least six genotypes of HCV and more than 50 subtypes; genotypes differ at 31% to 34% of nucleotide positions on pairwise comparisons of complete sequences, and there is a similar difference between encoded polyproteins. The major utility of the genotypes so far has been to characterize differential susceptibility to antiviral treatments, with genotypes I and IV being most resistant to interferon-based therapies.

PATHOGENESIS

HCV is not considered a cytopathic virus. Viral clearance and hepatic injury are related to the immune response to the virus. The antigen nonspecific arm is the first line of defense and consists of natural killer cells, neutrophils, and macrophages. Dendritic cells assume the role of professional antigen-presenting cells; these induce the virus-specific immune response from $CD4^+$ T helper cells, B cells, and $CD8^+$ cytotoxic T cells. The liver is the only known site of viral replication because negative RNA is detected only in the liver. The immunopathogenesis of HCV liver disease is still being elaborated, but cytokines and Fas ligand–induced apoptosis of hepatocytes probably play major roles. Extrahepatic manifestations of HCV include mixed cryoglobulinemia, membranoproliferative glomerulonephritis, diabetes mellitus, retinopathy, peripheral neuropathy, and lymphoma; pathogenesis of these entities is under current investigation.

PATHOLOGY

Several histologic features are characteristic of HCV, including bile duct damage, steatosis, and lymphoid follicles [79]. In a multicenter antiviral trial of children 5 to 18 years old, 121 liver biopsy specimens were reviewed at entry. Inflammation in the biopsy specimen was minimal in 42%, mild in 17%, moderate in 38%, and severe in only 3%. Five specimens had bridging fibrosis, and two had cirrhosis [80].

CLINICAL MANIFESTATIONS

Pergam and coworkers [81] reported more recently that infants of HCV-positive mothers were more likely to have low birth weight, to be small for gestational age, to need assisted ventilation, and to require admission to a neonatal intensive care unit. HCV-positive mothers with excess weight gain also had a greater risk of gestational diabetes [81]. Cholestasis of pregnancy is increased in HCV-infected mothers [82]. The European Paediatric Hepatitis C Virus Network reported the natural history of 266 children with vertical HCV infection; approximately 20% seemed to clear the infection, 50% had evidence of chronic asymptomatic infection, and 30% had evidence of chronic active infection [83]. Children with transfusion-acquired HCV also tend to have mild asymptomatic infection, although rarely infection may proceed to decompensated liver disease and liver transplantation [84]. In another large pediatric natural history study, 1.8% of children progressed to decompensated cirrhosis (mean age 9.6 years). These children were mostly perinatally infected with genotype 1a, and most of the mothers were intravenous drug users [85].

DIAGNOSIS

Diagnosis is usually made by screening of high-risk children for anti-HCV antibody. Infection is confirmed by HCV RNA by polymerase chain reaction (PCR) assay. The AAP recommends that infants born to HCV-infected mothers be screened by anti-HCV at 18 months postpartum because passively acquired maternal antibody can persist for 18 months [86].

TREATMENT

There are currently two FDA-approved antiviral therapies for children: interferon plus ribavirin given three times weekly, which is indicated for children 3 to 18 years old with HCV infection, and pegylated interferon plus ribavirin given once a week, which is indicated for children 5 to 18 years old; both regimens are given for 48 weeks for children with genotypes 1 and 4. Children with genotypes 2 and 3 may require only 24 weeks of therapy similar to adults, but this has not been well studied in children. Sustained viral response (e.g., negative HCV RNA 6 months after cessation of therapy) for thrice-weekly interferon plus ribavirin is 46% [87] and for weekly pegylated interferon plus ribavirin is 59% [88]. Many small molecule inhibitors of HCV replication, such as inhibitors of the NS3 serine protease and the RNA polymerase, are being studied in adults with positive preliminary results, although none have been approved by the FDA as yet. Such therapies will be tested in children after safety and efficacy are well established in adults.

PREVENTION

At present, there is no effective way to interrupt transmission of HCV from mother to infant. At present neither elective cesarean section nor avoidance of breast-feeding should be recommended to HCV-infected women [89], although scattered reports do show a higher risk of HCV transmission for infants whose mothers have HCV RNA in breast milk [90]. In one report, membrane rupture lasting 6 or more hours and internal fetal monitoring were associated with increased rates of transmission of HCV from mother to infant, suggesting there may be obstetric practices that can reduce transmission [37]. Others have reported an association of higher transmission rates with intrapartum exposure to virus-contaminated maternal blood secondary to a perineal or vaginal laceration [91].

HCV RNA is detectable in maternal colostrum. HCV transmission via breast-feeding has not been well documented, however. Inactivation of the virus by gastric acid and very low levels of virus in breast milk may explain this potential protective mechanism. The AAP and the American College of Obstetricians and Gynecologists support breast-feeding by mothers with HCV infection [86]. There is definitely a role for public education about risk avoidance for high-risk children and adolescents. Schwarz and colleagues [92] reported more recently that 19% of homeless caregivers were anti-HCV–positive, although no cases of HCV infection were found in the children, suggesting the importance of directing preventive education to the young.

HEPATITIS E VIRUS

Hepatitis E virus (HEV) is endemic in many developing countries, where it is responsible for more than 50% of cases of acute viral hepatitis [93]. More recent data have shown that HEV is more common worldwide than HAV [94]. HEV is an important public health concern as a major cause of enterically transmitted hepatitis worldwide. Cases of sporadic HEV in people with no history of recent travel (autochthonous infection) in developed countries are far more common than previously thought [94]. HEV is frequently misdiagnosed as drug-induced liver injury or hepatitis of unknown etiology. HEV has a poor prognosis in patients with preexisting chronic liver disease and pregnant women in their third trimester. Patients with unexplained hepatitis should be tested for HEV, regardless of their age, demographics, or travel history.

EPIDEMIOLOGY AND TRANSMISSION

HEV is spread through food or water contaminated by feces from an infected individual. Transmission of HEV is by the fecal-oral route. Water-borne outbreaks have often been reported in developing countries [94]. In contrast to the other agents of viral hepatitis, HEV commonly is found in wild and domestic animals, which may provide an important source of infections in humans [94]. Person-to-person transmission seems to be much less efficient than with HAV. HEV transmission is highly endemic in Asia, the Middle East, and Africa. Sporadic HEV infection has been reported in developing countries, particularly on the Indian subcontinent, where some studies have shown HEV to be the most common etiology of acute viral hepatitis [94]. In the United States, HEV infection is uncommon and generally occurs in travelers returning from countries with high endemicity. Autochthonous infection has been reported in developed regions such as North America, Europe, Japan, New Zealand, and Australia, and a porcine zoonosis has been suggested [94,95]. Compared with HEV infections in the developing world, in developed countries most autochthonous HEV infections are reported in middle-aged and elderly men [94].

Studies in endemic regions show high seroprevalence rates of HEV ranging from 15% to 60% [96–98]. The anti-HEV seroprevalence rate reaches more than 95% in children living in endemic areas by the age of 10 years. Anti-HEV antibodies are rarely detected in children. Anti-HEV seroprevalence increases to 40% in young adults without substantial increases later in life [96]. Maternal-to-fetal transmission of HEV ranges from 23.3% [99] to 50% [100]. Acute HEV infection is severe for the mother during the third trimester of pregnancy, resulting in a mortality rate of 15% to 25% [101]. In a large prenatal study in India, 28 of 469 pregnant women were positive for HEV RNA; 12 of these women had acute liver disease, and 2 died undelivered [102]. The remaining 16 women had mild disease with full recovery. Of 26 infants born, all were positive for HEV RNA and developed acute infection [102].

MICROBIOLOGY

HEV causing epidemic non-A, non-B hepatitis was identified in 1983 from a human challenge experiment and subsequently cloned in 1990. HEV is a spherical, nonenveloped, positive-strand RNA virus, classified as a member of the Caliciviridae family, that is approximately 32 to 34 nm in diameter [103]. Two major species of the virus are recognized: mammalian HEV, a virus that causes acute hepatitis in humans and has a reservoir in pigs and possibly a range of other mammals, and avian HEV. Four major genotypes of mammalian HEV have been reported. Genotype 1 HEV is the main cause of sporadic and epidemic HEV in developing regions of Asia, Africa, and South America. Genotype 2 has so far been identified in patients in Mexico, Chad, and Nigeria [104–106]. Genotype 3 HEV has been found in patients with autochthonous HEV in many developed regions and in pig populations worldwide [107]. Genotype 4 has been found in developed countries such as Japan, China, and Taiwan and in pig populations in those countries and India [108,109].

PATHOGENESIS

Peak viremia occurs during the incubation period and the early acute phase of disease. Immediately before the onset of clinical symptoms, HEV RNA can be detected in the blood and stool. The concentration of serum liver enzymes increases, with a marked elevation of serum aminotransferases, peaking at about 6 weeks after exposure coincident with anti-HEV in serum and decreasing HEV antigen in hepatocytes. Infiltrating lymphocytes in the liver have been found to be a cytotoxic/suppressor immunophenotype, and this supports the role of an immune-mediated response in the pathogenesis of liver injury [110].

A few days to weeks after the onset of clinical symptoms, HEV RNA is cleared from the blood; however, the virus continues to be shed in stool for another 2 weeks [111]. Researchers have been unable to explain the high HEV morbidity in pregnancy, why it is different from other hepatitis viruses such as HAV with similar epidemiologic features, and the difference in HEV morbidity in pregnant women in different geographic regions.

PATHOLOGY

Generally, individuals with HEV who travel from developing countries are diagnosed with serology without a liver biopsy. Few patients with autochthonous HEV require a liver biopsy because they have a self-limiting illness. In a few patients with more severe hepatitis, a liver biopsy may be required. The few data on hepatic histopathology of acute autochthonous HEV are limited to patients with severe disease. Liver histology in noncirrhotic liver is similar to that seen in other cases of acute viral hepatitis, with lobular disarray with reticulin framework distortion, portal tract expansion with severe mixed polymorphonuclear and lymphocytic inflammatory infiltrates, moderate to severe interface hepatitis, and cholangiolitis [112,113].

In patients with HEV who have underlying cirrhosis, the liver histology is nonspecific [114]. In the few transplant patients receiving immunosuppression who have developed chronic HEV infection, liver histology shows progressive fibrosis, portal hepatitis with lymphocytic infiltration, and piecemeal necrosis with progression to cirrhosis [115,116].

CLINICAL MANIFESTATIONS

In most individuals, HEV manifests as a self-limiting, acute, icteric hepatitis with symptoms including jaundice, malaise, anorexia, fever, abdominal pain, and arthralgia. Clinical disease is more common among adults than among children. Mortality rates associated with HEV are low and are thought to be about 1% in the general population [117]. HEV is more severe in pregnant women, however, in whom mortality rates can reach 20% [118,119].

The incubation period ranges from 2 to 9 weeks. The presentation of HEV in individuals infected in developed countries seems to be similar to individuals from endemic regions; however, the mortality rate is higher, ranging from 8% to 11%. Most autochthonous HEV infections are self-limiting [94]; 8% to 11% of infected individuals develop fulminant hepatitis and liver failure. Individuals with underlying chronic liver disease can have a poor outcome with mortality approaching 70% [120,121]. A study from India showed that patients with chronic liver disease and HEV superinfection have a 1-year mortality rate of 70% [122]. Chronic HEV infection has been documented in patients receiving immunosuppressive therapy after organ transplantation [115].

DIAGNOSIS

The antibody response to HEV infection follows a conventional course with specific IgM usually detectable at the onset of symptoms or deranged liver function, followed shortly by HEV-specific IgG [123]. Most primary serologic tests are enzyme immunoassays that use recombinant antigens derived from different strains of HEV. Conventional and real-time reverse transcriptase PCR assays have been used to detect HEV RNA in clinical specimens (mainly blood). Although reverse transcriptase PCR seems to be more sensitive than serology for HEV diagnosis, [124–126], the window of detectable HEV viremia is narrow [127]. Because patients might not present until sometime after the onset of illness, a negative result does not exclude infection.

TREATMENT

HEV illness usually is self-limiting over several weeks to months, and treatment is supportive. Patients with pre-existing chronic liver disease who develop hepatic failure as a result of HEV infection should be considered for liver transplant because such patients have a poor outcome. Administration of immunoglobulin has not been helpful in preventing the disease in HEV-endemic areas [110,128].

PREVENTION

The only way to prevent HEV disease is to reduce the risk of exposure to the virus. The risk for HEV transmission in infants born to asymptomatic anti-HEV–positive mothers seems to be low. No data suggest cesarean section prevents HEV transmission [129]. Given the low amount of HEV in colostrum (low infectivity), breast-feeding, an important nutrition source in endemic areas, should not be discouraged [129]. Mothers with symptomatic HEV with high viral loads should be advised not to breast-feed, however, because of potential risk of transmission [129]. Although there is no FDA-approved vaccine for HEV, several vaccines are under development, including a completed phase II randomized placebo-controlled trial in Nepal of a vaccine with efficacy of 95.5% [130]. At 2 years' follow-up, only 56% of vaccinated individuals had detectable anti-HEV, however. The most important issue is the safety and efficacy of the vaccine in women because mortality is high in pregnant women and individuals with chronic liver disease infected with HEV. Other issues include the durability of vaccine-induced immunity and its cost-effectiveness.

OTHER HEPATOTROPIC VIRUSES

Some cases of viral hepatitis cannot be attributed to the hepatitis A, B, C, D, or E viruses or even less common viruses that can infect the liver, such as cytomegalovirus, Epstein-Barr virus, herpesvirus, parvovirus, and adenovirus. These cases are called non-A–E hepatitis. Scientists continue to study the causes of non-A–E hepatitis. GB virus type C/hepatitis G virus (GBV-C/HGV) and TTV and its species variants such as SEN virus (SEN-V) have been a health care concern and received extensive investigation as possible agents of acute non-A–E hepatitis. Although they do not seem to be responsible for most sporadic acute non-A-E hepatitis cases, more research is needed.

GB VIRUS TYPE C/HEPATITIS G VIRUS

GBV-C/HGV was discovered in 1995 with relatively high prevalence in the general population of developed countries. GBV-C/HGV is transmitted by transfusion of blood and blood products, intravenous drug abuse, sexual contact, and maternal-to-fetal transmission. The potentially hepatotropic flavivirus-like virus has been detected in a few patients with acute and chronic hepatitis and in a certain proportion of blood donors and recipients of blood or blood components [131].

Epidemiology and Transmission

Approximately 1% to 5% of volunteer blood donors in developed countries are HGV viremic; however, the prevalence in the general population in some developing countries is 10% to 20%. GBV-C/HGV is transmitted parenterally. High-risk groups include intravenous drug users, patients with multiple transfusions, patients undergoing hemodialysis, and hemophiliacs. Transmission from mother to infant and sexual contact has been documented.

GBV-C/HGV is frequently transmitted from pregnant mothers to infants in the general population. The most critical factor is the titer of viral RNA in the maternal serum. In one study, the use of elective cesarean section in women with high titers of viral RNA resulted in decreased vertical transmission of the virus [131]. Until more is known about the pathogenesis of perinatal infection, cesarean section is not recommended for routine prevention of perinatal GBV-C/HGV infection, however.

Microbiology

GBV-C/HGV viruses, variants of the same viral species, belong to the Flaviviridae, distantly related to HCV, and are now classified into five genotypes (West Africa, North America, Asia). GBV-C/HGV has a positive-stranded, linear RNA genome with a large open reading frame that encodes a single large polyprotein [132].

Pathogenesis

Despite the described cases of acute and chronic hepatitis G, its hepatic tropism and the mechanism responsible for hepatitis are still unclear or controversial [132].

Pathology

GBV-C/HGV can cause persistent infection in young infants with unclear or insignificant evidence of liver disease [132].

Clinical Manifestations

There may be a rare association of GBV-C/HGV infection with transient elevation of aminotransferases in patients with jaundice. Only 0.3% of individuals with acute viral hepatitis are infected with GBV-C/HGV alone. Approximately 3% to 6% of individuals with non-A–E hepatitis are GBV-C/HGV viremic. GBV-C/HGV is not the major cause of acute viral hepatitis. To date, this virus has not been associated with acute or chronic hepatitis [133]. GBV-C/HGV has not been a cause of fulminant hepatic failure and it does not have an association with hepatocellular carcinoma.

Diagnosis

No commercial serologic tests are available. Indirect immunoassay to the envelope protein E2 is for research purposes only. E2-specific antibodies are associated with loss of detectable GBV-C/HGV RNA, which indicates recovery from GBV-C/HGV. Reverse transcriptase PCR is used for detecting GBV-C RNA in serum samples.

Treatment

Because the virus has never been shown to cause significant symptoms or liver damage, no treatment is indicated. HGV has been reported to respond to interferon therapy, but the infection recurs when the treatment is completed [134].

Prevention

Viral screening is not yet recommended before blood transfusion. Cesarean section is not a recommended practice to avoid maternal-to-fetal transmission of GBV-C/HGV.

TRANSFUSION-TRANSMITTED VIRUS

In 1997, a novel DNA virus was isolated from the serum of a Japanese patient who was diagnosed with hepatitis after blood transfusion of unknown etiology [135].

Epidemiology and Transmission

Epidemiologic studies suggest that TTV is mainly transmitted via the parenteral route and maternal-to-fetal transmission, although the fecal-oral route and sexual contact have been reported. Infection rate of TTV is higher in patients with liver diseases than in healthy donors. TTV is widespread throughout the world and can be detected in 50% to 95% of healthy persons [135]. Gerner and associates [136] suggested that TTV can be transmitted transplacentally. Transplacental transmission of TTV is possibly low and independent of viral load [135]. A study in the Republic of Congo showed that a significant number of infants acquired TTV infection at 3 months postpartum (61 [58%] of 105 women at a prenatal clinic and 36 [54%] of 68 infants); however TTV was detected in 43% of children with TTV-negative mothers (13 of 30). In addition, nucleotide sequences of TTV in these children were often unmatched with those in their mothers [137].

TTV may be transmitted early in childhood based on the evidence of higher viral copies of TTV and a high prevalence of TTV in children of all ages. Although the mechanism of postnatal transmission of TTV is unknown in some children, horizontal infection via breast-feeding could explain this because TTV was detected in breast milk from TTV-positive women whose infants were TTV-negative at both 5 days and 3 months of age, but shown to be TTV-positive at 6 months of age [138]. In addition, the breast-fed infants had an increased positive seroconversion rate of TTV with an increase in length of breast-feeding duration [139].

Microbiology

TTV is a nonenveloped, single-stranded, and circular DNA virus with the entire sequence of 3852 nucleotides and mostly resembles the members of the Circoviridae family. It is classified into 16 genotypes [140]. TTVs are extraordinarily diverse, spanning five groups including SANBAN and SEN viruses. Recombination between variants is frequent. The extremely high sequence divergence of TTV strains explains a mixed infection with different genotypes in the same individual. It is unclear how TTVs could be viable and why they require such genetic variation.

Pathogenesis

TTV can infect not only hepatocytes, but also extrahepatic tissues such as bone marrow. Although the pathogenicity of TTV is thought to be comparatively weak, it was postulated to cause liver damage in some studies [140].

Pathology

Histologic activity indices in patients with chronic HCV infection coinfected with TTV were higher than patients with HCV infection alone; however, the pathogenicity and clinical significance of TTV remain unclear at present [141].

Clinical Manifestations

TTV is a virus frequently isolated from patients with various types of viral hepatitis, from patients presenting with hepatitis of unknown etiology, and from healthy individuals. TTV has no effect on biochemical markers of associated viral hepatitis. It may be associated with a mild form of non-A–E hepatitis [142]. Although the mechanism of persistent TTV viremia is not well understood, a significant difference of liver biochemistry is not observed among healthy children with isolated TTV infection and children with HBV and HCV infection with TTV coinfection [143].

Diagnosis

No serologic test is currently available. The viral DNA has been detected by PCR.

Treatment

In cases of coinfection with HCV, TTV eradication was observed in some patients with interferon treatment, but the TTV DNA was detected again after the treatment [144]. Because there is substantial controversy regarding the disease-causing potential of TTV, interferon therapy for TTV is not routinely recommended.

Prevention

TTV screening is not yet recommended before blood transfusion. Cesarean section has not been a recommended practice to avoid maternal-to-fetal transmission of TTV.

CONCLUSION

Translational research has made many contributions to knowledge about the hepatotropic viruses, but knowledge gaps remain. The incidence and health care costs related to HAV should decrease dramatically with the use of the highly effective hepatitis A vaccine for all subjects 1 to 18 years old; universal vaccination for all adults as well may be a more practical strategy, rather than targeted immunization in high-risk groups. More effective strategies are needed to prevent maternal-to-fetal transmission of HBV because vaccine failures still occur in at least 10% of mother-infant pairs. New data have emerged in recent years on the natural history and treatment of chronic HBV infection in children, but antiviral resistance remains a main concern during long-term treatment of chronic HBV. Advances have been made in treatment of HCV in children, and promising results are seen with specifically targeted antiviral therapies. A novel hepatitis E vaccine was shown to be efficacious; however, more investigations to improve immunogenicity and safety are needed, especially for pregnant women, in whom morbidity and mortality are high. Close observations of HGV and TTV are needed to see if these viruses are truly of clinical significance.

REFERENCES

[1] A. Wasley, A. Fiore, B.P. Bell, Hepatitis A in the era of vaccination, Epidemiol. Rev. 28 (2006) 101–111.
[2] J.J. Berge, et al., The cost of hepatitis A infections in American adolescents and adults in 1997, Hepatology 31 (2000) 469–473.
[3] American Academy of Pediatrics, in: L.K. Pickering et al., (Ed.), Hepatitis A in Red Book: 2006 Report of the Committee on Infectious Diseases, twenty seventh ed., American Academy of Pediatrics, Elk Grove Village, IL, (2006) 326–335.
[4] A.E. Fiore, A. Wasley, B.P. Bell, Advisory Committee on Immunization Practices (ACIP). Prevention of hepatitis A through active or passive immunization: recommendations of the Advisory Committee on Immunization Practices (ACIP), MMWR Recomm. Rep. 55 (2006) 1–23.
[5] M.B. Koslap-Petraco, M. Shub, R. Judelsohn, Hepatitis A: disease burden and current childhood vaccination strategies in the United States, J. Pediatr. Health Care 22 (2008) 3–11.
[6] G.L. Armstrong, et al., The economics of routine childhood hepatitis A immunization in the United States: the impact of herd immunity, Pediatrics 119 (2007) e22–e29.
[7] C. Wheeler, et al., An outbreak of hepatitis A associated with green onions, N. Engl. J. Med. 353 (2005) 890–897.
[8] J.A. Cuthbert, Hepatitis A: old and new, Clin. Microbiol. Rev. 14 (2001) 38–58.
[9] L.S. Rosenblum, et al., Hepatitis A outbreak in a neonatal intensive care unit: risk factors for transmission and evidence of prolonged viral excretion among preterm infants, J. Infect. Dis. 164 (1991) 476–482.
[10] D.H. Hamer, B.A. Connor, Travel health knowledge, attitudes and practices among United States travelers, J. Travel Med. 11 (2004) 23–26.
[11] R. Steffen, Changing travel-related global epidemiology of hepatitis A, Am. J. Med. 118 (Suppl. 10A) (2005) 46S–49S.
[12] D.D. Chancellor, et al., Green onions: potential mechanism for hepatitis A contamination, J. Food Prot. 69 (2006) 1468–1472.
[13] H.B. Jenson, The changing picture of hepatitis A in the United States, Curr. Opin. Pediatr. 16 (2004) 89–93.
[14] J.C. Watson, et al., Vertical transmission of hepatitis A resulting in an outbreak in a neonatal intensive care unit, J. Infect. Dis. 167 (1993) 567–571.
[15] I. Tanaka, et al., Vertical transmission of hepatitis A virus, Lancet 345 (1995) 397.
[16] T. Erkan, et al., A case of vertical transmission of hepatitis A virus infection, Acta Paediatr. 87 (1998) 1008–1009.
[17] N. Urganci, et al., Neonatal cholestasis resulting from vertical transmission of hepatitis A infection, Pediatr. Infect. Dis. J. 22 (2003) 381–382.
[18] R.C. Noble, et al., Posttransfusion hepatitis A in a neonatal intensive care unit, JAMA 252 (1984) 2711–2715.
[19] R.M. Pinto, et al., Codon usage and replicative strategies of hepatitis A virus, Virus Res. 127 (2007) 158–163.
[20] J.T. Stapleton, Host immune response to hepatitis A virus, J. Infect. Dis. 171 (Suppl. 1) (1995) S9–S14.
[21] B. Fleischer, A. Vallbracht, Demonstration of virus-specific cytotoxic T lymphocytes in liver tissue in hepatitis A—a model for immunopathological reactions, Behring Inst. Mitt. (89) (1991) 226–230.
[22] P. Kryger, P. Christoffersen, Liver histopathology of the hepatitis A virus infection: a comparison with hepatitis type B and non-A, non-B, J. Clin. Pathol. 36 (1983) 650–654.
[23] G.L. Armstrong, B.P. Bell, Hepatitis A virus infections in the United States: model-based estimates and implications for childhood immunization, Pediatrics 109 (2002) 839–845.
[24] E. Elinav, et al., Acute hepatitis A infection in pregnancy is associated with high rates of gestational complications and preterm labor, Gastroenterology 130 (2006) 1129–1134.
[25] S.A. Gall, Expanding the use of hepatitis vaccines in obstetrics and gynecology, Am. J. Med. 118 (Suppl. 10A) (2005) 96S–99S.
[26] R.L. Renge, et al., Vertical transmission of hepatitis A, Indian J. Pediatr. 69 (2002) 535–536.
[27] E. Leikin, et al., Intrauterine transmission of hepatitis A virus, Obstet. Gynecol. 88 (1996) 690–691.
[28] R.S. McDuffie Jr., T. Bader, Fetal meconium peritonitis after maternal hepatitis A, Am. J. Obstet. Gynecol. 180 (1999) 1031–1032.
[29] S. Vento, et al., Fulminant hepatitis associated with hepatitis A virus superinfection in patients with chronic hepatitis C, N. Engl. J. Med. 338 (1998) 286–290.
[30] J.M. Lieberman, et al., Kinetics of maternal hepatitis a antibody decay in infants: implications for vaccine use, Pediatr. Infect. Dis. J. 21 (2002) 347–348.
[31] R. Dagan, et al., Immunization against hepatitis A in the first year of life: priming despite the presence of maternal antibody, Pediatr. Infect. Dis. J. 19 (2000) 1045–1052.
[32] G.W. Letson, et al., Effect of maternal antibody on immunogenicity of hepatitis A vaccine in infants, J. Pediatr. 144 (2004) 327–332.
[33] B.P. Bell, et al., Immunogenicity of an inactivated hepatitis A vaccine in infants and young children, Pediatr. Infect. Dis. J. 26 (2007) 116–122.
[34] S. Stojanov, et al., Administration of hepatitis A vaccine at 6 and 12 months of age concomitantly with hexavalent (DTaP-IPV-PRP approximately T-HBs) combination vaccine, Vaccine 25 (2007) 7549–7558.
[35] H.D. Nothdurft, Hepatitis A vaccines, Expert Rev. Vaccines 7 (2008) 535–545.
[36] N.S. Crowcroft, et al., PHLS Advisory Committee on Vaccination and Immunisation. Guidelines for the control of hepatitis A virus infection, Commun. Dis. Public Health 4 (2001) 213–227.
[37] E.E. Mast, M.J. Alter, H.S. Margolis, Strategies to prevent and control hepatitis B and C virus infections: a global perspective, Vaccine 17 (1999) 1730–1733.
[38] W.M. Lee, Hepatitis B virus infection, N. Engl. J. Med. 337 (1997) 1733–1745.
[39] S. Ramia, H. Bahakim, Perinatal transmission of hepatitis B virus-associated hepatitis D virus, Ann. Inst. Pasteur. Virol. 139 (1988) 285–290.
[40] W.H. Chen, et al., Neonatal gastric aspirates as a predictor of perinatal hepatitis B virus infections, Int. J. Gynaecol. Obstet. 60 (1998) 15–21.
[41] Z.J. Shao, et al., Maternal hepatitis B virus (HBV) DNA positivity and sexual intercourse are associated with HBV intrauterine transmission in China: a prospective case-control study, J. Gastroenterol. Hepatol. 22 (2007) 165–170.
[42] A. Soderstrom, G. Norkrans, M. Lindh, Hepatitis B virus DNA during pregnancy and post partum: aspects on vertical transmission, Scand. J. Infect. Dis. 35 (2003) 814–819.
[43] Z. Wang, et al., Quantitative analysis of HBV DNA level and HBeAg titer in hepatitis B surface antigen positive mothers and their babies: HBeAg passage through the placenta and the rate of decay in babies, J. Med. Virol. 71 (2003) 360–366.
[44] S.S. Plitt, A.M. Somily, A.E. Singh, Outcomes from a Canadian public health prenatal screening program for hepatitis B: 1997–2004, Can. J. Public Health 98 (2007) 194–197.
[45] J.B. Hill, et al., Risk of hepatitis B transmission in breast-fed infants of chronic hepatitis B carriers, Obstet. Gynecol. 99 (2002) 1049–1052.
[46] J.H. Kao, Diagnosis of hepatitis B virus infection through serological and virological markers, Expert Rev. Gastroenterol. Hepatol. 2 (2008) 553–562.
[47] Z. Zhang, et al., Severe dendritic cell perturbation is actively involved in the pathogenesis of acute-on-chronic hepatitis B liver failure, J. Hepatol. 49 (2008) 396–406.
[48] P. Arbuthnot, A. Capovilla, M. Kew, Putative role of hepatitis B virus X protein in hepatocarcinogenesis: effects on apoptosis, DNA repair, mitogen-activated protein kinase and JAK/STAT pathways, J. Gastroenterol. Hepatol. 15 (2000) 357–368.
[49] T.C. Wu, et al., Primary hepatocellular carcinoma and hepatitis B infection during childhood, Hepatology 7 (1987) 46–48.
[50] M. Woynarowski, et al., Inter-observer variability in histopathological assessment of liver biopsies taken in a pediatric open label therapeutic program for chronic HBV infection treatment, World J. Gastroenterol. 12 (2006) 1713–1717.
[51] E.K. Hsu, K.F. Murray, Hepatitis B and C in children, Nat. Clin. Pract. Gastroenterol. Hepatol. 5 (2008) 311–320.
[52] K. Shiraki, et al., Acute hepatitis B in infants born to carrier mother with the antibody to hepatitis B e antigen, J. Pediatr. 97 (1980) 768–770.
[53] F. Bortolotti, et al., An epidemiological survey of hepatitis C virus infection in Italian children in the decade 1990–1999, J. Pediatr. Gastroenterol. Nutr. 32 (2001) 562–566.

[54] T.I. Huo, et al., Sero-clearance of hepatitis B surface antigen in chronic carriers does not necessarily imply a good prognosis, Hepatology 28 (1998) 231–236.

[55] A.S. Lok, B.J. McMahon, Chronic hepatitis B, Hepatology 45 (2007) 507–539.

[56] G.G. Su, et al., Efficacy and safety of lamivudine treatment for chronic hepatitis B in pregnancy, World J. Gastroenterol. 10 (2004) 910–912.

[57] E.A. Belongia, et al., NIH Consensus Development Statement on Management of Hepatitis B: Draft, NIH Consens. State Sci. Statements (2008) 25.

[58] E.K. Hsu, K.F. Murray, Hepatitis B and C in children, Nat. Clin. Pract. Gastroenterol. Hepatol. 5 (2008) 311–320.

[59] M.M. Jonas, et al., Safety, efficacy, and pharmacokinetics of adefovir dipivoxil in children and adolescents (age 2 to <18 years) with chronic hepatitis B, Hepatology 47 (2008) 1863–1871.

[60] A. Mele, et al., Acute hepatitis delta virus infection in Italy: incidence and risk factors after the introduction of the universal anti-hepatitis B vaccination campaign, Clin. Infect. Dis. 44 (2007) e17–e24.

[61] V.H. Gonzalez-Quintero, et al., Assessing perinatal hepatitis B screening and neonatal prophylaxis in a large, multiethnic county, J. Reprod. Med. 51 (2006) 101–108.

[62] A. Soderstrom, G. Norkrans, M. Lindh, Hepatitis B virus DNA during pregnancy and post partum: aspects on vertical transmission, Scand. J. Infect. Dis. 35 (2003) 814–819.

[63] P. Sangfelt, et al., Serum ALT levels as a surrogate marker for serum HBV DNA levels in HBeAg-negative pregnant women, Scand. J. Infect. Dis. 36 (2004) 182–185.

[64] X.M. Xiao, et al., Prevention of vertical hepatitis B transmission by hepatitis B immunoglobulin in the third trimester of pregnancy, Int. J. Gynaecol. Obstet. 96 (2007) 167–170.

[65] J. Yuan, et al., Antepartum immunoprophylaxis of three doses of hepatitis B immunoglobulin is not effective: a single-centre randomized study, J. Viral Hepat. 13 (2006) 597–604.

[66] R. Vranckx, A. Alisjahbana, A. Meheus, Hepatitis B virus vaccination and antenatal transmission of HBV markers to neonates, J. Viral Hepat. 6 (1999) 135–139.

[67] Y. Bacq, Hepatitis B and pregnancy, Gastroenterol. Clin. Biol. 32 (2008) S12–S19.

[68] M. Gambarin-Gelwan, Hepatitis B in pregnancy, Clin. Liver Dis. 11 (2007) 945–963, x.

[69] N.L. Luban, et al., The epidemiology of transfusion-associated hepatitis C in a children's hospital, Transfusion 47 (2007) 615–620.

[70] R. Jhaveri, et al., The burden of hepatitis C virus infection in children: estimated direct medical costs over a 10-year period, J. Pediatr. 148 (2006) 353–358.

[71] E.A. Roberts, L. Yeung, Maternal-infant transmission of hepatitis C virus infection, Hepatology 36 (2002) S106–S113.

[72] J. Airoldi, V. Berghella, Hepatitis C and pregnancy, Obstet. Gynecol. Surv. 61 (2006) 666–672.

[73] K.A. Dowd, et al., Maternal neutralizing antibody and transmission of hepatitis C virus to infants, J. Infect. Dis. 198 (2008) 1651–1655.

[74] F. Bortolotti, et al., Epidemiological profile of 806 Italian children with hepatitis C virus infection over a 15-year period, J. Hepatol. 46 (2007) 783–790.

[75] A. Hayashida, et al., Re-evaluation of the true rate of hepatitis C virus mother-to-child transmission and its novel risk factors based on our two prospective studies, J. Obstet. Gynaecol. Res. 33 (2007) 417–422.

[76] J. Mok, et al., European Paediatric Hepatitis C Virus Network. When does mother to child transmission of hepatitis C virus occur, Arch. Dis. Child. Fetal Neonatal. Ed. 90 (2005) F156–F160.

[77] M. Thomson, T.J. Liang, Molecular Biology of Hepatitis C Virus in Hepatitis C: Biomedical Research Reports, in: T.J. Liang, J.H. Hoofnagle (Eds.), Academic Press, San Diego, CA, (2000), 1–24.

[78] T. Kato, T. Wakita, Production of infectious hepatitis C virus in cell culture, Uirusu 55 (2005) 287–295.

[79] N. Bach, S.N. Thung, F. Schaffner, The histological features of chronic hepatitis C and autoimmune chronic hepatitis: a comparative analysis, Hepatology 15 (1992) 572–577.

[80] Z.D. Goodman, et al., Pathology of chronic hepatitis C in children: Liver biopsy findings in the Peds-C Trial, Hepatology 47 (2008) 836–843.

[81] S.A. Pergam, et al., Pregnancy complications associated with hepatitis C: data from a 2003–2005 Washington state birth cohort, Am. J. Obstet. Gynecol. 199 (2008) 38.e1–38.e9.

[82] E.M. Berkley, et al., Chronic hepatitis C in pregnancy, Obstet. Gynecol. 112 (2008) 304–310.

[83] European Paediatric Hepatitis C Virus Network, Three broad modalities in the natural history of vertically acquired hepatitis C virus infection, Clin. Infect. Dis. 41 (2005) 45–51.

[84] P. Mohan, et al., Clinical spectrum and histopathologic features of chronic hepatitis C infection in children, J. Pediatr. 150 (2007) 168.e1–174.e1.

[85] F. Bortolotti, et al., Long-term course of chronic hepatitis C in children: from viral clearance to end-stage liver disease, Gastroenterology 134 (2008) 1900–1907.

[86] American, Academy of Pediatrics, in: L.K. Pickering et al., (Eds.), Hepatitis C in Red Book: 2006 Report of the Committee on Infectious Diseases, twenty seventh ed., American Academy of Pediatrics, Elk Grove Village, IL, (2006), 358.

[87] R.P. Gonzalez-Peralta, et al., Interferon alfa-2b in combination with ribavirin for the treatment of chronic hepatitis C in children: efficacy, safety, and pharmacokinetics, Hepatology 42 (2005) 1010–1018.

[88] S. Wirth, et al., Recombinant alfa-interferon plus ribavirin therapy in children and adolescents with chronic hepatitis C, Hepatology 36 (2002) 1280–1284.

[89] L. Pembrey, M.L. Newell, P.A. Tovo, EPHN Collaborators, The management of HCV infected pregnant women and their children European paediatric HCV network, J. Hepatol. 43 (2005) 515–525.

[90] A. Ruiz-Extremera, et al., Follow-up of transmission of hepatitis C to babies of human immunodeficiency virus-negative women: the role of breast-feeding in transmission, Pediatr. Infect. Dis. J. 19 (2000) 511–516.

[91] C. Steininger, et al., Increased risk of mother-to-infant transmission of hepatitis C virus by intrapartum infantile exposure to maternal blood, J. Infect. Dis. 187 (2003) 345–351.

[92] K.B. Schwarz, et al., Seroprevalence of HCV infection in homeless Baltimore families, J Health Care Poor Underserved. 19 (2007) 580–587.

[93] R. Aggarwal, S.R. Naik, Epidemiology of hepatitis E: past, present and future, Trop. Gastroenterol. 18 (1997) 49–56.

[94] H.R. Dalton, et al., Hepatitis E: an emerging infection in developed countries, Lancet Infect. Dis. 8 (2008) 698–709.

[95] R.H. Purcell, S.U. Emerson, Hepatitis E: an emerging awareness of an old disease, J. Hepatol. 48 (2008) 494–503.

[96] V.A. Arankalle, et al., Age-specific prevalence of antibodies to hepatitis A and E viruses in Pune, India, 1982 and 1992, J. Infect. Dis. 171 (1995) 447–450.

[97] E.T. Clayson, et al., Rates of hepatitis E virus infection and disease among adolescents and adults in Kathmandu, Nepal, J. Infect. Dis. 176 (1997) 763–766.

[98] H.T. Tran, et al., Prevalence of hepatitis virus types B through E and genotypic distribution of HBV and HCV in Ho Chi Minh City, Vietnam, Hepatol. Res. 26 (2003) 275–280.

[99] A. Kumar, et al., Hepatitis E in pregnancy, Int. J. Gynaecol. Obstet. 85 (2004) 240–244.

[100] S. Singh, et al., Mother-to-child transmission of hepatitis E virus infection, Indian J. Pediatr. 70 (2003) 37–39.

[101] S. Ranger-Rogez, S. Alain, F. Denis, Hepatitis viruses: mother to child transmission, Pathol. Biol. (Paris) 50 (2002) 568–575.

[102] R.M. Kumar, et al., Sero-prevalence and mother-to-infant transmission of hepatitis E virus among pregnant women in the United Arab Emirates, Eur. J. Obstet. Gynecol. Reprod. Biol. 100 (2001) 9–15.

[103] K.C. Hyams, New perspectives on hepatitis E, Curr. Gastroenterol. Rep. 4 (2002) 302–307.

[104] Y. Buisson, et al., Identification of a novel hepatitis E virus in Nigeria, J. Gen. Virol. 81 (2000) 903–909.

[105] H. van Cuyck-Gandre, et al., Characterization of hepatitis E virus (HEV) from Algeria and Chad by partial genome sequence, J. Med. Virol. 53 (1997) 340–347.

[106] A.W. Tam, et al., Hepatitis E virus (HEV): molecular cloning and sequencing of the full-length viral genome, Virology 185 (1991) 120–131.

[107] M. Banks, et al., Evidence for the presence of hepatitis E virus in pigs in the United Kingdom, Vet. Rec. 154 (2004) 223–227.

[108] L. Lu, C. Li, C.H. Hagedorn, Phylogenetic analysis of global hepatitis E virus sequences: genetic diversity, subtypes and zoonosis, Rev. Med. Virol. 16 (2006) 5–36.

[109] Y.C. Wang, et al., Prevalence, isolation, and partial sequence analysis of hepatitis E virus from domestic animals in China, J. Med. Virol. 67 (2002) 516–521.

[110] R. Aggarwal, K. Krawczynski, Hepatitis E: an overview and recent advances in clinical and laboratory research, J. Gastroenterol. Hepatol. 15 (2000) 9–20.

[111] E.T. Clayson, et al., Viremia, fecal shedding, and IgM and IgG responses in patients with hepatitis E, J. Infect. Dis. 172 (1995) 927–933.

[112] J.M. Peron, et al., Liver histology in patients with sporadic acute hepatitis E: a study of 11 patients from South-West France, Virchows Arch. 450 (2007) 405–410.

[113] P. Malcolm, et al., The histology of acute autochthonous hepatitis E virus infection, Histopathology 51 (2007) 190–194.

[114] G.L. Lockwood, et al., Hepatitis E autochthonous infection in chronic liver disease, Eur. J. Gastroenterol. Hepatol. 20 (2008) 800–803.

[115] E.B. Haagsma, et al., Chronic hepatitis E virus infection in liver transplant recipients, Liver Transpl. 14 (2008) 547–553.

[116] N. Kamar, et al., Hepatitis E virus and chronic hepatitis in organ-transplant recipients, N. Engl. J. Med. 358 (2008) 811–817.

[117] E.E. Mast, K. Krawczynski, Hepatitis E: an overview, Annu. Rev. Med. 47 (1996) 257–266.

[118] M.S. Khuroo, et al., Incidence and severity of viral hepatitis in pregnancy, Am. J. Med. 70 (1981) 252–255.

[119] M.S. Khuroo, S. Kamili, Aetiology and prognostic factors in acute liver failure in India, J. Viral Hepat. 10 (2003) 224–231.

[120] H.R. Dalton, et al., Locally acquired hepatitis E in chronic liver disease, Lancet 369 (2007) 1260.

[121] J.M. Peron, et al., Fulminant liver failure from acute autochthonous hepatitis E in France: description of seven patients with acute hepatitis E and encephalopathy, J. Viral Hepat. 14 (2007) 298–303.

[122] S. Kumar Acharya, et al., Hepatitis E virus (HEV) infection in patients with cirrhosis is associated with rapid decompensation and death, J. Hepatol. 46 (2007) 387–394.

[123] R. Bendall, et al., Serological response to hepatitis E virus genotype 3 infection: IgG quantitation, avidity, and IgM response, J. Med. Virol. 80 (2008) 95–101.

[124] C.C. Lin, et al., Diagnostic value of immunoglobulin G (IgG) and IgM anti-hepatitis E virus (HEV) tests based on HEV RNA in an area where hepatitis E is not endemic, J. Clin. Microbiol. 38 (2000) 3915–3918.

[125] M. El-Sayed Zaki, M.H. El-Deen Zaghloul, O. El Sayed, Acute sporadic hepatitis E in children: diagnostic relevance of specific immunoglobulin M and immunoglobulin G compared with nested reverse transcriptase PCR, FEMS Immunol. Med. Microbiol. 48 (2006) 16–20.

[126] N. Jothikumar, et al., A broadly reactive one-step real-time RT-PCR assay for rapid and sensitive detection of hepatitis E virus, J. Virol. Methods 131 (2006) 65–71.

[127] M. Takahashi, et al., Prolonged fecal shedding of hepatitis E virus (HEV) during sporadic acute hepatitis E: evaluation of infectivity of HEV in fecal specimens in a cell culture system, J. Clin. Microbiol. 45 (2007) 3671–3679.

[128] M.S. Khuroo, M.Y. Dar, Hepatitis E: evidence for person-to-person transmission and inability of low dose immune serum globulin from an Indian source to prevent it, Indian J. Gastroenterol. 11 (1992) 113–116.

[129] R.M. Chibber, M.A. Usmani, M.H. Al-Sibai, Should HEV infected mothers breast feed? Arch. Gynecol. Obstet. 270 (2004) 15–20.

[130] M.P. Shrestha, et al., Safety and efficacy of a recombinant hepatitis E vaccine, N. Engl. J. Med. 356 (2007) 895–903.

[131] H. Ohto, et al., Mother-to-infant transmission of GB virus type C/HGV, Transfusion 40 (2000) 725–730.

[132] V.I. Reshetnyak, T.I. Karlovich, L.U. Ilchenko, Hepatitis G virus, World J. Gastroenterol. 14 (2008) 4725–4734.

[133] J.M. Pawlotsky, D. Dhumeaux, The G virus: the orphan virus, Presse Med. 28 (1999) 1882–1883.

[134] J. Woelfle, et al., Persistent hepatitis G virus infection after neonatal transfusion, J. Pediatr. Gastroenterol. Nutr. 26 (1998) 402–407.

[135] D. Mutlu, H. Abacioglu, S. Altunyurt, Investigation of transplacental transmission of TT virus in mother-newborn pairs, Mikrobiyol. Bul. 41 (2007) 71–77.

[136] P. Gerner, et al., Mother-to-infant transmission of TT virus: prevalence, extent and mechanism of vertical transmission, Pediatr. Infect. Dis. J. 19 (2000) 1074–1077.

[137] F. Davidson, et al., Early acquisition of TT virus (TTV) in an area endemic for TTV infection, J. Infect. Dis. 179 (1999) 1070–1076.

[138] K. Iso, Y. Suzuki, M. Takayama, Mother-to-infant transmission of TT virus in Japan, Int. J. Gynaecol. Obstet. 75 (2001) 11–19.

[139] N. Inaba, et al., TTV materno-infantile infection—a study on the TTV frequency in Japanese pregnant women and the natural history of TTV mother-to-infant infection, Nippon. Rinsho 57 (1999) 1406–1409.

[140] S. Hino, H. Miyata, Torque teno virus (TTV): current status, Rev. Med. Virol. 17 (2007) 45–57.

[141] Z.J. Hu, et al., Clinicopathological study on TTV infection in hepatitis of unknown etiology, World J. Gastroenterol. 8 (2002) 288–293.

[142] M. Zaki, N.A. el-Hady, Molecular detection of transfusion transmitted virus coinfection with some hepatotropic viruses, Arch. Pathol. Lab. Med. 130 (2006) 1680–1683.

[143] A.R. Garbuglia, et al., TT virus infection: role of interferons, interleukin-28 and 29, cytokines and antiviral proteins, Int. J. Immunopathol. Pharmacol. 20 (2007) 249–258.

[144] J. Moreno, et al., Response of TT virus to IFN plus ribavirin treatment in patients with chronic hepatitis C, World J. Gastroenterol. 10 (2004) 143–146.

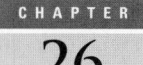

CHAPTER 26

HERPES SIMPLEX VIRUS INFECTIONS

Kathleen M. Gutierrez ⊛ Richard J. Whitley ⊛ Ann M. Arvin

CHAPTER OUTLINE

Herpes Simplex Virus   814
    Structure   814
    Replication   814
    Latency and Reactivation   815
Epidemiology and Transmission   815
    Maternal Infection   816
    Factors Influencing Transmission of Infection to the Fetus   816
    Incidence of Newborn Infection   818
    Times of Transmission of Infection   818
Immunologic Response   819
Neonatal Infection   820
    Pathogenesis and Pathology   820
    Clinical Manifestations   820

Diagnosis   824
    Clinical Evaluation   824
    Laboratory Assessment   825
Treatment   826
    Background   826
    Antiviral Drugs   826
    Other Issues in Acute Management   829
    Long-Term Management of Infected Infants   829
Prevention   829
    Background   829
    Management of Pregnant Women with Known Genital Herpes   830
    Management of Infants of Mothers with Genital Herpes   830
Conclusion   831

Neonatal herpes simplex virus (HSV) infection was identified as a distinct disease almost 75 years ago. The first written descriptions of neonatal HSV were attributed to Hass [1], who described the histopathologic findings of a fatal case, and to Batignani [2], who described a newborn infant with HSV keratitis. During subsequent decades, understanding of neonatal HSV infections was based on histopathologic descriptions of the disease, which indicated a broad spectrum of organ involvement in infants.

An important scientific breakthrough occurred in the mid-1960s, when Nahmias and Dowdle [3] showed two antigenic types of HSV. The development of viral typing methods provided the tools required to clarify the epidemiology of these infections. HSV infections "above the belt," primarily of the lip and oropharynx, were found in most cases to be caused by HSV type 1 (HSV-1). Infections "below the belt," particularly genital infections, were usually caused by HSV type 2 (HSV-2). The finding that genital HSV infections and neonatal HSV infections were most often due to HSV-2 suggested a cause-and-effect relationship between these two entities. This causal relationship was strengthened by detection of the virus in the maternal genital tract at the time of delivery, indicating that acquisition of the virus occurs by contact with infected genital secretions during birth.

DOI: 10.1016/B978-1-4160-6400-8.00026-2

Knowledge of HSV structure and function, epidemiology, natural history, and pathogenesis of neonatal HSV infection has increased during the past 3 decades [4]. The development of antiviral therapy represented a significant advance in the management of infected children and has substantially decreased the morbidity and mortality associated with neonatal HSV infections. Neonatal HSV infection is more amenable to prevention and treatment than many other pathogens because it is acquired most often at birth rather than in utero. Postnatal acquisition of HSV-1 has been documented from nonmaternal sources, and more cases caused by HSV-1 infections of the maternal genital tract have been identified recently. Perspectives on the changing presentations of neonatal HSV infection, the obstacles to diagnosis, and the value of antiviral therapy are addressed in this chapter.

HERPES SIMPLEX VIRUS
STRUCTURE

HSV-1 and HSV-2 are members of the large family of herpesviruses [4]. Other human herpesviruses include cytomegalovirus, varicella-zoster virus, Epstein-Barr virus, and human herpesviruses 6A, 6B, 7, and 8. Structurally, these viruses are virtually indistinguishable. The viral DNA genome is packaged inside an icosahedral capsid that is surrounded by a layer of proteins called the *tegument*. A lipid envelope that contains viral glycoproteins surrounds the capsid and tegument. These glycoproteins mediate virion attachment and entry into cells.

The HSV-1 and HSV-2 genomes consist of approximately 150,000 base pairs and encode more than 100 proteins [4]. The viral genomes consist of two components, L (long) and S (short), each of which contains unique sequences that can invert, generating four isomers. Viral genomic DNA extracted from virions or infected cells consists of four equal populations that differ in the relative orientation of these two unique components. Although the two viruses diverged millions of years ago, the order of genes in the HSV-1 and HSV-2 genomes follows the same linear pattern, and most genes have counterparts in both viruses. The nucleotide sequence of related genes and the amino acid residues of the proteins they encode often differ significantly, however [5,6]. The two viral types can be distinguished by using restriction enzyme analysis of genomic DNA or, more recently, by sequencing of selected genes or regions of the genome, which allows precise epidemiologic investigation of virus transmission.

REPLICATION

HSV replication is characterized by the transcription of three gene classes, α, β, and γ, that encode viral proteins made at immediate-early, early, and late times after virus entry into the cell [4]. Many of these genes can be removed from the viral genome without blocking the capacity of the virus to replicate in cultured cells, but most have important functions during infection of the host. The HSV genome can also be manipulated to insert foreign genes without inhibiting viral replication. Mutations that modify the virulence of HSV-1 and HSV-2 may provide an opportunity to design genetically engineered herpesviruses for use as vaccines [7].

HSV α genes are expressed at immediate-early times after infection and are responsible for the initiation of replication. These genes are transcribed in infected cells in the absence of viral protein synthesis. Products of the β genes, or early genes, include the enzymes necessary for viral replication, such as HSV thymidine kinase, which is targeted by acyclovir and related antiviral drugs, and other regulatory proteins. β genes require functional α gene products for expression. The onset of expression of β genes coincides with a decline in the rate of expression of α genes and an irreversible shutoff of host cellular macromolecular protein synthesis. Structural proteins, such as proteins that form the viral capsid, are usually of the γ, or late, gene class. The γ genes are heterogeneous and are differentiated from β genes by their requirement for viral DNA synthesis for maximal expression. Most glycoproteins are expressed predominantly as late genes. In addition to its regulatory and structural genes, the virus encodes genes that allow initial evasion of the innate host cell response, including gene products that block the interferon pathway. HSV-1 and HSV-2 also express proteins that interfere with adaptive immunity, as exemplified by an immediate-early protein, ICP47, that mediates the downregulation of major histocompatibility complex class I molecules, which are required for recognition of HSV-infected cells by HSV-specific CD8+ T cells [8,9].

Replication of viral DNA occurs in the nucleus of the cell. Assembly of the virus begins with formation of nucleocapsids in the nucleus, followed by egress across the nuclear membrane and envelopment at cytoplasmic locations. Virus particles are transported to the plasma membrane, where progeny virions are released. HSV glycoproteins have been designated as B, C, D, E, G, H, I, L, and M [4,5]. Glycoproteins B, D, and H (gB, gD, and gH) are required for infectivity and are targets of neutralizing antibodies against HSV; glycoprotein C (gC) binds to the C3b component of complement; and the glycoprotein E (gE) and glycoprotein I (gI) complex binds to the Fc portion of IgG.

The amino acid sequences of glycoprotein G (gG) produced by HSV-1 and HSV-2 are sufficiently different to elicit antibody responses that are specific for each virus type. The fact that the antibody response to the two G molecules exhibits minimal cross-reactivity has provided the basis for serologic methods that can be used to detect recent or past HSV-2 infection in individuals who have also been infected with HSV-1 [10–13]. The close antigenic relatedness between HSV-1 and HSV-2 interferes with the serologic diagnosis of these infections when using standard serologic assays, which do not distinguish between individuals who have had past infection with HSV-1 only, infection with HSV-2 only, or dual infection. Commercial type-specific tests based on gG must be used for diagnosis of HSV-2 infection [12]. Clinicians should be knowledgeable regarding the type of testing performed by the laboratory to interpret results correctly.

LATENCY AND REACTIVATION

All of the herpesviruses have a characteristic ability to establish latency, to persist in this latent state for various intervals of time, and to reactivate, causing virus excretion at mucosal or other sites. After primary infection, the HSV genome persists in sensory ganglion neurons for the lifetime of the individual. The biologic phenomenon of latency has been recognized and described since the beginning of the 20th century. In 1905, Cushing [14] observed that patients treated for trigeminal neuralgia by sectioning a branch of the trigeminal nerve developed herpetic lesions in areas innervated by the sectioned branch. This specific association of HSV with the trigeminal ganglion was suggested by Goodpasture [15]. Past observations have shown that microvascular surgery of the trigeminal nerve tract to alleviate pain associated with tic douloureux resulted in recurrent lesions in more than 90% of seropositive individuals [16,17].

Accumulated experience in animal models and from clinical observations suggests that inoculation of virus at the portal of entry, usually oral or genital mucosal tissue, results in infection of sensory nerve endings, and the virus is transported to the dorsal root ganglia [18]. Replication at the site of inoculation enhances access of the virus to ganglia, but is usually not associated with signs of mucocutaneous disease. Only a fraction of new infections with HSV-1 and HSV-2 cause clinically recognizable disease. When reactivation is triggered at oral or genital sites, virus is transported back down axons to mucocutaneous sites where replication and shedding of infectious HSV occurs.

Recognizing that excretion of infectious virus during reactivation is not usually associated with clinical signs of recurrent herpes lesions is essential for understanding the transmission of HSV to newborns. Clinically silent reactivations are much more common than recurrent lesions. Reactivation with or without symptoms occurs in the healthy host in the presence of HSV-specific humoral and cell-mediated immunity. Reactivation seems to be spontaneous, although symptomatic recurrences have been associated with physical or emotional stress, exposure to ultraviolet light, or tissue damage; immunosuppression is associated with an increased susceptibility to symptomatic HSV infections when reactivation occurs. Persistence of viral DNA has been documented in neuronal tissue of animal models and humans [4,19–21]. Because the latent virus does not multiply, it is not susceptible to drugs such as acyclovir that affect DNA synthesis and cannot be eradicated from the infected host. Understanding of the mechanisms by which HSV establishes a latent state and persists in this form remains limited.

EPIDEMIOLOGY AND TRANSMISSION

Transmission of HSV most often occurs as a consequence of intimate person-to-person contact. Virus must come in contact with mucosal surfaces or abraded skin for infection to be initiated.

The usual mode of HSV-1 transmission is through direct contact of a susceptible individual with infected secretions, although transfer in respiratory droplets is possible. Acquisition often occurs during childhood. Primary HSV-1 infection in a young child is usually asymptomatic, but clinical illness is associated with HSV gingivostomatitis. Primary infection in young adults has been associated with pharyngitis only or with a mononucleosis-like syndrome. Seroprevalence studies have shown that acquisition of HSV-1 infection, similar to that of other herpesvirus infections, is related to socioeconomic factors [22,23]. Antibodies, indicative of past infection, are found early in life among individuals of lower socioeconomic groups, presumably reflecting the crowded living conditions that provide a greater opportunity for direct contact with infected individuals. By the end of the 1st decade of life, 75% to 90% of individuals from lower socioeconomic populations develop antibodies to HSV-1 [24–26]. In middle and upper middle socioeconomic groups, 30% to 40% of individuals are seropositive by the middle of the 2nd decade of life.

A change in seroprevalence rates of HSV-1 has been recognized in the past few decades, which reflects a delay in acquisition of infection until later in life. An increase in the reported number of cases of genital herpes caused by HSV-2 may be related to a lower prevalence of prior HSV-1 infection in young adults. These individuals would not have the partial protection against HSV-2 infection that is probably conferred by cross-reactive HSV-1 immunity. In recent years, an increasing number of cases of genital HSV have been found to be caused by HSV-1 [27,28].

Because infection with HSV-2 is usually acquired through sexual contact, antibodies to this virus are rarely found until the age of onset of sexual activity [25]. A progressive increase in infection rates with HSV-2 in all populations begins in adolescence. In earlier studies, the precise seroprevalence of antibodies to HSV-2 had been difficult to determine because of cross-reactivity with HSV-1 antigens. During the late 1980s, seroepidemiologic studies performed using type-specific antigen for HSV-2 (glycoprotein G-2) identified this virus in approximately 25% to 35% of middle-class women in several geographic areas of the United States [11,29–31]. Based on national health surveys, the seroprevalence of HSV-2 in the United States from 1988–1994 was 21.9% for individuals 12 years and older [31]. Among individuals with serologic evidence of infection, less than 10% had a history of genital herpes symptoms. This seroprevalence represented a 30% increase compared with data collected from 1976–1980. There is evidence, however, from more recent national health surveys (1999–2004) that this trend of increasing HSV-2 seroprevalence is reversing [28]. HSV seroprevalence is highly variable and depends on geographic region, sex, age, race, and high-risk behaviors [32].

The molecular epidemiology of HSV infections can be determined by restriction enzyme analysis of viral DNA or polymerase chain reaction (PCR) and sequencing of regions of the HSV genome obtained from infected individuals. Viruses have essentially identical genetic profiles when they are from the same host or are epidemiologically related [33]. In a few circumstances, it has been shown, however, that superinfection or exogenous reinfection with a new strain of HSV is possible. Such occurrences are uncommon in a nonimmunocompromised host with recurrent genital HSV infection [33–35]. Differences in the genetic sequence of viral DNAs indicating exogenous infections are more common in immunocompromised individuals who are exposed to different HSVs, such as patients with acquired immunodeficiency syndrome (AIDS).

MATERNAL INFECTION

Infection with HSV-2, which reactivates and is shed at genital sites, is common in pregnant women. Using assays to detect type-specific antibodies to HSV-2, seroepidemiologic investigations have shown that approximately one in five pregnant women has had HSV-2 infection [23,30,36–40]. Given the capacity of HSV to establish latency, the presence of antibodies is a marker of persistent infection of the host with the virus. The incidence of infection in women of upper socioeconomic class was 30% or greater in three large studies [38,40,41]. These investigations have shown that most women with serologic evidence of HSV-2 infection have no history of symptomatic primary or recurrent disease. New HSV-2 infections are acquired during pregnancy with a frequency that is comparable to seroconversion rates among nonpregnant women, and these infections usually occur without clinical signs or symptoms [37–41].

Evaluation of pregnant women and their partners has shown that women can remain susceptible to HSV-2 despite prolonged sexual contact with a partner who has known genital herpes [39]. One in 10 women in this study were found to be at unsuspected risk for acquiring HSV-2 infection during pregnancy as a result of contact with a partner whose HSV-2 infection was asymptomatic. Most maternal infections are clinically silent during gestation. Infection during gestation may manifest in several clinical syndromes, however.

Widely disseminated disease is an uncommon problem encountered with HSV infections during pregnancy. As first reported by Flewett and coworkers [42] in 1969 and by others [43,44] subsequently, infection has been documented to involve multiple visceral sites in addition to cutaneous ones. In a few cases, dissemination after primary oropharyngeal or genital infection has led to severe manifestations of disease, including necrotizing hepatitis with or without thrombocytopenia, leukopenia, disseminated intravascular coagulopathy, and encephalitis. Although only a few patients have had disseminated infection, the mortality rate for these pregnant women is more than 50%. Fetal deaths were described in more than 50% of cases, although mortality did not correlate with the death of the mother. Surviving fetuses were delivered by cesarean section during the acute illness or at term; none of the surviving fetuses had evidence of neonatal HSV infection.

Earlier studies described an association of maternal primary infection before 20 weeks' gestation [45] with spontaneous abortion in some women. Although the original incidence of spontaneous abortion after a symptomatic primary infection during gestation was thought to be 25%, this estimate was not substantiated by prospective studies and was erroneous because of the small number of women followed. More precise data obtained from a prospective analysis of susceptible women showed that 2% or more acquired infection, but that acquisition of infection was not associated with a risk of spontaneous abortion [46]. With the exception of rare case reports, primary infection that develops later in gestation is not generally associated with premature rupture of membranes or premature termination of pregnancy [47].

Localized genital infection, whether it is associated with lesions or remains asymptomatic, is the most common form of HSV infection during pregnancy. Overall, prospective investigations using cytologic and virologic screening indicate that genital herpes occurs with a frequency of about 1% in women tested at any time during gestation [38,46]. Most genital infections were classified as recurrent when HSV-2–specific serologic testing was done. Transmission of infection to the infant is most frequently related to the actual shedding of virus at the time of delivery. Because HSV infection of the infant is usually the consequence of contact with infected maternal genital secretions at the time of delivery, the incidence of viral excretion at this time point has been of particular interest. The reported incidence of viral excretion at delivery is 0.01% to 0.39% for all women, regardless of their history of genital herpes [38,41].

Several prospective studies have evaluated the frequency and nature of viral shedding in pregnant women with a known history of genital herpes. These women represent a subset of the population of women with HSV-2 infection because they had a characteristic genital lesion from which virus was isolated. In a predominantly white, middle-class population, symptomatic recurrent infection occurred during pregnancy in 84% of pregnant women with a history of symptomatic disease [48]. Viral shedding from the cervix occurred in only 0.56% of symptomatic infections and 0.66% of asymptomatic infections. These data are similar to data obtained from other populations [29]. The incidence of cervical shedding in asymptomatic pregnant women has been reported to range from 0.2% to 7.4%, depending on the numbers of cultures that were obtained between symptomatic episodes. Overall, these data indicate that the frequency of cervical shedding is low, which may reduce the risk of transmission of virus to the infant when the infection is recurrent. The frequency of shedding does not seem to vary by trimester during gestation. No increased incidence of premature onset of labor was apparent in these prospective studies of women with known HSV-2 infection.

Most infants who develop neonatal disease are born to women who are completely asymptomatic for genital HSV infection during the pregnancy and at the time of delivery. These women usually have neither a past history of genital herpes nor a sexual partner reporting a genital vesicular rash and account for 60% to 80% of all women whose infants become infected [49,50].

FACTORS INFLUENCING TRANSMISSION OF INFECTION TO THE FETUS

The development of serologic assays that distinguish antibodies to HSV-1 from antibodies elicited by HSV-2 infection allowed an accurate analysis of risks related to perinatal transmission of HSV [10–13]. The category of maternal genital infection at the time of delivery influences the frequency of neonatal acquisition of infection. Maternal infections are classified as caused by HSV-1 or HSV-2 and as newly acquired or recurrent. These categories of maternal infection status are based on laboratory criteria and are independent of clinical signs.

Women with recurrent infections are those who have preexisting antibodies to the virus type that is isolated from the genital tract, which, until more recently, is usually HSV-2. Most women classified as having recurrent infection have no history of symptomatic genital herpes. Infections that are newly acquired, which have been referred to as first-episode infections, are categorized further as primary or first-episode nonprimary based on type-specific serologic testing. This differentiation is made whether clinical signs are present or not. Primary infections are infections in which the mother is experiencing a new infection with HSV-1 or HSV-2 and has not already been infected with the other virus type. These mothers are seronegative for any HSV antibodies (i.e., negative for HSV-1 or HSV-2) at the onset of infection. Nonprimary infections are infections in which the mother has a new infection with one virus type, usually HSV-2, but has antibodies to the other virus type, usually HSV-1, because of an infection that was acquired previously.

As transmission has been studied using type-specific serologic methods, it has become apparent that attempts to distinguish primary and recurrent disease by clinical criteria are unreliable. Serologic classification is an important advance because many "new" genital herpes infections in pregnancy represent the first symptomatic episode of infection acquired at some time in the past. In one study designed to evaluate acyclovir therapy, pregnant women who were thought to have recent acquisition of HSV-2 based on symptoms all had been infected previously. These women were experiencing genital symptoms, caused by reactivation of latent virus, for the first time [44]. A hierarchy of risk of transmission has emerged using laboratory tools to classify maternal infection. Infants born to mothers who have true primary infection at the time of delivery are at highest risk, with transmission rates of 50% or greater [46,49]. Infants born to mothers with new infections that are first episode but nonprimary seem to be at lower risk; transmission rates are estimated to be about 30%. The lowest risk of neonatal acquisition occurs when the mother has active infection caused by shedding of virus acquired before the pregnancy or at stages of gestation before the onset of labor. The estimated attack rate for neonatal herpes among these infants is less than 2%. This estimate is reliable because it is based on the cumulative experience from large, prospective studies of pregnant women in which viral shedding was evaluated at delivery, regardless of the mother's history of genital herpes or contact with a partner with suspected or documented genital herpes.

The higher risk of transmission to the infant when the mother has a new infection can be attributed to differences in the quantity and duration of viral shedding in the mother and in the transfer of passive antibodies from the mother to the infant before delivery. Primary infection is associated with larger quantities of virus replication in the genital tract ($>10^6$ viral particles per 0.2 mL of inoculum) and a period of viral excretion that may persist for an average of 3 weeks [51]. Many women with new infections have no symptoms, but shed virus in high titers. In some mothers, these infections cause signs of systemic illness, including fever, malaise, myalgias, dysuria, and headache. Viremia during primary HSV infection in women is common and is associated with systemic symptoms [52]. In a small percentage of cases, significant complications, such as urinary retention and aseptic meningitis, occur.

In contrast, virus is shed for an average of only 2 to 5 days and at lower concentrations (approximately 10^2 to 10^3 viral particles per 0.2 mL of inoculum) in women with symptomatic recurrent genital infections. Asymptomatic reactivation is also associated with short periods of viral replication, often less than 24 to 48 hours. One of the most important observations about HSV infections that has emerged from the evaluation of pregnant women is that new HSV-1 and HSV-2 infections often occur without any of the manifestations that were originally described as the classic findings in primary and recurrent genital herpes.

In parallel with the classification of maternal infection, the mother's antibody status to HSV at delivery seems to be an additional factor that influences the likelihood of transmission and probably affects the clinical course of neonatal herpes. Transplacental maternal neutralizing antibodies seem to have a protective, or at least an ameliorative, effect on acquisition of infection for infants inadvertently exposed to virus [53]. Maternal primary infection late in gestation may not result in significant passage of maternal antibodies across the placenta to the fetus. Based on available evidence, the highest risk of transmission from mothers with newly acquired genital herpes is observed when the infant is born before the transfer of passive antibodies to HSV-1 or HSV-2, when the infant is exposed at delivery or within the first few days of life [46,54].

The duration of ruptured membranes has also been described as an indicator of risk for acquisition of neonatal infection. Observations of a small cohort of women with symptomatic genital herpes indicated that prolonged rupture of membranes (>6 hours) increased the risk of acquisition of virus, perhaps as a consequence of ascending infection from the cervix [45]. It is recommended that women with active genital lesions at the time of onset of labor be delivered by cesarean section [55]. One study found that cesarean section significantly reduced the rate of HSV infection in infants born to women from whom HSV was isolated at the time of delivery (1.2% versus 7.7%, $P = .047$) [56]. This effect of cesarean delivery was established by postdelivery analysis of data on viral shedding at delivery for a large cohort of pregnant women. In the absence of a reliable rapid test for HSV in the birth canal, it is difficult at this time to apply this information in clinical practice. The benefit of cesarean section beyond 6 hours of ruptured membranes has not been evaluated. Although some protection may be expected, infection of the newborn has occurred despite delivery by cesarean section [50,57].

Certain forms of medical intervention during labor and delivery may increase the risk of neonatal herpes if the mother has active shedding of the virus, although in most instances, viral shedding is not suspected clinically. Fetal scalp monitors can be a site of viral entry through skin [56,58,59]. The benefits and risks of these devices should be considered for women with a history of recurrent genital HSV infections. Because most women with genital infections caused by HSV are asymptomatic during labor and have no history of genital herpes, it is usually impossible to make this assessment.

INCIDENCE OF NEWBORN INFECTION

A progressive increase in the number of cases of neonatal HSV infection to a rate of approximately 1 in 1500 deliveries was reported in King County, Washington, during the period from 1966–1983, when adult infection rates were also increasing [60]. Overall, the United States, with approximately 4 million deliveries each year, has an estimated 11 to 33 cases of neonatal infection per 100,000 live births. This estimate has been confirmed by a review of comprehensive hospital discharge data recorded in California for the years 1985, 1990, and 1995. The diagnosis of HSV infection in infants 6 weeks or younger was made in 11.7, 11.3, and 11.4 infants per 100,000 live births in each of these years [61]. A more recent study from California, using similar methods of analysis of hospital discharge data, found the incidence of HSV infection in infants to be 12.1 per 100,000 live births per year with no change from 1995–2003 [62]. The use of ICD-9 discharge diagnosis coding seems to be a sensitive but relatively nonspecific method for identifying neonatal HSV infections [63].

In studies in which maternal serologic status during pregnancy and virologic status at the time of delivery are evaluated prospectively, the rate of transmission leading to neonatal HSV infection ranges from 12 to 54 newborn infections per 100,000 births. Higher rates of transmission are seen in infants born to seronegative mothers and mothers infected with HSV-1 [56]. Based on seroprevalence studies, the highest risk HSV transmission would be expected to occur in infants born to non-Hispanic white mothers, whose HSV seroprevalence is the lowest [23]. Neonatal HSV infection occurs far less frequently than might be expected given the high prevalence of genital HSV infections in women of childbearing age in the United States. Some countries do not report a significant number of cases of neonatal HSV infection despite a similar high prevalence of antibodies to HSV-2 in women. In the United Kingdom, genital herpes infection is relatively common, but very few cases of neonatal HSV infection are recognized. Neonatal HSV infection in the Netherlands occurs in only 2.4 of 100,000 newborns [64].

Although underreporting of cases may explain some differences between countries, unidentified factors may account for these differences. The interpretation of incidence data must also include the potential for postnatal acquisition of HSV infection. Not all cases of neonatal infection are the consequence of intrapartum contact with infected maternal genital secretions, which alters the overall estimate of delivery-associated infection. The prevalence of neonatal HSV infection relative to serious bacterial infections in hospitalized neonates was evaluated more recently in a retrospective study and found to be 0.2% compared with 0.4% and 4.5% for infants with bacterial meningitis and serious bacterial infections [65].

TIMES OF TRANSMISSION OF INFECTION

HSV infection of the newborn can be acquired in utero, intrapartum, or postnatally. The mother is the most common source of infection for the first two of these three routes of transmission of infection. With regard to postnatal acquisition of HSV infection, the mother can be a source of infection from a genital or nongenital site. Other contacts or environmental sources of virus can lead to infection of the infant. A maternal source is suspected when maternal herpetic lesions are discovered shortly after the birth of the infant or when the infant's illness is caused by HSV-2. Although intrapartum transmission accounts for 85% to 95% of cases, in utero and postnatal infection must be recognized for public health and prognostic purposes.

In utero transmission is rare [66–69]. Although it was originally presumed that in utero acquisition of infection resulted in a totally normal infant or premature termination of gestation [45], it has become apparent that intrauterine acquisition of infection can lead to the clinical signs of congenital infection. When using stringent diagnostic criteria, more than 30 infants with symptomatic congenital disease have been described in the literature. These criteria include identification of infected infants with lesions present at birth; virologic confirmation of HSV; and exclusion of other infectious agents whose pathogenesis mimics the clinical findings of HSV infections, such as congenital cytomegalovirus infection, rubella, syphilis, or toxoplasmosis. Virologic diagnosis is a necessary criterion because no standard method for detection of IgM antibodies is available, and infected infants often fail to produce IgM antibodies detectable by research methods [54,70]. The manifestations of disease in this group of children range from the presence of skin vesicles at the time of delivery to the most severe neurologic abnormalities [50,68].

In utero infection can result from transplacental or ascending infection. The placenta can show evidence of necrosis and inclusions in the trophoblasts, which suggests a transplacental route of infection [71]. The situation can result in an infant who has hydranencephaly at the time of birth, or it may be associated with spontaneous abortion and intrauterine HSV viremia. Virus has been isolated from the products of conception under such circumstances. Histopathologic evidence of chorioamnionitis suggests ascending infection as an alternative route for in utero infection [72]. Risk factors associated with intrauterine transmission are unknown. Primary and recurrent maternal infections can result in infection of the fetus in utero. HSV DNA has been detected in the amniotic fluid of two women experiencing a first-episode nonprimary infection and in one woman during a symptomatic recurrent infection. All three infants were healthy at birth and showed no clinical or serologic evidence of HSV infection during follow-up [73].

The second and most common route of infection is intrapartum contact of the fetus with infected maternal genital secretions. Intrapartum transmission is favored by delivery of the infant to a mother with newly acquired infection.

Postnatal acquisition is the third route of transmission. Postnatal transmission of HSV-1 has been suggested as an increasing risk. Data from the National Institute of Allergy and Infectious Diseases (NIAID) Collaborative Antiviral Study Group (CASG) indicate that the frequency of infants with neonatal HSV-1 infection ranges from approximately 25% to 35% [50,74]. An increase in HSV-1 genital infections in the United States may account for some neonatal HSV-1 infections; however, some infants acquire nongenital HSV-1 from the mother after birth or from nonmaternal sources. Relatives and hospital personnel with orolabial herpes may be a reservoir of virus for infection of the newborn.

The documentation of postnatal transmission of HSV-1 has focused attention on sources of virus [75–79]. Postpartum transmission from mother to child has been reported as a consequence of nursing on an infected breast [80]. Transmission from fathers and grandparents has also been documented [79]. When the infant's mother has not had HSV infection, the infant may be inoculated with the virus from a nonmaternal contact in the absence of any possible protection from maternally derived passive antibodies. Because of the prevalence of HSV-1 infection in the general population, many individuals have intermittent episodes of asymptomatic excretion of the virus from the oropharynx and can provide a source of infection for the newborn. The occurrence of herpes labialis, commonly referred to as fever blisters or cold sores, has ranged from 16% to 46% in various groups of adults [81].

Population studies conducted in two hospitals indicated that 15% to 34% of hospital personnel had a history of nongenital herpetic lesions [81,82]. In both hospitals surveyed, at least 1 in 100 individuals documented a recurrent cold sore each week. As is true of genital herpes, many individuals have HSV-1 infection with no clinical symptoms at the time of acquisition or during episodes of reactivation and shedding of infectious virus in oropharyngeal secretions. Prospective virologic monitoring of hospital staff increased the frequency with which infection was detected by twofold; however, no cases of neonatal HSV infection were documented in these nurseries.

The risk of nosocomial infection in the hospital environment is a concern. Identification by restriction endonuclease or sequence analysis of virus recovered from an index case and a nursery contact leaves little doubt about the possibility of spread of virus in a high-risk nursery population [76,78]. The possible vectors for nosocomial transmission have not been defined. Whether personnel with herpes labialis should avoid working in the nursery while lesions are active remains a matter of debate. No cases of transmission of HSV from personnel to infants have been documented. Meticulous hand-washing procedures and continuing education of personnel in newborn nurseries can contribute to the low frequency of HSV transmission in this environment. Herpetic whitlow in a health care provider should preclude direct patient contact, regardless of the nursing unit. Because more infants are born to seronegative women now, our nursery practice is to exclude personnel with active herpes labialis from direct patient care activities until the lesion is crusted.

Because most mothers have antibodies to HSV, and these antibodies are transferred to their infants, exposures to the virus in the newborn period often may not result in neonatal disease. If the mother was seronegative, nosocomial exposure may pose a more significant risk to the infant, however.

IMMUNOLOGIC RESPONSE

The host response of the newborn to HSV is impaired compared with older children and adults [54,70,83–87]. There is no evidence for differences in virulence of particular HSV strains. The severity of the manifestations of HSV-1 and HSV-2 infections in the newborn can be attributed to immunologic factors. Relevant issues are protection by transplacental antibodies, the innate immune response of the exposed infant, and the acquisition of adaptive immunity by the infected newborn.

Passive antibodies to HSV influence the acquisition of infection and its severity and clinical signs [40,49,54,70]. Transplacentally acquired antibodies from the mother are not totally protective against newborn infection, but transplacentally acquired neutralizing antibodies correlate with a lower attack rate in exposed newborns [49,53,54]. Although the absence of any detectable antibodies has been associated with dissemination, the presence of antibodies at the time that clinical signs appear does not predict the subsequent outcome [50,70]. The most important example of the failure of passive antibodies to alter progression is the occurrence of encephalitis in untreated infants whose initial symptoms were limited to cutaneous lesions.

Most infected newborns eventually produce IgM antibodies, but the interval to detection is prolonged, requiring at least 2 to 4 weeks [54]. These antibodies increase rapidly during the first 2 to 3 months, but may be detectable for 1 year after infection. The quantity of neutralizing antibodies and antibodies that mediate antibody-dependent cellular cytotoxicity in infants with disseminated infection is lower than in infants with more limited disease [54,86]. Humoral antibody responses to specific viral proteins, especially glycoproteins, have been evaluated by assays for antibodies to gG and by immunoblot [10,70]. Immunoblot studies indicate that the severity of infection correlates directly with the number of antibody bands to defined polypeptides. Children with a more limited infection, such as infection of the skin, eye, or mouth, have fewer antibody bands compared with children with disseminated disease.

A vigorous antibody response to the ICP4 α gene product, which is responsible for initiating viral replication, has been correlated with poor long-term neurologic outcome, suggesting that these antibodies reflect the extent of viral replication. A regression analysis that compared neurologic impairment with the quantity of antibodies to ICP4 identified the child at risk for severe neurologic impairment [70].

Adaptive cellular immunity is a crucial component of the host response to primary herpetic infection. Newborns with HSV infections have a delayed T-lymphocyte proliferative response compared with older individuals [54,83,84]. Most infants have no detectable T-lymphocyte responses to HSV when evaluated 2 to 4 weeks after the onset of clinical symptoms [54]. The delayed T-lymphocyte response to viral antigens in infants whose initial disease is localized to the skin, eye, or mouth may be an important determinant of the frequent progression to more severe disease in infants [54,83]. The importance of interferon-γ may be related to its effect on the induction of innate immune mechanisms, such as natural killer cell responses [85]. Other mechanisms of the innate immune system of the newborn that may be deficient in controlling HSV include other nonspecific cytokine responses and complement-mediated effects. T lymphocytes from infected infants have decreased interferon-γ production during the 1st month of life. This defect can be predicted to limit the clonal expansion of helper and cytotoxic T lymphocytes specific for herpes viral antigens, allowing more extensive and prolonged viral replication.

Antibody-dependent cell-mediated cytotoxicity has been shown to be an important component of adaptive immunity to viral infection [86]. Lymphocytes, monocytes, macrophages, or polymorphonuclear leukocytes and antibodies and complement lyse HSV-infected cells in vitro [88]. However, newborns appear to have fewer effector lymphocytes than older individuals do. The immaturity of neonatal monocytes and macrophage function against HSV infection has been demonstrated in vitro and in animal models [89,90]. Additional information regarding the immune response to HSV is provided in Chapter 4.

NEONATAL INFECTON
PATHOGENESIS AND PATHOLOGY

After direct exposure, replication of HSV is presumed to occur at the portal of entry, which is probably the mucous membranes of the mouth or eye, or at sites where the skin has been damaged. Factors that determine whether the infection causes symptoms at the site of inoculation or disseminates to other organs are poorly understood. Sites of replication during the incubation period have not been well defined, but the virus evades the host response during this early stage, probably by mechanisms such as interfering with expression of the interferon response genes and blocking cell-mediated immune recognition of viral peptides by preventing major histocompatibility complex class I molecules from reaching the surface of infected cells.

Intraneuronal transmission of viral particles may provide a privileged site that is relatively inaccessible to circulating humoral and cell-mediated defense mechanisms, facilitating the pathogenesis of encephalitis. Transplacental maternal antibodies may be less effective under such circumstances. Disseminated infection seems to be the consequence of viremia. HSV DNA has been detected in peripheral blood mononuclear cells, even in infants who seem to have localized infection [91]. Extensive cell-to-cell spread could explain primary HSV pneumonia after aspiration of infected secretions.

After the virus has adsorbed to cell membranes, and penetration has occurred, viral replication proceeds, leading to release of progeny virus and cell death. The synthesis of cellular DNA and protein ceases as large quantities of HSV are produced. Many infants with disseminated HSV infection have high viral loads and higher concentrations of inflammatory cytokines compared with infants with central nervous system (CNS) infection alone or

skin, eye, or mouth disease [92]. Uncontrolled host immune responses may lead to the development of multiple organ dysfunction. Cell death in critical organs of the newborn, such as the brain, results in devastating consequences, as reflected by the long-term morbidity of herpes encephalitis. Cellular swelling, hemorrhagic necrosis, development of intranuclear inclusions, and cytolysis all result from the replication process and ensuing inflammatory response. Small, punctate, yellow-to-gray areas of focal necrosis are the most prominent gross lesions in infected organs. When infected tissue is examined by microscopy, there is extensive evidence of hemorrhagic necrosis, clumping of nuclear chromatin, dissolution of the nucleolus, cell fusion with formation of multinucleate giant cells, and, ultimately, a lymphocytic inflammatory response [93]. Irreversible organ damage results from ischemia and direct viral destruction of cells.

CLINICAL MANIFESTATIONS

Pediatricians must be prepared to consider the diagnosis of neonatal herpes in infants who have clinical signs consistent with the disease regardless of the maternal history or genital herpes. Only about 30% of mothers whose infants develop neonatal herpes have had symptomatic genital herpes or sexual contact with a partner who has recognized HSV infection during or before the pregnancy.

The clinical presentation of infants with neonatal HSV infection depends on the initial site and extent of viral replication. In contrast to human cytomegalovirus, neonatal infections caused by HSV-1 and HSV-2 are almost invariably symptomatic. Case reports of asymptomatic infection in the newborn exist, but are uncommon, and long-term follow-up of these children to document absence of subtle disease or sequelae was not described.

Classification of newborns with HSV infection is used for prognostic and therapeutic considerations [94]. Historically, infants with neonatal HSV infection were classified as having localized or disseminated disease, with the former group being subdivided into infants with skin, eye, or mouth disease versus infants with CNS infection. This classification system understates the significant differences in outcome within each category, however [95]. In a revised classification scheme, infants who are infected intrapartum or postnatally are divided into three groups: disease localized to the skin, eye, or mouth; encephalitis, with or without skin, eye, or mouth involvement; and disseminated infection that involves multiple organs, including the CNS, lung, liver, adrenals, skin, eye, or mouth. A few infants with intrauterine infection constitute a fourth category.

Knowledge of the patterns of clinical disease caused by HSV-1 and HSV-2 in the newborn is based on prospectively acquired data obtained through the NIAID CASG. These analyses have employed uniform case record forms from one study interval to the next. Of 186 infants enrolled in the NIAID CASG studies of neonatal herpesvirus infections from 1981–1997, 34% were classified with skin, eye, or mouth disease; 34% were classified with CNS disease; and 32% were classified with disseminated infection [74]. This analysis of the natural history of neonatal herpes infections likely underestimates the proportion of infants who present with skin, eye, or mouth disease. Patients with CNS or disseminated HSV infection were disproportionately enrolled in a high-dose acyclovir study conducted from 1989–1997. The presentation and outcome of infection, including the effect of antiviral therapy on prognosis, vary significantly according to the clinical categories [96]. Table 26–1 summarizes disease classification and outcome of 291 infants with neonatal HSV infections enrolled in NIAID CASG protocols.

Intrauterine Infection

Intrauterine infection is rare. The manifestations are seen in approximately 3 of every 100 infected infants [66]. When infection occurs in utero, severe disease follows acquisition of infection at virtually any time during gestation. In the most severely affected group of infants, evidence of infection is apparent at birth and is characterized by a triad of findings: skin vesicles or scarring, eye damage, and severe manifestations of microcephaly or hydranencephaly. CNS damage is caused by intrauterine encephalitis. Infants do not have evidence of embryopathy, such as cardiac malformations. Often, chorioretinitis combined with other eye findings, such as keratoconjunctivitis, is a component of the clinical presentation.

Serial ultrasound examination of the mothers of infants infected in utero has shown the presence of hydranencephaly, but cases are seldom diagnosed before delivery. Chorioretinitis alone should alert the pediatrician to the possibility of this diagnosis, although it is a common sign for other congenital infections. A few infants have been described who have signs of HSV infection at birth after prolonged rupture of membranes. These infants may have

no other findings of invasive multiorgan involvement—no chorioretinitis, encephalitis, or evidence of other diseased organs—and can be expected to respond to antiviral therapy. Antiviral therapy is ineffective for infants who are born with hydranencephaly. Intrauterine HSV infection has been reported as a cause of hydrops fetalis [97].

Disseminated Infection

Infants whose initial diagnosis is disseminated herpes have the worst prognosis for mortality. Many of these infants are born to mothers who are experiencing a new HSV-1 or HSV-2 infection and may lack any passively acquired antibodies against the infecting virus type [10,49,98]. Infants with disseminated infection have signs of illness within the 1st week of life, although the diagnosis may be delayed until the 2nd week. The onset of symptoms may occur less than 24 hours after birth, but most infants appear well at delivery. The short incubation period of disseminated herpes reflects an acute viremia, which allows transport of the virus to all organs; the principal organs involved are the adrenals and the liver, resulting in fulminant hepatitis in some cases [94,99–102]. Viremia is associated with infection of circulating mononuclear cells in these infants [91,99,101,103,104].

Infection can affect multiple organs, including the CNS, larynx, trachea, lungs, esophagus, stomach, lower gastrointestinal tract, spleen, kidneys, pancreas, and heart. Initial signs and symptoms are irritability, seizures, respiratory distress, jaundice, coagulopathy, and shock. The characteristic vesicular exanthem is usually not present when the symptoms begin. Untreated infants may develop cutaneous lesions resulting from viremia. More than one third of children with disseminated infection do not

TABLE 26–1 Demographic and Clinical Characteristics of Infants Enrolled in National Institute of Allergy and Infectious Diseases Collaborative Antiviral Study

Demographic Characteristics	Disease Classification		
	Disseminated	**Central Nervous System**	**Skin, Eye, or Mouth**
No. infants (%)	93 (32)	95 (33)	102 (35)
No. male/no. female	54/39	50/46	51/51
No. white race/other	60/33	73/23	76/26
No. premature, <36 wk (%)	33 (35)	20 (21)	24 (24)
Gestational age (wk)	36.5 ± 0.4	37.9 ± 0.4	37.8 ± 0.3
Enrollment age (days)	11.6 ± 0.7	17.4 ± 0.8	12.1 ± 1.1
Maternal age (yr)	21.7 ± 0.5	23.1 ± 0.5	22.8 ± 0.5
No. clinical findings (%)			
Skin lesions	72 (77)	60 (63)	86 (84)
Brain involvement	69 (74)	96 (100)	0 (0)
Pneumonia	46 (49)	4 (4)	3 (3)
Deaths at 1 yr* (%)	56 (60)	13 (14)	0 (0)
No. survivors with neurologic impairment/total no.† (%)			
Total	15/34 (44)	45/81 (56)	10/93 (11)
Adenine arabinoside	13/26 (50)	25/51 (49)	3/34 (9)
Acyclovir	1/6 (17)	18/27 (67)	4/51 (8)
Placebo	1/2 (50)	2/3 (67)	3/8 (38)

Regardless of therapy.
†*Denominators vary according to number with follow-up available.*

develop skin vesicles during the course of their illness [50,74,99]. Disseminated infections caused by HSV-1 and HSV-2 are indistinguishable by clinical criteria.

The diagnosis of disseminated neonatal herpes is exceedingly difficult because the clinical signs are often vague and nonspecific, mimicking signs of neonatal enteroviral disease or bacterial sepsis. The diagnosis of disseminated herpes should be pursued by obtaining specimens of oropharyngeal and respiratory secretions and a rectal swab to be tested by viral culture and by PCR testing if a qualified reference laboratory is available. Direct immunofluorescent methods are useful for rapid diagnosis of herpesvirus-infected cells in skin lesion specimens, but must not be used to test oropharyngeal or other secretions. If discrete lesions are unavailable for obtaining infected cells, the virus can also be detected in the peripheral blood of some infants by viral culture or PCR, but confirmation of viremia is unnecessary for clinical management.

Evaluation of the extent of dissemination is imperative to provide appropriate supportive interventions early in the clinical course. Infants should be assessed for hypoxemia, acidosis, hyponatremia, abnormal hepatic enzyme levels, direct hyperbilirubinemia, neutropenia, thrombocytopenia, and bleeding diathesis. Chest radiographs should be obtained. Depending on signs and whether the infant is stable enough, abdominal radiography, electroencephalography, and computed tomography (CT) or magnetic resonance imaging (MRI) of the head should be obtained to determine further the extent of disease. The radiographic picture of HSV lung disease is characterized by a diffuse, interstitial pattern, which progresses to a hemorrhagic pneumonitis and, rarely, a significant pleural effusion [105]. Frequently, necrotizing enterocolitis with pneumatosis intestinalis can be detected when gastrointestinal disease is present. Meningoencephalitis seems to be a common component of disseminated infection, occurring in about 60% to 75% of children. Usual examinations of cerebrospinal fluid (CSF), including viral culture and PCR, should be performed along with noninvasive neurodiagnostic tests to assess the extent of brain disease.

The mortality rate for disseminated HSV in the absence of therapy exceeds 80%, and many survivors are impaired. The most common causes of death of infants with disseminated disease are intravascular coagulopathy or HSV pneumonitis. Premature infants seem to at particularly high risk for disseminated disease with pneumonitis and have a high mortality rate, even with appropriate antiviral therapy [106]. There is evidence that the long-term neurologic outcome is better for infants who survive disseminated HSV-1 involving the CNS than for infants who are infected with HSV-2 [96,107].

Encephalitis

Almost one third of all infants with neonatal HSV infection have encephalitis only as the initial manifestation of disease [96,108]. These infants have clinical manifestations distinct from infants who have CNS infection associated with disseminated HSV. The pathogenesis of these two forms of brain infection is probably different. The virus is likely to reach brain parenchyma by a hematogenous route in infants with disseminated infection, resulting in multiple areas of cortical hemorrhagic necrosis. In contrast, neonates who present with only encephalitis are likely to develop brain disease because of retrograde axonal transport of the virus to the CNS.

The evidence for this hypothesis is twofold. First, newborns with disseminated disease have documented viremia. Second, infants with encephalitis are more likely to have received transplacental neutralizing antibodies from their mothers, which may allow only intraneuronal transmission of virus to the brain. Infants with localized HSV encephalitis as their initial manifestation of infection usually develop signs more than 1 week after birth, typically presenting in the 2nd or 3rd week, but sometimes not until 4 to 6 weeks. Clinical manifestations of encephalitis include seizures (focal and generalized), fever, lethargy, irritability, tremors, poor feeding, temperature instability, bulging fontanelle, and pyramidal tract signs. Similar signs are observed when disseminated herpesvirus is associated with encephalitis. As in cases of disseminated herpesvirus, many infants with encephalitis do not have skin vesicles when signs of illness begin. Some infants have a history or residual signs of lesions of the skin, eye, or mouth that were not recognized as herpetic. If untreated, infants with encephalitis may develop skin vesicles later in the disease course.

Anticipated findings on CSF examination include a mononuclear cell pleocytosis, moderately low glucose concentrations, and elevated protein. A few infants with CNS infection, proven by brain biopsy done immediately after the onset of seizures, have no abnormalities of CSF, but most infants have some pleocytosis and mild reduction of the glucose level. The hemorrhagic nature of the encephalitis may result in an apparent "bloody tap." Although initial protein concentrations may be normal or only slightly elevated, infants with localized brain disease usually show progressive increases in protein (≥1000 mg/dL). The importance of CSF examination in all infants is underscored by the finding that even subtle abnormalities have been associated with significant developmental sequelae [94].

Electroencephalography and CT or MRI can be very useful in defining the presence and extent of CNS abnormalities and should be obtained before discharge of all infants with this diagnosis [109,110]. Abnormalities may also be detected by ultrasound examination [110]. Typical abnormalities seen by neuroimaging include localized or multifocal areas of abnormal parenchymal attenuation, atrophy, edema, and hemorrhage involving the temporal, frontal, parietal, and subcortical regions of the brain (Fig. 26–1) [111]. Predominant brainstem involvement is rare but reported [112].

Localized CNS disease is fatal in approximately 50% of infants who are not treated. With rare exceptions, survivors are left with neurologic impairment [94]. The long-term prognosis is poor. Of surviving children, 50% have some degree of psychomotor retardation, often in association with microcephaly, hydranencephaly, porencephalic cysts, spasticity, blindness, chorioretinitis, or learning disabilities. Quantitative PCR methods show a greater amount of HSV-2 DNA in CSF from patients with more extensive

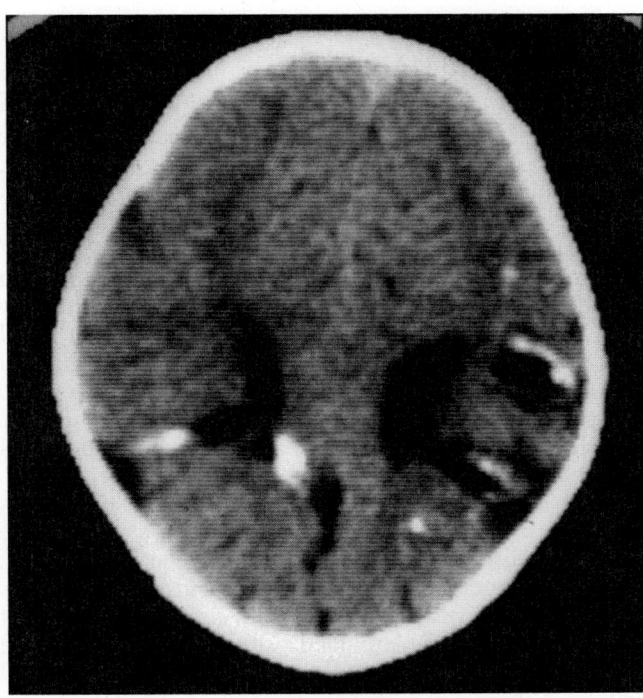

FIGURE 26–1　Herpes simplex encephalitis. Computed tomography scan of an infant with herpes simplex virus type 2 infection and severe sequelae.

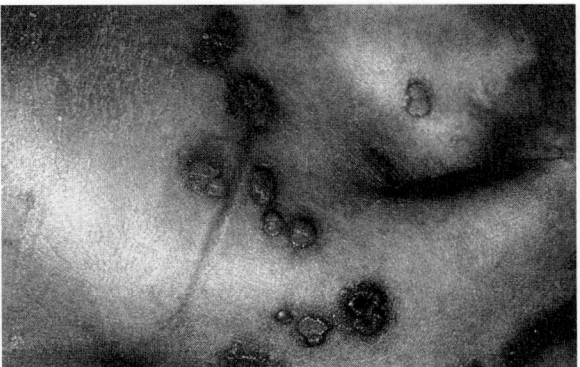

FIGURE 26–2　Cutaneous herpes simplex virus infection. Initial vesicular lesion in a premature infant with herpes simplex type 2 infection.

neurologic impairment [113]. There is evidence that progressive neurologic damage occurs after neonatal encephalitis; many infants have obvious severe sequelae within a few weeks after onset of HSV encephalitis [114,115].

Despite the presumed differences in pathogenesis, neurologic manifestations of disease in children with encephalitis alone are virtually identical to the findings for brain infection in disseminated cases. For infants with encephalitis, approximately 60% develop evidence of a vesicular rash characteristic of HSV infection. A newborn with pleocytosis and elevated protein in the CSF but without a rash can easily be misdiagnosed as having another viral or bacterial infection unless HSV infection is considered.

Skin, Eye, and Mouth Infections

Infection localized to the skin, eye, or mouth or some combination of these sites seems benign at the onset, but it is associated with a high risk of progression to serious disease. When infection is localized to the skin, the presence of discrete vesicles remains the hallmark of disease (Fig. 26–2). Vesicles occur in 90% of children with skin, eye, or mouth infection. The skin vesicles usually erupt from an erythematous base and are usually 1 to 2 mm in diameter. The formation of new lesions adjacent to the original vesicles is typical, creating a cluster that may coalesce into larger, irregular vesicles. In some cases, the lesions progress to bullae larger than 1 cm in diameter. Clusters of vesicles may appear initially on the presenting part of the body, presumably because of prolonged contact with infectious secretions during birth, or at sites of trauma (e.g., scalp monitor sites). Nevertheless, first herpetic lesions in infants with localized

cutaneous disease have been described on the trunk, extremities, and other sites.

Children with disease localized to the skin, eye, or mouth or some combination of these sites typically have symptoms within the first 7 to 10 days of life. Although discrete vesicles are usually encountered, crops and clusters of vesicles have been described, particularly before antiviral treatment was available or when the cause of the first lesions was not recognized. In these cases, the rash can progress to involve other cutaneous sites, presumably by viremia and hematogenous spread. The scattered vesicles resemble varicella. Although progression is expected without treatment, a few infants have had infection of the skin limited to one or two vesicles, with no further evidence of cutaneous disease. These infants may be identified after the newborn period and should have a careful evaluation because many are likely to have had neurologic disease that was not detected. A zosteriform eruption is another manifestation of herpetic skin disease reported in infants [116].

Infections involving the eye may manifest as keratoconjunctivitis. Ocular infection may be the only site of involvement in a newborn. When localized eye infection is observed in infants who also have microphthalmos and retinal dysplasia, intrauterine acquisition should be suspected, and a thorough neurologic evaluation should be done. Before antiviral therapy was available, persistent ocular disease resulted in chorioretinitis caused by HSV-1 or HSV-2 [117]. Keratoconjunctivitis can progress to chorioretinitis, cataracts, and retinal detachment despite therapy. Cataracts have been detected as a long-term consequence in infants with perinatally acquired HSV infections.

Localized infection of the oropharynx involving the mouth or tongue occurs, but newborns do not develop the classic herpetic gingivostomatitis caused by primary HSV-1 infection in older children. Overall, approximately 10% of patients have evidence of HSV infection of the oropharynx by viral culture. Many of these children did not undergo a thorough oral examination to determine whether the detection of infectious virus in oropharyngeal secretions was associated with lesions.

Long-term neurologic impairment has been encountered in children whose disease seemed to be localized to the skin, eye, or mouth during the newborn period

[50,94,115]. Significant findings include spastic quadri-plegia, microcephaly, and blindness. Important questions regarding the pathogenesis of delayed-onset neurologic debility are raised by these clinical observations. Despite normal clinical examination in these children, neurologic impairment became apparent between 6 months and 1 year of age. At this stage of the disease, the clinical presentation may be similar to that associated with congenitally acquired toxoplasmosis or syphilis.

Newborns who have skin lesions invariably experience recurrences for months or years. Continued recurrences are common, particularly when the infecting virus is HSV-2, whether or not antiviral therapy was administered.

Historically, although death was not associated with disease localized to the skin, eye, or mouth, approximately 30% of children eventually developed some evidence of neurologic impairment [50]. Table 26–2 shows morbidity and mortality 12 months after infection by HSV viral type and disease classification in patients enrolled in two studies conducted by the NIAID CASG from 1981–1997. With parenteral acyclovir therapy, virtually all children with HSV-1 and most children with HSV-2 disease of the skin, eye, or mouth who enrolled and who were available for follow-up at 12 months had normal development [74].

Subclinical Infection

A few cases of apparent subclinical infection with HSV proven by culture isolation of virus in the absence of symptoms have been described [118]. It has been difficult to document such cases in the course of prospective evaluations of several thousand infants from many centers around the United States. Conversely, infants who were exposed to active maternal infection at the time of delivery and who did not develop symptoms have been followed for the 1st year of life and did not have immunologic evidence of subclinical infection [49]. HSV-1 or HSV-2 may be recovered from the infant's oropharyngeal secretions transiently, without representing true infection. Because of the propensity of the newborn to develop severe or life-threatening disease, laboratory evidence of neonatal HSV infection requires careful follow-up for clinical signs and administration of antiviral therapy.

DIAGNOSIS
CLINICAL EVALUATION

The clinical diagnosis of neonatal HSV infection is difficult because the appearance of skin vesicles cannot be relied on as an initial component of disease presentation. Enteroviral sepsis is a major differential diagnostic possibility in infants with signs suggesting neonatal HSV. Bacterial infections of newborns can mimic neonatal HSV infection. Skin lesions may resemble lesions seen with bullous or crusted impetigo. Some infants infected by HSV have been described who had concomitant bacterial infections, including group b streptococci, *Staphylococcus aureus*, *Listeria monocytogenes*, and gram-negative bacteria. A positive culture for one of these pathogens does not rule out HSV infection if the clinical suspicion for neonatal herpes infection is present.

Many other disorders of the newborn can be indistinguishable from neonatal HSV infections, including acute respiratory distress syndrome, intraventricular hemorrhage, necrotizing enterocolitis, and various ocular or cutaneous diseases. When vesicles are present, alternative causes of exanthems should be excluded. Other diagnoses include enteroviral infection, varicella-zoster virus infection, and syphilis. Laboratory methods are available to differentiate these causes of cutaneous lesions in the newborn. Cutaneous disorders such as erythema toxicum, neonatal melanosis, acrodermatitis enteropathica, and incontinentia pigmenti often confuse physicians who suspect neonatal HSV infections. HSV lesions can be distinguished rapidly from lesions caused by these diseases using direct immunofluorescence stain of lesion scrapings or other methods for rapid detection of viral proteins and confirmation by viral culture.

HSV encephalitis is a difficult clinical diagnosis to make, particularly because many children with CNS infection do not have a vesicular rash at the time of clinical presentation. Infection of the CNS is suspected in a child who has evidence of acute neurologic deterioration, often associated with the onset of seizure, and in the absence of intraventricular hemorrhage and metabolic causes. PCR to detect viral DNA in CSF has become an important diagnostic method, largely replacing the need for diagnosis by brain biopsy [119]. Infants with localized

TABLE 26–2   Morbidity and Mortality among Patients after 12 Months by Viral Type, 1981-1997

| | No. Patients by Disease Classification (%)* | | | | | |
| | Skin, Eye, or Mouth | | Central Nervous System | | Disseminated | |
Outcome	HSV-1	HSV-2	HSV-1	HSV-2	HSV-1	HSV-2
Normal	24 (100)	19 (95)	4 (75)	7 (17.5)	3 (23)	14 (41)
Mild impairment	0 (0)	0 (0)	0 (0)	7 (17.5)	0 (0)	1 (3)
Moderate impairment	0 (0)	1 (5)	1 (14)	7 (17.5)	0 (0)	0 (0)
Severe impairment	0 (0)	0 (0)	2 (29)	13 (32.5)	1 (8)	3 (9)
Death	0 (0)	0 (0)	0 (0)	6 (15)	9 (69)	16 (47)
Unknown	Total of 20		Total of 16		Total of 16	

*Survival rate (by Cox regression analysis) of patients infected with HSV-2 was higher compared with patients infected with HSV-1; however, the difference was not statistically significant. Patients infected with HSV-2 were more likely to have neurologic abnormalities compared with patients infected with HSV-1 (borderline significance, P = .10).
HSV, herpes simplex virus.
Data from Kimberlin DW, et al. Natural history of neonatal herpes simplex virus infections in the acyclovir era. Pediatrics 108:223-229, 2001.

encephalitis usually have serial increases in CSF cell counts and protein concentrations and negative bacterial cultures of CSF. Noninvasive neurodiagnostic studies can be used to define sites of involvement.

LABORATORY ASSESSMENT

The appropriate use of laboratory methods is essential if a timely diagnosis of HSV infection is to be achieved. Virus isolation remains the definitive diagnostic method. If skin lesions are present, a swab of skin vesicles, done vigorously enough to obtain cells from the base of the lesion, should be made and transferred in appropriate virus transport media to a diagnostic virology laboratory. Rapid diagnosis should be attempted by preparing material from skin lesion scrapings for direct immunofluorescence testing to detect the presence of virus-infected cells or for testing by enzyme immunoassays for viral proteins. Because of the possibility of false-positive results using immunofluorescence or other antigen detection methods, specimens should also be obtained for confirmation by viral isolation. Direct immunofluorescence staining for virus-infected cells is unreliable unless the specimen is obtained from a skin lesion and adequate numbers of cells are collected. Cells from oropharyngeal swabs or from CSF should not be tested using this method.

Clinical specimens should be transported to the diagnostic virology laboratory without being frozen, and their processing should be expedited to permit rapid confirmation of the clinical diagnosis. In addition to skin vesicles, other materials or sites from which virus may be isolated include the CSF, stool, urine, throat, nasopharynx, and conjunctivae. Isolation of virus from swabs of superficial sites, such as the nasopharynx, may represent transient presence of the virus in secretions, when the culture is obtained within the first 24 hours after birth, and particularly when the specimen is taken immediately after birth.

Typing of an HSV isolate may be done by one of several techniques. Because the outcome of antiviral treatment and risk of late sequelae may be related to the virus type, typing is of prognostic and epidemiologic importance [94]. Results of viral cultures of the CSF may be positive for infants with disseminated HSV infections, but are usually negative for infants who have localized encephalitis.

Detection of HSV DNA in CSF by PCR can allow a rapid presumptive diagnosis of HSV encephalitis in the newborn [119–122]. PCR was used in the retrospective analysis of materials collected from 24 infants enrolled in the NIAID CASG antiviral studies [120]. HSV was detected by PCR assay of CSF in 71% of infants before antiviral therapy was initiated. At least one specimen was positive in 76% of infants, and all samples that were positive by viral culture were positive by PCR. Similar findings were reported by Swedish investigators when stored CSF specimens obtained from infants with neonatal HSV infection were tested for HSV by PCR. HSV DNA was detected from CSF in the acute phase of illness from 78% of patients with CNS disease [123].

Use of HSV PCR methods on CSF can potentially decrease the duration of time to diagnosis of some cases of HSV encephalitis; however, there are reports in older patients of initial negative HSV PCR results early in the course of illness. CSF obtained 4 to 7 days after the initial CSF samples was subsequently positive for HSV DNA in a few patients [124].

PCR tests of CSF were positive in 7 (24%) of 29 infants enrolled in the NIAID CASG antiviral studies whose clinical disease seemed to be limited to mucocutaneous lesions. Five of the six infants who were evaluated when 1 year old were developmentally normal [120]. The significance of this observation for disease classification and prognosis remains to be determined.

Most studies of PCR for the diagnosis of HSV CNS infections indicate the test is sensitive in approximately 75% to 100% of cases in small cohorts of infants [120–123]. Specificity of the test ranges from 71% to 100%. The broad range of values for sensitivity and specificity of HSV PCR probably results from different study methods and disease classifications [125].

Some studies have shown that HSV PCR may be used to detect HSV DNA in peripheral blood mononuclear cells and plasma of infants with proven neonatal HSV infection. Using a sensitive and well-standardized PCR method, investigators found HSV DNA in peripheral blood mononuclear cells of 6 of 10 infants tested and in plasma of 4 of 6 infants tested [91]. Other investigators have reported the presence of HSV DNA in serum of 67% (20 of 30) of infants with neonatal HSV infection [123].

In clinical practice, there is considerable interlaboratory variability in HSV PCR test performance. Diagnostic laboratories that perform HSV PCR testing must be able to validate their test and participate in national and in-house proficiency testing programs [126]. Interpretation of negative or positive HSV PCR results must depend on clinical findings. A negative PCR result for HSV in CSF in the setting of clinical, laboratory, or radiologic findings consistent with CNS infection does not rule out HSV infection. It is important to continue to use standard clinical and laboratory diagnostic methods for the evaluation of infants with possible neonatal HSV (Table 26–3).

Every effort should be made to confirm HSV infection by viral isolation. Cytologic examination of cells from the infant's lesions should not be used to diagnose HSV infection because reliable specific methods are available. Cytologic methods, such as Papanicolaou, Giemsa, or Tzanck staining, have a sensitivity of only approximately 60% to 70%. A negative result must not be interpreted as excluding the diagnosis of HSV and a positive result should not be the sole diagnostic determinant of HSV infection in the newborn. Intranuclear inclusions and multinucleated giant cells may be consistent with, but not diagnostic of, HSV infection.

In contrast to some other neonatal infections, serologic diagnosis of HSV infection has little clinical value. The interpretation of serologic assays is complicated by the fact that transplacentally acquired maternal IgG cannot be differentiated from endogenously produced antibodies, making it difficult to assess the neonate's antibody status during acute infection. Serial type-specific antibody testing may be useful for retrospective diagnosis if a mother without a prior history of HSV infection has a primary infection late in gestation and transfers little or no antibody to the fetus. Therapeutic decisions cannot await a diagnostic approach based on comparing acute phase and

TABLE 26–3　Initial Diagnostic Evaluation for Suspected Neonatal Herpes Simplex Virus Infection

Microbiologic Studies

Skin lesion: viral culture and direct viral examination

Cerebrospinal fluid: viral culture and HSV PCR*

Conjunctivae: viral culture

Nasopharynx and mouth: viral culture

Rectum: viral culture

Urine: viral culture

Ancillary Studies

Cerebrospinal fluid cell count, glucose and protein levels

Complete blood cell count with differential and platelet counts

Liver function studies

Coagulation studies

Electroencephalogram

Computed tomography or magnetic resonance imaging of head

Chest radiograph

Not Recommended

Direct viral examination of samples from conjunctivae, nasopharynx, mouth, rectum, urine, or cerebrospinal fluid

Herpes antibody from serum

Tzanck smear

*The diagnostic reliability of herpes simplex virus polymerase chain reaction (HSV PCR) results from blood or skin lesions performed outside of the research setting is unknown.

convalescent phase antibody titers. IgM production is delayed or does not occur in infected infants because of inherent immaturity in the immune response to systemic viral infections in the newborn, and commercially available assays for IgM antibodies to HSV have limited reliability. The results of specific laboratory tests for HSV should be used in conjunction with clinical findings and general laboratory tests, such as platelet counts, CSF analysis, and liver function tests, to establish a disease classification.

TREATMENT
BACKGROUND

The cumulative experience of the past 25 years shows that perinatally acquired HSV infections are amenable to treatment with antiviral agents. Acyclovir is the drug of choice [96]. Because most infants acquire infection at the time of delivery or shortly thereafter, antiviral therapy has the potential to decrease mortality and improve long-term outcome. The benefits that antiviral therapy can provide are influenced substantially by early diagnosis. The likelihood of disease progression in infants who acquire HSV infections is an established fact. Without treatment, approximately 70% of infants presenting with disease localized to the skin, eye, or mouth develop involvement of the CNS or disseminated infection. Treatment initiated after disease progression is not optimal because many of these children die or are left with significant neurologic impairment. Regardless of the apparently minor clinical

findings in some cases, the possibility of HSV infection in the newborn requires aggressive diagnostic evaluation, and likely or proven infection mandates the immediate initiation of intravenous acyclovir therapy.

ANTIVIRAL DRUGS

Historically, four nucleoside analogues have been used to treat neonatal herpes: idoxuridine, cytosine arabinoside, vidarabine, and acyclovir. Of these, the first three are nonspecific inhibitors of cellular and viral replication. The fourth, acyclovir, is monophosphorylated by HSV-specific thymidine kinases and then converted to its diphosphate and triphosphate forms by cellular enzymes. Acyclovir acts as a competitive inhibitor of HSV DNA polymerase and terminates DNA chain elongation [127]. Idoxuridine and cytosine arabinoside have no value as systemic therapy for any viral infection because of toxicity and equivocal efficacy. Vidarabine was the first drug shown to be efficacious; it decreased mortality and improved morbidity in cases of neonatal HSV infections [128]. A comparison of vidarabine with acyclovir suggests that these compounds have a similar level of activity for this disease; however, vidarabine is no longer available for clinical use [115]. Acyclovir is safe for use in newborns and is familiar to pediatricians from its other clinical uses.

Acyclovir has been established as efficacious for the treatment of primary genital HSV infection [129,130]. Oral and intravenous administration of acyclovir to the immunocompromised host decreases the frequency of reactivation after immunosuppression and the duration of disease [131]. Acyclovir has been established to be superior to vidarabine for the treatment of HSV encephalitis in older children and adults [132]. Because this compound is a selective inhibitor of viral replication, it has a low frequency of side effects. After pharmacokinetic and tolerance evaluation of acyclovir were done in infants [133,134], the NIAID CASG compared vidarabine and acyclovir for the treatment of neonatal HSV infection in a randomized trial [115]. The dose of vidarabine used was 30 mg/kg/day, and acyclovir was given at a dose of 10 mg/kg every 8 hours. The duration of therapy was 10 days. There were no significant differences in survival between the two treatment groups (Fig. 26–3). There were no differences in adverse effects or laboratory evidence of toxicity.

Survival with antiviral therapy depended on classification of the extent of disease at diagnosis (Fig. 26–4). Mortality and morbidity were also influenced by clinical status at the time of diagnosis and the virus type. Among infants with skin, eye, or mouth disease, those with HSV-1 infections were all normal developmentally at 1 year compared with 86% of infants with HSV-2 infections. Infants who were alert or lethargic when treatment was initiated had a survival rate of 91% compared with 54% for infants who were semicomatose or comatose; similar differences in survival rates related to neurologic status were observed in infants with disseminated infection. Prematurity, pneumonitis, and disseminated intravascular coagulopathy were poor prognostic signs [94].

Improved outcome compared with historical data probably reflects earlier diagnosis and institution of antiviral therapy, preventing progression of disease from skin, eye,

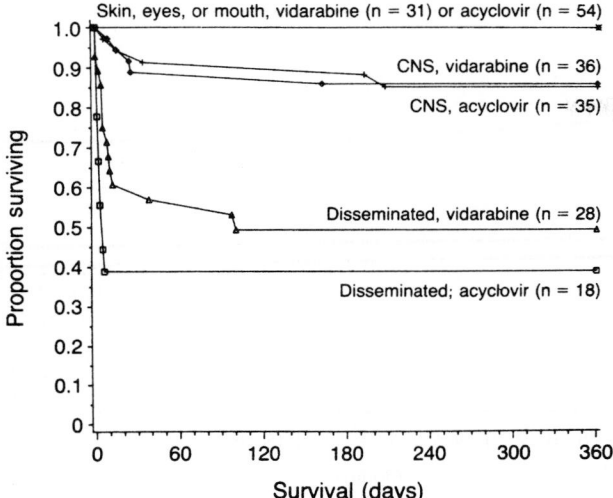

FIGURE 26–3 Survival of infants with neonatal herpes simplex virus infection according to treatment and extent of disease. The infection was classified as confined to skin, eyes, or mouth; affecting the central nervous system (CNS); or producing disseminated disease. After adjustment for extent of disease with use of a stratified analysis, overall comparison of vidarabine with acyclovir was not statistically significant ($P = .27$) by a log-rank test. No comparison of treatments within disease categories was statistically significant. *(From Whitley R, et al. A controlled trial comparing vidarabine with acyclovir in neonatal herpes simplex virus infection. N Engl J Med 324:444, 1991.)*

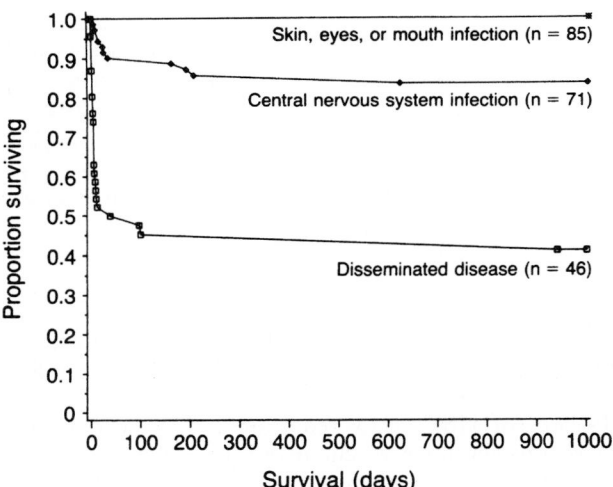

FIGURE 26–4 Survival of infants with neonatal herpes simplex virus infection according to extent of disease ($P < .001$ for all comparisons). *(From Whitley R, et al. Predictors of morbidity and mortality in neonates with herpes simplex infections. N Engl J Med 324:450, 1991.)*

or mouth to more severe disease. The mean duration of symptoms before treatment for all participants, regardless of disease classification, was 4 to 5 days, indicating that therapy might have been instituted even sooner. These observations suggested that further advances in therapeutic outcome might be achieved by earlier intervention. Despite advances in laboratory diagnosis and treatment of neonatal HSV, the mean time between onset of disease symptoms and initiation of antiviral therapy has not changed [74].

Despite the proven efficacy of antiviral therapy for neonatal HSV infection, the mortality rate remains high, and

many infants who survive disseminated or CNS disease have serious sequelae. This circumstance dictated the need to evaluate high doses of acyclovir and longer treatment regimens. Infants were enrolled in an NIAID CASG assessment of acyclovir given at an intermediate dose (45 mg/kg/day) or high dose (60 mg/kg/day). Mortality rates for infants with disseminated or CNS disease were lower for infants given high-dose acyclovir than observed in earlier studies (Fig. 26–5) [135]. There was no significant difference in morbidity status at 12 months of follow-up between high-dose and standard-dose acyclovir recipients for each of the three disease categories. Transient and reversible neutropenia occurred more frequently during high-dose therapy, but resolved during or after cessation of treatment. The dose of acyclovir used had no impact on the duration of viral shedding [135].

The current recommendation for treatment of neonatal HSV infection is acyclovir, 60 mg/kg/day in three doses (20 mg/kg/dose) given intravenously. Disseminated and CNS infections are treated at least 21 days. Duration of treatment for skin, eye, and mouth infection, after disseminated and CNS infection have been ruled out, is a minimum of 14 days [136]. The use of oral acyclovir is contraindicated for the treatment of acute HSV infections in newborns. Its limited oral bioavailability results in plasma and CSF concentrations of drug that are inadequate for therapeutic effects on viral replication. Other oral antiviral drugs, such as valacyclovir, have not been studied in infants and should not be used to treat acute HSV infection in newborns. The high risk of progression from localized mucocutaneous infections requires the administration of intravenous acyclovir to these infants, regardless of how well they seem at the time of diagnosis. In addition to intravenous therapy, infants with ocular involvement caused by HSV should receive one of the topical ophthalmic agents approved for this indication. Topical acyclovir is unnecessary for treatment of mucocutaneous lesions caused by HSV because parenteral drug reaches these sites.

Acyclovir treatment is based on clinical suspicion and laboratory diagnosis of neonatal HSV infection. Rapid methods, including direct antigen detection and PCR, should be used to facilitate early laboratory confirmation of suspected cases. Presumptive treatment is a reasonable option when circumstances prevent rapid laboratory diagnosis, and the clinical manifestations are those described for mucocutaneous infections, disseminated disease, or HSV encephalitis. These clinical manifestations could include skin lesions, seizures, hepatitis, hypothermia or fever, an ill-appearing infant, and CSF pleocytosis. Determining which infants admitted to the hospital with presumed sepsis should be treated empirically with acyclovir remains a topic of debate [137,138]. In all cases of presumptive therapy, specimens should be obtained for laboratory testing to guide the decision to continue treatment. During the course of therapy, careful monitoring is important to assess the therapeutic response. Even in the absence of clinical evidence of encephalitis, evaluation of the CNS should be done for prognostic purposes. Serial evaluations of hepatic and hematologic parameters may indicate changes caused by the viral infection or by drug toxicity.

Intravenous acyclovir is tolerated well by infants. Adequate hydration is necessary to minimize the risk of

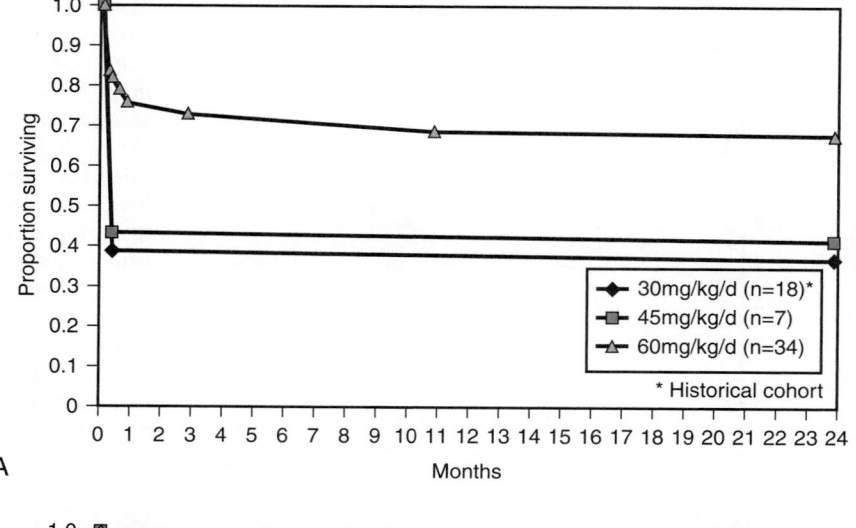

A

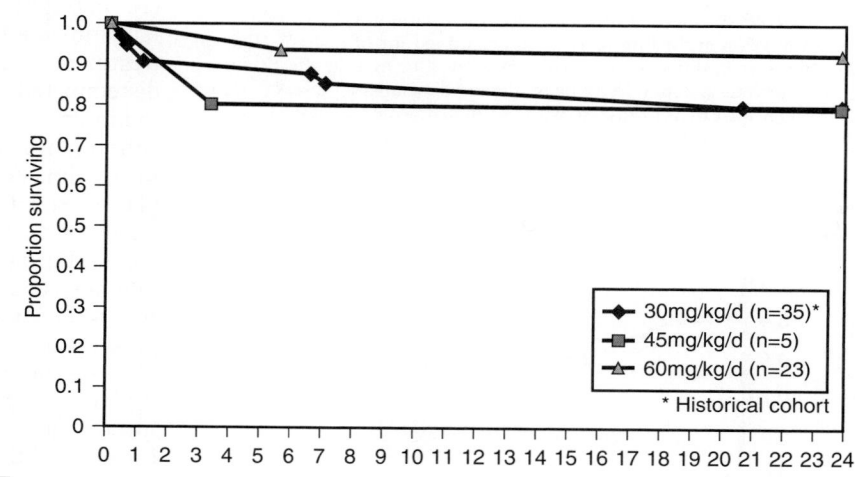

B

FIGURE 26–5 **A** and **B**, Mortality rates for patients with disseminated disease (**A**) and central nervous system disease (**B**) depending on dose of acyclovir. (*Data from Kimberlin DW, et al. Safety and efficacy of high-dose intravenous acyclovir in the management of neonatal herpes simplex virus infections. Pediatrics 108:230-238, 2001.*)

nephrotoxicity, and dosage adjustments are necessary if renal clearance is impaired. As for all drugs, the possibility of acute toxicity should be considered in any child receiving parenteral antiviral therapy and should be assessed by serially evaluating bone marrow, renal, and hepatic functions. The potential for long-term harm from these drugs remains to be defined; so far, no long-term adverse effects have been identified.

Acyclovir resistance has been reported in an infant with acute HSV infection of the larynx in the newborn period; in this case, the initial isolate was not inhibited by acyclovir, although the source of this infection could not be explained [139]. Acyclovir resistance has also been reported in a premature infant with cutaneous and CNS disease caused by an initially acyclovir-susceptible HSV. The infant developed recurrent disseminated HSV infection 8 days after a 21-day course of acyclovir. The virus isolated at the onset of recurrent symptoms was found to lack thymidine kinase activity on the basis of a frame-shift mutation in the thymidine kinase gene [140]. Another infant born to a mother with severe systemic primary HSV-2 infection developed an acyclovir-resistant mutant during acyclovir therapy for disseminated HSV

infection and eventually died. The use of steroids to treat blood pressure instability may have hampered this infant's immune response to infection further [141].

Isolates of HSV recovered from infants who received intravenous acyclovir for cutaneous disease in the newborn period and had subsequent recurrent cutaneous lesions typically remain sensitive to acyclovir [142]. Emergence of viral resistance to acyclovir has been described in patients requiring prolonged or repeated treatment with this drug. One infant who was given long-term oral acyclovir for suppression of recurrences during the first 6 months of life had a resistant HSV isolated from a lesion after therapy was discontinued, but subsequent isolates were susceptible [143].

Antiviral resistance does not generally explain the failure of infants with the disseminated or encephalitic form of the disease to respond well to antiviral therapy. Clinical deterioration, despite appropriate therapy and supportive care, can be attributed to virus-induced destruction of cells compromising infected organs, such as liver or brain, or irreversible changes, such as disseminated intravascular coagulopathy.

The observation of an association between late sequelae and frequent recurrences of skin lesions in infants who were treated for localized HSV-2 infections during the newborn period has raised questions about the potential efficacy of suppressive therapy with oral acyclovir. The NIAID CASG has undertaken an assessment of the safety and efficacy of suppression as an adjunct after the recommended treatment of mucocutaneous disease with intravenous acyclovir [143]. Infants were given 300 mg/m^2 two or three times per day for 6 months. Of 16 infants given the three daily doses, 13 (81%) had no recurrences of lesions while receiving therapy compared with 54% of infants from earlier studies who received intravenous acyclovir only. Of the 26 infants, 46% developed neutropenia. In one infant, suppressive therapy was associated with a transient recurrence of infection owing to an acyclovir-resistant isolate of HSV-2; subsequent recurrences were caused by susceptible isolates. Whether this effect on cutaneous recurrences, which was limited to periods of active oral suppressive therapy, has any effect on late neurologic sequelae is unknown.

A pilot study showed improved neurodevelopmental outcomes (compared with historical data) in a small group of infants treated with oral acyclovir for 2 years [144]. There was no comparative treatment group. Acyclovir therapy was relatively well tolerated in this small cohort of children; rare neutropenia and dental decay were reported. The dental decay was attributed to sugar in the acyclovir suspension.

Cases of breakthrough CNS HSV disease may occur despite oral acyclovir prophylaxis [145]. Until more published information becomes available regarding optimal dosing, duration, efficacy, and safety, oral acyclovir prophylaxis after neonatal HSV infection is not routinely recommended. Any decision to consider its use should be made in consultation with a pediatric infectious disease specialist or as part of a research protocol.

OTHER ISSUES IN ACUTE MANAGEMENT

Neonates with HSV infection should be hospitalized and managed with contact precautions if mucocutaneous lesions are present. Many infants with this infection have life-threatening problems, including disseminated intravascular coagulation, shock, and respiratory failure, and they require supportive care that is available only at tertiary medical centers.

There is no indication that administration of immunoglobulin or hyperimmunoglobulin is of value for the treatment of neonatal HSV infection. Although a series of studies have suggested that the quantity of transplacental neutralizing antibodies affects the attack rate among exposed infants and may influence the initial disease manifestations, the presence of antibodies may or may not influence the subsequent course of infection [49,50,53,54,86]. The administration of standard preparations of intravenous immunoglobulin does not enhance the titers of functional antibodies against HSV in infants with low birth weight [146]. The evaluation of virus-specific monoclonal antibodies in combination with antiviral therapy may become feasible as new technologies for deriving human or humanized antibody preparations are developed [147].

No other forms of adjunctive therapy are useful for treating neonatal HSV infections. Various experimental modalities, including interferon, immunomodulators, and immunization, have been attempted, but none has produced demonstrable effects.

LONG-TERM MANAGEMENT OF INFECTED INFANTS

With the advent of antiviral therapy, an increasing number of newborns with HSV infection are surviving and require careful long-term follow-up. The most common complications of neonatal HSV infection include neurologic and ocular sequelae that may be detected only on long-term follow-up. It is necessary that these children receive serial long-term evaluation from qualified pediatric specialists in these areas, which should include neurodevelopmental, ophthalmologic, and hearing assessments.

Recurrent skin vesicles are present in many children, including children who did not have obvious mucocutaneous disease during the acute phase of the clinical illness. Skin vesicles provide a potential source for transmission of infection to other children or adults who have direct contact with these infants. The use of day care for children, including children surviving neonatal HSV infections, stimulates many questions from day care providers about these children. There is some risk that children with recurrent HSV skin lesions would transmit the virus to other children in this environment. The most reasonable recommendation in this situation is to cover the lesions to prevent direct contact. HSV-1 is much more likely to be present in the day care environment in the form of asymptomatic infection or gingivostomatitis. In both cases, virus is present in the mouth and pharynx, and the frequent exchange of saliva and other respiratory droplets that occurs among children in this setting makes this route of transmission more likely. Education of day care workers and the general public about herpesvirus infections, their implications, and the frequency with which they occur in the population as a whole can calm fears and correct common misconceptions.

Parents of children with neonatal HSV infection often have significant guilt feelings. Parents often require support from psychologists, psychiatrists, or counselors. The family physician or pediatrician can provide a valuable supportive role to the family in this situation. Most parents and many physicians are unaware of the high prevalence of HSV-2 infection in the United States and of the lifelong persistence and subclinical nature of these infections. Concern about the risk of fetal and neonatal infection during subsequent pregnancies is often a major issue that can be addressed effectively based on the low risks as proven from large, prospective studies.

PREVENTION
BACKGROUND

Despite the progress that has been made in antiviral treatment of neonatal HSV infection, the ideal approach is to prevent the exposure of infants to active maternal infection at the time of delivery. Genital infections caused by HSV are often clinically silent when they are acquired as new infections and when the virus reactivates. With the high prevalence of HSV-2 infection in the U.S. population, women are at risk for acquiring new genital infections during pregnancy, and at least one in five becomes infected before pregnancy. The problem of asymptomatic genital HSV infection means that the transmission of HSV from mothers to infants cannot be eliminated even with the best obstetric management.

It is futile to obtain sequential genital cultures during the last weeks of gestation in women with a history of genital herpes in an effort to identify those who will have asymptomatic infection at the onset of labor [48]. These cultures do not predict the infant's risk of exposure at delivery because of the usually brief duration of asymptomatic shedding and the time required for the culture to become positive. Because of the attention of the lay press to the devastating outcome of neonatal HSV infections, many women who know that they have genital herpes experience severe anxiety about the potential risks to the fetus and the newborn. As a consequence these women may have an unnecessarily high frequency of cesarean deliveries. The risk of neonatal HSV infection in the newborn is approximately equivalent for women who have no prior history of genital herpes or a partner with known infection (Table 26–4).

MANAGEMENT OF PREGNANT WOMEN WITH KNOWN GENITAL HERPES

Women who have a history of recurrent genital herpes should be reassured that the risk of fetal or neonatal infection is very low. Intrauterine HSV infections are rare, with an estimated overall risk of 1 in 200,000 pregnancies [68]. Information about the risk of exposure to asymptomatic reactivation at delivery derived from six large-scale prospective studies is sufficient to conclude that the incidence of asymptomatic reactivation in these women is about 2% and that the attack rate for their exposed infants is approximately 3% or less; the risk of neonatal infection under these circumstances is less than 1 in 2000 deliveries.

Because laboratory methods cannot be used to detect asymptomatic infection in a timely manner, the current approach to management is to perform a careful vaginal examination at presentation and to elect cesarean delivery if the mother has signs or symptoms of recurrent genital

TABLE 26–4   Projected Risk of Transmission of Herpes Simplex Virus Type 2 (HSV-2) from Mothers to Infants at Delivery in a Cohort of 100,000 Pregnant Women

25% with Past HSV-2 Infection	75% Susceptible to HSV-2 Infection
25,000 women	75,000 women
1.5% reactivation at delivery	0.02% seroconversion/wk
375 women with reactivation	30 women with infection <2 wk before delivery
<5% risk of transmission to infant	50% risk of transmission
19 infected infants	15 infected infants

Data from Arvin AM. The epidemiology of perinatal herpes simplex infections. In Stanberry L (ed). Genital and Neonatal Herpes. New York, John Wiley & Sons, 1996, pp 179–192.

herpes at the onset of labor. Given the low probability of neonatal infection, it is appropriate to deliver infants of women who have a history of recurrent genital herpes but who have no active clinical disease at delivery by the vaginal route [55]. An analysis of the occurrence of HSV infections in infants in California showed no change from 1985–1995, despite a documented decrease in deliveries by cesarean section and an increase in the proportion of women with a previous diagnosis of genital herpes whose infants were delivered vaginally [61].

A culture for HSV obtained at the time of delivery may be useful in establishing whether the virus was present at delivery to facilitate recognition of neonatal infection if it occurs. The value of this approach has not been established, however. Alternative diagnostic approaches, such as those based on PCR to detect virus, may ultimately expedite identification of women at risk for delivering infected infants [148,149]. Evidence indicates that detection of viral presence in genital samples by PCR is more sensitive than culture methods. The significance of a positive PCR result in predicting risk of transmission of HSV to the infant is unknown, however [150]. Viral DNA can persist for a longer interval than infectious virus.

The utility of suppressive therapy of genital herpes in women with a known history of recurrent infection remains a question for clinical investigation because of risk-benefit considerations. Some studies indicate that prophylactic acyclovir reduces the number of genital lesions from HSV. Despite prophylaxis, a few women continue to have virus detectable by PCR [150]. Use of prophylactic valacyclovir also reduced clinical HSV recurrences, but did not decrease shedding of HSV within 7 days of delivery compared with placebo [151]. Even with suppressive therapy, the potential for neonatal HSV infection is not eliminated entirely. It is unknown whether acyclovir suppressive therapy late in pregnancy might alter the clinical presentation of neonatal HSV or compromise the interpretation of viral cultures [152].

The pharmacokinetics and metabolism of acyclovir in the human fetus are unknown. The possibility of fetal nephrotoxicity related to acyclovir is a potential risk that must be considered. Whether acyclovir treatment of mothers with primary genital herpes late in gestation can reduce the neonatal risk of these infections is a research issue. Signs of disseminated herpes in the mother warrant the administration of intravenous acyclovir, however.

Based on limited scientific evidence, the American College of Obstetricians and Gynecologists recommends that women with active recurrent genital herpes should be offered suppressive viral therapy at or beyond 36 weeks of gestation until delivery [55]. Universal antenatal type-specific HSV screening to prevent neonatal HSV is not recommended [153].

MANAGEMENT OF INFANTS OF MOTHERS WITH GENITAL HERPES

Infants of mothers with histories of genital herpes delivered vaginally or by cesarean section and whose mothers have no evidence of active genital herpetic infection are at low risk for acquiring neonatal HSV infection. These infants need no special evaluation during the newborn period. Infants delivered vaginally to mothers with an active genital HSV infection or who have genital cultures done at delivery that are positive for HSV should be isolated from other infants for the durations of their hospitalization up to age 4 weeks. Parents and primary care physicians should be notified about the exposure of the infant so that the infant can be observed for the occurrence of nonspecific signs consistent with possible neonatal herpes. The parents and responsible family members should be educated about the low risk of transmission to relieve anxiety and to ensure prompt return for care in the unlikely event that signs of infection appear. Information regarding infection should include a description of the risks associated with transmission of infection to the newborn, the common signs and symptoms of neonatal herpes, the necessity for careful monitoring for the onset of illness 4 to 6 weeks after birth, and the planned approach to treatment if symptoms occur.

It may be useful to obtain cultures from the exposed infant 24 to 48 hours after delivery and at intervals during the first 4 weeks of life. Sites from which virus may be recovered include the eye, oropharynx, and skin lesions that are suspected to be herpetic. Weekly viral cultures have been suggested for the surveillance of exposed infants; the utility of this approach has not been proved by prospective studies, and it should be considered an optional addition to clinical observation.

If cultures from any site in the infant are positive, a thorough diagnostic evaluation should be done, including obtaining additional specimens for viral culture from the site that was reported to be positive, the oropharynx, and the CSF, and treatment with intravenous acyclovir should be initiated. Viral cultures of urine and HSV PCR of peripheral blood mononuclear cells may also be considered to identify additional sites of viral infection. A positive HSV PCR result in addition to the initial positive culture can provide additional evidence to support the diagnosis of HSV infection. A negative HSV PCR result does not in itself rule out infection.

No data are available to support the administration of acyclovir to exposed infants who have no clinical signs or laboratory evidence of infection. Parameters for duration of such prophylaxis cannot be defined. The experience from other clinical settings is that the virus is suppressed only for the period the drug is given and is not eradicated. Careful clinical follow-up of these infants, with immediate institution of antiviral therapy if symptoms occur, is an appropriate approach.

An issue of frequent concern is whether the mother with an active genital HSV infection at delivery should be isolated from her infant after delivery. Women with recurrent orolabial HSV infection and cutaneous HSV infections at other sites (e.g., breast lesions) are at similar risk for transmission of virus to their newborns. Because transmission occurs by direct contact with the virus, appropriate precautions by the mother, including careful hand washing before touching the infant, should prevent any need to separate mother and child. In some cases, it is possible to have the exposed infant room-in with the mother as a means of isolating the infant from other newborns. Breast-feeding is contraindicated if the mother has vesicular lesions involving the breast.

CONCLUSION

Neonatal HSV infection is a life-threatening disease in the newborn. With an increasing prevalence of genital herpes and the recognition that many infections are completely asymptomatic in the mother, pediatricians, neonatologists, obstetricians, and family practitioners must continue to remain vigilant to infants whose symptoms may be compatible with HSV infections. Early identification leads to prompt treatment. It is hoped that the development of safe and efficacious vaccines and a better understanding of factors associated with transmission of virus from mother to infant will enable prevention of neonatal HSV infection.

ACKNOWLEDGMENTS

The databases on clinical presentations, diagnosis, and antiviral treatment of neonatal HSV infections have been generated through the efforts of the NIAID Collaborative Antiviral Study Group for more than 25 years, with support from the National Institute of Allergy and Infectious Diseases. The institute has also supported prognostic studies of HSV infection in pregnancy and newborns in the United States.

REFERENCES

[1] M. Hass, Hepataadrenal necrosis with intranuclear inclusion bodies: report of a case, Am. J. Pathol. 11 (1935) 127.

[2] A. Batignani, Conjunctivite da virus erpeticoin neonato, Boll. Ocul. 13 (1934) 1217.

[3] A. Nahmias, W.R. Dowdle, Antigenic and biological differences in herpesvirus hominis, Prog. Med. Virol. 10 (1968) 110–159.

[4] B. Roizman, D.M. Knipe, R.J. Whitley, Herpes simplex viruses, in: D.M. Knipe, P.M. Howley (Eds.), Fields Virology, Lippincott Williams & Wilkins, Philadelphia, 2007.

[5] P.G. Spear, Glycoproteins of herpes simplex virus, in: J. Bentz (Ed.), Viral Fusion Mechanisms, CRC Press, Boca Raton, FL, 1993.

[6] B. Roizman, et al., Identification and preliminary mapping with monoclonal antibodies of a herpes simplex virus 2 glycoprotein lacking a known type 1 counterpart, Virology 133 (1984) 242–247.

[7] B. Roizman, F.J. Jenkins, Genetic engineering of novel genomes of large DNA viruses, Science 229 (1985) 1208–1214.

[8] I.A. York, et al., A cytosolic herpes simplex virus protein inhibits antigen presentation to CD8+ T lymphocytes Cell 77 (1994) 525–535.

[9] P. Jugovic, et al., Inhibition of major histocompatibility complex class I antigen presentation in pig and primate cells by herpes simplex virus type 1 and 2 ICP47, J. Virol. 72 (1998) 5076–5084.

[10] W.M. Sullender, et al., Type-specific antibodies to herpes simplex virus type 2 (HSV-2) glycoprotein G in pregnant women, infants exposed to maternal HSV-2 infection at delivery, and infants with neonatal herpes, J. Infect. Dis. 157 (1988) 164–171.

[11] R.M. Coleman, et al., Determination of herpes simplex virus type-specific antibodies by enzyme-linked immunosorbent assay, J. Clin. Microbiol. 18 (1983) 287–291.

[12] A. Wald, R. Ashley-Morrow, Serological testing for herpes simplex virus (HSV)-1 and HSV-2 infection, Clin. Infect. Dis. 35 (Suppl. 2) (2002) S173–S182.

[13] R.L. Ashley, et al., Premarket evaluation of a commercial glycoprotein G-based enzyme immunoassay for herpes simplex virus type-specific antibodies, J. Clin. Microbiol. 36 (1998) 294–295.

[14] H. Cushing, Surgical aspects of major neuralgia of trigeminal nerve: report of 20 cases of operation upon the gasserian ganglion with anatomic and physiologic notes on the consequence of its removal, JAMA 44 (1905).

[15] E.W. Goodpasture, Herpetic infections with special reference to involvement of the nervous system, Medicine 8 (1929).

[16] C.A. Carton, E.D. Kilbourne, Activation of latent herpes simplex by trigeminal sensory-root section, N. Engl. J. Med. 246 (1952).

[17] G.J. Pazin, et al., Prevention of reactivated herpes simplex infection by human leukocyte interferon after operation on the trigeminal root, N. Engl. J. Med. 301 (1979) 225–230.

[18] A.L. Cunningham, et al., The cycle of human herpes simplex virus infection: virus transport and immune control, J. Infect. Dis. 194 (Suppl. 1) (2006) S11–S18.

[19] J.G. Stevens, M.L. Cook, Latent herpes simplex virus in spinal ganglia of mice, Science 173 (1971) 843–845.

[20] D.L. Rock, N.W. Fraser, Detection of HSV-1 genome in central nervous system of latently infected mice, Nature 302 (1983) 523–525.

[21] J.R. Baringer, Recovery of herpes simplex virus from human sacral ganglions, N. Engl. J. Med. 291 (1974) 828–830.

[22] F. Xu, et al., Seroprevalence of herpes simplex virus type 1 in children in the United States, J. Pediatr. 151 (2007) 374–377.

[23] F. Xu, et al., Seroprevalence of herpes simplex virus types 1 and 2 in pregnant women in the United States, Am. J. Obstet. Gynecol. 196 (2007) 43e1– 43e6.

[24] B.B. Wentworth, E.R. Alexander, Seroepidemiology of infectious due to members of the herpesvirus group, Am. J. Epidemiol. 94 (1971) 496–507.

[25] A.M. Arvin, The epidemiology of perinatal herpes simplex infections, in: L. Stanberry (Ed.), Genital and Neonatal Herpes, John Wiley & Sons, New York, 1996.

[26] A.J. Nahmias, et al., Antibodies to Herpesvirus hominis types 1 and 2 in humans. I. Patients with genital herpetic infections, Am. J. Epidemiol. 91 (1970) 539–546.

[27] W.E. Lafferty, et al., Herpes simplex virus type 1 as a cause of genital herpes: impact on surveillance and prevention, J. Infect. Dis. 181 (2000) 1454–1457.

[28] F. Xu, et al., Trends in herpes simplex virus type 1 and type 2 seroprevalence in the United States, JAMA 296 (2006) 964–973.

[29] A. Wald, et al., Virologic characteristics of subclinical and symptomatic genital herpes infections, N. Engl. J. Med. 333 (1995) 770–775.

[30] L.M. Frenkel, et al., Clinical reactivation of herpes simplex virus type 2 infection in seropositive pregnant women with no history of genital herpes, Ann. Intern. Med. 118 (1993) 414–418.

[31] D.T. Fleming, et al., Herpes simplex virus type 2 in the United States, 1976 to 1994, N. Engl. J. Med. 337 (1997) 1105–1111.

[32] J.S. Smith, N.J. Robinson, Age-specific prevalence of infection with herpes simplex virus types 2 and 1: a global review, J. Infect. Dis. 186 (Suppl. 1) (2002) S3–S28.

[33] T.G. Buchman, B. Roizman, A.J. Nahmias, Demonstration of exogenous genital reinfection with herpes simplex virus type 2 by restriction endonuclease fingerprinting of viral DNA, J. Infect. Dis. 140 (1979) 295–304.

[34] O.W. Schmidt, K.H. Fife, L. Corey, Reinfection is an uncommon occurrence in patients with symptomatic recurrent genital herpes, J. Infect. Dis. 149 (1984) 645–646.

[35] A.D. Lakeman, A.J. Nahmias, R.J. Whitley, Analysis of DNA from recurrent genital herpes simplex virus isolates by restriction endonuclease digestion, Sex. Transm. Dis. 13 (1986) 61–66.

[36] F.D. Boucher, et al., A prospective evaluation of primary genital herpes simplex virus type 2 infections acquired during pregnancy, Pediatr. Infect. Dis. J. 9 (1990) 499–504.

[37] Z.A. Brown, et al., Genital herpes in pregnancy: risk factors associated with recurrences and asymptomatic viral shedding, Am. J. Obstet. Gynecol. 153 (1985) 24–30.

[38] C.G. Prober, et al., Use of routine viral cultures at delivery to identify neonates exposed to herpes simplex virus, N. Engl. J. Med. 318 (1988) 887–891.

[39] J.A. Kulhanjian, et al., Identification of women at unsuspected risk of primary infection with herpes simplex virus type 2 during pregnancy, N. Engl. J. Med. 326 (1992) 916–920.

[40] Z.A. Brown, et al., Effects on infants of a first episode of genital herpes during pregnancy, N. Engl. J. Med. 317 (1987) 1246–1251.

[41] Z.A. Brown, et al., Neonatal herpes simplex virus infection in relation to asymptomatic maternal infection at the time of labor, N. Engl. J. Med. 324 (1991) 1247–1252.

[42] T.H. Flewett, R.G. Parker, W.M. Philip, Acute hepatitis due to Herpes simplex virus in an adult, J. Clin. Pathol. 22 (1969) 60–66.

[43] E.J. Young, A.P. Killam, J.F. Greene Jr., Disseminated herpesvirus infection: association with primary genital herpes in pregnancy, JAMA 235 (1976) 2731–2733.

[44] P.A. Hensleigh, et al., Genital herpes during pregnancy: inability to distinguish primary and recurrent infections clinically, Obstet. Gynecol. 89 (1997) 891–895.

[45] A.J. Nahmias, et al., Perinatal risk associated with maternal genital herpes simplex virus infection, Am. J. Obstet. Gynecol. 110 (1971) 825–837.

[46] Z.A. Brown, et al., The acquisition of herpes simplex virus during pregnancy, N. Engl. J. Med. 337 (1997) 509–515.

[47] Y.M. Dietrich, P.G. Napolitano, Acyclovir treatment of primary herpes in pregnancy complicated by second trimester preterm premature rupture of membranes with term delivery: case report, Am. J. Perinatol. 19 (2002) 235–238.

[48] A.M. Arvin, et al., Failure of antepartum maternal cultures to predict the infant's risk of exposure to herpes simplex virus at delivery, N. Engl. J. Med. 315 (1986) 796–800.

[49] C.G. Prober, et al., Low risk of herpes simplex virus infections in neonates exposed to the virus at the time of vaginal delivery to mothers with recurrent genital herpes simplex virus infections, N. Engl. J. Med. 316 (1987) 240–244.

[50] R.J. Whitley, Changing presentation of herpes simplex virus infection in neonates, J. Infect. Dis. 158 (1988) 109–116.

[51] L. Corey, et al., Genital herpes simplex virus infections: clinical manifestations, course, and complications, Ann. Intern. Med. 98 (1983) 958–972.

[52] C. Johnston, et al., Herpes simplex virus viremia during primary genital infection, J. Infect. Dis. 198 (2008) 31–34.

[53] A.S. Yeager, et al., Relationship of antibody to outcome in neonatal herpes simplex virus infections, Infect. Immun. 29 (1980) 532–538.

[54] W.M. Sullender, et al., Humoral and cell-mediated immunity in neonates with herpes simplex virus infection, J. Infect. Dis. 155 (1987) 28–37.

[55] ACOG Practice Bulletin, Clinical management guidelines for obstetrician-gynecologists. No. 82 June 2007. Management of herpes in pregnancy, Obstet. Gynecol. 109 (2007) 1489–1498.

[56] Z.A. Brown, et al., Effect of serologic status and cesarean delivery on transmission rates of herpes simplex virus from mother to infant, JAMA 289 (2003) 203–209.

[57] K.M. Stone, et al., National surveillance for neonatal herpes simplex virus infections, Sex. Transm. Dis. 16 (1989) 152–156.

[58] E.M. Kaye, E.C. Dooling, Neonatal herpes simplex meningoencephalitis associated with fetal monitor scalp electrodes, Neurology 31 (1981) 1045–1047.

[59] L.S. Parvey, L.T. Ch'ien, Neonatal herpes simplex virus infection introduced by fetal-monitor scalp electrodes, Pediatrics 65 (1980) 1150–1153.

[60] J. Sullivan-Bolyai, et al., Neonatal herpes simplex virus infection in King County, Washington: increasing incidence and epidemiologic correlates, JAMA 250 (1983) 3059–3062.

[61] K.M. Gutierrez, et al., The epidemiology of neonatal herpes simplex virus infections in California from 1985 to 1995, J. Infect. Dis. 180 (1999) 199–202.

[62] S.R. Morris, et al., Neonatal herpes morbidity and mortality in California, 1995–2003, Sex. Transm. Dis. 35 (2008) 14–18.

[63] F. Xu, et al., Incidence of neonatal herpes simplex virus infections in two managed care organizations: implications for surveillance, Sex. Transm. Dis. 35 (2008) 592–598.

[64] M.A. Gaytant, et al., [Incidence of herpes neonatorum in Netherlands], Ned. Tijdschr. Geneeskd. 144 (2000) 1832–1836.

[65] A.C. Caviness, et al., The prevalence of neonatal herpes simplex virus infection compared with serious bacterial illness in hospitalized neonates, J. Pediatr. 153 (2008) 164–169.

[66] S. Baldwin, R.J. Whitley, Intrauterine herpes simplex virus infection, Teratology 39 (1989) 1–10.

[67] A.L. Florman, et al., Intrauterine infection with herpes simplex virus: resultant congenital malformations, JAMA 225 (1973) 129–132.

[68] C. Hutto, et al., Intrauterine herpes simplex virus infections, J. Pediatr. 110 (1987) 97–101.

[69] M.A. South, et al., Congenital malformation of the central nervous system associated with genital type (type 2) herpesvirus, J. Pediatr. 75 (1969) 13–18.

[70] J. Kahlon, R.J. Whitley, Antibody response of the newborn after herpes simplex virus infection, J. Infect. Dis. 158 (1988) 925–933.

[71] A.G. Garcia, Maternal herpes-simplex infection causing abortion: histopathologic study of the placenta, Hospital (Rio J) 78 (1970) 1267–1274.

[72] A.M. Arvin, Fetal and neonatal infections, in: N. Nathanson, F. Murphy (Eds.), Viral Pathogenesis, Lippincott-Raven, New York, 1996.

[73] A. Alanen, V. Hukkanen, Herpes simplex virus DNA in amniotic fluid without neonatal infection, Clin. Infect. Dis. 30 (2000) 363–367.

[74] D.W. Kimberlin, et al., Natural history of neonatal herpes simplex virus infections in the acyclovir era, Pediatrics 108 (2001) 223–229.

[75] J. Douglas, O. Schmidt, L. Corey, Acquisition of neonatal HSV-1 infection from a paternal source contact, J. Pediatr. 103 (1983) 908–910.

[76] O. Hammerberg, et al., An outbreak of herpes simplex virus type 1 in an intensive care nursery, Pediatr. Infect. Dis. 2 (1983) 290–294.

[77] I.J. Light, Postnatal acquisition of herpes simplex virus by the newborn infant: a review of the literature, Pediatrics 63 (1979) 480–482.

[78] C.C. Linnemann Jr., et al., Transmission of herpes-simplex virus type 1 in a nursery for the newborn: identification of viral isolates by D.N.A. "fingerprinting" Lancet 1 (1978) 964–966.

[79] A.S. Yeager, R.L. Ashley, L. Corey, Transmission of herpes simplex virus from father to neonate, J. Pediatr. 103 (1983) 905–907.

[80] J.Z. Sullivan-Bolyai, et al., Disseminated neonatal herpes simplex virus type 1 from a maternal breast lesion, Pediatrics 71 (1983) 455–457.

[81] L.I. Hatherley, K. Hayes, I. Jack, Herpes virus in an obstetric hospital. II. Asymptomatic virus excretion in staff members, Med. J. Aust. 2 (1980) 273–275.

[82] L.I. Hatherley, K. Hayes, I. Jack, Herpes virus in an obstetric hospital. III. Prevalence of antibodies in patients and staff, Med. J. Aust. 2 (1980) 325–329.

[83] S.K. Burchett, et al., Diminished interferon-gamma and lymphocyte proliferation in neonatal and postpartum primary herpes simplex virus infection, J. Infect. Dis. 165 (1992) 813–818.

[84] B.A. Chilmonczyk, et al., Characterization of the human newborn response to herpesvirus antigen, J. Immunol. 134 (1985) 4184–4188.

[85] S. Kohl, M.W. Harmon, Human neonatal leukocyte interferon production and natural killer cytotoxicity in response to herpes simplex virus, J. Interferon. Res. 3 (1983) 461–463.

[86] S. Kohl, et al., Neonatal antibody-dependent cellular cytotoxic antibody levels are associated with the clinical presentation of neonatal herpes simplex virus infection, J. Infect. Dis. 160 (1989) 770–776.

[87] R.F. Pass, et al., Specific lymphocyte blastogenic responses in children with cytomegalovirus and herpes simplex virus infections acquired early in infancy, Infect. Immun. 34 (1981) 166–170.

[88] S. Kohl, Neonatal herpes simplex virus infection, Clin. Perinatol. 24 (1997) 129–150.

[89] L. Mintz, et al., Age-dependent resistance of human alveolar macrophages to herpes simplex virus, Infect. Immun. 28 (1980) 417–420.

[90] M.S. Hirsch, B. Zisman, A.C. Allison, Macrophages and age-dependent resistance to Herpes simplex virus in mice, J. Immunol. 104 (1970) 1160–1165.

[91] C. Diamond, et al., Viremia in neonatal herpes simplex virus infections, Pediatr. Infect. Dis. J. 18 (1999) 487–489.

[92] J. Kawada, et al., Evaluation of systemic inflammatory responses in neonates with herpes simplex virus infection, J. Infect. Dis. 190 (2004) 494–498.

[93] D.B. Singer, Pathology of neonatal Herpes simplex virus infection, Perspect. Pediatr. Pathol. 6 (1981) 243–278.

[94] R. Whitley, et al., Predictors of morbidity and mortality in neonates with herpes simplex virus infections. The National Institute of Allergy and Infectious Diseases Collaborative Antiviral Study Group, N. Engl. J. Med. 324 (1991) 450–454.

[95] A. Nahmias, Infection of the newborn with herpesvirus hominis, Adv. Pediatr. 17 (1970) 185–226.

[96] R.J. Whitley, D.W. Kimberlin, Infections in perinatology: antiviral therapy of neonatal herpes simplex virus infections, Clin. Perinatol. 24 (1997) 267–283.

[97] M.S. Anderson, M.J. Abzug, Hydrops fetalis: an unusual presentation of intrauterine herpes simplex virus infection, Pediatr. Infect. Dis. J. 18 (1999) 837–839.

[98] G. Malm, U. Berg, M. Forsgren, Neonatal herpes simplex: clinical findings and outcome in relation to type of maternal infection, Acta Paediatr. 84 (1995) 256–260.

[99] A.M. Arvin, et al., Neonatal herpes simplex infection in the absence of mucocutaneous lesions, J. Pediatr. 100 (1982) 715–721.

[100] D.S. Greenes, et al., Neonatal herpes simplex virus infection presenting as fulminant liver failure, Pediatr. Infect. Dis. J. 14 (1995) 242–244.

[101] W.S. Lee, et al., Neonatal liver transplantation for fulminant hepatitis caused by herpes simplex virus type 2, J. Pediatr. Gastroenterol. Nutr. 35 (2002) 220–223.

[102] A. Ford, et al., A 10-day-old neonate with fulminant hepatitis, J. Paediatr. Child Health 44 (2008) 471–472.

[103] S.E. Golden, Neonatal herpes simplex viremia, Pediatr. Infect. Dis. J. 7 (1988) 425–427.

[104] P. Gressens, J.R. Martin, HSV-2 DNA persistence in astrocytes of the trigeminal root entry zone: double labeling by in situ PCR and immunohistochemistry, J. Neuropathol. Exp. Neurol. 53 (1994) 127–135.

[105] C. Langlet, et al., An uncommon case of disseminated neonatal herpes simplex infection presenting with pneumonia and pleural effusions, Eur. J. Pediatr. 162 (2003) 532–533.

[106] D.P. O'Riordan, W.C. Golden, S.W. Aucott, Herpes simplex virus infections in preterm infants, Pediatrics 118 (2006) e1612–e1620.

[107] L. Corey, et al., Difference between herpes simplex virus type 1 and type 2 neonatal encephalitis in neurological outcome, Lancet 1 (1988) 1–4.

[108] D.W. Kimberlin, Herpes simplex virus infections of the central nervous system, Semin. Pediatr. Infect. Dis. 14 (2003) 83–89.

[109] E.M. Mizrahi, B.R. Tharp, A characteristic EEG pattern in neonatal herpes simplex encephalitis, Neurology 32 (1982) 1215–1220.

[110] M.A. O'Reilly, P.M. O'Reilly, R. de Bruyn, Neonatal herpes simplex type 2 encephalitis: its appearances on ultrasound and CT, Pediatr. Radiol. 25 (1995) 68–69.

[111] C. Toth, S. Harder, J. Yager, Neonatal herpes encephalitis: a case series and review of clinical presentation, Can. J. Neurol. Sci. 30 (2003) 36–40.

[112] G. Pelligra, et al., Brainstem involvement in neonatal herpes simplex virus type 2 encephalitis, Pediatrics 120 (2007) e442–e446.

[113] H. Kimura, et al., Quantitation of viral load in neonatal herpes simplex virus infection and comparison between type 1 and type 2, J. Med. Virol. 67 (2002) 349–353.

[114] L.T. Gutman, C.M. Wilfert, S. Eppes, Herpes simplex virus encephalitis in children: analysis of cerebrospinal fluid and progressive neurodevelopmental deterioration, J. Infect. Dis. 154 (1986) 415–421.

[115] R. Whitley, et al., A controlled trial comparing vidarabine with acyclovir in neonatal herpes simplex virus infection. Infectious Diseases Collaborative Antiviral Study Group, N. Engl. J. Med. 324 (1991) 444–449.

[116] S.I. Music, E.M. Fine, Y. Togo, Zoster-like disease in the newborn due to herpes-simplex virus, N. Engl. J. Med. 284 (1971) 24–26.

[117] A.J. Nahmias, W.S. Hagler, Ocular manifestation of herpes simplex in the newborn (neonatal ocular herpes), Int. Ophthalmol. Clin. 12 (1972) 191–213.

[118] J.D. Cherry, F. Soriano, C.L. Jahn, Search for perinatal viral infection: A prospective, clinical, virologic, and serologic study, Am. J. Dis. Child. 116 (1968) 245–250.

[119] R.J. Whitley, F. Lakeman, Herpes simplex virus infections of the central nervous system: therapeutic and diagnostic considerations, Clin. Infect. Dis. 20 (1995) 414–420.

[120] D.W. Kimberlin, et al., Application of the polymerase chain reaction to the diagnosis and management of neonatal herpes simplex virus disease. National Institute of Allergy and Infectious Diseases Collaborative Antiviral Study Group, J. Infect. Dis. 174 (1996) 1162–1167.

[121] H. Kimura, et al., Detection of viral DNA in neonatal herpes simplex virus infections: frequent and prolonged presence in serum and cerebrospinal fluid, J. Infect. Dis. 164 (1991) 289–293.

[122] J. Troendle-Atkins, G.J. Demmler, G.J. Buffone, Rapid diagnosis of herpes simplex virus encephalitis by using the polymerase chain reaction, J. Pediatr. 123 (1993) 376–380.

[123] G. Malm, M. Forsgren, Neonatal herpes simplex virus infections: HSV DNA in cerebrospinal fluid and serum, Arch. Dis. Child. Fetal. Neonatal. Ed. 81 (1999) F24–F29.

[124] A.A. Weil, et al., Patients with suspected herpes simplex encephalitis: rethinking an initial negative polymerase chain reaction result, Clin. Infect. Dis. 34 (2002) 1154–1157.

[125] D.W. Kimberlin, Neonatal herpes simplex infection, Clin. Microbiol. Rev. 17 (2004) 1–13.

[126] T.W. Smalling, et al., Molecular approaches to detecting herpes simplex virus and enteroviruses in the central nervous system, J. Clin. Microbiol. 40 (2002) 2317–2322.

[127] G.B. Elion, et al., Selectivity of action of an antiherpetic agent, 9-(2-hydroxyethoxymethyl) guanine, Proc. Natl. Acad. Sci. U. S. A. 74 (1977) 5716–5720.

[128] R.J. Whitley, et al., Vidarabine therapy of neonatal herpes simplex virus infection, Pediatrics 66 (1980) 495–501.

[129] Y.J. Bryson, et al., Treatment of first episodes of genital herpes simplex virus infection with oral acyclovir: a randomized double-blind controlled trial in normal subjects, N. Engl. J. Med. 308 (1983) 916–921.

[130] L. Corey, et al., Treatment of primary first-episode genital herpes simplex virus infections with acyclovir: results of topical, intravenous and oral therapy, J. Antimicrob. Chemother. 12 (Suppl. B) (1983) 79–88.

[131] R. Saral, et al., Acyclovir prophylaxis of herpes-simplex-virus infections, N. Engl. J. Med. 305 (1981) 63–67.

[132] R.J. Whitley, et al., Vidarabine versus acyclovir therapy in herpes simplex encephalitis, N. Engl. J. Med. 314 (1986) 144–149.

[133] M. Hintz, et al., Neonatal acyclovir pharmacokinetics in patients with herpes virus infections, Am. J. Med. 73 (1A) (1982) 210–214.

[134] A.S. Yeager, Use of acyclovir in premature and term neonates, Am. J. Med. 73 (1A) (1982) 205–209.

[135] D.W. Kimberlin, et al., Safety and efficacy of high-dose intravenous acyclovir in the management of neonatal herpes simplex virus infections, Pediatrics 108 (2001) 230–238.

[136] American Academy of Pediatrics, Herpes simplex, in: L.K. Pickering, C.J. Baker, D.W. Kimberlin, S.S. Long (Eds.), Red Book 2009 Report of the Committee on Infectious Diseases, 28th ed, American Academy of Pediatrics, Elk Grove Village, IL, 2009, pp. 363–373.

[137] S.S. Long, In defense of empiric acyclovir therapy in certain neonates, J. Pediatr. 153 (2008) 157–158.

[138] D.W. Kimberlin, When should you initiate acyclovir therapy in a neonate? J. Pediatr. 153 (2008) 155–156.

[139] A.C. Nyquist, et al., Acyclovir-resistant neonatal herpes simplex virus infection of the larynx, J. Pediatr. 124 (1994) 967–971.

[140] R.J. Oram, et al., Characterization of an acyclovir-resistant herpes simplex virus type 2 strain isolated from a premature neonate, J. Infect. Dis. 181 (2000) 1458–1461.

[141] M.J. Levin, et al., Development of acyclovir-resistant herpes simplex virus early during the treatment of herpes neonatorum, Pediatr. Infect. Dis. J. 20 (2001) 1094–1097.

[142] G.P. Rabalais, et al., Antiviral susceptibilities of herpes simplex virus isolates from infants with recurrent mucocutaneous lesions after neonatal infection, Pediatr. Infect. Dis. J. 8 (1989) 221–223.

[143] D. Kimberlin, et al., Administration of oral acyclovir suppressive therapy after neonatal herpes simplex virus disease limited to the skin, eyes and mouth: results of a phase I/II trial, Pediatr. Infect. Dis. J. 15 (1996) 247–252.

[144] K.F. Tiffany, et al., Improved neurodevelopmental outcomes following long-term high-dose oral acyclovir therapy in infants with central nervous system and disseminated herpes simplex disease, J. Perinatol. 25 (2005) 156–161.

[145] M. Fonseca-Aten, et al., Herpes simplex virus encephalitis during suppressive therapy with acyclovir in a premature infant, Pediatrics 115 (2005) 804–809.

[146] S. Kohl, et al., Effect of intravenously administered immune globulin on functional antibody to herpes simplex virus in low birth weight neonates, J. Pediatr. 115 (1989) 135–139.

[147] R.J. Whitley, Neonatal herpes simplex virus infections. Is there a role for immunoglobulin in disease prevention and therapy, Pediatr. Infect. Dis. J. 13 (1994) 432–438 discussion 438–439.

[148] R.W. Cone, et al., Frequent detection of genital herpes simplex virus DNA by polymerase chain reaction among pregnant women, JAMA 272 (1994) 792–796.

[149] D.A. Hardy, et al., Use of polymerase chain reaction for successful identification of asymptomatic genital infection with herpes simplex virus in pregnant women at delivery, J. Infect. Dis. 162 (1990) 1031–1035.

[150] D.H. Watts, et al., A double-blind, randomized, placebo-controlled trial of acyclovir in late pregnancy for the reduction of herpes simplex virus shedding and cesarean delivery, Am. J. Obstet. Gynecol. 188 (2003) 836–843.

[151] W.W. Andrews, et al., Valacyclovir therapy to reduce recurrent genital herpes in pregnant women, Am. J. Obstet. Gynecol. 194 (2006) 774–781.

[152] C.G. Prober, Management of the neonate whose mother received suppressive acyclovir therapy during late pregnancy, Pediatr. Infect. Dis. J. 20 (2001) 90–91.

[153] A.T. Tita, W.A. Grobman, D.J. Rouse, Antenatal herpes serologic screening: an appraisal of the evidence, Obstet. Gynecol. 108 (2006) 1247–1253.

HUMAN PARVOVIRUS

Stuart P. Adler ☉ William C. Koch

CHAPTER OUTLINE

Microbiology   835
General Aspects of Pathogenesis   836
Epidemiology and Transmission   837
    Overview   837
    Global Distribution   837
    Seasonality and Periodicity   837
    Seroprevalence by Age   838
    Seroprevalence by Gender   838
    Seroprevalence by Race   838
    Incidence   838
    Risk Factors for Acquisition   838
    Hospital Transmission   839
    Routes of Viral Spread   840
    Risk of Parvovirus B19 Acquisition for Women
      of Childbearing Age   840
Clinical Manifestations (Other than Intrauterine Infection)   841
    Erythema Infectiosum   841
    Transient Aplastic Crisis   841
    Arthropathy   842
    Infection in Immunocompromised Hosts   842
    Other Dermatologic Syndromes   843
    Central Nervous System Infection and Neurologic Disorders   843
    Renal Disease   844
    Myocardial Disease   844
General Aspects of Diagnosis   844
    Laboratory Diagnostic Methods   844
Epidemiology of Parvovirus B19 Infections and Risk of Acquisition
in Pregnant Women   845
    Prevalence and Incidence in the United States   845
    Prevalence and Incidence in Other Countries   845
Clinical Manifestations of Parvovirus B19 Infections in Pregnant
Women   846

Intrauterine Transmission Rates, Clinical Manifestations,
and Fetal Outcomes   847
    Overview   847
    Fetal Death   847
    Asymptomatic Fetal Infection   849
    Birth Defects   849
    Other Fetal Manifestations   849
    Fetal Hydrops   849
    Fetal Outcome in Relation to Maternal Manifestations   850
    Long-Term Outcomes   850
Pathogenesis of Infection in the Fetus   850
    Fetal Immune Responses to Parvovirus B19   850
    Pathogenesis of Parvovirus B19 Hydrops   850
Pathology in the Fetus   850
    Anatomic and Histologic Features   850
    Placenta   851
    Heart   851
    Other Organs   852
Diagnostic Evaluation and Management of the Woman and Fetus
Exposed to or Infected by Parvovirus B19 during Pregnancy   852
    Overview   852
    Prevalence of Erythema Infectiosum   852
    History of Exposure   852
    Clinical Features Suggesting Signs and Symptoms of Parvovirus
      B19 Infection in the Pregnant Woman   852
    Laboratory Diagnosis in the Pregnant Woman   852
    Fetal Monitoring   853
    Fetal Therapy   854
Differential Diagnosis   854
Prognosis   854
Prevention   855
    General Measures   855
    Vaccine Development   855

The parvoviruses are a family of single-stranded DNA viruses that have a wide cellular tropism and broad host range, causing infection in invertebrate species and vertebrates, from insects to mammals. Although many parvoviruses are important veterinary pathogens, there are only two human pathogens in the family: human parvovirus B19 and the more recently described human bocavirus [1,2]. Human bocavirus seems to be primarily a respiratory pathogen of young children and is not discussed further here. Human parvovirus B19 is most commonly referred to as parvovirus B19 or simply B19. A new genus and name have been proposed for this virus, *Erythrovirus* B19 [3], based on its cellular tropism for erythroid lineage cells and to distinguish it from the other mammalian parvoviruses. Compared with most other common human

viruses, B19 is a relatively new pathogen, but since its initial description B19 has come to be associated with a variety of seemingly diverse clinical syndromes in many different patient populations (Table 27–1). Although the list of clinical manifestations caused by B19 infection is probably not yet complete, some proposed relationships, such as to rheumatologic disease and neurologic disorders, remain controversial [4,5].

Parvovirus B19 was accidentally discovered by Cossart and associates [6] in 1975 as an anomalous band of precipitation while screening blood donor serum for hepatitis B antigen by counterimmunoelectrophoresis. The name *B19* refers to the donor unit from which it was originally isolated. Initial analysis of the new virus revealed it had physical features characteristic of the known parvoviruses [7],

TABLE 27–1 Clinical Manifestations Associated with Parvovirus B19 Infection

Diseases	Primary Patient Groups
Diseases Associated with Acute Infection	
Erythema infectiosum (fifth disease)	Normal children
Polyarthropathy	Normal adolescents and adults
Transient aplastic crisis	Patients with hemolytic anemia or accelerated erythropoiesis or both
Papular-purpuric "gloves and socks" syndrome	Normal adolescents and adults
Diseases Associated with Chronic Infection	
Persistent anemia (red blood cell aplasia)	Immunodeficient or immunocompromised children and adults
Nonimmune fetal hydrops	Intrauterine infection
Congenital anemia	Intrauterine infection
Chronic arthropathy	Rare patients with parvovirus B19–induced joint disease
Infection-associated hemophagocytosis	Normal or immunocompromised patients
Vasculitis or purpura	Normal adults and children
Myocarditis	Intrauterine infection, normal infants and children, immunocompromised patients

Adapted from Young NS, Brown KE. Parvovirus B19. N Engl J Med 350:586–597, 2004.

allowing classification in this family. Because the donors from whom it was originally isolated were asymptomatic, B19 infection was not initially associated with any illness, and for the next several years after its description it was a virus in search of a disease.

In 1981, Pattison and colleagues [8] noted a high prevalence of antibodies to this virus in the serum of children hospitalized with transient aplastic crisis of sickle cell disease and proposed B19 as the viral cause of this clinically well-described event. Serjeant and colleagues [9] later confirmed this association in population studies of sickle cell patients in Jamaica. In 1983, 8 years after its initial description, Anderson and coworkers [10] proposed B19 as the cause of the common childhood exanthem erythema infectiosum (EI), or fifth disease. The name *fifth disease* derives from the 19th century practice of numbering the common exanthems of childhood—EI was the fifth rash designated in this scheme, and it is the only one for which this numeric designation has persisted in clinical practice [11]. The others in the series included measles, scarlet fever, rubella, and Filatov-Dukes disease (a mild variant of scarlet fever that is no longer recognized).

The possibility of fetal disease associated with EI was considered long before the viral etiology was known primarily because of comparison with rubella and the incidence of congenital rubella syndrome after community epidemics [12–14]. Advances in knowledge of the virology of other animal parvoviruses and their known propensity to cause disease in the fetus and newborn animal further

fueled this concern [15]. This suspicion was confirmed in 1984 when two reports of B19 infection in pregnant women associated with adverse fetal outcomes appeared [16,17] and were later followed by a larger report of a series of cases of nonimmune hydrops fetalis caused by intrauterine infections with B19 [18]. Over the ensuing decade, various clinical manifestations associated with acute and chronic infection have since been attributed to this virus in different patient groups (see Table 27–1).

Since the initial reports of fetal infection, knowledge of the epidemiology, pathophysiology, and short-term outcome of fetal and neonatal infection with B19 has increased immensely based on numerous large population-based studies [19–23]. B19 infection during pregnancy has probably been the subject of more such studies than any of the other manifestations with the possible exception of transient aplastic crisis of sickle cell disease. There is still much to be learned, however, regarding the long-term outcome of fetal infection, unusual clinical manifestations of infection in neonates, and the immunologic response to infection. Lastly, the potential for prevention through vaccine development is a topic of current interest and ongoing research.

MICROBIOLOGY

Similar to other members of the family Parvoviridae, parvovirus B19 is a small, nonenveloped, single-stranded DNA virus. The taxonomy for this family has been revised to include two subfamilies, the Densovirinae, which are insect viruses, and the Parvovirinae, which infect vertebrates [24,25]. The Parvovirinae subfamily is composed of three genera: *Dependovirus*, *Parvovirus*, and *Erythrovirus*. Viruses of the *Dependovirus* genus require coinfection with another unrelated helper virus (adenovirus or herpesvirus) to complete their life cycle. Some *Dependovirus* strains infect humans (e.g., adeno-associated viruses), but the infection is asymptomatic and without consequence. In contrast to *Dependovirus* strains, members of the genera *Parvovirus* and *Erythrovirus* are able to replicate autonomously. Previously included in the genus *Parvovirus*, B19 is now classified as an *Erythrovirus*. At present, the genus *Erythrovirus* consists of only two members: B19 and a simian parvovirus that has a similar genomic organization as B19 and has a similar tropism for erythroid cells [26]. Although many parvoviruses are pathogenic to other mammals (e.g., canine parvovirus, feline panleukopenia virus), B19 and human bocavirus are the only parvoviruses proven to cause disease in humans.

There is only one recognized serotype of B19. Minor variations in the nucleotide sequence occur among different B19 viral isolates from different geographic areas, but these have not been definitely shown to affect clinical patterns of infection or pathogenicity [27–29]. Two isolates of human parvovirus whose nucleotide sequence differs significantly (>10%) from B19 have been described, V9 and V6 [30,31]. Both were isolated from patients with transient red blood cell aplasia indistinguishable clinically from typical B19-induced aplastic crisis. The clinical significance of these variants and whether they represent different genotypes or merely geographic variants of B19 remain topics of debate [29,32].

The B19 genome is very small (approximately 5.6 kb) and contained within an icosahedral protein capsid. The capsid structure and lack of an envelope make the virus very resistant to heat and detergent inactivation, features that seem to be important in transmission. The genome seems to encode only three proteins. Two are capsid proteins, designated VP1 and VP2. VP2 is smaller but more abundant and makes up approximately 96% of the capsid protein. VP1 is larger and makes up about 4% of the capsid, but contains a unique region that extends out from the capsid surface and serves as the attachment site for the cellular receptor [4]. VP2 has the unique ability to self-assemble into capsids that are morphologically and antigenically similar to B19 viruses when expressed in cell culture systems in vitro [33,34]. When present with VP1, the capsids incorporate proteins, but VP1 alone does not self-assemble [33].

The third gene product is a nonstructural protein designated NS1. The function of this protein is unclear, but it has been shown to be involved in regulation of the viral promoter and seems to have a role in DNA replication [25]. Studies of NS1 have been hampered by the observation that it seems to be toxic to cells by an unknown mechanism [35]. More recent studies have further suggested that production of NS1 can lead to programmed cell death (apoptosis) mediated by stimulation of cytokine production [36,37].

Because of its limited genomic complement, B19 requires a mitotically active host cell for replication. It can replicate only in certain erythroid lineage cells stimulated by erythropoietin, such as erythroid precursors found in bone marrow, fetal liver, umbilical cord blood, and a few erythroleukemic cell lines [25,38–42]. B19 cannot be propagated in standard cell cultures [43], a fact that had previously limited the availability of viral products for development of diagnostic assays. Much of this limitation has been overcome by the development of molecular methods for the detection of viral nucleic acid, but reliable commercial serologic assays are still limited.

The cellular receptor for the virus has been identified as globoside, a neutral glycosphingolipid that is present on erythrocytes where it represents the P blood group antigen [44]. The presence of this lipid is necessary for viral infection to occur, and individuals who lack this antigen (p phenotype) are naturally immune to B19 infection [45]. The P antigen is also present on other cells, such as endothelial cells, fetal myocardial cells, placenta, and megakaryocytes [44]. The tissue distribution of this receptor may explain some of the clinical manifestations of infection with this virus (see "Clinical Manifestations Other than Intrauterine Infection").

Although the P antigen is necessary for B19 viral infection, it is insufficient because some cells, particularly nonerythroid tissues, that express the receptor are incapable of viral infection [46]. More recently, a coreceptor has been described on human cells that are permissive for B19 infection [47]. The hypothesis is that the globoside is necessary for viral attachment, but the coreceptor somehow allows for viral entry into the cell where viral replication can occur. If confirmed, this hypothesis may provide an

alternative explanation of the pathogenesis of infection in nonerythroid tissues that express globoside without the coreceptor.

GENERAL ASPECTS OF PATHOGENESIS

Parvovirus B19 requires a mitotically active host cell to complete its full replicative life cycle. The primary target for B19 infection seems to be erythroid progenitor cells that are near the pronormoblast stage of development. The virus can be propagated only in human erythroid progenitor cells from bone marrow, umbilical cord blood, fetal liver, peripheral blood, and a few erythroid leukemic cell lines [48]. B19 lytically infects these cells with progressive loss of targeted cells as infection proceeds. In vitro hematopoietic assays show that B19 suppresses formation of erythroid colony-forming units, and this effect can be reversed by addition of serum containing anti-B19 IgG antibodies [49].

The virus has little to no effect on the myeloid cell line in vitro, but causes inhibition of megakaryocytopoiesis in vitro without viral replication or cell lysis [50]. Clinically, this is best illustrated in transient aplastic crisis of sickle cell disease. Patients have fever, weakness, and pallor on presentation, with a sudden and severe decrease in their reticulocyte count. This cessation of red blood cell production coupled with the shortened red blood cell survival because of chronic hemolysis produces a profound anemia. Examination of the bone marrow typically reveals hypoplasia of the erythroid cell line and a maturational arrest; giant pronormoblasts are often seen with intranuclear viral inclusions [49]. With development of specific antibodies, viral infection is controlled, and reticulocyte counts begin to increase.

Evaluation of infection in normal volunteers has shown similar hematologic changes, but because of the longer life of red blood cells, these changes are clinically insignificant [51]. Adult volunteers inoculated intranasally with B19 developed viremia after 5 to 6 days with a mild illness. Their reticulocyte counts decreased to undetectable levels, and this was accompanied by a modest decline in hemoglobin and hematocrit. Platelets and granulocyte counts also declined. Specific antibody production with IgM followed by IgG developed, and viremia was cleared rapidly. A second phase of illness developed at 17 to 18 days with rash and arthralgias but without fever, and hematologic indices had returned to normal.

The tissue distribution of the cellular receptor for the virus (P antigen) may explain the predominance of hematologic findings associated with B19 infection. Its presence on other tissues may help to explain other clinical manifestations, such as myocardial disease, congenital infection, and vasculitis syndromes. Although the cellular receptor is present and the virus can attach, in contrast to the erythroid cell, these cells are nonpermissive for viral replication; that is, the virus is unable to undergo a complete life cycle with the resultant lysis of the host cells, as described previously. Instead, interaction in these tissues leads to accumulation of the nonstructural protein NS1. This protein is essential for viral replication and has various proposed functions [25], but it seems to be toxic to most mammalian cell lines when present in excess [35]. NS1 has been associated with apoptosis and programmed cell death [37,42]. NS1 has also been linked to production of tumor necrosis factor-α and interleukin-6, a potent proinflammatory cytokine [36,42,52]. Cellular injury may occur through cytokine pathways and provide another mechanism aside from lytic infection for some of the clinical manifestations.

Chronic infections in immunocompromised patients develop when patients are unable to mount an adequate neutralizing antibody response. These infections are characterized by viral persistence in serum or bone marrow and lack of detectable circulating antibody. Clinical manifestations include chronic anemia or red blood cell aplasia and may include granulocytopenia and thrombocytopenia. The mechanism for leukopenia and thrombocytopenia is unknown, although it has been shown that B19 causes disturbances in megakaryocytic replication when infected in vitro [50].

EPIDEMIOLOGY AND TRANSMISSION
OVERVIEW

Parvovirus B19 is a highly contagious and common infection worldwide. In the United States, 60% or more of white adults are seropositive (have IgG antibodies to B19 in their sera). This seropositivity indicates a previous infection usually acquired in childhood. Among African Americans, the rate of seropositivity is about 30% [21]. Transmission of B19 from person to person is probably by droplets from oral or nasal secretions. This mode of transmission is suggested by the rapid transmission among individuals in close physical contact, such as schoolmates or family members, and from a study of healthy volunteers experimentally infected with B19, in whom virus was found in blood and nasopharyngeal secretions for several days beginning 1 or 2 days before symptoms appeared [51]. In the volunteer study, no virus was detected in urine or stool.

Given the highly contagious nature of B19 infections, it is not surprising that most outbreaks occur in elementary schools and occasionally child care centers. Susceptible seronegative adult school personnel are at high risk for acquiring the infection from students [21,53]. Some outbreaks in schools may be seasonal, often late winter and spring, and epidemic, with many children and staff acquiring the infection and developing symptoms of EI. At other times, the infection is endemic, with transmission occurring slowly and with only a few manifesting symptoms.

GLOBAL DISTRIBUTION

Parvovirus B19 infections occur worldwide. Serologic evidence of B19 infection has been found everywhere studied, including developed countries, undeveloped countries, urban and rural areas, and isolated island populations [54–59]. The diseases and associated signs and symptoms are the same worldwide. No clinically or epidemiologically important strain or antigenic differences have been detected, and serologic assays are independent of the source or location of patient serum. Disease resulting from B19 seems to be unrelated to specific viral genotypes, although analysis of the antigenic variation or nucleotide sequences of widely dispersed B19 isolates shows some heterogeneity of unknown significance [27,28,60–65].

SEASONALITY AND PERIODICITY

Transmission of parvovirus B19 continues throughout the year; however, there are seasonal variations in transmission rates. Outbreaks of EI most often occur in winter and spring in temperate climates and less frequently in fall and summer [66–68]. In schools or day care centers, outbreaks of EI may persist for months, usually starting in late winter or early spring and ending with summer vacation. Figure 27–1 highlights multiyear outbreaks of B19 exposure among pregnant women and the associated seasonal variation in Pittsburgh, Pennsylvania. Yearly, most cases occurred in late spring and summer.

In the island nation of Jamaica, careful studies of people with sickle cell disease showed that epidemics of transient aplastic crises occurred about every 5 years with little disease inside this interval [69]. Epidemics of B19 infections at 5-year intervals were also observed in

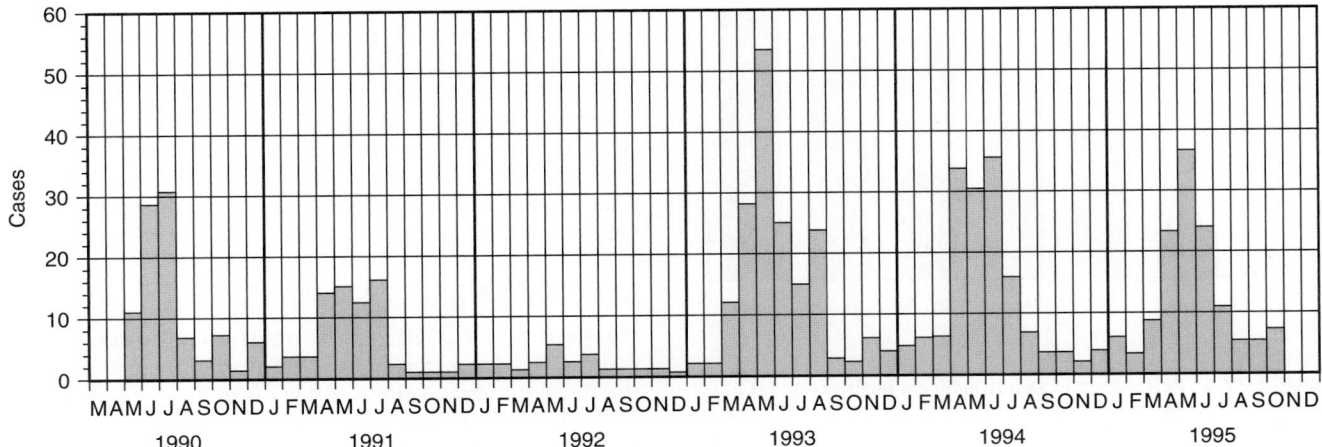

FIGURE 27–1 Seasonal variation in reported parvovirus B19 exposures in pregnant women. Each month is indicated by its first letter. (*Data from Harger J, Koch W, Harger GF. Prospective evaluation of 618 pregnant women exposed to parvovirus B19: risks and symptoms. Obstet Gynecol 91:413, 1998.*)

Rio de Janeiro, Brazil [70]. In Japan, age-related serologic evaluation of stored serum samples showed no evidence for B19 epidemics over a 10-year period [71]. The prevalence of IgG antibodies to B19 among three tribes of Amerindians living in remote regions of Brazil was very low (<11%), and in one tribe was zero for people younger than 30 years [57]. School nursing records in Iowa over 14 years identified cases of EI in all but one year [72].

SEROPREVALENCE BY AGE

In numerous studies of parvovirus B19 infection based on serologic testing, the seroprevalence of B19 infection increases with age [6,69,73–78]. Figure 27–2 shows the age-dependent increase in seroprevalence from Richmond, Virginia [79]. Transplacentally acquired maternal antibodies are undetectable by 1 year of age. In children younger than 5 years, the prevalence of IgG antibodies to B19 is usually less than 5%. The greatest increase in seroprevalence and B19 infection occurs between 5 and 20 years of age. By age 20 years, the seroprevalence of B19 infection increases from about 5% at 5 years of age to nearly 40%. Afterward, without regard to risk factors, B19 seroprevalence increases slowly. In adult blood donors, the seroprevalence of IgG antibodies to B19 ranges from 29% to 79% (median 45%) [76–82]. By age 50, the seroprevalence may be greater than 75%. Similar results on age-related seroprevalence of B19 infections were observed in India [80–86].

SEROPREVALENCE BY GENDER

In most studies, the prevalence of antibodies to parvovirus B19 in sera obtained from men and women is similar [59,74]. At least six studies have reported that women have a higher rate of B19 infection than men, however.*

*References [21,59,79,81,87,88].

study of adult blood donors, the proportion of women who were seropositive, 47.5%, was 1.5 times higher than in men. The prevalence of IgG antibodies averaged 51% for women of all ages compared with 38% for men in one of two family studies in Richmond, Virginia, and 64% for women and 50% for men in the other [21,79]. In Taiwan, the prevalence of IgG antibodies to B19 among women was significantly higher than among men (36.4% versus 29.4%; $P < .001$) [89]. The most likely explanation for the higher rates of B19 infection among women compared with men is that women are likely to have more frequent contact with children, especially school-age children who, because of school attendance, are the major sources of B19 transmission. For adults, contact with school-age children is the major risk factor for B19 infection [21].

SEROPREVALENCE BY RACE

In the United States, there are significant differences in the seroprevalence to parvovirus B19 between African Americans and whites. In Richmond, Virginia, approximately 60% of whites are seropositive compared with 45% of African Americans [21]. The reasons for the lower rate of infection among African Americans are unknown, but likely reflect the racial segregation of children in schools.

INCIDENCE

In tests of serum from random blood donors for evidence of a recent parvovirus B19 infection, the rate of infection using antigen detection is 0 to 2.6 per 10,000 individuals tested, with a median of 1 per 10,000, whereas using DNA detection, the rate is 0 to 14.5 per 10,000, with a median of 2 per 10 [90–95]. By contrast, when IgM antibodies to B19 were used to detect recent infection, the rate was zero, but all studies included less than 1000 patients [80,96,97]. As for seroprevalence, women may have a greater risk for infection during outbreaks of EI. During an epidemic of EI in Port Angeles, Washington, the attack rate for women was 15.6%, more than twice the rate of 7.4% for men [12].

In Spain and Chile, children have the highest rates of B19 infection, which is true for children ages 0 to 4 years and 5 to 9 years [98,99]. A study of 633 children with sickle cell disease followed at Children's Hospital in Philadelphia from 1996–2001 found that 70% were seronegative (susceptible), and during this period 110 of these patients developed B19 infections for an incidence of 11.3 per 100 patients per year [100]. Of the 110 patients infected, there were 68 episodes of transient aplastic crisis, characterized not only by an acute exacerbation of anemia, but also by acute chest syndrome, pain, and fever. The high incidence of disease among children with sickle cell disease emphasizes the need for a vaccine against B19.

RISK FACTORS FOR ACQUISITION

Parvovirus B19 is efficiently transmitted among persons residing in the same home, with attack rates, based on the development of signs and symptoms of EI, of 17% to 30% [12,101]. Using serologic testing to identify asymptomatic infection and to exclude immune individuals, the secondary attack rate for susceptible household contacts is 50%. Most secondary cases of EI or aplastic crisis in

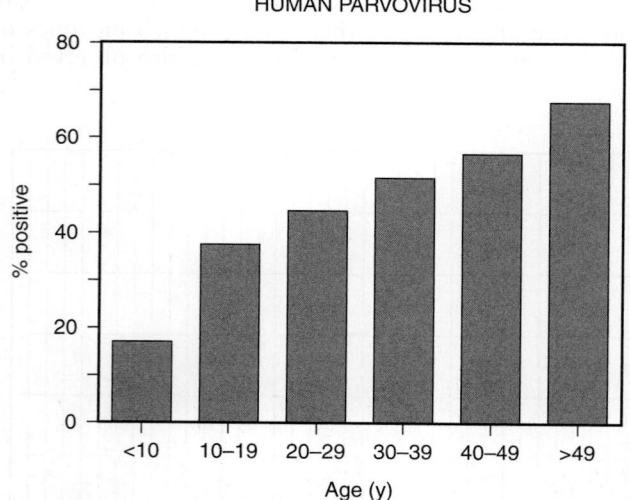

FIGURE 27–2 **Percentage of family subjects positive for IgG antibody to parvovirus B19 by age.** The sample includes 283 subjects from 111 families. Subjects were one twin of each twin pair, nontwin parents, and the oldest child of each family. *(Data from Adler SP, Koch W. Human parvovirus B19 infections in women of childbearing age and within families. J Pediatr Infect Dis 8:83, 1989.)*

the home occur 6 to 12 days after symptoms develop in the index case [10,12,101–104]. A serologic study of pregnant Danish women indicated that seropositivity was significantly correlated with increasing number of siblings, having a sibling of the same age, number of own children, and occupational exposure of children [105].

During epidemics, B19 transmission is widespread among school-age children. Studies of school or classroom outbreaks of EI with at least one serologically confirmed case of acute B19 infection revealed student infection rates of 1% to 62% based on the occurrence of a rash illness. The median infection rate for all studies was 23% [106–113]. Because asymptomatic infections are common, and other signs and symptoms of EI may be mild and overlooked, these studies undoubtedly underestimate the true incidence of infection. Studies of students using serologic assays to identify B19 infection during outbreaks report infection rates of 34% to 72% with most not associated with a rash illness [107,112,113]. Higher rates of infection occur in elementary schools and day care centers compared with secondary schools, and in students in boarding schools compared with students who live at home [12,75,111–113].

During school epidemics, employees in contact with children have the highest rates of infection compared with community controls. The attack rate based on detection of rash illness or arthropathy may be relatively low—12% to 25% [107,111]. The seroprevalence of B19 IgG antibodies to B19 in school employees is greater than adult community controls, however—50% to 75% [21,113,114]. When serologic testing is used to identify employees with asymptomatic infection and to exclude immune employees, the attack rate among the susceptible individuals is usually very high. In four school outbreaks where serologic testing was used, the attack rate among teachers ranged from 19% to 84%, and the frequency of asymptomatic infection was greater than 50% in all but one outbreak [107,110, 113,114]. The highest infection rates occurred among susceptible elementary school teachers compared with middle and high school teachers; this may reflect either exposure to more infected children or a greater likelihood of contact with respiratory secretions in younger children [113,114]. During a community-wide outbreak of EI in Connecticut in 1988, the infection rate among susceptible women was 16% for school teachers, 9% for day care workers and homemakers, but only 4% for other women working outside the home [113].

The risk of infection may be increased for school employees even in the absence of recognized epidemics of EI. In a study of 927 susceptible school employees conducted during a 3.5-year period when no community outbreaks were detected, the annual incidence of specific IgG seroconversion was 2.9% compared with 0.4% for a control population of 198 hospital employees [21]. The rate was higher, 3.4%, for school employees with jobs involving direct contact with children compared with only 0.6% observed for persons with jobs that did not involve contact with children [21]. Most (>50%) of the individuals who seroconverted did not recall an illness characterized by rash or arthropathy.

Salivary antibodies can be used to detect IgG and IgM antibodies to B19 because serum antibodies passively diffuse into saliva. Testing saliva for antibodies to B19 was useful in documenting outbreaks in schools and households. In an outbreak in England, school attack rates ranged from 8% to 50%, including an attack rate of 45% among the teaching staff [115]. The household transmission attack rate was 45% for 11 susceptible individuals. These rates are similar to what has been previously observed [115]. Crowding and low socioeconomic status are not proven risk factors for B19 infection. These risk factors are suggested, however, by the observation that in Rio de Janeiro, the seroprevalence of IgG antibodies to B19 is 35% in children age 5 years or younger, and in Niger it was 90% by 2 years of age [56,74].

HOSPITAL TRANSMISSION

Parvovirus B19 can be transmitted from infected patients to hospital workers [111]. Most, but not all, investigations reveal that hospital transmission of B19 to laboratory personnel is common and includes direct patient-to-patient transmission and indirect transmission from materials or specimens known to contain B19 [116–119]. One patient with sickle cell anemia became ill with aplastic crisis 9 to 11 days after contact in the hospital with a patient with hereditary spherocytosis hospitalized for aplastic crisis; B19 infection was confirmed in both patients [120]. An outbreak of EI occurred on a pediatric ward where 13 (26%) of 50 children developed a rash illness [121]. B19 seroconversion occurred in 5 (71%) of 7 children with rash illness and in 9 (35%) of 26 children who were asymptomatic.

Transmission from patient to health care worker occurred twice in one hospital after admission of patients with aplastic crisis [116]. In the first case, 4 (36%) of 11 susceptible employees with close contact had IgM antibodies to B19, indicating recent infection; in the second case, 10 (48%) of 21 employees either had specific IgM antibodies to B19 or seroconverted from IgG negative to positive. Eleven (79%) of 14 employees were symptomatic with rash or arthropathy. Another study of an outbreak of EI among health care workers on a pediatric ward found that 10 (33%) of 30 susceptible health care workers had serologic evidence of acute B19 infection, along with 2 (17%) of 12 immunocompromised patients being cared for on the ward [117,122]. The two infected patients were not symptomatic, but analysis of preexisting sera showed they acquired B19 while hospitalized. Onset of symptoms among the employees was temporally clustered, indicating a chronic source, such as an immunocompromised patient or person-to-person transmission.

Studies in Hong Kong identified three immunocompromised patients who seemed to transmit genetically identical strains of B19 from patient to patient [123]. At least one of these three patients seemed to be able to transmit the virus over many months. Immunocompromised patients often have chronic infections and may be infectious for long periods. DNA sequence analysis was also used in Japan to document B19 transmission between hospital staff members, including nursing staff, office workers and a physiotherapist [124].

Other investigations have observed little, if any, risk for hospital transmission. No evidence of patient-to-employee transmission was found among 10 susceptible health care workers with frequent contact with a chronically infected patient hospitalized for 24 days before institution of isolation precautions [125]. Transmission to hospital employees did not occur after exposure to a B19-infected mother, her infected stillborn fetus, and contaminated objects in the hospital room [126]. During a community outbreak of B19, none of 17 susceptible pregnant health care workers with possible exposure had serologic evidence (IgM antibodies to B19) of a recent infection [127]. In a case-control study of hospital transmission, serologic testing was used to determine the infection rates among personnel exposed to patients with sickle cell disease and transient aplastic crisis before the patients were placed in isolation [128]. Only 1 of 32 susceptible exposed hospital workers acquired a B19 infection compared with 3 of 37 susceptible workers not exposed. This study suggested that hospital workers who cared for patients with aplastic crisis were not at an increased risk for B19 acquisition.

Two prospective studies from one institution determined the incidence of infection in health care workers during endemic (nonepidemic) periods. The first study found the annual seroconversion rate to be 1.4% for 124 susceptible female health care workers followed for an average of 1.7 years. In a subsequent study of 198 susceptible hospital employees, the annual rate was 0.4% compared with 2.9% for school employees [21]. Taken as a whole, the evidence indicates that one must assume that B19 may be highly contagious in the hospital, although perhaps not in every circumstance. Many potential variables may affect rates of transmission from patients to staff, including the type of patient, immunocompromised status or nonimmunocompromised status, the duration of B19 infection at the time of hospitalization, and potentially the viral load of the infected patient. Patients with erythrocyte aplasia or others with suspected EI or B19 infection should be presumed to have a B19 infection until proven otherwise. These patients should receive respiratory and contact isolation while hospitalized.

ROUTES OF VIRAL SPREAD

Person-to-person spread of parvovirus B19 probably occurs through contact with respiratory secretions. Viral DNA is present in saliva [51,112,128,129] at levels similar to those in blood, and in a volunteer study infection was initiated by intranasal inoculation of B19 [51,130]. B19 cannot be detected in columnar epithelial cells of the large airways [131]. Indirect evidence suggests B19 is not transmitted by aerosols. Viruses transmitted by aerosols such as measles and influenza are rapidly spread during outbreaks, but new cases of EI are spread out over many months during school outbreaks, suggesting that B19 transmission is inefficient. B19 DNA may be found in the urine, but it is unlikely that this is associated with infectious virus.

The only well-documented route of spread for B19 is vertically from mother to fetus and from parenteral transfusion with contaminated blood products or needles. Vertical transmission is discussed later. Although transmission of B19 by transfusion occurs, it is rare because of the low prevalence of B19 viremia among donors of blood and blood

products; however, the risk increases for pooled blood products [130–135]. B19 DNA is frequently found in clotting factor concentrates, including products treated with solvents and detergents, steam, or monoclonal antibodies, and even treated products may be infectious [95,133,135–138]. Seroprevalence of IgG antibodies to B19 is high among hemophiliacs compared with age-matched controls and is higher for individuals who received frequent infusions of clotting factors prepared from large donor pools compared with infusions prepared from small donor pools [134].

Parvoviruses are resistant to chemical inactivation. In one hospital, B19 transmission occurred without recognized direct patient contact, suggesting possible transmission via fomites or environmental contamination [116]. That B19 is transmitted by fomites has not been directly established, but, considering the stability of related animal parvoviruses, this possibility exists. B19 DNA, not infectious virus, was found in a study of a suspected nosocomial outbreak in a maternity ward [127]. B19 DNA was detected by polymerase chain reaction (PCR) on the hands of the mother of a stillborn fetus infected with B19 and on the sink handles in her hospital room. Samples from countertops, an intravenous pump, and telephone were also positive by a sensitive nested PCR DNA technique. PCR is so sensitive that minute quantities of DNA can be detected via this technique, and the presence of B19 DNA on surfaces does not imply that these surfaces are sources of infection. Infected fetal tissues and placental or amniotic fluids are more likely sources of infection for health care workers than fomites.

RISK OF PARVOVIRUS B19 ACQUISITION FOR WOMEN OF CHILDBEARING AGE

We completed a large epidemiologic study to determine the relative risk of parvovirus B19 acquisition for women of childbearing age in daily contact with children, including nurses, day care employees, and teachers at all levels [21]. We identified risk factors for B19 infections for hospital and school employees during an endemic period. Serologic testing was employed to monitor 2730 employees of 135 schools in three school systems and 751 employees of a hospital, all in Richmond, Virginia. Of participants, 60% were initially seropositive. After adjusting for age, race, and gender, risk factors for seropositivity were contact with children 5 to 18 years old at home or at work and employment in elementary schools. Over 42 months, only 1 of 198 susceptible hospital employees seroconverted (0.42% annual rate) compared with 62 of 927 (2.93% annual rate) school employees (relative risk 6.9). Four factors associated with seroconversion were employment at elementary schools, contact with children 5 to 11 years old at home, contact with children 5 to 18 years old at work, and age younger than 30 years. Women in daily contact with school-age children had a fivefold increased annual occupational risk for B19 infection [21].

Several observations indicate that B19 infections were endemic, but not epidemic or pandemic in the Richmond area during the 42-month prospective evaluation [21]. First, few cases of B19 infection were reported by the school nurses, and no cluster of cases was observed at any single school or group of schools. Second, the seroconversion rates during each of three consecutive study periods were the same for all groups or subgroups. Third, for employees, B19 infections were not clustered at individual schools or groups of schools. Fourth, the infection rates that we observed in employees, even for elementary school teachers, were less than those observed for the 1988 Connecticut epidemic, where 46 infections occurred among 236 susceptible individuals exposed in the schools, for a minimum annual infection rate of 19% [113]. Also, in a study of secondary B19 infections among exposed household members, rates ranged from 30% to 50% [102].

B19 infections are often asymptomatic or without a rash, and low-level endemics go unnoticed. We observed that 28 of 60 infected employees were asymptomatic, and only 20 knew of a specific exposure. In a study of 52 household contacts of patients with B19 infections during an Ohio epidemic, infections without a rash occurred in 15 of 16 (94%) African Americans and 17 of 35 (47%) whites, and completely asymptomatic infections occurred in 11 of 16 (69%) African Americans and 6 of 30 (20%) whites [102]. During the Connecticut outbreak, 5 of 65 (8%) teachers who were never exposed to a child with a rash became infected [113]. The observations of high secondary attack rates during epidemics and the high rates of infections without a rash or asymptomatic infections provide strong evidence that even during periods when EI is inapparent in the community, school or hospital personnel in contact with children have a significant occupational risk for B19 infections.

Contact with elementary school–age children, whether at home or at work, may be the most important risk factor for B19 acquisition. When seropositivity for persons with children at home was stratified by the child's age, the association between seropositivity and children at home was significant ($P < .05$) when all children 5 to 18 years of age were included; for seroconversion, the significant association was with elementary school–age children at home [21]. The low seroprevalence and seroconversion rate among hospital employees without known contact with children indicates that this group has a low occupational risk for acquiring B19 infections.

The major conclusions from these studies were that when EI is inapparent in the community, school or hospital personnel in contact with children still have a significant occupational risk for B19 infections, and that school employees have an approximately twofold greater risk of acquiring B19 from children at work than from elementary school–age children at home. We also found that hospital employees without contact with children have a low risk for acquiring B19.

Using the Richmond data and assuming that on average 50% of pregnant women are immune, we estimate that in endemic periods 1% to 4% of susceptible women become infected during pregnancy. If the rate of fetal death after maternal infection is 5% to 10% (see "Intrauterine Transmission Rates, Clinical Manifestations, and Fetal Outcomes"), the occupational risk of fetal death for a pregnant woman with unknown serologic status is between 1 in 500 and 1 in 4000 These rates are so low that during endemic periods they do not justify intervention, such as serologic testing for pregnant women or furloughing or temporary transfer of pregnant seronegative

employees to administrative or other positions without child contact (see "Prevention").

Knowing B19 infection rates during endemic periods may be more important than knowing rates during epidemic periods. In the United States, B19 infections are endemic most of the time. Because greater than 75% of B19 infections are inapparent, most women who acquire B19 infection during pregnancy do so during endemic periods, not during epidemics. For establishing public health policy and assessing the potential importance of immunizing against B19, knowing that for seronegative women the endemic infection rate is 1% to 4% is more important than knowing epidemic rates, which vary widely depending on the frequency of susceptible individuals in a given population at a particular time.

CLINICAL MANIFESTATIONS (OTHER THAN INTRAUTERINE INFECTION)
ERYTHEMA INFECTIOSUM

The most common clinical manifestation of infection with parvovirus B19 is EI, or fifth disease, a well-known rash illness of children. EI begins with a mild prodromal illness consisting of low-grade fever, headache, malaise, and upper respiratory tract symptoms. This prodrome may be so mild as to go unnoticed. The hallmark of the illness is the characteristic exanthem. The rash usually occurs in three phases, but these are not always distinguishable [12,106,139]. The initial stage consists of an erythematous facial flushing described as a "slapped-cheek" appearance. In the second stage, the rash spreads quickly to the trunk and proximal extremities as a diffuse macular erythema. The third stage is central clearing of macular lesions, which occurs promptly, giving the rash a lacy, reticulated appearance. Palms and soles are usually spared, and the rash tends to be more prominent on the extensor surfaces. Affected children at this point are afebrile and feel well. Adolescents and adults often complain of pruritus or arthralgias concurrent with the rash. The rash resolves spontaneously, but typically may recur over 1 to 3 weeks in response to various environmental stimuli, such as sunlight, heat, exercise, and stress [140].

Lymphadenopathy is not a consistent feature, but has been reported in association with EI [101] and as a sole manifestation of infection [141–143]. A mononucleosis-like illness associated with confirmed B19 infections has occasionally been reported, but B19 does not typically cause a mononucleosis-like illness. Atypical rashes not recognizable as classic EI have also been associated with acute B19 infections; these include morbilliform, vesiculopustular, desquamative, petechial, and purpuric rashes [4].

Asymptomatic infection with B19 also occurs commonly in children and adults. In studies of large outbreaks, asymptomatic infection is reported in approximately 20% to 30% of serologically proven cases [101,102].

TRANSIENT APLASTIC CRISIS

As noted earlier, transient aplastic crisis was the first clinical illness to be definitively linked to infection with parvovirus B19. An infectious etiology had been suspected for this condition because it usually occurred only once in a given patient, had a well-defined course and duration of illness, and tended to occur in clusters within families and communities [140]. Attempts to link it to infection with any particular agent had repeatedly failed until 1981, when Pattison and colleagues [8] reported six positive tests for B19 (seroconversion or antigenemia) among 600 admissions to a London hospital—all six positive tests were in children with sickle cell anemia admitted with aplastic crisis. This association was confirmed by studies of an outbreak of aplastic crisis in the population with sickle cell disease in Jamaica [9].

Although such transient aplastic crises are most commonly associated with sickle cell anemia, any patient with a condition of increased red blood cell turnover and accelerated erythropoiesis can experience a similar transient red blood cell aplasia with B19 infection. B19-induced aplastic crises have been described in many hematologic disorders, including other hemoglobinopathies (e.g., thalassemia, sickle-C hemoglobin), red blood cell membrane defects (e.g., hereditary spherocytosis, stomatocytosis), enzyme deficiencies (e.g., pyruvate kinase deficiency, glucose-6-phosphate dehydrogenase deficiency), antibody-mediated red blood cell destruction (autoimmune hemolytic anemia), and decreased red blood cell production (e.g., iron deficiency, blood loss) [49,144]. B19 is not a significant cause of transient erythroblastopenia of childhood, another condition of transient red blood cell hypoplasia that usually occurs in younger, hematologically normal children and follows a more indolent course [4].

In contrast to EI, patients with a transient aplastic crisis are ill at presentation with fever, malaise, and signs and symptoms of profound anemia (e.g., pallor, tachypnea, tachycardia). Rash is rarely present in these patients [104,144]. The acute infection causes a transient arrest of erythropoiesis (see "General Aspects of Pathogenesis") with a profound reticulocytopenia. Given the short half-life of red blood cells in these patients and their dependence on active erythropoiesis to counterbalance their increased red blood cell turnover, this arrest of erythropoiesis leads to a sudden and potentially life-threatening decrease in serum hemoglobin. Children with sickle hemoglobinopathies may also develop a concurrent vaso-occlusive pain crisis, which may complicate the clinical picture further.

Leukopenia and thrombocytopenia may also occur during a transient aplastic crisis, but the incidence varies with the underlying condition. In a French study of 24 episodes of aplastic crisis (mostly in individuals with hereditary spherocytosis), 35% to 40% of patients were either leukopenic or thrombocytopenic compared with 10% to 15% reported in a large U.S. study of mostly sickle cell patients [104,145]. These transient declines in leukocyte count or platelets follow a similar time course as reticulocytopenia, although they are not as severe, and recovery occurs without clinical sequelae. The relative preservation of leukocyte and platelet counts in sickle cell anemia compared with other hereditary hemolytic anemias is presumably due to the functional asplenia associated with sickle cell disease [49].

As noted in experimental infection in human volunteers, B19 infection in normal subjects results in a decrease in the reticulocyte count, but owing to the normal red blood cell half-life, this is not clinically significant or noticeable. Varying degrees of leukopenia and

thrombocytopenia also occur after natural B19 infection in hematologically normal patients [51]. Some cases of idiopathic thrombocytopenic purpura and cases of childhood neutropenia have been reported in association with acute B19 infection [146,147]. Aside from these few anecdotal reports, larger studies have not confirmed B19 as a common cause of either idiopathic thrombocytopenic purpura or chronic neutropenia in children [48].

ARTHROPATHY

Joint symptoms are reported by 80% of adolescents and adults with parvovirus B19 infection, whereas joint symptoms are uncommon in children [12,106]. Arthritis or arthralgia may occur in association with the symptoms of typical EI or may be the only manifestation of infection. Women are more frequently affected with joint symptoms than men [12,106].

The joint symptoms of B19 infection usually manifest as the sudden onset of a symmetric peripheral polyarthropathy [148]. The joints most often affected are the hands, wrists, knees, and ankles, but the larger joints can also be involved [110,149]. The joint symptoms have a wide range of severity, from mild morning stiffness to frank arthritis with the classic combination of erythema, warmth, tenderness and swelling. Similar to the rash of EI, the arthropathy has been presumed to be immunologically mediated because the onset of joint symptoms occurs after the peak of viremia and coincides with the development of specific IgM and IgG antibodies [51]. Rheumatoid factor may also be transiently positive, leading to some diagnostic confusion with rheumatoid arthritis in adult patients [150]. There is no joint destruction, and in most patients joint symptoms resolve within 2 to 4 weeks. For some patients, joint discomfort may last for months or, in rare individuals, years. The role of B19 in these more chronic arthropathies is unclear.

The arthritis associated with B19 infection may persist long enough to satisfy clinical diagnostic criteria for rheumatoid arthritis or juvenile rheumatoid arthritis [89,97,149,151,152]. This finding has led some authors to suggest that B19 may be the etiologic agent of these conditions [5]. This speculation has been supported by the detection of B19 DNA in synovial tissue from patients with rheumatoid arthritis and reports of increased seropositivity among patients with these conditions [98,153–155]. The more recent findings of DNA from other viruses in addition to B19 in synovial tissue from patients with arthritis and B19 DNA in synovium from persons without arthritis suggest that this may be a nonspecific effect of inflammation [156,157]. A review of the accumulated evidence on this topic has concluded that B19 is unlikely to be a primary etiology in these rheumatic diseases, but it may be one of several viral triggers capable of initiating joint disease in genetically predisposed individiuals [158].

INFECTION IN IMMUNOCOMPROMISED HOSTS

Patients with impaired humoral immunity are at risk for developing chronic and recurrent infections with parvovirus B19. Persistent anemia, sometimes profound, with reticulocytopenia is the most common manifestation of such infections, which may also be accompanied by neutropenia, thrombocytopenia, or complete marrow suppression. Chronic infections with B19 occur in children with cancer who receive cytotoxic chemotherapy [159,160], children with congenital immunodeficiency states [161], children and adults with acquired immunodeficiency syndrome (AIDS) [162], and transplant recipients [163]. Chronic infections may even occur in patients with more subtle defects in immunoglobulin production, who are able to produce measurable antibodies to B19, but are unable to generate adequate neutralizing antibodies [164].

B19 has also been linked to viral-associated hemophagocytic syndrome [159,160], more generally referred to as infection-associated hemophagocytic syndrome. This condition of histiocytic infiltration of bone marrow and associated cytopenias usually occurs in immunocompromised patients. B19 is only one of several viruses that have been implicated as causing viral-associated hemophagocytic syndrome. Infection-associated hemophagocytic syndrome is generally considered to be a nonspecific response to various viral and bacterial insults, rather than a specific manifestation of a single pathogen.

Infections in immunocompromised hosts can lead to chronic infection; this is most often manifested as chronic anemia (red blood cell aplasia), but varying degrees of cytopenia have been described, ranging from thrombocytopenia or neutropenia to complete bone marrow failure [144]. Patients with an inability to produce neutralizing antibodies are at greatest risk, and this complication of B19 infection has been described in children with congenital immunodeficiency syndromes, patients receiving cytoreductive chemotherapy, transplant patients receiving immunosuppressive therapy, and adults and children with AIDS [144]. Increased recognition of B19 infection in solid organ transplant patients has led to many more recent reports [165–167]. Although most such infections are manifested as the typical persistent anemia, an association of B19 viremia with acute graft rejection has been described [168].

OTHER DERMATOLOGIC SYNDROMES
Vasculitis and Purpura

Various atypical skin eruptions have been described in association with parvovirus B19 infections. Most of these are petechial or purpuric in nature, often with evidence of vasculitis in descriptions of eruptions that report skin biopsy results, and may resemble the rash of other connective tissue diseases [4,169]. There are reports of confirmed acute B19 infections associated with nonthrombocytopenic purpura and vasculitis, including several cases clinically diagnosed as Henoch-Schönlein purpura [90,170], an acute leukocytoclastic vasculitis of unknown etiology in children. Chronic B19 infection has also been associated with a necrotizing vasculitis, including cases of polyarteritis nodosa and Wegener granulomatosis [171]. These patients had no underlying hematologic disorder and were generally not anemic at diagnosis. The pathogenesis is unknown, but could suggest an endothelial cell infection as occurs with some other viruses such as rubella.

Data from skin biopsy of rashes temporally associated with B19 infection are limited, although several reports have been published. B19 capsid antigens and DNA were found in a skin biopsy specimen from a patient with EI, and this observation lends support to a role for B19 in these vascular disorders [172]. Rashes resembling those of systemic lupus erythematosus, Henoch-Schönlein purpura, and other connective tissue disorders have been described [169,173]. In a controlled study of 27 children with Henoch-Schönlein purpura, B19 was not a common cause [174]. Only 3 of 27 children had detectable B19 IgM antibodies indicating a recent infection. The role of B19 in these conditions remains speculative.

Papular-Purpuric "Gloves and Socks" Syndrome

Papular-purpuric "gloves and socks" syndrome (PPGSS) is a distinctive, self-limited dermatosis first described in the dermatologic literature in 1990 [175]. PPGSS is characterized by fever, pruritus, and painful edema and erythema localized to the distal extremities in a distinct glove-and-sock distribution. The distal erythema is usually followed by petechiae or papules or purpura, and oral lesions often develop as well. Resolution of all symptoms usually occurs in 1 to 2 weeks. A search for serologic evidence of viral infection led to the discovery of an association with acute parvovirus B19 infection in many of these patients, based on demonstration of specific IgM or seroconversion. This association has been confirmed further with subsequent reports and demonstration of B19 DNA in skin biopsy samples and sera from these patients [175,176]. Initially described in adults, numerous children have now been described with this condition [177]. There seems to be sufficient evidence to suggest that PPGSS is a rare but distinctive manifestation of primary, acute infection with B19, occurring mainly in young adults, but also affecting children.

CENTRAL NERVOUS SYSTEM INFECTION AND NEUROLOGIC DISORDERS

Although various neurologic symptoms and disorders have been described in patients clinically diagnosed as having EI or laboratory-confirmed parvovirus B19 infection [4], the issue of whether B19 causes central nervous system (CNS) infection or is etiologic for other neurologic conditions remains unresolved. Cases of meningitis [178,179], encephalitis [180], and encephalopathy [181] secondary to B19 infection all have been reported. Many of these cases were reported during outbreaks of EI from older reports based on clinical diagnosis only, before reliable laboratory tests for B19 were available. In one study, headache was reported in 32% of children with rash illness [178].

There are no controlled comparative studies to evaluate the frequency of signs or symptoms suggestive of meningeal inflammation or CNS infection in B19 infection. Cerebrospinal fluid abnormalities such as pleocytosis and increased levels of cerebrospinal fluid protein have been reported in some, but not all, patients with meningismus or altered level of consciousness associated with EI [5]. B19 DNA has been detected in cerebrospinal fluid using PCR in several cases of serologically confirmed acute B19 infection with meningoencephalitis or encephalopathy [182–184]. Most of these reported patients were also viremic at the time, however, so the possibility that cerebrospinal fluid PCR was positive secondary to contamination from blood could not be completely excluded.

B19 infection has been associated with vasculitis and histopathologic changes in the CNS that potentially may lead to stroke [339]. Most cases of stroke in association with documented B19 infection have been reported in children; some of these children have had other concurrent medical conditions that could contribute to stroke, particularly sickle cell disease [340–342]. At least two cases of neonatal stroke have been reported in association with B19 infection: one related to maternal infection during gestation and the other associated with infection of the newborn infant [343,344].

Disorders of the peripheral nervous system have also been described, including brachial plexus neuropathy [185], carpal tunnel syndrome [188], extremity paresthesias and dysesthesias [186], and myasthenia-like weakness [187]. The onset of most of these peripheral nerve symptoms has been coincident with the onset of rash or joint pain or both at a time when the patient should have a brisk immune response, suggesting that the neurologic abnormalities could be immunologically mediated [5]. In the course of one well-described outbreak of EI among intensive care nurses, numbness and tingling of the fingers was reported in 54% of the 13 nurses infected with B19 [186]. The neurologic symptoms persisted for more than 1 year in three of the nurses, and one had low levels of B19 DNA in serum for more than 3 years in association with recurrent episodes of paresthesias. She was never anemic and had no demonstrable immunodeficiency [189]. Although these cases are suggestive, the role of B19 in neurologic disease, stroke, and CNS infection remains unresolved until the pathogenesis of the viral infection in these conditions can be elucidated [5,190].

RENAL DISEASE

Reports of renal disease after parvovirus B19 infection, previously rare, have increased [191–193]. Most have been case reports of glomerulonephritis or focal glomerulosclerosis temporally related to an acute B19 infection. Immune complex deposition has been shown in renal tissue, and B19 DNA can occasionally be found in renal tissue by PCR as well [194]. Renal failure is rarely reported. The virus is not known to infect kidney cells in vitro, and its presence in renal tissue could be secondary to filtration from the viremia of acute infection. B19 DNA has been detected in urine in studies of infants with evidence of intrauterine infections. It is possible that B19 antigens could trigger an immune complex–mediated nephritis, but this may be a nonspecific effect, and further study is necessary to define the relationship between B19 infection and the potential for renal disease.

MYOCARDIAL DISEASE

Parvovirus B19 is now a well-established, although infrequent, cause of myocarditis in children and adults. B19 DNA is often present within the myocardium of patients with myocarditis and idiopathic left ventricular failure [195–200]. B19 infection has also been associated with acute dilated cardiopathy, but the etiologic significance of B19 in the myocardium is unclear [201]. Myocarditis resulting from B19 infection usually resolves over several weeks, but is occasionally fatal [202–204].

GENERAL ASPECTS OF DIAGNOSIS

The diagnosis of EI (fifth disease) is usually based on the clinical recognition of the typical exanthem, benign course, and exclusion of other similar conditions. Laboratory confirmation is rarely necessary. A presumptive diagnosis of a parvovirus B19–induced transient aplastic crisis in a patient with known sickle cell disease (or other condition associated with chronic hemolysis) is based on an acute febrile illness, a sudden and severe decline in serum hemoglobin, and an absolute reticulocytopenia. Likewise, a clinical diagnosis of PPGSS can be based on the characteristic skin eruption in the distinct acral distribution.

LABORATORY DIAGNOSTIC METHODS

Specific laboratory diagnosis depends on identification of parvovirus B19 antibodies, viral antigens, or viral DNA. In an immunologically normal patient, determination of anti-B19 IgM is the best marker of recent or acute infection on a single serum sample. IgM antibodies develop rapidly after infection and are detectable for 6 to 8 weeks [205]. Specific IgG antibodies become detectable a few days after IgM and persist for years and probably for life. Seroconversion from IgG-negative to IgG-positive on paired acute and convalescent sera confirms a recent infection. Anti-B19 IgG primarily serves as a marker of past infection or immunity, however. Patients with EI or acute B19 arthropathy are almost always IgM-positive, so a diagnosis can generally be made from a single serum sample. Patients with B19-induced aplastic crisis may present before antibodies are detectable; however, IgM is detectable within 1 to 2 days of presentation, and detection of IgG follows within days [104].

The availability of serologic assays for B19 had previously been limited by the lack of a reliable and renewable source of antigen for diagnostic studies. The development of recombinant cell lines that express B19 capsid proteins has provided more reliable sources of antigen suitable for use in commercial test kits [206,207]. Several commercial kits are currently available for detection of B19 antibodies, but they employ a variety of different antigens (e.g., recombinant capsid proteins, fusion proteins, synthetic peptides), and their performance in large studies has varied [206]. Based on studies of the humoral immune response to the various B19 viral antigens, it seems to be important to have serologic assays based on intact capsids that provide conformational epitopes. Antibody responses to these antigens are more reliable and longer lasting than the responses to linear epitopes used in some assays [208].

At present, only one commercial assay based on such capsids has received approval from the U.S. Food and Drug Administration (FDA); other commercial assays for this purpose are considered research tests [209]. Until serologic tests are more standardized and results are more consistent, some knowledge of the assay and antigens used is necessary for proper interpretation of B19 antibody test results.

In immunocompromised or immunodeficient patients, serologic diagnosis is unreliable because humoral responses are impaired, so methods to detect viral particles or viral DNA are necessary to make the diagnosis of a B19 infection. As noted, the virus cannot be isolated on routine cell cultures, so viral culture is not useful. Detection of viral DNA by DNA hybridization techniques [210] or by PCR [211,212] is useful in these patients. Both techniques can be applied to various clinical specimens, including serum, amniotic fluid, fresh tissues, bone marrow, and paraffin-embedded tissues [148]. Histologic examination is also helpful in diagnosing B19 infection in certain situations. Examination of bone marrow aspirates in anemic patients typically reveals giant pronormoblasts or "lantern cells" against a background of general erythroid hypoplasia. The absence of such cells does not exclude B19 infection, however [213,214]. Electron microscopy has proven useful and may reveal viral particles in serum of some infected patients and in cord blood or tissues of hydropic infants (see "Pathogenesis of Infection in the Fetus").

EPIDEMIOLOGY OF PARVOVIRUS B19 INFECTIONS AND RISK OF ACQUISITION IN PREGNANT WOMEN
PREVALENCE AND INCIDENCE IN THE UNITED STATES

We completed three studies using complementary strategies to determine the incidence of parvovirus B19 infection during pregnancy. First, using the data from a study of school personnel, we estimated the average B19 infection rate among pregnant school personnel [21]. Of the 60 individuals who seroconverted in that study, 8 (13%) were pregnant. Not all pregnant women in the school system participated in the study. Although we had data on the pregnancy rates for the female school personnel who participated, these volunteers may have been biased toward younger women, raising the possibility that their pregnancy rates may not have been representative of all school employees. Of approximately 11,637 total school employees in Richmond, Virginia, we enrolled 2730 (24%) in our study. To determine if the sample enrolled was representative, we performed a random survey of 733 school employees at the schools studied. The results provided strong evidence that the seroprevalence and annual infection rates observed among study subjects were representative and applicable to the entire school employee population [21]. Assuming no seasonality to B19 infections, as none was observed, and that pregnancy does not affect susceptibility, we predicted that without regard to risk factors, seronegative pregnant personnel have an average annual infection rate of 3%, for a rate of 2.25% per pregnancy [21].

Second, in Richmond, Virginia, from 1989–1991, we collected sera from 1650 pregnant women from a lower socioeconomic group, who attended a high-risk pregnancy clinic for patients without medical insurance. This group was 80% African American with an average maternal age of 24 years. We randomly selected a subset of 395 women for serologic testing and monitoring, 35% of whom were seropositive. Of the 256 seronegative women, 2 (0.8%) seroconverted for an annual rate of 1.7%. This rate was similar to the rate observed among low-risk African American school personnel in Richmond [21].

Finally, we also obtained serial sera from a large group of private practice obstetric patients from Birmingham, Alabama [215]. From this serum bank, we randomly selected 200 patients per year over 4 years, 1987–1990. No significant differences in seroprevalence were observed by year among the 800 patients (average age 27 years and 88% white), and 46% were seropositive overall. Of 413 seronegative women serially tested over the 4 years, 5 seroconverted. Overall, the annual seroconversion rate was 2%. Combining data from the studies of pregnant women done in Richmond and Birmingham, we observed that 7 of 669 seronegative women seroconverted in pregnancy for a rate of 1% per pregnancy with a 95% confidence interval of 0.3% to 21%.

PREVALENCE AND INCIDENCE IN OTHER COUNTRIES

In numerous studies conducted worldwide, including pregnant women and women of reproductive age, the seroprevalence of IgG antibodies to parvovirus B19 has ranged from 16% to 81%, with most estimates between 35% and 55% [73,78,79,88,216–219]. In Denmark, a serologic survey of 31,000 pregnant Danish women found 65% had evidence of past infection [105]. The seroprevalence of IgG antibody among 1610 pregnant women in Barcelona was 35.03% [22]. Of pregnant Swedish women, 81% had parvovirus antibodies [220]. In Japan, the seroprevalence of IgG antibodies to B19 was 26% for women 21 to 30 years old and 44% for women 31 to 40 years old [78]. In Germany, 62.9% of 40,517 pregnant women had IgG antibodies to B19 [218]. The prevalence of IgG antibodies to B19 in cord blood from normal newborns also provides estimates of maternal immunity of 50% to 75% [19,221,222].

Without regard to maternal age or other potential risk factors, a South African study found that 64 (3.3%) of 1967 pregnant women acquired B19 infection during pregnancy, and another study in Barcelona found that 60 (3.7%) of 1610 pregnant women became infected with B19 during pregnancy [22,223]. Seroconversion rates among susceptible pregnant Danish women during endemic and epidemic periods were 1.5% and 13%. In Denmark, risk of infection increased with the number of children in the household, and having children ages 6 to 7 years resulted in the highest rate of seroconversion. Nursery school teachers had a threefold increased risk of acute infection [105]. Extrapolating to a 40-week period would place the infection rate during pregnancy among susceptible women at approximately 1.1%, with a range of 1% to 4% depending on risk factors. The Danish and Barcelona data are similar to data obtained in Richmond, Virginia [21].

A prospective study conducted from 1998–2000 of 2567 pregnant women found that 70% had IgG antibodies to B19 at the beginning of pregnancy, and of those seronegative, 2.4% acquired B19 during pregnancy [216]. A similar study of 13,449 women conducted in five European countries found that the risk of a seronegative woman acquiring B19 during pregnancy ranged from 0.61% in Belgium to 1.58% in Poland [217].

A few studies have tried to estimate the infection rate based on the prevalence of IgM antibodies to B19 in pregnancy or in women of reproductive age. Although B19-specific IgM is an accurate diagnostic test for recent infection, it is a poor test for epidemiology studies. B19 IgM persists for only a few months and underestimates the maternal infection rate because women who have had a B19 infection 6 to 9 months before testing would not be detected by this assay. Another problem with IgM surveys is that most studies have surveyed high-risk populations, such as women with rash illness, possible exposure to cases of EI, or recent diagnosis of adverse reproductive outcomes. Sampling high-risk populations biases the results toward rates higher than would be observed in population-based studies. A few studies have used B19-specific IgM to test pregnant women or women of reproductive age who did not have risk factors for infection. The observed range in these studies was 0 to 2.6% [19,221,224]. For susceptible women of reproductive age in populations known to be at increased risk for infection, the prevalence of IgM has ranged from 0 and 12.5% [19,78,128,225,226].

In countries other than the United States, the prevalence of IgG antibodies to B19 among pregnant women and women of reproductive age varies widely and is likely to reflect exposure during prior epidemics. Studies on infections during pregnancy are fraught with potentially confounding variables, such as use of IgM testing, which lacks sensitivity, and selection bias introduced by selection criteria for the population studied. Despite these problems, it is likely the risk for B19 infection during pregnancy in other countries is similar to that observed in the United States.

CLINICAL MANIFESTATIONS OF PARVOVIRUS B19 INFECTIONS IN PREGNANT WOMEN

The symptoms reported by pregnant women with a proven recent parvovirus B19 infection are usually vague and nonspecific, so serologic confirmation is essential to establish the diagnosis. The signs and symptoms of classic EI in children are significantly different in adults; the sunburned or slapped-cheek facial rash common in children rarely occurs in adults. Malaise is a common feature of B19 infection in children and in adults, but is nonspecific. In pregnant women and adolescents, the most characteristic symptom is symmetric arthralgias, occasionally with signs of arthritis, and usually involving the small distal joints of hands, wrists, and feet.

The proportion of pregnant women with serologically proven B19 infection who are asymptomatic varies with the inclusion criteria in the few studies that address symptoms. In a cohort of 1610 pregnant women studied in Barcelona, the sera of 30 women had IgM antibodies to B19 at the first prenatal visit, and another 30 seroconverted during pregnancy [22]. Of these 60 women, only

18 (30%) reported any combination of fever, rash, and arthralgias—70% were asymptomatic. The authors did not report when questions about symptoms were asked in relation to the serologic results, and no comment was made about the distribution of symptoms or about which joints were affected by the arthralgias [22]. Similarly, during an epidemic of EI in Connecticut, 69% of nonpregnant adults with serologically proven B19 infection were asymptomatic. In this study, symptoms were assessed by mailed questionnaires after the women were provided their serologic results [113,127]. In a British multicenter study, only 6 (3%) of 184 patients were asymptomatic, but the population was ascertained largely by recruiting women with typical symptoms, so this study is not comparable to the others [20].

We studied 618 pregnant women in Pittsburgh, Pennsylvania, with known exposure to someone with a rash illness highly suggestive of EI. Each exposed patient was questioned about symptoms before serologic testing. Only 33% of the 52 women with serologically proven B19 infection reported no symptoms, whereas the remaining 67% reported rash, fever, arthralgias, coryza, or malaise [227]. Malaise, although a very vague and nonspecific finding, was reported by 27 (52%) of the 52 infected women [227]. In contrast, only 5.5% of 307 exposed, but not susceptible (IgG seropositive, IgM seronegative), women reported this symptom. After malaise, symmetric arthralgias were the second most common symptom reported. Of the 618 pregnant women with known exposures, 24 (46%) of the 52 infected pregnant women reported arthralgias compared with 11 (3.6%) of 307 immune women and 12 (4.6%) of 259 susceptible, but uninfected women ($P < .0001$) [227]. Of the 24 women with arthralgias in this study, 23 also reported malaise, 16 reported rash, 7 reported coryza, and 7 reported fever. Among the 24 IgM-positive women with arthralgias, the symmetric joints most commonly affected by pain, swelling, and erythema were the knees (75%) followed by wrists (71%), fingers (63%), ankles (42%), feet (29%), elbows (29%), shoulders (17%), hips (13%), and back and neck (8%). Only 2 of the 24 women had only one set of joints involved, and very few other women reported monarticular pain or swelling. In most women, the arthralgias were easily controlled by anti-inflammatory drugs and lasted only 1 to 5 days. Arthralgias occasionally lasted 10 to 14 days, however, and in some women were so painful that they were incapacitated for 2 to 3 days.

The high frequency of arthralgia in pregnant women with B19 infection is consistent with reports that distal arthralgias and arthritis are the most frequent finding in adults with EI. The frequency of arthralgias among nonpregnant adults with proven B19 infection in the Torrington, Connecticut, epidemic was 24% (11 of 46 adults) compared with 12% (61 of 512 adults) in adults without B19 infection ($P < .05$) [113]. In another study in Connecticut, arthralgias occurred significantly more often (26%) in 19 adults with IgM antibodies to B19 than in 460 adults (7%) who lacked IgM antibodies to B19 ($P < .01$) [127]. Arthralgias were even more common during outbreaks in Ireland, occurring in 79% of 47 recently infected women and men. Of patients with arthralgias, 93% reported that their knees were involved [228].

Rash is less frequent in pregnant women than in children with EI, and the rash in pregnant women is not characteristic. In one report of the Connecticut epidemic, rashes occurred in 6 (13%) of 46 infected adults compared with 49 (10%) of 512 individuals who were uninfected. In another report, rashes occurred in 3 (16%) of 19 infected adults compared with 33 (7%) of 460 uninfected individuals. This difference was not significant ($P = .16$) and may represent random variation [113]. In contrast to the classic "curtain lace" rash in children, pregnant women (80%) often have a maculopapular rash that rarely involves the face and may be urticarial or morbilliform. In adults, these rashes are rarely pruritic and usually resolve within 1 to 5 days. A Japanese study reported that of 100 pregnant women with a confirmed B19 infection during pregnancy, 51 had a facial, body, or limb rash, and 49 were without symptoms [229]. In the Pittsburgh, Pennsylvania, series, coryza was reported by 23% of the 52 B19-infected pregnant women, but was reported in only 6.8% of the 307 previously infected women, and 5.8% of the 259 seronegative women [227]. This difference was significant ($P < .0001$), but the non-specific nature of coryza in pregnant women means this symptom alone is not diagnostically helpful.

In the Pittsburgh, Pennsylvania, series, a temperature 38° C or greater occurred in 19% of 52 IgM-seropositive, B19-infected women compared with 2.6% of 307 previously infected patients and 3.1% of 259 susceptible, non-infected patients ($P < .0001$) [227]. In 9 of 10 women with fever, at least one other symptom was present. No woman's temperature exceeded 38.9° C. In 16 uninfected women with fever, all had at least one other symptom, and temperatures ranged up to 40° C, suggesting that a temperature greater than 39° C in a pregnant woman indicates infections other than B19. In a London outbreak of B19 infection, 7 of the 10 infected adults had an elevated temperature [117]. In the Connecticut epidemic, fever was reported in 15% of the 46 infected individuals, but also in 16% of the 512 uninfected individuals [113]. Occasionally, pregnant women infected with B19 develop rapidly increasing fundal height, preterm labor, or pre-eclampsia. Such symptoms are nonspecific and rarely indicate B19 infection.

INTRAUTERINE TRANSMISSION RATES, CLINICAL MANIFESTATIONS, AND FETAL OUTCOMES
OVERVIEW

Primary maternal infection with parvovirus B19 during gestation has been associated with adverse outcomes, such as nonimmune hydrops fetalis, intrauterine fetal death, and asymptomatic neonatal infection, but also with normal delivery at term [16,17]. Initial reports of fetal hydrops related to maternal B19 infection were anecdotal and retrospective, suggesting rates of adverse outcomes of 26% and generating concern that B19 might be more fetotropic than rubella or CMV [230,231]. Subsequent reports of normal births after documented maternal B19 infection made clear the need for better estimates of the rate of intrauterine transmission and the risk of adverse outcomes [232,233].

FETAL DEATH

Parvovirus B19 was first linked to fetal death in 1984 [17]. As anticipated based on the epidemiology of B19 transmission, the percentage of all fetal deaths attributable to B19 varies probably depended on the frequency of B19 infections in the population being studied. Overall, the contribution of B19 infection to fetal death is variable.

Prospective studies report rates of intrauterine viral transmission ranging from 25% to 50% [20,234,235]. Initial studies indicated that the risk of an adverse fetal outcome after a recent maternal infection is less than 10% and probably much less, with greatest risk in the first 20 weeks of pregnancy [148]. A large British prospective study identified 186 pregnant women with confirmed B19 infections during an epidemic and followed these women to term [20]. There were 30 (16%) fetal deaths in all, with 17 (9%) estimated to be due to B19 on the basis of DNA studies of a sample of the abortuses. Most of the fetal deaths occurred in the first 20 weeks of gestation with an excess fetal loss in the second trimester [20]. The intra-uterine transmission rate was estimated at 33% based on analysis of the abortuses, fetal IgM in cord blood, and persistence of B19 IgG at 1-year follow-up of the infants. A smaller study of 39 pregnancies complicated by maternal B19 infection and followed to term found two fetal deaths (fetal loss rate of 5%), one (3%) of which was attributable to B19 and occurred at 10 weeks' gestation [234].

A prospective study conducted by the U.S. Centers for Disease Control and Prevention (CDC) identified 187 pregnant women with B19 infection and compared their outcomes with 753 matched controls [235]. The overall fetal loss rate in the infected group was 5.9% with 10 of 11 occurring before the 18th week of gestation compared with 3.5% fetal loss rate in the control group, suggesting a fetal loss rate of 2.5% attributable to B19. In a prospective Spanish study during an endemic period, 1610 pregnant women were screened for B19 infection, and 60 (3.7%) were identified [22]. There were five abortions among this group, but only one (1.7%) was caused by B19 based on histologic and virologic analysis of fetal samples. The incidence of vertical transmission was estimated at 25% based on serologic evaluation of the infants at delivery and at 1 year of age. In a similar prospective study of an obstetric population, 1967 pregnant women were screened, and 64 (3.3%) were identified as recently infected [223]. Among this group, no adverse effects were seen by serial ultrasound examinations, and no fetal hydrops was noted; one abortion occurred, but the fetus was not examined for evidence of B19 infection (maximal fetal loss attributable, 1.6%).

In a Japanese study of 100 women with a confirmed B19 infection during pregnancy, the fetal loss rate including hydrops and fetal death was 7% with all maternal infections occurring before the 20th week of gestation [229]. These results are similar to results from a larger study from Germany, where 1018 pregnant women with a confirmed B19 infection during pregnancy were studied [236]. The overall fetal death rate was 6.3%, with the highest death rate (11%) occurring among women infected before 20 weeks of gestation. The overall rate of hydrops was 3.9% [236]. In a case-control study of

192 women with fetal deaths, half occurring before 20 weeks' gestation and half after, there was serologic evidence of acute B19 infection in 1% of case and control groups [19]. The prevalence of IgG antibodies was also similar. In this study, the percentage of fetal deaths attributed to B19 infection was unlikely to exceed 3% in cases not selected for parvovirus exposure.

In another study, 5 (6.3%) of 80 women with spontaneous abortions between 4 and 17 weeks of gestation had IgM antibodies to B19 compared with 2 (2%) of 100 controls, but this difference was not statistically significant [226]. Additionally, these investigators studied the aborted fetuses from the five seropositive cases and found B19 DNA in only two.

In a prospective study of 39 pregnant women infected with B19 during a community-wide outbreak in Connecticut, there were two fetal deaths, and only one (3%) was attributable to B19 infection [234]. Among women followed prospectively and who acquired B19 infection during pregnancy, there was no evidence of fetal damage in 43 in Richmond, Virginia, and 52 in Pittsburgh, Pennsylvania, and one fetal loss among 56 pregnancies in women from Barcelona [22,23,227].

Two Chinese studies found fetal B19 infection frequently associated with fetal death [237,238]. The first study in China found that of 116 spontaneously aborted fetuses tested for B19 DNA, 27.3% were positive for parvovirus B19, but only 4% (1 of 25) of nonaborted fetal tissues in the control group tested positive [237]. This difference was significant. It was unknown when these samples were collected, or whether B19 was endemic or epidemic in the community. The second Chinese study examined 175 biopsy tissues from spontaneous abortions from 1994–1995 and found that 25% were positive for B19 DNA in the fetal tissues [238]. A control group of 20 fetal tissues came from induced abortions, and only 2 (5%) were positive. This difference was not statistically significant, but did support the observation that in China, B19 may be an important cause of fetal death, especially if B19 is epidemic in the community.

In contrast to the Chinese studies, a study from the Netherlands of fetal and placental tissue from 273 cases of first-trimester and second-trimester fetal loss were tested for serologic or virologic evidence of B19 infection [239]. Of the 273 cases, 149 were from seronegative women, and the fetal deaths for these women were considered unrelated to B19. The mothers had IgM antibodies to B19 at the time of abortion in only 2 of the remaining 124 cases (0.7% for all 273 cases). This study indicates that B19 infection was a rare cause of fetal loss during the first and second trimesters. No congenital anomalies were observed among the fetal tissues examined.

In a study of 1047 pregnant women in Kuwait, maternal blood samples were obtained in the first, second, and third trimesters and tested for serologic evidence of recent B19 infection [240]. Of the mothers, 47% were seronegative, and in these women the incidence of seroconversion was 16.5%. Among the women who seroconverted to B19, the rate of fetal loss was 5.4%. All the fetal deaths occurred in the first two trimesters, suggesting that fetal death after maternal B19 infection is common, particularly during the first and second trimesters.

A report from Toledo, Ohio, described five unexpected fetal deaths that occurred in the second trimester [241]. Only one of the fetuses was hydropic, but all five contained viral inclusions in the liver, and all five women were seropositive to B19.

Fetal deaths in the third trimester have also been reported (Table 27–2). A Swedish study of fetal deaths among 33,759 pregnancies found 93 cases of third-trimester fetal deaths, and of these, 7 (7.5%) had detectable B19 DNA in frozen placental tissue [242]. None of the seven fetuses was hydropic. The authors suggested B19 occasionally caused fetal death in the third trimester.

A study of 13 pregnant women who acquired B19 infection during pregnancy and in whom the time of acquisition was known was completed in Japan [243]. Nonimmune hydrops occurred in three fetuses whose mothers acquired B19 infection in the first half of pregnancy. Spontaneous abortion without hydrops and intrauterine growth restriction occurred in two fetuses whose mothers also developed B19 infection during the first half of pregnancy. The remaining eight fetuses, whose mothers acquired infection in the first and second half of pregnancy, were asymptomatic, although B19 DNA was detected in the immune serum of all of the infants. These results suggest that B19 transmission to the fetus is frequent, and fetal death may occur in almost half of the fetuses of infected mothers.

TABLE 27–2   Fetal Deaths from Parvovirus B19 Infection

Infection-to-Death Interval (wk)	Gestational Age at Death (wk)	Fetal Weight at Death (g)	Reference
1	39	3840	[17]
10	25	NR	[333]
13	22	409	[18]
4	20	161	[18]
4	24	420	[334]
4	26	695	[285]
9	24	580	[285]
7	18	300	[335]
8	19	236	[278]
1	4	NR	[336]
3	NR	NR	[336]
6	17	NR	[336]
10–19	23	NR	[337]
5	16	NR	[337]
(10)*	(11)†	Hydrops fetalis	[300]
(4)	(25)	Hydrops, 3320	[314]
(11)	(21)	Hydrops, 3111	[315]
(7)	(13)	Hydrops fetalis	[279]
(4)	(24)	Hydrops, 1495	[279]
(3)	(30)	Hydrops, 3550	[337]
(8)	(25)	Hydrops fetalis	[144]

*Numbers in parentheses in this column refer to intervals between exposure or onset of symptoms and diagnosis of hydrops fetalis.
†Numbers in parentheses in this column refer to gestational age at time of diagnosis of hydrops fetalis.
NR, not reported.

A Swedish study of 92 pregnancies with unexpected fetal death occurring after 22 weeks of gestation found B19 DNA in 13 (14%) of the 92 fetuses [244]. Only 2 of the 13 were hydropic. The Swedish study again suggests that B19 infection may infect the fetus in the third trimester and result in fetal death or hydrops. This observation was confirmed in a larger study also from Sweden, where 47 cases of fetal deaths occurring after 22 weeks of gestation were identified and compared with 53 normal pregnancies [245]. Seven of the 43 intrauterine fetal deaths were positive for parvovirus B19 DNA, whereas B19 DNA was not detected in any of the normal pregnancies.

Dichorionic twin pregnancies affected by maternal B19 infections have also been reported [246,247]. These reports indicate that one or both fetuses may be infected, and only one fetus may be symptomatic even if both are infected.

In two studies, the presence of IgM to B19 or B19 DNA or both in maternal sera of pregnant women with a history of unexplained recurrent abortions was significantly higher than in pregnant women without a history of recurrent abortion, suggesting that women who are prone to recurrent abortion may be more likely to abort after a B19 infection than others [248,249].

B19 is a likely cause of fetal death in the first, second, and third trimesters, and most infected infants are not hydropic. The estimates of fetal deaths attributable to B19 range from 0 to 27%, making it difficult to assess the precise increase in fetal mortality attributable to B19.

ASYMPTOMATIC FETAL INFECTION

Although published prospective studies of parvovirus B19 infection in pregnancy have varied in their estimates of adverse fetal outcome and rates of vertical transmission, most women infected during pregnancy deliver normal-appearing infants at term. Among these infants, some have asymptomatic infection [250]. A prospective study that combined serologic with virologic markers of infection suggested that intrauterine transmission is very high [23]. In this study, 43 pregnant women with a confirmed B19 infection were followed to delivery. The infants were tested at birth and at intervals throughout the 1st year of life for IgM and IgG to B19 and by PCR for viral DNA in serum, urine, or saliva. No fetal losses or cases of fetal hydrops were observed in this study; however, the rate of intrauterine viral transmission was 51% [23].

BIRTH DEFECTS

There is circumstantial evidence that intrauterine parvovirus B19 infection may occasionally cause birth defects. The first case was reported in 1987 [251]. An aborted fetus at 11 weeks' gestation was described with striking ocular abnormalities including microphthalmia; aphakia; and dysplastic changes of the cornea, sclera, and choroid of one eye, and retinal folds and degeneration of the lens in the other eye [252,253]. The mother had a history of a rash illness with arthropathy at 6 weeks that was serologically confirmed as B19 infection. There have been few additional reports of malformations or developmental abnormalities in aborted fetuses or live-born infants after

intrauterine infection, and the few cases that have been described could not be unequivocally attributed to infection with B19 [254–261].

There are no other data suggesting that B19 is an important cause of birth defects in live-born infants. In an uncontrolled study of 243 infants younger than 4 months with birth defects, none had IgM antibodies to B19 detected [221]. In a controlled study of 57 infants with structural abnormalities or stigmata of congenital infection, specific B19 IgM was not detected in cord blood of any of the affected infants or of the matched normal newborn controls [19]. There are also no data suggesting that structural defects are common in newborns after maternal B19 infection. After a large community-wide outbreak of EI, there was no increase in congenital malformations compared with the pre-epidemic and post-epidemic periods [262]. In the British study of maternal infections during pregnancy, outcomes were available for 186 patients; anencephaly was reported in 1 of the 30 fatal cases, but was not attributed to B19 infection, and hypospadias was present in 2 of the 156 live-born infants [20]. No new anomalies or serious neurodevelopmental problems were detected in the 114 infants followed clinically for at least 1 year [262]. In another prospective, but uncontrolled study of 39 pregnancies with maternal B19 infection, hypospadias was reported in 1 of the 37 live-born infants, and no abnormalities were reported in the one fatal case for which tissues were available [234].

OTHER FETAL MANIFESTATIONS

Meconium ileus and peritonitis has been associated with maternal parvovirus B19 infection in a few reports [144,259]. Three infants with congenital anemia after maternal infection and intrauterine hydrops have also been reported [16]. All three infants had abnormalities on bone marrow examination and B19 DNA detected in bone marrow by PCR. Hyperechogenic bowel, common in fetuses infected with cytomegalovirus, has also been observed in a fetus with intrauterine B19 infection [263].

FETAL HYDROPS

Although parvovirus B19 infection in utero may cause nonimmune hydrops fetalis, it is one of many causes of this syndrome and probably accounts for only 10% to 15% of fetal hydrops [144]. Hydrops fetalis is rare, occurring in only 1 in 3000 births; in 50% of cases, the etiology is unknown. In a study of 50 cases, B19 DNA was detected by in situ hybridization in the tissues of 4 fetuses; most of the cases were due to chromosomal or cardiovascular abnormalities [264]. In another study, B19 DNA was shown in 4 of 42 cases of nonimmune hydrops fetalis [265].

B19 infection is frequently associated with nonimmune fetal hydrops during local epidemics of EI. In a hospital series from England, 10 cases of B19-associated hydrops, representing 8% of all cases of nonimmune hydrops and 27% of anatomically normal cases of nonimmune hydrops, occurred over 17 years [255]. In a consecutive series of 72 patients with nonimmune hydrops from Germany, 3 (4.2%) had B19 infection [266]. In a series of 673 fetal and neonatal autopsies conducted over 6 years in Rhode Island, 32 (0.7%) cases of hydrops were identified, and 5 (16%) of these had histologic and laboratory evidence of B19 infection [267,268]. In the British study, 1 of the 156 live-born infants had been diagnosed with intrauterine hydrops and recovered after intrauterine transfusion; of the six fatal cases that were positive for B19 DNA, hydrops was present in one of three fatal cases with laboratory-confirmed intrauterine infection [20,255]. Postmortem examination may be unable to identify hydrops in fetal death occurring in early pregnancy. Published reports suggest that nonimmune hydrops is an uncommon manifestation of fetal infection with B19.

FETAL OUTCOME IN RELATION TO MATERNAL MANIFESTATIONS

No data suggest that the clinical manifestation of parvovirus B19 infection in the mother influences the pregnancy outcome. There is evidence for an association between a B19-affected fetus and maternal hypertension. Pregnancy-induced hypertension, preeclampsia, and eclampsia have been reported in some women with B19-associated fetal hydrops, and there is a record of improvement with spontaneous resolution of hydrops in one case [18,255,266,270–272,314]. Hypertension of pregnancy may be caused by poor fetal-placental perfusion, and there is an increased risk in pregnancies complicated by hydrops. It is unknown if there is an increased frequency of hypertensive disorders in B19-infected women compared with uninfected women, or if more careful monitoring of B19-infected women to detect findings of preeclampsia would be useful in identifying women at increased risk of B19-associated fetal hydrops.

LONG-TERM OUTCOMES

The long-term outcomes of live-born infants infected in utero with parvovirus B19 are discussed in "Prognosis."

PATHOGENESIS OF INFECTION IN THE FETUS
FETAL IMMUNE RESPONSES TO PARVOVIRUS B19

In studies in which serologic and virologic markers of infection have been examined, fetal immune responses to parvovirus B19 are variable [23,148,273]. B19-specific IgM in cord blood is a recognized marker of fetal infection, but sensitivity can be increased by adding other markers, such as IgA, PCR positivity, and persistence of B19 IgG at 1 year of age [23,148,273]. Infants exposed to B19 earlier in gestation may be less likely to show a positive IgM response owing to immaturity of the fetal immune system; for infants exposed later in gestation, the IgM response may be delayed because of interference by passively acquired maternal antibodies. In one study, only two of nine infected infants whose exposure occurred in the first 14 weeks of pregnancy were positive for B19 IgM at delivery, whereas all four infected infants exposed in the last trimester had B19-specific IgM in cord blood [23]. Serum IgA, similar to IgM, does not cross the

placenta, so for some other congenital viral infections (e.g., rubella and human immunodeficiency virus [HIV]), viral-specific IgA responses in cord blood have been used to provide evidence of intrauterine infection [274]. In the only study of B19 in which this response was examined, B19 IgA in cord blood was associated with maternal infection with B19, and for a few infants, this was the only marker of intrauterine infection [23].

The fetal immune response to B19 may be important for preventing B19-induced red blood cell aplasia in the fetus and is suggested by the observed decreased rates of fetal death after 20 weeks of gestation. Viral clearance by the fetus may be prolonged. IgM specific to B19 may be detected at 18 weeks of gestation [275]. Fetal serum collected at 21 weeks' gestational age neutralizes B19 virus in vitro [276].

PATHOGENESIS OF PARVOVIRUS B19 HYDROPS

Nonimmune hydrops is the best-characterized complication of fetal parvovirus B19 infection. Several mechanisms have been proposed, and more than one may contribute to hydrops [255]. Severe fetal anemia and thrombocytopenia is present in most cases [277]. Hemoglobin levels less than 2 g/dL are detected by cordocentesis of hydropic fetuses [269,278,279]. Hypoxic injury to tissues may result in increased capillary permeability. Severe anemia may also increase cardiac output, as evidenced by increases in umbilical venous pressure, and subsequently result in high-output heart failure [280]. Alternatively, myocarditis may precipitate heart failure. Reduced fetal myocardial function as shown by echocardiography occurs in some cases of fetal hydrops [270]. Regardless of the etiology, congestive heart failure could cause an increase in capillary hydrostatic pressure. Decreased venous return caused by massive ascites or organomegaly may lead to further cardiac decompensation. Hepatic function may be compromised by the extreme levels of extramedullary hematopoiesis, and lysis of B19-infected erythrocytes in the liver may cause hemosiderin deposition, fibrosis, and esophageal varices [271,272]. Impaired production of albumin could lead to a decrease in colloid osmotic pressure with transfer of fluid to the extravascular compartment. Placental hydrops may compromise further oxygen delivery to the fetus.

Finally, there is considerable evidence that fetal tissues other than erythroid cells may be susceptible to B19 infection. Virus has been shown in fetal myocytes, including cardiac myocytes, along with inflammatory changes; fetal myocarditis associated with B19 infection is well documented [131,257,281]. Histologic studies show vascular damage and perivascular infiltrates in other fetal tissues; it is unknown if this is due to B19 infection in endothelial cells or a nonspecific effect related to hypoxic damage.

PATHOLOGY IN THE FETUS
ANATOMIC AND HISTOLOGIC FEATURES

The hallmarks of fetal infection with parvovirus B19 are edema, anemia, and myocarditis, and these are reflected in the pathologic findings at autopsy, but otherwise portmortem reports of gross and histopathologic pathology reveal few features specific for intrauterine B19 infection.* At post mortem, B19-infected fetuses are often described as pale with subcutaneous edema. Rashes are almost always absent; however, a "blueberry muffin" rash caused by extramedullary hematopoiesis in the skin may occur [288].

Fetal anemia is common in fetal deaths caused by B19, but does not occur in all cases.* The histologic findings suggestive of B19 infection include erythroid hypoplasia or occasionally hyperplasia characteristic of recovery. Extramedullary hematopoiesis is common in many organs, especially the liver and spleen. Nucleated red blood cells with amphophilic intranuclear inclusions (Figs. 27–3 and 27–4) are highly suggestive of B19 infection. These nucleated red blood cells are often found in the lumens of vessels and at sites of extramedullary hematopoiesis [131]. When stained with hematoxylin and

---

*References [18,255,258,267,272,282–287].
*References [257,260,271,272,278,279,285,289].

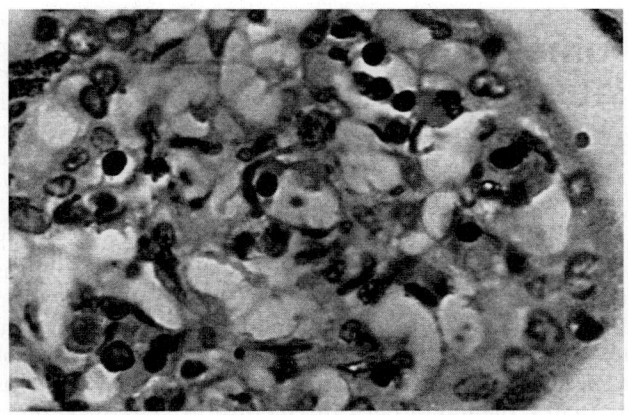

FIGURE 27–3 Placenta from a case of parvovirus B19–associated nonimmune hydrops shows fetal capillaries filled with erythroblasts, most with marginated chromatin and typical amphophilic intranuclear inclusions. (Hematoxylin & eosin stain.)

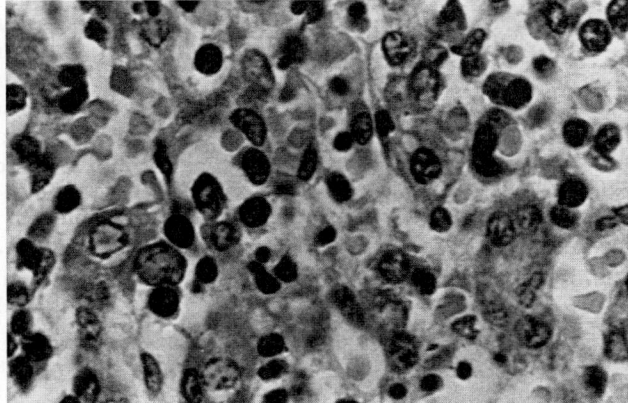

FIGURE 27–4 Fetal liver from a case of parvovirus B19–associated nonimmune hydrops shows extramedullary hematopoiesis, intranuclear inclusions in erythroblasts, and focal areas with hemosiderin and fibrosis. (Hematoxylin & eosin stain.)

eosin, the nuclei have an irregular band of dark chromatin. The center of the nucleus is lighter with a smooth texture. The specificity of intranuclear inclusions for fetal B19 infection is unknown, but it is probably high when associated with anemia and hydrops. Viral DNA or inclusions may also be present in macrophages and myocytes [131,281,290]. PCR to detect B19 DNA is the best method to diagnose B19 infection in a postmortem fetus. In one study, 6 of 34 cases of idiopathic nonimmune hydrops contained B19 DNA in either fetal or placenta tissues compared with no positive PCR results among 23 cases of hydrops that were noninfectious [338]. Histologic examination of these cases found no nucleated red blood cells with intranuclear inclusions.

PLACENTA

Parvovirus B19 infection of the placenta probably precedes fetal infection. The placenta is usually abnormal when associated with fetal death resulting from B19. Grossly, the placenta is often enlarged and edematous. Histologically, the placenta also contains nucleated red blood cells with typical intranuclear inclusions (see Fig. 27–4). Foci of red blood cell production also occur in the placenta, as does vascular inflammation [255,270,281]. In one study, vasculitis of villous capillaries or stem arteries occurred in 9 of 10 placentas [255]. There was swelling of endothelial cells, fragmentation of endothelial cell nuclei, and fibrin thrombi. B19 DNA occurs in endothelial cells of patients with myocarditis and in patients with cutaneous lesions, but has not been sought in placental endothelial cells.

The human placenta contains a B19 receptor, the neutral glycosphingolipid globoside, on the villous trophoblast layer of the placenta; the concentration of the globoside decreases with advancing pregnancy [291]. The highest concentration occurs in the first trimester with diminished reactivity in the second trimester. The presence of this globoside in the placenta provides a mechanism by which the virus infects the placenta and fetus. It also may explain why there is a difference in fetal outcome associated with gestational age. Maternal infections in late pregnancy have a better prognosis than infections occurring early in pregnancy. In addition to B19 receptors, there is also a B19-induced inflammatory response in the placenta, characterized by a significant number of CD3+ T cells and the inflammatory cytokine interleukin-2 [292].

HEART

The anemia associated with parvovirus B19 infection is due to a specific viral tropism for progenitor erythroid cells, specifically P antigen, which is found on these cells [293]. Clinical and laboratory evidence suggests, however, that B19 has a wider tropism than only erythroblasts [294]. Fetal myocardial cells contain P antigen [294]. Direct infection of myocardial cells after fetal B19 infection of extramedullary erythroid progenitor cells has been shown by in situ DNA hybridization or electron microscopy [60,72,131,295,296]. B19 myocarditis is also associated with acute lymphocytic infiltration. Case reports have described at least eight fetuses, five children, and four adults with myocarditis associated with a concurrent B19 infection [295,297–299,323–328]. B19 causes acute and chronic myocarditis in infants. This myocarditis and the cardiac enlargement present in some B19-infected fetuses with hydrops suggest that B19 is pathogenic for the myocardium.* In infected fetuses, the heart may be normal or symmetrically enlarged suggesting congestive heart failure. Pericardial effusions are common. Myocytes with intranuclear inclusions occur infrequently. Mononuclear cell infiltrates occur occasionally, and B19 DNA, not associated with cells, can be found in the lumens of large vessels. As a response to injury, focal areas with dystrophic calcification or fibroelastosis have been reported.

One case-control study examined the relationship between congenital heart disease and B19 infection [301]. Five of 29 cases of congenital heart disease had B19 DNA detected in cardiac tissue using PCR compared with none of 30 matched case controls. This difference was significant ($P < .02$). Other infections, including herpes simplex virus, cytomegalovirus, rubella, and toxoplasmosis, were excluded. Additional studies testing for B19 infection of congenital heart disease are appropriate.

OTHER ORGANS

Numerous other anatomic abnormalities have been described in association with parvovirus B19 infection of the fetus. The occurrence of these abnormalities is so infrequent, however, that it is unlikely that any are related to B19. These associated abnormalities include dystrophic calcification of the brain and adrenal glands, anencephaly and ventriculomegaly, pulmonary hypoplasia, hypospadias, cleft lip, meconium peritonitis, corneal opacification and angioedema, and thymic abnormalities.*

DIAGNOSTIC EVALUATION AND MANAGEMENT OF THE WOMAN AND FETUS EXPOSED TO OR INFECTED BY PARVOVIRUS B19 DURING PREGNANCY

OVERVIEW

Management of a pregnant woman exposed to parvovirus B19 requires knowledge of the prevailing status of EI in the community, a detailed history of the exposure, knowledge of characteristic symptoms and signs of maternal EI and B19 infection in the fetus, appropriate laboratory tests needed to confirm maternal and fetal infection, knowledge of the methods for monitoring the fetus at risk for nonimmune hydrops, knowledge of therapeutic approaches for treating the hydropic fetus, and information about the prognosis of maternal and fetal infection and the expected outcomes for the therapeutic intervention.

PREVALENCE OF ERYTHEMA INFECTIOSUM

The community health or school health departments may know if EI is endemic or epidemic in the community, increasing the probability of primary infection in susceptible pregnant women.

HISTORY OF EXPOSURE

Pregnant women who are potentially exposed to a person with EI should be asked about the type of exposure, including duration and location, brief or prolonged, household or workplace, indoor or outdoor, and contact with respiratory secretions. Exposure to a child within the household constitutes the highest risk.

Did the contact have symptoms typical of EI, including a low-grade fever and a typical slapped-cheek rash that soon spread to the trunk or limbs in a lacy pattern? Did the rash disappear and then reappear when the child was warm from exercise or bathing? Had the child been exposed to any known source of EI, such as an outbreak in school, preschool, or day care center; a family gathering; a play group; or church nursery? Was the child evaluated by a physician familiar with viral exanthems?

CLINICAL FEATURES SUGGESTING SIGNS AND SYMPTOMS OF PARVOVIRUS B19 INFECTION IN THE PREGNANT WOMAN

It should be determined if the mother's signs and symptoms are compatible with parvovirus B19 infection in adults, including at least one or more of the following: malaise, arthralgia, rash, coryza, or fever ($\geq 38°$ C). Pregnant women with such symptoms, especially malaise with symmetric arthralgias in the hands, wrists, knees, or feet, should be considered at high risk and tested for a recent B19 infection. In Barcelona, Gratacos and coworkers [22] found that only 30% of 60 IgM-positive women recalled any such symptoms. Pregnant women without such systemic symptoms but with a rapidly enlarging uterus (fundal height exceeding dates by >3 cm), an elevated serum alpha fetoprotein, preterm labor, or decreased fetal movement should be asked about B19 exposure. If ultrasonography reveals evidence of hydrops fetalis, or the fetus has ascites, pleural or pericardial effusion, skin thickening, polyhydramnios, or placentomegaly, maternal B19 testing is appropriate.

LABORATORY DIAGNOSIS IN THE PREGNANT WOMAN

With evidence of maternal parvovirus B19 exposure or maternal disease, maternal serum should be tested for IgG and IgM antibodies to B19. If there is probable or possible exposure, the first serum should be drawn at least 10 days after the exposure. Fetal morbidity is unlikely to occur within 2 weeks of exposure, so immediate serologic testing is appropriate for a woman or fetus with symptoms or signs of B19 infection.

If an initial serum sample is IgG-positive but IgM-negative, this indicates a previous maternal infection, and additional testing is usually unnecessary. The IgM assay is sensitive with few false-negative reactions. If an initial serum sample is negative for IgM and IgG, this indicates no previous maternal infection, and B19 is not responsible for maternal symptoms and signs or for hydrops fetalis.

If the IgM result is positive, a recent B19 infection is established regardless of the IgG titer. A concomitant

---

*References [131,255,257,258,267,275,281,297,300].
*References [18,20,131,254–256,258–261,273,286,302,303].

negative IgG titer indicates an early B19 infection without time for IgG to be detectable. If PCR is available, detection of maternal and fetal viremia by PCR for B19 DNA is also diagnostic of B19 infection. Viremia may precede the development of IgM antibodies by 7 to 14 days and may persist for several months after a primary infection.

A useful adjunct to IgM testing is measurement of IgG avidity to the VP1 capsid protein [304,305]. After a primary infection, initial IgG antibodies have low avidity for binding to the VP1 capsid. This avidity increases slowly over several weeks or months, and avidity can be used as a confirmatory test for the occasional patient for whom the diagnosis is initially unclear.

With a positive maternal IgM, the fetus must be examined for signs of hydrops fetalis by ultrasonography within 24 to 48 hours. If the gestational age is less than 18 weeks, the absence of hydrops may not be reassuring because hydrops could appear later. Several cases of severe hydrops fetalis spontaneously reverting to normal over 3 to 6 weeks have been reported, so advice about pregnancy termination is difficult [270,273,306].

Detection of maternal and fetal levels of B19 DNA (viral load) is a highly sensitive test for identifying B19 infection [305,307–309]. Peak maternal viral loads occur about 1 week after maternal infection, and fetal viral loads, approximately equal to maternal levels, occur 1 to 3 weeks after maternal infection. The prolonged persistence of B19 DNA in the blood means additional testing is required to establish the time of maternal infection. Viral loads are not predictive of the severity of fetal infection.

FETAL MONITORING

For a fetal gestational age of greater than 20 weeks, an initial negative ultrasound scan should be repeated weekly to detect hydrops. The number of weekly ultrasound scans that should be performed is controversial: Rodis and colleagues [256] originally suggested continuing weekly scans for 6 to 8 weeks after exposure; they reported a fetal death at 23 weeks of gestation, however, after maternal fever and arthralgias in the first trimester The interval between maternal B19 infection and fetal morbidity is uncertain. Based on this report, other authors recommended weekly ultrasound scans for 14 weeks after maternal B19 infection [306]. This monitoring often appeals to pregnant women fearful of fetal death, but it is time-consuming and expensive.

The duration of monitoring for hydrops fetalis might be best determined by examination of the interval between maternal exposure or symptoms of B19 infection and the appearance of hydrops fetalis or fetal death. Table 27–2 summarizes reports with adequate information to evaluate the interval, which include 14 intervals between maternal B19 exposure or infection and fetal death and 7 intervals between maternal exposure or infection and the first diagnosis of hydrops fetalis. The intervals range from 1 to 19 weeks (median 6 weeks). Between 3 and 11 weeks, 17 of 21 (81%) cases of hydrops fetalis developed. Because 11 of the 21 cases developed 4 to 8 weeks after maternal exposure or infection, this is the most common interval between infection and the detection of fetal hydrops.

Based on these observations, weekly ultrasound monitoring of the fetus for 12 weeks after maternal exposure is optimal, but does not detect all delayed cases and may be expensive. Such frequent scanning may not be considered cost-effective because the incidence of hydrops after maternal B19 infection is low in many studies. In our study, none of the 52 fetuses born to pregnant women positive for B19 IgM developed hydrops fetalis; however, the 95% confidence interval based on our sample size ranged from 0 to 8.6% risk for hydrops fetalis [227]. Using maternal symptoms as criteria for maternal B19 infection, other studies have suggested a 9% incidence of fetal death owing to B19 in women positive for B19 IgM [20].

The fetus in a B19-infected woman may be monitored with serial maternal serum alpha fetoprotein (MSAFP) measurements [310]. One report found elevated MSAFP in five B19 IgM–positive pregnancies associated with fetal death, but no fetal deaths in 11 IgM-positive women with B19 infection but normal MSAFP values [278]. A case of B19-associated fetal death discovered because of elevated MSAFP at 16 weeks in a routine test in an asymptomatic woman has also been described [18]. In adding a seventh case of fetal death associated with elevated MSAFP in women positive for B19 IgM, Bernstein and Capeless [310] suggested using MSAFP values to indicate a good fetal prognosis.

A German study found, however, that neither MSAFP nor human gonadotropin was a marker of B19-infected pregnancies, although both were frequently elevated when complications occurred [311]. The study included 35 pregnant women with fetal complications associated with B19; significant elevations of MSAFP occurred in 13 of 35 women, and elevations of human gonadotropin occurred in 25 of 35 women. The investigators tested 137 serum samples from 65 pregnant women without acute B19 infection and no fetal complications. Of the 30 women without fetal complications, there were significant elevations of MSAFP in only 2 women, and elevations of human gonadotropin occurred in only 5 women. Neither MSAFP nor human gonadotropin was a marker for a poor pregnancy outcome early on, but these proteins were frequently elevated when complications developed. Despite this study, there is insufficient experience using MSAFP, and MSAFP measurements at any gestational age are relatively nonspecific indicators of fetal well-being.

Electronic fetal monitoring is ineffective in detecting hydrops fetalis and predicting the outcome of pregnancy in women positive for B19 IgM. Contraction stress tests and nonstress tests are not accurate predictors of fetal well-being in cases of fetal anemia and hydrops fetalis. Similarly, fetal assessment with estriol measurements or other biochemical markers have no documented role in cases of hydrops fetalis.

Because fetal ultrasonography is readily available and provides rapid specific information about hydrops fetalis, it is the best method to monitor the fetus after maternal B19 infection. Doppler ultrasound of the middle cerebral artery may also be used to reveal increased peak systolic velocity suggestive of fetal anemia [312].

FETAL THERAPY

If hydrops fetalis is detected before 18 weeks, there is no effective intervention. Other causes of hydrops, such as chromosomal disorders or anatomic abnormalities, should be assessed. If the fetus is still viable via ultrasound at 18 weeks of gestation, percutaneous umbilical blood sampling, or cordocentesis, can be considered. At 18 weeks, the umbilical vein diameter is about 4 mm, the minimum size required for successful percutaneous umbilical blood sampling. Fetal blood should be obtained for hematocrit, reticulocyte count, platelet count, leukocyte count, anti-B19 IgM, karyotype, and tests for B19 DNA by PCR. The hematocrit must be determined immediately, and if fetal anemia is present, an intrauterine intravascular fetal transfusion is performed with the same needle puncture.

If the fetus is between 18 and 32 weeks of gestation when hydrops fetalis is detected, fetal transfusion should be considered. There are many successful reported cases of fetal transfusion for B19-induced hydrops fetalis, and some have long-term follow-up data, but the success rate of the procedure remains unknown [300,313–318]. Two or three separate transfusions are usually required before resolution of the fetal anemia and hydrops fetalis, increasing the 1% to 2% risk of each single percutaneous umbilical blood sampling procedure. Resolution of the hydrops usually occurs 3 to 6 weeks after the first transfusion. Although spontaneous resolution has been reported, it seems appropriate not to risk an uncertain outcome because the longer the fetal transfusion is delayed, the less likely it is to be successful, and the worse the potential harm to the fetus caused by continued fetal hypoxia.* Thrombocytopenia is also common and, if severe, may require intrauterine platelet transfusion [277]. There is also one report of a hydropic infant successfully treated with intraperitoneal γ-globulin high in titer to B19 [319]. For fetuses at 32 weeks' gestation or greater when hydrops is discovered, immediate delivery with neonatal exchange transfusion, thoracentesis, and paracentesis as indicated is usually the safest management.

DIFFERENTIAL DIAGNOSIS

Recalling that the hallmarks of fetal infection with parvovirus B19 are anemia, hydrops, and myocarditis helps in compiling a differential diagnosis. For infants with anemia, the differential diagnosis includes all the known causes of fetal anemia, such as fetal-maternal transfusion, intracranial bleeding, blood group incompatibilities, congenital anemias such as Diamond-Blackfan syndrome, nutritional deficiencies, and inborn metabolic errors. Fetal hydrops and fetal and placental edema may be associated with other congenital infections, particularly congenital syphilis, chromosomal abnormalities, immune hydrops associated with blood group incompatibilities, hypothyroidism, and heart and renal failure.

PROGNOSIS

Pregnant women can be reassured about the relatively low risk of fetal morbidity resulting from exposure to parvovirus B19. About half of women are already seropositive, and the seronegative maternal B19 infection rate ranges from about 29% for exposures by the woman's own children to 10% to 18% for other exposures. The expected fetal morbidity and mortality risk is around 2% (1 in 50). The overall risk of fetal death ranges from 0.3% ($\frac{1}{2} \times \frac{3}{10} \times \frac{1}{50} = \frac{3}{1000}$) to 0.1% ($\frac{1}{2} \times \frac{1}{10} \times \frac{1}{50} = \frac{1}{1000}$) [227]. Live-born infants infected in utero may die shortly after birth. There is one report of two infants born prematurely at 24 weeks and 35 weeks of age who developed an illness characteristic of congenital viral infection, including placentomegaly, petechial rash, edema, hepatomegaly, anemia, thrombocytopenia, and respiratory insufficiency; both died postnatally [320]. Both infants had nuclear inclusions in erythroid precursor cells, and PCR confirmed the presence of B19 DNA in one of the infants.

There is one report describing three live-born infants with severe CNS abnormalities after serologically confirmed maternal B19 infection [302,321]. Subsequent case reports have also identified CNS manifestations including mild to moderate hydrocephalus with CNS scarring associated with fetal B19 infection [322]. These reports suggest possible long-term neurologic sequelae in surviving infants that may not be apparent at birth.

Data regarding the long-term outcomes of live-born children infected in utero or born of mothers infected during pregnancy are very limited. In one study, 113 pregnant women with B19 infection during pregnancy and a control group of immune women were questioned about the health and development of their children when the median age of the children was 4 years for both groups [262]. The incidence of development delays in speech, language, information processing, and attention was similar between the study group and the controls (7.3% versus 7.5%). Two cases of cerebral palsy were found in the study group compared with none in the controls. Although not statistically significant, this 2% incidence of cerebral palsy in the infected group is 10-fold higher than the reported national incidence [262].

In a British study of 427 pregnant women with B19 infection and 367 of their surviving infants, 129 surviving infants were followed up at 7 to 10 years of age [329]. The follow-up included questionnaires to obstetricians and general practitioners on outcome of pregnancy and health of surviving infants. Maternal infection was confirmed by B19-specific IgM assay or IgG seroconversion or both. An excess rate of fetal loss was confined to the first 20 weeks of gestation and averaged 9%. There were seven cases of fetal hydrops with maternal infections between 9 and 20 weeks of gestation. There were no abnormalities attributable to B19 infection found at birth in surviving infants. There were no late effects observed between 7 and 10 years of age. The conclusions of this study were as follows: (1) Approximately 1 in 10 women infected before 20 weeks of gestation have a fetal loss owing to B19; (2) the risk of an adverse outcome of pregnancy beyond this stage is unlikely; and (3) infected women

---

*References [254,270,300,306,314,315].

can be reassured that the risk of congenital abnormality owing to B19 is less than 1%, and long-term development will be normal.

One study used IQ testing and standard neurodevelopmental tests to assess 20 children who had B19-induced fetal hydrops and intrauterine transfusion of packed red blood cells [313]. IQ testing of the 20 children between 13 months and 9 years of age revealed that all of the children ranged within 2 standard deviations of a population norm. There was no significant developmental delay. This study concluded that children who survived successful intrauterine transfusion from B19 anemia and hydrops had a good neurodevelopmental prognosis.

Another, more recent, study came to an opposite conclusion [330]. That study used Bayley scales of infant development to assess 16 transfused B19 hydropic fetuses who were live-born and survived. Assessments were done between 6 months and 8 years of age. Postnatal growth and health status were reported to be normal. Mild to severe developmental delay was observed in five of the children, suggesting that B19 infection may induce brain damage [330]. Most infants infected in utero with B19 survive and develop normally, but it is unlikely that all infected infants, whether owing to direct viral infection of the brain or as a consequence of intrauterine hypoxia, will develop normally.

PREVENTION
GENERAL MEASURES

Because parvovirus B19 is usually endemic in most communities, what is the appropriate management for pregnant women with daily contact with children? The prevalence of seropositivity (immunity) to B19 among pregnant women varies according to geographic location, sex, age, and race. Assuming that on average 50% of pregnant women are immune, that during endemic periods between 1% and 4% of susceptible women become infected during pregnancy, and that the rate of fetal death after maternal infection is 2%, the occupational risk of fetal death for a pregnant woman with unknown serologic status would be between 1 in 1000 and 1 in 2500. These rates are so low that they would not justify intervention such as serologic testing for pregnant women or furloughing or temporarily transferring pregnant seronegative employees to administrative or other positions without child contact. A detailed cost-benefit analysis for Germany reached the same conclusion [331]. During epidemic periods in specific schools, when the infection rates may be 5-fold to 20-fold higher, serologic testing or temporary transfer of pregnant employees may occasionally be appropriate, and some anxious women may choose to leave the workplace.

Given the low risk for individual pregnant women, seronegative women should not send their own children away. Schools and day care centers cannot stop B19 outbreaks by excluding children with rash illnesses because B19 is transmissible before the rash appears. Whether B19 can be transmitted via breast-feeding is unknown.

VACCINE DEVELOPMENT

For most women, fetal B19 infections during pregnancy do not occur from occupational exposure, but rather from exposure to school-age children at home. Given this factor, the highly communicable and endemic nature of the infection, the broad spectrum of illness that B19 causes, and the large portion of the population (30% to 50%) who are susceptible, an effective B19 vaccine, preferably administered in infancy, is appropriate, and at least one vaccine is being developed [332]. This vaccine comprises the major B19 capsid proteins VP1 and VP2 and is administered with a squalene adjuvant, MF59. After testing in a limited number of subjects, this vaccine seems safe and induces neutralizing antibodies. Studies using volunteers challenged with wild-type B19 should be able to assess efficacy. A vaccine that induces sustained neutralizing antibody IgG levels to B19 should be effective given that prior immunity to natural B19 infection protects against reinfection.

REFERENCES

[1] T. Allander, et al., Cloning of a human parvovirus by molecular screening of respiratory tract samples, Proc. Natl. Acad. Sci. U. S. A. 102 (2005) 12891–12896.
[2] D. Kesebir, et al., Human bocavirus infection in young children in the United States: molecular epidemiological profile and clinical characteristics of a newly emerging respiratory virus, J. Infect. Dis. 194 (2006) 1276–1282.
[3] F.A. Murphy et al., (Eds.), Virus Taxonomy. Sixth Report of the International Committee on Taxonomy of Viruses, Springer-Verlag, New York, 1995.
[4] N.S. Young, K.E. Brown, Parvovirus B19, N. Engl. J. Med. 350 (2004) 586–597.
[5] W.C. Koch, Fifth (human parvovirus B19) and sixth (herpesvirus 6) diseases, Curr. Opin. Infect. Dis. 14 (2001) 343–356.
[6] Y.E. Cossart, et al., Parvovirus-like particles in human sera, Lancet 1 (1975) 72–73.
[7] J. Summers, S.E. Jones, M.J. Anderson, Characterization of the genome of the agent of erythrocyte aplasia permits its classification as a human parvovirus, J. Gen. Virol. 64 (1983) 2527.
[8] J.R. Pattison, S.E. Jones, J. Hodgson, Parvovirus infections and hypoplastic crisis in sickle-cell anemia (letter), Lancet 1 (1981) 664–665.
[9] G.R. Serjeant, et al., Outbreak of aplastic crises in sickle cell anemia associated with parvovirus-like agent, Lancet 2 (1981) 595–597.
[10] M.J. Anderson, et al., Human parvovirus, the cause of erythema infectiosum (fifth disease) (letter), Lancet 1 (1983) 1378.
[11] J. Thurn, Human parvovirus B19: historical and clinical review, Rev. Infect. Dis. 10 (1988) 1005–1011.
[12] E.A. Ager, T.D.Y. Chin, J.D. Poland, Epidemic erythema infectiosum, N. Engl. J. Med. 275 (1966) 1326.
[13] J.E. Cramp, B.D.J. Armstrong, Erythema infectiosum: no evidence of teratogenicity, BMJ 2 (1977) 1031.
[14] J.R. Pattison, B19 virus infections in pregnancy, in: J.R. Pattison (Ed.), Parvoviruses and Human Disease, CRC Press, Boca Raton, FL, 1988.
[15] G. Siegel, Patterns of parvovirus disease in animals, in: J.R. Pattison (Ed.), Parvoviruses and Human Disease, CRC Press, Boca Raton, FL, 1988.
[16] T. Brown, et al., Intrauterine parvovirus infection associated with hydrops fetalis, Lancet 2 (1984) 1033.
[17] P.D. Knott, G.A.C. Welply, M.J. Anderson, Serologically proved intrauterine infection with parvovirus (letter), BMJ 289 (1984) 1960.
[18] A. Anand, et al., Human parvovirus infection in pregnancy and hydrops fetalis, N. Engl. J. Med. 316 (1987) 183.
[19] J.S. Kinney, et al., Risk of adverse outcomes of pregnancy after human parvovirus B19 infection, J. Infect. Dis. 157 (1988) 663.
[20] S.M. Hall, Public Health Laboratory Service Working Party on Fifth Disease. Prospective study of human parvovirus (B19) infection in pregnancy, BMJ 300 (1990) 1166–1170.
[21] S.P. Adler, et al., Risk of human parvovirus B19 infections among school and hospital employees during endemic periods, J. Infect. Dis. 168 (1993) 361.
[22] E. Gratacos, et al., The incidence of human parvovirus B19 infection during pregnancy and its impact on perinatal outcome, J. Infect. Dis. 171 (1995) 1360–1363.
[23] W.C. Koch, et al., Serologic and virologic evidence for frequent intrauterine transmission of human parvovirus B10 with a primary maternal infection during pregnancy, Pediatr. Infect. Dis. J. 17 (1998) 489–494.

[24] C.R. Pringle, Virus taxonomy update, Arch. Virol. 133 (1993) 491–495.

[25] C.R. Astell, et al., B19 parvovirus: biochemical and molecular features, in: L.J. Anderson, N.S. Young (Eds.), Monographs in Virology, vol. 20, Human Parvovirus B19, Karger, Basel, 1997.

[26] M.G. O'Sullivan, D.C. Anderson, J.D. Fikes, F.T. Bain, C.S. Carlson, S.W. Green, et al., Identification of a novel simian parvovirus from cynomolgus monkey with severe anemia: a paradigm for human B19 parvovirus infection, J. Clin. Invest. 93 (1994) 1571–1576.

[27] J. Mori, P. Beattie, D.W. Melton, B.J. Cohen, J.P. Clewley, Structure and mapping the DNA of human parvovirus B19, J. Gen. Virol. 68 (1987) 2797–2806.

[28] K. Umene, T. Nunoue, Genetic diversity of human parvovirus B19 determined using a set of restriction endonucleases recognizing four or five base pairs and partial nucleotide sequencing: use of sequence variability in virus classification, J. Gen. Virol. 72 (1997) 1991.

[29] G. Gallinella, et al., B19 virus genome diversity: epidemiological and clinical correlations, J. Clin. Virol. 76 (2003) 9124–9134.

[30] Q.T. Nguyen, et al., Novel human erythrovirus associated with transient aplastic crisis, J. Clin. Micro. 37 (1999) 2483–2487.

[31] Q.T. Nguyen, et al., Identification and characterization of a second human erythrovirus variant, A6, Virology 30 (2002) 374–380.

[32] A. Servant, et al., Genetic diversity within human erythroviruses: identification of three genotypes, J. Virol. 76 (2002) 9124–9134.

[33] C.S. Brown, et al., Assembly of empty capsids by using baculovirus recombinants expressing human parvovirus B19 structural proteins, J. Virol. 65 (1991) 2702–2706.

[34] S. Kajigay, et al., Self-assembled B19 parvovirus capsids, produced in a baculovirus system, are antigenically and immunogenically similar to native virions, Proc. Natl. Acad. Sci. U. S. A. 88 (1991) 4646–4650.

[35] K. Ozawa, et al., The gene encoding the nonstructural protein of B19 (human) parvovirus may be lethal in transfected cells, J. Virol. 62 (1988) 2884–2889.

[36] S. Moffat, et al., Human parvovirus B19 nonstructural protein NS1 induces apoptosis in erythroid lineage cells, J. Virol. 72 (1998) 3018–3028.

[37] N. Sol, et al., Possible interactions between the NS-1 protein and tumor necrosis factor alpha pathways in erythroid cell apoptosis induced by parvovirus B19, J. Virol. 73 (1999) 8762–8770.

[38] K. Ozawa, G. Kurtzman, N. Young, Replication of the B19 parvovirus in human bone marrow cell cultures, Science 233 (1986) 883–886.

[39] A. Srivastava, L. Lu, Replication of B19 parvovirus in highly enriched hematopoietic progenitor cells form normal human bone marrow, J. Virol. 62 (1988) 3059–3063.

[40] N. Yaegashi, et al., Propagation of human parovirus B19 in primary culture of erythroid lineage cells derived from fetal liver, J. Virol. 63 (1989) 2422–2426.

[41] T. Takahahsi, et al., B19 parvovirus replicates in erythroid leukemic cells in vitro, J. Infect. Dis. 160 (1989) 548–549.

[42] E. Miyagawa, et al., Infection of the erythroid cell line KU812Ep6 with human parvovirus B19 and its application to titration of B19 infectivity, J. Virol. Methods 83 (1999) 45–54.

[43] K.E. Brown, N.S. Young, J.M. Liu, Molecular, cellular and clinical aspects of parvovirus B19 infection, Crit. Rev. Oncol. Hematol. 16 (1994) 1–31.

[44] K.E. Brown, S.M. Anderson, N.S. Young, Erythrocyte P antigen: cellular receptor for B19 parvovirus, Science 262 (1993) 114–117.

[45] K.E. Brown, et al., Resistance to parvovirus B19 infection due to a lack of virus receptor (erythrocyte P antigen), N. Engl. J. Med. 330 (1994) 1192–1196.

[46] K.A. Weigel-Kelley, M.C. Yoder, A. Srivastava, Recombinant human parvovirus B19 vectors: erythrocyte P antigen is necessary but not sufficient for successful transduction of human hematopoietic cells, J. Virol. 75 (2001) 4110–4116.

[47] K.A. Weigel-Kelley, M.C. Yoder, A. Srivastava, Alpha5 beta 1 integrin as a cellular coreceptor for human parvovirus B19: requirement of functional activation of beta 1 integrin for viral entry, Blood 102 (2003) 3927–3933.

[48] K.E. Brown, N.S. Young, Parvovirus B19 infection and hematopoiesis, Blood Rev. 9 (1995) 176–182.

[49] N. Young, Hematologic and hematopoietic consequences of B19 infection, Semin. Hematol. 25 (1988) 159–172.

[50] A. Srivastava, et al., Parvovirus B19-induced perturbation of human megakaryocytopoiesis in vitro, Blood 76 (1990) 1997–2004.

[51] M.J. Anderson, et al., Experimental parvovirus infection in humans, J. Infect. Dis. 152 (1985) 257–265.

[52] S. Moffat, et al., A cytotoxic nonstructural protein, NS1, of human parvovirus B19 induces activation of interleukin-6 gene expression, J. Virol. 70 (1996) 8485–8491.

[53] N.L. Gilbert, et al., Seroprevalence of parvovirus B19 infection in daycare educators, Epidemiol. Infect. 133 (2005) 299–304.

[54] T. Teuscher, B. Baillod, B.R. Holzer, Prevalence of human parvovirus B19 in sickle cell disease and healthy controls, Trop. Geogr. Med. 43 (1991) 108.

[55] T.F. Schwarz, et al., Seroprevalence of human parvovirus B19 infection in São Tomé and Principe, Malawi and Mascarene Islands, Int. J. Med. Microbiol. 271 (1989) 231.

[56] P.H. Jones, et al., Human parvovirus infection in children and severe anaemia seen in an area endemic for malaria, J. Trop. Med. Hyg. 93 (1990) 67.

[57] R.B. de Freitas, et al., Prevalence of human parvovirus (B19) and rubellavirus infections in urban and remote rural areas in northern Brazil, J. Med. Virol. 32 (1990) 203.

[58] A. Gaggero, et al., Seroprevalence of IgG antibodies against parvovirus B19 among blood donors from Santiago, Chile, Rev. Med. Chil. 135 (2007) 443–448.

[59] C. Rohrer, et al., Seroprevalence of parvovirus B19 in the German population, Epidemiol. Infect. 16 (2008) 1–12.

[60] C.S. Brown, et al., Localization of an immunodominant domain on baculovirus-produced parvovirus B19 capsids: correlation to a major surface region on the native virus particle, J. Virol. 66 (1992) 69–89.

[61] A.L. Morey, et al., Immunohistological detection of human parvovirus B19 in formalin-fixed, paraffin-embedded tissues, J. Pathol. 166 (1992) 105.

[62] A.C. Loughrey, et al., Identification and use of a neutralizing epitope of parvovirus B19 for the rapid detection of virus infection, J. Med. Virol. 39 (1993) 97.

[63] F. Morinet, et al., Comparison of 17 isolates of the human parvovirus B19 by restriction enzyme analysis, Arch. Virol. 90 (1986) 165.

[64] K. Umene, T. Nunoue, The genome type of human parvovirus B19 strains isolated in Japan during 1981 differs from types detected in 1986 to 1987: a correlation between genome type and prevalence, J. Gen. Virol. 71 (1990) 983.

[65] K. Umene, T. Nunoue, Partial nucleotide sequencing and characterization of human parvovirus B19 genome DNAs from damaged human fetuses and from patients with leukemia, J. Med. Virol. 39 (1993) 333.

[66] A.L. Lawton, R.E. Smith, Erythema infectiosum: a clinical study of an epidemic in Branford, Connecticut, Arch. Intern. Med. 47 (1931) 28.

[67] L. Chargin, N. Sobel, H. Goldstein, Erythema infectiosum: report of an extensive epidemic, Arch. Dermatol. Syphilol. 47 (1943) 467.

[68] F.A.C. Galvon, An outbreak of erythema infectiosum—Nova Scotia, Can. Dis. Wkly. Rep. 9 (1983) 69.

[69] G.R. Serjeant, et al., Human parvovirus infection in homozygous sickle cell disease, Lancet 341 (1993) 1237.

[70] S.A. Oliveira, et al., Clinical and epidemiological aspects of human parvovirus B19 infection in an urban area in Brazil (Niteroi city area, State of Rio de Janeiro, Brazil), Mem. Inst. Oswaldo Cruz 97 (2002) 965–970.

[71] K. Yamashita, et al., A significant age shift of the human parvovirus B19 antibody prevalence among young adults in Japan observed in a decade, Jpn. J. Med. Sci. Biol. 45 (1992) 49.

[72] S.J. Naides, Erythema infectiosum (fifth disease) occurrence in Iowa, Am. J. Public Health 78 (1988) 1230.

[73] B.J. Cohen, M.M. Buckley, The prevalence of antibody to human parvovirus B19 in England and Wales, J. Med. Microbiol. 25 (1988) 151.

[74] J.P. Nascimento, et al., The prevalence of antibody to human parvovirus B19 in Rio de Janeiro, Brazil, Rev. Inst. Med. Trop. São Paulo 32 (1990) 41.

[75] R.N. Edelson, R.A. Altman, Erythema infectiosum: a statewide outbreak, J. Med. Soc. N. J. 67 (1970) 805.

[76] G.H. Werner, et al., A new viral agent associated with erythema infectiosum, Ann. N. Y. Acad. Sci. 67 (1957) 338.

[77] P. Greenwald, W.J. Bashe Jr., An epidemic of erythema infectiosum, Am. J. Dis. Child. 107 (1964) 30.

[78] N. Yaegashi, et al., Prevalence of anti-human parvovirus antibody in pregnant women, Nippon Sanka Fujinka Gakkai Zasshi 42 (1990) 162.

[79] W.C. Koch, S.P. Adler, Human parvovirus B19 infections in women of childbearing age and within families, Pediatr. Infect. Dis. J. 8 (1989) 83.

[80] B.J. Cohen, P.P. Mortimer, M.S. Pereira, Diagnostic assays with monoclonal antibodies for the human serum parvovirus-like virus (SPLV), J. Hyg. (Lond.) 91 (1983) 113.

[81] T.F. Schwarz, M. Roggendorf, F. Deinhardt, Häufigkeit der parvovirus-B19-infektionen. Seroepidemiologishe untersuchungen, Dtsch. Med. Wochenschr. 112 (1987) 1526.

[82] O. Bartolomei Corsi, et al., Human parvovirus infection in haemophiliacs first infused with treated clotting factor concentrates, J. Med. Virol. 25 (1988) 165.

[83] H. Eiffert, et al., Expression of an antigenic polypeptide of the human parvovirus B19, Med. Microbiol. Immunol. 179 (1990) 169.

[84] C.S. Brown, et al., An immunofluorescence assay for the detection of parvovirus B19 IgG and IgM antibodies based on recombinant viral antigen, J. Virol. Methods 29 (1990) 53.

[85] H. Rollag, et al., Prevalence of antibodies against parvovirus B19 in Norwegians with congenital coagulation factor defects treated with plasma products from small donor pools, Scand. J. Infect. Dis. 23 (1991) 675.

[86] M.M.M. Salimans, et al., Recombinant parvovirus B19 capsids as a new substrate for detection of B19-specific IgG and IgM antibodies by an enzyme-linked immunosorbent assay, J. Virol. Methods 39 (1992) 247.

[87] T.F. Schwarz, B. Hottenträger, M. Roggendorf, Prevalence of antibodies to parvovirus B19 in selected groups of patients and healthy individuals, Int. J. Med. Microbiol. Virol. Parasitol. Infect. Dis. 276 (1992) 437.

[88] A.J. Vyse, N.J. Andrews, L.M. Hesketh, The burden of parvovirus B19 infection in women of childbearing age in England and Wales, Epidemiol. Infect. 135 (2007) 1354–1362.

[89] K.H. Lin, et al., Seroepidemiology of human parvovirus B19 in Taiwan, J. Med. Virol. 57 (1999) 169–173.

[90] A.M. Couroucé, et al., Parvovirus (SPLV) et antigène Aurillac, Rev. Fr. Transfus. Immunohematol. 27 (1984) 5.

[91] Y. Cossart, Parvovirus B19 finds a disease (letter), Lancet 2 (1981) 988.

[92] H.J. O'Neill, P.V. Coyle, Two anti-parvovirus B19 IgM capture assays incorporating a mouse monoclonal antibody specific for B19 viral capsid proteins VP1 and VP2, Arch. Virol. 123 (1992) 125.

[93] B.J. Cohen, et al., Blood donor screening for parvovirus B19, J. Virol. Methods 30 (1990) 233.

[94] A. da Silva Cruz, et al., Detection of the human parvovirus B19 in a blood donor plasma in Rio de Janeiro, Mem. Inst. Oswaldo Cruz 84 (1989) 279.

[95] F. McOmish, et al., Detection of parvovirus B19 in donated blood: a model system for screening by polymerase chain reaction, J. Clin. Microbiol. 31 (1993) 323.

[96] N. Yaegashi, et al., Enzyme-linked immunosorbent assay for IgG and IgM antibodies against human parvovirus B19: use of monoclonal antibodies and viral antigen propagated in vitro, J. Virol. Methods 26 (1989) 171.

[97] S.J. Naides, et al., Rheumatologic manifestations of human parvovirus B19 infection in adults, Arthritis Rheum. 33 (1990) 1297.

[98] F. Martinez-Campillo, et al., Parvovirus B19 outbreak in a rural community in Alicante, Enferm. Infecc. Microbiol. Clin. 20 (2002) 376–379.

[99] K. Abarca, B.J. Cohen, P.A. Vial, Seroprevalence of parvovirus B19 in urban Chilean children and young adults, 1990 and 1996, Epidemiol. Infect. 128 (2002) 59–62.

[100] K. Smith-Whitley, et al., The epidemiology of human parvovirus B19 in children with sickle cell disease, Blood 103 (2003) 422.

[101] F.A. Plummer, et al., An erythema infectiosum-like illness caused by human parvovirus infection, N. Engl. J. Med. 313 (1985) 74.

[102] T. Chorba, et al., The role of parvovirus B19 in aplastic crisis and erythema infectiosum (fifth disease), J. Infect. Dis. 154 (1986) 383–393.

[103] P.P. Mortimer, Hypothesis: the aplastic crisis of hereditary spherocytosis is due to a single transmissible agent, J. Clin. Pathol. 36 (1983) 445.

[104] U.A. Saarinen, et al., Human parvovirus B19 induced epidemic red-cell aplasia in patients with hereditary hemolytic anemia, Blood 67 (1986) 1411.

[105] A. Valeur-Jensen, et al., Risk factors for parvovirus B19 infection in pregnancy, JAMA 281 (1999) 1099–1105.

[106] M.J. Anderson, et al., An outbreak of erythema infectiosum associated with human parvovirus infection, J. Hyg. (Lond.) 93 (1984) 85.

[107] J.G. Tuckerman, T. Brown, B.J. Cohen, Erythema infectiosum in a village primary school: clinical and virological studies, J. R. Coll. Gen. Pract. 36 (1986) 267.

[108] P. Morgan-Capner, et al., Sex ratio in outbreaks of parvovirus B19 infection (letter), Lancet 2 (1987) 98.

[109] F. Mansfield, Erythema infectiosum: slapped face disease, Aust. Fam. Physician 17 (1988) 737.

[110] A.D. Woolf, et al., Clinical manifestations of human parvovirus B19 in adults, Arch. Intern. Med. 149 (1989) 1153.

[111] A. Turner, O. Olojugba, Erythema infectiosum in a primary school: investigation of an outbreak in Bury, Public Health 103 (1989) 391.

[112] E.A. Grilli, M.J. Anderson, T.W. Hoskins, Concurrent outbreaks of influenza and parvovirus B19 in a boys' boarding school, Epidemiol. Infect. 103 (1989) 359.

[113] S.M. Gillespie, et al., Occupational risk of human parvovirus B19 infection for school and day-care personnel during an outbreak of erythema infectiosum, JAMA 263 (1990) 2061.

[114] L.J. Anderson, et al., Risk of infection following exposures to human parvovirus B19, Behring Inst. Mitt. 85 (1990) 60.

[115] P.S. Rice, B.J. Cohen, A school outbreak of parvovirus B19 infection investigated using salivary antibody assays, Epidemiol. Infect. 6 (1996) 331–338.

[116] L.M. Bell, et al., Human parvovirus B19 infection among hospital staff members after contact with infected patients, N. Engl. J. Med. 321 (1989) 485.

[117] D. Pillay, et al., Parvovirus B19 outbreak in a children's ward, Lancet 339 (1992) 107.

[118] B.J. Cohen, et al., Laboratory infection with parvovirus B19 (letter), J. Clin. Pathol. 41 (1988) 1027.

[119] H. Shiraishi, et al., Laboratory infection with human parvovirus B19 (letter), J. Infect. 22 (1991) 308.

[120] J.P.M. Evans, et al., Human parvovirus aplasia: case due to cross infection in a ward, BMJ 288 (1984) 681.

[121] K. Ueda, et al., Human parvovirus infection (letter), N. Engl. J. Med. 314 (1986) 645.

[122] D. Pillay, et al., Secondary parvovirus B19 infection in an immunocompromised child, Pediatr. Infect. Dis. J. 10 (1991) 623.

[123] S.L. Lui, et al., Nosocomial outbreak of parvovirus B19 infection in a renal transplant unit, Transplantation 71 (2001) 59–64.

[124] K. Miyamoto, et al., Outbreak of human parvovirus B19 in hospital workers, J. Hosp. Infect. 45 (2000) 238–241.

[125] D.E. Koziol, et al., Nosocomial human parvovirus B19 infection: lack of transmission from a chronically infected patient to hospital staff, Infect. Control Hosp. Epidemiol. 13 (1992) 343.

[126] S.F. Dowell, et al., Parvovirus B19 infection in hospital workers. Community or hospital acquisition, J. Infect. Dis. 172 (1995) 1076–1079.

[127] M.L. Carter, et al., Occupational risk factors for infection with parvovirus B19 among pregnant women, J. Infect. Dis. 163 (1991) 282.

[128] S.M. Ray, et al., Nosocomial exposure to parvovirus B19: low risk of transmission to healthcare workers, Infect. Control Hosp. Epidemiol. 18 (1997) 109–114.

[129] G. Patou, et al., Characterization of a nested polymerase chain reaction assay for detection of parvovirus B19, J. Clin. Microbiol. 31 (1993) 540.

[130] C.G. Potter, et al., Variation of erythroid and myeloid precursors in the marrow of volunteer subjects infected with human parvovirus (B19), J. Clin. Invest. 79 (1987) 1486.

[131] A.L. Morey, et al., Non-isotopic in situ hybridisation and immunophenotyping of infected cells in investigation of human fetal parvovirus infection, J. Clin. Pathol. 45 (1992) 673–678.

[132] P.P. Mortimer, et al., Transmission of serum parvovirus-like virus by clotting-factor concentrates, Lancet 2 (1983) 482.

[133] D.J. Lyon, et al., Symptomatic parvovirus B19 infection and heat-treated factor IX concentrate (letter), Lancet 1 (1989) 1085.

[134] M.D. Williams, et al., Transmission of human parvovirus B19 by coagulation factor concentrates, Vox Sang. 58 (1990) 177.

[135] M. Morfini, et al., Hypoplastic anemia in a hemophiliac first infused with a solvent/detergent treated factor VIII concentrate: the role of human B19 parvovirus (letter), Am. J. Hematol. 39 (1992) 149.

[136] K. Zakrzewska, et al., Human parvovirus B19 in clotting factor concentrates: B19 DNA detection by the nested polymerase chain reaction, Br. J. Haematol. 81 (1992) 407.

[137] T.F. Schwarz, et al., Removal of parvovirus B19 from contaminated factor VIII during fractionation, J. Med. Virol. 35 (1991) 28.

[138] A. Azzi, et al., Human parvovirus B19 infection in hemophiliacs infused with two high purity, virally attenuated factor VIII concentrates, Am. J. Hematol. 39 (1992) 228.

[139] M.J. Anderson, Rash illness due to B19 virus, in: J.R. Pattison (Ed.), Parvoviruses and Human Disease, CRC Press, Boca Raton, FL, 1988.

[140] L.J. Anderson, Role of parvovirus B19 in human disease, Pediatr. Infect. Dis. 6 (1987) 711–718.

[141] A.M. Garcia-Tapia, et al., Spectrum of parvovirus B19 infection: analysis of an outbreak of 43 cases in Cadiz, Spain, Clin. Infect. Dis. 21 (1995) 424–430.

[142] M. Zerbini, et al., Different syndromes associated with B19 parvovirus viraemia in paediatric patients: report of four cases, Eur. J. Pediatr. 151 (1992) 815–817.

[143] H. Tsuda, Y. Maeda, K. Nakagawa, Parvovirus B19-related lymphadenopathy, Br. J. Haematol. 85 (1993) 631–632.

[144] K.E. Brown, Human parvovirus B19 epidemiology and clinical manifestations, in: L.J. Anderson, N.S. Young (Eds.), Monographs in Virology, vol. 20, Karger, Basel, 1997, pp. 42–60.

[145] J.J. Lefrere, et al., Henoch-Schonlein purpura and human parvovirus infection, Pediatrics 78 (1986) 183–184.

[146] P.W. Saunders, M.M. Reid, B.J. Cohen, Human parvovirus induced cytopenias: a report of five cases, Br. J. Haematol. 63 (1986) 407–410.

[147] J.J. Lefrere, A.M. Courouce, C. Kaplan, Parvovirus and idiopathic thrombocytopenic purpura (letter), Lancet 1 (1989) 279.

[148] T.J. Török, Parvovirus B19 and human disease, Adv. Int. Med. 37 (1992) 431–455.

[149] D.G. White, et al., Human parvovirus arthropathy, Lancet 1 (1985) 419–421.

[150] S.J. Naides, E.H. Field, Transient rheumatoid factor positivity in acute human parvovirus B19 infection, Arch. Intern. Med. 148 (1988) 2587–2589.

[151] D.M. Reid, et al., Human parvovirus-associated with arthritis: a clinical and laboratory description, Lancet 1 (1985) 422–425.

[152] J.J. Nocton, et al., Human parvovirus B19-associated arthritis in children, J. Pediatr. 122 (1993) 186–190.

[153] B.A. Dijkmans, et al., Human parvovirus B19 DNA in synovial fluid, Arthritis Rheum. 31 (1998) 279–281.

[154] J.G. Saal, et al., Persistence of B19 parvovirus in synovial membranes of patients with rheumatoid arthritis, Rheumatology 12 (1992) 147–151.

[155] A. Mimori, et al., Prevalence of antihuman parvovirus B19 IgG antibodies in patients with refractory rheumatoid arthritis and polyarticular juvenile rheumatoid arthritis, Rheumatol. Int. 14 (1994) 87–90.

[156] M. Soderlund, et al., Persistence of parvovirus B19 DNA in synovial membranes of young patients with and without chronic arthropathy, Lancet 349 (1997) 1063–1065.

[157] H.D. Stahl, et al., Detection of multiple viral DNA species in synovial tissue and fluid of patients with early arthritis, Ann. Rheum. Dis. 59 (2000) 342–346.

[158] J.R. Kerr, Pathogenesis of human parvovirus B19 in rheumatic disease, Ann. Rheum. Dis. 59 (2000) 672–683.

[159] W.C. Koch, et al., Manifestations and treatment of human parvovirus B19 infection in immunocompromised patients, J. Pediatr. 116 (1990) 355–359.

[160] D.K. Van Horn, et al., Human parvovirus-associated red cell aplasia in the absence of hemolytic anemia, Am. J. Pediatr. Hematol-Oncol. 8 (1986) 235–239.

[161] G.J. Kurtzman, et al., Chronic bone marrow failure due to persistent B19 parvovirus infection, N. Engl. J. Med. 317 (1987) 287–294.

[162] N. Frickhofen, et al., Persistent B19 parvovirus infection in patients infected with human immunodeficiency virus type 1 (HIV-1): a treatable cause of anemia in AIDS, Ann. Intern. Med. 113 (1990) 926–933.

[163] H.T. Weiland, et al., Prolonged parvovirus B19 infection with severe anaemia in a bone marrow transplant recipient (letter), Br. J. Haematol. 71 (1989) 300.

[164] G. Kurtzman, et al., Pure red-cell aplasia of ten years' duration due to persistent parvovirus B19 infection and its cure with immunoglobulin therapy, N. Engl. J. Med. 321 (1989) 519–523.

[165] T.Y. Wong, et al., Parvovirus B19 infection causing red cell aplasia in renal transplantation on tacrolimus, Am. J. Kidney Dis. 34 (1999) 1119–1123.

[166] D. Geetha, et al., Pure red cell aplasia caused by parvovirus B19 infection in solid organ transplant recipients: a case report and review of the literature, Clin. Transplant. 14 (2000) 586–591.

[167] S. Pamidi, et al., Human parvovirus infection presenting as persistent anemia in renal transplant recipients, Transplantation 69 (2000) 2666–2669.

[168] Z.R. Zolnourian, et al., Parvovirus B19 in kidney transplant patients, Transplantation 69 (2000) 2198–2202.

[169] M. Seishima, H. Kanoh, T. Izumi, The spectrum of cutaneous eruptions in 22 patients with isolated serological evidence of infection by parvovirus B19, Arch. Dermatol. 135 (1999) 1556–1557.

[170] J.J. Lefrere, et al., Human parvovirus and aplastic crisis in chronic hemolytic anemias: a study of 24 observations, Am. J. Hematol. 23 (1986) 271–275.

[171] T.H. Finkel, et al., Chronic parvovirus B19 infection and systemic necrotising vasculitis. Opportunistic infeciton or aetiological agent, Lancet 343 (1994) 1255–1258.

[172] T.F. Schwarz, S. Wiersbitzky, M. Pambor, Case report: detection of parvovirus B19 in skin biopsy of a patient with erythema infectiosum, J. Med. Virol. 43 (1994) 171–174.

[173] C.M. Magro, M.R. Dawood, A.N. Crowson, The cutaneous manifestations of human parvovirus B19 infection, Hum. Pathol. 31 (2000) 488–497.

[174] P.J. Ferguson, et al., Prevalence of human parvovirus B19 infection in children with Henoch-Schonlein purpura, Arthritis Rheum. 39 (1996) 880–881.

[175] P.T. Smith, M.L. Landry, H. Carey, et al., Papular-purpuric gloves and socks syndrome associated with acute parvovirus B19 infection: case report and review, Clin. Infect. Dis. 27 (1997) 164–168.

[176] R. Grilli, et al., Papular-purpuric "gloves and socks" syndrome: polymerase chain reaction demonstration of parvovirus B19 DNA in cutaneous lesions and sera, J. Am. Acad. Dermatol. 41 (1999) 793–796.

[177] F.T. Saulsbury, Petechial gloves and socks syndrome caused by parvovirus B19, Pediatr. Dermatol. 15 (1998) 35–37.

[178] C. Brass, L.M. Elliott, D.A. Stevens, Academy rash: a probable epidemic of erythema infectiosum ("fifth disease"), JAMA 248 (1982) 568–572.

[179] A. Tsuji, et al., Aseptic meningitis with erythema infectiosum, Eur. J. Pediatr. 149 (1990) 449–450.

[180] H.H. Balfour Jr., G.M. Schiff, J.E. Bloom, Encephalitis associated with erythema infectiosum, JAMA 77 (1970) 133–136.

[181] C.B. Hall, F.A. Horner, Encephalopathy with erythema infectiosum, Am. J. Dis. Child. 131 (1977) 65–67.

[182] A. Okumura, T. Ichikawa, Aseptic meningitis caused by human parvovirus B19, Arch. Dis. Child. 68 (1993) 784–785.

[183] P. Cassinotti, et al., Persistent human parvovirus B19 infection following an acute infection with meningitis in an immunocompetent patient, Eur. J. Clin. Microbiol. Infect. Dis. 12 (1993) 701–704.

[184] T. Watanabe, M. Satoh, Y. Oda, Human parvovirus B19 encephalopathy, Arch. Dis. Child. 70 (1994) 71.

[185] K.J. Walsh, R.D. Armstrong, A.M. Turner, Brachial plexus neuropathy associated with human parvovirus infection, BMJ 296 (1988) 896.

[186] H. Faden, G.W. Gary Jr., M. Korman, Numbness and tingling of fingers associated with parvovirus B19 infection, J. Infect. Dis. 161 (1990) 354–355.

[187] O. Dereure, B. Montes, J.J. Guilhou, Acute generalized livedo reticularis with myasthenia-like syndrome revealing parvovirus B19 primary infection, Arch. Dermatol. 131 (1995) 744–745.

[188] K. Samii, et al., Acute bilateral carpal tunnel syndrome associated with human parvovirus B19 infection, Clin. Infect. Dis. 22 (1996) 162–164.

[189] H. Faden, G.W. Gary Jr., L.J. Anderson, Chronic parvovirus infection in a presumably immunologically healthy woman, Clin. Infect. Dis. 15 (1992) 595–597.

[190] F. Barah, et al., Neurological manifestations of human parvovirus B19 infection, Rev. Med. Virol. 13 (2003) 185–199.

[191] T. Nakazawa, et al., Acute glomerulonephritis after human parvovirus B19 infection, Am. J. Kidney Dis. 35 (2000) E31.

[192] A. Komatsuda, et al., Endocapillary proliferative glomerulonephritis in a patient with parvovirus B19 infection, Am. J. Kidney Dis. 36 (2000) 851–854.

[193] F. Diaz, J. Collazos, Glomerulonephritis and Henoch-Schoenlein purpura associated with acute parvovirus B19 infection, Clin. Nephrol. 53 (2000) 237–238.

[194] S. Tanawattanacharoen, et al., Parvovirus B19 DNA in kidney tissue of patients with focal segmental glomerulosclerosis, Am. J. Kidney Dis. 35 (2000) 1166–1174.

[195] R.M. Klein, et al., Frequency and quantity of the parvovirus B19 genome in endomyocardial biopsies from patients with suspected myocarditis or idiopathic left ventricular dysfunction, Z. Kardiol. 93 (2004) 300–309.

[196] K. Munro, et al., Three cases of myocarditis in childhood associated with human parvovirus (B19 virus), Pediatr. Cardiol. 24 (2003) 473–475.

[197] S. Lamparter, et al., Acute parvovirus B19 infection associated with myocarditis in an immunocompetent adult, Hum. Pathol. 34 (2003) 725–728.

[198] X. Wang, et al., Prevalence of human parvovirus B19 DNA in cardiac tissues of patients with congenital heart diseases indicated by nested PCR and in situ hybridization, J. Clin. Virol. 31 (2004) 20–24.

[199] B.D. Bultmann, et al., High prevalence of viral genomes and inflammation in peripartum cardiomyopathy, Am. J. Obstet. Gynecol. 195 (2006) 330–331.

[200] U. Kuhl, et al., Viral persistence in the myocardium is associated with progressive cardiac dysfunction, Circulation 112 (2005) 1965–1970.

[201] F. Kuethe, et al., Detection of viral genome in the myocardium: lack of prognostic and functional relevance in patients with acute dilated cardiomyopathy, Am. Heart J. 153 (2007) 850–858.

[202] F. Tavora, et al., Fatal parvoviral myocarditis: a case report and review of literature, Diagn. Pathol. 3 (2008) 21.

[203] T. Marton, W.L. Martin, M.J. Whittle, Hydrops fetalis and neonatal death from human parvovirus B19: an unusual complication, Prenat. Diagn. 7 (2005) 543–545.

[204] M. Nyman, L. Skjoldebrand-Sparre, K. Broliden, Non-hydropic intrauterine fetal death more than 5 months after primary parvovirus B19 infection, J. Perinat. Med. 33 (2005) 176–178.

[205] L.J. Anderson, et al., Detection of antibodies and antigens of human parvovirus B19 by enzyme-linked immunosorbent assay, J. Clin. Microbiol. 24 (1986) 522.

[206] B.J. Cohen, C.M. Bates, Evaluation of 4 commercial test kits for parvovirus B19-specific IgM, J. Virol. Methods 55 (1995) 11–25.

[207] W.C. Koch, A synthetic parvovirus B19 capsid protein can replace viral antigen in antibody-capture enzyme immunoassays, J. Virol. Methods 55 (1995) 67–82.

[208] J.A. Jordan, Comparison of a baculovirus-based VP2 enzyme immunoassay (EIA) to an *Escherichia coli*-based VP1 EIA for detection of human parvovirus B19 immunoglobulin M and immunoglobulin G in sera of pregnant women, J. Clin. Microbiol. 38 (2000) 1472–1475.

[209] S. Doyle, et al., Detection of parvovirus B19 IgM by antibody capture enzyme immunoassay: receiver operating characteristics analysis, J. Virol. Methods 90 (2000) 143–152.

[210] J.P. Clewly, Detection of human parvovirus using a molecularly cloned probe, J. Med. Virol. 15 (1985) 383–393.

[211] J.P. Clewly, Polymerase chain reaction assay of parvovirus B19 DNA in clinical specimens, J. Clin. Microbiol. 27 (1989) 2647.

[212] W.C. Koch, S.P. Adler, Detection of human parvovirus B19 DNA by using the polymerase chain reaction, J. Clin. Microbiol. 28 (1990) 65–69.

[213] E.D. Heegard, et al., Parvovirus B19 infection and Diamond-Blackfan anemia, Acta Pediatr. 85 (1996) 299–302.

[214] T.W. Crook, et al., Unusual bone marrow manifestations of parvovirus B19 infection in immunocompromised patients, Hum. Pathol. 31 (2000) 161–168.

[215] S.P. Adler, J.H. Harger, W.C. Koch, Infections due to human parvovirus B19 during pregnancy, in: M. Martens, S. Faro, D. Soper (Eds.), Infectious Diseases in Women, Saunders, Philadelphia, 2001.

[216] P.H. van Gessel, et al., Incidence of parvovirus B19 infection among an unselected population of pregnant women in the Netherlands: a prospective study, Eur. J. Obstet. Gynecol. Reprod. Biol. 128 (2006) 46–49.

[217] J. Mossong, et al., Parvovirus B19 infection in five European countries: seroepidemiology, force of infection and maternal risk of infection, Epidemiol. Infect. 24 (2007) 1–10.

[218] M. Enders, A. Weidner, G. Enders, Current epidemiological aspects of human parvovirus B19 infection during pregnancy and childhood in the western part of Germany, Epidemiol. Infect. 135 (2007) 563–569.

[219] D. Candotti, et al., Maternal-fetal transmission of human parvovirus B19 genotype 3, J. Infect. Dis. 194 (2006) 608–611.

[220] L. Skjoldebrand-Sparre, et al., A prospective study of antibodies against parvovirus B19 in pregnancy, Acta Obstet. Gynecol. Scand. 75 (1996) 336–339.

[221] P.P. Mortimer, et al., Human parvovirus and the fetus (letter), Lancet 2 (1985) 1012.

[222] V.S. Wiersbitzky, et al., Seroprävalenz von Antikörpern gegen das humane parvovirus B19 (Ringelröteln/erythema infectiosum) in der DDR-Bevölkerung, Kinderärztl. Prax. 58 (1990) 185.

[223] B.D. Schoub, et al., Primary and secondary infection with human parvovirus B19 in pregnant women in South Africa, S. Afr. Med. J. 83 (1993) 505–506.

[224] R. Barros De Freitas, et al., Survey of parvovirus B19 infection in a cohort of pregnant women in Belem, Brazil, Braz. J. Infect. Dis. 3 (1999) 6–14.

[225] G. Enders, M. Biber, Parvovirus B19 infections in pregnancy, Behring Inst. Mitt. 85 (1990) 74.

[226] B.B. Rogers, et al., Detection of human parvovirus B19 in early spontaneous abortuses using serology, histology, electron microscopy, in situ hybridization, and the polymerase chain reaction, Obstet. Gynecol. 81 (1993) 402.

[227] J.H. Harger, et al., Prospective evaluation of 618 pregnant women exposed to parvovirus B19: risks and symptoms, Obstet. Gynecol. 91 (1998) 413–420.

[228] J.R. Kerr, M.D. Curran, J.E. Moore, Parvovirus B19 infection—persistence and genetic variation, Scand. J. Infect. Dis. 27 (1995) 551–557.

[229] H. Chisaka, et al., Clinical manifestations and outcomes of parvovirus B19 infection during pregnancy in Japan, Tohoku J. Exp. Med. 209 (2006) 277–283.

[230] T.F. Schwarz, et al., Human parvovirus B19 infection in pregnancy (letter), Lancet 2 (1988) 566–567.

[231] E.S. Gray, A. Anand, T. Brown, Parvovirus infections in pregnancy (letter), Lancet 1 (1986) 208.

[232] T. Brown, L.D. Ritchie, Infection with parvovirus during pregnancy, BMJ 290 (1985) 559–560.

[233] J.S. Kinney, et al., Risk of adverse outcomes of pregnancy after human parvovirus B19 infection, J. Infect. Dis. 157 (1988) 663–667.

[234] J.F. Rodis, et al., Management and outcomes of pregnancies complicated by human B19 parvovirus infection: a prospective study, Am. J. Obstet. Gynecol. 163 (1990) 1168.

[235] T.J. Torok, et al., Reproductive outcomes following human parvovirus B19 infection in pregnancy (abstract 1374), in: Program and Abstracts of 31st ICAAC (Chicago), American Society for Microbiology, Washington, DC, 1991.

[236] M. Enders, et al., Fetal morbidity and mortality after acute human parvovirus B19 infection in pregnancy: prospective evaluation of 1018 cases, Prenat. Diagn. 24 (2004) 513–518.

[237] D. Xu, G. Zhang, R. Wang, The study on detection of human parvovirus B19 DNA in spontaneous abortion tissues, Zhonghua Shi Yan He Lin Chuang Bing Du Xue Za Zhi 12 (1998) 158–160.

[238] R. Wang, X. Chen, M. Han, Relationship between human parvovirus B19 infection and spontaneous abortion, Zhonghua Fu Chan Ke Za Zhi 32 (1997) 541–543.

[239] R.R. De Krijger, et al., Detection of parvovirus B19 infection in first and second trimester fetal loss, Pediatr. Pathol. Lab. Med. 18 (1998) 23–34.

[240] M. Makhseed, et al., Pattern of parvovirus B19 infection during different trimesters of pregnancy in Kuwait, Infect. Dis. Obstet. Gynecol. 7 (1997) 287–292.

[241] E. Lowden, L. Weinstein, Unexpected second trimester pregnancy loss due to maternal parvovirus B19 infection, South Med. J. 90 (1997) 702–704.

[242] L. Skjoldebrand-Sparre, et al., Parvovirus B19 infection: association with third-trimester intrauterine fetal death, Br. J. Obstet. Gynaecol. 107 (2000) 476–480.

[243] T. Nunoue, K. Kusuhara, T. Hara, Human fetal infection with parvovirus B19: maternal infection time in gestation, viral persistence and fetal prognosis, Pediatr. Infect. Dis. J. 21 (2002) 1133–1136.

[244] O. Norbeck, et al., Revised clinical presentation of parvovirus B19-associated intrauterine fetal death, Clin. Infect. Dis. 35 (2002) 1032–1038.

[245] T. Tolfvenstam, et al., Frequency of human parvovirus B19 infection in intrauterine fetal death, Lancet 357 (2001) 1494–1497.

[246] T.N. Leung, et al., Fetal parvovirus B19 infection in a twin pregnancy with 1 twin presenting with hydrops fetalis and the other asymptomatic: a case report, J. Reprod. Med. 5 (2007) 419–421.

[247] J.E. Dickinson, A.D. Keil, A.K. Charles, Discordant fetal infection for parvovirus B19 in a dichorionic twin pregnancy, Twin Res. Hum. Genet. 9 (2006) 456–459.

[248] M. el-Sayed Zaki, H. Goda, Relevance of parvovirus B19, herpes simplex virus 2, and cytomegalovirus virologic markers in maternal serum for diagnosis of unexplained recurrent abortions, Arch. Pathol. Lab. Med. 131 (2007) 956–960.

[249] J. Kishore, I. Gupta, Serological study of parvovirus B19 infection in women with recurrent spontaneous abortions, Indian J. Pathol. Microbiol. 49 (2006) 548–550.

[250] W.C. Koch, S.P. Adler, J. Harger, Intrauterine parvovirus B19 infection may cause an asymptomatic or recurrent postnatal infection, Pediatr. Infect. Dis. J. 12 (1993) 747–750.

[251] H.T. Weiland, et al., Parvovirus B19 associated with fetal abnormality (letter), Lancet 1 (1987) 682.

[252] N.G. Hartwig, et al., Embryonic malformations in a case of intrauterine parvovirus B19 infection, Teratology 39 (1989) 295.

[253] N.G. Hartwig, C. Vermeij-Keers, J. Versteeg, The anterior eye segment in virus induced primary congenital aphakia, Acta Morphol. Neerl. Scand. 26 (1988–1989) 283.

[254] M. Zerbini, et al., Symptomatic parvovirus B19 infection of one fetus in a twin pregnancy, Clin. Infect. Dis. 17 (1993) 262.

[255] A.L. Morey, et al., Clinical and histopathological features of parvovirus B19 infection in the human fetus, Br. J. Obstet. Gynaecol. 99 (1992) 566.

[256] J.F. Rodis, et al., Human parvovirus infection in pregnancy, Obstet. Gynecol. 72 (1988) 733.

[257] S.J. Naides, C.P. Weiner, Antenatal diagnosis and palliative treatment of non-immune hydrops fetalis secondary to fetal parvovirus B19 infection, Prenat. Diagn. 9 (1989) 105.

[258] V.L. Katz, N.C. Chescheir, M. Bethea, Hydrops fetalis from B19 parvovirus infection, J. Perinatol. 10 (1990) 366.

[259] M.C. Bloom, et al., Infection materno-foetale à parvovirus associée à une péritonite meconiale anétnatale, Arch. Fr. Pediatr. 47 (1990) 437.

[260] J.D. Bernard, et al., Infection materno-foetale à parvovirus humain B19: a propos de deux observations, J. Gynecol. Obstet. Biol. Reprod. 20 (1991) 855.

[261] T.F. Schwarz, et al., Parvovirus B19 infection of the fetus: histology and in situ hybridization, Am. J. Clin. Pathol. 96 (1991) 121.

[262] J.F. Rodis, et al., Long-term outcome of children following maternal human parvovirus B19 infection, Obstet. Gynecol. 91 (1998) 125–128.

[263] J.M. Jouannic, et al., Isolated fetal hyperechogenic bowel associated with intrauterine parvovirus B19 infection, Fetal Diagn. Ther. 20 (2005) 498–500.

[264] H.J. Porter, et al., Parvovirus as a cause of hydrops fetalis: detection by in situ DNA hybridisation, J. Clin. Pathol. 41 (1988) 381–383.

[265] N. Yaegashi, et al., The frequency of human parvovirus B19 infection in nonimmune hydrops fetalis, J. Perinat. Med. 22 (1994) 159–163.

[266] K.P. Gloning, et al., Successful intrauterine treatment of fetal hydrops caused by parvovirus B19 infection, Behring Inst. Mitt. 85 (1990) 79.

[267] B.B. Rogers, Y. Mark, C.E. Oyer, Diagnosis and incidence of fetal parvovirus infection in an autopsy series. I. Histology, Pediatr. Pathol. 13 (1993) 371.

[268] Y. Mark, B.B. Rogers, C.E. Oyer, Diagnosis and incidence of fetal parvovirus infection in an autopsy series. II. DNA amplification, Pediatr. Pathol. 13 (1993) 381.

[269] M.T. Peters, K.H. Nicolaides, Cordocentesis for the diagnosis and treatment of human fetal parvovirus infection, Obstet. Gynecol. 75 (1990) 501.

[270] P.G. Pryde, et al., Spontaneous resolution of nonimmune hydrops fetalis secondary to human parvovirus B19 infection, Obstet. Gynecol. 79 (1992) 859.

[271] R. Metzman, et al., Hepatic disease associated with intrauterine parvovirus B19 infection in a newborn premature infant, J. Pediatr. Gastroenterol. Nutr. 9 (1989) 112.

[272] R.A. Franciosi, P. Tattersall, Fetal infection with human parvovirus B19, Hum. Pathol. 19 (1988) 489.

[273] M. Zerbini, et al., Comparative evaluation of virological and serological methods in prenatal diagnosis of parvovirus B19 fetal hydrops, J. Clin. Microbiol. 34 (1996) 603–608.

[274] D.B. Lewis, C.B. Wilson, Developmental immunology and role of host defenses in neonatal susceptibility to infection, in: J.S. Remington, J.O. Klein (Eds.), Infectious Diseases of the Fetus and Newborn Infant, fourth ed., Saunders, Philadelphia, 1995.

[275] T.J. Török, et al., Prenatal diagnosis of intrauterine infection with parvovirus B19 by the polymerase chain reaction technique, Clin. Infect. Dis. 14 (1992) 149.

[276] A.L. Morey, et al., In vitro culture for the detection of infectious human parvovirus B19 and B19-specific antibodies using foetal haematopoietic precursor cells, J. Gen. Virol. 73 (1992) 3313.

[277] T.R. de Haan, et al., Thrombocytopenia in hydropic fetuses with parvovirus B19 infection: incidence, treatment and correlation with fetal B19 viral load, Br. J. Obstet. Gynaecol. 115 (2008) 76–81.

[278] D. Carrington, et al., Maternal serum alpha-fetoprotein-a marker of fetal aplastic crisis during intrauterine human parvovirus infection, Lancet 1 (1987) 433–435.

[279] M.J. Anderson, et al., Human parvovirus B19 and hydrops fetalis (letter), Lancet 1 (1988) 535.

[280] V. Sahakian, et al., Intrauterine transfusion treatment of nonimmune hydrops fetalis secondary to human parvovirus B19 infection, Am. J. Obstet. Gynecol. 164 (1991) 1090.

[281] H.J. Porter, A.M. Quantrill, K.A. Fleming, B19 parvovirus infection of myocardial cells (letter), Lancet 1 (1988) 535.

[282] A.G. Nerlich, et al., Pathomorphologie der fetalen parvovirus-B19-infektion, Pathologe 12 (1991) 204.

[283] P.J. Berry, et al., Parvovirus infection of the human fetus and newborn, Semin. Diagn. Pathol. 9 (1992) 4.

[284] E.O. Caul, M.J. Usher, P.A. Burton, Intrauterine infection with human parvovirus B19: a light and electron microscopy study, J. Med. Virol. 24 (1988) 55.

[285] H. Maeda, et al., Nonimmunologic hydrops fetalis resulting from intrauterine human parvovirus B19 infection: report of 2 cases, Obstet. Gynecol. 71 (1988) 482–485.

[286] A.M.W. van Elsacker-Niele, et al., Fetal pathology in human parvovirus B19 infection, Br. J. Obstet. Gynaecol. 96 (1989) 768.

[287] D. Bonneau, et al., L'infection à parvovirus B19 au cours de la grossesse, J. Gynecol. Obstet. Biol. Reprod. 20 (1991) 1109.

[288] C. Glaser, J. Tannenbaum, Newborn with hydrops and a rash, Pediatr. Infect. Dis. J. 11 (1992) 980–984.

[289] A. Nerlich, et al., Parvovirus B19-infected erythroblasts in fetal cord blood (letter), Lancet 337 (1991) 310.

[290] A.L. Morey, K.A. Fleming, Immunophenotyping of fetal hematopoietic cells permissive for human parvovirus B19 replication in vitro, Br. J. Haematol. 82 (1992) 302.

[291] J.A. Jordan, J.A. DeLoia, Globoside expression within the human placenta, Placenta 20 (1999) 103–108.

[292] J.A. Jordan, D. Huff, J.A. DeLoia, Placental cellular immune response in women infected with human parvovirus B19 during pregnancy, Clin. Diagn. Lab. Immunol. 8 (2001) 288–292.

[293] K.E. Brown, Human parvovirus B19 infections in infants and children, Adv. Pediatr. Infect. Dis. 13 (1998) 101–126.

[294] E.D. Heegaard, A. Hornsleth, Parvovirus: the expanding spectrum of disease, Acta Paediatr. 84 (1995) 109–117.

[295] M. Respondek, et al., Parvovirus particles in a fetal heart with myocarditis: ultrastructural and immunohistochemical study, Arch. Immunol. Ther. Exp. (Warsz) 45 (1997) 465–470.

[296] H.J. Porter, A.M. Quantrill, K.A. Fleming, B19 parvovirus infection of myocardial cells, Lancet (1988) 535–536.

[297] G. Nigro, et al., Acute and chronic lymphocytic myocarditis in infancy is associated with parvovirus B19 infection and high cytokine levels, Clin. Infect. Dis. 31 (2000) 65–69.

[298] E.D. Heegaard, et al., Parvovirus B19 infection associated with myocarditis following adult cardiac transplantation, Scand. J. Infect. Dis. 30 (1998) 607–610.

[299] N. Papadogiannakis, et al., Active, fulminant, lethal myocarditis associated with parvovirus B19 infection in an infant, Clin. Infect. Dis. 35 (2002) 1027–1031.

[300] B.W. Kovacs, et al., Prenatal diagnosis of human parvovirus B19 in nonimmune hydrops fetalis by polymerase chain reaction, Am. J. Obstet. Gynecol. 167 (1992) 461–466.

[301] X. Wang, et al., Investigation of parvovirus B19 in cardiac tissue from patients with congenital heart disease, Chin. Med. J. (Engl.) 112 (1999) 995–997.

[302] J.A. Conry, T. Török, P.I. Andrews, Perinatal encephalopathy secondary to in utero human parvovirus B-19 (HPV) infection (abstract 736S), Neurology 43 (Suppl.) (1993) A346.

[303] N. Plachouras, et al., Severe nonimmune hydrops fetalis and congenital corneal opacification secondary to human parvovirus B19 infection. A case report, J. Reprod. Med. 44 (1999) 377–380.

[304] M. Enders, et al., Human parvovirus B19 infection during pregnancy—value of modern molecular and serological diagnostics, J. Clin. Virol. 35 (2006) 400–406.

[305] M. Enders, et al., Improved diagnosis of gestational parvovirus B19 infection at the time of nonimmune fetal hydrops, J. Infect. Dis. 197 (2008) 58–62.

[306] A.U. Sheikh, J.M. Ernest, M. O'Shea, Long-term outcome in fetal hydrops from parvovirus B19 infection, Am. J. Obstet. Gynecol. 167 (1992) 337.

[307] T.R. de Haan, et al., Parvovirus B19 infection in pregnancy studies by maternal viral load and immune responses, Fetal Diagn. Ther. 22 (2007) 55–62.

[308] T.R. de Haan, et al., Parvovirus B19 infection in pregnancy: maternal and fetal viral load measurements related to clinical parameters, Prenat. Diagn. 27 (2007) 46–50.

[309] M. Dobec, A. Juchler, A. Flaviano, Prolonged parvovirus b19 viremia in spite of neutralizing antibodies after erythema infectiosum in pregnancy, Gynecol. Obstet. Invest. 63 (2007) 53–54.

[310] I.A. Bernstein, E.L. Capeless, Elevated maternal serum alpha-fetoprotein and hydrops fetalis in association with fetal parvovirus B19 infection, Obstet. Gynecol. 774 (1989) 456–457.

[311] K. Komischke, K. Searle, G. Enders, Maternal serum alpha-fetoprotein and human chorionic gonadotropin in pregnant women with acute parvovirus B19 infection with and without fetal complications, Prenat. Diagn. 17 (1997) 1039–1046.

[312] A. Kempe, et al., First-trimester treatment of fetal anemia secondary to parvovirus B19 infection, Ultrasound Obstet. Gynecol. 29 (2007) 226–228.

[313] J. Dembinski, et al., Neurodevelopmental outcome after intrauterine red cell transfusion for parvovirus B19-induced fetal hydrops, Br. J. Obstet. Gynaecol. 109 (2002) 1232–1234.

[314] W. Humphrey, M. Magoon, R. O'Shaughnessy, Severe nonimmune hydrops secondary to parvovirus B-19 infection: spontaneous reversal in utero and survival of a term infant, Obstet. Gynecol. 78 (1991) 900–902.

[315] A.L. Morey, et al., Parvovirus B19 infection and transient fetal ascites, Lancet 337 (1991) 496.

[316] T.F. Schwartz, et al., Human parvovirus B19 infection in pregnancy, Lancet 2 (1988) 566–567.

[317] P. Soothill, Intrauterine blood transfusion for non-immune hydrops fetalis due to parvovirus B19 infection, Lancet 356 (1990) 121–122.

[318] V. Sahakian, et al., Intrauterine transfusion treatment of nonimmune hydrops fetalis secondary to human parvovirus B19 infection, Am. J. Obstet. Gynecol. 164 (1991) 1090–1091.

[319] H. Matsuda, et al., Intrauterine therapy for parvovirus B19 infected symptomatic fetus using B19 IgG-rich high titer gammaglobulin, J. Perinat. Med 33 (2005) 561–563.

[320] H. Vogel, et al., Congenital parvovirus infection, Pediatr. Pathol. Lab. Med. 17 (1997) 903–912.

[321] T.T. Torok, Human parvovirus B19, in: J.S. Remington, J.O. Klein (Eds.), Infectious Diseases of the Fetus and Newborn Infant, fifth ed., Saunders, Philadelphia, 2001.

[322] V.L. Katz, et al., An association between fetal parvovirus B19 infection and fetal anomalies: a report of two cases, Am. J. Perinatol. 13 (1996) 43–45.

[323] G. Enders, et al., Life-threatening parvovirus B19-associated myocarditis and cardiac transplantation as possible therapy: two case reports, Clin. Infect. Dis. 26 (1998) 355–358.

[324] T. Orth, et al., Human parvovirus B19 infection associated with severe acute perimyocarditis in a 34-year-old man, Eur. Heart J. 18 (1997) 524–525.

[325] J.K.S. Chia, B. Jackson, Myopericarditis due to parvovirus B19 in an adult, Clin. Infect. Dis. 23 (1996) 200–201.

[326] C. Malm, E. Fridell, K. Jansson, Heart failure after parvovirus B19 infection, Lancet 341 (1993) 1408–1409.

[327] J. Saint-Martin, et al., Myocarditis caused by parvovirus, J. Pediatr. 116 (1990) 1007–1008.

[328] K.O. Schowengerdt, et al., Association of parvovirus B19 genome in children with myocarditis and cardiac allograft rejection: diagnosis using the polymerase chain reaction, Circulation 96 (1997) 3549–3554.

[329] E. Miller, et al., Immediate and long term outcome of human parvovirus B19 infection in pregnancy, Br. J. Obstet. Gynaecol. 105 (1998) 14–18.

[330] H.T. Nagel, et al., Long-term outcome after fetal transfusion for hydrops associated with parvovirus B19 infection, Obstet. Gynecol. 109 (2007) 42–47.

[331] B. Gartner, et al., Parvovirus B19 infections in pregnant women in day care facilities: health economic analysis of prohibition to employ seronegative women, Bundesgesundheitsblatt Gesundheitsforschung Gesundheitsschutz 50 (2007) 1369–1378.

[332] W.R. Ballou, et al., Safety and immunogenicity of a recombinant parvovirus B19 vaccine formulated with MF59C.1, J. Infect. Dis. 187 (2003) 675–678.

[333] P.R. Bond, et al., Intrauterine infection with human parvovirus (letter), Lancet 1 (1986) 448–449.

[334] C.H. Woernle, et al., Human parvovirus B19 infection during pregnancy, J. Infect. Dis. 156 (1987) 17–26.

[335] J.S. Samra, M.S. Obhrai, G. Constantine, Parvovirus infection in pregnancy, Obstet. Gynecol. 73 (1989) 832–834.

[336] P.P. Mortimer, et al., Human parvovirus and the fetus, Lancet 2 (1985) 1012.

[337] C.P. Weiner, S.J. Naides, Fetal survival after human parvovirus B19 infection: spectrum of intrauterine response in a twin gestation, Am. J. Perinatol. 9 (1992) 66.

[338] J.A. Jordan, Identification of human parvovirus B19 infection in idiopathic nonimmune hydrops fetalis, Am. J. Obstet. Gynecol. 174 (1996) 37–42.

[339] C.M. Magro, et al., Parvoviral infection of endothelial cells and its possible role in vasculitis and autoimmune diseases, J. Reumatol. 29 (2002) 1227–1235.

[340] M. Douvoyiannis, N. Litman, L. Goldman, Neurologic manifestations associated with parvovirus B19 infection, Clin. Infect. Dis. 48 (2009) 1713–1723.

[341] B. Guidi, et al., Case of stroke in a 7-year-old male after parvovirus B19 infection, Pediatr. Neurol. 28 (2003) 69–71.

[342] K.J. Wierenga, B.E. Serjeant, G.R. Serjeant, Cerebrovascular complications and parvovirus infection in homozygous sickle cell disease, J. Pediatr. 139 (2001) 438–442.

[343] J.L. Craze, A.J. Salisbury, M.G. Pike, Prenatal stroke associated with maternal parvovirus infection, Dev. Med. Child Neurol. 38 (1996) 84–85.

[344] T.R. De Haan, et al., Fetal stroke and congenital parvovirus B19 infection complicated by activated protein C resistance, Acta Paediatr. 95 (2006) 863–867.

CHAPTER
28

RUBELLA

Stanley A. Plotkin ⊗ Susan E. Reef ⊗ Louis Z. Cooper ⊗ Charles A. Alford, Jr.

CHAPTER OUTLINE

Virus 862
  Morphology and Physical and Chemical Composition 862
  Classification 864
  Antigen and Serologic Testing 864
  Growth in Cell Culture 865
  Pathogenicity for Animals 865
Epidemiology 865
Transmission In Utero 867
  Risk of Fetal Infection 868
  Risk of Congenital Defects 869
Natural History 869
  Postnatal Infection 869
  Congenital Infection 871
Pathogenesis 874
  Postnatal Infection 874
  Congenital Infection 874
Pathology 875
  Postnatal Infection 875
  Congenital Infection 875

Clinical Manifestations 876
  Postnatal Infection 876
  Congenital Infection 876
Laboratory Diagnosis 881
  Maternal Infection 881
  Congenital Infection 883
Management Issues 884
  Use of Immunoglobulin 884
  Termination of Pregnancy 884
  Clinical Management 885
  Chemotherapy 886
  Isolation 886
Prevention of Congenital Rubella 886
  Rubella Vaccine and Immunization Strategies 886
  Outbreak Control 889
  Surveillance 889
  Strategies for Elimination of Rubella and Congenital Rubella
    Syndrome 889

The impact of rubella virus infection and the progress made toward controlling congenital rubella infection have been well chronicled [1–9]. Rubella was first recognized in the mid-18th century as a clinical entity by German researchers, who called it *Rötheln*. They considered it to be a modified form of measles or scarlet fever [1]. Manton [10] first described it as a separate disease in the English literature in 1815. In 1866, Veale [11] gave it a "short and euphonious" name—*rubella*. The disease was considered mild and self-limited.

Rubella became a focus of major interest in 1941, after Gregg [12], an Australian ophthalmologist, associated intrauterine acquisition of infection with production of cataracts and heart disease. Although his findings were initially doubted, numerous reports of infants with congenital defects after maternal rubella infection soon appeared in the literature [1]. Subsequent investigations showed that the major defects associated with congenital rubella infection included congenital heart disease, cataracts, and deafness. Mental retardation and many defects involving almost every organ have also been reported [2–4,7,13,14]. Before the availability of specific viral diagnostic studies, the frequency of fetal damage after maternal infection in the first trimester was estimated to be greater than 20%, a figure now known to be much too low.

Recognition of the teratogenic potential of rubella infection led to increased efforts to isolate the etiologic agent. The viral cause of rubella was suggested by experimental infections in humans and monkeys in 1938, but was not confirmed until the isolation of the viral agent in cell cultures was reported independently in 1962 by Weller and Neva at Harvard University School of Public Health and by Parkman, Buescher, and Artenstein at Walter Reed Army Institute for Research [15–20]. This accomplishment paved the way for the development of serologic tests and a vaccine [2–4,21–23]. Efforts to develop a vaccine were hastened by events associated with a worldwide rubella pandemic in 1962–1964, which in the United States resulted in approximately 12.5 million cases of clinically acquired rubella, 11,000 fetal deaths, and 20,000 infants born with defects collectively referred to as congenital rubella syndrome (CRS); 2100 infants with CRS died in the neonatal period [24]. The estimated cost to the U.S. economy was approximately $2 billion. Routine use of rubella vaccine, in a two-dose schedule as measles-mumps-rubella vaccine (MMR), has not prevented importation-related infection, but it has eliminated endemic rubella in the United States [25]. CRS remains a problem in many countries, however, with current estimates of 110,000 new cases annually in developing countries [26].

In 1969, three strains of live-attenuated rubella vaccine were licensed in various countries: HPV-77 (high-passage virus, 77 times), grown in duck embryo for five passages (DE-5) or dog kidney for 12 passages (DK-12); Cendehill, grown in primary rabbit cells; and RA 27/3 (rubella abortus, 27th specimen, third explant), grown in human diploid fibroblast culture [27–29]. The RA 27/3 vaccine has been used exclusively in the United States since 1979 and is now the only strain in global use outside of Japan and China [2–4,7,30,31].

In addition to providing the impetus for vaccine research and development, the rubella pandemic provided the scientific community with a unique opportunity to gain knowledge about the nature of intrauterine and extrauterine infections and the immunity stimulated by both. The quest for more knowledge using the tools of molecular biology has continued since vaccine licensure and serves as a tribute to Gregg's historic contribution to our understanding of intrauterine infection.

Much interest has focused on the epidemiology of rubella and CRS in countries with immunization programs, the desirability of introducing vaccine in countries without a program, and the optimal strategy to control congenital rubella (i.e., universal immunization versus selective immunization of females versus combined strategy of universal vaccination and selective immunization) [3,5–7,32–38]. Vaccination of all children and of susceptible adolescents and young adults, particularly women, has had such a dramatic impact on the occurrence of rubella and congenital rubella in the United States that it has resulted in the elimination of endemic rubella and CRS from the United States [5,24,33,39,40]. Given the magnitude of international travel, the goal of eradication of rubella will remain elusive until similar goals are adopted by other countries. In 2003, the Pan American Health Organization (PAHO) adopted a resolution calling on all countries of the Western Hemisphere to eliminate rubella by 2010, a goal that appears to have now been achieved [41]. Among developing countries, rubella immunization has not yet been given priority, however.

Duration and quality of vaccine-induced immunity [5,8,42–61] and adverse events associated with immunization, particularly arthritis and the risk of the vaccine to the fetus [5,8,62–69], have been a concern, but the vaccine continues to confer long-lasting immunity, while placing the vaccinated person at minimal risk of adverse events. Success in eliminating endemic disease in the United States and the absence of teratogenicity observed after massive immunization programs (2001–2002) in Latin America offer considerable assurance about the long-term efficacy and safety of rubella vaccine. In Brazil, 28 million women were immunized in mass campaigns, and in Costa Rica, more than 2400 susceptible pregnant women were immunized. Although infants were infected, none had evidence of CRS.

Research on the characteristics of the rubella virus, its effect on the developing fetus, the host's immune response, and diagnostic methodology has yielded new information about the structural proteins of the virus and about the difference in the immune response to these proteins after congenital and acquired infections [70–90]. Differences in antibody profile may be useful in diagnosing congenital infection retrospectively and may provide further information on the pathogenesis of congenital infection [68,89,91]. Techniques that detect rubella-specific antibodies within minutes have been developed by using latex agglutination and passive hemagglutination

[92–98]. Studies to examine the subclass distribution of IgG and the kinetics of rubella-specific immunoglobulins (including IgA, IgD, and IgE) after acquired rubella, congenital infection, and vaccination may eventually lead to the development of additional diagnostic tools [99–103]. In particular, rubella IgG avidity testing can be helpful in distinguishing between recently acquired and remote infection [104–106].

Improved laboratory methods defined the risk of fetal infection and congenital damage in all stages of pregnancy [107–114]. The risk of fetal infection after first-trimester maternal infection and subsequent congenital anomalies after fetal infection may be higher than previously reported (81% and 85% in one study) [109]. The fetus may be at risk of infection throughout pregnancy, even near term, although the occurrence of defects after infection beyond 16 to 18 weeks of gestation is small. Sensitive laboratory assays have shown that subclinical reinfection after previous natural infection, as after vaccination, may be accompanied by an IgM response, making differentiation between subclinical reinfection and asymptomatic primary infection difficult sometimes [45,55,57,59]. IgG avidity testing may be helpful in this situation. Although reinfection usually poses no threat to the fetus, rare instances of congenital infection after maternal reinfection have been reported.*

Follow-up of patients with congenital rubella has provided information about the pathogenesis, immune status, interplay between congenital infection and human leukocyte antigen (HLA) haplotypes, and long-term outcome associated with congenital infection [121–138]. These studies have documented that congenital infection is persistent; that virtually every organ may be affected; and that autoimmunity and immune complex formation are probably involved in many of the disease processes, particularly in the delayed and persistent clinical manifestations. They also confirm earlier studies, noting an increased risk of diabetes mellitus and other endocrinopathies in patients with CRS compared with rates for the general population.

VIRUS
MORPHOLOGY AND PHYSICAL AND CHEMICAL COMPOSITION

Rubella virus is a generally spherical particle, 50 to 70 nm in diameter, with a dense central nucleoid measuring 30 nm in diameter. The central nucleoid is surrounded by a 10-nm-thick, single-layered envelope acquired during budding of the virus into cytoplasmic vesicles or through the plasma membrane [139–153]. Surface projections or spikes with knobbed ends that are 5 to 6 nm long have been reported. The specific gravity of the complete viral particle is 1.184 ± 0.004 g/mL, corresponding to a sedimentation constant of 360 ± 50 Svedberg units [139].

The wild-type virus contains within its core infectious positive strand RNA (molecular weight of 3 to 4×10^6)

*References 45, 47, 49, 51, 55–57, 59, 115–120.

containing 9800 nucleotides [124]. Full-length and subgenomic RNA are produced, and it is from the latter that viral structural proteins are translated. The rubella virus envelope contains lipids that differ quantitatively from lipids of the plasma membrane and are essential for infectivity [154,155]. Rubella virus is heat labile and has a half-life of 1 hour at 57° C [156]. In the presence of protein (e.g., 2% serum albumin), infectivity is maintained for 1 week or more at 4° C, however, and indefinitely at −60° C. Storage at freezer temperatures of −10° C to −20° C should be avoided because infectivity is rapidly lost [156,157]. Rubella virus can also be stabilized against heat inactivation by the addition of magnesium sulfate to virus suspensions [158]. Specimens for virologic examination should be transported to distant laboratories packed in ice rather than frozen, with the addition of stabilizer if possible. Infectivity is rapidly lost at pH levels less than 6.8 or greater than 8.1 and exhausted in the presence of ultraviolet light; lipid-active solvents; or other chemicals such as formalin, ethylene oxide, and β-propiolactone [156,159–161]. Infectivity of rubella in cell culture is inhibited by amantadine, but this drug seems to have no therapeutic effect [162–165].

Several laboratories have described the structural proteins of rubella virus and determined the nucleotide sequence of the genes coding for these proteins [70,85,139,166–169]. Originally, three structural proteins were identified and designated as VP-1, VP-2, and VP-3 [166]. These three major structural proteins now are designated E1, E2, and C, with relative molecular weights of 58,000, 42,000 to 47,000, and 33,000 [71–73]. E1 and E2 are envelope glycoproteins and make up the characteristic spikelike projections that are located on the viral membrane. Structural protein C, which is not glycosylated, is associated with the infectious 40S genomic RNA to form the nucleocapsid [75]. The E2 glycopeptide has been shown on polyacrylamide gels to be heterogeneous with two bands, which are designated E2a (relative molecular weight of 42,000) and E2b (relative molecular weight of 47,000) [71].

Monoclonal antibody studies have begun to delineate the functional activities of these structural proteins. E1 seems to be the viral hemagglutinin and binds hemagglutination-inhibiting and hemolysis-inhibiting antibody; E2 does not seem to be involved in hemagglutination [70,72,74,76–79]. Monoclonal antibodies specific for E1 and E2 have neutralizing activity because both proteins are involved in cell entry.*

Studies also indicate that there are multiple epitopes on the structural proteins that are involved in hemagglutination inhibition (HI) and neutralizing activities [79,82]. Molecular analyses of rubella viruses isolated during 1961–1997 from specimens obtained in North America, Europe, and Asia have documented the remarkable antigenic stability of the E1 envelope glycoprotein [84]. E1 amino acid sequences have differed by no more than 3%, indicating no major antigenic variation over the 36-year period that spanned the major worldwide pandemic of 1962–1964 and the 30 years since introduction of rubella vaccine. Two clades and 10 genotypes were evident, however [172]: Genotype I was isolated before 1970 and grouped into a single diffuse clade, indicating intercontinental circulation, whereas most of the post-1975 viruses segregated into geographic clades from each continent, indicating evolution in response to vaccination programs. Clade 2 seems to be Asian in origin [173].

Figure 28–1 shows the geographic distribution of the genotypes [174]. The availability of molecular analysis and the minor variations in amino acid sequences have provided an additional tool for monitoring the sources of infection in areas where indigenous rubella has been greatly reduced by high levels of immunization. As discussed in more detail later, the complexity of the

*References 74, 80, 89, 90, 170, 171.

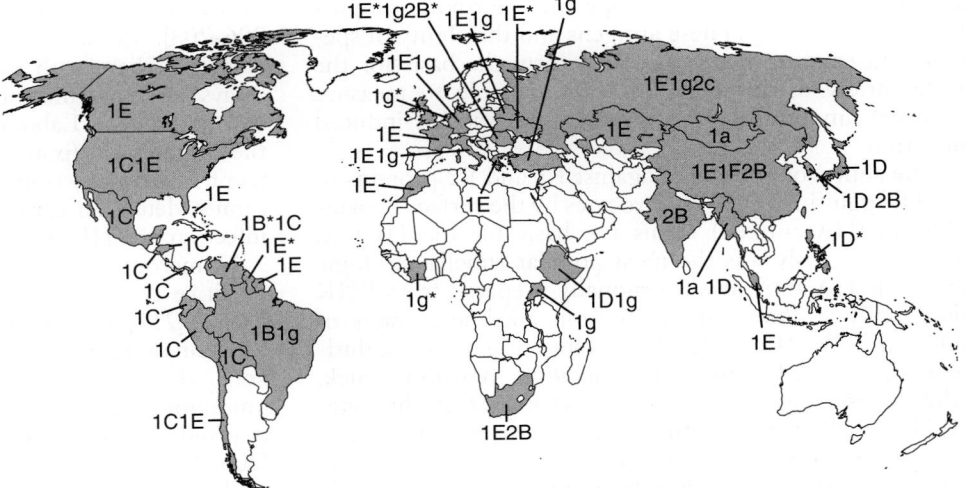

FIGURE 28–1 Global distribution of indigenous rubella viruses, 1995-2006. Data summarize information available as of the end of November 2006. *Shading* indicates countries where circulating rubella viruses have been identified. During this period, some countries reduced indigenous rubella transmission to low levels (e.g., Canada, the United Kingdom, and the United States).

*Viruses characterized after being imported into another country.

antigenic nature of the rubella virion affects the ability of the host to respond to the full complement of antigens and affects the various antibody assays required to detect all the corresponding antibody responses (see "Natural History").

CLASSIFICATION

Rubella has been classified as a member of the Togaviridae family (from the Latin word *toga*, meaning "cloak"), genus *Rubivirus* [175,176]. No serologic relationship exists between rubella and other known viruses. Minor biologic differences identified in different passaged strains of rubella virus are not reflected in the antigenic differences assessed by comparing protein composition or serologic reactions [139,169,177,178]. Differences in the immune response after immunization with the various vaccines now in use are not caused by inherent differences in the viral strain, but rather by modification of the viruses during their attenuation in cell culture [30]. The reported variation in the virulence of rubella epidemics does not seem to be explained by the molecular analyses described earlier, but it may result from differences in population susceptibility and underreporting of cases of congenital rubella [179–186].

ANTIGEN AND SEROLOGIC TESTING

Rubella virus may be isolated in cell culture from nasopharynx, serum, urine, cataracts, placenta, amniotic fluid, and fetal tissues. The nasopharynx is the best source because excretion is more persistent there. RK13 and Vero cells are the best substrates. Virus isolation takes many days to become positive and confirmed by neutralization, however. During pregnancy, it is important to attempt more rapid diagnosis through the use of reverse transcriptase polymerase chain reaction (PCR) [187]. Amniotic fluid is the best source, although chorionic villi and placenta may be positive. Primers come from nucleotides located between 731 and 854 of the E1 gene [188,189].

Purified rubella virus has many antigenic components associated with the viral envelope and the ribonucleoprotein core [161,167]. These antigens and the ability of specific antiserum to neutralize virus form the basis for the wide variety of serologic methods available to measure humoral immunity after natural and vaccine-induced infection.

The ability of antibodies against E1 and E2 proteins to inhibit agglutination of erythrocytes by the surface hemagglutinin (HA antigen) forms the basis for the HI test, which previously was the most popular rubella serologic test. The HA antigen was originally prepared from BHK tissue culture fluids and then from alkaline extracts of infected BHK-21 cells [23,190]. This antigen can agglutinate various red blood cells, including newborn chick, adult goose, pigeon, and human group O erythrocytes [191]. Rubella hemagglutinin is unique in its dependency on calcium ions to attach to red blood cell receptors [191,192]. After extraction from infected cells, rubella hemagglutinin is stable for months at −20° C, several weeks at 4° C, and overnight at 37° C, but is destroyed within minutes after heating to 56° C [190,192]. The HA

antigen can be protected from ether inactivation by pretreatment with polysorbate 80 (Tween 80).

Cells and serum contain heat-stable β-lipoproteins that can inhibit rubella hemagglutination and give rise to false-positive results [23,161]. Although it has been reported that nonspecific inhibitors do not interfere in the HI test if the HA antigen and erythrocytes are mixed before addition of serum, the recommended method is to pretreat the sera to remove these inhibitors [161,193]. Earlier test procedures used kaolin adsorption for removal of these nonspecific inhibitors; however, many faster and more specific methods are now used, such as treatment with heparin-$MnCl_2$ or dextran sulfate-$CaCl$ [194,195].

Cell-associated complement fixation antigen was first derived from infected rabbit kidney (RK-13) and African green monkey kidney cell cultures and later prepared from alkaline extracts of infected BHK-21 cells [22,196]. There are two complement fixation antigens: One is similar in size and weight to the hemagglutinin and infectious virus, and the other is smaller and "soluble" [170,197,198]. The antibody response as measured by the soluble antigen develops more slowly than the response to the larger antigen, which parallels the HI response. In contrast to the HA antigen, complement fixation antigens do not lose their antigenicity after either treatment [196,198].

Various precipitin antigens have been shown serologically; two of these, the theta and iota antigens, are associated with the viral envelope and core [199–201]. The antibody response to these two antigens is of interest. Antibodies to the theta antigen rise promptly and persist. Antibodies to the iota antigen are detectable later and for a shorter time [202]. The RA 27/3 vaccine seems to be unique among vaccine strains in its ability to elicit a response to the iota antigen, making its immune response more similar to natural infection. The significance of this observation is unclear [203].

Rubella virus antigen-antibody complexes (involving the envelope and the core antigens) cause aggregation of platelets [204,205]. The main platelet aggregation activity seems to reside with the viral envelope, however.

Antibody directed against the rubella virus can also be measured by virus neutralization in tissue culture [2–4,21, 206–208]. Although the presence of neutralizing antibodies correlates best with protective immunity, neutralization assays are time-consuming, expensive, and relatively difficult to perform. Laboratories have traditionally performed the complement fixation and HI tests. Because the complement fixation test is insensitive for screening purposes and cannot detect an early rise in antibody in acute acquired infection, the HI test has been the most widely used assay.*

Numerous more rapid, easily performed, reliable, and sensitive tests have replaced the HI test for routine use [92,210,211], including passive (or indirect) hemagglutination; single radial hemolysis (also known as hemolysis in gel), which is used widely abroad; radioimmunoassay; immunofluorescence; and enzyme immunoassay tests, also referred to as enzyme-linked immunosorbent assays [206,209–240]. Rapid latex agglutination and passive hemagglutination assays can provide results in minutes for

---

*References 2–4, 161, 202, 206, 209, 210.

screening and diagnostic purposes [92–98]. The numerous assays now available and their greater sensitivity compared with the HI test have led to some confusion about the level of antibody that should be considered indicative of immunity (see "Update on Vaccine Characteristics") [48,58,61, 210,238]. The HI test remains the reference test against which other assays are compared, however.

Immunoglobulin class-specific antibody can be measured in most of the serologic systems.* This most frequently involves detection of IgM in whole or fractionated sera. Numerous techniques are used to fractionate and then test the serum. An important consideration in any IgM assay is the possibility of false-positive results because of the presence of rheumatoid factor. Solid-phase IgM capture assays seem to be unaffected, however, by rheumatoid factor [103–106,221,236,247].

GROWTH IN CELL CULTURE

Rubella replicates in a wide variety of cell culture systems, primary cell strains, and cell lines [157,161,250]. The time required for virus recovery varies markedly, depending partly on the culture system being employed.

Generally, rubella growing in primary cell cultures (i.e., human, simian, bovine, rabbit, canine, or duck) produces interference to superinfection by a wide variety of viruses (especially enteroviruses, but also myxoviruses, papovaviruses, arboviruses, and to some extent herpesviruses), but no cytopathic effect [19,20,156]. In contrast, a cytopathic effect of widely varying natures results from infection of continuous cell lines (i.e., hamster, rabbit, simian, and human). Generally, primary cells, especially African green monkey kidney, have proved superior for isolation of virus from human material by the interference technique. The continuous RK-13 and Vero (vervet monkey kidney) cell lines are also used, however, because cytopathic effect is produced, and there is no problem with adventitious simian agents [157]. Continuous cell lines, such as BHK-21 and Vero, are best suited for antigen production because of the higher levels of virus produced.

All cell lines support chronic infection with serial propagation, but some are limited by the occurrence of cytopathic effect. These cells grow slowly and can be subcultivated fewer times than when not infected [157]. The mechanisms of rubella-induced interference and persistent infection in cell cultures are not completely understood. Although interferon production has been described after rubella infection of cell cultures, interference seems to be an intrinsic phenomenon [157,161,251–253]. As with other viruses, generation of defective interfering particles can be found in tissue culture [254]. These particles are thought to be nonessential for persistence, however.

Rubella virus can be plaqued in RK-13, BHK-21, SIRC (i.e., rabbit cornea), and Vero cells [161]. Plaquing forms the basis of neutralization assays, and differences in plaquing characteristics can be used as markers to differentiate strains [21,161,178,206–208].

---

*References 161, 217–221, 224, 226, 235–238, 241–249.

PATHOGENICITY FOR ANIMALS

Rubella virus grows in primates and in various small laboratory animals. The acquired or congenital disease has not been completely reproduced in any animal, however.

Vervet and particularly rhesus monkeys are susceptible to infection by the intranasal, intravenous, or intramuscular routes [255–257]. Although no rash develops, there is nasopharyngeal excretion of virus in all of the inoculated monkeys and demonstrable viremia in 50%. Attempts to produce transplacental infection in pregnant monkeys have been partially successful. Rubella virus has been recovered from the amnion and the placenta, but the embryo itself has not been shown to be consistently infected [258,259].

The ferret is the most useful of the small laboratory animals in rubella studies. Ferret kits are highly sensitive to subcutaneous and particularly to intracerebral inoculations. Virus has been recovered from the heart, liver, spleen, lung, brain, eye, blood, and urine for 1 month or longer after inoculation, and neutralizing and complement fixation antibodies have developed [260]. Ferret kits inoculated at birth develop corneal clouding. Virus appears in fetal ferrets after inoculation of pregnant animals [261].

Rabbits, hamsters, guinea pigs, rats, and suckling mice all have been infected with rubella virus, but none has proved to be a consistent and reliable animal model system for study of rubella infection [179,180,262–265]. Studies indicating that Japanese strains of rubella virus were less teratogenic to offspring of infected rabbits than U.S. strains have not been confirmed [179,180]. These experiments were conducted to examine further the hypothesis referred to earlier that there is a difference in the virulence among rubella virus strains circulating in Japan and other parts of the world [177,179–183,185].

EPIDEMIOLOGY

Humans are the only known host for rubella virus. Continuous cycling in humans is the only apparent means for the virus to be maintained in nature. Because rubella is predominantly a self-limited infection seen in late winter and spring, questions have arisen about how the virus persists throughout the remainder of the year. Person-to-person transmission probably occurs at very low levels in the general population throughout summer and winter and probably at much higher levels in closed populations of susceptible individuals [266–287]. Congenitally infected infants can shed virus from multiple sites and can serve as reservoirs of virus during periods of low transmission [165,288–293]. This is of particular concern in the hospital setting [165,285]. Efficiency of transmission may also vary among individuals, with some being better "spreaders" than others. This phenomenon may contribute to continued circulation of the virus [294].

Rubella has a worldwide distribution [295–301]. The virus circulates almost continually, at least in continental populations. In the continental temperate zones of the Northern Hemisphere, rubella is consistently more prevalent in the spring, with peak attack rates in March, April, and May; infection is much less prevalent during the remainder of the year, increasing or decreasing during the 2 months before or after the peak period [298,300]. Before widespread rubella immunization, sizable epidemics occurred every 5 to 9 years in temperate climates; however, the periodicity of rubella epidemics was highly variable in developed and developing countries, with major epidemics occurring at intervals ranging from 10 to 30 years. Epidemics usually built up and receded gradually over a 3- to 4-year interval, peaking at the midpoint [9,295,298,300].

The apparent increased infectivity and virulence of rubella as exemplified in the major epidemics have been the subject of considerable speculation. One popular thesis has been the unproven emergence of a more virulent strain of virus at widely separated intervals [177,179–183,185]. No convincing evidence exists concerning clinically different strains of rubella, however, and molecular analysis of the E1 envelope glycoprotein does not support the hypothesis of an epidemic versus endemic strain difference [84]. The apparent severity of the epidemic seems to be related to the number of susceptible adults, especially pregnant women, in any given population at the outset of an epidemic [184,186,300,302]. Host factors, such as the differences in the ability to transmit rubella, and still unknown factors may also be involved [294,302].

Attack rates in open populations have not been defined precisely for many reasons. Because rubella is such a mild disease, it is underreported, even in areas where reporting has been mandatory for years. Mandatory reporting did not begin in the United States until 1966 (Fig. 28–2) [298,303]. The high and variable rate of inapparent infection poses a major problem when attempting to interpret the recorded data, which are based usually on clinical findings [271,304–309].

In childhood, the most common time of infection, 50% or more of serologically confirmed infections result in inapparent illness. The ratio may be 6:1 or 7:1 in adults, perhaps as a result of silent reinfection in naturally immune individuals who have lost detectable antibody [271,307]. The frequent occurrence of infections that clinically mimic rubella makes it even more difficult to determine attack rates in open populations [310]. Attack rates undoubtedly depend on the number of susceptible individuals, which varies widely in different locations.

Serologic assessments of rubella attack rates have been performed in closed populations, such as military recruits, isolated island groups with small populations, boarding home residents, and household members [271–273,294, 306,309–317]. In such situations, individual exposure to the virus is more intense than encountered in open populations. Under these circumstances, 90% to 100% of children and adults who are susceptible may become infected. Attack rates in susceptible persons on college and university campuses and in other community settings range from 50% to 90% [9,302]. Similar to primary infection, reinfection probably is increased as exposure becomes more intense [271,307,315,316].

In most of the world, including the United States before the introduction of mass immunization of children in 1969, rubella was typically a childhood disease that was most prevalent in the 5- to 14-year-old age group [2,3,7,296–303]. It was rare in infants younger than 1 year of age. The incidence increased slowly for the first 4 years, increased steeply between 5 and 14 years, peaked around 20 to 24 years, and then leveled off. In developed countries before mass immunization, the incidence of infection did not reach 100% before the ages of 35 to 40 years; 5% to 20% of women of childbearing age remained susceptible to infection.

In the era before a rubella vaccine, in isolated or island populations, such as in Trinidad, some areas of Japan, Panama, rural Peru, and Hawaii, a relatively high rate of susceptibility was found among young adults [296,297, 299,300,313]; 26% to 70% of women of childbearing age remained susceptible. This situation existed even though rubella was endemic with ample opportunity for multiple introductions of virus from the outside. Low population density, tropical climate, low concentration of effective spreaders, and genetic factors all have been invoked to explain these low attack rates, but none can adequately account for this peculiar epidemiologic phenomenon by itself [294,299,300,302]. Later studies from 45 developing nations where rubella immunization efforts have been minimal have revealed a wide range of susceptibility (≤10% to approximately 25%) [314].

In other areas, particularly in South America, infections begin earlier in life, and peak incidence occurs before puberty [299]. Infection rates in most South American countries reach a plateau at approximately the same level as seen in Europe and North America, however, leaving 10% or more of young women who are susceptible, based on serologic tests. Chile seemed to be an exception, with almost all persons being infected before puberty [299]. The impact of major immunization programs in the PAHO countries to reach a goal of eliminating rubella by 2010 appears to have eliminated new infections to date. (http://new.paho.org/).

Initial mass vaccination of children with distribution of more than 29 million doses over the first year after licensure, followed by routine vaccination of 1-year-old children and vaccination of susceptible adolescents and adults, has been extremely successful in controlling rubella and CRS in the United States.* The characteristic 6- to 9-year epidemic cycle has been interrupted, and the reported incidence of rubella that ranged from approximately 200 to 400 cases annually during the period 1992–2000 decreased to less than 25 since 2001. For comparison,

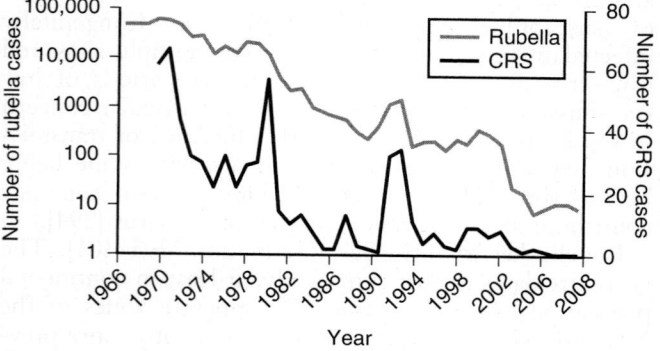

FIGURE 28–2 Cases of rubella and congenital rubella syndrome (CRS) in the United States, 1996-2008. (*Data from Centers for Disease Control and Prevention, courtesy of S. Reef, 2009.*)

*References 5, 24, 33, 39, 269, 303, 318.

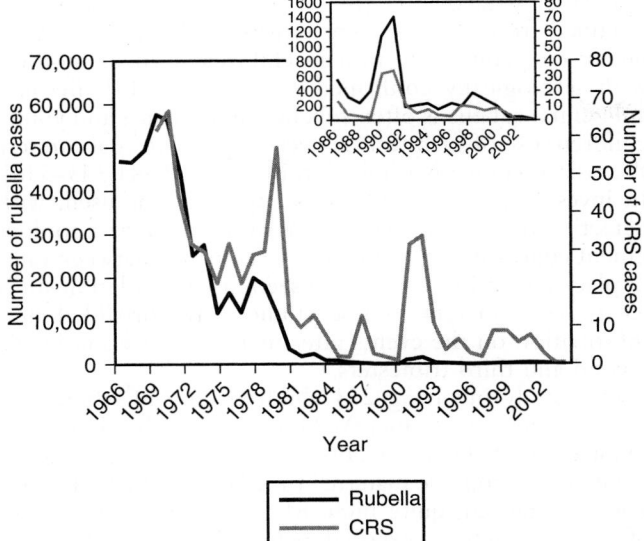

FIGURE 28–3 Incidence rates for reported cases of rubella and congenital rubella syndrome (CRS) in the United States, 1966-2003. *(Data from Centers for Disease Control and Prevention, courtesy of S. Reef, March 1, 2004.)*

there were approximately 58,000 cases reported in 1969, the year of vaccine licensure in the United States (Fig. 28–3).

Age-specific declines in the occurrence of rubella have been greatest in children, who, because they were the major reservoir of the virus, have been the primary target of the U.S. immunization program. The risk of rubella decreased by 99% in all age groups, however, after efforts to increase vaccination levels in older, susceptible persons, especially women of childbearing age (see "Prevention of Congenital Rubella") [266,268]. Until the late 1990s, serologic surveys documented susceptibility of 20% in this adult population; however, the National Health and Nutrition Examination Survey (NHANES) (1999–2004) documented susceptibility of less than 11% [319–322].

Adolescents and young adults now account for most reported cases, with more cases reported among individuals older than age 15 years than in children. Although there are fewer and smaller outbreaks since elimination was achieved, outbreaks are still reported in colleges, cruise ships, and other settings in which people live or work in proximity [277–279,282–287]. Outbreaks no longer occur among military recruits because they receive rubella vaccine as soon as they arrive for basic training [274].

Although the reported incidence of cases of CRS has decreased dramatically, the number of cases of rubella and congenital rubella reported in the United States increased in 1989–1991, documenting that the potential for cases will continue as long as immunization of children and women of childbearing age is not close to 100% [39]. The outbreak of rubella and subsequent clusters of congenital rubella among the Amish in Pennsylvania in 1991 and 1992 provided a reminder that there are still pockets of susceptible individuals in the United States [281]. The epidemiology of rubella is closely linked with the epidemiology of CRS. From 1997–1999, more than 90% of the mothers of infants with CRS were born outside the United States. Since 2000, the incidence of CRS

has been the lowest reported at a rate of less than 1 per 1 million live births and with most of the mothers of these infants born outside the United States and presumably unimmunized [323].

TRANSMISSION IN UTERO

In pregnant women with clinical or inapparent primary rubella, the virus infects the placenta during the period of viremia and subsequently infects the fetus [2,6,295, 310,324–339]. Intrauterine transmission of virus associated with maternal reinfection is rare. It is presumed that this difference is a reflection that viremia is absent or greatly reduced because of immunity induced by the primary infection (natural or vaccine induced).* Maternal infection may result in no infection of the conceptus, resorption of the embryo (seen only with infections occurring in the earliest stages of gestation), spontaneous abortion, stillbirth, infection of the placenta without fetal involvement, or infection of the placenta and fetus [6]. Infected infants can have obvious multiorgan system involvement or, as is frequently observed, no immediately evident disease [6,13,111,340–347]. After long-term follow-up, many of these seemingly unaffected infants have evidence of hearing loss or central nervous system (CNS) or other defects.†

Gestational age at the time of maternal infection is the most important determinant of intrauterine transmission and fetal damage [2–4,6,295,310,327]. The risk of fetal infection and congenital anomalies decreases with increasing gestational age. Fetal damage is rare much beyond the first trimester of pregnancy, as was shown in large British and American studies (Table 28–1).

Availability of more sensitive antibody assays has led to refinement of understanding of the risk of fetal infection and subsequent congenital defects throughout all stages of pregnancy [107,114]. Although the risk of defects does

---

*References 5, 6, 44, 46, 49, 51, 55–57, 59, 115, 120, 331–369.

†References 6, 13, 14, 116, 135, 136, 340, 341, 343–346.

TABLE 28–1 Fetal Abnormality Induced by Confirmed Rubella at Various Stages of Pregnancy

Stage of Pregnancy (wk)	United Kingdom Study (% Defective)*	United States Study (% Defective)†
≤4	—	70
5-8	—	40
≤10	90	—
11-12	33	—
9-12	—	25
13-14	11	—
15-16	24	—
13-16	—	40
≥17	—	8

*Data from Miller E, Cradock-Watson JE, Pollock TM. Consequences of confirmed maternal rubella at successive stage of pregnancy. Lancet 2:781-784, 1982.
†Data from South MA, Sever JL. Teratogen update: the congenital rubella syndrome. Teratology 31:297-307, 1985
From Plotkin SA, Orenstein WA, Offit PA (eds). Vaccines, 5th ed. Philadelphia, Saunders, 2008.

decrease with increasing gestational age, fetal infection can occur at any time during pregnancy. Data on the risk of fetal infection are inconsistent when maternal rubella infection occurs before conception [1,12,112,114, 348–351]. If some risk exists, it is small.

RISK OF FETAL INFECTION

Early attempts to define the risk of fetal infection relied on isolation of virus from products of conception [324–330]. Of products of conception obtained from women with clinical rubella during the first trimester, 40% to 90% were found to be infected. The higher rates were observed in serologically confirmed cases of maternal rubella and when improved isolation techniques were employed [329,330]. Attempts were made to refine the risk estimates by evaluating placental and fetal tissue separately. In some of these studies, equal rates of persistent placental and fetal infection were observed, ranging from 80% to 90% [329,330].

In other studies, persistent placental infection was found to be twice as frequent as fetal infection: 50% to 70% versus 20% to 30% [324,327]. High rates of fetal infection accompanied placental infection, however, when specimens obtained during the first 8 weeks of gestation were examined. Of 14 cases in which virus was cultured from placental tissue, six of seven fetuses were culture-positive when maternal rubella occurred during the first 8 weeks of pregnancy. In contrast, only one of seven fetal specimens was positive when infection occurred between 9 and 14 weeks of gestation [324]. In another similar study, fetal infection rates decreased sharply after the 8th week of gestation; placental infection rates decreased, but less rapidly [327]. After the 8th week, placental infection occurred in 36% (8 of 22) and fetal infection occurred in 10% (2 of 20) of cases. Although fetal infection was not documented beyond the 10th week of gestation, placental infections were identified up to the 16th week.

Further data on the risk of fetal infection have been obtained from studies using sensitive laboratory tests to detect congenital infection in children born to mothers with serologically confirmed rubella [107,114]. Because congenital rubella is often subclinical in infants and young children, use of such tests is necessary to assess accurately the risk of congenital infection [6,107–112,341,343–346]. In investigations in which this approach was used, with detection of rubella-specific IgM antibody in sera to document congenital infection, the discrepancy between rates of placental and fetal infection seen in viral isolation studies is less apparent. These studies have provided new information on the events after maternal infection in the second and third trimesters.

In a study involving 273 children (269 of whom had IgM antibody assessment), Miller and colleagues [109] reported that fetal infection after serologically documented symptomatic maternal rubella in the first trimester was, as expected, quite high: 81% (13 of 16), with rates of 90% for fetuses exposed before 11 weeks and 67% for fetuses exposed at 11 to 12 weeks (Table 28–2). Of greater interest is that the infection rate was 39% (70 of 178) after exposure in the second trimester (decreasing steadily from 67% at 13 to 14 weeks to 25% at 23 to 26 weeks), but increased to 53% (34 of 64) with third-trimester infection (with infection rates of 35%, 60%, and 100% during the last 3 months of pregnancy).

In another investigation of fetal infection after first-trimester maternal rubella infection based on IgM determination, Cradock-Watson and associates [107] found that 32% of 166 children were infected after exposure in the second trimester and that a comparable proportion (24% of 100) were infected after exposure in the third trimester. The rate of infection increased during the latter stages of gestation after initially decreasing to a low of 12% by the 28th week and was 58% (11 of 19) when maternal infection occurred near term. Even higher rates were observed when persistence of IgG antibody was used

---

TABLE 28–2 Risk of Serologically Confirmed Congenital Rubella Infection and Associated Defects in Children Exposed to Symptomatic Maternal Rubella Infection, by Weeks of Gestation

Weeks of Gestation	Infection		Defects*		Overall Risk of Defects (%)[†]
	No. Tested	Rate (%)	No. Followed	Rate (%)	
<11	10	90 (9)[‡]	9	100	90
11–12	6	67 (4)	4	50	33
13–14	18	67 (12)	12	17	11
15–16	36	47 (17)	14	50	24
17–18	33	39 (13)	10		
19–22	59	34 (20)			
23–26	32	25 (8)			
27–30	31	35 (11)	53		
31–36	25	60 (15)			
>36	8	100 (8)			
Total	258[§]	45 (117)	102	20	

*Defects in seropositive patients only.
[†]Overall risk of defects = rate of infection × rate of defects.
[‡]Numbers in parentheses are number of children infected.
[§]None of 11 infants whose mothers had subclinical rubella were infected.
Adapted from Miller E, Cradock-Watson JE, Pollock TM. Consequences of confirmed maternal rubella at successive stages of pregnancy. Lancet 2:781, 1982.

as the criterion for congenital infection. The true fetal infection rate probably lies between the rates calculated by using the IgM and persistent IgG data.

In both studies, the fetal infection rate declined between 12 and 28 weeks, suggesting that the placenta may prevent transfer of virus, although not completely [107]. Some of the infections recorded during the last weeks of pregnancy could have been perinatally or postnatally acquired (e.g., by means of exposure to virus in the birth canal or from breast milk), but the available evidence indicates that the placental barrier to infection may be relatively ineffective during the last month, perhaps to the same degree as that seen during the first trimester, and that the fetus is susceptible to infection throughout pregnancy, albeit to various degrees [352–354].

RISK OF CONGENITAL DEFECTS

Estimates of the risk of congenital anomalies in live-born infants after fetal infection have been affected by numerous factors. Early retrospective and hospital-based studies led to overestimates of the risk of congenital defects after first-trimester infection (up to 90%) [6,111,302]. The risk of abnormalities as determined by prospective studies relying on a clinical diagnosis of maternal rubella varied considerably (10% to 54% overall, with a 10% to 20% risk for major defects recognizable in children ≤3 years old) and tended to underestimate the risk because serologic evaluation of infants was not performed [111,348, 355–359]. The proportion of pregnancies electively terminated can affect observed malformation rates. The fact that fetal infection can occur during all stages of pregnancy also influences assessments of the risk of congenital defects.

Because most infants born with congenital rubella who were exposed after the 12th week of gestation do not have grossly apparent defects, long-term follow-up is necessary to detect subtle, late-appearing abnormalities, such as deafness and mental impairment.* This is especially true for infants infected beyond the 16th to 29th week of gestation, who seem to be at little, if any, risk of congenital anomalies [107,113]. Studies by Peckham [111,345] showed that estimates of the risk of defects are affected by the serologic status and age at evaluation of the child. The overall incidence of defects in 218 children studied when they were about 2 years old was 23%; it was 52% if maternal infection occurred before 8 weeks of gestation, 36% at 9 to 12 weeks, and 10% at 13 to 20 weeks. No defects were observed when maternal infection occurred after 20 weeks. When considering only seropositive children, the overall risk of defects increased to 38%, with increased risks of 75%, 52%, and 18% for the three gestational periods previously cited. At follow-up when the children were 6 to 8 years old, the overall risk of abnormalities in infected children who were seropositive when 2 years old increased from 38% to 59%; the risk after first-trimester infection increased from 58% to 82%.

Miller and colleagues [109] observed higher rates of defects in infected children observed for only 2 years (see Table 28–2). Defects were seen in 9 of 9 seropositive

children exposed during the first 11 weeks of gestation, 2 of 4 children exposed at 11 to 12 weeks, 2 of 12 children exposed at 13 to 14 weeks, and 7 of 14 children exposed at 15 to 16 weeks. Congenital heart disease and deafness were observed after infection before the 11th week; deafness was the sole defect identified after infection at 11 to 16 weeks of gestation. No defects were observed in 63 children infected after 16 weeks of gestation. Some children infected in the third trimester had growth restriction, however.

Although the number of subjects is small, results of the study of Miller and colleagues [109] indicate that the risk of damage is 85% in infants who were infected as fetuses during the first trimester and 35% after infection during weeks 13 to 16. These rates of defects are higher than previously reported, but they may be an accurate reflection of intrauterine events because all maternal cases were serologically confirmed, and sensitive antibody assays were used to detect congenital infection. With further follow-up, higher rates of defects may be observed.

These rates pertain to offspring known to be infected and are useful in evaluating the risk of defects given fetal infection. For counseling purposes, it is essential to know the risk of congenital defects after confirmed maternal infection. This risk can be derived by multiplying the rates of defects in infected fetuses by the rates of fetal infection. Based on the reported experience of Miller and colleagues [109], the risks are 90% for maternal infection before the 11th week of gestation, 33% for infection during weeks 11 to 12, 11% for weeks 13 to 14, and 24% for weeks 15 to 16 (see Table 28–2). The overall risk after maternal infection in the first trimester was 69%.

NATURAL HISTORY
POSTNATAL INFECTION
Virologic Findings

The pertinent virologic findings of postnatal infection are depicted in Figure 28–4. The portal of entry for rubella virus is believed to be the upper respiratory tract. Virus spreads through the lymphatic system, or by a transient viremia to regional lymph nodes, where replication first occurs. Virus is released into the blood 7 to 9 days after exposure and may seed multiple tissues, including the placenta. By the 9th to 11th day, viral excretion begins from the nasopharynx, kidneys, cervix, gastrointestinal tract, and various other sites.*

The viremia peaks at 10 to 17 days, just before rash onset, which usually occurs 16 to 18 days after exposure. Virus disappears from the serum in the next few days, as antibody becomes detectable [289,305,312,360]. Infection may persist, however, in peripheral blood lymphocytes and monocytes for 1 to 4 weeks [63,68,361,362]. Virus is excreted in high titers from nasopharyngeal secretions. Nasopharyngeal shedding rarely may be detected for 3 to 5 weeks. Although virus can usually be cultured from the nasopharynx from 7 days before to 14 days after rash onset, the highest risk of virus transmission is believed to be from 5 days before to 6 days after the appearance of

---

*References 6, 13, 14, 116, 135, 136, 340, 341, 343–346.

*References 9, 289, 305, 312, 352–354, 360.

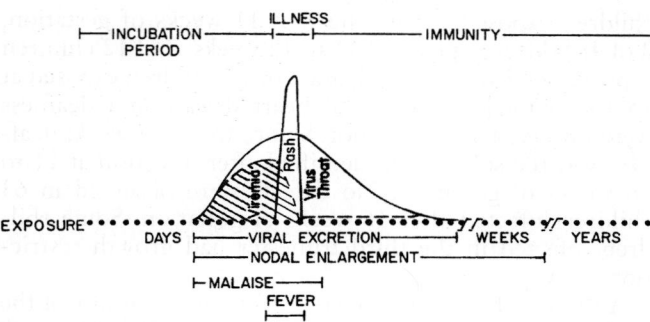

FIGURE 28–4 Relationship of viral excretion and clinical findings in postnatally acquired rubella. *(Data from Alford CA. Chronic congenital and perinatal infections. In Avery GB [ed]. Neonatology. Philadelphia, Lippincott, 1987.)*

rash. Viral shedding from other sites is not as consistent, intense, or prolonged [305,360]. Rubella virus has been cultured from skin at sites where rash was present and where it was absent [363,364].

Humoral Immune Response

In challenge studies conducted in the early 1960s, Green and coworkers [305] showed that neutralizing antibody was first detected in serum 14 to 18 days after exposure (usually 2 to 3 days after rash onset), peaked within 1 month, and persisted for the duration of the follow-up period of 6 to 12 months. The HI test soon became the standard method for detecting rubella antibodies after acute postnatal rubella infection because of its reliability and ease compared with the neutralization test. Several other methods for measuring rubella antibody responses have supplanted the HI test in popularity (see "Virus") [92,210,211]. Figure 28–5 depicts the kinetics of the immune response to acute infection detected by these

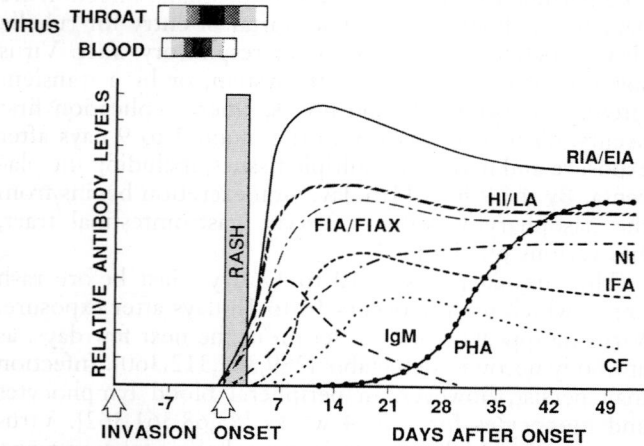

FIGURE 28–5 Schematic diagram of immune response in acute rubella infection. CF, complement fixation; EIA, enzyme immunoassay; FIA/FIAX and IFA, immunofluorescence assays; HI, hemagglutination inhibition; LA, latex agglutination; Nt, neutralization; PHA, passive agglutination; RIA, radioimmunoassay. *(Data from Herrmann KL. Rubella virus. In Lennette EH, Schmidt NJ [eds]. Diagnostic Procedures for Viral, Rickettsial and Chlamydial Infections. Washington, DC, American Public Health Association, 1979, p 725; and Herrmann KL. Available rubella serologic tests. Rev Infect Dis 7[Suppl 1]:S108, 1985.)*

various serologic assays, which have been exhaustively compared with the HI technique.*

There are generally three distinct patterns of antibody kinetics. Antibodies of the IgG class measured by HI, latex agglutination, neutralization, immunofluorescence, single radial hemolysis (or hemolysis in gel) (not shown in Fig. 28–5), radioimmunoassay, and enzyme-linked immunoassay theta precipitation (not shown) follow the first pattern. These IgG antibodies usually become detectable 5 to 15 days after rash onset, although they may appear earlier and may even be detected 1 or 2 days before the rash appears. The antibody titers rapidly increase to reach peak values at 15 to 30 days and then gradually decline over years to a constant titer that varies from person to person. In some patients with low levels of residual antibody, a second exposure to rubella virus may lead to low-grade reinfection of the pharynx. A booster antibody response can be detected with any of the assays. This antibody response rapidly terminates the new infection, which is most often subclinical, and little or no viremia occurs.†

A second pattern of immune response to rubella infection is seen when IgG antibodies are measured by passive hemagglutination. The peak titer of these antibodies is similar to that measured by HI, but the passive hemagglutination antibodies are relatively delayed in appearance, and levels increase only slowly to their maximal titers. They first become detectable 15 to 50 days after the onset of the rash and often take 200 days to reach peak titers. The antibodies probably persist for life. Booster responses may be seen with reinfections.

Studies indicate that the predominant IgG subclass detected by all these various assays is probably IgG1 [99,101]. Failure to detect IgG3 may be indicative of reinfection [102].

A third distinct pattern of antibody production is represented in Figure 28–5 by the IgM antibody class immune response. Rubella-specific IgM antibody can be measured by HI, immunofluorescence, radioimmunoassay, or enzyme immunoassay.‡ IgM antibodies are most consistently detectable 5 to 10 days after the onset of the rash, increase rapidly to peak values at around 20 days, and then decline so rapidly that they usually disappear by 50 to 70 days. In a few patients, low levels may persist for 1 year [365–367]. The booster IgG antibody response to reinfection described earlier does not usually involve the IgM class of antibody, and the presence of high-titer IgM antibodies usually indicates recent primary infection with rubella. More sensitive techniques, such as radioimmunoassay or enzyme immunoassay, may occasionally detect low levels of specific IgM antibodies in some patients with reinfections, which may cause some difficulty in differentiating subclinical reinfection, which is almost always of no consequence, from acute primary subclinical infection [45,55,57,59]. Determination of avidity of rubella-specific IgG may help resolve this problem [368–370]. Primary infection seems to be associated

---

*References 92–96, 202, 206–216, 218, 225–235, 237, 240.
†References 42, 48, 51, 54, 58, 60, 271, 316, 339.
‡References 103, 161, 217–221, 224, 226, 235, 236.

with low-avidity IgG, and reinfection seems to be associated with high-avidity IgG.

The kinetics of the immune response to rubella infection detected by other serologic assays is not as distinct as the three patterns just described, and marked variability among patients has been observed. Complement fixation antibodies or iota precipitins (not shown in Fig. 28–5) are lacking in the first 10 days after the rash and increase slowly to peak at 30 to 90 days [202]. These antibodies persist for several years in one third of patients and may reappear during reinfections. Iota precipitins do not persist for more than a few months and do not usually reappear with reinfections.

Antibodies of the IgA class appear within 10 days, but may disappear within another 20 days or persist for several years [100,103,217,242]. IgD and IgE antibodies appear rapidly (6 to 9 days) after infection, remain high for at least 2 months, and then decline slightly at 6 months [100]. IgE antibodies reach an early peak similar to that seen for IgM and IgA. In contrast, the IgD response is, delayed, similar to that of IgG.

The antibody response after infection is generally considered to confer complete and permanent immunity. Clinical reinfection is rare, and reinfections usually pose little risk to the fetus because placental exposure to the virus is minimal.* Some rare instances of fetal infection after maternal reinfection may be caused by an incomplete immune response to the various antigenic domains on each structural protein of the virus (see "Virus") [78–80,115,119,331,336–340]. Three cases after natural infection have been reported involving women who had positive HI results, but who had no detectable levels of neutralizing antibody [331,336,338]. The sensitivity of the neutralizing assay itself is an important determinant in interpreting these results [115,207]. This phenomenon also may account for the four reported cases of congenital infection that followed reinfection of women who had presumably been immunized previously [46,49,56,120]. Some reported instances of maternal reinfection probably (and in at least one case definitely) represent cases of primary acute infection [5,6,117,333–335].

Cellular Immune Response

Cellular immunity to rubella virus has been measured by lymphocyte transformation response, secretion of interferon, secretion of macrophage migration-inhibitory factor, induction of delayed hypersensitivity to skin testing, and release of lymphokines by cultured lymphocytes [371–382]. Peripheral blood lymphocytes from seropositive individuals respond better in each of these tests than do lymphocytes from uninfected persons, suggesting that these assays measure parameters of the cellular immune response to rubella virus. The results from other studies in which chromium 51 microcytotoxicity assays have been used are difficult to interpret because syngeneic cell lines have not been used to control for HLA-restricted responses [372,375].

In the first weeks after natural rubella infection, some degree of transient lymphocyte suppression may occur

[376,378]. Generally, cell-mediated immune responses precede the appearance of humoral immunity by 1 week, reach a peak value at the same time as the antibody response, and subsequently persist for many years, probably for life [341]. Acute infection may suppress skin reactivity to tuberculin testing for approximately 30 days [383].

Local Immune Response

The local antibody response at the portal of entry in the nasopharynx is essentially IgA in character, although IgG antibody from serum may diffuse into nasopharyngeal secretions. The nasopharyngeal IgA antibody persists at detectable levels for at least 1 year after infection. Its persistence apparently minimizes the tendency for reinfection after natural rubella infection. The lack of local IgA nasopharyngeal response after parenteral administration of live rubella vaccines (less so with the RA 27/3 strain than with other strains) probably plays a key role in the increased incidence of subclinical reinfection after vaccination.* Local antibody levels tend to be higher in individuals resistant to challenge with live virus, but no specific titer of antibody has been associated with complete protection.

A cell-mediated immune response in tonsillar cells has been detected by lymphocyte transformation and secretion of migration-inhibitory factor after natural rubella and after intranasal challenge with live RA 27/3 vaccine [388]. In guinea pigs, the response first becomes detectable 1 to 2 weeks after intranasal vaccination, peaks at 4 weeks, and disappears at about 6 weeks [389].

CONGENITAL INFECTION
Virologic Findings

An important feature that distinguishes congenital infection from postnatal infection is that the former is chronic.† During the period of maternal viremia, the placenta may become infected and transmit virus to the fetus (see "Transmission In Utero") [2,6,295,310,324–330]. Although virus may persist for months in the placenta, recovery of virus from the placenta at birth occurs infrequently [392]. In contrast, after the fetus is infected, the virus persists typically throughout gestation and for months postnatally. It can infect many fetal organs or only a few [327].

In infected infants, virus can be recovered from multiple sites (e.g., pharyngeal secretions, urine, conjunctival fluid, feces) and is detectable in cerebrospinal fluid, bone marrow, and circulating white blood cells.‡ Pharyngeal shedding of virus is more common, prolonged, and intense during the early months after delivery (Fig. 28–6). By 1 year of age, only 2% to 20% of infants shed virus [288–290]. Rarely, shedding may continue beyond the age of 2 years [291–293]. Virus can be isolated from the eye and cerebrospinal fluid, particularly when disease is evident in the corresponding organs and can persist for more than 1 year in the eye and CNS [393–396]. Virus has been isolated

---

*References 42, 45, 48, 51, 54, 55, 57–60, 339.

---

*References 42, 44, 48, 54, 58, 60, 384–387.
†References 2, 13, 295, 327, 390, 391.
‡References 2, 13, 165, 288–293, 295, 324, 325, 327, 329, 390–393, 396.

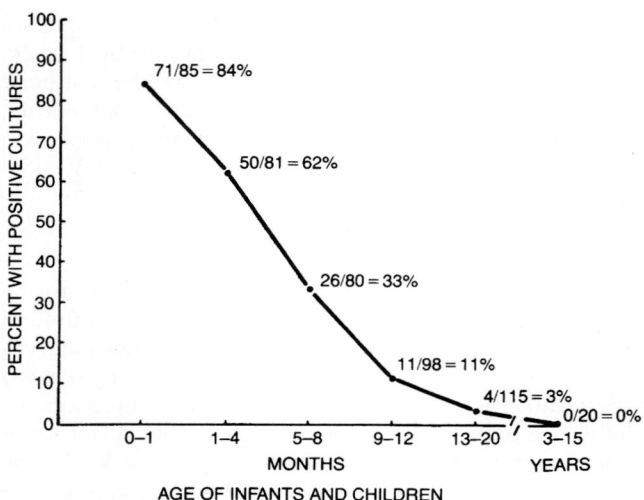

FIGURE 28–6 Rate of virus excretion by age in infants and children with congenital rubella infection. (*Data from Cooper LZ, Krugman S. Clinical manifestations of postnatal and congenital rubella. Arch Ophthalmol 77:434, 1967.*)

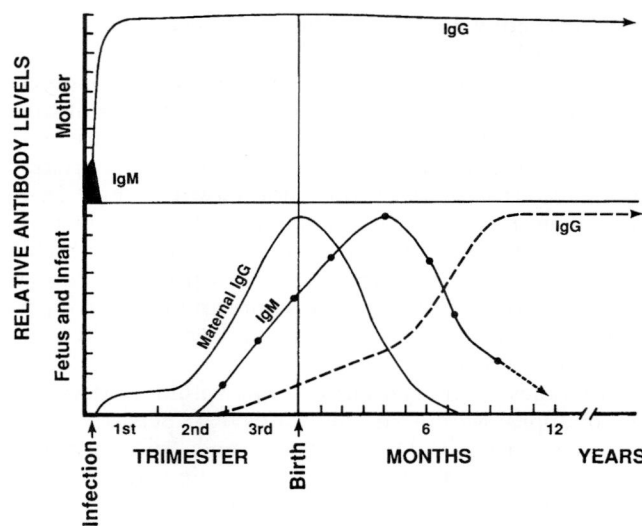

FIGURE 28–7 Schematic diagram of immune response in the mother, fetus, and infant after maternal and fetal rubella infections in the first trimester of pregnancy. (*Data from Alford CA. Immunology of rubella. In Friedman H, Prier JE [eds]. Rubella. Springfield, IL, Charles C Thomas, 1972.*)

from the brain of a 12-year-old boy with later appearing subacute panencephalitis occurring after congenital rubella infection [395,397,398].

Humoral Immune Response

Studies have shown that placental infection does not prevent passive transfer of maternal antibody and that the infected fetus can mount an immune response [295, 324–330,399–401]. Although the development and function of the other components of the immune response of the fetus may be important, critical factors that allow fetal infection to occur in the presence of antibody may be the timing when antibody is present in the fetal circulation, the quality of the antibody that the fetus produces, or both.

Although placental transfer of antibody occurs despite persistent infection, levels of antibody in fetal blood during the first half of gestation are only 5% to 10% of levels in maternal serum [402,403]. As the placental transfer mechanisms mature by mid-gestation (16 to 20 weeks), increasing levels of maternal IgG antibody are transferred to the fetus (Fig. 28–7) [404,405].

The development of the fetal humoral immune system apparently is too late to limit the effects of the virus. Cells with membrane-bound immunoglobulins of all three major classes—IgM, IgG, and IgA—appear in the fetus by 9 to 11 weeks of gestation [403]. Circulating fetal antibody levels remain low until mid-gestation, however, despite the presence of high titers of virus and the development of antigen receptors on the cell surface (see Fig. 28–7). At this time, levels of fetal antibody increase, with IgM antibody predominating [399,406–410]. Fetal IgA, IgD, and IgG also are made, although in lesser amounts [100,407,410]. As in the case with other chronic intrauterine infections, congenital rubella infection may lead to an increase in total IgM antibody levels [399,401,405,410]. Total IgA levels are also occasionally increased, but IgG levels seldom exceed levels of

uninfected infants [399,410–412]. At the time of delivery of infected infants, levels of IgG rubella antibodies in cord sera are equal to or greater than levels in maternal sera, even if the infant is born prematurely [399]. IgG is the dominant antibody present at delivery in rubella-infected infants and is mainly maternal in origin. In contrast, the IgM levels are lower, but are totally fetus derived.

In the first 3 to 5 months after birth, the levels of maternally derived IgG decrease as maternal antibody is catabolized (see Fig. 28–7) [399]. In contrast, IgM antibodies increase in titer and can predominate. Later, as viral excretion wanes and disappears, the IgM antibody levels diminish, and IgG becomes the dominant and persistent antibody type. Cradock-Watson and colleagues [410] found that total IgM was elevated in nearly all sera obtained from infected infants during the first 3 months of life and in half of sera from infected infants 3 to 6 months old. Rubella-specific IgM has been shown consistently to persist for 6 months, frequently for 1 year, and rarely longer when assayed by sensitive serologic procedures, such as radioimmunoassay and immunofluorescence [223,410]. Cradock-Watson and colleagues [410] also reported that IgM was detectable in 48 (96%) of 50 serum samples during the first 6 months of life and in 11 (29%) of 38 serum samples from children 6.5 months to 2 years old. The total level of antibody, as measured by various serologic tests, remains virtually unchanged throughout the 1st year of life, despite the fluctuations in immunoglobulin composition [399,410].

High levels of IgG antibody are usually maintained for several years after detectable virus excretion ends, suggesting that there may be continued antigenic stimulation. During the first few years of life, some patients have a relative hypergammaglobulinemia, particularly of the IgM and IgG classes of antibody, which results from the increased antigenic stimulus accompanying the chronic infection [405,410]. With increasing time, antibody levels may decrease and even become undetectable in 10% to 20% of patients [345,413–415]. Cooper and coworkers [415] found that the geometric mean HI titer decreased by a factor of 16 by age 5 years in 223 children with CRS. No HI antibodies were detected in 8 of 29 5-year-old children. In a study from Japan, only 3% of 381 children with congenital infection observed for more than 17 years had undetectable HI titers [416]. There was an initial rapid decline from a geometric mean titer of 1:416 ($2^{8.7}$) to 1:84 ($2^{6.4}$) over the first 2 years of follow-up. After this, there was a modest continuing decline, and the final geometric mean titer was 1:42 ($2^{5.4}$).

Cooper and coworkers [415] reported that congenitally infected children who have lost detectable rubella-specific antibody did not develop a boost in antibody titer after rubella vaccination. This finding may reflect some sort of immunologic tolerance that follows intrauterine exposure to rubella virus. None of the children with congenital rubella in Japan had evidence of significant boosts in antibody or a history of clinical disease when exposed during recent outbreaks of rubella [416,417]. RA 27/3 vaccine virus administered intranasally succeeded in inducing an immune response, however, so the problem may be less tolerance than low systemic levels of humoral or cellular immunity [415].

Hypogammaglobulinemia with low levels of all three major classes of immunoglobulins has been reported in a few instances of congenital rubella [137,165,418,419]. Usually, only IgA is affected; there may also be instances when IgG levels are low, whereas levels of IgM are two or three times the upper limit of normal for adults. These IgG and IgM abnormalities may occur with or without IgA abnormalities [418]. Over time, immunoglobulin development may become normal, and this can occur despite continued viral excretion, but is more likely if viral titers are decreasing [291].

In addition to defects in the immunoglobulin levels, defects in specific antibody production have been observed. One such defect is a complete lack of antibody response to any antigen, including the rubella virus itself. Response only to the virus, in the absence of a response to most other antigens, has also been reported [291]. This state of immunologic unresponsiveness resolves in many patients. Antibody production becomes normal as the patient's general condition improves and as immunoglobulin levels normalize.

Immunoprecipitation studies of sera from patients with CRS provide further information on defective antibody production. The studies indicate that the antibody profile to the three structural proteins of the rubella virus is qualitatively different from that observed in sera from persons with postnatally acquired infection (see "Virus") [88,89,91]. Little or no antibody to the core structural protein (C) is found, and the absolute and relative amounts of antibody to structural proteins E1 and E2 seem to vary with age [88,89]. These findings further suggest that the immune response of the infected fetus may be incomplete and may explain why detectable antibodies are not present in some serum samples [91,345,413–416]. If a serum sample contains relatively little antibody to structural protein E1 (i.e., hemagglutinin), assays that detect antibody to the whole virion are more likely to be positive than assays that detect antibody only to E1 (e.g., HI assay). It is unclear whether these abnormal antibody patterns persist for life.

Cellular Immune Response

Similar to the cells responsible for the humoral immune response (i.e., B cells), the cells involved in cellular immunity (i.e., T cells and macrophages) develop some of their functions early in gestation [420–422]. Little is known about their response in utero, however, because appropriate specimens have not been obtainable for study. The cellular immune response of the infected fetus has been inferred from studies of infected infants and children. Available evidence indicates that some infants with congenital rubella have impaired cellular immune responses.

Retarded development of the thymus and lymphocyte depletion have been reported, but these abnormalities may result from the stress of infection, rather than the virus itself [423]. Abnormal delayed hypersensitivity skin reactions to numerous antigens (e.g., diphtheria toxoid, *Candida*, dinitrofluorobenzene) have also been reported [291,424]. This defect has been associated with abnormalities in the humoral system and resolves as antibody production returns to normal.

Results of studies of in vitro lymphocyte blastogenesis in congenitally infected infants and children have been confusing. Early studies showed a poor response to phytohemagglutinin, vaccinia, and diphtheria toxoid [424–427]. Because rubella virus can depress the lymphocyte blastogenic response, and the virus can be isolated from lymphocytes of chronically infected infants, the abnormality may be a result of viral infection of the circulating blood cells, rather than an inherent defect in cell-mediated immunity [425,426,428,429]. This diminished cellular response may normalize over time because elevated lymphocyte responses have been detected in some older infected children [420,430].

Buimovici-Klein and colleagues [382,431] showed that lymphocytes from older children and adolescents with congenital rubella had no or very poor lymphocyte proliferative responses to rubella virus antigens and had markedly reduced interferon and migration-inhibition factor production. These studies indicated that these defects were greater in children exposed early in gestation than those exposed later, with the greatest degree of abnormality in children whose mothers had been infected during the first 8 weeks of pregnancy. The studies also pointed out that these defects could persist long after viral excretion had ceased. It remains unclear if these cellular immune defects are responsible for viral persistence or are yet another manifestation of intrauterine infection [431].

Other investigators have confirmed that patients with congenital rubella have defects in cell-mediated immunity [124,137,138]. Verder and colleagues [138] reported a decreased proportion of suppressor or cytotoxic (CD8+) T cells in an infant with congenital rubella. Rabinowe and coworkers [137] documented persistent T-cell abnormalities in patients with congenital infection who were 9 to 21 years old. Compared with normal subjects, congenitally infected patients had depressed ratios of T4 cells (helper or inducer) to T8 cells (from a decreased proportion of T4 and an increased percentage of T8 cells). Such findings persist for only 1 month after acute postnatal rubella infection [432].

Lymphocytes of infected children were unable to kill rubella-infected cells in a cytotoxicity assay [433]. These results were questioned because syngeneic target cells were not used, and these responses are known to be HLA restricted. Similar results have been reported by Verder and associates [138], however, who observed abnormal killer and natural killer cell activities.

Morag and associates [389] detected cytotoxic T lymphocytes in tonsillar lymphocytes after intranasal administration of RA 27/3 vaccine, but not after subcutaneous administration of another attenuated strain. Elevation of cytokines interleukin-4, interleukin-10, and tumor necrosis factor-α after vaccination has also been observed [434].

Interferon Response

It has long been suggested that the fetus has a deficient interferon response to viral infections, including rubella, but this evidence has been derived from indirect studies with in vitro cell systems or animal models [182,183, 329,435,436]. Technical difficulties have hampered direct studies of humans. Interferon that seemed to be specifically stimulated by the presence of rubella virus in rubella-infected human embryos has been shown, however [437]. The interferon was found at 7 weeks of gestation and persisted 12 weeks after symptoms ceased in the mothers. Direct study of fetal blood and amniotic fluid has also shown that the fetus can produce interferon in response to the virus [438].

Children with congenital infection have the capacity to make interferon on challenge. Desmyter and coworkers [439] reported that interferon could not be detected from the serum or urine of nine children 11 to 18 months old who were excreting virus. After vaccination with live measles vaccine (i.e., Edmonston B or Schwarz strains), all the children seroconverted, however, and produced detectable levels of interferon.

PATHOGENESIS
POSTNATAL INFECTION

The events leading to acute postnatal infection are relatively well known and have been discussed in detail in "Natural History." Available information indicates that viral replication and postinfection immune phenomena are involved in the clinical manifestations of the illness.

Viremia may lead to seeding of multiple organs, but few are clinically affected [6]. Speculation that the rash may be an immune phenomenon caused by circulating immune complexes has not been documented. Few persons with uncomplicated illness have immune complexes containing rubella virus, and virus has been isolated from involved and uninvolved skin [127,132,363,364]. Virus has been isolated from lymph nodes and conjunctiva, accounting for the lymph node enlargement and conjunctivitis observed in many patients [360,440]. Virus has been isolated from synovial fluid, but immune mechanisms may play a role in some cases of arthralgia and arthritis, particularly if symptoms are persistent [127,440–444].

Encephalitis is probably a manifestation of the immune response, but direct viral invasion may be involved, particularly in the rare case of progressive panencephalitis that has been reported to follow postnatal infection [125,445–447]. It has been suggested that pregnant women are at increased risk of serious complications because of the impaired immune response associated with pregnancy, but there are few data to support this claim [447–449]. There has also been interest, especially in Japan, in the influence of HLA type and other genetic factors on the incidence and severity of postnatal infection.* No consistent pattern has been reported.

CONGENITAL INFECTION

The outcome of maternal rubella infection follows a logical sequence of events, beginning with maternal infection, followed by viremia, placental seeding, and dissemination of infection to the fetus (see "Transmission In Utero" and "Natural History") [2,6,295,310,324–330]. The fetus may escape infection entirely, die in utero, be born with multiple obvious defects, or seem to be normal at birth only to develop abnormalities later in life [6,13,111,289, 340–347]. The variability in outcome is highlighted by the observation that one identical twin may be infected and the other spared [6,451,452].

The most important determinant of fetal outcome is gestational age at the time of infection.† The disease is more severe and has a greater tendency to involve multiple organs when acquired during the first 8 weeks of gestation. The factors that govern the influence of gestation are unknown. It is possible that immature cells are more easily infected and support the growth of virus better than older, more differentiated cells. It is also possible that the placenta becomes increasingly resistant to infection (or at least more able to limit infection) as it rapidly matures during the first trimester. A third possibility is that maturing fetal defense mechanisms become capable of confining and clearing the infection. This last explanation is probably important after 18 or 20 weeks of gestation, but seems unlikely in the latter half of the first trimester, when attenuation of fetal infection begins. It is likely that a combination of these and other factors are responsible for the decrease in virulence of fetal infection with increasing gestational age.

The hallmark of fetal infection is its chronicity, with the tendency for virus to persist throughout fetal life and after birth.‡ The fact that virus can be isolated long after birth also raises the possibility of reactivation, at least in brain tissue [398]. It is unclear why the virus has these properties because the fetus is not truly immunologically tolerant and seems to be able to produce interferon.§ In any case, chronic or reactivated infection can lead to ongoing pathologic processes.‖

The causes of cellular and tissue damage from congenital rubella infection are poorly defined [435,436]. Only a

---

*References 122, 123, 126, 128, 131, 450.
†References 2, 3, 6, 107, 114, 295, 310, 324, 327.
‡References 2, 13, 165, 288–293, 295, 310, 324–330, 382–398.
§References 223, 295, 341, 399, 400, 410, 435–439.
‖References 6, 13, 14, 111, 135, 136, 340, 341, 343–346.

variable, small number of cells are infected (1 per 1000 to 250,000) [330]. In tissue culture, infection with rubella virus has diverse effects, ranging from no obvious effect to cell destruction (see "Virus"); this is also likely to be the case in vivo [161], but cytolysis is uncommon (see "Pathology") [2,3,6,9,453–457]. Inflammation is minimal and consists mainly of infiltration of small lymphocytes. Polymorphonuclear leukocytes and plasma cells are lacking, particularly compared with other viral infections of the human fetus, in which inflammation and general necrosis are quite extensive. In contrast, vascular insufficiency seems to be more important than cell destruction or secondary inflammatory damage in the genesis of congenital defects [2,3,6,9,453–457]. This suggestion is supported by the observation that rubella virus has low destructive potential for cells growing in vitro, including those of human origin. Numerous investigators have maintained multiple types of rubella-infected human fetal cells in culture for years without loss of viability or evidence of cytopathic effect [458–460].

Other defects have been reported in chronically infected cells that might help explain the mechanism of congenital defects. These include chromosomal breaks, increased cellular multiplication time, and increased production of a protein inhibitor that causes mitotic arrest of certain cell types [390,458,461–466]. The mitotic arrest is presumably responsible for the reduced replication of infected cells.

A report by Bowden and associates [467] indicates that rubella virus may interfere with mitosis by having an adverse effect on actin microfilaments. Observations of Yoneda and coworkers [468] show that rubella virus may alter cell receptors to specific growth factors. All of these abnormalities, if occurring in vivo, may result in decreased cell multiplication because of slow growth rates and limited doubling potential during the period of embryogenesis, when cell division and turnover are normally very rapid. Naeye and Blanc [469] found histopathologic evidence for mitotic arrest and reduced cell numbers in infants who died of CRS. These observations have been offered to explain the increased incidence of intrauterine growth restriction seen in infants with congenital rubella, but this explanation probably represents an oversimplification of the actual mechanisms involved.

More recently, it has been shown that rubella virus capsid protein interacts with host cell proteins to inhibit translation [469a]. Although infection of adult human cells often results in apoptosis, infection of fetal cells does not [469b]. The reduction of apoptosis would favor the chronic infection that is the hallmark of congenital rubella. Excess cytokine stimulation from persistent infection may also play a role.

Immunologic responses also have been proposed as causes of cellular damage. Although cellular immune defects may be a result of chronic infection, it is possible that these defects contribute to ongoing tissue damage [382,427,431]. Excessive serum immunoglobulin development, persistent antibody production in the face of viral replication for prolonged periods, and production of rheumatoid factor, all indicative of overstimulation of the immune system, also may have a role in the pathogenesis of CRS [470,471]. The presence of immune complexes and autoantibodies and the influence of certain HLA types may contribute to the delayed expression of some signs of congenital rubella, such as pneumonitis, diabetes mellitus, thyroid dysfunction, and progressive rubella panencephalitis (see "Clinical Manifestations").* Some of these immunologic events may be directly involved in tissue damage (e.g., immune complexes, autoantibodies), whereas others may allow the virus to persist or reactivate.

PATHOLOGY
POSTNATAL INFECTION

Little is known about the pathology of postnatally acquired rubella because patients seldom die of this mild disease. As observed by Cherry [9], the histologic findings of tissues that have been examined (i.e., lymph nodes and autopsy specimens from patients dying with encephalitis) are unremarkable. Changes in lymphoreticular tissue have been limited to mild edema, nonspecific follicular hyperplasia, and some loss of normal follicular morphology. Examination of brain tissue has revealed diffuse swelling, nonspecific degeneration, and little meningeal and perivascular infiltrate.

CONGENITAL INFECTION

In contrast to the situation with postnatal rubella, much is known about the pathology of congenital rubella infection.† Generally, small foci of infected cells are seen in apparently normal tissue. Cellular necrosis and secondary inflammation are seldom obvious, although a generalized vasculitis predominates (see "Pathogenesis").

The pathologic findings of the placenta include hypoplasia, inflammatory foci in chorionic villi, granulomatous changes, mild edema, focal hyalinization, and necrosis [453,454,472,473]. Disease usually causes extensive damage to the endothelium of the capillaries and smaller blood vessels of the chorion. The vessel lesions consist mainly of endothelial necrosis, with fragmentation of intraluminal blood cells. Töndury and Smith [453] postulated that emboli of infected endothelial cells originating from the chorion might seed target organs in the fetus. These emboli may also contribute to organ damage by obstructing the fetal blood supply. Petechiae and the presence of hemosiderin-laden phagocytes in surrounding tissue are evidence of functional vascular damage [454].

Although not nearly as common as vascular lesions, specific cytolysis, presumably caused by direct viral effect on the cell, is also present in the placenta. This condition is characterized by cytoplasmic eosinophilia, nuclear pyknosis or karyorrhexis, and cellular necrosis. Specific nuclear and cytoplasmic cellular inclusion bodies are rare, but have been observed [473]. Although placentitis would be expected to be present in all affected placentas, regardless of when fetal infection occurred, Garcia and colleagues [473] found that placental lesions seemed to be more intense when infection occurred in the last trimester

---

*References 13, 14, 121, 124, 125, 127, 129, 130, 133–138, 398, 411.

†References 2, 3, 6, 9, 453–457, 472.

of pregnancy. This finding is consistent with the observation that the placenta is not a barrier to fetal infection in the latter stages of pregnancy [107,113,343,345].

Autopsies show that virtually every organ may be involved, with hypoplasia being a common finding. The necrotizing angiopathy of small blood vessels seen in the placenta is the most characteristic lesion in fetal organs. Cytolysis with tissue necrosis and accompanying inflammatory changes is also far less common, but has been found in the myocardium, brain, spinal cord, skeletal muscle, viscera, and epithelial cells of the developing lens, inner ear (organ of Corti), and teeth.

The overall pathologic process of congenital rubella, in keeping with its chronic nature, is progressive. Healing and new lesions can be found in specimens obtained in the later stages of gestation [453,454]. The pathologic changes vary among embryos in quantity and in organ distribution, and the location and nature of organ lesions depend on the gestational age at the time of infection [453]. The pathologic findings parallel the enormous variability of the clinical disease seen in infected newborns.

CLINICAL MANIFESTATIONS
POSTNATAL INFECTION
Rubella is usually a mild disease with few complications. Clinical illness may be more severe in adults.* Measles, varicella, and some enteroviruses acquired close to delivery may be associated with serious illness in the newborn, probably because of fetal exposure to transplacental viremia in the absence of protective levels of maternal antibody. One case report suggests that the same may be true in rubella. Sheinis and associates [475] reported the death of a neonate with rash onset when 12 days old; the mother developed rash on the day of delivery. This single observation needs to be confirmed. There are no conclusive data to indicate that infection in the immunocompromised host is associated with an increased risk of complications.

The first symptoms of rubella occur after an incubation period of 16 to 18 days (range 14 to 21 days). In a child, rash is often the first sign detected. In adolescents and adults, the eruption is commonly preceded by a 1- to 5-day prodromal period characterized by low-grade fever, headache, malaise, anorexia, mild conjunctivitis, coryza, sore throat, cough, and lymphadenopathy usually involving suboccipital, postauricular, and cervical nodes.

The constitutional symptoms often subside rapidly with the appearance of the rash. The rash can last 1 to 5 days or longer and can be pruritic in adults. Infection without a rash is quite common. The ratio of subclinical to clinical infections has varied from 1:9 to 7:1 [271,307]. Subclinical infection can lead to fetal infection, although it is unclear whether the risk is as great as that associated with clinically apparent infection.†

Arthralgia and frank arthritis with recrudescence of low-grade fever and other constitutional symptoms may appear after the rash fades. Joint involvement typically lasts 5 to 10 days, but may be more persistent. The frequency of these symptoms is variable, but they are more common in adults, particularly women [9]. In some studies of adult patients, the frequency has been 70% [476]. Thrombocytopenia (occurring in approximately 1 of 3000 patients) and acute postinfection encephalitis (occurring in 1 of 5000 to 6000 patients) are rare complications that usually occur 2 to 4 days after rash onset [9]. Rare complications associated with postnatal rubella include myocarditis, Guillain-Barré syndrome, relapsing encephalitis, optic neuritis, and bone marrow aplasia [9,477–481]. In a rubella outbreak in the Tongan islands, encephalitis was particularly frequent [482]. Two cases of a progressive panencephalitis, similar to measles-associated subacute sclerosing panencephalitis, have been reported [445,446]. This CNS disturbance is more likely to manifest in patients with CRS, although it still occurs infrequently [398,483,484]. Testalgia has also been reported in patients with rubella, but this may have been a coincidental finding [485,486].

An ophthalmic disease called Fuchs heterochromic cyclitis, a form of uveitis, has been associated more recently with rubella virus infection [487–491]. The disease usually affects only one eye with manifestations of chronic, low-grade anterior uveitis that may lead to cataract, glaucoma, vitreous opacities, and change of iris color. This condition is painless. All patients are seropositive for rubella, and intraocular antibody production of rubella (but not other pathogens) has been shown in adults and in a 13-year-old unvaccinated child [489,492].

CONGENITAL INFECTION
Gregg's original report [12] in 1941 defined CRS as a constellation of defects, usually involving some combination of congenital heart, eye, and hearing abnormalities, with or without mental retardation and microcephaly. After the extensive studies in the mid-1960s, in which virologic and serologic methods of assessment were used, the pathologic potential associated with intrauterine rubella infection had to be greatly expanded [2,3]. The recognition of various new defects associated with congenital rubella infection led to speculation that they had not existed before the 1962–1964 pandemic. A review of the abnormalities in infants born during previous nonepidemic periods indicated, however, that they were not new, but had not been appreciated previously because of the small number of affected infants studied [493].

The virus can infect one or virtually all fetal organs and, when established, can persist for long periods (see "Transmission In Utero," "Natural History," "Pathogenesis," and "Pathology").* Congenital rubella, a chronic infection, may kill the fetus in utero, causing miscarriage or stillbirth. At the other extreme, the infection may have no apparent effect clinically detectable at the delivery of a normal-appearing infant. Alternatively, severe multiple birth defects may be obvious in the newborn period. The wide spectrum of disease is discussed later and summarized in Tables 28–3 and 28–4.

---

*References 6, 9, 302, 305, 370, 474.
†References 2, 3, 6, 109, 112, 345, 351.

*References 6, 13, 14, 111, 135, 136, 165, 288–293, 295, 310, 324–330, 340–347, 390–398, 411.

TABLE 28-3 Abnormalities of Congenital Rubella Usually Not Detected until Second Year or Later

Defects	References
Hearing	
Peripheral	13, 333, 338, 515–518
Central	
Language	13, 510, 518, 519
Developmental	
Motor	13, 520, 521
Intellectual	13, 496, 520
Behavioral	13, 520
Psychiatric	13, 520
Autism	13, 446
Endocrine	
Diabetes	13, 116, 124, 129, 130
Precocious puberty	13, 14
Hypothyroidism	523–527
Thyroiditis	524–526
Hyperthyroidism	116, 529
Growth hormone deficiency	531, 532, 553
Addison disease	14
Visual	
Glaucoma (later onset)	533
Subretinal neovascularization	534, 535
Keratic precipitates	533
Keratoconus	536
Corneal hydrops	536
Lens absorption	537
Dental	511, 538
Progressive panencephalitis	392, 476, 477
Educational difficulties	13
Hypertension	539

during the neonatal period. Among infants who were followed, 71% developed manifestations of infection at various times in the first 5 years of life. Many important rubella defects can be undetectable or overlooked in the early months of life. Existing manifestations of infection can progress, and new manifestations may appear throughout life.* Some abnormalities of CRS usually are not detected until the 2nd year of life or later (see Table 28–3). The silent and progressive nature of congenital rubella infection has important implications for accurate, timely diagnosis and appropriate short-term and long-term management.

It is useful to group the clinical features of congenital rubella into three categories: transient manifestations in newborns and infants; permanent manifestations, which may be present at birth or become apparent during the 1st year of life; and developmental and late-onset manifestations, which usually appear and progress during childhood, adolescence, and early adult life [13,452,494]. These groupings overlap.

Transient Manifestations

Transient manifestations seem to reflect ongoing heavy viral infection, perhaps abetted by the newborn's emerging, often abnormal immune function [6,124,138]. Examples of these manifestations include hepatosplenomegaly, hepatitis, jaundice, thrombocytopenia with petechiae and purpura, discrete bluish red ("blueberry muffin") lesions of dermal erythropoiesis, hemolytic anemia, chronic rash, adenopathy, meningoencephalitis (in some cases), large anterior fontanelle, interstitial pneumonia, myositis, myocarditis, diarrhea, cloudy cornea, and disturbances in bone growth that appear as striated radiolucencies in the long bones. More than 50% of infants with these transient findings usually have evidence of intrauterine growth restriction and may continue to fail to thrive during infancy [289]. These transient abnormalities were referred to as the *expanded rubella syndrome* when widely reported after the pandemic of 1962–1964. Careful review of early observations during the 1940s and 1950s revealed that these were not new manifestations of congenital rubella.

These conditions usually are self-limiting and clear spontaneously over days or weeks [2]. These lesions are important from a diagnostic and prognostic standpoint.

Silent infections in the infant are much more common than symptomatic ones. Schiff and colleagues [344] prospectively examined 4005 infants born after the 1964 rubella epidemic. Based on virologic and serologic techniques to detect infection in the newborns, the overall rate of congenital rubella was greater than 2% compared with only approximately 0.1% in endemic years [344,351]. Of the infected newborns, 68% had subclinical infection

*References 6, 13, 14, 111, 135, 136, 340–347.

TABLE 28-4 Maximal Theoretical Risks of Congenital Rubella Syndrome (CRS) after Rubella Vaccination by Vaccine Strain, United States, 1971–1988*

Vaccine Strain	Susceptible Vaccinated Subjects	Normal Live Births	Risk of CRS Observed	Theoretical
RA 27/3	226	229†	0	0–1.8
Cendehill or HPV–77	94	94	—	0–3.8
Unknown	1	1	0	—
Total	*321*	*324*	*0*	*0–1.2*

*No women entered in the register after 1980 were vaccinated with Cendehill or HPV–77 vaccine.
†Includes three twin births.

They may be associated with other, more severe defects; this applies especially to thrombocytopenia and bone lesions [13,494]. The mortality rate was approximately 35% in one group of infants who presented with neonatal thrombocytopenia. Extreme prematurity, gross cardiac lesions or myocarditis with early heart failure, rapidly progressive hepatitis, extensive meningoencephalitis, and fulminant interstitial pneumonitis contributed to the mortality during infancy [452].

Permanent Manifestations

Permanent manifestations include heart and other blood vessel defects, eye lesions, CNS abnormalities, deafness, and various other congenital anomalies. These structural defects result from defective organogenesis (i.e., some cardiac, eye, and other organ defects) and from tissue destruction and scarring (i.e., hearing loss, brain damage, cataracts, chorioretinopathy, and vascular stenosis).

Relatively few defects result from gross anatomic abnormalities. It is uncertain that all of the malformations listed in Table 28–5 are associated with congenital rubella [13,325,391,465,493–521]. Because many of them occur in the absence of intrauterine rubella infection, their presence in affected infants may be coincidental [9].

Congenital heart disease is present in more than half of children infected during the first 2 months of gestation. The most common lesions, in descending order, are patent ductus arteriosus, pulmonary artery stenosis, and pulmonary valvular stenosis. Aortic valvular stenosis and tetralogy of Fallot have also been recorded. A patent ductus arteriosus occurs alone in approximately one third of cases; otherwise, it is frequently associated with pulmonary artery or valvular stenosis [13,494,506]. Stenosis of other vessels plays an important role in the spectrum of CRS [456,515,516]. These lesions may be related to coronary, cerebral, renal, and peripheral vascular disease seen in adults [135,522].

TABLE 28–5 Clinical Findings and Their Estimated Frequency of Occurrence in Young Symptomatic Infants with Congenitally Acquired Rubella

Clinical Findings	Frequency*	References
Adenopathies	++	480, 481
Anemia	+	481, 483
Bone		
Micrognathia	+	479
Extremities	+	479
Bony radiolucencies	++	480, 484–486, 493
Brain		
Encephalitis (active)	++	494, 495
Microcephaly	+	494, 495, 618
Brain calcification	Rare	495, 497, 498
Bulging fontanelle	+	384, 480
Cardiovascular system		
Pulmonary arterial hypoplasia	++	499
Patent ductus arteriosus	++	499
Coarctation of aortic isthmus	+	499
Interventricular septal defect	Rare	
Interauricular septal defect	Rare	
Others	Rare	13
Chromosomal abnormalities	?	458
Dermal erythropoiesis (blueberry muffin syndrome)	+	500, 501
Dermatoglyphic abnormalities	+	502, 503
Ear		
Hearing defects (severe)	+++	480
Peripheral	+++	480
Central	+	
Eye	++	480, 504–506
Retinopathy	+++	13
Cataracts	++	384, 479–481, 494, 504, 507, 618
Cloudy cornea	Rare	480
Glaucoma	Rare	481, 494, 504
Microphthalmos	+	480, 504

Continued

TABLE 28–5   Clinical Findings and Their Estimated Frequency of Occurrence in Young Symptomatic Infants with Congenitally Acquired Rubella—cont'd

Clinical Findings	Frequency	References
Genitourinary tract	+	480
Undescended testicle	+	480, 511
Polycystic kidney[†]	Rare	509
Bilobed kidney with reduplicated ureter[†]	Rare	509
Hypospadias	Rare	14, 510
Unilateral agenesis[†]	Rare	509
Renal artery stenosis with hypertension[†]	Rare	510
Hydroureter and hydronephrosis[†]	Rare	495
Growth restriction		
Intrauterine	+++	384, 479–481, 494, 507, 618
Extrauterine	++	511, 618
Hepatitis	Rare	479, 480, 494, 512
Hepatosplenomegaly	+++	384, 479, 481, 494, 507, 618
Immunologic dyscrasias	Rare	513
Interstitial pneumonitis (acute, subacute, chronic)	++	125, 480, 494, 514
Jaundice (regurgitative)	+	494, 507
Leukopenia	+	483
Myocardial necrosis	Rare	494, 495, 505, 512
Neurologic deficit	++	13, 496
Prematurity	+	384, 479–481, 494, 507, 512, 618
Thrombocytopenia with or without purpura	++	479–481, 494, 507, 618
Others[†]	Rare	
Esophageal atresia		618
Tracheoesophageal fistula		507
Anencephaly		507
Encephalocele		479, 507
Meningomyelocele		496
Cleft palate		507, 618
Inguinal hernia		
Asplenia		
Nephritis (vascular)		495
Clubfoot		507
High palate		511
Talipes equinovarus		511
Depressed sternum		511
Pes cavus		511
Clinodactyly		511
Brachydactyly		511
Syndactyly		511
Elfin facies		511

Frequency of occurrence is classified as follows: +, <20%; ++, 20%–50%; +++, 50%–75%.
[†]*Rarely associated with rubella syndrome (whether caused by infection is unknown). Incidence is seemingly increased in infants with congenital rubella.*

A "salt and pepper" retinopathy caused by disturbed growth of the pigmentary layer of the retina is the most common ocular finding [6,13,452,494]. Cataracts, often accompanied by microphthalmia, occur in approximately one third of all cases of congenital rubella. Bilateral cataracts are found in half of affected children. Primary glaucoma is uncommon; it does not affect a cataractous eye. Cataracts and infantile glaucoma may not be present or detectable at birth, but usually become apparent during the early weeks of life. Other ocular abnormalities occur later in life (see "Developmental and Late-Onset Manifestations").

Children with CRS exhibit numerous CNS abnormalities that follow widespread insult to the brain. Microcephaly can be a feature of this syndrome. Mental retardation and motor retardation are common and are directly related to the acute meningoencephalitis in 10% to 20% of affected children at birth [9]. Behavioral and psychiatric disorders have been confirmed in many patients [13,452].

Of particular interest is autism, which has been reported to occur with a frequency of approximately 6% [452]. Chronic encephalitis has been reported in young children [6]. Late-onset progressive panencephalitis may occur in the 2nd decade of life [398,483,484]. This condition is discussed later with other developmental manifestations.

The incidence of deafness has been underestimated because many cases had been missed in infancy and early childhood. Follow-up studies showed that deafness was the most common manifestation of congenital rubella, however, occurring in 80% or more of children infected.* In contrast to other serious defects, hearing impairment often is the only significant consequence of congenital rubella. Rubella-related defects of organogenesis (i.e., cataracts and some heart lesions) are uncommon after infection beyond 8 weeks of gestation. The organ of Corti is vulnerable to the effects of the virus up to the first 16 weeks, however, and perhaps up to the first 18 to 20 weeks. Deafness, ranging from mild to profound and from unilateral or bilateral, is usually peripheral (sensorineural) and is more commonly bilateral. Central auditory impairment and language delay may lead to a misdiagnosis of mental retardation [13,523–527].

Developmental and Late-Onset Manifestations

Developmental and late-onset manifestations have been reviewed by Sever and Shaver and their colleagues [135,136]. These manifestations include endocrinopathies, deafness, ocular damage, vascular effects, and progression of CNS disease (see Table 28–3).† Numerous mechanisms may be responsible for the continuing disease process that leads to these abnormalities, including persistent viral infection, viral reactivation, vascular insufficiency, and immunologic insult. The last problem may be mediated by circulating immune complexes and autoantibodies. Hyper-IgM syndrome with combined immunodeficiency and autoimmunity has been reported [528]. Abnormalities in cellular immunity and genetic factors have also been studied.

Insulin-dependent diabetes mellitus is the most frequent of all these manifestations, occurring in approximately 20% of patients by adulthood [13,121,129, 134–136,529]. This reported prevalence is 100 to 200 times that observed for the general population. A Japanese study of CRS patients with 40 years of follow-up reported only 1.1% diabetics, however [529a]. Studies of HLA type indicate that CRS patients with diabetes have the same frequencies of selected HLA haplotypes as diabetic patients without CRS (e.g., increased HLA-DR3 and decreased HLA-DR2). The presence of pancreatic islet cell and cytotoxic surface antibodies in children with CRS does not seem to be related to any specific HLA type. It has been postulated that congenital infection increases the penetrance of a preexisting susceptibility to diabetes in these patients [134]. Rabinowe and coworkers [137] also reported an elevation in the number of Ia-positive ("activated") T cells in patients with CRS.

They suggested that this T-cell abnormality may be related in these patients to the increased incidence of diabetes mellitus and other diseases associated with autoantibodies.

Thyroid dysfunction affects about 5% of patients and manifests as hyperthyroidism, hypothyroidism, and thyroiditis [121,133,530–535]. Autoimmune mechanisms seem to be responsible for these abnormalities. Clarke and colleagues [133] reported that 23% of 201 deaf teenagers with congenital infection had autoantibodies to the microsomal or globulin fraction, or both fractions, of the thyroid and that 20% of those with autoantibodies had thyroid gland dysfunction. Coexistence of diabetes and thyroid dysfunction has been reported, but the significance of the association is unknown [121,137].

Two cases of growth hormone deficiency have been reported [536]. The defect seems to be hypothalamic in origin. Among eight growth-restricted older children with CRS, Oberfield and associates [537] found no evidence, however, of functional abnormality in the hypothalamic-pituitary axis and normal or elevated levels of somatomedin C. Growth patterns in 105 subjects in late adolescence revealed three patterns: growth consistently below the fifth percentile; growth in the normal range, but early cessation of growth, usually with a final height below the fifth percentile; and normal growth. The magnitude of the cognitive deficits was closely correlated with growth failure [538]. Ziring [14] commented on a case with Addison disease, and precocious puberty has been observed [13,14].

The delayed diagnosis of preexisting deafness has already been mentioned. The hearing deficit can increase over time, however, and sudden onset of sensorineural deafness may occur after years of normal auditory acuity [356,539,540]. As reported by Sever and coworkers [135], the latter has been observed in a 10-year-old child.

Many late-onset ocular defects can occur. Glaucoma has been reported in patients 3 to 22 years old who did not previously have the congenital or infantile variety of glaucoma associated with CRS [541]. Other reported manifestations are keratic precipitates, keratoconus, corneal hydrops, and spontaneous lens absorption [542].

The retinopathy of congenital rubella, which was previously believed to be completely benign, has more recently been associated with the delayed occurrence of visual difficulties caused by subretinal neovascularization [543–545]. Another delayed manifestation associated with vascular changes is hypertension resulting from renal artery and aortic stenosis [522].

Mental retardation, autism, and other behavioral problems may be delayed in appearance and can be progressive [13,452]. The most serious delayed CNS manifestation is the occurrence of a progressive and fatal panencephalitis resembling subacute sclerosing panencephalitis, which manifests during the 2nd decade of life. The first cases were reported by Weil and Townsend and their coworkers [398,483]. At the time of their review, Waxham and Wolinsky [484] found that 10 cases of progressive rubella panencephalitis had been identified among patients with CRS. Two cases have been reported after postnatally acquired rubella [445,446]. Patients with this condition present with increasing loss of mental function, seizures, and ataxia. These symptoms continue to progress until the patient is in a vegetative state and ultimately dies.

---

*References 6, 9, 13, 14, 111, 135, 136, 340, 341, 343–346.

†References 13, 14, 121, 129, 134, 135, 137, 340, 345, 411, 484, 485, 503, 516, 522–527, 529–537, 540–546, 616, 617.

Rubella virus has been recovered from the brain of one congenitally infected patient [398]. Elevated serum and cerebrospinal fluid antibodies and increased amounts of cerebrospinal fluid protein and γ-globulin have been detected. Virus has also been isolated from lymphocytes, and rubella-specific immune complexes have been identified [125,546]. Although rare, this syndrome focuses attention on the ability of the virus to persist and to become reactivated after years of latency.

Long-Term Prognosis

Investigators examined 50 survivors of the congenital rubella epidemic of 1939–1943 in Australia at age 25, and their status was reviewed again in 1991 [547]. Seven subjects had died in the interval—three with malignancies, three with cardiovascular disease, and one with acquired immunodeficiency syndrome (AIDS). Among the survivors in 1991, 5 were diabetic, all 40 examined were deaf, 23 had eye defects, and 16 had cardiovascular defects. Despite these conditions, the group was characterized by remarkably good social adjustment. Most (29) were married, and they had 51 children—only 1 with a congenital defect (deafness presumed to be hereditary from his deaf father, who did not have congenital rubella). Most survivors were of normal stature, although 6 of the 40 were less than the third percentile for height.

The group of survivors from Australia is quite different from the approximately 300 survivors followed in New York since the rubella epidemic of 1963–1965 [39]. In their late 20s, approximately one third of these survivors were leading relatively normal lives in the community, one third were living with their parents with "noncompetitive" employment, and one third were residing in facilities with 24-hour care. Neither the Australian nor the New York group is a representative sample of all survivors of maternal rubella infection, but these groups do offer insight on long-term prognosis. The differences in outcome between the Australian group (survivors of Gregg's original patients) and the New York group probably reflect the different methods by which the groups were collected and the significant differences in the medical technology of the 1940s compared with the 1960s.

LABORATORY DIAGNOSIS

Timely, accurate diagnosis of acute primary rubella infection in a pregnant woman and congenital rubella infection in an infant is imperative if appropriate management is to be undertaken (see "Management Issues"). The diagnosis must be confirmed serologically or virologically because clinical diagnosis of postnatal and congenital rubella is unreliable. In any suspected exposure of a pregnant woman, every effort should be made to confirm rubella infection so that accurate counseling can be offered about the risks to the fetus. Laboratory proof of congenital infection facilitates proper treatment, follow-up, and long-term management.

MATERNAL INFECTION

All women of childbearing age should have been vaccinated against rubella as children or in gynecologic care before conception. In addition, they should be screened for rubella IgG antibodies at the first obstetric visit and tested further for IgM antibodies (see later) if they give a history of rash or exposure to rash illness earlier in pregnancy. Most experts accept an enzyme-linked immunosorbent assay titer of 10 IU or greater as an indication of immunity; however, some experts accept greater than 15 IU [548,549]. Women who are IgG antibody negative at the first visit should be retested 2 to 3 weeks later if the fetus is less than 16 weeks' gestational age to exclude intercurrent infection. All seronegative women should be vaccinated postpartum [550].

Because of inapparent infection, the variable clinical manifestations of rubella, and the mimicking of rubella by other viral exanthems, laboratory diagnosis is essential in managing potential rubella infection during pregnancy (see "Natural History" and "Clinical Manifestations") [161,210,237,238,551]. Although virus can be cultured from the nose and throat, isolation techniques are slow and labor-intensive. Reverse transcriptase PCR offers another reliable tool for confirming the diagnosis during acute rubella, but laboratory confirmation of acquired infection in nonpregnant persons is usually limited to serologic testing (see "Virus").

Acute primary infection can usually be documented by showing a significant increase in rubella IgG antibody level between acute and convalescent sera or the presence of rubella-specific IgM antibody. Appropriate timing of specimen collection with regard to rash onset (or exposure in the case of subclinical infection) is crucial for accurate interpretation of results. Diagnosis is greatly facilitated if the immune status is known before disease onset or exposure [270]. Women with laboratory evidence of immunity are not considered to be at risk. From a practical point of view, women with a history of vaccination on or after the first birthday should also be considered immune [267,268]. Because seroconversion is not 100% (see "Prevention of Congenital Rubella"), serologic testing may be indicated on an individual basis in vaccinated women who have a known exposure or a rash and illness consistent with rubella to rule out acute primary infection or reinfection.

Traditionally, a fourfold or greater increase in antibody titer (i.e., HI, complement fixation, or latex agglutination tests) has been considered a significant increase in antibody. With the advent of enzyme immunoassay, the diagnosis may be based on significant changes in optical density expressed as an index rather than a titer. The acute phase specimen should be obtained as soon as possible after onset of the rash, ideally within 7 days. If a positive titer is obtained for a specimen taken on the day of rash onset or 1 to 2 days later, the risk of acute infection is low, but cannot be excluded. The convalescent phase serum sample should be taken 10 to 14 days later. If the first serum sample is obtained more than 7 days after rash onset, some assays (e.g., HI) may be unable to detect a significant antibody increase because titers may have already peaked. In this situation, measurement of antibodies that appear later in the course of infection may be useful. A significant increase in complement fixation titer or a high HI, latex agglutination, or enzyme immunoassay titer and little or no antibody as measured by passive hemagglutination suggests recent infection.

When multiple serum samples are obtained in the course of the diagnostic work-up, all should be tested simultaneously in the same laboratory to avoid misinterpretation of laboratory-related variations in titer. Although a single high titer is consistent with recent infection, it is not specific enough to conclude that recent infection has occurred [270].

Detection of rubella-specific IgM is a very useful method for confirming acute recent infection. Although rubella-specific IgM testing is valuable, numerous factors can affect test results. Results must be interpreted with careful attention to the timing of the specimens. Samples obtained within the first several days after onset of rash may have low or undetectable levels of rubella-specific IgM, but a specimen obtained 7 to 14 days later invariably shows higher titers of antibody. The levels of rubella-specific IgM may decline promptly thereafter. Many of the methods previously described for detecting IgM have some limitations (see "Virus"). IgM antibody testing may involve pretreatment of the serum by various techniques to separate IgM from IgG, such as column chromatography, sucrose gradient centrifugation, or adsorption of IgG with staphylococcal protein A.

The serum IgM fraction can be assayed by HI, immunofluorescence, radioimmunoassay, or enzyme immunoassay.* A false-positive result may occur if the serum was pretreated with protein A because about 5% of IgG is not removed. The radioimmunoassay and enzyme immunoassay techniques can detect specific IgM antibodies directly in unfractionated sera, but false-positive results may be produced by the presence of rheumatoid factor [161,218,220]. A solid-phase, immunosorbent (i.e., capture) technique seems to be unaffected by rheumatoid factor [103,221,236,247]. A warning is necessary.

Although high or moderate titers provide very good evidence of recent infection, low rubella-specific IgM titers detected by sensitive assays must be interpreted cautiously. Low titers have been shown to persist for many months in a few patients after natural infection and can be detected in some immune patients with subclinical reinfection [45,55,57,59,365–370]. Diagnosis of subclinical infection is straightforward if the woman is known to be susceptible, the exposure is recognized, and a serum sample is obtained approximately 28 days after exposure.

The diagnosis of subclinical infection is more difficult if the immune status of the woman is unknown. It can be facilitated, however, if the acute-phase serum specimen is obtained as soon as possible after a recognized exposure that did not occur more than 5 weeks earlier [270]. The convalescent serum sample, if necessary, should be obtained approximately 3 weeks later. If the first specimen lacks detectable antibody, continued close clinical observance and serologic follow-up are necessary. If the first specimen has detectable antibody and was obtained within 7 to 10 days of exposure, there is no risk of infection, and further evaluation is unnecessary. A positive titer in a specimen obtained after this period indicates a need for further serologic investigation. If test results of paired serum specimens are inconclusive, rubella-specific IgM testing may be helpful, but a negative test result may be difficult to interpret. Dried blood spots have been useful in the detection of IgM antibodies because they show concordance with serum determinations [552,553].

More significant diagnostic difficulties arise when women of unknown immune status are exposed at an unknown time, were exposed more than 5 weeks earlier, or had rash onset more than 3 weeks earlier [270]. In these situations, expert consultation may be necessary if positive titers are obtained. Where available, avidity testing of rubella IgG may be used to help clarify the timing of infection. Recent rubella infection is characterized by antibody of low avidity. When such low-avidity antibody is found in the presence of rubella-specific IgM, it supports a diagnosis of recent rubella infection [368–370]. Avidity results, which relate to the binding of antibody to the E1 protein, can be crucial in distinguishing recent from past infection [554,555].

Table 28–6 gives information on the prevalence of IgM antibodies and positive reverse transcriptase PCR results in acquired infection according to time since onset of rash [556]. Figure 28–8 shows the pattern of test results according to the stage of infection [25].

Conclusive information about the timing of past infection and risk to the fetus is often unavailable, even when a combination of antibody assays is used. These situations

*References 161, 217–221, 224, 226, 235–239, 241–249.

TABLE 28–6   Percentage of Patients Testing Positive for Wild Measles and Rubella Virus Infection, by Time of Specimen Collection, Type of Specimen, and Type of Sampling Method Used—World Health Organization (WHO) Measles and Rubella Laboratory Network

	Time of Collection	Serum (%)	Dried Blood Spots (%)	Oral Fluid (%)
IgM				
	Early (day 0-3)	50	50	40
	Intermediate (day 4-14)	60-90	60-90	50-90
	Late (day 15-28)	100	100	100
Virus Detection (RT-PCR)				
	Early (day 0-3)	—	20	60-70
	Intermediate (day 4-14)	—	—	50
	Late (day 15-28)	—	—	—

RT-PCR, reverse transcriptase polymerase chain reaction.

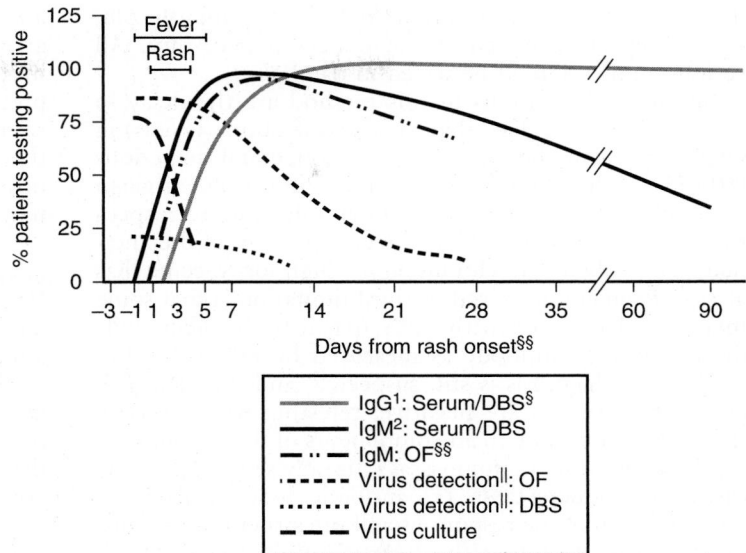

FIGURE 28–8 Pattern of test results among patients with mild rubella virus infection, by day from rash onset and type of sampling method used—World Health Organization (WHO) Measles and Rubella Laboratory Network. DBS, dried blood spots; OF, oral fluid.

* Illustrative schematic based on data presented at the Measles and Rubella Alternative Sampling Techniques Review Meeting, convened in Geneva, Switzerland, in June 2007.
† Immunoglobulin G.
‡ Dried blood spots.
§ Immunoglobulin M.
§§ Oral fluid.
‖ Virus RNA detection by conventional, nested, or real-time reverse transcription–polymerase chain reaction.
¶ Incubation period: 14–17 days.

can be minimized if prenatal rubella testing is done routinely. Laboratories performing prenatal screening should store these specimens until delivery in case retesting is necessary [267,551].

CONGENITAL INFECTION

A presumptive diagnosis of congenital rubella infection should be considered for any infant born to a mother who had documented or suspected rubella infection at any time during pregnancy (see "Transmission In Utero") [107,113]. The diagnosis should also be considered in any infant with evidence of intrauterine growth restriction and other stigmata consistent with congenital infection, regardless of maternal history (see "Clinical Manifestations"). Although such findings are sensitive for clinically apparent disease, they are nonspecific because many of them can be associated with other intrauterine infections, such as cytomegalovirus infection, syphilis, and toxoplasmosis. Many affected infants are asymptomatic. As with maternal rubella, congenital infection must be confirmed by laboratory tests.

In contrast to maternal rubella, attempting to isolate rubella virus in tissue culture is a valuable tool for diagnosing congenital rubella in newborns. The virus is most readily isolated from the posterior pharynx and less consistently from the conjunctivae, cerebrospinal fluid, or urine.* Virus isolation should be attempted as soon as

congenital rubella is suspected clinically because viral excretion wanes during infancy (see Fig. 28–7). In older children in whom virus shedding has ceased from other sites, virus may be isolated from cataractous lens tissue [395]. In children with encephalitis, virus may persist in the cerebrospinal fluid for several years [370–372,503].

There are two approaches for serologic diagnosis. First, cord serum can be assayed for the presence of rubella-specific IgM antibody [399,401,410,411]. Detectable IgM antibody is a reliable indicator of congenital infection because IgM is fetally derived. False-positive results may occur, however, because of rheumatoid factor or incomplete removal of IgG (largely maternal), depending on the techniques used. A few newborns with stigmata of congenital rubella may not have detectable levels of rubella-specific IgM in sera taken during the first days of life, and some infections may go undiagnosed if infection occurred late in pregnancy because it is theoretically possible that there was inadequate time for the fetus to produce detectable levels of specific IgM antibodies by the time of delivery [13,107,113].

A second approach is to monitor IgG levels in the infant over time to see if they persist. Maternally derived antibodies have a half-life of approximately 30 days [399,401,411]. As measured by the HI test, they usually decline at a rate of one twofold dilution per month and would be expected to disappear by 6 to 12 months of age (see Fig. 28–5). Persistence of IgG antibody at this age, especially in high titer, is presumptive evidence of intrauterine infection with rubella virus. Sera should be

---

*References 2, 13, 165, 288–293, 295, 324, 325, 327, 329, 393, 396.

drawn when the infant is 3 months and 5 to 6 months old, with a repeat specimen at 12 months if necessary. All serum samples should be tested in parallel.

Important limitations of this method are the delay in diagnosis and the fact that rubella infections occurring after birth may be mistaken for congenital infections [107,557]. The latter is usually more of a problem when attempting to diagnose congenital infection retrospectively in patients beyond infancy, especially if the incidence of rubella in childhood is high or vaccine has already been administered. A third limitation is that some infants and children with CRS (particularly older children) may lack antibody as measured by HI [345, 413–415]. If the diagnosis is still suspected, and the HI, IgM, and culture results are negative, retesting with an assay that detects antibody to all components of the virion, such as some enzyme immunoassays, is advised [91]. Some cases with undetectable HI antibody may be from an incomplete immune response to all the structural proteins of the virus, including the hemagglutinin (see "Virus") [86,87].

Other diagnostic methods, such as measurement of cellular immunity and response to vaccine (i.e., a failure to boost antibody titer), may also be helpful in this situation, but a definitive retrospective diagnosis often cannot be made [382,431,558,559]. Cerebrospinal fluid may also be examined for the presence of rubella-specific IgM [560]. As in the case for acquired infection, determination of avidity of IgG may be useful [368,370,561].

The availability of sensitive and specific tests for prenatal diagnosis of fetal infection after suspected or documented maternal rubella can greatly facilitate counseling. Although positive diagnoses were reported from examination of amniotic fluid, fetal blood, and chorionic villus sampling for virus isolation, rubella-specific IgM and antigens, interferon, and RNA [103,438,562–568], the low sensitivity of these assays added little to the counseling process. Reverse transcriptase nested PCR has been reported to offer a far more reliable and rapid tool and, where available, a valuable aid to counseling [189,569,570]. Timing of the specimen collection related to the timing of maternal infection may influence sensitivity, which reached 100% (eight of eight specimens) for amniotic fluid in one study and 83% (five of six specimens) for chorionic villus sampling in another study. Repeat testing may increase the yield of positive specimens [189,562].

Postnatal diagnosis of congenital rubella infection is based on one or more of the following tests: isolation of virus or positive reverse transcriptase PCR from fetal tissues or postnatal respiratory secretions, the demonstration of rubella-specific IgM antibodies in cord blood or neonatal serum, and persistence of rubella IgG antibodies beyond the 3 to 6 months required for elimination of maternally transmitted antibodies [187]. Figure 28–9 is an algorithm for diagnosis of maternal and congenital rubella proposed by Mendelson and colleagues [187].

MANAGEMENT ISSUES

The major management issues associated with postnatal infection arise when a pregnant woman is at risk of acquiring infection. Confirming the diagnosis, counseling about the risks of infection of and damage to the fetus, and discussing courses of action including the use of immunoglobulin and consideration of termination of pregnancy require a thorough understanding of the natural history and consequences of rubella in pregnancy. In the case of congenital infection, the emphasis is on diagnosis and acute and long-term management. Isolation may be important to reduce spread of infection.

USE OF IMMUNOGLOBULIN

The role of passive immunization with immunoglobulin after exposure to rubella is controversial.* Brody and co-workers [572] reported that large doses of immunoglobulin may have some efficacy, but immunoglobulin generally proved to be more useful when given prophylactically than when administered after exposure. This finding is not surprising because extensive viral replication is demonstrable 1 week or more before symptoms appear, with initial replication probably beginning even earlier. The amount of antirubella antibody in commercial immunoglobulin preparations is variable and unpredictable; specific hyperimmunoglobulin preparations are unavailable [574,575].

Theoretically, the role of circulating antibodies in rubella is mainly to limit the viremia and possibly to prevent replication at the portal of entry; antibody is less valuable after infection has begun. Fetal infection occurred when immunoglobulin was administered to the mother in what seemed to be adequate amounts soon after exposure. Another disadvantage of immunoglobulin is that it may eliminate or reduce clinical findings without affecting viral replication. Clinical clues of maternal infection would be masked without adequate protection of the fetus, resulting in a false sense of security.

It is recommended that use of immunoglobulin be confined to rubella-susceptible women known to have been exposed who do not wish to interrupt their pregnancy under any circumstances [266,268]. In this situation, large doses (20 mL in adults) should be administered. The patient should be advised that protection from fetal infection cannot be guaranteed.

TERMINATION OF PREGNANCY

A discussion of the complex issues involved in the decision about termination of pregnancy for maternal rubella is beyond the scope of this chapter. The decision must be carefully weighed by the physician and the prospective parents. The physician must have a thorough understanding of the known facts about the pathogenesis and diagnosis of congenital rubella and the risks to the fetus depending on the timing of maternal infection. Where available, analysis of amniotic fluid, fetal blood, or chorionic villus sampling by reverse transcriptase nested PCR may assist in antenatal diagnosis of infection [189, 569,570]. Expert consultation is desirable to ensure that the most current information is used in the decision-making process.

---

*References 2, 6, 9, 305, 311, 342, 345, 571–574.

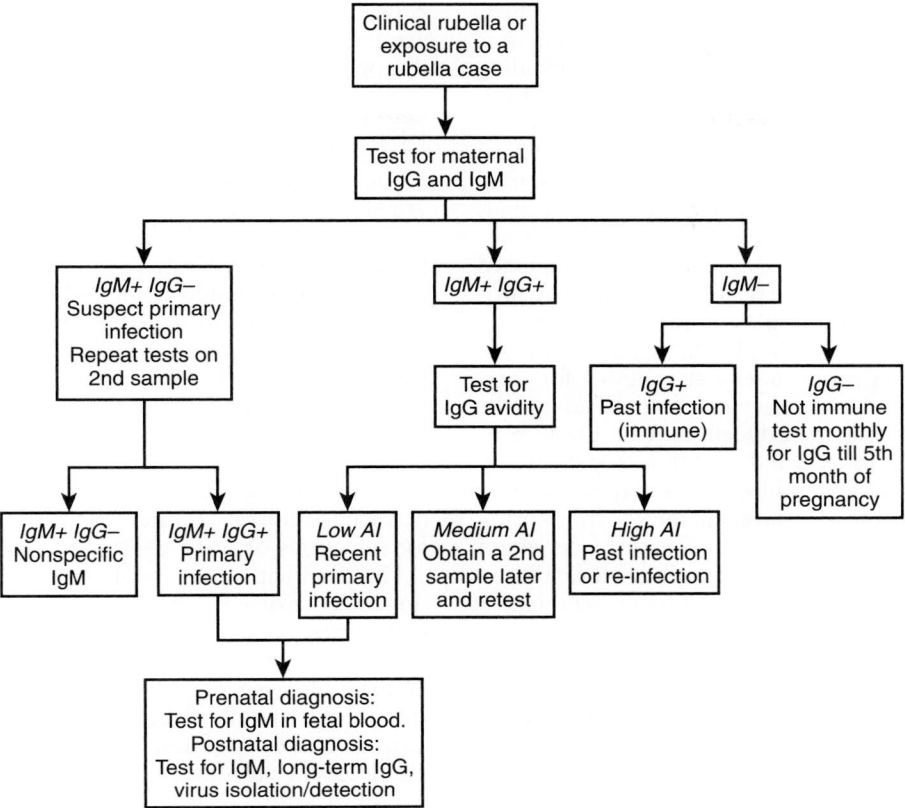

FIGURE 28–9 Algorithm for assessment of rubella infection in pregnancy shows a stepwise procedure beginning with testing of maternal blood for IgM and IgG. If maternal blood is negative for IgM (IgM−), the IgG results determine if the woman is seropositive (immune) or seronegative (not immune). If not immune, the woman should be retested monthly for seroconversion until the end of the 5th month of pregnancy. If the maternal blood is positive for IgM (IgM+) and IgG (IgG+), the next step would be an IgG avidity assay on the same blood sample to estimate the time of infection. Low avidity index (AI) indicates recent infection, whereas high AI indicates past positive and IgG negative (IgG−); recent primary infection is suspected, and the same tests should be repeated on a second blood sample obtained 2 to 3 weeks later. If the results remain the same (IgM+ IgG−), the IgM result is considered nonspecific, indicating that the woman has not been infected (however, she is seronegative and should be followed until the end of the 5th month). If the woman has seroconverted (IgM+ IgG+), recent primary infection is confirmed, and a prenatal diagnosis should be made if the woman wishes to continue her pregnancy. Determination of IgM in cord blood is the preferred diagnostic method with the highest prognostic value. Postnatal diagnosis is based on the newborn's serology (IgM for 6 to 12 months and IgG for >6 months) and on virus isolation from the newborn's respiratory secretions. (*Adapted from Mendelson E, et al. Laboratory assessment and diagnosis of congenital viral infections: rubella, cytomegalovirus [CMV], varicella-zoster virus [VZV], herpes simplex virus [HSV], parvovirus B19 and human immunodeficiency virus [HIV]. Reprod Toxicol 21:350-382, 2006.*)

CLINICAL MANAGEMENT

Acute rubella infection usually requires little clinical management. A patient with congenital infection may require medical, surgical, educational, and rehabilitative management, however. Many lesions are not apparent at birth because they have not yet appeared or cannot be detected. In keeping with its chronicity, congenital rubella must be managed as a dynamic rather than a static disease state. A continuing effort on the part of the physician must be made to define initially the extent of the problem and to detect evidence of progressive disease or emergence of new problems over time. Because of the broad range of problems, a multidisciplinary team approach to care is essential.

Complete pediatric, neurologic, cardiac, ophthalmologic, and audiologic examinations should be complemented by complete blood cell count, radiologic bone surveys, and often evaluation of cerebrospinal fluid for all newborns in whom the diagnosis is suspected, whether the infant is symptomatic or not. Some defects, such as interstitial pneumonitis, can be slowly progressive and apparently cause major functional difficulties months after birth. Infected infants require scrutiny during the first 6 months of life. Serial assessment for immunologic dyscrasias is necessary during this period because the humoral defects may be masked by the presence of maternal immunoglobulin.

Hearing defects and psychomotor difficulties are the most important problems because of their high incidence. Both often occur in infants who are initially asymptomatic. The new techniques for detection of hearing impairment in newborns and the state-mandated universal newborn hearing screening testing requirements have been initiated too recently to determine their utility in detection of unsuspected congenital rubella. Delay in diagnosis and therapeutic intervention has a profound impact on language development and skills acquisition and can magnify psychosocial adjustment problems within the entire family constellation.

Because many children with congenital rubella have multiple handicaps, early interdisciplinary treatment is warranted. Appropriate hearing aids; visual aids, including contact lenses; speech, language, occupational, and physical therapy; and special educational programs are frequently required for such children. Serial psychological and perceptual testing may be very helpful for ongoing management, particularly when performed by individuals experienced in assessing children with multiple handicaps who are sensorially deprived. In many cases, repeated testing is important because the problems seem to be progressive and require continuing assessment of the therapeutic approach. In the United States, most infants suspected to have congenital rubella are eligible for early intervention and habilitation services authorized by the Individuals with Disabilities Education Act. These programs offer services to affected children beginning in infancy, a critical time for children who may be hearing impaired. The impact of universal newborn hearing screening programs as another tool for early detection of congenital rubella and of cochlear implants for children with severe rubella deafness remains to be determined.

CHEMOTHERAPY

Because postnatal rubella is usually mild, there has been little need to pursue chemotherapeutic regimens, and the literature on this subject is sparse. Interferon has been used to treat chronic arthritis, and inosine pranobex (Isoprinosine) has been administered to a patient with postnatally acquired progressive rubella panencephalitis [446,546,576]. Chance temporal association between interferon administration and reported improvement in joint symptoms cannot be differentiated from potential therapeutic benefits of the interferon. In the trial of inosine pranobex, no improvement was observed.

Reports regarding treatment of infants with congenital rubella are limited. The course of congenital infection does not seem to be altered by any available chemotherapeutic agent. Because amantadine reduces the replication of rubella virus in vitro, it has theoretical possibilities as a chemotherapeutic agent [162–164]. Its use has been confined, however, to a 5-month-old infant with congenital infection [165]. Neither virus excretion nor clinical status was affected. Interferon has also been administered to a few infants with CRS. Arvin and associates [577] reported that nasopharyngeal excretion in three infants (3 to 5 months old) persisted throughout interferon administration, although at reduced titers compared with baseline. There was, however, no clinical effect. Larsson and coworkers [578] administered interferon to a 14-month-old child and reported regression of a cutaneous eruption resulting from vasculitis and disappearance of viremia. Viruria and other signs of viral persistence (e.g., rubella-specific IgM in the cerebrospinal fluid) were unaffected. It is also uncertain whether improvement in the rash was from interferon administration or was coincidental. A 10-month-old infant treated by Verder and coworkers [138] may have benefited from interferon, but improvement was also seen after exchange transfusions that preceded the interferon treatment. Inosine pranobex has been administered to some patients with progressive

rubella panencephalitis [546,579]. As for postnatally acquired disease, the results in this case have been disappointing.

ISOLATION

Patients with rubella are considered infectious from the 7th day before to the 5th to 7th day after the onset of the rash and should be placed in contact isolation [580,581]. Exposed rubella-susceptible patients confined to the hospital should be placed in contact isolation from the 7th through 21st day after exposure and tested appropriately to rule out asymptomatic infection [582]. Infectious patients with congenital rubella should also be in contact isolation [580]. Isolation precautions should be instituted as soon as rubella or congenital rubella is suspected. Only persons known to be immune (i.e., persons with serologic evidence of immunity or documentation of vaccination on or after the 1st birthday) should care for infectious or potentially infectious patients [266,268].

Children with CRS should be considered infectious for the 1st year of life unless repeated pharyngeal and urine culture results are negative [268,580]. Culture results are unlikely to become negative until the child is 3 to 6 months old (see Fig. 28–4). From a practical point of view, children older than 1 year are unlikely to be a significant source of infection. In the home situation, susceptible pregnant visitors should be informed of the potential risk of exposure.

PREVENTION OF CONGENITAL RUBELLA
RUBELLA VACCINE AND IMMUNIZATION STRATEGIES

Active immunization is the only practical means to prevent congenital rubella because passive immunization provides unreliable, transient protection (see "Management Issues"). There has been considerable debate, however, about the best way to use the vaccine [3,5–7,32, 37,583]. Because rubella vaccination is not aimed primarily at protecting the individual, but rather the unborn fetus, two basic strategies have been proposed: universal childhood immunization and selective vaccination of susceptible girls and women of childbearing age. The former approach is designed to interrupt transmission of virus by vaccinating the reservoir of infection; reduce the overall risk of infection in the general population; and provide indirect protection of unvaccinated, postpubertal women. The latter approach directly protects women at risk of being infected when pregnant, limits overall vaccine use, and allows virus to circulate and boost vaccine-induced immunity in the population. Experience gained during the past 30 years indicates that integration of both approaches is necessary to achieve maximum control in the shortest possible time [5,32,35,37].

At the time of licensure in 1969, available information indicated that the live-attenuated rubella vaccines were safe, noncommunicable, and highly effective [3,4,27–29]. Although information on the duration of vaccine-induced immunity was limited, public health policy makers in the

United States believed that vaccination of all children would provide protection into the childbearing years. The duration and quality of the immunity would have to be monitored continually. Because vaccine virus could cross the placenta and infect the fetus, cautious recommendations for vaccination of susceptible women of childbearing age were also proposed [343,584,585]. Vaccine was to be administered in this population only after susceptibility had been documented by serologic testing. Vaccinated women were also advised to avoid conception for 2 months after vaccination. After Fleet and colleagues [586] isolated virus from the fetus of a woman who had conceived 7 weeks before vaccination, this time interval was increased to 3 months as an extra precaution [266,268].

In some areas of the world, mass vaccination was considered undesirable because of concerns about the duration of vaccine-induced immunity [5–7,34,111]. Instead, vaccine was targeted for all girls 11 to 14 years of age and postpubertal women known to be seronegative. As with the U.S. program, pregnancy was to be avoided for 3 months after immunization. The goal was to immunize at least 90% of the women immediately at risk and simultaneously to provide a higher level of immunity throughout the group of women of childbearing age. It was recognized that this approach would take many years to have a significant effect on the incidence of congenital infection.

The U.S. strategy prevented epidemic disease, but initially had little effect on the occurrence of infection in young adults, particularly women of childbearing age (see "Epidemiology").* There was no evidence that infection was occurring in individuals who had been vaccinated years earlier (see "Update on Vaccine Characteristics"). Childhood vaccination decreased the overall risk of infection, but virus could still circulate in the community, especially wherever unvaccinated adolescents and adults congregated [271–279,282–287]. Although CRS could eventually be eliminated as vaccinated cohorts of children entered the childbearing years, this process would take many years, and potentially preventable cases of congenital infection would continue to occur [279]. Specific recommendations were made to increase vaccination levels in older individuals, particularly women of childbearing age (see "Vaccination Recommendations") [266,268].

Selective vaccination programs have not been successful because of the inability to immunize a sufficient proportion of the female population [7,35,36]. With this immunization approach, large-scale epidemics continue to occur, and the incidence of congenital rubella has not declined significantly since the introduction of vaccines. Because of these problems, in 1988, Great Britain implemented a program of MMR vaccination for all children in the 2nd year of life and initial catch-up in 2- to 4-year-olds. In 1994, a mass measles-rubella vaccine program for 5- to 16-year-old recipients was conducted to avert a measles epidemic. A preschool MMR booster was added in 1996 [35,37,587].

As highlighted in the previous paragraphs, the U.S. and UK programs adopted a combined approach to rubella control and elimination by the universal vaccination of children and selective vaccination of women of childbearing age. In 1997, as part of a regional initiative for rubella control and CRS prevention, PAHO developed a rubella and CRS control strategy that included introduction of a rubella-containing vaccine into routine childhood immunization programs, ensuring rubella vaccination of women of childbearing age to reduce the number of susceptible and to develop specific vaccination strategies for accelerated rubella control and CRS prevention. Two strategies for accelerated rubella control and CRS prevention were provided: Countries wishing to prevent and control CRS promptly were advised to conduct a one-time mass campaign to vaccinate all females 5 to 39 years of age with measles and rubella–containing vaccine, and countries wishing to prevent and control rubella and CRS promptly were advised to carry out a one-time mass campaign to vaccinate males and females 5 to 39 years of age with measles and rubella–containing vaccine [588].

Update on Vaccine Characteristics

Approximately 200 million doses of vaccine have been administered in the United States since rubella vaccines were licensed in 1969. The RA 27/3 strain of vaccine was licensed for use in Europe in 1971 and in the United States in 1979 and is now the only vaccine available. It was attenuated by serial passage in the WI-38 fetal human diploid cell strain with adaptation to growth at 30° C and is manufactured in the MRC-5 human diploid cell strain [387,586,589]. Although it has been used successfully by the intranasal and aerosol routes [590,591], it is licensed only for subcutaneous administration, usually as part of a combination with measles and mumps vaccines [592]. Compared with the Cendehill or HPV-77 strains of vaccines, the RA 27/3 vaccine elicits an immune response that more closely resembles the response occurring after natural infection [31,203,386,387]. There are no data to indicate the need for revaccination of persons who had previously received vaccine strains other than the RA 27/3.

Appropriate administration of the RA 27/3 vaccine induces an antibody response in 95% or more of persons 12 months old or older when vaccinated. Antibody is induced to the three major rubella virus structural proteins [86]. Vaccine efficacy and challenge studies indicate that more than 90% to 95% of vaccinated persons are protected against clinical illness or asymptomatic viremia. Although vaccine-induced titers are lower than titers after natural infection and are more likely to increase after reexposure, protection after a single dose of vaccine lasts for at least 18 years, if not for life.*

Detectable HI antibodies persist in almost all vaccinated subjects who initially seroconvert.† In current practice, most children receive two doses of a rubella-containing

*References 5, 24, 33, 39, 269, 303.

*References 42–44, 47, 48, 50, 52–54, 58, 60, 61, 271, 316, 603–606.
†References 43, 47, 50, 52, 58, 61, 322, 593–598.

vaccine, however, which does seem to improve seropositivity [599,600]. A survey of U.S. military recruits showed that 93% were seropositive for rubella [601]. Long-term studies of vaccinated persons who initially seroconverted and then lost detectable HI antibodies indicate that most of these individuals are also immune because they have detectable antibodies as measured by other, more sensitive assays or have a booster immune response (i.e., absence of IgM antibody and a rapid increase and decrease in IgG antibody) after revaccination [47,53,602].

Viremia and reinfection have been documented in some vaccinated persons and some naturally immune individuals who had very low titers of antibody [42,44, 48,54,60]. It is unknown how often this phenomenon occurs or places the fetus at risk, but the incidence of both events is believed to be low [8]. There are rare case reports of congenital infection after reinfection of mothers who had been previously infected or vaccinated (see "Virus" and "Natural History").* The lack of an international standard level of antibody considered to be protective frequently complicates the interpretation of serologic data when antibodies are detected only by tests more sensitive than the HI test. Cutoff levels ranging from 5 to 15 IU have been used.† Available information indicates that any appropriately measured level of detectable antibody should be considered presumptive evidence of past infection and immunity [266,268]. This applies to naturally acquired and vaccine-induced immunity.

Rubella vaccine is remarkably safe. Rash, low-grade fever, and lymphadenopathy are occasionally observed. The polyneuropathies, myositis, and vasculitis associated with the HPV-77 strain of vaccine have not been reported after administration of the RA 27/3 strain [9,604].

Vaccine-related arthralgia and arthritis remain a concern, particularly for susceptible women.‡ Although arthralgia has been reported in 3% of susceptible children, arthritis has been reported rarely in these vaccinated subjects. In contrast, joint pain occurs in 40% of susceptible vaccinated women, with arthritis-like signs and symptoms reported in 10% to 20% [5,68]. Persistent and recurring joint complaints have been reported, but most studies indicate that they occur infrequently. The high frequency (5%) of persistent joint symptoms reported by one group of investigators has not been confirmed [8,68]. This rate is still far less than that (30%) after natural infection, however, as reported by the same group of researchers [68]. Permanent disability and joint destruction have also been reported, but only rarely [65,68].

Most published data indicate that these and other adverse events associated with rubella vaccine occur only in susceptible vaccinated persons [5,8]. There is no conclusive evidence that there is an increased risk of reactions in persons who are already immune at the time of vaccination [8,68,127]. Vaccination programs of adults have not led to significant rates of absenteeism or disruption in everyday, work-related activities [8,282,284–287].

Although some vaccinated persons intermittently shed virus in low titers from the pharynx 7 to 28 days after vaccination, there is no evidence that vaccine virus is spread to susceptible contacts [5,482]. Vaccine virus can be recovered from breast milk, however, and may be transmitted to the breast-fed neonate [65,353,605,606]. The vaccine virus may elicit an immune response in some exposed neonates. There is no evidence of a significant alteration in the immune response or increased risk of reactions after vaccination at a later date [66,68]. Although a mild clinical infection from transmitted vaccine virus has been reported, infection with wild-type virus might have occurred [607].

The fetotropic and teratogenic potential of rubella vaccine virus has greatly influenced vaccination practices in the United States and worldwide. With the increased emphasis on vaccinating susceptible, postpubertal women in the United States, especially recent immigrants, the need to have accurate information on the risks of the vaccine virus on the fetus became even more important.

From 1971–1988, the U.S. Centers for Disease Control and Prevention (CDC) followed to term prospectively 321 pregnant women known to be susceptible to rubella by serologic testing who were vaccinated in the period from 3 months before to 3 months after conception (see Table 28–4) [69,266]. Approximately one third received vaccine during the highest risk period for viremia and fetal defects (1 week before to 4 weeks after conception) [62,69]. Of the women, 94 received HPV-77 or Cendehill vaccines, 1 received a vaccine of unknown strain, and 226 received RA 27/3 vaccine. None of the 229 offspring (three mothers who received RA 27/3 vaccine had twins) had malformations consistent with congenital rubella infection.

Although the observed risk of congenital defects is zero, from the obtained data in the United Kingdom, United States, Germany, and Sweden, a small theoretical risk of 0.5% (upper bound of 95% confidence limit 0.05%) cannot be ruled out. Limiting the analysis to the 293 infants born to susceptible mothers vaccinated 1 to 2 weeks before to 4 to 6 weeks after conception, the maximum theoretical risk is 1.3%. This risk is substantially less than the greater than 20% risk for CRS associated with maternal infection during the first 20 weeks of pregnancy and is no greater than the 2% to 3% rate of major birth defects in the absence of exposure to rubella vaccine [69,109,556].

These favorable data are consistent with the experience reported with Cendehill and RA 27/3 vaccines in the Federal Republic of Germany and the United Kingdom [64,67]. None of 98 infants in the Federal Republic of Germany and none of 21 infants in Great Britain whose mothers were known to be susceptible when vaccinated were born with congenital anomalies consistent with CRS. The most reassuring information comes from a rubella vaccine mass campaign involving 16 million women in Brazil during 2001–2002, among whom were 2327 susceptible, pregnant women. Follow-up studies on 76% of these women revealed an infection rate of 3.6% among their newborns, but no evidence of increased abortion, stillbirth, preterm birth, or CRS [608,609]. Similar negative data were reported from Costa Rica [610].

*References 47, 49, 56, 115, 120, 331, 336–338.
†References 58, 61, 210, 238, 602, 603.
‡References 5, 8, 63, 65, 66, 68.

Although fetal infection occurs, if rubella vaccine has any teratogenic potential, it must be rare.

Vaccination Recommendations

The control of rubella and congenital rubella in the United States has been predicated on universal immunization of children, with a single dose of vaccine given after the first birthday, and selective immunization of postpubertal and susceptible postpartum women. This approach remains the basis for current recommendations of the Advisory Committee on Immunization Practices (ACIP) of the Public Health Service and the American Academy of Pediatrics (AAP) [266,268]. Part of this success in control of rubella and congenital rubella has come from the recommended use of rubella vaccine as a component of the combined MMR vaccine, which in the United States is given routinely to 15-month-old children. As concerns arose about measles in adolescents and adults, attributed to the existence of a cohort of young adults representing the 2% to 10% failure rate for a single dose of measles vaccine and the theoretical possibility of waning immunity after successful immunization in early childhood, the ACIP and AAP added a second dose to the measles immunization schedule in 1989. The specific recommendation was that the second dose be given just before school entry or in the prepubertal period and that the vaccine be given as the MMR vaccine [266,268].

Rubella immunization (as MMR vaccine) should be offered to all women of childbearing age who do not have acceptable evidence of rubella immunity. Given the current data, routine screening of postpuberal women for susceptibility before rubella vaccination is no longer recommended. Women should understand the theoretical risk of fetal infection, however, and be advised not to become pregnant for at least 28 days after vaccination [276]. Known pregnancy is still considered a contraindication.

Missed opportunities should not be confused with bona fide contraindications for rubella immunization. These include the following:

1. Severe febrile illness
2. Altered immunity from congenital immunodeficiency; from acquired diseases such as leukemia, lymphoma, and generalized malignancy; and from therapy with radiation, corticosteroids, alkylating drugs, and antimetabolites
3. History of an anaphylactic reaction to neomycin (the vaccine does not contain penicillin)
4. Pregnancy, albeit because of theoretical concerns

Because vaccine virus is not transmitted through the nasopharynx, the presence of a susceptible pregnant woman in a household is not a contraindication for vaccination of other household members. Vaccine virus is present in breast milk and can infect the neonate, but breast-feeding also is not a contraindication to vaccination. Although vaccination is usually deferred for 8 to 12 weeks after receipt of immunoglobulin, receipt of anti-Rho (D) immunoglobulin (human) or blood products does not generally interfere with seroconversion and is not a contraindication to postpartum vaccination [611–614]. In this situation, 6- to 8-week postvaccination serologic testing should be performed, however, to ensure that seroconversion has occurred [613]. This is the only situation in which postvaccination testing is recommended as routine.

OUTBREAK CONTROL

Although outbreak control is an after-the-fact method of prevention, rapid, aggressive responses to outbreaks are necessary to limit the spread of infection and can serve as a catalyst to increase immunization levels. Although there is no conclusive evidence that vaccination after exposure prevents rubella, there are also no data to suggest that vaccinating an individual incubating rubella is harmful. Vaccination programs initiated in the middle of an outbreak serve to protect persons not adequately exposed in the current outbreak from future exposures.

Although laboratory confirmation of cases is important, control measures—including isolation of suspected cases or susceptible exposed persons, vaccination or exclusion of susceptible persons, and confirmation of the immune status of exposed pregnant women—should be implemented as soon as a suspected case has been identified (see "Management Issues"). Ideally, mandatory exclusion and vaccination of susceptible individuals should be practiced to ensure high rates of vaccination in the shortest possible period, particularly in the medical setting. Vaccination during an outbreak has not been associated with significant absenteeism in the workplace [8,282,284–287]. Vaccination before the occurrence of an outbreak is preferable, however, because vaccination causes far less disruption of routine work activities and schedules than rubella infection.

SURVEILLANCE

Surveillance of rubella and CRS is necessary for rubella prevention because the information can be used to evaluate the progress of the immunization program; to identify high-risk groups that would benefit from specific interventions; and to monitor the safety, efficacy, and durability of the vaccine. Surveillance can also draw attention to small numbers of cases before they develop into sizable outbreaks. Because rubella and CRS are reportable diseases, all suspected cases should be reported to local health officials.

STRATEGIES FOR ELIMINATION OF RUBELLA AND CONGENITAL RUBELLA SYNDROME

Elimination of rubella and CRS has been achieved in many countries (e.g., U.S., Sweden, Finland, Cuba), and two World Health Organization (WHO) regions have established elimination goals. As part of the strategy, integration with the measles elimination goal is critical. For all strategies for elimination, universal childhood vaccination is key with maintenance of high coverage. Although various elimination strategies have been used, the strategy that PAHO has recommended includes introduction of rubella-containing vaccines into routine vaccination programs for children 12 months of age and conducting a one-time mass campaign in adolescents and adults and periodic follow-up campaigns in children younger than 5 years. In the PAHO experience, it is necessary to vaccinate both males and females [25].

Given the frequency of international travel, all countries will remain at risk of imported disease during the foreseeable future. Maintaining high levels of immunization, ongoing surveillance (recognizing that the sporadic nature of new cases likely will add to delay in diagnosis), and prompt outbreak control measures remain critical for achieving and maintaining elimination of rubella. The efforts under way in the Western Hemisphere can be a global model that eventually will make rubella and CRS matters of historic interest [615].

REFERENCES

[1] C. Wesselhoff, Rubella (German measles), N. Engl. J. Med. 236 (1947) 943.

[2] S. Krugman (Ed.), Rubella symposium, Am. J. Dis. Child. 110 (1965) 345.

[3] S. Krugman (Ed.), Proceedings of the International Conference on Rubella Immunization, Am. J. Dis. Child. 118 (1969) 2.

[4] R.H. Regamy, et al. (Eds.), International Symposium on Rubella Vaccines, Symp. Ser. Immunobiol. Stand. 11 (1969) 1.

[5] S.R. Preblud, et al., Rubella vaccination in the United States: a ten-year review, Epidemiol. Rev. 2 (1980) 171.

[6] J.B. Hanshaw, J.A. Dudgeon, W.C. Marshall (Eds.), Viral Diseases of the Fetus and Newborn, second ed., Saunders, Philadelphia, 1985.

[7] S. Krugman (Ed.), International Symposium on Prevention of Congenital Rubella Infection, Rev. Infect. Dis. 7 (Suppl. 1) (1985) S1.

[8] S.R. Preblud, Some current issues relating to rubella vaccine, JAMA 254 (1985) 253.

[9] J.D. Cherry, Rubella, in: R.D. Feigin, J.D. Cherry (Eds.), Textbook of Pediatric Infectious Diseases, third ed., Saunders, Philadelphia, 1992.

[10] W.G. Manton, Some accounts of rash liable to be mistaken for scarlatina, Med. Trans. R. Coll. Physicians (Lond) 5 (1815) 149.

[11] H. Veale, History of epidemic Roetheln, with observations on its pathology, Edinb. Med. J. (1866) 12.

[12] N.M. Gregg, Congenital cataract following German measles in the mother, Trans. Ophthalmol. Soc. Aust. 3 (1941) 35.

[13] L.Z. Cooper, Congenital rubella in the United States, in: S. Krugman, A.A. Gershon (Eds.), Infections of the Fetus and the Newborn Infant, Alan R Liss, New York, 1975.

[14] P.R. Ziring, Congenital rubella: the teenage years, Pediatr. Ann. 6 (1977) 762.

[15] Y. Hiro, S. Tasaka, Die Rötheln sind eine Viruskrankheit, Monatsschr. Kinderheilkd. 76 (1938) 328.

[16] K. Habel, Transmission of rubella to *Macaca mulatta* monkeys, Public Health Rep. 57 (1942) 1126.

[17] S.B. Anderson, Experimental rubella in human volunteers, J. Immunol. 62 (1949) 29.

[18] S. Krugman, et al., Studies on rubella immunization. I. Demonstration of rubella without rash, JAMA 151 (1953) 285.

[19] T.H. Weller, F.A. Neva, Propagation in tissue culture of cytopathic agents from patients with rubella-like illness, Proc. Soc. Exp. Biol. Med. 111 (1962) 215.

[20] P.D. Parkman, E.L. Buescher, M.S. Artenstein, Recovery of rubella virus from army recruits, Proc. Soc. Exp. Biol. Med. 111 (1962) 225.

[21] P.D. Parkman, et al., Studies of rubella. II. Neutralization of the virus, J. Immunol. 93 (1964) 608.

[22] J.L. Sever, et al., Rubella complement fixation test, Science 148 (1965) 385.

[23] G.L. Stewart, et al., Rubella-virus hemagglutination-inhibition test, N. Engl. J. Med. 276 (1967) 554.

[24] W.A. Orenstein, et al., The opportunity and obligation to eliminate measles from the United States, JAMA 251 (1988) 1984.

[25] Progress toward elimination of rubella and congenital rubella syndrome—the Americas, 2003–2008, MMWR Morb. Mortal. Wkly. Rep. 57 (2008) 1176–1179.

[26] F.T. Cutts, E. Vynnycky, Modelling the incidence of congenital rubella syndrome in developing countries, Int. J. Epidemiol. 28 (1999) 1176–1184.

[27] H.M. Meyer Jr., P.D. Parkman, T.C. Panos, Attenuated rubella virus. II. Production of an experimental live-virus vaccine and clinical trial, N. Engl. J. Med. 275 (1966) 575.

[28] A. Prinzie, et al., Experimental live attenuated rubella virus vaccine: clinical evaluation of Cendehill strain, Am. J. Dis. Child. 118 (1969) 172.

[29] J.A. Plotkin, J.D. Farquhar, M. Katz, Attenuation of RA 27/3 rubella virus in WI-38 human diploid cells, Am. J. Dis. Child. 118 (1969) 178.

[30] F.T. Perkins, Licensed vaccines, Rev. Infect. Dis. 7 (Suppl. 1) (1985) S73.

[31] S.A. Plotkin, W.A. Orenstein, P.A. Offit (Eds.), Vaccines, fifth ed., Saunders, Philadelphia, 2008.

[32] A.R. Hinman, et al., Rational strategy for rubella vaccination, Lancet 1 (1983) 39.

[33] K.J. Bart, et al., Universal immunization to interrupt rubella, Rev. Infect. Dis. 7 (Suppl. 1) (1985) S177.

[34] J.A. Dudgeon, Selective immunization: protection of the individual, Rev. Infect. Dis. 7 (Suppl. 1) (1985) S185.

[35] D. Walker, H. Carter, I.J. Jones, Measles, mumps, and rubella: the need for a change in immunisation policy, BMJ 292 (1986) 1501.

[36] J.M. Best, et al., Maternal rubella at St. Thomas' Hospital in 1978 and 1986: support for augmenting the rubella vaccination programme, Lancet 2 (1987) 88.

[37] J. Badenoch, Big bang for vaccination: eliminating measles, mumps, and rubella, BMJ 297 (1988) 750.

[38] Recommendations from an ad hoc Meeting of the WHO Measles and Rubella Laboratory Network (LabNet) on use of alternative diagnostic samples for measles and rubella surveillance, MMWR Morb. Mortal. Wkly. Rep. 57 (2008) 657–660.

[39] Centers for Disease Control, Increase in rubella and congenital rubella in the United States, 1988–1990, MMWR Morb. Mortal. Wkly. Rep. 40 (1991) 93.

[40] Elimination of rubella and congenital rubella syndrome—United States, 1969–2004, MMWR Morb. Mortal. Wkly. Rep. 54 (2005) 279–282.

[41] Executive Committee of PAHO, New goal for vaccination programs in the region of the Americas: to eliminate rubella and congenital rubella syndrome, Pan Am. J. Public Health 14 (2003) 359.

[42] G.C. Harcourt, J.M. Best, J.E. Banatvala, Rubella-specific serum and nasopharyngeal antibodies in volunteers with naturally acquired and vaccine-induced immunity after intranasal challenge, J. Infect. Dis. 142 (1980) 145.

[43] R.E. Weibel, et al., Persistence of antibody in human subjects 7 to 10 years following administration of combined live attenuated measles, mumps, and rubella virus vaccines, Proc. Soc. Exp. Biol. Med. 165 (1980) 260.

[44] H.H. Balfour, et al., Rubella viraemia and antibody responses after rubella vaccination and reimmunisation, Lancet 1 (1981) 1078.

[45] J.E. Cradock-Watson, et al., Outcome of asymptomatic infection with rubella virus during pregnancy, J. Hyg. (Lond) 87 (1981) 147.

[46] L.M. Bott, D.H. Eizenberg, Congenital rubella after successful vaccination, Med. J. Aust. 1 (1982) 514.

[47] K.L. Herrmann, S.B. Halstead, N.H. Wiebenga, Rubella antibody persistence after immunization, JAMA 247 (1982) 193.

[48] S. O'Shea, J.M. Best, J.E. Banatvala, Viremia, virus excretion, and antibody responses after challenge in volunteers with low levels of antibody to rubella virus, J. Infect. Dis. 148 (1983) 639.

[49] G. Enders, A. Calm, J. Schaub, Rubella embryopathy after previous maternal rubella vaccination, Infection 12 (1984) 96.

[50] I.B. Hillary, A.H. Griffith, Persistence of rubella antibodies 15 years after subcutaneous administration of Wistar 27/3 strain live attenuated rubella virus vaccine, Vaccine 2 (1984) 274.

[51] R. Morgan-Capner, et al., Clinically apparent rubella reinfection, J. Infect. 9 (1984) 97.

[52] S. O'Shea, et al., Persistence of rubella antibody 8–18 years after vaccination, BMJ 288 (1984) 1043.

[53] M.K. Serdula, et al., Serological response to rubella revaccination, JAMA 251 (1984) 1974.

[54] J.E. Banatvala, et al., Persistence of rubella antibodies after vaccination: detection after experimental challenge, Rev. Infect. Dis. 7 (Suppl. 1) (1985) S86.

[55] J.E. Cradock-Watson, et al., Rubella reinfection and the fetus, Lancet 1 (1985) 1039.

[56] M. Forsgren, L. Soren, Subclinical rubella reinfection in vaccinated women with rubella-specific IgM response during pregnancy and transmission of virus to the fetus, Scand. J. Infect. Dis. 17 (1985) 337.

[57] L. Grangeot-Keros, et al., Rubella reinfection and the fetus, N. Engl. J. Med. 313 (1985) 1547.

[58] D.M. Horstmann, et al., Persistence of vaccine-induced immune responses to rubella: comparison with natural infection, Rev. Infect. Dis. 7 (Suppl. 1) (1985) S80.

[59] P. Morgan-Capner, et al., Detection of rubella-specific IgM in subclinical rubella reinfection in pregnancy, Lancet 1 (1985) 244.

[60] G.M. Schiff, et al., Challenge with rubella virus after loss of detectable vaccine-induced antibody, Rev. Infect. Dis. 7 (Suppl. 1) (1985) S157.

[61] S.Y. Chu, et al., Rubella antibody persistence after immunization: sixteen-year follow-up in the Hawaiian Islands, JAMA 259 (1988) 3133.

[62] S.W. Bart, et al., Fetal risk associated with rubella vaccine: an update, Rev. Infect. Dis. 7 (Suppl. 1) (1985) S95.

[63] J.K. Chantler, A.J. Tingle, R.E. Perry, Persistent rubella virus infection associated with chronic arthritis in children, N. Engl. J. Med. 313 (1985) 1117.

[64] G. Enders, Rubella antibody titers in vaccinated and nonvaccinated women and results of vaccination during pregnancy, Rev. Infect. Dis. 7 (Suppl. 1) (1985) S103.

[65] A.J. Tingle, et al., Postpartum rubella immunization: association with development of prolonged arthritis, neurological sequelae, and chronic rubella viremia, J. Infect. Dis. 152 (1985) 606.

[66] P.R. Preblud, et al., Postpartum rubella immunization. Letter to the editor, J. Infect. Dis. 154 (1986) 367.

[67] S. Sheppard, et al., Rubella vaccination and pregnancy: preliminary report of a national survey, BMJ 292 (1986) 727.

[68] A.J. Tingle, Postpartum rubella immunization (reply), J. Infect. Dis. 154 (1986) 368.

[69] Centers for Disease Control, Rubella vaccination during pregnancy—United States, 1971–1988, MMWR Morb. Mortal. Wkly. Rep. 38 (1989) 290.

[70] L. Ho-Terry, A. Cohen, Degradation of rubella virus envelope components, Arch. Virol. 65 (1980) 1.

[71] C. Oker-Blom, et al., Rubella virus contains one capsid protein and three envelope glycoproteins, E1, E2a, and E2b, J. Virol. 46 (1983) 964.

[72] M.N. Waxham, J.S. Wolinsky, Immunochemical identification of rubella virus hemagglutinin, Virology 126 (1983) 194.

[73] D.S. Bowden, E.G. Westway, Rubella virus: structural and non-structural proteins, J. Gen. Virol. 65 (1984) 933.

[74] L. Ho-Terry, A. Cohen, R.S. Tedder, Immunologic characterisation of rubella virion polypeptides, J. Med. Microbiol. 17 (1984) 105.

[75] C. Oker-Blom, et al., Rubella virus 40S genome RNA specifies a 24S subgenomic mRNA that codes for a precursor to structural proteins, J. Virol. 49 (1984) 403.

[76] P.H. Dorsett, et al., Structure and function of the rubella virus proteins, Rev. Infect. Dis. 7 (Suppl. 1) (1985) S150.

[77] R.F. Pettersson, et al., Molecular and antigenic characteristics and synthesis of rubella virus structural proteins, Rev. Infect. Dis. 7 (Suppl. 1) (1985) S140.

[78] M.N. Waxham, J.S. Wolinsky, A model of the structural organization of rubella virions, Rev. Infect. Dis. 7 (Suppl. 1) (1985) S133.

[79] M.N. Waxham, J.S. Wolinsky, Detailed immunologic analysis of the structural polypeptides of rubella virus using monoclonal antibodies, Virology 143 (1985) 153.

[80] K.Y. Green, P.H. Dorsett, Rubella virus antigens: localization of epitopes involved in hemagglutination and neutralization by using monoclonal antibodies, J. Virol. 57 (1986) 893.

[81] G. Vidgren, et al., Nucleotide sequence of the genes coding for the membrane glycoproteins E1 and E2 of rubella virus, J. Gen. Virol. 68 (1987) 2347.

[82] G.M. Terry, et al., Localization of the rubella E1 epitopes, Arch. Virol. 98 (1988) 189.

[83] D.M. Clarke, et al., Expression of rubella virus cDNA coding for the structural proteins, Gene 65 (1988) 23.

[84] T.K. Frey, L.D. Marr, Sequence of the region coding for virion proteins C and E2 and the carboxy terminus of the nonstructural proteins of rubella virus: comparison with alphaviruses, Gene 62 (1988) 85.

[85] K. Takkinen, et al., Nucleotide sequence of the rubella virus capsid protein gene reveals an unusually high G/C content, J. Gen. Virol. 69 (1988) 603.

[86] M.G. Cusi, et al., Antibody response to wild rubella virus structural proteins following immunization with RA 27/3 live attenuated vaccine, Arch. Virol. 101 (1988) 25.

[87] T.K. Frey, et al., Molecular analysis of rubella virus epidemiology across three continents, North America, Europe and Asia, 1961–1997, J. Infect. Dis. 178 (1998) 642.

[88] S. Katow, A. Sugiura, Antibody response to the individual rubella virus proteins in congenital and other rubella virus infections, J. Clin. Microbiol. 21 (1985) 449.

[89] A. de Mazancourt, et al., Antibody response to the rubella virus structural proteins in infants with the congenital rubella syndrome, J. Med. Virol. 19 (1986) 111.

[90] H. Chaye, et al., Localization of the virus neutralizing and hemagglutinin epitopes of E1 glycoprotein of rubella virus, Virology 189 (1992) 483.

[91] E.J. Hancock, et al., Lack of association between titers of HAI antibody and whole-virus ELISA values for patients with congenital rubella syndrome, J. Infect. Dis. 154 (1986) 1031.

[92] G.A. Castellano, et al., Evaluation of commercially available diagnostic kits for rubella, J. Infect. Dis. 143 (1981) 578.

[93] G.A. Storch, N. Myers, Latex-agglutination test for rubella antibody: validity of positive results assessed by response to immunization and comparison with other tests, J. Infect. Dis. 149 (1984) 459.

[94] J.W. Safford, G.G. Abbott, C.M. Diemier, Evaluation of a rapid passive hemagglutination assay for anti-rubella antibody: comparison to hemagglutination inhibition and a vaccine challenge study, J. Med. Virol. 17 (1985) 229.

[95] L.P. Skendzel, D.C. Edson, Latex agglutination test for rubella antibodies: report based on data from the College of American Pathologists surveys, 1983 to 1985, J. Clin. Microbiol. 24 (1986) 333.

[96] P. Vaananen, et al., Comparison of a simple latex agglutination test with hemolysis-in-gel, hemagglutination inhibition, and radioimmunoassay for detection of rubella virus antibodies, J. Clin. Microbiol. 21 (1985) 973.

[97] M.A. Chernesky, et al., Differences in antibody responses with rapid agglutination tests for the detection of rubella virus antibodies, J. Clin. Microbiol. 23 (1986) 772.

[98] R.C. Pruneda, J.C. Dover, A comparison of two passive agglutination procedures with enzyme-linked immunosorbent assay for rubella antibody status, Am. J. Clin. Pathol. 86 (1986) 768.

[99] G.A. Linde, Subclass distribution of rubella virus-specific immunoglobulin G, J. Clin. Microbiol. 21 (1985) 117.

[100] E.M. Salonen, et al., Kinetics of specific IgA, IgD, IgE, IgG, and IgM antibody responses in rubella, J. Med. Virol. 16 (1985) 1.

[101] A. Stokes, A. Mims, R. Grahame, Subclass distribution of IgG and IgA responses to rubella virus in man, J. Med. Microbiol. 21 (1986) 283.

[102] H.I.J. Thomas, P. Morgan-Capner, Specific IgG subclass antibody in rubella virus infections, Epidemiol. Infect. 100 (1988) 443.

[103] L. Grangeot-Keros, et al., Prenatal and postnatal production of IgM and IgA antibodies to rubella virus studied by antibody capture immunoassay, J. Infect. Dis. 158 (1988) 138.

[104] J. Nedeljkovic, T. Jovanovic, C. Oker-Blom, Maturation of IgG avidity to individual rubella virus structural proteins, J. Clin. Virol. 22 (2001) 47.

[105] N.M. Mehta, R.M. Thomas, Antenatal screening for rubella—infection or immunity? BMJ 325 (2002) 90.

[106] J.M. Best, et al., Interpretation of rubella serology in pregnancy—pitfalls and problems, BMJ 325 (2002) 147.

[107] J.E. Cradock-Watson, et al., Fetal infection resulting from maternal rubella after the first trimester of pregnancy, J. Hyg. (Lond.) 85 (1980) 381.

[108] M. Vejtorp, B. Mansa, Rubella IgM antibodies in sera from infants born after maternal rubella later than the twelfth week of pregnancy, Scand. J. Infect. Dis. 12 (1980) 1.

[109] E. Miller, J.E. Cradock-Watson, T.M. Pollock, Consequences of confirmed maternal rubella at successive stages of pregnancy, Lancet 2 (1982) 781.

[110] L. Grillner, et al., Outcome of rubella during pregnancy with special reference to the 17th-24th weeks of gestation, Scand. J. Infect. Dis. 15 (1983) 321.

[111] C. Peckham, Congenital rubella in the United Kingdom before 1970: the prevaccine era, Rev. Infect. Dis. 7 (Suppl. 1) (1985) S11.

[112] M. Bitsch, Rubella in pregnant Danish women 1975–1984, Dan. Med. Bull. 34 (1987) 46.

[113] N.D. Munro, et al., Temporal relations between maternal rubella and congenital defects, Lancet 2 (1987) 201.

[114] G. Enders, et al., Outcome of confirmed periconceptional maternal rubella, Lancet 1 (1988) 1445.

[115] J.W. Partridge, T.H. Flewett, J.E.M. Whitehead, Congenital rubella affecting an infant whose mother had rubella antibodies before conception, BMJ 282 (1981) 187.

[116] J.M. Best, et al., Congenital rubella affecting an infant whose mother had rubella antibodies before conception, BMJ 282 (1981) 1235.

[117] J.B. Levine, C.D. Berkowitz, J.W. St. Geme, Rubella virus reinfection during pregnancy leading to late-onset congenital rubella syndrome, J. Pediatr. 100 (1982) 589.

[118] G. Sibille, et al., [Reinfection after rubella and congenital polymalformation syndrome], J. Genet. Hum. 34 (1986) 305.

[119] L. Hornstein, U. Levy, A. Fogel, Clinical rubella with virus transmission to the fetus in a pregnant woman considered to be immune. Letter to the editor, N. Engl. J. Med. 319 (1988) 1415.

[120] H. Saule, et al., Congenital rubella infection after previous immunity of the mother, Eur. J. Pediatr. 147 (1988) 195.

[121] D. Floret, et al., Hyperthyroidism, diabetes mellitus and the congenital rubella syndrome, Acta Paediatr. Scand. 69 (1980) 259.

[122] H.E. Hansen, S.O. Larsen, J. Leerhoy, Lack of correlation between the incidence of rubella antibody and the distribution of HLA antigens in a Danish population, Tissue Antigens 15 (1980) 325.

[123] S. Kato, et al., HLA-linked genetic control in natural rubella infection, Tissue Antigens 15 (1980) 86.

[124] M. Tardieu, et al., Circulating immune complexes containing rubella antigens in late-onset rubella syndrome, J. Pediatr. 97 (1980) 370.

[125] P.K. Coyle, J.S. Wolinsky, Characterization of immune complexes in progressive rubella panencephalitis, Ann. Neurol. 9 (1981) 557.

[126] K. Ishii, et al., Host factors and susceptibility to rubella virus infection: the association of HLA antigens, J. Med. Virol. 7 (1981) 287.

[127] P.K. Coyle, et al., Rubella-specific immune complexes after congenital infection and vaccination, Infect. Immun. 36 (1982) 498.

[128] S. Kato, et al., HLA-DR antigens and the rubella-specific immune response in man, Tissue Antigens 19 (1982) 140.

[129] P. Rubinstein, et al., The HLA system in congenital rubella patients with and without diabetes, Diabetes 31 (1982) 1088.

[130] A. Boner, et al., Desquamative interstitial pneumonia and antigen-antibody complexes in two infants with congenital rubella, Pediatrics 72 (1983) 835.

[131] J. Ilonen, et al., HLA antigens in rubella seronegative young adults, Tissue Antigens 22 (1983) 379.

[132] B. Ziola, et al., Circulating immune complexes in patients with acute measles and rubella virus infections, Infect. Immun. 41 (1983) 578.

[133] W.L. Clarke, et al., Autoimmunity in congenital rubella syndrome, J. Pediatr. 104 (1984) 370.

[134] F. Ginsberg-Fellner, et al., Diabetes mellitus and autoimmunity in patients with congenital rubella syndrome, Rev. Infect. Dis. 7 (Suppl. 1) (1985) S170.

[135] J.L. Sever, M.A. South, K.A. Shaver, Delayed manifestations of congenital rubella, Rev. Infect. Dis. 7 (Suppl. 1) (1985) S164.

[136] K.A. Shaver, J.A. Boughman, W.E. Nance, Congenital rubella syndrome and diabetes: a review of epidemiologic, genetic, and immunologic factors, Am. Ann. Deaf 130 (1985) 526.

[137] S.L. Rabinowe, et al., Congenital rubella: monoclonal antibody-defined T cell abnormalities in young adults, Am. J. Med. 81 (1986) 779.

[138] H. Verder, et al., Late-onset rubella syndrome: coexistence of immune complex disease and defective cytotoxic effector cell function, Clin. Exp. Immunol. 63 (1986) 367.

[139] G. Bardeletti, N. Kessler, M. Aymard-Henry, Morphology, biochemical analysis and neuraminidase activity of rubella virus, Arch. Virol. 49 (1975) 175.

[140] J.M. Best, et al., Morphological characteristics of rubella virus, Lancet 2 (1967) 237.

[141] F.A. Murphy, P.E. Halonen, A.K. Harrison, Electron microscopy of the development of rubella virus in BHK-21 cells, J. Virol. 2 (1968) 1223.

[142] L.S. Oshiro, N.J. Schmidt, E.H. Lennette, Electron microscopic studies of rubella virus, J. Gen. Virol. 5 (1969) 205.

[143] G. Bardeletti, J. Tektoff, D. Gautheron, Rubella virus maturation and production in two host cell systems, Intervirology 11 (1979) 97.

[144] I.H. Holmes, M.C. Wark, M.F. Warburton, Is rubella an arbovirus? II. Ultrastructural morphology and development, Virology 37 (1969) 15.

[145] R. Maes, et al., Synthesis of virus and macromolecules by rubella-infected cells, Nature 210 (1966) 384.

[146] H.L. Nakhasi, et al., Rubella virus replication: effect of interferons and actinomycin D, Virus Res. 10 (1988) 1.

[147] M. Sato, et al., Evidence for hybrid formation between rubella virus and a latent virus of BHK21/WI-2 cells, Virology 69 (1976) 691.

[148] M. Sato, et al., Persistent infection of BHK21/WI-2 cells with rubella virus and characterization of rubella variants, Arch. Virol. 54 (1977) 333.

[149] M. Sato, et al., Isolation and characterization of a new rubella variant with DNA polymerase activity, Arch. Virol. 56 (1978) 89.

[150] M. Sato, et al., Persistent infection of primary human cell cultures with rubella variant carrying DNA polymerase activity, Arch. Virol. 56 (1978) 181.

[151] M. Sato, et al., Presence of DNA in rubella variant with DNA polymerase activity, Arch. Virol. 61 (1979) 251.

[152] K. Mifune, S. Matsuo, Some properties of temperature-sensitive mutant of rubella virus defective in the induction of interference to Newcastle disease virus, Virology 63 (1975) 278.

[153] M. Norval, Mechanism of persistence of rubella virus in LLC-MK2 cells, J. Gen. Virol. 43 (1979) 289.

[154] G. Bardeletti, D.C. Gautheron, Phospholipid and cholesterol composition of rubella virus and its host cell BHK21 grown in suspension cultures, Arch. Virol. 52 (1978) 19.

[155] A. Voiland, G. Bardeletti, Fatty acid composition of rubella virus and BHK21/13S infected cells, Arch. Virol. 64 (1980) 319.

[156] P.D. Parkman, et al., Studies of rubella. I. Properties of the virus, J. Immunol. 93 (1964) 595.

[157] K. McCarthy, C.H. Taylor-Robinson, Rubella, Br. Med. Bull. 23 (1967) 185.

[158] C. Wallis, J.L. Melnick, F. Rapp, Different effects of MgCl2 and MgSO4 on the thermostability of viruses, Virology 26 (1965) 694.

[159] A. Chagnon, P. Laflamme, Effect of acidity on rubella virus, Can. J. Microbiol. 10 (1964) 501.

[160] A. Fabiyi, et al., Rubella virus: growth characteristics and stability of infectious virus and complement-fixing antigen, Proc. Soc. Exp. Biol. Med. 122 (1966) 392.

[161] K.L. Herrmann, Rubella virus, in: E.H. Lennette, N.J. Schmidt (Eds.), Diagnostic Procedures for Viral, Rickettsial, and Chlamydial Infections, American Public Health Association, Washington, DC, 1979.

[162] K.W. Cochran, H.F. Maassab, Inhibition of rubella virus by 1-adamantanamine hydrochloride, Fed. Proc. 23 (1964) 387.

[163] S.A. Plotkin, Inhibition of rubella virus by amantadine, Arch. Gesamte Virusforsch. 16 (1965) 438.

[164] J.S. Oxford, G.C. Schild, In vitro inhibition of rubella virus by 1-adamantanamine hydrochloride, Arch. Gesamte Virusforsch. 17 (1965) 313.

[165] S.A. Plotkin, R.M. Klaus, J.A. Whitely, Hypogammaglobulinemia in an infant with congenital rubella syndrome: failure of 1-adamantanamine to stop virus excretion, J. Pediatr. 69 (1966) 1085.

[166] A. Vaheri, T. Hovi, Structural proteins and subunits of rubella virus, J. Virol. 9 (1972) 10.

[167] T. Vesikari, Immune response in rubella infection, Scand. J. Infect. Dis. 4 (Suppl.) (1972) 1.

[168] H. Liebhaber, P.A. Gross, The structural proteins of rubella virus, Virology 47 (1972) 684.

[169] J.K. Chantler, Rubella virus: intracellular polypeptide synthesis, Virology 98 (1979) 275.

[170] L. Ho-Terry, P. Londesborough, A. Cohen, Analysis of rubella virus complement-fixing antigens by polyacrylamide gel electrophoresis, Arch. Virol. 87 (1986) 219.

[171] C. Claus, et al., Rubella virus pseudotypes and a cell-cell fusion assay as tools for functional analysis of the rubella virus E2 and E1 envelope glycoproteins, J. Gen. Virol. 87 (Pt 10) (2006) 3029–3037.

[172] Y. Zhou, H. Ushijima, T.K. Frey, Genomic analysis of diverse rubella virus genotypes, J. Gen. Virol. 88 (Pt 3) (2007) 932–941.

[173] S. Katow, Molecular epidemiology of rubella virus in Asia: utility for reduction in the burden of diseases due to congenital rubella syndrome, Pediatr. Int. 46 (2) (2004).

[174] Global distribution of measles and rubella genotypes—update, Wkly. Epidemiol. Rec. 81 (2006) 474–479.

[175] F. Fenner, The classification and nomenclature of viruses, Intervirology 6 (1975) 1.

[176] J.L. Melnick, Taxonomy of viruses, Prog. Med. Virol. 22 (1976) 211.

[177] J.M. Best, J.E. Banatvala, Studies on rubella virus strain variation by kinetic hemagglutination-inhibition tests, J. Gen. Virol. 9 (1970) 215.

[178] A. Fogel, S.A. Plotkin, Markers of rubella virus strains in RK13 culture, J. Virol. 3 (1969) 157.

[179] R. Kono, Antigenic structures of American and Japanese rubella virus strains and experimental vertical transmission of rubella virus in rabbits, Symp. Ser. Immunobiol. Stand. 11 (1969) 195.

[180] R. Kono, et al., Experimental vertical transmission of rubella virus in rabbits, Lancet 1 (1969) 343.

[181] J.E. Banatvala, J.M. Best, Cross-serological testing of rubella virus strains, Lancet 1 (1969) 695.

[182] J.E. Potter, J.E. Banatvala, J.M. Best, Interferon studies with Japanese and U.S. rubella virus, BMJ 1 (1973) 197.

[183] J.E. Banatvala, J.E. Potter, M.J. Webster, Foetal interferon responses induced by rubella virus, Ciba Found. New Ser. 10 (1973) 77.

[184] K. Ueda, et al., An explanation for the high incidence of congenital rubella syndrome in Ryukyu, Am. J. Epidemiol. 107 (1978) 344.

[185] R. Kono, et al., Epidemiology of rubella and congenital rubella infection in Japan, Rev. Infect. Dis. 7 (Suppl. 1) (1985) S56.

[186] K. Ueda, et al., Incidence of congenital rubella syndrome in Japan (1965–1985): a nationwide survey of the number of deaf children with history of maternal rubella attending special schools for the deaf in Japan, Am. J. Epidemiol. 124 (1986) 807.

[187] E. Mendelson, et al., Laboratory assessment and diagnosis of congenital viral infections: rubella, cytomegalovirus (CMV), varicella-zoster virus (VZV), herpes simplex virus (HSV), parvovirus B19 and human immunodeficiency virus (HIV), Reprod. Toxicol. 21 (2006) 350–382.

[188] T.K. Frey, et al., Molecular cloning and sequencing of the region of the rubella virus genome coding for glycoprotein E1, Virology 154 (1986) 228–232.

[189] M.G. Revello, et al., Prenatal diagnosis of rubella virus infection by direct detection and semiquantitation of viral RNA in clinical samples by reverse transcription-PCR, J. Clin. Microbiol. 35 (1997) 708.

[190] P.E. Halonen, J.M. Ryan, J.A. Stewart, Rubella hemagglutinin prepared with alkaline extraction of virus grown in suspension culture of BHK-21 cells, Proc. Soc. Exp. Biol. Med. 125 (1967) 162.

[191] N.J. Schmidt, J. Dennis, E.H. Lennette, Rubella virus hemagglutination with a wide variety of erythrocyte species, Appl. Microbiol. 22 (1971) 469.

[192] T. Furukawa, et al., Studies on hemagglutination by rubella virus, Proc. Soc. Exp. Biol. Med. 126 (1967) 745.

[193] G. Haukenes, Simplified rubella haemagglutination inhibition test not requiring removal of nonspecific inhibitors, Lancet 2 (1979) 196.

[194] H. Liebhaber, Measurement of rubella antibody by hemagglutination inhibition. I. Variables affecting rubella hemagglutination, J. Immunol. 104 (1970) 818.

[195] H. Liebhaber, Measurement of rubella antibody by hemagglutination inhibition. II. Characteristics of an improved test employing a new method for the removal of non-immunoglobulin HA inhibitors from serum, J. Immunol. 104 (1970) 826.

[196] N.J. Schmidt, E.H. Lennette, Rubella complement-fixing antigens derived from the fluid and cellular phases of infected BHK-21 cells: extraction of cell-associated antigen with alkaline buffers, J. Immunol. 97 (1966) 815.

[197] N.J. Schmidt, E.H. Lennette, P.S. Gee, Demonstration of rubella complement-fixing antigens of two distinct particle sizes by gel filtration on Sephadex G-200, Proc. Soc. Exp. Biol. Med. 123 (1966) 758.

[198] N.J. Schmidt, E.H. Lennette, Antigens of rubella virus, Am. J. Dis. Child. 118 (1969) 89.

[199] N.J. Schmidt, B. Styk, Immunodiffusion reactions with rubella antigens, J. Immunol. 101 (1968) 210.

[200] A.A. Salmi, Gel precipitation reactions between alkaline extracted rubella antigens and human sera, Acta Pathol. Microbiol. Scand. 76 (1969) 271.

[201] G.L. LeBouvier, Precipitinogens of rubella virus infected cells, Proc. Soc. Exp. Biol. Med. 130 (1969) 51.

[202] R. Cappel, A. Schluederberg, D.M. Horstmann, Large-scale production of rubella precipitinogens and their use in the diagnostic laboratory, J. Clin. Microbiol. 1 (1975) 201.

[203] G.L. LeBouvier, S.A. Plotkin, Precipitin responses to rubella vaccine RA27/3, J. Infect. Dis. 123 (1971) 220.

[204] A. Vaheri, T. Vesikari, Small size rubella virus antigens and soluble immune complexes, analysis by the platelet aggregation technique, Arch. Gesamte Virusforsch. 35 (1971) 10.

[205] K. Penttinen, G. Myllyla, Interaction of human blood platelets, viruses, and antibodies. I. Platelet aggregation test with microequipment, Ann. Med. Exp. Biol. Fenn. 46 (1968) 188.

[206] E.H. Lennette, N.J. Schmidt, Neutralization, fluorescent antibody and complement fixation tests for rubella, in: H. Friedman, J.E. Prier (Eds.), Rubella, Charles C Thomas, Springfield, IL, 1973.

[207] A. Schluederberg, et al., Neutralizing and hemagglutination-inhibition antibodies to rubella virus as indicators of protective immunity in vaccinees and naturally immune individuals, J. Infect. Dis. 138 (1978) 877.

[208] H. Sato, et al., Sensitive neutralization test for rubella antibody, J. Clin. Microbiol. 9 (1979) 259.

[209] O.H. Meurman, Antibody responses in patients with rubella infection determined by passive hemagglutination, hemagglutination inhibition,

complement fixation, and solid-phase radioimmunoassay tests, Infect. Immun. 19 (1978) 369.

[210] K.L. Herrmann, Available rubella serologic tests, Rev. Infect. Dis. 7 (Suppl. 1) (1985) S108.

[211] L.P. Skendzel, K.R. Wilcox, D.C. Edson, Evaluation of assays for the detection of antibodies to rubella: a report based on data from the College of American Pathologists surveys of 1982, Am. J. Clin. Pathol. 80 (Suppl.) (1983) 594.

[212] G. Hauknes, Experience with an indirect (passive) hemagglutination test for the demonstration of rubella virus antibody, Acta Pathol. Microbiol. Scand. 88 (1980) 85.

[213] J.M. Kilgore, Further evaluation of a rubella passive hemagglutination test, J. Med. Virol. 5 (1980) 131.

[214] S. Inouye, K. Satoh, T. Tajima, Single-serum diagnosis of rubella by combined use of the hemagglutination inhibition and passive hemagglutination tests, J. Clin. Microbiol. 23 (1986) 455.

[215] G.B. Harnett, C.A. Palmer, E.M. Mackay-Scollay, Single-radial-hemolysis test for the assay of rubella antibody in antenatal, vaccinated, and rubella virus-infected patients, J. Infect. Dis. 140 (1979) 937.

[216] F.E. Nommensen, Accuracy of single radial hemolysis test for rubella immunity when internal reference standards are used to estimate antibody levels, J. Clin. Microbiol. 25 (1987) 22.

[217] P. Halonen, et al., IgA antibody response in acute rubella determined by solid-phase radioimmunoassay, J. Hyg. (Lond) 83 (1979) 69.

[218] H.O. Kangro, J.R. Pattison, R.B. Heath, The detection of rubella-specific IgM antibodies by radioimmunoassay, Br. J. Exp. Pathol. 59 (1978) 577.

[219] O.H. Meurman, M.K. Viljanen, K. Granfors, Solid-phase radioimmunoassay of rubella virus immunoglobulin M antibodies: comparison with sucrose density gradient centrifugation test, J. Clin. Microbiol. 5 (1977) 257.

[220] O.H. Meurman, B.R. Ziola, IgM-class rheumatoid factor interference in the solid-phase radioimmunoassay of rubella-specific IgM antibodies, J. Clin. Pathol. 31 (1978) 483.

[221] P.P. Mortimer, et al., Antibody capture radioimmunoassay for anti-rubella IgM, J. Hyg. (Lond.) 86 (1981) 139.

[222] G.C. Brown, et al., Rubella antibodies in human serum: detection by the indirect fluorescent-antibody technic, Science 145 (1964) 943.

[223] J.E. Cradock-Watson, et al., Comparison of immunofluorescence and radioimmunoassay for detecting IgM antibody in infants with the congenital rubella syndrome, J. Hyg. (Lond.) 83 (1979) 413.

[224] P.O. Leinikki, et al., Determination of virus-specific IgM antibodies by using ELISA: elimination of false-positive results with protein A-Sepharose absorption and subsequent IgM antibody assay, J. Lab. Clin. Med. 92 (1978) 849.

[225] M. Vejtorp, Enzyme-linked immunosorbent assay for determination of rubella IgG antibodies, Acta Pathol. Microbiol. Scand. 86 (1978) 387.

[226] M. Vejtorp, E. Fanoe, J. Leerhoy, Diagnosis of postnatal rubella by the enzyme-linked immunosorbent assay for rubella IgM and IgG antibodies, Acta Pathol. Microbiol. Scand. 87 (1979) 155.

[227] D. Bidwell, et al., Further investigation of the specificity and sensitivity of ELISA for rubella antibody screening, J. Clin. Pathol. 33 (1980) 200.

[228] L.P. Skendzel, D.C. Edson, Evaluation of enzyme immunosorbent rubella assays, Arch. Pathol. Lab. Med. 109 (1985) 391.

[229] P. Morgan-Capner, et al., A comparison of three tests for rubella antibody screening, J. Clin. Pathol. 32 (1979) 542.

[230] H. Champsaur, E. Dussaix, P. Tournier, Hemagglutination inhibition, single radial hemolysis, and ELISA tests for the detection of IgG and IgM to rubella virus, J. Med. Virol. 5 (1980) 273.

[231] R. Deibel, et al., Assay of rubella antibody by passive hemagglutination and by a modified indirect immunofluorescence test, Infection 8 (Suppl. 3) (1980) S255.

[232] M.V. Zartarian, et al., Detection of rubella antibodies by hemagglutination inhibition, indirect fluorescent-antibody test, and enzyme-linked immunosorbent assay, J. Clin. Microbiol. 14 (1981) 640.

[233] A.S. Weissfeld, W.D. Gehle, A.C. Sonnenworth, Comparison of several test systems used for the determination of rubella immune status, J. Clin. Microbiol. 16 (1982) 82.

[234] A.L. Truant, et al., Comparison of an enzyme-linked immunosorbent assay with indirect hemagglutination inhibition for determination of rubella virus antibody: evaluation of immune status with commercial reagents in a clinical laboratory, J. Clin. Microbiol. 17 (1983) 106.

[235] P.R. Field, C.M. Gong, Diagnosis of postnatally acquired rubella by use of three enzyme-linked immunosorbent assays for specific immunoglobulins G and M and single radial hemolysis for specific immunoglobulin G, J. Clin. Microbiol. 20 (1984) 951.

[236] H. Cubie, E. Edmond, Comparison of five different methods of rubella IgM antibody testing, J. Clin. Pathol. 38 (1985) 203.

[237] G. Enders, Serologic test combinations for safe detection of rubella infections, Rev. Infect. Dis. 7 (Suppl. 1) (1985) S113.

[238] M. Forsgren, Standardization of techniques and reagents for the study of rubella antibody, Rev. Infect. Dis. 7 (Suppl. 1) (1985) S129.

[239] L. Grillner, M. Forsgren, E. Nordenfelt, Comparison between a commercial ELISA, Rubazyme, and hemolysis-in-gel test for determination of rubella antibodies, J. Virol. Methods 10 (1985) 111.

[240] M.A. Chernesky, et al., Combined testing for antibodies to rubella nonstructural and envelope proteins sentinels infections in two outbreaks, Diagn. Microbiol. Infect. Dis. 8 (1987) 173.

[241] J. Ankerst, et al., A routine diagnostic test for IgA and IgM antibodies to rubella virus: absorption of IgG with Staphylococcus aureus, J. Infect. Dis. 130 (1974) 268.

[242] J.R. Pattison, J.E. Mace, Elution patterns of rubella IgM, IgA, and IgG antibodies from a dextran and an agarose gel, J. Clin. Pathol. 28 (1975) 670.

[243] J.R. Pattison, J.E. Mace, D.S. Dane, The detection and avoidance of false-positive reactions in tests for rubella-specific IgM, J. Med. Microbiol. 9 (1975) 355.

[244] J.R. Pattison, J.E. Mace, The detection of specific IgM antibodies following infection with rubella virus, J. Clin. Pathol. 28 (1975) 377.

[245] J.R. Pattison, et al., Comparison of methods for detecting specific IgM antibody in infants with congenital rubella, J. Med. Microbiol. 11 (1978) 411.

[246] E.O. Caul, et al., Evaluation of a simplified sucrose gradient method for the detection of rubella-specific IgM in routine diagnostic practice, J. Med. Virol. 2 (1978) 153.

[247] U. Krech, J.A. Wilhelm, A solid-phase immunosorbent technique for the rapid detection of rubella IgM by haemagglutination inhibition, J. Gen. Virol. 44 (1979) 281.

[248] P. Morgan-Capner, E. Davies, J.R. Pattison, Rubella-specific IgM detection using Sephacryl S-300 gel filtration, J. Clin. Pathol. 33 (1980) 1072.

[249] N. Kobayashi, et al., Separation of hemagglutination-inhibiting immunoglobulin M antibody to rubella virus in human serum by high-performance liquid chromatography, J. Clin. Microbiol. 23 (1986) 1143.

[250] A.L. Cunningham, J.R.E. Fraser, Persistent rubella virus infection of human synovial cells cultured in vitro, J. Infect. Dis. 151 (1985) 638.

[251] P.D. Parkman, et al., Attenuated rubella virus. I. Development and laboratory characterization, N. Engl. J. Med. 275 (1966) 569.

[252] J. Desmyter, et al., The mechanism of rubella virus interference, Symp. Ser. Immunobiol. Stand. 11 (1969) 139.

[253] M.B. Kleiman, D.H. Carver, Failure of the RA 27/3 strain of rubella virus to induce intrinsic interference, J. Gen. Virol. 36 (1977) 335.

[254] T.K. Frey, M.L. Hemphill, Generation of defective-interfering particles by rubella virus in Vero cells, Virology 164 (1988) 22.

[255] B. Sigurdardottir, et al., Association of virus with cases of rubella studied in Toronto: propagation of the agent and transmission to monkeys, Can. Med. Assoc. J. 88 (1963) 128.

[256] A.D. Heggie, F.C. Robbins, Rubella in naval recruits: a virologic study, N. Engl. J. Med. 271 (1964) 231.

[257] P.D. Parkman, et al., Experimental rubella virus infection in the rhesus monkey, J. Immunol. 95 (1965) 743.

[258] P.D. Parkman, P.E. Phillips, H.M. Meyer, Experimental rubella virus infection in pregnant monkeys, Am. J. Dis. Child. 110 (1965) 390.

[259] J.L. Sever, et al., Experimental rubella in pregnant rhesus monkeys, J. Infect. Dis. 116 (1966) 21.

[260] A. Fabiyi, G.L. Gitnick, J.L. Sever, Chronic rubella virus infection in the ferret (Mustela putorius fero) puppy, Proc. Soc. Exp. Biol. Med. 125 (1967) 766.

[261] L. Barbosa, J. Warren, Studies on the detection of rubella virus and its immunogenicity for animals and man, Semi-annual contract progress report to the National Institute for Neurological Diseases and Blindness, September 1, 1966 to March 1, 1967.

[262] R.J. Belcourt, F.C. Wong, M.J. Walcroft, Growth of rubella virus in rabbit foetal tissues and cell cultures, Can. J. Public Health 56 (1965) 253.

[263] J.S. Oxford, The growth of rubella virus in small laboratory animals, J. Immunol. 98 (1967) 697.

[264] E. Cotlier, et al., Pathogenic effects of rubella virus on embryos and newborn rats, Nature 217 (1968) 38.

[265] D.H. Carver, et al., Rubella virus replication in the brains of suckling mice, J. Virol. 1 (1967) 1089.

[266] Centers for Disease Control, Recommendation of the Immunization Practices Advisory Committee (ACIP). Rubella prevention, MMWR Morb. Mortal. Wkly. Rep. 39 (1990) 1.

[267] Centers for Disease Control revised ACIP recommendation for avoiding pregnancy after receiving a rubella containing vaccine, MMWR Morb. Mortal. Wkly. Rep. 50 (2001) 1117.

[268] Committee on Infectious Diseases, Rubella, in: G. Peter (Ed.), Report of the Committee on Infectious Diseases, twenty second ed., American Academy of Pediatrics, Elk Grove Village, IL, 1991.

[269] K.J. Bart, et al., Elimination of rubella and congenital rubella from the United States, Pediatr. Infect. Dis. 4 (1985) 14.

[270] J.M. Mann, et al., Assessing risks of rubella infection during pregnancy: a standardized approach, JAMA 245 (1981) 1647.

[271] D.M. Horstmann, et al., Rubella: reinfection of vaccinated and naturally immune persons exposed in an epidemic, N. Engl. J. Med. 283 (1970) 771.

[272] D.E. Lehane, N.R. Newberg, W.E. Beam Jr., Evaluation of rubella herd immunity during an epidemic, JAMA 213 (1970) 2236.

[273] R.B. Pollard, E.A. Edwards, Epidemic survey of rubella in a military recruit population, Am. J. Epidemiol. 101 (1975) 435.

[274] G.E. Crawford, D.H. Gremellion, Epidemic measles and rubella in Air Force recruits: impact of immunization, J. Infect. Dis. 144 (1981) 403.

[275] L.E. Blouse, et al., Rubella screening and vaccination program for US Air Force trainees: an analysis of findings, Am. J. Public Health 72 (1982) 280.

[276] J.H. Chretien, et al., Rubella: pattern of outbreak in a university, South Med. J. 69 (1976) 1042.

[277] Centers for Disease Control, Rubella in colleges—United States, 1983–1984, MMWR Morb. Mortal. Wkly. Rep. 34 (1985) 228.

[278] Centers for Disease Control, Rubella outbreaks in prisons—New York City, West Virginia, California, MMWR Morb. Mortal. Wkly. Rep. 34 (1985) 615.

[279] Centers for Disease Control, Rubella and congenital rubella syndrome—New York City, MMWR Morb. Mortal. Wkly. Rep. 35 (1986) 770 779.

[280] Centers for Disease Control, Increase in rubella and congenital rubella syndrome in the United States, MMWR Morb. Mortal. Wkly. Rep. 40 (1991) 93.

[281] Centers for Disease Control, Congenital rubella syndrome among the Amish—Pennsylvania, 1991–1992, MMWR Morb. Mortal. Wkly. Rep. 41 (1992) 468.

[282] A.K. Goodman, et al., Rubella in the workplace: the need for employee immunization, Am. J. Public Health 77 (1987) 725.

[283] M.C. McLaughlin, L.H. Gold, The New York rubella incident: a case for changing hospital policy regarding rubella testing and immunization, Am. J. Public Health 79 (1979) 287.

[284] B.F. Polk, et al., An outbreak of rubella among hospital personnel, N. Engl. J. Med. 303 (1980) 541.

[285] W.L. Greaves, et al., Prevention of rubella transmission in medical facilities, JAMA 248 (1982) 861.

[286] M.A. Strassburg, et al., Rubella in hospital employees, Infect. Control 5 (1984) 123.

[287] G.A. Storch, et al., A rubella outbreak among dental students: description of the outbreak and analysis of control measures, Infect. Control 6 (1985) 150.

[288] J.L. Sever, G. Monif, Limited persistence of virus in congenital rubella, Am. J. Dis. Child. 110 (1965) 452.

[289] L.Z. Cooper, S. Krugman, Clinical manifestations of postnatal and congenital rubella, Arch. Ophthalmol. 77 (1967) 434.

[290] W.E. Rawls, et al., Persistent virus infection in congenital rubella, Arch. Ophthalmol. 77 (1967) 430.

[291] R.H. Michaels, Immunologic aspects of congenital rubella, Pediatrics 43 (1969) 339.

[292] M.A. Menser, et al., Rubella viruria in a 29-year-old woman with congenital rubella, Lancet 2 (1971) 797.

[293] D.A. Shewmon, J.D. Cherry, S.E. Kirby, Shedding of rubella virus in a 41–2-year-old boy with congenital rubella, Pediatr. Infect. Dis. 1 (1982) 342.

[294] R.P. Hattis, et al., Rubella in an immunized island population, JAMA 223 (1973) 1019.

[295] T.H. Weller, C.A. Alford Jr., F.A. Neva, Changing epidemiologic concepts of rubella, with particular reference to unique characteristics of the congenital infection, Yale J. Biol. Med. 37 (1965) 455.

[296] W.E. Rawls, et al., WHO collaborative study on the seroepidemiology of rubella, Bull. World Health Organ. 37 (1967) 79.

[297] W.C. Cockburn, World aspects of the epidemiology of rubella, Am. J. Dis. Child. 118 (1969) 112.

[298] J.J. Witte, et al., Epidemiology of rubella, Am. J. Dis. Child. 118 (1969) 107.

[299] W.R. Dowdle, et al., WHO collaborative study on the seroepidemiology of rubella in Caribbean and Middle and South American populations in 1968, Bull. World Health Organ. 42 (1970) 419.

[300] D.M. Horstmann, Rubella: the challenge of its control, J. Infect. Dis. 123 (1971) 640.

[301] R. Assad, K. Ljungars-Esteves, Rubella—world impact, Rev. Infect. Dis. 7 (Suppl. 1) (1985) S29.

[302] D.M. Horstmann, Rubella, in: A.S. Evans (Ed.), Viral Infections of Humans: Epidemiologu and Control, second ed., Plenum Publishing, New York, 1985.

[303] S.E. Reef, et al., The changing epidemiology of rubella in the 1990s: on the verge of elimination and new challenges for control and prevention, JAMA 287 (2002) 464.

[304] E.L. Buescher, Behavior of rubella virus in adult populations, Arch. Gesamte Virusforsch. 16 (1965) 470.

[305] R.H. Green, et al., Studies of the natural history and prevention of rubella, Am. J. Dis. Child. 110 (1965) 348.

[306] D.M. Horstmann, et al., A natural epidemic of rubella in a closed population, Arch. Gesamte Virusforsch. 16 (1965) 483.

[307] J.A. Brody, The infectiousness of rubella and the possibility of reinfection, Am. J. Public Health 56 (1966) 1082.

[308] A.L. Bisno, et al., Rubella in Trinidad: seroepidemiologic studies of an institutional outbreak, Am. J. Epidemiol. 89 (1969) 74.

[309] J.L. Gale, et al., The epidemiology of rubella on Taiwan. III. Family studies in cities of high and low attack rates, Int. J. Epidemiol. 1 (1972) 261.

[310] F.A. Neva, C.A. Alford Jr., T.H. Weller, Emerging perspective of rubella, Bacteriol. Rev. 28 (1964) 444.

[311] J.A. Brody, et al., Rubella epidemic on St. Paul Island in the Pribilofs, 1963. I. Epidemiologic, clinical, and serologic findings, JAMA 191 (1965) 619.

[312] J.L. Sever, et al., Rubella epidemic on St. Paul Island in the Pribilofs, 1963. II. Clinical and laboratory findings for the intensive study population, JAMA 191 (1965) 624.

[313] S.B. Halstead, A.R. Diwan, A.I. Oda, Susceptibility to rubella among adolescents and adults in Hawaii, JAMA 210 (1969) 1881.

[314] A.R. Hinman, et al., Economic analyses of rubella and rubella vaccines: a global review, Bull. World Health Organ. 80 (2003) 264.

[315] J. Wilkins, et al., Reinfection with rubella virus despite live vaccine-induced immunity, Am. J. Dis. Child. 118 (1969) 275.

[316] T.W. Chang, S. DesRosiers, L. Weinstein, Clinical and serologic studies of an outbreak of rubella in a vaccinated population, N. Engl. J. Med. 283 (1970) 246.

[317] P.A. Gross, et al., A rubella outbreak among adolescent boys, Am. J. Dis. Child. 119 (1970) 326.

[318] S. Bloom, et al., Has the United States population been adequately vaccinated to achieve rubella elimination? Clin. Infect. Dis. 43 (Suppl. 3) (2006) S141–S145.

[319] K.A. Miller, Rubella susceptibility in an adolescent female population, Mayo Clin. Proc. 59 (1984) 31.

[320] S. Allen, Rubella susceptibility in young adults, J. Fam. Pract. 21 (1985) 271.

[321] C.A. Dykewicz, et al., Rubella seropositivity in the United States, 1988–1994, Clin. Infect. Dis. 33 (2001) 1279–1286.

[322] T.B. Hyde, et al., Rubella immunity levels in the United States population: has the threshold of viral elimination been reached? Clin. Infect. Dis. 43 (Suppl. 3) (2006) S146–S150.

[323] S.E. Reef, et al., The epidemiological profile of rubella and congenital rubella syndrome in the United States, 1998–2004: the evidence for absence of endemic transmission, Clin. Infect. Dis. 43 (Suppl. 3) (2006) S126–S132.

[324] C.A. Alford, F.A. Neva, T.H. Weller, Virologic and serologic studies on human products of conception after maternal rubella, N. Engl. J. Med. 271 (1964) 1275.

[325] D.J. Horstmann, et al., Maternal rubella and the rubella syndrome in infants, Am. J. Dis. Child. 110 (1965) 408.

[326] G.R.G. Monif, et al., Isolation of rubella virus from products of conception, Am. J. Obstet. Gynecol. 91 (1965) 1143.

[327] C.A. Alford Jr., Congenital rubella: a review of the virologic and serologic phenomena occurring after maternal rubella in the first trimester, South Med. J. 59 (1966) 745.

[328] A.D. Heggie, Intrauterine infection in maternal rubella, J. Pediatr. 71 (1967) 777.

[329] W.E. Rawls, J. Desmyter, J.L. Melnick, Serologic diagnosis and fetal involvement in maternal rubella, JAMA 203 (1968) 627.

[330] K.M. Thompson, J.O. Tobin, Isolation of rubella virus from abortion material, BMJ 2 (1970) 264.

[331] O. Strannegard, et al., Case of apparent reinfection with rubella, Lancet 1 (1970) 240.

[332] A. Boué, A. Nicholas, B. Montagnon, Reinfection with rubella in pregnant women, Lancet 2 (1971) 1251.

[333] G. Haukenes, K.O. Haram, Clinical rubella after reinfection, N. Engl. J. Med. 287 (1972) 1204.

[334] R.L. Northrop, W.M. Gardner, W.F. Geittman, Rubella reinfection during early pregnancy, Obstet. Gynecol. 39 (1972) 524.

[335] R.L. Northrop, W.M. Gardner, W.F. Geittman, Low-level immunity to rubella, N. Engl. J. Med. 287 (1972) 615.

[336] T. Eilard, O. Strannegard, Rubella reinfection in pregnancy followed by transmission to the fetus, J. Infect. Dis. 129 (1974) 594.

[337] J.A.M. Snijder, F.P. Schroder, J.H. Hoekstra, Importance of IgM determination in cord blood in cases of suspected rubella infection, BMJ 1 (1977) 23.

[338] M. Forsgren, G. Carlstrom, K. Strangert, Congenital rubella after maternal reinfection, Scand. J. Infect. Dis. 11 (1979) 81.

[339] A. Fogel, R. Handsher, B. Barnea, Subclinical rubella in pregnancy—occurrence and outcome, Isr. J. Med. Sci. 21 (1985) 133.

[340] M.D. Sheridan, Final report of a prospective study of children whose mothers had rubella in early pregnancy, BMJ 2 (1964) 536.

[341] N.R. Butler, et al., Persistence of rubella antibody with and without embryopathy: a follow-up study of children exposed to maternal rubella, BMJ 2 (1965) 1027.

[342] G.A. Phillips, et al., Persistence of virus in infants with congenital rubella and in normal infants with a history of maternal rubella, JAMA 193 (1965) 1027.

[343] J.B. Hardy, et al., Adverse fetal outcome following maternal rubella after the first trimester of pregnancy, JAMA 207 (1969) 2414.

[344] G.M. Schiff, J. Sutherland, I. Light, Congenital rubella, in: O. Thalhammer (Ed.), Prenatal Infections, International Symposium of Vienna, September 2–3, 1970. Georg Thieme Verlag, Stuttgart, 1971.

[345] G.S. Peckham, Clinical and laboratory study of children exposed in utero to maternal rubella, Arch. Dis. Child. 47 (1972) 571.

[346] M.A. Menser, J.M. Forrest, Rubella—high incidence of defects in children considered normal at birth, Med. J. Aust. 1 (1974) 123.

[347] J.A. Dudgeon, Infective causes of human malformations, Br. Med. Bull. 32 (1976) 77.

[348] R. Lundstrom, Rubella during pregnancy: a follow-up study of children born after an epidemic of rubella in Sweden, 1951, with additional investigations on prophylaxis and treatment of maternal rubella, Acta Paediatr. 51 (Suppl. 133) (1962) 1.

[349] W.L. Whitehouse, Rubella before conception as a cause of foetal abnormality, Lancet 1 (1963) 139.

[350] G.R.G. Monif, J.B. Hardy, J.L. Sever, Studies in congenital rubella, Baltimore 1964–65. I. Epidemiologic and virologic, Bull. Johns Hopkins Hosp. 118 (1966) 85.

[351] J.L. Sever, et al., Rubella in the Collaborative Perinatal Research Study. II. Clinical and laboratory findings in children through 3 years of age, Am. J. Dis. Child. 118 (1969) 123.

[352] M. Seppala, A. Vaheri, Natural rubella infection of the female genital tract, Lancet 1 (1974) 46.

[353] E. Buimovici-Klein, et al., Isolation of rubella virus in milk after postpartum immunization, J. Pediatr. 91 (1977) 939.

[354] E.B. Klein, T. Bryne, L.Z. Cooper, Neonatal rubella in a breast-fed infant after postpartum maternal infection, J. Pediatr. 97 (1980) 774.

[355] M.M. Manson, W.P.D. Logan, R.M. Loy, Rubella and other virus infections during pregnancy, in: Reports on Public Health and Medical Subjects, No. 101, Her Majesty's Stationery Office, London, 1960.

[356] M. Siegel, M. Greenberg, Fetal death, malformation and prematurity after maternal rubella: results of prospective study, 1949–1958, N. Engl. J. Med. 262 (1960) 389.

[357] G.C. Liggins, L.I. Phillips, Rubella embryopathy: an interim report on a New Zealand epidemic, BMJ 1 (1963) 711.

[358] D. Pitt, E.H. Keir, Results of rubella in pregnancy, III, Med. J. Aust. 2 (1965) 737.

[359] S.J. Sallomi, Rubella in pregnancy: a review of prospective studies from the literature, Obstet. Gynecol. 27 (1966) 252.

[360] A.D. Heggie, F.C. Robbins, Natural rubella acquired after birth: clinical features and complications, Am. J. Dis. Child. 118 (1969) 12.

[361] J.K. Chantler, A.J. Tingle, Isolation of rubella virus from human lymphocytes after acute infection, J. Infect. Dis. 145 (1982) 673.

[362] S. O'Shea, D. Mutton, J.M. Best, In vivo expression of rubella antigens on human leucocytes: detection by flow cytometry, J. Med. Virol. 25 (1988) 297.

[363] A.D. Heggie, Pathogenesis of the rubella exanthem: isolation of rubella virus from the skin, N. Engl. J. Med. 285 (1971) 664.

[364] A.D. Heggie, Pathogenesis of the rubella exanthem: distribution of rubella virus in the skin during rubella with and without rash, J. Infect. Dis. 137 (1978) 74.

[365] W. Al-Nakib, J.M. Best, J.E. Banatvala, Rubella-specific serum and nasopharyngeal immunoglobulin responses following naturally acquired and vaccine-induced infection: prolonged persistence of virus-specific IgM, Lancet 1 (1975) 182.

[366] J.R. Pattison, D.S. Dane, J.E. Mace, The persistence of specific IgM after natural infection with rubella virus, Lancet 1 (1975) 185.

[367] O.H. Meurman, Persistence of immunoglobulin G and immunoglobulin M antibodies after postnatal rubella infection determined by solid-phase radioimmunoassay, J. Clin. Microbiol. 7 (1978) 34.

[368] S. Rousseau, K. Hedman, Rubella infection and reinfection distinguished by avidity of IgG. Letter to the editor, Lancet 1 (1988) 1108.

[369] K. Hedman, I. Seppala, Recent rubella virus infection indicated by a low avidity of specific IgG, J. Clin. Immunol. 8 (1988) 214.

[370] P. Morgan-Capner, H.I.J. Thomas, Serological distinction between primary rubella and reinfection. Letter to the editor, Lancet 1 (1988) 1397.

[371] K.A. Smith, L. Chess, M.R. Mardiney Jr., The relationship between rubella hemagglutination inhibition antibody (HIA) and rubella induced in vitro lymphocyte triitated thymidine incorporation, Cell. Immunol. 8 (1973) 321.

[372] R.W. Steele, et al., A 52Cr microassay technique for cell-mediated immunity to viruses, J. Immunol. 110 (1973) 1502.

[373] M.C. Honeyman, J.M. Forrest, D.C. Dorman, Cell-mediated immune response following natural rubella and rubella vaccination, Clin. Exp. Immunol. 17 (1974) 665.

[374] L. McMorrow, et al., Suppression of the response of lymphocytes to phytohemagglutinin in rubella, J. Infect. Dis. 130 (1974) 464.

[375] R.W. Steele, et al., Development of specific cellular and humoral immune responses in children immunized with liver rubella virus vaccine, J. Infect. Dis. 130 (1974) 449.

[376] G.Y. Kanra, T. Vesikari, Cytotoxic activity against rubella-infected cells in the supernatants of human lymphocyte cultures stimulated by rubella virus, Clin. Exp. Immunol. 19 (1975) 17.

[377] T. Vesikari, et al., Cell-mediated immunity in rubella assayed by cytotoxicity of supernatants from rubella virus-stimulated human lymphocyte cultures, Clin. Exp. Immunol. 19 (1975) 33.

[378] R. Ganguly, C.L. Cusumano, R.H. Waldman, Suppression of cell-mediated immunity after infection with attenuated rubella virus, Infect. Immun. 13 (1976) 464.

[379] E. Buimovici-Klein, K.E. Weiss, L.Z. Cooper, Interferon production in lymphocyte cultures after rubella infection in humans, J. Infect. Dis. 135 (1977) 380.

[380] E. Rossier, et al., Absence of cell-mediated immunity to rubella virus 5 years after rubella vaccination, Can. Med. Assoc. J. 116 (1977) 481.

[381] E. Rossier, et al., Persistence of humoral and cell-mediated immunity to rubella virus in cloistered nuns and in schoolteachers, J. Infect. Dis. 144 (1981) 137.

[382] E. Buimovici-Klein, L.Z. Cooper, Cell-mediated immune response to rubella infections, Rev. Infect. Dis. 7 (Suppl. 1) (1985) S123.

[383] T. Mori, K. Shiozawa, Suppression of tuberculin hypersensitivity caused by rubella infection, Am. Rev. Respir. Dis. 131 (1985) 886.

[384] P.L. Ogra, et al., Antibody response in serum and nasopharynx after naturally acquired and vaccine-induced infection with rubella virus, N. Engl. J. Med. 285 (1971) 1333.

[385] W. Al-Nakib, J.M. Best, J.E. Banatvala, Detection of rubella-specific serum IgG and IgA and nasopharyngeal IgA responses using a radioactive single radial immunodiffusion technique, Clin. Exp. Immunol. 22 (1975) 293.

[386] S.A. Plotkin, J.D. Farquhar, Immunity to rubella: comparison between naturally and artificially induced resistance, Postgrad. Med. J. 48 (Suppl.) (1972) 47.

[387] S.A. Plotkin, J.D. Farquhar, P.L. Ogra, Immunologic properties of RA 27/3 rubella virus vaccine: a comparison with strains presently licensed in the United States, JAMA 225 (1973) 585.

[388] A. Morag, et al., Development and characteristics of in vitro correlates of cellular immunity to rubella virus in the systemic and mucosal sites in guinea pigs, J. Immunol. 113 (1974) 1703.

[389] A. Morag, et al., In vitro correlates of cell-mediated immunity in human tonsils after natural or induced rubella virus infection, J. Infect. Dis. 131 (1975) 409.

[390] G. Selzer, Virus isolation, inclusion bodies, and chromosomes in a rubella-infected human embryo, Lancet 2 (1963) 336.

[391] A.J. Rudolph, et al., Transplacental rubella infection in newly born infants, JAMA 191 (1965) 843.

[392] L.W. Catalano Jr., et al., Isolation of rubella virus from placentas and throat cultures of infants: a prospective study after the 1964–65 epidemic, Obstet. Gynecol. 38 (1971) 6.

[393] G.R.G. Monif, J.L. Sever, Chronic infection of the central nervous system with rubella virus, Neurology 16 (1966) 111.

[394] M.M. Desmond, et al., Congenital rubella encephalitis, J. Pediatr. 71 (1967) 311.

[395] M.A. Menser, et al., Persistence of virus in lens for three years after prenatal rubella, Lancet 2 (1967) 387.

[396] S.A. Plotkin, et al., Congenital rubella syndrome in late infancy, JAMA 200 (1967) 435.

[397] N.E. Cremer, et al., Isolation of rubella virus from brain in chronic progressive panencephalitis, J. Gen. Virol. 29 (1975) 143.

[398] M.L. Weil, et al., Chronic progressive panencephalitis due to rubella virus simulating subacute sclerosing panencephalitis, N. Engl. J. Med. 292 (1975) 994.

[399] C.A. Alford Jr., Studies on antibody in congenital rubella infections. I. Physicochemical and immunologic investigations of rubella-neutralizing antibody, Am. J. Dis. Child. 110 (1965) 455.

[400] T.H. Weller, C.A. Alford, F.A. Neva, Retrospective diagnosis by serologic means of congenitally acquired rubella infections, N. Engl. J. Med. 270 (1964) 1039.

[401] C.A. Alford Jr., et al., The diagnostic significance of IgM-globulin elevations in newborn infants with chronic intrauterine infections, in: D. Bergsma (Ed.), Birth Defects. Original Article Series, vol. 4, no. 5, National Foundation–March of Dimes, New York, 1968.

[402] D. Gitlin, The differentiation and maturation of specific immune mechanisms, Acta Paediatr. Scand. Suppl. 172 (1967) 60.

[403] A.R. Lawton, et al., Ontogeny of lymphocytes in the human fetus, Clin. Immunol. 1 (1972) 104.

[404] D. Gitlin, A. Biasucci, Development of gamma G, gamma A, beta IC-beta IA, CI esterase inhibitor, ceruloplasmin, transferrin, hemopexin, haptoglobin, fibrinogen, plasminogen, alpha 1-antitrypsin, orosomucoid, beta-lipoprotein, alpha 2-macroglobulin, and prealbumin in the human conceptus, J. Clin. Invest. 48 (1969) 1433.

[405] C.A. Alford Jr., Fetal antibody in the diagnosis of chronic intrauterine infections, in: O. Thalhammer (Ed.), Prenatal Infections, International Symposium of Vienna, September 2–3, 1970. Georg Thieme Verlag, Stuttgart, 1971.

[406] J.A. Bellanti, et al., Congenital rubella: clinicopathologic, virologic, and immunologic studies, Am. J. Dis. Child. 110 (1965) 464.

[407] J.V. Baublis, G.C. Brown, Specific response of the immunoglobulins to rubella infection, Proc. Soc. Exp. Biol. Med. 128 (1968) 206.

[408] S.M. Cohen, et al., Rubella antibody in IgG and IgM immunoglobulins detected by immunofluorescence, J. Lab. Clin. Med. 72 (1968) 760.

[409] T. Vesikari, et al., Congenital rubella: immune response of the neonate and diagnosis by demonstration of specific IgM antibodies, J. Pediatr. 75 (1969) 658.

[410] J.E. Cradock-Watson, M.K.S. Ridehalgh, S. Chantler, Specific immunoglobulins in infants with the congenital rubella syndrome, J. Hyg. (Lond.) 76 (1976) 109.

[411] C.A. Alford Jr., Immunoglobulin determinations in the diagnosis of fetal infection, Pediatr. Clin. North Am. 18 (1971) 99.

[412] G.H. McCracken Jr., et al., Serum immunoglobulin levels in newborn infants. II. Survey of cord and follow-up sera from 123 infants with congenital rubella, J. Pediatr. 74 (1969) 383.

[413] K.G. Kenrick, et al., Immunoglobulins and rubella-virus antibodies in adults with congenital rubella, Lancet 1 (1968) 548.

[414] J.B. Hardy, J.L. Sever, M.R. Gilkeson, Declining antibody titers in children with congenital rubella, J. Pediatr. 75 (1969) 213.

[415] L.Z. Cooper, et al., Loss of rubella hemagglutination-inhibition antibody in congenital rubella, Am. J. Dis. Child. 122 (1971) 397.

[416] K. Ueda, et al., Hemagglutination inhibition antibodies in congenital rubella: a 17-year follow-up in the Ryukyu Islands, Am. J. Dis. Child. 141 (1987) 211.

[417] K. Ueda, et al., Continuing problem in congenital rubella syndrome in southern Japan: its outbreak in Fukuoka and the surrounding areas after the 1965–1969 and 1975–1977 rubella epidemics, Fukuoka Acta Med. 77 (1986) 309.

[418] J.F. Soothill, K. Hayes, J.A. Dudgeon, The immunoglobulins in congenital rubella, Lancet 1 (1966) 1385.

[419] M.P. Hancock, C.C. Huntley, J.L. Sever, Congenital rubella syndrome with immunoglobulin disorder, J. Pediatr. 72 (1968) 636.

[420] A.R. Hayward, G. Ezer, Development of lymphocyte populations in the human foetal thymus and spleen, Clin. Exp. Immunol. 17 (1974) 169.

[421] M.D. Cooper, D.H. Dayton (Eds.), Development of Host Defenses, Raven Press, New York, 1977.

[422] M.E. Miller (Ed.), Host Defenses in the Human Neonate, Grune & Stratton, New York, 1978.

[423] C.L. Berry, E.N. Thompson, Clinicopathological study of thymic dysplasia, Arch. Dis. Child. 43 (1968) 579.

[424] L.R. White, et al., Immune competence in congenital rubella: lymphocyte transformation, delayed hypersensitivity and response to vaccination, J. Pediatr. 73 (1968) 229.

[425] J.R. Montgomery, et al., Viral inhibition of lymphocyte response to phytohemagglutinin, Science 157 (1967) 1068.

[426] G.B. Olson, M.A. South, R.A. Good, Phytohemagglutinin unresponsiveness of lymphocytes from babies with congenital rubella, Nature 214 (1967) 695.

[427] P.B. Dent, et al., Rubella-virus/leukocyte interaction and its role in the pathogenesis of the congenital rubella syndrome, Lancet 1 (1968) 291.

[428] G.B. Olson, et al., Abnormalities of in vitro lymphocyte responses during rubella virus infections, J. Exp. Med. 128 (1968) 47.

[429] J.J. Simmons, M.G. Fitzgerald, Rubella virus and human lymphocytes in culture, Lancet 2 (1968) 937.

[430] W.C. Marshall, et al., In vitro lymphocyte response in some immunity deficiency diseases and in intrauterine virus infections, Proc. R. Soc. Med. 63 (1970) 351.

[431] E. Buimovici-Klein, et al., Impaired cell-mediated immune response in patients with congenital rubella: correlation with gestational age at time of infection, Pediatrics 64 (1979) 620.

[432] T. Hyypia, et al., B-cell function in vitro during rubella infection, Infect. Immun. 43 (1984) 589.

[433] D.A. Fuccillo, et al., Impaired cellular immunity to rubella virus in congenital rubella, Infect. Immun. 9 (1974) 81.

[434] A.L. Pukhalsky, et al., Cytokine profile after rubella vaccine inoculation: evidence of the immunosuppressive effect of vaccination, Mediators Inflamm. 12 (4) (2003).

[435] C.A. Mims, Pathogenesis of viral infections in the fetus, Prog. Med. Virol. 10 (1968) 194.

[436] W.E. Rawls, Congenital rubella: the significance of virus persistence, Prog. Med. Virol. 10 (1968) 238.

[437] C.A. Alford Jr., Production of interferon-like substance by the rubella-infected human conceptus, Program and abstracts of the American Pediatric Society and Society of Pediatric Research Meeting, Atlantic City, April 29–May 2, 1970.

[438] P. Lebon, et al., Presence of an acid-labile alpha-interferon in sera from fetuses and children with congenital rubella, J. Clin. Microbiol. 21 (1985) 755.

[439] J. Desmyter, et al., Interferon in congenital rubella: response to live attenuated measles vaccine, J. Immunol. 99 (1967) 771.

[440] K. McCarthy, C.H. Taylor-Robinson, S.E. Pillinger, Isolation of rubella virus from cases in Britain, Lancet 2 (1963) 593.

[441] H.M. Hildebrandt, H.F. Maassab, Rubella synovitis in a 1-year-old patient, N. Engl. J. Med. 274 (1966) 1428.

[442] J.E. Yanez, et al., Rubella arthritis, Ann. Intern. Med. 64 (1966) 772.

[443] J.N. McCormick, et al., Rheumatoid polyarthritis after rubella, Ann. Rheum. Dis. 37 (1978) 266.

[444] R. Graham, et al., Isolation of rubella virus from synovial fluid in five cases of seronegative arthritis, Lancet 2 (1981) 649.

[445] P. Lebon, G. Lyon, Noncongenital rubella encephalitis, Lancet 2 (1974) 468.

[446] J.S. Wolinsky, B.O. Berg, C.J. Maitland, Progressive rubella panencephalitis, Arch. Neurol. 33 (1976) 722.

[447] F. Squadrini, et al., Rubella virus isolation from cerebrospinal fluid in postnatal rubella encephalitis, BMJ 2 (1977) 1329.

[448] Y.H. Thong, et al., Impaired in vitro cell-mediated immunity to rubella virus during pregnancy, N. Engl. J. Med. 289 (1973) 604.

[449] E.D. Weinberg, Pregnancy-associated depression of cell-mediated immunity, Rev. Infect. Dis. 6 (1984) 814.

[450] M.C. Honeyman, et al., HL-A antigens in congenital rubella and the role of antigens 1 and 8 in the epidemiology of natural rubella, Tissue Antigens 5 (1975) 12.

[451] R.M. Forrester, V.T. Lees, G.H. Watson, Rubella syndrome: escape of a twin, BMJ 1 (1966) 1403.

[452] L.Z. Cooper, The history and medical consequences of rubella, Rev. Infect. Dis. 7 (Suppl. 1) (1985) S1.

[453] G. Töndury, D.W. Smith, Fetal rubella pathology, J. Pediatr. 68 (1966) 867.

[454] S.G. Driscoll, Histopathology of gestational rubella, Am. J. Dis. Child. 118 (1969) 49.

[455] J.A. Dudgeon, Teratogenic effect of rubella virus, Proc. R. Soc. Med. 63 (1970) 1254.

[456] M.A. Menser, R.D.K. Reye, The pathology of congenital rubella: a review written by request, Pathology 6 (1974) 215.

[457] J.R. Esterly, E.H. Oppenheimer, Intrauterine rubella infection, in: H.S. Rosenberg, R.P. Bolande (Eds.), Perspectives in Pediatric Pathology, vol. 1, Year Book Medical Publishers, Chicago, 1973.

[458] A. Boué, J.G. Boué, Effects of rubella virus infection on the division of human cells, Am. J. Dis. Child. 118 (1969) 45.

[459] J.L. Smith, et al., Persistent rubella virus production in embryonic rabbit chondrocyte cell cultures (37465), Proc. Soc. Exp. Biol. Med. 143 (1973) 1037.

[460] A.D. Heggie, Growth inhibition of human embryonic and fetal rat bones in organ culture by rubella virus, Teratology 15 (1977) 47.

[461] W.E. Rawls, et al., Spontaneous virus carrier cultures and postmortem isolation of virus from infants with congenital rubella, Proc. Soc. Exp. Biol. Med. 120 (1965) 623.

[462] A. Boué, S.A. Plotkin, J.G. Boué, Action du virus de la rubéole sur différents systemes de cultures de cellules embryonnaires humaines, Arch. Gesamte Virusforsch. 16 (1965) 443.

[463] S.A. Plotkin, A. Boué, J.G. Boué, The in vitro growth of rubella virus in human embryo cells, Am. J. Epidemiol. 81 (1965) 71.

[464] T.H. Chang, et al., Chromosome studies of human cells infected in utero and in vitro with rubella virus, Proc. Soc. Exp. Biol. Med. 122 (1966) 236.

[465] J. Nusbacher, K. Hirschhorn, L.Z. Cooper, Chromosomal studies on congenital rubella, N. Engl. J. Med. 276 (1967) 1409.

[466] S.A. Plotkin, A. Vaheri, Human fibroblasts infected with rubella virus produce a growth inhibitor, Science 156 (1967) 659.

[467] D.S. Bowden, et al., Distribution by immunofluorescence of viral products and actin-containing cytoskeleton filaments in rubella virus-infected cells, Arch. Virol. 92 (1987) 211.

[468] T. Yoneda, et al., Altered growth, differentiation, and responsiveness to epidermal growth factor of human embryonic mesenchymal cells of palate by persistent rubella virus infection, J. Clin. Invest. 77 (1986) 1613.

[469] R.L. Naeye, W. Blanc, Pathogenesis of congenital rubella, JAMA 194 (1965) 1277.

[469a] C.S. Ilkow, V. Mancinelli, M.D. Beatch, T.C. Hobman, Rubella virus capsid protein interacts with poly(a)-binding protein and inhibits translation, J. Virol. 82 (2008) 4284–4294.

[469b] M.P. Adamo, M. Zapeta, T.K. Frey, Analysis of gene expression in fetal and adult cells infected with rubella virus, Virology 370 (2007) 1–11.

[470] C.B. Reimer, et al., The specificity of fetal IgM. Antibody or anti-antibody, Ann. N. Y. Acad. Sci. 254 (1975) 77.

[471] P.W. Robertson, V. Kertesz, M.J. Cloonan, Elimination of false-positive cytomegalovirus immunoglobulin M-fluorescent-antibody reactions with immunoglobulin M serum fractions, J. Clin. Microbiol. 6 (1977) 174.

[472] G. Altshuler, Placentitis with a new light on an old TORCH, Obstet. Gynecol. Ann. 6 (1977) 197.

[473] A.G.P. Garcia, et al., Placental pathology in congenital rubella, Placenta 6 (1985) 281.

[474] S. Krugman, et al., (Eds.), Rubella, in: Infectious Diseases of Children, Mosby, St. Louis, 1985.

[475] M. Sheinis, et al., Severe neonatal rubella following maternal infection, Pediatr. Infect. Dis. 4 (1985) 202.

[476] R.G. Judelsohn, S.A. Wyll, Rubella in Bermuda: termination of an epidemic by mass vaccination, JAMA 223 (1973) 401.

[477] T. Fujimoto, et al., Two cases of rubella infection with cardiac involvement, Jpn. Heart J. 20 (1979) 227.

[478] A.A. Saeed, L.S. Lange, Guillain-Barré syndrome after rubella, Postgrad. Med. J. 54 (1978) 333.

[479] N. Callaghan, M. Feely, B. Walsh, Relapsing neurological disorder associated with rubella virus infection in two sisters, J. Neurol. Neurosurg. Psychiatry 40 (1977) 1117.

[480] J.H. Connolly, et al., Carotid artery thrombosis, encephalitis, myelitis and optic neuritis associated with rubella virus infections, Brain 98 (1975) 583.

[481] P. Choutet, et al., Bone-marrow aplasia and primary rubella infection, Lancet 2 (1979) 966.

[482] S.A. Plotkin, Rubella vaccine, in: S.A. Plotkin, W.A. Orenstein, P.A. Offit (Eds.), Vaccines, fifth ed., Saunders, Philadelphia, 2008.

[483] J.J. Townsend, et al., Progressive rubella panencephalitis: late onset after congenital rubella, N. Engl. J. Med. 292 (1975) 990.

[484] M.N. Waxham, J.S. Wolinsky, Rubella virus and its effect on the nervous system, Neurol. Clin. 2 (1984) 267.

[485] D. Schlossberg, M.R. Topolosky, Military rubella, JAMA 238 (1974) 1273.

[486] S.R. Preblud, et al., Testalgia associated with rubella infection, South. Med. J. 73 (1980) 594.

[487] C.D. Quentin, H. Reiber, Fuchs heterochromic cyclitis: rubella virus antibodies and genome in aqueous humor, Am. J. Ophthalmol. 138 (2004) 46–54.

[488] L. Gordon, Fuch's heterochromic cyclitis: new clues regarding pathogenesis, Am. J. Ophthalmol. 138 (2004) 133–134.

[489] J.D. de Groot-Mijnes, et al., Rubella virus is associated with Fuchs heterochromic iridocyclitis, Am. J. Ophthalmol. 141 (2006) 212–214.

[490] A. Rothova, The riddle of Fuchs heterochromic uveitis, Am. J. Ophthalmol. 144 (2007) 447–448.

[491] R.N. Van Gelder, Idiopathic no more: clues to the pathogenesis of Fuchs heterochromic iridocyclitis and glaucomatocyclitic crisis, Am. J. Ophthalmol. 145 (2008) 769–771.

[492] M.J. Siemerink, et al., Rubella virus-associated uveitis in a nonvaccinated child, Am. J. Ophthalmol. 143 (2007) 899–900.

[493] L.R. White, J.L. Sever, F.P. Alepa, Maternal and congenital rubella before 1964: frequency, clinical features, and search for isoimmune phenomena, Pediatrics 74 (1969) 198.

[494] L.Z. Cooper, Rubella: a preventable cause of birth defects, in: D. Bergsma (Ed.), Birth Defects. Original Article Series, vol 4, no. 5. National Foundation–March of Dimes, New York, 1968.

[495] L.Z. Cooper, et al., Neonatal thrombocytopenic purpura and other manifestations of rubella contracted in utero, Am. J. Dis. Child. 110 (1965) 416.

[496] W.H. Zinkham, D.N. Medearis, J.E. Osborn, Blood and bone marrow findings in congenital rubella, J. Pediatr. 71 (1967) 512.

[497] A.J. Rudolph, Osseous manifestations of the congenital rubella syndrome, Am. J. Dis. Child. 110 (1965) 428.

[498] J.G. Rabinowitz, et al., Osseous changes in rubella embryopathy, Radiology 85 (1965) 494.

[499] W.L. Wall, et al., Roentgenological findings in congenital rubella, Clin. Pediatr. 4 (1965) 704.

[500] G.B. Reed Jr., Rubella bone lesions, J. Pediatr. 74 (1969) 208.

[501] S.B. Korones, et al., Congenital rubella syndrome: study of 22 infants, Am. J. Dis. Child. 110 (1965) 434.

[502] L.B. Rorke, A.J. Spiro, Cerebral lesions in congenital rubella syndrome, J. Pediatr. 70 (1967) 243.

[503] A.P. Streissguth, B.B. Vanderveer, T.H. Shepard, Mental development of children with congenital rubella syndrome: a preliminary report, Am. J. Obstet. Gynecol. 108 (1970) 391.

[504] M. Rowen, M.I. Singer, E.T. Moran, Intracranial calcification in the congenital rubella syndrome, AJR Am. J. Roentgenol. 115 (1972) 86.

[505] E.R. Peters, R.L. Davis, Congenital rubella syndrome: cerebral mineralizations and subperiosteal new bone formation as expressions of this disorder, Clin. Pediatr. (Phila) 5 (1966) 743.

[506] A.R. Hastreiter, et al., Cardiovascular lesions associated with congenital rubella, J. Pediatr. 71 (1967) 59.

[507] H.Z. Klein, M. Markarian, Dermal erythropoiesis in congenital rubella: description of an infected newborn who had purpura associated with marked extramedullary erythropoieses in the skin and elsewhere, Clin. Pediatr. (Phila) 8 (1969) 604.

[508] A.J. Brough, et al., Dermal erythropoieses in neonatal infants, Pediatrics 40 (1967) 627.

[509] R. Achs, K.G. Harper, M. Siegal, Unusual dermatoglyphic findings associated with the rubella embryopathy, N. Engl. J. Med. 274 (1966) 148.

[510] S.G. Purvis-Smith, P.R. Howard, M.A. Menser, Dermatoglyphic defects and rubella teratogenesis, JAMA 209 (1969) 1865.

[511] A.M. Murphy, et al., Rubella cataracts: further clinical and virologic observations, Am. J. Ophthalmol. 64 (1967) 1109.

[512] W.J. Collis, D.N. Cohen, Rubella retinopathy: a progressive disorder, Arch. Ophthalmol. 84 (1970) 33.

[513] B. Kresky, J.S. Nauheim, Rubella retinitis, Am. J. Dis. Child. 113 (1967) 305.

[514] G.M. Schiff, et al., Studies on congenital rubella, Am. J. Dis. Child. 110 (1965) 441.

[515] M.A. Menser, et al., Renal artery stenosis in the rubella syndrome, Lancet 1 (1966) 790.

[516] M.A. Menser, et al., Renal lesions in congenital rubella, Pediatrics 40 (1967) 901.

[517] G.W. Kaplan, A.P. McLaughlin III, Urogenital anomalies and congenital rubella syndrome, Urology 2 (1973) 148.

[518] J.M. Forrest, M.A. Menser, Congenital rubella in schoolchildren and adolescents, Arch. Dis. Child. 45 (1970) 63.

[519] S.B. Korones, et al., Congenital rubella syndrome: new clinical aspects with recovery of virus from affected infants, J. Pediatr. 67 (1965) 166.

[520] M.A. South, C.A. Alford Jr., The immunology of chronic intrauterine infections, in: E.R. Stiehm, V.A. Fulginiti (Eds.), Immunologic Disorders in Infants and Children, Saunders, Philadelphia, 1973.

[521] P. Phelan, P. Campbell, Pulmonary complications of rubella embryopathy, J. Pediatr. 75 (1969) 202.

[522] N.J. Fortuin, A.G. Morrow, W.C. Roberts, Late vascular manifestations of the rubella syndrome: a roentgenographic-pathologic study, Am. J. Med. 51 (1971) 134.

[523] G.S. Karmody, Subclinical maternal rubella and congenital deafness, N. Engl. J. Med. 278 (1968) 809.

[524] M.D. Ames, et al., Central auditory imperception: a significant factor in congenital rubella deafness, JAMA 213 (1970) 419.

[525] C.S. Peckham, et al., Congenital rubella deafness: a preventable disease, Lancet 1 (1979) 258.

[526] M. Rossi, A. Ferlito, F. Polidoro, Maternal rubella and hearing impairment in children, J. Laryngol. Otol. 94 (1980) 281.

[527] M.M. Weinberger, et al., Congenital rubella presenting as retarded language development, Am. J. Dis. Child. 120 (1970) 125.

[528] P.S. Palacin, et al., Congenital rubella syndrome, hyper-IgM syndrome and autoimmunity in an 18-year-old girl, J. Paediatr. Child Health 43 (2007) 716–718.

[529] M.A. Menser, J.M. Forrest, R.D. Bransby, Rubella infection and diabetes mellitus, Lancet 1 (1978) 57.

[529a] N. Takasu, T. Ikema, I. Komiya, G. Mimura, Forty-year observation of 280 Japanese patients with congenital rubella syndrome, Diabetes Care 28 (2005) 2331–2332.

[530] T.K. Hanid, Hypothyroidism in congenital rubella, Lancet 2 (1976) 854.

[531] P.I. Nieberg, L.I. Gardner, Thyroiditis and congenital rubella syndrome, J. Pediatr. 89 (1976) 156.

[532] A. Perez Comas, Congenital rubella and acquired hypothyroidism secondary to Hashimoto thyroiditis, J. Pediatr. 88 (1976) 1065.

[533] P.R. Ziring, et al., Chronic lymphocytic thyroiditis: identification of rubella virus antigen in the thyroid of a child with congenital rubella, J. Pediatr. 90 (1977) 419.

[534] T.W. AvRuskin, M. Brakin, C. Juan, Congenital rubella and myxedema, Pediatrics 69 (1982) 495.

[535] P.R. Ziring, B.A. Fedun, L.Z. Cooper, Thyrotoxicosis in congenital rubella, J. Pediatr. 87 (1975) 1002.

[536] M.A. Preece, P.J. Kearney, W.C. Marshall, Growth hormone deficiency in congenital rubella, Lancet 2 (1977) 842.

[537] S.E. Oberfield, et al., Growth hormone dynamics in congenital rubella syndrome, Brain Dysfunct. 1 (1988) 303.

[538] S. Chiriboga-Klein, et al., Growth in congenital rubella syndrome and correlation with clinical manifestations, J. Pediatr. 115 (1989) 251.

[539] M.M. Desmond, et al., The longitudinal course of congenital rubella encephalitis in nonretarded children, J. Pediatr. 93 (1978) 584.

[540] H. Anderson, B. Barr, E. Wedenberg, Genetic disposition—a prerequisite for maternal rubella deafness, Arch. Otolaryngol. 91 (1970) 141.

[541] W.P. Boger III, Late ocular complications in congenital rubella syndrome, Ophthalmology 87 (1980) 1244.

[542] W.P. Boger III, R.A. Petersen, R.M. Robb, Spontaneous absorption of the lens in the congenital rubella syndrome, Arch. Ophthalmol. 99 (1981) 433.

[543] A.F. Deutman, W.S. Grizzard, Rubella retinopathy and subretinal neovascularization, Am. J. Ophthalmol. 85 (1978) 82.

[544] K.E. Frank, E.W. Purnell, Subretinal neovascularization following rubella retinopathy, Am. J. Ophthalmol. 86 (1978) 462.

[545] D.H. Orth, et al., Rubella maculopathy, BMJ 64 (1980) 201.

[546] J.S. Wolinsky, et al., Progressive rubella panencephalitis: immunovirological studies and results of isoprinosine therapy, Clin. Exp. Immunol. 35 (1979) 397.

[547] E.D. McIntosh, M.A. Menser, A fifty-year follow-up of congenital rubella, Lancet 340 (1992) 414.

[548] J.L. Robinson, et al., Prevention of congenital rubella syndrome—what makes sense in 2006? Epidemiol. Rev. 28 (2006) 81–87.

[549] L.P. Skendzel, Rubella immunity. Defining the level of protective antibody, Am. J. Clin. Pathol. 106 (1996) 170–174.

[550] L. Dontigny, et al., Rubella in pregnancy, J. Obstet. Gynaecol. Can. 30 (2008) 152–168.

[551] S.R. Preblud, R. Kushubar, H.M. Friedman, Rubella hemagglutination inhibition titers, JAMA 247 (1982) 1181.

[552] R.F. Helfand, et al., Dried blood spots versus sera for detection of rubella virus-specific immunoglobulin M (IgM) and IgG in samples collected during a rubella outbreak in Peru, Clin. Vaccine Immunol. 14 (2007) 1522–1525.

[553] P. Hardelid, et al., Agreement of rubella IgG antibody measured in serum and dried blood spots using two commercial enzyme-linked immunosorbent assays, J. Med. Virol. 80 (2008) 360–364.

[554] K.M. Wilson, et al., Humoral immune response to primary rubella virus infection, Clin. Vaccine Immunol. 13 (2006) 380–386.

[555] C. Vauloup-Fellous, L. Grangeot-Keros, Humoral immune response after primary rubella virus infection and after vaccination, Clin. Vaccine Immunol. 14 (2007) 644–647.

[556] Revised ACIP recommendation for avoiding pregnancy after receiving a rubella-containing vaccine, MMWR Morb. Mortal. Wkly. Rep. 50 (2001) 1117.

[557] N.D. Munro, et al., Fall and rise of immunity to rubella, BMJ 294 (1987) 481.

[558] C.S. Hoskins, C. Pyman, B. Wilkins, The nerve deaf child—intrauterine rubella or not? Arch. Dis. Child. 58 (1983) 327.

[559] J.L. Iurio, C.S. Hoskins, C. Pyman, Retrospective diagnosis of congenital rubella, BMJ 289 (1984) 1566.

[560] T. Vesikari, O.H. Meurman, R. Maki, Persistent rubella-specific IgM-antibody in the cerebrospinal fluid of a child with congenital rubella, Arch. Dis. Child. 55 (1980) 46.

[561] M.G. Fitzgerald, G.R. Pullen, C.S. Hosking, Low affinity antibody to rubella antigen in patients after rubella infection in utero, Pediatrics 81 (1988) 812.

[562] K. Alestig, et al., Studies of amniotic fluid in women infected with rubella, J. Infect. Dis. 129 (1974) 79.

[563] M.J. Levine, et al., Diagnosis of congenital rubella in utero, N. Engl. J. Med. 290 (1974) 1187.

[564] L.L. Cederqvist, et al., Prenatal diagnosis of congenital rubella, BMJ 276 (1977) 615.

[565] F. Daffos, et al., Prenatal diagnosis of congenital rubella, Lancet 2 (1984) 1.

[566] G.M. Terry, et al., First trimester prenatal diagnosis of congenital rubella: a laboratory investigation, BMJ 292 (1986) 930.

[567] G. Enders, W. Jonatha, Prenatal diagnosis of intrauterine rubella, Infection 15 (1987) 162.

[568] L. Ho-Terry, et al., Diagnosis of fetal rubella infection by nucleic acid hybridization, J. Med. Virol. 24 (1988) 175.

[569] T.J. Bosma, et al., PCR for detection of rubella virus RNA in clinical samples, J. Clin. Microbiol. 33 (1995) 1075.

[570] M. Tanemura, et al., Diagnosis of fetal rubella infection with reverse transcription and nested polymerase chain reaction: a study of 34 cases diagnosed in fetuses, Am. J. Obstet. Gynecol. 174 (1996) 578.

[571] J.C. McDonald, Gamma-globulin for prevention of rubella in pregnancy, BMJ 2 (1963) 416.

[572] J.A. Brody, J.L. Sever, G.M. Schiff, Prevention of rubella by gamma globulin during an epidemic in Barrow, Alaska, in 1964, N. Engl. J. Med. 272 (1965) 127.

[573] P.F. McCallin, et al., Gammaglobulin as prophylaxis against rubella-induced congenital anomalies, Obstet. Gynecol. 39 (1972) 185.

[574] G.E.D. Urquhart, R.J. Crawford, J. Wallace, Trial of high-titre human rubella immunoglobulin, BMJ 2 (1978) 1331.

[575] G.M. Schiff, J.L. Sever, R.J. Huebner, Rubella virus: neutralizing antibody in commercial gamma globulin, Science 142 (1963) 58.

[576] R.D. Armstrong, et al., Interferon treatment of chronic rubella associated arthritis, Clin. Exp. Rheumatol. 3 (1985) 93.

[577] A.M. Arvin, et al., Alpha interferon administration to infants with congenital rubella, Antimicrob. Agents Chemother. 21 (1982) 259.

[578] A. Larsson, et al., Administration of interferon to an infant with congenital rubella syndrome involving persistent viremia and cutaneous vasculitis, Acta Paediatr. Scand. 65 (1976) 105.

[579] J.E. Jan, et al., Progressive rubella panencephalitis: clinical course and response to "Isoprinosine" Dev. Med. Child Neurol. 21 (1979) 648.

[580] J.S. Garner, B.P. Simmons, CDC guidelines for isolation precautions in hospitals, Infect. Control 4 (1983) 245.

[581] S.E. Reef, et al., Manual for the Surveillance of Vaccine-Preventable Diseases, Centers for Disease Control and Prevention, Atlanta, GA, 2008.

[582] W.W. Williams, CDC guidelines for infection control in hospital personnel, Infect. Control 4 (1983) 326.

[583] S.C. Schoenbaum, et al., Benefit-cost analysis of rubella vaccination policy, N. Engl. J. Med. 294 (1976) 306.

[584] T. Furukawa, et al., Clinical trials of RA 27/3 (Wistar) rubella vaccine in Japan, Am. J. Dis. Child. 118 (1969) 262.

[585] A. Vaheri, et al., Transmission of attenuated rubella vaccines to the human fetus: a preliminary report, Am. J. Dis. Child. 118 (1969) 243.

[586] W.F. Fleet Jr., et al., Fetal consequences of maternal rubella immunization, JAMA 227 (1974) 621.

[587] A.J. Vyse, et al., Evolution of surveillance of measles, mumps, and rubella in England and Wales: providing the platform for evidence-based vaccination policy, Epidemiol. Rev. 24 (2002) 125–136.

[588] C. Castillo-Solorzano, et al., New horizons in the control of rubella and prevention of congenital rubella syndrome in the Americas, J. Infect. Dis. 187 (Suppl. 1) (2003) S146–S152.

[589] S.A. Plotkin, D. Cornfeld, T.H. Ingalls, Studies of immunization with living rubella virus: trials in children with a strain cultured from an aborted fetus, Am. J. Dis. Child. 110 (1965) 381–389.

[590] D.S. Freestone, Clinical trials carried out to assess non-parenteral routes for administration of Wistar RA 27/3 strain live attenuated rubella vaccine, Dev. Biol. Stand. 33 (1976) 237–240.

[591] R. Ganguly, et al., Rubella immunization of volunteers via the respiratory tract, Infect. Immun. 8 (1973) 497–502.

[592] R.E. Weibel, et al., Clinical and laboratory studies of combined live measles, mumps, and rubella vaccines using the RA 27/3 rubella virus, Proc. Soc. Exp. Biol. Med. 165 (1980) 323–326.

[593] R. de Haas, et al., Prevalence of antibodies against rubella virus in The Netherlands 9 years after changing from selective to mass vaccination, Epidemiol. Infect. 123 (2) (1999).

[594] J. Mossong, et al., Seroprevalence of measles, mumps and rubella antibodies in Luxembourg: results from a national cross-sectional study, Epidemiol. Infect. 132 (1) (2004).

[595] Y.Y. Al Mazrou, et al., Serosurvey of measles, mumps and rubella antibodies in Saudi children, Saudi Med. J. 26 (10) (2005).

[596] D.M. Zanetta, et al., Seroprevalence of rubella antibodies in the State of Sao Paulo, Brazil, 8 years after the introduction of vaccine, Vaccine 21 (2003) 25–26.

[597] J.R. Kremer, et al., Waning antibodies to measles and rubella vaccinees—a longitudinal study, Vaccine 24 (14) (2006).

[598] J.M. Best, Rubella vaccines: past, present and future, Epidemiol. Infect. 107 (1) (1999).

[599] C. Vandermeulen, et al., Long-term persistence of antibodies after one or two doses of MMR-vaccine, Vaccine 25 (2007) 6672–6676.

[600] I. Davidkin, et al., Persistence of measles, mumps, and rubella antibodies in an MMR-vaccinated cohort: a 20-year follow-up, J. Infect. Dis. 197 (2008) 950–956.

[601] A.A. Eick, et al., Incidence of mumps and immunity to measles, mumps and rubella among US military recruits, 2000–2004, Vaccine 26 (2008) 494–501.

[602] P.P. Mortimer, et al., Are many women immunized against rubella unnecessarily? J. Hyg. (Lond.) 87 (1981) 131.

[603] W.A. Orenstein, et al., Prevalence of rubella antibodies in Massachusetts schoolchildren, Am. J. Epidemiol. 124 (1986) 290.

[604] S.L. Rutledge, O.C. Snead III, Neurologic complications of immunizations, J. Pediatr. 109 (1986) 917.

[605] G.A. Losonsky, et al., Effect of immunization against rubella on lactation products. I. Development and characterization of specific immunologic reactivity in breast milk, J. Infect. Dis. 145 (1982) 654.

[606] G.A. Losonsky, et al., Effect of immunization against rubella on lactation products. II. Maternal-neonatal interactions, J. Infect. Dis. 145 (1982) 661.

[607] R.D. Landes, et al., Neonatal rubella following maternal immunization, J. Pediatr. 97 (1980) 465.

[608] G.R. da Silva, et al., Seroepidemiological profile of pregnant women after inadvertent rubella vaccination in the state of Rio de Janeiro, Brazil, 2001–2002, Rev. Panam. Salud Publica 19 (2006) 371–378.

[609] L. Minussi, et al., Prospective evaluation of pregnant women vaccinated against rubella in southern Brazil, Reprod. Toxicol. 25 (2008) 120–123.

[610] X. Badilla, et al., Fetal risk associated with rubella vaccination during pregnancy, Pediatr. Infect. Dis. J. 26 (2007) 830–835.

[611] Centers for Disease Control, Immunization practices in colleges—United States, MMWR Morb. Mortal. Wkly. Rep. 36 (1987) 209.

[612] W.M. Edgar, M.H. Hambling, Rubella vaccination and anti-D immunoglobulin administration in the puerperium, Br. J. Obstet. Gynaecol. 84 (1977) 754.

[613] R.W. Watt, R.B. McGucken, Failure of rubella immunization after blood transfusion: birth of congenitally infected infant, BMJ 281 (1980) 977.

[614] N.A. Black, et al., Post-pubertal rubella immunisation: a controlled trial of two vaccines, Lancet 2 (1983) 990.

[615] S. Bloom, et al., Congenital rubella syndrome burden in Morocco: a rapid retrospective assessment, Lancet 365 (2005) 135–141.

[616] G.M. Schiff, M.S. Dine, Transmission of rubella from newborns: a controlled study among young adult women and report of an unusual case, Am. J. Dis. Child. 110 (1965) 447.

[617] W.P. Boger III, R.A. Petersen, R.M. Robb, Keratoconus and acute hydrops in mentally retarded patients with congenital rubella syndrome, Am. J. Ophthalmol. 91 (1981) 231.

[618] P.R. Preblud, et al., Assessment of susceptibility to measles and rubella, JAMA (1982) 247.

SMALLPOX AND VACCINIA

Julia A. McMillan

CHAPTER OUTLINE

Epidemiology and Transmission 899
    Variola 899
    Vaccinia 899
Microbiology 900
Pathogenesis, Pathology, and Prognosis 900
    Variola 900
    Vaccinia 901
Clinical Manifestations 901

    Variola 901
    Vaccinia 902
Diagnosis 903
Differential Diagnosis 903
Treatment 903
    Variola 903
    Vaccinia 904
Prevention 904

Smallpox is a severe exanthematous clinical disease caused by variola virus. Variola is a member of the genus *Orthopoxvirus* in the Poxviridae family; this genus also includes monkeypox, cowpox, rabbitpox, and vaccinia. Variola infection occurs only in humans, a fact that allowed eradication of this infection in the latter part of the 20th century in a global eradication program using preventive vaccine derived from the relatively benign vaccinia virus. The last case of smallpox in the United States occurred in 1949. In 1980, the world was declared free of smallpox by the World Health Organization (WHO); the last endemic case was diagnosed in Somalia in 1977. Routine vaccination of children and the general public was discontinued in the United States in 1972, and vaccination of health care workers was discontinued in 1976.

The U.S. Public Health Service accepted the recommendation of the Advisory Committee on Immunization Practices that routine smallpox vaccination in the United States be discontinued in 1971. This recommendation was based on two considerations: (1) the risk of contracting smallpox in the United States was small and (2) the risk of complications from immunization with vaccinia outweighed the potential benefits [1].

In 1986, international agreement led to destruction of all variola isolates except stocks to be maintained in WHO-designated laboratories in the United States and the Soviet Union. Concern that variola might be used as an agent of bioterrorism was raised during the 1990s, when it was learned that variola stored in the former Soviet Union had been sold to countries thought to be developing biologic weapons. It is in this context that smallpox and vaccinia virus and their potential effects on the pregnant woman and fetus have again become a matter of potential concern.

EPIDEMIOLOGY AND TRANSMISSION
VARIOLA

Variola was spread primarily through respiratory secretions in aerosolized droplets, and secondary infection required prolonged (6 to 7 hours) face-to-face contact.

Infection through direct contact with infected lesions, bedding, or clothing was thought to occur infrequently. The incubation period was 7 to 17 days (mean 12 days). Infected individuals were not generally contagious until the rash appeared after a 3- to 4-day prodrome of fever, malaise, backache, vomiting, and prostration. Because of the severity of the prodromal illness, infected individuals were usually confined to home or hospital by the time they presented a risk to others, and household contacts and health care professionals were the most frequent secondary cases. Infectivity persisted until all scabs had separated from the skin of the affected individual. The likelihood of spread to a susceptible individual was considered to be lower than that for measles and similar to the rate for varicella. Low temperature and dry conditions prolong virus survival, and outbreaks in the past were more common during dry winter months.

Past recorded experience regarding the frequency of transmission of variola from mother to fetus must be considered against the backdrop of near-universal childhood vaccination. Infection during the first half of gestation resulted in an increased likelihood of fetal death or prematurity. Overall, the rate of fetal loss or death after premature delivery ranged from 57% to 81% [2,3]. There are some documented cases of live-born infants infected in utero near term. In those instances, the likelihood of congenital or neonatal infection was greatest when the mother became ill during the period from 4 days before delivery to 9 days after delivery [4,5].

VACCINIA

Vaccinia virus transmission to the fetus after vaccination of pregnant women has been documented [6–8], although the frequency with which it occurs and the severity of resulting disease are difficult to determine from studies published during past decades [9,10]. Surveys that attempted to determine the rate of adverse effects of smallpox vaccination in the United States during the 20th century identified only one case of fetal vaccinia. In a retrospective study in

Scotland that depended on maternal recollection of timing of vaccination, MacArthur [6] found that fetal death occurred in 47% of pregnancies involving women vaccinated during the second or third trimesters and 24% of those vaccinated during the first trimester. Other studies have failed to find an increased risk of fetal death, miscarriage, or fetal malformations [11,12]. Primary vaccination during pregnancy in the years in which these studies were conducted was unusual, however, and the potential impact on the fetus after vaccination of nonimmune pregnant women cannot be extrapolated accurately.

For almost 30 years (1976–2002), vaccination against smallpox was available in the United States only for scientists who worked with vaccinia and related viruses in the laboratory setting. In 2002, the U.S. Department of Defense initiated a pre-event vaccination program to protect its personnel, and in 2003, the U.S. Public Health Service began vaccinating health care and public health workers who might be involved in caring for patients with smallpox or investigating circumstances surrounding the use of smallpox as an agent of bioterrorism. Criteria for exclusion of individuals at risk for adverse events (including pregnant women) were developed. Despite careful screening, military records indicate that during the calendar years 2003 and 2004, 7735 infants were born to women who inadvertently received smallpox vaccine (vaccinia) at some time during their pregnancy. Review of pregnancy outcomes for these women compared with military women who were pregnant during that same period and did not receive smallpox vaccine showed no statistically significant differences in frequency of birth defects or preterm delivery. When the comparison was limited to mothers who received vaccine during the first trimester, there was a small increase in the odds ratio for overall birth defects, but that finding also was not statistically significant [13].

In early 2003 the National Smallpox Vaccine in Pregnancy Registry was established by the U.S. Department of Defense and the Centers for Disease Control and Prevention (CDC) to enroll and follow prospectively women who had been inadvertently vaccinated while pregnant or within 4 weeks of conception as a part of the military or civilian public health preparedness effort. As of September 2006, 376 women had enrolled in the registry; 354 (94.1%) of these women had never received smallpox vaccine in the past. Most of the women in the registry (76.9%) were vaccinated during the first 4 weeks of pregnancy. There have been no cases of fetal vaccinia and no increase in fetal loss, prematurity, low birth weight, or major anomalies compared with the expected rates in the U.S. population [14]. Although these more recent studies offer reassurance that smallpox vaccination during pregnancy does not have adverse consequences for the fetus, caution must be used in extrapolating these results to a larger population whose overall health may be more variable.

MICROBIOLOGY

The poxviruses, including variola and vaccinia, are large, complex, double-stranded DNA viruses with a diameter of approximately 200 nm. The nucleotides of the two viruses are 96% homologous, as are 93% of the amino acids of the glycoproteins that make up the envelope of the two viruses. These envelope glycoproteins are important in antibody recognition. The virions have a characteristic brick shape on electron microscopy. Viral aggregates in infected host cells form intracytoplasmic inclusion bodies of approximately 10 μm. Both viruses can be grown on tissue culture derived from various mammalian cells, and cytopathic changes can be detected within 1 to 6 days.

PATHOGENESIS, PATHOLOGY, AND PROGNOSIS
VARIOLA

Introduction of variola onto respiratory mucosa is followed by local multiplication and spread to lymph nodes. An asymptomatic viremia occurs on about the 3rd or 4th day, distributing the virus to the spleen, bone marrow, and lymph nodes. Secondary viremia, occurring on about day 8, is followed on day 12 to 14 by systemic symptoms, including fever, malaise, headache, and prostration. During this secondary viremia, virus is carried by leukocytes to the dermis and oropharyngeal mucosa. Prodromal febrile illness is followed after about 3 days by development of enanthem and a maculopapular rash distributed at first primarily on the face, arms, and legs and then spreading to the trunk.

Mortality rates after smallpox varied depending on age, prior vaccination, and availability of supportive care. To some degree, mortality can be predicted by the characteristics of the rash (see "Clinical Manifestations"). Overall, the mortality rate was about 30%.

The mortality rate from smallpox among pregnant women was high. The more lethal hemorrhagic form of smallpox was more likely to occur in pregnant women. Rao and colleagues [3] followed 225 pregnant women in India from 1959–1962 and found a 75% mortality rate among previously unvaccinated pregnant women who developed smallpox compared with 24% to 25% among unvaccinated nonpregnant women and men. For vaccinated women, the mortality rate was 20.7% compared with 3% to 4% for men and nonpregnant women. Dixon [15] reported an overall mortality rate of 40% among pregnant women in a smallpox outbreak in North Africa in 1946.

Even when maternal infection is mild, transmission to the fetus can lead to increased rates of fetal death and premature delivery. Among 46 pregnancies followed by Lynch [2], 81% resulted in fetal death or early death after premature delivery. Other investigators reported much less frequent adverse effects on the fetus [4]. The sequence of events that lead to infection of the placenta and fetus in relation to maternal viremia has not been conclusively established. Development of symptomatic infection at 2 to 3 weeks of life in infants born to mothers whose illness began just before delivery suggests that placental infection and transmission to the fetus developed during the secondary viremic phase [4,11]. The consequences of fetal infection have been documented to involve widely disseminated foci of necrosis (i.e., skin, thymus, lungs, liver, kidneys, intestines, and adrenals) and characteristic intracytoplasmic inclusion bodies (i.e., Guarnieri bodies) in the decidual cells of the placenta [16,17].

It is thought that transplacental transmission of variola can occur at any time during gestation, and autopsy studies corroborate infection acquired during the second and third trimesters. Pathologic studies of fetuses lost during the first trimester are lacking; however, the increased frequency of miscarriage associated with maternal infection at that stage suggests a direct effect on the products of conception.

VACCINIA

Vaccinia infection after maternal vaccination is thought to result from transient viremia. The frequency with which inoculation of vaccinia virus through vaccination leads to viremia probably is related to the invasiveness of the vaccinia strain and the vaccination status (i.e., primary versus revaccination) of the individual being vaccinated. A report involving persons vaccinated from 1930–1953 described isolation of vaccinia 3 to 10 days after vaccination with a strain that is thought to be more invasive than the New York City Board of Health (NYCBOH) strain used during recent decades [18]. Viremia has been reported after NYCBOH strain vaccination [18,19], but the frequency with which it occurs is unknown. A study involving 28 healthy adults vaccinated using NYCBOH vaccine failed to detect viremia after successful vaccination [20]. Mihailescu and Petrovici [21] were able to isolate vaccinia from products of conception of 12 (3.2%) of 366 women who had been revaccinated during pregnancy and had undergone therapeutic abortion during the 1st or 2nd month of gestation.

In the past, pregnancy was not considered a contraindication to vaccination during periods of increased smallpox risk, and despite widespread use of vaccine during the past century, only 50 cases of fetal infection (3 in the United States) have been reported [22]. Levine and coworkers

[23] summarized 20 cases of fetal vaccinia infection reported from 1932–1972. At least 13 of the 20 women involved had received their first smallpox vaccination during the pregnancy. The time of vaccination ranged from 3 to 24 weeks of pregnancy, and delivery occurred an average of 8 weeks later; 10 infected infants were born alive, and 3 survived (Figs. 29–1 and 29–2).

CLINICAL MANIFESTATIONS
VARIOLA

Variola major is the form of smallpox that is of the greatest historical significance because of its high overall mortality rate (30%). Onset of rash was preceded by approximately 3 days of fever, myalgia, headache, and backache. Vomiting, diarrhea, abdominal pain, and seizures sometimes accompanied this prodromal period. The fever often was reduced as the rash appeared, only to recur and persist until skin lesions had scabbed. The appearance of the rash in patients with variola major was predictive of the severity of illness and of the associated mortality. The most common rash (90% of patients) was called *ordinary smallpox* and consisted of papules that progressed first to fluid-filled vesicles and then to firm, tense pustules that scabbed after 10 days to 2 weeks before separating from the underlying skin. The "pox" were distributed over the entire body, but predominated on the face and extremities, including the palms and soles. In contrast to the lesions of varicella, which appear in various stages (e.g., papules, vesicles, scabs) at one time, smallpox lesions all develop at the same rate. An enanthem involving painful lesions of the mouth and throat preceded the development of the rash by a day or less.

When the rash involved discrete lesions, it was referred to as *ordinary-discrete smallpox*. The case-fatality rate

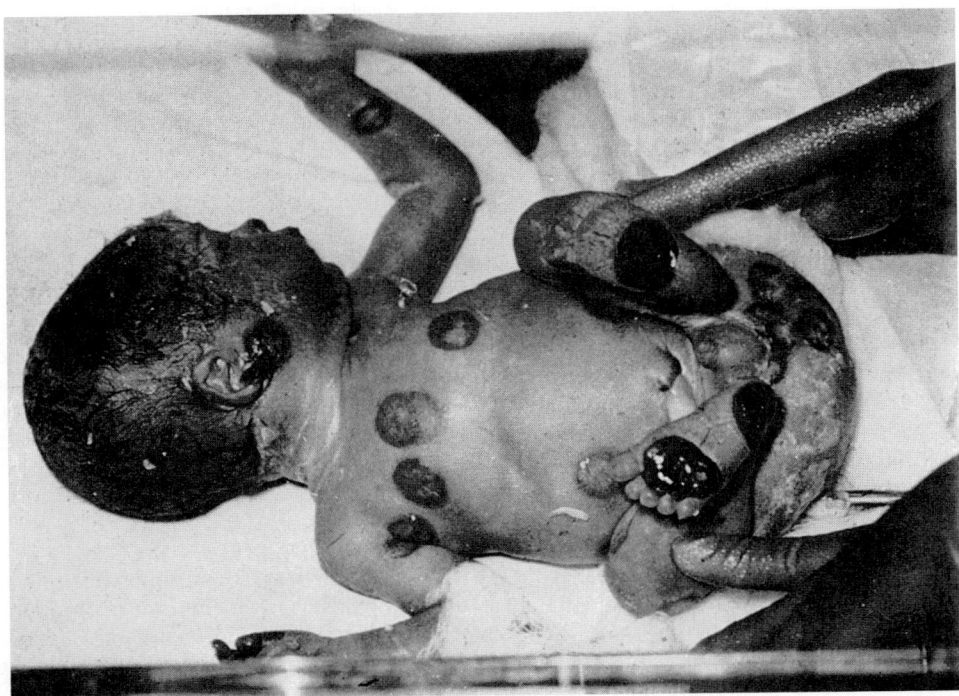

FIGURE 29–1 Generalized fetal vaccinia in an infant whose mother was immunized at 24 weeks of gestation. The infant was born at 30 weeks and survived. (*From Hanshaw JC, Dudgeon JA. Viral Diseases of the Fetus and Newborn. Philadelphia, Saunders, 1978, p 216.*)

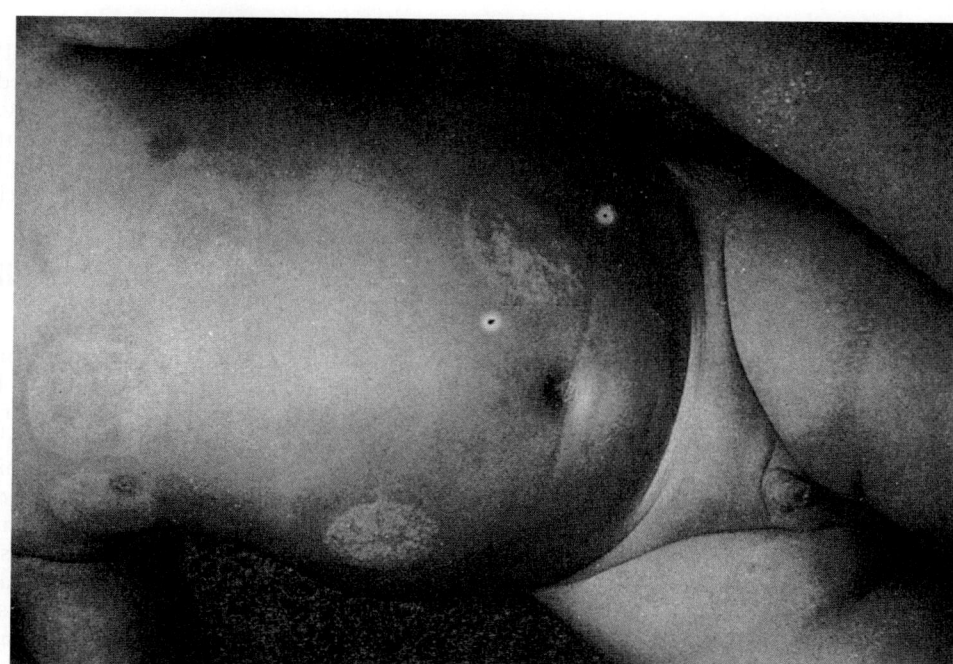

FIGURE 29–2 The same patient as in Figure 29–1 at 18 months of age. Scarring persists, but the lesions have healed. Smallpox vaccination was attempted without success. *(From Hanshaw JC, Dudgeon JA. Viral Diseases of the Fetus and Newborn. Philadelphia, Saunders, 1978, p 217.)*

associated with this form was less than 10%. When lesions were more numerous and less discrete (i.e., ordinary-semiconfluent and ordinary-confluent smallpox), the mortality rate was higher, approximating 50% to 75% for ordinary-confluent cases. Flat smallpox, in which lesions evolved more slowly and finally coalesced, accounted for about 7% of cases, but the mortality rate was greater than 90%. Hemorrhagic smallpox, or purpura variolosa, which was seen most commonly in pregnant women, was associated with an almost 100% mortality rate [24]. In the series of 255 pregnant women reported by Rao and colleagues [3], smallpox was least likely to take the hemorrhagic form during the first trimester of pregnancy, and the highest likelihood of the hemorrhagic form was during the 6th month. Modified smallpox, affecting previously vaccinated individuals, was a milder disease with fewer and smaller skin lesions. Death with this form was rare.

Alastrim, or variola minor, is virologically distinct from variola major. It was first recognized in the early 20th century in South Africa, spreading to the Americas and to Europe. As the name suggests, this form of smallpox was less severe, with a case-fatality rate of about 1%.

The increased likelihood of fetal death associated with maternal infection during pregnancy was described previously. When pathologic examination of the fetus and placenta in such cases has been reported, the fetus has exhibited well-circumscribed cutaneous and scalp lesions with maceration of internal organs, including the brain. Foci of necrosis and calcification have been seen in the thymus, lungs, liver, kidneys, intestines, and adrenals. Similar foci are seen in the placenta [16,17].

Marsden and Greenfield [4] described 34 infants whose mothers developed smallpox late in pregnancy or during the 2 weeks after delivery. Some newborns escaped symptomatic illness, although failed attempts at subsequent vaccination suggest that they were infected in utero. Based on the timing of illness in the newborns who developed smallpox compared with the appearance of rash in the mother, these investigators concluded that transmission of virus from mother to fetus occurs during the expected time of secondary maternal viremia. Other reports substantiate their conclusions. These and other researchers [2,15] describe great variability in severity of neonatal illness, including instances in which one twin escaped clinical disease, but the other developed smallpox [15].

The severity of fetal or neonatal involvement does not reflect the severity of maternal infection or her vaccination status. In his report of 47 cases of maternal-to-fetal transmission of variola, Lynch [2] described five infected infants born at term whose mothers had been exposed to smallpox during pregnancy, but had escaped clinical disease, presumably because of prior vaccination. Vaccination of newborns whose mothers developed clinical smallpox before or shortly after their birth did not always protect them from disease.

Details regarding the clinical findings and course associated with congenital variola are unavailable. Disease was acute and not associated with congenital anomalies. Some reports describe cutaneous lesions that are larger than the lesions usually associated with smallpox. Among the 22 infants with congenital and neonatal smallpox described by Marsden and Greenfield [4], 3 died, 1 of whom was born prematurely.

VACCINIA

Congenital vaccinia was rare, even during widespread vaccination programs. Reported mortality rate associated with congenital vaccinia was high, however. Of the 16 cases reviewed by Green and coworkers [8], six infants were born alive, but only one ultimately survived.

For at least 12 of the 16 women, vaccination during pregnancy had been their primary smallpox vaccination. Congenital vaccinia has been reported after vaccination between the 3rd and 24th weeks of pregnancy, but for most affected pregnancies, vaccination was in the second trimester. As is the case with congenital variola, large, discrete, circular necrotic lesions were seen on the skin of infected fetuses and newborns. Foci of necrosis studded multiple internal organs and the placenta.

In utero vaccinia infection has not been associated with serious birth defects or with other long-term adverse events in surviving infants. Infants of mothers vaccinated during pregnancy who escaped fetal infection were not at risk for sequelae.

DIAGNOSIS

Diagnosis of smallpox, whether in the pregnant woman, fetus, or newborn, was usually based on clinical findings along with a history of exposure to disease or vaccination. Today, suspicion that a patient may have smallpox would imply introduction of the disease through bioterrorism, and great care should be taken to prevent spread of the infection and to confirm the diagnosis in the laboratory. If skin lesions are scabbed, one or more scabs should be removed and included with other specimens. Local and state health authorities should be contacted immediately. State authorities should contact the CDC. Patient samples should be collected only by an individual wearing protective gown, mask, and gloves, and that individual should be someone who has been vaccinated, if possible. Throat swabs and swabs of vesicular fluid should be obtained. Blood samples and the swabs should be placed into a container sealed with adhesive tape and then placed into a second, watertight container. All samples should be sent directly to a Biological Safety Level 4 laboratory, where they can be processed safely. Laboratory confirmation can be performed by electron microscopy, nucleic acid identification, immunohistochemical studies, and tissue culture using cell culture or chorioallantoic egg membrane. Similar technique should be employed to confirm infection in the neonate. There is no known reliable intrauterine test for diagnosing congenital infection.

DIFFERENTIAL DIAGNOSIS

During the prodromal period, before the eruption of rash, maternal smallpox may be indistinguishable from other acute febrile illnesses. When the rash appears, the pattern of eruption and the characteristics of individual pox lesions should help distinguish it from other conditions, such as rubella, measles, meningococcemia, rickettsial diseases, rat-bite fever, and enteroviral infections. The widespread distribution of the lesions of variola major should distinguish it from localized papulovesicular rashes, such as impetigo, shingles, and insect bites. Varicella is the viral infection most likely to be confused with smallpox. Recommended routine vaccination of children against varicella leaves many younger clinicians without experience in recognizing this formerly common infection of childhood. Table 29-1 compares clinical characteristics of the two infections. In the past, smallpox sometimes

TABLE 29-1 Clinical Features Distinguishing Chickenpox from Smallpox

Clinical Features	Chickenpox	Smallpox
Fever onset	At the time of rash	2–4 days before rash
Rash characteristics	Pocks in different stages	Pocks in same stages
	Develops rapidly	Develops slowly
	More pocks on body	More pocks on face, arms, and legs
	Spares palms and soles	Affects palms and soles
Mortality	Rare	10%–30%, historically

was mistaken for drug eruptions and erythema multiforme, and hemorrhagic smallpox could be difficult to distinguish from meningococcemia, severe acute leukemia, or hemorrhagic varicella.

Congenital variola or vaccinia would be expected only in the context of a history of maternal smallpox or smallpox vaccination. In addition to careful consideration of prenatal maternal history, review of maternal postpartum course is important because historical reports suggest that neonatal smallpox may occur in association with maternal disease that manifests in the days after delivery [3]. In the absence of a maternal history of smallpox or vaccination, fetal or neonatal variola or vaccinia could be mistaken for congenital herpes simplex infection, congenital syphilis, or congenital dermatologic disease such as epidermolysis bullosa.

TREATMENT
VARIOLA

If maternal smallpox is suspected, contact and airborne isolation precautions, in addition to universal precautions, should be instituted immediately, and the patient should be cared for in a negative-pressure room if possible. Local and state health authorities should be notified immediately. Family and community contacts, emergency medical personnel, and health care workers who might have been exposed to the patient should be identified and immunized as soon as possible. Immunization within 4 days can ameliorate illness and, in some cases, prevent infection completely.

Patient management includes careful attention to fluid and electrolyte requirements and nutritional support. Antibiotic therapy, including an agent effective in treating infection caused by *Staphylococcus aureus*, should be provided if secondary infection is suspected. Cidofovir, a nucleoside analogue that inhibits DNA polymerase, has activity against variola. When used early in the course of infection, it has been effective in treating poxvirus infections in animals. Cidofovir is approved for use in treating cytomegalovirus infection, but it has not been used to treat smallpox. Adverse effects of cidofovir, primarily renal toxicity, would limit its use in treating suspected congenital variola.

VACCINIA

Adverse effects associated with administration of smallpox vaccine include inadvertent inoculation of sites beyond the vaccination site, including ocular inoculation, generalized vaccinia, eczema vaccinatum, progressive vaccinia (i.e., vaccinia necrosum), postvaccinal encephalitis, and fetal vaccinia. Vaccination programs have developed careful screening tools to prevent vaccination of individuals thought to be particularly susceptible to these adverse effects, including exclusion of women who are pregnant or intend to become pregnant within 4 weeks of vaccination. Congenital vaccinia among live-born infants is rare, and inadvertent vaccination during pregnancy should not be a reason to recommend termination of pregnancy. Vaccinia immunoglobulin (VIG) has been used to treat some complications associated with smallpox vaccination, including eczema vaccinatum and progressive vaccinia. It may be used for those same reasons during pregnancy, but VIG is not recommended as prophylaxis against congenital vaccinia. No data are available regarding appropriate dose or efficacy of VIG for treatment of congenital vaccinia. Treatment may be considered, however, for a viable infant born with lesions after a history of maternal vaccination. For information concerning availability, indications, and administration of VIG, physicians should contact the CDC Clinical Consultation Team (telephone: 877-554-4625).

Cidofovir is available for treatment of complications of smallpox vaccination only under the investigational new drug (IND) protocol administered by the CDC. It is released only as secondary treatment for complications that do not respond to treatment with VIG. An investigational agent, ST-246, was used more recently, along with VIG and cidofovir, to treat a 28-month-old boy who developed eczema vaccinatum after contact with his father, who had received smallpox vaccine 21 days before visiting his family while on leave from Iraq [25]. ST-246 has in vitro activity against multiple orthopoxviruses, and no serious adverse reactions were seen in human phase I studies. The combined treatment was successful in this single case, but the role of any single one of the three therapies could not be determined.

PREVENTION

After a remarkable, worldwide public health effort, smallpox was the first infectious disease to be eradicated in nature, during the latter part of the 20th century. Until concerns were raised regarding the potential use of smallpox as an agent of bioterrorism, protection from smallpox was thought to be unnecessary, and vaccination to protect against variola was discontinued. In the 21st century, inadvertent vaccination of pregnant military personnel, health care workers, and public health workers, many of whom are being vaccinated for the first time, poses the greatest risk for maternal and fetal infection. Careful screening of such individuals has been shown generally to be effective, but vaccination during pregnancy has occurred despite screening.

The National Smallpox Vaccine in Pregnancy Registry has been established to investigate instances of inadvertent smallpox vaccination during pregnancy. Civilian cases should be reported to state health departments or to the CDC (telephone: 404-639-8253 or 877-554-4625). Military cases should be reported to the Department of Defense (telephone: 619-553-9255; DSN: 619-553-9255; fax: 619-553-7601; e-mail: code25@nhrc.navy.mil). Health care providers are encouraged to save and forward products of conception from pregnancy losses associated with vaccination during pregnancy to the CDC or the Department of Defense. Specimens should be frozen at $-70°$ C, preferably in viral transport media before and during transport.

In September 2007, ACAM2000 replaced Dryvax as the only smallpox vaccine licensed by the U.S. Food and Drug Administration (FDA). Similar to Dryvax, which was initially approved in 1931, ACAM2000 is a live vaccinia virus vaccine; in contrast to Dryvax, ACAM2000 is produced in cell culture, allowing more rapid and uniform large scale production (*FDA News*) [26].

REFERENCES

[1] S. Krugman, S.L. Katz, Smallpox and Vaccinia, Mosby, St. Louis, 1981.
[2] F.W. Lynch, Dermatologic conditions of the fetus with particular reference to variola and vaccinia, Arch. Dermatol. Syphilis Chic. 26 (1932) 997.
[3] A.R. Rao, et al., Pregnancy and smallpox, J. Indian Med. Assoc. 40 (1963) 353.
[4] J.P. Marsden, C.R.M. Greenfield, Inherited smallpox, Arch. Dis. Child. 9 (1934) 309.
[5] R. Sharma, D.K. Jagdev, Congenital smallpox, Scand. J. Infect. Dis. 3 (1971) 245.
[6] P. MacArthur, Congenital vaccinia and vaccinia gravidarum, Lancet 2 (1952) 1104.
[7] G.J. Bourke, R.J. Whitty, Smallpox vaccination in pregnancy: a prospective study, BMJ 1 (1964) 1544.
[8] D.M. Green, S.M. Reid, K. Rhaney, Generalized vaccinia in the human foetus, Lancet 1 (1966) 1296.
[9] J.M. Lane, et al., Complications of smallpox vaccination, 1968: results of ten statewide surveys, J. Infect. Dis. 122 (1970) 303.
[10] J.M. Lane, et al., Complications of smallpox vaccination, 1968: national surveillance in the United States, N. Engl. J. Med. 281 (1969) 1201.
[11] M. Greenberg, et al., The effect of smallpox vaccination during pregnancy on the incidence of congenital malformations, Pediatrics 3 (1949) 456.
[12] M.T. Bellows, M.E. Hyman, K.K. Meritt, Effect of smallpox vaccination on the outcome of pregnancy, Public Health Rep. 64 (1949) 319.
[13] M.A. Ryan, et al., Evaluation of preterm births and birth defects to liveborn infants of U.S. military women who received smallpox vaccine, Birth Defects Res. A Clin. Mol. Teratol. 82 (2008) 533.
[14] M.A. Ryan, J.F. Seward, Pregnancy, birth, and infant health outcomes from the national smallpox vaccine in pregnancy registry, 2003–2006, Clin. Infect. Dis. 46 (Suppl. 3) (2008) S221.
[15] C.W. Dixon, Smallpox in Tripolitania, 1946: an epidemiological and clinical study of 500 cases, including trials of penicillin treatment, J. Hyg. 46 (1948) 351.
[16] A.G.P. Garcia, Fetal infection in chickenpox and alastrim, with histopathologic study of the placenta, Pediatrics 32 (1963) 895.
[17] J.P. Marsden, Metastatic calcification: notes on twins born shortly after an attack of smallpox in the mother, Br. J. Child. Dis. 28 (1930) 193.
[18] F. Fenner, et al., The Pathogenesis, Pathology and Immunology of Smallpox and Vaccinia, World Health Organization, Geneva, 1988.
[19] R.J. Blattner, et al., Antibody response to cutaneous inoculation with vaccinia virus: viremia and viruria in vaccinated children, J. Pediatr. 26 (1964) 176.
[20] J.F. Cummings, et al., Lack of vaccinia viremia after smallpox vaccination, Clin. Infect. Dis. 38 (2004) 456.
[21] R. Mihailescu, M. Petrovici, Effect of smallpox vaccination on the product of conception, Arch. Roum. Pathol. Exp. Microbiol. 34 (1975) 67–74.
[22] Centers for Disease Control and Prevention, Women with smallpox vaccine exposure during pregnancy reported to the National Smallpox Vaccine in Pregnancy Registry—United States, 2003, MMWR Morb. Mortal. Wkly. Rep. 52 (2003) 386.
[23] M.M. Levine, G. Edsall, L.J. Bruce-Chwatt, Live-virus vaccines in pregnancy: risks and recommendations, Lancet 2 (1974) 34.
[24] D. Paranjothy, I. Samuel, Pregnancy associated with haemorrhagic smallpox, J. Obstet. Gynaecol. Br. Emp. 67 (1960) 309.
[25] S. Vora, et al., Severe eczema vaccinatum in a household contact of a smallpox vaccinee, Clin. Infect. Dis. 46 (2008) 1555.
[26] Centers for Disease Control and Prevention, Notice to readers: newly licensed smallpox vaccine to replace old smallpox vaccine, 2008, MMWR Morb Mortal Wkly Rep 57 (2008) 207.

CHAPTER OUTLINE

Human Papillomavirus   905
Epstein–Barr Virus   906
Human Herpesvirus 6   907
Human Herpesvirus 7   908
Influenza A and B   908

Respiratory Syncytial Virus   910
Lymphocytic Choriomeningitis Virus   911
Molluscum Contagiosum   913
Rabies Virus   913
West Nile Virus   913

HUMAN PAPILLOMAVIRUS

Human papillomaviruses (HPV) are the cause of condyloma acuminatum (i.e., genital warts), cervical condylomata and cervical cancer [1–4]. More than 100 human HPV serotypes have been identified; approximately half of these have a predilection for anogenital infection [5,6]. Of these, serotypes 6 and 11 account for greater than 70% of cervical cancer worldwide, and serotypes 16 and 18 account for greater than 90% of anogenital warts [7,8]. The risk to an infant born to a mother with HPV infection is the development of juvenile laryngeal papillomatosis and possible development of anogenital warts, primarily owing to HPV serotypes 6 and 11 [9,10].

Hajek [11] associated the presence of condyloma acuminatum in a mother at the time of delivery with the subsequent development of laryngeal papilloma in her infant (Table 30–1). Cook and colleagues [12] described a similar association in five of nine children with laryngeal papilloma. All five of the children who developed laryngeal papilloma when younger than 6 months old were born to mothers who had condylomata acuminata at the time of delivery. The mothers of two of four other children with laryngeal papilloma had genital warts, but did not have them at the time of delivery. Seven (78%) of the nine children with laryngeal papilloma had mothers with condylomata acuminata. The expected incidence of condylomata acuminata in women in the population studied by Cook and colleagues [12] was 1.5%. Six of the nine children also had skin warts. Quick and coworkers [13] described a strong association between laryngeal papilloma in young children and maternal condylomata. Of the 31 patients with laryngeal papilloma they studied, 21 (68%) had been born to mothers who had had condylomata.

The basis for this epidemiologic relationship is evident from the detection of HPV DNA sequences in genital and laryngeal papilloma tissues [3]. Numerous studies have reported rates of newborn infection that ranged from 4% to 72% among infants born to HPV-infected mothers and 0.6% to 20% among infants born to mothers without detectable HPV DNA [14–20]. Smith and colleagues [21] investigated the risk of perinatal transmission based on concordance and sequence match to HPV types of both parents. Only 9 (1.6%) of 574 oral or genital specimens

from newborns were positive for HPV DNA, and of those, only one maternal-infant HPV match was detected, suggesting that perinatal transmission is rare [21]. Rare associations have been made between maternal genital HPV infections and neonatal giant cell hepatitis [22] and vulvar genital papillomas among stillborns [23]. Both associations were documented in only a few gestations, but were confirmed by HPV DNA polymerase chain reaction (PCR) or by electron microscopy.

HPV cannot be isolated by means of tissue culture, but HPV DNA sequences can be detected in cervical cells. Cervical infection is caused by several types of HPV, including types 6, 11, 16, 18, and 31, and is highly prevalent worldwide. HPV can be detected in epithelial cells that have a normal histologic appearance and from tissue samples of patients whose papillomatous lesions are in remission [24]. Clinically, most genital HPV infection is asymptomatic. The frequency of HPV detection has ranged from 5% to 15% in studies of women of childbearing age, with the highest incidence occurring among younger women [25–28]. Pregnancy was not associated with a higher rate of infection.

Although the incidence of cervical infection was 20% in women with a history of condyloma, most pregnant women with HPV infection do not have a history of genital warts. Infection of the infant probably occurs by exposure to the virus at delivery, although papillomatosis has been described in infants delivered by cesarean section. Tang and associates [29] described an infant who was born with condylomata acuminata around the anal orifice. The mother also had condylomata acuminata. It is unknown whether this case reflects transplacental hematogenous spread or direct extension across intact membranes.

Despite the prevalence of genital HPV infection, juvenile laryngeal papillomatosis remains a rare disease. The incidence of recurrent respiratory papillomatosis is approximately 3.96 per 100,000 in the pediatric population, with an incidence of 7 of every 1000 infants born to mothers with vaginal condyloma. The risk of subclinical transmission of HPV from mothers to infants is unknown. HPV-6 and HPV-16 DNA sequences were detected in the cells from foreskin tissue of 3 of 70 infants [30]. These HPV types are also found in genital warts. Because of the

DOI: 10.1016/B978-1-4160-6400-8.00030-4

TABLE 30-1   Effects of Other Viral Infections of the Fetus and Newborn

Infectious Agent	Increased Incidence of Abortion	Increased Risk of Prematurity	Major Clinical Manifestations in Infants
Human papillomavirus	No	No	Laryngeal papilloma, anogenital warts
Epstein-Barr virus	Possibly	Possibly	Unknown
Human herpesvirus 6	No	No	Febrile illness in postnatal period
Influenza viruses	No	No	Probably none
Respiratory syncytial virus	No	No	Pneumonia, bronchiolitis in postnatal period
Lymphocytic choriomeningitis virus	Yes	No	Hydrocephalus, chorioretinitis, viral meningitis, jaundice, thrombocytopenia (?)
Molluscum contagiosum virus	No	No	Rash
Rabies	No	No	None known

prevalence of asymptomatic HPV infection, the feasibility of preventing the rare cases of laryngeal papillomatosis by considering maternal condyloma acuminatum as an indication for cesarean delivery is uncertain.

Treatment of anogenital warts is not optimal, but podophyllum resin or podofilox is often used in older children and adults. Neither podophyllum resin nor podofilox has been tested for safety or efficacy in children, and both agents are contraindicated for use in pregnancy. Laryngeal papillomas recur even after repeated surgical removal. Interferon has been used with some success for treatment of laryngeal papillomas [31]. Although the mainstay of surgical management has traditionally been the CO_2 laser, newer surgical techniques have shown efficacy in the management of pediatric patients, including powered instrumentation and the pulsed dye laser. The traditional adjuvant medical therapies used for pediatric recurrent respiratory papillomatosis continue to be commonly used, including topical interferon alfa-2a, retinoic acid, and indole 3-carbinol/diindolylmethane (I3C/DIM). Topical cidofovir has shown efficacy in selected patients.

Currently, two HPV vaccines are available for the prevention, but not treatment, of HPV infection. One vaccine is protective against the two most common serotypes associated with cervical cancer (HPV serotypes 16 and 18) and the two most common serotypes associated with anogenital warts (HPV serotypes 6 and 11); this vaccine is licensed in the United States [32]. The second vaccine protects only against HPV serotypes 16 and 18 associated with cervical cancer; and is also licensed in the United States [33–35]. Although two approaches, preventive and therapeutic, have been pursued for HPV vaccines, to date only preventive vaccines that evoke a robust neutralizing antibody response to selected HPV serotypes have been successful. Further research to develop therapeutic vaccines that generate cytotoxic T lymphocytes and destroy HPV-infected neoplastic cells is under way [36].

EPSTEIN-BARR VIRUS

Epstein-Barr virus (EBV) is a human herpesvirus that is most familiar as the cause of infectious mononucleosis. Most women of childbearing age have been infected

asymptomatically in childhood. Because EBV cannot be isolated directly in tissue culture, serologic tests are used to detect recent primary or past infection.

Persons infected with EBV form IgG and IgM antibodies to viral capsid antigens (VCAs) soon after infection [37]. About 80% form antibodies to early antigens (EAs), which usually decrease to undetectable levels 6 months after infection. The presence of antibodies to EAs at later times after acute infection may indicate viral reactivation [38]. Antibodies to EBV-associated nuclear antigen (EBNA) develop 3 to 4 weeks after primary infection and probably persist for life, as do IgG antibodies to VCAs.

Prospective studies using antibodies to EAs as a marker of recent maternal EBV infection have yielded conflicting results. In a group of 719 women evaluated by Icart and Didier [39], pregnancies associated with early fetal death; birth of infants with a congenital abnormality, prematurity, or intrauterine growth restriction; and deaths or illnesses during the 1st week of life were more common in women who were positive for EA antibody during the first 3 months of pregnancy than in women who were not. Whether these women had a recent primary EBV infection or reactivation of an infection cannot be determined because EBV EA antibodies persist in some otherwise healthy adults and are associated with the reactivation of past EBV infection. In contrast, Fleisher and Bolognese [40] found that the frequency of antibodies to EA in pregnant women was 55% compared with 22% to 32% among nonpregnant adults, but the incidence of low birth weight, neonatal jaundice, or congenital anomalies was not increased among infants of women with anti-EA antibodies.

Primary EBV infection during pregnancy is unusual [41] because only 3% to 3.4% of pregnant women are susceptible [42,43]. Recent primary EBV infection is diagnosed by the presence of VCA IgG and IgM antibodies in the absence of antibodies to EBNA [44]. Six women were studied who had primary EBV infections during pregnancy as established by the presence of IgM antibody to VCA and the absence of antibody to EBNA in their sera [42]. Of these, only one woman had symptoms compatible with mononucleosis during pregnancy; she gave birth to a normal infant. Four of the remaining five pregnancies terminated abnormally. One woman had a spontaneous abortion, and the other three were delivered of premature infants. All three of the premature infants were abnormal. One was stillborn, one had multiple congenital anomalies, and one was small for gestational age. The products of abortion and the premature infants were not studied for evidence of an EBV infection. The abnormal infants in this study did not have a characteristic syndrome, but instead had a variety of abnormalities.

Fleisher and Bolognese [45] identified three infants born to women who had had silent EBV seroconversion during the first trimester. Two infants were normal; one infant had tricuspid atresia. EBV IgM was not detected in cord blood serum, and EBV was not recovered from the cord blood lymphocytes. Three infants of mothers with a primary EBV infection and infectious mononucleosis were normal at birth and had no serologic or virologic evidence of intrauterine infection [46].

Early reports implicated EBV as a cause of congenital anomalies, particularly congenital heart disease; however, Tallqvist and colleagues [47] were unable to detect an increase in incidence of antibodies to EBV in children 6 to 23 months old with congenital heart disease compared with normal, age-matched controls. EBV may cause congenital heart disease in an individual case, but this study suggests that it is an uncommon cause of cardiac defects. Brown and Stenchever [48] described an infant with multiple congenital anomalies who was born to a mother who had a positive monospot test result 4 weeks before conception and at 16 and 36 weeks of gestation. In addition to the anomalies, which involved many organs, the infant was small for gestational age. Normal chromosomal complements were found on standard and G-banded karyotypes. The total IgM level in the cord blood was not elevated. Studies were not performed for IgM VCA antibody or antibody to EA, and no attempts were made to isolate EBV. Although the evidence that the mother had mononucleosis near the time of conception is convincing, there is no virologic evidence that EBV was the cause of the anomalies.

Goldberg and associates [49] described an infant born with hypotonia, micrognathia, bilateral cataracts, metaphyseal lucencies, and thrombocytopenia. Immunologic evidence suggesting possible EBV infection included an elevated total IgM level, the presence of IgM anti-VCA antibody at 22 days of age, and a delay in development of anti-EBNA antibody until 42 days of age. Weaver and coworkers [50] described an infant with extrahepatic bile duct atresia and evidence of intrauterine EBV infection; EBV IgM was identified in serum obtained when the infant was 3 and 6 weeks old, and persistent EBV IgG was seen at 1 year.

Although EBV cannot be recovered by standard tissue culture methods, the virus can be detected by its capacity to transform B lymphocytes into persistent lymphoblastoid cell lines. In studies conducted to identify cases of intrauterine EBV infection, Visintine and colleagues [51] and Chang and Blankenship [52] observed spontaneous transformation of lymphocytes obtained from cord blood, but it was not associated with EBV. EBV-transformed cells were not found in any samples of cord blood from 2000 newborns studied by Chang and Seto [53] or from 25 newborns tested by Joncas and associates [54,55]. One study used nested PCR methods for amplifying EBV

DNA regions in circulating lymphocytes from 67 mother-infant pairs within 1 week of birth [56]. Approximately 50% of the women and two of the neonates were EBV PCR positive. Visintine and colleagues [51] studied 82 normal term infants, 28 infants with congenital anomalies, and 29 infants suspected to have congenital infections; they were unable to isolate EBV from any of these infants.

Two infants have been described in whom there was evidence of infection with EBV at birth [55,57]. A congenital cytomegalovirus (CMV) infection coexisted in both infants. Most of the clinical findings in the infants were compatible with usual findings in congenital CMV infections and included microcephaly, periventricular calcifications, hepatosplenomegaly, and inclusions characteristic of CMV in sections of tissues or cells in urinary sediments. One infant had deformities of the hands similar to those seen in arthrogryposis. Neither CMV nor EBV was isolated from the saliva or secretions of these infants. In the first infant, IgM antibody to EBV was present at birth, and EBNA-positive permanent lymphoblastoid cell lines were established on five occasions between 3 and 30 months of age. In the second infant, permanent lymphoblastoid cell lines were established from the peripheral blood at birth and from postmortem heart blood at 3 days of age. EBNA and EBV RNA were identified in these cells, and CMV DNA was identified in the cells from the liver of the same infant.

Attempts to isolate EBV from secretions obtained from the maternal cervix have been unsuccessful [51,53], but the virus can be detected at this site by DNA hybridization [58]. There is little evidence suggesting that natal transmission of EBV occurs. EBV was recovered, however, from genital ulcers in a young woman with infectious mononucleosis [59]. Fatal EBV infection was diagnosed by DNA hybridization of lymph node tissue from one infant who presented with failure to thrive, emesis, diarrhea, and a macular rash at 14 days of age, but this infection might have been acquired in utero [60].

EBV can be transmitted to newborns in the perinatal period by blood transfusion [51,54]. Permanent lymphoblastoid lines that contained EBV antigens were established by Joncas and coworkers [54] from the blood of two infants who had received transfusions. One of these infants did not develop permanent antibodies to EBV.

There is no evidence at present that EBV causes congenital anomalies. Because the early and the late serologic responses of young infants to a primary EBV infection differ from those found when a primary infection occurs at an older age [38,54,61], it would be difficult to screen large numbers of newborns for serologic evidence of an EBV infection sustained in utero.

HUMAN HERPESVIRUS 6

Human herpesvirus 6 (HHV-6) is a member of the herpesvirus family that has been identified as a cause of exanthema subitum (i.e., roseola) [62–64]. The virus exhibits tropism for T lymphocytes and is most closely related to human CMV by genetic analysis [65].

Seroepidemiologic studies have shown that HHV-6 is ubiquitous in the human population, regardless of geographic area, and that it infects more than 90% of infants during the first year of life [66–68]. IgG antibodies to HHV-6 are detected in almost all infants at birth, with a subsequent decline in seropositivity rates by 4 to 6 months of age as transplacentally acquired antibody is lost. The highest rate of acquisition of HHV-6 infection seems to occur during the first 6 months to 1 year of life as maternal antibodies wane. The seroepidemiologic evidence and restriction enzyme analysis of paired virus isolates from mothers and their infants suggest that the usual route of transmission is perinatal or postnatal [69].

No cases of symptomatic intrauterine HHV-6 infection have been confirmed since the agent was identified in 1986, although congenital infection has been documented and is estimated to occur at a frequency of 1% [70]. A case of intrauterine infection was documented by PCR in a fetus whose mother had human immunodeficiency virus (HIV) infection and HHV-6 in peripheral blood mononuclear cells [71], and 1 (0.28%) of 799 cord blood serum samples had IgM antibodies to HHV-6 [72]. Another study, using HHV-6 DNA PCR applied to cord blood specimens from 305 infants, showed a 1.6% (5 of 305) PCR positivity rate, suggesting in utero transmission [68]. Evidence of reinfection after presumed congenital HHV-6 infection also has been shown [73]. Primary HHV-6 infection, with its anticipated higher risk of transmission to the fetus, should be rare during pregnancy, however, because almost all women have been infected in childhood. Analogous to human CMV infection, the reactivation of maternal HHV-6, although it may be common during pregnancy, is not expected to cause symptomatic intrauterine infection.

In addition to the roseola syndrome, HHV-6 has been detected by PCR in peripheral blood lymphocytes obtained from infants younger than 3 months who had acute, nonspecific, febrile illnesses [74,75]. Two neonates who had fulminant hepatitis associated with HHV-6 infection have been described [76,77]. Other associations found among infants include a mononucleosis-like syndrome [78], pneumonitis [79], and one case report of possible immunodeficiency and pneumonitis associated with HHV-6 infection [80]. All clinical associations between disease in infants and HHV-6 infection must be evaluated with care, however, because of the evidence that most infants become infected with this virus within a few months after birth and that the virus persists after primary infection, as is characteristic of herpesviruses [71]. Clinicians also must be aware of the potential for false-positive results in serologic assays and in attempts to detect the virus by PCR [64].

HUMAN HERPESVIRUS 7

Human herpesvirus 7 (HHV-7) was discovered in the peripheral blood lymphocytes of a healthy adult in 1990 [81]. HHV-7 belongs to the *Roseolovirus* genus within the Betaherpesvirinae subfamily, along with HHV-6 and CMV. Similar to HHV-6, it causes primary infection in most individuals during childhood. Clinically symptomatic infection with HHV-7 seems to be significantly less common and occurs later than with HHV-6.

Based on seroepidemiologic studies [82–84], HHV-7 infection is ubiquitous in childhood and generally occurs

at a later age than HHV-6 infection. The average age at infection is about 2 years, and 75% of children are seropositive by 5 years of age. The primary mechanism of transmission is from contact with saliva of infected individuals. Because HHV-7 DNA has been detected in breast milk, breast-feeding may be another source of infection [85]. Antibodies to HHV-7 in breast milk may protect against infection, however, and in one study, breast-feeding was associated with a lower risk of early acquisition of HHV-7 infection [85,86]. HHV-7 DNA has been detected in 2.7% of cervical swabs obtained from women in their third trimester of pregnancy, but from none of the swabs of control women, suggesting that pregnancy may be associated with reactivation of HHV-7 [87]. Perinatal transmission from contact with infected maternal secretions is unknown, and neonatal infections with HHV-7 have not been reported [88]. Clinical symptoms are rarely associated with HHV-7 infection, but include nonspecific fever, with or without rash, which resembles exanthema subitum. Clinically apparent HHV-7 infections seem to have a high rate of central nervous system (CNS) involvement [89–92].

INFLUENZA A AND B

Early investigations of the teratogenic potential of influenza virus were epidemiologic studies in which the diagnosis of influenza was not confirmed serologically [93]. In 1959, Coffey and Jessup [93] reported an incidence of 3.6% of congenital defects in 664 Irish women who had histories of having had influenza during pregnancy compared with 1.5% of 663 women who did not have symptoms compatible with influenza. CNS anomalies were the most common type of defect, and of these, anencephaly was the most frequent. These investigators presented some evidence that women who had a history of having had influenza in the first trimester were more likely to give birth to infants who had congenital anomalies than women who had influenza later in the pregnancy. This evidence provided credence to the report.

In a similar study conducted in Scotland, Doll and Hill [94] were unable to confirm that congenital anomalies occurred with a higher frequency in infants of women who had histories of influenza during pregnancy than in infants of women who did not. After reviewing the reported incidence of stillbirth related to anencephaly recorded by the Registrar General for Scotland, they concluded that there was a small increase in risk of anencephaly if the mother had had influenza during the first 2 months of pregnancy. In performing this analysis, certain assumptions were made because of the lack of precise data. Record [95] and Leck [96] analyzed the same data and were unable to find an association between influenza and malformations of the CNS. An increase in congenital defects in infants of mothers who had influenza-like symptoms at 5 to 11 weeks of gestation was reported by Hakosalo and Saxen [97]. Most of these anomalies involved the CNS, but there was no increase in incidence of anencephaly in infants of women who had symptoms compatible with influenza compared with women who remained asymptomatic.

All of these studies were undertaken during influenza epidemics. It was assumed that, under these circumstances, there would be a high correlation between a history of influenza as elicited from the patient and infection with influenza virus. During the 1957 outbreak, Wilson and Stein [98] showed that 60% of pregnant women who denied symptoms of influenza had serologic evidence of having been recently infected. Conversely, 35% of women who stated that they had had influenza lacked serologic evidence of having been infected. Likewise, Hardy and coworkers [99] found that 24% of women who stated that they had had influenza lacked serologic evidence of past infection with the epidemic strain, and 39% of women with titers suggesting recent infection denied symptoms of influenza. MacKenzie and Houghton [100] summarized the reports implicating influenza virus as a cause of maternal morbidity and congenital anomalies and concluded that probably no association exists between maternal influenza infection and subsequent congenital malformations or neoplasms in childhood.

Several studies have been performed in which infection by influenza virus has been serologically confirmed. Hardy and coworkers [99] reported that the incidence of stillbirths was higher in 332 symptomatic pregnant women with serologically confirmed influenza infections than in 206 women with serologically confirmed infections who had remained asymptomatic or in 73 uninfected women. The control group of uninfected women was smaller than expected because the attack rate during the period of the study was very high. Major congenital anomalies occurred in 5.3% of women whose infections occurred during the first trimester compared with 2.1% of 183 women infected during the second trimester and 1.1% of 275 women infected during the third trimester. Supernumerary digits, syndactyly, and skin anomalies were excluded from these figures. Among infants of mothers infected during the first trimester, cardiac anomalies were the most common type of abnormality; none of these infants had anencephaly.

Griffiths and associates [101] observed a slight increase in congenital anomalies in infants born to women who had had serologically confirmed influenza during pregnancy compared with infants of women who had not; however, all of the infants with congenital anomalies were born to women who had had influenza in the second or third trimester, making it less likely that these anomalies were related to influenza. Monif and colleagues [102] did not document infection in any of eight infants born to mothers who had influenza A/Hong Kong infections in the second and third trimesters. Wilson and Stein [98] found no increase in congenital anomalies in women with serologic evidence of having been recently infected with influenza virus who had conceived during the 3-month period when influenza was epidemic.

Population-based epidemiologic studies have not shown that influenza infections during pregnancy are significantly associated with adverse perinatal outcomes. Influenza infections during pregnancy are more likely, however, to result in hospitalization for respiratory symptoms in pregnant women than in nonpregnant adults [103,104]. Hartert and associates [103] conducted a matched cohort study of pregnant women to determine pregnancy outcomes associated with respiratory hospitalizations during influenza seasons from 1985–1993. During those influenza seasons, 293 pregnant women were hospitalized for respiratory symptoms, at a rate of 5.1 per 1000 pregnant women. The prevalence of prematurity and low birth weight was not higher than a matched cohort of pregnant women hospitalized with nonrespiratory diagnoses. Pregnant women with asthma had higher rates of respiratory hospitalizations than those without asthma, and all of three fetal deaths in this cohort were singleton, late third trimester intrauterine fetal deaths in mothers who had asthma and were current smokers [103].

Intrauterine exposure to influenza virus does not cause a consistent syndrome. If there is a cause-and-effect association between influenza virus infections during pregnancy and congenital anomalies, the latter occur with low frequency. Hakosalo and Saxen [97] documented an increase in the use of nonprescription drugs during influenza outbreaks and suggested that drugs rather than infection with influenza virus may exert an erratic teratogenic influence. Many studies have investigated the possible association between influenza infection in pregnant women and subsequent development of bipolar affective disorders or schizophrenia among their offspring, with mixed results [105–107].

Viremia is rare during influenza infections, but it does occur. Few attempts have been made to show transplacental passage of the virus to the fetus. Ruben and colleagues [108] tested the cord sera of infants born to 22 mothers who had been pregnant during an influenza A/England/42/72 outbreak and who had had influenza hemagglutination inhibition titers to this virus of 1:16 or greater while pregnant. The investigators randomly collected 42 cord serum samples from infants who had been born on the same day as the selected infants. Of the 64 cord serum samples tested, a decrease in titer of fourfold or more was seen in four samples after treatment with 2-mercaptoethanol; this suggests that IgM antibody to influenza might have been present. Three of 16 cord blood samples tested gave positive lymphocyte transformation responses to influenza virus. All seven of the infants with evidence of antigenic recognition of influenza virus at birth had uncomplicated deliveries and remained healthy. Influenza A/Bangkok was isolated from the amniotic fluid of a mother with amnionitis and acute influenza infection at 36 weeks of gestation; the infant, who was born at 39 weeks, had serologic evidence of infection, but was asymptomatic [109].

Yawn and associates [110] studied a woman who developed influenza in the third trimester and died of pulmonary edema. A virus similar to the prototype strain A_2/Hong Kong/8/68 was isolated from the lung, hilar nodes, heart, spleen, liver, kidney, brain, and spinal cord of the mother and from the amniotic fluid and myocardium of the fetus. Ramphal and colleagues [111] studied another woman who died of complications of an influenza infection at term. A virus similar to strain A/Texas/77 was isolated from maternal tissues, but influenza virus was not isolated from any of the fetal tissues tested.

In contrast to intrauterine infections with influenza virus, which are rare, infections acquired by infants in the neonatal period are common. Passively transferred antibody to influenza virus may prevent symptomatic infections during the first few months of life if it is present in sufficient quantity [112,113]. Two cases of influenza A/Hong Kong/68 infection in infants who were younger than 1 month were described by Bauer and associates

[114]. The first infant developed high fever, irritability, and nasal discharge when 10 days old; the second infant, who was premature, developed fever and nasal congestion when 14 days old. Symptoms were restricted to the upper respiratory system, and both infants recovered within 4 days of onset of the illness. Influenza virus infection may be fatal in the neonatal period, however [115]. Several outbreaks of influenza virus infection have occurred in neonatal intensive care units. In general, illness has been mild [114,116]. Most of the eight infected neonates described by Meibalane and coworkers [116] had nonspecific symptoms, including apnea, lethargy, and poor feeding. Only two had cough or nasal congestion. None had tachypnea or respiratory distress, but three of five for whom chest radiographs were obtained had interstitial pneumonia.

Infants younger than 6 months cannot be protected by influenza vaccine. All health care professionals who care for high-risk newborns should receive the influenza A/influenza B vaccine annually in the fall. Pregnancy is not a contraindication for the administration of influenza vaccine [117,118].

During the 2009 H1N1 pandemic, pregnant women were found to be at high risk for severe influenza symptoms secondary to H1N1 infection, with up to 7.2 times higher risk of being hospitalized and 4.3 times more likely to be admitted to an ICU compared to non-pregnant women (MMWR 2010; 59:321-326). In a case series from New York City, in 2009, 16 pregnant and 1 postpartum women were admitted to an ICU or died. Nine of the women gave birth during their hospitalization; 8 of the infants were live-born, but one of those died shortly after birth, one infant was still-born, and 6 of the 8 live-born infants were admitted to a neonatal ICU. In California, all reported cases of pregnant women who were hospitalized or died due to H1N1 infection in 2009 were reviewed. Ninety-four pregnant and 8 postpartum women were identified, 95% were in their second or third trimester at the time of illness, one third had other underlying influenza complications besides pregnancy, 22 required intensive care and 8 died. The H1N1 maternal mortality ratio was 4.3 (NEJM 2010; 362:27-25). All 13 infants delivered during hospitalization survived and none had influenza.

RESPIRATORY SYNCYTIAL VIRUS

Although respiratory syncytial virus (RSV) is a common cause of upper respiratory tract infection in children and adults, there is no evidence that the virus causes intrauterine infection. Maternal infection has no known adverse effect on the fetus. RSV infections are frequently acquired by infants during the first few weeks of life and are associated with a high mortality rate. Two thirds of all infants become infected with RSV in the 1st year of life, and one third of them develop lower respiratory tract symptoms, 2.5% are hospitalized, and 1 in 1000 infants die as a result of RSV infection [119].

It was originally thought that passively transferred maternal antibody to RSV contributed to the severity of the infection in young infants by causing an immunopathologic reaction in the lung [120]. Later studies of the age-corrected incidence of symptomatic RSV infections showed a relative sparing of infants who were younger than 3 weeks [121,122]. This is the period during which maternal antibody is the highest. In subsequent studies, no evidence was found that the presence of maternal antibody adversely influenced the course of infection in the infant [123]. Lamprecht and colleagues [124] found an inverse relationship between the level of maternal neutralizing antibody and the severity of the RSV infection in the infant. Glezen and coworkers [125] found that the quantity of neutralizing antibody to RSV in cord sera was lower in infants with proven RSV infections than in randomly selected infants. None of the infected infants who had antibody titers of 1:16 or greater developed serious infections. Some authors have suggested that breastfeeding decreases the possibility that an infant will have a serious RSV infection early in life [126]; however, this has not been a consistent finding in every study. Because breast-feeding and crowded living conditions affect the incidence of RSV infection in infants, it has been difficult to define effects attributable solely to breast-feeding. Infection with RSV in infants who are younger than 4 weeks may be asymptomatic; consist of an afebrile upper respiratory syndrome; or be accompanied by fever, bronchiolitis or pneumonia, and apnea [127].

RSV accounted for 55% of cases of viral pneumonia in infants younger than 1 month in one study that evaluated hospitalized infants over a 5-year period [128]. Most infants who died had underlying medical conditions that involved the heart or lungs [129,130]. Premature infants who have recovered from hyaline membrane disease and who have bronchopulmonary dysplasia are especially likely to develop severe infections. The A subtype of RSV may have the potential to cause more severe disease than the B subtype [131].

Nosocomial outbreaks that have occurred in nurseries caring for premature and ill term infants have varied in severity. Neligan and colleagues [132] described an outbreak in which eight infants were infected. The first symptom in all infants was the development of a clear nasal discharge when 10 to 52 days old. Cough developed 2 to 7 days later. Three infants developed wheezing, and only one infant was seriously ill. In the outbreak described by Berkovich and Taranko [133], 14 infants in a premature nursery became ill when 11 to 184 days old. Of the 14 infants, 93% had coryza, 86% had dyspnea, 64% had pneumonia, and 36% had fever. Upper respiratory tract symptoms began 1 to 8 days before the first dyspnea in 11 infants. Changes compatible with pneumonia were visible on chest radiographs 3 to 5 days before clinical evidence of lower respiratory tract involvement developed. The degree of illness in the nine infants studied by Mintz and associates [134] was mild in four, moderate in two, and severe in two. One infant was asymptomatic. The infants who were the most seriously ill had fever, cyanosis, pulmonary infiltrates, and respiratory deterioration. Infants with RSV infections have developed respiratory arrest as a result of apnea [135,136].

Most infants infected during nosocomial outbreaks of RSV in nurseries were born prematurely, but had attained 4 weeks or more in chronologic age at the time they developed the infections [134,135]. Two nursery outbreaks were associated with dual infections caused by

RSV and rhinovirus or parainfluenza virus 3 [137,138]. A diffuse viral pneumonia, which is indistinguishable from severe RSV pneumonia, can be caused in rare instances by parainfluenza viruses alone or, rarely, by adenovirus [139]. Hall and coworkers [140] showed that infants who are younger than 3 weeks when they become infected with RSV have a greater incidence of nonspecific signs and a lesser incidence of lower respiratory tract infection than infants who are older than 3 weeks at the time of infection. RSV has been recovered from the oropharynx of infants who were younger than 48 hours [141]. It may be difficult to recognize the index case when RSV is introduced into the nursery [142].

Infants who are younger than 1 month have a higher mean maximal titer of virus in their secretions than older infants [143]. Of the infected infants studied by Hall and coworkers [143], 96% shed virus for 9 days. Objects contaminated with secretions from infected infants may be important sources of infection in nursery personnel. RSV in infected secretions is viable for 6 hours on countertops, for 45 minutes on cloth gowns and paper tissues, and for 20 minutes on skin [144]. Evidence suggests that personnel are at least as important in spreading the infection to infants as are other infected infants housed in the same area and that infection control measures can reduce the risk of transmission [145–147].

Any infant with rhinorrhea, nasal congestion, or unexplained apnea should be segregated and investigated for RSV infection. Personnel should be made aware that this agent, which causes only mild colds in adults, can cause fatal illnesses in infants. The specific diagnosis of RSV infection should be sought for infection control purposes and because ribavirin treatment has some effectiveness in infants with lower respiratory infection caused by this virus [148–151]. Methods have been described for administering aerosol ribavirin safely to infants receiving mechanical ventilation [152,153]. Questions concerning the benefits of ribavirin therapy for RSV pneumonia and the indications for its use remain [146,154]. Despite numerous studies in the United States and Canada regarding the use of aerosolized ribavirin, no clear improvement in clinical outcomes is consistent across all studies of ventilated and nonventilated infants with RSV infection [155,156]. Ribavirin aerosol therapy is not routinely recommended for RSV infection [157].

Although the benefit of treatment with ribavirin is controversial, there is clear evidence for the benefit of prophylaxis against RSV infection in infants at high risk for complications. Several studies showed the benefits of RSV intravenous immunoglobulin among selected infants at high risk for moderate to severe complications owing to RSV infection [158]. Such high-risk patients include infants and children younger than 2 years with chronic lung disease who have required medical therapy for lung disease within 6 months of the RSV season and premature infants who were 32 to 35 weeks' gestation at birth. RSV intravenous immunoglobulin is contraindicated for infants with cyanotic congenital heart disease because of possible safety concerns. Subsequently, a humanized anti-RSV monoclonal antibody preparation, palivizumab, was developed for intramuscular administration and shown to reduce by 55% hospitalizations resulting from RSV infection in these high-risk infants [158]. Initial concerns regarding the safety of palivizumab among infants with cyanotic congenital heart disease have been allayed based on clinical trials. Because of its greater uniformity and ease of administration and its efficacy in infants with cyanotic congenital heart disease, palivizumab is now the preferred method of RSV prophylaxis [159].

Improved survival of infants with RSV infection and underlying cardiopulmonary disease has been reported with advances in intensive care management [160,161]. Nevertheless, families of infants with medical conditions that predispose to severe RSV disease should be advised to avoid the higher risk of exposure associated with group daycare [162].

LYMPHOCYTIC CHORIOMENINGITIS VIRUS

Lymphocytic choriomeningitis virus (LCV) is spread from animals, primarily rodents, to humans. Person-to-person spread has not been described (Table 30–2) [163]. Mice and hamsters have been implicated most often as the source of human infections. When mice acquire LCV transplacentally or as newborns, they remain asymptomatic, but they shed the virus in their urine for months [164,165]. This phenomenon of "tolerance" has been extensively studied in laboratory-bred strains of mice. Domestic household mice also have been implicated as a source of human cases of infection with LCV [166].

Several outbreaks in animal handlers and in families have been traced to pet Syrian (or golden) hamsters (*Mesocricetus auratus*) [167,168]. Adult and newborn hamsters remain asymptomatic after infection with LCV and shed the virus in feces and urine for months [164]. In outbreaks in which human cases have been associated with contact with infected hamsters, the location of the hamster's cage correlated with attack rate. When the hamster's cage was in a common living area, 52% of 42

TABLE 30–2   Sources of Maternal or Neonatal Infection

Infectious Agent	Other People with Same Infection	Animal
Human papillomavirus	Yes	No
Epstein-Barr virus	Yes	No
Human herpesvirus 6	Yes	No
Influenza viruses	Yes	No
Respiratory syncytial virus	Yes	No
Lymphocytic choriomeningitis virus	No	House mice, pet Syrian hamsters, laboratory rats, rabbits
Molluscum contagiosum virus	Yes	No
Rabies	—	Yes

family members in contact with the hamster became infected [167]. In contrast, no one became infected when the cage was located in a more remote area, such as a basement or landing. LCV can be shed also by asymptomatic guinea pigs and rats [164,165,168].

Beyond the neonatal period, the illness caused by LCV is accompanied by fever, headache, nausea, and myalgia lasting 5 to 15 days [163,167,169]. In the outbreak of LCV described by Biggar and colleagues [167], fever occurred in 90% and headache occurred in 85% of patients. Myalgia occurred in 80% and was described as severe. The neck, shoulders, back, and legs were most often involved. Pain on eye movement occurred in 59%, nausea occurred in 53%, and vomiting occurred in 35%. About one fourth of the patients had a sore throat or photophobia. The illness was biphasic in 24% and was accompanied by swollen glands in 16%. A mononucleosis-like illness occurred in 6% of the patients characterized by intermittent fever, adenopathy, pharyngitis, extreme fatigue, and rash. Of patients with serologic evidence of having had an infection, 12% remained asymptomatic. Arthritis, encephalitis, and meningitis occurred in a few cases.

The diagnosis of infection with LCV can be made by isolation of the virus or by serology. The indirect fluorescent antibody titer may be positive the 1st day of symptoms [163,169]. The complement fixation titer generally does not increase until 10 days or longer after illness onset [163,168]. The neutralization titer increases late, usually after the 4th week, but persists the longest [163,168]. A positive indirect fluorescent antibody titer, a decreasing indirect fluorescent antibody or complement fixation titer, or an increasing neutralization titer suggests recent infection with LCV.

LCV infections during pregnancy may be underdiagnosed as causes of congenital infections and are associated with abortion, intrauterine infection, and perinatal infection. Ackermann and associates [170] described a 23-year-old woman who developed a febrile illness beginning 4 weeks after she assumed the care of a Syrian hamster. She was 7 months pregnant at the time of the illness and sustained a spontaneous abortion 4 weeks after onset of the fever. LCV was isolated from curettage material. Complement fixation antibodies to LCV were present initially, and neutralizing antibodies appeared later—a pattern compatible with recent infection. Diebel and coworkers [163] studied a pregnant woman who acquired LCV from a hamster and developed meningitis. One month after the onset of illness, a spontaneous abortion occurred. Biggar and coworkers [167] described a woman who acquired LCV during the first trimester of pregnancy. She had a spontaneous abortion 1 month after onset of the illness.

U.S. cases of 26 serologically confirmed congenital LCV infections identified from 1955–1996 were reviewed [171]; 85% (22 of 26) were in term infants with a median birth weight of 3520 g. The most common congenital abnormalities identified were chorioretinopathy (88%), macrocephaly (43%), and microcephaly (3%). There was a 35% (9 infants) mortality rate, with a 63% (10 of 16) rate of severe neurologic sequelae among reported survivors. One fourth of mothers had gestational exposure to rodents, and 50% of all women reported symptoms consistent with LCV infection.

Intrauterine infection of the fetus results in congenital hydrocephalus and chorioretinitis. In 1974, Ackermann and associates [172] reported that two children who were born to mothers who had been in contact with hamsters during the second half of pregnancy had hydrocephalus and chorioretinitis. Other problems included severe hyperbilirubinemia and myopia. The serologic pattern typical of recent infection was found in the mothers and infants and included a decreasing complement fixation titer and an increasing neutralization titer to LCV. Sheinbergas [169] found a statistically significant relationship between the presence of antibody to LCV and the occurrence of hydrocephalus in infants younger than 1 year. Thirty percent of 40 infants with hydrocephalus had indirect fluorescent antibody to LCV, whereas only 2.7% of 110 infants with other nervous system diseases had antibody to LCV. Fourteen (87.5%) of 16 infants who had serologically confirmed prenatal infection with LCV had hydrocephalus. Of these, six (37.5%) had been born with hydrocephalus, and the remaining eight developed it when 1 to 9 weeks old. Chorioretinal degeneration was found in 81%, and optic disk subatrophy was found in 56%. Mets and colleagues [173] performed ophthalmologic surveys among residents of a home for the severely mentally retarded, and sera from the 4 residents with chorioretinal scars and 14 residents with chorioretinitis were tested for *Toxoplasma gondii*, rubella virus, CMV, herpes simplex virus, and LCV. Two of the 4 residents with chorioretinal scars and 3 of the 14 residents with chorioretinitis had elevated antibody titers only to LCV [173].

Komrower and colleagues [166] described a mother who acquired LCV about 1 week before delivery. Despite segregation of the infant, LCV was acquired transplacentally or natally, and the infant subsequently became ill. The mother's initial symptoms included malaise, headache, fever, and cough. About 20 days after onset of symptoms and 12 days after delivery, increased numbers of cells and increased protein concentration occurred in the cerebrospinal fluid. The diagnosis of infection caused by LCV was confirmed by an increase in the mother's complement fixation titer from 1:2 to 1:64. The infant, who was probably premature, remained relatively stable until 11 days old, at which time seizures, stiff neck, and mild pleocytosis developed. The infant developed petechiae and died of a subarachnoid and intracerebral hemorrhage. LCV was isolated from the infant's cerebrospinal fluid and from mice caught in the home of the mother.

Because apparently healthy mice and hamsters may shed LCV chronically, pregnant women should avoid direct contact with these animals and with aerosolized excreta. Unless appropriate measures have been taken to ensure that laboratory animals are free of LCV, these precautions should apply to laboratory as well as domestic rodents. LCV causes spontaneous abortions. Hydrocephalus and chorioretinitis are common in infants who have survived intrauterine infection [169,172–174]. Women who acquire LCV infection during the weeks immediately before delivery may transmit the virus to their infants. Although the total number of intrauterine and perinatal infections from LCV is not large, the incidence of serious sequelae in the infant seems to be high. No treatment is available.

MOLLUSCUM CONTAGIOSUM

Molluscum contagiosum is a papular rash consisting of multiple discrete lesions that are acanthomas by histologic examination. The skin lesions are caused by a pox-like virus that has been difficult to study because it cannot be propagated in tissue culture. Epidemiologically, molluscum contagiosum is a disease of children and young adults. The virus may be transmitted by sexual conduct, given that the incidence increases among adolescents and young adults. Whether it is transmitted as a perinatal infection is unknown.

Wilkin [175] described five women who delivered infants at a time when they had the lesions of molluscum contagiosum in the genital area. None of the infants developed molluscum contagiosum. Mandel and Lewis [176] reported an infant who developed two papules on the thigh when 1 week old. These enlarged and were excised when the child was 1 year old. The results of histologic examination and the findings on electron microscopy were compatible with molluscum contagiosum. In 1926, Young [177] reported an infant with molluscum contagiosum of the scalp. The lesions appeared when the infant was 1.5 months old. No histologic studies were performed.

RABIES VIRUS

Transplacental transmission of rabies virus to the human fetus has not yet been described, although transplacental transmission occurs in experimental infections in many species [178–183]. Spence and associates [184] described an infant who was born 2 days before the onset of the mother's first symptom of encephalitis. The mother died of rabies on the 4th postpartum day. Rabies virus antigens were shown in the cornea, lacrimal gland, and various parts of the brain by fluorescent antibody stain. The child survived despite the fact that the mother and infant lacked neutralizing antibodies to rabies at the time of the birth.

Two reports described the successful administration of horse antirabies hyperimmune serum and duck embryo vaccine to pregnant women [178,184]. Unusual untoward effects did not occur, and the infants were delivered at term and were healthy. The mothers did not develop serum sickness, anaphylaxis, or neurologic complications, but if they had, the viability of the fetus might have been threatened. Horse antiserum to rabies virus has been replaced by human rabies immunoglobulin. The chance of an adverse reaction to administration of human immunoglobulin is very small. The vaccine that was previously grown in duck embryos has been replaced with an inactivated vaccine derived from virus grown in human diploid fibroblast cells [185]. No serious reactions have been reported after administration of this vaccine, and it is possible to achieve titers that are about 10-fold higher than titers found after administration of the duck embryo vaccine.

Because of the high likelihood of fatal disease after the bite of a rabid animal, postexposure prophylaxis should always be given. Pregnancy is not a contraindication. When it is necessary to administer prophylaxis to a pregnant woman, human rabies immunoglobulin and human diploid cell vaccine should be used to minimize potential adverse effects on the pregnancy. After reviewing the available data, the Advisory Committee on Immunization Practices of the U.S. Centers for Disease Control and Prevention (CDC) has recommended human diploid cell vaccine to rabies virus as a preexposure immunization that is safe for use in pregnant women who will likely be exposed to wild rabies virus before completion of pregnancy [186].

WEST NILE VIRUS

West Nile virus (WNV) is a mosquito-borne flavivirus that has caused epidemic infections in the United States since its introduction in 1999 [187]. Since then, three cases of intrauterine and breast-feeding transmission have been reported in the literature [188–190]. In 2002, a previously healthy woman at 27 weeks of gestation developed a febrile illness, followed by lower extremity paresis and meningoencephalitis. At 38 weeks of gestation, she delivered an infant with bilateral chorioretinitis and severe, bilateral white matter loss in the temporal and occipital lobes. Maternal, cord, and infant blood samples at birth were positive for WNV-specific IgM and neutralizing antibodies; cerebrospinal fluid from the infant was WNV IgM positive; and the placenta was WNV PCR positive [188]. A second reported case of intrauterine WNV infection occurring in the second trimester resulted in congenital chorioretinal scarring and severe CNS malformations of the newborn [189].

One case of probable breast-feeding transmission was reported in a woman who required red blood cell transfusions shortly after delivery. She began breast-feeding on the day of delivery and through the 2nd day of hospitalization. The woman had developed symptoms consistent with meningoencephalitis 6 days before delivery; subsequent evaluation of the units of transfused blood revealed 1 unit that was positive for WNV by PCR. Serum from the infant was positive for WNV-specific IgM at day 25 of life. The infant remained healthy at last report [190]. Although spontaneous abortions and stillbirths have been associated with flavivirus infections, these viruses have not previously been reported to be teratogenic. During 2002, the CDC investigated three other cases of maternal WNV infection in which the infants all were born at full term with no evidence of WNV infection or congenital sequelae; however, cranial imaging and ophthalmologic examinations were not performed on these infants [191].

No specific therapy is available for WNV infection, and the CDC does not recommend WNV screening of asymptomatic pregnant women. Pregnant women who have meningitis, encephalitis, acute flaccid paralysis, or unexplained fever in an area of ongoing WNV transmission should have serum and cerebrospinal fluid, if clinically indicated, tested for antibody to WNV. If WNV illness is diagnosed in the pregnant woman, ultrasound examination of the fetus should be considered no sooner than 2 to 4 weeks after maternal onset of illness, and fetal or amniotic testing can be considered. Infants born to women with known or suspected WNV infection during pregnancy should be evaluated for congenital WNV infection. Prevention of WNV infection should include application of insect repellant to skin and clothes when exposed to mosquitoes and avoidance of peak mosquito-feeding times at dawn and dusk [191].

REFERENCES

[1] S. Ono, H. Saito, M. Igarash, The etiology of papilloma of the larynx, Ann. Otol. 66 (1957) 1119.

[2] J.D. Almeida, J.D. Oriel, Wart virus, Br. J. Dermatol. 83 (1970) 698.

[3] L. Gissman, et al., Human papillomavirus types 6 and 11: DNA sequences in genital and laryngeal papillomas and in some cervical cancers, Proc. Natl. Acad. Sci. U. S. A. 80 (1983) 560.

[4] J.M. Walboomers, et al., Human papillomavirus is a necessary cause of invasive cervical cancer worldwide, J. Pathol. 189 (1999) 12–19.

[5] M. Schiffman, P.E. Castle, Human papillomavirus: epidemiology and public health, Arch. Pathol. Lab. Med. 127 (2003) 930–934.

[6] D.J. Wiley, et al., External genital warts: diagnosis, treatment, and prevention, Clin. Infect. Dis. 35 (Suppl 2) (2002) S210–S224.

[7] N. Munoz, et al., Epidemiologic classification of human papillomavirus types associated with cervical cancer, N. Engl. J. Med. 348 (2003) 518–527.

[8] G.M. Clifford, et al., Comparison of HPV type distribution in high-grade cervical lesions and cervical cancer: a meta-analysis, Br. J. Cancer 89 (2003) 101–105.

[9] A. Schaffer, J. Brotherton, R. Booy, Do human papillomavirus vaccines have any role in newborns and the prevention of recurrent respiratory papillomatosis in children? J. Paediatr. Child. Health 43 (2007) 579–580.

[10] A.L. Allen, E.C. Seigfried, The natural history of condyloma in children, J. Am. Acad. Dermatol. 39 (1998) 951.

[11] E.F. Hajek, Contribution to the etiology of laryngeal papilloma in children, J. Laryngol. 70 (1956) 166.

[12] T.A. Cook, et al., Laryngeal papilloma: etiologic and therapeutic considerations, Ann. Otol. 82 (1973) 649.

[13] C.A. Quick, et al., Relationship between condylomata and laryngeal papillomata, Ann. Otol. 89 (1980) 467.

[14] D.H. Watts, et al., Low risk of perinatal transmission of human papillomavirus: results from a prospective cohort study, Am. J. Obstet. Gynecol. 178 (1998) 365.

[15] M. Puranen, et al., Vertical transmission of human papillomavirus from infected mothers to their newborn babies and persistence of the virus in childhood, Am. J. Obstet. Gynecol. 174 (1996) 694.

[16] B.D. Fredericks, et al., Transmission of human papillomaviruses from mother to child, Aust. N. Z. J. Obstet. Gynaecol. 33 (1993) 30.

[17] E.M. Smith, et al., The association between pregnancy and human papilloma virus prevalence, Cancer Detect. Prev. 15 (1991) 397.

[18] F. Pakarian, et al., Cancer associated human papillomaviruses: perinatal transmission and persistence, Br. J. Obstet. Gynaecol. 101 (1994) 514.

[19] J. Cason, et al., Perinatal infection and persistence of human papillomavirus types 16 and 18 in infants, J. Med. Virol. 47 (1995) 209.

[20] T.V. Sedlacek, et al., Mechanism for human papillomavirus transmission at birth, Am. J. Obstet. Gynecol. 161 (1989) 55.

[21] E.M. Smith, et al., Human papillomavirus prevalence and types in newborns and parents: concordance and modes of transmission, Sex. Transm. Dis. 31 (2004) 57.

[22] R. Drut, et al., Human papillomavirus, neonatal giant cell hepatitis and biliary duct atresia, Acta Gastroenterol. Latinoam. 28 (1998) 27.

[23] E.P. Dias, et al., Congenital papillomas and papillomatoses associated with the human papillomavirus (HPV)—report on 5 cases, Rev. Paul. Med. 113 (1995) 957.

[24] B.M. Steinberg, et al., Laryngeal papillomavirus infection during clinical remission, N. Engl. J. Med. 308 (1983) 1261.

[25] U. Hording, et al., Prevalence of human papillomavirus types 11, 16 and 18 in cervical swabs: a study of 1362 pregnant women, Eur. J. Obstet. Gynecol. Reprod. Biol. 35 (1990) 191.

[26] T. Peng, et al., Prevalence of human papillomavirus infections in term pregnancy, Am. J. Perinatol. 7 (1990) 189.

[27] E.A. Kemp, et al., Human papillomavirus prevalence in pregnancy, Obstet. Gynecol. 79 (1992) 649.

[28] K.H. Fife, R.E. Rogers, B.W. Zwickl, Symptomatic and asymptomatic cervical infections with human papillomavirus during pregnancy, J. Infect. Dis. 156 (1987) 904.

[29] C.K. Tang, D.W. Shermeta, C. Wood, Congenital condylomata acuminata, Am. J. Obstet. Gynecol. 131 (1978) 912.

[30] A. Roman, K. Fife, Human papillomavirus DNA associated with foreskins of normal newborns, J. Infect. Dis. 153 (1986) 855.

[31] M.A. Avidano, G.T. Singleton, Adjuvant drug strategies in the treatment of recurrent respiratory papillomatosis, Otolaryngol. Head Neck Surg. 112 (1995) 197.

[32] L.E. Markowitz, et al., Quadrivalent human papillomavirus vaccine: recommendations of the Advisory Committee on Immunization Practices (ACIP), MMWR. Recomm. Rep. 56 (RR-2) (2007) 1–24.

[33] C.S. Derkay, Recurrent respiratory papillomatosis, Laryngoscope 111 (2001) 57.

[34] D.K. Chhetri, N.L. Shapiro, A scheduled protocol for the treatment of juvenile recurrent respiratory papillomatosis with intralesional cidofovir, Arch. Otolaryngol. Head Neck Surg. 129 (2003) 1081.

[35] D.M. Harper, et al., Sustained efficacy up to 4.5 years of a bivalent L1 virus-like particle vaccine against human papillomavirus types 16 and 18: follow-up from a randomised control trial, Lancet 367 (2006) 1247–1255.

[36] R. Roden, T.C. Wu, Preventative and therapeutic vaccines for cervical cancer, Expert. Rev. Vaccines 2 (2003) 495.

[37] W. Henle, G. Henle, C.A. Horwitz, Epstein-Barr virus-specific diagnostic tests in infectious mononucleosis, Hum. Pathol. 5 (1974) 551.

[38] G. Fleisher, et al., Primary Epstein-Barr virus infection in American infants: clinical and serological observations, J. Infect. Dis. 139 (1979) 553.

[39] J. Icart, J. Didier, Infections due to Epstein-Barr virus during pregnancy, J. Infect. Dis. 143 (1981) 499.

[40] G. Fleisher, R. Bolognese, Persistent Epstein-Barr virus infection and pregnancy, J. Infect. Dis. 147 (1983) 982.

[41] C.T. Le, S. Chang, M.H. Lipson, Epstein-Barr virus infections during pregnancy, Am. J. Dis. Child. 137 (1983) 466.

[42] J. Icart, et al., Etude prospective de l'infection à virus Epstein-Barr (EBV) au cours de la grossesse, Biomedicine 34 (1981) 160.

[43] F. Gervais, J.H. Joncas, Seroepidemiology in various population groups of the greater Montreal area, Comp. Immunol. Microbiol. Infect. Dis. 2 (1979) 207.

[44] C.A. Horowitz, et al., Long-term serologic follow-up of patients for Epstein-Barr virus after recovery from infectious mononucleosis, J. Infect. Dis. 151 (1985) 1150.

[45] G. Fleisher, R. Bolognese, Epstein-Barr virus infections in pregnancy: a prospective study, J. Pediatr. 104 (1984) 374.

[46] G. Fleisher, R. Bolognese, Infectious mononucleosis during gestation: report of three women and their infants studied prospectively, Pediatr. Infect. Dis. 3 (1984) 308.

[47] H. Tallqvist, et al., Antibodies to Epstein-Barr virus at the ages of 6 to 23 months in children with congenital heart disease, Scand. J. Infect. Dis. 5 (1973) 159.

[48] Z.A. Brown, M.A. Stenchever, Infectious mononucleosis and congenital anomalies, Am. J. Obstet. Gynecol. 131 (1978) 108.

[49] G.N. Goldberg, et al., In utero Epstein-Barr virus (infectious mononucleosis) infection, JAMA 246 (1981) 1579.

[50] L.T. Weaver, R. Nelson, T.M. Bell, The association of extrahepatic bile duct atresia and neonatal Epstein-Barr virus infection, Acta Paediatr. Scand. 73 (1984) 155.

[51] A.J. Visintine, P. Gerber, A.J. Nahmias, Leukocyte transforming agent (Epstein-Barr virus) in newborn infants and older individuals, J. Pediatr. 89 (1976) 571.

[52] R.S. Chang, W. Blankenship, Spontaneous in vitro transformation of leukocytes from a neonate, Proc. Soc. Exp. Biol. Med. 144 (1973) 337.

[53] R.S. Chang, D.Y. Seto, Perinatal infection by Epstein-Barr virus, Lancet 2 (1979) 201.

[54] J. Joncas, et al., Epstein-Barr virus in the neonatal period and in childhood, Can. Med. Assoc. J. 110 (1974) 33.

[55] J.H. Joncas, A. Wills, B. McLaughlin, Congenital infection with cytomegalovirus and Epstein-Barr virus, Can. Med. Assoc. J. 117 (1977) 1417.

[56] M.C. Meyohas, et al., Study of mother-to-child Epstein-Barr virus transmission by means of nested PCRs, J. Virol. 70 (1996) 6816.

[57] J. Joncas, et al., Dual congenital infection with the Epstein-Barr virus (EBV) and the cytomegalovirus (CMV), N. Engl. J. Med. 304 (1981) 1399.

[58] J.W. Sixbey, S.M. Lemon, J.S. Pagano, A second site for Epstein-Barr virus shedding: the uterine cervix, Lancet 2 (1986) 1122.

[59] J. Portnoy, et al., Recovery of Epstein-Barr virus from genital ulcers, N. Engl. J. Med. 311 (1984) 966.

[60] C.A. Horwitz, et al., Fatal illness in a 2 week old infant: diagnosis by detection of Epstein-Barr virus genomes from a lymph node biopsy, J. Pediatr. 103 (1983) 752.

[61] F. Gervais, J.H. Joncas, Correspondence-an unusual antibody response to Epstein-Barr virus during infancy, J. Infect. Dis. 140 (1979) 273.

[62] S.Z. Salahuddin, et al., Isolation of a new virus, HBLV, in patients with lymphoproliferative disorders, Science 234 (1986) 596.

[63] C. Lopez, et al., Characteristics of human herpesvirus-6, J. Infect. Dis. 157 (1988) 1271.

[64] C.T. Leach, C.V. Sumaya, N.A. Brown, Human herpesvirus-6: clinical implications of a recently discovered, ubiquitous agent, J. Pediatr. 1231 (1992) 173.

[65] G.L. Lawrence, et al., Human herpes virus 6 is closely related to human cytomegalovirus, J. Virol. 64 (1989) 287.

[66] J. Baillargeon, J. Piper, C.T. Leach, Epidemiology of human herpesvirus 6 (HHV-6) infection in pregnant and non-pregnant women, J. Clin. Virol. 16 (2000) 149.

[67] H. Dahl, et al., Reactivation of human herpesvirus 6 during pregnancy, J. Infect. Dis. 180 (1999) 2035.

[68] O. Adams, et al., Congenital infections with human herpesvirus 6, J. Infect. Dis. 178 (1998) 544.

[69] K. Yamaniski, et al., Exanthem subitum and human herpes virus 6, Pediatr. Infect. Dis. J. 12 (1993) 204.

[70] M.T. Caserta, et al., Human herpesvirus (HHV)-6 and HHV-7 infections in pregnant women, J. Infect. Dis. 196 (2007) 1296–1303.

[71] J.T. Aubi, et al., Intrauterine transmission of human herpes virus 6, Lancet 340 (1992) 482.

[72] W.M. Dunne, G.J. Demmler, Serologic evidence for congenital transmission of human herpesvirus 6, Lancet 340 (1992) 121.

[73] N.M. van Loon, et al., Direct sequence analysis of human herpesvirus 6 (HHV-6) sequences from infants and comparison of HHV-6 from mother/infant pairs, Clin. Infect. Dis. 21 (1995) 1017.

[74] P. Pruksananonda, et al., Primary human herpes virus 6 infection in young children, N. Engl. J. Med. 22 (1992) 1445.

[75] S. Kawaguchi, et al., Primary human herpesvirus 6 infection (exanthem subitum) in the newborn, Pediatrics 90 (1992) 628.

[76] H. Tajiri, et al., Human herpesvirus-6 infection with liver injury in neonatal hepatitis, Lancet 335 (1990) 863.

[77] Y. Asano, et al., Fatal fulminant hepatitis in an infant with human herpes-virus-6 infection, Lancet 335 (1990) 862.

[78] C. Kanegane, et al., Mononucleosis-like illness in an infant associated with human herpesvirus 6 infection, Acta Paediatr. Jpn. 37 (1995) 227.

[79] J.A. Hammerling, et al., Prevalence of human herpesvirus 6 in lung tissue from children with pneumonitis, J. Clin. Pathol. 49 (1996) 802.

[80] K.K. Knox, et al., Progressive immunodeficiency and fatal pneumonitis associated with human herpesvirus 6 infection in an infant, Clin. Infect. Dis. 20 (1995) 406.

[81] J.B. Black, P.E. Pellett, Human herpesvirus 7, Rev. Med. Virol. 3 (1993) 217.

[82] N. Frenkel, et al., Isolation of a new herpesvirus from human CD4+ T cells, Proc. Natl. Acad. Sci. U. S. A. 87 (1990) 748.

[83] G.R. Krueger, et al., Comparison of seroprevalences of human herpesvirus-6 and -7 in healthy blood donors from nine countries, Vox. Sang. 75 (1998) 193.

[84] D.A. Clark, et al., Prevalence of antibody to human herpesvirus 7 by age, J. Infect. Dis. 168 (1993) 251.

[85] H. Fujisaki, et al., Detection of human herpesvirus 7 (HHV-7) DNA in breast milk by polymerase chain reaction and prevalence of HHV-7 antibody in breast-fed and bottle-fed children, J. Med. Virol. 56 (1998) 275.

[86] B.P. Lanphear, et al., Risk factors for the early acquisition of human herpes-virus 6 and human herpesvirus 7 infections in children, Pediatr. Infect. Dis. J. 17 (1998) 792.

[87] T. Okuno et al., Human herpesviruses 6 and 7 in cervixes of pregnant women, J. Clin. Microbiol. 133 (1995) 1968.

[88] D. Boutolleau, et al., No evidence for a major risk of roseolovirus vertical transmission during pregnancy, Clin. Infect. Dis. 36 (2003) 1634.

[89] S. Torigoe, et al., Clinical manifestations associated with human herpesvirus 7 infection, Arch. Dis. Child. 72 (1995) 518.

[90] S. Torigoe, et al., Human herpesvirus 7 infection associated with central nervous system manifestations, J. Pediatr. 129 (1996) 301.

[91] D.A. Clark, et al., Diagnosis of primary human herpesvirus 6 and 7 infections in febrile infants by polymerase chain reaction, Arch. Dis. Child. 77 (1997) 42.

[92] M. Portolani, et al., Isolation of human herpesvirus 7 from an infant with febrile syndrome, J. Med. Virol. 45 (1995) 282.

[93] V.P. Coffey, W.J.E. Jessup, Maternal influenza and congenital deformities, Lancet 2 (1959) 935.

[94] R. Doll, A.B. Hill, Asian influenza in pregnancy and congenital defects, Br. J. Prev. Soc. Med. 14 (1960) 167.

[95] R.G. Record, Anencephalus in Scotland, Br. J. Prev. Soc. Med. 15 (1961) 93.

[96] I. Leck, Incidence of malformations following influenza epidemics, Br. J. Prev. Soc. Med. 17 (1963) 70.

[97] J. Hakosalo, L. Saxen, Influenza epidemic and congenital defects, Lancet 2 (1971) 1346.

[98] M.G. Wilson, A.M. Stein, Teratogenic effects of Asian influenza, JAMA 210 (1969) 336.

[99] J.M.B. Hardy, et al., The effect of Asian influenza on the outcome of pregnancy. Baltimore 1957–1958, Am. J. Public. Health 51 (1961) 1182.

[100] J.S. MacKenzie, M. Houghton, Influenza infections during pregnancy: association with congenital malformations and with subsequent neoplasms in children, and potential hazards of live virus vaccines, Bacteriol. Rev. 38 (1974) 356.

[101] P.D. Griffiths, C.J. Ronalds, R.B. Heath, A prospective study of influenza infections during pregnancy, J. Epidemiol. Commun. Health 34 (1980) 124.

[102] G.R.G. Monif, D.L. Soward, D.V. Eitzman, Serologic and immunologic evaluation of neonates following maternal influenza infection during the second and third trimesters, Am. J. Obstet. Gynecol. 114 (1972) 239.

[103] T.V. Hartert, et al., Maternal morbidity and perinatal outcomes among pregnant women with respiratory hospitalizations during influenza season, Am. J. Obstet. Gynecol. 189 (2003) 1705.

[104] J.A. Englund, Maternal immunization with inactivated influenza vaccine: rationale and experience, Vaccine 21 (2003) 3460.

[105] P.B. Mortensen, et al., Individual and familial risk factors for bipolar affective disorders in Denmark, Arch. Gen. Psychiatry 60 (2003) 1209.

[106] F. Limosin, et al., Prenatal exposure to influenza as a risk factor for adult schizophrenia, Acta Psychiatr. Scand. 107 (2003) 331.

[107] A.S. Brown, E.S. Susser, In utero infection and adult schizophrenia, Ment. Retard. Dev. Disabil. Res. Rev. 8 (2002) 51.

[108] F.L. Ruben, A. Winkelstein, R.E. Sabbagha, In utero sensitization with influenza virus in man, Proc. Soc. Exp. Biol. Med. 149 (1975) 881.

[109] J.A. McGregor, et al., Transplacental passage of influenza A/Bangkok (H3N2) mimicking amniotic fluid infection syndrome, Am. J. Obstet. Gynecol. 149 (1984) 856.

[110] D.H. Yawn, et al., Transplacental transfer of influenza virus, JAMA 216 (1971) 1022.

[111] R. Ramphal, W.H. Donnelly, P.A. Small, Fatal influenzal pneumonia in pregnancy: failure to demonstrate transplacental transmissions of influenza virus, Am. J. Obstet. Gynecol. 138 (1980) 347.

[112] J.M. Puck, et al., Protection of infants from infection with influenza A virus by transplacentally acquired antibody, J. Infect. Dis. 142 (1980) 844.

[113] P.D. Reuman, E.M. Ayoub, P.A. Small, Effect of passive maternal antibody on influenza illness in children: a prospective study of influenza A in mother-infant pairs, Pediatr. Infect. Dis. J. 6 (1987) 398.

[114] C.R. Bauer, et al., Hong Kong influenza in a neonatal unit, JAMA 223 (1973) 1233.

[115] V.V. Joshi, et al., Fatal influenza A2 viral pneumonia in a newborn infant, Am. J. Dis. Child. 126 (1973) 839.

[116] R. Meibalane, et al., Outbreak of influenza in a neonatal intensive care unit, J. Pediatr. 91 (1977) 974.

[117] C.V. Sumaya, R.S. Gibbs, Immunization of pregnant women with influenza A/New Jersey/76 virus vaccine: reactogenicity and immunogenicity in mothers and infants, J. Infect. Dis. 140 (1979) 141.

[118] J.V. Schmidt, A.T. Kroger, S.L. Roy, Report from the CDC. Vaccines in women, J. Womens Health (Larchmt) 13 (2004) 249.

[119] C.J. Holberg, Risk factors for respiratory syncytial virus-associated lower respiratory illnesses in the first year of life, Am. J. Epidemiol. 133 (1991) 1135.

[120] R.M. Chanock, et al., Influence of immunological factors in respiratory syncytial virus disease, Arch. Environ. Health 21 (1970) 347.

[121] J.W. Jacobs, et al., Respiratory syncytial and other viruses associated with respiratory disease in infants, Lancet 1 (1971) 871.

[122] R.H. Parrott, H.W. Kim, J.O. Arrobio, Epidemiology of respiratory syncytial virus infection in Washington, DC. II. Infection and disease with respect to age, immunologic status, race and sex, Am. J. Epidemiol. 98 (1973) 289.

[123] F.W. Bruhn, A.S. Yeager, Respiratory syncytial virus in early infancy, Am. J. Dis. Child. 131 (1977) 145.

[124] C.L. Lamprecht, H.E. Krause, M.A. Mufson, Role of maternal antibody in pneumonia and bronchiolitis due to respiratory syncytial virus, J. Infect. Dis. 134 (1976) 211.

[125] W.P. Glezen, et al., Risk of respiratory syncytial virus infection for infants from low-income families in relationship to age, sex, ethnic group, and maternal antibody level, J. Pediatr. 98 (1981) 708.

[126] M. Downham, et al., Breast-feeding protects against respiratory syncytial virus infections, BMJ 2 (1976) 274.

[127] F.W. Bruhn, S.T. Mokrohisky, K. McIntosh, Apnea associated with respiratory syncytial virus infection in young infants, J. Pediatr. 90 (1977) 382.

[128] M.J. Abzug, et al., Viral pneumonia in the first month of life, Pediatr. Infect. Dis. J. 9 (1990) 881.

[129] N.E. MacDonald, et al., Respiratory syncytial viral infection in infants with congenital heart disease, N. Engl. J. Med. 307 (1982) 397.

[130] S.H. Abman, et al., Role of respiratory syncytial virus in early hospitalizations for respiratory distress of young infants with cystic fibrosis, J. Pediatr. 113 (1988) 826.

[131] K.M. McConnochie, et al., Variation in severity of respiratory syncytial virus infections with subtype, J. Pediatr. 117 (1990) 52.

[132] G.A. Neligan, et al., Respiratory syncytial virus infection of the newborn, BMJ 3 (1970) 146.

[133] S. Berkovich, L. Taranko, Acute respiratory illness in the premature nursery associated with respiratory syncytial virus infection, Pediatrics 34 (1964) 753.

[134] L. Mintz, et al., Nosocomial respiratory syncytial virus infections in an intensive care nursery: rapid diagnosis by direct immunofluorescence, Pediatrics 64 (1979) 149.

[135] E.J. Goldson, et al., A respiratory syncytial virus outbreak in a transitional care nursery, Am. J. Dis. Child. 133 (1979) 1280.

[136] N.R. Church, C.A. Anas, C.B. Hall, Respiratory syncytial virus-related apnea in infants: demographics and outcome, Am. J. Dis. Child. 138 (1984) 247.

[137] W.M. Valenti, et al., Concurrent outbreaks of rhinovirus and respiratory syncytial virus in an intensive care nursery: epidemiology and associated risk factors, J. Pediatr. 100 (1982) 722.

[138] H.C. Meissner, et al., A simultaneous outbreak of respiratory syncytial virus and parainfluenza virus type 3 in a newborn nursery, J. Pediatr. 104 (1984) 680.

[139] D.F. Wensley, V.J. Baldwin, Respiratory distress in the second week of life, J. Pediatr. 106 (1985) 326.

[140] C.B. Hall, et al., Neonatal respiratory syncytial virus infection, N. Engl. J. Med. 300 (1979) 393.

[141] C.W. Wilson, D.K. Stevenson, A.M. Arvin, A concurrent epidemic of respiratory syncytial virus and echovirus 7 infections in an intensive care nursery, Pediatr. Infect. Dis. J. 8 (1989) 24.

[142] A. Unger, et al., Atypical neonatal respiratory syncytial virus infection, J. Pediatr. 100 (1982) 762.

[143] C.B. Hall, R.G. Douglas Jr., J.M. Geiman, Respiratory syncytial virus infections in infants: quantitation and duration of shedding, J. Pediatr. 89 (1976) 11.

[144] C.B. Hall, R.G. Douglas Jr., J.M. Geiman, Possible transmission by fomites or respiratory syncytial virus, J. Infect. Dis. 141 (1980) 98.

[145] D.R. Snydman, et al., Prevention of nosocomial transmission of respiratory syncytial virus in a newborn nursery, Infect. Control. Hosp. Epidemiol. 9 (1988) 105.

[146] J.M. Leclair, et al., Prevention of nosocomial respiratory syncytial virus infections through compliance with glove and gown isolation precautions, N. Engl. J. Med. 317 (1987) 329.

[147] R. Agah, et al., Respiratory syncytial virus (RSV) infection rate in personnel caring for children with RSV infections: routine isolation procedure vs routine procedure supplemented by use of masks and goggles, Am. J. Dis. Child. 141 (1987) 695.

[148] C.B. Hall, et al., Aerosolized ribavirin treatment of infants with respiratory syncytial viral infection: a randomized double-blind study, N. Engl. J. Med. 308 (1983) 1443.

[149] C.B. Hall, et al., Ribavirin treatment of respiratory syncytial viral infection in infants with underlying cardiopulmonary disease, JAMA 254 (1985) 3047.

[150] W.J. Rodriguez, et al., Aerosolized ribavirin in the treatment of patients with respiratory syncytial virus disease, Pediatr. Infect. Dis. J. 6 (1987) 159.

[151] D.A. Conrad, et al., Aerosolized ribavirin treatment of respiratory syncytial virus infection in infants hospitalized during an epidemic, Pediatr. Infect. Dis. J. 6 (1987) 152.

[152] K.M. Outwater, H.C. Meissner, M.B. Peterson, Ribavirin administration to infants receiving mechanical ventilation, Am. J. Dis. Child. 142 (1988) 512.

[153] L.R. Frankel, et al., A technique for the administration of ribavirin to mechanically ventilated infants with severe respiratory syncytial virus infection, Crit. Care Med. 15 (1987) 1051.

[154] E.R. Wald, B. Dashefsky, M. Green, In re ribavirin. A case of premature adjudication, J. Pediatr. 112 (1988) 154.

[155] C.G. Prober, E.E.L. Wang, Reducing the morbidity of lower respiratory tract infections caused by respiratory syncytial virus: still no answer, Pediatrics 99 (1997) 472.

[156] American Academy of Pediatrics, Committee on Infectious Diseases. Reassessment of the indications for ribavirin therapy in respiratory syncytial virus infections, Pediatrics 97 (1996) 137.

[157] Ribavirin therapy of respiratory syncytial virus, P.G. Lepow, M.L. McCrachen, C.F. Phillips (Eds.), Report of the Committee on Infectious Diseases, American Academy of Pediatrics, Elk Grove Village, IL, 1991.

[158] H.C. Meissner, S.S. Long, American Academy of Pediatrics Committee on Infectious Diseases and Committee on Fetus and Newborn. Revised indications for the use of palivizumab and respiratory syncytial virus immune globulin intravenous for the prevention of respiratory syncytial virus infections, Pediatrics 112 (2003) 1447.

[159] L.K. Pickering (Ed.), Red Book: Report of the Committee on Infectious Diseases, twenty seventh ed., American Academy of Pediatrics, Elk Grove Village, IL, 2006.

[160] F.W. Moler, et al., Respiratory syncytial virus morbidity and mortality estimates in congenital heart disease patients: a recent experience, Crit. Care Med. 20 (1992) 1406.

[161] L. Navas, et al., Improved outcome of respiratory syncytial virus infection in a high-risk hospitalized population of Canadian children, J. Pediatr. 121 (1992) 348.

[162] L.J. Anderson, et al., Day-care center attendance and hospitalization for lower respiratory tract illness, Pediatrics 82 (1988) 300.

[163] R. Diebel, et al., Lymphochytic choriomeningitis virus in man: serologic evidence of association with pet hamster, JAMA 232 (1975) 501.

[164] J.E. Smadel, M.J. Wall, Lymphocytic choriomeningitis in the Syrian hamster, J. Exp. Med. 75 (1942) 581.

[165] E. Traub, Persistence of lymphochoriomeningitis virus in immune animals and its relation to immunity, J. Exp. Med. 63 (1936) 847.

[166] G.M. Komrower, B.L. Williams, P.B. Stones, Lymphocytic choriomeningitis in the newborn, Lancet 1 (1955) 697.

[167] R.J. Biggar, et al., Lymphocytic choriomeningitis outbreak associated with pet hamsters: fifty-seven cases from New York state, JAMA 232 (1975) 494.

[168] J. Hotchin, The contamination of laboratory animals with lymphocytic choriomeningitis virus, Am. J. Pathol. 64 (1971) 747.

[169] M.M. Sheinbergas, Hydrocephalus due to prenatal infection with the lymphocytic choriomeningitis virus, Infection 4 (1974) 185.

[170] R. Ackermann, A. Stammler, B. Armbruster, Isolierung von Virus der lymphozytären Choriomeningitis aus Abrasionsmaterial nach Kontakt der Schwangeren mit einem Syrischen Goldhamster (Mesocricetus auratus), Infection 3 (1975) 47.

[171] R. Wright, et al., Congenital lymphocytic choriomeningitis virus syndrome: a disease that mimics congenital toxoplasmosis or cytomegalovirus infection, Pediatrics 100 (1997) E9.

[172] R. Ackermann, et al., Pränatale Infektion mit dem Virus der lymphozytären Choriomeningitis, Dtsch. Med. Wochenschr. 99 (1974) 629.

[173] M.B. Mets, et al., Lymphocytic choriomeningitis virus: an underdiagnosed cause of congenital chorioretinitis, Am. J. Ophthalmol. 130 (2000) 209.

[174] C. Chastel, et al., Infection transplacentaire par le virus de la choriomeningite lymphocytaire, Nouv. Presse Med. 71 (1978) 1089.

[175] J.K. Wilkin, Molluscum contagiosum venereum in a women's outpatient clinic: a venereally transmitted disease, Am. J. Obstet. Gynecol. 128 (1977) 531.

[176] M.J. Mandel, R.J. Lewis, Molluscum contagiosum of the newborn, Br. J. Dermatol. 84 (1970) 370.

[177] W.J. Young, Molluscum contagiosum with unusual distribution, Ky. Med. J. 24 (1926) 467.

[178] W. Cates Jr., Treatment of rabies exposure during pregnancy, Obstet. Gynecol. 44 (1974) 893.

[179] M.A. Martell, F.C. Montes, R.B. Alcocer, Transplacental transmission of bovine rabies after natural infection, J. Infect. Dis. 127 (1973) 291.

[180] J. Geneverlay, J. Dodero, Note sur un enfant né d'une mere en etat du rage, Ann. Inst. Pasteur Paris 55 (1935) 124.

[181] V.K. Viazhevich, A case of birth of a healthy baby to a mother during the incubation period of rabies, Zh. Mikrobiol. Epidemiol. Immunobiol. 28 (1957) 1022.

[182] C.G. Machada, et al., Observations sur un enfant né de mere atteinte de rage et soumis du traitement prophylactique par le serum et le vaccome amtorabiques, Bull. Soc. Pathol. Exp. 59 (1966) 764.

[183] R.N. Relova, The hydrophobia boy, J. Philipp. Med. Assoc. 39 (1963) 765.

[184] M.R. Spence, et al., Rabies exposure during pregnancy, Am. J. Obstet. Gynecol. 123 (1975) 655.

[185] H.M. Meyer, FDA: rabies vaccine, J. Infect. Dis. 142 (1980) 287.

[186] Public Health Service Advisory Committee on Immunization Practices, Human Rabies Prevention—United States, 1999 Recommendations of the Advisory Committee on Immunization Practices (ACIP), MMWR Morb. Mortal. Wkly. Rep. 48 (1999) 1.

[187] D. Nash, et al., The outbreak of West Nile infection in the New York City area in 1999, N. Engl. J. Med. 344 (2001) 1807.

[188] Centers for Disease Control and Prevention, Intrauterine West Nile virus infection—New York, 2002, MMWR Morb. Mortal. Wkly. Rep. 51 (2002) 1135.

[189] S.G. Alpert, J. Fergerson, L.P. Noel, Intrauterine West Nile virus: ocular and systemic findings, Am. J. Ophthalmol. 136 (2003) 733.

[190] Centers for Disease Control and Prevention, Possible West Nile virus transmission to an infant through breast-feeding—Michigan, 2002, MMWR Morb. Mortal. Wkly. Rep. 51 (2002) 877.

[191] Centers for Disease Control and Prevention, Interim guidelines for the evaluation of infants born to mothers infected with West Nile virus during pregnancy, MMWR Morb. Mortal. Wkly. Rep. 53 (2004) 154.

PROTOZOAN, HELMINTH, AND FUNGAL INFECTIONS

SECTION OUTLINE

31 Toxoplasmosis 918

32 Less Common Protozoan and Helminth Infections 1042

33 Candidiasis 1055

34 *Pneumocystis* and Other Less Common Fungal Infections 1078

TOXOPLASMOSIS

Jack S. Remington ⊛ Rima McLeod ⊛ Christopher B. Wilson ⊛ George Desmonts*

CHAPTER OUTLINE

The Organism   918
    Oocyst   919
    Tachyzoite   920
    Cyst   921
    Epidemiology   931
    Pathogenesis   936
    Pathology   939
    Clinical Manifestations   945
    Diagnosis   967

Guidelines for Evaluation of the Newborn with Suspected
    Congenital Toxoplasmosis   980
Differential Diagnosis   993
    Therapy   993
    Duration of Therapy   1000
Prevention   1017
    Food   1018
Resources   1028

Toxoplasma gondii is a protozoal parasite that can cause devastating disease in the fetus and newborn yet remain unrecognized in women who acquire the infection during gestation. In addition, in most countries, congenital infection and congenital toxoplasmosis in the newborn go undiagnosed, thereby predisposing to the occurrence of untoward sequelae of the infection, including decreased vision or blindness, decreased hearing or deafness, and mental and psychomotor retardation. The cost for special care of children with congenital toxoplasmosis born each year in the United States alone has been estimated to be in the hundreds of millions of dollars.

T. gondii is ubiquitous in nature and is the cause of a variety of illnesses that previously were thought to be due to other agents or to be of unknown cause. Toxoplasmic encephalitis has proved to be a significant cause of morbidity and mortality in immunodeficient patients, including infants, children, and adults with acquired immunodeficiency syndrome (AIDS). Toxoplasmosis in domestic animals is of economic importance in countries such as England and New Zealand, where it causes abortion in sheep, and in Japan, where it has caused abortion in swine. In a majority of infected infants, clinical signs are not recognized at birth, but sequelae of the congenital infection are recognized or develop later in life. In this chapter, the term congenital toxoplasmosis refers to cases in which signs of disease related to congenital infection are present.

The history of *T. gondii* began in 1908, when Nicolle and Manceaux observed a parasite in the spleen and liver of a North African rodent, the gundi (Ctenodactylus gundi) and proposed the name *Toxoplasma* (from the Greek toxon, "arc") *gondii* [1]. The organism soon attracted attention as a cause of disease in animals, and in 1923, Janku, an ophthalmologist in Prague, described the first recognized case in humans [2]. He found parasitic cysts in the retina of an 11-month-old child with congenital hydrocephalus and microphthalmia with large macular scars. The parasite noted by Janku was later recognized to be *T. gondii* by Levaditi, who suggested a possible connection between congenital hydrocephalus and toxoplasmosis [3].

It was not until 1937, however, that recognition of toxoplasmosis as a disease of humans had a real impact on medicine. In that year, Wolf and Cowen in the United States reported a fatal case of infantile granulomatous encephalitis, and along with their collaborators performed numerous studies, which established *T. gondii* as a cause of prenatally transmitted human disease [4,5]. (Case 4 in the report by Paige and coworkers [6] is of special interest because it established beyond question that the infantile form of the infection was prenatal in origin.)

The discovery of *T. gondii* as a cause of disease acquired later in life has been credited to Pinkerton and Weinman. In 1940, they described a generalized fatal illness in a young man that was caused by this organism [7]. In 1941, Pinkerton and Henderson provided a clinical description of two fatal cases of an acute febrile exanthematous disease in adults [8], and in the same year, Sabin described cases of toxoplasmic encephalitis in children [9].

In 1948, Sabin and Feldman originated a serologic test, the dye test, that allowed numerous investigators to study epidemiologic and clinical aspects of toxoplasmosis to demonstrate that *T. gondii* is the cause of a highly prevalent and widespread (most often asymptomatic) infection in humans, and to define the spectrum of disease in humans [10]. It was not until 1969, some 60 years after the discovery of the parasite, that *T. gondii* was found to be a coccidian and that the definitive host was found to be the cat.

THE ORGANISM

T. gondii is a coccidian and exists in three forms outside the cat intestine: an oocyst, in which sporozoites are formed [11,12]; a proliferative form, referred to as a tachyzoite; and a tissue cyst, which has an intracystic form termed a bradyzoite. (Because a single nomenclature has

---

*Deceased.

not been agreed on, the terms for each form are used as synonyms in this chapter.) For a more thorough discussion of the organism itself, including its cell biology, molecular biology, genetics, antigenic structure, and immunobiology, the reader is referred to reviews on these subjects [13–24].

OOCYST

The enteroepithelial cycle occurs in the intestines of members of the cat family (see "Transmission" section) and results in oocyst formation (Figs. 31–1 and 31–2). Schizogony and gametogony appear to take place throughout the small intestine but especially in the tips of the villi in the ileum. In cats, the prepatent period from the ingestion of cysts to oocyst production varies, ranging from 3 to 10 days after ingestion of tissue cysts, from 19 to 48 days

after ingestion of tachyzoites [25], and from 21 to 40 days after ingestion of oocysts [26].

Gametocytes appear throughout the small intestine from 3 to 15 days after infection. After zygote and oocyst formation, no further development occurs within the gut of the cat. Oocysts pass out of the gut with the feces; peak oocyst production occurs between days 5 and 8. Oocysts are shed in the feces for periods that range from 7 to 20 days. As many as 10 million oocysts may be shed in the feces in a single day. The fully sporulated oocyst is infective when ingested, giving rise to the extraintestinal forms. Within the cat, it also can give rise to the enteroepithelial cycle. Depending on the temperature and availability of oxygen, sporulation occurs in 1 to 21 days [27,28]. Sporulation takes place in 2 to 3 days at 24° C, 5 to 8 days at 15° C, and 14 to 21 days at 11° C [29]. Oocysts do not sporulate below 4° C or above 37° C [27].

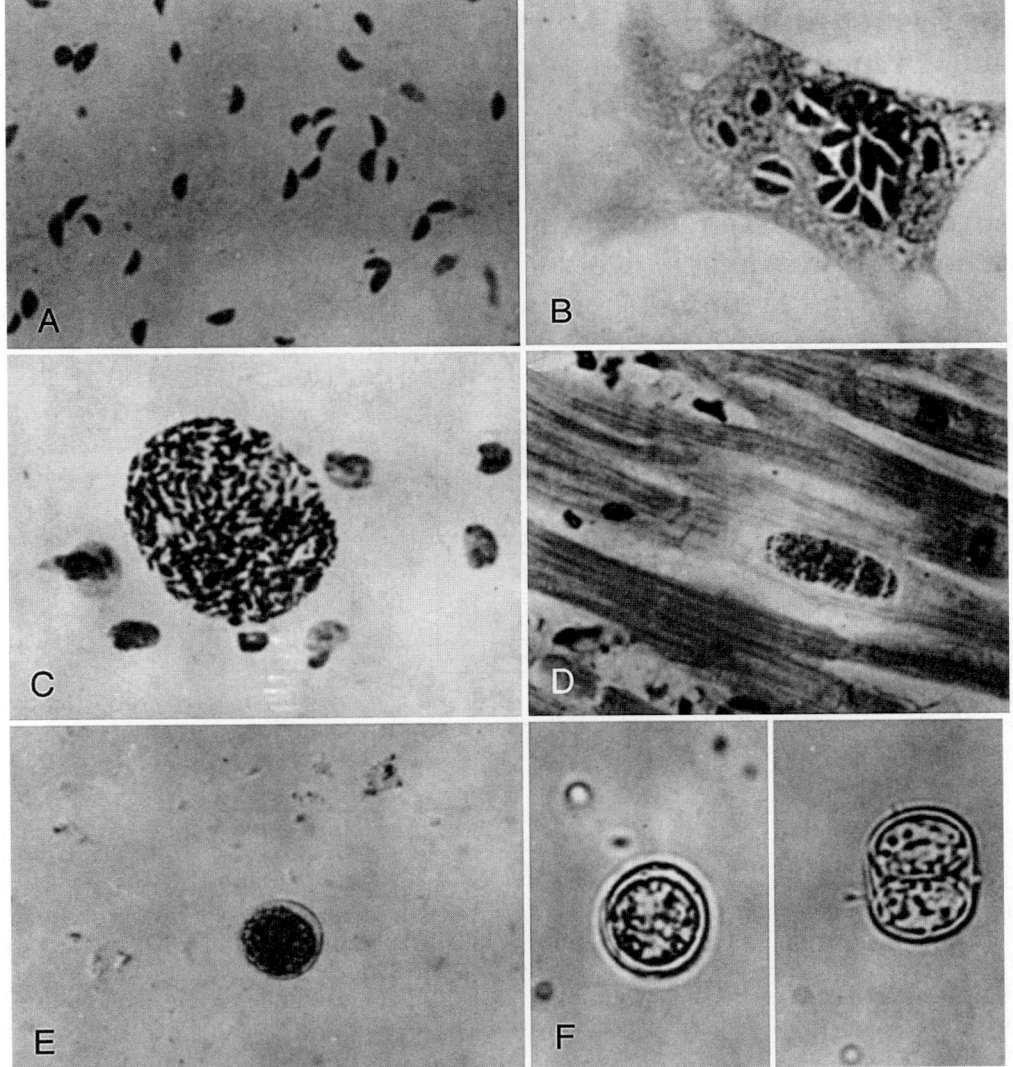

FIGURE 31–1 **The three forms of *Toxoplasma*. A**, Tachyzoites from peritoneal fluid of a 3-day infected mouse. **B**, Tachyzoite in cytoplasm of chick embryo fibroblast. **C**, Cyst in brain stained with periodic acid-Schiff. **D**, Cyst in myocardium of fatal human case. **E**, Microisolated cyst from brain in mouse. **F**, Unsporulated (left) and sporulated (right) oocysts. *(From Remington JS. Toxoplasmosis. In Kelly V [ed]. Brennemann's Practice of Pediatrics, vol 2. New York, Harper & Row, 1970.)*

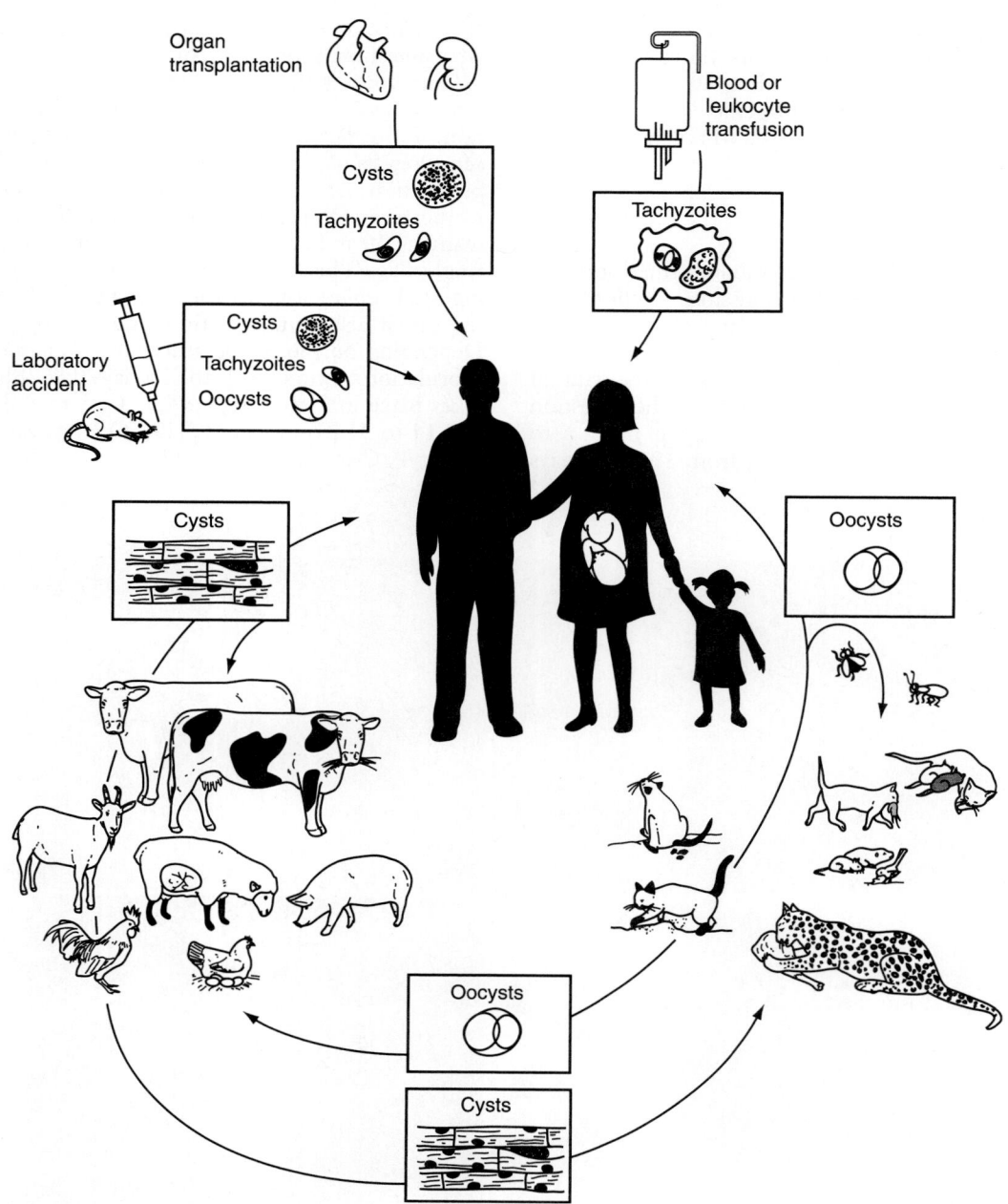

FIGURE 31–2 The life cycle of *Toxoplasma gondii*. The cat appears to be the definitive host. *(From Remington JS, McLeod R. Toxoplasmosis. In Braude AI [ed]. International Textbook of Medicine, vol II. Medical Microbiology and Infectious Disease. Philadelphia, WB Saunders, 1981.)*

TACHYZOITE

Tachyzoites are crescentic or oval, with one end attenuated (pointed) and the other end rounded (see Fig. 31–1, *A* and *B*); they are 2 to 4 μm wide and 4 to 8 μm long. The organisms stain well with either Wright or Giemsa stain. This form of the organism is employed in serologic tests (e.g., Sabin-Feldman dye test, fluorescent antibody methods, agglutination test).

The tachyzoite form requires an intracellular habitat to survive and multiply. It cannot survive desiccation, freezing and thawing, or action of the digestive juices of the human stomach [30]. This form of the parasite is destroyed within a few minutes in gastric juice, but a relatively small proportion of parasites can survive in tryptic digestive fluid for at least 3 hours but not as long as 6 hours. The organism is propagated in the laboratory in the peritoneum of mice [31] and in tissue cultures of mammalian cells [32].

The tachyzoites occur within vacuoles [33] in their host cells (see Fig. 31–1, *B*), and a definite space and an intravacuolar network are present between the parasite and the vacuole wall [34]. Host cell mitochondria and endoplasmic reticulum are concentrated in the host cell at the edge of the vacuole [35]. Reproduction in the tissues is by endodyogeny [36]. This is a process of internal budding in which two daughter cells are formed within the parent cell and are released with disruption of the parent cell. When additional nuclear divisions occur before the daughter organisms are completely separated, rosettes are formed; repeated endodyogeny results in a large collection of parasites within a cell.

The tachyzoite form is seen in the acute stage of the infection, during which it invades every kind of mammalian cell (see "Pathology," section). After host cell invasion, the organisms multiply within their vacuoles approximately every 4 to 6 hours and form rosettes. The cytoplasm becomes so filled with tachyzoites that ultimately the cell is disrupted, releasing organisms that then invade contiguous cells [37–39] or are phagocytosed [40]. Colonies of pseudocysts containing tachyzoites produced by endodyogeny may persist within host cells for prolonged periods without forming a true cyst. The duration of this type of infection *in vivo* is not known.

CYST

The tissue cyst (see Fig. 31–1, *C* and *D*) is formed within the host cell and may vary in size, ranging from cysts that contain only a few organisms to large cysts, 200 μm in size, that contain approximately 3000 organisms [41]. This form of *T. gondii* stains well with periodic acid-Schiff (PAS) stain, which causes it to stand out from the background tissue. The cyst wall is argyrophilic and weakly positive for PAS staining. Such cysts are demonstrable as early as the first week of infection in animals [42] and probably persist containing their viable parasites throughout the life of the host [25]. Although they may exist in virtually every organ, the brain and skeletal and heart muscles (see Fig. 31–1, *C* and *D*) appear to be the most common sites of latent infection [43]. Cysts are spherical in the brain and conform to the shape of muscle fibers in heart and skeletal muscles (see Fig. 31–1, *D*). Because of this persistence in tissues, the demonstration of cysts in histologic sections does not necessarily mean that the infection was recently acquired.

The cyst wall is disrupted by peptic or tryptic digestion, and the liberated parasites remain viable for at least 2 hours in pepsin-hydrochloric acid and for as long as 6 hours in trypsin [30], thereby allowing them to survive the normal digestive period in the stomach and even longer in the duodenum. In the presence of tissue, the liberated organisms remain viable for 3 hours in peptic digestive fluid and for at least 6 hours in tryptic digestive fluid. Freezing and thawing, heating above 66° C, and desiccation destroy this tissue cyst form; however, the organisms can survive as long as 2 months at 4° C [30]. Tissue cysts are rendered nonviable when internal temperatures have reached 68°C or −208°C [44]. Until more data are available, it appears that freezing at −20° C for 18 to 24 hours, followed by thawing, should be considered adequate for cyst destruction [30,45,46].

Like the tachyzoite, the cyst develops within a host cell vacuole [47,48]. Cysts may attain a relatively enormous size while still within the host cell. Tissue cysts in the brain are preferentially located within neurons and are retained within viable host cells irrespective of size or age [49]. This would explain the long-term survival of latent infection because the intracellular location could provide the minimal metabolic requirements of the resting stage (bradyzoite) [49]. A number of factors lead to bradyzoite differentiation and cyst formation, including arginine starvation, alkaline or acidic pH, and interferon-γ (IFN-γ) stimulation of inducible nitric oxide synthase (iNOS) and nitric oxide [50–52]. Cysts can form in tissue culture systems devoid of antibody and complement [53–55]. Immunity is of prime importance in regard to the presence of the different forms of the parasite during the extraintestinal cycle in the infected host. During the acute, initial state of the infection, parasites are present mainly as tachyzoites, which are responsible for parasitemia and systemic infection. When the host has developed an immune response, the infection usually reaches a latent or chronic stage, during which cysts are present in many tissues, and in the immunocompetent host, parasitemia and systemic infection with tachyzoites have subsided. These schematic definitions of the stages of the infection are important to the later discussion on congenital transmission. These two stages were defined by Frenkel and Friedlander in 1952 [56] as the first and third stages of *T. gondii* infection. They also described a second, subacute stage as a hypothesis to explain the pathogenesis of lesions observed in congenital toxoplasmosis. The existence of an intermediate stage of uncertain duration also seems likely in cases with subclinical infection, during which both encysted parasites and low-grade systemic infection with tachyzoites are present in the immune host. Whether "dormant" tachyzoites are present during chronic infection in addition to tissue cysts is not known.

Transmission

Congenital transmission of *T. gondii* from an infected mother to her fetus was the first form of transmission to be recognized [4]. Investigators in the reported cases raised two hypotheses in an attempt to explain congenital transmission. They considered that transmission might occur as a consequence of the acute, initial stage of the infection in a pregnant woman or as a consequence of a recrudescence (either local or systemic with recurrent parasitemia) of a chronic (latent) maternal infection during pregnancy.

Experimental studies of congenital infections in different animal species were helpful for understanding this form of transmission, but definitive data were not obtained until prospective studies were performed in humans in nations such as Austria, where screening for the diagnosis of *T. gondii* infection among pregnant women is routinely performed, and France, where screening is compulsory.

Congenital Transmission

The excellent correlation between isolation of *T. gondii* from placental tissue and infection of the neonate, along with results obtained at autopsy of neonates with congenital toxoplasmosis suggesting that the infection is acquired by the fetus *in utero* through the bloodstream, has led to the concept that infection of the placenta is an obligatory step between maternal and fetal infection. A likely scenario is that organisms reach the placenta during parasitemia in the mother. They then invade and multiply within cells of the placenta, and eventually some gain access to the fetal circulation.

Maternal Parasitemia

Acute Infection. From pathology studies in patients with toxoplasmosis, and from experiments in animals, it can be concluded that parasitemia occurs during the acute, initial stage of both subclinical and symptomatic infections. In an attempt to define the magnitude and duration of the parasitemia during subclinical infection, inoculation of mice was performed with clots of blood taken from women with recent subclinical infections (Desmonts G, unpublished data); these were the first seropositive blood samples obtained from pregnant women who were previously seronegative and who had been tested repeatedly during pregnancy. Approximately 50 patients were examined, and none of the samples were found to be seropositive. Because this method has proved to be valuable for isolation of *T. gondii* from patients with congenital toxoplasmosis (Table 31–1) and from newborns with subclinical infections, the absence of demonstrable organisms in these women suggests that parasitemia during the acute stage of acquired subclinical infection is no longer present, at least by the method employed, once serum antibodies are detectable. Attempts at isolation of *T. gondii* from blood of more than 30 patients with toxoplasmic lymphadenopathy were unsuccessful (Remington JS, unpublished data).

If it is accepted that transmission of *T. gondii* from a mother to her fetus reflects that parasitemia occurred in the mother, evidence indicates that parasitemia occurs at an early stage of the mother's infection before the appearance of serum antibodies [57] and clinical signs (if signs occur). We have observed this in several cases of acquired toxoplasmosis in pregnant women in whom lymphadenopathy appeared during the first month after they had been delivered of newborns with congenital *T. gondii* infection. Precise data are not available on the timing of events that occur after initial infection in humans. The delay between initial infection and occurrence of parasitemia is not known. Important considerations include the duration of parasitemia during the initial stage of the infection and the actual time between the initial infection and the earliest appearance of demonstrable specific antibodies.

TABLE 31–1 Parasitemia in Clinical Forms of Congenital Toxoplasmosis*

Clinical Form	No. of Infants	No. with Parasitemia (%)
Generalized	21	15 (71)
Neurologic or ocular	29	5 (17)
Subclinical	19	10 (52)
Total	69	30 (43)

Infants were studied during the first 2 months of life, but no infants had detectable parasitemia after 4 weeks of age.
Adapted from Desmonts G, Couvreur J. Toxoplasmosis: epidemiologic and serologic aspects of perinatal infection. In Krugman S, Gershon AA (eds). Infections of the Fetus and the Newborn Infant. Progress in Clinical and Biological Research, vol 3, New York, Alan R Liss, 1975, with permission.

Chronic Infection (Persistent or Recurrent Parasitemia). A systematic search for persistent parasitemia in humans, especially during pregnancy, has not been reported. Nevertheless, one case report bearing on this subject is pertinent here. Persistent parasitemia was evident in a clinically asymptomatic, otherwise healthy, 19-year-old primigravid woman during 14 months after she gave birth to a congenitally infected infant who died during delivery [58]. This parasitemia persisted despite treatment with pyrimethamine and sulfadiazine. During the period of parasitemia, the patient again became pregnant; the result of this second pregnancy was a healthy baby with no evidence of congenital toxoplasmosis. This case of persistent parasitemia is unique in our experience.

Huldt (Huldt G, personal communication to Remington JS, 1987) isolated *T. gondii* from the blood of an elderly but otherwise healthy woman 1 year after clinical lymphadenopathy. In another case, a woman 60 years of age with a suspected lymphoma had detectable parasitemia on several occasions during a period of 2 years. As has been observed in normal laboratory animals, parasitemia may be observed during chronic infection in the immunodeficient patient despite the presence of neutralizing antibodies in the serum [59].

Demonstration of *Toxoplasma gondii* in Placentas

Histologic Demonstration. *T. gondii* organisms have been demonstrated histologically in human placentas [60–63]. (See also "Placenta" section under "Pathology.")

In 1967, Sarrut reported histologic findings in the placentas of eight patients with congenital toxoplasmosis, with microscopic demonstration of the organism in four of them [64]. She noted a correlation between the clinical pattern of neonatal disease and the presence of histologically demonstrable parasites. Both cysts and tachyzoites were numerous and easily demonstrated in three patients with severe systemic fetal disease, whereas parasites were microscopically demonstrable in only one of five patients (see also under "Pathology") with milder disease. Parasites were not noted in cases in which clinical signs of the infection were delayed until weeks after birth. On the contrary, results following injection of placental tissue into mice were positive in patients with congenital toxoplasmosis, and in those with subclinical infection [65].

Isolation Studies

***Toxoplasma gondii* in Placentas During Acute Infection.** From the original studies performed in France in the 1960s, it was concluded that *T. gondii* frequently could be isolated from the placenta when acute infection occurred during pregnancy, but that such isolation was rarely if ever possible when infection occurred before conception [66]. This was true even for women with high antibody titers at the beginning of pregnancy, which suggested that infection might have been acquired shortly before conception. Similar results were obtained by Aspöck and colleagues [67]. These authors examined 2451 women who had decided on termination of their pregnancy. Of these women, 1139 (46%) were seropositive and 77 (3%) had a *T. gondii* indirect fluorescent antibody test titer of 1:256 or higher. The researchers injected the products of conception of 51 of these 77 women into mice. None of the results were positive. Because the researchers had used the whole product of conception after induced abortion, this negative result suggests that this conclusion—that placental infection is seldom if ever present at the time of delivery in women with high antibody titers at the beginning of pregnancy—might also be true for decidua, embryos, and placental tissues obtained early in pregnancy from such women.

When infection is acquired during pregnancy, the frequency of isolation of *T. gondii* from placentas obtained at the time of delivery is dependent on when seroconversion occurred during pregnancy. Table 31–2 shows the results obtained in 321 such cases. The frequency of positive isolation depended on the trimester of pregnancy in which maternal infection was acquired: the later it was acquired, the more frequently were parasites isolated. The frequency of isolation also depended on whether the women received treatment. Organisms were isolated less often if spiramycin was administered before delivery. These data were collected in the 1960s and 1970s during surveys carried out by Desmonts and Couvreur [68], which were feasibility studies of measures for prevention of congenital toxoplasmosis. The measures became compulsory in France in 1978. For many years (in the laboratory of one of us [GD]), placental tissue of women considered to be at risk of giving birth to a child with congenital *T. gondii* infection was routinely injected into mice for attempts at isolation of the parasite. (The number of placental inoculations performed in the Laboratoire de Serologie Neonatale et de Recherche sur la Toxoplasmose, Institut de Puériculture de Paris, averaged 800 per year.) The results support the conclusions of the initial surveys: *T. gondii* organisms frequently were present in the placenta on delivery when the acute infection occurred during pregnancy; the later the infection was acquired, the more frequently the placenta was involved. When infection occurred during the last few weeks of pregnancy, placental infection was demonstrable in more than 80% of cases.

A virtually perfect correlation was observed between neonatal and placental infection (see "Diagnosis" section) when the mother did not receive treatment during gestation or duration of the treatment was too brief or an inadequate dose of spiramycin (less than 3 g) was used [69]. Among 85 pregnancies ending in delivery of a child with congenital *T. gondii* infection, isolation of *T. gondii* from placental tissue was successful in 76 of 85 cases (89%). If the fact that only a relatively small portion of the placenta was digested for the inoculation into mice is taken into account, the high proportion of positive results supports the concept that placental infection is an obligatory occurrence between maternal and fetal infection. It also demonstrates that if the mother receives no or inadequate treatment, placental infection persists until delivery. Nevertheless, placental infection may not be demonstrable by mouse inoculation on delivery of a child with congenital *Toxoplasma* infection when the mother received treatment during pregnancy. In the series of cases reported by Couvreur and colleagues [69], the proportion of placentas from which *T. gondii* was isolated was 89 of 118 (75%) if the mothers had received treatment for more than 15 days with 3 g per day of spiramycin. This proportion was 10 of 20 (50%) if pyrimethamine plus sulfonamides was added to treatment during the last months of pregnancy.

***Toxoplasma gondii* in Placentas During Chronic Infection.** A study was performed by Remington and colleagues (in collaboration with Beverly Koops) in Palo Alto, Calif., to determine whether *T. gondii* can be isolated from placentas of women with stable dye test titers. Of the 499 placentas obtained consecutively, 112 (22%) were from women with positive dye test results. The digestion procedure (see "Isolation Procedures" later under "Diagnosis") was performed on 101 of these placentas. *T. gondii* organisms were not isolated from any of them. Thus in the population studied, chronic (latent) infection with *T. gondii* does not appear to involve the placenta significantly. By contrast, *T. gondii* has been isolated with relative ease from the adult human brain [43], skeletal muscle [43], and uterus [70].

Another study in which an attempt was made to isolate the organism from placental tissue is that of Ruiz and associates in Costa Rica [71]. Much smaller amounts of tissue were injected into mice, but isolation was successful in 1 of 100 placentas. The dye test titer in the mother from whose placenta the organism was isolated was 1:1024. Adequate clinical and serologic data for the offspring were not provided. The researchers stated that

TABLE 31–2 Attempts to Isolate *Toxoplasma** from Placenta at Delivery in Women Who Acquired *Toxoplasma* Infection During Pregnancy

Maternal Treatment During Pregnancy	Infection Acquired During First Trimester		Infection Acquired During Second Trimester		Infection Acquired During Third Trimester		Total	
	No. Examined	No. Positive (%)	No. Examined	No. Positive (%)	No. Examined	No. Positive (%)	No. Examined	No. Positive (%)
None	16	4 (25)	13	7 (54)	23	15 (65)	52	26 (50)
Spiramycin	89	7 (8)	144	28 (19)	36	16 (44)	269	51 (19)
Total	105	11 (10)	157	35 (22)	59	31 (53)	321	77 (24)

*By mouse inoculation.
Adapted from Desmonts G, Couvreur J. Congenital toxoplasmosis: a prospective study of the offspring of 542 women who acquired toxoplasmosis during pregnancy: pathophysiology of congenital disease. In Thalhammer O, Baumgarten K, Pollak A (eds). Perinatal Medicine, Sixth European Congress, Vienna. Stuttgart, Germany, Georg Thieme, 1979, with permission.

T. gondii organisms were not demonstrable in the placental tissue by microscopic examination. This finding is not surprising in view of the findings of Sarrut [64]. The high dye test titer in this case might have been due to an infection acquired during pregnancy. Ruoss and Bourne failed to isolate *T. gondii* from 677 placentas of mothers who were delivered of viable infants and who had low *T. gondii* antibody titers [72]. It can be concluded from these studies that placental infection is extremely rare in pregnant women with chronic *T. gondii* infection.

Fetal *Toxoplasma gondii* Infection and Congenital Toxoplasmosis

Acute Infection in the Mother. Direct data that demonstrate the frequency with which *T. gondii* is transmitted to the fetus during the period of acute infection in the mother come from prospective studies such as those performed by Desmonts and Couvreur [66], Kräubig [73], Kimball and colleagues [74], and Stray-Pedersen [75]. Fetal infection, the consequence of placental infection, depends on the time during gestation when maternal infection was acquired. Table 31–3 (which summarizes findings from the same group of cases as in Table 31–2, although the number of cases in both tables is not the same because placentas were available in only 321 of the 542 pregnancies) shows data collected in the 1960s and 1970s by Couvreur and Desmonts. In Table 31–4, children are classified into five groups: those with no congenital infection, subclinical congenital infection, mild congenital toxoplasmosis, severe congenital toxoplasmosis, and stillbirth or early death (shortly after birth). Children were considered to be free of congenital infection if they had no clinical manifestations suggesting congenital toxoplasmosis and if their results on *T. gondii* serologic testing became negative after disappearance of passively transmitted maternal antibodies. Congenital infection was classified as subclinical if no clinical signs of disease related to toxoplasmosis occurred during infancy. Clinical

TABLE 31–4 Frequency of Stillbirth, Clinical Congenital Toxoplasmosis, and Subclinical Infection Among Offspring of 500 Women Who Acquired *Toxoplasma* Infection During Pregnancy*

Outcome in Offspring	No. of Affected Infants (%) born to mothers whose:		
	Infection Acquired During First Trimester	Infection Acquired During Second Trimester	Infection Acquired During Third Trimester
No congenital *Toxoplasma* infection	109 (86)	173 (71)	52 (41)
Congenital toxoplasmosis			
Subclinical	3 (2)	49 (20)	68 (53)
Mild	1 (1)	13 (5)	8 (6)
Severe	7 (6)	6 (2)	0 (0)
Stillbirth or perinatal death[†]	6 (5)	5 (2)	0 (0)
Total	126 (100)	246 (100)	128 (100)

*Forty-two pregnancies are not included from Table 31–3 because it was not possible to ascertain the trimester during which infection occurred in the mother.
[†]See text.
Adapted from Desmonts G, Couvreur J. Congenital toxoplasmosis: a prospective study of the offspring of 542 women who acquired toxoplasmosis during pregnancy: pathophysiology of congenital disease. In Thalhammer O, Baumgarten K, Pollak A (eds). Perinatal Medicine, Sixth European Congress, Vienna. Stuttgart, Germany, Georg Thieme, 1979, with permission.

disease was considered to be mild if the infant was apparently normal, with normal development on follow-up evaluation. An example of mild disease is that of a child with no mental retardation or neurologic disorder on later examination but with isolated retinal scars discovered during a prospective eye examination (or, in one case, isolated intracranial calcifications on radiographic examination) performed because the child was at risk of having congenital *T. gondii* infection, having been born to a mother who acquired the infection during gestation. Cases were considered to be severe if both chorioretinitis and intracranial calcifications were present or if mental retardation or neurologic disorders were present. From the results shown in Table 31–3, the subclinical form was by far the most frequent presentation of congenital *T. gondii* infection; severe cases with survival of the fetus were infrequent.

In 500 pregnancies, it was possible to ascertain the trimester during which *T. gondii* infection had been acquired (See Table 31–4). *T. gondii* infection occurred in the fetus or was present in the newborn in 14%, 29%, and 59% of cases of maternal infection acquired during the first, second, and third trimesters, respectively. The proportion of cases of congenital toxoplasmosis was higher in the first- and second-trimester groups than in the third-trimester group. This was especially true for severe congenital toxoplasmosis (including cases with stillbirths, perinatal deaths, or severe neonatal disease). No case of severe toxoplasmosis was observed among the 76 offspring of mothers who had acquired *T. gondii* infection during their third trimester. Approach to detection and management of infection acquired during gestation determines and can modify severity of infection detected in

TABLE 31–3 Outcome of 542 Pregnancies in Which Maternal *Toxoplasma* Infection Was Acquired During Gestation: Incidence of Congenital Toxoplasmosis and Effect of Spiramycin Treatment in Mother During Pregnancy

Outcome in Offspring	No. of Affected Infants (%)	
	No Treatment	Treatment
No congenital *Toxoplasma* infection	60 (39)	297 (77)
Congenital toxoplasmosis		
Subclinical	64 (41)	65 (17)
Mild	14 (9)	13 (3)
Severe	7 (5)	10 (2)
Stillbirth or perinatal death*	9 (6)	3 (1)
Total	154 (100)	388 (100)

*See text.
Adapted from Desmonts G, Couvreur J. Congenital toxoplasmosis: a prospective study of the offspring of 542 women who acquired toxoplasmosis during pregnancy: pathophysiology of congenital disease. In Thalhammer O, Baumgarten K, Pollak A (eds). Perinatal Medicine, Sixth European Congress, Vienna. Stuttgart, Germany, Georg Thieme, 1979, with permission.

TABLE 31-5 Severity of Manifestations of Congenital Toxoplasmosis in Paris Before (1949–1960) and After (1984–1992) Introduction of Serologic Screening and Treatment Programs

Period	No. of Newborns	No. of Affected Infants (%)			
		CNS Disease	Hydrocephalus	Retinitis/Scar	Subclinical
1949 to 1960	147	93 (63%)	62 (67% of 93)	54 (33%)	0
1984 to 1992	234	8 (3%)*	—*	60 (26%)	166 (71%)

*Severe ocular or neurologic disease occurred only when infants were born to mothers from foreign countries where there was no screening during pregnancy (e.g., Morocco, Algeria, United Kingdom), they were not screened, or mothers were immunodeficient or erroneously considered immune. It also is noteworthy that in one hospital in France, in 1957, among 1085 premature infants, 7 had toxoplasmosis, whereas in this same hospital between 1980 and 1990, among approximately 10,000 premature infants, 2 had toxoplasmosis.
CNS, central nervous system.

infants and their later outcomes [76–79]. Of interest, after systematic serologic screening and treatment for *T. gondii* infection acquired in gestation was introduced in France in 1978, the frequency of severe toxoplasmosis diagnosed in newborns diminished remarkably (Table 31–5). This is discussed in more detail under "Effects of Systematic Screening of Pregnant Women at Risk on the Prevalence of Congenital *Toxoplasma gondii* Infection and of Congenital Toxoplasmosis."

Experience acquired since 1978 [80–83] has confirmed these earlier findings: Transmission of the parasite to the fetus was dependent on the time of acquisition of maternal infection during pregnancy. The proportion of cases that resulted in congenital *T. gondii* infection was very low if maternal infection was acquired during the first few weeks after conception. The later the maternal infection was acquired, the more frequent was transmission to the fetus. The frequency of congenital infection was 80% or higher if maternal infection was acquired during the last few weeks before delivery and if it was not treated. Table 31–6 shows the frequency of transmission by gestational age observed in a group of 930 women with acute *Toxoplasma* infection acquired during pregnancy who were referred to the Institut de Puériculture in Paris for prenatal diagnosis. The incidence of transmission rose from 1.2% when maternal infection occurred around the time of conception to 75% when it occurred close to term. These data were updated by Hohlfeld and coworkers [77], whose report includes the 2632 pregnant women for whom a prenatal diagnosis was performed between 1983 and 1992 (Table 31–7). The observed

TABLE 31-7 Incidence of Congenital *Toxoplasma gondii* Infection by Gestational Age at Time of Maternal Infection*

Week of Gestation	Infected Fetuses/Total No. Fetuses	Incidence (%)
0–2	0/100	0
3–6	6/384	1.6
7–10	9/503	1.8
11–14	37/511	7.2
15–18	49/392	13
19–22	44/237	19
23–26	30/116	26
27–30	7/32	22
31–34	4/6	67
Unknown	8/351	
Total	194/2632	7.4

*Maternal infection was treated with spiramycin in a dose of 9 million IU (3 g) daily.
Adapted from Hohlfeld P, et al. Prenatal diagnosis of congenital toxoplasmosis with polymerase-chain-reaction test on amniotic fluid. N Engl J Med 331:695–699, 1994.

TABLE 31-6 Fetal *Toxoplasma* Infection as a Function of Duration of Pregnancy*

Time of Maternal Infection	No. of Women	% Infected
Periconception	182	1.2
6–16 wk	503	4.5
17–20 wk	116	17.3
21–35 wk	88	28.9
Close to term	41	75

*Women were treated during gestation as soon as feasible after diagnosis of the acute acquired infection was established or strongly suspected. If prenatal diagnosis was made in the fetus, treatment was with pyrimethamine-sulfadiazine; otherwise it was spiramycin.
Adapted from Forestier F. Fetal diseases, prenatal diagnosis and practical measures. Presse Med 20:1448–1454, 1991, with permission.

incidence of transmission rose from 0% when maternal infection was acquired before week 2 of pregnancy to 67% when it was acquired between weeks 31 and 34. The incidence of transmission remained very low, less than 2%, when maternal infection was acquired during the first 10 weeks of gestation. It rose sharply when maternal infection was acquired during weeks 15 to 34.

To appropriately interpret the data provided by Hohlfeld and coworkers, a number of points deserve discussion. Their patients were referred to the Institut de Puériculture for prenatal diagnosis. Thus cases with fetal death in utero before the time of amniocentesis were not included. The consequence is that the incidence of congenital infection when maternal infection occurred during the first few weeks of pregnancy is slightly underestimated. For example, when Daffos and colleagues reported the first 746 cases from this same series, they [82] estimated the incidence of transmission to be 0.6% among 159 women with "periconceptional infection" and 3.7% among 487 women whose infection was acquired between weeks 6 and 16 of gestation. The observed incidence rates were 1.8% and 4.7%, respectively, if those fetuses that died in utero because of congenital toxoplasmosis before the time of blood sampling were included in the report. Another consequence of the recruitment of the cases reported by Hohlfeld and coworkers is that the number of cases with acquired maternal infection after week 26 of gestation is small because maternal infection acquired late during pregnancy was not discovered early enough to allow for performance of a prenatal diagnosis. The incidence of congenital infection was reported to be 194 of 2632 (7.4%). If, however, one excludes 100 cases of maternal infection acquired before week 2, and 351 in which gestational age at the time of maternal infection was unknown, the distribution of cases would be as follows: maternal infection acquired at gestational age 3 to 14 weeks, 1398 cases; 15 to 26 weeks, 745 cases; and 27 to 34 weeks, 38 cases. Most of the cases studied by Hohlfeld and coworkers occurred in women who acquired infection early in pregnancy. If cases of maternal acquired infection had been equally distributed through each of the weeks of gestation, from weeks 3 to 34, the adjusted mean transmission rate would have been 19.5%. The transmission rate observed by Jenum and associates in Norway [84] was 11 of 47 (23%).

A higher transmission rate, 65 of 190 (34%), was observed in a series of 190 consecutive cases of maternal acute *Toxoplasma* infection, each of whose sera was examined in a single laboratory in Paris (Thulliez P, personal communication to Desmonts G, 1999). These cases were more equally distributed in regard to gestational age at time of infection. The incidence rates of congenital infection in this series of 190 women were as follows: 4 to 16 weeks, 5 of 44 (11%); 17 to 28 weeks, 15 of 71 (21%); and 29 to 40 weeks, 45 of 75 (60%). In another series, reported by Dunn and associates [83], the mean rate of transmission was 29% in 603 cases studied in Lyon between 1987 and 1995.

A critical point to remember in reviewing the data obtained in the European countries where screening for *Toxoplasma* infection during pregnancy is routinely performed is that most patients are treated during pregnancy, which probably reduces the incidence of transmission of the parasite. The frequency of congenital toxoplasmosis (i.e., of fetal lesions or of clinical manifestations in the infant with congenital infection) also is highly dependent on the time of acquisition of maternal infection during pregnancy. The earlier maternal infection was acquired, the higher was the prevalence of fetal or neonatal disease among infants with congenital *T. gondii* infection.

A number of observations suggest that *T. gondii* may be present in the placenta but is transmitted to the previously uninfected fetus only after a delay. This delay has been termed the prenatal incubation period by Thalhammer [85,86]. Placental infection is a potential source of infection of the infant even long after maternal parasitemia has subsided. This has been documented in studies in which, after induced abortions, samples of fetal tissues and placentas were injected into mice in an attempt to isolate *T. gondii*. Table 31–8 shows the results obtained in 177 such cases in which no attempt at prenatal diagnosis of fetal infection had been made. Isolation attempts were successful from placentas in 10 cases (6%). In 8 of the 10 cases, placental and fetal tissues were injected separately and *T. gondii* organisms were isolated solely from the placentas and not from the fetus in four of those eight cases. The fetuses were not infected at the time the pregnancies were

TABLE 31–8 Isolation of *Toxoplasma* from Placental and Fetal Tissue after Termination of Pregnancy in 177 Women Who Acquired Infection Just Before or During Gestation

Maternal infection category I*	
No. of cases	115
No. of positive isolations	10 (9%)†
Maternal infection category II*	
No. of cases	62
No. of positive isolations	0

*Category I: Toxoplasma *infection was proved to have been acquired during pregnancy;* Category II: Toxoplasma *infection was noted to have been recently acquired; it occurred either before or soon after conception as judged by serologic test results obtained at the time of first examination, when patients were in their fourth to eighth week of gestation. No attempt at prenatal diagnosis was made in any of the cases.*
†Toxoplasma *was isolated in two cases from mixed placental and fetal tissues after curettage, in four cases from both placenta and fetal tissues injected separately, and in four cases solely from the placenta.*
Adapted from Desmonts G, et al. Prenatal diagnosis of congenital toxoplasmosis. Lancet 1:500–504, 1985, with permission.

terminated. In one of these cases, pregnancy was terminated at week 21 in a woman who had acquired her infection shortly before the fourth week of gestation. This case demonstrates that delay between maternal and fetal infection may be longer than 16 weeks. In other cases, the delay may be much shorter. Among 22 pregnancies terminated because congenital *T. gondii* infection had been demonstrated in the fetus by prenatal diagnosis (see "Prenatal Diagnosis of Fetal *Toxoplasma gondii* Infection" in "Diagnosis" section) (data not included in Table 31–8), the time that elapsed between maternal and fetal infection evidently was less than 8 weeks in 2 cases, less than 6 weeks in 2 cases, and less than 4 weeks in 1 case. The case histories also suggested that the later during gestation maternal infection occurred, the shorter was the delay between maternal and fetal *T. gondii* infection (Table 31–9). The data of Daffos demonstrate that it is almost always first- and second-trimester infections that are associated with substantial brain necrosis and hydrocephalus [82]. Recent data reveal that the magnitude of fetal involvement correlates with the amount of parasite DNA in amniotic fluid (see "Polymerase Chain Reaction Assay" ["Diagnosis"] and "Prevention") [87].

The severity of the disease depends on the age of the fetus at the time of transmission (see Table 31–9). This is determined both by the time during pregnancy when

TABLE 31–9 Frequency of Findings in the Fetus Correlated with Gestational Age When Infection Was Acquired

Fetal Gestational Age (wk) When Infected	Frequency of Ultrasound Evidence* of Infection	Frequency (%) of Cerebral Ventricular Dilation
<16	31 (60%) of 52	48
17–23	16 (25%) of 63	12
>24	1 (3%) of 33	0

Ascites, pericarditis, necrotic foci on brain.
Data from Daffos F, et al. Letter to the editor. Lancet 344:541, 1994.

maternal infection occurs and by the duration of the delay between maternal infection and transmission to the fetus (prenatal incubation period). The earlier the fetus is infected, the more severe the disease in the newborn. The likelihood that transmission will occur early in fetal life is greater when the mother acquires her infection during the first or second trimester of pregnancy.

Results of examination of fetuses after induced abortion agree with these conclusions. Among the 177 cases in which pregnancies were terminated without any prior attempt at prenatal diagnosis (see Table 31–8), results of inoculation tests of fetal tissues were positive in 4 cases. In each of these 4, macroscopic lesions were evident on gross examination of the aborted fetus at autopsy. The same was true for 22 fetuses of women in whom the decision to terminate the pregnancy was made after fetal infection was demonstrated by isolation of *T. gondii* from amniotic fluid or from cord blood samples obtained in an attempt at prenatal diagnosis [82]. Each of these 22 fetuses had multiple necrotic foci in the brain, even when appearance on a previous ultrasound examination (performed before the pregnancy was terminated) was normal.

Transmission during the third trimester almost always results in either subclinical infection or mild congenital toxoplasmosis. Exceptions have been noted: In two cases (Desmonts G, unpublished observations) in which maternal infection was acquired after 30 weeks of gestation, the offspring had severe systemic disease and died in the newborn period.

By collecting data from pregnancies that resulted in birth of severely damaged infants, it was possible to define more precisely the weeks of pregnancy during which infection produces the greatest risk of severe congenital toxoplasmosis in the newborn infant. The period of highest risk was weeks 10 to 24 [80]. Although the incidence of transmission to the fetus is highest during weeks 26 to 40, it results in milder infection in the newborn. Weeks 1 to 10 constituted a low-risk period because transmission to the fetus was infrequent. Although infrequent, cases have been observed in which infection was acquired before week 7, or even shortly before conception, which resulted in the birth of severely damaged infants. The attempt at prenatal diagnosis by Daffos and associates [82] in 159 cases of periconceptional maternal infection (i.e., infections that, as judged by serologic test results, had been acquired at the time of conception or within a few weeks after conception) revealed fetal infection in only 1.8% of cases (see earlier). Thus in these circumstances, transmission of parasites is infrequent.

A question that is frequently asked when toxoplasmic lymphadenopathy is diagnosed in women of childbearing age or when serologic test results in a sample of serum drawn for routine testing very early in pregnancy suggest recently acquired *T. gondii* infection is as follows: How long before pregnancy is acquisition of *T. gondii* infection to be considered a risk factor for transmission of the parasite to the fetus in a future pregnancy? The answer is that if toxoplasmic lymphadenopathy was already present at the time of conception, and/or if two samples of serum, the first drawn before the eighth week of gestation and the second 3 weeks later, are examined in parallel and have identical IgG titers, the initial stage of the infection probably occurred before conception. The avidity test also is helpful in this setting because high-avidity IgG antibodies develop at least 12 to 16 weeks (depending on the test kit used) after acquisition of infection. Thus the presence of high-avidity antibodies indicates that infection was acquired more than 12 to 16 weeks earlier (see also later discussions of serodiagnosis and avidity assays) [88–90]. In these conditions, the risk for congenital *T. gondii* infection is extremely low. Unfortunately, accumulated data do not allow for a more definitive answer. Cases that demonstrate that the exception does occur have been reported. Of special interest are cases in which the diagnosis of toxoplasmic lymphadenopathy was well established before pregnancy occurred because they provide reliable information in regard to the timing of events (clinical signs in the mother, beginning of pregnancy, and the development of signs, if any, in the infant). A summary of the history of the first reported case [80,91] appeared in the third and fourth editions of this book [92,93]. Another case was reported by Marty and coworkers in 1991 [94], and a third was reported by Vogel and associates in 1996 [95]. The time elapsed between the occurrence of lymphadenopathy and conception was 2 months for the first case and 3 and 2 months, respectively, for the next two cases. The patient described by Marty and coworkers received spiramycin for 6 weeks at the time of lymphadenopathy; however, she did not receive treatment during pregnancy. Neither the first (studied by Desmonts) [93] nor the third (Vogel) mother received any treatment. In the three cases, no specific sign of congenital toxoplasmosis was recognized in the newborn (except possibly in the case reported by Marty and coworkers, in which slight splenomegaly was noted in the neonate). Strabismus was noted at the age of 3 months in the first case. None of the infants was given treatment before the diagnosis of congenital toxoplasmosis infection was established. Definitive diagnosis was made in two infants when obstructive hydrocephalus developed at the ages of 4 months and 9 months, respectively. In the case described by Marty and coworkers, infection was still subclinical when the diagnosis was made at the age of 8 months because of an increase in the antibody load (see the "Diagnosis" section).

The clinical patterns and the delayed antibody response observed in the infants are highly suggestive that transmission of the parasite to the fetuses occurred after maternal IgG had reached a significant level in the fetal blood (i.e., after 17 to 20 weeks of gestation), and probably later in the patient (described by Marty and coworkers) whose infection remained subclinical, despite absence of treatment before the eighth month of life.

These three cases demonstrate that infection in the 3 months before conception does not always confer effective immunity against congenital transmission. Transmission rarely occurs in these conditions, however. In our experience [80], no other example of congenital infection has arisen among several hundred cases in which toxoplasmic lymphadenopathy occurred before pregnancy. The advice given (by G Desmonts) was that patients infected in the 6 months before conception should be treated with spiramycin. This intervention possibly reduced the incidence of congenital infection among the offspring of these patients.

That fetal infection is rare when maternal acquisition of *T. gondii* infection has occurred even a short time before pregnancy is in agreement with the observation first made by Feldman and Miller [96], and amply confirmed since, that congenital infection does not occur in siblings (except twins) of a child with congenital toxoplasmosis. Several exceptions have been reported. In one instance described by Garcia, congenital *T. gondii* infection affected offspring of two successive pregnancies [60]. The first infant, delivered by cesarean section for fetal distress at the seventh month of gestation, died at 24 hours with multiple organ involvement with *T. gondii*. About 5 months after delivery of this infant, the mother again became pregnant. This pregnancy ended in spontaneous abortion of a macerated fetus at about the sixth month of gestation. Microscopic examination revealed *T. gondii* infection in both cases, in fetal and placental tissue. Although the proof rests solely on histologic findings, the data presented in these cases appear incontrovertible. Silveira and colleagues [97] also reported that *T. gondii* had been transmitted from a Brazilian mother infected 20 years earlier. The mother had a chorioretinal macular scar and positive result on serologic tests for *T. gondii* infection over a 20-year period. She was without known immunocompromise and transmitted *T. gondii* to her fetus. Details of the evaluation for immunocompromise and clonal type of parasite were not available (Silveira, personal communication to J Remington, 2003). Manifestations in the infant included IgG and IgM specific for *T. gondii*, a macular scar, and a cerebral calcification.

Two cases of transmission to the fetuses of women with subclinical infection acquired before pregnancy also have been published in France. Time of infection was well established in both cases because sera drawn before conception were available for comparison with the mandatory sample taken at the beginning of pregnancy [98,99]. In both cases, sera were negative for *T. gondii* antibodies 7 months before pregnancy and found to be positive, with a high but stable titer of IgG antibodies at 3 and 4 weeks of gestation, respectively. Thus infection had occurred about 1 to 2 months before conception in both cases. In both, prenatal diagnostic testing proved positive, and severe fetal lesions were demonstrated after termination of the pregnancies. Therefore, it is well established that the acute subclinical infection in a pregnant woman can result in fetal infection and congenital toxoplasmosis, even when acquired by the mother before conception.

Serologic screening tests for acute *T. gondii* infection during pregnancy usually are performed at weeks 8 to 12 of gestation. If the results suggest a recently acquired infection, it formerly was difficult, even with the help of a second sampling of serum 3 weeks later, to decide whether infection occurred before or after the time of conception (see "Diagnosis" section). These cases were classified as "periconceptional," and in our practice (Desmonts G) [91,100], these women were managed as if they had been infected during gestation (spiramycin treatment and prenatal diagnosis). The transmission rate observed after "periconceptional" infection was 3 of 161 (1.8%) [82]. With the availability of the avidity assay, acquisition can be more readily dated regarding whether it occurred before conception if the test is performed during the first 12 to 16 weeks of gestation.

It is apparent that the rate of transmission of the parasite from a woman to her fetus after the acute infection rises from virtually zero, when *T. gondii* infection was acquired several months (the exact number is unclear) before pregnancy, to about 2% (or slightly less), when acquired at about the time of conception. An important point is that the transmission rate remains low for several weeks (approximately 10) after the beginning of pregnancy. After the tenth week of gestation, a shift occurs from this low transmission rate toward a steeply increasing incidence of congenital infection in relation to the gestational age. This shift was observed in the 11- to 14-week gestational age group in the series reported by Hohlfeld and coworkers [77] and after week 13 in the series reported by Dunn and associates [83]. Several hypotheses might explain this shift from a low toward a steeply rising risk of transmission. One relies on a truism: Congenital toxoplasmosis is a fetopathy, resulting from a placental infection. Thus a placenta and a fetus are necessary for the disease to develop. Hence, congenital *T. gondii* infection, when resulting from an infection acquired by the mother before the formation of the placenta, is the consequence of a recurrent parasitemia. The incidence of transmission in this situation depends on the frequency of recurrent parasitemia in a woman whose cell-mediated immunity with regard to *Toxoplasma* has not yet fully developed (see the "Pathogenesis" section). When maternal infection is acquired later during pregnancy, the parasite can reach the placenta during the initial parasitemia, which occurs in the mother before the development of any immune response. This mode of transmission is more effective for colonization of the placenta by the parasite. The later the infection occurs in the fetus, however, the less severe the disease because immunologic maturation has had time to develop.

A summary of the data just presented is shown in Figure 31–3, in which percentages of risk are given, to suggest a range in magnitude and not necessarily exact data. It also should be noted that the data used in this figure were obtained from women almost all of whom received spiramycin treatment during pregnancy. Hence, the outcome in the fetuses may have been more severe, both for transmission rates and for severity of infection, if results from untreated pregnancies had been used.

Chronic Maternal *Toxoplasma* Infection. Data obtained in prospective studies have established that chronic (or latent) maternal infection, per se, is not a risk for congenital infection [96]. Also, as a rule, evidence of previous chronic (latent) infection signifies that the future mother is not at risk of giving birth to a child with congenital *T. gondii* infection. These observations constitute the basis for the preventive measures that have been adopted by and have proved effective in countries such as Austria and France [100–102].

However, several reports suggest that chronically infected but immunocompromised mothers may rarely transmit the infection to their fetus [91,103–105]. Four of the cases were reported from France. This is not surprising because such cases usually are observed only in countries where screening for *Toxoplasma* infection during pregnancy is performed routinely.

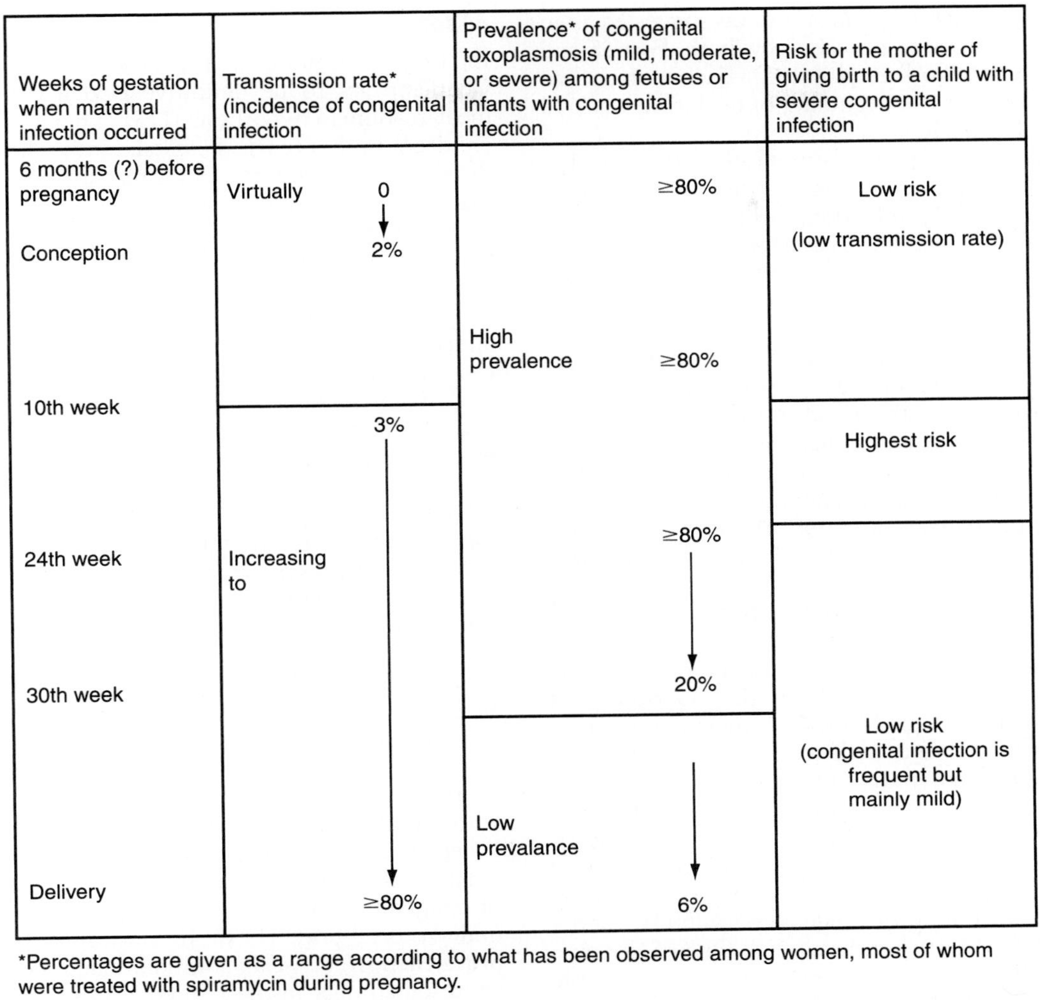

Weeks of gestation when maternal infection occurred	Transmission rate* (incidence of congenital infection)	Prevalence* of congenital toxoplasmosis (mild, moderate, or severe) among fetuses or infants with congenital infection	Risk for the mother of giving birth to a child with severe congenital infection
6 months (?) before pregnancy	Virtually 0	≥80%	Low risk
Conception	↓ 2%		(low transmission rate)
		High prevalence ≥80%	
10th week	3%		Highest risk
24th week	Increasing to	≥80%	
30th week		↓ 20%	Low risk (congenital infection is frequent but mainly mild)
		Low prevalance	
Delivery	↓ ≥80%	↓ 6%	

*Percentages are given as a range according to what has been observed among women, most of whom were treated with spiramycin during pregnancy.

FIGURE 31-3 Transmission rate and prevalence of congenital *Toxoplasma* infection or congenital toxoplasmosis among offspring of women with acute *Toxoplasma* infection in relation to gestational age at time of maternal infection.

A summary of the histories of the four cases follows: The women were known from previous pregnancies to have low and stable titers of IgG antibodies, which is characteristic of past infection and immunity. The same low titer of IgG was present at the beginning of the new pregnancy. Thus these women were considered to be immune, so that their fetus was judged not to be at risk. Treatment was therefore not given during gestation. Congenital *T. gondii* infection was demonstrated in each case: A subclinical infection was noted when the child was 12 months of age in one case (the history of which was published in previous editions of this book) [92,93]; spontaneous abortion occurred at 12 weeks of gestation, with demonstration of the parasite in fetal tissues in another case [103]; and congenital toxoplasmosis (chorioretinitis) was diagnosed at birth in the third case [104] and at 9 months of age in the fourth case [105]. In each of the four cases, a serologic relapse occurred during pregnancy, as evidenced by a significant increase in IgG antibodies that reached high titers in each woman. In three of the women, samples of sera drawn during pregnancy were available for retrospective examination. Of interest is that in these three cases, IgA

antibodies were present at the beginning of the serologic relapse. An IgM response was noted in only one woman. Serologic relapse had occurred between weeks 8 and 11 of gestation in the case ending in abortion and after weeks 10, 16, and 19, respectively, in the other three cases. Silveira and colleagues [97] also reported that *T. gondii* had been transmitted from a Brazilian mother infected 20 years earlier, as described.

Even if some cases have gone unpublished (Dr. Jacques Couvreur has data on two additional cases, as described in a personal communication to Desmonts G, 1999), the examples of offspring with congenital *T. gondii* infection born to mothers who, at the beginning of pregnancy, had serologic test results that established the presence of a chronic (latent) infection are exceptional. When this does occur, immunologic dysfunction must be suspected as having been the cause. The first case we observed [92,93] was that of a woman who had a low CD4+/CD8+ ratio associated with Hodgkin disease, from which she had recovered 2 years before becoming pregnant. She also previously underwent a splenectomy. No immunologic dysfunction was demonstrated in the other three women. Reinfection with oocysts of another *T. gondii* strain was suggested as an explanation for the cases observed by both Fortier and Gavinet and their coworkers [103,105]. Each woman had contact with kittens at the beginning of or during week 20 of gestation, respectively.

Transmission of *T. gondii* from mother to fetus has been observed in immunodeficient women owing to reactivation of the chronic infection, primarily in patients with AIDS (see "Congenital *Toxoplasma gondii* Infection and Acquired Immunodeficiency Syndrome" later, under "Clinical Manifestations"). It also has occurred as a consequence of other immunocompromised states that appear to have resulted in an active but subclinical infection in the chronically infected pregnant woman. One case was reported in the third and fourth editions of this book [92,93,106]. Two additional cases were published in 1990 [91], and a fourth in 1995 by d'Ercole and colleagues [107]. The immunologic dysfunction was associated with lupus erythematosus in three of the four patients and with pancytopenia in one. This last patient, and one of those with lupus, also previously had a splenectomy. Each of the four patients was given corticosteroids during gestation. Three [91] did not receive treatment for their *T. gondii* infection. The serologic evidence for (chronic) active infection was the unusually high IgG titers that had been present since childhood in two of the cases. One of these women gave birth to an infant with severe congenital toxoplasmosis that resulted in the death of the child at the age of 3 months. Congenital toxoplasmosis was diagnosed in the other case when chorioretinitis occurred in the infant at the age of 4 months. In one of the four mothers, the IgG titer rose from a relatively low titer at the beginning of pregnancy to 800 IU, and a weakly positive IgM test titer developed. One of her twin infants, a boy, died at the age of 9 days from toxoplasmic encephalomyelitis. His twin sister had subclinical congenital *T. gondii* infection.

The cases just described demonstrate conclusively that the presence of a chronic, yet active *T. gondii* infection in an immunocompromised pregnant woman results in a significant risk of congenital infection for the fetus and newborn. In addition to women with AIDS, this is especially true for women who must receive long-term treatment with corticosteroids during gestation [108]. Treatment of HIV infection in the woman chronically infected with *T. gondii* [109] also would be expected to substantially reduce or eliminate congenital *T. gondii* infection, although no data rigorously demonstrating this effect have been provided.

The significance of *T. gondii* infection as a cause of abortion has been a subject of considerable conjecture among workers in this field throughout the world [110,111]. A detailed review of this subject was presented in the first two editions of this book [92,112]; it is omitted from the present edition because no new data are available.

Transmission by Ingestion

Whether the mode of transmission consists of infective oocysts or meat that contains cysts, it appears that the natural route of transmission usually proceeds from animals (and contaminated soil or water) to humans by way of ingestion.

Meat

In 1965, Desmonts and colleagues in Paris published what appears to be definitive evidence in favor of the meat-to-human hypothesis [113]. They found that among children in a French hospital, antibodies to *T. gondii* developed at a rate five times that in the general population. Because it was the custom in this hospital to serve undercooked meat (mainly beef or horsemeat) as a therapeutic measure, these workers reasoned that this practice explained the higher incidence of infection among this hospitalized population. To test this hypothesis, they added undercooked mutton to the diet and observed that the yearly rate of acquisition of antibody to *T. gondii* doubled. Clinical signs of infection, mainly lymphadenopathy, developed in some of the children. Severe illness was not observed in any of them. Four years later, Kean and colleagues in New York reported a miniepidemic of toxoplasmosis in five medical students [114]. Epidemiologic evidence strongly implicated the ingestion of undercooked hamburgers, which the authors recognized might have been contaminated with mutton or pork, as the source of infection in these cases [115,116].

A number of isolated cases and recent miniepidemics of acute acquired *T. gondii* infection have been reported. Included were at least one case of congenital toxoplasmosis associated with consumption of undercooked venison or preparation of venison (McLeod R, personal observation), another that resulted in significant illness in adults who ingested undercooked lamb (Remington JS, unpublished data) [117], one in which undercooked kangaroo meat resulted in acute infection in 12 adults and a case of congenital toxoplasmosis [118], and another linked to undercooked pork [119]. In regard to venison, a high prevalence of *T. gondii* antibodies has been reported in white-tailed deer in the United States [120,121].

The prevalence rates in various countries indicate that the habits and customs of various populations in regard to the handling and preparation of meat products are an important factor in the spread of toxoplasmosis [122–125].

Oocysts

Although ingestion of undercooked meat (especially mutton or pork) explained one mode of transmission, such a hypothesis did not explain how herbivorous animals and vegetarian humans became infected. In humans, the prevalence of *T. gondii* antibodies was the same among vegetarian populations (e.g., Hindus) as among meat-eating populations in the same geographic area (e.g., Christians and Muslims in India) [126,127]. A possible explanation was forthcoming when Hutchison and associates [128], and several others working independently [129,130], described a new form of the parasite, the oocyst.

Oocyst formation has been found to occur only in members of the cat family (e.g., domestic cat, bobcat, mountain lion). Cats may excrete up to 10 million oocysts in a single day, and excretion may continue for 2 weeks. Once shed, the oocyst sporulates in 1 to 5 days and becomes infectious; it may remain so for more than 1 year under appropriate conditions (e.g., in warm, moist soil) [131,132]. This form of the parasite may be inactivated by freezing, heating to a temperature of 45° C to 55° C, drying, or treating with formalin, ammonia, or tincture of iodine. (For further information on the biology of the oocyst, the reader is referred to the works of Frenkel and Dubey [11,133]). Its buoyancy allows it to float to the top layers of soil after rain, a location more conducive to transmission than the deeper soil where cats usually bury their feces. Transport of the oocyst from the site of deposit may occur by a number of vectors. Coprophagous invertebrates such as cockroaches and flies may mechanically carry oocysts to food [134–136]. Earthworms also may play a role by carrying oocysts to the soil surface [28,137,138].

The relative importance of the oocyst versus undercooked or raw meat in transmission of *T. gondii* to humans remains to be defined. Whereas meat appeared to be of primary importance in most areas of the United States, as shown earlier by Etheredge and Frenkel [139], this was not true for other geographic areas and may not be true currently. Epidemics of toxoplasmosis associated with presumptive exposure to infected cats support the importance of this mode of transmission [140–143].

A cluster of cases of *T. gondii* in Panama [142] and another in a suburb of São Paulo, Brazil [144], appear to have been associated with oocyst-contaminated drinking water. An epidemic in Victoria, Canada, also was considered to be associated with oocysts from wild cats in reservoir water. This reservoir was thought to be contaminated with *T. gondii* oocysts excreted by cougars [145].

Illness and deaths of sea otters on the central coast of California have drawn attention to the presence of *T. gondii* in mussels [146,147]. Mussels appear to concentrate oocysts [146] that then can be consumed by the otters. Infections in aquatic mammals indicate contamination and survival of oocysts in seawater [146]. Lindsay and associates [146,148] demonstrated that oocysts can persist in seawater for many months, sporulate, and remain infectious. Kniel and coworkers [149] found that oocysts can persist and remain infective for up to 8 weeks on raspberries and that they also can adhere to raspberries and blueberries. Consumption of fresh produce with *T. gondii* oocysts could thus be a source of transmission to humans. Oocysts excreted by cats can directly contaminate produce and water used for agriculture. An epidemic in a riding stable in Atlanta raises the question of whether dust contaminated with oocysts with aerosolization could contribute to acquisition of oocysts in that setting [150].

Milk

Unpasteurized milk (goat milk has been especially implicated) has been implicated as a vehicle for transmission of *T. gondii* [151–153], but the process of pasteurization would kill all forms of the organism.

Chicken and Eggs

Prevalence of the infection in chickens reflects *T. gondii* strains in their environment because they feed from the ground [154]. Prevalence of *T. gondii* was determined in 118 free-range chickens from 14 counties in Ohio and in 11 chickens from a pig farm in Massachusetts. *T. gondii* antibodies were demonstrated in 20 of 118 chickens (17%) from Ohio and isolated from 11 of 20 seropositive chickens (55%). Parasites were not isolated from tissues of 63 seronegative chickens. Nineteen isolates were genotyped; five were type II and 14 were type III. Dubey et al isolated *T. gondii* from chickens in many countries [145,154]. In certain areas of Brazil, a high prevalence of infection in chickens and young children has been noted [155].

Other Means of Transmission
Blood Transfusion

Because prolonged parasitemia has been observed during latent toxoplasmosis in experimental animals [156] and in humans with asymptomatic acquired toxoplasmosis [58,157], transfused blood must be considered a potential vehicle for transmission of the infection. Siegal and colleagues described four patients with acute leukemia in whom overt toxoplasmosis developed after they were given leukocytes from donors with chronic myelogenous leukemia [158]. Three of the four patients died. Retrospective serologic analyses suggested that the transfused donor white cells were the source of the parasite. If a pregnant woman is to receive a whole blood transfusion, selection of a donor without antibodies to *T. gondii* is advisable whenever possible. Patients with chronic myelogenous leukemia and high titers of antibody to *T. gondii* should not be used as blood or blood cell donors [159,160].

Laboratory-Acquired Infections (Including Infections Acquired at Autopsy)

A number of cases of toxoplasmosis have been acquired by laboratory personnel who handle infected animals or contaminated needles and glassware [161–165]. We are aware of numerous cases of laboratory-acquired infection with *T. gondii* that have occurred in recent years. At the Palo Alto Medical Foundation laboratory and Stanford University, more than a dozen such instances have been identified. Some cases were in pregnant women (Remington JS, unpublished data). Certainly, this experience indicates that pregnancy is a contraindication to working with *T. gondii* for women who have no demonstrable *T. gondii* antibodies.

One instance has been reported of toxoplasmosis acquired during performance of an autopsy [166].

Arthropods

The data derived from studies of multiple potential insect vectors are negative and inconclusive [11]. Flies and cockroaches may serve as carriers of oocysts (see Fig. 31-2) [134,135,167].

EPIDEMIOLOGY
General Considerations

Toxoplasmosis is a zoonosis; the definitive host is the cat, and all other hosts are incidental. The organism occurs in nature in herbivorous, omnivorous, and carnivorous animals, including all orders of mammals, some birds, and probably some reptiles, although in reptiles this suggestion rests solely on interpretation of histologic preparations [168]. In regard to *T. gondii* in cold-blooded hosts, data suggest that natural infection might occur under suitable environmental conditions [169,170].

The organism is ubiquitous in nature, and toxoplasmosis is one of the most common infections of humans throughout the world. In humans, the prevalence of positive serologic test titers increases with age, indicating past exposure, and no significant difference in prevalence between men and women exists in reports from the United States.

Considerable geographic differences exist in prevalence rates. Differences in the epidemiology of the infection in various geographic locales and between population groups within the same locale may be explained by differences in exposure to the two main sources of the infection: the tissue cyst (in flesh of animals) and the oocyst (in soil and drinking water contaminated by cat feces). The high prevalence of infection in France has been attributed to a preference for consumption of undercooked meat [113]. A similarly high prevalence in Central America has been related to the frequency of stray cats in a climate favoring survival of oocysts and to the type of dwelling [131,171]. Of special note are reports of outbreaks of *T. gondii* infections among family members [132,172].

Among studies designed to identify the risk factors for *T. gondii* infection during pregnancy, results from France, Italy, Norway, and Yugoslavia were reported [123,125,173,174]. The conclusions were that ingestion of raw or undercooked meat, use of kitchen knives that have not been sufficiently washed, and ingestion of unwashed raw vegetables or fruits are factors associated with an increased risk. In a recent case-control study from Europe examining risk factors that predispose pregnant women to infection with *T. gondii* [175], the authors concluded that exposure to inadequately cooked or cured meat accounted for approximately 30% to 63% of infections; thus exposure to meat was interpreted to be the main risk factor for pregnant women in Europe. Other risk factors included contact with soil, which apparently accounted for approximately 6% to 17% of infections; travel outside Europe or the United States and Canada also apparently accounted for some infections. Although contact with soil would presumably reflect risk from cat excrement, the authors concluded that direct "contact with cats" was not a risk factor. They also concluded that mode of acquisition for a large proportion of infections (14% to 49%) remained unexplained.

In a recent study [176] exploring risk factors recognized by mothers of infants with congenital toxoplasmosis in the United States between 1981 and 1998, undercooked meat and possible cat excrement exposure, either one or both, were recognized by approximately 50% of the mothers, but the remainder of the mothers could not identify risk factors.

Consumption of meat that had been frozen was associated with a lower risk. Surprisingly, in Naples, Italy, Buffolano and colleagues [125] observed an increased risk associated with consumption of cured pork; this might be related to the fact that in southern Italy, cured pork usually contains only 1% salt to fresh weight, is stored at less than 12° C, and may be eaten within 10 days of slaughter. A pet cat at home was not associated with an increased risk in any of these studies, but cleaning the cat litter box was a significant risk factor among women in the study from Norway [123]. Health education was associated with a lower risk when it was provided using printed educational materials in a book or magazine [173]. This improved efficacy of print (versus oral) information was observed in the past in Saint Antoine Hospital in Paris; the yearly seroconversion rate decreased from 37 per 1000 to 11 per 1000 when explanatory drawings were given to every seronegative pregnant woman.

Prevalence of *Toxoplasma gondii* Antibodies Among Women of Childbearing Age

Knowledge of the prevalence of antibodies in women in the childbearing age group is important because of its relevance to the strategic approach for prevention of congenital toxoplasmosis. In evaluating results obtained in any serologic survey, the factors noted earlier under "General Considerations" (in "Epidemiology") must be examined, in addition to two potential causes of differences that may not be real: the serologic method used (and its accuracy) for collection of the data and the dates of collection of the sera.

The prevalence rate among pregnant women in Palo Alto has decreased remarkably, from 27% in 1964 and 24% in 1974 to 10% in 1987 and 1998. The prevalence among pregnant women in Malmo, Sweden, has diminished since 1983.

Relevant to the variability in prevalence of infection among populations within a given geographic area are the observations of Ades and associates [177]. They studied the prevalence of maternal antibody in an anonymous neonatal serosurvey in London in 1991. Among women born in the United Kingdom, the seroprevalence was estimated to be 12.7% in innercity London, 7.5% in suburban London, and 5.5% in nonmetropolitan areas. The prevalence in women from India was 7.6%; Africa, 15% to 41%; Pakistan and Bangladesh, 21%; Ireland, 31%; and the Caribbean, 33%. Thus much of the variation between districts might be explained by ethnic group or country-of-birth composition. Recent data from France are available from national surveys performed in 1995 and 2003 for the Direction Genérale de la Santé [178]. The seroprevalence was 54.3% in 1995, with considerable geographic differences, but had declined to 43.8% in 2003. In the 1995 survey, differences also were noted depending on the country of origin: France, 55%; other European countries, 46%; North Africa, 51%; and south Saharan Africa, 40%. A high prevalence (64%) was observed among women practicing, or whose husbands practiced, a "learned profession." In the Paris area, the seroprevalence has decreased from more than 80% in the 1960s to 72% in the 1970s and to 52% in 2003.

Cultural habits with regard to food probably are the major cause of the differences in frequency of *T. gondii* infection from one country to another, from one region to another in the same country, and from one ethnic group to another in the same region. The data just described all reveal a decrease in the prevalence rate of *T. gondii* antibodies in the United States and in Europe during the past 3 decades. This decrease is more striking in countries that had a high prevalence than in those in which it was low. Because meat probably is a main vector of infection in most developed countries, it seems logical to relate this decrease to a less frequent presence of *T. gondii* in meat, which probably results from improved methods in the way the animals are raised and in the processing of meat [179,180].

Data from one city or single population within that city may not accurately reflect the true prevalence or incidence of infection either in that city or elsewhere. The prevalence of the infection has decreased dramatically in the past 20 years or so but not necessarily in subpopulations, such as Los Angeles Hispanics, Floridians (Haitians), and Salvadorians.

What are the prevalence and incidence of congenital toxoplasmosis (and *T. gondii* infection) in the United States? We have no objective data to answer this question. It should be emphasized that the lack of systematic serologic screening of pregnant women in the United States for acute acquired *T. gondii* infections severely limits our ability to accurately assess the incidence of *T. gondii* infection among pregnant women in different populations and of congenital *T. gondii* infection.

Numerous variables influence whether congenital transmission will occur. Many of these factors are recognized but poorly understood. They include the strain and virulence of *T. gondii*, inoculum size, route of infection, time during gestation, and immunocompetence of the pregnant woman. All of these also pertain to infection of the fetus and its outcome in the newborn thereafter.

Incidence of Acquired Infection During Pregnancy

Estimates from Prevalence Rates: Mathematical Epidemiologic Models

Once seroconversion occurs, IgG antibodies essentially persist for the life of the affected person. Thus the prevalence of antibodies increases with increasing age and the proportion of uninfected persons decreases. If the hypothesis is accepted that the risk of acquiring *T. gondii* infection from the environment is the same at any age, and if this yearly seroconversion rate is known, the prevalence of antibodies in relation to age and the proportion of seronegative persons in this population at a given age can be computed easily [181]. Consider as an example a population of infants 1 year of age who are not infected and thus are seronegative: If their risk of acquiring *T. gondii* infection is 10% per year (i.e., for a yearly seroconversion rate of 10%), the probability that these infants will still be free of infection (seronegative) is 0.9 at 2 years of age, 0.81 at 3 years of age, 0.729 at 4 years of age, and so on. At age 20, the prevalence of antibodies will be 86.5%, and the proportion of seronegative persons will be 13.5%. The curves shown in Figure 31–4 depict the theoretical antibody prevalence rates, in relation to age, for a fixed yearly seroconversion rate ranging from 0.1% to 20% (representative of possible rates in various locations). The frequency of acquisition of *T. gondii* infection at a given age (the incidence of *T. gondii* infection at that age) is dependent on both the proportion of the population that is seronegative at that age and on the rate of seroconversion. In the example just given, in a population with a 10% yearly seroconversion rate from the age of

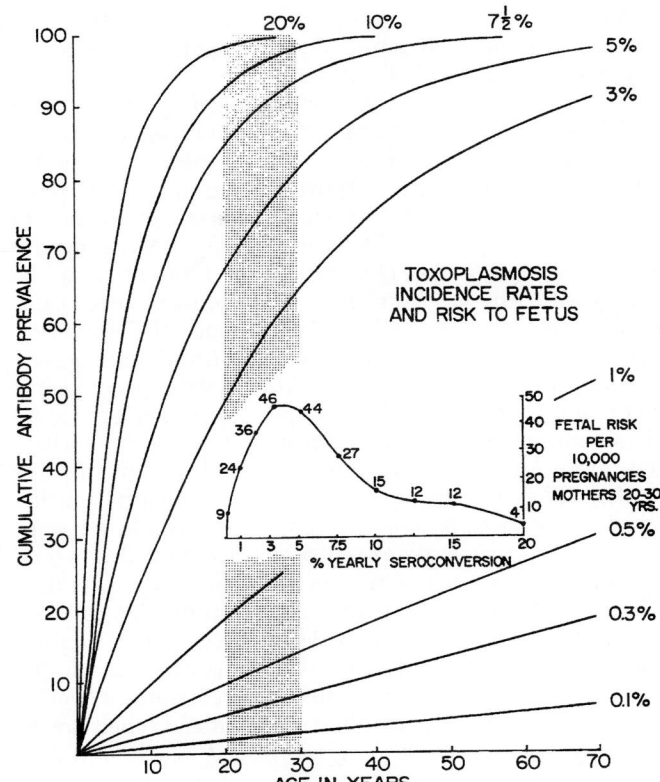

FIGURE 31–4 Incidence rates in mother and risk to fetus. (*Data from Frenkel JK.* Toxoplasma *in and around us. BioScience 23:343–352, 1973.*)

1 year, the incidence of acquired infection between 20 and 21 years of age will be 10% of 13.5% (i.e., 13.5 per 1000). The balance between the prevalence of immunity due to past infection and the risk of acquiring infection can result in apparently paradoxical findings when one examines the incidence of infection in the young adult. For example, in a population with a yearly seroconversion rate of 5% from the age of 1 year, the prevalence of antibodies will be 62% at age 20 and the incidence of infection between ages 20 and 21 will be 18.9 per 1000. Thus owing to the higher number of seronegatives, a lower constant risk of infection—5% instead of 10% per year—results in a higher frequency of infection acquired by the young adult.

Estimates from Prospective Studies of Acquired Infection During Pregnancy and Consequences of Health Education

During the early 1950s, congenital toxoplasmosis was recognized as a frequent cause of severe neonatal disease in France [65,182], and the feasibility of screening pregnant women for acquired infection during pregnancy was investigated. Serologic screening for *T. gondii* infection during pregnancy became common practice in France and in several European countries during those years. It also should be noted that the life cycle of the parasite was elucidated in the years 1970 to 1971, so that it became possible to instruct women about the mode of transmission of *T. gondii* and how they could avoid becoming infected. Whereas this health education was carefully attempted in some obstetric centers, no attempt at education was made in others.

The seroconversion rate was significantly lower when health education was attempted, especially when explanatory drawings were provided to seronegative women. Thoumsin and colleagues reported a summary of 22 years of screening for *T. gondii* infection during pregnancy in Liege, Belgium [183]. From 1966 to 1987, 20,901 pregnant women attending the Department of Obstetrics of the C.H.R. of Liege were screened. The numbers of seroconversions observed were 129 (6.4%) among 2027 seronegative women from 1966 to 1975 and 74 (2.8%) among 2601 women from 1976 to 1981. After 1981, prophylactic counseling was provided by a specially trained nurse to all seronegative pregnant women. From 1982 to 1987, the number of seroconversions observed was 48 of 3859 (1.2%). The authors do not state the mean time during which their patients were examined for possible seroconversion. If it was approximately 6 months, these data would suggest that the yearly seroconversion rate was greater than 120 per 1000 before 1975, 56 per 1000 from 1976 to 1981, and 24 per 1000 from 1982 to 1987. These values demonstrate a decrease in the risk of infection quite similar to the decrease observed in Paris, which was described above.

Since 1978, it has been obligatory under French law to test pregnant women for *T. gondii* infection acquired during gestation. The common practice is to perform a test for *T. gondii* antibodies at the first prenatal visit (usually at weeks 10 to 15). The result is reported to the patient; if it is negative, the laboratory that performed the test must send a letter to the woman describing hygienic measures she can practice to avoid infection with *T. gondii*. Serologic testing of seronegative women is repeated monthly until delivery to identify those who seroconvert. If the test performed at the first prenatal visit is suggestive of a recently acquired infection, an avidity assay should be performed. In some instances, a second sample of serum is obtained to attempt to determine whether the infection was acquired during the first few weeks of pregnancy or earlier. One consequence of this procedure is that the surveillance for acquired *T. gondii* infection now encompasses the entire pregnancy, including the first 10 weeks and not solely the last 30 weeks of gestation, as was the case during the first surveys performed in France.

Jeannel and associates [184] reported the results of a survey performed in the Paris area between 1981 and 1983. The prevalence of *T. gondii* antibodies was estimated to be 67.3% with a yearly seroconversion rate equal to 21 per 1000. In 1995, there was a yearly seroconversion rate of 19 per 1000 among patients who received health education. The incidence among primiparous women was twice that of multiparous women. This finding suggests that women who knew they were seronegative because they had been repeatedly tested for infection with *T. gondii* during a previous pregnancy tried to avoid acquiring this infection when they again became pregnant.

The differences in the frequency of *T. gondii* infection from one country to another can be illustrated by the differences in the incidence rates and in the prevalence rates. As an example, the yearly seroconversion rates calculated from the data from Norway [84] are nearly eight times lower than those calculated from the data obtained in 1995 in France [178], and the antibody prevalence rate at the age of pregnancy is five times lower in Norway than it is in France. In the Paris area, the yearly seroconversion rate observed during pregnancy was approximately 60 per 1000 during the late 1950s and early 1960s, and it was about 19 per 1000 in 1995. This lower seroconversion rate was observed as early as 1974, however, when instruction became available to pregnant women on how they could avoid becoming infected [185].

The seroconversion rates observed during these relatively recent surveys from France and from Norway can be used to calculate an expected prevalence rate according to the methods discussed earlier [181,186,187]. This calculated "expected" prevalence rate is lower than the observed prevalence rates in both surveys. This finding suggests that the risk of becoming infected with *T. gondii* is lower among pregnant women than in nonpregnant women, perhaps also the result of health care education provided at the first prenatal visit. Thus the timing of providing pregnant women with the appropriate information on prevention of infection with *T. gondii* at the first prenatal visit probably skews results of prospective studies of acquired *T. gondii* infection during pregnancy by selectively reducing the frequency of infection acquired during the second half of pregnancy.

Prevalence of Congenital *Toxoplasma gondii* Infection

At present, objective data are lacking on the prevalence of congenital *T. gondii* infection or congenital toxoplasmosis for the United States. Because screening of pregnant women in the United States is not systematic, our ability to accurately assess the incidence of *T. gondii* infection among pregnant women in different populations and of congenital *T. gondii* infection is limited. Data from one city or single population within that city may not accurately reflect the true prevalence or incidence of infection either in that city or elsewhere. Although the prevalence of the infection has decreased in some areas of the United States during the past 20 years or so, this is not necessarily the case in subpopulations even in those same areas.

Estimates from Studies at Birth or During Infancy

Estimates from clinical observations and from autopsy findings are based on data derived mainly from older studies [71,72], which underestimated the actual prevalence because congenital infection uncommonly results in stillbirth or neonatal death and frequently is not diagnosed during infancy because of subclinical infection in the infant and delayed occurrence of signs of infection [189,190].

Estimates from Serologic Screening of Neonates or Infants

The Commonwealth of Massachusetts began screening newborn sera in January 1986 to determine the incidence of congenital *T. gondii* infection. Newborn blood specimens are collected on filter paper and used to test for IgM antibodies by the sensitive IgM enzyme-linked immunosorbent assay (ELISA). From 1986 to 1999, 93 infants were detected who had IgM *T. gondii* antibodies, reflecting an incidence of approximately 1 in 12,000 births or perhaps 1 in 6,000 births if the sensitivity of the IgM test was 50% as found for some other IgM tests for newborn sera [191]. Although a careful follow-up evaluation was not performed for all seronegative infants, it is known that the diagnosis was missed in at least six infants in whom IgM antibodies were not detected but who were referred by local physicians. In one of these later-diagnosed children, *T. gondii* was isolated from cerebrospinal fluid; the infection was suspected on clinical grounds in this child, who was born prematurely with hydrocephalus, cerebral calcifications, and bilateral chorioretinitis. Thus this reported incidence is lower than the actual incidence despite the sensitivity of the method used to detect IgM antibodies of *T. gondii*. Nevertheless, if as many as 50% of cases were missed (which is unlikely) with the methodology used by the New England Regional Screening Program, an incidence of 1 per 10,000 births is strikingly different from the incidence of 1.3 per 1000 reported by Kimball and coworkers in 1971 from a prospective screening study of pregnant women in New York City [74]. With the discovery of the importance of detecting IgA and IgE antibodies (see "Diagnosis" section) in the newborn, serologic studies of newborns such as those being performed in Massachusetts should detect a higher percentage of infected infants.

Even if the prevalence of congenital infection is underestimated, however, the present data (at least from Massachusetts) suggest that the rate has significantly decreased during the last 2 decades in some populations in the United States [188]. This decrease in the prevalence rate of congenital *T. gondii* infection parallels the historical decrease in antibody prevalence rate observed in the adult. This would be expected from the epidemiologic models discussed earlier; in a population in which the seroprevalence rate was rather low (well below 50% in the adult, as it is in the United States), a decrease in the risk of acquiring infection immediately results in a decrease in the incidence of acquired infection in women in the childbearing age group.

The Danish Congenital Toxoplasmosis Study Group reported results of their feasibility study to determine the prevalence of the infection among live neonates and the maternofetal transmission rate in infected mothers who had received no treatment [192]. Secondarily, they assessed the feasibility and acceptability of neonatal screening using *T. gondii* IgM antibody testing on samples from phenylketonuria (PKU) cards. They reported a surprisingly low maternofetal transmission rate of 19.4% and estimated that a neonatal screening program based on detection of IgM *T. gondii* antibodies using PKU cards alone would identify 70% to 80% of cases of congenital toxoplasmosis; however, not all pregnancies and infants in their study were thoroughly evaluated, thus making the accuracy of this figure uncertain. Based on these findings, a two-step newborn screening program was initiated in Denmark in 1999. PKU card samples were screened for *T. gondii* IgM antibodies, and reactive samples were then evaluated by specific IgG, IgM, and IgA antibody testing. Screening between 1999

and 2007 identified 55 cases of congenital infection (1/4780); 12 of 47 infected infants had retinochoroidal and/or intracranial lesions. This screening program was terminated in 2007 because the incidence was lower than expected and they interpreted the high incidence of new retinal lesions in the first years of life following 3 months of treatment as lack of treatment efficacy, thus leading them to conclude that the program was not cost effective [Nielsen H, personal communication to R McLeod, 2010 and manuscript in press]. Whether outcome would have been more favorable and the conclusions different if these children had been treated for 1 year postnatally as is done in the US NCCTS studies (see section US National Collaborative Chicago-based treatment study below) is not known [193].

Effects of Systematic Screening of Pregnant Women at Risk on the Prevalence of Congenital *Toxoplasma gondii* Infection and of Congenital Toxoplasmosis

The purpose of the first attempts at systematic serologic screening was to identify pregnant women at risk, to try to prevent congenital toxoplasmosis or, if such infection was present, to allow for early instigation of treatment. Once the life cycle of the parasite was elucidated, primary preventive measures were possible through education of seronegative women (see "Prevention" section and Table 31–51). This is now currently done in several European countries and has proved moderately effective, as judged by the data discussed earlier; acquired *T. gondii* infection during pregnancy apparently is three times less frequent in France than it would be were no information provided to seronegative pregnant women in regard to the sources of infection and how they may reduce their risk of acquiring the infection. This estimation is very close to the conclusions of Foulon and colleagues [194], who calculated that in Brussels primary preventive measures reduced the seroconversion rates during pregnancy by 63%. Even better results are possible, however. One critical point is the time at which this education is provided. In most cases, this intervention occurs during the first prenatal visit, at approximately the tenth week of pregnancy. This timing does not reduce the number of infections acquired during the first 10 weeks of gestation or the number of seroconversions that occur within 2 weeks after the first prenatal visit because women whose seroconversion occurs at this time probably were in the initial stage of the infection (during which parasitemia occurs before antibodies become detectable in the serum) at the time they received the instruction. Thus the results of such an education program can only be a reduction in the number of infections that occur later during pregnancy. Because late acquired infections are those for which the rate of congenital transmission is the highest (resulting primarily in subclinical cases), it is understandable that in addition to a lower number of infections acquired during gestation, health education, if provided at first prenatal visit at about the tenth week of pregnancy, should result in a lower rate of transmission than observed in the previous surveys performed before the means by which *T. gondii* is horizontally transmitted to humans was known. In addition, the proportion of infected fetuses with the more severe form of congenital toxoplasmosis might be higher unless treatment during gestation is effective in the infected fetus. Health education, although useful, will not benefit those women who contract *T.gondii* infection during pregnancy from unrecognized sources which cannot be avoided. This appears to occur relatively commonly in the U.S. and in epidemics in North America (McLeod, Boyer and colleagues, unpublished observations 2010).

In France, congenital toxoplasmosis was the most frequent fetopathy in the years 1950 to 1960. For example, in this period, several cases of congenital toxoplasmosis were diagnosed each year among approximately 1000 premature infants admitted annually to l'Hôpital de l'Institut de Puériculture de Paris. In 1957, for instance, 7 cases were diagnosed among 1085 newborns. In the same hospital, however, only two cases have been observed between 1980 and 1990. Within 40 years the pediatrician has been witness to a dramatic change in the presenting signs of the disease (Couvreur J, written communication to Remington JS, 1998). In the past, patients were referred to the specialized toxoplasmosis clinic in Paris because they had clinical symptoms or often severe signs that suggested congenital toxoplasmosis. For instance, in a group of 147 neonates or infants with congenital *T. gondii* infection studied between 1949 and 1960, 62.5% had signs of central nervous system (CNS) involvement (with hydrocephalus in two thirds of the patients), and 32.5% had retinochoroiditis without clinical evidence of CNS involvement. Despite their being asymptomatic, most patients now attend the specialized clinic because they are suspected of having, or are diagnosed as having, congenital *T. gondii* infection. Congenital *T. gondii* infection is subclinical and remains subclinical in a majority of them. For example, congenital infection remained subclinical in 166 of 234 infants (71%) observed between 1984 and 1992. In this group, 60 of 234 (26%) had a retinal scar but no CNS involvement; CNS involvement with or without hydrocephalus was present in 8 of 234 (3%) of these infants. At present, severe neurologic or ocular involvement, or both, is observed only among infants born to women in the following patient groups: patients referred from foreign countries where screening is not performed during pregnancy (e.g., Morocco, Algeria, United Kingdom), mothers who for any reason were not screened during pregnancy, mothers who were immunodeficient, and mothers who were erroneously considered to be immune. With these exceptions, in which the clinical status may be considered abnormal (see "Chronic Maternal *Toxoplasma* Infection"), prenatal screening for maternal *T. gondii* infection during pregnancy appears to be an effective preventive measure for congenital toxoplasmosis in France, although the efficacy of this approach has not been formally tested in randomized controlled trials (see Table 31–5) [195,196].

Based on this evidence, mandatory prenatal screening is officially recommended in five European countries, with monthly testing recommended in France and Italy and every third month testing recommended in Austria, Lithuania, and Slovenia [197]. However, in the absence of evidence from randomized controlled clinical trials that prenatal screening and intervention reduces maternofetal transmission or severity of disease in children who are infected in utero (see section "Prevention"), the value of prenatal or neonatal screening has been questioned by some European authorities [195,197]. Given this uncertainty, in other European countries, where the seroprevalence among pregnant women, the incidence of congenital infection, and the numbers of cases of symptomatic congenital toxoplasmosis appear to be lower than in France, routine prenatal or neonatal screening is not, or is no longer, performed. However, it is acknowledged that the absence of evidence from controlled clinical trials is not evidence for the lack of benefit. For this reason, other authorities, including those in France [196] and in the United States [198,199]—although they agree that carefully designed studies are needed to determine the true benefit— believe that a program of screening, careful counseling, and treatment of the pregnant woman who acquires infection during pregnancy is appropriate. This is particularly true in countries such as Brazil, where the incidence of severe, symptomatic congenital toxoplasmosis appears to be much greater than in Europe and North America, perhaps reflecting the greater prevalence in Brazil of more virulent type I and atypical strains of *T. gondii* [200].

PATHOGENESIS

Factors Operative During Initial Infection
Genetics and Virulence of Toxoplasma gondii

Genetics of the parasite appear to influence outcome of the maternal infection (R. McLeod and colleagues, unpublished observations 2010). Also, the inoculum size influences the outcome of sporozoite infections in animal models (Dubey, personal communication to R McLeod, 2010) and it is likely that this is also true in human infections.

Not all *T. gondii* parasites are genetically identical. There are three clonal, archetypal lineages called type I, II, and III. Parasites within a lineage are genetically similar. Each lineage has distinct properties in cell culture systems and elicits different pathology in animal models.

Lehman and colleagues (2006) state that their findings suggest that *T. gondii* originated in South America, and that an early variant parasite was carried to Europe from South America, where it evolved into the archetypal type II lineage parasite. Archetypal clonal type II parasites currently cause the preponderance of *T. gondii* infections in Austria [201], France [202], and Poland [203]. There are also genetically variant or "atypical" parasites. Atypical *T. gondii* isolates have been found in Brazil along the Amazon and its tributaries, but have also been identified in other parts of the world, including the United States and Canada.

In a study by Ajzenberg and associates [204] of clonal types of isolates of *T. gondii* in France between 1987 and 2001, almost all (85% in the whole series, and 96% in 57 consecutive isolates from a laboratory in Limoges and a laboratory in Paris) of 86 congenitally infected children had clonal type II parasites. Type I and atypical isolates were not found in cases of asymptomatic or mild congenital toxoplasmosis. Three isolates with atypical genotypes, which were virulent in mice, were associated with severe congenital infection. In four cases, *T. gondii* was isolated only from the placenta, the infant was not infected, and all four were of clonal type I. Type II isolates occurred in persons with different levels of severity in their signs and symptoms. The main factor influencing severity was reported to be time of acquisition of the infection during gestation. This finding contrasts with that in a small series from Spain (where serologic screening during gestation is not the standard of care, as it is in France) in which all isolates were of clonal type I [205].

In a separate study by Romand [206], clonal types of parasites were not included in their analysis. Nonetheless, the highest amounts of parasite DNA detected in amniotic fluid by PCR assay were associated with the most severe disease in the newborn and most often were related to time in gestation when the infection was acquired (as discussed in "Polymerase Chain Reaction Assay" under "Diagnosis"). It is unclear at present whether any relationship exists between a specific clonal type(s) and either transmission or severity of the infection in the newborn or progression of disease in the congenitally infected infant.

In Brazil, atypical I/III recombinant parasites have been identified that appear to have different biologic behavior in mice and cause far more prominent eye infections in older children and adults [207,208]. Sixty percent of Brazilian children younger than 10 years of age in Minas Gerais state have serologic evidence of infection [155,207,209,210]. Eighty percent of adults are seropositive, and 20% of these have recurrent eye disease [209]. The greater prevalence of type I and atypical lineage *T. gondii* may also be an important factor in the greater severity of progressive eye disease during and following treatment of infants and children with congenital toxoplasmosis in Brazil [200]and Colombia [211,212]. However, severe congenital disease is not restricted to type I and atypical lineage parasites: archetypal type I, type II, and atypical parasites can cause both mild and severe congenital disease in the fetus and newborn infant and disease in older children and adults [202,213–215].

Host Genetics

Interactions of parasite genetics and host genetics are important in outcomes as well [200,216–218]. The frequency of the human leukocyte antigen (HLA) class II gene DQ3 was found to be increased in infants with congenital toxoplasmosis and hydrocephalus relative to the frequency of this gene in the U.S. population or in infants with congenital toxoplasmosis who did not have hydrocephalus [216,219]. Of interest is that this unique frequency of DQ3 also was noted to be a genetic marker of susceptibility to development of toxoplasmic encephalitis in patients with AIDS [219]. HLA class II DQ genes function in transgenic mice to protect against brain parasite burden. DQ1 protects better than DQ3. This observation is consonant with the observation that the DQ3 gene is more frequent in infants with congenital toxoplasmosis with hydrocephalus than in those without hydrocephalus, and than in the U.S. population [219].

Alleles of the collagen gene *col2a*, variants of which are associated with a genetic eye disease called Stickler disease, and of the lipid transporter gene *abc4r*, variants of which are associated with macular disease and hydrocephalus in a rat model, were associated with risk for eye disease and eye and brain disease, respectively, in children with congenital toxoplasmosis [216]. There was a parent of origin effect suggesting that epigenetic factors are also involved. It has also been demonstrated recently that in addition to these genes, alleles of TLR9, P2x7r, and ERAAP2 are associated with susceptibility to and manifestations of human congenital toxoplasmosis [219–223].

Role of Cells and Antibody

After local invasion (usually in the intestines), the organisms invade cells directly or are phagocytosed. They multiply intracellularly, causing host cell disruption, and then invade contiguous cells. Whereas human monocytes and neutrophils kill the vast majority of ingested *T. gondii* organisms, tachyzoites survive within macrophages derived in vitro from peripheral blood monocytes [224–226]. Data have shown that human peritoneal and alveolar macrophages kill *T. gondii* [227]. Cytotoxic T lymphocyte-mediated lysis of *T. gondii*-infected target cells did not lead to death of the intracellular parasites, however, indicating that intracellular *T. gondii* remains alive after lysis of host cells by cytolytic T cells [228,229]. The presence of persistent parasitemia observed in humans [58] and animals [230,231] can best be explained by the existence of intracellular parasites in the circulation.

T. gondii invades every organ and tissue of the human host except non-nucleated red blood cells, although evidence indicates that invasion of these cells may occur as well [232]. Termination of continued tissue destruction by *T. gondii* depends both on the development of cell-mediated immunity and on antibodies. Continued destruction may occur in those sites where ready access to circulating antibodies is impeded (e.g., CNS, eye). Despite the ability of antibodies in the presence of complement to kill extracellular *T. gondii* effectively *in vitro*, the intracellular habitat of this protozoon protects it from the effects of circulating antibodies.

Cyst formation can be demonstrated as early as the eighth day of experimental infection [42]. Cysts persist in multiple organs and tissues after immunity is acquired, probably for the life of the host.

The ability of the pregnant woman to control multiplication and spread of *T. gondii* depends not only on specific antibody synthesis but also on the time of appearance of cell-mediated immunity. In addition to the immunosuppression associated with pregnancy itself, cell-mediated immunity, at least as measured by antigen-specific lymphocyte transformation, may not be demonstrable for weeks or even months after acute infection with *T. gondii* in humans [233,234]. Although the importance of cellular immunity in the control of the initial acute infection in humans has not been defined, it is likely, from what is known about the immunology of toxoplasmosis in animal models [21,22] and studies with human immune cells [235–237], that cell-mediated immunity plays a major role. Susceptibility alleles of genes specifying innate and adaptive immunity also support this. The helper T-cell type 2 (T_H2) bias (toward humoral immunity and away from cellular immunity) established during normal gestation may compromise successful immunity against *T. gondii*, which requires a strong T_H1 response. In addition, it has been proposed that a strong T_H1 response against *T. gondii* may overcome the protective T_H2 cytokines at the maternal-fetal interface and result in fetal loss [238,239]. For a discussion of the immunoregulation of *T. gondii* infection and toxoplasmosis, the reader is referred to other sources [22,110,240–243].

Reinfection

Although survival from the acute stages of the initial *T. gondii* infection usually results in resistance to reinfection, the immunity associated with the chronic (latent) infection is only relative. Immunity to *T. gondii* in mice protects against but does not necessarily prevent reinfection [244–249]. Mice immunized with one strain of *T. gondii* and subsequently challenged with another strain have both strains encysted in their tissues. Reinfection may also be responsible for the rare human cases of apparent transmission from a chronically infected immunocompetent mother to her fetus [97,250,251]. Consistent with this possibility is a recent report, which suggested that infection by an atypical strain during pregnancy in a mother previously infected by an archetypal strain may result in infection in the fetus [252]. Disseminated congenital toxoplasmosis was observed in a newborn infant of an apparently immunocompetent mother who had evidence of infection before conception, and who likely became reinfected when she ingested raw horsemeat, likely imported from South America, during her pregnancy. This clinical occurance is exceptionally uncommon in France and therefore raised the possibility of the second infection being caused by a highly virulent *Toxoplasma* strain. The parasite isolated from the peripheral blood of her newborn infant was found to have an atypical genotype, which is very uncommon in Europe but had been described in South America. The investigators tested the hypothesis that reinfection may occur with a different genotype by using an experimental mouse model, which confirmed that acquired immunity against European *Toxoplasma* strains may not protect against reinfection by atypical strains acquired during travel outside Europe or by eating imported meat. With international travel and globalization of markets that involves products from Central and South America, and other continents being distributed throughout the world, the prior observation that once infected a pregnant women does not reacquire parasites that could be transmitted to her fetus may not always be accurate in the future.

Factors Operative During Latent Infection
Cyst Rupture

Factors that influence tachyzoite and bradyzoite interconversion are critical to understanding the pathogenesis of recrudescent infection.

Histologic evidence suggesting that cyst rupture concurs in humans has been reported [244,247]. In the brains of chronically infected mice, it is not unusual to find large and small cysts close together, suggesting the possibility that cyst rupture or "leakage" of bradyzoites has caused the satellite cysts [253]. It is not clear whether the satellite cysts are the result of cyst rupture or whether they simply developed at the same time as did the larger cysts in the same area.

Organisms that are intracellular and located within cysts are protected from antibody and cell-mediated immunity. Changes in the host cell membrane that may occur at the time of infection might predispose the infected cell to disruption by lymphokine-activated killer cells [22,236]. Cyst rupture would lead to release of viable organisms that can result in significant tissue damage.

Persistence of "Active" Infection

Frenkel has suggested that cyst rupture is responsible for underlying persistent immunity and antibody and that the encysted form of the organism causes localized or generalized relapse [11]. A persistent parasitemia has been demonstrated not only in laboratory animals [156,231,254] but also in humans [158,255,256]. In addition, a constant antigenic stimulus has been suggested to account for the persistence of *T. gondii* antibodies, which may remain at high titers for years after the acute infection and at lower titers for the life of the infected host. Antigen-specific lymphocyte proliferation has been demonstrated in persons who had acquired the infection as long ago as 30 years previously [234]. Another observation pointing to the persistence of active infection during chronicity in rodents is that despite having high levels of neutralizing antibody titers, hypergammaglobulinemia [257,258], and resistance to challenge with an ordinarily lethal dose of *T. gondii*, laboratory rats and mice chronically infected with *T. gondii* can transmit the organism to their offspring transplacentally (see "Transmission" section) [230,259].

"Immunologic Unresponsiveness" to Toxoplasma gondii Antigens

Results of studies in laboratory animals suggest that the maternal IgG antibody may inhibit formation of antibodies to *T. gondii* in the fetus [260].

The observation that *T. gondii* induces expansion of the particular V region, Vδ2, of the γδ T-cell response in acquired infection [261,262] led Hara and associates to examine Vδ2$^+$ γδ T-cell tolerance in infants with congenital *T. gondii* infection [263]. Important in this regard is the observation by Subauste and colleagues [237] that γδ T cells produce IFN-γ, a major mediator of resistance against *T. gondii* [264]. Hara and associates [263] noted that Vδ2$^+$ γδ T cells were anergic with or without clonal expansion during the newborn period in two infants with the congenital infection. Clonal expansion of Vδ2 was not observed to be associated with T-cell response downregulation, and no deletion of Vδ2$^+$ γδ T cells was observed. T-cell anergy was noted in the infants at the age of 1 month, and *T. gondii*-specific anergy was noted at 5 months.

Cord blood of infants with congenital toxoplasmosis has been reported to have increased numbers of CD45RO$^+$ T cells [265]. In the study by Hara and associates, most of the CD45RO$^+$ T cells were γδ T cells, and these T cell levels were not always elevated, especially in an infant with severe disease in the newborn period [263]. In their study, despite persistent αβ T-cell unresponsiveness in two infants with congenital toxoplasmosis, γδ T cells became reactive to live *T. gondii*-infected cells and produced IFN-γ after the infants reached 1 year of age.

Toxoplasma-specific memory CD4$^+$ T-cell responses may also be delayed in their appearance in congenital toxoplasmosis and may not be detectable until weeks or months after birth. McLeod and colleagues found that lymphocyte proliferation in response to *Toxoplasma* antigens, which detects responses by CD4$^+$ T cells, was below the limit of detection in 11 of 25 congenitally infected infants (usually those with the most severe manifestations) with congenital toxoplasmosis younger than 1 year of age [266]. The mechanism(s) for this absence of response and its restoration by 1 year of age remain to be determined. Furthermore, even when lymphocyte proliferation responses were first detected in congenitally infected children, production of IL-2 and IFN-γ assayed in parallel often was less than that by cells from adults with postnatal *Toxoplasma* infection. Results consistent with these were reported by another group. Fatoohi and colleagues [267] found that anti-*Toxoplasma* T-cell responses (determined using a different and less standardized assay) were lower in eight congenitally infected infants younger than 1 year of age than in persons with acquired *Toxoplasma* infection and congenitally infected children studied when they were older than 1 year of age. Nonetheless, anti-*Toxoplasma* T-cell responses were detectable in most of the congenitally infants younger than 1 year of age by this assay. Ciardelli and colleagues [268] also found that greater than 90% of congenitally infected infants less than 90 days of age had detectable T-cell proliferation and IFN-γ production in response to *Toxoplasma* antigen. The basis for the differences between these studies is unknown. Nonetheless, these data suggest that antigen-specific CD4$^+$ T-cell responses may develop more slowly or be diminished in some infants with congenital *Toxoplasma* infection.

Other aspects of immunologic unresponsiveness are discussed under "Special Problems Concerning Pathogenesis in the Eye" and in the "Diagnosis" section.

Special Problems Concerning Pathogenesis in the Eye and Brain

The plethora of data and the controversy that exists regarding immunity and hypersensitivity as they pertain to toxoplasmic chorioretinitis related to congenital toxoplasmosis preclude complete coverage of the subject here. The reader is referred to reviews of the relevant literature by O'Connor and colleagues [269–273] and to related work in the mouse model of congenital ocular toxoplasmosis [269–271,274–276]. Whereas Frenkel has been a proponent of the theory that toxoplasmic chorioretinitis in older children and adults is a hypersensitivity phenomenon [277], O'Connor and colleagues concluded that both the acute and the recurrent forms of necrotizing chorioretinitis are due to multiplication of *T. gondii* tachyzoites in the retina and that release of antigen into the retina of previously sensitized persons does not result in recurrence of the inflammatory response. *T. gondii* antigen and antibody have been detected in ocular fluids in experimental ocular toxoplasmosis [278]. The rapid resolution of inflammation that occurs with antimicrobial treatment in infants, children, and adults with congenital toxoplasmosis [279] suggests that parasite replication and the resulting destruction of retinal tissue causes the eye disease. Support for the role of the parasite per se also comes from studies in which results of PCR assay in samples of vitreous from adults with the acute acquired infection were positive [280,281]. Studies with PCR analysis also demonstrated that parasite DNA may be detected in aqueous fluid [282,283].

Data are not available in humans that clarify whether the pathogenesis of eye disease related to *T. gondii* in young children is the same as or different from that in adults. The immunologic parameters that may or may not operate in each situation constitute a major factor in determining the severity and outcome of eye infection and disease.

Although the peak incidence of chorioretinitis related to congenital *T. gondii* infection usually is between the ages of 12 and 20 years, chorioretinitis may not occur until late in adult life. Crawford and colleagues described a patient in whom the first eye symptoms occurred at the age of 61 years [284]. For the next 9 years, the inflammatory activity in the posterior segment of one eye continued relentlessly, causing pain and ultimately blindness. The severity of the pain necessitated enucleation. Masses of cysts were found in the retina. In such cases, it is impossible to determine whether the primary infection was congenital or acquired. Reports of significant numbers of cases of toxoplasmic chorioretinitis that occurred during the acute acquired infection in adults highlight the difficulties in attributing all of the cases of toxoplasmic chorioretinitis occurring later in life to the congenital infection [285,286].

The unique predilection of *T. gondii* for maculae, brain periaqueductal and periventricular areas, and basal ganglia in congenital toxoplasmosis remains unexplained. In the mouse model of Deckert-Schlüter and associates [287], it is of interest that congenitally infected mice have similar periventricular lesions, unlike in adult mice. It remains to be determined whether this difference is due to immaturity of the fetal immune system, unique interaction of *T. gondii* antigens with the fetal immune system, or development of the fetal brain at the time infection is initiated, or to some combination of these.

PATHOLOGY

In reviewing the literature on the pathology of congenital toxoplasmosis, it is immediately apparent that the genesis of the natural infection in the fetus is entirely comparable with that observed in experimental toxoplasmosis in animals. The position of necrotic foci and lesions in general suggests that the organisms reach the brain and all other organs through the bloodstream. Noteworthy is the remarkable variability in distribution of lesions and parasites among the different reported cases [288–291]. Age at the time of autopsy is a major modifying factor, but others include the virulence of the strain of *T. gondii*, the number of organisms actually transmitted from the mother to the fetus, the time during pregnancy when the infection occurred, the developmental maturity of the infant's immune system, and the number of organs and tissues carefully examined. After the appearance of early reports of cases of congenital toxoplasmosis, the prevailing impression was that the infection manifested itself in infants mainly as an encephalomyelitis and that visceral lesions were uncommon and insignificant. This view reflected the observation of a marked degree of damage to the CNS without a comparable degree of extraneural involvement in these infants. In some cases, however, extraneural lesions are severe and may even predominate [6,291,292]. Thus at autopsy, in some cases only the CNS and eyes may be involved, whereas in others wide dissemination of lesions and parasites may be noted. Between these two extremes are wide variations in the degree of organ and tissue involvement, but the CNS is never spared. The clinical importance of lesions in the CNS and eye is magnified by the limited ability of these tissues to regenerate, compared with the remarkable regenerative capacity of other tissues in the body. Active regeneration of extraneural tissues may be observed even in the most acute stages of infection in the infant [293]. Thus in extraneural organs, residual lesions may be so slight and insignificant that they are easily overlooked. In the CNS and eye, on the other hand, the lesser ability of nerve cells to regenerate leads to more severe permanent damage [293].

The presence of *T. gondii* in the cells lining alveoli and in the endothelium of pulmonary vessels led Callahan and coworkers to suggest that aspiration of infected amniotic fluid in the lungs may be a route of entry of the organism into the fetus [288]. That infection by this route may occur cannot be disputed. The diffuse character of the lung changes contrasts with the more focal lesions found in other organs and tissues. Zuelzer pointed out that this difference may be due to the position of the lungs in the route of circulation. Before dissemination to other tissues of the body all blood with parasites entering the venous circulation must first pass through the alveolar capillaries [293]. Thus the lungs are exposed to more parasites than any other single organ.

Placenta

The first description of *T. gondii* in placental tissues was by Neghme and coworkers [63]. Subsequently, a number of similar observations have been made [62,64,294–296]. Evidence for the likelihood of the hematogenous route of spread of *T. gondii* to the placenta is supplied by the fact that groups of tachyzoites can be found widely dispersed in the chorionic plate, decidua, and amnion, and organisms have been observed in the placental villi and umbilical cord without associated significant lesions (Fig. 31–5) [61–63,297–299]. The first description of the histopathologic features of a *T. gondii*-infected placenta of a woman with AIDS was by Piche and colleagues in 1997 [300]. The woman experienced a spontaneous abortion associated with fever and *T. gondii* pneumonia.

In five cases studied by Benirschke and Driscoll, the most consistent findings in the placentas were chronic inflammatory reactions in the decidua capsularis and focal reactions in the villi [296]. The lesions appeared to be

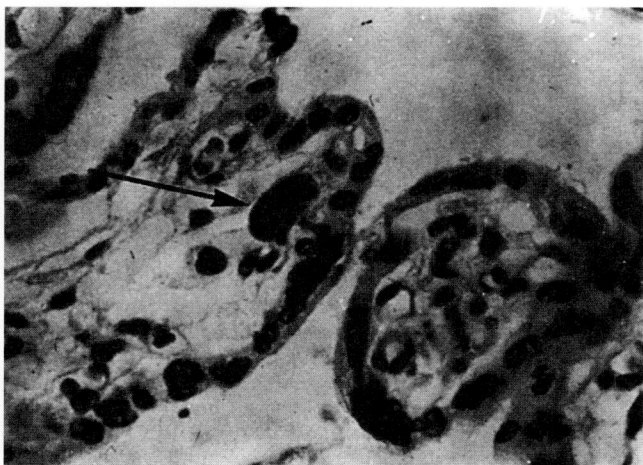

FIGURE 31–5 *Toxoplasma* cyst in the placenta of an infected fetus (*arrow*).

more severe in infants who died soon after birth. Villous lesions develop at random throughout the placenta. Single or multiple neighboring villi with low-grade chronic inflammation, activation of Hofbauer cells, necrobiosis of component cells, and proliferative fibrosis may be seen. Although villous lesions frequently are observed in placental toxoplasmosis, histologic examination of these foci does not reveal parasites; they occur in free villi and in villi attached to the decidua. Lymphocytes and other mononuclear cells, but rarely plasma cells, make up the intravillous and perivillous infiltrates. The decidual infiltrate consists primarily of lymphocytes. Inflammation of the umbilical cord is uncommon. When fetal hydrops is present, the placenta also is hydropic.

The organism is seen mainly in the tissue cyst form and may be present in the connective tissues of the amnionic and chorionic membranes and Wharton jelly and in the decidua. Benirschke and Driscoll observed one specimen from which the parasite was isolated in which contiguous decidua capsularis, chorion, and amnion contained organisms [296,294]. In a retrospective histologic examination of 13 placentas of newborns with serologic test results suggestive of congenital *T. gondii* infection, Garcia and associates observed organisms that had the morphology of *T. gondii* tachyzoites in four cases [301]. Of interest is that in 10 of their cases, on gross examination, the placenta was found to be abnormal, suggesting the diagnosis of prolonged fetal distress, hematogenous infection, or both.

In some cases, the diagnosis was made initially from examination of the placenta [61,302]. Altshuler made a premortem diagnosis by noting cysts in connective tissue beneath the amnion in a very hydropic placenta [302]. The fetal villi showed hydrops, an abundance of Hofbauer cells, and vascular proliferation. Numerous erythroblasts were present within the vessels of the terminal villi.

Elliott described lesions in a placenta following a third-month spontaneous abortion of a macerated fetus [295]. The placenta showed nodular accumulations of histiocytes beneath the syncytial layer. In villi that had pronounced histiocytic infiltrates, the syncytial layer was raised away from the villous stroma, and the infiltrate had spilled into the intervillous space. Disruption of the syncytium was associated with coagulation necrosis of the villous stroma and fibrinous exudate. Both encysted and free forms of *T. gondii* were present in the areas of histiocytic inflammation, in the zones of coagulation necrosis, and in the villi without either necrotizing inflammation or syncytial loss. The location of the organisms varied, but they seemed to be concentrated at the interface between the stroma and the trophoblast. This aggregation of histiocytes and organisms at the stroma-trophoblast interface suggested to Elliott that this is a favored site of growth for the parasite.

Central Nervous System

In infants who die in the newborn period, the severity of the cellular reaction in the leptomeninges of both brain and spinal cord reflects the amount of damage done to underlying tissue. The pia-arachnoid overlying destructive cortical or spinal cord lesions shows congestion of the vessels and infiltration of large numbers of lymphocytes, plasma cells, macrophages, and eosinophils. This type of change is particularly noticeable around small arterioles, venules, and capillaries. Complete obliteration of the gyri and sulci may be noted; the line of demarcation between the pia-arachnoid and brain substance is obscured. Parasites frequently are found within intimal cells of the arterioles, venules, and capillaries [288].

In the cerebral hemispheres, brainstem, and cerebellum, extensive diffuse and focal alterations of the parenchymal architecture are seen (Figs. 31–6 and 31–7)

[56,288,293,303,304]. The most characteristic change is the extensive necrosis of the brain parenchyma due to vascular involvement by lesions. The lesions are most intense in the cortex and basal ganglia and at times in the periventricular areas; they are marked by the formation of glial nodules [56], which Wolf and coworkers referred to as characteristic miliary granulomas [304]. Necrosis may progress to actual formation of cystic areas, which have a homogeneous eosinophilic material at the center of the cyst cavity. At the periphery of these cystic areas, focal calcification of necrotic, individual nerve cells may be evident. Calcification within zones of necrosis may be extensive, with the formation of broad bands of calcific material involving most of the cortical layers, or it may be scattered diffusely throughout the foci of necrosis. Calcium salts are deposited in coarse granules or in finely divided particles, which give the appearance of "calcium dust." Many cells become completely calcified, whereas others contain only a few particles of finely divided calcium. Some pathologists have suggested that the *T. gondii* organisms themselves become encrusted with calcium salts [5,293]. (Cells containing fine particles of calcium also are observed in cytomegalovirus infection of the fetus or newborn and may be mistakenly construed as evidence of *T. gondii*.) The extent of calcification appears to depend on the severity of the reaction and the duration of the infection [288]. *T. gondii* tachyzoites and cysts are seen in and adjacent to the necrotic foci, near or in the glial nodules, in perivascular regions, and in cerebral tissue uninvolved by inflammatory change (see Figs. 31–6, *D* and 31–7, *D*) [303].

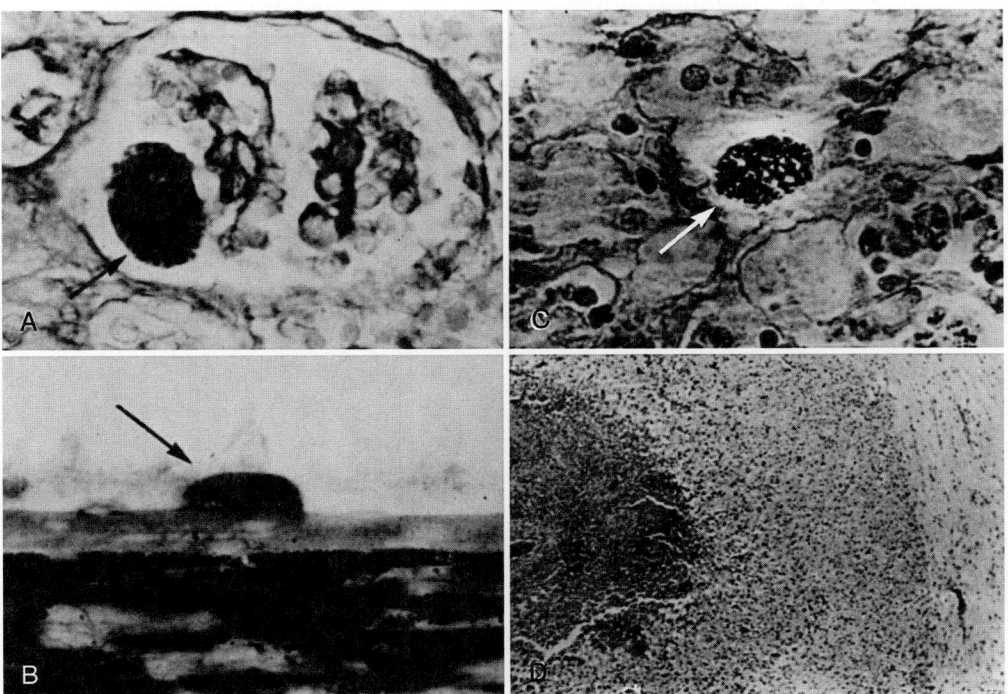

FIGURE 31–6 A, Large cyst (*arrow*) in glomerular space. **B**, *Toxoplasma* cyst (*arrow*) in the retina. Note incomplete pigmentation of the choroid. **C**, *Toxoplasma* cyst (*arrow*) in the cortex of the fetal adrenal gland. **D**, Section of brain showing abscess (*to the left*), normal brain (*on right*), and area of gliosis (*between*). Encysted parasites were abundant at the periphery of these areas. (*From Miller MJ, Seaman E, Remington JS. The clinical spectrum of congenital toxoplasmosis: problems in recognition. J Pediatr 70:714–723, 1967.*)

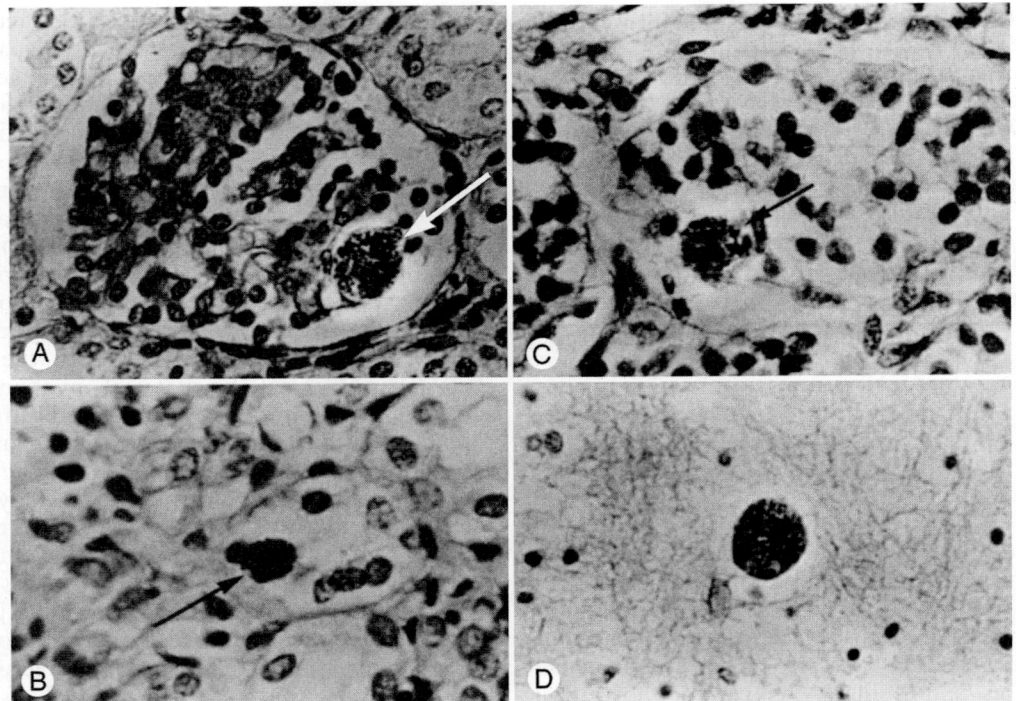

FIGURE 31-7 A, *Toxoplasma* cyst (*arrow*) within a glomerulus. Similar cysts were identified in endothelial cells of the glomeruli and free in the glomerular spaces. **B,** Encysted parasites (*arrow*) in a renal tubule cell. Other cysts were present within lumina of several tubules. **C,** *Toxoplasma* cyst (*arrow*) in immature testicular tissue. **D,** *Toxoplasma* cyst in cerebral cortex. Note lack of inflammatory response. *(From Miller MJ, Seaman E, Remington JS. The clinical spectrum of congenital toxoplasmosis: problems in recognition. J Pediatr 70:714–723, 1967.)*

Hervas and colleagues described an infant who developed progressive drowsiness, a weak cry, and grunting in the newborn period [305]. Computed tomography (CT) revealed cerebral calcifications, multiple ring-enhancing lesions mimicking brain abscesses, and moderate ventricular enlargement. At autopsy, *T. gondii* organisms were seen in the ventricular cerebrospinal fluid. Widespread necrosis and granulomatous lesions with mononuclear infiltrates also were noted.

The degree of change in the spinal cord is extremely variable. It may consist of local infiltration of lymphocytes and plasma cells or, on the other hand, almost complete disruption of the normal architecture, caused by the transformation of the gray and white matter into a mass of necrotic granulation tissue, may be seen. *T. gondii* cysts, which can be identified in the white matter, usually are unassociated with inflammatory reaction.

Periaqueductal and periventricular vasculitis with necrosis is a lesion that occurs only in toxoplasmosis [56]. The large areas of necrosis have been attributed to vascular thrombosis. The necrotic brain tissue autolyzes and gradually sloughs into the ventricles. The protein content of such ventricular fluid may be in the range of grams per deciliter, and the fluid has been shown to contain significant amounts of *T. gondii* antigens [306]. If the cerebral aqueduct of Sylvius becomes obstructed by the ependymitis, the lateral and third ventricles begin to resemble an abscess cavity containing accumulations of *T. gondii* and inflammatory cells [307]. Hydrocephalus develops in such children, and the necrotic brain tissue may calcify and become visible on radiographs. The fourth ventricle may show ulcers and ependymal nodules but is free from periventricular vasculitis and necrosis, apparently as a consequence of adequate drainage of its fluid through the foramina of Luschka and Magendie. The cerebrospinal fluid that communicates with the fourth ventricle often contains several hundred milligrams per deciliter of protein and fewer inflammatory cells than are seen in the lateral ventricle fluid [307]. Frequently, inflammation and necrosis are seen to involve the hypothalamus surrounding the third ventricle. Wolf and coworkers suggested that such lesions in the floor of the third ventricle probably cause the temperature lability observed in infants with congenital toxoplasmosis [304]. Destruction of brain tissue, especially intense periventricular necrosis, rather than obstruction of ventricular passages, appears to account for the development of hydrocephalus in some cases [293,304].

Eye

The histopathologic features of the ocular lesions depend on their stage of development at the time of the examination; a number of studies describing lesions in the earliest-recognized cases have been published [6,8,308–311], and were reviewed by Hogan in his classic thesis [312]. The description that follows is based on Hogan's summary of his and other cases.

The primary and principal lesions are found in the retina and choroid; secondary changes, such as iridocyclitis and cataracts [311], that occur in other portions of the eye are considered to represent complications of the chorioretinitis. Intraocular inflammation may cause microphthalmia, owing to arrest in development of the eye, or a secondary atrophy may result in shrinkage of the globe. The frequently reported failure of regression of the fetal pupillary vessels may indicate that an arrest in development occurred.

The inflammation commences in the retina (see Fig. 31–6, B), and a copious exudate in the vitreous produces a marked haze. Secondary involvement of the choroid causes marked elevation; small satellite foci are common. After healing, the lesions are atrophic and pale, with a variable amount of pigmentation at the margins.

The organisms first lodge in the capillaries of the inner layers of the retina, invade the endothelium, and extend into adjacent tissues. An intense focal inflammatory reaction results, with edema and infiltration of polymorphonuclear leukocytes, lymphocytes, plasma cells, mononuclear cells, and, in some cases, eosinophils. The reaction results in disruption and disorganization of the retinal layers. Cells are dislocated from the nuclear layers into the adjacent fiber layers. The external limiting membrane may be ruptured, displacing retinal cells into the subretinal space. The inner limiting membrane may also be interrupted, and cells from the inner nuclear layers are then displaced into the adjacent vitreous. Glial tissue, vascular connective tissue, and inflammatory exudate also extend through the interruptions in the inner and outer limiting membranes. In the zones of most acute inflammation, all retinal supporting and neural tissues are completely destroyed. The pigmentary epithelium shows extensive destruction. The retina may detach.

In the healing process, proliferation of the retinal pigment epithelial cells bordering the inflammatory foci occurs. Large lesions cause considerable necrosis and destruction, resulting in marked central atrophy of the retina and choroid. Disorganization of retinal cells has occurred [313].

Inflammation in the choroid is most acute beneath the retinal foci and is rather well demarcated. The Bruch membrane frequently is destroyed, and proliferation of connective tissue into the subretinal space may be seen. Retina and choroid thereby become fixed to each other by a scar. The choroidal vessels usually are engorged and show perivascular infiltration of lymphocytes, plasma cells, mononuclear cells, and eosinophils. Lymphocytes predominate, and both CD4+ and CD8+ lymphocytes are present [313].

Organisms are present in the retinal lesions and, in general, are most numerous where the lesions are most severe (see Fig. 31–6, B). Occasional parasites without an accompanying reaction are observed in relatively normal portions of the retina near the margins of inflammatory foci. The organisms may occur singly or in clusters, free or intracellularly, or in cysts (see Fig. 31–1, C and D). They are rarely seen in the choroid. They also have been found in the tissues of the optic papilla and in optic nerves associated with inflammatory cells in congenital cases [290,313].

Serofibrinous exudate and inflammatory cells extend into the vitreous through dehiscences in the inner limiting membrane of the retina. The exudate may be accompanied by masses of budding capillaries, and the vitreous becomes infiltrated with granulation tissue.

The optic disk may show papillitis, sometimes associated with optic neuritis and sometimes secondary to inflammation in the adjacent retina or papilledema caused by the hydrocephalus [313]. Leptomeningeal inflammation may be present around the optic nerve.

Ear

The presence of the parasite in the mastoid and inner ear and the accompanying inflammatory and pathologic changes have been considered to be causes of deafness in congenital toxoplasmosis [288,314]. Also, brainstem involvement affecting auditory nuclei can lead to inability to process auditory input.

Lungs and Heart

The alveolar septa may be widened, edematous, and infiltrated with mononuclear cells, occasional plasma cells, and rare eosinophils. The walls of small blood vessels may be infiltrated with lymphocytes and mononuclear cells, and parasites may be found in endothelial cells [288]. In many cases, some degree of bronchopneumonia, often caused by suprainfection with other agents, is present. T. gondii has been identified in the epithelial cells lining alveoli and within the endothelium of small blood vessels in such cases; in some affected patients, the pneumonic process was considered to be a prominent part of the general disease [288]. Single organisms have been found free in alveoli in the cases described by Zuelzer [293] and Paige and coworkers [6]. Of interest, their pathologic findings are identical to those described for adults in whom the lungs were particularly involved [8]. For a review of this subject in congenital and acquired cases, the reader is referred to the published articles by Couvreur [315] and Pomeroy and Filice [316].

T. gondii is almost always found in the heart in the form of cysts in myocardial fibers, accompanied by pathologic changes in the heart muscle. A focal infiltration with lymphocytes, plasma cells, mononuclear cells, and occasional eosinophils is seen. These foci usually do not contain organisms. In the focal areas of infiltration, the myocardial cells may undergo hyaline necrosis and fragmentation. Parasites are found in myocardial fibers in large aggregates and in cysts without any accompanying inflammatory reaction (see Fig. 31–1, D). Single parasites often may be present in areas of beginning necrosis and peripherally in larger areas of necrosis [288,293,303]. Extensive calcification of the heart, involving primarily the right ventricle and intraventricular septum, was observed in a 3-hour-old infant and was attributed to congenital toxoplasmosis [288]. Involvement of the heart has been demonstrated in a congenitally infected infant with AIDS who died of pneumocystis pneumonia and toxoplasmosis. Autopsy was limited to cardiac biopsy and revealed marked autolytic changes without evidence of inflammatory reaction or fibrosis. T. gondii organisms were identified in the muscle fibers [317].

Spleen, Liver, Ascites, and Kidney

Marked engorgement of the splenic pulp may be noted, along with erythropoiesis. In general, no significant pathologic changes that could be attributed to direct destruction by the parasite have been noted in the spleen. In some cases, an eosinophilic leukocytic infiltration has been described [56,293]. Organisms are rarely seen in the spleen.

In most cases, parasites are not identified in the liver, and neither necrosis nor inflammatory cell infiltrations are present. In some instances, in areas of marked hepatocellular degenerative changes do occur but without associated cellular infiltration [56,291,293]. The periportal spaces may be infiltrated with mononuclear cells, neutrophils, and eosinophils. Enlargement of the liver frequently is pronounced and is accompanied by erythropoiesis, as occurs also in the spleen. In a few cases, hepatic cirrhosis has been observed as a sequel to congenital toxoplasmosis [318]. Caldera and coworkers have described calcification in the liver seen both radiologically and at autopsy [319].

Congenital toxoplasmosis was diagnosed by exfoliative cytologic examination of ascitic fluid in a 7-week-old infant born at 38 weeks of gestation. Hepatomegaly and anemia developed shortly after birth, and liver failure and ascites during the first week of life. Because an extensive workup failed to reveal a cause, a paracentesis was performed that revealed tachyzoites both in Wright-stained smear preparations and in electron microscopy sections. This case is reminiscent of that of an adult patient with AIDS in whom the diagnosis of toxoplasmosis was first established on examination of Wright-Giemsa-stained smears of ascitic fluid obtained because of suspected bacterial peritonitis [320].

Numerous foci of hematopoiesis may be seen in the kidney. Focal glomerulitis often has been observed; in such cases, a majority of glomeruli remain intact [288,293]. In fully developed lesions, glomerular tufts undergo massive necrosis, and necrosis of adjacent tubules may be seen. In the earlier stages of the glomerular lesion, some capillary loops are still intact; in others, necrotic areas are observed in the basement membrane and epithelium, and the lumina are occluded by fibrin thrombi. In some of these partly preserved glomeruli, single parasites have been found in cells of the exudate within the capsular space or embedded in the necrotic remains of the capillary loop [293]. T. gondii cysts have been found in glomeruli and renal tubules of kidneys in which there were no other associated lesions (see Figs. 31–6, A and 31–7, A and B) [321,322]. In severely affected kidneys, focal areas of necrosis also are found in the collecting tubules in the medulla. The inflammatory infiltrations are predominantly mononuclear, although in some cases, numerous eosinophils also are seen scattered throughout. In 1966, Fediushina and Sherstennikova reported the pathologic findings in the kidneys in nine cases of congenital toxoplasmosis [323]. In three of these cases, distinct changes in the glomeruli were noted, and as described by these investigators, many of the changes appear to resemble those observed in glomerulonephritis from other causes, including streptococcal infection.

In 1972, Wickbom and Winberg reported a case of a 10-week-old boy with congenital toxoplasmosis who developed severe nephritis with the nephrotic syndrome [324]. In that same year, Shahin and associates reported a case of nephrotic syndrome in a 4-month-old infant with congenital toxoplasmosis [325]. Granular and pseudolinear glomerular deposits of IgM, fibrinogen, and T. gondii antigen and antibody were demonstrated in the glomeruli of the initial biopsy of renal tissue. After approximately 7 months of treatment, a second renal biopsy showed no evidence of the T. gondii antigen-antibody complexes previously noted, but IgM, fibrinogen, and the fourth component of complement (C4) were present. IgG and C3 were not demonstrable in the glomeruli in either biopsy specimen. Light microscopy of the first renal biopsy revealed glomeruli with a diffuse mild increase in mesangial cells and matrix. One glomerulus contained a segmented area of sclerosis that adhered to the Bowman capsule. Other findings included rare foci of tubular atrophy and associated interstitial fibrosis, occasional hyaline casts, focal tubular and interstitial calcification, and prominent tubular hyaline droplets. The second renal biopsy specimen, obtained after treatment with prednisone for 7 months and with pyrimethamine and sulfadiazine for 3 weeks, revealed glomeruli with varying degrees of damage, ranging from total hyalinization to partial collapse and segmental sclerosis. The tubulointerstitial changes were not significantly different from those observed in the first biopsy specimen. The results of electron microscopy also were reported.

Endocrine Organs

Parasites and numerous foci of necrosis have been identified in the adrenal cortex (see Fig. 31–6, C). Similar areas of necrosis have been found in the pancreas [6,288,292,293]. Parasites, usually without associated inflammation, have been found in the pituitary [288,292]. Large clusters of organisms, without accompanying inflammation or necrosis, have been found in the acini of the thyroid gland [6]. In the testes and ovaries, acute interstitial inflammation with focal areas of necrosis are frequently observed [6,56,288,292,293]. Necrosis of the seminiferous tubules with preservation of adjacent units is common, with infiltration with plasma cells, lymphocytes, mononuclear cells, and eosinophils. Parasites often are observed in the spermatogonia of intact tubules (see Fig. 31–7, C). Focal hematopoiesis has been observed in the interstitia of these organs.

Skeletal Muscle

Involvement varies, ranging in degree from parasitized fibers without pathologic changes to focal areas of infiltration or widespread myositis with necrosis. The organisms in parasitized fibers are found beneath the sarcolemmal sheaths. Hundreds of organisms may be present in a single long tubular space in a fiber, and T. gondii cysts frequently are seen in muscle fibers. The affected fibers are swollen and lose their striations, but as a rule, no inflammatory reactions are noted. By contrast, focal areas of inflammation and necrosis may be present in areas where only a few parasites or none can be identified. The cellular infiltrate consists mainly of mononuclear cells, but lymphocytes, plasma cells, and eosinophils also are present. In rare instances, focal inflammatory lesions may be found adjacent to heavily parasitized but unbroken muscle fibers [293]. Noteworthy is the description of severe involvement of the extraocular muscles in the case described by Rodney and coworkers [303].

Thymus

Sarrut observed a hypoplastic thymus in an infant who died of congenital toxoplasmosis at the age of 1 month (personal communication to Desmonts G, 1980). The disease was not diagnosed before autopsy. *T. gondii* organisms were isolated from the brain and heart. The histologic picture in this case was quite different from that described in experimental infection in newborn mice [326] in that in the former, hypoplasia involved both lymphocytes and Hassall corpuscles.

Skin

Torres found *T. gondii* tachyzoites without formation of lesions in the subcutaneous tissue of one infant [327]. In a case ("case 5") reported by Paige and associates, *T. gondii* organisms were present in the subcutaneous tissue, again with no associated inflammatory lesion or necrosis [6]. No rash was noted in the infant.

Bone

Milgram described osseous changes in a fatal case of congenital toxoplasmosis [292]. The infant died on day 17, and at autopsy widespread active infection was discovered. The parasite was found in almost all tissues of the body. Large numbers of inflammatory cells were found in the bone marrow, with deficient osteogenesis and remodeling in the primary spongiosa. Intracellular aggregates of *T. gondii* were present in macrophages in the bone marrow.

Immunoglobulin Abnormalities

Subtle abnormalities have been noted in the development of immunoglobulins in infants with subclinical congenital toxoplasmosis [328]. In several infants, retarded development of IgA for the first 3 years of life and excessive development of IgG and IgM were noted. The latter abnormality also is seen in congenital rubella, cytomegalic inclusion disease, and syphilis. In the *T. gondii*-infected children, the degree of increase in IgG and IgM appeared to be directly related to the severity of the infection.

Oxelius described monoclonal (M) immunoglobulins of the IgG class in the serum and cerebrospinal fluid of three newborns with severe clinical signs of congenital toxoplasmosis [329]. Because these M proteins were found in the sera of newborns but not in the sera of their mothers, Oxelius concluded that the M immunoglobulins were either selectively transferred or synthesized by the newborn. Reports by Van Camp and associates [330] and Griscelli and colleagues [331] suggest that the observation by Oxelius may not be uncommon. Griscelli and colleagues performed a survey of 27 newborns and older infants who had the severe form of congenital toxoplasmosis. In 11 of the infants, M IgG components were noted. These authors concluded that these components were synthesized by the fetus because they could be detected up to 75 days post partum and were absent in maternal serum. They were unable to define any anti-*T. gondii* antibody in isolated M IgG. Absorption of the hypergammaglobulinemic sera with antigens of *T. gondii* resulted in almost complete loss of anti-*Toxoplasma* antibodies detected using the dye test but did not affect the presence of the M component or significantly reduce the immunoglobulin levels. Similar results have been reported in *T. gondii*-infected mice; hypergammaglobulinemia and a condition that appeared to be a monoclonal spike was observed [258]. The underlying mechanism or the cause of the appearance of M components in infants with congenital toxoplasmosis is unknown. M components have also been described in congenital syphilis [332].

Toxoplasma gondii–Cytomegalovirus Infection

A number of reports of dual infection with *T. gondii*–cytomegalovirus have appeared [333–336]. In systematically searching for cytomegalovirus infection among nine autopsies in cases of congenital toxoplasmosis, Vinh and coworkers found these two diseases coexisting in two instances [335]. Sotelo-Avila and associates described a case of coexisting congenital toxoplasmosis and cytomegalovirus infection in a microcephalic infant who died at the age of 15 days [336]. Microscopically, numerous areas of calcification and necrosis and large cells with the characteristic nuclear inclusions of cytomegalovirus were seen. Aggregates of *T. gondii* were found in the cytoplasm of many of the cytomegalic inclusion cells in the CNS, lungs, retina, kidneys, and liver. Maszkiewicz and colleagues described a case of cytomegalic inclusion disease with toxoplasmosis in a premature infant [335].

CLINICAL MANIFESTATIONS
Infection in the Pregnant Woman

Because acute acquired *T. gondii* infection in the pregnant woman usually is unrecognized, the infection in such cases has been said to be asymptomatic. A diagnosis of asymptomatic infection is based largely on retrospective questioning of mothers who gave birth to infected infants and requires prospective clinical studies for documentation. Even if signs and symptoms are more frequently associated with the acute infection, they often are so slight as to escape the memory in the vast majority of women.

The most commonly recognized clinical manifestations of acquired toxoplasmosis are lymphadenopathy and fatigue without fever [163,337–339]. The groups of nodes most commonly involved are the cervical, suboccipital, supraclavicular, axillary, and inguinal. The adenopathy may be localized (e.g., most commonly a single posterior cervical node is enlarged), or it may involve multiple areas, including retroperitoneal and mesenteric nodes [340]. Palpable nodes usually are discrete, vary in firmness, and may or may not be tender; there is no tendency toward suppuration. The lymphadenopathy may occasionally have a febrile course accompanied by malaise, headache, fatigue, sore throat, and myalgia-features that closely simulate those of infectious mononucleosis. The spleen [341] and liver [342] also may be involved [343–345]. Atypical lymphocytes indistinguishable from those seen in infectious mononucleosis may be present in smears of peripheral blood. In some patients, lymphadenopathy may persist for as long as 1 year, and malaise also may be persistent, although this finding is more difficult to relate directly to the infection [346]. An exanthem may be present—it has been described in a pregnant patient [290]. An association of *T. gondii* infection and the clinical syndromes of polymyositis and dermatomyositis has been reported [347–350]. Chorioretinitis occurs in the acute acquired infection, and many such cases have been documented [351–355]. In São Paulo and Minais Gerais, Brazil, retinal disease has been reported to be common in the acute acquired infection [207,210].

Infection in the Infant
General Considerations

A diagnosis of congenital *T. gondii* infection usually is considered in infants who show signs of hydrocephalus, chorioretinitis, and intracranial calcifications. These signs, often described as the classic triad [356], were present in the first proven case of congenital toxoplasmosis described by Wolf and colleagues in 1939 [5]. Since this original observation was made, however, they, and other investigators, have seen and described congenitally infected infants who presented with a variety of clinical signs; the clinical spectrum may range from normal appearance at birth to a picture of erythroblastosis, hydrops fetalis, the classic triad of toxoplasmosis, or a variety of other manifestations [356,357]. Thus such wide variation in clinical signs precludes a diagnosis according to strict adherence to a set of specific clinical criteria. Such adherence may lead to misdiagnoses, especially in cases of congenital toxoplasmosis in which the signs mimic those of other disease states. Until the variability in the clinical picture of congenital *T. gondii* infection is appreciated by pediatricians and until the diagnosis is considered more often in infants with mild nonspecific illness, the blindness, mental retardation, and even death related to *T. gondii* infection will continue to go unrecognized.

Congenital *T. gondii* infection may occur in one of four forms: (1) a neonatal disease; (2) a disease (severe or mild) occurring in the first months of life; (3) sequelae or relapse of a previously undiagnosed infection during infancy, childhood, or adolescence; or (4) a subclinical infection. When clinically recognized in the neonate, the infection usually is severe. Symptoms and signs of generalized infection may be prominent, and signs referable to the CNS are almost always present. The neurologic signs frequently are more extensive than might be suspected at first.

In other neonates, neurologic signs (e.g., convulsions, bulging fontanelle, nystagmus, abnormal increase in head circumference) are the major indications of the diagnosis. Such manifestations are not always associated with gross cerebral damage; instead, they may be related to an active encephalitis not yet associated with irreversible cerebral necrosis or to obstruction of the cerebral aqueduct of Sylvius caused by edema or inflammatory cells, or both, rather than to extensive necrosis and irreversible brain parenchymal damage. In these latter infants who receive treatment, signs and symptoms may disappear and development may be normal thereafter.

Mild cases in the neonate usually are not recognized. Identification of the disease has been possible in prospective studies, however, when infants born to mothers known to have acquired *T. gondii* infection during pregnancy are examined. The most frequent signs include isolated chorioretinal scars. Such cases prove that the infection was active during fetal life without causing other detectable damage.

Most children with congenital *T. gondii* infection are thought to have been normal at birth, as signs or symptoms were not recognized and other signs become manifest weeks, months, or years later. Obviously, in many cases this clinical picture is not one of delayed onset of disease but one of late recognition of disease. Nevertheless, it has been possible to verify delayed onset of disease weeks or months or years after birth in children who at birth had no abnormalities that could be related to toxoplasmosis [61,182,328,358]. Disease with delayed onset may be severe and is most frequently seen in premature infants, in whom severe CNS and eye lesions appear during the first 3 months after birth. In the full-term infant with delayed onset of disease, manifestations arise mainly during the first 2 months of life. Clinical signs may be related to generalized infection (e.g., hepatosplenomegaly, delayed onset of icterus, lymphadenopathy); CNS involvement (e.g., encephalitis or hydrocephalus), which may occur after a more protracted period; or eye lesions, which may develop months or years after birth in infants and children whose fundi are checked repeatedly.

Sequelae most often are ocular (e.g., chorioretinitis occurring at school age or adolescence), but in some cases they are neurologic—for instance, convulsions may lead to the discovery of cerebral calcifications or retinal scars. Ocular lesions may recur during childhood, adolescence, or adulthood. In some instances, neurologic relapses (e.g., late obstruction of the aqueduct) have been observed.

Congenital *T. gondii* infection in the newborn in the series from France, and in a study performed in the United States [182,359], most frequently was a subclinical or inapparent infection, not, as had previously been thought, an obvious and fulminant one. In those infants who were clinically normal at birth, the infection was diagnosed by demonstration of persistent serologic test titers. Such asymptomatic infants may suffer no untoward sequelae of the infection, or more often, abnormalities such as chorioretinitis, strabismus, blindness, hydrocephaly or microcephaly, psychomotor and mental retardation, epilepsy, or deafness may develop or become apparent only months or even years later [245,360,361]. Such patients—asymptomatic at birth but demonstrating untoward sequelae later—were noted by Callahan and coworkers in the early 1940s (their cases 3 and 4) [288]. Frequently, neurologic signs or hydrocephalus appears between 3 and 12 months of life [362]. In patients with encephalitic lesions, CNS abnormalities that produce clinical signs rarely develop after the first year (see "Follow-up Studies" later on) [363].

At present, no parameters are available to use in predicting the precise outcome in a newborn with asymptomatic *T. gondii* infection who remains untreated. Hundreds of reports, however, attest to the crippling effects of infection when severe disease is apparent at birth.

Clinically Apparent Disease. One of the most complete studies was that of Eichenwald, who in 1947 initiated a study to discover the clinical forms of congenital toxoplasmosis and to determine the natural history of the infection and its effect on the infant [356]. The cases were referred by a group of cooperating hospitals in a systematic and prearranged manner. Sera were obtained from three groups of infants and their mothers. The first two groups consisted of 5492 infants examined because they had either undiagnosed CNS disease in the first year of life (neurologic disease group) or undiagnosed nonneurologic diseases during the first 2 months of life (generalized disease group). The third group consisted of 5761 normal infants. The incidence rates of serologically proven cases in the three groups were 4.9%, 1.3%, and 0.07%, respectively. Of the 11,253 infants studied, 156 had serologically proven congenital toxoplasmosis; 69% were in the neurologic disease group, and 28% were in the generalized disease group. The signs and symptoms in the infants in these two groups are shown in Table 31–10. Approximately one third showed signs and symptoms of an acute infectious process, with

TABLE 31–11   Major Sequelae of Congenital Toxoplasmosis Among 105 Patients Followed 4 Years or More

Condition	No. (%) with Neurologic Disease* (70 patients)	No. (%) with Generalized Disease† (31 patients)	No. (%) with Subclinical Disease (4 patients)
Mental retardation	69 (98)	25 (81)	2 (50)
Convulsions	58 (83)	24 (77)	2 (50)
Spasticity and palsies	53 (76)	18 (58)	0
Severely impaired vision	48 (69)	13 (42)	0
Hydrocephalus or microcephaly	31 (44)	2 (6)	0
Deafness	12 (17)	3 (10)	0
Normal	6 (9)	5 (16)	2 (50)

*Infants with otherwise undiagnosed central nervous system diseases in the first year of life.
†Infants with otherwise undiagnosed non-neurologic diseases during the first 2 months of life.
Adapted from Eichenwald HF. A study of congenital toxoplasmosis. In Siim JC (ed). Human Toxoplasmosis. Copenhagen, Munksgaard, 1960, with permission. Study performed in 1947.

TABLE 31–10   Signs and Symptoms Occurring Before Diagnosis or During the Course of Acute Congenital Toxoplasmosis

Signs and Symptoms	Frequency of Occurrence (%) in Infants with	
	Neurologic Disease* (108 Cases)	Generalized Disease† (44 Cases)
Chorioretinitis	94	66
Abnormal spinal fluid	55	84
Anemia	51	77
Convulsions	50	18
Intracranial calcification	50	4
Jaundice	29	80
Hydrocephalus	28	0
Fever	25	77
Splenomegaly	21	90
Lymphadenopathy	17	68
Hepatomegaly	17	77
Vomiting	16	48
Microcephaly	13	0
Diarrhea	6	25
Cataracts	5	0
Eosinophilia	4	18
Abnormal bleeding	3	18
Hypothermia	2	20
Glaucoma	2	0
Optic atrophy	2	0
Microphthalmia	2	0
Rash	1	25
Pneumonitis	0	41

*Infants with otherwise undiagnosed central nervous system diseases in the first year of life.
†Infants with otherwise undiagnosed non-neurologic disease during the first 2 months of life.
Adapted from Eichenwald HF. A study of congenital toxoplasmosis. In Siim JC (ed). Human Toxoplasmosis. Copenhagen, Munksgaard, 1960, with permission. Study performed in 1947.

splenomegaly, hepatomegaly, jaundice, anemia, chorioretinitis, and abnormal cerebrospinal fluid as the most common findings. The so-called classic triad of toxoplasmosis was demonstrated in only a small proportion of the patients. The fact that 98% of the infants had clinical evidence of infection can be explained by the manner in which the case material was collected for the study. Despite the fact that Eichenwald clearly defined this, his data for years have been misinterpreted to show that all infants with congenital T. gondii infection have signs and symptoms of infection, as set forth in Table 31–10. Most of the patients were evaluated over a period from birth to the age of 5 years or beyond. The overall mortality rate was 12% (no significant differences in mortality rate existed between the clinical groups), and approximately 85% of the survivors were mentally retarded. Convulsions, spasticity, and palsies developed in almost 75%, and about 50% had severely impaired vision (Table 31–11). It is noteworthy that deafness, usually attributed to congenital viral infections (e.g., cytomegalovirus infection, rubella), also occurs as a sequel to congenital T. gondii infection. The signs and symptoms in this series of patients differ in many respects from those recorded in reports published earlier, owing undoubtedly to the fact that the cases studied by Eichenwald were drawn from a relatively unselected group rather than from a limited survey based on infants tested solely because they showed most of the so-called classic signs of congenital toxoplasmosis.

Subclinical Infection. Studies of subclinical infection have been performed in an attempt to determine the following: how often congenital T. gondii infection is subclinical; whether it is really subclinical or whether, in fact, initial signs have gone unrecognized; and what the prognosis is for subclinical infection. For information on prognosis, see "Follow-up Studies," later on in this section.

TABLE 31-12 Data in 10 Newborns with Congenital *Toxoplasma* Infection Identified by the Presence of IgM *Toxoplasma* Antibodies

Finding	No. of Infants
Maternal illness ("flu")	2
Diagnosis suspected (neonate)	1
Gestational prematurity*	5
Intrauterine growth retardation†	2
Hepatosplenomegaly	1
Jaundice	1
Thrombocytopenia	1
Anemia	1
Chorioretinitis	2
Abnormal head size	0
Hydrocephalus	1
Microcephaly	0
Abnormal cerebrospinal fluid	8‡
Abnormalities on neurologic examination	1
Serum IgM elevated	9
Serum IgM *Toxoplasma* antibody	10

*<37 weeks of gestation.
†Lower tenth percentile (Grunewald).
‡Only eight were examined.
Adapted from Alford CA Jr, Stagno S, Reynolds DW. Congenital toxoplasmosis: clinical, laboratory, and therapeutic considerations, with special reference to subclinical disease. Bull N Y Acad Med 50:106–181, 1974, with permission.

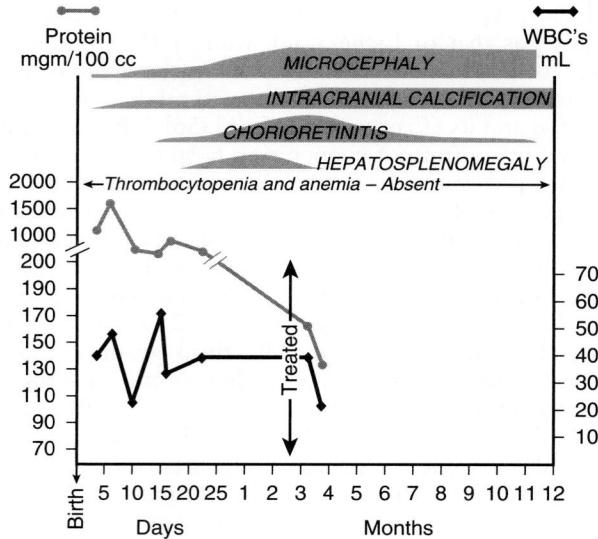

FIGURE 31–8 Severe form of congenital toxoplasmosis. Protein content and WBC count in cerebrospinal fluid, with clinical findings, over clinical course. *(From Alford CA, et al. Subclinical central nervous system disease of neonates: a prospective study of infants born with increased levels of IgM. J Pediatr 75:1167–1178, 1969.)*

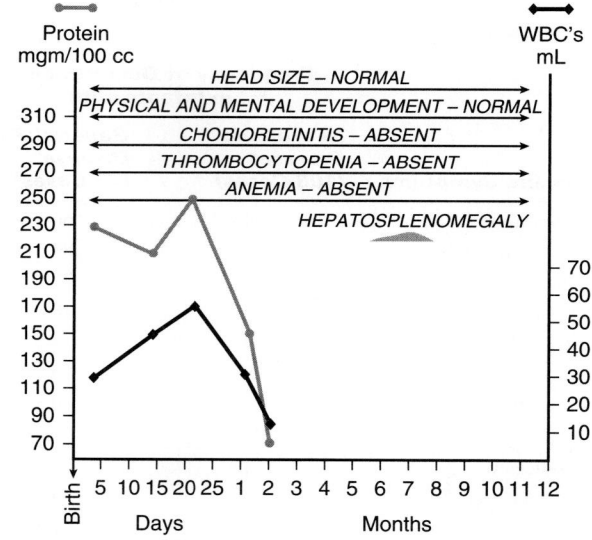

FIGURE 31–9 Mild form of congenital toxoplasmosis. Protein content and WBC count in cerebrospinal fluid, with clinical findings, over clinical course. *(Data from Alford CA, et al. Subclinical central nervous system disease of neonates: a prospective study of infants born with increased levels of IgM. J Pediatr 75:1167–1178, 1969.)*

Alford and colleagues performed a series of studies to determine the medical significance of the subclinical form of congenital *T. gondii* infection [328]. Their serologic screening program (see "Diagnosis" section) was performed in a moderately low-socioeconomic-status urban population in the southern United States, and 10 infants with congenital *T. gondii* infection were detected among 7500 newborns screened (1 proven case per 750 deliveries over a study period of 2.5 years). The findings in the 10 newborns are shown in Table 31–12. Only 1 infant had signs that suggested *T. gondii* infection (hepatosplenomegaly, chorioretinitis, cerebral calcification). Thus nine of the infected infants would have escaped detection were it not for the laboratory screening program. The investigators pointed out that, nevertheless, significant abnormalities were found in this group of newborns with so-called subclinical infection. Half were premature, and the average birth weight of the infected infants, 2664 g, was 349 g less than that of control infants (3013 g). Although no signs or symptoms referable to the nervous system were present in the nine infants, abnormalities in the cerebrospinal fluid were noted in each of the eight infants in whom this examination was performed. Cerebrospinal fluid lymphocytosis (10 to 110 cells per μL) and elevated protein levels (150 to 1000 mg/dL) persisted for 2 weeks to 4 months or more (average, at least 3 months for the group), even in infants who were given treatment in the first 4 weeks after birth. The findings in a severe case and a mild case are depicted graphically in Figures 31–8 and 31–9, respectively. The infant whose data are shown in Figure 31–8 was premature but demonstrated no signs of infection during the neonatal period. The elevated level of cerebrospinal fluid protein

suggested severe CNS involvement from birth onward. At 2.5 months of age, retarded growth of the head, generalized intracranial calcification, chorioretinitis, and hepatosplenomegaly first became evident; these abnormalities worsened despite treatment with pyrimethamine and sulfadiazine, which was, however, instituted late in the course of the infection. At the age of 4 years, this child had a developmental level of 2 years.

Figure 31–9 shows a representative example of the eight patients with milder disease, in six of whom cerebrospinal fluid abnormalities were present. Persistent lymphocytosis was detected in all, and elevations of cerebrospinal fluid protein levels were distinctly lower (150 to 285 mg/dL) in this group than in the two infants who proved to have severe disease.

Follow-up evaluation in infants who were asymptomatic at birth is discussed under "Follow-up Studies." The data indicate that nearly all children born with subclinical congenital *T. gondii* infection develop adverse sequelae.

How often is congenital infection subclinical? The only prospective data are from studies performed in France, where serologic examination of pregnant women for *T. gondii* infection is obligatory. Couvreur and colleagues reported on a series of 210 infants referred to them because acute acquired infection with *T. gondii* was diagnosed in the mothers before delivery [364]. The series includes all cases of congenital infection prospectively diagnosed from 1972 to 1981. Infants referred because of the presence of clinical signs but who were born to mothers in whom the diagnosis of acute acquired infection had not been previously made during pregnancy were not included (because diagnosis in these cases was retrospective). Among these 210 infants, 2 died during the first year of life; the cause of death in 1 was systemic congenital toxoplasmosis and in the other probably was not related to *T. gondii* infection. Twenty-one infants (10%) had severe congenital toxoplasmosis with CNS involvement. Eye lesions were present in most cases, and systemic disease was present in some. Seventy-one cases (34%) were mild, with normal findings on clinical examination except for the presence of peripheral retinal scarring or isolated intracranial calcifications in an asymptomatic child. Of the 210 infants, 116 (55%) had subclinical infections both at initial examination and at a subsequent examination at the age of 12 months. The frequency of the signs observed is shown in Table 31–13. As pointed out by the investigators, these figures for the respective frequencies of severe, mild, and subclinical cases are biased. Several biases probably decreased the relative frequency of severe congenital infection. The most severe cases with neonatal death were not referred to the investigators, nor probably were those in which congenital toxoplasmosis was so evidently severe that therapy did not appear worthwhile. In addition, an abortion often is performed when acquired infection is diagnosed sufficiently early during pregnancy. This intervention probably decreased the number of infected infants born alive despite early transmission of the parasites, which probably would have resulted in delivery of severely damaged infants (see "Transmission" section). Also, when diagnosis in the mother is made before delivery, treatment with spiramycin has resulted in fewer severely infected offspring and might have decreased the severity of infection in the fetus [78]. In the studies by Couvreur and colleagues [364], the numbers of severe cases were 16 (14%) among 116 infants born to untreated mothers and 3 (4%) in the 79 cases in which the mothers were known to have been treated.

This study [364] also allows for an estimation of the proportion of cases in which infection is really subclinical and of those in which initial signs have in fact not been recognized. Among 116 cases in which infection was considered to be subclinical by the referring physicians, 39 (33%) were discovered to have one or several signs of congenital toxoplasmosis; the most frequent sign was an abnormality on examination of the cerebrospinal fluid.

TABLE 31–13 Prospective Study of Infants Born to Women Who Acquired *Toxoplasma* Infection During Pregnancy: Signs and Symptoms in 210 Infants with Proven Congenital Infection

Finding	No. Examined	No. Positive (%)
Prematurity	210	
Birth weight <2500 g		8 (3.8)
Birth weight 2500–3000 g		5 (7.1)
Dysmaturity (intrauterine growth retardation)		13 (6.2)
Postmaturity	108	9 (8.3)
Icterus	201	20 (10)
Hepatosplenomegaly	210	9 (4.2)
Thrombocytopenic purpura	210	3 (1.4)
Abnormal blood count (anemia, eosinophilia)	102	9 (4.4)
Microcephaly	210	11 (5.2)
Hydrocephalus	210	8 (3.8)
Hypotonia	210	2 (5.7)
Convulsions	210	8 (3.8)
Psychomotor retardation	210	11 (5.2)
Intracranial calcifications on radiography	210	24 (11.4)
Abnormal ultrasound examination	49	5 (10)
Abnormal computed tomography scan of brain	13	11 (84)
Abnormal electroencephalographic result	191	16 (8.3)
Abnormal cerebrospinal fluid	163	56 (34.2)
Microphthalmia	210	6 (2.8)
Strabismus	210	11 (5.2)
Chorioretinitis	210	
Unilateral		34 (16.1)
Bilateral		12 (5.7)

Data adapted from Couvreur J, et al. A homogeneous series of 210 cases of congenital toxoplasmosis in 0- to 11-month-old infants detected prospectively. Ann Pediatr (Paris) 31:815–819, 1984.

In a newborn serologic screening program in Massachusetts, more thorough evaluations of the apparently asymptomatic newborns revealed 20% with eye disease and 20% with neurologic findings [365].

Prematurity

Prematurity and low Apgar scores are common among newborns with congenital *T. gondii* infection who have clinically apparent disease at birth [96,360,366,367]. In larger series, prematurity has been reported in 25% to more than 50% of the infants. When Lelong and co-workers searched for cases of congenital toxoplasmosis on a single ward of premature infants, they found 7 among 1085 infants (0.6%) [182].

Twins

In 1965, Glasser and Delta reviewed reports of congenital toxoplasmosis in twins that had appeared in the literature up to that year [61]. Later, Couvreur and colleagues reviewed this subject and added 14 of their own previously unpublished cases to the literature. Through 1980, we are aware of 35 cases of congenital toxoplasmosis in twins: 11 in monozygotic twins, 13 in dizygotic twins, and 11 whose type is undetermined [61,182,368–372], In 1986, Sibalic and associates reported on a series of 21 pairs of twins with congenital toxoplasmosis in 38 of the infants [373]. *T. gondii* was isolated from four infants. In the remainder, the diagnosis was made by serologic testing alone. Wiswell and coworkers reported congenital toxoplasmosis in triplets [374]. *T. gondii* was demonstrated in the cerebrospinal fluid of each infant; no mention was made of whether the infants were polyzygotic. Each of the three infants had severe disease.

The diagnosis of congenital toxoplasmosis probably would be missed in an asymptomatic twin were it not for specific lesions in the other twin that lead the physician to consider this diagnosis [322,368]. Thus variable clinical patterns have been noted in pairs of twins, and in some sets, one twin died and a subclinical infection existed in the other [322,357,371]. It is doubtful that the diagnosis of congenital toxoplasmosis would have been suspected in the surviving twins without benefit of the results of autopsy in their respective twins [322].

A distinct difference in clinical patterns has been observed between monozygotic and dizygotic twins. In nine pairs of monozygotic twins, the clinical pattern in each twin of a pair most often appears to be similar [61]. For example, chorioretinitis was found in each twin in seven pairs. In addition, with one exception [293], the lesions were either bilateral or unilateral in each twin of each pair considered. Each twin in four sets had hydrocephalus, in four sets cerebral calcification, in four sets convulsions, and in one set mental and motor retardation. In only two sets, in which each infant had hyperbilirubinemia, was there a marked variation from this similarity in clinical pattern in single sets. In each of these sets, one twin died and the other survived [293,322,368]. Among the monozygotic twins, a remarkable predominance of males (eight of nine pairs) was noted, a phenomenon as yet unexplained.

In dizygotic twins, on the other hand, discrepancies in clinical findings within single sets are frequent and marked. In 11 sets of dizygotic twins [368,371,372,375], chorioretinitis was present in 13 of the 22 twins but was observed in both twins of a set in only two instances [368,371,372], and even in these the lesions were not identical. Such discrepancies also were true for virtually all other clinical features in these twins. In many cases, one of the twins had a subclinical infection, whereas in the other it was severe [368,376]. In two sets of twins, one bichorial and biamniotic and the other monochorial and biamniotic, one infant in each set completely escaped infection [368]. An additional report confirms these findings [377].

Central Nervous System

Other clinical manifestations of CNS destruction are described later under "Mental Retardation," "Down Syndrome," and "Radiologic Abnormalities."

Although in infants with clinical manifestations the signs of congenital toxoplasmosis may vary considerably, widespread destruction of the CNS usually gives rise to the first clinical indications of disease. Among the most common manifestations are internal obstructive hydrocephalus [378], which often is present at birth or appears shortly thereafter and usually is progressive; seizures, which may range from muscular twitching and spasticity to major motor seizures; stiff neck with retraction of the head and, in some cases, opisthotonos; and spinal or bulbar involvement manifested by paralysis of the extremities, difficulty in swallowing, and respiratory distress. Thus the spectrum of neurologic manifestations is protean and may range from a massive acute encephalopathy to a subtle neurologic syndrome. That the infection can involve the spinal cord is highlighted by a case in a 4-week-old girl who had macrocephaly and paralysis of both legs. CT revealed hydrocephalus, and magnetic resonance imaging revealed numerous lesions in the cerebral parenchyma and spinal cord [379]. Eighty-four cases (6.5%) of toxoplasmosis were found among 1282 children younger than 1 year of age who had signs of neurologic disease without obvious underlying causative conditions [363]. (A similar frequency, 4.9%, was reported by Eichenwald [356]). The proportion of cases of congenital *T. gondii* infection was strikingly greater in infants with retinal lesions associated with CNS involvement (62 of 266 cases examined [23%]) than in those who had CNS lesions but no ocular lesions (22 of 1016 cases examined [2.2%]).

It is important to recognize that hydrocephalus due to aqueductal obstruction may be the sole clinical manifestation associated with congenital *T. gondii* infection. Occasionally, the hydrocephalus may be stable, but in most cases, management necessitates a neurosurgical shunt procedure [380]. In a significant number of infants, the prognosis is good, especially after shunt placement; the intelligence quotient (IQ) may be within the normal range. The performance of CT in the months after shunt placement is useful in determining long-term prognosis—which is good if the results of the CT are normal, even in some cases with clinically apparent encephalitis. The prognosis is less promising when there is little expansion of the cortical mantle in the months after ventriculoperitoneal shunt placement. Follow-up CT after shunt placement also is important to exclude subdural collections associated with bleeding from small vessels associated with reduction of pressure when the obstructive hydrocephalus is corrected.

Kaiser has presented a follow-up study of 10 children with hydrocephalus resulting from congenital toxoplasmosis [381]. Hydrocephalus was present at birth in only 3 of the 10 patients and was noted for the first time as late as 11 and 15 months in 2 patients, respectively. All children had progressive hydrocephalus, which required placement of a shunt. In the National Collaborative Chicago-based Congenital Toxoplasmosis Study (NCCCTS), hydrocephalus was present in 45 children. It usually was detected clinically at birth, occasionally prenatally, and after 2 weeks of age in 16 infants. Occasionally, hydrocephalus developed after birth. All children with substantial hydrocephalus, in which there was evidence of aqueductal obstruction and increased intracranial pressure, underwent placement of ventriculoperitoneal shunts.

From 1949 to 1960, Couvreur and Desmonts observed 300 cases of congenital toxoplasmosis [363]. These patients were found by clinical selection. Ocular disorders, particularly chorioretinitis (76%), and neurologic disturbances (51%) were present in most cases. Twenty-six percent had abnormalities in cranial volume, and 32% had intracranial calcifications.

Toxoplasmosis in children with abnormal cranial volume is uncommon without associated ocular lesions. Of 261 children younger than 2 years of age with hydrocephalus, 16 (6%) had congenital *T. gondii* infection; of 178 children of the same age group with microcephaly, only 3 (1.7%) had congenital *T. gondii* infection. (See also "Microcephaly.")

An interesting case of what appears to have been congenital *T. gondii* infection that manifested as a brain tumor at the approximate age of 1 year was reported by Tognetti and associates [382].

For information on the special problem of congenital toxoplasmosis in infants infected with human immunodeficiency virus (HIV), the reader is referred to "Congenital *Toxoplasma gondii* Infection and Acquired Immunodeficiency Syndrome" later in this section.

Microcephaly

Baron and coworkers examined the role of *T. gondii* in the pathogenesis of microcephaly and mental retardation [383]. Normal, normocephalic children served as controls, and adequate numbers of microcephalic children ranging in age from 5 months to 5 years were evaluated using the dye test. The data from this study did not reveal significant evidence of an association of *T. gondii* infection and microcephaly. Similar results were obtained by Thalhammer [384] and by Remington [385]. It should be remembered, however, that many microcephalic infants have died before the age of 5 years. Microcephaly in this infection usually reflects severe brain damage, but patients with microcephaly also have developed normally or near-normally.

Instability of Regulation of Body Temperature

As described in the "Central Nervous System" section under "Pathology," hypothermia may be present and may persist for weeks [6,56,386]. Wide fluctuations in temperature, from hypothermia to hyperthermia, have been reported [293].

Eye

Chorioretinitis

Because toxoplasmosis is one of the most common causes of chorioretinitis in the United States and much of the rest of the world, it is important to note that in the past, most workers had considered toxoplasmic chorioretinitis in older children and adults to be the result of a congenital infection rather than a manifestation of acquired toxoplasmosis. From data derived from extensive surveys of cases of uveitis, Perkins concluded that only about 1.5% of patients with toxoplasmic lymphadenopathy have chorioretinitis related to the acquired infection [387]. By contrast, in a study that attempted to determine the percentage of persons having ocular toxoplasmosis in childhood that were due to congenital infection versus infection acquired in childhood, among those with toxoplasmic chorioretinitis in Paris, patients with this disease were divided into groups where diagnosis was definitely congenital, definitely postnatally acquired or uncertain in terms of times of acquisition. In cases where origin of infection could be determined, acquired infections

were a more frequent cause of ocular toxoplasmosis than congenital infections. Cases of congenital ocular toxoplasmosis were more severe than acquired cases. Disease that was definitely congenital presented in younger children and was more severe [388].

Attesting to the potential severity of the outcome of congenital ocular toxoplasmosis are results of older studies such as those of Fair [389,390]. In a survey of almost 1000 children in state schools for the blind in the southern United States, Fair concluded that 51 (5%) of the students owed their visual disability to bilateral congenital central chorioretinitis, and of these, a diagnosis of congenital toxoplasmosis was certain or very probable in 40 (4%) [391]. All children showed the nystagmus and squint that always call for further examination. Kazdan and coworkers stated that the most common cause of posterior uveitis in children 15 years of age and younger at the Hospital for Sick Children in Toronto was congenital toxoplasmosis [392].

Congenital bilateral toxoplasmic macular scars, optic atrophy, and congenital cataracts were the major causes (43.5%) of low vision in a retrospective review of a population of 395 consecutive children younger than 14 years of age who attended the Low Vision Service of the State University of Campinas in São Paulo, Brazil, from 1982 to 1992 [393]. Previous studies have revealed similar results [394,395]. It was reported that use of low-magnification (telescopic prescriptions) eyeglasses significantly improved vision in these children and, in 63%, provided both social and personal benefits [393].

To assess the extent of ocular and systemic involvement in adolescent and adult patients with severe congenital toxoplasmosis, Meenken and coworkers [396] from the Netherlands reviewed clinical data, available since birth, in 15 patients whose severe toxoplasmosis was confirmed during the first year of life. The patients were residents of an institute for mentally and visually handicapped children and adults. Nine of them had received postnatal treatment for periods ranging from 2 to 10 months. Mean follow-up was 27 years. Although the diagnosis was made more than 25 years earlier, when more reliable serologic methods were not available, the serodiagnosis seems clear in 13 of the 15. Each of the 15 patients also had the combination of psychomotor retardation, epilepsy, and focal necrotizing retinitis diagnosed as being due to congenital toxoplasmosis. Intracerebral calcifications were present in 12 cases, and in 10 cases, obstructive hydrocephalus had been diagnosed in the first months of life; all received treatment, and all required repeated shunting procedures. In addition to chorioretinitis, the most common abnormal ocular features were optic nerve atrophy (83%), visual acuity of less than 0.1 (85%), strabismus (76%), and microphthalmos (53%). One half exhibited iridic abnormalities, and cataracts developed in approximately 40%. A majority of the cases of iris atrophy were in children aged 5 to 10 years. Of the 8 patients (16 eyes) with iridic atrophy, 12 (75%) had atrophic changes in the globe. In only one case was the chorioretinitis unilateral; it was bilateral in 97% of the remaining cases. In a majority of the cases, severe visual impairment was associated with optic nerve atrophy. The rate of documented recurrences was low (9%) when compared with the recurrence rate in patients who suffer solely from ocular involvement [397]. Some factors that appeared to account for this low documentation of recurrences were difficulties in examination, including the presence of cataract, extreme microphthalmos, band keratopathy, and lack of patient cooperation. The endocrinologic involvement in these patients is described later in the "Endocrine Disorders" section.

The risk of development of chorioretinitis in congenital cases appears to increase with increasing age during the early years of life. For example, in one case, unilateral (followed by bilateral) chorioretinitis developed between days 90 and 115 in a premature infant who received no treatment for *Toxoplasma* infection, in whom ophthalmoscopic examination was performed every 10 days [398]. By contrast, between 1981 and 1999 in 93 children in the NCCCTS who received treatment, no progression or development of new lesions was observed during the first year of life while treatment was ongoing, but later recurrence was noted in a small number of children [279]. Recurrences were documented in a subset of the children in the NCCCTS who received treatment during their first year of life. All of these children were examined by a single observer at specified intervals. The examinations are performed when they reach 1, 3.5, 5, 7.5, 10, and 15 years of age. The median age for the children who received treatment between 1981 and 1998 was approximately 5 years. The presence of new eye lesions was noted. Data for the children in this cohort in whom eye lesions have developed are presented in Table 31–14, along with various other clinical findings. Another group of children referred to the NCCCTS were designated historical "untreated" patients because they had not received treatment during their first year of life. They usually were referred because quiescent retinal disease was noted (See Table 31–14). Results are similar for over 200 children in the NCCCTS to 2010. New retinal lesions are not noted in the first year, during treatment and rarely occur before 5-7 years of age. The incidence of new lesions is low (10%) for treated children with no signs at birth and 35% for children with severe disease at birth. The most frequent time of recurrences is in adolescence. Children who were diagnosed after the first year of life, who were therefore not treated in the first year of life, had recurrences at the same ages, but had a much higher rate of development of recurrent retinal lesions [883, 884].

In a study by Parissi, among 47 patients with subclinical congenital toxoplasmosis at birth, the overall incidence of retinal lesions was 30% (Table 31–15) [399]. It was less in the first 4 years of life (approximately 23%) than after 5 years of age (40% to 50%). Thus localized ocular phenomena frequently develop as a late manifestation [245,359,361,400]. De Roever-Bonnet and colleagues [245] postulated that late development of eye lesions may be caused by second infections rather than by relapses, although supporting data for this hypothesis are lacking.

The occurrence of consecutive cases of ocular toxoplasmosis has been reported in siblings [401,402]. These cases may have been due to postnatally acquired infection.

Lappalainen and her colleagues observed typical retinal scars of congenital toxoplasmosis in three infants who were seronegative by the age of 1 year. They were born

to mothers who had seroconverted during the first trimester [403]. By the age of 5 years, one of these children had seroconverted. Seronegativity in congenital ocular disease also had been observed by Koppe and coworkers in two children who had become seronegative by the ages of 9 and 14 years [190]. Gross and coworkers [404] described the case of a congenitally infected child in whom attempts at diagnosis had failed with relatively insensitive serologic techniques (the CF test) but succeeded with immunoblot and PCR assay; one wonders if IgG antibody would indeed have been demonstrable had serologic testing been performed with more sensitive and specific serologic methods (e.g., the Sabin-Feldman dye test). This case raises the question of how frequently negative results on *T. gondii* serologic studies (and, correspondingly, missed diagnoses) actually occur in children with clinical features considered diagnostic of congenital toxoplasmic retinochoroiditis. In such cases, sera should be tested by multiple methods in a reference laboratory.

Clinical Findings on External Examination

Microphthalmia, small cornea, posterior cortical cataract, anisometropia, strabismus, and nystagmus may be present. Leukocoria has been reported [279, 405]. Nystagmus may result either from poor fixation related to the chorioretinitis or from involvement of the CNS. A history of "dancing eyes" should always raise the possibility of a bilateral congenital central chorioretinitis—a typical ocular lesion of congenital toxoplasmosis. Convergent or divergent strabismus may be caused by direct involvement of the retina or extraocular muscles or may result from involvement of the brain. The iris and ciliary body may be affected by foci of inflammation, with formation of synechiae. As a result, dilation of the pupils with mydriatics may be difficult.

Funduscopic Examination Findings

The characteristic lesion of ocular toxoplasmosis is a focal necrotizing retinitis (Fig. 31–10), which may be bilateral [406]. Such lesions in the acute or subacute stage of inflammation appear as yellowish white, cotton-like patches in the fundus. They may be solitary lesions that are about the same size as the optic disk or a little larger. More often, however, they appear in small clusters, among which lesions of various ages can be discerned. The more acute lesions are soft and cotton-like, with indistinct borders; the older lesions are whitish gray, sharply outlined, and spotted by accumulations of choroidal pigment. The inflammatory exudate that is cast off from the surface of the acute lesions often is so dense that clear visualization of the fundus is impossible. In such cases, the most that can be discerned is a whitish mass against the pale orange background of the fundus. The posterior hyaloid membrane often is detached, and precipitates of inflammatory cells—the equivalents of keratic precipitates in the anterior segment of the eye—are seen on the posterior face of the vitreous.

Retinal edema, which affects especially the macular and peripapillary areas, is commonly observed in the subacute phase of inflammation. Edema of the macula is almost

TABLE 31-14   New or Recrudescent Retinal Lesions in Treated and Historical Patients That Occurred after 1 Year of Age

Group	Patient Number	Age (yr) Noted*	Previous Eye Lesion	Active	Location	Visual Acuity Before; After	Serology During Relapse
Treated	7	6[A], 10[A]	No, Yes	Yes	Perimacular, peripheral[†]	20/20; 20/20[‡]	Not acute, N/A
	9	5[A]	No	No	Posterior pole	Nl; 20/50	N/A
	12	3[A], 10[A]	No, Yes	Yes	Peripheral, peripapillary[†]	20/20; 20/30	Not acute
	13	7[B]	Yes	Yes[§]	Perimacular[†]	6/400; 20/200	Not acute
	15	3[A]	Yes	No	Peripheral[†]	20/30; 20/30	N/A
	19	5[‡], 8[‡]	Yes	Yes[§]	Peripheral[†]	20/20; 20/20	Not acute
	21	4[A]	Yes	No	Perimacular[†]	Abnl; 1/30	N/A
Historical (untreated)	20	3[A]	Yes	Yes[§]	Peripheral	1/30; 20/400	Not acute
	25	10[A]	Yes	No	Peripheral	20/400; 18/200	Not acute
	27	7[A]	Yes	No	Perimacular	3/30; 5/30	N/A
	42	10[A]	Yes	Yes[§]	Perimacular[†]	20/30; 20/30	Not acute
	46	24[A]	Yes	Yes[§]	Perimacular[†]	20/60; 20/60	Not acute
	62	11[C], 13[C], 15[B]	Yes	Yes[§]	Perimacular, peripheral	20/20; 20/15	N/A
	82	16[A]	Yes	Yes[§]	Peripapillary	20/400; 20/400	Not acute
	89	12[B]	Yes	Yes[§]	Perimacular	20/100; N/A	Not acute

Data from the U.S. (Chicago) national collaborative treatment trial: patient numbers are those used in all prior publications. Recurrences were documented in a subset of the children in the U.S. (Chicago) National Collaborative Treatment Trial who received treatment during their first year of life. All of these children were examined in Chicago by a single observer at specified intervals. The examinations are when they reach 1, 3.5, 5, 7.5, 10, and 15 years of age. The median age for the children who received treatment is approximately 5 years old. The presence of new eye lesions was noted. Historical patients did not receive treatment in the first year of life and were referred after that time. There were 18 patients in the historical group and 76 in the treatment group.

[A]Recurrence documented at visit in Chicago (A), recurrence documented by history (B), photographs reviewed in Chicago, and recurrence documented by history only (C).
[†]Satellites of earlier lesion.
[‡]Quantitative visual acuity using Snellen chart or Allen cards.
[§]Symptoms present during active disease.
Abnl, abnormal; N/A, not available; Nl, normal.
From Mets MB, et al. Eye manifestations of congenital toxoplasmosis. Am J Ophthalmol 122:309–324, 1996.

TABLE 31–15 Results of Funduscopic Examination in 47 Patients with Congenital Toxoplasmosis Who Were Asymptomatic at Birth*

Age[†]	No. of Patients with Normal Fundi	No. of Patients with Chorioretinitis	Estimated Incidence of Ocular Lesions (%)
0–11 mo	8	3	27
1–4 yr	17	5	23
5–9 yr	6	4	40
>10 yr	2	2	50

*Children were selected who had congenital toxoplasmosis, either clinical or subclinical, with normal fundi at birth.
[†]Age = the age at the time of the last normal funduscopic examination or the first examination showing chorioretinitis, if chorioretinitis developed.
Adapted from Desmonts G. Some remarks on the immunopathology of toxoplasmic uveitis. In Böke W, Luntz MH (eds). Modern Problems in Ophthalmology. Ocular Immune Responses, vol 16. Basel, Switzerland, S Karger, 1976.

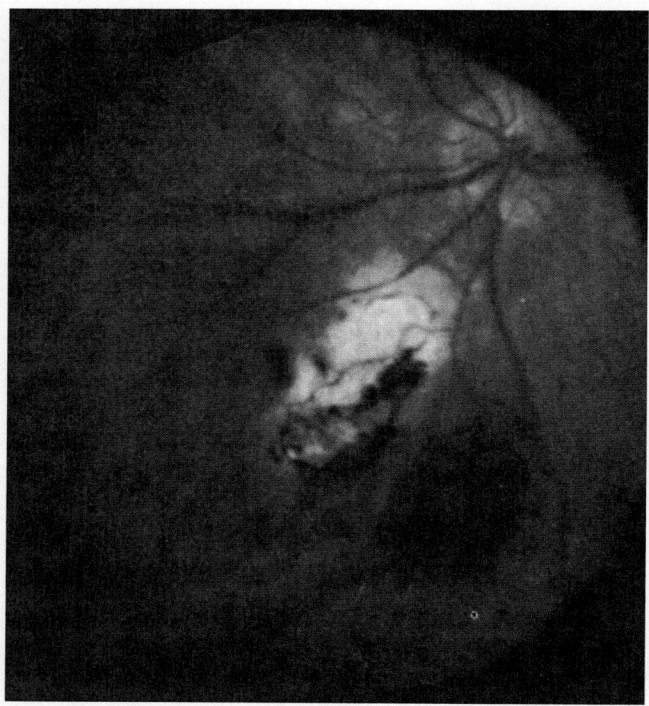

FIGURE 31–10 Chorioretinitis in congenital toxoplasmosis.

always present when acute inflammatory foci in the retina are situated within the macula. In older children, this edema is the principal cause of blurred vision when other causes, such as a central retinal lesion, involvement of the optic nerve, or extensive clouding of the vitreous, can be excluded. Macular edema usually is temporary, although cystic changes in the fovea sometimes occur as a result of long-standing edema. In this instance, central visual acuity may be permanently impaired despite the absence of central lesions or involvement of the optic nerve. Treatment with an antibody to Veg F can result in resolution of choroidal neovascular membranes [410].

The optic nerve may be affected either primarily, with damage resulting from destruction of the macula and other portions of the retina, or secondarily, with damage resulting from papilledema. Manschot and Daamen and others have described *T. gondii* in the optic nerve itself [290], or optic nerve inflammation [313].

What at first appears to be primary involvement of the optic nerve head, with papilledema and exudation of cells into the overlying vitreous, often turns out to be a juxtapapillary lesion. A retinal lesion contiguous to the head of the optic nerve can produce swelling and inflammation in the nerve, but when the acute lesion subsides, it becomes clear that the optic nerve itself has been spared and that a narrow rim of normal tissue separates the lesion from the nerve head.

Segmental atrophy of the optic nerve, characterized by pallor and loss of substance, especially of the temporal portion of the nerve head, may occur in association with macular lesions. In these cases, the prognosis is for limited vision.

Although a majority of lesions described in the older literature are at or near the posterior pole of the retina, peripheral lesions have been described. In one series of more than 100 children with congenital toxoplasmosis [279], more peripheral lesions were seen. With regard to the relative sizes of the macula and peripheral retina, however, macular lesions were predominant. These have roughly the same morphology as that of the more central lesions, but they tend to be less significant as a cause of central visual loss unless they are accompanied by massive contractures of the overlying vitreous. They can cause subsequent retinal detachment.

The anterior uvea often is the site of intense inflammation, characterized by redness of the external eye, cells and protein in the anterior chamber, large keratic precipitates, posterior synechiae, nodules on the iris, and, occasionally, neovascular formations on the surface of the iris. This reaction may be accompanied by steep rises in intraocular pressure and by formation of cataracts.

Isolated iritis should not be taken as an indication of toxoplasmosis. To be considered as a manifestation of toxoplasmosis, iritis should be preceded or at least accompanied by a posterior lesion. The same can be said of scleritis, which may be observed external to a focus of toxoplasmic chorioretinitis; it has no significance by itself as a sign of toxoplasmosis.

Ophthalmoscopic features of the intraocular lesions of congenital toxoplasmosis in infants are those listed in Table 31–26 (see later discussion) and have been reported [311] to include (1) unilateral or bilateral involvement of the macular region; (2) unilateral or bilateral occurrence of other lesions; (3) involvement of the periphery in one or more quadrants of the retina and choroid; (4) punched-out appearance of large and small lesions in the late phase; (5) occurrence of massive chorioretinal degeneration; (6) extensive connective tissue proliferation and heavy pigmentation, as contrasted with the dissociation of these changes in other chorioretinal lesions; (7) presence of an essentially normal retina and vasculature surrounding the lesions in all stages of the infection; (8) occurrence of associated congenital defects in the eyes; (9) rapid development of sequential optic nerve atrophy; and

(10) frequent clarity of the media in the presence of severe chorioretinitis or chorioretinal scars.

Hogan and coworkers tabulated the data from 22 cases of chorioretinitis in infants 6 months of age or younger with congenital toxoplasmosis (in 81%, the lesions were bilateral) from the literature published through 1949 [407]. A precise determination of prevalence cannot be gleaned from these reports because for many of the infants, the data were incomplete—for example, in some, no description of the fundus was provided, but other features such as microphthalmia were described. Of those infants for whom sufficient information was available, seven had only healed retinal lesions, five had only acute lesions, and four had both acute and healed lesions. Macular involvement was seen in 5, and peripheral retinal involvement in 10; diffuse retinal involvement was present in 3. Twelve infants had microphthalmia, 5 had optic nerve atrophy, 3 had papilledema, 8 had strabismus, 7 had nystagmus, 10 had anterior segment involvement, and 2 had cataracts; in 10, parasites were noted in the retina at autopsy.

Franceschetti and Bamatter reviewed the signs in 243 cases of congenital ocular toxoplasmosis and found the following percentages: bilateral involvement in 66%, unilateral involvement in 34%, microphthalmia in 23%, optic atrophy in 27%, nystagmus in 23%, strabismus in 28%, cataract in 8%, iritis and posterior synechiae in 8%, persistence of pupillary membrane in 4%, and vitreous changes in 11% [408].

The findings of Mets and colleagues [279] in congenitally infected children in the United States who were referred to the National Collaborative Chicago-based Congenital Toxoplasmosis Study (NCCCTS) are shown in Table 31–16. Other important features may be noted. For example, relatively normal visual acuity may occur in the presence of large macular scars either sparing or involving the fovea [279]. Synechiae and pupillary irregularities sometimes are present and reflect an especially severe intraocular inflammatory process. In the NCCCTS, we have noted the following (Noble G and coworkers, unpublished observations): In some patients with severe intraocular inflammation, retinal detachment may occur later in childhood. Intermittent occlusion (patching therapy) of the better-seeing eye may lead to substantial improvement in visual acuity even in the presence of large macular scars. Optical coherence tomography (OCT) may be useful in assessing depth of macular lesions, impact on optic nerve function, and differences over time and thus be of assistance in monitoring recurrences. In the NCCCTS, a small number of mothers had retinal scars, which indicates the importance of retinal examinations for mothers of congenitally infected infants.

A more recent report of eye findings in 173 children in the NCCCTS cohort identified cataracts in 27 eyes of 20 children (11.6%, 95% confidence interval [7.2%, 17.3%]) [409]. In the first year of life, 134 of these 173 children had been treated with pyrimethamine, sulfadiazine, and leucovorin, while the remaining 39 were not treated. Fourteen cataracts were present at birth and 13 developed postnatally. Locations of the cataracts included anterior polar (three eyes), anterior subcapsular (six eyes), nuclear (five eyes), posterior subcapsular (seven eyes), and unknown (six eyes). Thirteen cataracts were partial, nine

TABLE 31–16   Ophthalmologic Manifestations of Congenital Toxoplasmosis in Children in U.S. (Chicago) National Collaborative Treatment Trial*

Manifestation	Number with Finding (%)		
	Treatment Group N = 76	Historical Group N = 18	Total N = 94
Strabismus	26 (34)	5 (28)	31 (33)
Nystagmus	20 (26)	5 (28)	25 (27)
Microphthalmia	10 (13)	2 (11)	12 (13)
Phthisis	4 (5)	0 (0)	4 (4)
Microcornea	15 (20)	3 (17)	18 (19)
Cataract	7 (9)	2 (11)	9 (10)
Vitritis (active)	3 (4)†	2 (11)	5 (5)
Retinitis (active)	6 (8)	4 (22)	10 (11)
Chorioretinal scars	56 (74)	18 (100)	74 (79)
Macular	39/72 (54)‡	13/17 (76)	52/89 (58)
Juxtapapillary	37/72 (51)	9/17 (53)	46/89 (52)
Peripheral	43/72 (58)	14/17 (82)	57/89 (64)
Retinal detachment	7 (9)	2 (11)	9 (10)
Optic atrophy	14 (18)	5 (28)	19 (20)

*Children either received treatment with pyrimethamine and sulfadiazine during their first year of life (treatment group) or were referred after their first year of life when they had not been treated (historical group). In general, historical patients were referred because they had eye disease. Current mean ages of the children in these groups are in Table 31–34.
†Two additional patients, not included in this table, were receiving treatment, and retinochoroiditis had resolved but vitreous cells and veils persisted at time of examination.
‡Numerator represents number with finding. Denominator represents N, unless otherwise specified. Number in parentheses is percentage. Patients with bilateral retinal detachment in whom the location of scars was not possible were excluded from the denominator.
From Mets MB, et al. Eye manifestations of congenital toxoplasmosis. Am J Ophthalmol 122:309–324, 1996.

total, and five with unknown complexity. Twelve cataracts remained stable, 12 progressed, and progression was not known for 3. Five of 27 eyes had cataract surgery, with 2 of these developing glaucoma. Sixteen eyes of 11 patients had retinal detachment and cataracts. All eyes with cataracts had additional ocular lesions. Cataract removal in some cases led to improved visual function.

Choroidal neovascular membranes, which result in accumulation of fluid in the retina and can result in vision threatening bleeding into the retina, have been associated with toxoplasmic chorioretinitis [410].

Differential Diagnosis of Eye Lesions

Congenital Anomalies. The healed foci of toxoplasmic chorioretinitis may resemble a colobomatous defect (Fig. 31–11) [2]. The associated ocular, systemic, and serologic changes make toxoplasmosis the most likely diagnosis. Abnormal retinal morphology has been described in one fetal eye [313], and similar findings have been described in a variety of animal models of the congenital infection. Chromosome analysis was not available for the fetus, however.

Other Inflammatory Lesions. The differential diagnosis of eye lesions includes many of the inflammatory

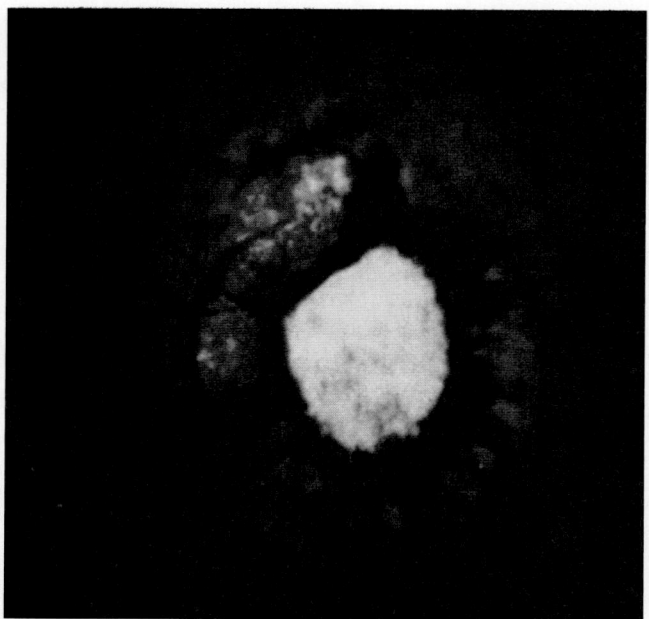

FIGURE 31–11 Macular scars (pseudocoloboma) of the retina in congenital toxoplasmosis.

lesions described in chapters 16, 23, 26, and 28. The lymphochoriomeningitis virus also can cause similar lesions.

Birth Injury. Intraocular hemorrhage may go unrecognized and may cause retinal damage with gliosis and fibrosis, potentially resulting in retinal detachment. The lesion usually is unilateral, associated cerebral damage is absent, and no serologic evidence is present to support a diagnosis of toxoplasmosis. Retinopathy of prematurity may occur in conjunction with toxoplasmic chorioretinitis.

Circulatory Disturbances. Congenital aneurysms and telangiectasia of retinal vessels may result in extensive retinal fibrosis, with pigmentation and detachment. The disease usually is unilateral and is not associated with cerebral involvement or other changes.

Neoplasms. Retinoblastoma rarely may have an appearance similar to that described for ocular toxoplasmosis. It most often is unilateral and is unassociated with visceral or cerebral damage unless an advanced stage has been reached. Pseudoglioma may be difficult to distinguish from a healed chorioretinitis lesion but usually is single and unilateral. Gliomas may be bilateral, progressing from a small nodule to a large polypoid mass protruding into the vitreous.

Mental Retardation

Numerous studies have attempted to establish a causal relationship between mental retardation and congenital toxoplasmosis. A prospective study on this subject is that of Alford and colleagues [328,411]. When these workers noted that changes in cerebrospinal fluid protein concentration and cell count were common in newborns with subclinical congenital toxoplasmosis, they set out to determine the significance of these changes in relation to later mental development. They compared the intellectual and social development of eight children, aged 2 to 4 years, who were identified at birth as having subclinical congenital toxoplasmosis, with those of eight matched controls. Their results revealed that varying degrees of intellectual impairment may be present in children who are asymptomatic at birth, reflecting the fact that brain damage does occur with subclinical congenital toxoplasmosis. These investigators concluded that although subclinical congenital toxoplasmosis does not necessarily cause overt mental retardation, it may be associated with some degree of intellectual impairment. Further studies along these lines have corroborated these findings (see "Follow-up Studies" later in this section), but until a much larger number of infants are examined over a longer time, these data can be considered only tentative.

The total contribution of congenital toxoplasmosis, including the less severe and clinically inapparent forms at birth, to mental retardation is uncertain. One of the earliest studies from Europe was that of Thalhammer in Vienna, who classified congenital toxoplasmosis into three broad categories: (1) generalized, with hepatomegaly, jaundice, myocarditis, pneumonitis, and similar effects; (2) cerebral, accompanied by at least one of the two characteristic signs, namely, chorioretinitis and intracerebral calcification; and (3) cerebral, accompanied by damage but without these signs [384]. Thalhammer concluded that the first type was rare, the second not common enough to be a problem, and the third a common condition creating serious medical and social problems. He studied 1332 children with congenital cerebral damage that could not be accounted for by postnatal encephalitic illness. The results of this study are summarized in Table 31–17. In children with cerebral defects of all types, the prevalence of *T. gondii* infection was about 17% higher than in normal children. Although the frequency of *T. gondii* infection in this series was not measurably greater in children with microcephaly, hydrocephalus, and cerebral palsy than it was in normal children, it was much greater in those with epilepsy and mental retardation. Thalhammer concluded from these statistics that in about 20% of the cases of mental retardation, the most important cerebral defects were due to congenital toxoplasmosis. Other investigators have similarly concluded from their data that congenital

TABLE 31–17 Frequency of *Toxoplasma* Infections in 1332 Children (Ages 1–14 Years) with Congenital Cerebral Defects Compared with 600 Normal Children

Type of Defect	No. Tested	No. Positive* (%)
Microcephaly	57	2 (3.5)
Hydrocephalus	191	17 (8.9)
Cerebral palsy	55	5 (9.1)
Epilepsy	344	73 (21.2)
Mental retardation	685	167 (24.4)
Cerebral defects (all types)	1332	264 (19.8)
None (normal)	600	20 (3.3)

*Dye test titers of 1:4 or higher were considered to be positive.
Adapted from Thalhammer O. Congenital toxoplasmosis. Lancet 1:23–24, 1962, with permission.

toxoplasmosis is or may be an important cause of mental retardation [412–415]. Through a series of computations from the data of others, Hume concluded that toxoplasmosis is the cause of impairment in at least 4% of the population composed of the "mentally retarded and [those with] cerebral dysfunction" [416].

Interpretation of many of these studies, and those by workers who found little or no significant difference between mentally retarded and control populations [363,383,417–421], is complicated by the high prevalence of acquired *Toxoplasma* infection among control subjects, which may mask the possible role of congenital toxoplasmosis in mental retardation (and other sequelae of encephalopathy, such as convulsions). For example, if the proportion of cases of mental retardation is small and the prevalence of *T. gondii* antibody titers in the control population is high, it is not possible with presently available diagnostic techniques to distinguish those cases in which *T. gondii* is the cause of mental retardation. Another cause of the variations in reported results is the choice of controls. In many studies, subjects were not properly matched, and any difference or lack of difference found was due solely to differences in populations from which the patients were chosen [420].

Only through large-scale prospective studies of infection with *T. gondii* acquired during the course of pregnancy, compiled by means of long-term observations of the infants, will accurate figures be obtained on the contribution of congenital *T. gondii* infection to mental deficiency (and epilepsy, blindness, and other disorders).

Down Syndrome

Although numerous investigators have interpreted their data as evidence of an association between toxoplasmosis in the mother and Down syndrome in the offspring [419,422–426], such an association has never been proved satisfactorily [426]. In a study of 71 such children, Thalhammer found a higher-than-normal prevalence of *T. gondii* antibodies [427]. He attributed the higher prevalence to their mental deficiency and suggested that their institutional environment probably favored a higher rate of acquired infection; the prevalence of *T. gondii* antibodies was no different from that in normal controls in the age group birth to 5 years and rose to levels higher than those demonstrated in controls only in the older age groups. Until adequate data to the contrary are furnished, the association between Down syndrome and toxoplasmosis in a newborn must be considered coincidental. Frenkel [428] points out that, in view of the chromosomal aberrations in Down syndrome, it would be necessary to demonstrate that toxoplasmosis is related to the nonhereditary or nondisjunction form of Down syndrome; if this is true, one would have to postulate an influence of *T. gondii* on the ovum, which thus far has not been demonstrated [423]. Much of the literature on this subject, and that on the relationship of toxoplasmosis to other entities in the newborn, is purely speculative.

Endocrine Disorders

The endocrine disorders that have been associated with congenital toxoplasmosis are nonspecific because they reflect the severity of the infection in those areas of the brain that are related to endocrine function. Two cases in which congenital toxoplasmosis and congenital myxedema occurred simultaneously have been reported [429,430]. Because each of these conditions is relatively uncommon, their concurrent appearance suggests more than mere coincidence. *T. gondii* has been demonstrated in histologic sections of the pituitary and thyroid glands of infants dying of toxoplasmosis, and it may be that such involvement contributed to or resulted in myxedema in these patients. Silver and Dixon described persistent hypernatremia in a congenitally infected infant who had evidence of vasopressin-sensitive diabetes insipidus without polyuria or polydipsia [386]. An associated finding was a marked eosinophilia in blood and bone marrow. A similar case was described by Margit and Istvan [431]. Diabetes insipidus has occurred in the perinatal period or developed later in childhood [431,432]. This disorder in such cases probably is secondary to pituitary-hypothalamic *T. gondii* infection. It has occurred in infants and children with severe brain damage and hydrocephalus, and in children who have only intracerebral calcifications [433–435].

Bruhl and colleagues reported sexual precocity in association with congenital toxoplasmosis in a male infant who, at the age of 2 years, showed rapid growth of the external genitalia and appearance of pubic hair, along with generalized convulsions, microcephaly, severe mental retardation, bilateral microphthalmia, and blindness (deafness was suspected because the child did not respond to noises) [436]. After 9 years of hospitalization, he died at the age of 13.5 years. The early onset of growth of the penis and testes and the development of pubic hair, and testicular biopsy and hormone assays, established the diagnosis of true precocity in this case. A cause-and-effect relationship between toxoplasmosis and precocious puberty could not be proved, but the presence of two rare disorders in the same patient suggested such a relationship. Also, a variety of lesions involving the hypothalamus have been associated with precocious puberty, and the third ventricle was dilated and the hypothalamus was distorted in the patient just described. The anterior pituitary appeared normal at autopsy—a prerequisite to development of precocious puberty in patients with lesions in or near the hypothalamus. Partial anterior hypopituitarism was observed in the infant reported by Coppola and coworkers [437]. Massa and colleagues described three children with growth hormone deficiency, two of whom were gonadotropin deficient and one of whom had precocious puberty, in addition to central diabetes insipidus [429].

In the study performed by Meenken and associates [396] (described previously in the "Chorioretinitis" section), overt endocrinologic disease was diagnosed in 5 of 15 patients with severe congenital toxoplasmosis, all of whom had serious eye disease due to the infection. Panhypopituitarism was observed in two, gonadal failure with dwarfism in one, precocious puberty with dwarfism and thyroid deficiency in one, and diabetes mellitus and thyroid deficiency in one. The investigators found that the major manifestations of the endocrine disease in these patients occurred at the mean age of 12 years (range, 9 to 16 years) and were associated with obstructive hydrocephalus and dilated third ventricle in each case.

Nephrotic Syndrome

In infants with congenital toxoplasmosis, generalized edema and ascites may reflect the presence of the nephrotic syndrome [324,438,439]. Protein and casts have been reported in the urine in such cases, as have hypoproteinemia, hypoalbuminemia, and hypercholesterolemia. In one case, there was a marked decrease in the serum IgG level, but IgM and IgA levels were normal [439]. Hypogammaglobulinemia has been reported to be associated with congenital toxoplasmosis in the absence of nephrosis [440].

Liver

Kove and coworkers described the pattern of serum transaminase activity in a newborn with cytomegalic inclusion disease and in another with congenital toxoplasmosis [441]. Jaundice developed in both. The patterns were unique and unlike those observed in infants with other causes of neonatal jaundice. The investigators pointed out that more studies are necessary to determine if serial measurements of serum transaminase will actually be a useful tool in the diagnosis of congenital toxoplasmosis and cytomegalic inclusion disease.

Jaundice, which occurs frequently, may reflect liver damage or hemolysis, or both. Among 225 infants with neonatal icterus studied by Couvreur and Desmonts, 5 (2.2%) were found to have congenital toxoplasmosis [363]. The conjugated hyperbilirubinemia and jaundice seen in infants with untreated congenital toxoplasmosis may persist for months [304]. In infants who receive treatment, hyperbilirubinemia and jaundice usually resolve in a few weeks.

Skin

Like almost all other signs of the infection, those referable to the skin are varied and nonspecific [442,443]. Thrombocytopenia may be associated with petechiae, ecchymoses, or even gross hemorrhages into the skin. Zuelzer described a fine punctate rash over the entire body of a 3-day-old infant [293]. Miller and colleagues noted albinism in one of the infants they studied but did not consider this to be caused by toxoplasmosis [322]. Wolf and associates noted a diffuse maculopapular rash in two infants with jaundice, beginning on the sixth day in one and on the ninth day in the other [304]. Reiss and Verron described a premature infant with a lenticular, deep blue-red, sharply defined macular rash over the entire body, including the palms and soles [444]. Diffuse blue papules [445] and "blueberry muffin" rash [446] (Fig. 31–12) have been observed in infants with congenital toxoplasmosis and those with congenital Rubella and other infections (see Chapter 1). Korovitsky and coworkers, in a discussion of skin lesions in toxoplasmosis, mentioned an exfoliative dermatitis in cases of congenital toxoplasmosis [447], but according to Justus, a cause-and-effect relationship between these two conditions was not shown in the infant he described [445]. In 1968, Justus reported complete calcification of the skin, except for the palms and soles, in a premature infant who died 10 minutes after birth [445]. The mother had experienced tetany during delivery and required supplemental calcium

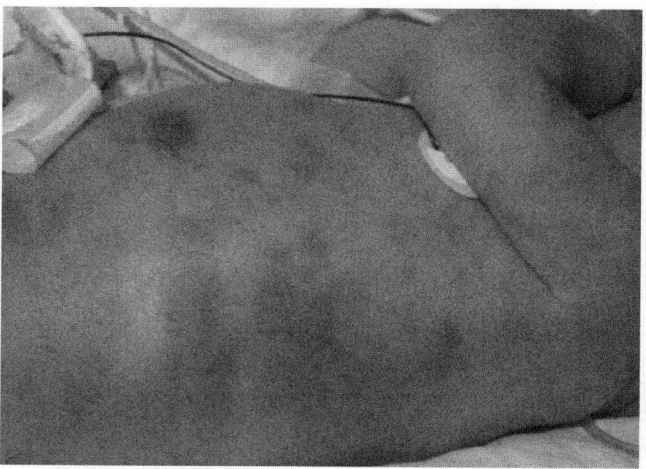

FIGURE 31–12 "Blueberry muffin" rash in an infant with congenital toxoplasmosis. *(From Mehta V, Balachandran C, Lonikar V. Blueberry muffin baby: a pictorial differential diagnosis. Dermatol Online J 14(2):8, 2008.)*

thereafter. Thus the calcifications may not have been due solely, or even in part, to congenital toxoplasmosis in the infant but rather may have been the result of a metabolic defect in calcium metabolism in the mother.

Malformations

The possibility that *T. gondii* can cause fetal malformations has been the subject of much conjecture. Thalhammer, commenting on the accumulated data on this subject, stated that he did not believe that *T. gondii* causes malformations [427]. He found 4 instances of malformations among 326 cases of congenital toxoplasmosis (1.2%), and this was less than the average incidence of malformations in his geographic area. Of 144 children with malformations, only 2 had *T. gondii* antibodies.

By contrast, workers in Germany [73,448–450], Greece [451], the former Czechoslovakia [452], and the former Soviet Union [453] interpret their data as proof that *T. gondii* causes fetal malformations. Most of these studies were performed in an uncontrolled and uncritical manner. For example, in the United States, Erdelyi suggested that some cases of palatal cleft malformations may be due to congenital toxoplasmosis [454]; a similar conclusion was reached by Jírovec and coworkers in Prague [454, 455]. The evidence in the study reported by Erdelyi consisted of dye test data, and in the study from Jírovec's group, skin test data drawn from investigations of mothers of children with cleft palate and harelip defects; the prevalence of positive results on skin testing in mothers of such children was found to be higher than that in controls from the general population. Carefully chosen controls should be a necessary feature of all such studies; results obtained from the general population are not applicable or valid.

Although involvement of the placenta by infection early in pregnancy might cause damage without direct infection of the developing embryo, the available data are insufficient either to support or to reject the hypothesis that *T. gondii* can cause fetal malformations. This problem is easily approached with existing epidemiologic methods and awaits careful controlled study.

Radiologic Abnormalities

Brain

Hydrocephalus characteristically is due to periaqueductal involvement. Obstruction of the aqueduct of Sylvius leads to enlargement of the third and lateral ventricles (Fig. 31–13, *A*). Obstruction of the foramen of Monro can lead to unilateral hydrocephalus (Fig. 31–14) (see also Fig. 31–13, *B*) [433]. Dramatic resolution and brain cortical expansion and growth can occur in conjunction with ventriculoperitoneal shunt placement and anti-*T. gondii* therapy (see Figs. 31–12, *C* and *D*). Calcifications may be single or multiple (Fig. 31–15; see also Fig. 31–13, *E* to *H*) and, surprisingly, in some cases have resolved with anti-*Toxoplasma* therapy during the first year of life (see Figs. 31–13, *E*) [456]. Contrast-enhancing lesions have been detected, indicating active encephalitis (see Fig. 31–13, *G*) [433]. Massive hydrocephalus, as

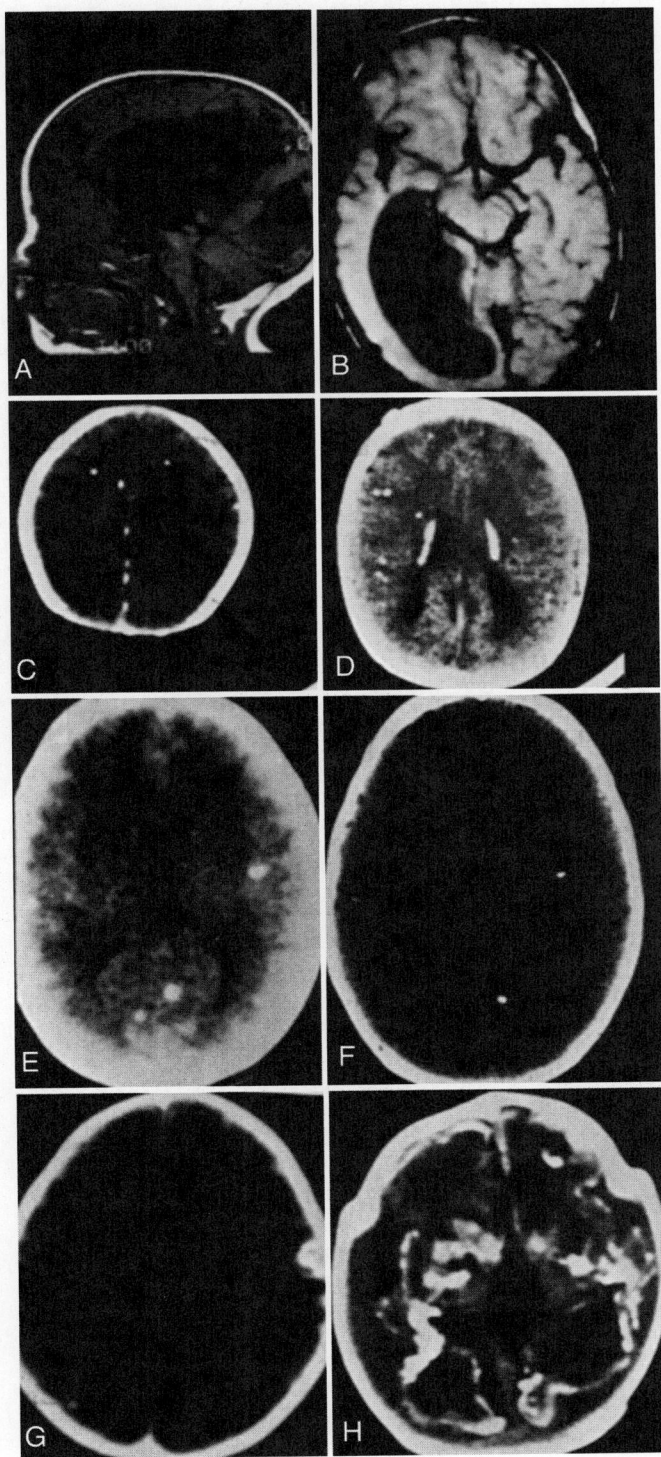

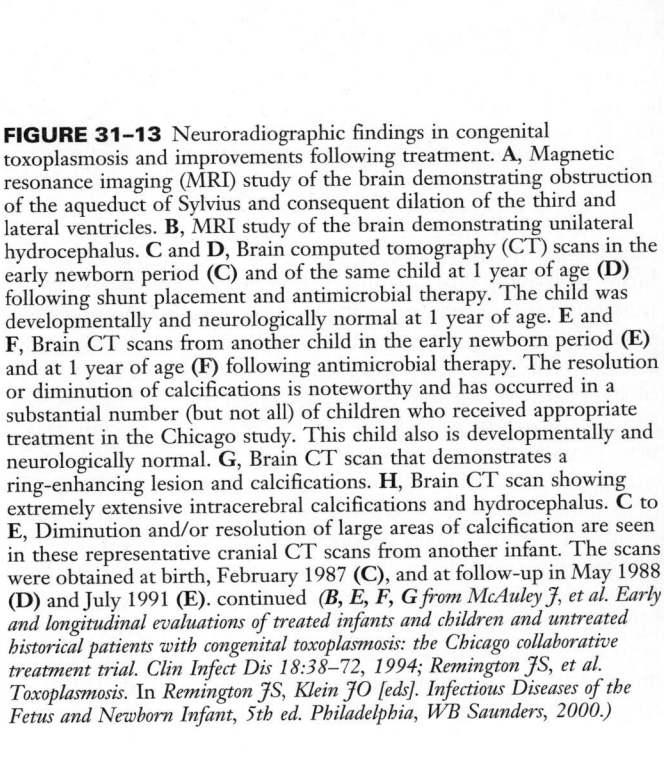

FIGURE 31–13 Neuroradiographic findings in congenital toxoplasmosis and improvements following treatment. **A**, Magnetic resonance imaging (MRI) study of the brain demonstrating obstruction of the aqueduct of Sylvius and consequent dilation of the third and lateral ventricles. **B**, MRI study of the brain demonstrating unilateral hydrocephalus. **C** and **D**, Brain computed tomography (CT) scans in the early newborn period (**C**) and of the same child at 1 year of age (**D**) following shunt placement and antimicrobial therapy. The child was developmentally and neurologically normal at 1 year of age. **E** and **F**, Brain CT scans from another child in the early newborn period (**E**) and at 1 year of age (**F**) following antimicrobial therapy. The resolution or diminution of calcifications is noteworthy and has occurred in a substantial number (but not all) of children who received appropriate treatment in the Chicago study. This child also is developmentally and neurologically normal. **G**, Brain CT scan that demonstrates a ring-enhancing lesion and calcifications. **H**, Brain CT scan showing extremely extensive intracerebral calcifications and hydrocephalus. **C** to **E**, Diminution and/or resolution of large areas of calcification are seen in these representative cranial CT scans from another infant. The scans were obtained at birth, February 1987 (**C**), and at follow-up in May 1988 (**D**) and July 1991 (**E**). continued (*B, E, F, G from McAuley J, et al. Early and longitudinal evaluations of treated infants and children and untreated historical patients with congenital toxoplasmosis: the Chicago collaborative treatment trial. Clin Infect Dis 18:38–72, 1994; Remington JS, et al. Toxoplasmosis. In Remington JS, Klein JO [eds]. Infectious Diseases of the Fetus and Newborn Infant, 5th ed. Philadelphia, WB Saunders, 2000.*)

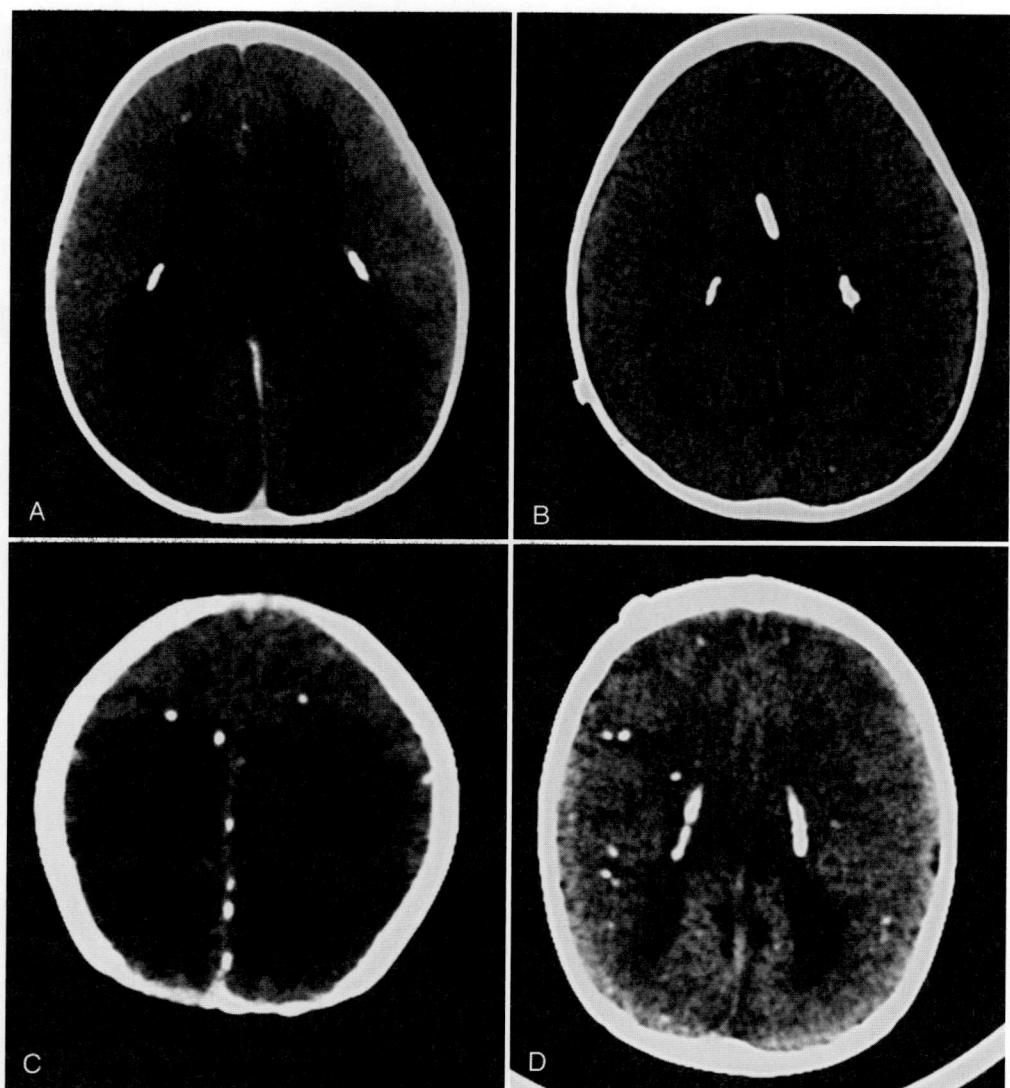

FIGURE 31–14 Cranial computed tomography (CT) scans of two infants, one represented in **A** and **B** and the other in **C** and **D**, before (A and C) and after (B and D) placement of ventriculoperitoneal shunts. CT scans and the subsequent normal development of such children indicate that it is not possible to predict ultimate cognitive outcome from the initial appearance of the CT scan. *(From Boyer KM, McLeod RL.* Toxoplasma gondii *[toxoplasmosis]. In* Long SS, Prober CG, Pickering LK [eds]. Principles and Practice of Pediatric Infectious Diseases. *New York, Churchill Livingstone, 1997.)*

documented by ultrasound examination, has been noted to develop in fetuses and newborns within a period as brief as 1 week and resolved in association with anti-*Toxoplasma* treatment in one fetus (Fig. 31–16) [457].

Radiologic signs in newborns exposed to primary *T. gondii* infection in utero were described by Virkola and colleagues [456]. The study included 42 mothers—37 were delivered of live-born infants and 5 experienced spontaneous abortions—with follow-up evaluation. The findings on brain ultrasonography associated with infection included calcifications, cysts, and the "candlestick sign"; those on abdominal ultrasonography were enlarged spleen and ascites. In some instances, these changes were associated with abnormalities in the newborn period.

Puri and coworkers described a 2-week-old infant with hydrocephalus [458]. A brain scan with ^{99m}Tc-pertechnetate showed an area of increased uptake in the left

temporoparietal region. A four-vessel angiogram showed large ventricles with a mass lesion in the left hemisphere pushing midline structures to the right. Findings on electroencephalography were abnormal, with sharp θ activity in the left parietotemporal area. A bubble ventriculogram showed obstruction of the left foramen of Monro. Because of the rapid deterioration of the patient's condition, a craniotomy was performed; it revealed a large granular infiltrating tumor in the left temporal region. Numerous *T. gondii* organisms were seen in the operative specimen of the brain. A similar cerebral mass lesion was described by Hervei and Simon in a case of congenital toxoplasmosis [459] and by Bobowski and Reed in a case of acquired toxoplasmosis [460]. Hervas and colleagues described a newborn with congenital toxoplasmosis whose cranial CT scan with contrast enhancement demonstrated calcifications and multiple ring-enhancing lesions not dissimilar to those seen in adult patients with AIDS, with multiple brain abscesses related to *T. gondii* [305]. McAuley and coworkers [433] also described enhancement around a lesion that resolved with antimicrobial treatment.

A CT scan, which allows for neuroanatomic localization of intracranial calcifications, delineation of ventricular size, and recognition of cortical atrophy, has proved to be valuable in evaluation of congenital toxoplasmosis [461–463]. Diebler and associates published results of CT scans in 32 cases of congenital toxoplasmosis [462]. They reported a clear relationship between the lesions observed on these scans, neurologic signs, and date of maternal infection. The destructive lesions were porencephalic cysts that when multiple may constitute multicystic encephalomalacia or even hydranencephaly. Dense and large calcifications were seen in the basal ganglia in seven cases, with or without periventricular calcifications. Hydrocephalus was always secondary to aqueductal stenosis. In one case, ocular calcification was noted. In a retrospective study of cases in which pachygyria-like changes were observed on CT or magnetic resonance imaging, a single case of congenital toxoplasmosis was noted [464]. Ultrasonography also has been suggested as useful for diagnosis of congenital

toxoplasmosis. CT scan of the brain detects calcifications not seen with ultrasonography of the brain [465,466]. Brief MRI (an axial single shot T2 MRI requiring 30-45 seconds) may be useful for following ventricular size when a child has had a VP shunt or otherwise requires follow-up of ventricular size. It can be performed with no sedation or contrast, lowering risks and complications (R. McLeod, unpublished observations).

Intracranial Calcification

With rare exceptions [319], the deposits of calcium noticed in congenital toxoplasmosis have been limited to the intracranial structures. The deposits are scattered throughout the brain and in some studies have been reported to have no characteristic distribution. In other studies, many children were observed to have prominent basal ganglia and periventricular califications [467–470]. Masherpa and Valentino described two types of calcifications: (1) multiple, dense round deposits 1 to 3 mm in diameter scattered in the white matter and, more frequently, in the periventricular areas of the occipitoparietal and temporal regions and (2) curvilinear streaks in the basal ganglia, mostly in the head of the caudate nucleus

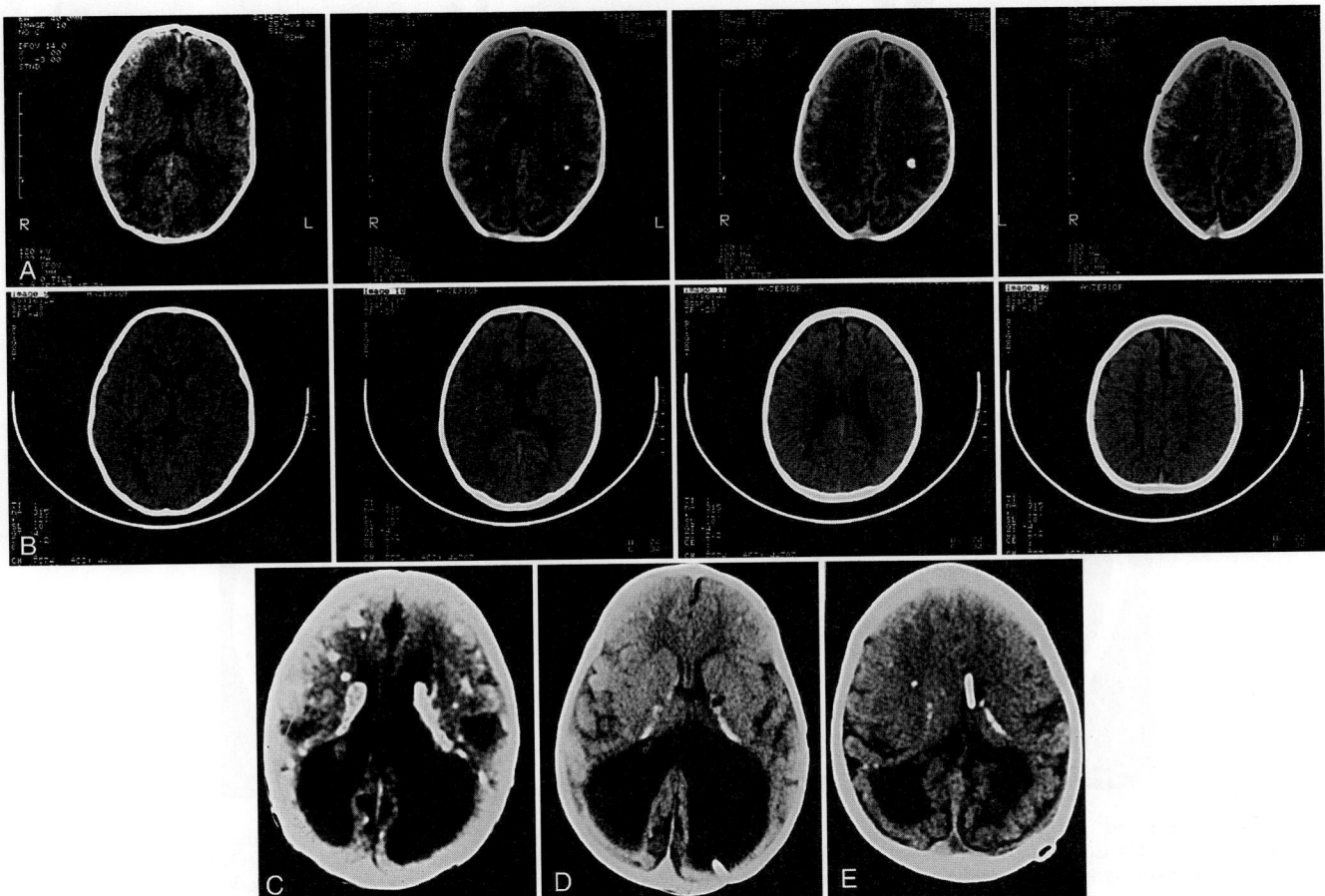

FIGURE 31–15 Additional examples of cranial computed tomography (CT) scans that demonstrate resolution of calcifications in children following treatment for congenital toxoplasmosis. **A** and **B**, CT scans in an infant obtained at birth, August 1992 (A), and in August 1993 (B). **C** to **E**, Diminution and/or resolution of large areas of calcification are seen in these representative cranial CT scans from another infant. The scans were obtained at birth, February 1987 (C), and at follow-up in May 1988 (D) and July 1991 (E).

Continued

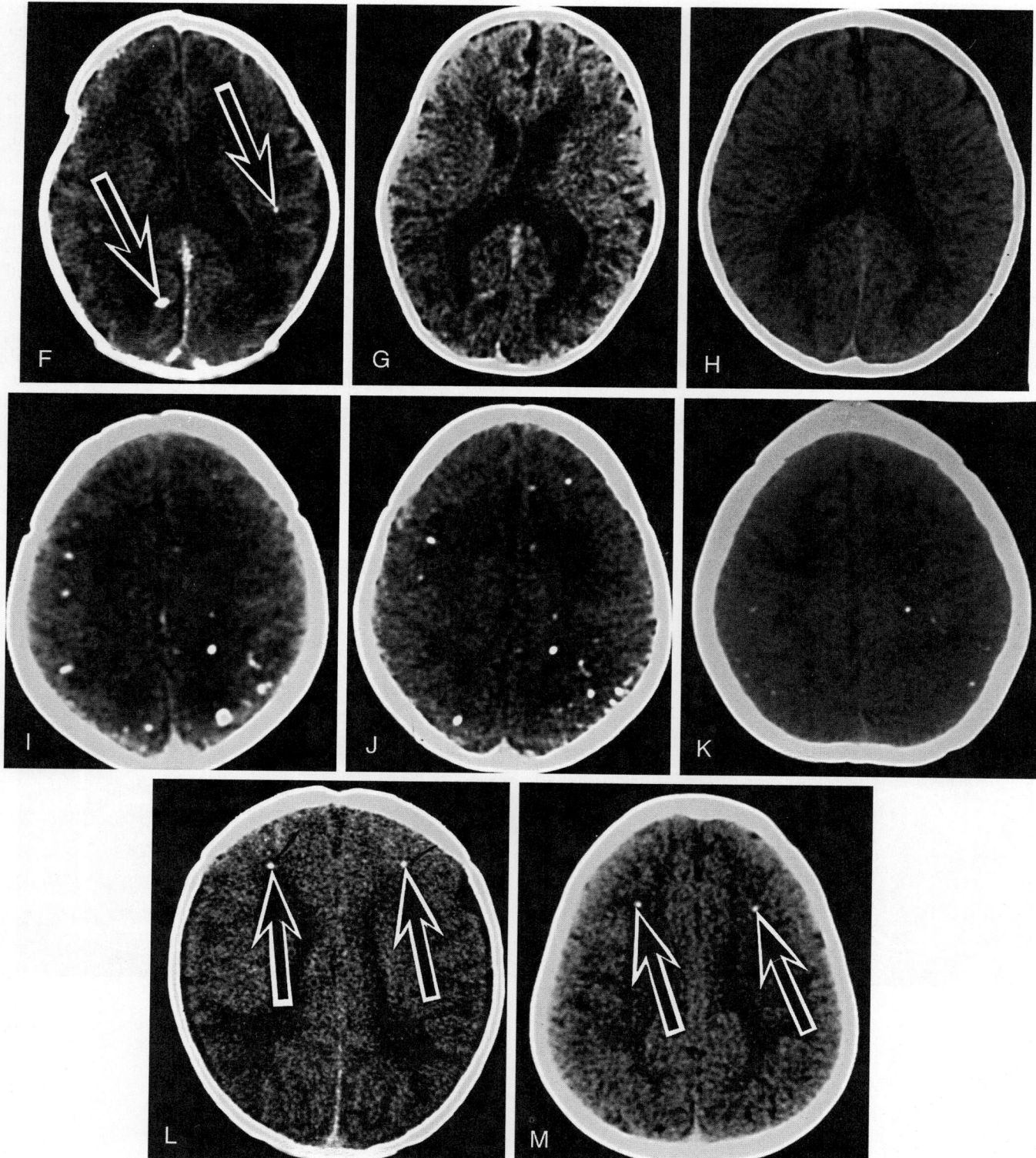

FIGURE 31–15—cont'd   F to H, Cranial CT scans of the dizygotic twin of the patient whose CT scans are shown in A and B. Newborn scan (F) was obtained August 1992. The calcifications (*arrows*) were seen to have resolved on follow-up scans obtained in November 1992 (G) and in August 1993 (H). Note: The patient whose scans are shown in A and B was randomized to receive initial higher dose therapy (6 months of 1 mg/kg/day of pyrimethamine), and the patient whose scans are shown in F to H was randomized to receive initial lower dose therapy (2 months of 1 mg/kg/day of pyrimethamine). Both infants completed 1 year of treatment with pyrimethamine 1 mg/kg each Monday, Wednesday, and Friday and sulfadiazine. Calcifications were seen to have resolved completely in cranial CT scans of both twins. **I to K,** Cranial CT scans obtained for another infant in the newborn period, January 1993 (I), and at follow-up in February 1993 (J) and January 1994 (K) demonstrate diminution and/or resolution of calcifications. This child has developed normally. **L** and **M,** Cranial CT scans obtained in the newborn period, May 1991 (L) and in August 1992 (M) in a different, noncompliant child who underwent treatment in our study for only 1 month. Arrows mark calcifications that remained the same size. (*From Patel DV, et al. Resolution of intracranial calcification in infants with treated congenital toxoplasmosis. Radiology 199:433–440, 1996, with minor modifications and permission.*)

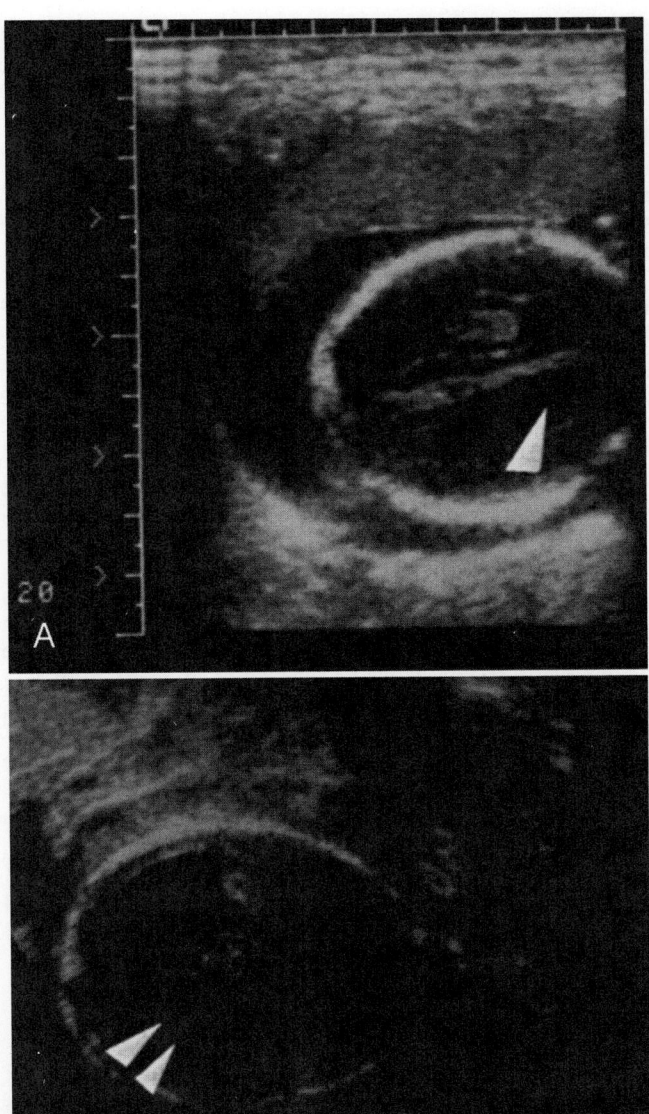

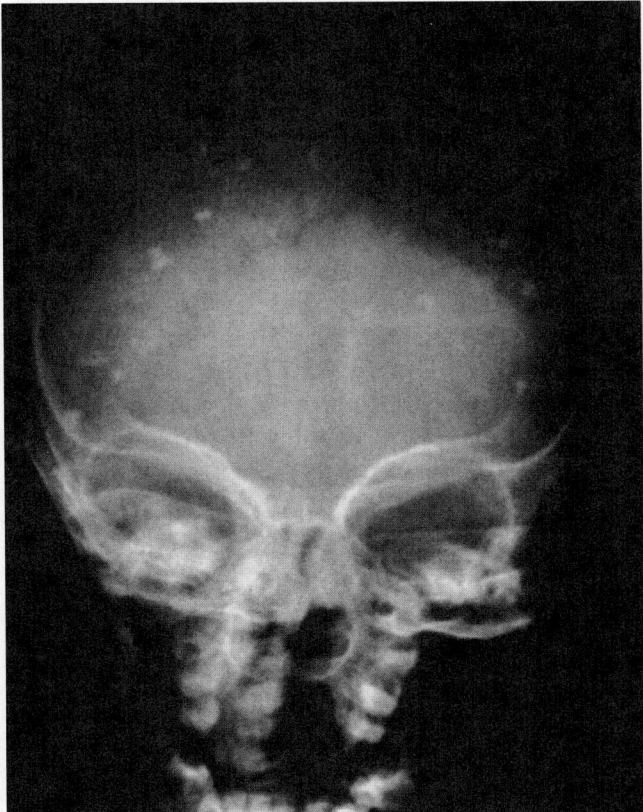

FIGURE 31–17 Cerebral calcifications in congenital toxoplasmosis in a 10-month-old infant; the infection was subclinical. *(Courtesy of J Couvreur, Paris.)*

FIGURE 31–16 Rapid development of massive hydrocephalus in a fetus between 20 **(A)** and 21 **(B)** weeks of gestation. Single arrowhead indicates cerebral ventricles in A, and double arrowheads indicate massively dilated ventricles in B.

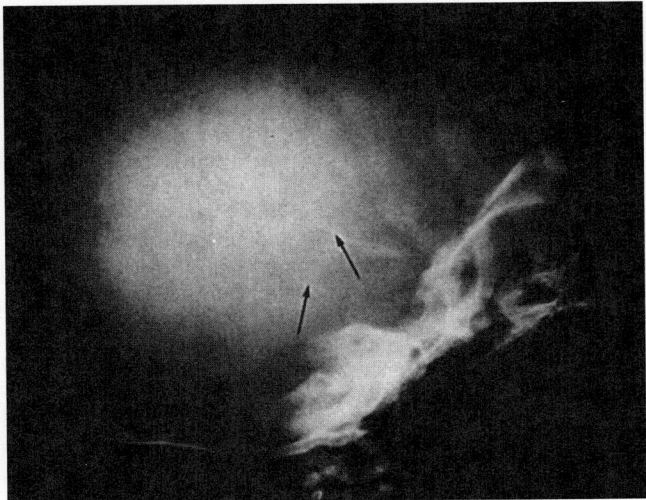

FIGURE 31–18 Cerebral calcifications in congenital toxoplasmosis in a neonate, with calcifications lining the ventricles (*arrows*). *(Courtesy of J Couvreur, Paris.)*

[471]. Some workers consider that evidence of both nodular calcifications and linear calcifications is pathognomonic of toxoplasmosis (Figs. 31–17 and 31–18).

Although in cytomegalic inclusion disease the calcifications are located chiefly subependymally and are bilaterally symmetrical, mostly in the walls of the dilated ventricles [469,470], these locations also are noted in congenital toxoplasmosis. The largest series of cases of cerebral calcification related to congenital toxoplasmosis are those of Dyke and colleagues [472] and of Mussbichler [473]. The latter reviewed material from 32 clinically well-documented cases. Approximately one third of the patients were 3 months of age or younger, and 80% were younger than 2 years of age. Mussbichler's findings—some original and others confirming the findings of

others—revealed that calcifications in the caudate nucleus, choroid plexuses, meninges, and subependyma are characteristic in toxoplasmosis, although some of these locations also have been described in cytomegalic inclusion disease. Because calcifications were present in multiple areas of the brain in the cases he reviewed, he concluded that calcifications found in the choroid plexuses alone should not be regarded as evidence of toxoplasmosis. Mussbichler found calcifications in the meninges that had not previously been described and attributed his ability to locate them to the use of appropriate projections that delineated them clearly. For those children who did not receive treatment, calcifications in the meninges and caudate nucleus were signs of a poor prognosis; they were found only in the youngest children, who died early. Conversely, disseminated nodular calcifications do not necessarily suggest a poor prognosis and have been discovered fortuitously in "normal" infants who were studied at approximately 1 year of age; in these children, a diagnosis of congenital toxoplasmosis had been made through a systematic survey. The increase in size and number of calcific lesions during a period of months or years in some cases suggests that the process of healing (and perhaps also of destruction) may occur long after the onset of the infection. Calcifications can diminish in size or resolve with treatment [456].

Osseous Changes

In 1974, Milgram described the radiographic signs present in an infant who died 17 days after birth with a severe clinical form of congenital toxoplasmosis [292]. Roentgenograms of several ribs and vertebrae and one femur revealed bands of metaphyseal lucency and irregularity of the line of provisional calcification at the epiphyseal plates. Periosteal reaction was not present. (Syphilis also may cause this same finding.)

Liver

Although it has been stated that calcifications do not occur outside the CNS in infants with congenital toxoplasmosis, Caldera and colleagues described cases of three infants with calcifications in the liver [319]. The calcifications were evident both radiologically and in the liver at autopsy.

Other Signs and Symptoms

Erythroblastosis and Hydrops Fetalis. Congenital toxoplasmosis may be confused with erythroblastosis related to isosensitization [299,423,474–479]. The peripheral blood picture and clinical course may be identical to those observed in other forms of erythroblastosis. This similarity is exemplified by cases such as those reported by Callahan and colleagues [288] and by Beckett and Flynn [62]. A negative Coombs test result is helpful in distinguishing erythroblastosis caused by congenital infection from that caused by blood group factor sensitization. In one case, fetal hydrops due to congenital toxoplasmosis resolved in association with treatment of toxoplasma infection with pyrimethamine, sulfadiazine with leucovorin between the 27th and 37th weeks of gestation (R. McLeod and colleagues, unpublished observation).

Cardiovascular Signs. Severe toxoplasmic myocarditis may be manifested clinically as edema [288].

Gastrointestinal Signs. In some cases, the first sign of the disease appears to be vomiting or diarrhea [288]. Feeding problems also are common.

Respiratory Difficulty. Respiratory difficulty [6,288], often with cyanosis, may be due to an interstitial toxoplasmic pneumonitis, to viral or bacterial suprainfection, or to CNS lesions affecting the respiratory control centers of the brain.

Deafness. From the follow-up studies of Eichenwald [356] and others [480], ample clinical and histologic [56,288,314,368,481] data are available to show that congenital infection with *T. gondii* can lead to deafness. The well-documented cases of profound hearing loss have been almost totally confined to infants with severe clinical disease, but in the series of children with subclinical infection at birth reported by Wilson and associates [480], 17% had significant hearing loss. In some instances, serologic and skin test surveys among deaf patients have suggested a cause-and-effect relationship [482], whereas in others, no such relationship has been found [483]. An association between epilepsy, cerebral palsy, and nerve deafness and the presence of antibodies to *T. gondii* in sera of Israeli children was noted (relative risk 2.5, $P = .03$; nerve deafness relative risk 7.1, $P = .01$) [484]. Such studies frequently are open to criticism, owing to the choice of controls. Thus no satisfactory data are available to support the contention that congenital toxoplasmosis may be a frequent cause of deafness [485]. In the NCCCTS, as of June 2010, no treated child with sensorineural hearing loss was identified (Table 31–18) [486]. One child with brainstem lesions involving the auditory nucleus had auditory perceptual difficulties.

Ascites. Vanhaesebrouck and coworkers described a preterm congenitally infected infant with isolated transudative ascites caused by *T. gondii* [487]. Neonatal [488] and fetal [77,489,490] ascites due to congenital toxoplasmosis have been reported.

Follow-up Studies

Adequate follow-up studies (see also the previous "Eye" section) to gain information on the natural course of congenital toxoplasmosis are lacking in most series of reported cases. In the vast majority, the original diagnosis was made in a retrospective manner, in most cases because of the presence of clinical signs of the infection. Most accumulated data, therefore, are from infants and older children with the most atypical form of congenital toxoplasmosis, that is, clinically apparent disease in the newborn period. It is in those infants who are actually in the majority—those who were asymptomatic at birth—that there is the greatest need for follow-up studies, such as those performed by Alford and colleagues [328,411], described previously. (See also the published studies by Hedenström and colleagues [491,492]). Findings on follow-up evaluation of the infants who were asymptomatic at birth in the Paris study are difficult to interpret because most were given treatment in the newborn period. In some, however, recognition of the first clinical finding

TABLE 31-18   Definitions of Hearing Impairment and Outcome in Reported Studies of Hearing in Cases of Congenital Toxoplasmosis [354,357,484]

Degree of Hearing Impairment	Definitions			Results		
	U.S. (Chicago) National Collaborative Treatment Trial [742]		Wilson et al [604].	Eichenwald [601]	U.S. (Chicago) National Collaborative Treatment Trial [792]	Wilson et al [604].	Eichenwald [601]
	ABR (dB/HL)	Audiogram (dB/HL)					
Normal	≤20	0–20	<25 dB*	NA	104	14	NA
Mild	>20–40	25–40	25–50 dB	NA	0	3	NA
Moderate	>40–60	>40	51–80 dB	NA	0	2	NA
Severe	>60	>70–90	Not found	NA	0	0	NA
Profound		>90	Not found	"Deaf"	0	0	15
Total					104	19	105

*Defined as "hearing reception threshold" by Wilson and McLeod [604].
ABR, auditory brain response; dB, decibels; HL, hearing level; NA, not available.
Adapted from McGee T, et al. Absence of sensorineural hearing loss in treated infants and children with congenital toxoplasmosis. Otolaryngol Head Neck Surg 106:75–80, 1992, with minor modifications and permission.

(usually chorioretinitis) was delayed until several weeks or months after birth, thereby illustrating an often reported observation in congenital toxoplasmosis: the normal appearance of a child for some months before overt disease is recognized [61,359,380,493].

Follow-up studies of those patients described by Eichenwald have already been mentioned. Two patients reported by Wolf and coworkers in 1942 [304] were still alive in 1959 and were being cared for in mental institutions [494]. One of them, first seen at the age of 3 years and 9 months, was about 22 years old at the time of the second report. She was mentally and physically retarded and oblivious to her environment, drooled constantly, was resistant to care and feeding, and was losing weight. She continued to have petit mal and grand mal seizures. Old chorioretinal scars were still present. The second patient was 2 years old when the diagnosis was made and about 18 years of age at the time of the last report. His IQ was only 40. He was said to have a pleasant personality and could engage in some project activities. Vision was 20/100 in one eye and 20/70 in the other.

Feldman and Miller analyzed 187 patients with congenital toxoplasmosis. Among 176 of these patients, 119 were 4 years of age or younger, 38 were 5 to 9 years of age, and 19 were 10 to 19 years of age [96]. Thirty-six had been delivered prematurely; 20% of the premature infants and 7% of those born at term died. Residual damage varied in degree, but most of the patients exhibited chorioretinitis, mental retardation, and abnormalities of head size. In this series, reported frequencies of abnormalities were as follows: intracerebral calcification, 59%; psychomotor retardation, 45%; seizures, 39%; chorioretinitis, 94%; microphthalmia, 36%; hydrocephalus, 22%; and microcephaly, 21% [357].

Puissan and coworkers observed the late onset of convulsions in an 8-year-old girl with congenital toxoplasmosis [495]. Of interest in this case was the demonstration of what appears to have been local production of T. gondii antibody in the cerebrospinal fluid when the convulsions began.

In the first report of the prospective study by Koppe and colleagues, follow-up data were obtained for 7 years for 12 congenitally infected children [360]. Four children had clinical signs (ocular only), and one was clinically normal but T. gondii had been isolated from the placenta and cerebrospinal fluid; these five were given pyrimethamine and sulfadiazine. No signs of cerebral damage or intracranial calcifications developed in any of the children, and all were said to be "mentally normal" at the age of 7 years [360]. Their development was judged by their performance in school, which was stated to be normal. In fact, in a later report, chorioretinal scars were present in 82% of these children [245], and because they were still younger than 15 years of age when last reported, they remained at risk for the development of additional sequelae. (See the "Amsterdam Study" section later for the final report.)

Congenital Toxoplasma Infection and Acquired Immunodeficiency Syndrome

Congenital transmission of T. gondii from pregnant women coinfected with T. gondii and HIV has been recognized as a unique problem [496–503] but fortunately a relatively

uncommon one [504–510]. Documentation of previous infection before conception and the absence of demonstrable IgM antibodies to T. gondii in many of these women suggests that transmission in HIV-infected women can occur in the context of chronic infection. However, Lago and colleagues [511] recently reported a case in which primary infection during pregnancy was documented in the absence of demonstrable IgM antibodies to T. gondii in the pregnant woman. This observation suggests that acute infection with T. gondii can occur in pregnant HIV-infected women in the absence of a detectable IgM antibody response to the parasite and does not constitute proof of chronic infection. Transmission of T. gondii from these chronically infected women would be most likely to occur in the setting of severe immunosuppression, but there are insufficient data at present to test this prediction. Such data would assist in determining the importance of this and other parameters of immunosuppression that place the fetus at risk for congenital T. gondii infection.

Noteworthy are the observations that most of the newborns did not have clinical signs of either infection at birth, even though in each case the infant was found to be dually infected with the parasite and HIV. In many of these infants, signs of severe disseminated infection developed within the first weeks or months of life.

Mitchell and colleagues described four young infants, two of whom were siblings, who were dually infected with HIV-1 and T. gondii [496]. Their mothers were similarly coinfected. The mother of the first infant had toxoplasmic encephalitis diagnosed at delivery. The other mothers had no clinical evidence of toxoplasmosis but did have T. gondii antibodies. The investigators concluded that the mother was the source of the infection in each of the infants. Of interest is that in three of the seven cases (three additional cases were diagnosed after the initial publication) documented at the University of Miami, the diagnosis was not suspected before the patient's death and was made only at autopsy (Mitchell C, personal communication to Remington JS, 1993). Three of the four cases from the original publication are briefly reviewed here as examples of the problem.

Case History: Infants 2 and 3

The mother of the siblings with congenital T. gondii infection had given birth to five children, four of whom were infected with HIV-1. The siblings with toxoplasmosis were the third and fifth born. AIDS developed in the mother 1 month after the birth of this fifth child, but she had no clinical or tomographic evidence of toxoplasmic encephalitis. She died 8 months later of tuberculosis and bacterial sepsis. An autopsy was not performed. One sibling, born at term and "appropriate for gestational age," was discharged from the hospital at 3 days of age in good condition, only to return at 3 months of age with complications of AIDS. He remained hospitalized until he died at age 6 months. At autopsy, he was found to have disseminated cytomegalovirus infection involving most visceral organs and all lobes of the lung, T. gondii pneumonitis, and diffuse CNS toxoplasmosis. The other sibling was a full-term female appropriate for gestational age. She had an unremarkable neonatal course. When seen at 5 weeks of age, she was in septic shock and emaciated and had severe oral thrush. She died within 1 hour after admission to the hospital. Blood cultures were positive for *Propionibacterium*; the autopsy revealed disseminated candidiasis involving the lungs and esophagus and diffuse intracerebral toxoplasmosis.

Case History: Infant 4

The patient was an appropriate-for-gestational-age, full-term female infant recognized at birth to be at risk for congenital toxoplasmosis and HIV-1 infection because her mother was known to be seropositive for *T. gondii* and had previously given birth to a child who died of AIDS. Results of examination at birth were normal, but the infant was given expectant treatment for toxoplasmosis with pyrimethamine and sulfadiazine because of the presence of IgM *T. gondii* antibodies in her serum. After an extended course of therapy complicated by hepatitis of unclear etiology, she died; permission for autopsy was denied. This child's mother died of AIDS 3 years later, never having developed clinical toxoplasmosis.

Marty and coworkers [512] described a 22-week pregnant, HIV-infected woman who was observed to have reactivation of her *T. gondii* serologic test titer (from an IgG dye test titer of 5 IU/mL to 400 IU at 1 year later). She had a CD4+ cell count of 90/mm³. An ultrasound examination revealed fetal hydrocephaly, and a therapeutic abortion was performed. The external morphology of the fetus was normal, but the autopsy revealed multiple abscesses in the brain and liver, and *T. gondii* was isolated from amniotic fluid, placenta, liver, spleen, heart, and brain.

Pathology

Information on pathologic changes in the CNS in fetuses or newborns coinfected with *T. gondii* and HIV-1 is relatively scarce. In three of the cases reported by Mitchell and coworkers, histologic evidence of meningitis included chronic leptomeningeal inflammatory cell infiltrates [496], *T. gondii* cysts, and microglial nodules that suggested an immune response against the parasite were seen in the brain in two cases. Examination of numerous slides from the brain of one infant, who had received treatment for toxoplasmosis, revealed only a single *T. gondii* cyst and no microglial nodules. The brain revealed chronic inflammation and widespread foci of necrosis surrounded by macrophages, lymphocytes, and plasma cells. Gliosis also was present. Immunoperoxidase staining demonstrated *T. gondii* in the CNS of this infant.

Insufficient data are available to estimate how frequently the diagnosis of congenital *T. gondii* infection in these dually infected infants might be suggested by serologic examination. IgM and IgG *T. gondii* antibodies have been demonstrable in some of these infants (Mitchell C and Kovacs A, personal communication to Remington JS, 1993) [498].

Treatment

Treatment of the Newborn. Data on the outcome of treatment of congenital *T. gondii* infection in these newborns are insufficient for any conclusions to be drawn. The diagnosis of coinfection with HIV usually has been made late and often a month or more after birth. Thus at least at present, whether to use drugs directed against HIV in combination with anti-*T. gondii* therapy in the early newborn period does not appear to be a major consideration. Of importance in this regard is that toxicity to the bone marrow may be considerably increased when, for example, zidovudine, pyrimethamine, and sulfadiazine are used together. When the diagnosis in the newborn is suspected or proved, we recommend that the pyrimethamine-sulfadiazine combination be used. Treatment is continued for the first year of life. Data from adults with HIV and *T. gondii* infections suggest that if the CD4+ cell count is maintained at greater than 200 cells/μL with antiretroviral treatment, it may be feasible, after the standard 1-year treatment, to discontinue treatment with pyrimethamine and sulfadiazine.

Treatment and Primary Prophylaxis in the Human Immunodeficiency Virus- and *Toxoplasma gondii*-Infected Pregnant Women. Treatment with pyrimethamine-sulfadiazine (and leucovorin) should be started in patients with active toxoplasmosis [513]. Clindamycin may be used as an alternative to sulfadiazine in the combination [514]. Use of pyrimethamine in the first trimester is contraindicated, as discussed earlier. The decision whether to use this drug should be made in consultation with experts.

Until more complete information becomes available on the special factors that predispose to congenital transmission of *T. gondii* in these women, we recommend that primary prophylaxis be used in those with CD4+ T-cell counts of fewer than 200 cells per mm³. The combination agent trimethoprim-sulfamethoxazole, commonly used in these patients to prevent *Pneumocystis* pneumonia, is effective in prevention of toxoplasmic encephalitis in patients with AIDS who can tolerate the drug. Use of this and other drug regimens for *T. gondii* primary prophylaxis is common practice for management of nonpregnant HIV-infected adults who also have chronic *T. gondii* infection [515]. More complete treatment of this subject is beyond the scope of this chapter. For a commentary on this issue in general, the reader is referred to reference [515]. It should be noted, however, that no data are available on whether pyrimethamine-sulfadiazine and pyrimethamine-clindamycin combinations are of comparable efficacy in preventing transmission of *T. gondii* to the fetus.

Of interest in regard to the transmission from mother to her fetus are two cases of CNS toxoplasmosis in HIV-infected pregnant women who gave birth to infants who were not infected with *T. gondii* [516,517].

DIAGNOSIS

The diagnosis of acute infection with *T. gondii* may be established by isolation of the organism from blood or body fluids, demonstration of the presence of cysts in the placenta or tissues of a fetus or newborn, demonstration of the presence of antigen or organisms or both in sections or preparations of tissues and body fluids, demonstration of antigenemia and antigen in serum and body fluids, specific nucleic acid sequences (e.g., using PCR methods), or serologic tests.

Diagnostic Methods
Laboratory Examination

Cerebrospinal Fluid. (See also "Serologic Diagnosis in the Newborn" and "Serologic Studies and Polymerase Chain Reaction Assay in Cerebrospinal Fluid; Polymerase Chain Reaction Assay in Urine" later on.) Approximately 4 decades ago, Callahan and colleagues, in reviewing the cerebrospinal fluid changes in 108 patients with congenital toxoplasmosis, stated, "Examination of the CSF affords the most constant significant laboratory examination for the presence of infantile toxoplasmosis [288]". Although the patients studied by these investigators had the most severe form of the disease, this statement is pertinent even today. Despite the fact that cerebrospinal fluid changes in infants with congenital toxoplasmosis are not specific for toxoplasmosis, the demonstration of these changes should lead the physician to consider a diagnosis of toxoplasmosis even in subclinical cases. The findings of xanthochromia and mononuclear pleocytosis in cases of congenital toxoplasmosis also are common in many other generalized infections of the newborn. Almost unique to infants with neonatal toxoplasmosis, however, is the very high protein content of the ventricular fluid. Although in some infants the protein level is just slightly above normal, in others it can be measured in grams per deciliter rather than in milligrams per deciliter [56,328,518]. Alford and associates considered that in most infants with congenital toxoplasmosis who appear clinically normal at birth, a "silent" CNS involvement is present as reflected by persistent cerebrospinal fluid pleocytosis and the elevated protein content (see also the "Central Nervous System" section under both "Pathology" and "Clinical Manifestations") [328].

Increases in protein levels and pleocytosis were not as common in a prospective study performed in France (Desmonts G, unpublished data). The difference probably is due to the difference in method of selection of cases. In the study reported by Alford and associates, only those infants in whom an elevated serum IgM was present at birth were screened for *T. gondii* antibody, and the development of the infection in these infants by the time of birth may have differed significantly from that in the French studies, in which infants were examined because of suspicion of maternal toxoplasmosis acquired during pregnancy. In the French study, the infants, who were infected very close to the time of labor or during labor, may not have had elevated serum IgM levels at birth and therefore would have been missed in the studies in which IgM screening alone was the criterion for case selection.

Persistence of IgM antibodies to *T. gondii* in the cerebrospinal fluid has been observed in some infected infants and may suggest continued active infection. Such persistence of IgM antibodies in the cerebrospinal fluid also has been reported in congenital rubella [519].

Specific IgG antibody formation in the CNS has been demonstrated in infants with congenital toxoplasmosis [520]. Two hundred forty-two examinations were performed in 206 congenitally infected infants as part of the routine cerebrospinal fluid workup. Only three cases

(1.8%) had demonstrable local IgG antibody formation in the CNS. *T. gondii* has been detected by PCR assay in cerebrospinal fluid of newborns with congenital toxoplasmosis (see "Polymerase Chain Reaction Assay," later on). Woods and Englund [521] described a newborn with severe congenital toxoplasmosis who had signs of brain destruction and whose cerebrospinal fluid was hazy and xanthochromic, with 302 white blood cells per mm^3 and 106 red blood cells per mm^3. The differential count revealed 1% neutrophils, 8% mononuclear cells, and 91% eosinophils. The cerebrospinal fluid glucose level was 23 mg/dL, and the cerebrospinal fluid protein level was 158 mg/dL. At the same time, the peripheral blood showed 16% eosinophils (absolute count 432 eosinophils per mm^3). Although peripheral blood eosinophilia is common in newborns with congenital toxoplasmosis, as are eosinophilic infiltrations of the pia-arachnoid overlying destructive cortical lesions, eosinophilia has not previously been reported in the cerebrospinal fluid of such newborns.

A newborn whose congenital toxoplasmosis caused hydrocephalus and cerebral atrophy and quadriparesis as a result of spinal cord atrophy had peripheral blood eosinophilia (40%) and markedly abnormal cerebrospinal fluid (13% of 98 white blood cells) (Barson W, personal communication to McLeod R, 1999). Treatment with pyrimethamine and sulfadiazine given to the mother during gestation may diminish manifestations, including cerebrospinal fluid pleocytosis or elevated cerebrospinal fluid protein in the infant [76].

Blood and Blood-Forming Elements. Leukocytosis or leukopenia may be present, and early in the course of the infection, lymphocytosis and monocytosis usually are found [6,288,386]. Marked polymorphonuclear leukocytosis frequently reflects suprainfection with bacteria.

Thrombocytopenia is common in infants who have other clinical signs of the infection and in subclinical cases [302,322,491,522], petechiae or ecchymoses may be the earliest clue to this congenital infection [288,293,299, 302,491]. Eosinophilia in the newborn period frequently has been observed, and the eosinophils may exceed 30% of the differential white blood cell count.*

Histologic Diagnosis
Demonstration of tachyzoites in tissues (e.g., brain biopsy, bone marrow aspirate) or body fluids (ventricular fluid or cerebrospinal fluid [289,305,526–529], aqueous humor [530], sputum [531]) establishes the diagnosis of active toxoplasmosis. Unfortunately, it frequently is difficult to visualize the tachyzoite form in tissues or impression smears stained by ordinary methods. Accordingly, the fluorescent antibody technique has been suggested for this purpose [75,532–534]. Because of its greater sensitivity and specificity, the peroxidase-antiperoxidase technique has largely supplanted the fluorescent antibody method [535]. Both methods are applicable to unfixed or formalin-fixed paraffin-embedded tissue sections. The pitfalls in interpretation of results with these methods have been discussed by Frenkel and Piekarski [536]. In

---

*References 6, 56, 288, 368, 386, 523–525.

the retina, because the retinal pigment epithelium is brown or black, a method that stains the parasites red, rather than brown, has proved useful for detection of the parasites [313]. Histologic demonstration of the cyst form establishes that the patient has toxoplasmosis but does not warrant the conclusion that the infection is acute unless there is associated inflammation and necrosis. On the other hand, because cysts may form early in infection, their demonstration does not exclude the possibility that the infection is still in the acute stages [537].

In the case of acute acquired toxoplasmosis in the pregnant patient, lymphadenopathy may reflect a variety of infectious agents [538]. Distinctive histologic changes in toxoplasmic lymphadenitis enable the pathologist to make a presumptive diagnosis of acute acquired toxoplasmosis [539]. These histologic changes represent the characteristic reaction of the host to the infection, but the organisms themselves are only rarely demonstrable. The histologic signs of infection in other tissues range from areas of no inflammation around cysts to acute necrotizing lesions associated with tachyzoites. The latter are seen almost solely in immunocompromised individuals. None of these changes confirms the diagnosis of toxoplasmosis unless the organism can be demonstrated.

Isolation Procedures

General Considerations

Isolation of the parasite from an infant provides unequivocal proof of infection, but unfortunately, such isolation usually takes too long to permit an early diagnosis. *T. gondii* is readily isolated from tissue obtained at autopsy (e.g., brain, skeletal muscle, or heart muscle); the organism may also be isolated from biopsy material from the neonate (e.g., skeletal muscle). In our experience, isolates from congenitally infected infants are most often avirulent for mice, and a period of 4 to 6 weeks is usually required for definitive demonstration of the parasite when this method is used. In cases in which the organism is virulent for mice, the parasite can often be demonstrated in the peritoneal fluid after 5 to 10 days. *T. gondii* has been isolated from body fluids (e.g., ventricular fluid or cerebrospinal fluid [304,516,527,540–546], subretinal fluid [547], and aqueous humor) [548] of infants and adults, and from amniotic fluid [544,549,550]. Isolation from tissues (e.g., skeletal muscle, lung, brain, or eye) obtained by biopsy or at autopsy from older children and adults may reflect only the presence of tissue cysts and thus does not constitute definitive proof of active acute infection. One possible exception is the isolation of *T. gondii* from lymph nodes in older children and adults; such evidence probably indicates relatively recently acquired infection because cysts are rarely found in lymph nodes. Attempts at isolation usually are performed by injection of suspect material into laboratory mice but also may be accomplished by inoculation into tissue culture preparations (see later discussion) [289,545,551,552]. One can observe plaque formation and both extracellular and intracellular parasites in unstained or stained preparations. Abbas found cell cultures less sensitive than mouse inoculation for isolation of the parasite [553]. Thus if cell cultures are used in attempts at primary isolation, it is advisable

also to use mouse inoculation when feasible. Tissue culture isolation is quite rapid (usually requiring 1 week or less) and should be used when early isolation is critical for the management of the patient. Because physicians often request that isolation procedures be performed, the following are offered as guidelines for the laboratory.

Specimens should be injected into animals and cell cultures as soon as possible after collection to prevent death of the parasite. Formalin kills the parasite, and freezing may result in death of both tachyzoite and cyst forms. If storage of specimens is necessary, refrigeration at 4° C is preferred. This can maintain the encysted form in tissues, if kept moist, for up to 2 months and prevents death of the tachyzoite for several days. The parasite can survive in blood for a week or longer (see "Transmission" section). For antibody determination, serum may be removed from clotted cord blood or blood obtained later in the newborn period; the clot should be stored at 4° C until the results of serologic tests are known. If results of serologic tests are not diagnostic and the reason for suspecting congenital toxoplasmosis remains, the blood clot should be injected into mice (or tissue culture) in the same way as for any other tissue specimen. Body fluids and heparinized blood can be injected directly, but we prefer to remove the plasma from the formed elements of blood and amniotic fluid, to eliminate the possibility of introducing a majority of *T. gondii* antibodies into the recipient animals. Passively transferred human antibody may interfere with infection of the mice, and thus with isolation of the organisms, and producing false-positive serologic test results in the inoculated animals for 6 weeks or longer [58]. Because the organisms are most likely to reside within white blood cells in patients with parasitemia, the buffy coat layer may be suspended in a small volume of sterile saline and inoculated into mice by the intraperitoneal or subcutaneous route or onto tissue culture.

Biopsy specimens and blood clots may be triturated with a mortar and pestle or tissue homogenizer in a small amount of normal saline before animal or tissue culture inoculation. After trituration, we generally add enough sterile saline so that the suspension can be drawn into a syringe. If connective tissue prevents aspiration through the needle, the suspension can be filtered through several layers of sterile gauze. Depending on the size of the mice, 0.5 to 2 mL is injected intraperitoneally, subcutaneously, or both. For isolation attempts from superficial enlarged lymph nodes, material can be obtained by needle aspiration of the node.

To isolate *T. gondii* from large amounts of tissue (e.g., placenta), we use trypsin digestion (0.25% trypsin in buffered saline, pH 7.2) [66]. The trypsin method makes it possible to isolate both tachyzoite and cyst forms. The former are killed more rapidly by pepsin-hydrochloric acid (HCl) [30]. The tissue is first minced with scissors and passed through a meat grinder or ground in a blender; it is then placed in a volume of trypsin solution (10 to 20 mL of trypsin solution per gram of tissue) and incubated with constant agitation for 1.5 to 2 hours at 37° C. (If the tissue is grossly contaminated, antibiotics may be added both to the digestion fluid and to the tissue digest before injection.) The suspension is passed through several layers of gauze to remove large particles and then is centrifuged. After the sediment has been washed three or four times in saline to remove trypsin, the digested material is resuspended in saline, and 0.5 to 1 mL is injected both intraperitoneally and subcutaneously into mice. If peptic digestion is desired, the solution is prepared by dissolving 4 g of pepsin (Difco 1:10,000), 7.5 g of sodium chloride, and 10.5 mL of concentrated HCl in water to a volume of 1500 mL. The method described by Dubey also may be used [554].

Mouse Inoculation

In most countries, it is not necessary to perform serologic testing in laboratory mice to determine if they are infected before they are used in isolation attempts. In areas of the world where normal laboratory mice have been found to be infected, serologic testing of individual mice must be performed before such use. Five to 10 days after intraperitoneal injection, the peritoneal fluid should be examined either fresh or in stained smears (Wright or Giemsa stain) for the presence of intracellular and extracellular tachyzoites (see Fig. 31–1, A). Demonstration of the organism is proof of the infection. Mice that die before 6 weeks have elapsed are examined for the presence of the organism in their peritoneal fluid; stained impression smears of liver and spleen also can be examined. If no organisms are found, suspensions of liver, spleen, and brain may be injected into fresh mice. Surviving mice are bled from the tail vein or orbital sinus for serologic testing after 6 weeks but may be bled from the tail vein more often (e.g., at 2-week intervals). (The dye test, agglutination test, IFA test, or ELISA can be used for this purpose.) We prefer to use the agglutination test as a screening method for this purpose because only a single drop of blood from the tail vein can be tested using microtiter plate wells. If antibodies are present, proof of infection must be obtained by demonstration of the parasite. This can be accomplished most easily by examining Giemsa-stained smears of fresh brain for demonstration of cysts (see Fig. 31–1, E). Examination of wet preparations of brain tissue may be misinterpreted if done by inexperienced workers; pine pollen has been confused with T. gondii cysts and has led to erroneous diagnosis of the infection. Examination is easier under phase microscopy. If cysts are not seen, injection into fresh mice of a suspension of brain, liver, and spleen should be performed to determine whether the parasite is present.

Tissue Culture

Isolation by tissue culture has been used routinely by Derouin and colleagues, with a high degree of success [549]. They use coverslip cultures of human embryonic fibroblasts (MRC5, bioMérieux, Lyon, France) in wells of 24-well plates (Nunc, Denmark) [552]. The sediment of approximately 10 mL of amniotic fluid is resuspended in 8 mL of minimum essential medium (MEM) supplemented with 10% fetal calf serum, penicillin (5 IU/mL), and streptomycin (50 mg/mL). One milliliter of the suspension is inoculated into each of six cell culture wells

and incubated for 72 to 96 hours at 37° C. Thereafter, they are washed with phosphate-buffered saline and fixed with cold acetone. Indirect immunofluorescence is then performed on the coverslip cultures, using rabbit anti-T. gondii IgG as the first antibody and fluorescein-labeled rabbit anti-IgG as the second antibody. After the coverslips are mounted onto slides, they are examined for the presence of T. gondii by fluorescence microscopy. Parasite division is readily observed in the cells, as is pseudocyst formation; if cells are heavily infected, foci of extracellular parasites may be present. Some workers stain the coverslips with Wright-Giemsa stain or use the immunoperoxidase method to demonstrate T. gondii in the cultures. These methods, however, are less sensitive than immunofluorescence for detection of low numbers of parasitized cells.

Special Considerations

Placenta. If congenital toxoplasmosis is suspected in a newborn, either because acute toxoplasmosis was diagnosed during pregnancy in the mother or because clinical signs raise suspicion of this diagnosis in the neonate, approximately 100 g of placenta should be kept without fixative and stored at 4° C until it can be injected into mice. Digestion with trypsin is preferable. This procedure resulted in isolation of T. gondii in 25% of placentas obtained from 123 mothers who acquired toxoplasmosis during pregnancy, and in each of these positive cases it was associated with a congenitally infected neonate [540]. Conversely, cases in which infants were proved to be infected, despite the inability to isolate T. gondii from their placentas, are rare unless mothers have received treatment during pregnancy [69,555].

Fricker-Hidalgo and colleagues [556] describe an increase in ability to diagnose congenital T. gondii infection at birth by combining polymerase chain reaction, study of the placenta, subinoculation of placenta, and serology. The placenta examination by polymerase chain reaction and mouse inoculation increased the sensitivity of the diagnosis of congenital toxoplasmosis at birth from 60% (use of serologic techniques on the newborn's blood only) to 75% (both serologic techniques and placental analysis). The specificity of Toxoplasma gondii detection in the placenta was 94.7%. It has been demonstrated in earlier studies that subinoculation studies of the placenta are useful to diagnose infection, and that prenatal treatment reduces the ability to isolate the parasite from the placenta.

Blood. T. gondii may be isolated from cord or peripheral blood of the newborn [526]. Such isolation should be attempted whenever possible because serologic diagnosis may be uncertain during the first weeks or months of life. In a study of 69 infants with congenital toxoplasmosis, Desmonts and Couvreur isolated T. gondii from peripheral blood in 30 (43%) of them (see Table 31–1) [557]. The high incidence (52%) of parasitemia in infants with subclinical infection is noteworthy, as is the overall frequency of parasitemia in congenital cases.

Relatively few positive results were obtained in infants with only neurologic or ocular signs of the disease. This might be related to the fact that these infants usually are not examined during the first days of life, unlike those with generalized disease or those in whom the possibility of disease is suspected because of prospective studies in their mothers. Seventy-one percent of the positive results were obtained from samples of blood taken during the first week of life. The percentage decreased to 33% when blood for isolation purposes was obtained during the following 3 weeks, and there were no positive results in infants older than 1 month of age [557].

Saliva. Levi and coworkers have reported the isolation of *T. gondii* from saliva of 12 of 20 patients, mostly with the lymphadenopathic form of the disease [531]. This report is interesting but requires confirmation. Whether the parasite can be isolated (or demonstrated by PCR assay) from sputum or saliva in the newborn period remains to be determined, but the presence of the organism in the alveoli of the lung suggests that attempts at isolation from such material might prove successful.

Postmortem Specimens. *T. gondii* is most easily isolated post mortem from brain specimens from infected infants and from infected infants who die months or years after birth, although it also has been isolated from virtually every organ and tissue of infants with congenital toxoplasmosis. Here again, digestion with either pepsin or trypsin is preferred because it allows for sampling of sufficiently large amounts of tissue. If necessary, brain specimens passed several times through a syringe and a 20-gauge needle can be injected into mice directly without prior digestion. It is noteworthy that isolation of *T. gondii* from the placenta is common in cases in which fetal death has occurred in utero. Although the organisms are regularly isolated from infected fetuses after induced abortion, they usually cannot be isolated from infected macerated fetal tissue that has remained in utero for an extended period of time after the fetus has died.

Tests of Cell-Mediated Immunity

Toxoplasmin Skin Test. At present, the skin test is not used in diagnosis of congenital infection, and no systematic study has been performed to define its potential usefulness for this purpose. It is discussed here for the sake of completeness.

Infection with *T. gondii* results in the development of cell-mediated immunity against the parasite. This may be demonstrated with the toxoplasmin skin test [558], which elicits delayed hypersensitivity. The large-scale use of the skin test, especially in population surveys, has yielded excellent agreement between the results of this test for delayed hypersensitivity and the presence or absence of antibody [558–563]. False-positive skin test results are rare [564]. Delayed skin hypersensitivity to *T. gondii* antigens in cases of acquired infection appears not to develop until months or years after the initial infection [70,168,560,565,566]. For this reason, the skin test appears to be most useful in the diagnosis of chronic (latent) infection; when results are positive, the possibility that the patient had a very recently acquired infection seems remote.

Antigen-Specific Lymphocyte Responses. Lymphocyte proliferation to *T. gondii* antigens has been shown to be a specific indicator of prior *T. gondii* infection in adults [233,234,567,568]. This technique has been found useful in establishing the diagnosis of congenital *T. gondii* infection in some infants [480,569,570]. Whereas depressed lymphocyte responsiveness to antigens of the infecting organisms has been reported in infants with congenital cytomegalovirus infection [571,572], congenital rubella [573,574], and congenital syphilis [575], specific cell-mediated immunity appears to develop for most infants with congenital *T. gondii* infection by 1 year of age, although the magnitude of the response is often less than that of their mothers [480]. In one series [480], lymphocyte proliferation to *T. gondii* antigen was both a sensitive (84%) and a specific (100%) indicator of congenital *T. gondii* infection; the sensitivity was similar in asymptomatic (82%) and in symptomatic (88%) infants [480]. Wilson and coworkers concluded that as a diagnostic tool, this method compared favorably with isolation of *T. gondii* and was superior in sensitivity to the IgM IFA test. In the study by Wilson and coworkers, a majority of the patients were not symptomatic or had mild infection, and tests of lymphocyte transformation were performed only once; it is possible that even greater sensitivity would be achieved with repeated testing (as was done with the IgM IFA test). Such repeated testing was done in the cases reported by McLeod and colleagues [570] and Yano and associates [576]. The patients described by McLeod and colleagues [521] had more severe involvement, and a substantial proportion of them did not exhibit lymphocyte blastogenic responses to *T. gondii* antigens in the first month of life. Similar results were reported by Fatoohi and colleagues [265] and by Gublietta and coworkers [577],whereas Ciardelli and colleagues [268] found that greater than 90% of congenitally infected infants less than 90 days of age had detectable T-cell proliferation and IFN-γ production in response to *Toxoplasma* antigen. The basis for the differences between these studies is unknown.

Lymphocyte Activation Markers in the Presence of *Toxoplasma gondii* Antigen. A study of increased expression of the marker of T-cell activation, CD25, with addition of *T. gondii* antigen to cultures of lymphocytes from congenitally infected infants described lymphocyte recognition in 38 (100%) of 38 congenitally infected infants in the first year of life (see also under "Immunologic Unresponsiveness to *T. gondii* Antigens") [522]. Nine (10%) of 89 uninfected infants, also had values of 7% or greater when tested initially but not when retested later.

Polymerase Chain Reaction Assay

In 1990, Grover and colleagues described the usefulness of PCR assay for rapid prenatal diagnosis of congenital *T. gondii* infection [578]. In a prospective study of 43 documented cases of acute maternal *T. gondii* infection acquired during gestation, PCR assay correctly identified the presence of *T. gondii* in all five samples of amniotic fluid from four proven cases of congenital infection and in three of five positive cases from a nonprospective group. Detection of IgM antibodies in fetal blood and inoculation of amniotic fluid into tissue cultures identified the infection in two and four of the nine infants with PCR-positive samples, respectively. Mouse inoculation of blood and amniotic fluid detected seven and six of the nine infants with PCR-positive samples, respectively. No false-positive results were obtained with any of the methods. PCR techniques have subsequently been used successfully on samples of ascitic fluid, amniotic fluid, cerebrospinal fluid, blood, urine, and tissues, including the placenta and brain of infants with congenital toxoplasmosis [75,404,579–592] (see discussion of PCR assay in amniotic fluid and effects of treatment, under "Prenatal Infection") [206,455,592]. Possible reasons for false-negative results include [593] mishandling of the sample before it is received by the laboratory and use of a single-copy target gene that limits the sensitivity and thus is not able to detect the *T. gondii* DNA in the sample. Because PCR assay in amniotic fluid is performed at 18 weeks of gestation by most investigators, reliability of this test performed earlier than 18 weeks of gestation is unknown.

Reischl and colleagues used real-time fluorescence PCR assays to compare results obtained with the more conventional 35-fold repeated B1 gene of *T. gondii* with a newly described multicopy genomic fragment, a 529-base-pair (bp) repeat element, that is repeated more than 300 times in the genome of *T. gondii* [594]. These investigators provided convincing evidence that the 529-bp repeat element provides the advantage of greater sensitivity than that with use of the B1 gene: this 529-bp element is being adopted by a number of reference laboratories using real-time PCR methods. This method is 92% sensitive and 100% specific (Figure 31-19).

Real-time PCR testing combines amplification and detection steps and use of a fluorescence-labeled oligonucleotide probe, making completion of the assay possible in less than 4 hours [175,595,596]. Real-time PCR analysis is useful to quantitate parasite concentration in amniotic fluid (Figure 31-19) [87]. Larger concentrations of parasites in amniotic fluid before 20 weeks of gestation have the greatest risks of severe outcome in the fetus and newborn (Figs. 31–20 and 31–21; Tables 31–19 and 31–20) [87,206].

Perhaps the greatest advance in prenatal diagnosis of *T. gondii* infection in the fetus has been the use of PCR on amniotic fluid without having to resort to a percutaneous umbilical blood sample [77]. PCR testing probably will replace many of the methods described in this section for diagnosis of the infection in the newborn.

Demonstration of Antigen in Serum and Body Fluids

The ELISA has been used to demonstrate *T. gondii* antigenemia in humans and animals with the acute infection [597–603], and antigen has been demonstrated in cerebrospinal fluid and amniotic fluid of newborns with congenital toxoplasmosis [597]. *T. gondii* antigens also have been demonstrated in urine of a congenitally infected infant by the ELISA [604]. Dot immunobinding also has been used for this purpose [605].

Demonstration of Antibodies in Serum and Body Fluids

The ultimate usefulness of tests for the diagnosis of toxoplasmosis depends on quality control of commercial kits,

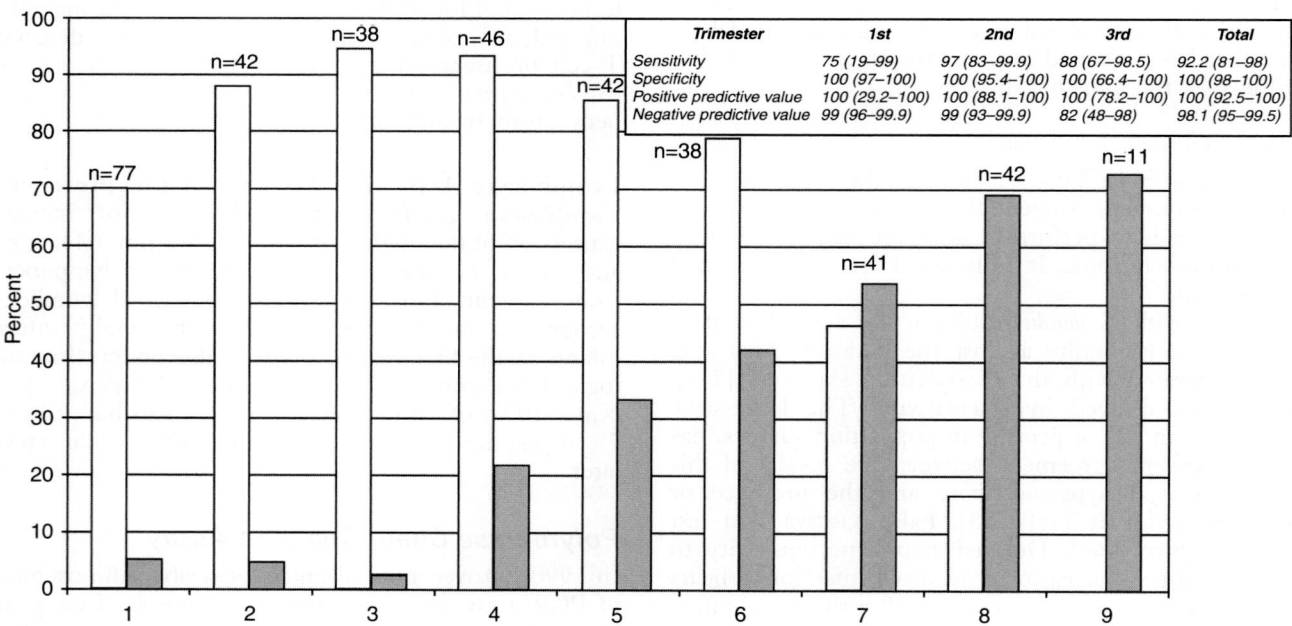

Trimester	1st	2nd	3rd	Total
Sensitivity	75 (19–99)	97 (83–99.9)	88 (67–98.5)	92.2 (81–98)
Specificity	100 (97–100)	100 (95.4–100)	100 (66.4–100)	100 (98–100)
Positive predictive value	100 (29.2–100)	100 (88.1–100)	100 (78.2–100)	100 (92.5–100)
Negative predictive value	99 (96–99.9)	99 (93–99.9)	82 (48–98)	98.1 (95–99.5)

FIGURE 31–19 Percentage of patients undergoing amniocentesis and cases of congenital *Toxoplasma* infection according to gestational age at maternal seroconverion. (Inset shows Sensitivity, Specificity, and Positive and Negative Predictive Value Estimates for Polymerase Chain Reaction Analysis). Inset data are percentage (95% confidence interval). Open histogram bar is Amniocentesis; Shaded histogram bar is Congenital toxoplasmosis. (*Adapted with permission from Wallon M, Franck J, Thulliez P, Huissoud C, Peyron F, Garcia-Meric P, Kieffer F. Accuracy of real-time polymerase chain reaction for Toxoplasma gondii in amniotic fluid. Obstet Gynecol 115(4):727–733, 2010.*)

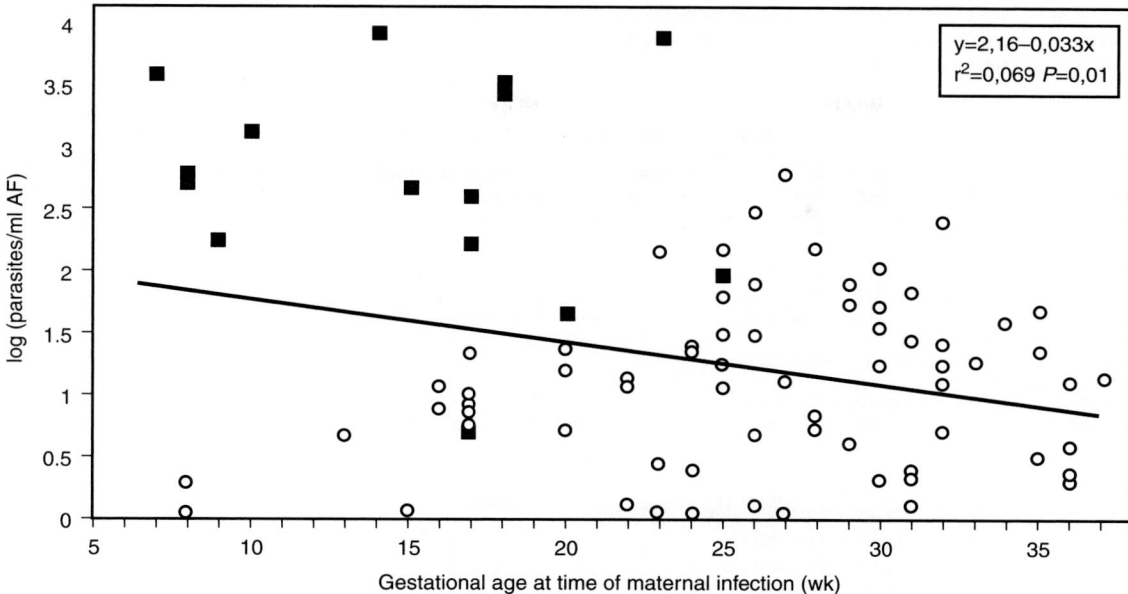

FIGURE 31–20 Correlation between *Toxoplasma* concentrations in amniotic fluid (AF) samples and gestational age at maternal infection for the 86 cases. Severity of the infection is represented in each case by ■ if severe signs of infection were recorded or by ○ if no or mild signs were observed. In general, the earlier the mother is infected, the higher the parasite numbers in amniotic fluid. Some babies who had relatively low numbers of parasites were severely infected, and many babies who had relatively high numbers of parasites were not severely infected. (*Data from Romand S, et al. Usefulness of quantitative polymerase chain reaction in amniotic fluid as early prognostic marker of fetal infection with* Toxoplasma gondii. *Am J Obstet Gynecol 190:797–802, 2004.*)

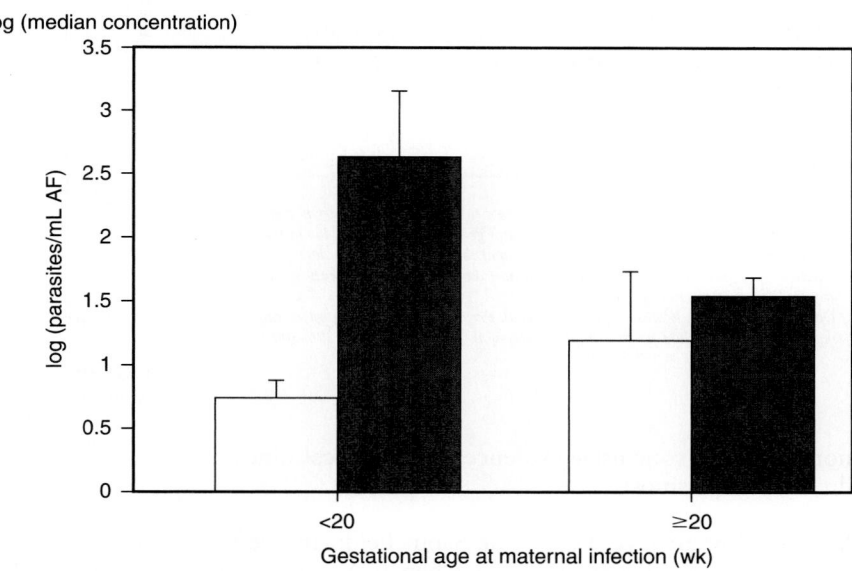

FIGURE 31–21 Comparison of median (interquartile range) parasite concentrations in AF between cases with subclinical infection (*unshaded bars*) and cases with infectious sequelae (*shaded bars*) for maternal infections acquired before or after 20 weeks of gestation. Clinical status was recorded either at birth or following fetal death (at fetopathologic examination). (*Data from Romand S, et al. Usefulness of quantitative polymerase chain reaction in amniotic fluid as early prognostic marker of fetal infection with* Toxoplasma gondii. *Am J Obstet Gynecol 190:797–802, 2004.*)

reliability of the laboratory performing the test, and accuracy and skill of persons interpreting results according to the specified clinical circumstance.

The most common serologic tests in use at present for diagnosis of *T. gondii* infection and toxoplasmosis are the Sabin-Feldman dye test [10], the indirect hemagglutination (IHA) test [127], the IFA test [606], the agglutination test [607], the ELISA [608–611], and the immunosorbent agglutination assay (ISAGA) [612–614]. Certain serologic methods are of little help in diagnosing congenital toxoplasmosis. This is especially true for some CF or IHA

tests [606]. Results with these tests may be weakly positive or even negative in a newborn with congenital toxoplasmosis, and in the infant's mother. The diagnosis of acute acquired toxoplasmosis may be established by the demonstration of rising serologic test titers [163]. A stable high titer, however, may have been reached by the time the patient is first seen by a physician. Because high titers (e.g., 300 to 1000 international units [IU]) may persist for many years after acute infection [96] (Figs. 31–22 and 31–23) and are present in the general population, a single high serologic test titer in any one method does

TABLE 31–19   Clinical Outcome of 88 Fetuses with Congenital Toxoplasmosis Diagnosed by PCR Assay in Amniotic Fluid According to Gestational Age at Maternal Infection

| Gestational Age (wk) When Mother Acquired Infection | No. of Newborns Affected at Birth | | | | | Number of Fetal Deaths | |
	Total	Subclinical Infection	Cerebral Calcifications	Retinochoroiditis Alone	Ventricular Dilation	Fetal Death	Medical Termination
<20	26	6	4	0	1	5‡	10§
≥20	62	52	6*	1	1	0	2
Total	88	58	10	1	2†	5	12

In association with retinochoroiditis in 1 case.
†*In association with cerebral calcifications and retinochoroiditis in 2 cases.*
‡*Four fetuses exhibited hydrops fetalis.*
§*Two fetuses revealed no sign of infection following fetopathologic examination.*
Data from Romand S, Chosson M, Frank J, et al. Usefulness of quantitative polymerase chain reaction in amniotic fluid as early prognostic marker of fetal infection with Toxoplasma gondii. Am J Obstet Gynecol 190:797-802, 2004.

TABLE 31–20   Maternal-Fetal Transmission Rates of *Toxoplasma gondii* Infection and Intervals Between Date of Maternal Infection and Amniocentesis According to Duration of Gestation at Maternal Infection

Duration of Gestation (wk) at Maternal Infection	Maternal-Fetal Transmission Rate	Intervals Between Date of Maternal Infection and Amniocentesis*
≤6	0/14 (0)	12.6 (11.3–14.6)
7–11	7/50 (14)	9.1 (7.2–11.1)
12–16	7/61 (11.5)	6.9 (5.3–8.7)
17–21	14/66 (21.2)	6.7 (5.3–7.6)
22–26	16/36 (44.4)	5.9 (5–7.4)
27–31	19/30 (63.3)	5.1 (4.4–6.1)
≥32	12/13 (92.3)	4.6 (2.5–5.3)

Mean (25th to 75th percentiles).
In considering the results of this study, it is important to note that the numbers of women with acute acquired infection differ substantially for each group. This is in part due to the time when women first seek prenatal care. Of note is that the intervals between date of maternal infection and amniocentesis also diminish with time during gestation at which infection was acquired, after 16 weeks of gestation.
Data from Romand S, Wallon M, Franck J, et al. Prenatal diagnosis using polymerase chain reaction on amniotic fluid for congenital toxoplasmosis. Obstet Gynecol 97:296–300, 2001.

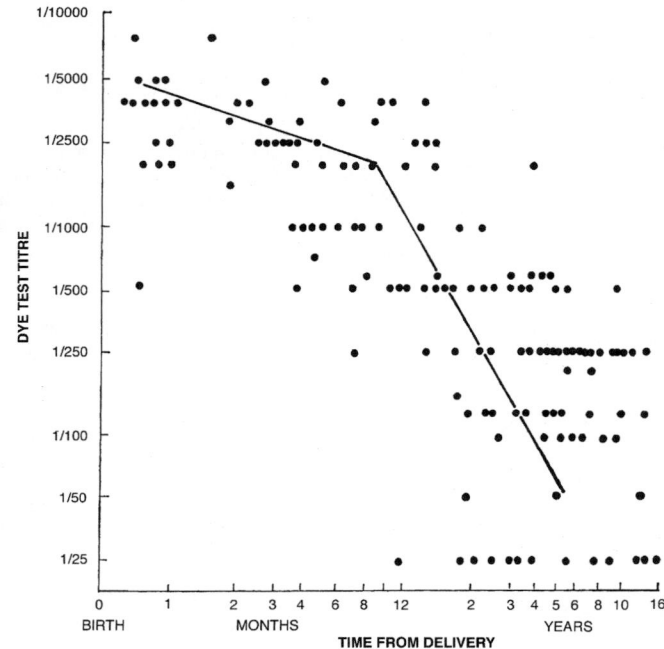

FIGURE 31–22   Dye test titers in 117 mothers of children with congenital toxoplasmosis in relation to time since delivery. *(Data from Couvreur J, Desmonts G. Congenital and maternal toxoplasmosis. A review of 300 congenital cases. Dev Med Child Neurol 4:519–530, 1962.)*

not constitute conclusive evidence that a clinical illness is due to toxoplasmosis.

Sabin-Feldman Dye Test. The Sabin-Feldman dye test is based on the observation that when living organisms (e.g., from the peritoneal exudate of mice) are incubated with normal serum, they become swollen and stain deeply blue when methylene blue is added to the suspension [10]. Parasites exposed to antibody-containing serum, under the same conditions, appear thin and distorted and are not stained when the dye is added. This is due to lysis of the organisms [615]. The membrane is disrupted because of activation of the complement system [616]. The titer reported is that dilution of serum at which half of the organisms are not killed (stained) and the other half are killed (unstained). (The stain is not required. Differentiation of lysed from nonlysed organisms may be readily accomplished under phase microscopy.) The World

Health Organization (WHO) has recommended that titers in most serologic tests be expressed in IU/mL of serum, compared with an international standard reference serum, which is available on request from the WHO [617].

Agglutination Test. The agglutination test [618,619] is available commercially in Europe and has been evaluated by a number of investigators [620–625]. The test employs whole parasites that have been preserved in formalin. The method is very sensitive to IgM antibodies. Nonspecific agglutination (apparently related to "naturally" occurring IgM *T. gondii* agglutinins) has been observed in persons devoid of antibody in the dye test and conventional IFA test [626]. These natural IgM antibodies do not cross the placenta but are detected at low titers as early as the second

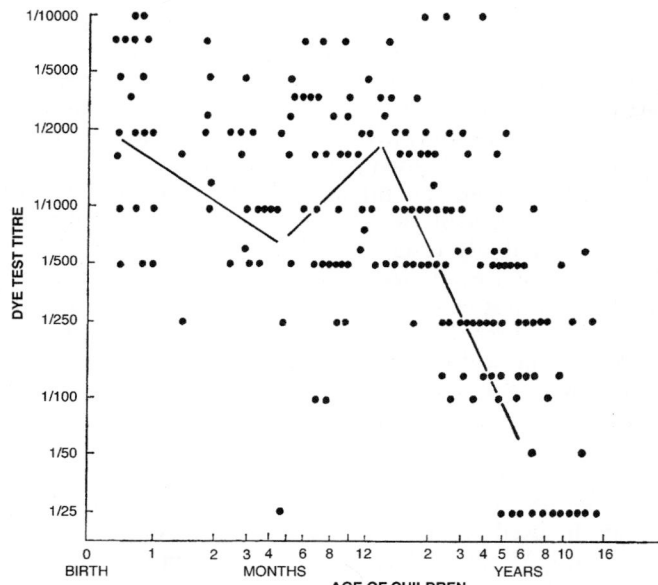

FIGURE 31–23 Dye test titers in 119 children with congenital toxoplasmosis in relation to age. (*Data from Couvreur J, Desmonts G. Congenital and maternal toxoplasmosis. A review of 300 congenital cases. Dev Med Child Neurol 4:519–530, 1962.*)

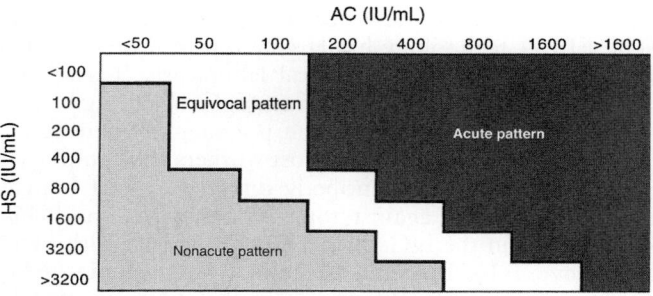

FIGURE 31–24 Interpretation of HS/AC test results. This differential agglutination test was performed as described in the text. (*Data from Dannemann BR, et al. Differential agglutination test for diagnosis of recently acquired infection with* Toxoplasma gondii. *J Clin Microbiol 28:1928–1933, 1990.*)

month of life. They do not develop in infants with maternal IgG antibody to *T. gondii*, however, so long as IgG antibody is present. False-positive results due to these natural antibodies may be avoided [627]. When they are, this test is excellent for wide-scale screening of pregnant women because it is accurate, simple to perform, and inexpensive [627,628]. A method that employs latex-tagged particles also may become available commercially [629–631].

Differential Agglutination Test. A chemical alteration of the outer membrane of the parasite led to the development of a unique differential agglutination method (HS/ AC test) that is very useful for helping to differentiate between acute and chronic infections in the pregnant patient [613,619,632,633]. The differential agglutination test compares titers obtained with formalin-fixed tachyzoites (HS antigen) with those obtained with acetone- or methanol-fixed tachyzoites (AC antigen) [613,619]. The AC antigen preparation contains stage-specific antigens that are recognized by IgG antibodies early during infection; these antibodies have different specificities from those found later in the infection [634]. Guidelines for interpretation of results for this test are shown in Figure 31–24. In the appropriate clinical setting, this method is useful for diagnosis of the acute infection using a single serum sample from the patient [613]. In practice, to assist with a clinical decision, it is important to take into consideration the results of other serologic tests along with those found in the HS/AC test. It is our practice to use the HS/AC test only in adults, and only in those who have IgG and IgM antibodies to *T. gondii* and in whom there is a question about whether the infection was recently acquired.

In the study by Dannemann and coworkers in which a single serum specimen was tested in each patient, the HS/AC test correctly identified all of the pregnant and almost all (31 of 33) of the nonpregnant patients with recently acquired toxoplasmic lymphadenopathy or asymptomatic infections [613]. Each of the seven women in their study who seroconverted during gestation had an acute pattern in the HS/AC test within 0 to 8 weeks after seroconversion in the dye test. Thirteen percent of 15 women who had been infected for at least 2 years had an acute pattern, but the wide range in duration of time from original infection (2 to 14 years) did not allow for an estimate of when the pattern in the HS/AC test changed from an acute to a nonacute pattern.

Conventional Indirect Fluorescent Antibody Test. In the conventional IFA test, slide preparations of killed *T. gondii* are incubated with serial dilutions of the patient's serum. If a specific reaction between the antigenic sites on the organisms and the patient's antibody occurs, it can be detected by a fluorescein-tagged antiserum prepared against serum immune globulins. A positive reaction is detected by the bright yellow-green fluorescence of the organisms seen on examination by fluorescence microscopy. In general, qualitative agreement with the dye test and IFA test has been excellent [606]. Despite the claims of many workers, reliable and reproducible quantitative titers frequently are difficult to obtain. To permit valid comparisons of results from different laboratories that express their titers as the last positive serum dilution, it should be noted that, depending on the laboratory, the dye test may vary in sensitivity, ranging between 0.1 and 0.5 IU/mL for the 50% endpoint. Thus a positive result for this test on a serum with a titer of 1000 IU/mL could be reported as 1:2000 or 1:10,000 in the dye test. The range is even greater with the IFA test.

Although most workers consider the IFA test to equal the dye test in specificity, false-positive results occur with some sera that contain antinuclear antibodies [635]. For this reason, in patients with connective tissue disorders (e.g., systemic lupus erythematosus), a dye test or ELISA can be performed to document a positive result on IFA testing.

To avoid misinterpretation of the polar staining of organisms that is due to naturally occurring IgM antibodies [636,637], the fluorescein-tagged conjugate should be only anti-IgG [638].

Conventional Enzyme-Linked Immunosorbent Assay.
The ELISA technology has largely replaced other methodologies in the routine clinical laboratory. It has been used successfully to demonstrate IgG, IgM, IgA, and IgE [639,640] antibodies in the pregnant woman, fetus, and newborn [610,641,642]. Most workers have employed an enzyme-conjugated antibody directed against human IgG [643–645] or against total immunoglobulins [646–650]. Titers in the IgG ELISA correlated well with titers in the dye, IHA, IFA, and CF tests in some studies [649] but not in others [650,651]. Commercial kits are widely available for detection of IgG or IgM antibodies. Their reliability for detection of IgM antibodies varies considerably, however, and false-positive results have been a serious problem [652,653].

Capture Enzyme-Linked Immunosorbent Assay. The capture ELISA is routinely employed by many laboratories for demonstration of IgM [158,608,624] and IgA [641,642,651] T. gondii antibodies in the fetus, newborn, and pregnant patient. In appropriately standardized methods (commercial kits), the IgA ELISA appears to be more sensitive than the IgM ELISA or IgM ISAGA for diagnosis of the infection in the fetus and newborn. IgA antibodies may persist for 8 months or longer in congenitally infected infants [610,642,608,640]. Demonstration of IgA T. gondii antibodies in an adult with early acute acquired infection is comparable to demonstration of IgM antibody, although IgA antibody may appear somewhat later than IgM antibody. In the adult, IgA T. gondii antibodies usually disappear earlier than do IgM antibodies, but as with the latter, IgA antibody titers may remain positive for a year or longer. Very high titers in either ELISA appear to correlate with more recent onset of the infection. Many cases in adults have been observed in which the IgM ELISA and HS/AC (see earlier) test results were positive and the IgA ELISA result was negative. We and others have not found the IgA test to be useful for diagnosis in most cases of acute infection in pregnant women [654].

IgG/IgM Western Blot Analysis for Mother-Infant Pairs. In the infected fetus, IgG and/or IgM serum antibodies produced against antigenic determinants of T. gondii may differ from those recognized by the IgG and/or IgM serum antibodies of the mother [283,655,656]. The fact that Western blot analysis can be used to demonstrate these differences in mother-baby pairs has led to the development of commercial kits for this purpose. The potential of this method for diagnosis of infection in the fetus and newborn is highlighted by the observations of Tissot-Dupont and colleagues, who prospectively studied IgG, IgM, and IgA Western blots in sera of 126 infants born to mothers who had acquired T. gondii infection during gestation [657]. Conventional serologic tests were performed during the first year of life, and Western blot analyses were performed on day 0 and/or day 5 and at 1 and 3 months of age. Serologic follow-up evaluation revealed that 23 of the infants had the congenital infection and that the remaining 103 infants were not infected. Although the Western blot method proved more sensitive than the IgM ISAGA (86.9% versus 69.6%,

respectively) (specificity of both methods was greater than 90%), the sensitivity increased to 91.3% when both tests were performed in combination. IgA blots were least sensitive. Similar results were reported by Pinon and associates in a collaborative study involving laboratories in the European Community Biomed 2 program [656].

Cases of congenital infection have been observed in the first months of life in infants in whom results of the IgM antibody tests were negative and the Western blot analysis result was positive. The Western blot method on mother-baby pairs may yield negative results during the first days of life in the infected newborn, however, and a demonstrable positive result in infected babies may not appear for weeks or even 2 or more months after birth [283]. Prenatal treatment during gestation and/or treatment of the infant may result in false-negative results on Western blot analysis. It is important that the Western blot method for mother-baby pairs always be used in combination with other serologic tests for IgG, IgM, and IgA antibodies. Western blot analysis for diagnosis of the congenital infection probably is most useful in those newborns in whom IgA and/or IgM T. gondii antibodies are not demonstrable in conventional serologic tests but whose mothers had a definite or highly likely diagnosis of acquired infection during gestation. It should be emphasized that no serologic test, performed singly or in combination, or the Western blot method allows for the diagnosis of the congenital infection in all cases. An example of IgG and IgM Western blots from a mother-baby pair is shown in Figure 31–25 [283]. Additional recent studies have suggested that comparisons of patterns of antibody response from mothers and their infants in Western blots are useful in establishing the diagnosis of congenital toxoplasmosis [658–660].

IgG Avidity Assay. The avidity assay should be used in conjunction with other serologic tests (i.e., T. gondii-specific IgG, IgM, IgA, IgE, and AC/HS) [88,89,283]. The method is most useful (and should be performed) in women in the first 16 weeks of gestation in whom IgM antibodies are found. It also is useful late in gestation to determine whether infection was acquired 4 or more months earlier, thereby allowing for an estimate of the rate of fetal infection at a given time during gestation. Testing for the avidity of antibodies against T. gondii stems from the knowledge that after primary antigenic stimulation, antibody-binding avidity (affinity) for an antigen is initially low but increases thereafter. IgG antibodies that are present owing to prior antigenic stimulus most often are of high avidity; this pertains to the secondary antibody response as well. (For a review, the reader is referred to the article by Hedman and colleagues) [661]. The most widely used method is one that employs the hydrogen bond-disrupting agent urea, which preferentially dissociates complexes formed by low-affinity antibodies. An avidity "index" may be determined as the percentage of antibodies that resist elution by 6M urea (e.g., in an ELISA plate). The method has been used by numerous investigators in an attempt to differentiate between recently acquired infection and infection acquired in the more distant past [662–666].Commercial

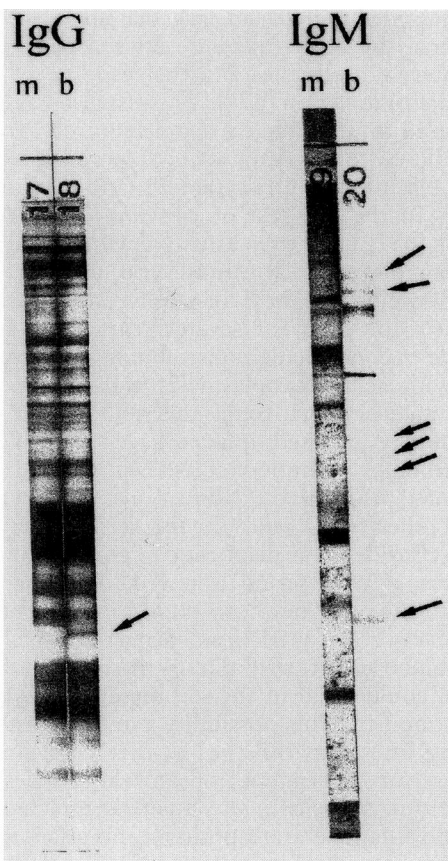

FIGURE 31–25 IgG and IgM Western blots of serum from a mother (m) and her newborn infant (b). Sera were drawn from mother and baby when the baby was 2 days of age. Arrows point to bands in the blot of the serum of the baby that were not present in the corresponding blot of the serum from the mother. Serologic test results in the mother were as follows (results in the baby are in parentheses): dye test, 600 IU (300 IU); IgM ELISA, 2.9 (IgM ISAGA, 3), both positive; IgA ELISA, 1.8 (1.3), both positive; IgE ELISA, negative (positive); PCR assay in placental tissue, negative. *Toxoplasma* was isolated from the placental tissue. *ELISA*, enzyme-linked immunosorbent assay; *IgA, IgG, IgM*, immunoglobulins A, G, M; *ISAGA*, immunosorbent agglutination assay; *PCR*, polymerase chain reaction. *(Adapted from Remington JS, Thulliez P, Montoya JG. Recent developments for diagnosis of toxoplasmosis. J Clin Microbiol 42:941–945, 2004.)*

kits are available in Europe and approval is currently under consideration in the U.S. [667].

At present, despite the many publications using the ELISA format, consensus on a standard procedure is lacking. Thus each investigator has had to define what constitutes a low-or high-avidity or equivocal result. What is generally agreed on is that a low avidity cannot be interpreted to mean that the patient has had a recently acquired infection because low-avidity antibodies may persist for more than 5 months, depending on the method used. A high-avidity result in the first trimester (or up to 16 weeks of gestation depending on the kit used), however, virtually rules out a recently acquired infection. Unfortunately, for all methods thus far reported, the equivocal range is broad, and a result in this range requires additional testing in a reference laboratory.

For diagnosis in the pregnant woman, the avidity method is most useful when used in the first 12 to 16 weeks of gestation because a high-avidity result late in gestation does not rule out an infection acquired in the first trimester or earlier. With the method used in their laboratory, Lappalainen and colleagues [668] reported that the predictive value of a high-avidity test result for excluding infection in the prior 5 months was 100%. In the Palo Alto laboratory, a high-avidity result obtained by an ELISA method during the first 16 weeks of gestation essentially excludes an infection acquired within the prior 4 months. Jenum and associates [669] concluded from their results with the avidity method that acquisition of *T. gondii* infection in early pregnancy can be excluded on the basis of results with a single serum sample collected in the first trimester. By confirming latent infection on the basis of a high-IgG avidity result early during gestation, the need to collect a second serum sample is eliminated. Antibiotic treatment has been suggested to affect the kinetics of IgG avidity maturation [670] and thereby prolong the duration of detectable low-avidity antibodies. It has been recently demonstrated, however, that treatment with spiramycin had no influence on the increase of the avidity index in pregnant women [671]. The avidity test is an excellent adjunctive method for ruling out infection acquired during the first 12 to 16 weeks of gestation [668,672–674].

The avidity assay is especially useful when only a single sample of serum has been obtained in which IgM *T. gondii* antibodies are present, and when the AC/HS test gives an acute or equivocal pattern. A recent study compared results obtained in an IgG avidity test with those obtained in the IgM ELISA and AC/HS test for sera that had equivocal or positive IgM ELISA or AC/HS test results [89]. A substantial proportion (e.g., 42 of 81 serum samples [52%] with high titers of *T. gondii* IgG antibodies) had high-avidity test results. Comparison of IgG avidity and differential agglutination test results also showed that 31 of 53 sera (59%) with equivocal and 4 of 33 sera (12%) with acute AC/HS test results had high avidity (i.e., were from women infected 4 or more months earlier). In 69 of 93 samples (74%) with positive or equivocal IgM ELISA results, 52 (56%) had high-avidity antibodies [88,89]. Of 87 (70%) samples with acute or equivocal AC/HS test results, 35 (40%) had high-avidity antibodies. Of 40 women given spiramycin in the first trimester in an attempt to prevent congenital transmission, 7 (8%) had high-avidity antibodies and thus did not require treatment. These women would not have required treatment with spiramycin if the avidity test result were known at the time.

Performance of the avidity test in the first 12 to 16 weeks of gestation has the potential to markedly decrease the need for obtaining follow-up sera and thereby reduce costs, to make unnecessary the need for PCR on amniotic fluid and for treatment of the mother with spiramycin, to remove the anxiety experienced by pregnant patients who are told that further testing is needed, and to decrease unnecessary abortions. Table 31–21 [283] shows results in the literature with avidity tests. In addition, it is important to note that confirmatory serologic testing in a reference laboratory with communication of results and correct interpretation of these results to the patient's physician by an expert decreased rates of unnecessary

TABLE 31–21   Usefulness of High-Avidity Test Results in IgM-Positive First-Trimester Pregnant Women

Patient No.*	Gestational Age (wk)	Dye Test (IgG)	IgM	Avidity
73	9	256	Positive	High
58	12	512	Positive	High
17	12	256	Positive	High
74	12	1024	Positive	High

*The high-avidity test result in each of these pregnant women reveals that they were infected before gestation. Without the avidity test results, the positive IgM antibody tests might have been interpreted as showing that the patients had acquired the infection during gestation. IgM, immunoglobulin M.

Adapted from Remington JS, Thulliez P, Montoya G. Recent developments for diagnosis of toxoplasmosis. J Clin Microbiol 42:941–945, 2004.

abortions by about 50% among women with positive IgM *Toxoplasma* antibody test results reported by outside laboratories [675].

Demonstration of Specific Immunoglobulin M Antibodies

A positive serum IgM test alone cannot be used to establish the diagnosis of any form of toxoplasmosis in the older child and adult. A positive result on IgM serologic testing in the fetus and in the newborn in the first days of life usually is diagnostic of the infection if contamination of fetal or newborn blood with maternal blood has not occurred. The validity of a positive IgM test result in this setting may be checked by repeating the test 3 to 4 days later. Because the half-life of IgM is short, the repeat testing will reveal either a highly significant drop in titer or, more commonly, a negative result that reveals the original positive titer to have been a "false positive." Also, isolated false-positive *T. gondii*-specific IgM test results have been noted with other fetal infections (Remington JS and McLeod R, unpublished data).

IgM Fluorescent Antibody Test. The IFA test has been adapted for the demonstration of IgM antibodies to *T. gondii*, and the method has been successfully used to establish acute congenital and acquired infections [328,618,676–682]. The use of IgM antibody for diagnosis of congenital infection stems from the discovery in 1963 by Eichenwald and Shinefield [683] that the fetus is able to produce IgM-specific antibody. Critical to this method is the choice of an antiserum that is specific for IgM [538,684]. Serious and misleading errors related to the use of antisera that have specificity not only for IgM but also for IgG have been reported in the literature.

Failure to demonstrate IgM antibodies in the IgM IFA test in sera from some patients with the acute acquired infection has been shown to be due to an inhibitory effect of high titers of IgG antibodies to *T. gondii* in these sera [685,686]. This problem may be avoided by removal of the IgG before performance of the IgM IFA test. Commercial kits are available for this purpose.

The presence of IgM antibodies in cord serum or in serum obtained from the neonate is evidence of specific antibody synthesis by the infected fetus *in utero*. Maternal IgM antibodies do not normally pass the placental barrier, as do maternal IgG antibodies. The IgM IFA test was the

first test designed to make an early diagnosis of congenital toxoplasmosis by distinguishing between passively transferred maternal antibodies and the response of the fetus and neonate to infection [677]. The test also has been successfully used to detect active acute acquired toxoplasmosis [163,539,687–689]. After acute acquired infection, the IgM IFA test titer may rise rapidly (and at times earlier than titers in the dye test or conventional IFA test) to high levels [687]. The titer usually declines, and the antibodies may disappear within several months; in some patients, however, the IgM IFA test result has remained positive at a low titer for several years. IgM antibodies to *T. gondii* may not be demonstrable in immunodeficient patients with acute toxoplasmosis and in patients with isolated active ocular toxoplasmosis. Only 25% to 50% of congenitally infected infants have *T. gondii*-specific IgM antibodies demonstrable by IgM IFA tests [480,608,684]. With two qualifications, demonstration of IgM antibodies to *T. gondii* in the serum of a newborn should be considered as diagnostic of congenital toxoplasmosis. First, if cord serum is tested, or if the serum is obtained in the early newborn period in an infant during whose delivery a placental "leak" occurred, which enabled maternal blood to mix with that of the infant, a false-positive result could occur in any serologic test for IgM, IgA, or IgE antibodies. This possibility can be investigated by performing the test on the mother's serum. If the mother's serum is negative for IgM antibodies and the infant's serum is positive, the infant is infected. If both mother and infant sera are positive, the infant should be tested again several days later; a marked fall in the IgM IFA test titer will have occurred if the IgM was maternally acquired because the half-life of IgM is only approximately 5 days [690,691]. If the IgM IFA test titer in the infant remains high or is rising, it is diagnostic of infection.

The second qualification is the presence of rheumatoid factor. False-positive IgM IFA test results may occur in sera that contain rheumatoid factor [692]. Rheumatoid factor may be present not only in adults but in infected newborns as well [329,693], purportedly as a result of an IgM immune response of the fetus in utero to passively transferred maternal IgG. After treatment of sera containing rheumatoid factor with heat-aggregated IgG, false-positive IgM IFA test titers become negative. By contrast, titers in cases of acute congenital or acquired toxoplasmosis are unaffected by this treatment. Thus treatment with heat-aggregated IgG or other commercially available adsorbent can be used to differentiate false-positive IgM IFA test titers related to rheumatoid factor from those related to specific IgM antibody to *T. gondii*. The incidence of rheumatoid factor in sera of infants with congenital toxoplasmosis is unknown. All infants who respond positively in the IgM IFA test should be tested for rheumatoid factor as well.

IgM Enzyme-Linked Immunosorbent Assay. The double-sandwich IgM ELISA for detection of IgM antibodies to *T. gondii* was developed by Naot and Remington and colleagues [158,608,609]. At present it is the most widely used method for demonstration of IgM antibodies to *T. gondii* in adults, the fetus, and newborns. In contrast with the conventional method in which the wells of microtiter plates are coated with antigen, the wells are coated with specific antibody to IgM. The IgM ELISA is more sensitive than the IgM IFA test for diagnosis of the recently acquired infection, and serum samples that test negative in the dye test but that contain either antinuclear antibodies or rheumatoid factor and thus cause false-positive results in the IgM IFA test also test negative in the double-sandwich IgM ELISA. This latter observation is attributed to the fact that serum IgM fractions are separated from IgG fractions during the initial step in the IgM ELISA procedure.

The double-sandwich IgM ELISA also is useful for diagnosis of congenital *T. gondii* infection [608]. Results of the double-sandwich IgM ELISA were positive in 43 of 55 serum samples (72.7%) from newborns with proven congenital *T. gondii* infection, whereas IgM IFA test results were positive in only 14 (25.4%) of these samples. Of the sera obtained from the infected newborns during the first 30 days of life, 81.2% were positive in the double-sandwich IgM ELISA, whereas only 25% were positive in the IgM IFA test. Use of the double-sandwich IgM ELISA avoids false-positive results related to rheumatoid factor and false-negative results related to competition from high levels of maternal IgG antibody that occur with the IgM IFA test. A number of modifications of the method have been described [365,694–703]. The double-sandwich IgM ELISA is superior to the IgM IFA test for diagnosis both of acute acquired and congenital *T. gondii* infections.

Immunosorbent Agglutination Assay for Demonstration of IgM, IgA, and IgE Antibodies. The ISAGA [612,614,652,701–703] is widely used by investigators because it combines the advantages of both the direct agglutination test and the double-sandwich (capture) ELISA in its specificity and sensitivity for demonstration of IgM, IgA, and IgE [614] antibodies to *T. gondii*. The ISAGA does not require use of an enzyme conjugate; it is as simple to perform as the direct agglutination test and is read in the same manner as for that test. Use of the ISAGA avoids false-positive results related to the presence of rheumatoid factor and/or antinuclear antibodies in serum samples. A commercial kit for IgM antibodies is available (bioMérieux).

The ISAGA is more sensitive and more specific than the IgM IFA and the IgM ELISA [704,705], and has been used effectively for diagnosis of congenital infection [706]. Specific IgA antibodies in the ISAGA test indicated congenital toxoplasmosis in three infants in the absence of associated IgM antibodies [707]. Pinon and coworkers found IgA antibodies in serum and cerebrospinal fluid of seven cases of congenital toxoplasmosis in the neonatal period [705,708].

Because of its high sensitivity, the ISAGA detects IgM antibodies earlier after the acute acquired infection (e.g., 1 to 2 weeks) than do other tests for IgM antibody. This sensitivity also results in the longest duration of detection of IgM antibody after infection. The method has been standardized by the recognition of this greater sensitivity to provide greater diagnostic power during early infections

in adults [704]. Pinon and coworkers [614] and Wong and associates [639] have found the IgE ISAGA to be useful for diagnosis of acute acquired infection in the pregnant woman and in the congenitally infected newborn. Its advantage is related to the early rise in titers of IgE antibodies and IgM and IgA antibodies and the much earlier disappearance of IgE antibodies. In the study by Pinon and coworkers, IgE antibodies in the adult persisted for less than 4 months. This test has been available in only a few specialty laboratories. As is true for appropriate interpretation of all other serologic tests for diagnosis of the acute infection, it should be used only in combination with other serologic methods [633,703].

The Problem of False-Positive *Toxoplasma gondii*-Specific IgM Tests. *Toxoplasma* IgM test kits are not subject to standardization in the United States, and a substantial proportion of them do not function reliably [653]. Not only is the lack of reliability of such test kits a problem, but use of results in the IgM assays to guide care of the pregnant woman by obstetricians in the United States, and probably elsewhere as well, is not always well informed. For example, Jones and associates [709] reported that 364 of 768 (47%) American College of Obstetrics and Gynecology (ACOG) members responded to a survey regarding their knowledge of toxoplasmosis in pregnant women and related OB-GYN practices. In the previous year, 7% diagnosed one or more cases of acute toxoplasmosis, and only 12% indicated that a positive *Toxoplasma* IgM test might be a false-positive result. Only 11% recalled an advisory sent to all ACOG members in 1997 by the FDA alerting them that some *Toxoplasma* IgM test kits have false-positive results. Sixty-seven percent of respondents were against universal screening of pregnant women for *T. gondii* infection [709]. If obstetricians are carefully educated on the subject, medical care offered to pregnant women would be greatly improved. A positive IgM test alone can never be used to establish the diagnosis of any form of toxoplasmosis.

Median and Variability of Duration of Positive *Toxoplasma gondii* IgM Antibody Results Measured by Immunofluorescence Testing and ISAGA. Gras and coworkers [710] from London and Lyon studied a cohort of 446 *Toxoplasma*-infected pregnant women to determine the median and variability of the duration of positive *T. gondii* IgM antibody results measured by an immunofluorescence test (IFT) and an immunosorbent agglutination assay (ISAGA). IgM antibodies were detected for longer using the ISAGA (median, 12.8 months; interquartile range [IQR], 6.9 to 24.9) than the IFT (median, 10.4; IQR, 7.1 to 14.4), but the variability among persons in the duration of IgM positivity was greatest with ISAGA. IgM-positive results persisted beyond 2 years in 27.1% (ISAGA), and 9.1% (IFT) of women. These investigators concluded that variation in the duration of IgM response measured by ISAGA and IFT limits their usefulness for predicting the timing of infection in pregnant women. Nonetheless, they concluded that measurement of IgM and IgG antibodies in cross-sectional serosurveys offers a useful method for estimating the incidence of *T. gondii* infection.

GUIDELINES FOR EVALUATION OF THE NEWBORN WITH SUSPECTED CONGENITAL TOXOPLASMOSIS

Guidelines for evaluation of the newborn of a mother who acquired her infection during gestation to confirm or rule out the diagnosis of congenital *T. gondii* infection are shown in Table 31–22.

Serologic Diagnosis of Acquired *Toxoplasma* Infection in the Pregnant Woman

The presence of a positive titer (except for the rare false-positive results mentioned earlier) in any of the serologic tests discussed earlier establishes the diagnosis of *T. gondii* infection. Because titers in each of these tests may remain elevated for years, a single high titer does not indicate whether the infection is acute or chronic, nor does it necessarily mean that the clinical findings are due to toxoplasmosis. Before a diagnosis of acute *T. gondii* infection or toxoplasmosis can be made by means of serologic tests, it is necessary to demonstrate a rising titer in serial specimens (either conversion from a negative to a positive titer or a rise from a low to a significantly higher titer) [163,711]. Because in the United States the diagnosis is frequently considered relatively late in the course of the patient's infection (Table 31–23), serologic test titers

TABLE 31–23 Trimester During Which Sera Were Drawn from Consecutive Pregnant Women for *Toxoplasma gondii* Serologic Testing

Trimester	2002		2003–2004	
	No. of Patients	%	No. of Patients	%
First	112	36	111	37
Second	132	43	146	49
Third	63	21	43	14
Total	307		300	

(e.g., dye test, IFA test, or ELISA) may have already reached their peak at the time the first serum is obtained for testing. The IgM IFA test, IgM ELISA, IgM ISAGA, and tests for IgA and IgE antibodies and IgG avidity appear to be of considerable help in these circumstances.* The most important fact for the clinician is that any patient with a positive IgG titer and a positive IgM IFA or IgM ELISA titer must be presumed to have recently acquired infection with *T. gondii* and be tested further in a reference laboratory [652,712]. Most mothers of children with congenital toxoplasmosis are unable to recall being ill during pregnancy. Some (10% to 20%) notice enlarged lymph nodes, mostly in the posterior cervical area, a sign that suggests relatively recently acquired infection. These enlarged nodes sometimes are still present at delivery. Clinical signs of infection in the pregnant woman are not necessarily associated with an increased predilection for transmission, as shown by the reports of cases in which, although the parasite was present in a lymph node biopsy performed as part of the diagnostic evaluation of lymphadenopathy, the offspring were uninfected [338,713,714]. Examples of similar cases of lymphadenopathy (with demonstration of the parasite in the nodes) in which congenital transmission did occur have been published [62,416,715,716].

Because a majority (greater than 80%) of cases of acquired *T. gondii* infection are subclinical, the diagnosis relies mainly on the results of serologic tests. To interpret serologic test results in the pregnant woman, it is important to understand how antibodies of different immunoglobulin classes and different specificities for antigenic determinants develop after the infection is acquired and which antibodies are detected in the different serologic methods used for diagnosis of this infection. In addition, the physician should have knowledge of the relationship of the time of acquisition of the infection to the onset of parasitemia (which results in infection of the placenta) and also to the onset of clinical manifestations (when present). The answers to many of these questions are unknown or only partly understood. What follows in this section is information and guidelines for interpretation of test results, as adopted from our personal experiences and supplemented by pertinent data from the literature. We have attempted whenever possible to distinguish between hypothesis and established fact.

TABLE 31–22 Guidelines for Evaluation of Newborn of Mother Who Acquired Her Infection During Gestation to Determine Whether Infant Has Congenital *Toxoplasma* Infection and to Assess Degree of Involvement

History and physical examination

Pediatric neurologic evaluation

Pediatric ophthalmologic examination

Complete blood cell count with differential, platelet count

Liver function tests (direct bilirubin, GGTP)

Urinalysis, serum creatinine

Serum quantitative immunoglobulins

Serum Sabin-Feldman dye test (IgG), IgM ISAGA, IgA ELISA, IgE ISAGA/ELISA* (with maternal serum, perform same tests as for infant except substitute IgM ELISA for the IgM ISAGA and also obtain AC/HS*)

Cerebrospinal fluid cell count, protein, glucose, and *T. gondii*–specific IgG and IgM antibodies and quantitative IgG to calculate antibody load

Subinoculate into mice or tissue culture 1 mL peripheral blood buffy coat or clot and digest of 100 g placenta (see "Diagnosis" section for method of digestion). Consider PCR of buffy coat from approximately 1 mL blood, cell pellet from approximately 1 mL cerebrospinal fluid, and cell pellet from 10 to 20 mL amniotic fluid (see "Diagnosis" section)

Brain computed tomography scan without contrast medium enhancement

Auditory brainstem response to 20 dB

When performed in combination in our laboratories, these tests have demonstrated a high degree of specificity and sensitivity in establishing the diagnosis of acute infection in the pregnant woman and congenital infection in the fetus and newborn.
ELISA, enzyme-linked immunosorbent assay; GGTP, γ-glutamyltranspeptidase; ISAGA, immunosorbent agglutination assay; IgA, IgE, IgG, IgM, immunoglobulins A, E, G, M; PCR, polymerase chain reaction.

---

*References 163, 538, 609, 612, 652, 689, 703.

TABLE 31–24 General Considerations Regarding IgM, IgG, IgA, and IgE Antibody Responses to Postnatally Acquired Infection with *Toxoplasma*

Antibodies	Uninfected Person	Recent (Acute) Infection	Chronic (Latent) Infection
IgM			
Directed toward antigens that cross-react	Present	Present	Present
Directed toward specific *Toxoplasma* antigens	Absent	Present in almost all cases. Period that IgM antibodies are present may vary from a few weeks to many months. Ability to detect these antibodies depends on serologic technique used.	Most often absent, but IgM antibodies may persist for years in some patients (about 5%). In such cases, titers are almost always low, but in some cases they remain high. Persistence of IgM antibodies is generally associated with low or medium titers of IgG antibodies.
IgG			
Directed toward antigens that cross-react	Absent	Absent (?)	Absent (?)
Directed toward specific *Toxoplasma* antigens	Absent (<2 IU/mL)*	Present. Rise from a low titer (2 IU/mL) to a high titer (300–6000 IU/mL). In a few patients, titers remain low (100–200 IU/mL). Duration of rise varies with patient and with serologic test used. Depending on serologic techniques, it may take from 2 to 6 mo for the IgG antibody titer to reach its peak.	Present. Stable or slowly decreasing titers (to a titer of 2–200 IU/mL). High titers (>300 IU/mL) persist for years in some patients (about 5%). A significant rise in titer is sometimes observed after a normal decrease in titer has occurred.
IgG avidity	Absent	Low	A high avidity test result reveals that the infection was acquired at least 12–16 weeks earlier. However, a low avidity test result may persist for more than 1 year.
IgA			
Directed toward antigens that cross-react	Absent	Absent (?)	Absent (?)
Directed toward specific *Toxoplasma* antigens	Absent	Present in almost all cases. Period that IgA antibodies are present may vary from several months to 1 year or more. They most commonly disappear by 7 months.	Most often absent
IgE			
Directed toward antigens that cross-react	Absent	Absent (?)	Absent (?)
Directed toward specific *Toxoplasma* antigens	Absent	Present	Absent

*Titers are expressed in international units (IU) to minimize technical differences that might occur among different laboratories.
IgA, IgE, IgG, IgM, *immunoglobulins A, E, G, M*; IU, *international units.*

The antigenic structure of *T. gondii* is complex; both cytoplasmic antigens, which are liberated when the organisms are lysed, and membrane antigens are involved in the immune response [717–723]. We know that certain antigens cross-react because normal human sera contain IgM antibodies that bind to these antigens [724–726]. It seems reasonable to suggest that antibodies formed in response to these different antigens differ both in their specificity and in their class and subclass of immunoglobulins [604]. These variations account for the fact that different antibodies may or may not be detected, depending on the serologic method employed.

In Table 31–24, we have attempted to describe the evolution of the IgM, IgG, IgA, and IgE antibody responses as they relate to interpretation of serologic test results in the diagnosis of *T. gondii* infection in the pregnant woman [610]. An example of the usefulness of these tests is shown in Table 31–25. The usefulness of the IgG avidity method is shown in Table 31–26 and discussed in an earlier

section. Agreement between the avidity test and the HS/AC test is 97% in the Palo Alto laboratory, as discussed previously.

Antibody Response in Relation to the Serologic Method Used

The methods for demonstration of specific IgM antibodies have been discussed earlier. They are valuable so long as it is possible to ascertain that a positive result is not due to the presence of "natural" IgM antibodies [727], rheumatoid factor, or antinuclear antibodies. For this reason, methods that rely on differences in titers after sera have been treated with 2-mercaptoethanol (e.g., the IHA and agglutination tests) are not satisfactory. Specific IgM antibodies may not be detectable within a few weeks after their first demonstration or may persist for years. In studies of women who seroconverted during gestation, IgA antibodies as measured by ELISA appeared at

TABLE 31-25 Serologic Test Results in Women Who Seroconverted During Pregnancy

Patient No.	Date	Dye Test: IgG (IU/mL)	IgM ELISA*	IgM ISAGA*	IgA ELISA*	AC/HS†	IgE ELISA‡	IgE ISAGA*
1	12/29/89	<2	0.4	0	0.6	NA	−	0
	02/23/90	200	5.0	12	1.8	A	+	6
	03/30/90	400	2.1	12	1.0	A	+	3
	04/30/90	800	1.3	12	0.8	A	+	3
	05/28/90	800	0.6	8	1.0	A	−	3
	06/26/90	800	1.1	6	1.0	A	+	3
2	02/17/89	<2	0.7	0	0.2	NA	−	0
	04/20/89	<2	0.2	0	0.0	NA	−	0
	05/18/89	160	6.4	12	2.8	NA	+	4
	08/23/89	200	2.7	12	0.8	A	±	0
3	03/09/82	Negative	0.0	QNS	QNS	QNS	−	6
	03/24/82	16	8.3	12	2.6	NA	+	9
	08/10/82	1000	4.9	12	2.6	A	+	6
	09/13/82	500	4.8	12	2.5	A	+	6
	12/07/82	200	4.1	12	1.0	A	+	3
	08/24/83	64	2.2	11	0.6	(A)	±	0

Positive results (in an adult): IgM ELISA = ≥1.7; IgM ISAGA = >3; IgA ELISA = 1.4; IgE ISAGA = 4 (3 is considered borderline).
†*AC/HS results: A, acute; NA, not acute; (A), borderline acute.*
‡*IgE ELISA: − negative; + positive; ±, equivocal (see 901).*
ELISA, *enzyme-linked immunosorbent assay;* IgA, IgE, IgG, IgM, *immunoglobulin A, E, G, M;* ISAGA, *immunosorbent agglutination assay;* IU, *international units;* QNS, *quantity not sufficient.*
Adapted from Wong SY, et al. Role of specific immunoglobulin E in diagnosis of acute Toxoplasma *infection and toxoplasmosis. J Clin Microb 31:2952–2959, 1993, with permission.*

TABLE 31-26 Usefulness of a High-Avidity Test Result in Women with a Positive IgM Test Titer in First 12 Weeks of Gestation

Patient No.	Duration of Gestation (wk)	Dye Test Titer (IU/mL)	IgM ELISA*	Percent Avidity†	Avidity Interpretation
1	10	51	4.7	44.4	High
2	9	51	2.3	41.6	High
3	11	102	2.6	31.2	High
4	8	102	5.8	33.8	High
5	12	410	2.9	47.3	High

Negative 0.0–1.6, equivocal 1.7–1.9, positive ≥2.0.
†*Low <15, borderline 15–30, high >30.*
IU, *international units.*

approximately the same time as for IgM antibodies [642]. Similar results have been observed with the IgE ISAGA [614,728]. Antibody titers in the IgE ISAGA decrease more rapidly than do IgA antibodies. In the study by Pinon and coworkers [614], they persisted for less than 4 months in 23 patients tested serially. In the study by Wong and associates, the IgE ISAGA results were similar to those reported by Pinon and coworkers, whereas IgE antibodies measured by ELISA persisted significantly longer in some seroconverters [639].

Titers in the dye test, the agglutination test, and the IHA test (when these latter two tests are performed with 2-mercaptoethanol) depend on the concentration of IgG antibodies; this is true also for the conventional IFA test when performed with a conjugate specific for IgG. Nevertheless, depending on which test is used, differences in the rise and fall of IgG antibody titers are noted; titers in the dye test rise more rapidly, whereas those measured in the agglutination and IHA tests in the presence of 2-mercaptoethanol rise slowly.

A summary of the IgG antibody responses to *T. gondii* infection, as measured by different serologic methods, is given in Table 31-27. For a discussion of the IgG avidity method, see earlier under "Demonstration of Antibodies in Serum and Body Fluids."

A special comment regarding the agglutination test is made here because of its commercial availability and increasing usefulness for screening and diagnosis of the acute infection in pregnant women. With the whole-cell agglutination test, agreement with the dye test was virtually 100%, except in some patients tested within a few days after they became infected, when only IgM antibodies were present [619]. With these serum samples, the dye test result was at times positive while the agglutination test result was still negative. By contrast, the agglutination test result may be positive at times when the dye test result is negative in chronically infected persons. This is due to the greater sensitivity of the agglutination test for detection of low titers of IgG antibodies. Because it takes more than 2 months (2 to 6 months) for IgG

TABLE 31–27 IgG Antibody Responses to *Toxoplasma* Infection as Measured by Different Serologic Methods*

Serologic Method	Uninfected Person	Recent (Acute) Infection	Chronic (Latent) Infection
Dye test	Negative (<1:4)	Rising from a negative or low titer (1:4) to a high titer (1:256 to 1:128,000).	Stable or slowly decreasing titer. Titers usually are low (1:4 to 1:256) but may remain high (≥1:1024) for years.
Agglutination test (after treatment of sera with 2-mercaptoethanol)	Negative (<1:4)	Rising slowly from a negative or low titer (1:4) to a high titer (1:512). If a high-sensitivity antigen is used, the titer may reach 1:128,000.	Stable or slowly decreasing titer. Titers usually are higher than in the dye test if a high-sensitivity antigen is used. Striking differences between dye test and agglutination test titers are observed in some patients.
IHA test (after treatment of sera with 2-mercaptoethanol)	Negative (<1:16)	Rising very slowly from a negative or low titer (1:16) to a high titer (1:1024). It may take 6 mo before a high titer is reached; in some patients, high titers are never observed	Stable or slowly decreasing titer. Titers usually are higher than in the dye test if a high-sensitivity antigen is used. Striking differences between dye test and agglutination test titers are observed in some patients.
Conventional IFA test (conjugated antiserum to IgG)	Negative (<1:20)	Rise in titer is parallel to rise in dye test titer, but decrease in titer might be slower than that in dye test.	Stable or slowly decreasing high or low titer.

Similar data for the IgG ELISA have not been published.
ELISA, *enzyme-linked immunosorbent assay;* IFA, *immunofluorescent antibody test;* IgG, *immunoglobulin G;* IHA, *indirect hemagglutination test.*

antibodies detected with the whole-cell agglutination test to reach a steady high titer, the existence of a steady high titer signifies that the infection was acquired more than 2 months earlier. As a consequence, if the first sample of serum has been obtained during the first 2 months of pregnancy, a stable agglutination test titer demonstrates that the infection occurred before the time of conception and that the risk of congenital infection in the infant is low [619].

It is exceedingly difficult to establish guidelines for interpretation of serologic methods that measure both IgM and IgG antibodies. For example, in examining paired sera that were stated to have high stable titers in the conventional IFA test (performed with a conjugate against total immunoglobulins), we frequently have observed a definite rise in titer between the samples when a method specific for IgG antibody was used (e.g., the dye test or the agglutination test performed with 2-mercaptoethanol). Although both samples had the same titer in the conventional IFA test, the titer in the first sample was the sum of the anti-IgM and anti-IgG antibody activities of the conjugate, whereas the titer in the second sample reflected only the anti-IgG antibody activity of the conjugate.

Establishing guidelines for the IHA and CF tests is made difficult by the fact that different antigen preparations cause markedly different results: Some preparations detect IgM antibodies, some detect IgG antibodies, and others detect both. Thus the evolution of the antibody response may differ not only when different tests are used but also when the same test is used in different laboratories. This problem has been paramount in the confusion surrounding the subject of the practical approach to diagnosing acute infection.

In a systematic screening program (Desmonts G and Thulliez P, unpublished data) in which follow-up sera from pregnant women are examined monthly, IgM antibodies are usually the first to appear, but low titers of IgG antibodies, as measured in the dye test, also appear early. Sera in which only IgM antibodies are detectable

are uncommon. A rise in IgM antibody titer is infrequently observed, suggesting that the IgM antibody titer rise is steep and that this rise does not last longer than 1 or 2 weeks before reaching its peak. By contrast, the rise in IgG antibody titer initially is slow. The titer, as measured in the dye test, usually remains relatively low (2 to 100 IU/mL or 1:10 to 1:100) for 3 to 6 weeks. Recognition of this fact is critical for proper interpretation of serologic test results when serum samples obtained 2 to 3 weeks apart are tested in parallel, especially if the dye test is performed with fourfold dilutions of the sera, which would require an eightfold (two-tube) rise in titer to be considered significant. In testing such sera in parallel, it is imperative to use twofold dilutions so that a fourfold (two-tube) rise can be detected. In our experience, this rise is difficult to detect in the IgG IFA test. After the initial 3 to 6 weeks, the rise in IgG antibody titer becomes steeper; high titers (greater than 400 IU/mL or 1:1000) usually are reached within an additional 3 weeks. Thereafter, the rise in titer is slower but may still be detectable over an additional 3 to 6 weeks if careful quantitative methodology is used (here again, this rise will be missed if fourfold dilutions of sera are used). Thus although the rise in IgG antibody titer as detected in the dye test differs from one case to another, it lasts for more than 2 months and sometimes as long as 3 months. The rise in IgG antibody titer, as detected in the agglutination test (in the presence of 2-mercaptoethanol), may parallel exactly the pattern described for the dye test, or the titer may rise more slowly; the peak may not occur earlier than 6 months after infection. As mentioned previously, by 6 months, titers in the IgM IFA test are no longer demonstrable in most cases. Titers in the capture IgM ELISA and in the IgM ISAGA, however, usually remain positive for this period, and in women who acquire the infection during pregnancy, the titers in these latter two tests are almost always positive at the time of parturition (the level of the titer depends on the duration of infection before delivery).

Although definitive data are not available, when specific treatment for *T. gondii* infection is administered early during the initial antibody response (when the IgG antibody titer is still low), it appears that the antibody response may be slowed and the titer (e.g., in the dye test, conventional IFA test, or ELISA) may remain relatively low so long as treatment is continued. A late (delayed) rise often is observed after cessation of treatment.

Practical Guidelines for Diagnosis of Infection in the Pregnant Woman

Guidelines for diagnosis of *Toxoplasma* infection are presented for three clinical scenarios: (1) that of a woman pregnant for a few weeks in whom a serologic test for *T. gondii* infection was performed on a routine basis by her physician or at her request; (2) that of a woman pregnant for a few months who is suspected of having acute toxoplasmosis; and (3) that of a woman who has just given birth to an infant suspected of having congenital toxoplasmosis. In almost all cases in the United States, the diagnosis in these situations must take into consideration two pieces of data: the results of a test for IgG antibodies (e.g., dye test, ELISA, IFA) and the results of a test for IgM antibody (e.g., IgM IFA, IgM ISAGA, or IgM ELISA). The accuracy of some ELISA kits being sold at present is unsatisfactory, and proper interpretation of the results of titers obtained for many of these kits has not been defined clearly. A number of studies attest to problem of false-positive and false-negative results obtained with certain kits that employ IFA or ELISA technology.*

Clinical Scenario 1: Very Early Pregnancy (first few weeks). If no antibody is demonstrable, the patient has not been infected and must be considered at risk of infection. A positive IgG test titer and a negative test result for IgM antibodies or high-avidity antibody test can be interpreted as reflecting infection that occurred months or years before the pregnancy, although very rarely IgM *T. gondii* antibodies may not be detected in recent infections. Essentially, there is no risk of the patient's giving birth to a congenitally infected child (unless she is immunosuppressed), regardless of the level of antibody titer. No matter how high the titer is, it should not be considered prognostically meaningful.

If IgM antibodies are present, the avidity test should be performed. If this is unavailable, the IgG test should be performed, with results compared with those for a second sample taken 3 weeks after the first. If no rise in IgG antibody test titer occurs, the infection was acquired before pregnancy, and almost no risk to the fetus exists. If a rise in IgG antibody test titer is observed, the infection probably was acquired less than 2 months previously, perhaps around the time of conception. In this situation, the risk of giving birth to an infected child is very low (see Table 31–8).

Clinical Scenario 2: Early Pregnancy (within a Few Months) plus Suspected Acute Infection. The diagnosis depends on three criteria: (1) the presence of lymphadenopathy in areas compatible with the diagnosis of acute acquired toxoplasmosis [346,538,539,592,731–742], (2) a high IgG test titer (300 IU/mL or greater), and (3)

presence of IgM antibody. If two of the three criteria are present, for purposes of management, the diagnosis of acute acquired toxoplasmosis should be considered likely. If, however, the IgG test titer is less than 300 IU/mL, a significant rise in titer should be demonstrable in a second serum sample obtained 2 to 3 weeks later. The avidity assay is particularly helpful in this setting. A high-avidity test result indicates acquisition of infection more than 12 to 16 weeks earlier (see earlier under "IgG Avidity Assay").

Important to consider in the pregnant patient in whom lymphadenopathy is observed is that high-avidity results were demonstrable only in those women whose lymphadenopathy had developed at least 4 months earlier [90]. Therefore, a high-avidity test result in a pregnant woman with recent development of lymphadenopathy (e.g., within 2 or 3 months of performing the avidity test) suggests a cause other than toxoplasmosis, and further workup is warranted to determine the cause of the lymphadenopathy. In that same study of the IgG avidity test in patients with lymphadenopathy, low-IgG avidity antibodies were observed in sera of patients whose lymphadenopathy had developed as long as 17 months before the time of serum sampling for testing. (This provides additional proof that low-IgG avidity test results should not be relied on for diagnosis of recently acquired infection.)

Clinical Scenario 3: Suspected Congenital Toxoplasmosis in a Newborn Infant. The diagnosis of the acute acquired infection in women who have just given birth to a child with suspected congenital toxoplasmosis is rarely difficult. As a rule, diagnosis of recent infection in the mother relies on the IgG test titer and the results of tests for IgM antibodies. Paradoxically, examination of maternal sera frequently is more useful for diagnosing subclinical or atypical congenital toxoplasmosis in a neonate than is examination of the child's serum. If IgM antibody is detected in the mother and no prior serologic test results are available, her newborn should be examined clinically and serologically to rule out congenital infection.

Because IgM antibodies as measured by ELISA or ISAGA may persist for many months or even years, their greatest value is in determining that a pregnant woman examined early in gestation has not recently been infected. A negative result virtually rules out recently acquired infection unless sera are tested late in gestation (in which case IgM antibodies may no longer be detectable), or so early after the acute infection that an antibody response has not yet occurred (in which case the acute infection would be identified in a screening program in which follow-up serologic testing is performed in seronegative pregnant women). A positive IgM test result is more difficult to evaluate, unless a significant rise in IgG or IgM titer can be demonstrated when sera are tested in parallel or when results of other tests (e.g., tests for IgA and IgE antibody and the HS/AC test) suggest recent infection. A very high IgM, IgA, or IgE titer is more likely to reflect recent infection, although such high titers may persist for months. Such positive sera should be confirmed with additional methods, such as the HS/AC or avidity test. In most cases, use of and consultation with a reference laboratory will be required. In the Palo Alto laboratory, a "chronic" pattern in the HS/AC test agrees virtually 100% with a "chronic" titer in the IgG avidity test.

---

*References 590, 652, 653, 712, 729, 730.

In the unusual situation in which a pregnant woman has a positive IgM antibody titer and a persistently negative IgG titer, a false-positive IgM result must be considered, and if feasible, all such patients should have IgG antibodies measured by a different method [57,733,734]. Examples of the serologic response in women who seroconverted during pregnancy are shown in Table 31–25.

Pinon and colleagues in France fortuitously diagnosed two cases of congenital toxoplasmosis in newborns whose mothers did not have detectable *T. gondii* antibodies at the time of birth. These cases prompted the investigators to perform a study over an 18-month period to determine by postnatal serologic follow-up whether they could detect women who were infected but whose results of serologic testing were negative at the time of delivery. They detected four cases of perinatal maternal infection, and two of these resulted in infected offspring. In view of these results, and to prevent missing maternal infection at the end of pregnancy, they suggest that serologic testing of seronegative women who have been screened monthly should continue such that the last blood sample is obtained approximately 30 days after they have given birth [57].

Prenatal Diagnosis of Fetal *Toxoplasma* Infection

Although PCR assay in amniotic fluid is now the method of choice, cordocentesis [735–737] may still be used when PCR methods are unavailable or in the rare instances in which the PCR assay result is negative and the ultrasonographic findings suggest fetal infection. For this reason, findings on clinical studies using this method are described here along with those for PCR analysis.

Amniocentesis: Polymerase Chain Reaction Assay in Amniotic Fluid

Results of PCR analysis performed in different laboratories may differ considerably; a result reported as positive or negative from one laboratory may even be the opposite of that from another laboratory. At present, no procedures for quality control in laboratories performing PCR assay for prenatal diagnosis are in place. PCR assay results from any laboratory must be reviewed with caution, and if possible, information or data on the reliability and validation data of the PCR tests from that laboratory should be requested.

In 1994, Hohlfeld and coworkers from Paris [77] published a follow-up to their cordocentesis study reported in 1988 [82]. Prenatal diagnosis, which included amniocentesis, ultrasonography, and fetal blood sampling, was performed in 2632 women who had acquired *T. gondii* infection during gestation. One hundred ninety-four cases of congenital toxoplasmosis were identified, and 178 of these were diagnosed by conventional methods of prenatal diagnosis. No false-positive results were reported. The overall sensitivity was 92%, the specificity was 100%, and the negative predictive value was 99%. The sensitivity of the IgM antibody test was 28%; of mouse inoculation with fetal blood, 72%; of mouse inoculation with amniotic fluid, 64%; and of tissue culture of amniotic fluid, 64%. The overall rate of spontaneous fetal loss was 1.3%. PCR assay was performed in the amniotic fluid

in 339 consecutive women, and the results were compared with those obtained by the conventional methods. By conventional testing, congenital infection was demonstrated in 34 fetuses, and in each the PCR test result also was positive. In three additional fetuses, only the PCR assay result was positive, and in each, the diagnosis of congenital infection was confirmed on follow-up investigation (autopsy in two and serologic study in one). One false-negative result was obtained with the PCR assay, and no false-positive results. The investigators concluded that the PCR assay is a more reliable, safer, simpler, and less expensive method than the conventional methods they had been using, and that it can be used from week 18 of gestation until term. They also concluded that fetal blood sampling is no longer necessary, and that amniocentesis together with the PCR test and inoculation of mice (tissue culture is less sensitive) is preferred (Table 31–28). The authors did not have data on the efficacy of testing amniotic fluid before 18 weeks of gestation. They stated that prenatal diagnosis should not be attempted until at least 4 weeks after the acute infection in the mother.

In 1998, Jenum and associates published the Norwegian experience with a nested PCR technique using amniotic fluid collected from 67 women diagnosed as having acquired the infection during gestation [590]. They also used mouse inoculation on each of the samples. They commented on the greater sensitivity of the PCR method because mouse inoculation results were affected by treatment in the mothers. Whereas Hohlfeld and coworkers [77] found a specificity of 100%, Jenum and associates [82] observed a specificity of only 94%, despite careful technical steps to avoid contamination of their samples. Their reported positive predictive value was 67%, with 10 true positives among 15 positive results. Three of eight infants with congenital toxoplasmosis diagnosed after birth had a negative result on PCR assay and mouse inoculation on prenatal examination. Thus in their study, a positive PCR assay result did not confirm infection in the fetus. For this reason, the researchers stated that

TABLE 31–28 Diagnostic Value of the Polymerase Chain Reaction (PCR) Assay Compared with Conventional Methods for Prenatal Diagnosis of Congenital *Toxoplasma gondii* Infection in 339 Pregnancies

Variable	PCR*	Conventional Methods*,†
Sensitivity	37/38 (97.4; 86.1–99.9)	34/38 (89.5; 72.2–97.0)‡
Specificity	301/301 (100; 98.8–100)	301/301 (100; 98.8–100)
Positive predictive value	37/37 (100; 90.5–100)	34/34 (100; 89.7–100)
Negative predictive value	301/302 (99.7; 98.7–100)	301/305 (98.7; 97.4–99.9)

*Positive tests/all tests (%; 95% confidence interval).
†Tissue culture of amniotic fluid, inoculation of mice with fetal blood and amniotic fluid, and determination of specific IgM in fetal blood.
‡The sensitivity of conventional methods in the study overall was somewhat higher (92%; 95% confidence interval, 88 to 96%).
IgM, immunoglobulin M.
Adapted from Hohlfeld P, et al. Prenatal diagnosis of congenital toxoplasmosis with polymerase-chain-reaction test on amniotic fluid. N Engl J Med 331:695–699, 1994.

positive results also require serologic follow-up testing for confirmation of the diagnosis. Prenatal diagnosis using PCR assay performed in amniotic fluid from each twin in a dizygotic pregnancy was recently reported by Tjalma and colleagues [740].

Because physicians must make decisions regarding management of a pregnancy after results of amniocentesis are obtained, it is of utmost importance that the PCR assay be specific insofar as there are no false-positive results. For example, according to a recent report, the use of a nested PCR technique [590] did not appear to yield results that fit this requirement; therefore, that nested PCR method cannot be considered to represent an improvement over conventional methods for prenatal diagnosis.

One shortcoming of the study reported by Hohlfeld and coworkers [77] is that the sensitivity and negative predictive value of the PCR assay in amniotic fluid were compared with those of conventional methods but were not analyzed relative to the status of the infection in the liveborn infants. The enthusiasm that has been generated for the reliability of the PCR assay should be tempered by the fact that because of the delay that can occur between the time of maternal infection and transmission of the parasite to the fetus (transmission may occur after the date of the amniocentesis), all congenital infections are not and cannot be identified by prenatal diagnosis. One case that suggests such a delay is reported in the publication by Hohlfeld and coworkers [76]. Before PCR testing was used for prenatal diagnosis, it was well recognized that not all cases of congenital T. gondii infection could be detected prenatally. Of 89 congenital infections, Hohlfeld and coworkers [77] reported 9 cases (10%) with a negative result on prenatal diagnostic testing. In other published series, the rate of congenital infections with no prenatally identified abnormal findings varied, ranging from 3% in the study by Pratlong and coworkers [741] to 8% in that by Berrebi and associates [742]. Actually, the number of infections that were not detected by the prenatal diagnostic procedures was underestimated in each of these studies, because a significant number of the offspring were lost to follow-up (50 of 211 [24%] [741]), or data were not provided by the investigators [77]. Before the use of PCR methods, it was not possible to define whether these discrepancies were due to a lack of sensitivity of the diagnostic procedures or to the fact that transmission of the parasite occurred after the amniocentesis or cordocentesis was performed. The higher sensitivity of PCR assay when compared with conventional methods explains why congenital infection had been missed in the past when the less sensitive conventional methods were used.

Nonetheless, a negative PCR test result in amniotic fluid does not rule out infection in the fetus.

In France, Kieffer and colleagues (2009) estimated the sensitivity, specificity, and positive and negative predictive values, per trimester and over all of pregnancy, for detection of T. gondii in amniotic fluid using real-time PCR. The cohort included 377 pregnant women identified as having Toxoplasma infection through prenatal screening. Available data included gestational age of maternal infection, details of maternal treatment, amniocentesis results, neonatal work-up and definitive infection status of the child. PCR analysis occurred in 261 (69%) of 377

patients. Except for 4 negative results for children who were infected, PCRs were accurate. Overall sensitivity was 92.2% (95% CI 87-98%) and the negative predictive value was 98.1% (95% CI 95-99%). Specificity and positive predictive values were 100%. A significant association did not occur with the trimester of maternal acquisition of infection. Thus, Real-time PCR for the 300 copy, 529 base pair T. gondii gene improves detection of T. gondii in amniotic fluid and is useful for determining whether there is fetal infection and for consequent proper treatment and monitoring. Neonatal evaluations are still necessary to determine manifestations of infection and for those who had negative PCR, to help to more definitively exclude infection.

In a study performed to determine whether quantification of PCR results would be helpful in predicting outcome of the infection in the fetus or newborn, parasite concentrations were estimated by real-time quantitative PCR assay in 88 consecutive positive amniotic fluid samples from 86 pregnant women [206]. Results were analyzed according to the gestational age at maternal infection and the clinical status in fetuses during pregnancy and at birth. A significant negative linear regression was observed between gestational age at maternal infection and parasite loads in amniotic fluid (see Fig. 31-20).

After adjustment for gestational age at maternal seroconversion, parasite concentration in amniotic fluid, and the total duration of prenatal treatment in the multivariate analysis, the two variables significantly and independently associated with most severe signs of infection (fetal death or cerebral ventricular dilation) were an early gestational age at maternal infection (odds ratio = 1.44/decreasing week gestation [95% CI, 1.12% to 1.85%]) and high parasite amniotic fluid concentrations (odds ratio = 15.4/log [parasites/mL of amniotic fluid] [95% CI, 2.45% to 97.7%]). In this series, each of the 11 cases in which parasite loads were greater than 100/mL, with onset of infection before 20 weeks, resulted in severe impairments in the offspring, indicating a 100% predictive value of poor prognosis (see Fig. 31-20).

The earlier in gestation infection occurs, the higher the parasite burden. Parasite burden in amniotic fluid as determined by quantitative PCR analysis also is a prenatal biologic marker of the severity of congenital infection. In a dizygotic twin pair, one had no parasites, and the other had greater than 600 parasites per milliliter. At pregnancy termination, the former infant had no signs of infection; the latter had disseminated multivisceral infection. Members of a second twin pair—one with clinical signs and the other without such signs—similarly were dicordant for parasite burden in amniotic fluid (3.2 versus 2800 parasites per milliliter), and both died. The twin with hydrocephalus and ventriculomegaly probably was the twin with amniotic fluid with the higher parasite burden (2800 parasites per milliliter).

Ultrasound examinations (Figure 31-26) are still required and should be performed each month following a negative PCR result on amniocentesis because congenital infections with extensive involvement and hydrocephalus have occurred in the setting of a negative PCR assay result. When the ultrasound appearance remains normal, it is still necessary to continue clinical and serologic follow-up

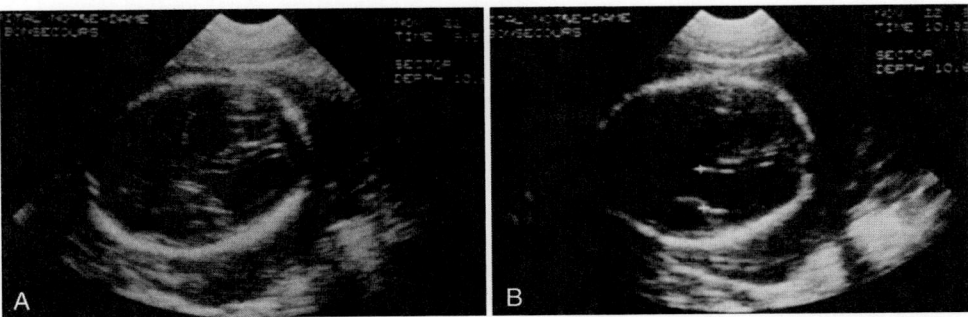

FIGURE 31–26 A and B, Ultrasound study of fetus with hydrocephalus resulting from toxoplasmosis. *(Courtesy of F Daffos, Paris.)*

evaluation of infants until congenital infection is definitively ruled out.

Immunoglobulin A Antibodies

The value of demonstration of IgA *T. gondii* antibodies in the fetus is now well recognized [642,647,741,743,744]. Therefore, testing for these antibodies for this purpose should be routine in all laboratories that test newborns for suspected congenital *T. gondii* infection.

Interferon

Interferon has been demonstrated in blood of fetuses infected with *T. gondii*, suggesting that the fetus is able to synthesize this cytokine as early as 26 weeks of gestation [745]. Its demonstration appears helpful when interferon level determination is used with other nonspecific tests for diagnosing *T. gondii* infection in the fetus. Interferon serum levels that were significantly higher than in controls also were demonstrated in sera of pregnant women during seroconversion for *T. gondii* antibodies [745].

T-Cell Subsets

T-cell subsets were evaluated in a group of uninfected and infected fetuses [746]. Significant differences from controls were noted in that the infected fetuses were characterized by a smaller percentage of CD3+ and CD4+ T cells and a decrease in absolute number of CD4+ cells and lower CD4+/CD8+ ratio. The mothers in this study were receiving treatment, and the possible results of this treatment on T cells could not be excluded. In addition, because the number of infected fetuses was small, it was not possible to analyze the values obtained relative to gestational age, as was done in the control, uninfected fetuses.

In another study, Lecolier and coworkers studied T lymphocyte subpopulations in normal and in six *T. gondii*-infected fetuses [743]. They noted a significant increase in number of CD8+ T cells in two cases investigated soon after maternal infection (3 and 6 weeks, respectively) and a significant decrease in number of CD4+ T cells in the four other cases that were investigated later (7 to 13 weeks after maternal infection). These observations suggest that alterations in T lymphocyte subsets in the infected fetus are similar to those that occur in the acute acquired infection in adults [257]. In another study by Foulon and associates, these results were not confirmed [551,550]. Thus further study is necessary to evaluate whether study of T-cell subsets will be a useful adjunct in prenatal diagnosis.

Complement

It appears that the C4 component of complement is significantly increased in fetuses congenitally infected with *T. gondii*. Gestational age is important in interpretation of results, but the measurement of C4 levels in the fetus may be a useful nonspecific adjunctive test for prenatal diagnosis [747].

Serologic Diagnosis in the Newborn

Because of the pleomorphism of congenital toxoplasmosis, because the infection most often is subclinical in the newborn, and because the infection may be mimicked by other infections and diseases of the neonate, the diagnosis of congenital *T. gondii* infection is far more complicated than is diagnosis of the acquired infection.

The serologic diagnosis of congenital *T. gondii* infection in the newborn is particularly difficult because of the high prevalence of antibodies to *T. gondii* among normal women of childbearing age in the United States and in much of the rest of the world. Thus a high antibody titer in a newborn may merely reflect past or recent infection in the mother (maternal IgG antibody having passed transplacentally to her fetus).

The fact that infection in the fetus may stimulate production of sufficient IgM to result in abnormally high levels of this immunoglobulin in the newborn has been shown in a variety of congenital infections by Stiehm and associates [690] and by Alford and coworkers [748,749]. Thus quantification of IgM in cord serum may be a valuable screening device for detecting infection in the newborn. At present, the consensus of those working on immunologic responses to perinatal infection is that enough "false-negative" results occur to suggest that quantification of IgM in the newborn may not be universally applicable for diagnosing infection [255,750,751]. Such false-negative results are not infrequent in premature infants with proven rubella [255]. For a nonspecific test to be beneficial as a screen, it seems that a slight excess in sensitivity resulting in overdiagnosis (false-positive results) can be accepted, but that lack of sensitivity in known cases, resulting in underdiagnosis (false-negative results) cannot be accepted.

As mentioned earlier, demonstration of IgM, IgA, or IgE antibodies to *T. gondii* in serum of the newborn is diagnostic of congenital *T. gondii* infection if contamination with maternal blood has not occurred. When an appropriate fluorescein-tagged antiserum to IgM has been employed, we have not had any false-positive results except for the qualifications mentioned earlier for the IgM IFA method. Because high levels of maternal IgG antibodies to *T. gondii* may compete for antigenic sites on the surface of the organisms [686] with the relatively low IgM antibody levels usually found in the fetus or neonate, weak reactions and low IgM antibody titers (1:2) indicate infection in the newborn. Even allowing for these weakly positive reactions, however, detectable specific IgM antibody is absent in the sera of most neonates with congenital toxoplasmosis (approximately 75%) when the IgM IFA test is used [480]. This false-negative result rate was only approximately 20% if the double-sandwich IgM ELISA method was used [608]. Because of the high incidence of false-negative results for the IgM IFA test, we recommend that the capture IgM ELISA or ISAGA method be used instead. It is noteworthy that the proportion of infants showing IgM antibody is the same whether illness is clinically manifest or subclinical. IgA antibodies have been demonstrated in as high as 90% of newborns with the congenital infection [642,752], which further attests to the great value of testing for these antibodies (Table 31–29). A number of investigators have reported greater sensitivity of IgA antibody determination for diagnosis in infected children than for IgM [611,641,642,753,754]. As emphasized by Foudrinier and coworkers, specificity of IgA detected at birth must be confirmed because equivocal and positive IgA test results were found in newborns during the first days of life, whereas subsequent sera became negative within less than 10 days [754]. They concluded that in a neonate born to a mother with IgA or IgM *T. gondii* antibodies, a positive IgA or IgM test result must be interpreted with caution and be confirmed after approximately 10 days of life, unless the diagnosis is established before this time. Additional data are needed to clarify whether all newborns with a positive IgA or IgM antibody titer at approximately 10 days of age are indeed infected, especially in those cases in which the maternal IgA or IgM antibody titers were very high. Determination of levels of β-human chorionic gonadotropin and of total IgA may prove to be of value as adjunctive tests.

Of note, however, we have never observed a false-positive result after the first day of life when the ISAGA was used for detection of IgM antibodies.

The value of demonstration of IgE antibodies also is clear. In one of our laboratories (Remington JS), 19 of 21 infants (90%) (ages birth to 5 weeks) with congenital toxoplasmosis and signs of CNS involvement tested positive for IgE antibodies (92% by ELISA and 62% by ISAGA) [639]; of the 10 tested in the first week of life, 9 had IgM antibody, and all 7 of those tested for IgA antibodies were seropositive. Seven of the 21 were first tested in the second week of life; 6 had IgM antibodies, and all 5 of those tested for IgA were seropositive. Of the 4 first tested at 3 to 5 weeks of life, 3 had both IgM and IgA antibody; 1 infant had neither [639]. In studies by Pinon and colleagues, 52 cases of congenital *T. gondii* infection (5 symptomatic and 47 "asymptomatic" cases) were studied; at birth or during the first month of life, none of the symptomatic and 13 (25%) of the "asymptomatic" infants were seropositive by IgE ISAGA. Thirty-five of the 52 infants (67%) were seropositive for IgA antibody by ISAGA [755,756].

If the infant is infected in utero at a time when it is immunologically competent to produce IgM antibodies but before the passage of maternal IgG *T. gondii* antibodies across the placenta has occurred, there is no reason to suspect competition for recognition of antigenic sites on the parasite. Data derived from studies of infants with very high IgM titers in the early newborn period support this hypothesis. Table 31–30 displays clinical and serologic data representing such an instance in a mother and her infant. The mother had had a high but stable dye test titer since the ninth week of pregnancy and a negative IgM IFA test titer. The same results were obtained during week 13. This finding suggests that infection occurred at about the time of conception or a few weeks earlier. She did not receive treatment and gave birth to a severely infected infant with generalized toxoplasmosis who died 8 days after delivery. This newborn had an unusually high IgM test titer. If, however, high titers of maternal antibody are present in the fetus before the organism reaches the fetus, as a consequence of delay by the placental barrier discussed earlier, it is possible that IgG antibody might compete (and "cover") for recognition sites [686] on the parasite or may by other means (e.g., feedback mechanism) suppress fetal IgM antibody synthesis. (This also might explain the paradoxical occurrence of an elevated IgM level in the serum of an infected infant in the presence of a negative IgM test titer.) That this may occur has been shown in an experimental animal model [757]. In our experience, IgM antibody titers usually decrease rapidly after the infant's own IgG antibodies have reached a high titer; at 1 year of age, IgM antibodies usually are not demonstrable or are present in very low titer.

In the absence of demonstration of the parasite, IgM or IgA antibodies to *T. gondii*, follow-up testing of infants with suspected toxoplasmosis is the only means of making a serologic diagnosis of subclinical toxoplasmosis. For proper interpretation of test titers in infants who are past the immediate newborn period, it is important to understand how passively transmitted maternal IgG decreases in the uninfected infant. Because the literature is replete

TABLE 31–29 Serologic Test Results for IgM and IgA Antibodies at Birth and During the Newborn Period in Sera of 23 Congenitally Infected and 49 Uninfected Offspring of Mothers Infected During Gestation*

Trimester Mother Acquired Infection (Time Test Performed)	IgM– IgA–	IgM+ IgA+	IgM+ IgA–	IgM– IgA+
Uninfected (at birth)	47	0	1	1
Infected (at birth)				
1st trimester	1	1	0	2
2nd trimester	1	0	0	5
3rd trimester	2	8	1	0
Infected (follow-up 1 wk to 3 mo)	3	11	0	9

*All mothers received spiramycin treatment during gestation from time seroconversion was noted.
IgA, IgM, *immunoglobulins A, M.*
Adapted from Decoster A, et al. Platelia-toxo IgA, a new kit for early diagnosis of congenital toxoplasmosis by detection of anti-P30 immunoglobulin A antibodies. J Clin Microbiol 29:2291–2295, 1991, with permission.

TABLE 31–30 Data in a Mother Who Acquired *Toxoplasma gondii* Infection at About the Time of Conception or a Few Weeks Earlier Who Had a Negative IgM Test Titer and Whose Infant Had a High IgM Test Titer

| Subject | Stage of Pregnancy or Age | Clinical Manifestations | Titer | | *T. gondii* Isolated |
			Dye Test* (IU/mL)	IgM Test†	
Mother	9 wk	None	2000	Negative	
	13 wk	None	2000	Negative	
	8 mo	Delivery			
	1 mo after delivery	None	2000	Negative	Blood negative
Infant	4 days	Hydrocephalus, microphthalmia, convulsions, abnormal cerebrospinal fluid	1000	Positive	Blood positive
	8 days	Death			Brain positive

*Dye test titers are approximately 8000 in the mother and 4000 in the infant if expressed as reciprocal of serum dilution.
†Titers are expressed as the reciprocal of the serum dilution.
IgM, *immunoglobulin M*; IU, *international units.*
Adapted from Desmonts G, Couvreur J. Toxoplasmosis in pregnancy and its transmission to the fetus. Bull N Y Acad Med 50:146–159, 1974, with permission. The mother was not treated.

with misinformation on the interpretation of *T. gondii* serologic studies in older infants, this important subject is dealt with here. In Figure 31–27, curve 1 shows the total serum IgG values in milligrams per deciliter in the newborn and infant to the age of 1 year. The values in the newborn at birth frequently are somewhat higher than they are in the mother and subsequently decrease. Minimal values (e.g., 300 to 400 mg/dL) are observed at about the third or fourth month, after which time the level increases with increasing production of IgG by the infant. Maternally transmitted antibodies (curve 2) progressively disappear because they are not synthesized by the infant. Their half-life is approximately 30 days; that is, they decrease by approximately one half per month (Fig. 31–28).

Figure 31–29 shows actual data from an uninfected infant plotted against the background of the theoretical decay curve for IgG maternal antibody (approximately one half the value every 30 days). Thus a titer of 1000 IU/mL at birth should drop to 1 IU/mL in 300

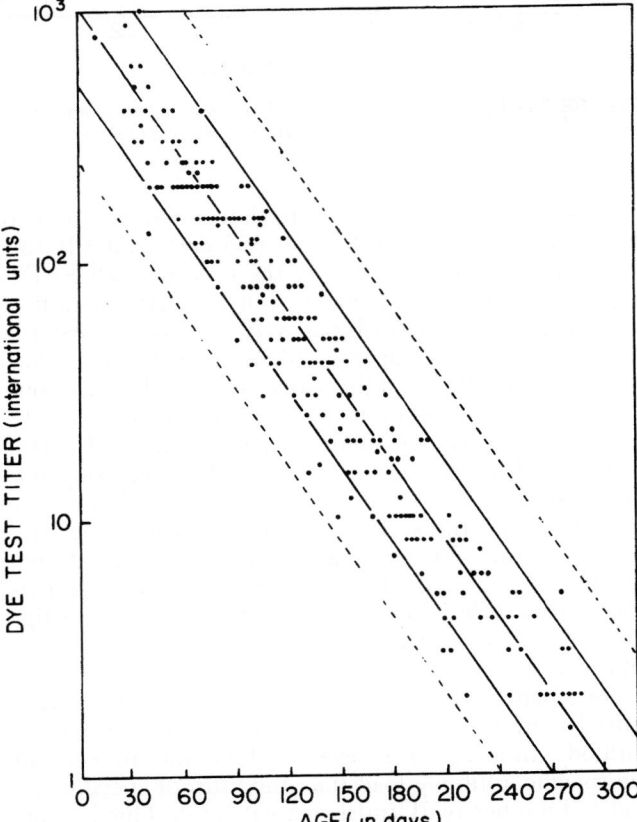

FIGURE 31–27 IgG and *Toxoplasma* antibodies: uninfected child. Curve 1, mg of IgG/dL; curve 2, IU of *Toxoplasma* antibody per ml; curve 3, IU of *Toxoplasma* antibody per mg of IgG. (*Data from Desmonts G, Couvreur J. Toxoplasmosis: epidemiologic and serologic aspects of perinatal infection. In Krugman S, Gershon AA [eds]. Infections of the Fetus and the Newborn Infant. Progress in Clinical and Biological Research, vol 3. New York, Alan R Liss, 1975.*)

FIGURE 31–28 Decrease in maternally transmitted *Toxoplasma* antibodies (dye test) in uninfected infants. The two parallel lines indicate one-half and twice the titer, plus or minus one twofold dilution. The result in one serum sample of each pair is on the theoretical line and is not represented by a dot. The result in the other serum sample of each pair is represented by a dot.

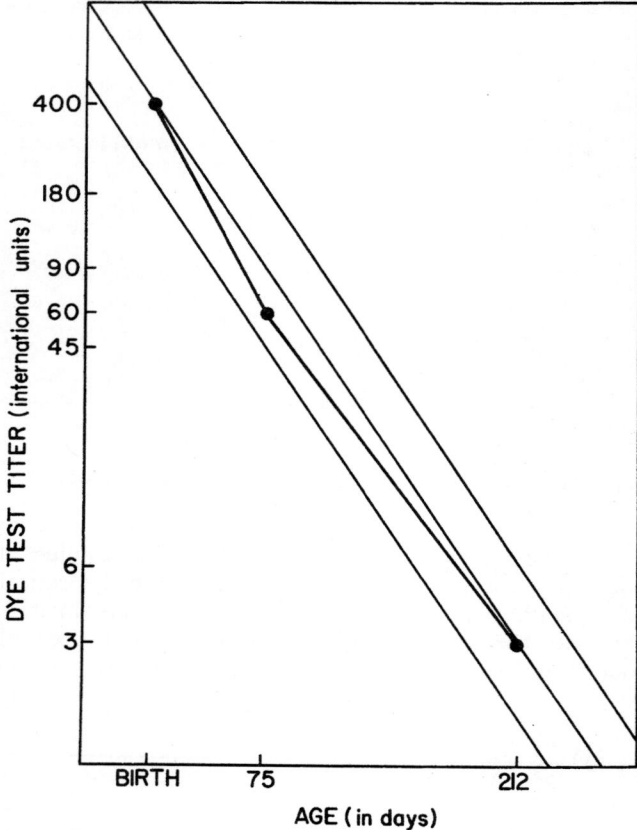

FIGURE 31–29 Evolution of maternally transmitted antibody (dye test) in an uninfected infant from birth to the age of 212 days.

remains constant. During the second and third months, the amount of IgG synthesized by the infant increases. Because this newly synthesized IgG does not contain antibodies to *T. gondii*, the antibody load decreases and will continue to decrease as IgG synthesis in the child progresses.

The production of antibody in infants with congenital toxoplasmosis varies considerably from one case to another and also is affected by treatment. Cases in which antibody production during fetal life can be demonstrated by antibody load are scarce. Early and delayed antibody production can, however, be demonstrated by the antibody load method. An example of early production is shown in Figure 31–30. During the first month of life, the titer in the infant decreases in proportion to the decrease in total IgG (curve 4). At 1 month of age, the situation is similar to that in an uninfected infant: The antibody titer and the total amount of IgG have diminished in the same proportions, and the antibody load is constant. During the second and third months, however, the antibody titer in the infected infant does not decrease at the rate expected, and the antibody load remains the same or may increase. This finding demonstrates that the IgG being synthesized by the infant contains at least as many specific antibodies to *T. gondii* as those in the maternal IgG, and this becomes obvious between the fourth and sixth months, when a definite increase in antibody titer and in antibody load occurs. In some cases, the rise in titer is not demonstrable until even later (Fig. 31–31).

The pattern observed in infants with a delayed onset of antibody response is shown in Figure 31–32. In this situation, the antibody titer remains parallel to the expected

days. The infant whose titers are shown here had titers of 400 IU/mL at birth, 60 IU/mL at 75 days, and 3 IU/mL at 212 days. These are exactly the expected values. Figure 31–28 shows results obtained in 430 paired sera from 93 uninfected infants with passively transmitted maternal antibodies plotted against their theoretical values. Ninety-three percent of the actual titers are less than onefold to twofold dilution different from the expected values. These data preclude acceptance that all infants with a positive titer at 4 to 6 months have congenital toxoplasmosis. The same rate of decrease applies to both high and low titers. It takes approximately the same amount of time for a decrease from 1000 to 250 IU/mL, a seemingly very significant variation, as for a decrease from 4 to 1 IU/mL, a titer difference that most investigators would consider negligible (i.e., no significant difference).

For a better estimate of this decrease in passively transmitted maternal antibodies, it is useful to compare the antibody titer and the level of IgG and to compute the specific antibody load (i.e., the ratio of specific antibodies [number of IU/mL] to total IgG). This is represented diagrammatically in Figure 31–27 by curve 3 and in Table 31–30. In Figure 31–27, as late as the fourth to sixth week of life, usually no change in the antibody load is observed; the IgG is still mainly maternal in origin. Although the titer of antibodies decreases, the total IgG decreases in a similar manner. As a result, the ratio

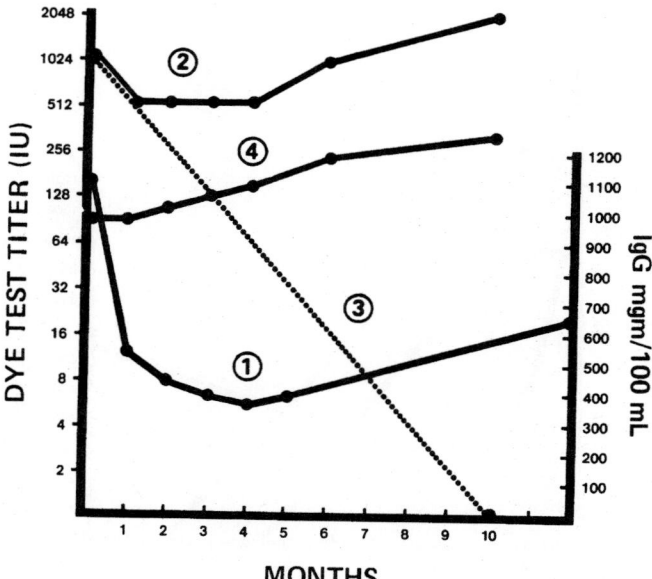

FIGURE 31–30 Antibodies in congenital toxoplasmosis (cases with early synthesis of antibodies). Curve 1, mg of IgG/dL; curve 2, IU of *Toxoplasma* antibody per mL; curve 3, expected titer if antibodies were maternal in origin; curve 4, IU of *Toxoplasma* antibody per milligram of IgG. (*Data from Desmonts G, Couvreur J. Toxoplasmosis: epidemiologic and serologic aspects of perinatal infection. In Krugman S, Gershon AA [eds]. Infections of the Fetus and the Newborn Infant. Progress in Clinical and Biological Research, vol 3. New York, Alan R Liss, 1975.*)

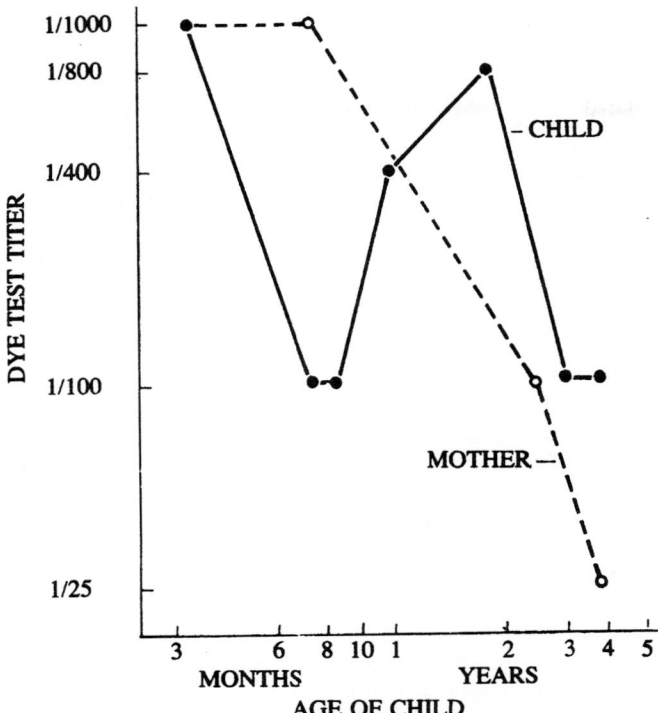

FIGURE 31–31 Example of antibody development (dye test) in a child with congenital toxoplasmosis in relation to time since birth. *(Data from Couvreur J, Desmonts G. Congenital and maternal toxoplasmosis. A review of 300 congenital cases. Dev Med Child Neurol 4:519–530, 1962.)*

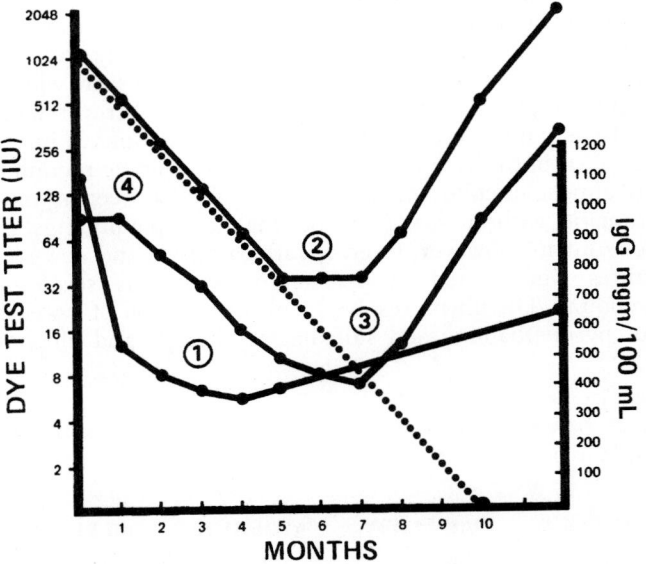

FIGURE 31–32 Antibodies in congenital toxoplasmosis (cases with delayed synthesis of antibodies). (Synthesis usually is not delayed more than 3 or 4 months if the child receives no treatment. It may be delayed up to the sixth or ninth months, if treatment is given.) Curve 1, mg of IgG per dL; curve 2, IU of *Toxoplasma* antibody per mL; curve 3, expected titer if antibodies were maternal in origin; curve 4, IU of *Toxoplasma* antibody per mg of IgG. *(Data from Desmonts G, Couvreur J. Toxoplasmosis: epidemiologic and serologic aspects of perinatal infection. In Krugman S, Gershon AA [eds]. Infections of the Fetus and the Newborn Infant. Progress in Clinical and Biological Research, vol 3. New York, Alan R Liss, 1975.)*

titer of passively transferred maternal antibodies. The antibody load decreases, proving that the infant has begun to synthesize IgG, which apparently does not contain significant amounts of antibodies to *T. gondii*. This situation may persist for several months before the onset of specific antibody production is demonstrable.

Another pattern of antibody development is that observed in infants born to mothers who acquire their infection very near the time of delivery. Such infants have been identified in prospective studies [66,68]. Serologic test titers may be negative in the cord blood or be very low, especially during the first weeks of life. In such cases, the diagnosis would usually be missed and, in fact, because of the low titer in the infant, probably never suspected.

Serologic Studies and Polymerase Chain Reaction Assay in Cerebrospinal Fluid; Polymerase Chain Reaction Assay in Urine

High titers of *T. gondii* antibodies often are observed in cerebrospinal fluid of newborns with congenital toxoplasmosis. This does not prove that antigenic stimulus or antibody formation has occurred within the CNS because the antibody load in the cerebrospinal fluid of these neonates, as a rule, is equal to that in their serum. High titers of *T. gondii* antibodies can be observed in the cerebrospinal fluid of newborns with other CNS diseases (e.g., congenital diseases due to syphilis [758] or cytomegalovirus), even when they are not infected with *T. gondii*. Because of passively transferred maternal *T. gondii* antibodies [752], and when the protein concentration is very high in the cerebrospinal fluid, the IgG concentration may reach the sensitivity level of the serologic test used. Thus demonstration of high titers of IgG antibodies in the cerebrospinal fluid in newborns is not useful diagnostically. Demonstration of IgM antibodies in the cerebrospinal fluid, especially in the absence of IgM antibodies in the serum, supports the diagnosis of *T. gondii* infection in the CNS. In contrast with this situation in the newborn, serologic testing of cerebrospinal fluid and determination of antibody load sometimes are diagnostic during infancy or childhood in patients with CNS toxoplasmosis. The diagnosis also is established if *T. gondii* antigens are demonstrable in the cerebrospinal fluid.

The method of choice for detection of the parasite in cerebrospinal fluid is PCR assay. It is both highly sensitive and specific for this purpose [435,759,760]. Fuentes and colleagues [759] detected the parasite by PCR assay in blood and cerebrospinal fluid from three of four newborns suspected of being congenitally infected with *T. gondii* and by PCR assay in urine from each of the four newborns. The investigators cautioned that because only urine from symptomatic newborns was examined, it will be necessary to assess the utility of PCR assay in urine from asymptomatic infants as well.

Effect of Treatment

T. gondii-specific IgM is rarely present in serum of an infant at birth who has received treatment with pyrimethamine and sulfadiazine in utero from week 17 of gestation until birth [76]. Data on the effects of treatment on production of IgM, IgA, and IgE antibodies are insufficient for comment [328,557,708]. Adequate data, however, are available on the effects of treatment on the dye test (IgG antibody) and antibody load method. These effects are described here. Alterations in antibody response vary among different cases and appear to depend in large part on the stage of synthesis of antibody in the child when treatment is begun.

If the infant does not begin producing antibody before treatment is started or if synthesis is at a low level, treatment apparently curbs the low-grade synthesis and prevents antibody formation. (This effect is not surprising because treatment kills the tachyzoite form, thereby halting the production of antigen.)

Data on the IgM antibody response and on the development of IgG antibody by the fetus and infant presented in this section support the hypothesis discussed earlier (see "Transmission" section) that some infants are not infected during intrauterine life but are infected during labor, from the infected placenta. The immune system of some newborns and fetuses can recognize *T. gondii* antigens with active synthesis of IgM and IgG antibodies. Once established, this synthesis of IgG and IgM antibodies does not appear to be affected by treatment. In other infants, production of *T. gondii* antibodies is delayed until maternally transmitted antibody decreases to a low titer or until specific treatment is discontinued, thereby allowing renewed proliferation of the organism. Thus in infants in whom a marked decrease in antibodies has occurred after birth, only to increase again at the age of 3 or 4 months, it seems plausible to suggest that the infection occurred not during fetal life but during labor.

The delay in antibody synthesis could be related solely to the late infection; this is substantiated by the fact that parasitemia frequently is demonstrable in cord blood or in the blood of the neonate during the first days of life (Table 31–31). Even if infection occurred during parturition, however, this explanation alone is insufficient for certain other observations. Antibodies develop readily during the first weeks of life in infants infected shortly before delivery so long as they received little or no maternal IgG antibody, whereas synthesis of antibody often is poor or completely lacking in infants whose early lesions prove that they were definitely infected during fetal life.

TABLE 31–31   Correlation of Age of Infant and Presence of Demonstrable Parasitemia

Age	No. of Infants	No. with Parasitemia (%)
Cord–1st wk	28	20 (71)
2nd wk	15	5 (33)
3rd–4th wk	15	5 (33)
2nd mo	11	9 (0)

Adapted from Desmonts G, Couvreur J. Toxoplasmosis: epidemiologic and serologic aspects of perinatal infection. In Krugman S, Gershon AA (eds). Infections of the Fetus and the Newborn Infant. Progress in Clinical and Biological Research, vol 3. New York, Alan R Liss, 1975, with permission.

Inhibition of fetal recognition of *T. gondii* antigen appears to offer the most satisfactory explanation for the delay in antibody synthesis observed in most infected infants. Maternal IgG is the most likely effector of this inhibitory effect. This is not solely of academic interest because such inhibition of antibody synthesis, whether by maternal IgG or by specific treatment, has important implications for the diagnosis of congenital toxoplasmosis. If treatment is begun early in these infants and is continued for some months, the diagnosis cannot be established serologically before 6 to 12 months of life.

Serologic Rebound After Treatment. Serologic rebound (Table 31–32) occurs commonly when pyrimethamine and sulfadiazine are discontinued [433,761,762]. In the study by Villena and associates, rebound occurred in 90% of the infants who received Fansidar, mainly 2 to 6 months after treatment was discontinued [763]. This serologic rebound suggests that although these antimicrobial agents eliminate active infection, probably through their effect on tachyzoites, not all organisms are eliminated despite 1 year of therapy. A small number of infants with very mild disease or minimal manifestations of infection, or both, have not exhibited such serologic rebound. In almost all children, serologic rebound has been asymptomatic, without changes in ophthalmoscopic findings. In one infant, however, fever, failure to thrive, and new seizures were noted in association with this serologic rebound. His illness resolved with resumption of 2 weeks of pyrimethamine and sulfadiazine therapy and did not

TABLE 31–32   Examples of Serologic Rebound in a Child Who Developed Symptoms (Patient 2) and in One Who Did Not (Patient 1)*

Patient	Age Serum Obtained (mo)	Dye Test	IgM ISAGA	IgM ELISA	IgA ELISA	IgE ISAGA	IgE ELISA
1	1	1 : 4096	9	Negative	Negative	Negative	Positive
	5†	1 : 128	Negative	Negative	Negative	Negative	Negative
	12‡	1 : 2048	12	7.8	Negative	Negative	Positive
2	1.5	1 : 8000	QNS	6.3	11.4	QNS	QNS
	15†	1 : 128	Negative	Negative	Negative	Negative	Negative
	17‡	1 : 8000	12	Negative	3.5	12	Positive

*Serologic tests were performed in the laboratory of Dr. Jack S. Remington.
†Sample obtained while patient was still taking pyrimethamine and sulfadiazine.
‡Sample obtained after pyrimethamine and sulfadiazine were stopped.
ELISA, enzyme-linked immunosorbent assay; IgA, IgE, IgG, IgM, Immunoglobulins A, E, G, M; ISAGA, immunosorbent agglutination assay; QNS, quantity not sufficient.

recur when these medications were discontinued. Thus it appears to be uncommon for symptomatic disease to develop at the time serologic rebound occurs in an infant.

These observations concerning serologic rebound have been confirmed recently in other cohorts of children [756]. Djurkovic-Djakovic and colleagues [764] found that serologic rebound occurred in 82 of 84 children (98%) without illness when medicines to treat their congenital toxoplasmosis were withdrawn at 1 year of age. The serologic profile in this rebound was IgG with a chronic-disease pattern in AC/HS and avidity tests, despite a high rate of detection of specific IgM and IgA. The serologic rebound occurred in 70% to 90% of congenitally infected children who received Fansidar/folinic acid [765]. Evidence of this phenomenon usually was noted 2 to 6 months after treatment was discontinued. Ophthalmologic surveillance during this time often did not identify recurrent chorioretinitis, although such identification has been reported [766]. It seems prudent to observe infants closely (especially by ophthalmologic examination), particularly during the months after therapy is discontinued. At present, no serologic markers have reliably been associated with recurrences of chorioretinitis in congenitally infected children. It was reported that the IgM level often was elevated with recurrences [767], but this association has not been found in the patients in the NCCCTS (see Table 31–14) [266]. More retinal lesions first identified after treatment was discontinued were noted by one group of investigators in the children infected earlier in gestation who had extraocular manifestations at birth [766].

DIFFERENTIAL DIAGNOSIS

The diseases to be considered in the differential diagnosis of toxoplasmosis are essentially the same as those described in Chapter 23 and also should include congenital lymphocytic choriomeningitis virus syndrome [768].

THERAPY
General Comments

We recommend specific therapy in every case of congenital toxoplasmosis or congenital *T. gondii* infection in infants younger than 1 year of age. Insufficient data are available to allow proper evaluation of treatment in the asymptomatic infected infant. Nevertheless, most investigators, including ourselves, consider that treatment for such infants should be undertaken in the hope of preventing the remarkably high incidence of late untoward sequelae seen in children who receive inadequate or no treatment [628].

Evaluation of the efficacy of treatment of congenital *T. gondii* infection is made difficult because of the high morbidity (both early and late) and mortality rates associated with this congenital infection; most workers are understandably reluctant to perform studies that would entail withholding specific therapy. Evaluation of treatment is difficult because of variations in severity and outcome of the infection and the disease. The parasite probably is never completely eliminated by specific therapy, and cure of disease (in contrast with infection) in humans apparently depends on the strain of parasite

involved, the organs infected, and the time during the course of infection when treatment is initiated. The agents that can be recommended for specific therapy at present are beneficial against the tachyzoite form, but none has been shown to effectively eradicate the encysted form, especially from the CNS and eye.

Neuroradiologic Follow-up Evaluation After Shunt Placement

Because it has not been possible to determine with certainty at the time of presentation what the response to shunt placement and antimicrobial therapy will be, a therapeutic approach expectant for good outcome is recommended for most infants with congenital toxoplasmosis. It often is difficult to predict whether such therapy will result in brain cortical growth and expansion. A follow-up CT scan in the perioperative period after shunt placement to assess adequacy of drainage and whether subdural collections have occurred is advisable and may be useful prognostically.

Specific Therapy
Pyrimethamine Plus Sulfonamides

Pyrimethamine, a substituted phenylpyrimidine antimalarial drug (Daraprim), brings about not only survival but also a radical cure of animals with experimental *T. gondii* infection. The persistence of this medicine in the blood was recognized many years ago in patients who received antimalarial prophylaxis with 25-mg weekly doses. The plasma half-life in adults is approximately 100 hours [769–772]. Pyrimethamine pharmacokinetics in newborns and those younger than 1.5 years of age have been reported (Fig. 31–33) [773]. Pyrimethamine serum half-life in infants is approximately 60 hours. Pyrimethamine dosages of 1 mg/kg per day yield serum drug levels of approximately 1000 to 2000 ng/mL 4 hours after a dose. Dosages of 1 mg/kg each Monday, Wednesday, and Friday yield serum levels of approximately 500 ng/mL 4 hours after a dose. Serum levels at intervals after these two dosages are shown in Figure 31–26. Cerebrospinal fluid levels are 10% to 20% of concomitant serum levels. Phenobarbital induces hepatic enzymes that degrade pyrimethamine, and phenobarbital therapy resulted in lower serum levels and shortened the half-life of pyrimethamine. Pyrimethamine plus sulfadiazine therapy has been associated with resolution of signs of active congenital toxoplasmosis, usually within the first weeks after initiation of therapy [773]. Favorable outcomes for newborns with substantial disease (e.g., microcephaly, multiple cerebral calcifications, hydrocephalus, meningoencephalitis, thrombocytopenia, hepatosplenomegaly, active chorioretinitis) have been associated with therapy during the first year of life, which resulted in pyrimethamine levels that ranged from 300 to 2000 ng/mL 4 hours after a dose [773]. Seizures have been reported in association with pyrimethamine serum levels of approximately 5000 ng/mL (Hoff R, personal communication to McLeod R, 1986). The inhibitory concentration (IC) and cidal concentration are dependent on the assay system used, the strain of parasite, and the time over which the assay is performed [773,774]. In a

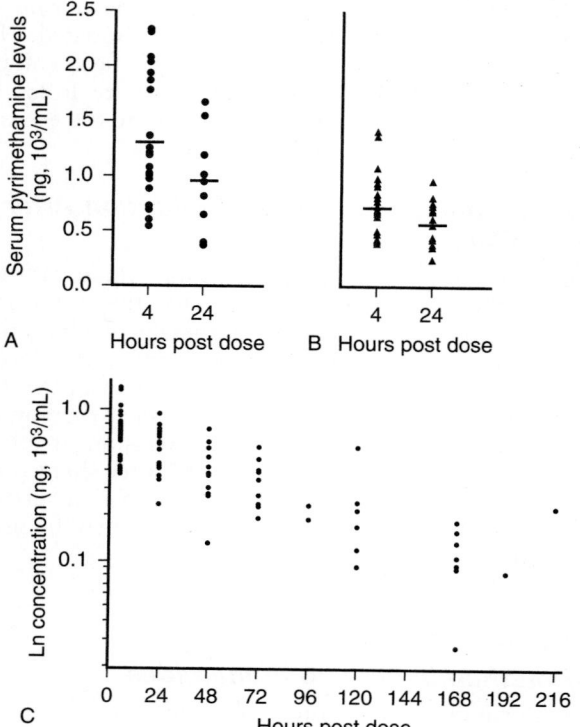

FIGURE 31–33 **Serum pyrimethamine levels obtained in infants with congenital *Toxoplasma* infection. A,** Pyrimethamine serum levels (4 and 24 hours after a dose) of children given 1 mg of pyrimethamine per kg daily. **B,** Pyrimethamine serum levels (4 and 24 hours after a dose) of children given 1 mg of pyrimethamine per kg on Monday, Wednesday, and Friday of each week. Values for children taking phenobarbital are not included. **C,** Pyrimethamine levels in sera of the entire population of infants taking 1 mg of pyrimethamine per kg on Monday, Wednesday, and Friday of each week. Values for children taking phenobarbital are not included. *(Data from McLeod R, et al. Levels of pyrimethamine in sera and cerebrospinal and ventricular fluids from infants treated for congenital toxoplasmosis. Antimicrob Agents Chemother 36:1040–1048, 1992.)*

study by McLeod and her colleagues, levels of pyrimethamine and sulfadiazine alone and in combination that inhibited growth of the type I RH strain of *T. gondii* in vitro after 24 hours were pyrimethamine IC_{50}, 100 ng/mL; sulfadiazine IC_{90}, 6.25 µg/mL; and pyrimethamine plus sulfadiazine IC_{90}, 25 ng/mL and 6.25 µg/mL [773].

Pyrimethamine and sulfadiazine act synergistically against *T. gondii*, with a combined activity eightfold that expected for merely additive effects [775–777]. Consequently, the simultaneous use of both drugs is indicated in all cases. Comparative tests have shown that sulfapyrazine, sulfamethazine, and sulfamerazine are about as effective as sulfadiazine [778,779]. All of the other sulfonamides tested (sulfathiazole, sulfapyridine, sulfadimidine, sulfisoxazole) are much less effective and are not recommended. For dosage recommendations, see Table 31–33. Sulfadiazine is used in addition to pyrimethamine. Appropriate dosing of pyrimethamine, sulfadiazine, and leucovorin in infants can be difficult because pediatric suspensions are not commercially available. The method shown in Figure 31–34 [433] was developed to facilitate administration of these medications to infants

in the NCCCTS. It is suggested that treating congenital toxoplasmosis in infants in the United States be done in conjunction with the NCCCTS to facilitate obtaining knowledge concerning optimal medication dosages and outcome of treatment of the congenital infection and disease. The NCCCTS treatment regimen is summarized in Tables 31–33 and 31–34, and in Figure 31–34. An alternative method, which incorporates pyrimethamine, sulfadiazine, and spiramycin, formerly was used extensively for treatment in infants in France. Treatment for the fetus in utero, by maternal therapy with pyrimethamine, sulfadiazine, and leucovorin (see "Outcome of Treatment of the Fetus in Utero," later on) (Fig. 31–35), has been followed by treatment during the first year of life.

Dorangeon and coworkers studied the transplacental passage of the combination pyrimethamine-sulfadoxine (Fansidar) by measuring drug levels in mother and neonate at time of delivery [780]. They noted that the levels of pyrimethamine in the newborn were 50% to 100% and those of sulfadoxine essentially 100% of the maternal levels, depending on when the drug was last administered to the mother. The authors recognized the limitations of their study; they did not evaluate levels in the fetus at different times during gestation, when adequate drug levels are especially critical.

Villena and colleagues, in France, have reported an extensive experience with pyrimethamine-sulfadoxine treatment of congenital toxoplasmosis in the infant and in the mother when prenatal diagnosis was positive [99,763]. Although in the United States pyrimethamine-sulfadoxine is at present not recommended for use in pregnant women, newborns, or children with *T. gondii* infection, this drug combination is increasingly being used in Europe. For this reason, the studies by Trenque and colleagues in Reims, France, are summarized here [781].

To evaluate the ratio of fetal to maternal concentrations of the drugs (F/M ratio), these investigators studied placental transfer of pyrimethamine and sulfadoxine at the end of gestation in 10 women who had seroconverted during pregnancy and had been taking the drug combination by mouth twice monthly along with folinic acid. Blood samples were collected at delivery from the mother and from the umbilical vein. The F/M ratios for pyrimethamine and sulfadoxine ranged from 0.43 to 1.03 (mean ± SD = 0.66 ± 0.22) and from 0.65 to 1.16 (mean ± SD = 0.97 ± 0.14), respectively. The patients had steady-state drug concentrations at the time of study. Concentrations of pyrimethamine in the fetus ranged from 50% to 100% (mean 66%) of simultaneous serum concentrations in the mothers. These results agree with those obtained in monkeys by Schoondermark-van de Ven and coworkers [782]. Trenque and colleagues concluded that the effective concentrations of both drugs at 14 days after the last dose justifies twice-monthly dosing of the drug combination in cases of documented fetal infection [781].

Preliminary follow-up studies [99,763,783] suggest that such treatment with Fansidar (1.25 mg/kg of pyrimethamine each 14 or each 10 days after treatment for the fetus in utero by treatment of the mother) may lead to a lower incidence of subsequent ocular disease with fewer

TABLE 31–33 Guidelines for Treatment of *Toxoplasma gondii* Infection in the Pregnant Woman and Congenital *Toxoplasma* Infection in the Fetus, Infant, and Older Child

Infection	Medication	Dosage	Duration of Therapy
In pregnant women infected during gestation			
First 18 wk of gestation or until term if fetus found not to be infected by amniocentesis at 18 wk	Spiramycin*	1 g every 8 hr without food	Until fetal infection is documented or until it is excluded at 18 wk of gestation (see also text)
If fetal infection confirmed after wk 18 of gestation and in all women infected after wk 24 (see text)	Pyrimethamine[†] *plus*	Loading dose: 50 mg each 12 hours for 2 days; then beginning on day 3, 50 mg per day	Until term[‡]
	Sulfadiazine *plus*	Loading dose: 75 mg/kg; then beginning 50 mg/kg each 12 hr (maximum 4 g/day)	Until term[‡]
	Leucovorin (folinic acid)[†]	10–20 mg daily[§]	During and for 1 wk after pyrimethamine therapy
Congenital *T. gondii* infection in the infant[§]	Pyrimethamine[†,§] *plus*	Loading dose: 1 mg/kg each 12 hours for 2 days; then beginning on day 3, 1 mg/kg per day for 2 or 6 mo[§]; then this dose every Monday, Wednesday, Friday[§]	1 yr[§]
	Sulfadiazine[‖] *plus*	50 mg/kg each 12 hr	1 yr[§]
	Leucovorin[†]	10 mg three times weekly	During and for 1 wk after pyrimethamine therapy
	Corticosteroids[¶] (prednisone) have been used when CSF protein is ≥1 g/dL and when active chorioretinitis threatens vision	0.5 mg/kg each 12 hr	Corticosteroids are continued until resolution of elevated (≥1 g/dL) CSF protein level or active chorioretinitis that threatens vision
Active chorioretinitis in older children	pyrimethamine[†] *plus*	Loading dose: 1 mg/kg each 12 hr (maximum 50 mg) for 2 days; then beginning on day 3, maintenance, 1 mg/kg per day (maximum 25 mg)	Usually 1–2 wk beyond the time that signs and symptoms have resolved
	Sulfadiazine[‖] *plus*	Loading dose: 75 mg/kg; then beginning 12 hr later, maintenance, 50 mg/kg every 12 hours	Usually 1–2 wk beyond the time that signs and symptoms have resolved
	Leucovorin[†]	10–20 mg three times weekly[†]	During and for 1 wk after pyrimethamine therapy
	Corticosteroids[¶] (prednisone)	1 mg/kg/day, divided bid; maximum 40 mg per day followed by rapid taper	Steroids are continued until inflammation subsides (usually 1–2 wk) and then tapered rapidly

Available only on request from the U.S. Food and Drug Administration (telephone number 301-443-5680), and then with this approval by physician's request to Aventis (908-231-3365).
[†]*Adjusted for megaloblastic anemia, granulocytopenia, or thrombocytopenia; blood cell counts, including platelets, should be monitored as described in text.*
[‡]*Subsequent treatment of the infant is the same as that described under treatment of congenital infection. When the diagnosis of infection in the fetus is established earlier, we suggest that sulfadiazine be used alone until after the first trimester, at which time pyrimethamine should be added to the regimen. The decision about when to begin pyrimethamine/sulfadiazine/leucovorin for the pregnant woman is based on an assessment of the risk of fetal infection, incidence of false-positive and false-negative results of amniocentesis with PCR assay, and risks associated with medicines. Although reliability of PCR assay results is laboratory dependent, results from the best reference laboratories, have a sensitivity for detection of the T. gondii 300 copy 529 base pair (bp) amniotic fluid PCR assay of 92% (see text). Thus PCR assay results reasonably determine therapeutic approach. (Data from reference (Wallon, et al, Obstet Gynecol, 2010)). With maternal acquisition of infection after 31 weeks of gestation, incidence of transmission exceeds 60%, and manifestations of infection are in general less severe. When infection is acquired between 21 and 29 weeks of gestation, management varies. After 24 weeks of gestation, we recommend that amniocentesis be performed and that pyrimethamine/leucovorin/sulfadiazine be used instead of spiramycin. Consultation with the reference laboratory is advised.*

In France, standard of care (until late in gestation) is to wait 4 weeks from the estimated time maternal infection is acquired until amniocentesis, to allow sufficient time for transmission to occur. Amniocentesis is not performed before 17 to 18 weeks of gestation. In some instances, when maternal infection is acquired between 12 and 16 weeks of gestation or after the 21st week of gestation, pyrimethamine and sulfadiazine treatment is initiated regardless of the amniotic fluid PCR result (see text for discussion). When this approach is used, a delay in amniocentesis when maternal infection is acquired between 12 and 16 weeks and after 21 weeks of gestation would not be logical.
[§]*Optimal dosage, feasibility, and toxicity currently are being evaluated in the ongoing Chicago-based National Collaborative Treatment Trial (NCTT) (telephone number 773-834-4131).*

These two regimens are currently being compared in a randomized manner in the NCTT. Data are not yet available to determine which, if either, is superior. Both regimens appear to be feasible and relatively safe.

The duration of therapy is unknown for infants and children, especially those with AIDS. See section on congenital Toxoplasma infection and AIDS.
[‖]*Alternative medicines for patients with atopy or severe intolerance of sulfonamides have included pyrimethamine and leucovorin with clindamycin, or azithromycin, or atovaquone, with standard dosages as recommended according to weight.*
[¶]*Corticosteroids should be used only in conjunction with pyrimethamine, sulfadiazine, and leucovorin treatment and should be continued until signs of inflammation (high CSF protein, ≥1 g/dL) or active chorioretinitis that threatens vision have subsided; dosage can then be tapered and the steroids discontinued.*
AIDS, acquired immunodeficiency syndrome; CI, confidence interval; CSF, cerebrospinal fluid.

TABLE 31-34   Oral Suspension Formulations for Pyrimethamine and Sulfadiazine in the United States

*Pyrimethamine, 2-mg/mL Suspension**

1. Crush four 25-mg pyrimethamine tablets in a mortar to a fine powder.
2. Add 10 mL of syrup vehicle.†
3. Transfer mixture to an amber bottle.
4. Rinse mortar with 10 mL of sterile water and transfer.
5. Add enough of the serum vehicle to make a final volume of 50 mL.
6. Shake very well until this is a fine suspension.
7. Label and give a 7-day expiration.
8. Store refrigerated.

Sulfadiazine, 100-mg/mL Suspension‡

1. Crush ten 500-mg sulfadiazine tablets in a mortar to a fine powder.
2. Add enough sterile water to make a smooth paste.
3. Slowly titrate the syrup vehicle† close to the final volume of 50 mL.
4. Transfer the suspension to a larger amber bottle.
5. Add sufficient syrup vehicle to make a final volume of 50 mL.
6. Shake well.
7. Label and give a 7-day expiration.
8. Store refrigerated.

*Pyrimethamine: 25-mg tablets (Daraprim, Glove Wellcome Inc.) NDC #0173-0201-55.
†Syrup vehicle: suggest 2% sugar suspension for pyrimethamine. If the infant is not lactose intolerant, 2% sugar suspension can be 2 g lactose per 100 mL distilled water. Suggest simple syrup or, alternatively, cherry syrup for sulfadiazine suspension.
‡Sulfadiazine: 500-mg tablets (Eon Labs Manufacturing, Inc.) NDC #00185-0757-01.

sequelae than described for untreated children in the earlier literature [356,784]. Randomization, statistical analysis, or long-term follow-up appears to be lacking in these studies, and whether there was consistency in the evaluations was not specified.

Issues of dosing, pharmacokinetics, serum and tissue levels, efficacy, toxicity, and safety are relevant to considerations concerning use of Fansidar to treat congenital toxoplasmosis [785]. Sulfadoxine was found to be less active than sulfadiazine when sulfonamides were tested in vitro either alone or in conjunction with pyrimethamine against a standard laboratory strain, the type I RH strain of *T. gondii*. Concentrations of pyrimethamine alone or in conjunction with sulfadiazine that were needed to inhibit *T. gondii* were greater than 25 ng/mL [773,786]. Although the clinical relevance of these in vitro tests is not known, it seems that brain and retinal tissue trough levels (i.e., minimum levels) should exceed this minimum amount, unless both other data correlating outcomes with lower tissue levels using a variety of strains of *T. gondii* and clinical trials were to demonstrate that lower levels are beneficial. The observation that cerebrospinal fluid levels of pyrimethamine were 10% to 25% of serum pyrimethamine levels in infants with congenital toxoplasmosis therefore is relevant [773]. The serum levels of pyrimethamine following 1.25 mg of Fansidar

Weigh baby *each* week.
Increase medications accordingly.

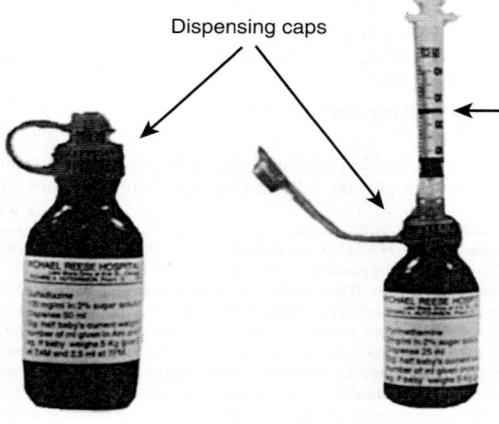

Dispensing caps

Medication syringe marked with number of mL to be given in each dose during that week.

	Sample label:	Sample label:	Sample label:
Medication:	Sulfadiazine	Pyrimethamine	Folinic acid (calcium leukovorin)
Concentration:	100mg/mL*	2mg/mL*	5mg tablets
Dispense:	50mL	25mL	30 tablets
Dosage:	Sig: half baby's current weight equals number of mL given in AM and PM. e.g., if baby weighs 5Kg give 2.5mL at 7AM and 2.5mL at 7PM.	Sig: half baby's current weight in Kg equals number of mL given once each day. e.g., if baby weighs 5Kg give 2.5mL daily.	Sig: 10mg (2 tablets) on Monday, Wednesday and Friday. Crush and give with formula or apple juice in one dosage.

* Suspended in 2% sugar solution. Suspension at usual concentration must be made up each week. Store refrigerated.

FIGURE 31-34   Preparation of pyrimethamine, sulfadiazine, and leucovorin in treatment of congenital toxoplasmosis. *(Adapted from McAuley J, et al. Early and longitudinal evaluations of treated infants and children and untreated historical patients with congenital toxoplasmosis: the Chicago collaborative treatment trial. Clin Infect Dis 18:38–72, 1994.)*

Diagnosis of mother:	Systematic serologic screening, before conception and intrapartum
Treatment of mother:	If acute serology, spiramycin reduces transmission Untreated 94 (60%) of 154 vs. treated 91 (23%) of 388*
Treatment of fetus:	Pyrimethamine, sulfadiazine, or termination N=54 livebirths; 34 terminations†
Diagnosis of fetus:	Ultrasounds; amniocentesis, PCR at 18 weeks' gestation Sensitivity 37 (97%) of 38: specificity 301 of 301‡
Outcome	All 54 normal development; initial report was 19% subtle findings: 7 (13%) intracranial calcifications, 3 (6%) chorioretinal scars§; follow up of 18 chilldren (median age 4.5 yr; range, 1-11 yr): 39% retinal scars, most scars were peripheral‖

*From Desmonts and Couvreur.[116]
†From Daffos, et al.[130]
‡From Hohlfeld, et al.; sensitivity is less before 17 and after 21 weeks' gestation.[125]
§From Hohlfeld, et al.[124]
‖From Brezin, et al.[1154]

FIGURE 31–35 Paris approach to prenatal prevention, diagnosis, and treatment. *(Adapted from Roberts F, McLeod R, Boyer K. Toxoplasmosis. In Katz S, Gershon A, Hotez P [eds]. Krugman's Infectious Diseases of Children, 10th ed. 2004 St Louis, CV Mosby, with minor modifications and permission.)*

administered every 14 days to infants were approximately 350 ng/mL peak and 25 ng/mL trough [780]. Thus cerebrospinal fluid, brain, and retinal levels may not exceed 25 ng/mL for much of the time during which this dosage regimen is administered. Consequently, potential therapeutic brain and retinal levels may not be achieved for substantial periods with twice-monthly dosing, and thus this regimen may not be effective for treatment.

Administration of Fansidar every 2 weeks is a more convenient regimen than daily administration of pyrimethamine and sulfadiazine and is routinely used in many areas of France [785]. No hematologic toxicity was reported when this regimen was administered [763], in contrast with relatively frequent but easily reversible neutropenia (requiring frequent hematologic monitoring) in children given 1 mg/kg of pyrimethamine daily or three times each week [433,773]. Serious and life-threatening toxicity has been reported with use of Fansidar in other clinical settings, and this finding has led to reluctance on the part of some investigators and physicians to recommend its use when other medicines, especially sulfonamides with shorter half-lives, are equally or potentially more effective [786]. No such serious side effects have been reported in the studies of congenital toxoplasmosis treated with Fansidar, but although the incidence of lethal hepatotoxicity [787] is estimated to be quite low, the numbers of women and children who have received treatment with this drug to date are not sufficient to exclude the possibility that it may occur [783,788,789].

Trenque and coworkers in Reims and Marseilles, France [790], studied population pharmacokinetics of pyrimethamine and sulfadoxine in 89 children between 1 week and 13.9 years of age (weighing 3 to 59 kg) with congenital toxoplasmosis treated with Fansidar two or three times a month. The authors report that influence of weight, but not age, on pyrimethamine pharmacokinetics was significant in young children.

Both pyrimethamine and the sulfonamides are potentially toxic. Because most physicians are familiar with untoward reactions to sulfonamides (e.g., crystalluria, hematuria and hypersensitivity, marrow suppression), only the toxic effects of pyrimethamine are considered here. Serum levels of sulfadiazine were similar when the drug was administered in two or four divided doses daily to eight patients infected with HIV (mean age, 43 years; range, 38 to 56 years) [791].

Toxic Effects of Pyrimethamine

Pyrimethamine inhibits dihydrofolate reductase, which is important in the synthesis of folic acid, thus producing reversible and usually gradual depression of the bone marrow [792,793]. Reversible neutropenia is the most frequent toxic effect, although platelet depression and anemia may occur as well. Other, less serious side effects are gastrointestinal distress, headaches, and a bad taste in the mouth. Accidental overdosing in infants has resulted in vomiting, tremors, convulsions, and bone marrow depression [794]. All patients who receive pyrimethamine should have a peripheral blood cell and platelet count twice each week. Folinic acid (in the form of leucovorin calcium) has been used to protect the bone marrow from toxic effects of pyrimethamine [162,795]. We usually administer 5 to 20 mg of leucovorin calcium each Monday, Wednesday, and Friday or even daily in infants or young children. The usual dosage in older children and adults is 10 to 20 mg/day orally.

Data suggesting that oral leucovorin calcium can be used to reverse the toxic effects of pyrimethamine have been presented. Nixon and Bertino clearly demonstrated that leucovorin calcium in tablet form was well absorbed (in adult subjects), thereby expanding the serum pool of reduced folates [796]. Under fasting conditions, the quantitative absorption of the orally administered preparation was close to 90%. The parenteral form (calcium leucovorin used for injection) may be ingested with equal effectiveness (Masur CJ, Lederle Laboratories, written communication to Remington JS, 1975). These substances, in contrast with folic acid, do not appear to inhibit the action of pyrimethamine on the proliferative form of *T. gondii* because of an active transport mechanism for folinic acid [797], and thus may be used in conjunction with the latter drug to allay toxicity.

Garin and colleagues used Fansidar in a small number of infants and consider this agent to be well tolerated, with a much simpler treatment regimen [798–800]. This antimicrobial combination is now widely used in Europe. The potential for serious toxicity of medication with a half-life as long as that of sulfadoxine has led others to avoid this regimen. Whether its potential for toxicity is as great in infants as in adults is not known.

Teratogenic Effects of Pyrimethamine

In experiments with pyrimethamine, Thiersch reported an effect on rat fetuses ranging from stunting to death, depending on the amount of pyrimethamine administered to the mothers during pregnancy [801]. The effect on the fetuses could be moderated, with a higher yield of live litters but also of stunted and malformed animals, when the mother was given leucovorin calcium at the time of drug administration. The malformations resulted from enormous doses (e.g., 12 mg/kg, compared with the usual dose in humans of 0.5 to 1 mg/kg) and were similar to those obtained with closely related folic acid analogues: general stunting of growth, general hydrops, cranial bone defects, incomplete cranial and brain development, rachischisis, internal hydrocephalus, ventral hernias, situs inversus, and combinations of all of these. An even more severe teratogenic effect was reported in the studies of Anderson and Morse, who similarly employed doses far higher than could ever be employed in humans [802]. Similar studies in rats are those of Dyban and associates [803,804]. In another study in rats, Krahe used doses more comparable to those employed in humans and noted fetal resorption but no teratogenic effects after large doses of pyrimethamine [805]. In 1971, Sullivan and Takacs pointed out the lack of comparative data on the teratogenic effects of pyrimethamine in different mammalian species [806]—a lack that adds to the difficulty in estimating the extent of teratogenic risk in humans. Their results in rats and hamsters emphasize the shortcomings of attempts to determine a safe clinical dose on the basis of tests limited to a single species of test animal. The drug was less teratogenic in golden hamsters than in Wistar rats. About 70% of rat fetuses were dead or malformed (the malformations included brachygnathia, cleft palate, oligodactyly, and phocomelia) as a result of administration of single oral doses of 5 mg (approximately 20 mg/kg) to pregnant females. Less than 10% of hamster fetuses died or were malformed after similar doses that on a milligram-per-kilogram basis were eight to nine times greater than those given to rats. Repeated doses nearer to those used in humans also were teratogenic in rats but not in hamsters. These investigators also demonstrated that folinic acid can significantly reduce the incidence of dead and malformed fetuses when administered during pyrimethamine treatment.

Puchta and Simandlova, using doses of 2, 5, and 10 mg/kg in rats, could demonstrate no malformations in rat fetuses [807]. Their results are in marked contrast with those of most other workers, and the differences remain to be explained.

In all of these studies, pyrimethamine was administered during the period of early organogenesis, which is the period of maximum susceptibility to damage by teratogenic agents.

Spiramycin

Spiramycin, a macrolide antibiotic that is available to physicians in the United States only by request to the FDA, has an antibacterial spectrum comparable to that of erythromycin and is active against *T. gondii*, as demonstrated in animal experiments [808,809]. In vitro studies also have been reported [810]. The actual concentration necessary to inhibit growth of or kill the organism is unknown. It has been described as having exceptional persistence in the tissues [811,812] in comparison with erythromycin, oleandomycin, or carbomycin. Such high tissue levels may account for the observations that spiramycin is much more active in vivo against susceptible bacteria than is erythromycin, despite higher serum levels attained with comparable doses of erythromycin and greater sensitivity of the bacteria to erythromycin in vitro [813]. A review of this antimicrobial agent has been published [814].

Spiramycin is supplied as a syrup and in capsules. The usual daily dose in adults is 1 g, three times a day. Garin and coworkers studied drug concentrations in serum, cord serum, and placenta in pregnant women [815]. On a daily regimen of 2 g by mouth, the average levels were 1.19 µg/mL (range, 0.50 to 2.0 µg/mL), 0.63 µg/mL (range, 0.20 to 1.8 µg/mL), and 2.75 µg/mL (range, 0.70 to 5.0 µg/mL), respectively. On a dosage schedule of 3 g daily, the results were 1.69 µg/mL (range, 1 to 4 µg/mL), 0.78 µg/mL (range, 0.75 to 2.0 µg/mL), and 6.2 µg/mL (range, 3.25 to 10 µg/mL), respectively. (These serum levels in the mother are similar to those obtained by Hudson and colleagues at 2 and 4 hours after a given dose in persons receiving 1 g every 6 hours [816]. Thus a total dose of 3 g daily resulted in levels in the placenta that were twice as high as those attained with a total dose of 2 g daily. (This is one reason for the recommendation of 3 g administered as a 1-g thrice-daily dose during gestation.) In both regimens, the concentration in cord serum was approximately one half and the placental levels approximately three to five times greater than the level in the corresponding maternal serum. The investigators stated that the levels achieved in the placenta are ample for treatment of *T. gondii* in that organ, but whether the levels in cord serum are sufficient for treatment of the fetus in utero remains to be verified. Forestier and associates published another study of spiramycin concentrations in the mother and the fetus (fetal blood sampling) [817].

Spiramycin pharmacokinetics exhibits individual variation. Fetomaternal concentrations were studied in 20 cases of maternal infection acquired between weeks 3 and 10 of pregnancy and treated with a daily dose of 3 g. The maternal plasma concentrations of spiramycin were 0.682 ± 0.132 mg/L in the first month of treatment; 0.618 ± 0.102 mg/L during weeks 20 to 24 of pregnancy; and 1.015 ± 0.22 mg/L in the sixth month. The mean fetal concentration was 0.290 mg/L during weeks 20 to

24 of pregnancy (i.e., 47% of maternal values), with a lack of correlation between mothers and fetuses. At birth, the placental concentration (2.3 µg/mL) was four times the average blood concentration in mothers (0.47 mg/L) and six and one half times the cord blood values (0.34 mg/L). A good correlation was found between maternal blood and placental values, and a fair correlation between cord blood and placental values. These facts suggest that monitoring of spiramycin treatment by measuring maternal spiramycin blood concentrations might be useful in determining effective individual dosage [69].

Very little definitive information is available on the efficacy of spiramycin in congenital toxoplasmosis in the newborn. In a study of 12 cases (mainly of severe clinical disease) by Martin and coworkers in which spiramycin was employed, the data are impossible to interpret because tetracyclines, pyrimethamine, sulfonamides, and corticosteroids frequently were also used in the same infants [818].

In a carefully designed study by Beverley and colleagues, congenitally infected mice were given spiramycin or a combination of sulfadimidine and pyrimethamine from the age of 4 to 8 weeks [819]. The levels of spiramycin in the heart, liver, kidney, and spleen were approximately 50 to 140 times greater than the serum levels after 4 weeks of treatment. Both treatment regimens were effective in preventing the histopathologic changes noted in congenitally infected mice not given treatment. Regardless of the form of treatment, a smaller number of cysts were found in the brains of mice that received treatment than in those of mice receiving no treatment (probably because treatment prevented the development of new cysts, rather than destroying cysts formed before initiation of therapy). The authors suggested that because spiramycin was as effective as the potentially toxic combination of pyrimethamine and sulfadimidine, it will be found to be preferable to the combination agent in treatment of congenital toxoplasmosis.

Because the optimal dose and route of administration of spiramycin in infants and adults have never been established for toxoplasmosis, the study by Back and coworkers on the pharmacology of parenteral spiramycin as an antineoplastic agent is pertinent [820]. Twelve patients with various types of far-advanced neoplastic diseases were given daily intravenous doses ranging from 5 to 160 mg/kg. Doses greater than 35 mg/kg produced local vasospasm, a feeling of coolness, strange taste, vertigo, dizziness, flushing of the face, tearing of the eyes, nausea, vomiting, diarrhea, and anorexia. No hematologic toxicity, electrocardiographic changes, or impairment of liver or kidney function were noticed. Of note, Q-T interval prolongation and life-threatening arrhythmias (cardiac arrest) were reported in two neonates receiving spiramycin (300,000 IU/kg per day by mouth) [821]. The infants recovered completely after immediate cardiopulmonary resuscitation maneuvers.

At present, the only indication for which we use spiramycin is in the actively infected mother to attempt to reduce transmission to her fetus [822]. It should be noted that spiramycin failed to prevent neurotoxoplasmosis in immunosuppressed patients [823]. Spiramycin may reduce the severity of infection in a fetus because it delays transmission to a later time in gestation when transmission is associated with less severe manifestations of infection. Lacking are data that conclusively demonstrate efficacy of spiramycin in treatment of the infected fetus. The controversy of whether spiramycin prevents transmission of *T. gondii* to the fetus is discussed later under "Serologic Screening" in the "Prevention" section. The subject has more recently been commented on by Montoya and Liesenfeld [824].

Other Drugs

At present, no clinical data are available to allow for recommendation of any of the drugs described next for treatment of the immunocompetent pregnant patient, fetus, or newborn.

Trimethoprim Plus Sulfamethoxazole. Despite reports of successful treatment of murine toxoplasmosis with a combination of trimethoprim and sulfamethoxazole (TMP-SMX) [825,826], trimethoprim alone has been found to have less effect against *T. gondii* both in vitro and in vivo [827–830]. The combination of this drug with sulfamethoxazole is synergistic in vitro [826] but is significantly less active in vitro and in vivo than the combination of pyrimethamine and sulfonamide. Previously, a number of reports have described use of the combination in human toxoplasmosis, but whether the effect of the combination was due solely to the sulfonamide component was unclear [831–833]. A recent, randomized trial of TMP-SMX versus pyrimethamine-sulfadiazine in toxoplasmic encephalitis in patients with AIDS by Torre and colleagues [834] revealed that TMP-SMX was a valuable alternative to pyrimethamine-sulfadiazine for that purpose. In Brazil, TMP-SMX was reported to reduce the incidence of recurrent toxoplasmic chorioretinitis in 61 patients, compared with that in 63 control patients (mean ages 26 ± 10 versus 27 ± 11 years [range, 7 to 53 years]) [209,835]. Nevertheless, we do not recommend its use in the infected fetus or newborn in the absence of carefully designed trials that reveal efficacy of TMP-SMX in congenital toxoplasmosis. When parenteral therapy is essential because of gastrointestinal disease, TMP-SMX may provide a temporizing alternative treatment.

Clindamycin. Clindamycin has been shown to be effective in treatment of murine toxoplasmosis [836,837] and ocular infection in rabbits [838]. Studies are needed, however, before it can be recommended for routine treatment of congenital infection in infants or pregnant women. When this antibiotic has been used in combination with pyrimethamine in patients with AIDS who have toxoplasmic encephalitis, results have been comparable to those with pyrimethamine-sulfadiazine treatment [839,840].

Tetracyclines. Both doxycycline [841] and minocycline [842,843] have efficacy in the treatment of murine toxoplasmosis. Doxycycline was used successfully in two patients with AIDS who had toxoplasmic encephalitis when it was administered at 300 mg per day intravenously in three divided doses [844]. When doxycycline was given orally at doses of 100 mg twice a day in six of the patients who were intolerant to pyrimethamine-sulfadiazine, five patients had associated neurologic and radiologic recurrences while receiving the drug [845]. Further study of the tetracyclines in the treatment of toxoplasmosis in adults is likely to involve their use in combination with other antimicrobial agents. No data are available on their use in the newborn or young children with toxoplasmosis, nor are they recommended for this purpose.

Rifampin. Rifampin in high doses was not effective against *T. gondii* in a murine model [846].

Macrolides. Macrolides-roxithromycin [847,848], clarithromycin [849], and the azalide azithromycin [850] have been shown to have activity against *T. gondii* in vivo in a mouse model. Stray-Pedersen studied levels of azithromycin in placental tissue, amniotic fluid, and maternal and cord blood [851]. Levels in maternal serum ranged from 0.017 to 0.073 mg/mL (mean, 0.028 mg/mL). Whole blood levels were higher (mean, 0.313 mg/mL). Mean levels in amniotic fluid and cord blood were 0.040 and 0.027 mg/mL, respectively. Placental levels were higher (mean, 2.067 mg/mL). It should be understood, however, that azithromycin is concentrated in tissues and intracellularly; thus, levels at these sites probably are of greater clinical importance than serum or blood levels. When used in combination with pyrimethamine, both clarithromycin and azithromycin have been successful in treating toxoplasmic encephalitis in adult patients with AIDS [515]. In non-AIDS patients, the combination of pyrimethamine plus azithromycin has been reported by Rothova and colleagues to be equal in efficacy to pyrimethamine plus sulfadiazine measured as time to resolution of active eye disease in patients with recurrent chorioretinitis [852,853]. Ketolides also are active both in vitro and in vivo in the mouse model of toxoplasmosis [244,854,855].

Atovaquone. Atovaquone has been reported to have potent in vitro activity against both tachyzoite and cyst forms [856,857]. It significantly reduced the mortality rate in murine toxoplasmosis and had remarkable, although differing, activity against different strains of *T. gondii* [856]. Atovaquone has been used in AIDS patients with toxoplasmic encephalitis with encouraging results [858,859]. Unfortunately, relapse occurred in approximately 50% of patients in whom atovaquone was used for acute therapy and continued alone as maintenance therapy [858,859]. Seventeen of 65 patients (26%) who received atovaquone as a single agent for maintenance therapy of toxoplasmic encephalitis experienced a relapse [860]. The combination of pyrimethamine and atovaquone may prove more useful [858]. Serum levels of atovaquone in patients with toxoplasmic encephalitis were not predictive of clinical response or failure [860]. Bioavailability of the drug is improved when medication is ingested with food. The reliability of absorption of this drug continues to be a problem. Survival time was significantly better among those patients with higher steady-state plasma concentrations of the drug [859,858]. Although a new formulation of atovaquone is reported to achieve higher plasma concentrations, prospective trials are needed to compare the efficacy of this drug with that obtained in standard drug regimens. This drug should never be used alone for the treatment of the acute infection, but rather it should be given in combination with drugs such as pyrimethamine. The adverse effects observed in these studies included hepatic enzyme abnormalities (50%), rash (25%), nausea (21%), and diarrhea (19%) [860]. Between 3% and 10% of patients receiving atovaquone were reported to discontinue the drug because of rash, hepatic enzyme abnormalities, nausea, or vomiting [858,860]. Leukopenia associated with the combination of pyrimethamine and atovaquone has responded to folinic acid (leucovorin) and granulocyte colony-stimulating factor therapy [858].

Recently, Meneceur and colleagues [861] demonstrated that the susceptibility in vitro to pyrimethamine, sulfadiazine, and atovaquone among 17 strains of *T. gondii* belonging to various genotypes varied.

Fluoroquinolones. A number of fluoroquinolones have been found to be active against *T. gondii* in vitro and in vivo in a mouse model of the acute infection. Their activity may be enhanced when used in combination with pyrimethamine, sulfadiazine, clarithromycin, or atovaquone [855,862,863].

DURATION OF THERAPY

The optimal duration of therapy in congenitally infected infants is not known. Among infants who were given the combination of pyrimethamine and sulfadiazine for relatively brief periods, untoward sequelae of the disease subsequently developed [864,865]. We, and other investigators (including our colleague J. Couvreur in Paris), recommend that therapy be continued for 1 year, as outlined in Tables 31–33 and 31–34. We recommend using the combination of pyrimethamine and sulfonamide for the entire 1-year period.

In some areas of Europe, treatment is continued for the first 2 years of life. We have not noted active disease or progression of signs or symptoms when treatment is discontinued when children are 1 year of age. For the special issue of treatment of the HIV- and *T. gondii*-infected newborn of an HIV-infected mother, see "Congenital *Toxoplasma gondii* Infection and Acquired Immunodeficiency Syndrome" earlier under "Clinical Manifestations."

Treatment of the Fetus Through Treatment of the Pregnant Woman

For additional pertinent information, see "Prevention of Congenital Toxoplasmosis Through Treatment of the Pregnant Woman" and Table 31–33. When the diagnosis of infection in the fetus is established earlier than 17 weeks, we suggest that sulfadiazine be used alone until after the first trimester, at which time pyrimethamine should be added to the regimen. The decision about when to begin pyrimethamine/sulfadiazine/leucovorin for the pregnant woman is based on an assessment of the risk of fetal infection, incidence of false-positive and false-negative results of amniocentesis with PCR, and risks of medicines. Although reliability of PCR results are laboratory dependent, results from the best reference laboratories, have a sensitivity for PCR of the *T. gondii* 300 copy 529 repeat gene with amniotic fluid of 92% (See earlier). Thus PCR results reasonably determine the therapeutic approach.

When the mother becomes infected between 22 and 29 weeks of gestation, the incidence of transmission exceeds 50%, manifestations of infection in the fetus are substantial. With maternal acquisition of infection after 31 weeks of gestation, incidence of transmission exceeds 60%, manifestations of infection are in general less severe.

When infection is acquired between 21 and 29 weeks of gestation, management varies. After 24 weeks of gestation, amniocentesis may be performed and pyrimethamine/leucovorin/sulfadiazine may be used instead of spiramycin. In the United States, Consultation with the Palo ALto reference laboratory (650-326-8120. *Toxoplasma* serology) or others with expertise is advised.

In France, standard of care (until late in gestation) is to treat women with newly acquired *T. gondii* infection as soon as the diagnosis is established, but to wait 4 weeks from the estimated time that maternal infection was acquired to perform amniocentesis to allow sufficient time for transmission to occur. Amniocentesis is not performed before 17 to 18 weeks of gestation. In some instances, when maternal infection is acquired between 12 and 16 weeks of gestation or after the 21st week of gestation, pyrimethamine and sulfadiazine treatment is initiated regardless of the amniotic fluid PCR result (see text for discussion). When this approach is used, a delay in amniocentesis when maternal infection is acquired between 12 and 16 weeks and after 21 weeks of gestation would not be logical.

With the advent of prenatal diagnosis (see earlier discussion), attempts are being made to provide treatment for the infected fetus of mothers who have decided to carry their pregnancy to term by treatment of the mother with pyrimethamine and sulfadiazine. Couvreur, in close cooperation with Daffos and colleagues, has made certain observations that should prove helpful [822]. Their data suggest that spiramycin, although effective in reducing the frequency of transmission of the organism from mother to fetus, does not alter significantly the pathology of the infection in the fetus. For this reason, after week 17 of gestation, they treat with pyrimethamine-sulfadiazine for the duration of pregnancy when fetal infection has been proved or is highly probable. (In a commentary, Jeannel and coworkers raise the question of whether spiramycin was of value in the pregnancies studied by Daffos and colleagues.) [866] During this treatment period, the mother is carefully monitored for development of hematologic toxicity. If significant toxicity appears despite treatment with folinic acid, the drug combination is discontinued until the hematologic abnormalities are corrected and the drug regimen is then restarted. In their opinion, pyrimethamine (in combination with sulfonamides) appears to be the most efficacious treatment for infection in the fetus and newborn. Whether it has untoward toxic effects on the fetus, even after organogenesis has occurred, is unknown. Of importance, use of this drug combination in pregnant women has been reported to substantially reduce the subsequent clinical manifestations of the infection in the newborn and the antibody response of the fetus. Therefore, it is critical to

understand that when the mother receives pyrimethamine and sulfadiazine, and the infant appears normal, that infant may or may not be infected. Thus if infection of the fetus was not established before in utero treatment was initiated, and the infant is clinically normal, determination of whether the infant should receive treatment throughout the first year of life is difficult. Following maternal treatment, no signs of infection may be detectable in the infant at birth, but untoward sequelae may develop in later months or years. In addition, the infected newborn may not have the typical clinical or serologic features of the congenital infection. This situation creates a serious dilemma in trying to determine whether such infants should receive treatment when they are born to mothers who received treatment during pregnancy. Thus use of pyrimethamine plus sulfadiazine cannot be recommended as routine in every woman who acquires the acute infection during pregnancy.

Because of the potential for this dilemma, if there is no contraindication to performing the procedure and diagnosis is uncertain we consider it important to employ amniocentesis to determine whether the fetus is infected in cases of *T. gondii* infection acquired before the last trimester of pregnancy. Demonstration of fetal infection will allow for this combination drug regimen to be chosen for the mother and the neonate. If, however, extenuating circumstances preclude prenatal diagnosis in a mother whose infection was proved to have occurred during the second or third trimester, the same course of treatment as that used for cases in which the diagnosis has been established in the fetus may be considered because infection acquired during the second trimester is associated with the highest risk for fetal disease, and in the third trimester, with the highest rate of transmission to the fetus.

The original report by Daffos and colleagues in 1988 was the first to highlight the importance of attempting to treat the infection in the fetus to improve clinical outcome [82]. In 24 of the 39 cases of proven infection, pregnancy was terminated at the request of the mother. Toxoplasmic encephalitis was noted in each of these 24 fetuses, including those in whom the findings on ultrasound examination were normal when the pregnancy was terminated. In every case, extensive necrotic foci were present, which suggested that sequelae might have been severe were the pregnancy not terminated. These findings also strongly suggest that early transmission (before week 24) usually results in severe congenital toxoplasmosis rather than subclinical infection (see Table 31–9).

In 15 of the 39 cases of diagnosed infection, the mother decided to continue her pregnancy. In these women, maternal infection was acquired between weeks 17 and 25 of gestation; in these cases, fetal ultrasound examination results were normal. Treatment with sulfonamides and pyrimethamine was begun as soon as the diagnosis of fetal infection was established, between 8 and 17 weeks after acquisition of the infection by the mother. After delivery, the presence of congenital *T. gondii* infection was demonstrated in the 15 newborns (in one infant, the serologic test result turned totally negative but became positive again a few weeks after treatment was discontinued, indicating that the infection was only suppressed, not eradicated). The 15 infants were asymptomatic despite the presence of cerebral calcifications in 4. Funduscopic appearance was normal, as were findings on the cerebrospinal fluid examination. Children were given pharmacologic treatment after birth, and all remained asymptomatic without neurologic signs or mental retardation. Ocular fundi remained normal in 13 children; retinal lesions were noted in 1 child at 4 months of age and in another at 18 months of age. The duration of follow-up was 3 to 30 months. Thus despite rather early (before week 26) transmission of parasites from mother to fetus, infection remained either subclinical or mild in those fetuses whose mothers received pyrimethamine and sulfonamide treatment during pregnancy. Positive findings at prenatal diagnosis should be considered an indication for this therapeutic regimen, which would not usually be considered because of its potential toxicity to both fetus and mother. It should be understood that for ethical reasons, controlled trials (with "treatment" and "no treatment" groups of patients) have not been performed and may not be performed if an untreated group is required. Thus one is left with studies in which historical data are used for comparison. Comparative trials likely will be performed in the future as newer therapies are developed or to contrast outcomes of the present approach with prompt initiation of treatment without amniocentesis, especially for early gestation infections.

Subsequent Studies

Couvreur and colleagues studied the outcome in 52 cases of congenital *T. gondii* infection diagnosed by prenatal examination in mothers who then were given the pyrimethamine, sulfadiazine, and spiramycin treatment regimen described by Daffos and colleagues [76,82]. Results in these infants were compared with those obtained in 51 infants with congenital toxoplasmosis whose mothers had received only spiramycin. Treatment for the infants after birth was the same in both groups. Although these two groups were not strictly comparable, valuable information can be gleaned from such a comparison so long as the focus remains on the qualitative direction of the results, rather than on the quantitative data. Remarkable were the lesser number of isolates from the placentas, the lower IgG antibody titers at birth and at 6 months of age, the lower prevalence of positive IgM antibody tests, and the higher number of subclinical infections in

the offspring of mothers who received the pyrimethamine-sulfadiazine regimen. These data further support those discussed earlier—that treatment of the fetus is possible and that such treatment may result in a more favorable outcome if pyrimethamine—sulfadiazine is in the regimen (Table 31–35) [822].

Boulot and colleagues [867] described two cases in which women with *Toxoplasma* infection diagnosed during pregnancy subsequently received treatment with pyrimethamine plus sulfadiazine alternated with spiramycin, as described by Daffos and coworkers. Despite prolonged maternal treatment, the infants born to these women had congenital toxoplasmosis; *T. gondii* was isolated from the placentas. Although the success of treatment in the fetus will depend on a number of variables, as discussed earlier, these results serve as a note of caution in regard to the information given to parents about the effectiveness of such prenatal treatment.

In 1989, Hohlfeld and colleagues [76] updated information published earlier by their same group [82]. Because these were the first such available data, and although only relatively short-term follow-up is provided, a reasonably comprehensive presentation of their data seems justified. They reported 89 fetal infections in 86 pregnancies (39 of these infected fetuses were included in the original report by Daffos and coworkers, discussed earlier). All of the women were given spiramycin, 3 g daily, throughout their pregnancy from the time maternal infection was proved or strongly suspected on the basis of serologic studies until fetal infection was documented or considered to be highly likely. Spiramycin treatment was instituted a mean of 36 ± 27 days after the estimated onset of infection. At prenatal examination, 80 of these women had had positive specific test results, and the remaining 9 had evidence of congenital *T. gondii* infection at birth. When fetal infection was confirmed, 34 terminations were performed at the request of the parents. The mean interval between infection and the beginning of therapy for continued pregnancies was remarkably and significantly shorter than for terminated pregnancies. The terminations were considered if severe lesions (marked hydrocephaly) were present on ultrasonogram at the time of prenatal diagnosis or when maternal infection had occurred very early in pregnancy. The main reason for termination was demonstration of cerebral lesions on ultrasonograms. Of interest is that the evolution

TABLE 31–35   Outcome of In Utero Treatment for Congenitally Infected Fetuses with Spiramycin or Spiramycin Followed by Pyrimethamine and Sulfadiazine

In Utero Treatment	No. of Patients	Dates of Study	Dates of Maternal Infection*	Duration of Follow-up	No. of Isolates from Placenta	Immune Load of IgG		IgM Prevalence	No. (%) of Subclinical Infections
						At Birth	At 6 Mo		
Spiramycin	51	1972–1982	22.8 (10–35)	46.7 mo (2 mo–11 yr)	23/30 (77%)	139	137	18/26 (69%)	17/51 (33%)
Spiramycin + pyrimethamine + sulfadiazine	52	1983–1989	22.6 (10–30)	76 wk (11–46 wk)	16/38[†] (42%)	86	70	8/46 (17%)[‡]	30/52 (57%)

*Weeks of gestation.
[†]P <0.01.
[‡]P <0.001.
IgG, IgM, Immunoglobulins G, M.
Adapted from Couvreur J, et al. In utero treatment of toxoplasmic fetopathy with the combination pyrimethamine-sulfadiazine. Fetal Diagn Ther 8:45–50, 1993.

of hydrocephalus was remarkably rapid in some of the cases, with ventricular dilation observed to develop within 10 days. (Ventricular dilation is an indirect sign of the presence of lesions due to *T. gondii*.) For most of the 52 pregnancies allowed to continue, treatment with pyrimethamine and sulfadiazine for 3 weeks alternating with spiramycin for 3 weeks was instituted, along with folinic acid (leucovorin). In 47 of 54 cases, postnatal treatment consisted of courses of pyrimethamine and sulfadiazine alternating with spiramycin, except in 3 infants, in whom only spiramycin was used. The mean period of follow-up was 19 months (range, 1 to 48 months).

In that study, subclinical infection was defined as complete absence of symptoms. The benign form included isolated subclinical signs, including intracerebral calcifications, normal neurologic status, and chorioretinal scars without visual impairment. This form was found mainly in older infants observed during the follow-up period and in younger infants when retinal scars were peripheral and did not involve the macular region (Hohlfeld P, personal communication to Remington JS, 1993). The severe form included hydrocephaly, microcephaly, bilateral chorioretinitis with impaired vision, and abnormal immunologic findings.

The overall risk of fetal infection was 7%, and this risk varied with time of maternal infection, as shown in Table 31–6. A more complete breakdown by week of gestation was published by the same group of investigators in 1994 (see Table 31–7) [77]. At prenatal diagnosis, the nonspecific signs were not predictive of the severity of the fetal lesions; they were not found to differ significantly when subsequently terminated pregnancies were compared with those pregnancies that were allowed to continue. Fifty-five infants were born of the 52 pregnancies that were allowed to continue; no intrauterine growth retardation was noted. The findings are shown in Table 31–36. Each of the seven infants with cerebral calcifications had normal findings on ophthalmologic and neurologic examinations (benign form).

Attempts at isolation of the parasite from the placenta were positive in 23 cases, negative in 20, and inconclusive in 3; isolation was not attempted in 9 cases. Cord blood was positive for IgM antibodies in 8 cases, negative in 46 cases, and not examined in 1 case.

TABLE 31–36 Findings at Birth in 55 Live Infants Born of 52 Pregnancies with Prenatal Diagnosis of Congenital Toxoplasmosis

Finding	No.*	%
Subclinical infection	44/54	81
Multiple intracranial calcifications	5/54	9
Single intracranial calcification	2/54	4
Chorioretinitis scar	3/54	6
Abnormal lumbar puncture	1/54	2
Evidence of infection on inoculation of placenta	23/46	50
Positive cord blood IgM antibody	8/53	15

Numerator = number of abnormalities present at birth; denominator = total number of infants examined for abnormalities.
Adapted from Hohlfeld P, et al. Fetal toxoplasmosis: outcome of pregnancy and infant follow-up after in utero treatment. J Pediatr 115:767, 1989, with permission.

Follow-up evaluation was for 6 months to 4 years in 54 of the infants. The overall subclinical infection rate was 76%. The outcomes are shown in Table 31–37, where they are compared with those in historical controls from a study performed from 1972 to 1981 [868].

The additional information provided by this publication [76] further supports and extends the indirect evidence these authors published earlier [82], that such treatment of the fetus reduces the number of biologic signs at birth and can reduce the likelihood of severe damage in the newborn. Thus prenatal management as discussed by Hohlfeld and colleagues and previously by Daffos and coworkers appears to have resulted in an increase in the proportion of subclinical infections in first- and second-trimester infections, and in a reduction of severe congenital toxoplasmosis and a shift from benign forms to subclinical infections. In the earlier study, a large percentage of the cases had been third-trimester infections, which are known to have a better prognosis. Hohlfeld and colleagues recognized that their superior results, at least in part, may have been due to accurate diagnosis and selective termination in the few cases in which the fetuses were severely affected (2.7% of all referred cases in their experience), and to the effect of spiramycin on prevention of congenital transmission and the apparent reduction in the severity of fetal infection associated with the regimen of pyrimethamine-

TABLE 31–37 Comparison with Historical Controls (1972–1981) of Outcome in Live-Born Infants Diagnosed with Congenital *Toxoplasma* Infection in a Study of Prenatal Diagnosis (1982–1988) in Which the Mothers Were Treated with a Regimen of Pyrimethamine-Sulfadiazine Alternated with Spiramycin

	Affected Infants											
	First Trimester				Second Trimester				Third Trimester			
	1972–1981		1982–1988		1972–1981		1982–1988		1972–1981		1982–1988	
Outcome	No.	%	No.	%	No.	%	No.	%	No.	%	No.*	
Subclinical	1	10	6	67	23	37	33	77	74	68	2	
Benign	5	50	2	22	28	45	10	23	31	29	0	
Severe	4	40	1	11	11	18	0	0	3	3	0	
Total	10		9		62		43		108		2	

See text.
Adapted from Hohlfeld P, et al. Fetal toxoplasmosis: outcome of pregnancy and infant follow-up after in utero treatment. J Pediatr 115:767, 1989, with permission.

sulfadiazine. In Hohlfeld and colleagues' series, only 4% were third-trimester infections because, in the first years of their experience, prenatal diagnosis was not performed for late infections during gestation. Now that more rapid methods are available for diagnosis, the authors consider that prenatal diagnosis and treatment also may be appropriate in the third trimester.

Outcome of Treatment of the Fetus in Utero

Outcome was not uniformly favorable [738] when the algorithm of Daffos and coworkers [82] and Hohlfeld and colleagues [76] for patient care was applied. As mentioned earlier, part of the favorable outcome of Hohlfeld and colleagues can be attributed to termination of pregnancies in which the fetus had severe involvement (e.g., hydrocephalus). Nonetheless, the individual outcomes reported are better than would have been expected for first-trimester and early second-trimester infections. Almost all of the infected children from pregnancies managed according to this algorithm have demonstrated normal development, and those who have had clinical signs do not appear to have manifestations associated with significant impairment of normal function [76]. Thus at present, the approach of Daffos and Hohlfeld and their coworkers [76] appears to provide the best possible outcome.

In this series, 148 fetal infections occurred in 2030 cases of maternal infection. The only predictive feature for fetal infection was fetal gestational age at onset of infection: For infection at less than 16 weeks, 31 of 52 (60%) fetuses had ultrasonographic evidence of infection. Possible abnormal findings included ascites, pericarditis, and necrotic foci; 48% had cerebral ventricular dilation. If pregnancy was terminated, large areas of necrosis in the fetal brain were noted at fetopathologic examination. For pregnancies terminated at 17 to 23 weeks of gestation, 16 of 63 (25%) infected fetuses had signs on ultrasonographic examination; 12% had ventricular dilation. For pregnancies terminated later than 24 weeks, 1 of 33 fetuses had signs on ultrasonographic evaluation. Hydrocephalus was not observed. Thus these investigators offer termination at less than 16 weeks of gestation (See Table 31–8).

In the Paris studies, when mothers were found to be infected well before 16 weeks of gestation (i.e., in the first weeks of gestation) and the fetus was found to be infected by amniocentesis at 17 to 18 weeks of gestation, many of the pregnancies were terminated. Almost uniformly the fetus was found to have brain necrosis; 48% had cerebral ventricular dilation (see Table 31–8) [82]. By contrast, Wallon and coworkers [869] do not terminate pregnancies of women who are acutely infected after 13 weeks of gestation, and who receive treatment, unless fetal brain ultrasonographic findings are markedly abnormal. Their approach is based on the fact that most infected children in their series were not severely impaired. In their experience with 116 congenitally infected children, only 2 children (2%) demonstrated some degree of visual impairment due to macular lesions, and these children had no neurologic or mental deficits. In this series, 31 (27%) were found to have cerebral calcifications or retinal lesions, but these children were neurologically and developmentally normal and without severe impairment of vision.

Mirlesse (personal communication to the authors, 1998 and 2004) described the outcome in 141 infected fetuses without cerebral dilation who received both prenatal and postnatal treatment. Neonatal data were available in 133 cases, and 104 children were observed for a mean of 31 months. Two children died of malignant hyperthermia, 1 child had seizures, 1 child had a psychiatric disorder, and 12 had new eye lesions that developed between 6 months and 2 years of age. Sixteen (12%) of 133 children had eye lesions when they were born (Table 31–38).

Prenatally, fetal ultrasound examinations were performed fortnightly, and head ultrasonographic evaluations and sometimes brain CT also were performed in the newborn period for some of the infants. The prenatal ultrasonographic evaluation was performed through the endovaginal route, using a 7-MHz probe, when there was a cephalic presentation of the fetus.

Of 133 children, hyperechogenic areas (HEAs) were present in 37 (26%), and HEAs were identified antenatally in 17 of 37 (46%). HEAs were never seen before 29 to 30 weeks of gestation. Ultrasound examinations underestimated lesions identified by CT at birth in 6 cases.

An important finding was that more fetuses demonstrated HEAs on CT scans if there was a longer interval between diagnosis of maternal and fetal infection (see Table 31–38). This finding could be explained in two alternative ways. It could be that longer delays in diagnosis and treatment were associated with infections acquired earlier in gestation when disease is more severe and thus there are more associated sequelae. Alternatively, more rapid diagnosis and treatment reduced sequelae.

Another important implication of these investigators' findings is that HEAs and their correlation with more frequent ophthalmologic disease demonstrate homogeneity of neurosensory involvement. In the NCCCTS, this frequent concordance of neurologic and ophthalmologic involvement also was noted. HEA predicts ophthalmologic abnormalities, but such abnormalities are not always present. Developmental outcome in these children who received treatment, whether HEAs were present or not, was normal (see Table 31–38).

Sequelae of Congenital Toxoplasmosis in Children Who Received No Treatment
Stanford-Alabama Study

Results of a collaborative study performed in the United States suggest that adverse sequelae develop in a very significant number of children born with subclinical congenital *T. gondii* infection [361]. In this study, the children were divided into two groups on the basis of indications for which serologic studies for toxoplasmosis were initially performed. Group I consisted of 13 children: Of these, 8 cases were detected as a result of routine screening of cord serum for IgM *T. gondii* antibodies [328] and as a result of testing for IgG and IgM antibodies to *T. gondii*. These tests were performed either because acute *T. gondii* infection was diagnosed during pregnancy or at term in the mother or because the children were screened for non-specific abnormalities in the newborn period. Although each of these 13 children was carefully evaluated, none

TABLE 31–38   Significant Correlations of Brain Hyperechogenic Areas in Fetal and Newborn Ultrasound Studies with Other Clinical Aspects of Congenital Toxoplasmosis

Clinical Feature	Cerebral Hyperechogenicity*		Total or [Significance of Difference]
	Present	Absent	
Interval between diagnosis of maternal and fetal infection	8.5 wk	6.5 wk	[P = .03]
Interval between maternal infection and institution of pyrimethamine-sulfadiazine treatment	9.5 wk	8.5 wk	[P = .06]
Ocular lesions	9/37 (24%)†	7/96 (7%)	16/133 (12%) [P <.008]
New eye lesions	7/37 (18%)	5/67 (7%)	12/104 (12%) [P <.058]

*See ultrasound for hyperechogenicity.
†Number with finding/number in group (%). Maximum duration of follow-up was until 2 years old. Note: delays in diagnosis and treatment were associated with cerebral hyperechogenicity on brain ultrasound and such hyperechogenicity was associated with more ocular lesions and development of new eye lesions.
From Mirlesse V, et al. Long-term follow-up of fetuses and newborn with congenital toxoplasmosis diagnosed and treated prenatally. (Personal communication to McLeod R, 2000).

had signs of neurologic, ophthalmologic, or severe generalized disease at birth or at the time of diagnosis of congenital *T. gondii* infection; they would not have been detected if screening tests for antibodies to *T. gondii* had not been performed. (Data regarding earlier clinical and laboratory evaluations of eight of the children from Alabama had been reported previously) [328,865,870].

Group II consisted of 11 children in whom neither their parents nor their physicians detected signs of congenital infection during the newborn period. The diagnosis was entertained only after they had ophthalmologic or neurologic signs suggestive of congenital *T. gondii* infection. Because these children were preselected as a result of having developed complications of their initially subclinical infection, and because it is possible that a more detailed evaluation during the newborn period might have detected abnormalities in some of them, they were analyzed separately from the children in group I. The characteristics of both groups are shown in Table 31–39.

Of the 24 children, 11 (5 in group I and 6 in group II) never received treatment (See Table 31–49). Four children (1 in group I and 3 in group II) were given treatment only

after adverse sequelae were noted or received treatment for less than 2 weeks, or both; for purposes of analysis, these children were referred to as "untreated." Nine children (7 in group I and 2 in group II) were given treatment for at least 3 weeks before 1 year of age and before the development of neurologic or intellectual deficits. Treatment in all cases consisted of regimens of pyrimethamine and sulfadiazine or pyrimethamine and trisulfapyrimidines.

All children were evaluated at least once. The results of the study revealed that untoward sequelae of their congenital infection ultimately developed in 22 of the 24 children (92%). The two children in whom sequelae did not develop were in group I; they were 8 and 10 years of age at the time of last examination.

Ophthalmologic Outcome. In group I, sequelae developed in 11 of 13 children (85%), and chorioretinitis was the initial manifestation of disease in all 11 (Table 31–40). The age at onset of eye disease ranged from 1 month to 9.3 years of age, with a mean of 3.7 years of age. At their most recent examination, three children had unilateral functional blindness, and the remaining eight had

TABLE 31–39 Characteristics of Children Born with Subclinical Congenital *Toxoplasma* Infection: Results of Stanford University–University of Alabama Study

Characteristic	Group I* (N = 13)	Group II* (N = 11)
Sex		
Male	4	9
Female	9	2
Race		
White	8	10
Black	5	0
Hispanic	0	1
Mean socioeconomic class†	4.08 ± 1.04	3.27 ± 1.19
Birth weight percentile		
<10	5	3
>10, <50	5	8
>50	3	0
Mean gestational age (wk)	37	38
Range	27.5–42.0	33.0–43.0
Mean age at diagnosis (wk)	2	34
Range	0.0–26.0	17.0–52.0
Mean age at most recent examination (yr)	8.26	8.68
Range	3.50–11.17	1.25–17.25
Treatment history for *Toxoplasma* infection‡		
Never treated	5	6
Treated after sequelae developed and/or for <2 wk	1	3
Treated	7	2

*Group I = children for whom serologic tests were performed either because Toxoplasma infection was diagnosed in the mother during pregnancy or at term or because the children were screened for nonspecific findings in the newborn period. Group II = children in whom no signs of congenital infection were found during the newborn period. Diagnosis was first entertained after these children presented with signs suggestive of congenital Toxoplasma infection.
†Hollingshead's classification, mean ± SD (Hollingshead AB. Social Class and Mental Illness: A Community Study. New York, John Wiley, 1958).
‡See text for definition and details of treatment.
Adapted from Wilson CB, et al. Development of adverse sequelae in children born with subclinical congenital Toxoplasma infection. Pediatrics 66:767–774, 1980, with permission.

TABLE 31–40 Ophthalmologic Outcome in Children Born with Subclinical Congenital *Toxoplasma* Infection: Results of Stanford University–University of Alabama Study

Ophthalmologic Finding	Group I* (N = 13)	Group II* (N = 10)†
No sequelae (7.6, 10)‡	2	0
Chorioretinitis		
Bilateral		
Bilateral blindness§	0	5
Unilateral blindness	3	3
Moderate unilateral visual loss	0	1‖
Minimal or no visual loss	5	1
Unilateral		
Minimal or no visual loss	3	0
Mean age at onset (yr)	3.67	0.42
Range	0.08–9.33	0.25–1.00
Recurrences of active chorioretinitis	3	2

*Group I = children for whom serologic tests were performed either because Toxoplasma infection was diagnosed in the mother during pregnancy or at term or because the children were screened for nonspecific findings in the newborn period. Group II = children in whom no signs of congenital infection were found during the newborn period. Diagnosis was first entertained after these children presented with signs suggestive of congenital Toxoplasma infection.
†One of the 11 children in group II was excluded because an adequate follow-up ophthalmologic examination was not performed.
‡Age (yr) at most recent examination.
§Blindness = vision not correctable to >20/200.
‖Macular involvement but vision correctable to 20/40.
Adapted from Wilson CB, et al. Development of adverse sequelae in children born with subclinical congenital Toxoplasma infection. Pediatrics 66:767–774, 1980, with permission.

chorioretinitis without loss of visual function. Subsequent to the initial episode of chorioretinitis, 3 of these 11 children had one or more additional episodes of active chorioretinitis at ages ranging from 1 to 8.7 years. Although temporarily decreased visual function was associated with the recurrent episodes of active chorioretinitis in some of these children, no permanent, additional loss of visual function has resulted.

In group II, eight children initially presented with ocular abnormalities (see Table 31–40). The age at onset of eye disease ranged from 3 months to 1 year of age, with a mean of 0.4 years of age. The two other children in group II in whom ophthalmologic examinations were performed had chorioretinitis at the time they had neurologic abnormalities. At their most recent examination, five children had bilateral functional blindness, three had unilateral functional blindness, one had moderate unilateral visual loss, and one had chorioretinitis without loss of visual function. Subsequent to the initial episode of

chorioretinitis, two of these children had recurrences of active chorioretinitis at 2.3 to 3.5 years of age. One child in group II did not have an adequate ophthalmologic evaluation at the time of last follow-up examination and is not included in the results of ophthalmologic outcome.

Neurologic Outcome. Neurologic sequelae (Table 31–41) developed less frequently than did chorioretinitis and were always associated with eye pathology. Five (38.5%) of 13 children in group I suffered neurologic sequelae. Major neurologic sequelae developed in 1 (8%) and minor neurologic sequelae developed in 4 (31%) children in group I. Two of the 4 children with minor neurologic sequelae in group I had delayed psychomotor development during the first 6 months of life, but their subsequent psychomotor development and neurologic status were normal when they were last examined at 3.7 and 8.7 years of age, respectively. Eight (73%) of 11 children in group II suffered neurologic sequelae—major neurologic sequelae developed in 2, and minor neurologic sequelae developed in 3.

Of the 16 children from both groups I and II for whom skull roentgenograms during infancy were available, 5 (mean age, 5.2 months) had intracranial calcifications and 11 (mean age, 4.8 months) did not. One of these children had normal findings on skull roentgenograms in the first month of life, but calcifications were noted on repeat roentgenograms at 3 months of age. Intracranial calcifications were noted on initial roentgenograms obtained between 3 and 10 months of age in the remaining 4 children. Of these 16 children, major neurologic sequelae developed in 3 of 5 children with intracranial

TABLE 31–41 Neurologic Outcome in Children Born with Subclinical Congenital *Toxoplasma* Infection: Results of Stanford University–University of Alabama Study

Neurologic Finding	Group I* (N = 13)	Group II* (N = 11)
No sequelae	8	3
Major sequelae[†]		
Hydrocephalus	0	1[‡]
Microcephaly	1[§]	1
Seizures	1	3[‖]
Severe psychomotor retardation	1	2[¶]
Minor sequelae		
Mild cerebellar dysfunction	2	4
Transiently delayed psychomotor development	2	2

Group I = children for whom serologic tests were performed either because Toxoplasma *infection was diagnosed in the mother during pregnancy or at term or because the children were screened for nonspecific findings in the newborn period. Group II = children in whom no signs of congenital infection were found during the newborn period. Diagnosis was first suspected when they presented with signs suggestive of congenital* Toxoplasma *infection.*
†*Microcephaly was diagnosed when the head circumference was below the third percentile; hydrocephalus was diagnosed on the basis of pneumoencephalography.*
‡*The same child had a seizure disorder and severe psychomotor retardation and was included in the figures under those categories in group II.*
§*The same child had a seizure disorder and severe psychomotor retardation and was included in the figures under those categories in group I.*
‖*One of these three children had mild cerebellar dysfunction and was included in the figures under that category in group II.*
¶*One of these two children first exhibited transiently delayed psychomotor development and was included in the figures under that category in group II.*
Adapted from Wilson CB, et al. Development of adverse sequelae in children born with subclinical congenital Toxoplasma *infection. Pediatrics 66:767–774, 1980, with permission.*

TABLE 31–42 Intelligence Testing in Children Born with Subclinical Congenital *Toxoplasma* Infection: Results of Stanford University–University of Alabama Study

Age and Intelligence Test Finding	Group I* (N = 13)	Group II* (N = 9)[†]
Mean age at most recent testing (yr)	7.40	10.20
Range	2.75–10.00	2.50–17.25
IQ[‡]	88.6 ± 23.4[§]	85.3 ± 25.6[‖]

Group I = children for whom serologic tests were performed either because Toxoplasma *infection was diagnosed in the mother during pregnancy or at term or because the children were screened for nonspecific findings in the newborn period. Group II = children in whom no signs of congenital infection were found during the newborn period. Diagnosis was first suspected when they had signs suggestive of congenital* Toxoplasma *infection.*
†*Two of 11 children in group II were excluded because they did not have intelligence formally evaluated.*
‡*Mean ± SD.*
§*Evaluation was performed with the Stanford-Binet Intelligence Scale, 6 children; Revised 1974 Wechsler Intelligence Scale for Children, 5 children; and McCarthy Scales of Children's Abilities, 2 children.*
‖*Evaluation was performed with the Stanford-Binet Intelligence Scale, 6 children; Revised 1974 Wechsler Intelligence Scale for Children, 1 child; McCarthy Scales of Children's Abilities, 1 child; and Cattell Infant Intelligence Scale, 1 child.*
Adapted from Wilson CB, et al. Development of adverse sequelae in children born with subclinical congenital Toxoplasma *infection. Pediatrics 66:767–774, 1980, with permission.*

calcifications and in 1 of 11 children without intracranial calcifications (P = .06). No correlation was found between neurologic outcome and birth weight, race, or age at the most recent examination. In eight children in group I, cerebrospinal fluid examinations were performed during the newborn period. In 7 of the children, abnormalities were detected; such abnormalities did not correlate with the development of any type of sequelae.

Intelligence Testing. The results of intelligence testing are presented in Table 31–42. IQ scores correlated directly with upper socioeconomic class (r = 0.37, P <.05). In addition, the 16 white children had a higher mean IQ (89.6 ± 26.3) than that of the 6 nonwhite children (81.2 ± 15), but this difference was not statistically significant. Two of the children in group I (one white, one African American) had moderately severe retardation (IQ scores of 36 and 62, respectively), as did two of the children (both white) in group II (IQ scores of 43 and 53). A tendency was identified for IQ scores to decrease on later testing among the seven children (six in group I and one in group II) who were tested more than once. The mean IQ score of these children fell from 96.9 to 74 over an average of 5.5 years, with all but one child showing a decrease on repeat testing.

No significant correlation was found between IQ scores and the finding of abnormal cerebrospinal fluid in the newborn period, intracranial calcifications on skull roentgenograms, age at time of testing, or birth weight below the tenth percentile. In fact, a trend toward higher IQ

scores (mean, 96.9) was identified in children with birth weight below the tenth percentile. These results of intelligence testing must be interpreted with caution. The range of IQ scores was wide, testing was performed by different persons, and different tests were employed.

Hearing Impairment. The incidence of sensorineural hearing loss in the study population also appeared to be excessive. In an earlier study in some of these children [865], the incidence of mild sensorineural hearing loss in 41 normal control children (mean age, 3.8 years) was 5%; no children with more severe sensorineural hearing loss were observed. In this study [361], the incidence of sensorineural hearing loss in children tested in group I was 30% and that in group II was 22%. One child in each group had moderate unilateral hearing loss.

Special Considerations. Because this study was not controlled and was only in part prospective, certain limitations must be considered in interpreting the data. Children in group II were detected because of the development of sequelae that were sufficiently significant to attract medical attention. Thus it would be inappropriate to use data from this group to determine the frequency of such sequelae among children born with subclinical infection. Nevertheless, data from group II do provide information regarding the potential seriousness of ocular disease in children born with subclinical congenital *T. gondii* infection and regarding the risk of subsequent neurologic sequelae in children in whom chorioretinitis developed previously. No data from this study or from other studies indicate that a significant bias toward more severe disease was introduced by the different screening methods employed in group I. It is likely, therefore, that the data from group I provide a reasonable estimate both of the seriousness and of the frequency of complications in children with initially subclinical congenital *T. gondii* infection. Because of the small sample size and the lack of a matched control group, these data must, however, be considered estimates. Moreover, whether postnatal therapy was beneficial cannot be determined from this study.

Paris Studies

Of 108 infants with congenital *T. gondii* infection who were diagnosed and evaluated prospectively by Couvreur and colleagues [364] and discussed by Szusterkac [871], 27 had chorioretinitis. In 26 of these infants, the lesions were present at the time of the first ophthalmoscopic examination after birth. In only one infant were findings on the eye examination normal at birth, with subsequent development of chorioretinitis. In three other infants, a retinal lesion was noted at the time of first examination, and a new lesion was discovered on follow-up examination. It is noteworthy that only 16 of the 108 infants were examined after the age of 2 years and only 3 were examined after the age of 5 years. Only 6 of these 19 children had chorioretinitis on initial examination. Of interest is the striking difference between the children who received treatment and those who did not during the first year of life. Among the children who received treatment, no lesions were discovered after the age of 2 years, whereas in 8% of the children given no treatment, chorioretinitis developed between 10 months and 4 years of age. It is possible to assume from the experience of Koppe and colleagues [245,360] and Wilson and coworkers [361] that careful follow-up evaluation in these 108 children would reveal additional cases of chorioretinitis and additional lesions in the 27 children who already had eye disease. Follow-up evaluation in such series is important because all of these children were identified prospectively and received treatment for approximately 1 year either from birth or from the time at which the diagnosis was established in the first months of life.

Additional data in children in whom congenital *T. gondii* infection was not recognized in the newborn period have been published by Briatte [872]. These data were obtained in collaboration with Couvreur, Hazemann, and Desmonts in Paris. Hazemann established a program at a number of medical centers in the Paris area in which any infant could be examined free of charge at the request of the mother. The first examination was performed when the infant was 10 months of age. Among the blood tests performed in this program was the dye test to detect cases of previously undiagnosed congenital *T. gondii* infection. Forty-eight infants with subclinical congenital *T. gondii* infection were detected among the 20,513 infants examined from 1971 through 1979. (The data were corrected for those cases in which the infection probably was acquired postnatally.) Infants with clinical toxoplasmosis probably were not examined in this program because these infants would already be under medical care, so that their mothers probably would not request their participation in this medical screening program. For the same reason, it is likely that the vast majority of infants screened had few or no problems during infancy.

The frequency of probable congenital *T. gondii* infection in the entire study population averaged 2.33 per 1000 (range, 0.38 to 5.2 per 1000 per study year). The frequency of chorioretinitis among the 48 infants is shown in Table 31–43. Of these 48 children (who, of course, did not receive treatment for their *T. gondii* infection during the first 10 months of life), chorioretinitis developed in 18% by the age of 4 years. In 8 of the children, chorioretinitis developed after the age of 10 months and before the age of 4 years. This latter finding differs considerably from that reported by Szusterkac [871] in infants who received treatment in the early weeks or months of life (see earlier discussion). Cerebral calcifications were present in 3 of the 48 infants previously unrecognized as having infection, which therefore had not been treated [872].

Interpretation of Stanford-Alabama and Paris Studies

For proper interpretation of the data presented for the Stanford-Alabama study [361] and the study reported by Briatte [872], it is important to understand how the data might be biased because of the method of case selection. The method used in the studies in Alabama for detection of subclinical congenital infection (detection of an increase in cord serum IgM) might have selected for the most "severe" (heavily infected) cases among subclinically infected newborns. In the studies performed by the Stanford group, some of the patients were selected because manifestations of the infection occurred during infancy. Thus in both of these studies, the method of selection might have predisposed to an increased frequency of more severe cases in the Stanford-Alabama study. By contrast, in the study reported by Briatte, it is probable that the most "benign" cases were selected among subclinically infected newborns because the investigators studied infants who had few or no medical problems during the first 10 months of life. Despite this bias toward "mild" infection, 18% of the infants whom the Paris group observed had ocular lesions by the age of 4 years.

TABLE 31–43 Frequency of Chorioretinitis in Infants with Subclinical Congenital *Toxoplasma* Infection First Discovered in a Systematic Serologic Screening Program

Age When Fundus Was Examined	No. of Children	Chorioretinitis Previously Recognized	New Cases of Chorioretinitis Discovered	Total No. of Children with Chorioretinitis in this Age Group (%)
10 mo	48	0	5	5 (10)
Examined again at 2 yr	31	5	3	8 (16)
Examined again at 4 yr	28	8	1	9 (18)

Data adapted from patients studied by Drs. J Couvreur, JJ Hazemann, and G Desmonts. Cases are discussed by Briatte.

Amsterdam Study

As mentioned earlier, in 1964 a prospective study was started in Amsterdam to determine the frequency of congenital toxoplasmosis [360]. Of 1821 pregnancies screened, 249 infants were enrolled in the study—21 because of seroconversion in the dye test, 42 because of a high baseline dye test titer, 183 because of a slight rise in dye test titer, and 3 because their mothers had toxoplasmosis shortly before gestation. At birth, four infants had chorioretinitis and parasites were isolated from placenta and cerebrospinal fluid of one other infant. Each of these five children received pharmacologic treatment. Seven children who were asymptomatic and whose dye test titer did not revert to negative received no treatment. Ten other questionably infected children who had no symptoms but whose dye test titer became negative 18 months after birth also received no treatment. These 22 children were evaluated annually for 5 years by physical examinations and dye and CF tests. No new abnormalities were detected, except in one patient with chorioretinitis, who required surgery to correct a squint at the age of 2 years [360]. The 12 congenitally infected children continued to be examined yearly until the age of 20 years.

The authors' original optimistic view was revised in their 1986 publication [190]. One of the five children who received treatment and one of the symptom-free children had new scars in their eyes at the age of 6 years. Additional new scars or acute lesions were observed in both the "treatment" and "no treatment" groups of children. In three children, scars appeared at ages 11, 12, and 13 years, respectively. One patient had a new scar in his right eye when examined for the first time at age 17, and another had no severe eye abnormalities until the age of 18 years, when an acute lesion appeared in the right macula that led to blindness in that eye. Another patient had a new acute lesion in her right eye at the age of 12 years and again in both eyes at the age of 13 years. Thus after a total of 20 years of follow-up, of 11 congenitally infected children, 9 had scars in one or both eyes. Four of these children had severely impaired vision in one eye, and three were blind in one eye. Among the 10 questionably infected children, 1 had a scar in the right macula at 5 years of age that led to severe visual impairment. Another child whose mother had toxoplasmosis during gestation remained persistently seropositive. He had not developed any scars in his eyes. The other eight children remained seronegative for 5 to 19 years, and some acquired toxoplasmosis during this time. The 11 congenitally infected children did not differ from controls in their school performance. None of the 11 was mentally retarded.

From the results of this prospective study, it is apparent that 9 of 11 children (82%) after 20 years of follow-up had significant sequelae of toxoplasmosis, and that 5 of these 11 had severely impaired vision (Fig. 31–36). Although the report by Wilson and associates described earlier demonstrated a similar percentage of untoward sequelae by the age of 10 years, theirs was not a prospective study [361].

U.S. National Collaborative Chicago-based Treatment Trial Study

A national, prospective study, the NCCCTS, is being carried out by a group of investigators based in Chicago

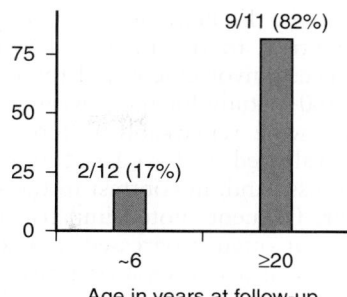

FIGURE 31–36 Visual outcome for 12 children who were asymptomatic at birth, untreated or treated less than once a month and evaluated when they were 6 and 20 years old. Percentage of children with retinal disease. Adverse outcomes in untreated congenital toxoplasmosis or when congenital toxoplasmosis was treated for only 1 month. (*Data from Koppe JG, Kloosterman GJ. Congenital toxoplasmosis: long-term follow-up. Padiatr Padol 17:171–179, 1982; Koppe JG, Loewer-Sieger DH, DeRoever-Bonnet H. Results of 20-year follow-up of congenital toxoplasmosis. Lancet 1:254–256, 1986.*)

(telephone number 773-834-4152/773-834-4131). This study is evaluating long-term outcome for infants given pyrimethamine (comparing two doses) in combination with leucovorin and sulfadiazine (100 mg/kg per day in two divided doses). Medications are begun when a child is younger than 2.5 months of age according to the method shown in Figure 31–34 and continued for 12 months. Therapy is monitored by parents with a nurse case manager and the primary physician, and compliance also has been documented with measurement of serum pyrimethamine levels. Children who have not received treatment during the first year of life and are referred to the study group when they are older than 1 year of age also are included in the study. Patients are evaluated comprehensively by the study group near the time of birth and at 1, 3.5, 5, 7.5, 10, and at 5-year intervals thereafter. The following parameters are evaluated: history; physical status; audiologic, ophthalmologic, neurologic, and cognitive function; and development; a number of other variables are measured by laboratory tests, including tests of hematologic status and serologic and lymphocyte response to *T. gondii* antigens, and neuroradiologic studies.

This ongoing study of the treatment of infants began in 1981. It continues to the present time and has provided an opportunity to determine and compare the manifestations, natural history, and outcomes in children with congenital toxoplasmosis who were treated with either one or another regimen.

This study began with a phase 1 clinical trial, which was conducted from 1981 to 1991. This phase demonstrated that it was feasible and safe to administer pyrimethamine and sulfadiazine to infants throughout the first year of life. Medicine preparation and administration were as shown in Figure 31–34 and Tables 31–33 and 31–34. Pharmacokinetics of pyrimethamine in infants were characterized. Twelve children took the recommended dosage of pyrimethamine and two children took a higher dose.

During phase 1, and in the subsequent phase that is still ongoing, many of the infants had severe involvement at the time of enrollment. The findings at presentation in infants in the NCCCTS were comparable to those in infants described by Eichenwald [356] at presentation. However, in contrast to the Eichenwald study for the children with severe involvement and the earlier Wilson and colleagues [604] study for those with milder involvement, outcomes were remarkably different when these children were evaluated at 1 to 10 years of life. There was no hearing loss. And, in contrast to the severe cognitive impairment, frequent motor impairments, seizures, and visual loss that often progressed in association with recurrent episodes of active chorioretinitis, most of the children were ambulatory without motor deficits. They were functioning normally in their families and school settings, without seizures, and without progression of their retinal disease, which often was already substantial at birth. These outcomes appeared to be considerably better than those described in any previously published study of comparable children who had been untreated or treated for only one month.

Based on these findings, demonstration of achievable blood levels of pyrimethamine, and documentation that these treatment regimens could be safely administered, a placebo controlled trial was considered as a next phase. However, after reviewing these data in 1990, the investigators and the Ethics (Institutional Review Boards and National Institutes of Health panels) and Data Safety Monitoring Boards, concluded that the outcomes for the children in the phase 1 study were markedly improved relative to all prior studies of comparably ill children. Based on this conclusion, a prospective, randomized, controlled efficacy trial with prespecified endpoints/outcomes of treatment was initiated with one group receiving a higher and the other group receiving a lower dose of pyrimethamine; the doses selected were those two doses that had been found to be safe in the initial 10 years of the phase 1 trial. This study has been criticized by some because there is no placebo control group, despite the fact that this group was not included because of the recommendations of the ethics boards. This is also a study of referred patients who choose to participate, which is a limitation of the design of this and most clinical trials. This reflects the lack of a systematic, standardized, mandated, or uniformly implemented serologic screening program for pregnant women and infants in the United States, in contrast to the program in place in France.

In this study, pyrimethamine has been administered with leucovorin and sulfadiazine to infants who are treated throughout their first year of life (Figure 31–34) [878]. Endpoints for outcomes were prespecified and based on a careful analysis of the literature and the phase 1 trial experience. Sample sizes were selected based on the predicted frequency of outcomes based on the earlier literature to be sufficient to detect significant differences in outcomes with the two treatment regimens with a beta error of 80%.

These two treatment regimes were not selected to be treatments that were widely disparate, with one expected to fail and one to succeed. Rather, they were based on two treatments that had been found to be feasible, safe, and that produced potentially therapeutic serum and CSF levels of pyrimethamine in the phase I trial. The underlying assumption was that there might be a dose-related effect for efficacy or safety but, even if there were

no differences in outcomes between the two treatment groups, if the improved outcomes observed in the phase 1 study compared to the outcomes described in the earlier literature were also present for the larger number of children in this randomized phase of the study, benefit and efficacy of treatment would be further supported by this comparative efficacy trial.

Infants are stratified on the basis of severity of disease at their first visit to the Chicago Center into the following categories: no disease, mild involvement, generalized disease, moderate or severe neurologic disease, with or without retinal disease, and with or without prenatal treatment. Children who were evaluated in the first two and a half months of life in Chicago were placed into these stratification categories and randomized to receive the higher or lower dose of pyrimethamine. This study has been supported by the U.S. National Institutes of Health and by donations of free transportation from airlines, which have allowed the evaluations to be performed by a single group of experienced observers, in a consistent, careful, and thoroughly documented manner. The periodic analyses of the data have provided information about the natural history of the treated infection in a detailed, rigorous, and consistent manner. Information has also been obtained regarding early or late side effects or toxicities of the medicines used, and the appearance of delayed sequelae. In the early phase, it was clear that this follow-up was important, since serologic test results after stopping the medicines showed a rebound in antibody titers specific to *T. gondii*, which suggested that bradyzoites were not eliminated by treatment and treated children therefore remained at risk for recrudescence of this disease.

During the 19 years since this randomized study was initiated, there have been some years in which the research grant support needed to bring children to Chicago for randomization and evaluation was not available. During those times, children were considered to be part of the feasibility/observational cohort and were evaluated as soon as research support was restored and travel to Chicago was possible. If infants could not be evaluated in Chicago by the time they had received 2.5 months of treatment, they were not randomized and were treated with the higher dose of pyrimethamine. Data for the randomized and observational cohorts have been analyzed separately and considered together throughout the study, and have been found to be comparable when reviewed by the Data Safety Monitoring Board each year. The prespecified enrollment targets for the severe stratification categories were met in 2008 and only those children who are in the no disease or mild categories are still randomized. All children in the moderate or severe categories now are treated with the higher dose of pyrimethamine.

Results for the period between 1981 and 2004 were reported in 2006 [878]. Outcomes, with comparisons between the lower and higher dosage and comparisons with data from earlier studies in which children were either untreated or treated for 1 month, are in Tables 31–18, 31–44, 31–45, 31–46, 31–48, 31–49.

In summary: Manifestations of active infection resolved in association with treatment [433,773,877–878]. Outcomes were markedly improved in this cohort relative to

TABLE 31–44 Ages (in Years) of Patients in U.S. (Chicago) National Collaborative Treatment Trial*

Patient Group	All Patients			Patients ≥5 Years of Age		
	Mean ± SD	Range	N	Mean ± SD	Range	N
Historical patients*	13.9 ± 8.9	5.4–33.4	28	15.3 ± 8.9	5.4–33.4	28
Treatment A: feasibility	11.7 ± 1.1	10.0–14.3	13	11.7 ± 1.1	10.0–14.3	13
Randomized	5.7 ± 1.9	1.9–8.8	38	6.7 ± 1.2	5.0–8.8	26
Treatment C: feasibility	3.5 ± 4.6	0.5–15	7	12.7 ± 3.2	10.5–15.0	2
Randomized	5.4 ± 2.0	0.9–10.0	28	6.7 ± 1.4	5.1–10.0	16

*Historical patients were patients who received no treatment and were diagnosed after 1 year of age. In the treatment groups, children received 2 months (Treatment A) or 6 months (Treatment C) of daily pyrimethamine and sulfadiazine, followed by pyrimethamine on Monday, Wednesday, and Friday and continued daily sulfadiazine for the remainder of the year of therapy.

those in children who were untreated or treated for 1 month with comparable severity at presentation. There was no sensorineural hearing loss (See Table 31–18). The incidence of recurrent eye lesions was approximately 10% into early adolescent years for those with no or mild symptoms at birth and approximately 30% for those with moderate or severe disease at birth. Cognitive and motor function was in the broad range of normal for 100% of the children categorized as having no or mild disease. Cognitive and motor functions were in the broad range

of normal for 73% and 80% of the children in the moderate and severe categories, respectively. There were no statistically significant differences in efficacy or toxicity between the treatment regimens (See Table 31– 47). The only substantial manifestation of toxicity was transient neutropenia, which responded to increased dosages of leucovorin or withholding of pyrimethamine (See Table 31–47). This appeared to occur primarily during the prodrome of concomitant viral infections. Dental caries occurred in one of the first children studied.

TABLE 31–45 Comparison of Ophthalmologic, Developmental, and Audiologic Outcomes with Postnatal Treatment

Study	Treatment	No. Studied	Mean Age (yr) When Data Tabulated (Range)	Percent with Finding of Impairment					
				Ophthalmologic			Neurologic		
				Lesions*	Vision[†]	New[‡]	Cognitive	Motor or Seizures	Audiologic
Eichenwald, 1959 [601]	0 or 1 mo P, S	104	4 (minimum)	NA	0, 42, 67[§]	NA	50, 81, 89[§]	0, 58, 76[§]	0, 10, 17[§]
Wilson et al, 1980 [604]	0 or 1 mo P, S	23	8.5 (1–17)	93	47	22	55 (20 severe)	20	22, 30[‖]
Koppe et al, 1986 [394]	0 or 1 mo P, S	12	20 (NA)	80	NA	NA	0	0	NA
Labadie and Hazemann, 1984 [400]	0	17	1 (NA)	28	NA	NA	NA	NA	NA
Couvreur et al, 1984 [559]	1 yr P, S, Sp	172	NA (2–11)	NA	NA	8	NA	NA	NA
Hohlfeld, 1989 [124]	Prenatal, 1 yr P, S, Sp	43	NA (0.5–4)	12	NA	NA	0	0	NA
Villena, 1998 [147]	F, Sp	47	NA (born 1980–89)	—	—	15/45 (33)[¶]	—	—	—
	1 yr F	19	NA (born 1990–96)	—	—	2/18 (11)	—	—	—
	2 yr F	12	NA (born 1990–97)	—	—	1/11 (9)	—	—	—
Peyron, 1996[778]	F□	121	12 (5–22)	—	—	37/121 (31)	—	—	—
Chicago study (historical patients)	0	7	5.6 (2–10)	100	86	29	25	25	14
Chicago study (treated patients)	Most for 1 yr P, S	37**	3.4 (0.3–10)	81	81	8	0, 24[h]	0, 24	0

*Any chorioretinal lesions.
[†]Vision impaired.
[‡]New lesions.
[§]Subclinical, generalized, neurologic.
[‖]Subclinical, generalized, neurologic.
[h]none, mild, moderate; severe neurologic.
[¶]Number with finding/number in group (%).
**These data are for the first 37 children studied before May 1991.
F, Fansidar (pyrimethamine 1.25 mg/kg each 14 days); F□, Fansidar (given in utero and postnatally—pyrimethamine 6 mg/5 kg each 10 days; small numbers also treated in utero; NA, not available; P, pyrimethamine; S, sulfonamides; Sp, spiramycin.
Adapted from McAuley J, et al. Early and longitudinal evaluations of treated infants and children and untreated historical patients with congenital toxoplasmosis: the Chicago collaborative treatment trial. Clin Infect Dis 18:38–72, 1994.

TABLE 31-46   Early Outcomes for Children ≥5 Years of Age in the U.S. (Chicago) National Collaborative Treatment Trial

| Untoward Sequela | % in Literature: 5 yr, 10 yr‡ | Historical Patients§ | Mild* | | | |
| | | | Treatment A† | | Treatment C† | |
			Feasibility	Randomized	Feasibility	Randomized
Vision <20/20	25, 50	11/14 (79) ‖	0/4	0/3	0/0	0/0
New retinal lesions	25, 85	5/9 (56)	0/4	1/3	0/0	0/0
Motor abnormality	10, 10	0/14 (0)	0/4	0/3	0/0	0/0
IQ <70	0–50, 0–50	0/13 (0)	0/4	0/3	0/0	0/0
δIQ ≥15	50, 50	0/5 (0)	0/4	1/3	0/0	0/0
Hearing loss	30, 30	0/14 (0)	0/4	0/3	0/0	0/0

| Untoward Sequela | % in Literature: 5 yr, 10 yr¶ | Historical Patients | Severe* | | | |
| | | | Treatment A | | Treatment C | |
			Feasibility	Randomized	Feasibility	Randomized
Vision <20/20	70, 70	10/10 (100)	7/9 (78)	8/9 (89)	1/2	6/9 (67)
New retinal lesions	50, 90	4/9 (44)	3/9 (33)	1/8 (13)	2/2	0/9 (0)
Motor abnormality	60, 60	1/10 (10)	3/9 (33)	2/9 (22)	0/2	1/9 (11)
IQ <70	90, >90	1/10 (10)	4/9 (44)	4/9 (44)	0/2	2/9 (22)
δIQ ≥15	95, 95	0/8 (0)	0/9 (0)	2/9 (22)	0/2	1/9 (11)
Hearing loss	30, 30	0/10 (0)	0/9 (0)	0/9 (0)	0/2	0/9 (0)

*Clinical disease considered "Mild" if infant is apparently normal and normal development is noted on follow-up evaluation (e.g., but has isolated nonmacular retinal scars or <3 intracranial calcifications on CT). Clinical disease considered "Severe" if neurologic signs or symptoms are present, symptomatic chorioretinitis has threatened vision, or if ≥3 intracranial calcifications are seen on CT.
†Treated children received 2 months (Treatment A) or 6 months (Treatment C) of daily pyrimethamine and sulfadiazine, followed by pyrimethamine on Monday, Wednesday, and Friday and continued daily sulfadiazine for the remainder of the year of therapy. Feasibility group patients underwent treatment in the early phase of the study before randomized study.
‡Data from Wilson et al [361].
§Historical patients were patients who received no treatment and were diagnosed after 1 year of age.
‖Number with abnormality/number in group (% affected). No differences between treatment regimens achieved statistical significance (P > 0.05 using Fisher Exact test).
¶Data from Eichenwald [356].
Note: Percentages not shown for groups with ≤4 patients.
CT, computed tomography; IQ, intelligence quotient.

TABLE 31-47   Episodes of Reversible Neutropenia Requiring Temporary Withholding of Medications for the U.S. National Collaborative Study*

| Regimen | No. of Episodes Medication Withheld (Mean ± S.D. [Range]) | No. Who Stopped Medication/No. in Group Who Have Completed 1 Year of Therapy (%) | No. of Children Who Stopped Medications Temporarily/No. in Group (%) | | Discontinued Medications Due to Neutropenia ≥4 times |
			Feasibility	Randomized	
Treatment A	1.8 ± 1.1 [1–4]	11/32 (34)	6/14 (43)	11/34 (32)	4
Treatment C	3.8 ± 3.1 [1–11]	17/48 (35)	1/4 (25)	10/28 (36)	5

*Children received 2 months (Treatment A) or 6 months (Treatment C) of daily pyrimethamine and sulfadiazine, followed by pyrimethamine on Monday, Wednesday, and Friday and continued daily sulfadiazine for the remainder of the year of therapy. Feasibility group patients received treatment in the early phase of the study before randomized study. Toxicity for Treatments A and C was measured as episodes of reversible neutropenia requiring temporary withholding of medications.

Thereafter, parents were cautioned to clean teeth of older infants because medications were administered in sugar suspensions. Pediatricians were cautioned to avoid using a second sulfonamide to treat concomitant infections such as otitis media because more prolonged neutropenia occurred in one child in conjunction with such therapy. There have been no late malignancies or hematologic dyscrasias in those who were treated [878].

These findings are similar to those reported in this NCCTS cohort at earlier times and in other studies in which children were treated in this manner.* Although the children in the NCCCTS study are largely children with moderate or severe disease [878], these outcomes

---

*References 14, 176, 198, 216, 224, 228, 266, 279, 409–410, 433, 456, 486, 570, 773, 786, 789, 873–875, 877–879, 881, 883–884, 893.

TABLE 31–48 Quantitative Visual Acuity in U.S. (Chicago) National Collaborative Treatment Trial in Patients with Macular Lesions (m) in at Least One Eye

Group	Patient No.	Right Eye	Left Eye
Treated*	7	20/20	0/20 (m)
	13	6/400 (m)	20/50 (m)[†]
	15	4/30 (m)	20/30 (m)[†]
	19	20/200[‡]	20/20 (m)
	21	1/30 (m)	1/30 (m)
	26	3/30 (m)	1/30 (m)
	28	20/30 (m)	15/30 (m)
	30	1/30 (m)	12/30[§]
	36	20/30	8/30 (m)
Historical*	20	20/400 (m)	20/25
	25	20/400 (m)	20/30
	27	5/30 (m)	1/30[‖]
	31	20/25	3/200 (m)
	38	20/400 (m)	20/25[‖]
	41	20/30	20/200 (m)
	42	20/70 (m)	20/30 (m)[†]
	46	20/200 (m)	20/60 (m)
	47	3/30 (m)	3/30[‖]
	82	20/400 (m)	20/15
	89	20/100 (m)	20/25

Treated: n = 39 (30 too young or with cognitive limitations that made it not possible for the child to cooperate with quantitative vision). Historical: n = 13 (2 too young for quantitative vision).
[†]*Surprisingly good vision in spite of foveal lesion.*
[‡]*Strabismus, microphthalmia, and amblyopia present.*
[§]*Poor cooperation, patient 4 years old.*
[‖]*Peripheral lesion with dragging of the macula.*
From Mets MB, et al. Eye manifestations of congenital toxoplasmosis. Am J Ophthalmol 122:309–324, 1996.

are considerably more favorable than those described for comparable children who were untreated or treated for shorter times in other studies.

All signs of active infection (i.e., thrombocytopenia, hepatitis, rash, meningitis, hypoglycorrhachia, active chorioretinitis, vitritis) resolved within weeks of initiation

of therapy [773]. Chorioretinitis did not progress or relapse during therapy.

Audiologic outcome was significantly better than that reported in the earlier literature (see Table 31–18) [486]. To the present time, no sensorineural hearing loss was noted in the 139 children who received treatment, in contrast with a 14% incidence of "deafness" [356] or 26% incidence of "hearing loss [361]" in earlier studies. Comparisons of outcomes in this and earlier studies are summarized in Table 31–18 (see also the next section, "Comparison of Outcomes").

Retinal disease became quiescent with therapy within weeks, with no recrudescence observed during therapy [773]. To the present time, new lesions (primarily those "satelliting" pre-existing lesions) occurred in older children. The oldest child who received treatment was 28 years in 2009. Lesions also occurred in previously normal-appearing retinae. These were noted first at study evaluations at 3.5, 5, or 7.5 years of age and had not been present at the preceding evaluation. To date, no loss in visual acuity has occurred when prompt treatment of active recurrent chorioretinitis was initiated. Comparison of early outcomes with 2 versus 6 months of 1 mg/kg/day of pyrimethamine, followed by this dosage administered on Monday, Wednesday, and Friday, both administered with sulfadiazine and leucovorin, is shown in Table 31–46. At present, no statistically significant differences have been noted. Thus treatment during the first year of life with pyrimethamine and sulfonamides, unfortunately, did not uniformly prevent recrudescent chorioretinitis. Determination of whether it reduces the incidence of recurrent or new chorioretinitis, compared with the almost uniform occurrence of this complication in children who did not receive treatment, who were diagnosed in earlier decades, requires longer follow-up evaluation of more children. It is especially important to try to determine whether treatment prevents subsequent chorioretinitis when no retinal lesions are present at birth.

Visual acuity that is adequate for all usual activities and reading has been noted in some children with large macular scars. Nonetheless, impairment of vision has been one of the two most prominent sequelae (Table 31–48).

TABLE 31–49 Comparison of Neurologic and Developmental Outcomes in the Chicago, Wilson et al, and Eichenwald Studies

	Chicago (1991)		Wilson et al (1980)		Eichenwald (1959)		
Outcome	Subclinical (N = 3)	Generalized/ Neurologic (N = 34)	Subclinical I (N = 13)	Subclinical II (N = 11)	Subclinical (N = 4)	Generalized (N = 31)	Neurologic (N = 70)
Seizures requiring therapy after first months	0 (0)*,[†]	4 (12)	1 (8)	3 (27)	2 (50)	24 (77)	58 (82)
Motor/tone permanent impairment	0 (0)	8 (24)	3 (23)	2 (18)	0 (0)	18 (58)	53 (76)
IQ <70	0 (0)	8 (24)	2 (15)	2 (18)	2 (50)	25 (81)	62 (89)
Sequentially lower IQ score	0/2 (0)	3[†]/13 (0)	6/6 (100)	0/1 (0)	NA	NA	NA

*Number affected/number tested if different from N (%).
[†]Three children had a >15-point diminution and 2 children had a >15-point increase in IQ score. The differences over time for the entire group were not statistically significant (P >.05)
IQ, intelligence quotient; NA, not available.
Data from references 356,361,433.

Visual impairment has presented a challenge in the care of children of school age; that is, special attention is needed to optimize their ability to read, and participation in learning activities must be ensured so that their visual impairments do not impair cognitive development. Retinal scars have been central, peripheral, unilateral, and bilateral in location and have resulted in partial and complete retinal detachment. Loss of sight at presentation (e.g., due to retinal detachment) usually has been associated with the most profound neurologic impairment. Visual outcomes to date are contrasted with those of earlier studies in the next section: "Comparison of Outcomes." Neurologic and cognitive function of most of these treated children has been significantly better than reported in earlier decades [433,873–875]. This is summarized in Table 31–49.

In the earlier report by Eichenwald [356], more than 80% of children who had substantial generalized and neurologic involvement at birth and who received no treatment or whose treatment was for 1 month had IQ scores below 70 at 4 years of age. In that report, initial involvement in the perinatal period appears to have been less severe or similar in severity to that of children in the NCCCTS. In contrast with the outcome in that earlier series, only 31% of the treated children who had substantial generalized or neurologic manifestations of infection or both in the perinatal period and who received treatment between 1982 and September 2008 in the NCCCTS had substantial cognitive impairments. The remaining 69% of the treated children in the NCCCTS who had substantial generalized or neurologic manifestations of infection or both in the perinatal period have to date demonstrated normal development and are likely to be capable of self-care. The relative contribution of shunt placement, antimicrobial therapy, and adjunctive supportive care to this improved outcome cannot be determined with certainty. The observation that almost all children without hydrocephalus in the NCCCTS have at least average cognitive function contrasts dramatically with the 81% incidence rate of mental retardation at 4 years of age in children having generalized disease in Eichenwald's series and who received no treatment or whose treatment was for 1 month [356]. This difference suggests that antimicrobial therapy may contribute significantly to the more favorable outcome. No deterioration of cognitive function has occurred over time in these children who received treatment, although visual impairment clearly has affected school performance and ability to acquire information and skills for some children [873]. This finding contrasts with earlier reports of diminished cognitive function over time for children not given treatment or those whose duration of treatment was less than 1 month who had subclinical disease in the perinatal period (described by Wilson and associates) [361]. Despite the remarkably good cognitive outcome for many of these children, the impact of the infection on their cognitive function is reflected in the fact that their IQ scores often are 15 points less than those of their nearest-age siblings ($P < .05$) [873].

Factors in the newborn period that often were associated with poorer prognosis in the NCCCTS study included apnea and bradycardia, hypoxia, hypotension, delays in shunt placement and/or initiation of therapy,

inability to perceive light retinal detachment, cerebrospinal fluid protein concentration greater than 1 g/dL, diabetes insipidus in the perinatal period, hypsarrhythmia, and markedly diminished size of the brain cortical mantle that did not increase after shunt placement [872]. Nevertheless, favorable outcomes also have been noted when some of these abnormalities were present [872,873,876].

The experiences in the NCCCTS (see CHAPTER 31–CHAPTER 31) indicate that initial appearance of the brain on CT scan is not necessarily predictive of poor outcomes. Therefore these investigators have approached this disease in infancy as one in which all aspects of care should be optimized because even when factors more frequently associated with adverse outcomes are present, adverse outcomes do not always occur.

It has been possible to discontinue antiepileptic medications in some infants who have had seizures (presumably due to active encephalitis) in the perinatal period, without recurrence of seizures. New-onset seizures have developed in a small number of treated children after the perinatal period. Hypsarrhythmia occurred in two children. One of these latter children responded dramatically and promptly to adrenocorticotropic hormone injections (pyrimethamine and sulfadiazine were administered concomitantly), and one responded to clonazepam treatment.

In many instances, a number of considerations may make it reasonable to withhold antiepileptic therapy after a short course of such medications. These considerations include the potential adverse interactions of many of the antiepileptic medications with the antimicrobial agents needed to treat *T. gondii* infection [877]. If antimicrobial therapy results in resolution of active encephalitis, which was the seizure focus, antiepileptic medications would no longer be needed. In the NCCCTS, a lack of recurrence of seizures when antiepileptic medications were discontinued in a number of cases [789,873,875] supports this approach. Levetiracetam has been used successfully for treatment of seizures and does not have the effect of inducing enzymes that degrade pyrimethamine as phenobarbital does and does not have the effect of displacing sulfonamides from albumin as does phenytoin.

Comparison of Outcomes. A comparison of the outcomes observed in the NCCCTS and in previous studies and their relationship to treatment is shown in Tables 31–45 and 31–49. Early treatment in the NCCCTS appeared to result in more favorable outcomes than were reported to occur for untreated infants or infants who received treatment for only 1 month [217,877–879]. This was the case although the severity of neurologic disease at birth in the NCCCTS was comparable to or greater than in those reported by Eichenwald and colleagues [356] in the same stratified disease categories.

Analysis of the full cohort is presently ongoing (McLeod R, unpublished). As of October 2008, 149 children who received treatment have been evaluated. Ages ranged from newborn to 26.8 years (mean age, 13.1 years). Forty-two historical (no treatment) patients also are being followed. They range in age from 5.8 to 61.8 years of age (mean age, 24.6 years). Outcomes appear to be similar to those reported in 2006 [878]; higher and lower dose regimens have remained similar in toxicity and in early outcomes for pre-established endpoints and active disease has continued to become quiescent with treatment. Enrollment in the NCCCTS is currently ongoing. Infants can be enrolled by phoning 773-834-4152 or 773-834-4131.

Current State of Knowledge Regarding the Effects of Postnatal Treatment on Outcome. Our review of available data and the experience presented above suggests that early postnatal treatment of infected infants improves long-term outcomes. We recognize that the current data suggesting benefit are not based on placebo-controlled clinical trials. Some argue that for this reason, despite the favorable results shown in other contexts, placebo-controlled studies are still needed to demonstrate efficacy [195,880]. Although we agree that such studies would be necessary to provide incontrovertible proof of efficacy, lack of evidence for benefit from placebo-controlled trials is not evidence that postnatal treatment is of no benefit. For this reason, until such placebo-controlled data with long-term follow-up and analyses as careful as those in the NCCCTS become available, we and others [196] continue to recommend that treatment be given following the regimens described for the NCCCTS study. Ideally, in the United States and Canada, when physicians feel this may be of benefit for their patients and in understanding the natural history of this disease, consideration should be given to referring cases to the NCCCTS.

Ophthalmologic Outcome in Children in the United States NCCCTS Study. In the NCCCTS study, recurrent toxoplasmic chorioretinitis was commonly observed in persons with apparent or proved congenital infection that was not treated in the perinatal period and during the first year of life [883,884]. Twenty-eight children were considered to have congenital *Toxoplasma* infection based on the presence of seropositivity by 24 months of age alone or in concert with central nervous system calcifications, hydrocephalus, or other clinical signs compatible with congenital *Toxoplasma* infection. However these children were not diagnosed in the first year of life and were therefore not treated; of these 28, 25 have returned for follow-up. Of these 25 patients with follow-up, 18 (72%) developed at least one new ocular lesion by the time of their most recent examination at 10.9 ± 5. 7 years of age, 7 (39%) had new lesions bilaterally, and 13 (52%) had new central lesions [884].

It is critical to note that the children who were untreated, although they presented with more mild disease and had more recurrent eye disease than occurred in those who were treated, are clearly a distinct group. They may not be comparable for many different reasons to those who were treated. Nonetheless, it is interesting to contrast the outcomes of children who were treated in the NCCCTS with those who were untreated. Of the 132 children who were diagnosed and treated in the first year of life or in utero and in the first year of life, and who were last examined at 10.8 ± 5.1 years of age, 108 returned for follow-up. Of the 108 followed-up patients, 34 (31%) developed at least one new ocular lesion, 13 (12%) had bilateral lesions, and 15 (14%) had new central lesions [883]. Development of new eye lesions and active chorioretinitis appeared to be more common around 5 to 7 years of age and in adolescence. In a substantial number from both groups, new lesions became

evident when they were 10 years of age or older, which indicates that long-term follow-up is important in assessing the efficacy of treatment given in early life.

This pattern of late recurrence in congenital toxoplasmic chorioretinitis is interesting in the context of recent observations in the Netherlands [885]. This is a study of a cohort of 153 persons, 11 of whom had congenital toxoplasmosis, and 82 of whom had ocular toxoplasmosis, which could not be categorized as either congenital or postnatally acquired. Specific treatment for episodes of recurrence and criteria for discontinuing treatment were not specified. In this study, 323 episodes of recurrence in first-affected eyes were detected in individuals followed-up from 0.3 to 41 years. Recurrence risk was greatest immediately following an episode and decreased with increasing disease-free intervals; recurrences often occurred in clusters. Relative risk of recurrence declined 72% with each 10-year interval after the first episode and declined 15% with each 10-year increase in age at the first episode. Patients more than 40 years of age were at higher risk of recurrence than younger patients. For the treated persons in the NCCCTS cohort, symptomatic recurrences have been relatively uncommon (878) and these have not occurred in clusters. For the persons not treated in their first year of life in the NCCCTS, there have been teenagers who had multiple recurrences prior to treatment and no further recurrences following treatment of the recurrence and then administration of suppressive medicine.

Treatment of Relapsing Chorioretinitis. The factors that lead to relapse of chorioretinitis are not known. An antimicrobial agent that eliminates encysted organisms in the eye is needed because it is clear that treatment with currently available antimicrobial agents does not uniformly prevent or eliminate relapsing chorioretinitis [433,881]. Longer follow-up of large numbers of treated infants (especially those who acquired their infection in the third trimester and have no retinal involvement at birth) is needed to determine whether treatment reduces the frequency of this sequela. After treatment during the first year of life, congenitally infected infants and young children remain at risk for relapse; for this reason, we and many other authorities currently recommend that they undergo ophthalmoscopy at 3- to 4-month intervals until they can reliably report visual symptoms. Studies are ongoing to determine whether continued frequent follow-up ophthalmologic evaluations and earlier treatment can prevent the devastating consequences of recurrent chorioretinitis. Careful evaluation, including retinal examination, should be performed whenever ocular symptoms suggestive of active chorioretinitis are present.

In infants and in the limited number of older children followed to date in the NCCCTS, active chorioretinitis appeared to resolve within 1 to 2 weeks of beginning treatment with pyrimethamine and sulfonamides as described in Table 31–33. Occasionally, particularly with relatively longer delays in initiating treatment, resolution of active lesions and vitritis was more prolonged. With recurrence of lesions after the first year of life, antimicrobial treatment has been continued 1 to 2 weeks beyond resolution of signs and symptoms. It is standard practice to administer prednisone (1 mg/kg daily in two divided doses [Table 31–33]) in conjunction with pyrimethamine and sulfonamides if inflammation threatens the macula, optic disk, or optic nerve. The efficacy of this practice is unknown. Some investigators have recommended clindamycin or tetracycline therapy [882]. No convincing data are available to allow determination of whether inclusion of these latter two medications would be beneficial.

In a randomized trial in Brazil that included 124 patients ranging in age from 7 to 53 years, prophylaxis with TMP/SMX in a dose of 160 mg/800 mg) given every 3 days for up to 20 months reduced the incidence of recurrent eye lesions from 23.8% (i.e., in 15 patients who received no treatment) to 6.6% (in 4 patients who received treatment) [209]. However, the high incidence of allergy to sulfonamides (25%) makes their use for prophylaxis a potential problem. If allergic reactions develop, treatment of active eye disease that occurs later may require use of other antimicrobials. A recent study demonstrates prevention of recurrences with intravitreal clindamycin (1.5 mg/0.1 ml) and dexamethasone (400 microgram/0.1 ml). Treatment was given weekly or every 4 weeks for pregnant patients and was associated with resolution of toxoplasmic retinochoroiditis (Lasave, et al, Ophthalmology, 2010).

Because transmission occurs frequently when acute infection is acquired in the latter part of the third trimester, we consider it reasonable to provide treatment for the fetus by administering pyrimethamine and sulfadiazine to the recently infected mother. A diagnostic procedure to detect infection in the fetus (see previous on "Prenatal Diagnosis of Fetal *Toxoplasma gondii* Infection") should be performed before this therapy is instituted because such treatment may obscure the diagnosis at birth. In such instances, decision making concerning treatment for the infant during the first year of life is significantly complicated by the lack of accurate diagnostic information.

When choroidal neovascular membranes have developed in the context of toxoplasmic chorioretinitis [410], especially with retinal hemorrhage, treatment with antibody to vascular endothelial growth factor has been curative. Such treatment has been used in infants and children.

Ophthalmologic Outcomes after Prenatal Followed by Postnatal Treatment of Congenital Toxoplasmosis. In a collaborative study by investigators in the United States (NCCCTS) and France, Brezin and colleagues [886] studied ophthalmologic outcome following treatment of congenital toxoplasmosis in utero and in the first year of life with pyrimethamine plus sulfadiazine and leucovorin. Ophthalmologic examinations were performed in 18 children born to mothers infected before 25 weeks of gestation. Both eyes were normal in 11 of the 18 children (61%) (mean age 4.5 years; range, 1 to 11). Only peripheral retinal disease was present in two children (both eyes in each). Four children had posterior pole scars in one eye; each of these four had normal visual acuity, and two of these four had peripheral retinal scars. The outcome was favorable for all but one child, in whom visual acuity was decreased and extensive, bilateral macular and peripheral lesions were present. In a similar, recent study in France [915], outcomes again were very favorable and shorter intervals between diagnosis and initiation of treatment were associated with improved visual outcomes.

These favorable results in France, especially the absence of central chorioretinitis, contrast markedly with the high prevalence of macular disease in the NCCCTS present at birth. The improved outcomes most likely reflect prenatal treatment of the French children. These French outcomes, including those of the Parisian center, suggest that a delay of > 8 weeks between maternal seroconversion and beginning of treatment is a risk factor for retinochoroiditis detected during the first two years of life in infants with treated congenital toxoplasmosis [915].

Prospective Ophthalmologic Follow-up Evaluation of a Cohort of Congenitally Infected Infants in Lyon, France. In an observational, prospective cohort study performed in Lyon, France by Binquet and her colleagues [766,887], maternal infections were identified through monthly testing of susceptible women. Most mothers became infected during the second trimester (89 [20%]) or third trimester (219 [68%]). Two hundred seventy-two (84%) were treated during pregnancy: 149 (46%) with spiramycin alone, 104 (32%) with spiramycin followed by pyrimethamine plus sulfadiazine, and 19 (6%) with pyrimethamine plus sulfadiazine. Treatment for the infant included a brief course (3 weeks) of pyrimethamine plus sulfadiazine followed by 1 year of treatment with Fansidar. In this cohort of 327 children (median duration of follow-up from birth was 6 years [interquartile range, 3 to 10], range, 6 months to 14 years), they [766] found that during a median follow-up period of 6 years, 79 (24%) had at least one retinochoroidal lesion, but bilateral visual impairment was not noted. Children who were diagnosed prenatally or at birth (rather than by an increase in specific IgG between 1 and 12 months of life), who had nonocular manifestations at the time of diagnosis, and who were premature had the highest likelihood of developing ophthalmologic manifestations. Thirteen (17%) of the 79 children had inactive lesions. The authors raise the possibility that the ophthalmologist may have observed those children with extraocular signs more closely. It also is possible that as examinations became easier with the increasing age of the children, more lesions that may have been easier to visualize were detected.

These same investigators recently reported that in this same cohort during a median follow-up period of 6 years after birth (interquartile range, 3 to 10 years), 238 (76%) of the 327 children (range, 6 months to 14 years) were free of any eye lesions. Sixty (18%) had no sequelae except for retinochoroiditis; 33 (11%) had at least one clinical sign of the infection (brain calcifications in 31, hydrocephalus in 6, microcephalus in 1). It is remarkable that in this cohort of 327 children, only 14 (4.3%) of 327 had visual impairment in one eye and none had bilateral visual impairment with a median follow-up of 6 years. Only 5 (1.5%) of 327 had neurologic symptoms. Thus, only 19 (5.8%) of 327 had apparent functional impairment due to congenital infection. Of the six with hydrocephalus, three had moderate psychomotor retardation, and two with calcifications had a single seizure. The investigators also reported that more than one lesion in the retina of the eye was predictive for involvement of the other eye. No association was found between new manifestations of infection and the age at which the initial

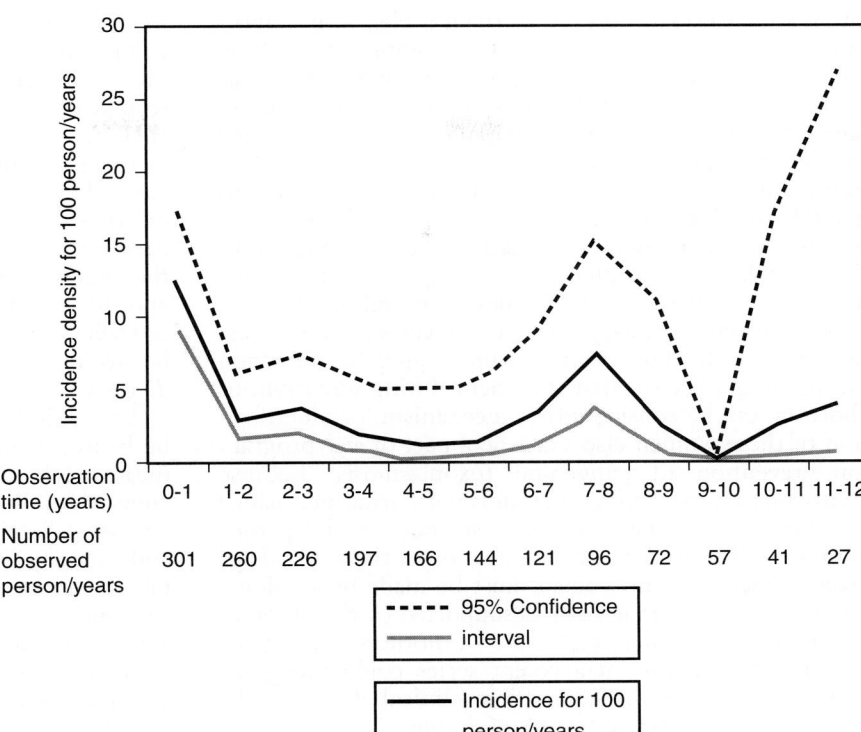

FIGURE 31–37 Incidence density of first ocular lesion after diagnosis of congenital toxoplasmosis in a cohort of children described by Wallon and coworkers. *(From Wallon M, et al. Long-term ocular prognosis in 327 children with congenital toxoplasmosis. Pediatrics 113:1567–1572, 2004.)*

lesion was detected, activity of retinal disease, or locations of retinal lesions [766]. Figure 31–37 shows the times at which the investigators noted new lesions [766].

PREVENTION

Congenital toxoplasmosis is a preventable disease. It is therefore the responsibility of health professionals who provide care for pregnant women to educate them on how they can prevent themselves from becoming infected (and thereby not place their fetus at risk). Lack of adoption of a systematic serologic screening program in the United States leaves primary prevention through education as the principal means of preventing this tragic disease. As a substantial proportion of infections are not associated with recognized risk factors, education concerning risk factors cannot eliminate the majority of infections. Nonetheless, a number of European studies suggest that educational materials can contribute to lowering numbers of infections and disease burden.

Seronegative pregnant women and immunodeficient patients are two populations in which avoidance of infection by *T. gondii* is most important. We consider that the data on morbidity, incidence, and cost of congenital toxoplasmosis warrant a major attempt to define and initiate means whereby congenital toxoplasmosis can be prevented [100]. Several methods for the prevention of congenital toxoplasmosis have been proposed. Attention to the specific hygienic measures outlined in Table 31–50 is the only method available for the primary prevention of congenital toxoplasmosis [181]. It is the responsibility

of all physicians caring for pregnant women and women attempting to conceive (women at risk) to inform them of these preventive measures so that they will not place their fetuses at risk. The impact of these measures on the incidence of acquired toxoplasmosis in a given population has been discussed earlier, in the "Epidemiology" section. A substantial effort to educate women at risk

TABLE 31–50   Methods for Prevention of Congenital Toxoplasmosis

Prevention of Infection in Pregnant Women

Women should take these precautions:
1. Cook meat to well done.
2. Avoid touching mucous membranes of mouth and eyes while handling raw meat. Wash hands thoroughly after handling raw meat.
3. Wash kitchen surfaces that come into contact with raw meat.
4. Wash fruits and vegetables before consumption.
5. Prevent access of flies, cockroaches, and so on to fruits and vegetables.
6. Avoid contact with materials that are potentially contaminated with cat feces (e.g., cat litter boxes) or wear gloves when handling such materials or when gardening.
7. Disinfect cat litter box for 5 minutes with nearly boiling water.

Prevention of Infection in Fetuses

1. Identify women at risk by serologic testing.
2. Treat during pregnancy, which results in an approximate 60% reduction in acquisition of infection among infants and a marked diminution in illness in the fetus and infant.

Adapted from Wilson CB, Remington JS. What can be done to prevent congenital toxoplasmosis? Am J Obstet Gynecol 138:357–363, 1980, with permission.

and the physicians who care for them is clearly an important aspect of any program for prevention [888–890]. Educational materials that indicate how infection can be avoided should be provided in written form, in different languages appropriate to the population, and integrated into existing prenatal programs, visits and classes [199]. For a cost-benefit analysis of preventive measures for congenital toxoplasmosis in the United States, the reader is referred to the article by Roberts and Frenkel [891]. Additional studies to test effectiveness of specific educational measures in different contexts may be useful [892].

In addition to primary preventive measures, it is necessary to identify those women who acquire the infection during pregnancy (so that treatment during gestation, or abortion, can be considered). A mechanism for identification of these women also must be a part of any program for prevention of congenital toxoplasmosis. Because approximately 90% of women infected during pregnancy have no clinical illness and because there are no pathognomonic clinical signs of the infection in the adult, diagnosis in the pregnant woman must be made by serologic methods. This approach also is supported by the observation that only approximately 50% of mothers of congenitally infected infants in a recent series could recognize known risk factors or compatible clinical illness [893]. This makes prospective testing desirable.

FOOD

The tissue cyst can be rendered noninfective by heating meat thoroughly to 66° C (150° F) or by having it smoked or cured. Curing may not eliminate the organism [46]. Freezing meat is a less reliable method of killing the cyst [46]; freezing meat at −20° C for 24 hours may be sufficient to destroy the tissue cyst [30], but not all freezers available in the United States can maintain this temperature even when new. To minimize the chance of infection resulting from handling raw meat, the hands should be thoroughly washed with soap and water after contact with the meat, and the mucous membranes of the mouth and eyes should not be touched with potentially contaminated hands while meat is handled. Eggs should not be eaten raw. Vegetables and fruits should be washed before they are eaten.

Oocysts and Cats

To avoid infection by oocysts, several measures can be suggested. Cat feces may be disposed of daily by burning or flushing down the toilet, and the empty litter pan may be made free of viable oocysts by pouring nearly boiling water into it (an exposure time of 5 minutes is sufficient) [894]. Strong ammonia (7%) also kills oocysts, but contact for at least 3 hours is necessary. Drying, disposing as part of ordinary garbage, surface burial, freezing, or using chlorine bleach, dilute ammonia, quaternary ammonium compounds, or any general disinfectant cannot be relied on [895]. Women who are seronegative during pregnancy and immunodeficient persons should avoid contact with cat feces altogether. For handling litter boxes or working in sand or soil that may have been contaminated by cat feces, disposable gloves should be worn. Because sandboxes often are used by cats as litter boxes, a cover should be placed over the sandbox when it is not

in use, and the hands should be washed after exposure to the sand. Flies, cockroaches, and probably other coprophagic animals serve as transport hosts for *T. gondii* and should be controlled and their access to food prevented [11]. Fruits and vegetables may have oocysts on their surfaces and should be washed before ingestion. Because the cat is the only animal known to produce the oocyst form, efforts should be directed toward preventing infection in cats. Feeding them dried, canned, or cooked food, rather than allowing them to depend on hunting (e.g., for birds and mice) as their source of food, reduces the likelihood of their becoming infected. Frozen raw meat also should be avoided because freezing may not always eliminate *T. gondii* [895].

Although it has been recommended that pet cats should be banished for the duration of pregnancy [896,897], this measure is hardly feasible and not necessary under most circumstances. Repeated requests for serologic testing of cats are being received by veterinarians in the United States, and in many instances, serologic test results are misinterpreted in respect to the danger of transmission. Patients are being misguided, unnecessary anxiety is being produced, and cats are being sacrificed without good reason. The fact is that cats with antibodies are safer pets than cats without antibodies because the presence of antibodies offers some degree of immunity to reinfection and thereby prevents or markedly decreases repetition of oocyst discharge [11]. Antibody determinations are not practical for the determination of infectivity of cats because the infectious oocysts usually are discharged before the development of antibodies in the animal [246,898]; routine serologic testing for this purpose should be discouraged.

Veterinarians and their lay staff caring for cats probably are at increased risk, and special precautionary measures must be exercised to protect pregnant personnel. Large numbers of cats are handled annually by animal practitioners and staff members, and as many as 1% of these cats may excrete oocysts. Feces from caged cats should be collected (preferably on a disposable tray or material) and discarded daily (preferably incinerated) before sporulation occurs. Care must be taken in handling feces for worm counts and similar procedures; samples should be examined within 24 hours of collection, and caution must be exercised to avoid contamination of hands, centrifuges, benches, and microscopes. Gloves should be worn at all times by those handling cat feces [896,899]. Pregnant veterinarians and their lay staff who are not seronegative may wish to consider having someone else handle materials potentially contaminated by oocysts.

Serologic Screening, Diagnosis, and Treatment in Pregnancy

Only a serologic screening program during gestation will detect the acute acquired infection and thereby facilitate diagnosis and treatment of the infected fetus and newborn.

The cost-effectiveness of systematic screening of women during pregnancy depends on a variety of factors, including the cost of tests and how frequently they are employed compared with the cost to society of caring for the diseased children who would be born in the absence of screening [403,628,900–905]. Wilson and

Remington [628] and McCabe and Remington [890] proposed that a screening program be considered in the United States. Such a program would include the performance of a serologic test equal in sensitivity, specificity, and reproducibility to the Sabin-Feldman dye test in all pregnant women. It is crucial that initial testing be performed as early as possible, but at least by 10 to 12 weeks of gestation. (Ideally, testing of all women just before pregnancy would identify those at risk.)

Discussion of all of the pros and cons of a systematic screening program for the United States is beyond the scope of this chapter. Of importance in this regard, however, is the fact that approximately 50% of women with children in the NCCCTS from 1981 to 1998 could not identify a risk factor for or illness consistent with toxoplasmosis [893]. Certain recent analyses of this subject warrant consideration. These analyses have been discussed by Boyer and colleagues [893] as follows:

There are economic analyses, Cochrane database reviews, and metareviews that address the value of screening programs and their outcomes. Some of these analyses and reviews have considered both well-performed studies and studies of dissimilar cohorts that have been inadequately designed, controlled, performed, or interpreted to be of equal value. Some authors of these analyses have noted that there are no perfectly designed and performed prospective, randomized, placebo-controlled studies that have follow-up and include economic analyses that clearly document savings in costs and efficacy of newborn or maternal screening.

Some investigators who have reviewed the available data concluded that without better prospective studies, it may be too costly or unwarranted to perform universal screening and treatment, even to prevent suffering, health care–related costs, loss of productivity and limitation in quality of life associated with untreated congenital toxoplasmosis. There are comments that such screening could cause unacceptable anxiety as a result of false-positive test results, or unnecessary pregnancy terminations due to serologic testing that was not confirmed in a high-quality reference laboratory or counseling that was suboptimal. In contrast, others have concluded that screening, in conjunction with careful confirmation in a high-quality reference laboratory and knowledgeable and caring counseling, is important to facilitate identification and treatment of this fetal and newborn parasitic encephalitis and retinitis.

We critically reviewed these analyses and the concerns they raise. Some important considerations are presented next. We conclude that a number of studies on this subject are seriously flawed. Fortunately, a number of carefully designed investigations on this subject have been performed as well. These latter works indicate that systematic detection of this infection in pregnant women and treatment of the infected fetus as described by Daffos and associates [906] result in better outcomes [893]. In the cohort described by Wallon and colleagues [765], improved outcomes for affected children were observed. Careful confirmation of serologic testing in a high-quality, reliable reference laboratory, and knowledgeable and empathetic medical care and counseling, is essential [893]. Another study performed by Gras and coworkers in a cohort of mothers in Lyon, France, examined the effect of prenatal treatment on the risk of intracranial and ocular lesions in

children with congenital toxoplasmosis [907]. This cohort included 181 infected children born to mothers who received treatment during gestation. The infants received 3 days of pyrimethamine and 3 weeks of sulfadiazine at approximately the time of birth, followed by 2 to 5 weeks of spiramycin therapy and then 12 or more months of Fansidar administered every 10 days. Thirty-eight children had hydrocephalus, intracranial calcifications on ultrasound study or skull film, or in one instance on CT scan, or ocular lesions detected by 3 years of age. These authors report the following percentages of retinal lesions detected over time: 4% (1 month), 9% (6 months), 11% (12 months, N = 157), 16% (3 years, N = 133), 19% (5 years, N = 96), 23% (7 years, N = 55). Because the locations of eye lesions that were apparently new were not clearly specified and not documented with photographs throughout the study, it is difficult to determine with certainty whether the lesions observed later were missed on initial examinations (which are more difficult in young infants and children) or truly were new lesions.

Gras and coworkers also state that, with one exception, outcomes were the same whether the mothers received no treatment, spiramycin, or pyrimethamine plus sulfadiazine before the infants were born. They [907] further reported an observation that is unusual and difficult to explain: They noted the best outcome (i.e., fewest intracranial lesions) with no treatment in utero or following the greatest delay in treatment in utero. The method of detection of intracranial lesions appears to have been by postnatal skull radiography or head ultrasound examination [907], both well known to be suboptimal in terms of sensitivity. The authors suggest that perhaps this result of improved outcome with less treatment could be due to immune suppression in the mother or fetus by pyrimethamine or sulfadiazine treatment, but they provide no supporting data for this hypothesis. The prenatal treatment modalities differed from those used in the cohorts reported by Hohlfeld and colleagues in Paris [77], and the treatment and methods of evaluation conducted postnatally differed from those described by the NCCCTS [433].

Hohlfeld and colleagues noted diminution of cerebrospinal fluid abnormalities indicative of active encephalitis when in utero treatment with pyrimethamine and sulfadiazine was used [76], and Couvreur and associates noted a reduction in isolation of *T. gondii* from placental tissue [69]. Without treatment, *T. gondii* can be isolated from approximately 90% of placentas. With treatment (initiated between 15 and 35 weeks of gestation; median, 23 weeks) *T. gondii* was isolated from placentas of approximately 77% of women given spiramycin [69] and approximately 42% of women given pyrimethamine plus sulfadiazine with leucovorin [69]. *T. gondii*-specific IgM antibody was present in fewer newborns born to mothers given pyrimethamine plus sulfadiazine than in the number of newborns born to mothers who received no treatment (17% versus 69%), and infection was more often subclinical in the newborns born to mothers who had treatment (33% versus 57%) [76].

Foulon's data [78] also are noteworthy: Effects of treatment on development of sequelae in the fetus and the infant up to 1 year were analyzed in 140 children. Sequelae were present in 7 (28%) of 25 children born to mothers who did not receive treatment and in 12 (10%) of 115 children born to mothers who did receive treatment. Multivariate analysis revealed that administration of antibiotic treatment was predictive of the absence of development of sequelae in children ($P = .026$; odds ratio 0.30; 95% confidence interval 0.104 to 0.86). Moreover, when antibiotics were used, a positive correlation was noted between development of sequelae and the time elapsed between when infection occurred and the start of treatment. More rapid instigation of antibiotic treatment after infection led to less frequent sequelae found in the newborn. ($P = .021$).

The NCCCTS investigators have noted resolution of a number of parameters including hepatitis, active chorioretinitis, meningoencephalitis, and no new eye lesions during sustained treatment for congenital toxoplasmosis during the first year of life [433].

Brezin and colleagues reported that 7 (39%) of 18 children with congenital toxoplasmosis treated in utero had eye lesions, with posterior pole lesions in four and with visual impairment in only one child [79]. The median duration of follow-up was 4.5 years (range 1 to 11 years). They were infected before 25 weeks of gestation. They had received in utero treatment before 35 weeks of gestation but not earlier than 22 weeks. Treatment was continued after birth until they were 1 year of age. Children in the NCCCTS also were infected early in gestation, but their mothers had not received treatment during gestation. In contrast with the French children who had received treatment in utero and had less severe eye disease, the children in the NCCCTS had a predominance of posterior pole eye lesions: 54% of children who received treatment in their first year of life, 82% of children with infection detected after their first year of life and therefore untreated, and 58% of the total.

Considerable discussion [908] is available on two recent studies of the efficacy of prenatal treatment in prevention and reduction of sequelae of the congenital infection. The commentary of Thulliez and coworkers is reproduced here in its entirety because of the importance of this analysis in understanding the strengths and weaknesses of the published data:

In their retrospective cohort study of 554 mother-child pairs, Gilbert and colleagues did not detect a significant effect from prenatal treatment on the risk of vertical transmission of toxoplasmosis [909]. This result is not surprising because there were very few untreated women and the analysis of no treatment versus pyrimethamine-sulphadiazine was restricted to half of the cohort who did not undergo amniocentesis. The confidence interval (0.37 to 3.03) for the odds ratio (1.06) for no treatment compared with pyrimethamine-sulphadiazine was therefore very wide and could include a doubling in the risk of transmission in untreated women. Thus an absence of evidence of prenatal treatment effect does not exclude a clinically important beneficial effect.

A further problem is that most of the untreated women were infected during the third trimester of pregnancy. Figure 31–4 shows that only three women infected before 28 weeks of gestation were not treated. The remaining 28 untreated women were infected after 28 weeks. The effect of treatment in the third trimester cannot be generalized to the whole of pregnancy. Finally, the authors explain their findings by suggesting that vertical transmission occurs soon after infection, during parasitemia. This hypothesis is not supported by any scientific studies in humans. On the contrary, one study found that the sensitivity of prenatal diagnosis was lower in early than midpregnancy, suggesting that vertical transmission may be delayed for some women infected in early pregnancy [206].

In the second report by Gras and colleagues [907], the authors unexpectedly found no evidence that prenatal treatment with pyrimethamine-sulphadiazine was more effective than spiramycin in reducing the risks of intracranial or ocular lesions in congenitally infected infants by 3 years of age. A potential explanation for this result is that mothers who transmitted the infection to their fetus soon after infection were more likely to be treated with pyrimethamine-sulphadiazine than mothers infected at the same gestation but in whom transmission was delayed until later in the pregnancy. These two groups may not be comparable because fetuses infected earlier in pregnancy have a higher risk of clinical signs. This explanation is suggested by the fact that mothers infected before 32 weeks were only given pyrimethamine-sulphadiazine if the diagnosis of fetal infection was positive (i.e., vertical transmission occurred between maternal infection and the date of fetal sampling). Other mothers infected before 32 weeks were treated with spiramycin until delivery, either because the prenatal diagnosis was negative or not attempted. In this latter group, transmission occurred either after amniocentesis or at some unknown time between the date of maternal infection and delivery; that is, later during gestation than in the group receiving pyrimethamine-sulphadiazine.

There are two further explanations for the lack of effect of pyrimethamine-sulphadiazine. First, there was a long delay before pyrimethamine-sulphadiazine was started. This was because the study was carried out more than 6 years ago, when mouse inoculation was the standard fetal diagnostic test [83] and pyrimethamine-sulphadiazine treatment would have been delayed for 3–6 weeks until results were known. Today, PCR analysis of amniotic fluid is widespread. Results are available in one day and women with infected fetuses are treated much earlier [522]. Secondly, women in the study given pyrimethamine-sulphadiazine actually received an alternating regimen with spiramycin. The periods of spiramycin treatment may have led to parasitic relapses in fetal tissues, as shown in experimental models (Piketty and colleagues, AAC, 1990). The current treatment policy for women with a positive prenatal diagnosis is to prescribe continuous treatment with pyrimethamine-sulphadiazine until delivery.

The data reported by Gilbert and colleagues [910] and Gras and coworkers [911] provide no convincing evidence that this policy should change.*

Each of us is in favor of a screening program for the United States similar to that being used at present in France (see Fig. 33–35). We recognize, however, that constraints of the present-day health care systems may not permit such screening on a monthly basis or, in some instances, screening of pregnant women per se. Cost-benefit analyses are especially relevant to mandated,

---

*Reproduced from Thulliez P, et al: Efficacy of prenatal treatment for toxoplasmosis: a possibility that cannot be ruled out. Int J Epidemiol 30:1315–1316, 2001. Reference numbers and cited figure refer to main text.

state-supported screening programs. Nevertheless, we believe that almost all parents, given the choice, would select a simple, not very costly, and direct measure that could prevent cognitive and ocular damage to their child as part of their health care coverage.

Introduction of prenatal screening and, in particular, use of PCR testing on amniotic fluid at 18 weeks of gestation has altered the approach to screening of women. The data that demonstrate a benefit of screening are from programs that screen on a monthly basis, as is done in France. In France, more than 90% of women now have their first prenatal visit (with testing to assess whether they are seropositive for *T. gondii* antibodies) in the first trimester. This early, first-trimester prenatal visit is a requirement for health care insurance coverage during gestation and at birth. This requirement considerably facilitates interpretation of results of serologic screening. Possible alternatives in locations where prevalence of antibody is low and resources are limited have not been studied systematically.

Available data indicate that better outcomes result with initiation of treatment within weeks after the diagnosis of recently acquired infection is made in the mother [78]. (This conclusion is also supported by the recent meta-analysis by the SYROCORT study group of 1438 mothers who were treated during pregnancy as part of 18 different European screening cohorts [912].) This analysis showed that the earlier prenatal treatment commenced following seroconversion the lower the risk of transmission with an odds ratio (adjusted for timing and type of prenatal treatment) of 0.48 in mothers treated less than 3 weeks after seroconversion, compared with odds ratio of 0.60 to 0.64 in mothers treated 3 to 8 weeks after seroconversion and to the reference value of 1.0 for mothers treated more than 8 weeks after seroconversion. This meta-analysis shows that early treatment following seroconversion is more effective than delayed treatment in preventing mother to infant transmission. Thus although no randomized controlled trials comparing treatment to no treatment have been performed, unless delayed treatment increases the risk of transmission compared to no treatment, a possibility we consider to be unlikely, then early treatment is beneficial. Accordingly, these findings support the notion that early testing would allow the detection of women whose fetuses are at greatest risk of being infected and appropriate management decisions to be made regarding treatment.

If the diagnosis of newly acquired maternal infection has been made, it becomes important to determine as early as possible whether the fetus has been infected because treatment of the fetus through administration of specific therapy to the pregnant woman may be indicated (see later discussion). PCR analysis of amniotic fluid allows fetal infection to be detected. Therefore, women must be informed of the importance of a visit to their physician as early as possible in pregnancy to allow for early serologic testing. Under optimal circumstances, if a pregnant woman is seronegative at the time of her first prenatal evaluation, serologic follow-up testing should be performed monthly thereafter to allow for timely recognition of newly acquired infection. This is the approach with the greatest potential for benefit. We recognize that such frequent testing may not be feasible. If it is not, blood for the second serum

sample should be drawn at a time in the second trimester such that if recently acquired infection is confirmed, PCR analysis in the amniotic fluid can be performed at 18 to 21 weeks of gestation. If that second serum does not reveal recently acquired infection, a third serum sample can be obtained in the early third trimester. If seroconversion is observed at that time, we recommend PCR on amniotic fluid; if the PCR assay reveals infection in the fetus, the mother should receive pyrimethamine-sulfadiazine in an attempt to treat the fetus. A final serum sample is obtained at the time of parturition to detect those mothers who acquired their infection very late in gestation but whose fetuses are at greatest risk of infection. Luyasu and associates [913] reported seven cases of subclinical congenital *T. gondii* infection in infants born to mothers who acquired their infection between 2 and 4 weeks before delivery. They emphasized that because children born to mothers who become infected close to term are at greatest risk for development of the congenital infection and must be given appropriate treatment to attempt to prevent untoward sequelae of the infection, it is important to screen seronegative pregnant women until the time of delivery.

A woman whose is seropositive on initial testing ideally then undergoes testing for IgM antibodies. If the IgM test result is positive, an avidity test should be performed on the same serum sample. If a high-avidity test result is observed in a woman in her first trimester, acute infection during the first trimester is essentially excluded. For further decisions regarding patient management and desirability of confirmatory testing if the IgM test result is positive and the avidity test titer is low or equivocal, the reader is referred to the discussion in the "Avidity Assay" section and the section "Practical Guidelines for Diagnosis of Infection in the Pregnant Women." In patients with a positive IgG test result and a negative result on testing for IgM antibodies in the first trimester, with no clinical signs of acute toxoplasmosis, no further testing would be performed because in the United States the probability that these women are acutely infected is remote.

In addition to the data described above that show the importance of early, monthly serologic screening, if the risk of maternofetal transmission is to be reduced by antenatal treatment, early detection and antenatal treatment may reduce the risk of subsequent sequelae in those who do become infected. The data of Brézin and associates indicate that subsequent retinal disease is less frequent, and also less severe, in the infants born to mothers managed according to the method used by the group in Paris [886]. Similarly, Foulon and colleagues showed that earlier initiation of antenatal treatment was associated with a decreased risk of sequelae by 1 year of age [78]. However, reports by Gras and colleagues [911] and the meta-analyses done by the SYROCOT [912] study group concluded that antenatal treatment did not reduce the risk of ocular sequelae even when started within 5 weeks of seroconversion, although there was a trend suggesting that early antenatal treatment may reduce the risk of intracranial lesions; neurologic follow-up is still in progress [195].

The basis for these conflicting conclusions regarding the impact of antenatal treatment on ocular sequelae is unclear. However, comparison of two recent reports that reached contrasting conclusions [914,915] raises the possibility that studies like SYROCOT, which group together cases from multiple centers whose approaches to prenatal diagnosis and treatment vary substantially, may obscure significant findings observed at centers whose frequency of screening and approach to intervention are done according to the method used in Paris. Freeman and coworkers [914] analyzed 281 cases from multiple centers throughout Europe and concluded that prenatal treatment did not decrease the incidence of retinochoroiditis. Among these 281 cases were 129 from three centers in France whose approach to antenatal management paralleled the method used in Paris, whereas the remaining cases came from centers in multiple countries with quite different approaches. By contrast to the conclusions reached by Freeman and coworkers, when Kieffer and colleagues [915] analyzed the 129 cases from the three centers in France and an additional 171 cases from these centers, they found that when antenatal therapy was not administered within 8 weeks of seroconversion, the risk of retinochoroiditis was significantly greater (hazard ratio 2.54; 95% confidence interval 1.14 to 5.65) than when therapy was administered within 8 weeks of seroconversion. While there are other possible explanations for the discordant conclusions in these two and other studies, these findings are compatible with the interpretation that early detection of infection permits prompt treatment of infection that otherwise causes irreversible destruction of ocular and CNS tissue in utero.

We agree with Kieffer and coworkers [915] that while a randomized, controlled trial would be required to conclusively resolve these discordant conclusions, the evidence cited above suggests that monthly screening and early antenatal therapy may be warranted to reduce the risk of eye disease attributable to congenital toxoplasmosis. Although postnatal treatment can lead to rapid resolution of active infection and improve outcome [433] some children given treatment do not experience significant improvement; and even for those who function normally, the in utero infection is not without late consequences because cognitive outcomes for children who receive treatment are in some instances less favorable than for their uninfected siblings [873]. For these reasons, we currently consider that antenatal diagnosis and management is preferred when possible.

At present in the United States, *T. gondii* serology is performed haphazardly by laboratories and with kits of varying quality for physicians who may understand little of the disease or the tests, and unfortunately, in many cases inappropriate decisions are made on the basis of unreliable information [631,652]. For these reasons, our present lack of systematic screening—in a setting of sporadic screening that is inadequately supervised—may result in more harm than good. We and the FDA recommend that any serologic test results suggesting that infection was acquired during pregnancy be confirmed and interpreted by a reference laboratory before decisions regarding treatment, prenatal diagnosis, or therapeutic abortion are made [652,712].

We recently proposed guidelines [199] for serologic screening and management of women who are suspected or confirmed to have acquired toxoplasmosis during pregnancy in the United States. These guidelines are outlined in the form of management algorithms in Figures 31–38 and 31–39. Serologic testing for both IgG and IgM antibodies should be performed initially at clinical, nonreference laboratories. In most cases, testing in early gestation will confirm that the mother has not previously been infected, as indicated by the absence of IgG and IgM antibodies, and in other cases, that infection was acquired in the distant past, as indicted by the presence of IgG antibodies in the absence of IgM antibodies. Additional testing at a reference laboratory is required primarily in those women with IgG seroconversion or positive or equivocal IgM antibody test results. It is important to recognize that a positive IgM antibody test at any time during gestation does not necessarily indicate recently acquired infection. The greatest value of a positive IgM test is that it indicates the necessity for performing confirmatory testing in a reference laboratory before any conclusions regarding the presence or absence of recently acquired infection and risk to the fetus can be made.

Special Usefulness of the Avidity Assay Earlier in Gestation

Recently, several tests for avidity of *Toxoplasma* IgG antibodies have been introduced to help discriminate between recently acquired and distant infection [88,283]. The commercial tests are available in Europe but are not licensed in the United States. Results are based on the measurement of functional affinity of specific IgG antibodies [88,283]. IgG affinity, which initially is low after primary antigenic challenge, increases during subsequent weeks and months by antigen-driven B cell selection. Protein-denaturing reagents, including urea, are used to dissociate the antibody-antigen complex. The avidity result is determined by using the ratios of antibody titration curves of urea-treated and untreated samples.

The use of the avidity test in the acutely infected woman during the first 12 to 16 weeks of gestation was recently described [88]. The usefulness of testing for IgG avidity was evaluated in a reference laboratory in the United States. European investigators have reported that high-avidity IgG *T. gondii* antibodies exclude acute infection in the preceding 3 months. In this U.S. study, 125 serum samples taken from 125 pregnant women in the first trimester were chosen retrospectively because either the IgM or differential agglutination (AC/HS) test in the *Toxoplasma* Serologic Profile suggested or was equivocal for a recently acquired infection. Of 93 (74.4%) serum samples with either positive or equivocal results in the IgM ELISA, 52 (55.9%) had high-avidity antibodies, which suggests that the infection probably was acquired before gestation. Of 87 (69.6%) serum samples with an acute or equivocal result in the AC/HS test, 35 (40.2%) had high-avidity antibodies. Forty women were given spiramycin in an attempt to prevent congenital transmission, and 7 (17.5%) had high-avidity antibodies. These findings highlight the value of IgG avidity testing of a single serum sample obtained in the first trimester of pregnancy for IgG avidity.

The avidity test does not establish the diagnosis of the acute infection. At present, definitive serologic diagnosis of acute infection during gestation can be made only if paired serum samples reveal a significant increase in titer, most often of IgG antibodies [88,283]. Such increasing

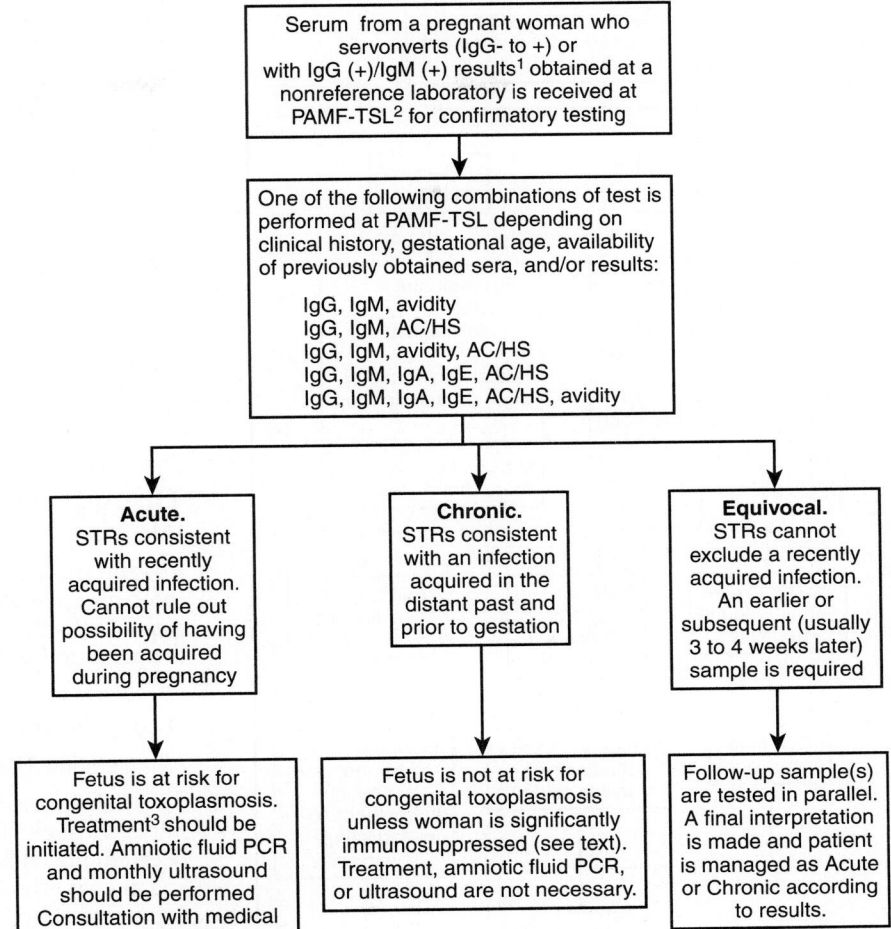

FIGURE 31–38 Serologic testing and management of toxoplasmosis during pregnancy on the basis of results obtained at the Palo Alto Medical Foundation Toxoplasma Serology Laboratory (PAMF-TSL), telephone number (650) 853–4828. **A,** A serum sample with positive results of IgG and IgM antibody tests is the most common reason for requesting confirmatory testing at PAMF-TSL. **B,** PAMF-TSL or US (Chicago, IL) National Collaborative Treatment Trial Study, telephone number (773) 834–4152. **C,** Treatment with spiramycin or with pyrimethamine, sulfadiazine, and folinic acid (see text and table 6). *AC/HS,* differential agglutination test; *STRs,* serologic test results at PAMF-TSL; *TSP, Toxoplasma* serologic panel. *(From Montoya JG, Remington JS. Management of* Toxoplasma gondii *infection during pregnancy. Clin Infect Dis 47:554–566, 2008.)*

titers are not commonly seen in pregnant women in the United States because no systematic serologic screening to detect seroconversion is done. Although successful screening programs have been used in France and Austria for many years, in the United States, usually only a single serum sample is submitted for testing, frequently late in gestation (see Table 31–23). It is noteworthy that more than 57% of these sera were obtained from pregnant patients after the first trimester of gestation, and 14% to 21%, after the second trimester of gestation. Use of such relatively late-gestation serum samples clearly demonstrates the difficulty in attempts to prevent transmission to the fetus in the United States. Results have not changed in the past several years. As noted, almost all women in France (95%) seek prenatal care in the first trimester because government medical benefits are then made available for the remainder of the pregnancy. Early prenatal care permits initiation of serologic screening early in gestation. This approach contrasts remarkably with that used in the United States.

Because IgM antibodies may persist for months or even years after acute infection, their greatest value is in determining that a pregnant woman was not infected recently. A negative result virtually rules out recent infection, unless serum samples are tested so late after onset of infection that

IgM antibody has disappeared or so early in acute infection that an antibody response has not occurred or is not yet detectable. When results are positive, a number of additional serologic tests, including those for the detection of IgG, IgA, and IgE antibodies, and a combination of these tests, the *Toxoplasma* Serologic Profile (TSP), can help discriminate between recently acquired and distant infection. The differential agglutination (AC/HS) test most closely approaches a single reference standard test for the discrimination of recently acquired and distant infection. At present in the United States, however, this test is done only by the *Toxoplasma* Serology Laboratory at the Palo Alto Medical Foundation (TSL-PAMF) in Palo Alto because the required antigen preparations are not commercially available. In addition, as is true for IgM antibodies, an acute pattern in the AC/HS test may persist for longer than 1 year.

Liesenfeld and coworkers investigated the usefulness of testing for avidity of IgG antibodies in a *Toxoplasma* serology reference laboratory in the United States that processes serum samples primarily from pregnant women [88]. In most cases, the physician requests information about the time of onset of the infection on the basis of results obtained from a single serum sample. The goal of these investigators was to compare results obtained in an IgG avidity test with those obtained in the IgM ELISA and AC/HS tests.

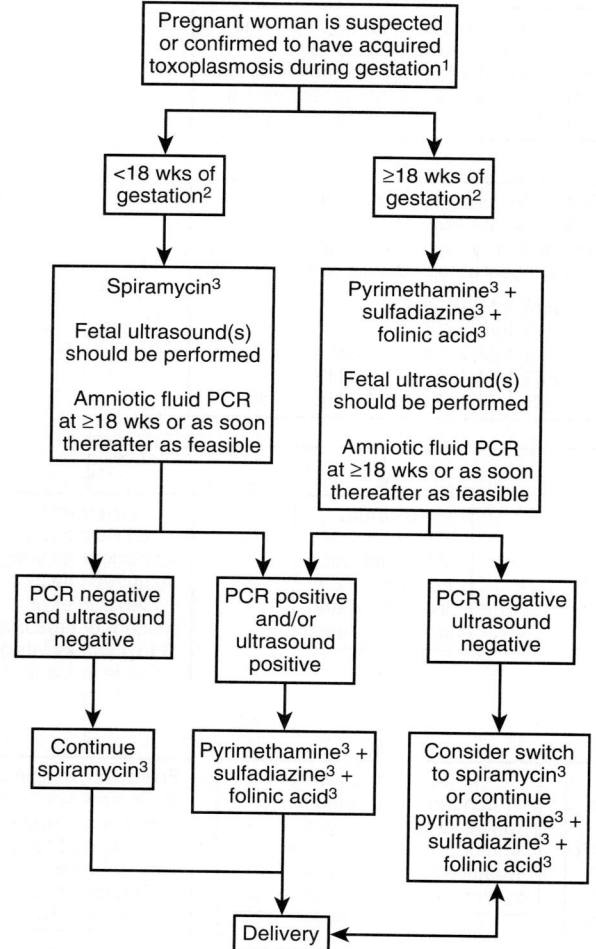

FIGURE 31–39 Approach for pregnant women who are suspected or confirmed to have toxoplasmosis acquired during gestation. **1**, Consultation with a reference laboratory or physician expert in toxoplasmosis is suggested (i.e., Palo Alto Medical Foundation Toxoplasma Serology Laboratory, telephone number (650) 853–4828, or US [Chicago, IL] National Collaborative Treatment Trial Study, telephone number (773) 834–4152). **2**, Gestational age at which maternal infection was suspected or confirmed to have been acquired (or the best estimate); this is not the gestational age at which the patient consulted with or was seen by the health care provider. **3**, For dosages and comments, see Table 31–6. Folic acid should not be used as a substitute for folinic acid. *wks,* Weeks. *(From Montoya JG, Remington JS. Management of* Toxoplasma gondii *infection during pregnancy.* Clin Infect Dis *47:554–566, 2008.)*

All pregnant women who have a positive result on IgM *T. gondii* serologic testing should have an IgG avidity test performed. This test is most valuable in the first 12 to 16 weeks of gestation (see under "Diagnosis"). In two reference laboratories, the results from the AC/HS test complement the information provided by the avidity assay. The avidity assay is particularly useful in the first 4 months of gestation when IgM is present and the AC/HS test result is acute or equivocal. Time of conversion from low or equivocal to high avidity is highly variable among persons tested. Once a high-avidity test result is obtained, it can be concluded that the patient was infected at least 3 to 5 months earlier. Low-avidity test results should not be interpreted to mean recently acquired infection. The reason is that low-avidity antibodies may persist for as long as 1 year, and borderline or low-avidity antibodies can persist in the presence or absence of *T. gondii*-specific IgM antibodies. Forty percent of women with *T. gondii*-specific IgG but no IgM antibodies had borderline or low-avidity antibodies in one study [89].

The avidity test is best used in conjunction with a panel of tests, for example, *T. gondii*-specific IgG, IgM, IgA, and AC/HS tests. The avidity test should not be used alone; results should be interpreted in the context of other serologic tests that indicate acute infection in the first 12 to 16 weeks of gestation. The avidity test can be used to assess whether acute acquired infection in the mother that is first detected late in gestation was acquired more than 12 to 16 weeks earlier. This provides information about risk to the fetus.

Prevention of Congenital Toxoplasmosis Through Treatment of the Pregnant Woman

For the special instance of the pregnant woman with HIV infection, see earlier section on "Congenital *Toxoplasma gondii* Infection and Acquired Immunodeficiency Syndrome," under "Clinical Manifestations."

Acute Infection

Antimicrobial Therapy

Treatment during pregnancy (see also "Treatment of the Fetus through Treatment of the Pregnant Woman") has been employed in an attempt to decrease both the incidence and the severity of congenital infection. This treatment is administered to a pregnant woman with a recently acquired (acute) infection in the hope that such treatment will prevent spread of infection to the fetus. The rationale for such treatment is based on the observation that there is a significant lag period between the onset of maternal infection and infection of the fetus. In the first such study, performed in Germany, Kräubig used a combination of sulfonamides and pyrimethamine [73,916]. Because of its potential teratogenic effects, pyrimethamine was not administered during the first 12 to 14 weeks of gestation. Kräubig noted a definite reduction in incidence of congenitally acquired infection in infants born to mothers who received treatment (5%) versus those who did not (16.6%)—a 70% reduction (prevention). Kräubig considered these data an indication that treatment is necessary if a diagnosis of acute acquired toxoplasmosis is made during pregnancy. Thalhammer, who closely collaborated in these studies with Kräubig, agreed with this statement because it appears that all cases of congenital toxoplasmosis might be prevented by such an approach [917,918]. In 1982, Hengst from Berlin reported similar results in a prospective study [919].

In a separate and independent study performed in France [68], daily oral doses of 2 to 3 g of spiramycin in four divided doses were administered for 3 weeks to women who acquired toxoplasmosis during pregnancy. Such courses of treatment were arbitrarily repeated at 2-week intervals up to the time of delivery. Only women who completed at least one such course were considered to have undergone treatment. Cases of congenital *T. gondii* infection were significantly more frequent among

154 women who received no treatment (58%) than among 388 women who received treatment (23%). Clinically apparent disease in the newborns, however, was just as frequent among children born with congenital *T. gondii* infection from both groups of women (28% and 27% of infected offspring, respectively). This finding suggests that spiramycin treatment in the pregnant woman might have reduced by 60% the frequency of transmission of *T. gondii* to the offspring but did not apparently modify the pattern of infection in the infected fetus. Although the difference between treated and untreated groups is highly significant, however, the pregnant women in this study who received no treatment do not represent a good control group for several reasons. Most women diagnosed in their first trimester received treatment, whereas the proportion of women who received no treatment is rather low among women who acquired *T. gondii* infection during the last months of pregnancy. Thus more infections occurred earlier in the treated group than in the untreated group, a fact that of itself might have led to fewer congenital infections and to a higher proportion of cases with clinical disease among infected infants, if untreated. Nevertheless, congenital infections were less frequent in the treated group in each trimester of pregnancy. Consequently, the decrease in fetal infections could be assumed to reflect bias not only in the selection of cases but in treatment as well.

Variability in the clinical aspects of congenital infection also must be considered. Table 31–51 shows the comparison between treated and untreated groups of pregnant women. No difference in the proportion of mild and subclinical cases was found. By contrast, the number of stillbirths decreased and the proportion of children born alive with severe disease increased slightly in the treated group. The numbers are too small to be significant, but the reason for the increase in incidence of severe disease despite treatment during fetal life is that the treatment, although undertaken too late to prevent severe damage, might sometimes have prevented fetal death.

A prospective study that compares the efficacy of spiramycin versus pyrimethamine plus sulfonamide for prevention of congenital transmission has not been performed. When compared with data obtained from historical controls, the more recent studies suggest the importance of

the pyrimethamine plus sulfonamide regimen. Each of the studies involved an attempt to isolate the organism from placentas. In one such study of 32 women, each of whose fetuses was diagnosed as being infected by isolation of the parasite from amniotic fluid or blood between weeks 24 and 30 of gestation (update of originally published data [69]), infection in the mothers was documented to have occurred between weeks 10 and 29 of gestation. The mothers were given 3 g of spiramycin daily as soon as the diagnosis of their acute acquired infection was made. Pyrimethamine plus sulfonamide was given during the last 2 months of gestation. Because of the potential hazard for mother or fetus, use of the combination of pyrimethamine plus sulfonamide was restricted by Couvreur and colleagues to the last 2 months of gestation and to a high-risk group in which fetal infection was documented during pregnancy. *T. gondii* was isolated from 47% of the placentas (examined after delivery) from these 32 cases. In marked contrast, *T. gondii* was isolated from 71.5% of placentas of 21 infants born to mothers who received spiramycin alone and, using historical controls, from 89% of placentas of 85 infants born to mothers who received an inadequate spiramycin regimen (duration of treatment less than 2 weeks or daily dose of only 2 g, which is considered by the investigators to be too low) or who received no treatment.

In Austria, Aspöck and colleagues routinely used spiramycin before week 16 of gestation and pyrimethamine plus a sulfonamide after week 15 of gestation. In their prospective study, this treatment regimen was highly successful [900].

Together, these data strongly suggest that treatment is effective, although a placebo controlled randomized trial demonstrating such effectiveness has not been performed.. In addition, because spiramycin also may delay transmission of the parasite to the fetus, it should have the added benefit of reducing the severity of the disease in the fetus and newborn because of the increased maturity of the maternal immune response and of the fetus at the time infection occurs. Critically designed studies are needed to clarify this question. Nevertheless, until such data become available—and in view of the prevention rate of congenital infection of 60% to 70% achieved in the two studies mentioned earlier—it would appear prudent to advise treatment in women who acquire the infection during pregnancy. The dose of spiramycin is 3 g per day. Toxicity has not proved to be a problem with spiramycin in such cases. This drug is at present available in the United States only by request to the FDA. Pyrimethamine plus sulfadiazine can be employed in the second and third trimesters of pregnancy with the precautionary measures mentioned earlier in the "Therapy" section (see also "Treatment of the Fetus In Utero"). Whether sequelae in infected children who received treatment in utero are as frequent or as serious as those in children who received no treatment is a question that can be answered only by long-term observation.

Repeated here are our recommendations made previously in "Treatment of the Fetus through Treatment of the Pregnant Woman."

When the diagnosis of infection in the fetus is established earlier than 17 weeks, we suggest that sulfadiazine be used alone until after the first trimester, at which time pyrimethamine should be added to the regimen. The

TABLE 31–51 Effect of Spiramycin Treatment on Relative Frequency of Stillbirth and on Different Aspects of Congenital Toxoplasmosis

Outcome in Offspring	No. (%) of Affected Offspring	
	No Treatment	*Treatment*
Congenital toxoplasmosis		
Subclinical	64 (68)	65 (72)
Mild	14 (15)	13 (14)
Severe	7 (7)	10 (11)
Stillbirth or perinatal death†	9 (10)	3 (3)
Total	94 (100)	91 (100)

†See text.
Adapted from Desmonts G, Couvreur J. Congenital toxoplasmosis: a prospective study of the offspring of 542 women who acquired toxoplasmosis during pregnancy: pathophysiology of congenital disease. In Thalhammer O, Baumgarten K, Pollak A (eds). Perinatal Medicine, Sixth European Congress, Vienna. Stuttgart, Germany, Georg Thieme, 1979, with permission.

decision about when to begin pyrimethamine/sulfadiazine/leucovorin for the pregnant woman is based on an assessment of the risk of fetal infection, incidence of false-positive and false-negative results of amniocentesis with PCR, and risks of medicines. Although reliability of PCR results are laboratory dependent, results from the best reference laboratories, have a sensitivity for PCR of the *T. gondii* 300 copy 529 bp gene with amniotic fluid of 92%. Thus PCR results reasonably determine the therapeutic approach.

When the mother becomes infected between 22 and 31 weeks of gestation, the incidence of transmission exceeds 50% and manifestations of infection in the fetus are substantial, 92% for 22 to 26 weeks and for 27 to 31 weeks. With maternal acquisition of infection after 31 weeks of gestation, incidence of transmission exceeds 60% and, manifestations of infection are in general less severe. Sensitivity of PCR in amniotic fluid is 92%.

When infection is acquired between 21 and 29 weeks of gestation, management varies. After 24 weeks of gestation, we recommend that amniocentesis be performed and that pyrimethamine/leucovorin/sulfadiazine be used instead of spiramycin. Consultation with the reference laboratory is advised.

In France, standard of care (until late in gestation) is to wait 4 weeks from the estimated time that maternal infection is acquired until amniocentesis to allow sufficient time for transmission to occur. Amniocentesis is not performed before 17 to 18 weeks of gestation. In some instances, when maternal infection is acquired between 12 and 16 weeks of gestation or after the 21st week of gestation, pyrimethamine and sulfadiazine treatment is initiated regardless of the amniotic fluid PCR result. This is because of concerns about the confidence intervals and reliability of negative amniotic fluid PCR results. When this approach is used, a delay in amniocentesis when maternal infection is acquired between 12 and 16 weeks and after 21 weeks of gestation would not be logical.

Termination of Pregnancy

Confirmatory serologic testing in a reference laboratory and communication of the results and their correct interpretation by an expert to the patient's physician decreased the rate of unnecessary pregnancy terminations by approximately 50% among women with positive IgM *Toxoplasma* antibody test results reported by outside laboratories [88].

The decision whether to treat with antimicrobial agents or to perform an abortion in a woman suspected of acquiring *T. gondii* infection during pregnancy should ultimately be made by the patient in conjunction with her physician after careful consideration of the potential results with each of these two modalities of intervention. Therapeutic abortion may be considered in women who are known to have acquired acute *T. gondii* infection early during gestation or in whom the likelihood of their having acquired acute infection early during gestation is very high. Only approximately 22% of women who acquire primary *T. gondii* infection during the first 22 to 24 weeks of gestation transmit the infection to their offspring. Even if all women who acquire the infection during the first two trimesters were to elect abortion, less than one half of all

cases of congenital toxoplasmosis would be prevented because more than 50% of infected offspring result from maternal infection acquired in the last trimester.

Prenatal examination has for the first time allowed for an objective decision by the pregnant woman in regard to abortion and whether her aborted fetus would indeed be congenitally infected. Such a decision was previously based on a statistical estimation of the risk to the fetus. Considerable controversy has arisen in regard to whether and under what circumstances abortion might be considered. The controversy appears to have stemmed from the publication by Berrebi and colleagues in *The Lancet* [736], who concluded that only ultrasonographic evidence of hydrocephalus indicates a poor outcome; for this reason they no longer use the gestational age-related statistics that Daffos and colleagues propose [82] to counsel affected couples. Berrebi's group [742] studied 163 mothers who acquired their infection with *T. gondii* before 28 weeks of gestation. All were given spiramycin treatment, and 23 also received pyrimethamine and sulfadiazine. Each underwent cordocentesis and regular ultrasound examinations. Their 162 live-born infants were evaluated over 15 to 71 months. Three fetuses died in utero, and 27 of 162 live-born infants had congenital toxoplasmosis: 10 had clinical signs of the infection, 5 with isolated or multiple intracranial calcifications, 7 with peripheral chorioretinitis, and two with moderate ventricular dilation. Because each of the 27 was free of symptoms and demonstrated normal neurologic development at 15 to 71 months of age, the investigators concluded that acute fetal infection identified in first- and second-trimester pregnancies need not be an indication for interruption of the pregnancy if fetal ultrasonographic evaluation results are normal (no evidence of fetal death or hydrocephalus) and treatment of the fetus is instigated.

In a letter to the editor of *The Lancet* commenting on the results of Berrebi and associates, Wallon and coworkers [869] also were conservative in their conclusions. From the results of their studies, they recommend that termination not be performed unless fetal ultrasonographic examination reveals morphologic abnormalities. In a simultaneously published letter to the editor of *The Lancet*, Daffos and colleagues [906] concurred that too many pregnancies are terminated because congenital toxoplasmosis is diagnosed prenatally, but these authors were far less optimistic than Berrebi and associates about the outcome for the fetus infected early in gestation. Daffos and colleagues stated that in a study of 148 fetal infections diagnosed by prenatal examination, "the best (and perhaps the only) factor with predictive value for the severity of the fetal infection is gestational age at the time of maternal infection." In their study, they noted that if the infection occurred before 16 weeks of gestation, 31 of 52 fetuses (60%) had ultrasonographic evidence of infection, including ascites, pericarditis, or necrotic foci in the brain, and 48% had cerebral ventricular dilation. If infection had occurred between 17 and 23 weeks, 16 of 63 fetuses (25%) had ultrasonographic signs, and only 12% had ventricular dilation. In those cases of infection after 24 weeks, only 1 of 33 fetuses (3%) had ultrasonographic signs, and none had hydrocephalus. Thus the approach that Daffos and his colleagues had recommended 6 years earlier [82] appeared to remain valid. These workers accept parental requests for termination in those cases in which infection occurs before 16 weeks because of the severe prognosis for the fetus. In such instances, they have always found large areas of brain necrosis at necropsy, even when there was no evidence of ventricular dilation on ultrasound evaluation. They conclude that such dilation of the ventricles would have developed in many of these cases if the pregnancy had been allowed to continue, even if treatment with pyrimethamine and sulfadiazine was used.

Recently, Kieffer and coworkers [915] reported findings similar to the work of Berrebi and colleagues, that not all fetuses infected early in gestation had severe abnormalities when they were born. Like Berrebi and coworkers, they no longer concluded that early gestation infection of the pregnant woman uniformly had poor outcomes.

It is hoped that in the near future this issue will be resolved by a collaborative effort to review all pertinent data by interested investigators and, if necessary, to design studies aimed at formulating a consensus and guidelines for providing the patient with objective information during counseling about termination of pregnancy. In one study [206] in which real-time PCR analysis was evaluated, quantitation of the PCR revealed that higher parasite burden in amniotic fluid is associated with more damage to the fetus (see also section on "PCR").

Despite the fact that IgM tests do not differentiate between acute and chronic infection, a positive IgM test result strongly influences pregnant women in their choice to terminate or continue the pregnancy. In the United States, such decisions often are made on the basis of results for a single serum specimen in which the result of IgM antibody testing is positive and confirmatory testing is not done. We previously estimated that approximately 20% of women who are told that they have a positive result on IgM antibody testing will request therapeutic abortion [920]. In that study, approximately 60% of the results of IgM tests reported as positive by commercial laboratories were negative in the IgM test in the Palo Alto reference laboratory. In the cases with reported positive IgM test results, evidence of recently acquired infection, as determined by the *Toxoplasma* Serologic Profile, also was absent. Thus at a minimum, 12 of every 20 fetuses that were not infected were aborted. In a more recent study, Liesenfeld and associates [920] from the same laboratory determined the accuracy of *T. gondii* serologic test results obtained in commercial laboratories and the role of confirmatory testing in preventing unnecessary abortion. Congenital toxoplasmosis is a preventable disease. It is therefore the responsibility of health professionals who provide care for pregnant women to educate them on how they can prevent themselves from becoming infected (and thereby not place their fetus at risk). Lack of adoption of a systematic serologic screening program in the United States leaves education as the principal means of preventing this tragic disease.

Physicians who recommend or perform an abortion must be knowledgeable about the subject so that an intelligent decision can be made. Because abortions are performed as late as 22 to 24 weeks of gestation in the United States, the practitioner has time to obtain an initial serologic specimen early in gestation and a follow-up specimen later in gestation to define those women at risk of transmitting *T. gondii* to their offspring (see "Serologic Screening" section). Guidelines for the interpretation of serologic tests on specimens obtained during pregnancy have been given previously in the "Diagnosis" section. If tests for IgM antibodies to *T. gondii* are unavailable to assist in establishing the diagnosis of acute infection, it should be understood that the risk of congenital toxoplasmosis is almost zero in a patient whose serum shows a high IgG test titer in the second month of pregnancy. A high IgG test titer at that time indicates an infection that occurred at least 2 months before (and perhaps much earlier) in all but rare exceptions in which the serologic test titer rises steeply for several weeks. On the contrary, women who will later give birth to a congenitally infected infant, when examined during the second or third month of pregnancy, either have no antibody (i.e., they are not yet infected) or may have a low titer (associated with IgM antibody) as a result of an infection acquired during the past few days or weeks. A careful follow-up examination and confirmatory testing in a reference laboratory along with amniocentesis for PCR assay and mouse inoculation may reveal infection in the fetus in time to allow for consideration of termination of the pregnancy in these cases. Treatment for the infected mother to attempt to prevent transmission of the infection to the fetus appears more worthy of consideration in such circumstances.

Chronic (Latent) Infection

The controversial subjects of congenital transmission, repeated abortion, and perinatal fetal mortality during chronic (latent) infection have already been discussed. A review of the pertinent literature on this controversy is available [921]. In an attempt to prevent infection and reduce fetal wastage, a series of women who had had previous abortions, premature births, or similar misfortunes were given pyrimethamine treatment by Cech and Jirovec of Prague [452]. A marked reduction in perinatal fetal mortality rate was observed in those women who received treatment. The investigators interpreted their results as showing a remarkable effect of pyrimethamine on the outcome of pregnancy in the skin test-positive women. Their results appear to be very favorable, but because the study was uncontrolled, these results must be interpreted with caution. Studies along the same line are those of Eckerling and associates in Israel [922] and others [923–925]. Results reported by Sharf and coworkers in Israel [926] suggested an etiologic relationship between latent maternal toxoplasmosis and spontaneous abortions, premature deliveries, and stillbirths. A number of such women were given pyrimethamine and triple sulfonamides before their next pregnancy and sulfonamides alone during pregnancy. The researchers interpreted their results as evidence that such treatment significantly increased the chance of a successful outcome of the pregnancy. Unfortunately, their controls were poorly defined and appear inadequate for statistical analysis.

Kimball and colleagues stated that, despite the association of antibodies to *T. gondii* with sporadic abortion noted by them, there is no evidence that therapy to prevent abortion should be administered routinely to

TABLE 31–52 Some Pertinent Resources and Telephone Numbers/Internet Sites

Reference laboratory for serology, isolation, and PCR assay (U.S.)	650-853-4828
Paris laboratory for serology, isolation, and PCR assay (France)	33-1-58-41-22-51
FDA for IND number to obtain spiramycin for treatment for a pregnant woman (U.S.)	301-827-2335
FDA Public Health Advisory	301-594-3060
Spiramycin (Aventis) for treatment for a pregnant woman (U.S.)	908-231-3365
Congenital Toxoplasmosis Study Group (U.S.)	773-834-4152/ 773-834-4131
Educational pamphlet/The March of Dimes (U.S.): "Prevention of Congenital Toxoplasmosis"	312-435-4007
Educational pamphlet: "Congenital Toxoplasmosis: The Hidden Threat"	1-800-323-9100
Educational pamphlet: "Toxoplasmosis," NIH publication No. 83-308	301-496-5717 www.naid.nih.gov
Information concerning AIDS and congenital toxoplasmosis (U.S.)	305-243-6522
Educational information on the Internet	www.toxoplasmosis.org

AIDS, *acquired immunodeficiency syndrome*; FDA, *U.S. Food and Drug Administration*; IND, *Investigational New Drug*; NIH, *National Institutes of Health*; PCR, *polymerase chain reaction.*

pregnant women with antibodies to *T. gondii*—even those with high titers [927]. In their series, there was a significantly greater incidence of abortions in patients with CF test titers of 1:8 or higher than in those with titers 1:4 or lower ($P < .01$). But they considered it unwarranted to recommend therapy to a group of pregnant women of whom only 10% could be expected to abort without therapy. Whether therapy for toxoplasmosis in patients with CF test titers of 1:8 or higher who are threatening to abort would be beneficial is unknown.

The question must now be raised whether there is sufficient evidence to warrant the routine prophylactic use of a drug with toxic and teratogenic potential against *T. gondii* in pregnant women who have positive serologic titers and a history of chronic abortion. Until the controversy is resolved by further evidence justifying the risk of therapy, the only conclusion that can be made is that pyrimethamine must not be used in such cases [928,929]. There are continued reports of use of such treatment [930].

RESOURCES

A summary of useful resources with means to contact the relevant agencies is presented in Table 31–52.

ACKNOWLEDGMENTS

We are sincerely grateful to Drs. Jacques Couvreur, Fernand Daffos, J. P. Dubey, Jose G. Montoya, Oliver Liesenfeld, and Kenneth Boyer for their advice and help in the preparation of this chapter.

We thank Drs. F. Daffos, and A.G. Noble for providing their data for inclusion in this chapter. We appreciate the assistance of Lara Kallal, Diana Chamot, Mari Sautter, and Peggy Wakeman.

The work on which this chapter is based was supported by grants AI 04717, AI 302230, AI 27530, and AI 16945 from the National Institutes of Health and the Research to Prevent Blindness Foundation.

REFERENCES

[1] C. Nicolle, L. Manceaux, Sur un protozoaire nouveau de gondi, *Toxoplasma*, Arch. Inst. Pasteur. (Tunis) 2 (1909) 97–103.

[2] J. Janku, Pathogenesa a patologicka anatomie tak nazvaneho vrozeneho kolobomu zlute skvrny v oku normalne velikem a mikrophthalmickem s nalezem parazitu v sitnici, Cas. Lek. Cesk. 62 (1923) 1021–1027.

[3] C. Levaditi, Au sujet de certaines protozooses hereditaires humaines à localization oculaires et nerveuses, C. R. Soc. Biol. (Paris) 98 (1928) 297–299.

[4] A. Wolf, D. Cowen, B. Paige, Human Toxoplasmosis: Occurrence in Infants as an Encephalomyelitis Verification by Transmission to Animals, Science 89 (1939) 226–227.

[5] A. Wolf, D. Cowen, B. Paige, Toxoplasmic encephalomyelitis, Trans. Am. Neurol. Assoc. 65 (1939) 76–79.

[6] B.H. Paige, D. Cowen, A. Wolf, Toxoplasmic encephalomyelitis. V. Further observations of infantile toxoplasmosis; intrauterine inception of the disease; visceral manifestations, Am. J. Dis. Child. 63 (1942) 474–514.

[7] H. Pinkerton, D. Weinman, *Toxoplasma* infection in man, Archives of Pathology 30 (1940) 374–392.

[8] H. Pinkerton, R.G. Henderson, Adult toxoplasmosis, JAMA 116 (1941) 807–814.

[9] A.B. Sabin, Toxoplasmic encephalitis in children, JAMA 116 (1941) 801–807.

[10] A.B. Sabin, H.A. Feldman, Dyes as microchemical indicators of a new immunity phenomenon affecting a protozoan parasite (*Toxoplasma*), Science 108 (1948) 660–663.

[11] J.K. Frenkel, Toxoplasmosis: Parasite life cycle pathology and immunology, in: L.P.L. Hammond Dm (Ed.), University Park Press, Baltimore, 1973.

[12] N. Levine, Sarcocystis, Toxoplasma, and Related Protozoa, Burgess Publishing, Minneapolis, 1973.

[13] M. Beaman, J. Remington, Cytokines and resistance against *Toxoplasma gondii*: evidence from in vivo and in vitro studies, in: C.C.N.C. Sonnenfeld G et al., (Ed.), Biomedical Press, New York, 1992.

[14] R. McLeod, D. Mack, C. Brown, *Toxoplasma gondii*–new advances in cellular and molecular biology, Exp. Parasitol. 72 (1991) 109–121.

[15] S.Y. Wong, J.S. Remington, Biology of *Toxoplasma gondii*, in: B.D. Broder Smt (Ed.), Williams & Wilkins, Baltimore, 1994.

[16] M.F. Cesbron, J.F. Dubremetz, A. Sher, The immunobiology of toxoplasmosis, Res. Immunol. 144 (1993) 7–8.

[17] J.P. Dubey, D.S. Lindsay, C.A. Speer, Structures of *Toxoplasma gondii* tachyzoites, bradyzoites, and sporozoites and biology and development of tissue cysts, Clin. Microbiol. Rev. 11 (1998) 267–299.

[18] C. Mercier, M.F. Cesbron-Delauw, L.D. Sibley, The amphipathic alpha helices of the *Toxoplasma* protein GRA2 mediate post-secretory membrane association, J. Cell Sci. 111 (1998) 2171–2180.

[19] L.D. Sibley, D.K. Howe, Genetic basis of pathogenicity in toxoplasmosis, Curr Top Microbiol Immunol. 219 (1996) 3–15.

[20] C.A. Hunter, C.S. Subauste, J.S. Remington, The role of cytokines in toxoplasmosis, Biotherapy 7 (1994) 237–247.

[21] J. Alexander, C.A. Hunter, Immunoregulation during toxoplasmosis, Chem. Immunol. 70 (1998) 81–102.

[22] E.Y. Denkers, R.T. Gazzinelli, Regulation and function of T-cell-mediated immunity during *Toxoplasma gondii* infection, Clin. Microbiol. Rev. 11 (1998) 569–588.

[23] L.D. Sibley, *Toxoplasma gondii*: perfecting an intracellular life style, Traffic 4 (2003) 581–586.

[24] E.Y. Denkers, From cells to signaling cascades: manipulation of innate immunity by *Toxoplasma gondii*, FEMS Immunol. Med. Microbiol. 39 (2003) 193–203.

[25] J.P. Dubey, J.K. Frenkel, Feline toxoplasmosis from acutely infected mice and the development of *Toxoplasma* cysts, J. Protozool. 23 (1976) 537–546.

[26] A. Freyre, et al., Oocyst-induced *Toxoplasma gondii* infections in cats, J. Parasitol. 75 (1989) 750–755.

[27] J.P. Dubey, N.L. Miller, J.K. Frenkel, Characterization of the new fecal form of *Toxoplasma gondii*, J. Parasitol. 56 (1970) 447–456.

[28] J.P. Dubey, N.L. Miller, J.K. Frenkel, The *Toxoplasma gondii* oocyst from cat feces, J. Exp. Med. 132 (1970) 636–662.

[29] J.K. Frenkel, J.P. Dubey, N.L. Miller, *Toxoplasma gondii* in cats: faecal stages identified as coccidian oocysts, Science 167 (1970) 893–896.

[30] L. Jacobs, J.S. Remington, M.L. Melton, The resistance of the encysted form of *Toxoplasma gondii*, J. Parasitol. 46 (1960) 11–21.

[31] L. Jacobs, The biology of *Toxoplasma*, Am. J. Trop. Med. Hyg. 2 (1953) 365–389.

[32] M.K. Cook, L. Jacobs, Cultivation of *Toxoplasma gondii* in tissue cultures of various derivations, J. Parasitol. 44 (1958) 172–182.

[33] E. Suss-Toby, J. Zimmerberg, G.E. Ward, *Toxoplasma* invasion: the parasitophorous vacuole is formed from host cell plasma membrane and pinches off via a fission pore, Proc. Natl. Acad. Sci. U. S. A. 93 (1996) 8413–8418.

[34] L.D. Sibley, et al., *Toxoplasma* modifies macrophage phagosomes by secretion of a vesicular network rich in surface proteins, J. Cell Biol. 103 (1986) 867–874.

[35] A.P. Sinai, P. Webster, K.A. Joiner, Association of host cell endoplasmic reticulum and mitochondria with the *Toxoplasma gondii* parasitophorous vacuole membrane: a high affinity interaction, J. Cell Sci. 110 (1997) 2117–2128.

[36] M. Goldman, R.K. Carver, A.J. Sulzer, Similar internal morphology of *Toxoplasma gondii* and *Besnoitia jellisoni* stained with silver protein, J. Parasitol. 43 (1957) 490–491.

[37] W. Bommer, K.H. Hofling, H.H. Heunert, Multiplication of *Toxoplasma* in cell cultures, Dtsch. Med. Wochenschr. 94 (1969) 1000–1002.

[38] E. Lund, E. Lycke, P. Sourander, A cinematographic study of *Toxoplasma gondii* in cell cultures, Br. J. Exp. Pathol. 42 (1961) 357–362.

[39] K. Hirai, K. Hirato, R. Yanagwa, A cinematographic study of the penetration of cultured cells by *Toxoplasma gondii*, Jpn. J. Vet. Res. 14 (1966) 83–90.

[40] T.C. Jones, S. Yeh, J.G. Hirsch, The interaction between *Toxoplasma gondii* and mammalian cells. I. Mechanism of entry and intracellular fate of the parasite, J. Exp. Med. 136 (1972) 1157–1172.

[41] J. Remington, Discussion in Laison R. Observations on the nature and transmission of *Toxoplasma* in the light of its wide host and geographical range, Surv. Ophthalmol. 6 (1961) 721–758.

[42] R. Lainson, Observations on the development and nature of pseudocysts and cysts of *Toxoplasma gondii*, Trans. R. Soc. Trop. Med. Hyg. 52 (1958) 396–407.

[43] J.S. Remington, E.N. Cavanaugh, Isolation of the encysted form of *Toxoplasma gondii* from human skeletal muscle and brain, N. Engl. J. Med. 273 (1965) 1308–1310.

[44] A.W. Kotula, et al., Effect of freezing on infectivity of *Toxoplasma gondii* tissue cysts in pork, J. Parasitol. 54 (1991) 687–690.

[45] J.P. Dubey, Effect of freezing on the infectivity of *Toxoplasma* cysts to cats, J. Am. Vet. Med. Assoc. 165 (1974) 534–536.

[46] K. Work, Resistance of *Toxoplasma gondii* encysted in pork, Acta Pathol. Microbiol. Scand. 73 (1968) 85–92.

[47] W. Bohne, J. Hessemann, U. Gross, Reduced replication of *Toxoplasma gondii* is necessary for induction of bradyzoite-specific antigens: a possible role for nitric oxide in triggering stage conversion, Infect. Immun. 62 (1994) 1761–1767.

[48] M. Soete, D. Camus, J. Dubremetz, Experimental induction of bradyzoite-specific antigen expression and cyst formation by the RH strain of *Toxoplasma gondii* in vitro, Exp. Parasitol. 78 (1994) 361–370.

[49] D.J. Ferguson, W.M. Hutchison, The host-parasite relationship of *Toxoplasma gondii* in the brains of chronically infected mice, Vichows Arch A Pathol Anat Histopathol 411 (1987) 39–43.

[50] B.A. Fox, J.P. Gigley, D.J. Bzik, *Toxoplasma gondii* lacks the enzymes required for de novo arginine biosynthesis and arginine starvation triggers cyst formation, Int. J. Parasitol. 34 (2004) 323–331.

[51] U. Gross, et al., Developmental differentiation between tachyzoites and bradyzoites of *Toxoplasma gondii*, Parasitol. Today 12 (1996) 30–33.

[52] L.M. Weiss, K. Kim, The development and biology of bradyzoites of *Toxoplasma gondii*, Front. Biosci. 5 (2000) D391–D405.

[53] L. Jacobs, New knowledge of *Toxoplasma* and toxoplasmosis, Adv. Parasitol. 11 (1973) 631–669.

[54] M.J. Hogan, et al., Morphology and culture of *Toxoplasma*, Arch. Ophthalmol. 64 (1960) 655–667.

[55] D.S. Lindsay, et al., Examination of tissue cyst formation by *Toxoplasma gondii* in cell cultures using bradyzoites, tachyzoites, and sporozoites, J. Parasitol. 77 (1991) 126–132.

[56] J.K. Frenkel, S. Friedlander, Toxoplasmosis: Pathology of Neonatal Disease, US Government Printing Office, Washington, DC, 1952.

[57] C. Marx-Chemla, et al., Should immunologic monitoring of toxoplasmosis seronegative pregnant women stop at delivery? Presse Med. 19 (1990) 367–368.

[58] M.J. Miller, W.J. Aronson, J.S. Remington, Late parasitemia in asymptomatic acquired toxoplasmosis, Ann. Intern. Med. 71 (1969) 139–145.

[59] F. Derouin, et al., Detection of circulating antigens in immunocompromised patients during reactivation of chronic toxoplasmosis, Europ. J. Clin. Micro. 6 (1987) 44–48.

[60] A.G. Garcia, Congenital toxoplasmosis in two successive sibs, Arch. Dis. Child. 43 (1968) 705–710.

[61] L. Glasser, B.G. Delta, Congenital toxoplasmosis with placental infection in monozygotic twins, Pediatrics 35 (1965) 276–283.

[62] R.S. Beckett, F.J. Flynn Jr., Toxoplasmosis: report of two new cases, with a classification and a demonstration of the organisms in the human placenta, N. Engl. J. Med. 249 (1953) 345–350.

[63] A. Neghme, E. Thiermann, F. Pino, Toxoplasmosis humana en Chile, Bol. Inf. Parasit. Chil. 7 (1952) 6–8.

[64] S. Sarrut, Histological study of the placenta in congenital toxoplasmosis, Ann. Pediatr. (Paris) 14 (1967) 2429–2435.

[65] G. Desmonts, J. Couvreur, The clinical expression of infection in the newborn. 3. Congenital toxoplasmosis, 21e Congrès des Pédiatres de Langue Française 3 (1967) 453–488.

[66] G. Desmonts, J. Couvreur, Toxoplasmosis in pregnancy and its transmission to the fetus, Bull. N. Y. Acad. Med. 50 (1974) 146–159.

[67] H. Aspöck, et al., Attempts for detection of *Toxoplasma gondii* in human embryos of mothers with preconceptional *Toxoplasma* infections, Mitt. Osterr. Ges. Tropenmed. Parasitol. 5 (1983) 93–97.

[68] G. Desmonts, J. Couvreur, Congenital toxoplasmosis. A prospective study of the offspring of 542 women who acquired toxoplasmosis during pregnancy, With letter to the editor in: P.A.B.K. Thalhammer O (Ed.), Georg Thieme Verlag, Stuttgart, Germany, 1979.

[69] J. Couvreur, G. Desmonts, P. Thulliez, Prophylaxis of congenital toxoplasmosis. Effects of spiramycin on placental infection, J. Antimicrob. Chemother. 22 (b) (1988) 193–200.

[70] J.S. Remington, M.L. Melton, L. Jacobs, Chronic *Toxoplasma* infection in the uterus, J. Lab. Clin. Med. 56 (1960) 879–883.

[71] A. Ruiz, M. Flores, E. Kotcher, The prevalence of *Toxoplasma* antibodies in Costa Rican postpartum women and their neonates, Am. J. Obstet. Gynecol. 95 (1966) 817–819.

[72] C.F. Ruoss, G.L. Bourne, Toxoplasmosis in pregnancy, J. Obstet. Gynaecol. Br. Commonw. 79 (1972) 1115–1118.

[73] H. Kräubig, Preventive method of treatment of congenital toxoplasmosis, in: K.H. Kirchhoff H (Ed.), G Thieme Verlag, Stuttgart, Germany, 1966.

[74] A.C. Kimball, B.H. Kean, F. Fuchs, Congenital toxoplasmosis: a prospective study of 4,048 obstetric patients, Am. J. Obstet. Gynecol. 111 (1971) 211–218.

[75] B. Stray-Pedersen, A prospective study of acquired toxoplasmosis among 8,043 pregnant women in the Oslo area, Am. J. Obstet. Gynecol. 136 (1980) 399–406.

[76] P. Hohlfeld, et al., Fetal toxoplasmosis: outcome of pregnancy and infant follow-up after in utero treatment, J. Pediatr. 115 (1989) 765–769.

[77] P. Hohlfeld, et al., Prenatal diagnosis of congenital toxoplasmosis with polymerase-chain-reaction test on amniotic fluid, N. Engl. J. Med. 331 (1994) 695–699.

[78] W. Foulon, et al., Treatment of toxoplasmosis during pregnancy: a multicenter study of impact on fetal transmission and children's sequelae at age 1 year, Am. J. Obstet. Gynecol. 180 (1999) 410–415.

[79] A. Brézin, et al., Ophthalmic outcome after pre- and post-natal treatment of congenital toxoplasmosis, Am. J. Ophthalmol. 135 (2003) 779–784.

[80] G. Desmonts, Acquired toxoplasmosis in pregnant women. Evaluation of the frequency of transmission of *Toxoplasma* and of congenital toxoplasmosis, Lyon Med. 248 (1982) 115–123.

[81] G. Desmonts, et al., Prenatal diagnosis of congenital toxoplasmosis, Lancet 1 (1985) 500–504.

[82] F. Daffos, et al., Prenatal management of 746 pregnancies at risk for congenital toxoplasmosis, N. Engl. J. Med. 318 (1988) 271–275.

[83] D. Dunn, et al., Mother-to-child transmission of toxoplasmosis: risk estimates for clinical counselling, Lancet 353 (1999) 1829–1833.

[84] P.A. Jenum, et al., Incidence of *Toxoplasma gondii* infection in 35,940 pregnant women in Norway and pregnancy outcome for infected women, J. Clin. Microbiol. 36 (1998) 2900–2906.

[85] O. Thalhammer, Fetale und angeborene Cytomegalie: zur Bedeutung die prantalen Inkubationszeit, Monatsschr. Kinderheilkd. 116 (1968) 209–211.

[86] O. Thalhammer, Prenatal incubation period, in: O. Thalhammer (Ed.), Georg Thieme Verlag, Stuttgart, Germany, 1971.

[87] S. Romand, et al., Usefulness of quantitative polymerase chain reaction in amniotic fluid as early prognostic marker of fetal infection with *Toxoplasma gondii*, Am. J. Obstet. Gynecol. 190 (2004) 797–802.

[88] O. Liesenfeld, et al., Effect of testing for IgG avidity in the diagnosis of *Toxoplasma gondii* infection in pregnant women: experience in a U.S. reference laboratory, J. Infect. Dis. 183 (2001) 1248–1253.

[89] J.G. Montoya, et al., VIDAS test for avidity of *Toxoplasma*-specific immunoglobulin G for confirmatory testing of pregnant women, J. Clin. Microbiol. 40 (2002) 2504–2508.

[90] J.G. Montoya, H.B. Huffman, J.S. Remington, Evaluation of the immunoglobulin G avidity test for diagnosis of toxoplasmic lymphadenopathy, J. Clin. Microbiol. 42 (2004) 4627–4631.

[91] G. Desmonts, J. Couvreur, P. Thulliez, Congenital toxoplasmosis: five cases with mother-to-child transmission of pre-pregnancy infection, Presse Med. 19 (1990) 1445–1449.

[92] J.S. Remington, J.O. Klein, Infectious Diseases of the Fetus and Newborn Infant, second ed., WB Saunders, Philadelphia, 1983.

[93] J.S. Remington, J.O. Klein, Infectious Diseases of the Fetus and Newborn Infant, fourth ed., WB Saunders, Philadelphia, 1995.

[94] P. Marty, et al., Toxoplasmose congénitale et toxoplasmose ganglionnaire maternelie préconceptionnelle, Presse Med. 20 (1991) 387.

[95] N. Vogel, et al., Congenital toxoplasmosis transmitted from an immunologically competent mother infected before conception, Clin. Infect. Dis. 23 (1996) 1055–1060.

[96] H.A. Feldman, L.T. Miller, Congenital human toxoplasmosis, Ann. N. Y. Acad. Sci. 64 (1956) 180–184.

[97] C. Silveira, et al., Toxoplasmosis transmitted to a newborn from the mother infected 20 years earlier, Am. J. Ophthalmol. 136 (2003) 370–371.

[98] J. Pons, et al., Congenital toxoplasmosis: mother-to-fetus transmission of pre-pregnancy infection, Presse Med. 24 (1995) 179–182.

[99] I. Villena, C. Quereux, J.M. Pinon, Congenital toxoplasmosis: value of prenatal treatment with pyrimethamine-sulfadoxine combination, Prenat. Diagn. 18 (1998) 754–756 (letter).

[100] G. Desmonts, Prevention de la toxoplasmosis: remarques sur l'experience poursuivie en France, in: M. Marois (Ed.), Alan R Liss, New York, 1985.

[101] H. Aspöck, H. Flamm, O. Picher, Toxoplasmosis surveillance during pregnancy–10 years of experience in Austria, Mitt. Osterr. Ges. Tropenmed. Parasitol. 8 (1986) 105–113.

[102] H. Flamm, H. Aspöck, Toxoplasmosis surveillance during pregnancy in Austria–results and problems, Padiatr. Grenzgeb. 20 (1981) 27–34.

[103] B. Fortier, et al., Spontaneous abortion and reinfection by *Toxoplasma gondii*, Lancet 338 (1991) 444 (letter).

[104] C. Hennequin, et al., Congenital toxoplasmosis acquired from an immune woman, Pediatr. Infect. Dis. 16 (1997) 75–76.

[105] M.F. Gavinet, et al., Congenital toxoplasmosis due to maternal reinfection during pregnancy, J. Clin. Microbiol. 35 (1997) 1276–1277.

[106] B. Wechsler, et al., Toxoplasmosis and disseminated lupus erythematosus: four case reports and a review of the literature, Ann. Med. Interne (Paris) 137 (1986) 324–330.

[107] C. D'Ercole, et al., Recurrent congenital toxoplasmosis in a woman with lupus erythematosus, Prenat. Diagn. 15 (1995) 1171–1175.

[108] O. Falusi, et al., Prevalence and predictors of *Toxoplasma* seropositivity in women with and at risk for human immunodeficiency virus infection, Clin. Infect. Dis. 35 (2002) 1414–1417.

[109] J.P. Ioannidis, et al., Perinatal transmission of human immunodeficiency virus type 1 by pregnant women with RNA virus loads <1000 copies/ml, J. Infect. Dis. 183 (2001) 539–545.

[110] C.A. Hunter, J.S. Remington, Immunopathogenesis of toxoplasmic encephalitis, J. Infect. Dis. 170 (1994) 1057–1067.

[111] J.S. Remington, et al., Studies on toxoplasmosis in El Salvador. Prevalence and incidence of toxoplasmosis as measured by the Sabin-Feldman dye test, Trans. R. Soc. Trop. Med. Hyg. 64 (1970) 252–267.

[112] J.S. Remington, *Toxoplasmosis*, in: K.B.M. Gellis Ss (Ed.), WB Saunders, Philadelphia, 1976.

[113] G. Desmonts, et al., Etude epidemiologique sur la toxoplasmose: L'influence de la cuisson des viandes de boucherie sur la frequence de l'infection humaine, Rev Fr Etud Clin Biol 10 (1965) 952–958.

[114] B.H. Kean, A.C. Kimball, W.N. Christenson, An epidemic of acute toxoplasmosis, JAMA 208 (1969) 1002–1004.

[115] P.M. Schantz, D.D. Juaranek, M.G. Schultz, Trichinosis in the United States, 1975: increase in cases attributed to numerous common-source outbreaks, J. Infect. Dis. 136 (1977) 712–715.

[116] J.P. Dubey, Toxoplasmosis, J. Am. Vet. Med. Assoc. 189 (1986) 166–170.

[117] A.M. Bonametti, et al., Outbreak of acute toxoplasmosis transmitted thru the ingestion of ovine raw meat, Rev Soc Bras Med Trop 30 (1996) 21–25.

[118] M.B. Robson, et al., A probable foodborne outbreak of toxoplasmosis, Commun. Dis. Intell. 19 (1995) 517–522.

[119] W.Y. Choi, et al., Foodborne outbreaks of human toxoplasmosis, J. Infect. Dis. 175 (1997) 1280–1282.

[120] J.A. Vanek, et al., Prevalence of *Toxoplasma gondii* antibodies in hunter-killed white-tail deer (Odocoileus virginianus) in four regions of Minnesota, J. Parasitol. 82 (1996) 41–44.

[121] J.G. Humphreys, R.L. Stewart, J.P. Dubey, Prevalence of *Toxoplasma gondii* antibodies in sera of hunter-killed white-tailed deer in Pennsylvania, Am. J. Vet. Res. 56 (1995) 172–173.

[122] M. Guebre-Xabier, et al., Sero-epidemiological survey of *Toxoplasma gondii* infection in Ethiopia, Ethiop. Med. J. 31 (1993) 201–208.

[123] G. Kapperud, et al., Risk factors for *Toxoplasma gondii* infection in pregnancy, Am. J. Epidemiol. 144 (1996) 405–412.

[124] R. Raz, et al., Seroprevalence of antibodies against *Toxoplasma gondii* among two rural populations in Northern Israel, Isr. J. Med. Sci. 29 (1993) 636–639.

[125] W. Buffolano, et al., Risk factors for recent *Toxoplasma* infection in pregnant women in Naples, Epidemiol. Infect. 116 (1996) 347–351.

[126] B.D. Rawal, Toxoplasmosis: a dye-test survey on sera from vegetarians and meat eaters in Bombay, Trans. R. Soc. Trop. Med. Hyg. 53 (1959) 61–63.

[127] L. Jacobs, The interrelation of toxoplasmosis in swine, cattle, dogs and man, Public Health Rep. 72 (1957) 872–882.

[128] W.M. Hutchison, J.F. Dunachie, K. Work, The fecal transmission of *Toxoplasma gondii* (brief report), Acta Pathol. Microbiol. Scand. 74 (1968) 462–464.

[129] H.G. Sheffield, M.L. Melton, *Toxoplasma gondii*: transmission through feces in absence of Toxocara cati eggs, Science 164 (1969) 431–432.

[130] J.K. Frenkel, J.P. Dubey, N.L. Miller, *Toxoplasma gondii*: fecal forms separated from eggs of the nematode Toxocara cati, Science 164 (1969) 432–433.

[131] J.K. Frenkel, A. Ruiz, M. Chinchilla, Soil survival of *Toxoplasma* oocysts in Kansas and Costa Rica, Am. J. Trop. Med. Hyg. 24 (1975) 439–443.

[132] S.G. Coutinho, R. Lobo, G. Dutra, Isolation of *Toxoplasma* from the soil during an outbreak of toxoplasmosis in a rural area in Brazil, J. Parasitol. 68 (1982) 866–868.

[133] J.P. Dubey, J.K. Frenkel, Cyst-induced toxoplasmosis in cats, J. Protozool. 19 (1972) 155–177.

[134] G.D. Wallace, Experimental transmission of *Toxoplasma gondii* by filth-flies, Am. J. Trop. Med. Hyg. 20 (1971) 411–413.

[135] G.D. Wallace, Experimental transmission of *Toxoplasma gondii* by cockroaches, J. Infect. Dis. 126 (1972) 545–547.

[136] D.D. Smith, J.K. Frenkel, Cockroaches as vectors of Sarcocystis muris and of other coccidia in the laboratory, J. Parasitol. 64 (1978) 315–319.

[137] M.B. Markus, Earthworms and coccidial oocysts, Ann. Trop. Med. Parasitol. 68 (1974) 247–248.

[138] A. Ruiz, J.K. Frenkel, Intermediate and transport hosts of *Toxoplasma gondii* in Costa Rica, Am. J. Trop. Med. Hyg. 29 (1980) 1161–1166.

[139] G.D. Etheredge, J.K. Frenkel, Human *Toxoplasma* infection in Kuna and Embera children in the Bayano and San Blas, Eastern Panama, Am. J. Trop. Med. Hyg. 53 (1995) 448–457.

[140] S.M. Teutsch, et al., Epidemic toxoplasmosis associated with infected cats, N. Engl. J. Med. 300 (1979) 695–699.

[141] S. Stagno, et al., An outbreak of toxoplasmosis linked to cats, Pediatrics 65 (1980) 706–712.

[142] M.W. Benenson, et al., Oocyst-transmitted toxoplasmosis associated with ingestion of contaminated water, N. Engl. J. Med. 307 (1982) 666–669.

[143] W.R. Bowie, et al., Outbreak of toxoplasmosis associated with municipal drinking water, Lancet 350 (1997) 173–177.

[144] L.M. Bahia-Oliveira, et al., Highly endemic, waterborne toxoplasmosis in north Rio de Janeiro State, Brazil, Emerg. Infect. Dis. 9 (2003) 55–62.

[145] J.P. Dubey, et al., Biological and genetic characterisation of *Toxoplasma gondii* isolates from chickens (Gallus domesticus) from Sao Paulo, Brazil: unexpected findings, Int. J. Parasitol. 32 (1) (2002) 99–105.

[146] D.S. Lindsay, et al., Removal of *Toxoplasma gondii* oocysts from sea water by eastern oysters (Crassostrea virginica), J. Eukaryot. Microbiol. vol. 48 (2001) 197S–198S.

[147] M.A. Miller, et al., An unusual genotype of *Toxoplasma gondii* is common in California sea otters (Enhydra lutris nereis) and is a cause of mortality, Int. J. Parasitol. 34 (2004) 275–284.

[148] D.S. Lindsay, et al., Sporulation and survival of *Toxoplasma gondii* oocysts in seawater, J. Eukaryot. Microbiol. 50 (b) (2003) 687–688.

[149] K.E. Kniel, et al., Examination of attachment and survival of *Toxoplasma gondii* oocysts on raspberries and blueberries, J. Parasitol. 88 (2002) 790–793.

[150] J.P. Dubey, S.P. Sharma, D.D. Juranek, A.J. Sulzer, S.M. Teutsch, Characterization of *Toxoplasma gondii* isolates from an outbreak of toxoplasmosis in Atlanta, Georgia. Am J Vet Res. 42 (1981) 1007–1010.

[151] H.P. Riemann, et al., Toxoplasmosis in an infant fed unpasteurized goat milk, J. Pediatr. 87 (1975) 573–576.

[152] C.D.A. Chiari, D.P. Neves, Human toxoplasmosis acquired by ingestion of goat's milk, Mem. Inst. Oswaldo Cruz 79 (1984) 337–340.

[153] J.J. Sacks, R.R. Roberto, N.F. Brooks, Toxoplasmosis infection associated with raw goat's milk, JAMA 248 (1982) 1728–1732.

[154] J.P. Dubey, et al., *Toxoplasma gondii* isolates of free-ranging chickens from Rio de Janeiro, Brazil: mouse mortality, genotype, and oocyst shedding by cats, J. Parasitol. 89 (4) (2003) 851–853.

[155] D. Hill, J.P. Dubey, *Toxoplasma gondii*: transmission, diagnosis and prevention, Clin. Microbiol. Infect. 8 (2002) 634–640.

[156] J.S. Remington, M.L. Melton, L. Jacobs, Induced and spontaneous recurrent parasitemia in chronic infections with avirulent strains of *Toxoplasma gondii*, J. Immunol. 87 (1961) 578–581.

[157] E.A. Shevkunova, L.A. Rokhina, M.F. Nugumanova, A case of chronic acquired toxoplasmosis with positive agents detectable in the blood, Med. Parazitol. (Mosk) 44 (1975) 235–238.

[158] S.E. Siegel, et al., Transmission of toxoplasmosis by leukocyte transfusion, Blood 37 (1971) 388–394.

[159] B. Beauvais, et al., Toxoplasmosis and transfusion, Ann. Parasitol. Hum. Comp. 51 (1976) 625–635.

[160] B. Beauvais, et al., Toxoplasmosis and chronic myeloid leukemia, Nouv. Rev. Fr. Hematol. 16 (1976) 169–184.

[161] D.E. Kayhoe, et al., Acquired toxoplasmosis. Observations on two parasitologically proved cases treated with pyrimethamine and triple sulfonamides, N. Engl. J. Med. 257 (1957) 1247–1254.

[162] J.K. Frenkel, R.W. Weber, M.N. Lunde, Acute toxoplasmosis. Effective treatment with pyrimethamine, sulfadiazine, leucovorin, calcium, and yeast, JAMA 173 (1960) 1471–1476.

[163] J.S. Remington, L.O. Gentry, Acquired toxoplasmosis: infection versus disease, Ann. N. Y. Acad. Sci. 174 (1970) 1006–1017.

[164] N.L. Miller, J.K. Frenkel, J.P. Dubey, Oral infections with *Toxoplasma* cysts and oocysts in felines, other mammals, and in birds, J. Parasitol. 58 (1972) 928–937.

[165] K. Markvart, M. Rehnova, A. Ostrovska, Laboratory epidemic of toxoplasmosis, J. Hyg. Epidemiol. Microbiol. Immunol. 22 (1978) 477–484.

[166] H.C. Neu, Toxoplasmosis transmitted at autopsy, JAMA 202 (1967) 844.

[167] H. Mayer, Investigaciones sobre toxoplasmosis, Bol. Of. Sanit. Panam. (Engl) 58 (1965) 485–497.

[168] L. Jacobs, Propagation, morphology and biology of *Toxoplasma*, Ann. N. Y. Acad. Sci. 64 (1956) 154–179.

[169] W.B. Stone, R.D. Manwell, Toxoplasmosis in cold-blooded hosts, J. Protozool. 16 (1969) 99–102.

[170] N.D. Levine, R.R. Nye, A survery of blood and other tissue parasites of leopard frogs Rana pipiens in the United States, J Wildl Dis 13 (1977) 17–23.

[171] A. Ruiz, J.K. Frenkel, *Toxoplasma gondii* in Costa Rican cats, Am. J. Trop. Med. Hyg. 29 (1980) 1150–1160.

[172] B.J. Luft, et al., Functional and quantitative alterations in T lymphocyte subpopulations in acute toxoplasmosis, J. Infect. Dis. 150 (1984) 761–767.

[173] L. Baril, et al., Facteurs de risque d'acquisition de la toxoplasmose chez les femmes enceintes en 1995 (France), *Bulletin épidémiologique hebdoma-daire*, 16 (1996) 73–75.

[174] B. Bobic, et al., Risk factors for *Toxoplasma* infection in a reproductive age female population in the area of Belgrade, Yugoslavia, Eur. J. Epidemiol. 14 (1998) 605–610.

[175] A.J. Cook, et al., Sources of *Toxoplasma* infection in pregnant women: European multicentre case-control study. On behalf of the European Research Network on Congenital Toxoplasmosis, BMJ 321 (2000) 142–147.

[176] K. Boyer, et al., Risk factors for *Toxoplasma gondii* infection in mothers of infants with congenital toxoplasmosis: implications for prenatal treatment and screening, Am. J. Obstet. Gynecol. 192 (2005) 564–571.

[177] A. Ades, et al., Maternal prevalence of *Toxoplasma* antibody based on anonymous neonatal serosurvey: a geographical analysis, Epidemiol. Infect. 110 (1993) 127–133.

[178] T. Ancelle, et al., La toxoplasmose chez la femme enceinte en France en 1995, Bull. Epidemiol. Hebdom. Direct Gen. 51 (1996) 227–228.

[179] J.P. Dubey, et al., Sources and reservoirs of *Toxoplasma gondii* infection on 47 swine farms in Illinois, J. Parasitol. 81 (1995) 723–729.

[180] R. Edelhofer, H. Aspöck, Modes and sources of infections with *Toxoplasma gondii* in view of the screening of pregnant women in Austria, Mitt. Osterr. Ges. Tropenmed. Parasitol. 18 (1996) 59–70.

[181] J.K. Frenkel, *Toxoplasma* in and around us, BioScience 23 (1973) 343–352.

[182] M. Lelong, et al., Thoughts on 7 cases of congenital toxoplasmosis. Different clinical aspects of this infirmity, Arch. Fr. Pediatr. 15 (1959) 433–448.

[183] H. Thoumsin, J. Senterre, R. Lambotte, Twenty-two years screening for toxoplasmosis in pregnancy: Liege, Belgium, Scand. J. Infect. Dis. 84 (b) (1992) 84–85.

[184] D. Jeannel, et al., Epidemiology of toxoplasmosis among pregnant women in the Paris area, Int. J. Epidemiol. 17 (1988) 595–602.

[185] R. Bronstein, Toxoplasmose et grossesse, Concours Med. 104 (1982) 4177–4186.

[186] S.O. Larsen, M. Lebech, Models for prediction of the frequency of toxoplasmosis in pregnancy in situations changing infection rates, Int. J. Epidemiol. 23 (1994) 1309–1314.

[187] L. Papoz, et al., A simple model relevant to toxoplasmosis applied to epidemiologic results in France, Am. J. Epidemiol. 123 (1986) 154–161.

[188] J.L. Jones, D. Kruszon-Moran, M. Wilson, *Toxoplasma gondii* infection in the United States, 1999–2000, Emerg. Infect. Dis. 9 (2003) 1371–1374.

[189] J.G. Koppe, G.J. Kloosterman, Congenital toxoplasmosis: long-term follow-up, Padiatr. Padol. 17 (1982) 171–179.

[190] J.G. Koppe, D.H. Loewer-Sieger, H. De Roever-Bonnet, Results of 20-year follow-up of congenital toxoplasmosis, Am. J. Ophthalmol. 101 (1986) 248–249.

[191] M. Jara, et al., Epidemiology of congenital toxoplasmosis identified by population-based newborn screening in Massachusetts, Pediatr. Infect. Dis. J. 20 (12) (2001) 1132–1135.

[192] M. Lebech, et al., Feasibility of neonatal screening for *Toxoplasma* infection in the absence of prenatal treatment. Danish congenital toxoplasmosis study group, Lancet 353 (1999) 1834–1837.

[193] A. Benard, et al., Survey of European programmes for the epidemiological surveillance of congenital toxoplasmosis, Euro. Surveill. 13 (15) (2008) pii: 18834.

[194] W. Foulon, A. Naessens, M.P. Derde, Evaluation of the possibilities for preventing congenital toxoplasmosis, Am. J. Perinatol. 11 (1) (1994) 57–62.

[195] R. Gilbert, Treatment for congenital toxoplasmosis: finding out what works, Mem. Inst. Oswaldo Cruz 104 (2) (2009) 305–311.

[196] F. Peyron, When are we going to celebrate the centenary of the discovery of efficient treatment for congenital toxoplasmosis? Mem. Inst. Oswaldo Cruz 104 (2) (2009) 316–319.

[197] K. Boubaker, et al., Toxoplasmosis during pregnancy and infancy. A new approach for Switzerland, Swiss Med. Wkly. 138 (49–50 Suppl. 168) (2008) 1–8.

[198] R. McLeod, et al., Why prevent, diagnose and treat congenital toxoplasmosis? Mem. Inst. Oswaldo Cruz 104 (2) (2009) 320–344.

[199] J.G. Montoya, J.S. Remington, Management of *Toxoplasma gondii* infection during pregnancy, Clin. Infect. Dis. 47 (4) (2008) 554–566.

[200] R.E. Gilbert, et al., Ocular sequelae of congenital toxoplasmosis in Brazil compared with Europe, PLoS Negl. Trop. Dis. 2 (8) (2008) e277.

[201] T. Lehmann, et al., Globalization and the population structure of *Toxoplasma gondii*, Proc. Natl. Acad. Sci. U. S. A. 103 (30) (2006) 11423–11428.

[202] F. Peyron, et al., Serotyping of *Toxoplasma gondii* in chronically infected pregnant women: predominance of type II in Europe and types I and III in Colombia (South America), Microbes Infect. 8 (9–10) (2006) 2333–2340.

[203] D. Nowakowska, et al., Genotyping of *Toxoplasma gondii* by multiplex PCR and peptide-based serological testing of samples from infants in Poland diagnosed with congenital toxoplasmosis, J. Clin. Microbiol. 44 (4) (2006) 1382–1389.

[204] D. Ajzenberg, et al., Genotype of 86 *Toxoplasma gondii* isolates associated with human congenital toxoplasmosis, and correlation with clinical findings, J. Infect. Dis. 186 (5) (2002) 684–689.

[205] I. Fuentes, et al., Genotypic characterization of *Toxoplasma gondii* strains associated with human toxoplasmosis in Spain: direct analysis from clinical samples, J. Clin. Microbiol. 39 (4) (2001) 1566–1570.

[206] S. Romand, et al., Prenatal diagnosis using polymerase chain reaction on amniotic fluid for congenital toxoplasmosis, Obstet. Gynecol. 97 (2001) 296–300.

[207] R.W. Portela, et al., A multihousehold study reveals a positive correlation between age, severity of ocular toxoplasmosis, and levels of glycoinositolphospholipid-specific immunoglobulin A, J. Infect. Dis. 190 (2004) 175–183.

[208] C. Su, et al., Recent expansion of *Toxoplasma* through enhanced oral transmission, Science 299 (2003) 414–416.

[209] C. Silveira, et al., The effect of long-term intermittent trimethoprim/sulfamethoxazole treatment on recurrences of toxoplasmic retinochoroiditis, Am. J. Ophthalmol. 134 (2002) 41–46.

[210] A.L. Vallochi, et al., Ocular toxoplasmosis: more than just what meets the eye, Scand. J. Immunol. 55 (2002) 324–328.

[211] J.E. Gomez-Marin, M.T. Montoya-de-Londono, J.C.A. Castano-Osorio, maternal screening program for congenital toxoplasmosis in Quindio, Colombia and application of mathematical models to estimate incidences using age-stratified data, Am. J. Trop. Med. Hyg. 57 (2) (1997) 180–186.

[212] M.E. Grigg, et al., Unusual abundance of atypical strains associated with human ocular toxoplasmosis, J. Infect. Dis. 184 (5) (2001) 633–639.

[213] J.C. Boothroyd, M.E. Grigg, Population biology of *Toxoplasma gondii* and its relevance to human infection: do different strains cause different disease? Curr. Opin. Microbiol. 5 (4) (2002) 438–442.

[214] M.L. Darde, et al., Severe toxoplasmosis caused by a *Toxoplasma gondii* strain with a new isoenzyme type acquired in French Guyana, J. Clin. Microbiol. 36 (1) (1998) 324.

[215] E.C. Neto, et al., High prevalence of congenital toxoplasmosis in Brazil estimated in a 3-year prospective neonatal screening study, Int. J. Epidemiol. 29 (5) (2000) 941–947.

[216] S.E. Jamieson, et al., Genetic and epigenetic factors at COL2A1 and ABCA4 influence clinical outcome in congenital toxoplasmosis, PLoS ONE 3 (6) (2008) e2285.

[217] J.S. Remington, R. McLeod, P. Thulliez, G. Desmonts, Toxoplasmosis, in: G. K.J. Remington, C. Wilson, C. Baker (Eds.), sixth ed., WB Saunders, Philadelphia, 2006.

[218] M. Demar, et al., Fatal outbreak of human toxoplasmosis along the Maroni River: epidemiological, clinical, and parasitological aspects, Clin. Infect. Dis. 45 (7) (2007) e88–e95.

[219] D.G. Mack, et al., HLA-Class II genes modify outcome of *Toxoplasma gondii* infection, Int J Parasitol 29 (1999) 1351–1358.

[220] S.E. Jamieson, et al., Host genetic and epigenetic factors in toxoplasmosis, Mem Inst Oswaldo Cruz 104 (2009) 162–169.

[221] S.E. Jamieson, et al., Evidence for associations between the purinergic receptor P2X(7)(P2RX7) and toxoplasmosis, Genes Immun, 2010 June 10 [Epub ahead of print].

[222] M.P. Lees, et al., P2X7 receptor-mediated killing of an intracellular parasite, *Toxoplasma gondii*, by human and murine macrophages, J Immunol 184 (2010) 7040–7046.

[223] T.G. Tan et al., Identification of T. gondii epitopes, adjuvants, and host genetic factors that influence protection of mice and humans Vaccine, 28 (2010) 3977-3989.

[224] R. McLeod, et al., Effects of human peripheral blood monocytes, monocyte-derived macrophages, and spleen mononuclear phagocytes on *Toxoplasma gondii*, Cell. Immunol. 54 (1980) 330–350.

[225] C.B. Wilson, J.S. Remington, Activity of human blood leukocytes against *Toxoplasma gondii*, J. Infect. Dis. 140 (1979) 890–895.

[226] C.B. Wilson, V. Tsai, J.S. Remington, Failure to trigger the oxidative metabolic burst by normal macrophages: possible mechanism for survival of intracellular pathogens, J. Exp. Med. 151 (1980) 328–346.

[227] J.R. Catterall, et al., Nonoxidative microbicidal activity in normal human alveolar and peritoneal macrophages, Infect. Immun. 55 (1987) 1635–1640.

[228] C. Brown, R. Estes, R. McLeod, Fate of an intracellular parasite during lysis of its host cell by cytotoxic T cells (unpublished, 1995).

[229] K. Yamashita, Cytotoxic T-lymphocyte-mediated lysis of *Toxoplasma gondii*-infected target cells does not lead to death of intracellular parasites, Infect. Immun. 66 (1998) 4651–4655.

[230] J.S. Remington, L. Jacobs, M.L. Melton, Congenital transmission of toxoplasmosis from mother animals with acute and chronic infections, J. Infect. Dis. 108 (1961) 163–173.

[231] G. Huldt, Experimental toxoplasmosis. Parasitemia in guinea pigs, Acta Pathol. Microbiol. Scand. 58 (1963) 457–470.

[232] J.M. Jadin, J. Creemers, Ultrastructure and biology of *Toxoplasma*. 3. Observations on intraerythrocytic *Toxoplasma* in a mammal, Acta Trop. 25 (1968) 267–270.

[233] S.E.J. Anderson, J.L. Krahenbuhl, J.S. Remington, Longitudinal studies of lymphocyte response to *Toxoplasma* antigen in humans infected with T. gondii, J. Clin. Lab. Immunol. 2 (1979) 293–297.

[234] J.L. Krahenbuhl, J.D. Gaines, J.S. Remington, Lymphocyte transformation in human toxoplasmosis, J. Infect. Dis. 125 (1972) 283–288.

[235] C.S. Subauste, et al., Preferential activation and expansion of human peripheral blood γδ T cells in response to *Toxoplasma gondii* in vitro and their cytokine production and cytotoxic activity against T. *gondii*-infected cells, J. Clin. Invest. 96 (1995) 610–619.

[236] C.S. Subauste, L. Dawson, J.S. Remington, Human lymphokine-activated killer cells are cytotoxic against cells infected with *Toxoplasma gondii*, J. Exp. Med. 176 (1992) 1511–1519.

[237] C.S. Subauste, et al., Alpha beta T cell response to *Toxoplasma gondii* in previously unexposed individuals, J. Immunol. 160 (1998) 3403–3411.

[238] R.G. Lea, A.A. Calder, The immunology of pregnancy, Curr. Opin. Infect. Dis. 10 (1997) 171–176.

[239] R. Raghupathy, Th1-type immunity is incompatible with successful pregnancy (see comments), Immunol. Today 18 (1997) 478–482.

[240] E.Y. Denkers, et al., Neutrophils, dendritic cells and *Toxoplasma*, Int. J. Parasitol. 34 (2004) 411–421.

[241] J. Aliberti, et al., Molecular mimicry of a CCR5 binding-domain in the microbial activation of dendritic cells, Nat. Immunol. 4 (2003) 485–490.

[242] L. Kasper, et al., *Toxoplasma gondii* and mucosal immunity, Int. J. Parasitol. 34 (2004) 401–409.

[243] S. Shapira, et al., The NF-kappaB signaling pathway: immune evasion and immunoregulation during toxoplasmosis, Int. J. Parasitol. 34 (2004) 393–400.

[244] F. Araujo, T. Slifer, S. Kim, Chronic infection with *Toxoplasma gondii* does not prevent acute disease or colonization of the brain with tissue cysts following reinfection with different strains of the parasite, J. Parasitol. 83 (1997) 521–522.

[245] H. De Roever-Bonnet, J.G. Koppe, D.H. Loewer-Sieger, Follow-up of children with congenital *Toxoplasma* infection and children who become serologically negative after 1 year of age, all born in 1964–1965, in: B.K.P. A. Thalhammer O (Ed.), Georg Thieme Verlag, Stuttgart, Germany, 1979.

[246] J.P. Dubey, J.K. Frenkel, Experimental *Toxoplasma* infection in mice with strains producing oocysts, J. Parasitol. 59 (1973) 505–512.

[247] I. Nakayama, Persistence of the virulent RH strain of *Toxoplasma gondii* in the brains of immune mice, Keio J. Med. 13 (1964) 7–12.

[248] J. Rodhain, Formation de pseudokystes au cours d'essais d'immunité croisée entre souches différentes de toxoplasmes, CR Seances Soc Biol Fil (Paris) 144 (1950) 719–722.

[249] H. Werner, I. Egger, Protective effect of *Toxoplasma* antibody against re-infection (author's transl), Trop. Med. Parasitol. 24 (1973) 174–180.

[250] C. Bachmeyer, et al., Congenital toxoplasmosis from an HIV-infected woman as a result of reactivation, J. Infect. 52 (2) (2006) e55–e57.

[251] F. Lebas, et al., Congenital toxoplasmosis: a new case of infection during pregnancy in a previously immunized and immunocompetent woman, Arch. Pediatr. 11 (8) (2004) 926–928.

[252] A. Elbez-Rubinstein, et al., Congenital toxoplasmosis and reinfection during pregnancy: case report, strain characterization, experimental model of reinfection, and review, J. Infect. Dis. 199 (2) (2009) 280–285.

[253] D. van der Waaij, Formation, growth and multiplication of *Toxoplasma gondii* cysts in mouse brains, Trop. Geogr. Med. 11 (1959) 345–370.

[254] S. Ito, et al., Demonstration by microscopy of parasitemia in animals experimentally infected with *Toxoplasma gondii*, Natl. Inst. Anim. Health Q. (Tokyo) 6 (1966) 8–23.

[255] M.J. Miller, P.J. Sunshine, J.S. Remington, Quantitation of cord serum IgM and IgA as a screening procedure to detect congenital infection: results in 5,006 infants, J. Pediatr. 75 (1969) 1287–1291.

[256] J.K.A. Beverley, A rational approach to the treatment of toxoplasmic uveitis, Trans. Ophthalmol. Soc. 78 (1958) 109–121.

[257] J.S. Remington, R. Hackman, Changes in serum proteins of rats infected with *Toxoplasma gondii*, J. Parasitol. 51 (1965) 865–870.

[258] J.S. Remington, R. Hackman, Changes in mouse serum proteins during acute and chronic infection with an intracellular parasite (*Toxoplasma gondii*), J. Immunol. 95 (1966) 1023–1033.

[259] J.K.A. Beverley, Congenital transmission of toxoplasmosis through successive generations of mice, Nature 183 (1959) 1348–1349.

[260] F.G. Araujo, J.S. Remington, Immune response to intracellular parasites: suppression by antibody, Proc. Soc. Exp. Biol. Med. 139 (1972) 254–258.

[261] P. de Paoli, et al., Phenotypic profile and functional characteristics of human gamma and delta T cells during acute toxoplasmosis, J. Clin. Microbiol. 30 (1992) 729–731.

[262] F. Scalise, et al., Lymphocytes bearing the gamma delta T-cell receptor in acute toxoplasmosis, Immunology 76 (1992) 668–670.

[263] T. Hara, et al., Human V delta 2+ gamma delta T-cell tolerance to foreign antigens of *Toxoplasma gondii*, Proc. Natl. Acad. Sci. U. S. A. 93 (1996) 5136–5140.

[264] Y. Suzuki, et al., Interferon-gamma: the major mediator of resistance against *Toxoplasma gondii*, Science 240 (1988) 516–518.

[265] C. Michie, D. Harvey, Can expression of CD45RO, a T-cell surface molecule, be used to detect congenital infection? Lancet 343 (1994) 1259–1260.

[266] R. McLeod, et al., Phenotypes and functions of lymphocytes in congenital toxoplasmosis, J. Lab. Clin. Med. 116 (5) (1990) 623–635.

[267] A.F. Fatoohi, et al., Cellular immunity to *Toxoplasma gondii* in congenitally infected newborns and immunocompetent infected hosts, Eur. J. Clin. Microbiol. Infect. Dis. 22 (3) (2003) 181–184.

[268] L. Ciardelli, et al., Early and accurate diagnosis of congenital toxoplasmosis, Pediatr. Infect. Dis. J. 27 (2) (2008) 125–129.

[269] G.N. Dutton, The causes of tissue damage in toxoplasmic retinochoroiditis, Trans. Ophthalmol. Soc. U. K. 105 (1986) 404–412.

[270] G.N. Holland, K.G. Lewis, An update on current practices in the management of ocular toxoplasmosis, Am. J. Ophthalmol. 134 (2002) 102–114.

[271] G.N. Holland, et al., Toxoplasmosis, in: H.G.N.W.K.R. Pepose Js (Ed.), Mosby-Year Book, St Louis, 1996.

[272] G.R. O'Connor, The influence of hypersensitivity on the pathogenesis of ocular toxoplasmosis, Trans. Am. Ophthalmol. Soc. 68 (1970) 501–547.

[273] G.R. O'Connor, Ocular toxoplasmosis, Trans. New Orleans Acad. Ophthalmol. 31 (1983) 108–121.

[274] J. Hay, et al., Congenital neuro-ophthalmic toxoplasmosis in the mouse, Ann. Trop. Med. Parasitol. 81 (1987) 25–28.

[275] J. Hay, et al., Congenital toxoplasmic retinochoroiditis in a mouse model, Ann. Trop. Med. Parasitol. 78 (1984) 109–116.

[276] W.M. Hutchison, et al., A study of cataract in murine congenital toxoplasmosis, Ann. Trop. Med. Parasitol. 76 (1982) 53–70.

[277] J.K. Frenkel, Pathogenesis of toxoplasmosis and of infections with organisms resembling *Toxoplasma*, Ann. N. Y. Acad. Sci. 64 (1956) 215–251.

[278] D.F. Rollins, et al., Detection of toxoplasmal antigen and antibody in ocular fluids in experimental ocular toxoplasmosis, Arch. Ophthalmol. 101 (1983) 455–457.

[279] M.B. Mets, et al., Eye manifestations of congenital toxoplasmosis, Am. J. Opthalmol. 122 (1996) 309–324.

[280] C.C. Chan, et al., Diagnosis of ocular toxoplasmosis by the use of immunocytology and the polymerase chain reaction, Am. J. Ophthalmol. 117 (1994) 803–805.

[281] J.G. Montoya, et al., Use of the polymerase chain reaction for diagnosis of ocular toxoplasmosis, Ophthalmology 106 (1999) 1554–1563.

[282] J.G. Montoya, J.S. Remington, Toxoplasmic chorioretinitis in the setting of acute acquired toxoplasmosis, Clin. Infect. Dis. 23 (1996) 277–282.

[283] J.S. Remington, P. Thulliez, J.G. Montoya, Recent developments for diagnosis of toxoplasmosis, J. Clin. Microbiol. 42 (2004) 941–945.

[284] J.B. Crawford, *Toxoplasma* retinochoroiditis, Arch. Ophthalmol. 76 (6) (1966) 829–832.

[285] L. Jacobs, M.J.R. Fair, M.J.H. Bickerton, Adult ocular toxoplasmosis. A preliminary report of a parasitologically proved case, Arch. Ophthalmol. 51 (1954) 287.

[286] K. Norose, T. Tokushima, A. Yano, Quantitative polymerase chain reaction in diagnosing ocular toxoplasmosis, Am. J. Ophthalmol. 111 (1996) 441–442.

[287] P.F. Kohler, Maturation of the human complement system. I. Onset time and site of fetal C1q, C4, C3, and C5 synthesis, J. Clin. Invest. 52 (1973) 671–677.

[288] W.P. Callahan Jr., W.O. Russell, M.G. Smith, Human toxoplasmosis, Medicine 25 (1946) 343–397.

[289] K. Hayes, et al., Cell culture isolation of *Toxoplasma gondii* from an infant with unusual ocular features, Med. J. Aust. 1 (1973) 1297–1299.

[290] W.A. Manschot, C.B. Daamen, Connatal ocular toxoplasmosis, Arch. Ophthalmol. 74 (1965) 48–54.

[291] H.R. Pratt-Thomas, W.M. Cannon, Systemic infantile toxoplasmosis, Am. J. Pathol. 22 (1946) 779–795.

[292] J.W. Milgram, Osseous changes in congenital toxoplasmosis, Arch. Pathol. 97 (1974) 150–151.

[293] W.W. Zuelzer, Infantile toxoplasmosis, with a report of three cases, including two in which the patients were identical twins, Arch. Pathol. 38 (1944) 1–19.

[294] J. Mellgren, L. Alm, A. Kjessler, The isolation of *Toxoplasma* from the human placenta and uterus, Acta Pathol. Microbiol. Scand. 30 (1952) 59–67.

[295] W.G. Elliott, Placental toxoplasmosis: a report of a case, Am. J. Clin. Pathol. 53 (1970) 413–417.

[296] K. Benirschke, S.G. Driscoll, The Pathology of the Human Placenta, Springer-Verlag, New York, 1967.

[297] R.A. Cardoso, et al., Congenital toxoplasmosis, in: J.C. Siim (Ed.), Munksgaard, Copenhagen, 1960.

[298] S.G. Driscoll, Fetal infections in man, in: K. Benirschke (Ed.), Comparative aspects of reproductive failure, Springer-Verlag, New York, 1967, 279–295.

[299] S. Farber, J.M. Craig, Clinical Pathological Conference (Children's Medical Center, Boston, Mass), J. Pediatr. 49 (1956) 752–764.

[300] M. Piche, et al., Placental toxoplasmosis in AIDS. Immunohistochemical and ultrastructural study of a case, Ann. Pathol. 17 (1997) 337–339.

[301] A.G. Garcia, et al., Placental morphology of newborns at risk for congenital toxoplasmosis, J. Trop. Pediatr. 29 (1983) 95–103.

[302] G. Altshuler, Toxoplasmosis as a cause of hydranencephaly, Am. J. Dis. Child. 125 (1973) 251–252.

[303] M.B. Rodney, et al., Infantile toxoplasmosis: report of a case with autopsy, Pediatrics 5 (1950) 649–663.

[304] A. Wolf, D. Cowen, B.H. Paige, Toxoplasmic encephalomyelitis. VI. Clinical diagnosis of infantile or congenital toxoplasmosis; survival beyond infancy, Arch. Neurol. Psychiatry. 48 (1942) 689–739.

[305] J.A. Hervas, et al., Central nervous system congenital toxoplasmosis mimicking brain abscesses, Pediatr. Infect. Dis. J. 6 (1987) 491–492.

[306] J.K. Frenkel, Pathology and pathogenesis of congenital toxoplasmosis, Bull. N. Y. Acad. Med. 50 (1974) 182–191.

[307] J.K. Frenkel, Toxoplasmosis. Mechanisms of infection, laboratory diagnosis and management, Curr. Top. Pathol. 54 (1971) 27–75.

[308] F. Bamatter, La choriorétinite toxoplasmique, Ophthalmologica 114 (1947) 340–358.

[309] C.D. Binkhorst, Toxoplasmosis. Report of four cases, with demonstration of parasites in one case, Ophthalmologica 115 (1948) 65–67.

[310] P. Heath, W.W. Zuelzer, Toxoplasmosis (report of eye findings in infant twins), Trans. Am. Ophthalmol. Soc. 42 (1944) 119–131.

[311] F.L. Koch, et al., Toxoplasmic encephalomyelitis. VII. Significance of ocular lesions in the diagnosis of infantile or congenital toxoplasmosis, Arch. Ophthalmol. 29 (1943) 1–25.

[312] M.J. Hogan, Ocular Toxoplasmosis, Columbia University Press, New York, 1951.

[313] F. Roberts, et al., Histopathological features of ocular toxoplasmosis in the fetus and infant, Arch Ophthalmol 119 (1999) 51–58.

[314] G. Kelemen, Toxoplasmosis and congenital deafness, Arch. Ophthalomol. 68 (1958) 547–561.

[315] J. Couvreur, The lungs in toxoplasmosis, Rev. Mal. Respir. 3 (1975) 525–532.

[316] C. Pomeroy, G.A. Filice, Pulmonary toxoplasmosis: a review, Clin. Infect. Dis. 14 (1992) 863–870.

[317] M.D. Medlock, J.T. Tilleli, G.S. Pearl, Congenital cardiac toxoplasmosis in a newborn with acquired immunodeficiency syndrome, Pediatr. Infect. Dis. J. 9 (1990) 129–132.

[318] M. Lelong, et al., Toxoplasmose du nouveau-né avec ictére et cirrhose du foie, Arch. Fr. Pediatr. 10 (1953) 530–536.

[319] R. Caldera, S. Sarrut, A. Rossier, Hepatic calcifications in the course of congenital toxoplasmosis, Arch. Fr. Pediatr. 19 (1962) 1087–1093.

[320] D.M. Israelski, et al., Toxoplasma peritonitis in a patient with acquired immunodeficiency syndrome, Arch. Intern. Med. 148 (1988) 1655–1657.

[321] B.H. Kean, R.G. Grocott, Sarcosporidiosis or toxoplasmosis in man and guinea pig, Am. J. Pathol. 21 (1945) 467–483.

[322] M.J. Miller, E. Seaman, J.S. Remington, The clinical spectrum of congenital toxoplasmosis: problems in recognition, J. Pediatr. 70 (1967) 714–723.

[323] N.A. Fediushina, G.E. Sherstennikova, Damage of the kidneys in congenital toxoplasmosis, Vrach. Delo 4 (1966) 121–122.

[324] B. Wickbom, J. Winberg, Coincidence of congenital toxoplasmosis and acute nephritis with nephrotic syndrome, Acta Paediatr. Scand. 61 (1972) 470–472.

[325] G. Huldt, Studies on experimental toxoplasmosis, Ann. N. Y. Acad. Sci. 177 (1971) 146–155.

[326] G. Huldt, S. Gard, S.G. Olovson, Effect of Toxoplasma gondii on the thymus, Nature 224 (1973) 301–303.

[327] C.M. Torres, Affinité de l'Encephalitozoon chagasi agent étiologique d'une méningoencephalomyélitis congénitale avec myocardité et myosité chez l'homme, C. R. Soc. Biol. 86 (1927) 797–1799.

[328] C.J. Alford, S. Stagno, D.W. Reynolds, Congenital toxoplasmosis: clinical, laboratory, and therapeutic considerations, with special reference to subclinical disease, Bull. N. Y. Acad. Med. 50 (1974) 160–181.

[329] V.A. Oxelius, Monoclonal immunoglobulins in congenital toxoplasmosis, Clin. Exp. Immunol. 11 (1972) 367–380.

[330] B. Van Camp, P. Reynaert, D. Van Beers, Congenital toxoplasmosis associated with transient monoclonal IgGl-lambda gammopathy, Rev. Infect. Dis. 4 (1982) 173–178.

[331] C. Griscelli, et al., Congenital toxoplasmosis. Fetal synthesis of oligoclonal immunoglobulin G in intrauterine infection, J. Pediatr. 83 (1973) 20–26.

[332] F. Koch, et al., Symptomatische Makroglobulinamie bei Lues connata, Z. Kinderheilkd. 78 (1956) 283–300.

[333] F. De Zegher, et al., Concomitant cytomegalovirus infection and congenital toxoplasmosis in a newborn, Eur. J. Pediatr. 147 (1988) 424–425.

[334] W. Maszkiewicz, et al., Coexistence of cytomegalic inclusion disease, toxoplasmosis and in a premature infant, Pediatr. Pol. 57 (1982) 821–826.

[335] L.T. Vinh, et al., Association of congenital toxoplasmosis and cytomegaly in infants. Study of two anatomo-clinical cases, Arch. Fr. Pediatr. 27 (1970) 511–521.

[336] C. Sotelo-Avila, et al., Coexistent congenital cytomegalovirus and toxoplasmosis in a newborn infant, J. Tenn. Med. Assoc. 67 (1974) 588–592.

[337] J.K.A. Beverley, C.P. Beattie, Glandular toxoplasmosis. A survey of 30 cases, Lancet 1 (1958) 379–384.

[338] M.F. Stanton, H. Pinkerton, Benign acquired toxoplasmosis with subsequent pregnancy, Am. J. Clin. Pathol. 23 (1953) 1199–1207.

[339] A. Tenhunen, Glandular toxoplasmosis: occurrence of the disease in Finland, Copenhagen: Munksgaard, 72. S. Acta Pathol. Microbiol. Scand. (Suppl. 172) (1964) S1–S72.

[340] R. Joseph, et al., Abdominal lymphadenopathy as first localization of acquired toxoplasmosis, in: J.C. Siim (Ed.), Munksgaard, Copenhagen, 1960.

[341] T.C. Jones, B.H. Kean, A.C. Kimball, Acquired toxoplasmosis, N. Y. State J. Med. 69 (1969) 2237–2242.

[342] T.L. Vischer, C. Bernheim, E. Engelbrecht, Two cases of hepatitis due to Toxoplasma gondii, Lancet 2 (1967) 919–921.

[343] J.K. Frenkel, J.S. Remington, Hepatitis in toxoplasmosis, N. Engl. J. Med. 302 (1980) 178–179, (letter).

[344] H. Masur, T.C. Jones, Hepatitis in acquired toxoplasmosis, N. Engl. J. Med. 301 (1979) 613, (letter).

[345] A.B. Weitberg, et al., Acute granulomatous hepatitis in the course of acquired toxoplasmosis, N. Engl. J. Med. 300 (1979) 1093–1096.

[346] J.D. Siim, Clinical and diagnostic aspects of human acquired toxoplasmosis, 1960; (reprinted from Human Toxoplasmosis, Copenhagen, Munksgaard, 1960), 53–79.

[347] J.E. Greenlee, et al., Adult toxoplasmosis presenting as polymyositis and cerebellar ataxia, Ann. Intern. Med. 82 (1975) 367–371.

[348] P.E. Phillips, S.S. Kassan, L.J. Kagen, Increased Toxoplasma antibodies in idiopathic inflammatory muscle disease. A case-controlled study, Arthritis Rheum. 22 (1979) 209–214.

[349] J.L. Pollock, Toxoplasmosis appearing to be dermatomyositis, Arch. Dermatol. 115 (1979) 736–737.

[350] B.S. Samuels, R.L. Rietschel, Polymyositis and toxoplasmosis, JAMA 235 (1976) 60–61.

[351] D.W. Gump, R.A. Holden, Acquired chorioretinitis due to toxoplasmosis, Ann. Intern. Med. 90 (1979) 58–60.

[352] H. Masur, et al., Outbreak of toxoplasmosis in a family and documentation of acquired retinochoroiditis, Am. J. Med. 64 (1978) 396–402.

[353] J.B. Michelson, et al., Retinitis secondary to acquired systemic toxoplasmosis with isolation of the parasite, Am. J. Ophthalmol. 86 (1978) 548–552.

[354] M. Saari, et al., Acquired toxoplasmic chorioretinitis, Arch. Ophthalmol. 94 (1971) 1485–1488.

[355] B.J. Luft, J.S. Remington, Acute Toxoplasma infection among family members of patients with acute lymphadenopathic toxoplasmosis, Arch. Intern. Med. 144 (1) (1984) 53–56.

[356] H.F. Eichenwald, A study of congenital toxoplasmosis, with particular emphasis on clinical manifestations, sequelae and therapy, in: J.C. Siim (Ed.), Munksgaard, Copenhagen, 1960.

[357] H.A. Feldman, Toxoplasmosis, Pediatrics 22 (1958) 559–574.

[358] G. Desmonts, T.C. Jones, Congenital toxoplasmosis, N. Engl. J. Med. 291 (1974) 365–366.

[359] C.J. Alford, et al., Subclinical central nervous system disease of neonates: a prospective study of infants born with increased levels of IgM, J. Pediatr. 75 (1969) 1167–1178.

[360] J.G. Koppe, et al., Toxoplasmosis and pregnancy, with a long-term follow-up of the children, Eur. J. Obstet. Gynecol. Reprod. Biol. 4 (1974) 101–110.

[361] C.B. Wilson, et al., Development of adverse sequelae in children born with subclinical congenital Toxoplasma infection, Pediatrics 66 (1980) 767–774.

[362] A. Rossier, et al., Toxoplasmose congénitale á manifestation retardée. Effet du traitement, Sem. Hop. 37 (1961) 1266–1268.

[363] J. Couvreur, G. Desmonts, Congenital and maternal toxoplasmosis. A review of 300 congenital cases, Dev. Med. Child Neurol. 4 (1962) 519–530.

[364] J. Couvreur, et al., A homogeneous series of 210 cases of congenital toxoplasmosis in 0- to 11-month-old infants detected prospectively, Ann. Pediatr. (Paris) 31 (1984) 815–819.

[365] N. Guerina, et al., Neonatal serologic screening and early treatment for congenital Toxoplasma gondii infection, N. Engl. J. Med. 330 (1994) 1858–1863.

[366] J. Paul, Fr-ngeburt und Toxoplasmose, Urban v. Schwarzenberg, München, 1962.

[367] J.L. Sever, Perinatal infections affecting the developing fetus and newborn, in: H. Eichenwald (Ed.), US Government Printing Office, Washington, DC, 1968.

[368] J. Couvreur, G. Desmonts, J.Y. Girre, Congenital toxoplasmosis in twins: a series of 14 pairs of twins: absence of infection in one twin in two pairs, J. Pediatr. 89 (1976) 235–240.

[369] W.F. Murphy, J.L. Flannery, Congenital toxoplasmosis occurring in identical twins, Am. J. Dis. Child. 84 (1952) 223–226.

[370] B. Benjamin, H.F. Brickman, A. Neaga, A congenital toxoplasmosis in twins, Can. Med. Assoc. J. 80 (1958) 639–643.

[371] H.G. Farquhar, Congenital toxoplasmosis. Report of two cases in twins, Lancet 259 (1950) 562–564.

[372] R.E. Yukins, F.C. Winter, Ocular disease in congenital toxoplasmosis in nonidentical twins, Am. J. Ophthalmol. 62 (1966) 44–46.

[373] D. Sibalic, O. Djurkovic-Djakovic, R. Nikolic, Congenital toxoplasmosis in premature twins, Folia Parasitol. (Praha) 33 (1986) 7–13.

[374] T.E. Wiswell, et al., Congenital toxoplasmosis in triplets, J. Pediatr. 105 (b) (1984) 59–61.

[375] C.D. Binkhorst, Toxoplasmosis: A Clinical, Serological Study with Special Reference to Eye Manifestations, HE Stenfert, Leiden, Netherlands, 1948.

[376] P. Tolentino, A. Bucalossi, Due casi di encefalomielite infantile di natura toxoplasmica, Policlin. Infant 16 (1948) 265–284.

[377] F. Peyron, et al., Congenital toxoplasmosis in twins: a report of fourteen consecutive cases and a comparison with published data, Pediatr. Infect. Dis. J. 22 (2003) 695–701.

[378] J. Martinovic, et al., Frequency of toxoplasmosis in the appearance of congenital hydrocephalus, J. Neurosurg. 56 (1982) 830–834.

[379] R. Wende-Fischer, et al., Toxoplasmosis, Monatsschr. Kinderheilkd. 141 (1993) 789–791.

[380] M. Ribierre, J. Couvreur, J. Canetti, Les hydrocéphalies par sténose de l'aqueduc de sylvius dans la toxoplasmose congenitale, Arch. Fr. Pediatr. 27 (1970) 501–510.

[381] G. Kaiser, Hydrocephalus following toxoplasmosis, Z. Kinderchir. 40 (b) (1985) 10–11.

[382] F. Tognetti, E. Galassi, G. Gaist, Neurological toxoplasmosis presenting as a brain tumor. Case report, J. Neurosurg. 56 (1982) 716–721.

[383] J. Baron, et al., The incidence of cytomegalovirus, herpes simplex, rubella, and Toxoplasma antibodies in microcephalic, mentally retarded, and normocephalic children, Pediatrics 44 (1969) 932–939.

[384] O. Thalhammer, Congenital toxoplasmosis, Lancet 1 (1962) 23–24.

[385] J.S. Remington, (cited by Frenkel, J.K.). Some data on the incidence of human toxoplasmosis as a cause of mental retardation, in: H.F. Eichenwald (Ed.), The Prevention of Mental Retardation Through Control of Infectious Diseases, Public Health Service Publication No. 1962, U.S. Government Printing Office, Washington, DC, 1968, 89–97.

[386] H.K. Silver, M.S. Dixon, Congenital toxoplasmosis: report of case with cataract, "atypical" vasopressin-sensitive diabetes insipidus, and marked eosinophilia, Am. J. Dis. Child. 88 (1954) 84–91.

[387] E.S. Perkins, Ocular toxoplasmosis, Br. J. Ophthalmol. 57 (1973) 1–17.

[388] E. Delair, et al., Respective roles of acquired and congenital infections in presumed ocular toxoplasmosis, Am. J. Ophthalmol. 146 (6) (2008) 851–855.

[389] J.R. Fair, Congenital toxoplasmosis–diagnostic importance of chorioretinitis, JAMA 168 (1958) 250–253.

[390] J.R. Fair, Congenital toxoplasmosis. III. Ocular signs of the disease in state schools for the blind, Am. J. Ophthalmol. 48 (1959) 165–172.

[391] J.R. Fair, Congenital toxoplasmosis. V. Ocular aspects of the disease, J. Med. Assoc. Ga. 48 (1959) 604–607.

[392] J.J. Kazdan, J.C. McCulloch, J.S. Crawford, Uveitis in children, Can. Med. Assoc. J. 96 (1967) 385–391.

[393] K.M. de Carvalho, et al., Characteristics of a pediatric low-vision population, J. Pediatr. Ophthalmol. Strabismus. 35 (1998) 162–165.

[394] B.P.C. Buchignani, M.R.B.M. Silva, Levantamento das causes e resultados, Brasileiros de Oftalmologia. 50 (1991) 49–54.

[395] N. Kara-José, et al., Estudos retrospectivos dos primeiros 140 caves atendidos na Clinica de Visao Subnormal do Hospital das Clinicas da UNICAMP, Arq. Bras. Oftalmol. 51 (1988) 65–69.

[396] C. Meenken, et al., Long term ocular and neurological involvement in severe congenital toxoplasmosis, Br. J. Ophthalmol. 79 (1995) 581–584.

[397] A. Rothova, Ocular involvement in toxoplasmosis, Br. J. Ophthalmol. 77 (1993) 371–377.

[398] M.J. Hogan, et al., Early and delayed ocular manifestations of congenital toxoplasmosis, Trans. Am. Ophthalmol. Soc. 55 (1957) 275–296.

[399] G. Parissi, Essai d'évaluation du risque de poussée évolutive secondaire de choriorétinite dans la toxoplasmose congénitale, Thèse Paris-Saint-Antoine, Paris, 1973.

[400] M. De Vroede, et al., Congenital toxoplasmosis: late appearance of retinal lesions after treatment, Acta Paediatr. Scand. 68 (1979) 761–762.

[401] P. Lou, J. Kazdan, P.K. Basu, Ocular toxoplasmosis in three consecutive siblings, Arch. Ophthalmol. 96 (1978) 613–614.

[402] G.A. Stern, P.E. Romano, Congenital ocular toxoplasmosis. Possible occurrence in siblings, Arch. Ophthalmol. 96 (1978) 615–617.

[403] M. Lappalainen, et al., Cost-benefit analysis of screening for toxoplasmosis during pregnancy, Scand. J. Infect. Dis. 27 (1995) 265–272.

[404] U. Gross, et al., Possible reasons for failure of conventional tests for diagnosis of fatal congential toxoplasmosis: report of a case diagnosed by PCR and Immunoblot, Infection 20 (1992) 149–152.

[405] M.C. Pettapiece, D.A. Hiles, B.L. Johnson, Massive congenital ocular toxoplasmosis, J. Pediatr. Ophthalmol. 13 (1976) 259–265.

[406] G.R. O'Connor, Manifestations and management of ocular toxoplasmosis, Bull. N. Y. Acad. Med. 50 (1974) 192–210.

[407] M.J. Hogan, S.J. Kimura, G.R. O'Connor, Ocular toxoplasmosis, Arch. Ophthalmol. 72 (1964) 592–600.

[408] A. Francescheti, F. Bamatter, Toxoplasmose oculaire. Diagnostic clinique, anatomique et histopharsitologique des affections toxoplasmiques, Acta I Congr. Lat. Ophthalmol. 1 (1953) 315–437.

[409] V. Arun, et al., Cataracts in congenital toxoplasmosis, J. AAPOS 11 (6) (2007) 551–554.

[410] J.D. Benevento, et al., Toxoplasmosis-associated neovascular lesions treated successfully with ranibizumab and antiparasitic therapy, Arch. Ophthalmol. 126 (8) (2008) 1152–1156.

[411] S.A. Saxon, et al., Intellectual deficits in children born with subclinical congenital toxoplasmosis: a preliminary report, J. Pediatr. 82 (1973) 792–797.

[412] A. Berengo, et al., Serological research on diffusion of toxoplasmosis. Study of 1720 patients hospitalized in a psychiatric hospital, Minerva Med. 57 (1966) 2292–2305.

[413] W. Caiaffa, et al., Toxoplasmosis and mental retardation–report of a case-control study, Mem. Inst. Oswaldo Cruz 88 (1993) 253–261.

[414] Z. Kozar, et al., Toxoplasmosis as a cause of mental deficiency, Neurol. Neurochir. Pol. 4 (1954) 383–396.

[415] V.V. Kvirikadze, I.A. Yourkova, On the role of congenital toxoplasmosis in the origin of oligophrenia and of its certain other forms of mental ailments, Zh. Nevropatol. Psikhiatriia 61 (1961) 1059–1062.

[416] O.S. Hume, Toxoplasmosis and pregnancy, Am. J. Obstet. Gynecol. 114 (1972) 703–715.

[417] I. Cook, E.H. Derrick, The incidence of Toxoplasma antibodies in mental hospital patients, Australas. Ann. Med. 10 (1961) 137–141.

[418] O.D. Fisher, Toxoplasma infection in English children. A survey with toxoplasmin intradermal antigen, Lancet 2 (1951) 904–906.

[419] E. Hoejenbos, M.G. Stronk, In quest of toxoplasmosis as a cause of mental deficiency, Psychiatr. Neurol. Neurochir. 69 (1966) 33–41.

[420] M.J. Mackie, A.J. Fiscus, P. Pallister, A study to determine causal relationships of toxoplasmosis to mental retardation, Am. J. Epidemiol. 94 (1971) 215–221.

[421] H. Stern, et al., Microbial causes of mental retardation. The role of prenatal infections with cytomegalovirus, rubella virus, and Toxoplasma, Lancet 2 (1969) 443–448.

[422] N.A. Labzoffsky, et al., A survey of toxoplasmosis among mentally retarded children, Can. Med. Assoc. J. 92 (1965) 1026–1028.

[423] G. Macer, Toxoplasmosis in obstetrics, its possible relation to mongolism, Am. J. Obstet. Gynecol. 87 (1963) 66–70.

[424] H. Thiers, G. Romagny, Mongolisme chez une enfant atteinte de toxoplasmose; discussion du rapport étiologique, Lyon Med. 185 (1951) 145–151.

[425] H.O. Kleine, Toxoplasmose als Ursache von Mongolismus, Z. Geburtschilfe Gynaekol. 147 (1956) 13–27.

[426] L. Hostomská, et al., Mongolismus und latente Toxoplasmose der Mutter, Endokrinologie 34 (1957) 296–304.

[427] O. Thalhammer, Die angeborene Toxoplasmose, in: K.H. Kirchhoff H (Ed.), Georg Thieme Verlag, Stuttgart, Germany, 1966.

[428] J.K. Frenkel, Toxoplasmosis, in: K. Benirschke (Ed.), Springer, New York, 1966.

[429] K. Aagaard, J. Melchior, The simultaneous occurrence of congenital toxoplasmosis and congenital myxoedema, Acta Paediatr. 48 (1959) 164–168.

[430] H. Andersen, Toxoplasmosis in a child with congenital myxoedema, Acta Paediatr. 44 (1955) 98–99.

[431] T. Margit, E.R. Istvan, Congenital toxoplasmosis causing diabetes insipidus, Orv. Hetil. 124 (1983) 827–829.

[432] G. Massa, et al., Hypothalamo-pituitary dysfunction in congenital toxoplasmosis, Eur. J. Pediatr. 148 (1989) 742–744.

[433] J. McAuley, et al., Early and longitudinal evaluations of treated infants and children and untreated historical patients with congenital toxoplasmosis: the Chicago collaborative treatment trial, Clin. Infect. Dis. 18 (1994) 38–72.

[434] N. Oygür, et al., Central diabetes insipidus in a patient with congenital toxoplasmosis, Am. J. Perinatol. 15 (1998) 191–192.

[435] R. Yamakawa, et al., Congenital toxoplasmosis complicated by central diabetes insipidus in an infant with Down syndrome, Brain Dev. 18 (1996) 75–77.

[436] H.H. Bruhl, R.C. Bahn, A.B. Hayles, Sexual precocity associated with congenital toxoplasmosis, Mayo Clin. Proc. 33 (1958) 682–686.

[437] A. Coppola, et al., Partial anterior hypopituitarism caused by toxoplasmosis congenita. Description of a clinical case, Minerva Med. 78 (1987) 403–410.

[438] J. Couvreur, et al., The kidney and toxoplasmosis, Ann. Pediatr. (Paris) 31 (1984) 847–852.

[439] J.P. Guignard, A. Torrado, Interstitial nephritis and toxoplasmosis in a 10-year-old child, J. Pediatr. 85 (1974) 381–382.

[440] E. Farkas-Bargeton, Personal communication cited by Rabinowicz T. Acquired cerebral toxoplasmosis in the adult, in: D. Hentsch (Ed.), Hans Huber, Bern, Switzerland, 1971.

[441] S. Kove, et al., Pattern of serum transaminase activity in neonatal jaundice due to cytomegalic inclusion disease and toxoplasmosis with hepatic involvement, J. Pediatr. 63 (1963) 660–662.

[442] E. Freudenberg, Akute infantile Toxoplasmosis-Enzephalitis, Schweiz. Med. Wochenschr. 77 (1947) 680–682.

[443] T. Hellbrügge, Über Toxoplasmose, Dtsch. Med. Wochenschr. 74 (1949) 385–389.

[444] H.J. Reiss, T. Verron, Beiträge zur Toxoplasmose, Dtsch. Gesundheitsw. 6 (1951) 646–653.

[445] J. Justus, Cutaneous manifestations of toxoplasmosis, Curr. Probl. Dermatol. 4 (1972) 24–47.

[446] V. Mehta, C. Balachandran, V. Lonikar, Blueberry muffin baby: a pictorial differential diagnosis, Dermatol. Online J. 14 (2) (2008) 8.

[447] L.K. Korovitsky, et al., Skin lesions in toxoplasmosis, Vestn. Dermatol. Venerol. 38 (1962) 28–32.

[448] H. Langer, The significance of a latent Toxoplasma infection during gestation [Die bedeutung der latenten mutterlichen toxoplasma-infection fur die gestation], in: K.H. Kirchhoff (Ed.), G. Thiene VErlag, Stutgart, Germany, 1966, 123–138.

[449] W. Mohr, Toxoplasmose, vol 1, Springer-Verlag, Berlin, 1952.

[450] L. Schmidtke, On toxoplasmosis, with special reference to care in pregnancy, Monatsschr. Gesundheitsw. Sozialhyg. 23 (1961) 587–591.

[451] P.A. Georgakopoulos, Etiologic relationship between toxoplasmosis and anencephaly, Int. Surg. 59 (1974) 419–420.

[452] J.A. Cech, O. Jirovec, The importance of latent maternal infection with Toxoplasma in obstetrics, Bibl. Gynaecol. 11 (1961) 41–90.

[453] L.K. Korovickij, et al., Toksoplazmoz, Gosmedizdat Kkr SSR, Kiev, Ukraine, 1962.

[454] R. Erdelyi, The influence of toxoplasmosis on the incidence of congenital facial malformations: preliminary report, Plast. Reconstr. Surg. 20 (1957) 306–310.

[455] O. Jírovec, et al., Studien mit dem toxoplasmintest. I. Bereitung des toxoplasmins. Technik des intradermalen Testes. Frequenz der Positivitat bei normaler Bevolkerung und bei einigen Krankengruppen, Zentralb. Bakteriol. [Orig] 169 (1957) 129–159.

[456] D.V. Patel, et al., Resolution of intracranial calcifications in infants with treated congenital toxoplasmosis, Radiology 199 (1996) 433–440.

[457] S. Friedman, et al., Congenital toxoplasmosis: prenatal diagnosis, treatment and postnatal outcome, Prenat. Diagn. 19 (1999) 330–333.

[458] S. Puri, R.P. Spencer, M.E. Gordon, Positive brain scan in toxoplasmosis, J. Nucl. Med. 15 (1974) 641–642.

[459] S. Hervei, K. Simon, Congenital toxoplasmosis mimicking a cerebral tumor. Special aspects in serodiagnostics of connatal toxoplasmosis (author's transl), Monatsschr. Kinderheilkd. 127 (1979) 43–47.

[460] S.J. Bobowski, W.G. Reed, Toxoplasmosis in an adult, presenting as a space-occupying cerebral lesion, Arch. Pathol. Lab. Med. 65 (1958) 460–464.

[461] A.T. Collins, L.D. Cromwell, Computed tomography in the evaluation of congenital cerebral toxoplasmosis, J. Comput. Assist. Tomogr. 4 (1980) 326–329.

[462] C. Diebler, A. Dusser, O. Dulac, Congenital toxoplasmosis. clinical and neuroradiological evaluation of the cerebral lesions, Neuroradiology 27 (1985) 125–130.

[463] D. Dunn, L.A. Weisberg, Serial changes in a patient with congenital CNS toxoplasmosis as observed with CT, Comput. Radiol. 8 (1984) 133–139.

[464] D.S. Titelbaum, J.C. Hayward, R.A. Zimmerman, Pachygyric-like changes: topographic appearance at MR imaging and CT and correlation with neurologic status, Radiology 173 (1989) 663–667.

[465] A. Calabet, et al., Congenital toxoplasmosis and transfontanelle brain echography. Apropos of 8 cases observed in newborn infants and infants, J. Radiol. 65 (1984) 367–373.

[466] S. Neuenschwander, M.D. Cordier, J. Couvreur, Congenital toxoplasmosis: contribution of transfontanelle echotomography and computed tomography, Ann. Pediatr. (Paris) 31 (1984) 837–839.

[467] A.E. Brodeur, Radiologic Diagnosis in Infants and Children, CV Mosby, St Louis, 1965.

[468] E.R. Lindgren, Einschliesslich Kontrastmethoden. in: T.W. Olivecrona H (Ed.), Springer-Verlag, Berlin, 1954.

[469] K.H. Potter, Pathology of the Fetus and Infant, Year Book Medical, Chicago, 1961.

[470] J.M. Traveras, E.H. Wood, Diagnostic Neuroradiology, Williams & Wilkins, Baltimore, 1964.

[471] F. Masherpa, V. Valentino, Intracranial Calcifications, Charles C Thomas, Springfield, Ill, 1959.

[472] C.G. Dyke, et al., Toxoplasmic encephalomyelitis. VIII. Significance of roentgenographic findings in the diagnosis of infantile or congenital toxoplasmosis, AJR Am. J. Roentgenol. 47 (1942) 830–844.

[473] H. Mussbichler, Radiologic study of intracranial calcifications in congenital toxoplasmosis, Acta Radiol. Diagn. (Stockh) 7 (1968) 369–379.

[474] A. Bain, et al., Congenital toxoplasmosis simulating haemolytic disease of the newborn, Br. J. Obstet. Gynaecol. 63 (1956) 826–832.

[475] E.G. Hall, et al., Congenital toxoplasmosis in newborn, Arch. Dis. Child. 28 (1953) 117–124.

[476] W. Schubert, Fruchttod und Hydrops universalis durch Toxoplasmose, Virchows Arch. 330 (1957) 518–524.

[477] N.F. Siliaeva, A case of congenital toxoplasmic meningoencephalitis complicated by an edematous form of symptomatic erythroblastosis, Arkh. Patol. 27 (1965) 67–70.

[478] L.G. Nelson, J.E. Hodgman, Congenital toxoplasmosis with hemolytic anemia, Calif. Med. 105 (1966) 454–457.

[479] H.P. Roper, A treatable cause of hydrops fetalis, J. R. Soc. Med. 79 (1986) 109–110.

[480] C.B. Wilson, et al., Lymphocyte transformation in the diagnosis of congenital Toxoplasma infection, N. Engl. J. Med. 302 (1980) 785–788.

[481] F. Koch, J. Schorn, G. Ule, über Toxoplasmose, Dtsch. Z. Nervenheilkd. 166 (1951) 315–348.

[482] S. Tós-Luty, H. Chrzastek-Spruch, J. Uminski, Studies on the frequency of a positive toxoplasmosis reaction in mentally deficient, deaf and normally developed children, Wiad. Parazytol. 10 (1964) 374–376.

[483] W. Ristow, On the problem of the etiological importance of toxoplasmosis in hearing disorders, especially in deaf-mutism, Z. Laryngol. Rhinol. Otol. 45 (1966) 251–264.

[484] I. Potasman, et al., Congenital toxoplasmosis: a significant cause of neurological morbidity in Israel? Clin. Infect. Dis. 20 (1995) 259–262.

[485] I. Wright, Congenital toxoplasmosis and deafness. An investigation, Pract. Otorhinolaryngol. (Basel) 33 (1971) 377–387.

[486] T. McGee, et al., Absence of sensorineural hearing loss in treated infants and children with congenital toxoplasmosis, Otolaryngol. Head Neck Surg. 106 (1992) 75–80.

[487] P. Vanhaesebrouck, et al., Congenital toxoplasmosis presenting as massive neonatal ascites, Helv. Paediatr. Acta 43 (1988) 97–101.

[488] N.T. Griscom, et al., Diagnostic aspects of neonatal ascites: report of 27 cases, AJR Am. J. Roentgenol. 128 (1977) 961–969.

[489] J. Blaakaer, Ultrasonic diagnosis of fetal ascites and toxoplasmosis, Acta Obstet. Gynecol. Scand. 65 (1986) 653–654.

[490] F. Daffos, Technical aspects of prenatal samplings and fetal transfusion, Curr. Stud. Hematol. Blood Transfus. 55 (1986) 127–129.

[491] G. Hedenström, G. Huldt, R. Lagercrantz, Toxoplasmosis in children. A study of 83 Swedish cases, Acta Paediatr. 50 (1961) 304–312.

[492] G. Hedenström, The variability of the course of congenital toxoplasmosis on some relatively mild cases, in: J.C. Siim (Ed.), Munksgaard, Copenhagen, 1960.

[493] J. Couvreur, G. Desmonts, Les poussées évolutives tardives de la toxoplasmose congénitale, Cah. Coll. Med. Hop. Paris 5 (1964) 752–758.

[494] A. Wolf, D. Cowen, Perinatal infections of the central nervous system, J. Neuropathol. Exp. Neurol. 18 (1959) 191–243.

[495] C. Puissan, G. Desmonts, P. Mozziconacci, Evolutivité neurologique tardive d'une toxoplasmose congénitale démontrée par l'étude du L.C.R, Ann. Pediatr. (Paris) 18 (1971) 224–227.

[496] C.D. Mitchell, et al., Congenital toxoplasmosis occurring in infants perinatally infected with human immunodeficiency virus 1, Pediatr. Infect. Dis. J. 9 (1990) 512–518.

[497] N.E. Cohen-Addad, et al., Congenital acquired immunodeficiency syndrome and congenital toxoplasmosis: pathologic support for a chronology of events, J. Perinatol. 8 (1988) 328–331.

[498] P. Velin, et al., Double contamination materno-foetale par le VIH 1 et le toxoplasme, Presse Med. 20 (1991) 960 (letter).

[499] J.M. O'Donohoe, M.J. Brueton, R.E. Holliman, Concurrent congenital human immunodeficiency virus infection and toxoplasmosis, Pediatr. Infect. Dis. J. 10 (1991) 627–628.

[500] A. Taccone, et al., An unusual CT presentation of congenital cerebral toxoplasmosis in an 8-month-old boy with AIDS, Pediatr. Radiol. 22 (1992) 68–69.

[501] P.A. Tovo, et al., Prognostic factors and survival in children with perinatal HIV-1 infection, Lancet 339 (1992) 1249–1253.

[502] M.J. Miller, J.S. Remington, Toxoplasmosis in infants and children with HIV infection or AIDS, in: W.C.M. Pizzo Pa (Ed.), Williams & Wilkins, Baltimore, 1990.

[503] G. Castelli, et al., Toxoplasma gondii infection in AIDS children in Italy, Int Conf AIDS 9 (1993) 419.

[504] H. Minkoff, et al., Vertical transmission of Toxoplasma by human immunodeficiency virus-infected women, Am. J. Obstet. Gynecol. 176 (1997) 555–559.

[505] European Collaborative Study, Low incidence of congenital toxoplasmosis in children born to women infected with human immunodeficiency virus, Eur. J. Obstet. Gynecol. Reprod. Biol. 68 (1996) 93–96.

[506] G.D. Shanks, R.R. Redfield, G.W. Fischer, Toxoplasma encephalitis in an infant with acquired immunodeficiency syndrome, Pediatr. Infect. Dis. J. 6 (1987) 70–71.

[507] L.J. Bernstein, et al., Defective humoral immunity in pediatric acquired immune deficiency syndrome, J. Pediatr. 107 (1985) 352–357.

[508] G.B. Scott, et al., Mothers of infants with the acquired immunodeficiency syndrome. Evidence for both symptomatic and asymptomatic carriers, JAMA 253 (1985) 363–366.

[509] G. Desmonts, Central nervous system toxoplasmosis, Pediatr. Infect. Dis. J. 6 (1987) 872–873 (letter).

[510] S.E. O'Riordan, A.G. Farkas, Maternal death due to cerebral toxoplasmosis, Br. J. Obstet. Gynaecol. 105 (1998) 565–566.

[511] E.G. Lago, et al., Toxoplasma gondii antibody profile in HIV-infected pregnant women and the risk of congenital toxoplasmosis, Eur. J. Clin. Microbiol. Infect. Dis. 28 (4) (2009) 345–351.

[512] P. Marty, et al., Prenatal diagnosis of severe fetal toxoplasmosis as a result of toxoplasmic reactivation in an HIV-1 seropositive woman, Prenat. Diagn. 14 (1994) 414–415.

[513] B.J. Luft, J.S. Remington, Toxoplasmic encephalitis in AIDS. AIDS commentary, Clin. Infect. Dis. 15 (1992) 211–222.

[514] M. Beaman, B. Luft, J. Remington, Prophylaxis for toxoplasmosis in AIDS, Ann. Intern. Med. 117 (1992) 163–164.

[515] O. Liesenfeld, S.Y. Wong, J.S. Remington, Toxoplasmosis in the setting of AIDS, in: M.T.C.B.D. Bartlett Jg (Ed.), Williams & Wilkins, Baltimore, 1999.

[516] H. Hedriana, et al., Normal fetal outcome in a pregnancy with central nervous system toxoplasmosis and human immunodeficiency virus infection, J. Reprod. Med. 38 (1993) 747–750.

[517] P. Vanhems, O. Irion, B. Hirschel, Toxoplasmic encephalitis during pregnancy, AIDS 7 (1992) 142–143.

[518] M. Wallon, et al., Value of cerebrospinal fluid cytochemical examination for the diagnosis of congenital toxoplasmosis at birth in France, Pediatr. Infect. Dis. J. 17 (1998) 705–710.

[519] T. Vesikari, O.H. Meurman, R. Mäki, Persistent rubella-specific IgM-antibody in the cerebrospinal fluid of a child with congenital rubella, Arch. Dis. Child. 55 (1980) 46–48.

[520] J. Couvreur, et al., Increased local production of specific G immunoglobulins in the cerebrospinal fluid in congenital toxoplasmosis, Ann. Pediatr. (Paris) 31 (1984) 829–835.

[521] C.R. Woods, J. Englund, Congenital toxoplasmosis presenting with eosinophilic meningitis, Pediatr. Infect. Dis. J. 12 (1993) 347–348.

[522] P. Hohlfeld, et al., Fetal thrombocytopenia: a retrospective survey of 5,194 fetal blood samplings, Blood 84 (1994) 1851–1856.

[523] I.D. Riley, G.C. Arneil, Toxoplasmosis complicated by chickenpox and smallpox, Lancet 2 (1950) 564–565.

[524] J.H. Magnusson, F. Wahlgren, Human toxoplasmosis: an account of twelve cases in Sweden, Acta Pathol. Microbiol. Scand. 25 (1948) 215–236.

[525] G.A. Schwarz, E.K. Rose, W.E. Fry, Toxoplasmic encephalomyelitis (clinical report of 6 cases), Pediatrics 1 (1948) 478–494.

[526] J.D. Verlinde, O. Makstenieks, Repeated isolation of Toxoplasma from the cerebrospinal fluid and from the blood, and the antibody response in four cases of congenital toxoplasmosis, Ant. van Leeuwen. 16 (1950) 366–372.

[527] A.F. Dorta, et al., Congenital toxoplasmosis (second case parasitologically proved during life, in Venezuela), Arch. Venez. Pueric. Pediatr. 27 (1964) 332–339.

[528] J.A. Embil, et al., Visualization of Toxoplasma gondii in the cerebrospinal fluid of a child with a malignant astrocytoma, Can. Med. Assoc. J. 133 (1985) 213–214.

[529] J.J. Coffey, Congenital toxoplasmosis 38 years ago, Pediatr. Infect. Dis. 4 (1985) 214 (letter).

[530] H. Habegger, Toxoplasmose humaine; mise en évidence des parasites dan les milieux intra-oculaires; humeur aquese, exudat rétrorétinien, Arch. Ophthalmol. (Paris) 14 (1954) 470–488.

[531] G.C. Levi, et al., Presence of Toxoplasma gondii in the saliva of patients with toxoplasmosis. Eventual importance of such verification concerning the transmission of the disease (preliminary report), Rev. Inst. Med. Trop. Sao Paulo 10 (1968) 54–58.

[532] Y. Tsunematsu, K. Shioiri, N. Kusano, Three cases of lymphadenopathia toxoplasmotica–with special reference to the application of fluorescent antibody technique for detection of Toxoplasma in tissue, Jpn. J. Exp. Med. 34 (1964) 217–230.

[533] K. Shioiri-Nakano, Y. Aoyama, Y. Tsuenmatsu, The application of fluorescent-antibody technique to the diagnosis of glandular toxoplasmosis, Rev. Med. (Paris) 8 (1971) 429–436.

[534] G. Khodr, R. Matossian, Hydrops fetalis and congenital toxoplasmosis. Value of direct immunofluorescence test, Obstet. Gynecol. 51 (Suppl. 1) (1978) 74S–75S.

[535] F.K. Conley, K.A. Jenkins, J.S. Remington, Toxoplasma gondii infection of the central nervous system. Use of the peroxidase-antiperoxidase method to demonstrate Toxoplasma in formalin fixed, paraffin embedded tissue sections, Hum. Pathol. 12 (1981) 690–698.

[536] J.K. Frenkel, G. Piekarski, The demonstration of Toxoplasma and other organisms by immunofluorescence: a pitfall, J. Infect. Dis. 138 (1978) 265–266 (editorial).

[537] E.H. Kass, et al., Toxoplasmosis in the human adult, Arch. Intern. Med. 89 (1952) 759–782.

[538] J.S. Remington, Toxoplasmosis in the adult, Bull. N. Y. Acad. Med. 50 (1974) 211–227.

[539] R.F. Dorfman, J.S. Remington, Value of lymph-node biopsy in the diagnosis of acute acquired toxoplasmosis, N. Engl. J. Med. 289 (1973) 878–881.

[540] G. Desmonts, J. Couvreur, Isolation of the parasite in congenital toxoplasmosis: its practical and theoretical importance, Arch. Fr. Pediatr. 31 (1974) 157–166.

[541] A.R. Deutsch, M.E. Horsley, Congenital toxoplasmosis, Am. J. Ophthalmol. 43 (1957) 444–448.

[542] A. Ariztía, et al., Toxoplasmose connatal activa en un recién nacido con demonstracion del parasito in vivo: primer caso en Chile, Rev. Chil. Pediatr. 25 (1954) 501–510.

[543] H. De Roever-Bonnet, Congenital toxoplasmosis, Trop. Geogr. Med. 13 (1961) 27–41.

[544] L. Schmidtke, Demonstration of Toxoplasma in amniotic fluid: preliminary report, Dtsch. Med. Wochenschr. 82 (1957) 1342.

[545] C.H. Chang, et al., Isolation of Toxoplasma gondii in tissue culture, J. Pediatr. 81 (1972) 790–791.

[546] J.G. Dos Santos Neto, Toxoplasmosis: a historical review, direct diagnostic microscopy, and report of a case, Am. J. Clin. Pathol. 63 (1975) 909–915.

[547] H. Matsubayashi, et al., A case of ocular toxoplasmosis in an adult, the infection being confirmed by the isolation of the parasite from subretinal fluid, Keio J. Med. 10 (1961) 209–224.

[548] R. Frezzotti, et al., A case of congenital toxoplasmosis with active chorioretinitis. Parasitological and histopathological findings, Ophthalmologica 169 (1974) 321–325.

[549] F. Derouin, Early prenatal diagnosis of congenital toxoplasmosis using amniotic fluid samples and tissue culture, Eur. J. Clin. Microbiol. Infect. Dis. 7 (1988) 423–425.

[550] S.M. Teutsch, et al., Toxoplasma gondii isolated from amniotic fluid, Obstet. Gynecol. 55 (Suppl. 3) (1980) 2S–4S.

[551] W. Foulon, et al., Detection of congenital toxoplasmosis by chronic villus sampling and early amniocentesis, Am. J. Obstet. Gynecol. 163 (1990) 1511–1513.

[552] F. Derouin, M.C. Mazeron, Y.J. Garin, Comparative study of tissue culture and mouse inoculation methods for demonstration of Toxoplasma gondii, J. Clin. Microbiol. 25 (1987) 1597–1600.

[553] A.M. Abbas, Comparative study of methods used for the isolation of Toxoplasma gondii, Bull. World Health Organ. 36 (1967) 344–346.

[554] J.P. Dubey, Refinement of pepsin digestion method for isolation of Toxoplasma gondii from infected tissues, Vet. Parasitol. 74 (1998) 75–77.

[555] F. Philippe, et al., Why monitor infants born to mothers who had a seroconversion for toxoplasmosis during pregnancy? Reality and risk of subclinical congenital toxoplasmosis in children. Review of 30,768 births, Ann. Pediatr. (Paris) 35 (1988) 5–10.

[556] H. Fricker-Hidalgo, et al., Value of Toxoplasma gondii detection in one hundred thirty-three placentas for the diagnosis of congenital toxoplasmosis, Pediatr. Infect. Dis. J. 26 (9) (2007) 845–846.

[557] G. Desmonts, J. Couvreur, Toxoplasmosis: epidemiologic and serologic aspects of perinatal infection, in: G.A.A. Krugman S (Ed.), Alan R Liss, New York, 1975.

[558] J.K. Frenkel, Dermal hypersensitivity to Toxoplasma antigens (toxoplasmins), Proc. Soc. Exp. Biol. Med. 68 (1948) 634–639.

[559] J. Mayes, et al., Transmission of Toxoplasma gondii infection by liver transplantation, Clin. Infect. Dis. 21 (1995) 511–515.

[560] J.K. Frenkel, Uveitis and toxoplasmin sensitivity, Am. J. Ophthalmol. 32 (1949) 127–135.

[561] J.K.A. Beverley, C.P. Beattie, C. Roseman, Human Toxoplasma infection, J. Hyg. 52 (1954) 37–46.

[562] L. Jacobs, et al., A comparison of the toxoplasmin skin tests, the Sabin-Feldman dye tests, and the complement fixation tests for toxoplasmosis in various forms of uveitis, Bull. Johns Hopkins Hosp. 99 (1956) 1–15.

[563] J.K. Frenkel, L. Jacobs, Ocular toxoplasmosis. Pathogenesis, diagnosis and treatment, AMA Arch. Ophthalmol. 59 (1958) 260–279.

[564] H.E. Kaufman, Uveitis accompanied by a positive Toxoplasma dye test, Arch. Ophthalmol. 63 (1960) 767–773.

[565] J.S. Remington, et al., Toxoplasma antibodies among college students, N. Engl. J. Med. 269 (1963) 1394–1398.

[566] L. Jacobs, Toxoplasmosis, N. Z. Med. J. 61 (1962) 2–9.

[567] L. Tremonti, B.C. Walton, Blast transformation and migration-inhibition in toxoplasmosis and leishmaniasis, Am. J. Trop. Med. Hyg. 19 (1970) 49–56.

[568] S.E. Maddison, et al., Lymphocyte proliferative responsiveness in 31 patients after an outbreak of toxoplasmosis, Am. J. Trop. Med. Hyg. 28 (1979) 955–961.

[569] B. Stray-Pedersen, Infants potentially at risk for congenital toxoplasmosis. A prospective study, Am. J. Dis. Child. 134 (1980) 638–642.

[570] R. McLeod, M.O. Beem, R.G. Estes, Lymphocyte anergy specific to Toxoplasma gondii antigens in a baby with congenital toxoplasmosis, J. Clin. Lab. Immunol. 17 (1985) 149–153.

[571] R.C. Gehrz, et al., Specific cell-mediated immune defect in active cytomegalovirus infection of young children and their mothers, Lancet 2 (1977) 844–847.

[572] D.W. Reynolds, P.H. Dean, Cell mediated immunity in mothers and their offspring with cytomegalovirus (CMV) infection, Pediatr. Res. 12 (1978) 498.

[573] C.A. Alford Jr., Rubella (Ed.), KJO Remington JS. WB Saunders, Philadelphia, 1976.

[574] D.A. Fuccillo, et al., Impaired cellular immunity to rubella virus in congenital rubella, Infect. Immun. 9 (1974) 81–84.

[575] P.S. Friedmann, Cell-mediated immunological reactivity in neonates and infants with congenital syphilis, Clin. Exp. Immunol. 30 (1977) 271–276.

[576] A. Yano, et al., Immune response to Toxoplasma gondii. I. Toxoplasma-specific proliferation response of peripheral blood lymphocytes from patients with toxoplasmosis, Microbiol. Immunol. 27 (1983) 455–463.

[577] S. Guglietta, et al., Age-dependent impairment of functional helper T cell responses to immunodominant epitopes of Toxoplasma gondii antigens in congenitally infected individuals, Microbes. Infect. 9 (2) (2007) 127–133.

[578] C.M. Grover, et al., Rapid prenatal diagnosis of congenital Toxoplasma infection by using polymerase chain reaction and amniotic fluid, J. Clin. Microbiol. 28 (1990) 2297–2301.

[579] E. van de Ven, et al., Identification of Toxoplasma gondii infections by BI gene amplification, J. Clin. Microbiol. 19 (1991) 2120–2124.

[580] J. Cazenave, et al., Contribution of a new PCR assay to the prenatal diagnosis of congenital toxoplasmosis, Prenat. Diagn. 12 (1992) 119–127.

[581] U. Gross, et al., Improved sensitivity of the polymerase chain reaction for detection of Toxoplasma gondii in biological and human clinical specimens, Eur. J. Clin. Microbiol. 11 (1992) 33–39.

[582] J. Dupouy-Camet, et al., Comparative value of polymerase chain reaction and conventional biological tests, Ann. Biol. Clin. 50 (1992) 315–319.

[583] T. Bergstrom, et al., Congenital Toxoplasma gondii infection diagnosed by PCR amplification of peripheral mononuclear blood cells from a child and mother, Scand. J. Infect. Dis. 30 (1998) 202–204.

[584] I. Fuentes, et al., Urine sample used for congenital toxoplasmosis diagnosis by PCR, J. Clin. Microbiol. 34 (1996) 2368–2371.

[585] B. Knerer, et al., Detection of Toxoplasma gondii with polymerase chain reaction for the diagnosis of congenital toxoplasmosis, Wien. Klin. Wochenschr. 107 (1995) 137–140.

[586] Liesenfeld O, et. al. Use of the polymerase chain reaction on amniotic fluid for prenatal diagnosis of congenital infection with Toxoplasma gondii, in: 97th General Meeting of the American Society of Microbiology (ASM), May 4-8, 1997, Miami, FL. Abstract C-484, p 204.

[587] H. Pelloux, et al., A new set of primers for the detection of Toxoplasma gondii in amniotic fluid using polymerase chain reaction, FEMS Microbiol. Lett. 138 (1996) 11–15.

[588] A. Paugam, et al., Seroconversion toxoplasmique pendant la grossesse, Presse Med. 11 (1993) 1235.

[589] H. Fricker-Hidalgo, et al., Detection of Toxoplasma gondii in 94 placentae from infected women by polymerase chain reaction, in vivo, and in vitro cultures, Placenta 19 (1998) 545–549.

[590] P.A. Jenum, et al., Diagnosis of congenital Toxoplasma gondii infection by polymerase chain reaction (PCR) on amniotic fluid samples. The Norwegian experience, APMIS 106 (1998) 680–686.

[591] R. Gratzl, et al., Follow-up of infants with congenital toxoplasmosis detected by polymerase chain reaction analysis of amniotic fluid, Eur. J. Clin. Microbiol. Infect. Dis. 17 (1998) 853–858.

[592] M. Lelong, et al., Acquired toxoplasmosis (study of 227 cases), Arch. Fr. Pediatr. 17 (1960) 1–51.

[593] H. Pelloux, et al., A second European collaborative study on polymerase chain reaction for Toxoplasma gondii, involving 15 teams, FEMS Microbiol. Lett. 165 (1998) 231–237.

[594] U. Reischl, et al., Comparison of two DNA targets for the diagnosis of toxoplasmosis by real-time PCR using fluorescence resonance energy transfer hybridization probes, BMC Infect. Dis. 3 (1) (2003) 7.

[595] E.A. Ferro, et al., Effect of Toxoplasma gondii infection kinetics on trophoblast cell population in Calomys callosus, a model of congenital toxoplasmosis, Infect. Immun. 70 (2002) 7089–7094.

[596] M.D. Cleary, et al., Toxoplasma gondii asexual development: identification of developmentally regulated genes and distinct patterns of gene expression, Eukaryot. Cell 1 (2002) 329–340.

[597] F.G. Araujo, E. Handman, J.S. Remington, Use of monoclonal antibodies to detect antigens of Toxoplasma gondii in serum and other body fluids, Infect. Immun. 30 (1980) 12–16.

[598] F. van Knapen, S.O. Panggabean, Detection of circulating antigen during acute infections with Toxoplasma gondii by enzyme-linked immunosorbent assay, J. Clin. Microbiol. 6 (1977) 545–547.

[599] E.G. Lindenschmidt, Enzyme-linked immunosorbent assay for detection of soluble Toxoplasma gondii antigen in acute-phase toxoplasmosis, Eur. J. Clin. Microbiol. 4 (1985) 488–492.

[600] T. Asai, et al., Detection of nucleoside triphosphate hydrolase as a circulating antigen in sera of mice infected with Toxoplasma gondii, Infect. Immun. 55 (1987) 1332–1335.

[601] H.J. Turunen, Detection of soluble antigens of Toxoplasma gondii by a four-layer modification of an enzyme immunoassay, J. Clin. Microbiol. 17 (1983) 768–773.

[602] A. Hassl, O. Picher, H. Aspöck, Studies on the significance of detection of circulation antigen (cag) for the diagnosis of a primary infection with T. gondii during pregnancy, Mitt. Osterr. Ges. Tropenmed. Parasitol. 9 (1987) 91–94.

[603] J. Hafid, et al., Detection of circulating antigens of Toxoplasma gondii in human infection, Am. J. Trop. Med. Hyg. 52 (1995) 336–339.

[604] J. Huskinson, P. Stepick-Biek, J.S. Remington, Detection of antigens in urine during acute toxoplasmosis, J. Clin. Microbiol. 27 (1989) 1099–1101.

[605] R.G. Brooks, S.D. Sharma, J.S. Remington, Detection of Toxoplasma gondii antigens by a dot-immunobinding technique, J. Clin. Microbiol. 21 (1985) 113–116.

[606] B.C. Walton, B.M. Benchoff, W.H. Brooks, Comparison of the indirect fluorescent antibody test and methylene blue dye test for detection of antibodies to *Toxoplasma gondii*, Am. J. Trop. Med. Hyg. 15 (1966) 149–152.

[607] Sérologie de l'Infection Toxoplasmique en Particulier á Son Début: Méthodes et Interprétation des Résultants, Foundation Mérieux, Lyon, France, 1975.

[608] Y. Naot, G. Desmonts, J.S. Remington, IgM enzyme-linked immunosorbent assay test for the diagnosis of congenital *Toxoplasma* infection, J. Pediatr. 98 (1981) 32–36.

[609] Y. Naot, J.S. Remington, An enzyme-linked immunosorbent assay for detection of IgM antibodies to *Toxoplasma gondii*: use for diagnosis of acute acquired toxoplasmosis, J. Infect. Dis. 142 (1980) 757–766.

[610] M.H. Bessieres, et al., IgA antibody response during acquired and congenital toxoplasmosis, J. Clin. Pathol. 45 (1992) 605–608.

[611] A. Decoster, et al., IgA antibodies against P30 as markers of congenital and acute toxoplasmosis, Lancet 2 (1988) 1104–1106.

[612] G. Desmonts, Y. Naot, J.S. Remington, Immunoglobulin M-immunosorbent agglutination assay for diagnosis of infectious diseases: diagnosis of acute congenital and acquired *Toxoplasma* infections, J. Clin. Microbiol. 14 (1981) 486–491.

[613] B.R. Dannemann, et al., Differential agglutination test for diagnosis of recently acquired infection with *Toxoplasma gondii*, J. Clin. Microbiol. 28 (1990) 1928–1933.

[614] J.M. Pinon, et al., Detection of specific immunoglobulin E in patients with toxoplasmosis, J. Clin. Microbiol. 28 (1990) 1739–1743.

[615] M. Lelong, G. Desmonts, Sur la nature de phénomene de Sabin et Feldman, C R Seances Soc Biol Fil 146 (1952) 207–209.

[616] H.A. Feldman, To establish a fact: Maxwell Finland lecture, J. Infect. Dis. 141 (1980) 525–529.

[617] G.A. Hansen, J. Lyng, E. Petersen, Calibration of a replacement preparation for the second international standard for anti-*Toxoplasma* serum, human, WHO Expert Committee on Biological Standardization BS/94 (1994) 1761.

[618] M.E. Camargo, P.G. Leser, M.H. Kiss, N.V. Amato, Serology in early diagnosis of congenital toxoplasmosis, Rev. Inst. Med. Trop. Sao Paulo 20 (1978) 152–160.

[619] P. Thulliez, et al., A new agglutination test for the diagnosis of acute and chronic *Toxoplasma* infection, Pathol. Biol. 34 (1986) 173–177.

[620] G. Niel, M. Gentilini, Immunofluorescence quantitative, test de Remington et agglutination directe: confrontation et apport de leur pratique simultanée dans le diagnostic sérologique de la toxoplasmose, Foundation Mérieux, Lyon, France, 1975.

[621] P. Couzineau, La réaction d'agglutination dans le diagnostic sérologique de la toxoplasmose, Foundation Mérieux, Lyon, France, 1975.

[622] H. Baufine-Ducrocq, Les anticrops naturels dans de serodiagnostic de la toxoplasmose par agglutination directe, Foundation Mérieux, Lyon, France, 1975.

[623] J.P. Garin, et al., Immunofluorescence et agglutination dans le diagnostic serologique de la toxoplasmose valeur comparative de la recherche de IgM et du test au 2-mercapto-éthanol, Foundation Mérieux, Lyon, France, 1975.

[624] M. Laugier, Notre experience du depistage de la toxoplasmose congenitale dans la region Marseillaise (méthodes-interprétation des résultats), Foundation Mérieux, Lyon, France, 1975.

[625] G. Desmonts, P. Thulliez, The *Toxoplasma* agglutination antigen as a tool for routine screening and diagnosis of *Toxoplasma* infection in the mother and infant, Dev. Biol. Stand. 62 (1985) 31–35.

[626] G. Desmonts, et al., Natural antibodies against *Toxoplasma*, Nouv. Presse Med. 3 (1974) 1547–1549.

[627] G. Desmonts, J.S. Remington, Direct agglutination test for diagnosis of *Toxoplasma* infection: method for increasing sensitivity and specificity, J. Clin. Microbiol. 11 (1980) 562–568.

[628] C.B. Wilson, J.S. Remington, What can be done to prevent congenital toxoplasmosis? Am. J. Obstet. Gynecol. 138 (1980) 357–363.

[629] R.A. Payne, J.M. Francis, W. Kwantes, Comparison of a latex agglutination test with other serological tests for the measurement of antibodies to *Toxoplasma gondii*, J. Clin. Pathol. 37 (1984) 1293–1297.

[630] J. Nagington, A.L. Martin, A.H. Balfour, Technical method. A rapid method for the detection of antibodies to *Toxoplasma gondii* using a modification of the Toxoreagent latex test, J. Clin. Pathol. 36 (1983) 361–362.

[631] M. Wilson, D.A. Ware, K.W. Walls, Evaluation of Commercial Serology Kits for Toxoplasmosis, in: Joint Meeting of the Royal and American Societies of Tropical Medicine and Hygiene. 33rd Annual Meeting of the American Society of Tropical Medicine, 1984 Baltimore.

[632] S. Wong, J.S. Remington, Toxoplasmosis in pregnancy, Clin. Infect. Dis. 18 (1994) 853–862.

[633] O. Liesenfeld, et al., Study of Abbott toxo IMx system for detection of immunoglobulin G and immunoglobulin M *Toxoplasma* antibodies: value of confirmatory testing for diagnosis of acute toxoplasmosis, J. Clin. Microbiol. 34 (1996) 2526–2530.

[634] Y. Suzuki, et al., Antigen(s) responsible for immunoglobulin G responses specific for the acute stage of *Toxoplasma* infection in humans, J. Clin. Microbiol. 26 (1988) 901–905.

[635] F.G. Araujo, et al., False-positive anti-*Toxoplasma* fluorescent-antibody tests in patients with antinuclear antibodies, Appl. Microbiol. 22 (1971) 270–275.

[636] K.M. Hobbs, E. Sole, and K.A. Bettelheim, Investigation into the immunoglobulin class responsible for the polar staining of *Toxoplasma gondii* in the fluorescent antibody test, Zentralbl. Bakteriol. Mikrobiol. Hyg. A 239 (1977) 409–413.

[637] A.J. Sulzer, M. Wilson, E.C. Hall, *Toxoplasma gondii*: polar staining in fluorescent antibody test, Exp. Parasitol. 29 (1971) 197–200.

[638] F. De Meuter, H. De Decker, Indirect fluourescent antibody test in toxoplasmosis. Advantage of the use of fluorescent anti-IgG conjugate (author's transl), Zentralbl. Bakteriol. Mikrobiol. Hyg. A. 233 (1975) 421–430.

[639] S.Y. Wong, et al., The role of specific immunoglobulin E in diagnosis of acute *Toxoplasma* infection and toxoplasmosis, J. Clin. Microbiol. 31 (1993) 2952–2959.

[640] J.M. Pinon, et al., Evaluation of risk and diagnostic value of quantitative assays for anti-*Toxoplasma gondii* immunoglobulin A (IgA), IgE, and IgM and analytical study of specific IgG in immunodeficient patients, J. Clin. Microbiol. 33 (1995) 878–884.

[641] A. Decoster, et al., Platelia-toxo IgA, a new kit for early diagnosis of congenital toxoplasmosis by detection of anti-P30 immunoglobulin A antibodies, J. Clin. Microbiol. 29 (1991) 2291–2295.

[642] P. Stepick-Biek, et al., IgA antibodies for diagnosis of acute congenital and acquired toxoplasmosis, J. Infect. Dis. 162 (1990) 270–273.

[643] A. Balsari, et al., ELISA for *Toxoplasma* antibody detection: a comparison with other serodiagnostic tests, J. Clin. Pathol. 33 (1980) 640–643.

[644] A. van Loon, J. van der Veen, Enzyme-linked immunosorbent assay for quantitation of *Toxoplasma* antibodies in human sera, J. Clin. Pathol. 33 (1980) 635–639.

[645] E.J. Ruitenberg, F. van Knapen, The enzyme-linked immunosorbent assay and its application to parasitic infections, J. Infect. Dis. 136 (Suppl.) (1977) S267–S273.

[646] Y. Carlier, et al., Evaluation of the enzyme-linked immunosorbent assay (ELISA) and other serological tests for the diagnosis of toxoplasmosis, Bull. World Health Organ. 58 (1980) 99–105.

[647] J.R. Denmark, B.S. Chessum, Standardization of enzyme-linked immunosorbent assay (ELISA) and the detection of *Toxoplasma* antibody, Med. Lab. Sci. 35 (1978) 227–232.

[648] A. Capron, et al., Application of immunoenzyme methods in diagnosis of human parasitic diseases, Ann. N. Y. Acad. Sci. 254 (1975) 331.

[649] K.W. Walls, S.L. Bullock, D.K. English, Use of the enzyme-linked immunosorbent assay (ELISA) and its microadaptation for the serodiagnosis of toxoplasmosis, J. Clin. Microbiol. 5 (1977) 273–277.

[650] A. Voller, et al., A microplate enzyme-immunoassay for *Toxoplasma* antibody, J. Clin. Pathol. 29 (1976) 150–153.

[651] D. Milatovic, I. Braveny, Enzyme-linked immunosorbent assay for the serodiagnosis of toxoplasmosis, J. Clin. Pathol. 33 (1980) 841–844.

[652] O. Liesenfeld, et al., False-positive results in immunoglobulin M (IgM) *Toxoplasma* antibody tests and importance of confirmatory testing: the Platelia toxo IgM test, J. Clin. Microbiol. 35 (1997) 174–178.

[653] M. Wilson, et al., Evaluation of six commercial kits for detection of human immunoglobulin M antibodies to *Toxoplasma gondii*, J. Clin. Microbiol. 35 (1997) 3112–3115.

[654] M. Gorgievski-Hrisoho, D. Germann, L. Matter, Diagnostic implications of kinetics of immunoglobulin M and A antibody responses to *Toxoplasma gondii*, J. Clin. Microbiol. 34 (1996) 1506–1511.

[655] J.S. Remington, F.G. Araujo, G. Desmonts, Recognition of different *Toxoplasma* antigens by IgM and IgG antibodies in mothers and their congenitally infected newborns, J. Infect. Dis. 152 (1985) 1020–1024.

[656] J.M. Pinon, et al., Strategy for diagnosis of congenital toxoplasmosis: evaluation of methods comparing mothers and newborns and standard methods for postnatal detection of immunoglobulin G, M, and A antibodies, J. Clin. Microbiol. 39 (2001) 2267–2271.

[657] D. Tissot Dupont, et al., Usefulness of Western blot in serological follow-up of newborns suspected of congenital toxoplasmosis, Eur. J. Clin. Microbiol. Infect. Dis. 22 (2003) 122–125.

[658] I. Canedo-Solares, et al., Congenital toxoplasmosis: specific IgG subclasses in mother/newborn pairs, Pediatr. Infect. Dis. J. 27 (5) (2008) 469–474.

[659] V. Meroni, F. Genco, Toxoplasmosis in pregnancy: evaluation of diagnostic methods, Parassitologia 50 (1–2) (2008) 51–53.

[660] E. Tridapalli, et al., Congenital toxoplasmosis: the importance of the western blot method to avoid unnecessary therapy in potentially infected newborns, Acta Paediatr. 97 (9) (2008) 1298–1300.

[661] K. Hedman, et al., Avidity of IgG in serodiagnosis of infectious diseases, Rev. Med. Microbiol. 4 (1993) 123–129.

[662] G.J.N. Cozon, et al., Estimation of the Avidity of Immunoglobulin G for Routine Diagnosis of Chronic *Toxoplasma gondii* Infection in Pregnant Women, Eur J Clin Microbiol Infect Dis 17 (1998) 32–36.

[663] C.L. Rossi, A simple, rapid enzyme-linked immunosorbent assay for evaluating immunoglobulin G antibody avidity in toxoplasmosis, Diagn. Microbiol. Infect. Dis. 30 (1998) 25–30.

[664] D. Ashburn, et al., Do IgA, IgE, and IgG avidity tests have any value in the diagnosis of *Toxoplasma* infection in pregnancy, J. Clin. Pathol. 51 (1998) 312–315.

[665] H. Pelloux, et al., Determination of anti-Toxoplasma gondii immunoglobulin G avidity: adaptation to the Vidas system, Diagn Microbiol Infect Dis 32 (1998) 69–73.

[666] G.J. Cozon, et al., Estimation of the avidity of immunoglobulin G for routine diagnosis of chronic *Toxoplasma gondii* infection in pregnant women, Eur. J. Clin. Microbiol. Infect. Dis. 17 (1998) 32–36.

[667] H. Pelloux, et al., Determination of anti-*Toxoplasma gondii* immunoglobulin G avidity: adaptation to the VIDAS system (bioMerieux), Diagn. Microbiol. Infect. Dis. 32 (1998) 69–73.

[668] M. Lappalainen, et al., Toxoplasmosis acquired during pregnancy: improved serodiagnosis based on avidity of IgG, J. Infect. Dis. 167 (1993) 691–697.

[669] P.A. Jenum, B. Stray-Pedersen, A.G. Gundersen, Improved diagnosis of primary Toxoplasma gondii infection in early pregnancy by determination of antitoxoplasma immunoglobulin G activity, J. Clin. Microbiol. 35 (1997) 1972–1977.

[670] A. Sensini, et al., IgG avidity in the serodiagnosis of acute Toxoplasma gondii infection: a multicenter study, Clin. Microbiol. Infect. 2 (1996) 25–29.

[671] P. Flori, et al., Reliability of immunoglobulin G antitoxoplasma avidity test and effects of treatment on avidity indexes of infants and pregnant women, Clin. Diagn. Lab. Immunol. 11 (2004) 669–674.

[672] K. Hedman, et al., Recent primary Toxoplasma infection indicated by a low avidity of specific IgG, J. Infect. Dis. 159 (1989) 736–739.

[673] M.E. Camargo, et al., Avidity of specific IgG antibody as a marker of recent and old Toxoplasma gondii infections, Rev. Inst. Med. Trop. Sao Paulo 33 (1991) 213–218.

[674] D.H.M. Joynson, R.A. Payne, B.K. Rawal, Potential role of IgG avidity for diagnosing toxoplasmosis, J. Clin. Pathol. 43 1032–1033.

[675] O. Liesenfeld, et al., Confirmatory serologic testing for acute toxoplasmosis and rate of induced abortions among women reported to have positive Toxoplasma immunoglobulin M antibody titers, Am. J. Obstet. Gynecol. 184 (2001) 140–145.

[676] K.A. Karim, G.B. Ludlam, The relationship and significance of antibody titres as determined by various serological methods in glandular and ocular toxoplasmosis, J. Clin. Pathol. 28 (1975) 42–49.

[677] J.S. Remington, M.J. Miller, I. Brownlee, IgM antibodies in acute toxoplasmosis. I. Diagnostic significance in congenital cases and a method for their rapid demonstration, Pediatrics 41 (1968) 1082–1091.

[678] J.S. Remington, M.J. Miller, I. Brownlee, IgM antibodies in acute toxoplasmosis. II. Prevalence and significance in acquired cases, J. Lab. Clin. Med. 71 (1968) 855–866.

[679] M.N. Lunde, Laboratory methods in the diagnosis of toxoplasmosis, Health Lab. Sci. 10 (1973) 319–328.

[680] S. Stagno, E. Thiermann, Value of indirect immunofluorescent test in the serological diagnosis of acute toxoplasmosis, Bol. Chil. Parasitol. 25 (1970) 9–15.

[681] G.J. Aparicio, B.I. Cour, Application of immunofluorescence to the study of immunoglobulin fractions in the diagnostic of acquired and congenital toxoplasmosis. Clinical value, Rev. Clin. Esp. 125 (1972) 37–42.

[682] G. Dropsy, J. Carquin, J.C. Croix, Technics of demonstration of IgM type antibodies in congenital infections, Ann Bio Clin (Paris) 29 (1971) 67–73.

[683] H.F. Eichenwald, H.R. Shinefield, Antibody production by the human fetus, J. Pediatr. 63 (1963) 870.

[684] J.S. Remington, G. Desmonts, Congenital toxoplasmosis: variability in the IgM-fluorescent antibody response and some pitfalls in diagnosis, J. Pediatr. 83 (1973) 27–30.

[685] N. Pyndiah, et al., Simplified chromatographic separation of immunoglobulin M from G and its application to Toxoplasma indirect immunofluorescence, J. Clin. Microbiol. 9 (1979) 170–174.

[686] G.A. Filice, A.S. Yeager, J.S. Remington, Diagnostic significance of immunoglobulin M antibodies to Toxoplasma gondii detected after separation of immunoglobulin M from immunoglobulin G antibodies, J. Clin. Microbiol. 12 (1980) 336–342.

[687] P.C. Welch, et al., Serologic diagnosis of acute lymphadenopathic toxoplasmosis, J. Infect. Dis. 142 (2) (1980) 256–264.

[688] M.N. Lunde, et al., Serologic diagnosis of active toxoplasmosis complicating malignant diseases, vol. 25, 1970.

[689] G. Desmonts, et al., Early diagnosis of acute toxoplasmosis. Critical study of Remington's test, Nouv. Presse. Med. 1 (1972) 339–342.

[690] E.R. Stiehm, A.J. Amman, J.D. Cherry, Elevated cord macroglobulins in the diagnosis of intrauterine infections, N. Engl. J. Med. 275 (1966) 971–977.

[691] W.F. Barth, et al., Metabolism of human gamma macroglobulins, J. Clin. Invest. 43 (1964) 1036–1048.

[692] B. Hyde, E.V. Barnett, J.S. Remington, Method for differentiation of nonspecific from specific Toxoplasma IgM fluorescent antibodies in patients with rheumatoid factor, Proc. Soc. Exp. Biol. Med. 148 (1975) 1184–1188.

[693] C.B. Reimer, et al., The specificity of fetal IgM: antibody or anti-antibody? Ann. N. Y. Acad. Sci. 254 (1975) 77–93.

[694] G. Filice, et al., Detection of IgM-anti-Toxoplasma antibodies in acute acquired and congenital toxoplasmosis, Boll. Ist. Sieroter. Milan. 76 (1984) 271–273.

[695] P. Pouletty, et al., An anti-human immunoglobulin M monoclonal antibody for detection of antibodies to Toxoplasma gondii, Eur. J. Clin. Microbiol. 3 (1984) 510–515.

[696] F. Santoro, et al., Serodiagnosis of Toxoplasma infection using a purified parasite protein (P30), Clin. Exp. Immunol. 62 (1985) 262–269.

[697] P. Pouletty, et al., An anti-human M chain monoclonal antibody: use for detection of IgM antibodies to Toxoplasma gondii by reverse immunosorbent assay, J. Immunol. Methods 76 (1985) 289–298.

[698] J.Y. Cesbron, et al., A new ELISA method for the diagnosis of toxoplasmosis. Assay of serum IgM by immunocapture with an anti-Toxoplasma gondii monoclonal antibody, Presse Med. 19 (1986) 737–740.

[699] E.G. Lindenschmidt, Demonstration of immunoglobulin M class antibodies to Toxoplasma gondii antigenic component P3500 by enzyme-linked antigen immunosorbent assay, J. Clin. Microbiol. 24 (1986) 1045–1049.

[700] P. Herbrink, et al., Interlaboratory evaluation of indirect enzyme-linked immunosorbent assay, antibody capture enzyme-linked immunosorbent assay, and immunoblotting for detection of immunoglobulin M antibodies to Toxoplasma gondii, J. Clin. Microbiol. 25 (1987) 100–105.

[701] G. Filice, et al., IgM-IFA, IgM-ELISA, DS-IgM-ELISA, IgM-ISAGA, performed on whole serum and IgM fractions, for detection of IgM anti-Toxoplasma antibodies during pregnancy, Boll. Ist. Sieroter. Milan. 65 (1986) 131–137.

[702] M. Saathoff, H.M. Seitz, Detection of Toxoplasma-specific IgM antibodies–comparison with the ISAGA (immunosorbent agglutination assay) and immunofluorescence results, Z. Geburtshilfe Perinatol. 189 (1985) 73–78.

[703] J.G. Montoya, J.S. Remington, Studies on the serodiagnosis of toxoplasmic lymphadenitis, Clin. Infect. Dis. 20 (1995) 781–790.

[704] P. Thulliez, et al., Evaluation de trois réactifs de détection par immunocapture des IgM spécifiques de la toxoplasmose, Fevfrlab 169 (1988) 25–31.

[705] J.M. Pinon, et al., Detection of IgA specific for toxoplasmosis in serum and cerebrospinal fluid using a non-enzymatic IgA-capture assay, Diagn. Immunol. 4 (1986) 223–227.

[706] D. Plantaz, et al., Value of the immunosorbent agglutination assay (ISAGA) in the early diagnosis of congenital toxoplasmosis, Pediatrie 42 (1987) 387–391.

[707] Y. Le Fichoux, P. Marty, H. Chan, Contribution of specific serum IgA assay to the diagnosis of toxoplasmosis, Ann. Pediatr. (Paris) 34 (1987) 375–379.

[708] J.M. Pinon, et al., Early neonatal diagnosis of congenital toxoplasmosis: value of comparative enzyme-linked immunofiltration assay immunological profiles and anti-Toxoplasma gondii immunoglobulin M (IgM) or IgA immunocapture and implications for postnatal therapeutic strategies, J. Clin. Microbiol. 34 (1996) 579–583.

[709] J.L. Jones, et al., Survey of obstetrician-gynecologists in the United States about toxoplasmosis, Infect. Dis. Obstet. Gynecol. 9 (1) (2001) 23–31.

[710] L. Gras, et al., Duration of the IgM response in women acquiring Toxoplasma gondii during pregnancy: implications for clinical practice and cross-sectional incidence studies, Epidemiol. Infect. 132 (2004) 541–548.

[711] D.J. Krogstad, D.D. Juranek, K.W. Walls, Toxoplasmosis. With comments on risk of infection from cats, Ann. Intern. Med. 77 (1972) 773–778.

[712] FDA, Public health advisory: limitations of Toxoplasma IgM commercial test kits, (1997).

[713] S. Gard, J.H. Magnusson, A glandular form of toxoplasmosis in connection with pregnancy, Acta Med. Scand. 141 (1951) 59–64.

[714] E. Jeckeln, Lymph node toxoplasmosis, Z. Frankf. Path 70 (1960) 513–522.

[715] J.C. Siim, Toxoplasmosis acquisita lymphonodosa: clinical and pathological aspects, Ann. N. Y. Acad. Sci. 64 (1956) 185–206.

[716] J. Couvreur, Prospective study of acquired toxoplasmosis in pregnant women with a special reference to the outcome of the fetus, in: D. Hentsch (Ed.), 1971.

[717] E. Handman, J.S. Remington, Serological and immunochemical characterization of monoclonal antibodies to Toxoplasma gondii, Immunology 40 (1980) 579–588.

[718] E. Handman, J.S. Remington, Antibody responses to Toxoplasma antigens in mice infected with strains of different virulence, Infect. Immun. 29 (1980) 215–220.

[719] S. Li, et al., Serodiagnosis of recently acquired Toxoplasma gondii infection with a recombinant antigen, J. Clin. Microbiol. 38 (2000) 179–184.

[720] A.M. Johnson, H. Roberts, A.M. Tenter, Evaluation of a recombinant antigen ELISA for the diagnosis of acute toxoplasmosis and comparison with traditional antigen ELISAs, J. Med. Microbiol. 37 (1992) 404–409.

[721] V. Martin, et al., Detection of human Toxoplasma-specific immunoglobulins A, M, and G with a recombinant Toxoplasma gondii rop2 protein, Clin. Diagn. Lab. Immunol. 5 (1998) 627–631.

[722] A. Redlich, W.A. Muller, Serodiagnosis of acute toxoplasmosis using a recombinant form of the dense granule antigen GRA6 in an enzyme-linked immunosorbent assay, Parasitol. Res. 84 (1998) 700–706.

[723] A.M. Tenter, A.M. Johnson, Recognition of recombinant Toxoplasma gondii antigens by human sera in an ELISA, Parasitol. Res. 77 (1991) 197–203.

[724] S.D. Sharma, et al., Western Blot analysis of the antigens of Toxoplasma gondii recognized by human IgM and IgG antibodies, J. Immunol. 131 (1983) 977–983.

[725] H.A. Erlich, et al., Identification of an antigen-specific immunoglobulin M antibody associated with acute Toxoplasma infection, Infect. Immun. 41 (1983) 683–690.

[726] I. Potasman, et al., Toxoplasma gondii antigens recognized by sequential samples of serum obtained from congenitally infected infants, J. Clin. Microbiol. 25 (1987) 1926–1931.

[727] I. Potasman, F.G. Araujo, J.S. Remington, Toxoplasma antigens recognized by naturally occurring human antibodies, J. Clin. Microbiol. 24 (1986) 1050–1054.

[728] U. Gross, O. Keksel, M.L. Dardé, The value of detecting immunoglobulin E (IgE) antibodies for the serological diagnosis of Toxoplasma gondii infection, Clin. Diagn. Lab. Immunol. 4 (1997) 247–251.

[729] J.C. Petithory, et al., Performance of European laboratories testing serum samples for Toxoplasma gondii, Eur. J. Clin. Microbiol. Infect. Dis. 15 (1996) 45–49.

[730] W.T. Hofgartner, J.J. Plorde, T.R. Fritsche, Detection of IgG and IgM antibodies to Toxoplasma gondii: evaluation of 4 newer commercial immunoassays, J Clin Microbiol 35 (1997) 3313–3315.

[731] A. Terragna, Toxoplasmic lymphadenitis, in: D. Hentsch (Ed.), 1971.

[732] T.C. Jones, B.H. Kean, A.C. Kimball, Toxoplasmic lymphadenitis, JAMA 192 (1965) 87–91.

[733] N. Gussetti, R. D'Elia, Natural immunoglobulin M antibodies against Toxoplasma gondii during pregnancy, Am. J. Obstet. Gynecol. 51 (1990) 1359–1360.

[734] E. Konishi, A pregnant woman with a high level of naturally occurring immunoglobulin M antibodies to Toxoplasma gondii, Am. J. Obstet. Gynecol. 157 (1987) 832–833.

[735] N. Hezard, et al., Prenatal diagnosis of congenital toxoplasmosis in 261 pregnancies, Prenat. Diagn. 17 (1997) 1047–1054.

[736] A. Berrebi, et al., Termination of pregnancy for maternal toxoplasmosis, Lancet 344 (1994) 36–39.

[737] F. Pratlong, et al., Fetal diagnosis of toxoplasmosis in 190 women infected during pregnancy, Prenat. Diagn. 14 (1994) 191–198.

[738] P. Boulet, et al., Pure fetal blood samples obtained by cordocentesis: technical aspects of 322 cases, Prenat. Diagn. 10 (1990) 93–100.

[739] B. Legras, et al., Blood chemistry of human fetuses in the second and third trimesters, Prenat. Diag. 10 (1990) 801–807.

[740] W. Tjalma, et al., Discordant prenatal diagnosis of congenital toxoplasmosis in a dizygotic pregnancy, Eur. J. Obstet. Gynecol. Reprod. Biol. 79 (1998) 107–108.

[741] F. Pratlong, et al., Antenatal diagnosis of congenital toxoplasmosis: evaluation of the biological parameters in a cohort of 286 patients, Br. J. Obstet. Gynaecol. 103 (1996) 552–557.

[742] A. Berrebi, W. Kobuch, Toxoplasmosis in pregnancy, Lancet 344 (1994) 950.

[743] B. Lecolier, et al., T-cell subpopulations of fetuses infected by *Toxoplasma gondii*, Eur. J. Clin. Microbiol. Infect. Dis. 8 (1989) 572–573.

[744] A. Decoster, et al., Anti-P30 IgA antibodies as prenatal markers of congenital *Toxoplasma* infection, Clin. Exp. Immunol. 87 (1992) 310–315.

[745] J. Raymond, et al., Presence of gamma interferon in human acute and congenital toxoplasmosis, J. Clin. Microbiol. 28 (1990) 1434–1437.

[746] P. Hohlfeld, et al., *Toxoplasma gondii* infection during pregnancy: T lymphocyte subpopulations in mothers and fetuses, Pediatr. Infect. Dis. J. 9 (1990) 878–881.

[747] Y. Cohen-Khallas, et al., La fraction C4 du complement: un nouveau marqueur indirect pour le diagnostic antenatal de la toxoplasmose, Presse Med. 21 (1992) 908.

[748] C.A. Alford, et al., A correlative immunologic, microbiologic and clinical approach to the diagnosis of acute and chronic infections in newborn infants, N. Engl. J. Med. 277 (1967) 437–449.

[749] C.A. Alford, Immunoglobulin determinations in the diagnosis of fetal infection, Pediatr. Clin. North Am. 18 (1971) 99–113.

[750] G.H. McCracken Jr., et al., Evaluation of a radial diffusion plate method for determining serum immunoglobulin levels in normal and congenitally infected infants, J. Pediatr. 75 (1969) 1204–1210.

[751] S.B. Korones, et al., Neonatal IgM response to acute infection, J. Pediatr. 75 (1969) 1261–1270.

[752] J.D. Thorley, et al., Passive transfer of antibodies of maternal origin from blood to cerebrospinal fluid in infants, Lancet 1 (1975) 651–653.

[753] B. Patel, et al., Immunoglobulin-A detection and the investigation of clinical toxoplasmosis, J. Med. Microbiol. 38 (1993) 286–292.

[754] F. Foudrinier, et al., Value of specific immunoglobulin A detection by two immunocapture assays in the diagnosis of toxoplasmosis, Eur. J. Clin. Microbiol. Infect. Dis. 4 (1995) 585–590.

[755] I. Villena, et al., Detection of specific immunoglobulin E during maternal, fetal, and congenital toxoplasmosis, J. Clin. Microbiol. 37 (1999) 3487–3490.

[756] F. Foudrinier, et al., Clinical value of specific immunoglobulin E detection by enzyme-linked immunosorbent assay in cases of acquired and congenital toxoplasmosis, J. Clin. Microbiol. 41 (2003) 1681–1686.

[757] F.G. Araujo, J.S. Remington, IgG antibody suppression of the IgM antibody response to *Toxoplasma gondii* in newborn rabbits, J. Immunol. 115 (1975) 335–338.

[758] G.H. McCracken Jr., J.M. Kaplan, Penicillin treatment for congenital syphilis. A critical reappraisal, JAMA 228 (1974) 855–858.

[759] I. Fuentes, Urine as sample for congenital toxoplasmosis diagnosis by polymerase chain reaction (unpublished), 1996.

[760] S.F. Parmley, F.D. Goebel, J.S. Remington, Detection of *Toxoplasma gondii* DNA in cerebrospinal fluid from AIDS patients by polymerase chain reaction, J. Clin. Microbiol. 30 (1992) 3000–3002.

[761] B. Fortier, et al., Study of developing clinical outbreak and serological rebounds in children with congenital toxoplasmosis and follow-up during the first 2 years of life, Arch. Pediatr. 4 (1997) 940–946.

[762] S. Kahi, et al., Circulating *Toxoplasma gondii*-specific antibody-secreting cells in patients with congenital toxoplasmosis, Clin. Immunol. Immunopathol. 89 (1998) 23–27.

[763] I. Villena, et al., Pyrimethamine-sulfadoxine treatment of congenital toxoplasmosis: follow-up of 78 cases between 1980 and 1997. Reims toxoplasmosis group, Scand. J. Infect. Dis. 30 (1998) 295–300.

[764] O. Djurkovic-Djakovic, et al., Serologic rebounds after one-year-long treatment for congenital toxoplasmosis, Pediatr. Infect. Dis. J. 19 (2000) 81–83.

[765] M. Wallon, et al., Serological rebound in congenital toxoplasmosis: long-term follow-up of 133 children, Eur. J. Pediatr. 160 (2001) 534–540.

[766] M. Wallon, et al., Long-term ocular prognosis in 327 children with congenital toxoplasmosis, Pediatrics 113 (2004) 1567–1572.

[767] D. Sibalic, O. Djurkovic-Djakovic, B. Bobic, Onset of ocular complications in congenital toxoplasmosis associated with immunoglobulin M antibodies to *Toxoplasma gondii*, Eur. J. Clin. Microbiol. Infect. Dis. 9 (1990) 671–674.

[768] R. Wright, et al., Congenital lymphocytic choriomeningitis virus syndrome: a disease that mimics congenital toxoplasmosis or cytomegalovirus infections, Pediatrics 100 (1997) E91–E100.

[769] C.C. Smith, J. Ihrig, Persistent excretion of pyrimethamine following oral administration, Am. J. Trop. Med. Hyg. 8 (1959) 60–62.

[770] D.R. Stickney, et al., Pharmacokinetics of pyrimethamine (PRM) and 2,4-diamino-5-(3′,4′-dichlorophenyl) -6- methylpyrimidine (DMP) relevant to meningeal leukemia, Proc. Am. Assoc. Cancer Res. 14 (1973) 52.

[771] E. Weidekamm, et al., Plasma concentrations of pyrimethamine and sulfadoxine and evaluation of pharmacokinetic data by computerized curve fitting, Bull. World Health Organ. 60 (1982) 115–122.

[772] R.A. Ahmad, H.J. Rogers, Pharmacokinetics and protein binding interactions of dapsone and pyrimethamine, Br. J. Clin. Pharmacol. 10 (1980) 519–524.

[773] R. McLeod, et al., Levels of pyrimethamine in sera and cerebrospinal and ventricular fluids from infants treated for congenital toxoplasmosis. Toxoplasmosis study group, Antimicrob. Agents Chemother. 36 (5) (1992) 1040–1048.

[774] M.J. Gubbels, C. Li, B. Striepen, High-throughput growth assay for *Toxoplasma gondii* using yellow fluorescent protein, Antimicrob. Agents Chemother. 47 (2003) 309–316.

[775] D.E. Eyles, N. Coleman, An evaluation of the curative effects of pyrimethamine and sulfadiazine, alone and in combination, on experimental mouse toxoplasmosis, Antibiot. Chemother. 5 (1955) 529–539.

[776] H.G. Sheffield, M.L. Melton, Effect of pyrimethamine and sulfadiazine on the fine structure and multiplication of *Toxoplasma gondii* in cell cultures, J. Parasitol. 61 (1975) 704–712.

[777] D.E. Eyles, N. Coleman, Synergistic effect of sulfadiazine and Daraprim against experimental toxoplasmosis in the mouse, Antibiot. Chemother. 3 (1953) 483–490.

[778] D.E. Eyles, N. Coleman, The relative activity of the common sulfonamides against toxoplasmosis in the mouse, Am. J. Trop. Med. Hyg. 2 (1953) 54–63.

[779] D.E. Eyles, N. Coleman, The effect of sulfadimetine, sulfisoxazole, and sulfapyrazine against mouse toxoplasmosis, Antibiot. Chemother. 5 (1955) 525–528.

[780] P.H. Dorangeon, et al., Passage transplacentaire de l'association pyriméthamine-sulfadoxine lors du traitement anténatal de la toxoplasmose congénitale, Presse Med. 19 (1990) 2036.

[781] T. Trenque, et al., Human maternofoetal distribution of pyrimethamine-sulphadoxine, Br. J. Clin. Pharmacol. 45 (1998) 179–180 (letter).

[782] E. Schoondermark-van de Ven, et al., Study of treatment of congenital *Toxoplasma gondii* infection in Rhesus monkeys with pyrimethamine and sulfadiazine, Antimicrob. Agents Chemother. 39 (1995) 137–144.

[783] F. Peyron, M. Wallon, C. Bernardoux, Long-term follow-up of patients with congenital ocular toxoplasmosis, N. Engl. J. Med. 334 (1996) 993–994 (letter).

[784] C.B. Wilson, Treatment of congenital toxoplasmosis during pregnancy, J. Pediatr. 116 (1990) 1003–1005.

[785] S. Corvaisier, et al., Population pharmacokinetics of pyrimethamine and sulfadoxine in children treated for congenital toxoplasmosis, Antimicrob. Agents Chemother. 48 (2004) 3794–3800.

[786] D.G. Mack, R. McLeod, New micromethod to study the effect of antimicrobial agents on *Toxoplasma gondii*: comparison of sulfadoxine and sulfadiazine individually and in combination with pyrimethamine and study of clindamycin, metronidazole, and cyclosporin A, Antimicrob. Agents Chemother. 26 (1984) 26–30.

[787] B.J. Zitelli, et al., Fatal hepatic necrosis due to pyrimethamine-sulfadoxine (Fansidar), Ann. Intern. Med. 106 (1987) 393–395.

[788] D. Matsui, Prevention, diagnosis, and treatment of fetal toxoplasmosis, Clin. Perinatol. 21 (1994) 675–689.

[789] R. McLeod, Treatment of congenital toxoplasmosis, in: Plenary Symposium: Advances in Therapy of Protozoal Infections, Orlando, FL, October 6, 1994.

[790] T. Trenque, et al., Population pharmacokinetics of pyrimethamine and sulfadoxine in children with congenital toxoplasmosis, Br. J. Clin. Pharmacol. 57 (1997) 735–741.

[791] M.K. Jordan, et al., Plasma pharmacokinetics of sulfadiazine administered twice daily versus four times daily are similar in human immunodeficiency virus-infected patients, Antimicrob. Agents Chemother. 48 (2004) 635–637.

[792] R.W. Ryan, et al., Diagnosis and treatment of toxoplasmic uveitis, Trans. Am. Acad. Ophthalmol. Otolaryngol. 58 (1954) 867–884.

[793] E.S. Perkins, C.H. Smith, P.B. Schofield, Treatment of uveitis with pyrimethamine (Daraprim), Br. J. Ophthalmol. 40 (1956) 577–586.

[794] J. Elmalem, et al., Severe complications arising from the prescription of pyrimethamine for infants being treated for toxoplasmosis, Therapie 40 (1985) 357–359.

[795] J.K. Frenkel, G.H. Hitchings, Relative reversal by vitamins (p-aminobenzoic, folic and folinic acids) of the effects of sulfadiazine and pyrimethamine on *Toxoplasma*, mouse and man, Antibiot. Chemother. 7 (1957) 630–638.

[796] P.F. Nixon, J.R. Bertino, Effective absorption and utilization of oral formyltetrahydrofolate in man, N. Engl. J. Med. 286 (1972) 175–179.

[797] C.J. Allegra, et al., Potent in vitro and in vivo anti-*Toxoplasma* activity of the lipid-soluble antifolate trimetrexate, J. Clin. Invest. 79 (1987) 478–482.

[798] H. Maisonneuve, et al., Congenital toxoplasmosis. Tolerability of the sulfadoxine-pyrimethamine combination. 24 cases, Presse Med. 13 (1984) 859–862.

[799] J.P. Garin, et al., Effect of pyrimethamine sulfadoxine (Fansidar) on an avirulent cystogenic strain of *Toxoplasma gondii* (Prugniaud strain) in white mice, Bull. Soc. Pathol. Exot. Filiales 78 (1985) 821–824.

[800] J.P. Garin, B. Paillard, Experimental toxoplasmosis in mice. Comparative activity of clindamycin, midecamycin, josamycin, spiramycin, pyrimethamine-sulfadoxine, and trimethoprim-sulfamethoxazole, Ann. Pediatr. (Paris) 31 (1984) 841–845.

[801] J.B. Thiersch, Effect of certain 2,4-diaminopyrimidine antagonists of folic acid on pregnancy and rat fetus, Proc. Soc. Exp. Biol. Med. 87 (1954) 571–577.

[802] S.I. Anderson, L.M. Morse, The influence of solvent on the teratogenic effect of folic acid antagonist in the rat, Exp. Mol. Pathol. 5 (1966) 134–145.

[803] A.P. Dyban, I.M. Akimova, Characteristic features of the action of chloridine on various stages of embryonic development (experimental investigation), Akush. Ginekol. (Mosk) 41 (1965) 21–38.

[804] A.P. Dyban, I.M. Akimova, V.A. Svetlova, Effects of 2,4-diamino-5-chlorphenyl-6-ethylpyrimidine on embryonic development of rats, Dokl. Akad. Nauk SSSR 163 (1965) 1514–1517.

[805] M. Krahe, Investigations on the teratogen effect of medicine for the treatment of toxoplasmosis during pregnancy, Arch. Gynakol. 202 (1965) 104–109.

[806] G.E. Sullivan, E. Takacs, Comparative teratogenicity of pyrimethamine in rats and hamsters, Teratology 4 (1971) 205–210.

[807] V. Puchta, E. Simandlova, On the question of fetal injury due to pyrimethamine (Daraprim), in: L.H. Kirchhoff H (Ed.), Georg Thieme Verlag, Stuttgart, Germany, 1971.

[808] J.P. Garin, D.E. Eyles, Spiramycin therapy of experimental toxoplasmosis in mice, Presse Med. 66 (1958) 957–958.

[809] P. Mas Bakal, Deferred spiramycin treatment of acute toxoplasmosis in white mice, Ned. Tijdschr. Geneeskd. 109 (1965) 1014–1017.

[810] Niel G, Videau D. Activité de la spiramycine in vitro sur *Toxoplasma gondii*, in: Réunion Inter Discipl. Chimioth. Antiinfect. 3–12, Paris, France; 1981.

[811] J.A. Macfarlane, et al., Spiramycin in the prevention of postoperative staphylococcal infection, Lancet 1 (1968) 1–4.

[812] F. Benazet, M. Dubost, Apparent paradox of antimicrobial activity of spiramycin, Antibiot. Ann. 6 (1958) 211–224.

[813] R. Sutherland, Spiramycin: a reappraisal of its antibacterial activity, Br. J. Pharmacol. 19 (1962) 99–110.

[814] S. Kernbaum, Spiramycin; therapeutic value in humans (author's transl), Sem. Hop. Paris 58 (1982) 289–297.

[815] J.P. Garin, et al., Theoretical bases of the prevention by spiramycin of congenital toxoplasmosis in pregnant women, Presse Med. 76 (1968) 2266.

[816] D.G. Hudson, G.M. Yoshihara, W.M. Kirby, Spiramycin: clinical and laboratory studies, AMA Arch. Intern. Med. 97 (1956) 57–61.

[817] F. Forestier, et al., Suivi therapeutique foetomaternel de la spiramycine en cours de grossesse, Arch. Fr. Pediatr. 44 (1987) 539–544.

[818] C. Martin, et al., The course of congenital toxoplasmosis. Critical study of 12 treated cases, Ann. Pediatr. (Paris) 16 (1969) 117–128.

[819] J.K.A. Beverley, et al., Prevention of pathological changes in experimental congenital *Toxoplasma* infections, Lyon Med. 230 (1973) 491–498.

[820] N. Back, et al., Clinical and experimental pharmacology of parenteral spiramycin, Clin. Pharmacol. Ther. 3 (1962) 305–313.

[821] M. Stramba-Badiale, et al., QT interval prolongation and risk of life-threatening arrhythmias during toxoplasmosis prophylaxis with spiramycin in neonates, Am. Heart. J. 133 (1997) 108–111.

[822] J. Couvreur, et al., In utero treatment of toxoplasmic fetopathy with the combination pyrimethamine-sulfadiazine, Fetal Diagn. Ther. 8 (1993) 45–50.

[823] C. Leport, et al., Failure of spiramycin to prevent neurotoxoplasmosis in immunosuppressed patients, Med. Clin. North Am. 70 (1986) 677–692 (letter).

[824] J.G. Montoya, O. Liesenfeld, Toxoplasmosis, Lancet 363 (2004) 1965–1976.

[825] S. Stadtsbaeder, M.C. Calvin-Preval, The trimethoprim-sulfamethoxazole association in experimental toxoplasmosis in mice, Acta Clin. Belg. 28 (1973) 34–39.

[826] P.L. Grossman, J.S. Remington, The effect of trimethoprim and sulfamethoxazole on *Toxoplasma gondii* in vitro and in vivo, Am. J. Trop. Med. Hyg. 28 (1979) 445–455.

[827] H.A. Feldman, Effects of trimethoprim and sulfisoxazole alone and in combination on murine toxoplasmosis, J. Infect. Dis. 128 (Suppl.) (1973) S774–S776.

[828] J. Remington, Trimethoprim-sulfamethoxazole in murine toxoplasmosis, Antimicrob. Agents Chemother 9 (1976) 222–223.

[829] J. Sander, T. Midtvedt, The effect of trimethoprim on acute experimental toxoplasmosis in mice, Acta Pathol. Microbiol. Scand. B 78 (1970) 664–668.

[830] R. Brus, et al., Antitoxoplasmic activity of sulfonamides with various radicals in experimental toxoplasmosis in mice, Z. Tropenmed. Parasitol. 22 (1971) 98–103.

[831] R. Norrby, et al., Treatment of toxoplasmosis with trimethoprim-sulfamethoxazole, Scand. J. Infect. Dis. 7 (1975) 72–75.

[832] A. Domart, M. Robineau, C. Carbon, Acquired toxoplasmosis: a new chemotherapy: the sulfamethoxazole-trimethoprim combination, Nouv. Presse Med. 2 (1973) 321–322.

[833] G. Mossner, Klinische ergebnisse mit dem kombination-spraparat sulfamethoxazole + trimethoprim, in: Progress in Antimicrobial and Anticancer Chemotherapy, University Press, 1970, 966–970.

[834] D. Torre, et al., Randomized trial and trimethoprim-sulfamethoxazole versus pyrimethamine-sulfadiazine for therapy of toxoplasmic encephalitis in patients with AIDS, Antimicrob. Agents Chemother. 42 (1998) 1346–1349.

[835] R.B. Nussenblatt, et al., Strategies for the treatment of intraocular inflammatory disease, Transplant. Proc. 30 (1998) 4124–4125.

[836] F.G. Araujo, J.S. Remington, Effect of clindamycin on acute and chronic toxoplasmosis in mice, Antimicrob. Agents Chemother. 15 (1974) 647–651.

[837] P.R. McMaster, et al., The effect of two chlorinated lincomycin analogues against acute toxoplasmosis in mice, Am. J. Trop. Med. Hyg. 22 (1973) 14–17.

[838] K.F. Tabbara, R.A. Nozik, G.R. O'Connor, Clindamycin effects on experimental ocular toxoplasmosis in the rabbit, Arch. Ophthalmol. 92 (1974) 244–247.

[839] B.R. Dannemann, D.M. Israelski, J.S. Remington, Treatment of toxoplasmic encephalitis with intravenous clindamycin, Arch. Intern. Med. 148 (1988) 2477–2482.

[840] B.R. Dannemann, et al., Treatment of toxoplasmic encephalitis in patients with AIDS: a randomized trial comparing pyrimethamine plus clindamycin to pyrimethamine plus sulfadiazine, Ann. Intern. Med. 116 (1992) 33–43.

[841] H.R. Chang, R. Comte, J.C. Pechere, In vitro and in vivo effects of doxycycline on *Toxoplasma gondii*, Antimicrob. Agents Chemother. 34 (1990) 775–780.

[842] K.F. Tabbara, S. Sakuragi, G.R. O'Connor, Minocycline in the chemotherapy of murine toxoplasmosis, Parasitology 84 (1982) 297–302.

[843] H.R. Chang, et al., Activity of minocycline against *Toxoplasma gondii* infection in mice, J. Antimicrob. Chemother. 27 (1991) 639–645.

[844] Pope-Pegram L., et. al., Abstract: Treatment of Presumed Central Nervous System Toxoplasmosis with Doxycycline. In Program and Abstracts of VII Int'l Conference on AIDS; Florence, Italy; June 16-21,1991; Vol 1:188.

[845] Turett, G., et. al. (Abstract) Failure of doxycycline in the treatment of cerebral toxoplasmosis, in: Sixth International Conference on AIDS; San Francisco, California; Th.B.479; June 20–24, 1990.

[846] J.S. Remington, T. Yagura, W.S. Robinson, The effect of rifampin on *Toxoplasma gondii*, Proc. Soc. Exp. Biol. Med. 135 (1970) 167–172.

[847] J. Chan, B.J. Luft, Activity of roxithromycin (RU 28965), a macrolide, against *Toxoplasma gondii* infection in mice, Antimicrob. Agents Chemother. 30 (1986) 323–324.

[848] B.J. Luft, In vivo and in vitro activity of roxithromycin against *Toxoplasma gondii* in mice, Eur. J. Clin. Microbiol. 6 (1987) 479–481.

[849] F.G. Araujo, et al., Activity of clarithromycin alone or in combination with other drugs for treatment of murine toxoplasmosis, Antimicrob. Agents Chemother. 36 (1992) 2454–2457.

[850] F.G. Araujo, D.R. Guptill, J.S. Remington, Azithromycin, a macrolide antibiotic with potent activity against *Toxoplasma gondii*, Antimicrob. Agents Chemother. 32 (1988) 755–757.

[851] B. Stray-Pedersen, The European Research Network on Congenital Toxoplasmosis Treatment Group. Azithromycin levels in placental tissue, amniotic fluid and blood, in: 36th Interscience conference on Antimicrobial Agents and Chemotherapy, American Society for Microbiology, Washington, DC, 1996.

[852] A. Rothova, et al., Azithromycin for ocular toxoplasmosis, Br. J. Ophthalmol. 82 (1998) 1306–1308.

[853] L.H. Bosch-Driessen, et al., A prospective, randomized trial of pyrimethamine and azithromycin vs pyrimethamine and sulfadiazine for the treatment of ocular toxoplasmosis, Am. J. Ophthalmol. 134 (2002) 34–40.

[854] F.G. Araujo, et al., Use of ketolides in combination with other drugs to treat experimental toxoplasmosis, J. Antimicrob. Chemother. 42 (1998) 665–667.

[855] A.A. Khan, et al., Activity of gatifloxacin alone or in combination with pyrimethamine or gamma interferon against *Toxoplasma gondii*, Antimicrob. Agents Chemother. 45 (1) (2001) 48–51.

[856] F.G. Araujo, J. Huskinson, J.S. Remington, Remarkable in vitro and in vivo activities of the hydroxynaphthoquinone 566C80 against tachyzoites and tissue cysts of *Toxoplasma gondii*, Antimicrob. Agents Chemother. 35 (2) (1991) 293–299.

[857] J. Huskinson-Mark, F.G. Araujo, J.S. Remington, Evaluation of the effect of drugs on the cyst form of *Toxoplasma gondii*, J. Infect. Dis. 164 (1) (1991) 170–171.

[858] J.A. Kovacs, Efficacy of atovaquone in treatment of toxoplasmosis in patients with AIDS, Lancet 340 (1992) 637–638.

[859] R. Torres, et al., Atovaquone for salvage treatment and suppression of toxoplasmic encephalitis in patients with AIDS, Clin. Infect. Dis. 24 (1997) 422–429.

[860] C. Katlama, et al., Atovaquone as long-term suppressive therapy for toxoplasmic encephalitis in patients with AIDS and multiple drug intolerance, AIDS 10 (1996) 1107–1112.

[861] P. Meneceur, et al., In vitro susceptibility of various genotypic strains of *Toxoplasma gondii* to pyrimethamine, sulfadiazine, and atovaquone, Antimicrob. Agents Chemother. 52 (4) (2008) 1269–1277.

[862] A.A. Khan, et al., Trovafloxacin is active against *Toxoplasma gondii*, Antimicrob. Agents Chemother. 40 (1996) 1855–1859.

[863] A.A. Khan, et al., Activity of trovafloxacin in combination with other drugs for treatment of acute murine toxoplasmosis, Antimicrob. Agents Chemother. 41 (1997) 893–897.

[864] P. Pointud, et al., Positive toxoplasmic serology in polymyositis, Ann. Med. Interne (Paris) 127 (1976) 881–885.

[865] S. Stagno, et al., Auditory and visual defects resulting from symptomatic and subclinical congenital cytomegaloviral and *Toxoplasma* infections, Pediatrics 59 (1977) 669–678.

[866] D. Jeannel, et al., What is known about the prevention of congenital toxoplasmosis? Lancet 336 (1990) 359–361.

[867] P. Boulot, et al., Limitations of the prenatal treatment of congenital toxoplasmosis with the sulfadiazine-pyrimethamine combination, Presse Med. 19 (1990) 570.

[868] J. Couvreur, et al., Etude d'une serie homogene de 210 cas de toxoplasmose congénitale chez des nourrissons ages de 0 à 11 mois et depistes de facon prospective, Sem. Hop. Paris 61 (1985) 3015–3019.

[869] M. Wallon, et al., Letter to the editor, Lancet 344 (1994) 541.

[870] C.A. Alford Jr., D.W. Reynolds, S. Stagno, L. Gluck (Ed.), Current concepts of chronic perinatal infections, 1975.

[871] M. Szusterkac, A propos de 124 cas de toxoplasmose congénitale: aspects cliniques et paracliniques en fonction des circonstances du diagnostic retrospectif ou prospectif; resultats du traitement, Faculté de Médecine Saint-Antoine, Paris, 1980.

[872] C. Briatte, Etude de 55 cas de toxoplasmose congenitale depistes lors de bilans de santé systematiques après l'age de 10 mois. Centre de bilans de

santé de la securité sociale de la Region Parisienne, Faculté de Médecine Saint-Antoine, Paris, 1980.

[873] N. Roizen, et al., Developmental and neurologic function in treated congenital toxoplasmosis, Pediatr. Res. 31 (1992) 353A.

[874] A.G. Noble, et al., Chorioretinal lesions in mothers of children with congenital toxoplasmosis in the National Collaborative Chicago-based, Congenital Toxoplasmosis Study, Scientia Medica 20 (2010), Epub ahead of print.

[875] C.N. Swisher, K. Boyer, R. McLeod, The toxoplasmosis study group. Congenital toxoplasmosis, Semin. Pediatr. Neurol. 1 (1994) 4–25.

[876] J.L. Sever, et al., Toxoplasmosis: maternal and pediatric findings in 23,000 pregnancies, Pediatrics 82 (1988) 181–192.

[877] R. McLeod, et al., Levels of pyrimethamine in sera and cerebrospinal and ventricular fluids from infants treated for congenital toxoplasmosis, Antimicrob. Agents Chemother. 36 (1992) 1040–1048.

[878] R. McLeod, et al., Outcome of treatment for congenital toxoplasmosis, 1981–2004: the national collaborative Chicago-based, congenital toxoplasmosis study, Clin. Infect. Dis. 42 (10) (2006) 1383–1394.

[879] K. Boyer, J. Marcinak, R. McLeod, Toxoplasma gondii (Toxoplasmosis), in: S. Long, L.K. Pickering, C.G. Prober (Eds.), Principles and Practice of Pediatric Infectious Diseases, third ed., Churchill Livingstone, New York, section 274, 2007.

[880] M.R. Stanford, et al., Antibiotics for toxoplasmic retinochoroiditis: an evidence-based systematic review, Ophthalmology 110 (5) (2003) 926–931, quiz 931–932.

[881] M.G. Mets, D.G. Mack, K. Boyer, Congenital ocular toxoplasmosis, in: G.T.T.S. Mets Mb (Ed.), 1992, 1094.

[882] R.E.J. Engstrom, et al., Current practices in the management of ocular toxoplasmosis, Am. J. Ophthalmol. 111 (1991) 601–610.

[883] L. Phan, et al., Longitudinal study of new eye lesions in treated congenital toxoplasmosis, Ophthalmology 115 (3) (2008) 553–559, e8.

[884] L. Phan, et al., Longitudinal study of new eye lesions in children with toxoplasmosis who were not treated during the first year of life, Am. J. Ophthalmol. 146 (3) (2008) 375–384.

[885] G.N. Holland, et al., Analysis of recurrence patterns associated with toxoplasmic retinochoroiditis, Am. J. Ophthalmol. 145 (6) (2008) 1007–1013.

[886] A.P. Brezin, et al., Ophthalmic outcomes after prenatal and postnatal treatment of congenital toxoplasmosis, Am. J. Ophthalmol. 135 (2003) 779–784.

[887] C. Binquet, et al., Prognostic factors for the long-term development of ocular lesions in 327 children with congenital toxoplasmosis, Epidemiol. Infect. 131 (2003) 1157–1168.

[888] J.K. Frenkel, Congenital toxoplasmosis: prevention or palliation? Am. J. Obstet. Gynecol. 141 (1981) 359–361.

[889] J.B. Henderson, et al., The evaluation of new services: possibilities for preventing congenital toxoplasmosis, Int. J. Epidemiol. 13 (1984) 65–72.

[890] R. McCabe, J.S. Remington, Toxoplasmosis: the time has come, N. Engl. J. Med. 318 (1988) 313–315 (editorial).

[891] T. Roberts, J.K. Frenkel, Estimating income losses and other preventable costs caused by congenital toxoplasmosis in people in the United States, J. Am. Vet. Med. Assoc. 196 (1990) 249–256.

[892] E.L. Gollub, et al., Effectiveness of health education on Toxoplasma-related knowledge, behaviour, and risk of seroconversion in pregnancy, Eur. J. Obstet. Gynecol. Reprod. Biol. 136 (2) (2008) 137–145.

[893] K.M. Boyer, et al., Risk factors for Toxoplasma gondii infection in mothers of infants with congenital toxoplasmosis: implications for prenatal management and screening, Am. J. Obstet. Gynecol. 192 (2) (2005) 564–571.

[894] J.K. Frenkel, Breaking the transmission chain of Toxoplasma: a program for the prevention of human toxoplasmosis, Bull. N. Y. Acad. Med. 50 (1974) 228–235.

[895] J.K. Frenkel, Toxoplamosis in cats and man, Feline Pract. 5 (1975) 28–41.

[896] W.J. Hartley, B.L. Munday, Felidae in the dissemination of toxoplasmosis to man and other animals, Aust. Vet. J. 50 (1974) 224–228.

[897] W.M. Hutchison, et al., The life cycle of the coccidian parasite, Toxoplasma gondii, in the domestic cat, Trans R Soc Trop Med Hyg 65 (1971) 380–399.

[898] J.K. Werner, B.C. Walton, Prevalence of naturally occurring Toxoplasma gondii infections in cats from U.S. military installations in Japan, J. Parasitol. 58 (1972) 1148–1150.

[899] J.K. Frenkel, J.P. Dubey, Rodents as vectors for feline coccidia, Isospora felis and Isospora rivolta, J. Infect. Dis. 125 (1972) 69–72.

[900] H. Aspock, A. Pollak, Prevention of prenatal toxoplasmosis by serological screening of pregnant women in Austria, Scand. J. Infect. Dis. Suppl 84 (1992) 32–37.

[901] T. Roos, et al., Systematic serologic screening for toxoplasmosis in pregnancy, Obstet. Gynecol. 81 (2) (1993) 243–250.

[902] Z. Szenasi, et al., Prevention of congenital toxoplasmosis in Szeged, Hungary Int. J. Epidemiol. 26 (2) (1997) 428–435.

[903] A. Hassl, Efficiency analysis of toxoplasmosis screening in pregnancy: comment, Scand. J. Infect. Dis. 28 (1996) 211–212 (letter).

[904] M. Lappalainen, et al., Screening of toxoplasmosis during pregnancy, Isr. J. Med. Sci. 30 (1994) 362–363.

[905] T.J. Bader, G.A. Macones, D.A. Asch, Prenatal screening for toxoplasmosis, Obstet. Gynecol. 90 (1997) 457–464.

[906] F. Daffos, et al., Letter to the editor, Lancet 344 (1994) 541.

[907] L. Gras, et al., Effect of prenatal treatment on the risk of intracranial and ocular lesions in children with congenital toxoplasmosis, Int. J. Epidemiol. 30 (6) (2001) 1309–1313.

[908] A. Eskild, P. Magnus, Little evidence of effective prenatal treatment against congenital toxoplasmosis–the implications for testing in pregnancy, Int. J. Epidemiol. 30 (6) (2001) 1314–1315 (commentary).

[909] R.E. Gilbert, et al., Effect of prenatal treatment on mother to child transmission of Toxoplasma gondii: retrospective cohort study of 554 mother-child pairs in Lyon, France, Int. J. Epidemiol. 30 (6) (2001) 1303–1308.

[910] R.E. Gilbert, et al., Effect of prenatal treatment on mother to child transmission of Toxoplasma gondii: retrospective cohort study of 554 mother-child pairs in Lyon, France, Int. J. Epidemiol. 30 (6) (2001) 1303–1308.

[911] L. Gras, et al., Effect of prenatal treatment on the risk of intracranial and ocular lesions in children with congenital toxoplasmosis, Int. J. Epidemiol. 30 (2001) 1309–1313.

[912] R. Thiebaut, et al., Effectiveness of prenatal treatment for congenital toxoplasmosis: a meta-analysis of individual patients' data, Lancet 369 (9556) (2007) 115–122.

[913] V. Luyasu, et al., Congenital toxoplasmosis and seroconversion at the end of pregnancy: clinical observations, Acta Clin. Belg. 52 (1997) 381–387.

[914] K. Freeman, et al., Predictors of retinochoroiditis in children with congenital toxoplasmosis: European, prospective cohort study, Pediatrics 121 (5) (2008) e1215–e1222.

[915] F. Kieffer, et al., Risk factors for retinochoroiditis during the first 2 years of life in infants with treated congenital toxoplasmosis, Pediatr. Infect. Dis. J. 27 (1) (2008) 27–32.

[916] H. Kräubig, Erste praktische Erfahrungen mit der Prophylaze der konnatalen Toxoplasmose, Med. Klin. 58 (1963) 1361–1364.

[917] O. Thalhammer, Congenital toxoplasmosis in Vienna. Summering [sic] findings and opinions, in: L. Specia (Ed.), 1969.

[918] O. Thalhammer, Prevention of congenital toxoplasmosis, Neuropediatrie 4 (1973) 233–237.

[919] V.P. Hengst, Effectiveness of general testing for Toxoplasma gondii infection in pregnancy, Zentralbl. Gynakol. 104 (1982) 949–956.

[920] O. Liesenfeld, et al., False-positive results in immunoglobuline M (IgM) toxoplasma antibody tests and importance of confirmatory testing: the Platelia Toxo IgM test, J Clin Microbiol 35 (1997) 174–178.

[921] J.S. Remington, Toxoplasmid and human abortion, in: S.S.H. Meigs Jv (Ed.), 1963.

[922] B. Eckerling, A. Neri, E. Eylan, Toxoplasmosis: a cause of infertility, Fertil. Steril. 19 (1968) 883–891.

[923] H. Langer, Toxoplasma infection during pregnancy, Zentralbl. Gynakol. 86 (1964) 745–750.

[924] S. Vlaev, Opyt profilaktiki vrozdennogo toksoplazmoza, Vop Okrany Materin Dets 10 (1965) 78–82.

[925] V.F. Isbruch, Contributions to the problem of toxoplasmosis. I. Should we, at the present state of knowledge, treat pregnant women with positive toxoplasmosis titers, with Daraprim and Supronal? Zentralbl. Gynakol. 82 (1960) 1522–1544.

[926] M. Sharf, I. Eibschitz, E. Eylan, Latent toxoplasmosis and pregnancy, Obstet. Gynecol. 42 (1973) 349–354.

[927] A.C. Kimball, B.H. Kean, F. Fuchs, The role of toxoplasmosis in abortion, Am. J. Obstet. Gynecol. 111 (1971) 219–226.

[928] J.S. Remington, Toxoplasma and chronic abortion, Obstet. Gynecol. 24 (1964) 155–157, (editorial).

[929] H. Feldman, Congenital toxoplasmosis, N. Eng. J. Med. 26 (1963) 1212, (letter).

[930] S.D. Cengir, F. Ortac, F. Soylemez, Treatment and results of chronic toxoplasmosis. Analysis of 33 cases, Gynecol. Obstet. Invest. 33 (2) (1992) 105–108.

CHAPTER OUTLINE

Ascaris 1042
Giardiasis 1043
American Trypanosomiasis: Chagas Disease 1043
    The Organism 1043
    Epidemiology and Transmission 1043
    Pathology 1043
    Biopsy and Autopsy Studies 1043
    Clinical Manifestations 1044
    Abortions and Stillbirths 1044
    Congenital Infections 1044
    Diagnosis 1044
    Prognosis for Recurrence 1045
    Therapy 1045
    Prevention 1045

African Trypanosomiasis: African Sleeping Sickness 1045
Entamoeba histolytica 1045
Malaria 1046
    The Organisms 1046
    Epidemiology and Transmission 1046
    Pathology 1046
    Congenital Malaria 1048
Schistosomiasis 1052
Trichomonas vaginalis 1052
Trichinosis 1052
Babesiosis 1052
Pneumocystis jiroveci 1052

Parasitic infections are highly prevalent in many developing areas of the world and may be common among pregnant women in developed countries. The placenta serves as an effective barrier, even in infections such as malaria and schistosomiasis in which systemic involvement and hematogenous spread are common. Although transplacental infections of the fetus are uncommon, the prevalence of parasitic infections among infants younger than 1 month is high in developing countries, and infections occur primarily through transmission during or shortly after birth.

In a study conducted in Guatemala, Kotcher and colleagues [1] found that 30% of newborns had acquired a protozoal infection by 2 weeks of age. Although these infants were infected with *Entamoeba histolytica* and *Entamoeba coli*, *Endolimax nana*, and *Iodamoeba buetschlii*, they remained asymptomatic. *Giardia lamblia* was found by the fifth week of life and *Trichuris trichiura* by the 16th week of life. A study conducted in a regional hospital in Togo revealed that 55% of infants and children from birth to 16 years old demonstrated evidence of parasitic infections in stool or urine, with obvious neonatal infections occurring as well [2].

Pneumocystis jiroveci (previously classified as *Pneumocystis carinii*) is considered in Chapter 34 [3].

ASCARIS

Ascaris lumbricoides is the most prevalent parasitic infection worldwide, affecting up to 1 billion people. In humans, *Ascaris* eggs are ingested through fecal-oral contamination, hatch in the small intestine, and then penetrate the intestinal lumen to migrate extensively through blood and lymphatics. Larvae eventually reach the pulmonary circulation, where they migrate into the alveolar sacs, through the respiratory tree to the esophagus, and into the small intestine. Because *Ascaris* may migrate to many organs, worms are occasionally found in the uterus and the fallopian tubes [4].

Human fetuses apparently can mount an immune response to maternal *Ascaris* infection, and congenital infections are rare. Sangeevi and associates [5] studied the IgG and IgM responses to *Ascaris* antigens from matched maternal and cord bloods in south India and found evidence of fetal IgM directed against *Ascaris* antigens in 12 of 28 samples. Clinical status of the infants was not reported. Chu and coworkers [6], however, described an infant whose delivery was complicated by the simultaneous delivery of 12 adult *A. lumbricoides* worms. During preparations for a cesarean section, which was being undertaken because of prolonged premature labor and fetal distress, one worm passed from the vagina, and another was found in the vagina. When the placenta was removed, 10 worms were found on the maternal side of the placenta. The infant was delivered in good condition. The infant passed two female worms, which were 28 and 30 cm long, on the second and sixth days of life. He was treated with piperazine citrate, but no other worms were passed, and no eggs were seen after the 11th day of life. Fertilized ova of *A. lumbricoides* were found in the amniotic fluid and in the newborn's feces. An adhesion connected the mother's intestine and uterus, but it is uncertain whether the worms passed directly from the mother's intestine to the placenta and amniotic fluid, and were swallowed by the fetus; whether larvae passed hematogenously from the mother's lung to the placenta and thereby reached the fetal circulation, lung, and gastrointestinal tract; or whether female worms in the placenta produced fertile eggs that reached the amniotic fluid and were swallowed by the fetus.

Other investigators have reported fetal evidence of Ascaris infection in infants as young as 1 to 2 weeks old and in one infant with failure to thrive and bloody diarrhea at 3 weeks who responded to levamisole therapy [7].

GIARDIASIS

G. lamblia causes a localized intestinal infection, with no systemic involvement, and *G. lamblia* infection in pregnancy has not been associated with fetal infection. Severe maternal infection that compromises nutrition can affect fetal growth, but such a severe illness is rare [8]. Neonatal *G. lamblia* infection can result from fecal contamination at birth. Infected infants are usually asymptomatic [9]. Treatment of pregnant women with giardiasis is generally deferred until after the first trimester unless symptoms are severe. There is some evidence that maternal antibody may be protective against neonatal giardiasis [10].

AMERICAN TRYPANOSOMIASIS: CHAGAS DISEASE

Millions of people in Central and South America are infected by *Trypanosoma cruzi* and related protozoa. Because of the chronicity of these infections, they have a significant impact on public health. One estimate suggests that approximately 40,000 women and 2000 newborns may be infected on an annual basis in North America, primarily in Mexico, although up to 3780 infected pregnant women and 189 congenitally infected infants could be born among Hispanic populations in the United States [11].

THE ORGANISM

The form of the organism that circulates in human blood is the trypomastigote. Cell division does not occur in the bloodstream. In tissue, the flagellum and undulating membrane are lost, and the organism differentiates into a leishmanial form, the amastigote [12,13]. Amastigotes multiply by binary fission, and masses of amastigotes are grouped into pseudocysts. The amastigotes in pseudocysts may evolve into trypanomastigotes and, on rupture of the pseudocyst, can gain access to the bloodstream or to new cells. Two strains of *T. cruzi* that cause human infections have been identified by biochemical differences among nine enzymes produced by the parasite [14].

EPIDEMIOLOGY AND TRANSMISSION

T. cruzi infects primates, marsupials, armadillos, bats, and many rodents, including guinea pigs, opossums, and raccoons; birds are not infected [15]. Infection of insects and mammals with *T. cruzi* is most common between the latitudes 398N (i.e., northern California and Maryland) and 438S (i.e., southern Argentina and Chile) and on the islands of Aruba and Trinidad [1]. The usual vectors are in the family Reduviidae, subfamily Triatominae. The main vector in Venezuela is *Rhodnius prolixus*; in Brazil, *Panstrongylus megistus*; and in Argentina, *Triatoma infestans* (conenosed bug) [15]. These species are well adapted to human dwellings. Triatominae are hematophagous insects. They acquire and transmit the infection by biting infected

vertebrates, including humans. The life span of the insect is not shortened by infection with *T. cruzi*; infected insects live up to a year after the onset of infection. In North America, the sylvatic habitat of the vector and the low virulence of the strains of *Trypanosoma* are responsible for the relative rarity of the disease. Colloquial terms used for the usual vector include the kissing or assassin bug in the southwestern United States; pito, hito, or vinchuca in Spanish America; and barbeiro in Portuguese America [16].

The vector is most commonly found in huts of mud and sticks and in other housing containing cracks. In vectors infected with *T. cruzi*, metacyclic trypomastigotes congregate in the rectum. Bites become contaminated when defecation occurs. The infective form reaches the bloodstream through the site of the bite or by penetrating mucous membranes, conjunctivae, or abraded skin [12]. *Trypanosoma rangeli* is spread by a few species of the triatomid bug. These metacyclic trypanosomes develop, divide, and multiply in the salivary gland. They are injected directly into the site of the bite.

Infections can also be acquired by blood transfusion [17] and transplacentally. The isoenzyme patterns of *T. cruzi* recovered from congenitally infected infants and their mothers are identical, but transplacental transmission may not always follow maternal infection with enzymatically similar strains [18].

PATHOLOGY

Placenta

The placenta is a relatively effective barrier to the spread of infection to the fetus [13]. The organism reaches the placenta by the hematogenous route and traverses the placental villi to the trophoblasts. After differentiation into amastigotes, the organism remains within Hofbauer (phagocytic) cells of the placenta until it is liberated into the fetal circulation [19–21].

Maternal parasitemia is greatest in the acute phase of infection; however, the period of intense parasitemia is short. Of the reported cases of congenital Chagas disease, only four have originated during the acute phase of infection [13]. Most congenital infections occur in infants born to women with the chronic form of the disease.

Infected placentas are pale, yellow, and bulky. They have an appearance similar to the placentas of infants with erythroblastosis fetalis. Infection of the placenta is much more common than infection of the fetus.

BIOPSY AND AUTOPSY STUDIES

Two histologic types of lesions are recognized: those that contain parasites and those that do not [13]. In tissue sections, the parasite assumes the morphology of *Leishmania* bodies, which are round and contain an ovoid nucleus and a rodlike blepharoplast. Inflammation usually does not occur unless a pseudocyst ruptures. Tissue reactions induced by an antibody are believed to be responsible for lesions in which the parasite cannot be demonstrated. After infection, an antibody that cross-reacts with the endocardium, the interstitium, and the blood vessels of the heart is formed and is referred to as an endocardial-vascular-interstitial antibody [22–24]. This antibody has an affinity for the plasma membranes of the endocardium, endothelial cell, and striated muscle, and for *T. cruzi*. Endocardial-vascular-interstitial antibody is present in 95% of persons with Chagas heart disease and in 45% of asymptomatic patients with serologic evidence of having had Chagas disease [24].

Tissue replication of the organism causes damage to the ganglia of the autonomic nervous system and to muscle [15]. Injury to the Auerbach plexus results in megaesophagus, megacolon, and dilation of other parts of the gastrointestinal tract and gallbladder. Similarly, the conducting system of the heart and the myocardium may be infected. Sudden death from arrhythmias can occur.

CLINICAL MANIFESTATIONS

In the mother, urticaria is often present at the site of the bite, regardless of whether the insect was infected [12]. The favored site for the bite is the face, presumably because this is the part of the body that is most often exposed during sleep. In acute infections, an inflammatory nodule, referred to as a chagoma, may develop at the site of the bite. If the bite is on the face, it is often associated with a unilateral, nonpurulent edema of the palpebral folds and an ipsilateral regional lymphadenopathy (i.e., Romaña sign). Between 2 and 3 weeks after the bite, parasitemia, fever, and a moderate local and general lymphadenopathy develop. The infection can extend and involve the myocardium, resulting in tachycardia, arrhythmia, hypotension, distant heart sounds, cardiomegaly, and congestive heart failure. The latter feature is more severe in pregnant and postpartum women than in nonpregnant women. Hepatosplenomegaly and encephalitis also occur. The mortality rate during the acute phase is 10% to 20%. Death is usually attributed to cardiac dysfunction. Many survivors have abnormal electrocardiograms.

In the chronic phase, the placenta and fetus may be infected despite the fact that the mother is asymptomatic [12]. Chronic Chagas disease often comes to medical attention because of the occurrence of an arrhythmia. These patients often do not have signs or symptoms of congestive heart failure [15]. Of 503 patients with myocardiopathy of chronic Chagas disease studied by Vasquez [25], 19.8% died during an observation period of 6 years—37.5% suddenly and 55.2% with congestive heart failure.

ABORTIONS AND STILLBIRTHS

Of 300 abortions in Argentina, 3 (1%) were performed because of Chagas disease [26]. In Chile and Brazil, 10% of all abortions are attributed to Chagas disease [12]. When the fetus is aborted, massive infection of the placenta is usually found.

CONGENITAL INFECTIONS

Bittencourt and coworkers [27] found *T. cruzi* antibodies in 226 of 2651 pregnant women; 28.3% of seropositive mothers had parasitemia. Nevertheless, the risk of transmission to the fetus is low, and live births of infants congenitally infected with *T. cruzi* are rare. It is postulated that upregulation of fetal or neonatal immunity might

be important in preventing vertical infection [28]. Congenital infections occur in 1% to 4% of women with serologic evidence of having had Chagas disease [1,12, 13,21,29,30]. Among infants with a birth weight of 2500 g or more, congenital infections are rare [19,31–34]. Among low-birth-weight infants, congenitally infected infants can be premature or small for gestational age, or both. Congenital infections were found in 10 (2.3%) of 425 infants by Saleme and associates in Argentina [26], in 10 (2%) of 500 infants weighing less than 2000 g by Bittencourt and coworkers in Brazil [27], and in 3 (1.6%) of 186 infants with birth weights of more than 2000 g and in 1 (0.5%) of 200 premature infants with birth weights of 2000 g or less by Howard in Chile [35].

Congenitally infected infants may develop symptoms at birth or during the first few weeks of life. Early-onset jaundice, anemia, and petechiae are common. These symptoms are similar to those associated with erythroblastosis fetalis [13]. As occurs in older patients, congenitally infected infants may have hepatosplenomegaly, cardiomegaly, and congestive heart failure and have involvement of the esophagus leading to dysphagia, regurgitation, and megaesophagus [24,36]. Some infants have myxedematous edema. Pneumonitis has been associated with infection of the amnionic epithelium [37]. Congenitally infected infants can be born with encephalitis or can develop it postnatally. It is generally associated with hypotonia, a poor suck, and seizures [12]. The cerebrospinal fluid shows mild pleocytosis, which consists primarily of lymphocytes. Cataracts and opacification of the media of the eye have also been observed [29]. Both twins may be congenitally infected, or one may escape infection [38].

Of 64 congenitally infected infants for whom follow-up results were known, Bittencourt [13] reported that 7.8% died the first day, 35.9% died when younger than 4 months, 9.3% died between the ages of 4 and 24 months, and 42.2% survived for more than 24 months. Of those who survived for 2 years or longer, 74% had no serious clinical symptoms despite continued parasitemia. However, subclinical abnormalities might have been found if electrocardiography or radiography had been performed.

As with other congenital infections, the immune system of the fetus is stimulated. IgM antibody to *T. cruzi* and endocardial-vascular-interstitial antibody are formed [13,24].

DIAGNOSIS

The diagnosis should be suspected at the time of abortions and stillbirths, and in infants who develop symptoms compatible with congenital infection. An easy, but often omitted, means of making a diagnosis of congenital infection is to examine the placenta for the amastigote of *T. cruzi*. The gross appearance of the placenta is similar to that seen in erythroblastosis fetalis. It appears that examination of infected amniotic fluid by PCR is not useful in diagnosing congenital infection [39].

Motile trypomastigotes can also be demonstrated by examining blood under a coverslip [13]. The number of parasites is low initially but increases subsequently.

Thin and thick smears can be examined after being stained with Giemsa stain. Microhematocrit concentration and examination of the buffy coat enhance the detection of parasites in congenital Chagas disease [40]. If more than 10 parasites/mm³ are found, the infant generally dies [26].

Xenodiagnosis is performed by allowing laboratory-bred uninfected insects to feed and ingest the patient's blood. The fecal contents of the insects are examined for trypomastigotes 30 to 60 days later. Blood may also be injected into mice. In mothers with acute Chagas disease, the parasites are found in blood smears beginning 3 weeks after onset of the infection, and they persist for several months. Parasites can be demonstrated for years by xenodiagnosis.

In the chronic stages of the disease, the diagnosis can be made histologically by sampling skeletal muscle. The histologic appearance of the parasite in tissue sections is similar to that of toxoplasmosis. However, the amastigotes in Chagas disease contain a blepharoplast that is lacking in toxoplasmosis.

Several tests for antibody are available. Complement-fixing antibody crosses the placenta from mother to infant. This test, referred to as the Machado-Guerreiro reaction, demonstrates antibodies that exhibit a cross-reaction with *Leishmania donovani* and with sera from patients with lepromatous leprosy. In uninfected infants, complement-fixing antibodies are no longer demonstrable after the 40th day of life; in infected infants, these antibodies persist [13].

Agglutinating antibodies may also be demonstrable. Uninfected infants with titers of agglutinating antibody of 1:512 or less at birth have negative titers by 2 months of age [29]. The titer of agglutinating antibody in uninfected infants with initial titers of 1:1024 or higher becomes negative by 6 months of age. IgM fluorescent antibodies can be demonstrated in some infants, but infected infants do not always have a positive test result [24,38]. Data suggest that fetal IgG to specific acute-phase antigens may be useful in the diagnosis of congenital Chagas disease, but maternal and neonatal serologic tests using the microhematocrit, direct parasitologic visualization, and indirect hemagglutination or enzyme-linked immunosorbent assay have proved to be reliable [41,42].

PROGNOSIS FOR RECURRENCE

Congenital infections can recur during subsequent pregnancies [43]. The same mother, however, often has healthy children before and after the affected one [24].

THERAPY

In the past, various drugs, including nitrofurans, 8-aminoquinolines, and metronidazole, were thought to have some effect on the blood-borne form of the parasite. They were ineffective in eliminating the tissue form, the amastigote. There is no therapy available for prevention of congenital infection, but early detection of neonatal infection and treatment with nifurtimox has resulted in cure rates of up to 90% [44]. Information regarding treatment can be obtained from the Parasitic Disease Drug Service, Centers for Disease Control and Prevention, Atlanta.

PREVENTION

The main means of prevention is to improve housing so that the vector cannot reach the inhabitants, especially during sleep. In endemic areas, potential blood donors should be tested, and only those who lack serologic evidence of having had Chagas disease should be permitted to donate blood. The addition of gentian violet (1:4000 solution) to blood has been useful as a means of preventing transmission of the infection to the recipient of the blood [15].

AFRICAN TRYPANOSOMIASIS: AFRICAN SLEEPING SICKNESS

Whereas few cases of congenital disease have been reported, infection with *Trypanosoma brucei gambiense* and *T. brucei rhodesiense* in adults is severe and often fatal, and congenital infection is most likely underreported. Humans are infected by the bite of an infected male or female tsetse fly, which injects trypomastigotes into the host. Humans are the primary reservoir for *T. gambiense* and large, wild game the hosts for *T. rhodesiense*. Once injected, the organism disseminates throughout the bloodstream. Signs and symptoms of infection appear after 2 to 4 weeks, and a chronic infection develops 6 months to 1 to 2 years later. The chronic stage includes a progressive meningoencephalitis, which is often fatal if left untreated. Infection with *T. gambiense* is associated with lymphadenopathy and is slowly progressive, whereas infection with *T. rhodesiense* is rapidly progressive.

The parasite can be transmitted transplacentally, but few cases have been reported [45,46]. Transplacental infection can cause prematurity, abortion, and stillbirth. Transplacental infection has been proved in infants who were born in nonendemic areas to infected mothers or if the parasite was identified in the peripheral blood in the first 5 days of life. Central nervous system involvement is common in congenital infection and, in some infants, may be slowly progressive.

The diagnosis should be suspected in an infant with unexplained fever, anemia, hepatosplenomegaly, or progressive neurologic symptoms whose mother is from an endemic area. The parasite can be identified in thick smears from peripheral blood or in the cerebrospinal fluid. In infants, treatment with suramin or melarsoprol has been reported with good results; however, in a case report of congenital trypanosomiasis [45], severe neurologic symptoms persisted after delayed diagnosis and treatment when the child was 22 months old.

ENTAMOEBA HISTOLYTICA

There is some evidence that amebiasis during pregnancy may be more severe and have a higher fatality rate than that expected in nonpregnant women of the same age [47,48]. Abioye [48] found that 68% of fatal cases of amebiasis in females 15 to 34 years old occurred in pregnant women, whereas only 17.1% and 12.5% of fatal cases of typhoid or other causes of enterocolitis, respectively, in women in this age group occurred during pregnancy. Czeizel and coworkers [49] found a significantly higher incidence of positive stool cultures for *E. histolytica* among women who had spontaneous abortions than among those who gave birth to living infants at term.

Amebiasis has been reported in infants as young as 3 to 6 weeks old [50–52]. In most instances, person-to-person transmission was considered likely, and the mother was the probable source of the infant's infection [50]. In one fatal case, the father had cysts of *E. histolytica* in his stool, whereas no evidence of infection with *E. histolytica* was found in the mother [51]. Perinatal infections have occurred in countries such as the United States in which the disease is rare.

Most infants reported with amebiasis in the perinatal period had illnesses with sudden, dramatic onset and were seriously ill. Bloody diarrhea was followed by development of hepatomegaly and hepatic abscess, rectal abscess, and gangrene of the appendix and colon with perforation and peritonitis. Persistent bloody diarrhea that is complicated by the development of a mass in or around the liver should lead to a thorough investigation about whether infection with *E. histolytica* could be the cause. Maternal amebiasis has also been associated with low birth weight [53].

Routine stool examinations for ova and parasites may be negative. Despite this, trophozoites of *E. histolytica* can usually be found in biopsy specimens of gastrointestinal ulcers and of the wall of the liver abscesses. The organisms cannot always be demonstrated in pus aspirated from the center of the abscess. An elevated indirect hemagglutination titer to *E. histolytica* can be helpful in diagnosing extraintestinal amebiasis. However, high titers are not usually seen until 2 weeks or more after onset of the infection in older patients and are not always present in neonates with severe extraintestinal infections [50]. Infants have been successfully treated with oral metronidazole [52]. Critically ill children should receive intravenous therapy with dehydroemetine or metronidazole.

MALARIA

It is estimated that about half a billion malaria infections resulting in 1 million deaths a year occur worldwide [54]. Although malaria is recognized as the major health problem of many countries, its impact on pregnancy and infant mortality has probably been underestimated.

THE ORGANISMS

Of the four species of malaria, *Plasmodium vivax* has the widest distribution, but *Plasmodium falciparum* tends to predominate in tropical areas. Malaria is spread to humans by the bite of anopheline mosquitoes. Of the many species of anopheline mosquito capable of becoming infected with malarial parasites, those that enter houses are more important than those preferring an outdoor habitat [55]. Mosquitoes that feed at night on human blood while the victim is asleep are the most important vectors.

After the bite of the mosquito, sporozoites are injected into the bloodstream but are cleared within one-half hour. The parasites mature in the parenchymal cells of the liver and form a mature schizont, which contains 7500 to 40,000 merozoites, depending on the species.

The release of the merozoites results in the appearance of the ring stage in erythrocytes in the peripheral blood. Within hours, the parasite assumes an ameboid form and is referred to as a trophozoite. The sexual form is called a gametocyte. In infections with *P. vivax*, *Plasmodium malariae*, and *Plasmodium ovale*, all forms are seen in the peripheral blood from early ring forms through mature schizonts and gametocytes. In infections with *P. falciparum*, usually only rings and gametocytes are found in the peripheral blood.

EPIDEMIOLOGY AND TRANSMISSION

In addition to transmission by the bite of mosquitoes, malaria can be transmitted by transfusion of blood products. In infants, this has occurred after simple transfusion and after exchange transfusion [56–59]. The onset of symptoms in neonates infected by blood products has varied from 13 to 21 days.

Malaria parasites survive in blood for weeks. Relapses can occur from *P. vivax* for up to 2 years and rarely for up to 4 years. Relapses from *P. malariae* have occasionally occurred 5 years or more after infection, but low-grade chronic parasitemia that is unassociated with symptoms is more common.

Malaria may be transmitted by reuse of syringes and needles and has spread by this route among heroin addicts. Infection in heroin addicts who become pregnant can result in congenital infections [60].

PATHOLOGY
Effect of Pregnancy on Malaria

The density and the prevalence of parasitemia are increased in pregnant women compared with women who are not pregnant but who reside in the same geographic area [61–65]. For *P. falciparum*, Campbell and colleagues [66] found a parasite density of 6896/mm³ in pregnant women and 3808/mm³ in nonpregnant women; for *P. vivax*, the parasite density was 3564/mm³ for pregnant women and 1949/mm³ for nonpregnant women. The prevalence and the density of the parasitemia decrease with increasing parity. Reinhardt and associates [62] found that the placenta was infected in 45% of primiparous women compared with 19% of women with a parity of five. This trend toward an increase in resistance to malaria with parity has been attributed by some to the increase in immunity that would be expected with an increase in age. However, the prevalence and the density of parasitemia are increased in pregnant women of all parities compared with those in nonpregnant women of the same parity [61–63]. This suggests that pregnancy, as well as age, is an important factor in determining susceptibility to malaria [61].

Infection of the Placenta

The intervillous spaces of infected placentas are packed with lymphoid macrophages, which contain phagocytosed pigment in large granules. Lymphocytes and immature polymorphonuclear leukocytes are also present in large numbers. Numerous young and mature schizonts are present. Trophozoites and gametocytes are uncommon [67,68]. Jelliffe [69] has suggested that the intensity of the infection in the placenta is related to the severity of the effect on the fetus. In general, the inflammatory response in placentas infected with *P. falciparum* is more intense than that in those infected with *P. malariae*.

Effect of Malaria on Fetal Survival and Birth Weight

Up to 40% of the world's pregnant women are exposed to malaria infection during pregnancy. In those with little or no preexisting immunity, malaria may be associated with a high risk for maternal and perinatal mortality. Fetal and perinatal loss may be as high as 60% to 70% in non-immune women with malaria [70]. In 1941, Torpin [71] reviewed 27 cases of malaria that had occurred in pregnant women during the preceding 20 years in a city in the United States. The maternal mortality rate was 4%, and the fetal mortality rate was 60%. In 1951, in Vietnam, Hung [72] found a fetal death rate of 14% among women who had infected placentas. Many of these women had had severe attacks of malaria during the first trimester and had sustained spontaneous abortions at that time.

Low birth weight is more common when the placenta is infected by parasites than when the mother is infected but the placenta is not [62,63,69,73,74]. The mean birth weight is lower if the placenta is infected with *P. falciparum* than if it is infected with *P. malariae*. Maternal anemia and placental insufficiency probably affect the fetus. It has been postulated that heavy infiltrations of parasites, lymphocytes, and macrophages interfere with the circulation of maternal blood through the placenta and result in diminished transport of oxygen and nutrients to the fetus [63]. The transport through the placenta of antibody to malaria may also be decreased when placental inflammation is severe [61].

Bruce-Chwatt [67] found that when the placenta was infected, infant weight at birth was an average of 145 g less than the weight of infants born to women with uninfected placentas. Similarly, Archibald [75] found infant weight at birth to be 170 g less, and Jelliffe [69,74] found it to be 263 g less in infants of women with infected placentas than in infants of women with uninfected placentas. In the studies performed by Bruce-Chwatt [67] and Jelliffe [69,74], 20% of the infants born to mothers with infected placentas weighed 2500 g or less, whereas 10% and 11%, respectively, of those born to mothers with uninfected placentas weighed 2500 g or less. Cannon [63] found that 37% of women who had infected placentas gave birth to infants weighing 2500 g or less, compared with 12% of those who had uninfected placentas. For primiparous women, 44% of those with infected placentas and 27% of those with uninfected placentas gave birth to infants weighing 2500 g or less [76]. Infants who have parasites demonstrable in their cord blood appear to be more severely affected than those who do not have parasitemia at the time of delivery; the mean weight gain of the mothers of these infants and the head and chest circumferences of the infants at birth are lower than expected [62]. Larkin [77] studied the prevalence of *P. falciparum* infection among 63 pregnant women and

their newborns in southern Zambia and found peripheral parasitemia in 63% (40 of 63) of mothers and 29% (19 of 65) of newborns. Infected newborns had a mean average birth weight 469 g lower than uninfected newborns but did not have a higher incidence of preterm delivery.

Using the method developed by Dubowitz and associates [78] for scoring gestational age, Reinhardt and colleagues [62] found no evidence that the incidence of infants who were small for gestational age was increased when the placenta was infected. This finding suggested that low birth weight resulted from prematurity of infants born to women with malaria.

Jelliffe [69] observed that because malaria influences birth weight, it has an important effect on infant survival in countries in which it is endemic. In 1925, Blacklock and Gordon [79] found that 35% of infants born to mothers with infected placentas died within the first 7 days of life, whereas only 5% of those born to mothers with uninfected placentas died during this period. In 1958, Cannon [63] found that the mortality rate among infants 7 days old or younger was 6.9% for those whose mothers' placentas were infected, compared with 3.4% for those whose mothers' placentas were uninfected.

The data suggesting that malaria has an important influence on birth weight and therefore on infant survival have been given further credence by the demonstration by MacGregor and Avery [76] that control of malaria in a region is followed by an increase in mean birth weight of infants born there. After DDT spraying on the island of Malaita in the British Solomon Islands, the mean birth weight for infants of mothers of all parities increased by 165 g. For infants of primiparous women, the mean birth weight increased by 252 g [76]. There was a concomitant decrease in the number of infants with birth weights of 2500 g or less; the incidence of births in this weight range fell by 8% for all births and by 20% for infants of primiparous women [76].

Steketee and colleagues [80] reviewed studies between 1985 and 2000 and summarized the population attributable risk (PAR) of malaria on anemia, low birth weight, and infant mortality in malaria endemic areas. Approximately 3% to 15% of anemia, 8% to 14% of low birth weight, 8% to 36% of preterm low birth weight, 13% to 70% of intrauterine growth retardation and low birth weight, and 3% to 8% of infant mortality were attributable to malaria. Maternal anemia was associated with low birth weight, and fetal anemia was associated with increased infant mortality. It was estimated that 75,000 to 200,000 annual infant deaths are associated with malaria infection in pregnancy [80]. Malaria therefore contributes to fetal loss, stillbirth, prematurity, and neonatal death [74,81].

Influence of Maternal Antibody on Risk of Infection

Antimalarial antibodies are transferred from the mother to the infant. The prevalence of precipitating antibody to *P. falciparum* within 24 hours of birth in Gambia was 87% in newborns and 87.5% in their mothers [82]. The prevalence of antibody in these newborns reflected the extent to which malaria had been controlled in the area in which their mothers lived. In infants born in the provinces with more malaria, 97% had antibodies to malaria, whereas 75.8% of infants born in an urban area had antibodies to malaria.

Antibodies to malaria can be detected by complement fixation, indirect hemagglutination, and indirect fluorescence. Agglutinating and precipitating antibodies are also formed [83]. Levels of precipitating antibodies and antibodies detected by indirect hemagglutination decrease from birth to 25 weeks of age [84,85]. Subsequently, as a result of postnatal acquisition of infection, endogenous antibody synthesis begins and antibody levels rise.

Bray and Anderson [61] have suggested that the amount of IgG transferred to the fetus is decreased when the placenta is heavily infested with parasites. They found that women who were pregnant during the wet season in Gambia had higher mean antibody titers to *P. falciparum* than those who were pregnant during the dry season. This pattern reflected the mothers' serologic responses to the increase in exposure to malaria during the wet season. The antibody titers of the infants born to women who were pregnant during the wet season were not higher than those of infants born to women who had been pregnant during the dry season. The infants born to women who had been pregnant during the wet season had lower mean titers of antibody to malaria at birth than infants born during other seasons. In infants 2 to 3 months old, parasitemia was found in 32% born during the wet season but in only 3% to 15% born in other seasons.

Other Factors Influencing Risk of Infection

Infants younger than 3 months have a lower than expected incidence of clinical disease, death from malaria, and parasitemia [82,84]. This has been attributed to a variety of factors, including the possibility that infants of this age are less exposed to and therefore less often bitten by mosquitoes. However, the two most important causes are probably the fact that the level of serologic immunity is high at this age and that fetal hemoglobin is present in the circulating red blood cells. Sehgal and associates [86] studied the role of humoral immunity in acquired malaria infection among newborns in Papua New Guinea. Among 104 newborns, there was a 3.8% incidence of congenital malaria and a cumulative incidence of acquired malaria of 3% at 12 weeks, 16% by 24 weeks, 24% by 36 weeks, and 38% by 48 weeks of age. Ninety-six percent of infants lost maternal antibody between 4 and 7 months, and most cases of asymptomatic malaria occurred among infants with detectable malaria antibody.

Although there were seasonal fluctuations in the overall incidence of parasitemia, Gilles [87] showed that the corrected rates were always lower for infants from birth to 2 months old than for infants 3 to 4 or 5 to 6 months old. He did not find differences in sleeping habits or in the amount of exposure to mosquitoes among infants in these age groups. In June to October, parasitemia was found in 10% of those from birth to 2 months old, 42% of those 3 to 4 months old, and 53% of those 5 to 6 months old; in May, parasitemia was found in 0% of infants from birth to 2 months old, 11% of those 3 to 4 months old, and 16% of those 5 to 6 months old. The rise

in prevalence of parasitemia corresponded with a fall in the amount of fetal hemoglobin in the red blood cells [87]. The fact that cells containing fetal hemoglobin are poor hosts for the malarial parasite had been previously suggested by Allison [88,89] as one of the reasons for the selective advantage of sickle cell anemia and sickle cell trait in areas in which malaria is endemic. Although antibody is undoubtedly important in protecting newborns from malaria, Campbell and coworkers [6] and Reinhardt and associates [66] pointed out that antibody levels in infants from birth to 2 months old might be low or absent even when the mother has had parasitemia and placental infection. The presence of fetal hemoglobin in the red cells may serve as a source of protection for infants who do not derive high levels of antibody from their mothers.

Placental infection as a risk for congenital malaria was studied in 197 infants in Cameroon. Infants born to placenta-infected mothers were more likely to develop malaria than infants born to women without placental infection [90]. Rates of infant infection and parasitemia were not related to maternally derived malaria antibodies.

CONGENITAL MALARIA
Occurrence

There has been no consistently accepted definition of congenital malaria. Some have taken the position that parasites must be demonstrable in the peripheral blood of the infant during the first day of life; others have accepted cases that were confirmed within the first 7 days of life [81]. In areas in which malaria is endemic, infants are exposed to mosquitoes and may become infected by this route at a very young age. It may be difficult to distinguish congenital cases from acquired cases. However, a sufficient number of cases of congenital malaria have been reported from countries that are free of malaria, thereby eliminating the possibility of postnatal transmission, to establish the fact that the clinical onset of disease in a congenitally infected infant can be delayed for weeks and rarely even for months [59,60,91,92]. The prevalence of parasitemia in infants younger than 3 months was 0.7% among those born during the dry season in the rural part of Gambia, compared with 11.4% among those born during the wet season, which suggests that postnatal infection is a more common event than congenital malaria [65]. It is probable that IgG antibody transmitted from the mother to the infant is an important factor in determining whether parasites that reach the fetal circulation establish an infection. The presence of passively transferred antibody in the neonate may lengthen the incubation period beyond that which would be expected in the nonimmune host.

The frequency of placental infection varies according to the prevalence of malaria in the population, the vigor of measures of control, and the availability of nonprescription antimalarial drugs. However, among Nigerian women who did not receive antimalarial agents, three studies suggested that the frequency of infection of the placenta remained relatively stable over a 30-year period. In 1948 through 1950, Bruce-Chwatt [67] found that 20% of the placentas from 228 pregnancies were infected.

One (0.4%) of the 235 neonates had the trophozoites of *P. falciparum* in a peripheral smear obtained on the fifth day of life. In 1958 Cannon [63] found that 26% of the placentas were infected; in 1970 Williams and McFarlane [93] found that 37% of the placentas were infected. None of the cord blood samples of the infants in these latter studies contained parasites. In 1964 through 1965 in Uganda, Jelliffe found that 16% of the 570 placentas were infected but only one (0.18%) infant was infected at birth [69].

The studies of Kortmann [94], Reinhardt, and colleagues [62], and Schwetz and Peel [95] suggest that parasitemia in cord blood may be more common than had been previously believed and that the presence of parasites does not necessarily indicate that the infant will become infected. Reinhardt and colleagues [62] found 33% of 198 placentas to be infected. Thick smears of the cord blood were positive for 21.7% of the 198 infants and 55% of the infants of mothers who had had parasitemia during the pregnancy. Thin smears were negative for all 198 infants. Kortmann [94] was able to demonstrate parasites in 19.7% of the placentas of 1009 women but in only 3.8% of cord blood from their infants. Eleven infants who had parasites in their cord blood also had peripheral smears performed; parasites were demonstrable in the peripheral blood of only two (18%). Lehner and associates [94] found a 14.6% incidence of cord parasitemia and a 7.7% incidence of peripheral parasitemia among 48 newborns in Papua New Guinea. Whereas all maternal and cord samples had malaria antibodies, low levels of cord malaria antibody were found to correlate with cord parasitemia. Schwetz and Peel [96] demonstrated parasites in 6% of cord blood samples and 3.6% of peripheral blood samples of infants born to mothers in Central Africa. Because the rate of infection of the placenta was 74%, this study demonstrates that the placenta, although frequently infected, serves as a relatively effective barrier and that parasites infrequently reach the fetus. The relative importance of transplacental infection or transmission by transfer from mother to infant during labor as mechanisms by which the infant acquires malaria remains uncertain [95].

Despite massive involvement of the placenta, it is generally agreed that clinically apparent congenital infections are rare in areas in which malaria is endemic and levels of maternal immunity are high. Covell [82] reviewed cases of congenital malaria that had been reported up to 1950 and estimated the incidence at 16 (0.3%) infections per 5324 live births. This rate pertained to areas of the world in which malaria was endemic. For women having an overt attack of malaria during pregnancy, the rate of congenital infection was higher and was estimated to be 1% to 4% [82]. Congenital malaria is more common among infants of women who have clinical attacks of malaria during pregnancy than in those with chronic subclinical infections; however, congenital malaria may occur in infants of mothers who are asymptomatic throughout their pregnancies [81,92,97]. Often, parasitemia is not demonstrable in the mother; splenomegaly occurs frequently [72]. Congenital malaria is more common in infants of women who have immigrated to areas in which malaria is endemic than in women who have been raised to maturity

in such areas because their levels of immunity are lower than those of the native population. Conversely, congenital malaria is also more common among women who immigrate from areas in which malaria is endemic to areas that are free of malaria. Loss of immunity results from lack of frequent exposure. Although rare, congenital malaria may also occur as a result of maternal infection by chloroquine-resistant *P. falciparum*. A number of reported cases of chloroquine-resistant congenital malaria in Africa and Indonesia responded to treatment with intravenous quinine [98–100].

Clinical Presentation

Cases of congenital malaria have been identified in countries in which malaria is endemic and in countries in which it is not, including Great Britain and the United States. Most infants with congenital malaria have had the onset of the first sign or symptom when 10 to 28 days old [59,101,102]. However, onsets occurring as early as 8 hours and as late as 8 weeks of age have been reported [81,91,92,103–106]. Keitel and coworkers [60] described a case of malaria in a 15-month-old child who had been separated from her mother when 6 weeks old but who was breast-fed during this 6-week period. The infection was caused by *P. malariae*. The source of the mother's infection was probably contaminated needles and syringes used to inject heroin. The infant must have derived the infection from her mother because she had always lived in an area that was free of malaria. Hulbert [102] reviewed the 49 cases of congenital malaria reported in the United States since 1950 and found that the mean age at onset of symptoms was 5.5 weeks (range, 0 to 60 weeks) and that 96% of these children had signs or symptoms when 2 to 8 weeks old. There was no association found between age of symptom onset and *Plasmodium* species.

Most cases of congenital infection have occurred in infants of mothers who had overt attacks of malaria during pregnancy. However, Harvey and associates [92] and McQuay and colleagues [104] reported cases of congenital infection with *P. malariae* in which the mother had lived in an area that was free of malaria for 3 years or more. In these cases, it is likely that the mothers had had onset of their infection many years before their move from an endemic area.

The most common clinical findings in cases of congenital malaria are fever, anemia, and splenomegaly, which occur in more than 80% of cases [59,107]. The anemia, which may be accompanied by pallor, is associated with a reticulocytosis in about one half of the cases. Jaundice and hyperbilirubinemia are found in about one third of the cases. The direct or the indirect bilirubin level may be elevated, depending on whether liver dysfunction or hemolysis is the most important process in an individual case [59]. Hepatomegaly may occur but is less common than splenomegaly. Nonspecific findings include failure to thrive, poor feeding, regurgitation, and loose stools. In developing countries, when malaria occurs during the first few months of life, it is frequently complicated by other illness, such as pneumonia, septicemia, and diarrhea [105].

Of the 107 cases of congenital malaria summarized by Covell [82], 40% were caused by *P. falciparum*, 32% were caused by *P. vivax*, and 1.9% were caused by *P. malariae*. The clinical findings of congenital malaria are not distinguishable from the signs and symptoms of malaria that has been acquired by the bite of a mosquito. IgM antibody to *P. falciparum* was found in the cord blood of one infant [103]. The mother had probably had her first attack of malaria during that pregnancy and had high fever and parasitemia at delivery. Reinhardt and colleagues [62] found that the total IgM levels in the cord blood of infants of infected mothers were similar to those of infants of uninfected mothers. Although fever and parasitemia may occur within 24 hours of birth, hepatosplenomegaly and anemia at birth as a result of a chronic intrauterine infection have not been described. Normal red blood cells can cross from the maternal to the fetal circulation [62]. If parasitized cells cross, however, they must usually be destroyed by the immune defenses of the fetus and by the maternal antimalarial antibodies that have passed transplacentally.

Treatment

Chloroquine is the drug of choice for sensitive strains of *P. falciparum* and for *P. malariae*. For these infections, chloroquine phosphate should be administered orally in an initial dose of 10 mg/kg of chloroquine base (maximum, 600 mg of base), followed in 6 hours by a dose of 5 mg/kg of chloroquine base (maximum, 300 mg of base). Subsequent doses of 5 mg/kg of chloroquine base should be given 24 and 48 hours after the first dose (maximum, 300 mg of base). Parenteral therapy consists of quinidine gluconate at a dose of 10 mg/kg as a loading dose (maximum, 600 mg) in normal saline given over 1 to 2 hours and then 0.02 mg/kg per minute until oral therapy can be given. Infections with *P. vivax* may be treated with chloroquine alone because sporozoite forms are not transmitted, and there is no exoerythrocytic phase in congenital infections; administration of primaquine is unnecessary. The treatment of transfusion-acquired infections is the same as that for congenital infections because there is no exoerythrocytic phase in these infections.

In serious infections in infants of mothers who may have been exposed to chloroquine-resistant strains of *P. falciparum*, alternate therapy should be considered. In adults, combinations of quinine, pyrimethamine, and a sulfonamide or quinine and tetracycline have been used with success [108]. Intravenous quinidine in combination with exchange transfusion has been used in a severe case of maternal *P. falciparum* malaria [109]. Intravenous quinidine or the combination of quinine and trimethoprim-sulfamethoxazole has been suggested for treatment of infants with resistant *P. falciparum* infection [110]. Intravenous quinine is no longer available in the United States, but in adults, oral quinine may be useful in less severe cases of chloroquine-resistant *P. falciparum*. Mefloquine is an oral antimalarial effective against most *P. falciparum* strains. Recommended therapy for *P. falciparum* infection in areas with known chloroquine resistance is variable, depending on ability to appropriately diagnose resistant *P. falciparum*, the percentage of parasitemia, signs of

organ involvement (especially of the central nervous system), and other systemic manifestations of malaria. Severe malaria may require intensive care, and exchange transfusion may be necessary if the degree of parasitemia is greater than 10%. Sequential smears should be monitored to ensure adequacy of therapy. The treatment regimen of choice is quinine sulfate given as 25 mg/kg (maximum dose, 2000 mg) in three doses for 3 to 7 days in addition to tetracycline given as 5 mg/kg four times each day for 7 days (maximum individual dose, 250 mg). The risk of dental staining in children younger than 8 years of age must be weighed against the risks of malaria-related morbidity and mortality. Pyrimethamine-sulfadoxine and mefloquine are not licensed for use in infants and pregnant women by the U.S. Food and Drug Administration; data regarding use of mefloquine during pregnancy do not indicate a risk of adverse outcomes during pregnancy. Inadvertent use of mefloquine during the first trimester of pregnancy should be reported to the Centers for Disease Control and Prevention Malaria Center (phone: 770-488-7760). Current recommendations regarding treatment can also be obtained from the Malaria Branch, Centers for Disease Control and Prevention, Atlanta. Recent clinical trials using an artemisinin combination treatment compared with intravenous quinine in Asian adults have demonstrated improved outcomes; trials among African populations are underway but consideration for use among pregnant women have been hampered by safety concerns in animal studies [54].

Prevention

Because malaria chemoprophylaxis may not be 100% effective, decreasing or eliminating exposure to mosquitoes is an important strategy for preventing malaria during pregnancy. Exposure to mosquitoes should be avoided by use of mosquito netting around beds, wire mesh screening on windows, insecticides, and mosquito repellants.

Although the possible toxicity of administering prophylactic antimalarial agents to women during pregnancy has been much discussed, controlled trials have shown that there is little risk and much to gain from such a practice. Treatment only for identified cases of maternal malaria, rather than the administration of malaria prophylaxis, failed to reduce the incidence of malaria-related low birth weight because only 12 of 65 women who had plasmodial pigmentation of the placenta had symptoms leading to an antenatal diagnosis of malaria [98–100,111]. Morley and associates [112] showed that administration of a prophylactic monthly dose of 50 mg of pyrimethamine during pregnancy resulted in improved maternal weight gain and in an increase in the mean birth weight of 157 g compared with administration of antimalarial drugs only for febrile episodes. Pyrimethamine prophylaxis is avoided in pregnant women because of concern that this dihydrofolate reductase inhibitor may cause abnormalities by interference with folic acid metabolism. Congenital defects have occurred in the offspring of animals ingesting pyrimethamine during pregnancy [113]. One possible case of pyrimethamine teratogenicity in a human fetus has been described [114], and evidence of embryo resorption has been documented in pregnant Wistar rats given sulfadoxine-pyrimethamine [115].

A retrospective review of 1627 reports of women exposed to mefloquine before or during pregnancy revealed a 4% prevalence of congenital malformations among infants of these women, reportedly similar to that observed in the general population [116]. A second report demonstrated a high rate of spontaneous abortions, but not congenital malformations, among 72 female U.S. soldiers who inadvertently received mefloquine during pregnancy [117]. Sufficient data do not exist to recommend the use of mefloquine in pregnant women, although its use in these women may be considered when exposure to chloroquine-resistant *P. falciparum* is unavoidable. The dose is 250 mg of the salt taken orally once each week, beginning 1 week before travel and ending 4 weeks after the last exposure. The combination of pyrimethamine and sulfadoxine for prophylaxis against chloroquine-resistant strains of *P. falciparum* is no longer recommended because the risk of Stevens-Johnson syndrome or neutropenia outweighs the potential benefit. Prophylaxis with chloroquine and proguanil is an alternative if a pregnant woman from a nonendemic area must risk exposure to resistant *P. falciparum* [118].

Chloroquine alone also has been used as prophylaxis during pregnancy and has been shown to be of benefit [119]. Gilles [64] found that parasitemia developed in more than 75% of pregnant women who received no prophylactic drug or who received folic acid but no antimalarial drugs. Sixty-three percent of these women developed anemia at 16 to 24 weeks' gestation. In contrast, only 2 (17%) of 12 pregnant women who received a dose of 600 mg of chloroquine base followed by a weekly dose of 25 mg of pyrimethamine developed parasitemia, and only one developed anemia. Although anemia may be an important cause of low birth weight, as Harrison and Ibeziako maintained [120], malaria appears to be an important cause of anemia in pregnant women [120,121].

Chloroquine and the other 4-aminoquinolines, such as amodiaquine and hydroxychloroquine, have similar activities and toxicities. The safety of administering chloroquine during pregnancy has been questioned. The usual recommendation for prophylaxis is 300 mg of chloroquine base once each week. Hart and Naunton [122] attributed the abnormal outcome of four pregnancies in a single patient to the administration of chloroquine during the pregnancies. This patient, who had systemic lupus erythematosus (SLE), took 150 to 300 mg chloroquine base daily. Two of the children who had had intrauterine exposures to chloroquine had severe cochleovestibular paresis and posterior column defects. Another had a Wilms tumor and hemihypertrophy. The fourth pregnancy ended in a spontaneous abortion at 12 weeks' gestation. As pointed out by Jelliffe [123] and Clyde [124], the dose given to this pregnant patient was three to seven times higher than the dose recommended for prophylaxis against malaria. Two other studies reported pregnancy outcomes after exposure to antimalarials. Parke [125] described 14 pregnancies among eight patients with SLE who took chloroquine or hydroxychloroquine during pregnancy. Three pregnancies ended in spontaneous abortion or neonatal death during periods of increased

SLE activity; of the remaining 11 pregnancies, 6 were normal full-term deliveries, 1 ended in stillbirth, and 4 ended in spontaneous abortion. No congenital deformities occurred. Levy and coworkers [126] reviewed the cases of 24 women who took chloroquine or hydroxychloroquine during a total of 27 pregnancies. Eleven women had SLE, three had rheumatoid arthritis, and four were taking malaria prophylaxis. There were 14 normal deliveries, 6 abortions attributed to severe underlying disease or social conditions, 3 stillbirths, and 4 spontaneous abortions. No congenital abnormalities were identified. The risk of poor outcome was higher among women with connective tissue disease, for which chloroquine and hydroxychloroquine doses are much higher than for malaria prophylaxis. Despite widespread use of weekly doses of chloroquine in pregnant women, teratogenic effects have not been confirmed in controlled trials [127].

The consequences of an attack of malaria during pregnancy are serious. Hindi and Azimi [91] described a woman who became pregnant while living in Nigeria but who stopped taking prophylactic doses of pyrimethamine at the onset of pregnancy. At 6 months' gestation, she had a febrile illness and was treated with chloroquine for 2 weeks. At 8 months' gestation, she had a second attack of malaria and was delivered of an infant who was 4 weeks premature and small for gestational age. The infant developed malaria during the first few weeks of life and was treated with chloroquine. The total exposure of this infant to chloroquine would have been less if the mother had been taking it weekly in prophylactic doses.

Women living in or returning from areas in which malaria is endemic should continue to take prophylactic antimalarial agents. Although primaquine is not known to have teratogenic effects, experience with its use during pregnancy is limited; it is therefore recommended that treatment with primaquine to eradicate the exoerythrocytic phase in *P. vivax* infections be deferred until after delivery [114,128].

Some investigators think the widespread use of prophylaxis may lower the level of maternal immunity and increase the severity of cases of malaria seen in children who are younger than 1 year. There is no evidence that administration of antimalarial drugs prophylactically to pregnant women has changed the expected incidence of infection during the first few months of life.

Because of the tremendous global burden of disease imposed by malaria infections, a key initiative in the prevention of malaria is the emphasis on development of malaria vaccines. The cloning of the *P. falciparum* receptor protein, which allows red blood cell attachment, should facilitate the development of a malarial vaccine [129,130]. Vaccine candidates are in development, but no effective vaccine will be immediately available [131–133]. Other techniques for malaria prevention include use of improved chemoprophylactic regimens and development of animal models for malaria infection in which to test vaccines and antimalarial drugs. A rhesus monkey model mimicking human infection after exposure to *Plasmodium coatneyi* has been tested with potential for use in animal studies [134]. Recommendations for malaria prophylaxis in pregnant women may be obtained from the Malaria Branch, Centers for Disease Control and Prevention, Atlanta.

SCHISTOSOMIASIS

Schistosomiasis (i.e., bilharziasis) contributes to infertility by causing sclerosis of the fallopian tubes or cervix [135]. It is estimated that 9 to 13 million women may be afflicted by genital schistosomiasis in Africa alone [136]. The placenta usually does not become infected until the third month of pregnancy or thereafter [137]. Although the frequency of placental infection is as high as 25% in endemic areas, the infestations are light and cause little histologic reaction [137,138]. In their study of the impact of placental infection on the outcome of pregnancy, Renaud and coworkers [137] concluded that there was little evidence that the size or weight of the infant was affected and that placental bilharziasis was not an important cause of intrauterine growth retardation or prematurity.

TRICHOMONAS VAGINALIS

Infection of the vagina of the pregnant woman with *Trichomonas vaginalis* is not uncommon, but no adverse effect on the fetus has been documented [139–141]. There are six reports in the literature of *T. vaginalis* recovered from a respiratory source among neonates, all with respiratory illness whose viral and bacterial cultures revealed no other pathogens, but a causal relationship was not certain [142,143]. During the first 2 weeks of life, female newborns may be particularly susceptible to infection because of the influence of maternal estrogens on the vaginal epithelium. By 3 to 6 weeks of age, the vaginal pH is no longer acid [144]. *T. vaginalis* has been found in 0% to 4.8% of sequentially studied female newborns [144–146]. Among infants younger than 3 weeks who had vaginal discharges, *T. vaginalis* was the probable cause of the discharge in 17.2% [147]. In addition to causing a vaginal discharge [148], infection of the newborn with *T. vaginalis* may aggravate candidal infections and may be associated with urinary tract infections [144]. In most infants, the white blood cells found in the urine originate from the vagina rather than from the bladder [149]. However, several reports suggest that a bacterial urinary tract infection can be present concomitantly [150,151]. In symptomatic cases, metronidazole has been used at a dosage of 500 mg twice daily or 15 mg/kg/day divided in 3 doses for 5 to 7 days [144,149,152].

TRICHINOSIS

Prenatal transmission of trichinosis from mother to infant is rare. Four larvae, however, were found in the diaphragm of a fetus by Kuitunen-Ekbaum [153]. No evidence of infection with trichinosis was found in 25 newborns studied by McNaught and Anderson [154]. Despite this, *Trichinella spiralis* has been found in the placenta, in the milk of nursing women, and in the tissue from the mammary gland [155]. In 1939, Hood and Olson [156] found *T. spiralis* in pressed muscle preparations from 4 (8.3%) of 48 infants from birth to 12 months of age. Although transplacental transmission is rare, *T. spiralis* is present in the placenta of women with acute trichinosis and can be passed to the infant by means of breast milk.

BABESIOSIS

Babesia microti is a tick-borne protozoan that infects erythrocytes and causes a malaria-like illness. Most cases in the United States have occurred in the Northeast. Raucher and colleagues [157] described a *B. microti* infection in a pregnant woman that began in the 19th week of gestation; the infant was born at term without evidence of infection. Ten neonatal cases have been reported in the literature. Of those, seven were transfusion-related, two were congenital, and one was secondary to tick transmission [158].

PNEUMOCYSTIS JIROVECI

P. jiroveci is an infectious agent with a history. In 1988, DNA analysis demonstrated that *Pneumocystis* was not a protozoan, but a fungus [159,160]. Subsequent DNA analysis has led to the change in nomenclature of *P. carinii* to *P. jiroveci*, a name chosen in honor of the parasitologist Otto Jirovec, who is credited by some with the original description of this organism [159,160]. *P. carinii* as a fungus has been defined based on molecular analysis [161,162]. Previous controversy over the classification *Pneumocystis* existed because of the difficulty in cultivating and further characterizing the biochemical nature of the organism. Questions remained until polymerase chain reaction techniques established that *P. jiroveci* was not found in lung samples from any other mammals [163]. However, genetic analysis clearly demonstrated differences between human and nonhuman *Pneumocystis* isolates [164]. This organism is covered in detail in Chapter 34: "Pneumocystis and Other Less Common Fungal Infections."

REFERENCES

[1] E. Kotcher, et al., Acquisition of intestinal parasites in newborn infants, Fed. Proc. 24 (1965) 442.
[2] A.D. Agbere, et al., Gastrointestinal and urinary parasitic infection in children at a regional hospital center in Togo: some epidemiological aspects, Med. Trop. 55 (1995) 65.
[3] J.R. Stringer, et al., A new name (*Pneumocystis jiroveci*) for Pneumocystis from humans, Emerg. Infect. Dis. 8 (2002) 891.
[4] R. Sterling, A.J.L. Guay, Invasion of the female generative tract by *Ascaris lumbricoides*, JAMA 107 (1936) 2046.
[5] C.B. Sanjeevi, S. Vivekanandan, P.R. Narayanan, Fetal response to maternal ascariasis as evidenced by anti-*Ascaris lumbricoides* IgM antibodies in the cord blood, Acta Paediatr. Scand. 80 (1991) 1134.
[6] W. Chu, et al., Neonatal ascariasis, J. Pediatr. 81 (1972) 783.
[7] L.M. Costa-Macedo, L. Rey, *Ascaris lumbricoides* in neonate: evidence of congenital transmission of intestinal nematodes, Rev. Soc. Bras. Med. Trop. 33 (1991) 371.
[8] N.S. Roberts, et al., Intestinal parasites and other infections during pregnancy in Southeast Asian refugees, J. Reprod. Med. 30 (1985) 720.
[9] A.K. Kreutner, V.E. Del Bene, M.S. Amstey, Giardiasis in pregnancy, Am. J. Obstet. Gynecol. 140 (1981) 895.
[10] A. Tellez, et al., Antibodies in mother's milk protect children against giardiasis, Scand. J. Infect. Dis. 35 (2003) 322.
[11] P. Buekens, et al., Mother-to-child transmission of Chagas' disease in North America: why don't we do more? Matern. Child Health J. 12 (3) (2008) 283–286.
[12] J.H. Edgcomb, C.M. Johnson, American trypanosomiasis (Chagas' disease), in: C.H. Binford, O.H. Connor (Eds.), Pathology of Tropical and Extraordinary Disease, vol. 1, Armed Forces Institute of Pathology, Washington, DC, 1976, pp. 244–251.
[13] A. Bittencourt, Congenital Chagas' disease, Am. J. Dis. Child. 130 (1976) 97.
[14] M.A. Miles, The epidemiology of South American trypanosomiasis—biochemical and immunological approaches and their relevance to control, Trans. R. Soc. Trop. Med. Hyg. 77 (1983) 5.
[15] P.D. Marsden, South American trypanosomiasis (Chagas' disease), Int. Rev. Trop. Med. 4 (1981) 97.

[16] C.A. Santos-Buch, American trypanosomiasis: Chagas' disease, Int. Rev. Exp. Pathol. 19 (1979) 63.

[17] V. Amato Neto, et al., Rev. Inst. Med. Trop. Sao Paulo 10 (1968) 46.

[18] A.L. Bittencourt, E. Mota, Isoenzyme characterization of *Trypanosoma cruzi* from congenital cases of Chagas' disease, Ann. Trop. Med. Parasitol. 4 (1985) 393.

[19] A.L. Bittencourt, M. Sadigursky, H.A. Barbosa, Doenca de Chagas congenita: estudo de 29 caspiatos, Rev. Inst. Med. Trop. Sao Paulo 17 (1975) 146.

[20] A. Rassi, et al., Sobre a transmissão congenita da doenca de Chagas, Rev. Goiana Med. 4 (1958) 319.

[21] M.A. Delgado, C.A. Santos Buch, Transplacental transmission and fetal parasitosis of *Trypanosoma cruzi* in outbred white Swiss mice, Am. J. Trop. Med. Hyg. 27 (1978) 1108.

[22] P.M. Cossio, et al., Chagasic cardiopathy: demonstration of a serum gamma globulin factor which reacts with endocardium and vascular structures, Circulation 49 (1974) 13.

[23] P.M. Cossio, et al., Antibodies reacting with plasma membrane of striated muscle and endothelial cells, Circulation 50 (1974) 1252.

[24] A. Szarfman, et al., Immunologic and immunopathologic studies in congenital Chagas' disease, Clin. Immunol. Immunopathol. 4 (1975) 489.

[25] A.D. Vasquez, Doctoral thesis, Universidad del los Andes, Venezuela, 1959.

[26] A. Saleme, et al., Enfermedad de Chagas-Mazza congenita en Tucuman, Arch. Argent. Pediatr. 59 (1971) 162.

[27] A.L. Bittencourt, et al., Incidence of congenital Chagas' disease in Bahia, Brazil J. Trop. Pediatr. 31 (1985) 242.

[28] J. Bekemans, et al., Maternal *Trypanosoma cruzi* infection upregulated capacity of uninfected neonate cells to produce pro- and anti-inflammatory cytokines, Infect. Immun. 68 (2000) 5430.

[29] A.P. Barousse, et al., Enfermedad de Chagas congenita en area no endemica, Medicina (B. Aires) 38 (1978) 611.

[30] S.B. Blanco, E.L. Segura, R.E. Gurtler, Control of congenital transmission of *Trypanosoma cruzi* in Argentina, Medicina (B. Aires) 59 (Suppl. 2) (1999) 138.

[31] S. Stagno, R. Hurtado, Enfermedad de Chagas congenita: studio immunologico y diagnostico mediante immunofluorescencia con anti IgM, Bol. Chil. Parasitol. 26 (1971) 20.

[32] A.L. Bittencourt, et al., Incidencia da transmissão congenita da doenca de Chagas em partos a termo, Rev. Inst. Med. Trop. Sao Paulo 16 (1974) 197.

[33] M. Rubio, B.J. Howard, Enfermedad de Chagas congenita. II. Halazgo anatomopatologico en 9 casos, Bol. Chil. Parasitol. 23 (1968) 113.

[34] E. Azogue, C. LaFuente, C. Darras, Congenital Chagas' disease in Bolivia: epidemiological aspects and pathological findings, Trans. R. Soc. Trop. Med. Hyg. 79 (1985) 176.

[35] J.E. Howard, La enfermedad de Chagas congenita, thesis. Universidad de Chile, Santiago, Chile, 1962.

[36] A.L. Bittencourt, et al., Esophageal involvement in congenital Chagas' disease, Am. J. Trop. Med. Hyg. 33 (1984) 30.

[37] A.L. Bittencourt, et al., Pneumonitis in congenital Chagas' disease: a study of ten cases, Am. J. Trop. Med. Hyg. 30 (1981) 38.

[38] R. Hoff, et al., Congenital Chagas' disease in an urban population: investigation of infected twins, Trans. R. Soc. Trop. Med. Hyg. 72 (1978) 247.

[39] M. Virreira, et al., Amniotic fluid is not useful for diagnosis of congenital *Trypanosoma cruzi* infection, Am. J. Trop. Med. Hyg. 75 (6) (2006) 1082–1084.

[40] H. Feilij, L. Muller, S.M. Gonzalez Cappa, Direct micromethod for diagnosis of acute and congenital Chagas' disease, J. Clin. Microbiol. 18 (1983) 327.

[41] M.B. Reyes, et al., Fetal IgG specificities against *Trypanosoma cruzi* antigens in infected newborns, Proc. Natl. Acad. Sci. U. S. A. 87 (1990) 2846.

[42] S.B. Blanco, et al., Congenital transmission of *Trypanosoma cruzi*: an operational outline for detecting and treating infected infants in north-western Argentina, Trop. Med. Int. Health 5 (2000) 293.

[43] A.L. Bittencourt, M.C. Gomes, Gestacoes sucessivas de uma paciente chagasica com ocorrencia de casos de transmissao congenita da doenca, Rev. Med. Bahia 67 (1967) 166.

[44] P.R. Moya, et al., Tratamiento de la enfermedad de Chagas con Nifurtimox durante los primeros meses de vida, Medicina (B Aires) 45 (1985) 553.

[45] S. Lingam, et al., Congenital trypanosomiasis in a child born in London, Dev. Med. Child Neurol. 27 (1985) 664.

[46] M.C. Reinhardt, C.L. Macleod, Parasitic Infections in Pregnancy and the Newborn, Oxford University Press, New York, 1988.

[47] P.J. Armon, Amoebiasis in pregnancy and the puerperium, Br. J. Obstet. Gynaecol. 85 (1978) 264.

[48] A.A. Abioye, Fatal amoebic colitis in pregnancy and puerperium: a new clinico-pathological entity, J. Trop. Med. Hyg. 76 (1973) 97.

[49] E. Czeizel, et al., Possible relation between fetal death and *E. histolytica* infection of the mother, Am. J. Obstet. Gynecol. 96 (1966) 264.

[50] A.C. Dykes, et al., Extraintestinal amebiasis in infancy: report of three patients and epidemiologic investigations of their families, Pediatrics 65 (1980) 799.

[51] T. Botman, P.J. Ruys, Amoebic appendicitis in a newborn infant, Trop. Geogr. Med. 15 (1963) 221.

[52] J.H.M. Axton, Amoebic proctocolitis and liver abscess in a neonate, S. Afr. Med. J. 46 (1972) 258.

[53] M.L. Dreyfuss, et al., Determinants of low birth weight among HIV-infected pregnant women in Tanzania, Am. J. Clin. Nutr. 74 (2001) 814.

[54] D.A. Milner Jr., et al., Severe malaria in children and pregnancy: an update and perspective, Trends Parasitol. 24 (12) (2008) 590–595.

[55] M.D. Young, Malaria, in: G.W. Hunter III, J.C. Schwartzwelder, F. Clyde (Eds.), Tropical Medicine, Philadelphia, WB Saunders, 1976, pp. 353–396.

[56] I.A. Shulman, et al., Neonatal exchange transfusions complicated by transfusion-induced malaria, Pediatrics 73 (1984) 330.

[57] D.A. Piccoli, S. Perlman, M. Ephros, Transfusion-acquired *Plasmodium malariae* infection in two premature infants, Pediatrics 72 (1983) 560.

[58] S. Sinclair, S.K. Mittal, M. Singh, Neonatal transfusion malaria, Indian Pediatr. 8 (1971) 219.

[59] S. Ghosh, et al., Clinical and hematologic peculiarities of malaria in infancy, Clin. Pediatr. (Phila) 17 (1978) 369.

[60] H.G. Keitel, et al., Nephrotic syndrome in congenital quartan malaria, JAMA 161 (1956) 521.

[61] R.S. Bray, M.J. Anderson, Falciparum malaria and pregnancy, Trans. R. Soc. Trop. Med. Hyg. 73 (1979) 427.

[62] M.C. Reinhardt, et al., Malaria at delivery in Abidjan, Helv. Paediatr. Acta 33 (Suppl. 41) (1978) 65.

[63] D.S.H. Cannon, Malaria and prematurity in the western region of Nigeria, BMJ 2 (1958) 877.

[64] H.M. Gilles, et al., Malaria, anaemia and pregnancy, Ann. Trop. Med. Parasitol. 63 (1969) 245.

[65] I. McGregor, Epidemiology, malaria and pregnancy, Am. J. Trop. Med. Hyg. 33 (1984) 517.

[66] C.C. Campbell, J.M. Martinez, W.E. Collins, Seroepidemiological studies of malaria in pregnant women and newborns from coastal El Salvador, Am. J. Trop. Med. Hyg. 29 (1980) 151.

[67] L.J. Bruce-Chwatt, Malaria in African infants and children in southern Nigeria, Ann. Trop. Med. Parasitol. 46 (1952) 173.

[68] T. Taufa, Malaria and pregnancy, P. N. G. Med. J. 21 (1978) 197.

[69] E.F.P. Jelliffe, Low birth-weight and malarial infection of the placenta, Bull. World Health Organ. 38 (1968) 69.

[70] C.E. Shulman, E.K. Dorman, Importance and prevention of malaria in pregnancy, Trans. R. Soc. Trop. Med. Hyg. 97 (2003) 30.

[71] R. Torpin, Malaria complicating pregnancy with a report of 27 cases, Am. J. Obstet. Gynecol. 41 (1941) 882.

[72] L.V. Hung, Paludisive at grossesse a Saigon, Rev. Palud. Med. Trop. 83 (1951) 75.

[73] A.J. Spita, Malaria infection of the placenta and its influence on the incidence of prematurity in eastern Nigeria, Bull. World Health Organ. 21 (1959) 242.

[74] E.F.P. Jelliffe, Placental malaria and foetal growth, in: Nutrition and Infection: CIBA Foundation Study Group No 31, xxx, J&A Churchill, 1967, pp. 18–40.

[75] H.M. Archibald, The influence of malarial infection of the placenta on the incidence of prematurity, Bull. World Health Organ. 15 (1956) 842.

[76] J.D. MacGregor, J.G. Avery, Malaria transmission and fetal growth, BMJ 3 (1974) 433.

[77] G.L. Larkin, P.E. Thuma, Congenital malaria in a hyperendemic area, Am. J. Trop. Med. Hyg. 45 (1991) 587.

[78] L.M.S. Dubowitz, V. Dubowitz, G. Goldberg, Clinical assessment of gestational age in the newborn infant, J. Pediatr. 77 (1970) 1.

[79] D.B. Blacklock, R.M. Gordon, Malaria parasites in the placental blood, Ann. Trop. Med. Parasitol. 19 (1925) 37.

[80] R.W. Steketee, et al., The burden of malaria in pregnancy in malaria-endemic areas, Am. J. Trop. Med. Hyg. 64 (1-2 Suppl) (2001) 28–35.

[81] R. Meno, Pregnancy and malaria, Med. J. Malaysia. 27 (1972) 115.

[82] G. Covell, Congenital malaria, Trop. Dis. Bull. 47 (1950) 1147.

[83] I.A. McGregor, Immunity to plasmodial infections; consideration of factors relevant to malaria in man, Int. Rev. Trop. Med. 4 (1971) 1.

[84] L. Molineaux, et al., Longitudinal serological study of malaria in infants in the West African savanna, Bull. World Health Organ. 56 (1978) 573.

[85] H.M. Mathews, H.O. Lobel, J.G. Breman, Malarial antibodies measured by the indirect hemagglutination test in West African children, Am. J. Trop. Med. Hyg. 25 (1976) 217.

[86] V.M. Sehgal, W.A. Siddiqui, M.P. Alpers, A seroepidemiological study to evaluate the role of passive maternal immunity to malaria in infants, Trans. R. Soc. Trop. Med. Hyg. 83 (1989) 105–106.

[87] H.M. Gilles, The development of malarial infection in breast-fed Gambian infants, Ann. Trop. Med. Parasitol. 51 (1957) 58.

[88] A.C. Allison, Genetic factors in resistance to malaria, Ann. N. Y. Acad. Sci. 91 (1961) 710.

[89] A.C. Allison, Malaria in carriers of the sickle cell trait and in newborn children, Exp. Parasitol. 6 (1957) 418.

[90] J.Y. Le Hesran, et al., Maternal placental infection with *Plasmodium falciparum* and malaria morbidity during the first two years of life, Am. J. Epidemiol. 146 (1997) 826.

[91] R.D. Hindi, P.H. Azimi, Congenital malaria due to *Plasmodium falciparum*, Pediatrics 66 (1980) 977.

[92] B. Harvey, J.S. Remington, A.J. Sulzer, IgM malaria antibodies in a case of congenital malaria in the United States, Lancet 1 (1969) 333.

[93] A.I.O. Williams, H. McFarlane, Immunoglobulin levels, malarial antibody titres and placental parasitaemia in Nigerian mothers and neonates, Afr. J. Med. Sci. 1 (1970) 369.

[94] H.F. Kortmann, Malaria and pregnancy, thesis. Manuel Drukkrig Elinkwijk, Utrecht, Netherlands, 1972.

[95] J. Schwetz, M. Peel, Congenital malaria and placental infections amongst the Negroes of Central Africa, Trans. R. Soc. Trop. Med. Hyg. 28 (1934) 167.

[96] P.J. Lehner, C.J. Andrews, Congenital malaria in Papua New Guinea, Trans. R. Soc. Trop. Med. Hyg. 82 (1988) 822.

[97] H.D. Davies, et al., Congenital malaria in infants of asymptomatic women, Can. Med. Assoc. J. 146 (1992) 1755.

[98] R.T.H. Dianto, Congenital falciparum malaria with chloroquine resistance type II, Paediatr. Indones. 29 (1989) 237.

[99] D. Chabasse, et al., Chloroquine-resistant *Plasmodium falciparum* in Mali revealed by congenital malaria, Trans. R. Soc. Trop. Med. Hyg. 82 (1988) 547.

[100] A.I. Airede, Congenital malaria with chloroquine resistance, Ann. Trop. Paediatr. 11 (1991) 267.

[101] Centers for Disease Control and Prevention, Congenital malaria infection in an infant born to a Kampuchean refugee, MMWR Morb. Mortal. Wkly Rep. 29 (1980) 3.

[102] T.V. Hulbert, Congenital malaria in the United States: report of a case and review, Clin. Infect. Dis. 14 (1992) 922.

[103] V. Thomas, C. Wing Chit, A case of congenital malaria in Malaysia with IgM malaria antibodies, Trans. R. Soc. Trop. Med. Hyg. 74 (1980) 73.

[104] R.M. McQuay, et al., Congenital malaria in Chicago: a case report and a review of published reports (U.S.A.), Am. J. Trop. Med. 16 (1967) 258.

[105] P.S. Dhatt, et al., A clinicopathological study of malaria in early infancy, Indian Pediatr. 26 (1979) 331.

[106] W.A. Olowu, S.E. Torimiro, Congenital malaria in 8 hours old newborn: case report, Niger. J. Med. 11 (2002) 81.

[107] D. Subramanian, K.J. Moise, A.C. White, Imported malaria in pregnancy: report of four cases and review of management, Clin. Infect. Dis. 15 (1992) 408.

[108] D.M. Zarou, H.C. Lichtman, L.M. Hellman, The transmission of chromium 51 tagged maternal erythrocytes from mother to fetus, Am. J. Obstet. Gynecol. 88 (1964) 565.

[109] L.H. Malaria, in: P.D. Hoeprich (Ed.), Infection Diseases: A Modern Treatise of Infectious Processes, 2nd edition, Harper & Row, Hagerstown, MD, 1977, pp. 1075–1087.

[110] R.D. Wong, et al., Treatment of severe falciparum malaria during pregnancy with quinidine and exchange transfusion, Am. J. Med. 92 (1992) 561.

[111] T.C. Quinn, et al., Congenital malaria: a report of four cases and a review, J. Pediatr. 101 (1982) 229.

[112] M. Watkinson, D.I. Rushton, Plasmodial pigmentation of placenta and outcome of pregnancy in West African mothers, BMJ 287 (1983) 251.

[113] D. Morley, M. Woodland, W.F.J. Cuthbertson, Controlled trial of pyrimethamine in pregnant women in an African village, BMJ 1 (1964) 667.

[114] Centers for Disease Control and Prevention, Chemoprophylaxis of malaria, MMWR Morb. Mortal. Wkly Rep. 27 (Suppl) (1978) 81.

[115] J.P. Harpy, Y. Darbois, G. Lefebvre, Teratogenicity of pyrimethamine, Lancet 2 (1983) 399.

[116] E.O. Uche-Nwachi, Effect of intramuscular sulfadoxine-pyrimethamine on pregnant Wistar rats, Anat. Rec. 250 (1998) 426.

[117] B. Vanhauwere, H. Maradi, L. Kerr, Post-marketing surveillance of prophylactic mefloquine (Lariam) use in pregnancy, Am. J. Trop. Med. Hyg. 58 (1998) 17–21.

[118] B.L. Smoak, et al., The effects of inadvertent exposure of mefloquine chemoprophylaxis on pregnancy outcomes and infants of US Army servicewomen, J. Infect. Dis. 176 (1997) 831.

[119] C.J. Ellis, Antiparasitic agents in pregnancy, Clin. Obstet. Gynecol. 13 (1986) 269.

[120] K.A. Harrison, P.A. Ibeziako, Maternal anaemia and fetal birthweight, J. Obstet. Gynaecol. Br. Commonw. 80 (1973) 798.

[121] F.D. Schofield, A.D. Parkinson, A. Kelly, Changes in hemoglobin values and hepatosplenomegaly produced by control of holoendemic malaria, BMJ 1 (1964) 587.

[122] C.W. Hart, R.F. Naunton, The ototoxicity of chloroquine phosphate, Arch. Otolaryngol. 80 (1964) 407.

[123] E.F.P. Jelliffe, Letter to the editor, J. Pediatr. 88 (1976) 362.

[124] D.F. Clyde, Letter to the editor, J. Pediatr. 88 (1976) 362.

[125] A. Parke, Antimalarial drugs and pregnancy, Am. J. Med. 85 (Suppl. 4A) (1988) 30.

[126] M. Levy, et al., Pregnancy outcome following first trimester exposure to chloroquine, Am. J. Perinatol. 8 (1991) 174.

[127] M.S. Wolfe, J.F. Cordero, Safety of chloroquine in chemosuppression of malaria during pregnancy, BMJ 290 (1985) 1466.

[128] M. Katz, Treatment of protozoan infections: malaria, Pediatr. Infect. Dis. 2 (1983) 475.

[129] J.B. Dame, et al., Structure of the gene and coding the immunodominant surface antigen of the sporozoite of the human malarial parasite, Science 225 (1984) 593.

[130] V. Enea, et al., DNA cloning of *Plasmodium falciparum* circumsporozoite gene: amino acid sequence of repetitive epitope, Science 225 (1984) 628.

[131] I.S. Soares, M.M. Rodrigues, Malaria vaccine: roadblocks and possible solutions, Braz. J. Med. Biol. Res. 31 (1998) 317.

[132] P.M. Graves, Comparison of the cost-effectiveness of vaccines and insecticide impregnation of mosquito nets for the prevention of malaria, Ann. Trop. Med. Parasitol. 92 (1996) 399.

[133] V.S. Moorthy, M.F. Good, A.V. Hill, Malaria vaccine developments, Lancet 363 (2004) 150.

[134] B.B. Davison, et al., *Plasmodium coatneyi* in the rhesus monkey (*Macaca mulatta*) as a model of malaria in pregnancy, Am. J. Trop. Med. Hyg. 59 (1998) 189.

[135] C.H.W. Bullough, Infertility and bilharziasis of the female genital tract, Br. J. Obstet. Gynaecol. 83 (1976) 819.

[136] G. Poggensee, et al., Schistosomiasis of the lower reproductive tract without egg excretion in urine, Am. J. Trop. Med. Hyg. 59 (1998) 782.

[137] R. Renaud, et al., Placental bilharziasis, Int. J. Gynaecol. Obstet. 10 (1972) 25.

[138] A.L. Bittencourt, et al., Placental involvement in *Schistosomiasis mansoni*, Am. J. Trop. Med. Hyg. 29 (1980) 571.

[139] S.M. Ross, A. Van Middelkoop, Trichomonas infection in pregnancy–does it affect perinatal outcome? S. Afr. Med. J. 63 (1983) 566.

[140] R.T. Franjola, et al., *Trichomonas vaginalis* en embarazadas y en recien nacidos, Rev. Med. Chil. 117 (1989) 142.

[141] J.E. Carter, K.C. Whithaus, Neonatal respiratory tract involvement by *Trichomonas vaginalis*: a case report and review of the literature, Am. J. Trop. Med. Hyg. 78 (1) (2008) 17–19.

[142] L.C. McLaren, et al., Isolation of *Trichomonas vaginalis* from the respiratory tract of infants with respiratory disease, Pediatrics 71 (1983) 888.

[143] I. Hiemstra, F. Van Bel, H.M. Berger, Can *Trichomonas vaginalis* cause pneumonia in newborn babies? BMJ 289 (1984) 355.

[144] F.L. Al-Salihi, J.P. Curran, J.S. Wang, Neonatal *Trichomonas vaginalis*: report of three cases and review of the literature, Pediatrics 53 (1974) 196.

[145] L.G. Feo, The incidence of *Trichomonas vaginalis* in the various age groups, Am. J. Trop. Med. 5 (1956) 786.

[146] R.E. Trussell, et al., Vaginal trichomoniasis: complement fixation, puerperal morbidity and early infection of newborn infants, Am. J. Obstet. Gynecol. 44 (1942) 292.

[147] A. Komorowska, A. Kurnatowska, J. Liniecka, Occurrence of Trichomonas vaginalis (Donne) in girls in relation to hygiene conditions, Wiad. Parazytol. 8 (1962) 247.

[148] I.S. Danesh, J.M. Stephen, J. Gorbach, Neonatal *Trichomonas vaginalis* infection, J. Emerg. Med. 13 (1995) 1.

[149] J.M. Littlewood, H.G. Kohler, Urinary tract infection by *Trichomonas vaginalis* in a newborn baby, Arch. Dis. Child. 41 (1966) 693.

[150] R.J. Postlethwaite, *Trichomonas vaginalis* and *Escherichia coli* urinary infection in a newborn infant, Clin. Pediatr. (Phila) 14 (1975) 866.

[151] P. Dagenais-Perusse, et al., Vaginite á trichomonas du nourrison, Union Med. Can. 93 (1964) 1228.

[152] I.A. Crowther, *Trichomonas vaginitis* in infancy, Lancet 1 (1962) 1074.

[153] E. Kuitunen-Ekbaum, The incidence of trichinosis in humans in Toronto: findings in 420 autopsies, Can. Public Health J. 32 (1941) 569.

[154] J.B. McNaught, E.V. Anderson, The incidence of trichinosis in San Francisco, JAMA 107 (1936) 1446.

[155] B.F. Salzer, A study of an epidemic of 14 cases of trichinosis with cures by serum therapy, JAMA 67 (1916) 579.

[156] M. Hood, S.W. Olson, Trichinosis in the Chicago area, Am. J. Hyg. 29 (1939) 51.

[157] H.S. Raucher, H. Jaffin, J.L. Glass, Babesiosis in pregnancy, Obstet. Gynecol. 63 (1984) 75.

[158] L.M. Fox, et al., Neonatal babesiosis: case report and review of the literature, Pediatr. Infect. Dis. J. 25 (2) (2006) 169–173.

[159] W.T. Hughes, *Pneumocystis carinii* vs. *Pneumocystis jiroveci*: another misnomer (response to Stringer et al), Emerg. Infect. Dis. 9 (2003) 276.

[160] A.E. Wakefield, et al., Molecular probes for the detection of *Pneumocystis carinii*, Trans. R. Soc. Trop. Med. Hyg. 84 (Suppl 1) (1990) 17–18.

[161] J. Li, T. Edlind, Phylogeny of *Pneumocystis carinii* based on ß-tubulin sequence, J. Eukaryotic. Microbiol. 41 (1994) 97S.

[162] E. Mazars, et al., Polymorphism of the thymidylate synthase gene of *Pneumocystis carinii* from different host species, J. Eukaryot. Microbiol. 42 (1995) 26.

[163] L. Ma, J.A. Kovacs, Expression and characterization of recombinant human-derived *Pneumocystis carinii* dihydrofolate reductase, Antimicrob. Agents Chemother. 44 (2000) 3092.

[164] S. Banerji, et al., Analysis of genetic diversity at the arom locus in isolates of *Pneumocystis carinii*, J. Eukaryot. Microbiol. 42 (1995) 675.

CHAPTER OUTLINE

Introduction 1055
Epidemiology and Transmission 1055
Microbiology 1056
Pathogenesis 1058
Pathology 1060
Clinical Manifestations 1060
    Oropharyngeal Candidiasis 1060
    Diaper Dermatitis 1060
    Congenital Candidiasis 1062

Invasive Fungal Dermatitis 1062
    Catheter-Related Candidal Infections 1062
Candidemia and Disseminated Candidiasis 1063
Diagnosis 1065
Treatment 1067
    Antifungal Agents 1068
Prevention 1072
    Fluconazole Prophylaxis 1072

INTRODUCTION

Candida species are important pathogens in the neonate. Over the past 2 decades, there has been a significant increase in the incidence of systemic candidiasis in neonatal intensive care (NICU) patients, particularly among the very low birth weight (VLBW; birth weight ≤1500 g) infants [1–5]. Infections range from superficial colonization to widely disseminated, life-threatening disease. Unfortunately, the most dramatic rise has been in the incidence of invasive or systemic candidiasis. With improvements in technology, more aggressive approaches to the treatment of VLBW infants have become the standard of care. Concomitantly, there has been an increase in risk factors for neonates to develop candidemia, most notably the prolonged use of indwelling intravascular catheters and multiple courses of broad-spectrum antimicrobial agents [6,7].

Candida albicans remains the most frequently isolated yeast species among infected neonates; however, the incidence of infection with other species, particularly *Candida parapsilosis* and *Candida glabrata*, has increased exponentially over the past 10 years [8–12]. The importance of *Candida* as a pathogen in VLBW infants is reflected by a mortality rate approaching 30% in this fragile group of immunocompromised patients, even among those who receive appropriate antifungal therapy, and a significant accompanying morbidity among survivors [5,13,14].

EPIDEMIOLOGY AND TRANSMISSION

Infections with *Candida* species afflict immunocompromised hosts, diabetics, trauma patients, postoperative patients (particularly after gastrointestinal procedures), and neonates; and are most often nosocomially acquired [1,15,16]. The SENTRY Antimicrobial Surveillance Program, monitoring bloodstream infections (BSI) due to both *Candida* spp. and bacteria among all patients in participating hospitals, reports *Candida* species as the fourth most common nosocomial BSI overall, with *C. albicans*

the most common single pathogen [15]. In neonates, the numbers are equally striking. Approximately 1.4% of early-onset neonatal infections result from *Candida* species, for late-onset sepsis the incidence varies from 2.6% to 16.7% among the very low birth weight infants (VLBW, ≤ 1500 g) and up to 20% for the extremely low birth weight infants (ELBW, ≤ 1000 g) [5,6,17–19]. Among hospitals participating in the Neonatal Institute of Child Health and Human Development (NICHD) Neonatal Research Network, *C. albicans* was the third most frequent single organism isolated among all pathogens responsible for late onset sepsis [20].

Although *C. albicans* remains the leading cause of disseminated fungal infection among hospitalized patients, the isolation of other yeast species, including *C. glabrata, C. parapsilosis, Candida tropicalis, Candida krusei, Candida lusitaniae, Candida dubliniensis,* and even *Saccharomyces cerevisiae,* is occurring more frequently [4,9,15,21]. Table 33–1 displays the relative distribution of *Candida* species recovered from the bloodstream of all NICU patients in the National Nosocomial Infection Surveillance (NNIS) system compared with the overall population reported in the SENTRY program [9,15]. Among neonates *C. albicans* and *C. parapsilosis* remain the predominant species compared with adults in whom the predominant species isolated are *C. albicans, C. parapsilosis,* and *C. glabrata,* each of which accounts for approximately 15% of yeast infections [12]. Historically, *C. albicans* has been considered the most virulent species. A retrospective study of neonatal candidiasis in the 1980s revealed a 24% mortality rate among infants infected with *C. albicans,* but no deaths among those infected with *C. parapsilosis* [11]. Later case series have shown an increase in infections with non-*Candida albicans Candida* (NCAC) species and mortality for neonates infected with *C. glabrata* and *C. parapsilosis* equivalent to that for *C. albicans* infections [8,22–24]. Although *C. albicans* may be responsible for more infections than NCAC species, almost all *Candida* species have been implicated in disease and any candidal infection in the neonate can be life threatening.

TABLE 33–1 Frequency of Isolation of *Candida* Species Causing Candidemia Sepsis

	Percent of Blood Culture Isolates	
Candida Species	**Neonates***	**All Patients†**
C. albicans	58	55
C. parapsilosis	34	15
C. glabrata	2	15
C. tropicalis	4	9
Other species	2	6

*Data from Fridkin SK, et al. Changing incidence of Candida bloodstream infections among NICU patients in the United States: 1995–2004. Pediatrics 117:1680–1687, 2006;
†Pfaller MA, et al. International surveillance of bloodstream infections due to Candida species: frequency of occurrence and in vitro susceptibilities to fluconazole, ravuconazole, and voriconazole of isolates collected from 1997 through 1999 in the SENTRY antimicrobial surveillance program. J Clin Microbiol 39:3254–3259, 2001 [9,15].

Candida species are commensal organisms, colonizing the human skin, gastrointestinal tract, and female genitourinary tract [16,25–27]. Studies evaluating gastrointestinal tract colonization document approximately 5% of neonates are colonized with *Candida* on admission to the NICU; up to 50% are colonized by the end of the first week and almost three fourths by the end of the first month of life [25,28–30]. A variety of *Candida* species colonize the human gastrointestinal tract, including *C. albicans, C. tropicalis, C. glabrata,* and *C. parapsilosis* in neonates [28,30,31]. More than one species may be recovered from a single host, but there is usually a predominant colonizing species [32]. The *Candida* strain colonizing the infant most often is acquired by vertical transmission from the maternal vaginal mucosa after passage through the birth canal [32–34]. Using molecular typing techniques, vertical transmission of *C. albicans, C. parapsilosis,* and *C. glabrata* has been documented in term and preterm infants [32,33,35]. Heavy maternal colonization or maternal *Candida* vaginitis is an important risk factor for efficient transmission, resulting in increased neonatal colonization and the potential for disease [33,34,36]. Intrauterine fetal infections occur rarely, but they have been attributed to ascending infection from the vagina of the mother and transplacental transmission [37,38]. Breast-feeding can result in transmission of yeast present on the maternal skin to the infant's oral mucosa, and *Candida* species have been recovered from expressed breast milk [39]. Candidal mastitis increases the risk of transmission. Perinatal transmission can result in colonization, congenital candidiasis, or mucocutaneous infections in the term infant, whereas the result can be disseminated or systemic candidiasis in the preterm infant [40,41].

Although maternal vertical transmission is more common, acquisition of *Candida* from care providers may occur and is the primary mode of transmission for *C. parapsilosis* [22,32,33]. In one study evaluating 19 mother-infant pairs; no maternal reservoir could be demonstrated among infants colonized with *C. parapsilosis* [32]. Although different from the typical transmission route seen with *C. albicans* and *C. glabrata* (the two species found most often in the maternal gastrointestinal or genitourinary tract), this observation is not surprising. Given

that maternal gastrointestinal or genitourinary colonization with *C. parapsilosis* is uncommon, the risk of perinatal exposure and transmission is equally low [42]. After birth, NICU personnel, rather than the mother, have the greatest contact with the preterm or sick infant. Because *C. parapsilosis* is the most common *Candida* species recovered from the hands of health care providers, transmission can be expected and may be a contributing factor to the increased incidence of *C. parapsilosis* catheter-associated infections in high-risk neonates [43,44].

Colonization is important in the development of disease because the *Candida* strain recovered in infection usually is identical to the colonizing strain [45–47]. Disseminated infections result from translocation across the gastrointestinal tract epithelium of commensal *Candida* species [16,45,48]. However, colonization does not inevitably lead to disease, and infection does occur in the absence of apparent colonization [49]. Direct transmission of *Candida* to NICU infants has been documented from exogenous yeast carried by hands of hospital personnel or found on equipment [44,50,51]. This emphasizes the need for proper hand hygiene among health care workers in the NICU—although most of the antimicrobial soaps available are not fungicidal, and it is primarily the mechanical action of washing that decreases the burden of *Candida* species present [52,53]. Vaudry and colleagues described an outbreak of candidemia in seven infants without central intravascular catheters, and molecular typing of the *C. albicans* strains grouped the isolates into two cohorts corresponding with the timing of infections and the geographic location of babies in the nursery [54]. The use of intravascular pressure-monitoring devices has been associated with *C. parapsilosis* fungemia in an NICU [55]. *Candida* infections have resulted from retrograde administration of medications by multiple-use syringes in infants receiving total parenteral nutrition; in these cases, the responsible organisms, *C. albicans, C. tropicalis,* and *C. parapsilosis,* were isolated from the blood of the infants and the medication syringe [44]. The outbreak subsided with a change to single-use syringes. A nursery outbreak of *Candida guilliermondii,* a typically nonpathogenic NCAC, was traced to contaminated heparin vials used for flushing needles for blood drawing [55]. All of these examples point to the ubiquitous nature of *Candida* species and the need for stringent infection control practices on the NICU to decrease the acquisition of nosocomial infections [56,57].

MICROBIOLOGY

The name *Candida* comes from the Latin term candidus, meaning "glowing white," which refers to the smooth, glistening white colonies formed by these yeasts when grown on culture media. The taxonomy of the genus *Candida* is somewhat challenging and incomplete because of the reclassification of certain species (e.g., Torulopsis glabrata has been correctly identified as *C. glabrata*) and the discovery of new species such as *C. dubliniensis, Candida orthopsilosis,* and *Candida metapsilosis* (the last two previously classified as part of the *C. parapsilosis* complex) [58–60]. Previously used terms, such as Fungi Imperfecti, *Oidium,* and *Monilia,* are no longer used in classifying the genus *Candida*. Fungi Imperfecti, or Deuteromycetes, refers to the class of fungi that reproduce asexually. This was the prevailing theory regarding *Candida*; however, a teleomorph, or sexual stage, has been described for certain *Candida* species (e.g., *C. krusei*, *C. guilliermondii*), eliminating this characteristic as a useful tool in classification [61]. *Oidium* and *Monilia* were 19th century terms that are no longer used to refer to the genus *Candida*, although the term monilial is still commonly used to describe the characteristic rash observed in cutaneous *Candida* infections [61,62].

Although more than 150 species of *Candida* have been described, relatively few species infect humans. Most exist as environmental saprophytes, and more than one half the *Candida* species described cannot even grow at 37° C, making them unlikely candidates to be successful human pathogens [63]. *C. albicans* is the most prevalent species causing human disease, but other pathogenic species include *C. parapsilosis*, *C. glabrata*, *C. tropicalis*, *Candida pseudotropicalis*, *C. paratropicalis*, *C. krusei*, *Candida lusitaniae*, *C. guilliermondii*, *C. dubliniensis*, and *C. orthopsilosis*. The primary pathogens among neonates are *C. albicans* and *C. parapsilosis* (see Table 33–1).

Members of the genus *Candida* are ubiquitous and form a heterogeneous group of eukaryotic, dimorphic, or polymorphic organisms. All *Candida* species grow as yeast cells or blastoconidia under general culture conditions between 25° C and 35° C, and growth is augmented by increased sugar or fat content in the media. Yeast cells are approximately 2 to 10 μm in the largest dimension, round to oval, and reproduce by budding. *C. albicans* is among the larger yeast at 4 to 6 × 6 to 10 μm, whereas *C. glabrata* and *C. parapsilosis* are among the smallest at 1 to 4 μm × 2 to 9 μm and 2 to 4 × 2 to 9 μm, respectively [61]. Figure 33–1, *A* shows *C. albicans* single blastoconidia and budding yeast cells. Most members of the genus also produce a filamentous form: pseudohyphae (see Fig. 33–1, *B*) or true hyphae (see Fig. 33–1, *C*). *C. glabrata* is the only pathogenic species that does not produce filamentous forms, existing exclusively as blastoconidia [61]. *C. parapsilosis* forms pseudohyphae but not true hyphae. Only *C. dubliniensis* and *C. albicans* form true hyphae (see Fig. 33–1, *C*), distinguishing these two species as polymorphic rather than dimorphic. Formation of a germ tube precedes the development of true hyphae, and this change in morphology can be induced by growth in serum or other specialized media or by incubation at 37° C. The clinical diagnostic microbiology laboratory has exploited this distinction by use of the germ tube formation test to rapidly identify *C. albicans* over other *Candida* species [64].

The ability to form true hyphae is considered one of the prime virulence factors for *C. albicans* [65]. Microscopic examination of infected human and animal tissue usually demonstrates the presence of *C. albicans* hyphae [66–70]. Conversely, nonfilamentous yeast, such as *S. cerevisiae*, rarely cause human disease, and genetically altered strains of *C. albicans*, which cannot filament normally, are generally less virulent in animal models of fungemia. [71–75] Other commonly recognized virulence factors for *C. albicans* include the production of proteinases and phospholipases, hydrophobicity, the presence of various

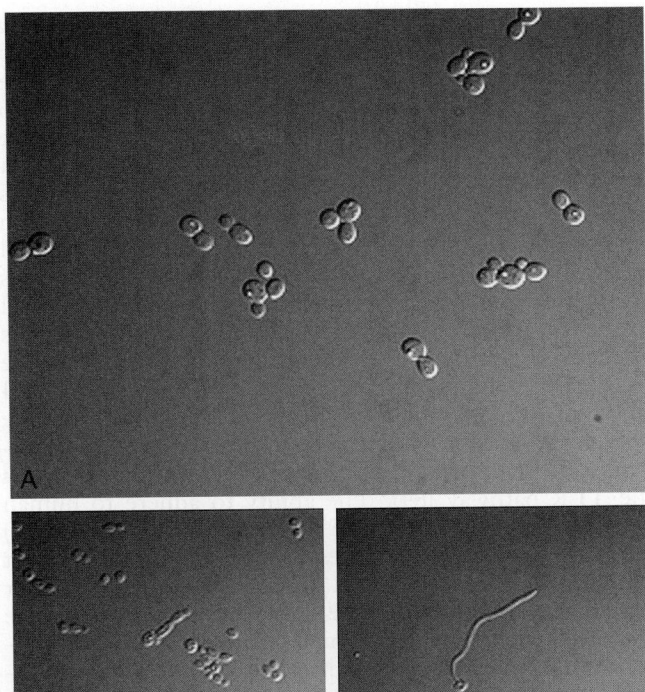

FIGURE 33–1 Light microscopy photographs of *Candida albicans* blastoconidia or yeast cells (**A**), pseudohyphae (**B**), and true hyphae (**C**). *(Courtesy Cheryl A. Gale, MD, University of Minnesota Medical School, Minneapolis.)*

surface molecules (e.g., receptors, adhesions), and the production of biofilm (which may be particularly important in catheter-associated infections) [66,70,74,76–80].

A variety of surface molecules of *C. albicans* are responsible for modulating epithelial adhesion by interacting with host ligands on the epithelial or endothelial surface [71,81,82]. Ligands include sugar residues on human buccal epithelial cells and a wide variety of extracellular matrix proteins, such as fibronectin, fibrinogen, types I and IV collagen, laminin and the complement components iC3b and C3d [83]. Reciprocally, human cells recognize yeast cell ligands via pattern recognition receptors (PRRs), such as Toll-like receptors (TLR) or the β-glucan receptor (βGR) Dectin-1 [84,85]. In tissue culture assays, *C. albicans* is more adherent than other *Candida* species to every form of human epithelium and endothelium available, including cultured buccal epithelium, enterocytes (adult and fetal), cervical epithelium, and human umbilical vein endothelial cells [36,86–88]. The adhesive molecules responsible for epithelial and endothelial adhesion may also facilitate binding between individual *Candida* cells and the subsequent development of "fungus balls" found in infected organs [83,89]. No single adhesin molecule is completely responsible for the adherence of *C. albicans* to human epithelium, and multiple methods of interacting with the host surface are postulated for this commensal organism [83]. *C. albicans* and *C. parapsilosis* both adhere well to the surface of catheters and, in the process, form a biofilm—although the biofilms formed by *C. albicans* are more dense and complex than those formed by other *Candida* spp [90–93]. The biofilm microenvironment promotes fungal growth with hyphal transformation and may confer relative drug resistance because of poor penetration of antimicrobial agents into this mass of extracellular matrix, yeast cells, and hyphae [78,94]. In vitro studies of *C. albicans* biofilms document the development of fluconazole resistance within 6 hours of formation [91]. Biofilm formation is associated with persistent fungemia and with co-infection by nosocomial bacterial pathogens, such as *Staphylococcus* species [90,95,96]. *Candida* spp. induce a strong TLR-mediated pro-inflammatory response in cultured oral epithelial cells resulting in profound IL-8 secretion [97]. In addition, the βGR dectin-1 and toll-like receptors TLR2 and TLR4 (thought to be the main receptors for the innate immune system recognition of *C. albicans*) appear to work synergistically, with dectin-1 amplifying TNF-α production via the TLR pathway [84]. The ability to adhere to human epithelium and endothelium (and to itself and catheters) resulting in microenvironmental changes, is a significant virulence factor setting *C. albicans* apart from other *Candida* species, and may be a prominent reason for the increased frequency with which *C. albicans* is found colonizing the host and causing disease at epithelial and endothelial sites.

Virulence factors of other *Candida* species have not been well studied. A fibronectin receptor that facilitates epithelial adhesion has been described in *C. tropicalis* [98,99]. *C. glabrata* colonizes the gastrointestinal tract, but no specific virulence factors have been identified in this nonfilamentous *Candida* species [100]. *C. parapsilosis* has been recovered from the alimentary tract of neonates, but no work has been done to implicate or exclude the gastrointestinal tract as a possible source of infection among neonates, and no specific virulence factors have been identified in this *Candida* species [24,28,35,93]. *C. glabrata* and *C. parapsilosis* produce biofilms; however, this area has not been well investigated for either of these pathogenic NCAC species [78,93]. Overall *Candida* species exhibit relatively low-level virulence factors compared with organisms that typically cause disease in an immunocompetent host. Candidal virulence factors serve to differentiate the more virulent from the less virulent *Candida* species, rather than to distinguish *Candida* from other more pathogenic microbes.

PATHOGENESIS

The pathogenesis of invasive candidiasis involves a common sequence of events in all at-risk hosts: colonization, resulting from adhesion of the yeast to the skin or mucosal epithelium (particularly the gastrointestinal tract); penetration of the epithelial barriers; and locally invasive or widely disseminated disease. Dissemination to deep visceral organs results from hematogenous spread [101]. However, not every colonized patient develops a *Candida* infection. The unique combination of host factors and yeast virulence mechanisms results in the persistence of benign colonization or the progression to infection among high-risk neonatal patients, as outlined in Figure 33–2. Yeast virulence factors were described in the preceding section. Host risk factors, listed in Table 33–2,

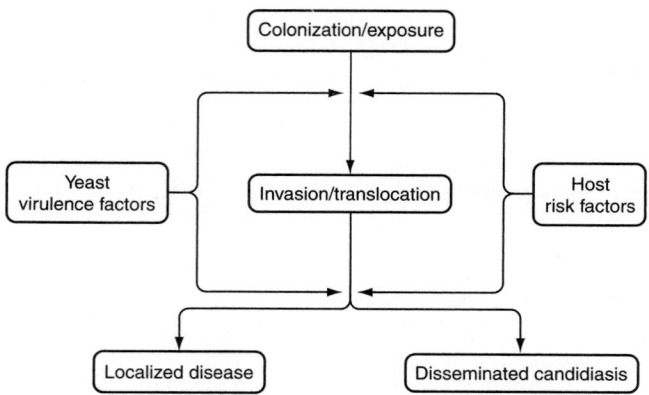

FIGURE 33–2 The pathogenesis of neonatal candidiasis follows a pathway from colonization to infection, modified by multiple host factors and yeast virulence factors.

TABLE 33–2   Host Factors Enhancing Risk for Candidiasis in Neonates

High burden of colonization with *Candida* species
Prematurity, especially gestational age <28 weeks
Very low birth weight (<1500 g)
Apgar score <5 at 5 minutes
Prolonged broad-spectrum antimicrobial therapy
Third generation cephalosporin exposure
Indwelling catheters, especially central intravascular catheters
Total parenteral hyperalimentation >5 days
Intravenous lipid emulsion >7 days
Intubation
Exposure to an H2 blocker
Abdominal surgery
Necrotizing enterocolitis
Spontaneous intestinal perforation
Cardiac surgery
Prolonged hospitalization >7 days
Steroid therapy
Neutropenia
Hyperglycemia

are potentially more important in the development of neonatal candidal infections [14,48,102]. Limitation of exposure to all predisposing conditions for candidal infection is highly desirable but rarely feasible, especially in the VLBW infant.

Indiscriminate, frequent, or prolonged use of broad-spectrum antimicrobial agents, resulting in alterations of the normal skin and intestinal microbial flora, allows for overgrowth of the colonizing strain of *Candida* and a concomitant increased risk for translocation and hematogenous spread [48]. The greater the density of organisms in the neonatal gastrointestinal tract, the greater is the chance of dissemination [103]. High levels of *Candida* colonization found in certain nurseries are linked to patterns of antibiotic usage, including a particularly strong association with third generation cephalosporin use [8,47,104].

The immunocompromised state predisposes an infant to candidal infection, whether caused by the developmentally immature immune system of the newborn, a congenital immunodeficiency, or the immunosuppression accompanying steroid therapy. No single defect in the immune system appears to be solely responsible for an increased susceptibility of premature neonates to candidal infections. Healthy adults have circulating IgG antibodies to Candida antigens, which effectively opsonize the organism and activate the alternative complement pathway [105–107]. Neonatal IgG levels depend on maternal exposure to the yeast accompanied by transplacental transmission of candidal antibodies, and the ability for the infant to respond to a new challenge with a Candida species, which may be slow and inadequate [105,108,109]. Polymorphonuclear leukocytes ingest and kill Candida; therefore, neutropenia is an important risk factor [70,110]. Disseminated candidiasis in neonates is associated with the intravenous administration of dexamethasone and hydrocortisone [111–113]. Steroid therapy results in immunosuppression and may have direct effects on colonization and translocation from the gastrointestinal tract. In vitro studies have shown that C. albicans is more adherent to monolayers of cultured enterocytes treated with dexamethasone than to untreated control monolayers, whereas mice injected with dexamethasone demonstrate higher levels of gastrointestinal tract colonization with C. albicans and increased rates of dissemination to the kidney [68]. Steroids may have a direct effect on the yeast by regulation of gene expression, including multidrug resistance genes and other modulators of virulence [114]. The presence of indwelling catheters is a significant predisposing risk factor for neonatal candidiasis. Endotracheal tubes, urinary catheters, peritoneal catheters, chest tubes, mediastinal tubes, and ventriculoperitoneal shunts can all become infected, but the greatest risk lies with intravascular catheters, particularly central venous catheters [5,50]. All catheters in the vascular space for more than a day begin to develop a thrombin sheath with a matrix-like substance, providing an optimal site for accumulation of micro-organisms [76]. Candida species adhere extremely well to the inert surface of the catheter, and electron microscopy studies have shown that Candida species are able to burrow into the catheter and form a surrounding biofilm [76,82,115]. This sequence results in a unique microenvironment, providing a barrier to host defenses and offering optimal conditions for growth and proliferation of the Candida organism, often resulting in the development of an infected mural thrombus extending from the tip of the catheter [116–118]. The "fungal mass" adherent to the catheter can then serve as a source for persistent fungemia or embolic spread of Candida species to distant organs [1,48]. The original source of the yeast that "sticks" to the line may be from hematogenous spread of endogenous gastrointestinal tract Candida strains or from nosocomial transmission through placement or handling of the catheter itself [44,54,101]. Use of the catheter for hyperalimentation is an additional risk, especially with the infusion of high dextrose-containing total parenteral solutions and intralipids [5,6,48,119]. Any compromise of epithelial barriers can predispose the neonate to candidal infections. Abdominal surgery and cardiac surgery are associated with an increased risk for disseminated candidiasis, especially among term infants [48,95]. Necrotizing enterocolitis (NEC) is strongly associated with Candida fungemia [5,16,120]. The loss of mucosal integrity after mesenteric ischemia and NEC provides a portal of entry for the dissemination of endogenous gastrointestinal flora [101]. Spontaneous intestinal perforation, occurring most often in the extremely preterm infant, is highly associated with candidemia [19,121]. As with any nosocomially acquired organism, prolonged hospitalization is a significant risk factor for the development of candidiasis [5].

Prematurity is a key risk factor for candidiasis, especially infants born at less than 28 weeks' gestation or VLBW neonates [4,5,48]. With improvements in technology, the current standard of care in the NICU includes an aggressive approach to the treatment of VLBW infants such that life for an extremely premature infant combines nearly all the risk factors for candidiasis in one patient [48,122]. The premature infant is born with immature epithelial barriers and an immature immune system. The skin and mucosal epithelium of these very tiny infants are minimally protective, readily breaking down with exposure to air and routine nursing procedures [123]. Preterm infants have the lowest levels of circulating maternal IgG of all neonates, having lost the opportunity for transplacental transfer that occurs during the third trimester of pregnancy [124]. Even if specific anti-Candida IgG is present, opsonization and complement activation are diminished [125]. Complement levels are extremely low in preterm infants, with biochemical abnormalities of C3 resulting in inadequate activation of this pathway for fighting infections [126]. Neutropenia is common among infants born at less than 28 weeks' gestation [127]. Virtually every premature infant begins life with a course of empirical broad-spectrum antibiotics, leading to an interruption in the process of establishing the normal gastrointestinal microflora and the potential for unchecked proliferation of Candida [50,128,129]. Endotracheal and intravascular catheters are true lifelines for the VLBW premature infant needing respiratory, inotropic agent, and nutritional support. Because venous access is often difficult to obtain and maintain in these infants, intravascular access lines are not automatically rotated and frequently remain in place for weeks. Even the fairly healthy VLBW infant often displays feeding intolerance that can require prolonged central total parenteral nutrition (TPN) rather than enteral feeds [5]. As reported by the National Institute of Child and Human Development (NICHD) Neonatal Research Network, the adjusted odds ratio for any episode of late-onset sepsis is 3.1 in VLBW infants receiving TPN for 8 to14 days, rising to 4.0 for an infant receiving TPN for more than 22 days [20]. Saiman and colleagues reported odds ratios for developing candidemia of 2.93 for infants less than 1000 g receiving TPN more than 5 days and 2.91 for IV intralipid use for more than 7 days [48]. Unfortunately, NEC may also accompany feeding intolerance, leading to an additional risk for disseminated candidiasis [130–132]. Corticosteroid use is also common in these patients [132]. Multiple reviews report that almost one half of the infants with a birth weight of less than 750 g are postnatally exposed to corticosteroids: hydrocortisone used to treat hypotension; dexamethasone, methylprednisolone or hydrocortisone used for severe lung disease [112,132,133]. Hyperglycemia and hyperlipidemia are common in these immature patients receiving TPN, steroids, or both [113,119]. Prolonged length of stay is the rule rather than the exception for the NICU infant, with or without a nosocomially acquired infection. The average corrected gestational age at discharge from the NICU is between 35 and 36 weeks, and the average NICU hospitalization is approximately 62 days; however, the length of stay to achieve 36 weeks' gestational age is even longer for the infant born at less than 28 weeks' gestation [20,48]. Each of these factors especially in combination, make the VLBW preterm infant an extremely high-risk candidate for the development of candidiasis.

PATHOLOGY

The tissue pathology observed in *Candida* species infections depends on the site of involvement and the extent of invasion or dissemination. Histologic evaluation of mucosal or epithelial lesions reveals superficial ulcerations with the presence of yeast and filamentous forms of *Candida* species, including a prominent polymorphonuclear (PMN) leukocyte infiltration [134]. Extremely low birth weight (ELBW; birth weight $\leq$ 1000 g) infants can develop invasive fungal dermatitis with erosive lesions; biopsy of these lesions reveals invasion of fungal elements through the epidermis into the dermis [123,134]. In disseminated neonatal infections, *Candida* species can invade virtually any tissues. Microabscesses are commonly found in the kidney, retina, and brain, but they also have been described in the liver, spleen, peritoneum, heart, lungs, and joints [11,134–137]. When *C. albicans* is the infecting organism, abscesses contain a predominance of hyphal elements with a significant accompanying infiltration of PMNs and prominent tissue necrosis, especially in the kidney [66,136,138]. Mycelia are frequently found invading the walls of blood vessels within infected tissues [15,67,136]. Retinal lesions, vitreal fungal lesions, and even lens abscesses with cataract formation have been described in neonates [139,140]. Evaluation of brain material shows significant inflammation with seeding of the meninges and may include parenchymal lesions, ventriculitis, perivasculitis, and ependymal inflammation [137,141–143]. Macroscopic fungus balls can form in fluid-filled spaces lined with epithelial or endothelial cells, such as the urinary tract, the central nervous system (CNS), and the intravascular space (particularly the right atrium) [117,144]. Fungus balls are large collections of intertwined hyphae, pseudohyphae, and yeast cells that presumably grow from *Candida* species initially adherent to the epithelial or endothelial surface of the involved organ [138,145,146]. Foreign bodies present in these fluid-filled spaces, such as urinary catheters, ventricular shunts, or central venous catheters, can also serve as the nidus for infection and precipitate the formation of a fungus ball [117,135,138,145,146].

In intrauterine candidal infections, macroscopic chorioamnionitis is evident, and histologic examination of the fetal membranes and the chorionic plate often reveal fungal elements with an extensive PMN infiltration [147,148]. Along with diffuse placental inflammation, focal granulomatous lesions can be present in the umbilical cord [140,149]. The detection of placental pathology consistent with candidal chorioamnionitis can lead to the early detection of congenital candidiasis in the infant [150].

CLINICAL MANIFESTATIONS

Candida species are responsible for a variety of infections in neonates with a broad spectrum of clinical presentations, ranging from mild, irritating thrush and diaper dermatitis in the healthy term infant to life-threatening systemic disease in the extremely premature infant. The primary forms of candidiasis among infants are mucocutaneous infections, congenital candidiasis, catheter-related candidemia, and systemic or disseminated candidiasis. Individual organ system involvement (e.g., urinary tract infection, isolated meningitis, endophthalmitis) can occur, but infection occurs much more often as a component of disseminated infection, especially in the premature infant. Table 33–3 lists features of the various presentations of neonatal candidiasis.

OROPHARYNGEAL CANDIDIASIS

Oropharyngeal candidiasis (i.e., thrush) can occur at any time during infancy. Among hospitalized infants, the overall incidence is reported as 3%, with a median age of onset of 9 to 10 days in NICU patients [151,152]. Specific risk factors include vaginal delivery, maternal vaginal *Candida* species infection, and birth asphyxia [152,153]. In a study of more than 500 mother-infant pairs, an eight-fold increase was observed in the incidence of thrush among infants born to mothers with symptomatic candidal vaginitis compared with infants born to asymptomatic mothers [153]. A multivariate analysis of factors among NICU infants reported that birth asphyxia was the only event significantly associated with the development of thrush [152]. Although *Candida* species can be transmitted from mother to infant during breast-feeding, thrush occurs more often among formula-fed infants [154]. *C. albicans* is the most common species isolated from infants with thrush, but other NCAC species, such as *C. parapsilosis* and *C. glabrata*, increasingly are found as commensals and infecting agents [154–156].

Thrush manifests as irregular white plaques on the oral mucosa, including the buccal and lingual surfaces and the palate. The underlying mucosa may appear normal or erythematous and may have an ulcerative base to the white lesion. Physical removal of the plaques usually is difficult and often results in mucosal damage. Infected infants can be healthy or quite irritable, with disinterest in oral feedings and obvious discomfort with any care involving contact with the oral lesions.

DIAPER DERMATITIS

Diaper dermatitis can occur any time during infancy, with a peak incidence at age 7 to 9 months in term infants (10% incidence) and approximately 10 to 11 weeks among VLBW infants (28% incidence) [46,157]. Most infants

TABLE 33-3 Features of Neonatal Candidiasis

Clinical Syndrome	Age at Onset	Host Risk Factors*	Presentation	Diagnosis	Treatment	Multiorgan Involvement	Prognosis
Mucocutaneous Infections							
Thrush	Throughout infancy	Birth asphyxia	White plaques on oral mucosa	Physical examination	Topical or oral antifungal therapy	None	Excellent
Diaper dermatitis	Throughout infancy; peak at 7–9 mo (term) and 10–11 wk (preterm)	Gastrointestinal colonization	Intense erythema of perineal area with satellite lesions	Physical examination	Topical antifungal therapy	None in term infants	Excellent
Congenital candidiasis	Birth	Premature rupture of membranes or uterine foreign body	Widespread erythematous maculopapular rash ± vesicles Pneumonia in preterm infants	Physical examination Culture of lesions for *Candida* spp	Topical antifungal therapy Systemic antifungal therapy for pneumonia	Uncommon Dissemination can occur in preterm infants	Excellent in term infants; excellent in preterm infants without dissemination
Invasive fungal dermatitis	<2 weeks	<1000 g Vaginal delivery Postnatal steroids Hyperglycemia	Erosive, crusting lesions in dependent areas	Physical examination Biopsy and culture of lesions	Systemic antifungal therapy	Common	Good if localized without dissemination
Systemic Infections							
Catheter-related infections	>7 days	Intravascular catheters	Sepsis	Blood culture by catheter grows *Candida* spp but peripheral blood cultures sterile	Catheter removal and systemic antifungal therapy	Rare Endocarditis or right atrial mass or thrombus	Good without dissemination or complication
Candidemia	>7 days		Sepsis	Only blood cultures grow *Candida* spp	Systemic antifungal therapy	Common in VLBW infants	Good to fair Risk of ROP in VLBW infants
Disseminated candidiasis	>7 days		Severe sepsis Multiorgan involvement	Blood and urine, CSF or other sites grow *Candida* spp Clinical and/or radiographic evidence for multiorgan involvement	Systemic antifungal therapy	Always (sites most often involved are kidneys, CNS, eyes, heart)	Fair to poor
Renal candidiasis	>7 days	Congenital urinary tract anomalies Neurogenic bladder	Sepsis Urinary tract obstruction	Urine culture grows *Candida* spp Ultrasound evidence of renal fungal lesions	Systemic antifungal therapy	Uncommon with isolated UTI	Good
CNS candidiasis	>7 days	Neural tube defects Indwelling CSF shunt or catheter	Sepsis None to focal neurologic signs	CSF culture grows *Candida* spp CSF culture grows *Candida* spp ± signs of inflammation; lesions by cranial imaging	Systemic antifungal therapy	Common	Poor

*Factors, in addition to those listed in Table 33–2, pertaining to the specific clinical syndrome listed.
CNS, central nervous system; CSF, cerebrospinal fluid; ROP, retinopathy of prematurity; UTI, urinary tract infection; VLBW, very low birth weight.

with candidal diaper dermatitis have gastrointestinal colonization, with stool cultures positive for a *Candida* species [157]. Some infants also have oropharyngeal candidiasis. *C. albicans* is the most common species isolated, but there has been an increase in the recovery of other NCAC species, particularly *C. glabrata* and *C. parapsilosis*, when cultures are obtained [19].

The characteristic rash of candidal diaper dermatitis is confluent and intensely erythematous with satellite lesions and pustules [157,158]. As with oral thrush, the lesions can be very irritating to the infant, especially during normal perineal care. In the term infant, the rash resolves rapidly after treatment with an appropriate topical antifungal agent [154]. The preterm infant has a greater risk for spread beyond the diaper area. In a prospective study, Faix and colleagues found mucocutaneous disease in 7.8% of all preterm infants, and most had diaper dermatitis [151]. Among preterm infants with dermatitis and an associated change in clinical status, 32% developed systemic disease, compared with 2.1% of healthy infants [151]. Therefore, it is prudent to monitor the preterm infants with candidal diaper dermatitis for signs of systemic infection.

CONGENITAL CANDIDIASIS

Congenital candidiasis typically presents at birth or within the first 24 hours of life, resulting from a maternal intrauterine infection or from massive exposure to maternal vaginal colonization with *Candida* during labor and delivery [19]. Hematogenous dissemination from mother to fetus, direct invasion of intact membranes, and ascending infection after ruptured membranes have been postulated as mechanisms for intrauterine infection [19,147,159]. Recognized risk factors for congenital candidiasis differ from those associated with postnatal infection and include prolonged rupture of membranes and the presence of an intrauterine foreign body, most commonly a cerclage suture [159,160]. Infants with the latter risk factor are more likely to be born prematurely and to have more severe skin involvement with disseminated disease [159]. While *C. albicans* is the predominant species responsible for congenital candidiasis, cases of congenital infections with *C. glabrata* and *C. parapsilosis* have been described [19,160,161].

Although there are rare case reports of infants with congenital candidiasis without skin involvement, the classic presentation is one of diffuse cutaneous disease [37,162,163]. Dermatologic findings include a widespread erythematous maculopapular rash, often with well-demarcated borders, that evolves into vesicles or pustules with eventual desquamation [160,162,163]. Any part of the skin may be involved, including the palms and soles, but the lesions typically are more prominent in the skin folds or intertriginous areas [19,164]. Preterm infants can have a diffuse, widespread, intensely erythematous dermatitis that resembles a mild burn or the early stages of staphylococcal scalded skin syndrome [165]. This form of congenital candidiasis often leads to massive desquamation, often accompanied by a prominent leukocytosis [37,162]. Extensive desquamation can lead to severe fluid and electrolyte imbalances in the extremely premature infant [37].

In term infants, clinical findings usually are limited to the skin, and recovery is uneventful after topical antifungal therapy. However, meningitis has been reported in the term infant with congenital candidiasis, and some infants may have nonspecific clinical signs of sepsis, such as poor perfusion, hypotonia, and temperature instability, suggesting systemic disease [162,166]. In preterm infants, cutaneous findings can be coupled with pulmonary invasion and early respiratory distress. In this circumstance, the chest radiograph is atypical for surfactant deficiency and the expected ground-glass appearance is replaced by a nodular or alveolar infiltrate [164]. Hematogenous dissemination is uncommon, but it can occur more frequently among preterm neonates and infants with widespread cutaneous involvement, pulmonary disease, and central intravascular catheters [160]. Every attempt should be made to avoid placing central intravascular catheters through the infected skin of patients with congenital candidiasis.

INVASIVE FUNGAL DERMATITIS

Invasive fungal dermatitis is a unique clinical entity described in the ELBW infant occurring during the first 2 weeks of life [134,167]. *Candida* species are frequently isolated, but infection with other filamentous non-*Candida* fungi, including species of *Aspergillus*, *Trichosporon*, *Curvularia*, and *Bipolaris*, can result in this clinical presentation [134,168,169]. Specific risk factors for invasive fungal dermatitis include a gestational age less than 26 weeks, vaginal birth, postnatal steroid administration, and hyperglycemia [134]. The immature skin of the extremely preterm infant is not an efficient barrier to the external invasion of *Candida*, making these neonates more susceptible to invasive cutaneous disease. The stratum corneum of the preterm infant is extremely thin, and keratinization with maturation of the barrier properties typically occurs beyond the second week of life [160].

Neonates with invasive fungal dermatitis have characteristic skin lesions with severe erosions, serous drainage, and crusting, often occurring on dependent surfaces such as the back or abdomen [134]. Biopsy of the affected area shows invasion of fungal elements through the epidermis into the dermis [134]. Without prompt and appropriate therapy, dissemination with resulting widespread systemic disease is a frequent complication. As with congenital candidiasis, infants with extensive erosive lesions are at risk for the development of fluid and electrolyte abnormalities and secondary infections with other skin microorganisms.

CATHETER-RELATED CANDIDAL INFECTIONS

Catheter-related candidal infections are disease processes of the sick, hospitalized preterm or term infant requiring prolonged use of intravascular catheters or other invasive means of support [40,48,122]. Almost any type of indwelling foreign body can become infected, but vascular catheter-related candidemia is the most frequent and serious infection. The incidence increases after a central vascular catheter has been in place for more than 7 days. These infections have been associated with umbilical venous and arterial catheters and with percutaneously placed arterial or central venous catheters (i.e., femoral venous, subclavian, Broviac, or Silastic lines) [3,170]. Peripheral venous catheters have the same potential for fungemia in the premature infant, especially when used for the delivery of hyperalimentation fluid, and have been associated with the development of skin abscesses at the insertion site [171,172]. Catheter-related candida infection can occur in the absence of cutaneous infection in neonates with one or more of the predisposing conditions listed in Table 33–2, and the infection can arise from endogenous gastrointestinal organisms or from nosocomial transmission. Infected neonates exhibit nonspecific signs of sepsis, including feeding intolerance, apnea, hyperglycemia, and temperature instability, but no evidence of multiorgan involvement. Preterm infants also may exhibit hemodynamic instability or respiratory distress. Thrombocytopenia is a common presenting feature [4,173]. The vascular catheter tip provides an excellent nidus for growth of *Candida* and affords a source of ongoing fungemia. An infected thrombus or fungus ball can form on the catheter tip, serving as a source of platelet consumption or embolic dissemination [116,117]. By definition, catheter-related candidemia is infection of the catheter only; there is no dissemination or multiorgan involvement. Prompt catheter removal at the earliest sign of infection, although often impractical in the management of many of the highest-risk neonates, is necessary to contain the infection and prevent persistent candidemia with the attendant risk of developing disseminated infection or other complications. Candidal infections of right atrial catheters are associated with endocarditis and intracardiac fungal masses; the latter may result in cardiac dysfunction because of the enlarging right atrial mass [117,174].

Although infected intravascular catheters provide the greatest concern for dissemination, infection can occur with almost any type of catheter used in the treatment of the VLBW infant. Prolonged endotracheal intubation for mechanical ventilation can be required in the extremely premature infant with respiratory distress and in the sick term infant after cardiac or other extensive surgery. The concurrent ongoing presence of the endotracheal tube can lead to candidal colonization with the potential for development of pneumonia, although invasive lung infection is uncommon [25,95,175]. Candidal cystitis can accompany the prolonged use of indwelling bladder catheters by facilitating ascending infection, and cystic fungal masses can form, resulting in urethral obstruction [176–178]. Infants with vesicoureteral reflux and a candidal bladder infection are at increased risk for renal parenchymal infection [145,176]. Candidal peritonitis can develop with the prolonged use of peritoneal catheters placed intraoperatively for drainage or, more often, placed for peritoneal dialysis [135]. Peritoneal dialysis catheters are at extremely high risk for infection because of the frequent handling required and the high dextrose concentration of the indwelling dialysis fluid [135]. *Candida* species have been recovered from the pleural fluid draining from thoracic tubes and from the fluid draining through surgically placed mediastinal tubes [164]. With cystitis, dissemination and widespread disease can be complications, but *Candida* peritonitis or pleuritis rarely leads to fungemia [25,135].

CANDIDEMIA AND DISSEMINATED CANDIDIASIS

Candidemia and disseminated or systemic candidiasis usually are associated with multiple invasive infection enhancing factors and are infections of the sick preterm or term infant who is in the NICU more than 7 days [122,136,179]. However, most cases occur among ELBW infants, who have an incidence of candidemia ranging from 5.5% to 20% [5,8,48]. The source of the infecting *Candida* species can be the infant's endogenous flora or from nosocomial transmission, and all the *Candida* species listed in Table 33–1 have been implicated in systemic disease [20,48,175]. While candidemia without organ involvement can occur, *Candida* spp. have such high affinity for certain organs (e.g., kidney, eye, heart, CNS) that dissemination appears to be the rule rather than the exception, particularly in the neonate with persistent fungemia [2,136,137]. The clinical presentation of the infant with candidemia can vary greatly depending upon the extent of systemic disease. The most common presentation is one with clinical features typical of bacterial sepsis, including lethargy, feeding intolerance, hyperbilirubinemia, apnea, cardiovascular instability, and the development or worsening of respiratory distress. The preterm infant can become critically ill, requiring a significant escalation in cardiorespiratory support. Fever rarely occurs, even with widespread disease. New-onset glucose intolerance and thrombocytopenia are common presenting findings that can persist until adequate therapy has been instituted and the infection contained [25,113,119,173]. This association is so strong that the presence of persistent hyperglycemia with thrombocytopenia in a neonate cared for in the NICU is almost diagnostic for untreated candidemia [173]. Leukocytosis with either a neutrophil predominance or neutropenia can be seen [102]. Neutropenia is more often associated with overwhelming systemic disease. Skin abscesses have been described with systemic disease and are attributed to the deposition of septic emboli in end vessels of the skin [180]. Infants also can have specific organ involvement, such as renal insufficiency, meningitis, endophthalmitis, endocarditis, or osteomyelitis, confirming dissemination. Complex multiorgan involvement is the hallmark of disseminated candidiasis, especially among VLBW premature infants, and results from diffuse hematogenous spread [8,181,182]. The suspicion or diagnosis of candidemia or the diagnosis of candidal infection of any single organ system should prompt a thorough examination and survey of the infant for additional organ involvement [2,182,183]. Almost any organ can become infected, but the most common sites for candidal dissemination are the urinary tract, the CNS, and the eye [2,137,181,182]. The specific clinical presentation for each of these systems is described separately in the following sections. For the infant with disseminated candidiasis, complications can be extensive, multiorgan system failure common, and the need for escalated intensive support frequent and prolonged [136,183].

Renal Candidiasis

Renal involvement occurs in most infants with candidemia, because each of the same risk factors that predispose to disseminated disease specifically increase the risk for renal disease [184]. Every infant with candidemia should have an evaluation of the urinary tract for candidal infection. Infants with congenital urinary tract anomalies and those requiring frequent catheterization for neurologic reasons are at increased risk for an isolated *Candida* species urinary tract infection (UTI) [144,145]. Congenital urinary tract anomalies, such as cloacal exstrophy, can provide a portal of entry for *Candida* species present on the skin. Urinary stasis, whether caused by a congenital anatomic obstruction or a functional obstruction (e.g., in the neurogenic bladder with myelomeningocele), increases the risk of candidal bladder infections [185]. Regardless of the underlying cause, candidal UTIs generally manifest with the same nonspecific systemic signs as with candidemia, whereas specific renal findings can be silent or manifest as urinary tract obstruction, hypertension, or renal failure [144,145,186–190]. Acute renal insufficiency or failure is a common clinical presentation and may be nonoliguric, oliguric, or anuric. In the nonoliguric form, urine output remains normal or near normal, but elevation of the serum creatinine level may be quite dramatic [144]. Renal ultrasonography often reveals parenchymal abnormalities suggestive of single or multiple abscesses; however, lesions may not be obvious at initial presentation, becoming evident only later in the disease process [145,186]. With oliguria, obstruction of the urinary tract by a discrete fungus ball or balls must be considered [187,188]. These fungal masses commonly are found in the ureteropelvic junction and usually are diagnosed by ultrasonography, but are found rarely by physical examination as a palpable flank mass [66,190]. Hypertension may be the only initial clinical feature in neonatal renal candidiasis [189].

Central Nervous System Candidiasis

CNS candidiasis most often accompanies disseminated candidiasis, with up to 50% of VLBW infants having some form of CNS infection [191,192]. Neonates with neural tube defects and those requiring indwelling cerebrospinal fluid (CSF) shunts are at increased risk for isolated candidal infections of the CNS. Meningitis is the most frequently reported form of CNS infection, but parenchymal abscesses, ventriculitis, vasculitis and perivasculitis, ependymal inflammation, osteomyelitis of the skull or vertebral bodies, and even fungus balls within the subarachnoid space have been described, although rarely [2,137,146,193–196]. The specific clinical presentation is extremely variable but typically occurs when infants are older than 1 week [197,198]. The initial presentation is similar to that of disseminated candidiasis, subtle or quite severe, with cardiorespiratory instability and rapid overall deterioration [137]. Less frequently, an infant may have only neurologic signs, such as seizures, focal neurologic changes, an increase in head circumference, or a change in fontanelle quality [137,192]. Because clinical findings may be limited or nonexistent, the possibility of CNS involvement with *Candida* must always be considered in neonates with candidemia or evidence for invasive candidal disease at other sites.

Candidal Ophthalmologic Infections

Endophthalmitis results from hematogenous spread of *Candida* species to the eye of the infant and is a diagnosed complication in approximately 6% of infants with systemic candidiasis [139]. Overall risk factors for ophthalmologic infection are the same as factors predisposing to disseminated disease. Infants with prolonged candidemia (i.e., blood cultures positive for more than 4 days) are significantly more likely to develop end-organ involvement of the eye, kidney, or heart [181]. Ophthalmic infections have been reported with all *Candida* species listed in Table 33–1 [181,199]. Because the clinical presentation of candidal chorioretinitis is frequently silent, an indirect ophthalmoscopic examination should be performed on all infants diagnosed with or suspected of having candidemia or systemic candidiasis. Lesions can be unilateral or bilateral, and these appear as individual yellow-white, elevated lesions with indistinct borders in the posterior fundus [139,199]. Vitreous lesions occasionally occur, and some infants show vitreal inflammation or a nonspecific choroidal lesion with hemorrhage or Roth spots in the posterior retina [141,182]. Infection of the lens occurs rarely; five case reports of lens abscesses in preterm infants exist, and each infant presented with a unilateral cataract [141,200–202].

In addition to the ophthalmologic infections caused by *Candida* species, an association between candidemia and retinopathy of prematurity (ROP) has been described in neonates with no previous evidence for chorioretinitis or endophthalmitis [203–209]. Early reports suggested a significant increase in the incidence of any stage ROP among infants with *Candida* sepsis compared with those without candidiasis (95% versus 69%) and an increased probability of severe ROP requiring laser surgery (41% versus 9%) [203]. Subsequent retrospective studies have demonstrated a greater incidence of threshold ROP and need for laser surgery among infants with *Candida* sepsis but no greater overall incidence of ROP of any severity [205,206,208–210]. Data are inconclusive as to cause and effect, but an association clearly is documented [140]. Premature infants of any gestational age who develop candidal sepsis should be followed closely by an ophthalmologist for the late development of severe ROP.

Spontaneous Intestinal Perforation

Invasive disseminated candidiasis is associated with the occurrence of spontaneous intestinal perforation in preterm infants [135,211–214]. This syndrome is distinct from NEC, occurring predominantly during the first 2 to 3 weeks of life among the smallest, most premature infants on the NICU (median gestational age, 24 weeks; median birth weight, 634 g) [121]. Specific predisposing factors identified for spontaneous intestinal perforation include umbilical arterial catheterization, hypothermia, indomethacin therapy (prophylactic or treatment), and cyanotic congenital heart disease [135,214,215]. Neonates typically have bluish discoloration of the abdomen and a gasless pattern on abdominal radiographs, without pneumatosis intestinalis, often accompanied by systemic signs such as hypotension [121]. Disseminated candidiasis frequently is diagnosed in association with this syndrome; one series reported up to 33% of affected infants with cultures of blood, peritoneal fluid, CSF, or urine positive for *Candida* species [121]. Pathologic examination of the involved intestinal area demonstrates mucosal invasion by yeast and filamentous forms of *Candida* species

[126,211,214,215]. It is not clear from these specimens, nor from the clinical picture, whether the perforation is a result of primary candidal invasion of the intestinal mucosa or the colonizing *Candida* strain merely invades bowel damaged by another insult. Whatever the cause, the association exists; suggesting that clinicians should consider extensive evaluation for disseminated candidiasis with the diagnosis of a spontaneous intestinal perforation in the extremely premature infant.

DIAGNOSIS

The diagnosis of most mucocutaneous disease is based on the characteristic clinical findings described earlier. Culture of the lesions of oral thrush or diaper dermatitis usually is not indicated. However, in an infant refractory to therapy, culture with susceptibility determination of the recovered organism may identify a NCAC species with a susceptibility pattern requiring modification of specific therapy [156]. In congenital candidiasis, a presumptive diagnosis can be made by Gram stain of vesicular contents of an individual lesion or by potassium hydroxide preparations of skin scrapings, with confirmation by culture of discrete lesions or swabs of skin folds or intertriginous areas. Cultures of blood, urine, and CSF are indicated for term infants with systemic signs of infection and for all affected preterm infants, healthy or ill appearing [37]. In the infant with change in respiratory or radiographic status, endotracheal aspirate cultures that grow *Candida* species are difficult to interpret because most often this represents colonization rather than pulmonary invasion [25]. The characteristic skin lesions of invasive fungal dermatitis often are diagnostic, but a skin biopsy provides a definitive diagnosis and tissue for culture and species determination. Biopsy is more sensitive than skin swabs in identifying other non-*Candida* filamentous fungi included in the differential diagnosis for this disease process [134].

Given the increasing incidence of invasive candidiasis among premature infants, clinicians caring for these infants must be alert to the possibility of *Candida* in any infant who develops signs of systemic infection, especially neonates with predisposing conditions (see Table 33–2). The differential diagnosis includes primarily other microorganisms responsible for nosocomial sepsis [175]. At a minimum, any infant with systemic signs of infection should have blood cultures obtained from a peripheral venipuncture and from all indwelling intravascular catheters. Most *Candida* species are identified by growth on standard bacteriologic culture media with aerobic processing, and requesting separate fungal cultures does not increase the yield of *Candida* species [8,64]. Previous recommendations were to monitor such cultures for up to 10 days to ensure adequate growth of the slower-growing *Candida* species [64,164]. However, in one report, 90% of cultures for *Candida* species were positive by 72 hours, before and immediately after the initiation of antifungal therapy [216]. Multiple or repeat blood cultures increase the likelihood of obtaining a positive result [217,218]. For infants with an indwelling intravascular catheter or catheters, samples obtained through each catheter and from a peripheral vessel are recommended for culture.

Recovery of a *Candida* species from the culture sample obtained from an intravascular catheter and not from the peripheral blood supports the diagnosis of catheter-related candidemia without dissemination. However, caution should be used in making this distinction in neonates. First, the sensitivity of a single blood culture in diagnosing candidiasis is low; a single sterile peripheral blood culture does not exclude disseminated candidiasis [217]. Second, by the time the culture results are known (usually 24 to 48 hours after collection), dissemination might have occurred, especially in the preterm infant. Disparate results do indicate that the catheter tip is infected, and prompt removal of the catheter is indicated to prevent dissemination and other complications.

If disseminated candidiasis is suspected based on the clinical picture, or a positive blood culture is obtained from a peripheral vessel, additional studies are indicated. Even after the initiation of appropriate antifungal therapy, daily blood samples should be collected until culture results are negative, as the risk for multiorgan involvement increases the longer fungemia persists [181]. Because renal and CNS candidiasis can be clinically silent at presentation, urine and CSF should be obtained for analyses and culture. The presence of budding yeast or filamentous fungal forms by microscopic examination of the urine or CSF suggests invasive disease. Because *Candida* species are frequent contaminants of nonsterilely collected urine samples, urine should be obtained by sterile urethral catheterization or suprapubic aspiration [179,184]. In clinical practice, suprapubic aspiration is infrequently performed in many NICUs, and sterile urethral catheterization is reported to be an efficient method for obtaining urine cultures from infants younger than 6 months [219]. The current consensus is that a *Candida* species UTI in neonates be defined as 10^4 or more colony-forming units of *Candida* species per mL in a culture obtained by sterile urethral catheterization [184,185]. Cultures of the CSF are more likely to be positive if the volume of CSF obtained is at least 1 mL [137]. Even when an optimal volume of CSF is cultured, a negative result does not eliminate the possibility of CNS disease because infection can occur in areas of the brain not in communication with the CSF [137,143,220]. Analysis of the CSF for abnormalities suggestive of inflammation, including an elevated white blood cell count or protein level or a decreased glucose level, suggests meningitis, but normal values do not exclude CNS infection [221]. Interpretation of CSF values can be complicated by the presence of blood due to a traumatic lumbar puncture or pre-existing intracranial hemorrhage in the preterm infant. Cultures of other clinically suspicious sites, such as peritoneal fluid or a skin abscess or vesicle, can help to confirm the diagnosis in an ill infant. However, cultures of healthy-appearing skin and mucous membranes or cultures of endotracheal secretions without the presence of pulmonary symptoms are not helpful in diagnosing systemic infections. Endotracheal tube secretion cultures may not be helpful in the infant with respiratory symptoms because *Candida* pneumonia is more often a result of hematogenous spread [46,179]. If any other catheters are present, such as chest or mediastinal tubes, cultures of the fluid drainage also should be obtained.

A culture from a usually sterile body site that grows *Candida* species confirms the diagnosis of candidiasis. Determination of the *Candida* species involved is equally important. Historically, because most infections were caused by *C. albicans*, many laboratories did not go beyond the initial identification of a yeast in culture as *Candida* [69,130,222]. Today, the incidence of infections with the NCAC species has increased dramatically, and identification of the species involved is important for epidemiologic and therapeutic reasons [164,223]. Knowledge of the infecting *Candida* species can help to determine whether the source of the infection is endogenous or from nosocomial transmission. This can be especially important in determining whether an apparent outbreak of candidiasis in a particular NICU is a coincidence or caused by a common source [50,54,55,222]. From the therapeutic perspective, when comparing the various pathogenic *Candida* species, variations exist in susceptibility to the common antifungal agents (Table 33–4), and defining the infecting *Candida* species is important in determining appropriate antifungal therapy [35].

To determine the extent and severity of candidiasis, additional laboratory tests are indicated when evaluating the infant with suspected disseminated candidiasis, including a complete blood count with differential and platelet counts and determinations of the levels of serum glucose, creatinine, blood urea nitrogen, bilirubin, liver transaminases, and C-reactive protein. The white blood cell count may be normal, high, or low; however, in the neonate, neutropenia may suggest a severe, overwhelming infection [127]. Thrombocytopenia is strongly associated with systemic candidiasis and may be an early indicator of this disease [161,173]. Elevations in the blood urea nitrogen and creatinine levels may indicate renal infection. Mild elevations in the serum bilirubin levels may be a part of the sepsis syndrome, but marked elevations in the serum bilirubin concentration or liver enzymes indicate extensive liver involvement [3]. Elevation of the C-reactive protein level is a nonspecific indicator of systemic infection [17,100]. Unfortunately, obtaining normal values for any or all of these ancillary laboratory tests does not completely exclude the possibility of candidiasis, especially CNS disease, in the high-risk neonate [137].

Because of the predilection of *Candida* for certain organs, specific imaging studies are indicated to diagnose the extent of dissemination. Renal ultrasonography, echocardiography, and cranial imaging are recommended for all infants with candidemia or systemic candidiasis [181]. Renal and bladder ultrasonography are extremely sensitive, but nonspecific, in their ability to define abnormalities resulting from *Candida* infections. The ultrasonographic appearance of a nonshadowing echogenic focus strongly suggests a renal fungus ball, particularly when the infant has a urine culture that grows *Candida* [224]. However, blood clots, fibrinous deposits, and nephrocalcinosis may have the same ultrasound appearance, confounding interpretation [225]. Another common ultrasonographic finding is renal parenchymal infiltration characterized by enlarged kidneys with diffusely increased echogenicity [224]. In any given infant with renal candidiasis, one or both of these ultrasound findings can be seen. Limited information exists about the accuracy of computed tomography (CT) or magnetic resonance imaging (MRI) in diagnosing renal candidiasis [226]. Echocardiography is useful in neonates with central venous catheters when the primary concern is for endocarditis with an infected thrombus at the catheter tip site or a right atrial mass [117,174]. Cranial ultrasonography easily can reveal enlarged ventricles, calcifications, cystic changes, and intraventricular fungus balls in infants with CNS candidiasis [142,186]. Ventriculitis can be diagnosed by the appearance of intraventricular septations or debris [137]. Interpretation of the cranial ultrasonography can be difficult in the preterm neonate who has experienced an intraventricular hemorrhage in the past or has developed periventricular leukomalacia. Intracranial abscesses due to *Candida* species reportedly have been mistaken for intracranial hemorrhage [227]. Cranial CT and MRI offer certain advantages over ultrasonography, including superior imaging of the posterior fossa and infratentorial and non-midline structures [228]. Calcifications are seen best with CT and the addition of intravenous contrast can aid in the identification of intracranial abscesses. However, as a practical matter, cranial ultrasonography is more frequently used because it can be performed at the bedside of a critically ill infant. In addition to these imaging studies, all neonates with confirmed or suspected candidemia should have a dilated ophthalmologic examination, preferably by a pediatric ophthalmologist

TABLE 33–4   General Patterns of Susceptibility of *Candida* Species to Antifungal Agents

Candida Species	Amphotericin B	Flucytosine*	Fluconazole	Voriconazole	Caspofungin
C. albicans	S	S	S	S	S
C. parapsilosis	S	S	S	S	S to I[†]
C. glabrata	S to I[‡]	S	I to R[§]	S	S
C. tropicalis	S	S	S	S	S
C. krusei	S to I[‡]	R	R[‖]	S	S
C. lusitaniae	I to R	—	S	S	S

*Resistance develops rapidly when used as monotherapy.
[†]Isolates of C. parapsilosis have slightly higher minimal inhibitory concentrations (MIC).
[‡]A significant proportion of clinical isolates of C. glabrata and C. krusei have reduced susceptibility to amphotericin B.
[§]Between 30% and 65% of clinical isolates of C. glabrata are resistant to fluconazole.
[‖]C. krusei are intrinsically resistant to fluconazole.
I, intermediately resistant; R, resistant; S, susceptible.
Data from references [48,131,238,241,248,251,284,315].

[139,199]. The infant who has characteristic lesions of *Candida* endophthalmitis has a confirmed diagnosis of disseminated disease.

Despite heightened awareness of the more subtle presentations of disseminated candidiasis and improvements in the ancillary and imaging studies available to clinicians, an accurate and timely diagnosis of candidal infections in the neonate remains a challenge. This largely reflects continued reliance on a positive culture for *Candida* species from a normally sterile body fluid (e.g., blood, urine, CSF, peritoneal fluid) or a potentially infected site to confirm the diagnosis and guide therapy. Autopsy studies suggest that the specificity of blood cultures for candidiasis approaches 100%; however, the sensitivity in the diagnosis of disseminated candidiasis is low, ranging from 30% with single organ involvement up to 80% with four or more organs involved [217]. The situation in the neonate is further complicated by the fact that fluid volumes as low as 1 mL may be obtained for culture, additionally diminishing the sensitivity especially if the total burden of organisms in the fluid is low [228]. The development of techniques for more sensitive, reliable, and rapid diagnosis of candidal infections is a priority and is an active area of investigation [229,230]. A number of molecular diagnostic assays that exploit recognition of small amounts of *Candida* species proteins or DNA, including the β-glucan antigen assay, scanning electron microscopy of fluid containing yeast, and polymerase chain reaction (PCR) testing, are being evaluated in adults and older children [230–232]. None of these assays has been rigorously evaluated in a population of neonates [183]. β-1,3-D-Glucan is a major component of the fungal cell wall found in all clinically relevant *Candida* species. Various assays are reported to have 85% sensitivity and 95% specificity for candidemia by detecting very small amounts of this fungal cell wall antigen [233,234]. PCR amplification of an area of the genome common to *C. albicans* and other pathogenic *Candida* species can be successfully performed, again using very small volumes of blood, urine, or CSF; this assay appears to be the best hope for rapid diagnosis [231]. Extensive use of PCR assays has previously been limited by unacceptably high rates of fungal contamination resulting in false-positive tests, but newer assays are more specific and sensitive [231,235–237]. Each of these assays holds promise for the rapid detection of fungus in small volumes of body fluids and does not require the presence of live *Candida* species. One major drawback to many early PCR assays, compared with culture, was the lack of differentiation between pathogenic *Candida* species; the diagnosis they provided was simply candidiasis. However, newer PCR assays are able to distinguish between various yeast species [235,237]. With specific culture or PCR results, the clinician knows which *Candida* species is causing the infection and can tailor the therapeutic plan accordingly. Without specific results, more generic management plans must be employed. However, because the institution of therapy often is delayed due to the lack of a positive culture when clinical deterioration begins, which may lead to systemic complications from persistent fungemia, knowing the neonate has a *Candida* species may lead to improved therapeutic management.

TREATMENT

Therapy and management of candidiasis in the neonate require an effective antifungal agent coupled with appropriate supportive care and measures to eliminate factors favoring ongoing infection. In the NICU, the first two objectives are easier to achieve than the last. Multiple antifungal therapies are available, but few have been studied for determination of appropriate dose and interval, safety, and efficacy in neonates, especially VLBW infants. Amphotericin B has been the mainstay of antifungal therapy for more than 40 years, but newer agents may be indicated in certain settings [238–241]. Table 33–4 summarizes the antimicrobial susceptibility pattern of pathogenic *Candida* species to the most common antifungal agents, and Table 33–5 and the following discussion outline important features regarding use of each agent in the neonate with candidiasis. Because candidiasis often is a nosocomially acquired infection, most infected infants are already in the NICU, where appropriate intensive care to support these critically ill infants is readily available. If the hospital nursery is unable to address the needs of a critically ill neonate, transfer to a higher-level NICU should be considered. Unfortunately, the elimination of all risk factors for ongoing candidemia often is an unattainable goal, and the clinician frequently must settle for a less than optimal reduction of risk factors.

With the diagnosis of candidemia or disseminated candidiasis, immediate consideration should be given to the removal of all potentially contaminated medical hardware-especially central intravascular catheters [242]. For ongoing fungemia, successful medical treatment of *Candida* species infections while the catheters remain in place is rare [22,116,136]. The risk of dissemination also increases with every day the infant remains fungemic, as does the rate of infection of previously uninfected intravascular lines [136,243]. The clinician must face the reality that most preterm infants with systemic candidiasis require central access because of the clinical instability directly attributable to the ongoing candidemia, which in large part is caused by the ongoing presence of the infected catheter. If all lines cannot be removed, removal of a potentially infected catheter with insertion of a new line at a different site or a sequential reduction in the number of catheters is preferable to inaction. Infants with more than one catheter may not have all lines infected at the time of diagnosis, and removal of the catheter known or most likely to be infected may resolve the problem and allow continued therapy through the remaining line [118]. Antifungal therapy should be administered through the remaining central catheter to maximize drug delivery to a potential site of ongoing infection. Daily blood cultures to determine whether fungemia is persistent and whether additional infected catheters should be removed are necessary. Consideration should be given to surgical resection of infected tissue if antifungal therapy does not achieve sterilization (e.g., urine) or if mechanical complications caused by the presence of a fungus ball arise (e.g., right atrial mass). Although successful medical therapy for endocarditis caused by *Candida* species can often be achieved, large right atrial masses are almost impossible to sterilize and may also compromise hemodynamic function, necessitating surgical removal [117,118,174,227,244].

TABLE 33–5 Systemic Antifungal Agents for the Treatment of Invasive Candidiasis in Neonates

Drug	Dose	Interval	Route	Indications	Toxicities	Toxicity Monitoring	Comments
Amphotericin B	0.5–1.0 mg/kg/day	q24h	IV	Candidemia, invasive candidiasis	Renal, hematologic, hepatic	Urine output, creatinine, potassium, magnesium, liver enzymes	Not indicated to treat C. lusitaniae Dose adjustments may be required for renal failure
Lipid-associated amphotericin B preparations	3–5 mg/kg/day	q24h	IV	Invasive candidiasis with severe preexisting renal insufficiencies	Similar to amphotericin B	Urine output, creatinine, potassium, magnesium, liver enzymes	May be indicated in patients failing therapy or requiring higher doses
Flucytosine	50–100 mg/kg/day	q12-24h	PO	For therapy in combination with amphotericin B with CNS infection	Renal, cardiac, hematologic, gastrointestinal, hepatic	Serum levels of liver enzymes, complete blood cell count with differential count	Desired serum levels 40–60 µg/mL; bone marrow toxicity can be severe; excellent CSF penetration
Fluconazole	6–12 mg/kg/day	<7 d,[†] q72h 7–14 d, q48h >14 d, q24h	PO, IV	Alternative therapy to amphotericin B for localized urinary tract infection, mucocutaneous disease	Hepatic, gastrointestinal	Liver enzymes	Excellent CSF penetration; oral formulation well absorbed; not indicated to treat C. krusei or C. Glabrata
Echinocandins*							
Caspofungin	1–2 mg/kg/day	q24 hr	IV	Severe &/or refractory systemic infections hepatic & renal	Minimal, potential	Creatinine, urine output, liver enzymes	CSF penetration variable
Micafungin	0.75–3 mg/kg/day	q24 hr	IV	Severe &/or refractory systemic infections hepatic & renal	Minimal, potential	Creatinine, urine output, liver enzymes	CSF penetration variable

[†]*Age in days.*
CNS, *central nervous system;* CSF, *cerebrospinal fluid;* IV, *intravenous;* PO, *oral.*
Data from references [238,248–251,295,296,315].
Note: Recommendations are not included for the use of voriconazole due to concerns for potential toxicities and lack of adequate published trial in neonates (see text for further details). From Sabo JA, Abdel-Rahman SM. Voriconazole: a new triazole antifungal. Ann Pharmacother 34:1032–1043, 2000.[286]
Published reports on echinocandin use in neonates include small studies of patients with caspofungin and micafungin – neither of which is currently licensed for use in neonates. However, the data suggests safety and efficacy (see text for further details). We recommend verifying dosage and indications based on most current publications.
From references [248,250,251,295,296].

Surgical removal of an enlarging right atrial candidal mass in the face of ongoing fungemia and hemodynamic instability may be lifesaving for the premature infant [174]. Most renal fungal balls can be treated medically because of the high levels of most antifungal agents attained in the urine [176,185]. However, in an infant with complete obstruction of urinary flow caused by the presence of one or more fungal balls, surgical removal is indicated [187–189]. Hyperglycemia can be avoided by judicious administration of dextrose and insulin therapy if glucose intolerance persists. Corticosteroid therapy should be avoided or tapered as tolerated.

ANTIFUNGAL AGENTS
Topical Antifungal Therapy

Topical antifungal agents are indicated for thrush, diaper dermatitis, and uncomplicated congenital candidiasis in the term infant [19]. Nystatin, the most commonly used topical therapy, is a polyene drug that is not absorbed by the gastrointestinal tract, making it a topical agent in any of the three common formulations: oral suspension, ointment, or powder. The oral suspension is indicated for the treatment of thrush in patients of all ages. However, because of the high osmolality of the oral suspension (caused by the added sucrose expedient), care should be taken and use limited in the very premature infant or the neonate with compromise of the gastrointestinal tract [154]. Reports of clinical cure vary widely, from as low as 30% to as high as 85% [154,155]. Nystatin should be applied directly to the lesions of oral thrush. If swallowed rapidly, there is minimal contact with the lesions and little efficacy. Nystatin ointment or powder, when applied to diaper dermatitis, has an 85% cure rate [154]. Because thrush often accompanies diaper dermatitis, many clinicians add oral nystatin when prescribing perineal therapy, even if no oral lesions exist. Data suggest no added efficacy with this practice, which should be discouraged [154,245]. If oral lesions are present, treatment is indicated. However, if oral lesions are not present, the source of the *Candida* species probably is the lower gastrointestinal tract, in which nystatin is not an optimal agent.

Miconazole gel is a nonabsorbable formulation of this azole, developed particularly for treatment of thrush, which is not available in the United States [154,246]. The gel formulation is said to offer more prolonged contact with the oral lesions and has a reported efficacy of greater than 90% [154]. Side effects predominantly are gastrointestinal, similar to nystatin, but use of this agent has been evaluated only in a limited number of preterm infants [154]. Miconazole creams and ointments, and other topical azole formulations, frequently are prescribed for diaper dermatitis with excellent results [154,247].

Gentian violet, the first topical therapy for oral thrush, has become the treatment of last resort. Although effective, the liquid treatment must be applied directly to the lesions, and it causes unsightly dark purple stains on the infant's mouth, clothes, bedclothes, and often on the hands and clothes of the care provider. Complications include local irritation and ulceration from the direct application of the treatment to adjacent normal mucosa [154]. Given these inconveniences, most clinicians avoid gentian violet in favor of administering systemic therapy when topical treatments fail [155].

Systemic Antifungal Therapy
Amphotericin B

Amphotericin B deoxycholate is a polyene antifungal agent available since the 1960s. The American Academy of Pediatrics Committee on Infectious Diseases, the Pediatric Infectious Disease Society (PIDS), and the Infectious Disease Society of America (IDSA) recommend amphotericin B as the primary antifungal agent for the treatment of candidemia, disseminated candidiasis, and any form of invasive candidiasis in the neonate [248–251]. Most pathogenic *Candida* species are susceptible to amphotericin B (see Table 33–4). However, reports suggest a proportion of *C. glabrata* and *C. krusei* isolates have a somewhat reduced susceptibility to amphotericin B, which can be overcome by using higher dose therapy, and resistance has been described for isolates of *C. lusitaniae.** Very occasional resistance with *C. parapsilosis* has been reported [254].

Amphotericin B acts by binding to ergosterol in the fungal cell membrane, altering cell permeability with subsequent depolarization and leakage of cytoplasmic contents, eventually leading to cell death. Although amphotericin B has a higher affinity for ergosterol than the cholesterol in human cell membranes, toxicity is a risk with this drug. Neonates tolerate the drug well with minimal toxicity [255,256]. Toxicities reported in neonates receiving amphotericin B include renal insufficiency with occasional renal failure, hypokalemia, and hypomagnesemia caused by excessive renal losses, bone marrow suppression with anemia and thrombocytopenia, and abnormalities in hepatic enzymes [221,257]. Most toxicities are dose dependent and reversible on cessation of therapy [257]. Nephrotoxicity is the most common and worrisome toxic effect. A substantial rise in creatinine and decrease in urine output can be observed; however, it is frequently difficult to differentiate between renal insufficiency caused by inadequately treated systemic

renal candidiasis and that due to amphotericin B. Amphotericin B-induced nephrogenic diabetes insipidus has been described in adults, but not in neonates [258]. Although there is a potential for renal failure, most infants display no or mild nephrotoxicity that resolves with decreasing the dose of amphotericin B or after completion of therapy. A common and very uncomfortable side effect in adults and older children receiving amphotericin B is an infusion-related reaction consisting of fever, chills, nausea, headache, and occasional hypotension [256]. No such toxicity has been described in neonates [238,255,256]. Any neonate receiving amphotericin B should have serial monitoring of serum potassium and magnesium levels and of renal, liver, and bone marrow function.

Amphotericin B is not water soluble and is available only as an intravenous preparation. In neonates, there is a tremendous variability in the half-life, clearance, and peak serum concentrations after dosing [238,255,256]. Treatment success in neonates has been documented at doses of 0.5 to 1.5 mg/kg/day [193,255,259,260]. Most clinicians initiate therapy with a dose of 0.5 mg/kg and increase it to 1.0 mg/kg given once daily if no significant toxicity occurs. Dosing may need to be adjusted in the infant with pre-existing renal insufficiency [248]. Doses greater than 1.0 mg/kg daily rarely are needed for treating *Candida* species infections. The test dose, historically given to adults to determine the need for medication to ameliorate infusion-related symptoms, is not required in neonates. The risk for dissemination is so high among infants that no delay should occur in delivering treatment doses.

Although excellent plasma levels and tissue penetration occur with this dosing regimen for amphotericin B, CSF penetration is variable. In adults, CSF concentrations of amphotericin B are only 5% to 10% of plasma levels [248]. Neonatal CSF concentrations of amphotericin B generally are higher but more variable, ranging from 40% to 90% of plasma levels in one study of preterm infants [261]. The higher CSF concentrations achieved in neonates compared with adults may be related to the immature blood-brain barrier. However, the variability in concentrations suggests to some clinicians that amphotericin B as a single agent for the treatment of neonatal CNS infections may be ineffective. Fluconazole and 5-flucytosine penetrate the CSF well and can provide synergy with amphotericin B in killing some *Candida* species, especially *C. albicans*. Combinations of one or both of these agents with amphotericin B have resulted in successful treatment of CNS candidiasis in infants where single therapy alone was unsuccessful [193,262,263]. Successful treatment of CNS disease with amphotericin monotherapy also has been reported [221,255,259]. Systemic amphotericin may not be necessary in the few infants with isolated bladder candidal infection. In rare cases, bladder instillation of amphotericin B, alone or in combination with fluconazole, has been successfully used to treat infants with isolated cystitis or urinary tract fungal balls [185,264].

Amphotericin B Lipid Formulations

As an alternative to standard amphotericin B, three lipid-associated formulations are approved for use in adults: liposomal amphotericin B (L-AmB), amphotericin B lipid

---
*References 12, 131, 241, 248, 252, 253.

complex (ABLC), and amphotericin B cholesterol sulfate complex (ABCD). Fungal susceptibility patterns for these lipid-associated formulations are the same as for conventional amphotericin B deoxycholate [265–267]. Each is significantly more expensive than conventional amphotericin B [239]. The main purported advantage to these amphotericin B preparations is the ability to deliver a higher dose of medication with lower levels of toxicity. In adults and older children receiving a lipid-formulation of amphotericin B, significantly lower rates of infusion-related reactions and creatinine elevations are reported compared with conventional amphotericin B [268]. Several case reports of successful use of these preparations in neonates have been published, but almost no controlled studies have been performed [266,267,269,270]. Three studies of liposomal amphotericin B that have included neonates demonstrated no major adverse events, diminished toxicities associated with conventional amphotericin (i.e., hypokalemia and hyperbilirubinemia), and treatment success rates of 70% to 100% [265,271,272]. Two studies of ABLC in pediatric patients have included small numbers of neonates and demonstrated efficacy rates of 75% to 85%, with no significant toxicities [266,267]. CNS penetration may be better with these preparations in adult patients, but there are no data for neonates to support this claim [267]. Renal penetration of the lipid-associated formulations is poor compared with conventional amphotericin, and treatment failure at this site of infection has been reported [177,263,268].

Although randomized, controlled trials of the lipid-associated preparations in neonates are lacking, available information suggests that they may be safe and effective, although not superior to conventional amphotericin B. Treatment with amphotericin B deoxycholate remains the most appropriate therapy for infants with invasive infections with *Candida* species, especially for those with renal infection [239,248,249]. The amphotericin B lipid formulations may have a role in the treatment of invasive candidiasis in neonates with pre-existing severe renal disease or infants who fail to respond to conventional amphotericin B after removal of all intravascular catheters, but more data are needed.

Fluorocytosine

5-Flucytosine (5-FC) is a fluorine analogue of cytosine. The antifungal activity of 5-FC is based on its conversion to 5-fluorouracil, which inhibits thymidylate synthetase, disrupting DNA synthesis. This mechanism of action is not fungal specific, and significant host toxicities are reported in adults [239]. All pathogenic *Candida* species are susceptible to this agent, but resistance develops rapidly when used as monotherapy (see Table 33–4) [252]. 5-FC has excellent CNS penetration and is used primarily in combination with amphotericin B in the treatment of neonatal CNS candidiasis because early studies demonstrated synergy with these two agents [193,252,262]. However, other reports suggest no added therapeutic benefit when 5-FC is combined with amphotericin B [239,255,273]. The potential benefit of 5-FC added to amphotericin B must be weighed against potentially significant toxicities when considering the use of this agent.

Flucytosine is available only in an enteral preparation, limiting its use in most critically ill neonates with systemic candidiasis.

Azoles

The azoles are a class of synthetic fungistatic agents that inhibit fungal growth through inhibition of the fungal cytochrome P-450 system [274]. This action is not fungal specific, and interactions with the host cytochrome P-450 system can cause alterations in the pharmacokinetics of concomitant medications the infant is receiving and produce hepatotoxicity. Clinical hepatotoxicity is rare with use of the newer azoles, such as fluconazole and voriconazole, in adults and older children, and their overall safety profile is favorable [275]. However, monitoring of transaminases in patients receiving azoles is recommended [238]. Adverse endocrine and metabolic effects have been attributed to the use of azoles in adults [276]. The development of fungal resistance is a significant concern with this class of antifungal agents (see Table 33–4) [12].

Fluconazole, the azole used most frequently in neonates, is water soluble, available in oral or intravenous preparations, and highly bioavailable in the neonate [238,277]. Fluconazole has a long plasma half-life, with excellent levels achieved in the blood, CSF, brain, liver, spleen, and especially the kidneys, where it is excreted unchanged in the urine [278]. The pharmacokinetics of fluconazole in neonates change dramatically over the first weeks of life, presumably because of increased renal clearance with maturity; therefore, the dosing interval is based on both postnatal and postconceptual age (see Table 33–5) [278,279]. Transient thrombocytopenia, elevations in creatinine, mild hyperbilirubinemia, and transient increases in liver transaminases have been documented in neonates [31,278,280].

Several studies have shown fluconazole to be efficacious in the treatment of invasive candidiasis in the neonate. In one prospective, randomized trial versus amphotericin B, rates of survival and clearance of the organism were equivalent for both treatment groups [281–283]. Infants treated with fluconazole had less renal and hepatic toxicity and had a shorter time to the complete removal of central intravascular catheters, which was attributed to the ability to convert to oral therapy for completion of the treatment course [281]. Although these features make the use of fluconazole appear quite attractive, the primary concern with fluconazole is the potential for fungi to develop resistance [15,252]. Although most pathogenic *Candida* species are susceptible to fluconazole, *C. krusei* is intrinsically resistant to this azole, as are up to 65% of *C. glabrata* isolates (see Table 33–4) [131,240,284,285]. Both of these NCAC species can cause neonatal disease; therefore, the use of fluconazole as empirical single therapy is not recommended. The IDSA guidelines recommend the administration of fluconazole as an alternative therapy to amphotericin B for disseminated, invasive neonatal candidiasis or congenital candidiasis with systemic signs after the pathogenic *Candida* species is identified and susceptibility determination completed [248]. Because of its unaltered renal clearance, fluconazole is an excellent choice for the treatment of isolated urinary tract infections resulting from susceptible

Candida species, and oral fluconazole is an alternative therapy in refractory mucocutaneous disease [155,277,279]. Combination therapy with amphotericin B was evaluated in a multicellular trial of nonneutropenic adults with candidemia with excellent results [243]. Due to the excellent CSF preparation of fluconazole, combination therapy with amphotericin has been suggested when CNS disease is present [137].

Voriconazole is a second-generation azole, derived from fluconazole, with increased potency and a broader spectrum of activity (see Table 33–4) [286–288]. Voriconazole is active in vitro against all clinically relevant *Candida* species, including *C. krusei* and *C. glabrata*, and no resistance by fluconazole-resistant strains has been seen [12,289]. Voriconazole is metabolized by the liver, and the only clinically significant adverse event reported in adults is the occurrence of visual disturbances [286]. For this reason concerns have been raised about the possibility of unknown interactions with the developing retina, discouraging therapeutic trials in neonates [250]. The neonatal literature is limited, but one case report does describe successful combination therapy with voriconazole and liposomal amphotericin B in a premature infant with disseminated fluconazole resistant *C. albicans* infection [290]. A more recent report showed safety and efficacy in a very small group of neonates treated with voriconazole [291]. Although this agent appears to be safe and effective in children, further trials in neonates are indicated before routine recommendation can be established. Posaconazole and ravuconazole are the two newest triazoles and there is no data available on their use in either pediatric or neonatal patients.

Echinocandins

Echinocandins are a novel class of antifungal drugs that act by a unique and completely fungal-specific mechanism—inhibition of the synthesis of β-1,3-D-glucan, an essential component of the fungal cell wall [292]. Because there is no mammalian equivalent to the fungal cell wall, the safety profile for the echinocandins is excellent and significantly better than the polyenes or azoles [240,292]. Three drugs in this class, anidulafungin, caspofungin, and micafungin, are currently only licensed for use in the United States as intravenous formulations because of poor oral availability [250]. Echinocandins are fungicidal against all pathogenic *Candida* species [241,293]. Concerns have been raised that *C. parapsilosis* may be less susceptible to this drug based on in vitro testing, but clinical response to invasive disease in adults has been excellent [294]. Because the mechanism of action is completely different from the other antifungal agents currently in use, the echinocandins are excellent candidates for use in combined therapy, especially for refractory infections. Pharmacokinetic studies in the neonatal population are limited, but those completed show caspofungin and micafungin are well tolerated, but have a shorter serum half-life and more rapid clearance, emphasizing the importance of evaluating the neonatal population separate from older children and adults [250,295]. Recommendations for optimal dosage in the neonate, especially preterm, for either of these agents remain unclear [250].

Multiple case reports suggest safety and efficacy [296–300]. One multicenter trial of micafungin in pediatric, adult, and neonatal patients demonstrated an overall greater than 80% success rate in treating refractory candidemia, either alone or in combination with other antifungal agents, but the number of neonates enrolled was small [301]. A review of the use of caspofungin in pediatric patients was also favorable, as was a recent pharmacokinetic study among infants less than 3 months of age [300,302]. No data has been published regarding the use of anidulafungin in neonates. The most current guidelines from the IDSA recommend caspofungin as a second-line agent for neonatal candidemia without dissemination [248]. Development of this novel class of truly fungicidal agents against *Candida* spp. has greatly expanded our options for treating invasive candidiasis in adults. If the echinocandins prove to be as safe and effective for neonates, clinicians could have the ability to combine antifungal agents with different general mechanisms of action (i.e., amphotericin B + an echinocandin, or an azole + an echinocandin) to optimize therapeutic efficacy.

Length of Therapy

No matter which antifungal therapy is chosen, the length of therapy to adequately treat invasive neonatal candidiasis is prolonged (see Table 33–3). There are no controlled clinical trials to provide the optimal length of therapy for any of the antifungal agents and no consensus among neonatologists and pediatric infectious disease specialists [263]. The IDSA recommends a minimum of 14 to 21 days of systemic therapy after negative blood, urine, and CSF culture results have been obtained along with the resolution of clinical findings [248]. Case series employing amphotericin B suggest that a cumulative dose of 25 to 30 mg/kg be administered (estimated at a mean of 4 weeks) [3,255]. Therapy for endocarditis typically lasts 6 weeks [248]. In neonates with isolated *Candida* cystitis, treatment for 7 days appears to be adequate. Therapy must be administered intravenous initially, but in an infant who responds to fluconazole, completion of the course with oral therapy is acceptable [279]. Infants with fungal abscesses, renal lesions, intracranial lesions, or right atrial fungal masses should have sonographic or radiographic evidence of resolution before completing therapy [144,224,238]. Close monitoring for relapse after the cessation of therapy is necessary given the high rate of recurrence, especially in infants with CNS disease [2,137,200].

Prognosis

Despite the current advances in neonatal care and antifungal therapy, the prognosis for the infant who develops an invasive fungal infection is still quite variable, but generally poor. Mortality rates range from 20% to 50%, with significant accompanying morbidity [151,170,303]. Factors determining the final prognosis include the degree of prematurity, extent of dissemination, severity of illness, and the rapidity of institution of appropriate antifungal and supportive therapy [304]. Infants with isolated catheter-related candidal infections, uncomplicated urinary tract infections, or candidemia without dissemination tend to have a good outcome with the potential for complete recovery without sequelae. Infants with extreme prematurity, widely disseminated disease, multiorgan involvement, renal or hepatic failure, and ophthalmologic or CNS infection have a much worse prognosis. In studies of VLBW infants surviving candidemia, disseminated candidiasis, or candidal meningitis, candidiasis survivors were significantly more likely to have a major neurologic abnormality (40% to 60% versus 11% to 25%) and a subnormal (<70) Mental Developmental Index (40% versus 14%) than noninfected infants of the same gestational age and birth weight [141,170]. In a series of ELBW neonates with disseminated candidiasis, including meningitis, Friedman and colleagues found a higher incidence of chronic lung disease (100% versus 33%), periventricular leukomalacia (26% versus 12%), severe ROP (22% versus 9%), and adverse neurologic outcomes at 2 years' corrected age (60% versus 35%) for infected infants than for gestational age- and birth weight-matched, noninfected controls [304]. Among the infected neonates with adverse neurologic outcomes, 41% had severe disabilities compared with 12% of the control infants, and all infants with parenchymal brain lesions diagnosed by cranial ultrasonography at the time of candidiasis had poor neurologic outcomes [22]. The visual outcome following endophthalmitis is generally good after provision of appropriate systemic antifungal therapy. Only a small percentage of infants have significant visual impairment, although most have some decrease in visual acuity [139]. Severe ROP has developed in preterm infants who recovered from candidiasis but never had endophthalmitis [204,207]. These infants may require laser surgery and may be at significant risk for vision loss [204]. Great strides have been made in our ability to diagnose and treat invasive candidiasis, but we must strive to continue to improve therapeutic management and address the issues of morbidity.

PREVENTION

The old adage that "an ounce of prevention is worth a pound of cure" could never be truer than when considering neonatal candidiasis. Treatment is difficult, prolonged, and prevents mortality and morbidity little more than one half of the time. The development of strategies to prevent neonatal candidal infections should be a priority on the NICU. Many of the factors listed in Table 33–2 that enhance the risk for candidiasis are unavoidable, such as prematurity and low birth weight, but every attempt should be made to address conditions that can be reduced, starting with exposure to the yeast itself. Appropriate diagnosis and treatment of maternal candidal vaginosis and urinary tract infections during pregnancy may decrease vertical transmission [248]. Prevention of horizontal transmission from caregivers by the use of good hand hygiene and gloves has resulted in limited success [49,50,305]. In studies of health care workers, appropriate hand hygiene is helpful in reducing superficial and transient flora, but it does not affect deep and permanent flora overall, with no significant reduction in the recovery of *C. albicans* detected after antimicrobial or alcohol washes [53,306–309]. Elimination of artificial fingernails among care providers and the judicious use of gloves may reduce

exposure and transmission [50]. The meticulous care of long-term indwelling catheters is recommended, especially if used to administer hyperalimentation.

Reduction in exposures to medications associated with neonatal candidiasis is an important part of prevention. Broad-spectrum antibiotic therapy and the postnatal use of hydrocortisone and dexamethasone are associated with fungal sepsis [48,111,203,305]. Two separate multicenter trials have shown an association between heavy levels of gastrointestinal tract colonization with *Candida* species and exposure to third-generation cephalosporins or H2 antagonists [48,305]. Both medications alter the enteric microenvironment, favoring fungal colonization and potential dissemination. The use of topical petrolatum ointment in skin care of the ELBW infant is associated with a significantly increased incidence of invasive candidal infections [310]. Although attempts at providing good skin care to prevent epidermal breakdown in the ELBW infant are laudable, the use of petrolatum ointment does not appear to be the best choice, and the increased risk of infection appears to outweigh any potential benefits.

FLUCONAZOLE PROPHYLAXIS

Chemoprophylaxis with antifungal agents such as oral nystatin and especially fluconazole has been a major area for investigation in recent years, with the goal of reducing candidal colonization and the accompanying potential for invasive disseminated disease. The cardinal rule of antimicrobial prophylaxis is to use one agent with minimal toxicities for prophylaxis and others for therapy. The use of oral nystatin to prevent systemic candidiasis has been practiced in many NICUs for decades, is tolerated well by neonates, with no fungal resistance documented, but efficacy in preventing invasive infection is not consistently achieved [171,311–313]. The development of multiple new antifungal agents (as described in the preceding section on treatment) has lead to the selection of fluconazole as the best new agent for anticandidal prophylaxis in the neonate [314,315]. Meta-analysis of four published randomized controlled trials of systemic antifungal prophylaxis with fluconazole in VLBW infants showed a significantly lower incidence of invasive fungal infection in the fluconazole group (RR 0.23), reduced mortality (RR 0.61), and an estimated number needed to treat (NNT) to prevent one extra case of invasive fungal infection of 130 in the overall VLBW population or 62 for ELBW infants [23,31,315–317]. All studies demonstrated safety, with no emergence of fungal resistance [314]. However, when looked at individually, the significance of the reduction in infection is dependent upon the baseline rate of systemic candidiasis in the participating nurseries. The most impressive reduction, NNT of 5, was reported in the study with the highest incidence of disease in the placebo group [31]. Institutional variability exists with respect to overall rates of infection, and discrepancies within subpopulations—such as ELBW infants, or those with multiple risk factors as listed in Table 33–2. These observations indicate that the NNT may vary dramatically based on the baseline incidence of systemic candidiasis for an individual NICU, suggesting that the basis for recommendations regarding fluconazole prophylaxis should be specific

NICU characteristics, rather than be universal guidelines [318]. Alternatively, targeted prophylaxis for the highest risk patents may be the best approach. Subsequent studies evaluating this approach for the preterm infant less than 1000 g or less than 27 weeks or those with specific accompanying risk factors (central venous catheter or >3 days of antibiotics) over a more limited period of time have shown a reduction in both invasive disease and mortality [314]. The targeted prophylaxis approach also limits drug exposure, reducing concerns for the emergence of drug resistance [35,289,319]. Widespread fluconazole prophylaxis in adult patients has clearly been associated with the development of resistant microorganisms and it would be naïve to ignore this concern in the nursery [320]. While the majority of published studies do not report the emergence of resistant *Candida*, follow-up to date is short term and fluconazole-resistant *C. parapsilosis* isolates colonizing neonates were reported by one group after the institution of a fluconazole prophylaxis program for ELBW infants [280,321]. The role for fluconazole prophylaxis, targeted or not, requires further clarification. Additional studies are indicated to explore the use of novel therapies for the prevention of *Candida* species colonization and systemic disease.

REFERENCES

[1] M.A. Pfaller, Nosocomial candidiasis: emerging species, reservoirs, and modes of transmission, Clin. Infect. Dis. 22 (1996) S89–S94.

[2] R.L. Chapman, R.G. Faix, Invasive neonatal candidiasis: an overview, Semin. Perinatol. 27 (2003) 352–356.

[3] K.M. Butler, C.J. Baker, *Candida*-An increasingly important pathogen in the nursery, Pediatr. Clin. North Am. 35 (1988) 543–563.

[4] M.S. Rangel-Frausto, et al., National epidemiology of mycoses survey (NEMIS): variations in rates of bloodstream infections due to *Candida* species in seven surgical intensive care units and six neonatal intensive care units, Clin. Infect. Dis. 29 (1999) 253–258.

[5] B.J. Stoll, N. Hansen, Infections in VLBW infants: studies from the NICHD Neonatal Research Network, Semin. Perinatol. 27 (2003) 293–301.

[6] R.L. Chapman, Prevention and treatment of *Candida* infections in neonates, Semin. Perinatol. 31 (2007) 39–46.

[7] K.N. Feja, et al., Risk factors for candidemia in critically ill infants: a matched case-control study, J. Pediatr. 147 (2005) 156–161.

[8] E.H. Kossoff, E.S. Buescher, M.G. Karlowicz, Candidemia in a neonatal intensive care unit: trends during fifteen years and clinical features of 111 cases, Pediatr. Infect. Dis. J. 17 (1998) 504–508.

[9] S.K. Fridkin, et al., Changing incidence of *Candida* bloodstream infections among NICU patients in the United States: 1995–2004, Pediatrics 117 (2006) 1680–1687.

[10] M.Y. Lin, et al., Prior antimicrobial therapy and risk for hospital-acquired *Candida glabrata* and *Candida krusei* fungemia: a case-case-control study, Antimicrob. Agents Chemother. 49 (2005) 4555–4560.

[11] R.G. Faix, Invasive neonatal candidiasis-comparison of *albicans* and *parapsilosis* infection, Pediatr. Infect. Dis. J. 11 (1992) 88–93.

[12] M.A. Pfaller, et al., Trends in antifungal susceptibility of *Candida* spp. isolated from pediatric and adult patients with bloodstream infections: SENTRY antimicrobial surveillance program, 1997 to 2000, J. Clin. Microbiol. 40 (2002) 852–856.

[13] P.B. Smith, et al., Excess costs of hospital care associated with neonatal candidemia, Pediatr. Infect. Dis. J. 26 (2007) 197–200.

[14] D.K. Benjamin, et al., Neonatal candidiasis among extremely low birth weight infants: risk factors, mortality rates, and neurodevelopmental outcomes at 18 to 22 months, Pediatrics 117 (2006) 84–92.

[15] M.A. Pfaller, et al., International surveillance of bloodstream infections due to *Candida* species: frequency of occurrence and in vitro susceptibilities to fluconazole, ravuconazole, and voriconazole of isolates collected from 1997 through 1999 in the SENTRY antimicrobial surveillance program, J. Clin. Microbiol. 39 (2001) 3254–3259.

[16] G.T. Cole, A.A. Halawa, E.J. Anaissie, The role of the gastrointestinal tract in hematogenous candidiasis: from the laboratory to the bedside, Clin. Infect. Dis. 22 (1996) S73–S88.

[17] R.A. Polin, The "ins and outs" of neonatal sepsis, J. Pediatr. 143 (2003) 3–4.

[18] B.J. Stoll, et al., Changes in pathogens causing early-onset sepsis in very-low-birth-weight infants, N. Engl. J. Med. 347 (2002) 240–247.

[19] J.L. Rowen, Mucocutaneous candidiasis, Semin. Perinatol. 27 (2003) 406–413.

[20] B.J. Stoll, et al., Late-onset sepsis in very low birth weight neonates: the experience of the NICHD Neonatal Research Network, Pediatrics 110 (2002) 285–291.

[21] V.P. Baradkar, M. Mathur, S. Kumar, Neonatal septicaemia in a premature infant due to Candida dubliniensis, Indian J. Med. Microbiol. 26: 382–389, 2008.

[22] D.K. Benjamin, et al., When to suspect fungal infection in neonates: a clinical comparison of *Candida albicans* and *Candida parapsilosis* fungemia with coagulase-negative staphylococcal bacteremia, Pediatrics 106 (2000) 712–718.

[23] L. Clerihew, N. Austin, W. McGuire, Systemic antifungal prophylaxis for very low birthweight infants: a systematic review, Arch. Dis. Child. Fetal. Neonatal Ed. 93 (2008) F198–F200.

[24] D. Trofa, A. Gacser, J.D. Nosanchuk, *Candida parapsilosis*, an. emerging. fungal. pathogen, Clin. Microbiol. Rev. 21 (2008) 606–625.

[25] J.L. Rowen, et al., Endotracheal colonization with *Candida* enhances risk of systemic candidiasis in very low birth weight infants, J. Pediatr. 124 (1994) 789–794.

[26] E. Farmaki, et al., Fungal colonization in the neonatal intensive care unit: risk factors, drug susceptibility, and association with invasive fungal infections, Am. J. Perinatol. 24 (2007) 127–135.

[27] Y. Kai-Larsen, et al., Antimicrobial components of the neonatal gut affected upon colonization, Pediatr. Res. 61 (2007) 530–536.

[28] A.E. El-Mohandes, et al., Incidence of *Candida parapsilosis* colonization in an intensive care nursery population and its association with invasive fungal disease, Pediatr. Infect. Dis. J. 13 (1994) 520–524.

[29] D. Kaufman, et al., Patterns of fungal colonization in preterm infants weighing less than 1000 grams at birth, Pediatr. Infect. Dis. J. 25 (2006) 733–737.

[30] V. Vendettuoli, et al., The role of *Candida* surveillance cultures for identification of a preterm subpopulation at highest risk for invasive fungal infection, Pediatr. Infect. Dis. J. 27 (2008) 1114–1118.

[31] D. Kaufman, R. Boyle, K.C. Hazen, Fluconazole prophylaxis against fungal colonization and infection in preterm infants, N. Engl. J. Med. 345 (2001) 1660–1666.

[32] L.A. Waggoner-Fountain, et al., Vertical and horizontal transmission of unique *Candida* species to premature newborns, Clin. Infect. Dis. 22 (1996) 803–808.

[33] J.M. Bliss, et al., Vertical and horizontal transmission of *Candida albicans* in very low birth weight infants using DNA fingerprinting techniques, Pediatr. Infect. Dis. J. 27 (2008) 231–235.

[34] X.D. She, et al., Genotype comparisons of strains of *Candida albicans* from patients with cutaneous candidiasis and vaginal candidiasis, Chin. Med. J. 121 (2008) 1450–1455.

[35] J.L. Rowen, et al., *Candida* isolates from neonates: frequency of misidentification and reduced fluconazole susceptibility, J. Clin. Microbiol. 37 (1999) 3735–3737.

[36] C.M. Bendel, Colonization and epithelial adhesion in the pathogenesis of neonatal candidiasis, Semin. Perinatol. 27 (2003) 357–364.

[37] D.E. Johnson, T.R. Thompson, P. Ferrieri, Congenital candidiasis, Am. J. Dis. Child. 135 (1981) 273–275.

[38] A.M. Dvorak, B. Gavaller, Congenital systemic candidiasis, Report of a case, N. Engl. J. Med. 274 (1966) 540–543.

[39] A. Gonzalez Ochoa, L. Dominguez, Various epidemiological and pathogenic findings on oral moniliasis in newborn infants, Rev. Inst. Salubr. Enferm. Trop. 17 (1957) 1–12.

[40] J.E. Baley, Neonatal candidiasis-the current challenge, Clin. Perinatol. 18 (1991) 263–280.

[41] P. Manzoni, et al., Type and number of sites colonized by fungi and risk of progression to invasive fungal infection in preterm neonates in neonatal intensive care unit, J. Perinat. Med. 35 (2007) 220–226.

[42] P.L. Fidel, J.A. Vazquez, J.D. Sobel, *Candida glabrata*: review of epidemiology, pathogenesis, and clinical disease with comparison to *C. albicans*, Clin. Microbiol. Rev. 12 (1999) 80–87.

[43] S.A. Hedderwick, et al., Epidemiology of yeast colonization in the intensive care unit, Eur. J. Clin. Microbiol. Infect. Dis. 19 (2000) 663–670.

[44] R.J. Sheretz, et al., Outbreak of *Candida* blood stream infections associated with retrograde medication administration in a neonatal intensive care unit, J. Pediatr. 120 (1992) 455–461.

[45] B.C. Fox, H.L. Mobley, J.C. Wade, The use of a DNA probe for epidemiological studies of candidiasis in immunocompromised hosts, J. Infect. Dis. 159 (1989) 488–494.

[46] J.E. Baley, et al., Fungal colonization in the very low birth weight infant, Pediatrics 78 (1986) 225–232.

[47] M.H. White, Epidemiology of invasive candidiasis: recent progress and current controversies, Int. J. Infect. Dis. 1 (1997) S7–S10.

[48] L. Saiman, et al., Risk factors for candidemia in neonatal intensive care unit patients, The national epidemiology of mycosis survey study group, Pediatr. Infect. Dis. J. 19 (2000) 319–324.

[49] Y.C. Huang, et al., Outbreak of *Candida albicans* fungaemia in a neonatal intensive care unit, Scand. J. Infect. Dis. 30 (1998) 137–142.

[50] S.E. Reef, et al., Nonperinatal nosocomial transmission of *Candida albicans* in a neonatal intensive care unit: prospective study, J. Clin. Microbiol. 36 (1998) 1255–1259.

[51] L.R. Asmundsdottir, et al., Molecular epidemiology of candidemia: evidence of clusters of smoldering nosocomial infections, Clin. Infect. Dis. 47 (2008) E17–E24.

[52] J.M. Boyce, D. Pittet, Guideline for hand hygiene in health-care settings: recommendations of the healthcare infection control practices advisory committee and the HICPAC/SHEA/APIC/IDSA hand hygiene task force, Infect. Control. Hosp. Epidemiol. 23 (2002) S3–S40.

[53] J.P. Burnie, Candida and hands, J. Hosp. Infect. 8 (1986) 1–4.

[54] W.L. Vaudry, A.J. Tierney, W.M. Wenman, Investigation of a cluster of systemic Candida albicans infections in a neonatal intensive care unit, J. Infect. Dis. 158 (1988) 1375–1379.

[55] S.L. Solomon, et al., Nosocomial fungemia in neonates associated with intravascular pressure-monitoring devices, Pediatr. Infect. Dis. J. 5 (1986) 680–685.

[56] D. Kaufman, Strategies for prevention of neonatal invasive candidiasis, Semin. Perinatol. 27 (2003) 414–424.

[57] D.A. Kaufman, Prevention of invasive Candida infections in preterm infants: the time is now, Exp. Rev. Anti. Infect. Ther. 6 (2008) 393–399.

[58] G. St Germain, M. Laverdiere, Torulopsis Candida, a new opportunistic pathogen, J. Clin. Microbiol. 24 (1986) 884–885.

[59] S.R. Lockhart, et al., Geographic distribution and antifungal susceptibility of the newly described species Candida orthopsilosis and Candida metapsilosis in comparison to the closely related species Candida parapsilosis, J. Clin. Microbiol. 46 (2008) 2659–2664.

[60] D. Sullivan, D. Coleman, Candida dubliniensis: characteristics and identification, J. Clin. Microbiol. 36 (1998) 329–334.

[61] R.A. Calderone, Taxonomy and Biology of Candida, ASM Press, Washington, DC, 2002.

[62] G.P. Moran, D.J. Sullivan, D.C. Colema, Emergence of Non-Candida albicans Candida Species as Pathogens, ASM Press, Washington, DC, 2002.

[63] F. Schauer, R. Hanschke, Taxonomy and ecology of the genus Candida, Mycoses 42 (1999) 12–21.

[64] T.G. Emori, R.P. Gaynes, An overview of nosocomial infections, including the role of the microbiology laboratory, Clin. Microbiol. Rev. 6 (1993) 428–442.

[65] G. San-Blas, et al., Fungal morphogenesis and virulence, Med. Mycol. 38 (2000) 79–86.

[66] C.M. Bendel, et al., Comparative virulence of Candida albicans yeast and filamentous forms in orally and intravenously inoculated mice, Crit. Care Med. 31 (2003) 501–507.

[67] C.M. Bendel, et al., Systemic infection following intravenous inoculation of mice with Candida albicans int1 mutant strains, Mol. Genet. Metab. 67 (1999) 343–351.

[68] C.M. Bendel, et al., Cecal colonization and systemic spread of Candida albicans in mice treated with antibiotics and dexamethasone, Pediatr. Res. 51 (2002) 290–295.

[69] F.C. Odds, Candida species and virulence, ASM News 60 (1994) 313–318.

[70] R.A. Calderone, In vitro and ex vivo assays of virulence in Candida albicans, Methods Mol. Biol. 56 (2009) 85–93.

[71] C.A. Gale, et al., Linkage of adhesion, filamentous growth, and virulence in Candida albicans to a single gene, INT1, Science 279 (1998) 1355–1358.

[72] B.R. Braun, A.D. Johnson, Control of filament formation in Candida albicans by the transcriptional repressor TUP1, Science 277 (1997) 105–109.

[73] J.F. Staab, P. Sundstrom, Genetic organization and sequence analysis of the hypha-specific cell wall protein gene HWPl of Candida albicans, Yeast 14 (1998) 681–686.

[74] H.J. Lo, et al., Nonfilamentous C. albicans mutants are avirulent, Cell 90 (1997) 939–949.

[75] L.L. Hoyer, The ALS gene family of Candida albicans, Trends Microbiol. 9 (2001) 176–180.

[76] I.A. Critchley, L.J. Douglas, Differential adhesion of pathogenic Candida species to epithelial and insert surfaces, FEMS Microbiol. Lett. 28 (1985) 199–203.

[77] J.E. Cutler, Punitive virulence factors of Candida albicans, Annu. Rev. Microbiol. 45 (1991) 187–218.

[78] C.J. Seneviratne, L. Jin, L.P. Samaranayake, Biofilm lifestyle of Candida: a mini review, Oral. Dis. 14 (2008) 582–590.

[79] H. Badrane, et al., The Candida albicans phosphatase Inp51p interacts with the EH domain protein Irs4p, regulates phosphatidylinositol-4, 5-bisphosphate levels and influences hyphal formation, the cell integrity pathway and virulence, Microbiology 154 (2008) 3296–S3308.

[80] F.C. Odds, Secreted proteinases and Candida albicans virulence, Microbiology 154 (2008) 3245–3246.

[81] R.A. Calderone, et al., Identification of C3D receptors on Candida albicans, Infect. Immun. 56 (1988) 252–258.

[82] Y. Fukazawa, K. Kagaya, Molecular bases of adhesion of Candida albicans, J. Med. Vet. Mycol. 35 (1997) 87–99.

[83] M.K. Hostetter, Adhesions and ligands involved in the interaction of Candida spp. with epithelial and endothelial surfaces, Clin. Microbiol. Rev. 7 (1994) 29–42.

[84] G. Ferwerda, et al., Dectin-1 synergizes with TLR2 and TLR4 for cytokine production in human primary monocytes and macrophages, Cell. Microbiol. 10 (2008) 2058–2066.

[85] K.M. Dennehy, G.D. Brown, The role of the beta-glucan receptor Dectin-1 in control of fungal infection, J. Leukoc. Biol. 82 (2007) 253–258.

[86] C.M. Bendel, et al., Epithelial adhesion in yeast species: correlation with surface expression of the integrin analog, J. Infect. Dis. 171 (1995) 1660–1663.

[87] S.M. Wiesner, et al., Adherence of yeast and filamentous forms of Candida albicans to cultured enterocytes, Crit. Care. Med. 30 (2002) 677–683.

[88] K.S. Gustafson, et al., Molecular mimicry in Candida albicans-role of an integrin analog in adhesion of the yeast to human endothelium, J. Clin. Invest. 87 (1991) 1896–1902.

[89] M.K. Hostetter, New insights into candidal infections, Adv. Pediatr. 43 (1996) 209–230.

[90] S.P. Hawser, L.J. Douglas, Biofilm formation by Candida species on the surface of catheter materials in vitro, Infect. Immun. 62 (1994) 915–921.

[91] D.M. Kuhn, et al., Comparison of biofilms formed by Candida albicans and Candida parapsilosis on bioprosthetic surfaces, Infect. Immun. 70 (2002) 878–888.

[92] G. Ramage, et al., Candida biofilms: an update, Eukaryot. Cell 4 (2005) 633–638.

[93] T. Rossignol, et al., Correlation between biofilm formation and the hypoxic response in Candida parapsilosis, Eukaryot. Cell 8(4) (2009) 550–559.

[94] L.J. Douglas, Penetration of antifungal agents through Candida biofilms, Methods. Mol. Biol. 499 (2009) 37–44.

[95] P.J. Eubanks, et al., Candida sepsis in surgical patients, Am. J. Surg. 166 (1993) 617–620.

[96] R.G. Faix, S.M. Kovarik, Polymicrobial sepsis among intensive care nursery infants, J. Perinatol. 9 (1989) 131–136.

[97] L. Li, A. Dongari-Bagtzoglou, Oral epithelium-Candida glabrata interactions in vitro, Oral. Microbiol. Immunol. 22 (2007) 182–187.

[98] S.A. Klotz, R.L. Smith, A fibronectin receptor on Candida albicans mediates adherence of the fungus to extracellular matrix, J. Infect. Dis. 163 (1991) 604–610.

[99] C.M. Bendel, M.K. Hostetter, M. McClellan, Distinct mechanisms of epithelial adhesion for Candida albicans and Candida tropicalis identification of the participating ligands and development of inhibitory peptides, J. Clin. Invest. 92 (1993) 1840–1849.

[100] J. Brieland, et al., Comparison of pathogenesis and host immune responses to Candida glabrata and Candida albicans in systemically infected immunocompetent mice, Infect. Immun. 69 (2001) 5046–5055.

[101] G.T. Cole, A.A. Halawa, E.J. Anaissie, The role of the gastrointestinal tract in hematogenous candidiasis: from the laboratory to the bedside, Clin. Infect. Dis. 22 (1996) S73–S88.

[102] I.R. Makhoul, et al., Review of 49 neonates with acquired fungal sepsis: further characterization, Pediatrics 107 (2001) 61–66.

[103] L.D. Pappu-Katikaneni, K.P.P. Rao, E. Banister, Gastrointestinal colonization with yeast and Candida septicemia in very low birth weight infants, Mycoses 33 (1990) 20–23.

[104] C.M. Cotten, M.S., et al., The association of third-generation cephalosporin use and invasive candidiasis in extremely low birth-weight infants, Pediatrics 118 (2006) 717–722.

[105] D.W. Warnock, J.D. Milne, A.M. Fielding, Immunoglobulin classes of human serum antibodies in vaginal candidiasis, Mycopathologia 63 (1978) 173–175.

[106] Y.H. Thong, A. Ferrante, Alternative pathway of complement activation by Candida albicans, Aust. N. Z. J. Med. 8 (1978) 620–622.

[107] D.L. Gordon, G.M. Johnson, M.K. Hostetter, Characteristics of iC3b binding to human polymorphonuclear leucocytes, Immunology 60 (1987) 553–558.

[108] V.C. Stanley, C.J. Carroll, R. Hurley, Distribution and significance of Candida precipitins in sera from pregnant women, J. Med. Microbiol. 5 (1972) 313–320.

[109] C.H. Kirkpatrick, et al., Inhibition of growth of Candida albicans by iron-saturated lactoferrin: relation to host defense mechanisms in chronic mucocutaneous candidiasis, J. Infect. Dis. 124 (1971) 539–545.

[110] R.D. Diamond, R. Krzesicki, W. Jao, Damage to pseudohyphal forms of Candida albicans by neutrophils in the absence of serum in vitro, J. Clin. Invest. 61 (1978) 349–359.

[111] C.M. Botas, et al., Disseminated candidal infections and intravenous hydrocortisone in preterm infants, Pediatrics 95 (1995) 883–887.

[112] N.N. Finer, et al., Postnatal steroids: short-term gain, long-term pain? J. Pediatr. 137 (2000) 9–13.

[113] A.R. Stark, et al., Adverse effects of early dexamethasone in extremely-low-birth-weight infants, National Institute of Child Health and Human Development Neonatal Research Network, N. Engl. J. Med. 344 (2001) 95–101.

[114] D. Banerjee, et al., A genome-wide steroid response study of the major human fungal pathogen Candida albicans, Mycopathologia 164 (2007) 1–17.

[115] D. Andes, et al., Development and characterization of an in vivo central venous catheter Candida albicans biofilm model, Infect. Immun. 72 (2004) 6023–6031.

[116] S.C. Eppes, J.L. Troutman, L.T. Gutman, Outcome of treatment of candidemia in children whose central catheters were removed or retained, Pediatr. Infect. Dis. J. 8 (1989) 99–104.

[117] D.E. Johnson, et al., Candida septicemia and right atrial mass secondary to umbilical vein catheterization, Am. J. Dis. Child. 135 (1981) 275–277.

[118] R.G. Faix, Nonsurgical treatment of Candida endocarditis, J. Pediatr. 120 (1992) 665–666.

[119] M.K. Hostetter, Handicaps to host defense-effects of hyperglycemia on C3 and Candida albicans, Diabetes 39 (1990) 271–275.

[120] J.A. Lemons, et al., Very low birth weight outcomes of the National Institute of Child Health and Human Development Neonatal Research Network, January 1995 through December 1996, Pediatrics 107(1) (2001) E1.

[121] E.E. Adderson, A. Pappin, A.T. Pavia, Spontaneous intestinal perforation in premature infants: a distinct clinical entity associated with systemic candidiasis, J. Pediatr. Surg. 33 (1998) 1463–1467.

[122] D.E. Weese-Mayer, et al., Risk factors associated with candidemia in the neonatal intensive care unit: a case-control study, Pediatr. Infect. Dis. J. 6 (1987) 190–196.

[123] G.L. Darmstadt, J.G. Dinulos, Neonatal skin care, Pediatr. Clin. North Am. 47 (2000) 757–782.

[124] M. Ballow, et al., Development of the immune system in very low birth weight (less than 1500 g) premature infants: concentrations of plasma immunoglobulins and patterns of infections, Pediatr. Res. 20 (1986) 899–904.

[125] D.L. Gordon, M.K. Hostetter, Complement and host defense against microorganisms, Pathology 18 (1986) 365–375.

[126] T.L. Zach, M.K. Hostetter, Biochemical abnormalities of the third component of complement in neonates, Pediatr. Res. 26 (1989) 116–120.

[127] Z.S. al-Mulla, R.D. Christensen, Neutropenia in the neonate, Clin. Perinatol. 22 (1995) 711–739.

[128] P. Manzoni, et al., Early-onset neutropenia is a risk factor for *Candida* colonization in very low-birth-weight neonates, Diagn. Microbiol. Infect. Dis. 57 (2007) 77–83.

[129] M.J. Kennedy, P.A. Volz, Effect of various antibiotics on gastrointestinal colonization and dissemination by *Candida albicans*, Sabouraudia 23 (1985) 265–273.

[130] M.A. Pfaller, et al., Bloodstream infections due to *Candida* species: SENTRY antimicrobial surveillance program in North America and Latin America, 1997–1998, Antimicrob. Agents Chemother. 44 (2000) 747–751.

[131] D.J. Diekema, et al., Epidemiology of candidemia: 3-year results from the emerging infections and the epidemiology of Iowa organisms study, J. Clin. Microbiol. 40 (2002) 1298–1302.

[132] A.A. Fanaroff, M. Hack, M.C. Walsh, The NICHD Neonatal Research Network: changes in practice and outcomes during the first 15 years, Semin. Perinatol. 27 (2003) 281–287.

[133] H.J. Helbock, R.M. Insoft, F.A. Conte, Glucocorticoid responsive hypotension in extremely low birth weight newborns, Pediatrics 92 (1993) 715–717.

[134] J.L. Rowen, et al., Invasive fungal dermatitis in the less-than-or-equal-to 1000 gram neonate, Pediatrics 95 (1995) 682–687.

[135] D.E. Johnson, et al., *Candida* peritonitis in the newborn infant, J. Pediatr. 97 (1980) 298–300.

[136] D.K. Benjamin, et al., Neonatal candidemia and end-organ damage: a critical appraisal of the literature using meta-analytic techniques, Pediatrics 112 (2003) 634–640.

[137] R.G. Faix, R.L. Chapman, Central nervous system candidiasis in the high-risk neonate, Semin. Perinatol. 27 (2003) 384–392.

[138] R.L. Chapman, R.G. Faix, Persistently positive cultures and outcome in invasive neonatal candidiasis, Pediatr. Infect. Dis. J. 19 (2000) 822–827.

[139] J.E. Baley, F. Ellis, Neonatal candidiasis: ophthalmologic infection, Semin. Perinatol. 27 (2003) 401–405.

[140] L. Drohan, et al., Candida (amphotericin-sensitive) lens abscess associated with decreasing arterial blood flow in a very low birth weight preterm infant, Pediatrics 110 (2002) e65.

[141] B.A. Doctor, et al., Clinical outcomes of neonatal meningitis in very-low-birth-weight infants, Clin. Pediatr. 40 (2001) 473–480.

[142] M. Marcinkowski, et al., Fungal brain abscesses in neonates: sonographic appearances and corresponding histopathologic findings, J. Clin. Ultrasound 29 (2001) 417–421.

[143] J.E. Carter, et al., Neonatal *Candida parapsilosis* meningitis and empyema related to epidural migration of a central venous catheter, Clin. Neurol. Neurosurg. 110 (2008) 614–618.

[144] D.K. Benjamin, R.G. Fisher, R.E. McKinney, Candidal mycetoma in the neonatal kidney, Pediatrics 104 (1999) 1126–1129.

[145] K. Bryant, C. Maxfield, G. Rabalais, Renal candidiasis in neonates with candiduria, Pediatr. Infect. Dis. J. 18 (1999) 959–963.

[146] W.D. Winters, D.W.W. Shaw, E. Weinberger, *Candida* fungus balls presenting as intraventricular masses in cranial sonography, J. Clin. Ultrasound. 23 (1995) 266–270.

[147] R.K. Whyte, Z. Hussain, D. Desa, Antenatal infections with *Candida* species, Arch. Dis. Child. 57 (1982) 528–535.

[148] I.C. Hood, et al., Fetal inflammatory response in second trimester candidal chorioamnionitis, Early Hum. Dev. 11 (1985) 1–10.

[149] N. Rudolph, et al., Congenital cutaneous candidiasis, Arch. Dermatol. 113 (1977) 1101–1103.

[150] D.A. Schwartz, S. Reef, *Candida albicans* placentitis and funisitis-early diagnosis of congenital candidemia by histopathologic examination of umbilical cord vessels, Pediatr. Infect. Dis. J. 9 (1990) 661–665.

[151] R.G. Faix, et al., Mucocutaneous and invasive candidiasis among very low birth weight (less than 1, 500 grams) infants in intensive care nurseries: a prospective study, Pediatrics 83 (1989) 101–107.

[152] P. Gupta, et al., Clinical profile and risk factors for oral candidosis in sick newborns, Indian Pediatr. 33 (1996) 299–303.

[153] S.S. Daftary, et al., Oral thrush in the new-born, Indian Pediatr. 17 (1980) 287–288.

[154] J.E. Hoppe, Treatment of oropharyngeal candidiasis and candidal diaper dermatitis in neonates and infants: review and reappraisal, Pediatr. Infect. Dis. J. 16 (1997) 885–894.

[155] R.A. Goins, et al., Comparison of fluconazole and nystatin oral suspensions for treatment of oral candidiasis in infants, Pediatr. Infect. Dis. J. 21 (2002) 1165–1167.

[156] C.L. Kleinegger, et al., Frequency, intensity, species, and strains of oral *Candida* vary as a function of host age, J. Clin. Microbiol. 34 (1996) 2246–2254.

[157] J.J. Leyden, Diaper dermatitis, Dermatol. Clin. 4 (1986) 23–28.

[158] J.J. Leyden, A.M. Kligman, The role of microorganisms in diaper dermatitis, Arch. Dermatol. 114 (1978) 56–59.

[159] H. Roque, Y. Abdelhak, B.K. Young, Intra amniotic candidiasis, Case report and meta-analysis cases, J. Perinat. Med. 27 (1999) 253–262.

[160] G.L. Darmstadt, J.G. Dinulos, Z. Miller, Congenital cutaneous candidiasis: clinical presentation, pathogenesis, and management guidelines, Pediatrics 105 (2000) 438–444.

[161] K.D. Fairchild, et al., Neonatal *Candida glabrata* sepsis: clinical and laboratory features compared with other *Candida* species, Pediatr. Infect. Dis. J. 21 (2002) 39–43.

[162] V.K. Pradeepkumar, V.S. Rajadurai, K.W. Tan, Congenital candidiasis: varied presentations, J. Perinatol. 18 (1998) 311–316.

[163] S.M. Wang, C.H. Hsu, J.H. Chang, Congenital candidiasis, Pediatr. Neonatol. 3 (2008) 94–96.

[164] C.M. Bendel, M.K. Hostetter, Systemic candidiasis and other fungal infections in the newborn, Semin. Pediatr. Infect. Dis. 5 (1994) 35–41.

[165] J.E. Baley, R.A. Silverman, Systemic candidiasis: cutaneous manifestations in low birth weight infants, Pediatrics 82 (1988) 211–215.

[166] S.R. Barone, L.R. Krilov, Neonatal candidal meningitis in a full-term infant with congenital cutaneous candidiasis, Clin. Pediatr. (Phila) 34 (1995) 217–219.

[167] C. Melville, et al., Early onset systemic *Candida* infection in extremely preterm neonates, Eur. J. Pediatr. 155 (1996) 904–906.

[168] M. Fernandez, et al., Cutaneous phaeomycosis caused by *Curvularia lunata* and a review of *Curvularia* infections in pediatrics, Pediatr. Infect. Dis. J. 18 (1999) 727–731.

[169] M.G. Bryan, et al., Phaeohyphomycosis in a premature infant, Cutis 65 (2000) 137–140.

[170] B.E. Lee, et al., Comparative study of mortality and morbidity in premature infants (birth weight, < 1,250 g) with candidemia or candidal meningitis, Clin. Infect. Dis. 27 (1998) 559–565.

[171] E. Leibovitz, et al., Systemic candidal infections associated with use of peripheral venous catheters in neonates: a 9-year experience, Clin. Infect. Dis. 14 (1992) 485–491.

[172] O.J. Hensey, C.A. Hart, R.W.I. Cooke, *Candida albicans* skin abscesses, Arch. Dis. Child. 59 (1984) 479–480.

[173] M.P. Dyke, K. Ott, Severe thrombocytopenia in extremely low birth weight infants with systemic candidiasis, J. Paediatr. Child Health 29 (1993) 298–301.

[174] J.E. Foker, et al., Management of intracardiac fungal masses in premature infants, J. Thorac. Cardiovasc. Surg. 87 (1984) 244–250.

[175] M.J. Richards, et al., Nosocomial infections in pediatric intensive care units in the United States, National nosocomial infections surveillance system, Pediatrics 103 (1999) e39.

[176] P.O. Gubbins, S.A. McConnell, S.R. Penzak, Current management of funguria, Am. J. Health. Syst. Pharm. 56 (1999) 1929–1935.

[177] R.J. Hitchcock, et al., Urinary tract candidiasis in neonates and infants, Br. J. Urol. 76 (1995) 252–256.

[178] J.W. Ruderman, A clue (tip-off) to urinary infection with *Candida*, Pediatr. Infect. Dis. J. 9 (1990) 586–588.

[179] J.E. Baley, Neonatal candidiasis: the current challenge, Clin. Perinatol. 18 (1991) 263–280.

[180] G.P. Bodey, M. Luna, Skin lesions associated with disseminated candidiasis, JAMA 229 (1974) 1466–1468.

[181] D.E. Noyola, et al., Ophthalmologic, visceral, and cardiac involvement in neonates with candidemia, Clin. Infect. Dis. 32 (2001) 1018–1023.

[182] J.E. Baley, R.M. Kligman, A.A. Fanaroff, Disseminated fungal infections in very low-birth-weight infants: clinical manifestations and epidemiology, Pediatrics 73 (1984) 144–152.

[183] D.K.J. Benjamin, H. Garges, W.J. Steinbach, Candida bloodstream infections in neonates, Semin. Perinatol. 27 (2003) 375–383.

[184] J.R. Phillips, M.G. Karlowicz, Prevalence of *Candida* species in hospital-acquired urinary tract infections in a neonatal intensive care unit, Pediatr. Infect. Dis. J. 16 (1997) 190–194.

[185] M.G. Karlowicz, Candidal renal and urinary tract infections in neonates, Semin. Perinatol. 27 (2003) 393–400.

[186] K.T. Tung, L.M. MacDonald, J.C. Smith, Neonatal systemic candidiasis diagnosed by ultrasound, Acta Radiol. 31 (1990) 293–295.

[187] C.W. Eckstein, E.J. Kass, Anuria in a newborn secondary to bilateral ureteropelvic fungus balls, J. Urol. 127 (1982) 109–110.

[188] M.Y. Khan, Anuria from *Candida* pyelonephritis and obstructing fungal balls, Urology 21 (1983) 421–423.

[189] D. Sirinelli, et al., Urinoma and arterial hypertension complicating neonatal renal candidiasis, Pediatr. Radiol. 17 (1987) 156–158.

[190] M. McDonnell, A.H. Lam, D. Isaacs, Nonsurgical management of neonatal obstructive uropathy due to *Candida albicans*, Clin. Infect. Dis. 21 (1995) 1349–1350.

[191] R.G. Faix, et al., Genotypic analysis of a cluster of systemic *Candida albicans* infections in a neonatal intensive care unit, Pediatr. Infect. Dis. J. 14 (1995) 1063–1068.

[192] R.G. Faix, Systemic *Candida* infections in infants in intensive care nurseries-high incidence of central nervous system involvement, J. Pediatr. 105 (1984) 616–622.

[193] C. Glick, G.R. Graves, S. Feldman, Neonatal fungemia and amphotericin B, South Med. J. 86 (1993) 1368–1371.

[194] L.S. Goldsmith, et al., Cerebral calcifications in a neonate with candidiasis, Pediatr. Infect. Dis. J. 9 (1990) 451–453.

[195] P.W. Brill, et al., Osteomyelitis in a neonatal intensive care unit, Radiology 131 (1979) 83–87.

[196] M.E. Bozynski, R.A. Naglie, E.J. Russell, Real-time ultrasonographic surveillance in the detection of CNS involvement in systemic *Candida* infection, Pediatr. Radiol. 16 (1986) 235–237.

[197] S. Levin, L. Zaidel, D. Bernstein, Intra-uterine infection of fetal brain by *Candida*, Am. J. Obstet. Gynecol. 130 (1978) 597–599.

[198] S. Sood, et al., Disseminated candidosis in premature twins, Mycoses 41 (1998) 417–419.

[199] J.E. Baley, W.L. Annable, R.M. Kliegman, *Candida* endophthalmitis in the premature infant, J. Pediatr. 98 (1981) 458–461.

[200] J.H. Stern, C. Calvano, J.W. Simon, Recurrent endogenous candidal endophthalmitis in a premature infant, J. AAPOS. 5 (2001) 50–51.

[201] W. Todd Johnston, M.S. Cogen, Systemic candidiasis with cataract formation in a premature infant, J. AAPOS. 4 (2000) 386–388.

[202] G.K. Shah, J. Vander, R.C. Eagle, Intralenticular *Candida* species abscess in a premature infant, Am. J. Ophthalmol. 129 (2000) 390–391.

[203] M. Mittal, R. Dhanireddy, R.D. Higgins, *Candida* sepsis and association with retinopathy of prematurity, Pediatrics 101 (1998) 654–657.

[204] D.E. Noyola, et al., Association of candidemia and retinopathy of prematurity in very low birthweight infants, Ophthalmology 109 (2002) 80–84.

[205] M.G. Karlowicz, et al., Does candidemia predict threshold retinopathy of prematurity in extremely low birth weight (<= 1000 g) neonates? Pediatrics 105 (2000) 1036–1040.

[206] L.C. Gago, A. Capone, M.T. Trese, Bilateral presumed endogenous *Candida* endophthalmitis and stage 3 retinopathy of prematurity, Am. J. Ophthalmol. 134 (2002) 611–613.

[207] M.F. Haroon Parupia, R. Dhanireddy, Association of postnatal dexamethasone use and fungal sepsis in the development of severe retinopathy of prematurity and progression to laser therapy in extremely low-birth-weight infants, J. Perinatol. 21 (2001) 242–247.

[208] M. Tadesse, et al., Race, *Candida* sepsis, and retinopathy of prematurity, Biol. Neonate 81 (2002) 86–90.

[209] P. Manzoni, et al., Fungal and bacterial sepsis and threshold ROP in preterm very low birth weight neonates, J. Perinatol. 26 (2006) 23–30.

[210] I. Kremer, et al., Systemic candidiasis in babies with retinopathy of prematurity, Graefes Arch. Clin. Exp. Ophthalmol. 230 (1992) 592–594.

[211] N.J. Robertson, et al., Spontaneous intestinal perforation and *Candida* peritonitis presenting as extensive necrotizing enterocolitis, Acta Paediatr. 92 (2003) 258–261.

[212] S. Bond, D.L. Stewart, R.W. Bendon, Invasive *Candida* enteritis of the newborn, J. Pediatr. Surg. 35 (2000) 1496–1498.

[213] C.L. Meyer, N.R. Payne, S.A. Roback, Spontaneous, isolated intestinal perforations in neonates with birth weight less than 1, 000 g not associated with necrotizing enterocolitis, J. Pediatr. Surg. 26 (1991) 714–717.

[214] A.C. Mintz, H. Applebaum, Focal gastrointestinal perforations not associated with necrotizing enterocolitis in very low birth weight neonates, J. Pediatr. Surg. 28 (1993) 857–860.

[215] M. Kaplan, et al., Necrotizing bowel disease with *Candida* peritonitis following severe neonatal hypothermia, Acta Paediatr. Scand. 79 (1990) 876–879.

[216] R.L. Schelonka, S.A. Moser, Time to positive culture results in neonatal *Candida* septicemia, J. Pediatr. 142 (2003) 564–565.

[217] J. Berenguer, et al., Lysis-centrifugation blood cultures in the detection of tissue-proven invasive candidiasis, Disseminated versus single-organ infection, Diagn. Microbiol. Infect. Dis. 17 (1993) 103–109.

[218] R.L. Schelonka, et al., Volume of blood required to detect common neonatal pathogens, J. Pediatr. 129 (1996) 275–278.

[219] C.V. Pollack Jr., E.S. Pollack, M.E. Andrew, Suprapubic bladder aspiration versus urethral catheterization in ill infants: success, efficiency and complication rates, Ann. Emerg. Med. 23 (1994) 225–230.

[220] R.G. Faix, *Candida parapsilosis* meningitis in a premature infant, Pediatr. Infect. Dis. J. 2 (1983) 462–464.

[221] M. Fernandez, et al., Candidal meningitis in neonates: a 10-year review, Clin. Infect. Dis. 31 (2000) 458–463.

[222] P. Villari, et al., Molecular epidemiology as an effective tool in the surveillance of infections in the neonatal intensive care unit, J. Infect. 37 (1998) 274–281.

[223] M.A. Pfaller, Epidemiology of nosocomial candidiasis: the importance of molecular typing, Braz. J. Infect. Dis. 4 (2000) 161–167.

[224] L.H. Berman, et al., An assessment of sonography in the diagnosis and management of neonatal renal candidiasis, Clin. Radiol. 40 (1989) 577–581.

[225] A.M. Krensky, J.M. Reddish, R.L. Teele, Causes of increased renal echogenicity in pediatric patients, Pediatrics 72 (1983) 840–846.

[226] A. Erden, et al., Radiological findings in the diagnosis of genitourinary candidiasis, Pediatr. Radiol. 30 (2000) 875–877.

[227] S.C. Johnson, N.J. Kazzi, *Candida* brain abscess-a sonographic mimicker of intracranial hemorrhage, J. Ultrasound Med. 12 (1993) 237–239.

[228] C.C. Huang, et al., Central nervous system candidiasis in very low-birth-weight premature neonates and infants: US characteristics and histopathologic and MR imaging correlates in five patients, Radiology 209 (1998) 49–56.

[229] A.N Ellepola, Laboratory diagnosis of invasive candidiasis, J. Microbiol. 43 (2005) 65–84.

[230] A. Lain, et al., Diagnosis of invasive candidiasis by enzyme-linked immunosorbent assay using the N-terminal fragment of *Candida albicans* hyphal wall protein I. BMC Microbiol. 7 (2007) 35.

[231] L. Metwally, et al., Improving molecular detection of *Candida* DNA in whole blood: comparison of seven fungal DNA extraction protocols using real-time PCR, J. Med. Microbiol. 57 (2008) 296–303.

[232] G. Naja, et al., Rapid detection of microorganisms with nanoparticles and electron microscopy, Microsc. Res. Tech. 71 (2008) 742–748.

[233] S. Fujita, et al., Evaluation of a newly developed down-flow immunoassay for detection of serum mannan antigens in patients with candidaemia, J. Med. Microbiol. 55 (2006) 537–543.

[234] A. Kedzierska, et al., Current status of fungal cell wall components in the immunodiagnostics of invasive fungal infections in humans: galactomannan, mannan and (1→3)-beta-D-glucan antigens, Eur. J. Clin. Microbiol. Infect. Dis. 26 (2007) 755–766.

[235] X.Y. Zhou, et al., Practical method for detection and identification of Candida, Aspergillus, and Scedosporium spp. by use of rolling-circle amplification, J. Clin. Microbiol. 46 (2008) 2423–2427.

[236] S. Gebert, D. Siegel, N. Wellinghausen, Rapid detection of pathogens in blood culture bottles by real-time PCR in conjunction with the pre-analytic toot MolYsis, J. Infect. 57 (2008) 307–316.

[237] A. Lau, et al., Multiplex tandem PCR: a novel platform for rapid detection and identification of fungal pathogens from blood culture specimens, J. Clin. Microbiol. 46 (2008) 3021–3027.

[238] J.M. Bliss, M. Wellington, F. Gigliotti, Antifungal pharmacotherapy for neonatal candidiasis, Semin. Perinatol. 27 (2003) 365–374.

[239] S.D. Kicklighter, Antifungal agents and fungal prophylaxis in the neonate, NeoReviews (2002) e249–e254.

[240] A. Gafter-Gvili, et al., Treatment of invasive candidal infections: systematic review and meta-analysis, Mayo Clin. Proc. 83 (2008) 1011–1021.

[241] L. Ostrosky-Zeichner, et al., Antifungal susceptibility survey of 2, 000 bloodstream *Candida* isolates in the United States, Antimicrob. Agents Chemother. 47 (2003) 3149–3154.

[242] M.G. Karlowicz, et al., Should central venous catheters be removed as soon as candidemia is detected in neonates? Pediatrics 106 (2000) e63.

[243] J.H. Rex, P.G. Pappas, A.W. Karchmer, A randomized and blinded multicenter trial of high-dose fluconazole plus placebo versus fluconazole plus amphotericin B as therapy for candidemia and its consequences in nonneutropenic subjects, Clin. Infect. Dis. 36 (2003) 1221–1228.

[244] R.G. Faix, et al., Successful medical treatment of *Candida parapsilosis* endocarditis in a premature infant, Am. J. Perinatol. 7 (1990) 272–275.

[245] D. Munz, K.R. Powell, C.H. Pai, Treatment of candidal diaper dermatitis: a double-blind placebo-controlled comparison of topical nystatin with topical plus oral nystatin, J. Pediatr. 101 (1982) 1022–1025.

[246] S. Wainer, et al., Prophylactic oral gel for the prevention of neonatal fungal rectal colonization and systemic infection, Pediatr. Infect. Dis. J. 11 (1992) 713–716.

[247] P. Concannon, et al., Diaper dermatitis: a therapeutic dilemma. Results of a double-blind placebo controlled trial of miconazole nitrate 0.25%, Pediatr. Dermatol. 18 (2001) 149–155.

[248] P.G. Pappas, et al., Guidelines for treatment of candidiasis, Clin. Infect. Dis. 38 (2004) 161–189.

[249] L.K. Pickering, Red Book, 2006 Report of the Committee on Infectious Diseases (Candidiasis), twentyseventh ed., American Academy of Pediatrics, Elk Grove Village, IL, 2006.

[250] B. Almirante, D. Rodriguez, Antifungal agents in neonates: issues and recommendations, Pediatr. Drugs. 9 (2007) 311–321.

[251] T. Zaoutis, T.J. Walsh, Antifungal therapy for neonatal candidiasis, Curr. Opin. Infect. Dis. 6 (2007) 592–597.

[252] M.A. Pfaller, et al., In vitro activities of 5-fluorocytosine against 8,803 clinical isolates of *Candida spp.*: global assessment of primary resistance using national committee for clinical laboratory standards susceptibility testing methods, Antimicrob. Agents Chemother. 46 (2002) 3518–3521.

[253] N.B. McClenny, et al., Change in colony morphology of *Candida lusitaniae* in association with development of amphotericin B resistance, Antimicrob. Agents Chemother. 46 (2002) 1325–1328.

[254] N. Linder, G. Klinger, I. Shalit, Treatment of candidaemia in premature infants: comparison of three amphotericin B preparations, J. Antimicrob. Chemother. 52 (2003) 663–667.

[255] K.M. Butler, M.A. Rench, C.J. Baker, B. Amphotericin, as a single agent in the treatment of systemic candidiasis in neonates, Pediatr. Infect. Dis. J. 9 (1990) 51–56.

[256] A.R. Kingo, J.A. Smyth, D. Waisman, Lack of evidence of amphotericin B toxicity in very low birth weight infants treated for systemic candidiasis, Pediatr. Infect. Dis. J. 16 (1997) 1002–1003.

[257] J.E. Baley, R.M. Kliegman, A.A. Fanaroff, Disseminated fungal infections in very low-birth-weight infants: therapeutic toxicity, Pediatrics 73 (1984) 153–157.

[258] E. Spath-Schwalbe, et al., Successful use of liposomal amphotericin B in a case of amphotericin B-induced nephrogenic diabetes insipidus, Clin. Infect. Dis. 28 (1999) 680–681.

[259] J. Hall, et al., Amphotericin B dosage for disseminated candidiasis in premature infants, J Perinatol. 1987 Summer;7(3):194–198.

[260] G. Serra, P. Mezzano, W. Bonacci, Therapeutic treatment of systemic candidiasis in newborns, J. Chemother. 3(Suppl. 1) (1991) 240–244.

[261] J.E. Baley, et al., Pharmacokinetics, outcome of treatment, and toxic effects of amphotericin B and 5-fluorocytosine in neonates, J. Pediatr. 116 (1990) 791–797.

[262] P.J. Chesney, R.A. Justman, W.M. Bogdanowicz, *Candida* meningitis in newborn infants-review and report of combined amphotericin B flucytosine therapy, Johns. Hopkins. Med. J. 142 (1978) 155–160.

[263] J.L. Rowen, J.M. Tate, N.C.S. Group, Management of neonatal candidiasis, Pediatr. Infect. Dis. J. 17 (1998) 1007–1011.

[264] B. Baetz-Greenwalt, B. Debaz, M.L. Kumar, Bladder fungus ball: a reversible cause of neonatal obstructive uropathy, Pediatrics 81 (1988) 826–829.

[265] A. Juster-Reicher, et al., Liposomal amphotericin B (AmBisome) in the treatment of neonatal candidiasis in very low birth weight infants, Infection 28 (2000) 223–226.

[266] F. Adler-Shohet, H. Waskin, J.M. Lieberman, Amphotericin B lipid complex for neonatal invasive candidiasis, Arch. Dis. Child. Fetal Neonatal Ed. 84 (2001) F131–F133.

[267] T.J. Walsh, et al., Amphotericin B lipid complex in pediatric patients with invasive fungal infections, Pediatr. Infect. Dis. J. 18 (1999) 702–708.

[268] B. Dupont, Overview of the lipid formulations of amphotericin B, J. Antimicrob. Chemother. 49 (2002) 31–36.

[269] P. Ferrari, et al., Favorable course of cerebral candidiasis in a low-birth weight newborn treated with liposomal amphotericin B, Pediatr. Med. Chir. 23 (2001) 197–199.

[270] H. Al Arishi, et al., Liposomal amphotericin B in neonates with invasive candidiasis, Am. J. Perinatol. 15 (1998) 643–648.

[271] A. Scarcella, et al., Liposomal amphotericin B treatment for neonatal fungal infections, Pediatr. Infect. Dis. J. 17 (1998) 146–148.

[272] J.H. Weitkamp, et al., *Candida* infection in very low birth-weight infants: outcome and nephrotoxicity of treatment with liposomal amphotericin B (AmBisome), Infection 26 (1998) 11–15.

[273] R.A. Smego, J.R. Perfect, D.T. Durack, Combined therapy with amphotericin B and 5-fluorocytosine for *Candida* meningitis, Rev. Infect. Dis. 6 (1984) 791–801.

[274] E.M. Johnson, M.D. Richardson, D.W. Warnock, In vitro resistance to imidazole antifungals in *Candida albicans*, J. Antimicrob. Chemother. 13 (1984) 547–558.

[275] V. Novelli, H. Holzel, Safety and tolerability of fluconazole in children, Antimicrob. Agents Chemother. 43 (1999) 1955–1960.

[276] M.S. Lionakis, G. Samonis, D.P. Kontoyiannis, Endocrine and metabolic manifestations of invasive fungal infections and systemic antifungal treatment, Mayo Clin. Proc. 83 (2008) 1046–1060.

[277] V. Triolo, et al., Fluconazole therapy for *Candida albicans* urinary tract infections in infants, Pediatr. Nephrol. 17 (2002) 550–553.

[278] H. Saxen, K. Hoppu, M. Pohjavuori, Pharmacokinetics of fluconazole in very low birth weight infants during the first two weeks of life, Clin. Pharmacol. Ther. 54 (1993) 269–277.

[279] T.G. Wenzl, et al., Pharmacokinetics of oral fluconazole in premature infants, Eur. J. Pediatr. 157 (1998) 661–662.

[280] S.D. Kicklighter, et al., Fluconazole for prophylaxis against candidal rectal colonization in the very low birth weight infant, Pediatrics 107 (2001) 293–298.

[281] M. Driessen, et al., Fluconazole vs. amphotericin B for the treatment of neonatal fungal septicemia: a prospective randomized trial, Pediatr. Infect. Dis. J. 15 (1996) 1107–1112.

[282] S. Wainer, et al., Prospective study of fluconazole therapy in systemic neonatal fungal infection, Pediatr. Infect. Dis. J. 16 (1997) 763–767.

[283] C. Fasano, J. O'Keeffe, D. Gibbs, Fluconazole treatment of neonates and infants with severe fungal infections not treatable with conventional agents, Eur. J. Clin. Microbiol. Infect. Dis. 13 (1994) 351–354.

[284] P. Ferrieri, D. Guse, L. Phillip, 2002–2003 Antibiotic susceptibilities at Fairview-University Medical Center, Clin Microbiol Lab Newslett 25 (2008) 1–2.

[285] M.A. Pfaller, et al., Trends in species distribution and susceptibility to fluconazole among blood stream isolates of *Candida* species in the United States, Diagn. Microbiol. Infect. Dis. 33 (1999) 217–222.

[286] J.A. Sabo, S.M. Abdel-Rahman, Voriconazole: a new triazole antifungal, Ann. Pharmacother. 34 (2000) 1032–1043.

[287] T.J. Walsh, T. Driscoll, Pharmacokinetics and safety of intravenous voriconazole in children after single- or multiple-dose administration, Antimicrob. Agents Chemother. 48 (2004) 2166–2172.

[288] T.J. Walsh, I. Lutsar, T. Driscoll, Voriconazole in the treatment of aspergillosis and other invasive fungal infections in children, Pediatr. Infect. Dis. J. 21 (2002) 240–248.

[289] F.M.C. Muller, et al., Azole cross-resistance to ketoconazole, fluconazole, itraconazole and voriconazole in clinical *Candida albicans* isolates from HIV-infected children with oropharyngeal candidosis, J. Antimicrob. Chemother. 46 (2000) 338–341.

[290] K.M. Muldrew, H.D. Maples, C.D. Stowe, Intravenous voriconazole therapy in a preterm infant, Pharmacotherapy 25 (2005) 893–898.

[291] V. Kohli, et al., Voriconazole in newborns, Indian Pediatr. 45 (2008) 236–238.

[292] E.A. Stone, H.B. Fung, H.L. Kirschenbaum, Caspofungin: an echinocandin antifungal agent, Clin. Ther. 24 (2002) 351–377.

[293] E.E. Roling, et al., Antifungal activities of fluconazole, caspofungin (MK0991), and anidulafungin (LY 303366) alone and in combination against *Candida spp.* and *Cryptococcus neoformans* via time-kill methods, Diagn. Microbiol. Infect. Dis. 43 (2002) 13–17.

[294] J. Mora-Duarte, et al., Comparison of caspofungin and amphotericin B for invasive candidiasis, N. Engl. J. Med. 347 (2002) 2020–2029.

[295] G.P. Heresi, D.R. Gerstmann, M.D. Reed, The pharmacokinetics and safety of micafungin, a novel echinocandin, in premature infants, Pediatr. Infect. Dis. J. 25 (2006) 1110–1115.

[296] C.M. Odio, et al., Caspofungin therapy of neonates with invasive candidiasis, Pediatr. Infect. Dis. J. 23 (2004) 1093–1097.

[297] M. Yalaz, M. Akisu, S. Hilmiogul, Successful caspofungin treatment of multidrug resistant *Candida parapsilosis* septicaemia in an extremely low birth weight neonate, Mycoses 49 (2006) 242–245.

[298] N. Belet, et al., Caspofungin treatment in two infants with persistent fungaemia due to *Candida lipolytica*, Scand. J. Infect. Dis. 38 (2006) 559–562.

[299] S. Manzar, M. Kamat, S. Pyati, Caspofungin for refractory candidemia in neonates, Pediatr. Infect. Dis. J. 25 (2006) 282–283.

[300] X. Saez-Llorens, et al., Pharmacokinetics and safety of caspofungin in neonates and infants less than 3 months of age, Antimicrob. Agents Chemother. 53 (2008) 869–875.

[301] L. Ostrosky-Zeichner, D.P. Kontoyiannis, J. Raffalli, International, open-label, noncomparative, clinical trial of micafungin alone and in combination for treatment of newly diagnosed and refractory candidemia, Eur. J. Clin. Microbiol. Infect. Dis. 24 (2005) 654–661.

[302] T. Lehrnbecher, A.H. Groll, Experiences with the use of caspofungin in paediatric patients, Mycoses 51 (2008) 58–64.

[303] H.W. Boucher, et al., Newer systemic antifungal agents: pharmacokinetics, safety and efficacy, Drugs 64 (2004) 1997–2020.

[304] S. Friedman, S.E. Richardson, K. O'Brien, Systemic *Candida* infection in extremely low birth weight infants: short term morbidity and long term neurodevelopmental outcome, Pediatr. Infect. Dis. J. 19 (2000) 499–504.

[305] M.G. Karlowicz, et al., Should central venous catheters be removed as soon as candidemia is detected in neonates? Pediatrics 106 (2000) e63.

[306] J.H. Rex, et al., Practice guidelines for the treatment of candidiasis, Clin. Infect. Dis. 30 (2000) 662–678.

[307] L. Saiman, et al., Risk factors for *Candida* species colonization of neonatal intensive care unit patients, Pediatr. Infect. Dis. J. 20 (2001) 1119–1124.

[308] Y.C. Huang, et al., Outbreak of *Candida parapsilosis* fungemia in neonatal intensive care units: clinical implications and genotyping analysis, Infection 27 (1999) 97–102.

[309] E. Larson, et al., Assessment of alternative hand hygiene regimens to improve skin health among neonatal intensive care unit nurses, Heart Lung 29 (2000) 136–142.

[310] J.R. Campbell, E. Zaccaria, C.J. Baker, Systemic candidiasis in extremely low birth weight infants receiving topical petrolatum ointment for skin care: a case-control study, Pediatrics 105 (2000) 1041–1045.

[311] M.A. Ozturk, et al., Oral nystatin prophylaxis to prevent invasive candidiasis in neonatal intensive care unit, Mycoses 6 (2006) 484–492.

[312] D. Isaacs, Fungal prophylaxis in very low birth weight neonates: nystatin, fluconazole or nothing? Curr. Opin. Infect. Dis. 3 (2008) 246–250.

[313] M.E. Sims, Y. Yun, H. You, Prophylactic oral nystatin and fungal infections in very-low-birthweight infants, Am. J. Perinatol. 5 (1988) 33–36.

[314] D.A. Kaufman, Fluconazole prophylaxis: can we eliminate invasive *Candida* infections in the neonatal ICU? Curr. Opin. Pediatr. 20 (2008) 332–340.

[315] C.M. Healy, C.J. Baker, Fluconazole prophylaxis in the neonatal intensive care unit, Pediatr Infect Dis J. 2009 Jan;28(1):49–52.

[316] P. Manzoni, et al., A multicenter, randomized trial of prophylactic fluconazole in preterm neonates, N. Engl. J. Med. 356 (2007) 2483–2495.

[317] C. Cabrera, M. Frank, D. Carter, Fluconazole prophylaxis against systemic candidiasis after colonization: a randomized, double blinded study, J. Perinatol. 22 (2002) 603.

[318] S.L. Long, D.K. Stevenson, Reducing *Candida* infections during neonatal intensive care: management choices, infection control, and fluconazole prophylaxis, J. Pediatr. 147 (2005) 896–900.

[319] J.H. Weitkamp, et al., Fluconazole prophylaxis for prevention of invasive fungal infections in targeted highest risk preterm infants limits drug exposure, J. Perinatol. 28 (2008) 405–411.

[320] J.H. Rex, M.G. Rinaldi, M.A. Pfaller, Resistance of *Candida* species to fluconazole, Antimicrob. Agents Chemother. 39 (1995) 1–8.

[321] P. Manzoni, et al., Routine use of fluconazole prophylaxis in a neonatal intensive care unit does not select natively fluconazole-resistant *Candida* subspecies, Pediatr. Infect. Dis. J. 27 (2008) 731–737.

CHAPTER OUTLINE

Pneumocystis jiroveci (Formerly Known as *Pneumocystis carinii*)
Infection   1079
   History   1079
   The Organism   1080
   Epidemiology and Transmission   1081
   Pathology   1085
   Pathogenesis   1086
   Clinical Manifestations   1088
   Diagnosis   1090
   Treatment   1092
   Prognosis   1093
   Prevention   1094
Aspergillosis   1095
   The Organism   1095
   Epidemiology and Transmission   1095
   Pathogenesis   1096
   Pathology   1096
   Clinical Manifestations   1096
   Diagnosis and Differential Diagnosis   1097
   Therapy   1097
   Prognosis   1098
   Prevention   1098
Blastomycosis   1098
   The Organism   1098
   Epidemiology and Transmission   1098
   Pathology   1098
   Clinical Manifestations   1099
   Diagnosis and Differential Diagnosis   1099
   Therapy   1099
   Prognosis   1099
   Prevention   1099
Coccidioidomycosis   1099
   The Organism   1100
   Epidemiology and Transmission   1100
   Pathogenesis   1100
   Pathology   1101
   Clinical Manifestations   1101
   Diagnosis and Differential Diagnosis   1101
   Therapy   1102
   Prognosis   1102
   Prevention   1102

Cryptococcosis   1103
   The Organism   1103
   Epidemiology and Transmission   1103
   Pathogenesis   1104
   Pathology   1104
   Clinical Manifestations   1104
   Diagnosis and Differential Diagnosis   1105
   Therapy   1105
   Prognosis   1105
   Prevention   1105
Malassezia Infections   1105
   The Organism   1106
   Epidemiology and Transmission   1106
   Pathogenesis   1106
   Clinical Manifestations   1106
   Diagnosis   1106
   Therapy   1107
   Prognosis   1107
   Prevention   1107
Phycomycosis   1107
   The Organism   1107
   Epidemiology and Transmission   1108
   Pathogenesis   1108
   Pathology   1108
   Clinical Manifestations   1108
   Diagnosis and Differential Diagnosis   1108
   Therapy   1109
   Prognosis   1109
   Prevention   1109
Dermatophytoses   1109
   The Organism   1109
   Epidemiology and Transmission   1109
   Pathogenesis   1110
   Pathology   1110
   Clinical Manifestations   1110
   Diagnosis and Differential Diagnosis   1111
   Therapy   1111
   Prognosis   1111
   Prevention   1112
Antifungal Therapy in Neonates and Young Infants   1112

Fungal infections, other than those caused by *Candida* species, rarely are considered in the differential diagnosis for an acutely ill newborn infant because disorders of bacterial and viral etiology are vastly more common. Nevertheless, fungal infections do occur in neonates, especially in premature infants and those of very low birth weight (less than 1500 g), and can cause serious and frequently fatal disease. The number of cases of invasive infection attributed to fungi among all patients in the United States quadrupled between 1990 and 2000. With advances in neonatal care, the epidemiology of fungal infections in the neonatal intensive care unit (NICU) has changed dramatically, with an estimated tenfold increase in the past decade. As with any other infectious disease, the risk of fungal infection depends on the host and risk of exposure. The neonate has some risk of exposure to either *Malassezia furfur* or *Pneumocystis jiroveci* (previously *Pneumocystis carinii*, classified as a fungus on the basis of DNA sequence analysis), has a limited risk of exposure to *Aspergillus* species, and has an extremely low risk of exposure to other fungi—especially in the NICU setting. Therefore, it is not surprising that the most common fungal infection in neonates is candidiasis, followed by infections with *P. jiroveci* and *M. furfur*, whereas case reports or small series constitute the literature on aspergillosis and other fungal infections.

Mycotic infections, whether confined to epidermal structures or involving deep tissues, are caused by fungi free-living in soil or present in bird or mammal excreta or in decaying organic matter. In instances of fungal infection in newborns, organisms most often are acquired in utero through the hematogenous route, from the mother during birth, or from the environment on postnatal exposure. When inhaled, ingested, or inoculated directly into tissue, these saprophytic micro-organisms can cause infection after birth in infants with undue susceptibility. Although much has been learned regarding the pathogenesis, immune response, and treatment of fungal infections in older children and adults, studies to determine the cause of increased susceptibility or resistance to infection with fungi, especially in neonates, are incomplete. Limited published studies that prophylactic antifungal therapy of hospitalized high risk neonates, primarily with fluconazole, may decrease the rate of systemic fungal infections. In these studies the primary outcome has generally been the prevention of systemic candidiasis [1]. Advances have been made in the diagnosis and treatment of neonatal fungal infections, however.

PNEUMOCYSTIS JIROVECI (FORMERLY KNOWN AS PNEUMOCYSTIS CARINII) INFECTION

P. jiroveci, a fungus with a history of unsettled taxonomy, was discovered in the lungs of small mammals and humans in Brazil more than 80 years ago. Today it is a cause of often fatal pneumonia in patients with immunodeficiencies, hematologic malignancy, collagen-vascular disorders, or organ allografts and in those who receive corticosteroids and immunosuppressive drug therapy. Although congenital or neonatal infection with *Pneumocystis* is uncommon, it can occur in infants younger than 1 year of age in two well-defined epidemiologic settings: (1) in epidemics in nurseries located in impoverished areas of the world and (2) in isolated cases in which the infected child has an underlying primary immunodeficiency disease [2] or acquired immunodeficiency syndrome (AIDS).

This section of the chapter reviews the problem of *Pneumocystis* infection in the newborn. Much of our knowledge of the epidemiologic, pathologic, and clinical features of pneumocystosis, however, is drawn from observations of the infection in older children and adults.

As a result, we have elected to include data derived from such observations to present a more complete picture of the infectious process caused by this unique organism.

HISTORY

In 1909, Chagas [3] in Brazil first described the morphologic forms of *Pneumocystis* in the lungs of guinea pigs infected with *Trypanosoma cruzi*. He believed the forms to represent a sexual stage in the life cycle of the trypanosome and not a different organism. Carini [4], an Italian working in Brazil, saw the same organism-like cysts in the lungs of rats experimentally infected with *Trypanosoma lewisi*. His slide material subsequently was reviewed by the Delanoës and their colleagues [5] at the Pasteur Institute in Paris. They recognized that these alveolar cysts were present in the lungs of local Parisian sewer rats and thereby established that the "organisms" were independent of trypanosomes. They proposed the name *P. carinii* for the new species.

At about this time, Chagas may have unwittingly described the first human case of pneumocystosis when he reported the presence of similar organisms in the lungs of a patient with interstitial pneumonia who had died of American trypanosomiasis [6]. Nevertheless, no definite etiologic connection was made between *P. carinii* and human pneumonic disease for another 30 years. The reason for this delay was the belief during this period that infantile syphilis was responsible for virtually all instances of interstitial plasma cell pneumonia. In 1938, Benecke [7] and Ammich [8] identified a histologically similar pneumonic illness in nonsyphilitic children that was characterized by a peculiar honeycombed exudate in alveoli. Subsequent scrutiny of photomicrographs in their reports revealed the presence of *P. carinii* organisms [9], but it was not until 1942 that Van der Meer and Brug [10] in the Netherlands unequivocally recognized the organism in lungs from two infants and one adult. The first epidemics of interstitial plasma cell pneumonia were reported shortly thereafter among premature debilitated babies in nurseries and foundling homes in central Europe. In 1952 Vanek and Jirovec [9] in Czechoslovakia provided the most convincing demonstration of the etiologic relationship of *P. carinii* to this disease in an autopsy study of 16 cases.

Pneumocystosis was first brought to the attention of pediatricians in the United States in 1953 by Deamer and Zollinger [11], who reviewed the pathologic and epidemiologic features of the European disease. Lunseth and associates [12] generally are credited for the initial case report of interstitial plasma cell pneumonia occurring in an infant born in the United States. Curiously, the latter authors neither identified *Pneumocystis* organisms in their histologic sections nor even alluded to the organism in their discussion of causation of the disease. During the next year, the presence of *Pneumocystis* pneumonia in the United States was documented in several published studies [13–15].

In 1957 Gajdusek [16] presented an in-depth perspective on the history of the infection that included an extensive bibliography. This review was particularly timely because the next decade was to see the disturbing emergence of *P. carinii* pneumonia in the Western world—even while the epidemic disease in central Europe was waning—to the degree that it would become pre-eminent among the so-called opportunistic pulmonary infections in the immunosuppressed host. In 1988, DNA analysis demonstrated that *Pneumocystis* was not a protozoan but a fungus [17,18]. Subsequent DNA analysis has led to the change in nomenclature from *P. carinii* to *P. jiroveci*, a name chosen in honor of the parasitologist Otto Jirovec, who now is credited by some with the original description of this organism [19,20].

THE ORGANISM

The precise taxonomic status of *P. jiroveci* as a fungus has been defined on the basis of molecular analysis [17,18]. Because the organism has only recently been propagated in vitro, efforts to classify it and to elucidate its structure and life cycle have been based exclusively on morphologic observations of infected lungs from animals and humans. The earliest of these investigations was performed by parasitologists; accordingly, the terminology applied to the forms of *Pneumocystis* seen in diseased tissue has been that reserved for protozoal organisms.

Three developmental forms of this presumably unicellular microbe [21] have been described: a thick-walled cyst, an intracystic sporozoite, and a thin-walled trophozoite [4,22,23]. The form of *Pneumocystis* that assists with diagnosis is the cyst, which may contain up to eight sporozoites. Each sporozoite is round to crescent shaped, measures 1 to 2 μm in diameter, and contains an eccentric nucleus. This cystic unit with its intracystic bodies is seen well in Giemsa-stained imprint smears of infected fresh lung [16,24]. Giemsa stain, however, results in staining of background alveoli and host cell fragments and does not stain empty cysts. Gomori methenamine silver stain, which highlights only the cyst wall of *Pneumocystis*, is preferable to Giemsa stain when tissues must be screened for the presence of organisms [25–27]. The cysts stained with silver have a thin, often wrinkled black capsule that may be round, crescentic, or disk shaped. Cysts measure 4 to 6 μm in diameter and must be distinguished from erythrocytes. The cysts often occur in clusters within an alveolus.

The typical honeycombed intra-alveolar exudate of *Pneumocystis* pneumonia is largely a collection of interlocking cysts whose walls flatten at points of contact, so that each cyst assumes a hexagonal shape. The internal structure of the silver-stained cyst is variable. In the lighter staining round cysts, a pair of structures about 1 μm long resembling opposed commas or parentheses often are seen; these occasionally are connected end to end by thin, delicate strands [25]. Other cysts contain only a marginal nodule (Fig. 34–1). Whether these intracystic details correspond to the sporozoite-like bodies seen in Giemsa-stained preparations is not clear. Evidence from both light and electron microscopy, however, suggests that they may not be located within cyst cytoplasm at all; instead, they may be thickened portions of the cyst wall [28–30].

Staining procedures, other than those using Giemsa and methenamine silver, have been employed less frequently to delineate the cyst form of the organism. The cyst wall stains red with periodic acid-Schiff stain [31].

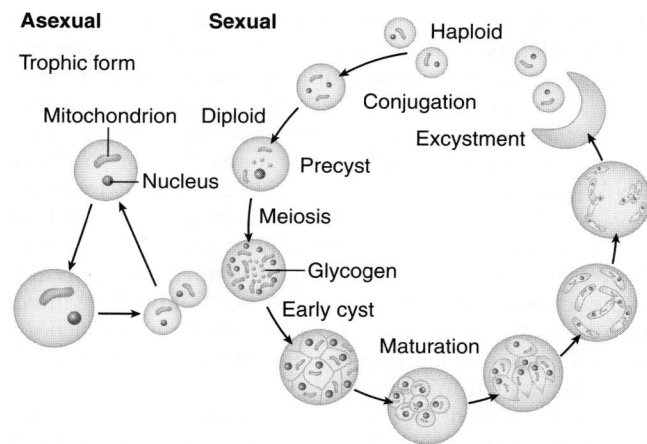

FIGURE 34–1 Imprint smear of fresh lung tissue stained with methenamine silver shows a cluster of cysts of *Pneumocystis jiroveci*. Typical comma-shaped bodies and marginal nodules are visible within cysts ∞625. *(From Ruskin J, Remington JS. The compromised host and infection. JAMA 202:1070, 1967.)*

A modified Gram-Weigert method stains both the cyst wall and the intracystic sporozoites [32]. Gridley fungus stain may identify cyst outlines. More reliable stains for this purpose are the modified toluidine blue stain of Chalvardjian and Grawe [33] and the crystal violet stain [34], which color the cyst wall purple. Electron microscopy has been an invaluable tool in morphologic studies of *P. jiroveci* [22,29,35–43]. It has helped to confirm that the structures regarded as *Pneumocystis* under light microscopy are, in fact, typical micro-organisms and not just degradation products of host cells [44].

Both trophozoite and cystlike stages have been delineated [43]. The trophozoite is thin walled and measures between 1.5 and 2.0 μm in diameter. It has numerous evaginations or pseudopodia-like projections that appear to interdigitate with those of other organisms in the alveolar space [38,43]. It has been postulated that the pseudopodia make up the reticular framework within which organisms reside in an alveolus, accounting for the fact that organisms remain clumped in lung imprints [24,33]. It also has been suggested that the pseudopodia anchor *Pneumocystis* to the alveolar septal wall [41]. The prevailing opinion, however, is that no specialized organelle of attachment exists. Rather, the surfaces of *P. jiroveci* and alveolar cells (specifically, type I pneumonocytes) are closely opposed, without fusion of cell membranes [45]. This adherence of *P. jiroveci* to alveolar lining cells may explain why organisms are not commonly found in expectorated mucus or tracheal secretions [38].

The classic cystic unit of *P. jiroveci* is thick walled and measures 4 to 6 μm in diameter. The intracystic bodies measure 1.0 to 1.7 μm across and bear a marked similarity to small trophozoites (Figure 34–2) [43]. In addition, thick-walled cysts rich in glycogen particles but without intracystic bodies ("precysts"), partly empty cysts, and collapsed cystic structures have been identified. The collapsed cysts are crescentic and presumably are the same crescentic forms seen frequently in silver-stained specimens under light microscopy. They commonly have defects in their walls.

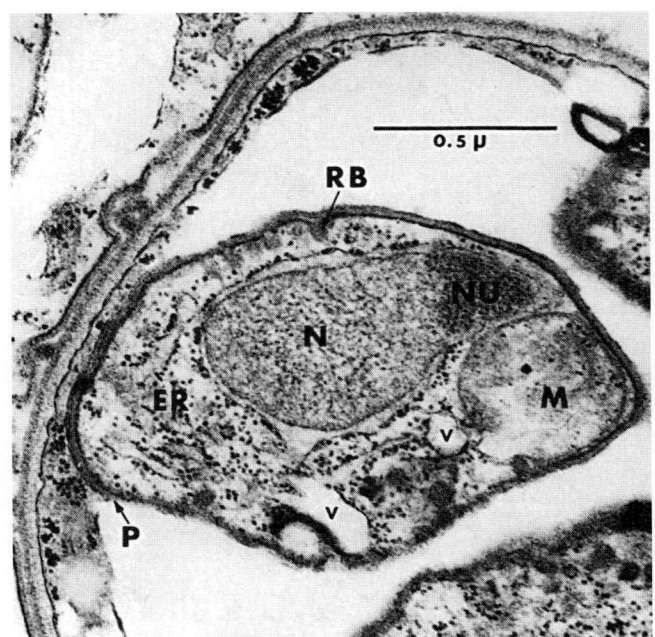

FIGURE 34–2 Intracystic body within mature cyst. Six-layer effect of cyst wall occurs only where there is contact with adjacent organisms. Note unit-membrane character of undulating membranes that form innermost layer of cyst wall and outer and inner membranes of pellicle (P). Round bodies (RB) appear to arise from pellicle (*arrow*). Rough endoplasmic reticulum (ER) is well developed. Ribosomes are attached to the external membrane of nucleus, and this membrane appears to communicate with membranes of rough endoplasmic reticulum. Cytoplasm also contains vacuoles (v). Nucleus (N) contains nucleolus (NU). Mitochondrion (M) is at the right. ×80,000. *(From Campbell WG Jr. Ultrastructure of* Pneumocystis *in human lung. Life cycle in human pneumocystosis. Arch Pathol 93:312, 1972.)*

Life cycles for *P. jiroveci* have been proposed. They have been based on the variant forms of the fungus detected by light [29,30,46–48] and electron microscopy [43,49]. One scheme suggests that the thick-walled round cyst undergoes dissolution or "cracking," whereupon the intracystic bodies pass through tears in the wall (Figure 34–3) [43]. It is not known whether the bodies escape from the cyst by active motility or whether they are extruded passively as a consequence of cyst collapse. At this stage, the intracystic bodies resemble free thin-walled trophozoites. It had been suggested that division of the intracystic body must occur soon after its expulsion from the mature, thick-walled cyst, to account for the large numbers of small trophozoites (1 μm in diameter) seen in the infected lung [29]. Electron microscopic observations, however, indicate that another source for the smaller trophozoite is the immature, thin-walled *Pneumocystis* cyst [49]. In any case, the small trophozoites evolve to larger forms, their walls thicken, and a precyst develops that is devoid of intracystic bodies. The cyclic process is completed when formation of the mature cyst, containing eight daughter cysts, is achieved.

Previous controversy over the classification of *Pneumocystis* as a protozoan [50,51] or as a fungus [52] resulted because of the difficulty in cultivating and further characterizing the biochemical nature of the organism. Arguments in favor of a protozoan taxonomy were based

mainly on the resemblance of its structural features to those of other protozoa. The organism has cystic and trophozoite stages, pseudopodia in cell walls, and pellicles around intracystic sporozoites [41,53]. In addition, the disease caused by *Pneumocystis* responds to antiprotozoal—namely, antitrypanosomal or antitoxoplasmal—chemotherapy. On the other hand, like fungi, *P. jiroveci* contains a paucity of cellular organelles, its nucleus is not visibly prominent, its cell membrane is layered throughout an entire life cycle, and its cell wall stains vividly with silver [29].

The question of species specificity of *Pneumocystis* remained similarly unanswered until recent polymerase chain reaction (PCR) techniques established that *P. jiroveci* is not found in lung samples from any other mammals [53]. Although most workers concur that human and rodent forms of the organism are morphologically indistinguishable by light and electron microscopy [22,30,43], serologic studies designed to demonstrate identity between human and animal species [28,50] or even between human strains from diverse geographic locales [54,55] yield conflicting results. Genetic analysis, however, clearly demonstrated differences between human and nonhuman *Pneumocystis* isolates [53,56–59].

Successful propagation of *P. jiroveci* in vitro was first reported in 1977 by Pifer and colleagues [60] at the St. Jude Children's Research Hospital. This group of investigators serially passed organisms in primary embryonic chick epithelial lung cells over 12 days and noted a 100-fold increase in the number of cysts. Inoculation of trophozoites alone yielded modest numbers of cyst forms, with typical cytopathogenic effects. Continuing cultivation of *Pneumocystis*, however, was not achieved. In addition, the organisms could not be grown in cell-free media employed commonly for the propagation of other organisms [60]. Limited replication of *Pneumocystis* since has been accomplished in more widely available tissue culture cell lines (Vero, Chang liver, MRC 5, WI 38) [61–64]. These tissue culture systems have not been used to isolate *P. jiroveci* from the lungs of animals or humans with suspected infection. Examination of the organism in tissue culture, however, has confirmed the existence of each of its morphologic forms and has provided insight into the biologic interaction between the organism and the host cells [64].

EPIDEMIOLOGY AND TRANSMISSION

The natural habitat of *P. jiroveci* is unknown. The distribution of human infection is worldwide [65–90], and a variety of wild and domestic animal species harbor the organism without demonstrable pulmonary disease. Rarely, clinically evident *Pneumocystis* pneumonitis, not unlike the disease in humans, arises spontaneously in the animal host [91–96].

The prevalence of infection with *Pneumocystis* remains to be determined because studies to detect latent carriage of the organism in large populations have not been performed. Serologic surveys, however, indicate that infection is widespread and acquired in early life. Meuwissen and colleagues [97] in the Netherlands noted that immunofluorescent antibodies to *P. jiroveci* are first detectable in

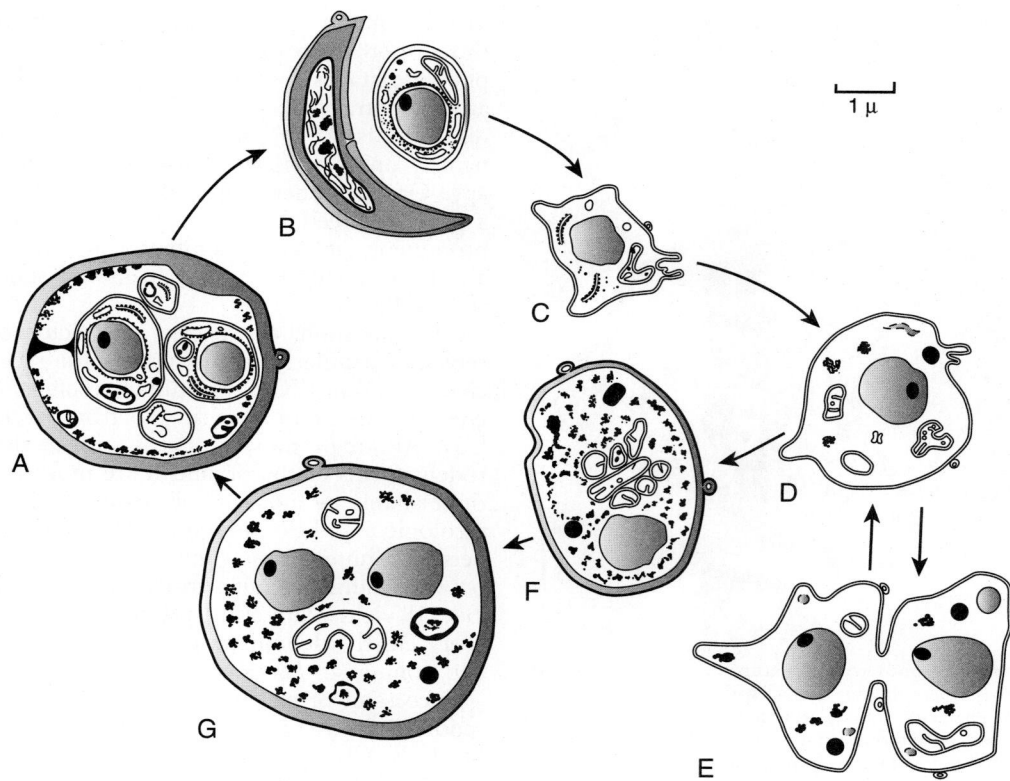

FIGURE 34–3 **Probable life cycle of *Pneumocystis* within pulmonary alveoli. A,** Mature cyst with intracystic bodies; **B,** empty cyst and recently escaped intracystic body; **C,** small trophozoite; **D,** larger trophozoite; **E,** possible budding or conjugating form; **F,** large trophozoite undergoing thickening of pellicle; **G,** precyst. *(From Campbell WG Jr. Ultrastructure of* Pneumocystis *in human lung. Life cycle in human pneumocystosis. Arch Pathol 93:312, 1972.)*

healthy children at 6 months of age, and by age 4 years, nearly all children are seropositive. Pifer and associates [98] in the United States found significant titers of antibody to *Pneumocystis* in healthy 7-month-old infants and in two thirds of normal children by age 4 years. Gerrard and coworkers [99] in England detected *P. jiroveci* antibodies in serum from 48% of 94 young healthy children. Pifer and associates [100] also found that serologic evidence of *Pneumocystis* infection is present before immunosuppressive therapy with corticosteroids elicits *Pneumocystis* pneumonia in healthy rats. Authors of a number of autopsy reviews have attempted to determine the incidence of *Pneumocystis* infection, but the results have been divergent, owing to the heterogeneity of the populations studied [87,101–107]. Those studies conducted in central Europe after World War II [102] or in cancer referral centers in the United States [107] have yielded higher rates of infection.

Few published reports have been devoted exclusively to the descriptive epidemiology of *Pneumocystis* pneumonia in the United States. In a literature review of the subject, Le Clair [108] accumulated 107 accounts of the disease recorded from 1955 through 1967. The male-to-female ratio of infected persons was in excess of 2:1, but ethnic distribution was even. The disease was reported from diverse geographic locales (21 of the 50 states). The largest number of cases (33) occurred in infants younger than 1 year of age. Proved or presumptive congenital

immunodeficiencies were identifiable in virtually all of the children in this group. In patients 1 to 10 years of age, who constituted the next largest group (26), only six had a primary immune deficit, whereas most of the other children had an underlying hematologic malignancy. The remaining patients, ranging in age from 10 to 81 years, were persons with assorted malignancies or renal allografts who almost always had had prior exposure to corticosteroids, radiation, or cytotoxic drugs. The mortality rate for the entire group of patients was 95%.

The Centers for Disease Control and Prevention (CDC) updated Le Clair's study by investigating the epidemiologic, clinical, and diagnostic aspects of all confirmed cases of pneumocystosis reported to its Parasitic Disease Drug Service between 1967 and 1970 [109,110]. The first of these reports has particular relevance because it focused only on the infectious episodes in infants and young children [109]. A total of 194 documented cases of *P. jiroveci* pneumonia were analyzed, and 29 occurred in infants younger than 1 year of age. The attack rate for this group (8.4 per million) was more than five times higher than that for other age groups. Eighty-three percent of these infants had an underlying primary immunodeficiency disease. Moreover, because the inheritance of the primary immunodeficiency state often was sex linked, the preponderance of infection (88%) occurred in males. The mean age at diagnosis in the immunodeficient infants was 7.5 months, whereas the epidemic form of the infection in European and Asian infants was associated with peak morbidity in the third and fourth months of life [16,24]. Twenty-four percent of the infected children with immunodeficiencies had at least one sibling with an identifiable immune deficiency in whom *P. jiroveci* pneumonia also developed [109].

After this analysis of cases indigenous to the United States was complete, it became evident that infantile pneumocystosis could be introduced into the United States from epidemics abroad. The first such case was reported in 1966 when a 3-month-old Korean infant died of *Pneumocystis* infection after being brought to the United States from an orphanage in Korea [111]. The potential for imported pneumocystosis received renewed publicity with the cessation of the war in Vietnam. Surveillance for *Pneumocystis* infection in American-adopted Vietnamese orphans was urged when it was recognized that large numbers of infants exposed to the hardships of war and malnutrition in Indochina had experienced fulminant *Pneumocystis* pneumonia [112,113]. In quick succession, multiple cases of *Pneumocystis* infection among these refugee Vietnamese were reported [114–117]. Most of the affected infants were approximately 3 months of age; this was exactly the age at which pneumocystosis had emerged in the marasmic children infected during the earlier nursery epidemics in central Europe and Asia.

The epidemiology of *P. jiroveci* infection has changed as cases of human immunodeficiency virus (HIV) infection have occurred in infants [118]. As is true in adults with acquired immunodeficiency syndrome (AIDS), infants with AIDS are at high risk for this opportunistic infection. Among children with perinatally acquired HIV infection, *P. jiroveci* pneumonitis occurs most often among infants 3 to 6 months of age [119].

It has been suggested [120–124] that *P. jiroveci* may be an important cause of pneumonitis in immunologically intact infants. In a prospective study of infant pneumonia, Stagno and coworkers [124] detected *Pneumocystis* antigenemia in 10 (14%) of 67 infants. None of these 10 infants with serologic evidence of *Pneumocystis* infection had a primary immunodeficiency, nor had any received immunosuppressive medication. Antigenemia did not occur in control infants or in infants with pneumonitis caused by *Chlamydia trachomatis*, respiratory syncytial virus, cytomegalovirus, adenovirus, or influenza A and B viruses. Histopathologic confirmation of *Pneumocystis* pneumonia was possible in the only one of these infants who underwent open lung biopsy. *P. jiroveci* also causes pneumonia in infants living in resource-limited countries, even when the child is not malnourished. Shann and associates [125] found *P. jiroveci* antigen in serum from 23 of 94 children in Papua New Guinea, who were hospitalized with pneumonia. Nevertheless, more cases need to be confirmed histologically before it is established that *Pneumocystis* infection produces morbidity in previously healthy infants.

The mode of transmission of *P. jiroveci* remains unclear. Sporadic cases of pneumocystosis serve as poor models of infection transmission because they may not become clinically manifest until long after the host has acquired the organism. That person-to-person spread of *Pneumocystis* could occur was first suggested by the European nursery epidemics. Even in these institutional outbreaks,

however, it was readily appreciated that direct interpatient transfer of the organism happened rarely [16]. Rather, seroepidemiologic investigation indicated that healthy, subclinically infected nursery personnel transmitted the infection [46,54,55]. The mode of spread of *Pneumocystis* from infected asymptomatic persons to susceptible infants in the closed nursery environment is not known. Airborne droplet transmission was suspected when "sterilization of air with ionizing radiation [126]" and isolation of uninfected infants from infected infants and their seropositive attendants [127] reduced the frequency of clinical disease. The hypothesis that *Pneumocystis* is transmissible through the air presupposes that the organism can be found in respiratory secretions. Although, as emphasized earlier, the intra-alveolar histopathologic features of pneumocystosis mitigate against this occurrence, *Pneumocystis* occasionally is detected in tracheal aspirates and sputum [32,47,128–132].

Epidemiologic investigation of sporadic pneumocystosis indicates that person-to-person transmission of the infection is possible. The sequential development of *Pneumocystis* pneumonia in immunosuppressed adults occupying adjoining hospital beds has been recorded [132,133]. Jacobs and associates [134] described a cluster of cases of *P. jiroveci* pneumonia in previously healthy adults who all were hospitalized between July and October 1989. Whereas all five patients were on different floors of this hospital on three different services, two of the patients were briefly in the intensive care unit at the same time. Immunologic evaluation in three of the five patients revealed normal CD4+, CD8+, and CD4+/CD8+ ratios but depressed responses to T-cell lectin phytohemagglutinin and T cell-dependent B-cell pokeweed mitogen. Occurrence of pneumocystosis among family members also has been reported [121,135,136]. Pneumonia developed in three family members in a strikingly related time sequence [121]. More commonly, cases within a family emerge over a period of several years, and affected members almost always are infant siblings with either proven or suspected underlying immunodeficiencies. In at least three family studies, no fewer than three siblings succumbed to the infection [135,137,138]. It is unlikely, however, that direct patient-to-patient transfer of the organism occurred in any of these settings because in almost all instances, development of disease in the sibling occurred months or years later, often long after the death of the initially infected child [109].

Contagion could still be implicated in the family milieu if a reservoir of asymptomatic infection with *P. jiroveci* existed among healthy family members. Supporting evidence comes from two published accounts of infants with primary immunodeficiencies and pneumocystosis: The parents were deemed to be possible sources of the infection because their sera contained specific anti-*Pneumocystis* antibody [138,139].

Maternal transfer of *Pneumocystis* to infants from colostrum or from the genital tract at parturition also might maintain *Pneumocystis* within a family, but screening of breast milk [136] and cervical secretions [137] with Giemsa and methenamine silver stains has failed to reveal the presence of the organism. Alternatively, acquisition of *P. jiroveci* by infants in utero could occur. Unfortunately, it is difficult to test this hypothesis in the absence of reliable serologic tools to detect subclinical infection in the newborn. The paucity of documented cases of overt *Pneumocystis* pneumonia in stillborn infants or in the early neonatal period, however, argues against frequent intrauterine passage of the organism.

In 1962 Pavlica [140], in Czechoslovakia, recorded the first instance of congenital infection. The infant described was stillborn. The parents and a female sibling were in good health. The mother's serum had complement-fixing antibodies against *Pneumocystis*. Subsequently, in a report detailing experience with *Pneumocystis* infection in southern Iran, a male child who had died at 2 days of age was described; autopsy examination revealed scattered although definite alveolar foci of typical *Pneumocystis* infection [141]. The authors reasoned that this represented congenital infection rather than an acquired disease with an untenably short incubation period. Bazaz and colleagues [137] in the United States described the striking development of *Pneumocystis* pneumonia in three otherwise healthy female siblings who died at 3 months, 2 months, and 3 days of age, respectively; again, an in utero source for their infections was considered to be most likely. In none of these cases of presumptive congenital pneumocystosis, however, was the placenta examined histologically for the presence of the organism. One infant, born to a mother with AIDS and documented *P. jiroveci* pneumonia in the fourth month of gestation, did not have *P. jiroveci* infection in the newborn period [142]. Beach and coworkers [143] described an HIV-positive newborn with meconium aspiration and pneumonia who had *P. jiroveci* identified in lung biopsy material at 19 days of age. Despite the infant's positive HIV status, serum from the infant's mother was HIV negative, and the serum from the father was HIV positive. Because the parents disappeared shortly after the infant's birth, follow-up evaluation was not possible; however, the parents had no previous history of *P. jiroveci* pneumonia, and the mother had been noted to be markedly wasted.

The mode of transmission of *Pneumocystis* in older children was first explored in the United States at the University of Minnesota Hospitals [144] and at St. Jude Children's Research Hospital [107], where an unusually high number of cases was recorded. At neither center was it possible to reconstruct the spread of pneumocystosis from one patient to another. In most cases, the onset of illness appeared to antedate admission to the hospital. No attempt was made to incriminate healthy carriers as point sources for seemingly isolated episodes of infection. At Memorial Hospital in New York, *Pneumocystis* pneumonia developed in 11 patients, including 6 children, over a 3-month period [145]. Although no definite evidence of communicability could be discerned in this statistically significant cluster of cases, several of the *Pneumocystis*-infected children had had contact with each other and had shared rooms at various times; in addition, results of serologic tests for *Pneumocystis* infection were positive in two physicians caring for these patients. Similar outbreaks have since occurred in two pediatric hospitals in Indianapolis [146] and Milwaukee, Wis [147]. At these centers, the increased rates of pneumocystosis were

clearly related, as they were at St. Jude Children's Research Hospital [107,148], to the use of more intensive cancer chemotherapy regimens. In a seroepidemiologic investigation of the cases in the Indianapolis outbreak, however, it was found that transmission of *Pneumocystis* probably occurred within the hospital environment. A direct association was noted between duration of hospitalization and risk of subsequent *Pneumocystis* infection. Furthermore, a significantly higher prevalence of positive results on serologic testing for *Pneumocystis* was detected among staff members who had close contact with infected children than among personnel whose duties did not include such patient contact. Precisely how *Pneumocystis* was originally introduced into the hospital was not determined.

The possibility that *Pneumocystis* pneumonia is a zoonotic disease and that infestation of rodents or even domesticated pets could provide a sizable reservoir for human infection has been investigated to a limited degree. Abundant infection of rodents with *Pneumocystis* was discovered in patients' homes in many of the index cases in ward epidemics in Czechoslovakia [149]. At St. Jude Children's Research Hospital, a high rate of exposure to pets was noted among the *Pneumocystis*-infected children with malignancy [150]. Of course, these findings would have epidemiologic significance only if the species of *Pneumocystis* infecting both animals and humans was the same. This remains to be shown. Experimental attempts to produce clinical pneumocystosis in multiple animal species by inoculation of infected human lung suspensions have not been successful [151–153] unless the animal was congenitally athymic [154] or immunosuppressed by treatment with corticosteroids [155].

Airborne transmission of *Pneumocystis* was first presumptively demonstrated by Hendley and Weller in 1971 [153]. These investigators observed that in cesarean section-obtained, barrier-sustained (COBS) rats given corticosteroids, infections with *Pneumocystis* developed following exposure to a common air supply from standard infected rats, whereas control COBS animals that received corticosteroids remained free of infection. One potential flaw in this experimental design was that the corticosteroid therapy could have reactivated previously latent *Pneumocystis* infection in any of the challenged animals. To circumvent this problem, Walzer and coworkers [151] challenged congenitally athymic (nude) mice. These animals received no exogenous immunosuppressants and still contracted pneumocystosis after exposure to air from infected rats. Thus, these studies documented airborne transmission of *P. jiroveci* and spread of the organism between different animal species. Of note is that soon after these experiments were published, a natural epizootic of *Pneumocystis* pneumonia was uncovered in a colony of nude mice [154]. Other studies using the murine model of pneumocystosis have suggested that subclinical transmission of the infection also can occur. Healthy rats exposed to animals with *Pneumocystis* pneumonia remain well but are found to have titers of anti-*Pneumocystis* antibodies consistent with acute acquisition of the infection [155]. In addition, rats with pre-existing *Pneumocystis* antibodies may become antigenemic on comparable exposure to overt infection; these animals may be experiencing subclinical reinfection [100].

PATHOLOGY

The gross and microscopic pathologic features of *P. jiroveci* pneumonia have been elucidated in a number of excellent reviews.* At autopsy in typically advanced infection, both lungs are heavy and diffusely affected. The most extensive involvement often is seen in posterior or dependent areas. At the lung margins anteriorly, a few remaining air-filled alveoli may constitute the only portion of functioning lung at the time of death [11]. Subpleural air blebs not infrequently are seen in these anterior marginal areas. Occasionally, prominent mediastinal emphysema or frank pneumothorax can be noted. The color of the lungs is variously described as dark bluish purple [24,141], yellow-pink [25], or pale gray-brown [11,27]. The pleural surfaces are smooth and glistening, with little inflammatory reaction. Hilar adenopathy is uncommon. Necrosis of tissue is not a feature of the disease.

Although these gross features of widespread infection are strikingly characteristic, focal or subclinical pneumocystosis presents a less recognizable picture. In this condition, the lung has tiny 3- to 5-mm reddish brown retracted areas contained within peribronchial and subpleural lobules, where hypostasis is greatest [24,31]. Even these features, however, may be absent because of variable involvement of adjacent lung tissue by concomitant pathologic processes.

The microscopic appearance of both the contents and the septal walls of pulmonary alveoli in *Pneumocystis* pneumonia are virtually pathognomonic of the infection. The outstanding histologic finding with hematoxylin and eosin stain is an intensely eosinophilic, foamy, or honeycomb-like material uniformly filling the alveolar sacs (Figure 34–4). This intra-alveolar material is composed largely of packets of *P. jiroveci* [126,159]. Typical cysts or trophozoite forms of the organism within alveoli are visible only after application of special stains such as methenamine silver.

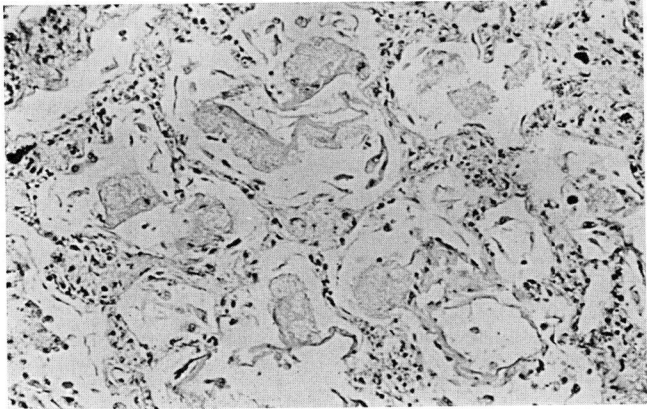

FIGURE 34–4 Section of lung tissue obtained at autopsy showing the amorphous, proteinaceous intra-alveolar infiltrate characteristic of pneumonitis caused by *Pneumocystis jiroveci*. Hematoxylin and eosin stain, ×160. *(From Remington JS. The compromised host. Hosp Pract 7:59–70, 1972.)*

*References [11,16,24,27,32,126,144,156–158].

The type and degree of cellular inflammatory response provoked by the intra-alveolar cluster of *Pneumocystis* organisms vary in different hosts [126]. The descriptive histologic term for pneumocystosis—interstitial plasma cell pneumonia—is derived from the pronounced plasma cellular infiltration of the interalveolar septa observed almost exclusively in newborns in European nursery epidemics. Distention of alveolar walls to 5 to 10 times the normal thickness, with resultant compression of alveolar spaces and capillary lumens, typically is noted in this form of the disease. Hyaline membranes develop occasionally [11], often when the foamy honeycomb pattern within alveoli is least prominent [144]. Septal cell hyperplasia is apparently a nonspecific reaction of lung tissue to injury induced by infections of diverse etiology [160].

Hughes and colleagues [150] studied the histologic progression of typical *Pneumocystis* pneumonia based on the number and location of organisms and the cellular response in pulmonary tissue. The lung samples were from children with underlying malignancy who had received intensive chemotherapy. The authors categorized three sequential stages in the course of the disease. In the first stage, no septal inflammatory or cellular response is seen, and only a few free cyst forms are present in the alveolar lumen; the remainder are isolated in the cytoplasm of cells on the alveolar septal wall. The second stage is characterized by an increase in the number of organisms within macrophages fixed to the alveolar wall and desquamation of these cells into the alveolar space; again, only minimal septal inflammatory response is seen at this time. Finally, a third stage is identified in which extensive reactive and desquamative alveolitis can be seen. Such diffuse alveolar damage may be the major pathologic feature in certain cases [161]. Variable numbers of cysts of the organism, presumably undergoing dissolution, are present within the alveolar macrophages. These findings underscore an earlier claim [162] that the so-called foamy exudate within alveoli is neither foamy edema fluid nor the product of an exudative inflammatory reaction but largely a collection of coalesced alveolar cells and macrophages that contain sizable digestive vacuoles and remnant organisms.

The mechanism of spread of *Pneumocystis* throughout pulmonary tissue is not completely understood. Direct invasion by the organism through septal walls into the interstitium or the lymphatic or blood vascular spaces of the lung is considered unlikely [31,144,150], except in rare instances when systemic dissemination of the organism occurs (see later discussion). Instead, it is probable that coughing expels cysts from the alveoli into larger airways and that the organisms are then inhaled into previously uninvolved alveolar areas [126]. This hypothesis of interairway transfer of *Pneumocystis* is supported by the fact that the heaviest concentration of organisms usually is found in dependent portions of the lung parenchyma.

Interstitial fibrosis is a distinct but infrequently reported complication of *Pneumocystis* pneumonia in older children and adults but has been reported in infants only rarely [12,144,157,158,163–169]. Nowak [166], in Europe, first emphasized that fibrosis was not unusual in the lungs of infants at autopsy who had especially protracted infection with *P. jiroveci*. *Pneumocystis*-infected lungs sometimes demonstrate, in addition to fibrosis, other pathologic features compatible with a more chronic destructive inflammatory process. Multinucleate alveolar giant cells occasionally accompany alveolar cell proliferation [24,27,31,158]. Whether presence of these cells is more often a response to undetected concomitant viral infection is unknown. Typical granulomatous reactions with organisms visible in the granulomas also have been described [158,170,171]. Extensive calcification of *Pneumocystis* exudate and adjacent lung tissue may ultimately develop [27,144,158].

PATHOGENESIS

The clinical conditions that predispose patients to the development of *Pneumocystis* pneumonia are associated with impaired immune responses, leading to the presumption that *Pneumocystis* causes disease not because it is intrinsically virulent but because the host's immune mechanisms fail to contain it (Table 34–1). The severity of *P. jiroveci* pneumonia in infants with AIDS illustrates this phenomenon dramatically. The primary role of immunocompromise also would explain in part why *Pneumocystis* pneumonia did not emerge as a serious health problem until more than 30 years after the disease was first recognized. European epidemics of *Pneumocystis* arose out of the devastation of World War II and widespread use of antibacterial drugs. Each of these two seemingly unrelated events served ultimately to disrupt the normal host-organism immunologic interaction in favor of the organism. The war resulted in institutionalization of inordinate numbers of orphans under conditions of overcrowding and malnutrition. At the same time, antibacterial therapy dramatically enhanced survival rates of these institutionalized infants, who would otherwise have succumbed to bacterial sepsis during the first days or

weeks of life. In addition, it was realized that *Pneumocystis* infection appeared in these marasmic children at an age when their immunoglobulin G levels reached a physiologic nadir. By 1960, the orphanage epidemics had abated in Europe as environmental conditions improved, but they persisted in Asia, where poverty and overcrowding continued [141,172]. Subsidence of the epidemic disease and more widespread antibacterial drug therapy, along with sophisticated immunosuppressive drug treatment, contributed thereafter to awareness in Europe and North America of isolated instances of *Pneumocystis* infection among children suffering from a variety of identifiable immunodeficiencies.

Weller, in Europe, was among the first to experimentally induce *Pneumocystis* pneumonia in animals [173,174]. His crucial observation relative to pathogenesis of the infection was that in rats pretreated with cortisone (and penicillin) and exposed to suspensions of *Pneumocystis*-containing lung tissue, *Pneumocystis* pneumonia develops with the same frequency and severity as in corticoid-treated animals that were not subsequently inoculated with organisms. The intensity of such artificially induced animal infection also was noted to be less marked than that in spontaneous human pneumocystosis of the epidemic variety. Comparable observations in the rabbit model were made by Sheldon in the United States [152]. He showed that cortisone and antimicrobial agents were sufficient to induce *Pneumocystis* infection without direct exposure of animals to an exogenous source of organisms. The inescapable conclusion of these carefully designed studies was that *Pneumocystis* infection is latent in rats and rabbits and becomes clinically manifest only when host resistance is altered.

In 1966, Frenkel and colleagues [175] published a hallmark study of rat pneumocystosis. They showed that clinical and histopathologically significant involvement with *Pneumocystis* is regularly inducible in rats by "conditioning" them with parenteral cortisone over a period of 1 to 2 months. Premature death from complicating bacterial infection was prevented by simultaneous administration of antibacterial agents. Of interest is their finding that regression of established interstitial pneumonitis occurs if cortisone conditioning is stopped early enough; on the other hand, rats continuing to receive cortisone die of coalescent alveolar *Pneumocystis* infiltration, and the infiltrate is almost devoid of inflammatory cells. These histologic changes are, in fact, an exact replica of those observed in sporadic cases of human *Pneumocystis* infection developing in congenitally immunodeficient and exogenously immunosuppressed patients. Those authors attempted to precipitate clinical pneumocystosis with a variety of immunosuppressants other than cortisone. Of eight cytotoxic agents and antimetabolites tested, only cyclophosphamide was shown to activate latent infection. Total-body irradiation and lymphoid tissue ablation (splenectomy, thymectomy) by themselves were incapable of inducing overt *Pneumocystis* pneumonia.

The clinical association between pneumocystosis and protein-calorie malnutrition also has been reproduced in a rat model [176]. Healthy rats given either a regular or a low-protein diet gain weight and exhibit little to no evidence of pneumocystosis post mortem. By contrast,

TABLE 34–1 Conditions Associated with *Pneumocystis jiroveci* Pneumonia

1. Premature infants aged 2 to 4 months with marasmus and malnutrition, usually living in foundling homes in geographic locales endemic for pneumocystosis
2. Infants and children with congenital (primary) immunodeficiency disease
   a. Severe combined immunodeficiency
   b. X-linked agammaglobulinemia
   c. X-linked immunodeficiency
   d. Variable immunodeficiency
   e. Immunodeficiency with hyperimmunoglobulinemia
   f. Immunodeficiency associated with Wiskott-Aldrich syndrome
3. Children and adults with acquired immunodeficiency
   a. Disease-related: lymphoreticular malignancies; multiple myeloma; dysproteinemias
   b. Drug-related (corticosteroids, cyclophosphamide, busulfan, methotrexate, colloidal gold); organ transplantation; lymphoreticular malignancies; solid tumors; collagen vascular disorders; miscellaneous diseases treated with immunosuppressants
   c. Acquired immunodeficiency syndrome (human immunodeficiency virus infection)

Adapted from Burke BA, Good RA. Pneumocystis carinii *infection. Medicine 52:23, 1972; Walzer PD, et al.* Pneumocystis carinii *pneumonia in the United States; epidemiologic, diagnostic and clinical features. Ann Intern Med 80:83, 1974, with permission.*

in rats fed a protein-free diet, which produces weight loss and hypoalbuminemia, fatal infection regularly developed; administration of corticosteroid only foreshortened their median survival time [170].

None of the experimental models described thus far permit a precise appraisal of the relative importance of the cellular and humoral components of host defense against *Pneumocystis*. Although corticosteroids, cytotoxic drugs, and starvation interfere primarily with cell-mediated immunity, they do not always induce purely functional cellular defects. For example, it is known from in vitro cell culture studies that corticosteroids do not inhibit the uptake of *Pneumocystis* by alveolar macrophages [64]. Rather, the immunosuppressive effects of chemotherapeutic agents or of malnutrition are far more complex, and ultimately both cellular and humoral arms of the immune system may be impaired by them.

The production of pneumocystosis in the nude mouse without the use of exogenous immunosuppressants implies that susceptibility to the infection relates most to a defect in thymic-dependent lymphocytes [151]. Antibody deficiency must be less important because certain strains of nude mice are resistant to pneumocystosis, yet neither these animals nor their susceptible littermates produce measurable antibodies. These findings do not exclude a role for antibody in control of established infection with the organism; indeed, it has been shown in vitro that *P. jiroveci* organisms adherent to rat alveolar macrophages become interiorized only after anti-*Pneumocystis* serum is added to the culture system [155].

That primary immune deficits could predispose to sporadic pneumocystosis was first reported, unwittingly, by Hutchison in England in 1955 [85]. He described male siblings with congenital agammaglobulinemia who died of pneumonia of "similar and unusual" histology. *P. jiroveci* was implicated as the etiologic agent of these fatal infections only when the pathologic sections were reviewed by Baar [177], who had reported the first case of *Pneumocystis* pneumonia in England earlier that year [71]. In one of the first such reports from the United States, Burke and her colleagues [178] stressed what was to be regarded as a typical histologic finding in *Pneumocystis*-infected agammaglobulinemic children—namely, the absence or gross deficiency of plasma cells in pulmonary lesions (and in hematopoietic tissues). This deficiency contrasted sharply with the extensive plasmacytosis seen in epidemic infections. In addition, sera from some of these hypogammaglobulinemic children did not contain antibody to a *Pneumocystis* antigen derived from lung tissue in "epidemic" European cases [55].

None of these *Pneumocystis*-infected patients with a primary humoral immunodeficiency disease had evidence of an isolated impairment of cellular immunity. (Indeed, only once has pneumocystosis been reported in association with a pure T cell deficiency—namely, in DiGeorge's syndrome [179]). Most of the *Pneumocystis* infections, however, did occur in the infants with severe combined immunodeficiency, a state characterized by profound depression of both cellular and humoral immunity.

That the integrity of the cellular immune system is critical for resistance to *Pneumocystis* may be inferred from the steroid-induced and congenitally athymic animal models of pneumocystosis described earlier and from clinical experience with the infection in older children with lymphoreticular malignancies, collagen-vascular disorders, or organ allografts. These individuals receive broad immunosuppressive therapy designed to inhibit mainly the cellular arm of the immune system. Indeed, the incidence of *Pneumocystis* infection in these patients is related less to the nature of the underlying condition than to the intensity of immunosuppressive chemotherapy given for it [126,144,148,160,180–182].

For many years it had not been possible to study in vitro the cellular immune response to *P. jiroveci* because of the impurity of available antigens. Preliminary experiments with an antigen derived from a cell culture suggested that specific cell-mediated immunity may be depressed in children with active *Pneumocystis* pneumonia. Lymphocytes from two such children failed to transform in the presence of the antigen [183], whereas lymphocytes from healthy, seropositive adults were in most cases stimulated specifically to undergo blastogenesis [183,184].

The humoral immune response to pneumocystosis has been measured in a variety of infected populations.* The most detailed serosurveys have been conducted in Iran [24,187] and central Europe [188–190] in infants with typical epidemic interstitial plasma cell pneumonia. Infants in Iranian orphanages had elevated levels of all immunoglobulins presumably because of the abundance of infective organisms in their institutional environments compared with values recorded in age-matched healthy U.S. infants [187]. No statistical difference was detectable in immunoglobulin concentrations between *Pneumocystis* carriers (those with "focal pneumocystosis") and uninfected infants within an orphanage. Prominent elevation in serum IgM levels correlated with the intensity of *Pneumocystis* disease as measured by clinical, radiographic, and histologic (e.g., plasma cell infiltration) criteria. The peak values of IgM persisted for only a short "crisis" period and then rapidly decreased toward normal. Serum IgG concentrations reached significantly depressed values of less than 200 mg/dL only in infants with massive interstitial pneumonitis. A precipitous drop in serum IgA level was recorded in three *Pneumocystis*-infected children 2 to 3 days before onset of marked respiratory impairment; the complete absence of alveolar IgA also was documented by fluorescent antibody techniques.

Iranian workers have proposed a provocative hypothesis relating these alterations in immunoglobulin levels to the pathogenesis of infant pneumocystosis. The level of transplacentally transferred maternal anti-*Pneumocystis* IgG decreases during the infant's first months of life. This reduction may be accentuated and occur earlier in premature infants, owing in part to malnutrition, diarrhea, and inordinate gastrointestinal protein loss [24,187,191,192]. This low IgG concentration probably predisposes these infants to intra-alveolar proliferation of *P. jiroveci*. Normally, IgA prevents surface spread of the organism. If serum IgA levels also are low, so that bronchoalveolar IgA secretion ceases (this remains to be proved), surface spread of the infection proceeds. Subsequently, progression of

---

*References [109,144,150,157,185,186].

focal pneumocystosis to clinically evident pneumonia occurs. Increased IgM antibody formation reflects a humoral response to the highly antigenic cyst walls of the organism. If the infant survives, active production of *Pneumocystis*-specific IgG occurs during the fifth to ninth month of life. Patients with "hypoimmune pneumocystosis," so named by Dutz [24], with underlying congenital immunodeficiency (or acquired immune defects from immunosuppressive chemotherapy) would not exhibit such an IgG response and thus would be subject to recurrence of clinically manifest pneumonic disease. An obstacle to complete acceptance of this hypothesis is that it assigns a major role to IgG and IgA in host defense against *P. jiroveci* infection. Yet *Pneumocystis* pneumonia has not been reported in children who produce little or no IgA, such as those with ataxia-telangiectasia [144].

Brzosko and his colleagues [188–190,193] in Poland have studied the immunopathogenesis of *Pneumocystis* pneumonia at the tissue level by immunofluorescent methodology. These investigators first reported that γ-globulin is present in the intra-alveolar exudate of *Pneumocystis* infection [193]. Subsequently, they demonstrated that this collection of γ-globulin represents the specific antibody component of *Pneumocystis* antigen-antibody complexes [189]. Direct immunofluorescent staining of infected lung tissue with fluorescein-conjugated antihuman globulin or rheumatoid factor revealed a large amount of "immune" globulins bound to packets of *Pneumocystis*. In the same infected tissue blocks, immunofluorescent complement fixation reactions also resulted in marked fluorescence of *Pneumocystis*-γ-globulin complexes. The avidity of these conglomerates for rheumatoid factor and complement supports the assumption that the tissue-bound γ-globulin deposits are specific immune reactants to *P. jiroveci* [189]. The most intense fluorescence coincided with periodic acid-Schiff-positive structures (presumably glycoproteins or mucoproteins) on the outer aspect of thick-walled cysts, suggesting that the major antigenicity of the organism resides in its mucoid envelope [188].

Polish workers attempted to reconstruct the immuno-morphologic events in typical epidemic pneumocystosis [190]. In the earliest stage of infection, the antigenic constituents of *P. jiroveci* induce the formation of IgM and IgG anti-*Pneumocystis* antibodies, possibly in hilar and mediastinal lymph nodes. These antibodies bind to aggregates of alveolar *Pneumocystis* to form immune complexes. The latter then bind complement, with resultant gradual disintegration of the masses of organisms and their eventual phagocytosis by alveolar macrophages. Immunoglobulin-forming plasma cells proliferate in the interstitium and, conceivably, contribute additional antibody to the *Pneumocystis* aggregates. Clearly, no impairment in immunoglobulin synthesis is recorded in this analysis of epidemic pneumocystosis, but retarded binding of complement components to the immune complexes is regularly observed. Because the ultimate destruction and removal of the *Pneumocystis*-antibody conglomerates are complement dependent and the complement system is, in general, physiologically deficient in the first few months of life, survival of a particular infant with epidemic *Pneumocystis* pneumonia may depend on the stage of development and relative functional competency of the complement system.

CLINICAL MANIFESTATIONS
General Considerations

No clinical features are pathognomonic for *P. jiroveci* infection. Organisms residing in scattered intra-alveolar foci may evoke no illness [31,194,195], whereas histologically advanced infection may provoke variable symptoms and signs in different hosts. Features attributable to *Pneumocystis* infection per se may be obfuscated by concomitant infection with other opportunistic pathogens or by dramatic complications of an underlying condition [27,185]. Furthermore, clinical syndromes ascribable to *Pneumocystis* may be simulated by other infections (cytomegalovirus [16], or by inflammatory processes (drug-induced pulmonary toxicity [196], radiation fibrosis [197] and neoplasia (pulmonary leukemia [198] capable of producing interstitial pulmonary infiltrates in older children and adults. Thus, recognition of pneumocystosis on clinical grounds requires above all a high index of suspicion whenever interstitial pneumonia occurs in settings known to predispose to infection with the organism.

Despite these caveats, *Pneumocystis* is distinguishable from other opportunistic microbes by the fact that infection with this organism commonly surfaces when underlying disorders are quiescent. For example, in the case of severe combined immunodeficiency disease, pneumocystosis can develop only after immunologic competence has been at least partially restored by bone marrow transplantation [109,144,199]. Reversal of immune paralysis apparently elicits sufficient inflammation to convert subclinical infection to overt pneumonitis. Similarly, in children with lymphocytic leukemia, pneumocystosis most often occurs during periods of clinical and hematologic remission [145,150,200–203]. It may be inferred from these observations that pneumocystosis is not merely an end-stage infection in a host with a preterminal illness but, on the contrary, often represents a potentially treatable cause of death in patients whose primary immunodeficiency or malignancy has been controlled or effectively cured.

Symptoms and Signs
Epidemic Infection in Infants

The onset of epidemic types of infection in infants is reported to be slow and insidious. Initially, nonspecific signs of restlessness or languor, poor feeding, and diarrhea are common. Tachypnea and periorbital cyanosis gradually develop. Cough productive of sticky mucus, although not prominent, may appear later [16,31]. Respiratory insufficiency progresses over 1 to 4 weeks, and patients exhibit increasingly severe tachypnea, dyspnea, intercostal retractions, and flaring of the nasal alae. Fever is absent or of low grade [204]. Physical findings are strikingly minimal and consist primarily of fine crepitant rales with deep inspiration. Chest roentgenograms, however, typically demonstrate pulmonary infiltrates early in the illness. The duration of untreated disease is 4 to 6 weeks, but it often is difficult to determine an exact date of onset of illness. Before the introduction of pentamidine therapy, the mortality rate for such epidemic infant infection is estimated to have been between 20% and 50% [72,186].

Sporadic Infection in Infants

The typical clinical syndrome is less evident in sporadic cases of pneumocystosis occurring in infants with acquired or congenital immunodeficiency and in older children with acquired immunodeficiency. In infants with primary immunodeficiency diseases, the onset of clinical infection can be insidious, and illness can extend over weeks or possibly months [144], a course not unlike that seen in epidemic pneumocystosis. By contrast, in most infants with congenital immunodeficiency or AIDS and in older children with acquired immune deficits, *Pneumocystis* pneumonia manifests abruptly and is a more symptomatic, short-lived disease [42,105,110,144,150]. Among infants with HIV infection, the median age at onset is 4 to 5 months, and the mortality rate is between 39% and 59% [205]. High fever and nonproductive cough are initial findings, followed by tachypnea, coryza, and, later, cyanosis. Death may supervene within a week or so. If no treatment is given, essentially all patients with this form of pneumocystosis die.

Radiologic Findings

Because the extent of pulmonary involvement in *P. jiroveci* pneumonia rarely is detectable by physical examination, a chest roentgenogram showing diffuse infiltrative disease is the most useful indicator of infection in a susceptible host [42,206]. Although certain characteristic patterns of radiographic involvement have been ascribed to *Pneumocystis* pneumonitis, it is worth emphasizing that the findings may vary depending on the presence of coincident pulmonary infection and on the nature of the underlying disease state.

Epidemic Infection in Infants

Ivady and colleagues [186] in Hungary studied the radiographic progression of epidemic infantile *Pneumocystis* pneumonia and identified five stages. The first three stages are recognizable when the infant is virtually symptom free and are defined by the presence of perivascular and peribronchial peripheral shadows extending toward the pleura. The two later stages more closely coincide with respiratory insufficiency and reveal changes resembling "butterfly" pulmonary edema and peripheral emphysematous blebs. The radiographic findings of mild ("focal") *Pneumocystis* pneumonia described by Vessal and associates [207] in infants from an Iranian orphanage included hilar interstitial infiltrate, thymic atrophy, pulmonary hyperaeration, and scattered lobular atelectasis. Although none of these signs is specific for *Pneumocystis* infection, they persist longer (3 weeks to 2 months) in serologically proven cases. Indeed, surviving infants may exhibit focal interstitial infiltrates after organisms are cleared from the lung [208] and for as long as 1 year [204,209].

Sporadic Infection in Infants

A majority of radiologic characterizations of *Pneumocystis* pneumonia have emphasized the sporadic form of the infection. Minor differences in descriptive details usually reflect differences in the populations studied [144,169,210–214]. In infants, especially those with immunodeficiency

syndromes, the initial roentgenogram often shows haziness spreading from the hilar regions to the periphery, which assumes a finely granular, interstitial pattern. An antecedent gross alveolar infiltrate usually is not seen [144]. The peripheral granularity may progress to coalescent nodules. These changes resemble the "atelectatic" radiographic abnormalities of hyaline membrane disease. In both conditions, aeration is absent peripherally. Pneumothorax with subcutaneous and interstitial emphysema and pneumomediastinum are not uncommon and are associated with a poor prognosis [215]. Even with therapy, radiographic clearing can lag far behind clinical improvement.

As experience with *Pneumocystis* has broadened, especially in older children and adults, a number of atypical roentgenographic abnormalities have been described [42,213,214,216–223]. These atypical findings include hilar and mediastinal adenopathy, pleural effusions, parenchymal cavitation, pneumatoceles, nodular densities, and unilateral or lobar distribution of infiltrates. By contrast, the chest roentgenographic appearance can remain essentially normal well after the onset of fever, dyspnea, and hypoxemia. The presence of such roentgenographically silent lung disease can be visualized as abnormal findings by pulmonary computed tomography.

Laboratory Studies

Routine laboratory studies yield little diagnostic information in *Pneumocystis* infection. Abnormalities in hemoglobin concentration or white blood cell count are more likely to result from an underlying disease of the hematopoietic system or cytotoxic drug effect. Neither laboratory value is consistently altered by secondary pneumocystosis. Nevertheless, a subgroup of infants with primary immunodeficiency disease and infection caused by *P. jiroveci* can exhibit significant eosinophilia [31,72,138,144]. Jose and associates [138] first emphasized the association of peripheral blood eosinophilia and pneumocystosis in a report describing three infected male siblings with infantile agammaglobulinemia. In one of the infants, eosinophilia developed very early in the course of the illness, and the differential eosinophil count peaked at 42% as the respiratory disease worsened. Accordingly, it has been suggested that the combination of cough, tachypnea, diffuse haziness on chest roentgenograms, and eosinophilia in an infant with immunodeficiency can be indicative of *Pneumocystis* pneumonia [138,144]. Hypercalcemia with or without nephrocalcinosis has been reported in infants with epidemic pneumocystosis [72]. Measurement of serum calcium levels in other patients with *Pneumocystis* infection, however, has revealed normal values whether or not coincident foci of pulmonary or renal parenchymal calcification existed [105,144,150].

A constant pathophysiologic finding in pneumocystosis, and in other interstitial pulmonary diseases, is that of ventilation and perfusion defects most compatible with an "alveolar-capillary block" syndrome.* Arterial blood gas determinations in infected patients show severe hypoxemia and hypocapnia, often before profound subjective respiratory insufficiency or even radiologic abnormalities

---

*References [120,125,144,180,185,224–227].

[228] supervene. Less commonly, modest hypercapnia with respiratory acidosis is recorded [224]. This respiratory pathophysiology correlates well with the anatomic pulmonary lesion in *Pneumocystis* pneumonia. Concentration of organisms within alveoli and inflammation of the surrounding alveolar septa not unexpectedly lead to interference in gas transfer, whereas persistence of areas of normal lung parenchyma and lack of significant airway obstruction account for the usual absence of carbon dioxide retention.

Concurrent Infection

The clinical presentation of pneumocystosis may be altered by simultaneous infection with other organisms. Certainly, infection with a variety of opportunistic pathogens is not surprising in patients with broadly compromised immunologic defense mechanisms. Infection with one or more organisms was found in 56% of *Pneumocystis*-infected infants and children with primary immunodeficiency disease reported to the CDC [109]. Comparable rates of multiple infections also have been noted in several large series of patients with acquired immune defects and pneumocystosis [21,144,160,229].

Infection with cytomegalovirus appears to be the most common "unusual" infection associated with pneumocystosis. Indeed, in his 1957 review, Gajdusek [16] already was able to cite numerous published studies referring to the "unexpectedly high frequency of association" of the two infections. He conceded that one infection most probably predisposed the affected patient to the other. On the basis of electron micrographic observations of cytomegalovirus-like particles within pneumocysts, Wang and coworkers [39] hypothesized that *P. jiroveci* may even serve as an intermediate host or reservoir of the virus. The possibility of viral parasitism of (or symbiosis with) *Pneumocystis* also was explored by Pliess and Seifert [230] and by Vawter and colleagues [40], who were impressed by the resemblance of the outer membranes of *P. jiroveci* to an imperfect form of myxovirus. It is still unclear, however, whether this inordinate concurrence of *Pneumocystis* and cytomegalovirus is caused by a specific and unique relationship between the two organisms or by coincidental infection of highly susceptible hosts with ubiquitous microbes [160,231]. Histopathologic examination of lung biopsy specimens from infants with AIDS often demonstrates concomitant cytomegalovirus and *P. jiroveci* infections [232,233].

DIAGNOSIS

The diagnosis of *Pneumocystis* pneumonia remains difficult. The organism must be visualized in the respiratory tract of ill persons, and often this can be accomplished only by bronchoalveolar lavage (BAL) or, in infants, a lung biopsy. Recently, PCR assay has been used for diagnosis in fluid specimens obtained by BAL. Nevertheless, this technique is still not sensitive and specific enough for routine clinical use. Attempts to isolate *Pneumocystis* from clinical specimens on synthetic media or in tissue culture have not been successful, and serologic techniques to detect active infection have been too insensitive.

Examination of Pulmonary Secretions

During the European epidemics, parasitic forms were recognized in mucus from infected infants [32,48,129]. Specimens usually were obtained through a catheter or laryngobronchoscope passed into the hypopharynx, and smears of the aspirated secretions were fixed in ether-alcohol and stained by the Gram-Weigert technique. By this method, Le Tan-Vinh and associates [32] in France reported antemortem diagnosis of *Pneumocystis* pneumonia in eight of nine infants. Toth and coworkers [129] in Hungary recovered *P. jiroveci* from tracheopharyngeal and gastric aspirates of 22 infants whose illness had just begun; in some cases, organisms were observed 7 to 10 days before the appearance of symptoms. The mere presence of organisms in hypopharyngeal secretions, however, did not always presage acute pneumonic disease in these environments, where pneumocystosis was endemic. Rather, it often reflected chronic subclinical carriage of the organism [24].

Diagnosis of sporadic cases of pneumocystosis by examination of sputum or tracheal and gastric aspirates has never been as rewarding. The rate of recovery of *Pneumocystis* from upper airway secretions in the cases compiled by the CDC was estimated to be only about 6% [110]. Japanese investigators have described a method of concentrating sputum samples with acetyl-L-cysteine in 0.2N sodium hydroxide solution, which permits filtration and centrifugation of a pellet of *Pneumocystis* [234]. Ognibene and associates [235] reported the use of induced sputa in the diagnosis of pneumonia in 18 children with HIV infection or malignancy. Nine sputum samples were positive for *P. jiroveci* by immunofluorescent antibody testing. Four of the patients with negative findings by examination of sputum samples subsequently underwent BAL; BAL fluid was negative for *P. jiroveci* in all four. The remaining five patients received treatment for bacterial pneumonia and responded to therapy. This technique required ultrasonic nebulization in the children, and the youngest patient in this report was 2 years of age.

Percutaneous Lung Aspiration

The need to obtain lung tissue for a more accurate assessment of the presence of *Pneumocystis* pneumonia has been appreciated for some time. Percutaneous needle aspiration of the lung was already of proven value by the late 1950s in diagnosis of epidemic pneumocystosis in infants [16]. Subsequently, it was successfully employed in infected infants and children with underlying primary and acquired immunodeficiencies [81,150,236,237]. The procedure is performed without general anesthesia so that the child's respiratory function is not further compromised. Under fluoroscopy, a 20-gauge spinal needle with syringe in place is guided into the midportion of the lung. The resultant aspirate (usually less than 0.1 mL in amount) may be transferred directly to slides as unsmeared drops or first cytocentrifuged to increase the concentration of organisms in the sample [238]. Slides are allowed to air dry and then are stained with Gram, Gomori methenamine silver, and toluidine blue O stains. The residual material in the syringe is diluted with 2 mL of sterile saline and cultured for bacteria and fungi.

Children with platelet counts of less than 60,000/mm³ receive fresh whole blood or platelet transfusions before the procedure. Pneumothorax appears to be the major complication encountered. In one series, it occurred in 37% of the patients, and evacuation of air by thoracotomy tube was required in 14% [237].

Lung Biopsy

It has been argued that aspiration is inferior to biopsy in that the former does not permit histologic examination of lung tissue. Open lung biopsy has been proposed as the most reliable method for identifying and estimating the extent of *Pneumocystis* infection, and for demonstrating the presence of complicating pathologic conditions such as coexistent infection, malignancy, or interstitial fibrosis [144,225,229,239–241]. It may be hazardous, however, to perform a thoracotomy using general anesthesia in patients with marginal pulmonary reserve [242]. Although the procedure has been associated with an acceptably low incidence of serious complications in critically ill children [243–246], determination of its risk-to-benefit ratio based on the infant's underlying disease, expected life span, and clinical condition is appropriate in individual cases [247,248]. Unfortunately, these analyses have not yet been applied rigorously to infants and young children with suspected pneumocystosis. Technical modification in the performance of open biopsy that would avoid general anesthesia and endotracheal intubation (e.g., using thoracoscopy) may be particularly advantageous for diagnosis of *Pneumocystis* pneumonia in small children [249].

Whichever invasive technique is employed for retrieval of tissue to test for the presence of *P. jiroveci*, it is generally agreed that immediate examination and staining of frozen sections or imprints of fresh lung (or alveolar secretions) are critical.* Processing of paraffin-embedded tissue incurs an unnecessary delay of one or more days in diagnosis, and the sections may actually reveal fewer organisms than the imprint smears. Although techniques using Giemsa stain are rapid and specific for the intracystic bodies of *P. jiroveci*, organisms are more readily located and identified against a background of tissue cells with a methenamine silver stain. It should be appreciated that other silver-positive organisms, such as *Torulopsis* [252] and zygomycete spores [253], can mimic the cystic structure of *P. jiroveci* and that smears of *Pneumocystis* rather than fungi should be employed as controls for the stain [254].

Unfortunately, the standard methenamine silver stain technique is slow (3 to 4 hours) and requires expertise usually found only in special histopathology laboratories. To circumvent these problems, several rapid (less than 30 minutes) and simple modifications of the silver stain have been developed [255–258]. Because the results with these stains have not been as consistent as those achieved with the standard, more lengthy procedure, many laboratories have chosen not to use silver for rapid screening of specimens but prefer instead toluidine blue O [33,259–262] and cresyl echt violet [34,263] for this purpose.

Serologic Tests

It is clear that sensitive and specific serologic methods are desirable to detect active *Pneumocystis* infection. It is disappointing that despite extensive investigation, no method has been proved to be entirely satisfactory.

Serodiagnosis of *P. jiroveci* infection in infants by detection of immunofluorescent antibodies was first reported in 1964 in Europe [264]. It was found that IgM and IgG anti-*Pneumocystis* immunofluorescent antibodies appear sequentially in sera during the course of clinical infection. Both classes of antibodies are present in sera of diseased infants during the first weeks of pneumonia, but only IgG antibodies persist during convalescent periods or in cases of protracted infection [265].

The worth of immunofluorescent antibody tests in the diagnosis of sporadic pneumocystosis was examined subsequently in the United States by Norman and Kagan [266] at the CDC. They observed low rates of serologic reactivity among patients with suspected and confirmed cases, positive results in sera from patients who seemed to have only cytomegalovirus and other fungal infections, and negative results in sera from six infants with primary immunodeficiency diseases and documented pneumocystosis. Although it is possible to increase the specificity and sensitivity of these tests for *Pneumocystis* [267,268], such tests detect background levels of *Pneumocystis* antibody in clinically healthy persons [97,98,268] and, as a result, fail to discriminate between patients with active disease and those who are latently infected with the organism.

The performance of the immunofluorescent antibody test has been hampered for years by the crude *Pneumocystis* antigens employed. Impure antigen results in autofluorescence of uninfected lung tissue, and extensive absorption of sera risks undue reduction in intensity of staining of organisms. For this reason, several laboratories have attempted to prepare a *Pneumocystis* antigen that is isolated as nearly as possible from the lung parenchyma, to which it characteristically clings. Techniques designed to extract free *P. jiroveci* from infected lung include bronchoalveolar saline lavage [30,229], enzymatic digestion of lung homogenates [263], and differential centrifugation of lung homogenates on sucrose [269] or Ficoll-Hypaque density gradients. These purified antigens have been used to generate immune sera that have been applied in immunofluorescent staining of *Pneumocystis* in lung tissue [270,271] and in upper airway secretions [272,273].

To avoid the problem posed by the insensitivity of antibody determinations per se in pneumocystosis, Pifer and colleagues [98] developed a counterimmunoelectrophoretic assay for detecting circulating *Pneumocystis* antigen in suspected cases. In an initial evaluation of the test, antigenemia was demonstrated in up to 95% of children with *Pneumocystis* pneumonia and was absent in normal control children. Antigen also was found in the sera of 15% of oncology patients who did not have pneumonia, however. Thus, although antigenemia appears to be superior to circulating antibody as a serologic correlate of *Pneumocystis* infection, antigenemia alone cannot be equated with a diagnosis of pneumocystosis without corroborating clinical data.

---

*References [16,42,237,239,244,250,251].

TREATMENT
Specific Therapy

Hughes and coworkers [274] in 1974 first demonstrated that the combination of trimethoprim and sulfamethoxazole (TMP-SMX) was effective in treatment of cortisone-induced rat pneumocystosis. This combination was shown to be as efficacious as pentamidine in children infected with *Pneumocystis* who also had underlying malignancy [275]. Several uncontrolled trials of TMP-SMX in congenitally immunodeficient infants [276,277] and in older immunosuppressed children and adults [276,277] confirmed the efficacy and low toxicity of this combination agent. The dosage employed was 20 mg of TMP and 100 mg of SMX per kg of body weight per day, given orally in four divided doses for 14 days. This daily dose was two to three times that used in treatment of bacterial infections. The equivalent efficacy of TMP-SMX and of pentamidine has been confirmed in pediatric cancer patients with *P. jiroveci* pneumonia [278].

TMP-SMX is the drug of choice for treatment of *P. jiroveci* pneumonia in infants and children. The oral route of administration can be used in mild cases, for which the recommended dosage is 20 mg TMP plus 100 mg SMX per kg per day in divided doses every 6 to 8 hours apart. Infants with moderate or severe disease require treatment by the intravenous route with 15 to 20 mg TMP plus 75 to 100 mg SMX per kg per day in divided doses 6 to 8 hours apart. Generally, treatment is given for 3 weeks. Adverse reactions to TMP-SMX will develop in approximately 5% of infants and children without HIV infection and 40% of children with HIV infection; most commonly seen is a maculopapular rash that clears after discontinuation of the drug. Other adverse reactions are uncommon and include neutropenia, anemia, renal dysfunction, and gastrointestinal symptoms or signs.

In infants who do not respond to TMP-SMX or in whom serious adverse reactions develop, pentamidine isethionate in a single daily dose of 4 mg/kg given intravenously may be used. Other drugs have been tested in limited studies in infants and young children with HIV infection and *P. jiroveci* pneumonia, including atovaquone, trimetrexate-leucovorin, oral TMP-dapsone, pyrimethamine-sulfadoxine, clindamycin plus primaquine, and aerosolized pentamidine.

The ease with which TMP-SMX can be administered and its lack of adverse side effects make it an attractive combination for empirical therapy for suspected pneumocystosis. Such treatment is reasonable in infants who are gravely ill and whose outlook for recovery from underlying disease is bleak. Several objections to the universal adoption of this approach have been raised. In at least half of the immunosuppressed children with typical clinical and roentgenographic features of *Pneumocystis* pneumonia, the illness is in fact not related to infection with *P. jiroveci* [279]. Identification of the etiologic agent and proper management of the disorder can be accomplished only by first performing appropriate diagnostic procedures.

Until 1958, no therapy specific for *P. jiroveci* infection was available. In that year, Ivady and Paldy [280] in Hungary recorded the first successful use of several aromatic diamidines, including pentamidine isethionate, in

16 of 19 infected infants. By 1962 the Hungarian investigators had used pentamidine therapy in 212 patients with epidemic *Pneumocystis* pneumonia [189]. During the next several years, favorable responses to this drug were observed in infants and children with both the epidemic and the sporadic forms of the infection [139,144,150]. Treatment produced a dramatic reduction in the mortality rate for the epidemic disease from 50% to less than 4% [278,281]. In the cases of sporadic infection reported to the CDC [110,282,283], survival rates ranged from 42% to 63% for those patients who received the drug for 9 or more days. In cases confined largely to young children and managed at a single institution, cure rates were noted to be as high as 68% to 75% [150,275]. Because spontaneous recovery from *Pneumocystis* pneumonia in immunodepressed persons is rare [284], it is clear that pentamidine therapy reduced the mortality rate in such patients to nearly 25%.

The recommended dose of the drug is 4 mg/kg intravenously once daily for 14 days. Clinical improvement becomes evident 4 to 6 days after initiation of therapy, but radiographic improvement may be delayed for several weeks.

Pentamidine toxicity from intravenous and intramuscular use has been reported. Although toxicity from pentamidine apparently was not a significant problem in the marasmic infants with *Pneumocystis* infection treated during the European epidemics [285], the CDC determined that 189 (47%) of 404 children and adults given the drug for confirmed or suspected *Pneumocystis* infection suffered one or more adverse effects [110]. Immediate systemic reactions, such as hypotension, tachycardia, nausea, vomiting, facial flushing, pruritus, and subjective experience of unpleasant taste in the mouth, were noted particularly after intravenous administration of the drug. Herxheimer's reactions, although described for patients given pentamidine for leishmaniasis [286], occurred rarely [287]. Local reactions at injection sites—namely, pain, erythema, and frank abscess formation—developed in 10% to 20% of patients [110,283]. Elevation in serum glutamic-oxaloacetic transaminase levels was frequently recorded and may have resulted partly from this local trauma. Hypoglycemia ensued not uncommonly after the fifth day of pentamidine therapy but often was asymptomatic [282]. (Hypoglycemia also was observed in pediatric patients with AIDS who were given pentamidine for treatment of *P. jiroveci* pneumonia [288]). Pentamidine-associated pancreatitis also has been reported in children and adults with HIV infection [289–291]. Although overt anemia was rare, megaloblastic bone marrow changes or depressed serum folate levels were noted [282].

Supportive Care

A critical component in the management of *Pneumocystis* pneumonia is oxygen therapy. Because hypoxemia can be profound, the fraction of inspired oxygen should be adjusted to maintain the arterial oxygen tension at 70 mm Hg or above. The inspired oxygen concentration should not exceed 50% to avoid oxygen toxicity. Assisted or controlled ventilation may be required. Methods of ventilatory support have been a volume-regulated positive-pressure respirator [292] at either low or high frequency and membrane lung bypass [293]. Other ancillary measures, such as administration of γ-globulin [144,276,294] to infected congenitally immunodeficient children, warrant further study.

The use of early adjunctive corticosteroid therapy in the treatment of *P. jiroveci* pneumonia in adults with AIDS can increase survival and reduce the risk of respiratory failure [295,296]. A national consensus panel has recommended the use of corticosteroids in adults and adolescents with HIV infection and documented or suspected *P. jiroveci* pneumonia [297]. Two studies have supported the use of corticosteroids in decreasing the morbidity and mortality associated with *P. jiroveci* pneumonia [298,299].

PROGNOSIS
Chronic Sequelae

Little is known about the residual effects of successfully treated *Pneumocystis* pneumonia on pulmonary function. Patients may suffer additional "pulmonary" morbidity from other opportunistic infections or from noninfectious complications of underlying disease or its therapy. Robbins and associates [165] were fortunate enough to be able to follow the course of a hypogammaglobulinemic child with *Pneumocystis* infection treated with pentamidine in 1964; during the ensuing 5 years, despite intercurrent episodes of otitis media and bacterial pneumonia, she exhibited normal exercise tolerance and pulmonary function without evidence of reactivation of her *Pneumocystis* infection [242]. Hughes and coworkers [150] evaluated 18 children with underlying malignancies over periods of 1 to 4 years after surviving *Pneumocystis* infection. Although pulmonary function tests were not performed, none of the subjects demonstrated clinical or roentgenographic evidence of residual pulmonary disease. In a subsequent study from the same institution, pulmonary function was assessed serially in surviving children [148]. Significant improvement in function was noted within 1 month of the infection, and all abnormalities resolved by 6 months. This finding is in contrast with the observation of recurrent wheezing episodes and abnormal pulmonary function on follow-up evaluation of infants who had pneumonitis during the first 3 months of life [300,301]. Although later morbidity was independent of the original etiologic agent, 17% of these patients were thought to have *P. jiroveci* infection.

It seems inevitable that respiratory dysfunction can result from severe episodes of *Pneumocystis* pneumonia that provoke interstitial fibrosis or extensive calcification (as discussed earlier under "Pathology"). Cor pulmonale has been observed in infants with such protracted infection [144]. In one notably well-studied patient, an adult with biopsy-proven fibrosis that appeared 4 months after curative pentamidine therapy, serial tests of pulmonary function revealed persistent ventilatory defects of the restrictive type and impairment of carbon monoxide–diffusing capacity [167]. Although a possible link between pentamidine therapy per se and lung fibrosis was suggested by earlier observations in rat pneumocystosis

[175,302], healthy animals given the drug exhibit no histologic abnormalities [150]. Moreover, pulmonary fibrosis has been described after *Pneumocystis* pneumonia in patients who received treatment with pyrimethamine and sulfonamide [169] and TMP-SMX [303].

Recurrent Infection

Recurrence of *Pneumocystis* pneumonia after apparently curative courses of therapy has been documented in infants and children with underlying congenital immunodeficiency or malignancy. As early as 1966, Patterson and colleagues [304] reported the case of an infant with probable severe combined immunodeficiency who experienced one presumptive and two substantiated bouts of pneumocystosis at approximately 5-month intervals; treatment with pentamidine resulted in "cure" on each occasion, although radiographic abnormalities persisted [305]. A few years later, Richman and associates [306] and then Saulsbury [294] described recurrent pneumocystosis in two children with hypogammaglobulinemia; in the first case, three proven attacks responded to pentamidine; and in the second child, two separate episodes of infection were treated successfully with TMP-SMX. At St. Jude Children's Research Hospital, a study of 28 children with malignancy whose pneumocystosis was treated with pentamidine revealed that 4 (14%) suffered a second infection [150,168]. The clinical manifestations, roentgenographic findings, and response to therapy were similar for each child in both infectious episodes. In addition, no differences in host factors were discernible in those patients who had recurrent infection and those who did not. Other examples of recurrent pneumocystosis emerging rather soon after clinical recovery have been observed in patients given either pentamidine or TMP-SMX [307]. Whether recurrences of *Pneumocystis* pneumonia result from reinfection or from relapse of previously treated infection is not known.

Clinical and morphologic studies provide conflicting views on the completeness of *Pneumocystis* killing by specific drugs. The Hungarian workers, who first used pentamidine in epidemic pneumocystosis among infants, witnessed progressive degeneration of *P. jiroveci* in tracheal mucus from the sixth day of therapy; by the tenth day, the organisms had almost entirely disintegrated [186]. In their review of sporadic pneumocystosis in the United States, Western and associates [282] similarly concluded that pentamidine probably eliminates organisms from the lung. In two patients, no microscopically visible *P. jiroveci* organisms were present at 5 and 14 days, respectively, after initiation of therapy. Also, none of 11 patients who died more than 20 days after receiving pentamidine had demonstrable organisms in their lungs, even though they survived an average of 189.5 days after administration of the drug. In ultrastructural studies, Campbell [43] detected what he believed to be the destructive effects of pentamidine on the organisms. In a lung biopsy specimen obtained surgically 16 hours after onset of therapy, structurally normal trophozoites or mature cysts with intracystic bodies were absent. A few apparent "ghosts" of trophozoites were noted within phagosomes of intra-alveolar macrophages.

By contrast, pentamidine does not promptly eradicate potentially viable forms of the organism. Hughes and coworkers [150] identified intact *P. jiroveci* in lung aspirates (or autopsy material) 10 to 20 days after institution of drug treatment. Richman and associates [306] demonstrated normal-appearing *Pneumocystis* organisms in a lung aspirate from a clinically cured patient 3 days after completion of his 14-day course of pentamidine. Similarly, Fortuny and colleagues [130] recovered organisms from induced sputa on each of 11 days of pentamidine injections.

TMP-SMX appears to have only a limited and non-lethal effect on organisms. Experiments have shown that short-term treatment with the drug combination ultimately fails to prevent emergence of recrudescent *Pneumocystis* infection. In one study, a therapeutic dosage of TMP-SMX was given prophylactically to children with acute lymphocytic leukemia for a 2-week period beginning 28 days after initiation of antineoplastic treatment [308]. Although the incidence of *Pneumocystis* infection in these children after TMP-SMX was discontinued was not different from that observed in persons who did not receive the drug, the time interval to development of infection was lengthened. Reinfection rather than relapse may have accounted for the late infections, but relapse seems more likely in view of the following results in experimental animals [309]. Immunocompetent rats were given TMP-SMX for as long as 6 weeks and then placed in individual isolator cages to exclude the possibility of acquisition of new organisms from the environmental air. After 12 weeks of immunosuppressive therapy with prednisone, *P. jiroveci* was still found in the lungs of at least 90% of both the animals given TMP-SMX and the control animals, given no treatment. These human and animal data are particularly relevant to the design of prophylactic regimens to prevent *Pneumocystis* infection in humans. They provide a compelling argument for the need to continue prophylaxis for as long as host defenses are considered to be too compromised to keep latent *Pneumocystis* infection in check.

Reactivation of pneumocystosis is not surprising in light of the pathogenesis and pathology of the infection in the immunodeficient subject. Frenkel and colleagues [19] showed clearly in the earliest experimental animal models of *Pneumocystis* pneumonia that anti-*Pneumocystis* therapy alone was not completely curative and that relapse was to be anticipated unless factors provoking the infection (namely, corticosteroid administration) were minimized. Long-term ultrastructural studies of *Pneumocystis* pneumonia in the rat confirmed that even with tapering of corticosteroid and apparent restoration of immune function, focal clusters of *P. jiroveci* are detectable in surviving animals for at least 21 weeks. Furthermore, in humans, drugs might not reach organisms residing within the foci of fibrosis and calcifications formed during especially severe infection [310]. Indeed, Dutz [24] contended that drugs play no therapeutic role in epidemic pneumocystosis once the chronic plasma cellular infiltrate is established. Radiographic resolution is slow, and survival and permanent immunity to reinfection relate not to chemotherapy but to specific anti-*Pneumocystis* immunoglobulin production in the affected infants.

Unfortunately, the congenitally immunodeficient or exogenously immunosuppressed child does not possess such normal immune responsiveness and thus is subject to recurrent infection.

PREVENTION

The first successful attempts to prevent pneumocystosis with drugs were reported in infants with the epidemic form of the infection. In a controlled trial conducted in an Iranian orphanage where the infection was endemic (attack rate of 28%), the biweekly administration of a pyrimethamine and sulfadoxine combination to marasmic infants before the second month of life entirely eradicated *Pneumocystis* pneumonia from the institution [24]. In a children's hospital in Budapest, Hungary, pentamidine given every other day for a total of seven doses to premature infants from the second week of life provided equally effective prophylaxis. During the 6 years of the study, *Pneumocystis* infection did not develop among 536 premature babies who received this treatment, whereas 62 fatal cases were recorded elsewhere in the city [311].

On the basis of promising results in a rat model of infection, TMP-SMX was evaluated in a randomized double-blind controlled trial in children with cancer who were at extremely high risk for *Pneumocystis* pneumonitis [312]. The daily dosage for prophylaxis was 5 mg of TMP plus 20 mg of SMX per kg of body weight, administered orally in two divided doses. Seventeen (21%) of 80 children receiving placebo acquired pneumocystosis, whereas the infection developed in none of 80 patients given TMP-SMX. No adverse effects of TMP-SMX administration were observed, although oral candidiasis was more prevalent among the patients in the treatment group than among the control patients. In a subsequent uncontrolled trial, the prophylactic efficacy of TMP-SMX was confirmed; cases of infection developed only in those children in whom the TMP-SMX was discontinued while they were still receiving anticancer chemotherapy [313]. More recently, a regimen of TMP-SMX prophylaxis given 3 days a week was shown to be as effective as daily administration [314].

The gratifying success of TMP-SMX prophylaxis in prevention of *Pneumocystis* infection has been duplicated in other medical centers caring for children with underlying malignancy [315]. Administration of the drug for the duration of antineoplastic therapy has become standard practice. It would seem prudent to reserve TMP-SMX prophylaxis for persons at relatively high risk for *Pneumocystis* pneumonitis. Congenitally immunodeficient children and infants with AIDS who have had a prior episode of *Pneumocystis* pneumonia would appear to be prime candidates for preventive therapy. The CDC issued a set of guidelines for chemoprophylaxis against *P. jiroveci* pneumonia in children with HIV infection in 1991 [147,315,316] and updated these guidelines in accordance with the most recent epidemiologic surveillance data demonstrating that despite recommendations established for *P. jiroveci* prophylaxis, no substantial decrease in *P. jiroveci* pneumonitis has occurred [317]. The surveillance data indicated that continued cases were the result of failure to identify HIV-infected infants and the poor sensitivity of CD4 [318] counts to determine infants' risk for development of *P. jiroveci* pneumonitis, rather than because of treatment failures [319]. These updated guidelines recommend promptly identifying infants and children born to HIV-infected women, initiating prophylaxis at 4 to 6 weeks of age for all of these children, and continuing prophylaxis through 12 months of age for HIV-infected children and offer new algorithms based on clinical and immunologic status to continue prophylaxis beyond 12 months of age. Although no chemoprophylactic regimens for *P. jiroveci* pneumonia among HIV-infected children have been approved as labeling indications by the U.S. Food and Drug Administration (FDA), TMP-SMX currently is recommended as the drug of choice in children with HIV infection. This recommendation is based on the known safety profile of TMP-SMX and its efficacy in adults with HIV infection and in children with malignancies. Alternative regimens recommended for HIV-infected children who cannot tolerate TMP-SMX include aerosolized pentamidine in children more than 5 years of age, oral dapsone, and oral atovaquone. One study suggests that TMP-SMX use is associated with a decreased incidence of *P. jiroveci* pneumonitis and an increased incidence of HIV encephalopathy, both as initial AIDS-defining conditions in infants and children [320].

ASPERGILLOSIS

Invasive aspergillosis is a disease of the immunocompromised host, including the premature infant in the neonatal intensive care unit (NICU). Although aspergillosis is uncommon among neonates, its incidence in this age group appears to have increased during the past 2 decades, coinciding with the increased survival of infants who are increasingly more immature at birth. Rapid progression from either primary cutaneous aspergillosis or pulmonary aspergillosis to dissemination is common in these immature infants. Thus early recognition with appropriate antifungal therapy is critical for an optimal outcome.

Aspergillosis has been reported in infants who range in age from 1 to 7 weeks. In 1955 Zimmerman [321] described a 13-day-old neonate who became febrile in association with formation of a subcutaneous abscess caused by *Staphylococcus*. Despite antimicrobial therapy for the abscess, pneumonia and hepatosplenomegaly subsequently developed, and the infant died at 1 month of age. *Aspergillus sydowii* was isolated from the lung, brain, pericardial, and pleural fluid. Allan and Andersen [322] reported disseminated aspergillosis in an infant who showed the first signs of disease on the second day of life and who died at 18 days of age. At autopsy, *Aspergillus* was identified in the lung, liver, spleen, heart, thyroid, bowel, and skin of this infant; *Aspergillus* fumigatus grew from cultures of the liver, spleen, and bowel. Luke and coworkers [323] reported disseminated aspergillosis in a debilitated infant who died at 7 weeks of age. At autopsy, *A. fumigatus* was isolated from the blood, heart, and kidneys, and the fungus was identified on microscopic examination in the endocardium, brain, and kidneys. Akkoyunlu and Yücell [324] reported a case of aspergillosis in an infant in whom onset of respiratory and central

nervous system (CNS) disease occurred at 2 weeks of age. This infant died at 20 days of age with pneumonia and meningitis. *Aspergillus* was cultured from lung and brain tissue obtained at autopsy. The source of infection was thought to be infected grain on the farm where the infant lived. Infection in two of these four infants was considered secondary to prematurity or to antibiotic or corticosteroid therapy [325,326], but predisposing causes for disseminated aspergillosis were not found in the others [327,328]. Thirty-one additional cases of cutaneous or disseminated aspergillosis in infants have been reported [329–350], and only 11 infants survived [331,333,338–342]. The diagnosis seldom was made before death, and in most cases, the infant died despite institution of antifungal therapy. Infants who survived were more likely to have primary cutaneous infection without dissemination. As in previously reported cases, *Aspergillus* infection was secondary to prematurity [328,344,346,348–350], antibiotic therapy [334], or serious underlying disease [330,331,343,345,347].

THE ORGANISM

The genus *Aspergillus* contains about 900 distinct species [351], but only 8 have been shown to be pathogenic for humans. Identification of species of *Aspergillus* is made on the basis of morphology and structural details of the conidia-producing structures when grown on specialized media. These fungi reproduce by asexual spores or conidia, developing characteristic branching, septate hyphae as they grow. *Aspergillus* species produce a variety of mycotoxins in nonhuman hosts, but none have been identified in isolates from infected adults. Reported virulence factors include production of protease, phospholipases, and hemolysin, each of which may function to promote invasion of damaged skin [352]. Fibrinogen and laminin receptors are present on the conidia of *A. fumigatus*, and they may augment infection of traumatized skin by interaction with exposed extracellular matrix ligands [353,354]. The species that are pathogenic in humans and animals are *A. fumigatus* (which is the most common), *Aspergillus flavus, Aspergillus nidulans, Aspergillus niger,* and *Aspergillus terreus,* and less frequently, *Aspergillus glaucus, Aspergillus restrictus, Aspergillus versicolor,* and *A. sydowii* [352]. Most cases of neonatal aspergillosis are caused by *A. fumigatus*.

EPIDEMIOLOGY AND TRANSMISSION

Aspergillus species are ubiquitous and abundant in the environment. These fungi are found throughout the world in grains and decaying vegetation, soil, and other organic matter. Infection with *Aspergillus* is common in animals [355]. *Aspergillus* spores frequently are isolated from the air because they are easily dispersed, lightweight, and resistant to destruction. Although it has been reported that infection is more common in persons exposed to large numbers of conidia [356–360], occupational predisposition has been questioned [361–365], and a history of inordinate exposure is infrequent. No racial or gender predisposition has been found in the infection rate, but clinical disease in adults is more common in men than in women [366].

Species of *Aspergillus* most often are acquired by humans through inhalation of spores into the respiratory tract, but saprophytic infection with *Aspergillus* may be found in the external auditory canal, skin, nails, nasal sinuses, and vagina [367–370]. Although infection in newborns may result from inhalation of conidia from the environment, the fungus also can be acquired, albeit rarely, during gestation or at the time of birth from an infection in the mother. None of the mothers in one study showed evidence of disseminated infection during pregnancy, and studies of vaginal flora were performed in only one [322]. In the infant of that mother, onset of infection was at 2 days of age; studies were not performed in the mother until 1 month postpartum. Results of culture of vaginal secretions for *Aspergillus* were negative, and appearance by chest roentgenogram was normal. Although person-to-person transmission has not been reported, another source of infection suggested by Allan and Andersen [322] was a second infant in the same nursery. That infant died, but because an autopsy was not performed, the diagnosis of *Aspergillus* infection could not be confirmed.

Aspergillus species are found in the hospital setting; thus it is not surprising that infants in the NICU are exposed to this fungus, and that invasive disease results because of the immaturity of their immune system and skin barriers. Sources within the hospital include packaged gauze, tape, limb boards, adhesive monitor leads, and pulse oximetry probes [322,323,371]. Contaminated hyperalimentation fluid has been associated with neonatal aspergillosis. Hospital outbreaks have been associated with airborne contamination during hospital renovation or nearby road construction and from bird droppings in the air ducts [372,373]. Hospital water systems harboring fungi have resulted in airborne transmission from sinks and restrooms. The most common mode of transmission in the neonate is contamination of skin breakdown sites, abrasions, or open wounds [374]. The skin of the premature infant is extremely fragile, does not provide an adequate barrier to the environment, and is prone to breakdown or abrasion even with usual handling.

PATHOGENESIS

Four morphologic forms of the fungus representing stages of development from germination of conidia to fructification have been identified in humans infected with *Aspergillus* [375]. The progressive changes in morphology may reflect the host's susceptibility or resistance to the fungus. After inhalation, ingestion, or inoculation of the spore, primary hyphae form from the germinating conidia, evoking an intense polymorphonuclear leukocyte response. As infection continues, unbranched, straight, or spiraling hyphae may be seen. Later, characteristic branching occurs, and vegetative forms of *Aspergillus* may be identified in devitalized tissue. In infants, the most common microscopic findings are acute inflammation, hemorrhagic infarction, and subsequent necrosis, and invasion of tissue by characteristic hyphae. Vegetative forms apparently are not found in infants because the disease progresses so rapidly that death occurs first.

Aspergillosis results when the immunocompromised infant with an appropriate portal of entry is exposed to this fungus, resulting in either locally invasive or widely disseminated infection. The primary host defense in humans is the phagocyte, so with inhalation of *Aspergillus* spores, macrophages act by rapidly killing conidia. Neutrophils are involved when conidia escape the reticuloendothelial system and begin the mycelial phase [352]. Oxidative killing is an important host defense [375]. Corticosteroid therapy impairs macrophage and neutrophil killing of *Aspergillus* spores and hyphae [376]. Neutropenia, a common predisposing condition in adults and children with aspergillosis, rarely accompanies neonatal aspergillosis [377,378]. Rather, the underlying problem in neonates appears to be a qualitative defect in neutrophil function [375]. The mechanical disruption of skin by minor trauma, such as removal of adhesive tape securing devices (e.g., intravenous catheters or endotracheal tubes), can allow invasion by *Aspergillus* [379,380].

PATHOLOGY

Increasingly, *Aspergillus* infection in premature infants in the NICU first manifests as primary cutaneous aspergillosis. In this circumstance, skin biopsy of the lesions reveals extensive disruption of the epidermis, with invasion of the dermis by the septate, 45-degree branching hyphae characteristic of this fungus [341,380]. In infants with aspergillosis, prematurity or antibiotic or corticosteroid therapy may contribute to the risk of infection. In two reported cases of aspergillosis in infants [321,324], however, no predisposing causes were identified. In infants, dissemination of the infection appears to be more common than locally invasive infection [321–324,381].

Aspergillus can invade tissue by direct extension, as in orbital or nasal sinus infection into the brain, or it may be widely disseminated by the hematogenous route. In young infants, dissemination appears to result from the primary focus of infection in the lung or skin. The organs most often involved in invasive or disseminated infection are the lung, gastrointestinal tract, brain, liver, kidney, thyroid, and heart [382]. Skin and subcutaneous areas, genital tract, and adrenal glands are sometimes involved. One of the infants with primary cutaneous aspergillosis in the reported cases had skin infection also, and at autopsy *Aspergillus* was identified in the spleen [323]. In disseminated aspergillosis, invasion of blood vessels results in infarction and necrosis. Because the fungus invades and occludes the vessels, hemorrhagic necrosis is frequently seen in the lung and gastrointestinal tract in both infants and adults. Microscopic examination of infected tissues reveals extensive involvement, with dichotomous branching of septate hyphae and the presence of conidial heads in air-containing tissues such as the lung [352]. Necrotizing bronchitis with pseudomembrane formation, invasive tracheitis, and necrotizing bronchopneumonia are found by examination of lung tissue from infants [339,377]. Although granulomatous lesions occasionally are seen throughout an infected organ, suppuration with polymorphonuclear leukocytes and abscess formation are more common.

CLINICAL MANIFESTATIONS

The number of reports of neonatal infection with *Aspergillus* limited to the skin has been increasing [334,336, 338–342,346,349]. Premature infants have a unique predisposition to primary cutaneous aspergillosis as a result of their poor skin barrier function. Nine infants have been reported, and all survived with medical or surgical treatment, or both. The cutaneous lesions typically begin as multiple erythematous or violaceous papules that rapidly progress to hemorrhagic bullae, followed by the development of purpuric ulcerations and black eschar formation within 24 hours [344,382]. Lesions often begin on the back or other dependent areas and may be mistaken for pressure sores, but they can occur anywhere on the body where trauma has occurred [339,379]. The lesions of primary cutaneous aspergillosis have been mistaken for bullous impetigo and thermal burns from cutaneous CO_2 probe placement [378]. New skin lesions in a premature infant that are black or brown in appearance are suspicious for aspergillosis, but other fungi can give this appearance; therefore, biopsy and culture are necessary to establish an early diagnosis.

Most of the infants with disseminated aspergillosis in reported cases had signs of pulmonary infection that were thought to be pneumonia, not pulmonary infarction. One infant had a cutaneous infection that appeared as a maculopapular rash on the second day of life [322]. Skin lesions became scaly and later pustular. In this infant, enlargement of the liver became apparent, and the infant failed to gain weight. The case reported by Luke and associates [323] was characterized by jaundice, hepatosplenomegaly, heart murmur, ascites, and melena. Cerebrospinal fluid in the affected infant contained white blood cells, but further details were not reported. Jaundice and enlargement of liver and spleen were prominent in the case reported by Zimmerman [326], and the infant described by Akkoyunlu and Yücell [324] had pneumonia and meningitis. Liver disease also was dominant in the cases reported by Mangurten and coworkers [328] and Gonzalez-Crussi and colleagues [329]. Widespread dissemination to the large and small bowel, liver, pancreas, peritoneum, and lung was demonstrated in the infant with aspergillosis and leukemia [330].

DIAGNOSIS AND DIFFERENTIAL DIAGNOSIS

Diagnostic considerations in patients with cutaneous aspergillosis include infections due to other fungi, particularly *Candida* and Phycomycetes organisms. In infants with disseminated aspergillosis without skin involvement, diagnosis is difficult. Although *Aspergillus* can be identified by direct microscopic examination or culture of secretions, its presence does not necessarily indicate infection even in the presence of clinical disease. Demonstration of *Aspergillus* by culture or by microscopic examination of tissue obtained by biopsy or from body fluids establishes the diagnosis. *Aspergillus* species grow readily on almost all laboratory media, and characteristic conidiophores usually are present within 48 hours of incubation. Fungal blood and other body fluid cultures yield *Aspergillus* in less than 75% of cases, however [352].

Hematoxylin-eosin, periodic acid-Schiff, Schwartz-Lamkins, and Grocott and Gomori methenamine silver stains can be used to visualize septate hyphae in tissue. Spores and branching septate hyphae measuring 4 μm in diameter may be seen. The presence of conidiospores in tissue is infrequent, but they may be seen in specimens of saprophytic infection. Mycelia of *Aspergillus* may be confused with pseudohyphae of *Candida*, which usually are smaller and have no branching; yeast forms usually are present. Phycomycetes can be distinguished from *Aspergillus* by their large size, irregularity, and absence of septa. The greatest difficulty is encountered in distinguishing *Aspergillus* in tissue from *Penicillium*, which also can cause infection in humans [383]. The hyphae of *Penicillium* are broader and contain fewer septa. Culture of tissue establishes the diagnosis. Potassium hydroxide smear of the contents of a papule or blister may reveal characteristic hyphae, allowing for a rapid presumptive diagnosis until culture results are available [339]. PCR techniques may be useful in detecting *Aspergillus* species in serum, cerebrospinal fluid, or other potentially infected body fluids [384]. The detection of *Aspergillus* antigen can be helpful in diagnosis, but no data on antigenemia are available for infants [383,385]. The use of galactomannan assays has been demonstrated to have acceptable sensitivity and specificity in adults and in some high risk pediatric populations, such as oncology patients, but few data have been reported in neonates and young infants, and these data suggest poor specificity. Additional diagnostic modalities useful for detecting the extent of involvement in neonates with suspected dissemination infection include lumbar puncture; chest radiography; computed tomography of the brain and chest; abdominal ultrasound examination of liver, spleen, and kidneys; and funduscopic examination. Even if CNS involvement is present, the cerebrospinal fluid may not show an inflammatory response.

THERAPY

Intravenous amphotericin B deoxycholate remains the drug of choice for treatment for all forms of neonatal aspergillosis (Table 34–2) [386,387]. Amphotericin B should be administered at a dose of 1.5 mg/kg of body weight once daily and infused over a 1- to 2-hour period. This drug is very well tolerated in neonates, and infusion-related adverse effects are rare. Although nephrotoxicity is

TABLE 34–2 Susceptibility of Fungi to Amphotericin B

Fungus	Very Susceptible	Moderately Susceptible	Resistant
Aspergillus species		+	
Blastomyces dermatitidis	+		
Cryptococcus neoformans	+		
Coccidioides immitis	+		
Malassezia furfur		+	
Phycomycetes			
Fusarium species			+
Mucorales		+	
Scedosporium species			+

possible, it is quite uncommon in neonates and young infants. The optimal duration of therapy is not known, but courses up to 10 weeks are not uncommon. Lipid-associated preparations of amphotericin B have had limited use in neonates but have been used to successfully treat invasive aspergillosis in older children. Daily doses of 5 mg/kg apparently are well tolerated. No studies suggesting either safety or efficacy for azoles, often used in older patients with primary cutaneous aspergillosis, have been published. One study, however, evaluated itraconazole in a few neonates [388]. Other antifungal agents, such as voriconazole and caspofungin, have not been evaluated in neonates for pharmacokinetics, safety, or efficacy, and these drugs should not be employed [210,211]. Complete surgical resection of infected, necrotic tissue, in conjunction with amphotericin B therapy, is necessary to treat cutaneous aspergillosis, but preterm infants with extensive cutaneous lesions occasionally may not be able to tolerate full excision. Vitrectomy and intravitreous amphotericin B can be considered the preferred treatment for endophthalmitis caused by *Aspergillus* species [387].

PROGNOSIS

The prognosis for primary cutaneous aspergillosis in infants is poor because of rapid dissemination, and a high mortality rate is reported even with institution of amphotericin B therapy. Nevertheless, a high index of suspicion—coupled with prompt biopsy of a skin lesion and institution of empirical therapy with amphotericin B continued until results of diagnostic tests including culture become available—has allowed a good outcome in some infants [339].

PREVENTION

Because the risk of death associated with neonatal aspergillosis remains high, attempts to reduce exposure to *Aspergillus* species are of primary importance in preventing this infection. Filtration systems reduce the airborne transmission of *Aspergillus* spores, and rooms equipped with high-efficiency particulate air (HEPA) filters are virtually fungus free. Construction on or near the NICU should be avoided. Excellent skin care, including the judicious use of adhesive tape, monitor probes, and wound dressing material, is indicated for the prevention of skin breakdown with potential exposure to environmental *Aspergillus* species.

BLASTOMYCOSIS

Infection with *Blastomyces* has been reported in only four newborns [212–214], although infection with this fungus occurred in 19 women during pregnancy [214,216–221]. In all but three of these nine women, the infection was diagnosed and treated before delivery. The three women who received no treatment had disseminated infection. Two of the infants born to these three mothers were healthy at birth, but one of them died at 3 weeks of age when *Blastomyces* was identified in lung tissue [212]. The second infant presented at 18 days of age with respiratory distress, and infection with *Blastomyces dermatitidis* was

diagnosed by lung biopsy. He received amphotericin B but died 3 weeks after initiation of therapy [213]. The third infant was not infected. Two additional pregnancies ended in stillbirths. Infection with *Blastomyces* was not identified in any of the other infants in the reported cases.

THE ORGANISM

Blastomyces is a dimorphic fungus that has a mycelial form at room temperature and a yeast form at 378° C [222]. The mycelial form is found in soil, where it may exist for long periods [223,389,390]. Conidiophores arise at right angles to the hyphae and are believed to be infectious for humans when mycelia are disturbed. When inhaled, the fungus converts to the yeast form, which is multinucleate, containing 8 to 12 nuclei. It has a thick wall and reproduces by single budding with a broad connection to the parent [390].

EPIDEMIOLOGY AND TRANSMISSION

Blastomycosis is endemic in the Mississippi and Ohio river valleys in the United States and in parts of Canada [391–401]. Sporadic cases have been reported in Central and South America and in Africa [402]. The infection is more common in middle-aged men [391,400,401], particularly those who are employed outdoors in rural areas [401].

Blastomyces is acquired by inhalation of contaminated soil, and the lung is the initial focus of infection [403]. Primary cutaneous blastomycosis by direct inoculation of the organism into skin has been reported [403–405]. It has been suggested that human-to-human transmission does not occur, but Craig and colleagues [406] reported probable human-to-human transmission through sexual intercourse. In addition, mother-to-fetus transmission has been suggested.

Pulmonary infection has been identified as the initial site of infection due to *Blastomyces dermatitidis* [403]. In some instances, the pulmonary disease is self-limited and may resolve without therapy [407]. In some instances, however, both progressive pulmonary disease and dissemination can occur. Although no extensive studies in immunocompromised patients have been conducted, both corticosteroid therapy and other immunosuppressive therapy may increase the risk not only of acquisition of the fungus but also dissemination as well [398,408]. It has been suggested by some studies that a relatively immunosuppressed state occurs during pregnancy, which may account for this increased risk of dissemination [402,409,410]. When dissemination occurs, the skin, bones, and genitourinary system are most commonly involved. The CNS, liver, spleen, and lymph nodes are not commonly affected. Cell-mediated immunity appears to decrease the risk of disseminated blastomycosis [411].

PATHOLOGY

The inflammatory response in the lung consists of proliferation of polymorphonuclear leukocytes followed by formation of noncaseating granuloma with epithelioid and giant cells. Extrapulmonary sites of infection show a similar histologic pattern, with the exception of the skin, which shows pseudoepitheliomatous hyperplasia and microabscesses.

CLINICAL MANIFESTATIONS

Acute symptomatic pulmonary infection in children and adults with *Blastomyces* is associated with abrupt onset of chills and fever, myalgias, and arthralgias. Pleuritic pain is common early, and cough is prominent and may become productive of purulent sputum late in the course of the disease. Resolution of symptoms without therapy is common. Pulmonary infection, however, may become chronic and slowly progressive, with chronic cough, hemoptysis, pleuritic chest pain, and weight loss.

When dissemination occurs, skin infections are reported in as many as 80% of adult cases [403,412–415]. These infections are most common on exposed surfaces, and lesions have a verrucous appearance, particularly in the later stages. Abscesses may occur at the periphery of the lesions. In some patients, the skin lesions appear as shallow ulcerations with central granulation tissue that bleeds easily. Other sites of infection include subcutaneous tissue, bone, and joints and the genitourinary system, particularly the epididymis and prostate. CNS infection is uncommon; however, it usually is associated with headache, confusion, and meningismus [416]. Involvement of the liver and spleen is uncommon.

Of nine women with blastomycosis during pregnancy, seven had disseminated infection; in three of the four in whom studies were done, no evidence of placental infection could be found [216–220]. One of these women had received amphotericin B for 35 days before the birth of her infant. *B. dermatitidis* was cultured from the placenta in the fourth woman, and the organism was visualized in both the fetal and the maternal placental tissue [220]. None of their infants, however, were infected. In one woman in whom placental studies were not done, the fungus was isolated from urine, and her infant died at 3 weeks of age with pulmonary blastomycosis [212]. At autopsy, the infant had no evidence of extrapulmonary infection, suggesting that the fungus may have been acquired by aspiration of infected secretions during birth rather than by hematogenous spread in utero. In the other infant, although the original site of infection was the lung, the fungus was found at autopsy in the kidneys as well [213].

DIAGNOSIS AND DIFFERENTIAL DIAGNOSIS

Because of the rarity of neonatal blastomycosis, enumeration of specific signs that may lead to its diagnosis is difficult. As suggested by findings in the four cases reviewed here, and by extrapolated data in infants with other nonopportunistic fungal infections, the diagnosis should be considered in an infant born in an endemic area for *Blastomyces* who has signs of indolent, progressive pulmonary disease and whose chest radiograph demonstrates bilateral nodular densities. In older children and adults, the clinical picture in acute pulmonary infection with *Blastomyces* appears similar to that in acute bacterial, mycoplasmal, and viral infections. Radiographic findings also are nonspecific. Chronic infection can simulate

infection with *Mycobacterium tuberculosis* and other fungi, and mass lesions can suggest carcinoma. Few specific signs are associated with extrapulmonary blastomycosis. The skin lesions may be mistaken for squamous cell carcinoma.

Diagnosis of blastomycosis is made by visualization of fungus in culture of secretions or tissue. Serologic studies to determine the presence of complement-fixing antibodies lack sensitivity [392], but results of immunodiffusion tests for precipitating antibody may be positive in as many as 80% of adult cases [417,418]. No data regarding skin test reactivity or serologic studies in infants with blastomycosis have been reported.

THERAPY

In view of the rarity of this infection and the limited (or lack of) information regarding pharmacokinetics and safety of antifungal drugs other than amphotericin B in neonates, it appears prudent to treat *Blastomyces* infections in infants with amphotericin B deoxycholate, presumably for a minimum of 6 weeks. Itraconazole and fluconazole have been shown to be safe and efficacious in adults and older children.

PROGNOSIS

Each of the two reported neonates with blastomycosis died [216,217]. In one the diagnosis was not suspected, and in the other the infection progressed despite antifungal therapy.

PREVENTION

Data that address prevention of blastomycosis in neonates are lacking. In pregnant women who reside in or travel through endemic areas, however, a respiratory illness should suggest this diagnosis. Prompt diagnosis and therapy for pregnant women have been associated with prevention of illness in young infants [216–221].

COCCIDIOIDOMYCOSIS

Clinically apparent infection with *Coccidioides immitis* in infants in the first month of life has been reported infrequently despite the high incidence of infection in children living in areas where the fungus is endemic [419]. Most affected infants have been born at term, even when transmission was congenital. The first case of coccidioidomycosis in a neonate was reported by Cohen in 1949 [420]. Although the diagnosis was not established until the infant was 15 weeks of age, signs of pulmonary disease were present at 1 week of age. Dactylitis was evident at 2 weeks of age; the infected finger was the site from which the fungus finally was isolated. Coccidioidomycosis has been reported in 11 other infants; each had clinical onset by 10 weeks of age [421–429]. Although pulmonary disease was prominent in each infant, disseminated infection was found at autopsy in all who died. Two of the infants had signs of meningitis [421,422], but the fungus was isolated from cerebrospinal fluid in only one of them [422]. In two additional reported cases, the infants survived. In one the diagnosis was made by serologic testing [428], and in the other the diagnosis was established when the fungus was identified in tracheal secretions [429].

THE ORGANISM

C. immitis is the only species of *Coccidioides*; it is found below the surface of the soil. *C. immitis* exists in two phases: saprophytic and parasitic. Saprophytic *Coccidioides* exists in a mycelial form in nonliving material, only rarely in tissue [430]. Hyphae have regularly spaced septa with alternating infectious spores and sterile cells. Arthrospores are infectious components of hyphae and are barrel shaped, measuring 2 to 10 μm in width. Spores may be round or ovoid, in which case they are more typically chlamydospores. An annual rainfall of 5 to 20 inches in alkaline soil and a prolonged hot, dry season followed by precipitation favor the formation of spores [431]. Infectious spores become airborne with minimal disturbance during the hot, dry season and may remain infectious for several weeks. Arthrospores, which have been known to be transported on clothes or other inanimate objects containing contaminated dust, may cause infection great distances from endemic areas [432].

The parasitic form of *C. immitis* is the spherule. The spherule forms in tissue from inhaled or inoculated arthrospores. It measures 10 to 80 μm in diameter and contains endospores, which form within the spherule by cleavage of cytoplasm. Mature spherules rupture, liberating a few hundred to several hundred endospores, which subsequently develop into new spherules [430].

EPIDEMIOLOGY AND TRANSMISSION

C. immitis is found in soil 12 to 14 cm below the surface. Sunlight appears to destroy the fungus. *Coccidioides* is endemic in the Western Hemisphere in the San Joaquin Valley and southern counties of California, southern Arizona, New Mexico, and western Texas, and in Mexico, Guatemala, Honduras, Venezuela, Paraguay, Colombia, and Argentina. In endemic areas, naturally occurring infection has been reported in a variety of wild and domestic animals, including cattle [433], sheep [434,435], dogs [436], horses and burros [437], and rodents [438].

Epidemiologic studies have estimated that approximately 10 million persons currently residing in endemic areas have been infected with *C. immitis* [439]. The rate of infection in susceptible persons arriving in an endemic area is 15% to 50% within the first year [440]. After residence in an endemic area for 5 years, 80% of susceptible persons will become infected. In more than 50% of these, infection is asymptomatic and can be demonstrated only by the presence of delayed hypersensitivity to coccidioidin skin test antigen. The incidence of infection is highest in the early summer and remains high until the first rains of winter. The rate of infection also is higher in dry seasons that follow a season of heavy rainfall [441,442].

No racial or gender difference in incidence of primary coccidioidomycosis has been noted. Primary infection is recognized more frequently in women, however, because they are more likely than men to have cutaneous hypersensitivity reactions [443,444]. Considerable racial differences have been reported in the risk of disseminated disease. Mexican Indian men are three times more likely to disseminate the fungus than white men; black men are 14 times more prone to dissemination than white men; and Filipino men are reported to be 175 times more susceptible than white men [439,445,446]. In women, dissemination is more common during pregnancy [447–451]. Before puberty, no gender difference in clinical manifestations or extent of disease is seen.

Studies to determine explanations for increased susceptibility in men, nonwhite races, and pregnant women have not been performed. Patients with lymphomas, leukemia, and diabetes mellitus are reported to have no higher incidence of clinically significant or disseminated coccidioidal infection than in other persons [452], but disseminated infection may be more common in patients with AIDS [453] and in those receiving corticosteroids or immunosuppressive therapy [454].

Coccidioidomycosis in infants has been considered to result from inhalation of arthrospores. Transmission of coccidioidomycosis from mother to infant in utero has been reported by Shafai [437], who described twins born to a woman who died 24 hours post partum with disseminated coccidioidomycosis. Both infants died with widespread disease. Christian and associates [423] described one case in which onset of disease was at 3 weeks of age in an infant living in a nonendemic area. The infant's mother had inactive coccidioidal osteomyelitis but did not have pulmonary or cutaneous disease, suggesting that infection in the infant may have been acquired in utero or at the time of birth. An infant described by Cohen [420] was born to a mother with active coccidioidomycosis during pregnancy; pulmonary disease was evident in the infant at the age of 1 week, again suggesting that the infection may have been acquired in utero. Respiratory symptoms developed at 2 weeks of age in one infant born to a woman who subsequently died of disseminated coccidioidomycosis, but the infant became clinically well after 3 weeks of therapy with intravenous amphotericin B [422]. Bernstein and co-workers [427] reported onset of disease in an infant at 5 days of age, and although no evidence of disease was noted in the mother, disease onset in the infant shortly after birth suggested in utero transmission of the fungus. By contrast, in the several reported cases of disseminated coccidioidomycosis in pregnant women, only three instances of placental infection were noted, with no evidence of infection in any of the infants [455–459].

Human-to-human transmission of *C. immitis* is rare. Even though infectious arthrospores can be found in residual pulmonary cavities and benign pulmonary granulomas in humans [419], secondary cases within families are unusual. Eckmann and coworkers [447] reported six cases of coccidioidomycosis acquired at the bedside of a patient with coccidioidal osteomyelitis whose cast was contaminated with spherule-containing exudate.

PATHOGENESIS

The respiratory tract is the initial focus of infection by *C. immitis* in most infants and adults. Direct inoculation of fungus into the skin, reported rarely in adults and older children [448], has not been described in neonates.

After arthrospores are inhaled, mature spherules develop in the bronchial mucosa 4 to 7 days later [449,450]. Granulomas form rapidly, involving pulmonary lymphatics and tracheobronchial lymph nodes. In adults with mild disease, a few scattered lesions may be present; however, when pulmonary involvement is extensive, an outpouring of polymorphonuclear leukocytes fill alveoli, and a radiographic appearance of bronchopneumonia is noted. Ulceration of bronchi and bronchioles can occur, with later development of bronchiectasis. Hematogenous dissemination with multiple organ involvement occurs frequently in neonates, and severe CNS infection is a frequent complication.

PATHOLOGY

The typical histologic appearance of lesions in *Coccidioides* infection is that of a granuloma with epithelioid cells and Langhans' giant cells. Granulomas occur in infants and older patients. In immunocompromised hosts, suppuration can be prominent, but with adequate host response, hyalinization, fibrosis, and calcification occur.

Coccidioides can disseminate by blood flow to any organ in the body. The most significant focus of infection after dissemination is the CNS; the brain, meninges, or spinal cord can be involved. Dissemination to the CNS is most common in children and in white males and is the most common cause of death in patients with coccidioidomycosis [428,451]. In cases of meningitis, presence of a thick exudate encasing the brain invariably results in noncommunicating hydrocephalus. Involvement around the base of the brain usually is more extensive than that above the cerebral cortex. On microscopic examination, the meninges are seen to be studded with small granulomas; similar lesions may be present in the underlying brain substance. In the spinal cord, infection may result in compression by the thick, tough inflammatory membrane, with subsequent loss of motor and sensory functions.

Other organs involved when the infection becomes disseminated include the skin, lungs and pleura, spleen, liver, kidneys, heart, genital tract, adrenal glands, and, occasionally, skeletal muscle. In infants, cutaneous infection most often makes its appearance as a papular rash in the diaper area. The gastrointestinal tract is almost always spared in infants, although the peritoneum and bowel serosa frequently are studded with granulomas. In each of three infants who died of disseminated coccidioidomycosis, the lungs and spleen were involved. One infant had infection in the liver, and one had documented meningitis. Skin infection was present in only one infant [355]. One of the surviving infants had pulmonary infection and osteomyelitis [420], and another had pulmonary infection and chorioretinitis [428].

CLINICAL MANIFESTATIONS

Although primary pulmonary coccidioidal infection is asymptomatic in 60% of older children and adults [452], and only 25% have an illness severe enough to seek medical attention, each of the infected newborns in the reported cases had signs of pulmonary disease. After an incubation period of 10 to 16 days, signs of a mild lower respiratory tract disorder appear, characterized by a dry, nonproductive cough. Findings can include low-grade fever, anorexia, and malaise, and significant respiratory distress. Physical examination of the chest may demonstrate few abnormalities, but roentgenograms typically show evidence of bronchopneumonia or segmental or peribronchial disease in infants. Hilar nodes often are enlarged, and small pleural effusions are common.

Cavitary lesions became apparent in one infant several months after birth and cleared by the age of 30 months [420]. It is in such chronic lesions that the saprophytic form of *Coccidioides* has been demonstrated [430].

In infants, dissemination of infection is frequent, and when dissemination to the CNS occurs, infection in brain and meninges can be overlooked [453]. Signs, which are vague and nonspecific, include anorexia and lethargy. Nuchal rigidity is infrequent. As the infection progresses, other CNS manifestations include confusion, obtundation, coma, and seizures. Papilledema is a late finding.

DIAGNOSIS AND DIFFERENTIAL DIAGNOSIS

Granulomatous pulmonary disease caused by *C. immitis* in adults can mimic tuberculosis, Q fever, psittacosis, ornithosis, viral pneumonias, or other fungal infections, particularly histoplasmosis. In infants, pulmonary coccidioidomycosis may appear to be similar to bacterial infection. In patients with coccidioidal meningitis, considerations in the differential diagnosis include tuberculous meningitis, cryptococcosis, histoplasmosis, blastomycosis, candidiasis, and partially treated bacterial meningitis [427]. In coccidioidal meningitis, the cerebrospinal fluid usually is under increased pressure. Pleocytosis with mononuclear cells is characteristic, but in cases discovered early, a preponderance of polymorphonuclear cells may be found. Eosinophils are common in cerebrospinal fluid in patients with coccidioidal meningitis. The cerebrospinal fluid glucose level is decreased, and the protein level may be markedly elevated.

The diagnosis of coccidioidomycosis must be suspected in infants with unexplained pulmonary disease who are born to mothers who reside in endemic areas. In addition, a history of travel to an endemic area or an occupational hazard involving exposure to contaminated dust may be important clues leading to suspicion of coccidioidal infection [454,460,461]. Establishing a diagnosis of coccidioidomycosis in an infant is difficult. Identification of spherules in pus, sputum, or tissue is diagnostic of infection with *C. immitis*. Direct microscopic examination is best performed if the infected material is partially digested with 10% sodium or potassium hydroxide. Specimens treated by alkalinization are unsatisfactory for culture.

Spherules may be easier to identify if equal parts of iodine and Sudan IV are used. Iodine is absorbed into the wall of the spherule, and Sudan IV differentiates fat globules from spherules [462]. Because spherule-like artifacts are commonly found in sputum and pus, however, direct examination may be misleading. Direct microscopic examination of gastric aspirate and cerebrospinal fluid usually is unrewarding, and even results of culture of cerebrospinal fluid in cases of coccidioidal meningitis can be negative [453]. Identification of spherules in tissue obtained by biopsy or at autopsy is best accomplished with use of Gridley or Gomori methenamine silver stain. Hematoxylin-eosin may be used but often fails to give enough contrast between spherules and host tissue.

Coccidioides can be grown on Sabouraud glucose agar; specimens submitted for culture should include sputum, pus from cutaneous lesions, cerebrospinal fluid, and urine. Because the morphology of mycelia is variable, the fungus can be injected into mice for demonstration of characteristic endosporulating spherules. Culture and animal inoculation are time-consuming and dangerous for laboratory personnel; accordingly, most investigational studies employ immunologic and serologic tests for demonstration of infection with *Coccidioides*.

Studies of development of delayed hypersensitivity in adults, with intradermal injections of 0.1 mL of coccidioidin, have demonstrated that positive reactions may occur 3 days to 2 weeks after the onset of symptoms and may persist for years [430]. In adults without erythema nodosum or erythema multiforme, a dilution of 1:100 of skin test antigen has been used. A positive reaction is manifested 24 to 48 hours after injection as induration of 5 mm or more. Cross-reactions may occur with coccidioidin in patients with histoplasmosis, and coccidioidin can evoke an antibody response to yeast-phase *Histoplasma* but not to *Coccidioides*. False-negative reactions can occur in patients with disseminated infection or in those in whom skin testing is performed before development of cellular immune response to the fungus. Cohen and Burnip [458] performed coccidioidin skin tests in newborns in an endemic area. Among 220 infants studied, positive reactions occurred in 2, but neither had evidence of disease. Two infants born to women with coccidioidal meningitis during pregnancy had negative results on skin testing and no clinical or serologic evidence of infection. Thus skin tests are not useful in establishing a diagnosis of coccidioidomycosis in infants.

Precipitin and complement fixation tests for antibodies to *Coccidioides* have been important in the diagnosis of coccidioidomycosis [463,464]. The complement fixation test has been useful in determining the extent of infection and the prognosis [463]. Precipitating antibodies appear to belong to the IgM class of immunoglobulins and are present in 90% of adults within 4 weeks of onset of symptoms [464]. In most instances, precipitins disappear in 4 to 6 weeks [465]. Coccidioidal antibodies demonstrated by complement fixation tests appear more slowly and only in cases of severe infection. Antibody titers of greater than 1:16 may indicate disseminated infection. The presence of complement-fixing antibodies in cerebrospinal fluid is diagnostic of coccidioidal meningitis; however, only 75% of patients with active meningeal infection have demonstrable antibody in cerebrospinal fluid [463].

A test for detection of coccidioidal antibody using an immunodiffusion technique is available and appears to correlate with the complement fixation test [466,467]. Huppert and associates [468] also have described a latex particle agglutination test that measures antibody paralleling precipitin titers. It is recommended that tests for precipitins and complement-fixing antibodies both be employed for best results in diagnosing coccidioidomycosis [468]. Other serologic tests for coccidioidal antibodies include counterimmunoelectrophoresis [469] and radioimmunoassay [470]; however, results of these techniques in neonates have not been reported.

THERAPY

Coccidioidal infection appears to be less responsive to amphotericin B than other fungal infections and frequently requires prolonged treatment for control. Intravenous amphotericin B deoxycholate at a daily dose of 1 mg/kg of body weight, however, is the drug of choice for the acute treatment of coccidioidomycosis. Because only 5% to 10% of serum levels of amphotericin B is distributed to the CNS, intrathecal administration of amphotericin B also is necessary. The duration of intrathecal amphotericin B therapy may be monitored by coccidioidal complement fixation titer in cerebrospinal fluid. In patients in whom antibodies never develop in cerebrospinal fluid despite coccidioidal meningitis, the duration of therapy is guided by the cerebrospinal fluid findings.

Although amphotericin B has been used in the long-term treatment of adults with CNS disease, no data on use of this drug in young infants have been reported. Prolonged therapy (for more than 1 year) is almost always necessary. In adults and older children, prolonged therapy with itraconazole or fluconazole rather than amphotericin B has been shown to be useful. In patients with CNS disease complicated by noncommunicating hydrocephalus, cerebrospinal fluid shunting may be necessary.

PROGNOSIS

The mortality rate among infants with coccidioidomycosis is high. With three exceptions, all of the infants in whom coccidioidal infection was identified died, with infection recognized only at autopsy.

PREVENTION

Although dust control has been shown to reduce the incidence of infection in persons who are transients in endemic areas [442,471], evidence that such control reduces frequency of infection among long-term residents in these areas is limited. In persons at risk for the development of severe or disseminated infection, attempting to control dust may be beneficial. Cohen [420] suggested that in one case, an infant acquired the infection from inhalation of dust blown into the nursery. Use of air conditioning, filters, and respirators in areas where persons are at risk has been encouraged [472]. Masks have been recommended for persons working in heavily contaminated areas [460]. Other investigators have suggested spraying soil with fungicides [473], but such treatment reaches a depth of only 0.6 cm, which allows the fungus to survive below that level. Careful handling of heavily contaminated dressings by hospital personnel is recommended to prevent acquisition of infection. Isolation or segregation of patients with coccidioidomycosis, however, does not appear to be necessary.

Levine and coworkers [474] have employed a vaccine that has been effective in preventing disease in animals, but results in humans as measured by serologic and skin tests have been erratic [440] and have not shown protection from infection [475].

CRYPTOCOCCOSIS

The occurrence of cryptococcosis in the neonate is rare, with fewer than a dozen cases reported, most before 1990 [476–481]. All but one infant died, and in each case, organisms with the morphologic appearance of *Cryptococcus* were identified by microscopic examination of tissue obtained at autopsy or by culture. The youngest patient in the reported cases of cryptococcal infection was 20 minutes old [476]. This infant, with obvious in utero onset of infection, had hydrocephalus and an enlarged liver and spleen and died at 40 minutes of age. Encapsulated, yeast-like organisms were identified in the brain, liver, and spleen. Neuhauser and Tucker [477], in their description of three infants with cryptococcosis, noted that one had the disease at birth and died at 19 days of age. At autopsy, organisms with the appearance of *Cryptococcus* were identified in the brain, liver, spleen, and bone. Morphologically similar organisms were recovered in specimen cultures from the infant and from the endocervix of the mother. Nassau and Weinberg-Heiruti [478] reported one case of cutaneous and disseminated cryptococcosis in an infant; Heath [479] described a newborn with endophthalmitis associated with widespread cryptococcal infection. Gavai and associates [480] reported the case of the only surviving infant; blood cultures grew *Cryptococcus neoformans*, and amphotericin B therapy was administered.

In adults, the respiratory tract in most instances has been considered to be the primary focus of infection with *Cryptococcus* [473,482–484], but the fungus appears to have a special predilection for the brain and meninges [485,486]. Dissemination of infection to the CNS is common [486] and is more likely to occur in patients whose defenses against infection are compromised by disease or certain therapeutic agents [487–489].

THE ORGANISM

The genus *Cryptococcus* is limited to spherical or oval encapsulated cells that reproduce by multilateral budding. Yeast cells vary in size, but most measure 5 to 10 μm in diameter exclusive of the mucinous capsule, which may be one half to five times the size of the cell. Although *Cryptococcus* usually appears on microscopic examination as encapsulated yeast, some strains of *C. neoformans* may produce true hyphae [490]. Of the seven species of *Cryptococcus*, only *C. neoformans* is pathogenic for humans, and it also is the only species that produces hyphae. A saprophytic species, *C. neoformans* var. innocuous, is culturally and morphologically identical to *C. neoformans* and frequently is confused with it.

Three serologic types of *C. neoformans* have been identified using type-specific capsular polysaccharide antisera [491]. Cross-reactions have been noted with *C. albicans*, *Trichophyton* extract, and other antigens [492].

EPIDEMIOLOGY AND TRANSMISSION

C. neoformans has been isolated from all areas of the world. The original isolate was made by San Felice from peaches [493], and Klein [494] recovered the fungus from cow's milk. Emmons [495] isolated *C. neoformans* from soil and later reported that the milk probably had

been contaminated with soil that contained excreta from pigeons [496]. Although natural cryptococcal infection in pigeons has not been demonstrated, many authors have suggested that pigeons may be the primary source of pathogenic *Cryptococcus* [497–499]. Others believe the soil to be the primary source, with pigeon excreta merely enhancing growth of *Cryptococcus* [500,501].

Some authors have reported recovery of *C. neoformans* from areas inhabited by birds other than pigeons [502–504], but Fragner [505] was able to isolate *C. neoformans* only from pigeon roosts and nonpathogenic species from roosts of other birds. Nevertheless, it is generally accepted that avian habitats, particularly of feral pigeons, represent the major source of *C. neoformans* for humans and animals.

Sources of *C. neoformans* other than pigeon roosts have been reported. Clarke and colleagues [506] isolated the fungus from apples, and McDonough and associates [507] recovered the organism from wood. Cryptococcus also has been found occasionally in soil not contaminated with bird excreta [508]. *C. neoformans* may cause disease in animals [509], and epidemics of cryptococcal mastitis have occurred in dairy cows [510,511]. None of the personnel caring for the cows acquired the infection.

Human cryptococcosis can occur at any age, but approximately 60% of patients are between the ages of 30 and 50 years [512]. Infection is three times more common in men than in women and is particularly frequent in white men. It has been suggested that this gender difference is related at least in part to the enhanced phagocytic activity of leukocytes for *Cryptococcus* in the presence of estrogen [513].

Infection with *C. neoformans* has been thought to result primarily from inhalation of the fungus from an exogenous source, and the respiratory tract is the primary focus of infection [514]. Direct inoculation into the skin and ingestion of the fungus, however, have been suggested as alternative routes of infection [515–517]. Tonsils also have been reported as a possible initial focus of infection [518]. Littman and Zimmerman [484] along with other investigators have suggested that *Cryptococcus* can be isolated from the oropharynx, normal skin, vagina, and intestinal tract of humans with no apparent disease [519]. Whether isolates are actually *C. neoformans* has been questioned. Tynes and coworkers [520] suggested that pathogenic *Cryptococcus* can be present in sputum as a saprophyte, although before their report, isolation of *C. neoformans* from humans had been considered indicative of disease.

Only one of the mothers giving birth to infected offspring [476–479,481] had any illness during pregnancy that could be attributed to infection with *Cryptococcus* [476–479], and although inhalation of *Cryptococcus* cannot be excluded in newborns infected with this organism, the onset of disease at birth suggests that the transmission of the fungus occurred in utero. Isolation of encapsulated yeast from the endocervix of the mother of one affected infant [477] suggested that transmission in this case may have occurred from an ascending vaginal infection. In no other reported instance of cryptococcal infection during pregnancy has transmission to the infant occurred [519,521]. Kida and colleagues [522] reported the case of a woman with HIV infection and AIDS who died with disseminated cryptococcal infection 2 days after the birth of her infant, who was uninfected.

Transmission from person to person, except for isolated cases of possible congenital transmission, has not been reported.

PATHOGENESIS

The presence of pathogenic *Cryptococcus* in humans has been considered to be an indication of disease related to that fungus. The possibility of saprophytic colonization of the skin, sputum, mucous membranes, and feces of healthy persons with *C. neoformans* has been suggested, however [493,523,524]; such colonization would indicate an endogenous source of the fungus. The isolation of encapsulated yeast from the endocervix of an asymptomatic, apparently healthy mother lends support to this contention. Although clinically apparent infection with *C. neoformans* can occur in the normal host, a high incidence of infection has been reported in patients with Hodgkin disease, lymphosarcoma, leukemia, and diabetes mellitus [487–489,524–526], and in those with HIV infection and AIDS. The use of corticosteroids or other immunosuppressive therapy has been associated with a higher incidence of cryptococcosis [527]. Mechanisms of enhanced susceptibility in patients with these underlying disorders or associated with such treatments are similar to those discussed earlier in connection with candidiasis. Cryptococcal infections in these patients, however, have not increased as strikingly as some of the other opportunistic fungal infections [528].

No data specific to infants are available regarding increased susceptibility or resistance to infection with *Cryptococcus*. In the review by Siewers and Cramblett [529] of cryptococcal infections in children, only one of four patients showed evidence of underlying disease. Although gestational age was unknown in two of the eight infants with neonatal cryptococcosis, five of these were born prematurely. Only the surviving infant received antibiotics, and none received corticosteroids. The surviving infant also was receiving hyperalimentation through a central venous catheter.

Presence of a factor in normal human serum that inhibits growth of *C. neoformans* has been demonstrated and may explain the low incidence of clinically apparent cryptococcal infections [530–532]. Alterations in this factor due to disease or therapy may account for the high incidence of cryptococcal infection in patients with diseases of the reticuloendothelial system and in those who are receiving treatment with immunosuppressive drugs. No data are available regarding inhibitory factors in the serum of newborns.

PATHOLOGY

In infants and adults, the respiratory tract appears to be the primary focus of infection, and follows inhalation of the fungus. In some instances, the skin (by direct inoculation) or the gastrointestinal tract (by ingestion) may be the initial route of infection. In adults, respiratory infection usually is subacute or chronic, and the lesion most commonly encountered is a solitary nodule measuring 2 to 7 cm in diameter and located at the periphery of the lung, at the hilar area, or in the middle of a lobe [484]. Hilar lymphadenopathy usually is minimal. In infants and occasionally in adults, diffuse infiltration [533] or miliary disease similar to that typical of tuberculosis may be evident in the lung [534]. Fibrosis and calcification are rare, but cavitary disease may be found in 10% of adults with pulmonary cryptococcal infection [512]. Small subpleural nodules frequently are found at autopsy in these patients [535], but pleuritic reaction is rare.

Microscopically, pulmonary lesions of cryptococcal infection may give the appearance of nonspecific granulomas. If tissue reaction is minimal, the mass has a mucoid appearance—a finding more common in infants. In most instances, an aggregate of encapsulated budding cells with intertwining loose connective tissue can be seen. Granulomatous reaction may occur, with infiltration of lymphocytes and epithelioid cells but without caseation necrosis. Diffuse pneumonic infiltration seen in infants is characterized by accumulation of fungus in alveoli, and an outpouring of histiocytes and tissue macrophages with ingested organisms may be seen.

Cutaneous cryptococcal infection occurs in about 15% of adult cases [536] but has not been reported in infants. Dissemination can occur through the bloodstream to any organ in the body, including the liver, spleen, kidneys, adrenal glands, bone, and eyes, but the CNS is the most common site of infection after dissemination. Lesions outside the CNS in both adults and infants may appear densely granulomatous, similar to tuberculous lesions [483]. CNS evidence of meningitis includes a gray adherent exudate in the subarachnoid space. More extensive involvement can be present around the base of the brain in older patients. In some instances, small granulomas are present in the meninges and along the blood vessels. The underlying surface of the brain can show small, cystlike lesions consisting of fungal or mucinous material. The cellular reaction can be minimal or extensive, with mononuclear inflammatory cells. The infection can extend along the vessels into the brain substance to a variable depth, resulting in pinpoint cysts in gray matter. Parenchymatous lesions may result from embolization and are found in periventricular gray matter and basal ganglia and in white matter of the cerebral hemispheres. Such lesions are found more often in adults than in infants and appear as nonspecific granulomas or as cysts containing mucinous material from capsules of cryptococci. On occasion, discrete granulomas can be found in any part of the brain, spinal cord, or meninges and may act like space-occupying lesions.

CLINICAL MANIFESTATIONS

Infants with cryptococcosis have multisystem involvement characterized by enlargement of the liver or spleen or both, jaundice, hydrocephalus, and, in many instances, chorioretinitis. Roentgenologically, Neuhauser and Tucker [477] found intracranial calcifications scattered over the cortex and within the brain substance in three newborns. It is noteworthy that these findings are compatible with those found in many congenital infections, including toxoplasmosis, rubella, syphilis, and cytomegalovirus infection.

One infant was thought to have had toxoplasmosis and cryptococcal infection [477].

Dissemination of *Cryptococcus* to other organs in infants usually produces signs of disease in one or more sites, most commonly the CNS. Signs vary with the location and extent of CNS involvement. Cryptococcal granulomas in the brain may produce signs similar to those of space-occupying lesions caused by other diseases. Meningitis most often manifests as headache, which can become progressively worse, and is accompanied by nausea, vomiting, and lethargy. As infection continues, seizures can occur. On examination, papilledema may be noted, but nuchal rigidity is uncommon. When the brain is extensively involved, obtundation and coma often result. Cranial nerves can be involved, and amblyopia, diplopia, and optic atrophy are frequent findings. The infant who survived had no evidence of cryptococcosis beyond positive blood cultures. No meningitis, ophthalmic, or pulmonary involvement was present.

DIAGNOSIS AND DIFFERENTIAL DIAGNOSIS

Neonatal cryptococcal infection can appear similar to congenital infection with *Toxoplasma gondii*, rubella virus, cytomegalovirus, and *Toxoplasma pallidum*. Pulmonary cryptococcal infection can be confused with congenital or neonatal tuberculosis or infections with fungi other than *Cryptococcus*.

CNS infection in infants can be confused with tuberculous meningitis. In cases of localized granulomatous disease, considerations in the differential diagnosis must include brain abscess caused by bacteria, cerebrovascular thromboses, and hemorrhage.

Diagnosis of infection with *Cryptococcus* is made by visualization of encapsulated yeasts in sputum or in cerebrospinal fluid, by culture, or by animal inoculation. Microscopic examinations of pus, sputum, exudates, and cerebrospinal fluid are best performed by using India ink, which is displaced by the capsule. Thick specimens of sputum or pus can be mixed with an equal volume of 10% sodium or potassium hydroxide to dissolve tissue and cellular debris before addition of fresh India ink.

In cryptococcal meningitis, the cerebrospinal fluid usually is under increased pressure, and pleocytosis may be present, with a predominance of mononuclear cells. The cerebrospinal fluid glucose level is decreased in only 55% of adult cases, and protein content is increased in 90% [477]. Direct microscopic examination of cerebrospinal fluid using an equal volume of India ink may show encapsulated yeasts in 50% of culture-proven cases. If yeast is found, the diagnosis is established because *Cryptococcus* is the only encapsulated yeast that infects the CNS in humans.

Specimens submitted for culture when diagnosis of cryptococcal infection is suspected should include sputum, cerebrospinal fluid, blood, urine, and bone marrow. If cutaneous lesions are present, pus also should be submitted.

Microscopic examination of tissue obtained by biopsy or at autopsy may strongly support the diagnosis of cryptococcal infection. Although Gridley and methenamine silver stains demonstrate the fungus very well, other fungi also are visualized with these stains. Specific stains for capsular mucin such as mucicarmine [537] and the

Rinehart-Abdul-Haj technique for detection of acid mucopolysaccharide [538] are beneficial, especially for distinguishing *Cryptococcus* from *Histoplasma*.

Immunologic and serologic tests have been proposed as aids in diagnosing infection with *Cryptococcus*. Delayed hypersensitivity to cryptococcal antigens has been noted in adults, but dermal response has not been useful as a diagnostic test [539]. No studies of response to cryptococcal skin test antigens in infants have been reported.

Serum agglutinins, complement-fixing hemagglutination, and indirect fluorescent methods have been described [483,540–545]. Latex and complement fixation tests for detection of cryptococcal antigen in serum and body fluids also have been reported [546–550]. Circulating cryptococcal antigen has been demonstrated in serum and cerebrospinal fluid in patients with meningeal and disseminated infections [551–554]; titers of antigen decrease with recovery. It also has been noted that cryptococcal antibody in serum can increase during recovery from infection with *Cryptococcus*. The latex particle agglutination test has proved to be valuable for detection of cryptococcal antigen in the cerebrospinal fluid of patients in whom findings on culture and microscopic examination of cerebrospinal fluid are negative [552,553,555–557]. No data are available on serologic studies in newborns with cryptococcal infection.

THERAPY

The drugs of choice for treatment of cryptococcal meningitis are intravenous amphotericin B and oral flucytosine. The amphotericin B dose is 1 mg/kg given once daily, and the flucytosine dose is 100 to 150 mg/kg divided into four oral doses. This dosage should be continued for 4 to 8 weeks. In adults, the combination is given for 2 weeks and is followed by either fluconazole or itraconazole administered orally, but no data exist on the appropriate dose, route, safety, or efficacy of these two antifungal agents in young infants.

PROGNOSIS

All of the newborns with cryptococcal infection reported who did not receive treatment died within days to weeks of onset of the disease. One infant survived without apparent sequelae after receiving amphotericin B for 6 weeks.

PREVENTION

Preventive measures should be directed at elimination of exogenous sources of *Cryptococcus*. A solution containing hydrated lime and sodium hydroxide has been shown to be effective in eradicating cryptococci from contaminated pigeon roosts when sprayed on soil containing the organism [558].

MALASSEZIA INFECTIONS

Redline and Dahms [559] in 1981 provided the first description of systemic infection with *Malassezia* species in a very low birth weight infant who was receiving long-term intravenous hyperalimentation including intralipids. Since that first publication, this infection has been described in patients of all ages, but preterm neonates receiving intralipid therapy constitute the patient population with the highest incidence of fungemia [560].

THE ORGANISM

The genus *Malassezia* consists of seven distinct species of yeast sharing common morphologic characteristics, nutritional requirements, and molecular features. All members of the genus cause skin disease in humans, but only *Malassezia furfur*, *Malassezia pachydermatis*, *Malassezia globus*, and *Malassezia sympodialis* are associated with neonatal infections [561–564]. Individual yeast cells are 2.5 to 6.0 μm and round, oval, or cylindrical, depending on the species. Each species demonstrates monopolar budding, whereas in certain species, pseudomycelia also may develop [561]. All *Malassezia* species except *M. pachydermatis* are obligatory lipophiles. This requirement for a source of lipid for growth and development explains the concordance of neonatal systemic disease with the infusion of intravenous lipid emulsions.

EPIDEMIOLOGY AND TRANSMISSION

Malassezia is best known as the fungus responsible for tinea versicolor, a common skin infection among adults [565]. *M. furfur* and *M. pachydermatis* also are responsible for catheter-related bloodstream infections, occurring primarily in neonates or older immunocompromised hosts [565]. *M. sympodialis* and *M. globus* are associated with neonatal pustulosis, also known as neonatal acne [562–564]. Skin colonization with *Malassezia* species is nearly universal among adults, and direct transmission from caregivers to infants is the most common route of acquisition in the neonate [565,566]. These organisms persist on the hands of caregivers, despite appropriate hand hygiene, and on many hospital surfaces [561,567]. *Malassezia* organisms can be recovered from contaminated plastic surfaces for up to 3 months, and this persistence may facilitate nursery transmission [568]. *M. pachydermatis* causes infection in dogs, primarily otitis externa, and nursery outbreaks have been associated with colonization in pets of health care providers [569].

The prevalence of colonization with *Malassezia* species among neonates in the NICU ranges from 30% to 100%, with fully half of the infants in some nurseries colonized by the end of the second week of life [570]. Colonization of catheters is thought to occur secondary to skin colonization or direct nosocomial transmission, as seen with clusters or outbreaks of *Malassezia* infections in an NICU [566,569,571,572]. Catheter-associated infections typically occur in infants older than 7 days of age, with the peak incidence in the third week of life [562,573,574]. Neonatal pustulosis typically develops between 5 days and 3 weeks of age [575,576].

PATHOGENESIS

The pathogenesis of neonatal *Malassezia* infections requires colonization of the skin, followed either by the development of localized neonatal pustulosis or colonization of an indwelling vascular catheter leading to systemic infection. Factors increasing colonization rates among neonates in the NICU include extreme prematurity (gestational age less

than 26 weeks), prolonged time in an isolette, the use of occlusive dressings, and prolonged length of NICU stay [566]. Sebum on the skin, especially that of the face, provides the required source of fat in the case of neonatal pustulosis [561]. Catheter-related infections are always associated with the administration of intravenous lipid emulsions, whether Broviac central intravenous or percutaneously placed Silastic catheters are used [566]. Intravascular catheters used only for hyperalimentation (without intralipids) or medication administration and other types of indwelling catheters do not become infected because the infusate they deliver does not provide the lipid nutritional support necessary for *Malassezia* organisms to proliferate. Intravascular catheters frequently develop thrombi or fibrin sheaths that become adherent to the vascular wall, which then may become infected [564,576,577]. The infected thrombus then serves as a source for ongoing fungemia or dissemination to visceral organs through microembolism [576,578,579]. Persistent fungemia is common with neonatal *Malassezia* infections, yet disseminated disease rarely occurs. Rare cases of meningitis, renal infection, liver abscess, and severe pulmonary or cardiac involvement have been reported [573]. Additional predisposing conditions for the development of neonatal systemic *Malassezia* infections include short-gut syndrome, gastroschisis, necrotizing enterocolitis, and complex congenital heart disease [560,570,580,581]. The need for prolonged parenteral, rather than enteral, nutrition is the common denominator in all of these predisposing conditions. Although less common than infections due to spread of the skin-colonizing organisms, infections due to direct nosocomial transmission of *Malassezia* species are documented [561,582].

CLINICAL MANIFESTATIONS

In neonatal pustulosis, or neonatal acne, the classic lesions are pinpoint erythematous papules that develop into overt pustules, most commonly seen over the chin, cheeks, and forehead, with occasional extension to the neck or scalp [570,580]. Lesions are not irritating to the infant, do not disseminate, and typically resolve over time without therapy—yet the appearance of neonatal pustulosis often is disturbing to parents.

Infants with catheter-related *Malassezia* fungemia typically have any combination of the following nonspecific findings: lethargy, poor feeding, temperature instability, hepatosplenomegaly, hemodynamic instability, and worsening or new respiratory distress [565]. Fever occurs in 53% of cases, and thrombocytopenia, which may be severe, is observed in 48% of cases. Most infants do not become critically ill but have the clinical picture of an ongoing indolent infection. Infants also may have a malfunctioning catheter following occlusion by a *Malassezia*-infected thrombus [561].

DIAGNOSIS

The diagnosis frequently is made by noting the appearance of a fluffy white precipitate visible in the clear connecting tubing of the infected catheter [578,583,584]. Gram stain of this material reveals the characteristic appearance of *M. furfur* or *M. pachydermatis*, and culture of this material will allow isolation of the organism.

In the absence of any sign of catheter infection, results of culture of blood drawn directly from the catheter may be positive, whereas those obtained from peripheral vessels will be sterile. When *Malassezia* infection is suspected, the laboratory should be notified because these yeasts are not recovered from routine culture media, and special lipid supplementation is required for their growth and identification [583]. Newer methods of fungal identification including PCR techniques may be advantageous in diagnosing this organism but are not yet universally available [585]. Echocardiography is indicated in infants who have persistent fungemia, so that an infected thrombus on the catheter tip can be excluded [586].

THERAPY

Prompt removal of the infected catheter is the optimal treatment for neonatal *Malassezia* infections. Although dissemination is rare, antifungal therapy usually is provided to ensure clearance of the organism from the bloodstream. Amphotericin B is the most frequently used agent, although in vitro testing suggests only moderate susceptibility of *Malassezia* species to this agent [580]. With removal of the catheter, and thereby the high concentration of lipid, the organism will no longer survive. Vascular catheter complications, including retained catheters and catheter breakage, have been reported with *Malassezia* infections, with one series suggesting *M. furfur* contributes directly to catheter fragility and breakage [587]. Thrombolytic therapy with urokinase and tissue plasminogen activator has been used to facilitate the removal of adherent *M. furfur*-infected catheters and avoid surgical extraction [578,583]. If a large thrombus remains after catheter removal, serial monitoring for dissolution by echocardiography is indicated, and some authorities believe that antifungal therapy should be continued until complete resolution is achieved, although this approach is controversial [584]. Although therapy usually is not indicated with neonatal pustulosis, severe, extensive involvement has been treated with topical ketoconazole ointment [580].

PROGNOSIS

Prognosis generally is excellent with prompt diagnosis and removal of the infected catheter. Rarely reported complications include severe CNS, pulmonary, and liver disease, with only an occasional death in the extremely low birth weight preterm infant [565].

PREVENTION

The prevention of *Malassezia* infections in neonates has not been studied. The judicious use of intralipids may significantly limit the risk. In patients in whom intralipid therapy cannot be avoided, this fungal infection should be suspected if the central venous catheter malfunctions or if mild, nonspecific signs of infection are noted.

PHYCOMYCOSIS

Infection with Phycomycetes organisms occurs infrequently in newborns, but 24 cases have been reported in the literature [588–607]. Sixteen of the infants died; in eight of these, the diagnosis was not suspected during life. One infant died 3 days after the diagnosis was established and therapy was initiated. The gastrointestinal tract was the focus of infection in 8 of 18 cases. Two neonates had only CNS infection, and a third had CNS infection and intestinal involvement. In none of these three was clinical evidence of nasopharyngeal or orbital infection documented. One infant described by Miller and coworkers [595] had rhinocerebral infection and survived, and Lewis and colleagues [599] reported a fatal case in which the affected infant had methylmalonic aciduria and rhinocerebral mucormycosis. White and associates [596] described an infant with cellulitis of the abdominal wall who also survived. In a case reported by Ng and Dear [598], the affected infant had multiple abscesses due to *Rhizopus* infection and survived following treatment. Three additional reports have described infants with cutaneous phycomycosis [601–603]. Two of the three died despite medical and surgical therapy. One of the infants who died had progressive infection that involved the gastrointestinal and respiratory tracts [602]. Four infants had cutaneous infections that developed at intravenous catheter sites [604–607].

Although infection with Phycomycetes is common in adults receiving immunosuppressive therapy and in those with neoplastic diseases, particularly hematologic or reticuloendothelial malignancies [608], none of the infants described in these reports received such drugs or had neoplasia. In adults, acidosis resulting from uncontrolled diabetes mellitus or from hepatic or renal failure appears to contribute significantly to infection with Phycomycetes organisms [608–614]. Although none of the infants in the reported cases had diabetes mellitus or hepatic failure, diarrhea was a prominent finding in 6 of 10 infants; however, acidosis as a complication of diarrhea was not commented on in any of the case reports. One patient had renal failure and acidosis [597], and four others were acidotic, including the infant with methylmalonic aciduria [599,601]. Five of the 24 infants were born prematurely, and 1 term neonate had underlying congenital heart disease and had undergone complex cardiac surgery; intensive antimicrobial therapy was given to all but 1 infant. Two infants were receiving nasogastric feedings [592,599], and in one, cellulitis developed beneath a jejunostomy dressing [596]. In another infant, cutaneous infection developed under an abdominal adhesive tape that attached a radiant thermosensor [603].

THE ORGANISM

Some confusion regarding the taxonomy of Phycomycetes exists in the literature [615]. For purposes of simplicity, we shall consider Phycomycetes as the class and Mucorales as the order of the three most common genera causing phycomycosis—*Mucor*, *Absidia*, and *Rhizopus* [616]. Phycomycosis, however, also includes infection with species of *Mortierella*, *Basidiobolus*, *Hyphomyces*, and *Entomophthora* [615].

Hyphae are best stained by hematoxylin-eosin, for which they have an affinity; methenamine silver stains are inferior for this fungus. Characteristically, hyphae are randomly branched, are rarely septate, and appear empty. The diameter of hyphae is variable even within the length of the same mycelium. Because these fungi are not sufficiently pathogenic for laboratory animals, attempts at isolation by inoculation are not useful as a diagnostic procedure.

EPIDEMIOLOGY AND TRANSMISSION

Phycomycetes organisms are found throughout the world in soil, in animal manure, and on fruits. Fungi of this class frequently are found in refrigerators and are commonly known as bread molds [617–619]. *Basidiobolus* and *Entomophthora* can be isolated from decaying organic matter. Infection with Phycomycetes has been reported in humans and animals [620].

In infants with phycomycosis, the infection may have been the result either of ingestion of the fungus into the gastrointestinal tract or of inhalation into the nasopharynx or lung after birth, but saprophytic colonization in the vagina of the mothers and intrapartum acquisition cannot be excluded. Little is known regarding the presence of Phycomycetes on the skin, in the feces, or in pharyngeal or vaginal secretions in the absence of clinical disease. Emmons [620] noted that after exposure to Phycomycetes patients with bronchiectasis may cough up spores for several days in the absence of clinical infection. Isolation of these fungi from other sites without evidence of disease has not been reported, but data from newborns suggest that saprophytic colonization with Phycomycetes may be similar to the commensalism with *Candida*. No evidence is available to suggest that human-to-human transmission occurs. In one case reported by Dennis and coworkers [593], *Rhizopus oryzae* was isolated from the Elastoplast that was used as an adhesive for the abdominal dressing. In another infant described by White and coworkers [596], abdominal wall cellulitis developed beneath the adhesive dressing of a jejunostomy. Linder and colleagues [603] isolated *Rhizopus* from the adhesive tape used to attach the thermosensor. In each of these infants, cultures of similar dressings and of tape used in the same units failed to grow the fungi [596,603].

PATHOGENESIS

The bowel is a frequent site of infection in infants; disease in this location appears to be associated with malnutrition or diarrhea [590,601]. Underlying medical conditions seem to play a major pathogenic role in most cases of phycomycosis. The high incidence of rhinocerebral infection in adults with diabetes mellitus has been noted, but the biochemical abnormality that increases susceptibility is considered to be acidosis, rather than endocrine dysfunction [592,610]. Straatsma and coworkers [608] have suggested that acidosis from any cause, including hepatic or renal failure, may increase susceptibility to phycomycosis. Of interest are the reported infants and adults with gastrointestinal phycomycosis. Most had diarrhea, which may be accompanied by severe acidosis, especially in infants. Whether diarrhea preceded or was a complication of gastrointestinal phycomycosis in these cases cannot be determined. The mechanism of increased susceptibility to infection with Phycomycetes in an acidotic state is incompletely understood. Although optimal growth of Phycomycetes occurs at pH 4.0 in vitro but not at pH 2.7 or 7.3 [621], acidification is not suitable for the sexual cycle of Phycomycetes. In the host, acidosis may delay polymorphonuclear response and limit fibroblastic reaction [610,614]. Prematurity, antibiotics, and diarrhea may have been some of the predisposing factors in the infants who died of this infection.

PATHOLOGY

The characteristic histopathologic features of infection with this class of fungi include vascular invasion with necrosis or hemorrhage. Necrotic and suppurative lesions demonstrating massive infiltration by polymorphonuclear leukocytes are seen in invasive or disseminated phycomycosis. In patients with subcutaneous infection, lesions usually are granulomatous with epithelioid and Langhans' giant cells. Conspicuous infiltration with eosinophils occurs in subcutaneous infection, particularly with species of *Basidiobolus*. Vascular invasion in such cases is rare.

CLINICAL MANIFESTATIONS

The clinical manifestations of phycomycosis in neonates and young infants depend on the site or sites of infection. With cutaneous disease, the appearance is similar to that in cutaneous aspergillosis, and involved sites include surgical wounds, intravascular catheter insertion sites, and areas of skin breakdown. The usual symptoms of gastrointestinal phycomycosis in adults are bloody diarrhea and cramping abdominal pain. Because vascular invasion and necrosis occur, perforation and peritonitis with a rapidly fatal course are common. In seven of eight infants with phycomycosis, diarrhea and abdominal distention or signs of peritoneal irritation, or both, were prominent findings. Two infants had free air in the peritoneal cavity from perforation. One infant without abdominal signs had CNS infection without other organ involvement. In extremely premature and low-birth-weight neonates, invasive fungal dermatitis has been reported to be caused by Phycomycetes [622].

DIAGNOSIS AND DIFFERENTIAL DIAGNOSIS

The clinical picture in infants with phycomycosis appears to be very similar to that in children with aspergillosis. Phycomycetes have the same affinity for vascular invasion, hemorrhage, necrosis, and suppuration. Bacterial infection in the lung may be indistinguishable from phycomycosis on clinical grounds. Hemorrhagic infarction of the lung or bowel from other causes has the same presenting signs as those due to infection with Phycomycetes. The cerebrospinal fluid in infants with CNS infection does not show a consistent pattern. Glucose and protein levels often are normal. Xanthochromia with small numbers of red blood cells is common, and a few mononuclear or polymorphonuclear cells may be present [614].

The diagnosis of phycomycosis should be considered in debilitated infants, particularly those with acidosis related to diarrhea, or with hepatic or renal failure, who do not respond to correction of the acidotic state. Sinus or orbital abnormalities in such patients should be investigated for the presence of Phycomycetes. Adults receiving immunosuppressive therapy or antimetabolites for hematologic diseases in whom pulmonary or gastrointestinal symptoms develop must be evaluated for possible Phycomycetes infection.

The diagnosis of infection with these fungi can be difficult because culture results frequently are negative [623]. Demonstration of the fungus is best accomplished by microscopic examination of tissue and visualization of the broad, branching, nonseptate hyphae. A 10% solution of potassium hydroxide is used, although hematoxylin-eosin staining is preferred for specimens of tissue. Exudates from the nasopharynx or necrotic tissue obtained by débridement should be cultured on Sabouraud glucose agar. Because of the ubiquity of these fungi, demonstration of the organism in tissue is necessary to establish a diagnosis of phycomycosis.

Although normal human serum contains substances that inhibit growth of *Rhizopus* in vitro [624], serologic and immunologic tests have not been extensively studied as diagnostic aids for patients with phycomycosis. Bank and associates [625], using an extract of *Rhizopus* isolated from a patient, produced a cutaneous reaction with an intradermal injection in the patient but not in control subjects. They also found complement-fixing antibodies in the serum of the patient but not in controls, although the same extract was used. Jones and Kaufman [626] demonstrated antibodies to a homogenate of the fungus by an immunodiffusion technique in 8 of 11 patients with mucormycosis.

THERAPY

Of paramount importance in the treatment of phycomycosis is correction of metabolic derangement; cessation of antibiotics, corticosteroids, or immunosuppressive agents whenever possible; and débridement or excision of necrotic tissue [627–631]. In conjunction with these measures, various antifungal agents in addition to amphotericin B have been employed, but no data are available that allow recommendations for specific drugs, doses, or duration.

PROGNOSIS

The diagnosis of phycomycosis in infants most often is made at autopsy. The diagnosis was not considered before death in nine patients in the reported cases. In 13 patients, the organism was identified and therapy was given; 6 of the 13 recovered [588–607].

PREVENTION

Measures to protect the fragile skin of immature extremely low birth weight infants should limit the ability of these fungi to invade. As with *Aspergillus* infection, activities that would allow exposure to Phycomycetes such as construction, should be limited in or near the NICU.

DERMATOPHYTOSES

The dermatophytes—*Epidermophyton*, *Microsporum*, and *Trichophyton*—often are responsible for infection of keratinized areas of the body, including skin, hair, and nails. Superficial infection with these "ringworm" fungi has been reported infrequently in newborns, although infants have been considered susceptible to infection with these specialized fungi [632]. In 1876 Lynch [633] reported the case of an infant with tinea faciei who was only 6 hours of age. Unfortunately, the diagnosis was made clinically, and no documentation of dermatophyte infection by microscopic examination or culture was obtained. More recently, Jacobs and colleagues [634] described an 8-day-old infant with tinea faciei due to *Microsporum canis*. An outbreak of neonatal ringworm in five infants in an NICU was linked to the index case in a nurse who was infected with *M. canis* by her cat [635]. Dermatophyte

infections in infants from a few weeks of age to several months of age have been described [636–648].

Because of the infrequent reports of dermatophyte infections in infants, few investigative studies defining factors contributing to increased infantile susceptibility or resistance to infection by dermatophytes have been performed [642,643]. Wyre and Johnson [644] suggested that increased humidity in the incubator may have contributed to the risk of infection in an infant with pityriasis versicolor, and Lanska and associates [646] indicated that prolonged exposure to humidified oxygen by hood may have increased susceptibility to the cutaneous fungal infection observed in three infants.

THE ORGANISM

Dermatophytes have been placed in the class of imperfect fungi, Deuteromycetes, in the order Moniliales [616]. Because of a sexual stage in some dermatophytes, however, some authors have preferred to classify certain genera as belonging to the class Ascomycetes [649,650].

Hyphae of dermatophytes are long, undulant, and branching. Many septa are present along the length of hyphae. Hyphae break at the septa into barrel-shaped arthrospores. In culture, dermatophytes form conidiophores, with resulting microconidia and macroconidia. Genera and species identification is based on gross characteristics of colony and microscopic morphology of conidia. A complete review of distinguishing features may be found in standard mycology textbooks [651].

EPIDEMIOLOGY AND TRANSMISSION

Dermatophytes are distributed throughout the world in humans and animals; many also are found in soil, water, vegetation, and animal excrement [652]. The fungus can contaminate combs, hairbrushes, shoes, and shower floors and has been isolated from air [653,654]. Contamination of soil with dermatophytes has been thought to occur in keratinous debris from infected animals and humans [652], and no evidence is available to suggest that these fungi are free-living saprophytes in soil.

Dermatophyte infection most often is acquired from contact with infected persons or animals. Infections with *Microsporum gypseum* can result from contact with soil contaminated with the fungus. Human-to-human transmission can occur with *Epidermophyton floccosum*, *Microsporum audouinii*, *Trichophyton mentagrophytes*, *Trichophyton rubrum*, *Trichophyton schoenleinii*, *Trichophyton tonsurans*, and *Trichophyton violaceum* [655]. Zoophilic dermatophytes include *M. canis*, *Trichophyton gallinae*, *T. mentagrophytes*, and *Trichophyton verrucosum*. Although *M. canis* usually is transmitted to humans from young animals, particularly kittens, transmission between persons is suggested in the case of an infant reported by Bereston and Robinson [636]. Pinetti and coworkers [656] isolated *M. canis* and *M. gypseum* from flies, which suggests an additional mode of transmission.

In newborns with dermatophyte infection, the fungus probably is acquired after birth from contact with infected nursery personnel, household members, or animals. In the case reported by Lynch [633] of clinically apparent infection at 6 hours of age, the fungal infection probably was acquired in utero. In this case, evidence of infection in the mother was lacking, but the fungus has been demonstrated on skin in the absence of clinical disease [657,658].

PATHOGENESIS

Despite worldwide distribution of dermatophytes and frequency of exposure of humans to these fungi, the incidence of clinically apparent infection in infants and adults is considerably lower than would be expected. Few studies defining host factors responsible for protection have been performed. Although Knight [659] has shown in experimental studies in humans that macerated moist skin is more susceptible to the infection than dry skin, the role of immunologic factors in the control of dermatophyte infection remains obscure. Repeated infection may occur at identical sites as long as 2 years after primary infection [659,660], despite reports that infection may offer partial immunity to reinfection [661,662].

Roth and colleagues [336] along with others [663–667] have demonstrated antidermatophyte activity in normal human serum and have suggested that this substance may restrict dermatophyte infection to superficial layers of skin. No studies investigating the role of antifungal activity in sweat have been reported, although immunoglobulins and antibodies have been demonstrated in sweat [668]. Although antidermatophyte activity has been reported in serum at birth [667], no specific studies have been performed in infants to define other host factors or to determine immunologic consequences of dermatophyte infection.

Most infected neonates weigh less than 1000 g at birth and have a gestational age of less than 26 weeks.

PATHOLOGY

Dermatophyte infection generally is confined to keratinized areas of the body and only rarely invades deeper tissues. Lesions may be vesicular and contain serous fluid. Inflammatory reaction with polymorphonuclear leukocyte infiltration is minimal and usually represents secondary bacterial infection. Occasionally, intense inflammatory reactions may occur in the absence of bacterial infection, especially in children with tinea capitis resulting from *T. mentagrophytes*. These pustular lesions, or kerions, surround infected hair follicles and appear to be reactions to virulent strains of fungus.

Favus is a chronic infection usually caused by *T. schoenleinii* or *T. mentagrophytes*. Granulomatous formation occurs, with giant cells and masses of hyphae around the hair follicle. Overlying the infection is a crust of cellular debris and degenerating hyphae. This lesion is convex, and scarring and alopecia appear after healing.

In infants of extremely low birth weight, invasive dermatitis can occur with *Trichosporon* species. Skin biopsies reveal invasion of the epidermis with this yeast, often with spread along hair follicles and then into the dermis (Fig. 34–5), similar to the histologic picture of invasive fungal dermatitis caused by *Candida* species, *Aspergillus* species, or Phycomycetes organisms [652].

CLINICAL MANIFESTATIONS

Dermatophytosis is classified generally by focus of infection and less commonly by species of infecting fungus. Tinea capitis is a fungal infection of the scalp and hair caused by

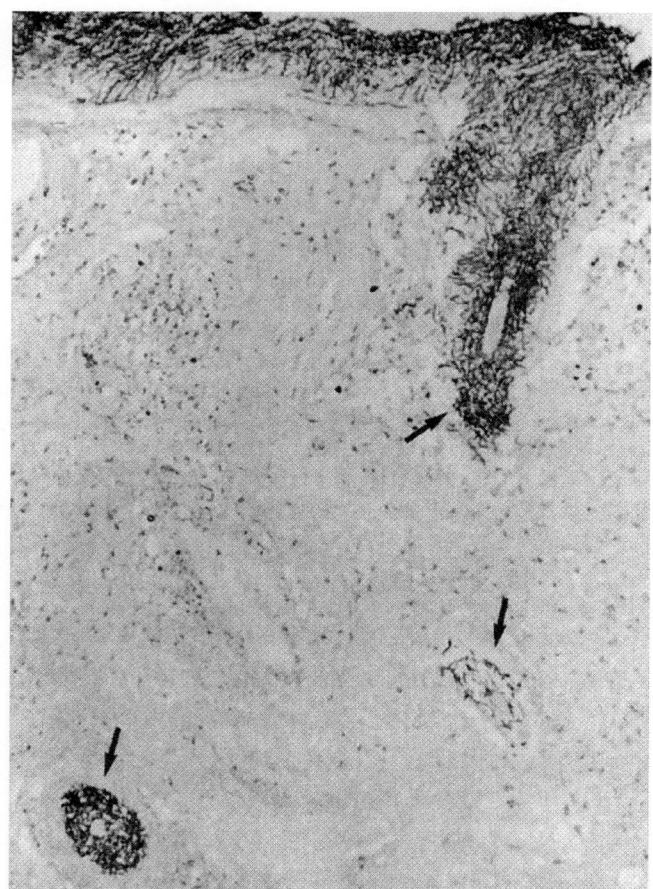

FIGURE 34–5 Skin biopsy specimen from extremely low birth weight infant with invasive fungal dermatitis caused by *Candida albicans*. Intense involvement of the epidermis with pseudohyphae extending along hair follicles (*arrows*) is demonstrated following staining with Grocott methenamine silver. ×10.

Microsporum and *Trichophyton*. It occurs most often in infants, older children, and adults. Alteras [663] reported that in a group of 7000 patients, 70 infants between 2 and 12 months of age had tinea capitis. In this study, *M. audouinii* was the most common fungus in infants. Other fungi reportedly causing tinea capitis include *M. canis*, *T. violaceum*, *T. tonsurans*, *T. mentagrophytes*, *T. schoenleinii*, *Microsporum ferrugineum*, *E. floccosum*, and *T. rubrum*. Infection begins with small scaling papules that spread peripherally, forming circular pruritic patches. Both kerion and favus formation can occur.

Tinea corporis, or ringworm of smooth skin, can result from infection with species of *Microsporum*, *Trichophyton*, or *Epidermophyton*, although infections with *Microsporum* species are the most common (Fig. 34–6). Infants and children appear to be more susceptible to tinea corporis than adults. King and coworkers [637] described five infants with tinea corporis who ranged in age from 3 weeks to 7 months. *Microsporum* species predominated in that study, but one infant, who was 8 weeks of age, was infected with *E. floccosum*. In older children, *M. canis* and *T. mentagrophytes* are more common causes of tinea corporis. Lesions, which may be single or multiple, are round or oval scaling, erythematous patches. As infection spreads peripherally, the center of the

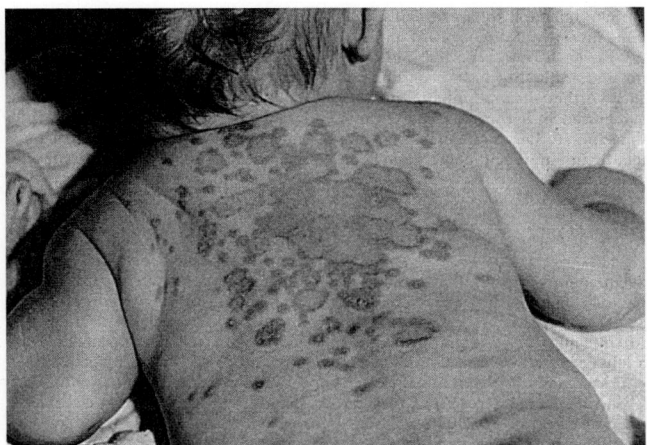

FIGURE 34–6 Tinea corporis caused by *Microsporum* species in a 4-month-old infant.

lesion may show some clearing. In some instances, an intense inflammatory reaction with vesiculation at the margins, accompanied by severe pruritus, may be noted. Patches of infected areas may coalesce, forming extensive plaques with serpiginous borders. Deep granulomas or nodules may form, especially when the infection is caused by *T. rubrum*.

Tinea cruris is a fungal infection of the groin, perineum, or perianal area and most often is caused by *E. floccosum* (Fig. 34–7). *T. mentagrophytes* and *T. rubrum* are unusual causes of infection at these sites. Although *Candida* species account for a majority of fungal infections in the diaper area, King and coworkers [637] described one infant with *E. floccosum* infection in the perineum. Infection with this fungus is characterized by brownish areas of scaly dermatitis with small, superficial pustules at the periphery of the lesion. Infection with *T. mentagrophytes*, which usually spreads from the feet, is associated with marked inflammation. Tinea cruris caused by *T. rubrum* may be unilateral and may be only one part of a generalized scaly, erythematous, plaquelike eruption. Tinea pedis, or athlete's foot, is the most common dermatophyte infection in adults but is rare in infants.

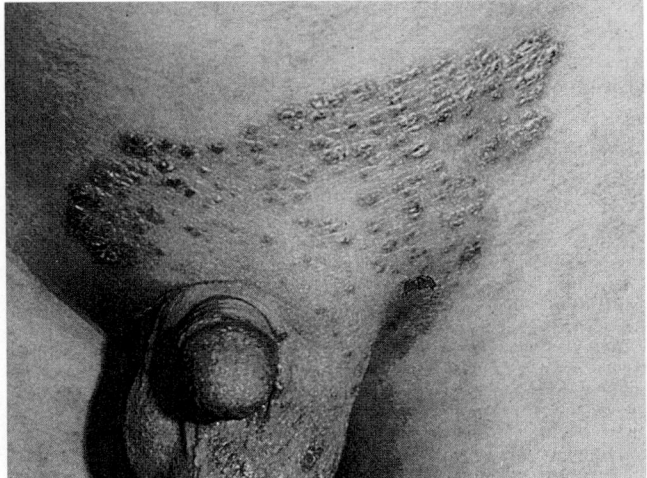

FIGURE 34–7 Tinea cruris infection with *Epidermophyton floccosum* in a young infant.

In extremely immature premature neonates, invasive fungal dermatitis can occur in areas of skin breakdown (Fig. 34–8) [652].

DIAGNOSIS AND DIFFERENTIAL DIAGNOSIS

Dermatophyte infection may be mistaken for seborrhea, impetigo, or psoriasis. Tinea capitis may appear similar to alopecia areata, but scaling usually is absent in the latter. The presumptive diagnosis is made by direct microscopic examination of infected material. Areas to be examined should be cleansed with 70% alcohol, and scrapings should be made with a scalpel or scissors from the active periphery of the lesion. If vesicles are present, the tops should be removed for examination. Hairs infected with *M. audouinii* or *M. canis* may be identified by using Wood's light, which emits monochromatic ultraviolet rays. Infected hairs show a green-yellow fluorescence and may be removed for examination. Scrapings from nails, obtained from deep layers, should be thin. Specimens are placed on a glass slide, and a few drops of 10% sodium or potassium hydroxide are added. A coverslip is added, and the specimen is gently heated over a low flame. Microscopic examination under low power should take place immediately. The presence of hyphae confirms the diagnosis of fungal infection. Young hyphae appear as long, thin threads, and older hyphae have many spores. Spores may be found either within the hair follicle or around its base. Shelley and Wood [669] have described a technique of crushing the hair. They found it to be superior to the use of potassium hydroxide for identifying the fungus in the hair. Identification of the genus and species of dermatophyte can be made only by culture. Infected material should be cultured on a Sabouraud glucose agar slant, and microscopic examination of hyphae and conidia performed.

In premature infants with brown- or black-appearing lesions at areas of skin trauma, the diagnosis of invasive fungal dermatitis should be determined by skin biopsy and culture (see under "Aspergillosis" and "Phycomycosis"). Blood cultures also may yield *Trichosporon beigelii* if this etiologic agent is responsible for the skin lesions.

THERAPY

Topical therapy with keratolytic or fungicidal medications may be beneficial in some cases of dermatophyte infection, especially tinea pedis, in which results with use of griseofulvin are not encouraging. Whitfield's ointment, 1% solution of tolnaftate, or an ointment with 3% each of sulfur and salicylic acid may be used. Topical therapy should be continued until culture specimens and scrapings are negative for fungus. For invasive fungal dermatitis in premature infants, amphotericin B deoxycholate administered intravenously is the agent of choice. Some studies, however, have suggested tolerance of *Trichosporon* species to amphotericin, and fluconazole has been shown to be effective in the treatment of trichosporonosis.

PROGNOSIS

Untreated dermatophyte infection is slowly progressive and can be disfiguring, especially in cases of kerion and favus reactions. Secondary bacterial infections are common, particularly in cases of tinea pedis. Deep tissue

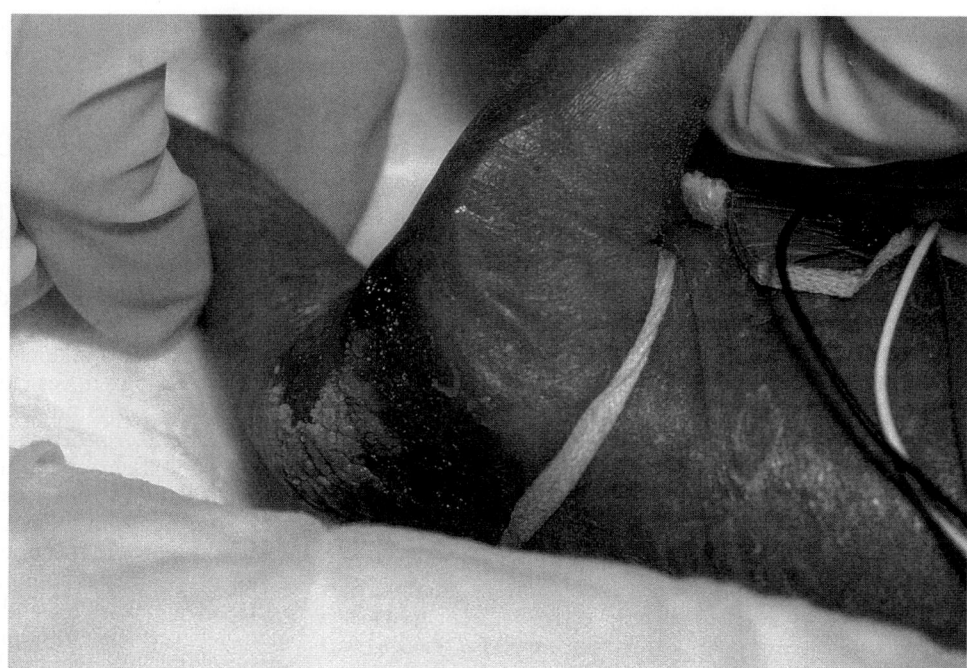

FIGURE 34–8 Diffuse involvement of the buttocks by invasive fungal dermatitis, caused by *Trichosporon* species, in an extremely low birth weight infant. The lesion is a tightly adherent white-and-buff-colored crust.

invasion occurs in extremely low birth weight neonates, typically with *T. beigelii* infections, and most reported cases have had a fatal outcome [652].

PREVENTION

Separate combs, hairbrushes, and clippers should be available for the newborn and should not be shared with others in the household. Infected animals and household contacts should be promptly treated [670].

ANTIFUNGAL THERAPY IN NEONATES AND YOUNG INFANTS

Amphotericin B deoxycholate is the mainstay of therapy for invasive fungal infections in neonates. For certain infections, flucytosine or fluconazole may be useful (Table 34–3). Although newer azoles, lipid formulations of amphotericin B, and echinocandins have been studied and shown to be useful in adults and older children with some invasive fungal infections, limited or no information regarding the pharmacokinetics, safety, and efficacy of these new antifungals in neonates is available. For many

invasive infections in adults (e.g., candidiasis, aspergillosis), these agents have been demonstrated to have similar efficacy but reduced toxicity, especially the dose-limiting toxicity often noted with conventional amphotericin B in adults and older children. For some fungal infections, however, amphotericin B has limited in vitro activity, and use of alternative agents may be necessary.

AMPHOTERICIN B

Amphotericin B is a polyene antimicrobial that reacts with sterols in cell membranes, resulting in cellular damage and lysis. Serum levels in adults average 1.5 μg/mL 1 hour after intravenous injection of 0.6 to 1 mg/kg; the half-life is approximately 24 hours, but levels of 0.14 μg/mL have been detected in serum for at least 3 weeks [671]. Only one tenth to one twentieth of the serum levels is distributed into the cerebrospinal fluid.

Few studies have been performed of the clinical pharmacology of amphotericin B in newborns or older infants from which an accurate recommendation for dosage can be extrapolated. McCoy and coworkers [672] reported peak serum concentrations at 1 hour of 2.6 μg/mL in the

TABLE 34–3 Antifungal Drugs for Infants with Systemic Fungal Infection

Agent	Metabolism/Excretion	CSF/Serum Concentration	Dose Change in Renal Failure	Daily Dose (mg/kg)
Amphotericin B		40–90%	None	0.5–1.5
Liposomal amphotericin B	Hepatic	?	None	3–6
Flucytosine	Renal	>75%	Yes	100–150
Fluconazole	Renal	>60%	Yes	2–12
Itraconazole	Hepatic	<1%	None	2–5

CSF, cerebrospinal fluid.

mother and in arterial cord blood after a maternal infusion of 0.6 mg of amphotericin B. The amphotericin B concentration in the amniotic fluid was 0.08 µg/mL. Ismail and Lerner [217] reported that levels of amphotericin B in cord blood were 33% of the maternal serum concentrations. Hager and associates [220] obtained simultaneous amphotericin B levels in maternal blood, cord blood, and amniotic fluid 26 hours after an infusion of 20 mg. The levels were 1.9, 1.3, and 0.3 µg/mL, respectively. Ward and co-workers [673] reported that serum levels of amphotericin B in a premature infant were similar to those found in older children and adults, and those levels persisted for at least 17 days after amphotericin B had been discontinued.

The toxicity of amphotericin B in humans can be significant. Adults and older children frequently experience nausea, vomiting, headache, chills, and fever during infusion of this agent [674]. Infusion-related adverse events are rare in neonates, however [675]. Hypokalemia can develop, but often concomitant drugs being administered with amphotericin B to the neonate may account for this association. Serum electrolytes should be carefully monitored, and hypokalemia can be corrected with potassium replacement. Nephrotoxicity is the most important toxic effect in adults and older children. This adverse effect has been shown to correlate with the total dose of amphotericin B [676] and results from drug-induced renal vasoconstriction, and from direct action of amphotericin B on renal tubules [677]. Other findings can include a rise in serum creatinine and blood urea nitrogen levels and a decrease in creatinine clearance, and cylindruria, renal tubular acidosis, tubular necrosis, and nephrocalcinosis. Nephrotoxicity from amphotericin B is rare in neonates; when it occurs, it often is the result of infection rather than an adverse drug effect and is reversible with a reduction in daily dose from 1.0 to 0.5 mg/kg [675,678].

The effect of amphotericin B on the fetus has not been extensively studied. Several reports of the use of amphotericin B in pregnant women have now been published [216–221,522,672,679–685]. In no instance was there evidence of teratogenicity or fetal toxicity related to this antifungal agent. Amphotericin for use during pregnancy is a category B drug. Systemic fungal infections have been successfully treated in pregnant women without obvious effects on the fetus, but the number of cases reported has been small. Adequate and well-controlled studies have not been conducted; therefore, use of this drug during pregnancy is indicated only if it is clearly needed [686].

The initial intravenous dose of amphotericin B in neonates should be 0.5 to 1.0 mg/kg, and the drug should be suspended in sterile water in a concentration of no greater than 0.1 mg/mL. The maximum daily dose and duration of therapy depends on the focus and extent of fungal disease [687], and on the minimal inhibitory concentration (MIC) of amphotericin B for the organism [688]. The neonatal dose is 0.5 to 1.5 mg/kg per day. Although some authors have suggested monitoring serum levels of amphotericin B [689,690], others disagree because of the predictable pharmacokinetics of this drug [691,692]. Rate of administration varies, but typically the dose can be given over 1 to 2 hours, and no longer than 4 hours.

Intrathecal administration of amphotericin B can be necessary in patients with coccidioidomycosis meningitis. Few data are available on the ideal intrathecal dose of amphotericin B in children with fungal meningitis. The initial intrathecal dose in infants should be 0.01 mg, gradually increased over a period of 5 to 7 days to 0.1 mg given every other day or every third day. Amphotericin B for intrathecal administration should not exceed a concentration of 0.25 mg/mL of diluent, and further dilution with cerebrospinal fluid is recommended. Complications of intrathecal amphotericin B administration include cerebrospinal fluid pleocytosis (arachnoiditis), transient radiculitis, and sensory loss.

Three lipid formulations of amphotericin B are commercially available: amphotericin B lipid complex (ABLC), amphotericin B cholesteryl sulfate complex (i.e., amphotericin B colloidal dispersion [ABCD]), and liposomal amphotericin B (L-AmB). These formulations differ in the amount of amphotericin B and lipids, vesicle size and structure, and pharmacokinetic properties. These lipid formulations have demonstrated comparable clinical efficacy, and reduced nephrotoxicity, in comparison with conventional amphotericin B in adults; none is superior in effectiveness to conventional amphotericin B. No studies have compared the safety and effectiveness of lipid preparations with conventional amphotericin B in neonates.

Lackner and coworkers [338] reported successful use of a lipid formulation of amphotericin B, in a daily dose of 5 mg/kg, in two premature infants with disseminated fungal infections. In addition, Weitkamp and associates reported use of this preparation in a daily dose of 1 to 5 mg/kg in 21 low birth weight infants with *Candida* infections and demonstrated its efficacy without apparent nephrotoxicity [693]. Scarcella and colleagues [694] also reported using a lipid formulation of amphotericin B in 44 infants with severe fungal infections. Using a daily dose of 1 to 5 mg/kg, they reported transient hypokalemia but successful outcomes in 32 infants, but 12 infants of very low birth weight died.

5-FLUCYTOSINE

5-Flucytosine, a fluoropyrimidine, has been shown to have in vitro activity against some fungi [674,695–697]. It has been used in combination with conventional amphotericin B for an additive antifungal effect for the treatment of disseminated candidiasis and cryptococcosis. The drug is absorbed well from the gastrointestinal tract, and, with doses of 100 to 150 mg/kg, serum levels vary, ranging from 17 to 44 µg/mL [698]. In the cerebrospinal fluid, levels of 5-flucytosine may be as high as 88% of serum concentrations [699]. The drug is administered orally in a total daily dose of 50 to 150 mg/kg, given in four divided doses, for 2 to 6 weeks in adults. Experience with this agent in infants is increasing. Rapid emergence of resistance of fungi after initiation of flucytosine therapy has been reported for *Candida* and for *C. neoformans* [695–700]. Flucytosine has been used extensively in infants and children receiving amphotericin B [701–704]. Few untoward side effects have been noted, even with prolonged use. Toxic effects of flucytosine include transient neutropenia and hepatocellular damage [705]. Because the drug is cleared by the kidneys, the dose should be reduced and serum levels determined in infants with impaired renal function. Accumulation of flucytosine in the blood can result in serious toxicity to the bone marrow.

FLUCONAZOLE AND ITRACONAZOLE

Fluconazole is an azole antifungal agent and is available in an intravenous and an oral preparation. This agent has been shown to achieve good penetration into cerebrospinal fluid, ocular fluid, and skin [706]. It is effective against many fungi, including *Candida, Coccidioides,* and dermatophytes. Its use in neonates has been limited. Wiest and associates [707] used fluconazole in a premature infant with disseminated candidiasis unresponsive to amphotericin B and flucytosine. The infant received 6 mg/kg per day intravenously, with peak and trough serum levels of 10.3 and 6.98 mg/mL, respectively. Gürses and Kalayci [708] reported successful use of fluconazole alone in a premature infant with candidal meningitis. Dreissen and coworkers [709,710] in two reports indicated that fluconazole was effective and associated with fewer side effects than those observed with amphotericin B. A review of 62 episodes of neonatal candidemia revealed that fluconazole was used as the first-line agent in 6 episodes, with successful eradication of infection in five of the episodes. Fluconazole was used as an alternative agent in another 13 episodes, with eradication of infection in 8 of the 13. Fluconazole was well tolerated [711]. Fluconazole also has been used in pregnancy without harmful effects on the fetus [712].

Itraconazole, another azole antifungal agent, has had limited use in neonates. Bhandari and Narange [713] reported its use in two premature infants with disseminated candidiasis. Each received 10 mg/kg per day in two divided doses for 3 and 4 weeks, respectively. Both infants did well without any evidence of toxicity. A pharmacokinetic study of oral itraconazole in infants and children 6 months to 12 years of age demonstrated potentially therapeutic concentrations with a daily dose of 5 mg/kg. Itraconazole was well tolerated [714]. Only limited data are available on use of itraconazole in neonates.

VORICONAZOLE

Voriconazole is a second-generation antifungal triazole with a broad spectrum of activity, excellent oral bioavailability, and a good safety profile in adults [210]. Voriconazole is approved by the FDA for use in adults for treatment of invasive aspergillosis and in salvage therapy for infections caused by *Scedosporium* and *Fusarium* species. Voriconazole has been successfully used to treat disseminated infection caused by *Trichosporon* species. Data are available that support the safety and efficacy of voriconazole for the treatment of invasive fungal infections in children 9 months to 15 years of age. Only one study, however, has reported pharmacokinetic data in young infants [211].

Treatment with voriconazole in 69 children with aspergillosis, scedosporiosis, and other invasive fungal infections resulted in favorable outcomes in patients who were intolerant of or refractory to conventional antifungal therapy [715]. The dosage was 6 mg/kg administered every 12 hours intravenously on day 1, followed by 4 mg/kg every 12 hours, until clinical improvement allowed a change to oral therapy at a dose of 100 or 200 mg twice a day for patients weighing less than 40 kg or 40 kg or greater, respectively.

ECHINOCANDINS: CASPOFUNGIN

Echinocandins are cyclic hexapeptides with an N-acyl aliphatic or aryl side chain that expands the antifungal spectrum to include *Candida* species, *Aspergillus* species, and *P. jiroveci,* but not *C. neoformans.* Echinocandins are administered only parenterally because of their large molecular size. They inhibit the biosynthesis of 1,3-beta-glucans, which are key constituents of the fungal cell wall. The enzyme system for 1,3-beta-glucan synthesis is absent in mammalian hosts.

Echinocandins that currently are in use include caspofungin, micafungin, and anidulafungin. Caspofungin has been approved by the FDA for salvage therapy in adults with invasive aspergillosis. The echinocandins have demonstrated in vivo activity against esophageal candidiasis and disseminated candidiasis in adults. Hepatotoxicity has been observed at very high doses. Data on use in infants are very limited, however, and studies are needed to determine the pharmacokinetics, optimal doses, and indications for echinocandins, and their effectiveness, in infants and children [716].

GRISEOFULVIN

Griseofulvin has significantly altered the morbidity associated with dermatophyte infection. This drug is deposited in epidermal structures before keratinization. As keratinized areas are exfoliated, they are replaced by noninfected tissue. In patients with tinea capitis, it may be necessary to clip the hair frequently because as growth occurs, the ends of hairs may continue to harbor viable fungus. The oral dose of griseofulvin is 10 mg/kg per day for 7 to 10 days. Occasionally, a daily dose of 20 to 40 mg/kg is necessary for cure. In some instances, therapy must be continued for 3 weeks. Data on the use of griseofulvin in newborns are limited. Ross [717] reported use of griseofulvin in an infant 1 month of age at a daily dose of 10 mg/kg for 4 weeks without untoward effects.

Griseofulvin is derived from a species of *Penicillium,* and cross-sensitivity may exist between penicillin and griseofulvin. The incidence of hypersensitivity reactions to griseofulvin in patients allergic to penicillin, however, has not been reported. The most common untoward reaction to griseofulvin is rash. Urticaria and angioneurotic edema are occasional findings, and elevation of transaminases may occur. In one report, griseofulvin was shown to cross the placenta in low concentrations, but fetal effects were not discussed [718]. A study comparing griseofulvin with terbinafine [719], and case reports of successful treatment of tinea capitis with itraconazole and fluconazole, suggest that all of these antifungal agents can be used as alternative agents with better tolerability and fewer side effects [720].

REFERENCES

[1] L. Clerihew, N. Austin, W. McGuire, Prophylactic systemic antifungal agents to prevent mortality and morbidity in very low birth weight infants, Cochrane Database Syst. Rev. (4) (2007) CD003850.
[2] H. Fudenberg, et al., Primary immunodeficiencies: report of a World Health Organization committee, Pediatrics 47 (1971) 927.
[3] C. Chagas, Nova *Trypanomiazaea humana,* Mem. Inst. Oswaldo Cruz 1 (1909) 159.
[4] A. Carini, Formas de eschizogonia do *Trypanosoma lewisii,* Soc. Med. C. São Paulo 16 Aoakut. Bull Inst Pasteur 9 (1911) 937.
[5] P. Delanoe, M. Delanoe, Sur les rapports des kystes de carini du poumon des rats avec le *Trypanosoma lewisii,* Présenté par *M. Laveran.* Note de Delanoe et Delanoe. C. R. Acad. Sci. 155 (1912) 658.

[6] C. Chagas, Nova entidade morbida do homen; rezumo geral de estudos etiologicos e clinicos, Mem. Inst. Oswaldo Cruz 3 (1911) 219.

[7] E. Benecke, Eigenartige Bronchiolenerkrankung im ersten Lebensjahr, Verh. Dtsch. Ges. Pathol. 31 (1938) 402.

[8] O. Ammich, Über die nichtsyphilitische interstitielle Pneumonie des ersten Kindesalters, Virchows Arch. Pathol. Anat. 302 (1938) 539.

[9] J. Vanek, O. Jirovec, Parasitäre Pneumonie. "Interstitielle" plasmazellen Pneumonie der Frühgeborenen, verursacht durch *Pneumocystis carinii*, Zentralbl. Bakteriol. Orig. 158 (1952) 120.

[10] G. Van der Meer, S.L. Brug, Infection par *Pneumocystis* chez l'homme et chez les animaux, Ann. Soc. Belg. Med. Trop. 22 (1942) 301.

[11] W.C. Deamer, H.U. Zollinger, Interstitial "plasma cell" pneumonia of premature and young infants, Pediatrics 12 (1953) 11.

[12] J.H. Lunseth, et al., Interstitial plasma cell pneumonia, J. Pediatr. 46 (1955) 137.

[13] G. Dauzier, T. Willis, R.N. Barnett, *Pneumocystis carinii* pneumonia in an infant, Am. J. Clin. Pathol. 26 (1956) 787.

[14] H. Hamperl, *Pneumocystis* infection and cytomegaly of the lungs in the newborn and adult, Am. J. Pathol. 32 (1956) 1.

[15] H.T. Russell, B.M. Nelson, *Pneumocystis* pneumonitis in American infants, Am. J. Clin. Pathol. 26 (1956) 1334.

[16] D.C. Gajdusek, *Pneumocystis carinii*-etiologic agent of interstitial plasma cell pneumonia of premature and young infants, Pediatrics 19 (1957) 543.

[17] J.C. Edman, et al., Ribosomal RNA sequence shows *Pneumocystis carinii* to be a member of the fungi, Nature 334 (1988) 519.

[18] S.L. Stringer, et al., *Pneumocystis carinii*: sequence from ribosomal RNA implies a close relationship with fungi, Exp. Parasitol. 68 (1989) 450.

[19] J.K. Frenkel, *Pneumocystis* pneumonia, an immunodeficiency-dependent disease (IDD): a critical historical overview, J. Eukaryot. Microbiol. 46 (1999) 89S.

[20] W.T. Hughes, *Pneumocystis carinii* vs. *Pneumocystis jiroveci*: another misnomer (response to Stringer et al), Emerg. Infect. Dis. 9 (2003) 276.

[21] R.A. LeClair, *Pneumocystis carinii* and interstitial plasma cell pneumonia: a review, Am. Rev. Respir. Dis. 16 (1967) 1131.

[22] E.G. Barton, W.G. Campbell, *Pneumocystis carinii* in lungs of rats treated with cortisone acetate, Am. J. Pathol. 54 (1969) 209.

[23] J. Vavra, K. Kucera, N.D. Levine, An interpretation of the fine structure of *Pneumocystis carinii*, J. Protozool. 15 (1968) 12.

[24] W. Dutz, *Pneumocystis carinii* pneumonia, Pathol. Annu. 5 (1970) 309.

[25] J.A. Esterly, N.E. Warner, *Pneumocystis carinii* pneumonia, Arch. Pathol. 80 (1965) 433.

[26] K.K. Sethi, *Pneumocystis carinii* pneumonia, Lancet 1 (1967) 1387 (letter).

[27] J.A. Minielly, S.D. Mills, K.E. Holley, *Pneumocystis carinii* pneumonia, Can. Med. Assoc. J. 100 (1969) 846.

[28] J.E. McNeal, R.G. Yaeger, Observations on a case of *Pneumocystis* pneumonia, Arch. Pathol. 70 (1960) 397.

[29] J. Vavra, K. Kucera, *Pneumocystis carinii* Delanoë, its ultrastructure and ultrastructural affinities, J. Protozool. 17 (1970) 463.

[30] H.K. Kim, W.T. Hughes, S. Feldman, Studies of morphology and immunofluorescence of *Pneumocystis carinii*, Proc. Soc. Exp. Biol. Med. 141 (1972) 304.

[31] W.H. Sheldon, Pulmonary *Pneumocystis carinii* infection, J. Pediatr. 61 (1962) 780.

[32] T.V. Le, et al., Diagnostic "in vivo" de la pneumonie á "*Pneumocystis*", Arch. Fr. Pediatr. 20 (1963) 773.

[33] A.M. Chalvardjian, L.A. Grawe, A new procedure for the identification of *Pneumocystis carinii* cysts in tissue sections and smears, J. Clin. Pathol. 16 (1963) 383.

[34] M.C. Bowling, I.M. Smith, S.L. Wescott, A rapid staining procedure for *Pneumocystis carinii*, Am. J. Med. Tech. 39 (1973) 267.

[35] W. Bommer, *Pneumocystis carinii* from human lungs under electron microscope, Am. J. Dis. Child. 104 (1962) 657.

[36] H.C. Huneycutt, W.R. Anderson, W.S. Hendry, *Pneumocystis carinii* pneumonia: case studies with electron microscopy, Am. J. Clin. Pathol. 41 (1964) 411.

[37] E.G. Barton Jr., W.G. Campbell Jr., Further observations on the ultrastructure of *Pneumocystis*, Arch. Pathol. 83 (1967) 527.

[38] S.N. Huang, K.G. Marshall, *Pneumocystis carinii* infection: a cytologic, histologic and electron microscopic study of the organism, Am. Rev. Respir. Dis. 102 (1970) 623.

[39] N.S. Wang, S.N. Huang, W.M. Thurlbeck, Combined *Pneumocystis carinii* and cytomegalovirus infection, Arch. Pathol. 90 (1970) 529.

[40] G.F. Vawter, B.G. Uzman, A. Nowoslawski, Pneumocystis carinii, Ann. N.Y. Acad. Sci. 174 (1970) 1048.

[41] E.K. Ham, et al., Ultrastructure of *Pneumocystis carinii*, Exp. Mol. Pathol. 14 (1971) 362.

[42] M.A. Luna, et al., *Pneumocystis carinii* pneumonitis in cancer patients, Tex. Rep. Biol. Med. 30 (1972) 1.

[43] W.G. Campbell Jr., Ultrastructure of *Pneumocystis* in human lung: life cycle in human pneumocystosis, Arch. Pathol. 93 (1972) 312.

[44] A. Nietschke, Zur Frage des histologischen Nachweises von Pneumocysten bei der interstitiellen Pneumonie, Monatsschr. Kinderheilkd. 108 (1960) 142.

[45] K. Yoneda, P.D. Walzer, Attachment of *Pneumocystis carinii* to type I alveolar cells studied by freeze-fracture electron microscopy, Infect. Immun. 40 (1983) 812.

[46] J. Vanek, O. Jirovec, J. Lukes, Interstitial plasma cell pneumonia in infants, Ann. Paediatr. 180 (1953) 1.

[47] K. Kucera, On the morphology and developmental cycle of *Pneumocystis carinii* of human and rat origin, Folia Parasitol 13 (1966) 113.

[48] K. Kucera, T. Valousek, The direct proof of *Pneumocystis carinii* in alive nurslings and a new evolutive stage of *Pneumocystis*, Folia Parasitol 13 (1966) 113.

[49] M. Vossen, et al., Developmental biology of *Pneumocystis carinii*, an alternative view on the life cycle of the parasite, Z. Paracitesmnkd. 55 (1978) 101.

[50] O. Goetz, Die Ätiologie der interstitiellen sogenannten plasmazellularen Pneumonie des jungen Säuglings, Arch. Kinderheilk. 163 (1960) 1.

[51] O. Jirovec, Das Problem der *Pneumocystis* Pneumonien vom parasitologischen Standpunkte, Monatsschr. Kinderheilkd. 108 (1960) 136.

[52] W. Giese, Die Ätiologie der interstitielle plasmazellulären Säuglingspneumonie, Monatsschr. Kinderheilkd. 101 (1953) 147.

[53] A.E. Wakefield, et al., Molecular probes for the detection of *Pneumocystis carinii*, Trans. R. Soc. Trop. Med. Hyg. 84 (Suppl. 1) (1990) 17.

[54] O. Vivell, Die Serologie der interstitiellen Pneumonie, Monatsschr. Kinderheilkd. 108 (1960) 146.

[55] O. Goetz, Serologische Befunde interstitieller Pneumonien aus den vereinigten Staaten, Arch. Kinderheilk. 170 (1964) 60.

[56] J. Li, T. Edlind, Phylogeny of *Pneumocystis carinii* based on ß-tubulin sequence, J. Eukaryot. Microbiol. 41 (1994) 97S.

[57] E. Mazars, et al., Polymorphism of the thymidylate synthase gene of *Pneumocystis carinii* from different host species, J. Eukaryot. Microbiol. 42 (1995) 26.

[58] L. Ma, J.A. Kovacs, Expression and characterization of recombinant human-derived *Pneumocystis carinii* dihydrofolate reductase, Antimicrob. Agents Chemother. 44 (2000) 3092.

[59] S. Banerji, et al., Analysis of genetic diversity at the arom locus in isolates of *Pneumocystis carinii*, J. Eukaryot. Microbiol. 42 (1995) 675.

[60] M.J. Murphy, L.L. Pifer, W.T. Hughes, *Pneumocystis carinii* in vitro: a study by scanning electron microscopy, Am. J. Pathol. 86 (1977) 387.

[61] C.R. Latorre, A.J. Sulzer, L. Norman, Serial propagation of *Pneumocystis carinii* in cell line cultures, Appl. Environ. Microbiol. 33 (1977) 1204.

[62] L.L. Pifer, D. Woods, W.T. Hughes, Propagation of *Pneumocystis carinii* in Vero cell culture, Infect. Immun. 20 (1978) 66.

[63] M.S. Bartlett, P.A. Verbanac, J.W. Smith, Cultivation of *Pneumocystis carinii* with WI-38 cells, J. Clin. Microbiol. 10 (1979) 796.

[64] H. Masur, T.C. Jones, The interaction in vitro of *Pneumocystis carinii* with macrophages and L-cells, J. Exp. Med. 147 (1978) 157.

[65] R.D.K. Reye, R.E.J. Ten Seldam, *Pneumocystis* pneumonia, J. Pathol. Bacteriol. 72 (1956) 451.

[66] G.R. da Silva, M.C. Gomes, R.F. Santos, *Pneumocystis* pneumonia in the adult: report of a case associated with corticosteroid therapy for rheumatoid arthritis, Rev. Inst. Med. Trop. Sao Paulo 7 (1965) 31.

[67] F. Gagne, F. Hould, Interstitial plasmacellular (parasitic) pneumonia in infants, Can. Med. Assoc. J. 74 (1956) 620.

[68] T. Pizzi, M. Diaz, Neumonia intersticial plasmocelular: II. Investigacion parasitologia del *Pneumocystis carinii*, Rev. Chil. Pediatr. 27 (1956) 294.

[69] A. Thijs, P.G. Janssens, Pneumocystosis in Congolese infant, Trop. Geogr. Med. 15 (1963) 158.

[70] S. Jarnum, et al., Generalized *Pneumocystis carinii* infection with severe idiopathic hypoproteinemia, Ann. Intern. Med. 68 (1968) 138.

[71] H.S. Baar, Interstitial plasmacellular pneumonia due to *Pneumocystis carinii*, J. Clin. Pathol. 8 (1955) 19.

[72] E.K. Ahvenainen, Interstitial plasma cell pneumonia, Pediatr. Clin. North Am. 4 (1957) 203.

[73] J. Vlachos, Necropsy findings in six cases of *Pneumocystis carinii* pneumonia, Arch. Dis. Child. 45 (1970) 146.

[74] A.B. Desai, R.C. Shak, K.N. Schgal, *Pneumocystis carinii* pneumonia, Indian. Pediatr. 8 (1971) 129.

[75] S.F. Cahalane, *Pneumocystis carinii* pneumonia: report of a case and review of the literature, J. Ir. Med. Assoc. 50 (1962) 133.

[76] J.K. Kaftori, et al., *Pneumocystis carinii* pneumonia in the adult, Arch. Intern. Med. 109 (1962) 114.

[77] G. Fontana, O. Tamburello, Epidemiologia della polmonite interstiziale plasmacellulare nell' I.P.A.I. di Roma, Minerva Nipiol. 19 (1969) 20.

[78] R.M. Nakamura, et al., Coexistent cytomegalic inclusion disease and *Pneumocystis carinii* infection in adults, Acta Pathol. Jpn. 14 (1964) 45.

[79] S.K. Lim, C.S. Moon, Studies on *Pneumocystis carinii* pneumonia: epidemiological and clinical studies of 80 cases, Jonghap Med. 6 (1960) 69.

[80] B. Ryan, *Pneumocystis carinii* infection in Melanesian children, J. Pediatr. 60 (1962) 914.

[81] D.M.O. Becroft, J.M. Costello, *Pneumocystis carinii* pneumonia in siblings: diagnosis by lung aspiration, N. Z. Med. J. 64 (1965) 273.

[82] O.D. Laerum, et al., *Pneumocystis carinii* pneumonia in Norway, Scand. J. Respir. Dis. 53 (1972) 247.

[83] Z. Byhosko, Pneumonia caused by *Pneumocystis carinii*, Pediatr. Pol. 31 (1956) 493.

[84] G. Mikhailov, Pneumocystic pneumonia, Arch. Patol. (Moscow) 21 (1959) 46.

[85] J.H. Hutchison, Congenital agammaglobulinemia, Lancet 2 (1955) 844.

[86] W.J. Pepler, *Pneumocystis* pneumonia, S. Afr. Med. J. 32 (1958) 1003.

[87] A. Moragas, M.T. Vidal, *Pneumocystis carinii* pneumonia: first autopsy series in Spain, Helv. Paediatr. Acta 26 (1971) 71.

[88] G. Nathorst-Windahl, et al., Massive fatal *Pneumocystis* pneumonia in leukemia: report of two cases, Acta Pathol. Microbiol. Scand. 62 (1964) 472.

[89] K. Salfelder, et al., Neumocistosis, Merida, Venezuela, 1966 Universidad de los Andes, Facultad de Medicina.

[90] A.A. Abioye, Interstitial plasma cell pneumonia (*Pneumocystis carinii*) in Ibadan, W. Afr. Med. J. 16 (1967) 130.

[91] B.R.H. Farrow, et al., *Pneumocystis* pneumonia in the dog, J. Comp. Pathol. 82 (1972) 447.

[92] J.N. Shively, et al., *Pneumocystis carinii* pneumonia in two foals, J. Am. Vet. Med. Assoc. 162 (1973) 648.

[93] S. Van den Akker, E. Goldbloed, Pneumonia caused by *Pneumocystis carinii* in a dog, Trop. Geogr. Med. 12 (1960) 54.

[94] C.N. Nikolskii, A.N. Shchetknin, *Pneumocystis* in swine, Veterinaria 44 (1967) 65.

[95] F.W. Chandler, et al., Pulmonary pneumocystosis in nonhuman primates, Arch. Pathol. Lab. Med. 100 (1976) 163.

[96] C.V. Richter, G.L. Humason, J.H. Godbold, Endemic *Pneumocystis carinii* in a marmoset colony, J. Comp. Pathol. 88 (1978) 171.

[97] J. Meuwissen, et al., Parasitological and serologic observations of infection with *Pneumocystis* in humans, J. Infect. Dis. 136 (1977) 43.

[98] L.L. Pifer, et al., *Pneumocystis carinii* infection: evidence for high prevalence in normal and immunosuppressed children, Pediatrics 61 (1978) 35.

[99] M.P. Gerrard, et al., Serological study of *Pneumocystis carinii* infection in the absence of immunosuppression, Arch. Dis. Child. 62 (1987) 177.

[100] L.L. Pifer, et al., Subclinical *Pneumocystis carinii* infection: implications for the immunocompromised patient, Program and Abstracts of the 20th Interscience Conference on Antimicrobial Agents and Chemotherapy, New Orleans, September 22-24, 1980 (Abstract 340).

[101] J.J. Robinson, Two cases of pneumocystosis: observation in 203 adult autopsies, Arch. Pathol. 71 (1961) 156.

[102] K. Weisse, E. Wedler, Über das Vorkommen der sogenannten "*Pneumocystis carinii*" Klin. Wochenschr. 32 (1954) 270.

[103] W.B. Hamlin, Pneumocystis carinii, JAMA 204 (1968) 173.

[104] J.A. Esterly, *Pneumocystis carinii* in lungs of adults at autopsy, Am. Rev. Respir. Dis. 97 (1968) 935.

[105] C.L. Vogel, et al., *Pneumocystis carinii* pneumonia, Ann. Intern. Med. 68 (1968) 97.

[106] M.R. Sedaghatian, D.B. Singer, *Pneumocystis carinii* in children with malignant disease, Cancer 29 (1972) 772.

[107] D.R. Perera, et al., *Pneumocystis carinii* pneumonia in a hospital for children: epidemiologic aspects, JAMA 214 (1970) 1074.

[108] R.A. Le Clair, Descriptive epidemiology of interstitial pneumocystic pneumonia, Am. Rev. Respir. Dis. 99 (1969) 542.

[109] P.D. Walzer, et al., *Pneumocystis carinii* pneumonia and primary immune deficiency diseases of infancy and childhood, J. Pediatr. 82 (1973) 416.

[110] P.D. Walzer, et al., *Pneumocystis carinii* pneumonia in the United States: epidemiologic, diagnostic and clinical features, Ann. Intern. Med. 80 (1974) 83.

[111] B.H. Hyun, C.F. Varga, L.J. Thalheimer, *Pneumocystis carinii* pneumonitis occurring in an adopted Korean infant, JAMA 195 (1966) 784.

[112] Z. Danilevicius, A call to recognize *Pneumocystis carinii* pneumonia, JAMA 231 (1975) 1168, (editorial).

[113] A. Eidelman, A. Nkongo, R. Morecki, *Pneumocystis carinii* pneumonitis in Vietnamese infant in U.S, Pediatr. Res. 8 (1974) 424.

[114] J.C. Redman, *Pneumocystis carinii* pneumonia in an adopted Vietnamese infant: a case of diffuse fulminant disease, with recovery, JAMA 230 (1974) 1561.

[115] W.A. Gleason Jr., V.J. Roden, F. DeCastro, *Pneumocystis* pneumonia in Vietnamese infants, J. Pediatr. 87 (1975) 1001.

[116] A.I. Eidelman, et al., *Pneumocystis carinii* pneumonia in Vietnamese orphans, MMWR Morb. Mortal. Wkly. Rep. 25 (1976) 15.

[117] G.S. Giebink, et al., *Pneumocystis carinii* pneumonia in two Vietnamese refugee infants, Pediatrics 58 (1976) 115.

[118] Centers for Disease Control, Update: acquired immunodeficiency syndrome–United States, MMWR Morb. Mortal. Wkly. Rep. 35 (1986) 757.

[119] R.J. Simonds, et al., *Pneumocystis carinii* pneumonia among U.S. children with perinatally acquired HIV infection, JAMA 270 (1993) 470.

[120] H.A. Lyons, K. Vinijchaikul, G.R. Hennigar, *Pneumocystis carinii* pneumonia unassociated with other disease, Arch. Intern. Med. 108 (1961) 929.

[121] J.M. Watanabe, et al., *Pneumocystis carinii* pneumonia in a family, JAMA 193 (1965) 685.

[122] A.G. Weinberg, et al., Monoclonal macroglobulinemia and cytomegalic inclusion disease, Pediatrics 51 (1973) 518.

[123] M. Rao, et al., *Pneumocystis carinii* pneumonia: occurrence in a healthy American infant, JAMA 238 (1977) 2301.

[124] S. Stagno, et al., *Pneumocystis carinii* pneumonitis in young immunocompetent infants, Pediatrics 66 (1980) 56.

[125] F. Shann, et al., Pneumonia associated with infection with *Pneumocystis*, respiratory syncytial virus, *Chlamydia, Mycoplasma*, and cytomegalovirus in children in Papua New Guinea, BMJ 292 (1986) 314.

[126] J.B. Robbins, *Pneumocystis carinii* pneumonitis, a review, Pediatr. Res. 1 (1967) 131.

[127] G.A. Von Harnack, Organisatorische Probleme bei der Bekämpfung der interstitiellen Pneumonie, Monatsschr. Kinderheilkd. 108 (1960) 159.

[128] J.W. Erchul, L.P. Williams, P.P. Meighan, *Pneumocystis carinii* in hypopharyngeal material, N. Engl. J. Med. 267 (1962) 926.

[129] G. Toth, E. Balogh, M. Belay, Demonstration in tracheal secretion of the causative agent of interstitial plasma cell pneumonia, Acta Paediatr. Acad. Sci. Hung. 7 (1966) 25.

[130] I.E. Fortuny, K.F. Tempero, T.W. Amsden, *Pneumocystis carinii* pneumonia diagnosed from sputum and successfully treated with pentamidine isethionate, Cancer 26 (1970) 911.

[131] J.A. Smith, C.M. Wiggins, Identification of *Pneumocystis carinii* in sputum, N. Engl. J. Med. 289 (1973) 1254, (letter).

[132] W.K. Lau, L.S. Young, J.S. Remington, *Pneumocystis carinii* pneumonia: diagnosis by examination of pulmonary secretions, JAMA 236 (1976) 2399.

[133] J.H. Brazinsky, J.E. Phillips, *Pneumocystis* pneumonia transmission between patients with lymphoma, JAMA 209 (1969) 1527, (letter).

[134] J.L. Jacobs, et al., A cluster of *Pneumocystis carinii* pneumonia in adults without predisposing illnesses, N. Engl. J. Med. 324 (1991) 246.

[135] J.D. Robbins, T. Fodor, *Pneumocystis carinii* pneumonia, MMWR Morb. Mortal. Wkly. Rep. 17 (1968) 51.

[136] L.O. Gentry, J.S. Remington, *Pneumocystis carinii* pneumonia in siblings, J. Pediatr. 76 (1970) 769.

[137] G.R. Bazaz, et al., *Pneumocystis carinii* pneumonia in three full-term siblings, J. Pediatr. 76 (1970) 767.

[138] D.G. Jose, R.A. Gatti, R.A. Good, Eosinophilia with *Pneumocystis carinii* pneumonia and immune deficiency syndromes, J. Pediatr. 79 (1971) 748.

[139] H.J. Meuwissen, et al., Diagnosis of *Pneumocystis carinii* pneumonia in the presence of immunological deficiency, Lancet 1 (1970) 1124.

[140] F. Pavlica, Erste Beobachtung von angeborener pneumozysten Pneumonie bei einem reifen, ausgetragenen Totgeborenen, Zentralbl. Allg. Pathol. 103 (1962) 236.

[141] C. Post, W. Dutz, I. Nasarian, Endemic *Pneumocystis carinii* pneumonia in South Iran, Arch. Dis. Child. 39 (1964) 35.

[142] P. Brock, et al., AIDS in two African infants born in Belgium, Acta Paediatr. Scand. 76 (1987) 175.

[143] R.S. Beach, et al., *Pneumocystis carinii* pneumonia in a human immunodeficiency virus 1-infected neonate with meconium aspiration, Pediatr. Infect. Dis. J. 10 (1991) 953.

[144] B.A. Burke, R.A. Good, *Pneumocystis carinii* infection, Medicine 52 (1973) 23.

[145] C. Singer, et al., *Pneumocystis carinii* pneumonia: a cluster of eleven cases, Ann. Intern. Med. 82 (1975) 772.

[146] T.K. Ruebush, et al., An outbreak of *Pneumocystis* pneumonia in children with acute lymphocytic leukemia, Am. J. Dis. Child. 132 (1978) 143.

[147] M.J. Chusid, K.A. Heyrman, An outbreak of *Pneumocystis carinii* pneumonia at a pediatric hospital, Pediatrics 62 (1978) 1031.

[148] W.T. Hughes, et al., Intensity of immunosuppressive therapy and the incidence of *Pneumocystis carinii* pneumonitis, Cancer 36 (2004) 1975.

[149] K. Kucera, Some new views on the epidemiology of infections caused by *Pneumocystis carinii*, in: A. Corradetti (Ed.), Procedings of the First International Congress of Parasitology, Rome, Italy, September 26-28, 1964, Pergamon Press, Oxford, 1964, p. 452.

[150] W.T. Hughes, et al., *Pneumocystis carinii* pneumonitis in children with malignancies, J. Pediatr. 82 (1973) 404.

[151] P.D. Walzer, et al., Nude mouse: a new experimental model for *Pneumocystis carinii* infection, Science 197 (1977) 177.

[152] W.H. Sheldon, Experimental pulmonary *Pneumocystis carinii* infection in rabbits, J. Exp. Med. 110 (1959) 147.

[153] J.O. Hendley, T.H. Weller, Activation and transmission in rats of infection with *Pneumocystis*, Proc. Soc. Exp. Biol. Med. 137 (1971) 1401.

[154] K. Ueda, et al., Chronic fatal pneumocystosis in nude mice, Jpn. J. Exp. Med. 47 (1977) 475.

[155] P.D. Walzer, M.E. Rutledge, Humoral immune responses in experimental *Pneumocystis carinii* pneumonia, Clin. Res. 28 (1980) 381.

[156] R.A. Price, W.T. Hughes, Histopathology of *Pneumocystis carinii* infestation and infection in malignant disease in childhood, Hum. Pathol. 5 (1974) 737.

[157] P. Rosen, D. Armstrong, C. Ramos, *Pneumocystis carinii* pneumonia: a clinicopathologic study of 20 patients with neoplastic diseases, Am. J. Med. 53 (1972) 428.

[158] W.R. Weber, F.B. Askin, L.P. Dehner, Lung biopsy in *Pneumocystis carinii* pneumonia: a histopathologic study of typical and atypical features, Am. J. Clin. Pathol. 67 (1977) 11.

[159] H. Hamperl, Zur Frage des Organismnnachweises bei der interstitiellen plasmacellularen Pneumonie, Klin. Wochenschr. 30 (1952) 820.

[160] D. Rifkind, T.D. Faris, R.B. Hill, *Pneumocystis carinii* pneumonia: studies on the diagnosis and treatment, Ann. Intern. Med. 65 (1966) 943.

[161] F.B. Askin, A.A. Katzenstein, *Pneumocystis* infection masquerading as diffuse alveolar damage: a potential source of diagnostic error, Chest 79 (1981) 420.

[162] R.I. Kramer, V.C. Cirone, H. Moore, Interstitial pneumonia due to *Pneumocystis carinii* and cytomegalic inclusion disease and hypogammaglobulinemia occurring simultaneously in an infant, Pediatrics 29 (1962) 816.

[163] G.R. Hennigar, et al., *Pneumocystis carinii* pneumonia in an adult, Am. J. Clin. Pathol. 35 (1961) 353.

[164] A.D. Nicastri, R.V.P. Hutter, H.S. Collins, *Pneumocystis carinii* pneumonia in an adult: emphasis on antemortem morphologic diagnosis, N. Y. State J. Med. 65 (1965) 2149.

[165] J.B. Robbins, et al., Successful treatment of *Pneumocystis carinii* pneumonitis in a patient with congenital hypogammaglobulinemia, N. Engl. J. Med. 272 (1965) 708.

[166] J. Nowak, Late pulmonary changes in the course of infection with *Pneumocystis carinii*, Acta Med. Pol. 7 (1966) 23.

[167] M.E. Whitcomb, et al., Interstitial fibrosis after *Pneumocystis carinii* pneumonia, Ann. Intern. Med. 73 (1970) 761.

[168] W.T. Hughes, W.W. Johnson, Recurrent *Pneumocystis carinii* pneumonia following apparent recovery, J. Pediatr. 79 (1971) 755.

[169] H.B. Kirby, B. Kenamore, J.C. Guckian, *Pneumocystis carinii* pneumonia treated with pyrimethamine and sulfadiazine, Ann. Intern. Med. 75 (1971) 505.

[170] K.O. Schmid, Studien zur Pneumocystis-erkrankung des Menschen: I. Mitteilung, das wechselnde Erscheinungsbild der *Pneumocystis* Pneumonie beim Säugling: konkordante und discordante Form, Pneumocystosis granulomatose, Frankf. Z. Pathol. 74 (1964) 121.

[171] B. Cruickshank, Pulmonary granulomatous pneumocystosis following renal transplantation: report of a case, Am. J. Clin. Pathol. 63 (1975) 384.

[172] W. Dutz, et al., Marasmus and *Pneumocystis carinii* pneumonia in institutionalized infants: observations during an endemic, Z. Kinderheilkd. 117 (1974) 241.

[173] R. Weller, Zur Erzeugung der Pneumocystosen im Tierver-such, Z. Kinderheilkd. 76 (1955) 366.

[174] R. Weller, Weitere Untersuchungen über experimentele Rattenpneumocystose in Hinblick auf die interstitielle Pneumonie der Frühgeborenen, Z. Kinderheilkd. 78 (1956) 166.

[175] J.K. Frenkel, J.T. Good, J.A. Shultz, Latent *Pneumocystis* infection of rats, relapse and chemotherapy, Lab. Invest. 15 (1966) 1559.

[176] W.T. Hughes, et al., Protein-calorie malnutrition: a host determinant for *Pneumocystis carinii* infection, Am. J. Dis. Child. 128 (1974) 44.

[177] Baar, cited in J.H. Hutchison, Congenital agammaglobulinemia, Lancet 2 (1955) 1196 (letter).

[178] B.A. Burke, L.J. Krovetz, R.A. Good, Occurrence of *Pneumocystis carinii* pneumonia in children with agammaglobulinemia, Pediatrics 28 (1961) 196.

[179] A.M. DiGeorge, Congenital absence of the thymus and its immunologic consequences: occurrence with congenital hypoparathyroidism, in: R.A. Good, D. Bergsman (Eds.), Immunologic Diseases in Man, Birth Defects, Original Article Series, National Foundation Press, New York, 1968.

[180] D. Rifkind, et al., Transplantation pneumonia, JAMA 189 (1964) 808.

[181] V.A. Fulginiti, et al., Infections in recipients of liver homografts, N. Engl. J. Med. 279 (1968) 619.

[182] R.A. Le Clair, Transplantation pneumonia, associated with *Pneumocystis carinii*, among recipients of cardiac transplants, Am. Rev. Respir. Dis. 100 (1969) 874.

[183] L.M. Quittell, M. Fisher, C.M. Foley, *Pneumocystis carinii* pneumonia in infants given adrenocorticotropic hormone for infantile spasms, J. Pediatr. 110 (1987) 901.

[184] H.G. Herrod, et al., The in vitro response of human lymphocytes to *Pneumocystis carinii*, Clin. Res. 27 (1979) 811.

[185] J. Ruskin, J.S. Remington, *Pneumocystis carinii* infection in the immunosuppressed host, Antimicrob. Agents Chemother. 7 (1967) 70.

[186] G. Ivady, et al., *Pneumocystis carinii* pneumonia, Lancet 1 (1967) 616, (letter).

[187] E. Kohout, et al., Immunoglobulin levels in infantile pneumocystosis, J. Clin. Pathol. 25 (1972) 135.

[188] W.J. Brzosko, A. Nowoslawski, Identification of *Pneumocystis carinii* antigens in tissues, Bull. Acad. Pol. Sci. Biol. 13 (1965) 49.

[189] W.J. Brzosko, A. Nowoslawski, K. Madalinski, Identification of immune complexes in lungs from *Pneumocystis carinii* pneumonia cases in infants, Bull. Acad. Pol. Sci. Biol. 12 (1964) 137.

[190] W.J. Brzosko, et al., Immunohistochemistry in studies on the pathogenesis of *Pneumocystis* pneumonia in infants, Ann. N. Y. Acad. Sci. 177 (1971) 156.

[191] B. Creamer, W. Dutz, C. Post, The small intestinal lesion of chronic diarrhea and marasmus in Iran, Lancet 1 (1970) 18.

[192] W. Dutz, et al., Bowel mucosal patterns and immunoglobulins in 100 infants from birth to one year of age, Pahlavi Med. J. 1 (1970) 234.

[193] W.J. Brzosko, A. Nowoslawski, Immunohistochemical studies on *Pneumocystis* pneumonia, Bull. Acad. Pol. Sci. Biol. 11 (1963) 563.

[194] W.H. Sheldon, Subclinical *Pneumocystis* pneumonitis, Am. J. Dis. Child. 97 (1959) 287.

[195] M.A. Charles, M.I. Schwarz, *Pneumocystis carinii* pneumonia, Postgrad. Med. 53 (1973) 86.

[196] R.B. Weiss, F.M. Muggia, Cytotoxic drug-induced pulmonary disease: update 1980, Am. J. Med. 68 (1980) 259.

[197] M.J.S. Richards, W.M. Wara, Radiation pneumonitis complicated by *Pneumocystis carinii*, Int. J. Radiat. Oncol. Biol. Phys. 4 (1978) 287.

[198] R.J. Wells, et al., Pulmonary leukemia in children presenting as diffuse interstitial pneumonia, J. Pediatr. 96 (1980) 262.

[199] C.O. Solberg, et al., Infectious complications in bone marrow transplant patients, BMJ 1 (1971) 18.

[200] W.F. White, H.M. Saxton, I.M.P. Dawson, *Pneumocystis* pneumonia: report of three cases in adults and one in a child with a discussion of the radiological appearances and predisposing factors, BMJ 2 (1961) 1327.

[201] W.T. Hughes, Infections during continuous complete remission of acute lymphocytic leukemia: during and after anticancer therapy, Int. J. Radiat. Oncol. Biol. Phys. 1 (1976) 305.

[202] J.J. Iacuone, et al., Acute respiratory illness in children with acute lymphoblastic leukemia, J. Pediatr. 90 (1977) 915.

[203] S.E. Siegel, et al., Pneumonia during therapy for childhood acute lymphoblastic leukemia, Am. J. Dis. Child. 134 (1980) 28.

[204] S.F. Thomas, W. Dutz, E.J. Khodadad, *Pneumocystis carinii* pneumonia (plasma cell pneumonia): roentgenographic, pathologic and clinical correlations, AJR Am. J. Roentgenol. 98 (1966) 318.

[205] S.B. Hauger, Approach to the pediatric patient with HIV infection and pulmonary symptoms, J. Pediatr. 119 (1991) S25.

[206] J. Ruskin, J.S. Remington, The compromised host and infection: I. *Pneumocystis carinii* pneumonia, JAMA 202 (1967) 1070.

[207] K. Vessal, et al., Roentgenologic changes in infantile *Pneumocystis carinii* pneumonia, AJR Am. J. Roentgenol. 120 (1974) 254.

[208] K. Vessal, et al., Verlaufskontrolle der Pneumocystose im Röntgenbild, Radiologe 16 (1976) 38.

[209] K.H. Falkenbach, K.D. Bachmann, B.J. O'Laughlin, *Pneumocystis carinii* pneumonia, AJR Am. J. Roentgenol. 85 (1961) 706.

[210] D.W. Denning, et al., Efficacy and safety of voriconazole in the treatment of acute invasive aspergillosis, Clin. Infect. Dis. 34 (2002) 563.

[211] R. Herbrecht, et al., Voriconazole versus amphotericin B for primary therapy of invasive aspergillosis, N. Engl. J. Med. 347 (2002) 408.

[212] E.A. Watts, P.D. Gard Jr., S.W. Tuthill, First reported case of intrauterine transmission of blastomycosis, Pediatr. Infect. Dis. 2 (1983) 308.

[213] S. Maxson, et al., Perinatal blastomycosis: a review, Pediatr. Infect. Dis. J. 11 (1992) 760.

[214] L.B. Lemos, M. Soofi, E. Amir, Blastomycosis and pregnancy, Ann. Diagn. Pathol. 6 (2002) 211.

[215] G. Robillard, et al., Plasma cell pneumonia in infants: review of 51 cases, J. Can. Assoc. Radiol. 16 (1965) 161.

[216] A.D. Neiberg, et al., *Blastomyces dermatitidis* treated during pregnancy: report of a case, Am. J. Obstet. Gynecol. 128 (1977) 911.

[217] M.D. Ismail, S.A. Lerner, Disseminated blastomycosis in a pregnant woman: review of amphotericin B usage during pregnancy, Am. Rev. Respir. Dis. 126 (1982) 350.

[218] I. Cohen, Absence of congenital infection and teratogenesis in three children born to mothers with blastomycosis and treated with amphotericin B during pregnancy, Pediatr. Infect. Dis. 6 (1987) 76.

[219] L. Daniel, I.E. Salit, Blastomycosis during pregnancy, Can. Med. Assoc. J. 131 (1984) 759.

[220] H. Hager, et al., Disseminated blastomycosis in a pregnant woman successfully treated with amphotericin-B: a case report, J. Reprod. Med. 33 (1988) 485.

[221] C.T. King, et al., Antifungal therapy during pregnancy, Clin. Infect. Dis. 27 (1998) 1151.

[222] J.W. Rippon, Medical Mycology: the Pathogenic Fungi and the Pathogenic Actinomycetes, second ed., WB Saunders, Philadelphia, 1982.

[223] J.F. Denton, et al., Isolation of *Blastomyces dermatitidis* from soil, Science 133 (1961) 126.

[224] E. Kerpel-Fronius, F. Varga, G. Bata, Blood gas and metabolic studies in plasma cell pneumonia and in newborn prematures with respiratory distress, Arch. Dis. Child. 39 (1964) 473.

[225] E. Smith, I.A. Gaspar, Pentamidine treatment of *Pneumocystis carinii* pneumonitis in an adult with lymphatic leukemia, Am. J. Med. 44 (1968) 626.

[226] P.B. Doak, et al., *Pneumocystis carinii* pneumonia: transplant lung, Q. J. Med. 165 (1973) 59.

[227] W.T. Hughes, S.K. Sanyal, R.A. Price, Signs, symptoms, and pathophysiology of *Pneumocystis carinii* pneumonitis, Natl. Cancer Inst. Monogr. 43 (1976) 77.

[228] B.A. Friedman, et al., Roentgenographically atypical *Pneumocystis carinii* pneumonia, Am. Rev. Respir. Dis. 111 (1975) 89.

[229] L.O. Gentry, J. Ruskin, J.S. Remington, *Pneumocystis carinii* pneumonia: problems in diagnosis and therapy in 24 cases, Calif. Med. 116 (1972) 6.

[230] G. Pliess, K. Seifert, Elektronenoptische Untersuchung bei experimenteller Pneumocystose, Beitr. Pathol. Anat. 120 (1959) 399.

[231] F. Von Lichtenberg, Enigmatic organisms of man and animal models: summation, Ann. N. Y. Acad. Sci. 174 (1970) 1052.

[232] A. Rubenstein, et al., Pulmonary disease in children with acquired immunodeficiency syndrome and AIDS-related complex, J. Pediatr. 108 (1986) 498.

[233] V.V. Joshi, et al., Pathology of opportunistic infections in children with acquired immunodeficiency syndrome, Pediatr. Pathol. 6 (1986) 145.

[234] Y. Yoshida, et al., Studies of *Pneumocystis carinii* and *Pneumocystis carinii* pneumonia: V. Diagnosis by cyst concentration from sputum, Jpn. J. Parasitol. 27 (1978) 473.

[235] F.P. Ognibene, et al., Induced sputum to diagnose *Pneumocystis carinii* pneumonia in immunosuppressed pediatric patients, J. Pediatr. 115 (1989) 430.

[236] H.D. Johnson, W.W. Johnson, *Pneumocystis carinii* pneumonia in children with cancer: diagnosis and treatment, JAMA 214 (1970) 1067.

[237] S. Chaudhary, et al., Percutaneous transthoracic needle aspiration of the lung: diagnosing *Pneumocystis carinii* pneumonitis, Am. J. Dis. Child. 131 (1977) 902.

[238] H.M. Clink, et al., *Pneumocystis carinii* pneumonitis, Lancet 2 (1975) 1265, (letter).

[239] P.P. Rosen, N. Martini, D. Armstrong, *Pneumocystis carinii* pneumonia: diagnosis by lung biopsy, Am. J. Med. 58 (1975) 794.

[240] D.H. Tyras, et al., The role of early open lung biopsy in the diagnosis and treatment of *Pneumocystis carinii* pneumonia, Ann. Thorac. Surg. 18 (1974) 571.

[241] L.L. Michaelis, et al., *Pneumocystis* pneumonia: the importance of early open lung biopsy, Ann. Surg. 183 (1976) 301.

[242] M. Bradshaw, et al., *Pneumocystis carinii* pneumonitis, Ann. Intern. Med. 73 (1970) 775.

[243] S.A. Roback, et al., Diagnostic open lung biopsy in the critically ill child, Pediatrics 52 (1973) 605.

[244] L.J. Wolff, et al., The causes of interstitial pneumonitis in immunocompromised children: an aggressive systematic approach to diagnosis, Pediatrics 60 (1977) 41.

[245] T.V.N. Ballantine, et al., Interstitial pneumonitis in the immunologically suppressed child: an urgent surgical condition, J. Pediatr. Surg. 12 (1977) 501.

[246] W.H. Mason, S.E. Siegel, B.L. Tucker, Diagnostic open lung biopsy in immunosuppressed pediatric patients, Clin. Res. 27 (1979) 114.

[247] G.S. Leight Jr., L.L. Michaelis, Open lung biopsy for the diagnosis of acute, diffuse pulmonary infiltrates in the immunosuppressed patient, Chest 73 (1978) 477.

[248] S.J. Rossiter, et al., Open lung biopsy in the immunosuppressed patient: is it really beneficial? J. Thorac. Cardiovasc. Surg. 77 (1979) 338.

[249] B.M. Rodgers, F. Moazam, J.L. Talbert, Thoracoscopy: early diagnosis of interstitial pneumonitis in the immunologically suppressed child, Chest 75 (1979) 126.

[250] H.K. Kim, W.T. Hughes, Comparison of methods for identification of *Pneumocystis carinii* in pulmonary aspirates, Am. J. Clin. Pathol. 60 (1973) 462.

[251] P.P. Rosen, Frozen section management of a lung biopsy for suspected *Pneumocystis carinii* pneumonia, Am. J. Surg. Pathol. 1 (1977) 79.

[252] R.C. Young, J.E. Bennett, E.W. Chu, Organisms mimicking *Pneumocystis carinii*, Lancet 2 (1976) 1082, (letter).

[253] D.J. Reinhardt, W. Kaplan, F.W. Chandler, Morphologic resemblance of Zygomycetes spores to *Pneumocystis carinii* cysts in tissue, Am. Rev. Respir. Dis. 115 (1977) 170.

[254] W.A. Demicco, et al., False-negative biopsy in *Pneumocystis carinii* pneumonia, Chest 75 (1979) 389.

[255] J.W. Smith, W.T. Hughes, A rapid staining technique for *Pneumocystis carinii*, J. Clin. Pathol. 25 (1972) 269.

[256] C.J. Churukian, E.A. Schenk, Rapid Grocott's methenamine-silver nitrate method for fungi and *Pneumocystis carinii*, Am. J. Clin. Pathol. 68 (1977) 427.

[257] C.T. Mahan, G.E. Sale, Rapid methenamine-silver stain for *Pneumocystis* and fungi, Arch. Pathol. Lab. Med. 102 (1978) 351.

[258] R.L. Pintozzi, Modified Grocott's methenamine-silver nitrate method for quick staining of *Pneumocystis carinii*, J. Clin. Pathol. 31 (1978) 803.

[259] L.L. Pifer, D.R. Woods, Efficacy of toluidine blue "O" stain for *Pneumocystis carinii*, Am. J. Clin. Pathol. 69 (1978) 472.

[260] O.P. Settnes, P.E. Larsen, Inhibition of toluidine blue O stain for *Pneumocystis carinii* by additives in the diethyl ether, Am. J. Clin. Pathol. 72 (1979) 493.

[261] R.L. Pintozzi, L.J. Blecka, S. Nanos, The morphologic identification of *Pneumocystis carinii*, Acta Cytol. 23 (1979) 35.

[262] R.B. Cameron, J.C. Watts, B.L. Kasten, *Pneumocystis carinii* pneumonia: an approach to rapid laboratory diagnosis, Am. J. Clin. Pathol. 72 (1979) 90.

[263] J. Meuwissen, et al., New method for study of infections with *Pneumocystis carinii*, J. Infect. Dis. 127 (1973) 209, (letter).

[264] A. Nowoslawski, W.J. Brzosko, Indirect immunofluorescent test for serodiagnosis of *Pneumocystis carinii* infection, Bull. Acad. Pol. Sci. Biol. 12 (1964) 143.

[265] W. Brzosko, K. Madalinski, A. Nowoslawski, Fluorescent antibody and immuno-electrophoretic evaluation of the immune reaction in children with pneumonia induced by *Pneumocystis carinii*, Exp. Med. Microbiol. 19 (1967) 397.

[266] L. Norman, I.G. Kagan, A preliminary report of an indirect fluorescent antibody test for detecting antibodies to cysts of *Pneumocystis carinii* in human sera, Am. J. Clin. Pathol. 58 (1972) 170.

[267] W.K. Lau, L.S. Young, Immunofluorescent antibodies against *Pneumocystis carinii* in patients with and without pulmonary infiltrates, Clin. Res. 25 (1977) 379.

[268] V. Shepherd, B. Jameson, G.K. Knowles, *Pneumocystis carinii* pneumonitis: a serological study, J. Clin. Pathol. 32 (1979) 773.

[269] P.D. Walzer, et al., *Pneumocystis carinii*: new separation method from lung tissue, Exp. Parasitol. 47 (1979) 356.

[270] J.A. Minielly, F.C. McDuffie, K.E. Holley, Immunofluorescent identification of *Pneumocystis carinii*, Arch. Pathol. 90 (1970) 561.

[271] S.K. Lim, R.H. Jones, W.C. Eveland, Fluorescent antibody studies on experimental pneumocystosis, Proc. Soc. Exp. Biol. Med. 136 (1971) 675.

[272] S.K. Lim, W.C. Eveland, R.J. Porter, Development and evaluation of a direct fluorescent antibody method for the diagnosis of *Pneumocystis carinii* infections in experimental animals, Appl. Microbiol. 26 (1973) 666.

[273] S.K. Lim, W.C. Eveland, R.J. Porter, Direct fluorescent antibody method for the diagnosis of *Pneumocystis carinii* pneumonitis from sputa or tracheal aspirates from humans, Appl. Microbiol. 27 (1974) 144.

[274] W.T. Hughes, et al., Efficacy of trimethoprim and sulfamethoxazole in the prevention and treatment of *Pneumocystis carinii* pneumonitis, Antimicrob. Agents Chemother. 5 (1974) 289.

[275] W.T. Hughes, et al., Comparison of pentamidine isethionate and trimethoprim-sulfamethoxazole in the treatment of *Pneumocystis carinii* pneumonia, J. Pediatr. 92 (1978) 285.

[276] A. Lipson, W.C. Marshall, A.R. Hayward, Treatment of *Pneumocystis carinii* pneumonia in children, Arch. Dis. Child. 52 (1977) 314.

[277] W.E. Larter, et al., Trimethoprim-sulfamethoxazole treatment of *Pneumocystis carinii* pneumonitis, J. Pediatr. 92 (1978) 826.

[278] S.E. Seigel, et al., Treatment of *Pneumocystis carinii* pneumonitis: a comparative trial of sulfamethoxazole-trimethoprim vs pentamidine in pediatric patients with cancer: report from the children's cancer study group, Am. J. Dis. Child. 138 (1984) 1051.

[279] G.D. Overturf, Use of trimethoprim-sulfamethoxazole in pediatric infections: relative merits of intravenous administration, Rev. Infect. Dis. 9 (Suppl. 2) (1987) 168.

[280] G. Ivady, L. Paldy, Ein neues Behandlungsverfahren der interstitiellen plasmazelligen Pneumonie Frühgeborener mit fünfwertigen Stibium und aromatischen Diamidien, Monatsschr. Kinderheilkd. 106 (1958) 10.

[281] K. Lörinczi, J. Mérth, K. Perényi, Pentaminnel szerzett tapasztalatink az interstitialis plasmasejtes pneumonia kezelésében, Gyermekgyogyaszat 15 (1964) 207.

[282] K.A. Western, D.R. Perera, M.G. Schultz, Pentamidine isethionate in the treatment of *Pneumocystis carinii* pneumonia, Ann. Intern. Med. 73 (1970) 695.

[283] Parasitic Disease Drug Service, Pentamidine releases for *Pneumocystis* pneumonia, MMWR Morb. Mortal. Wkly. Rep. 25 (1976) 365.

[284] J.C. Shultz, S.W. Ross, R.S. Abernathy, Diagnosis of *Pneumocystis carinii* pneumonia in an adult with survival, Am. Rev. Respir. Dis. 93 (1966) 943.

[285] G. Ivady, L. Paldy, Treatment of *Pneumocystis carinii* pneumonia in infancy, Natl. Cancer Inst. Monogr. 43 (1976) 201.

[286] E.B. Schoenbach, E.M. Greenspan, The pharmacology, mode of action and therapeutic potentialities of stilbamidine, pentamidine, propamidine and other aromatic diamidines: a review, Medicine 27 (1948) 327.

[287] F.R. Stark, et al., Fatal Herxheimer reaction after pentamidine in *Pneumocystis* pneumonia, Lancet 1 (1976) 1193 (letter).

[288] C.M. Stahl-Bayliss, C.M. Kalman, O.L. Laskin, Pentamidine-induced hypoglycemia in patients with the acquired immune deficiency syndrome, Clin. Pharmacol. Ther. 39 (1986) 271.

[289] A. Pauwels, et al., Pentamidine-induced acute pancreatitis in a patient with AIDS, J. Clin. Gastroenterol. 12 (1990) 457.

[290] G. Wood, et al., Survival from pentamidine induced pancreatitis and diabetes mellitus, N. Z. J. Med. 21 (1991) 341.

[291] T.L. Miller, et al., Pancreatitis in pediatric human immunodeficiency virus infection, J. Pediatr. 120 (1992) 223.

[292] G.W. Geelhoed, et al., The diagnosis and management of *Pneumocystis carinii* pneumonia, Ann. Thorac. Surg. 14 (1972) 335.

[293] G.W. Geelhoed, P. Corso, W.L. Joseph, The role of membrane lung support in transient acute respiratory insufficiency of *Pneumocystis carinii* pneumonia, J. Thorac. Cardiovasc. Surg. 68 (1974) 802.

[294] F.T. Saulsbury, M.T. Bernstein, J.A. Winkelstein, *Pneumocystis carinii* pneumonia as the presenting infection in congenital hypogammaglobulinemia, J. Pediatr. 95 (1979) 559.

[295] S. Gagnon, et al., Corticosteroids as adjunctive therapy for severe *Pneumocystis carinii* pneumonia in the acquired immunodeficiency syndrome, N. Engl. J. Med. 323 (1990) 1444.

[296] S.A. Bozzette, et al., A controlled trial of early adjunctive treatment with corticosteroids for *Pneumocystis carinii* pneumonia in the acquired immunodeficiency syndrome, N. Engl. J. Med. 323 (1990) 1451.

[297] NIH-University of California Expert Panel for Corticosteroids as Adjunctive Therapy for *Pneumocystis* Pneumonia, Special report: consensus statement on the use of corticosteroids as adjunctive therapy for *Pneumocystis* pneumonia in the acquired immunodeficiency syndrome, N. Engl. J. Med. 323 (1990) 1500.

[298] G.E. McLaughlin, et al., Effect of corticosteroids on survival of children with acquired immunodeficiency syndrome and *Pneumocystis carinii*-related respiratory failure, J. Pediatr. 126 (1995) 821.

[299] M.R. Bye, A.M. Cairns-Bazarian, J.M. Ewig, Markedly reduced mortality associated with corticosteroid therapy of *Pneumocystis carinii* pneumonia in children with acquired immunodeficiency syndrome, Arch. Pediatr. Adolesc. Med. 148 (1994) 638.

[300] S.K. Sanyal, et al., Course of pulmonary dysfunction in children surviving *Pneumocystis carinii* pneumonitis, Am. Rev. Respir. Dis. 124 (1981) 161.

[301] D.M. Brasfield, et al., Infant pneumonitis associated with cytomegalovirus, *Chlamydia*, *Pneumocystis* and *Ureaplasma*: follow-up, Pediatrics 79 (1987) 76.

[302] R.M. Kluge, D.M. Spaulding, A.J. Spain, Combination of pentamidine and trimethoprim-sulfamethoxazole in the therapy of *Pneumocystis carinii* pneumonia in rats, Antimicrob. Agents Chemother. 13 (1978) 975.

[303] J. Ruskin, Parasitic diseases in the immunocompromised host, in: R.H. Rubin, L.S. Young (Eds.), Clinical Approach to Infection in the Compromised Host, Plenum Publishing, New York, 1981.

[304] J.H. Patterson, *Pneumocystis carinii* pneumonia; pentamidine therapy, Pediatrics 38 (1966) 926, (letter).

[305] J.G.B. Russell, *Pneumocystis* pneumonia associated with agammaglobulinemia, Arch. Dis. Child. 34 (1959) 338.

[306] D.D. Richman, L. Zamvil, J.S. Remington, Recurrent *Pneumocystis carinii* pneumonia in a child with hypogammaglobulinemia, Am. J. Dis. Child. 125 (1973) 102.

[307] L. Ross, et al., Recurrent *Pneumocystis carinii* pneumonia, Clin. Res. 25 (1977) 183.

[308] L.J. Wolff, R.L. Baehner, Delayed development of *Pneumocystis* pneumonia following administration of short-term high-dose trimethoprim-sulfamethoxazole, Am. J. Dis. Child. 132 (1978) 525.

[309] W.T. Hughes, Limited effect of trimethoprim-sulfamethoxazole prophylaxis on *Pneumocystis carinii*, Antimicrob. Agents Chemother. 16 (1979) 333.

[310] D.P. LeGolvan, K.P. Heidelberger, Disseminated, granulomatous *Pneumocystis carinii* pneumonia, Arch. Pathol. 95 (1973) 344.

[311] C. Post, et al., Prophylaxis of epidemic infantile pneumocystosis with a 20:1 sulfadoxine and pyrimethamine combination, Curr. Ther. Res. 13 (1971) 273.

[312] P. Kemeny, et al., Prevention of interstitial plasma-cell pneumonia in premature infants, Lancet 1 (1973) 1322, (letter).

[313] W.T. Hughes, et al., Successful chemoprophylaxis for *Pneumocystis carinii* pneumonitis, N. Engl. J. Med. 297 (1977) 1419.

[314] R.B. Wilber, et al., Chemoprophylaxis for *Pneumocystis carinii* pneumonitis: outcome of unstructured delivery, Am. J. Dis. Child. 134 (1980) 643.

[315] W.T. Hughes, et al., Successful intermittent chemoprophylaxis for *Pneumocystis carinii* pneumonitis, N. Engl. J. Med. 316 (1987) 1627.

[316] R.E. Harris, et al., Prevention of *Pneumocystis* pneumonia: use of continuous sulfamethoxazole-trimethoprim therapy, Am. J. Dis. Child. 134 (1980) 35.

[317] U.S. Department of Health and Human Services, Guidelines for prophylaxis against *Pneumocystis carinii* pneumonia for children infected with human immunodeficiency virus, MMWR Morb. Mortal. Wkly. Rep. 40 (RR-2) (1991) ii–113.

[318] Centers for Disease Control and Prevention, 1999 USPHS/IDSA guidelines for the prevention of opportunistic infections in persons infected with human

immunodeficiency virus, MMWR Morb. Mortal. Wkly. Rep. 48 (RR-10) (1999) 1.

[319] R.J. Simonds, et al., Prophylaxis against *Pneumocystis carinii* pneumonia among children with perinatally acquired HIV infection in the United States, N. Engl. J. Med. 332 (1995) 786.

[320] Y.A. Maldonado, R.G. Araneta, A. Hersh, *Pneumocystis carinii* pneumonia prophylaxis and early clinical manifestations of severe perinatal human immunodeficiency virus type 1 infection. Northern California pediatric IIIV consortium, Pediatr. Infect. Dis. J. 17 (1998) 398.

[321] L.E. Zimmerman, Fatal fungus infections complicating other diseases, Am. J. Clin. Pathol. 25 (1955) 46.

[322] G.W. Allan, D.H. Andersen, Generalized aspergillosis in an infant 18 days of age, Pediatrics 26 (1960) 432.

[323] J.L. Luke, R.P. Bolande, S. Grass, Generalized aspergillosis and *Aspergillus* endocarditis in infancy, Pediatrics 31 (1963) 115.

[324] A. Akkoyunlu, F.A. Yücell, Aspergillose bronchopulmonaire et encéphalomeningel chez un nouveau-né de 20 jours, Arch. Fr. Pediatr. 14 (1957) 615.

[325] L. Matturi, S. Fasolis, L'aspergillosi generalizzata neonatale, Folia Hered. Pathol. 12 (1962) 87.

[326] A.J. Paradis, L. Roberts, Endogenous ocular aspergillosis: report of a case in an infant with cytomegalic inclusion disease, Arch. Ophthalmol. 69 (1963) 765.

[327] K. Brass, Infecciones hospitalarias asporgilosas bronco-pulmonares en lactantes y ninos menores, Mycopathologia 57 (1975) 149.

[328] H.H. Mangurien, B. Fernandez, Neonatal aspergillosis accompanying fulminant necrotizing enterocolitis, Arch. Dis. Child. 54 (1979) 559.

[329] F. Gonzalez-Crussi, et al., Acute disseminated aspergillosis during the neonatal period: report of an instance of a 14-day-old infant, Clin. Pediatr. 18 (1979) 137.

[330] J.H. Raaf, et al., *Aspergillus*-induced small bowel obstruction in a leukemic newborn, Surgery 81 (1977) 111.

[331] R. Mouy, et al., Granulomatose septique chronique revelée par une aspergillose pulmonaire neonatale, Arch. Pediatr. 2 (1995) 861.

[332] A. Bruyere, et al., Entérocolite ulcéro-nécrotique néonatale et aspergillose, Pediatrie 38 (1983) 185.

[333] W.D. Rhine, A.A. Arvin, D.K. Stevenson, Neonatal aspergillosis: a case report and review of the literature, Clin. Pediatr. 25 (1986) 400.

[334] R.D. Granstein, L.R. First, A.J. Sober, Primary cutaneous aspergillosis in a premature neonate, Br. J. Dermatol. 103 (1980) 681.

[335] R. Shiota, et al., *Aspergillus* endophthalmitis, Br. J. Ophthalmol. 71 (1987) 611.

[336] J.G. Roth, J.L. Troy, N.B. Esterly, Multiple cutaneous ulcers in a premature neonate, Pediatr. Dermatol. 8 (1991) 253.

[337] D.A. Schwartz, M. Jacquette, H.S. Chawla, Disseminated neonatal aspergillosis: report of a fatal case and analysis of risk factors, Pediatr. Infect. Dis. J. 7 (1988) 349.

[338] H. Lackner, et al., Liposomal amphotericin-B (AmBisome) for treatment of disseminated fungal infections in two infants of very low birth weight, Pediatrics 89 (1992) 1259.

[339] J.L. Rowen, et al., Invasive aspergillosis in neonates: report of five cases and literature review, Pediatr. Infect. Dis. J. 11 (1992) 576.

[340] R.W. Perzigian, R.G. Faix, Primary cutaneous aspergillosis in a preterm infant, Am. J. Perinatol. 10 (1993) 269.

[341] M. Gupta, B. Weinberger, P.N. Whitley-Williams, Cutaneous aspergillosis in a neonate, Pediatr. Infect. Dis. J. 15 (1996) 464.

[342] M. Papouli, et al., Primary cutaneous aspergillosis in neonates: case report and review, Clin. Infect. Dis. 22 (1996) 1102.

[343] A.H. Scroll, et al., Invasive pulmonary aspergillosis in a critically ill neonate: case report and review of invasive aspergillosis during the first 3 months of life, Clin. Infect. Dis. 27 (1998) 437.

[344] N.E. Meessen, K.M. Oberndorff, J.A. Jacobs, Disseminated aspergillosis in a premature neonate, J. Hosp. Infect. 40 (1998) 249.

[345] F.K. van Landeghem, et al., Aqueductal stenosis and hydrocephalus in an infant due to *Aspergillus* infection, Clin. Neuropathol. 19 (2000) 26.

[346] F.C. Amod, et al., Primary cutaneous aspergillosis in ventilated neonates, Pediatr. Infect. Dis. J. 19 (2000) 482.

[347] M. Marcinkowski, et al., Fatal aspergillosis with brain abscesses in a neonate with DiGeorge syndrome, Pediatr. Infect. Dis. 19 (2000) 1214.

[348] V. Richardson, et al., Disseminated and cutaneous aspergillosis in a premature infant: a fatal nosocomial infection, Pediatr. Dermatol. J. 18 (2001) 366.

[349] C.A. Woodruff, A.A. Hebert, Neonatal primary cutaneous aspergillosis: case report and review of the literature, Pediatr. Dermatol. 19 (2002) 439.

[350] M.D. Herron, et al., Aspergillosis in a 24-week newborn: a case report, J. Perinatol. 23 (2003) 256.

[351] K.B. Raper, D.I. Fennell (Eds.), The Genus Aspergillus, Williams & Wilkins, Baltimore, 1965.

[352] D.W. Denning, Invasive aspergillosis, Clin. Infect. Dis. 26 (1998) 781.

[353] P. Coulot, et al., Specific interaction of *Aspergillus fumigatus* with fibrinogen and its role in cell adhesion, Infect. Immun. 62 (1994) 2169.

[354] G. Tronchin, et al., Expression and identification of a laminin-binding protein in *Aspergillus fumigatus* conidia, Infect. Immun. 65 (1997) 9.

[355] S. Walmsley, et al., Invasive *Aspergillus* infections in a pediatric hospital: a ten-year review, Pediatr. Infect. Dis. J. 12 (1993) 673.

[356] P.K.C. Austwick, M. Gitter, C.V. Watkins, Pulmonary aspergillosis in lambs, Vet. Rec. 72 (1960) 19.

[357] R.K. Merchant, et al., Fungal endocarditis: a review of the literature and report of three cases, Ann. Intern. Med. 48 (1958) 242.

[358] L. Renon, Recherches cliniques et expérimentales sur la pseudotuberculose aspergillaire, These No 89. G Steinheil, Paris, 1893.

[359] L. Renon, L'Étude sur l'Aspergillose chez les Animaux et chez l'Homme, Masson, Paris, 1897.

[360] G. Dieulafoy, A. Chantemesse, G.F.I. Widal, Une pseudotuberculose myosique, Congres. Int. Berlin Gaz. Hop. (Paris) 63 (1890) 821.

[361] E.F. Wahl, M.J. Erickson, Primary pulmonary aspergillosis, J. Med. Assoc. Ga. 17 (1928) 341.

[362] K.P.W. Hinson, A.J. Moon, N.S. Plummer, Bronchopulmonary aspergillosis: a review and a report of eight new cases, Thorax 7 (1952) 317.

[363] J.M. Macartney, Pulmonary aspergillosis: a review and description of three new cases, Thorax 19 (1964) 287.

[364] D. Hunter, K.M.A. Perry, Bronchiolitis resulting from the handling of bagasse, Br. J. Ind. Med. 3 (1946) 64.

[365] F.C. Stallybrass, A study of *Aspergillus* spores in the atmosphere of a modern mill, Br. J. Ind. Med. 18 (1961) 41.

[366] N.F. Conant, et al., Aspergillosis, in: N.F. Conant, D.T. Smith, R.D. Baker et al., (Eds.), Manual of Clinical Mycology, 3rd ed, WB Saunders, Philadelphia, 1971, pp. 699–724.

[367] A. Castellani, Fungi and fungous diseases, Arch. Derm. Syphilol. 17 (1928) 61.

[368] S.M. Finegold, J.F. Murray, Aspergillosis: a review and report of twelve cases, Am. J. Med. 27 (1959) 463.

[369] A. Sartory, R. Sartory, Un cas d'onychomycose dû à l'*Aspergillus fumigatus* Fresenius, Bull. Acad. Med. (Paris) 109 (1945) 482.

[370] A.E.W. Gregson, C.J. La Touche, Otomycosis: a neglected disease, J. Laryngol. Otol. 75 (1961) 45.

[371] J.M. McCarty, et al., Outbreak of primary cutaneous aspergillosis related to intravenous arm boards, J. Pediatr. 108 (1986) 721.

[372] A.G. Dewhurst, et al., Invasive aspergillosis in immunocompromised patients: potential hazard of hospital building work, BMJ 301 (1990) 802.

[373] P.W. Collins, et al., Invasive aspergillosis in immunosuppressed patients, BMJ 301 (1990) 1046.

[374] T.J. Walsh, D.M. Dixon, Nosocomial aspergillosis: environmental microbiology, hospital epidemiology, diagnosis and treatment, Eur. J. Epidemiol. 5 (1989) 131.

[375] P.K.C. Austwick, Pathogenicity, in: K.B. Raper, D.I. Fennell (Eds.), The Genus *Aspergillus*, Williams & Wilkins, Baltimore, 1965, p. 82.

[376] I. Theobald, et al., Pulmonary aspergillosis as initial manifestation of septic granulomatosis (chronic granulomatous disease, CGD) in a premature monozygotic female twin and FDG-PET diagnosis of spread of the disease, Radiologe 42 (2002) 42.

[377] A.H. Groll, et al., Invasive pulmonary aspergillosis in a critically ill neonate: case report and review of invasive aspergillosis during the first 3 months of life, Clin. Infect. Dis. 27 (1998) 437.

[378] M.D. Herron, et al., Aspergillosis in a 24-week newborn: a case report, J. Perinatol. 23 (2003) 256.

[379] F.C. Amod, et al., Primary cutaneous aspergillosis in ventilated neonates, Pediatr. Infect. Dis. J. 19 (2000) 482.

[380] J.A. van Burik, R. Colven, D.H. Spach, Cutaneous aspergillosis, J. Clin. Microbiol. 36 (1998) 3115.

[381] E.P. Cawley, Aspergillosis and the aspergilli: report of a unique case of the disease, Arch. Intern. Med. 80 (1947) 423.

[382] R.C. Young, et al., Aspergillosis: the spectrum of disease in 98 patients, Medicine 49 (1970) 147.

[383] S. Huang, L.S. Harris, Acute disseminated penicilliosis, Am. J. Clin. Pathol. 39 (1963) 167.

[384] M.J. James, et al., Use of a repetitive DNA probe to type clinical and environmental isolates of *Aspergillus flavus* from a cluster of cutaneous infections in a neonatal intensive care unit, J. Clin. Microbiol. 38 (2000) 3612.

[385] M.H. Weiner, Antigenemia detected by radioimmunoassay in systemic aspergillosis, Ann. Intern. Med. 92 (1980) 793.

[386] D.W. Denning, D.A. Stevens, Antifungal and surgical treatment of invasive aspergillosis: review of 2,121 published cases, Rev. Infect. Dis. 12 (1990) 1147.

[387] D.A. Stevens, et al., Practice guidelines for diseases caused by *Aspergillus*. Infectious Diseases Society of America, Clin. Infect. Dis. 30 (2000) 696.

[388] J.A. van Burik, R. Colven, D.H. Spach, Itraconazole therapy for primary cutaneous aspergillosis in patients with AIDS, Clin. Infect. Dis. 27 (1998) 643.

[389] J.F. Denton, A.F. DiSalvo, Isolation of *Blastomyces dermatitidis* from natural sites at Augusta, Georgia, Am. J. Trop. Med. 13 (1964) 716.

[390] M.J. Tenenbaum, J. Greenspan, T.M. Kerkering, Blastomycosis, CRC Crit. Rev. Microbiol. 3 (1982) 139.

[391] Blastomycosis Cooperative Study of the Veterans Administration. Blastomycosis: I. A review of 198 collected cases in Veterans Administration hospitals, Am. Rev. Respir. Dis. 89 (1964) 659.

[392] M.L. Furcolow, et al., Prevalence and incidence studies of human and canine blastomycosis: I. Cases in the United States, 1885–1968, Am. Rev. Respir. Dis. 102 (1970) 60.

[393] M.L. Furcolow, et al., Prevalence and incidence studies of human and canine blastomycosis: II. Yearly incidence studies in three selected states, 1960–1967, Am. J. Epidemiol. 92 (1970) 121.

[394] M.D. Kepron, et al., North American blastomycosis in central Canada, Can. Med. Assoc. J. 106 (1972) 243.

[395] A.S. Sekhon, M.S. Bogorus, H.V. Sems, Blastomycosis: report of three cases from Alberta with a review of Canadian cases, Mycopathologia 68 (1979) 53.

[396] A.S. Sekhon, F.L. Jackson, H.J. Jacobs, Blastomycosis: report of the first case from Alberta, Canada, Mycopathologica 79 (1982) 65.

[397] S.A. Robertson, P.L. Kimball, L.Z. Magtibay, Pulmonary blastomycosis diagnosed by cytologic examination of sputum, Can. Med. Assoc. J. 126 (1982) 387.

[398] J. Kane, et al., Blastomycosis: a new endemic focus in Canada, Can. Med. Assoc. J. 129 (1983) 728.

[399] E.W. Chick, The epidemiology of blastomycosis, in: Y. Al-Doory (Ed.), The Epidemiology of Human Mycotic Disease, Charles C Thomas, Springfield, Ill, 1975, p. 103.

[400] P. Witorsch, J.P. Utz, North American blastomycosis: a study of 40 patients, Medicine 47 (1968) 169.

[401] E. Habte-Gabr, I.M. Smith, North American blastomycosis in Iowa: review of 34 cases, J. Chronic Dis. 26 (1973) 585.

[402] E.D. Weinberg, Pregnancy associated depression of cell-mediated immunity, Rev. Infect. Dis. 6 (1984) 814.

[403] J.F. Denton, A.F. DiSalvo, Additional isolations of Blastomyces dermatitidis from natural sites, Am. J. Trop. Med. Hyg. 28 (1979) 697.

[404] J. Schwartz, G.L. Baum, Blastomycosis, Am. J. Clin. Pathol. 11 (1951) 999.

[405] J.W. Gnann Jr., et al., Human blastomycosis after a dog bite, Ann. Intern. Med. 98 (1983) 484.

[406] M.W. Craig, W.N. Davey, R.A. Green, Conjugal blastomycosis, Am. Rev. Respir. Dis. 102 (1970) 86.

[407] L.D. Recht, et al., Self-limited blastomycosis: a report of thirteen cases, Am. Rev. Respir. Dis. 120 (1979) 1109.

[408] L.D. Recht, et al., Blastomycosis in immunocompromised patients, Am. Rev. Respir. Dis. 125 (1982) 359.

[409] S.A. Gall, Maternal adjustments in the immune system in normal pregnancy, Clin. Obstet. Gynecol. 26 (1983) 521.

[410] V. Sridama, et al., Decreased levels of helper T cells: a possible cause of immunodeficiency in pregnancy, N. Engl. J. Med. 307 (1982) 352.

[411] G.C. Cozad, C.T. Chang, Cell mediated immunoprotection in blastomycosis, Infect. Immun. 28 (1980) 398.

[412] E.I. Cherniss, B.A. Wisbren, North American blastomycosis: a clinical study of 40 cases, Ann. Intern. Med. 44 (1956) 105.

[413] R.S. Abernathy, Clinical manifestation of pulmonary blastomycosis, Ann. Intern. Med. 51 (1959) 707.

[414] W.R. Lockwood, et al., The treatment of North American blastomycosis: ten years' experience, Am. Rev. Respir. Dis. 100 (1969) 314.

[415] M.J. Duttera, S. Osterhout, North American blastomycosis: a survey of 63 cases, South Med. J. 62 (1969) 295.

[416] G.R. Kravitz, et al., Chronic blastomycotic meningitis, Am. J. Med. 71 (1981) 501.

[417] L. Kaufman, et al., Specific immunodiffusion test for blastomycosis, Appl. Microbiol. 26 (1973) 244.

[418] J.E. Williams, et al., Serologic response in blastomycosis: diagnostic value of double immunodiffusion assay, Am. Rev. Respir. Dis. 123 (1981) 209.

[419] W.T. Hughes, The deep mycoses, in: V.C. Kelley (Ed.), Brennemann's Practice of Pediatrics, Harper & Row, Hagerstown, Md, 1970, p. 1.

[420] R. Cohen, Coccidioidomycosis: case report in children, Arch. Pediatr. 66 (1949) 241.

[421] H.W. Hyatt, Coccidioidomycosis in a three week old infant, Am. J. Dis. Child. 105 (1963) 127.

[422] T.E. Townsend, R.W. McKey, Coccidioidomycosis in infants, Am. J. Dis. Child. 86 (1953) 51.

[423] J.R. Christian, et al., Pulmonary coccidioidomycosis in a 21 day old infant, Am. J. Dis. Child. 92 (1956) 66.

[424] C.R. Westley, W. Haak, Neonatal coccidioidomycosis in a Southwestern Pima Indian, South Med. J. 67 (1974) 855.

[425] T. Shafai, Neonatal coccidioidomycosis in premature twins, Am. J. Dis. Child. 132 (1978) 634.

[426] T.R. Larwood, Transactions of the 7th Annual Meeting of the Veterans Administration and Armed Forces Coccidioidomycosis Study Group, San Francisco, 1962.

[427] D.I. Bernstein, et al., Coccidioidomycosis in a neonate; maternal-infant transmission, J. Pediatr. 99 (1981) 752.

[428] S.E. Golden, et al., Disseminated coccidioidomycosis with chorioretinitis in early infancy, Pediatr. Infect. Dis. J. 5 (1986) 272.

[429] D.D. Child, et al., Radiographic findings of pulmonary coccidioidomycosis in neonates and infants, AJR Am. J. Roentgenol. 145 (1985) 261.

[430] M.J. Fiese, Coccidioidomycosis, Charles C Thomas, Springfield, Ill, 1958.

[431] K.T. Maddy, The geographic distribution of Coccidioides immitis and possible ecologic implications, Ariz. Med. 15 (1958) 178.

[432] B.L. Albert, T.F. Sellers, Coccidioidomycosis from fomites, Arch. Intern. Med. 123 (1963) 253.

[433] L.T. Giltner, Occurrence of coccidioidal granuloma (coccidioidomycosis) in cattle, J. Agric. Res. 14 (1918) 533.

[434] M.D. Beck, Occurrence of Coccidioides immitis in lesions of slaughtered animals, Proc. Soc. Exp. Biol. Med. 26 (1929) 534.

[435] C.L. Davis, G.W. Stiles Jr., A.N. McGregor, Pulmonary coccidioidal granuloma: a new site of infection in cattle, J. Am. Vet. Med. Assoc. 91 (1937) 209.

[436] R.E. Reed, Diagnosis of disseminated canine coccidioidomycosis, J. Am. Vet. Med. Assoc. 128 (1956) 196.

[437] R.E. Reed, C.J. Prchal, K.T. Maddy, Veterinary aspects of coccidioidomycosis: panel discussion, Proceedings of a symposium on coccidioidomycosis. US Government Printing Office, Washington, DC, 1957.

[438] C.W. Emmons, Isolation of Coccidioides from soil and rodents, Public Health Rep. 57 (1942) 109.

[439] J.P. Rhoads, Coccidioidomycosis, J. Okla. State Med. Assoc. 58 (1965) 410.

[440] D. Pappagianis, Coccidioidomycosis, in: P.D. Hoeprich (Ed.), Infectious Diseases, Harper & Row, Hagerstown, MD, 1972.

[441] C.E. Smith, An epidemiological study of acute coccidioidomycosis with erythema nodosum, Proc. Sixth Pacific Science Congress 5 (1939) 797.

[442] C.E. Smith, et al., Effect of season and dust control on coccidioidomycosis, JAMA 132 (1946) 833.

[443] E.L. Overholt, R.B. Hornick, Primary cutaneous coccidioidomycosis, Arch. Intern. Med. 114 (1964) 14.

[444] W.A. Winn, Coccidioidomycosis and amphotericin, Med. Clin. North Am. 47 (1963) 1131.

[445] M.A. Gifford, W.C. Buss, R.J. Douds, Coccidioides fungus infection, Kern County, 1900–1936, Kern County Health Department Annual Report, 1936–1937, p. 39.

[446] M.D. Beck, Epidemiology, coccidioidal granuloma, Calif. State Dept. Public Health Special Bull. 57 (1931) 19.

[447] B.H. Eckmann, G.L. Schaefer, M. Huppert, Bedside interhuman transmission of coccidioidomycosis via growth on fomites: epidemic involving 6 persons, Am. Rev. Respir. Dis. 89 (1964) 175.

[448] J.M. Wilson, C.E. Smith, O.A. Plunkett, Primary cutaneous coccidioidomycosis: the criteria for diagnosis, Calif. Med. 79 (1953) 233.

[449] H.K. Faber, C.E. Smith, E.C. Dickson, Acute coccidioidomycosis with erythema nodosum in children, J. Pediatr. 15 (1939) 163.

[450] J.W. Birsner, The roentgen aspects of five hundred cases of pulmonary coccidioidomycosis, AJR Am. J. Roentgenol. 72 (1954) 556.

[451] H.D. Riley, Systemic mycoses in children, Curr. Probl. Pediatr. 2 (1972) 3.

[452] C.E. Smith, et al., Varieties of coccidioidal infection in relation to epidemiology and control of the disease, Am. J. Public Health 36 (1946) 1394.

[453] R.G. Caudill, C.E. Smith, J.A. Reinarz, Coccidioidal meningitis: a diagnostic dilemma, Am. J. Med. 49 (1970) 360.

[454] O.A. Plunkett, Ecology and spread of pathogenic fungi, in: N.V. Sternberg Th, V.D. Newcomer (Eds.), Therapy of Fungus Diseases, an International Symposium, Little, Brown, Boston, 1955, p. 18.

[455] L.E. Smale, J.W. Birsner, Maternal deaths from coccidioidomycosis, JAMA 140 (1949) 1152.

[456] C.M. Peterson, et al., Coccidioidal meningitis and pregnancy: a case report, Obstet. Gynecol. 73 (1989) 835.

[457] R. Cohen, Placental Coccidioides: proof that congenital Coccidioides is nonexistent, Arch. Pediatr. 68 (1951) 59.

[458] R. Cohen, R. Burnip, Coccidioidin skin testing during pregnancy and in infants and children, Calif. Med. 72 (1950) 31.

[459] M.A. McCaffree, G. Altshuler, K. Benirschke, Placental coccidioidomycosis without fetal disease, Arch. Pathol. Lab. Med. 102 (1978) 512.

[460] S.B. Werner, et al., An epidemic of coccidioidomycosis among archeology students in Northern California, N. Engl. J. Med. 286 (1972) 507.

[461] S.H. Gehlbach, J.D. Hamilton, N.F. Conant, Coccidioidomycosis: an occupational disease in cotton-mill workers, Arch. Intern. Med. 131 (1973) 254.

[462] J.R. Creitz, J.F. Puckett, A method for cultural identification of Coccidioides immitis, Am. J. Clin. Pathol. 24 (1954) 1318.

[463] C.E. Smith, M.T. Saito, S.A. Simons, Pattern of 39,500 serologic tests in coccidioidomycosis, JAMA 160 (1956) 546.

[464] Y. Swaki, et al., Patterns of human antibody reactions in coccidioidomycosis, J. Bacteriol. 91 (1966) 422.

[465] C.C. Campbell, Use and interpretation of serologic and skin tests in the respiratory mycoses: current considerations, Dis. Chest 54 (Suppl. 1) (1968) 49.

[466] M. Huppert, J.W. Bailey, The use of immunodiffusion tests in coccidioidomycosis: I. The accuracy and reproducibility of the immunodiffusion test which correlates with complement fixation, Am. J. Pathol. 44 (1965) 364.

[467] M. Huppert, J.W. Bailey, The use of immunodiffusion tests in coccidioidomycosis: II. An immunodiffusion test as a substitute for the tube precipitin test, Am. J. Clin. Pathol. 44 (1965) 369.

[468] M. Huppert, et al., Evaluation of a latex particle agglutination test for coccidioidomycosis, Am. J. Clin. Pathol. 49 (1968) 96.

[469] A.R. Graham, K.J. Ryan, Counter immunoelectrophoresis employing coccidioidin in serologic testing for coccidioidomycosis, Am. J. Clin. Pathol. 73 (1980) 574.

[470] A. Cotanzaro, F. Flatauer, Detection of serum antibodies in coccidioidomycosis by solid-phase radioimmunoassay, J. Infect. Dis. 147 (1983) 32.

[471] W. Drips, C.E. Smith, Epidemiology of coccidioidomycosis, JAMA 190 (1964) 1010.

[472] L.L. Schnelzer, I.R. Tabershaw, Exposure factors in occupational coccidioidomycosis, Am. J. Public Health 52 (1968) 107.

[473] M.J. Khan, R. Myers, R. Koshy, Pulmonary cryptococcosis: a case report and experimental study, Dis. Chest 36 (1959) 656.

[474] H.B. Levine, J.M. Cobb, C.E. Smith, Immunogenicity of spherule-endospore vaccines of Coccidioides immitis for mice, J. Immunol. 85 (1961) 218.

[475] D. Pappagianis, Evaluation of the Protective Efficacy of the Killed Coccidioides immitis Vaccine in Man, American Society for Microbiology, Washington, DC, 1986.

[476] J. Oliverio Campos, Congenital meningoencephalitis due to Torulopsis neoformans: preliminary report, Bol. Clin. Hosp. Civis Lisb. 18 (1954) 609.

[477] E.B.D. Neuhauser, A. Tucker, The roentgen changes produced by diffuse torulosis in the newborn, AJR Am. J. Roentgenol. 59 (1948) 805.

[478] E. Nassau, C. Weinberg-Heiruti, Torulosis of the newborn, Harefuah 35 (1948) 50.

[479] P. Heath, Massive separation of retina in full-term infants and juveniles, JAMA 144 (1950) 1148.

[480] M. Savai, S. Gaur, L.D. Frenkel, Successful treatment of cryptococcosis in a premature neonate, Pediatr. Infect. Dis. J. 14 (1995) 1009.

[481] R. Kaur, et al., Cryptococcal meningitis in a neonate, Scand. J. Infect. Dis. 34 (2002) 542.

[482] W. Freeman, *Torula* infection of central nervous system, J. Psychol. Neurol. 43 (1931) 236.

[483] L.B. Cox, J.C. Tolhurst, Human Torulosis, Melbourne University Press, Melbourne, 1946.

[484] M.L. Littman, L.E. Zimmerman, Cryptococcosis (Torulosis), Grune & Stratton, New York, 1956.

[485] C.A. Carton, Treatment of central nervous system cryptococcosis: a review and report of four cases treated with Actidione, Ann. Intern. Med. 37 (1952) 123.

[486] C.A. Carton, L.A. Mount, Neurosurgical aspects of cryptococcosis, J. Neurosurg. 8 (1951) 143.

[487] L.E. Zimmerman, H. Rappaport, Occurrence of cryptococcosis in patients with malignant disease of the reticuloendothelial system, Am. J. Clin. Pathol. 24 (1954) 1050.

[488] W.T. Butler, et al., Diagnostic and prognostic value of clinical and laboratory findings in cryptococcal meningitis, a follow-up study of forty patients, N. Engl. J. Med. 270 (1964) 59.

[489] J.G. Gruhn, J. Sanson, Mycotic infection in leukemic patients at autopsy, Cancer 16 (1963) 61.

[490] J.J. Shadomy, J.P. Utz, Preliminary studies on a hyphae-forming mutant of *Cryptococcus neoformans*, Mycologia 58 (1966) 383.

[491] E.E. Evans, The antigenic composition of *Cryptococcus neoformans*: I. A serologic classification by means of the capsular and agglutination reactions, J. Immunol. 64 (1950) 423.

[492] E.E. Evans, L.J. Sorensen, K.W. Walls, The antigenic composition of *Cryptococcus neoformans*: V. A survey of cross-reactions among strains of *Cryptococcus* and other antigens, J. Bacteriol. 66 (1953) 287.

[493] F. San Felice, Contributo alla morfologia e biologia del blastomiceti che si sviluppano nei succhi di alcuni frutti, Annali dell'Instituto d'Igrene Sperimentale della R Universita di Roma 4 (1894) 463.

[494] E. Klein, Pathogenic microbes in milk, J. Hyg. 1 (1901) 78.

[495] C.W. Emmons, The significance of saprophytism in the epidemiology of the mycoses, Trans. N. Y. Acad. Sci. 17 (1954) 157.

[496] C.W. Emmons, Saprophytic source of *Cryptococcus neoformans* associated with the pigeon (*Columbia livia*), Am. J. Hyg. 62 (1955) 227.

[497] C.J. Kao, J. Schwartz, The isolation of *Cryptococcus neoformans* from pigeon nests, with remarks on the identification of virulent cryptococci, Am. J. Clin. Pathol. 27 (1957) 652.

[498] M.L. Littman, R. Borok, Relation of the pigeon to cryptococcosis: natural carrier state, host resistance and survival of *Cryptococcus neoformans*, Mycopathol. Mycol. Appl. 36 (1968) 329.

[499] M.L. Littman, S.S. Schneierson, *Cryptococcus neoformans* in pigeon excreta in New York City, Am. J. Hyg. 69 (1959) 49.

[500] L. Ajello, Comparative ecology of respiratory mycotic disease agents, Bacteriol. Rev. 31 (1967) 6.

[501] J.D. Schneidau Jr., Pigeons and cryptococcosis, Science 143 (1964) 525.

[502] M. Hajsig, Z. Curoija, Kriptokoki u fekalijama fazana golubova s osvrlom na nalaze *Cryptococcus neoformans*, Vet. Arch. 35 (1965) 115.

[503] E. Tsubura, Experimental studies in cryptococcosis: I. Isolation of *Cryptococcus neoformans* from avian excreta and some considerations on the source of infection, Fungi Fungous Dis. 3 (1962) 50.

[504] F. Staib, Vorkommen von *Cryptococcus neoformans* in vogelmist, Zentralbl. Bakteriol. 182 (1961) 562.

[505] P. Fragner, The findings of cryptococci in excrements of birds, Cesk. Epidemiol. Mikrobiol. Imunol. 11 (1962) 135.

[506] D.S. Clarke, R.H. Wallace, J.J. David, Yeasts occurring on apples and in apple cider, Can. J. Microbiol. 1 (1954) 145.

[507] E.S. McDonough, et al., Human pathogenic fungi recovered from soil in an area endemic for North American blastomycosis, Am. J. Hyg. 73 (1961) 75.

[508] L. Ajello, Occurrence of *Cryptococcus neoformans* in soils, Am. J. Hyg. 67 (1968) 72.

[509] J.T. McGrath, Cryptococcosis of the central nervous system in domestic animals, Am. J. Pathol. 30 (1954) 651.

[510] J. Simon, R.E. Nichols, E.V. Morse, An outbreak of bovine cryptococcosis, J. Am. Vet. Med. Assoc. 122 (1953) 31.

[511] W.D. Pounden, J.M. Amberson, R.F. Jaeger, A severe mastitis problem associated with *Cryptococcus neoformans* in a large dairy herd, Am. J. Vet. Res. 13 (1952) 121.

[512] G.D. Campbell, Primary pulmonary cryptococcosis, Am. Rev. Respir. Dis. 94 (1966) 236.

[513] J.A. Mohr, et al., Estrogen-stimulated phagocytic activity in human cryptococcosis, Am. Rev. Respir. Dis. 99 (1969) 979.

[514] M.L. Littman, J.E. Walter, Cryptococcosis: current status, Am. J. Med. 45 (1968) 922.

[515] W.M. Gandy, Primary cutaneous cryptococcosis, Arch. Derm. Syphilol. 62 (1950) 97.

[516] R.L. Brier, C. Mopper, J. Stone, Cutaneous cryptococcosis, Arch. Dermatol. 75 (1957) 262.

[517] M.J. Takos, Experimental cryptococcosis produced by the ingestion of virulent organisms, N. Engl. J. Med. 254 (1956) 598.

[518] W. Freeman, Torula meningo-encephalitis: comparative histopathology in seventeen cases, Trans. Am. Neurol. Assoc. 56 (1930) 203.

[519] A. Kida, C.A. Abramowsky, C. Santoscoy, Cryptococcosis of the placenta in a woman with acquired immunodeficiency syndrome, Hum. Pathol. 20 (1989) 920.

[520] B. Tynes, et al., Variant forms of pulmonary cryptococcosis, Ann. Intern. Med. 69 (1968) 1117.

[521] P.M. Silberfarb, G.A. Sarosi, F.E. Tosh, Cryptococcosis and pregnancy, Am. J. Obstet. Gynecol. 112 (1972) 714.

[522] D.N. Curole, Cryptococcal meningitis in pregnancy, J. Reprod. Med. 26 (1981) 317.

[523] F. Reiss, G. Szilagyi, Ecology of yeast-like fungi in a hospital population: detailed investigation of *Cryptococcus neoformans*, Arch. Dermatol. 91 (1965) 611.

[524] V.P. Collins, A. Gellborn, J.R. Trimble, The coincidence of cryptococcosis and disease of the reticulo-endothelial and lymphatic systems, Cancer 4 (1951) 883.

[525] B. Burrows, W.R. Barclay, Combined cryptococcal and tuberculous meningitis complicating reticulum cell sarcoma, Am. Rev. Tuberc. Pulm. Dis. 78 (1958) 760.

[526] Annual report of the Division of Epidemiology, Bureau of Preventable Diseases, Department of Health, New York, NY, 1963–1964.

[527] E. Goldstein, O.N. Rambo, Cryptococcal infection following steroid therapy, Ann. Intern. Med. 56 (1962) 114.

[528] A.S. Levine, R.G. Graw Jr., R.C. Young, Management of infections in patients with leukemia and lymphoma: current concepts and experimental approaches, Semin. Hematol. 9 (1972) 141.

[529] C.M.F. Siewers, H.G. Cramblett, Cryptococcosis (torulosis) in children: a report of four cases, Pediatrics 34 (1964) 393.

[530] G.L. Baum, D. Artis, Growth inhibition of *Cryptococcus neoformans* by cell-free human serum, Am. J. Med. Sci. 241 (1961) 613.

[531] H.J. Igel, R.P. Bolande, Humoral defense mechanisms in cryptococcosis: substances in normal human serum, saliva and cerebrospinal fluid affecting the growth of *Cryptococcus neoformans*, J. Infect. Dis. 116 (1966) 75.

[532] G. Szilagyi, F. Reiss, J.C. Smith, The anticryptococcal factor of blood serum: a preliminary report, J. Invest. Dermatol. 46 (1966) 306.

[533] J.B. Hamilton, G.R. Tyler, Pulmonary torulosis, Radiology 47 (1946) 149.

[534] R.R. Greening, L.J. Menville, Roentgen findings in torulosis: report of four cases, Radiology 48 (1947) 381.

[535] R.K. Haugen, R.D. Baker, The pulmonary lesions in cryptococcosis with special reference to subpleural nodules, Am. J. Clin. Pathol. 24 (1954) 1381.

[536] M. Moore, Cryptococcosis with cutaneous manifestations, J. Invest. Dermatol. 28 (1957) 159.

[537] A. Spickard, Diagnosis and treatment of cryptococcal disease, South Med. J. 66 (1973) 26.

[538] R.D. Lillie, Histopathologic Technique, Blakiston, Philadelphia, 1954.

[539] J.F. Rhinehart, S.K. Abdul-Haj, An improved method for histologic demonstration of acid mucopolysaccharides in tissues, Arch. Pathol. 52 (1951) 189.

[540] O. Berghausen, Torula infection in man, Ann. Intern. Med. 1 (1927) 235.

[541] J.F. Kessel, F. Holtzwart, Experimental studies with *Torula* from a knee infection in man, Am. J. Trop. Med. 15 (1935) 467.

[542] R.B. Dienst, *Cryptococcus histolyticus* isolated from subcutaneous tumor, Arch. Derm. Syphilol. 37 (1938) 461.

[543] S.B. Salvin, R.F. Smith, An antigen for detection of hypersensitivity to *Cryptococcus neoformans*, Proc. Soc. Exp. Biol. Med. 108 (1961) 498.

[544] J.E. Bennett, H.F. Hasenclever, G.L. Baum, Evaluation of a skin test for cryptococcosis, Am. Rev. Respir. Dis. 91 (1965) 616.

[545] W.H. Newberry, et al., Epidemiologic study of *Cryptococcus neoformans*, Ann. Intern. Med. 67 (1967) 724.

[546] B.Z. Rappaport, B. Kaplan, Generalized *Torula* mycosis, Arch. Pathol. Lab. Med. 1 (1926) 720.

[547] A.Q. Pollock, L.M. Ward, A hemagglutination test for cryptococcosis, Am. J. Med. 32 (1962) 6.

[548] R.A. Vogel, T.F. Seelers, P. Woodward, Fluorescent antibody techniques applied to the study of human cryptococcosis, JAMA 178 (1961) 921.

[549] R.A. Vogel, The indirect fluorescent antibody test for the detection of antibody in human cryptococcal disease, J. Infect. Dis. 116 (1966) 573.

[550] J.E. Walter, R.W. Atchison, Epidemiological and immunological studies of *Cryptococcus neoformans*, J. Bacteriol. 92 (1966) 82.

[551] N. Bloomfield, M.A. Gordon, D.F. Elmendorf Jr., Detection of *Cryptococcus neoformans* antigen in body fluid by latex particle agglutination, Proc. Soc. Exp. Biol. Med. 114 (1963) 64.

[552] M.A. Gordon, D.K. Vedder, Serologic tests in diagnosis and prognosis of cryptococcosis, JAMA 197 (1966) 961.

[553] J.E. Walter, R.D. Jones, Serodiagnosis of clinical cryptococcosis, Am. Rev. Respir. Dis. 97 (1968) 275.

[554] E.J. Young, et al., Pleural effusions due to *Cryptococcus neoformans*: a review of the literature and report of two cases with cryptococcal antigen determination, Am. Rev. Respir. Dis. 121 (1980) 743.

[555] J.E. Bennett, H.F. Hasenclever, B.S. Tynes, Detection of cryptococcal polysaccharide in serum and spinal fluid: value in diagnosis and prognosis, Trans. Assoc. Am. Physicians 77 (1964) 145.

[556] L. Kaufman, S. Blumer, Value and interpretation of serological tests for the diagnosis of cryptococcosis, Appl. Microbiol. 16 (1968) 1907.

[557] D.D. Bindschadler, J.E. Bennett, Serology of human cryptococcosis, Ann. Intern. Med. 69 (1968) 45.

[558] J.S. Goodman, L. Kaufman, M.G. Koenig, Diagnosis of cryptococcal meningitis: value of immunologic detection of cryptococcal antigen, N. Engl. J. Med. 285 (1971) 434.

[559] J.E. Walter, E.G. Coffee, Control of *Cryptococcus neoformans* in pigeon coops by alkalinization, Am. J. Epidemiol. 87 (1968) 173.

[560] R.W. Redline, B.B. Dahms, *Malassezia* pulmonary vasculitis in an infant on long-term intralipid therapy, N. Engl. J. Med. 305 (1981) 1395.

[561] M.J. Marcon, D.A. Powell, Human infections due to *Malassezia spp*, Clin. Microbiol. Rev. 5 (1992) 101.

[562] J.G. Long, H.L. Keyserling, Catheter-related infection in infants due to an unusual lipophilic yeast: *Malassezia furfur*, Pediatrics 76 (1985) 896.

[563] W.M. Dankner, et al., *Malassezia fungemia* in neonates and adults: complication of hyperalimentation, Rev. Infect. Dis. 9 (1987) 743.

[564] S.J. Weiss, P.E. Schoch, B.A. Cunha, *Malassezia furfur* fungemia associated with central venous catheter lipid emulsion infusion, Heart Lung 20 (1991) 87.

[565] V.C. Erchiga, V.D. Florencia, *Malassezia* species in skin disease, Curr. Opin. Infect. Dis. 15 (2002) 133.

[566] V. Bernier, et al., Skin colonization by *Malassezia* species in neonates, Arch. Dermatol. 138 (2002) 215.

[567] K.E. Shattuck, et al., Colonization and infection associated with *Malassezia* and *Candida* species in a neonatal unit, J. Hosp. Infect. 34 (1996) 123.

[568] E. Larson, et al., Assessment of alternative hand hygiene regimens to improve skin health among neonatal intensive care nurses, Heart Lung 29 (2000) 136.

[569] A. van Belkum, T. Boekhout, R. Bosboon, Monitoring spread of *Malassezia* infections in a neonatal intensive care unit by PCR-mediated genetic typing, J. Clin. Microbiol. 32 (1994) 2528.

[570] H.J. Chang, et al., An epidemic of *Malassezia pachydermatis* in an intensive care nursery associated with colonization of health care workers' pet dogs, N. Engl. J. Med. 338 (1998) 706.

[571] P. Ahtonen, et al., *Malassezia furfur* colonization of neonates in an intensive care unit, Mycoses 33 (1990) 543.

[572] D.A. Powell, et al., *Malassezia furfur* skin colonization of infants hospitalized in intensive care units, J. Pediatr. 111 (1987) 217.

[573] V. Hruszkewycz, et al., Complications associated with central venous catheters inserted in critically ill neonates, Infect. Control Hosp. Epidemiol. 12 (1991) 544.

[574] H.M. Richet, et al., Cluster of *Malassezia furfur* pulmonary infections in infants in a neonatal intensive-care unit, J. Clin. Microbiol. 27 (1989) 1197.

[575] J.M. Nicholls, K.Y. Yuen, H. Saing, *Malassezia furfur* infection in a neonate, Br. J. Hosp. Med. 49 (1993) 425.

[576] D.A. Powell, et al., Broviac catheter-related *Malassezia furfur* sepsis in five infants receiving intravenous fat emulsions, J. Pediatr. 105 (1984) 987.

[577] J.L. Aschner, et al., Percutaneous central venous catheter colonization with *Malassezia furfur*: incidence and clinical significance, Pediatrics 80 (1987) 535.

[578] E.H. Kim, et al., Adhesion of percutaneously inserted Silastic central venous lines to the vein wall associated with *Malassezia furfur* infection, JPEN J. Parenter. Enteral Nutr. 17 (1993) 458.

[579] D.A. Powell, et al., Scanning electron microscopy of *Malassezia furfur* attachment to Broviac catheters, Hum. Pathol. 18 (1987) 740.

[580] M.J. Marcon, D.A. Powell, Epidemiology, diagnosis, and management of *Malassezia furfur* systemic infection, Diagn. Microbiol. Infect. Dis. 7 (1987) 161.

[581] C.A. Doerr, et al., Solitary pyogenic liver abscess in neonates: report of three cases and review of the literature, Pediatr. Infect. Dis. J. 13 (1994) 64.

[582] B.E. Carey, *Malassezia furfur* infection in the NICU, Neonatal Netw. 9 (1991) 19.

[583] P.H. Azimi, et al., *Malassezia furfur*: a cause of occlusion of percutaneous central venous catheters in infants in the intensive care nursery, Pediatr. Infect. Dis. J. 7 (1988) 100.

[584] S.T. Nguyen, C.H. Lund, D.J. Durand, Thrombolytic therapy for adhesion of percutaneous central venous catheters to vein intima associated with *Malassezia furfur* infection, J. Perinatol. 21 (2001) 331.

[585] M.J. Marcon, D.A. Powell, D.E. Durrell, Methods for optimal recovery of *Malassezia furfur* from blood culture, J. Clin. Microbiol. 24 (1986) 696.

[586] U.H. Tirodker, et al., Detection of fungemia by polymerase chain reaction in critically ill neonates and children, J. Perinatol. 23 (2003) 117.

[587] M.J. Marcon, et al., In vitro activity of systemic antifungal agents against *Malassezia furfur*, Antimicrob. Agents Chemother. 31 (1987) 951.

[588] S.E. Levin, C. Isaacson, Spontaneous perforation of the colon in the newborn, Arch. Dis. Child. 35 (1960) 378.

[589] R.R. Gatling, Gastric mucormycosis in a newborn infant, Arch. Pathol. 67 (1959) 249.

[590] P. Neame, D. Raaner, Mucormycosis, Arch. Pathol. 70 (1960) 261.

[591] J.R. Jackson, P.N. Karnauchow, Mucormycosis of the central nervous system, Can. Med. Assoc. J. 76 (1957) 130.

[592] C. Isaacson, S.E. Levin, Gastrointestinal mucormycosis in infancy, S. Afr. Med. J. 35 (1961) 582.

[593] J.E. Dennis, et al., Nosocomial *Rhizopus* infection (zygomycosis) in children, J. Pediatr. 96 (1980) 824.

[594] D.M. Michalak, et al., Gastrointestinal mucormycosis in infants and children: a cause of gangrenous intestinal cellulitis and perforation, J. Pediatr. Surg. 15 (1980) 320.

[595] R.D. Miller, P.G. Steinkuller, D. Naegele, Nonfatal maxillocerebral mucormycosis with orbital involvement in a dehydrated infant, Ann. Ophthalmol. 12 (1980) 1065.

[596] C.B. White, P.J. Barcia, J.W. Bass, Neonatal zygomycotic necrotizing cellulitis, Pediatrics 78 (1986) 100.

[597] F. Varricchio, A. Wilks, Undiagnosed mucormycosis in infants, Pediatr. Infect. Dis. J. 8 (1989) 660.

[598] P.C. Ng, P.R.F. Dear, Phycomycotic abscesses in a preterm infant, Arch. Dis. Child. 64 (1989) 862.

[599] L.L. Lewis, H.K. Hawkins, M.S. Edwards, Disseminated mucormycosis in an infant with methylmalonic aciduria, Pediatr. Infect. Dis. J. 9 (1990) 851.

[600] P.F. Crim 3rd, D. Demello, W.J. Keenan, Disseminated zygomycosis in a newborn, Pediatr. Infect. Dis. J. 3 (1984) 61.

[601] A.E. Arisoy, et al., *Rhizopus* necrotizing cellulitis in a preterm infant: a case report and review of the literature, Pediatr. Infect. Dis. J. 12 (1993) 1029.

[602] N.M. Craig, et al., Disseminated *Rhizopus* infection in a premature infant, Pediatr. Dermatol. 11 (1994) 346.

[603] N. Linder, et al., Primary cutaneous mucormycosis in a premature infant: case report and review of the literature, Am. J. Perinatol. 15 (1998) 35.

[604] S.B. Amin, et al., *Absidia corymbifera* infections in neonates, Clin. Infect. Dis. 26 (1998) 990.

[605] D. Oh, D. Notrica, Primary cutaneous mucormycosis in infants and neonates: case report and review of the literature, J. Pediatr. Surg. 37 (2002) 1607.

[606] V. Buchta, et al., Primary cutaneous *Absidia corymbifera* infection in a premature newborn, Infection 31 (2003) 57.

[607] E. Scheffler, G.G. Miller, D.A. Classen, Zygomycotic infection of the neonatal upper extremity, J. Pediatr. Surg. 38 (2003) E16.

[608] B.R. Straatsma, L.E. Zimmerman, J.D.M. Gass, Phycomycosis: a clinicopathologic study of fifty-one cases, Lab. Invest. 11 (1962) 963.

[609] W.H. Sheldon, H. Bauer, Activation of quiescent mucormycotic granulomas in rabbits by induction of acute alloxan diabetes, Am. J. Pathol. 34 (1958) 575.

[610] H. Bauer, J.F. Flanagan, W.H. Sheldon, Experimental cerebral mucormycosis in rabbits with alloxan diabetes, Yale J. Biol. Med. 28 (1955) 29.

[611] T.D. Elder, R.D. Baker, Pulmonary mucormycosis in rabbits with alloxan diabetes: increased invasiveness of fungus during acute toxic phase of diabetes, Arch. Pathol. 61 (1956) 159.

[612] R.A. Schofield, R.D. Baker, Experimental mucormycosis (*Rhizopus* infection) in mice, Arch. Pathol. 61 (1956) 407.

[613] J.E. Johnson, Infection and diabetes, in: M. Ellenberg, H. Rifkin (Eds.), Diabetes Millitus: Theory and Practice, McGraw-Hill, New York, 1969.

[614] W.H. Sheldon, H. Bauer, The development of the acute inflammatory response to experimental cutaneous mucormycosis in normal and diabetic rabbits, J. Exp. Med. 110 (1959) 845.

[615] C.W. Emmons, C.H. Binford, J.P. Utz, Medical Mycology, second ed., Lea & Febiger, Philadelphia, 1970.

[616] C.J. Alexopoulos, Introductory Mycology, second ed., John Wiley, New York, 1962.

[617] R.H. Whittaker, New concepts of kingdoms of organisms, Science 163 (1969) 150.

[618] C.W. Dodge, Phycomycetes, in: C.W. Dodge (Ed.), CV Mosby, St Louis, 1935, p. 97.

[619] N.F. Conant, et al., Mucormycosis, in: N.F. Conant et al., (Ed.), WB Saunders, Philadelphia, 1971, pp. 403–416.

[620] C.W. Emmons, Phycomycosis in man and animals, Riv. Patol. Veg. 4 (1964) 329.

[621] P.R. Burkholder, I. McVeigh, Growth of *Phycomyces blakesleeanus* in relation to varied environmental conditions, Am. J. Bot. 27 (1940) 634.

[622] M. Fernandez, et al., Cutaneous phaeohyphomycosis caused by *Curvularia lunata* and a review of *Curvularia* infections in pediatrics, Pediatr. Infect. Dis. J. 18 (1999) 72731.

[623] R.D. Meyer, M.D. Rosen, D. Armstrong, Phycomycosis complicating leukemia and lymphoma, Ann. Intern. Med. 77 (1972) 871.

[624] G.R. Gale, A.M. Welch, Studies of opportunistic fungi: I. Inhibition of *Rhizopus oryzae* by human serum, Am. J. Med. Sci. 241 (1961) 604.

[625] H. Bank, et al., Mucormycosis of head and neck structures: a case with survival, BMJ 1 (1962) 766.

[626] K.W. Jones, L. Kaufman, Development and evaluation of an immunodiffusion test for diagnosis of systemic zygomycosis (mucormycosis): preliminary report, J. Clin. Microbiol. 7 (1978) 97.

[627] H.J. Roberts, Cutaneous mucormycosis: report of a case with survival, Arch. Intern. Med. 110 (1962) 108.

[628] M.L. Dillon, W.C. Sealy, B.L. Fetter, Mucormycosis of the bronchus successfully treated by lobectomy, J. Thorac. Cardiovasc. Surg. 35 (1958) 464.

[629] J.S. Harris, Mucormycosis: report of a case, Pediatrics 16 (1955) 857.

[630] W. McCall, R.R. Strobos, Survival of a patient with central nervous system mucormycosis, Neurology 7 (1957) 290.

[631] H. Oswald, H.P.R. Seeliger, Tierexperimentelle Untersuchungen mit antimycotischen Mitteln, Arzneimittelforschung 8 (1958) 370.

[632] L.A. Duhring, Diseases of the Skin, third ed., JB Lippincott, Philadelphia, 1988.

[633] J.R. Lynch, Case of ringworm occurring in an infant within 6 hours of birth, Med. Press Circ. 21 (1876) 235.

[634] A.H. Jacobs, P.H. Jacobs, N. Moore, Tinea faciei due to *Microsporum canis*, JAMA 219 (1972) 1476.

[635] L.M. Drusin, et al., Nosocomial ringworm in a neonatal intensive care unit: a nurse and her cat, Infect. Control Hosp. Epidemiol. 21 (2000) 605.

[636] E.W. Bereston, H.M. Robinson, Tinea capitis and corporis in an infant 4 weeks old, Arch. Derm. Syphilol. 68 (1953) 582.

[637] W.C. King, I.K. Walter, C.S. Livingood, Superficial fungus infections in infants, Arch. Dermatol. 68 (1953) 664.

[638] L.F. Hubener, Tinea capitis (*Microsporum canis*) in a 30 day old infant, Arch. Dermatol. 76 (1957) 242.

[639] E.R. Alden, D.A. Chernila, Ringworm in an infant, Pediatrics 44 (1969) 261.

[640] W.L. Weston, E.G. Thorne, Two cases of tinea in the neonate treated successfully with griseofulvin, Clin. Pediatr. 16 (1977) 601.

[641] C.M. Ross, Ringworm of the scalp at 4 weeks, Br. J. Dermatol. 78 (1966) 554.

[642] P. Yesudian, A. Kamalam, *Epidermophyton floccosum* infection in a three week old infant, Trans. St. Johns Hosp. Dermatol. Soc. 59 (1973) 66.

[643] K. Kleibl, H.A. Al-Ghareer, M.F. Sakr, Neonatal tinea circinata, Mykosen 26 (1982) 152.

[644] H.W. Wyre Jr., W.T. Johnson, Neonatal pityriasis versicolor, Arch. Dermatol. 117 (1981) 752.

[645] H.M. Gondim Goncalves, et al., Tinea capitis caused by *Microsporum canis* in a newborn, Int. J. Dermatol. 31 (1992) 367.

[646] M.J. Lanska, R. Silverman, D.J. Lansaka, Cutaneous fungal infections associated with prolonged treatment in humidified oxygen hoods, Pediatr. Dermatol. 4 (1987) 346.

[647] A. Kamalan, A.S. Thambish, Tinea faciei caused by *Microsporum gypseum* in a two day old infant, Mykosen 24 (1981) 40.

[648] E.B. Smith, G.L. Gellerman, Tinea versicolor in infancy, Arch. Dermatol. 93 (1984) 362.

[649] L. Ajello, A taxonomic review of the dermatophytes and related species, Sabouraudia 6 (1968) 147.

[650] C.O. Dawson, J.C. Gentles, Perfect stage of *Keratinomyces ajelloi*, Nature 183 (1959) 1345.

[651] G. Rebell, D. Taplin, H. Blank, Dermatophytes, Dermatology Foundation of Miami, Miami, 1964.

[652] J.L. Rowen, et al., Invasive fungal dermatitis in the £1000 gram neonate, Pediatrics 95 (1995) 682.

[653] M.P. English, M.D. Gibson, Studies in epidemiology of tinea pedis, BMJ 1 (1959) 1442.

[654] S. Rothman, G. Knox, D. Windhourst, Tinea pedis as a source of infection in the family, Arch. Dermatol. 75 (1957) 270.

[655] L. Ajello, Geographic distribution and prevalence of the dermatophytes, Ann. N. Y. Acad. Sci. 89 (1960) 30.

[656] P. Pinetti, A. Lostia, F. Tarentino, The role played by flies in the transmission of the human and animal dermatophytic infection, Mycopathologia 54 (1974) 131.

[657] R.L. Baer, S.A. Rosenthal, D. Furnari, Survival of dermatophytes applied on the feet, J. Invest. Dermatol. 24 (1955) 619.

[658] R.L. Baer, et al., Experimental investigations on mechanism producing acute dermatophytosis of feet, JAMA 160 (1956) 184.

[659] A.G. Knight, A review of experimental fungus infections, J. Invest. Dermatol. 59 (1972) 354.

[660] D.W.R. Mackenzie, The extra human occurrence of *Trichophyton tonsurans var. sulfureum* in a residential school, Sabouraudia 1 (1961) 58.

[661] G. Hildick-Smith, H. Blank, I. Sarkany, Tinea capitis, Little, Brown, Boston, 1964.

[662] M.A. Roig, J.M.T. Rodriguez, The immune response in childhood dermatophytoses, Mykosen 30 (1987) 574.

[663] I. Alteras, Tinea capitis in suckling infants, Mykosen 13 (1970) 567.

[664] F.D. Weidman, Laboratory aspects of epidermophytosis, Arch. Dermatol. 15 (1929) 415.

[665] R.S. Goodman, D.E. Temple, A. Lorinez, A miniaturized system for extracorporeal hemodialysis with application to studies on serum antidermophyte activity, J. Invest. Dermatol. 37 (1961) 535.

[666] S.S. Greenbaum, Immunity in ringworm infections, Arch. Dermatol. 10 (1924) 279.

[667] A.L. Lorincz, J.O. Priestly, P.H. Jacobs, Evidence for humoral mechanism which prevents growth of dermatophytes, J. Invest. Dermatol. 31 (1958) 15.

[668] C.O. Page, J.S. Remington, Immunologic studies in normal human sweat, J. Lab. Clin. Med. 69 (1967) 634.

[669] W.B. Shelley, M.G. Wood, New technic for instant visualization of fungi in hair, J. Am. Acad. Dermatol. 2 (1980) 69.

[670] R.C. Burke, Tinea versicolor: susceptibility factors and experimental infection in human beings, J. Invest. Dermatol. 36 (1961) 389.

[671] B.T. Fields Jr., J.H. Bates, R.S. Abernathy, Amphotericin B serum concentrations during therapy, Appl. Microbiol. 19 (1970) 955.

[672] M.J. McCoy, J.F. Ellenberg, A.P. Killum, Coccidioidomycosis complicating pregnancy, Am. J. Obstet. Gynecol. 137 (1980) 739.

[673] R.M. Ward, F.R. Sattler, A.S. Dotton Jr., Assessment of antifungal therapy in an 800-gram infant with candidal arthritis and osteomyelitis, Pediatrics 72 (1983) 234.

[674] R.S. Abernathy, Treatment of systemic mycoses, Medicine 52 (1973) 385.

[675] K.M. Butler, M.A. Rench, C.J. Baker, B. Amphotericin, as a single agent in the treatment of systemic candidiasis in neonates, Pediatr. Infect. Dis. J. 9 (1990) 51.

[676] R.P. Miller, J.H. Bates, Amphotericin B toxicity, Ann. Intern. Med. 71 (1969) 1089.

[677] D.K. McCurdy, M. Frederic, J.R. Elkington, Renal tubular acidosis due to amphotericin B, N. Engl. J. Med. 278 (1968) 124.

[678] J.E. Baley, R.M. Kliegman, A.A. Fanaroff, Disseminated fungal infections in very low-birth-weight infants: therapeutic toxicity, Pediatrics 73 (1984) 153.

[679] R. Feldman, Cryptococcosis (torulosis) of the central nervous system treated with amphotericin B during pregnancy, South Med. J. 52 (1959) 1415.

[680] G.W.E. Aitken, E.M. Symonds, Cryptococcal meningitis in pregnancy treated with amphotericin B: a case report, J. Obstet. Gynaecol. Br. Commonw. 69 (1962) 677.

[681] D. Kuo, A case of torulosis of the central nervous system during pregnancy, Med. J. Aust. 49 (1962) 558.

[682] W.G. Sanford, J.R. Rosch, R.B. Stonehill, A therapeutic dilemma: the treatment of disseminated coccidioidomycosis with amphotericin B, Ann. Intern. Med. 56 (1962) 553.

[683] R.E. Harris, Coccidioidomycosis complicating pregnancy: report of 3 cases and review of the literature, Obstet. Gynecol. 28 (1966) 401.

[684] L.E. Smale, K.G. Waechter, Dissemination of coccidioidomycosis in pregnancy, Am. J. Obstet. Gynecol. 107 (1970) 356.

[685] F.J. Hadsall, J.J. Acquarelli, Disseminated coccidioidomycosis presenting as facial granulomas in pregnancy: a report of two cases and a review of the literature, Laryngoscope 83 (1973) 51.

[686] V.V. Moudgal, J.D. Sobel, Antifungal drugs in pregnancy: a review, Expert Opin. Drug Saf. 2 (2003) 475.

[687] R.F. Jacobs, et al., Laryngeal candidiasis presenting as inspiratory stridor, Pediatrics 69 (1982) 234.

[688] R.G. Faix, *Candida parapsilosis* meningitis in a premature infant, Pediatr. Infect. Dis. J. 2 (1983) 462.

[689] J.D. Cherry, et al., Amphotericin B therapy in children, J. Pediatr. 75 (1969) 1063.

[690] D.J. Drutz, et al., Treatment of disseminated mycotic infections: new approach to therapy with amphotericin B, Am. J. Med. 45 (1968) 405.

[691] K.J. Christiansen, et al., Distribution and activity of amphotericin B in humans, J. Infect. Dis. 152 (1985) 1037.

[692] D.J. Drutz, In vitro antifungal susceptibility testing and measurement of levels of antifungal agents in body fluids, J. Infect. Dis. 9 (1987) 392.

[693] J.H. Weitkamp, et al., *Candida* infection in very low-birth-weight infants: outcome and nephrotoxicity of treatment with liposomal amphotericin B (AmBisome), Infection 26 (1998) 11.

[694] A. Scarcella, et al., Liposomal amphotericin B treatment for neonatal fungal infections, Pediatr. Infect. Dis. J. 17 (1998) 146.

[695] S. Shadomy, In vitro studies with 5-fluorocytosine, Appl. Microbiol. 17 (1969) 871.

[696] S. Shadomy, Further in vitro studies with 5-fluorocytosine, Infect. Immun. 2 (1970) 484.

[697] S. Shadomy, What's new in antifungal chemotherapy, Clin. Med. 79 (1972) 14.

[698] P.L. Steer, et al., 5-Fluorocytosine: an oral antifungal compound: a report on clinical and laboratory experience, Ann. Intern. Med. 76 (1972) 15.

[699] G.A. Sarosi, et al., Amphotericin B in cryptococcal meningitis, Ann. Intern. Med. 70 (1969) 1079.

[700] I.I.R. Harrison, et al., Amphotericin B and imidazole therapy for coccidioidal meningitis in children, Pediatr. Infect. Dis. 2 (1983) 216.

[701] P.N. McDougall, et al., Neonatal systemic candidiasis: a failure to respond to intravenous miconazole in two neonates, Arch. Dis. Child. 57 (1982) 884.

[702] A. Sutton, Miconazole in systemic candidiasis, Arch. Dis. Child. 58 (1983) 319.

[703] P. Duffty, D.J. Lloyd, Neonatal systemic candidiasis, Arch. Dis. Child. 58 (1983) 318.

[704] L.D. Lilien, R.S. Ramamurthy, R.S. Pildes, *Candida albicans* with meningitis in a premature neonate successfully treated with 5-flucytosine and amphotericin B: a case report and review of the literature, Pediatrics 61 (1978) 57.

[705] J.E. Bennett, Therapy of cryptococcal meningitis with 5-fluorocytosine, Antimicrob. Agents Chemother. 10 (1970) 28.

[706] K.W. Brammer, P.R. Farrow, J.K. Faulkner, Pharmacokinetics and tissue penetration of fluconazole in humans, Rev. Infect. Dis. 12 (Suppl. 3) (1990) S318.

[707] D.B. Wiest, et al., Fluconazole in neonatal disseminated candidiasis, Arch. Dis. Child. 66 (1991) 1002.

[708] N. Gürses, A.G. Kalayci, Fluconazole monotherapy for candidal meningitis in a premature infant, Clin. Infect. Dis. 23 (1996) 645.

[709] M. Driessen, et al., Fluconazole vs amphotericin B for the treatment of neonatal fungal septicemia: a prospective randomized trial, Pediatr. Infect. Dis. J. 15 (1996) 1107.

[710] M. Driessen, et al., The treatment of systemic candidiasis in neonates with oral fluconazole, Ann. Trop. Paediatr. 17 (1997) 263.

[711] Y.C. Huang, et al., Fluconazole therapy in neonatal candidemia, Am. J. Perinatol. 17 (2000) 411.

[712] E.C. Wiesinger, et al., Fluconazole in *Candida albicans* sepsis during pregnancy: case report and review of the literature, Infection 24 (1996) 263.

[713] V. Bhandari, A. Narange, Oral itraconazole therapy for disseminated candidiasis in low birth weight infants, J. Pediatr. 120 (1992) 330.

[714] L. de Repentigny, et al., Repeated-dose pharmacokinetics of an oral solution of itraconazole in infants and children, Antimicrob. Agents Chemother. 42 (1998) 404.

[715] T.J. Walsh, et al., Voriconazole in the treatment of aspergillosis, scedosporiosis and other invasive fungal infections in children, Pediatr. Infect. Dis. J. 21 (2002) 240.

[716] J.A. Franklin, J. McCormick, P.M. Flynn, Retrospective study of the safety of caspofungin in immunocompromised pediatric patients, Pediatr. Infect. Dis. J. 22 (2003) 747.

[717] C.M. Ross, Ringworm of the scalp at four weeks, Br. J. Dermatol. 78 (1966) 554.

[718] A. Rubin, D. Dvornik, Placental transfer of griseofulvin, Am. J. Obstet. Gynecol. 92 (1965) 882.

[719] B.E. Elewski, Treatment of tinea capitis: beyond griseofulvin, J. Am. Acad. Dermatol. 40 (1999) S27.

[720] H. Caceres-Rios, et al., Comparison of terbinafine and griseofulvin in the treatment of tinea capitis, J. Am. Acad. Dermatol. 42 (2000) 80.

SECTION V

DIAGNOSIS AND MANAGEMENT

SECTION OUTLINE

35 Healthcare–Associated Infections in the Nursery 1126

36 Laboratory Aids for Diagnosis of Neonatal Sepsis 1144

37 Clinical Pharmacology of Anti-Infective Drugs 1160

38 Prevention of Fetal and Early Life Infections through Maternal–Neonatal Immunization 1212

HEALTHCARE–ASSOCIATED INFECTIONS IN THE NURSERY

Susan E. Coffin ⊛ Theoklis E. Zaoutis

CHAPTER OUTLINE

Special Issues for Neonates 1126
Epidemiology 1127
    Incidence 1127
    Maternally Acquired Infections 1127
    Nonmaternal Routes of Transmission 1127
    Risk Factors for Health Care–Associated Infections 1128
Etiologic Agents 1128
    Coagulase-Negative Staphylococci 1129
    Other Gram-Positive Bacteria 1129
    Gram-Negative Bacteria 1130
    Multidrug-Resistant Organisms 1130
    Fungi 1131
    Viral Pathogens 1131
Device-Related Infections 1132

Catheter-Associated Bloodstream Infections 1132
Ventilator-Associated Pneumonia 1134
Catheter-Associated Urinary Tract Infections 1135
Ventricular Shunt–Associated Infections 1135
Preventing Transmission of Health Care–Associated Infections 1135
    Surveillance 1135
    Standard and Transmission-Based Precautions in the Nursery 1136
Other Related Issues 1138
    Health Care Workers 1138
    Family-Centered Care 1138
    Breast-Feeding 1138
    Visitors 1139
    Skin and Cord Care 1139

Neonates, especially premature neonates who require intensive medical care, are among the patients at highest risk for nosocomial or health care–associated infections (HAIs). Although the rate of HAIs varies with the specific patient population and institution, some series have reported that more than 20% of critically ill neonates who survive more than 48 hours acquire a nosocomial infection [1-3]. Neonatal HAIs are associated with significant morbidity, mortality, and excessive direct health care costs [3]. Prevention of these infections should be a major priority in all neonatal intensive care units (NICUs) and nurseries. The most important risk factors for HAIs in neonates, gestational age and birth weight, cannot be modified. Close attention to clinical practice and the patient care environment is mandatory to minimize the risk of infections. This chapter reviews the epidemiology, microbiology, pathogenesis, and prevention of neonatal HAIs.

SPECIAL ISSUES FOR NEONATES

The innate and adaptive arms of the neonatal immune system are functionally less mature than that of older infants, children, and adults (see Chapter 4). Compared with term infants, preterm infants have less developed specific components of the innate immune system, particularly factors that maintain physiologic barriers. Immature and easily damaged skin is a major factor in the relative immunocompromised state of preterm infants. Iatrogenic breeches in skin integrity, such as those caused by percutaneous medical devices and surgical wounds, also constitute a significant risk.

Although the cellular precursors of the human immune system are present around the beginning of the second trimester, T cells, neutrophils, monocytes, and the complement pathways are functionally impaired at this time. Neonatal neutrophils show decreased chemotaxis, diminished adherence to the endothelium, and impaired phagocytosis (see Chapter 4) [4,5]; neonatal complement levels and opsonic capacity also are reduced, particularly in premature neonates. In addition, immature T-cell function results in diminished production of cytokines, T-cell killing of virally infected cells, and B-cell differentiation and maturation.

Passively acquired maternal IgG is the sole source of neonatal IgG. Because transplacental transfer of maternal IgG occurs primarily in the third trimester, the serum IgG levels of many preterm neonates are very low. Soon after birth, maternal IgG levels begin to decline, and neonatal production of antigen-specific immunoglobulins begins. Serum IgG concentrations reach about 60% of adult levels by 1 year of age in term neonates [6]. Given the incomplete transfer of maternal IgG and an impaired ability to produce antigen-specific immunoglobulins, premature infants typically have significantly lower levels of serum IgG than their term counterparts, a difference that can persist throughout the 1st year of life. Developmental issues of other organ systems can also affect the risk of HAIs. The immature gastrointestinal tract, characterized by reduced acidification of gastric contents and the fragile integrity of the intestinal epithelium, provides another potential portal of entry for pathogens.

Colonization resistance, the incomplete passive protection associated with colonization of skin and mucous membranes with "normal flora," also provides protection from invasive infections caused by pathogenic or commensal bacteria. The in utero environment is sterile; however, colonization begins within the first few days of life. The acquisition of normal colonizing flora is disrupted in hospitalized newborns for various reasons, including the presence of pathogenic bacteria in the hospital environment and on the hands of health care workers, the frequent use of antimicrobial agents, and exposure to invasive procedures. As a result, the microflora of infants in the NICU can be markedly different from healthy term infants [7,8]. Multidrug-resistant coagulase-negative staphylococci (CoNS) and *Klebsiella*, *Enterobacter*, and *Citrobacter* species colonize the skin and the respiratory and gastrointestinal tracts of a high proportion of NICU neonates by the 2nd week of hospitalization [9–12]. In addition, hospitalized neonates can become colonized with *Candida* and other yeasts [13–16].

EPIDEMIOLOGY
INCIDENCE

The incidence of HAIs varies markedly by birth weight, gestational age, underlying conditions, and exposure to medical devices [17]. Reported rates of specific infections in similar patient populations differ dramatically by institution. In the past, much of this variation likely arose from differences in patient populations and clinical practices. The patient safety movement has resulted in marked reductions in the rates of many specific HAIs in numerous NICU settings, however. The risk of HAIs previously reported is likely greater than that currently experienced by many neonatal patients.

In 1999, a nationwide multicenter surveillance study, the Pediatric Prevention Network (PPN) Point Prevalence Survey, was undertaken to determine the point prevalence of and to define risk factors associated with nosocomial infections in NICU patients [18]. This study included 827 infants from 29 NICUs. Of the 827 infants, 94 (11.4%) had an active nosocomial infection on the day of the survey. Bacteremia accounted for 53% of infections. Lower respiratory tract infections; ear, nose, or throat infections; and urinary tract infections accounted for 13%, 9%, and 9% (Table 35–1).

In contrast to the NICU setting, the frequency of nosocomial infection in well-infant nurseries has been estimated to be 0.3% to 1.7% [19–21]. Generally, non–life-threatening infections such as conjunctivitis account for most infections in the well-infant population. The remainder of this chapter focuses almost entirely on nosocomial infections in NICUs.

MATERNALLY ACQUIRED INFECTIONS

Differentiating maternally acquired and hospital-acquired infections can be difficult. Surveillance definitions typically describe nosocomial infections as infections that arise 2 or more days after initial admission to a nursery or NICU. No precise time point or definition perfectly discriminates infections that clinically were likely attributable to vertical transmission from infections transmitted within the NICU. Approximately 90% of hospitalized neonates with an infection presumed to be of maternal origin had onset of symptoms within 48 hours of birth. Maternally acquired bloodstream infections were more likely to be caused by group B streptococci, other streptococci, and *Escherichia coli* and were rarely caused by CoNS [22].

NONMATERNAL ROUTES OF TRANSMISSION

Nonmaternal routes of transmission generally can be divided into three categories: contact (from either direct or indirect contact from an infected person or a contaminated source), droplet (from large respiratory droplets that fall out of the air at a maximum distance of 3 feet), and airborne (from droplet nuclei, which can remain suspended in air for long periods and as a result travel longer distances). Specific microorganisms can be spread by more than one mechanism; in most instances, a single mode of spread predominates, however. The U.S. Centers for Disease Control and Prevention (CDC) has developed a system of precautions to prevent the spread of HAIs that is based on these modes of transmission [23].

Most neonatal HAIs are caused by the infant's own flora. The "abnormal flora" of the neonate residing in the NICU is determined at least in part, however, by the NICU environment and the hands of health care workers. Contact transmission of bacteria, viruses, and fungi on the hands of health care workers is arguably the most important, yet seemingly preventable mechanism by which potentially

TABLE 35–1   Distribution of Infections Acquired in the Neonatal Intensive Care Unit by Birth Weight and Site

| Birth Weight | No. Patients | | No. Infections | | | | | |
	Total Surveyed	With Infections (%)	Total	Bacteremia (%)	Respiratory Infections (%)	ENT Infections (%)	UTIs (%)	Other Infections (%)
<500	13	1/13 (7.7)	1	1/1 (100)	0	0	0	0
501–1000	246	43/246 (17.5)	58	31/58 (53.4)	9/58 (15.5)	5/58 (8.6)	4/58 (7)	9/58 (15.5)
1001–1500	147	21/147 (14.3)	26	15/26 (57.7)	2/26 (7.7)	2/26 (7.7)	1/26 (3.8)	6/26 (23.1)
1501–2000	74	2/74 (2.7)	2	2/2 (100)	0	0	0	0
2001–2500	74	5/74 (6.8)	5	2/5 (40)	1/5 (20)	1/5 (20)	1/5 (20)	0
>2500	239	16/239 (6.7)	17	7/17 (41.2)	2/17 (11.8)	2/17 (11.8)	3/17 (17.6)	3/17 (17.6)
Unknown	34	6/347 (1.7)	7	3/7 (42.8)	1/7 (14.3)	0	1/7 (14.3)	2/7 (28.6)
Total	*827*	*94/827 (11.4)*	*116*	*61/116 (52.6)*	*15/116 (12.9)*	*10/116 (8.6)*	*10/116 (8.6)*	*20/116 (17.2)*

ENT, ear, nose, or throat; UTIs, urinary tract infections.
Adapted from Sohn AH, et al. Prevalence of nosocomial infections in neonatal intensive care unit patients: results from the first national point-prevalence survey. J Pediatr 139:821–827, 2001.

pathogenic organisms are spread. Poor compliance with hand hygiene has been repeatedly shown as a cause of outbreaks and transmission of resistant microorganisms [24–27]. With use of molecular techniques, even organisms typically considered to originate solely from normal flora (e.g., CoNS) have been shown to have clonal spread in the hospital setting, suggesting contact transmission by means of the hands of health care workers [28,29].

Transmission via contaminated inanimate objects also occurs and has been described as a potential mechanism of spread of pathogens in multiple NICU outbreaks [27,30,31]. Implicated items have included linens, medical devices, soap dispensers, and breast pumps. These observations highlight the need for careful attention to disinfecting items shared among infants.

Spread of infection through large respiratory droplets is an important mode of transmission for pertussis and certain respiratory viruses. The early identification and appropriate use of precautions for suspected cases are particularly important for nurseries that admit infants from the community. In addition, an ill adult, either a health care worker or a parent, can be the source of these infections in the NICU. Measles, varicella, and pulmonary tuberculosis are usually spread via the airborne route by means of droplet nuclei, but are not typical risks in a nursery or NICU.

Other sources of HAIs include contaminated infusions, medications, and feeding powders or solutions, which can be either intrinsically or extrinsically contaminated and have been reported as the source of outbreaks caused by a variety of different pathogens. It is important when possible to mix infusions in a controlled environment (usually the pharmacy), to avoid multiuse sources of medication, and to use bottled or sterilized feeding solutions when breast milk is unavailable.

RISK FACTORS FOR HEALTH CARE–ASSOCIATED INFECTIONS

Patient-Related Factors

As discussed earlier, infants in NICUs have intrinsic factors that predispose them to infection, such as an immature immune system and compromised skin or mucous membranes. In addition, multiple extrinsic factors play important roles in the development of infection, such as presence of indwelling catheters; performance of invasive procedures; and administration of certain medications, such as steroids and antimicrobial agents.

Although the relationship between birth weight and HAIs is likely confounded by multiple other unmeasured factors, such as immune system immaturity, birth weight remains one of the strongest risk factors for HAIs. Data from the CDC show an inverse association between birth weight and the risk of developing either bloodstream infections or ventilator-associated pneumonia (VAP), even after adjusting for central venous catheter (CVC) and ventilator use [22]. Similarly, in the PPN Point Prevalence Survey, infants weighing 1500 g or less at birth were 2.69 (95% confidence interval 1.75 to 4.14; $P < .001$) times more likely to have an infection than infants weighing more than 1500 g [18].

Severity of illness scores have been developed to derive risk-adjusted rates of morbidity and mortality in NICU patients. Stratification by birth weight is the most common strategy used to risk-adjust NICU infection data. Other scores used by some institutions include the Score for Neonatal Acute Physiology (SNAP) [32] and the Clinical Risk Index for Babies (CRIB) [33]. Risk adjustment using these scores can provide more accurate predictions of neonatal mortality and nosocomial infections, although they are not universally used, even within narrow birth weight strata.

Medical Devices

The presence of indwelling intravascular or transmucosal medical devices has been identified repeatedly as one of the greatest risk factors for HAIs in neonates. Importantly, these associations persist after adjustment for birth weight [18]. The epidemiology of HAIs related to medical devices is discussed in more detail later.

Therapeutic Agents

Numerous medications and other therapeutic agents crucial to the survival of infants in the NICU increase risk of infection. The widespread use of broad-spectrum antimicrobial agents has been associated with increased colonization with resistant organisms in many settings, including NICUs [8,17]. In addition to increasing colonization, use of antimicrobial agents increases the risk of invasive infection with resistant bacteria [34] and with fungal pathogens [35]. Other medications can also be associated with the development of HAIs. Infants who receive corticosteroids after delivery are at approximately 1.3 to 1.6 times higher risk for nosocomial bacteremia in the subsequent 2 to 6 weeks than infants who do not receive this intervention [36,37]. In addition, colonization and infection with bacterial and fungal pathogens have been shown to increase with the use of H_2 blockers [13,38].

Parenteral alimentation and intravenous fat emulsion have been shown in some studies to increase risk of bloodstream infection in premature infants even after adjustment for other covariables, such as birth weight and CVC use; the pathogenesis of this possible association remains unclear [39,40]. Investigators have suggested that fat emulsions could have a direct effect on the immune system [41]. Alternatively, as with any intravenous fluids, parenteral alimentation has the potential for intrinsic and extrinsic contamination, and fat emulsion especially may serve as a growth medium for certain bacteria and fungi. Finally, total parenteral alimentation and intravenous administration of fats likely delay the normal development of gastrointestinal mucosa because of lack of enteral feeding, encouraging translocation of pathogens across the gastrointestinal mucosa. Other risk factors related to infection include poor hand hygiene and environmental issues, such as understaffing and overcrowding [42–44].

ETIOLOGIC AGENTS

The microbiology of neonatal HAIs is diverse (Table 35–2). Detailed discussions of the microbiology of sepsis and meningitis and of specific organisms can be found in other chapters.

TABLE 35–2   Most Common Nosocomial Pathogens in Neonatal Intensive Care Unit Patients: Distribution by Site

Pathogen	No. Infections (%)				
	Bloodstream	EENT	GI	Pneumonia	Surgical Site
CoNS	3833 (51)	787 (29.3)	102 (9.6)	434 (16.5)	119 (19.2)
Staphylococcus aureus	561 (7.5)	413 (15.4)	—	440 (16.7)	138 (22.3)
Group B streptococci	597 (7.9)	—	—	150 (5.7)	—
Enterococcus	467 (6.2)	92 (3.4)	—	120 (4.6)	55 (8.9)
Candida	518 (6.9)	—	—	—	—
Escherichia coli	326 (4.3)	163 (6.1)	147 (13.9)	152 (5.8)	74 (12)
Other streptococci	205 (2.7)	199 (7.4)	—	86 (3.3)	—
Enterobacter	219 (2.9)	120 (4.5)	58 (5.5)	215 (8.2)	47 (7.6)
Klebsiella pneumoniae	188 (2.5)	76 (2.8)	104 (9.8)	152 (5.8)	39 (6.3)
Pseudomonas aeruginosa	—	178 (6.6)	—	308 (11.7)	—
Haemophilus influenzae	—	72 (2.7)	—	38 (1.4)	—
Viruses	—	136 (5.1)	317 (30*)	—	—
Gram-positive anaerobes	—	—	99 (9.4)	—	—
Other enteric bacilli	—	—	8 (0.8)	—	—
Miscellaneous organisms	607 (8.1)	449 (26.7)	223 (21)	570 (21.7)	147 (23.7)
Total	*7521 (100)*	*2685 (100)*	*1058 (100)*	*2665 (100)*	*619 (100)*

Rotavirus constituted 96.4% of viruses isolated from gastrointestinal infections.
CoNS, coagulase-negative staphylococci; EENT, eye, ear, nose, or throat; GI, gastrointestinal; NICU, neonatal intensive care unit.
Adapted from Gaynes RP, et al. Nosocomial infections among neonates in high-risk nurseries in the United States. National Nosocomial Infections Surveillance System. Pediatrics 98:357–361, 1996.

COAGULASE-NEGATIVE STAPHYLOCOCCI

Since the early 1980s, CoNS have been the most common cause of HAIs in the NICU [43]. National Nosocomial Infections Surveillance (NNIS) and PPN surveillance data estimate that 32% of total pathogens and 48% to 51% of bloodstream infections are caused by these organisms [18,22]. Although an infrequent cause of fatal infection, bacteremia caused by CoNS has been associated with prolonged NICU stay and increased hospital charges, even after adjustment for birth weight and severity of illness on admission [45]. A 10-year, prospective, multicenter Australian study found that 57% of all late-onset infections during the study period were due to CoNS. Molecular techniques suggest that infections caused by *Staphylococcus epidermidis* can result from clonal dissemination and that there is often concordance between the strains infecting infants and strains carried on the hands of health care workers [28,46,47]. In one study, four clones accounted for 43 of 81 study strains (53%) [28]. This finding suggests that a significant proportion of CoNS infections may be preventable by strict adherence to infection control practices. The fact that a hand hygiene campaign was associated with increased hand hygiene compliance and a lower rate of CoNS-positive cultures further supports this contention [48].

OTHER GRAM-POSITIVE BACTERIA

Enterococcus accounts for approximately 10% of all neonatal HAIs, 6% to 15% of bloodstream infections, 0% to 5% of cases of pneumonia, 17% of urinary tract infections, and 9% of surgical site infections [18,22]. Sepsis and meningitis are common manifestations of enterococcal infection during NICU outbreaks [48–50].

The presence of a nonumbilical CVC, prolonged presence of a CVC, and bowel resection all have been identified as independent risk factors for enterococcal infections in NICU patients [50]. Because *Enterococcus* colonizes the gastrointestinal tract and can survive for long periods on inanimate surfaces, the patient's environment may become contaminated and, along with the infant, serve as a reservoir for ongoing spread of the organism.

Historically, before the recognized importance of hand hygiene and the availability of antimicrobial agents, group A streptococci were a major cause of puerperal sepsis and fatal neonatal sepsis. Although less common now, group A streptococci remain a cause of outbreaks in nurseries and NICUs [51–54]. Group A streptococci–associated clinical manifestations include severe sepsis and soft tissue infections. Molecular techniques have enhanced the ability to define outbreaks, and use of these techniques has suggested that transmission can occur between mother and infant, between health care worker and infant, and between infants—probably indirectly on the hands of health care workers [52,53]. In one recurring outbreak, inadequate laundry practices seemed to be a contributing factor [55].

Data from the CDC have shown that group B streptococci infections account for less than 2% of non–maternally acquired nosocomial bloodstream and pneumonia infections [22]. Numerous studies from the 1970s and 1980s showed nosocomial colonization of infants born to women negative for group B streptococci [56–60]. These studies suggested a rate of transmission to infants born to seronegative mothers of 12% to 27% [57,58]. A case-control study evaluating risk factors for late-onset infection caused by group B streptococci showed that premature birth was a strong predictor [61]. In that study, 50% of the infants with late-onset infection caused by group B streptococci were born at less than 37 weeks of gestation (compared with 15% of controls), and only 38% of the mothers of these infants were colonized with group B streptococci, suggesting possible nosocomial transmission of group B streptococci during the NICU stay.

GRAM-NEGATIVE BACTERIA

Organisms from the Enterobacteriaceae family have long been recognized as an important cause of HAIs, including sepsis, pneumonia, urinary tract infections, and soft tissue infections; morbidity and mortality rates frequently are high [62]. *Enterobacter* species, *Klebsiella pneumoniae*, *E. coli*, and *Serratia marcescens* are the members of Enterobacteriaceae most commonly encountered in the NICU. Many outbreaks owing to gram-negative bacteria have been reported. Underlying causes of these outbreaks include contaminated equipment [63–66], formula or breast milk [66–71], and intravenous fluids [72–74]; understaffing; overcrowding; and poor hand hygiene practices [75–78]. The origins of these organisms are often unclear, although many authors hypothesize that at least some episodes of gram-negative bacteremia are a consequence of intestinal translocation. This hypothesis is consistent with the observation that enteric feedings have been associated with a reduced risk of gram-negative infections [79].

Pseudomonas aeruginosa, an opportunistic pathogen that can persist in relatively harsh environments, frequently has been associated with HAIs and outbreaks in NICUs. Nosocomial *P. aeruginosa* infections vary in their clinical presentation, but the most common manifestations are respiratory; ear, nose, or throat; and bloodstream infections [18]. *P. aeruginosa* infections, particularly bloodstream infections, have been associated with a very high mortality rate [80]. Risk factors for infection include feeding intolerance, prolonged parenteral alimentation, and long-term intravenous antimicrobial therapy [80]. Outbreaks owing to *P. aeruginosa* have been linked to contaminated hand lotion [81], respiratory therapy solution [82], a water bath used to thaw fresh frozen plasma [83], a blood gas analyzer [84], and bathing equipment [85]. Health care workers and their contaminated hands also have been linked with *Pseudomonas* infections in the NICU. In a study of a New York outbreak, recovery of *Pseudomonas* species from the hands of health care workers was associated with older age and history of use of artificial nails [86]. This and other studies suggest that the risk of transmission of *Pseudomonas* to patients is higher among health care workers with onychomycosis or who wear long artificial or long natural nails [86,87]. As a result of these and other findings, the CDC revised its 2002 hand hygiene recommendations to include a recommendation against the presence of health care workers with artificial fingernails in intensive care units [88].

MULTIDRUG-RESISTANT ORGANISMS

Staphylococcus aureus has frequently been identified as a cause of nosocomial infection and outbreaks in well-infant nurseries and NICUs. Methicillin-resistant *S. aureus* (MRSA) has become a serious nosocomial pathogen, and outbreaks have been reported in many areas of hospitals, including nurseries [89–91]. With the emergence of community strains of MRSA, nosocomial transmission of MRSA with the molecular phenotype of either community-associated or hospital-associated strains has been shown [92,93]. In addition to the usual manifestations of neonatal nosocomial infection, *S. aureus* HAIs (caused by methicillin-sensitive strains or MRSA strains) can manifest as skin infections [94], bone and joint infections [95], parotitis [96], staphylococcal scalded skin syndrome [97,98], toxic shock syndrome [89], and disseminated sepsis.

Direct contact is the presumed mechanism of most instances of *S. aureus* transmission. Several distinct reservoirs of MRSA have been identified and associated with MRSA outbreaks, including parents, visitors, and health care workers [90,97,99,100]. Understaffing and overcrowding have been associated with *S. aureus* outbreaks in NICUs [90,101]. The potential for airborne transmission has been suggested by "cloud babies," described by Eichenwald and colleagues [102], in which the respiratory secretions or desquamated skin from a colonized infant carry *S. aureus* over relatively long distances. "Cloud" health care workers also have been described; in such cases, the point source of an outbreak was determined to be a colonized health care worker with a viral respiratory infection [94,103]. Parents can also transmit MRSA to their newborn infants on passage through a colonized birth canal or postpartum handling [104,105].

The emergence of vancomycin-resistant enterococci (VRE) is a concern in all hospital settings, and several VRE outbreaks have been reported in NICUs [106,107]. In neonates, VRE seem to cause clinical syndromes indistinguishable from syndromes caused by susceptible enterococci [50]. Vancomycin use, which is especially prevalent in the NICU, has increased markedly and has probably contributed to the growing prevalence of resistant gram-positive organisms in neonatal patients [108]. More recent observations suggest that clinical infections caused by VRE may signal the presence of a larger reservoir of VRE among asymptomatic colonized infants, and some authors have suggested that active surveillance may be required to interrupt ongoing transmission [109,110].

Over the past decade, the array and prevalence of resistant gram-negative organisms have rapidly expanded. Extended-spectrum β-lactamases (ESBLs) are plasmid-mediated resistance factors produced by members of the Enterobacteriaceae family. ESBLs inactivate third-generation cephalosporins and aztreonam. *K. pneumoniae* and *E. coli* are the organisms most commonly recognized as ESBL-producing organisms, but other ESBL-producing gram-negative bacilli are being increasingly identified. NICU outbreaks caused by other ESBL-producing organisms have been identified; transfer of ESBL-carrying plasmids to other Enterobacteriaceae organisms has been shown in several NICU outbreaks [111,112]. Two mechanisms of acquisition of resistant gram-negative organisms have been shown through molecular epidemiologic investigations: patient-to-patient transfer (presumably via contaminated health care worker hands or medical equipment) and de novo emergence as a consequence of antibiotic exposure [113,114].

FUNGI

Candida species are the third most common pathogen identified in patients with late-onset sepsis and are associated with morbidity and mortality rates similar to those observed with sepsis from gram-negative bacteria [115]. More recent reports have also linked neonatal candidiasis to increased neurodevelopmental impairment in infancy [116] and retinopathy of prematurity [117] and have quantified the cost of an episode of candidemia in the NICU to be $28,000 to $39,000 [118,119].

Fridkin and colleagues [120] reported on data from the NNIS network, including 128 NICUs covering 130,523 patients over a 10-year period ending in 2004. Of 1997 cases of candidemia in these patients, 57.9% were *Candida albicans*, 33.7% were *Candida parapsilosis*, 3.8% were *Candida tropicalis*, 2% were *Candida glabrata*, and 0.2% were *Candida krusei*. Over time, there was an overall decrease in candidemia in neonates weighing less than 1000 g, but no change in the distribution of *Candida* species. The combined mortality rate for neonates with candidemia was 13%, which did not significantly differ among infecting species. There was variability, however, with respect to the incidence of candidemia in different NICUs, ranging from 2.4% to 20.4%.

A retrospective cohort study of neonatal candidiasis using the 2003 Kids Inpatient Database reported the incidence of candidiasis at 15 per 10,000 NICU admissions [119]. Two thirds of the cases occurred in neonates with a birth weight of less than 1000 g. Of these patients, neonates with extremely low birth weight were twice as likely to die as propensity-matched neonates with extremely low birth weight without candidiasis. The overall mortality attributable to candidiasis in neonates with extremely low birth weight was 11.9%.

Many risk factors have been associated with neonatal candidemia. Colonization likely precedes infection, and this can occur either vertically (via the maternal genitourinary tract) or horizontally (nosocomial spread). The relative roles of gastrointestinal tract colonization and enteric translocation versus skin surface colonization and catheter-related infection are unclear and not mutually exclusive [121]. A prospective study, including 35 infected neonates, suggested that risk factors for candidemia included gestational age 32 weeks or younger, Apgar score less than 5, shock, disseminated intravascular coagulation, intralipid use, parenteral nutrition, CVCs, H_2 blockers, intubation, and length of stay more than 7 days [35]. Various other studies have largely confirmed or expanded on these results, including two more recent reports. A prospective, multicenter study by Benjamin and coworkers [116] analyzed data from 320 infants with extremely low birth weight and invasive candidiasis and found birth weight less than 750 g, male gender, delayed enteral feeding, and cephalosporin use all to be associated with disease. Cotten and associates [122] reported on 3702 infants with extremely low birth weight in 12 NICUs, linking candidiasis with third-generation cephalosporin use.

Fluconazole prophylaxis at dosage at 3 mg/kg or 6 mg/kg twice weekly reduces rates of candidemia in premature neonates in NICUs that have a high incidence of candidemia [123,124]. Because there are limited safety data on the prolonged use of fluconazole in neonates, the Infectious Diseases Society of America recommends routine fluconazole prophylaxis only for premature infants and infants with the extremely low birth weights in nurseries that have a high incidence of invasive candidiasis [125].

Malassezia species, which are lipophilic yeasts, frequently colonize NICU patients. In one French study, 30 of 54 preterm neonates (56%) became colonized with *Malassezia furfur* [126]. *Malassezia pachydermatis*, a zoonotic organism present on the skin and in the ear canals of healthy dogs and cats, also has been associated with nosocomial outbreaks in NICUs [126,127]. In one report, the outbreak seemed to be linked to colonization of health care workers' pet dogs [126].

Invasive mold infections are a rare cause of nosocomial infection in neonates, but when they occur, they are associated with a high mortality rate. *Aspergillus* infections may manifest as pulmonary, central nervous system, gastrointestinal, or disseminated disease. A cutaneous presentation, with or without subsequent dissemination, seems to be the most common presentation for hospitalized premature infants without underlying immunodeficiency [128,129]. Often, skin maceration is the presumed portal of entry. In a series of four patients who died of disseminated *Aspergillus* infection that started cutaneously, a contaminated device used to collect urine from the male infants was implicated [129]. Similarly, contaminated wooden tongue depressors, used as splints for intravenous and arterial cannulation sites, were associated with cutaneous infection owing to *Rhizopus microsporus* in four premature infants [130]. In addition to preterm birth, use of broad-spectrum antimicrobial agents, steroid therapy, and hyperglycemia are thought to be risk factors for mold infection.

Even zoophilic dermatophytes have been described as a source of nosocomial infection in neonates. In one report, five neonatal cases in one unit were traced to an infected nurse and her cat [131]. Prolonged therapy for the nurse and her cat was necessary to clear their infections.

VIRAL PATHOGENS

Nosocomial viral infections can be a significant problem for neonates [132]. Introduction of common viral pathogens into the NICU can be associated with (1) admission of infants from the community, (2) health care workers who work while ill or infectious, and (3) visitors.

Enteric Viruses

Although many pathogens can cause nosocomial gastroenteritis, rotavirus is responsible for 95% or more of viral infections in high-risk nurseries, including the NICU [22,133]. The clinical picture of rotavirus infections in newborns can vary markedly; there are many reports of asymptomatic rotavirus infection in nurseries [134]. In addition, rotavirus can be manifested as frequent and watery stools in term infants and as abdominal distention and bloody, mucoid stools in preterm neonates [133,135]. A high titer of virus is excreted in stool of infected persons, and the organism is viable on hands and in the environment for relatively prolonged periods [136,137].

Attention to hand hygiene and disinfection of potential fomites are crucial in preventing spread of infection. Rotavirus outbreaks in NICUs have been associated with poor hand hygiene, ill health care workers, and ill visitors [137]. Rotaviruses [138] and other enteric viruses, including norovirus [139], astrovirus [140], and toroviruses [141], have been associated with necrotizing enterocolitis.

Respiratory Viruses

Respiratory viruses, including influenza A virus, parainfluenza virus, coronavirus, respiratory syncytial virus, and adenovirus, have been reported to cause nosocomial infections in NICU patients [142–145]. Associated clinical findings include rhinorrhea, tachypnea, retractions, nasal flaring, rales, and wheezing, but illness can also be manifested as apnea, sepsis-like illness, and gastrointestinal symptoms [137,145–147]. Identified risk factors for acquisition vary from study to study, but have included low birth weight, low gestational age, twin pregnancy, mechanical ventilation, and high CRIB score [143–146]. Contact and droplet transmission are the most common modes of spread of infection—highlighting the importance of scrupulous hand hygiene and adherence to transmission-based precautions.

Enteroviruses

Numerous nursery and NICU outbreaks of enteroviral infection have been reported [148–150]. In a neonate with enteroviral infection, clinical manifestations can range from mild gastroenteritis to a severe and fulminant sepsis-like syndrome or meningitis and encephalitis. The latter presentation can be associated with a high mortality rate [149]. Several outbreak investigations have shown the introduction of enterovirus into a nursery via vertical transmission to an index case, with subsequent horizontal spread [149,151]. Enteroviruses are typically shed in the stool of infected neonates for long periods, providing a reservoir of organisms that can be transmitted when breaches of infection control practices occur.

Cytomegalovirus

Congenital cytomegalovirus (CMV) infection can be asymptomatic or fulminant. Postnatally acquired CMV infections almost always follow a benign course in healthy term infants. Postnatal CMV infection in premature infants can be severe, however, and associated with hepatitis, bone marrow suppression, or pneumonitis [152–154]. The incidence of postnatal CMV infections in preterm infants has decreased significantly with the routine use of CMV-seronegative blood products. At present, most postnatal CMV infections are acquired through breast milk [155]. Approximately one third of infants who are breastfed by mothers with CMV detected in breast milk can develop infection [156]. In one study, approximately 50% of these infants had clinical features of infection, and 12% presented with a sepsis-like syndrome. At present, no proven, highly effective method is available for removing CMV from breast milk without destroying its beneficial components. Some data suggest, however, that freezing breast milk before use may decrease the CMV

titer, limiting subsequent transmission [157]. Person-to-person transmission within the NICU has also been documented [158,159], but the extent to which this occurs is controversial [160]. More detailed information on the clinical features and management of CMV is presented in Chapter 23.

Herpes Simplex Virus

Most neonates with herpes simplex virus (HSV) acquire the infection from their mother, although nursery transmission of HSV infection has been described [161–163]. Although the precise mechanism of transmission remains unclear in some cases, contact transmission has been commonly implicated. Presumed patient-to-patient transmission apparently via the hands of health care workers has been described [163]. Additionally, HSV can frequently be recovered from the hands of parents and health care worker with herpes labialis [164]. Strict attention to hand hygiene is critical to prevent nursery spread of HSV. Health care workers with herpetic whitlow are typically restricted from patient contact until the lesion is healed. An in-depth discussion of the clinical features and management of HSV is provided in Chapter 26.

Varicella-Zoster Virus

With the adoption of varicella vaccine and health care worker screening for varicella immunity, nosocomial transmission of varicella-zoster virus has become rare [165]. Infants at greatest risk are premature infants born at less than 28 weeks of gestation who did not receive transplacental maternal antibodies. Transmission is most likely to occur from an adult with early, unrecognized symptoms of varicella because the virus is excreted in respiratory secretions 24 to 48 hours before onset of the characteristic rash. Management of neonates exposed to and infected with varicella-zoster virus is discussed in Chapter 22.

Hepatitis A

NICU outbreaks of hepatitis A have been reported and have typically been recognized after diagnosis of a symptomatic adult [166–168]. Transmission has been documented via blood transfusion from a donor with acute infection [168]. In addition, indirect patient-to-patient transmission through fomites or health care worker hands can occur when there are subclinical cases (as is typical in neonatal hepatitis A infection) and lapses in the adherence to standard precautions. Neonatal hepatitis is discussed in depth in Chapter 25.

DEVICE-RELATED INFECTIONS
CATHETER-ASSOCIATED BLOODSTREAM INFECTIONS
Epidemiology and Pathogenesis

Bloodstream infections account for a large proportion of all HAIs in NICU patients [18], and most are related to the use of an intravascular catheter [169]. Peripheral intravenous catheters are the most frequently used devices for neonatal patients. When a longer duration of access is necessary, nontunneled CVCs such as umbilical catheters or peripherally inserted central catheters are commonly used [170].

The CDC has tracked rates of HAIs for many years, originally in the NNIS system and more recently in the National Healthcare Safety Network (NHSN). Using standardized definitions, NHSN reported rates of HAIs among 127 participating level III NICUs. Data from 2006–2007 that were published by NHSN revealed that the mean rate of central catheter–associated bloodstream infections ranged from 3.7 per 1000 catheter days for infants with birth weights less than 750 g to 2 per 1000 catheter days for infants with birth weights greater than 2500 g. Rates of umbilical catheter–associated bloodstream infections were 4.7 per 1000 catheter days for infants with birth weights less than 750 g and 1 per 1000 catheter days for infants with birth weights greater than 2500 g (Table 35–3) [171].

The origins of invasive organisms in neonates with catheter-associated bloodstream infections are often debated. Molecular analysis has show that most CoNS isolated from neonates with catheter-associated bloodstream infections are concordant with isolates recovered from lumens of catheter hubs, suggesting that many of these episodes of infection may be a consequence of intraluminal contamination, potentially associated with inadequate disinfection before catheter access [172]. Contamination of the catheter exit site has also been identified as a mechanism of infection in pediatric and adult patients. Finally, infusion of contaminated fluids, medications, or blood products can also give rise to catheter-associated bloodstream infections.

Prevention and Control

Several advisory groups, including the CDC, the Vermont-Oxford Collaborative, and the Infectious Diseases Society of America, have published detailed recommendations of strategies to reduce the incidence of catheter-associated bloodstream infections that strike a balance between patient safety and cost-effectiveness [169,173,174]. A compendium of strategies to prevent specific HAIs has been endorsed

TABLE 35–4 Evidence-Based Strategies to Prevent Catheter-Associated Bloodstream Infections

Conduct surveillance for catheter-associated bloodstream infections (B-II)
Educate health care workers who insert and maintain catheters (A-II)
Use checklist to ensure adherence to proper practices during insertion (B-II)
Perform hand hygiene before catheter insertion (B-II)
Use a catheter cart or kit that contains all necessary materials for catheter insertion (B-II)
Adhere to maximal sterile barrier precautions during catheter insertion (A-I)
Disinfect skin with appropriate antiseptic before catheter insertion and during dressing changes (A-I)
Povidone-iodine solution recommended for infants <2 mo and for infants with nonintact skin
2% chlorhexidine-based preparation preferred for all infants >2 mo
Disinfect catheter hubs and needleless connectors before accessing catheter (B-II)
Remove nonessential catheters promptly (A-II)
Perform dressing changes every 7 days or more frequently if dressing loose or soiled (A-I)

Adapted from Marschall J, et al. Strategies to prevent central line-associated bloodstream infections in acute care hospitals. Infect Control Hosp Epidemiol 29(Suppl 1):S22–S30, 2008.

by the Society of Healthcare Epidemiologists of America and the Infectious Diseases Society of America and includes detailed information on strategies to prevent catheter-associated bloodstream infections (Table 35–4) [174]. A key strategy to minimize the risk of catheter-associated bloodstream infections is the prompt removal of indwelling catheters when no longer medically necessary. Practices such as early enteral feeding and rapid conversion to oral medications whenever possible can shorten the length of time a patient requires a catheter. Finally, participation in quality improvement activities focused on improved hand hygiene and better adherence to best practices for catheter placement and maintenance has been shown to reduce the rate of catheter-associated bloodstream infections in NICUs [175].

Evidence-based guidelines for the prevention catheter-associated bloodstream infections in all patient populations recommend to avoid catheter placement in the groin because of a higher risk of infection [169]. More recent data in neonatal patients have shown, however, that catheter placement in the lower extremity is not associated with an increased risk of infection in neonates [176]. Umbilical veins and arteries are available for CVC insertion only in neonates. The umbilicus provides a site that can be cannulated easily, allowing for collection of blood specimens and hemodynamic measurements, but soon after birth, the umbilicus becomes heavily colonized with skin flora and other microorganisms. Nonetheless, rates of catheter colonization and catheter-associated bloodstream infections attributable to umbilical catheters are similar to rates associated with other types of CVC. Colonization rates for umbilical artery catheters are estimated to be 40% to 55%; the estimated rate for umbilical artery catheter–related bloodstream infection is 5% [169].

TABLE 35–3 Rates of Catheter-Associated Bloodstream Infection by Birth Weight Category*

	Pooled Mean	
Birth Weight (g)	**Umbilical CA-BSI[†]**	**Non–Umbilical CA-BSI[‡]**
≤750	4	3.7
751–1000	2.6	3.3
1001–1500	1.9	2.6
1501–2500	0.9	2.4
>2500	1	1

Neonatal intensive care unit component of reported data, 2006–2007
[†]*No. umbilical catheter–associated (CA) bloodstream infections (BSIs) × 1000/No. umbilical and catheter days.*
[‡]*No. non–umbilical central catheter–associated (CA) bloodstream infections (BSIs) × 1000/No. umbilical and catheter days.*
Adapted from Edwards JR, et al. National Healthcare Safety Network (NHSN) Report, data summary for 2006 through 2007, issued November 2008. Am J Infect Control 36:609–626, 2008.

Colonization rates are 22% to 59% for umbilical vein catheters; rates for umbilical vein catheter–related bloodstream infections are 3% to 8% [169].

Careful skin antisepsis before insertion of an intravascular catheter is crucial to prevention of intravascular device–related bacteremia. The CDC recommends chlorhexidine-based preparations because these products have been found to be superior to povidone-iodine in reducing the risk of catheter colonization (a recognized surrogate marker of catheter-associated bloodstream infections). Although not approved by the U.S. Food and Drug Administration (FDA) for use in infants younger than 2 months of age, some NICUs have reported the off-label use of this product [177].

Antiseptic solutions "locked" into a catheter lumen have been investigated as a strategy to prevent or treat catheter-associated bloodstream infections in adult patients; only a few studies have been performed in patients younger than 1 year of age. In a study performed in a community level III nursery, high-risk infants (infants with very low birth weight and others with critical illnesses) were randomly assigned to have a newly placed peripherally inserted central catheter "locked" several times a day with either a vancomycin-heparin solution or a heparin-only solution. The investigators noted a significant reduction in the incidence of catheter-related bloodstream infections (relative risk 0.13; 95% confidence intervals 0.01 to 0.57) [178]. A single-center randomized clinical trial of fusidic acid–heparin solutions infused and held within a catheter lumen was associated with a significant reduction in the incidence of catheter-associated bloodstream infections (6.6 versus 24.9 per 1000 catheter days; $P < .01$; relative risk 0.28; 95% confidence interval 0.13 to 0.60). The high rate of catheter-associated bloodstream infections in the control group of infants suggests that this intervention might not be beneficial in settings that have already achieved low infection rates [179]. Because many NICUs achieve substantial reductions in the rates of catheter-associated bloodstream infections through application of other evidence-based practices, the role of antiseptic lock solutions needs further investigation.

In 2008, a Cochrane review examined whether prophylactic systemic antibiotics prevented neonatal infection or death. Through systematic review of the published literature, the investigators found only three small studies that evaluated this question. Although the authors observed that use of prophylactic systemic antibiotics was associated with a decreased risk of bloodstream infections, they concluded that this practice could not be recommended because there was no significant difference in overall mortality, and there were significant safety concerns related to the possible selection of resistant organisms [180].

Other strategies that are commonly used by clinicians caring for adult patients are not commonly used to prevent catheter-associated bloodstream infections in NICU patients. Although antiseptic-impregnated catheters are recommended for adult patients [169], these catheters are not available in sizes small enough for neonates. In addition, although the CDC recommends changing the insertion site of peripheral intravenous catheters at least every 72 to 96 hours in adults, data suggest that leaving peripheral intravenous catheters in place in pediatric patients does not increase the risk of complications [181]. The 2002 CDC guidelines recommend that peripheral intravenous catheters be left in place in children until therapy is completed, unless complications occur [169].

VENTILATOR-ASSOCIATED PNEUMONIA

Epidemiology and Pathogenesis

Health care–associated pneumonia is the second most common HAI in NICU patients; most of these cases are VAP. Neonatal VAP has been associated with increased direct costs and prolonged length of hospitalization [182]. Gram-negative organisms are the most commonly recovered pathogens from tracheal specimens of patients with VAP [182].

The pathogenesis of VAP is most commonly attributed to one of three different mechanisms: aspiration of secretions, colonization of the aerodigestive tract, or use of contaminated equipment [183]. Specific risk factors for VAP are associated with these basic pathogenic mechanisms and include host characteristics (prematurity, low birth weight, sedation, or use of paralytic agents), exposure to medical devices (endotracheal intubation, mechanical ventilation, orogastric or nasogastric tube placement), and factors that increase bacterial colonization of the aerodigestive tract (broad-spectrum antimicrobial agents, antacids, or H_2 blockers) [182,184–186].

Prevention and Control

Few studies have been performed to assess the effectiveness of VAP prevention strategies in pediatric patients; most commonly used strategies to prevent VAP in NICU patients are based on studies performed in adults. In 2008, infectious disease experts and hospital epidemiologists published a broad review entitled, "Strategies to Prevent Ventilator-Associated Pneumonia in Acute Care Hospitals." This document should serve as a guideline for NICUs working to reduce the rate of VAP in their patients; Table 35–5 provides a summary of these recommendations [183]. The core recommendations are designed to interrupt the three most common mechanisms by which VAP typically develops. An obvious, but key, component of VAP prevention is to minimize the use of invasive mechanical ventilation. This can be accomplished

TABLE 35–5   Evidence-Based Strategies to Prevent Ventilator-Associated Pneumonia

Conduct surveillance for ventilator-associated pneumonia (A-II)
Educate health care workers who care for ventilated patients (A-II)
Implement practices for disinfection, sterilization, and maintenance of respiratory equipment (A-II)
Perform regular oral care (A-I)
Ensure patients are maintained in semirecumbent position, unless medical contraindication exists (B-II)
Promote use of noninvasive ventilation when possible (B-III)

Adapted from Coffin SE, et al. Strategies to prevent ventilator-associated pneumonia in acute care hospitals. Infect Control Hosp Epidemiol 29(Suppl 1):S31–S40, 2008.

by the use of weaning protocols, daily sedation vacations to assess readiness to wean, and increased use of noninvasive ventilation [187,188].

Practices designed to minimize aspiration of pathogenic organisms include performing regular oral care (even in the absence of teeth), patient positioning in a semirecumbent angle, avoiding gastric overdistention, and avoiding unplanned extubations. A single-center study showed delayed onset of tracheal colonization in intubated infants who were positioned on their side; however, no studies have shown a clear reduction in neonatal VAP associated with strict adherence to this practice [189]. Appropriate placement of enteral feeding tubes should be verified before their use [190,191]. To prevent regurgitation and potential aspiration of stomach contents by a sedated patient, overdistention of the stomach should be avoided by regular monitoring of the patient's intestinal motility, serial measurement of residual gastric volume or abdominal girth, reducing the use of narcotics and anticholinergic agents, and adjusting the rate and volume of enteral feedings [190,191]. Oral decontamination, with the intent of decreasing oropharyngeal colonization, has been studied in adults and seems to reduce the incidence of VAP [192,193]. Many NICUs have already adopted regular oral care as a component of their VAP prevention activities.

Finally, avoidance of H_2 blocking agents and proton pump inhibitors in patients without a high risk of stress gastritis may reduce the risk of VAP by minimizing the density of bacterial colonization of the stomach [194]. Two small studies performed in pediatric patients failed to show a significant benefit; however, the authors stressed that additional studies with larger sample sizes are needed to confirm these findings [195,196]. Further studies are needed to define the most important VAP prevention strategies for young infants and to determine the relative contribution of each of these strategies in neonates.

Careful attention to the appropriate disinfection and reprocessing of reusable components of respiratory care equipment is also important [197]. In addition, circuits should be monitored for the accumulation of condensate and drained periodically, with care taken to avoid allowing the condensate, a potential reservoir for pathogens, to drain toward the patient [191]. Other basic infection control measures, such as hand hygiene and standard precautions, can also reduce the risk of VAP and other types of nosocomial pneumonia and are generally recommended for all ventilated patients [183].

CATHETER-ASSOCIATED URINARY TRACT INFECTIONS

Nosocomial urinary tract infections are commonly identified as the most common cause of HAIs in adults [198]; however, data from NHSN and single-center studies suggest that the incidence of catheter-associated urinary tract infections among hospitalized neonates is significantly lower than observed in adults [171,199]. Gram-negative organisms, yeast, and enterococci are the most frequently reported pathogens [199]. Risk factors that have been specifically identified in young children include prolonged catheterization and young age [199,200]. Although few studies have prospectively evaluated strategies to prevent catheter-associated urinary tract infections in neonates, implementation of the strategies outlined in the document "Strategies to Prevent Catheter-Associated Urinary Tract Infections" is recommended [198].

VENTRICULAR SHUNT–ASSOCIATED INFECTIONS

Premature infants are at significant risk of intraventricular hemorrhage and may require temporary or permanent diversion of cerebrospinal fluid to manage obstructive hydrocephalus. Placement of cerebrospinal fluid shunts is associated with a significant risk of postoperative infections, either ventriculitis or more superficial surgical site infections. Premature births, prior shunt placement, breeches in aseptic technique during shunt placement, and use of a neuroendoscope have been identified as risk factors for shunt infections [201,202]. Use of antimicrobial-impregnated suture material and shunt catheters are currently being evaluated as possible strategies to reduce the risk of these infections [203–205].

PREVENTING TRANSMISSION OF HEALTH CARE–ASSOCIATED INFECTIONS

An effective infection control program that focuses on reducing risk on a prospective basis can decrease the incidence of HAIs [206,207]. The principal function of such a program is to protect the infant and the health care worker from risk of HAI in a manner that is cost-effective. Activities crucial to achieving and maintaining this goal include collection and management of critical data relating to surveillance for nosocomial infection and direct intervention to interrupt the transmission of infectious diseases [19].

SURVEILLANCE

Surveillance is an essential component of infection prevention programs. The definitions provided by the CDC have been widely adopted and provide specific definitions and data collection for the NICU population [208–210]. These definitions do not distinguish, however, late-onset infections caused by transplacentally acquired organisms (e.g., group B streptococcus infections) from more typical nosocomial infections [210]. Distinction between maternal and hospital sources of infection is important, although difficult at times, because control measures designed to prevent acquisition from hospital sources would be ineffective in preventing perinatal acquisition of pathogens [211]. Surveillance for infections in healthy newborns also is challenging because of the typically short length of stay. Infections can develop after discharge, and these are more difficult for infection control practitioners to capture. Methods for postdischarge surveillance have been developed, but because most neonatal infections that occur after discharge are noninvasive [212], such surveillance has not been widely implemented owing to concerns about the cost-effectiveness of these labor-intensive processes.

Surveillance data must be analyzed and presented in a way that facilitates interpretation, comparison directed internally and with comparable external benchmarks, and dissemination within the organization. Quality improvement tools (e.g., control and run charts) can be useful for these purposes. Statistical tools should be used to determine the significance of findings, although statistical significance should always be balanced with the evaluation of clinical significance [213]. External benchmarking through interhospital comparison is a valuable tool for improving quality of care [214,215], but should be performed only when surveillance methodologies (e.g., case definitions, case finding, data collection methods, intensity of surveillance) [213] can reasonably be assumed to be consistent between facilities.

Infection data must be shared with personnel who can effect change and implement infection control interventions. Written reports summarizing the data and appropriate control charts should be provided to the facility's infection control committee, unit leaders, and members of the hospital administration on an ongoing basis. The interval between reports is determined by the needs of the institution. In addition to formal written reports, face-to-face reports are appropriate in the event of identification of a serious problem or an outbreak. Infection control practitioners can serve as consultants to assist NICU or neonatology service leaders in addressing infection rate increases or outbreak management.

More recently, controversy has emerged over the use of active surveillance cultures to identify infants colonized with multidrug-resistant organisms. Although many adult ICUs have begun to screen all patients routinely on admission for carriage of various multidrug-resistant organisms, this practice has not yet been consistently adopted by NICUs. Factors such as the perceived low rate of carriage of resistant organisms by infants have undoubtedly led some neonatologists to question the need for universal screening on NICU admission. Data have shown, however, that a significant reservoir of resistant organisms can exist in hospitalized neonates. After two patients developed clinical infections owing to VRE, surveillance cultures revealed that more than 15% of other patients in the same unit had unsuspected VRE colonization [109,110].

Some units have adopted regularly scheduled point prevalence surveys as an alternative strategy to universal surveillance. Point prevalence surveys are most useful in units with a known low prevalence of multidrug-resistant organisms and can be used for early detection of increasing rates of carriage of multidrug-resistant organisms. Some NICUs have used active surveillance for carriage of multidrug-resistant organisms to guide programs that have led to the successful eradication of MRSA [216].

STANDARD AND TRANSMISSION-BASED PRECAUTIONS IN THE NURSERY

The most widely accepted guideline for preventing the transmission of infections in hospitals was developed by the CDC [217]. Updated in 2007, the guideline recommends using two tiers of precautions. The first and most important, standard precautions, was designed for the management of all hospitalized patients regardless of their diagnosis or presumed infection status. The second,

transmission-based precautions, is intended for patients documented or suspected to be infected or colonized with highly transmissible or epidemiologically important pathogens for which additional precautions to interrupt transmission are needed.

Standard Precautions

Standard precautions are designed to reduce the risk of transmission of microorganisms from recognized and unrecognized sources and are to be followed for the care of all patients, including neonates. They apply to blood; all body fluids, secretions, and excretions except sweat; nonintact skin; and mucous membranes. Components of standard precautions include hand hygiene and wearing gloves, gowns, and masks and other forms of eye protection.

Hand Hygiene

Hand hygiene plays a key role for caregivers in the reduction of nosocomial infection for patients [26,218] and in prevention of HAIs. Hand hygiene should be performed before and after all patient contacts; before donning sterile gloves to perform an invasive procedure; after contact with blood, body fluids or excretions, mucous membranes, nonintact skin, and wound dressings; in moving from a contaminated body site to a clean body site during patient care (i.e., from changing a diaper to performing mouth care); after contact with inanimate objects in the immediate vicinity of the patient; after removing gloves; and before eating and after using the restroom [88]. When hands are visibly soiled or contaminated with proteinaceous materials, blood, or body fluids and after using the restroom, hands should be washed with soap and water.

When hands are not visibly soiled, alcohol-based hand rubs, foams, or gels are an important tool for hand hygiene. Compared with washing with soap and water, use of the alcohol-based products is at least as effective against a variety of pathogens and requires less time, and these agents are less damaging to skin. The CDC "Guideline for Hand Hygiene in the Health Care Setting" calls for use of alcohol hand rubs, foams, or gels as the primary method to clean hands except when hands are visibly soiled [88]. Specific activities that have been independently associated with increased density of pathogens on health care worker hands include skin contact, respiratory care, and diaper changes. Additionally, investigators have shown that the use of gloves during these activities does not fully protect health care workers' hands from bacterial contamination [219]. Programs that have been successful in improving hand hygiene and decreasing nosocomial infection have used multidisciplinary teams to develop interventions focusing on use of the alcohol rubs in the setting of institutional commitment and support for the initiative [26,220,221].

Health care workers should wash hands and forearms to the elbows on arrival in the nursery. A 3-minute scrub has been suggested [67], but consensus on optimal duration of initial hand hygiene is lacking. At a minimum, the initial wash should be long enough to ensure thorough washing and rinsing of all parts of the hands and forearms. Routine hand washing throughout care delivery should consist of wetting the hands, applying product, rubbing all surfaces of the hands and fingers vigorously for at least 15 seconds, rinsing, and patting dry with disposable towels [88]. Wearing hand jewelry has been associated with increased microbial load on hands; whether this results in increased transmission of pathogens is unknown. Many experts recommend, however, that hand and wrist jewelry not be worn in the nursery [222,223]. In addition, the CDC guideline states that staff who have direct contact with infants in NICUs should not wear artificial fingernails or nail extenders [88]. Only natural nails kept less than ¼ inch long should be allowed; at least one outbreak in an NICU was associated with a health care worker who wore artificial nails [224].

Gloves

Clean, nonsterile gloves are to be worn whenever contact with blood, body fluids, secretions, excretions, and contaminated items is anticipated. The health care worker should change gloves when moving from dirty to clean tasks performed on the same patient, such as after changing a diaper and before suctioning a patient, and whenever they become soiled. Because hands can become contaminated during removal of gloves, and because gloves may have tiny, unnoticeable defects, wearing gloves is not a substitute for hand hygiene. Hand hygiene must be performed immediately after glove removal [23].

Gowns

Personnel in nurseries including the NICU historically have worn cover gowns for all routine patient contact. The practice has not been found to reduce infection or colonization in neonates and is unnecessary [225,226]. Instead, CDC guidelines recommend nonsterile, fluid-resistant gowns to be worn as barrier protection when soiling of clothing is anticipated and in performing procedures likely to result in splashing or spraying of body substances [23]. Possible examples of such procedures in the NICU are placing an arterial line and irrigating a wound. The Perinatal Guidelines of the American Academy of Pediatrics and the American College of Obstetricians and Gynecologists recommend that a long-sleeved gown be worn over clothing when a neonate is held outside the bassinette by nursery personnel [67].

Masks

Nonsterile masks, face shields, goggles, and other eye protectors are worn in various combinations to provide barrier protection and should be used during procedures and patient care activities that are likely to generate splashes or sprays of body substances and fluids [23].

Other Standard Precautions

Standard precautions also require that reusable patient care equipment be cleaned and appropriately reprocessed between patients; that soiled linen be handled carefully to prevent contamination of skin, clothing, or the environment; that sharps (i.e., needles, scalpels) be handled carefully to prevent exposure to blood-borne pathogens; and that mouthpieces and other resuscitation devices be used rather than mouth-to-mouth methods of resuscitation [23].

Transmission-Based Precautions

In addition to standard precautions, which must be used for every patient, the CDC recommends transmission-based precautions when the patient is known or suspected to be infected or colonized with epidemiologically important or highly transmissible organisms. Always used in addition to standard precautions, transmission-based precautions comprise three categories: contact precautions, droplet precautions, and airborne precautions.

Contact Precautions

Contact precautions involve the use of barriers to prevent transmission of organisms by direct or indirect contact with the patient or contaminated objects in the patient's immediate environment [23]. Sources of indirect contact transmission in nurseries include monitor leads, thermometers, isolettes, breast pumps [227], toys, and contaminated hands [208].

Ideally, a patient requiring contact precautions should be placed in a private room. Many nurseries have few if any isolation rooms, however. Cohorting of patients infected with the same microorganism can be a safe and effective alternative [23]. The American Academy of Pediatrics states that infected neonates requiring contact precautions can be safely cared for without an isolation room if staffing is adequate to allow appropriate hand hygiene, a 4- to 6-foot-wide space can be provided between care stations, adequate hand hygiene facilities are available, and staff members are well trained regarding infection transmission modes [67].

Health care workers should wear clean, nonsterile gloves when entering the room or space of a patient requiring contact precautions and should wear a cover gown when their clothing will have contact with the infant, environmental surfaces, or items in the infant's area. A cover gown also should be worn when the infant has excretions or secretions that are not well contained, such as diarrhea or wound drainage, which may escape the diaper or dressing. Infant care equipment should be dedicated to the patient if possible so that it is not shared with others [23]. Examples of conditions in the neonate that require contact precautions include neonatal mucocutaneous HSV infection, respiratory syncytial virus infection, varicella (also see airborne precautions), and infection or colonization with a resistant organism such as MRSA.

Droplet Precautions

Droplet precautions are intended to reduce the risk of transmission of infectious agents in large-particle droplets from an infected person. Such transmission usually occurs when the infected person generates droplets during coughing, sneezing, or talking or during procedures such as suctioning. These relatively large droplets travel only short distances and do not remain suspended in the air and can be deposited on the conjunctiva, nasal mucosa, or mouth of persons working within 3 feet of the infected patient [23]. Patients requiring droplet precautions should be placed in private rooms (see earlier discussion of isolation rooms in nurseries in the section on contact precautions), and staff should wear masks when working within 3 feet of the patient [23]. Examples of conditions in the neonate that necessitate droplet precautions are pertussis and invasive *Neisseria meningitidis* infection.

Airborne Precautions

Airborne precautions are designed to reduce the risk of airborne transmission of infectious agents [23]. Because of their small size, airborne droplet nuclei and dust particles containing infectious agents or spores can be widely spread on air currents or through ventilation systems and inhaled by or deposited on susceptible hosts. Special air-handling systems and ventilation are required to prevent transmission. Patients requiring airborne precautions should be placed in private rooms in negative air-pressure ventilation with 6 to 12 air changes per hour. Air should be externally exhausted or subjected to high-efficiency particulate air (HEPA) filtration if it is recirculated [208].

Examples of conditions in neonates for which airborne precautions are required are varicella-zoster virus infections and measles. Susceptible health care workers should not enter the rooms of patients with these viral infections. If assignment cannot be avoided, susceptible staff members should wear masks to deliver care. If immunity has been documented, staff members need not wear masks [208]. Airborne precautions also are required for active pulmonary tuberculosis, and although neonates are rarely contagious, the CDC recommends isolating patients while they are being evaluated [228]. A more important consideration is the need to isolate the family of a suspected tuberculosis patient until an evaluation for pulmonary tuberculosis has been completed because the source of infection frequently is a member of the child's family [229,230].

OTHER RELATED ISSUES
HEALTH CARE WORKERS

Health care workers caring for neonates have the potential to transmit or to acquire infections while providing care to infant patients. Health care workers are at high risk of acquiring respiratory syncytial virus when caring for infected children and can subsequently spread infection to other patients [231–233]. Generally, health care workers with respiratory, cutaneous, mucocutaneous, or gastrointestinal infections should not deliver direct patient care to neonates [234]. In addition, nonimmune staff members exposed to highly communicable diseases, such as varicella and measles, should not work during the contagious portion of the incubation period [235]. In contrast, staff members with HSV infection rarely have been implicated in transmission of HSV to infants and do not need to be routinely excluded from direct patient care. Lesions should be covered, and health care workers should be instructed not to touch their lesions and to practice excellent hand hygiene.

Acquisition of CMV often is a concern of pregnant health care workers because of the potential effect on the fetus. The prevalence of asymptomatic CMV secretion is approximately 1% among infants in most nurseries [208]. Because the risk of acquiring CMV infection is the same for health care workers compared with the general population, pregnant caregivers can safely provide care to neonates who are shedding CMV.

Nurse-to-patient ratios have been inversely correlated with the rates of nosocomial infections and mortality [42,236,237]. Although optimal staffing ratios have not been established for NICUs and vary according to characteristics of individual units and patients, one study showed that the incidence of clustered *S. aureus* infections was 16 times higher after periods when the infant-to-nurse ratio exceeded 7:1. Decreased compliance with hand hygiene during a period of understaffing has been associated with increased rates of nosocomial infection [75].

FAMILY-CENTERED CARE

Family-centered care has emerged as a guiding principle of pediatric health care. In the NICU, health care workers often encourage parents to become involved in the nonmedical aspects of their infant's care. Principles of family-centered care also include liberal NICU visitation for relatives, siblings, and family friends and the involvement of parents in the development of nursery policies and programs that promote parenting skills [238]. The benefits of family-centered care can be undermined by an increased risk of infection for the neonatal patient. Mothers can transmit infections to neonates postpartum, although separation of mother and newborn rarely is indicated. To ensure the risk of postpartum transmission is minimal, all mothers should wash their hands before handing their infants. For mothers with postpartum fever, care should be taken to ensure that the infant does not come into contact with contaminated dressings, linen, clothing, or pads [234].

Mothers with other infections can also safely visit their infants. Mothers with active herpes labialis should not kiss or nuzzle their infants until lesions have cleared; lesions should be covered, and a surgical mask may be worn until the lesions are crusted and dry. The importance of hand hygiene should be emphasized. Mothers with viral respiratory infections should be educated about how to interrupt transmission of these pathogens. Strategies such as covering a cough, prompt disposal of used tissues, and scrupulous hand hygiene should be taught before visiting. In addition, masks can be worn to reduce the risk of droplet transmission [234,235].

As previously mentioned, a few infections do require brief separations of mother and infant. Women with untreated active pulmonary tuberculosis should be separated from their infants until they no longer are contagious. Mothers with group A streptococcal infections, especially if a draining wound is present, also should be isolated from their infants until they are no longer contagious.

BREAST-FEEDING

Numerous studies support the value of human milk for infants (see Chapter 5). Breast milk provides optimal nutritional content for infants, and breast-fed infants experience fewer episodes of infection and sepsis during the 1st year of life [15,239]. There are, however, several infectious contraindications to breast-feeding; mothers who have active untreated tuberculosis, human immunodeficiency virus (HIV) infection (except in countries where the risk of not breast-feeding outweighs the potential risk of HIV transmission [see Chapters 5 and 21]), breast abscesses (as opposed to simple mastitis that is being treated with antimicrobial therapy), or HSV lesions around the nipples should not breast-feed. In contrast, mothers who are positive for hepatitis B surface antigen may safely breast-feed their infants because ingestion of infected milk has not been shown to increase the risk of transmission to an infant who has received hepatitis B virus immunoglobulin and vaccine immediately after birth [240].

Transmission of CMV has been observed in preterm infants who receive breast milk of CMV-seropositive mothers, presumably owing to the infant's low titers of anti-CMV antibody. Decisions regarding breast-feeding should weigh the benefits of human milk and the risk of CMV transmission. Freezing breast milk has been shown to decrease viral titers, but does not eliminate CMV; pasteurization of human milk can inactivate CMV (see Chapter 5). Either method may be considered in attempts to decrease risk of transmission for breast-feeding NICU neonates [241].

Neonates in the NICU frequently are incapable of breast-feeding because of maternal separation, unstable respiratory status, and immaturity of the sucking reflex. For these reasons, mothers of such infants must use a breast pump to collect milk for administration through a feeding tube. Pumping, collection, and storage of breast milk create opportunities for contamination of the milk and for cross-infection if equipment is shared among mothers. Several studies have shown contamination of breast pumps, contamination of expressed milk that had been frozen and thawed, and higher levels of stool colonization with aerobic bacteria in infants fed precollected breast milk [15,179,242,243]. Mothers who are able to pump or express their breast milk should be taught optimal collection, storage, and administration techniques. Cleaning and disinfection of breast pumps should be included in educational material provided to nursing mothers. In addition, mothers should be instructed to perform hand hygiene and cleanse nipples with cotton and plain water before expressing milk in sterile containers [211,241].

Expressed breast milk can be refrigerated for 48 hours and can be safely frozen ($-20°$ C $\pm 2°$ C [$-4°$ F $\pm 3.6°$ F]) for 6 months [211]. Vessels containing frozen breast milk can be thawed quickly under warm running water (avoiding contamination with tap water) or gradually in a refrigerator. Exposure to high temperatures, as may be experienced in a microwave, can destroy valuable components of the milk. Thawed breast milk can be stored in the refrigerator for 24 hours before it must be discarded. To avoid proliferation of microorganisms, milk administered through a feeding tube by continuous infusion should hang no longer than 4 to 6 hours before replacement of the milk, container, and tubing [234].

VISITORS

The principles of family-centered care encourage liberal visitation policies in the well-infant nursery (or rooming-in scenario) and in the NICU. Parents, including fathers, should be allowed unlimited visitation to their newborns, and siblings should be allowed liberal visitation. Expanding the number of visitors to neonates may increase the risk of disease exposure, however, if education and screening for symptoms of infection are not implemented. Written policies should be in place to guide sibling visits, and parents should be encouraged to share the responsibility of protecting their newborn from contagious illnesses.

Adult visitors to neonates, including parents, have been implicated in outbreaks of infections including *P. aeruginosa* infection, pertussis, and *Salmonella* infection [236,244,245]. The principles for sibling visitation should be applied to adult visitors as well. Visitors should be screened for symptoms of contagious illness, should be instructed to perform hand hygiene before entering the NICU and before and after touching the neonate, and should interact only with the family member they came to the hospital to visit. Families of neonates who have lengthy NICU stays may come to know each other well and serve as sources of emotional support to one another. Nevertheless, they should be educated about the potential of transmitting microorganisms and infections between families if standard precautions and physical separation are not maintained, even though they may be sharing an inpatient space.

SKIN AND CORD CARE

Bathing the newborn is standard practice in nurseries, but very little standardization in frequency or cleansing product exists. If not performed carefully, bathing can be detrimental to the infant, resulting in hypothermia, increased crying with resulting increases in oxygen consumption, respiratory distress, and instability of vital signs [177]. Although the initial bath or cleansing should be delayed until the neonate's temperature has been stable for several hours, removing blood and drying the skin immediately after delivery may remove potentially infectious microorganisms such as hepatitis B virus, HSV, and HIV, minimizing risk to the neonate from maternal infection [234]. When the newborn requires an intramuscular injection in the delivery room, infection sites should be cleansed with alcohol to prevent transmission of organisms that may be present in maternal blood and body fluids [170]. For routine bathing in the first few weeks of life, plain warm water should be used. This is especially important for preterm infants and full-term infants with barrier compromise such as abrasions or dermatitis. If a soap is necessary for heavily soiled areas, a mild pH-neutral product without additives should be used, and duration of soaping should be restricted to less than 5 minutes no more than three times per week [177].

Few randomized studies comparing cord care regimens and infection rates have been performed, and consensus has not been reached on best practice regarding care of the umbilical cord stump. A review published in 2003 described care regimens used for more than 2 decades, including combinations of triple dye, chlorhexidine, 70% alcohol, bacitracin, hexachlorophene, povidone-iodine, and "dry care" (soap and water cleansing of soiled periumbilical skin), and found variable impact on colonization of the stump [246]. The study authors suggested that dry cord care alone may be insufficient and that chlorhexidine seemed to be a favorable antiseptic choice for cord care because of its activity against gram-positive and gram-negative bacteria. They went on to stress, however, that large, well-designed studies were required before firm conclusions could be drawn. The current Perinatal Guidelines do not recommend a specific regimen, but warn that use of alcohol alone is not an effective method of preventing umbilical cord colonization and omphalitis [241]. The Perinatal Guidelines further recommend that diapers be folded away from and below the stump and that emollients not be applied to the stump [177].

REFERENCES

[1] N. Zafar, et al., Improving survival of vulnerable infants increases neonatal intensive care unit nosocomial infection rate, Arch. Pediatr. Adolesc. Med. 155 (2001) 1098–1104.

[2] E. Nagata, A.S. Brito, T.L. Matsuo, Nosocomial infections in a neonatal intensive care unit: incidence and risk factors, Am. J. Infect. Control 30 (2002) 26–31.

[3] N.R. Payne, et al., Marginal increase in cost and excess length of stay associated with nosocomial bloodstream infections in surviving very low birth weight infants, Pediatrics 114 (2004) 348–355.

[4] S. Bektas, B. Goetze, C.P. Speer, Decreased adherence, chemotaxis and phagocytic activities of neutrophils from preterm neonates, Acta Paediatr. Scand. 79 (1990) 1031–1038.

[5] J. Kallman, et al., Impaired phagocytosis and opsonisation towards group B streptococci in preterm neonates, Arch. Dis. Child. Fetal. Neonatal. Ed. 78 (1998) F46–F50.

[6] E.R. Stiehm, The physiologic immunodeficiency of immaturity, in: E.R. Stiehm (Ed.), Immunologic Disorders in Infants and Children, Saunders, Philadelphia, 1986.

[7] D.A. Goldmann, J. Leclair, A. Macone, Bacterial colonization of neonates admitted to an intensive care environment, J. Pediatr. 93 (1978) 288–293.

[8] K. Sprunt, Practical use of surveillance for prevention of nosocomial infection, Semin. Perinatol. 9 (1985) 47–50.

[9] R. Bennet, et al., Fecal bacterial microflora of newborn infants during intensive care management and treatment with five antibiotic regimens, Pediatr. Infect. Dis. 5 (1986) 533–539.

[10] S.L. Hall, et al., Evaluation of coagulase-negative staphylococcal isolates from serial nasopharyngeal cultures of premature infants, Diagn. Microbiol. Infect. Dis. 13 (1990) 17–23.

[11] B. Fryklund, et al., Importance of the environment and the faecal flora of infants, nursing staff and parents as sources of gram-negative bacteria colonizing newborns in three neonatal wards, Infection 20 (1992) 253–257.

[12] C.L. Pessoa-Silva, et al., Extended-spectrum beta-lactamase-producing *Klebsiella pneumoniae* in a neonatal intensive care unit: risk factors for infection and colonization, J. Hosp. Infect. 53 (2003) 198–206.

[13] L. Saiman, et al., Risk factors for *Candida* species colonization of neonatal intensive care unit patients, Pediatr. Infect. Dis. J. 20 (2001) 1119–1124.

[14] W.R. Jarvis, The epidemiology of colonization, Infect. Control Hosp. Epidemiol. 17 (1996) 47–52.

[15] A.E. el-Mohandes, et al., Use of human milk in the intensive care nursery decreases the incidence of nosocomial sepsis, J. Perinatol. 17 (1997) 130–134.

[16] K.E. Shattuck, et al., Colonization and infection associated with *Malassezia* and *Candida* species in a neonatal unit, J. Hosp. Infect. 34 (1996) 123–129.

[17] R.S. Baltimore, Neonatal nosocomial infections, Semin. Perinatol. 22 (1998) 25–32.

[18] A.H. Sohn, et al., Prevalence of nosocomial infections in neonatal intensive care unit patients: results from the first national point-prevalence survey, J. Pediatr. 139 (2001) 821–827.

[19] W.E. Scheckler, et al., Requirements for infrastructure and essential activities of infection control and epidemiology in hospitals: a consensus panel report. Society for Health Care Epidemiology of America, Am. J. Infect. Control 26 (1998) 47–60.

[20] P.W. Neumann, M. O'Shaughnessy, M. Garnett, Laboratory evidence of human immunodeficiency virus infection in Canada in 1986, Can. Med. Assoc. J. 137 (1987) 823.

[21] Bureau of Communicable Disease Epidemiology, Laboratory Centre for Disease Control, Health and Welfare, Canada, Canadian nosocomial infection surveillance program: annual summary, June 1984-May 1985, Can. Dis. Wkly. Rep. 12 (1986) S1.

[22] R.P. Gaynes, et al., Nosocomial infections among neonates in high-risk nurseries in the United States. National Nosocomial Infections Surveillance System, Pediatrics 98 (1996) 357–361.

[23] J.S. Garner, Guideline for isolation precautions in hospitals. The Hospital Infection Control Practices Advisory Committee, Infect. Control Hosp. Epidemiol. 17 (1996) 53–80.

[24] D. Pittet, et al., Bacterial contamination of the hands of hospital staff during routine patient care, Arch. Intern. Med. 159 (1999) 821–826.

[25] E.L. Larson, et al., A multifaceted approach to changing handwashing behavior, Am. J. Infect. Control 25 (1997) 3–10.

[26] D. Pittet, et al., Effectiveness of a hospital-wide programme to improve compliance with hand hygiene. Infection Control Programme, Lancet 356 (2000) 1307–1312.

[27] D.M. Nguyen, et al., Risk factors for neonatal methicillin-resistant *Staphylococcus aureus* infection in a well-infant nursery, Infect. Control Hosp. Epidemiol. 28 (2007) 406–411.

[28] P. Villari, C. Sarnataro, L. Iacuzio, Molecular epidemiology of *Staphylococcus epidermidis* in a neonatal intensive care unit over a three-year period, J. Clin. Microbiol. 38 (2000) 1740–1746.

[29] C.C. Carlos, et al., Nosocomial *Staphylococcus epidermidis* septicaemia among very low birth weight neonates in an intensive care unit, J. Hosp. Infect. 19 (1991) 201–207.

[30] A.B. Zafar, L.K. Sylvester, S.O. Beidas, *Pseudomonas aeruginosa* infections in a neonatal intensive care unit, Am. J. Infect. Control 30 (2002) 425–429.

[31] V. Rabier, et al., Hand washing soap as a source of neonatal *Serratia marcescens* outbreak, Acta Paediatr. 97 (2008) 1381–1385.

[32] D.K. Richardson, et al., Score for Neonatal Acute Physiology: a physiologic severity index for neonatal intensive care, Pediatrics 91 (1993) 617–623.

[33] The CRIB (Clinical Risk Index for Babies) score: a tool for assessing initial neonatal risk and comparing performance of neonatal intensive care units, The International Neonatal Network, Lancet 342 (1993) 193–198.

[34] D. Sirot, Extended-spectrum plasmid-mediated beta-lactamases, J. Antimicrob. Chemother. 36 (1995) 19–34.

[35] L. Saiman, et al., Risk factors for candidemia in Neonatal Intensive Care Unit patients. The National Epidemiology of Mycosis Survey study group, Pediatr. Infect. Dis. J. 19 (2000) 319–324.

[36] B.J. Stoll, et al., Dexamethasone therapy increases infection in very low birth weight infants, Pediatrics 104 (1999) e63.

[37] L.A. Papile, et al., A multicenter trial of two dexamethasone regimens in ventilator-dependent premature infants, N. Engl. J. Med. 16 (1998) 1112–1118.

[38] C.M. Beck-Sague, et al., Bloodstream infections in neonatal intensive care unit patients: results of a multicenter study, Pediatr. Infect. Dis. J. 13 (1994) 1110–1116.

[39] S.B. Brodie, et al., Occurrence of nosocomial bloodstream infections in six neonatal intensive care units, Pediatr. Infect. Dis. J. 19 (2000) 56–65.

[40] A. Holmes, et al., Risk factors and recommendations for rate stratification for surveillance of neonatal healthcare-associated bloodstream infection, J. Hosp. Infect. 68 (2008) 66–72.

[41] L. Sirota, et al., Effect of lipid emulsion on IL-2 production by mononuclear cells of newborn infants and adults, Acta Paediatr. 86 (1997) 410–413.

[42] J. Tucker, Patient volume, staffing, and workload in relation to risk-adjusted outcomes in a random stratified sample of UK neonatal intensive care units: a prospective evaluation, Lancet 359 (2002) 99–107.

[43] D.A. Goldmann, W.A. Durbin Jr., J. Freeman, Nosocomial infections in a neonatal intensive care unit, J. Infect. Dis. 144 (1981) 449–459.

[44] J.P. Cimiotti, et al., Impact of staffing on bloodstream infections in the neonatal intensive care unit, Arch. Pediatr. Adolesc. Med. 160 (2006) 832–836.

[45] J.E. Gray, et al., Coagulase-negative staphylococcal bacteremia among very low birth weight infants: relation to admission illness severity, resource use, and outcome, Pediatrics 95 (1995) 225–230.

[46] C.C. Carlos, et al., Nosocomial *Staphylococcus epidermidis* septicaemia among very low birth weight neonates in an intensive care unit, J. Hosp. Infect. 19 (1991) 201–207.

[47] V. Milisavljevic, et al., Genetic relatedness of *Staphylococcus epidermidis* from infected infants and staff in the neonatal intensive care unit, Am. J. Infect. Control 33 (2005) 341–347.

[48] P.J. Sharek, et al., Effect of an evidence-based hand washing policy on hand washing rates and false-positive coagulase negative staphylococcus blood and cerebrospinal fluid culture rates in a level III NICU, J. Perinatol. 22 (2002) 137–143.

[49] P.E. Coudron, et al., *Streptococcus faecium* outbreak in a neonatal intensive care unit, J. Clin. Microbiol. 20 (1984) 1044–1048.

[50] L.M. Luginbuhl, et al., Neonatal enterococcal sepsis: case-control study and description of an outbreak, Pediatr. Infect. Dis. J. 6 (1987) 1022–1026.

[51] C.C. Geil, W.K. Castle, E.A. Mortimer Jr., Group A streptococcal infections in newborn nurseries, Pediatrics 46 (1970) 849–854.

[52] J.R. Campbell, et al., An outbreak of M serotype 1 group A streptococcus in a neonatal intensive care unit, J. Pediatr. 129 (1996) 396–402.

[53] E. Bingen, et al., Mother-to-infant vertical transmission and cross-colonization of *Streptococcus pyogenes* confirmed by DNA restriction fragment length polymorphism analysis, J. Infect. Dis. 165 (1992) 147–150.

[54] H.D. Isenberg, et al., Clinical laboratory and epidemiological investigations of a *Streptococcus pyogenes* cluster epidemic in a newborn nursery, J. Clin. Microbiol. 19 (1984) 366–370.

[55] W.A. Brunton, Infection and hospital laundry, Lancet 345 (1995) 1574–1575.

[56] A. Paredes, et al., Nosocomial transmission of group B streptococci in a newborn nursery, Pediatrics 59 (1977) 679–682.

[57] R.C. Aber, et al., Nosocomial transmission of group B streptococci, Pediatrics 58 (1976) 346–353.

[58] B.F. Anthony, D.M. Okada, C.J. Hobel, Epidemiology of the group B streptococcus: maternal and nosocomial sources for infant acquisitions, J. Pediatr. 95 (1979) 431–436.

[59] C.S. Easmon, et al., Nosocomial transmission of group B streptococci, BMJ 283 (1981) 459–461.

[60] F.J. Noya, et al., Unusual occurrence of an epidemic of type Ib/c group B streptococcal sepsis in a neonatal intensive care unit, J. Infect. Dis. 155 (1987) 1135–1144.

[61] F.Y. Lin, et al., Prematurity is the major risk factor for late-onset group B streptococcus disease, J. Infect. Dis. 188 (2003) 267–271.

[62] M. Ayan, et al., Analysis of three outbreaks due to *Klebsiella* species in a neonatal intensive care unit, Infect. Control Hosp. Epidemiol. 24 (2003) 495–500.

[63] R.W. van den Berg, et al., *Enterobacter cloacae* outbreak in the NICU related to disinfected thermometers, J. Hosp. Infect. 45 (2000) 29–34.

[64] S.H. Jeong, et al., Neonatal intensive care unit outbreak caused by a strain of *Klebsiella oxytoca* resistant to aztreonam due to overproduction of chromosomal beta-lactamase, J. Hosp. Infect. 48 (2001) 281–288.

[65] M.B. Macrae, et al., A simultaneous outbreak on a neonatal unit of two strains of multiply antibiotic resistant *Klebsiella pneumoniae* controllable only by ward closure, J. Hosp. Infect. 49 (2001) 183–192.

[66] P. Berthelot, et al., Investigation of a nosocomial outbreak due to *Serratia marcescens* in a maternity hospital, Infect. Control Hosp. Epidemiol. 20 (1999) 233–236.

[67] Centers for Disease Control and Prevention, *Enterobacter sakazakii* infections associated with the use of powdered infant formula—Tennessee, 2001, MMWR Morb. Mortal. Wkly. Rep. 51 (2002) 298–300.

[68] L.G. Donowitz, et al., Contaminated breast milk: a source of *Klebsiella* bacteremia in a newborn intensive care unit, Rev. Infect. Dis. 3 (1981) 716–720.

[69] F. Fleisch, et al., Three consecutive outbreaks of *Serratia marcescens* in a neonatal intensive care unit, Clin. Infect. Dis. 34 (2002) 767–773.

[70] W.R. Gransden, et al., An outbreak of *Serratia marcescens* transmitted by contaminated breast pumps in a special care baby unit, J. Hosp. Infect. 7 (1986) 149–154.

[71] A.C. Moloney, et al., A bacteriological examination of breast pumps, J. Hosp. Infect. 9 (1987) 169–174.

[72] L.K. Archibald, et al., *Enterobacter cloacae* and *Pseudomonas aeruginosa* polymicrobial bloodstream infections traced to extrinsic contamination of a dextrose multidose vial, J. Pediatr. 133 (1998) 640–644.

[73] N.S. Matsaniotis, et al., *Enterobacter* sepsis in infants and children due to contaminated intravenous fluids, Infect. Control 5 (1984) 471–477.

[74] M.K. Lalitha, et al., Identification of an IV-dextrose solution as the source of an outbreak of *Klebsiella pneumoniae* sepsis in a newborn nursery, J. Hosp. Infect. 43 (1999) 70–73.

[75] S. Harbarth, et al., Outbreak of *Enterobacter cloacae* related to understaffing, overcrowding, and poor hygiene practices, Infect. Control Hosp. Epidemiol. 20 (1999) 598–603.

[76] W.L. Yu, et al., Outbreak investigation of nosocomial *Enterobacter cloacae* bacteraemia in a neonatal intensive care unit, Scand. J. Infect. Dis. 32 (2000) 293–298.

[77] L.K. Archibald, et al., *Serratia marcescens* outbreak associated with extrinsic contamination of 1% chlorxylenol soap, Infect. Control Hosp. Epidemiol. 18 (1997) 704–709.

[78] M.L. van Ogtrop, et al., *Serratia marcescens* infections in neonatal departments: description of an outbreak and review of the literature, J. Hosp. Infect. 36 (1997) 95–103.

[79] M. Dalben, et al., Investigation of an outbreak of *Enterobacter cloacae* in a neonatal unit and review of the literature, J. Hosp. Infect. 70 (2008) 7–14.

[80] L. Leigh, et al., *Pseudomonas aeruginosa* infection in very low birth weight infants: a case-control study, Pediatr. Infect. Dis. J. 14 (1995) 367–371.

[81] V.E. Becks, N.M. Lorenzoni, *Pseudomonas aeruginosa* outbreak in a neonatal intensive care unit: a possible link to contaminated hand lotion, Am. J. Infect. Control 23 (1995) 396–398.

[82] M.M. McNeil, et al., Nosocomial *Pseudomonas pickettii* colonization associated with a contaminated respiratory therapy solution in a special care nursery, J. Clin. Microbiol. 22 (1985) 903–907.

[83] G. Muyldermans, et al., Neonatal infections with *Pseudomonas aeruginosa* associated with a water-bath used to thaw fresh frozen plasma, J. Hosp. Infect. 39 (1998) 309–314.

[84] S.M. Garland, et al., *Pseudomonas aeruginosa* outbreak associated with a contaminated blood-gas analyser in a neonatal intensive care unit, J. Hosp. Infect. 33 (1996) 145–151.

[85] M. Vochem, M. Vogt, G. Doring, Sepsis in a newborn due to *Pseudomonas aeruginosa* from a contaminated tub bath, N. Engl. J. Med. 345 (2001) 378–379.

[86] M. Foca, et al., Endemic *Pseudomonas aeruginosa* infection in a neonatal intensive care unit, N. Engl. J. Med. 343 (2000) 695–700.

[87] R.L. Moolenaar, et al., A prolonged outbreak of *Pseudomonas aeruginosa* in a neonatal intensive care unit. Did staff fingernails play a role in disease transmission? Infect. Control Hosp. Epidemiol. 21 (2000) 80–85.

[88] J.M. Boyce, D. Pittet, Guideline for hand hygiene in healthcare settings. Recommendations of the Health Care Infection Control Practices Advisory Committee and the HICPAC/SHEA/APIC/IDSA Hand Hygiene Task Force. Society for Health Care Epidemiology of America/Association for Professionals in Infection Control/Infectious Diseases Society of America, MMWR Recomm. Rep. 51 (2002) 1–45.

[89] M. Nakano, et al., An outbreak of neonatal toxic shock syndrome-like exanthematous disease (NTED) caused by methicillin-resistant *Staphylococcus aureus* (MRSA) in a neonatal intensive care unit, Microbiol. Immunol. 46 (2002) 277–284.

[90] B.M. Andersen, et al., Spread of methicillin-resistant *Staphylococcus aureus* in a neonatal intensive unit associated with understaffing, overcrowding and mixing of patients, J. Hosp. Infect. 50 (2002) 18–24.

[91] Y. Saito, et al., Epidemiologic typing of methicillin-resistant *Staphylococcus aureus* in neonate intensive care units using pulsed-field gel electrophoresis, Microbiol. Immunol. 42 (1998) 723–729.

[92] C. Eckhardt, et al., Transmission of methicillin-resistant *Staphylococcus aureus* in the neonatal intensive care unit from a patient with community-acquired disease, Infect. Control Hosp. Epidemiol. 24 (2003) 460–461.

[93] U. Seybold, et al., Emergence of and risk factors for methicillin-resistant *Staphylococcus aureus* of community origin in intensive care nurseries, Pediatrics 122 (2008) 1039–1046.

[94] A. Belani, et al., Outbreak of staphylococcal infection in two hospital nurseries traced to a single nasal carrier, Infect. Control 7 (1986) 487–490.

[95] M.R. Ish-Horowicz, P. McIntyre, S. Nade, Bone and joint infections caused by multiply resistant *Staphylococcus aureus* in a neonatal intensive care unit, Pediatr. Infect. Dis. J. 11 (1992) 82–87.

[96] G. Sabatino, et al., Neonatal suppurative parotitis: a study of five cases, Eur. J. Pediatr. 158 (1999) 312–314.

[97] L. Saiman, et al., Molecular epidemiology of staphylococcal scalded skin syndrome in premature infants, Pediatr. Infect. Dis. J. 17 (1998) 329–334.

[98] J. Dave, et al., A double outbreak of exfoliative toxin-producing strains of *Staphylococcus aureus* in a maternity unit, Epidemiol. Infect. 112 (1994) 103–114.

[99] J.A. Otter, et al., Identification and control of an outbreak of ciprofloxacin-susceptible EMRSA-15 on a neonatal unit, J. Hosp. Infect. 67 (2007) 232–239.

[100] L. James, et al., Methicillin-resistant *Staphylococcus aureus* infections among healthy full-term newborns, Arch. Dis. Child. Fetal. Neonatal. Ed. 93 (2008) F40–F44.

[101] R.W. Haley, D.A. Bregman, The role of understaffing and overcrowding in recurrent outbreaks of staphylococcal infection in a neonatal special-care unit, J. Infect. Dis. 145 (1982) 875–885.

[102] H.F. Eichenwald, O. Kotsevalov, L.A. Fasso, The "cloud baby": an example of bacterial-viral interaction, Am. J. Dis. Child. 100 (1960) 161–173.

[103] R.J. Sheretz, et al., A cloud adult: the *Staphylococcus aureus*-virus interaction revisited, Ann. Intern. Med. 124 (1996) 539–547.

[104] A.S. Morel, et al., Nosocomial transmission of methicillin-resistant *Staphylococcus aureus* from a mother to her preterm quadruplet infants, Am. J. Infect. Control 30 (2002) 170–173.

[105] M. Reusch, et al., Prevalence of MRSA colonization in peripartum mothers and their newborn infants, Scand. J. Infect. Dis. 40 (2008) 667–671.

[106] D.F. McNeeley, F. Saint-Louis, G.J. Noel, Neonatal enterococcal bacteremia: an increasingly frequent event with potentially untreatable pathogens, Pediatr. Infect. Dis. J. 15 (1996) 800–805.

[107] Y. Golan, et al., Transmission of vancomycin-resistant enterococcus in a neonatal intensive care unit, Pediatr. Infect. Dis. J. 24 (2005) 566–567.

[108] C. Arnold, et al., Variability in vancomycin use in newborn intensive care units determined from data in an electronic medical record, Infect. Control Hosp. Epidemiol. 29 (2008) 667–670.

[109] N. Singh, et al., Control of vancomycin-resistant enterococci in the neonatal intensive care unit, Infect. Control Hosp. Epidemiol. 26 (2005) 646–649.

[110] J. Duchon, et al., Epidemiology of enterococci in a neonatal intensive care unit, Infect. Control Hosp. Epidemiol. 29 (2008) 374–376.

[111] R.A. Venezia, et al., Molecular epidemiology of an SHV-5 extended-spectrum beta-lactamase in Enterobacteriaceae isolated from infants in a neonatal intensive care unit, Clin. Infect. Dis. 21 (1995) 915–923.

[112] K. Shannon, et al., A hospital outbreak of extended-spectrum beta-lactamase-producing *Klebsiella pneumoniae* investigated by RAPD typing and analysis of the genetics and mechanisms of resistance, J. Hosp. Infect. 39 (1998) 291–300.

[113] B. Anderson, et al., Molecular and descriptive epidemiology of multidrug-resistant Enterobacteriaceae in hospitalized infants, Infect. Control Hosp. Epidemiol. 29 (2008) 250–255.

[114] P.C. Chan, et al., Control of an outbreak of pandrug-resistant *Acinetobacter baumannii* colonization and infection in a neonatal intensive care unit, Infect. Control Hosp. Epidemiol. 28 (2007) 423–429.

[115] B.J. Stoll, et al., Late-onset sepsis in very low birth weight neonates: the experience of the NICHD Neonatal Research Network, Pediatrics 110 (2 Pt 1) (2002) 285–291.

[116] D.K. Benjamin Jr., et al., Neonatal candidiasis among extremely low birth weight infants: risk factors, mortality rates, and neurodevelopmental outcomes at 18 to 22 months, Pediatrics 117 (2006) 84–92.

[117] P. Manzoni, et al., Fungal and bacterial sepsis and threshold ROP in preterm very low birth weight neonates, J. Perinatol. 26 (2006) 23–30.

[118] P.B. Smith, et al., Excess costs of hospital care associated with neonatal candidemia, Pediatr. Infect. Dis. J. 26 (2007) 197–200.

[119] T.E. Zaoutis, et al., Outcomes attributable to neonatal candidiasis, Clin. Infect. Dis. 44 (2007) 1187–1193.

[120] S.K. Fridkin, et al., Changing incidence of *Candida* bloodstream infections among NICU patients in the United States: 1995–2004, Pediatrics 117 (2006) 1680–1687.

[121] D.A. Kaufman, et al., Patterns of fungal colonization in preterm infants weighing less than 1000 grams at birth, Pediatr. Infect. Dis. J. 25 (2006) 733–737.

[122] C.M. Cotten, et al., The association of third-generation cephalosporin use and invasive candidiasis in extremely low birth-weight infants, Pediatrics 118 (2006) 717–722.

[123] D. Kaufman, et al., Fluconazole prophylaxis against fungal colonization and infection in preterm infants, N. Engl. J. Med. 345 (2001) 1660–1666.

[124] P. Manzoni, et al., A multicenter, randomized trial of prophylactic fluconazole in preterm neonates, N. Engl. J. Med. 356 (2007) 2483–2495.

[125] P.G. Pappas, et al., Clinical practice guidelines for the management of candidiasis: 2009 update by the Infectious Diseases Society of America, Clin. Infect. Dis. 48 (2009) 503–535.

[126] E. Chryssanthou, U. Broberger, B. Petrini, *Malassezia pachydermatis* fungaemia in a neonatal intensive care unit, Acta Paediatr. 90 (2001) 323–327.

[127] H.J. Chang, et al., An epidemic of *Malassezia pachydermatis* in an intensive care nursery associated with colonization of health care workers' pet dogs, N. Engl. J. Med. 338 (1998) 706–711.

[128] A.H. Groll, et al., Invasive pulmonary aspergillosis in a critically ill neonate: case report and review of invasive aspergillosis during the first 3 months of life, Clin. Infect. Dis. 27 (1998) 437–452.

[129] S. Singer, et al., Outbreak of systemic aspergillosis in a neonatal intensive care unit, Mycoses 41 (1998) 223–227.

[130] S.J. Mitchell, et al., Nosocomial infection with *Rhizopus microsporus* in preterm infants: association with wooden tongue depressors, Lancet 348 (1996) 441–443.

[131] L.M. Drusin, et al., Nosocomial ringworm in a neonatal intensive care unit: a nurse and her cat, Infect. Control Hosp. Epidemiol. 21 (2000) 605–607.

[132] S.E. Gelber, A.J. Ratner, Hospital-acquired viral pathogens in the neonatal intensive care unit, Semin. Perinatol. 26 (2002) 346–356.

[133] R. Sharma, et al., Clinical manifestations of rotavirus infection in the neonatal intensive care unit, Pediatr. Infect. Dis. J. 21 (2002) 1099–1105.

[134] J. Flores, et al., Serological response to rotavirus infection in newborn infants, J. Med. Virol. 42 (1994) 97–102.

[135] C.N. Lee, et al., Genetic characterization of the rotaviruses associated with a nursery outbreak, J. Med. Virol. 63 (2001) 311–320.

[136] S.A. Sattar, et al., Interruption of rotavirus spread through chemical disinfection, Infect. Control Hosp. Epidemiol. 15 (1994) 751–756.

[137] M.A. Widdowson, et al., An outbreak of diarrhea in a neonatal medium care unit caused by a novel strain of rotavirus: investigation using both epidemiologic and microbiological methods, Infect. Control Hosp. Epidemiol. 23 (2002) 665–670.

[138] R. Herruzo, et al., Identification of risk factors associated with nosocomial infection by rotavirus P4G2 in a neonatal unit of a tertiary-care hospital, Clin. Microbiol. Infect. 15 (2009) 280–285.

[139] R.M. Turcios-Ruiz, et al., Outbreak of necrotizing enterocolitis caused by norovirus in a neonatal intensive care unit, J. Pediatr. 153 (2008) 339–344.

[140] S. Bagci, et al., Detection of astrovirus in premature infants with necrotizing enterocolitis, Pediatr. Infect. Dis. J. 27 (2008) 347–350.

[141] A. Lodha, et al., Human torovirus: a new virus associated with neonatal necrotizing enterocolitis, Acta Paediatr. 94 (2005) 1085–1088.

[142] E. Birenbaum, et al., Adenovirus type 8 conjunctivitis outbreak in a neonatal intensive care unit, Arch. Dis. Child. 68 (1993) 610–611.

[143] J. Sizun, et al., Neonatal nosocomial respiratory infection with coronavirus: a prospective study in a neonatal intensive care unit, Acta Paediatr. 84 (1995) 617–620.

[144] R.J. Cunney, et al., An outbreak of influenza A in a neonatal intensive care unit, Infect. Control Hosp. Epidemiol. 21 (2000) 449–454.

[145] S.E. Moisiuk, et al., Outbreak of parainfluenza virus type 3 in an intermediate care neonatal nursery, Pediatr. Infect. Dis. J. 17 (1998) 49–53.

[146] X. Sagrera, et al., Outbreaks of influenza A virus infection in neonatal intensive care units, Pediatr. Infect. Dis. J. 21 (2002) 196–200.

[147] N.B. Halasa, et al., Medical and economic impact of a respiratory syncytial virus outbreak in a neonatal intensive care unit, Pediatr. Infect. Dis. J. 24 (2005) 1040–1044.

[148] V.P. Syriopoulou, et al., Clinical and epidemiological aspects of an enterovirus outbreak in a neonatal unit, J. Hosp. Infect. 51 (2002) 275–280.

[149] B. Jankovic, et al., Severe neonatal echovirus 17 infection during a nursery outbreak, Pediatr. Infect. Dis. J. 18 (1999) 393–394.

[150] K. Kusuhara, et al., An echovirus type 18 outbreak in a neonatal intensive care unit, Eur. J. Pediatr. 167 (2008) 587–589.

[151] M. Chambon, et al., An outbreak due to echovirus type 30 in a neonatal unit in France in 1997: usefulness of PCR diagnosis, J. Hosp. Infect. 43 (1999) 63–68.

[152] M.P. Griffin, et al., Cytomegalovirus infection in a neonatal intensive care unit: subsequent morbidity and mortality of seropositive infants, J. Perinatol. 10 (1990) 43–45.

[153] M. Vochem, et al., Transmission of cytomegalovirus to preterm infants through breast milk, Pediatr. Infect. Dis. J. 17 (1998) 53–58.

[154] M.H. Sawyer, D.K. Edwards, S.A. Spector, Cytomegalovirus infection and bronchopulmonary dysplasia in premature infants, Am. J. Dis. Child. 141 (1987) 303–305.

[155] J. Maschmann, et al., Cytomegalovirus infection of extremely low-birth weight infants via breast milk, Clin. Infect. Dis. 33 (2001) 1998–2003.

[156] K. Hamprecht, et al., Epidemiology of transmission of cytomegalovirus from mother to preterm infant by breastfeeding, Lancet 357 (2001) 513–518.

[157] M. Sharland, M. Khare, A. Bedford-Russell, Prevention of postnatal cytomegalovirus infection in preterm infants, Arch. Dis. Child. Fetal. Neonatal. Ed. 86 (2002) F140.

[158] C. Aitken, et al., Molecular epidemiology and significance of a cluster of cases of CMV infection occurring on a special care baby unit, J. Hosp. Infect. 34 (1996) 183–189.

[159] S.A. Spector, Transmission of cytomegalovirus among infants in hospital documented by restriction-endonuclease-digestion analyses, Lancet 1 (1983) 378–381.

[160] G.J. Demmler, et al., Nosocomial cytomegalovirus infections within two hospitals caring for infants and children, J. Infect. Dis. 156 (1987) 9–16.

[161] C.C. Linnemann Jr., et al., Transmission of herpes-simplex virus type 1 in a nursery for the newborn: identification of viral isolates by D.N.A. "fingerprinting" Lancet 1 (1978) 964–966.

[162] O. Hammerberg, et al., An outbreak of herpes simplex virus type 1 in an intensive care nursery, Pediatr. Infect. Dis. 2 (1983) 290–294.

[163] H. Sakaoka, et al., Two outbreaks of herpes simplex virus type 1 nosocomial infection among newborns, J. Clin. Microbiol. 24 (1986) 36–40.

[164] R. Turner, et al., Shedding and survival of herpes simplex virus from "fever blisters" Pediatrics 70 (1982) 547–549.

[165] M. Hayakawa, et al., Varicella exposure in a neonatal medical centre: successful prophylaxis with oral acyclovir, J. Hosp. Infect. 54 (2003) 212–215.

[166] B.S. Klein, et al., Nosocomial hepatitis A: a multinursery outbreak in Wisconsin, JAMA 252 (1984) 2716–2721.

[167] J.C. Watson, et al., Vertical transmission of hepatitis A resulting in an outbreak in a neonatal intensive care unit, J. Infect. Dis. 167 (1993) 567–571.

[168] L.S. Rosenblum, et al., Hepatitis A outbreak in a neonatal intensive care unit: risk factors for transmission and evidence of prolonged viral excretion among preterm infants, J. Infect. Dis. 164 (1991) 476–482.

[169] N.P. O'Grady, et al., Guidelines for the prevention of intravascular catheter-related infections. Centers for Disease Control and Prevention, MMWR Morb. Mortal. Wkly. Rep. 51 (2002) 1–26.

[170] J.D. Siegel, The newborn nursery, in: J. Bennet, P.S. (Eds.), Hospital Infections, 5th ed., B.P., Lippincott-Raven, Philadelphia, 1998.

[171] J.R. Edwards, et al., National Healthcare Safety Network (NHSN) Report, data summary for 2006 through 2007, issued November 2008, Am. J. Infect. Control 36 (2008) 609–626.

[172] J.S. Garland, et al., Cohort study of the pathogenesis and molecular epidemiology of catheter-related bloodstream infection in neonates with peripherally inserted central venous catheters, Infect. Control Hosp. Epidemiol. 29 (2008) 243–249.

[173] J.D. Horbar, et al., Collaborative quality improvement for neonatal intensive care. NIC/Q Project Investigators of the Vermont Oxford Network, Pediatrics 107 (2001) 14–22.

[174] J. Marschall, et al., Strategies to prevent central line-associated bloodstream infections in acute care hospitals, Infect. Control Hosp. Epidemiol. 29 (Suppl. 1) (2008) S22–S30.

[175] M.G. Capretti, et al., Impact of a standardized hand hygiene program on the incidence of nosocomial infection in very low birth weight infants, Am. J. Infect. Control 36 (2008) 430–435.

[176] V. Hoang, et al., Percutaneously inserted central catheter for total parenteral nutrition in neonates: complications rates related to upper versus lower extremity insertion, Pediatrics 121 (2008) e1152–e1159.

[177] G.L. Darmstadt, J.G. Dinulos, Neonatal skin care, Pediatr. Clin. North Am. 47 (2000) 757–782.

[178] J.S. Garland, et al., A vancomycin-heparin lock solution for prevention of nosocomial bloodstream infection in critically ill neonates with peripherally inserted central venous catheters: a prospective, randomized trial, Pediatrics 116 (2005) e198–e205.

[179] L. Filippi, et al., Fusidic acid and heparin lock solution for the prevention of catheter-related bloodstream infections in critically ill neonates: a retrospective study and a prospective, randomized trial, Pediatr. Crit. Care Med. 8 (2007) 556–562.

[180] L.A. Jardine, G.D. Inglis, M.W. Davies, Prophylactic systemic antibiotics to reduce morbidity and mortality in neonates with central venous catheters, Cochrane Database Syst. Rev. (1) (2008) CD006179.

[181] J.S. Garland, et al., Peripheral intravenous catheter complications in critically ill children: a prospective study, Pediatrics 89 (1992) 1145–1150.

[182] T.M. Yuan, L.H. Chen, H.M. Yu, Risk factors and outcomes for ventilator-associated pneumonia in neonatal intensive care unit patients, J. Perinat. Med. 35 (2007) 334–338.

[183] S.E. Coffin, et al., Strategies to prevent ventilator-associated pneumonia in acute care hospitals, Infect. Control Hosp. Epidemiol. 29 (Suppl. 1) (2008) S31–S40.

[184] W. Petdachai, Nosocomial pneumonia in a newborn intensive care unit, J. Med. Assoc. Thai. 83 (2000) 392–397.

[185] J.Y. Kawagoe, et al., Risk factors for nosocomial infections in critically ill newborns: a 5-year prospective cohort study, Am. J. Infect. Control 29 (2001) 109–114.

[186] R. Pepe, Nosocomial pneumonia, in: R. Carrico (Ed.), Association for Professionals in Infection Control and Epidemiology, Washington, DC, 2002.

[187] W. Lesiuk, et al., Non-invasive mandatory ventilation in extremely low birth weight and very low birth weight newborns with failed respiration, Przegl. Lek. 59 (2002) 57–59.

[188] M.I. Fernandez-Jurado, M. Fernandez-Baena, Use of laryngeal mask airway for prolonged ventilatory support in a preterm newborn, Paediatr. Anaesth. 12 (2002) 369–370.

[189] H. Aly, et al., Randomized, controlled trial on tracheal colonization of ventilated infants. Can gravity prevent ventilator-associated pneumonia, Pediatrics 122 (2008) 770–774.

[190] Centers for Disease Control and Prevention, Guidelines for prevention of nosocomial pneumonia, MMWR Morb. Mortal. Wkly. Rep. 46 (1997) 1–79.

[191] M.H. Kollef, The prevention of ventilator-associated pneumonia, N. Engl. J. Med. 340 (1999) 627–634.

[192] D.C. Bergmans, et al., Prevention of ventilator-associated pneumonia by oral decontamination: a prospective, randomized, double-blind, placebo-controlled study, Am. J. Respir. Crit. Care Med. 164 (2001) 382–388.

[193] J. Pugin, et al., Oropharyngeal decontamination decreases incidence of ventilator-associated pneumonia: a randomized, placebo-controlled, double-blind clinical trial, JAMA 265 (1991) 2704–2710.

[194] D.J. Cook, et al., Stress ulcer prophylaxis in critically ill patients: resolving discordant meta-analyses, JAMA 275 (1996) 308–314.

[195] K. Ildizdas, H. Yapicioglu, H. Yilmaz, Occurrence of ventilator-associated pneumonia in mechanically ventilated pediatric intensive care patients during stress ulcer prophylaxis with sucralfate, ranitidine, and omeprazole, J. Crit. Care 17 (2002) 240–245.

[196] E. Lopriore, D.G. Markhorst, R.J. Gemke, Ventilator-associated pneumonia and upper airway colonisation with gram negative bacilli: the role of stress ulcer prophylaxis in children, Intensive Care Med. 28 (2002) 763–767.

[197] O.C. Tablan, et al., Guidelines for preventing health-care-associated pneumonia, 2003: recommendations of CDC and the Healthcare Infection Control Practices Advisory Committee, MMWR Recomm. Rep. 53 (RR-3) (2004) 1–36.

[198] E. Lo, et al., Strategies to prevent catheter-associated urinary tract infections in acute care hospitals, Infect. Control Hosp. Epidemiol. 29 (Suppl. 1) (2008) S41–S50.

[199] J.M. Langley, M. Hanakowski, J.C. Leblanc, Unique epidemiology of nosocomial urinary tract infection in children, Am. J. Infect. Control 29 (2001) 94–98.

[200] J.A. Lohr, et al., Hospital-acquired urinary tract infections in the pediatric patient: a prospective study, Pediatr. Infect. Dis. J. 13 (1994) 8–12.

[201] M.J. McGirt, et al., Risk factors for pediatric ventriculoperitoneal shunt infection and predictors of infectious pathogens, Clin. Infect. Dis. 36 (2003) 858–862.

[202] A.V. Kulkarni, J.M. Drake, M. Lamberti-Pasculli, Cerebrospinal fluid shunt infection: a prospective study of risk factors, J. Neurosurg. 94 (2001) 195–201.

[203] C.J. Rozzelle, J. Leonardo, V. Li, Antimicrobial suture wound closure for cerebrospinal fluid shunt surgery: a prospective, double-blinded, randomized controlled trial, J. Neurosurg. Pediatr. 2 (2008) 111–117.

[204] R. Eymann, et al., Clinical and economic consequences of antibiotic-impregnated cerebrospinal fluid shunt catheters, J. Neurosurg. Pediatr. 1 (2008) 444–450.

[205] A. Pattavilakom, et al., Reduction in shunt infection using antibiotic impregnated CSF shunt catheters: an Australian prospective study, J. Clin. Neurosci. 14 (2007) 526–531.

[206] R.W. Haley, et al., The efficacy of infection surveillance and control programs in preventing nosocomial infections in US hospitals, Am. J. Epidemiol. 121 (1985) 182–205.

[207] I. Adams-Chapman, B.J. Stoll, Prevention of nosocomial infections in the neonatal intensive care unit, Curr. Opin. Pediatr. 14 (2002) 157–164.

[208] Centers for Disease Control and Prevention, Division of Health Care Quality Promotion. National Nosocomial Infections Surveillance (NNIS) System Report, data summary from January 1992 through June 2003, issued August 2003, Am. J. Infect. Control 30 (2003) 481–498.

[209] T.G. Emori, et al., National nosocomial infections surveillance system (NNIS): description of surveillance methods, Am. J. Infect. Control 19 (1991) 19–35.

[210] J.S. Garner, et al., CDC definitions for nosocomial infections, 1988, Am. J. Infect. Control 16 (1988) 128–140.

[211] D. Moore, Nosocomial infections in newborn nurseries and neonatal intensive care units, in: C. Mayhall (Ed.), Hospital Epidemiology and Infection Control, Lippincott Williams & Wilkins, Philadelphia, 1999.

[212] A. Sinha, D. Yokow, R. Platt, Epidemiology of neonatal infections: experience during and after hospitalization, Pediatr. Infect. Dis. J. 22 (2003) 244–250.

[213] T. Lee, O. Baker-Montgomery, Surveillance, in: R. Carrico (Ed.), Association for Professionals in Infection Control and Epidemiology, Washington, DC, 2002.

[214] R.P. Gaynes, S. Solomon, Improving hospital-acquired infection rates: the CDC experience, J. Comm. J. Qual. Improv. 22 (1996) 457–467.

[215] L.K. Archibald, R.P. Gaynes, Hospital-acquired infections in the United States: the importance of interhospital comparisons, Infect. Dis. Clin. North Am. 11 (1997) 245–255.

[216] J. Khoury, et al., Eradication of methicillin-resistant *Staphylococcus aureus* from a neonatal intensive care unit by active surveillance and aggressive infection control measures, Infect. Control Hosp. Epidemiol. 26 (2005) 616–621.

[217] J.D. Siegel, et al., 2007 Guideline for isolation precautions: preventing transmission of infectious agents in health care settings, Am. J. Infect. Control 35 (10 Suppl. 2) (2007) S65–S164.

[218] E.L. Larson, et al., An organizational climate intervention associated with increased handwashing and decreased nosocomial infections, Behav. Med. 26 (2000) 14–22.

[219] C.L. Pessoa-Silva, et al., Dynamics of bacterial hand contamination during routine neonatal care, Infect. Control Hosp. Epidemiol. 25 (2004) 192–197.

[220] D. Pittet, Improving adherence to hand hygiene practice: a multidisciplinary approach, Emerg. Infect. Dis. 7 (2001) 234–240.

[221] S.P. Won, et al., Handwashing program for the prevention of nosocomial infections in a neonatal intensive care unit, Infect. Control Hosp. Epidemiol. 25 (2004) 742–746.

[222] D.M. Salisbury, et al., The effect of rings on microbial load of health care workers' hands, Am. J. Infect. Control 25 (1997) 24–27.

[223] W.E. Trick, et al., Impact of ring wearing on hand contamination and comparison of hand hygiene agents in a hospital, Clin. Infect. Dis. 36 (2003) 1383–1390.

[224] A. Gupta, et al., Outbreak of extended-spectrum beta-lactamase-producing *Klebsiella pneumoniae* in a neonatal intensive care unit linked to artificial nails, Infect. Control Hosp. Epidemiol. 25 (2004) 210–215.

[225] S. Pelke, et al., Gowning does not affect colonization or infection rates in a neonatal intensive care unit, Arch. Pediatr. Adolesc. Med. 148 (1994) 1016–1020.

[226] H.J. Birenbaum, et al., Gowning on a postpartum ward fails to decrease colonization in the newborn infant, Am. J. Dis. Child. 144 (1990) 1031–1033.

[227] T.B. Lee, et al., Recommended practices for surveillance. Association for Professionals in Infection Control and Epidemiology, Inc. Surveillance Initiative working group, Am. J. Infect. Control 26 (1998) 277–288.

[228] C.B. Bridges, et al., Prevention and control of influenza: recommendations of the Advisory Committee on Immunization Practices (ACIP), MMWR Recomm. Rep. 49 (RR-3) (2000) 1–38; quiz CE1-CE7.

[229] D. Bozzi, et al., Guideline for preventing the transmission of *Mycobacterium tuberculosis* in health care facilities, MMWR Mortal. Morb. Wkly. Rep. 43 (1994) 1–132.

[230] F.M. Munoz, et al., Tuberculosis among adult visitors of children with suspected tuberculosis and employees at a children's hospital, Infect. Control Hosp. Epidemiol. 23 (2002) 568–572.

[231] C.B. Hall, et al., Nosocomial respiratory syncytial virus infections, N. Engl. J. Med. 293 (1975) 1343–1346.

[232] C.B. Hall, et al., Control of nosocomial respiratory syncytial viral infections, Pediatrics 62 (1978) 728–732.

[233] C.B. Hall, et al., Neonatal respiratory syncytial virus infection, N. Engl. J. Med. 300 (1979) 393–396.

[234] American Academy of Pediatrics and American College of Obstetricians and Gynecologists, Inpatient perinatal care services, in: L.C. Gilstrap, W. Oh (Eds.), Guidelines for Perinatal Care, fifth ed., American Academy of Pediatrics, and Washington, DC, American College of Obstetricians and Gynecologists, Elk Grove Village, IL, 2002.

[235] D. Moore, Newborn nursery and neonatal intensive care unit, in: R. Carrico (Ed.), Association for Professionals in Infection Control and Epidemiology, Washington, DC, 2002.

[236] N.M. Spearing, R.L. Horvath, J.G. McCormack, Pertussis: adults as a source in healthcare settings, Med. J. Aust. 177 (2002) 568–569.

[237] S.K. Fridkin, et al., The role of understaffing in central venous catheter-associated bloodstream infections, Infect. Control Hosp. Epidemiol. 17 (1996) 150–158.

[238] H. Harrison, The principles for family-centered neonatal care, Pediatrics 92 (1993) 643–650.

[239] M.E. Fallot, J.L. Boyd 3rd, F.A. Oski, Breast-feeding reduces incidence of hospital admissions for infection in infants, Pediatrics 65 (1980) 1121–1124.

[240] American Academy of Pediatrics, Infection control for hospitalized children, in: L.K. Pickering (Ed.), Red Book: Report of the Committee on Infectious Diseases, twenty sixth ed., American Academy of Pediatrics, Elk Grove Village, IL, 2003.

[241] American Academy of Pediatrics and American College of Obstetricians and Gynecologists, Perinatal infections, in: L.C. Gilstrap, W. Oh (Eds.), Guidelines for Perinatal Care, fifth ed., American Academy of Pediatrics, and Washington, DC, American College of Obstetricians and Gynecologists, Elk Grove Village, IL, 2002.

[242] A.E. el-Mohandes, et al., Bacterial contaminants of collected and frozen human milk used in an intensive care nursery, Am. J. Infect. Control 21 (1993) 226–230.

[243] C.J. D'Amico, C.A. DiNardo, S. Krystofiak, Preventing contamination of breast pump kit attachments in the NICU, J. Perinat. Neonatal Nurs. 17 (2003) 150–157.

[244] B. Wittrock, et al., Parents as a vector for nosocomial infection in the neonatal intensive care unit, Infect. Control Hosp. Epidemiol. 22 (2001) 472.

[245] G.L. Cartolano, et al., A parent as a vector of *Salmonella brandenburg* nosocomial infection in a neonatal intensive care unit, Clin. Microbiol. Infect. 9 (2003) 560–562.

[246] L.C. Mullany, G.L. Darmstadt, J.M. Tielsch, Role of antimicrobial applications to the umbilical cord in neonates to prevent bacterial colonization and infection: a review of the evidence, Pediatr. Infect. Dis. J. 22 (2003) 996–1002.

LABORATORY AIDS FOR DIAGNOSIS OF NEONATAL SEPSIS

Geoffrey A. Weinberg ✺ Carl T. D'Angio

CHAPTER OUTLINE

Diagnostic Utility of Laboratory Tests   1144
In Search of the Ideal Laboratory Test   1145
Complete Blood Counts and White Blood Cell Ratios   1146
    Total Leukocyte Count, Differential Leukocyte Count, and
        Morphology   1146
    Total Neutrophil Count   1146
    Total Nonsegmented Neutrophil Count   1148
    Neutrophil Ratios   1148
    Platelet Count   1149
Acute Phase Reactants   1149
    C-Reactive Protein   1150
    Procalcitonin   1151

Erythrocyte Sedimentation Rate   1151
Other Acute Phase Reactants   1151
Additional Laboratory Studies   1152
    Cytokines and Chemokines   1152
    Adhesion Molecules and Cellular Receptors   1152
    Lymphocyte and Neutrophil Marker Analysis   1152
    Miscellaneous Analytes   1152
    Microscopic Examination of Placenta, Umbilical Cord, Gastric
        Aspirates, and External Ear Canal Fluid   1153
    Screening Panels   1154
Perspectives and Conclusions   1156

For years, investigators have sought a test or panel of tests able to diagnose neonatal sepsis accurately and more rapidly than is possible with the isolation of microorganisms from specimens of sterile body fluids or tissues. Although results of some studies have been encouraging, the isolation of microorganisms from sources such as the blood, cerebrospinal fluid (CSF), urine, other body fluids (peritoneal, pleural, joint, middle ear), or tissues (bone marrow, liver, spleen) remains the most valid method of diagnosing bacterial sepsis. Many advances in non–culture-based methods, which may nevertheless remain microorganism specific, such as tests employing polymerase chain reaction (PCR) amplification technology, are promising for more rapid diagnosis of infection. This chapter discusses nonspecific laboratory aids for the diagnosis of invasive bacterial infections. Specific microbiologic techniques are discussed in Chapter 6 and in chapters addressing specific pathogens.

DIAGNOSTIC UTILITY OF LABORATORY TESTS

In establishing the usefulness of any laboratory determination, a balance must be reached between sensitivity and specificity [1]. For a clinician needing to decide whether to institute or withhold therapy on the basis of a test result, the predictive values (and perhaps likelihood ratios) [2] of that test are also important. In relation to neonatal infection, these terms can be defined as follows (Fig. 36–1):

Sensitivity: If infection is present, how often is the test result abnormal?
Specificity: If infection is absent, how often is the test result normal?

Positive predictive value: If the test result is abnormal, how often is infection present?
Negative predictive value: If the test result is normal, how often is infection absent?
Likelihood ratio, positive test result: If the test result is abnormal, how much does that result increase the pretest probability of disease?
Likelihood ratio, negative test result: If the test result is normal, how much does that result decrease the pretest probability of disease?

In attempting to discover the presence of a serious illness such as neonatal bacteremia, which is life-threatening yet treatable, diagnostic tests with maximal (100%) sensitivity and negative predictive value are desirable. In other words, if infection were present, the result would always be abnormal; if the result were normal, infection would always be absent. The reduced specificity and positive predictive value that this combination may engender usually are acceptable because overtreatment with antibiotics on the basis of a false-positive result is likely to be of limited harm compared with withholding therapy on the basis of a false-negative result. Some authorities prefer the use of likelihood ratios because predictive values vary with the prevalence of a disease, while likelihood ratios relate only to the test performance (sensitivity, specificity) [3,4]. Large likelihood ratios (>10) imply that a test result would conclusively increase the probability of the disease being present, whereas small likelihood ratios (<0.1) minimize the probability of the disease being present.

In reviewing a report of a new laboratory aid for the diagnosis of neonatal sepsis, the first consideration is to determine what reference standard was used to evaluate the new test (i.e., what was the gold standard applied). In one study of infants who died with unequivocal

Laboratory Test Result		**Bacterial Infection Present**		
		Yes	**No**	
	Positive	TRUE POSITIVES (a)	FALSE POSITIVES (b)	POSITIVE PREDICTIVE VALUE (a)/(a+b)
	Negative	FALSE NEGATIVES (c)	TRUE NEGATIVES (d)	NEGATIVE PREDICTIVE VALUE (d)/(c+d)
		SENSITIVITY (a)/(a+c)	SPECIFICITY (d)/(b+d)	PREVALENCE (a+c)/(a+b+c+d)
		LIKELIHOOD RATIO, POSITIVE sensitivity/(1–specificity)	LIKELIHOOD RATIO, NEGATIVE (1–sensitivity)/specificity	

FIGURE 36–1 Diagnostic test characteristics. Sensitivity, specificity, positive predictive value, and negative predictive value are commonly expressed as percentages; likelihood ratios represent -fold increases or -fold decreases in probability [1–3].

evidence of infection at autopsy, bacteria were grown from 32 of 39 antemortem blood cultures (sensitivity of only 82%) [5]. Among 50 infants without pathologic findings of infection at autopsy, 48 had negative blood culture results (specificity of 96%). A positive blood or CSF culture result had a 94% chance of being associated with serious neonatal infection (positive predictive value of 94%), whereas a negative blood culture result indicated absence of serious infection only 87% of the time (negative predictive value of 87%). It is likely that the predictive values cited in this study already are different from the values that may be observed in practice because of the high prevalence (44%) of positive bacterial culture results in the autopsy cases reviewed [5]. (High prevalence inflates the positive predictive value and depresses the negative predictive value; low prevalence depresses the positive predictive value and inflates the negative predictive value.)

The lack of perfection of the generally accepted gold standard of bacterial culture complicates the search for new laboratory aids in the diagnosis of neonatal sepsis; it may be unclear whether a new test is truly functioning better than culture, which itself may not be "perfect." Interpretation of bacterial culture results may become even more complicated as intrapartum antibiotic prophylaxis to prevent early-onset group B streptococcal sepsis becomes more common [6–9]. It may not be clinically necessary to require detection of only *bacterial* sepsis. Tests that yield results considered "falsely positive" in the absence of bacterial disease may still be clinically useful in assigning normal versus abnormal status if the results register positive because of *serious viral disease* that may require antiviral therapy (e.g., neonatal enterovirus or herpes simplex infections).

Two additional points warrant consideration in this context. First, unless the report is generated from an unselected cohort or prospective study, the predictive values given in the report may be misleading. Prevalence of sepsis may vary greatly if certain groups of newborns are preselected, which would alter the predictive values

of the test being studied. The most useful test in one population of infants with very low birth weight may function quite differently in another population of older infants with larger birth weights who are growing normally. Second, because the body's response to an infection necessarily begins after the invasion of a pathogen, it may never be possible to diagnose an infection immediately—there may always be a lag in the physiologic response on which the diagnostic test is based. Each report of a new test claiming superiority to bacterial culture must be critically evaluated in the extended clinical setting, and standardization within clinical laboratories and among institutions is required.

IN SEARCH OF THE IDEAL LABORATORY TEST

Even bacterial blood cultures performed with modern, continuously computer-monitored detection technology do not reach 100% sensitivity for the diagnosis of neonatal infection. Incubation of bacteria may take several days, and genuine bacteremia may be missed because of the small volume of blood taken from infants with very low birth weight. A set of properties of the ideal or perfect diagnostic test has been proposed [10,11]. These characteristics should be kept in mind as the different laboratory tests for neonatal infection are discussed in this chapter.

First, the laboratory analyte would be biochemically stable (to ease transport requirements), easy to analyze (quick laboratory turnaround time), and obtainable from a small volume of blood. Second, the analyte would have clear diagnostic cutoffs between normal and abnormal, across various gestational ages, and across birth weights. Third, the test would be inexpensive and comparable among different laboratories, so that it could be widely applied.

In addition, the ideal laboratory test for the diagnosis of neonatal infection would be maximally sensitive (no false-negative results) and highly specific (few false-positive results) and have a physiologic window of opportunity for sampling. More precisely, the test would become abnormal just as infection was present and remain abnormal for some time, to allow for clinicians to use it as a diagnostic aid even if the clinical symptoms of infection were initially missed.

Finally, the ideal marker would correlate well with progress of infection, perhaps even predicting outcome [10,11]. As we review each test in this chapter, it will become apparent that none of the currently available laboratory aids for the diagnosis of infection fulfill these ideal properties. Although new tests are continually being studied, it is uncertain that any will ever achieve perfection.

COMPLETE BLOOD COUNTS AND WHITE BLOOD CELL RATIOS
TOTAL LEUKOCYTE COUNT, DIFFERENTIAL LEUKOCYTE COUNT, AND MORPHOLOGY

Total leukocyte counts are of limited value in the diagnosis of septicemia in newborns [12–16]. Total leukocyte counts are particularly unreliable indicators of infection during the first several hours of early-onset (within 48 hours of birth) sepsis because they are normal at the time of initial evaluation in more than one third of infants with proven bacteremia [5,17–28]. Conversely, among neonates evaluated for suspected sepsis, far less than half of neonates with reduced (<5000 cells/mm³) or elevated (>20,000 cells/mm³) cell counts are ultimately identified to be infected [5,20,22,29].

Differential leukocyte counts also have not functioned well as markers for infectious disease in the newborn period. Increased percentages of lymphocytes have been described in association with pertussis and congenital syphilis, whereas minor changes of little diagnostic value have been noted in infants with ABO incompatibility, in sepsis, and in maternal hypertension [30,31]. Monocyte counts, normally higher in neonates than in older children or adults, may be elevated further in some cases of congenital syphilis, perinatal listeriosis, ABO incompatibility, and recovery from sepsis [27,31–36]. Eosinophilia, a common finding in premature infants, has been related to numerous factors, including low birth weight, immaturity, establishment of positive nitrogen balance, improved nutritional status, and use of total parenteral nutrition or blood transfusions [36–41]. A dramatic decrease in the absolute number of eosinophils, detectable only if serial counts have been performed, frequently accompanies sepsis or serious infection [31,38,42]. Basophil counts tend to follow the fluctuations in eosinophil numbers in ill or healthy newborns [40]. Conflicting data have been reported for the utility of differential leukocyte counts for identifying neonates with bacterial meningitis [43,44].

Several investigators have shown that significant changes in neutrophil morphology occur in association with serious bacterial infection, with the appearance of toxic granules, Döhle bodies, and vacuolization [25,42–47]. These features are of limited value in establishing a diagnosis; their presence has at best a positive predictive value for sepsis of only slightly more than 50% [5,25,45–47] and at worst a positive predictive value of 33% to 37% [48,49]. Identical

morphologic features can occur as artifacts in citrate-anticoagulated blood samples stored for longer than 1 hour before smears are made [50].

TOTAL NEUTROPHIL COUNT

Recognizing the low predictive value of total leukocyte counts in serious neonatal bacterial disease, several investigators have studied the dynamics of neutrophil counts during the 1st month of life [35,42,45,51–56]. These researchers and others uncovered patterns of change sufficiently constant to establish limits of normal variation (Fig. 36–2) and defined noninfectious conditions involving the mother or the infant that might have significant effects on neutrophil values (Tables 36–1 and 36–2). Largely on the basis of these data, it was suggested that calculation of the absolute number of circulating neutrophils (polymorphonuclear plus immature forms) might provide a useful index of neonatal infection. Clinical experience has only partly supported this premise.

Most series of consecutive cases of neonatal sepsis have shown abnormal neutrophil counts at the *time of onset of symptoms* in only about two thirds of infants.* In some series, 80% to 90% of infected infants have had abnormal values [23,48,51,71], whereas in other series, initial neutrophil counts were reduced or elevated in only one fourth to one third of infants with bacteremia, particularly when counts were determined early in the course of illness [28,57,72]. The neutrophil count, although slightly more sensitive than the total leukocyte count, is too often normal in the face of serious infection to be used as a guide for treatment.

Baley and associates [52] investigated the causes of neutropenia among consecutive admissions to a neonatal intensive care unit. Low neutrophil counts were found in 6% of these infants, most of whom were premature and of low birth weight. Less than half of the episodes of neutropenia could be attributed to infection (bacterial, viral, necrotizing enterocolitis). Rather, most were of unknown cause or occurred in infants with perinatal complications. Similar findings have been described by Rodwell and coworkers [59] among 1000 infants evaluated for sepsis in the first 24 hours of life.

The neutrophil count can be of value in specific clinical situations. The association of neutropenia, respiratory distress, and early-onset (<48 hours) sepsis caused by group B streptococci is well documented [18,23,63,73–76], although the recognition that a similar association exists for early sepsis caused by other microorganisms has not been adequately emphasized. Several authors have described infants with septicemia related to *Haemophilus influenzae* [77,78], pneumococci [79–81], *Escherichia coli* [78], or nonenterococcal group D streptococci [82] whose clinical course was similar to that described for group B streptococcal infection. Because all infants were noted to be ill at birth or shortly thereafter, when neutrophil counts normally are increasing, a low count (0 to 4000 cells/mm³) in this clinical setting is a highly significant finding. In many cases, the low number of circulating neutrophils reflects a depletion of bone marrow

---

*References [5,15–18,26,45,46,65–70].

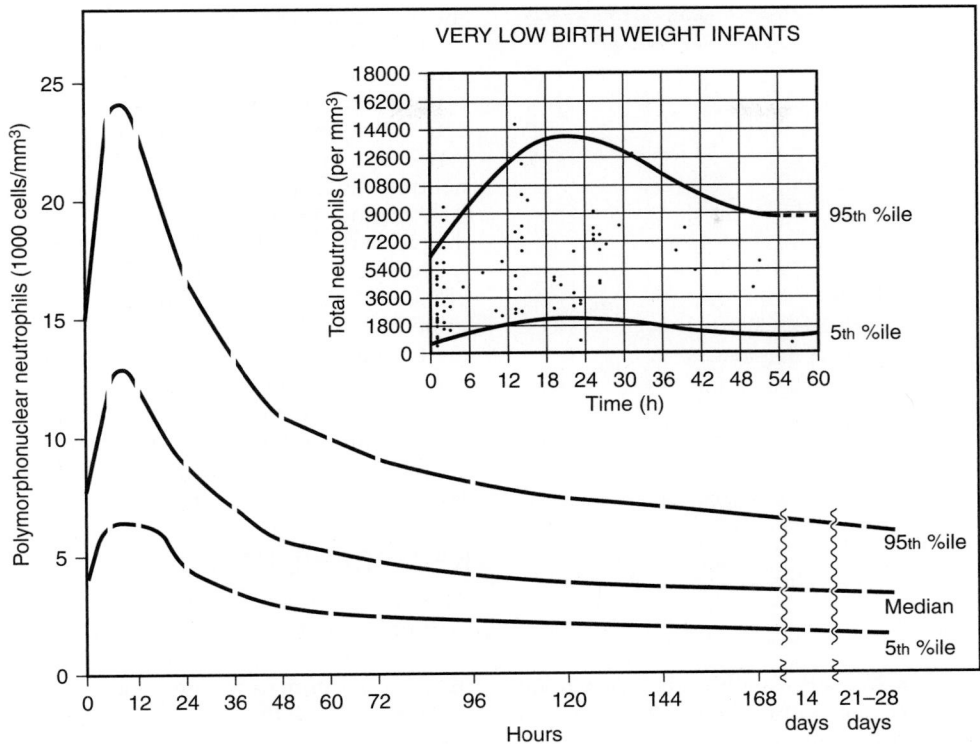

FIGURE 36–2 **Total neutrophil counts in normal term infants and in very low birth weight infants (*inset*).** The limits for term infants are close to those defined by Xanthou [35], Marks and colleagues [53], and Schelonka and associates [55], but are significantly higher during the first 18 hours of life than the reference values of Manroe and coworkers [45]. (*Data from Gregory J, Hey E. Blood neutrophil response to bacterial infection in the first month of life. Arch Dis Child 47:747–753, 1972; inset, data from Mouzinho A, et al. Revised reference ranges for circulating neutrophils in very-low-birth-weight neonates. Pediatrics 94:76–82, 1999.*)

TABLE 36–1   Clinical Factors Affecting Neutrophil Counts in Newborn Infants

| Factor | Neutrophil Counts* | | | | |
	Decrease	Increase	Total Immature Increase	Increased I: T Ratio[†]	Approximate Duration (hr)
Maternal hypertension [57–59]	++++	0	+	+	72
Maternal fever, neonate healthy	0	++	+++	++++	24
≥6 hours intrapartum oxytocin administration	0	++	++	++++	120
Asphyxia (5-min Apgar score ≤5) [57,60]	+	++	++	+++	24–60
Meconium aspiration syndrome [60]	0	++++	+++	++	72
Pneumothorax with uncomplicated hyaline membrane disease	0	++++	++++	++++	24
Seizures—no hypoglycemia, asphyxia, or central nervous system hemorrhage	0	+++	+++	++++	24
Prolonged (≥4 min) crying [61]	0	++++	++++	++++	1
Asymptomatic blood glucose ≤30 mg/dL	0	++	+++	+++	24
Hemolytic disease [42]	++	++	+++	++	7–28 days
Surgery [51]	0	++++	++++	+++	24
High altitude [62]	0	++++	++++	0	6[‡]

*+, 0%-25% of neonates affected; ++, 25%-50%; +++, 50%-75%; ++++, 75%-100%.
[†]*Ratio of immature forms to total neutrophils.*
[‡]*Not tested after 6 hours.*
Data from Manroe BL, et al. The neonatal blood count in health and disease. I. Reference values for neutrophilic cells. J Pediatr 95:89–98, 1979, with additions as noted.

TABLE 36-2   Clinical Factors with No Effect on Neutrophil
Counts in Newborn Infants

Race
Gender
Maternal diabetes
Fetal bradycardia
Mode of delivery*
Premature rupture of membranes, mother afebrile
Meconium staining, no lung disease
Uncomplicated hyaline membrane disease [63]
Uncomplicated transient tachypnea of the newborn
Hyperbilirubinemia, physiologic, unexplained [18]
Phototherapy
Diurnal variation [35,51]
Brief (≤3 min) crying [64]

*Total neutrophil counts in cord blood of infants delivered vaginally or by cesarean section after
labor (2–14 hr) are twice those of infants delivered by cesarean section without labor [64].
Data from Manroe BL, et al. The neonatal blood count in health and disease. I. Reference
values for neutrophilic cells. J Pediatr 95:89–98, 1979, with additions as noted.

granulocyte reserves [78,83] and usually indicates a poor prognosis.* The absolute neutrophil count may be useful for screening infants with symptomatic illness including respiratory distress in the first few hours of life, if not for asymptomatic infants [29,85].

TOTAL NONSEGMENTED NEUTROPHIL COUNT

The blood smear and differential cell count during the newborn period are strikingly different from values seen at any other time of life. Immature forms are present in relatively large numbers, particularly among premature infants and during the first few days of life [35,45,46,86]. The number of immature neutrophils, mostly nonsegmented (band, stab) forms, increases from a maximal normal value of 1100 cells/mm³ in cord blood to 1500 cells/mm³ at 12 hours of life and gradually decreases to 600 cells/mm³ by 60 hours of life. Between 60 and 120 hours, the maximum count decreases from 600 to 500 cells/mm³ and remains unchanged through the 1st month of life [45]. For unexplained reasons, possibly related to differences in the definition of a nonsegmented neutrophil [65], higher counts have been recorded by other authors [16,61]. Metamyelocytes and myelocytes also are often present in significant numbers during the first 72 hours after delivery, but disappear almost entirely toward the end of the 1st week of life [35]. Even occasional promyelocytes and blast cells may be seen during the early days of life in healthy infants [35].

As neutrophils are released from the bone marrow in response to infection, an increasing number of immature cells enter the bloodstream, producing a differential cell count with a "shift to the left" even greater than that normally present in the neonate [71]. This response is so inconstant, however, that, with few exceptions [18,65,66],

the absolute band or immature (bands, metamyelocytes) neutrophil count has been found to be of little diagnostic value.* In many infants with infection, despite an increased proportion of immature cell types in the differential leukocyte count, exhaustion of the bone marrow reserves prevents an increase in the absolute number of band neutrophils in the circulation [83,87,88]. This is particularly common in more seriously ill patients, in whom early diagnosis is most critical [5,71,78,83].

Despite its relative insensitivity, the immature neutrophil count has been found to have good positive predictive value in some [5,46,49,71,75], although not all [48], studies. In infants with clinical evidence of sepsis and high band counts in whom culture results remain negative, follow-up cultures and investigation for a history of perinatal events that might explain the discrepancy (see Table 36–1) or for the possibility of infection related to other causes, such as enteroviruses, are indicated [89].

NEUTROPHIL RATIOS

The unreliability of absolute band counts led to the investigation of neutrophil ratios as an index of neonatal infection. Determinations have included the ratio of either bands or all immature neutrophils (e.g., bands, metamyelocytes, and myelocytes) to either segmented neutrophils (the immature-to-mature neutrophil ratio [I:M ratio]) or to all neutrophils (the immature-to-total neutrophil ratio [I:T ratio]). Despite the early enthusiasm of researchers, the clinical studies that include these determinations have failed to show a consistent correlation with the presence of serious bacterial disease. As might be expected, low band counts caused by exhaustion of marrow can produce misleadingly low ratios in the presence of serious or overwhelming infection [46,75,82,83].

Clinical experience with I:M ratios [46,71] is insufficient to verify their accuracy. Initial studies in which the I:M ratio was used have been disappointing, however, with normal values recorded in more than one third of infected infants. Band-to-total neutrophil ratios, although more extensively studied, also have proved to be too unpredictable to be diagnostically helpful. The most favorable report would have missed 10% of neonates with sepsis, while recording falsely abnormal values in almost 20% of uninfected infants [20]. The sensitivity of this determination in other series varies, ranging from 70% to 30%, which precludes its use in a clinical setting [24–26,70,71].

The I:T ratio is the best studied of the ratios [70,90]. Inclusion in the numerator of all immature forms, rather than just band cells, heightens accuracy by accounting for the increase in metamyelocytes that is sometimes seen with accelerated release from the neutrophil storage pool [71]. Use of total rather than segmented neutrophils in the denominator has the advantage of always yielding a value between 0 and 1 inclusive. The maximum ratio for the first 24 hours is 0.16 [45,60]. It gradually declines to around 0.12 by 60 hours of age and remains unchanged for the remainder of the 1st month [45]. A normal value up to 0.2, with age unspecified, has been found in some laboratories [20]. I:T ratios during the first 5 days of life are less than 0.2 in 96% of healthy premature infants with a gestational age of 32 weeks or less [86].

Numerous clinical studies have evaluated the I:T ratio. Results have been widely disparate, but in most series, they indicate that this ratio is too unreliable to achieve more than limited usefulness by itself. Sensitivities ranging from more than 90%* to 70% [22,92], 60% [57,69,72], or less [93,94] have been reported. Elevated ratios caused by various perinatal conditions have been seen in 25% to 50% of uninfected ill infants (see Table 36–1) [21,22]. Perhaps the greatest value of the I:T ratio lies in its good negative predictive value: If the I:T ratio is normal, the likelihood that infection is absent is extremely high (99%).[†]

Serial determinations of the I:T ratio may lead to increased sensitivity [49,90,95]. Some authors have found, however, that interreader variability leads to enough bias to limit the usefulness of leukocyte ratios for general use [96].

PLATELET COUNT

Several extensive studies have established that the normal platelet count in newborns, regardless of birth weight, is rarely less than 100,000/mm^3 during the first 10 days of life or less than 150,000/mm^3 during the next 3 weeks [18,69,97–100]. Although it would behoove the clinician to perform a work-up for sepsis in any infant with unexplained thrombocytopenia [100–102], a reduction in the number of circulating platelets has been shown to be an insensitive, nonspecific, and relatively late indicator of serious bacterial infection during the neonatal period. Automated measurements of mean platelet volume have added little to the platelet count as a diagnostic aid [103,104].

Only 10% to 60% of newborns with proven bacterial invasion of the bloodstream or meninges have platelet counts of less than 100,000/mm^3.* The average duration of thrombocytopenia is about 1 week, but can be 2 to 3 weeks. The nature of the organism involved (whether gram-positive, gram-negative, or fungal) has been reported in some, but not all, studies to correlate with the platelet count nadir and duration of thrombocytopenia [18,72,99,103]. Although platelet counts may begin to decrease several days before the onset of clinical signs of infection, in most cases values remain elevated until 1 to 3 days after serious illness is already apparent [19,26,41,65,99]. Thrombocytopenia accompanying bacterial infection is thought to be caused by a direct effect of bacteria or bacterial products on platelets and vascular endothelium, leading to increased aggregation and adhesion, or by increased platelet destruction caused by immune mechanisms [46,65,99–101].

In addition to the widely known association between thrombocytopenia and intrauterine infections related to syphilis, toxoplasmosis, rubella, and cytomegalovirus infection, reduced platelet counts also have been described with postnatal viral infections with enteroviruses and herpes simplex virus, each of which can cause an illness clinically indistinguishable from bacterial sepsis [101–106]. Conditions that predispose the infant to sepsis, such as placement of an umbilical catheter, birth asphyxia, mechanical ventilation, meconium aspiration, multiple exchange transfusions, and necrotizing enterocolitis, have independently caused thrombocytopenia in the absence of positive blood culture results [41,102,107–109]. Nonspecific neonatal thrombocytopenia also has been reported with various conditions causing maternal thrombocytopenia, including pregnancy-induced hypertension [41]. Infants with moderate to severe Rh hemolytic disease also are thrombocytopenic [110].

ACUTE PHASE REACTANTS

In the presence of inflammation caused by infection, trauma, or other cellular destruction, the liver, under the influence of proinflammatory cytokines interleukin (IL)-1β, IL-6, and tumor necrosis factor (TNF)-α, rapidly synthesizes large amounts of certain proteins collectively known as *acute phase reactants* [111–114]. Serum levels of these proteins usually increase together, and generally the degree of change in one is proportional to the degree of change in the others (two important exceptions are albumin and transferrin, which decrease together) (Fig. 36–3). Acute phase reactants are produced very early in fetal life, beginning in the 4th to 5th week of gestation [115]. Their exact role in the inflammatory process is unknown; most seem to be part of a primitive nonspecific (innate) defense mechanism. Several acute phase reactants have been extensively evaluated in neonatal sepsis, including C-reactive protein (CRP), fibrinogen, and other proteins that influence the erythrocyte sedimentation rate; haptoglobin; and α$_1$-acid glycoprotein (orosomucoid). Measurement of proinflammatory cytokines and their receptors, chemokines, cell markers, and anti-inflammatory cytokines also

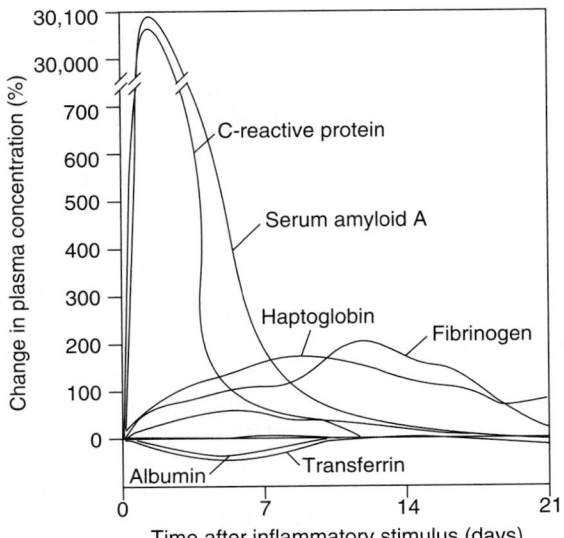

FIGURE 36–3 Acute phase reactants in patients with inflammatory illnesses. The response of C-reactive protein is greater than that of all other acute phase proteins except serum amyloid A. Levels of certain plasma proteins decrease during the acute phase response. (*Data from Gabay C, Kushner I. Acute-phase proteins and other systemic responses to inflammation. N Engl J Med 340:448–454, 1999.*)

---

*References [18,21,45,48,75,91].

[†]References [3,20–22,48,69,75,76].

*References [17–19,23,25,48,72,99].

involved in the immune cascade following infection holds promise to increase diagnostic accuracy further; these tests are discussed later.

C-REACTIVE PROTEIN

The most useful of the acute phase reactants seems to be CRP. CRP is a globulin that forms a precipitate when combined with the C-polysaccharide of *Streptococcus pneumoniae* [113,114]. Because the appearance of CRP in the blood has been closely associated with tissue injury, particularly when caused by an acute inflammatory process, it has been suggested that the primary function of CRP is to act as a carrier protein, binding and facilitating clearance of potentially toxic foreign or altered materials released from invading microorganisms or damaged tissues. Its roles in activation of the classic complement pathway, promotion of phagocytosis, regulation of lymphocyte function, and platelet activation are unclear [70,111–114].

Differences in laboratory techniques and in the interpretation of what constitutes a positive result for CRP assay have been partly responsible for conflicting opinions about the reliability of this test during the neonatal period [70,113,116,117]. Early clinical reports must be interpreted in light of the knowledge that the capillary tube precipitation and gel immunodiffusion techniques used for assay of CRP in those studies were less sensitive and specific than more modern immunochemical methods [70,117]. A comparison of reactions obtained by different investigators using the capillary tube method revealed widely disparate results, depending on the sensitivity of the commercial antiserum used in the assay.

Newer rapid and reliable quantitative methods have been developed in which monoclonal CRP-specific antibody is used [117–120]. Fully automated turbidimetric and nephelometric methods can provide quantitative results in 30 to 60 minutes, whereas enzyme immunoassays, such as the enzyme-multiplied immunoassay technique, can give results in less than 10 minutes. Determination of CRP levels in serum by numerous authors using many techniques (radial immunodiffusion, electroimmunodiffusion, spot immunoprecipitate assay, enzyme-multiplied immunoassay technique, and nephelometry) has shown the upper limit of normal to be 10 mg/L (1 mg/dL) during the neonatal period [49,113,114,118,121]. Analysis of paired serum specimens obtained from mothers and their infants (fetuses and premature infants and full-term neonates) has shown that CRP crosses the placenta either only in very low concentrations or not at all [113]. Gestational age does not seem to influence the validity of results [23,113]. CRP normal ranges may vary with time over the first 48 hours of life, however, with 95th percentile values of 5 mg/dL, 14 mg/dL, and 10 mg/dL at 0, 24, and 48 hours of age [117,122].

Most surveys in sera of neonates with systemic bacterial infections have shown significant elevations of CRP levels *at the time of onset of signs* (i.e., diagnostic test sensitivity) in 50% to 90% of cases.* A poor response is particularly frequent among infants whose infection occurs during the first 12 to 24 hours of life and among infants with infection caused by gram-positive bacteria, including group B

streptococci [23,91,124]. Although the intensity of the response does not always reflect the severity of the infection, the relationship between formation of CRP and the degree of tissue injury indicates that infants who show a positive response usually have systemic infections or involvement of deeper tissues [23,130].

Measurement of CRP levels is not completely specific. The response of CRP to nonbacterial infections is variable; increased serum levels have been found in infants with viral infections [131]. A strong correlation between elevated CRP levels and chorioamnionitis has been described in women with premature rupture of membranes and in the cord blood of their infants [132,133]. Increases of CRP levels in neonates also have been associated with noninfectious conditions causing tissue injury or inflammation, such as fetal asphyxia, respiratory distress syndrome, intracerebral hemorrhage, and meconium aspiration pneumonitis [121,124,134]. Because these conditions often are confused or associated with newborn bacterial infection, such false-positive elevations greatly reduce the positive predictive value of CRP determinations and their usefulness in diagnosis. The mean incidence of falsely elevated CRP values in ill but not septic neonates is approximately 5% to 15% [91,94,123,134,135].

The reported overall sensitivity of CRP at the onset of signs of sepsis ranges from 50% to 90%, and the specificity ranges from 85% to 95%. The positive and negative predictive values may range from 30% to greater than 95%. It is clear from the foregoing discussion that despite new technology permitting more rapid and precise measurement, reliance on CRP levels *alone* as an early indicator of neonatal bacterial infection cannot be recommended. Although CRP levels possibly are helpful in combination with other tests as part of a sepsis screening panel (see later discussion), when CRP assay is used alone as an initial test for infection, even if the most favorable results are assumed, approximately 10% of cases would be missed, and 5% of uninfected infants would be incorrectly diagnosed as having infection.

Nevertheless, determination of serial CRP levels does seem to be of some value in excluding serious infection [70,113,114,135]. Although assay results in a few infants are normal at the onset of invasive bacterial disease, CRP levels increase rapidly and usually are abnormal within 1 day (CRP doubling time is 8 hours). CRP levels peak at 2 to 3 days and remain elevated until infection is controlled and resolution of the inflammatory process begins [21,23,91,113,136]. Thereafter, by virtue of a relatively short serum half-life of about 19 hours, CRP levels decline promptly and return to normal within 5 to 10 days in most infants who have a favorable outcome [23,24,114,135].

Serial measurements of CRP levels over 1 to 3 days after onset of possible neonatal bacterial infection may help determine the duration of antibiotic therapy and identify the occurrence of relapse or complications during or after treatment of known infection. Several studies document that serial determination of CRP levels in this fashion yields diagnostic sensitivity of 75% to 98%; specificity of 90%; and, perhaps most notably, negative predictive value of 99% [49,124–127,135–138]. These studies suggest that although the relatively low sensitivity of initial CRP

---

*References [21,23,49,70,113,114,122–129].

determination precludes the firm diagnosis of bacterial infection, the very high negative predictive value of several normal CRP determinations in combination allows the early cessation of empirical 7- to 10-day courses of intravenous antibiotics. It is less likely, however, that serial CRP determinations would allow cessation of empirical 2- to 3-day courses of antibiotics. Also, the kinetics of increase and decrease of elevated CRP levels does not differ sufficiently to allow distinction between newborns with positive bacterial blood cultures and newborns with negative bacterial blood cultures [136].

PROCALCITONIN

Several authors have described an early and specific elevation in serum levels of procalcitonin in infants with invasive bacterial disease [139–143]. Procalcitonin concentrations naturally fluctuate during the first 48 hours of life, however, mandating careful (perhaps hourly) adjustments in the normal reference ranges and complicating use of procalcitonin as a diagnostic aid [122,143–145]. In addition, the normal reference ranges seem to depend on the estimated gestational age of the premature newborn [146]. Elevation of procalcitonin levels was only modestly reliable (75% to 80% sensitivity and specificity) even for the diagnosis of late-onset sepsis in older neonates in whom the fluctuations after birth had resolved [147].

ERYTHROCYTE SEDIMENTATION RATE

The development more than 50 years ago of an erythrocyte sedimentation rate, by use of a microhematocrit tube and a few drops of capillary blood, permitted the application of this test in very small infants [148,149]. Attempts at standardization have shown that the microerythrocyte sedimentation rate increases slowly during the first weeks of life, perhaps as a result of increasing fibrinogen and decreasing hematocrit levels. Maximal normal rates have varied so widely, however, that any laboratory attempting to use this test in neonates must establish its own normal values [150–152].

Sedimentation rates do not vary significantly with gestational age, birth weight, or gender, but are related inversely to the hematocrit level, particularly in infants with hematocrit readings of less than 0.40 [150,151]. Comparisons between the microerythrocyte sedimentation rate and standard methods have shown good correlation in simultaneous analyses of samples obtained from cord blood, from infants with physiologic jaundice, and from healthy older children [150]. Rapid alternative methods, such as determination of the zeta sedimentation ratio [153] and plasma viscosity [154], compared well with standard erythrocyte sedimentation rate assays and were thought to reflect a change in the same plasma proteins; however, they have not been evaluated in newborns. The microerythrocyte sedimentation rate generally is normal or only mildly elevated in noninfectious conditions, such as respiratory distress syndrome, aspiration pneumonia, and asphyxia, and in superficial infections [150,152]. Significant elevations are unusual in healthy infants, but can occur in the presence of Coombs-positive hemolytic disease and physiologic hyperbilirubinemia [21,150,152].

Although extensive clinical experience has shown that sedimentation rates eventually become elevated in most infants with systemic bacterial infections, this increase may not have occurred at the time of the initial evaluation in 30% to 70% of infants with proven sepsis, particularly when disseminated intravascular coagulopathy is present.* When the sedimentation rate is elevated, its return to normal can be exceedingly slow despite clinical recovery, sometimes taking several weeks from the time of onset of illness [150]. Use of the microerythrocyte sedimentation rate is of little value in either diagnosing or monitoring serious bacterial infection during the newborn period.

OTHER ACUTE PHASE REACTANTS
Fibrinogen

The increase in plasma fibrinogen level associated with infection has been recognized for many years through its effects on the erythrocyte sedimentation rate. Clinical experience with the use of fibrinogen levels is limited, but generally disappointing. Median fibrinogen concentrations in infected infants overlapped to a great extent with levels obtained from normal infants, and low values despite severe infection also have been reported [155,156]. Concentrations may be affected by birth weight and test methodology and decrease dramatically in the presence of disseminated intravascular coagulopathy.

Haptoglobin

Haptoglobin is an α_2-glycoprotein that reacts with free hemoglobin to form a complex, which is removed by the reticuloendothelial system. Gestational age, neonatal asphyxia, gender, and hemolytic ABO/Rh disease have no significant influence on haptoglobin levels in cord blood or during the postnatal period; however, elevated levels usually persist for several days after exchange transfusion, probably as a result of passive transfer of blood with adult concentrations of the protein. Inaccuracies related to phenotypic variants of haptoglobin, although seen when levels are measured by radial immunodiffusion, have not presented a problem when concentrations are determined by laser nephelometry. Clinical studies have raised serious doubts about the reliability of haptoglobin concentrations in the prediction of neonatal sepsis [20,24,121,157,158].

α_1-Acid Glycoprotein

α_1-Acid glycoprotein (orosomucoid) is produced by lymphocytes, monocytes, neutrophils, and hepatocytes. It exists as an integral membrane protein of leukocytes and is liberated into the plasma as the cells disintegrate [112]. The function of α_1-acid glycoprotein is unknown, but it may have a role in forming collagen, binding steroid hormones, and modifying lymphocyte responsiveness [138,159]. Although early studies suggested that α_1-acid glycoprotein might be a specific and sensitive indicator

---

*References [21,23,84,128,150,152].

of neonatal bacterial infection, subsequent surveys have been unable to confirm this favorable experience [20,121,130,138,159–164].

Others

Other acute phase proteins evaluated for the early diagnosis of neonatal sepsis include α_1-proteinase inhibitor (α_1-antitrypsin) [24,164], the complex of elastase and α_1-proteinase inhibitor [165,166], α_1-antichymotrypsin [164], inter-α-inhibitor proteins [167], ceruloplasmin [168], and secretory phospholipase A_2 [169]. No definitive clinical studies suggest that any of these reactants are helpful for diagnosis or management in the neonate suspected to have a bacterial infection. Serum amyloid A protein, another acute phase reactant, seemed to be slightly more sensitive than CRP in predicting early-onset sepsis in full-term infants, although the differences were not maintained after 24 hours of symptoms, and few normal controls were studied to define specificity [170].

ADDITIONAL LABORATORY STUDIES
CYTOKINES AND CHEMOKINES

Cytokines such as IL-1β, IL-6, IL-10, and TNF-α and chemokines such as IL-8 and others are endogenous mediators of the innate immune response to inflammation, including (but not limited to) inflammation caused by bacterial infections. Cord and postnatal blood cytokine concentrations may vary as a result of clinical complications during the perinatal period. IL-1β is elevated in cord plasma specimens from infants born after induced vaginal or urgent cesarean delivery, whereas IL-6 is elevated in the presence of chorioamnionitis and delivery room intubation, yet depressed in the presence of pregnancy-induced hypertension [123,171,172]. Because of the confounding effects of maternal complications, differences in chronologic age from the first hours to days of life, and illness severity, the reported performance of various cytokine markers must be viewed with some caution [4,117,123]. Also, it is not always clear that the first available laboratory method of measuring a cytokine is the most sensitive; it has been reported that the sensitivity and specificity of IL-8 assays are improved markedly by measuring detergent-lysed whole-blood samples, rather than by using plasma samples as reported in earlier studies [173].

Nevertheless, several studies suggest that elevated levels of IL-6 detected after birth may provide an early and sensitive parameter for the diagnosis of neonatal bacterial infection [121–123,172,174–179]. Elevated concentrations have also been correlated with a fatal outcome in older children [180]. Similarly, levels of IL-8 were found to be elevated in cord blood from infants in whom histologic evidence of chorioamnionitis was noted and in infants with sepsis [129,175,181,182]. Because of variations in study design and methodology, estimates of diagnostic sensitivity and specificity for IL-6 and IL-8 levels range from 60% to greater than 95% for each [129,183–185]. In addition, although plasma and tracheal aspirate IL-8 and IL-10 levels correlate with bacterial sepsis, they are nonspecific in neonates with necrotizing enterocolitis [186].

ADHESION MOLECULES AND CELLULAR RECEPTORS

Upregulation of adhesion molecules such as E-selectin, L-selectin, and intercellular adhesion molecule-1 has been suggested as a discriminating feature of bacterial sepsis [125,178,187–189]. Genetic polymorphisms in mannose-binding lectins seem to underlie susceptibility to infection in some premature neonates; it is unknown whether this analyte could be used for diagnostic purposes [190]. Cytokine receptors and receptor antagonists such as soluble TNF-α and IL-2 receptors and IL-1 receptor antagonist have been explored as potential aids in the laboratory diagnosis of neonatal sepsis [129,176,183,191,192]. Further clinical data are needed to determine whether measurement of these analytes is truly useful for the diagnosis and follow-up evaluation of neonatal sepsis.

LYMPHOCYTE AND NEUTROPHIL MARKER ANALYSIS

Another component of the inflammatory response to infection is the change in surface markers of white blood cell populations as measured by flow cytometry. Activation of T lymphocytes after infection results in upregulation of the lymphocyte surface marker CD45RO isoform coupled to loss of the CD45RA isoform. Sequential analysis of the distribution of early CD45RA-CD45RO dual expression and later CD45RO expression alone discriminated bacterial (and viral) infection from respiratory distress or erythrocyte incompatibility in a few infants [193]. The surface expression of the neutrophil surface marker CD11b yielded good sensitivity, specificity, and predictive values in diagnosing neonatal bacterial and fungal infection in several studies [188,194,195]. The expression of CD11b and other markers such as soluble CD40 ligand may be affected by duration of labor and chronologic age; further studies are required to define normal ranges and clinical utility [188,196,197]. Expression of another neutrophil surface marker, CD64, has been found to correlate with early-onset and late-onset nosocomial newborn sepsis in some studies [198–200].

MISCELLANEOUS ANALYTES

Fibronectin is an adhesive, high-molecular-weight glycoprotein of 450,000 kDa that has been identified on cell surfaces and in extracellular fluids. It is thought, by virtue of its stickiness, to act as an intercellular cement and maintain microvascular integrity and to act as an opsonin and aid in the phagocytic function of neutrophils and macrophages [112,201]. Generally, the concentration of fibronectin in fetal plasma increases with gestational age to concentrations at term of approximately half the concentrations found in healthy adults [201–203]. Plasma concentrations usually decrease significantly during the course of neonatal sepsis, probably as a result of clearance by the reticuloendothelial system of products of the inflammatory response. The rate of recovery of fibronectin concentrations as infection resolves is relatively rapid, occurring over 5 to 7 days [201,202]. Attempts to characterize a decrease in fibronectin concentrations as a specific marker for sepsis have been disappointing, however [21].

Demonstration of increased amounts of total IgM in umbilical cord sera previously was thought to be helpful in identifying infants with infections acquired in the intrauterine environment, particularly infections caused by rubella virus, cytomegalovirus, *Treponema pallidum*, and *Toxoplasma gondii* [204]. On the basis of this experience, several studies, mainly in the late 1960s and early 1970s, attempted to use serially determined IgM concentrations in the evaluation of infants suspected to have acute postnatal bacterial infections. The sensitivity of IgM concentrations in infants with bacterial sepsis, meningitis, pneumonia, or urinary tract infection is low; specificity was low as well in that viral infections, minor localized bacterial infections, and meconium aspiration were associated with a significant increase in IgM concentrations [21,204–208]. Determination of IgM concentrations as an index of neonatal bacterial infection has largely been abandoned.

The discovery that neutrophils that have phagocytized bacteria reduce nitroblue tetrazolium (NBT) dye to purple formazan led to development of several tests using this leukocyte enzyme activity for detection of bacterial infections involving the systemic circulation [209]. It was shown that in most cases, most peripheral neutrophils reduce nitroblue tetrazolium during the course of an untreated or ineffectively treated infection, whereas only a small proportion of neutrophils do so in the absence of infection. Attempts to incorporate this assay into the newborn period were hampered by difficulty in establishing standard techniques and normal values, and the predictive value of the test was found to be lower than expected [210–215]. The NBT test now is rarely used in the diagnosis of neonatal infection [93]. Many years ago, changes in leukocyte lactate dehydrogenase [216] and in alkaline phosphatase [217] concentrations were thought to be potentially useful indices of neonatal infection. These determinations have received little further attention since that time.

Bacterial infections are known to alter carbohydrate metabolism in neonates. Although hypoglycemia [218] and hyperglycemia [219] have been described in infants with sepsis, the association between changes in blood glucose concentrations and neonatal infection is of limited value as a diagnostic aid.

An exciting discovery in the field of immunology is that multicellular organisms share many evolutionarily conserved aspects of their innate immune systems. Innate immunity depends on molecules such as specialized cellular receptors and binding proteins (e.g., toll-like receptors and mannose-binding proteins), serum complement proteins, and several substances produced and released at the site of infection by neutrophils [220,221]. This last group includes the antimicrobial peptides of the defensin and cathelicidin classes, bactericidal/permeability-increasing protein, lysozyme, and lactoferrin [220–222]. Some of these substances are found in vernix caseosa, the lipid-rich substance covering the skin of the fetus and newborn infant [223]. Further studies on the kinetics of these molecules in health and disease may lead to diagnostic aids for newborn sepsis [222–224].

Finally, sepsis or, more properly, the systemic inflammatory response to sepsis causes hemodynamic changes in regional blood flow. Early in sepsis, peripheral vasoconstriction is seen, whereas in advanced sepsis, generalized vasodilation and shock occur. An interesting concept in diagnostic techniques for neonatal sepsis is to attempt to measure noninvasively deviations in peripheral vascular reactivity or heart rate characteristics. In one small study, newborns with early-onset sepsis (clinical or bacteriologic) had lower degrees of mean peripheral skin perfusion and a higher amount of postocclusion reactive hyperemia as measured by a laser Doppler instrument [175]. The sensitivity and specificity for the measurement of reactive hyperemia were equivalent to or greater than those for measurement of IL-6, IL-8, and TNF-α in this study [175]. A computerized index of reductions in heart rate variability and transient decelerations in heart rate seemed to correlate with late-onset clinical and proven sepsis and, in some cases, predicted sepsis [225].

MICROSCOPIC EXAMINATION OF PLACENTA, UMBILICAL CORD, GASTRIC ASPIRATES, AND EXTERNAL EAR CANAL FLUID

Microscopic examination of tissues or body fluids is a time-honored but insensitive and nonspecific aid in the diagnosis of neonatal sepsis. An association of neonatal sepsis with pathologic changes in the placenta and umbilical cord was suggested more than 40 years ago [226,227]. Neonatal infection acquired at or about the time of birth often is associated with chorioamnionitis or funisitis [228–230]. Histologic sections of the placenta show acute inflammatory changes, with infiltration of the umbilical vein by neutrophils and gross or microscopic evidence of chorioamnionitis. The probability of finding inflammatory changes in these tissues is inversely related to birth weight and directly related to the duration of rupture of membranes before delivery, the presence of meconium in amniotic fluid, and fetal distress and hypoxia [231–233]. Some inflammatory changes are apparent in the placenta and its membranes or the umbilical cord in 30% of live-born infants [228]. The presence of chorioamnionitis and placentitis does not automatically imply significant neonatal infection.

The stomach of the newborn contains fluid swallowed before and during delivery. The presence of neutrophils and bacteria in a stained smear of the gastric aspirate indicates inflammation of the amniotic fluid, placenta, and other tissues of the birth canal [234,235]. The neutrophils in the gastric aspirate obtained during the 1st day of life are from the mother and do not indicate a fetal inflammatory response [236]. The presence of these maternal leukocytes indicates exposure to possible infection and does not identify an infectious disease in the newborn. After the 1st day, the gastric aspirate contains swallowed bronchial secretions, and examination of a stained preparation may suggest pneumonia in the neonate if inflammatory cells are present [237]. The presence of neutrophils in the aspirated ear canal fluid also indicates exposure to an infected environment. Stained smears and bacterial cultures of neonatal gastric aspirate or external ear canal fluid reflect the flora of the birth canal, and results parallel those of cultures of specimens obtained from the maternal vagina, endocervix, endometrium, and placenta [238–242]. The information obtained does not greatly influence decision making regarding antimicrobial therapy [239].

Pathogens frequently are isolated when daily tracheal aspirates for intubated infants are cultured. Because many (if not all) intubated newborns eventually become colonized with potentially pathogenic microbes, however, the positive predictive value of this test is less than 30% [243]. Similar to gastric aspirates or external ear canal fluid, tracheal aspirates reflect environmental influences, but do not imply sepsis.

Molecular detection tests for bacteria or bacterial products have been applied to amniotic fluid and neonatal blood. The limulus lysate assay for the detection of endotoxin did not prove to be clinically useful [244]. PCR amplification of bacterial DNA from blood seems promising, but is not ready for general clinical use [245,246].

SCREENING PANELS

The inability of any single laboratory test to provide rapid, reliable, and early identification of neonates with bacterial sepsis has led to efforts to devise a panel of screening tests, combining data from several different determinations, as a means of increasing predictive value.* The results generally have shown little increase in positive predictive value (if a test result is abnormal, disease is present) compared with most individual screening tests, although negative predictive value (if a result is normal, disease is absent) has been remarkably good, approaching 100% in some studies. Performance characteristics of some screening panel tests are summarized in Table 36–3 and compared with single tests.

One attempt to diagnose neonatal sepsis through multiple, simple, standard laboratory determinations involved more than 500 infants younger than 7 days of age studied by Philip and colleagues [20,69,249]. The authors devised a "sepsis screen" for use with infants believed to be at risk for, or showing clinical evidence of, serious bacterial infection. In addition to the standard procedures (blood, CSF, and urine cultures and chest film), the evaluation included a screening panel consisting of total leukocyte count, determination of the I:M ratio, CRP and haptoglobin assays, and microerythrocyte sedimentation rate. An abnormality in any two or more of these items was considered to reflect a "positive sepsis screen," and no abnormality or an abnormality in one item reflected a "negative sepsis screen"; the test turnaround time was 1 hour.

Analysis of the results [20,69] showed a 39% probability that serious bacterial infection was present if two or more test results were positive (positive predictive value) and a 99% probability that infection was not present if only one or no result was positive (negative predictive value). In actual numbers, as a result of the sepsis screen, 60 of 524 infants with clinically suspected sepsis received unnecessary treatment with antimicrobial agents (false positives; specificity of 88%), and 3 with subsequently proven bacterial infection were missed (false negatives; sensitivity of 93%) [69]. Comparable results have been reported by Gerdes and Polin [21], who used a sepsis screen similar to that used by Philip, and by others who used only hematologic or clinical indices [17,45,47,59,95]. Panels of screening tests have not always functioned better than

relying solely on the I:T neutrophil ratio, however, particularly in the 1st week of life [20–22,48,59,69,75].

By virtue of its high negative predictive value, the screening panel used by Philip [249] in an intensive care nursery resulted in a significant decrease in the use of antimicrobial agents. Not only did fewer neonates receive antimicrobial agents, but also treatment could be discontinued earlier with greater confidence in the infants who were being administered these agents. Philip [249] was careful to emphasize, however, that screening tests are intended only to augment clinical evaluation. When the evidence obtained by history or physical examination conflicts with a negative screen result, antimicrobial therapy should be started. Similarly, a screening panel combining clinical evaluation and IL-8 and CRP assays led to fewer antibiotic courses being administered compared with neonates treated with standard clinical diagnosis [248]. Neither the IL-8 nor the CRP assays detected all bacteremic neonates at the time of the first evaluation, but when used together as a panel with clinical judgment, greater sensitivity was achieved [248].

An increasingly important area in which a screening test panel might be useful is in the evaluation of asymptomatic infants whose mothers have been given intrapartum antibiotics to decrease the risk of early-onset neonatal group B streptococcal sepsis [6–9]. The American Academy of Pediatrics and the U.S. Centers for Disease Control and Prevention (CDC) recommend that a "limited evaluation," consisting of complete blood cell count and a blood culture, be performed in infants whose mothers met the criteria for intrapartum antibiotic prophylaxis, but who did not receive a complete course of prophylactic treatment [8,9]. The goal is to identify infants with sepsis, including infants whose blood cultures may have been sterilized temporarily by maternal antibiotic prophylaxis.

Ottolini and colleagues [29] tested the utility of a complete blood count screening panel in 1665 infants whose mothers met the criteria for intrapartum antibiotic prophylaxis, but did not receive a full course of treatment. These investigators found that the diagnostic test sensitivity and specificity of an abnormal white blood cell count (i.e., total white blood cell count of $\leq 5000/mm^3$ or $\geq 30,000/mm^3$, absolute neutrophil count of $<1500/mm^3$, or I:M ratio of >0.2) were 41% and 73% [29]. Because of the low incidence of true sepsis, even after only partial maternal antibiotic prophylaxis, the positive predictive value of the complete blood count panel was only 1.5%, and the positive likelihood ratio only 1.5. A positive test result was not indicative of newborn sepsis. The negative predictive value of the screen was 99%, implying that a normal test result would at least reassure the clinician that sepsis was not present. The negative predictive value of an infant's appearing asymptomatic also was 99%, however; the complete blood count panel did not add any diagnostic information beyond that gained simply by obtaining a careful history and physical examination of the infant. Similar conclusions were reached by Escobar and associates [85]. The ineffectiveness of the screening panel in these studies may have been due to the low rates of culture-proven sepsis, but many U.S. centers where group B streptococcal sepsis prophylaxis is employed now have such low rates of sepsis.

---

*References [4,117,125,150,151,247,248].

TABLE 36-3   Performance Characteristics of Tests and Screening Panels for Early-Onset Neonatal Bacteremia: Selected Reports

Source, Test (Test Cutoff*)	No. Newborns Evaluated	Prevalence of Culture-Documented Bacterial Sepsis (%)	Sensitivity (%)	Specificity (%)	Positive Predictive Value (%)	Negative Predictive Value (%)	Positive Likelihood Ratio	Positive Likelihood Ratio
Philip [20]	376	8						
Any ≥2 abnormalities in I:T ratio, total WBC, CRP, microerythrocyte sedimentation rate, haptoglobin			93	88	39	99	7.8	0.08
Rodwell [48]	298	9						
Any ≥3 abnormalities in I:T ratio, total neutrophils, total WBC, I:M ratio, platelet count, degenerative changes of neutrophils			96	78	31	99	4.4	0.05
Chiesa [122]	134	8						
CRP: At birth (4 mg/L)			73	83	28	97	4.3	0.33
CRP: At 24 hr (of life) (10 mg/L)			91	87	38	99	7	0.10
IL-6: At birth (200 ng/L)			73	89	36	97	6.6	0.30
IL-6: At 24 hr (30 ng/L)			64	71	16	96	2.2	0.50
PCT: At birth (1 µg/L)			82	95	60	98	16.4	0.19
PCT: At 24 hr (100 µg/L)			100	96	69	100	2.5	~0
Døllner [123]	166	14.5						
CRP (10 mg/L)			63	89	48	93	5.7	0.42
IL-6 (20 ng/L)			78	64	27	95	2.2	0.34
CRP, IL-6, or both			96	58	28	99	3.7	0.07
Franz [248]	1291	1						
Clinical signs, plus CRP (10 mg/L), IL-8 (70 ng/L), or both			80	87	68	93	6.2	0.23
Benitz [126]	999	1.5						
Serial CRP levels: Any of 3 tests performed over 48 hr (10 mg/L)			89	70	5	99	3	0.16

*Test cutoff refers to the value above which the test result is considered abnormal.
CRP, C-reactive protein; IL-6, interleukin-6; I:M ratio, immature-to-mature neutrophil ratio (see text); I:T ratio, immature-to-total neutrophil ratio; PCT, procalcitonin; WBC, white blood cell (total leukocyte) count.

PERSPECTIVES AND CONCLUSIONS

As discussed previously, on examining all of the data published to date, it is difficult to choose one cytokine, acute phase reactant, or screening panel for current use as the "best" test (see Table 36–3) [117,183,184,247,248]. Why is this still the case in the 21st century, after so many advances in medical science and biotechnology, and with the plethora of studies of newborn sepsis, or, why has the "ideal test" not been discovered? [10,11] Besides the difficulties in constructing a quick, easy-to-analyze, stable, analytic test with clear diagnostic cutoffs across gestational ages and birth weights and optimal sensitivity and specificity [10,11], there are further clinical epidemiologic constraints in study design that are limiting.

First, some authors do not differentiate between perinatal (early-onset) and postnatal (late-onset) sepsis. This omission can lead to bias because different neonatal pathogens cause early-onset and late-onset disease. Second, because the normal ranges of many analytes vary across gestational and chronologic age, results are again confounded [117,122]. Third, not all reports of neonatal sepsis diagnostic tests include healthy controls, and consequently construction of the normal range of results for an analytic test poses difficulties. Another problem is the lack of universal agreement on the definition of newborn sepsis or systemic inflammatory response syndrome. Some studies restrict the analyses to culture-proven sepsis, although false-negative cultures owing to low blood sample volume or maternal antibiotic therapy may lead to bias. Other studies analyze clinical septicemia, although no universal definition of this entity exists, which also may lead to diagnostic bias; very few studies separately analyze data using proven and clinically diagnosed sepsis [123]. A fifth problem is that the current neonatal illness severity scores (e.g., Score for Neonatal Acute Physiology [SNAP], SNAP-Perinatal Extension [SNAP-PE], Clinical Risk Index for Babies [CRIB]), which theoretically could lead to better stratification of patients and more accurate interstudy comparisons, are cumbersome to use [117,123].

Finally, Chiesa and colleagues [117] noted that "the usefulness of a test will depend, above all, on the clinical condition of the baby. If the baby is really very sick, the test will not give very much additional information . . . if the baby is evidently well . . . a positive test result [will] not dramatically increase the probability that the baby is infected. . . ." In other words, it is essential for the clinician to heed bayesian statistical theory—one must consider the pretest (prior) probability (essentially, the disease prevalence) of infection and the test characteristics (sensitivity, specificity) to interpret and apply diagnostic test results properly. Many of these confounding effects can be seen in the data of Table 36–3, in which various studies have used different populations of infants, definitions of sepsis, and laboratory cutoff points, leading to different estimates of the utility of any one laboratory test.

Faced with the imperfection of currently available laboratory aids for the diagnosis of neonatal sepsis, what is today's practitioner to do? History, physical examination, and clinical impression still constitute a large part of clinical medicine, even in the era of molecular diagnostics and therapeutics. A single normal laboratory test should not sway a clinician against empirical therapy for a newborn if it seems to be clinically indicated, and an isolated abnormal test result should not be enough for the clinician to demand therapy. This concept may be restated in diagnostic test statistical terminology as follows: At present, there is no one test or test panel with a high enough positive likelihood ratio or a low enough negative likelihood ratio to recommend it uniquely over all others. The negative predictive values of available tests are not yet high enough, when results are normal, to lead to the withholding of therapy for an uncommon, but possibly life-threatening disease (neonatal sepsis). Conversely, the positive predictive values of available tests are not yet high enough when results are abnormal to lead to routine institution of antimicrobial therapy.

When laboratory testing is combined with clinical impression (and perhaps serial laboratory monitoring), predictive values may increase enough to help the clinician make decisions. When the risk of an uncommon disease with a poor outcome is high, however, and the risk of antimicrobial therapy is low, it may be difficult ever to find a test with predictive values high enough to "rule in" or "rule out" disease with complete confidence.

Clinical judgment, using standardized definitions of historical risk factors, signs, and symptoms, may sometimes perform as well as laboratory screening panels [29,85]. This point may be especially important to remember in resource-poor settings in developing countries [250]. Much future work is needed in the area of rapid diagnosis of neonatal sepsis to move beyond the current best menu of simple, rapid, and inexpensive (albeit imperfect) tests such as total neutrophil counts, total leukocyte counts, I:T ratios, and CRP assay. Continued improvements in blood culture technology are decreasing the time to positivity of neonatal blood cultures, which may at least speed up bacteriologic confirmation of septicemia [251–253].

REFERENCES

[1] A.R. Feinstein, Clinical biostatistics: XXXI. On the sensitivity, specificity, and discrimination of diagnostic tests, Clin. Pharmacol. Ther. 17 (1975) 104–116.

[2] R. Jaeschke, et al., Users' guides to the medical literature. III. How to use an article about a diagnostic test. B. What are the results and will they help me in caring for my patients? JAMA 271 (1994) 703–707.

[3] M. Radetsky, The laboratory evaluation of newborn sepsis, Curr. Opin. Infect. Dis. 8 (1995) 191–199.

[4] G.J. Escobar, Effect of the systemic inflammatory response on biochemical markers of neonatal bacterial infection: a fresh look at old confounders, Clin. Chem. 49 (2003) 21–22.

[5] E. Squire, B. Favara, J. Todd, Diagnosis of neonatal bacterial infection: hematologic and pathologic findings in fatal and nonfatal cases, Pediatrics 64 (1979) 60–64.

[6] B.J. Stoll, et al., Changes in pathogens causing early-onset sepsis in very-low-birth-weight infants, N. Engl. J. Med. 347 (2002) 240–247.

[7] T.B. Hyde, et al., Trends in incidence and antimicrobial resistance of early-onset sepsis: population-based surveillance in San Francisco and Atlanta, Pediatrics 110 (2002) 690–695.

[8] Centers for Disease Control and Prevention, Prevention of perinatal group B streptococcal disease, MMWR Morb. Mortal. Wkly. Rep. 51 (2002) 1–22.

[9] American Academy of Pediatrics, Group B streptococcal infections, in: L.K. Pickering (Ed.), Red Book: Report of the Committee on Infectious Diseases, twenty eighth ed., American Academy of Pediatrics, Elk Grove Village, IL, 2009.

[10] P.C. Ng, H.S. Lam, Diagnostic markers for neonatal sepsis, Curr. Opin. Pediatr. 18 (2006) 125–131.

[11] H.S. Lam, P.C. Ng, Biochemical markers of neonatal sepsis, Pathology 40 (2008) 141–148.

[12] E.C. Dunham, Septicemia in the newborn, Am. J. Dis. Child. 45 (1933) 229–253.

[13] W.L. Nyhan, M.D. Fousek, Septicemia of the newborn, Pediatrics 22 (1958) 268–278.

[14] K.C. Buetow, S.W. Klein, R.B. Lane, Septicemia in premature infants, Am. J. Dis. Child. 110 (1965) 29–41.

[15] R.S. Moorman Jr., S.H. Sell, Neonatal septicemia, South Med. J. 54 (1961) 137–141.

[16] P. Hänninen, P. Terho, A. Toivanen, Septicemia in a pediatric unit: a 20-year study, Scand. J. Infect. Dis. 3 (1971) 201–208.

[17] S.A. Spector, W. Ticknor, M. Grossman, Study of the usefulness of clinical and hematologic findings in the diagnosis of neonatal bacterial infections, Clin. Pediatr. 20 (1981) 385–392.

[18] H. Kuchler, H. Fricker, E. Gugler, La formule sanguine dans le diagnostic précoce de la septicémie du nouveau-né, Helv. Paediatr. Acta 31 (1976) 33–46.

[19] U. Töllner, F. Pohlandt, Septicemia in the newborn due to gram-negative bacilli: risk factors, clinical symptoms, and hematologic changes, Eur. J. Pediatr. 123 (1976) 243–254.

[20] A.G.S. Philip, J.R. Hewitt, Early diagnosis of neonatal sepsis, Pediatrics 65 (1980) 1036–1041.

[21] J.S. Gerdes, R.A. Polin, Sepsis screen in neonates with evaluation of plasma fibronectin, Pediatr. Infect. Dis. J. 6 (1987) 443–446.

[22] J.C. King Jr., E.D. Berman, P.F. Wright, Evaluation of fever in infants less than 8 weeks old, South Med. J. 80 (1987) 948–952.

[23] A.G.S. Philip, Response of C-reactive protein in neonatal group B streptococcal infection, Pediatr. Infect. Dis. J. 4 (1985) 145–148.

[24] C.H. Speer, A. Bruns, M. Gahr, Sequential determination of CRP, alpha-1 antitrypsin and haptoglobin in neonatal septicaemia, Acta Paediatr. Scand. 72 (1983) 679–683.

[25] C.H. Liu, et al., Degenerative changes in neutrophils: an indicator of bacterial infection, Pediatrics 74 (1984) 823–827.

[26] S. Jahnke, G. Bartiromo, M.J. Maisels, The peripheral white blood cell count in the diagnosis of neonatal infection, J. Perinatol. 5 (1985) 50–56.

[27] H.J. Rozycki, G.E. Stahl, S. Baumgart, Impaired sensitivity of a single early leukocyte count in screening for neonatal sepsis, Pediatr. Infect. Dis. J. 6 (1987) 440–442.

[28] R.D. Christensen, et al., Fatal early onset group B streptococcal sepsis with normal leukocyte counts, Pediatr. Infect. Dis. J. 4 (1985) 242–245.

[29] M.C. Ottolini, et al., Utility of complete blood count and blood culture screening to diagnose neonatal sepsis in the asymptomatic at risk newborn, Pediatr. Infect. Dis. J. 22 (2003) 430–434.

[30] M.I. Marks, T. Stacy, H.F. Krous, Progressive cough associated with lymphocytic leukemoid reaction in an infant, J. Pediatr. 97 (1980) 156–160.

[31] A.G. Weinberg, et al., Neonatal blood cell count in health and disease. II. Values for lymphocytes, monocytes, and eosinophils, J. Pediatr. 106 (1985) 462–466.

[32] P. Roth, Colony stimulating factor 1 levels in the human newborn infant, J. Pediatr. 119 (1991) 113–116.

[33] G. Karayalcin, et al., Monocytosis in congenital syphilis, Am. J. Dis. Child. 131 (1977) 782–783.

[34] A.M. Visintine, J.M. Oleske, A.J. Nahmias, *Listeria monocytogenes* infection in infants and children, Am. J. Dis. Child. 131 (1977) 393–397.

[35] M. Xanthou, Leucocyte blood picture in healthy full-term and premature babies during neonatal period, Arch. Dis. Child. 45 (1970) 242–249.

[36] R. Lawrence Jr., et al., Eosinophilia in the hospitalized neonate, Ann. Allergy 44 (1980) 349–352.

[37] J.M. Burrell, A comparative study of the circulating eosinophil level in babies. II. In full term infants, Arch. Dis. Child. 28 (1953) 140–142.

[38] E.L. Gibson, Y. Vaucher, J.J. Corrigan Jr., Eosinophilia in premature infants: relationship to weight gain, J. Pediatr. 95 (1979) 99–101.

[39] T. Gunn, et al., Peripheral total parenteral nutrition for premature infants with the respiratory distress syndrome: a controlled study, J. Pediatr. 92 (1978) 608–613.

[40] A.M. Bhat, J.W. Scanlon, The pattern of eosinophilia in premature infants: a prospective study in premature infants using the absolute eosinophil count, J. Pediatr. 98 (1981) 612–616.

[41] D.S. Chudwin, et al., Posttransfusion syndrome: rash, eosinophilia, and thrombocytopenia following intrauterine and exchange transfusions, Am. J. Dis. Child. 136 (1982) 612–614.

[42] M. Xanthou, Leucocyte blood picture in ill newborn babies, Arch. Dis. Child. 47 (1972) 741–746.

[43] W.A. Bonadio, D.S. Smith, CBC differential profile in distinguishing etiology of neonatal meningitis, Pediatr. Emerg. Care 5 (1989) 94–96.

[44] M. Metrov, E.F. Crain, The complete blood count differential ratio in the assessment of febrile infants with meningitis, Pediatr. Infect. Dis. J. 10 (1991) 334–335.

[45] B.L. Manroe, et al., The neonatal blood count in health and disease. I. Reference values for neutrophilic cells, J. Pediatr. 95 (1979) 89–98.

[46] A. Zipursky, et al., The hematology of bacterial infections in premature infants, Pediatrics 57 (1976) 839–853.

[47] M. Amato, H. Howald, G. von Muralt, Qualitative changes of white blood cells and perinatal diagnosis of infection in high-risk preterm infants, Pädiatr. Pädol. 23 (1988) 129–134.

[48] R.L. Rodwell, A.L. Leslie, D.I. Tudehope, Early diagnosis of neonatal sepsis using a hematologic scoring system, J. Pediatr. 112 (1988) 761–767.

[49] C. Berger, et al., Comparison of C-reactive protein and white blood cell count with differential in neonates at risk for septicemia, Eur. J. Pediatr. 154 (1995) 138–144.

[50] R.D. Christensen, Morphology and concentration of circulating neutrophils in neonates with bacterial sepsis, Pediatr. Infect. Dis. J. 6 (1987) 429–430.

[51] J. Gregory, E. Hey, Blood neutrophil response to bacterial infection in the first month of life, Arch. Dis. Child. 47 (1972) 747–753.

[52] J.E. Baley, et al., Neonatal neutropenia: clinical manifestations, cause, and outcome, Am. J. Dis. Child. 142 (1988) 1161–1166.

[53] J. Marks, D. Gairdner, J.D. Roscoe, Blood formation in infancy. III. Cord blood, Arch. Dis. Child. 30 (1955) 117–120.

[54] A. Mouzinho, et al., Revised reference ranges for circulating neutrophils in very-low-birth-weight neonates, Pediatrics 94 (1999) 76–82.

[55] R.L. Schelonka, et al., Peripheral leukocyte count and leukocyte indexes in healthy newborn term infants, J. Pediatr. 125 (1994) 603–606.

[56] L. Coulombel, et al., The number of polymorphonuclear leukocytes in relation to gestational age in the newborn, Acta Paediatr. Scand. 68 (1979) 709–711.

[57] W.D. Engle, C.R. Rosenfeld, Neutropenia in high-risk neonates, J. Pediatr. 105 (1984) 982–986.

[58] J.E. Brazy, J.K. Grimm, V.A. Little, Neonatal manifestations of severe maternal hypertension occurring before the thirty-sixth week of pregnancy, J. Pediatr. 100 (1982) 265–271.

[59] R.L. Rodwell, D.I. Tudehope, P.H. Gray, Hematologic scoring system in early diagnosis of sepsis in neutropenic newborns, Pediatr. Infect. Dis. J. 12 (1993) 372–376.

[60] P. Merlob, et al., The differential leukocyte count in full-term newborn infants with meconium aspiration and neonatal asphyxia, Acta Paediatr. Scand. 69 (1980) 779–780.

[61] R.D. Christensen, G. Rothstein, Pitfalls in the interpretation of leukocyte counts of newborn infants, Am. J. Clin. Pathol. 72 (1979) 608–611.

[62] C. Carballo, et al., Effect of high altitude on neutrophil counts in newborn infants, J. Pediatr. 119 (1991) 464–466.

[63] J.A. Menke, G.P. Giacoia, H. Jockin, Group B beta hemolytic streptococcal sepsis and the idiopathic respiratory distress syndrome: a comparison, J. Pediatr. 94 (1979) 467–471.

[64] J.P. Frazier, et al., Leukocyte function in healthy neonates following vaginal and cesarean section deliveries, J. Pediatr. 101 (1982) 269–272.

[65] A. Zipursky, H.M. Jaber, The haematology of bacterial infection in newborn infants, Clin. Haematol. 7 (1978) 175–193.

[66] G.I. Akenzua, et al., Neutrophil and band counts in the diagnosis of neonatal infections, Pediatrics 54 (1974) 38–42.

[67] J.C. Rooney, D.J. Hill, D.M. Danks, Jaundice associated with bacterial infection in the newborn, Am. J. Dis. Child. 122 (1971) 39–41.

[68] I. Benuck, R.J. David, Sensitivity of published neutrophil indexes in identifying newborn infants with sepsis, J. Pediatr. 103 (1983) 961–963.

[69] A.G.S. Philip, Detection of neonatal sepsis of late onset, JAMA 247 (1982) 489–492.

[70] O. Da Silva, A. Ohlsson, C. Kenyon, Accuracy of leukocyte indices and C-reactive protein for diagnosis of neonatal sepsis: a critical review, Pediatr. Infect. Dis. J. 14 (1995) 363–366.

[71] R.D. Christensen, P.P. Bradley, G. Rothstein, The leukocyte left shift in clinical and experimental neonatal sepsis, J. Pediatr. 98 (1981) 101–105.

[72] C.P. Speer, et al., Neonatal septicemia and meningitis in Göttingen, West Germany, Pediatr. Infect. Dis. J. 4 (1985) 36–41.

[73] H.S. Faden, Early diagnosis of neonatal bacteremia by buffy-coat examination, J. Pediatr. 88 (1976) 1032–1034.

[74] J.C. Leonidas, et al., Radiographic findings in early onset neonatal group B streptococcal septicemia, Pediatrics 59 (1977) 1006–1011.

[75] B.L. Manroe, et al., The differential leukocyte count in the assessment and outcome of early-onset neonatal group B streptococcal disease, J. Pediatr. 91 (1977) 632–637.

[76] N.R. Payne, et al., Correlation of clinical and pathologic findings in early onset neonatal group B streptococcal infection with disease severity and prediction of outcome, Pediatr. Infect. Dis. J. 7 (1988) 836–847.

[77] S.E. Courtney, R.T. Hall, *Haemophilus influenzae* sepsis in the premature infant, Am. J. Dis. Child. 132 (1978) 1039–1040.

[78] R.D. Christensen, et al., Granulocyte transfusions in neonates with bacterial infection, neutropenia, and depletion of mature marrow neutrophils, Pediatrics 70 (1982) 1–6.

[79] R. Bortolussi, T.R. Thompson, P. Ferrieri, Early-onset pneumococcal sepsis in newborn infants, Pediatrics 60 (1977) 352–355.

[80] H. Johnsson, et al., Neonatal septicemia caused by pneumococci, Acta Obstet. Gynecol. Scand. 71 (1992) 6–11.

[81] J. Jacobs, et al., Neonatal sepsis due to *Streptococcus pneumoniae*, Scand. J. Infect. Dis. 22 (1990) 493–497.

[82] J.B. Alexander, G.P. Giacoia, Early onset nonenterococcal group D streptococcal infection in the newborn infant, J. Pediatr. 93 (1978) 489–490.

[83] R.D. Christensen, G. Rothstein, Exhaustion of mature marrow neutrophils in neonates with sepsis, J. Pediatr. 96 (1980) 316–318.

[84] R.J. Boyle, Early identification of sepsis in infants with respiratory distress, Pediatrics 62 (1978) 744–750.

[85] G.J. Escobar, et al., Neonatal sepsis workups in infants >2000 grams at birth: a population-based study, Pediatrics 106 (2000) 256–263.

[86] B.W. Lloyd, A. Oto, Normal values for mature and immature neutrophils in very preterm babies, Arch. Dis. Child. 57 (1982) 233–235.

[87] J.G. Wheeler, et al., Neutrophil storage pool depletion in septic, neutropenic neonates, Pediatr. Infect. Dis. 3 (1984) 407–409.

[88] R.D. Christensen, T.E. Harper, G. Rothstein, Granulocyte-macrophage progenitor cells in term and preterm neonates, J. Pediatr. 109 (1986) 1047–1051.

[89] A.M. Lake, et al., Enterovirus infections in neonates, J. Pediatr. 89 (1976) 787–791.

[90] J.S. Gerdes, Clinicopathologic approach to the diagnosis of neonatal sepsis, Clin. Perinatol. 18 (1991) 361–381.

[91] N.J. Mathers, F. Pohlandt, Diagnostic audit of C-reactive protein in neonatal infection, Eur. J. Pediatr. 146 (1987) 147–151.

[92] M.P. Sherman, K.H. Chance, B.W. Goetzman, Gram's stains of tracheal secretions predict neonatal bacteremia, Am. J. Dis. Child. 138 (1984) 848–850.

[93] P. Kite, et al., Comparison of five tests used in diagnosis of neonatal bacteraemia, Arch. Dis. Child. 63 (1988) 639–643.

[94] B.K. Schmidt, et al., Coagulase-negative staphylococci as true pathogens in newborn infants: a cohort study, Pediatr. Infect. Dis. J. 6 (1987) 1026–1031.

[95] D.N. Greenberg, B.A. Yoder, Changes in the differential white blood cell count in screening for group B streptococcal sepsis, Pediatr. Infect. Dis. J. 9 (1990) 886–889.

[96] R.L. Schelonka, et al., Differentiation of segmented and band neutrophils during the early newborn period, J. Pediatr. 127 (1995) 298–300.

[97] W.J. Appleyard, A. Brinton, Venous platelet counts in low birth weight infants, Biol. Neonate 17 (1971) 30–34.

[98] A.J. Aballi, Y. Puapondh, F. Desposito, Platelet counts in thriving premature infants, Pediatrics 42 (1968) 685–689.

[99] H.D. Modanlou, O.B. Ortiz, Thrombocytopenia in neonatal infection, Clin. Pediatr. 20 (1981) 402–407.

[100] M. Andrew, J. Kelton, Neonatal thrombocytopenia, Clin. Perinatol. 11 (1984) 359–390.

[101] D.Y. Tate, et al., Immune thrombocytopenia in severe neonatal infections, J. Pediatr. 98 (1981) 449–453.

[102] P. Mehta, et al., Thrombocytopenia in the high-risk infant, J. Pediatr. 97 (1980) 791–794.

[103] J.D. Guida, et al., Platelet count and sepsis in very low birth weight neonates. Is there an organism-specific response, Pediatrics 111 (2003) 1411–1415.

[104] C.H. Patrick, J. Lazarchick, The effect of bacteremia on automated platelet measurements in neonates, Am. J. Clin. Pathol. 93 (1990) 391–394.

[105] J.F. Modlin, Fatal echovirus 11 disease in premature neonates, Pediatrics 66 (1980) 775–780.

[106] R.A. Ballard, et al., Acquired cytomegalovirus infection in preterm infants, Am. J. Dis. Child. 133 (1979) 482–485.

[107] A. Ballin, et al., Reduction of platelet counts induced by mechanical ventilation in newborn infants, J. Pediatr. 111 (1987) 445–449.

[108] C.C. Patel, Hematologic abnormalities in acute necrotizing enterocolitis, Pediatr. Clin. North Am. 24 (1977) 579–584.

[109] J.J. Hutter Jr., W.E. Hathaway, E.R. Wayne, Hematologic abnormalities in severe neonatal necrotizing enterocolitis, J. Pediatr. 88 (1976) 1026–1031.

[110] J.M. Koenig, R.D. Christensen, Neutropenia and thrombocytopenia in infants with Rh hemolytic disease, J. Pediatr. 114 (1989) 625–631.

[111] C. Gabay, I. Kushner, Acute-phase proteins and other systemic responses to inflammation, N. Engl. J. Med. 340 (1999) 448–454.

[112] M.B. Pepys, M.L. Baltz, Acute phase proteins with special reference to C-reactive protein and related proteins (pentaxins) and serum amyloid A protein, Adv. Immunol. 34 (1983) 141–212.

[113] D.L. Jaye, K.B. Waites, Clinical applications of C-reactive protein in pediatrics, Pediatr. Infect. Dis. J. 16 (1997) 735–747.

[114] L.O. Hansson, L. Lindquist, C-reactive protein: its role in the diagnosis and follow-up of infectious diseases, Curr. Opin. Infect. Dis. 10 (1997) 196–201.

[115] D. Gitlin, A. Biasucci, Development of IgG, IgA, IgM, β1C/β1A, Cv'1 esterase inhibitor, ceruloplasmin, transferrin, hemopexin, haptoglobin, fibrinogen, plasminogen, α_1-antitrypsin, orosomucoid, β-lipoprotein, α_2-macroglobulin, and prealbumin in the human conceptus, J. Clin. Invest. 48 (1969) 1433–1446.

[116] R.M. Nakamura, Nephelometric immunoassays, in: R.C. Boguslaski, E.T. Maggio, R.M. Nakamura (Eds.), Clinical Immunochemistry: Principles of Methods and Applications, Little, Brown, Boston, 1984.

[117] C. Chiesa, et al., Diagnosis of neonatal sepsis: a clinical and laboratory challenge, Clin. Chem. 50 (2004) 279–287.

[118] L.A. Hanson, et al., The diagnostic value of C-reactive protein, Pediatr. Infect. Dis. J. 2 (1983) 87–90.

[119] A. Wassunna, et al., C-reactive protein and bacterial infection in preterm infants, Eur. J. Pediatr. 149 (1990) 424–427.

[120] H. Vallance, G. Lockitch, Rapid, semi-quantitative assay of C-reactive protein evaluated, Clin. Chem. 37 (1991) 1981–1982.

[121] M. Pourcyrous, et al., Acute phase reactants in neonatal bacterial infection, J. Perinatol. 11 (1991) 319–325.

[122] C. Chiesa, et al., C-reactive protein, interleukin-6, and procalcitonin in the immediate postnatal period: influence of illness severity, risk status, antenatal and perinatal complications, and infection, Clin. Chem. 49 (2003) 60–68.

[123] H. Døllner, L. Vatten, R. Austgulen, Early diagnostic markers for neonatal sepsis: comparing C-reactive protein, interleukin-6, soluble tumour necrosis factor receptors and soluble adhesion molecules, J. Clin. Epidemiol. 54 (2001) 1251–1257.

[124] M. Pourcyrous, et al., Significance of serial C-reactive protein responses in neonatal infection and other disorders, Pediatrics 92 (1993) 431–435.

[125] P.C. Ng, et al., Diagnosis of late onset neonatal sepsis with cytokines, adhesion molecule, and C-reactive protein in preterm very low birthweight infants, Arch. Dis. Child. 77 (1997) F221–F227.

[126] W.E. Benitz, et al., Serial C-reactive protein levels in the diagnosis of neonatal infection, Pediatrics 102 (1998) e41.

[127] S. Ehl, et al., C-reactive protein is a useful marker for guiding duration of antibiotic therapy in suspected neonatal bacterial infection, Pediatrics 99 (1997) 216–221.

[128] D.B. Shortland, et al., Evaluation of C-reactive protein values in neonatal sepsis, J. Perinat. Med. 18 (1990) 157–163.

[129] C. Santana Reyes, et al., Role of cytokines (interleukin-1beta, 6, 8, tumour necrosis factor-alpha, and soluble receptor of interleukin-2) and C-reactive protein in the diagnosis of neonatal sepsis, Acta Paediatr. 92 (2003) 221–227.

[130] D. Isaacs, et al., Serum acute phase reactants in necrotizing enterocolitis, Acta Paediatr. Scand. 76 (1987) 923–927.

[131] J. Saxstad, L.Å. Nilsson, L.Å. Hanson, C-reactive protein in serum from infants as determined with immunodiffusion techniques. II. Infants with various infections, Acta Paediatr. Scand. 59 (1970) 676–680.

[132] P. Hawrylyshyn, et al., Premature rupture of membranes: the role of C-reactive protein in the prediction of chorioamnionitis, Am. J. Obstet. Gynecol. 147 (1983) 240–246.

[133] H.R. Salzer, et al., C-reactive protein: an early marker for neonatal bacterial infection due to prolonged rupture of amniotic membranes and/or amnionitis, Acta Obstet. Gynecol. Scand. 66 (1987) 365–367.

[134] N.Y.N. Schouten-Van Meeteren, et al., Influence of perinatal conditions on C-reactive protein production, J. Pediatr. 120 (1992) 621–624.

[135] H.N. Bomela, et al., Use of C-reactive protein to guide duration of empiric antibiotic therapy in suspected early neonatal sepsis, Pediatr. Infect. Dis. J. 19 (2000) 531–535.

[136] S. Ehl, B. Gehring, F. Pohlandt, A detailed analysis of changes in serum C-reactive protein levels in neonates treated for bacterial infection, Eur. J. Pediatr. 158 (1999) 238–242.

[137] A.R. Franz, et al., Reduction of unnecessary antibiotic therapy in newborn infants using interleukin-8 and C-reactive protein as markers of bacterial infections, Pediatrics 104 (1999) 447–453.

[138] A.G.S. Philip, Acute-phase proteins in neonatal infection, J. Pediatr. 105 (1984) 940–942.

[139] M. Assicot, et al., High serum procalcitonin concentrations in patients with sepsis and infection, Lancet 1 (1993) 515–518.

[140] D. Gendrel, et al., Procalcitonin as a marker for the early diagnosis of neonatal infection, J. Pediatr. 128 (1996) 570–573.

[141] G. Monneret, et al., Procalcitonin and C-reactive protein levels in neonatal infections, Acta Paediatr. 86 (1997) 209–212.

[142] D. Gendrel, C. Bohuon, Procalcitonin as a marker of bacterial infection, Pediatr. Infect. Dis. J. 19 (2000) 679–687.

[143] A.M.C. Van Rossum, R.W. Wulkan, A.M. Oudesluys-Murphy, Procalcitonin as an early marker of infection in neonates and children, Lancet Infect. Dis. 4 (2004) 620–630.

[144] C. Chiesa, et al., Reliability of procalcitonin concentrations for the diagnosis of sepsis in critically ill neonates, Clin. Infect. Dis. 26 (1998) 664–672.

[145] A. Lapillone, et al., Lack of specificity of procalcitonin for sepsis diagnosis in premature infants, Lancet 351 (1998) 1211–1212.

[146] D. Turner, et al., Procalcitonin in preterm infants during the first few days of life: introducing an age related nomogram, Arch. Dis. Child. Fetal Neonatal. Ed. 91 (2006) F283–F286.

[147] J.B. López Sastre, et al., Procalcitonin is not sufficiently reliable to be the sole marker of neonatal sepsis of nosocomial origin, BMC Pediatr. 6 (2006) 16.

[148] B.A. Barrat, P.I. Hill, A micromethod for the erythrocyte sedimentation rate suitable for use on venous or capillary blood, J. Clin. Pathol. 33 (1980) 1145.

[149] A.D. Lascari, The erythrocyte sedimentation rate, Pediatr. Clin. North Am. 19 (1972) 1113–1121.

[150] S.M. Adler, R.L. Denton, The erythrocyte sedimentation rate in the newborn period, J. Pediatr. 86 (1975) 942–948.

[151] H.E. Evans, L. Glass, C. Mercado, The micro-erythrocyte sedimentation rate in newborn infants, J. Pediatr. 76 (1970) 448–451.

[152] K.K. Ibsen, et al., The value of the micromethod erythrocyte sedimentation rate in the diagnosis of infections in newborns, Scand. J. Infect. Dis. 23 (1980) 143–145.

[153] M. Bennish, J. Vardiman, M.C. Beem, The zeta sedimentation ratio in children, J. Pediatr. 104 (1984) 249–251.

[154] J. Stuart, J.T. Whicher, Tests for detecting and monitoring the acute phase response, Arch. Dis. Child. 63 (1988) 115–117.

[155] E.J. Sell, J.J. Corrigan Jr., Platelet counts, fibrinogen concentrations, and factor V and factor VIII levels in healthy infants according to gestational age, J. Pediatr. 82 (1973) 1028–1032.

[156] A.H. Jensen, et al., Evolution of blood clotting factor levels in premature infants during the first 10 days of life: a study of 96 cases with comparison between clinical status and blood clotting factor levels, Pediatr. Res. 7 (1973) 638–644.

[157] T.T. Salmi, Haptoglobin levels in the plasma of newborn infants with special reference to infections, Acta Paediatr. Scand. 241 (1973) 7–55.

[158] F. Kanakoudi, et al., Serum concentrations of 10 acute-phase proteins in healthy term and preterm infants from birth to age 6 months, Clin. Chem. 41 (1995) 605–608.

[159] S.K. Lee, D.W. Thibeault, D.C. Heiner, α_1-Antitrypsin and α_1-acid glycoprotein levels in the cord blood and amniotic fluid of infants with respiratory distress syndrome, Pediatr. Res. 12 (1978) 775–777.

[160] P. Boichot, et al., L'orosomucoide à la période néonatale: étude chez le nouveau-né sain et le nouveau-né infecté, Pédiatrie 35 (1980) 577–588.

[161] J. Bienvenu, et al., Laser nephelometry of orosomucoid in serum of newborns: reference intervals and relation to bacterial infections, Clin. Chem. 27 (1981) 721–726.

[162] A.G.S. Philip, J.R. Hewitt, $\alpha_1\beta$-Acid glycoprotein in the neonate with and without infection, Biol. Neonate 43 (1983) 118–124.

[163] J.M. Treluyer, et al., Septicémies néonatales: diagnostic biologique et antibiothérapie: à propos d'une série de 46 cas, Arch. Fr. Pédiatr. 48 (1991) 317–321.

[164] T.J. Gutteberg, B. Haneberg, T. Jergensen, Lactoferrin in relation to acute phase proteins in sera from newborn infants with severe infections, Eur. J. Pediatr. 142 (1984) 37–39.

[165] R.L. Rodwell, et al., Capillary plasma elastase alpha-1-proteinase inhibitor in infected and non-infected neonates, Arch. Dis. Child. 67 (1992) 436–439.

[166] C.P. Speer, M. Rethwilm, M. Gahr, Elastase-α1-proteinase inhibitor: an early indicator of septicemia and bacterial meningitis in children, J. Pediatr. 111 (1987) 667–671.

[167] Y.W. Baek, et al., Inter-alpha inhibitor proteins in infants and decreased levels in neonatal sepsis, J. Pediatr. 143 (2003) 11–15.

[168] M. Suri, V.K. Sharma, S. Thirupuram, Evaluation of ceruloplasmin in neonatal septicemia, Indian Pediatr. 28 (1991) 489–493.

[169] A.J.J. Schrama, et al., Secretory phospholipase A$_2$ in newborn infants with sepsis, J. Perinatol. 28 (2008) 291–296.

[170] S. Arnon, et al., Serum amyloid A: an early and accurate marker of neonatal early-onset sepsis, J. Perinatol. 27 (2007) 297–302.

[171] L.C. Miller, et al., Neonatal interleukin-1α, interleukin-6, and tumor necrosis factor: cord blood levels and cellular production, J. Pediatr. 117 (1990) 961–965.

[172] F. Kashlan, et al., Umbilical vein interleukin 6 and tumor necrosis factor alpha plasma concentrations in the very preterm infant, Pediatr. Infect. Dis. J. 19 (2000) 238–243.

[173] T.W. Orlikowsky, et al., Evaluation of IL-8 concentrations in plasma and lysed EDTA-blood in healthy neonates and those with suspected early onset bacterial infection, Pediatr. Res. 56 (2004) 804–809.

[174] C. Buck, et al., Interleukin-6: a sensitive parameter for the early diagnosis of neonatal bacterial infection, Pediatrics 93 (1994) 54–58.

[175] H. Martin, B. Olander, M. Norman, Reactive hyperemia and interleukin 6, interleukin 8, and tumor necrosis factor-α in the diagnosis of early-onset neonatal sepsis, Pediatrics 108 (2001) e61.

[176] J. Messer, et al., Evaluation of interleukin-6 and soluble receptors of tumor necrosis factor for early diagnosis of neonatal infection, J. Pediatr. 129 (1996) 574–580.

[177] R. Gomez, et al., The fetal inflammatory response syndrome, Am. J. Obstet. Gynecol. 179 (1998) 194–202.

[178] T. Lehrnbecher, et al., Immunologic parameters in cord blood indicating early-onset sepsis, Biol. Neonate 70 (1996) 206–212.

[179] A. Panero, et al., Interleukin-6 in neonates with early and late onset infection, Pediatr. Infect. Dis. J. 16 (1997) 370–375.

[180] J.S. Sullivan, et al., Correlation of plasma cytokine elevations with mortality rate in children with sepsis, J. Pediatr. 120 (1992) 510–515.

[181] K. Shimoya, et al., Interleukin-8 in cord sera: a sensitive and specific marker for the detection of preterm chorioamnionitis, J. Infect. Dis. 165 (1992) 957–960.

[182] I. Nupponen, et al., Neutrophil CD11b expression and circulating interleukin-8 as diagnostic markers for early-onset neonatal sepsis, Pediatrics (2001) 108: e12.

[183] A. Malik, et al., Beyond the complete blood cell count and C-reactive protein: a systematic review of modern diagnostic tests for neonatal sepsis, Arch. Pediatr. Adolesc. Med. 157 (2003) 511–516.

[184] S. Mehr, L.W. Doyle, Cytokines as markers of bacterial sepsis in newborn infants: a review, Pediatr. Infect. Dis. J. 19 (2000) 879–887.

[185] M.A. Verboon-Maciolek, et al., Inflammatory mediators for the diagnosis and treatment of sepsis in early infancy, Pediatr. Res. 59 (2006) 457–461.

[186] M.C. Harris, et al., Cytokine elaboration in critically ill infants with bacterial sepsis, necrotizing enterocolitis, or sepsis syndrome: correlation with clinical parameters of inflammation and mortality, J. Pediatr. 147 (2005) 462–468.

[187] J. Figueras-Aloy, et al., Serum soluble ICAM-1, VCAM-1, L-selectin, and P-selectin levels as markers of infection and their relation to clinical severity in neonatal sepsis, Am. J. Perinatol. 24 (2007) 331–338.

[188] S.K. Kim, et al., Comparison of L-selectin and CD11b on neutrophils of adults and neonates during the first month of life, Pediatr. Res. 53 (2003) 132–136.

[189] H. Kuster, K. Degitz, Circulating ICAM-1 in neonatal sepsis, Lancet 1 (1993) 506.

[190] A.B. Dzwonek, et al., The role of mannose-binding lectin in susceptibility to infection in preterm neonates, Pediatr. Res. 63 (2008) 680–685.

[191] E. De Bont, et al., Increased plasma concentrations of interleukin-1 receptor antagonist in neonatal sepsis, Pediatr. Res. 37 (1995) 626–629.

[192] M.L. Spear, et al., Soluble interleukin-2 receptor as a predictor of neonatal sepsis, J. Pediatr. 126 (1995) 982–985.

[193] S. Hodge, et al., Surface activation markers of T lymphocytes: role in the detection of infection in neonates, Clin. Exp. Immunol. 113 (1998) 33–38.

[194] E. Weirich, et al., Neutrophil CD11b expression as a diagnostic marker for early-onset neonatal infection, J. Pediatr. 132 (1998) 445–451.

[195] R. Turunen, et al., Increased CD11b-density on circulating phagocytes as an early sign of late-onset sepsis in extremely low-birth-weight infants, Pediatr. Res. 57 (2005) 270–275.

[196] N.P. Weinschenk, A. Farina, D.W. Bianchi, Neonatal neutrophil activation is a function of labor length in preterm infants, Pediatr. Res. 44 (1998) 942–945.

[197] J.M. Cholette, et al., Developmental changes in soluble CD40 ligand, J. Pediatr. 152 (2008) 50–54.

[198] P.C. Ng, et al., Neutrophil CD64 expression: a sensitive diagnostic marker for late-onset nosocomial infection in very low birthweight infants, Pediatr. Res. 51 (2002) 296–303.

[199] P.C. Ng, et al., Neutrophil CD64 is a sensitive diagnostic marker for early-onset neonatal infection, Pediatr. Res. 56 (2004) 796–803.

[200] V. Bhandari, et al., Hematologic profile of sepsis in neonates: neutrophil CD64 as a diagnostic marker, Pediatrics 121 (2008) 129–134.

[201] K.D. Yang, J.F. Bohnsack, H.R. Hill, Fibronectin in host defense: implications in the diagnosis, prophylaxis and therapy of infectious diseases, Pediatr. Infect. Dis. 12 (1993) 234–239.

[202] J.M. Koenig, et al., Role of fibronectin in diagnosing bacterial infection in infancy, Am. J. Dis. Child. 142 (1988) 884–887.

[203] M.H. McCafferty, et al., Normal fibronectin levels as a function of age in the pediatric population, Pediatr. Res. 17 (1982) 482–485.

[204] C.A. Alford Jr., Immunoglobulin determinations in the diagnosis of fetal infection, Pediatr. Clin. North Am. 18 (1971) 99–113.

[205] B.M. Kagan, V. Stanincova, N. Felix, IgM determination in neonate and infants for diagnosis of infection, J. Pediatr. 77 (1970) 916.

[206] W.N. Khan, et al., Immunoglobulin M determinations in neonates and infants as an adjunct to the diagnosis of infection, J. Pediatr. 75 (1969) 1282–1286.

[207] W.J. Blankenship, et al., Serum gamma-M globulin responses in acute neonatal infections and their diagnostic significance, J. Pediatr. 75 (1969) 1271–1281.

[208] S.B. Korones, et al., Neonatal IgM response to acute infection, J. Pediatr. 75 (1969) 1261–1270.

[209] R.L. Baehner, Use of the nitroblue tetrazolium test in clinical pediatrics, Am. J. Dis. Child. 128 (1974) 449–451.

[210] P. Cocchi, S. Mori, A. Becattini, Nitroblue-tetrazolium reduction by neutrophils of newborn infants in in vitro phagocytosis test, Acta Paediatr. Scand. 60 (1971) 475–478.

[211] B.H. Park, B. Holmes, R.A. Good, Metabolic activities in leukocytes of newborn infants, J. Pediatr. 76 (1970) 237–241.

[212] G.H. McCracken Jr., H.F. Eichenwald, Leukocyte function and the development of opsonic and complement activity in the neonate, Am. J. Dis. Child. 121 (1971) 120–126.

[213] D.C. Anderson, L.K. Pickering, R.D. Feigin, Leukocyte function in normal and infected neonates, J. Pediatr. 85 (1974) 420–425.

[214] A.O. Shigeoka, J.I. Santos, H.R. Hill, Functional analysis of neutrophil granulocytes from healthy, infected, and stressed neonates, J. Pediatr. 95 (1979) 454–460.

[215] A.O. Shigeoka, et al., Defective oxidative metabolic responses of neutrophils from stressed neonates, J. Pediatr. 98 (1981) 392–398.

[216] D.W. Powers, E.M. Ayoub, Leukocyte lactate dehydrogenase in bacterial meningitis, Pediatrics 54 (1974) 27–33.

[217] H. Donato, et al., Leukocyte alkaline phosphatase activity in the diagnosis of neonatal bacterial infections, J. Pediatr. 94 (1979) 242–244.

[218] R.D. Leake, R.H. Fiser Jr., W. Oh, Rapid glucose disappearance in infants with infection, Clin. Pediatr. 20 (1981) 397–401.

[219] T. James III, M. Blessa, T.R. Boggs Jr., Recurrent hyperglycemia associated with sepsis in a neonate, Am. J. Dis. Child. 133 (1979) 645–646.

[220] M. Zasloff, Vernix, the newborn, and innate defense, Pediatr. Res. 53 (2003) 203–204.

[221] O. Levy, Impaired innate immunity at birth: deficiency of bactericidal/permeability-increasing protein (BPI) in the neutrophils of newborns, Pediatr. Res. 51 (2002) 667–669.

[222] N.J. Thomas, et al., Plasma concentrations of defensins and lactoferrin in children with severe sepsis, Pediatr. Infect. Dis. J. 21 (2002) 34–38.

[223] H. Yoshio, et al., Antimicrobial polypeptides of human vernix caseosa and amniotic fluid: implications for newborn innate defense, Pediatr. Res. 53 (2003) 211–216.

[224] I. Nupponen, et al., Extracellular release of bactericidal/permeability-increasing protein in newborn infants, Pediatr. Res. 51 (2002) 670–674.

[225] M.P. Griffin, et al., Heart rate characteristics and clinical signs in neonatal sepsis, Pediatr. Res. 61 (2007) 222–227.

[226] K. Benirschke, Routes and types of infection in the fetus and the newborn, Am. J. Dis. Child. 99 (1960) 714–721.

[227] W.A. Blanc, Pathways of fetal and early neonatal infection: viral placentitis, bacterial and fungal chorioamnionitis, J. Pediatr. 59 (1961) 473–496.

[228] G.R.H. Kelsall, R.A. Barter, C. Manesss, Prospective bacteriological studies in inflammation of the placenta, cord and membranes, J. Obstet. Gynaecol. Br. Commonw. 74 (1967) 401–411.

[229] A.M. Overbach, S.J. Daniel, G. Cassady, The value of umbilical cord histology in the management of potential perinatal infection, J. Pediatr. 76 (1970) 22–31.

[230] M.G. Wilson, et al., Prolonged rupture of fetal membranes: effect on the newborn infant, Am. J. Dis. Child. 107 (1964) 138–146.

[231] J.E. Morison, Foetal and Neonatal Pathology, third ed., Butterworth, Washington, DC, 1970.

[232] H. Fox, F.A. Langley, Leukocytic infiltration of the placenta and umbilical cord: a clinico-pathologic study, Obstet. Gynecol. 37 (1971) 451–458.

[233] R. Dominguez, A.J. Segal, J.A. O'Sullivan, Leukocytic infiltration of the umbilical cord: manifestation of fetal hypoxia due to reduction of blood flow in the cord, JAMA 173 (1960) 346–349.

[234] G.S. Anderson, et al., Congenital bacterial pneumonia, Lancet 2 (1962) 585–587.

[235] A. Ramos, L. Stern, Relationship of premature rupture of the membranes to gastric fluid aspirate in the newborn, Am. J. Obstet. Gynecol. 105 (1969) 1247–1251.

[236] U. Vasan, et al., Origin of gastric polymorphonuclear leukocytes in infants born after prolonged rupture of membranes, J. Pediatr. 91 (1977) 69–72.

[237] C.Y. Yeung, A.S.Y. Tam, Gastric aspirate findings in neonatal pneumonia, Arch. Dis. Child. 47 (1972) 735–740.

[238] J. Scanlon, The early detection of neonatal sepsis by examination of liquid obtained from the external ear canal, J. Pediatr. 79 (1971) 247–249.

[239] T.J. Zuerlein, J.C. Butler, T.D. Yeager, Superficial cultures in neonatal sepsis evaluations: impact on antibiotic decision making, Clin. Pediatr. 29 (1990) 445–447.

[240] H.H. Handsfield, W.A. Hodson, K.K. Holmes, Neonatal gonococcal infection. I. Orogastric contamination with *N. gonorrhoeae*, JAMA 225 (1973) 697–701.

[241] R.R. MacGregor, W.W. Tunnessen Jr., The incidence of pathogenic organisms in the normal flora of the neonate's external ear and nasopharynx, Clin. Pediatr. 12 (1973) 697–700.

[242] L.C. Mims, et al., Predicting neonatal infections by evaluation of the gastric aspirate: a study in two hundred and seven patients, Am. J. Obstet. Gynecol. 114 (1972) 232–238.

[243] Y.L. Lau, E. Hey, Sensitivity and specificity of daily tracheal aspirate cultures in predicting organisms causing bacteremia in ventilated neonates, Pediatr. Infect. Dis. J. 10 (1991) 290–294.

[244] Y. Hazan, et al., The diagnostic value of amniotic Gram stain examination and limulus amebocyte lysate assay in patients with preterm birth, Acta Obstet. Gynecol. Scand. 74 (1995) 275–280.

[245] N. Laforgia, et al., Rapid detection of neonatal sepsis using polymerase chain reaction, Acta Paediatr. 86 (1997) 1097–1099.

[246] J.A. Jordan, M.B. Durso, Comparison of 16S rRNA gene PCR and BACTEC 9240 for detection of neonatal bacteremia, J. Clin. Microbiol. 38 (2000) 2574–2578.

[247] P.W. Fowlie, B. Schmidt, Diagnostic tests for bacterial infection from birth to 90 days—a systematic review, Arch. Dis. Child. Fetal Neonatal. Ed. 78 (1998) F92–F98.

[248] A.R. Franz, et al., Measurement of interleukin 8 in combination with C-reactive protein reduced unnecessary antibiotic therapy in newborn infants: a multicenter, randomized, controlled trial, Pediatrics 114 (2004) 1–8.

[249] A.G.S. Philip, Decreased use of antibiotics using a neonatal sepsis screening technique, J. Pediatr. 98 (1981) 795–799.

[250] M.W. Weber, et al., Predictors of neonatal sepsis in developing countries, Pediatr. Infect. Dis. J. 22 (2003) 711–717.

[251] J.A. Garcia-Prats, et al., Rapid detection of microorganisms in blood cultures of newborn infants utilizing an automated blood culture system, Pediatrics 105 (2000) 523–527.

[252] Y. Kumar, et al., Time to positivity of neonatal blood cultures, Arch. Dis. Child. Fetal Neonatal. Ed. 85 (2001) F182–F186.

[253] J. Jardine, et al., Incubation time required for neonatal blood cultures to become positive, J. Paediatr. Child Health 42 (2006) 797–802.

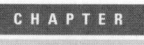

CHAPTER 37

CLINICAL PHARMACOLOGY OF ANTI-INFECTIVE DRUGS

Kelly C. Wade ⊙ Daniel K. Benjamin, Jr.

CHAPTER OUTLINE

Introduction   1160

Basic Principles of Clinical Pharmacology   1161
    Optimizing Antimicrobial Therapy Using PK-PD Principles   1163

Placental Transport of Antibiotics   1165

Excretion of Antibiotics in Human Milk   1166

Penicillin   1168

Antistaphylococcal Treatment   1171

Aminoglycosides   1177

Broad-Acting Agents with Activity Against Pseudomonas   1188

Antiviral Medications   1194

Antifungal Medications   1195

References   1202

INTRODUCTION

Effective antimicrobial treatment typically begins with empirical therapy at a dose that is most likely to cure the infection with the minimum risk of toxic effects. To select the correct dosage, clinicians need to understand and apply the principles of pharmacokinetics (PK) and pharmacodynamics (PD). This chapter will focus on basic pharmacology and the application of PK and PD principles to the most commonly used anti-infective drugs to guide optimal therapy of common infections in the newborn and young infant.

This chapter proceeds from the exhaustive review of the pharmacology of antimicrobial agents provided by Drs. Sáez-Llorens and McCracken in the previous edition. In areas in which information remains relevant and unchanged, I acknowledge their efforts and permission to use a previous text. Since the previous edition of this book was published, more relevant PK data have been reported. Additional studies have supported an integrated PK and PD (PK-PD) approach to antibiotic therapy. Finally, the range of antimicrobial drugs discussed has been expanded to include antifungal and non-HIV antiviral medications. Information on antimicrobial drugs that are no longer used

or rarely used has been omitted to make room for new information.

The clinical pharmacology, indication, dosing, and toxicity of licensed drugs are included in the label and available through the Physicians' Desk Reference (www.pdr. net) [1] and the Federal Drug Administration (FDA) Center for Drug Evaluation and Research (www.fda.gov/cder/) [1]. However, the use of many drugs remains off-label in term and premature neonates due to inadequate PK and efficacy studies. In this chapter drugs are organised into the following five categories of efficacy: (1) gram-positive infections including MRSA, (2) gram-negative infections, (3) polymicrobial or complicated serious infections, (4) viral infections, and (5) fungal infections. The pharmacology of drugs in neonates is unique and should not be extrapolated from data derived from studies in older patients whenever possible. Few drugs have been adequately studied in the extremely preterm infant so many of the dosing guidelines in this high-risk patient group remain empirical. In such cases, we will review the mechanism of action and dosing relative to known PK-PD properties and safety.

TABLE 37–1 Drugs Not Routinely Used in Neonates

Drug	Potential Adverse Effect	References
Tetracycline	Depressed bone growth and teeth abnormalities	[90,117,662]
Chloramphenicol	Circulatory collapse, impaired mitochondrial protein synthesis, bone marrow aplasia; gray baby syndrome	[2,3,5,6,663]
Sulfonamide	Bilirubin displacement with rare but possible kernicterus; increased risk of hemolysis in G6PD-deficient infants	[21,664]
Trimethoprim-sulfamethoxazole (available in 1:5 ratio)	Same as sulfonamide; bilirubin displacement with rare but possible kernicterus; increased risk of hemolysis in G6PD-deficient infants	[1,665]
Ceftriaxone	Highly protein bound, potential to displace bilirubin; cannot be coadministered with calcium containing fluids	[1,20]

A few antimicrobial drugs have been associated with serious toxicity (Table 37–1) and therefore their use in neonates is discouraged in developed countries. The most notable on this list is chloramphenicol. Chloramphenicol has been associated with circulatory collapse, otherwise known as gray baby syndrome, and death in infants due to drug accumulation following excessive dosages. This complication can be traced to immaturity of the glucuronyl transferase activity in the fetus and young newborn infants, coupled with diminished renal function [2–6]. Chloramphenicol toxicity appears to be related to impaired mitochondrial

protein synthesis and to direct inhibition of myocardial contractile activity. Since this toxicity results from free drug accumulation, multiple exchange transfusions or charcoal hemoperfusion may reverse the clinical syndrome by removing the free drug from the blood [7–9]. Anemia due to dose related marrow suppression is the most common untoward reaction to chloramphenicol; however, severe idiosyncratic bone marrow aplasia occurs in approximately 1 in 40,000 patients of all ages receiving the antibiotic [3].

BASIC PRINCIPLES OF CLINICAL PHARMACOLOGY

The rapidly changing physiologic processes characteristic of fetal and neonatal development profoundly affect the PK properties of antibiotics [10–12]. Maturation affects total body water, drug metabolism, and drug elimination. Gastric absorption is highly variable. These changes can result either in subtherapeutic drug concentrations, thereby delaying bacterial eradication, or in toxic drug concentrations that cause morbidity. Common PK terms and abbreviations are defined in Table 37–2.

The PK of a drug describes the relationship between drug dose and subsequent concentration in the blood over time. Four basic components explain the PK of a drug: absorption, distribution, metabolism, and excretion. Absorption of drugs administered at extravascular sites typically occurs by passive diffusion across biologic membranes. This process is affected by chemical properties of the drug, such as its molecular weight, ionization, and lipid solubility, and by physiologic factors, such as local pH and blood flow, which undergo developmental changes as the newborn matures. The severity of infections and the inconsistent absorption after extravascular administration warrant most antimicrobial therapy to be delivered by the intravenous route in developed countries.

TABLE 37–2 Common Pharmacokinetic Terms

PK Term	Abbreviation	Definition	Units
Maximum concentration	C_{max}	Maximal drug concentration at end of infusion. Alternatively, for drugs that are rapidly distributed (α-phase), the peak concentrations may be evaluated 30 minutes after end of infusion to give the concentration after the initial rapid phase of distribution	μg/mL or mg/L
Minimum concentration	C_{min}	Minimal drug concentration just before subsequent dose	μg/mL or mg/L
Clearance	Cl	The amount of blood from which all drug is removed per unit of time through both renal and nonrenal mechanisms	(mL/min)/kg (L/hr)/kg
Volume of distribution	Vd	Hypothetical volume of fluid through which a drug is dispersed	L/kg
Elimination rate constant	k_e $k_e = Cl/Vd$	For drugs with first order kinetics, the ratio of clearance to volume of distribution (Cl/Vd)	1/hr or hr^{-1}
Half-life	$t_{1/2}$ of β-phase = (0.693)/ke	Time it takes to clear half of the drug from plasma. It is directly proportional to the Vd and inversely proportional to Cl.	hr
Bioavailability	F	The fraction of the administered dose that reaches the systemic circulation. F = 1 for intravenous administration. After oral administration, F is reduced by incomplete absorption, first-pass metabolism, and distribution into other tissue.	%
Area under the concentration time curve	AUC	Measure of total drug exposure, typically over 24-hour period	mg * L/hr

Oral absorption of antimicrobial agents is difficult to predict and can only be determined by carefully executed experiments. Bioavailability describes the fraction of an administered dose of a drug that reaches the systemic circulation. By definition, intravenous medications have 100% bioavailability. However, oral medications have decreased bioavailability due to incomplete absorption and first-pass hepatic metabolism. Unique neonatal features that impact absorption changes with gestational and chronologic age include the alkaline gastric pH, slow gastric emptying, high gastrointestinal-to-whole body surface area ratio, increased permeability of bowel mucosa, irregular peristalsis, prolonged intestinal transit time, differences in first pass hepatic metabolism, and the deconjugational activity of the intestinal enzyme β-glucuronidase [10].

Intramuscular absorption of antimicrobial agents is generally comparable to intravenous administration; however, substantial differences can exist because intramuscular antibiotic absorption is dependent upon regional blood flow [13,14]. Intramuscular absorption can be profoundly reduced in infants with hypoxia, hypotension, or poor tissue perfusion.

After drug absorption into the bloodstream, the dose of a drug is distributed into all of the body compartments and tissues that the product is physically able to penetrate, including water compartments and adipose tissue. This distributive phase is typically rapid, and the drug is said to distribute into its volume of distribution or Vd. This volume is considered hypothetical because it is based on sampling drug concentrations in serum or plasma after dosing. Interpretation of these samples requires the assumption that the drug is uniformly distributed throughout the body. However, drugs do not distribute in a uniform fashion. Drugs that are water soluble or highly bound to plasma proteins have a high plasma concentration and a low volume of distribution because the drug tends to remain in the blood. Drugs that are lipid soluble or bind extensively to tissue are present in the plasma in low concentrations and therefore have large volumes of distribution. Volume of distribution in the neonate is usually larger than in children (and premature infants larger than in term infants) due to the larger extracellular water compartment in neonates.

The extracellular fluid volume in newborns is considerably greater than that in children and adults. In the first 3 months of life, it decreases from 7.3 to 5.8 L/m^2 and then remains nearly constant throughout infancy and early childhood [15]. Extracellular fluid volume is also increased with prematurity, so that peak serum concentrations are lower in preterm infants compared with term infants after similar dosages. Expanded extracellular volumes prolong drug elimination and lead to longer half-lives. The clinical application of these concepts is particularly relevant to aminoglycosides because the efficacy is associated with the peak concentration whereas toxicity is associated with trough concentrations.

Protein binding can also impact drug distribution and elimination. Quantitative and qualitative differences exist between the serum proteins of newborns and those of older infants [16]. These differences affect the degree to which antimicrobial agents are protein bound. Variables that impact protein binding include concentrations of plasma proteins (such as albumin), concentration of drug, drug affinity for protein-binding sites, presence of competing substances for protein-binding sites (e.g., furosemide, bilirubin), and plasma pH. Protein-bound drug has negligible antibacterial activity and remains in the intravascular space with limited distribution into tissue and limited excretion. Because only free drug is active and available for elimination, changes in protein binding can dramatically affect exposure and efficacy. Protein binding for some antibiotics is lower in neonates than in adults so extrapolation is not advised [17] and the PK of the free drug needs to be determined.

Some antibacterial agents are capable of displacing bilirubin from albumin-binding sites, including the sulfonamides, moxalactam, cefoperazone, and ceftriaxone [18–20]. Theoretically, jaundiced neonates receiving these antibiotics are at increased risk of developing kernicterus. This complication, however, has been documented only for sulfonamides [21]. Most antimicrobial drugs do not displace bilirubin because most have a much lower binding affinity for albumin than bilirubin [22], and thus the extent of protein binding by an antibiotic does not necessarily correlate with bilirubin displacement [19,23–25].

Drugs start to be eliminated from the body as soon as they are delivered. If doses are given at a rate that balances the drug clearance rate, then target steady state drug concentrations can be maintained. Drug clearance is the volume of blood, serum, or plasma completely cleared of drug per unit of time and is expressed units of volume/time, for example L/hour or mL/min. Clearance is not only related to infant size (L/hour/kg), but also to clinical characteristics such as renal disease, hepatic disease, and drug interactions. Clearance of water soluble drugs usually occurs via excretion into the urine; while lipid soluble drugs are often metabolized to water-soluble metabolites by the liver before they can be excreted.

Drug elimination occurs through hepatic metabolism, renal excretion, or both, and is affected by physiologic maturation [10,12]. Hepatic metabolism involves chemical transformation of the drug into a form that is more fat-soluble for elimination in the bile and feces, or a form more water-soluble for elimination by the kidneys. The ontogeny of the cytochrome P450 metabolizing enzymes in newborn development has been evaluated and reviewed [12,26]. Newborns are at risk for toxicity from drug accumulation due to deficiencies in hepatic glucuronyl transferase or hepatic esterases. Drugs can also induce enzyme production leading to drug interaction. Phenobarbital stimulates hepatic enzyme production, thereby increasing the clearance and lowering serum concentrations of some drugs including anticoagulants, corticosteroids, phenytoin, metronidazole, and theophylline.

Renal elimination of active drug or metabolites occurs via glomerular filtration and/or tubular secretion. Some drugs are reabsorbed in renal tubules, thus further altering their elimination rate. Renal function varies with gestational age, chronologic age, and disease state. The constant state of renal function fluctuation has a profound impact on antibiotic PK. In newborns, the glomerular filtration rate is 30% to 60% of adult levels. A remarkable increase in renal function occurs over the first 2 weeks of life [12,27]. As a result, sustained serum concentrations and prolonged half-life values of many drugs eliminated through the kidneys are observed in the first days of life. After birth, renal function improves more slowly in premature infants, leading to prolonged drug elimination over the first few weeks of life. Drug elimination is also reduced in sick infants due to decreased renal blood flow resulting from respiratory insufficiency, hypotension, or dehydration. For example, hypoxemic infants have a prolonged serum half-life of aminoglycosides [28]. Because renal function is constantly changing in the first month of life, a PK profile is determined on multiple occasions during this period to define the proper dosage and frequency of administration of an antibiotic.

Most drugs are cleared through first order elimination. This means that a constant proportion of drug is cleared per unit of time. Initially, there is a steep fall in concentration, after which the decline becomes shallower as the amount of drug remaining decreases. When the concentration time profile is plotted on a log-linear scale, the decline is linear because the shape of the relationship between concentration and time is described by an exponential function. The elimination rate constant (k_e) is the ratio of clearance to volume of distribution and is usually expressed in units of L/hour.

Each patient has a unique elimination rate constant that reflects the clearance and volume of distribution of the drug. The elimination rate constant can be converted into the clinically meaningful concept of drug half-life, the time it takes for the concentration of a drug to fall to half. The half-life of a drug is estimated by the equation $t_{1/2} = 0.693/k_e$ because the exponential log of 0.5 is 0.693. Half-life estimates are patient specific. For drugs eliminated by first order kinetics, the elimination rate constant represents the ratio of drug clearance and volume of distribution. For patients with renal insufficiency, delayed renal clearance of gentamicin will result in a half-life that can be three times as long as patients with normal renal function. Patients with fluid overload have a large volume of distribution and a longer half-life, and therefore may need to receive a higher dose of medication less frequently.

OPTIMIZING ANTIMICROBIAL THERAPY USING PK-PD PRINCIPLES

Optimizing antimicrobial therapy in neonates requires a thorough understanding of the relationship between dose and exposure (PK) and between exposure and optimal response to therapy (PD) [29,30]. Our goal is an integrative approach using knowledge from microbiology (MIC, MBC), PK, and PD such that we can have a high probability that a specific dose of an antibiotic can cure a particular infection in a defined population of infants. Carefully designed clinical trials can then be performed to confirm the results of such an integrative modeling and simulation approach.

Minimal Inhibitory Concentration

The in vitro drug susceptibilities of commonly encountered bacterial pathogens allow comparison of potencies for eradication. Ideally both the minimal inhibitory concentration (MIC) and the minimal bactericidal concentration (MBC) should be determined. To account for the great variation in pathogens and susceptibilities in different nurseries and geographic regions, this knowledge can be generated for each specific newborn unit. The higher the MIC, the more difficult it is to eradicate a pathogen with that drug, even if the MIC falls within the established sensitive range.

Pharmacokinetic Data

New analytical techniques and the computer algorithms for population PK model analysis have made PK evaluation of drugs in infants more feasible. PK explains the relationship between drug dose and the concentration of drug in the plasma or serum over time. PK studies are performed after a single dose and after multiple doses to determine concentrations at steady state. Drug levels can now be measured using mass spectroscopy in as little as 0.1 mL volume obtained by heel stick. For drugs that exhibit protein binding, it is important to measure the quantity of total and nonprotein bound drug. Subsequently, multiple serum samples are obtained to determine concentrations of the drug at a given time after the dose. The serum half-life and volume of distribution are calculated by plotting the serum concentration-time curves and calculating the clearance, a measure of the disappearance of drug from serum [31]. Population PK analysis allows investigators to study a medication in a diverse group of preterm and term infants of different ages so that changes in drug clearance and volume of distribution can be explained by maturational covariates (gestational age at birth, chronologic age, weight, or renal function) in a mathematical model. Monte Carlo simulation using these models of drug clearance and volume of distribution is used to predict and compare drug exposure from different dosing regimens to provide dose adjustments for maturational changes in an infant.

It is clinically important to determine the active drug concentrations in the cerebrospinal fluid (CSF) [32]. CNS penetration of drugs is usually expressed as the fraction of cerebrospinal fluid (CSF) drug concentrations divided by the plasma or serum concentrations since most studies link a single CSF sample with a simultaneous blood sample. In the 1980s, new antibiotics were tested in a rabbit model of meningitis before use in infants to determine the CSF penetration and bactericidal activity of the drug against commonly encountered meningeal pathogens [33–35]. More data are needed to understand the CSF penetration of antimicrobial drugs in the presence or absence of meningitis in neonates. Some current antimicrobial trials attempt to collect CSF from standard of care sampling to measure drug levels in CSF.

Pharmacodynamics

PD equations describe the relationships between the drug concentration-time profile and the ability to eradicate the organism, prevent emerging resistance, and minimize adverse effects. Dose and time of infusion determine the maximum drug concentration achieved. Dose and dosing interval determine the overall drug exposure per 24-hour interval (24-hour area under the concentration curve [AUC]) and the minimum concentration between dosing intervals. Bacterial eradication is typically evaluated in relation to the maximum drug concentration, the AUC, and the percent of time that the drug concentration is above a minimum threshold, as determined by the MIC of the target organism.

Pharmacokinetic/Pharmacodynamic Approach

To achieve the best therapeutic response, drug dose should be related to antimicrobial effect through an integrated PK-PD approach, in which a dose is chosen to target a therapeutic drug concentration relative to the MIC of the offending organism [30]. Three important PK parameters are the peak serum level (C_{max}), the trough level (C_{min}), and the AUC (Tables 37–2, 37–3). These PK-PD parameters are used to quantify the activity of an antibiotic. Antimicrobial agents are typically associated with one of three patterns of activity (Table 37–3, Figure 37–1) [29,30,36,37]: (1) those that exhibit concentration-dependent killing and prolonged persistent postantibiotic effects, and thus achieve optimal killing when the maximal concentration exceeds a threshold Peak/MIC ratio. These products have additional impact related to the total drug exposure AUC/MIC ratio; (2) agents that exhibit time-dependent killing patterns and therefore achieve optimal killing when the duration of drug exposure above a MIC exceeds a percent of time greater than MIC; (3) agents that are most effective when the maximal total drug exposure exceeds a threshold AUC/MIC ratio. Threshold PK-PD therapeutic exposure targets are determined through in vitro experiments, animal models, and human studies that relate drug exposure to MIC and efficacy.

TABLE 37–3   PK-PD Relationships for Optimal Antimicrobial Treatment

Antimicrobial Activity	PK-PD Parameter and Goal of Therapy	Definition	Drug Class	Dosing Goal
Concentration-dependent killing with postantibiotic effect	C_{max}/MIC	Bacterial killing is proportional to maximal concentration achieved relative to MIC of offending organism	Aminoglycosides Fluoroquinolones Daptomycin	Enhance peak concentration
Time-dependent killing	T>MIC	Bacterial killing is proportional to the amount of time the drug concentration is maintained above the MIC of offending organism	β-lactams: Penicillins Cephalosporins Carbepenems	Enhance duration of exposure by short dosing intervals
Time-dependent killing with postantibiotic effect	AUC/MIC	Bacterial killing is proportional to the amount of total drug exposure relative to MIC of offending organism	Vancomycin Clindamycin Linezolid Azoles	Enhance amount of drug using both dose and interval

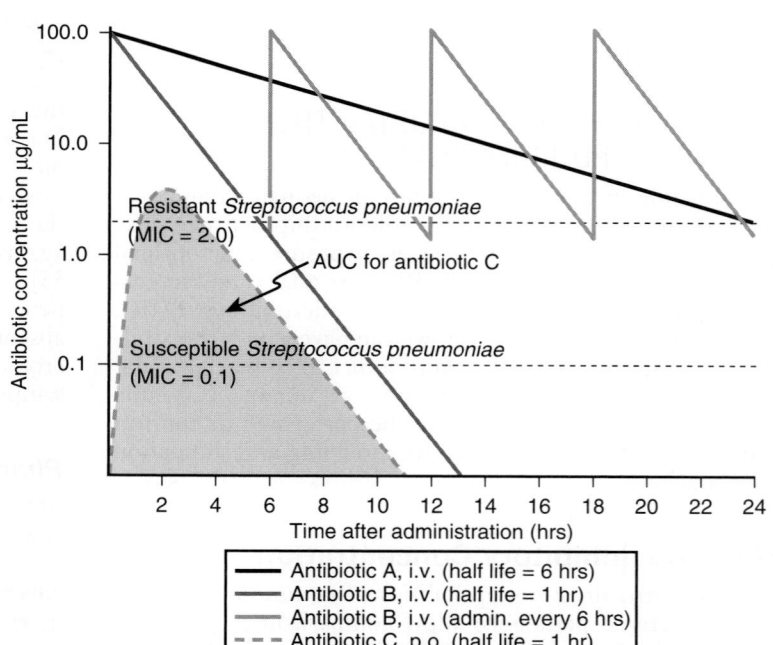

FIGURE 37–1 Effects of dose (mg/kg), dosing interval, and route of administration on total drug exposure as defined by the AUC and its relationship to the MIC of the pathogen being treated. Antibiotics administered intravenously with a long serum half-life of 6 hours (antibiotic A) achieve a relatively large AUC compared with antibiotics with a shorter half-life of 1 hour (antibiotic B), which require more frequent dosing (every 6 hours in this example) to achieve similar drug exposure to the pathogen. Orally administered antibiotics (antibiotic C) generally produce a much lower AUC than those administered intravenously. The MICs for penicillin-susceptible and penicillin-resistant *S. pneumoniae* are superimposed on the graph. *(From Bradley JS, Dudley MN, Drusano GL. Predicting efficacy of antiinfectives with pharmacodynamics and Monte Carlo simulation. Pediatr Infect Dis J 22:982–992, 2003, quiz 993–995.) [36]*

PLACENTAL TRANSPORT OF ANTIBIOTICS

Antimicrobial agents are prescribed for approximately 20% of pregnant women [38,39], and many of these drugs are given at the end of pregnancy for amnionitis or intrauterine bacterial infections. Understanding placental transport is therefore an important component of antimicrobial therapy in the neonate.

Drugs may be transported across the placenta either passively, by simple diffusion, or actively, by energy-dependent processes [40]. Factors influencing transplacental passage include lipid solubility, degree of ionization, molecular weight, protein-binding affinity, surface area of the fetalmaternal interface, placental blood flow, stage of pregnancy, and placental metabolism. Placental drug biotransformation

ensues by oxidation, reduction, hydrolysis, or conjugation with endogenous chemicals. In addition, antibiotics concentrate to various degrees in fetal tissues, depending on lipid solubility, specific binding to biologic constituents, changes in fetal circulation, and gestational age.

Ratios of infant to maternal serum concentrations of commonly-used antimicrobial agents are shown in Table 37–4 [2,41–84]. Maternal serum concentrations are usually lower than those reported in nonpregnant women because of a larger plasma volume and an increased renal plasma clearance during pregnancy [85,86]. Due to differences in maternal dosage, route of administration, gestational age, timing of sample collection, and methods of measuring antimicrobial activity, a wide range of serum values for pregnant women and infants and of percentages of transplacental penetration is obtained for most drugs.

TABLE 37–4 Transplacental Passage of Antimicrobial Agents

Antimicrobial Agent	Trimester	Serum Infant-to-Maternal Ratio(s) (%)	Potential Adverse Effects on Fetus or Infant	Reference
Amikacin	1, 2	8–16	Ototoxicity	[43]
	3	30–50		[44]
Amoxicillin	3	30	None	[45]
Ampicillin	1, 2	50–250	None	[46]
	3	20–200		
Cefazolin	1, 2	2–27	None	[48–50]
	3	36–69		
Cefoperazone	3	33–48	None	[51,52]
Cefotaxime	2	80–150	None	[53]
Ceftriaxone	3	9–120	None	[54]
Cefuroxime	3	18–108	None	[55,56]
Cephalexin	3	33	None	[58]
Chloramphenicol	3	30–106	Circulatory collapse	[2,60,61]
Clindamycin	2	10–25	None	[41,48]
	3	30–50		[62]
Cloxacillin	3	20–97	None	[48,63]
Dicloxacillin	3	7–12	None	[48,64,66]
Erythromycin	2, 3	1–20	None	[41,67]
Gentamicin	2, 3	21–44	Ototoxicity; potentiation of MgSO$_4$-induced neuromuscular weakness	[68,69]
Imipenem	3	14–52	Seizure activity	[70]
Kanamycin	3	26–48	Ototoxicity	[48,71]
Nafcillin	3	16	None	[48]
Nitrofurantoin	3	38–92	Hemolysis in G6PD deficiency	[73]
Penicillin G	1, 2	26–70	None	[46,48]
	3	15–100		[46,48,74]
Sulfonamides	3	13–275	Hemolysis in G6PD deficiency; jaundice and potential kernicterus	[75–80]
Tetracyclines	3	10–90	Depressed bone growth; abnormal teeth; possible inguinal hernia	[48,50,81–83, 90,91,662,666]
Tobramycin	1, 2	20	Ototoxicity	[42,48]
Trimethoprim	1, 2	27–131	Teratogenic in animals	[83,84,665]

G6PD, *glucose-6-phosphate dehydrogenase;* MgSO$_4$, *magnesium sulfate.*

From Table 37–4 it can be seen that infant serum concentrations of some antibiotics, such as ampicillin [46], cefotaxime [53], chloramphenicol [60,61], and sulfonamides [75,76,80,87], approach or even exceed those in maternal serum. These high and rapidly attainable fetal ampicillin serum concentrations explain, in part, the benefit of intrapartum administration of ampicillin to pregnant women colonized with group B streptococci in reducing early-onset neonatal sepsis. The ratio of infant to maternal serum values for methicillin [66,72] is considerably higher than that for dicloxacillin [64,66]; this may be a result of differences in serum protein binding (37% and 98%, respectively). Antibiotics with low transplacental penetration include cephalothin [59,65], dicloxacillin [64,66], erythromycin [41,67], nafcillin [48], and tobramycin [42,48].

Complete evaluation of the possible adverse effects of drugs on the developing fetus must be performed before the drug is used during pregnancy. Some reported adverse events associated with antibiotics [88,89] include kernicterus (sulfonamides), ototoxicity (streptomycin), inhibition of infant bone growth (tetracyclines), and discoloration of teeth (tetracyclines). Anecdotal clinical experience is not sufficient to assess properly the safety of antibiotic administration during pregnancy. Rather, carefully planned prospective toxicity studies in the fetus and neonate, first in animals and then in humans, are warranted.

Due to the ease of transplacental passage of sulfonamides and their significant bilirubin-displacing capabilities, with the associated theoretical risk for development of kernicterus in the infant, these drugs should not be given to pregnant women near term [78]. Jaundice and hemolytic anemia have been noted in newborns with G6PD deficiency after maternal sulfonamide administration near term.

The tetracyclines readily cross the placental barrier and concentrate in many tissues of the developing fetus [83]. Of particular interest is the deposition of tetracycline in fetal bones and deciduous teeth [81–83,90,91]. Calcification of deciduous teeth begins during the fourth month of gestation, and crown formation of the anterior teeth is almost complete at term. Tetracycline administered during this gestational period produces yellow discoloration, enamel hypoplasia, and abnormal development of those teeth. These effects have been documented for tetracycline, oxytetracycline, and demethylchlortetracycline. One report found a possible association between ciprofloxacin therapy given to young infants and teeth discoloration [92], but this association has not been confirmed in other studies.

Chloramphenicol has been associated with circulatory collapse (gray baby syndrome) and death in premature infants who received the drug during the first weeks of life [2]. Chloramphenicol should not be administered to pregnant women near term because of the absence of glucuronyl transferase activity in the fetal liver and the potential danger of serum drug accumulation and shock in the newborn [93].

EXCRETION OF ANTIBIOTICS IN HUMAN MILK

Approximately 20% of postpartum women are prescribed an antibiotic; [94] however, the concentration of antimicrobial agents in breast milk is typically so low that neither therapeutic nor harmful effects are likely to occur. The amount of drug could be significant if the drug accumulates in breast milk, the infant ingests a large volume of milk, infant feeding times correlate with maximal maternal plasma concentrations, or the drug has reasonable bioavailability in the infant [95,96]. Assessment of the safety of antibiotics in milk has relied primarily on anecdotal clinical experience, rather than on carefully controlled long-term studies.

Most drugs are transferred into breast milk by passive diffusion, exocytosis, or reverse pinocytosis [95]. Factors influencing the transfer of antibiotics from plasma to milk include maternal serum concentration of unbound drug and the physiochemical properties of the drug (e.g., molecular weight, lipid solubility, degree of ionization, and protein-binding capability) [95–98]. Small, lipid-soluble, nonionized drugs traverse the lipid bilayers into breast milk more readily than larger, ionized, water soluble drugs. Although drugs with high lipid solubility tend to accumulate in milk, the extent varies with the fat content of the milk. The ionization power of drugs depends on the pH of the milk and the drug dissociation constant (pKa). Weak bases become more ionized with decreasing pH. Early postpartum human milk has a pH of 7.0 to 7.1, while mature milk after 2 weeks has a pH of approximately 7.3 to 7.4, each compared with the normal serum pH of 7.35 to 7.45. Therefore, drugs that are weak bases (pKa greater than pH), such as erythromycin, isoniazid, metronidazole, and tetracyclines, would be expected to ionize and accumulate in the lower pH environment of colostrum. Weak acids, such as ampicillin, are more likely to be ionized in maternal serum and therefore not transfer at high levels into breast milk. Drugs that are highly serum protein-bound, such as ceftriaxone, tend to remain in the intravascular space in the maternal circulation. Data pertaining to antibiotic concentrations in the colostrum are not available. Because blood flow and permeability are increased during the colostral phase [97], it is possible that these drugs are present in concentrations equal to or greater than those found in mature milk.

The maternal serum and breast milk concentrations of commonly used antimicrobial agents have been reviewed [52,95,99,100]. Milk to plasma ratios show considerable variability due to the extremely small number of women studied and the differences in age, gestation, dosing regimen, and underlying pathophysiology. In general, the concentrations of metronidazole, sulfonamides, and trimethoprim in breast milk are similar to those in maternal serum (milk-to-serum ratio of 1.0), whereas those of chloramphenicol, erythromycin, and tetracycline are 50% to 75% of maternal serum values. The concentrations of penicillins, oxacillin, various cephalosporins, and aminoglycosides in milk are low.

Although the milk-to-plasma ratio is frequently quoted to predict drug distribution into breast milk, its utility for those drugs with higher milk-to-serum ratios is suspect. The milk-to-plasma ratio is typically obtained at a single point in time. However, the concentration of drug in breast milk and plasma is not constant and the ratio of milk-to-plasma concentrations varies greatly over time. Most studies are not performed at steady state. Furthermore, most studies usually do not expose the infant to the breast milk and cannot comment on infant systemic exposure. Instead, Chung et al recommend that the milk-to-plasma ratio be used as a qualitative estimate of the possible magnitude of infant drug exposure [95]. By taking the peak breast milk concentration and an assumed ingestion of breast milk intake (150 mL/kg/day), they have derived an estimated potential infant dose correlated with predicted infant exposure (Table 37–5 modified with permission from Chung and coworkers) [95]. In addition, infant maturity, developmental characteristics of drug disposition, and tolerance of drug when given directly to the infant, and the possible extent to which the drug may modify the infant's intestinal gut flora need to be taken into consideration.

Most drugs are predicted to yield breast milk concentrations that produce limited exposure to newborns

(Table 37–5). Single dose PK studies describe very limited breast milk concentrations after maternal administration of penicillin, amoxicillin, ticarcillin, cephalosporins [54, 101–108]. For mother's receiving ampicillin, additional studies confirmed minimal concentration of ampicillin in breast milk concentration and minimal to no infant exposure [105,109,110]. Clavulanic acid was not detected in breast milk [105]. One study observed higher than expected concentrations of ceftazidime in breast milk from women receiving a high dose regimen at steady state [111]. The predicted infant ceftazidime exposure remains limited especially given the poor bioavailability of ceftazidime. The overall tolerability profile of penicillin and cephalosporins, along with the low concentration of these drugs in breast milk, support their use in breast-feeding infants [112].

TABLE 37–5   Summary of Reported Breast Milk Concentrations of Selected Antibiotic and Estimated Maximal Potential Infant Daily Dose for Medications That Distribute into Breast Milk*

Drug (No. mothers studied)	Maternal Dose Regimen†	Peak Milk [mg/L]‡	Corresponding Potential Infant Dose§(mg/kg/day)	Infant Clinical Dose (mg/kg/day)	Theoretical Safety Concerns	Reference
Drugs for which the effect on nursing infants is unknown but may be of concern, consider discarding breast milk in most circumstances						
Metronidazole	2 g once	45.8	6.87	7.5–30	In vitro mutagen	[120,667,668]
Metronidazole	400 mg tid for 3–4 days	15.5	2.44	7.5–30		
Chloramphenicol	250 mg q6h for 7–10 days	2.8	0.43	50–75	Idiosyncratic bone marrow suppression.	[669–671]
Chloramphenicol	500 mg q6h for 7–10 days	6.1	0.92	50–75	Extremely unlikely to achieve levels to cause gray baby syndrome	[5,6]
Maternal medication usually compatible with breast-feeding with ongoing observation of infant						
Erythromycin	2 g/day	3.2	0.48	15–50	GI distress, pyloric stenosis	[52,118]
Azithromycin	1g then 48 hr later 500 mg/day for 3 days	2.8	0.42	5–10	GI distress	[672]
Clindamycin	600 mg q6h	3.8	0.57	25–40	C. difficile colitis	[119,673]
Clindamycin	150 mg tid for at least 7 days	3.1	0.47	25–40	C. difficile colitis	[119,674]
Cotrimoxazole (trimethoprim/sulfamethoxazole)	3 tablets bid for 5 days (80 mg trimethoprim/ 400 mg sulfamethoxazole)	2.0 (trim) 5.3 (sulf)	0.3 (trim) 0.8 (sulf)	6–10 (trim) 75–150 (sulf)	Hemolytic anemia with sulfa drugs in infants with G6PD deficiency	[116,675–677]
Nitrofurantoin	100 mg tid for 4 doses	2.2	0.33	5–7	Hemolytic anemia in infants with G6PD deficiency	[678,679]
Tetracycline	2 g/day	0.4–2	0.3	25–50	Typically none reported. Teeth staining	[666,680] [90,117]
Ciprofloxacin	750 mg q12h for 3 doses	8.2	1.23	100–150	Arthropathy, none reported	[114,115]
Ofloxacin	400 mg q12h for 3 doses	2.4	0.36	none	Arthropathy, none reported	[114]

*Adapted with permission from Chung AM, Reed MD, Blumer JL. Antibiotics and breast-feeding: a critical review of the literature. Paediatr Drugs 4:817–837, 2002 [95] and including supplemental references from Academy of Pediatrics CoD. Transfer of drugs and other chemicals into human milk. Pediatrics 108:776–789, 2001 [112].
†Highest possible concentration was used.
‡Assuming infant consumes approximately 150 mL/kg/day of breast milk.
§Varies with detail given in citation.
bid, twice daily; tid, three times daily; qxh, every x hours; trim, trimethoprim; sulf, sulfamethoxazole; GI, gastrointestinal.

The rare possibility of hypersensitivity reactions or altered intestinal flora–associated diarrhea in breast feeding infants remains a theoretical concern.

Broad-acting agents should be reserved for the most serious infections. The most recent review of antibiotics in breast-feeding [95] reported personal communication with Merck of limited data on detectable low levels of imipenem in breast milk of women, typically 0.2 to 0.5 mg/L. Cilastin was not detected. Despite this low exposure in breast milk, infant exposure would be further limited by poor bioavailability and drug inactivation at alkaline or acidic pH. The similarities in drug characteristics of meropenem and imipenem suggest that breast milk exposure from meropenem would be minimal. The physiochemical properties of aztreonam suggest limited transfer into breast milk since it is inactivated in acidic solutions and exhibits moderate protein binding and low lipid solubility [1]. Single dose PK studies confirmed a minimal amount of aztreonam in breast milk of women [113].

The physiochemical properties of fluoroquinolones (weak acid, low molecular weight, high lipid solubility, low protein binding, and good bioavailability) suggest that fluoroquinolones can accumulate in breast milk; [1,114] however, the predicted infant dose exposure is limited (see Table 37–5) and a case report of one infant revealed negligible ciprofloxacin infant serum concentrations (<0.03 mg/L) despite accumulation in breast milk after 10 days of maternal exposure (maternal serum 0.21 mg/mL, breast milk 0.98 mg/L) [115]. This report highlighted the difficulty of predicting infant exposure from maternal plasma and milk concentrations. The risk of fluoroquinolone-induced arthropathies or cartilage erosion in neonates has not been explored. Although the predicted fluoroquinolone exposure to an infant is predicted to be negligible, most recommend against the use of a fluoroquinolone while breast-feeding due to theoretical concerns for adverse events.

Sulfonamides and tetracycline both distribute relatively poorly into breast milk yet have theoretical concerns for associated adverse events in neonates [52]. The amount of sulfamethoxazole and tetracyclines in breast milk is low and of unclear clinical significance. One breast-fed infant with G6PD deficiency experienced hemolytic anemia while the mother was receiving sulfamethoxypyridazine [116]. The adverse effects of tetracyclines on developing teeth and bones are well documented when the drug is given directly to infants and children; however, the limited exposure in breast milk has not been directly associated with abnormalities [82,90,117]. Although many use these theoretical concerns to discourage breast-feeding during maternal exposure to sulfonamides or tetracyclines, the American Academy of Pediatrics states that sulfapyridine, sulfafurazole, and sulfamethoxazole (with trimethoprim), tetracycline, doxycycline, and minocycline are compatible with breast-feeding. Caution is advised for infants with jaundice, G6PD deficiency, severe illness, or significant prematurity [112].

Macrolides, azithromycin, and clindamycin distribute into breast milk. However, the actual amount the infant would receive from breast-feeding remains very small (see Table 37–5). Neonatal exposure may be further limited by bioavailability. One case report of erythromycin-induced pyloric stenosis during breast-feeding exposure in a 3-week-old infant has been reported [118]. One report incriminated the administration of clindamycin to a mother in the development of antibiotic-induced colitis in her breast-fed infant [119]. The American Academy of Pediatrics has described erythromycin and clindamycin as usually compatible with breast-feeding [112]. Azithromycin is likely to be compatible with breast-feeding as well [95].

Metronidazole effectively distributes into breast milk and achieves infant plasma concentrations approximately one-fifth the exposure observed in the mother's plasma [120]. Breast-fed infants whose mothers were administered metronidazole therapy had no difference in adverse events compared with infants whose mothers received ampicillin or no antibiotics. Metronidazole has been detected in infant plasma and has potential carcinogenesis or mutagenesis properties in vitro and in mice [121–123]. Although the extrapolation of mutagenesis properties in humans remain unknown [124,125], clinicians often consider withholding breast-feeding during maternal metronidazole exposure [112].

The decision to allow or stop breast-feeding is based on the likelihood that high milk concentrations are attained for a particular antibiotic, whether the drug is expected to be absorbed into neonatal plasma, and whether significant adverse events are commonly associated with this agent. The American Academy of Pediatrics Committee on Drugs recommends that breast-feeding be transiently discontinued during the course of treatment with metronidazole (an in vitro mutagen) or chloramphenicol (associated with a theoretical risk of idiosyncratic bone marrow suppression), and cautions with the use of nalidixic acid, nitrofurantoin, and sulfa drugs, which can cause hemolysis in G6PD-deficient infants [112]. In general, the severity of the woman's infection, rather than the drug that she is receiving, most often is the more important contraindication to breast-feeding.

PENICILLIN

Penicillin has been used for treatment of neonatal bacterial infections for more than 3 decades. It is safe and well tolerated. However, efficacy is limited by resistance. Many species of streptococci, *Listeria monocytogenes*, meningococci, and *Treponema pallidum* remain susceptible to penicillin whereas most species of staphylococci, pneumococci, and gonococci have become resistant.

Microbiologic Activity

Penicillin and other β-lactam derivatives interfere with bacterial cell wall synthesis by reacting with one or more penicillin-binding proteins (PBPs) to inhibit transpeptidation [126]. The transpeptidase activity of PBPs is essential for cross-linking adjacent peptides and for incorporating newly-formed peptidoglycan into an already existing strand. Subsequently, this event promotes bacterial cell lysis.

Several mechanisms of bacterial resistance to penicillin and other β-lactams have been identified. The most important is by inactivation through enzymatic hydrolysis of the β-lactam ring by β-lactamases [127]. These enzymes are produced by most staphylococci and enteric gram-negative bacilli and by many *Neisseria gonorrhoeae* strains. Another mechanism of resistance involves decreased permeability of the outer membrane of gram-negative bacteria, which can prevent this drug from reaching its target site [128]. In addition, by poorly defined mechanisms, some group B streptococci are inhibited but not killed by penicillin, a phenomenon termed tolerance [129]. The first group B streptococcus isolates with elevated MIC to ß-lactamase antibiotics by a mutation in the penicillin-binding protein have recently been described [130]. Usual MICs of penicillin against streptococci are between 0.005 and 0.1 µg/mL. For *T. pallidum*, the corresponding concentration ranges are between 0.02 and 0.2 µg/mL. Many pneumococcal strains isolated around the world are considered to be relatively (MICs of 0.1 to 1 µg/mL) or highly (MICs of 2 µg/mL or greater) resistant to multiple antibiotics, including penicillins, macrolides, and third-generation cephalosporins [131].

Pharmacokinetic Data

Most of the penicillin dose is excreted in the urine in unchanged form. Tubular secretion accounts for approximately 90% of urinary penicillin, whereas glomerular filtration contributes the remaining 10%. Biliary excretion also occurs, and this may be an important route of elimination in newborns with renal failure.

Aqueous Penicillin G

A mean peak serum concentration of 24 µg/mL (range, 8 to 41 µg/mL) is observed after a dose of 25,000 units/kg of penicillin G is given intramuscularly to infants with birth weights of less than 2000 g [132]. The peak values do not change appreciably with increasing birth weight or chronologic age up to 14 days. After a dose of 50,000 units/kg, peak serum values of 35 to 40 µg/mL were detected in neonates of different ages. The concentrations at 4 and 8 hours after the dose were not substantially different from those after a dose of 25,000 units/kg. The half-life of penicillin in serum becomes longer in smaller and younger infants. Half-life values of 1.5 to 10 hours are observed in the first week of life; the longer half-lives are in smallest infants with birth weights less than 1500 g. A shorter half-life of 1.5 to 4 hours was observed after 7 days of age. The half-life of penicillin also decreases as creatinine clearance improves.

Procaine Penicillin G

In the first week after birth, a 50,000 unit/kg intramuscular dose of procaine penicillin G produces mean serum values of 7 to 9 µg/mL for up to 12 hours and a 24-hour trough concentration of 1.5 µg/mL [132]. Older neonates have lower 24-hour trough concentrations, 0.4 µg/mL, due to their increased clearance and shorter half-lives. These serum values are approximately twice those obtained in the original study of 22,000 units/kg, suggesting a linear relationship between dose and serum concentration [133]. No accumulation of penicillin in serum is observed after 7 to 10 days of daily doses of procaine penicillin G. The drug was well tolerated without evidence of local reaction at the site of injection.

Benzathine Penicillin G

Penicillin can be detected in serum and urine for up to 12 days after a single intramuscular injection of 50,000 units/kg of benzathine penicillin G in newborns. Peak serum concentrations of 0.4 to 2.5 µg/mL (mean, 1.2 µg/mL) are observed 12 to 24 hours after administration, and levels of 0.07 to 0.09 µg/mL are present at 12 days [134,135]. This preparation has been well tolerated by infants. Muscle damage from intramuscular injection as judged from creatinine values does not appear to be appreciably different from that after intramuscular administration of the other penicillins.

Cerebrospinal Fluid Penetration

Penicillin does not penetrate CSF well, even when meninges are inflamed. Peak concentrations of 1 to 2 µg/mL are measured 30 minutes to 1 hour after an intravenous dose of 40,000 units/kg of penicillin G is given to infants and children with bacterial meningitis [136]. Although these values are 2% to 5% of concomitant serum concentrations, the concentrations exceed the MIC values for streptococci and susceptible pneumococci by 50- to 100-fold. CSF concentrations of penicillin are not optimal to treat neonatal meningitis caused by penicillin-resistant pneumococci. CSF concentrations decrease as meningeal inflammation is reduced. Concentrations of penicillin in CSF during the first several days of therapy are maintained in the range of 0.5 to 1 µg/mL; thereafter, the values are 0.1 µg/mL or less by 4 hours after the dose.

Procaine penicillin G administered by intramuscular injection in newborns provides sufficient CSF exposure for the treatment of congenital neurosyphilis. Procaine penicillin G administered intramuscularly at a dose of 50,000 units/kg provides mean CSF concentrations ranging from 0.12 to 0.7 µg/mL between 4 and 24 hours after a dose [137,138]. These CSF values are at least several fold greater than the required minimum spirocheticidal concentration [139]. Benzathine penicillin G does not provide adequate CSF exposure and is not recommended for the treatment of congenital neurosyphyllis [135].

Safety

All forms of penicillin are typically well tolerated in newborns. Cutaneous allergic manifestations to penicillin are rare in the newborn and young infant.

PK-PD and Clinical Implications for Dosing

Penicillin remains effective for therapy for infections caused by group B streptococci and *T. pallidum*. The dosage recommended for neonatal sepsis or pneumonia is 50,000 to 100,000 units/kg per day administered in two to four divided doses, whereas that for meningitis is 250,000 to 450,000 units/kg per day in two to four divided doses, depending on birth weight and chronologic age [140]. The pharmacodynamic target for β-lactam antibiotics is the T>MIC [30]. The trough penicillin concentrations remain above the MIC for streptococci.

Penicillin remains effective therapy for congenital syphilis. However, because central nervous system involvement in congenital syphilis is difficult to exclude with certainty, benzathine penicillin G should not be used for therapy. Its use is acceptable for asymptomatic infants with normal findings on CSF examination and roentgenologic studies, but who have positive results on treponemal serologic studies (presumably from maternal origin), if follow-up can be ensured. For symptomatic infants, and for asymptomatic infants with laboratory or radiologic evidence suggestive of congenital syphilis, the recommended regimen is either aqueous crystalline penicillin G, 100,000 to 150,000 units/kg daily for 10 to 14 days administered intravenously every 12 hours during the first 7 days of life, and every 8 hours thereafter, for a total of at least 10 days. Alternatively, procaine penicillin G, 50,000 units/kg daily administered intramuscularly for at least 10 days [140].

Ampicillin

Antimicrobial Activity

Ampicillin remains the preferred penicillin for initial empirical therapy for neonatal septicemia and meningitis because it provides broader antimicrobial activity without sacrificing safety. Ampicillin is commonly used in combination with aminoglycosides. Compared with penicillin G, ampicillin has increased in vitro efficacy against most strains of enterococci and *L. monocytogenes*, and against some gram-negative pathogens, such as *Haemophilus influenzae, Escherichia coli, Proteus mirabilis, and Salmonella* species. It is only rarely active against *Staphylococcus aureus*. Approximately 90% of group B streptococci and *L. monocytogenes* organisms are inhibited by 0.06 µg/mL or less of ampicillin. Almost two thirds of the gram-negative enteric bacilli isolated from CSF cultures of infants enrolled in the Second Neonatal Meningitis Cooperative Study (1976 to 1978) were inhibited by 10 µg/mL or less of ampicillin [141]. Recently, however, an increased rate of ampicillin-resistant gram-negative bacilli has been reported and possibly linked to the frequent use of intrapartum prophylaxis with ampicillin to prevent early-onset group B streptococcal neonatal infection [142].

Pharmacokinetic Data

Ampicillin, similar to many β-lactam antibiotics, is cleared by renal elimination. Therefore, drug clearance and half-life are dependent on renal maturation [10,12,143]. Plasma drug clearance increases (and half-life decreases) with increasing birth weight, gestational age, and chronologic age. Despite its frequent use, the PK of ampicillin in extremely low birth weight infants remains sparse.

Serum ampicillin concentration-time curves have been determined after intramuscular doses in newborns [144–146]. The mean peak serum concentrations 0.5 to 1 hour after 5, 10, 20, and 25 mg/kg doses were 16, 25, 54, and 57 µg/mL, respectively, whereas the values at 12 hours were from 1 to 15 µg/mL (mean, 5 µg/mL). After 50 mg/kg doses, the mean peak values were higher in low birth weight infants (100 to 130 µg/mL) compared with larger term infants (80 to 85 µg/mL). Peak serum concentrations as high as 300 µg/mL (mean values, 180 to 216 µg/mL) are observed 1 to 2 hours after a 100 mg/kg dose [147]. These latter values exceed the MIC90 values of group B streptococci by at least 3000-fold. Half-life decreases with advancing age from 3 to 6 hours in the first week of life to 2 to 3.5 hours thereafter.

Serum ampicillin concentration-time curves after intravenous doses have been characterized for preterm and term infants. After a 100 mg/kg intravenous dose,

premature infants 26 to 33 weeks gestation had a lower mean peak serum concentration (135 µg/mL) compared with more mature 34 to 40 week infants (153 µg/mL) [148]. When the loading dose was followed by maintenance ampicillin doses of 50 mg/kg intravenously at 12- to 18-hour intervals, the mean peak and trough serum concentrations in steady-state conditions were 113 and 30 µg/mL, respectively, for premature neonates, and 140 and 37 µg/mL for full-term neonates. Despite the lower peak concentration in premature infants, the trough value was maintained likely given the longer half-life in the premature newborn (9.5 hours) compared with full-term newborns (7 hours). Trough values of 30 µg/mL exceed the MIC90 value for group B streptococci by 300-fold.

Cerebrospinal Fluid Penetration

Concentrations of ampicillin in CSF vary greatly. The largest concentrations (3 to 18 µg/mL) occur approximately 2 hours after a 50 mg/kg intravenous dose and exceed the MIC90 values for group B streptococci and *L. monocytogenes* by 50- to 300-fold [147]. By contrast, these peak concentrations equal or exceed the MIC values against many *E. coli* strains by only several fold. The values in CSF are lower later in the course of meningitis, when meningeal inflammation subsides.

Safety

Ampicillin is well tolerated when administered parenterally to newborns. Nonspecific rashes and urticaria are rarely observed, and diarrhea is uncommon. Elevations of serum glutamic-oxaloacetic transaminase and creatinine values frequently are detected in neonates and probably represent local tissue destruction at the site of intramuscular injection. Mild eosinophilia may be noted in newborns and young infants. Alteration of the microbial flora of the bowel may occur after parenteral administration of ampicillin, but overgrowth of resistant gram-negative organisms and *Candida albicans* occurs more frequently after oral administration [149]. Diarrhea usually subsides on discontinuation of therapy.

PK-PD and Clinical Implications for Dosing
(See Table 37–11)

Vast clinical experience has demonstrated that ampicillin is a safe and effective drug for therapy for neonatal bacterial infections caused by susceptible organisms. Combined ampicillin and aminoglycoside therapy is appropriate initial empirical management of suspected bacterial infections of neonates because it provides broad antimicrobial activity and potential synergism against many strains of group B streptococci, *L. monocytogenes*, and enterococci [150–152]. ß-lactam antibiotics exhibit time-dependent killing therefore the PK-PD target is T>MIC [30]. Frequent dosing intervals are used to maintain drug exposure over each dosing interval. For systemic bacterial infections other than meningitis, a dosage of 25 to 50 mg/kg per dose given two to three times a day in the first week of life, and then three to four times a day thereafter, is recommended [153]. For therapy for bacterial meningitis, we recommend a dosage of at least

200 mg/kg per day, although some consultants use dosages as high as 300 mg/kg per day. Premature infants may continue to receive ampicillin 2 to 3 times a day for up to 4 weeks depending on gestational age, chronologic age, and renal function (see Table 37–11).

ANTISTAPHYLOCOCCAL TREATMENT

S. aureus infections occur in nurseries either as sporadic cases or in the form of disease outbreaks. In recent years, multiply-resistant strains, especially methicillin-resistant *S. aureus* (MRSA) and coagulase-negative staphylococcal species such as methicillin-resistant *Staphylococcus epidermidis* (MRSE) have been responsible for an increasing number of nosocomially acquired staphylococcal infections in many neonatal care units.

Antistaphylococcal Penicillins (Table 37–6)
Antimicrobial Activity

Nafcillin and oxacillin are the mainstays of methicillin-sensitive staphylococcal therapy. These semisynthetic agents are engineered to be resistant to hydrolysis by most staphylococcal β-lactamases by virtue of a substituted side chain that acts by steric hindrance at the site of enzyme attachment. Most penicillinase-producing staphylococci are inhibited by less than 0.5 μg/mL of nafcillin and oxacillin [154].

Pharmacokinetic Data *(Table 37–6)*

Nafcillin

Unlike other penicillins, nafcillin exhibits primarily *hepatic* clearance rather than renal clearance. Only 8% to 25% of this drug is excreted in the urine in a 24-hour period [155]. The administration of 5-, 10-, 15-, and 20-mg/kg intramuscular doses of nafcillin to full-term newborns in the first 4 days of life produces mean peak serum concentrations 1 hour later of 10, 25, 30, and 37 μg/mL, respectively [144,155]. These concentrations are significantly higher than those obtained in older children receiving comparable amounts of this drug [155]. Preterm infants weighing less than 2000 g had higher steady state peak concentrations, 100 to 160 μg/mL, after receiving 33- to 50-mg/kg intravenous doses [156]. In these preterm infants, the half-life ranged from 2.2 to 5.5 hours.

Oxacillin

Oxacillin exhibits primarily renal clearance. Despite this difference in clearance mechanism, the PK of oxacillin in neonates is similar to that of nafcillin. Mean peak serum concentrations of approximately 50 and 100 μg/mL are produced by 20- and 50-mg/kg intramuscular doses, respectively [145,157]. The serum half-life of oxacillin in premature infants is about 3 hours in the first week of life and 1.5 hours thereafter.

Safety

The antistaphylococcal penicillins are well tolerated in newborn and young infants. Repeated intramuscular injections can result in muscle damage, sterile muscle abscess, and elevation of creatinine concentrations. Nephrotoxicity (interstitial nephritis or cystitis) is rare in newborns, but occurs in 3% to 5% of children who receive large doses of methicillin and possibly the other antistaphylococcal penicillins, with the exception of nafcillin [158,159]. Reversible hematologic abnormalities such as neutropenia or eosinophilia commonly are observed in children undergoing treatment with these drugs, but their incidence in newborns is unknown [159–162]. Because nafcillin has a predominant biliary excretion, accumulation of this drug in serum can occur in jaundiced neonates, and potential adverse effects can develop. Extravasation of nafcillin at the injection site can result in necrosis of local tissue.

PK-PD and Clinical Implications for Dosing
(See Tables 37–6, 37–11)

Nafcillin and oxacillin are the antistaphylococcal drugs most often used for treatment of methicillin-sensitive staphylococcal infections in neonates. Like other ß-lactam antibiotics, it is important to maintain the drug concentrations over the dosing interval (T>MIC). Therefore, as infants mature, drug clearance improves, and dosing intervals shorten. The dosage of oxacillin is 25 to 50 mg/kg every 12 hours (50 to 150 mg/kg per day) in the first week of life and every 6 to 8 hours (75 to 200 mg/kg per day) thereafter. The larger dosage is indicated for infants with disseminated staphylococcal disease or meningitis. For nafcillin, the dosage is 25 mg/kg (50 mg/kg for meningitis) per dose given every 12 hours in the first week of life and every 6 to 8 hours thereafter. Depending on gestational age at birth and chronologic age, extremely preterm infants may have delayed clearance and therefore should continue twice daily dosing for 2 to 4 weeks (Table 37–11). If an infant does not respond to antimicrobial therapy as anticipated, one should consider an occult site of staphylococcal disease (e.g., abscess, osteomyelitis, endocarditis), pathogen resistance, or the need to shorten the dosing interval to maintain time above MIC. Appropriate drainage of purulent foci, addition of an aminoglycoside or rifampin to the regimen, and use of vancomycin are among several options to consider in management of unresponsive infections.

Methicillin Resistant Staphylococcal Infections (MRSE and MRSA) (See Table 37–6)

MRSA now constitute a relatively common cause of infection outbreaks in some nurseries, and methicillin-resistant *S. epidermidis* (MRSE) strains are an important cause of catheter-associated disease, particularly among low birth weight premature infants. Glycopeptide antibiotics such as vancomycin or teicoplanin (in Europe) are the drugs of choice for infections caused by these resistant strains. Infections may be treated with combination therapy: a glycopeptide with an aminoglycoside or rifampin. More recently, the use of linezolid, clindamycin, and daptomycin are being explored for the treatment of MRSA infections.

Vancomycin (See Table 37–6)
Antimicrobial Activity

Vancomycin is bactericidal against most aerobic and anaerobic gram-positive cocci and bacilli but is ineffective against most gram-negative bacteria. The drug interferes

TABLE 37-6 Drugs Used in Treatment of *Staphylococcus aureus*

Drug	Route of Elimination	Mean C$_{max}$ (µg/mL)	Mean Half-life (hr)	CLSI Sensitivity Breakpoint MIC	PK-PD Target [188,681]	CSF Penetration	Safety and Clinical Pearls
MRSA							
Vancomycin 15 mg/kg	Renal	25–30	Day 0–7 6.7 (<2 kg) 5.9 (>2 kg) 4.1≈3 months	≤2	AUC/MIC >100–400 Trough 10 (15 if MRSA pneumonia) Keep level above the MIC	30%–50% inflamed [682] 0%–20% non-inflamed	• Check levels in renal insufficiency or changing renal function. • 10%–20% penetration epithelial lung fluid • Consider increased trough target (15–20) with difficult or difficult-to-treat infection
Clindamycin 5–7.5 mg/kg	Hepatic	10	6	≤0.5	AUC/MIC	Poor	Good bone penetration, often effective against MRSA (check D-test)
Linezolid 10 mg/kg	Renal 30% Nonrenal 65% Metabolites renally excreted	12	5.6 (<7 days and <34 wk) 2.8 (<80 days and 25–40 wk)	<4	AUC/MIC >80	27%–100%	• Monitor blood counts to evaluate for rare thrombocytopenia and anemia if used >14 days. • Enhanced lung penetration with accumulation in epithelial lung lining fluid • CSF penetration unreliable
Rifampin 10 mg/kg/day	Hepatic	4	Not defined	<1	Not defined	5%–20%	• Light sensitive • Used in combination therapy due to induction of resistance
Daptomycin 6 mg/kg	Hepatic	36–41	Not defined	≤1	C$_{max}$/MIC AUC/MIC	Not defined	• Myopathy, elevated CPK • Awaiting further PK, safety evaluation. • No lung penetration
MSSA							
Nafcillin 50 mg/kg	Hepatic	160	4 (days 0–7) 3 (days >7)	≤2	T>MIC >50%	10%–30%	• Bone marrow suppression • Monitor CBC
Oxacillin 50 mg/kg	Renal	100	3 (days 0–7) 1.5 (days > 7)	≤2	T>MIC >50%	Not defined	• Bone marrow suppression • Monitor CBC

MRSA, *methicillin-resistant* S. aureus; MSSA, *methicillin-sensitive* S. aureus; T, *time*; MIC, *minimum inhibitory concentration*; AUC, *area under the concentration time curve*.

with the phospholipid cycle of cell wall synthesis, alters plasma membrane function, and inhibits RNA synthesis [1,163]. There is no cross-resistance between vancomycin and other antibiotics. Synergistic bacterial killing has been demonstrated for vancomycin with aminoglycosides.

Pharmacokinetic Data *(See Table 37–6)*

Vancomycin is not metabolized by the body and is excreted unchanged in the urine by glomerular filtration [1]. Vancomycin clearance reflects renal maturation and increases with gestational and chronologic age. Vancomycin is approximately 55% protein bound.

The PK of vancomycin has been studied in preterm and term infants. Vancomycin clearance improves and elimination half-life shortens with gestational age and chronologic age. Serum creatinine remains an important predictor of renal clearance, even after gestational age and postchronologic age are accounted for. Although vancomycin and gentamicin exhibit similar changes in drug clearance with renal maturation, vancomycin clearance is more delayed likely due to protein binding.

In the first week after birth, peak concentrations of 17 to 30 µg/mL are produced at the end of a 30-minute infusion of a 15-mg/kg dose given to neonates weighing less than 2000 g. Slightly higher values are observed in larger infants. In infants up to 12 months of age, doses of 10 mg/kg produce similar peak serum concentrations.

Population PK studies have attempted to explain the observed variability of vancomycin with chronologic age, maturity, and renal function. In the largest population PK study of 1103 vancomycin concentrations from 374 newborns and infants less than 2 years of age, creatinine levels were strongly correlated with vancomycin elimination, while chronologic age and prematurity (<28 weeks) were significant but less important predictors of vancomycin clearance [164]. Vancomycin clearance for a typical 27 day old, 1.8 kg, ex-33 week gestational age infant with a creatinine of 0.6 mg/dL is estimated to be 0.10 to 0.12 L/hr [164–166]. The volume of distribution (0.5 to 0.8 L/kg) varies with weight and is larger than that reported in older children.

Traditional and population PK studies consistently report improved clearance and shorter half-lives with advancing gestational age and chronologic age [164–171]. The half-life decreases from 6 to 7 hours in the first week of life, to 4 hours in early infancy, then to 2 to 2.5 hours in childhood. In preterm infants, serum half-life of vancomycin is prolonged and variable. The half-life in 1-month old premature infants who weighed less than 1000 g at birth is approximately 10 hours; older premature infants have shorter half-lives of approximately 4 to 5 hours [167,168].

Neonates undergoing extracorporeal membrane oxygenation (ECMO) receiving vancomycin have a larger volume of distribution, lower clearance, and longer half-life [172–175]. However, since infants on ECMO typically have renal insufficiency, some of the delayed vancomycin clearance may be explained by elevated serum creatinine [164].

Vancomycin does not readily penetrate the CSF unless the meninges are inflamed. The CSF concentrations of vancomycin are 10% to 15% of the concomitant serum concentrations in infants with minimal meningeal inflammation,

for example, as seen in ventriculoperitoneal shunt infections [176]. The degree of CSF penetration of vancomycin is similar to that for nafcillin. In premature infants born at 26 to 31 weeks of gestational age, dosages of 20 mg/kg every 18 to 24 hours were associated with CSF vancomycin concentrations of 2.2 to 5.6 µg/mL, 26% to 68% of their corresponding serum values [177].

Safety

Initial experience with vancomycin in the 1950s suggested a moderate incidence of ototoxicity and nephrotoxicity. These adverse effects were presumably related to the impurities found in early preparations of the drug [178]. Further studies have indicated that vancomycin is well-tolerated and safe when administered intravenously, particularly in newborns and young infants [176,179]. Rare cases of ototoxicity and nephrotoxicity typically involved excessive doses, underlying hearing loss or renal disease, and concomitant therapy with other ototoxic or nephrotoxic agents [180]. To minimize risk of nephrotoxicity or ototoxicity, vancomycin trough levels are monitored in patients with underlying renal dysfunction or those receiving concomitant therapy with aminoglycoside [181,182]. Renal function should be monitored during vancomycin therapy. After rapid administration, some patients develop a histamine reaction characterized by an erythematous pruritic rash that can persist for several hours but tends to resolve with antihistamine medications. Use of a slower infusion rate (i.e., over 45 to 60 minutes) usually avoids this adverse event. Vancomycin is irritating to tissue and is thus always administered through the intravenous route.

PK-PD and Clinical Implications for Dosing *(See Tables 37–6, 37–11)*

The primary indication for vancomycin therapy in newborns is for infections caused by MRSA and by ampicillin-resistant enterococci. Vancomycin is the initial drug of choice for documented infections caused by *S. epidermidis* because most strains are resistant to penicillin, methicillin, cephalosporins, and aminoglycosides. The rate of killing of staphylococci is slow for vancomycin compared with β-lactams. If susceptibility data for staphylococcal infections reveals methicillin sensitivity, then the antibiotic regimen should be adjusted. For β-lactam sensitive staphylococci and enterococci, vancomycin was inferior to nafcillin and ampicillin when comparing bactericidal rate and rapidity of blood sterility [183,184].

Vancomycin is a concentration-independent, time-dependent antibiotic with moderate postantibiotic effect (PAE) [185]. The continued suppression of bacterial growth against gram-positive bacteria can persists for several hours depending on the organism and initial antibiotic concentration, typically ranging from 0.6 to 2 hours for *S. aureus* and 4 to 6 hours for *S. epidermidis* [186]. Both increased AUC/MIC and increased Time>MIC have been shown to promote bacterial clearance [187,188]. MRSA and *S. epidermidis* are typically sensitive to vancomycin with MIC<2 mg/L. Serum bactericidal titers of 1:8 (approximate serum concentrations of 12 mg/L) have been associated with clinical cures in children [176]. Animal models of endocarditis have correlated outcome with trough serum concentrations [189]. In these studies, the vancomycin concentrations exceed the MIC for 100% of the dosing interval, bactericidal activity was maintained [190]. Bactericidal activity has also been shown when vancomycin trough concentrations were greater than 10 mg/L [191]. Keeping the trough level above the MIC is likely to be necessary for effective vancomycin treatment.

Several vancomycin dosing regimens have been proposed [164,165,192]. Traditional dosage schedule for vancomycin in neonates is typically 10 to 15 mg/kg every 12 hours (20 to 30 mg/kg/day) in the first week of life and every 8 hours (30 to 45 mg/kg/day) thereafter. Extremely premature infants have unique dosing requirements to account for changes in body water composition and postnatal maturation in renal function. Recently, analysis of population PK studies suggest that vancomycin dosage can be dependent on serum creatinine and independent of postmenstrual age [164]. Beyond the newborn period, daily administration of 40 to 60 mg/kg (divided into three or four doses) is recommended. The larger dosage (15 mg/kg) is used for treatment of central nervous system infection or pneumonia.

Historically, vancomycin dosing has been designed to achieve peak serum concentrations between 20 to 40 mg/L and serum trough concentrations of 5 to 10 mg/L. In light of advances in our understanding the PK-PD relationship for vancomycin, peak levels are rarely useful since they are not associated with efficacy [192]. There is no clear relationship between peak concentration and nephrotoxicity, except possibly when peak levels exceed 60 mg/L [181,182]. The relationship between serum levels and efficacy or toxicity have not been determined in neonates.

Therapeutic drug monitoring is now focused on trough serum concentrations to optimize PK-PD efficacy targets. Trough values of at least 10 ensure that the non-protein-bound vancomycin concentration will typically remain above the MIC of the offending organism. Many infectious disease experts advocate for higher trough concentrations (i.e., 10 to 20 μg/mL, when treating serious MRSA infections) [193,194]. The safety of these higher exposures has not been evaluated in children. Extremely preterm infants, infants with renal insufficiency or variable renal function, and infants on ECMO are likely to need more frequent monitoring.

The dramatic increase in worldwide prevalence of vancomycin-resistant enterococci (VRE) and the serious threat posed by the spread of vancomycin resistant staphylococci has discouraged the use of vancomycin for antimicrobial prophylaxis or empirical therapy.

Linezolid (See Table 37–6)
Antimicrobial Activity

Linezolid is a synthetic oxazolidinone antibiotic that inhibits bacterial protein synthesis in a broad range of gram-positive organisms [1,195–198]. In kill curve experiments, linezolid is bacteriostatic against staphylococci and enterococci but can be bacteriocidal against streptococci [199–201]. Linezolid has a unique mechanism of action and therefore does not exhibit cross-resistance with antistaphylococcal penicillins

or vancomycin. It is FDA-approved for treatment of infections caused by glycopeptide-resistant strains of *Enterococcus faecium*, *S. aureus*, and *S. pneumoniae* in neonates [1,195,196].

Pharmacokinetic Data (Table 37–6)

Linezolid is known for its rapid and nearly complete absorption after oral dosing [1,195]. Bioavailability is approximately 100% in adults but has not been well characterized in neonates. Only 30% of linezolid is eliminated via the kidneys as active drug in the urine. Nonrenal pathways account for approximately 65% of total body clearance for linezolid. Linezolid is oxidized on the morpholine ring resulting in two inactive metabolites that are then excreted in the urine. The specific biotransformation pathways in children have not been defined. Linezolid is not a cytochrome P450 substrate. Single dose PK for intravenous linezolid has been assessed in 42 neonates (25 to 40 weeks of gestation) in the first 80 days of life [202–204]. Linezolid clearance increases rapidly in the first week of life and is relatively constant from day 8 to 79 after birth. The increases in clearance are likely related to the development of biotransformation pathways after birth and age associated increases in glomerular filtration for the residual renal elimination of the drug. Linezolid volume of distribution varies inversely with gestational age. In the first week of life, preterm infants have a slower clearance and longer half-life (2.0 (mL/min)/kg and 5.6 hours) compared with more mature infants (3.8 (mL/min)/kg and 3 hours). Beyond the first week of life, clearance and half-life estimates are similar (5.1 (mL/min)/kg and 1.5 hours) in preterm and term infants up to 90 days of age. Linezolid trough concentrations at 11 hours are 0 to 4 μg/mL. Infants receiving 10 mg/kg dose are predicted to have a mean area under the concentration curve (AUC) of 54.9 mg*h/L. Infants have faster clearance and shorter half lives than older infants such that infants (>7 days old) dosed every 8 hours achieve similar AUC as older children. CSF penetration by linezolid is inconsistent; children with ventricular peritoneal shunts receiving the drug did not consistently achieve or maintain therapeutic concentrations in the CSF. In adults, moderate hepatic or renal insufficiency does alter the pharmacokinetics of linezolid. The drug's metabolites accumulate in adults with renal insufficiency; however, the clinical significance of these metabolites is unknown.

Safety

Linezolid has been well tolerated in the small number of infants and children in PK and efficacy trials. In pediatric comparator trials, the most common drug-related adverse events in children treated with linezolid were diarrhea, nausea, vomiting, anemia, and thrombocytopenia [205–207]. Drug-related adverse events rarely led to discontinuation of therapy. Linezolid is a reversible, nonselective inhibitor of monoamine oxidase [1,196]; therefore, it has the potential for interaction with adrenergic and serotonergic agents. Patients receiving linezolid may have an enhanced pressor response to sympathomimetic agents including dopamine. Myelosuppression has been reported and therefore complete blood counts should be monitored weekly in patients on linezolid therapy, particularly for therapy beyond 2 weeks [1,196]. One noncomparative study found good therapeutic outcomes, but a high rate of adverse reactions, in adults with serious gram-positive infections treated with linezolid for a mean of 28 days [208].

PK-PD and Clinical Implications for Dosing
(See Tables 37–6, 37–11)

Linezolid is indicated for the treatment of vancomycin resistant *E. faecium* (VRE) infections, pneumonia due to MRSA or *S. pneumoniae*, and severe, complicated skin infections due to susceptible organisms [197,198]. Linezolid penetrates respiratory secretions and epithelial lining fluid better than vancomycin [209]. Linezolid exhibits time-dependent killing with moderate to prolonged persistent antimicrobial effects [201]. The primary PD determinant associated with efficacy in the neutropenic thigh infection model for *S. pneumoniae* and *S. aureus* is an AUC/MIC ratio of 50 and 80, respectively [210]. Susceptible strains of *Enterococcus* and *Streptococcus* species have MIC of 2 µg/mL, whereas the susceptible strains of staphylococci have MIC of 4 µg/mL. In adults with MRSA or VRE favorable outcomes were experienced in 97% of those who achieved a linezolid AUC/MIC ratio of greater than 95 compared with 75% of those who had lower AUC/MIC ratios [211]. Administration of continuous linezolid infusions, such that drug concentrations are maintained above the MIC for entire dosing interval, has been associated with bacteriocidal activity [212,213]. For adults with MRSA infections, there appears to be no significant difference in clinical cure or microbiologic cure between linezolid and vancomycin [214]. However, linezolid was superior to vancomycin in one adult comparator trial of complicated skin and soft tissue infections [215].

Linezolid clinical trials have been performed in hospitalized young infants and children with documented gram-positive infections [195,206,216]. Linezolid was well tolerated at a dosage of 10 mg/kg every 8 hours and as effective as vancomycin for treatment of resistant gram-positive infections. Infants require dosing every 8 hours to maintain AUCs similar to those achieved in adolescents and adults dosed every 12 hours [1,196]. An AUC of 100 would achieve AUC/MIC ratios of 50 if the MIC of organism was 2, as would be expected for most enterococcal or streptococcal infections. Higher doses may be needed to achieve this AUC/MIC target in infants with faster drug clearance or infants with MRSA infections where the MIC may be between 2 to 4 µg/mL; PD targets have not been confirmed in clinical trials. In the first few days of life, infants may accumulate linezolid as clearance is rapidly changing. For extremely preterm infants younger than 7 days of chronologic age, we would consider a dose of 10 mg/kg every 12 hours [153,195]. The risk of drug accumulation is balanced with the need to rapidly achieve and maintain adequate plasma and tissue concentrations of drug during a developmental period of rapidly improving clearance. The potential for linezolid resistance has been documented; further emergence and spread of such resistance may depend on its prudent use.

Clindamycin (See Table 37–6)
Antimicrobial Activity

Clindamycin replaced its parent compound lincomycin because it is more completely absorbed from the gut, has fewer adverse effects, and has greater antibacterial activity in vitro [1,217,218]. Clindamycin is primarily a bacteriostatic agent that acts by inhibiting protein synthesis through reversible binding to bacterial ribosomes, thus inhibiting bacterial protein synthesis. Clindamycin is active against gram-positive cocci such as *S. aureus*, *S. pneumoniae* (including many multidrug-resistant strains), and *Streptococcus pyogenes*. It also maintains notable activity against anaerobic bacteria, especially members of the *Bacteroides* group. Aerobic gram-negative bacteria are not usually susceptible to this antibiotic. Resistance to clindamycin appears to be related to alterations of its target site and not to reduced uptake or to breakdown of the drug by the resistant bacteria.

Pharmacokinetic Data

Clindamycin pharmacology has been recently reviewed; however there is a paucity of information in neonates [1,217,218]. Clindamycin exhibits significant (94%) protein binding. The drug is eliminated primarily by the liver, with only about 10% excreted in unchanged form in the urine. Clindamycin is reported to be a cytochrome P-450 substrate that may increase the neuromuscular blocking action of tubocurarine and pancuronium. Clindamycin has been shown to accumulate in patients with hepatic dysfunction. It is widely distributed throughout the body including pleural fluid, ascites, bone, and bile. However, no significant levels (~20%) are seen in the CSF, even in setting of meningitis. Experimental meningitis animal models have demonstrated CSF penetration after parenteral administration [219]. In adults, clindamycin exhibits excellent bioavailability after oral administration.

When intravenous clindamycin was administered to infants in the first 4 weeks after birth, in a dosage schedule of 6.5 mg/kg every 8 hours (preterm) or 5 mg/kg every 6 hours (term), the mean peak serum concentrations was 10 µg/mL and trough values ranged from 2.8 to 5.5 µg/mL [220]. The serum elimination half-life was inversely related to gestational age and birth weight. Premature neonates demonstrated a mean serum half-life of 8.7 hours, compared with 3.6 hours for term newborns [220]. Another study of 12 neonates demonstrated a serum elimination half-life of 3.5 to 9.8 hours (mean, 6.3 hours) [221]. Neonates have longer elimination half-lives for clindamycin than the 3 hour half-life observed in infants 1 month to 1 year.

Safety

Adverse effects of clindamycin include diarrhea, rashes, elevated levels of hepatic enzymes, granulocytopenia, thrombocytopenia and, rarely, Stevens-Johnson syndrome. The most serious potential complication to consider is pseudomembranous colitis. Many asymptomatic neonates are colonized with *C. difficile*, the presumed etiologic agent of pseudomembranous colitis [222]. However, evidence for an association of *C. difficile* colonization with colitis in newborns is lacking and pseudomembranous colitis is rare in both newborns and young infants. This adverse effect also is observed with the use of ß-lactam and other antimicrobial agents.

PK-PD and Clinical Implications for Dosing
(See Tables 37–6, 37–11)

Recent clinical information suggests that clindamycin can be effectively used to treat MRSA infections [223–225]. Caution is advised, however, because resistance to clindamycin can be induced after selective antimicrobial pressure, particularly in MRSA organisms that initially are clindamycin-susceptible and erythromycin-resistant. Use of clindamycin in selected MRSA-infected newborn patients can obviate the need for vancomycin therapy. For treatment of the rare *B. fragilis* infections in newborns, especially those involving the central nervous system, metronidazole or clindamycin have been used. Clindamycin is said to have poor penetration into the CSF [226] albeit good penetration into brain tissue [227].

Considerable debate exists regarding the optimal dose of clindamycin. Antibacterial activity is concentration-independent and time-dependent with considerable post-antibiotic effect [185,228]. Clindamycin has antibacterial activity that appears to be maximized as drug concentrations approach 1 to 4 times the MIC and also has a considerable postantibiotic effect (4 to 6 hours) [229–231]. In the murine thigh infection model, clindamycin has been effective against clindamycin-susceptible (and noninducible) MRSA [232]. One proposed PK-PD target is to maintain the clindamycin concentration above the MIC for 50% of the dosing interval. Most staphylococcal species have a low MIC (<1 mg/L) for the drug. Much lower dosing than is currently used in adults was shown to achieve equivalent killing and maintain the clindamycin concentration above the MIC for 100% of the dosing interval [229]. Empirical dosing information based upon the limited PK information available is 5 mg/kg/dose administered every 12 hours in the first week of life and every 6 to 8 hours thereafter. Preterm infants may have decreased clindamycin clearance, therefore dosing interval is typically maintained at 8 to 12 hours for the first 2 to 4 weeks after birth. These doses are less than recommended in infants and young children (25 to 40 mg/kg/day divided every 6 to 8 hours). More neonatal PK data is needed, especially in extremely low birth weight infants with serious bacterial infections in the first 90 days after birth. Because clindamycin is highly protein bound, assays need to clearly quantify the molecularly active nonprotein bound exposure to clindamycin.

Rifampin

In selected neonates with persistent, systemic staphylococcal infections, rifampin has been used to provide a synergistic effect when given with other antistaphylococcal drugs [1,233–237]. Resistance rapidly emerges with rifampin monotherapy. In adults, rifampin is widely distributed throughout the body including the CSF [1,238–240]. Rifampin is 80% protein-bound and is eliminated in bile after progressive deacetylation to metabolites that remain microbiologically active. No dose adjustment is needed for renal insufficiency. Rifampin is bacteriocidal through the inhibition of bacterial-specific DNA-dependent RNA polymerase activity. It is active against most strains of *Neisseria meningitidis*, *Mycobacterium tuberculosis*, and aerobic gram-positive bacteria including MSSA, MRSA, and *S. epidermidis*. Safety concerns regarding rifampin are focused on thrombocytopenia, liver dysfunction and jaundice; liver function and blood count monitoring is recommended. Rifampin has been found to compete with bilirubin for biliary excretion and increased bilirubin has been observed. Rifampin is also known to induce cytochrome P-450 enzymes and therefore drug interactions are possible [241]. Rifampin has been shown to accelerate elimination of drugs that are used in the neonatal population, including phenytoin, azole antifungal agents, narcotic analgesics, diazepam, and corticosteroids.

Neonatal PK information for intravenous rifampin is sparse and dosing remains empiric [234,237,242,243]. In one small study, infants (mean age of 23 days) received rifampin 10 mg/kg/day and had a mean peak concentration of 4.02 µg/mL and a mean 12-hour trough concentration of 1.11 µg/mL [243]. In children, rifampin clearance is induced after 8 days of therapy. As rifampin clearance increases and half-life decreases, the dosing interval may need to be shortened to accommodate induced clearance in prolonged therapy [244]. Uncontrolled clinical case series suggest that rifampin used as an adjunct to vancomycin therapy can provide prompt clearance of persistent staphylococcal bacteremia or ventriculitis in high risk neonates [234,237,242,243].

Teicoplanin

Teicoplanin is a glycopeptide antibiotic that is almost identical to vancomycin with regard to its antibacterial spectrum of activity. It is used frequently in Europe where it is approved for the treatment of gram-positive infections [245,246]; however, it is not approved for use in the United States. Teicoplanin may have some advantages over vancomycin in terms of tolerability, with a lower propensity to cause nephrotoxicity and histaminic-type reactions. Teicoplanin also has a longer elimination half-life allowing for longer dosing intervals. It rapidly penetrates into tissue and reaches high concentrations in the kidney, trachea, lungs, and adrenals but does not penetrate well into the cerebrospinal fluid. It is excreted unchanged in the urine after a prolonged elimination phase.

Despite these potential advantages, teicoplanin PK data adequate to formulate dosage regimens in neonates are lacking. In one study, four neonates received a single dose of 6 mg/kg, and the mean peak serum teicoplanin concentration was 19.6 µg/mL, with a mean half-life of 30 hours [247]. In several noncomparative trials, the clinical and bacteriologic response rates ranged between 80% and 100% in 173 infected neonates given teicoplanin 8 to 10 mg/kg intravenously once daily, after a loading dose of 10 to 20 mg/kg [248]. A recent study of 37 episodes of staphylococcal bacteremia in neonates treated with a loading dose of 16 mg/kg teicoplanin followed by a maintenance dose of 8 mg/kg/day achieved bacterial eradication in 89% and survival of 94% with no documented drug-related adverse events [249]. One neonate was reported to have tolerated teicoplanin overdose (20 mg/kg/day for 5 days) [250].

Daptomycin

Daptomycin is the first-in-class of the cyclic lipopeptide family [251–254]. Lipopeptides have a unique mechanism of action. They insert into bacteria membranes and cause a rapid membrane depolarization leading to inhibition of protein, DNA and RNA synthesis, cell leakage, and ultimately cell death. Daptomycin exhibits rapid, concentration-dependent, bacteriocidal activity against MRSA, MRSE, vancomycin-resistant *S. aureus*, and VRE. The product is approved in the United States for the treatment of complicated skin and skin structure infections, and *S. aureus* bacteremia [232,251,255–258]. Daptomycin is not indicated for the treatment of pneumonia due to its inactivation by surfactant [259]. Daptomycin exhibits a high degree of protein binding, and is primarily excreted unchanged by the kidney. In clinical trials, a few adults receiving daptomycin had elevated creatine phosphokinase (CPK) enzyme and, rarely, myopathy [251,260]. The manufacturer recommends monitoring CPK weekly while on therapy and discontinuing therapy for myopathy, myalgia, or CPK greater than 1000 mg/dL [251].

Daptomycin is not approved for use in children or neonates. One single dose PK study in 25 children with suspected or proven gram-positive infections revealed more rapid clearance in younger children with adolescents [261]. Two infants with complicated MRSA infections who received 6 mg/kg dose every 12 hours had peak and trough concentrations that were consistent with concentrations observed in adults treated with a 4 mg/kg daily dose [262]. These infants achieved microbiologic and clinical cure; however, their exposure was less than that achieved in adults receiving daptomycin at the approved dose of 6 mg/kg/day for treatment of MRSA bacteremia.

AMINOGLYCOSIDES (See Table 37–7)

History

For more than 3 decades, the aminoglycosides have been relied upon for therapy for neonatal sepsis because of their broad-spectrum antibacterial activity against gram-negative bacilli. However, their use in some centers is decreasing because of the emergence of resistant strains. Currently, gentamicin, tobramycin, and amikacin are the aminoglycosides of choice in most nurseries. Because amikacin is resistant to degradation by most of the plasmid-mediated bacterial enzymes that inactivate gentamicin and tobramycin, some centers have held amikacin in reserve for treatment of nosocomially acquired infections due to multidrug-resistant gram-negative organisms. Gentamicin resistance occurs frequently enough in some European, Latin American, and U.S. centers to warrant use of amikacin as a first-line drug for therapy of life-threatening gram-negative infections. Thus far, its routine use has not resulted in emergence of resistant strains.

The history of aminoglycoside usage in the late 1950s and 1960s is an excellent example of the inherent problems of adapting dosages derived from studies in adults to newborns. Irreversible ototoxicity in neonates was caused by excessive doses of streptomycin or kanamycin. By contrast, the PK of gentamicin, tobramycin, amikacin, and netilmicin were carefully defined in the neonate before routine use of these drugs; appropriate studies thus provided a scientific basis for safe and effective dosage regimens. The risk of aminoglycoside toxicity is minimal when these agents are administered to infants in the proper dosage and when serum concentrations are closely monitored and kept within the recommended therapeutic range.

The evolution of gentamicin dosing over recent years is also an excellent example of dosing modifications that target PD to achieve optimal therapeutic exposure. Aminoglycoside administration using extended dosing intervals appears to be at least as safe and effective as giving these drugs in two or three divided doses. The extended dosing interval schedule provides a higher peak concentration to maximize the concentration-dependent bacterial killing and take advantage of the prolonged postantibiotic effect (PAE) of the aminoglycosides [263–265].

Antimicrobial Activity

Aminoglycosides act on microbial ribosomes to irreversibly inhibit protein synthesis. In general, gentamicin, tobramycin, and amikacin have good antibacterial activity against most gram-negative strains isolated in many hospitals worldwide. Tobramycin has the greatest antipseudomonal activity [266], while amikacin is the only drug of this class that reliably provides activity against *Serratia* species and other coliforms with nosocomially-acquired resistance. Although staphylococci are susceptible in vitro to aminoglycosides, infections caused by these pathogens usually do not respond satisfactorily to aminoglycoside therapy alone. Synergistic bactericidal activity between aminoglycosides and the penicillins has been demonstrated in vitro and in animals against *S. aureus* [267], group B streptococci [268,269], *L. monocytogenes* [151], and enterococci [152], in spite of low-level resistance of each microorganism to the aminoglycoside alone.

Possible mechanisms of bacterial resistance to these drugs include alteration of the ribosomal binding site, changes in the cell surface proteins to prevent entrance of drug into the cell, and induction of aminoglycoside-inactivating enzymes. Antibiotic resistance in clinical situations is most often a result of extrachromosomally controlled (R-factor) enzymes. Phosphorylation, adenylation, and acetylation are the three most common enzymatic mechanisms encountered [270–272]. High concentrations of aminoglycosides may reduce the emergence of resistance by targeting resistant subpopulations.

Some gram-negative organisms, notably *Pseudomonas aeruginosa* and *Enterobacter* species, demonstrate reduced uptake of aminoglycosides after initial exposure [273,274]. Such reduced uptake can decrease bacterial killing and is referred to as adaptive resistance; it may last for several hours after initial antibiotic exposure but appears to be reversible after a duration of low plasma aminoglycoside concentrations [275].

Pharmacokinetic Data (See Table 37–7)

Gentamicin

Gentamicin is the most methodically studied aminoglycoside in newborns; however, there is considerable interpatient variability in gentamicin concentrations achieved in neonates. This variability is typically due to changes in renal function and body water composition with

TABLE 37-7 Aminoglycosides and Aztreonam for the Treatment of Gram-negative Infections

Drug	Route of Elimination	Peak µg/mL	Half-life (hours)	PK:PD Target	Protein Binding %0	CSF%‡	CLSI MIC§ E. coli, Klebsiella	CLSI MIC§ P. aeruginosa	Safety and Clinical Pearls
Gentamicin 2.5 mg/kg q12 4 mg/kg q24 5 mg/kg q24	Renal	6 7–8 9–12	PNA <7 days 8–11 (<2000 g) 5 (>2000 g) 3–4 (PNA >7 days)	Peak/MIC >8–10 TDM Goal Peak 6–12 Trough <2	0%–30%	5%	≤4	≤4	FOR AMINOGLYCOSIDES Daily dosing a strong option, but "daily" may require dosing every 36 or 48 hours TDM especially if PNA <7 days and treatment >48 hr Follow urine output, creatinine Consider hearing screen
Amikacin 7.5 mg/kg q12 15 mg/kg q24	Renal	15 25	PNA <7 days 6–8 (<2000 g) 5–6 (>2000 g) 5 (PNA >7 days)	Peak/MIC Peak 20–30 Trough <5	0%–10%	20%–34%	≤16	≤16	
Tobramycin 2 mg/kg	Renal	4–6	PNA <7 days 9–17 (<1500 g) 8–9 (<2500 g) 3–4.5 (>2500 g)	Peak/MIC Peak 6–12 Trough <2	0%–10%	0	≤4	≤4	
Aztreonam 30 mg/kg 50 mg/kg	Renal	75* 100 200	5–7 hr (preterm)* 2.5 hr (term) 1.7 hr >28 days	Peak/MIC	56%	17%–33%	≤8	≤8	Measure glucose 1 hr after dose Rare AE: rash, diarrhea Monitor CBC, LFT

Data from references 32, 389, 438, 439, 683.
Preterm, <7 days of age, lower concentrations and longer half-life.
‡*Proportion of product found in CSF relative to serum.*
§*Higher dosing for meningitis or infections due to P. aeruginosa.*
TDM, therapeutic drug monitoring; CBC, complete blood count; LFT, liver function tests.

advancing gestational age, chronologic age, and creatinine clearance [276–292].

Gentamicin is administered via intramuscular or intravenous injection. Early PK studies of gentamicin demonstrated that the serum concentration-time curves after an intramuscular injection and after a 20-minute intravenous infusion were nearly superimposable [276,293]. Aminoglycosides such as gentamicin cannot be administered orally for treatment of systemic infection because they are not absorbed from the intact gastrointestinal tract [294].

Analysis of peak and trough concentrations reveal significant interpatient variability within and between studies. Recent clinical trials have compared gentamicin concentrations using traditional and extended-interval dosing regimens in primarily term and near-term neonates in the first week after birth: traditional 2.5 mg/kg dosing is associated with mean peak concentrations of 6.5 µg/mL and 12-hour trough concentration near 2 µg/mL [295–297]; extended interval regimens of 4, 5, or 8 mg/kg dosing yields peak concentrations of 8, 10, and 11 µg/mL, respectively, and 24-hour trough concentrations near 1 µg/mL for the 4 to 5 mg/kg regimen and "next day" trough values of 0.3 to 6.2 µg/mL for the 8 mg/kg regimen [295–299,300].

Neonates have reduced gentamicin clearance and increased volume of distribution compared with older patients. Neonatal population PK studies of gentamicin have attempted to explain the variability of gentamicin disposition with demographic and clinical variables [301–305]. Volume of distribution is consistently associated with infant weight and ranges from 0.45 to 0.69 L/kg. The mean relative clearance is between 0.04 to 0.06 (L/h)/kg typically depending on how many premature infants were included in the model and their chronologic age. Clearance improves with advancing gestational age, chronologic age, postmenstrual age, and creatinine clearance as expected for improved renal maturation [305]. Extended dosing intervals are often warranted in extremely premature infants and those with elevated creatinine or decreased urine output. In a traditional dosing regimen (2.5 mg/kg/dose), preterm infants often required 18 to 24 hour dosing intervals to achieve trough concentrations less than 2 µg/mL [281,287,306–309].

The serum half-life of gentamicin is longer in younger, smaller, more immature infants and those with reduced creatinine clearance [276,278,280,281,285,286]. During the first week of life, very low birth weight (800 to 1500 g) infants have long gentamicin half-lives, up to 14 hours, compared with 4.5 hours in term infants. More recent studies have reported elimination half lives of 8 to 9 hours in the first week after birth, and 5 hours in 12- to 24-day-old infants [303,304]. Both perinatal asphyxia and patent ductus arteriosus (or its treatment) are associated with prolonged serum gentamicin half-life likely due to decreased renal clearance [291,310].

CSF concentrations of gentamicin in infants with meningitis are from 0.3 to 3.7 µg/mL (mean, 1.6 µg/mL) 1 to 6 hours after a 2.5-mg/kg dose [141]. Peak values are observed 4 to 6 hours after the dose and are correlated with the degree of meningeal inflammation and dosage. During the 1970s, the Neonatal Meningitis Cooperative Study Group evaluated lumbar intrathecal and intraventricular gentamicin administration in comparative studies with systemic antibiotic therapy alone [141]. Despite higher CSF and intraventricular fluid concentrations, neither route of administration of therapy was associated with a better outcome in infants with meningitis caused by gram-negative enteric organisms. In fact, case-fatality rates were significantly greater in intraventricular gentamicin recipients. Poor outcomes may in part be explained by the rapid lysis of gram-negative bacteria associated with high ventricular fluid gentamicin concentrations, the subsequent release of significantly larger amounts of endotoxin into the ventricular fluid, and greater meningeal inflammation [311].

Serum concentrations are altered by exchange transfusion and ECMO; after a two volume exchange transfusion, serum aminoglycoside concentrations are reduced by 19% to 62% [312,313]. Whenever possible, such procedures are best timed to precede the next scheduled dose of gentamicin. Therapeutic drug monitoring is needed to guide dosing for infants on ECMO because gentamicin, and probably other aminoglycosides, exhibit a higher volume of distribution, a lower clearance, and a longer half-life [314].

Tobramycin

Tobramycin (see Table 37–7) offers two theoretical advantages over gentamicin for therapy for neonatal infections: increased in vitro activity against *P. aeruginosa* and decreased nephrotoxicity [315]. The lower incidence of nephrotoxicity for tobramycin has been documented in laboratory animals and human adults but not in neonates [316]. Because of the relative resistance of neonates to aminoglycoside nephrotoxicity, the applicability of such advantages in young infants is uncertain.

After a 2 mg/kg dose of tobramycin, mean peak serum concentrations of 4 to 6 µg/mL are observed at 30 to 60 minutes [317]. When an identical dose is given to low birth weight neonates, mean peak serum values are 8 µg/mL. Predose trough concentrations are higher in smaller and more premature infants; trough concentrations are often greater than 2 µg/mL in premature neonates receiving 2.5 mg/kg doses every 12 hours [318–320]. The serum tobramycin half-life is also prolonged in smaller, younger, and more premature infants and in those infants with delayed creatinine clearance [317,318,320]. In the first week after birth, very low birth weight infants (<1500 g) have half-life values as long as 9 to 17 hours, compared with values of 3 to 4.5 hours for larger infants (>2500 g) and older infants who are 1 to 4 weeks old. Premature infants born at less than 30 weeks of gestation, often require dosage intervals of 18 to 24 hours [318,320,321]. Therapeutic drug monitoring and individualization of the dosage schedule are often needed to provide the optimal therapy for very low birth weight infants.

Amikacin

Neonatal amikacin (see Table 37–7) PK data are limited. Mean peak serum concentrations of 15 to 20 µg/mL occur 30 minutes to 1 hour after 7.5-mg/kg doses of amikacin. Mean trough concentrations of 3 to 6 µg/mL are detected 12 hours after administration [322,323]. Doses of 10 mg/kg at 12-hour intervals were required to achieve a mean peak value of 21.5 μg/mL and a trough concentration of 3.3 μg/mL. By contrast, investigators in another study [324] noted that subtherapeutic serum concentrations of amikacin given to premature infants in 7.5 mg/kg intravenous doses every 12 hours were present in only 10% of infants younger than 2 weeks of age. As many as 38% of infants 29 days of age or older had peak serum concentrations below 15 μg/mL.

Serum half-life of amikacin is longer in younger and more premature infants [322,323]. Half-life values of 7 to 8 hours occur in low birth weight infants 1 to 3 days of age, and half-life values of 4 to 5 hours in term infants who are older than 1 week of age. The serum half-life is prolonged in hypoxemic newborns [28]. More recently, neonatal population PK studies of amikacin have explored the wide variability of disposition. In a study of one day old, preterm and term infants (24 to 41 weeks), amikacin clearance increased with gestational age and volume of distribution increased with body weight [325]. In more mature infants (mean GA 35 weeks) treated with amikacin in the first week of life, clearance and volume of distribution varied with weight [326].

Reports of CSF concentrations of amikacin are scarce [327–330]. In the presence of uninflamed meninges in 1-day-old infants, CSF values ranged from 0.2 to 2.7 μg/mL when measured at 1 to 4 hours after a single 10-mg/kg dose administered by slow intravenous infusion [328]. Simultaneous concentrations in serum ranged from 15 to 29 μg/mL. The highest CSF concentration reported has been 9.2 μg/mL after a 7.5 mg/kg dose was administered intramuscularly to an infant with meningitis [322]. Amikacin concentration in ventricular fluid 12 hours after 1 or 2 mg intraventricular doses and 2 to 8 hours after intramuscular doses varies, ranging from 4.5 to 11.6 μg/mL (mean, 7.3 μg/mL). In the largest and most recent study of 43 preterm and term infants (mean postmenstrual age 36 weeks, range, 26 to 41 weeks) the median amikacin CSF concentration was 1.09 μg/mL (range, 0.34 to 2.65 μg/mL) and the mean peak and trough serum concentration were 35.7 μg/mL and 3.8 μg/mL, respectively [327]. Concentrations in CSF were low likely because the CSF sampling occurred at a median of 25 hour after amikacin administration; no correlation between CSF white blood cell count and CSF amikacin levels was identified.

Safety

The major adverse effects of aminoglycoside antibiotics are renal toxicity, ototoxicity, and, rarely, neuromuscular blockade [331–334]. Aminoglycosides are eliminated through glomerular filtration, but some drug is reabsorbed in the proximal tubule. Aminoglycosides may accumulate in renal tubular cells where they fuse with cytoplasmic lysosomes and inhibit phospholipases, with the resultant accumulation of phospholipid aggregates and release of lysosomal contents within the renal tubular cells. The potential for nephrotoxicity varies among the aminoglycosides because of differences in the rate of uptake and amount of drug accumulation in the renal cortex. This renal cortical uptake is saturable in rats [335]. Human nephrectomy studies have

also demonstrated saturable uptake: higher renal cortical aminoglycoside (amikacin, gentamicin but not tobramycin) concentrations when doses were administered by continuous infusion or twice daily compared with once daily [336,337]. Toxicity is correlated with elevated drug trough concentrations and prolonged therapy, but not with high peak concentrations. Extended aminoglycoside dosing intervals produce longer periods at low drug concentration, thereby lessening the potential for renal drug accumulation and toxicity.

Meta-analysis of adult trials of extended interval aminoglycoside administration compared with conventional multidose daily administration showed that the rate of nephrotoxicity with extended interval dosing was less than or equal to that observed with traditional regimens [338–344]. In addition to drug dose and administration regimen, the risk factors for nephrotoxicity also include the concomitant medications and the patient's clinical condition.

The reported incidence of aminoglycoside nephrotoxicity ranges from 5% to 25% and is thought to be lower in children than adults [334]. It has been suggested that the immature kidney of the neonate may be protected from major toxic effects of aminoglycosides. Transient cylindruria and proteinuria may occur after prolonged administration of any of these drugs, but significant elevations in blood urea nitrogen and creatinine values are rarely observed [345–352]. In neonatal comparative trials of once-daily extended-interval dosing compared with multi-dose standard dosing of aminoglycosides, nephrotoxicity was rare and there was no significant difference noted between the two dosing administration groups [339]. Because renal excretion accounts for the elimination of approximately 80% of an aminoglycoside dose, the risk of toxicity is greatest when drug elimination is impaired by reduction in renal function for any reason. Therapeutic drug monitoring is often helpful in neonates. The criteria of maintaining peak and trough serum aminoglycoside concentrations within recommended values for older children and adults to prevent nephrotoxicity [353] have not been systematically assessed in newborns and should be considered as a guide rather than an established rule for formulating dosages of aminoglycosides in this age group. Factors that may be associated with increased risk for aminoglycoside nephrotoxicity include acidosis, hypovolemia, hypoalbuminemia, sodium depletion, duration of therapy, increased total aminoglycoside dose, and frequency of administration and co-administration of furosemide, vancomycin, or prostaglandin synthesis inhibitors such as indomethacin [348,350,354,355].

Neomycin [356,357], streptomycin [358], kanamycin [359], and gentamicin [141] each have been implicated as a cause of sensorineural hearing loss in infants and children. Gentamicin and streptomycin also have been associated with vestibular impairment. However, it is difficult to incriminate the aminoglycosides as the single causative agent of hearing loss in most studies because of the high-risk conditions present in affected patients such as asphyxia, hyperbilirubinemia, and incubator/ventilator noise exposure that have been independently associated with ototoxicity [360]. Although animal studies have demonstrated a synergistic effect of noise combined with neomycin or kanamycin administration on development of ototoxicity, such an effect has not been substantiated in the human neonate exposed to both incubator noise and kanamycin [360,361].

In a prospective evaluation of long-term toxicity of kanamycin and gentamicin, neither was incriminated as the sole agent responsible for hearing impairment [362]. Ototoxicity has been related primarily to very high total aminoglycoside dosages: high-frequency sensorineural hearing loss in infants with normal renal function is more likely if the total dosage exceeds 500 mg/kg [362]. Data from the first Neonatal Meningitis Cooperative Study [141] indicated that profound deafness potentially related to gentamicin exposure developed in only 1 (1.3%) of 79 infants who received a minimum of 5 to 7.5 mg/kg/day of the drug for 3 weeks or longer. Auditory toxicity was reported in only three infants in the four studies that have evaluated once daily gentamicin compared with standard interval dose regimen [339]. Vestibular toxicity is difficult to assess in neonates and has not been evaluated. The precise mechanism involved in ototoxicity is unknown. Some evidence suggests that point mutations in mitochondrial DNA are relevant to explain hearing loss in selected persons following aminoglycoside treatment [298]. Even for the rare hospitalized infant with ototoxicity after receiving concurrent dosages of aminoglycosides, it is difficult to establish a direct causal relationship in many of the published studies because of their complicated clinical histories.

In recent years, the introduction of brainstem response audiometry has facilitated assessment of hearing during the neonate's hospital stay [363]. A blinded study of auditory brainstem responses in neonates who received amikacin or netilmicin showed a high incidence of transient abnormalities, but permanent bilateral sensorineural hearing loss occurred in 2% of infants in each of the amikacin, netilmicin, and control group [364]. In another study, significant delayed auditory brainstem responses were detected in 14 control infants and 15 neonates who received a daily dose of 5 to 7.5 mg/kg for 6 to 10 days of either gentamicin or tobramycin [365]. Long-term follow-up of these infants was not performed to document whether the abnormalities were transient or permanent. Other investigators failed to demonstrate permanent vestibular damage in 37 children aged 2 to 4 years who received netilmicin during the neonatal period [366].

Aminoglycoside-associated neuromuscular blockade has been reported only rarely [367–369]. The underlying mechanism appears to be inhibition of acetylcholine release at the neuromuscular junction by these drugs [370]. The aminoglycoside may act alone or synergistically with other neuromuscular blocking agents. Hypermagnesemia in newborns, often due to antenatal exposure to maternal magnesium administered for preeclampsia, may potentiate the neuromuscular blocking effects of aminoglycosides. Diagnosis is made by nerve conduction studies, which reveal a progressive fatigue and posttetanic facilitation characteristic of a nondepolarizing, curare-like neuromuscular block. Reversal of this block is achieved by neostigmine or calcium or both. Potentiation of neuromuscular blockade can be observed in infant botulism when aminoglycosides are administered

to treat suspected sepsis [371]. Prophylactic treatment with calcium is not indicated because this cation may interfere with the antimicrobial activity of aminoglycosides against certain organisms. Newborns who require early surgical intervention and have large fluctuations in fluid volume and renal function are likely at the highest risk for this rare adverse event.

PK-PD and Clinical Implications for Dosing
(Table 37–8; see Tables 37–7, 37–11)

Aminoglycosides still remain effective for the initial empirical therapy in newborns with suspected gram-negative sepsis. The choice of the aminoglycoside to be routinely used is mainly dependent on the patterns of microbial resistance within a nursery. Amikacin remains one option for empirical treatment when multiply-resistant coliforms are frequently isolated within an individual neonatal unit. The aminoglycosides are usually safe to use in the newborn when administered according to the recommended dosage and with careful monitoring, particularly in premature infants of very low birth weight or infants with hypoxemia, renal dysfunction, or anesthetic effects. Therapeutic drug monitoring is needed to guide dosing in infants on ECMO.

Systemic aminoglycoside therapy remains an acceptable initial empirical treatment choice when meningitis is present because in combination with ampicillin, this agent offers potential synergistic activity against group B streptococci and *L. monocytogenes*. Aminoglycosides have been demonstrated to be effective for therapy for meningitis caused by susceptible gram-negative bacteria. However, if gram-negative bacilli are seen on CSF smears or later isolated as the causative agent of meningitis, third-generation cephalosporins or carbapenems should be considered. Combined therapy with a cephalosporins and an aminoglycoside is often used for the first 7 to 10 days of therapy for possible synergistic bacterial killing, and to prevent emergence of bacterial resistance during the treatment, especially for meningitis caused by *Serratia*, *Pseudomonas*, *Acinetobacter*, *Citrobacter*, and *Enterobacter* species.

Aminoglycosides demonstrate concentration-dependent bactericidal activity (see Table 37–7) [37]. In vitro time-kill curves and animal studies both demonstrate the increased rate and extent of killing with increasing concentration of aminoglycosides [372]. Early studies in gram-negative infections showed clinical response was associated with peak serum concentrations of greater than 7 μg/mL for gentamicin and tobramycin and 28 μg/mL for amikacin [373,374]. Subsequently, adult studies demonstrated effective response to therapy near 90% for a ratio of more than 8:1 for *E. coli* bacteremia [375] or 10:1 for gram-negative pneumonia [376]. The PD of aminoglycosides in the treatment of gram-negative infections has not been evaluated in infants.

In addition to therapeutic killing, high concentrations of aminoglycosides also provide a postantibiotic effect (PAE) (i.e., the sustained suppression of bacterial growth even after the antibiotic concentration is below the MIC of the target organism) [231]. In vitro, aminoglycosides demonstrate a PAE of 1 to 3 hours against *P. aeruginosa*

TABLE 37-8 Serum Peak and Trough Concentrations of Gentamicin in Preterm and Term Neonates*

Study	GA (wk)	N	ODD Regimen Daily Dose (mg/kg)	Peak (µg/mL)	Trough (µg/mL)	N	SDD Regimen Daily Dose (mg/kg)†	Peak (µg/mL)	Trough (µg/mL)	Reference
Gentamicin										
Skopnik et al	≥38	10	4	10.9	0.8 ± 0.2	10	4	7.4	1.0 ± 0.4	[298]
Hayani et al	≥34	11	5	10.7 ± 2.1	1.7 ± 0.4	15	5	6.6 ± 1.3	1.7 ± 0.5	[295]
De Alba-Romero	≥38	13	5	9.2 ± 1.5	1.1 ± 0.4	15	5	5.7 ± 1.3	1.5 ± 0.6	[296]
De Alba-Romero	29–37	20	5	9.7 ±1.8	1.6 ± 0.8	17	5	7.1 ± 1.7	2.7 ± 0.9	[296]
Skopnik‡	32–38	28	4	7.9 ± 1.6	1.0 ± 0.5	27	5	6.1 ± 1.1	2.0 ± 1.1	[684]
Miron	32–37	17	5	9.9 ± 4.6	1.5 ± 0.5	18	5	5.9 ± 1.7	2.4 ± 0.9	[685]
Agrawal	≥2500 g	20	4	8.2 ± 1.7	0.9 ± 0.4	21	5	6.2 ± 1.5	1.9 ± 0.5	[380]
Chotigeat	≥34	27	4–5	8.9 ± 1.6	0.9 ± 0.4	27	4–5	5.9 ± 1.6	1.4 ± 0.5	[686]
Kosalaraksa	≥2000 g	33	5	10.1 ± 3.0	1.6 ± 1.1	31	5	7.8 ± 2.0	2.6 ± 1.2	[687]
Krishnan	32–36	9	4	5.9 ± 1.1	1.96 ± 0.6	9	5	3.9 ± 0.8	2.8 ± 0.7	[688]
Solomon	32–36	13	4	7.4 ± 2.3	1.8 ± 0.9	12	5	6.7 ± 2.4	2.0 ± 1.1	[689]
Solomon	≥37	24	4	7.1 ± 2.6	1.3 ± 1.0	24	5	7.0 ± 2.8	1.5 ± 1.0	[689]
Thureen	≥34	27	4	7.9 ± 0.2	1.0 ± 0.5	28	5	6.7 ± 0.3	2.1 ± 1.1	[297]
Amikacin										
Langhendries	>34	10	15	23.6 ± 3.3	2.7 ± 1.2	12	15	13.6 ± 3.3	3.5 ± 1.4	[383]
Kotze	≥38	20	15	30.6 ± 2.8	1.7 ± 0.8	20	15	18.5 ± 4.0	3.5 ± 2.4	[384]

*Neonates who received SDD or ODD dosing in several randomized comparison trials included in Cochrane review [339].
†Twice daily.
‡Not included in Cochrane review.
GA, gestational age; ODD, once-daily dosing; SDD, standard daily dosing.

and 1 to 2 hours against Enterobacteriaceae [377]. Animal models suggest an even longer period of PAE, 2 to 7.5 hours [377,378]. The PAE is prolonged by increasing aminoglycoside concentration and in the presence of neutrophils [379]. PAE has not been demonstrated in clinical trials given ethical restraints of such studies. The duration of PAE is unknown in neonates but given the immature immunity of neonates, it may be less than calculated in animal models.

Ideally, dosing regimens for aminoglycosides would attempt to maximize killing, take advantage of the PAE, minimize adaptive resistance, reduce emergence of resistance, and diminish the potential for toxicity. Therapeutic drug monitoring is used to individualize dosage regimens. Peak serum concentrations should be maintained at 8 to 12 µg/mL for gentamicin and tobramycin, and at 20 to 30 µg/mL for amikacin to achieve the PD target (i.e., a peak (Cmax)/MIC ratio of >8 to 10). To potentially minimize the rare risk of toxicity, trough values are typically kept less than 2 µg/mL for the former drugs and less than 5 µg/mL for amikacin. To determine peak serum concentrations, blood samples are obtained 30 minutes after completion of the intravenous infusion or 45 to 60 minutes after an intramuscular administration. Trough serum concentrations are measured just before the next dose of the aminoglycoside.

In traditional or "standard" neonatal dosing regimens, gentamicin is administered at a dose of 2.5 mg/kg typically every 12 hours, with extended dosing intervals (18 to 24 hours) in preterm infants. The amikacin dosage is a 7.5 mg/kg dose to be used for infants weighing less than 2000 g and a 10 mg/kg dose for all other infants. For amikacin, a 12-hour dosing interval is recommended in the first week of life and an 8-hour interval used thereafter. Therapeutic drug monitoring is often used to individualize dosage schedules for infants weighing less than 1500 g at birth or born at less than 30 weeks of gestation.

Use of Extended Dosing Intervals to Achieve PD Exposure Targets (Tables 37–8, 37–11)

The rationale for use of extended dosing intervals is based on several PK, pharmacodynamic, and microbiologic principles of aminoglycosides [263–265,339]: (1) Aminoglycosides exhibit concentration-dependent bacterial killing in which higher peak/MIC ratios are associated with improved bactericidal response; C_{max}/MIC ratios greater than 10 have been linked to superior efficacy of aminoglycosides against gram-negative bacteria, including *Pseudomonas*. (2) Aminoglycosides exhibit a postantibiotic effect (PAE) in which bacterial growth is suppressed despite serum concentrations below the MIC; drug concentrations, therefore, can remain below the pathogen's MIC for a period without compromising efficacy. (3) Nephrotoxicity is associated with aminoglycoside uptake into renal cells and possibly into the cochlea and vestibular membrane, but cellular uptake is more efficient with low sustained concentrations and (in animals) uptake is a saturable process so that transient high peak levels do not lead to excessive drug accumulation. (4) Gram-negative bacteria have been shown to exhibit adaptive resistance after continuous exposure to aminoglycosides, a property that may be minimized by providing high bacteriocidal exposures minimizing time for bacterial growth in presence of antibiotic. (5) The lower glomerular filtration rate in neonates, especially the first few days of life and in preterm infants, suggest that more time for clearance may be needed to prevent toxic accumulation of aminoglycosides, and (6) once daily dosing is associated with less hospital cost. Although increased peak concentrations lengthen the duration of PAE, no research has been conducted in neonates to define the pharmacodynamics of this phenomenon in this age group.

Considerable evidence generated in adults with extended dosing intervals of aminoglycoside administration prompted studies in the pediatric and neonatal populations. Several comparison trials have been conducted in neonates to evaluate peak and trough gentamicin or amikacin concentrations after administration of "standard dosing" and "once-daily dosing" regimens (see Table 37–8) [296,380–384]. Mean peak concentrations in each study were higher in the once-daily regimen (5.9 to 10.7 µg/mL) than in the twice-daily group (3.9 to 7.4 µg/mL); and mean trough concentrations were lower in the daily group (0.8 to 1.9 µg/mL) than in the standard (1.0 to 2.8 µg/mL). Dose adjustment was indicated more often in the standard dosing groups. One study compared 2.5 to 3 mg/kg dosing every 24 hours and 4.5 to 5 mg/kg dosing every 48 hours in 58 very low birth weight infants (600 to 1500 g) [381]. The 48-hour dosing schedule achieved therapeutic serum concentrations and higher peak/MIC ratios for infecting microorganisms. Nearly one third of these infants, however, had extremely low serum gentamicin concentrations before the next dose, suggesting that a 36-hour interval might be more appropriate for very low birth weight infants. Another study evaluated single doses of 5 mg/kg of tobramycin and gentamicin administered at extended intervals and found that only 1.3% of these infants had subtherapeutic concentrations, compared with 26.8% of those given the traditional 2.5 mg/kg doses [382].

Once daily interval dosing was also explored for amikacin (see Table 37–8) [383–385]. In term infants, 15 mg/kg daily amikacin therapy in the first 3 days of life leads to significantly increased peak levels. Both regimens yield trough levels less than 5 µg/mL. Langhendries and colleagues then extended their study to include preterm infants, which received 15.5 to 20 mg/kg at a dosage interval of 24 to 42 hours depending on gestational age group. Dosage interval was also extended by 6 hours for infants with a history of hypoxia or who were receiving concurrent indomethacin therapy. In these preterm infants receiving extended interval amikacin dosing, the mean peak level was 27.8 µg/mL and mean trough level was 3.7 µg/mL. Amikacin-associated nephrotoxicity was not observed and results of BAERs evaluation were similar in study participants and nonstudy controls. No ototoxicity was reported in either study.

More recently, the Cochrane Collaboration performed a review of "standard multiple-doses a day" and "once-daily"

dosing regimens of gentamicin for the treatment of suspected or proven sepsis in neonates in 11 trials and a total of 574 neonates [339]. All 36 infants with proven sepsis, regardless of treatment regimen, showed adequate clearance of sepsis. Once-daily dosing of gentamicin was superior in its ability to achieve a peak level of at least 5 µg/mL and a trough level less than 2 µg/mL. Ototoxicity and nephrotoxicity were not noted with either treatment regimen. They conclude that based on PK properties and PD targets, the once a day regimen may be superior in treating sepsis in neonates more than 32 weeks gestation. Based on these data and on proposed dosing guidelines to date, therapeutic recommendations for once daily or extended interval aminoglycosides are presented in Table 37–11.

Aztreonam

Aztreonam is the first synthetic monocyclic β-lactam (monobactam) antibiotic approved for use in clinical medicine. Its aminoglycoside-like activity, good CSF penetration, and absence of nephrotoxic or ototoxic side effects make aztreonam potentially useful when combined with ampicillin for initial empirical therapy in newborns with severe, suspected sepsis.

Antimicrobial Activity

Aztreonam has good activity against a broad spectrum of aerobic gram-negative bacteria, but its activity against gram-positive or anaerobic organisms is poor [1,386,387]. Most E. coli, Klebsiella pneumoniae, and Citrobacter species are inhibited by less than 1 µg/mL of aztreonam. Serratia and Enterobacter are less susceptible (MIC_{90} of 1 to 4 µg/mL), whereas H. influenzae and N. gonorrhoeae are more susceptible (MIC_{90} of 0.2 µg/mL or less). Higher concentrations of aztreonam are needed to inhibit growth of P. aeruginosa (MIC 8 to 12 µg/mL) [386,388]. Like other β-lactams, aztreonam exerts its antimicrobial activity by interfering with bacterial cell wall synthesis by binding to PBPs, especially PBP-3 of aerobic gram-negative bacteria. This drug is stable to hydrolysis by chromosome- or plasmid-mediated β-lactamases of the Enterobacteriaceae and does not induce chromosomal β-lactamase production.

Pharmacokinetic Data

PK of intravenous aztreonam (20 to 30 mg/kg per dose of body weight) has been evaluated in a limited number of neonates [389]. Several small studies evaluated the pharmacokinetics following a 20 mg/kg per dose in neonates [390–396]. Serum concentrations and half-life decreased with chronologic age. The mean serum aztreonam concentration was 54 µg/mL in the first week of life and 45 µg/mL in infants 2 to 22 days of age. The half-life decreased from 3.5 to 6.6 hours in up to 3-day-old neonates, to 2.0 to 4.0 hours thereafter. Small premature infants weighing less than 1500 g have longer half-lives compared with larger preterm infants, 5.3 versus 4.1 hours, respectively [397]. A larger 30-mg/kg intravenous dose of aztreonam administered to infants weighing less than 2000 g during their first week of life resulted in peak serum concentrations from 65 to 79 µg/mL after the first dose and 77 to 83 µg/mL after 3 to 6 days of therapy [388]. Trough values were highly variable and ranged between

8.2 and 70.7 μg/mL. The half-life decreased from 7.6 to 5.5 hours after 3 to 6 doses. Older infants and young children have a shorter mean half-life of 1.7 hours [398].

Aztreonam has good penetration into the CSF of newborns with bacterial meningitis [399]. In a 7-day-old infant with newly diagnosed bacterial meningitis, a CSF concentration of 13.3 μg/mL was obtained 1.3 hours after an aztreonam dose, representing 18.8% of a simultaneously measured serum concentration. Pediatric patients with acute bacterial meningitis have concentrations of aztreonam in CSF that are 17% to 33% of serum values [400].

Safety

Aztreonam appears to be well tolerated with no apparent side effects when given intravenously to newborns in PK studies. Adverse reactions described in adults include rashes, nausea, diarrhea, and eosinophilia, but their incidence is low [1,386,387]. Aztreonam effects on bowel flora are limited to a reduction in coliforms without significant changes in anaerobic bacteria. Colonization by resistant bacteria resulting from aztreonam therapy does not appear to be as much of a problem as that encountered with the use of the third-generation cephalosporins. Because aztreonam contains 780 mg of arginine per gram of antibiotic, concern has been raised regarding possible arginine-induced hypoglycemia [401]. Arginine is rapidly metabolized and can be transformed to glucose leading to transient hyperglycemia. As a result of this transient hyperglycemia, insulin concentrations can immediately rise, with the subsequent induction of hypoglycemia. These fluctuations in blood glucose and subsequent variation in insulin concentration can be potentially important in premature infants exposed to a metabolic stress. A study addressing this safety issue indicated that aztreonam was well tolerated and safe in premature infants when a glucose solution was concomitantly infused (at a glucose infusion rate greater than 5 mg/kg per minute) [402].

PK-PD and Clinical Implications for Dosing

Aztreonam is still considered an investigational drug for neonates and infants younger than 3 months of age. Data from a prospective, randomized study of 58 neonates with infections caused by gram-negative bacilli, including *P. aeruginosa*, suggest that the use of aztreonam in combination with ampicillin is as effective as treatment with ampicillin and amikacin [401]. Individual aztreonam doses of 30 mg/kg given two to four times daily can achieve median peak serum bactericidal titers of about 1:16 and can maintain trough serum concentrations that exceed the MIC_{90} for most gram-negative bacteria.

CEPHALOSPORINS

Cephalosporins are semisynthetic derivatives of a 7-aminocephalosporanic acid nucleus [403,404]. The individual derivatives differ chemically by the addition of various side chains. The cephalosporins exert their antibacterial action in a manner similar to that described earlier for penicillin.

It has become customary to group cephalosporins into generations of agents on the basis of their antibacterial spectrum of activity. First-generation cephalosporins

include cefazolin, cephalothin, cephalexin, and cefadroxil. Second-generation agents include cefaclor, cefprozil, cefamandole, cefuroxime, and loracarbef; and third-generation agents include cefoperazone, cefotaxime, ceftizoxime, ceftriaxone, and ceftazidime. A fourth-generation, cephalosporin and cefepime, has recently undergone PK evaluation in neonates. Cefepime has been shown to be effective for therapy for meningitis in children and should be useful for treatment of multiresistant gram-negative bacillary infections in pediatric patients. In the following section, we have focused on the most well-studied cephalosporins in neonates.

Antimicrobial Activity

The *first-generation* cephalosporins such as cefazolin have good activity against gram-positive organisms but limited activity against gram-negative bacteria. Susceptible pathogens include streptococci, penicillin-susceptible and penicillin-resistant staphylococci, and penicillin-susceptible pneumococci. Although typically the activity against coliforms is good, other antibiotics are often preferred for treatment of infections caused by these organisms. *P. aeruginosa*, *Serratia marcescens*, *Enterococci*, MRSA, *L. monocytogenes*, *Enterobacter* species, indole-positive *Proteus* species, and *B. fragilis* all are resistant to these antibacterial agents [404].

Compared to first-generation cephalosporins, *second generation* agents have improved stability to hydrolysis by β-lactamases and therefore have increased activity against many gram-negative bacteria. Cefuroxime is more active than cephalothin against group B streptococci, pneumococci, and gram-negative enteric bacilli and also is active against *H. influenzae*, meningococci, gonococci, and staphylococci [405]. The second-generation agents have very poor activity against *P. aeruginosa*, enterococci, and *L. monocytogenes*.

The *third-generation* cephalosporins, such as cefotaxime and ceftazidime, have excellent in vitro activity against *H. influenzae*, gonococci, meningococci, and many gram-negative enteric bacilli. Ceftazidime and cefoperazone, however, are the only ones with adequate anti-*Pseudomonas* activity. *L. monocytogenes* and enterococci are uniformly resistant to these agents. Susceptibility of gram-positive organisms to these agents is variable but generally is lower than that to either first- or second- generation cephalosporins.

The *fourth-generation* cephalosporins demonstrate activity against gram-positive and gram-negative bacterial pathogens, including *P. aeruginosa*. Evidence also indicates that isolates of ceftazidime- and cefotaxime-resistant *Enterobacter* species are susceptible to cefepime [406]. Resistant organisms include enterococci, *L. monocytogenes*, MRSA, MRSE, and anaerobes.

Resistance to the cephalosporins develops through several mechanisms. Cephalothin and cefazolin can be inactivated by β-lactamases [407]. Exposure of some gram-negative bacteria, such as *P. aeruginosa* or *E. cloacae*, to second- or third-generation agents can induce the production of chromosomally mediated potent β-lactamases by these bacteria, which can hydrolyze even the β-lactamase-stable cephalosporins [407]. Several plasmid-mediated β-lactamases have been shown to play a role in the resistance of certain gram-negative enteric bacilli to third-generation cephalosporins [408]. Other mechanisms of resistance include alterations in the permeability of the outer membranes of gram-negative bacteria to these drugs that limit their ability to reach the PBP target sites. Mutations leading to functional or quantitative changes in PBPs constitute an additional means by which bacteria can resist the antimicrobial action of these drugs [407,408].

Pharmacokinetic Data

Cefazolin

The intramuscular administration of 25 mg/kg doses of cefazolin (Table 37–9) produces serum concentrations of 55 to 65 μg/mL, respectively, 1 hour after the dose. The concentrations at 12 hours drop to 13 to 18 μg/mL, respectively [409]. Intravenous doses of 25 mg/kg administered to six premature infants 2 to 12 days of age resulted in mean serum concentrations of 92, 79, 48, and 12 μg/mL at 0.5, 1, 4, and 12 hours, respectively, after the end of the infusion [410]. The drug is excreted in the urine in unchanged form [411]. The serum half-life of cefazolin decreases from 4.5 to 5 hours in the first week of life to approximately 3 hours by 3 to 4 weeks of age. CSF penetration of cefazolin is poor.

Cefuroxime

The intramuscular administration of 10 mg/kg doses of cefuroxime (see Table 37–9) produces serum concentrations that range between 15 and 25 μg/mL 30 to 60 minutes after the injection [412]. Intramuscular doses of 25 mg/kg given to neonates weighing less than 2.5 kg during their first week of life produce mean serum concentrations of 49, 30, and 15 μg/mL at 2, 4, and 8 hours after the injection, respectively [413]. For larger newborns, the corresponding values were lower (34, 21, and 9 μg/mL, respectively). In a study of preterm and term infants receiving cefuroxime 25 mg/kg every 12 hours, median steady state serum concentrations were 45, 26, and 11 μg/mL after 0.5, 5 and 12 hours respectively [414]. Repeated administration of the drug did not result in serum accumulation. About 70% of the daily cefuroxime dose could be recovered in urine in a 24-hour period. Half-life times have been reported to range from 2 to 11 hours (mean, 6 hours). CSF cefuroxime concentrations of 2.3 to 5.3 μg/mL were measured in three newborns with meningitis [412]. These values represented 12% to 25% of the corresponding serum concentrations. In three other neonates without meningeal inflammation, concentrations were lower and ranged from 0.4 to 1.5 μg/mL.

Cefotaxime

About 80% of the cefotaxime (see Table 37–9) dose is excreted in urine; however, only a third of the drug is eliminated in unchanged form [415]. Cefotaxime is rapidly metabolized in the body to desacetyl-cefotaxime through the action of esterases found in the liver, erythrocytes, and other tissues [415]. This metabolite is biologically active, but its antibacterial activity is generally lower than that of cefotaxime. Synergistic interactions against many organisms can be demonstrated when these two compounds are combined in vitro [416]. Desacetyl-cefotaxime accounts for 15% to 45% of the peak and 45% to 70% of the trough concentrations of total cefotaxime [417–419].

Several investigators have evaluated the PK properties of cefotaxime in newborns [417–422]. About 80% of the cefotaxime dose is excreted in urine; however, only a third of the drug is eliminated in unchanged form [415]. A 25 mg/kg intravenous dose produces concentrations of 60 to 80 μg/mL immediately after the end of drug infusion, which decreases to 35 to 50 μg/mL 30 minutes later [419,421]. Serum cefotaxime concentrations are higher in premature newborns and in those younger than 1 week of age. The administration of a 50 mg/kg intravenous dose during the first week of life results in peak serum concentrations of 116 μg/mL (range, 46 to 186 μg/mL) in low birth weight infants, compared with 133 μg/mL (range, 76 to 208 μg/mL) in term neonates [417]. Values decline thereafter to approximately 34 to 38 μg/mL 6 hours after the dose. The mean half-life is 4.6 hours for low birth weight neonates and 3.4 hours for larger newborns [417].

Both cefotaxime and its metabolite penetrate well into the CSF of infants with meningitis [421,423,424]. Concentrations of 7.1 to 30 μg/mL are detected 1 to 2 hours after a 50 mg/kg intravenous dose and represented 27% to 63%, respectively, of simultaneously measured serum values. CSF concentrations as high as 20 μg/mL in neonates with or without meningitis have been reported [423].

Ceftazidime

Numerous reports on the PK of ceftazidime (see Table 37–9) in neonates have been published [13,422,425–434]. Peak serum concentrations of 35 to 269 μg/mL (mean, 77 μg/mL) have been observed after intravenous administration of 25- to 30-mg/kg doses of ceftazidime to newborns of various gestational ages during their first week of life [432,434]. Mean trough values measured 9 to 12 hours after the dose are from 15 to 19 μg/mL [426,429–432]. These concentrations are higher than those detected in older infants receiving identical ceftazidime dosages. When the dose is increased to 50 mg/kg intravenously, mean peak serum concentrations are 102 to 118 μg/mL and mean trough values 8 hours after the dose are from 29 to 41 μg/mL [13,428]. Most of the ceftazidime dose is excreted in the urine. Not surprisingly, the mean elimination half-life is inversely related to gestational age and varies from 4.2 to 6.7 hours. The peak serum concentrations 1 to 2 hours after the intramuscular administration of 50 mg/kg of ceftazidime are about 67% lower than those observed with intravenous infusion [13,429]. Neonatal exposure to indomethacin or to asphyxia decreases the glomerular filtration rate and clearance of ceftazidime.

Ceftazidime penetrates well into the CSF, especially when meningitis is present [431,435]. In infants with bacterial meningitis, CSF concentrations of 1.8 to 7.9 μg/mL are obtained 2 to 7 hours after a 50-mg/kg dose, corresponding to 6% to 46% of a simultaneous serum concentration [436]. The extent of penetration is lower in patients with aseptic meningitis and relatively poor in those with uninflamed meninges [431,437].

Cefepime (Table 37–9)

Recent PK studies in neonates given a 50 mg/kg intravenous dose every 12 hours have shown a mean C_{max} of 89 [438] and 121 [439] μg/mL, half-life of 4.9 [438] and 4.3 [439] hour, and clearance of 1.2 mL/min/kg [438,439].

TABLE 37-9 Pharmacology of Cephalosporins

Drug Dose	Route of Elimination	Infant Characteristics	C_{max} (μg/mL)	Half-life (hr)	PK:PD Target	Protein Binding	CSF* Penetration with Meningitis	CLSI MIC* E. coli Klebsiella	CLSI MIC* P. aeruginosa	Clinical Pearls‡
Cefazolin 25 mg/kg	Renal	PNA <14 days	55–80	4–5 hr <7 days 3 hr >14 days	T>MIC >60%–70%	80%	Poor	≤8	Resistant	Perioperative prophylaxis
Cefotaxime 50 mg/kg	Liver and RBC esterase† Renal 30%	0–7 days	116–132	0.8–1.5	T>MIC >60%–70%	30%	27%–63%	≤8	Resistant	Does not cover P. aeruginosa
Ceftazidime 50 mg/kg	Renal	32–40 wk GA	111–102	4–6.7	T>MIC >60%–70%	15%	6%–46%	≤8	≤8	Covers P. aeruginosa
Cefepime 50 mg/kg	Renal	PNA 0–14 days PNA >14 days	90–120	4.5 hr < 14 days 1.8 hr >14 days	T>MIC >60%–70%	18%	9%–67%	≤8	≤8	Covers P. aeruginosa

*From references 32, 683.
†Metabolites maintain antimicrobial activity but less than cefotaxime.
‡Safety considerations for cephalosporins: Hypersensitivity, diarrhea, eosinophilia, BM suppression, risk factor for candidiasis in extremely preterm infants, seizures related to massive exposure.

Penetration into CSF appears to be good, with CSF concentrations averaging 3.3 to 5.7 μg/mL at 0.5 and 8 hours after drug administration [440].

Safety

In general, cephalosporins are well tolerated by neonates. Adverse reactions that have been observed, mostly in older patients, include hypersensitivity reactions, diarrhea, thrombophlebitis, pain on intramuscular injection, eosinophilia, leukopenia, granulocytopenia, and seizures related to the administration of massive doses of these drugs [441,442]. Falsely elevated serum creatinine concentrations have been observed in patients who received cefoxitin or cephalothin. Alterations of the bowel bacterial flora are most pronounced with the third-generation agents, especially ceftriaxone and cefoperazone, and can lead to intestinal colonization by resistant organisms such as *Candida, Pseudomonas, Enterobacter,* or *Enterococcus* species. Subsequent superinfections by these drug-resistant pathogens have been described in neonates [441,443]. Another potential adverse effect related to disruption of bacterial intestinal flora by potent cephalosporins is the induction of antibiotic-associated colitis, presumably caused by overgrowth of toxin-producing *C. difficile.*

Bleeding disorders occurring with the use of cephalosporins have been well documented, mostly in adults. Hemostatic abnormalities associated with the use of cephalosporins can be mediated by several mechanisms. Immune-mediated platelet destruction with resultant thrombocytopenia is very rare but has been associated with the administration of cephalothin, cefazolin, cefamandole, cefaclor, and cefoxitin in older patients [444]. A second rare mechanism involves the development of antibodies, usually immunoglobulin G (IgG), against certain clotting factors such as factor V or VIII. Platelet dysfunction can be observed after several days of therapy with any of the cephalosporins. These drugs may inhibit adenosine diphosphate (ADP)-induced platelet aggregation, with resultant prolongation of the bleeding time. The effect is slowly reversible after discontinuation of the drug [445]. Another mechanism is defective fibrinogen-to-fibrin conversion, which has been observed with drugs such as cefazolin and cefamandole, particularly in patients with renal failure, who have very high serum antibiotic concentrations [444,445].

The most important mechanism is hemostatic abnormalities involving interference with the production of vitamin K-dependent clotting factors (II, VII, IX, and X), with resultant hypoprothrombinemia [445]. This effect-observed most commonly with moxalactam and cefamandole therapy and rarely with cefotaxime and ceftriaxone therapy—is believed to be related to, but not necessarily caused by, the presence of the N-methylthiotetrazole side chain in moxalactam, cefamandole, and cefoperazone. In patients with inadequate dietary intake, inhibition of colonic bacteria such as *E. coli* or *Bacteroides*, which are capable of vitamin K production, may lead to hypoprothrombinemia secondary to vitamin K deficiency. This side effect usually is avoidable or reversible by the administration of supplemental vitamin K.

An immune-mediated severe hemolytic reaction to ceftriaxone has been described in children and adults.

Because ceftriaxone has a high avidity for protein binding, a theoretical concern is that its use in the neonatal period can be associated with a significant displacement of bilirubin from albumin-binding sites, thereby inducing a hyperbilirubinemia. Ceftriaxone, when given to neonates in the first days of life, has been associated with an immediate and prolonged decrease in the reserve albumin concentration, which could predispose a vulnerable infant to bilirubin encephalopathy.

Clinical Implications

Cephalosporins, like other β-lactams, have time dependent bacterial killing properties [29,30,36]. Therefore, the pharmacodynamic target associated with bacterial killing is time>MIC. For most of these drugs, clearance occurs through renal elimination. As neonatal kidneys mature, dosing intervals need to decrease to provide therapeutic drug concentrations above the MIC of target organisms.

The usefulness of first-generation cephalosporins for therapy for neonatal bacterial infections is restricted. Their activity against gram-negative bacteria is limited and unpredictable, and their penetration into the CSF is relatively poor; thus, these drugs are not indicated for initial therapy for suspected neonatal bacterial infections. Cefazolin dosing is typically 25 mg/kg given intravenously every 12 hours for newborns weighing less than 2000 g in the first 2 weeks of life and every 8 hours for older infants. Extremely preterm infants may continue twice a day dosing for up to 28 days of life. For infants weighing more than 2000 g, the dose is given every 8 to 12 hours in the first week of life and every 8 hours thereafter. Use in neonates is generally limited to prophylaxis of perioperative infections, and treatment of urinary tract and soft tissue infections caused by susceptible organisms.

Although second-generation cephalosporins have been successfully used to treat neonatal infections caused by susceptible bacteria, these antibiotics are not typically recommended for routine use because of limited experience in newborns and because of their inferior activity to that of third-generation agents against gram-negative bacteria. With the advent of multidrug-resistant pneumococci, other antibiotics, such as amoxicillin-clavulanate, are preferred for treatment of neonatal otitis media.

As a group, third-generation cephalosporins are useful agents for the treatment of suspected or proven bacterial infections in newborns. Their advantages include excellent in vitro activity against the major pathogens for newborns, including aminoglycoside-resistant gram-negative bacilli, adequate CSF penetration with resultant high bactericidal activity in CSF of infants with meningitis, and a proven record of safety and tolerability [446]. Indications for use of individual agents vary in accordance with their pharmacologic properties.

The clinical efficacy and safety of cefotaxime in the treatment of neonatal infections have been well documented in several studies [421,443,447,448]. Cefotaxime is typically not used alone for initial therapy in suspected sepsis because of its poor activity against *L. monocytogenes* and enterococci. The addition of ampicillin provides antibacterial coverage against these organisms. One potential problem associated with the routine use of this drug is the possible emergence of cefotaxime-resistant gram-negative bacteria in the nursery [443]. Some nurseries, however, have not documented this problem even after 2 years of continuous use of this antibiotic [447]. Cefotaxime reaches CSF concentrations that are 50 to several hundred times greater than the MIC_{90} of susceptible gram-negative enteric bacilli or group B streptococci isolated from newborns with meningitis, and has therefore been shown to be effective for the treatment of neonatal meningitis caused by susceptible bacteria [449]. The dosage of cefotaxime in newborns is 50 mg/kg every 12 hours during the first week of life and every 8 hours thereafter. In full-term infants older than 3 weeks, a 6-hour regimen can be used for treatment of meningitis [450].

I do not recommend using ceftazidime alone for initial therapy for suspected neonatal sepsis because this antibiotic is not active against enterococci and *L. monocytogenes* and because of the possibility for emergence of cephalosporin-resistant gram-negative organisms. Several treatment failures have occurred when the offending organism proved to be a gram-positive bacterium [431]. Increased colonization and superinfection by resistant organisms such as enterococci and *C. albicans* have been encountered in patients receiving ceftazidime [433,451]. The use of ceftazidime is typically reserved for situations in which gram-negative bacteria, notably *P. aeruginosa*, have been isolated or are strongly suspected of being the causative microorganisms in neonates with sepsis, meningitis, or other invasive infections. The dosage is 100 mg/kg/day in two (in infants born weighing less than 2000 g) or three (in those born at 2000 g or greater) divided doses during the first week of life and 150 mg/kg/day in three divided doses for older neonates.

Cefepime has been evaluated in young children with serious bacterial infections, including meningitis, and has been comparable in safety and efficacy to third-generation cephalosporins [452]. Recent PK information supports the typical dosing regimen, 30 mg/kg every 12 hours during first two weeks of life and 50 mg/kg every 12 hours thereafter. Meningitis or severe infections due to *Pseudomonas* or *Enterobacter* species may require dosing every 8 hours to maintain the concentrations above the MIC of the offending organism. Although data on the use of cefepime in the neonatal period are lacking because of its extended activity and stability against β-lactamase-producing bacteria, cefepime can be used for treatment of multidrug-resistant gram-negative infections. In a small randomized trial of 90 infants, cefepime was safe and therapeutically equivalent to cefotaxime for treatment of bacterial meningitis in infants and children [453].

BROAD-ACTING AGENTS WITH ACTIVITY AGAINST PSEUDAMONAS
(See Table 37–9)
β-Lactam/β-lactamase Inhibitor Antibiotics
Antimicrobial Activity

Combination β-lactam and β-lactamase inhibitor antibiotics (piperacillin/tazobactam, ticarcillin/clavulanate) offer broad spectrum activity and have re-emerged as an

alternative to extended spectrum cephalosporins and the emergence of cephalosporin-induced pathogen resistance [454]. These drugs are bactericidal against many organisms with the exception of methicillin resistant staphylococcus and enterococcus (ticarcillin/clavulanate). Recently, the use of ß-lactam/ß-lactamase combination antibiotics have become appealing in neonates because of their safety profiles and their decreased likelihood to propagate bacterial resistance compared with extended-spectrum cephalosporins. However, more PK and PD knowledge in neonates is needed to optimize dosing guidelines. These agents are not typically recommended for treatment of central nervous system infections because penetration of β-lactamase inhibitors has not been well defined.

Piperacillin-Tazobactam
Antimicrobial Activity

Piperacillin is formulated with the β-lactamase inhibitor tazobactam in an 8:1 ratio for intravenous preparation [455]. Piperacillin is an acylampicillin, a semisynthetic penicillin that is a piperazine derivative of ampicillin. Piperacillin is active against a broad range of gram-positive and gram-negative bacteria including *S. aureus*, streptococci, *H. influenzae*, *N. meningitidis*, *L. monocytogenes*, *K. pneumoniae*, *P. mirabilis*, *S. marcescens*, and many anaerobes. In contrast to ticarcillin, piperacillin has better activity against enterococci and *P. aeruginosa*. In vitro synergistic activity with gentamicin has been demonstrated against *P. aeruginosa*, coliforms, and susceptible *S. aureus* strains. Synergy and antagonism has been demonstrated with cephalosporins perhaps due to the ability of some cephalosporins to induce β-lactamase production [456–458]. Because piperacillin is susceptible to hydrolysis by β-lactamase, it is now manufactured with a β-lactamase inhibitor, tazobactam. Piperacillin-tazobactam is not approved by the FDA for use in infants less than 2 months of age. However, it has been considered for neonates with proven bacterial infections, particularly those infected with difficult to treat polymicrobial sepsis or infections due to *P. aeruginosa* or *K. pneumoniae*.

Pharmacokinetic Data (Table 37–9)

Piperacillin and tazobactam are widely distributed into tissue and body fluids, including the intestinal mucosa and biliary system; however, distribution into cerebrospinal fluid is low in adults with noninflamed meninges as with most penicillins [1,454,455,459–461]. Protein binding is estimated to be 30% for both piperacillin and tazobactam. Each drug is eliminated primarily through the kidneys via glomerular filtration and tubular secretion with approximately 70% excreted as unchanged, active drug in the urine in children and adults. The primary nonrenal route of elimination is biliary excretion [460,462]. Piperacillin metabolite desethyl piperacillin maintains some microbiologic activity, whereas the single metabolite of tazobactam does not.

Piperacillin/tazobactam is approved for use in children and infants older than 2 months [463–465]. Elimination is dependent on renal function and therefore improves with age until adult clearance is achieved around 2 years of age. Children receiving piperacillin/tazobactam have somewhat reduced piperacillin elimination and prolonged half-life (0.7 hour vs. 0.5 hour) compared with piperacillin alone likely because of competitive antagonism for renal tubular secretion [465,466].

The PK of piperacillin has been evaluated in 98 neonates (29 to 40 weeks of gestation) in the first 2 weeks of life [467,468]; however, the PK of piperacillin/tazobactam has not been described. Preterm neonates have lower peak piperacillin concentrations due to their higher volume of distribution. In the first week after birth, the mean peak serum concentration after an intravenous 75 mg/kg dose is 180 µg/mL, 233 µg/mL, and 207 µg/mL for infants 29 to 31 weeks, 33 to 35 weeks, or 38 to 40 weeks of gestation. Immature renal function leads to prolonged half-life and delayed clearance, thus allowing preterm infants to maintain concentrations over the dosing interval. The mean 12-hour trough concentrations ranged from 20 µg/mL in 29- to 31-week gestational infants to 5 µg/mL in term infants [468]. In the second week of life, 8-hour trough concentrations ranged from 19 µg/mL for less than 33-week-gestation infants to 6 µg/mL for term infants [468]. Piperacillin half-life similarly decreases with advanced gestational age, chronologic age, and birth weight consistent with renal maturation. The prolonged half-life in neonates decreases from 6 hours in the first 2 days after birth, to 4 hours in the first week, and to 2 hours by the second week [467,468]. Infants with septic shock and significant renal insufficiency have prolonged half-life up to 14 hours. In older infants, the reported half-life of piperacillin is 0.75 hours in 1- to 6-month-old infants [464] and for piperacillin/tazobactam is 1.4 hours for 2- to 6-month-old infants [463].

CSF piperacillin concentrations of 2.6 to 6 µg/mL were measured in three neonates without meningitis within 7 hours of the intravenous administration of a 100-mg/kg dose [467]. In one infant with *Pseudomonas* meningitis, piperacillin reached a concentration of 19 µg/mL in the CSF 2.5 hours after administration of a 200 mg/kg intravenous dose [467]. Human and animal models suggest that modest CSF penetration is expected for β-lactamase inhibitors [469].

Safety

In a prospective, randomized, comparative, open-label trial of children with severe intra-abdominal infections, patients receiving piperacillin/tazobactam had a similar rate of adverse reactions when compared with those receiving cefotaxime and metronizdazole [1,470,471]. Adverse events reported in more than 1% of children in this study including diarrhea, fever, vomiting, local reaction, abscess, sepsis, abdominal pain, infection, bloody diarrhea, pharyngitis, constipation, and elevated SGOT enzyme. These adverse events were infrequent compared with transient complications encountered in adult trials. Bleeding manifestations, neuromuscular excitability, and seizures have occurred in patients receiving β-lactam antibiotics, including piperacillin. Impaired hemostasis secondary to platelet dysfunction occurs less frequently than with carbenicillin and ticarcillin [445]. The sodium content in piperacillin is less than half that in ticarcillin, which may be important in some newborns with cardiac or renal disease.

PK-PD and Clinical Implications for Dosing

Piperacillin-tazobactam, either alone or combined with aminoglycosides, has been used successfully for the treatment of bacteriologically proven neonatal infections [454]. Neonatal PK knowledge and clinical experience is limited and dosing recommendations remain empirical. Piperacillin and tazobactam are both mainly eliminated through the kidney by glomerular filtration and tubular secretion. Therefore it is rational to have initial dosage regimens for piperacillin-tazobactam based upon the PK of piperacillin; however, PK studies of piperacillin-tazobactam are still needed.

The PD of efficacy for β-lactam antibiotics depends on the time that the drug concentration exceeds the MIC for the pathogen. To maintain piperacillin concentrations above the MIC, the dosing interval may need to be shortened for susceptible pathogens with MICs greater than 4 to 8 µg/mL, such as can be seen for *Pseudomonas, Enterobacter,* or *Klebsiella* [463]. Given the modest CSF penetration, higher dosages may be considered for meningitis.

Dosing recommendations are variable and hindered by the paucity of PK data. One study suggested that piperacillin doses of 100 mg/kg every 12 hours may be appropriate and that a dose of 200 mg/kg every 12 hours should be used for meningitis [467]. In another PK study [468], a dosage schedule of 75 mg/kg given every 12 hours during the first week after birth and every 8 hours thereafter for infants less than 36-week gestation was recommended. For full-term infants, a 75-mg/kg dose given every 8 hours during the first week after birth and every 6 hours thereafter was recommended. Neonatal trough concentrations at 8 to 12 hours would help ensure that levels can be maintained above the MIC for at least 60% of the dosing interval.

Ticarcillin-Clavulanate (See Table 37–9)

Ticarcillin is a semisynthetic penicillin with pharmacologic and toxic properties virtually identical to those of other semisynthetic penicillin [472,473]. The coadministration of clavulanic acid with ticarcillin significantly enhances the antibacterial activity of the latter drug against several organisms, including some ticarcillin-resistant strains of *E. coli, K. pneumoniae, P. mirabilis,* and staphylococci [474,475]. *Enterococcus* species are resistant to ticarcillin. Clavulanate is a β-lactam with weak antibacterial activity, but it has the property of being a potent irreversible inhibitor of several ß-lactamases produced by gram-positive and gram-negative bacteria. Current ticarcillin-clavulanate combination formulation (Timentin R) is approved for children greater than 3 months of age for the treatment of bacterial sepsis, respiratory infections, urinary tract infections, and intra-abdominal infections [1]. Information regarding the use of this compound in newborns is limited. Ticarcillin activity against *P. aeruginosa* and its formulation with the ß-lactamase inhibitor clavulanate make it attractive for serious bacterial disease of neonates [476]. Synergy with aminoglycosides has been demonstrated for the treatment of some strains of *Pseudomonas.*

Pharmacokinetic Data

Ticarcillin-clavulanate is available for intravenous administration in a 30:1 ticarcillin-clavulanate ratio [1,472,473]. Like piperacillin, ticarcillin is eliminated via glomerular filtration and renal tubular secretion. Approximately 60% to 70% of ticarcillin is excreted unchanged in urine during the first 6 hours after administration. However, only 30% to 40% of clavulanic acid is excreted unchanged in the urine while the remainder undergoes nonrenal metabolism. Ticarcillin is approximately 45% protein bound whereas clavulanic acid is approximately 25% protein bound. Ticarcillin penetrates well into bile and pleural fluid.

PK data for ticarcillin-clavulanic acid has been assessed in 64 preterm and term neonates; however, the ratio of ticarcillin/clavulanate was not consistent between reports [477–480]. In a study of 24 newborns (25 to 39 weeks of gestation) who received 80 mg/kg ticarcillin and 3.5 mg/kg clavulanate, the ticarcillin peak serum concentrations (mean 183 µg/mL, range 100 to 400) and half-life (mean 4.5 hours, range 1.2 to 9.5) are similar to those observed after administration of ticarcillin alone [480]. The ticarcillin and clavulanate half-lives were shorter in term infants (ticarcillin 2.7 hours, clavulanate 1.4 hours) than in preterm infants (ticarcillin 4.2 hours, clavulanate 2.6 hours) [479]. Similar results were reported for the one PK study that evaluated the commercially available product with a 30:1 ratio of ticarcillin:clavulanate [478].

Ticarcillin and clavulanate have different PK profiles. Ticarcillin is renally eliminated and clearance improves with renal maturation and chronologic age. Alternatively, clavulanate is eliminated through nonrenal mechanisms and is more rapid [454]. Ticarcillin accumulates in young neonates due to renal immaturity; however, clavulanate does not and therefore the ticarcillin:clavulanate ratio observed in older patient is not likely maintained in neonates. Simulation of ticarcillin and clavulanate exposure using a population PK model [478] suggested that a lower dose (50 mg/kg ticarcillin) administered more frequently (i.e., every 6 hours) was needed to maintain both ticarcillin and clavulanate levels. The significance of altered ticarcillin:clavulanate ratios is unclear [481] since we do not know the optimal duration or concentration for serum clavulanate.

Safety

Ticarcillin-clavulanate possesses the characteristic safety profile of other penicillin antibiotics. Adverse reactions include anaphylaxis, bleeding disorders, seizures, headache, gastrointestinal disturbances, transient elevation hepatic enzymes, hypernatremia, and hypokalemia. Ticarcillin-clavulanate has been studied in 296 children (>3 months old) in controlled trials and another 408 children in uncontrolled clinical trials [1]. Clinical trials in neonates are lacking. Anecdotal reports and small case-series suggest that ticarcillin-clavulanate is well tolerated in neonates.

PK-PD and Clinical Implications for Dosing
(Table 37–10)

Ticarcillin-clavulanate is typically used along with an aminoglycoside for infants with severe gram-negative enteric infections or *Pseudomonas* sepsis, anecdotally with satisfactory safety and effectiveness. The most consistent dosing recommendation for neonates is 50 mg/kg every 6 hours, the same dose as recommended in infants greater than 3 months of age with moderate infections. Frequent dosing is needed to maintain clavulanic acid levels since

clavulanic acid clearance is more rapid than ticarcillin in infants. Clavulanic acid CSF penetration is only modest and is inconsistent in adult and animal models; therefore its use in treatment of CNS infections is discouraged. Ticarcillin-clavulanate should not be mixed in the same container or administered simultaneously with an aminoglycoside because of the physical and chemical incompatibilities between these two drug classes.

Carbapenems

Carbapenems (see Table 37–9) are β-lactam antibiotics known for their exceptionally broad activity and activity against extended spectrum ß-lactamase-producing gram-negative organisms [1,482]. *Imipenem* was the first drug in this new class. However, imipenem is susceptible to degradation by the enzyme dehydropeptidase-1 in the kidney and therefore imipenem is now formulated with cilastatin, a dehydropeptidase inhibitor. The coadministration of both imipenem/cilastatin (1:1 ratio) increases the urinary concentration of imipenem, prolongs the imipenem serum half-life, and appears to prevent the nephrotoxicity induced by high doses of imipenem. Cilastatin itself has no intrinsic antimicrobial activity. *Meropenem* is a newer carbapenem that is not susceptible to dehydropeptidase degradation. Meropenem is structurally different from imipenem in two ways: the carbapenem ring structure of meropenem includes an additional ß-methyl group in the C-1 position, providing stability against the human renal tubular enzyme dehydropeptidase and a long, substituted pyrrolidine side chain present in the C-2 position allows greater activity against intracellular target sites in organisms such as *P. aeruginosa* [483]. Meropenem was approved by the FDA for use in children older than 3 months on the basis of extensive pediatric investigations across a wide range of infections, including meningitis and complicated abdominal infections [484]. Meropenem is being increasingly studied in neonates for the treatment of complicated intra-abdominal infections\infections due to *Pseudomonas* or extended spectrum ß-lactamase producing bacterial infections. The newest carbepenems, ertapenem and doripenem, have yet to be studied in infants.

Antimicrobial Activity

Imipenem and meropenem have an exceptionally broad spectrum of activity. The bacterial species considered resistant to these drugs are MRSA, methicillin-resistant *S. epidermidis*, *Stenotrophomonas maltophilia*, *Burkholderia cepacia*, and *E. faecium* [482]. These drugs maintain activity against extended spectrum ß-lactamase (ESBL) producing organisms. It has been estimated that approximately 98% of unselected bacterial pathogens isolated from humans are susceptible to carbapenems at concentrations of 8 µg/mL or less [485,486]. Carbepenems produce in vitro MIC_{90} values of 1 µg/mL against the most commonly isolated species of gram-positive and enteric gram-negative aerobic bacteria including group B streptococci, penicillin-susceptible and penicillin-resistant *S. pneumoniae*, MSSA, *L. monocytogenes*, *Citrobacter freundii*, *E. coli*, *H. influenzae*, *Klebsiella*, *Proteus*, *Serratia*, *and Acinetobacter* species. The MIC_{90} values are typically less than 2 µg/mL for anaerobic bacteria [482,485]. *P. aeruginosa* has an MIC_{50} and MIC_{90} of 1 and greater than

8 for imipenem/cilastatin and of 0.5 and 16 for meropenem, respectively. Meropenem is consistently more active against *P. aeruginosa* than imipenem. These inhibitory concentrations against *P. aeruginosa* are comparable to those of ceftazidime. Synergistic interactions between carbapenems and aminoglycosides can be demonstrated in vitro against *P. aeruginosa* and *S. aureus* isolates. Antagonistic interactions usually are observed when imipenem is combined with other ß-lactams, probably as a result of chromosomal ß-lactamase induction by imipenem [485].

Carbapenem's unusually broad antibacterial spectrum is related to its ability to penetrate efficiently the outer membrane of gram-negative bacteria, its high binding affinity for PBP-2, and its resistance to hydrolysis by both plasmid- and chromosomally mediated ß-lactamases [486,487]. Some ß-lactamases produced by *S. maltophilia*, *Aeromonas hydrophila*, and *B. fragilis*, however, are capable of hydrolyzing imipenem and meropenem. Emergence of carbapenem-resistant strains during therapy with this drug is rare except in the case of *P. aeruginosa*, in which resistance occurs in as many as 17% of isolates [482].

Pharmacokinetic Data

Imipenem-Cilastatin

For both imipenem and cilastatin (Table 37–10), serum concentration is directly proportional to the administered dose [483,488,489]. Higher serum concentrations are achieved with cilastatin than with identical doses of imipenem. Imipenem when co-administered with cilastatin is eliminated as active drug through the kidneys [485]. Cilastatin is excreted primarily in unchanged form in the urine, but about 12% of the drug appears as the metabolite N-acetylcilastatin [485].

In neonatal studies, the intravenous administration of 10-, 15-, 20- and 25-mg/kg doses of both drugs results in mean peak imipenem concentrations of 11, 21, 30, and 55 µg/mL, respectively, compared with mean cilastatin values of 28, 37, 57, and 69 µg/mL, respectively [488,489]. After 3 to 4 days of treatment with 20-mg/kg intravenous doses of imipenem-cilastatin every 12 hours, peak serum concentrations are 35 and 86 µg/mL for imipenem and cilastatin, respectively. The mean serum half-life of imipenem is about 2 hours, whereas that of cilastatin is 5 to 6.4 hours [488]. The half-life for both drugs is inversely related to birth weight and gestational age and is considerably longer than the 1-hour half-life reported for both drugs in older infants and in healthy adult volunteers [488–491]. During the neonatal period, the plasma clearance of cilastatin is only about 25% of that of imipenem [488].

Although both imipenem and cilastatin penetrate well into the CSF in the presence of meningeal inflammation [492,493], data derived from neonatal studies are scant. In one newborn who received a 15-mg/kg intravenous dose, concentrations of 1.1 and 0.8 µg/mL were noted for imipenem and cilastatin, respectively, at 1.5 hours after injection. In a second neonate who received a 25-mg/kg dose, CSF values of 5.6 and 1.8 µg/mL were found for imipenem and cilastatin, respectively [489].

Meropenem

Meropenem (Table 37–10) was approved by the FDA for use in children older than 3 months of age on the basis of extensive pediatric investigations across a wide range of infections, including meningitis and complicated abdominal infections [1,494]. Small PK studies have been published in infants born at 23 to 40 weeks of gestation and up to 60 days of age [483,495,496]. Meropenem exhibits dose-proportional linear PK properties with dosages of meropenem from 10 to 40 mg/kg. A 20 mg/kg dose of meropenem results in peak serum concentrations of about 50 µg/mL. Meropenem clearance increases with gestational age and chronologic age as the kidneys mature. In the most recent population PK study of meropenem in preterm and term infants, serum creatinine and postmenstrual age were the best overall predictor of meropenem clearance [495]. Half-life, volume of distribution, and total drug clearance of meropenem were 3 hours, 0.46 to 0.74 L/kg, and 1.8 to 2.6 mL/min/kg, respectively, for premature infants and 2 hours, 0.48 L/kg, and 3.15 mL/min/kg for full-term neonates. The half-life decreases to 1.6 hours at 2 to 5 months of age as renal maturation occurs.

Safety

Both imipenem-cilastatin and meropenem appear to be well tolerated when administered intravenously to newborns in relatively small PK studies. In a review of studies conducted worldwide including thousands of patients, most of whom were adults, it was observed that the nature and frequency of side effects were similar to those of other ß-lactam antibiotics; these adverse effects consisted mainly of nausea, vomiting, diarrhea, thrombophlebitis, thrombocytosis, eosinophilia, and elevation of hepatic enzyme concentrations [497]. Colonization by *Candida* or imipenem-resistant bacteria occurred in about 16% of patients, and secondary superinfection was noted in about 6% [497]. Alterations of bowel flora in children given imipenem-cilastatin have been minimal in the few patients studied in detail [493]. A worrisome report suggests that imipenem treatment in infants with bacterial meningitis was possibly associated with drug-related seizure activity [498]. In infants with bacterial meningitis, seizures developed in 7 of 21 infants (33%), aged 3 to 48 months following imipenem therapy. In this study [498], CSF imipenem and cilastatin peak concentrations ranged from 1.4 to 10 µg/mL and 0.8 to 7.2 µg/mL, respectively. It is believed that interference of ß-lactam antibiotics with the inhibitory effects of the neurotransmitter gamma-aminobutyric acid (GABA) can result in epileptiform bursts [499,500]. In mice, imipenem has been shown to induce seizure activity at serum concentrations two to three times lower than those of penicillin and cefotaxime [501]. Meropenem has less affinity than imipenem for the gamma-aminobutyric acid receptor and consequently has demonstrated a lower propensity to cause seizures in animal models [502]. In infants and children with meningitis, treatment with meropenem was well tolerated, and no drug-related seizure activity was observed [494].

PK-PD and Clinical Implications for Dosing
(Table 37–10)

Imipenem-cilastatin and meropenem are not recommended for routine use in the treatment of suspected or proven neonatal infections with rare exceptions. Both agents should be primarily reserved to treat infections caused by multidrug-resistant microorganisms. Data in

TABLE 37–10 Broad-Acting Agents with Activity Against *Pseudomonas*

Drug	Infant Characteristics	C_{max} µg/mL (mean)	Half-life (hr)	Route of Elimination	Protein Binding	PD Target‡	CSF Penetration for Antibiotic Only	ESBL	CLSI MIC* Klebsiella E. coli	CLSI MIC* P. aeruginosa	Clinical Pearls†
Piperacillin/ tazobactam (PK Pip only) 75 mg/kg	<14 days 29–31 wk 33–40 wk	180 230	6 @ 2 days 4 @ 7 days 2 @ 14 days	Renal Biliary	30%	T/MIC >50%	5%–30% (pip)	No	≤16	≤16	2.8 mEq Na/g Superior to Ticar for Pseudomonas and anaerobes
Ticarcillin/ clavulanate 75 mg/kg tic	<2200 g ≤34 wk ≤19 days old	≈200 (75 mg/kg)	5 @ 4 days 4 @ 9 days 3 @ 18 days 2 @ >30 days	(T) Renal (C) nonrenal	45%	T/MIC >50%	40% (tic)	No	≤16	<16	5 mEq Na/g Resistant to enterococci, Klebsiella
Imipenem/ Cilastatin 25 mg/kg	Preterm (mean 29 wk) Full term	75 97	2.5 1.9 (Cil 5 hr)	Renal metabolism (inhibited by cilastatin)	20%	T/MIC >40–60%	15%–27% (imip)	Yes	≤4	≤4	Rare incidence seizures in pt with CNS disease
Meropenem 20 mg/kg	Preterm Full term	44 40	2.9 2	Renal	2%	T/MIC >40–60%	6%–10%	yes	≤4	≤4	Possibly lower risk seizures

*From references 32, 683.

†Safety considerations similar to β-lactams: hypersensitivity, diarrhea, seizures (notably in patients with CNS disease and imipenem), rare risk of bleeding.

‡Neonatal PD has not been performed. Neonates may need longer T>MIC to account for immune deficiencies.

Pip, piperacillin; Ticar or tic, ticarcillin; C, clavulanate; (imip), imipenem; ESBL, extended spectrum β-lamase producing organism; CLSI, clinical laboratory standards institute; MIC, minimal inhibitory concentration; PK pip, pharmacokinetics derived from piperacillin alone; Na, sodium; CNS, central nervous system; CSF, cerebrospinal fluid; PD, pharmacodynamic target for efficacy.

TABLE 37–11 Suggested Dosage Schedules for Systemic Antibiotics Used in Newborns*

Antibiotics	Route	Dosage (mg/kg) and Interval of Administration by Weight				
		<1200 g*	1200–2000 g		>2000 g	
		Age 0–4 Wk	Age 0–7 Days	Age >7 Days	Age 0–7 Days	Age >7 Days
Amikacin† (SDD)	IV, IM	7.5 q12h	7.5 q12h	7.5 q8h	10 q12h	10 q8h
Amikacin† (ODD)	IV, IM	18 q48h	15 q36h	15 q24h	15 q24-36h	15 q24h
Ampicillin	IV, IM					
Meningitis		100 q12h	100 q12h	100 q8h	100 q8h	100 q6-8h
Other infections		50 q12h	50 q12h	50 q8h	50 q8h	50 q6-8h
Aztreonam	IV, IM	30 q12h	30 q12h	30 q8h	30 q8-12h	30 q6-8h
Cefazolin	IV, IM	20 q12h	20 q12h	20 q12h	20 q12h	20 q8h
Cefepime	IV, IM	50 q12h	50 q12h	50 q8h	50 q12h	50 q8h
Cefotaxime	IV, IM	50 q12h	50 q12h	50 q8h	50 q12h	50 q8h
Ceftazidime	IV, IM	50 q12h	50 q12h	50 q8h	50 q8h	50 q8h
Clindamycin	IV, IM	5–7.5 q12h	5–7.5 q12h	5–7.5 q8h	5–7.5 q8h	5–7.5 q6h
Gentamicin† (SDD)	IV, IM	2.5 q18h	2.5 q12h	2.5 q8h	2.5 q12h	2.5 q8h
Gentamicin† (ODD)	IV, IM	5 q48h	4 q36h	4 q24h	4 q24h	4 q24h
Imipenem	IV, IM	20 q12h	20 q12h	20 q12h	20 q12h	20 q8h
Linezolid	IV	10 q8h	10 q12h	10 q8h	10 q12h	10 q8h
Metronidazole	IV	7.5 q48h	7.5 q24h	7.5 q12h	7.5 q12h	15 q12h
Meropenem	IV, IM	20 q12h	20 q12h	20 q8-12h	20 q8-12h	20 q8h
Nafcillin	IV	25 q12h	25 q12h	25 q8h	25 q8h	25–50 q6h
Oxacillin	IV, IM	25 q12h	25 q12h	25 q8h	25 q8h	25–50 q6h
Penicillin G (units)	IV					
Meningitis		50,000 q12h	50,000 q12h	50,000 q8h	50,000 q8h	50,000 q6h
Other infections		25,000 q12h	25,000 q12h	25,000 q8h	25,000 q8h	25,000 q6h
Piperacillin/tazobactam	IV, IM	50–75 q12	50–75 q12h	50–75 q8h	50–75 q8h	50–75 q6h
Rifampin	IV	5–10 q12	5–10 q12h	5–10 q12h	5–10 q12h	5–10 q12h
Ticarcillin-clavulanate		75 q12h	75 q12h	75 q8h	75 q8h	75 q6h
Tobramycin† (SDD)	IV, IM	2.5 q18h	2 q12h	2 q8h	2 q12h	2 q8h
Tobramycin (ODD)		5 q48h	4 q36h	4 q24h	4 q24h	4 q24h
Vancomycin†	IV	15 q24h	10–15 q12h	10–15 q8-12h	10–15 q8h	10–15 q8h

*Based upon anecdotal clinical experience, neonatal and hospital formularies and notable references [153,690,691,692].
Dosing for infants <1200 g is typically based upon limited PK information. Use of most of these drugs remain off-label in neonates due to need for more pharmacokinetic and safety information. Higher dosing may be indicated for treatment of meningitis or micro-organism with higher MIC, such as Pseudomonas. In the absence of complete pharmacokinetic information across gestation age and postnatal ages, interhospital variability in dosing guidance is expected.
†Adjustments of further dosing intervals should be based on aminoglycoside half-lives calculated after serum peak and trough concentrations measurements.
IM, intramuscular; IV, intravenous; ODD, once-daily dosing; PO, oral; SDD, standard daily dosing.

25 neonates with proven bacterial infections suggest that single-drug therapy with imipenem-cilastatin using a 25-mg/kg dose given two to four times daily is both efficacious and safe [503]. Because newborns have lower renal clearance capability and somewhat greater blood-brain permeability than those in older infants and children, high concentrations of imipenem-cilastatin could be achieved in the CSF of neonates, especially those with bacterial meningitis, potentially resulting in drug-related seizure activity. Evidence from case reports suggests that meropenem also is safe and effective for treatment of neonatal infections. Because meropenem is more active against *P. aeruginosa*, not metabolized in the kidney, and has not been linked to the potential induction of seizures, we believe that if a carbapenem is selected for therapy in a newborn, meropenem should be the agent of choice.

Meropenem, like other β-lactam antibiotics, exhibits time-dependent killing, so the goal of therapy is to keep meropenem serum concentrations above the MIC for at least 40% of the dosing interval for immunocompetent patients [30]. Some authors have recommended higher T>MIC intervals in immunocompromised patients and particularly those with *Pseudomonas* infections due to the higher MIC_{50} of 4 and MIC_{90} of 32. The meropenem dose exposure relationship has been evaluated using Monte Carlo simulation and the population PK model. In the first 2 weeks after birth, 20 mg/kg of meropenem administered every 8 hours can maintain the PK-PD target of 60% T>MIC in more than 99% of preterm and term infants if the pathogen is susceptible with a MIC value of less than 8 μg/mL [495]. NICU-specific sensitivities for nosocomial pathogens must be considered when considering appropriate exposure. Higher dosing will need to be determined for meningitis and for the treatment of the more resistant organisms such as *P. aeruginosa*. Further studies are required before these drugs can be recommended for use in select newborns and before an appropriate dosage schedule can be formulated.

ANTIVIRAL MEDICATIONS

Viral infections in the neonate are fortunately rare yet associated with significant morbidity and mortality. Viral therapy is available for the treatment of HIV, HSV, CMV, and VZV. The pharmacology of medications used to treat or prevent HIV infections is discussed in Chapter 21 and has been recently reviewed [504–506]. The pharmacology of acyclovir, ganciclovir, and oseltamivir will be reviewed here [1]. These drugs need further PK investigation in neonates.

Acyclovir for the Treatment of HSV

Acyclovir is a nucleoside analogue used against herpes simplex virus (HSV) and varicella-zoster virus. The PK of acyclovir in neonates requires further investigation. PK is limited to 3 infants (less than 60 days old) receiving oral acyclovir (300 mg/m²) for 3 doses [507]. The maximum concentration (1.88 µg/mL) was higher than observed in adults receiving a larger dose (400 mg/m²) and suggests adequate bioavailability. The elimination half-life of 3 hours was longer than the 2.4 hours observed in adults. Mortality was reduced in infants with neonatal HSV disease who received high dose, 60 mg/kg/day, compared with infants receiving 45 mg/kg/day (given every 8 hours) for 21 days [508,509]. The survival rate was similar for infants with CNS disease. Neutropenia was the most significant adverse event reported; however, there were no reported adverse sequelae and the neutropenia was transient. The dosing interval may need to be increased in premature infants who are expected to have decreased creatinine clearance [510].

Ganciclovir for the Treatment of Congenital CMV

Antimicrobial Activity

Ganciclovir is approved for the prevention or treatment of cytomegalovirus virus in adults [1].

Ganciclovir is a synthetic guanine derivative that specifically inhibits viral DNA synthesis by inhibiting viral DNA polymerase resulting in termination of viral DNA elongation [511,512]. Ganciclovir is active against CMV and, to a lesser extent, HSV.

Pharmacokinetic Data

Ganciclovir is phosphorylated by viral protein kinases to ganciclovir triphosphate, the active metabolite that persists for days in CMV-infected cells [512]. To a lesser degree, normal, uninfected cells can generate monophosphorylated ganciclovir, thus possibly explaining its cytotoxic side effects [513]. Ganciclovir exhibits low protein binding. CSF penetration is 24% to 70% of the respective plasma concentrations. Renal excretion of unchanged drug occurs by glomerular filtration and active tubular secretion. Half-life in adults is 3.5 hours. Dose adjustment is advised in renal insufficiency. Ganciclovir exhibits linear kinetics with dose escalation.

Single dose, intravenous ganciclovir PK has been evaluated in 27 neonates less than 50 days old. After a 4 mg/kg or 6 mg/kg intravenous dose, the peak concentration was 5.5 and 7.0 µg/mL, respectively; systemic clearance was 3.14 and 3.56 mL/kg/min, respectively; and the half-life was 2.4 hours for both doses [514]. Clearance was less than the 4.7 mL/kg/min reported in children but the half-life was similar; neonates had high interpatient variability. Population PK analysis of these newborns showed that ganciclovir clearance was associated with body weight and creatinine clearance [515]. The mean population clearance was 0.4 L/hr and the volume of distribution was 1.73 L. A recent population PK analysis in young infants receiving intravenous ganciclovir or oral valganciclovir showed similar results, namely a mean clearance of 0.32 L/hr and volume of distribution of 1.78 L [516]. Because ganciclovir is eliminated through the kidney, we would expect a delay in drug clearance during the first week of life and in extremely premature infants.

Valganciclovir is the oral prodrug of ganciclovir. Valganciclovir is rapidly hydrolyzed to ganciclovir. PK studies of valganciclovir are limited [516–520]. A recent study of 24 neonates reported that 16 mg/kg oral valganciclovir administered twice daily achieves similar exposure to the 6 mg/kg per dose intravenous ganciclovir regimen and the target AUC_{0-12} of 27 mg*hr/L [520]. The median bioavailability was 41%. Ganciclovir clearance doubled over the 6 weeks of therapy and the AUC was reduced nearly 50%. However, infants receiving valganciclovir had more consistent AUC over 6 weeks of therapy, likely because bioavailability increased by 32% over the course of treatment. This dose was consistent with the 15 mg/kg dose recommended in smaller studies [519]. Viral load decreased in all infants (median 0.7 log viral DNA copies per milliliter); however, this decrease in viral load was not associated with C_{max} or AUC. Neutropenia remained the most significant adverse effect and grade 3 to 4 neutropenia occurred in 38% of infants, and was correlated with higher C_{max} and higher AUC.

Safety

Ganciclovir label contains a black box warning for risk of granulocytopenia, anemia, and thrombocytopenia, and the drug should be avoided in patients with cytopenia or history of cytopenia. Dose reduction is also indicated in renal impairment. Additional reported adverse events include fever, anorexia, and vomiting. Ganciclovir has important drug interactions: it should not be combined with imipenem-cilastin due to concern for seizures and caution is required when combined with other nucleoside analogues, cyclosporine, and amphotericin B due to potential additive toxicity.

In a placebo-controlled trial of ganciclovir in infants, neutropenia occurred in 63% of infants receiving ganciclovir compared with 21% in the control infants [521]. Adverse events in infants participating in a phase 2 study of 8 versus 12 mg/kg/day included retinal detachment, neutropenia, and a moderate increase in creatinine and liver enzymes [522]. It remains unclear if these adverse events were attributed to either progression of CMV disease, adverse drug effect, or both. Periodic monitoring of blood counts, serum creatinine, and liver function is recommended, and hematologic manifestations are typically transient.

PK-PD and Clinical Indications

Ganciclovir is indicated for the treatment of CMV retinitis in immunocompromised patients or the prevention of CMV disease in transplant recipients. The relationship between ganciclovir exposure and clinical response has not been established. In vitro studies have shown that median inhibitory concentrations ranged from 0.02 to 3.48 µg/mL. A placebo-controlled trial in neonates with central nervous system manifestations, demonstrated a reduction of hearing deterioration in infants receiving intravenous ganciclovir 12 mg/kg/day for 6 weeks [521]. Safety and efficacy of ganciclovir has not been established for congenital CMV disease. There was a higher incidence of neutropenia in infants receiving ganciclovir compared with placebo. Controversy exists regarding the potential benefits of prolonged ganciclovir therapy to neonates given the prolonged duration of intravenous access required and risk of adverse drug events [523]. Oral valganciclovir, a prodrug that is rapidly hydrolyzed to ganciclovir and approved for use in adults, is under investigation in children and neonates.

Oseltamivir for the Treatment of Influenza

The CDC estimates that each year more than 200,000 hospitalizations and 36,000 deaths are attributable to influenza in the United States [524,525]. In the 2003–2004 influenza seasons, the CDC reported 153 influenza-related deaths in children with a median age of 3 years. The highest mortality rate in children was among children younger than 6 months of age. In addition to mortality, children are known to have high rates of hospitalization and can suffer chronic neurologic or neuromuscular conditions [526–530]. Neonates and young infants are particularly vulnerable because vaccination is ineffective and antiviral treatment is not recommended in infancy. Immunization of pregnant mothers and all adults who contact infants is the best means of preventing influenza infection in infants. Neuraminidase inhibitors are effective in the treatment of sensitive influenza species in infants older than 1 year of age if initiated within 48 hours of symptoms.

Antimicrobial Activity

Neuraminidase inhibitors inhibit influenza virus type A and type B by binding to a highly conserved region of the neuraminidase protein on the viral surface to inhibit viral penetration, replication, and disease [531]. The only neuraminidase inhibitor available for oral treatment in children younger than 6 years is oseltamivir [1,532] because this drug has been shown to be safe and effective at reducing both the duration and severity of influenza symptoms in adult and pediatric patients over the age of 1 year [533–538]. However, neuraminidase inhibitor resistance among circulating influenza strains is increasing.

Pharmacokinetic Data

Oseltamivir PK has been established in adults and children more than 1 year of age [532,539], but infant PK is unknown. Oseltamivir has excellent bioavailability after oral dosing and is extensively converted by hepatic esterases to oseltamivir carboxylate. At least 75% of an oral dose reaches the systemic circulation as the active form oseltamivir carboxylate. This active form is then renally excreted. Oseltamivir carboxylate is not a substrate for, nor an inhibitor of, cytochrome P450 enzymes. PK analysis in children revealed that younger patients cleared both the prodrug and the active metabolite faster than adult patients, resulting in a lower exposure for a given milligram per kilogram dose.

Safety

Oseltamivir has been well tolerated in adult and pediatric clinical trials [1,535,536,540,541]. The most common reported adverse events are related to gastrointestinal disturbances, particularly nausea and vomiting, but its safety has not been determined in infants under 1 year of age. Roche Laboratory, Inc. issued an alert in 2003 that oseltamivir should not be used in infants younger than 1 year old because one animal study showed high mortality in 7-day-old rats treated with 500 times the typical human dose [542]. Interestingly, rats treated with 250 times the typical human dose did not experience side effects or mortality. These young rats had higher plasma levels of prodrug and higher drug concentrations in the CNS than older rats; however, levels far exceeded those experienced in human studies. The relevance to humans remains unknown and there is great uncertainty in extrapolating juvenile animal data to human infants. The Better Pharmaceutics for Children Act (BPCA) executive summary states that it was considered unlikely that infants older than 3 to 6 months of age would be at significant risk [543]. Two case series of oseltamivir treatment in a total of 154 infants under 1 year of age revealed no serious complications [544,545].

In response to the H1N1 epidemic, the FDA in October 2009 issued an Emergency Use Authorization for Oseltamivir to include dosing recommendations for infants less than 1 year of age. In light of the limited data on safety and dosing, health care providers are encouraged to limit use to infants with confirmed H1N1 influenza or infant that have been exposed to a confirmed 2009 H1N1 influenza case and to carefully monitor for adverse events [546].

Clinical Implication

Infants are at high risk for influenza associated morbidity and mortality. In infants hospitalized with influenza, the possible benefit of therapy may outweigh the risks. An ongoing clinical trial supported by the NICHD funded Collaborative Antiviral Study Group will provide safety and PK information for oseltamivir in neonates and young infants.

ANTIFUNGAL MEDICATIONS

In the extremely premature infant, invasive candidiasis is common, often fatal, and frequently results in severe neurodevelopmental impairment. The therapeutic agents of choice in the nursery have been fluconazole and amphotericin products. Echinocandins are emerging as first-line therapy in older patients and their PK, safety, and efficacy are under investigation in young infants.

A hallmark of neonatal candidiasis is (CNS) infection. The incidence of CNS involvement is higher in the young infant than older patients; and invasive candidiasis (isolation of *Candida* from normally sterile body fluids) from any source has been associated with neurodevelopmental impairment. The diagnosis of CNS disease is very difficult, such that CNS involvement should be presumed in the young, premature infant.

Meningoencephalitis

CNS infection is not limited to meningitis; CNS infection with *Candida* is more accurately described as meningoencephalitis. Because the infection is based in brain tissue, it is likely that brain tissue penetration is more important to management of CNS infection with *Candida* rather than a strict assessment of penetration into the cerebrospinal fluid. This helps explain why amphotericin B deoxycholate and the echinocandins are likely to be effective in treating invasive candidiasis in young infants, provided that the levels of these products in the blood are sufficiently high to drive the product into the brain.

Amphotericin B

Amphotericin B (approved in 1958) is so named because it is amphoteric, forming soluble salts in both acidic and basic environments [547]. However, because of its insolubility in water, amphotericin B for clinical use is actually amphotericin B mixed with the detergent deoxycholate in a 3:7 mixture [547,548].

Antimicrobial Activity

Amphotericin products bind to ergosterol, the major sterol found in fungal cytoplasmic membranes [549,550]. The lipophilic amphotericin B acts by preferential binding to fungal membrane ergosterols, creating transmembrane channels, which result in an increased permeability to monovalent cations. The fungicidal activity is believed to be due to a damaged barrier and subsequent cell death through leakage of essential nutrients from the fungal cell. Amphotericin B also has oxidant activity, which disrupts cellular metabolism, inhibits proton ATPase pumps, depletes cellular energy reserves, and promotes lipid peroxidation to result in an increase in membrane fragility and ionized calcium leakage [549,550].

Pharmacokinetic Data

Amphotericin B is released from its carrier and is distributed very efficiently (greater than 90%) with lipoproteins. The antifungal drug is taken up preferentially by organs of the reticuloendothelial system, and follows a three-compartment distribution model. There is an initial 24- to 48-hour half-life reflecting uptake by host lipids, very slow release, and excretion into urine and bile, and a subsequent terminal half-life of up to 15 days [551]. In a small series (n = 13) evaluating the pharmacokinetics of amphotericin B among premature infants (27.4 ± 5 weeks), nine subjects showed elimination of amphotericin B at steady state with an estimated elimination half-life of 14.8 hours. The rest of the infants, however, showed minimal drug elimination during the dosing interval suggesting substantial drug accumulation and interindividual variability [552]. In a small series of premature infants born at 27.4 (± 5) weeks gestational age (n = 5), CSF amphotericin B concentrations were 40% to 90% of serum concentrations obtained simultaneously [552].

Safety

Tolerance to amphotericin B deoxycholate is limited by its acute and chronic toxicities. In addition to fungal ergosterol, the drug also interacts with cholesterol in human cell membranes; this likely accounts for its toxicity [553]. Amphotericin B also has a constrictive effect on renal arterioles, leading to a reduction in the glomerular filtration rate [554]. Up to 80% of older patients receiving amphotericin B develop either infusion-related toxicity or nephrotoxicity [547]; however, the product is likely better tolerated in young infants. Renal function usually returns to normal after cessation of amphotericin B, although permanent renal impairment is common after larger doses in older patients [555].

PK-PD and Clinical Implications

Experimental in vitro and in vivo studies support concentration-dependent killing with a prolonged post-antifungal effect, suggesting large daily doses will be most effective and that achieving optimal peak concentrations is important [556]. Peak levels are achieved 1 hour after a 4-hour infusion and reach a plateau at the third consecutive day of a constant dose. (4). The total dose administered over time correlates with increased tissue concentrations, suggesting a progressive accumulation with continued drug administration [557]. However, there is no evidence of a clinical dose effect [558] to support higher doses (greater than 1 mg/kg/day) of amphotericin B [559]. Cerebrospinal fluid (CSF) values are only 2% to 4% of serum concentrations and sometimes difficult to detect [560]. Yet, a small case series completed in young infants suggests that the penetration of the product may be greater in this population. As the drug penetrates well into brain tissue, 1 mg/kg dosing should be sufficient for central nervous infections (see "Meningoencephalitis").

Amphotericin B Lipid-Associated Formulations

In addition to conventional amphotericin B deoxycholate, three fundamentally different lipid-associated formulations have been developed that offer the advantage of an increased daily dose of the parent drug, better delivery to the primary reticuloendothelial organs (lungs, liver, spleen), and reduced toxicity: amphotericin B lipid complex (ABLC), amphotericin B colloidal dispersion (ABCD), and liposomal amphotericin B (L-amphotericin B) [561–563].

ABLC is a tightly packed, ribbon-like structure of a bilayered membrane formed by combining dimyristoylphosphatidylcholine, dimyristoyl phosphatidylglycerol, and amphotericin B in a ratio of 7:3:3. ABCD is composed of disklike structures of cholesteryl sulfate complexed with amphotericin B in an equimolar ratio. L-amphotericin B consists of small, uniformly sized unilamellar vesicles of a lipid bilayer of hydrogenated soy phosphatidylcholine-distcaryl phosphatidylglycerol-cholesterol-amphotericin B in the ratio 2:0.8:1:0.4 [564,565].

Pharmacokinetic Data

Lipid formulations of amphotericin B generally have a slower onset of action and are less active than amphotericin B alone in time-kill studies, presumably due to the required disassociation of free amphotericin B from the lipid vehicle [566]. It is postulated that activated monocytes/macrophages take up drug-laden lipid formulations and transport them to the site of infection, where phospholipases release the free drug [563]. The different PK and toxicities of the lipid formulations are reflected in the dosing recommendations: ABLC is recommended at 5 mg/kg/day, ABCD at 3 to 5 mg/kg/day, and L-amphotericin B at 1 to 5 mg/kg/day. However, most clinical data have been obtained with the use of these preparations at 5 mg/kg/day.

The dosage of 5 mg/kg/day is especially pertinent to the young infant given the frequency of CNS disease (see previous "Meningoencephalitis" section). Animal studies suggest that on a similar dosing schedule, the lipid products are almost always not as potent as amphotericin B, but that the ability to safely administer higher daily doses of the parent drug improves their efficacy [560], such that they compare favorably with the amphotericin B deoxycholate preparation with less toxicity. A multicenter maximum-tolerated-dose study of L-amphotericin B using doses from 7.5 to 15 mg/kg/day found a nonlinear plasma pharmacokinetic profile with a maximal concentration at 10 mg/kg/day and no demonstrable dose-limiting nephrotoxicity or infusion-related toxicity [567].

Lipid formulations have the added benefit of increased tissue concentration compared with conventional amphotericin B, specifically in the liver, lungs, and spleen. However, it is not entirely clear whether these higher concentrations in tissue are truly available to the microfoci of infection. L-amphotericin B has a comparatively higher peak plasma level and prolonged circulation in plasma [565], while ABCD has a lower plasma level than amphotericin B after infusion but a longer half-life and larger volume of distribution [568].

Safety Data

Lipid formulations appear to stabilize amphotericin B in a self-associated state so that it is not available to interact with the cholesterol of human cellular membranes [565,569]. Another theory for the decreased nephrotoxicity of lipid formulations is the preferential binding of amphotericin B to serum high-density lipoproteins compared with amphotericin B's binding to low-density lipoproteins [570]. The high-density lipoprotein-bound amphotericin B appears to be released to the kidney more slowly, or to a lesser degree. For infusion-related toxicity there is a general agreement that L-amphotericin B has less toxicity than ABLC, whereas ABCD appears closer in toxicity to conventional amphotericin B [571,572].

Several reviews have focused on amphotericin B PK in children. In one study of five premature infants and five older children, the volume of distribution was smaller and the elimination clearance more rapid than previously reported in adults. Serum levels were approximately half of those in adults with comparable doses, and interpatient variability was marked in the premature infants [573].

PK-PD and Clinical Implications for Dosing

Antifungal efficacy is dependent on the AUC_{0-24}. The key target organ is the brain, even if the lumbar puncture is normal. Killing of the organism in the brain depends not only on AUC_{0-24} but also total AUC exposure during

therapy. That is, CNS disease usually requires extended therapy [574]. So while many sources suggest 1 or 2 weeks of antifungal therapy, we suggest at least 21 days. We acknowledge that optimal length of therapy is not known as of this writing.

There are no data or consensus opinions among authorities indicating improved efficacy of any new amphotericin B lipid formulation over conventional amphotericin B [561,563,567,571,575]. This fact leaves the clearest indication for a lipid formulation over amphotericin B to be reducing nephrotoxicity; however, nephrotoxicity in the young infant is thought to be uncommon.

Pyrimidine Analogues: 5-Fluorocytosine

5-Fluorocytosine (5-FC) is a fluorinated analogue of cytosine synthesized as a potential antitumor agent and initially approved for use in 1972 [561]. Unfortunately, most reports detail clinical failure with monotherapy for yeast infections [576]. The antimycotic activity of the drug results from the rapid conversion of 5-FC into 5-fluorouracil (5-FU) within susceptible fungal cells [577,578]. The two mechanisms of action of 5-FU are incorporation into fungal RNA in place of uridylic acid to inhibit fungal protein synthesis, and inhibition of thymidylate synthetase to inhibit fungal DNA synthesis [578]. The latter appears to be the dominant mechanism. Clinical and microbiologic antifungal resistance appears to develop quickly to 5-FC monotherapy.

Pharmacokinetic Data

Fungistatic 5-FC is thought to enhance the antifungal activity of amphotericin B, especially in anatomic sites where amphotericin B penetration is often suboptimal, such as cerebrospinal fluid (CSF), heart valves, and the vitreal body [558]. 5-FC penetrates well into most body sites because it is small, highly water soluble, and not bound by serum proteins to any great extent [578]. In a study involving 33 neonates in the UK treated with intravenous or oral 5-FC that underwent therapeutic drug monitoring, drug concentrations were low (trough, <20 mg/L or peak, <50 mg/L) in 40.5%; undetectable in 5.1%; high (trough level >40 mg/L or peak >80 mg/L) in 38.9%; and potentially toxic (>100 mg/L) in 9.9% [579].

Safety

The mechanism of toxicity for 5-FC is unknown; but toxicity is common and substantial. 5-FC may exacerbate myelosuppression; toxic levels may develop when in combination with amphotericin B due to nephrotoxicity of the amphotericin B and the decreased renal clearance of 5-FC [580]. If 5-FC is used, routine serum level monitoring is warranted because peak serum concentrations of 100 μg/mL or greater are associated with bone marrow aplasia. Approximately 50% of patients who receive the product experience substantial toxicity, including azotemia, renal tubular acidosis, and myelosuppression [581]. The product is also known to cause gastrointestinal complications and in the premature infant at risk for necrotizing enterocolitis, its use should be undertaken with extreme caution. Given the narrow therapeutic range and need for therapeutic drug monitoring and the need for oral administration in the United States, this drug is seldom used in neonates.

Clinical Implications

Nearly all clinical studies involving 5-FC are combination antifungal protocols for cryptococcal meningitis due to the inherently rather weak antifungal activity of 5-FC monotherapy. The use of 5-FC in premature neonates is discouraged. A study evaluating risk factors and mortality rates of neonatal candidiasis among extremely premature infants showed that infants with *Candida* meningitis who received amphotericin B in combination with 5-FC experiences a prolonged time to sterilization of the CSF compared with those receiving amphotericin B monotherapy (median of 17.5 versus 6 days, respectively) [582].

Azoles: Fluconazole and Voriconazole

The azoles are subdivided into imidazoles and triazoles on the basis of the number of nitrogens in the azole ring [549,583], with the structural differences resulting in different binding affinities for the cytochrome P-450 (CYP) enzyme system. The triazoles are the products used in young infants and will be covered here. Of the older first-generation triazoles, fluconazole is effective against most *Candida* species, but it is unreliable for the treatment of *Candida glabrata* and it is ineffective against the very rare cases of neonatal *Aspergillus* infections. Newer, second-generation triazoles (voriconazole, posaconazole, and ravuconazole) are modifications of prior triazoles with an expanded antifungal spectrum of activity and generally lower MIC values than the older compounds [584]. Only voriconazole has been investigated in children younger than 12 years.

Antimicrobial Activity

The azole antifungals are heterocyclic synthetic compounds that inhibit the fungal cytochrome P-450$_{14DM}$ (also known as lanosterol 14a-demethylase), which catalyzes a late step in ergosterol biosynthesis [583]. The drugs bind to the heme group in the target protein and block demethylation of the C-14 of lanosterol, leading to substitution of methylated sterols in the membrane and depletion of ergosterol. The result is an accumulation of precursors with abnormalities in fungal membrane permeability, membrane-bound enzyme activity, and lack of coordination of chitin synthesis [585,586].

Fluconazole

Fluconazole (Diflucan; Pfizer Inc., New York) is a bis-triazole approved by the FDA for use in treating cryptococcosis and *Candida* infections in 1990. An in vitro time-kill study showed that the rate of fluconazole fungistatic activity was not influenced by concentration once the maximal fungistatic concentration was surpassed, which is in contrast to the concentration-dependent fungicidal activity of amphotericin B [587] or caspofungin [588]. Fluconazole is well absorbed from the gastrointestinal tract and is cleared predominantly by the renal route as unchanged drug, whereas metabolism accounts for only a minor proportion of fluconazole clearance [589]. Binding to plasma proteins is low (12%) [590]. Gastric absorption of oral fluconazole is virtually unaffected by pH or the presence of food in the stomach.

Fluconazole is available as either an oral or an intravenous form, and oral fluconazole has a high bioavailability of approximately 90% relative to its intravenous administration. Fluconazole passes into tissues and fluids very rapidly, probably due to its relatively low lipophilicity and limited degree of binding to plasma proteins. Concentrations of fluconazole are 10- to 20-fold higher in the urine than in blood, and drug concentrations in the CSF and vitreous humor of the eye are approximately 80% of those found simultaneously in blood [590]. The concentrations of fluconazole in body fluids such as vaginal secretions, breast milk, saliva, and sputum are also similar to those in blood, and the fluid to blood ratio remains stable after multiple doses. There is a linear plasma concentration-dose relationship.

Simple conversion of the corresponding adult dosage of fluconazole on a weight basis is inappropriate for young infants. A recent population PK study in premature infants suggests that maintenance fluconazole doses of 12 mg/kg/day are necessary to achieve exposures similar to older children and adults [591]. In addition, a loading dose of 25 mg/kg would achieve steady state concentrations sooner than the traditional dosing scheme. This strategy is currently being evaluated in a phase I clinical trial.

Safety

Side effects of fluconazole are uncommon. In one study of 24 immunocompromised children, elevated transaminases were observed in only two cases [592]. A large review of 78 reports that used fluconazole in a total of 726 children younger than the age of 1 year showed it was generally well tolerated [593]. Another review of 562 children from 12 clinical studies confirmed that pediatric results mirror the excellent safety profile seen in adults. The most common side effects were gastrointestinal upset (7.7%) (vomiting, diarrhea, nausea) and a skin rash (1.2%) [594]. Fluconazole affects the metabolism of cyclosporine, leading to its increased concentration when they are used together [595].

PK-PD and Clinical Implications for Dosing

Fluconazole may be used as monotherapy for treatment of candidiasis in the nursery. It should be given 12 mg/kg daily. There does not appear to be antagonism if the product is used with amphotericin B. In a multicenter trial of 236 patients with invasive candidiasis, those treated with fluconazole plus amphotericin B versus fluconazole alone trended toward better success and more rapid resolution of *Candida* fungemia with the combination [596]. Fluconazole is particularly appropriate for urinary tract infections due to its concentrating effect in the bladder. Fluconazole is also effective for superficial skin infections because the stratum corneum:serum ratio is high [597].

Some centers use fluconazole for prophylaxis; however, this is not yet considered standard of care. In a single-center blind trial over a 30-month period 100 infants with birth weights less than 1000 g, those infants who received fluconazole for 6 weeks had a decrease in the development of invasive fungal infection compared with the placebo (0% vs. 20%) [598]. A larger prospective, randomized double-blind, controlled trial conducted in 8 NICUs in Italy among 322 infants with birth weight less than 1500 g showed that a fluconazole prophylaxis regimen of 3 to 6 mg/kg several times per week for 4 to 6 weeks reduced the incidence of *Candida* colonization [9.8% in the 6 mg group, 7.7% in the 3 mg group, and 29.2% in the placebo group ($P<.001$)] and invasive fungal infections [2.7% in the 6 mg group (P=0.005), 3.8% in the 3 mg group (P=0.02), and 13.2% in the placebo group] [599]. A retrospective study evaluating the incidence of invasive candidiasis and *Candida*-related mortality among infants with birth weights less than 1000 g who received fluconazole prophylaxis (3 mg/kg several times per week) for 6 weeks showed that the incidence of invasive candidiasis and *Candida*-associated mortality decreased. In the group receiving fluconazole, no increase in fluconazole resistant *Candida* strains was observed [600]. Similarly, another report demonstrated that the use of fluconazole prophylaxis for 4 to 6 weeks in infants with birth weights less than 1500 g did not increase the incidence of fungal colonization and infections caused by natively fluconazole-resistant *Candida* species [601].

Results of fluconazole prophylaxis studies in premature infants are encouraging; however, the universal implementation of such a strategy across nurseries has not been broadly used because: (1) the rate of *Candida* infections vary greatly among centers [602] and (2) there are insufficient neurodevelopmental follow-up data in these infants to justify prophylaxis [603]. A multicenter international trial is underway to answer questions regarding the need of prophylaxis based on rates of systemic *Candida* infections in individual nurseries.

Voriconazole

Voriconazole (VFend; Pfizer Inc., New York) is a second-generation triazole and a synthetic derivative of fluconazole. Voriconazole has activity against most *Candida* species and against *Aspergillus* [604–608].

Pharmacokinetic Data

Voriconazole is extensively metabolized by the liver and its bioavailability in adults is approximately 90%. It appears that CYP2C19 plays a major role in the metabolism of voriconazole, and this enzyme exhibits genetic polymorphism, dividing the population into poor and extensive metabolizers as a result of a point mutation in the gene encoding the protein CYP2C19 [609]. About 5% to 7% of the white population has a deficiency in expressing this enzyme, so genotype plays a key role in the pharmacokinetics of voriconazole [610]. As many as 20% of non-Indian Asians have low CYP2C19 activity and can achieve voriconazole levels as much as fourfold greater than those homozygous subjects who metabolize the drug more extensively [611].

Voriconazole is 44% to 67% plasma bound with nonlinear pharmacokinetics, has a variable half-life of approximately 6 hours [612] with large interpatient variation in blood levels [613] and good CSF penetration [584,585,614–618]. Time-kill studies against *Candida* species and *Cryptococcus neoformans* revealed in vitro non-concentration-dependent fungistatic activity, similar to that of fluconazole [587].

Oral absorption is nonlinear and rapid, with an approximately fivefold accumulation over 14 days in one study of

hematologic malignancy patients [618]. In a study assessing voriconazole levels after intravenous-to-oral switching, mean voriconazole levels did fall following oral administration compared with intravenous administration, but most subjects achieved steady state 4 days after dosing began. Maximum plasma voriconazole levels occurred at the end of the 1-hour intravenous infusion and between 1.4 and 1.8 hours after oral administration [611]. A PK study in six cirrhosis patients demonstrated hepatic-impaired patients should receive the same oral loading dose, but half the maintenance dose [619]. In contrast to adults, elimination of voriconazole follows linear kinetics in children. They have a higher elimination capacity and therefore require a larger (4 mg/kg twice daily vs. 3 mg/kg twice daily) maintenance dose [124,125] after a 6-mg/kg load for two doses the first day of therapy [620,621]. The kinetics of the product in young infants are not known.

Safety

Voriconazole's main side effects include reversible dose-dependent visual disturbances (increased brightness, blurred vision) [618,622] in as many as one third of treated patients, elevated hepatic transaminases with increasing doses [622], and occasional skin reactions likely due to photosensitization [585,605,623]. The visual side effects have resulted in great caution in the use of the product in premature infants because of the concern of the developing retina as a target organ for toxicity. No such long-term effects have been observed nor studied in the young infant; however, most clinicians reserve this product for the occasional case of aspergillosis [624] and as a third-line agent for candidiasis.

PK-PD and Clinical Implications

A multicenter trial of voriconazole versus fluconazole for treating esophageal candidiasis in 391 immunocompromised patients showed similar success rates with voriconazole (98.3%) and fluconazole (95.1%) [625], although overall safety and tolerability of both antifungals were acceptable. In an open-label evaluation of 58 children with a proven or probable invasive fungal infection (most had aspergillosis). 45% percent of children had a complete or partial response, and only 7% were discontinued from voriconazole because of intolerance. The most commonly reported adverse events in these children included elevation in hepatic transaminases, skin rash, and photosensitivity reaction, and abnormal vision. Intravenously administered voriconazole has been used successfully in preterm infants of very low birth weight with primary cutaneous aspergillosis [626].

Echinocandins
Antimicrobial Activity

A relatively new class of antifungals, the echinocandins and the amino-containing pneumocandin analogues, are cyclic hexapeptide agents that interfere with cell wall biosynthesis by noncompetitive inhibition of 1,3-β-D-glucan synthase, an enzyme present in fungi but absent in mammalian cells [584,585]. This 1,3-β-d-glucan, an essential cell wall polysaccharide, forms a fibril of three helically entwined linear polysaccharides and provides structural integrity for the fungal cell wall [627,628].

Echinocandins inhibit hyphal tip growth, converting the mycelium into small clumps of cells, but the older septated cells with little glucan synthesis are not killed [629]. Therefore the echinocandin activity endpoint is morphologic change, not in vitro medium clearing. Echinocandins are generally fungicidal in vitro against *Candida* species, although not as rapidly as amphotericin B [556,584], but appear to be fungistatic against *Aspergillus* [630]. As a class these agents are not metabolized through the CYP enzyme system, but through a presumed *O*-methyltransferase, lessening some of the drug interactions and side effects seen with the azole class. The echinocandins appear to have a prolonged and dose-dependent fungicidal antifungal effect on *C. albicans* compared with the fungistatic fluconazole [631].

Three compounds in this class (caspofungin, micafungin, and anidulafungin) are FDA-approved for use in adults. Few studies have evaluated the use of echinocandins in children; most constitute early phase I/II safety and pharmacokinetic studies. Because neonates with candidemia often suffer from disseminated disease in the central nervous system, which is associated with neurodevelopmental impairment, dosing of antifungal agents in this population should target the central nervous system.

An experimental rabbit model of hematogenous *Candida* meningoencephalitis in which micafungin was used as a prototype echinocandin suggests that doses of 8 mg/kg/day are necessary to achieve maximal microbicidal activity in the central nervous system parenchyma of rabbits [574]. When these data are extrapolated to the neonatal population using simulation techniques, the lowest fungal burden in the neonatal central nervous system parenchyma is achieved with micafungin doses of 10 to 15 mg/kg/day [574].

Caspofungin
Pharmacokinetic Data

Caspofungin (Cancidas; Merck Co., Whitehouse Station, N.J.) is a fungicidal, water-soluble, semisynthetic derivative of the natural product pneumocandin B_0 [632]. It has linear pharmacokinetics [633], is hepatically excreted with a β-phase half-life of 9 to 10 hours in adults [634], and has uncommon adverse effects [615]. Parenteral administration is preferred due to the low bioavailability when administered orally. It is not metabolized by the CYP isozyme system, and the rate of killing for caspofungin in time-kill studies is greater than that of amphotericin B, which does not require cell growth for activity [627].

There is no known maximal tolerated dose and no toxicity-determined maximal length of therapy. The usual course is to begin with a "load" followed by a lesser daily dose. PK appears slightly different in children compared with adults, with caspofungin levels lower in smaller children and with a reduced half-life [635]. PK projections suggest that dosing at 50 mg per m^2 appears to be more appropriate in children rather than using 1 mg/kg/day [636]. The kinetics in young infants are not well described, especially at dosages that should be used to clear central nervous system infections. Caspofungin given 25 mg/m^2 is thought to provide similar exposure to 50 mg/m^2 given to adults; however, this exposure is unlikely to clear central nervous system infections in young infants. Thus a recommended dosage cannot be provided from these data [637].

Safety

1,3-β-D-glucan is a selective target present only in fungal cell walls and not in mammalian cells; therefore, the echinocandins are rarely toxic in humans [627]. There appears to be no apparent myelotoxicity or nephrotoxicity with the agent [636,638,639].

PK-PD and Clinical Implications

Caspofungin was approved by the FDA in February 2001 for refractory aspergillosis or intolerance to other therapies, and in January 2003 was approved for candidemia and various other sites of invasive *Candida* infections in adults. In a multicenter trial of 239 patients with invasive candidiasis, 73.4% of patients who received caspofungin had a favorable response at the end of therapy, compared with 61.7% in the amphotericin B group [640]. Mortality was similar in both groups, and the proportion of patients with drug-related adverse events was higher in the amphotericin B group.

Caspofungin in newborns has been used off-label as single or adjuvant therapy for refractory cases of disseminated candidiasis. A study from Costa Rica reported the use of caspofungin (0.5 to 1 mg/kg/day for the first 2 to 3 days and 1 to 2 mg/kg/day for the remaining of the course) among 10 neonates (mean gestational age 33.5 ±1.77) with refractory disseminated candidiasis; all patients had a sterile blood culture within 3 to 7 days of starting caspofungin and the drug was well tolerated [641]. Through a retrospective chart review, another center identified 13 cases of neonates [median gestational age 27 weeks (range, 24 to 28)] treated with caspofungin (1 to 1.5 mg/kg/day) for refractory disseminated candidiasis; 11 of the infants achieved blood sterilization within a median of 3 days (range, 1 to 21). However, all but 3 patients had their intravascular lines removed before the onset of caspofungin therapy [642]. In this cohort, two patients died within 2 days of starting caspofungin; one patient developed severe thrombophlebitis after the initial dose; two patients had hypokalemia while on caspofungin; and four patients had a greater than three-fold elevation of alanine aminotransferase (ALT) and aspartate aminotransferase (AST) [642].

Additional studies of caspofungin in the pediatric population are necessary to assess its efficacy. In addition, pharmacokinetic studies in neonates are needed before the widespread use of this antifungal agent in the nursery.

Micafungin
Pharmacokinetic Data

Micafungin (Fujisawa Healthcare, Inc., Deerfield, Ill.) is an echinocandin lipopeptide compound [643] with a half-life of approximately 12 hours. There are dose-independent linear plasma pharmacokinetics with the highest drug concentrations detected in the lung, followed by the liver, spleen, and kidney. Micafungin (like the other echinocandins) does not penetrate the CSF [644], but levels were detected in the brain tissue, choroidal layer, meninges, and cerebellum in an experimental rabbit animal model [574]. The product therefore can be considered in premature and young infants (see "Meningoencephalitis" section). Time-kill study of micafungin against

Candida species demonstrated potent fungicidal activity against most isolates, including a concentration-dependent postantifungal effect [645].

The pharmacokinetics of micafungin have been well studied in young infants, perhaps more thoroughly than any other antifungal agent as of this writing. A phase I, sequential and single-dose (0.75, 1.5, and 3.0 mg/kg) study of intravenous micafungin in 18 premature infants (mean gestational age 26.4 ± 2.4 weeks) weighing more than 1000 g showed that micafungin pharmacokinetics in preterm infants was linear; premature infants displayed a shorter half-life (8 hours) and a more rapid rate of clearance (approximately 39 (mL/hr)/kg) compared with published data in older children and adults [646]. In this study, an additional 4 infants weighing less than 1000 g received 0.75 mg/kg/day of micafungin and demonstrated shorter mean half-life (5.5 hours) and more rapid mean clearance per body weight (79.3 ±12.5 (mL/hr)/kg) when compared with the heavier infants [646]. These results suggest that young infants may require higher micafungin doses when compared with older children and adults. Data from 12 premature infants (mean birth weight and gestational age 851 g and 27 weeks, respectively) suggests that a micafungin dose of 15 mg/kg/day achieves similar exposures (mean area under the curve 437.5 (±99.4) mg*hr/L) to adults receiving 5 mg/kg/day [647]. Micafungin doses of 7 to 10 mg/kg/day administered to 13 premature infants (mean birth weight and gestational age 1449 (±1211) g 27.3 (±4.68) weeks, respectively) provided adequate exposure (median area under the curve of 258.1 to 291.2 mg/hr/L) to treat central nervous system candidiasis [648].

Safety

The safety profile of micafungin is optimal when compared with other antifungal agents [1]. In clinical trials of micafungin, patients have demonstrated fewer adverse events compared with liposomal amphotericin B and fluconazole. The most common adverse events were related to the gastrointestinal tract (i.e., nausea, diarrhea). Hypersensitivity reactions associated with micafungin have been reported and 5% of patients receiving the product may develop liver enzyme elevation. Hyperbilirubinemia, renal impairment, and hemolytic anemia related to micafungin use have also been identified in postmarketing surveillance of the drug. The most common adverse events in a phase I micafungin study of 77 children (2 to 17 years of age) with fever and neutropenia were diarrhea (19.5%), epistaxis (18.2%), abdominal pain (16.9%), and headache (16.9%) [649]. Micafungin has very few drug interactions; however, when administered simultaneously it increases overall exposure (AUC) of sirolimus (21%), nifedipine (18%), and itraconazole (22%).

PK-PD and Clinical Implications

A pediatric substudy (n = 106, ages 0 to 16 years including 14 neonates) was conducted between 2003 and 2005 as part of a double-blind, randomized, multinational trial comparing micafungin (2 mg/kg/day) with liposomal amphotericin B (3 mg/kg/day) for first-line treatment for invasive candidiasis [650]. Treatment success was defined as clinical and mycologic response at the end of therapy. The median duration of study drug administration was 15 days for micafungin (range, 3 to 42 days) and 14.5 days for liposomal amphotericin B (range, 2 to 34 days). In a modified intent-to-treat analysis, the rate of overall treatment success was similar for micafungin (72.9%, 35/48) when compared with liposomal amphotericin B (76.0%, 38/50), with an adjusted difference between treatment groups of −2.4 (95% CI 20.1, 15.3) when stratified by neutropenic status. However, when stratified by age group, liposomal amphotericin B outperformed micafungin in all age groups except for the neonatal group [650]. This observation could be related to the low micafungin dose used in this trial. In general, micafungin was better tolerated than liposomal amphotericin B as evidenced by the fewer adverse events that led to discontinuation of therapy [650].

Anidulafungin
Pharmacokinetic Data

Anidulafungin (Pfizer) is a semisynthetic terphenyl-substituted antifungal derived from echinocandin B, a lipopeptide fungal product [651]. It has linear pharmacokinetics with the longest half-life of all the echinocandins (approximately 18 hours) [652] and has shown fungistatic or fungicidal activity in different settings [653]. Analysis in healthy rabbits revealed linear PK with dose-proportional increases in AUC [654]. Neither end-stage renal impairment, dialysis, nor mild to moderate hepatic failure changes the pharmacokinetics of anidulafungin in patients [655].

Tissue concentrations after multiple dosing were highest in lung and liver, followed by spleen and kidney, with measurable concentrations in the brain tissue. The PK showed approximately sixfold lower mean peak concentrations in plasma, and twofold lower AUC values compared with values with similar doses of caspofungin and micafungin.

There is only one study evaluating the PK of anidulafungin in children 2 to 17 years, and none in young infants [656]. The current anidulafungin formulation requires reconstitution with 20% dehydrated alcohol, therefore, its safety and PK profile in infants younger than 2 years is being evaluated in a new formulation that does not contain alcohol.

Safety

Anidulafungin has an excellent safety profile and appears to be well tolerated [657]. A phase I study reported anidulafungin to be well tolerated in 29 healthy volunteers, with the highest dose cohort experiencing transient liver function test elevations that exceeded twice the upper limit of normal [658]. In a separate study, 12 subjects with mild or moderate hepatic impairment did not cause clinically significant changes in the PK parameters of anidulafungin [659]. However, in patients with severe hepatic impairment, the plasma concentrations of anidulafungin are decreased and plasma clearance increased [660]. In a study of 25 neutropenic children receiving anidulafungin as empirical therapy, rare adverse events included facial erythema and rash, elevation in serum blood urea nitrogen, and fever and hypotension [656].

PK-PD and Clinical Implications

Clinical trials with anidulafungin are ongoing. A phase III, randomized, double-blind study in adult patients with invasive candidiasis showed that anidulafungin was not inferior to fluconazole in the treatment of invasive candidiasis [661]. The frequency and types of adverse events were similar in the two groups [661]. Neonatal and pediatric formulations and subsequent studies are needed.

REFERENCES

[1] Drug Label. Federal Drug Administration (FDA) Center for Drug Evaluation and Research. Available at www.accessdata.fda.gov/scripts/cder/drugsatfda/. Accessed Physicians' Desk Reference, Medical Economics. Available at www.pdr.net. Accessed 5/25/2010.
[2] L.E. Burns, J.E. Hodgman, A.B. Cass, Fatal circulatory collapse in premature infants receiving chloramphenicol, N. Engl. J. Med. 261 (1959) 1318–1321.
[3] A. Mulhall, J. de Louvois, R. Hurley, Chloramphenicol toxicity in neonates: its incidence and prevention, Br. Med. J. (Clin. Res. Ed.) 287 (1983) 1424–1427.
[4] O. Ramilo, B.T. Kinane, G.H. McCracken Jr., Chloramphenicol neurotoxicity, Pediatr. Infect. Dis. J. 7 (1988) 358–359.
[5] J.M. Sutherland, Fatal cardiovascular collapse of infants receiving large amounts of chloramphenicol, AMA J. Dis. Child. 97 (1959) 761–767.
[6] C.F. Weiss, A.J. Glazko, J.K. Weston, Chloramphenicol in the newborn infant. A physiologic explanation of its toxicity when given in excessive doses, N. Engl. J. Med. 262 (1960) 787–794.
[7] B. Chavers, C.M. Kjellstrand, S.M. Mauer, Exchange transfusion in acute chloramphenicol toxicity, J. Pediatr. 101 (1982) 652.
[8] S.M. Mauer, B.M. Chavers, C.M. Kjellstrand, Treatment of an infant with severe chloramphenicol intoxication using charcoal-column hemoperfusion, J. Pediatr. 96 (1980) 136–139.
[9] D.L. Kessler Jr., A.L. Smith, D.E. Woodrum, Chloramphenicol toxicity in a neonate treated with exchange transfusion, J. Pediatr. 96 (1980) 140–141.
[10] J.V. Aranda, S.J. Yaffe (Eds.), Neonatal and Pediatric Pharmacology: Therapeutic Principles in Practice, third ed. Lippincott, Williams, & Wilkins, Philadelphia, 2005.
[11] K. Allegaert, et al., Developmental pharmacology: neonates are not just small adults, Acta Clin. Belg. 63 (2008) 16–24.
[12] G.L. Kearns, et al., Developmental pharmacology: drug disposition, action, and therapy in infants and children, N. Engl. J. Med. 349 (2003) 1157–1167.
[13] A. Boccazzi, et al., Comparison of the concentrations of ceftazidime in the serum of newborn infants after intravenous and intramuscular administration, Antimicrob. Agents Chemother. 24 (1983) 955–956.
[14] A. Mulhall, Antibiotic treatment of neonates: does route of administration matter? Dev. Pharmacol. Ther. 8 (1985) 1–8.
[15] B. Friis-Hansen, Body water compartments in children: changes during growth and related changes in body composition, Pediatrics 28 (1961) 169–181.
[16] R. Wise, The clinical relevance of protein binding and tissue concentrations in antimicrobial therapy, Clin. Pharmacokinet. 11 (1986) 470–482.
[17] H. Kurz, A. Mauser-Ganshorn, H.H. Stickel. Differences in the binding of drugs to plasma proteins from newborn and adult man, Eur. J. Clin. Pharmacol. 11 (1977) 463–467.
[18] W.J. Cashore, W. Oh, R. Brodersen, Bilirubin-displacing effect of furosemide and sulfisoxazole. An in vitro and in vivo study in neonatal serum, Dev. Pharmacol. Ther. 6 (1983) 230–238.
[19] H.R. Stutman, K.M. Parker, M.I. Marks, Potential of moxalactam and other new antimicrobial agents for bilirubin-albumin displacement in neonates, Pediatrics 75 (1985) 294–298.
[20] J.M. Gulian, et al., Bilirubin displacement by ceftriaxone in neonates: evaluation by determination of "free" bilirubin and erythrocyte-bound bilirubin, J. Antimicrob. Chemother. 19 (1987) 823–829.
[21] W.A. Silverman, et al., A difference in mortality rate and incidence of kernicterus among premature infants allotted to two prophylactic antibacterial regimens, Pediatrics 18 (1956) 614–625.
[22] R. Brodersen, B. Friis-Hansen, L. Stern, Drug-induced displacement of bilirubin from albumin in the newborn, Dev. Pharmacol. Ther. 6 (1983) 217–229.
[23] A. Robertson, W. Karp, R. Brodersen, Bilirubin displacing effect of drugs used in neonatology, Acta Paediatr. Scand. 80 (1991) 1119–1127.
[24] A. Robertson, S. Fink, W. Karp, Effect of cephalosporins on bilirubin-albumin binding, J. Pediatr. 112 (1988) 291–294.
[25] P.C. Walker, Neonatal bilirubin toxicity. A review of kernicterus and the implications of drug-induced bilirubin displacement, Clin. Pharmacokinet. 13 (1987) 26–50.
[26] M.J. Blake, et al., Ontogeny of drug metabolizing enzymes in the neonate, Semin. Fetal. Neonatal. Med. 10 (2005) 123–138.
[27] K. Allegaert, et al., Renal drug clearance in preterm neonates: relation to prenatal growth, Ther. Drug. Monit. 29 (2007) 284–291.
[28] M.G. Myers, R.J. Roberts, N.J. Mirhij, Effects of gestational age, birth weight, and hypoxemia on pharmacokinetics of amikacin in serum of infants, Antimicrob. Agents Chemother. 11 (1977) 1027–1032.
[29] G.L. Drusano, Pharmacokinetics and pharmacodynamics of antimicrobials. Clin. Infect. Dis. 45 (Suppl. 1) (2007) S89–S95.
[30] G.L. Drusano, Antimicrobial pharmacodynamics: critical interactions of "bug and drug". Nat. Rev. Microbiol. 2 (2004) 289–300.
[31] R.H. Levy, L.A. Bauer, Basic pharmacokinetics, Ther. Drug. Monit. 8 (1986) 47–58.
[32] D.R. Andes, W.A. Craig, Pharmacokinetics and pharmacodynamics of antibiotics in meningitis, Infect. Dis. Clin. North. Am. 13 (1999) 595–618.
[33] U.B. Schaad, et al., Pharmacokinetics and bacteriological efficacy of moxalactam (LY127935), netilmicin, and ampicillin in experimental gram-negative enteric bacillary meningitis, Antimicrob. Agents Chemother. 17 (1980) 406–411.
[34] C. Odio, M.L. Thomas, G.H. McCracken Jr., Pharmacokinetics and bacteriological efficacy of mezlocillin in experimental Escherichia coli and Listeria monocytogenes meningitis, Antimicrob. Agents Chemother. 25 (1984) 427–432.
[35] G.H. McCracken Jr., Y. Sakata, K.D. Olsen, Aztreonam therapy in experimental meningitis due to Haemophilus influenzae type b and Escherichia coli K1, Antimicrob. Agents Chemother. 27 (1985) 655–656.
[36] J.S. Bradley, G.L. Drusano, Predicting efficacy of antiinfectives with pharmacodynamics and Monte Carlo simulation, Pediatr. Infect. Dis. J. 22 (2003) 982–992, quiz 993–995.
[37] W.A. Craig, Pharmacokinetic/pharmacodynamic parameters: rationale for antibacterial dosing of mice and men, Clin. Infect. Dis. 26 (1998) 1–10, quiz 11–12.
[38] U. Amann, et al., Antibiotics in pregnancy: analysis of potential risks and determinants in a large German statutory sickness fund population, Pharmacoepidemiol. Drug Saf. 15 (2006) 327–337.
[39] J.R. Niebyl, Antibiotics and other anti-infective agents in pregnancy and lactation, Am. J. Perinatol. 20 (2003) 405–414.
[40] M.R. Syme, J.W. Paxton, J.A. Keelan, Drug transfer and metabolism by the human placenta, Clin. Pharmacokinet. 43 (2004) 487–514.
[41] A. Philipson, L.D. Sabath, D. Charles, Transplacental passage of erythromycin and clindamycin, N. Engl. J. Med. 288 (1973) 1219–1221.
[42] B. Bernard, et al., Tobramycin: maternal-fetal pharmacology, Antimicrob. Agents. Chemother. 11 (1977) 688–694.
[43] B. Bernard, et al., Maternal-fetal pharmacological activity of amikacin, J. Infect. Dis. 135 (1977) 925–932.
[44] S. Matsuda, et al., Evaluation of amikacin in obstetric and gynecological fields (author's transl), Jpn. J. Antibiot. 27 (1974) 633–636.
[45] M. Buckingham, et al., Gastro-intestinal absorption and transplacental transfer of amoxicillin during labour and the influence of metoclopramide, Curr. Med. Res. Opin. 3 (1975) 392–396.
[46] H. Nau, Clinical pharmacokinetics in pregnancy and perinatology. II. Penicillins, Dev. Pharmacol. Ther. 10 (1987) 174–198.
[47] D.A. Kafetzis, D.C. Brater, J.E. Fanourgakis, Materno-fetal transfer of azlocillin, J. Antimicrob. Chemother. 12 (1983) 157–162.
[48] D. Charles, B. Larsen (Eds.), Placental Transfer of Antibiotics, Raven Press, New York, 1984.
[49] B. Bernard, et al., Maternal-fetal transfer of cefazolin in the first twenty weeks of pregnancy, J. Infect. Dis. 136 (1977) 377–382.
[50] A. Dekel, et al., Transplacental passage of cefazolin in the first trimester of pregnancy, Eur. J. Obstet. Gynecol. Reprod. Biol. 10 (1980) 303–307.
[51] K. Shimizu, Cefoperazone: absorption, excretion, distribution, and metabolism, Clin. Ther. 3 (1980) 60–79.
[52] G.G. Briggs, R.K. Freeman, S.J. Yaffe (Eds.), Drugs in Pregnancy and Lactation: a Reference Guide to Fetal and Neonatal Risk, Williams & Wilkins, Baltimore, 1998.
[53] D.A. Kafetzis, et al., Transfer of cefotaxime in human milk and from mother to foetus, J. Antimicrob. Chemother. 6 (Suppl. A) (1980) 135–141.
[54] D.A. Kafetzis, et al., Ceftriaxone distribution between maternal blood and fetal blood and tissues at parturition and between blood and milk postpartum, Antimicrob. Agents Chemother. 23 (1983) 870–873.
[55] I. Craft, B.M. Mullinger, M.R. Kennedy, Placental transfer of cefuroxime, Br. J. Obstet. Gynaecol. 88 (1981) 141–145.
[56] P. Bousfield, et al., Cefuroxime: potential use in pregnant women at term, Br. J. Obstet. Gynaecol. 88 (1981) 146–149.
[57] D.E. Holt, et al., Transplacental transfer of cefuroxime in uncomplicated pregnancies and those complicated by hydrops or changes in amniotic fluid volume, Arch. Dis. Child. 68 (1993) 54–57.
[58] G. Creatsas, et al., A study of the kinetics of cephapirin and cephalexin in pregnancy, Curr. Med. Res. Opin. 7 (1980) 43–46.
[59] S. Morrow, P. Palmisano, G. Cassady, The placental transfer of cephalothin, J. Pediatr. 73 (1968) 262–264.
[60] W.C. Scott, R.F. Warner, Placental transfer of chloramphenicol (Chloromycetin), JAMA 142 (1950) 1331–1332.
[61] S. Ross, et al., Placental transmission of chloramphenicol (Chloromycetin), JAMA 142 (1950) 1361.
[62] A.J. Weinstein, R.S. Gibbs, M. Gallagher, Placental transfer of clindamycin and gentamicin in term pregnancy, Am. J. Obstet. Gynecol. 124 (1976) 688–691.
[63] L. Herngren, M. Ehrnebo, L.O. Boreus, Drug binding to plasma proteins during human pregnancy and in the perinatal period. Studies on cloxacillin and alprenolol, Dev. Pharmacol. Ther. 6 (1983) 110–124.
[64] M.A. MacAulay, S.R. Berg, D. Charles, Placental transfer of dicloxacillin at term, Am. J. Obstet. Gynecol. 102 (1968) 1162–1168.
[65] M.A. MacAulay, D. Charles, Placental transfer of cephalothin, Am. J. Obstet. Gynecol. 100 (1968) 940–946.

[66] R. Depp, et al., Transplacental passage of methicillin and dicloxacillin into the fetus and amniotic fluid, Am. J. Obstet. Gynecol. 107 (1970) 1054–1057.

[67] L. Kiefer, et al., The placental transfer of erythromycin, Am. J. Obstet. Gynecol. 69 (1955) 174–177.

[68] H. Yoshioka, T. Monma, S. Matsuda, Placental transfer of gentamicin, J. Pediatr. 80 (1972) 121–123.

[69] C.S. L'Hommedieu, et al., Potentiation of magnesium sulfate–induced neuromuscular weakness by gentamicin, tobramycin, and amikacin, J. Pediatr. 102 (1983) 629–631.

[70] A. Heikkila, O.V. Renkonen, R. Erkkola, Pharmacokinetics and transplacental passage of imipenem during pregnancy, Antimicrob. Agents Chemother. 36 (1992) 2652–2655.

[71] H.C. Jones, Intrauterine ototoxicity. A case report and review of literature, J. Natl. Med. Assoc. 65 (1973) 201–203.

[72] M.A. MacAulay, W.B. Molloy, D. Charles, Placental transfer of methicillin, Am. J. Obstet. Gynecol. 115 (1973) 58–65.

[73] J.E. Perry, A.L. Leblanc, Transfer of nitrofurantoin across the human placenta, Tex. Rep. Biol. Med. 25 (1967) 265–269.

[74] J.H.E. Woltz, H.A. Zintel, The transmission of penicillin to amniotic fluid and fetal blood in the human, Am. J. Obstet. Gynecol. 50 (1945) 330.

[75] M. Ziai, M. Finland, Placental transfer of sulfamethoxypyridazine, N. Engl. J. Med. 257 (1957) 1180–1181.

[76] R.A. Sparr, J.A. Pritchard, Maternal and newborn distribution and excretion of sulfamethoxypyridazine (Kynex), Obstet. Gynecol. 12 (1958) 131–134.

[77] H.I. Kantor, et al., Effect on bilirubin metabolism in the newborn of sulfisoxazole administered to the mother, Obstet. Gynecol. 17 (1961) 494–500.

[78] A.K. Brown, N. Cevik, Hemolysis and jaundice in the newborn following maternal treatment with sulfamethoxypyridazine (Kynex), Pediatrics 36 (1965) 742–744.

[79] R.P. Perkins, Hydrops fetalis and stillbirth in a male glucose-6-phosphate dehydrogenase-deficient fetus possibly due to maternal ingestion of sulfisoxazole: a case report, Am. J. Obstet. Gynecol. 111 (1971) 379–381.

[80] A.K. Khan, S.C. Truelove, Placental and mammary transfer of sulfasalazine, Br. Med. J. 2 (1979) 1553.

[81] A.H. Kline, R.J. Blattner, M. Lunin, Transplacental effect of tetracyclines on teeth, JAMA 188 (1964) 178–180.

[82] A.H. Kutscher, et al., Discoloration of teeth induced by tetracycline administered ante partum, JAMA 184 (1963) 586–587.

[83] A.L. Leblanc, J.E. Perry, Transfer of tetracycline across the human placenta, Tex. Rep. Biol. Med. 25 (1967) 541–545.

[84] L.M. McEwen, Trimethoprim-sulfamethoxazole mixture in pregnancy, BMJ 4 (1971) 490–491.

[85] A. Philipson, Pharmacokinetics of antibiotics in pregnancy and labour, Clin. Pharmacokinet. 4 (1979) 297–309.

[86] J.C. Mucklow, The fate of drugs in pregnancy, Clin. Obstet. Gynaecol. 13 (1986) 161–175.

[87] E. Esbjorner, G. Jarnerot, L. Wranne, Sulfasalazine and sulfapyridine serum levels in children to mothers treated with sulfasalazine during pregnancy and lactation, Acta Paediatr. Scand. 76 (1987) 137–142.

[88] V. Apgar, Drugs in pregnancy, JAMA 190 (1964) 840–841.

[89] J.M. Sutherland, I.J. Light, The effect of drugs upon the developing fetus, Pediatr. Clin. North Am. 12 (1965) 781–806.

[90] E.R. Grossman, Tetracycline and staining of the teeth, JAMA 255 (1986) 2442–2443.

[91] A.H. Kutscher, et al., Discoloration of deciduous teeth induced by administration of tetracycline antepartum, Am. J. Obstet. Gynecol. 96 (1966) 291–292.

[92] P. Lumbiganon, K. Pengsaa, T. Sookpranee, Ciprofloxacin in neonates and its possible adverse effect on the teeth, Pediatr. Infect. Dis. J. 10 (1991) 619–620.

[93] K. Krasinski, R. Perkin, J. Rutledge, Gray baby syndrome revisited, Clin. Pediatr. (Phila) 21 (1982) 571–572.

[94] S. Ito, et al., Prospective follow-up of adverse reactions in breast-fed infants exposed to maternal medication, Am. J. Obstet. Gynecol. 168 (1993) 1393–1399.

[95] A.M. Chung, M.D. Reed, J.L. Blumer, Antibiotics and breast-feeding: a critical review of the literature, Paediatr. Drugs 4 (2002) 817–837.

[96] J.T. Wilson, Determinants and consequences of drug excretion in breast milk, Drug Metab. Rev. 14 (1983) 619–652.

[97] C.S. Catz, G.P. Giacoia, Drugs and breast milk, Pediatr. Clin. North Am. 19 (1972) 151–166.

[98] J.T. Wilson, et al., Drug excretion in human breast milk: principles, pharmacokinetics and projected consequences, Clin. Pharmacokinet. 5 (1980) 1–66.

[99] S. Ito, Drug therapy for breast-feeding women, N. Engl. J. Med. 343 (2000) 118–126.

[100] J.T. Wilson, et al., Pharmacokinetic pitfalls in the estimation of the breast milk/plasma ratio for drugs, Annu. Rev. Pharmacol. Toxicol. 25 (1985) 667–689.

[101] D.A. Kafetzis, et al., Passage of cephalosporins and amoxicillin into the breast milk, Acta Paediatr. Scand. 70 (1981) 285–288.

[102] A. Dresse, et al., Transmammary passage of cefoxitin: additional results, J. Clin. Pharmacol. 23 (1983) 438–440.

[103] H. Yoshioka, et al., Transfer of cefazolin into human milk, J. Pediatr. 94 (1979) 151–152.

[104] B. Fulton, L.L. Moore, Antiinfectives in breast milk. Part I: Penicillins and cephalosporins, J. Hum. Lact. 8 (1992) 157–158.

[105] S. Matsuda, Transfer of antibiotics into maternal milk, Biol. Res. Pregnancy Perinatol. 5 (1984) 57–60.

[106] P. Bourget, V. Quinquis-Desmaris, H. Fernandez, Ceftriaxone distribution and protein binding between maternal blood and milk postpartum, Ann. Pharmacother. 27 (1993) 294–297.

[107] M. Dubois, et al., A study of the transplacental transfer and the mammary excretion of cefoxitin in humans, J. Clin. Pharmacol. 21 (1981) 477–483.

[108] W.C. Shyu, et al., Excretion of cefprozil into human breast milk, Antimicrob. Agents Chemother. 36 (1992) 938–941.

[109] I. Matheson, M. Samseth, H.A. Sande, Ampicillin in breast milk during puerperal infections, Eur. J. Clin. Pharmacol. 34 (1988) 657–659.

[110] P.E. Branebjerg, L. Heisterberg, Blood and milk concentrations of ampicillin in mothers treated with pivampicillin and in their infants, J. Perinat. Med. 15 (1987) 555–558.

[111] J.D. Blanco, et al., Ceftazidime levels in human breast milk, Antimicrob. Agents Chemother. 23 (1983) 479–480.

[112] Academy of Pediatrics CoD, Transfer of drugs and other chemicals into human milk, Pediatrics 108 (2001) 776–789.

[113] P.M. Fleiss, et al., Aztreonam in human serum and breast milk, Br. J. Clin. Pharmacol. 19 (1985) 509–511.

[114] H. Giamarellou, et al., Pharmacokinetics of three newer quinolones in pregnant and lactating women, Am. J. Med. 87 (1989) 49S–51S.

[115] D.K. Gardner, S.G. Gabbe, C. Harter, Simultaneous concentrations of ciprofloxacin in breast milk and in serum in mother and breast-fed infant, Clin. Pharm. 11 (1992) 352–354.

[116] H.C. Atkinson, E.J. Begg, B.A. Darlow, Drugs in human milk. Clinical pharmacokinetic considerations, Clin. Pharmacokinet. 14 (1988) 217–240.

[117] D.J. Stewart, Teeth discoloured by tetracycline bleaching following exposure to daylight, Dent. Pract. Dent. Rec. 20 (1970) 309–310.

[118] H. Stang, Pyloric stenosis associated with erythromycin ingested through breast milk, Minn. Med. 69 (1986) 669–670 682.

[119] C.F. Mann, Clindamycin and breast-feeding, Pediatrics 66 (1980) 1030–1031.

[120] L. Heisterberg, P.E. Branebjerg, Blood and milk concentrations of metronidazole in mothers and infants, J. Perinat. Med. 11 (1983) 114–120.

[121] M. Rustia, P. Shubik, Experimental induction of hepatomas, mammary tumors, and other tumors with metronidazole in noninbred Sas:MRC(WI) BR rats, J. Natl. Cancer Inst. 63 (1979) 863–868.

[122] M. Rustia, P. Shubik, Induction of lung tumors and malignant lymphomas in mice by metronidazole, J. Natl. Cancer Inst. 48 (1972) 721–729.

[123] M.S. Legator, T.H. Connor, M. Stoeckel, Detection of mutagenic activity of metronidazole and niridazole in body fluids of humans and mice, Science 188 (1975) 1118–1119.

[124] C.M. Beard, et al., Cancer after exposure to metronidazole, Mayo Clin. Proc. 63 (1988) 147–153.

[125] C.M. Beard, et al., Lack of evidence for cancer due to use of metronidazole, N. Engl. J. Med. 301 (1979) 519–522.

[126] H.C. Neu, Penicillin-binding proteins and beta-lactamases: their effects on the use of cephalosporins and other new beta-lactams, Curr. Clin. Top. Infect. Dis. 8 (1987) 37–61.

[127] H.C. Neu, Contribution of beta-lactamases to bacterial resistance and mechanisms to inhibit beta-lactamases, Am. J. Med. 79 (1985) 2–12.

[128] J.H. Nayler, Resistance to beta-lactams in gram-negative bacteria: relative contributions of beta-lactamase and permeability limitations, J. Antimicrob. Chemother. 19 (1987) 713–732.

[129] E. Tuomanen, D.T. Durack, A. Tomasz, Antibiotic tolerance among clinical isolates of bacteria, Antimicrob. Agents Chemother. 30 (1986) 521–527.

[130] S. Dahesh, et al., Point mutation in the group B streptococcal pbp2x gene conferring decreased susceptibility to beta-lactam antibiotics, Antimicrob. Agents Chemother. 52 (2008) 2915–2918.

[131] F. Van Bambeke, et al., Multidrug-resistant *Streptococcus pneumoniae* infections: current and future therapeutic options, Drugs 67 (2007) 2355–2382.

[132] G.H. McCracken Jr., et al., Clinical pharmacology of penicillin in newborn infants, J. Pediatr. 82 (1973) 692–698.

[133] N.N. Huang, R.H. High, Comparison of serum levels following the administration of oral and parenteral preparations of penicillin to infants and children of various age groups, J. Pediatr. 42 (1953) 657–658.

[134] J.O. Klein, et al., Levels of penicillin in serum of newborn infants after single intramuscular doses of benzathine penicillin G, J. Pediatr. 82 (1973) 1065–1068.

[135] J.M. Kaplan, J.G.H. McCracken, Clinical pharmacology of benzathine penicillin G in neonates with regard to its recommended use in congenital syphilis, J. Pediatr. 82 (1973) 1069–1072.

[136] J.P. Hieber, J.D. Nelson, A pharmacologic evaluation of penicillin in children with purulent meningitis, N. Engl. J. Med. 297 (1977) 410–413.

[137] G.H. McCracken Jr., J.M. Kaplan, Penicillin treatment for congenital syphilis. A critical reappraisal, JAMA 228 (1974) 855–858.

[138] M.E. Speer, et al., Cerebrospinal fluid levels of benzathine penicillin G in the neonate, J. Pediatr. 91 (1977) 996–997.

[139] M.E. Speer, E.O. Mason, J.T. Scharnberg, Cerebrospinal fluid concentrations of aqueous procaine penicillin G in the neonate, Pediatrics 67 (1981) 387–388.

[140] American Academy of Pediatrics. Committee on Infectious Diseases. Red Book: Report of the Committee on Infectious Diseases, American Academy of Pediatrics, Elk Grove Village, Ill, 2007.

[141] G.H. McCracken Jr., S.G. Mize, N. Threlkeld, Intraventricular gentamicin therapy in gram-negative bacillary meningitis of infancy. Report of the second neonatal meningitis cooperative study group, Lancet 1 (1980) 787–791.

[142] T.A. Joseph, S.P. Pyati, N. Jacobs, Neonatal early-onset *Escherichia coli* disease. The effect of intrapartum ampicillin, Arch. Pediatr. Adolesc. Med. 152 (1998) 35–40.

[143] J.N. van den Anker, R. de Groot, Assessment of glomerular filtration rate in preterm infants by serum creatinine: comparison with inulin clearance, Pediatrics 96 (1995) 1156.

[144] M. Grossman, W. Ticknor, Serum levels of ampicillin, cephalothin, cloxacillin, and nafcillin in the newborn infant, Antimicrob. Agents Chemother. (Bethesda) 5 (1965) 214–219.

[145] S.G. Axline, S.J. Yaffe, H.J. Simon, Clinical pharmacology of antimicrobials in premature infants. II. Ampicillin, methicillin, oxacillin, neomycin, and colistin, Pediatrics 39 (1967) 97–107.

[146] R.W. Boe, et al., Serum levels of methicillin and ampicillin in newborn and premature infants in relation to postnatal age, Pediatrics 39 (1967) 194–201.

[147] J.M. Kaplan, et al., Pharmacologic studies in neonates given large dosages of ampicillin, J. Pediatr. 84 (1974) 571–577.

[148] L.B. Dahl, et al., Serum levels of ampicillin and gentamycin in neonates of varying gestational age, Eur. J. Pediatr. 145 (1986) 218–221.

[149] J.W. Bass, et al., Adverse effects of orally administered ampicillin, J. Pediatr. 83 (1973) 106–108.

[150] M.D. Cooper, et al., Synergistic effects of ampicillin-aminoglycoside combinations on group B streptococci, Antimicrob. Agents Chemother. 15 (1979) 484–486.

[151] W.M. Scheld, et al., Response to therapy in an experimental rabbit model of meningitis due to *Listeria monocytogenes*, J. Infect. Dis. 140 (1979) 287–294.

[152] G.H. McCracken Jr., J.D. Nelson, M.L. Thomas, Discrepancy between carbenicillin and ampicillin activities against enterococci and *Listeria*, Antimicrob. Agents Chemother. 3 (1973) 343–349.

[153] T. Young, B. Magnum, NeoFax 2008, Thomson Reuters, Montvale, NJ, 2008.

[154] H.C. Neu, Antistaphylococcal penicillins, Med. Clin. North Am. 66 (1982) 51–60.

[155] W.J. O'Connor, et al., Serum concentration of nafcillin in newborn infants and children, Antimicrob. Agents Chemother. (Bethesda) 10 (1964) 188–191.

[156] W.J. Banner, et al., Pharmacokinetics of nafcillin in infants with low birth weights, Antimicrob. Agents Chemother. 17 (1980) 691–694.

[157] L.E. Burns, J.E. Hodgman, P.F. Wehrle, Treatment of premature infants with oxacillin, Antimicrob. Agents Chemother. (Bethesda) 10 (1964) 192–199.

[158] L.D. Sarff, G.H. McCracken, Methicillin-associated nephropathy or cystitis, J. Pediatr. 90 (1977) 1031–1032.

[159] W. Kitzing, J.D. Nelson, E. Mohs, Comparative toxicities of methicillin and nafcillin, Am. J. Dis. Child. 135 (1981) 52–55.

[160] G.R. Greene, E. Cohen, Nafcillin-induced neutropenia in children, Pediatrics 61 (1978) 94–97.

[161] M.C. Nahata, S.L. DeBolt, D.A. Powell, Adverse effects of methicillin, nafcillin and oxacillin in pediatric patients, Dev. Pharmacol. Ther. 4 (1982) 117–123.

[162] A.A. Mallouh, Methicillin-induced neutropenia, Pediatr. Infect. Dis. 4 (1985) 262–264.

[163] C. Watanakunakorn, Mode of action and in-vitro activity of vancomycin, J. Antimicrob. Chemother. 14 (Suppl. D) (1984) 7–18.

[164] E.V. Capparelli, et al., The influences of renal function and maturation on vancomycin elimination in newborns and infants, J. Clin. Pharmacol. 41 (2001) 927–934.

[165] M. de Hoog, et al., Vancomycin population pharmacokinetics in neonates, Clin. Pharmacol. Ther. 67 (2000) 360–367.

[166] R.E. Seay, et al., Population pharmacokinetics of vancomycin in neonates, Clin. Pharmacol. Ther. 56 (1994) 169–175.

[167] J.R. Gross, et al., Vancomycin pharmacokinetics in premature infants, Pediatr. Pharmacol. (New York) 5 (1985) 17–22.

[168] S.H. Naqvi, et al., Vancomycin pharmacokinetics in small, seriously ill infants, Am. J. Dis. Child. 140 (1986) 107–110.

[169] M.B. Leonard, et al., Vancomycin pharmacokinetics in very low birth weight neonates, Pediatr. Infect. Dis. J. 8 (1989) 282–286.

[170] G. Koren, A. James, Vancomycin dosing in preterm infants: prospective verification of new recommendations, J. Pediatr. 110 (1987) 797–798.

[171] A. James, et al., Vancomycin pharmacokinetics and dose recommendations for preterm infants, Antimicrob. Agents Chemother. 31 (1987) 52–54.

[172] H. Mulla, S. Pooboni, Population pharmacokinetics of vancomycin in patients receiving extracorporeal membrane oxygenation, Br. J. Clin. Pharmacol. 60 (2005) 265–275.

[173] M.L. Buck, Vancomycin pharmacokinetics in neonates receiving extracorporeal membrane oxygenation, Pharmacotherapy 18 (1998) 1082–1086.

[174] R.D. Amaker, J.T. DiPiro, J. Bhatia, Pharmacokinetics of vancomycin in critically ill infants undergoing extracorporeal membrane oxygenation, Antimicrob. Agents Chemother. 40 (1996) 1139–1142.

[175] E.B. Hoie, et al., Vancomycin pharmacokinetics in infants undergoing extracorporeal membrane oxygenation, Clin. Pharm. 9 (1990) 711–715.

[176] U.B. Schaad, G.H. McCracken Jr., J.D. Nelson, Clinical pharmacology and efficacy of vancomycin in pediatric patients, J. Pediatr. 96 (1980) 119–126.

[177] P.D. Reiter, M.W. Doron, Vancomycin cerebrospinal fluid concentrations after intravenous administration in premature infants, J. Perinatol. 16 (1996) 331–335.

[178] M.C. McHenry, T.L. Gavan, Vancomycin, Pediatr. Clin. North Am. 30 (1983) 31–47.

[179] M. de Hoog, et al., Newborn hearing screening: tobramycin and vancomycin are not risk factors for hearing loss, J. Pediatr. 142 (2003) 41–46.

[180] J.E. Geraci, Vancomycin, Mayo Clin. Proc. 52 (1977) 631–634.

[181] W.J. Tissing, M.A. Umans-Eckenhausen, J.N. van den Anker, Vancomycin intoxication in a preterm neonate, Eur. J. Pediatr. 152 (1993) 700.

[182] V. Bhatt-Mehta, et al., Lack of vancomycin-associated nephrotoxicity in newborn infants: a case-control study, Pediatrics 103 (1999) e48.

[183] P.M. Small, H.F. Chambers, Vancomycin for *Staphylococcus aureus* endocarditis in intravenous drug users, Antimicrob. Agents Chemother. 34 (1990) 1227–1231.

[184] H.F. Chambers, R.T. Miller, M.D. Newman, Right-sided *Staphylococcus aureus* endocarditis in intravenous drug abusers: two-week combination therapy, Ann. Intern. Med. 109 (1988) 619–624.

[185] C.H. Nightengale, et al., (Ed.), Antimicrobial Pharmacodynamics in Theory and Clinical Practice, 2nd ed. Informa Healthcare, New York, 2007.

[186] E. Lowdin, I. Odenholt, O. Cars, In vitro studies of pharmacodynamic properties of vancomycin against *Staphylococcus aureus* and *Staphylococcus epidermidis*, Antimicrob. Agents Chemother. 42 (1998) 2739–2744.

[187] P.A. Moise-Broder, et al., Pharmacodynamics of vancomycin and other antimicrobials in patients with *Staphylococcus aureus* lower respiratory tract infections, Clin. Pharmacokinet. 43 (2004) 925–942.

[188] M.J. Rybak, The pharmacokinetic and pharmacodynamic properties of vancomycin, Clin. Infect. Dis. 42 (Suppl. 1) (2006) S35–S39.

[189] G.W. Kaatz, et al., The emergence of resistance to ciprofloxacin during treatment of experimental *Staphylococcus aureus* endocarditis, J. Antimicrob. Chemother. 20 (1987) 753–758.

[190] M.K. Lacy, et al., Comparison of vancomycin pharmacodynamics (1 g every 12 or 24 h) against methicillin-resistant staphylococci, Int. J. Antimicrob. Agents 15 (2000) 25–30.

[191] M.E. Klepser, et al., Comparison of bactericidal activities of intermittent and continuous infusion dosing of vancomycin against methicillin-resistant *Staphylococcus aureus* and *Enterococcus faecalis*, Pharmacotherapy 18 (1998) 1069–1074.

[192] M. de Hoog, J.W. Mouton, J.N. van den Anker, Vancomycin: pharmacokinetics and administration regimens in neonates, Clin. Pharmacokinet. 43 (2004) 417–440.

[193] American Thoracic Society and The Infectious Disease Society of America. Guidelines for the management of adults with hospital-acquired, ventilator-associated, and healthcare-associated pneumonia, Am. J. Respir. Crit. Care Med. 171 (2005) 388–416.

[194] S. Yee-Guardino, et al., Recognition and treatment of neonatal community-associated MRSA pneumonia and bacteremia, Pediatr. Pulmonol. 43 (2008) 203–205.

[195] K.A. Lyseng-Williamson, K.L. Goa, Linezolid: in infants and children with severe gram-positive infections, Paediatr. Drugs 5 (2003) 419–429, discussion 430–431.

[196] Pharmacia & Upjohn Company, Zyvox: linezolid injection, linezolid tablets, linezolid for oral suspension package insert, Pharmacia & Upjohn, Kalamazoo, Mich, 2002.

[197] D.L. Stevens, B. Dotter, K. Madaras-Kelly, A review of linezolid: the first oxazolidinone antibiotic, Expert. Rev. Anti. Infect. Ther. 2 (2004) 51–59.

[198] R.C. Moellering, Linezolid: the first oxazolidinone antimicrobial, Ann. Intern. Med. 138 (2003) 135–142.

[199] T. Zaoutis, et al., In vitro activities of linezolid, meropenem, and quinupristin-dalfopristin against group C and G streptococci, including vancomycin-tolerant isolates, Antimicrob. Agents Chemother. 45 (2001) 1952–1954.

[200] M.J. Rybak, et al., Comparative in vitro activities and postantibiotic effects of the oxazolidinone compounds eperezolid (PNU-100592) and linezolid (PNU-100766) versus vancomycin against *Staphylococcus aureus*, coagulase-negative staphylococci, *Enterococcus faecalis*, and *Enterococcus faecium*, Antimicrob. Agents Chemother. 42 (1998) 721–724.

[201] W.A. Craig, Basic pharmacodynamics of antibacterials with clinical applications to the use of beta-lactams, glycopeptides, and linezolid, Infect. Dis. Clin. North Am. 17 (2003) 479–501.

[202] G.L. Kearns, et al., Single dose pharmacokinetics of linezolid in infants and children, Pediatr. Infect. Dis. J. 19 (2000) 1178–1184.

[203] G.L. Kearns, et al., Impact of ontogeny on linezolid disposition in neonates and infants, Clin. Pharmacol. Ther. 74 (2003) 413–422.

[204] G.L. Jungbluth, I.R. Welshman, N.K. Hopkins, Linezolid pharmacokinetics in pediatric patients: an overview, Pediatr. Infect. Dis. J. 22 (2003) S153–S157.

[205] B.A. Jantausch, et al., Linezolid for the treatment of children with bacteremia or nosocomial pneumonia caused by resistant gram-positive bacterial pathogens, Pediatr. Infect. Dis. J. 22 (2003) S164–S171.

[206] S.L. Kaplan, et al., Linezolid versus vancomycin for treatment of resistant gram-positive infections in children, Pediatr. Infect. Dis. J. 22 (2003) 677–686.

[207] S.L. Kaplan, et al., Linezolid for the treatment of community-acquired pneumonia in hospitalized children. Linezolid pediatric pneumonia study group, Pediatr. Infect. Dis. J. 20 (2001) 488–494.

[208] E. Bishop, et al., Good clinical outcomes but high rates of adverse reactions during linezolid therapy for serious infections: a proposed protocol for monitoring therapy in complex patients, Antimicrob. Agents Chemother. 50 (2006) 1599–1602.

[209] J.E. Conte Jr., et al., Intrapulmonary pharmacokinetics of linezolid, Antimicrob. Agents Chemother. 46 (2002) 1475–1480.

[210] D. Andes, et al., In vivo pharmacodynamics of a new oxazolidinone (linezolid), Antimicrob. Agents Chemother. 46 (2002) 3484–3489.

[211] C.R. Rayner, et al., Clinical pharmacodynamics of linezolid in seriously ill patients treated in a compassionate use programme, Clin. Pharmacokinet. 42 (2003) 1411–1423.

[212] C. Adembri, et al., Linezolid pharmacokinetic/pharmacodynamic profile in critically ill septic patients: intermittent versus continuous infusion, Int. J. Antimicrob. Agents 31 (2008) 122–129.

[213] C. Jacqueline, et al., In vivo efficacy of continuous infusion versus intermittent dosing of linezolid compared to vancomycin in a methicillin-resistant *Staphylococcus aureus* rabbit endocarditis model, Antimicrob. Agents Chemother. 46 (2002) 3706–3711.

[214] D.L. Stevens, et al., Linezolid versus vancomycin for the treatment of methicillin-resistant *Staphylococcus aureus* infections, Clin. Infect. Dis. 34 (2002) 1481–1490.

[215] J. Weigelt, et al., Linezolid versus vancomycin in treatment of complicated skin and soft tissue infections, Antimicrob. Agents Chemother. 49 (2005) 2260–2266.

[216] J.G. Deville, et al., Linezolid versus vancomycin in the treatment of known or suspected resistant gram-positive infections in neonates, Pediatr. Infect. Dis. J. 22 (2003) S158–S163.

[217] D. Guay, Update on clindamycin in the management of bacterial, fungal and protozoal infections, Expert. Opin. Pharmacother. 8 (2007) 2401–2444.

[218] J. Spizek, J. Novotna, T. Rezanka, Lincosamides: chemical structure, biosynthesis, mechanism of action, resistance, and applications, Adv. Appl. Microbiol. 56 (2004) 121–154.

[219] M.M. Paris, et al., Clindamycin therapy of experimental meningitis caused by penicillin- and cephalosporin-resistant *Streptococcus pneumoniae*, Antimicrob. Agents Chemother. 40 (1996) 122–126.

[220] M.J. Bell, et al., Pharmacokinetics of clindamycin phosphate in the first year of life, J. Pediatr. 105 (1984) 482–486.

[221] G. Koren, et al., Pharmacokinetics of intravenous clindamycin in newborn infants, Pediatr. Pharmacol. 5 (1986) 287–292.

[222] S.T. Donta, M.G. Myers, *Clostridium difficile* toxin in asymptomatic neonates, J. Pediatr. 100 (1982) 431–434.

[223] J.G. Newland, G.L. Kearns, Treatment strategies for methicillin-resistant *Staphylococcus aureus* infections in pediatrics, Paediatr. Drugs 10 (2008) 367–378.

[224] G. Martinez-Aguilar, et al., Clindamycin treatment of invasive infections caused by community-acquired, methicillin-resistant and methicillin-susceptible *Staphylococcus aureus* in children, Pediatr. Infect. Dis. J. 22 (2003) 593–598.

[225] A.L. Frank, et al., Clindamycin treatment of methicillin-resistant *Staphylococcus aureus* infections in children, Pediatr. Infect. Dis. J. 21 (2002) 530–534.

[226] W.E. Feldman, *Bacteroides fragilis* ventriculitis and meningitis. Report of two cases, Am. J. Dis. Child. 130 (1976) 880–883.

[227] J. de Louvois, Bacteriological examination of pus from abscesses of the central nervous system, J. Clin. Pathol. 33 (1980) 66–71.

[228] P.G. Ambrose, et al., Pharmacokinetics-pharmacodynamics of antimicrobial therapy: it's not just for mice anymore, Clin. Infect. Dis. 44 (2007) 79–86.

[229] R.E. Lewis, et al., Evaluation of low-dose, extended-interval clindamycin regimens against *Staphylococcus aureus* and *Streptococcus pneumoniae* using a dynamic in vitro model of infection, Antimicrob. Agents Chemother. 43 (1999) 2005–2009.

[230] M.E. Klepser, et al., Bactericidal activity of low-dose clindamycin administered at 8- and 12-hour intervals against *Staphylococcus aureus*, *Streptococcus pneumoniae*, and *Bacteroides fragilis*, Antimicrob. Agents Chemother. 41 (1997) 630–635.

[231] W.A. Craig, Post-antibiotic effects in experimental infection models: relationship to in-vitro phenomena and to treatment of infections in man, J. Antimicrob. Chemother. 31 (Suppl. D) (1993) 149–158.

[232] K.L. LaPlante, et al., Activities of clindamycin, daptomycin, doxycycline, linezolid, trimethoprim-sulfamethoxazole, and vancomycin against community-associated methicillin-resistant *Staphylococcus aureus* with inducible clindamycin resistance in murine thigh infection and in vitro pharmacodynamic models, Antimicrob. Agents Chemother. 52 (2008) 2156–2162.

[233] G. Acocella, Clinical pharmacokinetics of rifampicin, Clin. Pharmacokinet. 3 (1978) 108–127.

[234] A. Shama, S.K. Patole, J.S. Whitehall, Intravenous rifampicin in neonates with persistent staphylococcal bacteraemia, Acta Paediatr. 91 (2002) 670–673.

[235] G.L. Archer, M.J. Tenenbaum, H.B. Haywood III, Rifampin therapy of *Staphylococcus epidermidis*. Use in infections from indwelling artificial devices, JAMA 240 (1978) 751–753.

[236] R.J. Faville Jr., et al., *Staphylococcus aureus* endocarditis. Combined therapy with vancomycin and rifampin, JAMA 240 (1978) 1963–1965.

[237] J.C. Ring, et al., Rifampin for CSF shunt infections caused by coagulase-negative staphylococci, J. Pediatr. 95 (1979) 317–319.

[238] Rifampin, for Injection Only. Label, 1997. Available at http://www.accessdata.fda.gov/drugsatfda_docs/anda/99/64-217_rifampin_prntlbl.pdf. Accessed 5/25/10.

[239] C.A. Jamis-Dow, et al., Rifampin and rifabutin and their metabolism by human liver esterases, Xenobiotica 27 (1997) 1015–1024.

[240] T. Mindermann, W. Zimmerli, O. Gratzl, Rifampin concentrations in various compartments of the human brain: a novel method for determining drug levels in the cerebral extracellular space, Antimicrob. Agents Chemother. 42 (1998) 2626–2629.

[241] M. Niemi, et al., Pharmacokinetic interactions with rifampicin: clinical relevance, Clin. Pharmacokinet. 42 (2003) 819–850.

[242] T.V. Stanley, V. Balakrishnan, Rifampicin in neonatal ventriculitis, Aust. Paediatr. J. 18 (1982) 200–201.

[243] T.Q. Tan, et al., Use of intravenous rifampin in neonates with persistent staphylococcal bacteremia, Antimicrob. Agents Chemother. 37 (1993) 2401–2406.

[244] J.R. Koup, et al., Pharmacokinetics of rifampin in children. I. Multiple dose intravenous infusion, Ther. Drug. Monit. 8 (1986) 11–16.

[245] Sanofi-aventis. Teicoplanin Drug Label. Available at http://pk.sanofi-aventis.com/products/targocid.pdf Accessed 5/25/2010.

[246] R.D. Pryka, K.A. Rodvold, J.C. Rotschafer, Teicoplanin: an investigational glycopeptide antibiotic, Clin. Pharm. 7 (1988) 647–658.

[247] E. Tarral, et al., Pharmacokinetics of teicoplanin in children, J. Antimicrob. Chemother. 21 (Suppl. A) (1988) 47–51.

[248] V. Fanos, N. Kacet, G. Mosconi, A review of teicoplanin in the treatment of serious neonatal infections, Eur. J. Pediatr. 156 (1997) 423–427.

[249] M. Yalaz, et al., Experience with teicoplanin in the treatment of neonatal staphylococcal sepsis, J. Int. Med. Res. 32 (2004) 540–548.

[250] V. Fanos, et al., Renal tolerability of teicoplanin in a case of neonatal overdose, J. Chemother. 10 (1998) 381–384.

[251] Cubicin, Daptomycin for injection. Full prescribing information, Cubist Pharmaceuticals, Lexington, Mass, 2006.

[252] S.K. Straus, R.E. Hancock, Mode of action of the new antibiotic for gram-positive pathogens daptomycin: comparison with cationic antimicrobial peptides and lipopeptides, Biochim. Biophys. Acta 1758 (2006) 1215–1223.

[253] M.I. Ardura, et al., Daptomycin therapy for invasive gram-positive bacterial infections in children, Pediatr. Infect. Dis. J. 26 (2007) 1128–1132.

[254] F. Weis, A. Beiras-Fernandez, G. Schelling, Daptomycin, a lipopeptide antibiotic in clinical practice, Curr. Opin. Investig. Drugs 9 (2008) 879–884.

[255] S.N. Leonard, C.M. Cheung, M.J. Rybak, Activities of ceftobiprole, linezolid, vancomycin, and daptomycin against community-associated and hospital-associated methicillin-resistant *Staphylococcus aureus*, Antimicrob. Agents Chemother. 52 (2008) 2974–2976.

[256] J. Brauers, et al., Bactericidal activity of daptomycin, vancomycin, teicoplanin and linezolid against *Staphylococcus aureus*, *Enterococcus faecalis* and *Enterococcus faecium* using human peak free serum drug concentrations, Int. J. Antimicrob. Agents 29 (2007) 322–325.

[257] B.M. Diederen, et al., In vitro activity of daptomycin against methicillin-resistant *Staphylococcus aureus*, including heterogeneously glycopeptide-resistant strains, Antimicrob. Agents Chemother. 50 (2006) 3189–3191.

[258] M.J. Rybak, et al., In vitro activities of daptomycin, vancomycin, linezolid, and quinupristin-dalfopristin against staphylococci and enterococci, including vancomycin-intermediate and -resistant strains, Antimicrob. Agents Chemother. 44 (2000) 1062–1066.

[259] J.A. Silverman, et al., Inhibition of daptomycin by pulmonary surfactant: in vitro modeling and clinical impact, J. Infect. Dis. 191 (2005) 2149–2152.

[260] B.H. Dvorchik, et al., Daptomycin pharmacokinetics and safety following administration of escalating doses once daily to healthy subjects, Antimicrob. Agents Chemother. 47 (2003) 1318–1323.

[261] S.M. Abdel-Rahman, et al., Single-dose pharmacokinetics of daptomycin in children with suspected or proved gram-positive infections, Pediatr. Infect. Dis. J. 27 (2008) 330–334.

[262] M. Cohen-Wolkowiez, et al., Daptomycin use in infants: report of two cases with peak and trough drug concentrations, J. Perinatol. 28 (2008) 233–234.

[263] D.M. Kraus, M.P. Pai, K.A. Rodvold, Efficacy and tolerability of extended-interval aminoglycoside administration in pediatric patients, Paediatr. Drugs 4 (2002) 469–484.

[264] C.A. Knoderer, J.A. Everett, W.F. Buss, Clinical issues surrounding once-daily aminoglycoside dosing in children, Pharmacotherapy 23 (2003) 44–56.

[265] D.N. Fisman, K.M. Kaye, Once-daily dosing of aminoglycoside antibiotics, Infect. Dis. Clin. North Am. 14 (2000) 475–487.

[266] R.M. Kluge, et al., Comparative activity of tobramycin, amikacin, and gentamicin alone and with carbenicillin against *Pseudomonas aeruginosa*, Antimicrob. Agents Chemother. 6 (1974) 442–446.

[267] C. Watanakunakorn, T. Bannister, Comparison of the in vitro activity of BL-P1654 with gentamicin and carbenicillin against *Pseudomonas aeruginosa*, Antimicrob. Agents Chemother. 6 (1974) 471–473.

[268] H.M. Swingle, R.L. Bucciarelli, E.M. Ayoub, Synergy between penicillins and low concentrations of gentamicin in the killing of group B streptococci, J. Infect. Dis. 152 (1985) 515–520.

[269] S.A. Calderwood, et al., Resistance to six aminoglycosidic aminocyclitol antibiotics among enterococci: prevalence, evolution, and relationship to synergism with penicillin, Antimicrob. Agents Chemother. 12 (1977) 401–405.

[270] S. Shakil, et al., Aminoglycosides versus bacteria: a description of the action, resistance mechanism, and nosocomial battleground, J. Biomed. Sci. 15 (2008) 5–14.

[271] J.E. Davies, Aminoglycosides: ancient and modern, J. Antibiot. (Tokyo) 59 (2006) 529–532.

[272] L.P. Kotra, J. Haddad, S. Mobashery, Aminoglycosides: perspectives on mechanisms of action and resistance and strategies to counter resistance, Antimicrob. Agents Chemother. 44 (2000) 3249–3256.

[273] G.L. Daikos, et al., Adaptive resistance to aminoglycoside antibiotics from first-exposure down-regulation, J. Infect. Dis. 162 (1990) 414–420.

[274] G.L. Daikos, V.T. Lolans, G.G. Jackson, First-exposure adaptive resistance to aminoglycoside antibiotics in vivo with meaning for optimal clinical use, Antimicrob. Agents Chemother. 35 (1991) 117–123.

[275] L.B. Gilleland, et al., Adaptive resistance to aminoglycoside antibiotics in *Pseudomonas aeruginosa*, J. Med. Microbiol. 29 (1989) 41–50.

[276] J.W. Paisley, A.L. Smith, D.H. Smith, Gentamicin in newborn infants. Comparison of intramuscular and intravenous administration, Am. J. Dis. Child. 126 (1973) 473–477.

[277] D.B. Haughey, et al., Two-compartment gentamicin pharmacokinetics in premature neonates: a comparison to adults with decreased glomerular filtration rates, J. Pediatr. 96 (1980) 325–330.

[278] G.H. McCracken Jr., D.F. Chrane, M.L. Thomas, Pharmacologic evaluation of gentamicin in newborn infants, J. Infect. Dis. 124 (Suppl.) (1971) S214–S223.

[279] G.H. McCracken, N.R. West, L.J. Horton, Urinary excretion of gentamicin in the neonatal period, J. Infect. Dis. 123 (1971) 257–262.

[280] J.C. Miranda, et al., Gentamicin kinetics in the neonate, Pediatr. Pharmacol. (New York) 5 (1985) 57–61.

[281] K.W. Hindmarsh, et al., Pharmacokinetics of gentamicin in very low birth weight preterm infants, Eur. J. Clin. Pharmacol. 24 (1983) 649–653.

[282] C. Kildoo, et al., Developmental pattern of gentamicin kinetics in very low birth weight (VLBW) sick infants, Dev. Pharmacol. Ther. 7 (1984) 345–356.

[283] S. Landers, et al., Gentamicin disposition and effect on development of renal function in the very low birth weight infant, Dev. Pharmacol. Ther. 7 (1984) 285–302.

[284] D. Zoumboulakis, et al., Gentamicin in the treatment of purulent meningitis in neonates and infants, Acta Paediatr. Scand. 62 (1973) 55–58.

[285] C. Husson, et al., Pharmacokinetic study of gentamicin in preterm and term neonates, Dev. Pharmacol. Ther. 7 (Suppl. 1) (1984) 125–129.

[286] J.W. Kasik, et al., Postconceptional age and gentamicin elimination half-life, J. Pediatr. 106 (1985) 502–505.

[287] S.J. Szefler, et al., Relationship of gentamicin serum concentrations to gestational age in preterm and term neonates, J. Pediatr. 97 (1980) 312–315.

[288] J.O. Klein, et al., Gentamicin in serious neonatal infections: absorption, excretion, and clinical results in 25 cases, J. Infect. Dis. 124 (Suppl.) (1971) S224–S231.

[289] R.D. Milner, et al., Clinical pharmacology of gentamicin in the newborn infant, Arch. Dis. Child. 47 (1972) 927–932.

[290] M.J. Chang, et al., Kanamycin and gentamicin treatment of neonatal sepsis and meningitis, Pediatrics 56 (1975) 695–699.

[291] C.A. Friedman, B.R. Parks, J.E. Rawson, Gentamicin disposition in asphyxiated newborns: relationship to mean arterial blood pressure and urine output, Pediatr. Pharmacol. (New York) 2 (1982) 189–197.

[292] B. Edgren, et al., Gentamicin dosing in the newborn. Use of a one-compartment open pharmacokinetic model to individualize dosing, Dev. Pharmacol. Ther. 7 (1984) 263–272.

[293] G.H. McCracken Jr., N. Threlkeld, M.L. Thomas, Intravenous administration of kanamycin and gentamicin in newborn infants, Pediatrics 60 (1977) 463–466.

[294] J. Black, et al., Pharmacology of gentamicin, a new broad-spectrum antibiotic, Antimicrob. Agents Chemother. (Bethesda) 161 (1963) 138–147.

[295] K.C. Hayani, et al., Pharmacokinetics of once-daily dosing of gentamicin in neonates, J. Pediatr. 131 (1997) 76–80.

[296] C. de Alba Romero, et al., Once daily gentamicin dosing in neonates, Pediatr. Infect. Dis. J. 17 (1998) 1169–1171.

[297] P.J. Thureen, et al., Once- versus twice-daily gentamicin dosing in neonates >/=34 weeks' gestation: cost-effectiveness analyses, Pediatrics 103 (1999) 594–598.

[298] H. Skopnik, et al., Pharmacokinetics and antibacterial activity of daily gentamicin, Arch. Dis. Child. 67 (1992) 57–61.

[299] F.S. Lundergan, et al., Once-daily gentamicin dosing in newborn infants, Pediatrics 103 (1999) 1228–1234.

[300] A.H. Thomson, et al., Population pharmacokinetics of intramuscular gentamicin administered to young infants with suspected severe sepsis in Kenya, Br. J. Clin. Pharmacol. 56 (2003) 25–31.

[301] A.H. Thomson, et al., Population pharmacokinetics of gentamicin in neonates, Dev. Pharmacol. Ther. 11 (1988) 173–179.

[302] P.D. Jensen, B.E. Edgren, R.C. Brundage, Population pharmacokinetics of gentamicin in neonates using a nonlinear, mixed-effects model, Pharmacotherapy 12 (1992) 178–182.

[303] M.L. Vervelde, et al., Population pharmacokinetics of gentamicin in preterm neonates: evaluation of a once-daily dosage regimen, Ther. Drug Monit. 21 (1999) 514–519.

[304] J.H. Botha, M.J. du Preez, M. Adhikari, Population pharmacokinetics of gentamicin in South African newborns, Eur. J. Clin. Pharmacol. 59 (2003) 755–759.

[305] B. Garcia, et al., Population pharmacokinetics of gentamicin in premature newborns, J. Antimicrob. Chemother. 58 (2006) 372–379.

[306] A. Mulhall, J. de Louvois, R. Hurley, Incidence of potentially toxic concentrations of gentamicin in the neonate, Arch. Dis. Child. 58 (1983) 897–900.

[307] G. Koren, et al., Optimization of gentamicin therapy in very low birth weight infants, Pediatr. Pharmacol. (New York) 5 (1985) 79–87.

[308] B.J. Zarowitz, et al., High gentamicin trough concentrations in neonates of less than 28 weeks gestational age, Dev. Pharmacol. Ther. 5 (1982) 68–75.

[309] C.K. Charlton, et al., Gentamicin dosage recommendations for neonates based on half-life predictions from birthweight, Am. J. Perinatol. 3 (1986) 28–32.

[310] K.L. Watterberg, et al., Effect of patent ductus arteriosus on gentamicin pharmacokinetics in very low birth weight (less than 1,500 g) babies, Dev. Pharmacol. Ther. 10 (1987) 107–117.

[311] M.M. Mustafa, et al., Increased endotoxin and interleukin-1 beta concentrations in cerebrospinal fluid of infants with coliform meningitis and ventriculitis associated with intraventricular gentamicin therapy, J. Infect. Dis. 160 (1989) 891–895.

[312] R.M. Kliegman, et al., Pharmacokinetics of gentamicin during exchange transfusions in neonates, J. Pediatr. 96 (1980) 927–930.

[313] J.S. Bertino Jr., et al., Alterations in gentamicin pharmacokinetics during neonatal exchange transfusion, Dev. Pharmacol. Ther. 4 (1982) 205–215.

[314] P. Cohen, et al., Gentamicin pharmacokinetics in neonates undergoing extracorporeal membrane oxygenation, Pediatr. Infect. Dis. J. 9 (1990) 562–566.

[315] C.R. Smith, et al., Double-blind comparison of the nephrotoxicity and auditory toxicity of gentamicin and tobramycin, N. Engl. J. Med. 302 (1980) 1106–1109.

[316] S. Itsarayoungyuen, et al., Tobramycin and gentamicin are equally safe for neonates: results of a double-blind randomized trial with quantitative assessment of renal function, Pediatr. Pharmacol. (New York) 2 (1982) 143–155.

[317] J.M. Kaplan, et al., Clinical pharmacology of tobramycin in newborns, Am. J. Dis. Child. 125 (1973) 656–660.

[318] M.C. Nahata, et al., Effect of gestational age and birth weight on tobramycin kinetics in newborn infants, J. Antimicrob. Chemother. 14 (1984) 59–65.

[319] L. Cordero, et al., Serum tobramycin levels in low- and very-low-birthweight infants, Am. J. Perinatol. 1 (1984) 242–246.

[320] A.M. Arbeter, et al., Tobramycin sulfate elimination in premature infants, J. Pediatr. 103 (1983) 131–135.

[321] M.C. Nahata, et al., Tobramycin pharmacokinetics in very low birth weight infants, Br. J. Clin. Pharmacol. 21 (1986) 325–327.

[322] J.B. Howard, et al., Amikacin in newborn infants: comparative pharmacology with kanamycin and clinical efficacy in 45 neonates with bacterial diseases, Antimicrob. Agents Chemother. 10 (1976) 205–210.

[323] J.B. Howard, G.H. McCracken Jr., Pharmacological evaluation of amikacin in neonates, Antimicrob. Agents Chemother. 8 (1975) 86–90.

[324] C.G. Prober, A.S. Yeager, A.M. Arvin, The effect of chronologic age on the serum concentrations of amikacin in sick term and premature infants, J. Pediatr. 98 (1981) 636–640.

[325] N. Bleyzac, et al., Population pharmacokinetics of amikacin at birth and interindividual variability in renal maturation, Eur. J. Clin. Pharmacol. 57 (2001) 499–504.

[326] J.H. Botha, et al., Determination of population pharmacokinetic parameters for amikacin in neonates using mixed-effect models, Eur. J. Clin. Pharmacol. 53 (1998) 337–341.

[327] K. Allegaert, et al., Cerebrospinal fluid compartmental pharmacokinetics of amikacin in neonates, Antimicrob. Agents Chemother. 52 (2008) 1934–1939.

[328] M.D. Yow, An overview of pediatric experience with amikacin, Am. J. Med. 62 (1977) 954–958.

[329] H. Trujillo, et al., Clinical and laboratory studies with amikacin in newborns, infants, and children, J. Infect. Dis. 134 (Suppl.) (1976) S406–S411.

[330] J.B. Philips, G. Cassady, Amikacin: pharmacology, indications and cautions for use, and dose recommendations, Semin. Perinatol. 6 (1982) 166–171.

[331] T. Nakashima, et al., Vestibular and cochlear toxicity of aminoglycosides: a review, Acta Otolaryngol. 120 (2000) 904–911.

[332] M.P. Mingeot-Leclercq, P.M. Tulkens, Aminoglycosides: nephrotoxicity, Antimicrob. Agents Chemother. 43 (1999) 1003–1012.

[333] G.J. Matz, Aminoglycoside cochlear ototoxicity, Otolaryngol. Clin. North Am. 26 (1993) 705–712.

[334] S.K. Swan, Aminoglycoside nephrotoxicity, Semin. Nephrol. 17 (1997) 27–33.

[335] R.A. Giuliano, et al., In vivo uptake kinetics of aminoglycosides in the kidney cortex of rats, J. Pharmacol. Exp. Ther. 236 (1986) 470–475.

[336] G.A. Verpooten, et al., Once-daily dosing decreases renal accumulation of gentamicin and netilmicin, Clin. Pharmacol. Ther. 45 (1989) 22–27.

[337] M.E. De Broe, L. Verbist, G.A. Verpooten, Influence of dosage schedule on renal cortical accumulation of amikacin and tobramycin in man, J. Antimicrob. Chemother. 27 (Suppl. C) (1991) 41–47.

[338] A.R. Smyth, K.H. Tan, Once-daily versus multiple-daily dosing with intravenous aminoglycosides for cystic fibrosis, Cochrane. Database. Syst. Rev. 3 (2006) CD002009.

[339] S.C. Rao, M. Ahmed, R. Hagan, One dose per day compared to multiple doses per day of gentamicin for treatment of suspected or proven sepsis in neonates, Cochrane Database Syst. Rev. (2006) Jan 25;(1):CD005091.

[340] M.Z. Ali, M.B. Goetz, A meta-analysis of the relative efficacy and toxicity of single daily dosing versus multiple daily dosing of aminoglycosides, Clin. Infect. Dis. 24 (1997) 796–809.

[341] T.C. Bailey, et al., A meta-analysis of extended-interval dosing versus multiple daily dosing of aminoglycosides, Clin. Infect. Dis. 24 (1997) 786–795.

[342] R. Ferriols-Lisart, M. Alos-Alminana, Effectiveness and safety of once-daily aminoglycosides: a meta-analysis, Am. J. Health Syst. Pharm. 53 (1996) 1141–1150.

[343] W.J. Munckhof, M.L. Grayson, J.D. Turnidge, A meta-analysis of studies on the safety and efficacy of aminoglycosides given either once daily or as divided doses, J. Antimicrob. Chemother. 37 (1996) 645–663.

[344] M. Barza, et al., Single or multiple daily doses of aminoglycosides: a meta-analysis, BMJ 312 (1996) 338–345.

[345] B.M. Assael, R. Parini, F. Rusconi, Ototoxicity of aminoglycoside antibiotics in infants and children, Pediatr. Infect. Dis. 1 (1982) 357–365.

[346] R. Parini, et al., Evaluation of the renal and auditory function of neonates treated with amikacin, Dev. Pharmacol. Ther. 5 (1982) 33–46.

[347] G. Heimann, Renal toxicity of aminoglycosides in the neonatal period, Pediatr. Pharmacol. (New York) 3 (1983) 251–257.

[348] G.P. Giacoia, J.J. Schentag, Pharmacokinetics and nephrotoxicity of continuous intravenous infusion of gentamicin in low birth weight infants, J. Pediatr. 109 (1986) 715–719.

[349] P. Rajchgot, et al., Aminoglycoside-related nephrotoxicity in the premature newborn, Clin. Ther. 35 (1984) 394–401.

[350] Y. Aujard, et al., Gentamicin, nephrotoxic risk and treatment of neonatal infection, Dev. Pharmacol. Ther. 7 (Suppl. 1) (1984) 109–115.

[351] I. Tessin, et al., Enzymuria in neonates during treatment with gentamicin or tobramycin, Pediatr. Infect. Dis. J. 6 (1987) 870–871.

[352] J.B. Gouyon, et al., Urinary excretion of N-acetyl-glucosaminidase and beta-2-microglobulin as early markers of gentamicin nephrotoxicity in neonates, Dev. Pharmacol. Ther. 10 (1987) 145–152.

[353] J.G. Dahlgren, E.T. Anderson, W.L. Hewitt, Gentamicin blood levels: a guide to nephrotoxicity, Antimicrob. Agents Chemother. 8 (1975) 58–62.

[354] L. Gagliardi, Possible indomethacin-aminoglycoside interaction in preterm infants, J. Pediatr. 107 (1985) 991–992.

[355] Y. Zarfin, et al., Possible indomethacin-aminoglycoside interaction in preterm infants, J. Pediatr. 106 (1985) 511–513.

[356] J.T. King, Severe deafness in an infant following oral administration of neomycin, J. Med. Assoc. Ga. 51 (1962) 530–531.

[357] M.M. De Beukelaer, et al., Deafness and acute tubular necrosis following parenteral administration of neomycin, Am. J. Dis. Child. 121 (1971) 250–252.

[358] G.C. Robinson, K.G. Cambon, Hearing loss in infants of tuberculous mothers treated with streptomycin during pregnancy, N. Engl. J. Med. 271 (1964) 949–951.

[359] G.H. McCracken Jr., Changing pattern of the antimicrobial susceptibilities of *Escherichia coli* in neonatal infections, J. Pediatr. 78 (1971) 942–947.

[360] S. Winkel, et al., Possible effects of kanamycin and incubation in newborn children with low birth weight, Acta Paediatr. Scand. 67 (1978) 709–715.

[361] S.A. Falk, N.F. Woods, Hospital noise: levels and potential health hazards, N. Engl. J. Med. 289 (1973) 774–781.

[362] T. Finitzo-Hieber, et al., Ototoxicity in neonates treated with gentamicin and kanamycin: results of a four-year controlled follow-up study, Pediatrics 63 (1979) 443–450.

[363] A. Starr, et al., Development of auditory function in newborn infants revealed by auditory brainstem potentials, Pediatrics 60 (1977) 831–839.

[364] T. Finitzo-Hieber, G.H. McCracken Jr., K.C. Brown, Prospective controlled evaluation of auditory function in neonates given netilmicin or amikacin, J. Pediatr. 106 (1985) 129–136.

[365] P.A. Bernard, J.C. Pechere, R. Hebert, Altered objective audiometry in aminoglycosides-treated human neonates, Arch. Otorhinolaryngol. 228 (1980) 205–210.

[366] A.M. Hauch, B. Peitersen, E. Peitersen, Vestibular toxicity following netilmicin therapy in the neonatal period, Dan. Med. Bull. 33 (1986) 107–109.

[367] C.R. Ream, Respiratory and cardiac arrest after intravenous administration of kanamycin with reversal of toxic effects by neostigmine, Ann. Intern. Med. 59 (1963) 384–387.

[368] C.B. Pittinger, Y. Eryasa, R. Adamson, Antibiotic-induced paralysis, Anesth. Analg. 49 (1970) 487–501.

[369] W.A. Warner, E. Sanders, Neuromuscular blockade associated with gentamicin therapy, JAMA 215 (1971) 1153–1154.

[370] S. Yamada, Y. Kuno, H. Iwanaga, Effects of aminoglycoside antibiotics on the neuromuscular junction: part I, Int. J. Clin. Pharmacol. Ther. Toxicol. 24 (1986) 130–138.

[371] J.I. Santos, P. Swensen, L.A. Glasgow, Potentiation of *Clostridium botulinum* toxin aminoglycoside antibiotics: clinical and laboratory observations, Pediatrics 68 (1981) 50–54.

[372] M.K. Lacy, et al., The pharmacodynamics of aminoglycosides, Clin. Infect. Dis. 27 (1998) 23–27.

[373] R.D. Moore, C.R. Smith, P.S. Lietman, Association of aminoglycoside plasma levels with therapeutic outcome in gram-negative pneumonia, Am. J. Med. 77 (1984) 657–662.

[374] R.D. Moore, C.R. Smith, P.S. Lietman, The association of aminoglycoside plasma levels with mortality in patients with gram-negative bacteremia, J. Infect. Dis. 149 (1984) 443–448.

[375] R.D. Moore, P.S. Lietman, C.R. Smith, Clinical response to aminoglycoside therapy: importance of the ratio of peak concentration to minimal inhibitory concentration, J. Infect. Dis. 155 (1987) 93–99.

[376] A.D. Kashuba, et al., Optimizing aminoglycoside therapy for nosocomial pneumonia caused by gram-negative bacteria, Antimicrob. Agents Chemother. 43 (1999) 623–629.

[377] B. Fantin, et al., Factors affecting duration of in-vivo postantibiotic effect for aminoglycosides against gram-negative bacilli, J. Antimicrob. Chemother. 27 (1991) 829–836.

[378] B. Vogelman, et al., In vivo postantibiotic effect in a thigh infection in neutropenic mice, J. Infect. Dis. 157 (1988) 287–298.

[379] J.E. Kapusnik, et al., Single, large, daily dosing versus intermittent dosing of tobramycin for treating experimental *Pseudomonas* pneumonia, J. Infect. Dis. 158 (1988) 7–12.

[380] G. Agarwal, et al., Comparison of once-daily versus twice-daily gentamicin dosing regimens in infants > or = 2500 g, J. Perinatol. 22 (2002) 268–274.

[381] A. Rastogi, et al., Comparison of two gentamicin dosing schedules in very low birth weight infants, Pediatr. Infect. Dis. J. 21 (2002) 234–240.

[382] M.L. Avent, et al., Gentamicin and tobramycin in neonates: comparison of a new extended dosing interval regimen with a traditional multiple daily dosing regimen, Am. J. Perinatol. 19 (2002) 413–420.

[383] J.P. Langhendries, et al., Once-a-day administration of amikacin in neonates: assessment of nephrotoxicity and ototoxicity, Dev. Pharmacol. Ther. 20 (1993) 220–230.

[384] A. Kotze, P.R. Bartel, D.K. Sommers, Once versus twice daily amikacin in neonates: prospective study on toxicity, J. Paediatr. Child. Health 35 (1999) 283–286.

[385] J.P. Langhendries, et al., Adaptation in neonatology of the once-daily concept of aminoglycoside administration: evaluation of a dosing chart for amikacin in an intensive care unit, Biol. Neonate 74 (1998) 351–362.

[386] A.R. Tunkel, W.M. Scheld, Aztreonam, Infect. Control Hosp. Epidemiol. 11 (1990) 486–494.

[387] M.H. Lebel, G.H. McCracken Jr., Aztreonam: review of the clinical experience and potential uses in pediatrics, Pediatr. Infect. Dis. J. 7 (1988) 331–339.

[388] S. Likitnukul, et al., Pharmacokinetics and plasma bactericidal activity of aztreonam in low-birth-weight infants, Antimicrob. Agents Chemother. 31 (1987) 81–83.

[389] H.R. Stutman, Clinical experience with aztreonam for treatment of infections in children, Rev. Infect. Dis. 13 (Suppl. 7) (1991) S582–S585.

[390] H. Tanaka, et al., Pharmacokinetics and clinical studies of aztreonam in neonates and premature infants, Jpn. J. Antibiot. 43 (1990) 524–527.

[391] S. Arai, et al., Pharmacokinetics and clinical studies on aztreonam in neonates, Jpn. J. Antibiot. 43 (1990) 479–486.

[392] S. Azagami, et al., Pharmacokinetics and clinical safety of aztreonam in neonates, Jpn. J. Antibiot. 43 (1990) 405–412.

[393] R. Fuji, et al., Pharmacokinetics and clinical studies on aztreonam in neonates and premature infants (the second report). Study on effectiveness and safety in combination therapy using aztreonam and ampicillin. A study of aztreonam in the perinatal co-research group, Jpn. J. Antibiot. 43 (1990) 563–578.

[394] R. Fuji, et al., Pharmacokinetics and clinical studies in neonates and premature infants (the first report). Study on effectiveness and safety in mono-therapy with aztreonam. A study of aztreonam in the perinatal co-research group, Jpn. J. Antibiot. 43 (1990) 543–562.

[395] K. Sunakawa, et al., Pharmacokinetic and clinical studies on aztreonam in neonates and premature infants, Jpn. J. Antibiot. 43 (1990) 413–423.

[396] Y. Toyonaga, et al., Pharmacokinetic and clinical evaluation of aztreonam in neonates and premature infants, Jpn. J. Antibiot. 43 (1990) 425–443.

[397] L. Cuzzolin, et al., Pharmacokinetics and renal tolerance of aztreonam in premature infants, Antimicrob. Agents Chemother. 35 (1991) 1726–1728.

[398] M.R. Millar, et al., Pharmacokinetics of aztreonam in very low birthweight neonates, Eur. J. Clin. Microbiol. 6 (1987) 691–692.

[399] R.L. Greenman, et al., Penetration of aztreonam into human cerebrospinal fluid in the presence of meningeal inflammation, J. Antimicrob. Chemother. 15 (1985) 637–640.

[400] H.R. Stutman, M.I. Marks, E.A. Swabb, Single-dose pharmacokinetics of aztreonam in pediatric patients, Antimicrob. Agents Chemother. 26 (1984) 196–199.

[401] M.A. Umana, et al., Evaluation of aztreonam and ampicillin vs. amikacin and ampicillin for treatment of neonatal bacterial infections, Pediatr. Infect. Dis. J. 9 (1990) 175–180.

[402] R. Uauy, et al., Metabolic tolerance to arginine: implications for the safe use of arginine salt-aztreonam combination in the neonatal period, J. Pediatr. 118 (1991) 965–970.

[403] J. Elks, Structural formulae and nomenclature of the cephalosporin antibiotics, Drugs 34 (Suppl. 2) (1987) 240–246.

[404] J.S. Bertino Jr., W.T. Speck, The cephalosporin antibiotics, Pediatr. Clin. North Am. 30 (1983) 17–26.

[405] J.D. Nelson, Cefuroxime: a cephalosporin with unique applicability to pediatric practice, Pediatr. Infect. Dis. 2 (1983) 394–396.

[406] J. Garau, The clinical potential of fourth-generation cephalosporins, Diagn. Microbiol. Infect. Dis. 31 (1998) 479–480.

[407] D. Milatovic, I. Braveny, Development of resistance during antibiotic therapy, Eur. J. Clin. Microbiol. 6 (1987) 234–244.

[408] C.C. Sanders, C. Watanakunakorn, Emergence of resistance to beta-lactams, aminoglycosides, and quinolones during combination therapy for infection due to *Serratia marcescens*, J. Infect. Dis. 153 (1986) 617–619.

[409] N. Chang, et al., (Ed), Studies on Cefazolin in Obstetrics and Gynecology With Special Reference to Its Clinical Pharmacology in the Neonate, University Park Press, Baltimore, 1972.

[410] Y. Sakata, The pharmacokinetic studies of cephalothin, cefazolin and cefmetazole in the neonates and the premature babies, Kurume Med. J. 27 (1980) 275–298.

[411] K.I. Plaisance, C. Nightingale, R. Quintiliani (Eds.), Pharmacology of the Cephalosporins, Marcel Dekker, New York, 1986.

[412] M. Renlund, O. Pettay, Pharmacokinetics and clinical efficacy of cefuroxime in the newborn period, Proc. R. Soc. Med. 70 (Suppl. 9) (1977) 183.

[413] C.H. Dash, M.R. Kennedy, S.H. Ng. Cefuroxime in the First Week of Life, Proceedings of the 19th Interscience Conference of Antimicrobial Agents and Chemotherapy, Washington, DC, American Society for Microbiology, 1980.

[414] J. de Louvois, A. Mulhall, R. Hurley, Cefuroxime in the treatment of neonates, Arch. Dis. Child. 57 (1982) 59–62.

[415] J. Chamberlain, et al., Metabolism of cefotaxime in animals and man, J. Antimicrob. Chemother. 6 (Suppl. A) (1980) 69–78.

[416] R.N. Jones, A.L. Barry, C. Thornsberry, Antimicrobial activity of desacetyl-cefotaxime alone and in combination with cefotaxime: evidence of synergy, Rev. Infect. Dis. 4 (Suppl.) (1982) S366–S373.

[417] G.H. McCracken Jr., N.E. Threlkeld, M.L. Thomas, Pharmacokinetics of cefotaxime in newborn infants, Antimicrob. Agents Chemother. 21 (1982) 683–684.

[418] J. de Louvois, A. Mulhall, R. Hurley, The safety and pharmacokinetics of cefotaxime in the treatment of neonates, Pediatr. Pharmacol. (New York) 2 (1982) 275–284.

[419] J. Crooks, et al., Pharmacokinetics of cefotaxime and desacetyl-cefotaxime in neonates, J. Antimicrob. Chemother. 14 (Suppl. B) (1984) 97–101.

[420] H.M. von Hattingberg, et al., Pharmacokinetics of cefotaxime in neonates and children: clinical aspects, J. Antimicrob. Chemother. 6 (Suppl. A) (1980) 113–118.

[421] D.A. Kafetzis, et al., Treatment of severe neonatal infections with cefotaxime. Efficacy and pharmacokinetics, J. Pediatr. 100 (1982) 483–489.

[422] P. Begue, et al., Comparative pharmacokinetics of four new cephalosporins: moxalactam, cefotaxime, cefoperazone and ceftazidime in neonates, Dev. Pharmacol. Ther. 7 (Suppl 1) (1984) 105–108.

[423] V. von Loewenich, et al., Cefotaxime and desacetylcefotaxime in cerebrospinal fluid of newborn and premature infants, Padiatr. Padol. 18 (1983) 361–366.

[424] T.G. Wells, et al., Cefotaxime therapy of bacterial meningitis in children, J. Antimicrob. Chemother. 14 (Suppl. B) (1984) 181–189.

[425] B.M. Assael, et al., Clinical pharmacology of ceftazidime in paediatrics, J. Antimicrob. Chemother. 12 (Suppl. A) (1983) 341–346.

[426] P. Begue, et al., Multicenter clinical study and pharmacokinetics of ceftazidime in children and newborn infants, Pathol. Biol. (Paris) 34 (1986) 525–529.

[427] J. de Louvois, A.B. Mulhall, Ceftazidime in neonatal infections, Arch. Dis. Child. 60 (1985) 891–892.

[428] G.H. McCracken Jr., N. Threlkeld, M.L. Thomas, Pharmacokinetics of ceftazidime in newborn infants, Antimicrob. Agents Chemother. 26 (1984) 583–584.

[429] E.M. Padovani, et al., Ceftazidime pharmacokinetics in preterm newborns on the first day of life, Biol. Res. Pregnancy. Perinatol. 7 (1986) 71–73.

[430] J.G. Prinsloo, et al., Pharmacokinetics of ceftazidime in premature, newborn and young infants, S. Afr. Med. J. 65 (1984) 809–811.

[431] D.C. Low, J.G. Bissenden, R. Wise, Ceftazidime in neonatal infections, Arch. Dis. Child. 60 (1985) 360–364.

[432] A. Mulhall, J. de Louvois, The pharmacokinetics and safety of ceftazidime in the neonate, J. Antimicrob. Chemother. 15 (1985) 97–103.

[433] J. de Louvois, A. Mulhall (Eds.), Ceftazidime in the Treatment of Neonates, Elsevier, Amsterdam, 1986.

[434] W.M. Gooch, E. Swensen (Eds.), Neonatal Pharmacokinetic Characteristics of Ceftazidime, American Society for Microbiology, Washington, DC, 1983.

[435] J.L. Blumer, et al., Pharmacokinetics and cerebrospinal fluid penetration of ceftazidime in children with meningitis, Dev. Pharmacol. Ther. 8 (1985) 219–231.

[436] J. Blumer, M. Reed, S. Aronoff (Eds.), CSF Penetration and Pharmacokinetics of Ceftazidime in Children With Bacterial Meningitis, American Society for Microbiology, Washington, DC, 1983.

[437] I.W. Fong, K.B. Tomkins, Penetration of ceftazidime into the cerebrospinal fluid of patients with and without evidence of meningeal inflammation, Antimicrob. Agents Chemother. 26 (1984) 115–116.

[438] E. Capparelli, et al., Population pharmacokinetics of cefepime in the neonate, Antimicrob. Agents Chemother. 49 (2005) 2760–2766.

[439] V. Lima-Rogel, et al., Population pharmacokinetics of cefepime in neonates with severe nosocomial infections, J. Clin. Pharm. Ther. 33 (2008) 295–306.

[440] J.L. Blumer, M.D. Reed, C. Knupp, Review of the pharmacokinetics of cefepime in children, Pediatr. Infect. Dis. J. 20 (2000) 337–342.

[441] U.B. Schaad, The cephalosporin compounds in severe neonatal infection, Eur. J. Pediatr. 141 (1984) 143–146.

[442] R. Roos (Ed.), New Beta-Lactams, Elsevier, Amsterdam, 1986.

[443] C.S. Bryan, et al., Gentamicin vs cefotaxime for therapy of neonatal sepsis. Relationship to drug resistance, Am. J. Dis. Child. 139 (1985) 1086–1089.

[444] N.U. Bang, R.B. Kammer, Hematologic complications associated with B-lactam antibiotics, Rev. Infect. Dis. 5 (1983) S380.

[445] G.J. Johnson (Ed.), Antibiotic-Induced Hemostatic Abnormalities, Elsevier, Amsterdam, 1986.

[446] G.H. McCracken Jr., Use of third-generation cephalosporins for treatment of neonatal infections, Am. J. Dis. Child. 139 (1985) 1079–1080.

[447] M.A. Hall, R.C. Beech, D.V. Seal, The use of cefotaxime for treating suspected neonatal sepsis: 2 years' experience, J. Hosp. Infect. 8 (1986) 57–63.

[448] N.V. Parshina, Clinical effectiveness and pharmacokinetic characteristics of cefotaxime in premature infants with pneumonia, Antibiot. Med. Biotekhnol. 31 (1986) 298–301.

[449] J.A. Hoogkamp-Korstanje, Activity of cefotaxime and ceftriaxone alone and in combination with penicillin, ampicillin and piperacillin against neonatal meningitis pathogens, J. Antimicrob. Chemother. 16 (1985) 327–334.

[450] M.A. Hall, et al., A randomised prospective comparison of cefotaxime versus netilmicin/penicillin for treatment of suspected neonatal sepsis, Drugs 35 (Suppl. 2) (1988) 169–177.

[451] C.M. Odio, et al., Comparative efficacy of ceftazidime vs. carbenicillin and amikacin for treatment of neonatal septicemia, Pediatr. Infect. Dis. J. 6 (1987) 371–377.

[452] X. Saez-Llorens, M. O'Ryan, Cefepime in the empiric treatment of meningitis in children, Pediatr. Infect. Dis. J. 20 (2001) 356–361.

[453] X. Saez-Llorens, et al., Prospective randomized comparison of cefepime and cefotaxime for treatment of bacterial meningitis in infants and children, Antimicrob. Agents Chemother. 39 (1995) 937–940.

[454] C.M. Rubino, P. Gal, J.L. Ransom, A review of the pharmacokinetic and pharmacodynamic characteristics of beta-lactam/beta-lactamase inhibitor combination antibiotics in premature infants, Pediatr. Infect. Dis. J. 17 (1998) 1200–1210.

[455] A. Gin, et al., Piperacillin-tazobactam: a beta-lactam/beta-lactamase inhibitor combination, Expert. Rev. Anti. Infect. Ther. 5 (2007) 365–383.

[456] G.L. Drusano, S.C. Schimpff, W.L. Hewitt, The acylampicillins: mezlocillin, piperacillin, and azlocillin, Rev. Infect. Dis. 6 (1984) 13–32.

[457] J.D. Allan, G.M. Eliopoulos, R.C. Moellering Jr., The expanding spectrum of beta-lactam antibiotics, Adv. Intern. Med. 31 (1986) 119–146.

[458] J.A. Moody, L.R. Peterson, D.N. Gerding, In vitro activities of ureidopenicillins alone and in combination with amikacin and three cephalosporin antibiotics, Antimicrob. Agents Chemother. 26 (1984) 256–259.

[459] L.L. Schoonover, et al., Piperacillin/tazobactam: a new beta-lactam/beta-lactamase inhibitor combination, Ann. Pharmacother. 29 (1995) 501–514.

[460] H.M. Bryson, R.N. Brogden, Piperacillin/tazobactam. A review of its antibacterial activity, pharmacokinetic properties and therapeutic potential, Drugs 47 (1994) 506–535.

[461] C.M. Perry, A. Markham, Piperacillin/tazobactam: an updated review of its use in the treatment of bacterial infections, Drugs 57 (1999) 805–843.

[462] J.A. Giron, B.R. Meyers, S.Z. Hirschman, Biliary concentrations of piperacillin in patients undergoing cholecystectomy, Antimicrob. Agents Chemother. 19 (1981) 309–311.

[463] M.D. Reed, et al., Single-dose pharmacokinetics of piperacillin and tazobactam in infants and children, Antimicrob. Agents Chemother. 38 (1994) 2817–2826.

[464] M.C. Thirumoorthi, et al., Pharmacokinetics of intravenously administered piperacillin in preadolescent children, J. Pediatr. 102 (1983) 941–946.

[465] C.B. Wilson, et al., Piperacillin pharmacokinetics in pediatric patients, Antimicrob. Agents Chemother. 22 (1982) 442–447.

[466] R. Wise, et al., Pharmacokinetics and tissue penetration of tazobactam administered alone and with piperacillin, Antimicrob. Agents Chemother. 35 (1991) 1081–1084.

[467] M. Placzek, et al., Piperacillin in early neonatal infection, Arch. Dis. Child. 58 (1983) 1006–1009.

[468] N. Kacet, et al., Pharmacokinetic study of piperacillin in newborns relating to gestational and postnatal age, Pediatr. Infect. Dis. J. 11 (1992) 365–369.

[469] W. Kern, et al., Evaluation of piperacillin-tazobactam in experimental meningitis caused by a beta-lactamase-producing strain of K1-positive *Escherichia coli*, Antimicrob. Agents Chemother. 34 (1990) 697–701.

[470] H.C. Maltezou, et al., Piperacillin/tazobactam versus cefotaxime plus metronidazole for treatment of children with intra-abdominal infections requiring surgery, Eur. J. Clin. Microbiol. Infect. Dis. 20 (2001) 643–646.

[471] A. Arguedas, et al., An open, multicenter clinical trial of piperacillin/tazobactam in the treatment of pediatric patients with intra-abdominal infections, J. Chemother. 8 (1996) 130–136.

[472] J.D. Nelson, G.H. McCracken Jr., Use of ticarcillin/clavulanate (Timentin) in the management of pediatric infections. Introduction, Pediatr. Infect. Dis. J. 17 (1998) 1183–1184.

[473] J.L. Blumer, Ticarcillin/clavulanate for the treatment of serious infections in hospitalized pediatric patients, Pediatr. Infect. Dis. J. 17 (1998) 1211–1215.

[474] R. Sutherland, et al., Antibacterial activity of ticarcillin in the presence of clavulanate potassium, Am. J. Med. 79 (1985) 13–24.

[475] G. Pulverer, G. Peters, G. Kunstmann, In-vitro activity of ticarcillin with and without clavulanic acid against clinical isolates of gram-positive and gram-negative bacteria, J. Antimicrob. Chemother. 17 (Suppl. C) (1986) 1–5.

[476] H.C. Neu, Carbenicillin and ticarcillin, Med. Clin. North Am. 66 (1982) 61–77.

[477] P. Begue, F. Quiniou, B. Quinet, Efficacy and pharmacokinetics of Timentin in paediatric infections, J. Antimicrob. Chemother. 17 (Suppl. C) (1986) 81–91.

[478] A.H. Burstein, et al., Ticarcillin-clavulanic acid pharmacokinetics in preterm neonates with presumed sepsis, Antimicrob. Agents Chemother. 38 (1994) 2024–2028.

[479] G. Fricke, et al., The pharmacokinetics of ticarcillin/clavulanate acid in neonates, J. Antimicrob. Chemother. 24 (Suppl. B) (1989) 111–120.

[480] S.B. Fayed, et al., The prophylactic use of ticarcillin/clavulanate in the neonate, J. Antimicrob. Chemother. 19 (1987) 113–118.

[481] S.M. Abdel-Rahman, G.L. Kearns, The beta-lactamase inhibitors: clinical pharmacology and rational application to combination antibiotic therapy, Pediatr. Infect. Dis. J. 17 (1998) 1185–1194.

[482] G.G. Zhanel, et al., Comparative review of the carbapenems, Drugs 67 (2007) 1027–1052.

[483] J.L. Blumer, Pharmacokinetic determinants of carbapenem therapy in neonates and children, Pediatr. Infect. Dis. J. 15 (1996) 733–737.

[484] J.S. Bradley, et al., Carbapenems in clinical practice: a guide to their use in serious infection, Int. J. Antimicrob. Agents 11 (1999) 93–100.

[485] S.P. Clissold, P.A. Todd, D.M. Campoli-Richards, Imipenem/cilastatin. A review of its antibacterial activity, pharmacokinetic properties and therapeutic efficacy, Drugs 33 (1987) 183–241.

[486] M.O. Santos-Ferreira, J.O. Vital, In-vitro antibacterial activity of imipenem compared with four other beta-lactam antibiotics (ceftazidime, cefotaxime, piperacillin and azlocillin) against 828 separate clinical isolates from a Portuguese hospital, J. Antimicrob. Chemother. 18 (Suppl. E) (1986) 23–26.

[487] R.J. Williams, Y.J. Yang, D.M. Livermore, Mechanisms by which imipenem may overcome resistance in gram-negative bacilli, J. Antimicrob. Chemother. 18 (Suppl. E) (1986) 9–13.

[488] B.J. Freij, et al., Pharmacokinetics of imipenem-cilastatin in neonates, Antimicrob. Agents Chemother. 27 (1985) 431–435.

[489] W.C. Gruber, et al., Single-dose pharmacokinetics of imipenem-cilastatin in neonates, Antimicrob. Agents Chemother. 27 (1985) 511–514.

[490] R.F. Jacobs, et al., Single-dose pharmacokinetics of imipenem in children, J. Pediatr. 105 (1984) 996–1001.

[491] J.D. Rogers, et al., Pharmacokinetics of imipenem and cilastatin in volunteers, Rev. Infect. Dis. 7 (Suppl. 3) (1985) S435–S446.

[492] R.F. Jacobs, et al., Cerebrospinal fluid penetration of imipenem and cilastatin (Primaxin) in children with central nervous system infections, Antimicrob. Agents Chemother. 29 (1986) 670–674.

[493] J. Modai, et al., Penetration of imipenem and cilastatin into cerebrospinal fluid of patients with bacterial meningitis, J. Antimicrob. Chemother. 16 (1985) 751–755.

[494] J.S. Bradley, Meropenem: a new, extremely broad spectrum beta-lactam antibiotic for serious infections in pediatrics, Pediatr. Infect. Dis. J. 16 (1997) 263–268.

[495] J.S. Bradley, et al., Meropenem pharmacokinetics, pharmacodynamics, and Monte Carlo simulation in the neonate, Pediatr. Infect. Dis. J. 27 (2008) 794–799.

[496] J.G. van Enk, D.J. Touw, H.N. Lafeber, Pharmacokinetics of meropenem in preterm neonates, Ther. Drug Monit. 23 (2001) 198–201.

[497] G.B. Calandra, et al., Review of adverse experiences and tolerability in the first 2,516 patients treated with imipenem/cilastatin, Am. J. Med. 78 (1985) 73–78.

[498] V.K. Wong, et al., Imipenem/cilastatin treatment of bacterial meningitis in children, Pediatr. Infect. Dis. J. 10 (1991) 122–125.

[499] S.R. Snavely, G.R. Hodges, The neurotoxicity of antibacterial agents, Ann. Intern. Med. 101 (1984) 92–104.

[500] S. Hori, et al., Inhibitory effect of cephalosporins on gamma-aminobutyric acid receptor binding in rat synaptic membranes, Antimicrob. Agents Chemother. 27 (1985) 650–651.

[501] R.H. Eng, et al., Seizure propensity with imipenem, Arch. Intern. Med. 149 (1989) 1881–1883.

[502] I.P. Day, et al., Correlation between in vitro and in vivo models of proconvulsive activity with the carbapenem antibiotics, biapenem, imipenem/cilastatin and meropenem, Toxicol. Lett. 76 (1995) 239–243.

[503] M.A. Collins, M. Tolpin, Group atcI-Cs, Clinical evaluation of imipenem-cilastin as a single agent therapy for sepsis neonatorum, Program and abstracts of the 27th Interscience Conference on Antimicrobial Agents and Chemotherapy 1987, American Society for Microbiology, Washington, DC, 1987 (abstract).

[504] G.M. Pacifici, Pharmacokinetics of antivirals in neonate, Early Hum. Dev. 81 (2005) 773–780.

[505] G.M. Pacifici, Transfer of antivirals across the human placenta, Early Hum. Dev. 81 (2005) 647–654.

[506] E. Capparelli, N. Rakhmanina, M. Mirochnick, Pharmacotherapy of perinatal HIV, Semin. Fetal. Neonatal. Med. 10 (2005) 161–175.

[507] W.M. Sullender, et al., Pharmacokinetics of acyclovir suspension in infants and children, Antimicrob. Agents Chemother. 31 (1987) 1722–1726.

[508] D.W. Kimberlin, Management of HSV encephalitis in adults and neonates: diagnosis, prognosis and treatment, Herpes 14 (2007) 11–16.

[509] D.W. Kimberlin, et al., Safety and efficacy of high-dose intravenous acyclovir in the management of neonatal herpes simplex virus infections, Pediatrics 108 (2001) 230–238.

[510] J.A. Englund, C.V. Fletcher, H.H. Balfour Jr., Acyclovir therapy in neonates, J. Pediatr. 119 (1991) 129–135.

[511] C.S. Crumpacker, Ganciclovir, N. Engl. J. Med. 335 (1996) 721–729.

[512] J.K. McGavin, K.L. Goa, Ganciclovir: an update of its use in the prevention of cytomegalovirus infection and disease in transplant recipients, Drugs 61 (2001) 1153–1183.

[513] P. Wutzler, R. Thust, Genetic risks of antiviral nucleoside analogues: a survey, Antiviral. Res. 49 (2001) 55–74.

[514] J.M. Trang, et al., Linear single-dose pharmacokinetics of ganciclovir in newborns with congenital cytomegalovirus infections. NIAID collaborative antiviral study group, Clin. Pharmacol. Ther. 53 (1993) 15–21.

[515] X.J. Zhou, et al., Population pharmacokinetics of ganciclovir in newborns with congenital cytomegalovirus infections. NIAID collaborative antiviral study group, Antimicrob. Agents Chemother. 40 (1996) 2202–2205.

[516] E.P. Acosta, et al., Ganciclovir population pharmacokinetics in neonates following intravenous administration of ganciclovir and oral administration of a liquid valganciclovir formulation, Clin. Pharmacol. Ther. 81 (2007) 867–872.

[517] C.F. Meine Jansen, et al., Treatment of symptomatic congenital cytomegalovirus infection with valganciclovir, J. Perinat. Med. 33 (2005) 364–366.

[518] S. Schulzke, C. Buhrer, Valganciclovir for treatment of congenital cytomegalovirus infection, Eur. J. Pediatr. 165 (2006) 575–576.

[519] L. Galli, et al., Valganciclovir for congenital CMV infection: a pilot study on plasma concentration in newborns and infants, Pediatr. Infect. Dis. J. 26 (2007) 451–453.

[520] D.W. Kimberlin, et al., Pharmacokinetic and pharmacodynamic assessment of oral valganciclovir in the treatment of symptomatic congenital cytomegalovirus disease, J. Infect. Dis. 197 (2008) 836–845.

[521] D.W. Kimberlin, et al., Effect of ganciclovir therapy on hearing in symptomatic congenital cytomegalovirus disease involving the central nervous system: a randomized, controlled trial, J. Pediatr. 143 (2003) 16–25.

[522] R.J. Whitley, et al., Ganciclovir treatment of symptomatic congenital cytomegalovirus infection: results of a phase II study. National Institute of Allergy and Infectious Diseases collaborative antiviral study group, J. Infect. Dis. 175 (1997) 1080–1086.

[523] K. Smets, et al., Selecting neonates with congenital cytomegalovirus infection for ganciclovir therapy, Eur. J. Pediatr. 165 (2006) 885–890.

[524] W.W. Thompson, et al., Influenza-associated hospitalizations in the United States, JAMA 292 (2004) 1333–1340.

[525] W.W. Thompson, et al., Mortality associated with influenza and respiratory syncytial virus in the United States, JAMA 289 (2003) 179–186.

[526] H.S. Izurieta, et al., Influenza and the rates of hospitalization for respiratory disease among infants and young children, N. Engl. J. Med. 342 (2000) 232–239.

[527] K.M. Neuzil, et al., The effect of influenza on hospitalizations, outpatient visits, and courses of antibiotics in children, N. Engl. J. Med. 342 (2000) 225–231.

[528] K.M. Neuzil, et al., The burden of influenza illness in children with asthma and other chronic medical conditions, J. Pediatr. 137 (2000) 856–864.

[529] K.M. Neuzil, et al., Burden of interpandemic influenza in children younger than 5 years: a 25-year prospective study, J. Infect. Dis. 185 (2002) 147–152.

[530] Center for Disease Control and Prevention. Severe morbidity and mortality associated with influenza in children and young adults: Michigan, 2003. MMWR 52 (2003) 837–840.

[531] D.E. Noyola, Neuraminidase inhibitors in pediatric patients: potential place in influenza therapy, Paediatr. Drugs 5 (2003) 125–131.

[532] G. He, J. Massarella, P. Ward, Clinical pharmacokinetics of the prodrug oseltamivir and its active metabolite Ro 64-0802, Clin. Pharmacokinet. 37 (1999) 471–484.

[533] S.L. Johnston, et al., Oral oseltamivir improves pulmonary function and reduces exacerbation frequency for influenza-infected children with asthma, Pediatr. Infect. Dis. J. 24 (2005) 225–232.

[534] J.W. Massarella, et al., The pharmacokinetics and tolerability of the oral neuraminidase inhibitor oseltamivir (Ro 64-0796/GS4104) in healthy adult and elderly volunteers, J. Clin. Pharmacol. 40 (2000) 836–843.

[535] K.G. Nicholson, et al., Efficacy and safety of oseltamivir in treatment of acute influenza: a randomised controlled trial. Neuraminidase inhibitor flu treatment investigator group, Lancet 355 (2000) 1845–1850.

[536] J.J. Treanor, et al., Efficacy and safety of the oral neuraminidase inhibitor oseltamivir in treating acute influenza: a randomized controlled trial. US oral neuraminidase study group, JAMA 283 (2000) 1016–1024.

[537] F.G. Hayden, et al., Use of the selective oral neuraminidase inhibitor oseltamivir to prevent influenza, N. Engl. J. Med. 341 (1999) 1336–1343.

[538] F.G. Hayden, et al., Use of the oral neuraminidase inhibitor oseltamivir in experimental human influenza: randomized controlled trials for prevention and treatment, JAMA 282 (1999) 1240–1246.

[539] C. Oo, et al., Pharmacokinetics of anti-influenza prodrug oseltamivir in children aged 1–5 years, Eur. J. Clin. Pharmacol. 59 (2003) 411–415.

[540] R. Dutkowski, et al., Safety and pharmacology of oseltamivir in clinical use, Drug. Saf. 26 (2003) 787–801.

[541] R.J. Whitley, et al., Oral oseltamivir treatment of influenza in children, (erratum appears in Pediatr. Infect. Dis. J. 20 (4) (2001) 421, Pediatr. Infect. Dis. J. 20:127–133, 2001.

[542] Hoffman-La-Roche. Dear Healthcare Professional Letter, 2003. Available at http://www.fda.gov/downloads/Safety/MedWatch/SafetyInformation/SafetyAlertsforHumanMedicalProducts/UCM169493.pdf Accessed 5/25/2010.

[543] L.L. Lewis, BPCA Executive Summary NDA 21-087/NDA21-246, 2004. Available at http://www.fda.gov/downloads/Drugs/DevelopmentApprovalProcess/DevelopmentResources/UCM163346.pdf. Accessed 5/25/2010.

[544] D. Tamura, T. Miura, Y. Kikuchi, Oseltamivir phosphate in infants under 1 year of age with influenza infection, Pediatr. Int. 47 (2005) 484.

[545] S. Okamoto, et al., Experience with oseltamivir for infants younger than 1 year old in Japan, Pediatr. Infect. Dis. J. 24 (2005) 575–576.

[546] US Food and Drug Administration. Available at http://www.fda.gov/Drugs/DrugSafety/PostmarketDrugSafetyInformationforPatientsandProviders/ucm183870.htm and http://www.fda.gov/downloads/Drugs/DrugSafety/InformationbyDrugClass/UCM143872.pdf. Accessed on 5/25/2010.

[547] H.A. Gallis, R.H. Drew, W.W. Pickard, Amphotericin B: 30 years of clinical experience, Rev. Infect. Dis. 12 (1990) 308–329.

[548] J.P. Latge, Aspergillus fumigatus and aspergillosis, Clin. Microbiol. Rev. 12 (1999) 310–350.

[549] J.F. Meis, P.E. Verweij, Current management of fungal infections, Drugs 61 (Suppl. 1) (2001) 13–25.

[550] J. Brajtburg, et al., Amphotericin B: current understanding of mechanisms of action, Antimicrob. Agents Chemother. 34 (1990) 183–188.

[551] A.J. Atkinson Jr., J.E. Bennett, B. Amphotericin, pharmacokinetics in humans, Antimicrob. Agents Chemother. 13 (1978) 271–276.

[552] J.E. Baley, et al., Pharmacokinetics, outcome of treatment, and toxic effects of amphotericin B and 5-fluorocytosine in neonates, J. Pediatr. 116 (1990) 791–797.

[553] B.E. De Pauw, New antifungal agents and preparations, Int. J. Antimicrob. Agents 16 (2000) 147–150.

[554] E. Albengres, H. Le Louet, J.P. Tillement, Systemic antifungal agents. Drug interactions of clinical significance, Drug. Saf. 18 (1998) 83–97.

[555] B.J. Kullberg, B.E. de Pauw, Therapy of invasive fungal infections, Neth. J. Med. 55 (1999) 118–127.

[556] A.H. Groll, S.C. Piscitelli, T.J. Walsh, Antifungal pharmacodynamics: concentration-effect relationships in vitro and in vivo, Pharmacotherapy 21 (2001) 133S–148S.

[557] K.J. Christiansen, et al., Distribution and activity of amphotericin B in humans, J. Infect. Dis. 152 (1985) 1037–1043.

[558] D.W. Denning, D.A. Stevens, Antifungal and surgical treatment of invasive aspergillosis: review of 2,121 published cases, Rev. Infect. Dis. 12 (1990) 1147–1201.

[559] M. Ellis, Amphotericin B preparations: a maximum tolerated dose in severe invasive fungal infections? Transpl. Infect. Dis. 2 (2000) 51–61.

[560] B. Luna, R.H. Drew, J.R. Perfect, Agents for treatment of invasive fungal infections, Otolaryngol. Clin. North Am. 33 (2000) 277–299.

[561] W.E. Dismukes, Introduction to antifungal drugs, Clin. Infect. Dis. 30 (2000) 653–657.

[562] R.T. Proffitt, et al., Pharmacology and toxicology of a liposomal formulation of amphotericin B (AmBisome) in rodents, J. Antimicrob. Chemother. 28 (Suppl. B) (1991) 49–61.

[563] A. Wong-Beringer, R.A. Jacobs, B.J. Guglielmo, Lipid formulations of amphotericin B: clinical efficacy and toxicities, Clin. Infect. Dis. 27 (1998) 603–618.

[564] J. Brajtburg, J. Bolard, Carrier effects on biological activity of amphotericin B, Clin. Microbiol. Rev. 9 (1996) 512–531.

[565] J.W. Hiemenz, T.J. Walsh, Lipid formulations of amphotericin B: recent progress and future directions, Clin. Infect. Dis. 22 (Suppl. 2) (1996) S133–S144.

[566] E.D. Ralph, et al., Comparative in vitro effects of liposomal amphotericin B, amphotericin B-deoxycholate, and free amphotericin B against fungal strains determined by using MIC and minimal lethal concentration susceptibility studies and time-kill curves, Antimicrob. Agents Chemother. 35 (1991) 188–191.

[567] T.J. Walsh, et al., Safety, tolerance, and pharmacokinetics of high-dose liposomal amphotericin B (AmBisome) in patients infected with *Aspergillus* species and other filamentous fungi: maximum tolerated dose study, Antimicrob. Agents Chemother. 45 (2001) 3487–3496.

[568] R.M. Fielding, et al., Comparative pharmacokinetics of amphotericin B after administration of a novel colloidal delivery system, ABCD, and a conventional formulation to rats, Antimicrob. Agents Chemother. 35 (1991) 1208–1213.

[569] H.J. Schmitt, New methods of delivery of amphotericin B, Clin. Infect. Dis. 17 (Suppl. 2) (1993) S501–S506.

[570] K.M. Wasan, et al., Influence of lipoproteins on renal cytotoxicity and antifungal activity of amphotericin B, Antimicrob. Agents Chemother. 38 (1994) 223–227.

[571] J.R. Graybill, et al., Antifungal compounds: controversies, queries and conclusions, Med. Mycol. 38 (Suppl. 1) (2000) 323–333.

[572] O. Ringden, et al., Severe and common side-effects of amphotericin B lipid complex (Abelcet), Bone Marrow Transplant. 22 (1998) 733–734.

[573] J.R. Starke, et al., Pharmacokinetics of amphotericin B in infants and children, J. Infect. Dis. 155 (1987) 766–774.

[574] W.W. Hope, et al., The pharmacokinetics and pharmacodynamics of micafungin in experimental hematogenous *Candida* meningoencephalitis: implications for echinocandin therapy in neonates, J. Infect. Dis. 197 (2008) 163–171.

[575] S.P. Dix, V.T. Andriole, Lipid formulations of amphotericin B, Curr. Clin. Top. Infect. Dis. 20 (2000) 1–23.

[576] R.C. Young, et al., Aspergillosis. The spectrum of the disease in 98 patients, Medicine (Baltimore) 49 (1970) 147–173.

[577] J.E. Bennet, Flucytosine, Ann. Intern. Med. 86 (1977) 319–321.

[578] A. Vermes, H.J. Guchelaar, J. Dankert, Flucytosine: a review of its pharmacology, clinical indications, pharmacokinetics, toxicity and drug interactions, J. Antimicrob. Chemother. 46 (2000) 171–179.

[579] A.C. Pasqualotto, et al., Flucytosine therapeutic monitoring: 15 years experience from the UK, J. Antimicrob. Chemother. 59 (2007) 791–793.

[580] D.A. Stevens, et al., Practice guidelines for diseases caused by *Aspergillus*. Infectious Diseases Society of America, Clin. Infect. Dis. 30 (2000) 696–709.

[581] A.M. Stamm, et al., Toxicity of amphotericin B plus flucytosine in 194 patients with cryptococcal meningitis, Am. J. Med. 83 (1987) 236–242.

[582] D.K. Benjamin Jr., et al., Neonatal candidiasis among extremely low birth weight infants: risk factors, mortality rates, and neurodevelopmental outcomes at 18 to 22 months, Pediatrics 117 (2006) 84–92.

[583] D.A. Frattarelli, et al., Antifungals in systemic neonatal candidiasis, Drugs 64 (2004) 949–968.

[584] E.J. Ernst, Investigational antifungal agents, Pharmacotherapy 21 (2001) 165S–174S.

[585] T.J. Walsh, et al., New targets and delivery systems for antifungal therapy, Med. Mycol. 38 (Suppl. 1) (2000) 335–347.

[586] K. De Beule, J. Van Gestel, Pharmacology of itraconazole, Drugs 61 (Suppl. 1) (2001) 27–37.

[587] M.E. Klepser, et al., Evaluation of voriconazole pharmacodynamics using time-kill methodology, Antimicrob. Agents Chemother. 44 (2000) 1917–1920.

[588] E.J. Ernst, et al., In vitro pharmacodynamic properties of MK-0991 determined by time-kill methods, Diagn. Microbiol. Infect. Dis. 33 (1999) 75–80.

[589] K.W. Brammer, P.E. Coates, Pharmacokinetics of fluconazole in pediatric patients, Eur. J. Clin. Microbiol. Infect. Dis. 13 (1994) 325–329.

[590] A. Wildfeuer, et al., Fluconazole: comparison of pharmacokinetics, therapy and in vitro susceptibility, Mycoses 40 (1997) 259–265.

[591] K.C. Wade, et al., Population pharmacokinetics of fluconazole in young infants, Antimicrob. Agents Chemother. 52 (2008) 4043–4049.

[592] C. Viscoli, et al., Fluconazole in the treatment of candidiasis in immunocompromised children, Antimicrob. Agents Chemother. 35 (1991) 365–367.

[593] R. Schwarze, A. Penk, L. Pittrow, Administration of fluconazole in children below 1 year of age, Mycoses 42 (1999) 3–16.

[594] V. Novelli, H. Holzel, Safety and tolerability of fluconazole in children, Antimicrob. Agents Chemother. 43 (1999) 1955–1960.

[595] D. Debruyne, Clinical pharmacokinetics of fluconazole in superficial and systemic mycoses, Clin. Pharmacokinet. 33 (1997) 52–77.

[596] J.H. Rex, et al., A randomized and blinded multicenter trial of high-dose fluconazole plus placebo versus fluconazole plus amphotericin B as therapy for candidemia and its consequences in nonneutropenic subjects, Clin. Infect. Dis. 36 (2003) 1221–1228.

[597] J. Faergemann, H. Laufen, Levels of fluconazole in serum, stratum corneum, epidermis-dermis (without stratum corneum) and eccrine sweat, Clin. Exp. Dermatol. 18 (1993) 102–106.

[598] D. Kaufman, et al., Fluconazole prophylaxis against fungal colonization and infection in preterm infants (see comment), N. Engl. J. Med. 345 (2001) 1660–1666.

[599] P. Manzoni, et al., A multicenter, randomized trial of prophylactic fluconazole in preterm neonates (see comment), N. Engl. J. Med. 356 (2007) 2483–2495.

[600] C.M. Healy, et al., Fluconazole prophylaxis in extremely low birth weight neonates reduces invasive candidiasis mortality rates without emergence of fluconazole-resistant *Candida* species, Pediatrics 121 (2008) 703–710.

[601] P. Manzoni, et al., Routine use of fluconazole prophylaxis in a neonatal intensive care unit does not select natively fluconazole-resistant *Candida* subspecies, Pediatr. Infect. Dis. J. 27 (2008) 731–737.

[602] C.M. Cotten, et al., The association of third-generation cephalosporin use and invasive candidiasis in extremely low birth-weight infants, Pediatrics 118 (2006) 717–722.

[603] D.K. Benjamin Jr., First, do no harm, Pediatrics 121 (2008) 831–832.

[604] E.K. Manavathu, J.L. Cutright, P.H. Chandrasekar, Organism-dependent fungicidal activities of azoles, Antimicrob. Agents Chemother. 42 (1998) 3018–3021.

[605] J.A. Sabo, S.M. Abdel-Rahman, Voriconazole: a new triazole antifungal, Ann. Pharmacother. 34 (2000) 1032–1043.

[606] E. Johnson, et al., Activity of voriconazole, itraconazole, fluconazole and amphotericin B in vitro against 1763 yeasts from 472 patients in the voriconazole phase III clinical studies, Int. J. Antimicrob. Agents 32 (2008) 511–514.

[607] E.M. Johnson, A. Szekely, D.W. Warnock, In-vitro activity of voriconazole, itraconazole and amphotericin B against filamentous fungi, J. Antimicrob. Chemother. 42 (1998) 741–745.

[608] E.K. Manavathu, et al., A comparative study of the in vitro susceptibilities of clinical and laboratory-selected resistant isolates of *Aspergillus spp.* to amphotericin B, itraconazole, voriconazole and posaconazole (SCH 56592), J. Antimicrob. Chemother. 46 (2000) 229–234.

[609] J.A. Goldstein, S.M. de Morais, Biochemistry and molecular biology of the human CYP2C subfamily, Pharmacogenetics 4 (1994) 285–299.

[610] L. Purkins, et al., Pharmacokinetics and safety of voriconazole following intravenous- to oral-dose escalation regimens, Antimicrob. Agents Chemother. 46 (2002) 2546–2553.

[611] L.B. Johnson, C.A. Kauffman, Voriconazole: A new triazole antifungal agent, Clin. Infect. Dis. 36 (2003) 630–637.

[612] M.A. Ghannoum, D.M. Kuhn, Voriconazole - Better chances for patients with invasive mycoses, Eur. J. Med. Res. 7 (2002) 242–256.

[613] D.W. Denning, et al., Efficacy and safety of voriconazole in the treatment of acute invasive aspergillosis, Clin. Infect. Dis. 34 (2002) 563–571.

[614] A.H. Groll, T. Lehrnbecher, New antifungal drugs and the pediatric cancer patient: current status of clinical development, Klin. Padiatr. 217 (2005) 158–168.

[615] C.C. Chiou, A.H. Groll, T.J. Walsh, New drugs and novel targets for treatment of invasive fungal infections in patients with cancer, Oncologist 5 (2000) 120–135.

[616] C.J. Clancy, M.H. Nguyen, In vitro efficacy and fungicidal activity of voriconazole against *Aspergillus* and *Fusarium* species, Eur. J. Clin. Microbiol. Infect. Dis. 17 (1998) 573–575.

[617] D.J. Sheehan, C.A. Hitchcock, C.M. Sibley, Current and emerging azole antifungal agents, Clin. Microbiol. Rev. 12 (1999) 40–79.

[618] H.M. Lazarus, et al., Safety and pharmacokinetics of oral voriconazole in patients at risk of fungal infection: a dose escalation study, J. Clin. Pharmacol. 42 (2002) 395–402.

[619] K.K.C. Tan, N. Wood, A. Weil, Multi-dose pharmacokinetics of voriconazole in chronic hepatic impairment, in: Program and Abstracts of the 41st Interscience Conference on Antimicrobial Agents and Chemotherapy, American Society of Microbiology, Washington DC, Chicago, Ill, 2001 (abstract).

[620] T.J. Walsh, et al., Pharmacokinetics and safety of intravenous voriconazole in children after single- or multiple-dose administration, Antimicrob. Agents Chemother. 48 (2004) 2166–2172.

[621] T.J. Walsh, et al., Voriconazole in the treatment of aspergillosis, scedosporiosis and other invasive fungal infections in children, Pediatr. Infect. Dis. J. 21 (2002) 240–248.

[622] K. Tan, et al., Investigation of the potential relationships between plasma voriconazole concentrations and visual adverse events or liver function test abnormalities, J. Clin. Pharmacol. 46 (2006) 235–243.

[623] D.W. Denning, C.E. Griffiths, Muco-cutaneous retinoid-effects and facial erythema related to the novel triazole antifungal agent voriconazole, Clin. Exp. Dermatol. 26 (2001) 648–653.

[624] R.P. Santos, et al., Successful medical treatment of cutaneous aspergillosis in a premature infant using liposomal amphotericin B, voriconazole and micafungin, Pediatr. Infect. Dis. J. 26 (2007) 364–1346.

[625] R. Ally, et al., A randomized, double-blind, double-dummy, multicenter trial of voriconazole and fluconazole in the treatment of esophageal candidiasis in immunocompromised patients, Clin. Infect. Dis. 33 (2001) 1447–1454.

[626] K. Frankenbusch, et al., Severe primary cutaneous aspergillosis refractory to amphotericin B and the successful treatment with systemic voriconazole in

two premature infants with extremely low birth weight, J. Perinatol. 26 (2006) 511–514.

[627] K. Bartizal, et al., In vitro preclinical evaluation studies with the echinocandin antifungal MK-0991 (L-743,872), Antimicrob. Agents Chemother. 41 (1997) 2326–2332.

[628] M.B. Kurtz, C.M. Douglas, Lipopeptide inhibitors of fungal glucan synthase, J. Med. Vet. Mycol. 35 (1997) 79–86.

[629] J.R. Graybill, The echinocandins, first novel class of antifungals in two decades: will they live up to their promise? Int. J. Clin. Pract. 55 (2001) 633–638.

[630] D.P. Kontoyiannis, A clinical perspective for the management of invasive fungal infections: focus on IDSA guidelines. Infectious Diseases Society of America, Pharmacotherapy 21 (2001) 175S–187S.

[631] E.J. Ernst, M.E. Klepser, M.A. Pfaller, Postantifungal effects of echinocandin, azole, and polyene antifungal agents against *Candida albicans* and *Cryptococcus neoformans*, Antimicrob. Agents Chemother. 44 (2000) 1108–1111.

[632] T. Chiller, et al., Influence of human sera on the in vitro activity of the echinocandin caspofungin (MK-0991) against *Aspergillus fumigatus*, Antimicrob. Agents Chemother. 44 (2000) 3302–3305.

[633] A.H. Groll, et al., Compartmental pharmacokinetics of the antifungal echinocandin caspofungin (MK-0991) in rabbits, Antimicrob. Agents Chemother. 45 (2001) 596–600.

[634] J.A. Stone, et al., Single- and multiple-dose pharmacokinetics of caspofungin in healthy men, Antimicrob. Agents Chemother. 46 (2002) 739–745.

[635] T. Lehrnbecher, A.H. Groll, Experiences with the use of caspofungin in paediatric patients, Mycoses 51 (Suppl. 1) (2008) 58–64.

[636] T.J. Walsh, et al., Pharmacokinetics, safety, and tolerability of caspofungin in children and adolescents, Antimicrob. Agents Chemother. 49 (2005) 4536–4545.

[637] X. Saez-Llorens, et al., Pharmacokinetics and safety of caspofungin in neonates and infants less than 3 months of age, Antimicrob. Agents Chemother. 53 (2009) 869–875.

[638] A.H. Groll, T.J. Walsh, Caspofungin: pharmacology, safety and therapeutic potential in superficial and invasive fungal infections, Expert. Opin. Investig. Drugs 10 (2001) 1545–1558.

[639] C.A. Sable, et al., Safety and tolerability of caspofungin acetate in the treatment of fungal infections, Transpl. Infect. Dis. 4 (2002) 25–30.

[640] J. Mora-Duarte, et al., Comparison of caspofungin and amphotericin B for invasive candidiasis, N. Engl. J. Med. 347 (2002) 2020–2029.

[641] C.M. Odio, et al., Caspofungin therapy of neonates with invasive candidiasis, Pediatr. Infect. Dis. J. 23 (2004) 1093–1097.

[642] G. Natarajan, et al., Experience with caspofungin in the treatment of persistent fungemia in neonates, J. Perinatol. 25 (2005) 770–777.

[643] A.H. Groll, et al., Micafungin: pharmacology, experimental therapeutics and clinical applications, Expert. Opin. Investig. Drugs 14 (2005) 489–509.

[644] S. Okugawa, et al., A case of invasive central nervous system aspergillosis treated with micafungin with monitoring of micafungin concentrations in the cerebrospinal fluid, Scand. J. Infect. Dis. 39 (2007) 344–346.

[645] E.J. Ernst, et al., In vitro activity of micafungin (FK-463) against *Candida spp.*: microdilution, time-kill, and postantifungal-effect studies, Antimicrob. Agents Chemother. 46 (2002) 3846–3853.

[646] G.P. Heresi, et al., The pharmacokinetics and safety of micafungin, a novel echinocandin, in premature infants, Pediatr. Infect. Dis. J. 25 (2006) 1110–1115.

[647] P. Smith, et al., Pharmacokinetics of an elevated dosage of micafungin in premature neonates, Pediatr. Infect. Dis. J. 28 (2009) 412–415.

[648] D.K. Benjamin Jr., et al., Safety and pharmacokinetics of repeat-dose micafungin in young infants, Clin Pharmacol. Ther. 87 (2010) 93–99.

[649] N.L. Seibel, et al., Safety, tolerability, and pharmacokinetics of micafungin (FK463) in febrile neutropenic pediatric patients, Antimicrob. Agents Chemother. 49 (2005) 3317–3324.

[650] F. Queiroz-Telles, et al., Micafungin versus liposomal amphotericin B for pediatric patients with invasive candidiasis: substudy of a randomized double-blind trial, Pediatr. Infect. Dis. J. 27 (2008) 820–826.

[651] J.M. Joseph, R. Kim, A.C. Reboli, Anidulafungin: a drug evaluation of a new echinocandin, Expert. Opin. Pharmacother. 9 (2008) 2339–2348.

[652] R. Lucas, et al., LY303366 single dose pharmacokinetics and safety in healthy volunteers, in: Program and Abstracts of the 36th Annual Interscience Conference on Antimicrobial Agents and Chemotherapy, 1996, New Orleans, American Society of Microbiology, Washington, DC, 1996.

[653] V. Petraitis, et al., Antifungal efficacy, safety, and single-dose pharmacokinetics of LY303366, a novel echinocandin B, in experimental pulmonary aspergillosis in persistently neutropenic rabbits, Antimicrob. Agents Chemother. 42 (1998) 2898–2905.

[654] A.H. Groll, et al., Pharmacokinetic and pharmacodynamic modeling of anidulafungin (LY303366): reappraisal of its efficacy in neutropenic animal models of opportunistic mycoses using optimal plasma sampling, Antimicrob. Agents Chemother. 45 (2001) 2845–2855.

[655] J.A. Dowell, et al., Anidulafungin does not require dosage adjustment in subjects with varying degrees of hepatic or renal impairment, J. Clin. Pharmacol. 47 (2007) 461–470.

[656] D.K. Benjamin Jr., et al., Safety and pharmacokinetics of intravenous anidulafungin in children with neutropenia at high risk for invasive fungal infections, Antimicrob. Agents Chemother. 50 (2006) 632–638.

[657] J.A. Vazquez, The safety of anidulafungin, Expert. Opin. Drug. Saf. 5 (2006) 751–758.

[658] D. Thye, et al., Anidulafungin: a phase 1 study to identify the maximum tolerated dose in healthy volunteers, in: Program and Abstracts of the 41st Interscience Conference on Antimicrobial Agents and Chemotherapy, 2001, Dec 16–19, 2001, Chicago, Ill. American Society of Microbiology, Washington, DC, 2001.

[659] D. Thye, et al., Anidulafungin: pharmacokinetics in subjects with mild and moderate hepatic impairment, in: Program and Abstracts of the 41st Interscience Conference on Antimicrobial Agents and Chemotherapy, 2001. Dec 16–19, 2001, Chicago, Ill. American Society of Microbiology, Washington, DC, 2001.

[660] D. Thye, et al., Anidulafungin: pharmacokinetics in subjects with severe hepatic impairment, in: Program and Abstracts of the 42nd Annual Interscience Conference on Antimicrobial Agents and Chemotherapy, 2002, San Diego. American Society of Microbiology, Washington, DC, 2002.

[661] A.C. Reboli, et al., Anidulafungin versus fluconazole for invasive candidiasis, N. Engl. J. Med. 356 (2007) 2472–2482.

[662] G.H. McCracken, H.F. Einchenwald, J.D. Nelson, Tetracyclines, J. Pediatr. 76 (1970) 803–804.

[663] A. Mulhall, D.J. Berry, J. de Louvois, Chloramphenicol in paediatrics: current prescribing practice and the need to monitor, Eur. J. Pediatr. 147 (1988) 574–578.

[664] E. Beutler, L. Luzzatto, Hemolytic anemia, Semin. Hematol. 36 (1999) 38–47.

[665] R. Gleckman, S. Alvarez, D.W. Joubert, Drug therapy reviews: trimethoprim-sulfamethoxazole, Am. J. Hosp. Pharm. 36 (1979) 893–906.

[666] A.C. Posner et al., (Eds.), Further Observations on the Use of Tetracycline Hydrochloride in Prophylaxis and Treatment of Obstetric Infections, Medical Encyclopedia, New York, 1955.

[667] S.H. Erickson, G.L. Oppenheim, G.H. Smith, Metronidazole in breast milk, Obstet. Gynecol. 57 (1981) 48–50.

[668] C.M. Passmore, et al., Metronidazole excretion in human milk and its effect on the suckling neonate, Br. J. Clin. Pharmacol. 26 (1988) 45–51.

[669] J. Havelka, A. Frankova, Adverse effects of chloramphenicol in newborn infants, Cesk. Pediatr. 27 (1972) 31–33.

[670] J. Havelka, et al., Excretion of chloramphenicol in human milk, Chemotherapy 13 (1968) 204–211.

[671] J.E. Smadel, et al., Chloramphenicol in the treatment of tsutsugamushi disease, J. Clin. Invest. 28 (1949) 1196–1215.

[672] J.J. Kelsey, et al., Presence of azithromycin breast milk concentrations: a case report, Am. J. Obstet. Gynecol. 170 (1994) 1375–1376.

[673] J.A. Smith, J.R. Morgan, A.R. Rachlis, Clindamycin in human breast milk, Can. Med. Assoc. J. 112 (1975) 806.

[674] B. Steen, A. Rane, Clindamycin passage into human milk, Br. J. Clin. Pharmacol. 13 (1982) 661–664.

[675] R.E. Kauffman, C. O'Brien, P. Gilford, Sulfisoxazole secretion into human milk, J. Pediatr. 97 (1980) 839–841.

[676] R. Arnauld, Etude du passage de la trimethoprime dans le lait maternel, Ouest. Med. 25 (1972) 959.

[677] R.D. Miller, A.J. Salter, The passage of trimethoprim/sulfamethoxazole into breast milk and its significance. Proceedings of the 8th International Congress of Chemotherapy, Hellenic Soc. Chemother. 1 (1974) 687–691.

[678] G. Pons, et al., Nitrofurantoin excretion in human milk, Dev. Pharmacol. Ther. 14 (1990) 148–152.

[679] I. Varsano, J. Fischl, S.B. Shochet, The excretion of orally ingested nitrofurantoin in human milk, J. Pediatr. 82 (1973) 886–887.

[680] Tetracycline in breast milk, BMJ 4 (1969) 791 (letter).

[681] M.J. Rybak, Therapeutic options for gram-positive infections, J. Hosp. Infect. 49 (Suppl. A) (2001) S25–S32.

[682] J. Albanese, et al., Cerebrospinal fluid penetration and pharmacokinetics of vancomycin administered by continuous infusion to mechanically ventilated patients in an intensive care unit, Antimicrob. Agents Chemother. 44 (2000) 1356–1358.

[683] S. Chamberland, et al., Antibiotic susceptibility profiles of 941 gram-negative bacteria isolated from septicemic patients throughout Canada. The Canadian study group, Clin. Infect. Dis. 15 (1992) 615–628.

[684] H. Skopnik, G. Heimann, Once daily aminoglycoside dosing in full term neonates, Pediatr. Infect. Dis. J. 14 (1995) 71–72.

[685] D. Miron, et al., Tolerability of once-daily-dosing of intravenous gentamicin in preterm neonates born at 32–37 weeks of gestation, Harefuah 142 (2003) 413–415, 487.

[686] U. Chotigeat, A. Narongsanti, D.P. Ayudhya, Gentamicin in neonatal infection: once versus twice daily dosage, J. Med. Assoc. Thai. 84 (2001) 1109–1115.

[687] P. Kosalaraksa, et al., Once versus twice daily dose of gentamicin therapy in Thai neonates, J. Med. Assoc. Thai. 87 (2004) 372–376.

[688] L. Krishnan, S.A. George, Gentamicin therapy in preterms: a comparison of two dosage regimens, Indian Pediatr. 34 (1997) 1075–1080.

[689] R. Solomon, et al., Randomized controlled trial of once vs. twice daily gentamicin therapy in newborn, Indian Pediatr. 36 (1999) 133–137.

[690] Lexi-Comp's Pediatric Lexi-Drugs, Available at www.lexi.com Accessed 12/30/2008.

[691] C.G. Prober, D.K. Stevenson, W.E. Benitz, The use of antibiotics in neonates weighing less than 1200 grams (see comment), Pediatr. Infect. Dis. J. 9 (1990) 111–121.

[692] M. de Hoog, J.W. Mouton, J.N. van den Anker, New dosing strategies for antibacterial agents in the neonate, Semin. Fetal. Neonatal. Med. 10 (2005) 185–194.

PREVENTION OF FETAL AND EARLY LIFE INFECTIONS THROUGH MATERNAL–NEONATAL IMMUNIZATION

James E. Crowe, Jr.

CHAPTER OUTLINE

Overall Principles   1212
    Obstacles to Neonatal Vaccination   1212
    Vaccine Strategies for Protecting Neonates Against
      Infection   1216
    Passive Immunization   1218

Active Immunization   1220
Specific Vaccines for Infants   1223
Premature Infants   1228
Regulation of Vaccines and Advisory Bodies   1228

OVERALL PRINCIPLES

Vaccination has been the most effective medical intervention in the modern era. Historically, the focus on vaccine development and implementation programs has been on preventing infectious diseases during infancy and early childhood. The current vaccine schedule for early childhood is replete with dozens of inoculations with an array of safe and effective vaccines that have dramatically reduced the incidence of many previously formidable childhood infectious diseases. Close review of the schedule, however, reveals that most vaccines are clustered in the 2 months to 15 months age group, while there is a paucity of approved vaccines for the neonatal period (Figure 38–1). Safe and effective vaccination of pregnant women and neonates is difficult to achieve, but clearly is now an important target of development. Some of the major pathogens of the neonatal period, such as Group B streptococcus sepsis and meningitis and respiratory syncytial virus bronchiolitis and pneumonia, remain neonatal plagues that can only be addressed by new strategies.

A number of fundamental general principles have been defined through our experience in childhood vaccination programs. First, the usual goal of vaccination is to prevent disease, rather than to induce sterilizing protection against infection. In fact, most licensed vaccines do not completely prevent infection. Eradication of microorganisms in the population is a very difficult goal, whereas excellent protection against severe disease is often achievable. Second, while vaccines generally benefit the individual being immunized, additional public health benefits are often observed when herd immunity is induced in a previously susceptible population. This is especially important for protecting neonates, since there often is insufficient time to induce an adequate immune response for protection in the early weeks of life, and vaccines may not be safe, tested, or immunogenic in this age group. Protecting all of the household contacts and caregivers against infection is currently the most feasible approach for protection of neonates against most diseases. Third, the mechanism by which many vaccines induce protection is poorly understood. Generally current vaccine development programs are accomplished using correlates of protection rather than definitive knowledge of mechanism. A correlate of protection is typically a serologic test with an estimated cutoff of protection that allows comparison of the relatively common data on immunogenicity for different vaccines or vaccine preparations, in contrast to efficacy data, which are difficult to achieve without large numbers of subjects. Examples of correlates of protection that have been established by historical practice are summarized in Table 38–1. Finally, there is significant variation in response to vaccines among individuals that is poorly understood. Responses are affected by many factors such as age, immune status, nutritional status, genetic polymorphisms, and environmental exposures.

Disclosure: This chapter is meant to review the principles of vaccination, and many specific indications, practices, and recommendations are discussed below that were current at the time of writing. Vaccine practice is, however, a constantly changing enterprise. Practitioners should consult the vaccine package inserts for FDA-approved uses, and the relevant current documents of the regulatory and advisory bodies for up-to-date information. The recommendations and guidelines of the Advisory Committee on Immunization Practices (ACIP) of the Centers for Disease Control and Prevention (CDC) are regularly updated on the website www.cdc.gov. The ACIP is the only entity in the federal government that makes such recommendations. The American Academy of Pediatrics also issues guidelines, as published in notices in the Academy journal *Pediatrics*, and in the periodic handbook called the *Red Book*.

OBSTACLES TO NEONATAL VACCINATION

To date, there are many vaccines for infancy and early childhood; however, very few vaccines have been successfully implemented in the neonatal period. A large number of obstacles make it difficult to establish a safe and effective neonatal vaccination program (Table 38–2).

Recommended Immunization Schedule for Persons Aged 0 Through 6 Years—United States • 2010

For those who fall behind or start late, see the catch-up schedule

Vaccine ▼ Age ►	Birth	1 month	2 months	4 months	6 months	12 months	15 months	18 months	19–23 years	2–3 years	4–6 years
Hepatitis B[1]	HepB	HepB			HepB						
Rotavirus[2]			RV	RV	RV[2]						
Diphtheria, Tetanus, Pertussis[3]			DTaP	DTaP	DTaP	see footnote[3]	DTaP				DTaP
Haemophilus influenzae type b[4]			Hib	Hib	Hib[4]	Hib					
Pneumococcal[5]			PCV	PCV	PCV	PCV				PPSV	
Inactivated Poliovirus[6]			IPV	IPV	IPV						IPV
Influenza[7]					Influenza (Yearly)						
Measles, Mumps, Rubella[8]						MMR		see footnote[8]			MMR
Varicella[9]						Varicella		see footnote[9]			Varicella
Hepatitis A[10]						HepA (2 doses)			HepA Series		
Meningococcal[11]									MCV		

Range of recommended ages for all children except certain high-risk groups

Range of recommended ages for certain high-risk groups

This schedule includes recommendations in effect as of December 15, 2009. Any dose not administered at the recommended age should be administered at a subsequent visit, when indicated and feasible. The use of a combination vaccine generally is preferred over separate injections of its equivalent component vaccines. Considerations should include provider assessment, patient preference, and the potential for adverse events. Providers should consult the relevant Advisory Committee on Immunization Practices statement for detailed recommendations: http://www.cdc.gov/vaccines/pubs/acip-list.htm. Clinically significant adverse events that follow immunization should be reported to the Vaccine Adverse Event Reporting System (VAERS) at http://www.vaers.hhs.gov or by telephone, 800-822-7967.

1. **Hepatitis B vaccine (HepB).** (Minimum age: birth)
   At birth:
   - Administer monovalent HepB to all newborns before hospital discharge.
   - If mother is hepatitis B surface antigen (HBsAg)-positive, administer HepB and 0.5 mL of hepatitis B immune globulin (HBIG) within 12 hours of birth.
   - If mother's HBsAg status is unknown, administer HepB within 12 hours of birth. Determine mother's HBsAg status as soon as possible and, if HBsAg-positive, administer HBIG (no later than age 1 week).

   After the birth dose:
   - The HepB series should be completed with either monovalent HepB or a combination vaccine containing HepB. The second dose should be administered at age 1 or 2 months. Monovalent HepB vaccine should be used for doses administered before age 6 weeks. The final dose should be administered no earlier than age 24 weeks.
   - Infants born to HBsAg-positive mothers should be tested for HBsAg and antibody to HBsAg 1 to 2 months after completion of at least 3 doses of the HepB series, at age 9 through 18 months (generally at the next well-child visit).
   - Administration of 4 doses of HepB to infants is permissible when a combination vaccine containing HepB is administered after the birth dose. The fourth dose should be administered no earlier than age 24 weeks.

2. **Rotavirus vaccine (RV).** (Minimum age: 6 weeks)
   - Administer the first dose at age 6 through 14 weeks (maximum age: 14 weeks 6 days). Vaccination should not be initiated for infants aged 15 weeks 0 days or older.
   - The maximum age for the final dose in the series is 8 months 0 days
   - If Rotarix is administered at ages 2 and 4 months, a dose at 6 months is not indicated.

3. **Diphtheria and tetanus toxoids and acellular pertussis vaccine (DTaP).** (Minimum age: 6 weeks)
   - The fourth dose may be administered as early as age 12 months, provided at least 6 months have elapsed since the third dose.
   - Administer the final dose in the series at age 4 through 6 years.

4. ***Haemophilus influenzae* type b conjugate vaccine (Hib).** (Minimum age: 6 weeks)
   - If PRP-OMP (PedvaxHIB or Comvax [HepB-Hib]) is administered at ages 2 and 4 months, a dose at age 6 months is not indicated.
   - TriHiBit (DTaP/Hib) and Hiberix (PRP-T) should not be used for doses at ages 2, 4, or 6 months for the primary series but can be used as the final dose in children aged 12 months through 4 years.

5. **Pneumococcal vaccine.** (Minimum age: 6 weeks for pneumococcal conjugate vaccine [PCV]; 2 years for pneumococcal polysaccharide vaccine [PPSV])
   - PCV is recommended for all children aged younger than 5 years. Administer 1 dose of PCV to all healthy children aged 24 through 59 months who are not completely vaccinated for their age.
   - Administer PPSV 2 or more months after last dose of PCV to children aged 2 years or older with certain underlying medical conditions, including a cochlear implant. See *MMWR* 1997;46(No. RR-8).

6. **Inactivated poliovirus vaccine (IPV)** (Minimum age: 6 weeks)
   - The final dose in the series should be administered on or after the fourth birthday and at least 6 months following the previous dose.
   - If 4 doses are administered prior to age 4 years a fifth dose should be administered at age 4 through 6 years. See *MMWR* 2009;58(30):829–30.

7. **Influenza vaccine (seasonal).** (Minimum age: 6 months for trivalent inactivated influenza vaccine [TIV]; 2 years for live, attenuated influenza vaccine [LAIV])
   - Administer annually to children aged 6 months through 18 years.
   - For healthy children aged 2 through 6 years (i.e., those who do not have underlying medical conditions that predispose them to influenza complications), either LAIV or TIV may be used, except LAIV should not be given to children aged 2 through 4 years who have had wheezing in the past 12 months.
   - Children receiving TIV should receive 0.25 mL if aged 6 through 35 months or 0.5 mL if aged 3 years or older.
   - Administer 2 doses (separated by at least 4 weeks) to children aged younger than 9 years who are receiving influenza vaccine for the first time or who were vaccinated for the first time during the previous influenza season but only received 1 dose.
   - For recommendations for use of influenza A (H1N1) 2009 monovalent vaccine see *MMWR* 2009;58(No. RR-10).

8. **Measles, mumps, and rubella vaccine (MMR).** (Minimum age: 12 months)
   - Administer the second dose routinely at age 4 through 6 years. However, the second dose may be administered before age 4, provided at least 28 days have elapsed since the first dose.

9. **Varicella vaccine.** (Minimum age: 12 months)
   - Administer the second dose routinely at age 4 through 6 years. However, the second dose may be administered before age 4, provided at least 3 months have elapsed since the first dose.
   - For children aged 12 months through 12 years the minimum interval between doses is 3 months. However, if the second dose was administered at least 28 days after the first dose, it can be accepted as valid.

10. **Hepatitis A vaccine (HepA).** (Minimum age: 12 months)
    - Administer to all children aged 1 year (i.e., aged 12 through 23 months). Administer 2 doses at least 6 months apart.
    - Children not fully vaccinated by age 2 years can be vaccinated at subsequent visits
    - HepA also is recommended for older children who live in areas where vaccination programs target older children, who are at increased risk for infection, or for whom immunity against hepatitis A is desired.

11. **Meningococcal vaccine.** (Minimum age: 2 years for meningococcal conjugate vaccine [MCV4] and for meningococcal polysaccharide vaccine [MPSV4])
    - Administer MCV4 to children aged 2 through 10 years with persistent complement component deficiency, anatomic or functional asplenia, and certain other conditions placing them at high risk.
    - Administer MCV4 to children previously vaccinated with MCV4 or MPSV4 after 3 years if first dose administered at age 2 through 6 years. See *MMWR* 2009;58:1042–3.

The Recommended Immunization Schedules for Persons Aged 0 through 18 Years are approved by the Advisory Committee on Immunization Practices (http://www.cdc.gov/vaccines/recs/acip), the American Academy of Pediatrics (http://www.aap.org), and the American Academy of Family Physicians (http://www.aafp.org).
Department of Health and Human Services • Centers for Disease Control and Prevention

FIGURE 38–1 Recommended Immunization Schedule for Persons Aged 0 Through 6 Years-United States, 2010 This schedule indicates the recommended ages for routine administration of currently licensed vaccines, as of December 15, 2 for children aged 0 through 6 years. Any dose not administered at the recommended age should be administered at a subsequent visit, when indicated and feasible. Licensed combination vaccines may be used whenever any component of the combination is indicated and other components are not contraindicated and if approved by the Food and Drug Administration for that dose of the series. Providers should consult the relevant Advisory Committee on Immunization Practices statement for detailed recommendations, including high-risk conditions: http://www.cdc.gov/vaccines/pubs/acip-list.htm. Clinically significant adverse events that follow immunization should be reported to the Vaccine Adverse Event Reporting System (VAERS). Guidance about how to obtain and complete a VAERS form is available at http://www.vaers.hhs.gov or by telephone, 800-822-7967. The Recommended Immunization Schedule for Persons Aged 0 Through 18 Years are approved by the Advisory Committee on Immunization Practices (www.cdc.gov/vaccines/recs/acip), the American Academy of Pediatrics (http://www.aap.org), and the American Academy of Family Physicians (http://www.aafp.org). Department of Health and Human Services, Centers for Disease Control and Prevention.

TABLE 38-1   Selected Correlates of Protection for Common Childhood Vaccines*

Vaccine	Type of Test	Correlate of Protection	Reference(s)
Diphtheria	Toxin neutralization	0.01–0.1 International Units (IU)/mL	[101]
Hepatitis A	Enzyme-linked immunosorbent assay (ELISA)	10 mIU/mL	[102]
Hepatitis B	ELISA	10 mIU/mL	[103]
Haemophilus influenzae type b polysaccharides	ELISA	1 μg/mL	[104]
H. influenzae type b conjugate	ELISA	0.15 μg/mL	[105]
Influenza virus	Hemagglutination inhibition	1:40 dilution	[106]
Measles	Microneutralization	120 mIU/mL	[107]
Pneumococcus	ELISA; opsonophagocytosis	0.20–0.35 μg/mL (for children); 1:8 dilution	[108,109]
Polio	Serum neutralizing	1:4 to 1:8 dilution	[110]
Rubella	Immunoprecipitation	10–15 mIU/mL	[111,112]
Tetanus	Toxin neutralization	0.1 IU/mL	[113]
Varicella	Serum neutralizing; ELISA	1:64 dilution; 5 IU/mL	[114,115]

*Modified from Table 4 in reference 116, Plotkin SA. Vaccines: correlates of vaccine-induced immunity. Clin Infect Dis 47:401–409, 2008.

TABLE 38-2   Obstacles to Safe and Effective Vaccination of Neonates and Young Infants

Safety Concerns

Occult or late presentation of congenital immunodeficiency

Occurrence of sudden infant death syndrome during this period

Presentation of developmental delay and neurologic syndromes during this period

Increased risk of intussusception with gut inflammation at young age

Increased risk of wheezing with provocation due to high-resistance airways

Need for medical workup for sepsis/meningitis when neonates present with fever without localizing symptoms

Immunologic Immaturity

Antibody genes lacking somatic mutations

Poor magnitude of antibody immune responses

Poor quality of antibody immune responses

Poor durability of antibody responses

Cytokine bias in response to infection (low Th1/Th2 ratio)

Low levels of complement

Inability to respond to polysaccharides

Concern for inducing tolerance

Antibody-mediated suppression of humoral responses caused by transplacentally-acquired maternal antibodies

Interference by concomitant exposure to antigens from other infections, environmental antigens, or vaccine antigens

Safety Concerns

The Hippocratic principle *primo non nocere*, first do no harm, is the supreme driving principle in all vaccination programs, but even more so in the development of neonatal vaccines. Many events and factors that occur during the neonatal period can complicate the interpretation of vaccine safety at this age. The population at risk for birth defects is estimated to be about 3% or 4%, and not all of these defects are fully apparent at the time of birth. There is a strong trend in the United States to discharge neonates from hospitals and birthing centers before 24 hours of age. If a defect was present at birth but not detected until later, it might be falsely linked to a vaccine given to the neonate. Many if not most congenital immunodeficiencies do not declare themselves this early in life. In some areas of the world, a high percentage of infants are infected with HIV, but this status is not known at the time of birth. Live virus vaccines and the live mycobacterium BCG, while generally effective, are usually contraindicated in immunodeficient individuals. Other types of congenital defects MANIFEST during early infancy, a time in which many vaccinations are given. For instance, many neurologic disorders, including seizure disorders and neurodegenerative diseases, MANIFEST in the first few months of life. Many cardiopulmonary disorders, for instance cyanotic heart disease or cystic fibrosis, do not cause symptoms in the neonatal period. Sudden infant death syndrome also occurs early in life during the target period of vaccination. The cause of this fatal disorder is not well understood; therefore it is very difficult to assess the risk of exacerbation of SIDS by infection or vaccination. A large number of physiologic changes occur during the first few months of life. Young infants possess airways with very small diameters, which exhibit very high resistance especially during airway inflammation. Therefore, young infants are prone to wheezing with relatively minor provocation. Infants are obligate nose breathers. Therefore, a vaccine that has the potential to cause an increase in nasal secretions leading to nasal obstruction, such as live attenuated respiratory virus vaccines, can interfere with feeding, which is a significant problem at this age. Also, infants are susceptible to intestinal intussusception during inflammation of the gastrointestinal tract.

There are also medical factors that complicate the evaluation of vaccines in this age group. Infants in the first two months of life who exhibit fever without localizing symptoms generally undergo a complete medical workup for sepsis and meningitis. A vaccine that causes even a low rate of fever in this age group will be associated with a large number of expensive and unnecessary medical workups.

Immunologic Immaturity

Neonates are clearly in transition in their immunologic development as they move from a sterile environment enveloped in the placenta, through the birth canal, into a world with vast numbers of environmental and microbial exposures. Generally it is thought that fetal immune systems are regulated in utero to avoid robust innate and adaptive immune responses to self-antigens or to maternal antigens that cross the placenta. Mouse models suggest that fetuses can be tolerized to antigens following in utero exposure, while human studies are more limited. Suppressive T regulatory cells in the fetus are generated against noninherited maternal antigens, and these cells establish functional tolerance to foreign antigens present during development in utero. For instance, one study observed T regulatory cells in the lymph nodes of fetal products of conception at 18 to 22 weeks of gestation that promoted maternal microchimerism (presence of maternal cells in the fetus) in 15 out of 18 lymph node samples [1]. Foreign antigens clearly do cross the placenta [2,3]. Some human studies suggest that fetal adaptive immune responses to nonself antigens are relatively intact [4–7]. Overall, the evidence suggests that the fetal immune system promotes a relatively high level of tolerance, but it is not devoid of functional activity.

Following parturition, a rapid transition must be made to deal with new antigens from food, the environment, and commensal bacteria, and to differentiate them from harmful micro-organisms. It is likely that this transition takes time, and that human neonates still exhibit some features of predisposition to tolerance, associated with persistence of long-lived T regulatory cells [1] and significant evidence of B cell tolerance [8]. Theoretical concerns are sometimes raised that exposure to antigens early in life during a phase when the immune milieu exhibits a residual tolerogenic status might result in the infant becoming *less* well able to respond to the antigen rather than achieving immunologic priming for memory.

Neonates tend to make poor immune responses following infection or vaccination, both in terms of quantity and quality. The magnitude of antibody responses, as measured by serology, is reduced. The time to peak titer is often delayed by a month or more, compared with the response of older children. The function of the antibodies is low, for example the neutralizing activity of antiviral antibody responses, suggesting that neonates secrete antibodies that bind but do not kill viruses. And the durability of the antibody response made early in life is poor. Young infants who are demonstrated to be infected with a virus early in life, as evidenced by disease and virus shedding, may seroconvert in the months following infection, but then appear to be seronegative the year following. It is likely that this suggests a neonatal B cell response characterized by differentiation of naïve antigen-specific cells to antibody secreting plasma cells without induction of long-lived plasma cells or significant numbers of memory B cells. The B cells of neonates are markedly predisposed to apoptosis following stimulation, compared with adult cells, because of reduced expression of IL-4 receptor and higher levels of gene expression related to proapoptotic programs [9].

Neonatal mice exhibit skewed antibody gene segment usage compared with adult mice; however, most evidence in human infants suggests that the antibody variable gene repertoire is very similar to that of adults, including microbial-specific B-cell repertoires. The antibody sequences of B cells of infants exhibit mature levels of junctional diversity, including N and P type of insertions, and the lengths of the antibody variable loops (complementarity determining regions) are similar to those of adults [10]. The distinguishing molecular difference between adult and infant antibodies is the striking lack of somatic mutations in infant antibody sequences [10]. The use of germline sequences to encode antibodies to microorganisms early in life leads to the generation of low affinity antibodies [11]. Somatic mutations, which occur in the germinal center during antigen exposure, are the driving molecular force behind antibody affinity maturation and increases in antibody function. It is not clear currently whether the lack of mutations stems from the fact that neonatal B cells are encountering antigen for the first time (as opposed to the secondary responses made by older previously exposed individuals), or whether there are intrinsic B cell defects in affinity maturation. Following stimulation with the CD40 ligand and cytokines (mimicking T helper cell interaction), human cord blood B cells do upregulate the transcription of genes involved in somatic hypermutation including activation-induced cytidine deaminase (AID) and error-prone DNA polymerases [12].

There are also factors extrinsic to B cells that affect antibody responses early in life. T cell responses, while perhaps more robust than B cell responses early in life, exhibit some altered features compared with adult T cells. In particular, neonatal responses generally appear to be reduced in the magnitude of Th1 type cytokines, with relatively preserved levels of Th2 cytokines, leading to an overall Th2-biased response. Undoubtedly the model of Th1 versus Th2 biases in this age group is a gross oversimplification of very complex and highly regulated responses that are skewed early in life in various ways. In addition, professional antigen presenting cells such as dendritic cells and macrophages may exhibit developmental programs that affect the outcome of humoral responses.

There are also extrinsic factors that affect the function of the antibody proteins themselves. For instance, complement protein levels are low in neonates, especially terminal elements of the complement cascade. Complement-fixing antibodies may not be able to induce effective formation of membrane attack complexes when terminal complement components are in short supply. Complement also is necessary for optimal antigen presentation in many cases.

Infants exhibit a particular deficiency in responding to capsular polysaccharides, such as those of pathogenic bacteria including *Neisseria meningitides*, *Haemophilus influenzae*, *Streptococcus pneumoniae*, and others. A functional response to the small repeating units of these carbohydrates is usually not observed until the age of two years, although this deficiency has been overcome with conjugate vaccines, discussed later. (For a more detailed discussion of fetal and neonatal immunity, see Chapter 4.)

Maternal Antibodies

Antibodies from the mother cross the placenta into the fetus, beginning at about 32 weeks, and increasing until term. The transfer appears to be an active process, mediated by a receptor (FcRn) that specifically transports immunoglobulin G (IgG) but not other immunoglobulin isotypes. In some cases, the IgG titer of antibodies at birth exceeds those of the mother. The transfer is beneficial because the infant becomes effectively passively immunized against all of the pathogens to which the mother had mounted an effective response. Acquisition of these antibodies affords protection against severe disease in many cases, but the antibodies are lost over time. Passively acquired maternal antibodies may, however, interfere with the response of neonates to infection or immunization, a phenomenon termed antibody-mediated immune suppression.

Interference

In some cases, the suboptimal responses exhibited by neonates may be due to interference caused when multiple exposures, infections, or immunizations occur simultaneously. Combination vaccines have been carefully developed, with an eye toward adding new vaccine antigens in such a way as to maintain effective responses to existing vaccines. However, it is common to observe that addition of new antigens can affect the quantitative response to other components of the vaccine. Forcing multiple exposures early in life could lead to interference [13]. It should be remembered that vaccines are not the only exposures, as neonates are also exposed to a myriad of naturally acquired infections, food and environmental antigens, and allergens. Vaccine antigens, in fact, represent a very small component of the antigen exposures early in life.

Logistics of Immunization Programs

Immunization programs have to be implemented in the context of an overall public health approach. In many areas of the world, children have the highest rate of access to medical interventions in the newborn period. Investigators interested in global health have often dreamed of a single efficacious vaccination given at birth for all major childhood infections because access to children is highest at birth. However, this goal is not really realistic, given the obstacles outlined above. Therefore, each country has to develop an approach to vaccinating infants that achieves the highest feasible coverage based on local resources, infrastructure, financial commitments, cold chain, and other practical considerations. Even if a vaccine has been shown in definitive clinical trials to be efficacious, the effectiveness of a vaccine in the field often is determined by practical considerations of cost/benefit, adverse event profile, and the clinical relevance to the experience of the practitioner and of parents. While pediatricians in the outpatient setting in the United States generally are strong advocates of proper vaccination, hospital physicians and staff who manage the peripartum period are less acculturated to routine vaccination of neonates. Administration of multiple vaccines to all newborns before discharge after birth would require an infrastructure and culture that is not currently present. Parents play a major role in decision making too, appropriately so. Parents will need to be convinced of the clinical benefit and the safety of any vaccines offered shortly after birth.

VACCINE STRATEGIES FOR PROTECTING NEONATES AGAINST INFECTION

There are four major vaccination strategies for protecting neonates: (1) maternal immunization during pregnancy, (2) passive immunization with antibodies or immune globulins, (3) active immunization of neonates, and (4) immunization of contacts to prevent transmission.

Maternal Immunization

Immunization of mothers during pregnancy is an attractive strategy for several reasons. Pregnant women typically are easy to identify, and in many areas of the world there is a high level of access to prenatal care. The principle of maternal immunization is to induce or boost the levels of antibodies against micro-organisms in the mother's serum, causing a quantitative or qualitative enhancement of the IgG isotype antibodies that cross the placenta and circulate in the blood of the fetus. Maternal immunization has been shown to be safe and effective for several diseases, especially tetanus [14–16] and influenza [16–20], has been tested for respiratory syncytial virus [21], and is being tested for pertussis (ClinicalTrials.gov Identifier: NCT00553228).

In 1979, the U.S. Food and Drug Administration (FDA) introduced a classification of fetal risks due to pharmaceuticals given during pregnancy. Pregnancy category A is applied when adequate and well-controlled studies have failed to demonstrate a risk to the fetus in the first trimester of pregnancy (and there is no evidence of risk in later trimesters). Pregnancy category B pertains when animal reproduction studies have failed to demonstrate a risk to the fetus and there are no adequate and well-controlled studies in pregnant women *or* animal studies have shown an adverse effect, but adequate and well-controlled studies in pregnant women have failed to demonstrate a risk to the fetus in any trimester. Pregnancy category C is assigned when animal reproduction studies have shown an adverse effect on the fetus and there are no adequate and well-controlled studies in humans, but potential benefits may warrant use of the drug in pregnant women despite potential risks. All vaccines that have been licensed by the FDA are categorized as pregnancy category C, except for the quadrivalent human papillomavirus vaccine, which is category B.

Maternal Immunization to Prevent Tetanus, Diphtheria, and Pertussis

In developed countries tetanus and diphtheria are essentially controlled or eliminated. In the 1970s there was a worldwide push to deliver tetanus diphtheria (Td) vaccine to a broad segment of the population by targeting susceptible pregnant women. These campaigns were highly effective in markedly reducing or eliminating tetanus of the mother and infant in some areas. Still, in the 47 poorest countries in Africa and Asia, an estimated 128,250 babies and up to 30,000 mothers died of tetanus in 2004, according to UNICEF [22]. That agency has set a goal to deliver nearly 400 million doses of vaccine in mothers and infants in an effort to eliminate the disease in these groups by 2012. There does not seem to be any problem with performance or safety of the vaccine in these groups; the shortfall stems simply from implementation.

Pertussis on the other hand has been much more difficult to address. Major reductions in numbers of pertussis cases were accomplished by childhood pertussis vaccination through the middle of the 20th century; however, the disease has been rising in incidence for several decades. It is estimated that hundreds of thousands of cases occur in adults in the United States each year, which places infant contacts at risk. Many feel that the durability of solid vaccine-induced immunity may not extend beyond early adolescence, leaving a susceptible adult and older adolescent population.

Pregnant mothers can be infected with *Bordetella pertussis* and suffer symptomatic respiratory tract disease, spanning from mild to severe. Surprisingly, there is little evidence in the literature that pregnant women are more susceptible to severe disease than other healthy adults. Also, there is little evidence that infection of pregnant mothers is associated with adverse outcomes for the fetus, such as fetal demise or altered development. Therefore the focus of maternal immunization against pertussis is on preventing severe disease in young infants *after* birth.

Most of the deaths due to pertussis occur in infants less than 2 months of age, at a time before routine immunization is initiated. The optimal strategy to protect these young infants is not entirely clear. Immunization of women postpartum could maximize immunity in the mother to prevent the mother from acquiring a new infection and transmitting it to newborns. However, data suggest that mothers are the source of pertussis in less than a quarter of cases [23]. Therefore this strategy may have minimal effect on reducing risk in the first months of life. Immunization in the second or third trimester of pregnancy is of potential benefit to the mother by prevention of disease in her, and induces higher levels of antibodies that can be transferred across the placenta. In the first half of the 20th century, pregnant mothers were commonly immunized with whole-cell pertussis vaccine, and it was clear that third trimester vaccination raised the level of antibodies in infants. Efficacy was not studied or proven in a rigorous way, however. There is the suggestion in clinical and epidemiology surveillance studies that maternal immunization reduces the incidence of disease in infants [24–26]. Tetanus, reduced-diphtheria, acellular pertussis vaccine (TdaP) was licensed for use in adolescents and adults in the United States in 2005. This vaccine is commonly given to pregnant women without evidence of harm to mothers or fetuses. Recent changes in policies of the ACIP recommend that adolescents and adults should receive a single dose of TdaP (instead of a single dose of Td), if their last dose of Td was greater than 2 years ago (instead of greater than 10 years ago). The American College of Obstetricians and Gynecologists (ACOG) and the American Academy of Pediatrics now recommend that women should receive TdaP before pregnancy if possible. However, if immunization is not accomplished before pregnancy, TdaP should be given in the second or third trimester, preferably before 32 weeks gestation, to protect the mothers and to transfer immunity to the fetus [27].

Maternal Immunization to Prevent Influenza

Immunization of pregnant women against influenza is important for the health of both the mother and the infant. The risk of influenza during pregnancy continues to be underappreciated. Seasonal influenza poses a significant risk to the health of pregnant women during annual winter seasonal epidemics [28,29]. Both the ACIP and the (ACOG) recommend that all pregnant women be immunized during the influenza season. Vaccination is recommended at any gestational age. The indicated vaccine is conventional trivalent inactivated vaccine, given by the intramuscular route in the deltoid muscle. Although an intranasal live attenuated trivalent vaccine is available, that vaccine is not recommended during pregnancy. Immunization during pregnancy has been shown to be safe for both the infant and the mother. Pregnant mothers appear to respond well to inactivated influenza virus vaccination, in a similar manner to nonpregnant women, achieving elevated antiviral antibody titers in both maternal serum and umbilical cord serum [18]. A careful prospective trial in 158 mother/infant pairs suggested that immunization of pregnant women could delay onset or reduce severity of disease in infants [30]. Influenza antibody titers in umbilical cord blood of immunized mothers do achieve protective levels; in fact they can be higher than those of the mother. Higher levels of maternal anti-influenza antibodies are associated with greater and longer protection of infants.

Maternal Immunization to Prevent RSV Infection

Respiratory syncytial virus (RSV) causes hospitalization of infants for wheezing, pneumonia, or apnea, with a peak incidence at about 6 weeks of age. There appears to be some relative sparing of disease in the first weeks of life, possibly associated with maternal antibodies. It is difficult to contemplate inducing immunity in neonates before this age; therefore investigators have investigated maternal immunization against RSV to increase the titer of virus neutralizing maternal antibodies that cross the placenta. The rationale is that, for every twofold rise in maternal antibodies that could be achieved, infants might be protected for an additional 3 weeks if a conventional IgG antibody half-life of 21 days is observed. A small experimental trial of an RSV subunit protein vaccine has been conducted in pregnant women. The vaccine, an immunoaffinity-purified protein isolated from infected cell culture designated purified protein 2 (PFP-2), was safe but minimally immunogenic in a small trial [21]. The promise of this strategy remains unresolved.

Measles-Mump-Rubella (MMR) Vaccine During Pregnancy

Women are advised not to receive the MMR vaccine during pregnancy because all components are live viruses. Rubella virus is of particular concern since there is the theoretical possibility of this live virus vaccine causing congenital rubella syndrome. A number of women have inadvertently received this vaccine while pregnant or soon before conception. The CDC collected data about the outcomes of their births. From 1971–1989, 324 infants were born to 321 women who received rubella vaccine while pregnant and continued pregnancy to term, and no cases of congenital rubella syndrome were identified [31]. Given that the risk to the fetus appears to be negligible, a recommendation suggesting termination of pregnancy following inadvertent immunization is not warranted.

PASSIVE IMMUNIZATION

Antibodies in the blood of otherwise healthy previously infected adults can be collected in the form of plasma or serum, which can also be fractionated to isolate polyclonal immune globulins. If the collections are performed from large numbers of randomly selected healthy donors and pooled, then the resulting preparation of gamma globulin will contain an average titer of antibodies to microorganisms that is found in the donor population. Administration of antibodies to naïve recipients to confer temporary humoral immunity is termed passive immunization.

A large number of hyperimmune and conventional immune globulins and a monoclonal antibody have been licensed for use in humans (See Table 38–3). Conventional immune globulin is used to treat a number of conditions, including congenital or acquired immunodeficiency, Kawasaki disease, and idiopathic thrombocytopenic purpura, and to provide postexposure prophylaxis for hepatitis A and measles. Donors can be screened by serology to identify subsets of individuals with high functional titers of specific antibodies, enabling polyclonal antibody preparations that are enriched in activity for a specific organism, termed hyperimmune globulin (for example RSV immune globulin) [32]. A large number of immune globulins have been produced, such as preparations for botulism, hepatitis B, tetanus, cytomegalovirus, varicella-zoster virus, rabies virus, and vaccinia-virus. Most of these have been used in neonates.

Immunoglobulins are derived from human blood products, so there is the theoretical risk of transmission of adventitious infectious agents. These products are prepared from plasma by a process called Cohn fractionation, which removes most of the potential adventitious agents and purifies the product. Plasma is treated with ethanol in increasing concentrations up to 40%. The pH is progressively reduced over the course of the fractionation, as is the temperature. Five major fractions are recovered, each containing a specific precipitate. In recent years, preparations have also been treated with a solvent-detergent viral inactivation process that is highly effective [33].

RSV Immune Globulin and Monoclonal Antibodies

RSV immune globulin was partially effective in preventing hospitalization due to severe RSV [34–36]; however the intravenous route and large volumes needed brought challenges for administration. Subsequently, a neutralizing humanized mouse monoclonal antibody to the RSV fusion protein (palivizumab) was developed and licensed that allowed for intramuscular administration. The efficacy of palivizumab was assessed in a randomized, double-blind, placebo-controlled trial (designated the Impact-RSV Study) in high risk infants, with a 55% reduction in hospitalizations [37]. This antibody is the only monoclonal antibody licensed to date for any infectious disease. An affinity-matured second generation RSV monoclonal antibody (motavizumab) is in late-stage clinical trials [38].

Hepatitis B Immune Globulin

This immune globulin for intramuscular administration is used to treat babies born to mothers who test positive for hepatitis B surface antigen (HBsAg) (or who have not been screened) with or without hepatitis B e antigen (HBeAg). Infants born to mothers known to be HBsAg-positive should receive hepatitis B immune globulin after physiologic stabilization of the infant and preferably within 12 hours of birth. The hepatitis B vaccine series should be initiated simultaneously, if not contraindicated, with the first dose of the vaccine given concurrently with the hepatitis B immune globulin, but at a different site.

TABLE 38–3   FDA-Approved Products for Passive Immunization and Immunotherapy

Disease	Product	Indication
Infant botulism	Botulism immune globulin (BabyBIG)	Treatment of infant botulism
Cytomegalovirus	CMV immune globulin	Prevention or treatment in immunocompromised
Hepatitis B Ig	Hepatitis B immune globulin	Postexposure prophylaxis
Tetanus	Tetanus immune globulin	Treatment of tetanus infection
Varicella (chickenpox)	Varicella-zoster virus immune globulin	Postexposure prophylaxis in high-risk individuals
Rabies	Rabies immune globulin	Postexposure prophylaxis (administered with rabies vaccine)
Vaccinia (smallpox vaccine)	Vaccinia immune globulin	Treatment of progressive infection
Hepatitis A	Pooled human immune globulin	Prevention of hepatitis A infection
Measles	Pooled human immune globulin	Prevention of measles infection
Congenital/acquired immunodeficiency	Pooled human immune globulin	Treatment of immunodeficiency
ITP/Kawasaki disease	Pooled human immune globulin	Treatment of inflammatory state
Respiratory syncytial virus	Palivizumab (humanized mouse monoclonal antibody)	Prevention of respiratory syncytial virus disease in high-risk infants

Women admitted for delivery, who were not screened for HBsAg during the prenatal period, should be tested. While test results are pending, the newborn infant should receive hepatitis B vaccine within 12 hours of birth. If the mother is later found to be HBsAg-positive, the infant should receive hepatitis B immune globulin as soon as possible and within seven days of birth; however, the efficacy of hepatitis B immune globulin administered after 48 hours of age is not known [39]. Testing for HBsAg and anti-hepatitis B surface antigen antibodies is recommended at 12 to 15 months of age for infants who were born to HBsAg-positive mothers and who were immunized and given HBIg at birth. If HBsAg is not detectable and surface antigen specific antibodies are present, the child is considered protected [40].

Varicella-Zoster Immune Globulin (VZIG)

This hyperimmune globulin has been used to protect high-risk individuals following exposure. VZIG treatment is expected to be most effective when it is initiated as soon as possible after exposure, but it may be effective if administered as late as 96 hours after exposure. Treatment after 96 hours is of uncertain value. Small particle aerosols transmit varicella, so assessing exposure is complex. The CDC has defined what constitutes a "substantial" varicella exposure, with the central concept that direct contact exposure is defined as greater than 1 hour of direct contact with an infectious person while indoors [41]. The onset of varicella in pregnant women from 5 days before to 2 days after delivery is estimated to result in severe varicella infection in about a quarter of those newborn infants, with a high risk of death [42–44]. Although numbers of treated infants are not adequate to determine a rigorous efficacy, VZIG reduced disease. In the UK, surveillance studies suggested the proportion of deaths among neonates infected with varicella decreased from 7% to none after the onset of routine use of VZIG in this setting [45]. In October 2004, Massachusetts Public Health Biologic Laboratories, the only U.S.-licensed manufacturer of VZIG, discontinued manufacturing this product. In February 2006, an investigational VZIG product, VariZIG (made by Cangene in Canada) became available under an investigational new drug application with an expanded access protocol. VariZIG can be requested from an authorized U.S. distributor. Intravenous immune globulin (IVIG) should be the primary means of postexposure prophylaxis among persons at high risk of severe varicella complications if VZIG or VariZIG is not available, according to the CDC's Advisory Committee on Immunization Practices (ACIP).

The uses in infants of VZIG in the past, or VariZIG currently, are outlined in the following, which is excerpted from the former VZIG package insert [46] and the VariZIG recommendations of the CDC ACIP, available at www.cdc.gov.

Immunocompromised Children

VZIG is recommended for passive immunization of susceptible, immunocompromised children after significant exposure to chickenpox or zoster. These children include those with primary cellular immune deficiency disorders or neoplastic diseases and those currently receiving immunosuppressive treatments.

Newborns of Mothers with Varicella Shortly Before or After Delivery

VZIG is indicated for newborns of mothers who develop chickenpox within 5 days before or within 48 hours after delivery.

Premature Infants

Although the risk of postnatally acquired varicella in the premature infant is unknown, it is wise to administer varicella zoster immune globulin to exposed premature infants of 28 weeks of gestation or more if their mothers have a negative or uncertain history of varicella. Premature infants of less than 28 weeks of gestation or birth weight of less than 1000 grams should be considered for VZIG regardless of maternal history since they may not yet have acquired transplacental maternal antibodies.

Full-Term Infants Less than 1 Year of Age

Mortality from varicella in the first year of life is four times higher than that in older children, but lower than mortality in immunocompromised children or normal adults. The decision to administer VZIG to infants less than 1 year of age should be evaluated on an individual basis. After careful evaluation of the type of exposure, susceptibility to varicella including maternal history of varicella and zoster, and presence of underlying disease, VZIG may be administered to selected infants.

VZIG does not appear to significantly alter the attack rate in healthy neonates who are exposed in utero within 5 days of delivery (30% to 40%), but the rate of complications and fatal outcomes appears to be substantially lower for neonates who are treated with VZIG.

Cytomegalovirus Immune Globulin

This preparation is a purified immunoglobulin for intravenous administration derived from pooled adult human plasma selected for high titers of antibody for cytomegalovirus (CMV) [47]. It is generally used for the prophylaxis of cytomegalovirus disease associated with transplantation of kidney, lung, liver, pancreas, and heart in older subjects. Only limited information is available about the use of CMV-IGIV in pregnancy or the neonatal period, and more study is needed to more fully evaluate the possible benefits and risks of passive immunization with CMV-IGIV in such situations. This hyperimmune globulin has been given to a limited number of pregnant women with primary CMV infection in an attempt to treat or prevent congenital CMV infection. There is some evidence from a prospective, uncontrolled study that administration of CMV-IGIV to pregnant women with confirmed primary CMV infection and with CMV-positive amniotic fluid may decrease the risk of symptomatic congenital CMV disease in their infants; however, this treatment is considered experimental at this time.

Botulinum Immune Globulin

Infant botulism is a form of human botulism caused by ingestion of *Clostridium botulinum* spores that colonize and grow in the infant's large intestine, resulting in the secretion of botulinum neurotoxin into the intestine. The toxin can cause flaccid paralysis with respiratory and feeding failure. Botulinum immune globulin is an orphan drug product with high titers of antibodies against botulinum toxin for intravenous administration that is indicated for the treatment of patients below 1 year of age with infant botulism caused by toxin type A or B. The approach, using isolation of immune globulin from the plasma of donors immunized with pentavalent (ABCDE) botulinum toxoid, was developed by the California Department of Health Services. Treatment within 3 days of admission to hospital shortened mean hospital stay of all (type A and type B) infant botulism patients by several weeks, significantly shortened length of ICU stay, duration of mechanical ventilation, and length of tube feedings [48].

ACTIVE IMMUNIZATION

Immunization of individuals directly to stimulate adaptive immune responses characterized by memory is termed active immunization. This approach is preferred when feasible because long-lasting responses can be induced by brief medical encounters, without further intervention, or in some cases with periodic boosting.

The general approach to developing an effective vaccine starts with an understanding of pathogenesis and correlates of immunity. For instance, tetanus is caused by a toxin secreted by a bacterium, not by the organism itself, so the licensed vaccine was designed to induce antibodies to the toxin rather than the bacterium. Once the fundamentals of the disease are understood through epidemiology studies and animal model experiments, vaccine candidates are developed and tested in preclinical models, usually including small animals such as mice and then nonhuman primates. Human studies are conducted in phases, with increasing numbers of subjects. Phase I trials establish safety (typically in several dozen subjects), phase II trials investigate dose and expanded safety data collection (typically in hundreds of subjects), phase III trials establish efficacy (typically in many thousands of subjects), and phase IV surveillance is sometimes conducted after licensure. There are a large number of strategies for development of vaccines that have been successful to date (Table 38–4).

Jennerian Vaccines

The simplest approach, pioneered by Jenner, uses an animal micro-organism to infect humans to induce cross-protective immune responses. This approach was used to develop the smallpox vaccine vaccinia, which was also multiply passaged. BCG is a live mycobacterial strain that is used in many parts of the world as a tuberculosis vaccine during the neonatal period.

In recent years, a modified Jennerian approach has been used in which virus genes from animal viruses have been combined with genes from the matching human virus to create chimeric viruses that retain the authentic human protective antigens, but incorporate animal genes that perform suboptimally during virus replication resulting in attenuation. Since these organisms often replicate in the recipients to some degree, they can often induce both T- and B-cell responses and can be very immunogenic. There are two principal ways that the chimeric

---

TABLE 38-4   Major Types of Vaccines

- Jennerian approach (use of inoculation with a naturally occurring animal pathogen to induce a cross-protective immune response to a human pathogen); e.g., vaccinia virus (the smallpox vaccine), rhesus rotavirus (withdrawn), human-bovine rotavirus reassortant viruses, Bacillus Calmette-Guérin (BCG; a vaccine against tuberculosis)
- Live attenuated viruses
  - Naturally occurring avirulent isolates; e.g., the Jeryl Lynn strain of mumps virus, poliovirus
  - Cell culture passaged mutants (with in vitro marker, such as cold-adapted, temperature-sensitive, small plaque, or other phenotype); e.g., rubella virus Wistar Institute RA 27/3 strain, influenza, poliovirus, measles and mumps viruses, varicella virus, rotavirus
- Inactivated (killed or disrupted) virus; e.g., influenza, inactivated poliovirus, hepatitis A virus, rabies virus
- Toxoid, a bacterial toxin whose toxicity has been reduced; e.g., diphtheria and tetanus toxoids
  - Chemical treatment
  - Genetic manipulation of toxin sequence
- Subunit proteins
  - Purified from serum, cell or egg culture, or recombinant expression systems such as yeast; e.g., hepatitis B surface antigen, papillomavirus
  - Purified from bacterial culture, *Bordetella pertussis*
- Polysaccharides; e.g., *Haemophilus influenzae* type B, *Streptococcus pneumoniae*, *Neisseria meningitidis*
  - Plain, or conjugated to a protein
- Combined vaccines, e.g., MMR/V, DTaP/Hib/IPV, HepA/B, and others
- Experimental approaches
  - Vectored vaccines, DNA, peptides, mimotopes

---

vaccines are made. If the virus genome is segmented, then the animal virus and the human virus are used to coinfect cells in culture, and viruses with various combinations of gene origins arise, a process termed reassortment. If the genome is nonsegmented, then the viral genomes are cloned by molecular biology techniques to make a cDNA copy of each genome. By molecular means, these genomes can be manipulated to make chimeras, point mutations, or gene deletions or gene order shuffling. Once the altered cDNA is made, plasmid DNA is used to transfect mammalian cells and generate a live mutant virus, a process termed "virus rescue." The modified Jennerian approach has been successful using genes from nonhuman primate and bovine rotaviruses by reassortment. Bovine parainfluenza virus type 3 has been tested in infants as young as two months [49], and chimeric experimental vaccines for respiratory syncytial virus or human parainfluenza virus type 3 have been developed by rescue from cDNA using the bovine virus backbone [50,51].

Attenuation of Live Human Viruses

Live viruses have been attenuated in additional ways. Typically, viruses can be multiply-passaged in cell culture, during which attenuated viral variants arise as a consequence of viral polymerase error. Mutation rate (or selection for survival of mutants in culture) can be accelerated by passaging and adapting in cells from a different species (resulting in "host range restriction" mutations), passaging in the presence of chemical mutagens that cause missense mutations in the virus genomes, or selecting for an in vitro phenotype such as cold-adaptation, temperature sensitivity, or small plaque phenotype (for instance the live attenuated trivalent influenza vaccine). Vaccines for poliovirus, measles, rotavirus, rubella, and others have been derived in this way. In some cases, investigators have isolated naturally attenuated or avirulent virus strains from human subjects that can be used as vaccines with their native sequence. Vaccines for mumps and polio virus have been derived in this manner. Six experimental live attenuated vaccine candidates for respiratory syncytial virus made in this way have been tested in clinical trials [52–57]. A live attenuated vaccine candidate for parainfluenza type 3 (the main cause of croup in infants) was developed by multiple passaging in cell culture (designated *cp*45, because it had been cold-passaged 45 times in culture) and has been studied in infants and found to be immunogenic [58]. A phase II trial has been conducted with combined experimental vaccines for respiratory syncytial virus and for parainfluenza type 3 [59].

Inactivated Vaccines

Growing organisms in culture in the laboratory followed by inactivation is a simple approach that has been dramatically successful for some organisms. Organisms can be inactivated by beta propiolactone, formalin, UV irradiation, and other techniques. The Salk polio vaccine had a dramatic effect on polio epidemiology when implemented. Similar efforts with influenza led to the development of the inactivated trivalent influenza vaccine that is the mainstay of current prevention against influenza disease. Excellent inactivated vaccines also have been developed for hepatitis A and rabies virus. This approach is not without its potential problems, however. If a virulent strain is used to produce the virus stock, inadequate inactivation can lead to iatrogenic disease such as occurred in the so-called Cutter incident. A number of children immunized with an inactivated poliovirus vaccine preparation containing inadequately inactivated Mahoney poliovirus developed paralytic poliomyelitis [60]. Also, unexpected adverse events have followed immunization with inactivated vaccines. In the 1960s, a formalin-inactivated RSV vaccine induced enhanced disease in children when they were later exposed to natural infection, resulting in several deaths [61,62]. Similarly, an inactivated measles vaccine induced a response known as "atypical" measles that was associated with giant cell pneumonia and an unusual rash on exposure to wild-type virus.

Toxoids

Diseases caused by bacterial toxins (generally exotoxins) have been successfully addressed by the development of toxoids. In some manner, the virulence of the toxin is reduced or removed, while preserving the immunogenicity of the resulting protein. Detoxification can be achieved by treating wild-type toxins with chemicals to alter them, or by creating genetic mutant forms of toxin that can be expressed in the laboratory. These vaccines tend to be very immunogenic and effective. Tetanus toxoid and diphtheria toxoid are the prototypes for this approach. Toxoids are also used sometimes as the carrier protein to which polysaccharides are attached in conjugate vaccines.

Subunit Proteins

The success of inactivated virus vaccines led to the idea that nonreplicating materials could induce protective responses as long as the materials contained the protective antigens (usually the target of protective antibodies) in a conformationally intact presentation. Microbial proteins can be partially or highly purified from whole organism cultures by extraction and purification, or individual proteins can be expressed in a recombinant fashion from DNA copies of the coding region of the protein. Hepatitis B surface antigen (HBsAg), a highly effective vaccine, was originally isolated from the plasma of naturally infected subjects, but now is expressed in *Saccharomyces cerevisiae*. The use of nonreplicating proteins has the advantage that the antigen will not likely cause the disease produced by the microbe; however, inoculation with proteins usually does not induce MHC Class I restricted cytolytic T cells, and the response to subunit proteins is often weak in the absence of adjuvants.

Polysaccharide Vaccines

Encapsulated bacteria are some of the major pathogens of infancy. Immunity to most of these organisms is mediated by type-specific capsular polysaccharide antibodies. Therefore, immunization with polysaccharides purified from the organism is immunogenic and protective in older individuals. For instance, there is a 23-valent polysaccharide vaccine for protection against invasive disease caused by the pneumococcus. Infants less than 2 years of age, however, do not respond to polysaccharides. Investigators found, however, that conjugation of these polysaccharides to carrier proteins enabled young infants to respond to the immunizations with robust antibody responses to the polysaccharides. The intellectual concept was that the carrier protein would facilitate coupled T helper cell induction by B cells specific for the polysaccharides that process and present peptides from the associated protein, thus inducing T cell help for the response. Interestingly, different carrier proteins exhibit differing performance levels. Now we know that some of these carrier proteins also work in part by stimulating pattern recognition receptors such as Toll-like receptors.

The first conjugate vaccines were aimed at *H. influenzae* type B (Hib), a former major cause of sepsis and meningitis in infancy. The polysaccharide Hib vaccine worked poorly in young children, while the conjugate vaccine has virtually eliminated the disease in the United States. Conjugated vaccines have been developed for *S. pneumoniae* that are effective, but a challenge is to incorporate as many type-specific polysaccharides as possible to cover circulating field strains. The frequency of strains varies in different geographic locations. The current pneumococcal conjugate vaccine, designated PCV7 or Prevnar and containing antigens from serotypes 4, 6B, 9V, 14, 18C, 19F, and 23F, was licensed in 2000 and can be used in children under the age of 2 years. This conjugate vaccine has been incorporated into the childhood immunization schedule in the United States for infants aged 2 to 23 months. Subjects older than 2 years of age at high risk of disease can be given the 23-valent polysaccharide vaccines (designated PPV23 or PPSV), marketed as Pneumovax or Pnu-Immune. Additional conjugate vaccines are being studied; a 9-valent (PCV9) vaccine provides coverage of the serotypes in PCV7 plus coverage of serotypes 1 and 5, while an 11-valent (PCV11) vaccine provides PCV9 coverage plus serotypes 3 and 7F. A conjugate strategy for a vaccine for older subjects has been developed for four meningococcus subtypes. Quadrivalent meningococcal polysaccharide vaccine (designated MPSV4, Menomune, Sanofi Pasteur) was the only meningococcal vaccine available in the United States until a quadrivalent meningococcal conjugate vaccine (designated MCV4, Menactra, Sanofi Pasteur) was approved for young children in 2007. This vaccine is approved now in subjects aged 2 to 55 years, but is being studied in younger children. Experimental meningococcal conjugate vaccines are being further developed to cover as many types as possible.

Combination Vaccines

The relatively large number of successful childhood vaccines resulted in an inordinate number of needle injections to deliver all recommended vaccines. Therefore a push has been made over the years to combine vaccines to reduce injections, visits, and administration costs. Most childhood vaccines in use today are in fact combination vaccines. Various combinations are possible, and depend in part on the intellectual property and the clinical experience of the manufacturer. Diphtheria and pertussis toxoids are routinely coadministered with pertussis antigens, but Hib conjugate vaccine and trivalent inactivated poliovirus can be added to this combination. Measles, mumps, rubella, and varicella live attenuated viruses can be coadministered as a single inoculation. Even live or killed poliovirus and live or killed influenza virus vaccines can be considered to be combination vaccines because they each contain three different viruses representing antigenic variants.

When converting vaccines from a monovalent form to a combined form, manufacturers must demonstrate that the combination does not result in interference that reduces the efficacy of any of the components. For instance, the dose of each of the three live poliovirus vaccine strains was adjusted to achieve optimal immunogenicity for each without interference. Often serologic correlates of protection are followed for the purpose of analyzing whether interference occurs. Interpretation of these serologic tests is definitive only when a solid quantitative correlate of protection has been established, which is often lacking.

Experimental Approaches

A number of additional technologies are being explored for the development of new vaccines. Insertion of heterologous sequences into an attenuated organism is termed using a vectored approach. This approach is common in preclinical development today, using viral vectors

such as poxviruses, adenoviruses, alphaviruses, and other organisms. Bacterial vectors such as *Salmonella* and BCG are also under investigation. DNA immunization using plasmid DNAs that encode microbial antigens that are expressed under the control of mammalian promoters is administered by needle injection or by "gene-gun" gold particle-mediated inoculation. These and other approaches are common in the preclinical arena and in phase I healthy adult trials, but they face significant regulatory hurdles before neonatal vaccine trials could be contemplated.

Adjuvants

Immunologic adjuvants are substances that enhance the magnitude, induction, or durability of antigen-specific immune responses when used in combination with specific vaccine antigens. Typically adjuvants are not antigenic when administered in the absence of vaccine antigens. Historically, there has only been one type of adjuvant licensed for human use, aluminum salts (alum). These inorganic compounds, such as aluminum hydroxide and aluminum phosphate, mediate aggregation and physical deposition effects for the complexed antigens, but they also have additional effects. These and other adjuvants cause inflammatory responses, sometimes mediated by Toll-like receptors and other pattern recognition molecules. This mechanism is a two-edged sword, as untoward effects of inflammation may occur, and alum may skew the cytokine responses to antigen toward a Th2-dominated profile.

Many newer adjuvants are under development; a large number has been tested in adults in the context of experimental HIV vaccine trials. Various classes of new adjuvants include oil-based products, virosomes, and organic molecules such as squalene—QS21 and MF59 adjuvants are being investigated closely. Toll-like receptor agonists are being investigated in an attempt to stimulate the innate immune system in a controlled fashion. Despite the explosion of knowledge of innate immune mechanisms in recent years, incorporation of adjuvants into vaccine development programs is still largely an empirical exercise.

Route of Inoculation

Various routes of inoculation are used for immunization, depending on the mechanism of action, convenience, and the technology used. Live attenuated viruses intended to induce gastrointestinal tract mucosal immunity (such as rotavirus and poliovirus vaccines) are fed orally. Live attenuated viruses intended to induce respiratory tract mucosal immunity, such as live attenuated influenza vaccine, can be administered as intranasal drops or spray. Live viruses designed to induce high levels of systemic immunity marked by elevated serum levels of antibody, such as measles, mumps, rubella, and varicella, are given by a parenteral route such as intramuscular or subcutaneous. This strategy makes sense because the pathogenesis of systemic diseases such as measles often involves a viremia during which the circulating viruses are susceptible to serum antibodies. Interestingly, the site of intramuscular inoculation (deltoid, gluteus, quadriceps) can affect the immunogenicity of vaccination, so providers should follow the vaccine package insert to most closely replicate the conditions used in the successful efficacy trials.

Timing

The age of vaccine recipients and presence or absence of passively acquired maternal antibodies greatly affects response to vaccination. The antibody response to measles virus vaccine, for instance, is highly susceptible to inhibition by small amounts of maternal antibodies. Administration of vaccine before 12 months of age is associated with diminished responses in infants due to the presence of passively derived maternal antibodies, and administration before 6 months of age is associated with diminished responses even in infants lacking passively acquired maternal antibodies [63]. Therefore vaccination is optimally initiated after 12 months of life [63]. This plan represents a major problem in developing world environments because the disease often occurs in infants less than 1 year of age. It was reasoned that one effective approach might be to deliver an increased dose of attenuated virus in young infants in an attempt to overcome suppression mediated by maternal antibodies. In 1989, high-titer measles vaccine using the Edmonston-Zagreb strain was recommended by the WHO for use in areas with a high incidence of measles in children younger than 9 months [64]. Three years later, that recommendation was withdrawn because reports from Haiti, Senegal, and Guinea-Bissau suggested an increased incidence of female mortality occurring after administration of the high-titered vaccine [65,66]. The pathogenesis of this process is not fully understood, and the association was not observed in all areas where high-titered vaccine was used. Nevertheless, high-titered vaccine is no longer used.

Many childhood vaccines are initiated in the first weeks or months of life, including DPT and DTaP, polio, Hib, and hepatitis B vaccines. Multiple doses of these vaccines are often required to achieve sufficient immunogenicity and protection early in life. The interval between doses also may significantly affect the immunogenicity of particular vaccines. Often the optimal interval is not known, or cannot be implemented, because most countries develop a standard infant vaccine administration schedule. Having done so, the introduction of new vaccines early in life is typically designed to fit the established visit schedule, such as 2, 4, and 6 months of life in the United States.

Birth Dosing

Most infant vaccines are not actually administered during the neonatal period; however, there are a few notable exceptions. BCG is given in many countries of the world shortly after birth. A series of hepatitis B inoculations can begin shortly after birth as well. Universal immunization with hepatitis B vaccine is principally aimed at preventing sexually transmitted or blood borne disease later in life; however, initiating the series near the time of birth can contribute to the interruption of mother-child transmission in the setting of maternal infection. If a mother is known to be infected, a combination of hepatitis B immune globulin and hepatitis B vaccine is administered at the time of birth.

SPECIFIC VACCINES FOR INFANTS
Bacille Calmete Guerin

This organism is a live attenuated *Mycobacterium bovis* vaccine. It is given soon after birth in most countries in sub-Saharan Africa. It is estimated that approximately three quarters of the global birth cohort is immunized near the time of birth with this vaccine. It is not routinely used in the United States. Various substrains and preparations are used in different countries, and the efficacy of the vaccine against infection is questionable. However, there is a consensus that vaccination reduces the most severe forms of tuberculosis, disseminated processes marked by miliary disease or tuberculous meningitis, which among otherwise healthy individuals most commonly occur in children of less than 2 to 4 years of age. There are a large number of studies whose numbers conflict; however, meta-analysis suggests that vaccination prevents about 75% of miliary disease and tuberculous meningitis [67,68]. In contrast, it is not clear that BCG affects pulmonary tuberculosis disease.

The vaccine causes a significant local inflammatory reaction in many cases, but is safe in immunocompetent children. It is estimated that less than 5 in a million healthy children develop disseminated disease with BCG [69], and many of these children prove to have congenital immunodeficiencies. In contrast, a special concern with this live vaccine is that the geographic areas in which it is most used also are areas where HIV infection is especially common and often undiagnosed. As a consequence, universal vaccination of infants results in inoculation of a significant number of infants who will develop HIV infection and AIDS. The risk of disseminated BCG infection and disease is several hundred fold increased in infants with HIV infection (estimated incidence 401 to 1300 per 100,000) [69]. The WHO has now made HIV infection in infants a full contraindication to BCG vaccination [70].

Diphtheria

Corynebacterium diphtheriae is an aerobic gram-positive bacterium which secretes a toxin that inactivates human elongation factor eEF-2, thus inhibiting translation during protein synthesis by human cells. The site of infection, generally the throat, becomes sore and swollen. The toxin can cause damage to the myelin sheaths in the central and peripheral nervous system leading to loss of motor control or sensation. Immunization with diphtheria toxoid has been in widespread use since the 1930s; the vaccine is one of the safest in use. The toxoid can be manufactured from diphtheria toxin treated with formalin to inactivate the toxicity but maintain immunogenicity, and is administered as part of the DPT vaccine beginning at about 2 months. Pertussis toxin (PT) and diphtheria toxin (DT) also have been detoxified genetically by introduction of point mutations that cause a loss of enzymatic activity but retention of binding activity. One mutant DT protein that is a toxoid with a single amino acid mutation at the enzymatic active site, designated CRM_{197}, is the protein carrier for a licensed *H. influenzae* type B vaccine.

Pertussis

B. pertussis is a gram-negative coccobacillus which causes an acute respiratory illness with multiple protracted phases. The organism secretes a number of toxins that affect respiratory tract epithelial cells, and also some that have systemic effects such as the promotion of lymphocytosis. The disease is most severe in the youngest infants [71]; however, routine vaccination typically does not begin until age 6 to 8 weeks. The need for inducing herd immunity to reduce disease in the contacts of infants through immunizing healthy adults, adolescents, and pregnant mothers was discussed above. There are two principal types of pertussis vaccines, inactivated organisms ("whole-cell," often abbreviated P) and a formulation that uses antigen fragments derived from the organism ("acellular," often abbreviated aP). Both vaccines are immunogenic and protective, but the acellular vaccine causes about a tenfold lower rate of side effects such as fever or injection site pain and erythema. Most developed countries use acellular pertussis vaccine, but many countries continue to use the whole-cell vaccine because it is cheaper and equally efficacious. The WHO Expanded Program on Immunization (EPI) uses the whole cell vaccine in its vaccination efforts.

It seems to be intuitive that if the most severe disease caused by pertussis occurs in the first months of life, then adding a dose of vaccine near the time of birth might be effective in reducing disease early in life, and indeed this approach has been investigated recently in three relatively small studies of neonatal acellular pertussis vaccination in the United States and Europe [72–74]. Although the protocols and vaccines differed somewhat, it is not clear that adding a birth dose of acellular pertussis vaccine increases immunity to pertussis without interfering with other vaccine responses or the long-term immunogenicity of pertussis vaccine. An Italian study showed that a birth dose of aP vaccine followed by the standard Italian schedule for DTaP vaccination at 3, 5 and 11 months resulted in earlier antibody responses but lower PT IgG levels at 7 to 8 months of age [74]. A U.S. trial studied DTaP administered at birth plus the conventional vaccination schedule at 2, 4, and 6 months. Pertussis antibody levels were similar at 6 months of age in the two groups, but at 7-month levels were significantly lower in the group vaccinated at birth, an effect that was still noted at 18 months of age [72]. A German study of aP vaccine at birth revealed induction of a higher response to pertussis antigens at 3 months of age compared with controls and equivalent pertussis antibody titers at 8 months of age with or without a birth dose [73]. Previous trials with whole-cell pertussis vaccine in this age group also generated data that raised the question of whether inhibition of response is caused by an early dose. More study is needed in this area.

Tetanus

Clostridium tetani, the bacterial cause of tetanus, enters through open wounds from environmental sources and produces a toxin that causes prolonged spasms and tetani. The tetanus toxoid vaccine was developed in 1926. The vaccine is a solution of formaldehyde-deactivated toxin isolated from the bacterium. It also is one of the safest vaccines in use, and is perhaps the most immunogenic vaccine in use in children. Immunization of infants is routinely initiated at 2 months of age.

Neonatal tetanus (tetanus neonatorum) is caused by contamination of the stump of the umbilical cord. The symptoms of the disease often begin in the first 2 weeks of life, well before routine vaccination is initiated at 2 months, and the disease is often fatal. Maternal immunization and clean treatment of the umbilical cord stump are the best approaches to prevention of this disease.

Tetanus of mothers can occur during pregnancy following wound contamination. Most cases of obstetric tetanus occur in the puerperal or postpartum period, however, often after complicated deliveries or surgical or spontaneous abortions [75].

Poliovirus

There are two types of poliovirus vaccines in use. The first is a trivalent live attenuated vaccine developed by Albert Sabin in the 1950s and licensed in 1961, containing attenuated poliovirus, types I, II, and III, grown in monkey kidney cell tissue culture. This vaccine is administered orally, replicates in the intestine, but does not invade neurons, thus it induces long-lasting intestinal and humoral immunity. Shedding of vaccine viruses in the stool results in transmission of vaccine viruses to close contacts, which has both benefits and risks. The benefit is that many naïve contacts who were not vaccinated themselves become inoculated and immune, thus achieving a high level of herd immunity. For this reason, the live vaccine is preferred in most large-scale eradication efforts in areas where disease still occurs.

Attenuated polioviruses do mutate during replication, however, and lose aspects of attenuation. Rarely (about one case per million doses), these partial revertant viruses cause vaccine-associated paralytic poliomyelitis. The last case of wild-type poliovirus disease acquired in the United States occurred in 1979. For this reason, the United States discontinued use of the live vaccine in 2000. The live vaccine is contraindicated in pregnant women and subjects with HIV infection, other serious immunodeficiencies, or their household contacts.

The other vaccine, inactivated polio vaccine (IPV) is a killed virus preparation, first developed by Salk and licensed in 1955. Killed vaccine induces principally humoral immunity, but still exhibits excellent efficacy against disease. IPV does not have the benefit of causing herd immunity, but also does not transmit virus to contacts and does not cause vaccine-associated paralysis. The enhanced potency IPV vaccine that is in current use has been in use since 1998. It is a component of some combination vaccine formulations.

Varicella Zoster Virus

Varicella zoster virus (VZV) is spread by the respiratory route by small particle aerosol, and is one of the most infectious agents that affect humans. Before implementation of vaccination, infection was universal in childhood, consisting of a febrile syndrome with vesicular rash. The disease, though often relatively mild, was sometimes complicated by pneumonia, central nervous system effects (including encephalitis), secondary infection such as bacterial cellulitis or fasciitis, and hemorrhagic conditions. Varicella during pregnancy can have adverse consequences for the fetus and infant of a nonimmune mother, including congenital varicella syndrome. It has been estimated that several dozen cases of this syndrome occurred each year before universal immunization. There was close consideration for many years whether universal vaccination was warranted in the United States because there were only about 100 varicella-associated deaths a year, and it was expected that the vaccine strain would persist, dormant in the sensory-nerve ganglia like the wild-type virus. Further, the durability of protection was not known. Since varicella disease is often more severe in older subjects, concern was raised about the possibility of waning immunity during adulthood leading to more severe disease. Nevertheless, based on an extended experience in Japan and excellent safety and efficacy data, the virus was licensed for universal immunization in the United States in 1995 [76].

This vaccine contains the Oka strain of live, attenuated VZV. The Oka strain was isolated in Japan in the early 1970s from vesicular fluid in a healthy child who had natural varicella and was attenuated through sequential propagation in cell monolayer cultures in the laboratory [77]. The virus in the Oka/Merck vaccine in use in the United States was further passaged in MRC-5 human diploid-cell cultures for a total of 31 passages. The combination MMRV vaccine was licensed in 2005 on the basis of noninferiority of immunogenicity of MMRV compared with MMR and varicella vaccine given at different sites [78]. The ACIP recommends the use of either MMRV vaccine or the separate MMR and varicella vaccines for children at 12 to 15 months of age, and expressed a preference for the MMRV vaccine for the second dose, given at 4 to 6 years of age.

Measles Virus

The current measles vaccine is a live attenuated strain given subcutaneously. There are numerous strains of attenuated virus that have been developed, and the strains used in the vaccine have varied between countries and over the years in the United States. The live attenuated Edmonston B strain was licensed in 1963 and used until 1975. A further attenuated vaccine called the Schwarz strain was introduced in 1965 and used for a number of years. Finally, a live, further attenuated preparation of the Enders-Edmonston virus strain was developed and licensed in 1968 (designated the "Moraten" strain because it was more attenuated). This is the only measles virus vaccine currently used in the United States. The vaccine is highly immunogenic in seronegative subjects. Maternal antibodies inhibit vaccine immunogenicity in the first year of life. Therefore, vaccination is delayed until 12 to 15 months of age in the United States and other countries of the developed world.

Mumps Virus

Mumps virus causes a febrile illness most commonly associated with parotitis, but also sometimes more severe conditions including aseptic meningitis. Pregnant women who contract mumps infection during the first trimester of pregnancy suffer an increased risk for fetal death [79], but pregnancies not resulting in fetal demise are not associated

with congenital malformations [80]. In the early 1960s, an inactivated vaccine was used, but live attenuated virus has been used exclusively since 1978. The current vaccine strain has an interesting history. The noted virologist Maurice Hilleman isolated the virus from the throat of his daughter, Jeryl-Lynn, and developed it as the vaccine strain. Later studies revealed the vaccine strain is actually a mixture of two strains that have differing genetics and in vitro growth characteristics [81]. The vaccine is typically given as a component of MMR or MMRV vaccine at 12 to 15 months of age. The incidence of mumps in the United States has been remarkably reduced by universal vaccination since the 1960s, especially notable after the widespread use of a second dose of mumps vaccine among U.S. schoolchildren began in 1990. Recent outbreaks in the United States, however, raise the question of whether a new strain or strategy is needed [82].

Rubella Virus

Rubella virus is a member of the Togaviridae family that is spread by respiratory droplets, causing a mild infection with viremia. The rubella virus vaccine is a live attenuated virus first licensed in 1969. It is given subcutaneously, now usually as a component of MMR or MMRV vaccine, beginning between 12 and 15 months of age. The live rubella virus vaccine currently distributed in the United States, prepared using the RA 27/3 strain grown in human diploid cell culture, was licensed in the United States in 1979. Several strains used previously, including the HPV-77 and Cendehill strains, induced more adverse events and less durable immunity.

The main goal of rubella immunization is prevention of congenital rubella syndrome. There are several approaches that have been used to achieve immunity in women of childbearing age. For many years in the UK, girls were inoculated against rubella in their early teens, as the childhood disease in boys and girls is typically mild and the focus was on prevention of congenital rubella syndrome. In the United States, an alternate strategy was used, that of immunizing all children in an effort to reduce circulation of the virus in the population, and thus the risk of exposure of pregnant women to children with virus shedding. Both strategies showed some effectiveness, but universal immunization proved more effective. Rubella and congenital rubella syndrome have been eliminated in the United States because of high vaccine coverage and high rates of immunity in the population [83].

Rubella vaccine has long been incorporated into the MMR or MMRV combination vaccines for universal immunization of both boys and girls starting at 12 to 15 months, followed by a booster dose at school entry. The WHO also recommends that countries undertaking measles elimination should also take the opportunity to eliminate rubella through the use of measles-rubella (MR) or MMR vaccine in their childhood immunization programs.

Hepatitis B

Hepatitis B virus causes a potentially life-threatening liver disease that in many cases becomes chronic. Hepatitis B virus is transmitted between people by contact with blood or other body fluids. Children typically acquire hepatitis B infection in one of three ways: (1) Perinatal transmission from an infected mother at birth, (2) early childhood infections through close interpersonal contact with infected household contacts, or (3) blood transfusion. Hepatitis B vaccines have been available since 1982. The strategy in the United States initially was to target vaccine to health care workers and patients at high risk; however, that strategy was not adequately effective because of poor compliance. Currently, the strategy is that all infants should receive the hepatitis B vaccine. This approach has several benefits. First, universal vaccination typically achieves higher coverage of those later at risk than targeted programs. Second, initiation of immunization near the time of birth interrupts vertical transmission from mother to child. In areas where mother-to-infant spread of hepatitis is common, the first dose of vaccine should be given within 24 hours of birth. When it is known that a mother is actively infected at the time of birth, the baby is treated with both hepatitis B immune globulin and vaccine. The original vaccine was prepared from the plasma of patients infected with hepatitis B, but now the protective antigen, hepatitis B surface antigen, is produced in a recombinant form in yeast.

Apart from the direct metabolic effects of liver dysfunction, chronic infection with hepatitis B also is associated with liver cancer. Therefore the hepatitis vaccine was the first licensed vaccine to prevent cancer.

Hepatitis A

Hepatitis A is transmitted by the fecal-oral route and causes acute liver disease. Transmission is relatively common in day-care settings. This inactivated vaccine is recommended for all children, starting at 1 year of age. Two single-antigen vaccines are licensed in the United States, and one hepatitis vaccine combined with hepatitis B vaccine. The vaccine is given as a two-dose series.

Influenza Virus Vaccine

Influenza virus is a respiratory virus spread by large particle aerosol and fomites. This orthomyxovirus circulates in humans in two major types (A and B), with two distinct A subtypes currently causing disease in humans, designated H1N1 and H3N2. Therefore, current seasonal influenza vaccines are trivalent, including A/H1N1, A/H3N2, and B antigens. The virus uses an RNA dependent RNA polymerase to replicate that is error-prone, and each year point mutations occur in the major antigenic proteins hemagglutinin and neuraminidase, a process called antigenic drift. This constant variation in circulating strains requires that new antigens be considered for incorporation into influenza vaccines on an annual basis. Periodically, the segmented genome of this RNA virus reassorts (mixes segments genetically) with a heterologous influenza strain (typically of animal origin), causing a complete change in the hemagglutinin and/or neuraminidase, a process termed antigenic shift. When these shifts occur with a virus that replicates well and transmits well in humans, then pandemics occur. Pandemics are declared by the WHO when a new influenza virus subtype emerges that infects humans, causing serious illness, and the virus spreads easily among humans in more than one world region. Major worldwide pandemics occurred in 1918 (H1N1), 1957 (H2N2), 1968 (H3N2), and most recently in 2009 (novel H1N1).

Two types of influenza vaccines are currently licensed. The first is an inactivated preparation prepared by inactivating wild-type viruses prepared in eggs. The effectiveness of this trivalent vaccine is not entirely clear, but in general is estimated by most experts to be about 70% [84]. The efficacy varies year-to-year based on the accuracy of the match of the prepared vaccine strain antigens (chosen based on prior year data) and the eventual circulating antigens of the current year. The vaccine is most effective against severe disease and hospitalization, but probably also reduces the absolute number of infections.

Seasonal influenza vaccines are indicated for pregnant women of any gestation, and children as young as 6 months of age. Although the vaccine is not licensed for use in neonates, young infants and newborns can benefit greatly from a comprehensive influenza vaccination program if all of the intimate contacts of the infant, such as household contacts and caregivers, can be immunized, achieving a herd immunity effect. Some inactivated influenza vaccines still contain a preservative related to mercury called thimerosal. Concern was raised in the past that thimerosal might be causally related to developmental disorders. In 2004 the Institute of Medicine published a comprehensive review of the question and concluded that there is no evidence of such a relationship [85]. Thimerosal-free inactivated influenza vaccine is available now, however.

The second type of influenza vaccine is a trivalent live attenuated virus suspension that is delivered by nasal spray device. This approach was initially developed in 1960, but took several decades to bring to licensure. The attenuating genes and mutations have been defined, enabling scientists to coinfect new wild-type antigenic variants (drifted strains) in the laboratory with the attenuated strains. Selection methods have been developed to isolate new strains that arise from reassortment of the segmented genomes, such that the new vaccine strains possess the new surface proteins for immunogenicity but the established virus genes encoding the internal attenuating virus proteins. New vaccines need to be prepared each year to address antigenic drift. Live attenuated vaccine has been shown to be highly efficacious, leading to its licensure in 2003 [86,87]. Initially the vaccine was licensed for persons 5 to 49 years of age. In 2007 the FDA approved an expanded label to include children 2 to 5 years of age. A comparative trial of inactivated vaccine and live attenuated vaccine in children 6 to 59 months of age showed that 54.9% fewer cases of cultured-confirmed influenza occurred in the group that received live attenuated vaccine than in the group that received inactivated vaccine [88]. Respiratory tract infection with wild-type influenza virus can cause wheezing. Current studies are investigating whether or not there will be a minor association of live attenuated virus vaccination and wheezing. If safe, this vaccine would benefit younger infants who suffer a high burden of serious disease caused by influenza.

Streptococcus pneumoniae Vaccines

S. pneumoniae is a gram-positive encapsulated organism that causes invasive diseases in infants and young children, including meningitis, bacteremia and sepsis, and pneumonia. Disease is caused by dozens of different types, which are based on the capsular polysaccharide. Immunity is mediated by type-specific antibodies that bind the polysaccharides. Two types of vaccines are available to prevent pneumococcal disease (polysaccharide and conjugate vaccines), but only the conjugate vaccine is used in infants. The polysaccharide vaccine was developed first, with 14-valent vaccine in 1977 and 23-valent vaccine in 1983. Long chains of capsular polysaccharides are collected from inactivated bacteria. Polysaccharide vaccine is indicated for children and adults at high risk, but the vaccine is not effective in children less than 2 years of age. The safety of the vaccine for pregnant women has not been studied carefully; however, adverse consequences have not been reported in newborns whose mothers were vaccinated with pneumococcal polysaccharide vaccine during pregnancy.

A conjugate vaccine was developed that shows a high level of safety and efficacy against invasive disease [89]. The seven serotypes of *S. pneumoniae* that are included in the vaccine (designated types 4, 6B, 9V, 14, 18C, 19F, and 23F) were chosen because they are the strains that most commonly cause serious invasive disease in children. Routinely, the vaccine is given at 2, 4, 6, and 12 to 15 months of age, but it can be given as early as 6 weeks of age. Efforts are underway to increase the number of serotypes in conjugate vaccines, as discussed previously.

Rotavirus

Rotavirus is the most common cause of dehydrating diarrhea in infants throughout the world. The infection, which is acute and can be treated by rehydration, causes a large number of hospitalizations in the United States and deaths in developing countries. Interestingly, rotavirus infection in healthy full-term neonates often is asymptomatic or results in only mild disease, suggesting a possible short-lived protective effect from passively transferred maternal antibodies [90].

Ongoing worldwide surveillance has revealed a wide diversity of strains causing disease, but it is clear that four or five types are the most common causes of severe disease. Scientists at the National Institutes of Health developed a tetravalent live attenuated vaccine based on a modified Jennerian approach. One of the vaccine components was a rhesus monkey rotavirus (RRV), and the other strains were made by reassorting the genes that determine type with RRV to generate three additional strains. This vaccine showed efficacy against severe disease and was licensed in 1998 [91]. The vaccine was recommended for universal childhood vaccination at ages 2, 4, and 6 months [92]; however, it was withdrawn within a year [93] due to a temporal association with intussusception [94]. There is a sense that the age of immunization may be critical for association with intussusception, with older infants being more susceptible. This rhesus rotavirus tetravalent vaccine has also been tested in neonates, with a 0-, 2-, 4-month three-dose schedule, where it did not cause fever or other serious adverse events [95]. It appeared to induce rotavirus antibodies adequately in this setting, although with lower magnitude and kinetics than in infants starting at 2 months of age. This vaccine is not under further development, however.

Subsequently, two similar vaccines were developed that appear to be safe and immunogenic. The first, another modified Jennerian approach vaccine, a pentavalent human-bovine reassortant rotavirus vaccine was licensed in the United States in 2006 (RotaTeq). It is a live, oral vaccine that contains five reassortant rotaviruses developed from human and bovine parent rotavirus strains [96]. The parental bovine virus strain, Wistar Calf 3 (WC3), was isolated in 1981 from a calf with diarrhea in Pennsylvania, and then reassortants were made. The REST efficacy trial studied the vaccine in nearly 70,000 infants and found a high level of safety and efficacy against severe disease [97]. This vaccine is administered in a three-dose schedule, at 2, 4, and 6 months of age.

A third live attenuated rotavirus vaccine was licensed in the United States in 2008 for oral administration, which is based on a single attenuated human strain (Rotarix). Five phase III clinical trials were conducted worldwide to assess the safety and efficacy of the monovalent vaccine in support of United States licensure. The biologic license application included data from nearly 75,000 infants [98], and showed safety and efficacy against severe disease using a two-dose schedule, beginning at 2 months of age. The use of this vaccine was temporarily suspended by the FDA for several months during 2010 after it was found that the vaccine contained porcine circovirus type-1 (PCV-1). However, PCV-1 is commonly found in pigs and pork products and is not known to cause illness in humans or animals. Therefore, use of Rotarix was resumed in May 2010.

Current recommendations are that rotavirus vaccines be used for universal immunization during infancy, with care to keep the initiation of the two- or three-dose series at a young age. The ACIP also recommends immunization of premature infants, unless they are still hospitalized (to avoid nosocomial transmission to other vulnerable patients in the hospital).

Haemophilus influenzae Type B (Hib) Vaccine

H. influenzae was a major cause of serious invasive bacterial disease before institution of vaccine programs, and there are still many areas of the world where disease occurs because vaccine is not available. The principal life-threatening diseases are meningitis, bacteremia with sepsis, buccal, preseptal and orbital cellulitis, and epiglottitis. Immunity to the disease is conferred by antipolysaccharide polyribosylribitol phosphate (PRP) antibodies directed to the capsular polysaccharide. A purified polysaccharide vaccine was licensed in 1985; however, it was not effective in children less than about 18 months of age because of their inability to mount robust antibody responses to polysaccharides. The vaccine was only marketed for 3 years. Subsequently, Hib polysaccharide-protein conjugate vaccines were developed that are effective in young infants.

The Hib polysaccharide has been successfully conjugated to several proteins, the meningococcal group B outer membrane protein C (vaccine designated PRP-OMPC), tetanospasmin (toxoid of the *C. tetani* neurotoxin, vaccine designated PRP-T), or the mutant diphtheria protein

(CRM$_{197}$, vaccine designated HbOC). The vaccines all exhibit a high level of safety and immunogenicity. Hib conjugate vaccine is expensive to manufacture, limiting worldwide implementation, and occasional supply problems have limited full use in the developed world. Nevertheless, the vaccine has virtually eliminated the disease in countries where universal vaccination is used. Furthermore, it has been observed that widespread immunization reduces not only disease but also nasal carriage, resulting in extended benefits due to herd immunity and lack of transmission to even those not vaccinated.

Neisseria meningitidis Vaccines

N. meningitidis is also a significant cause of invasive bacterial disease in childhood, causing sepsis and meningitis. Again, antibodies to the capsular polysaccharide mediate protection against invasive disease. The first meningococcal vaccine was a monovalent polysaccharide vaccine first used in the early 1970s. A quadrivalent polysaccharide vaccine has been licensed since 1981, which protects against four subtypes of meningococcus—A, C, Y, and W-135. Children less than 2 years of age do not mount an adequate response to the polysaccharide, so this vaccine is used only in older children. A tetravalent meningococcal conjugate vaccine, also containing the A, C, Y, and W-135 subtypes, has now been developed and was licensed in the United States in 2005. The conjugate is expected to induce more durable immunity in vaccinees. Currently it is licensed for use in persons 2 to 55 years of age, although clinical trials are ongoing to determine the safety in younger populations. Neither the polysaccharide nor the conjugate vaccine protects against subtype B, which causes about one third of all the meningococcus cases in the United States.

PREMATURE INFANTS

Premature infants are at special risk for many infectious diseases for several reasons. First, if birth occurs before about 32 weeks, very little maternal antibody is transferred to the baby before birth. Second, the physiology of the airways, gastrointestinal tract, and other organ systems is not fully mature, and severe disease is more common on that basis. Third, premature infants are even more immature immunologically than term infants, who themselves mount immune responses to infection that are less robust than those of older children and adults. Therefore, premature infants are an especially vulnerable population who should be the focus of high compliance with vaccination recommendations. Studies reveal, however, that immunizations are not being given in a timely manner to many of these infants [99].

There are specific data on the use of a number of licensed vaccines in premature infants, especially for hepatitis B vaccine. The response of infants weighing less than 2000 g to this vaccine is lower than that of term infants [100]; however, there may be benefit to early vaccination. Current guidelines recommend that the initial vaccine dose be given as usual, but if the infant weighs less than 2 kg on initial immunization, this dose is not considered part of the routine three-dose vaccination series.

Rotavirus

Rotavirus vaccine should be given to premature infants, if the recommended schedule can be accomplished in a timely manner. In the phase III trials of RotaTeq, vaccine or a placebo was administered to 2070 preterm infants (25 to 36 weeks of gestational age; median: 34 weeks) [97]. The ACIP considers the benefits of rotavirus vaccine vaccination of premature infants to outweigh the theoretical risks of horizontal transmission by shedding. Given this recommendation, premature infants should be immunized with rotavirus vaccine upon discharge from the neonatal intensive care unit if between 6 and 12 weeks of chronologic age.

Influenza

Vaccinating all household contacts and caregivers of premature infants against seasonal influenza is indicated, as discussed previously. Neonates are not eligible for vaccination themselves.

TdaP

Again, all close contacts should be up to date on these immunizations, as discussed previously. Mothers should be offered postpartum immunization, if needed.

REGULATION OF VACCINES AND ADVISORY BODIES

Vaccines are regulated by national governments. The United States Food and Drug Administration's Vaccines and Related Biological Products Advisory Committee (VRBPAC) reviews and approves use of vaccines in the United States. Just because a vaccine is licensed by a regulatory agency, however, does not mean that it will automatically be used in practice. Various advisory boards review the feasibility and appropriateness of implementing vaccination, especially universal vaccination.

The Advisory Committee on Immunization Practices (ACIP) of the Centers for Disease Control and Prevention provides advice and guidance on effective control of vaccine-preventable diseases in the U.S. civilian population. The ACIP develops written recommendations for routine administration of vaccines to the pediatric and adult populations, and suggests details of vaccination schedules in terms of dosage, frequency, and contraindications. ACIP statements are considered official U.S. federal recommendations for the use of vaccines and immune globulins.

The Committee on Infectious Diseases of the American Academy of Pediatrics (AAP) publishes *The Red Book*, the official publication of the academy containing guidelines pertaining to infectious diseases. It is updated every 2 to 3 years; interim policy updates are issued in the academy's journal. The guidelines from these regulatory and advisory bodies occasionally vary from one another for a time, but in general there is an effort to harmonize recommendations.

REFERENCES

[1] J.E. Mold, et al., Maternal alloantigens promote the development of tolerogenic fetal regulatory T cells in utero, Science 322 (2008) 1562–1565.
[2] D. Gitlin, et al., The selectivity of the human placenta in the transfer of plasma proteins from mother to fetus, J. Clin. Invest. 43 (1964) 1938–1951.

[3] K.M. Adams, J.L. Nelson, Microchimerism: an investigative frontier in auto-immunity and transplantation, JAMA 291 (2004) 1127–1131.

[4] L.S. Rayfield, L. Brent, C.H. Rodeck, Development of cell-mediated lympholysis in human foetal blood lymphocytes, Clin. Exp. Immunol. 42 (1980) 561–570.

[5] C. Granberg, T. Hirvonen, Cell-mediated lympholysis by fetal and neonatal lymphocytes in sheep and man, Cell. Immunol. 51 (1980) 13–22.

[6] A. Marchant, et al., Mature CD8(+) T lymphocyte response to viral infection during fetal life, J. Clin. Invest. 111 (2003) 1747–1755.

[7] D. Rastogi, et al., Antigen-specific immune responses to influenza vaccine in utero, J. Clin. Invest. 117 (2007) 1637–1646.

[8] F.H. Claas, et al., Induction of B cell unresponsiveness to noninherited maternal HLA antigens during fetal life, Science 241 (1988) 1815–1817.

[9] C. Tian, et al., Low expression of the interleukin (IL)-4 receptor alpha chain and reduced signalling via the IL-4 receptor complex in human neonatal B cells, Immunology 119 (2006) 54–62.

[10] J.H. Weitkamp, et al., Natural evolution of a human virus-specific antibody gene repertoire by somatic hypermutation requires both hotspot-directed and randomly-directed processes, Hum. Immunol. 66 (2005) 666–676.

[11] N.L. Kallewaard, et al., Functional maturation of the human antibody response to rotavirus, J. Immunol. 180 (2008) 3980–3989.

[12] A.L. Bowen, et al., Transcriptional control of activation-induced cytidine deaminase and error-prone DNA polymerases is functionally mature in the B cells of infants at birth, Hum. Immunol. 67 (2006) 43–46.

[13] C.A. Siegrist, Blame vaccine interference, not neonatal immunization, for suboptimal responses after neonatal diphtheria, tetanus, and acellular pertussis immunization, J. Pediatr. 153 (2008) 305–307.

[14] J.P. Stanfield, D. Gall, P.M. Bracken, Single-dose antenatal tetanus immunisation, Lancet 1 (1973) 215–219.

[15] M.A. Koenig, et al., Duration of protective immunity conferred by maternal tetanus toxoid immunization: further evidence from Matlab, Bangladesh, Am. J. Public Health 88 (1998) 903–907.

[16] J.A. Englund, et al., Maternal immunization with influenza or tetanus toxoid vaccine for passive antibody protection in young infants, J. Infect. Dis. 168 (1993) 647–656.

[17] D.L. Murray, et al., Antibody response to monovalent A/New Jersey/8/76 influenza vaccine in pregnant women, J. Clin. Microbiol. 10 (1979) 184–187.

[18] C.V. Sumaya, R.S. Gibbs, Immunization of pregnant women with influenza A/New Jersey/76 virus vaccine: reactogenicity and immunogenicity in mother and infant, J. Infect. Dis. 140 (1979) 141–146.

[19] A.S. Deinard, P. Ogburn Jr., A/NJ/8/76 influenza vaccination program: effects on maternal health and pregnancy outcome, Am. J. Obstet. Gynecol. 140 (1981) 240–245.

[20] O.P. Heinonen, et al., Immunization during pregnancy against poliomyelitis and influenza in relation to childhood malignancy, Int. J. Epidemiol. 2 (1973) 229–235.

[21] F.M. Munoz, P.A. Piedra, W.P. Glezen, Safety and immunogenicity of respiratory syncytial virus purified fusion protein-2 vaccine in pregnant women, Vaccine 21 (2003) 3465–3467.

[22] UNICEF, Participate, vaccinate, eliminate: together against maternal and newborn tetanus, UNICEF, Geneva, 2008.

[23] K.M. Bisgard, et al., Infant pertussis: who was the source? Pediatr. Infect. Dis. J. 23 (2004) 985–989.

[24] P. Cohen, S.J. Scadron, The effects of active immunization of the mother upon the offspring, J. Pediatrics. 29 (1946) 609–619.

[25] P. Cohen, H. Schneck, E. Dubow, Prenatal multiple immunization, J. Pediatr. 38 (1951) 696–704.

[26] M.M. Cortese, et al., Pertussis hospitalizations among infants in the United States, 1993 to 2004, Pediatr. 121 (2008) 484–492.

[27] CDC, Preventing tetanus, diphtheria, and pertussis among adults: use of tetanus Toxoid, reduced diphtheria toxoid and acellular pertussis vaccine: recommendations of ACIP and recommendation of ADIP, supported by the healthcare infection control practices advisory committee (HICPAC), for use of Tdap among health-care personnel, MMWR Morb. Mortal. Wkly. Rep. 55 (2006) 1–37.

[28] K.M. Neuzil, et al., Impact of influenza on acute cardiopulmonary hospitalizations in pregnant women, Am. J. Epidemiol. 148 (1998) 1094–1102.

[29] W.L. Irving, et al., Influenza virus infection in the second and third trimesters of pregnancy: a clinical and seroepidemiological study, BJOG 107 (2000) 1282–1289.

[30] P.D. Reuman, E.M. Ayoub, P.A. Small, Effect of passive maternal antibody on influenza illness in children: a prospective study of influenza A in mother-infant pairs, Pediatr. Infect. Dis. J. 6 (1987) 398–403.

[31] CDC, Current trends rubella vaccination during pregnancy-United States, 1971–1988, MMWR Morb. Mortal. Wkly. Rep. 38 (1989) 289–293.

[32] G.R. Siber, et al., Protective activity of a human respiratory syncytial virus immune globulin prepared from donors screened by microneutralization assay, J. Infect. Dis. 165 (1992) 456–463.

[33] B. Horowitz, et al., Inactivation of viruses in labile blood derivatives. I. Disruption of lipid-enveloped viruses by tri(n-butyl)phosphate detergent combinations, Transfusion 25 (1985) 516–522.

[34] J.R. Groothuis, et al., Prophylactic administration of respiratory syncytial virus immune globulin to high-risk infants and young children. The respiratory syncytial virus immune globulin study group, N. Engl. J. Med. 329 (1993) 1524–1530.

[35] Group TPS, Reduction of respiratory syncytial virus hospitalization among premature infants and infants with bronchopulmonary dysplasia using respiratory syncytial virus immune globulin prophylaxis. The PREVENT study group, Pediatrics 99 (1997) 93–99.

[36] J.R. Groothuis, Role of antibody and use of respiratory syncytial virus (RSV) immune globulin to prevent severe RSV disease in high-risk children, J. Pediatr. 124 (1994) S28–S32.

[37] Group TI-RS, Palivizumab, a humanized respiratory syncytial virus monoclonal antibody, reduces hospitalization from respiratory syncytial virus infection in high-risk infants, Pediatrics 102 (1998) 531–537.

[38] K. Abarca, et al., Safety, tolerability, pharmacokinetics, and immunogenicity of motavizumab, a humanized, enhanced-potency monoclonal antibody for the prevention of respiratory syncytial virus infection in at-risk children, Pediatr. Infect. Dis. J. 28 (2009) 267–272.

[39] R.P. Beasley, et al., Efficacy of hepatitis B immune globulin for prevention of perinatal transmission of the hepatitis B virus carrier state: final report of a randomized double-blind, placebo-controlled trial, Hepatology 3 (1983) 135–141.

[40] E.E. Mast, et al., A comprehensive immunization strategy to eliminate transmission of hepatitis B virus infection in the United States: recommendations of the advisory committee on immunization practices (ACIP) part 1: immunization of infants, children, and adolescents, MMWR Recomm. Rep. 54 (2005) 1–31.

[41] CDC, Prevention of varicella: recommendations of the advisory committee on immunization practices (ACIP), MMWR Morb. Mortal. Wkly. Rep. 45 (RR11) (1996) 1–26.

[42] P.A. Brunell, Fetal and neonatal varicella-zoster infections, Semin. Perinatol. 7 (1983) 47–56.

[43] J.D. Meyers, Congenital varicella in term infants: risk reconsidered, J. Infect. Dis. 129 (1974) 215–217.

[44] A.L. Pastuszak, et al., Outcome after maternal varicella infection in the first 20 weeks of pregnancy, N. Engl. J. Med. 330 (1994) 901–905.

[45] E. Miller, J.E. Cradock-Watson, M.K. Ridehalgh, Outcome in newborn babies given anti-varicella-zoster immunoglobulin after perinatal maternal infection with varicella-zoster virus, Lancet 2 (1989) 371–373.

[46] Laboratories MPHB, Varicella-zoster immune globulin (human) (package insert), Massachusetts Public Health Biologic Laboratories, Boston, 2000.

[47] D.R. Snydman, et al., A pilot trial of a novel cytomegalovirus immune globulin in renal transplant recipients, Transplantation 38 (1984) 553–557.

[48] S.S. Arnon, et al., Human botulism immune globulin for the treatment of infant botulism, N. Engl. J. Med. 354 (2006) 462–471.

[49] R.A. Karron, et al., Evaluation of a live attenuated bovine parainfluenza type 3 vaccine in two- to six-month-old infants, Pediatr. Infect. Dis. J. 15 (1996) 650–654.

[50] A.A. Haller, et al., Expression of the surface glycoproteins of human parainfluenza virus type 3 by bovine parainfluenza virus type 3, a novel attenuated virus vaccine vector, J. Virol. 74 (2000) 11626–11635.

[51] A.C. Schmidt, et al., Recombinant bovine/human parainfluenza virus type 3 (B/HPIV3) expressing the respiratory syncytial virus (RSV) G and F proteins can be used to achieve simultaneous mucosal immunization against RSV and HPIV3, J. Virol. 75 (2001) 4594–4603.

[52] W.T. Friedewald, et al., Low-temperature-grown RS virus in adult volunteers, JAMA 204 (1968) 690–694.

[53] P.F. Wright, et al., Administration of a highly attenuated, live respiratory syncytial virus vaccine to adults and children, Infect. Immun. 37 (1982) 397–400.

[54] R.A. Karron, et al., Identification of a recombinant live attenuated respiratory syncytial virus vaccine candidate that is highly attenuated in infants, J. Infect. Dis. 191 (2005) 1093–1104.

[55] R.A. Karron, et al., Respiratory syncytial virus (RSV) SH and G proteins are not essential for viral replication in vitro: clinical evaluation and molecular characterization of a cold-passaged, attenuated RSV subgroup B mutant, Proc. Natl. Acad. Sci. U. S. A. 94 (1997) 13961–13966.

[56] R.A. Karron, et al., Evaluation of two live, cold-passaged, temperature-sensitive respiratory syncytial virus vaccines in chimpanzees and in human adults, infants, and children, J. Infect. Dis. 176 (1997) 1428–1436.

[57] P.F. Wright, et al., Evaluation of a live, cold-passaged, temperature-sensitive, respiratory syncytial virus vaccine candidate in infancy, J. Infect. Dis. 182 (2000) 1331–1342.

[58] R.A. Karron, et al., A live human parainfluenza type 3 virus vaccine is attenuated and immunogenic in young infants, Pediatr. Infect. Dis. J. 22 (2003) 394–405.

[59] R.B. Belshe, et al., Evaluation of combined live, attenuated respiratory syncytial virus and parainfluenza 3 virus vaccines in infants and young children, J. Infect. Dis. 190 (2004) 2096–2103.

[60] N. Nathanson, A.D. Langmuir, The Cutter incident. Poliomyelitis following formaldehyde-inactivated poliovirus vaccination in the United States during the spring of 1955. II. Relationship of poliomyelitis to Cutter vaccine, Am. J. Hyg. 78 (1963) 29–60.

[61] A.Z. Kapikian, An epidemiologic study of altered clinical reactivity to respiratory syncytial (RS) virus infection in children previously vaccinated with an inactivated RS virus vaccine, Am. J. Epidemiol. 89 (1969) 405–421.

[62] H.W. Kim, et al., Respiratory syncytial virus disease in infants despite prior administration of antigenic inactivated vaccine, Am. J. Epidemiol. 89 (1969) 422–434.

[63] H.A. Gans, et al., Deficiency of the humoral immune response to measles vaccine in infants immunized at age 6 months, JAMA 280 (1998) 527–532.

[64] Group EPoIGA, Expanded programme on immunization, Wkly. Epidemiol. Rec. 65 (1990) 5–11.

[65] P. Aaby, et al., Sex-specific differences in mortality after high-titre measles immunization in rural Senegal, Bull. World Health Organ. 72 (1994) 761–770.

[66] P. Aaby, et al., Five year follow-up of morbidity and mortality among recipients of high-titre measles vaccines in Senegal, Vaccine 14 (1996) 226–229.

[67] B.B. Trunz, P. Fine, C. Dye, Effect of BCG vaccination on childhood tuberculous meningitis and miliary tuberculosis worldwide: a meta-analysis and assessment of cost-effectiveness, Lancet 367 (2006) 1173–1180.

[68] L.C. Rodrigues, V.K. Diwan, J.G. Wheeler, Protective effect of BCG against tuberculous meningitis and miliary tuberculosis: a meta-analysis, Int. J. Epidemiol. 22 (1993) 1154–1158.

[69] A. Lotte, et al., Second IUATLD study on complications induced by intradermal BCG-vaccination, Bull. Int. Union Tuberc. Lung Dis. 63 (1988) 47–59.

[70] A.C. Hesseling, et al., Consensus statement on the revised World Health Organization recommendations for BCG vaccination in HIV-infected infants, Int. J. Tuberc. Lung Dis. 12 (2008) 1376–1379.

[71] K.M. Farizo, et al., Epidemiological features of pertussis in the United States, 1980–1989, Clin. Infect. Dis. 14 (1992) 708–719.

[72] N.B. Halasa, et al., Poor immune responses to a birth dose of diphtheria, tetanus, and acellular pertussis vaccine, J. Pediatr. 153 (2008) 327–332.

[73] M. Knuf, et al., Neonatal vaccination with an acellular pertussis vaccine accelerates the acquisition of pertussis antibodies in infants, J. Pediatr. 152 (2008) 655–660, 660.e1.

[74] C. Belloni, et al., Immunogenicity of a three-component acellular pertussis vaccine administered at birth, Pediatrics 111 (2003) 1042–1045.

[75] V. Fauveau, et al., Maternal tetanus: magnitude, epidemiology and potential control measures, Int. J. Gynaecol. Obstet. 40 (1993) 3–12.

[76] R.E. Weibel, et al., Live attenuated varicella virus vaccine. Efficacy trial in healthy children, N. Engl. J. Med. 310 (1984) 1409–1415.

[77] M. Takahashi, et al., Live vaccine used to prevent the spread of varicella in children in hospital, Lancet 2 (1974) 1288–1290.

[78] Merck & Co, I. ProQuad (measles, mumps, rubella, and varicella [Oka/Merck] virus vaccine live) (package insert). Merck, Whitehouse Station, NJ, 2005.

[79] M. Siegel, H.T. Fuerst, N.S. Peress, Comparative fetal mortality in maternal virus diseases. A prospective study on rubella, measles, mumps, chicken pox and hepatitis, N. Engl. J. Med. 274 (1966) 768–771.

[80] M. Siegel, Congenital malformations following chickenpox, measles, mumps, and hepatitis. Results of a cohort study, JAMA 226 (1973) 1521–1524.

[81] G. Amexis, et al., Sequence diversity of Jeryl Lynn strain of mumps virus: quantitative mutant analysis for vaccine quality control, Virology 300 (2002) 171–179.

[82] G.H. Dayan, et al., Recent resurgence of mumps in the United States, N. Engl. J. Med. 358 (2008) 1580–1589.

[83] CDC, Elimination of rubella and congenital rubella syndrome - United States, 1969–2004, MMWR Morb. Mortal. Wkly. Rep. 54 (2005) 279–282.

[84] P.F. Wright, The use of inactivated influenza vaccine in children, Semin. Pediatr. Infect. Dis. 17 (2006) 200–205.

[85] Medicine Io, Immunization safety review: vaccines and autism, National Academies Press, Washington, DC, 2004.

[86] R.B. Belshe, et al., The efficacy of live attenuated, cold-adapted, trivalent, intranasal influenzavirus vaccine in children, N. Engl. J. Med. 338 (1998) 1405–1412.

[87] R.B. Belshe, et al., Efficacy of vaccination with live attenuated, cold-adapted, trivalent, intranasal influenza virus vaccine against a variant (A/Sydney) not contained in the vaccine, J. Pediatr. 136 (2000) 168–175.

[88] R.B. Belshe, et al., Live attenuated versus inactivated influenza vaccine in infants and young children, N. Engl. J. Med. 356 (2007) 685–696.

[89] S. Black, et al., Efficacy, safety and immunogenicity of heptavalent pneumococcal conjugate vaccine in children. Northern California Kaiser Permanente vaccine study center group, Pediatr. Infect. Dis. J. 19 (2000) 187–195.

[90] R.F. Bishop, et al., Clinical immunity after neonatal rotavirus infection. A prospective longitudinal study in young children, N. Engl. J. Med. 309 (1983) 72–76.

[91] A.Z. Kapikian, et al., Efficacy of a quadrivalent rhesus rotavirus-based human rotavirus vaccine aimed at preventing severe rotavirus diarrhea in infants and young children, J. Infect. Dis. 174 (Suppl. 1) (1996) S65–S72.

[92] CDC, Rotavirus vaccine for the prevention of rotavirus gastroenteritis among children, MMWR Morb. Mortal. Wkly. Rep. 48 (RR-2) (1999) 1–23.

[93] CDC, Withdrawal of rotavirus vaccine recommendation, MMWR Morb. Mortal. Wkly. Rep. 48 (1999) 1007.

[94] T.V. Murphy, et al., Intussusception among infants given an oral rotavirus vaccine, N. Engl. J. Med. 344 (2001) 564–572.

[95] T. Vesikari, et al., Neonatal administration of rhesus rotavirus tetravalent vaccine, Pediatr. Infect. Dis. J. 25 (2006) 118–122.

[96] P.M. Heaton, et al., Development of a pentavalent rotavirus vaccine against prevalent serotypes of rotavirus gastroenteritis, J. Infect. Dis. 192 (Suppl. 1) (2005) S17–S21.

[97] T. Vesikari, et al., Safety and efficacy of a pentavalent human-bovine (WC3) reassortant rotavirus vaccine, N. Engl. J. Med. 354 (2006) 23–33.

[98] G.M. Ruiz-Palacios, et al., Safety and efficacy of an attenuated vaccine against severe rotavirus gastroenteritis, N. Engl. J. Med. 354 (2006) 11–22.

[99] D.L. Langkamp, et al., Delays in receipt of immunizations in low-birth-weight children: a nationally representative sample, Arch. Pediatr. Adolesc. Med. 155 (2001) 167–172.

[100] N. Linder, et al., Hepatitis B vaccination: long-term follow-up of the immune response of preterm infants and comparison of two vaccination protocols, Infection 30 (2002) 136–139.

[101] J. Ipsen, Circulating antitoxin at the onset of diphtheria in 425 patients, J. Immunol. 54 (1946) 325–347.

[102] A.E. Fiore, S. Feinstone, B. Bell, Hepatitis A vaccines, in: S.A. Plotkin, W.A. Orenstein, P.A. Offit (Eds.), Vaccines, fifth ed., Saunders-Elsevier, London, 2008.

[103] A.D. Jack, et al., What level of hepatitis B antibody is protective? J. Infect. Dis. 179 (1999) 489–492.

[104] P. Anderson, The protective level of serum antibodies to the capsular polysaccharide of *Haemophilus influenzae* type b, J. Infect. Dis. 149 (1984) 1034–1035.

[105] P.A. Denoel, et al., Quality of the *Haemophilus influenzae* type b (Hib) antibody response induced by diphtheria-tetanus-acellular pertussis/Hib combination vaccines, Clin. Vaccine Immunol. 14 (2007) 1362–1369.

[106] W.R. Dowdle, et al., Inactivated influenza vaccines. 2. Laboratory indices of protection, Postgrad. Med. J. 49 (1973) 159–163.

[107] R.T. Chen, et al., Measles antibody: reevaluation of protective titers, J. Infect. Dis. 162 (1990) 1036–1042.

[108] G.R. Siber, et al., Estimating the protective concentration of anti-pneumococcal capsular polysaccharide antibodies, Vaccine 25 (2007) 3816–3826.

[109] L. Jodar, et al., Serological criteria for evaluation and licensure of new pneumococcal conjugate vaccine formulations for use in infants, Vaccine 21 (2003) 3265–3272.

[110] S.A. Plotkin, E. Vidor, Poliovirus vaccine-inactivated, in: S.A. Plotkin, W.A. Orenstein, P.A. Offit (Eds.), Vaccines, fifth ed., Elsevier, London, 2008.

[111] L. Matter, K. Kogelschatz, D. Germann, Serum levels of rubella virus antibodies indicating immunity: response to vaccination of subjects with low or undetectable antibody concentrations, J. Infect. Dis. 175 (1997) 749–755.

[112] L.P. Skendzel, Rubella immunity. Defining the level of protective antibody, Am. J. Clin. Pathol. 106 (1996) 170–174.

[113] J.A. McComb, The prophylactic dose of homologous tetanus antitoxin, N. Engl. J. Med. 270 (1964) 175–178.

[114] D.L. Krah, et al., Comparison of gpELISA and neutralizing antibody responses to Oka/Merck live varicella vaccine (Varivax) in children and adults, Vaccine 15 (1997) 61–64.

[115] S. Li, et al., Inverse relationship between six week postvaccination varicella antibody response to vaccine and likelihood of long term breakthrough infection, Pediatr. Infect. Dis. J. 21 (2002) 337–342.

[116] S.A. Plotkin, Vaccines: correlates of vaccine-induced immunity, Clin. Infect. Dis. 47 (2008) 401–409.

INDEX

Note: Page numbers followed by *f* indicate figures and *t* indicate tables.

A

ABCD. *See* Amphotericin B cholesterol sulfate complex
ABLC. *See* Amphotericin B lipid complex
Abortion, 6–7.
　See also Spontaneous abortion
　coxsackie virus, 770
　echoviruses, 770
　gestational chickenpox, 671–672
　gestational measles and, 690
　gestational mumps, 697
　poliovirus and, 770
　septic, 609–610
　T. gondii and, 927, 1027
　Trypanosoma cruzi, 1044
　viruses and, 770
Abrupto placentae, 64
Abscess, 5. *See also* Brain abscess;
　Neonatal brain abscess
　adrenal, 444
　liver, 230, 324
　lung, 287
　metaphyseal, 300
　metastatic, bone and joint infection, 299
　perirectal, 347
　pneumonia and, 292
　retropharyngeal, 276–277
　of skin, 346
　UTI, 315
Absolute band counts, 1148
ACAM 2000, 904
Acellular pertussis vaccine with diphtheria and tetanus toxoids, 154–155
ACIP. *See* Advisory Committee on Immunization Practices
Acquired immunodeficiency syndrome. *See* AIDS
Acquired *Toxoplasma*
　antibody response, 981*t*
　pregnancy, 980–985
　　health education consequences, 933–934
　　prevalence rates, mathematic epidemiologic models, 933
Actin polymerization, *listeria monocytogenes*, 474
Active immunization, 1220–1223
　human studies, 1220
　measles, 693
Acute demyelinating encephalitis, 688

Acute hemorrhagic leukoencephalitis, 688
Acute inflammatory response, 96
Acute necrotizing fasciitis, 347
Acute phase proteins, 1152
Acute phase reactants, 1149–1152
　inflammatory illnesses and, 1149*f*
Acute respiratory infections, 29
Acute toxoplasmosis, 169–170
Acyclovir, 18, 679–680, 831
　herpes simplex virus, 791
　for HSV, 1194
　neonatal herpes and, 826
　for pregnant women, 680
　resistance, 828
　varicella during pregnancy, 670
Adaptive immune system, 81
Adaptive immunity, 101–103, 165–168
Adenitis, 500
　Bacille Calmette-Guérin vaccines, 592
　group B streptococcal infection, 443–444
Adenopathy, 247–248
Adhesion molecules, 91, 96, 1152
Adjunctive therapy, 259–260
　HSV and, 168–169
　neonatal sepsis, 259–260
　pyogenic infections, 161–162
Adjuvants, 1222
Adrenal abscess, 444
Adrenal gland, 637
Advisory Committee on Immunization Practices (ACIP), 889, 1212, 1228
Aeromonas hydrophila, 392
　clinical manifestations, 392
　diagnosis and therapy, 392
　nature of organism, epidemiology pathogenesis, 392
African sleeping sickness, 1045
African trypanosomiasis, 1045
Agglutinating antibodies, 1045
Agglutination test, 970, 974–975, 982–983
AIDS (Acquired immunodeficiency syndrome), 253, 516, 621–660, 632*t*, 639*t*, 651, 707, 843, 918, 1079, 1084.
　See also HIV/AIDS; Joint United Nations Program on HIV/AIDS

C. neoformans, 1104
CMV and, 721
congenital Toxoplasmosis, 966–967
　case histories, 966–967
AIDS indicator diseases, children, younger than 13 years, 624
AIDS-defining conditions, 628, 638
Airborne precautions, 1138
Airway surface liquid, 84–85
Alastrim, 902
Allergies, 692
Allograft
　recipients, 710–711
　transplantation, 718
Altastaph. *See* anti-*S. aureus* immunoglobulin
Alternative complement pathway activity, 87–88
Alternative pathway, 86
Amantadine, congenital rubella infection, 886
Amastigotes, 1043
Amebiasis transmission, 1046
American trypanosomiasis, 1043–1045
Amikacin, 256, 1179–1183
　clinical dosing implications, 1178*t*, 1181–1182, 1182*t*, 1193*t*
　CSF concentrations, 1180
　M. avium-intracellulare complex, with HIV, 633
　nurseries and, 239
　PD exposure targets, extended dosing intervals for, 1181, 1182–1183, 1182*t*
　PK-PD dosing, 1181–1182
　postantibiotic effect, 1181
　safety, 1180–1181
　serum half-life, 1180
8-amino-quinolines, *Trypanosoma cruzi*, 1045
Aminoglycoside nephrotoxicity, 1180
Aminoglycoside-associated neuromuscular blockade, 1181
Aminoglycosides, 256, 1177–1188, 1178*t*
　antimicrobial activity, 1177
　Campylobacter, 389
　Citrobacter sp. and, 231
　endocarditis, 340
　history, 1177–1179

mediastinitis, 342
NEC, 337
neonatal sepsis, 260
nurseries and, 239
pericarditis, 341
pharmacokinetic data, 1177–1179
Pseudomonas species, eye infections, 350
salmonellosis, 381
skin infections, 348
solitary hepatic abscess, 325
UTI, 319
yersinia enterocolitica, 392
Amniocentesis, 1001, 1026
　fetal *Toxoplasma* infection, 985–987
　IAI and, 65
Amnionic inflammation, *Ureaplasma* species, 609*f*
Amnionitis, 67, 439
Amniopatch, 66–67
Amniotic cavity, 430–431
Amniotic fluid
　Ascaris, 1042–1043
　cultures
　　in preterm labor, 61–62
　　studies of, 611
　examination, 52
　glucose, IAI, 52
　HSV-2, 818
　IL-6, 52–53
　infection, 239, 430–432, 608–609, 609*f*
　isolates, 53
　microbes in, 53*t*
　neonatal GBS, 430–431
　PCR assay in, fetal *Toxoplasma* infection, 985–987
　testing, diagnostic values, 66, 68*t*
　Toxoplasma gondii in, 973*f*
　　gestational age and, 973*f*
Amoxicillin
　breast milk, 1167–1168
　measles, 693
　otitis media, 285
　Shigella infection, 385
Amoxicillin-clavulanate
　otitis media, 285
　yersinia enterocolitica, 392
Amphotericin B, 1069, 1112–1113, 1196
　antimicrobial activity, 1196
　candidiasis, 1067

Amphotericin B (*Continued*)
  Coccidioides immitis organism, 1102
  cryptococcosis infection, 1105
  dose, 1113
  effect on fetus, 1113
  endophthalmitis and, 1097–1098
  intrathecal administration, 1113
  lipid formulations, 1113
  Malassezia infections, 1107
  pharmacokinetic data, 1196
  PK-PD, clinical implication and, 1196
  safety, 1196
  toxicity, 1113
Amphotericin B cholesterol sulfate complex (ABCD), 1069–1070, 1113
Amphotericin B deoxycholate, 1112
  Aspergillus organism, 1097–1098
  dermatophytoses, 1111
  fungi susceptibility, 1097*t*
Amphotericin B lipid complex (ABLC), 1069–1070, 1113, 1196–1197
  dosing implications, 1197
  pharmacokinetic data, 1196–1197
  PK-PD dosing, 1197
  safety data, 1197
Ampicillin, 17–18, 229, 1170–1171
  antimicrobial activity, 1170
  appendicitis, 329
  breast milk concentrations, 1167–1168
  Campylobacter, 389
  cerebrospinal fluid penetration, 1170
  chorioamnionitis and, 55
  clinical dosing implications, 1170–1171
  concentrations, in maternal and fetal sera, 54, 56*f*
  GBS, 447
  group B streptococcal disease, 255
  Listeria, 482
  mediastinitis, 342
  to mother, fetal drug concentrations and, 257
  NEC, 337
  neonatal group B streptococcal sepsis, 160
  nurseries and, 239
  osteomyelitis, 305
  peritonitis, 333
  pharmacokinetic data, 1170
  PK-PD, 1170–1171
  pneumonia, 292
  S. aureus, 255–256
  safety, 1170
  salmonellosis, 380
  serum concentrations, 1165*t*, 1166

Shigella infection, 385
skin infections, 348
Ampicillin and aminoglycoside, 256
Ampicillin and cefotaxime combination, 449–450
Ampicillin and gentamicin combination, 256
  GBS, 255
  group B streptococcal infection, 449–450
Ampicillin and sulbactam, solitary hepatic abscess, 325
Ampicillin and tobramycin, 256
Ampicillin-resistant *Citrobacter* species, 231
Ampicillin-resistant organisms, 287
Amsterdam study, toxoplasmosis, 1009
Anaerobes, 233
Anaerobic bacteria, 233–234
Anaerobic infections, 259
Analytes, 1152–1153
Androgens, 192
Anemia, 637
Anergy, 122
Anidulafungin, 1071, 1201–1202
  pharmacokinetic data, 1201
  PK-PD, and clinical implications, 1202
  safety, 1201
  tissue concentrations, 1201
Animal models
  CMV and, 726
  rubella virus, pathogenicity for, 865
Anogenital warts, 906
Anoxia, 298
Antenatal care, 41–42
Antenatal hydronephrosis, 314
Antibacterial agents, bilirubin and, 1162
Antibiotics, 18.
  See also Prophylactic antibiotics; specific antibiotics
  appendicitis, 329
  breast milk concentrations, infant daily dose, 1167*t*
  breast-feeding, 210
  cessation, phycomycosis, 1109
  EAEC, 376
  EPEC gastroenteritis, 373
  in human milk, 1166–1171
  in labor, adverse outcomes, 63*t*
  lock solution, catheter-associated bloodstream infections, 261
  NICUs, 256
  osteomyelitis, 305
  placental transport, 1165–1166
  pneumonia, 292
  preterm birth, 64*t*
  PROM, 70–71
    adverse outcomes, 63*t*
  prophylaxis
    GBS, 454, 454*f*
    staphylococcal infection, 509

resistance, 41
Staphylococcus aureus infection, 506–509
  therapy, 44
    chorioamnionitis and, 54–55
  treatment, neonates with infection, 43–44
  trials, 62–64
Antibodies
  complement interactions, GBS, 438
  in congenital *T. gondii*, 990*f*
  placental transfer of, 157
  T. gondii, 170
Antibody kinetics, patterns of, rubella virus, 870, 870*f*, 871
Antibody production, 148–150
  CD4 effector T-cell and, 125–126
Antibody responsiveness, 151–152, 151*t*
Antibody tests, Chagas disease, 1045
Antibody-dependent cellular cytotoxicity, 168, 820
Antifungal agents, 1068–1072, 1195–1202
  Candida spp. and, 1066*t*
  candidiasis, 1067
  invasive candidiasis in neonates, 1068*t*
  neonates and young infants, 1112–1114
    systemic fungal infection in, 1112*t*
  systemic, 1069–1071
  topical, 1068–1069
Antifungal therapies.
  See Antifungal agents
Antigen
  detection, GBS, 447
  presentation
    in fetus, 110
    intracellular pathways of, 109*f*
    in neonate, 110
    T-cells and, 107–141
  testing, rubella virus, 864–865
Antigenemia, 739
Antigen-independent naïve T-cell proliferation, 120–121
Antigen-presenting cells, 147–148
Antigen-specific immune mechanisms, 102*f*
Antigen-specific lymphocyte responses, 971
Antigen-specific major histocompatibility complex (MHC) cytotoxicity, 131–132, 131*f*
Antigen-specific T-cell function, in fetus and neonate, 138–139
  responses, 171
Anti-hepatitis B surface antigen antibodies, testing for, 1218–1219

Anti-infective drugs, clinical pharmacology of, 1161–1211
  introduction, 1160
Antimalarial antibodies, 1047–1048
Antimalarial drugs, prophylaxis and treatment, 38–39
Antimetabolites, *Pneumocystis* pneumonia, rat study, 1086
Antimicrobial agents, 14–15, 223, 242. *See also* Antimicrobial prophylaxis
  bloodstream and, 1162
  brain abscess, 258–259
  breast-feeding, 210
  Citrobacter sp. and, 231
  congenital toxoplasmosis in pregnancy, 1024–1026
  EPEC gastroenteritis, 370–371, 373
  GBS, 449–450
  group B streptococcal infection, 449*t*
  infant to maternal serum concentrations, ratios, 1165, 1165*t*
  intramuscular absorption, 1162
  measles, 693
  mediastinitis, 342
  for neonatal sepsis, 255–256
  nurseries and, 238–239
  optimizing, using PK-PD principles, 1163–1164
  oral absorption, 1162
  osteomyelitis, 305
  pneumonia, 292
  resistance, 18
  salmonellosis, 380
  sepsis in fetus and, 257
  Shigella infection, 384–385
  toxicity, 1161, 1161*t*
  trials, 613
  UTI, 319
  Yersinia enterocolitica, 392
Antimicrobial peptides, 83
Antimicrobial prophylaxis, 314
Antimicrobial therapy.
  See Antimicrobial agents
Antioxidants, 205
Antiparasitic lipids, 204
Antipicornavirus drugs, 791
Antipseudomonal penicillin, 350
Antiretroviral drugs, 645, 648–651. *See also* specific drug
  challenges, 649–651
  classes, 649
  early treatment, 648
  initial, choice of, 649
  recommended dosages, 650*t*
Antiretroviral prophylaxis regimens (ARV)
  perinatal HIV transmission
    breast-feeding infants, 642*t*
    non-breast-feeding infants, 641*t*
  safety and toxicity of, 645–646
Antiretroviral resistance, 646

anti-*S. aureus* immunoglobulin (Altastaph), 509–510
Antistaphylococcal penicillins, 1171–1177, 1172*t*
  antimicrobial activity, 1171
  clinical dosing implications, 1171, 1172*t*, 1193*t*
  pharmacokinetic data, 1171, 1172*t*
  PK-PD, 1171
  safety, 1171
Antituberculosis drugs, 589
Antiviral agents, 18, 1194–1195
  congenital cytomegalovirus, 743
  HCV, 807
  HSV, 826–829
Aortic valvular stenosis, 878
APC. *See* T cell-antigen-presenting cell
Apgar score, 236, 243–244
Apoptosis, 132–133
Appendicitis, 327–329
  clinical manifestations, 327–328
  diagnosis, 328
  microbiology, 327
  pathogenesis, 327
  prognosis, 328–329
  signs of, 328*t*
  treatment, 329
Aqueous penicillin G, 1169
Arthropathy, 842
Arthropods, 931
ARV. *See* Antiretroviral prophylaxis regimens
Ascaris eggs, life cycle, 1042
Ascaris lumbricoides, 1042–1043
Ascites, 336
  Toxoplasma gondii, 943–944, 964
Ascitic fluid, *Toxoplasma gondii*, 944
Aseptic meningitis, infectious/noninfectious causes, 259*t*
Aseptic technique, 28–29
Aspergillosis, 1095–1098
Aspergillus organism, 1095, 1131
  clinical manifestations, 1096–1097
  diagnosis and differential diagnosis, 1097
  epidemiology and transmission, 1095–1096
  pathogenesis, 1096
  pathology, 1096
  prevention, 1097–1098
  therapy, 1097–1098
Assassin bug, 1043
Atovaquone
  fluoroquinolones and, 1000
  Toxoplasma gondii, 1000
Attenuated vaccines
  polio, 1224
  respiratory syncytial virus, 1220–1221
  rotavirus, 1227
  viral, 792, 1220–1221

Attenuated virus, 1225
Attenuated virus vaccination, 1226
Atypical measles, 693
Autoimmune regulator gene (AIRE gene), 117
Autologous blood, 202*t*
Autopsy
  microbiology, 251
  Toxoplasma gondii, 931
Autoreactive B cells, 144
Avidity assay, early gestation and, 1022–1024
Azithromycin
  breast milk, 1168
  breast milk concentrations, infant daily dose, 1168
  Campylobacter, 389
  EAEC, 376
  Toxoplasma gondii, 1000
Azole antifungals, 1070–1071, 1198
  hepatotoxicity, 1070
Aztreonam, 392, 1183–1184
  antimicrobial activity, 1183
  clinical dosing implications, 1184
  pharmacokinetic data, 1183–1184
  PK-PD dosing, 1184
  safety, 1184

B

B. pertussis, 1224
B-1 cells, IgM isotype and, 151
Babesia microti, 1052
Babesiosis, 1052
Bacille Calmette-Guérin-induced lymphadenitis, 592
Bacille Calmette-Guérin-induced osteitis, 592
Bacillus Calmette-Guérin, 72, 276, 285, 290, 343, 1223
  vaccination, HIV in children and, 1223
Bacillus Calmette-Guérin vaccines, 40, 41, 59, 591–593
  adverse reactions, 592
  effectiveness, 593
  history and development, 591
  preparation and administration, 591–592
  tuberculin skin test results, 592–593
Bacillus cereus, 233
Bacitracin disk susceptibility testing, 420
BACTEC, 578
Bacteremia, 251–255, 289–290, 379, 441, 442, 480–481, 497–499
  animal models, 255
  birth weight, 226*t*
  multiple organisms and, 234
  onset of signs, mortality v, 225*t*
Bacterial agents, 393–394
  gastroenteritis, 393–394

Bacterial antigens, detection of, body fluid specimens and, 251
Bacterial culture, negative, infant treatment, 258
Bacterial infections
  causing neonatal sepsis, 224*t*
  of fetal liver, 323
  HIV in children, 632–633
  human milk and, 211–212
  respiratory tract, 210, 276–296
  screening panels, 1154
Bacterial meningitis, 224, 253–254
Bacterial pathogens, 361–393
  breast milk transmission, 20
  geographic regions, 26–27
  uncommon, 234, 235*t*
Bacterial peptides, 474
Bacterial resistance, 255–256
Bacterial sepsis, 221–275, 222, 791
  pathogenesis, 239–243
Bacterioides fragilis, 233
Bacteriuria, 61
BAL. *See* Bronchoalveolar lavage
BALT. *See* Bronchus-associated lymphoid tissue
Bayley score, 56
B-cell
  activation, 144–145
  development, early, 142–144
  differentiation, into plasma cells, 149
  early life and, 1215
  immature, of bone marrow, 144
  immunity, Antibody-dependent cellular cytotoxicity and, 168
  immunoglobin and, 141–159
  marginal zone and, 150–151
  maturation, 144–145
  overview, 141–142
  preimmune selection, 144–145
  selection, naïve follicular B cells and, 147
  signaling, negative regulation of, 146
  T cell-dependent responses, 151–153
Bcl-2 family members, 132
BCR engagement, 146
Bell staging criteria, 335*t*
Benzathine penicillin G, 1169
Benzyl penicillin and aminoglycoside, 43
Bilirubin, 1162
Biofilm formation, *Staphylococcus epidermidis*, 495*f*
Birth
  DCs, 103
  defects, parvovirus B19, 849
  G-CSF levels, 90
  infections acquired during, 15–19
  neutrophil counts, 89
  process, enteroviruses, 762

Birth weight, 224
  bacteremia and, 226*t*
  Group B streptococcal disease, incidence and mortality of, 235*t*
  malaria, 1047
  neonatal sepsis, 236
  VAP and, 1128
Blastomyces, 1098
Blastomyces dermatitidis, 1098
Blastomycosis, 1098–1099
  clinical manifestations, 1099
  diagnosis and differential diagnosis, 1099
  epidemiology and transmission, 1098
  organism, 1098
  pathology, 1098–1099
  prevention, 1099
  prognosis, 1099
  therapy, 1099
Bleeding disorders, cephalosporins, 1187
Blood
  examination, UTI, 318
  optimal volume of, 249
  products, cytomegalovirus, 745
  screening, 20
  supply, neonatal epiphysis, 299*f*
  Toxoplasma gondii, 968, 970–971
Blood culture
  contamination, bacteremia v, 249–250
  neonatal sepsis and, 249–250
  positive, 249
  from umbilical vessels, 249
  UTI, 316–317
Blood patch, PROM and, 66
Blood smear, during newborn period, 1148
Blood transfusions
  CMV, 718, 719
  EBV, 907
  GB virus type C/Hepatitis G virus, 809
  HBV, 1225–1226
  malaria, 1046
  Toxoplasma gondii, 931
  Trypanosoma cruzi, 1043
Blood-brain barrier, 435–436
Blood-forming elements, *Toxoplasma gondii*, 968
Bloodstream
  group B streptococcal infection, 432
  Staphylococci, 496
Bloodstream infections (BSI), 1055, 1132–1133
  ureaplasmas, 614
"Bloody tap,", 255
Blueberry muffin rash, 958*f*
B-lymphocytes, 360
Body fluid specimens, bacterial antigens in, 251
Body temperature, congenital *Toxoplasma gondii*, 951

Bone
  changes, viral lesions and, 304
  Toxoplasma gondii, 945
Bone and joint bacterial
  infections, 297–310
  GBS, clinical features, 440*t*
Bone marrow
  examination, parvovirus B19,
    836
  phagocyte production by,
    88–89
  transplant, VZV, 681
Botulinum immune globulin,
  1219–1220
Bradyzoite, 169–170, 918–919
Brain
  coxsackievirus B strains, 769
  radiologic abnormalities of,
    Toxoplasma gondii infections,
    959–961, 959*f*, 960*f*
Brain abscess, 240, 248, 250–251,
  504. *See also* Neonatal brain
  abscess
  group B streptococcal
    infection, 444
  infant management, 258–259
  pathology of, 243
Brain calcifications, 1016–1017
Brain injury, *T. gondii*, 171
Brainstem response audiometry,
  1181
Breast abscess, 211–212
Breast feeding
  cellular elements, 201
  diarrhea, 360, 360*t*
  IgE antibody concentration,
    201
  IgG antibody, 200–201
  IgM antibodies, 201
  mucosal immune system, 200
  poliovirus antibody, 200–201
Breast infection, 500, 501*f*
Breast milk
  alimentary tract, 204
  antibiotics in, 1166–1171
  antibodies, boosting, 40
  anti-inflammatory agents, 205
  antioxidants, 205
  antiparasitic lipids, 204
  antiviral lipids, 204
  chemokines in, 207
  concentrations, amoxicillin,
    1167–1168
  cytomegalovirus, 745–746
  diarrheal disease, 207–208
  expressed, 1139
  HAV, 802–803
  HBV, 803
  HCV, 807
  interleukin-6, 206, 206*t*
  interleukin-7, 207
  interleukin-10, 205
  Lactobacillus species, 203–204
  lysozyme, 204
  monosialoganoglioside and,
    203
  NEC, 338
  storage of, 745–746

transmission
  bacterial pathogens, 20
  HIV infection, 19, 625
Breast-fed infants, otitis media
  and, 281
Breast-feeding, 42–43, 191,
  209–210, 281, 288–289, 792.
  See also Weaning
  antimicrobial agents, 210
  asthma and, 209–210
  bacterial respiratory infections,
    210
  carnitine deficiency, 211
  clostridium difficile, 390
  CMV, 712–713
  demographics of, 213
  diarrhea and, 360
  HCV, 807
  HIV
    infection, 624–625
    transmission, 645
      antiretroviral prophylaxis
        regimens, 642*t*
  hyperbilirubinemia, 211
  infectious risks, 211–213,
    1138–1139
  inherited metabolic diseases,
    210
  Klebsiella pneumoniae, 208
  necrotizing enterocolitis,
    208–209
  neonate
    immunoglobin levels in, 200*t*
    infection and, 261
  NICU, 1139
  nutrient deficiencies, 211
  pneumonia and, 288–289
  traditional v. artificial forms,
    214–215
  viral respiratory infections, 210
  WNV, 913
Broad spectrum β-lactam
  antibiotics, 258
Broad-acting agents
  breast milk concentrations,
    infant daily dose, 1168
  pseudomonas and, 1186*t*,
    1188–1193, 1192*t*
Broad-spectrum antibiotic
  therapy, 1072
Broad-spectrum antimicrobial
  agents
  Candida and, 1058
  HAIs and, 1128
Bronchitis, 774
Bronchoalveolar lavage (BAL),
  Pneumocystosis, 1090
Bronchus-associated lymphoid
  tissue (BALT), 198, 199
BSI. *See* Bloodstream infections
Buffy-coat examination, 250
Bullae, 348
Bullous impetigo, 502

C

C. fetus infection, 386
  differential diagnosis, 389
  epidemiology, 387

C. jejuni, 386
  diagnosis, 388–389
  epidemiology, 387
  therapy, 389
C. koseri, 231
C. neoformans, 1103
C. perfringens, 233–234
C. tetani, 234
C. tetani-contaminated clay
  powder, 234
C. trachomatis, 32, 53, 61
  eye infections and, 349
Calcineurin, 122
CAMP (Christie-Atkins-Munch-
  Petersen) testing, group B
  streptococcal infection, 420
Campylobacter, β-lactam, 389
Campylobacter species, 385–389
  affecting humans, 386*t*
  clinical manifestations, 388
  diagnosis, 388–389
  epidemiology, 387–388
  infection, 389
  nature of organism, 385–386
  pathogenesis, 386–387
  pathology, 387
  therapy, 389
CA-MRSA. *See* Community-
  acquired MRSA
Candida albicans, 83, 250, 256,
  393–394, 1055
  light microscopy photographs,
    1057*f*
  milk macrophage, 201
Candida endophthalmitis,
  1066–1067
Candida enteritis, 393–394
Candida sepsis, 1064
Candida species, 1055,
  1078–1079, 1131
  abdominal surgery, 1059
  antifungal agents and, 1066*t*
  bone and joint infection, 298
  cardiac surgery, 1059
  cerebrospinal fluid, 1065
  infections, 346, 1113
  isolation of, frequency of,
    1056*t*
  maternal vertical transmission,
    1056
  organisms, 304
  pneumonia, 1065
  UTIs and, 311
Candidal chorioretinitis, 1064
Candidal cystitis, 1063
Candidal infections, intrauterine,
  1060
Candidal ophthalmologic
  infections, 1064
Candidal peritonitis, 1063
Candidemia, 1063–1065
Candidemia sepsis, 1056*t*
Candidiasis, 1055–1077.
  See also Neonatal candidiasis
  central nervous system, 1064
  infection, 1195
  clinical manifestations,
    1060–1063

diagnosis, 1066
epidemiology and
  transmission, 1055–1056
introduction, 1055
invasive, 1068*t*
microbiology, 1056–1058
in neonates, host factors, 1058*t*
pathogenesis, 1058–1060
pathology, 1060
treatment, 1067–1072
Capsular polysaccharides, 1228
  antibody to, 437
  immune resistance and, 432–433
  neonates and, 1215
Capture ELISA (Enzyme-linked
  Immunosorbent assay), 976
Carbapenems, 1186*t*, 1190–1193
  antimicrobial activity,
    1190–1191
  appendicitis, 329
  dosing implications,
    1191–1193, 1192*t*
  pharmacokinetic data, 1191,
    1192*t*
  PK-PD dosing, 1191–1193
  safety, 1191
  third-generation, 256
Carbohydrate(s)
  antigens, 150
  components, breast milk and,
    203–204
  metabolism in neonates, 1153
  of milk, 195
Carnitine deficiency, 211
Carrier proteins, 197
Case-fatality rate (CFR),
  infections, 25*t*
Casein, human, 196
CASG. *See* Collaborative
  Antiviral Study Group
Caspofungin, 1071, 1097–1098,
  1114, 1200
  pharmacokinetic data, 1200
  PK-PD, and clinical
    implications, 1200
  safety, 1200
Cat
  feces, 1018
  oocysts and, 1018
Catalase
  production, 494
  test, 470–471
Catheter
  neonatal sepsis and, 238
  removal, 508–509
    bacteremia and, 508–509
    Malassezia infections, 1107
Catheter-associated bacteremia,
  498
Catheter-associated infections,
  258, 1106
  bloodstream, 1132–1134
    antibiotic lock solution, 261
    epidemiology and
      pathogenesis, 1132–1133
    prevention, evidence-based
      strategies, 1133–1134,
      1133*t*

prevention and control, 1133–1134
rates of, by birthweight category, 1133t
candidal, 1062–1063
CoNS, treatment, 498–499
Malassezia infections, 1106
urinary tract infections, 1135
Cationic antimicrobial peptides, 493–494
Cats, serologic testing of, 1018
CCR7 chemokine receptor, 101
CD1 locules, 111
CD4 effector T-cell
    antibody production and, 125–126
    subset differentiation, regulation of, 125
CD4 monitoring, HIV-exposed infants, 634t
CD4 T cells, 124, 139, 140–141
    alloantigen and, 124
    HSV, 166–167
    naïve B cell activation and, 146–147
    recent thymic emigrants, 117–118
CD4+ T-lymphocyte count, 628–631
CD5 expression, 151
CD8+ cytotoxic T lymphocytes, 627
CD8 T cells, 140, 141
    chemokine production, 128
    cytokine production, 128
    HSV, 167
    recent thymic emigrants, 117–118
CD22 expression, 153
CD28, 122
CD31, 119
CD38, 119
CD40 ligand, 128–129, 147
CD45 isoform, 119–120
CDC (Centers for Disease Control and Prevention)
    enterovirus surveillance, 765
    National Smallpox Vaccine in Pregnancy Registry, 900
    pneumocystosis and, 1082–1083
cDCs. *See* Myeloid dendric cells
CDR3
    diversity, mechanisms, 113–114
    length (of immunoglobulin heavy chain), 143–144
    region (of immunoglobulin heavy chain), 143–144
Cefaclor, 385
Cefamandole, 385
Cefazolin, 1185
    dosing, 1187
    GBS, 454
    group B streptococcal disease, 255
Cefepime, 1185–1187, 1186t

Cefixime, 521
    N. gonorrhoeae, 521
    Shigella infection, 385
Cefoperazone, 381, 1162
Cefotaxime, 17–18, 256, 381, 1185
    neonatal meningitis, 258
    serum concentrations, 1165t, 1166
    skin infections, 348
Ceftazidime, 256, 1185
    breast milk concentrations, 1167–1168
    neonatal meningitis, 258
    Pseudomonas species, eye infections, 350
    skin infections, 348
Ceftriaxone, 33, 256, 381, 1162
    gonococcal ophthalmia neonatorum, 521
    N. gonorrhoeae, 521
    S. pneumonia sepsis, 228
    skin infections, 348
    in vitro susceptibility, 448
Cefuroxime, 1185
Cell activation, *Listeria* species and, 476–477
Cell culture
    growth in, rubella virus, 865
    Toxoplasma gondii, 969
Cell-associated complement fixation antigen, rubella virus, 864
Cell-associated viremia, CMV and, 719–720
Cell-mediated immunity
    fetal rejection and, 476
    tests for, *Toxoplasma gondii*, 971
Cellular elements
    breast feeding and, 201
    functions of, breast milk and, 203
Cellular immune responses
    breast milk and, 205
    Listeria monocytogenes, 474
    Pneumocystis jiroveci, 1087
    rubella infection, 873–874
    rubella virus, 871
Cellular immune system, 1087
Cellulitis, 500
    group B streptococcal infection, 443–444, 446
Central memory CD4 T cells, 126–127
Central nervous system (CNS)
    African sleeping sickness, 1045
    candidiasis, 1064
    CMV and, 729
    Coccidioides immitis organism, 1101
    congenital *Toxoplasma gondii*, 949, 950–951
    infected infants, congenital cytomegalovirus, 724–725
    infection
        adults, 480, 584
        candidiasis and, 1195
        cryptococcosis, 1105

parvovirus B19, 843–844
    phycomycosis, 1107
    ureaplasmas, 614–615
    Toxoplasma gondii, 939–940, 941–942
Central venous catheter (CVC), HAIs and, 1128
Cephalexin
    osteomyelitis, 305
    Shigella infection, 385
Cephalhematoma, 346
Cephalosporin plus aminoglycoside, 231
Cephalosporins, 18, 229, 1184–1188
    Aeromonas hydrophila, 392
    antimicrobial activity, 1184–1185
    appendicitis, 329
    breast milk concentrations, 1167–1168
    Campylobacter, 389
    Candida and, 1058
    clinical implications, 1187–1188
    first-generation, 255–256, 1184, 1187
    fourth-generation, 1184
    group B streptococcal disease, 255
    Listeria, 482
    N. gonorrhoeae, 521
    NEC, 337
    nurseries and, 239
    otitis media, 285
    pericarditis, 341
    pharmacokinetic data, 1185–1187, 1186t
    pneumonia, 292
    PROM and, 67–68
    resistance, 1184–1185
    safety, 1187–1188
    second-generation, 1184, 1187
    skin infections, 348
    solitary hepatic abscess, 325
    third-generation, 256, 1184, 1187
    UTI, 319
    vitamin K-dependent factors, 1187
    in vitro susceptibility, 448
    Yersinia enterocolitica, 392
Cerclage, 73
Cerebral palsy, 59
Cerebral tissue necrosis, 243
Cerebrospinal fluid (CSF), 163, 1144
    amikacin, 1180
    amphotericin B, 1196
    ampicillin, 1170
    Candida spp. and, 1065
    congenital toxoplasmosis, 1019
    drug concentration, 1163
    examination, 251–255, 253t, 264
        chemical characteristics, 253t
        congenital tuberculosis, 586, 586f

low birth weight infants, 253t
    osteomyelitis, 304–305
    Toxoplasma gondii, 968
    UTI, 316–317
    gentamicin, 1179
    HSV, 163
    PCR assay, 991
    penicillin, 1169
    serologic screening, 991
    serologic studies of, *T. gondii* in, 991
Cerebrospinal fluid lymphocytosis, 948
Cerebrospinal glucose levels, 253
Cervical cancer, 905
Cervical condylomata, 905
Cervical plugging, 66
Cervical ureaplasma infection, preterm birth, 610–611
Cesarean delivery, 246
    chorioamnionitis, 55
    HSV-2, 817
    maternal HIV transmission prevention, 35
    sepsis and, 241
CFR. *See* Case-fatality rate
CFU-GM. *See* Colony-forming unit-granulocyte-monocyte
Chagas disease, 1043–1045
    agglutinating antibodies, 1045
    antibody tests, 1045
    congenital infections, 1044
    diagnosis, 1044–1045
    mothers with, 1045
    prevention, 1045
    recurrence, prognosis for, 1045
    therapy, 1045
Chagas heart disease, 1043–1044
Chagoma, 1044
Charcoal hemoperfusion, circulatory collapse, 1161
Chemical conjunctivitis, 349
Chemokines, 95–96
    in breast milk, 206t, 207
    immunoregulatory effects of, 82t
    neonatal sepsis, 1152
    production, 127–131
        CD8 T-cells and, 128
        decreased, by neonatal T cells, 129–130
        NK cells, 106
Chemoprophylaxis, 19, 38–39
    group B streptococcal infection, 452–457
        historical precedents, 452
    neonatal sepsis, 261
    for neonate, 456–457
    tuberculosis in nurseries, 594
Chemotactic factors, 91
Chemotaxis inhibitory protein of staphylococci, 494
Chemotherapy
    congenital cytomegalovirus, 743
    congenital rubella infection, 886
    tuberculosis and, 577

Chest radiograph
  congenital tuberculosis, 586f
  tuberculosis in pregnancy, 583
Chicken, *Toxoplasma gondii*, 931
Chickenpox, 661–705, 662
  active immunization against,
      684–685
  clinical manifestations, 668–678
  complications, 669
  cutaneous lesions, 667
  diagnosis, 678–679
  diagnostic technique, 678–679
  differential diagnosis, 678–679
  immunocompromised
      children, 669
  incidence and distribution, 663
  maternal effects, 669
  in nursery, isolation
      procedures, 683–684, 684t
  pathogenesis, 667
  pathology, 667–668
  postnatally acquired, 677
  preventive measures, 683–684
  smallpox v, 903t
  and zoster, 661–685
  zoster v, 663
Chickenpox in pregnancy,
    incidence, 664
Chickenpox pneumonia, 669
Chickenpox rash, 668–669
Childhood vaccination programs,
    1212
Childhood vaccines, correlates of
    protection, 1214t
Chlamydia conjunctivitis, 602, 603f
Chlamydia infections, 601–606
Chlamydia trachomatis, 3, 32, 169,
    520
  clinical manifestations, 603
  developmental cycle, 602,
      602f
  epidemiology and
      transmission, 601
  microbiology, 601–602
  pathogen, 601–602
  pathogenesis, 602–603
  conjunctivitis, 602
  pathology, 603
  pneumonia, 603
  prenatal infections, 603
Chlamydial conjunctivitis
  diagnosis, 604
  differential diagnosis, 604–605
  NAATs, 604
  prognosis, 605
  therapy, 605
Chlamydial pneumonia
  diagnosis, 604
  differential diagnosis, 604–605
  prognosis, 605
  therapy, 605
Chlamydial trachomatis
  prevention, 605–606
  therapy, 605
Chlamydial trachomatis screening,
    pregnant woman, 605
Chlamydial trachomatis vaccine,
    606

Chloramphenicol, 1166
  Aeromonas hydrophila, 392
  breast-feeding, 210
  Campylobacter, 389
  circulatory collapse and, 1161
  EPEC gastroenteritis, 373
  Listeria, 482
  neonatal sepsis, 260
  salmonellosis, 380
  serum concentrations, 1165t,
      1166
  Yersinia enterocolitica, 392
Chlorhexidine, omphalitis and, 31
Chloroquine
  congenital malaria, 1050
  pregnancy an, 1051
Chloroquine-resistant *P.
    falciparum*, 1050
Cholera, during pregnancy, 391
Cholera toxin, 390
Cholesterol, 195
Chorioamnionitis, 62–63, 65, 69,
    608–610
  antibiotic therapy for, 54–55
  histologic, 608
  prematurity and, 60
Chorioamnionitis studies
  long-term outcomes, 58–59
  short-term outcomes, 57–58
Chorionic villus sampling, HIV
    infection, 627
Chorioretinitis, 930, 1005–1006,
    1013
  congenital toxoplasmosis, 954f
  external examination, 951, 952
  frequency of, subclinical
      congenital toxoplasma
      infection, 1008t
  relapsing, treatment for,
      1015–1016
  toxoplasmosis, 951–952
Christie-Atkins-Munch-Petersen
    testing. *See* CAMP
Chromosomal aberrations,
    gestational varicella and, 671
chromosomal aberrations,
    gestational measles and, 689
Chronic disease syndromes,
    CMV, 719
Chronic granulomatous disease,
    497
Chronic intra-amniotic infection,
    55
  management, 55–57
Chronic lung disease (CLD),
    perinatal, 612–614
Chronic maternal *Toxoplasma*
    infection, 928–930
Chronic pulmonary disease in
    infancy, 292
CID. *See* Cytomegalic inclusion
    disease
Cidofovir
  respiratory papillomatosis, 906
  variola, 903
Ciprofloxacin
  M. avium-intracellulare
      complex, with HIV, 633

neonatal meningitis, 258
Circulatory collapse,
    chloramphenicol and, 1161
Circumcision, bacillus Calmette-
    Guérin, 343
Circumcision infection, 343
  tuberculosis, 585
Citrobacter species, 231
Clarithromycin
  fluoroquinolones and, 1000
  M. avium-intracellulare
      complex, with HIV, 633
  Toxoplasma gondii, 1000
Classic pathway activation, 86
Classic pathway complement
    activity, 87, 87t
Clavulanate, PK profile, 1190
Clavulanic acid, breast milk
    concentrations, 1167–1168
CLD. *See* Chronic lung disease
Cleft palate, otitis media and, 281
Clindamycin, 18, 1172t, 1175–1176
  antimicrobial activity, 1175
  appendicitis, 329
  breast milk, 1168
  GBS, 72, 454
  IAI, 54
  mediastinitis, 342
  NEC, 337
  peritonitis, 333
  pharmacokinetic data, 1175
  PK-PD dosing, 1172t, 1176,
      1193t
  safety, 1175–1176
  Toxoplasma gondii, 999
  in vitro susceptibility, 448
Clindamycin and erythromycin,
    507
Clinical amnionitis, 608–610
Clinical intra-amniotic infection.
    See Intra-amniotic infection
Clinical pharmacology, basics of,
    1161–1164
Clinical Risk Index for Babies
    (CRIB), 1128, 1156
Clofazimine, *M. avium-
    intracellulare* complex, with
    HIV, 633
Clonal anergy, 144
Clonal deletion, 144
Clostridial sepsis, 233–234
Clostridium botulinum spores,
    1219–1220
Clostridium difficile, 389–390
  clinical manifestations, 390
  diagnosis, 390
  epidemiology, 389–390
  nature of organism,
      pathophysiology and, 389
  prevention, 390
  therapy, 390
Clostridium species, 233–234
Clostridium tetani, 31, 1224
Cloud baby, 774
CMV. *See* Cytomegalovirus
CNS. *See* Central nervous system
CO_2 laser, condyloma
    acuminatum, 906

Coagulase-negative staphylococci
    (CoNS), 222, 223–224, 225,
    226, 229–230, 256, 490–491,
    492, 1133
  HAIs, 1129
  virulence mechanisms of,
      495–496
Co-amoxiclav, PROM and, 68
Coccidioidal antibody test, 1102
Coccidioides immitis, 1099–1100
Coccidioides immitis organism, 1100
  clinical manifestations, 1101
  dessimination, 1101
  diagnosis and differential
      diagnosis, 1101–1102
  epidemiology and
      transmission, 1100
  organ systems, 1101
  pathogenesis, 1100–1101
  pathology, 1101
  Precipitin, 1102
  prevention, 1102
  prognosis, 1102
  respiratory tract, 1100–1101
  therapy, 1102
Coccidioidomycosis, 1099–1102
Coccidioidomycosis meningitis,
    amphotericin B, 1113
Cochrane Library, PROM and,
    68
Cochrane Pregnancy and
    Childbirth Group Trials
    register, 242
Cochrane Review, neonatal
    infection, prophylactic
    systemic antibiotics, 1134
Cochrane Update on antenatal
    corticosteroids, 67
Cognate T-cell-B-cell
    interaction, 151–152
Coitus, PROM and, 62–63
Coliform organisms, 368
  human milk donors, 368
Colistin, EPEC gastroenteritis,
    373
Collaborative Antiviral Study
    Group (CASG), 743
Collaborative Perinatal Research
    Study, 236–237
Collectins, 85–86
Colonic flora, 83
Colonization
  Candida spp., 1056
  group B streptococcal
      infection, 424–425
  Neisseria gonorrhoeae, 518
  Staphylococcus epidermidis, 495
Colonization rates, umbilical vein
    catheters and, 1133–1134
Colonization resistance, neonatal
    immune system, 1126–1127
Colony-forming unit-
    granulocyte-monocyte
    (CFU-GM), 88–89, 88f
Colony-stimulating factors
    (CSFs), 88–89, 95–96
  in breast milk, 206t, 207
  pyogenic infections, 161–162

Colostral cells, 201
Colostrum, human
  antibodies, 199t
  cell-mediated immunologic
    reactivity, 199t
  components and hormones, 198t
  HCV, 807
  immunoglobulin levels, 199f
  nutritional components,
    194–197, 194t
Combination antimicrobial
  therapy
  MRSA, 508
  MRSA infections, 1171
Combination therapy, HIV and,
  costs, 651
Combination vaccines, 1222
Combinatorial receptor
  engagement, 98
Committee on Infectious
  Diseases of American Academy
  of Pediatrics, 1228
Communicability, period of,
  measles, 687
Community-acquired infections,
  20–21
  CMV and, 719
Community-acquired MRSA
  (CA-MRSA), 490
Community-acquired neonatal
  sepsis, etiology of, 26t
Community-acquired staphylococcus
  aureus (CA-MRSA), 503
Complement, 85–88
  fetal Toxoplasma infection, 987
  in fetus and neonate, 87
Complement activation, 87t
  biologic consequences, 86–87
Complement components, breast
  milk and, 204
Complement fixation
  antimalarial antibodies, 1048
  neonates and, 1215
Complement fixation tests,
  Coccidioides immitis organism,
  1102
Complementarity-determining
  regions (CDRs)
  immunoglobin molecules,
    113–114
  of TCR molecules, 113–114
Complete blood count, white
  blood cell ratios and,
  1146–1149
Condyloma acuminatum, 905,
  906
Congenital aneurysms, 956
Congenital anomalies
  EBV, 907
  influenza and, 908
Congenital candidiasis, 1062
  diagnosis, 1065
Congenital cerebral defects,
  Toxoplasma gondii infections,
  956t
Congenital chickenpox, 691
  maternal infection near term,
    677–678

Congenital cytomegalovirus
  central nervous system and,
    infected infants, 724–725
  chemotherapy, 743
  differential diagnosis, 742
  ganciclovir, 1194–1195
  passive immunization, 743
  prevention, 744–746
  treatment, 743–744
  vaccines, 743–744
Congenital defects
  gestational measles and,
    690–691
  rubella virus, 869
Congenital disease, 8
Congenital enterovirus
  infections, pathology, general
  considerations, 768
Congenital heart disease, CRS, 878
Congenital hemorrhagic
  varicella, 668f
Congenital human
  cytomegalovirus (HCMV), 10
  asymptomatic infection,
    734–735
  clinical manifestations,
    730–736, 730t
  diagnosis, 737–742, 737t
    viral detection, 737–738
  ganciclovir, 18
  long-term outcome, 733–734
  manifestations after, 733t
  maternal immunity and,
    714–716, 714t
  natural history of, 736f
  perinatal infection, 736–737
  during pregnancy, 715
  public health significance, 706
  symptomatic infection,
    731–734
    acute manifestations, 731–733
Congenital infection, 19, 263
  fetal antibody response,
    153–154
  neonate syndromes caused, 9t
  T-cell response to, 139–140
Congenital listeriosis, 323
Congenital malaria, 38,
  1048–1051
  clinical presentation,
    1049–1050
  mefloquine, 1050
  occurrence, 1048–1049
  prevention, 1050–1051
  treatment, 1050
Congenital malformations,
  672–675
  gestational mumps and, 697
  viruses, 770–771
Congenital measles, 691–692
Congenital neutropenia, 262
Congenital ocular toxoplasmosis,
  951
Congenital Pneumocystis jiroveci,
  1084
Congenital pneumonia, 276–296
  pathogenesis and pathology,
  286

Congenital rubella infection, 861,
  871–874
  clinical management, 885–886
  diagnosis, 883–884
  management issues, 884–886
  prevention, 886–890
  virologic findings, 871–872
  virus excretion rate, 872f
Congenital rubella syndrome
  (CRS), 8, 742, 1225
  clinical findings/occurrence
    frequency, 878t
  developmental manifestations,
    880–881
  elimination strategies, 889–890
  laboratory diagnosis, 881–884
  late-onset manifestations,
    880–881
  long-term prognosis, 881
  maternal infection, 881–883
  permanent manifestations,
    878–880
  after rubella vaccination, 877t
  transient manifestations,
    877–878
  United States cases, 866, 866f
    incidence rates, 867f
Congenital syphilis, 8, 632, 742,
  1169–1170
Congenital T. gondii infection,
  154
Congenital toxoplasmosis, 742
  acute infection, 1024–1026
    antimicrobial therapy,
      1024–1026
  antibody development, no
    treatment, 991f
  cerebrospinal fluid, 1019
  cerebrospinal fluid
    lymphocytosis, 948
  chorioretinitis in, 954f
  fetal/newborn ultrasound
    studies, 1005t
  funduscopic examination, 954t
  by gestational age, 925t
  macular pseudocoloboma of
    retina, 956f
  mild form, 948–949, 948f
  newborns with, IgM
    Toxoplasma antibodies, 948t
  no treatment, sequelae of,
    1004–1017
  ophthalmologic
    manifestations, 955t
  ophthalmologic outcomes,
    prenatal/postnatal
    treatment, 1016
  parasitemia, 922t
  pregnancy, 949t, 1025
    approach to patient, 1024f
    gestational time and, 1026
    latent infection, 1027–1028
    outcomes, 1019
    pregnancy termination,
      1026–1027
    resources/telephone
      numbers/internet sites,
      1028t

Congenital rubella infection, 861,
  screening of, 935–936
  seroconversion, 1021
  untreated women, 1020
  prenatal diagnosis of
    findings at birth, 1003t
    pyrimethamine-sulfadiazine
      alternated with
      spiramycin, 1003t
  prevalence of, 934–935
    at birth/during infancy, 934
    serologic screening, 934–935
  prevention, 1017–1028, 1017t
    food and, 1018–1028
    maternal treatment,
      1024–1028
    in pregnancy, 1018–1024
    serologic screening,
      1018–1024
  severe form, 948f
  severity of manifestations, 925t
  since birth, antibody
    development, 991f
  subclinical, untreated children,
    1004–1017, 1006f
  treatment programs, 925t
Congenital tuberculosis, 583–586
  chest radiograph, 586f
  clinical features, 585–586
  diagnosis, 585–586
    criteria for, 585
  of ear, 284
  prognosis, 590–591
  signs and symptoms, 586t
Congenital vaccinia, 902–903
Congenital varicella, rash v., date
  of onset, 678t
Congenital varicella syndrome,
  672–673
  diagnosis of, 675
  incidence of, 676t
Congenitally infected infants,
  ophthalmologic follow-up,
  Lyon, France, 1016–1017, 1017f
Conidiospore, 1097
Conjugate vaccines, 1227
  GBS, 457
Conjugated pneumococcal
  vaccine, 647
Conjunctivitis, 349–350
  Chlamydia trachomatis, 603f
  group B streptococcal
    infection, 445
CoNS. See Coagulase-negative
  staphylococci
Contraception, natural, breast-
  feeding and, 210
Conventional IFA test.
  See Conventional indirect
  fluorescent antibody test
Conventional indirect fluorescent
  antibody test, interpretation,
  Toxoplasma gondii, 975
Conventional indirect fluorescent
  antibody test (Conventional
  IFA test), interpretation,
  Toxoplasma gondii, 975
Cord blood, 102, 154, 675
  IgA isotype, 158

Cord blood (*Continued*)
  parasitemia, 992
  response, 153
  tregs, 135
Cord care regimens, 348
  infection and, 1139–1140
  studies, 1139–1140
Cord serum
  congenital rubella infection,
    883
  IgM antibodies in, 978
Corticosteroids, 680, 999
  cessation, 1109
  enteroviruses and, 791
  HAIs and, 1128
  HIV-associated encephali, 635
  Pneumocystosis, 1093
  preterm labor and, 242
  PROM and, 67–68
  use, *Candida* and, 1059–1060
  varicella during pregnancy, 670
Corynebacterium diphtheriae, 278,
    1223
Coryza, 774
COS type distribution, GBS, 427
Counterimmunoelectrophoresis,
    251
Coxsackie virus, 756
  A16, mouse myocardium,
    760*f*
  abortion and, 770
  B strain
    clinical and pathologic
      findings, 779*t*
    pathology, 768–769
  B1, 778–780
    mouse myocardium, 760*f*
  B2, 780
  B3, 780
  B4, 780
  B5, 780–781
  congenital malformations,
    770–771
  neonatal infections, 763
  pregnancy and, 762
  prematurity and stillbirth, 771
  A strains, 778
    pathology, 768
  transplacental transmission,
    761–762
Coxsackie virus B4 encephalitis,
    769*f*
Coxsackie virus B4 myocarditis,
    768*f*
Cranial computed tomography,
    outcomes, CMV infection, 734
C-reactive protein (CRP), 85,
    505–506, 1149–1151
  group B streptococcal
    infection, 447
  levels, measurement of,
    1150–1151
  neonatal sepsis, 244
  onset of infectious signs, 1150
  PROM and, 66
CRIB. *See* Clinical Risk Index for
    Babies
CRP. *See* C-reactive protein

CRS. *See* Congenital rubella
    syndrome
Cryptococcal meningitis, 1105
Cryptococcosis, 1103–1105
  clinical manifestations,
    1104–1105
  diagnosis and differential
    diagnosis, 1105
  dissemination of, 1105
  epidemiology and
    transmission, 1103–1104
  latex particle agglutination
    test, 1105
  organism, 1103
  pathogenesis, 1104
  pathology, 1104
  prevention, 1105
  prognosis, 1105
  therapy, 1105
Cryptosporidium, 395
CSF. *See* Cerebrospinal fluid
CSFs. *See* Colony-stimulating
    factors
CT, osteomyelitis, 303
C-type lectin receptors, 98
Culture-based screening
  Group B streptococcal
    infection, maternal
    colonization, 454*f*
  Mycobacterium tuberculosis, 578
Cultures
  optimal number, 249
  therapy and, 256–257
Cutaneous abscess, 500
Cutaneous aspergillosis, 1096,
    1097
Cutaneous lesions
  chickenpox, 667
  in zoster, 668
Cutaneous listeriosis, 478*f*
Cutter incident, 1221
Cyclophosphamide, *Pneumocystis*
    pneumonia, rat study, 1086
Cyst
  formation, *Toxoplasma gondii*,
    937
  rupture, 938
Cystic fibrosis, 292
Cystlike stages, *Pneumocystis
    jiroveci*, 1080, 1081*f*
Cysts, 243
  atovaquone and, 1000
  Pneumocystis jiroveci, 1080*f*
  T. gondii, 919*f*, 920*f*, 921–931
Cytokines, 81, 81*t*, 127–131,
    157–158, 170
  in breast milk, 193, 206*t*
  circulating/cerebrospinal fluid
    levels of, HSV, 163
  CMV and, 720
  HSV and, 162–163
  immunoglobulin and, 125–126
  immunoregulatory effects of,
    82*t*
  intracellular pathogens, 102*f*
  Listeria and, 475–476
  neonatal sepsis, 1152
  newborns and, 477

production, 96–100, 122
  CD8 T-cell and, 128
  decreased, by neonatal T
    cells, 129–130
  after long-term in vitro
    differentiation, of effector
    CD4 T cells, 130–131
  by neonatal T cells, after
    short-term in vitro
    differentiation, 130
  NK cells, 106
  NK-mediated cytotoxicity
    and, 107
  postnatal ontogeny of, 128
  after short-term in vitro
    differentiation, by
    neonatal T cells, 130
Cytolytic cell mechanisms,
  activation of, 476*f*
Cytomegalic inclusion disease
  (CID), 706
Cytomegalovirus (CMV), 3, 8,
    9–10, 171–172, 253, 604–605,
    706–755, 1132
  acute infection, pathogenesis
    of, 724
  breast-feeding, 712–713, 713*t*,
    1139
  cell-associated viremia and,
    719–720
  chronic viral excretion,
    727–728, 728*f*
  clinical manifestations,
    730–737
  epidemiology, 711–719, 712*f*
    overview, 711–712
  hospital workers and, 718–719
  host immune response,
    723–724, 723*t*
  human milk and, 211, 212
  intrauterine transmission,
    715–716, 715*t*
  isolation of, 12
  maternal excretion of, infant
    infection v, 717*t*
  maternal infection, and vertical
    transmission, 714–717
  maternal seroimmunity, rate
    of, 715*t*
  modes of transmission, 712
  nosocomial transmission,
    717–718
  organ systems and, 728–730
  pathogenesis, 719–728
    host immunity and, 722–723
  pathology, 728–730
  perinatal infection, 716–717
  reinfection of, 715–716
  replication, 709–711
  sexual transmission, 717
  as source of, young children,
    713–714, 713*t*
  study, pregnant women, 723
  T cell response to, 141
Cytomegalovirus cellular
  tropism, 711
Cytomegalovirus during
  pregnancy

  clinical signs and symptoms,
    740
  diagnosis of, 740–741
  diagnostic tests, 741
  fetal infection, maternal
    laboratory tests, 741
  IgG avidity assay, 740–741
  IgM assays, 740
  laboratory markers, 740
  prenatal diagnosis, 741–742
  prevention, 744–745
  viral cultures, 741
Cytomegalovirus (CMV) IgM
  serology, 737–738
Cytomegalovirus immune
  globulin, 1219
Cytomegalovirus transmission,
    713–714
Cytomegalovirus (CMV) virion
  envelope of, 709
  regions of, 707, 708*f*
  tegument of, 709
Cytomegalovirus (CMV) virus,
    707–711
Cytomegalovirus (CMV) virus
  genome, 707
Cytomegalovirus-affected teeth,
    732, 733*f*
Cytomegalovirus-encoded
  pathogenic functions, 720–722
Cytosine arabinoside, neonatal
  herpes and, 826
Cytotoxicity, 126

D
Dacryocystitis, 350
Dactylitis, 1099–1100
Danish Congenital
    Toxoplasmosis Study Group,
    prevalence study, 935
Daptomycin, 508, 1177
DCs. *See* Dendritic cells
Deafness, 964
  congenital CMV, 732–733
  CRS, 880
Deaths, pertussis, 1217
Defense agents, features of,
    breast milk and, 203
Defense factors, breast milk and,
    203–207
Defense system, mechanisms of,
    human milk and, 198
Dehydroemetine, *Entamoeba
    histolytica*, 1046
Delayed cutaneous
    hypersensitivity, 138
Delayed-type hypersensitivity
    (DTH), 94
Delivery, 817–818.
  See also Cesarean delivery
  acquired infections at, 9*t*, 19
  care, neonatal infection
    and, 42
  EPEC, 366
  genital herpes, 830*t*
  group B streptococcal infection
    and, 426
  HSV, 830–831

HSV type 2, 817–818
infections, 19
N. gonorrhoeae, 519
premature, neonatal GBS, 430
prior drug administration, 242–243
UTIs and, 310
Dendritic cells (DCs), 101–103, 109
HSV and, 164
properties and functions, 101–102
Dental defects, congenital CMV, 732
Dermatologic syndromes, parvovirus B19, 843
Dermatophytes, 1109
Dermatophytoses, 1109–1112
clinical manifestations, 1110–1111
diagnosis and differential diagnosis, 1111
epidemiology and transmission, 1109–1110
keratolytic medications, 1111
lesions, 1110
organism, 1109
pathogenesis, 1110
pathology, 1110
prevention, 1112
prognosis, 1111–1112
therapy, 1111
Developmental anomalies, 8
Developmental immunology, host defenses in, infection and, 80–191
Device-related infections, 1132–1135
Dexamethasone
neonatal meningitis, 258
to neonates, 243
Dextran-conjugated anti-immunoglobulin mAbs, 153
Diagnostic needle aspiration, 251
Diagnostic test, characteristics, 1145*f*
Diaper dermatitis, 1060–1062
Diaper rash, 348
Diarrhea, 30, 774–775, 964
breast feeding and, 360, 360*t*
differential diagnosis, 399–400, 400*t*
micro-organisms responsible, 359–418
Diarrheal disease, 636
prevention, in breast milk, 207–208
Diarrhea-related HUS, 375
Dicloxacillin
infant to maternal serum concentrations, ratios, 1165
osteomyelitis, 305
Differential agglutination test (HS/AC test)
interpretation, *Toxoplasma gondii*, 975*f*
Toxoplasma gondii, 975

Differential cell count, during newborn period, 1148
Differential leukocyte count, 1146
Diffuse hepatitis, 324
Diphtheria, 278, 1223
maternal immunization, 1216–1217
neonatal, 278
respiratory, 278
Diphtheria toxoid (DT), 1221, 1223
Direct acid-fast bacilli smear, congenital tuberculosis, 586
Direct-acting antimicrobial agents
breast milk and, 203–204
general features of, breast milk and, 203
Disseminated aspergillosis, 1097
Disseminated candidiasis, 1063–1065
diagnosis, 1065
treatment, 1067–1068
Disseminated neonatal herpes, 821–822
Disseminated vaccinia, 679
DNA amplification based typing methods, 471
DNA hybridization, HCMV, 738
DNA hybridization techniques, parvovirus B19, 845
DNA macro restriction pattern analysis, PFGE, 471
DNA recombination, 113
DNA vaccine platform, congenital cytomegalovirus, 744
DNA-based technology, gonococcal ophthalmia neonatorum, 519–520
DNA-dependent protein kinase, 113
DNAemia, 741, 744–745
Dorsal root ganglia, HSV and, 815
Dosing, drugs, 1163–1164
Down syndrome, *Toxoplasma gondii* infections, 957
Doxycycline, *Toxoplasma gondii*, 999–1000
Drinking water, *Toxoplasma gondii*, 931
Droplet infection, measles by, incubation period for, 687
Droplet infection precautions, 1137–1138
Drug(s). *See also specific drugs*
absorption, into bloodstream, 1162
administration, delivery and, 242–243
administration (non-antibiotic), to neonate, 243
antituberculosis, 587*t*
under concentration curve, 1163–1164
developing fetus, 1166

distribution, 1162
protein binding and, 1162
dosing, 1163–1164
PK/PD approach, 1164
elimination, 1162
eruptions, 692
half-life of, 1163
milk to plasma ratios, 1166
not routinely used, in neonates, 1161*t*
PK of, 1161
for *T. gondii*, 999–1000
Drug susceptibility testing, mycobacteria and, 578
Dryvax, 904
DT. *See* Diphtheria toxoid
DTH. *See* Delayed-type hypersensitivity
Duck embryo vaccine, rabies, 913
Ductus arteriosus, CRS, 878
Duranavir, 649–651
Dye test, maternally transmitted *T. gondii* antibody, uninfected infants, 990*f*

E
E. coli, 208, 223, 239, 240, 241, 250
milk macrophage, 201
UTIs and, 311
E. faecium, 229
EAEC. *See* Enteroaggregative *E. coli*
Early life infection prevention, through maternal-neonatal immunization, 1212–1230
overall principles, 1212–1228
Early pregnancy loss, 610
Toxoplasma gondii in, 943
EBNA. *See* EBV-associated nuclear antigen
EBV. *See* Epstein-Barr virus
EBV-associated nuclear antigen (EBNA), 906
E-cadherin, 471
Echinocandins, 1071, 1114, 1199–1200
antimicrobial activity, 1199–1200
Echovirus 1, 781
Echovirus 2, 781
Echovirus 3, 781
Echovirus 4, 781
Echovirus 5, 782
Echovirus 6, 782
Echovirus 7, 782
Echovirus 8, 782
Echovirus 9, 782–783
neonatal infection with, 782*t*
Echovirus 11, 784–785
neonatal infection with, 783*t*
nursery outbreaks, 775
Echovirus 13, 785
Echovirus 14, 785
Echovirus 16, 785
Echovirus 17, 785–786
Echovirus 18, 786
Echovirus 19, 786

Echovirus 20, 786
Echovirus 21, 786
Echovirus 25, 786
Echovirus 30, 786
Echovirus 31, 787
Echovirus 33, 787
Echoviruses, 756–757, 769, 781–787
abortion and, 770
congenital malformations, 771
neonatal infections, 763–764
prematurity and stillbirth, 771
transplacental transmission, 762
Ecthyma gangrenosum, 346
Effector T cells, 122, 123*f*, 126
CMV and, 722
migration, 132
naïve T cell and, 124–127
Eggs, *Toxoplasma gondii*, 931
EHEC. *See* Enterohemorrhagic *E. coli*
Ehlers-Danlos syndrome, preterm PROM and, 62
EI. *See* Erythema infectiosum
EIEC. *See* Enteroinvasive *E. coli*
ELBW infant. *See* Extremely low birth weight infant
Electrolytes, 903
Elementary body (EB), 602
ELISA (Enzyme-linked immunosorbent assay), 364, 788, 789
enterovirus antibodies, 759
HCMV, 739
measles virus, 686
mumps organism, 695
rotavirus, 398
Toxoplasma gondii, 972, 976, 977
varicella zoster virus antibody, 678–679
ELISPOT assays, T cell detection, 138–139
Embryo, infection of, 6–10
Embryonic death, and resorption, 6
Empyema, 287, 292
Encapsulated bacteria, 1221
Encephalitis, 688. *See also* Herpes simplex encephalitis
coxsackievirus B5, 780–781
Endocardial fibroelastosis, gestational mumps and, 697
Endocarditis, 338–340, 499
group B streptococcal infection, 445
maternal GBS, 446
Endocrine disorders, *Toxoplasma gondii* infections, 957
Endocrine glands, CMV and, 729
Endocrine organs
pathology of, 637
Toxoplasma gondii, 944
Endophthalmitis, 1064, 1097–1098
Endothelial cells, CMV and, 720
Endotracheal intubation, catheter-related candidal infections, 1063

Energy, of milk, 195
Entamoeba histolytica, 394,
    1045–1046
Enteral feeding tubes, 1135
Enteric cytopathogenic human
    orphan viruses, 756–757
Enteric fever, 379–380
Enteric host defense mechanisms,
    359–360
Enteric viruses, 208, 395,
    1131–1132
Enteritis, 386
Enteroaggregative *E. coli*
    (EAEC), 361–362, 375–376
    clinical manifestations, 376
    diagnosis and therapy, 376
    epidemiology and
        transmission, 375–376
Enterobacter sakazakii, 393
Enterobacter septicemia, 231
Enterobacter species, 231
Enterobacteriaceae family, HAIs,
    1130
Enterococcal sepsis, 229
Enterococcus, 256
    neonatal HAIs, 1129
    UTIs and, 311
Enterococcus faecalis, 223, 277
Enterococcus species, 229, 256
Enterohemorrhagic *E. coli*
    (EHEC), 361–362, 374–375
Enteroinvasive *E. coli* (EIEC),
    361–362, 365
Enteropathogenic *E. coli* (EPEC)
    classic serotypes, 365–374
    epidemiology and
        transmission, 365–368
    gastroenteritis, 366
        antimicrobial susceptibility
            patterns, 374
        clinical manifestations,
            370–371
        complications of, 369
        diagnosis, 371–372
        infection-control measures,
            374
        nursery epidemic, 367
        pathogenesis, 368–369
        pathology, 369–370
        prevention, 374
        prognosis, 372–373
        therapy, 373–374
    gastroenteritis with *Salmonella*,
        372
    gastroenteritis with *Shigella*,
        372
Enterotoxigenic *Escherichia coli*
    (ETEC), 362–365
    clinical manifestations, 364
    diagnosis, 364
    epidemiology and
        transmission, 363–364
    pathology, 364
    therapy and prevention,
        364–365
Enterovirus, 756–799, 1132
    antipicornavirus drugs, 791

ascending infection, during
    birth, 762
classification, genomic, 758*t*
clinical manifestations,
    769–787
geographic distribution and
    season, 764–765
host range, 764
host systems, 759
human, classification of, 757,
    757*t*
IgM antibody tests, 789
infections, 756–799, 768, 787
    differential diagnosis, 789
    histology, 789
    isolations in U.S., nonpolio,
        766*t*
    morphology, 758–759
    neonatal infections, 762
    pathogenesis, 765–768, 767*f*
        events during, 765–766
        factors affecting, 767–768
    prematurity and stillbirth,
        771
    replication, 758–759, 758*t*
    transplancental transmission,
        762
Enteroviruses, nonpolio
    manifestations of, 778–787
    neonatal infection, 772–776,
        773*t*
    prognosis, 790
    therapy
        meningoencephalitis, 791
        mild, nonspecific febrile
            illness, 791
        myocarditis, 791
        non-specific, 791
        paralytic poliomyelitis, 791
        sepsis-like illness, 791
        specific, 790–791
env gene, 626
Environmental antigens, T-cell
    reactivity to, 138
Environmental macromolecules,
    human milk and, 198, 198*t*
Enzyme-linked immunosorbent
    assay. *See* ELISA
Enzymes, human milk, 197
Eosinophilic pustular folliculitis,
    349
Eosinophils, 93
EPEC. *See* Enteropathogenic
    E. coli
Epidemics, 238–239
Epidermal necrolysis, 637
Epiglottitis, 277
Epiphysitis, 299–300
Epithelial adhesion, *Candida
    albicans*, 1057–1058
Epithelial barriers, against
    infection, 83–85
Epithelial cells
    breast milk and, 203
    human milk and, 213–214
Epithelial lesions, *Candida* and,
    1060

Epithelium, group B
    streptococcal infection, 429
Epstein-Barr virus (EBV), 637,
    719, 906–907
    during pregnancy, 906–907
Equipment screening, 20
Erysipelas, 241–242
Erythema infectiosum (EI), 841
    exposure history, 852
    prevalence of, 852
Erythema toxicum, 348
Erythroblastosis, *Toxoplasma
    gondii* infections, 964
Erythrocyte sedimentation rate,
    1151
Erythromycin, 33
    breast milk, 1168
    Campylobacter, 389
    GBS and, 72
    gonococcal ophthalmia
        neonatorum, 521–522
    infant to maternal serum
        concentrations, ratios, 1165
    ocular trachoma, 606
    pertussis, 280
    vaginal *Ureaplasma urealyticum*
        infection, 62*t*
    in vitro susceptibility, 448
Erythromycin-resistant *S. aureus*
    conjunctivitis, 349
Escherichia coli, 230, 277,
    361–376, 362*t*
    immunoglobulin antibody and,
        199
    pathotypes, 376
Esophagitis, 342
    in HIV, 636
Estrogens, 192*t*
ETEC. *See* Enterotoxigenic
    Escherichia coli
Ethambutol (EMB)
    M. avium-intracellulare
        complex, with HIV, 633
    tuberculosis and, 587–588,
        587*t*, 589–590
Ethnic groups, breast-feeding,
    213
Ethnicity, neonatal sepsis and,
    236–237
Exanthem, 781
Exfoliative toxins, 495
Exogenous cytokines, HSV and,
    169
Exonuclease activity, 115
Expanded rubella syndrome, 877
Extended spectrum β-lactamase
    nurseries and, 239
    UTI, 319
External ear canal fluid,
    microscopic examination,
    1153–1154
Extracellular fluid volume,
    newborns, 1162
Extracellular microbial
    pathogens, 159–160
Extracorporeal membrane
    oxygenation (ECMO), GBS, 450

Extremely low birth weight
    infant (ELBW infant),
    neonatal candidiasis, 1072
Eye
    Toxoplasma gondii, 939, 941*f*,
        942–943
    toxoplasmosis, 951–956
Eye infections, 349–350
    antipseudomonal penicillin,
        350
    ceftazidime, 350
    HSV and, 823–824
Eye lesions
    birth injury, 956
    circulatory disturbances, 956
    congenital anomalies, 955,
        956*f*
    congenital toxoplasmosis, 1020
    differential diagnosis, 955–956
    inflammatory, 955–956
    neoplasms, 956
Eye prophylaxis, 33

F

Facial cellulitis, group B
    streptococcal infection,
    443–444
Failure to thrive, 637
Fallopian tubes, tuberculosis, 583
FAMA test, 677–678
    varicella zoster virus antibody,
        678–679
Famciclovir, pregnant women,
    680
Family-centered care, 1138–1140
    infection risk, 1138
Fansidar, 994–996
    administration of, 997
    congenital toxoplasmosis,
        996–997
Fas molecules, 132
Favus, 1110
FDA (Federal Drug
    Administration) Center for
    Drug Evaluation and Research,
    1160
Fecal IgA content, human milk
    feeding and, 200
Federal Drug Administration.
    See FDA
Femoral venipuncture,
    osteomyelitis and, 298
Fetal anemia, 851
Fetal antibody response
    congenital infection, 153–154
    maternal immunization,
        153–154
Fetal B cells, 149–150
Fetal blood, maternal IgG and,
    927
Fetal CD7+ prothymocytes, 112
Fetal chickenpox, lesions in,
    frequency of, 668*t*
Fetal conventional dendritic cells,
    102–103
Fetal death, parvovirus B19,
    847–849, 848*t*

Fetal defenses, *T. gondii*, 170–172
Fetal extrathymic T-cell differentiation, 134
Fetal growth restriction, congenital CMV, 732
Fetal hemoglobin, malaria, 1048
Fetal hydrops, parvovirus B19, 849
Fetal immunization response, in animal models, 153–154
Fetal infection, 5–6
  absence of, 6
  rubella virus, 867–869, 868*t*
Fetal infection prevention, through maternal-neonatal immunization, 1212–1230
  overall principles, 1212–1228
Fetal life, monocytes and macrophages, 100–101
Fetal liver, 134
  pre-B cells in, 143
Fetal lung maturity, determining, 72
Fetal malformations, 676–677
Fetal membranes, 5
  infiltrates, preterm birth v, 60*f*
Fetal natural killer cell-mediated cytotoxicity, 107
Fetal parvovirus B19
  anatomic and histologic features, 850–851
  diagnostic evaluation and management, 852–854
  differential diagnosis, 854
  pathology in, 850–852
  of placenta, 851
  prognosis, 854–855
Fetal regulatory T cells, 134–135
Fetal rubella infection, immune response, first trimester (of pregnancy), 872, 872*f*
Fetal spleen tissue, 150–151
Fetal surveillance, PROM and, 72
Fetal survival, malaria, 1047
Fetal tachycardia, 243
Fetal T-cell compartment, phenotype and function of, 133–134
Fetal T-cell sensitization, 138
Fetal to maternal concentrations of drugs (F/M ratios), 994
Fetal *Toxoplasma gondii*
  acute maternal infection, 924–930
  gestational age, 926*t*
  during pregnancy, 925*t*
  prenatal diagnosis, 985–987
  transmission, third trimester, 927
Fetal transfusion, hydrops fetalis and, 854
Fetal tregs, 135
Fetal triple-negative thymocytes, 113
Fetal viability, PROM, treatment before, 68–69
Fetal *Toxoplasma gondii*, 929

Fetus
  Ascaris, 1042–1043
  gestational measles and, 689–691
  gestational varicella and, 671–677
  immune responses, parvovirus B19 infection, 850
  infection of, 6–10
  modes of inoculation, 584*t*
  neonatal GBS, 430
  parvovirus B19 infection, pathogenesis of, 850
  treatment effects, congenital toxoplasmosis, 1019–1020
  tuberculosis, 580
  visceral lesions in, chickenpox, 667–668
Fetus in utero, *T. gondii*
  treatment, 994
  treatment outcome, 1004
Fever
  causes, 52
  first month of life, 264
  neonatal sepsis and, 246–247
  UTI, 315
Fibrinogen, 1149–1150, 1151
Fibroblasts, CMV and, 711
Fibronectin, 1152
  breast milk and, 204
  GBS, 439
Flavobacterium species, nurseries and, 238
Flucloxacillin, osteomyelitis, 305
Fluconazole, 1070, 1114, 1198–1199
  candidemia, 1131
  dosing implications, 1198–1199
  PK-PD dosing, 1198–1199
  safety, 1198
  trichosporonosis, 1111
Fluconazole prophylaxis, 1072–1073
Fluconazole-resistant *C. parapsilosis*, 1072–1073
5-Flucytosine (5-FC), 1070, 1113
  fungi and, 1113
Fluid reservoirs, infection, 29
Fluids, 903
  GBS, 450
  Shigella infection, 384–385
Fluorescent antibody procedures, EPEC gastroenteritis, 374
Fluorocytosine, 1070
5-Fluorocytosine, 1197–1198
  clinical implications, 1198
  pharmacokinetic data, 1197
  safety, 1197
Fluorogenic RT-PCR, GBS, 452
Fluoroquinolones
  EAEC, 376
  physiochemical properties, 1168
  Toxoplasma gondii, 1000
  tuberculosis in pregnancy, 589

F/M ratios. *See* Fetal to maternal concentrations of drugs
Focal bacterial infections, 322–358
Focal infection, neonatal sepsis, 244
Follicle, germinal centers of, 147
Fomites
  decontamination of, 263
  measles virus, 686
Fontanelle, bulging, 248
Food
  congenital toxoplasmosis and, 1018–1028
  Toxoplasma gondii, 930–931
Food handling, HAV, 800
Foscarnet, congenital cytomegalovirus, 743
Fucidic acid, osteomyelitis, 305
Fulminant sepsis, 260
Fungal dermatitis, 1108, 1112*f*
Fungal infections
  HIV and, 633–634
  less common, 1078–1124
Fungal meningitis, amphotericin B, 1113
Fungal products, 161
Fungi, 1131
  5-flucytosine and, 1113
  amphotericin B deoxycholate and, 1097*t*
  gastroenteritis, 393–394
Fungicidal medications, dermatophytoses, 1111
Funisitis, 500–501
Furazolidone, *Shigella* infection, 385

G

gag genes, 625
Galactosemia, 210, 240, 263
Gallium-67 bone imaging, osteomyelitis, 303
GALT. *See* Gut-associated lymphoid tissue
Gametocytes, *Toxoplasma gondii*, 920*f*
Ganciclovir
  antimicrobial activity, 1194
  congenital CMV infection, 18, 1194–1195
  congenital cytomegalovirus, 743
  pharmacokinetic data, 1194
  PK-PD, and clinical indication, 1195
  safety, 1194
Gardnerella vaginalis, 53
Gas gangrene, 241–242
Gastric acid barrier, 360
Gastric acidification, 83
Gastric acidity, *Salmonella* species, 378
Gastric aspirates, microscopic examination, 1153–1154
Gastroenteritis, bacterial agents, 393–394
Gastroenteritis studies, 367, 379

Gastrointestinal disorders, sepsis and, 247–248
Gastrointestinal homeostasis, in breast milk, 207–208
Gastrointestinal signs, sepsis and, 248
Gastrointestinal tract, 83
  CMV and, 729
  micafungin and, 1201
  pathology of, 636
Gatifloxacin, in vitro susceptibility, 448
GAVI. *See* Global Alliance for Vaccines and Immunization
GB virus type C/Hepatitis G virus, 809–810
  clinical manifestations, 809–810
  diagnosis, 810
  epidemiology and transmission, 809
  microbiology, 809
  pathogenesis, 809
  pathology, 809
  prevention, 810
  treatment, 810
GBS. *See* Group B streptococci
G-coupled protein receptor-like molecules, CMV and, 721–722
Gender, neonatal sepsis, 237, 237*t*
Genes, CMV and, 721
Genital colonization, GBS, 437
Genital cytomegalovirus excretion, rate of, 716
Genital herpes
  delivery transmission, 830*t*
  pregnant women, management of, 830
Genital herpes simplex virus, 169
Genital tract, group B streptococcal infection, 429
Genital tract organisms, 5
Genitourinary tract infection, preterm birth v, 60*t*
Genitourinary tuberculosis, 578, 580–581
Genome-wide phage display technique, 429
Genotypes, 863, 863*f*
Gentamicin, 43, 256, 1177–1179, 1178*t*, 1180–1181
  appendicitis, 329
  Campylobacter, 389
  cerebrospinal fluid concentrations, 1179
  chorioamnionitis, 55
  NEC, 337
  neonatal sepsis, 260
  nurseries and, 239
  peritonitis, 333
  Pseudomonas species, eye infections, 350
  serum half-life, 1179
  solitary hepatic abscess, 325
  tuberculosis in pregnancy, 589
Gentamicin clearance, neonates, 1179
Gentian violet, 1069

Geographic regions
bacterial pathogens, 26–27
neonatal sepsis, 237–238
Germinal center B cells, 147
Gestation
maternal *Toxoplasma gondii*,
spiramycin treatment and,
924*t*
pyrimethamine and
sulfadiazine, 1026
Gestational age
congenital toxoplasmosis, 925*t*
fetal *Toxoplasma gondii*, 926*t*
rubella virus, transmission in
utero, 867–869
Gestational chickenpox, abortion
and prematurity, 671–672
Gestational measles
chromosomal aberrations, 689
congenital defects, 690–691
fetal effects, 689–691
Gestational mumps, fetus
abortion and, 697
Gestational varicella, 672
fetal effects, 671–677
pneumonia, with and without,
670, 670*t*
Giardia lamblia, 394–395, 1043
Gliomas, 956
Global Alliance for Vaccines and
Immunization (GAVI), 41
Global neonatal deaths, 44
Global public health, 24
Gloves, 1137
Glucose intolerance, new-onset,
disseminated candidiasis, 1063
Glutamine, 262
Glycoconjugates, breast milk
and, 203
Glycopeptide antibiotics, 1171
Glycoprotein B, CMV, 716
Glycoprotein G, HSV and, 814
Gold standard, 1145
Gonococcal infection, 516–523
epidemiology and
transmission, 516–518
eye infections and, 349
numbers of cases, 519*f*
Gonococcal ophthalmia
neonatorum, 491*f*, 519–520,
521
ceftriaxone, 521
prophylaxis for, 521–522
Gonococcal sepsis, 298
Gowns, 1137
Graft rejection, 138
Graft-*versus*-host disease, 138
Gram-negative bacteria, HAIs
and, 1130
Gram-negative enteric bacilli
osteomyelitis and, 297
otitis media, 284
Gram-negative infections, 17–18
Gram-positive bacteria, HAIs,
1129–1130
Granulocyte colony-stimulating
factor, neonatal sepsis, 259
Granulocytes, 89

Granuloma
Coccidioides immitis organism,
1101
formation, listeriosis, 477
Granulomatous pulmonary
disease, 1101
Granzyme cytotoxins, 131, 131*f*
Griseofulvin, 1114
Group A streptococci, 226–228
NICUs, 1129
Group B streptococcal sepsis, 297
Group B streptococcal
septicemia, 446
Group B streptococci (GBS),
159–162, 222, 224, 225,
419–469
adjunctive therapies, 451
adrenal abscess, 444
antenatal detection of, rapid
assays for, 452
antimicrobial agents, 449–450,
449*t*
asymptomatic infection
in adults, 424–429
infants and children, 425–426
bacteriuria, during pregnancy,
447
bloodstream, 432
bone and joint infections, 443
clinical features, 440*t*
capsular polysaccharide, 423*f*
antibody to, 437
type Ia, 423*f*
type Ib, 423*f*
types II through VIII, 423*f*
cellular invasion, 432
classification, 420–421
clinical manifestations and
outcome, 440–447
early-onset, 440–442, 441*f*
late-late-onset, 442
late-onset infection, 442
colonial morphology and
identification, 420
diagnosis, 447–448
organism isolation/
identification, 447–448
differential diagnosis, 448
early v. late-onset, incidence
of, 453*f*
early-onset
pathology, 439–440
risk factors and, 436–437,
442*t*
fatality rates, 436*t*
features of, 443*t*
genome analysis, 421
hydrolysis of bile esculin agar,
420
immunology and pathogenesis,
429–439
incidence of
in neonates, 428–429
parturients, 428–429
infection, 2, 229, 236, 251,
257, 260, 301, 632
antimicrobial agents, 255
attack rates v. fatalities, 236*t*

by birth weight, incidence
and mortality of, 235*t*
colonization and infection,
incidence of, 27–28
management algorithms, 257
intrapartum antimicrobial
prophylaxis, 18
isolates, serotype distribution,
426–427
laboratory tests, 447–448
maternal colonization, 429–430
culture-based screening, 454*f*
maternal infection, 446–447
molecular epidemiology, 428
mucosal immune response, 437
neonatal sepsis, 244
neonates, transmission to, 426
NICUs, 1129–1130
pathogenesis
host factors and, 436–439
host-bacterial interactions
and, 429–436
prevention, 452–458
prognosis, 451–452
pulmonary and bloodstream
entry, 432
relapse, 446
sepsis and, 238
serotypes, 427*f*
strains, 422*f*
bacterial products, 422–424
epidemiology and
transmission, 424–429
growth requirements,
422–424
human and bovine origin, 420
virulence factors, 430*t*
supportive management, 450
testing for, 420
treatment, 448–451
in vitro susceptibility,
448–449
ultrastructure, 421
unusual manifestations,
444–446, 445*t*
UTIs and, 310
vaccine, 457
Group C streptococci, 228
Group G streptococci, 228
Growth factors, breast milk, 197,
205
Growth hormone deficiency, 880
Gut flora, 84
Gut-associated lymphoid tissue
(GALT), 199
human milk and, 198

H

H. influenzae, 251
H. influenzae type B (Hib)
breast milk and, 205
polysaccharide vaccine, 155
polysaccharide-tetanus vaccine,
156
H$_2$ blockers, 1128, 1135
HAART (Highly active
antiretroviral therapy), 622,
627, 648, 649, 651

indications for, 648*t*
during pregnancy, 644–645
treatment recommendations,
630
Haemophilus influenzae, 224, 233,
281, 282, 1215
Haemophilus influenzae type B
(Hib) polysaccharide,
1227–1228
Haemophilus influenzae type B
(Hib) vaccine, 1227–1228
HAIs. *See* Health care-associated
infections
HA-MRSA. *See* Hospital-
acquired methicillin-resistant
S. aureus
Hand hygiene, 20, 28, 1136–1137
Hand-foot-and mouth syndrome,
679
Haptoglobin, 1151
HAV. *See* Hepatitis A virus
HBsAg. *See* Hepatitis B surface
antigen
HBV. *See* Hepatitis B virus
HCMV. *See* Congenital human
cytomegalovirus
HCV. *See* Hepatitis C virus
Health care workers, infections
and, 1138–1140
Health care-associated infections
(HAIs)
epidemiology, 1127–1128
incidence, 1127
etiologic agents, 1128–1132,
1129*t*
in nursery, 1078–1124
preventing transmission,
1135–1138
surveillance, 1135–1136
risk factors for, 1128
medical devices, 1128
patient-related, 1128
therapeutic agents, 1128
Health care-associated
pneumonia, 1134
Hearing
deficit, congenital rubella
infection, 885
Toxoplasmosis, 965*t*
Hearing loss-associated
cytomegalovirus, 733–734
pathogenesis, 725–726
Heart
coxsackievirus B strains, 768,
768*f*
parvovirus B19 infection of,
851
Toxoplasma gondii in, 943
Helminth infections, 1042–1054
Hemagglutination, rubella virus,
864
Hemagglutination inhibition,
rubella virus, 863
Hematogenous transplacental
infections, pathogenesis of, 5*f*
Hematogenously acquired
measles, incubation period,
687

Hematopoiesis, 88
Hematopoietic system, CMV and, 729
Hematoxylin-eosin, hyphae, 1107
Hemochromatosis, listeriosis and, 472–473
β-hemolysin, 495
β-hemolysin/cytolysin, 435
γ-hemolysin, 494
Hemolytic-uremic syndrome (HUS), 361–362
Hemorrhagic disease, breast-feeding, 211
Hemorrhagic meningoencephalitis, 243
HEPA filters, 1138
 aspergillus organism, 1097–1098
Hepatitis, 775, 800–813, 801*t*.
 See also Hepatitis A virus; Hepatitis B virus; Hepatitis C virus; Hepatitis D virus; Hepatitis E virus
vaccine, 1225–1226
Hepatitis A virus (HAV), 633, 800–803, 801*f*, 1226
 clinical manifestations, 802
 diagnosis, 802
 epidemiology and transmission, 800–801
 microbiology, 801
 NICU outbreaks, 1132
 pathogenesis, 801
 pathology, 802
 prevention, 802–803
 treatment, 802
 vaccines, 802
Hepatitis B immune globulin, 1218–1219
Hepatitis B surface antigen (HBsAg), 1218–1219
Hepatitis B virus (HBV), 633, 801, 803–806, 1225–1226
 clinical manifestations, 804
 diagnosis, 804
 epidemiology and transmission, 803
 host and viral serologic markers, 805*f*
 human milk and, 212
 microbiology, 803–804, 803*f*
 particles, 803*f*
 pathogenesis, 804
 pathology, 804
 prevention, 805–806
 treatment, 804–805
 vaccination, 41
 vaccine, 805
  infant response, 1228
 vaccine schedules, 805, 805*t*
Hepatitis C virus (HCV), 633, 806–807
 clinical manifestations, 807
 diagnosis, 807
 epidemiology and transmission, 806
 HIV and, 633

human milk and, 212
microbiology, 806
pathogenesis, 806
pathology, 807
prevention, 807
treatment, 807
Hepatitis D virus (HDV), 803–806
Hepatitis E virus (HEV), 807–809
 clinical manifestations, 808
 diagnosis, 809
 epidemiology and transmission, 807–808
 microbiology, 808
 pathogenesis, 808
 pathology, 808
 prevention, 809
 treatment, 809
Hepatomegaly, 247, 731
Hepatotoxicity, 587
 azoles and, 1070
Hepatotropic viruses, 809–810, 811
Heroin addicts, malaria, 1046
Herpangina, 774
Herpes simplex encephalitis, 823*f*
 HSV, 822–823, 823*f*
Herpes simplex virus (HSV), 13, 162–169, 661–662, 706, 814–833, 814–815, 1132
 acyclovir, 1194
 adaptive immunity, 165–168
 adjunctive therapy and vaccination, 168–169
 antigen presentation, viral inhibition of, 165–166
 antivirals, 826–829
 β genes, 814
 breast-feeding and, 210
 concomitant bacterial infections, 824
 cutaneous infection, 823, 823*f*
 cytokines and chemokines, circulating/cerebrospinal fluid levels of, 163
 diagnosis, 824–826, 826*t*
  clinical evaluation, 824–825
 disseminated infection, 821–822
  survival and, 828*f*
 epidemiology and transmission, 815–819
 γ genes, 814
 α genes, 814
 human milk and, 212
 immunologic response, 819–820
 innate immunity, 162
 intrauterine infection, 821
 laboratory assessment, 825–826
 latency and reactivation, 815
 neonatal infection, 820–824
  acute management, 829
  classification system, 820
  clinical manifestations, 820–824
  long-term management, 829
  pathogenesis and pathology, 820
  prevention, 829–831
   background, 829–830
 postnatal infection, 140

PROM and, 73
replication, 814
structure, 814
subclinical infection, 824
treatment, 826–829
 background, 826
 neonatal survival and, 826*t*, 830*t*
typing of, 825
vaginal delivery, 830–831
viral type, morbidity and mortality among, 824*t*
Herpes simplex virus type 2.
 See HSV type 2
Herpesvirus family, 706, 814
Herpesviruses.
 See also Herpesvirus family; HSV; HSV type 1; HSV type 2
latency, 710
Herxheimer's reactions, 1092
HEV. *See* Hepatitis E virus
Hexachlorophene bathing, 348
HHV type 6 (Human herpes virus-6), 907–908
HHV-7 (Human herpesvirus 7), 908
Hib. *See* H. influenzae type B
High-avidity test, positive IgM test titer, 12 week gestation, 982*t*
Highly sensitive nucleic acid amplification tests (NAATs), *Chlamydial* conjunctivitis, 604
HIV (Human immunodeficiency virus), 2, 3, 8, 9–10, 12, 17, 41, 43, 253, 516, 579, 580, 621–660, 693, 1084.
 See also Mother to infant HIV transmission
 amikacin, 633
 associated encephali, 635
 Bacille Calmette-Guérin vaccines, 592
 breast milk and, 203–204
 C. neoformans, 1104
 cardiovascular complications, 636
 child survival, 35
 in children
  bacterial infections, 632–633
  BCG vaccination and, 1223
  CDC definition of, younger than 13 years, 629*t*
  CDC revised definition, younger than 13 years, 630*t*
  classification of, 628–632
 clinical manifestations and pathology, 632–637
 infectious complications, 632–634
 co-infection *congenital Toxoplasmosis*, newborn, treatment of, 967
 and comorbid *congenital Toxoplasmosis*
  case histories, 966–967
  newborn, treatment of, 967
  pregnant woman, treatment of, 967

 congenital Toxoplasmosis and,
  pathology of, 967
 diagnosis, 627–628
  early infancy, 627–628
 encephalopathy, 635*f*, 637
 epidemiology, 623
 exposed infants
  CD4 monitoring, 634*t*
  treatment, 646–651
   supportive care and general management, 646–647
   vaccination of, 646–647
 future goals, 651
 gene expression, 625
 hematologic problems, 637
 human milk and, 211
 immune abnormalities in, 626
 in infants
  evaluation and management of, 629*t*
  mycobacterial infections, 632
  P. jiroveci infection and, 1083
 listeriosis and, 472–473
 malaria and, 39
 measles, 689
 morbidity, mortality, prognosis, 637–638
 mucocutaneous disease, 637
 ophthalmologic pathology, 635
 pentamidine-associated pancreatitis, 1092
 prevention, 638–646
  low/middle income countries, 35
 PROM and, 73
 testing, 593–594
  Pregnant woman, 627
 transmission, 623–625
  breast milk, 19
  disparity of, 33–34, 33*t*
  intrapartum infection, 624
  intrauterine, 623–624
  postpartum infection, 624–625
 tuberculosis in pregnancy, 590
 viral infections with, 633
HIV-1 (Human immunodeficiency virus type 1)
 DNA PCR assay, 627–628
 human milk and, 212–213
 infected cells, 107
 infection, 141
  early infant infection, pathogenesis of, 626–627
  molecular biology, 625–626
HIV/AIDS, 33–35, 729
 N. gonorrhoeae, 519
HIVNET 012, 644
HIV-specific immune response, 626–627
HLA-E. *See* Human leukocyte antigen E
HLA-G. *See* Human leukocyte antigen G
Holder pasteurization, 211
Homing receptor expression, 167–168

Horner syndrome, 675
Horse antirabies hyperimmune serum, 913
Hospital
  infection control, 28–29
  workers, CMV, 718–719
Hospital discharge, recent, neonatal sepsis, 263–264
Hospital transmission, parvovirus, 839–840
Hospital-acquired methicillin-resistant *S. aureus* (HA-MRSA), 491–492, 506
Host antibody, *Toxoplasma gondii*, 937–938
Host cells, *Toxoplasma gondii*, 937–938
Host defenses, 100
  developmental immunology, infection and, 80–191
  mechanisms
    HSV, 162
    overview, 159–160
    zoster, 678
  neonatal pathogens, classes of, 159–172
  Staphylococcus epidermidis, 496–497
Host factors, neonatal bacterial sepsis and, 240–241
Host genetics, *Toxoplasma gondii*, 937
Host immune response
  CMV modulation of, 723–724, 723t
  listeriosis, normal adults, 473–476
  N. gonorrhoeae, 519
Host immunity, CMV and, pathogenesis, 722–723
Host serologic markers, HBV, 805f
Household contacts
  HIV infection, 625
  infections in, 263–264
Household transmission, parvovirus, 839
HPV. *See* Human papillomavirus
HS/AC test. *See* Differential agglutination test
HSV. *See* Herpes simplex virus
HSV type 1 (Herpes simplex virus type 1), 813
HSV type 2 (Herpes simplex virus type 2), 813, 818.
  See also Genital herpes
  intrapartum transmission, 818
  labor and delivery, 817–818
  maternal infection, 816
  newborn infection, 818
  nosocomial infection, 819
  postnatal acquisition, 819
  transmission of infection
    to fetus, 816–818
    times of, 818–819
    in utero, 818
HTLV-1. *See* Human T-lymphotropic virus 1
HTLV-2. *See* Human T-lymphotropic virus 2

Human α-defensins, 83
Human cytokine family ligands, 81t
Human effector CD8 T cells, 126
Human herpes virus-6. *See* HHV type 6
Human herpesvirus 7. *See* HHV-7
Human immunodeficiency virus. *See* HIV
Human immunodeficiency virus type 1. *See* HIV-1
Human leukocyte antigen E (HLA-E), 110
Human leukocyte antigen G (HLA-G), 106, 111
Human milk, 192–220, 207–213
  antibiotics in, 1166–1171
  antibodies, 199t
  bacterial infections, 211–212, 211t
  BALT, 198
  benefits, 207–210
  bioactive peptides, 196–197
  carrier proteins, 197
  cell-mediated immunologic reactivity, 199t
  components and hormones, 198t
  hormones, 197, 198t
  immunoglobulin levels, 199f
  nucleotides in, 196t
  nutritional proteins, 196
  potential risks, 210–213
    noninfectious, 210–211
  protective factors in, 360–361
  soluble and cellular factors in, role of, 214t
  summary, 213–215
  viral infections, 212–213
Human Milk Banking Association of North America, 211
Human milk donors, coliform organisms, 368
Human neutrophil proteins (HNP), 83
Human papillomavirus (HPV), 905–906
  infected mothers, 905
  vaccines, 906
Human parvovirus, 834–860.
  See also Parvovirus B19
Human serum globulin, enteroviruses and, 790
Human T-lymphotropic virus 1 (HTLV-1), 213
Human T-lymphotropic virus 2 (HTLV-2), 213
Humeral immune responses
  breast milk and, 205
  Pneumocystis jiroveci, 1052
  rubella virus, 870–871, 870f
HUS. *See* Hemolytic-uremic syndrome
Hyaline membrane disease, 291–292
Hydrocephalus, 963f
  congenital *Toxoplasma gondii*, 950
  fetal *Toxoplasma* infection, 987f

Hydrolysis of sodium hippurate broth, group B streptococcal infection, 420
Hydrops fetalis, 852–853
  fetal monitoring, 853
  fetal therapy, 854
  Toxoplasma gondii infections, 964
Hygienic measures, staphylococcal infection, 509
Hyper-IgM syndrome, 148
Hyperbilirubinemia, 318, 1201
  breast-feeding and, 211
Hyperglycemia with thrombocytopenia, candidemia and, 1063
Hyperimmune group B streptococcal globulin, group B streptococcal infection, 451
Hyperimmune plasma, 743
Hyperthermia, 789
Hyphae
  hematoxylin-eosin, 1107
  light microscopy photographs, 1057f
Hypogammaglobulinemia, 873
Hyponatremia, 248
Hypotension, 441
Hypothermia, 497, 789, 951
Hypothermia in newborns, 240, 246–247

I
IAI. *See* Intra-amniotic infection
Ibuprofen with indomethacin, 243
ICN. *See* Inclusion conjunctivitis of newborn
ICOS, 125
Idoxuridine, 826
IFN. *See* Interferon
IFN-γ, 107, 126–127, 169, 170, 206–207
IgA antibodies
  serologic test results, 988t
  Toxoplasma, 981t
  to *Toxoplasma* infection, 987–988
IgA isotype (Immunoglobulin), 158, 198–201
IgA1 protease, 518–519
IgD, 158
IgD antibody concentration, 201
IgE, 158
IgE antibodies, 987–988
  Toxoplasma, 981t
IgE antibody concentration, breast feeding and, 201
IgG. *See* Immunoglobulin
IgG antibody(ies)
  concentration, 281–282
    breast feeding and, 200–201
    at one year, 158
    parvovirus B19, 844
  detection, HCMV, 739
  patterns of, 870
  responses, serologic test measurements, 983t
  rubella infection, 871
  Toxoplasma, 981t, 984

IgG avidity assay
  cytomegalovirus during pregnancy, 740–741
  kinetics of, 740f
  Toxoplasma gondii, 976–978, 978t
IgG/IgM Western Blot Analysis, for mother-infant pairs, *Toxoplasma gondii*, 976, 977f
IgM antibodies
  concentration, 819
    breast feeding and, 201
  in cord serum, 978
  detection, 739–740
  patterns of, rubella virus, 870–871
  serologic test results, to *Toxoplasma* infection, 988t
  testing
    pregnancy termination, 1027
    toxoplasmosis, 1021
    Toxoplasma gondii, 968, 981t, 984, 987–988
IgM assays
  cytomegalovirus during pregnancy, 740
  ELISA, 1023
  HCMV, 739–740
  Toxoplasma gondii, 978–979, 987–988
IgM fluorescent antibody test, 978
IgM isotype, 151, 158
IgM *Toxoplasma* antibodies, congenital *Toxoplasma gondii* and, 948t
IgM+IgD+CD27+ B-cell subset, 150–151, 153
Imaging, *Candida* spp. and, 1066–1067
Imipenem, 1190–1191
  Aeromonas hydrophila, 392
  in vitro susceptibility, 448
  Yersinia enterocolitica, 392
Imipenem-cilastatin, 1191, 1192t
  dosing implications, 1191–1193
  safety, 1191
Immature neutrophil count, 1148
Immune clearance, noncapsular factors and, 433–434
Immune exclusion, breast-feeding and, 209–210
Immune globulins, 1218
Immune resistance, capsular polysaccharide and, 432–433
Immune response
  fetal rubella infection, first trimester (of pregnancy), 872, 872f
  group B streptococcal infection, 425
  maternal rubella infection, first trimester (of pregnancy), 872, 872f
  T cell antigen-presenting cell, 121–122, 121f
Immune response detection, HCMV, 739–740

Immune system, 81
  modulators of, breast milk and,
    205–207
Immunity, 157–158
Immunization, 14, 791–792.
  See also Active immunization;
    Global Alliance for Vaccines
    and Immunization
  antibody responses, premature
    infant, 155–156
  birth dosing, 1223
  route of inoculation, 1222–1223
  schedule, ages 0-6yrs, 1213*f*
  strategies, rubella vaccine and,
    886–889
  timing of, 1223
Immunocompetent cells,
  lactational hormones, 200
Immunocompetent hosts, CMV
  and, 707
Immunocompromised hosts, 1219
  chickenpox in, 669
  CMV and, 721
  parvovirus B19, 837, 842–843
Immunodeficient patients,
  congenital toxoplasmosis, 1017
Immunofluorescent antibody
  test, 1091
Immunoglobulin (IgG), 14,
  157–158, 157*t*, 509–510, 1218.
  See also IgE antibodies; IgE
    antibody concentration; IgG
    antibody(ies); IgG avidity
    assay; IgG/IgM Western Blot
    Analysis; IgM antibodies; IgM
    assays; IgM fluorescent
    antibody test; IgM isotype;
    IgM *Toxoplasma* antibodies
  antibody
      Escherichia coli and, 199
      rubella virus, 868
  B cells and, 141–159
      overview, 141–142
  cells, 150–151
  congenital cytomegalovirus, 743
  congenital rubella infection, 884
  cytokines and, 125–126
  genes, 114*f*
      loci, 143
  HEV, 809
  levels
      in breast-feeding neonate,
        200*t*
      first year of life, 156*f*
      infant pneumocystosis,
        1087–1088
      milk and colostrum, 199*f*
  measles, 693, 695
  molecules
      CDRs of, 113–114
      structure, 141*f*
  repertoire formation, 142–144
  secretion, molecular basis for,
    148–149
  Staphylococcus aureus and, 494
  synthesis, by fetus and neonate,
    157–158
  Toxoplasma gondii, 945
  viral infections, 792

Immunoglobulin A *T. gondii*
  antibodies, 987
Immunoglobulin class-specific
  antibody, 865
Immunoglobulin isotype
  switching, 148–150
Immunoglobulin-secreting
  plasma cells, 149
Immunologic adjuvants, 1222
Immunomodulator, 93
Immunoprecipitation studies,
  rubella infection, 873
Immunoprophylaxis, 18
  GBS, 457–458
  neonatal infection, 261–263
  staphylococcal infection,
    509–510
Immunosorbent agglutination
  assay (ISAGA)
  positive *T. gondii* IgM antibody
    test, duration of, 979
  Toxoplasma gondii, 979,
    987–988
Immunosuppressants,
  Pneumocystis pneumonia, rat
  study, 1086
Immunosuppressive
  chemotherapy
  phycomycosis, 1107
  Pneumocystis pneumonia, 1087
Immunosuppressive therapy
  cessation, 1109
  myocarditis of unknown
    origin, 791
Immunotherapy, FDA approved
  products, 1218*t*
Impetigo, 679
In utero diagnosis, 5
In utero infection, 9–10
  T. gondii, 988, 989*t*
  vaccinia, 903
Inactivated polio vaccines (IPV),
  1221, 1224
Incision and drainage,
  osteomyelitis, 305
Inclusion conjunctivitis of
  newborn (ICN), 600
Incubation period, mumps
  organism, 696
Indirect fluorescence,
  antimalarial antibodies, 1048
Indirect hemagglutination,
  antimalarial antibodies, 1048
Indole 3-carbinol/
  diindolylmethane, respiratory
  papillomatosis, 906
Indomethacin, to neonate, 243
Indwelling catheters, *Candida*
  and, 1059
Infant(s)
  death, 67*t*
  healthy, 8–10
  infection, pets and, 264
  influenza and, 909–910
  management of, maternal
    genital herpes and, 830–831
  Toxoplasma gondii, 946–967
    forms of, 946
  vaccination, obstacles to, 1214*t*

Infections, 693. *See also* Mixed
  infections
  acquired during delivery, 19
  of adrenal glands, 326–327
  of biliary tract, 325–326
  breast-feeding and, 211–213
  cytologic/histologic diagnosis,
    12
  data, 1136
  endocrine organs, 342
  of fetus, 1–23
    pathogenesis, 3–15
  of gastrointestinal tract, 505
  health care workers,
    1138–1140
  human milk and, 198–207
  migration to, mononuclear
    phagocytes and, 94
  newborn infant, 1–23
    associated obstetric factors,
      52–79
    first month of life, 19–21
    oral cavity, 276–280
    pathogenesis and
      microbiology, 19–21
  preterm birth and, 59–64
  prevention, 18–19
  PROM, diagnosis of, 67–68
  risk, family-centered care, 1138
  salivary glands, 342
  serologic diagnosis, 12–13
  skin, 342–348
  subcutaneous tissue, 342–348
  in twins, 241
  umbilical cord and, 241–242
  underlying abnormalities with,
    21
Infectious agents. *See also specific
  infectious agents*
  human milk and, 198*t*
  isolation and identification,
    11–13
Infectious diseases
  epidemiology and
    management, changes in, 3*t*
  premature infants, 1228
Inflammation, congenital
  cytomegalovirus, 725
Inflammation regulation, 157–158
Inflammatory diarrhea, 399–400
Inflammatory illnesses, 1149*f*
Inflammatory mediators, sepsis
  and, 434–435
Inflammatory responses, 146–147
  age-related, GBS, 440
Influenza, 1228
  maternal immunization, 1217
  oseltamivir and, 1195
Influenza A, 908–910
Influenza B, 908–910
Influenza vaccination, 40
Influenza virus vaccine, 910, 1226
INH. *See* Isoniazid
Inherited metabolic diseases, 210,
  241
Inhibitors of NS3 serine
  protease, 807
Innate antibacterial immunity,
  510

lactoferrin, 510
Innate immune mechanisms, 102*f*
Innate immune pattern
  recognition receptors, 96–98
Innate immune resistance,
  Staphylococcus aureus, 493–494
Innate immune response, CMV
  and, 722
Innate immune system, 81–83
Innate immunity, 101–103, 722,
  1153
  HSV, 162–165
  humoral mediators of, 85–88
Innate immunity regulation,
  98–100
Inosine pranobex (Isoprinosine),
  886
Insecticide-treated bednets, 39
Insulin-dependent diabetes
  mellitus, CRS, 880
Integrated health care programs,
  maternal HIV transmission
  prevention, 35
Intelligence testing, Stanford-
  Alabama study, 1007*t*
Interference, neonatal
  vaccination and, 1216
Interferon (IFN)
  congenital rubella infection, 886
  fetal *Toxoplasma* infection, 987
  HSV and, 162–163
  Listeria and, 475–476, 475*f*
  newborns, 477
  plus ribavirin, HCV, 807
  rubella infection, 874
α-interferon
  HBV, 804–805
  respiratory papillomatosis,
    906
Interferon-γ release assay,
  582–583
Interleukin-2 production, infants
  6-12 months, 140
Interleukin-6, 7, 54
  in breast milk, 206, 206*t*
Interleukin-7, 120–121, 207
Interleukin-10, 205
Interleukin-15, 120–121
Internet, 2
Internet sites, infectious disease, 3*t*
Interocular hemorrhage, 956
Interstitial fibrosis, 1085–1086
Interstitial lung disease, 635–636
Intestinal epithelial cells, 84
Intestinal epithelium, 84, 360
Intra-amniotic infection (IAI),
  51, 52–59. *See also* Chronic
  intra-amniotic infection
  antepartum criteria, 54–55
  diagnosis, 54–55
  maternal antibiotic therapy,
    intrapartum v. postpartum,
    56*t*
  microbiology of, 53–54, 53*t*
  neonatal criteria, 55
  pathogenesis of, 52–53
  preterm, 58*t*
  prevention strategies, 59, 59*t*
  stages of, 52*f*

Intracranial calcifications, 1006–1007
  Toxoplasma gondii infections, 961–964, 961*f*, 963*f*
Intrapartum antibiotic prophylaxis, 1154
  GBS, 453–455
  neonatal sepsis and, 455
Intrapartum antimicrobial prophylaxis, 18
Intrapartum care, neonatal infection and, 42
Intrapartum chemoprophylaxis, 2
  neonatal group B streptococcal sepsis, 160
Intrauterine bacterial hepatitis, 323
Intrauterine growth restriction, low birth weight and, 8
Intrauterine infection
  antibody response to, 154
  of fetus, LCV, 912
  influenza and, 909–910
Intrauterine pneumonia, 276–296
  pathogenesis and pathology, 286
Intrauterine tuberculosis, 323
Intravascular catheters
  blood cultures, 249
  bone and joint infection, 299
  catheter-related candidal infections, 1063
  endocarditis, 340
Intravenous fluids, HAIs and, 1128
Intravenous immunoglobulin (IVIG), 262
  birth weight and, 224
  CMV and, 730
  enteroviruses and, 790
  group B streptococcal infection, 451
  HIV and, 647
  neonatal group B streptococcal sepsis, 160
  neonatal sepsis, 259–260, 508
  salmonellosis, 381
Invasive candidiasis in neonates, systemic antifungal agents, 1068*t*
Invasive devices.
  See also Catheter-associated bacteremia
  osteomyelitis and, 298
Invasive fungal dermatitis, 1062, 1110, 1110*f*, 1111
IPEX syndrome, 134
IPV. *See* Inactivated polio vaccines
IQ testing, parvovirus B19, 855
Iron, neonate sepsis and, 241
ISAGA. *See* Immunosorbent agglutination assay
Isolation
  congenital rubella infection, 886
  microorganisms, 248–249
Isolation rates, group B streptococcal infection, 424

Isolation rooms, mumps, 699
Isoniazid (INH), 594
  tuberculosis and, 586
  tuberculosis in pregnancy, 583, 588
Isoprinosine. *See* Inosine pranobex
Isotype switching, 148
  immunoglobulin production and, 149–150
  postnatal regulation, 158
Itraconazole, 1114
IV broad-spectrum antibiotics, 43
IVIG. *See* Intravenous immunoglobulin

J

Jaundice, 247, 731
  UTI, 315
Jennerian vaccines, 1220.
  See also Modified Jennerian approach
Joint United Nations Program on HIV/AIDS (UNAIDS), 623

K

Kanamycin, 1180–1181
  Shigella infection, 385
Kawasaki disease, 692
Keratolytic medications, dermatophytoses, 1111
Ketoconazole ointment, *Malassezia* infections, 1107
Kidneys
  CMV and, 729
  Toxoplasma gondii, 943–944
Killer cell lectin-like receptor G1 (KLRG1), 120
Killer cells (KCs), source of, 131
Kissing bug, 1043
Klebsiella oxytoca, 230, 393
Klebsiella pneumoniae, 230
  breast-feeding, 208
Klebsiella species, 223, 230–231, 238
KLRG1. *See* Killer cell lectin-like receptor G1
Koplik spots, 687

L

L. monocytogenes, 230, 256
Labor and delivery, HSV-2, 817–818
Laboratory markers, cytomegalovirus during pregnancy, 740
Laboratory tests
  diagnostic utility of, 1144–1145
  ideal, 1145–1146
  rubella virus, 864–865
Laboratory-acquired infections, 931
α-Lactalbumin, breast milk and, 204
β-lactam, 506, 1188
  Campylobacter, 389

group B streptococcal disease, 255
  mediastinitis, 342
  NEC, 337
  peritonitis, 333
  in vitro susceptibility, 449
β-lactam antibiotics/B-lactamase inhibitor combination, 1188
  antimicrobial activity, 1188
β-lactam inhibitors
  mediastinitis, 342
  NEC, 337
  peritonitis, 333
Lactation
  initiation and maintenance of, 193
  performance, 193
  physiology of, 192–197
  secretory products of, 194–197
Lactational hormones
  immunocompetent cells, 200
  immunologic reactivity and, 199–200
Lactobacillus species, 203–204
Lactoferrin, 207, 262–263, 360–361
  breast milk and, 204
  innate antibacterial immunity, 510
  supplementation, low birth weight neonates, 261
Lactose, 193
β-lactamase inhibitor, 1188
β-lactam, 228, 1168–1169
L-AmB. *See* Liposomal amphotericin B
Lamivudine, 646
Lancefield group B β-hemolytic streptococci, 419
Language delays, CMV infection, 733–734
Laryngeal papilloma, 905
Laryngitis, 277
Laryngotracheobronchitis, 774
Latency, herpesviruses, 710
Latex agglutination detection, 251
  group B streptococcal infection, 420
  rotavirus, 398
Latex particle agglutination test, cryptococcosis infection, 1105
LCV. *See* Lymphocytic choriomeningitis virus
Leiomyomas, 637
Leishmaniasis, pentamidine for, 1092
Leucine-rich repeat-containing receptors, 97–98
Leucovorin, 994, 1002–1003
  preparation of, 996*f*
Leukocytosis, 968
Leukopenia, 968
Levofloxacin, in vitro susceptibility, 448
Likelihood ratio, 1144
Limulus, 251

Linezolid, 507–508, 1172*t*, 1174–1175
  antimicrobial activity, 1174
  clinical dosing implications, 1172*t*, 1175, 1193*t*
  clinical trials, 1175
  pharmacokinetic data, 1172*t*, 1174
  PK-PD dosing, 1175
  pneumonia, 292
  safety, 1174–1175
  in vitro susceptibility, 448
Lipids
  of milk, 195
  to neonates, 243
Liposomal amphotericin B (L-AmB), 1069–1070, 1113, 1201
Listeria
  antigenic structure and typing systems, 471
  bacterial peptides, 474
  clinical forms of, 481
  clinical reports, 482
  management, 483
  pathology, 477–478
  severe meningitis, 480, 480*f*
  therapy, 482–483
  virulence factors, 471–472
  in vitro studies, 482
  in vivo studies, 482
Listeria DNA, 471
Listeria hominis, 470
Listeria monocytogenes, 13, 52, 169, 222, 230, 276, 393, 470
  cellular invasion by, 474*f*
  cellular response, 474
  occurrence, 472–473
  organism, 470–472
    culture and identification, 470–471
    morphology, 470
    motility, 470
  during pregnancy, 479
Listeria placentitis, 478, 478*f*
Listeria species
  cell activation and, 476–477
  clinical manifestations, 478–481
  epidemiology and transmission, 472–473
  host response, neonates, 476–477
  natural reservoir and human transmission, 472
Listeria-infected infants, 481–482
Listeriolysin O (LLO), 471–472
Listerioma, 477
Listeriopod, 471–472
Listeriosis, 470–488
  diagnosis, 481
  high-risk individuals, 473*t*
  host response, normal adults, 473–476
  nosocomial transmission, 473
  pathogenesis, 473–477
  during pregnancy, 478–479, 483

prevention and outbreak management, 483–484
risk, reducing, 483t
serology, 481
Listeriosis monocytogenes, organism isolation of, 481
molecular detection, 481
prognosis, 482
Live virus vaccines, 14, 646–647
Live-attenuated measles virus, 694
Live-attenuated mumps virus, 698
Live-attenuated oral poliovirus vaccines (OPV), 757
Live-attenuated vaccines
congenital cytomegalovirus, 744
measles, 686, 693–694
varicella, 684
Liver, 477
CMV and, 729
dysfunction, 636
listeriosis and, 473
Toxoplasma gondii, 943–944, 958, 964
transplant, 809
Liver infections, 322–325
clinical manifestations, 324
diagnosis, 324
microbiology, 322–323
pathogenesis, 323–324
prognosis, 324
LLO. *See* Listeriolysin O
Local immune response, rubella virus, 871
Lopinavir plus ritonavir, 649
Lopinavir-ritonavir combination, 649
Low birth weight infants, 243, 252
cerebrospinal fluid examination, 253t
dermatophytoses, 1110
gestational chickenpox and, 671, 671t
intrauterine growth restriction and, 8
Invasive fungal dermatitis, 1062
malaria, 1047
maternal varicella, 675
neonatal meningitis, 258
neonatal sepsis, 238
Low birth weight neonates, lactoferrin supplementation, 261
Lower genital tract infections, premature birth v, 61, 61t
Lower genital tract organisms, premature birth v, 61
Lower respiratory tract infections, 605
Lumbar puncture, 251–255
GBS, 447
method, 252
not performed, 252
ureaplasmas, 615
Lung biopsy
congenital tuberculosis, 586
Pneumocystosis, 1046
Lung parenchymal cells, 85
Lungs
CMV and, 730

coxsackievirus B strains, 769
Toxoplasma gondii in, 943
Lymph nodes, 247–248
Lymphadenopathy, 841, 945–946
Lymphocyte(s), 141–142
human milk and, 213–214
rubella infection, 873
subpopulations
in autologous blood, 202t
in human milk, 202t
Lymphocyte activation markers, *Toxoplasma gondii*, 971
Lymphocyte marker analysis, 1152
Lymphocytic choriomeningitis virus (LCV), 911–912, 955–956
Lymphocytic interstitial pneumonitis, 635, 636f
Lymphoid differentiation, 88f
Lymphoid organs, 637
Lymphoid tissue, naïve T cell and, 118
Lysozyme, 204, 207

M

M. avium-intracellulare complex, 633, 637
with HIV, 633
M. fermentans, 615–616
M. genitalium, 615–616
M. pneumoniae, 615–616
M. tuberculosis, 169
Macrolide, in vitro susceptibility, 448
Macrolides
breast milk, 1168
Toxoplasma gondii, 1000
Macrolides-roxithromycin, *Toxoplasma gondii*, 1000
Macrophages, 170
CMV and, 720
human milk and, 213–214
Macular edema, 952–954
Macular pseudocoloboma of retina, 956f
Major histocompatibility complex (MHC)
class Ia, 108–109
class II, 109–110
class I-related chain A, 111
class I-related chain B, 111
molecule expression
in fetus, 110
in neonate, 110
molecules, antigen presentation by, 108–110
neonatal B cells and, 148
Major outer membrane protein (MOMP), 601–602
Malaria, 37–39, 1046–1051
anopheline mosquitoes, 1046
birth weight, 1047
control, strategies and challenges, 39
epidemiology and transmission, 1046
fetal survival, 1047
and HIV, 39
organisms, 1046

pathology, 1046–1048
placental infection, 1046–1047
pregnancy, 37–38, 1046
prevention and treatment, 38–39
prophylaxis, 1050–1051
risk of infection and factors affecting, 1048
maternal antibody and, 1047–1048
Malaria parasitemia, 37–38
Malassezia, 1105–1107
catheter-related, 1106
clinical manifestations, 1106
diagnosis, 1106–1107
epidemiology and transmission, 1106
Ketoconazole ointment, 1107
organism, 1106
pathogenesis, 1106
prevention, 1107
prognosis, 1107
therapy, 1107
vascular catheter complications, 1107
Malassezia furfur, 1078–1079
Malassezia species, NICU patients, 1131
Malassezia-infected thrombus, 1106
Malignancies, 637
Mammary barrier, 193
Mammary gland
cellular reactions in, 203
developmental anatomy, 192, 192t
function, endocrine control of, 192–193
homing mechanism for, 200
Mannose-binding lectin (MBL), 85
Mannose-binding lectin pathways (of activation), 82f, 86
Mantoux tuberculin skin test, 582, 632–633
Maraviroc, 649–651
Marginal zone B cells, 150
of fetus and neonate, 150–151
Marker, ideal, 1146
Masks, 1137
Mastitis, 211–212
Mastoiditis, 285
Maternal antibiotic therapy, intrapartum v. postpartum studies, IAI, 56t
Maternal antibodies
neonatal antibody responses, inhibition, 157
neonatal vaccination, 1216
Maternal bacterial vaginosis, 54
Maternal birth canal, agents in, microbiology of, 16, 16t
Maternal bloodstream, microbial invasion, 5–6
Maternal *Candida* vaginitis, 1055–1056
Maternal care, essential services, 36t

Maternal chickenpox, 683
Maternal colonization, GBS, culture-based screening, 454f
Maternal congenital cytomegalovirus infection, symptoms and long-term outcome, 735–736, 735t
Maternal cytomegalovirus, 726–727
perinatal infection, 727
recurrent infection, 727
symptoms and long-term outcome, 735–736, 735t
Maternal decidua, NK cells of, 106
Maternal education, socioeconomic status and, 45
Maternal exposure, breast-feeding, 210
Maternal FcRn expression, 156
Maternal fever, neonatal sepsis and, 236
Maternal genital herpes, infants and, management of, 830–831
Maternal group B streptococcal bacteriuria, 436
Maternal history, neonatal sepsis and, 248
Maternal HIV transmission prevention, 35
cesarean section, 35
integrated health care programs, 35
Maternal immunity
congenital malaria, 1049
malaria prophylaxis and, 1051
rate of, congenital cytomegalovirus and, 714t
Maternal immunization, 1216
antibody response to, 154
fetal antibody response, 153–154
influenza, 1217
pertussis, 1216–1217
RSV, 1217
tetanus, diphtheria, pertussis, 1216–1217
Maternal immunoglobulin, fetal blood and, 927
Maternal infection, 43
GBS, 446–447
Giardiasis lamblia, 1043
transmission, 10
transplacental spread, 4
and vertical transmission, CMV, 714–717
viral sources of, 911t
Maternal intrapartum antibiotic prophylaxis, neonates and, management of, 455–456, 456f
Maternal intrapartum antimicrobial agents, infant management and, 257–258
Maternal membrane rupture, 239
Maternal microbial flora, developing fetus and, 239

Maternal parasitemia, 922, 1043
  acute toxoplasmosis, 922
  chronic toxoplasmosis, 922
Maternal plasma viral load, 639
Maternal rash, 692
Maternal rubella infection,
  immune response, first
  trimester (of pregnancy), 872,
  872f
Maternal septicemia, 608–610
Maternal seroimmunity, CMV,
  rate of, 715t
Maternal smallpox, fetal
  transmission, 900
Maternal sulfonamide
  administration, 1166
Maternal systemic infection
  during pregnancy, 516
Maternal *Toxoplasma gondii*
  case studies, 929
  to fetus, incidence rates, 933f
  gestation and, spiramycin
    treatment and, 924t
  transmission rate, 926, 928
Maternal varicella, 673, 674f
  limb abnormalities, 675
  low birth weight, 675
  neurologic involvement, 674
  ocular abnormalities, 673–674
Maternal viremia, enterovirus,
  765
Maternal zidovudine, 644
Maternal-fetal tolerance, 4
Maternal-fetal transmission rates
  fetal *Toxoplasma* infection, 986
  Toxoplasma gondii, 974t
Maternally acquired infections,
  1127
Maternally acquired *T. gondii*
  infection, IgM titer test and,
  989t
Maternally derived antigens,
  maternally administered,
  138–139
Maternally derived IgG antibody,
  156–157
Maternally transmitted *T. gondii*
  evolution of, uninfected
    infants, 990f
  uninfected infants, 989f
Maternal-neonatal
  immunization, infection
  prevention, 1212–1230
Maternal-to-fetal transmission,
  HAV, 801
Maternity wards
  chickenpox in, horizontal
    transmission, 665
  measles, 694t
Matrix metalloproteinase
  (MMP), 57
MBL. *See* Mannose-binding
  lectin
MBL pathways (of activation).
  See Mannose-binding lectin
  pathways
MDR tuberculosis. *See* Multi-
  drug resistant tuberculosis

Measles (Rubeola), 661–705,
  685–695. *See also* Nosocomial
  infections
  active immunization, 693
  clinical manifestations,
    688–692
  communicability of, 687
  complications and mortality,
    688–689
  death rates, 689
  diagnosis and differential
    diagnosis, 692–693
  droplet infection, incubation
    period, 687
  maternal effects, 689
  passive immunization, 693–695
  pathology, 687–688
  in pregnancy, incidence, 664
  prevention, 693–695
  prodrome and rash, 688
  prodrome or rash, 694t
  therapy, 693
  vaccine, 686
    antibody response, 155
Measles encephalitis, 688
Measles virus, 1225
  antigenic properties and, 686
  genomic data on, 685
  propagation of, 685–686
  serologic tests, 686
  transmission and
    epidemiology, 686
Measles virus replication, 687
Measles-mumps-rubella (MMR)
  vaccine, 861–862, 1225
  HIV, 647
  during pregnancy, 1217–1218
Measles-rubella vaccine, 1225
Meat
  frozen, 932
  oocysts, 930–931
  Toxoplasma gondii, 930
  undercooked, 932
Mediastinitis, 341–342
Mefloquine, 1051
  congenital malaria, 1048–1051
Membrane attack complex,
  86–87
Memory B cells, 147
Memory CD4 T-cell subsets,
  postnatal ontogeny of, 127
Memory CD8 T-cells, 126
Memory cells, 124–127
Memory T-cells
  activation, 127
  overview, 126–127
Meningitis, 221–275, 231, 241,
  248, 251–255, 419, 441, 442,
  449, 504
  epidemiology of, 235–239
  GBS penetration, 435–436
  mortality rate, 260
  negative bacterial cultures and,
    259
  neurologic sequelae, 260, 261
Meningococcemia, 692
Meningoencephalitis, 1196
  therapy, 791

Menstrual cycle, mammary gland
  response, 192–193
Mental retardation, 861, 880–881
  congenital toxoplasmosis,
    956–957
Meropenem, 256, 1190–1191,
  1192t
  Aeromonas hydrophila, 392
  breast milk concentrations,
    infant daily dose, 1168
  dosing implications, 1191–1193
  neonatal meningitis, 258
  safety, 1191
  in vitro susceptibility, 448
Mesenteric lymph nodes, EPEC,
  369–370
Metastatic abscess, bone and
  joint infection, 299
Methemoglobinemia, UTI, 315
Methicillin, infant to maternal
  serum concentrations, ratios,
  1165
Methicillin-resistant *S. aureus*
  (MRSA), 255–256, 276, 343,
  490, 491–492, 500, 1130, 1171,
  1172t
  combination antimicrobial
    therapy, 508
  endocarditis, 340
  osteomyelitis, 296, 297, 305
  skin infection and, 344
  solitary hepatic abscess, 325
Methicillin-resistant *S.
  epidermidis* (MRSE), 1171
  combination antimicrobial
    therapy, 1171
Metronidazole
  appendicitis, 329
  breast milk, 1168
  breast-feeding, 210
  Entamoeba histolytica, 1046
  mediastinitis, 342
  milk to plasma ratios, 1166
  solitary hepatic abscess, 325
  T. vaginalis infection, 60
  Trypanosoma cruzi, 1045
MIC. *See* Minimal inhibitory
  concentration
Micafungin, 1071, 1200–1201
  gastrointestinal tract and, 1201
  pharmacokinetic data,
    1200–1201
  PK-PD, and clinical
    implications, 1201
  safety, 1201
Miconazole gel, 1069
Microbes
  in amniotic fluid, 53t
  neutrophil killing of, 92–93
Microbicidal oxygen, 156–157
Microbiologic techniques,
  neonatal sepsis and, 248
Microcephaly
  congenital CMV, 731–732
  congenital *Toxoplasma gondii*,
    951
Microorganisms, 4–5, 4t
  isolation of, 248–249

Microphthalmia, 952
Middle ear, lateral section, 284f
Middle ear effusion, 280–281, 284
Milia, 348
Miliary tuberculosis, 580, 581f
Milk. *See also* Breast milk; Human
  milk; Human milk donors
  altered pregnancy and, 207
  immunoglobulin, 214
  lymphocytes, 201
  macrophage, 201
  minerals of, 195
  nonprotein nitrogen, 195–196
  nutritional components,
    194–197, 194t
  production, phases, 194
  proteins, 196
  secretion, 193
  Toxoplasma gondii, 931
  transitional, 194
  vitamins of, 195
Milk to plasma ratios, drugs and,
  1166
Milk-born outbreaks, *C. jejuni*, 388
Milk-specific proteins, 193
Minimal inhibitory concentration
  (MIC), 1163–1164
  pharmacodynamics,
    1163–1164
  pharmacokinetic data, 1163
Minocycline, 999–1000
MIRIAD study, 640
Mixed infections, 234
MMR vaccine. *See* Measles-
  Mumps-Rubella vaccine;
  Mumps-measles-rubella
  vaccine
Modified Jennerian approach, 1220
Mold infections, 1131
Molecular detection tests, 1154
Molecular diagnostic assays,
  Candida spp. and, 1067
Mollicutes, 607
Molluscum contagiosum, 913
MOMP. *See* Major outer
  membrane protein
Monoclonal antibodies
  respiratory syncytial virus
    immune globulin and, 1218
  staphylococcal epitopes and,
    510
Monoclonal antibody studies,
  rubella virus, 863
Monocytes, production and
  differentiation, 93–94
Monocytosis, 472
Mononuclear phagocytes,
  93–101, 157–158
  HSV and, 100–101, 163–164
  migration of, 94
Mononucleosis, 906
Monosialoganglioside, 203
Morphology, 1146
Mortality
  infections, 25, 25t
  neonatal peritonitis, 333
  neonatal sepsis, 223–224
  osteomyelitis of maxilla, 307

Mortality rate
  meningitis, 260
  smallpox, 900
Mosquitoes, anopheline, malaria, 1046
Mother to infant HIV transmission, risk factors, 34t
Mouse study
  inoculation, 969, 970
  neonatal vaccination, 1215
Mouth infections, HSV and, 823–824
Moxalactam, 1162
MRI, osteomyelitis, 303
MRSA. *See* Methicillin-resistant *S. aureus*
MRSE. *See* Methicillin-resistant *S. epidermidis*
MSCRAMMs, 492–493, 496
Mucocutaneous disease, 637
Mucosa-associated lymphoid tissue (MALT), 105
Mucosal immune response, GBS, 437
Mucosal immune system, breast feeding and, 200
Mucosal injury, pathogenesis of, 334f
Mucosal lesions, 1060
Multi-drug resistant (MDR) tuberculosis, 579
Multi-drug resistant viridans streptococci, 228–229
Multidrug-resistant coagulase-negative staphylococci (CoNS), 1126–1127
Multidrug-resistant organisms, HAIs and, 1130
Multilocus enzyme electrophoresis, 428
Multi-locus sequence typing (MLST), 490
Mumps, 661–705, 695–699. *See also* Nosocomial infections
  active immunization, 698
  clinical manifestations, 696–698
  diagnosis and differential diagnosis, 698
  immunoglobulin, 699
  maternal effects of, 696–697
  organism, 695
    communicability, 695–696
    epidemiology and transmission, 695–696
    incubation period, 696
    properties and propagation, 695
  passive immunization, 698
  pathogenesis, 696
  pathology, 696
  in pregnancy, incidence, 664, 696
  prevention, 698–699
  therapy, 698
  virus, 1225
Mumps organism, communicability, 695–696
Mumps pancreatitis, 696

Mumps-measles-rubella vaccine (MMR vaccine), 887, 1222
Muscle necrosis, coxsackievirus B strains, 768
Mussels, *Toxoplasma gondii*, 931
Mycobacterial infections, HIV-infected infants, 632
Mycobacterium bovis vaccine, 1223
Mycobacterium tuberculosis, 37, 222
Mycoplasma hominis, 607, 608, 615f
  colonization, 607–608
  diagnosis, 616–617
  sites of infection, 615
  transmission of, 611
Mycoplasmal infections, 607–620
Mycoplasmas, 607, 615–616
Mycotic infections, 1078–1079
Myeloid dendric cells (cDCs), 101
Myeloid differentiation, 88f
Myelosuppression, 1174–1175
Myocardial disease, 844
Myocarditis
  related to enteroviruses, 775
  therapy, 791

N

N. gonorrhoeae, 32, 53, 61
  Ceftriaxone, 521
  preterm birth and, 61
N. meningitidis, 230, 251, 1228
NAATs. *See* Highly sensitive nucleic acid amplification tests
Nafcillin, 255–256, 1171
  infant to maternal serum concentrations, ratios, 1165
  osteomyelitis, 305
Naïve B cells
  activation, CD4 T-cell help for, 146–147
  fully mature, 144–145
  new emigrant, 144–145
Naïve CD4+T cells
  differentiation, 123f
  memory T cells v, 126
Naïve follicular B cells, B-cell selection and, 147
Naïve T cell surface phenotype, ontogeny of, 118–120
Naïve T cells, 117–118, 124–127
  activated, differentiation of, 124–127
  activation, 121–124
  anergy, 121–124
  costimulation, 121–124
  homeostatic proliferation, 120–121
  survival of, 118
NALP3, 97–98
Nasopharynx infections, 276–280
National Collaborative Chicago-based Treatment Trial Study, U.S. (NCCCTS)
  congenital toxoplasmosis, 955, 955t
  ophthalmologic outcomes, prenatal/postnatal treatment, 1016

outcomes, 965t, 1010, 1011t, 1012t, 1013t
  audiologic, 1013
  comparison of, 1014–1015
  neurologic and cognitive, 1013–1014, 1013t
  neutropenia, 1012t
  ophthalmologic, 1015
  postnatal treatment and, 1015
  retinal disease, 1013
  visual acuity, 1012t, 1013–1014
pyrimethamine with leucovorin and sulfadiazine, 1010, 1011t
toxoplasmosis, 1009–1017
National Nosocomial Infection Surveillance (NNIS) system, 1055
National Smallpox Vaccine in Pregnancy Registry, 900, 904
Natural killer cells (NK cells), 103–107
  cytokine and chemokine production and, 106
  cytokine responsiveness and dependence, 105
  cytotoxicity, 104, 104f, 105, 106f
  HSV, 164
  Listeria species and, 477
  overview and development, 103–104
  receptors, 104–105
    families of, 104–105
Natural killer T cells (NKT), 135–136
  of neonate, 136
  overview, 135–136
NCCCTS. *See* National Collaborative Chicago-based Trial Study, U.S.
NEC. *See* Necrotizing enterocolitis
Necrotic bone sequestration, 302
Necrotizing enterocolitis (NEC), 262, 333–338, 394, 775
  Bell staging criteria, 335t
  breast-feeding, 208–209
  clinical manifestations, 335–336
  diagnosis, 336–337
  microbiology, 334–335
  pathogenesis of, 334f
  pathology and pathogenesis, 334
  prevention, 337–338
  prognosis, 338
  treatment, 337
Necrotizing fasciitis, 500–501
Necrotizing retinitis, 952
Needle aspiration
  osteomyelitis, 303–304, 305
  pericarditis, 341
Negative predictive value, 1144
Neisseria gonorrhoeae, 277, 516
  clinical manifestations, 519
  diagnosis, 519–520
  differential diagnosis, 520, 520t
  microbiology, 518
  neonatal, treatment for, 521t

pathogenesis, 518–519
pathology, 519
prevention, 521–522
prognosis, 521
treatment, 520–521
UTIs and, 310
Neisseria meningitidis, 224, 232–233
  neonates and, 1215
  vaccines, 1228
Nelfinavir, 646, 649
Neoantigen, 124
Neomycin, 1180–1181
  EPEC gastroenteritis, 373
  salmonellosis, 380
  tuberculosis in pregnancy, 589
Neonatal antibody responses, inhibition of, by maternal antibodies, 157
Neonatal B cells, 149–150
  CD22 expression and, 153
  circulating MHC II, 148
  differentiation of, 149–150
Neonatal bacteremia
  incidence of, 25
  surveys, 225t
Neonatal bacterial meningitis, 244t
Neonatal bacterial sepsis
  clinical signs, 244, 244t
  host factors and, 240–241
  management of, 17–18
Neonatal brain abscess, pathology of, 243
Neonatal candidiasis
  broad-spectrum antibiotic therapy, 1072
  cohort study, 1131
  features, 1061t
  length of therapy, 1071
  pathogenesis, 1058f
  prevention, 1072–1073
  prognosis, 1071–1072
Neonatal chickenpox, lesions in, frequency of, 668t
Neonatal death
  infection as cause, 24–25
  maternal rash, date of onset, 692t
  measles at parturition, 692t
  related to infection, indirect causes, 39
Neonatal defenses, 160, 162
  T. gondii, 170–172
Neonatal disease, 230
Neonatal enterococcal bacteremia, 239–240
Neonatal enterovirus infections, pathology, general considerations, 768
Neonatal epiphysis, blood supply in, 299f
Neonatal group B streptococcal infection
  ascending amniotic infection, 430–432
  incidence, 428–429
  pathologic mechanisms, 431f

Neonatal group B streptococcal sepsis
  capsular polysaccharide-protein conjugate vaccines, 160
  immunologic interventions, 160–162
  intrapartum chemoprophylaxis, 160
  prevention, 160–161
Neonatal herpes simplex virus infection, 742
Neonatal IgG, 1126–1127
Neonatal illness, integrated management, 44
Neonatal illness severity scores, 1156
Neonatal immune response
  neonatal vaccination, 1215
  studies, 152
Neonatal immune system, innate and adaptive arms, 1126
Neonatal immunization, 41
  programs, logistics of, 1216
Neonatal infections, 29–39, 45
  diagnosis, 16–17
  enteroviruses, 762
  global burden of, 24–29
  global perspective, 24–51
  intrapartum care, 42
  management, 43
  prevention, 39–45
  prophylactic systemic antibiotics, 1134
  protection from, vaccine strategies for, 1216–1218
  reduction of, strategies for, 40t
  twins, 241
  viruses, 772–787
Neonatal infectious diseases
  diagnosis of, 787–789
  clinical, 787–788
  differential diagnosis, 787–789
Neonatal intensive care unit (NICU)
  antibiotics, 256
  Aspergillus organism, 1096
  breast-feeding, 1139
  chickenpox in, 665
  Clostridium difficile, 389–390
  CoNS infections, 1129
  distribution of infections, 1127t, 1128
  fungal infections, 1078–1079
  GBS, 1129–1130
  Group A streptococci, 1129
  HAIs, 1127
  HAV, 1132
  Malassezia, 1106, 1131
  staphylococcal infection, 509
  vertical transmission, 1127
  visitors to, infection, 1139
Neonatal listeriosis
  early-onset, 479, 479t, 483
  late-onset, 479–480, 479t
  rash of, 480f
Neonatal macrophages, 98–100
  activation, 95

Neonatal meningitis, 240
  bacteria, 227t
  broad spectrum β-lactam antibiotics, 258
  CFR of, 25t
  incidence of, 25
  pathology of, 243
  treatment, 258
Neonatal monocytes, 98–100
Neonatal monocytes activation, antimicrobial activity and, 95
Neonatal natural killer cell-mediated cytotoxicity, 107
Neonatal neutrophils
  adhesion of, 91
  migration of, 91–92
Neonatal pathogens, antimicrobial resistance in, 28
Neonatal regulatory T cells, 134–135
Neonatal sepsis, 17, 51, 59, 71–72, 1146. *See also* Neonatal bacterial sepsis; Neonatal sepsis syndrome
  acute phase reactants and, 1149–1150
  adhesion molecules, 1152
  adjunctive therapies, 259–260
  antimicrobial agents for, 255–256
  Apgar score, 236
  bacterial infections causing, 224t
  bacteriology, 223–234
  birth weight, 236
  breast-feeding, 209
  cellular receptors, 1152
  CFR of, 25t
  clinical manifestations, 243–248
  diagnosis, 248–255
  differential diagnosis, 245t
  early-onset, 53, 222–223, 223t
  epidemiologic surveillance, 263
  epidemiology of, 235–239
  ethnicity, 236–237
  fever and hypothermia, 246–247
  geographic regions, 237–238
  incidence of, 25
  by sex, 237t
  infant and mother, risk factors, 236
  infants developing, characteristics of, 235–238
  intrapartum antibiotic prophylaxis and, 455
  IVIG, 508
  laboratory aids, 255, 1144–1160
  laboratory studies, 1152–1155
  late-onset, 222–223, 223t
  clinical signs, 244
  management, 255–260
  maternal characteristics, 237t
  maternal factors, 261

  maternal risk factors, 243
  microbiology, 226t
  pathogenesis, 239–243
  pathology of, 243
  perspectives and conclusions, 1156
  prevention, 261–263
  obstetric factors, 261
  procedures, 238
  prognosis, 260–261
  rare causes, 234, 235t
  socioeconomic status, 238
Neonatal sepsis syndrome, 498
Neonatal sera, 87
Neonatal T-cells, 127–131, 149
  activation, 122–124
  anergy, 122–124
  costimulation, 122–124
Neonatal tetanus, 234, 1224
Neonatal vaccination
  immunologic immaturity, 1215
  interference, 1216
  maternal antibodies, 1216
  obstacles to, 1212–1216, 1214t
  safety concerns, 1220t
Neonatal vaccination program, 1212, 1214t
Neonates
  drugs not used in, 1161t
  immunologic development, 1215
  with infection
    antibiotic treatment of, 43–44
    identification of, 43
  special issues for, 1126–1127
Neoplasms, eye lesions and, 956
Nephropathy, 636–637
Nephrotic syndrome, 958
Nephrotoxicity, 1097–1098
  of amphotericin B, 1069
Netilmicin, 256
Neuroepithelium, 726
Neutralization, viral identification by, 759–760
Neutropenia, 1059
Neutrophil(s), 89–93
  breast milk and, 202
  clearance, of neutrophilic inflammation, 93
  marker analysis, 1152
  migration, to injury sites/infection sites, 90–91
  number of, 104f
  precursors, 89
  production of, 89–90
  ratios, 1148–1149
  resolution, of neutrophilic inflammation, 93
  response, GBS, 434
  Staphylococci and, 496
  transfusions, pyogenic infections, 161
  values, in mother/infant, 1146, 1147t
Neutrophilic inflammation, 93
Nevirapine regimen, 646
  antiretroviral regimens, 644

Newborn
  congenital *Toxoplasma gondii*, IgM *Toxoplasma* antibodies, 948t
  evaluation guidelines, for congenital toxoplasmosis, 980–993, 980t
  first month of life, infections, 19–21
  health, vital statistics, 4t
  infection in, diagnosis of, 13
  modes of inoculation, 584–585, 584t
  serologic diagnosis, 987–993
NIAID CASG antiviral studies, 820–821, 821t, 825, 826, 827, 828–829
NICHD Maternal-Fetal Medicine Units Network study, 68
NICU. *See* Neonatal intensive care unit
Nitric oxide, antimicrobial activity of, 94–95
Nitrofurans, *Trypanosoma cruzi*, 1045
NK cells. *See* Natural killer cells
NKT. *See* Natural killer T cells
NNIS system. *See* National Nosocomial Infection Surveillance system
NOD1, 97–98
NOD2, 97–98
Noma (cancrum oris), 277
Non hematopoietic cells, 81
Non-Candida filamentous fungi, 1065
Nonclassic antigen presentation molecules, 110–111
Non-Hodgkin lymphoma, 637
Noninfectious conditions, differential diagnosis, 245t
Nonmaternal routes of transmission, categories of, HAIs, 1127–1128
Nonviral intracellular pathogens, 169–172
Nosocomial infections, 28
  chickenpox, 666, 683
  newborn nursery, 666, 666t
  in nursery, 664–666
  cytomegalovirus, 745–746
  HSV type 2, 819
  measles, prevention guidelines, 693–695
  mumps, 698–699
  RSV, 910
Nosocomial urinary tract infections, 1135
NTHANES III (Third National Health and Nutrition Examination Survey)
  CMV and, 711
  rubella, 867
Nucleic acid amplification, 578
Nucleoside analogues, neonatal herpes and, 826
Nucleotide binding domain-containing receptors, 97–98

Nucleotides
 in human milk, 196t
 of mature milk, 196
 in supplemental formula,
  196t
Nulliparas, 70
Nursery
 amikacin, 239
 aminoglycosides and, 239
 cefotaxime-resistant gram-
  negative bacteria, 1187–1188
 chickenpox, 666
  isolation procedures,
   683–684, 684t
 CMV, 718
 fluconazole, 1198
 gastroenteritis, 367
 HAIs, 1078–1124
 HIAs, 1125–1143
 infection control, 792
 Klebsiella species, 238
 measles, 694t
 nosocomial chickenpox,
  664–666
 nosocomial measles, prevention
  guidelines, 693–695
 nosocomial mumps, 698–699
 nosocomial RSV, 910
 outbreaks, 238–239
  echovirus 11, 775
 personnel, tuberculosis, 594
 precautions
  standard, 1136–1138
  transmission-based,
   1136–1138
 Proteus species, 238
 school teachers, parvovirus
  B19, epidemiology of, 845
 VZV, incidence and
  distribution, 664–666
 workers, tuberculosis, 594
Nursery-acquired infections,
 19–20. *See also* Nosocomial
 infections
Nystatin, 1068, 1072–1073

O

Obstetric patients, GBS, 447
Obstetric tetanus, 1224
"Occult HBV," 803–804
Ocular abnormalities, 1006
 congenital CMV, 732
 maternal varicella and,
  673–674, 673f
Ocular toxoplasmosis
 external eye examination,
  952
 funduscopic examination,
  952–955
Ocular trachoma, 601
 prophylaxis, 606
Oka/Merck vaccine, 1225
Oligohydramnios, 66
Oligosaccharides, 203
Omphalitis, 30–31, 241–242,
 242f, 346, 500–501
Oocysts, 919, 919f, 930–931
 cats and, 1018
Oophoritis, 696

Ophthalmia neonatorum, 32–33,
 516, 519
Opsonins, 92
Optic disk, *Toxoplasma gondii* in,
 943
Optic nerve, 952–954
OPV. *See* Live-attenuated oral
 poliovirus vaccines; Oral
 poliovirus vaccine
ORACLE II study, 60, 613
ORACLE trial, 613
 PROM and, 68
Oral poliovirus vaccine (OPV),
 778
 T cell-specific response, 140
Orchitis, 696
Ordinary smallpox, 901
Ordinary-discrete smallpox,
 901–902
Organ systems
 aspergillosis and, 1095
 Candida spp. and, 1066–1067
 candidemia, 1063
 CMV, 728–730
 Coccidioides immitis organism,
  1101
 parvovirus B19 infection and,
  852
Organ transplantation, 745
Organisms
 causing peritonitis, 329
 Streptococcus agalactiae, 419–424
 umbilical cord and, 242f
Organomegaly, 247–248
Organs, coxsackievirus B strains,
 769
Oropharyngeal candidiasis,
 1060
Orosomucoid, 1149–1150,
 1151–1152
Orphan viruses, 756–757
Orthomyxovirus, 1226
Oseltamivir
 antimicrobial activity, 1195
 clinical implication, 1195
 influenza and, 1195
 pharmacokinetic data, 1195
 safety, 1195
Osteoarticular infection, 504–505
Osteomyelitis, 296
 bone involvement, distribution
  of, 301t
 clinical manifestations, 300–301
 diagnosis, 302–304
 differential diagnosis, 304
 group B streptococcal
  infection, 443, 444f
 of maxilla, 306–307
 microbiology, 297–298
 Mycoplasma, 298
 pathogenesis, 298–300
 prognosis, 301–302
 therapy, 304–305
 white blood cell count, 304
Otitis externa, 347
Otitis media, 280–285, 688
 breast-feeding and, 210
 diagnosis, 283t
 epidemiology, 282

group B streptococcal
 infection, 445
 microbiology, 282–284, 283t
 pathogenesis and pathology,
  281–282
 prognosis, 285
 treatment, 285
Oxacillin, 1171
 osteomyelitis, 305
 solitary hepatic abscess, 325
Oxacillin-resistant *Staphylococcus
 aureus*, 296
Oxygen therapy, *Pneumocystosis*,
 1092–1093
Oxygen-dependent microbicidal
 mechanisms, 92
Oxytocin induction, 193
 PROM and, 71

P

P. aeruginosa, eye infections and,
 349
P. carinii, 1052
PACTG 076 study, 639
PAHO. *See* Pan American Health
 Organization
Pan American Health
 Organization (PAHO), rubella,
 862
Pancreatitis, 775
Panosteitis, 301
Panton-Valentine leukocidin
 (PVL), 494
Papular cutaneous lesions, 481
Papular-purpura "gloves and
 socks" syndrome, 843
Paracentesis, 336
Paralysis, viruses and, 776
Paralytic poliomyelitis, 791
Paramyxovirus organism,
 685–686
 classification and morphology,
  685
Paranasal sinuses, infection of,
 277–278
Parasitemia
 age of infant and, 992t
 congenital toxoplasmosis, 922t
 persistent, 922
Parasites, 394–395
Parasitic infections, 1042
Parechovirus(es), 756–799, 787
 geographic distribution and
  season, 764–765
 host systems, 759
 neonatal infection, 772–776
  inapparent infection, 772
  manifestations of, 773t
  mild, nonspecific febrile
   illness, 772
  sepsis-like illness, 772–773
 neonatal infections, 763–764
 prognosis, 790
 replication, 758–759
 transplacental transmission, 762
Parechovirus 1, 787
Parechovirus 2, 787
Parechovirus 2A protein, 758
Parechovirus 3, 787

Parechovirus 4, 787
Parenteral feeding, 20
Paris study, toxoplasmosis,
 1008–1017
 interpretation of, 1008
Paronychia, 346
Parotitis, 500, 696
Parturition, predisposition to
 tolerance, 1215
Parvovirus B19, 834, 835t,
 844–845
 asymptomatic fetal infection,
  849
 birth defects, 849
 childbearing women and, risk
  for, 840–841
 clinical manifestations, 841–844
 CNS infection, 843–844
 dermatologic syndromes, 843
 diagnosis
  general aspects, 844–845
  laboratory methods, 844–845
 epidemiology, pregnant
  women and, 845–846
 epidemiology and
  transmission, 837–841
  acquisition, risk factors for,
   838–839
  global distribution, 837
  incidence, 838
  overview, 837
  seasonality and periodicity,
   837–838, 837f
  seroprevalence
   by age, 838
   by gender, 838
   by race, 838
 fetal hydrops, 849
 fetal immune responses, 850
 fetal manifestations, 849
 fetal monitoring, 853
 fetal outcomes, 847–850
 fetus, pathology in, 850–852
 hospital transmission, 839–840
 hydrops, pathogenesis of, 850
 intrauterine transmission,
  847–850
 maternal manifestations
  fetal outcome v, 850
  long-term outcomes, 850
 microbiology, 835–836
 neurologic disorders, 843–844
 pathogenesis, 836–837
  in fetus, 850
 placenta, 851f
 pregnancy
  clinical manifestations,
   846–847
  diagnostic evaluation of,
   852–854
  epidemiology of, 845–846
  prevalence/incidence
   other countries, 845–846
   United States, 845
 prevention, 855
  general measures, 855
 school-age children, 841
 vaccine development, 855
 viral spread, routes of, 840

Passive antibody, pyogenic
infections, 161
Passive immunization,
1218–1220
FDA approved products, 1218t
measles, 693–695
Pathogens. *See also specific
pathogens*
human milk and, 211–212
UTIs, 313t
PBPs. *See* Penicillin-binding
proteins
PCR assay (Polymerase chain
reaction assay), 12, 741, 788–789
in amniotic fluid, 973f, 974t
fetal *Toxoplasma* infection,
985–987
of amniotic fluid, congenital
toxoplasmosis in pregnancy,
1021
Candida spp. and, 1067
in cerebrospinal fluid, 991
conventional methods v., fetal
Toxoplasma infection, 989f
EBV, 907
gonococcal ophthalmia
neonatorum, 519–520
HCMV, 737–739
HIV infection, intrapartum
infection, 624
HSV, 815–816, 824–825
M. hominis, 616–617
Mycobacterium tuberculosis, 578
parvovirus B19, 845
Pneumocystis jiroveci, 1081
Pneumocystosis, 1090
real-time, 255
rubella virus infection, 864, 882
Toxoplasma gondii antigens,
971–979, 974t
Ureaplasma species, 616–617
in urine, *T. gondii*, 991
varicella zoster virus antibody,
678
VZV, 663
PCR-based technology, *Listeriosis
monocytogenes* organism, 481
PD. *See* Pharmacodynamics
Pediatric Prevention Network
(PPN) Point Prevalence
Survey, 1127
Pelvic inflammatory disease, 608
Penicillin, 18, 1168–1170.
See also Antipseudomonal
penicillin; Aqueous penicillin
G; Benzyl penicillin and
aminoglycoside; Penicillin G;
Penicillinase-resistant
penicillins; Penicillin-binding
proteins; Procaine penicillin G
breast milk concentrations,
1167–1168
cerebrospinal fluid
penetration, 1169
chorioamnionitis, 55
clinical dosing applications,
1169–1170
endocarditis, 340

GBS, 255, 454
Listeria, 482
microbiologic activity,
1168–1169
to mother, group B
streptococcal disease, 257
N. gonorrhoeae, 521
neonatal group B streptococcal
sepsis, 160
osteomyelitis of maxilla, 307
otitis media, 285
pharmacokinetic data, 1169
PK-PD, 1169–1170
pneumonia, 292
PROM and, 67–68
S. pneumonia sepsis, 228
safety, 1169
UTI, 319
in vitro susceptibility, 448
Penicillin G, 229
GBS, 447
neonatal meningitis, 258
nurseries and, 239
osteomyelitis, 305
pneumonia, 292
S. aureus, 255–256
skin infections, 348
Penicillin plus aminoglycoside,
Citrobacter sp. and, 231
Penicillin resistance,
N. gonorrhoeae, 519
Penicillinase-resistant penicillins,
255–256
endocarditis, 340
measles, 693
osteomyelitis, 305
pericarditis, 341
skin infections, 348
Penicillin-binding proteins
(PBPs), 1168
Pentamidine, 1092
Pentamidine isethionate
Pneumocystosis and, 1092
toxicity, 1092
Pentamidine-associated
pancreatitis, HIV infection
and, 1092
Pentoxifylline, neonatal sepsis, 259
Pentraxin, 85–86
Percutaneous lung aspiration,
Pneumocystosis, 1046
Perforated amebic appendicitis,
327
Perforation
causes of, 331f
sites of, 331f
Perforin cytotoxins, 131, 131f
Pericarditis, 340–341
Perinatal chickenpox, 677–678
Perinatal cytomegalovirus
infection, 736–737
diagnosis, 742
Perinatal group B streptococcal
infection, 455
Perinatal HIV prevention
experience in, 638–640
international experience in,
640–645

Perinatal HIV transmission, 622
guidelines for, 640t
Perinatal measles, 691–692, 695
Perinatal mumps, 697–698
Perinatal *Mycoplasma hominis*,
611–615
Perinatal outcome, placental
malaria, 38
Perinatal sepsis onset, postnatal
sepsis v, 1156
Perinatal tuberculosis,
conclusions on, 595
Perinatal *ureaplasma* infection,
611–615
Periodontal disease, premature
birth, 61
Peripartum sepsis, 17
Peripheral blood cell count,
mumps, 696
Perirectal abscesses, 347
Peritonitis, 329–333
clinical manifestations, 331–332
diagnosis, 332
etiology of, 330t
group B streptococcal
infection, 444
microbiology, 329–330
pathogenesis, 330
prognosis, 332–333
signs of, 332t
treatment, 333
Periventricular leukomalacia
(PVL), 56
Person-to-person transmission,
Pneumocystis jiroveci, 1083
Pertussis, 278–280, 1224
antibody to, 279
clinical presentation of, 279
complications, 279–280
diagnostic methods, 280
maternal immunization,
1216–1217
Pertussis toxin (PT), 1223
Pertussis vaccines, 280
Petechiae, 731
congenital CMV, 732f
Petrolatum ointment, neonatal
candidiasis, 1072
Pets, infant infection and, 264
PFGE. *See* Pulsed-field gel
electrophoresis
Phage-display technology,
495–496
Phagocyte cells, *Staphylococcus
aureus* and, 493–494, 493f
Phagocyte production, by bone
marrow, 88–89
Phagocytes, 88–89
GBS, 438–439
of infant, 246
Phagocytosis, 92
Pharmacodynamic equations,
1163–1164
Pharmacodynamics (PD), 1160
MIC and, 1163–1164
Pharmacokinetic (PK), 1160
data
aztreonam, 1183–1184

minimal inhibitory
concentration, 1163
of drug, 1161
terms, 1161t
Pharyngitis, 276–277, 774
Pharynx cultures, 250–251
Phenobarbital, 993–994
Phenylketonuria, 210
Phorbol ester, 123
Phycomycosis, 1107–1109
clinical manifestations, 1108
diagnosis and differential
diagnosis, 1108–1109
epidemiology and
transmission, 1108
pathogenesis, 1108
pathology, 1108
prevention, 1109
prognosis, 1109
therapy, 1109
Phycomycosis organism, 1107
Physicians' Desk Reference, 1160
Pilus island-based vaccines, GBS,
458
Piperacillin, 1172
appendicitis, 329
mediastinitis, 342
solitary hepatic abscess, 325
Yersinia enterocolitica, 392
Piperacillin-tazobactam regimen,
1188–1189
antimicrobial activity, 1188
dosing implications, 1189
pharmacokinetic data, 1186t,
1188–1189
PK-PD dosing, 1189
safety, 1189
PK. *See* Pharmacokinetic
Placenta
CMV and, 730
congenital rubella infection, 871
infection of, 6
malaria and, 1047
microscopic examination,
1153–1154
mumps virus and, 698
neonatal GBS, 430
parvovirus B19 infection, 851,
851f
Toxoplasma gondii, 922,
940–941, 940f, 970
during chronic infection,
923–924
Trypanosoma cruzi, 1043
visceral lesions in, chickenpox,
667–668
Placental drug
biotransformation, 1165
Placental infection, 5–6
absence of, 6
congenital malaria, 1048–1049
rubella virus, 868
Placental malaria, perinatal
outcome, 38
Plain film radiographs,
osteomyelitis, 302
Plasma cell generation, 148–149
Plasma cells, 148–149

Plasma HIV RNA levels, 648
Plasma HIV-1 DNA PCR assay, 628
Plasmablasts, 148
Plasmacytoid dendritic cells, adult v. neonatal, 103
Plasmodium falciparum, 1046
Plasmodium falciparum antigens, adaptive immune response, 139
Plasmodium vivax, 1046
Platelet count (in newborns), 1149
Pleconaril, enteroviruses and, 791
Pleiotropic anti-inflammatory cytokine IL-10, breast milk and, 205
Pleocytosis, 1101
Plesiomonas shigelloides, 392–393
Pleural effusions, 292
Pleural fluid, 291
Pneumococcal infections, 228
Pneumococcal polysaccharide vaccines, 40–41
Pneumocystis, 1078–1124.
    See also Pneumocystosis
Pneumocystis carinii infection.
    See Pneumocystis jiroveci
Pneumocystis infection, 1085
Pneumocystis jiroveci, 628, 1052, 1078–1095
    airborne transmission, 1084
    cellular immune responses, 1087
    cystlike stages, 1081*f*
    cysts, 1080*f*
    epidemiology and transmission, 1081–1084
    history, 1079–1080
    HIV, 1083
    HIV-exposed infants, 634*t*
    humeral immune responses, 1087
    intracystic body, 1081*f*
    life cycles for, 1081
    maternal transfer, to infants, 1083–1084
    mode of transmission, 1083
    organism, 1080–1081
    pathology, 1085–1086
    PCR assay, 1081
    person-to-person transmission, 1083
    pulmonary alveoli, life cycle of, 1082*f*
    within pulmonary alveoli, life cycle of, 1082*f*
    staining procedures, 1080
    in vitro, 1081
    in vitro cellular immune response to, 1087
Pneumocystis pneumonia, 1080, 1082
    in animals, 1086
    cellular immune system, 1087
    conditions associated, 1086*t*
    pathogenesis, 1086–1088
    rat study, 1086
Pneumocystis-infected children with malignancy, 1084

Pneumocystis-infected lungs, 1085–1086
Pneumocystosis, 1079
    bronchoalveolar lavage, 1090
    clinical manifestations, 1043
    concurrent infection, 1045
    with cytomegalovirus, clinical manifestations, 1090
    diagnosis, 1045–1046
    epidemic infection, signs and symptoms, 1044
    laboratory studies, 1045
    lung biopsy, 1046
    percutaneous lung aspiration, 1046
    prevention, 1048–1049
    prognosis, 1047–1048
        chronic sequelae, 1048
        recurrent infection, 1048–1051
    pulmonary secretions, examination of, 1046–1051
    radiologic findings, 1044–1045
        epidemic infection, 1045
        sporadic infection, 1045
    serologic tests, 1046–1048
    signs and symptoms, 1043–1044
    sporadic infection, signs and symptoms, 1044
    supportive care, 1047
    treatment, 1046
        specific therapy, 1046–1047
Pneumonia, 29, 250–251, 285–292, 441, 502–503, 774.
    See also Health care-associated pneumonia
    categories of, 285
    Chlamydia trachomatis, 603
    clinical manifestations, 289
    diagnosis, 289–291
        clinical, 289
        histologic and cytologic, 290
        immunologic, 290–291
        microbiologic, 289–290
        radiologic, 289
    differential diagnosis, 291–292
    epidemiology, 288–289
        developing countries, 288–289
        epidemic disease, 288
        incidence, 288, 288*t*
        race and socioeconomic status, 288
    GBS, 439–440, 441*f*
    management, 292
    microbiology, 287
    pathogenesis and pathology, 286–287
    perinatal, 612
    prognosis, 292
Pneumonia acquired after birth, 276–296
    causes, 285–286
Pneumonia acquired during birth, 276–296
    causes, 285

and first month, pathogenesis and pathology, 286–287
Pneumonia prophylaxis, HIV-exposed infants, 634*t*
Pneumonitis
    congenital CMV, 732
    intra-alveolar cluster, stain of, 1085*f*
    intra-alveolar cluster of, 1085
Podophyllum resin, 906
Polio vaccine, 789, 791–792, 1220–1221
Poliomyelitis, 756
    clinical findings, 777*t*
    inapparent infection, 777
    infection acquired in utero, 777
    postnatally acquired infection, 777–778
    prevention, 791–792
Poliovirus, 1224
    abortion and, 770
    congenital malformations, 770
    manifestations of, 776–778
        general considerations, 776–777
    neonatal infections, 763
    pathology, 768
    prematurity and stillbirth, 771
    prognosis, 789
    transplacental transmission, 761
Poliovirus antibody, breast feeding and, 200–201
Polofilox, 906
Polymerase chain reaction assay.
    See PCR assay
Polymorphonuclear leukocytes, 89
    human milk and, 213–214
Polymorphonuclear neutrophils (PMNs), CMV and, 720
Polysaccharide, antibody response to, 155
Polysaccharide antigens, immunochemistry of, 421–422
Polysaccharide Hib vaccine, 1221–1222
Polysaccharide vaccine, salmonellosis, 381
Polysaccharide vaccines, 1221–1222
Polysaccharide-protein conjugates, antibody response to, 155
Polysaccharides, 1226–1227
Population pharmacokinetic analysis, 1163
Positive predictive value, 1144
Postabortal fever, 609–610
Postmortem specimens, *Toxoplasma gondii*, 971
Postnatal care, neonatal infection and, 42
Postnatal infection
    persistent, 10
    T-cell response, 140–141
Postnatal sepsis, perinatal sepsis onset v, 1156
Postnatally acquired chickenpox, 677

Postnatally acquired measles, 691
Postnatally acquired *Toxoplasma gondii*, antibody response, 981*t*
Postnatally acquired varicella, premature infant, 1219
Postnatal-specific antibody responses, 154–156
Postpartum fever, 609–610
Postpartum period, tuberculosis effect on, 581
Potassium, *Yersinia enterocolitica*, 392
Poultry, *C. jejuni*, 387
Povidone-iodine, gonococcal ophthalmia neonatorum, 521–522
Poxviruses, microbiology, 900
pp65, 744
Pre-B cell maturation, 142–143
Pre-BCR complex, 142
Precipitin, *Coccidioides immitis* organism, 1102
Precipitin antigens, rubella virus, 864
Predictive values, of test, 1145
Prednisone, chorioretinitis, treatment for, 1015–1016
Pregnancy. *See also Toxoplasma gondii*
    acquired *T. gondii*, 980–985
        health education consequences, 933–934
        incidence of, 933–934
        prevalence rates, mathematic epidemiologic models, 933
    acyclovir, 680
    antibiotics, 1165
    Bordetella pertussis, 1217
    Chlamydial trachomatis screening, 605
    chloroquine and, 1051
    cholera during, 391
    chronic infection, diagnosis of, 11
    CMV study, 723
    congenital cytomegalovirus, 715
    congenital *Toxoplasma gondii*, 949*t*
    congenital toxoplasmosis, 1017
    effect of tuberculosis on, 582
    famciclovir, 680
    GBS, 425, 429, 447
    genital herpes, management of, 830
    gonococcal infections, 516–518
    HAART during, 644–645
    HAV, 802, 803
    HBV, 806
    HIV and comorbid *congenital Toxoplasmosis*, 967
    HIV testing, 627
    HSV-2, 816
    infection in
        diagnosis of, 10–13
        cytologic/histologic, 12
        prevention and management, 13–15

Pregnancy (*Continued*)
serologic, 12–13
skin test, 13
management of, 11*t*
influenza and, 908, 909
influenza vaccine and, 910
LCV, 912
live vaccines and, 14
measles in
incidence of, 686
pathogenesis, 686–687
mefloquine, 1050, 1051
MMR vaccine, 1217–1218
Neisseria gonorrhoeae, 521
outcome, adverse, 610–611
parvovirus
clinical features, 852
laboratory diagnosis,
852–853
parvovirus B19
epidemiology of, 845–846
prevalence/incidence
other countries, 845–846
United States, 845
periconceptional infection,
diagnosis of, 11
rabies, 913
rubella and, fetal abnormality
and, 867*t*
rubella vaccine, 888
seasonal influenza vaccines,
1226
seroconverting during, 982*t*
subclinical infection, diagnosis
of, 10–11
substance abuse during,
242–243
successful, 4
symptomatic infection,
diagnosis of, 10
T. gondii in, 923
termination
congenital rubella infection,
884
congenital toxoplasmosis in
pregnancy, 1026–1027
T. gondii, 1002–1003, 1004
tuberculosis and, 577, 581–582
tuberculosis treatment,
588–590
vaccinia virus, 899–900
valacyclovir, 680
with Varicella-Zoster virus
infection, 676–677
zoster in, incidence of, 664
Pregnancy-related hormones,
199–200
Pregnant woman. *See* Pregnancy
Premature birth, 7–8
Candida and, 1059–1060
chorioamnionitis and, 60
clinical infection and, 60–61
congenital *Toxoplasma gondii*,
949
gestational measles and, 690
gestational mumps and, 697
infection and, biochemical
links of, 62

lower genital tract infections v,
61, 61*t*
viruses, 771
Premature infants
infectious diseases, 1228
mother's milk and, 200
Premature labor, preterm PROM
and, 62
Premature neonate, human milk
and, 197
Premature rupture of membranes
(PROM), 52–59, 60, 69–72.
See also Preterm PROM
antibiotic for, adverse
outcomes, 63*t*
complications, 66–67, 66*t*
definition, 52–53
diagnosis, 65–66
early third trimester,
treatment, 69–72
etiology, 65
fetal viability, treatment
before, 68–69
incidence, 65
infant death with, 67*t*
infection, diagnosis of, 67–68
investigational treatment, 69
management plans, 69*t*
natural history, 66
predictors of, tests as, 65
preterm, trials, 61
prevention, 72–73
recurrence of, 72–73
special situations, 73
term neonate, treatment, 54–55
PREMET study, 60
Prenatal screening, 936, 1020–1021
Prenatal sensitization, 138
Prepatellar bursitis, 444*f*
Preterm birth
antibiotics, 64*t*
cervical ureaplasma infection,
610–611
infections and, 59–64, 60*t*
Preterm induction, mid-third
trimester, 72
Preterm labor
amniotic fluid cultures in, 61–62
corticosteroids and, 242
Preterm PROM, 53, 58
Primary ciliary dyskinesia, 290
Primary immune response,
isotype switching and, 148
Primary pulmonary coccidioidal
infection, 1101
Primary septic arthritis, 305–306
bacterial organisms, 306*t*
organisms isolated, 306*t*
Pro-B cell maturation, 142–143
Probiotics, 337
Procaine penicillin G, 1169
Procalcitonin, 1151
Prodrome, 688, 694*t*
Progenitor cells, 836
Proinflammatory cytokines,
excess production of, 96
Proinflammatory mediators, 205
Prokaryotes, 607

Prolactin, 192*t*
PROM. *See* Premature rupture of
membranes
Prophylactic antibiotics, 1134
Prostaglandin, PROM and, 71
Protease inhibitors, 649
HIV and, costs, 651
Protein antigens
antibody responses, neonate
and young infant, 154–155
of mature milk, 195–196
Protein binding sites, 1162
Protein C, 863
Protein-calorie malnutrition,
Pneumocystis pneumonia, rat
study, 1086–1087
Proteins, breast milk and, 204
Proteins 2B4 (CD244), 105
Prothymocytes, 111–112, 112*f*
thymocyte differentiation and,
111–113
Protozoan infections, 633–634,
1042–1054
Pseudohyphae, light microscopy
photographs, 1057*f*
Pseudomonal eye infections, 349
Pseudomonas, broad-acting agents
and, 1186*t*, 1188–1193, 1192*t*
Pseudomonas aeruginosa, 232
HAIs, 1130
UTIs and, 311
Pseudomonas sepsis, 232, 1190
Pseudomonas species
eye infections, 350
nurseries and, 238
Psychomotor retardation,
733–734
PT. *See* Pertussis toxin
Public health, HCMV, 736*t*
Pulmonary alveoli, *Pneumocystis
jiroveci* within, life cycle of,
1082*f*
Pulmonary artery stenosis, 878
Pulmonary hypoplasia, PROM
and, 64
Pulmonary secretions,
examination of, *Pneumocystosis*,
1046–1051
Pulsed dye laser, respiratory
papillomatosis, 906
Pulsed-field gel electrophoresis
(PFGE), 490
DNA macro-restriction
pattern analysis, 471
group B streptococcal
infection, 428
Purpura, 731, 843
Pustulosis, 500
PVL. *See* Panton-Valentine
leukocidin; Periventricular
leukomalacia
Pyarthrosis, 299–300
Pyelonephritic isolates, 314
Pyelonephritis, 315
Pyogenic infections, adjunctive
therapy, 161–162
Pyrazinamide (PZA)
tuberculosis and, 587

tuberculosis in pregnancy,
589–590
Pyridoxine, tuberculosis and,
586–587
Pyrimethamine, 993–994, 999
congenital toxoplasmosis,
996–997
fluoroquinolones and, 1000
F/M ratios for, 994
oral suspension formulations,
996*t*
preparation of, 996*f*
teratogenic effects of, 998
toxicity, 997–998
Pyrimethamine and sulfonamide
regimen
chorioretinitis, treatment for,
1015–1016
spiramycin v., congenital
toxoplasmosis in pregnancy,
1025
Toxoplasma gondii, 999
toxoplasmosis, 993–998
Pyrimethamine with leucovorin
and sulfadiazine, 1010, 1011*t*
Pyrimethamine-sulfadiazine,
1005, 1009
congenital toxoplasmosis in
pregnancy, 1020
fetal treatment, through
maternal treatment, 1001
gestation and, 1026
Toxoplasmic encephalitis, 999
Pyrimethamine-sulfadiazine, and
spiramycin
congenital toxoplasmosis,
prenatal diagnosis of,
1003*t*
T. gondii, 1002
Pyrimidine analogues,
1197–1198
PZA. *See* Pyrazinamide

Q

Quinidine, congenital malaria,
1048–1051
Quinine and tetracycline
regimen, congenital malaria,
1048–1051
Quinolones
Campylobacter, 389
N. gonorrhoeae, 519
salmonellosis, 380
Shigella infection, 385
in vitro susceptibility, 448
Quinupristin-dalfopristin, 508
in vitro susceptibility, 448
Quorum sensing, *S. aureus* and, 495

R

Rabies virus, 913
Radiologic abnormalities,
Toxoplasma gondii infections,
959–964
Radiologic skeletal surveys,
osteomyelitis, 302
Radiologic tests, tuberculosis,
578

RAG activity, 144
RAG protein expression, 114, 143
RAG proteins, 113
Random-amplified polymorphic DNA assay, group B streptococcal infection, 428
Ranitidine therapy, neonates and, 243
RANTES, 128, 721–722
Rapid assays, GBS, antenatal detection of, 452
Rapid HIV testing, 627
Rapid virus identification, 788–789
RAS signaling pathway, 123
Rash, 776, 881
  measles, 688, 694t
  neonatal listeriosis, 480f
  rubella virus, 869–870
  Toxoplasma gondii infections, 958
  variola, 901
RDS. *See* Respiratory distress syndrome
Receptor editing, 144
Recirculation, naïve T cell and, 118
Recombinant G-CSF, neonatal group B streptococcal sepsis, 161
Recombinant GM-CSF, neonatal group B streptococcal sepsis, 161
Recombinant human cytokine molecules, group B streptococcal infection, 451
Recombinant virus vaccine, congenital cytomegalovirus, 744
Regulatory T cells, 134–135
  overview, 134
Reinfection, *Toxoplasma gondii*, 938
Renal candidiasis, 1063–1064
Renal cortical scintigraphy, 318
Renal disease
  HIV, 636–637
  parvovirus B19, 844
Renal pyelectasis, 314
Renal scintigraphy, UTI, 319
Reproductive tract, *Mycoplasma hominis*, 608
Reproductive tract diseases, 607–608
Resistance plasmids, salmonellosis, 381
Respiratory difficulty, 964
Respiratory distress, 229, 247, 291t
Respiratory distress syndrome (RDS), 51
  PROM and, 64
  tocolytics and, 71–72
Respiratory droplets
  HSV, 815
  measles virus, 686
  VZV, 663
Respiratory illness, 774
  echovirus 11, 785
  enteroviruses and, 774

Respiratory papillomatosis, 906
Respiratory syncytial virus (RSV), 910–911.
  See also Nosocomial infections attenuated vaccines, 1220–1221
  breast-feeding and, 210
  maternal immunization, 1217
Respiratory syncytial virus immune globulin, monoclonal antibodies and, 1218
Respiratory tract, 84–85
  bacterial infections, 210, 276–296
  Coccidioides immitis organism, 1100–1101
Respiratory viruses, 1132
Restriction enzyme fragment length polymorphism analysis, group B streptococcal infection, 428
Restriction fragment length polymorphism analysis, of mycobacterial DNA, 579
Retina, *Toxoplasma gondii* in, 943
Retinal edema, 952–954
Retinal lesions, ocular toxoplasmosis, 953t
Retinoblastoma, 956
Retinochoroiditis, 1016–1017
Retinoic acid, respiratory papillomatosis, 906
Retinopathy of congenital rubella, 880
Retinopathy of prematurity (ROP), 1064
Retropharyngeal abscess, 276–277
Retropharyngeal cellulitis, 276–277
Rhesus monkey rotavirus (RRV), 1227
Rheumatoid factor, 978
Rhizopus in vitro, 1109
Ribavirin, 911
RIF. *See* Rifampin
Rifampin, 1176
Rifampin (RIF)
  Toxoplasma gondii, 1000
  tuberculosis and, 587
  tuberculosis in pregnancy, 589
Rifaximin, EAEC, 376
Ringworm. *See* Tinea capitis
Ritonavir, 649
RNA replication, HAV, 801
RNA viruses, 757
Rochester criteria, febrile infants, 264
ROP. *See* Retinopathy of prematurity
Roseola, 692
Roseola syndrome, 908
Rotavirus, 30, 208, 395–399, 1227, 1228
  clinical manifestations, 397–398
  diagnosis, 398
  differential diagnosis, 399–400
  epidemiology, 397
  infection and immunity, 396–397

pathogenesis, 396
  therapy and prevention, 398–399
  vaccines, 399
RRV. *See* Rhesus monkey rotavirus
RSV. *See* Respiratory syncytial virus
Rubella vaccination, CRS after, 877t
Rubella vaccine
  characteristics, 887–889
  immunization strategies and, 886–889
  recommendations, 889
Rubella virus, 171–172, 604–605, 692, 861–898, 862–865, 889–890, 1217–1218, 1225
  animals and, pathogenicity for, 865
  antibody kinetics, 870f
  antigen testing, 864–865
  cell culture, growth in, 865
  cellular immune responses, 871
  classification, 864
  clinical manifestations, 876–881
    congenital infection, 876–881
    postnatal infection, 876
  congenital abnormalities, after second year/later, 877t
  congenital defects, 869
  elimination strategies, 889–890
  epidemiology, 865–867
  fetal infection risk, 868–869, 868t
  global distribution, 863f
  human milk and, 213
  IgG antibodies, 881
  immunization, 1225
    contraindications, 889
  isolation of, 12
  local immune response, 871
  morphology and physical/chemical composition, 862–864
  natural history, 869–874
  outbreak control, 889
  pandemic, 862
  pathogenesis, 874–875
    congenital infection, 874–875
    postnatal infection, 874
  pathology, 875–876
    congenital infection, 875–876
    postnatal infection, 875
  postnatal infection, 869–871
    virologic findings, 869–870
  postnatally acquired, viral excretion v. clinical findings, 870f
  pregnancy
    assessment algorithm, 885f
    fetal abnormality and, 867t
  serologic testing, 864–865
  surveillance, 889
  transmission in utero, 865
  United States cases, 866f
    incidence rates, 867f

Rubella virus infection, positive status for, 882t
Rubella virus vaccine, 1225
Rubeola. *See* Measles
Rudimentary mammary tissue, 192

S
S. aureus, 229–230, 250, 255–256, 290, 292
S. aureus bacteremia, 499
S. aureus-α-toxin, 494
S. dysenteriae serotype 1, 383
S. epidermidis, 229–230, 250
S. marcescens, nurseries and, 238
S. pneumoniae sepsis, Ceftriaxone, 228
S. pneumoniae, 251, 277, 281, 282
Sabin-Feldman dye test, *Toxoplasma gondii*, 974, 974f, 975f
Saliva, *Toxoplasma gondii*, 971
Salivary antibodies, 839
Salmonella enterica, 376
Salmonella gastroenteritis, 380
Salmonella infection
  extraintestinal complications, 379
  UTIs and, 310
Salmonella meningitis, 379
Salmonella species, 169, 222, 232, 376–381
  breast-feeding, 208
  clinical manifestations, 378–380
  epidemiology and transmission, 377–378
  nature of organism, 376–377
  serotypes and serogroups, 377t
Salmonellosis
  diagnosis, 380
  prevention, 381
  therapy, 380–381
Salt and pepper retinopathy, 879
Scarlet fever, 692
Schistosomiasis, 1052
School epidemics, 839, 841
Sclerema neonatorum, 347–348
Score for Neonatal Acute Physiology (SNAP), 1128, 1156
Screening panels, 1154–1155
  asymptomatic infants, 1154
  performance characteristics, early-onset neonatal bacteremia, 1155t
Screening system, congenital toxoplasmosis in pregnancy, 1020–1021
Seasonal influenza vaccines, 1226
Secondary lymph node tissues, 118
Seizures, 248, 441
  pyrimethamine, 993–994
Sensitivity, laboratory tests and, 1144
SENTRY Antimicrobial Surveillance Program, 1055

Sepsis, 497–499.
See also Neonatal group B streptococcal sepsis; Neonatal sepsis; Pseudomonas sepsis
early-onset, 497
in fetus, maternal antimicrobial agents, 257
hypothermia in newborns, 246–247
inflammatory mediators and, 434–435
late-onset disease, 263
neonate neurologic signs, 248
umbilical, 324
Sepsis-like illness, therapy, 791
Septic abortion, 609–610
Septic arthritis
group B streptococcal infection, 443
parenteral therapy and, 450
therapy, 304–305
Septic shock, GBS, 159–160, 438
Septicemia, 297, 419
Seroconversion
antenatal therapy and, congenital toxoplasmosis in pregnancy, 1021–1022
congenital toxoplasmosis in pregnancy, 1021
rate, acquired *Toxoplasma gondii*, health education consequences, 934
Serologic assays
congenital rubella infection, 883
congenital *Toxoplasma gondii*, 935–936
cryptococcosis infection, 1105
LCV, 912
maternal *Toxoplasma gondii*, 928
newborn, *Toxoplasma* infection, 987–993
parvovirus B19, 844
pregnancy, seroconverting during, *Toxoplasma*, 982t
Toxoplasma infection, IgG antibody responses to, 983t
Serologic rebound, *Toxoplasma gondii*, 945, 992t
Serologic screening
cerebrospinal fluid, *T. gondii*, 991
congenital *Toxoplasma gondii*, 934–935
severity of manifestations, 925t
guidelines, congenital toxoplasmosis in pregnancy, 1022, 1023f
HAV, 802
measles virus, 686
Pneumocystosis, 1046–1048
rubella virus, 864–865
VZV, 662
Serologic testing, *Toxoplasma gondii*
method used, antibody response v, 981–984
pregnant women, 980t
Serology, 789
Serratia marcescens, 232

Serum agglutinins, cryptococcosis infection, 1105
Serum ampicillin concentration-time curves
newborns and, 1172
preterm/term infants, 1172
Serum factors, *Listeria*, 477
Serum HIV RNA, 624
Serum IgM antibody, HAV, 802
Serum IgM fraction, 882
Serum pyrimethamine levels, toxoplasmosis, 994f
Severe meningitis, *Listeria*, 480f
Sexual intercourse
HBV, 803
HSV, 815
Sexually transmitted diseases (STDs), 32, 41–42, 520
CMV as, 717
Shiga toxin, 374–375
Shigella, 381–385
nature of organism, 381–382
Shigella dysenteriae serotype 1, 375
Shigella infection
age-related incidence, 383f
antimotility agents, 385
Cefaclor, 385
Cefamandole, 385
clinical manifestations, 383–384
diagnosis, 384
kanamycin, 385
prevention, 385
therapy, 384–385
Shigella serogroups, 382, 382t
Shigellosis
incubation period, 383
sepsis during, 384
Shingles, 661
Shunt placement, neuroradiologic follow-up, toxoplasmosis, 993
Siderophore iron, 241
Signaling pathway inhibition, *Toxoplasma gondii*, 103
Silver nitrate, gonococcal ophthalmia neonatorum, 521–522
Skeletal deformity, PROM and, 65
Skeletal muscle, *Toxoplasma gondii*, 944
Skin
Aspergillus organism, 1096–1097
barrier function of, 83
group B streptococcal infection and, 446
HIV, 637
Toxoplasma gondii, 945, 958
Skin (of neonates), 85
Skin antisepsis, 1134
Skin care, infection and, 1139–1140
Skin infections, 342–348
ceftazidime, 348
ceftriaxone, 348
clinical manifestations, 344–347, 345t
diagnosis, 324
differential diagnosis, 324

epidemiology, 344
HSV and, 823–824
microbiology, 344
pathogenesis, 343–344
prevention, 348
treatment, 348
Skin inflammation, hygienic care, 348
Skin lesions
HSV-2 and, 823
Invasive fungal dermatitis, 1062
sepsis and, 248
Skin test antigen
Coccidioides immitis organism, 1100
cryptococcosis infection, 1105
Skin tests, 13
Slide agglutination tests, enteropathogenic *E. coli* (EPEC) gastroenteritis, 371–372
Smallpox, 679, 899–904
chickenpox v, 903t
diagnosis, 903
differential diagnosis, 903
mortality rate, 900
prevention, 904
SNAP. *See* Score for Neonatal Acute Physiology
Socioeconomic status
maternal education and, 45
neonatal sepsis, 238
Solitary abscess, 322–323
Solitary hepatic abscess
prognosis, 324
treatment, 325
vancomycin, 325
Soluble products, human milk and, 198–201
Somatic hypermutation, 147
Specific IgM serologic testing, *Toxoplasma gondii*, 978–979
Spectinomycin, *N. gonorrhoeae*, 519, 521
Spherules, 1100
identifying, 1101–1102
Sphingosine 1-phosphate receptors, 118
Spinal cord, coxsackievirus B strains, 769
Spinal cord disease, 635
Spiramycin, 998–1000, 1002
Austria study, 1025
congenital toxoplasmosis in pregnancy, 1020, 1024–1025, 1025t
fetomaternal concentrations, 998–999
gestation, 924t
maternal *Toxoplasma gondii*, gestation and, 924t
pyrimethamine plus sulfonamide v, 1025
T. gondii and, 998
Spleen, 150
Toxoplasma gondii in, 943–944
Splenic abscess, 325
Splenic marginal zone B cells, 150

Splenomegaly, 247, 731
Spontaneous abortion, 610
HSV-2, 816
Spontaneous apoptosis, neonatal T cells and, 133
Spontaneous intestinal perforation, 1064–1065
Spontaneous naïve peripheral T-cell, proliferation, 120–121
Spontaneous preterm birth, 61
Sputum collection, 578
Squamous cell carcinoma, 1099
Standard precautions, 1136–1138
Stanford-Alabama study, 1004–1008
hearing impairment, 1007
intelligence testing, 1007, 1007t
neurologic outcome in, 1006–1007, 1007t
ophthalmologic outcome in, 1005–1006, 1006t
special considerations, 1007–1008
toxoplasmosis, 1006t
interpretation of, 1008
Staphylococcal infection, 241–242, 489–515
nurseries and, 238
prevention, 509–510
Staphylococcal osteomyelitis, 303
Staphylococcal peptidoglycan, 491–492
Staphylococcal pulmonary infections, 502
Staphylococcal scalded skin syndrome (SSSS), 497, 502, 502f, 503f
Staphylococcal teichoic acid, 491–492
Staphylococci
laboratory media, 491
microbiology, 491–492
Staphylococcus, aspergillosis and, 1095
Staphylococcus aureus, 83, 222, 223, 229–230, 276, 491–492, 903, 1171
cell wall, 491
clinical manifestations, 497–505
epidemiology and transmission, 489–491
epithelial attachment and invasion, 492–493
HAIs and, 1130
host compliment-mediated clearance, 494
IgG, 494
innate immune resistance, 493–494
milk macrophage, 201
pathogenesis of disease, 492–497
pathology, 497
resistance to oxacillin, 296
secreted toxins, 494–495
UTIs and, 310, 311
virulence mechanisms of, 492, 493f

Staphylococcus aureus infection, diagnosis, 505–506
Staphylococcus epidermidis, 223
biofilm formation, 495*f*
Staphylococcus epidermidis biofilm, 495*f*, 496, 496*f*
Stavudine, 646
Stavudine and zidovudine, 649
STDs. *See* Sexually transmitted diseases
Stem cell factor, 89
Sterile cord cutting, 28–29
Steroid therapy, immunosuppression with, 1059
Stillbirth, 6–7
congenital toxoplasmosis in pregnancy, 1025*t*
Toxoplasma gondii during pregnancy, in offspring, 924*t*
Trypanosoma cruzi, 1044
viruses, 771
STM. *See* Streptomycin
Stool cultures
amebiasis, 1046
enteropathogenic *E. coli* (EPEC) gastroenteritis, 371
Shigella infection, 384
Stool flora, 83
Streptococcus agalactiae, 276
organism, 419–424
Streptococcus mitis, 228
Streptococcus pneumoniae, 224, 228, 688
CRP and, 1150
Streptococcus pneumoniae vaccines, 1226–1227
Streptococcus pyogenes, 276, 688
Streptomycin (STM), 1166, 1180–1181
Listeria, 482
neonatal sepsis, 260
tuberculosis and, 588
Subcutaneous tissue, infections, 342–348
Substance abuse, during pregnancy, 242–243
Subunit proteins, 1221
Subunit vaccines, congenital cytomegalovirus, 744
Sudden infant death syndrome, 776
breast-feeding and, 210
group B streptococcal infection and, 446
Sulfadiazine, 994
fluoroquinolones and, 1000
oral suspension formulations, 996*t*
preparation of, 996*f*
Sulfadimidine, 994
Sulfadoxine, toxoplasmosis, 996–997
Sulfadoxine-pyrimethamine, malaria and, 1050–1051
Sulfamethoxazole-trimethoprim disk susceptibility testing, 420
Sulfapyridine, 994
Sulfathiazole, 994

Sulfisoxazole, 994
Sulfonamides, 223, 999, 1162, 1166
breast milk, 1168
milk to plasma ratios, 1166
serum concentrations, 1165*t*, 1166
Shigella infection, 385
toxicity, 997
Supplemental formula, nucleotides in, 196*t*
Supportive treatment, HAV, 802
Suppurative arthritis, 298
Suppurative parotitis, 500
Supraglottis, group B streptococcal infection, 445–446
Surface immunoglobulin, 146
Surgical intervention, appendicitis, 329
Syphilis, 253
transplacental bacterial bone infection and, 298
SYROCOT study, 1021
System antibiotics, for newborns, dosage schedules, 1193*t*
Systematic screening program, congenital toxoplasmosis, 1018–1019
Systemic antifungal agents, invasive candidiasis in neonates, 1068*t*
Systemic candidiasis, 1063
Systemic fungal infection, antifungal agents for, 1112*t*
Systemic inflammatory response, to sepsis, 1153

T

T. gondii, 10, 13
antigen-specific CD4 T-cell responses, 171
CSF, 991
immune response, 170–172
immunologic intervention, 172
T. gondii-specific memory CD4+ T-cell responses, 171
T. pallidum, 10, 12, 171–172
T. vaginalis infection
metronidazole and, 60
preterm birth and, 61
αβ TCR-positive thymocyte, 115
development of, 112*f*
γδ TCR gene rearrangements, ontogeny of, 137
αβ T-cell, 111
T cell-antigen-presenting cell (APC), 108
immune response and, 121*f*
surface molecules and, 90*t*
T cell-dependent antigens, response to, 152
T cell-derived cytokines, immunomodulatory effects, 90*t*, 124
γδ T cell, 136–138
HSV, 165
phenotype and function, 136–137

T cell-independent antigens, response to, 152–153
γδ T-cell function, ontogeny of, 137
T helper type 2 cells, 95
T lymphocytes
breast milk and, 202
HAV, 801
Tachyzoites, 169–170, 919*f*, 920–921, 920*f*, 968–969
atovaquone and, 1000
Toxoplasma gondii, 919, 920*f*
Tazobactam
mediastinitis, 342
solitary hepatic abscess, 325
T-cell, 105
activated, 122
activation, 101
antigen presentation and, 107–141, 108*f*
circulating, 119
effector response, termination of, 132–133
expansion
apoptosis, 132–133
regulation of, 132–133
function, in fetus, 141
immune response, HSV, 165–166
immunity, maternal transfer of, 139
reactivity, to environmental antigens, 138
response, 161
postnatal infection, 140–141
vaccination, 140–141
responses, neonates and, 1215
Staphylococcus, 497
subsets, fetal *Toxoplasma* infection, 987
T-cell mediated cytotoxicity, 131–132
T-cell mediated immunity, *T. gondii*, 171
T-cell receptor. *See* TCR
T-cell receptor excision circles (TRECs), 115–116, 116*f*
T-cell-specific response, oral poliovirus vaccine, 140
TCR α gene sequence, 113
rearrangement of, 115
TCR β gene sequence, 113
TCR diversity, intrathymic generation of, 113–115
TCR genes, 114*f*
TCR molecules, CDRs of, 113–114
TCR repertoire, fetal and neonatal, 115
Technetium-99m bone imaging, osteomyelitis, 303
Teicoplanin, 1171, 1176
in vitro susceptibility, 448
Telangiectasia of retinal vessels, 956
Temperature, of infant, 246
Temporal bone pathology, CMV and, 726

Teratogenesis, 8
Terminal components, 86–87
Terminal deoxytransferase, 143–144
Tetanus, 31–32, 241–242, 1224
maternal immunization, 1216–1217
Tetanus immunization, 41–42
Tetanus toxoid, 280, 1221
maternal immunization with, 154
Tetracycline, 999, 1166
breast milk, 1168
Campylobacter, 389
gonococcal ophthalmia neonatorum, 521–522
Listeria, 482
N. gonorrhoeae, 519
Toxoplasma gondii, 999–1000
Tetracycline resistant gonococci, 349
Tetralogy of Fallot, CRS, 878
Third National Health and Nutrition Examination Survey, CMV and. *See* NTHANES III
Thrombocytopenia, 336
candidiasis, 1066
Thrombolytic therapy, *Malassezia* infections, 1107
Thymic cellularity, 113
Thymic ontogeny, 111–113
Thymic rudiment, 111
Thymocyte, 113
differentiation, 111–113
growth, and differentiation factors, 117
post-selection maturation, 117
Thymocyte selection
late maturation and, 116–117
positive v. negative, late maturation and, 116–117
Thymus
HIV, 637
rubella infection, 873
Toxoplasma gondii, 945
Thyroid dysfunction, CRS, 880
Ticarcillin
breast milk concentrations, 1167–1168
PK profile, 1190
Ticarcillin-clavulanate, 1186*t*, 1189–1190
clinical dosing implications, 1190
mediastinitis, 342
pharmacokinetic data, 1189–1190
PK-PD dosing, 1190
safety, 1190
T-independent type II antigens, 152
Tinea capitis, 1110
Tinea corporis (Ringworm), 1110–1111, 1111*f*
Tinea cruris, 1111, 1111*f*
Tissue biopsy, 251
Tissue culture
congenital rubella infection, 883

Tissue culture (*Continued*)
  EBV, 907
  HCMV, 738
  Toxoplasma gondii, 970
Tissue culture systems, viruses, 759, 759*f*
Tissue macrophages, production and differentiation, 93–94
TLRs. *See* Toll-like receptors
T-lymphocytes, 360
  CMV and, 722
TMP-SMX. *See* Trimethoprim-sulfamethoxazole
TNF family ligands. *See* Tumor necrosis factor family ligands
TNF-α. *See* Tumor necrosis factor-α
TNFR. *See* Tumor necrosis factor-α receptors
TNFR-associated death domain (TRADD), 133
TNF-related apoptosis-inducing ligand (TRAIL), 105
Tobramycin, 256, 1178*t*, 1179
  infant to maternal serum concentrations, ratios, 1165
Tocolytics
  PROM and, 67–68
  RDS and, 71–72
Toll-like receptor 2, breast milk and, 206
Toll-like receptors (TLRs), 84, 96–100, 97*t*
  CMV and, 721
  HSV and, 162–163
  Listeria and, 475–476
  newborns and, 477
Toll-like receptors-induced cytokine production, adult v. neonatal cells, 99*t*
Topical therapy, dermatophytoses, 1111
TORCH acronym, 4–5, 4*t*
Total leukocyte count, 1146
Total neutrophil count, 1146–1148
  factors affecting, 1147*f*
  newborn infants, 1149*f*
  in normal term infants, 1147*f*
  very low birth weight infants, 1147*f*
Total non-segmented neutrophil count, 1148
Total parenteral nutrition (TPN), *Candida* and, 1059–1060
Total protein concentration, 253
Toxic shock syndromes, 499, 499*f*
Toxicity, antimicrobial drugs, 1161, 1161*t*
Toxins, 494–495
Toxoids, 1221
Toxoplasma gondii, 169–172, 604–605, 918, 1000
  "active" infection, 938
  in amniotic fluid, 973*f*
  antigenic structure of, 981*t*

antigen-specific lymphocyte responses, 971
arthropods, 931
clinically apparent disease, 947
congenital cerebral defects and, 956*t*
congenital transmission, 921–930, 933
cyst, glomerulus, 942*f*
diagnosis, 967–979
diagnostic methods, 968–979
drugs for, 999–1000
epidemiology, 931–936
  general considerations, 931–932
eye, 939
fetal treatment, through maternal treatment, 1000–1004
in fetus, treatment guidelines, 995*t*
follow-up studies, 964–966
genetics and virulence, 936–937
histologic demonstration, 922
histologic diagnosis, 968–969
host defense mechanisms, 169–170
host genetics, 937
infant, 946–967
  treatment guidelines, 995*t*
initial infection, 936–938
isolation of, placental and fetal tissue, 926*t*
isolation procedures, 969–971
isolation studies, 922–924, 923*t*
kidneys, 943–944
laboratory examination, 968
latent infection, factors operative during, 938–939
life cycle of, 919
major sequelae, 947*t*
malformations, 958
meat, 930
in older child, treatment guidelines, 995*t*
in optic disk, 943
the organism, 918–993
osseous changes, 964
pathogenesis of, 936–939
pathology, 939–945
in placenta, 922
  during acute infection, 922–923
  during chronic infection, 923–924
during pregnancy
  clinical manifestations, 945–967
  diagnosis guidelines, 984–985
    clinical scenarios, 984
  stillbirth and subclinical infection, in offspring, 924*t*
  treatment guidelines, 995*t*
prenatal diagnosis, 1001
prevention, diagnosis, and treatment, Paris approach, 1002*t*

reinfection, 938
serologic testing, method used, antibody response v, 981–984
signs and symptoms, 947*t*, 964
subclinical infection, 947–949
therapy, duration of, 1000–1017
transmission of, 921–930
  by ingestion, 930–931
treatment
  effect of, 991–993
  serologic rebound after, 992–993, 992*t*
treatment studies, 1002–1004, 1002*t*
Toxoplasma gondii antibodies
  childbearing-age women, 932–933
  in serum and body fluids, 972–978
  uninfected child, 989*f*
Toxoplasma gondii antigens
  "immunologic unresponsiveness," 938–939
  lymphocyte activation markers and, 971
  in serum and body fluids, 972
Toxoplasma gondii cyst
  within glomerulus, 942*f*
  in placenta, 940*f*
  in retina, 941*f*
Toxoplasma gondii-Cytomegalovirus infection, 945
Toxoplasma gondii-specific IgM tests, false-positive, 979
Toxoplasma Serologic Profile (TSP), 1023
Toxoplasma Serology Laboratory at Palo Alto Medical Foundation (TSL-PAMF), 1023
Toxoplasmic encephalitis, 918, 1001
  atovaquone and, 1000
  pyrimethamine-sulfadiazine, 999
Toxoplasmic lymphadenopathy, 927
Toxoplasmic myocarditis, 964
Toxoplasmin skin test, 971
Toxoplasmosis, 253, 917–1041
  Amsterdam study, 1009
  differential diagnosis, 993–1017
  therapy, 993–1000
    general comments, 993
    specific, 993–1000
TPN. *See* Total parenteral nutrition
Tracheal aspirates, 250–251
TRADD. *See* TNFR-associated death domain
TRAIL. *See* TNF-related apoptosis-inducing ligand
Transfusion-acquired perinatal cytomegalovirus infection, 737, 745
Transfusion-transmitted virus (TTV), 800, 810
  clinical manifestations, 810
  diagnosis, 810

epidemiology and transmission, 810
microbiology, 810
pathogenesis, 810
pathology, 810
prevention, 810
treatment, 810
Transient aplastic crisis, 841–842
Transient bacteremia, 240
Transmission
  genital herpes, 830*t*
  by ingestion, *Toxoplasma gondii*, 930–931
  Toxoplasma gondii, mother to fetus, 930
Transmission rate, maternal *Toxoplasma gondii*, 928, 929*f*
Transmission-based precautions, 1136–1138
Transplacental bacterial bone infection, syphilis and, 298
Transplacental fetal infection, 323
  effects of, 7*t*
Transplacental transmission, 913. *See also* Viruses
  African sleeping sickness, 1045
  of variola, 901
  VZV organism, 663
Traumatic lumbar puncture, 254–255
TRECs. *See* T-cell receptor excision circles
Tregs, 134, 135
  HSV, 167
Treponema pallidum, 276, 323
Triatoma infestans, 1043
Trichinosis, 1052
Trichomonas vaginalis, 1052
Trigeminal nerve, HSV and, 815
Trimethoprim
  milk to plasma ratios, 1166
  Toxoplasma gondii, 999
Trimethoprim-sulfamethoxazole (TMP-SMX), 634
  Aeromonas hydrophila, 392
  chorioretinitis, treatment for, 1015–1016
  HIV infected children and, 1094–1095
  Listeria, 482
  neonatal meningitis, 258
  Pneumocystosis, 1092, 1094
    recurrent infection, 1093–1094
  pneumonia and, 288–289
  salmonellosis, 381
  Toxoplasma gondii, 999
  Yersinia enterocolitica, 392
Trophozoite, 1080
Truant auramine-rhodamine stain, 588–590
Trypanosoma brucei gambiense, 1045
Trypanosoma brucei rhodesiense, 1045
Trypanosoma cruzi, 1043
  abortions and stillbirths, 1044

biopsy and autopsy studies, 1043–1044
clinical manifestations, 1044
congenital infections, 1044
diagnosis, 1044–1045
epidemiology and transmission, 1043
pathology, 1043
placenta, 1043
prevention, 1045
recurrence, prognosis for, 1045
therapy, 1045
Trypomastigote organism, 1043
TSL-PAMF. *See* Toxoplasma Serology Laboratory at Palo Alto Medical Foundation
TSP. *See* Toxoplasma Serologic Profile
TTV. *See* Transfusion-transmitted virus
Tuberculin skin test, 13
Bacille Calmette-Guérin vaccines, 592–593
positive mother, infant born of, 593–594
Tuberculosis, 35–37, 577–600
case rates, 579
epidemiology, 579–580
human milk and, 212
modes of inoculation, fetus and newborn, 584–585, 584t
in mother, 583–584
mycobacteriology, 578–579
postnatal exposure, 594–595
pregnancy, 580–583
INH, 588
screening for, 582–583
treatment, 588–590
pyridoxine, 586–587
routes of transmission, 584–585
stages of, 577
terminology, 577–578
treatment, 586–591
general principles, 588
infants on, following, 590
neonates and infants, 590
vaccination, 591–593
Tumor necrosis factor (TNF) family ligands, 81t, 90t, 123f, 129
immunoregulatory effects of, 82t
Tumor necrosis factor-2 (TNF-2), 61
Tumor necrosis factor-α (TNF-α), 82t, 95–96, 100, 124, 170–171
in breast milk, 206
Tumor necrosis factor-α receptors (TNFR), 132
Tumor necrosis factor-ligand proteins, 127–131
decreased, by neonatal T cells, 129–130
Tumor target cells, NK cells, 103–104
Twins
congenital *Toxoplasma gondii*, 949
dizygotic, 950
infection in, 241

neonatal infections in, 241
Tympanic membrane, 284, 284f
Type 1 IFN, 102, 162–163
Type V isolates, 426–427
Typhoid fever, 379–380

U
U. urealyticum, 292
Ultrasonography
fetal, 1004
pregnancy termination, 1026–1027
fetal abnormalities and, 676
fetal *Toxoplasma* infection, 986–987
fetal/newborn, congenital toxoplasmosis, 1005t
osteomyelitis, 303
UTI, 318
Umbilical cord, 31
aseptic necrosis of, 242
developing countries, 234
microscopic examination, 1153–1154
organisms and, 242f
Umbilical cord sera, 1153
Umbilical discharge, 242
Umbilical sepsis, 324
Umbilical tissue cultures, 501
Umbilical vein, 584
Umbilical vein catheterization, 20
Umbilical vessels, blood cultures from, 249
UNAIDS. *See* Joint United Nations Program on HIV/AIDS
Under concentration curve (AUC), drugs, 1163–1164
UNICEF, 31–32, 44
HIV/AIDS and, 34–35
Universal screening, prenatal care, 13
Ureaplasma species, 607
amnionic inflammation, 609f
diagnosis, 616–617
osteomyelitis and, 298
transmission of, 611
Ureaplasma urealyticum, 607–608
colonization, 607–608
Ureaplasmal infection, 610
bloodstream infections, 614
central nervous system infection, 614–615
CLD and, 612
vertical transmission, 611
Urinary calculi, 608
Urinary cytomegalovirus excretion, rate of, 716
Urinary tract, 608, 675
diseases, 607–608
imaging, 318–319
Urinary tract bacterial infections. *See* Urinary tract infections
Urinary tract infections (UTIs), 311–321. *See also* Nosocomial urinary tract infections
chemical determinations, 318
clinical manifestations, 315–316, 315t

diagnosis, 316–319
epidemiology, 311
incidence of, 312t
first year of life, 313t
management and prevention, 319
microbiology, 311
pathogenesis, 311–315
pathogens responsible, 313t
pathology, 315
prognosis, 319–320
Urine culture, 250, 316
Urine sediment, 317–318
Urokinase, 1107
Urticaria, *Trypanosoma cruzi*, 1044
US28, CMV and, 721–722
UTIs. *See* Urinary tract infections
Uvea, congenital toxoplasmosis, 954

V
Vaccination, 1212.
See also Immunization
genital HSV and, 169
HIV-exposed infants, 646–647
HSV and, 168–169
strategies, 1216–1218
T-cell response, 140–141
Vaccine(s), 40, 1212.
See also Immunization; specific vaccines
congenital cytomegalovirus, 743–744
development, parvovirus B19, 855
evaluation of, medical factors, 1214–1215
experimental approaches, 1222–1223
HAV, 802
HBV, 805
HEV, 809
for infants, 1223–1228
live-attenuated varicella, 684
major types, 1220t
maternally administered, 138–139
neonatal infection, 1216–1218
regulation, advisory bodies and, 1228
response to, 155f
Vaccine regulation, advisory bodies, 1228
Vaccine viral infections, 778
Vaccine-induced immunity
rubella, 862
rubella vaccine and, 887
Vaccinia, 899–904, 902–903, 904
clinical manifestations, 901–903
epidemiology and transmission, 899–900
after maternal vaccination, 901, 901f, 902f
treatment, 903–904
Vaccinia immunoglobulin (VIG), 904

Vacuole, 473–474
Vagina, *Ureaplasma* colonization, 607–608
Vaginal delivery
HSV and, 830–831
N. gonorrhoeae, 519
Vaginal *Ureaplasma urealyticum* infection, erythromycin and, 62t
Valacyclovir, 680
Vancomycin, 506–507, 1171–1174, 1172t
antimicrobial activity, 1171–1173
catheter-associated CoNS infections, 498–499
clinical dosing implications, 1173–1174
dosing regimens, 1174
GBS, 454
group B streptococcal disease, 255
NEC, 337
neonatal sepsis, 261
osteomyelitis, 305
osteomyelitis of maxilla, 307
pharmacokinetic data, 1172t, 1173
PK-PD, 1173–1174
pneumonia, 292
safety, 1173
skin infections, 348
UTI, 319
Vancomycin plus aminoglycoside and cefotaxime, neonatal meningitis, 258
Vancomycin plus rifampin combination therapy, 508
Vancomycin-resistant enterococci (VRE), 229, 1130
VAP. *See* Ventilator-associated pneumonia
Varicella, 661–662
passive immunity, 681–683
during pregnancy, 1224–1225
acyclovir, 670
vaccine, 14, 661
Varicella-zoster immune globulin (VZIG), 1219
full-term infants, 1 year or less, 1219
for newborns, 1219
postnatally acquired, 1219
Varicella-zoster virus (VZV), 637, 1132, 1224–1225
antibody, 678–679, 682f
immunity to, 680–685
immunization, 647
organism, 662
antigenic properties of, 662
chickenpox v, 663
classification and morphology, 662
communicability, 663
epidemiology and transmission, 662–666
incidence and distribution, 664

Varicella-zoster virus (VZV) (*Continued*)
    newborn nursery, 664–666
    incubation period, 663
    pathogenesis of, 666–667
    propagation, 662
    serologic tests, 662
    transplacental transmission, 663
    prevention, 680–685
    therapy, 679–680
    of mother, 679–680
    transmission of, 682*f*
Variola, 900–902, 903
    clinical manifestations, 901–903
    epidemiology and transmission, 899–900
    pathogenesis, pathology, and prognosis, 900–901
    treatment, 903–904
VARIVAX Pregnancy Registry, 14
VariZIG, 1219
Vascular catheter complications, 1107
Vasculitis, 843
Ventilator-associated pneumonia (VAP), 286–287, 1134–1135
    birth weight and, 1128
    epidemiology and pathogenesis, 1134
    prevention, evidence-based strategies, 1134*t*
    prevention and control, 1134
Ventricular shunt-associated infections, 1135
Vertical transmission
    congenital toxoplasmosis, 1020
    NICU, 1127
Very-low birth weight infants (VLBW), 223
    Candida and, 1059–1060
    total neutrophil count, 1147*f*
Vesicoureteral reflux (VUR), 311–313
    antimicrobial prophylaxis, 314
    urinary tract imaging, 318
Vibrio cholerae, 390–391
    clinical manifestations, 391
    diagnosis, 391
    epidemiology, 391
    nature of organism, 390
    pathogenesis, 390
    therapy and prevention, 391
Vidarabine, neonatal herpes and, 826
Viral antigen specific T cells
    chemotactic receptor expression, 167–168
    homing receptor expression, 167–168
Viral capsid antigens (VCAs), 906
Viral cultures, cytomegalovirus during pregnancy, 741

Viral diagnostic laboratory, 788–789
Viral double-stranded DNA (dsDNA), cytomegalovirus virion, 707–709, 708*f*
Viral excretion, CMV and, 727–728
Viral genes, CMV and, 721
Viral infections
    effects, 906*t*
    HIV and, 633
    human milk and, 212–213
    less common, 905–916
    NK cells, 104
    prevention, 791–792
    prognosis, 789–790
Viral lesions, bone changes and, 304
Viral pathogens, 1131–1132
Viral replication, 722
    CMV, 709–711, 719
Viral respiratory infections, 210
Viral serologic markers, 805*f*
Viral shedding, 716
    CMV, 712
    HSV-2, 816, 817
Viral types, genotypes of, 764
Viral typing methods, 813
Viral-associated hemophagocytic syndrome, 843
Viremia, 909
Viridans streptococci, 228–229
Virions, heat treatment, 759
Virulence factor
    group B streptococcal strains, 430*t*
    Listeria, 471–472
    mechanisms, CoNS, 495–496
    Shigella, 382
Virulence factor expression
    Candida spp., 1058
    regulation of, *S. aureus* and, 495
Virulence gene expression, 472
Virus isolation, 788
Viruses, 162–169, 395–399, 661, 757–761
    antigenic characteristics, 759–760
    cardiovascular manifestations, 775
    classification of, 757–758
    clinical manifestations, 769–787
    congenital malformations, 770–771
    epidemiology and transmission, 761–765
    general considerations, 761
    exanthem, 775–776
    gastrointestinal manifestations, 774–775
    host range, 761
    host systems, 759
    IAI, 51

maternal/neonatal infection, 911*t*
    neonatal infection, 772–787
    neurologic manifestations, 776
    pathology, 768–769
    prematurity and stillbirth, 771
    replication, 759
    respiratory illness and, 774
    tissue culture systems, 759
    transplacental transmission, 761–762
        coxsackie viruses, 761–762
        echoviruses, 762
        enteroviruses, 762
        parechoviruses, 762
        polio viruses, 761
Visceral lesions, in mother, chickenpox, 668
Vision, toxoplasmosis and, 1009*f*
Visitors (to nursery), infection and, 1139
Visual loss, 1006
Vital statistics, newborn health, 4*t*
Vitamins, of milk, 195
Vitamin A, measles, 693
Vitamin K, breast-feeding, 211
Vitamin K-dependent factors
    cephalosporins, 1187
    deficiency, 637
Vitrectomy, 1097–1098
Vitreous, 943
V(D)J recombination, 113, 115
    of immunoglobulin gene loci, 143
V(D)J segment usage, of fetus and neonate, 143
VLBW. *See* Very-low birth weight infants
Voiding cystourethrography, 318–319
Vomiting, 774–775, 964
Voriconazole, 1071, 1097–1098, 1114, 1198, 1199
    pharmacokinetic data, 1199
    PK-PD, and clinical implications, 1199
    safety, 1199
VRE. *See* Vancomycin-resistant enterococci
VUR. *See* Vesicoureteral reflux
VZIG. *See* Varicella-zoster immune globulin
VZV. *See* Varicella-zoster virus

W
Water, *C. jejuni*, 388
Weaning, 193
West Nile virus (WNV), 913–914
Whey-protein fraction, 196
White blood cell count
    HIV infection, 637

    osteomyelitis, 304
Whitfield's ointment, dermatophytoses, 1111
WHO, 44
    antiretroviral drugs, 645
    Bacille Calmette-Guérin vaccines, 591
    HIV infection, 623
WHO Measles and Rubella laboratory network
    sampling methods, 882*t*
    test results from, 882*t*
Whole-blood interferon-γ, tuberculosis in pregnancy, 582–583
Whole-cell agglutination test, *Toxoplasma*, 982–983
Whole-cell pertussis vaccine, 157
    antibody response, 154
WHO-sponsored multicenter Young Infant Study, 27
WIC programs, 213
Wild measles, positive status for, 882*t*
Witch's milk, 192
WNV. *See* West Nile virus

Y
Yeast cells, light microscopy photographs, 1057*f*
Yersinia enterocolitica, 391–3(
    clinical manifestations, 392
    nature of organism, epidemiology, pathogenesis, 391
    therapy, 392
Youth education, *Neisseria gonorrhoeae*, 521

Z
Zalcitabine and didanosine, 649
Zalcitabine and stavudine, 649
Zidovudine regimen, 14–15, 635, 644, 646
    intrapartum, 644
    pediatric AIDS clinical trials, 639*t*
ZIG. *See* Zoster immunoglobulin
Zoophilic dermatophytes, 1131
Zoster, 661
    after congenital varicella syndrome, 675
    cutaneous lesions in, 668
    diagnosis, 679
    differential diagnosis, 679
    neonates/older children, 678
    in pregnancy, incidence of, 664
Zoster immunoglobulin (ZIG), 681